TE LINDE'S
OPERATIVE GYNECOLOGY

Eleventh Edition

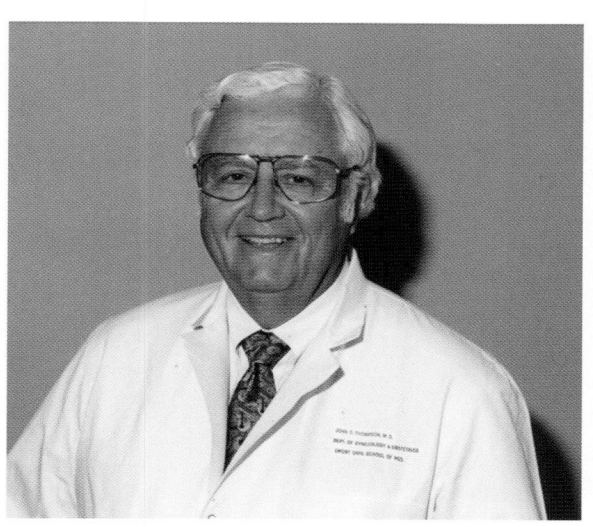

DR. THOMPSON

We are honored to pay tribute to our friend and colleague, John Daniel Thompson, MD, in this eleventh edition of *Te Linde's Operative Gynecology*. Dr. Thompson coedited three editions of *Te Linde's Operative Gynecology* in 1985, 1992, and 1997, and his attention to detail is apparent in meticulous descriptions of surgical techniques and his eloquent expression of the meaning of our work. He is credited with redefining our combined specialties:

- Obstetrics is concerned with the quality of human reproduction and all the factors and functions that affect the quality adversely or favorably.
- Gynecology is concerned with all aspects of human femaleness in health and disease.

Dr. Thompson's distinguished career spans many decades and is highlighted by numerous accolades. Among his greatest accomplishments is his role in training and mentoring hundreds of residents and fellows during his 25 years as Chairman of the Department of Gynecology and Obstetrics at Emory University School of Medicine and Chief of Gynecology and Obstetrics at Grady Memorial Hospital in Atlanta, Georgia. By example, Dr. Thompson instilled in his trainees the belief that "any definition of a successful life must include service to others." This commitment to serving others is, indeed, an honorable legacy that will benefit generations to come.

CONTRIBUTORS

Nadeem R. Abu-Rustum, MD
Professor
Department of Obstetrics and Gynecology
Weill Cornell Medical Center
Director, Minimally Invasive Surgery
Gynecology Service, Department of Surgery
Memorial Sloan-Kettering Cancer Center
New York, New York

Rony A. Adam, MD
Professor
Division of Female Pelvic Medicine and Reconstructive
    Surgery
Department of Obstetrics and Gynecology
Vanderbilt University Medical Center
Nashville, Tennessee

Marisa R. Adelman, MD
Assistant Professor
Department of Obstetrics and Gynecology
University of Utah
Salt Lake City, Utah

Kaled Alektiar, MD
Member, Attending Physician
Department of Radiation Oncology
Memorial Sloan-Kettering Cancer Center
New York, New York

Paul M. Allen, MD, MHA, MPH, FACOG
Consultant in Health Care Management, Accreditation,
    and Medicare ASC Certification for Ambulatory Surgery
    Centers
Los Angeles, California

Ted L. Anderson, MD, PhD
Betty and Lonnie S. Burnett Professor
Vice Chair for Gynecology
Department of Obstetrics and Gynecology
Vanderbilt University Medical Center
Nashville, Tennessee

Alicia Armstrong, MD, MHSCR
Professor
Department of Obstetrics and Gynecology
Uniformed Services University of the Health Sciences
Bethesda, Maryland
Adjunct Professor
Department of Obstetrics and Gynecology
Howard University School of Medicine
Washington, District of Columbia
Chief, Gynecologic Services
National Institute of Child Health and Human Development
National Institute of Health
Bethesda, Maryland

Richard R. Barakat, MD
Professor
Department of Obstetrics and Gynecology
Weill Cornell Medical College
Chief, Gynecology Service
Department of Surgery
Ronald O. Perelman Chair in Gynecologic Surgery
Vice Chairman, Clinical Activities
Department of Surgery
Memorial Sloan-Kettering Cancer Center
New York, New York

Matthew D. Barber, MD, MHS
Professor
Department of Obstetrics and Gynecology
Cleveland Clinic Lerner College of Medicine
Vice Chair for Clinical Research
Department of Obstetrics, Gynecology, and Women's Health
    Institute
Cleveland Clinic
Cleveland, Ohio

Jack B. Basil, MD
Chairman
Department of Obstetrics and Gynecology
Good Samaritan Hospital
Cincinnati, Ohio

Kelly A. Bennett, MD
Associate Professor
Department of Obstetrics and Gynecology
Vanderbilt University Medical Center
Director, Junior League Fetal Center at Vanderbilt
Department of Obstetrics and Gynecology
Monroe Carell Junior Children's Hospital at Vanderbilt
Nashville, Tennessee

Eric J. Bieber, MD, MSHCM
President, Community Hospitals—West Region
President, University Hospitals Accountable Care
    Organization
Clinical Professor of Reproductive Biology
Case Western Reserve University School of Medicine
Shaker Heights, Ohio

Lesley L. Breech, MD
Associate Professor
Department of Pediatric and Adolescent Gynecology
Department of Obstetrics and Gynecology
University of Cincinnati
Division Director
Pediatric and Adolescent Gynecology Department
Cincinnati Children's Hospital Medical Center
Cincinnati, Ohio

Diana Broomfield, MD, MBA, FACOG, FACS
Chief, Division of Reproductive Endocrinology and
   Infertility
Department of Obstetrics and Gynecology
Howard University
Washington, District of Columbia
Medical Director
Department of Reproductive Endocrinology and
   Infertility
Maryland IVF
Columbia, Maryland

Joseph Buscema, MD
Clinical Associate Professor
Department of Obstetrics and Gynecology
University of Arizona
Tucson, Arizona

James J. Burke II, MD
The Donald G. Gallup, MD, Scholar of Gynecologic
   Oncology
Associate Professor and Director, Gynecologic
   Oncology
ACI Surgical Associates
Mercer University School of Medicine
Savannah, Georgia

William J. Butler, MD
Professor and Chairman
Department of Obstetrics and Gynecology
Mercer University School of Medicine
Director
Central Georgia Fertility Institute
Medical Center of Central Georgia
Macon, Georgia

David Carnovale, MD
Associate Professor
Clerkship Director
Mercer University School of Medicine
Department of Obstetrics and Gynecology
Director of Assisted Reproductive Technologies
Central Florida Fertility Institute
The Medical Center of Central Georgia
Macon, Georgia

Dennis S. Chi, MD
Professor
Department of Obstetrics and Gynecology
Weill Cornell Medical Center
Deputy Chief
Gynecology Service
Department of Surgery
Memorial Sloan-Kettering Cancer Center
New York, New York

Chi Chiung Grace Chen, MD
Assistant Professor
Department of Gynecology and Obstetrics
Johns Hopkins University School of Medicine
Baltimore, Maryland

Mindy S. Christianson, MD
Assistant Professor
Division of Reproductive Endocrinology and Infertility
Department of Gynecology and Obstetrics
Johns Hopkins University School of Medicine
Baltimore, Maryland

William A. Cliby, MD
Professor
Department of Obstetrics and Gynecology
Mayo Clinic College of Medicine
Chair, Division of Gynecologic Surgery
Department of Obstetrics and Gynecology
Mayo Clinic
Rochester, Minnesota

Kristin Coppage, MD
Maternal Fetal Medicine Faculty
Department of Obstetrics and Gynecology
Good Samaritan Hospital
Cincinnati, Ohio

Marta Ann Crispens, MD, FACOG
Associate Professor and Director
Division of Gynecologic Oncology
Department of Obstetrics and Gynecology
Vanderbilt University Medical Center
Nashville, Tennessee

Carrie Cwiak, MD, MPH
Associate Professor
Department of Gynecology and Obstetrics
Emory University School of Medicine
Medical Director
Family Planning Clinic
Grady Health System
Atlanta, Georgia

Mark A. Damario, MD
Associate Professor
Department of Obstetrics, Gynecology,
   and Women's Health
University of Minnesota School of Medicine
Medical Director
Reproductive Medicine Center
University of Minnesota Physicians
Minneapolis, Minnesota

John O. L. DeLancey, MD
Norman F. Miller Professor of Gynecology
Department of Obstetrics and Gynecology
University of Michigan
Ann Arbor, Michigan

Jed Delmore, MD
Professor
Department of Obstetrics and Gynecology
University of Kansas School of Medicine, Wichita
Wichita, Kansas

Mark J. Dougherty, MD
President
Lexington Infectious Disease Consultants
Hospital Epidemiologist
Division of Infectious Diseases
Baptist Hospital Lexington
Lexington, Kentucky

Alexander Duncan, MD
Assisting Professor
Pathology and Laboratory Medicine
Emory University School of Medicine
Director Special Consultation Lab
Emory Medical Labs
Emory University Hospital
Atlanta, Georgia

Tola B. Fashokun, MD
Assistant Professor
Department of Gynecology and Obstetrics
Johns Hopkins University
Faculty Attending
Department of Gynecology and Obstetrics
Johns Hopkins Bayview Medical Center
Baltimore, Maryland

Jeffrey M. Fowler, MD
Professor
Department of Obstetrics and Gynecology
The Ohio State University Medical School
Vice-Chair
Department of Obstetrics and Gynecology
Wexner Medical Center
Columbus, Ohio

David M. Gershenson, MD
Professor of Gynecologic Oncology
Department of Gynecologic Oncology and Reproductive
    Medicine
The University of Texas M.D. Anderson Cancer Center
Professor of Gynecologic Oncology
Department of Gynecologic Oncology and Reproductive
    Medicine
The University of Texas M.D. Anderson Cancer Center
Houston, Texas

Victor Gomel, MD, FRCSC, FACOG
Professor
Department of Obstetrics and Gynecology
University of British Columbia
BC Women's Hospital and Health Centre
Vancouver, British Columbia, Canada

W. David Hager, MD, FACOG
Department of Obstetrics and Gynecology
Central Baptist Hospital
Lexington, Kentucky

Victoria L. Handa, MD, MHS
Professor
Department of Gynecology and Obstetrics
Johns Hopkins University School of Medicine
Baltimore, Maryland

Oz Harmanli, MD
Associate Professor
Department of Obstetrics and Gynecology
Tufts University School of Medicine
Director
Division of Urogynecology and Pelvic Surgery
Department of Obstetrics and Gynecology
Baystate Medical Center
Springfield, Massachusetts

John S. Hesla, MD
Medical Director
Oregon Reproductive Medicine
Portland, Oregon

Gerald B. Hickson, MD
Assistant Vice Chancellor for Health Affairs
Associate Dean for Faculty Affairs
Director, Clinical Risk and Loss Prevention
The Center for Patient and Professional Advocacy
Vanderbilt University Medical Center
Nashville, Tennessee

Mitchel Hoffman, MD
Professor and Director, Division of Gynecologic Oncology
Department of Obstetrics and Gynecology
Morsani College of Medicine
University of South Florida
Tampa, Florida

Ira R. Horowitz, MD, SM, FACOG, FACS
John D. Thompson Professor and Chairman
Department of Gynecology and Obstetrics
Emory University School of Medicine
Chief Medical Officer
Emory University Hospital
Atlanta, Georgia

Howard W. Jones III, MD
Professor of Obstetrics and Gynecology
Director of Gynecologic Oncology
Vanderbilt University School of Medicine
Nashville, Tennessee

Keisha Jones, MD, MSC
Assistant Professor
Division of Urogynecology and Pelvic Surgery
Department of Obstetrics and Gynecology
Tufts University School of Medicine
Baystate Medical Center
Springfield, Massachusetts

Hey-Joo Kang, MD
Assistant Professor
Department of Reproductive Endocrinology and Infertility
Weill Cornell Medical College
Attending
Department of Obstetrics and Gynecology
New York Presbyterian Hospital, Cornell
New York, New York

Jennifer F. Kawwass, MD
Reproductive Endocrinology and Infertility Fellow
Division of Reproductive Endocrinology and Infertility
Department of Gynecology and Obstetrics
Emory University
Atlanta, Georgia

Joseph L. Kelley III, MD
Professor
Department of Obstetrics, Gynecology, and Reproductive Sciences
University of Pittsburgh
Director
Department of Gynecologic Oncology
Magee Women's Hospital of the University of Pittsburgh
    Medical Center
Pittsburgh, Pennsylvania

Lindsay M. Kuroki, MD
Resident
Department of Obstetrics and Gynecology
Washington University School of Medicine
Postgraduate Year 4
Department of Obstetrics and Gynecology
Barnes Jewish Hospital
St. Louis, Missouri

Eva Lathrop, MD, MPH
Assistant Professor
Department of Gynecology and Obstetrics
Emory University School of Medicine
Atlanta, Georgia

Mario M. Leitao Jr, MD
Associate Professor
Department of Obstetrics and Gynecology
Weill Cornell Medical College
Associate Member, Division of Gynecology
Co-Director, Robotic Surgery Program
Department of Surgery
Memorial Sloan-Kettering Cancer Center
New York, New York

Barbara S. Levy, MD
Vice President, Health Policy
Department of Advocacy
American College of Obstetricians and Gynecologists
Washington, District of Columbia

Gary H. Lipscomb, MD
Professor
Departments of Obstetrics and Gynecology, Family Medicine
University of Tennessee Health Science Center
Memphis, Tennessee

Jaime B. Long, MD
Chief, Section of Urogynecology
Department of Obstetrics and Gynecology
Reading Health System
West Reading, Pennsylvania

Bhagirath Majmudar, MD
Professor of Pathology
Associate Professor of Gynecology–Obstetrics
Department of Pathology
Emory University
Pathologist
Department of Pathology
Grady Health Systems
Atlanta, Georgia

Mark G. Martens, MD, FACOG
Vice-Chair and Clinical Professor
Department of Obstetrics and Gynecology
Rutgers Robert Wood Johnson Medical School
Chair
Department of Obstetrics and Gynecology
Jersey Shore University Medical Center
Neptune, New Jersey

L. Stewart Massad, MD
Professor
Department of Obstetrics and Gynecology
Washington University School of Medicine
St. Louis, Missouri

Kellie L. Mathis, MD
Assistant Professor
Senior Associate Consultant
Department of Surgery
Mayo Clinic
Rochester, Minnesota

Addison K. May, MD, FACS, FCCM
Professor of Surgery and Anesthesiology
Department of Trauma and Surgical Critical Care
Vanderbilt University School of Medicine
Director, Surgical Intensive Care
Department of Trauma and Surgical Critical Care
Vanderbilt University Medical Center
Nashville, Tennessee

Kevin E. Miller, MD
Clinical Assistant Professor
Department of Obstetrics and Gynecology
University of Kansas School of Medicine, Wichita
Wichita, Kansas

Ilene N. Moore, MD, JD, FCLM
Assistant Professor of Medical Education and Administration
The Center for Patient and Professional Advocacy
Vanderbilt University Medical Center
Nashville, Tennessee

David G. Mutch, MD
Ira & Judy Gall Professor of Gynecologic Oncology
Director, Division of Gynecology Oncology
Washington University School of Medicine
Medical Doctor
Department of Obstetrics and Gynecology
Barnes Jewish Hospital
St. Louis, Missouri

Devin D. Namaky, MD
TriHealth Obstetrics and Gynecology Residency Faculty
Department of Obstetrics and Gynecology
Good Samaritan Hospital
Cincinnati, Ohio

James Pavelka, MD
Division Director—Gynecologic Oncology
Department of Obstetrics and Gynecology
TriHealth
Cincinnati, Ohio

Herbert B. Peterson, MD
Kenan Distinguished Professor
Department of Obstetrics and Gynecology
University of North Carolina at Chapel Hill
Chapel Hill, North Carolina

Amy E. Pollack, MD, MPH
Senior Lecturer
Population and Family Health
Columbia University Mailman School of Public Health
New York, New York

Pedro T. Ramirez, MD
Professor
Department of Gynecologic Oncology and Reproductive
  Medicine
University of Texas MD Anderson Cancer Center
Houston, Texas

Carla P. Roberts, MD, PhD
Associate Professor
Division of Reproductive Endocrinology and
    Infertility
Department of Gynecology and Obstetrics
Emory University School of Medicine
Chief of Service
Department of Obstetrics and Gynecology
Emory University Hospital—Midtown
Atlanta, Georgia

John A. Rock, MD
Senior Vice President, Health Affairs
Dean, Herbert Wertheim College of Medicine
Professor of Obstetrics and Gynecology
Department of Obstetrics and Gynecology
Florida International University
Miami, Florida

Zev Rosenwaks, MD
Director and Physician-in-Chief, Ronald O. Perelman and
    Claudia Cohen Center for Reproductive Medicine
Revlon Distinguished Professor of Reproductive Medicine in
    Obstetrics and Gynecology
Professor of Obstetrics and Gynecology and Reproductive
    Medicine
Department of Reproductive Medicine and Obstetrics and
    Gynecology
Weill Cornell Medical College
Attending Physician
Department of Reproductive Medicine and Obstetrics and
    Gynecology
New York-Presbyterian Hospital/Weill Cornell Medical
    Center
New York, New York

Ritu Salani, MD, MBA
Assistant Professor
Department of Obstetrics and Gynecology
The Ohio State University Wexner Medical Center
Columbus, Ohio

Joseph S. Sanfilippo, MD, MBA
Professor
Department of Reproductive, Endocrinology, and
    Infertility
University of Pittsburgh
Director
Department of Reproductive, Endocrinology, and Infertility
Magee-Women's Hospital
Pittsburg, Pennsylvania

Jonathan E. Sevransky, MD, MHS
Assistant Professor of Medicine
Department of Medicine
Emory University
Director, Medical Intensive Care Unit
Center for Critical Care
Emory University Hospital
Atlanta, Georgia

Howard T. Sharp, MD
Professor and Vice Chair
Department of Gynecology and Obstetrics
University of Utah Health Sciences
Salt Lake City, Utah

Matthew T. Siedhoff, MD, MSCR
Assistant Professor
Department of Obstetrics and Gynecology, Division of
    Advanced Laparoscopy and Pelvic Pain
University of North Carolina at Chapel Hill
Chapel Hill, North Carolina

Betty Ruth Speir, MD, FACOG
Adjunct Professor of Obstetrics and Gynecology
Department of Obstetrics and Gynecology
University of South Alabama College of Medicine
Mobile, Alabama

Xiaomang B. Stickles, MD
Assistant Professor
Division of Gynecologic Oncology
Department of Obstetrics and Gynecology
Vanderbilt University Medical Center
Department of Obstetrics and Gynecology
Vanderbilt University Hospital
Nashville, Tennessee

Y. Hernandez Suarez, MD, MBA
Associate Professor
Department of Obstetrics and Gynecology
FIU Herbert Wertheim College of Medicine
Miami, Florida

Paniti Sukumvanich, MD
Assistant Professor
Department of Obstetrics, Gynecology, and Reproductive
    Sciences
University of Pittsburgh School of Medicine
Department of Obstetrics, Gynecology, and Reproductive
    Sciences
Magee-Womens Hospital of the University of Pittsburgh
    Medical Center
Pittsburgh, Pennsylvania

May S. Thomassee, MD
Assistant Professor of Obstetrics and
    Gynecology
Department of Obstetrics and Gynecology
Vanderbilt University Medical Center
Nashville, Tennessee

Pankaj Tiwari, MD
Assistant Professor
Department of Plastic Surgery
The Ohio State University
Attending Physician
Department of Plastic Surgery
The Wexner Medical Center
Columbus, Ohio

Kyle J. Tobler, MD
Clinical Fellow, Reproductive Endocrinology and
    Infertility
Department of Gynecology and Obstetrics
Johns Hopkins University School of
    Medicine
Baltimore, Maryland

Laszlo Ungar, MD
Private Professor
Department of Obstetrics and Gynecology
University of Szeged Medical School
Szeged, Hungary
Head of Metropolitan Gynecologic Oncology Service
Department of Obstetrics and Gynecology
Jahn Ferenc Hospital
Budapest, Hungary

James Unger, MD
Associate Professor
Department of Obstetrics and Gynecology
Louisiana State University Health Sciences Center
Chief of Gynecology
Department of Obstetrics and Gynecology
Louisiana State University Health Sciences Center
Shreveport, Louisiana

Edward E. Wallach, MD
J. Donald Woodruff Professor of Gynecology
Department of Obstetrics and Gynecology
Johns Hopkins University School of Medicine
Baltimore, Maryland

Mark D. Walters, MD
Professor
Department of Surgery
Cleveland Clinic
Vice Chair, Gynecology
Department of Obstetrics and Gynecology
Women's Health Institute
Cleveland Clinic
Cleveland, Ohio

Jeffrey S. Warshaw, MD
Assistant Professor
Department of Obstetrics and Gynecology
University of Minnesota
Urogynecologist
Department of Obstetrics and Gynecology
Hennepin County Medical Center
Minneapolis, Minnesota

E. James Wright, MD
Associate Professor
Director of Reconstructive and Neurological
    Urology
Department of Urology
Johns Hopkins University
Baltimore, Maryland

Amanda C. Yunker, DO, MSCR
Assistant Professor
Department of Obstetrics and Gynecology
Vanderbilt University Medical Center
Nashville, Tennessee

Howard A. Zacur, MD, PhD
Professor, Reproductive Endocrinology and
    Infertility
Department of Obstetrics and Gynecology
Johns Hopkins University School of Medicine
The Johns Hopkins Hospital
Baltimore, Maryland

Emmanuel Zervos, MD, FACS
Vice Chairman, Professor, and Chief
Division of Surgical Oncology
Department of Surgery
East Carolina University
Medical Director
Department of Surgical Oncology
Vidant Medical Center
Greenville, North Carolina

Carl W. Zimmerman, MD
Frances and John B. Burch Chair
Department of Obstetrics and Gynecology
Vanderbilt University School of Medicine
Division Director
Female Pelvic Medicine and Reconstructive
    Surgery
Vanderbilt University Medical Center
    Nashville, Tennessee

FOREWORD

In the early 1940s, Richard Te Linde hand wrote, page by page, in longhand the first edition of *Te Linde's Operative Gynecology*. His week was full. Two days spent in the operating room with usually five or six major cases scheduled, 3 days in the office, and grand rounds on Saturday morning until noon made for a busy week. At home after a long day's work and in a half-reclining position necessitated by a hip fracture while ice skating in earlier years, he wrote a description of the operations he himself had used to correct various gynecologic disorders.

The first edition, published in 1946 following the end of World War II, comprised 725 pages, all written by Dr. Te Linde himself. The present eleventh edition, 70 years later, has more than twice the number of pages and involves 50 authors.

Times have changed and Te Linde's text has changed with it.

The first edition in 1946 was widely read. Enhancing its attractiveness were the illustrations and the superb line drawings by artists trained under Max Brödel, the German medical artist brought to Baltimore by Howard A. Kelly (Kelly clamp), the founding gynecologic chairman at Johns Hopkins.

The use of drawings rather than photographs has continued through the various editions, including the eleventh edition. In this latest edition, most of the drawings have been colorized to even more clearly portray the location of blood vessels, ligaments, other structures, and surgical techniques. The text and illustrations are also supplemented by on line access to video demonstrations of selected vaginal surgeries.

The frequency of gynecologic operations per unit of population is declining. This is due to a number of factors, including alternate treatments for myomas, hormonal control of abnormal bleeding, alternatives to surgical treatment for infertility, and the decrease in the number of children per family, as well as the relatively high incidence of cesarean sections, all of which preserve the pelvic structures and therefore greatly reduce the need for surgical repair of musculofascial pelvic defects.

In today's environment, the gynecologic surgeon, particularly the young gynecologic surgeon, may have less personal experience with the many surgical procedures now available and the complications that can occur. This requires advanced preoperative preparation by discussions with colleagues, residents, and fellows considering the indications for surgery, choice of techniques, and potential problems, all supplemented by an authoritative volume at hand. This, of course, is the *Te Linde*.

In the eleventh edition, there has been one entirely new chapter concerning robotic surgery, which is becoming more and more frequently used. This chapter is by Jed Delmore and Kevin E. Miller.

But even though the titles of the other chapters remain largely unchanged, the freshness and contemporary aspect of the book has been maintained by having 82% of the chapters written by new and authoritative contemporary specialists.

Finally, the long experience in the operating room of John Rock and Howard Jones III ensures that the 50-odd authors speak from practical experience. It is this personal, vast surgical experience which Richard Te Linde expressed in the first edition and which has continued to the present day that makes *Te Linde's Operative Gynecology* such a valuable text for every gynecologic surgeon.

Howard W. Jones Jr
Norfolk, Virginia
September 2014

PREFACE

Even as surgical techniques continue to evolve and new techniques are introduced, basic surgical principles remain. With this new eleventh edition of *Te Linde's Operative Gynecology*, the reader will find an increased emphasis on minimally invasive techniques of gynecologic surgery, but there remains a strong surgical foundation based on the correct diagnosis of the clinical condition, a complete and careful preoperative evaluation and counseling, a thorough understanding of the anatomy and physiology, and a thoughtful plan for postoperative recovery with appropriate expectations. The authors are all skilled and experienced surgeons who have had careers of surgical instruction, who not only guide the reader through the well-illustrated technique of surgery but also discuss the foundations of surgery.

In this new edition, we have included a new chapter on robotic surgery, and the chapter on electrosurgical techniques has been extensively updated to include vessel sealing instruments. The chapter on professional liability has been completely redone with new authors and an emphasis on risk prevention. The eleventh edition also boasts many new authors who have brought some fresh, new ideas and approaches to this classic text. Thirty-five of the fifty-one chapters have new authors who have reorganized and updated much of the diagnostic evaluation and management approaches to various gynecologic conditions. The editors have taken pains to select the best surgeons and the best teachers so that the textbook continues to maintain Richard Te Linde's comfortable reading style and the helpful, practical "surgical pearls," which will improve the skills of both the junior resident and the experienced gynecologic surgeon.

Definitions, summary, questions/answers, and best surgical practices continue to be an important component of each chapter. In addition, where appropriate, contributing authors have added a "stepwise approach" to the performance of a specific gynecologic operation.

Illustrations have always been an important aspect of *Te Linde's Operative Gynecology*, and the excellent line drawing of Leon Schlossberg, P. L. Malone, John Deutch, and Jennifer Smith have contributed much to success of previous editions. In the eleventh edition, 167 new surgical illustrations have been added to the text and both old and new drawings have been colorized to add to the clarity and contrast of the illustrations and to provide a brighter, more modern look to the book. The compact disc that accompanies the textbook features good teaching examples of both a standard abdominal and vaginal hysterectomy—surgical techniques that are all too often neglected in today's market-driven push to perform surgery using the robot or through a single laparoscopic trocar.

All of the techniques discussed and illustrated in this text are based on the extensive experience of the authors and editors, but it is important to appreciate that every patient and every situation is unique. Readers must exercise good clinical judgment. The authors, editors, and publisher are not responsible for errors or omissions or for any consequences from application or any other information in this book and make no warranty, expressed or implied, with respect to the contents of this publication.

Such a text requires enormous contributions from many experts. The authors and editors sincerely thank all the contributors. Special acknowledgment to the Lippincott Williams & Wilkins editorial team of Rebecca Gaertner, Executive Editor; Jamie Elfrank, Senior Acquisitions Editor; and Tom Conville, Development Editor. We also commend Rob Flewell, Certified Medical Illustrator, whose artistic skills significantly enhance this edition. A special thanks to Maria Medranda, Sandra Allen, Laura Creel, Lynne Black, and Julie Smith for their editorial assistance.

As always, we are deeply indebted to the many authors who labored so hard to incorporate their experience into the previous editions of this text. This eleventh edition would not be possible without their contributions. We cannot help but include a special work of thanks to Dr. Richard W. Te Linde who we were both fortunate to know and to the previous editors, Drs. Richard F. Mattingly and John D. Thompson from whom we learned so much. We sincerely hope that you and your patients will benefit from the combined experience and dedication of the many contributors to this and the many previous editions of *Te Linde's Operative Gynecology*.

Howard W. Jones III, MD
John A. Rock, MD

PREFACE FROM FIRST EDITION

Gynecology has become a many-sided specialty. No longer is it simply a branch of general surgery. In order to practice this specialty in its broad sense, the gynecologist must be trained in a comprehensive field. He must be a surgeon, expert in his special field, he must be trained in the fundamentals of obstetrics, he must have the technical skill to investigate female urologic conditions, he must have an understanding of endocrinology as it applies to gynecology, he should be well grounded in gynecologic pathology, and finally, he must be able to recognize and deal successfully with minor psychiatric problems that arise so commonly among gynecologic patients. With this concept of the specialty in mind, this book has been written. It then becomes apparent, when one seeks training in gynecology beyond the simplest fundamentals such as are taught to undergraduates, that special works are necessary for training those who intend to practice it. The author is a firm believer in the system of long hospital residencies for training young men in the various surgical specialties when their minds are quick to grasp ideas and their fingers are nimble. This volume has been written particularly for this group of men. Unfortunately, there is a paucity of good gynecologic residencies in the United States in the sense that the author has in mind. Many positions bear the name of residency but fail to give the resident sufficient operative work to justify the name. Another excellent method of development of the young gynecologist is an active assistantship to a well-trained, mature gynecologist. If the assistant is permitted to stand at the operating table opposite his chief day after day, eventually he will acquire skill and judgment which he himself will be able to utilize as an operator. When such a preceptor system is practiced, it is important that the assistant be given some surgery of his own to do while he is still young. If a man is forced to think of himself only as a perennial assistant, this frame of mind will kill his ability to accept responsibility of his own. However, many must learn their operative gynecology under less favorable circumstances than those of the fortunate resident or assistant. This volume should be of value to those who, by self-instruction, must acquire a certain degree of operative skill. Finally, it must be admitted that more gynecology is practiced today by general surgeons in this country than by gynecologists. Although this is not ideal, circumstances make it necessary, and much of this gynecologic surgery is well done. It is hoped that many general surgeons will use this volume as a reference book.

In connection with general surgery, it is only fair to say that much has come to gynecology by way of general surgeons of the old school, who practiced general surgery in the broadest sense. Now that gynecology and/or obstetrics has become a specialty unto itself, it is well in our training of men not to swing too far from general abdominal surgery. In spite of the most careful preoperative investigation, mistakes in diagnosis will be made, and at times, the gynecologist will be called upon to take care of general surgical conditions in the region of lower abdomen and the rectum. With this in mind, the author has included in this volume a consideration of a few of the commoner general surgical conditions occasionally encountered incidentally with gynecology or by mistaken diagnosis.

Operative Gynecology is written with the primary purpose of describing the technique of the usual and some of the rare operative procedures. It also includes indications for and against operations as well as pre- and postoperative care of patients. Although gynecology is divided into several fields, these fields interlock so that it has been found impossible to compose a volume on gynecologic surgery to the exclusion of the other divisions of the specialty.

Gynecologic pathology, for instance, is the bedrock upon which good gynecologic surgery is practiced. Without an understanding of it, surgery becomes merely a mechanical job, and errors in surgical judgment are inevitable. Hence, it has become necessary to include in this volume a minimum of gross and microscopic pathology, as it applies directly to the surgical subject under consideration. Also, some consideration is given to psychology and psychiatry in relation to gynecologic surgery. The author believes that getting the young woman on whom a hysterectomy must be done into the proper frame of mind to accept it is as important as possessing the technical skill to perform the operation.

Richard W. Te Linde
Baltimore, Maryland, 1946

CONTENTS

SECTION VI ■ SURGERY FOR OBSTETRICS

SECTION VII ■ SURGERY FOR CORRECTIONS OF DEFECTS IN PELVIC SUPPORT AND PELVIC FISTULAS

SECTION VIII ■ RELATED SURGERY

SECTION IX ■ GYNECOLOGIC ONCOLOGY

CHAPTER 1
Operative Gynecology Before the Era of Laparoscopy: A Brief History

Paul M. Allen

DEFINITIONS

Cadaveric particles—Elements associated with the transmission of puerperal sepsis as described by Dr. Ignaz Semmelweis before the development of germ theory by Robert Koch and Louis Pasteur later in the 19th century. Dr. Semmelweis hypothesized that medical students were transmitting disease to parturient patients by carrying cadaveric particles on their hands from the anatomical dissection room to the First Obstetrical Clinic of the Vienna General Hospital in 1847.

Humors and dyscrasias—Before the development of germ theory, disease conditions were thought to result from an imbalance of the four bodily humors resulting in dyscrasias.

Kelly air cystoscope—An instrument designed in 1893 by Dr. Howard Kelly to allow visualization of the female urinary bladder and catheterization of the ureters by placing the patient in the knee–chest position to allow distention of the bladder from gravity and posture. Dilatation of the urethra is generally required prior to introduction of this instrument into the urethra and bladder.

Knee–chest position—Dr. J. Marion Sims and later Dr. Howard Kelly realized the value of placing the patient in this position to allow distention of the vagina as well as the urinary bladder from the effects of gravity and posture.

Miasmas—Before the development of germ theory, diseases were thought to be transmitted through miasmas (bad air).

Modified Kelly air cystoscope—An instrument designed by Drs. Paul Allen and Gordon Davis in 1992 similar to the Kelly air cystoscope in which the shaft of the speculum is shortened, widened, and brazened to prevent reflection of a laser beam off the surface of the speculum. This instrument is used for urethral colposcopy, a technique previously undescribed. Use of this instrument requires dilatation of the urethra prior to introduction into the female urethra.

Ovariotomy—The term used by Dr. Ephraim McDowell to describe the first successful abdominal operation involving a laparotomy with drainage of the contents of an ovarian tumor followed by an oophorectomy.

Stereo clinics and stereograms—Teaching tools developed by Dr. Howard Kelly to demonstrate surgical techniques and procedures. Stereograms were photographs taken by Anthony Murray, a Baltimore photographer, showing all aspects of a surgical procedure stepwise.

Gynecology, also spelled *gynaecology*, is defined by the Oxford English Dictionary as "that department of medical science which treats of the functions and diseases peculiar to women." The word was first used as such in the middle of the 19th century. In 1867, gynecology represented the physiology and pathology of the nonpregnant state. Although most histories of gynecology trace its roots back to antiquity, the field of medicine we call by that name today really has had a fairly recent origin. The successful removal of an ovarian tumor by Ephraim McDowell in 1809 was as rare an event as it was a spectacular one. In the preceding centuries, the history of gynecologic surgery was closely tied to the history of general surgery, and the obstacles that had to be overcome were the same. Infection, hemorrhage and shock, and pain were all effective barriers to any but emergency surgical procedures in the days before anesthesia.

"The history of gynecology," Howard Kelly wrote in 1912, "seems to me more full of dramatic interest than the evolution of any other medical or surgical specialty." Himself an accomplished historian of medicine, Kelly noted that, "It was, notably, anesthesia which robbed surgery of its horrors, asepsis which robbed it of its dangers, and cellular pathology which came as a godsend to enable the operator to discriminate between malignant and non-malignant growths." Here, in a nutshell, we have the landmarks of much of the history of gynecology of the last 150 years. Ann Dally was correct when she noted that until recently, much of what has been written about the history of gynecology was written by gynecologists themselves, who picked their own heroes. With the rise of the new history of women and the social history of medicine since the 1970s, a much more balanced view has emerged.

There are many ways to approach the history of a medical and surgical specialty such as gynecology. The usual practice in textbooks that make an attempt to include some history is to tell the story in terms of who discovered what and who did which operation first. These facts are of interest but hardly constitute the history of the field. Besides the surgical operations of gynecology, the techniques devised, and the instruments to carry them out, there is much to be learned from the changing picture of diseases and their diagnoses; from the professionalization of the field, including the societies, journals, and textbooks that have been created; and from the education required to master the science and practice of operative gynecology. It is in these terms, rather than in tracing simply the great ideas and their creators, that this historical introduction proceeds.

Any major medical textbook can itself serve as a convenient window through which we can see history unfold. Robert Hahn has vividly described the changing world view of obstetrics by examining the succeeding editions of *Williams*

Obstetrics since its first edition in 1903. Likewise, the 50 years that have elapsed since the first edition of Richard Wesley Te Linde's *Operative Gynecology* provide an equal opportunity to describe the major developments in the companion field of gynecology.

In recounting the history of the development of operative gynecology in the United States, we can appreciate that the highly energetic pioneers of the 19th century who successfully completed theretofore unprecedented surgical procedures all manifested extraordinary personal and professional attributes of courage, persistence, tenacity, dedication, and commitment, on the scale manifested by Navy SEAL and Special Forces commandoes in contemporary times.

Capturing the inventive and imaginative spirit of these pioneer gynecologic surgeons is of salient importance to understanding our heritage as pelvic surgeons for women. Despite being embroiled repeatedly in controversy surrounding their discoveries and their respective work, they all ultimately emerged from the shadow of doubt and criticism into the light of acclaim as successful pelvic surgeons with enormous contributions of epochal surgical impact. They paved the way for the development of lifesaving and life-enhancing surgical procedures for women patients. These pioneers modeled for us the professional lives we live today as surgical gynecologists. For all of us that are, will be, or ever have been gynecologic surgeons, facing our own daunting challenges and dealing with our own controversies, the stories of these Herculean historical figures offer a deep, if not bottomless, cornucopia of inspiration and strength.

Offsetting this are the equally dramatic and moving stories of patients who endured the pain and suffering of their pathologic conditions. These were their compelling motivations for undergoing early attempts at selected surgical procedures. They endured the consequent pain and suffering of withstanding these operations without the benefit of anesthesia and without the benefit of antiseptic measures for infection prevention and control as we know them today. The travails of these patients matched the drama of a Greek tragedy, and should touch us deeply as surgeons, not only to feel compassion and sympathy for these vulnerable women patients, but also to celebrate their ultimate victories in realizing the successful outcomes of the surgical procedures they had undergone in the hope of a cure.

BARRIERS TO SURGICAL PROGRESS

In ancient times, the lack of real anatomic knowledge was a barrier to the development of surgery. It is sometimes said that because the ancient Egyptians had effective techniques for the evisceration of bodies for mummification, they must have had a good knowledge of the body. However, removal of the internal organs during the embalming process was performed by technicians who did not concern themselves with the structure of the bodies they were preparing.

Anatomy was pursued in Alexandria during the Hellenistic period, but it had few, if any, practical applications until a later time. By the end of the 13th century, anatomic dissection again became more common, but often, it was limited to one or two public dissections a year or the study of animals. Surgeons were responsible for the few autopsies that were performed to determine the cause of death. This was especially important if a crime was suspected or drowning had to be established.

Soranus, the Roman physician and writer who practiced in the reigns of the Emperors Trajan (98–117) and Hadrian (117–138), is perhaps best known for his text entitled *Gynecology*. This book is somewhat mistitled because it is mostly devoted to what we would call obstetrics. Soranus wrote about

prenatal and postnatal problems, as well as those associated with delivery itself. This ancient text has been translated and has an excellent introduction by Owsei Temkin. Recently, it has been reissued in a paperback edition.

Although Soranus' *Gynecology* still makes interesting reading, it hardly qualifies as an early text on the subject of operative gynecology. However, like other physicians of his time, Soranus clearly noted that the best midwife was one who was trained in all branches of therapy, "… for some cases must be treated by diet, others by surgery, while still others must be cured by drugs."

In the 1840s, the Hungarian obstetrician Ignaz Semmelweis showed clearly that puerperal fever could be prevented by disinfecting the hands of doctors before they examined their patients during the course of delivery. Despite good statistical evidence, his method of washing hands in chlorinated lime solution was not widely adopted. In fact, it met with outright resistance from most physicians.

Another obstacle to the development of operative gynecology was the understanding of principles of antisepsis and infection control and prevention. Ignaz Semmelweis (1818–1865) was a Hungarian physician born in Budapest. He began studying law at the University of Vienna in 1837 and then switched to studying medicine at that institution the following year. After receiving his doctorate in medicine degree there in 1844, he decided to specialize in obstetrics, after failing to receive an appointment to an internal medicine clinic in Vienna. He was appointed assistant to Professor Johann Klein at the First Obstetrical Clinic at Vienna General Hospital on July 1, 1846. His responsibilities in this position included examining patients each morning before the professor made rounds, teaching obstetrics to medical students, supervising difficult deliveries, and being the clerk of records. Dr. Semmelweis was quite disturbed to know that the puerperal sepsis mortality rate was considerably higher on his service than on the second service staffed by midwives. In his publication, he said that "it made me so miserable that life seemed worthless." Dr. Semmelweis searched fastidiously for predictor variables that might account for the outcome variable, eliminating such factors as crowding, climate, and even religious factors. He realized that the only difference in operating the two clinics was the staffing pattern.

In 1847, his friend and colleague, Dr. Jakob Kolletschka, a professor of Forensic Medicine, died after an accidental puncture with a student's scalpel in performing a postmortem examination. Dr. Kolletschka's own autopsy revealed the findings similar to those of patients with mortality from childbed fever. Dr. Semmelweis concluded that he and the medical students carried "cadaveric particles" from the autopsy table to the First Obstetrical Clinic, unlike the midwives staffing the Second Obstetrical Clinic.

It is important to understand that at this juncture in history, the germ theory of disease had not been discovered by Louis Pasteur and Robert Koch and subsequently applied to antisepsis in the operating room by Dr. Joseph Lister.

Dr. Semmelweis instituted a policy on his service of using a solution of chlorinated lime for medical students and physicians to wash their hands between conducting autopsies and subsequently examining patients in labor. He selected the chlorinated lime solution because it effectively removed the putrid smell of infected autopsy tissue. As a result of implementing this policy, the mortality rate in the First Obstetrical Clinic dropped 90%. This then became equivalent to the mortality rate in the Second Obstetrical Clinic staffed by midwives.

Dr. Semmelweis' conclusions were not consonant with established medical and scientific opinions of that era. Disease states were thought at that time to be caused by an imbalance of bodily *humors* that resulted in *dyscrasias* and were often treated with bloodletting. Factors thought to be causative of the spread of disease were *miasmas*. Thus, Semmelweis' findings were contrary to such thought. Consequently, his ideas were rejected. Physicians felt that their social status as gentleman was inconsistent with the idea that their hands could be unclean. Dr. Semmelweis did not publish his findings until 1858, although they were reported by his colleagues. In this country, the Harvard anatomist and writer Oliver Wendell Holmes (1809–1894) met similar disbelief and resistance when he suggested in 1842 that it was the physicians themselves who were carrying the dreaded puerperal infections to their patients.

Although there were instances of anatomical study in earlier times, we generally begin the story with the work of Andreas Vesalius and the publication of his *De humani corporis fabrica* in 1543. Before this time, anatomic knowledge was not tied to the teaching and practice of medicine. The tradition of the surgeon–anatomists, of whom Vesalius was a stellar example, culminated in the late 18th century with the work of the English surgical teacher John Hunter (1728–1793) and his older brother William (1718–1783). It was William's classic book about the gravid uterus with its detailed engravings that shed new light on the structures of the female pelvis.

In the 19th century, for all types of surgery, the problems of pain, hemorrhage, and infection had to be solved before operations could be undertaken safely. The problems of surgical dressings and postoperative infections were generally a matter of trial and error. The Scottish surgeon and gynecologist Sir James Simpson (1811–1870) urged his surgical colleagues to perform their operations on the kitchen tables of their patients to avoid the dangers of hospital infections, or "hospitalism" as it came to be called.

In the middle 1860s, Joseph Lister (1827–1912), while working in Glasgow, began experiments using carbolic acid, a phenol derivative, to clean the instruments, sutures, and dressings he was using in his operations. He based his work on an understanding of the germ theory of disease, which was then just in its infancy as a major theory of disease causation. Lister believed it was important to prevent the germs present in the air or on instruments and sutures from entering the wound, which would prevent the formation of the heretofore much desired laudable pus. Lister, too, met much opposition to his method of antisepsis. Partly because of the frequent changes in the system he was developing, which made it difficult for others to follow him, and because of the inadequate understanding of the germ theory by most surgeons, it took nearly two decades for antiseptic surgery to become routine. In Lister's case, as was also true for Holmes and Semmelweis, some of the resistance undoubtedly stemmed from the fact that doctors never like being told that what they are doing is actually causing harm to their patients.

Lister encountered a great deal of opposition, particularly in his own country. Lawson Tait (1845–1899), an active and polemical gynecologist who settled in Birmingham, was staunchly opposed to Lister's system of antisepsis. Tait paid much attention to general cleanliness when he was operating, and he actually achieved quite good results. However, his older colleague, Spencer Wells (1818–1897) of London, was a devoted follower of the antiseptic system in his many ovarian operations, perhaps because he had a clear grasp of the role of microbes. In 1864, the year before Lister began using carbolic acid in Glasgow and 3 years before he published his first results, Wells published a paper in the *British Medical Journal* entitled "Some Causes of Excessive Mortality after Surgical Operations." Wells clearly described the recent work on germs by Louis Pasteur (1822–1895) in France. There is no definite proof that Lister was aware of the paper, but it is hard to imagine that he did not know what was appearing in the national medical journal. Thus, gynecologists probably had a much greater hand in the development of safe surgery in the last century than is usually acknowledged.

Dr. Crawford W. Long was a graduate of the University of Pennsylvania School of Medicine. Practicing in his native Jefferson, Georgia, this young dandy bachelor doctor hosted ether-sniffing parties for his friends at his office. Dr. Long noticed that his frolicking, partygoing friends, when intoxicated, would sustain without wincing falls and blows that would ordinarily cause pain. He noticed his own painless bruises sustained during his ether jags. James Venables, an intimate in Dr. Long's circle of friends, complained of two small tumors on the back of his neck. Mr. Venables winced and procrastinated when Dr. Long offered to excise the tumors surgically. Visiting his patient and friend in March 1842, he offered to excise the tumors while Mr. Venables sniffed ether, and the patient was amenable to such an offer. Dr. Long had procured the bottle of ether from his friend, Robert Goodman, of Athens, Georgia.

> "Dear Bob: I am under the necessity of troubling you a little. I am entirely out of ether, and wish some by tomorrow night. We have some girls in Jefferson who are anxious to see it taken, and nothing could afford me more pleasure than to take it in their presence and to get a few sweet kisses. You will please hand the order below to Dr. Reece, and if you can meet with the opportunity to send the medicines to me tomorrow, you will confer a great favor by doing so. If you cannot send them tomorrow, get Dr. Reece to send them by the stage on Wednesday. I can persuade the girls to stay until Wednesday night, but would prefer receiving the ether sooner. Your friend, Crawford W. Long."

It was in such a spirit of simplicity, good fellowship, and joy of living without pretense that Dr. Crawford Long set the stage for his revolutionary discovery at the age of 26 years. On March 30, 1842, Dr. Long invited his friend and patient to position himself on a table in his office and poured ether on a towel as he was accustomed to doing at his parties. James Venables' classmates and the headmaster at the Academy were spectators. Feeling his patient's pulse and testing sensation with pinpricks, he incised and then excised the tumor in about five minutes. The patient sat up after the towel was removed from his face and had to be shown the tumor to believe that it had been excised.

Long's discovery was not received well with his medical colleagues, who believed his claims were ridiculous and that he might kill a patient using ether for anesthesia. Dr. Long's practice dwindled because of this. We acknowledge Dr. Long and his discovery annually on Doctors Day, March 30.

Known as the Father of Modern Pathology, Rudolf Virchow (1821–1902) introduced the concept that the cell was the basic unit that had to be studied to understand disease. He founded the field of cellular pathology and pathologic histology. He was the first to discover leukemia cells. Like Dr. Howard Kelly, who studied with Dr. Virchow in Berlin on one of his trips to Europe, Dr. Virchow was an ardent civic reformer and the founder of social medicine. Here is his direct quote on this topic:

> "Medicine is a social science, and politics is nothing else but medicine on a large scale. Medicine, as a social science, as the science of human beings, has the obligation to point out problems and to attempt their theoretical solution: the politician, the practical anthropologist, must find the means for their actual solution... The physicians are the natural attorneys of the poor, and social problems fall to a large extent within their jurisdiction."

The pioneering works of Andreas Vesalius, Ignaz Semmelweis, Crawford Long, and Rudolf Virchow launched the processes of removing obstacles to the development of operative gynecology. Each of them was subjected to considerable criticism professionally, because they were ahead of their times with their ideas. Ultimately, each of them prevailed, and all of them are honored today for their watershed contributions.

BEGINNINGS OF GYNECOLOGIC SURGERY IN 19TH-CENTURY AMERICA

Opening the abdominal cavity to remove extrauterine pregnancies was successfully accomplished several times in the later 18th century but did not become routine until the advent of anesthesia and antisepsis/asepsis. Ephraim McDowell (1771–1830) (Fig. 1.1) made surgical history with his successful removal of a large ovarian cyst in his patient Jane Todd Crawford, who in 1809 rode 60 miles to her doctor's house in Danville, Kentucky, to undergo an untried operation without any assurance of cure and without the benefit of anesthesia. Although McDowell is often referred to as a backwoods physician, he was in fact a well-trained surgeon. His Edinburgh training probably gave him confidence in his diagnosis and courage to attempt a surgical cure rather than have his patient face certain death from her relentlessly growing tumor. During his study tour in Scotland, he probably heard that in the previous century, the popular surgical teacher John Hunter had suggested such an operation, believing that "women could bear spaying just as well as did animals."

The drama of McDowell's case is best described in the words of the surgeon himself:

"In December, 1809, I was called to see a Mrs. Crawford, who had for several months thought herself pregnant. She was affected with pains similar to labor pains, from which she could find no relief. So strong was the presumption of her being in the last stage of pregnancy, that two physicians, who were consulted on her case, requested my aid in delivering her. The abdomen was considerably enlarged, and had the appearance of pregnancy, though the inclination of the tumor was to one side, admitting of an easy removal to the other. Upon examination, per vaginum, I found nothing in the uterus; which induced the conclusion that it must be an enlarged ovarium. Having never seen so large a substance extracted, nor heard of an attempt, or success attending any operation, such as this required, I gave to the unhappy woman information of her dangerous situation. She appeared willing to undergo an experiment, which I promised to perform if she would come to Danville. ... With the assistance of my nephew and colleague, James McDowell, M.D., I commenced the operation, which was concluded as follows: Having placed her on a table of the ordinary height, on her back, and removed all her dressing which might in any way impede the operation, I made an incision about three inches from the musculus rectus abdominis, on the left side, continuing the same nine inches in length, parallel with the fibers of the above named muscle, extending into the cavity of the abdomen, the parietes of which were a good deal contused, which we ascribed to the resting of the tumor on the horn of the saddle during her journey. The tumor then appeared in full view, but was so large that we could not take it away entire. We put a strong ligature around the fallopian tube near to the uterus; we then cut open the tumor, which was the ovarium and fibrinous part of the fallopian tube very much enlarged. We took out fifteen pounds of a dirty, gelatinous looking substance. After which we cut through the fallopian tube, and extracted the sack, which weighed seven pounds and one half. As soon as the external opening was made, the intestines rushed out upon the table; and so completely was the abdomen filled by the tumor, that they could not be replaced during the operation, which was terminated in about twenty-five minutes. We then turned her upon her left side, so as to permit the blood to escape; after which, we closed the external opening with the interrupted suture, leaving out, at the lower end of the incision, the ligature which surrounded the fallopian tube. Between every two stitches we put a strip of adhesive plaster, which, by keeping the parts in contact, hastened the healing of the incision. We then applied the usual dressing, put her to bed, and prescribed a strict observance of the antiphlogistic regimen. In five days I visited her, and much to my astonishment found her engaged in making up her bed. I gave her particular caution for the future; and in twenty five days, she returned home as she came, in good health, which she continues to enjoy."

McDowell's patient long outlived her surgeon. He did not publish his feat until 1816, by which time he had performed several more oophorectomies. McDowell is sometimes cited as a pioneer of early ambulation, unwitting as it was in his case. If his sturdy patient had not recovered so well, her failure would surely have been blamed on rising too early from her bed after such extensive surgery. McDowell also did not mention the intense drama of this Christmas day operation. When the townsfolk of Danville heard about his plan, they were incensed. They gathered in a tense group outside his house, with a rope slung over a tree, ready to lynch the surgeon if his "experiment" proved a failure. McDowell certainly had the nature of a true pioneer.

T. G. Thomas, in his 1876 centennial review of obstetrics and gynecology, reported that Alexander Dunlap of Springfield, Ohio, claimed he did his first ovarian operation in 1843. Dunlap said he sent the report of this case to a medical journal, which sent it back to him saying that they "could not publish the case of such an unjustifiable operation."

By 1876, Thomas wrote, "It is to estimate the amount of good this operation has bestowed upon humanity. Practiced today in every civilized country in the world, yielding the statistics of seventy to seventy-five per cent of recoveries, and daily being improved in its various steps, it may be regarded as one of the greatest surgical triumphs of the century."

In the middle decades of the 19th century, another American surgeon working in the South helped to popularize gynecologic surgery by another set of pioneering feats. James Marion

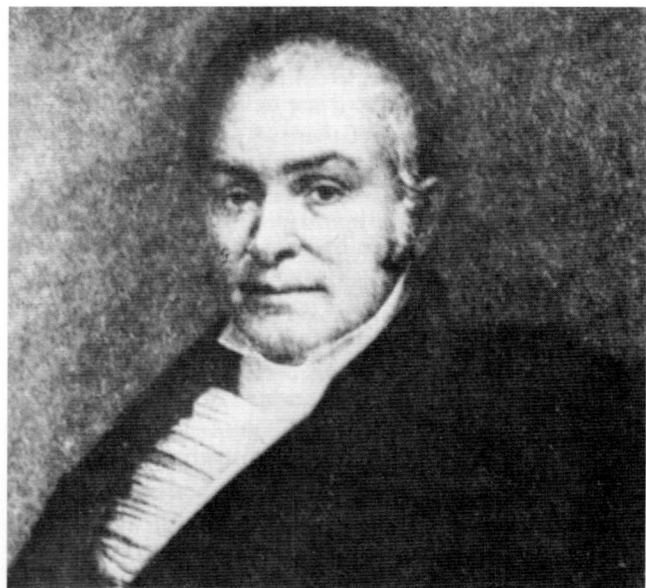

FIGURE 1.1 Ephraim McDowell (1771–1830), one of the earliest abdominal surgeons.

Sims (1813–1883) (Fig. 1.2) told the dramatic tale of his development of a successful technique to repair vesicovaginal fistulas in his widely read autobiography *The Story of My Life*, which was published the year after his death. He described his repeated attempts to achieve a permanent closure of these fistulas in a few of his young slave-women patients. Sims began his experiments in 1845 and continued them for 4 years. In these preanesthesia and preantiseptic days, Sims produced remarkable results. He had had no experience in pelvic surgery, and in fact claimed that he disliked it. It was his custom to turn away patients with pelvic disorders, referring them to other doctors in his Alabama neighborhood. Many of his planter friends owned slaves, some of whom suffered from vesicovaginal fistulas as a result of traumatic births. These wounds were considered incurable and made the young women unacceptable for household work. After several entreaties to help one of his planter friends who had such a slave, Sims began with a small group of women, operating on some of them repeatedly over the course of 4 years.

Sims' many failures only increased his determination to succeed. The colleagues who at first assisted him at the operations abandoned him, and his friends, he claimed, begged him to give up what was considered to be a hopeless effort. He trained other young slave patients to assist him, and on his 29th operation on one of the patients, he finally succeeded. In reviewing his work in 1852, Sims did cite several successful cases by other American surgeons between 1839 and 1849. He claimed originality for:

> "1st. for the discovery of a method by which the vagina can be thoroughly explored, and the operation easily performed [the Sims, or lateral, position]. 2nd. For the introduction of a new suture apparatus, which lies imbedded in the tissues for an indefinite period without danger of cutting its way out, as do silk ligatures. And 3rd. For the invention of a self-retaining catheter, which can be worn with the greatest comfort by the patient during the whole process of treatment."

The new "suture apparatus" used silver wire. This provided the breakthrough needed for the successful repair of vesicovaginal fistulas. Sims used silver in many of his other operations. In a 10th anniversary lecture at the New York Academy

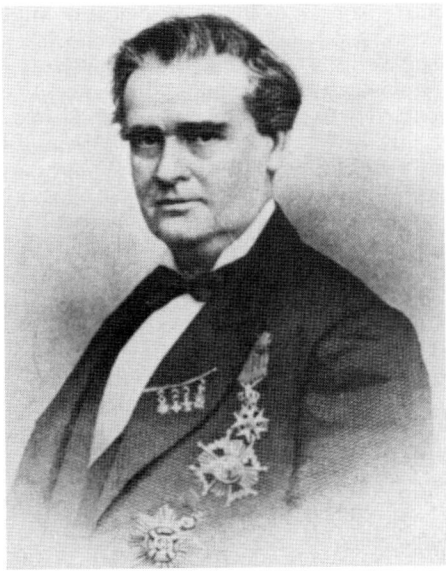

FIGURE 1.2 James Marion Sims (1813–1883).

of Medicine in 1857, Sims somewhat immodestly told his august audience that the use of silver suture was one of the great achievements of 19th-century surgery. Sims wrote and spoke frequently about his development of a successful procedure for the definitive cure of vesicovaginal fistula, but never more eloquently than in his Anniversary Address in November 1857, in which he described his work with silver sutures over the previous 12 years. The audience included several past presidents of the academy and most of the distinguished colleagues at the Woman's Hospital. After 4 years of fruitless effort, Sims proclaimed a new dawn on June 21, 1849. Since that day, he claimed, he had used no other suture in any of his surgical work.

It is worth noting that Sims' early patients—the slave women of Montgomery, Alabama, and the poor Irish servant girls who were predominant patients of the Woman's Hospital in New York—were equally vulnerable, so it is not hard to see why some recent historians have been very critical of Sims and his coworkers. Yet with the advent of anesthesia and the use of antiseptic techniques, such surgery became increasingly routine. The repair of vesicovaginal fistulas and the removal of ovaries for a wide variety of indications were the beginning of the field of operative gynecology as it is known today. The story is, of course, not purely an American one. The English, French, and German contributions were important and can be found in any general history of medicine or of obstetrics and gynecology. In 1876, Sims became president of the American Medical Association, and in the same year, he and others founded the American Gynecological Association.

Even with the advent of effective and relatively safe anesthesia after 1846, it was several decades before surgeons were ready to increase the number of their operations. At midcentury and during the Civil War in the 1860s, surgery was generally confined to amputations after accidents; hernia repair when the intestine became incarcerated in the hernia sac, thus threatening life; an occasional ligation of a major vessel for aneurysm; and cystotomy for bladder stones. Therefore, Sims, operating in the 1840s, was truly a pioneer.

Also pioneers in the field of gynecologic surgery by midcentury were the Atlee brothers of Lancaster, Pennsylvania. They rediscovered oophorectomy, which was also being done in England by the 1860s, and were among the early leaders who performed myomectomy for fibroid tumors of the uterus.

Of semantic interest is the changing terminology for ovarian surgery. *Ovariotomy*, often used imprecisely to refer to removal of the ovary, actually was first used in that way in the 1850s by James Simpson and other British gynecologists. Ovariotomy means to cut into the ovary for removal of a cyst or tumor. In the 1870s, gynecologists such as Edmund Peaslee of New York, in his book on ovarian tumors, stated that *oophorectomy* was a more precise and distinctive term for removal of the ovary.

John Light Atlee (1799–1885) actively practiced medicine for 65 years, during which time he performed more than 2,000 operations and attended 3,200 births. John Atlee performed 78 ovarian operations between 1843 and 1883, with 64 recoveries and only 14 deaths. Thus, he validated McDowell's work of the early part of the 19th century. Atlee's younger brother, Washington Lemuel Atlee (1808–1878) (Fig. 1.3), also was involved in some of the ovarian cases but deserves separate credit for being one of the first to successfully treat the problem of uterine leiomyomata.

The Atlee brothers were relatively conservative gynecologic surgeons. It was their careful approach coupled with their obvious successes that gave other surgeons increasing confidence to operate. Thus, they played an important role in the early stages of operative gynecology as it developed into the

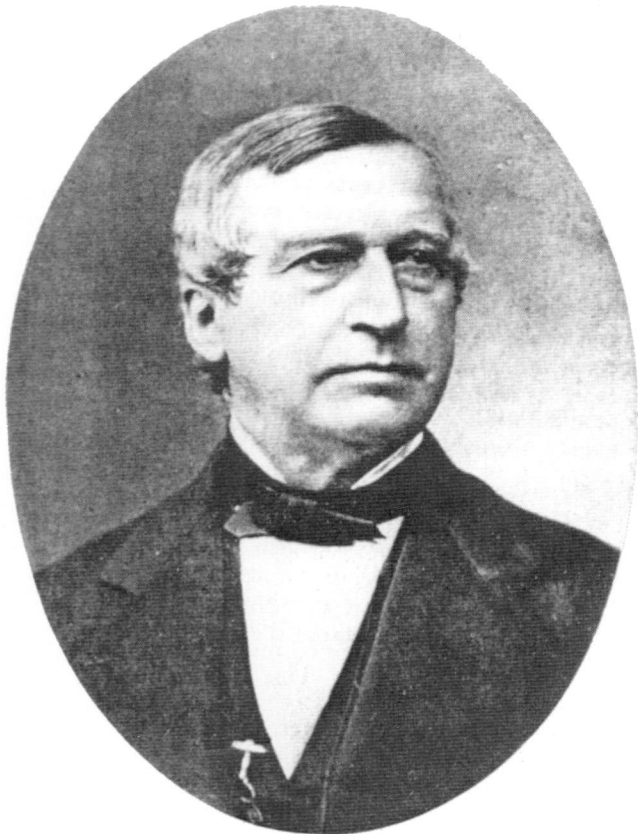

FIGURE 1.3 Washington Lemuel Atlee (1808–1878).

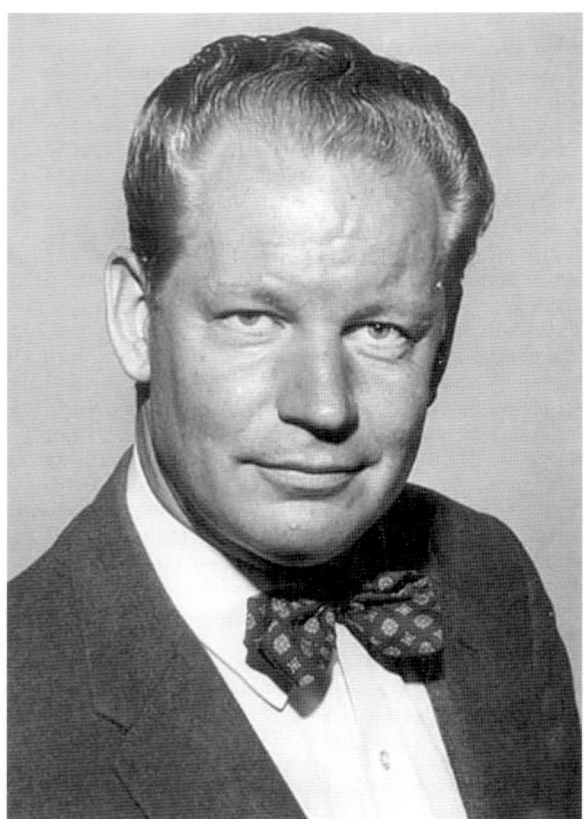

FIGURE 1.4 Jack Rodney Robertson (1917–)

specialty it would become in the next generation. Ovariotomy, the most controversial of gynecologic procedures, was also the key to making it a surgical specialty. Indeed, some gynecologists claimed that operating for ovarian cysts and tumors laid the groundwork for all abdominal surgery in the last decades of the 19th century.

By the 1880s, the specialty of gynecology, or the science of women, as some historians have called it, was well on its way to being established as one of the subdivisions of medical labor. Ornella Moscucci, in her perceptive history of gynecology in Britain, quotes the eminent surgeon from Birmingham, Lawson Tait, in his aptly entitled book of 1889, *Diseases of Women and Abdominal Surgery*:

> "The great function of woman's life has for years made her the subject of specialists, male and female, the obstetricians. The subsidiary relations of her special organs and the special requirements of her physique, based upon these, have necessitated the establishment of another class of specialist, the gynecologist."

The evolving settings in which these surgical procedures were performed have a captivating history as well, from the table in the surgeon's home in which the first ovariotomy was completed on Christmas Day in 1809; through the operating rooms in the earliest Women's Hospitals in New York, Philadelphia, and Baltimore; and more recently to the safe, sanitary, and secure environment of an accredited, office-based gynecologic surgical facility, such as the one of the earliest of these venues developed by the author of this chapter some 20 years ago.

The scope of operative gynecology has evolved in a paradoxically undulating and intriguing manner as well. As the

discipline of operative gynecology was unfolding in the 19th century, urogynecologic procedures were developed to treat vesicovaginal fistulas that defined and distinctively characterized the emerging discipline of surgical gynecology. These fistulas were sustained as complications of childbirth and were consequent to dystocia resulting from fetopelvic disproportion with protracted labor patterns, intrapartal fetal demise, and subsequent postpartal necrosis and sloughing of the vaginal and bladder walls prior to the development of modern operative obstetrics. As time passed, the operative urogynecology that heralded the early definition of surgical gynecology fell away from the discipline for more than 50 years in the 20th century, only to be reintegrated into operative gynecology by Dr. Jack Robertson (Fig. 1.4) more than 35 years ago. Although Dr. Robertson encountered considerable resistance on many fronts in his efforts to reintegrate urogynecology into operative gynecology, the overarching theme beyond technology that justified his efforts and sustained him through these controversies was his repeated and enduring emphasis on the historical aspects of the development of techniques for vesicovaginal fistula repair and for air cystoscopy by Drs. J. Marion Sims and Howard Kelly, respectively.

WOMEN AS PATIENTS IN THE 19TH CENTURY

The growth of interest in women's diseases began long before the 19th century. In the Renaissance, for instance, the publication of a large, encyclopedic work entitled *Gynaecia*, by Caspar Wolf (1532–1601), and later similar collections represented what had been written since antiquity. The mere existence of such texts, however, does not mean that much attention was given to the treatment of women, except as it related to childbirth.

Any discussion of the treatment of women's diseases since the latter half of the 19th century must take into account a variety of interpretations of women's role in society and both professional and lay views of women's health. Historical assessments in our own time have contributed to the furthering of interest in the issues of women's health. Today's discussions are best understood in the light of their historical roots.

Historians of the family and the role of women in the 19th century have written much about the separate spheres for women and the cult of domesticity in which there was a rigid distinction between the home, where it was thought women belonged, and the economic world outside. Thus, the "cult of true womanhood," as historians have called it, made sharp distinctions between women's place in the family and the working world of men. As the social role of woman was increasingly defined, they were, in a sense, held hostage in the home. Women were judged by the male world and themselves according to four cardinal virtues: piety, purity, submissiveness, and domesticity.

To these social distinctions between men and women were added the biologic differences. The biologic notions of women in the 19th century ranged widely, but they included the idea that women were not only physically weaker than men (although morally superior) but inherently diseased or pathologic. Their cyclical physiology was believed to make women unsuitable for sustained work or learning. Feminist historians of recent times have taken doctors of an earlier era to task for casting women as frail creatures entirely dependent on their biology, destined to be kept from the male world of education, politics, the professions, and any but domestic work. As Ornella Moscucci points out, however, the medical ideas about the social destiny of women were far more complex than has been assumed.

On both sides of the Atlantic, the view of Victorian women was influenced by the writings of eminent physicians. In Boston, a Harvard Medical School professor, Edward H. Clarke (1820–1877), wrote a book in 1873 entitled *Sex in Education; or, A Fair Chance for the Girls*. This book was widely reviewed and discussed. Similarly, Henry Maudsley (1835–1918) in England, an influential psychiatrist and medical teacher, also wrote about the supposed harm of higher education on the physiologic development of postpubescent girls. Clarke's book, which has become known as a uterine manifesto, clearly set the brain and the uterus in opposition. Higher education, Clarke claimed, might be good for developing the intellect, but that occurred at the expense of the reproductive organs, thus dooming the woman to a state of stunted womanhood and lifelong invalidism.

Sex in Education went through 17 printings and editions in the space of a few years. Because of its popularity and notoriety, it is worth citing one of Clarke's case reports:

"Miss D—went to college in good physical condition. During the four years of her college life, her parents and the college faculty required her to get what is popularly called an education. Nature required her, during the same period, to build and put in working order a large and complicated reproductive mechanism a matter that is popularly ignored—shoved out of sight like a disgrace. She naturally obeyed the requirements of the faculty, which she could see, rather than the requirements of the mechanism within her, that she could not see. Subjected to the college regimen, she worked four years in getting a liberal education. Her way of work was sustained and continuous, and out of harmony with the rhythmical periodicity of the female organization. The stream of vital and constructive force evolved within her was turned steadily to the brain, and away from the ovaries and their accessories. The result of this sort of education was, that these last-mentioned organs, deprived of sufficient opportunity and nutriment, first began to perform their functions with pain, a warning of error that was unheeded; then, to cease to grow;... And so Miss D—spent the few years next succeeding her graduation in conflict with dysmenorrhea, headache, neuralgia, and hysteria."

Many writings in the 1870s and 1880s attempted to refute the medical notions of physicians such as Clarke and Maudsley. In this country, Mary Putnam Jacobi (1842–1906), a physician and future champion of women in higher education and the professions, submitted a prizewinning essay that refuted Clarke's contentions that work by the brain interfered with uterine function and the menses. In Britain, the pioneer woman-physician Elizabeth Garrett Anderson (1836–1917) claimed that it was boredom that caused the medical symptoms of middle-class women, not higher education.

By the middle of the 19th century, even the use of the speculum as a diagnostic instrument stirred controversy. The speculum was known to the ancients, but it fell into disuse by the early modern period. Early in the 19th century, Joseph Recamier (1774–1852) reintroduced it in Paris, and soon the speculum was routinely used in treating inflammatory disease. It was also used in the routine examination of prostitutes in France and England.

In the Victorian climate of concern about women and their diseases, as well as their moral sensibilities, vaginal examinations were not routine. When they were performed, great efforts were made to preserve the patient's privacy and dignity, as the accompanying illustrations show (Figs. 1.5 and 1.6). A battle over the morality of the use of the speculum also ensued. The speculum, opponents of its use believed, could lead to sexual stimulation and sexual excesses. The term "speculum rape" was used in the debates over the Contagious Disease Acts in England in the 1860s.

Meanwhile, the surgeons went about debating the advisability of oophorectomy. One of the most prominent proponents of ovarian surgery for symptoms not just associated with demonstrable ovarian disease was an American surgeon named Robert Battey (1828–1895) of Georgia. In 1872, he removed the ovaries of a 32-year-old woman who had claimed invalidism for 16 years. Battey reported that his patient was cured after the bilateral oophorectomy. (Cured of *what* remains the intriguing question.) In succeeding years, the Battey operation became popular with some surgeons. Battey himself tried a vaginal approach to the ovaries but soon reverted to abdominal section. He advocated bilateral removal of the ovaries, whether or not they revealed any sign of disease, to ameliorate menstrual difficulties or psychological symptoms.

With historical examples such as the Battey operation, it is no surprise that feminist historians today level charges of male physicians' exploitation of their female patients. One of the most drastic charges claimed that most of the gynecologic surgery of the late 19th century was a calculated plot against women, a tacit conspiracy between insecure husbands and anxious gynecologists.

Ann Douglas, a literary historian and feminist, was one of the earliest to invoke the notion of a conspiracy of male physicians to subject their female patients to mutilating, harmful, and unnecessary surgery. She simply dismissed 19th-century doctors as ignorant because they did not receive the kind of medical training we have now come to take for granted. However, because the physician of 1870 did not yet have the understanding of physiology or pathophysiology enjoyed by his colleagues a century later, calling most earlier doctors ignorant, callous, or worse was not warranted.

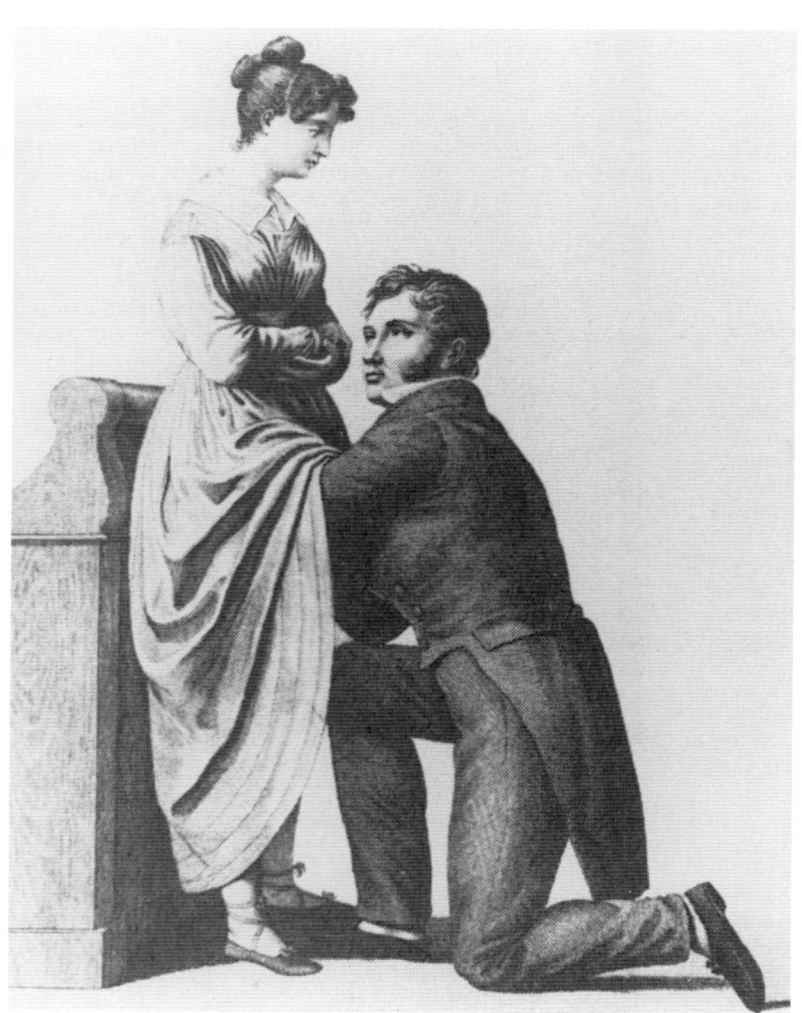

FIGURE 1.5 This famous illustration of "the touch" in a gynecologic examination is from a 19th-century French text frequently used in America. Note the avoidance of eye contact between doctor and patient and the dress shielding the woman's body from view. (From Wertz RW, Wertz DC. *Lying-in: a history of childbirth in America, expanded edition.* New Haven, CT: Yale University Press, 1989:78, with permission.)

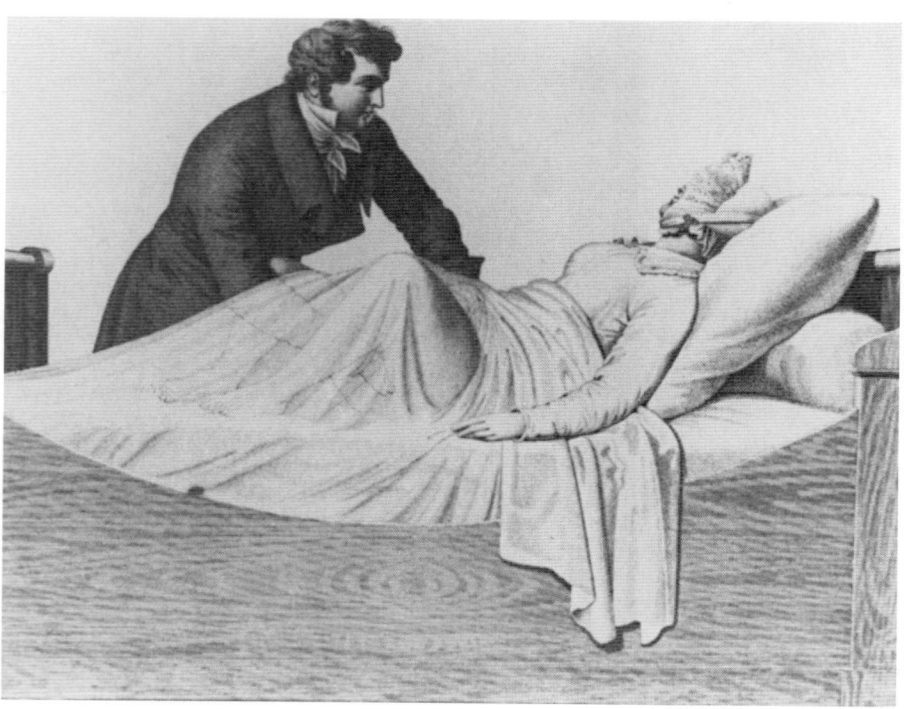

FIGURE 1.6 This 19th-century drawing illustrates another technique for preserving the patient's modesty: The doctor conducting a gynecologic examination looks directly into the woman's eyes to assure her that her private parts are safe from his gaze. (From Wertz RW, Wertz DC. *Lying-in: a history of childbirth in America, expanded edition.* New Haven, CT: Yale University Press, 1989:84, with permission.)

Those with a less conspiratorial view of history have shown that other views of both husbands and male physicians existed in the late part of the last century. The economist Thorstein Veblen, for instance, believed that nonworking wives served as status symbols for their husbands rather than as threats or temptations to eager surgeons.

Women learned and taught surgery, including gynecologic procedures, at the Women's Medical College of Pennsylvania from its founding in 1850. But it is also fair to say that there were few women actively practicing gynecologic surgery until well into this century. A notable exception was Mary Dixon Jones of Brooklyn, who by the 1890s had won respect from her male colleagues. Her story has recently been told by Regina Morantz-Sanchez, whose observations of Dixon Jones' career help us to understand how a woman made it in a man's world. Morantz-Sanchez, in her book about the libel trial of Dixon Jones in the early 1890s, charts the development of gynecologic surgery as a specialty. Dixon Jones was unusual because she was a successful woman-surgeon, but also because she was on the cusp of the developments in gynecology and its evolution from a field that viewed women in their social as well as their biologic roles to a 20th-century surgical specialty that concentrated on the pathology of diseased organs and the most appropriate and effective surgical techniques.

Morantz-Sanchez nicely illustrates this evolution of gynecology by framing the developments by the textbooks of Thomas Addis Emmet and J. C. Skene of the 1880s, still using the language of women as "other" than men, with the 1909 text of Howard Kelly and Charles Noble, *Gynecology and Abdominal Surgery*, in which there is no discussion of women's social roles because the focus is on surgical technique. Thus, the language of medicine can be used to trace the changes in medicine itself.

THE RELATION BETWEEN SURGERY AND GYNECOLOGY

The complex relation between general surgery and gynecology played a continuing role in the professional definition of gynecology as a 20th-century specialty. Moreover, several important contributions to surgery, such as chloroform anesthesia, rubber gloves, and early ambulation, were influenced by gynecologists as well as surgeons. The latter two items are discussed subsequently.

By 1905, the Chicago gynecologist Franklin H. Martin (1857–1935) was convinced that the three closely allied fields—surgery, gynecology, and obstetrics—were making sufficient progress to warrant a new journal. There was a shared feeling, Martin wrote in the opening editorial of *Surgery, Gynecology, and Obstetrics*, "… that the field of the three allied specialties represented by its title is not over-cultivated, and that there is already a place for a creditable magazine representing in one publication these three divisions of surgery."

Another of the founding editors of the journal, the gynecologist J. Clarence Webster, wrote a provocative editorial in the first issue on "The Future of Gynecology." Webster firmly laid to rest an idea that had gained some acceptance by 1905—that gynecology was doomed to extinction, to be gradually merged with the practice of the general surgeon. Webster assured his readers that contrary to what some had claimed, much advance had occurred in the preceding decades, and, moreover, "… it is very evident that almost all the important advances have resulted from the work of men who have given their entire energies to the specialty. At the present day the leading authorities everywhere are those who still limit their attention to this sphere of work."

In a programmatic statement to the American Gynecological Society in 1920, Robert L. Dickinson (1861–1950) contended that gynecologists promote surgery. "But if we be just surgeons, by surgeons we may be displaced." In this presidential address to the society, Dickinson claimed that gynecologic procedures constituted one fourth of all surgery, but this hardly accounted for the extent of the field, "… since operation is needed by less than one-tenth of the patients that come to the doctor for ailments peculiar to women (childbearing not included)." It was true, of course, that for much of the preceding century, gynecology was a medical rather than a surgical discipline, often taught in medical schools as part of the course on diseases of women and children.

In the early decades of the 20th century, the professional battles between the general surgeons (who increasingly dominated the field of abdominal surgery) and the gynecologists (who wished to lay claim to the same territory) waxed and waned. Dr. Howard Longyear of Detroit noted in 1917 that general surgeons tended to scorn the area of the pelvis, whereas this area was being increasingly perfected by gynecologists. These surgeons wanted to move upward in the body from surgery of the female genitalia and the pelvis to the abdomen. Longyear also noted that the Sims operation for vesicovaginal fistula did more to establish operative gynecology as a specialty than did any other single procedure or development.

The complex relations between surgery and gynecology also can be traced by following the name changes in the American Medical Association specialty section. In 1903, at its founding, it was called Section on Obstetrics and Gynecology. From 1912 until 1936, it was called Section on Obstetrics, Gynecology, and Abdominal Surgery. Then the name was changed once again, dropping the abdominal surgery component.

One area of joint progress forged by surgeons and gynecologists was the introduction of the use of rubber gloves, which helped to expand the work of all surgeons. The idea of using some form of protective covering for the surgeon's hands occasionally appeared in the medical literature in the early decades of the 19th century, but it was not until the end of the century that some of the associates of Dr. William S. Halsted (1852–1922) at the Johns Hopkins Hospital in Baltimore began to use gloves routinely. About two decades after their introduction, Dr. Halsted recalled the story:

> In the winter of 1889 and 1890—I cannot recall the month—the nurse in charge of my operating room complained that the solutions of mercuric chloride produced a dermatitis of her arms and hands. As she was an unusually efficient woman, I gave the matter my consideration and one day in New York requested the Goodyear Rubber Company to make as an experiment two pair of thin rubber gloves with gauntlets. On trial these proved to be so satisfactory that additional gloves were ordered. In the autumn, on my return to town, the assistant who passed the instruments and threaded the needles was also provided with rubber gloves to wear at the operations. At first the operator wore them only when exploratory incisions into joints were made. After a time the assistants became so accustomed to working in gloves that they also wore them as operators and would remark that they seemed to be less expert with the bare hands than with the gloved hands.
>
> I think it was Dr. Bloodgood, my house surgeon, who first made this comment and that he was the first to wear them invariably, when operating. … Dr. Hunter Robb in 1894, in his book on aseptic technic recommended that the operator wear rubber gloves. Dr. Robb was, at that time, resident gynecologist of the Johns Hopkins Hospital and had frequent opportunities to observe the technic of the surgical clinic.

Gynecologists were also closely involved in the form of postoperative care we have now come to take for granted: early ambulation after surgery. With the change from 2 or 3 weeks of enforced bed rest after surgery to active ambulation within a few hours of the operation, we have improved recovery, shortened hospital stays, and reduced costs, as well as postoperative complications. But like all new techniques or practices, early rising after surgery did not win rapid acceptance.

Ephraim McDowell's patient in 1809 not only was ambulant early but also engaged in physical tasks such as making her own bed. Her surgeon clearly was not pleased with her activity, which was not in keeping with customary and usual practices of the day.

What we call early ambulation was not found again in the medical literature until the very last year of the 19th century, when Emil Ries, a professor of gynecology in Chicago, published a landmark paper, which soon disappeared from view. It was rediscovered four decades later. Ries noted in his 1899 paper that he wanted to change treatment radically by freeing patients from "... many irksome and disagreeable features of convalescence following vaginal and abdominal surgery." Ries found that his patients could be fed and allowed out of bed much sooner than was the usual custom. "Very soon I found," he wrote, "that the period for which it was advisable to confine such cases to bed could be counted by hours instead of days, so that of late I have allowed my patients to get up within twenty-four to forty-eight hours and to leave the hospital four to six days after their vaginal celiotomy." These patients, Ries also noted, did not have the listlessness or muscular weakness that was usually seen after 2 or 3 weeks in bed.

In the preoperative preparation of his patients, Ries also went against the usual custom of completely emptying the bowel. Most textbooks, he said, claimed that early action of the bowels helped to prevent peritonitis. However, in most patients with an empty intestinal tract, regular movements did not resume until after they were eating a regular diet. Ries maintained that cause and effect were confused because it was not movement of the bowels that prevented peritonitis, but freedom from inflammation that allowed the bowels to move.

At the meeting of the Southern Surgical and Gynecological Society in Baltimore in 1906, H. J. Boldt described 384 cases of early ambulation that he had accumulated since 1890. All recovered well. Ironically, Boldt reported, the most serious objection raised by his colleagues was that early ambulation increased the risk of thrombosis. This was clearly wrong, he said, from both a theoretic and an empirical point of view, because his patients had better circulation from exercising.

Early ambulation was discussed repeatedly in the succeeding decade, but it received far from universal acceptance. Even Howard Kelly, the country's leading teacher of gynecology, noted in 1911 that great progress was made as a result of Boldt's and Ries' work, but that it was far from standard practice. Early ambulation really became a routine practice with the exigencies of World War II (which resulted in a shortage of hospital personnel) and with the work of Daniel J. Leithauser, a general surgeon from Detroit who rediscovered Boldt and Ries. Although doctors may not have prescribed early ambulation, as in the case of McDowell, patients probably were up and about far more often than we realize. Dr. Bert Dunphy of San Francisco told me that when he had a hernia repair while he was a house officer at the Peter Bent Brigham Hospital in 1938, his surgeon prescribed strict bed rest after the operation. Dunphy was up on the first day and thereafter and felt perfectly well, if a bit guilty.

GYNECOLOGY IN THE 20TH CENTURY AND DR. TE LINDE'S BOOK

In the 1890s, when Thomas Cullen (1868–1953) was a medical student in Toronto, he recalled that "... there were anteversions, anteflexions, retroversions, and retroflexions and that

some of the displacements might be relieved by appropriate pessaries." Abdominal gynecologic operations, Cullen continued, "... were limited almost entirely to the removal of large ovarian cysts. An occasional myomatous uterus was removed, but the fatality in this class of cases was so high that the operation was rarely attempted." Cullen also said that he did hear of cancers of the uterus in his student days, but only cauterization or curettage was performed. Entire removal of the uterus was not yet being done.

By the turn of the 20th century, the leadership of gynecology in this country had clearly moved to the new Johns Hopkins Hospital, where Howard A. Kelly (1858–1943) (Fig. 1.7) began to train a series of young men who put gynecology on a strong academic footing in the next two generations. Kelly received both his bachelor's and medical degrees from the University of Pennsylvania. After his medical graduation in 1882, Kelly spent some time in Germany learning the latest surgical and pathologic techniques.

Like President Theodore Roosevelt, who, for similar reasons, journeyed to the North Dakota Badlands to invigorate himself and to regain his health, he journeyed west to Colorado and worked as a ranch hand and cowboy on the OZ Ranch in Elbert County.

While at the ranch, he had an intense religious experience and life-defining moment, one that his medical and surgical colleagues could not understand, which he later described in *A Scientific Man and the Bible*:

> "In the midst of the cold and lonely winter far out in the plains, I had a never-to-be-forgotten experience one day during one of Colorado's three-day blizzards, while I was bedfast with snow blindness from glare of the sun on the snow striking unprotected eyes. There came, as I sat propped up in my bed, an overwhelming sense of a great light in the room and the certainty of the near presence of God, lasting perhaps a few minutes and then fading away, leaving a realization and a conviction never afterwards to be questioned in all the vicissitudes of life, whatever they might be, a certainty above and beyond the process of human reason" (Fig. 1.8).

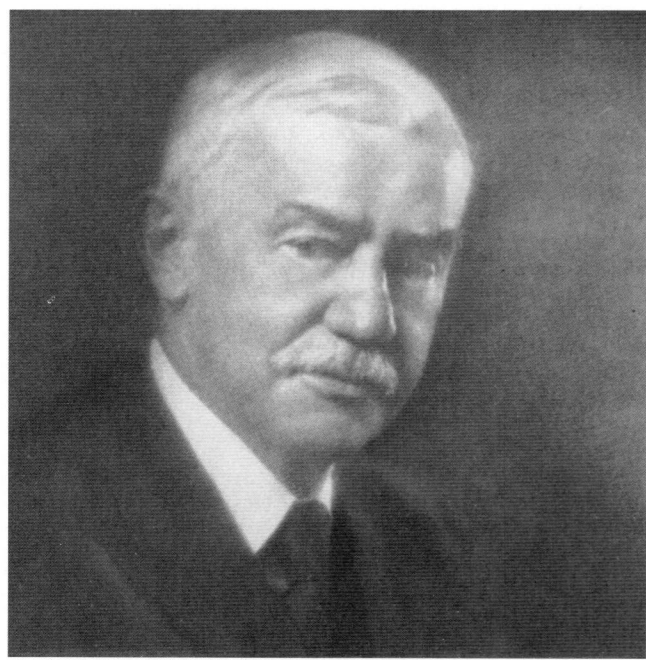

FIGURE 1.7 Howard A. Kelly (1858–1943). (From Davis AW. *Dr. Kelly of Hopkins*. Baltimore, MD: The Johns Hopkins Press, 1959.)

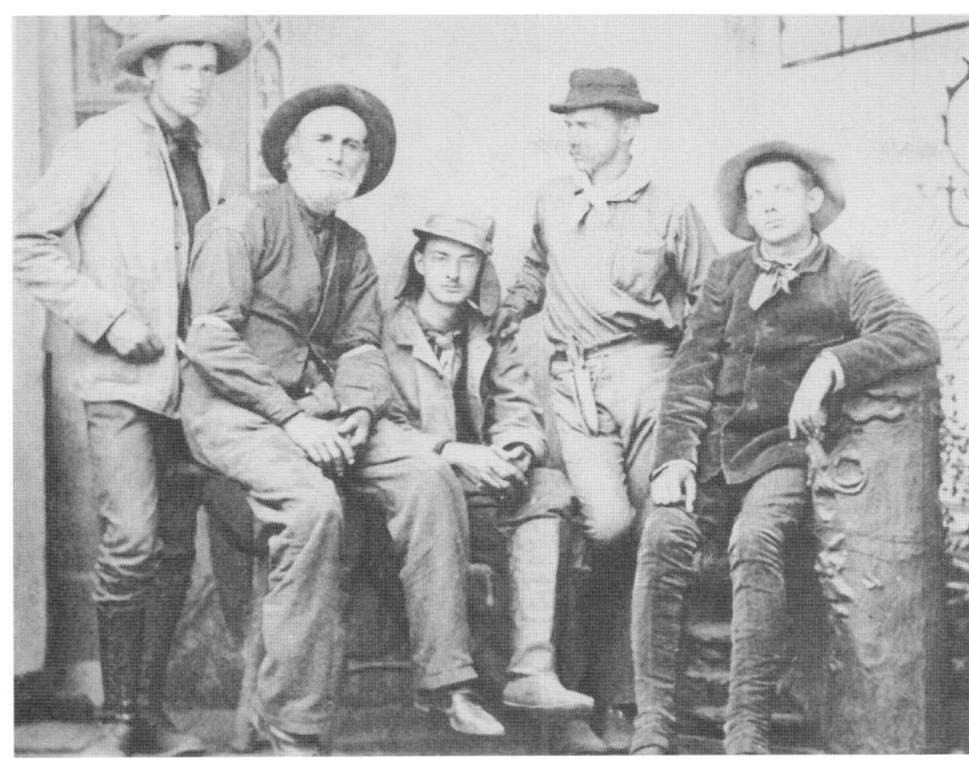

FIGURE 1.8 Dr. Howard A. Kelly and other ranch hands at OZ Ranch in Elbert County, CO, 1880. (From Allen P, Setze T. Howard Atwood Kelly, M.D. (1858–1943): his life and his enduring legacy. *South Med J* 1991:84;361.)

After a year in Colorado, his health restored, Kelly returned to Philadelphia to complete his medical studies. He was awarded the Doctor of Medicine degree on March 15, 1882. He took his internship in the Episcopal Hospital in Kensington, a working-class district of Philadelphia, and subsequently established his practice there. He founded the Women's Hospital of Philadelphia there in Kensington. It was during this period that he first attracted the attention of Sir William Osler. When a woman in the medical ward died of nephritis, Kelly, being doubtful of obtaining permission for autopsy, stealthily went to the morgue and extracted the kidneys through the vaginal vault. Osler, himself a pathologic anatomist in Montreal, heard about the method and thereafter followed with interest the career of the young surgeon.

By this time, Dr. William Osler had moved from Montreal and accepted a position at the University of Pennsylvania in Philadelphia, providing an opportunity for closer observation of Kelly. Osler often visited the Kensington Hospital to watch Kelly operate, and he is said to have remarked that he had never seen a more skillful surgeon. When the position of assistant professor of obstetrics and gynecology came open at the University of Pennsylvania, Osler recommended Kelly and at that time dubbed him the "Kensington colt" because he was only 31 years old and was a "dark horse" to obtain the appointment. The trustees did accept Osler's recommendation and give Kelly the position, but he was there only about a year before events led him elsewhere.

Meanwhile, plans were being made in Baltimore to use the millions left by a wealthy philanthropist, Johns Hopkins, to establish a university and hospital. In 1884, Dr. William Welch was called from Bellevue in New York to take the chair of pathology. At his urging, Dr. William Osler was brought down from Philadelphia to head the department of medicine, and Dr. William Halsted was appointed to the chair of general surgery. Again, Dr. Osler used his influence with the trustees of the new institution to insist that Kelly be offered the position of professor of obstetrics and gynecology. Kelly was enthusiastic about working with those renowned physicians and starting his own department, but he had misgivings about a department of obstetrics and gynecology. Kelly did not like the practice or teaching of obstetrics, and his goal was to divide the chair so that he would become professor of gynecology.

In 1886, Kelly made the first of many trips to Europe to study under the great physicians there. In Leipzig, Max Saenger demonstrated the practicability of palpating female ureters in their lower pelvic portions. In 1888, Kelly dissected cadavers under the direction of Dr. Rudolf Virchow in Berlin to study the anatomic relations of the ureters and to attempt to determine the most efficacious method of ureteral catheterization.

At age 31, the youthful-appearing Kelly, who many patients thought was still a student or resident, initiated a residency program in gynecology with a strong link to the pathology department. Even more than half a century later, the leading texts in the field—*Eastman's (Williams') Obstetrics*, *Te Linde's Operative Gynecology*, and *Novak's Gynecologic and Obstetric Pathology*—were written by professors in Baltimore who had received their training at Hopkins with Kelly and his assistants.

Kelly soon found that his interests and skills were in gynecologic surgery; therefore, he turned the obstetric service over to J. Whitridge Williams (1866–1931), who became a leader in that field and the author of the most widely used textbook of the time. Kelly had a great interest in the female urinary system, realizing that the symptomatology of urinary tract disease is often intertwined with that of the reproductive organs. He invented the air cystoscope and devised ureteral

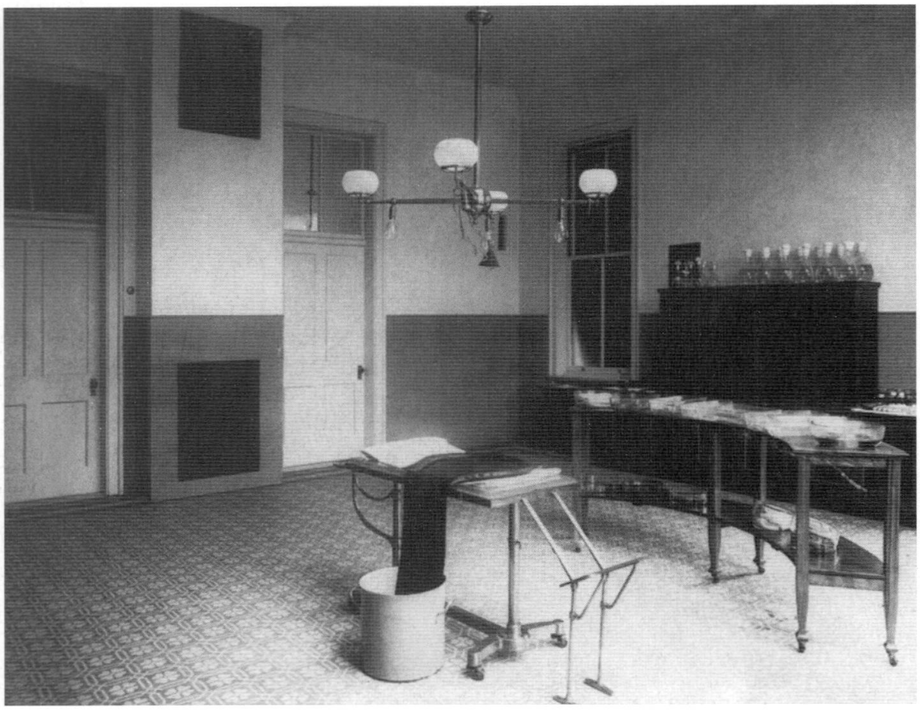

FIGURE 1.9 Dr. Howard A. Kelly's operating room at the Johns Hopkins Hospital. To the left is the door to the corridor. In the center is the door to the ether room. The rubber pad was used for drainage during irrigation of the abdomen. A similar pad was developed by Dr. Kelly for drainage of blood and amniotic fluid during and after a vaginal delivery.

catheters. He was the first to plicate the vesical sphincter for stress incontinence of urine. Physicians from all over the world came to Baltimore to watch him operate (Figs. 1.9 and 1.10).

Kelly's legendary operative skill was well described by Cullen, who later became one of Kelly's outstanding residents and successors to the chair at Hopkins. Kelly and Hunter Robb, his earlier resident, went to the Toronto General Hospital not long after Kelly became chief at Hopkins. Cullen was an intern in Toronto at the time and handled the instruments during an operation that Kelly and Robb had agreed to perform. Cullen's description speaks for itself:

> I turned around to thread a needle and when I turned back found to my amazement that the operator had the abdomen open. Operators in the General often took ten minutes to get that far. After cutting through the skin, fat and fascia they were apt to get

lost in the muscles. Kelly and Robb working together used dissecting forceps as I had never seen them used. One man pulling each way, the cleavage between the muscles was seen at once and the opening in the abdomen could be completed without difficulty. I watched, fascinated, while Kelly went ahead and finished that operation and did the second, working with clock-like precision and at a speed I had not imagined possible. By the time he had finished, the course of my professional life was decided. Up to that afternoon I had intended to be a physician. From that afternoon I knew I had to be a surgeon.

Chance often determines the course of one's life, so it was fortunate for Cullen that he had to wait 6 months for his residency with Kelly to start. He used this time to begin the study of pathology with William H. Welch at Hopkins, and it was the close alliance of gynecology and pathology, begun by Kelly and continued by Cullen, that shaped the careers

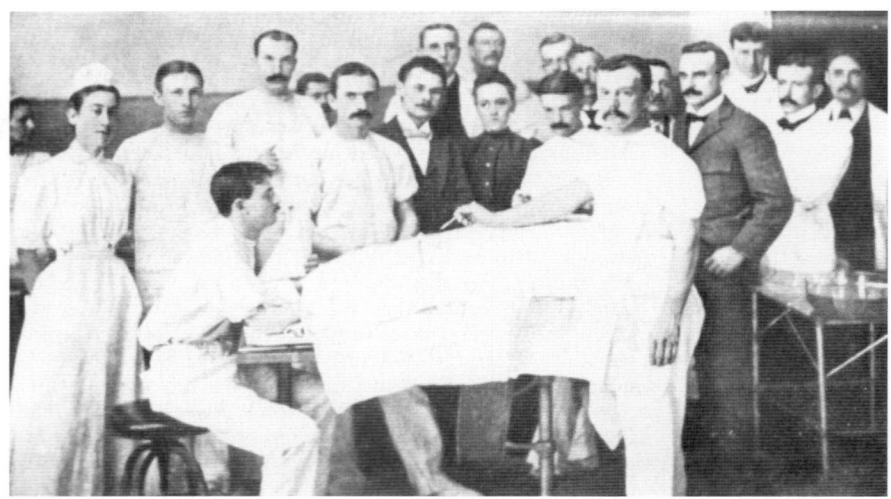

FIGURE 1.10 Howard Kelly operates. Grouped about the operating table, left to right, are Emma Beckwith, head nurse, Jay Durkee (*seated*), Thomas S. Cullen, Max Brödel (*center*), Elisabeth Hurdon, J. E. Stokes, and John G. Clark. (From Davis AW. *Dr. Kelly of Hopkins*. Baltimore, MD: The Johns Hopkins Press, 1959.)

of many future gynecologists at Hopkins and elsewhere and determined the course of the field itself.

In 1898, Kelly published a two-volume textbook called *Operative Gynecology*, certainly the direct ancestor of the volume you have in your hands. Kelly wrote in the preface, "My aim in writing this book has been to place in the hands of the many friends who have from time to time visited me and followed my work, a convenient summary of the various gynecological operations I have found best in my own practice."

Although gynecology at the end of the last century was still a very young science, in Kelly's words, change was at hand: "Although I have spent several years in the preparation of my book, so rapid have been the changes in the gynecological field that I have found it necessary to rewrite some of the chapters two and even three times." A little more than a dozen years later, in the preface to his text entitled *Medical Gynecology*, Kelly reiterated the pace of the changes: "What a transformation two generations have witnessed in the field of gynecology! From modest beginnings, as a sort of minor specialty coupled with diseases of children and often professed by general practitioners with no special training, it has grown to the dignity of a major surgical specialty, so extensive that many gynecologists of today (1912) claim the entire field of abdominal surgery as their proper domain by right of discovery and conquest." This was also a time when radical or complete removal of tumors and repair of hernias became increasingly common. Kelly and his residents were pioneers in radical hysterectomy when Hugh Young of Hopkins introduced radical prostatectomy.

Summarizing Kelly's surgical innovations, Audrey Davis wrote:

> "In the first place, he developed a combined vaginal and abdominal method of examination, perfected and carried out with unusual expertness the common plastic repairs, and successfully operated through the abdomen. His suspension of the retroflexed uterus was a signal innovation of the day and of this period of his development in surgical methods. Second, he early turned his attention to the urinary tract and began what he later considered his most important contributions to his specialty."

When Kelly heard about the discovery of radium by the Curies in Paris in 1898, he associated this with the problem of malignancy, and he determined to obtain some of the material for the treatment of cancer. In 1904, he bought a small tube containing a few milligrams of radium and began to use it in the treatment of small external lesions. He continued to experiment with the treatment and determined to acquire more radium. In 1913, he went to Colorado to study methods of extracting radium from carnotite deposits there.

His rapid acceptance of the new treatment brought him much criticism, and he was called a quack not only by the lay public but also by some of his medical colleagues. In 1913, his friend Dr. William Mayo defended him in a letter:

> "Don't you fret about what they are saying about you and radium. Your friends know what you are trying to accomplish and with your energy, persistence, and great intelligence you will succeed. But no man has tried to do something that is different from that of the average man without being subjected to abuse and criticism. It is a curious phase of human nature to attack what it does not understand. So do not think about it again."

From 1917 on, the Howard A. Kelly Hospital on Eutaw Street in Baltimore had 5 1/2 g of radium, said to be the largest amount available at that time in any clinic in the world. That hospital was the first to use radium in packs at appreciable skin distances, the first to use a teleradium apparatus, the first to establish a large radon plant, and the first in Baltimore and

one of the first in America to install an apparatus for deep x-ray therapy. For years, the Kelly Hospital administered all of the radiation for patients at Johns Hopkins and did most of the radiation work in Baltimore and the state of Maryland.

Remembering the dry lectures of his medical school days, Kelly determined to teach by demonstration and by allowing his residents the widest possible latitude in caring for their patients under his supervision. According to Harvey:

> "Kelly's postgraduate discipline by means of this long-term residency was an entirely new concept in surgical training at that time. Each year the assistant residents were given increasing responsibilities in the care of patients and in procedures in the operating room. Surgery upon the ward patients was done almost exclusively by the resident and his assistants, subject to consultation and help when necessary by the senior staff. … Judging by the quality of his many residents, one may wonder whether this was not his greatest contribution to his specialty" (Fig. 1.10).

Dr. William T. Howard, Jr., one of Kelly's residents, described his method of instruction in the operating room:

> "In the new B operating room, while assistants looked after anesthetizing and otherwise preparing the patient for operation, Kelly gave the history of the patient's illness, the results of the physical examination and laboratory tests, the diagnosis, and proposed procedure. When all was in readiness, operator and assistants in position, Kelly, glancing at the large wall clock, announced the time and began. Throughout operation, in a running talk, he described each procedure, and in abdominal cases what he found, and what he intended doing at each step and why. Whenever practicable, he let the students and visitors view each step. The operation completed, Kelly again glanced at the clock and announced the time. Often after operation, he would go to the blackboard and using both hands rapidly sketch and describe just what he had found and what he had done."

Because he did so much medical writing, Kelly saw the need for photographs to illustrate the procedures he wanted to teach. In Baltimore, he found an excellent photographer, Anthony Murray, who filled a large folio with some 1,500 photographs of operations. Kelly then devised what he termed the "stereogram," a photograph of each step in an operation with the written text describing it. He and his photographers then took great pains to make the stereograms as complete and as perfect as possible. He traveled to Europe to photograph the procedures of the great surgeons there. Often, it was necessary to wait for years for a particular operation. He published the stereograms in book form starting in 1908 and titled them *The Stereo Clinic.*

At times, however, the nature of the subject demanded a drawing rather than a photograph. Kelly had had a facility for sketching since childhood, and he always used his own drawings for teaching his students. When he saw the need for more elaborate illustrations for his publications, Kelly determined to obtain a medical artist for Hopkins. He heard about an artist, Max Brödel, then working in Germany. After a campaign of several years' duration, he succeeded in 1894 in bringing Brödel to Baltimore and installing him as a resident at the Johns Hopkins Hospital (Fig. 1.11).

The spectacular results of the collaboration between Kelly and Brödel are described by Davis: Four years after Brödel began work at Hopkins, Kelly's two-volume work *Operative Gynecology* (1898) appeared. Not only did these volumes proclaim to the world Dr. Kelly's leadership in gynecology, but they introduced to medical circles the illustrations that revolutionized medical illustration.

Some years later, the Department of Art as Applied to Medicine was established in the Johns Hopkins University School

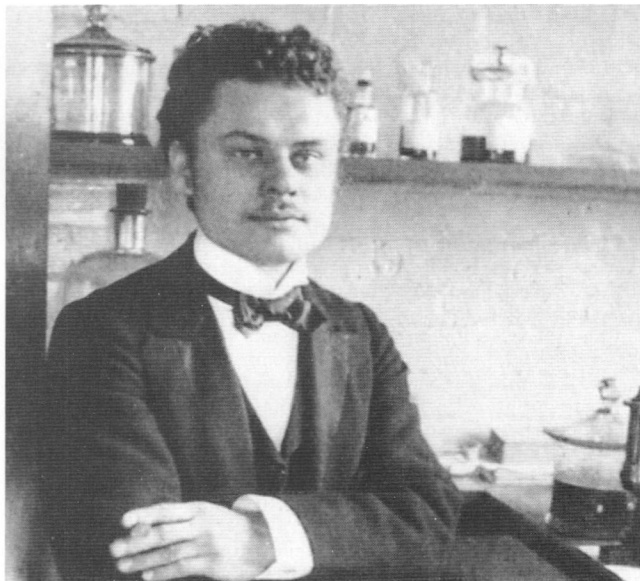

FIGURE 1.11   Max Brödel. (From Robinson J. *Tom Cullen of Baltimore*. New York: Oxford University Press, 1949, with permission.)

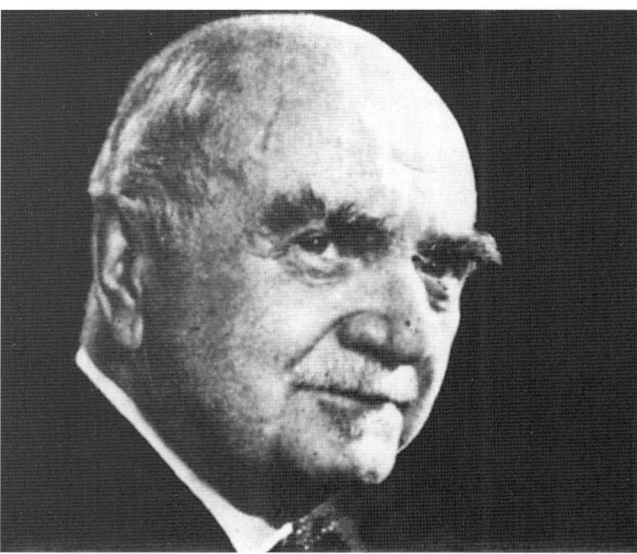

FIGURE 1.12   Thomas S. Cullen (1868–1953). (From Robinson J. *Tom Cullen of Baltimore*. New York: Oxford University Press, 1949, with permission.)

of Medicine. It was the first department of its kind in the world and continues to the present.

At a testimonial dinner on Kelly's 75th birthday, Brödel described Kelly's method of teaching the illustrators:

"A clear and vivid mental picture always must precede the actual picture on paper. The planning of the picture therefore is the all-important thing, not the execution. This is where we learned from Dr. Kelly. He had a way of making little modest outline sketches when he explained his operative procedure to his illustrators.... He invented diagrams to show variations of form and relationship, motion, pressure, tension, rupture, the development of a pathological process, the sequence of operative steps, the placing of ligatures, sutures, etc.; in short, every clinical phenomenon, every operative procedure flowed in simple, eloquent lines from the end of his pencil. ... Dr. Kelly always permitted the artists to make original investigation to clear up the obscure point. ... Without his sympathetic attitude we could not have learned our trade as we did."

Kelly's brilliant 30-year career as the head of gynecology at Hopkins was equaled by his prominence in other fields of endeavor. He became a civic leader in Baltimore, at one time running for public office. His special crusades were against alcohol, tobacco, prostitution, and political corruption. He was a devout Christian and Bible scholar, reading the Bible in the original Greek and Hebrew. He never lost his early interest in natural history, and he became an authority on herpetology, mycology, and lichenology. He was ahead of his time as an environmentalist and bought wilderness land in Florida and Canada for preservation. He gave the land in Florida to the state, and it is now Kelly Park in Orange County.

As long ago as 1900, in his classic text, *Cancer of the Uterus*, Thomas Cullen, student of and successor to Kelly (**Fig. 1.12**), wrote that "The number of cases of cancer of the genital tract coming too late for operation is so appalling that the surgeon is ever seeking to devise ways and means by which the dread malady may be more generally detected at the earliest possible moment—at a time when complete removal of the malignant tissue is still possible. ... But since it is the general practitioner who, as a rule, is the first consulted, upon him largely falls the responsibility of arriving at a timely diagnosis."

One of the greatest advances in gynecology in this century has been the improvement in the early detection and cure rate of cancer of the uterine cervix that has resulted from the development of cytology and the recognition of carcinoma in situ. In 1943, George N. Papanicolaou (1883–1962) and Herbert Traut (1894–1963) published their seminal monograph entitled *Diagnosis of Uterine Cancer by the Vaginal Smear*. Papanicolaou had worked on this technique since the 1920s, but, like many other innovations in medicine, it took years to find widespread acceptance. Further publications by Papanicolaou and others, notably Ruth Graham, demonstrated beyond a doubt that cytologic studies could almost infallibly detect cervical cancer.

Cancer in situ was recognized early in the century by Cullen and in 1912 by J. Schottlander and F. Kermauner, but its relation to invasive cancer was not well understood. This relation was more clearly described in 1944 by G. A. Galvin and Te Linde in several reports. Since then, the relation has been amply confirmed, and early cervical cancer has become a detectable and curable disease. Since its inception by Hans Hinselmann in Germany in the 1920s, colposcopy has given a new dimension to the assessment of cervical carcinoma, making blind, random cervical biopsies unnecessary and providing more accuracy in finding and treating localized lesions.

By the early 1970s, the editor of a new journal, *Gynecologic Oncology*, pointed out that "... the scientific importance of gynecologic oncology may be gained from the observation that the tumors that we study and treat are prototypes for cancer in other areas of the body, for the histogenesis of the two principal uterine cancers is probably understood better than that of any other tumor in the body."

The immediate post–World War II years were a period of truly astounding medical developments and saw the explosive growth of medical research funding and new hospital construction. After 1945, penicillin became available for civilian use, and this was soon followed by other antibiotics. Hormone replacement became increasingly possible, and in 1946, the year that Richard Te Linde published the first edition of this textbook, Congress passed the Hill-Burton Act, making federal funds available to localities for the construction of new hospitals. These and other developments of the time greatly changed and expanded the work of medicine.

THE BEGINNING OF THE ERA OF LAPAROSCOPY

Although the emphasis of this historical chapter is on developments before the introduction of laparoscopy, the ability to visualize and subsequently to intervene by the less invasive laparoscopic technique surely represents an important milestone in the history of operative gynecology. The details of the history of the various endoscopic possibilities are discussed in the chapters devoted to these techniques, but a few general historical reflections may be in order at this point.

Laparoscopy seems to have been developed more or less independently in the United States and in various countries in Europe. In 1911, Bertram Bernheim, a general surgeon at Johns Hopkins, reported two cases in which, through a small abdominal incision, he introduced a proctoscope to examine the upper abdomen in a procedure he called organoscopy. The source of the illumination was an incandescent light on a band around his head. The experience must not have been satisfactory, as there were no follow-up reports.

In the mid-1930s at the same Johns Hopkins, in a trial of a small series of patients that was never published, Richard Te Linde introduced a Kelly air cystoscope into the abdomen through a small subumbilical incision with the patients in a deep Trendelenburg position. The Kelly air cystoscope was simply a 10-cm-long tube, which came in various diameters up to 2 cm, with a flange at the distal end and a suitable handle. It was routinely used at Hopkins to examine the bladder. The patient was in the knee–chest position for the cystoscopic examination. The bladder distended with air and when the obturator, which normally was also a part of the instrument, was removed. The light source was an incandescent bulb placed just above the patient's buttocks and a conical head mirror with a central hole to direct the light along the line of site. The illumination was very good with this technique. Although the pelvic organs could be seen with the introduction of the cystoscope into the abdomen, the area of inspection was so small that the concept was abandoned.

It is curious indeed that Te Linde apparently did not think of introducing the cystoscope through the posterior fornix with the patient in the knee–chest position, especially as this was the exact position used to cystoscope the bladder with the Kelly cystoscope and was a technique commonly and frequently used at Johns Hopkins during this era. At that time, female urology was part of the division of gynecology.

It remained for Albert Decker with T. H. Cherry to use the knee–chest position to introduce a lens cystoscope with a miniaturized incandescent bulb at the tip through the posterior fornix to visualize the pelvic organs. Thus, culdoscopy was born and was widely used in the United States during the era of 1950 to 1970, especially after the adoption of the fiberoptic cold light system, which gave far better illumination than the miniaturized incandescent bulb. During this era, it was not unusual at Johns Hopkins to have five or six patients per day listed in the operating room for a culdoscopic examination.

After about 1970, laparoscopy, with its fiberoptic cold light system, superseded the culdoscopic approach. About this time, operative laparoscopy blossomed, and one of the first widely used procedures was the ligation of the fallopian tubes by various techniques.

In Europe, in contrast to the United States, there was no great use of the culdoscope. The development of observational and operative laparoscopy continued uninterruptedly from about 1912, when, according to Cohen, the Swedish Hans Christian Jacobaeus described 109 laparoscopies in 69 patients using an electric cystoscope.

As previously mentioned, the historical details of procedures are included in the appropriate chapters. However, two general observations may be made.

First, developmental progress in endoscopy of the abdominal cavity has been a function of development of the physical sciences: optics, mechanics, electronics, etc. Thus, the current popular robotic laparoscopic procedures result not only from medical ingenuity but from the participation of the capitalistic industrial complex. The consequence of this is that the use of the laparoscopic instrumentation is greatly encouraged by commercial interests. The danger is—if there is a danger—that physicians may be unduly influenced by commercial as opposed to scientific priorities.

Second, the laparoscopic operative procedures have been widely adopted, often without randomized clinical trials to scientifically define and evaluate their role in operative gynecology.

These two points are made as an observation and not necessarily as a criticism, as the advantages of a shortened hospital stay and less patient discomfort are obvious. However, the fact is that there are few data on the short- and long-term results that are designed to evaluate results from laparoscopy with alternate procedures. The adoption of laparoscopic operative procedures progressed in spite of the recent emphasis on the importance of evidence-based medicine. Rock and Warshaw have elaborated on this aspect of operative laparoscopy.

Knowledge of the history of operative gynecology is not only of intrinsic interest but also allows us to appreciate our innovative predecessors and may stimulate some of us to be the subject of future historians.

OPERATIVE GYNECOLOGY, FIRST EDITION, 1946

Richard Wesley Te Linde was born in Wisconsin in 1894, and, except for the years that he attended a small liberal arts college in Holland, Michigan, he spent all his formative years in Wisconsin. When he was ready to go to medical school, he went to Madison, but in 1916, the University of Wisconsin had only a 2-year school. Te Linde completed the 2 preclinical years and then transferred to Johns Hopkins for the final 2 years. He graduated with the class of 1920 and spent the rest of his professional career associated with Hopkins, where he became chief of the gynecology division of the department of surgery and then chair of the separate department of gynecology in 1939. He held that post until his retirement in 1960, when the newly reunified department of obstetrics and gynecology was reestablished.

Just as his teacher Howard Kelly had felt the need to compile a textbook of operative gynecology half a century earlier, Te Linde believed that the many-sided specialty that gynecology had become by World War II required a new text. With Kelly's earlier text as a model, Te Linde wished to incorporate the vast changes that had occurred in the period separating the two books. During this 50-year span, there were changes in our knowledge of hormones, new surgical techniques, and the ability to visualize the abdominal and pelvic organs.

Te Linde chose the same simple title for his own text. Although Kelly's had been published by Appleton in New York, Te Linde chose Lippincott in Philadelphia. Gynecology, Te Linde wrote in the preface in 1946, was no longer to be considered simply a branch of general surgery. The gynecologist, he stressed, must still be a good surgeon but must also master the pathology of gynecologic disorders and the newly burgeoning field of endocrinology. New books were appearing in all these fields except gynecologic surgery, and it was this void that Te Linde wished to fill.

Te Linde wrote his text with the "… primary purpose of describing the technique of the usual and some of the rarer operative procedures. It also includes indications for and against operations as well as pre- and postoperative care of patients." Gynecologic pathology, Te Linde stressed in the Hopkins tradition, is the bedrock of good gynecologic surgery. "Without an understanding of it, surgery becomes merely a mechanical job, and errors in surgical judgment are inevitable." In the organization of his text and in the subsequent editions over the succeeding half century to the present edition, one can readily see important landmarks in the history of operative gynecology. Some of these were discussed in a previous section.

The 751-page first edition of 1946, all of it written by Te Linde, had a first printing of 5,000 copies, which quickly sold out. A second printing was equally successful. The reviews have always been laudatory. Of the sixth edition of 1985, edited by Richard Mattingly and John Thompson, the *Journal of the American Medical Association* reviewer ended by saying, "I cannot imagine any gynecologist who performs surgery doing without it, first as a primer and then as a reminder." By 1962, when the third edition appeared and Te Linde had retired from the chairmanship of his department, he decided that, like all the other major medical textbooks of the time, his book needed a group of authors to bring out new revisions. In the preface to that edition, he states that his book has never been simply a manual of surgical technique—that surgical philosophy is equally important. "What does it profit a woman if the operation is technically perfect and the procedure unnecessary or even harmful?" One reason unnecessary procedures still prevailed, Te Linde noted, was the lack of knowledge of gynecologic pathology, still the "bedrock upon which good surgery is done." Therefore, Te Linde justified including a considerable amount of pathology in his text. Pathology is what has differentiated gynecologic surgery from general surgery since Howard Kelly's years at the turn of the 20th century. Surgical texts, and by implication their surgical readers, have generally not devoted nearly as much attention to pathology as have gynecologists, some of whose leaders have actually been very well versed in pathology.

The fact that Te Linde could produce three editions, each larger than the first, is a testament to his broad knowledge of his field, his ability as a writer, and his stamina for hard work. He died in Baltimore in 1989 at the age of 95.

In the decades since the third edition of 1962, the world of medicine and the society in which it is practiced have seen much change. By the mid-1960s, when significant advances in the treatment of infections, malignancies, and hormonal disorders had become evident, these successes had an impact on gynecology just as they did in other areas of medicine. The reduction in mastoid infections, for instance, has changed the practice of the otolaryngologist considerably. In gynecology, the reduction in major pelvic inflammatory disease forced gynecologists to focus more of their attention on other disorders. Also affecting gynecologic surgery by the middle of this century were significant improvements in obstetric practices, which sharply reduced injuries to the bladder and rectum. Hysterectomies and suspensory operations were not performed for vague symptoms of illness as often as they had been.

We have also lived through social revolutions that have changed the way our society carries on its business and dispenses its social prerogatives. Especially prominent in the 1960s, a civil rights movement, greater concern for our environment, a resurgence of consumer rights, and a revitalized women's movement profoundly affected our social institutions, including medicine. Within medicine, no specialty has been more touched by these trends than obstetrics and gynecology.

The new feminism viewed abortion, childbirth, contraception, and gynecologic surgery as a means of social control of female patients by doctors, most of whom were men. The feminist movement challenged not only the domination of doctors but also the supposed benevolence of their knowledge and practices.

As the world has changed, so have our expectations. In the decades after the first edition of Te Linde's book appeared, when wonder drugs were touted as curing previously untreatable illnesses, the public began to expect much from its doctors, and we were not shy in claiming that ever-greater investments in medical research would lead to more cures. It is hardly surprising, then, that in these last few decades, as we began to spend increasing amounts of our gross national product for health, those who paid the bill became increasingly interested in seeing just what their money was actually buying. Like most other social institutions, medicine lost much of the autonomy it had for so long taken for granted. Although as a profession we did not always get all we wanted, we were for decades amazingly adept at preventing those things we did not want. Now, that, too, has changed, as has the practice of medicine.

The division of labor in all areas of medicine grew as the 20th century progressed. In the last decades of the century, what used to be called general practice became the specialty of family practice. In the Anglo-American world of the late 20th century, both obstetrics and gynecology were caught in the middle of the battles between specialists and generalists. Likewise, they became involved in the tensions among primary, secondary, and tertiary medical care. Similar strife occurred in earlier centuries among those vying for a place and for status among physicians caring for women in childbirth and in disease. If one looks at the table of contents of this edition and compares it with a simpler period of half a century or a century ago, one will see what great breadth the field of operative gynecology continues to enjoy.

BEST SURGICAL PRACTICES

- As Dr. Ignaz Semmelweis taught us, hand hygiene was and still is an important principle of antisepsis and infection control and prevention. Hand hygiene surveillance studies continue to show that there are opportunities for improvement in following nationally recognized guidelines for hand hygiene in all health care professionals, including gynecologic surgeons.
- Controversy and criticism inevitably follow the discovery of pioneering surgical principles and procedures. Bringing forth a new idea by publishing it in a peer-reviewed journal can bring balance and support to the introduction of a novel concept or other tangible contribution. Whereas Drs. Semmelweis, Long, and McDowell delayed publishing their discoveries, thus sometimes antagonizing those whom they might have convinced of the merits of their work, Drs. Sims, Kelly, Vesalius, and Virchow were quicker to publish their discoveries and accordingly were met with less resistance and more acceptance.
- Development and maintenance of an accredited office-based surgical facility can provide a safe, sanitary, and secure environment for performing many gynecologic procedures, thus avoiding scheduling problems and nosocomial infections that may be inherent in operating in an acute care facility.
- Involvement in community affairs and volunteerism, as practiced by Drs. Howard Kelly, Rudolf Virchow, and Andreas Vesalius, adds balance and fulfillment to the professional life of the operative gynecologist.

BIBLIOGRAPHY

Accreditation sought by growing number of Ob-Gyns for Ambulatory Surgery Centers. *ACOG Today* 2001;45:9.

Allen PM, Rock JA. *Social contract of academic medical centers to the community: an historical perspective*. 2013 [in press].

Allen P, Setze T. Howard Atwood Kelly, M.D. (1858–1943): his life and his enduring legacy. *South Med J* 1991;84:361.

Anderson EG. Sex in mind and education: a reply. *Fortn Rev* 1874; 15:582.

Beacham WD. The American Academy of Obstetrics and Gynecology: first presidential address. *Obstet Gynecol* 1953;1:115.

Bender GA. *Great moments in medicine: a history of medicine in pictures: Vesalius and the anatomy of man, 195–203, conquerors of pain: 202–215, Semmelweis: defender of motherhood 216–225, Rudolf Virchow and cellular pathology: 238–253, J. Marion Sims: gynecologic surgeon 254–263*. Detroit, MI: Parke-Davis, 1961.

Bernheim BM. Organoscopy. *Ann Surg* 1911;53:764.

Boldt HJ. The management of laparotomy patients and their modified after-treatment. *New York Med J* 1907;85:145.

Brieger GH. The development of surgery: historical aspects important in the origin and development of modern surgical science. In: Sabiston DC, ed. *Christopher's textbook of surgery*, 14th ed. Philadelphia, PA: WB Saunders, 1991:1.

Brieger GH. Early ambulation: a study in the history of surgery. *Ann Surg* 1983;197:443.

Brunschwig A. Whither gynecology? *Am J Obstet Gynecol* 1968; 100:122.

Cohen MR. *Laparoscopy, culdoscopy and gynecography*. Philadelphia, PA: WB Saunders, 1970:112.

Cullen TS. *Cancer of the uterus: its pathology, symptomatology, diagnosis, and treatment*. New York: Appleton, 1900.

Cullen TS. The evolution of gynecology. *Ohio State Med J* 1924; 20:484.

Cullen TS. The relation of obstetrics, gynecology and abdominal surgery to the public welfare. *JAMA* 1916;66:239.

Dally A. *Women under the knife: a history of surgery*. London, UK: Hutchinson Radius, 1991.

Davis A. *Dr. Kelly of Hopkins*. Baltimore, MD: The Johns Hopkins Press, 1959.

Decker A, Cherry TH. Culdoscopy: new method in diagnosis of pelvic disease—a preliminary report. *Am J Surg* 1944;64:40.

Dickinson RL. Original communications: a program for American Gynecology Society presidential address. *Am J Obstet Gynecol* 1921;1:2.

Ehrenreich B, English D. *For her own good: 150 years of the experts' advice to women*. Garden City, NY: Anchor Press/Doubleday, 1978.

Flexner JT. *Doctors on horseback, pioneers of American medicine. Chapter 3: A backwoods Galahad: Ephraim McDowell and Chapter 6: The Death of Pain: Crawford W. Long*. New York: Dover Publications, 1969.

Gusberg SB. An introduction to volume 1. *Gynecol Oncol* 1972;1:i.

Hahn R. *Sickness and health: an anthropological perspective*. New Haven, CT: Yale University Press, 1995:209.

Halsted WS. The employment of fine silk in preference to catgut and the advantages of transfixing tissues and vessels in controlling haemorrhage. *JAMA* 1913;60:1119.

Harris S. *Woman's surgeon: the life story of J. Marion Sims*. New York: Macmillan, 1950.

Jacobi MP. *A question of rest for women during menstruation*. London, UK: Smith & Elder, 1878.

Jones HW Jr, Jones GS, Ticknor WE. *Richard Wesley Te Linde*. Baltimore, MD: Williams & Wilkins, 1986.

Kelly HA. Getting up early after grave surgical operations. *Surg Gynecol Obstet* 1911;13:78.

Kelly HA. *History of gynecology in America: a cyclopedia of American medical biography*, 2 vols. Philadelphia, PA: WB Saunders, 1912:xxxix.

Kelly HA. *Medical gynecology*. New York: Appleton, 1912.

Kelly HA. *A scientific man and the bible*. New York: Harper and Bros, 1925.

Kelly HA. *Operative gynecology*. New York: Appleton, 1898.

Long ER. *A history of pathology, Chapter IX: Virchow and cellular pathology*. New York: Dover Publications, 1965:114.

Longo LD. The rise and fall of Battey's operation: a fashion in surgery. *Bull Hist Med* 1979;53:244.

Longyear HW. The relations of gynecology to general surgery, past and present. *JAMA* 1917;69:501.

Martin FH. Surgery, gynecology, and obstetrics. *Surg Gynecol Obstet* 1905;1:62.

Maudsley H. Sex in mind and on education. *Fortn Rev* 1874;15:466.

McDowell E. Extirpation of diseased ovaria. *Eclectic Repertory* 1817;7:742 [reprinted in Brieger GH, ed. *Medical America in the nineteenth century*. Baltimore: The Johns Hopkins Press, 1972].

McGregor DK. *From midwives to medicine: the birth of American gynecology*. New Brunswick, MJ: Rutgers University Press, 1989.

Meigs JV. *Progress in gynecology: fifty years of surgical progress, 1905–1955*. Chicago: The Franklin H. Martin Memorial Foundation, 1955 [reprinted from Davis L, ed. *Surgery: gynecology and obstetrics with international abstracts of surgery*].

Morantz R. The lady and her physician. In: Hartman M, Banner L, eds. *Clio's consciousness raised: new perspectives on the history of women*. New York: Harper & Row, 1974:38.

Morantz-Sanchez R. *Conduct unbecoming a woman: medicine on trial in turn-of-the-century Brooklyn*. New York: Oxford University Press, 1999.

Morantz-Sanchez R. Making it in a man's world: the late nineteenth-century surgical career of Mary Amanda Dixon Jones. *Bull Hist Med* 1995;69:542.

Moscucci O. *The science of woman: gynaecology and gender in England 1800–1929*. Cambridge: Cambridge University Press, 1990:30.

O'Dowd MJ, Philipp EE. *The history of obstetrics and gynecology*. New York: Parthenon Publishing Group, 1994.

Ricci JV. *The development of gynaecological surgery and instruments*. Philadelphia, PA: Blakiston, 1949.

Ries E. Some radical changes in the after-treatment of celiotomy cases. *JAMA* 1899;33:454.

Robinson J. *Tom Cullen of Baltimore*. London, UK: Oxford University Press, 1949.

Rock JA, Jeffrey RW. The history and future of operative laparoscopy. *Am J Obstet Gynecol* 1994;170:7.

Rock JA, Johnson TRB, Woodruff JD, eds. *The first 100 years: Department of Gynecology and Obstetrics of the Johns Hopkins Hospital*. Baltimore, MD: The Johns Hopkins University Press, 1991.

Russett CE. *Sexual science: the Victorian construction of womanhood*. Cambridge, MA: Harvard University Press, 1989.

Sims JM. On the treatment of vesico-vaginal fistula. *Am J Med Sci* 1852;23:59.

Sims JM. *Silver sutures in surgery*. The Anniversary Discourse, the New York Academy of Medicine. New York: S&W Wood, 1858.

Sims JM. *The story of my life*. New York: Appleton, 1884 [reprinted by Dacapo Press, 1968].

Simpson JY. *Hospitalism: its effects on the results of surgical operations*. Edinburgh: Oliver Boyd, 1869.

Speert H. *Obstetrics and gynecology in America*. Chicago, IL: American College of Obstetricians and Gynecologists, 1980.

Temkin O, trans. *Soranus' gynecology*. Baltimore, MD: The Johns Hopkins Press, 1956.

Thomas TG. A century of American medicine, 1776–1876: obstetrics and gynecology. *Am J Med Sci* 1876;72:138.

Webster JC. The future of gynecology. *Surg Gynecol Obstet* 1905;1:63.

Wells TS. Some causes of excessive mortality after surgical operations. *BMJ* 1864;2:384 [see also Brieger G. American surgery and the germ theory of disease. *Bull Hist Med* 1966;40:135].

Wertz RW, Wertz DC. *Lying-in: a history of childbirth in America*, expanded edition. New Haven, CT: Yale University Press, 1989.

Wood AD. The fashionable diseases: women's complaints and their treatment in nineteenth century America. *J Interdisc Hist* 1973;4:25 [reprinted in Hartman M, Banner L, eds. *Clio's consciousness raised: new perspectives on the history of women*. New York: Harper & Row, 1974:1].

CHAPTER 2
The Ethics of Pelvic Surgery

Mindy S. Christianson and Edward E. Wallach

DEFINITIONS

Autonomy—The concept describing an individual's self-determination and the right to direct his or her own life through his or her own decisions, actions, and beliefs.

Beneficence—The duty to do good on the behalf of others through an active promotion of the good of the patient and shelter from harm.

Informed consent—A process of communication between a physician and a patient that addresses the risks, benefits, and alternatives of a proposed medical intervention while meeting the core criteria of competence, exchange of information, understanding of exchanged information, and voluntary authorization.

Nonmaleficence—Literally translated as "do no harm," this concept describes the need both to prevent harm and to refrain from harmful acts.

THEORY AND PRACTICE OF ETHICS IN MEDICINE

The practice of medicine is governed by a system of beliefs that guide the actions of physicians and other health care professionals to act and make decisions that are regarded as ethically acceptable. Throughout the practice of medicine, different sets of standards and concepts of ethically acceptable behavior have existed as the predominant code for health care professionals. Codes such as those set by the Hippocratic oath served as the mainstay of professional behavior for centuries until a different system took its place in the first half of the 20th century. This transition reflects changing societal values of health and well-being that evolved over time as a result of political, cultural, scientific, and technologic advancement.

The field of bioethics emerged in the 1950s. Before that time, ethical principles of the Hippocratic oath were regarded as the ethical standards for medicine. The guiding principle of physician action was primum non nocere—first do no harm. In the Hippocratic tradition, the model of paternalism structured the therapeutic relationship. The physician was designated as the most qualified person to make decisions about treatment options for a patient. As such, it was the physician's judgment that determined what was to be considered as harm or benefit resulting from a medical procedure, not that of the patient or the patient's family. This convention was based on the belief that only an expert in science and medicine was qualified enough to make the best choice among treatment options for patients. During a time when medical therapies were limited and choices were few, this approach was not viewed as problematic to patient care. However, as changes in society, science, and medicine unfolded, patients and the general public began to question these traditional views of the physician–patient relationship.

With the introduction of significant scientific and cultural revolutions that characterized the post–World War II period in the United States, these standards set by the Hippocratic oath were considered to be ineffectual to meet the growing demands of medicine and ethics. Movements advancing civil rights, women's issues, and the growing recognition of individual rights and autonomy dominated the social climate. Carried over into medicine and science, a new set of health care innovations introduced new moral debates to society and the medical profession about the purpose of medical care, the definition of health, and the ability of mankind to regulate the physiology of the human body. The birth control pill, organ transplant, and dialysis are just a few examples of the significant life-altering innovations of the time. The ethical questions raised in response to the cultural and scientific climate challenged the previous notions of ethical behavior of physicians. In particular, the notion that physicians were the most appropriate members in the therapeutic relationship to make choices for the patient was rejected. Decisions about the vast array of available medical therapies and choices seemed inherently incongruent with the concept of paternalism. With the rise in the importance of autonomy and individual rights, society campaigned to replace the paternalistic structure of medicine with a model that established the patient as the primary decision maker.

This movement resulted in the establishment of a system of principle-based ethics as the driving force behind modern medicine. In 1977, the Belmont Report outlined what these principles or standards should be. This massive effort to reshape modern bioethics resulted in the establishment of the following principles as the cornerstone of contemporary medical ethics: autonomy, beneficence, nonmaleficence, and justice.

Autonomy—The concept of autonomy embodies the ideal of self-determination—that a person shapes his or her own life through his or her own decisions, actions, and beliefs. As such, individuals have the right to make decisions about their lives that reflect their own beliefs of well-being and values. Inherent in the principle of autonomy is the requirement that others (i.e., physicians) must respect a patient's right of self-determination.

Nonmaleficence—Nonmaleficence, defined as "do no harm," has its origins in the original tenets of the Hippocratic oath. This principle encompasses the need both to prevent harm and to refrain from harmful acts.

Beneficence—The definition of the principle of beneficence is to do good on the behalf of others. In the case of the principle of beneficence, physicians are expected to actively promote the good of the patient, not just shelter him or her from harm. Though this may seem to be a subtle distinction from the principle of nonmaleficence, it is critical to the principle-based theory of ethics, as it requires the performance of positive acts to advance the well-being of others.

Justice—The principle of justice addresses the need to treat all persons fairly. In the case of health care, this pertains to both the physician–patient relationship and the public health obligations of physicians in the allocation of scarce medical resources.

In this principle-based ethics model, all four core elements hold, in theory, equal importance. In many of the clinical situations that physicians routinely address, these elements may seem to be in conflict with one another. The solution to complex ethical dilemmas requires the balancing of these principles and, oftentimes, a prioritization of one over the others. An example of this is in an emergent medical situation when the principle of beneficence may temporarily overrule autonomy. However these principles are weighted, they must ultimately be used in a way that results in medical choices serving the good of the patient by reflecting his or her values and beliefs.

Though the system of principle-based ethics as established by the Belmont Report is the forerunner of ethical standards of behavior in modern medicine, other legitimate models of bioethical theory exist. They are broad in nature and are guiding principles, but all come from the view that the system of principle-based ethics does not offer enough to guide behavior in the complex setting of health care. Two examples of this are feminist ethics and casuistry. Feminist ethics is based on the notion that decisions are made in the context of relationships and personal virtues, such as compassion, friendship, and love. Principle-based ethics does not take these factors into consideration, neglecting the problems raised in a society in which men and women are not viewed as equals, and, as a result, does not serve the true interests of the patient. A second example is casuistry, or case-based ethics. This theory is founded on the principle that moral lessons gained from the resolution of actual cases in medicine have more value than do a set of theoretic and unchanging principles. Using this model, ethical reasoning results from weighing the outcomes of real cases as examples and forming a set of modifiable principles from those conclusions. These are just two examples of the diversity of ethical theories that guide medicine and serve as solutions to ethical puzzles that cannot be solved using the standard principle-based ethics commonly in place today.

The very nature of the field of obstetrics and gynecology sets the stage for a variety of ethical dilemmas. Issues surrounding the beginnings of human life and reproductive function naturally facilitate profound and often controversial questions and debate. In addition, the women's rights movement has raised other issues specific to the care of women, such as subjugation and control of women's bodies through society and medicine. Despite this broad range of issues, ethical discussions in obstetrics and gynecology have often been perceived in terms of a single controversial issue: abortion. Yet, the field of bioethics in women's health has a rich and broad set of important implications for the practice of medicine and the health of women. Recent advances in medicine and science have introduced novel therapeutic options to many of the conditions that gynecologists face, such as cervical cancer, uterine fibroids, and infertility. Genetic and pharmaceutical therapies, new diagnostic modalities, noninvasive surgical options, and the emergence of assisted reproductive technologies, including in vitro fertilization, set the stage for a multitude of multifaceted ethical questions and debates. This chapter will present some of the foundational concepts in bioethics and women's health that serve as a launching point for addressing the more complex and novel ethical issues as they arise in the present setting of medicine and the future.

AUTONOMY AND INFORMED CONSENT

Informed consent is a mechanism whereby the autonomy of a patient is recognized, respected, and preserved in health care decisions. It is the result of a process whereby a patient makes a voluntary decision to proceed with a medical intervention with a sound understanding of the benefits and risks of the procedure, as well as alternative therapies if the procedure is declined. The respect of informed consent has two purposes. On the one hand, the process of achieving informed consent respects and recognizes the patient's autonomy. On the other hand, patients benefit when they make decisions on their own behalf because they themselves are most familiar with their own values, beliefs, and ideas of well-being and health. When patients make informed and voluntary decisions about their health care, they can make choices that meet their own concept of what's good and what's beneficial.

The term *informed consent* has legal and ethical dimensions. Legally, informed consent can be viewed as an end point. The legal requirements of informed consent are met when the conversation between the physician and the patient is documented, either on an informed consent form or in the medical record. Often, getting a signature on a form is synonymous with achieving informed consent, but informed decision making goes well beyond the legal form. Ethically, informed decision making involves a process of communication between the physician and the patient through which the patient is able to make an autonomous decision either to authorize the intervention (informed consent) or reject it (informed refusal).

The legal and ethical dimensions of informed consent are often used interchangeably but can have very different meanings and implications. Unfortunately, the function and meaning of informed consent is often misinterpreted, and it is viewed primarily as a legal document with a patient's signature denoting full understanding and authorization. It is important to keep in mind that both the legal and ethical requirements of informed consent are essential in health care. However, as important legal documentation is, it should not be placed before the ethical duties to the patient. Legal documentation in a chart or on a form does not substitute for the process of communication and autonomous decision making. Not all legal documents with a patient's signature reflect that an adequate informed consent process has taken place.

A valid informed consent is both informed and autonomously authorized. To achieve this, the physician must ensure that five core components are met in the decision-making process: (a) competence, (b) voluntariness, (c) disclosure, (d) understanding, and (e) authorization or refusal. These core components serve as a guide for physicians when discussing medical interventions with patients to ensure that a patient makes the most appropriate decision possible. Without satisfying all five of these core components, an adequate informed consent process has not been achieved.

Competence

In the usual clinical setting, other than situations involving formal psychiatric evaluation, the determination of competence tends to be more of a working judgment than a formal assessment. Beauchamp and Childress describe decision-making capacity as follows: "Although the properties most crucial to the determination of competence are controversial, in biomedical contexts a person has generally been viewed as competent if able to understand a therapy or research procedure, to deliberate regarding major risks and benefits, and to make a decision in light of this deliberation."

Voluntariness

Ethically valid informed consent can only be obtained through the voluntary authorization by a patient for a medical intervention. It is not sufficient merely to meet the criteria of decision-making capacity, disclosure, and understanding. The patient must be able to use this information to formulate a decision that is not controlled by others. If a patient is manipulated or coerced into making a decision, then valid informed consent will not have been achieved.

Disclosure

Autonomous decision making must be made in the context of information about the medical intervention. The physician must disclose sufficient information that allows the patient to make an informed decision reflecting his or her beliefs and values, including the risks, benefits, and alternatives of the proposed medical intervention. The core of ethical disclosure is about facilitating the patient's autonomous choice to accept or reject health care. Although there is no definitive rule about how much information should be given to the patient, a valid informed consent does not require that the patient be informed of every conceivable risk that could occur, no matter how remote or how trivial. Listing risks, either verbally or in writing, that do not have applicability to the patient does not promote autonomy. Instead, a balance must be achieved between the patient and the physician to determine how much information and detail is necessary for the patient to make a meaningful decision.

Understanding

The patient must make a decision based on an understanding of the information provided. It is not sufficient to mention or list the possible risks to an intervention. The patient must comprehend the ramifications of these risks when considering whether to proceed with an intervention. The physician must be certain to convey information about the risks, including the possible procedures involved to address a bad outcome if it occurs. The patient should then be able to weigh the risks and the benefits of the procedure in his or her own terms.

Authorization

The corollary of informed consent is informed refusal. Informed refusal is the decision of the patient to decline the proposed medical intervention. The respect for the patient's autonomy that is implicit in informed consent extends to the choice to refuse treatment, even when the decision is made against the recommendation of the physician. Informed refusal can be as minor as refusing a simple elective procedure to refusing life-saving treatments. A patient may refuse treatment for a variety of reasons. One reason may be that the intervention or the outcome is misaligned with his or her concept of good. For example, a patient may refuse a medical therapy because he or she believes it to be harmful or incongruous with his or her personal beliefs (e.g., blood transfusion refusal for a Jehovah's Witness).

A balance must be met between respect for the autonomy of the patient and the physician's duty to beneficence. It is the job of the physician to be as certain as possible that this decision is informed and consistent with the values and beliefs of the patient. In situations when the refusal may result in significant impairment, pain, or death, the physician should make every attempt to ensure that these decisions are consistent with the patient's beliefs and have been so over time. Physicians may still be considering their patient's best interest by giving preference to his or her spiritual or personal convictions over the medical good. Another important aspect of informed refusal is that it can occur either at the initiation of a treatment or later during the course of the treatment. This becomes apparent when a patient refuses to continue a treatment or undergo a similar or identical intervention. The willingness of the patient to undergo a therapy in the past does not mean that consent is implied in the future.

Under certain circumstances, a physician must proceed with a medical intervention without the informed consent of the patient. Generally, these circumstances involve emergent situations. For example, the patient may be suddenly incapacitated or unconscious and therefore incapable of providing any sort of autonomous authorization. Alternatively, the patient may be conscious and otherwise able to make decisions but, because of the emergent and critical nature of her condition, it is medically necessary to initiate an immediate intervention,

and there is no time to engage in a discussion with the patient. In the first situation, there may be time to obtain authorization from an appropriate family member or designated medical decision maker. In the second situation (and sometimes in the first), there is no time, and the physician must make a decision on behalf of the patient. This decision should be made based on what is judged to be in the best medical interest of the patient and usually assumes most people would opt on the side of instituting lifesaving measures.

Informed consent plays a vital role in the practice of obstetrics and gynecology because this field of medicine pertains to the anatomy and function of a woman's reproductive system and sexuality. Issues specific to women's health have been brought to the forefront because of concerns of historical control and subjugation of women and their bodies through society and medicine. In addition, there is a growing trend to recognize the vital role of relationships in a patient's medical decision making with respect to reproductive issues. Patients rarely make decisions about their sexuality and reproduction in a vacuum but instead do so within the context of relationships with others, whether friends, partners, or families. It is critical to recognize these qualities inherent in obstetrics and gynecology when obtaining informed consent for a medical therapy or procedure to maximize the autonomous expression of the patient's personal preferences.

ETHICAL ISSUES IN SURGICAL TRAINING

Competence of the surgeon is a moral commitment to the patient, especially before undertaking a novel surgical procedure. Adequate preparation in the basic and clinical sciences and training in surgical techniques must have been accomplished before any new surgical procedure is introduced into clinical medicine. An overenthusiastic rush into the use of a procedure is exemplified by the sudden popularity of cardiac transplantation in the 1960s. The preparatory laboratory work in cardiac transplantation started in 1905, but the first successful replacement of the heart in a dog took place in 1960. Immune suppression, which is crucial to the procedure, was introduced in 1958, and longtime survival of grafts occurred by 1965. Christian Barnard reported the first successful human heart transplantation in December 1967 in South Africa. By the end of 1968, 101 human heart transplantations had been performed by 64 surgical groups in 22 countries. Most patients improved briefly and then died of rejection of the transplant or infections. In 2 years, the procedure was largely discredited, and it took more than 10 additional years to reestablish wide acceptance of the operation. This experience illustrates the need to limit difficult and complex procedures to specialized centers that have the resources and adequately trained surgeons to perform them.

This is equally true for complex pelvic surgery. The adoption of subspecialty boards by the American Board of Obstetrics & Gynecology, each with requirements for postresidency fellowship training and evaluation standards for certification, has helped to emphasize the need for specialized training in surgical techniques for pelvic surgeons. The rapid expansion of the use of robotic surgery training procedures prompts the responsibility for providing future gynecologists who are technically skilled to serve society effectively and safely. In addition to underlying knowledge, clinical experience, training, and practice, the competent surgeon operates with the attentiveness and focus commensurate with the surgical theater. Indeed, legitimate concerns regarding the potential impairment of overfatigued house staff managing and operating on patients have led to changes in house staff work hours and training.

Training programs are now charged with the simultaneous challenge of vigilantly protecting the welfare of their patients from potentially suboptimal care while ensuring that their surgeons, after completion of training, operate competently under emergent and suboptimal conditions.

Many surgeons trained before World War II participated in residency programs affiliated with large inner-city hospitals where patients without adequate resources or health insurance received care. It was accepted that these patients would receive treatment or even surgery by physicians-in-training (including senior medical students, interns, and residents), preferably under the supervision of skilled volunteers or paid clinical faculty and only when the trainee had reached the necessary level of competence. When health care became an entitlement under Medicare and Medicaid government-funded health insurance became more prevalent, many patients sought the services of private physicians. The so-called free care or resident services were often unable to recruit sufficient patients to provide adequate training for new surgeons. This was particularly true in pelvic surgery; given the choice, these patients sought refuge from the clinic, where privacy and dignity were hard to maintain, and fled in large numbers to private doctors' offices. Surgical teaching thereafter often involved the private patient, with the resident now performing complete procedures under the supervision and assistance of the patient's private physician. This arrangement potentially left patients either poorly informed or uninformed about the participation of physicians-in-training. This arrangement often became apparent when complications arose or the medical records were reviewed during litigation. Although patients are typically better informed now, it remains ethically necessary to inform them about teaching or training in each case so that objections can be dealt with before the planned procedure. Most surgeons involved in teaching programs inform their patients that surgery demands a team effort and that residents may be involved in assisting or operating with them, but that, as the private surgeons of record, they not only will be present but also will be in charge and responsible for everything that takes place during the procedure. Teaching should not take place in the operating room without such a disclosure and the patient's informed consent in this regard. The resident's role, status, and experience should be clear to the patient. We are long past the era of introducing medical students to patients as doctors rather than revealing their actual status.

Because of the limitation on the number of hours a doctor-in-training may work, producing competent surgeons today has become even more challenging than in the past. This situation has necessitated approaches to supplement and amplify the residency program specifically as it affects surgical training. Novel training methods designed to accelerate the learning curve have been devised. These are directed at familiarizing the trainee with instrumentation and the handling of surgical instruments, improving manual dexterity, sharpening hand–eye coordination, and heightening awareness of pelvic anatomy. In addition, decision-making skills and essentials of emergency management need to be developed during the course of residency training. One valuable approach in use is the animal surgical laboratory, for instance, using pigs for training in laparoscopic surgery. Obviously, the size of structures in laboratory animals does not precisely simulate that in humans, and anatomic relationships do not reflect those of a human patient. Simulation training has expanded in residency training. For example, computer simulators have been developed to enhance resident training in laparoscopic and robotic surgery. Simulators for endoscopic surgical procedures use mannequins or human models. Fabricated pelvic models are also frequently used to heighten skills for practicing maneuvers for normal and operative delivery. These innovative exercises assist in preparing the student for experiences encountered in the operating room and may even succeed in refreshing the already practicing surgeon in performance of specific techniques. Simulated programs have also been developed that incorporate computerized lessons for improving history-taking skills and for simulating emergency management in the form of skill stations. The final arbiter for gaining surgical skills is the surgical procedure itself, carried out in actual patients under the guidance and supervision of an accomplished surgeon who has the ability to communicate effectively about both the procedure and techniques. The only way to learn to manage surgical complexities adroitly is through personal experience while under the direct tutelage of a preceptor who has previously experienced unplanned occurrences. In addition to foundational medical and surgical knowledge, clinical experience, training, and practice, the competent physicians must act in a responsible and professional manner, whether in the clinical or surgical setting. Impairment of a physician's skills must be fully evaluated so that he or she may be given assistance to improve and injury to his or her patients is avoided. Health care institutions must have peer-accessible mechanisms in place to facilitate this process.

EXAMINATION UNDER ANESTHESIA

Concern arose several years ago that medical students were performing preoperative pelvic examinations on anesthetized patients without having obtained specific prior consent. Because of public concern, both the American Congress of Obstetricians and Gynecologists (ACOG) and the Association of American Medical Colleges (AAMC) released statements emphasizing the predominance of patient autonomy and appropriate informed consent over the exigencies of medical education.

In actual practice, examination under anesthesia (EUA) is routinely performed only by members of the surgical team to enable better appreciation of the patient's pelvic anatomy. The surgical team typically numbers between one to four members; at its largest, it includes an attending surgeon, senior resident, junior resident/intern, and medical student. Although the major portions of the surgery are performed by the senior experienced surgeons, the junior assistants, such as the medical student, perform the essential and ancillary tasks of retraction, exposure, and minor suturing.

An ACOG committee opinion issued in 2011 noted: "If a pelvic examination that is planned for an anesthetized woman undergoing surgery offers her no personal benefit and is performed solely for teaching purposes, it should be performed only with her specific informed consent, obtained when she has full decision-making capacity." One can legitimately argue that all surgeons and surgical assistants, including the medical student, require maximum appreciation of the surgical field to optimize their performances during the procedure. Accordingly, the pelvic examinations should not be construed as offering "no personal benefit" to the patient. Furthermore, the EUA should not be considered as separate from the procedure itself but as a necessary adjunct. This ability of the members of the house staff, who provide intraoperative and postoperative assistance, should not be curtailed by exclusion from an essential component of the gynecologic procedure.

At least three steps can be taken to ensure that the rights of the patient are respected while ensuring appropriate surgical care: (a) explicitly incorporating the EUA on the operative consent form, (b) openly discussing with the patient the importance and participation of all team members in the EUA, and (c) ensuring an atmosphere of patient respect and dignity by agreeing in advance to a specific, limited number of pelvic examinations.

MEDICAL LEGAL ASPECTS OF GYNECOLOGIC CARE

Obstetricians and gynecologists pay among the highest premiums for professional liability insurance of all medical specialties. In many states, this factor has led to early retirement, elimination of obstetrical and/or surgical procedures from practice, or relocation to another state. Being named in a malpractice suit leads to endless hours of effort unrelated to medical practice, undesired anxiety, and, in some instances, withdrawal from practice. A number of factors contribute to the cost of insurance coverage. Obstetricians and gynecologists can exercise control over some of these factors to minimize the chances of being cited in a claim. Two simple principles are helpful in preventing a legal claim or in providing a defense should a claim be filed. These two concepts form the basis of all risk-management and loss-prevention strategies. Plaintiff and defense attorneys have reached consensus that these two factors, documentation and communication, improve the odds that a lawsuit will not be filed or that a lawsuit, once filed, can be successfully defended.

By way of documentation, the following basic and simple initiatives should be a component of each physician's protocol for charting and record keeping.

1. Recording of date and time of each entry in the chart
2. Legible handwriting
3. Contemporary entry of all notes in the chart
4. Appropriate correction of inaccurate entries
5. Avoidance of conflict among physicians and nurses in the charting of patient information
6. When using electronic medical records, individualization of each entry instead of "cutting and pasting" prior notes, especially when using templates, which are becoming more commonly utilized

The alacrity with which a physician responds to a patient's symptom or concerns can be established with certainty if notes are complete, properly dated, and timed. This chronology is instrumental in establishing a timeline for a patient's care and will be more credible in a courtroom or in a hearing than a plaintiff's client's recollection weeks or months after the fact. Because an adverse surgical outcome is not synonymous with negligence, expression of reasons for clinical judgment in choice of a diagnosis or treatment plan demonstrates that alternatives have been considered by the physician. The physician should document these alternatives in the chart and indicate that they were each discussed with the patient before treatment.

Entries in the chart should clearly demonstrate the course of care rendered and rationale underlying the choice of a specific treatment plan. If handwritten, notes should be legible and interpretable by anyone who reviews the chart. An inability to read one's own handwriting can only negatively affect the physician's credibility. The time frame of management is crucial, and prompt recording of events will prevent doubt when events occurring before a complication are documented only after the complication has occurred. Notations regarding telephone conversations with consulting physicians or family members should also be entered in the chart with the date and time of contact. Similarly, electronic mail correspondences

with patients should be part of the medical record. An incorrect entry in the chart should be corrected properly by striking out the erroneous entry and initialing and dating the changes. If a supplemental note is written, it should be listed as an addendum. A patient's chart should not be used as a vehicle for expressing opinions on the intelligence of or decision rendered by another health care provider or for the purpose of criticism.

When an unanticipated adverse event occurs, the insurance company or risk-management representative should be notified promptly. The communication of a physician with legal and/or insurance representatives and health care providers is important in anticipating legal problems. However, a cornerstone of medical care is the physician's sensitivity in communicating with the patient with understanding and compassion. She should be given ample time to ask questions, and these inquires should be answered truthfully. Breakdown of communications in the patient–physician relationship is a recurring theme in the pathway leading to litigation.

A physician may appear in court to testify in three possible scenarios: as a *defendant*, as a *material witness*, or as an *expert witness* on behalf of either the plaintiff or the defendant. Although each instance has its unique aspects, in all cases, the physician will have an opportunity to prepare the testimony with the attorney who is representing him/her. As a *defendant* at either a sworn deposition or in a courtroom, the physician will have received general and specific instructions from the attorney representing him/her with regard to how to respond to questions. Each response should be concise, to the point, and directed only at the specific question raised by the plaintiff's attorney. Most of all, the answers must be honest and forthright, as well as accurate with respect to the patient's clinical course and management as described in the medical records. The defendant should request the opportunity to view the medical record at any time should there be need to recall specific details such as dates, times, and sequences of events.

A physician may be called as a *material witness* because of his/her association with the specific case as a participant or observer, but not as a defendant. The same principles of deportment apply as for an appearance as a defendant. The material witness testifies on the facts of the case and should not express opinions that require personal expertise.

The physician who chooses to serve as an *expert witness* is called on to do so because of his/her personal experience and training with the particular clinical situation under consideration. The role of an expert witness carries with it significant responsibilities. First and foremost is the possession of knowledge, skills, and experience to fulfill this role. Second, the expert witness should be objective and unbiased and able to discuss standards of care on a broad scale rather than be constrained by his/her personal approach. It is clearly unethical for an expert witness to lack the appropriate credentials and/or to misrepresent the standard of care reflected in the case for which he/she is testifying. Fundamentally, *standard of care* refers to a level of care that is generally thought to represent the norm. Standard of care rendered in specific conditions may differ from one locale or group of physicians to another, simply because standards are arbitrarily developed and not universally held. If an adverse event occurs, a distinction must be made between a bad outcome that is independent of the quality of rendered care and a bad outcome that is clearly due to negligence or to substandard care.

A number of safeguards exist to protect patients from faulty or unethical clinical practice. At the local level, hospital credentials committees, as required by the Joint Commission on Accreditation of Hospitals and Health Care Organizations, are given the responsibility for reviewing the credentials of applicants for initial and continuing staff privileges. This responsibility mandates attention to the volume of cases attended per annum and the quality of care rendered. Privileges can be curtailed for performance of specific procedures or may be suspended for practice in general in cases in which the physician provides inappropriate care or exhibits ethical infractions. The American Board of Obstetrics & Gynecology (ABOG) credentials specialists and subspecialists on the basis of training, experience, and performance on examinations. Over the past three decades, a periodic reexamination is required for maintenance of specialty certification. This maintenance-of-certification (MOC) process involves evaluation of performance on didactic examinations and assessment of cognitive skills. In addition, physicians take MOC tests to maintain board certification and earn continuing medical education (CME) credits. Recently, the Accreditation Council for Graduate Medical Education or ACGME and the American Board of Medical Specialties (ABMS) have stressed the importance of education and achievement of six core competencies (patient care, medical knowledge, communication skills, professionalism, practice-based learning and improvement, and systems-based practice). In addition, certifying boards require proof of licensure in good standing for certification and recertification. State medical societies are empowered to review patients' complaints and charges of unethical behavior of licensees. The National Practitioner Data Bank receives and makes available data regarding infractions of practice standards. This device was established by Congress to prevent physicians with past disciplinary action and malpractice awards from relocating from one state to another without detection.

Unfortunately, there are too few safeguards aside from collegial observation that can monitor surgical technique and/or interaction with patients. The responsibility of the physician requires introspection and candor, especially when factors such as physical and mental impairment or substance abuse infringe on the physician's ability to practice safely and effectively. Currently, there is no formal assessment of surgical skills. Professionalism is implicit in day-to-day behavior and self-assessment. A *New England Journal of Medicine* report (Papadakis et al., 2005) addressed the association of disciplinary action against physicians with unprofessional behavior in medical school and emphasized the importance of professionalism as a core competency. The report's conclusion was that disciplinary action among practicing physicians by state medical licensing boards correlated strongly with a history of unprofessional behavior in medical school. The strongest association was in those who had demonstrated irresponsible behavior or diminished ability to improve their behavior as students earlier on.

PRIVACY AND THE HEALTH INSURANCE PORTABILITY AND ACCOUNTABILITY ACT

In 1996, Congress passed the Health Insurance Portability and Accountability Act (HIPAA), establishing minimal national standards to ensure confidentiality of protected health information (also referred to as *individually identifiable health information*). This move was due, in part, to the mainstream use of electronic technology in health care, which promoted concern over patient confidentiality. The subsequent additions to the original HIPAA provisions included the Privacy Rules, extending jurisdiction to health plans, billing services, hospitals, and individual health care providers. At the time of compliance deadlines, all of these covered entities were required to implement the established standards to protect patients' individually identifiable health information. The caveat to

the Privacy Rules was that the protection of patients' privacy could not negatively interfere with the quality of care or create unnecessary burdens to patient care.

Quoting from the guidelines published by the Centers for Disease Control and Prevention and the U.S. Department of Health and Human Services (DHHS), the HIPAA Privacy Rule:

- Gives patients more control over their health information
- Sets boundaries on the use and release of health records
- Establishes appropriate safeguards that the majority of health care providers and others must achieve to protect the privacy of health information
- Holds violators accountable with civil and criminal penalties that can be imposed if they violate patients' privacy rights
- Strikes a balance when public health responsibilities support disclosure of certain forms of data
- Enables patients to make informed choices based on how individual health information may be used
- Enables patients to find out how their information may be used and what disclosures of their information have been made
- Generally limits release of information to the minimum reasonably needed for the purpose of the disclosure
- Generally gives patients the right to obtain a copy of their own health records and request corrections
- Empowers individuals to control certain uses and disclosures of their health information

The complexity of the HIPAA regulations has made their implementation challenging and controversial. Specific confusion regarding disclosures to family members abounds, particularly in cases when the patient has authorized his or her family to be an active participant in health care. This also arises among health care providers when seeking information about their patients to provide continuity of care. Ultimately, HIPAA does afford latitude for professional judgment as to the "best interests" of the particular patient, so long as the disclosures conform to the "minimum necessary standards." In addition, the Privacy Rule does not replace federal or state laws and makes an allowance for individual institutions to adopt more stringent policies to protect patients' privacy.

CONFIDENTIALITY

The foundation of the physician–patient relationship is trust. This is based on two premises: that a patient has the right to privacy and respect of privacy allows for patients to disclose the necessary information to their physician. This is particularly relevant in gynecology, in which patients share sensitive information with their physicians about intimacy and sexuality. For this reason, confidentiality is one of the most essential aspects to the successful therapeutic relationship.

It is the exception, more than the rule, for patient confidentiality to be violated. Tension and ambiguity, however, have long surrounded the parameters wherein breaches of patient confidentiality are justified. The Code of Ethics of the American Medical Association (AMA), revised in 1957, stated: "A physician may not reveal the confidences entrusted to him in the course of medical attendance, or the deficiencies he may observe in the character of patients, unless he is required to do so by law or unless it becomes necessary to protect the welfare of the individual or of the community." Exceptions to the breach of confidentiality include times when the withholding of information may harm a third party or threaten public health. Mandatory exceptions include cases of violence and violent crime and the negligence and abuse of individuals, including women, children, and the elderly. Some states also require mandatory reporting of infectious diseases that may pose a serious public health risk, such as certain sexually transmitted diseases and tuberculosis. A notable case of the need to violate patient confidentiality is *Tarasoff v. Regents of the University of California*. In this case, a court found the University of California negligent for failing to forewarn murder victim Tatiana Tarasoff and her family after Prosenjit Poddar confided in one of his therapists that he intended to kill her. Two months after the temporary detainment of Poddar for this initial threat, he acted on it by murdering Tarasoff. As the majority opinion in the 1976 Tarasoff case emphasized: "The protective privilege ends where the public peril begins."

Gynecologists are confronted with a variety of complex and difficult scenarios in the clinical and surgical arenas when it comes to maintaining or breaking patient confidentiality. In this setting, physicians must balance their legal obligations with their medical obligations of trust to the patient. Challenging and not uncommon conflicts of patient confidentiality occur in obstetrics. An example is when a woman seeks a pregnancy termination or sterilization procedure while requesting confidentiality from her partner. Counseling such a patient, especially after having attained her trust and confidence, may help defuse the situation. Yet, physicians must keep their duty to the patient and her confidentiality in mind before acting in situations such as this. When in doubt, either over personal convictions or professional duties, a hospital ethics committee may be required to intervene. Ultimately, however, in the absence of a countervailing public health or legal mandate, the obligation of patient confidentiality predominates.

ETHICAL ISSUES IN RESEARCH ON HUMAN SUBJECTS

Although the Nuremberg medical war crimes trials of Nazi doctors and the ensuing Nuremberg Code in 1949 represent a landmark in research ethics involving human subjects, they made little impact on research practices in the United States. Biomedical research expanded exponentially after World War II without significant regulation or oversight. The Nuremberg Code established the need for the "voluntary consent of the human subject." It covered such other matters as the need to justify a study in terms of expected beneficial results and risks, avoiding harm and injury to subjects, freedom for the subject to withdraw, and obligation of the investigator to stop a study if continuation would likely cause injury, disability, or death.

In 1966, the U.S. Public Health Service introduced the requirement that all human subject research funded by the government must be peer-reviewed by a local institutional review board (IRB). The objective was to protect the rights of the individuals involved and review the quality of the informed consent and the risks and benefits of the study. This regulation was the result of a growing awareness that these kinds of safeguards often were not followed even in the best academic institutions in the United States.

Several unethical studies reached the attention of the public during the 1960s and 1970s. Of highest notoriety was the Tuskegee study, which was organized by the U.S. Public Health Service to follow the natural history of syphilis in a cohort of 400 rural African American men. The lack of meaningful informed consent in 1932, when the study began, and the subsequent withholding of penicillin treatment until the study was exposed and halted in 1972 shocked the public and spurred Congress into action. The end result, as described above, was

the issuance of the Belmont Report and its articulation of the prevailing principles of bioethics: autonomy, justice, and beneficence.

Federal regulations mandate the creation of ongoing IRBs with appropriate oversight of human subject research. Pursuant to the doctrine of autonomy, informed consent procurement is now a formalized process. In randomized controlled trials, potential participants must be notified of the risks, benefits, and alternatives to the care provided by the study. Beneficence and justice dictate that equipoise exists between the alternative treatments and between these treatments and the standard of care and that potentially beneficial findings of the study will be meaningful and relevant for the study population.

This evolution of research ethics is applicable for students of surgery as well. Although federal regulations cover research funded by the government, their ethical underpinnings should apply to all research involving human subjects, regardless of the source of funding. Surgeons continually try to innovate and improve their skills and the procedures used, but they must be mindful of the possible need for antecedent work in basic science and the animal laboratory and the need for informed consent and peer review when significant deviation from standard practice is contemplated. In most instances, new surgical procedures should be developed in appropriately controlled research trials with all the safeguards needed for the protection of human subjects. Most institutions require anyone investigating and co-investigating to complete a curriculum that includes research ethics.

INFORMED REFUSAL AND THE JEHOVAH'S WITNESS PATIENT

Founded in the late 19th century, the Jehovah's Witness community is governed by the Watchtower Society, which issues doctrinal positions via its official journal, the *Watchtower*. On July 1, 1945, an article in that journal established the familiar Jehovah's Witness prohibition against blood transfusions. The biblical sources cited—Genesis 9:4, Leviticus 17:13–14, and Acts 15:19–21—are understood by conventional Judeo–Christian theology as proscriptions against consuming the blood of animals. Nevertheless, Jehovah's Witnesses forbid transfusions of whole blood or its constituents: plasma, packed red blood cells, platelets, and white blood cells. The penalty for transgression is severe: eternal damnation and, more immediately, social ostracism and "disfellowshipping" by other Witnesses. In the June 15, 2004, edition of the *Watchtower*, however, explicit clarifications were issued revealing that transfusion of fractionated components of plasma, packed red blood cells, platelets, and white blood cells was permissible and subject to the individual's discretion.

The wrenching ethical quandary arises when a Jehovah's Witness patient asserts her autonomy to refuse transfusion, thereby risking exsanguination during surgery or from medical conditions such as dysfunctional uterine bleeding. Could or should physician beneficence override a competent patient's refusal of treatment? When locked in conflict, which bioethical principle prevails: autonomy or beneficence? In these instances, it is also important for physicians to consider the concept of good and well-being from the perspective of the patient. Physicians often are in situations in which they cannot provide medical beneficence, but that does not prevent them from assisting in spiritual or emotional beneficence. In the case of a Jehovah's Witness, a physician may appeal to the principle of beneficence while withholding treatment at the request of a competent patient.

American courts have not reached consensus concerning the withholding of blood products for Jehovah's Witnesses, but several dominant trends appear. Surgeons who choose to respect the wishes of a competent Jehovah's Witness patient to refuse blood products in the face of imminent exsanguination are, in general, protected from wrongful death liability. Likewise, courts generally endorse a patient's right to refuse treatment. However, when the patient has dependents who would be otherwise abandoned, or in obstetric situations in which the fetal well-being will be placed in jeopardy, courts have intervened to order transfusions.

From an ethical perspective, a gynecologist contemplating a surgical procedure for a Jehovah's Witness should take the following steps to ensure that the patient and surgical team are prepared for the potential decision to withhold blood products:

- Extensive, confidential preoperative counseling to ascertain informed consent. Specifically, the surgeon should verify the patient's understanding and acceptance of Watchtower Society doctrine, understanding of the potential repercussions of refusing transfusion, and awareness of the views of dissident Jehovah's Witnesses. This should be thoroughly documented in the chart. In cases in which the patient's decision-making capacity may be in question, the physicians should request additional professional input from a psychiatrist.
- Consultation, as needed, with the hospital ethics committee.
- Preoperative consultation with the anesthesiologist.

There are several prophylactic steps that can be taken to avoid the likelihood of a transfusion. These include preoperative iron and/or recombinant erythropoietin therapy and intraoperative use of vasopressin, volume expanders, hypotensive anesthesia, hypothermia, and ligation of major vessels. An intraoperative cell salvage machine, commonly referred to as a "cell saver," is also a viable alternative for patients with religious objections to receiving blood transfusions. These devices suction, wash, and filter blood so it can be given back to the patient's body as needed.

ADVANCED PLANNING AND END-OF-LIFE DECISION MAKING

Policies and regulations regarding death and dying have been set largely by the courts on a case-by-case basis when intractable controversies have arisen with doctors, patients, patients' families, or hospital administrators that must be resolved before a judge. The introduction of life-sustaining technology, such as the respirator that can keep the human body functioning biologically even in cases when the prospect of a return to normalcy is unlikely, has introduced a host of new dilemmas and questions about medical decisions at the end of life. When terminally ill patients, their families, and their health care teams all agree on the use and withholding of treatment at the end of life, there is usually no overt dilemma, except the question of the prudent use of scarce resources. When there is agreement among all parties, there is seldom a need to go to court, and courts discourage bringing these cases before them. When there is disagreement among the patient, the patient's family, the physician or team of physicians, and/or the hospital, the stage is set for conflict that often must be decided by an arbitrator. The courts have traditionally provided guidance in such cases. These rulings, however, often are not universal and are influenced by contemporary public attitudes. Although each case and its outcome is not comparable, the general consensus is that the patient's autonomous choices are binding and that the ultimate goal of medicine is not to preserve life at any cost, but to relieve pain and suffering in keeping with the patient's wishes.

A recent ACOG committee opinion statement in 2007 addressed the issue of medical futility for today's obstetrician–gynecologist. The statement described the concept of medical futility to justify a physician's unilateral refusal to provide treatment requested by a patient or a patient's family. This decision may be based on the physician's perception that further treatment will not obtain a specific physiologic goal or will not achieve a reasonable quality of life. The statement also recommends that physicians and health care institutions develop policies dealing with conflicts relating to the concept of medical futility and patient care.

Since the development of these life-sustaining interventions, there have been several landmark cases: Karen Ann Quinlan, Nancy Cruzan, and Terri Schiavo. Each of these cases represents a different scenario in which physicians and family members struggle to make difficult decisions in surrogate for their loved one. The situation of Karen Ann Quinlan is one example of the type of disagreement that can occur between a patient's family and the providing health care institution. Karen Ann Quinlan was a 21-year-old woman who had been in a prolonged coma and sustained on a respirator. When the likelihood of recovery disappeared, her family's request to remove the respirator was challenged by the hospital. The courts ultimately ordered the removal of the respirator, and she died 10 years later.

In the case of Nancy Cruzan, a difficult decision had to be made when the wishes of the patient were unknown. Nancy Cruzan was in a prolonged coma, and her parents wanted to withdraw food and fluid. There was no record of her prior stated or documented wishes, and, as a result of a Missouri state law forbidding withdrawal without such evidence, this did not take place. The case was taken to the U.S. Supreme Court, which ultimately found the Missouri statute constitutional and, therefore, did not grant the request to the parents. This case is landmark because, in the course of handing down this decision, the U.S. Supreme Court established the right of competent patients to refuse any kind of treatment, also including life-sustaining treatment. In addition, the Supreme Court determined that no distinction was necessary between artificial feeding and other forms of therapy. Ultimately, evidence was found of Nancy Cruzan's prior wishes that she would not be kept alive in a permanent coma, and she was allowed to die after treatment was withdrawn.

The Terri Schiavo case is another example of the complexity of surrogate decision making. In contrast to the two previous cases, this one represents disagreement between the family members of the patient. On February 1990, Terri Schiavo suffered a myocardial infarction resulting in severe brain damage leaving only minimal brain stem function intact. At the time of this initial event, Schiavo did not have a living will or written documentation of her medical care wishes. Her husband and parents worked together to care for her with the hope that she would recover all or part of her cerebral functions, having a feeding tube inserted and placing her in a skilled nursing facility. Eight years later, Terri's husband came to the conclusion that her status had not and would not improve. Stating that his wife had previously expressed her wishes not to live under such circumstances, he appealed to the courts to take on the role of the ward's surrogate to remove the feeding tube and allow her to die. A court order to remove the feeding tube in April 2001 was immediately followed by an appeal by her parents claiming that they had evidence that Schiavo would want to live. Furthermore, they believed that novel medical therapies would be able to improve Schiavo's condition and restore some of her ability to function. They felt that Schiavo was conscious and responsive and, given the ability to speak for herself, would express her desire to live.

In response to this new information, the court reversed its ruling and, 2 days later, the tube was reinserted. Over the course of 15 years, Schiavo's feeding tube was placed and removed a total of three times in response to different court rulings. After several attempts for appeal, the final ruling ordered the removal of the feeding tube in March 2005, and, less than 2 weeks later, Terri Schiavo passed away.

Many such cases did not deal directly with the issues pertaining to terminal illness, but they provided the moral and legal environment in which such requests can more readily be honored by the physician. Sufficient consensus among patient advocacy groups and professional medical organizations led to the Patient Self-Determination Act, passed by Congress in 1990. This act required hospitals to promote the use of advance directives by their patients to qualify for federal funds for Medicare and Medicaid. Almost every state in the country has enacted laws that allow for advanced-care planning to direct the care of and protect the rights of patients who are terminally ill and suddenly incapacitated. These are referred to as *advanced directives*, and they include a variety of different mechanisms whereby a patient can direct his/her medical care in the case of his/her sudden or gradual decline in decisional capacity. The different forms of advanced directives include:

Durable power of attorney for health care—A legal document in which a patient designates a specific individual to make health care decisions in the setting of loss of decisional capacity

Living will—A legal document in which the patient describes his/her treatment preferences in the setting of loss of decision-making capacity, such as the continuation of nutrition, hydration, or ventilator support

Health care proxy (attorney-in-fact for health care)—The individual designated by the patient to make surrogate decisions in the case of loss of decision-making capacity

Do not resuscitate (DNR)—A type of advanced directive that specifically directs the withholding of lifesaving procedures in the case of cardiopulmonary arrest, such as cardiopulmonary resuscitation and defibrillation

Gynecologists should familiarize themselves with different forms of advance directives and the applicable laws. They should also discuss these issues with their patients and their families to ensure that the best arrangement can be made. The ideal time to do this is preferably before such decisions are actually needed for implementation, such as before significant illness or surgery.

RELATIONSHIPS WITH INDUSTRY

While development of pharmaceutical agents and medical devices is important for improving health care, the goals of industry may conflict with a physician's duty to his/her patients. ACOG has recognized this challenge in recent years and has produced several committee opinions regarding this since 1985. The most recent update was issued in 2012. Specifically, ACOG warns that gifts tied to promotional material may influence professional behavior and are therefore discouraged. Use of samples should be limited to those patients with a true financial need. Training on the proper use of medical devices should ideally be provided through professional societies with CME accreditation. When this is not possible, industry-provided training should be limited to FDA-approved indications for using the equipment or device for the shortest time possible. ACOG provides specific guidelines for industry sponsorship of research.

ETHICAL CHALLENGES SPECIFIC TO GYNECOLOGIC CARE

Several issues specific to the care of women and their reproductive health represent ethical dilemmas unique to gynecology. These include abortion, assisted reproductive technologies, and sterilization of women. In each case, the nuances of addressing the health care issues of women require additional consideration to ethical topics mentioned above.

Abortion

Termination of pregnancy is entertained in a variety of settings in obstetrics and gynecology. A patient may seek an abortion for a broad spectrum of circumstances, ranging from an unintended and undesired pregnancy (failure or nonuse of birth control, sexual assault, failure of emergency contraception), severe fetal anomalies (aneuploidy, congenital abnormalities incompatible with life), or threatened maternal health (preeclampsia, severe hyperemesis gravidarum, cardiomyopathy). Because of the many diverse clinical scenarios for the termination of a pregnancy, it benefits physicians to be aware of the issues relating to abortion, regardless of whether or not they have personal objections to the procedure.

The core ethical and legal issues surrounding abortion include the right of the woman to control her own body and reproduction, the moral and legal status of the fetus, the rights and interests of the fetus to be protected from harm, and the degree to which outside parties such as national and state governments have authority to protect or restrict these rights. These issues tend to polarize the general public and government into two camps: prolife or prochoice. Because of the two extremes of positions that exist in the debate about abortion, little headway has been made to reach a common ground since legalization of abortion in the United States in 1973.

The two major legal cases that have shaped most abortion law in the United States in the past century are *Roe v. Wade* and *Planned Parenthood v. Casey*. Although these decisions do not encompass all laws pertaining to abortion, they are the two most well known and influential. In 1973, *Roe v. Wade* recognized the following rights: the fundamental right of privacy, protection of an individual's bodily integrity, and protection of an individual's decisional autonomy. The rights outlined in *Roe v. Wade* were weighed against the interests of the state in terms of the protection of a potential human life and the health of the mother. However, *Roe v. Wade* did not address questions such as the moral or legal status of the fetus. Under these three rights, the Supreme Court interpreted the Constitution as granting significant protections to an individual's right not to have a child. As such, a woman's choice to terminate a pregnancy was given specifically to her and not to the government. At the same time, the Supreme Court recognized the states' interests in protecting both women's health and the potential life of the fetus, giving the individual states the authority to enact laws imposing strict safeguards and even restricting procedures.

Roe v. Wade also accomplished several other legal milestones. It intended to limit states' restrictions on a woman's right to terminate a pregnancy by establishing a "strict scrutiny standard." By this standard, individual states that proposed laws, such as mandatory husband consent requirements and mandatory waiting periods, were determined to be unconstitutional. In addition, *Roe v. Wade* established a trimester framework for outlining the degree of the state's interests in abortion law. During the first trimester, the woman's interests had precedence above the interests of the state to protect the potential life. During the second trimester, a woman's privacy interests and the state's interest in the protection of the woman's life and the potential life of the fetus were balanced. After the time of viability, the state's interest in protecting the potential life had priority unless the life of the woman was at stake. Minors were also addressed under the Roe framework. Under *Roe v. Wade*, minors were required to inform or involve their parent or guardian in the decision to terminate the pregnancy. In cases when this was not possible, either because of fear of the consequences of disclosure or when the guardian was unavailable, minors were required to obtain a waiver of parental involvement mandate from the court, also known as a judicial bypass. Finally, *Roe v. Wade* placed federal and state limitations for the use of public funding of abortions for Medicaid patients.

Planned Parenthood v. Casey (1992) reaffirmed the central tenets of *Roe v. Wade* but changed the law significantly by removing the trimester framework based on the notion that it did not adequately recognize the state's interest in the potential life before viability. Under Casey, the states' interests take priority from the outset of pregnancy, not just during later gestations, and, as such, states were permitted to make laws to restrict abortion in the process of protecting their interests. These individual state-by-state laws were constitutional only if they met the "undue burden" standard. Under this standard, the state's restrictions could not place an undue burden on the woman in deciding to terminate her pregnancy. Such a restriction had the effect of placing a substantial obstacle in the path of a woman seeking an abortion of a nonviable fetus. Many states have interpreted "undue burden" in different ways, creating restrictions—such as increased parental involvement, mandatory waiting periods, unwieldy requirements for abortion centers, and counseling biased toward continuing the pregnancy—that are deemed constitutional. A more recent example of such an obstacle is the requirement for a woman to undergo transvaginal sonography prior to voluntary pregnancy termination.

Abortion is one of the few medical procedures from which physicians may opt out in nonemergent situations because of ethical or religious objections. Under this situation, legislatures have recognized that professionals may legally refuse to provide abortion services. "Conscience" or "refusal" clauses make abortion services one of the few areas in which a physician legally may opt out of performing a medically indicated procedure because of personal objections; however, the scope of the right to opt out differs from state to state. Legally, under the protections of conscientious objection, no physician is required to do a procedure if it is in conflict with his or her ethical, moral, or religious beliefs. This principle applies only in situations in which the patient's life is not at stake. In cases when the life of the woman is threatened by the ongoing pregnancy and no other providers are immediately available, a physician cannot refuse to treat the woman.

The statutes of conscientious objection do not exempt physicians from making a responsible, truthful, and timely referral to another practitioner or health care facility that provides the service or from rendering care in a life-threatening emergency when an alternate health care provider is not available. Failure to provide an appropriate referral can constitute malpractice (i.e., fall below the legal standard of care) and also may violate ethical standards of care. Many states have patient abandonment laws that put specific burdens on physicians to refer or transfer care of patients before terminating a relationship. At minimum, the physician is expected to guide the patient to valid resources to identify an abortion provider.

The most recent debates about abortion pertain to the issues of partial birth abortion (D&X) and RU-486. Many professional organizations for women's health have rebuked the validity of the partial birth bans. Legislation addressing partial birth abortion has been described by ACOG as "inappropriate, ill advised, and dangerous" because "intact D&X may be the best or most appropriate procedure in a particular circumstance to save the life or preserve the health of a woman, and only the doctor, in consultation with the patient, based upon the woman's particular circumstances, can make this decision." Arguments against partial birth abortion have been criticized for being a rhetorical strategy to place greater restrictions on the present abortion statutes.

Special Issues for Assisted Reproductive Technology Patients

The rapidity of developments in the field of assisted reproductive technology (ART) continues to raise ethical dilemmas. Basic to all is whether the preimplantation embryo has special significance and when personhood is established. The variety of technologic advances highlights this concept. All of the new offshoots of ART, including embryo cryopreservation, preimplantation genetic diagnosis and screening with discarding of embryos, and new approaches to fertility preservation, raise ethical issues, most of which focus on the sanctity of the embryo. The principles of autonomy, beneficence, nonmaleficence, and justice all enter into the equation and have been addressed by the American Society for Reproductive Medicine Ethics Committee in its reports beginning in 1986 and by ongoing publications in its journal.

Sterilization of Women

Sterilization of the female patient is subject to the same ethical principles as any other surgical procedure. Unique to the issue of sterilization is that it is often a social choice rather than a medical necessity. It is critical that the physician address nonmedical factors associated with sterilization without bias, particularly when a patient seeks counsel in deciding whether or not to pursue sterilization. A 2007 ACOG committee opinion specifically addresses special issues related to sterilization. For instance, hysterectomy for the sole purpose of sterilization is deemed inappropriate. Women with mental disabilities, who have an impaired ability to participate in the informed consent process, are not automatically justified to undergo sterilization. However, these women should not necessarily be denied the procedure, if desired. In these situations, the physician should consult with the patient's family and her caregivers to devise a plan that suits the best interest of the patient while respecting her autonomy.

CONCLUSION

This chapter has presented a sample of the issues pertinent to the practice of gynecology. As a field that combines the challenges of medicine, surgery, and the complex issues specific to the care of women and their reproductive health, several other important ethical aspects may not have been addressed here. Moreover, innovative technologies and therapeutic procedures present new dilemmas to the practicing physician on a regular basis. Physicians have many resources with which to approach some of the difficult questions that may arise in their own practices. Institution or individual practice ethics committees, oversight committees, and ethics consult services are available for multidisciplinary and peer review of challenging ethical cases. Physicians at all levels of practice should feel confident to turn to these mechanisms for guidance in the case of difficult ethical situations.

BEST SURGICAL PRACTICES

- Informed consent is a mechanism whereby the patient's autonomy is respected.
- Physicians are responsible for maintaining medical and surgical competence.
- The confidentiality of the patient should be protected. Only in special circumstances can it be overridden.
- Physicians should be familiar with the different forms of advance directives and discuss end-of-life decision making with their patients.
- Gynecologists should be aware that several issues specific to the care of women and their reproductive health present ethical dilemmas that are often unique to gynecology.

BIBLIOGRAPHY

American College of Obstetricians and Gynecologists Department of Professional Liability/Risk Management. *2003 ACOG survey on professional liability: national ACOG statistics*. Washington, DC: American College of Obstetricians and Gynecologists, 2004.

American Fertility Society. Ethics Committee. Ethical considerations of the new reproductive technologies. *Fertil Steril* 1986;46(3 suppl 1): 1S.

Beauchamp TL, Childress JF. *Principles of biomedical ethics*, 4th ed. New York: Oxford University Press, 1994.

Beecher HK. Ethics and clinical research. *N Engl J Med* 1966; 274:1354.

Centers for Disease Control and Prevention (CDC). HIPAA privacy rule and public health. Guidance from CDC and the U.S. Department of Health and Human Services. *MMWR Morb Mortal Wkly Rep* 2003;52(suppl 1–17):19.

Sterilization of women, including those with mental disabilities. ACOG Committee Opinion No. 371. American College of Obstetrics and Gynecologists. *Obstet Gynecol* 2007;110: 217.

Committee on Ethics. American College of Obstetricians and Gynecologists. ACOG Committee Opinion No. 362. Medical futility. *Obstet Gynecol* 2007;109:791.

Department of Health, Education and Welfare, Ethics Advisory Board. *Report and conclusions: HEW support of research involving human in vitro fertilization and embryo transfer*. Washington, DC: Government Printing Office, 1979.

Faden RR, Beauchamp TL. *A history and theory of informed consent*. New York: Oxford University Press, 1986.

Gillon R. Refusal of potentially life-saving blood transfusions by Jehovah's Witnesses: should doctors explain that not all JWs think it's religiously required? *J Med Ethics* 2000;26:299.

Gostin LO. Deciding life and death in the courtroom. *JAMA* 1997;278:1523.

Hodgson CS. Disciplinary action by medical boards and prior behavior in medical school. *N Engl J Med* 2005;353:2673.

Jacox A, Carr DB, Payne R. New clinical-practice guidelines for the management of pain in patients with cancer. *N Engl J Med* 1994; 330:651.

Jonsen AR. *The birth of bioethics*. New York: Oxford University Press, 1998.

King NMP. *Making sense of advance directives*. Dordrecht, The Netherlands: Kluwer Academic Publishers, 1993.

LaFollette H, ed. *Ethics in practice: an anthology*. Cambridge, MA: Blackwell, 1997.

Moreno-Hunt C, Gilbert WM. Current status of obstetrics and gynecology resident medical-legal education. *Obstet Gynecol* 2005;106:1382.

Papadakis MA, Teherani A, Banach MA, et al. Introduction. In: Reich WT, ed. *The encyclopedia of bioethics*, revised ed. New York: Simon & Schuster Macmillan, 1995.

Papadakis MA, Teherani A, Ranach MA, et al. Disciplinary action by medical boards and prior behavior in medical school. *N Engl J Med* 2005;25:2673.

Professional relationships with industry. Committee Opinion No. 541. American College of Obstetrics and Gynecologists. *Obstet Gynecol* 2012;120:1243.

Professional responsibilities in obstetric-gynecologic medical education and training. ACOG Committee Opinion No. 500. American College of Obstetricians and Gynecologists. *Obstet Gynecol* 2011;118:400.

Robertson JA. *Children of choice: freedom and the new reproductive technologies*. Princeton, NJ: Princeton University Press, 1994.

Rothman DJ. *Strangers at the bedside*. New York: Basic Books, 1991.

Ryan KJ. Abortion or motherhood, madness and suicide. *Am J Obstet Gynecol* 1992;160:1415.

United States Department of Health and Human Services. *The Belmont report: ethical principles and guidelines for the protection of human subjects of research*. Washington, DC: Government Printing Office, 1979.

Veatch RM. *Medical ethics*. Boston, MA: Jones & Bartlett, 1989.

CHAPTER 3
Psychological Aspects of Pelvic Surgery

Betty Ruth Speir

DEFINITIONS

Anxiety—A feeling of apprehension, uncertainty, and fear without apparent stimulus and associated with physiologic changes (tachycardia, sweating, tremor, etc.).

Grief—The normal emotional response to an external and consciously recognized loss; it is self-limited, gradually subsiding within a reasonable time.

Insanity—Mental derangement or disorder. The term is a social and legal rather than medical one and indicates a condition that renders the affected person unfit to enjoy liberty of action because of the unreliability of his or her behavior with concomitant danger to self and others.

Regression—A return to a former or earlier state; a subsidence of symptoms or of a disease process; the turning backward of the libido to an early fixation at infantile levels because of inability to function in terms of reality.

Ethnicity—Ethnicity is a socially defined category based on common culture or nationality. Ethnicity can, but does not have to, include common ancestry.

Iatrogenic injury—An inadvertent adverse effect or complication resulting from medical treatment or "originating from a physician."

Gender identity—Gender identity refers to a person's private sense of, and subjective experience of, the person's own gender.

Psychodynamics—Psychodynamics is the theory and systematic study of the psychological forces that underlie human behavior.

Vaginismus—Vaginismus is vaginal tightness causing discomfort, burning, pain, penetration problems, or complete inability to have intercourse.

Robotics—Robotic surgery is a technique in which a surgeon performs surgery using a computer that remotely controls very small instruments attached to a robot.

INTRODUCTION

Neuroscientific research over the past decade continues to validate the oneness of the psyche and the soma (Fig. 3.1). Gynecologic surgery, in particular, does not simply alter the soma, but temporarily and sometimes permanently alters the psyche of the patient. The modern gynecologist needs to be more than a skilled technician: he or she must be willing and able to identify the potential psychological effects of the surgery performed and must be prepared with the knowledge and skills to address these effects with the patient.

Sir William Osler taught,
   "The good physician knows the disease the patient has.
   The great surgeon knows the patient who has the disease."

The technologic revolution has presented today's surgeon with a vast array of sophisticated equipment. In capable hands, miraculous surgical feats can be performed on a woman's body, but at what cost to her psychological self? The removal or reconstruction of diseased or dysfunctional anatomy may set off a chain reaction of parallel events in a woman's psyche.

For a surgeon, the gynecologic operation may be a quotidian event of usually simple dimension. For the patient, however, each procedure is a unique and intimidating experience. Her sense of well-being and health may be threatened. She may lose control over her body for some indefinite period of time. She may perceive the planned procedure as temporarily or even permanently affecting her sexual identity.

As complicated procedures become routine, the surgeon risks losing perspective about the impact of surgery on the life of the individual woman. The patient who experiences ablative genital (or breast) surgery is strongly influenced by her emotions. These vary in degree but are usually cumulative. As the patient passes through the presurgical, surgical, and postsurgical experiences, she may be stressed beyond her capacity to compensate. If help is not available to facilitate emotional healing and rehabilitation, permanent psychological damage may result.

The majority of women do heal and take up their lives, raise their children, work at their jobs, and relate well to their husbands or lovers. For them, the healing interval is relatively quick, and the stress is modest. Do not underestimate what can be learned from this psychologically healthy segment of women patients. In the 1940s, Abraham Maslow studied people with exceptional mental health to develop his hierarchy of needs theory. He discovered that these people's potential had never been weakened by negative thinking, a defeatist outlook, or a destructive self-image. "The rest of us," he declared, "fixate at a lower level because someone or something has implanted notions of limitations."

Once you become cognizant of the success statistics in your own patient population, you may discover why most women recover after gynecologic surgery to zestfully reembrace life, whereas others begin to slowly turn away from its possibilities.

It will never be enough for a surgeon to be a trained mechanic, able only to diagnose and repair. He or she must also be prepared to predict, recognize, and begin treatment of the psychological consequences of gynecologic disorders. This chapter is designed to help surgeons and other physicians better understand the female perspective and to use that knowledge to facilitate multidimensional healing.

ANKH

The ansate cross, Egyptian emblem of generation, symbol for life and soul and eternity, is a mark universally designated to depict femaleness (Fig. 3.2). By using this hieroglyph, modern scientists continue an ancient tradition of respect and reverence for women. Within the inner sanctum of every woman's mind lie symbols that are powerful and personal. These feminine

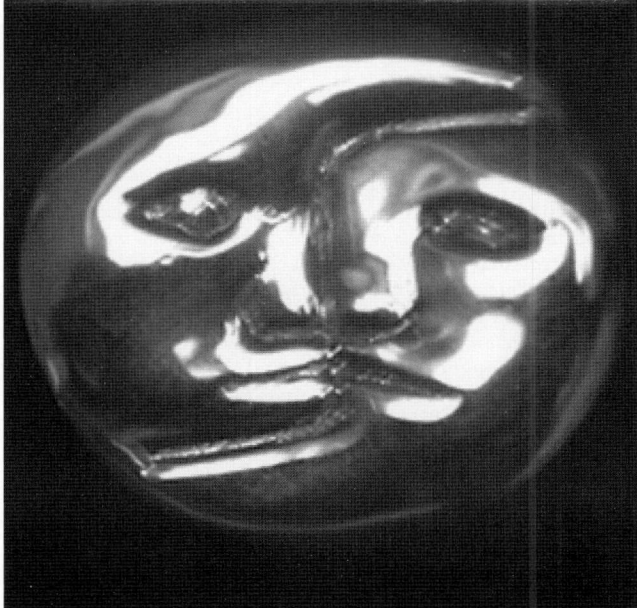

FIGURE 3.1 *Inseparable psyche–soma*: Sculpture and photo by James Sardonis—http://www.sardonis.com.

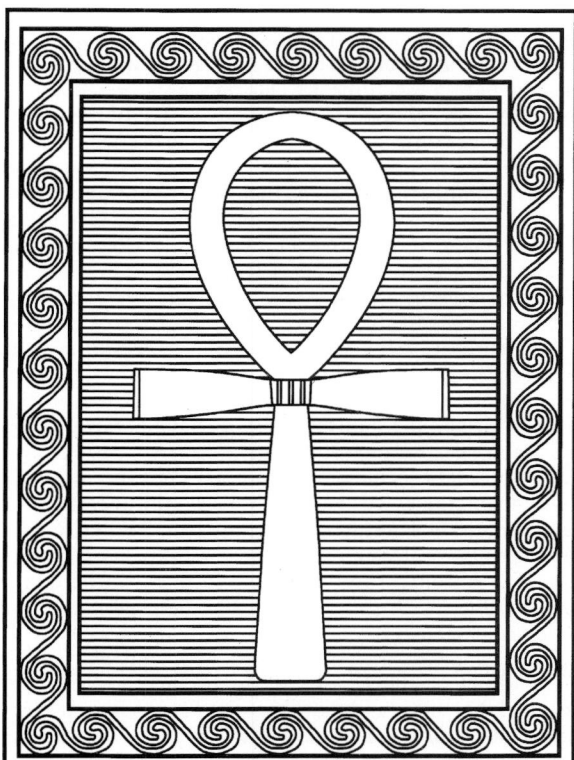

FIGURE 3.2 The ansate cross, or ankh amulet, is an ancient Egyptian symbol of life and sexuality.

identity markers are guarded and guided by her instincts, and no surgeon can successfully maneuver in this labyrinth of psychological and psychosexual emotion and cause no harm unless the female patient acts as a guide.

Egyptian writings from almost 4,000 years ago in the Kahun Papyrus depict the uterus as having an important and powerful effect on mental life. Current research tends to agree with the ancient scribes. The uterus has great symbolic value for many modern women, too. Beginning with the rite of passage called menstruation, a strong invisible bond is formed between a woman and her body. Her biologic clock has been set. For the next 40 years or so, she will be reminded each month that she is a woman, and menstruation is regarded by many as palpable proof of their femininity.

Others believe that menstruation is part of a natural cleansing cycle that purges the body of poisons that accumulate during the month. They know from experience that the premenstrual symptoms of edema, bloating, headaches, and emotional tension will be washed away in the tide of their monthly flow.

For some, the rhythm of the menstrual cycle is used as a way to time and order their lives. Like the phases of the moon, this cycle bestows a sense of routine, regularity, and predictability that has emotional significance. With the onset of menstruation, a woman is forever changed. Surgical removal of any of the reproductive organs will change her again, but how?

The effect of a woman's menstrual cycle on many medical conditions is well documented. Medical suppression of ovulation is commonly used as a way to evaluate and treat such chronic conditions as migraine, epilepsy, asthma, rheumatoid arthritis, irritable bowel syndrome, and diabetes. Research at the National Institutes of Health (NIH) and other leading institutions has shown "how nerves, molecules and hormones connect the brain and immune system, how the immune system signals the brain and affects our emotions, and documents how our brain can signal the immune system, making us more vulnerable to illnesses." What we have known intuitively is now understood scientifically. Hormones secreted during a woman's menstrual cycle affect her mood. Could the decline of these hormones during the natural aging process contribute to dementia? The future is alive with fascinating neuroscientific and neuroimmunomodulation elucidation, but today's woman is backlit by the skepticism of some scientists. Her concerns about her body and the way it will work after surgery are immediate and quite often, heart wrenching.

A woman about to undergo a hysterectomy might wonder if her lover will be able to detect the absence of her uterus. After the surgery, will she be thought of as less of a woman? Will her partner abandon her for someone who is still complete, either in the sense of being able to offer the possibility of a child or complete in the sense of having experienced no unnatural surgical transformations?

Will orgasm be as pleasurable for her after the surgery? For many women, the uterus has symbolic significance as a sexual organ. The uterus contracts during orgasm. Some women perceive this as most pleasurable. If the patient believes the uterus is essential to sexual response, then, in fact, it often becomes so, and women with this mindset may become sexually dysfunctional when it is removed.

Once the procedure is accomplished, will she still look and sound like a woman, or will she become noticeably more masculine? For others, the uterus is closely tied to feelings of attractiveness and sexual desirability. To a few women, removal of the uterus or ovaries or both constitutes a desexing, a permanent destruction of female identity and function. Sadly, certain members of the medical community as well as the feminist community perpetuate this notion and increase the attendant fear when they refer to women who must have their ovaries removed as "castrates."

Some women become distressed when they learn they must deal with the certainty of absolute sterility. For those who choose motherhood, the uterus, ovaries, breasts, and vagina work in harmony with other factors to attract a necessary mate and get down to the business of creating new life. These organs are vital to the sexual and reproductive aspects of a woman's life; thus, impending loss of these physical structures because of disease or dysfunction sometimes creates deep angst that must be resolved before surgery is attempted. Many women who have all the children they want and who do not wish to get pregnant again are still sometimes disturbed by the finality of the decision. The gynecologist should assure these maternal women that, although they will no longer be able to conceive a child, the powerful urge to create will never leave them. In time, they will learn to direct this primal energy into other areas of their lives and be immensely satisfied with the results. Studies such as the Ethnicity, Needs, and Decisions of Women project (ENDOW), a 5-year, three-phase, multicenter collaboration, are focusing on many of these issues and will help the gynecologist better understand the patient.

Today's modern woman, for the most part, is an avid information seeker. She surfs the Internet, buys the latest books, reads magazine articles, and conducts in-depth interviews with peers who have experienced similar gynecologic problems. A certain proportion of the harvested material is useful to her and perhaps even illuminating for the physician, but unfortunately, some of the sources are inherently flawed, prejudicial, illogical, or without scientific basis. It is the physician's responsibility to separate the grains of truth from the chaff. All the information the patient has gathered represents her attempt to prepare herself psychologically for the ordeal ahead, and she must never be condemned or made to feel small for trying to protect herself.

For the gynecologist, it is not necessary, or even possible, to change a patient's basic attitude or feelings. It is, however, vital to acknowledge them. The right information, reassurance, and support usually quickly modify many negative factors and lead to a healthier attitude and understanding of the surgical process. It is crucial that the patient be allowed to vent her anxiety and give voice to her fears.

COMMUNICATION

Patients in General

Diplomats the world over understand the significance of effective communication. Indeed, the prospect for world peace depends on their ability to interact efficiently. A female patient's psychological bearing before, during, and after the gynecologic procedure can depend on the communication techniques used by her physician. You must establish rapport, speak of the real and present danger to her health, and then elaborate on your plans to protect her.

Whenever possible, provide pleasant surroundings where you and your patient can comfortably hold a private conversation. Push all other thoughts out of your mind. These few minutes belong exclusively to her, and the quality of the time you spend actively communicating will pay healthy dividends for you both.

Whether explaining the simplicity of a needle-directed breast biopsy or the intricacies of hysterectomy, you must be able to highlight the technical details of the procedure and its postsurgical realities in a nonthreatening but utterly truthful manner. Begin the presentation using simple but thorough explanations and examples of the procedures. Your patient will let you know how much information she can or wishes to process by the questions she asks.

Your patient needs confidence in your technical ability, to know that her problem is being taken seriously and that you are qualified to competently help her cope with all of the ramifications of this new experience.

Dealing with the patient's feelings is not usually difficult if the surgeon accepts the viewpoint that many of the patient's emotions are part of the gynecologic situation. To the physician, the presurgical tension is predictable, familiar, transient, and simply comes with the territory; but to each new patient, it epitomizes an unfamiliar, dramatic, and life-altering experience.

To interpret the patient's true feelings, simply listen to her. Listening well is both an art and a skill, and the surgeon who cares about the patient's complete health as well as her quick recovery works diligently to hone a sharp edge on this valuable tool. Listen and you will hear the woman give a name to her most profound doubts and fears. Repeat her words so that you are absolutely certain you understand what she said, and so that she is absolutely assured that you are listening to her.

Begin the communication process by finding out what the patient perceives will be done to her body and why the procedure is necessary. Find out what she believes the consequences of the surgery will be. How does she think the surgery will impact her life? As she discusses the implications of her decision, her knowledge, fears, and biases will emerge. At this point, you should be able to supplement the patient's perspective with appropriate explanations about anatomy, physiology, and pathology. After this, it is time to describe in detail the usual preoperative, operative, and postoperative routines. Address the patient's questions and fears in as many ways as it takes for her to become confident that she understands what will happen to her.

Carefully explain what you are going to do to help her. If she wants or needs to know, describe the common physical sensations, bandages, incisions, catheters, tubing, and medications that are associated with her particular procedure. Define the patient's role in her own convalescence and recovery. Give her a general timetable for how long she will feel discomfort and need to use pain medication, when she will be ambulatory, and finally, when she will be discharged from the hospital or outpatient center.

Relate the most common complications that might occur as the result of her surgery. Injuries that might affect the quality of her life, even temporarily, should never come as a postsurgical surprise, nor should they be glossed over during the signing of the consent forms. Every patient wants to trust the doctor.

Informed Consent/Ethical Issues

Tell a patient that she has the option of robotic surgery and you'll probably get an exuberant response. "A robot! How cool is that! What's its name?" Angelos, who runs the first surgical ethics program in the United States, understands that most people automatically think new anything is better than old everything and that robots are magnificent manifestations of technology. He knows that many surgeons prefer to walk on the cutting edge, too, but in reality, is this a slippery ethical slope?

Before a proper informed decision can be made, the patient should know that in the beginning, a new procedure or system has fewer data on outcomes on which to base a decision, and the patient's surgeon should be honest about his or her level of experience. The ultimate decision must be based on what

benefits the patient is expecting from the procedure and which choice is the most likely to produce that benefit.

Iatrogenic injury remains the most common cause of lower urinary tract trauma. An understanding of the prevention, recognition, and treatment of urologic complications is important for every surgeon performing major pelvic surgery. Injury to a woman's genitourinary system may take 10 to 20 years to develop full-blown symptoms, about the same time line as from multiple childbirths, but it remains a possibility. Physicians, however, disagree on whether or not to tell the patient that, because of damage to the pelvic nerves or pelvic supportive structures, urinary incontinence after hysterectomy could be a long-term adverse effect. Only 4% of the hysterectomies performed are for relief from symptoms of incontinence.

Complications such as the formation of adhesions may occur in as many as 55% of patients after gynecologic surgery. These adhesions can become a critical issue from the standpoint of reproductive potential. Their presence is also strongly associated with pelvic pain, abnormal bowel function, and small bowel obstruction.

The mentally competent patient has a moral, legal, and ethical right to make an intelligent informed decision and can only do it if she is privy to all of the available facts concerning her situation. It is essential for her to be involved in the decision-making processes, because the more committed she is to the proposed treatment, the more invested she will become in her own preparation and rehabilitation. This point is supported by the findings of the ENDOW Study.

The art of touching, the therapeutic laying on of the hands, is important. Being lonely, frightened, and sick is a reason for the patient to be touched by her physician, especially if she seems particularly overwhelmed by her situation. To touch the patient's shoulder or hold her hand while talking to her is therapeutic. Even a comforting hug is appropriate if it fits the circumstances and the patient reaches out to you. Before fetal monitoring, quality of labor was evaluated by sitting at the patient's bedside with the physician's hand on her abdomen to feel uterine contractions. Often, the presence of the physician and a warm hand on her abdomen made the patient relax, rest, and become calmer during active labor. Cancer patients, especially, on hearing bad news need immediate human-to-human contact to stay grounded enough to face that terrible moment. The professional boundaries of roles, time, place, space, gifts and services, chaperoned examinations, physical contact, money, and formal language were never intended to be an impermeable membrane separating a doctor's ability to administer human kindness. A healer's touch can often comfort a distressed patient when words are inadequate.

A patient's family is a vital part of her support system and can be a potent ally, or not, to the health care team. If your patient requests that family members be present during her consultation, allow it, but speak directly to her whenever possible.

Once the initial presurgical discussions are complete, your patient may need some time to digest all the new information she has received. After assimilation, allow her to contact you for clarification or to ask more questions. This is especially important if the procedure involves new techniques or technologies.

Patients have the right to know the physician's level of experience regarding surgical techniques, as well as a thorough description and performance history of any device that will be used or implanted in their bodies. Rosen believes this is especially important because different procedures have different risks, and the patient should know why her physician prefers one method or product over another. Other countries have government registries that track the outcomes and complications of medical devices so surgeons can quickly determine superior and inferior performers. A physician expert in a Swedish hip registry disclosed, "The risk in the United States that a patient will need a replacement procedure because of a flawed product or technique can be double the risk of countries with databases... and doctors in Sweden are much less likely than American doctors to embrace new devices until registry data show they work." The American patient should know the status of Food and Drug Administration (FDA) surveillance and whether the physician and device manufacturer have any financial connection.

Patient–clinician communication has never been more important. Paget et al. list seven basic principles as a starting point:

- Mutual respect
- Harmonized goals
- A supportive environment
- Appropriate decision partners
- The right information
- Transparency and full disclosure
- Continuous learning

Patients from Other Cultures

In the United States, the number of patients from other cultures is increasing dramatically. In many cases, these patients are situated in dense clusters, and physicians in these areas are either multilingual or have assistants who are able to act as interpreters. However, no matter where your practice is located, chances are that at some point during your career as a physician, an individual from another culture will need your help.

Mull makes the following suggestions for communicating effectively with a person whose language you do not speak and whose culture is foreign to you: Make sure that your office staff are courteous and respectful. Show the genuine concern you feel. Be friendly and helpful to build rapport and develop a repertoire of knowledge. Familiarize yourself with the general principles of their traditional medicine. Whenever possible, have an interpreter present. Learn a few key phrases in their language, and use these for initial greeting and during examinations. Electronic linguistic assistants, such as the Franklin devices, are available in most languages. Include, at least in discussion, any family members your patient considers influential. Always ask what they have done to treat themselves. Have they consulted an influential family member? A healer? Have they used home or herbal remedies?

Physicians should be aware of common themes that exist in cross-cultural medicine, including the following:

- Fear of blood loss
- Fear of cold
- Tradition of male dominance
- Conservatism in sexual matters relative to teenage girls
- Poorly developed concept of preventive medicine
- Intolerance of side effects from medication
- Expectation of expeditious wellness
- Reluctance to discuss emotions with people who are not family members

Diaz-Gilbert cautions health care professionals to check their prejudices at the door and not to assume that a non–English-speaking person is uneducated. The following are some guidelines for effective communication with patients from other cultures:

- Allot extra time for the patient from another culture.
- Address every patient initially in English.
- Ask if the patient carries a bilingual dictionary.
- Gesture or write down simple words or phrases.
- Use visual cues, such as insurance forms, calendars, medication bottles, or anatomical sketches. If necessary, draw a picture to convey what you mean.

If the patient needs to perform a specific task, such as disrobing, carefully pantomime each step. Remain aware that direct eye contact, certain hand or finger gestures, and physical touch are offensive, are disrespectful, or can be construed as sexually suggestive in certain cultures.

When a cultural language barrier exists, reliance on body language becomes crucially important. Work at learning to read it. These patients experience the same emotional responses to surgery and need the same education and reassurances. Having to use the services of a foreign doctor in an alien land makes the surgical process even more frightening for them.

PSYCHOLOGICAL PREPARATION FOR SURGERY

Massler and Devansan said that there is an emotional response to any physical assault on the body. The magnitude of the response is expected to be proportional to the degree of emotional investment one has in the part of the body under siege. Among women, anatomic entities most vulnerable to this emotional reaction are the face, hair, breasts, genitalia, and abdominal wall.

Second only to cesarean birth, hysterectomy is the most frequently performed major surgical procedure done on reproductive-aged women. Over 600,000 women a year have hysterectomies in the United States. Newer, minimally invasive procedures have shortened hospital stays and have lessened visible disfigurement of the body. Schwartz and Williams of the Mayo Clinic concluded that detrimental psychological effects reported to occur after hysterectomy are not supported by prospective studies. Indeed, in most patients, mood was elevated.

The majority recover quickly from the procedure and enjoy the new freedom that comes to an individual when a chronic health problem has been resolved. Your patients, however, are not always older, wiser women, and they do not always recover quickly. If you know the signs to look for, you will be able to help that patient who is having a harder time adjusting to pelvic surgery, especially if it was a radical, life-threatening, or unexpected event.

In his book, *Matters of Life and Death*, Daniel Bruns writes, "Even the strongest person can be shaken by the horrors of some medical cures. Beyond this, life anxiety is even more common in persons with pre-existing emotional difficulties or characterologic disorders. These persons may go through life like eggshells, intact and functioning, but with psychological fragility. When faced with an extreme life stressor, such a person may simply shatter." How will you, as the physician, recognize the vulnerable?

Roeske researched 13 factors related to poor prognosis for excellent mental health after hysterectomy. The following factors begin to define the patient who might react negatively to genital surgical stress:

- Gender identity
- Previous adverse reactions to stress
- Previous depressive episodes
- Family history of mental illness
- History of multiple physical complaints, especially lower back pain

- Numerous hospitalizations or surgeries
- Age less than 35 years at time of hysterectomy
- Desire for a child or more children
- Fear of loss of libido
- Significant other's negative attitude toward procedure
- Marital dissatisfaction or instability
- Cultural or religious disapproval
- Lack of vocation or hobbies

Barnes and Tinkham's research also indicates that patients tend to react to current stress in much the same way as they reacted to past crises and personal losses. Well-established patterns of behavior repeat themselves. By taking a patient's history, the surgeon can be forewarned about which patients are likely to have the most difficulty handling the emotional aspects of gynecologic surgery. Equipped with this information, the surgeon can prepare to offer extra support in the form of reassurance, educational information, and—if indicated or requested—the names of psychotherapists who are trained to deal with women's health issues.

The Psychology of Pelvic Pain

Andrews said the problem of chronic pelvic pain (CPP) is very common. "About one in ten outpatient gynecologist appointments, up to 40 percent of laparoscopies, and up to 12 percent of hysterectomies are for chronic pelvic pain. We spend over a billion dollars just on outpatient management of chronic pelvic pain."

Singh, Rivlin, et al. list the following psychophysiologic therapies as possible interventions to reduce the severity of the symptoms: reassurance, counseling, relaxation therapy, stress management, and biofeedback techniques. They caution that consultation with a psychologist, urologist, neurologist, and gastrointestinal or other specialist is very important before considering invasive or aggressive management.

Management of the pain is difficult because there could be so many possible causes: Endometriosis, pelvic inflammatory disease, adhesive disease, pelvic congestion syndrome, ovarian retention syndrome, ovarian remnant syndrome, adenomyosis, and leiomyomas, and the list goes on. Benjamin-Pratt and Howard believe the best approach may be to use a combination approach that treats the disease and also teaches pain management.

Chronic or constant pain causes immense suffering because the patient cannot escape it or never knows when it will strike. Acute pain, like that of childbirth, has a beginning and a real end. The woman knows that no matter how much she hurts, there will be relief soon. While awaiting diagnosis or surgical treatment, the patient should be encouraged to keep a pain diary.

Pelvic Pain Support Network lists helpful suggestions to describe pain. These are useful for self-illumination for the patient as well as a diagnostic aid to present to the doctor:

- On a scale of 0 to 10, how bad is the pain?
- How long have you been having the pain?
- Where is the pain?
- Has the pain ever been diagnosed? If so, what was the diagnosis?
- What investigations have you had in the past?
- Describe the pain in your own words (burning, stabbing).
- What makes the pain worse? What makes it better?
- Is there a pattern? Diaries are useful for this.
- Have you been prescribed medication? Did it help or not?
- What activities does the pain prevent you from doing?
- How long can you do a certain thing before you have to rest?

Common Emotional Responses to Surgery

Insecurity

Giving up control of one's body, even temporarily, is uncomfortable for all of us, but it is terrifying for people who feel generally insecure. One of the most common defense mechanisms against feelings of insecurity is to institute rigid controls over all aspects of life. These patients may have no control over getting sick. They will have little if any control during the surgical procedures. The postsurgical setting will be a hospital room where the staff tell the patient when to awake, take medicine, eat, bathe, walk, have visitors, and have blood drawn. The health care workers will probe such personal matters as urination, defecation, and passage of flatus. Anxiety, anger, and feelings of being assaulted combine with insecurity to produce an unhappy, fearful, and sometimes raging patient.

These feelings are greatly diminished when the patient believes the surgery will improve her quality of life. There will eventually be relief from pain, removal of cancer, an end to heavy bleeding, restoration of fertility, or some other positive result. She will be better than she was before the surgery. The transition to becoming this healthier person is made easier when she trusts and believes in her physician.

Anxiety or Fear

Anxiety or fear associated with surgery is essentially universal. Most common is fear of the unknown or of what the patient imagines she will be forced to endure during hospitalization. Factual information about the surgical and recovery process and competent care by a compassionate hospital staff help to diminish this fear. Surgeons should assume responsibility for the behavior of the hospital staff toward their patients. When a patient complains of ill treatment by any of the health care providers, the physician should deal with the situation personally to decrease the probability of a future recurrence of the offensive or thoughtless behavior.

Patients may fear the loss of economic competence. A woman who has worked for many years may lose her sense of usefulness when disabled for some length of time. Whether she plays a major or minor role, the contribution she makes to her family's economic stability will be important to her. The sense of identity and self-esteem she derives from her job may also be threatened by the outcome of her surgery.

Fear of anesthesia is often a thinly disguised fear of dying as well as a fear of loss of control. It may be appropriate to confront the fear of dying directly so that the patient has the opportunity to express why she is afraid. Is the fear general or specific? Did a close relative suffer from the same affliction and die during or shortly after surgery? Does the patient have a strong intuitive feeling that something will go wrong? If so, ask her what you can do to modify the surgical situation. Determine whether the scheduled date of surgery or the particular hospital is significant. The fact that you consider her feelings an important issue and a normal part of the gynecologic disease process may be enough to calm her fears.

Regression and Dependency

In most people who are ill or who undergo surgery, regression to a more dependent state is fairly common. Dealing with a woman who is no longer self-sufficient or emotionally stable is difficult for the patient's family and friends. These members of her supporting cast are accustomed to her presurgical roles as wage earner, wife, mother, friend, cook, adviser, shopper, housekeeper, taxi driver, entertainer, and more. When she becomes ill and can no longer function to make their lives easier, family members and friends often become frustrated and angry. They may apply overt or subtle pressure to try to force the woman to exert herself and fulfill her usual roles. A change in roles is difficult, but often the illness teaches family and friends why this particular woman is valuable to them. In many cases, those who temporarily assume her normal duties or help her cope with the surgical experience discover strengths of hers of which they were previously unaware.

When the disease and prospect of surgery are new to the patient, all these factors, as well as a feeling of ill health, contribute to an emotional fragility that yields extremely labile emotions, including feelings of sadness, despondency, tearfulness, and irritability. The usual defense mechanisms are often temporarily weakened or destroyed. The woman is vulnerable to attack on all personal and professional fronts. She needs time with people she cares about, and she needs time alone to sort out her thoughts and emotions.

Grief

Grief is a normal, natural reaction to illness or loss of any kind; it is essential to emotional healing. Recognizing the various stages of grief allows the surgeon to help the female patient understand what is happening to her.

Denial is the first and most primitive emotional response to loss, and it can take many forms. The patient may demonstrate denial by not going to the doctor when she finds a lump in her breast or when she notices abnormal bleeding. She may pretend the symptoms do not exist or are a temporary nuisance. Not remembering instructions the physician gave her could be a manifestation of denial. She may forget important facts or deny the seriousness of the problem. Denial allows people to function for a little while in a make-believe world. With this primitive mechanism, they survive emotional stresses they might otherwise be unable to handle.

Bargaining with a higher power is the second stage of grief. Many patients feel they have carte blanche to bargain when they are experiencing a loss. "Make this bad thing that has happened to me go away, and I swear I will become a better person."

Guilt can surface before or after a loss. Most guilt feelings are completely inappropriate, in that the focus of the guilt rarely is directly related to the cause of the loss. When they are sick, many people feel that they are being punished for not being perfect. Explain to your guilt-ridden patients that their feelings are normal under the circumstances. Although guilt can sometimes deliver devastating, incapacitating blows, the good news is that it is usually transitory.

Depression comes in varying degrees to most people experiencing grief; it is characterized by feelings of helplessness, hopelessness, and worthlessness. Other symptoms include middle-of-the-night insomnia, nightmares, loss of appetite or excessive eating, lethargy, difficulty making decisions, psychosomatic symptoms, and fatigue unexplained by activity.

Ask the patient if she has any of these symptoms. Postsurgical depression is common. Depressed patients usually admit that the sad feelings are routine and occur daily. When prolonged, they indicate the patient has been unable to work through the grief process. Something emotional has yet to be resolved.

Rage turned inward often manifests as depression. When the patient is able to identify what she is angry about, to ventilate the rage, the depression usually begins to lift. When she takes charge of her life again and makes decisions, even small ones, she begins to feel better, and feelings of helplessness, hopelessness, and worthlessness abate. However, when the depressed patient becomes suicidal, stringent intervention must occur. The suicidal patient presents serious challenges and will be discussed in specific detail later in this chapter.

The stage at which the patient ventilates her anger can be difficult for those providing care, but it should be accepted as healthy. The patient may go to extremes, writing letters to the newspaper or speaking of suing her physician. She may complain bitterly about the nursing staff and the hospital. Such actions are a form of protest at the stress that has been dealt to her body and mind. In most instances, this behavior means that the depression is lifting and the patient is beginning to move toward the resolution of her grief. The depressed patient should be encouraged to ventilate by talking, to establish an enjoyable form of physical exercise, and to begin to take charge of her own life.

Resolution and integration eventually occur. The stressful experience of loss finally becomes an accepted part of her life. The memory causes sadness and regret, but no longer the devastating immobilization found in the earlier stages of grief. Integration does not mean the experience is forgotten, only that it has less trauma associated with it. After integration, certain stimuli can provoke flashback grief. The painful emotional tapes begin to play again, but the patient learns that the bad time is a rerun and will not last long.

The stages of grief do not always occur in order. The patient may feel fragments of several of them at the same time. If a female patient's behavior seems bizarre, excessive, or out of the realm of what would usually be anticipated during her particular surgical experience, look for the role grief might be playing in her life.

PSYCHODYNAMICS SPECIFIC TO DIAGNOSIS AND SURGERY

Patient–Physician Bonding

Neither scalpel nor laser can divide the psyche from the soma. As technical skills have improved and multiplied, robotic surgery has become commonplace, and comprehensive care of the gynecologic patient has declined. However, a knowledgeable and compassionate PA (physician's assistant) can be invaluable to both the surgeon and the patient. Increased emphasis on scientific and procedural care usually means less time in the consultation room and more time in the examining or procedure rooms. This is unfortunate for all concerned, because it takes time to explore the concepts, fears, and psychological wellbeing of the individual patient both before and after surgery.

It takes time to scan the books and magazines women read, to search the same Internet sites, to listen to the voices of their advocates, and to evaluate, critique, and learn from their sources of information; but it is important to make the effort. Otherwise, you run the risk of being out of touch, or worse still, appearing arrogant and condescending. Women in general have a sixth sense about these attitudes, and women about to undergo surgery or those recovering from surgical trauma to their bodies are hypersensitive to all manner of psychological stimuli.

The medicolegal climate has also potentiated perioperative anxiety. When you inform your patient, as she prepares for surgery, that she can bleed to death, be subjected to blood transfusions, have an adverse reaction to anesthesia, or sustain bowel or urinary tract injuries, you augment her innate fear of surgery. Some patients experience strong pressure from extreme feminist groups to seek and maintain a controlling role in her life, over her destiny, and over the surgeon. Under these circumstances, it is more necessary than ever for the pelvic surgeon to take the time to explore the patient's psyche in the preoperative and postoperative periods in order to avoid undesirable psychological sequelae. Having personable, competent health care workers in your office who assist in preparing your patient for surgery is also indispensable. Anatomical charts have become works of art, and they, as well as videos and other teaching aids, are useful in explaining the technical details; however, despite all the educational tools and staff assistance, the most important person remains you, the doctor. Unless you sit and answer questions on a one-to-one basis, you are neglecting your responsibility to her.

Much of the time, the questions will deal with information the patient has gleaned from literature, popular talk shows, and the Internet. Some of the opinions she reads or hears will frighten her or make her suspicious, and a few patients may initially come to your office thinking of you as a potential enemy. A staunch feminist may express the belief that you are just another insistently prosurgical doctor out to highjack her womb and add it to your trophy collection.

Popular literature today often stresses sexism, ageism, and greed on the part of doctors. *The Silent Passage* and *Our Bodies, Ourselves* were among the first widely read books on which patients depended for their gynecologic information. In these, they read that "for well over a century in the United States, women's uteri and ovaries have been subject to routine medical abuse," and "one should not be railroaded into hysterectomy nor onto hormones." Hysterectomy is described as "devastating" surgery, and for some women, it certainly can be. These books found a wide audience and led to the publication of other books, which took an even more radical approach, all in the name of protecting women from castrating medical experts who might use their position of authority to hurt, not help, them.

The Ultimate Rape: What Every Woman Should Know About Hysterectomies and Ovarian Removal was inspired after the author underwent a hysterectomy. She suffered extreme physical and emotional trauma following the surgery, but when she complained to her physicians, they advised her to go see a psychiatrist, because all her symptoms were in her head. The book's title is evidence of the rage she felt at their pronouncement. Now her voice is joined by others who believe every woman has the right to be thoroughly informed about procedures and consequences before consenting to gynecologic modifications. And certainly, a woman should.

In *No More Hysterectomies*, touted as the first living textbook on the Web, the reader learns how the male-dominated medical profession and the insurance industry have sanctioned millions of unwarranted hysterectomies. One testimonial to the ideas presented in the book describes the current medical environment as a "woman's hormonal holocaust."

The enlightening news is that interest generated by these sources and their legions of followers has had a positive and direct effect on women's health research. Global studies are numerous and are concentrating on traditional as well as alternative methods of treatment for menopause, hysterectomy, hormone replacement therapy (HRT), cancer, endometriosis, fibroids, and dementia. For the first time in the history of medical science, research is being conducted on a large scale to determine how women of various ethnicities and cultures and with differences in their physiology react to menopause, gynecologic surgery, hormone therapy, and sexual function. The ENDOW Study has found ethnic/racial differences in women's perceptions of hysterectomy and their decision making regarding elective surgery. Negative connotations were found to be more prevalent among African-American women, thus indicating a need for added support and preoperative information. Future generations of women will reap

the benefits from this research, but the overwhelming aura that prevails in today's gynecologic patient is one of confusion.

After reading just a sampling of the lay literature, some women feel that surgical removal of their female organs and commencement of hormonal therapy constitutes an unnatural, chemotherapy-like assault on their physical bodies. It is the task of the physician to admit into evidence the medical facts necessary to correct any gross misconceptions that could affect patient care. Sometimes, it may seem as if the patient, armed with advice about natural remedies for her severe pelvic pain, heavy bleeding, or hot flashes, wants to drag you with her back into the Dark Ages. Be patient and also prepared, if necessary, to explain the medically sound benefits of life lived outside the cave.

Be compassionate. No matter how routine the job becomes, compassion is a vital requisite to becoming an exceptional communicator and healer. Empathy often follows experience, and those times when you are able to make a noticeably positive difference in your patient's life are inspirational. To try the one new thing that might help many patients in the future, it is necessary to earn the trust of a single patient in the present.

The days are gone when a doctor was considered omnipotent, when he—and rarely, she—received a hock of ham for the birth of a child or had to tell a woman that she would have to live with the eventual hump on her back because it was a natural process of aging. Patients know about osteoporosis and heart disease and about reproductive technology and brain neurotransmitters. The media have turned every living room into a medical school. Some patients present videos and clippings detailing current research and experimental treatments relative to their specific diagnoses. They know a little, and they want to know more. Many patients want to participate in their health care and absolutely should be encouraged to do so. Unlike the doctors of old, who, for the most part, had to contend with an uneducated populace, the modern physician must form a partnership with the modern patient. Mutual responsibility, respect, and trust eventually strengthen this bond.

The cornerstone of the initial work is truth. Use good judgment about when to tell all the facts, particularly those that point to a devastating diagnosis, but never lie. In 1961, 90% of physicians surveyed in a single, large urban hospital stated that they withheld the diagnosis of cancer from their patients. Today, the position has been totally reversed, with 97% reporting that they reveal the true diagnosis of cancer.

Doctors, however, are not the only members of the team with ethical obligations. Patients also have the responsibility to tell the physician the truth relative to their symptoms, medications, allergies, and past medical histories and to relate any significant traumas or family history that could affect their current situations.

Question your patient specifically about stressful life events. Did she respond to these in a positive or negative way? Of all inquiries, this is the most important indicator of how the patient will respond to any current stress. Once the physician knows the answer, psychological preparation for diagnosis or surgery can begin in earnest.

Researchers in the United Kingdom have compiled data from multiple trial studies confirming that psychological preparation for surgery is effective. The general hypothesis was that communication and counseling are important determinants of numerous factors, including the following:

- Accuracy of the diagnosis
- Effectiveness of disease management
- Disease or problem prevention
- Patient satisfaction

- Adherence to treatment
- Psychological well-being
- Patient understanding of procedures
- Professional satisfaction and levels of stress

Information about each of these parameters was compiled, and considerable evidence existed to support all the hypotheses. In review, Davis and Johnston reported that psychological preparation is effective in reducing negative effect, pain, medication, and length of hospital stay and in improving behavioral recovery and physiologic functioning.

Surgical Whispers

The surgeon should make it a point to be with the patient while anesthesia is administered. Knowing that you are there with her from the beginning will help her feel safe. At the end of each surgical procedure, whisper into your patient's ear, "You're going to be well very soon." You may be surprised to find she needs less pain medication and recovers more quickly than do patients without the benefit of this positive prophecy. The mind itself is a powerful force, as evidenced by neuroscientific research. Dr. Esther M. Sternberg, Director of Integrative Neural Immune Program and Chief of the Section on Neuroendocrine Immunology and Behavior at the National Institute of Mental Health and National Institutes of Health, says that "With stress reduction endogenous opiates are produced that decrease pain. These come from the same cells in the hypothalamus that make the stress hormone CRH." Understanding these brain-immune connections will help the surgeon understand how his or her support and encouragement can decrease the patient's pain. Youngs et al. believe the surgeon or a familiar associate should also be present immediately after surgery to reassure the patient, orient her to her surroundings, and make certain she has adequate pain relief. Even if the patient appears unresponsive during the immediate postoperative phase, a familiar voice and reassuring word can be immensely beneficial.

Immediate Postoperative Care

Hospital stays have become much shorter. Some hysterectomies are being performed as outpatient procedures. These factors are having a positive psychological effect on patients. She knows that she is getting well when she no longer requires needles and is able to ambulate and urinate without assistance. It has long been known that early ambulation significantly reduces morbidity as well as the incidence of phlebitis and pneumonia. As long as intravenous therapy and urethral catheterization are maintained, the patient remains immobile and consequently at higher risk for venous stasis, ileus, and pulmonary complications. The incidence of pulmonary embolus in the postoperative hysterectomy patient has decreased in the past decades with shortened stays and early ambulation.

Crisis Intervention

It is important to recognize a patient who is overwhelmed by stress. A stress crisis can occur during any phase between diagnosis and recuperation. A crisis has been described as an obstacle to important life goals that becomes insurmountable when the individual employs customary methods of problem solving. Kaplan highlighted the following four phases of crisis:

1. Arousal occurs, and attempts are made at problem solving.
2. Increased tension leads to distress and disorganization, because arousal hinders rather than promotes coping behavior. Insomnia and fatigue frequently result.

3. Internal and external emergency resources are mobilized. Novel methods of coping are tried.
4. A state of progressive deterioration, exhaustion, and decompensation ensues as the problems drag on and on without resolution.

Dennerstein and van Hall report that the types of problems dealt with in crisis therapy include loss, change in status or role, interpersonal problems, and problems of choice between two or more alternatives. As an advocate, encourage your patient to communicate her feelings and to understand the problem enough to identify and define it; then help her rehearse alternative ways of coping.

One of the best concepts to apply during any stressful situation is to give the assurance that this particular moment, no matter how painful, is temporary. The surgical procedure and all the stages of mending that follow will have a beginning, a middle, and an end.

PSYCHOSEXUAL REHABILITATION

Goal

The goal of psychosexual rehabilitation after gynecologic or breast surgery is to restore sexual function, sexual identity, body image, and self-esteem. Most of the work must be done by the patient herself, but she may need assistance from her doctor and other health care providers because the experience is new to her. She has no gauge to measure what is normal for her particular situation and what is aberrant. You do.

Improving Communication

Even women who are not gynecologic surgery patients sometimes have sexual difficulties and find it embarrassing to talk about the difficulties with a doctor. Combine this intrinsic modesty with the stress of disease and not knowing how her surgery will affect her sexual life, and broaching the topic can be very difficult for a woman. When women do seek help, they are confronted with the barriers of mutual embarrassment, lack of research, limited treatment options, stereotypes, ageism, clinician reluctance to pursue the subject matter, and clinician misinformation or lack of training.

Many women and their physicians, who sometimes fear they are not qualified to help, are reluctant to speak of personal problems such as libido, arousal, coital pain, or past traumatic sexual events. Much of this reluctance can be overcome if the gynecologist knows what questions to ask when taking a sexual history, preferably during an initial or annual examination prior to any body-altering surgery. It is incumbent on the surgeon to begin this conversation.

Simon conducts personal sexual history interviews using questions he divides into the following broad categories:

- Biologic and hormonal
- Lack of appropriate stimuli
- Intrapersonal relationship
- Interpersonal history
- Contextual—lack of privacy, safety, and emotional rapport

The patient will elaborate on the areas of most concern to her.

Davis suggests that the physician ask the following open-ended questions to obtain a sexual history: Are you sexually active? Are you or your partner having any sexual difficulties at this time? Has there been any change in your sexual activity? Have you ever experienced any unwanted or harmful sexual activity? Another good question is: What sort of sexual problems do you have?

Even if the patient is initially reluctant to discuss such personal issues, she will have learned that you are willing to discuss them should the need arise. Davis also believes that a physician's confidence in dealing with sexual issues increases when the cycles of sexual response discussed below are learned and when the factors that affect them (e.g., psychological, environmental, and physiologic) are understood.

Sexual Cycle Primer

One of the ways to broach the subject of sexual function is to educate the patient about the cycle of normal female sexual response. In a sexual and sexual dysfunction tutorial, Davis describes the following stages: desire, arousal, plateau phase, orgasm, and resolution phase.

Desire is the motivation and inclination to be sexual. It is dependent on internal (fantasies) and external sexual cues and also on adequate neuroendocrine functioning.

Arousal is characterized by erotic feelings and vaginal lubrication as blood flow increases to the vagina. In addition to feelings of sexual tension, the sexually excited woman may experience tachycardia, rapid breathing, elevated blood pressure, breast engorgement, muscle tension, nipple erection, and other physical signs of arousal such as a flush. This is the stage where the vagina lengthens, distends, and dilates, and the uterus elevates partially out of the pelvis.

During the plateau phase, sexual tension, erotic feelings, and vasocongestion reach maximum intensity. The labia become more swollen and turn dark red, and the lower third of the vagina swells and thickens to form the orgasmic platform. The clitoris becomes more swollen and elevated, and the uterus elevates fully out of the pelvis. Eventually, women reach the threshold point of orgasmic inevitability. Orgasm is a myotonic response mediated by the sympathetic nervous system and is experienced as a sudden release of the tension built up during previous phases. Women, unlike men, experience no refractory period but can experience multiple orgasms during a single cycle. They can also experience orgasms before, during, and after intercourse provided they receive enough clitoral stimulation.

The last phase is called the resolution phase. Women experience a feeling of relaxation and well-being. The body returns to a resting state. Complete uterine descent, detumescence of the clitoris and orgasmic platform, and decongestion of the vagina and labia take about 5 to 10 minutes.

Sexual Dysfunction

Over 50% of *all* women are affected at one time or another by female sexual dysfunction (FSD). The Women's Health Foundation lists seven classifications for FSD disorders:

- Hypoactive sexual desire
- Sexual aversion
- Sexual arousal
- Orgasmic
- Dyspareunia
- Vaginismus
- Noncoital sexual pain

Feldhaus-Dahir reports on the many barriers to helping patients with sexual dysfunction, which is multifactorial and abysmally misunderstood. Since the FDA has approved nothing to treat premenopausal or postmenopausal women's sexual dysfunction, the menopausal woman and her physician have limited choices, but they do have a few.

A well-estrogenized vagina is essential for normal sexual function, but many women still believe estrogen therapies (discussed in more detail below) will harm them. Clinicians in the United States who prescribe androgen therapy use testosterone marketed for hypogonadal men, but at 10% of the dosage. A premenopausal woman naturally produces 10% of the amount produced by a normal male.

Some neurotransmitters, widely in use for other reasons, show promise treating sexual dysfunction. Simon lists bupropion, nefazodone, and buspirone as effective agents for desire, arousal, and orgasm. SSRIs have a negative effect on sexual desire.

Sexual Function after Surgery

Patients who talk about their sex lives frequently describe four pleasures associated with sexuality. These universal elements are touching, genital caressing, orgasm, and gratifying a partner. When a patient is recovering from surgery or has experienced surgical loss of coital function, genital caressing as a receiver or giver can be satisfying. Once a woman learns early in life how to be orgasmic, she can often learn to be so again despite major genital loss, including of her clitoris. When the ability to experience orgasm by one favorite means is destroyed by disease, the patient can be encouraged to experiment with alternative methods that do not conflict with her value system. Women who will never experience vaginal intercourse again can discover they are able, with education and imagination, to fulfill their feminine role as givers of pleasure if they choose to do so.

When a patient's psychosexual rehabilitation after surgery seems to be impaired and she fails to make steady progress toward resumption of her usual role, appropriate self-esteem, energy, identity, and ability to handle stress, she should be offered help. Help should be offered as soon as she mentions the problem. Early intervention is often easy and brief. The surgeon should be the first person to help the patient, with counseling and, if necessary, suitable medications.

A postsurgical patient may expect too much too soon from herself, or she may head off in the opposite direction and begin to assume the role of invalid. In most cases, however, she will be caught somewhere in between these two extremes. Once she begins to exhibit her normal patterns of relating to others, you will know she has officially begun the process of genuine healing.

You will be able to tell when she enters the healing phase because she will become less dependent on you, the nurses, and even her family members. As her strength increases, she will want to resume her usual activities. The inevitable, normal, uncomfortable grief process will commence. Encourage the patient to talk about her feelings rather than repressing them or brooding, because worry and rumination are forms of repetitive thought that are concomitant with and predictive of depressed mood. Dreary thoughts fuel a depressed mood and turn it into something ugly and dangerous; this has the potential to cause long-term or permanent psychological damage.

The patient has the power within to effect change in herself. Family members and friends should be cautioned, at this point, to allow verbal ventilation. It's a form of healthy discontent that frequently provides the impetus to hurry up and lose the sick image and begin to see herself as well and strong again.

Cosmetics, dress, and grooming are important parts of the rehabilitation process. When a postoperative patient combs her hair, puts on lipstick, and demands her own nightgown instead of hospital garb, she has begun to heal. When a patient feels that the surgery was disfiguring, she needs to compensate by learning new ways to dress or groom. She needs to feel whole and complete and responsible again as quickly as possible.

Most of the time, the mate or lover of the woman is caring and considerate of her. There is genuine concern for her health, hope for a quick recovery, and the willingness to assume many aspects of her role until she is well. Often there is a deepening of affection between the partners as gifts of love and concern are given and received. That special someone is in the waiting room during the surgical ordeal and by the patient's bedside when she awakes. There are flowers and gifts and promises made and kept. There is an abundance of reciprocal love. Adjustment to new roles is relatively smooth, causing new bonds to form and old ones to strengthen.

The surgical patient begins to see herself as a sexual person when her sexual identity is validated by her sexual partner, friends, family, and even admiring strangers she passes on the street. The woman who has had a mastectomy or other body-altering surgery needs to know her partner still finds her attractive and desirable. Without this affirmation, she may have a great deal of trouble seeing herself as a sexual being.

A potential roadblock to healing, however, is the fact that some sexual partners cannot accept an incomplete person. Some surgical procedures result in the loss of vulva, clitoris, or vagina. Radical pelvic surgery can leave a woman with a colostomy or urinary diversion. A severely altered body image concurrent with loss of health and vigor poses a serious threat to a woman's self-esteem. The woman who has lost her sexual identity feels damaged beyond repair. Some complain of continuing pelvic pain without obvious structural cause. Interest in sex vanishes, and the patient may actually leave her sexual partner or force the partner to abandon her. As she terminates her sexual identity, she feels old before her time and begins to draw in the edges of her life. These women need intense psychosexual therapy if they are ever to heal emotionally. Table 3.1 outlines the major factors that occur with psychosexual dysfunction.

In some cases, the woman's partner becomes a bigger problem than her physical disability. It is possible her significant other constructed a fragile emotional bond with body parts rather than with the actual woman. If she had or has cancer, the partner may irrationally feel that the cancer is contagious. If she is receiving radiation treatment, he may feel that if he resumes sexual relations with her, he, too, might absorb radiation from her body and be burned. The couple may be accustomed to frequent sex, and any change in the woman's availability stresses the relationship. The fear of causing pain also has an inhibiting effect. Emotional isolation and loss of nurturing occur in both partners when the woman experiences physical disability. As surgeon to the postoperative patient, you are her first line of psychosexual defense, and yours will not be an easy job.

Sexual adjustment is often significantly impaired in women after pelvic exenteration and gracilis myocutaneous vaginal reconstruction. In one of the few studies that exist, 84% of the patients resumed sexual activity within the first year after surgery. A modified version of the Sexual Adjustment Questionnaire was used; the responses outlined the most common problems patients face after the surgery: self-consciousness about a urostomy or colostomy, being seen in the nude by their partner, vaginal dryness, and vaginal discharge. It is hoped that future modifications in surgical technique, more realistic patient counseling, and aggressive postoperative support will minimize these problems in the future. Less serious matters can cause self-esteem and body image problems, too, if their aftermath includes or leads to bowel incontinence, urinary incontinence, vaginal vault prolapse, and scarring.

Bowel incontinence is rarely discussed even with a woman's physician because it is so embarrassing. Whether from obstetric injuries, injury to the anal muscles, infections, or diminished muscle strength from aging, once the cause and severity are determined, treatment can begin. This might include dietary changes, constipating medications, muscle strengthening exercises, biofeedback techniques, and sometimes surgical repair of the muscle. Some or all of these remedies help the woman control the discharge of embarrassing gas or stool. It is most important to discuss possible remedies because many women feel there is nothing that can be done for them but the frightening colostomy, when in actual fact, colostomy is a procedure that is rarely required.

As many as 50% of all women experience occasional urinary incontinence. In an attempt to lessen the blow to a woman's ego and make the event more socially acceptable, manufacturers hire movie stars to make commercials about the effectiveness of diapers for grown women. Diapers do treat the symptoms and allow for more freedom of movement, but not in an intimate setting. For many years, gynecologists have instructed patients about Kegel exercises to tighten the muscles of the pelvic floor, but this may not be enough to stop the embarrassing leakage of urine. The patient needs to know that there are tests that can determine the exact cause of the problem, and treatments using bladder retraining therapy, medications, and surgery. Urinary incontinence may be more socially acceptable today, but it is never normal, no matter what the woman's age.

Both bowel and urinary incontinence can be caused by vaginal vault prolapse, and this condition must be ruled out because it drastically affects sexual functioning. The presence of a mass can cause painful intercourse, difficulty accepting penetration, and a great deal of psychological anxiety when the tissue can be seen in the vaginal opening. This condition, if left untreated, only worsens with time, but techniques that correct female organ–supporting defects in the pelvis can restore sexual functioning and with it, a woman's sense of vitality and feminine allure.

Hormonal Therapy

HRT remains a controversial issue. It is imperative that HRT be discussed preoperatively with the patient facing surgery and the loss of her ovaries. Initial misinterpretation of the results of the Women's Health Initiative (WHI) Study has created much

TABLE 3.1 Major Factors in Psychosexual Dysfunction
Symptomatic
Interpersonal (discord with significant other)
Organic (disease, malnutrition, malfunction of body organs)
Psychiatric (anxiety, depression, schizophrenia)
Alcohol or drug abuse
Iatrogenic (suggestions, medication, surgery)
Learned
Family (childhood negative sexual associations, experiences)
Religion (imposed prohibitions internalized)
Early unpleasant sexual experiences
Gynecologic disorders (damaged genitalia, loss of breasts, uterus)
Intrapsychic conflict
Failure to develop psychosexually
Restrictive childrearing
Religious influences

fear and angst for both the gynecologist and the patient. The harmful effects were overestimated, and the media created undue alarm regarding breast cancer.

Pines et al., in careful evaluation of the data in the estrogen–progestin arm, show the risk for breast cancer and cardiovascular events to be most minute, about 0.1% for every year of use. No risk was observed for women younger than 60 years of age. It must be remembered that the WHI Study recruited women in their late 60s. Even so, the trees of thought planted during this and other massive studies continue to bear fruit.

Davey's analysis reveals there are multiple risks for breast cancer, not just HRT. In the Nurse's Health Study, HRT used continuously from age 50 to 60, benign breast disease, and family history played equal triplet roles in determining who was at risk for breast cancer.

With WHI, the incidence of breast cancer was increased in the women who currently used estrogen plus progestin HRT, but the incidence progressively *decreased* after stopping HRT. When placebo was compared to women taking estrogen-only HRT, the incidence of breast cancer was reduced and *stayed reduced for 10.7 years* after stopping HRT. Also in the placebo arm, the incidence was reduced if they had *ever* taken HRT.

Good things appear in the near future of menopausal women who use the 10-year window of opportunity after menopause to protect themselves with HRT. The development of micronized progesterone and transdermal estrogen seem to promise more good than harm.

The Kronos Early Estrogen Prevention Study of 727 recently menopausal women over 4 years found that hormone therapy improved symptoms of depression and anxiety without loss of cognition or increase in blood pressure.

Another 16-year study that involved 60,000 postmenopausal female nurses found that those who took HRT for 10 years reduced their risk of dying from all causes by 37%, with the most dramatic reduction being death from cardiac disease. After 10 years, the reduced risk for all causes was 16% because of the increased risk of dying from breast cancer. That risk rose to 43%, but the women who contracted breast cancer during the first 10 years had a lower death rate from the disease than did women who had never taken hormones, probably because of early detection. Chances of early detection of breast cancer are probably better for hormone users because they receive regular checkups.

In an extensive review of current literature on the subject, dubbed "the New Science of Estrogen," Hammond provides an overview of the risks and benefits of HRT and also includes information on therapeutic alternatives. Cardiovascular benefits of estrogen outweigh the risks. With combined estrogen–progestin therapy, studies have shown some increase in stroke and venous thromboembolism. Hammond feels that steroid hormonal therapy should be considered an integral part of the appropriate and necessary care of American women after menopause. The anticipated reduction of cardiovascular disease (CVD) and osteoporotic fractures by nearly 50% should be laudable goals for any health care system.

Statistics show overwhelmingly that CVD—not cancer—is the leading cause of mortality for postmenopausal women. In fact, 1 in 2 women will eventually die of heart disease or stroke, whereas only 1 in 25 women will die of breast cancer. Although the incidence of heart disease, including coronary artery disease and stroke, is low in premenopausal women, heart disease is the most frequent cause of death in women over the age of 50. Since 1984, the death rate from CVD in men has decreased, whereas the death rate for women has increased. Numerous epidemiologic studies support the long-term benefit

of estrogen in preventing CVD. Observational studies, such as the Postmenopausal Estrogen/Progestin Intervention Study sponsored by the National Institutes of Health, revealed that HRT can increase high-density lipoprotein cholesterol and decrease low-density lipoprotein cholesterol. The Nurses' Health Study demonstrated a reduction in the risk of CVD of up to 50% among current HRT users. Women who use estrogen have significantly less coronary artery stenosis than do women who do not use it. Takahashi et al. found that long-term HRT (for more than 2 years) may delay carotid intimal–medial thickness in healthy postmenopausal women.

Moreover, patients with the most advanced coronary artery disease experience the most benefit from HRT. Only 35% of women surveyed were aware of the connection between heart disease and menopause.

Current theories indicate that estrogen has extraordinarily complex biologic effects that translate into a variety of actions in diverse tissues. There is growing scientific evidence that estrogen exerts its beneficial actions on tissues of the skeletal, urogenital, digestive, cardiovascular, ocular, and nervous systems.

HRT is also first-line therapy for osteoporosis for most women, and treatment should begin as soon as possible after the menopause. Enough time has elapsed since the WHI media scare and cessation of estrogen therapy by users that a marked and rapid loss of bone density is being noted in those who stopped their replacement therapy. Yates and Barrett-Connor studied the association between HRT cessation and hip fracture risk. Concurrent with WHI, women in National Osteoporosis Risk Assessment currently on HRT had a 40% lower incidence of hip fracture compared to those who had never used HRT. Women who stopped using HRT more than 5 years earlier had similar hip fracture use to women who had never used HRT. Preliminary data suggest that even the elderly respond to estrogen replacement. However, there are therapeutic alternatives and lifestyle modifications (diet and routine exercise) that perimenopausal women must be counseled about to create a comprehensive prevention program. Such an effort can have a significant impact on long-term morbidity and mortality associated with osteoporosis.

Because one of their jobs is to find every needle that gets lost in the proverbial haystacks of their homes, women have phenomenal memories. When they become less adept at remembering where they and other people put their things, they fear the worst—that they are losing their minds—and this fear is not illogical. Women constitute 72% of the population over the age of 85 years, and roughly half of this group has Alzheimer disease (AD). Not only do women constitute a greater proportion of this older population, but AD is expressed earlier in women than men. This may be related to the estrogen loss that occurs with menopause. Hammond cites a study that found women who took estrogen for more than a year experienced a dramatic delay in AD onset. But even the group of women who averaged only 4 months of estrogen therapy, and most likely took the medication to control symptoms such as hot flashes, experienced a delay in AD onset. It has been speculated that a brief exposure to estrogen influenced AD expression 20 to 30 years later by preventing an irreversible loss of neurons associated with the occurrence of hot flashes. Research is ongoing, but one study found that estrogen replacement therapy in postmenopausal women is associated with a 50% reduction in the risk of developing AD because it slows the decline of visual memory. Lebrun's study in clinical endocrinology supports findings that endogenous estrogens protect against cognitive decline with aging.

Colon cancer occurs more often in women than men and is a leading cause of cancer incidence and deaths in women.

Even though mortality rates for colon cancer have decreased 25% among women in the last 20 years, it remains the third leading cause of cancer deaths in this group. The concept that postmenopausal estrogen replacement therapy may decrease the risk of colorectal cancer has received considerable attention, even though the hormone has no indication for this use. Multiple epidemiologic studies have been published that examined this relationship. The majority of these suggest an inverse, protective effect for estrogen, particularly with current use. Although the precise mechanism by which estrogen reduces colon cancer risk is unknown, it has been hypothesized that it affects bile acid metabolism or promotes tumor suppressor activity. The inclusion of estrogen as a measure to prevent colon cancer should be part of the discussions between menopausal women and their physicians. Counseling should include the American Cancer Society recommendations for annual digital rectal examination and fecal occult blood testing as well as a flexible sigmoidoscopy every 5 years or colonoscopy every 10 years.

Age-related macular degeneration (AMD) may be reduced by estrogen administration. This disease is the leading cause of legal blindness in the United States, accounting for as many as 60% of all new cases. There is no medical treatment, and surgical management in the form of photocoagulation is effective in only a small percentage of patients with the wet type of the disease. In the Rotterdam study, women who experienced menopause at an earlier age had a 90% increased risk of exhibiting signs of late AMD compared with those who experienced menopause at a later age. These data suggest that HRT reduces the risk of developing AMD.

Counseling women about replacement therapy must be combined with discussions about the importance of lifestyle changes, including the following:

- Normalization of weight
- Dietary intervention
- Smoking cessation
- Regular exercise
- Control of hypertension
- Control of diabetes
- Control of alcohol consumption
- Control of lipid elevations

Routinely, HRT counseling should go beyond simple symptom control to include both short- and long-term benefits, contraindications, common patient concerns, and misconceptions.

The contraindications to estrogen replacement that have been established by the FDA include known or suspected pregnancy or breast cancer, estrogen-dependent neoplasia, undiagnosed abnormal genital bleeding, and active thromboembolic disorders. However, ongoing research suggests that some of these contraindications may not be absolute. In the meantime, all of the relative contraindications must be carefully discussed and weighed against the risk of not prescribing HRT. This is also a good time to discuss the common concerns and misconceptions that women have about estrogen, even if patients do not raise them. For example, many women are concerned that estrogen may bring on the return of monthly bleeding, restore fertility, or produce weight gain.

When bilateral oophorectomy is anticipated in a premenopausal patient, HRT should be discussed before surgery, because one of the greatest fears of younger women is surgery-induced menopause. Patients should be told that estrogen therapy can be started immediately after surgery and that hot flashes and other menopausal symptoms can be avoided. The natural conjugated estrogens do not cause hypercoagulability and are safe during the immediate convalescent period.

Parker et al., in a recent lead study in *Obstetrics and Gynecology*, recommend ovarian conservation until at least age 65 because of their benefit to long-term survival. With ovarian preservation, the need for exogenous hormones is delayed.

The long-term benefits of HRT in preventing osteoporosis, CVD, and colon cancer are well established. The health of the vagina and lower urinary tract is also maintained. *The Journal of the British Menopause Society* says that various studies have demonstrated the efficacy of estrogen replacement in improving urinary and stress incontinence. The vagina lubricates more easily with sexual arousal, and intercourse is more comfortable with an estrogenic vaginal mucosa. Many women report an increased interest in and enjoyment of sex.

For women who do experience a loss of libido, even while taking estrogenic hormones, the new androgen therapies look promising as a way to improve sexual function and psychological well-being. Testosterone delivered via transdermal patches or gel bypasses the liver and has no negative effect on cholesterol. The skin serves as a constant reservoir; therefore, blood levels show fewer fluctuations.

However, there are physicians who believe hormonal balances induced by prescription medications should only be offered for relief of extreme menopausal symptoms and only for a short while. The author of *Dr. Susan Love's Hormone Book* and *Dr. Susan Love's Breast Book* is one such physician. She is a staunch supporter of eating soybean products and using herbal remedies such as black cohosh to maintain estrogen levels, the use of acupuncture and paced respiration for hot flashes, exercise, and using vitamin and calcium supplements. But even she admitted in an interview, "If my symptoms [for menopause] worsen, I may feel that I want to take some kind of drug. I certainly would be open to that."

By 2030, 1.2 billion women will be menopausal or postmenopausal. Wu et al. reported that if the surgery rates for pelvic floor disorders remain unchanged, the number of women expected to undergo inpatient and outpatient procedures for stress urinary incontinence (SUI) and pelvic organ prolapse (POP) will significantly increase. In 2010, records show 210,700 SUI surgeries performed. This number will increase over 47% by 2050. During the same time frame, POP surgeries will increase from 166,000 to 245,970.

The National Institutes of Health recommends human sexuality courses for all health care professionals in graduate schools. A majority of medical schools offer 3 to 10 hours of human sexuality instruction, usually embedded in other courses; this is not nearly enough to help a sexually dysfunctional patient. Even trained professionals who are members of the American Urogynecologic Society underestimated the prevalence of the problem. Only 22% of urogynecologists reported they had developed the habit of screening their patients for sexual dysfunction.

Professionals don't realize the tremendous societal burdens that the angst resulting from sexual dysfunction creates, as reflected in divorce, domestic violence, single-parent families, quality of life issues, and problems in forming enduring relationships. A few in the medical community are working for international standardization and continuing education and training in the area of sexual dysfunction. If successful, this will directly translate into greater competency and help for 50 million women in the United States alone.

SPECIAL CASES

Every patient is special and deserves to be treated with compassion and sensitivity. Women who are already in tumultuous life situations at the time of surgery present the greatest challenge.

The Teenager

Bluestein and Starling report that one million teenagers a year conceive. Of these million pregnancies, 400,000 end in abortion and 100,000 in miscarriage. Childbearing teenagers face a 60% excess in maternal mortality compared with adults and are most likely to suffer toxemia, anemia, hemorrhage, cervical trauma, cephalopelvic disproportion, excessive weight gain, and premature labor. These complications are due more to social and behavioral correlates than inherent adolescent aspects. Correlates include inadequate prenatal care, poor nutrition, substance abuse, and emotional distress.

Among 1,000 teenagers who have first-trimester abortions, one or two will experience fever, hemorrhage, and emergency abdominal surgical procedures. These numbers are lower than for older women, but the rate for cervical injury, which could affect future childbearing, is 5.5 per 1,000 teenagers, notably higher than the 1.7 to 3.1 per 1,000 for adults. Bluestein and Starling recommend the following communication techniques for the teenage patient:

- Guarantee confidentiality to build trust. Conduct the initial interview alone. Teenage girls may want to relate private information to the physician but not in the presence of a parent.
- Be patient. Gear communication to the patient's emotional and intellectual development.
- Be nonjudgmental. Gently explore the teenager's family and social environments. Will family members and friends support or harm your patient?
- Discuss the teenager's long-term plans. Be aware of ethnic differences in health-related matters.

Female patients who belong to local or national gangs come into the health care system with a unique set of problems and values. It is imperative that the surgeon not add to the patient's stress more than is absolutely necessary. Sometimes, the simple act of being treated like a human being worthy of consideration is a novel and humbling experience.

The Senior Woman

The new kid on the block for the next many years will be the senior woman. Kuzmarov et al. caution family doctors that they will need to be able to evaluate and manage sexual problems in the senior couple. Of spouses over the age of 76, 24% reported having sex within the last month. This same group averaged 2.75 episodes per month. The numbers soar upward relative to younger more active seniors.

The study found many women take a cerebral, cognitive approach and respond to their partners for reasons of intimacy, bonding, commitment, love, affection, and the acceptance of it all rather than simply to scratch a vascular itch.

It is easy to imagine a grandmother baking cookies or rocking a new baby in the family. Our culture makes it a little more difficult to imagine this same woman flushed and happy from an energetic romp in the sack with her favorite beau. Sex after 60 is a reality for many women and men. These people enjoyed sex when they were young, they perfected it as the years flowed by, and the thought of doing without expression of the natural urges, even temporarily, is discomfiting.

When an older woman faces gynecologic surgery, therefore, do not assume she is asexual. She may simply view her sex life as her private business and be loath to discuss it. Do not antagonize or humiliate the senior patient by assuming her sexuality is a thing of the past (Table 3.2).

TABLE 3.2 Excerpted from "Communicating with Seniors/Advice Techniques and Tips" Your Attitude Is Showing!

- Avoid stereotyping or reinforcing incorrect perceptions about seniors. Show older people as you know them to be; active participants, using a full range of abilities in a full range of roles and activities.
- Shun ageism, racism, and sexism in conversation, text, illustrations, and photographs. They are prohibited by law.
- Especially avoid ageist language (that categorizes seniors negatively), such as "the aged," "the elderly," "oldsters," "senile," "feeble," etc.
- Use "seniors," "older persons," or "older adults" if you need to indicate the age group.
- Beware of patronizing, condescending, or childish expressions and tone when talking with or about seniors.
- Keep in mind that seniors are generally wise shoppers whose lifelong experience comes in handy in detecting flattery and insincere deference.
- Remember that the way you use language reflects your attitudes and your respect for the audience.

Source: Communicating with Seniors, Health Canada, 2001. Reproduced with the permission of the Minister of Public Works and Government Services Canada, 2013.

If the surgical procedure will affect her sexually, explain the consequences. Assure her that the surgery will leave her as whole and as functional as possible. Give this woman the opportunity to express her anxieties and to ask questions. If her mate or lover is present, include this person in the discussion. In the senior woman who has a large cystocele, rectocele, or uterine or vault prolapse, every effort should be made to avoid colpocleisis. Sacrospinous colpopexy and vaginal reconstructive surgery are indicated. The fact that a woman is older and sexually inactive at the time of surgery does not mean that she will never be active again. Much preparation and explanation must be given to evaluate and prepare her for the closing off of her vagina or its subsequent reconstruction should that become necessary.

Butler et al. advise that, when taking a sexual history, ask if the symptoms started after a period of sexual activity. Excretory urogram and cystoscopy can sometimes be avoided with a diagnosis of postcoital cystitis and subsequent antibiotic treatment. A history of traumatic intercourse in the presence of an atrophic vagina may indicate a need for estrogen therapy and lubricants rather than dilation and curettage. Butler et al. also caution physicians not to assume an older woman is sexually inactive. They advise checking for sexually transmitted diseases in older women as you would in younger ones.

When surgery is indicated, perform it as if the senior woman was still young and had many years of sexuality ahead of her, because she probably does. If the surgery occurs in the genital area, do not shave her pubic hair. The procedure is archaic and microbiologically unnecessary if competent sterilization procedures are followed. As men age, they sometimes lose hair on the head. As women age, the pubic hair sometimes thins, and once shaved, it may never grow back.

Many older women have had to curb their sexual appetites to compensate for physiologic changes that have occurred in a mate. Removal of excessive vaginal mucosa during pelvic surgery compromises the vagina, which is already losing elasticity.

This inhibits penetration during coitus and can cause painful intercourse. Be understanding and helpful if solutions are possible. If the dysfunction resulting from the surgery will be permanent, encourage the couple to experiment with various ways to please each other or seek the advice of a sex therapist that is knowledgeable about creative sexual play.

Butler instructs physicians to educate themselves about the effects of medications on sexuality. More than 200 medications have sexual dysfunction as a side effect. Many are effective in lower doses that do not harm the libido or the patient's physical ability.

The positive benefits of a healthy sex life are multiple. Emotional intimacy and the ability to connect physically with another human being bring great joy and satisfaction. This need to connect intensifies rather than diminishes with age.

The Sexually Assaulted Patient

According to FBI statistics, reported rapes and sexual assaults in the United States are up nearly 5% since the year 2000. It is estimated that only about 16% of rapes that occur are ever reported. One third of sexually assaulted victims are under the age of 12. Convicted rape and sexual assault offenders testify that two thirds of their victims are younger than 18. Two thirds of the victims older than 18 knew their attacker prior to the rape. A sad fact is that almost one fifth of the women who are raped before the age of 18 are raped again after the age of 18. Many require medical attention: Up to 22% suffer genital trauma, up to 40% incur sexually transmitted disease, and 1% to 5% become pregnant as a result of the rape. Rape survivors are 13 times more likely than the general population to attempt suicide.

Most hospital emergency rooms have strict protocols to follow when treating sexually assaulted patients. The proper collection of evidence and initial treatment of injuries is a priority. The surgeon who repairs the gynecologic damage done to these female patients should be aware of the general characteristics of psychological trauma associated with rape.

The symptoms of rape trauma syndrome compiled by Blair and Warner can be found in Table 3.3.

Many of these symptoms are the same as seen in posttraumatic stress disorder (PTSD). These authors also outlined the

TABLE 3.3 Symptoms of Rape Trauma Syndrome

Recurrent, painful recollections or dreams of the event
Suddenly acting or feeling as if the event were recurring
Demonstrations of fear, anger, or anxiety
Crying, restlessness, or tenseness
Controlled feelings masked by a false demeanor of calmness, composure, or subdued attitude
Matter-of-fact answering of questions
Inappropriate smiles or laughter
Inability to remember parts of the event because reexposure to stimuli present during the traumatic moment reinvokes the associated pain
Decreased interest in important activities
Lack of future plans
Limited range of affect
Detachment toward others
Sleep disorders
Difficulty concentrating
Hypervigilance
Irritability
Angry outbursts

necessary skills that any caregivers attempting to help a sexually assaulted victim should possess:

- Understand rape and sexual assault.
- Assess how the patient perceives the act.
- Identify and reinforce the patient's ability to cope.
- Assist significant others.
- Coordinate care and help if the victim needs assistance.
- Mobilize community resources.

The rape patient, from the youngest child to the oldest adult, has survived an attack on her physical body. Most gynecologists are familiar with the legacy of these attacks (up to 75% of patients seen with CPP were physically or emotionally abused). The assaulted patient now needs reassurance from her surgeon and other health care workers that she will also survive the damage done to her psyche.

Hensley reported for National Public Radio that Naval researchers studied 800 soldiers who had been traumatized by atrocities like roadside bombs and gunshot wounds. While 61% of the soldiers who received morphine did develop PTSD, 79% of those who did not experience PTSD *also* received morphine. Dr. Matthew Friedman at the Department of Veteran Affairs National Center for PTSD writes that the findings add to the evidence already collected that "rapid pain reduction" after a traumatic injury may lower the risk of PTSD.

Could it also help the sexually assaulted if they received the morphine within hours of the trauma?

The Cancer Patient

In 2009, 84,155 women in the United States were diagnosed with gynecologic cancer. (This figure covers 90% of the population.) That same year, 27,813 women in the United States died from a gynecologic cancer. (This figure covers 100% of the population.)

Bloch cautions physicians that the manner in which the diagnosis of cancer is disclosed to the patient can determine whether the patient lives or dies. It is imperative to instill hope and the desire to fight the disease. A diagnosis of cancer by telephone can be devastating and is viewed by many physicians and patients as a form of cruelty.

In her book, *The Balance Within: The Science Connecting Health and Emotions*, Dr. Esther M. Sternberg presents evidence that relief from stress can make you less vulnerable to illness. The cancer patient shares the same fears common to all surgical patients. She may be psychologically attached to the body part that must be removed. She may fear anesthesia, disfigurement, the unknown, the hospital experience and staff, debility, loss of economic competence, and sexual dysfunction.

In addition to the normal realm of anxiety associated with surgery, a diagnosis of cancer brings special stresses to a woman's life. Schain describes universal concerns experienced by people diagnosed with cancer no matter where in the body the cancer is located. These people fear death, postoperative adjuvant treatment, and recurrence.

The cancer patient is concerned about dying or being injured during the operation. Preoperative anxiety can manifest as anorexia, insomnia, tachycardia, fear, and panic. Acute depression is not uncommon and can lead to suicidal tendencies.

The patient is afraid of becoming unable to take care of her family members. Will she be sick for long? Who will raise her children if she dies? Who will care for her parents? Will her loved ones be supportive, or will they begin to back away from her? If the woman is alone, without mate or family, she fears becoming unable to care for herself.

The treating surgeon can ease some of the cancer patient's fear by free and open communication. Educate the patient about exactly what to expect, and offer reassurance if possible. Explain the procedure she is about to undergo and the positive benefits that you both hope will result. Help her understand your commitment to her is long term. The best facilities have a team of helpers that include specialists as well as volunteers. The following study illustrates the results one group of patients obtained after a few lifestyle lessons.

Breast cancer patients ($n = 227$) who had undergone mastectomy and chemotherapy were randomized to a program of psychological intervention. They were trained in coping skills for stress, lifestyle changes, exercise, and advice on how to talk to their physicians.

A *year* later, these patients experienced better quality of life than did the controls. Psychological help at 4 months continued to yield positive results at 12. There was a reduction in symptoms and cancer treatment toxicities. Also, patients who exercised the most were able to receive significantly higher relative doses of taxane-based chemotherapy than did those patients who exercised some or not at all.

Surgery and cancer in the urogenital region can be consciously or unconsciously interpreted as mutilation. The possibility of some degree of postoperative sexual dysfunction can create a fear of abandonment by the sexual partner. If possible, assure both the patient and her partner that they will continue to be able to bring joy, pleasure, and comfort to each other.

The psychological effect of cancer on a woman is largely determined by whether the malignancy is primary, recurrent, or terminal. The surgeon is usually the patient's first big gun aimed at the cancer, as well as the patient's greatest hope for a complete cure. The surgeon is most likely the first physician to learn the stage of growth of the cancer, and the family will be waiting to hear the results of the surgical experience. How advanced is the cancer? What is the prognosis? What happens next?

If the news is good, the patient recovers and has routine checkups to monitor her health for the rest of her life. If the news is not good, the results should be revealed with as much sensitivity and hope as possible. Although no patient should ever be given an absolute death sentence, it is the surgeon's job to foster courage in the terminal patient.

The surgeon must wrestle with personal, ethical, and moral conflicts when the surgery for the cancer patient is palliative. Should procedures be performed that extend death and not life? If she is able, the patient herself must make the choice.

If the cancer patient elects to have a palliative procedure, her postoperative care may be shared by radiologists, chemotherapists, and others who specialize in cancer treatment. However, as her gynecologist, you should maintain contact and assist in trying to get the patient well or to at least enhance the quality of the remainder of her life. Meaningful psychosocial support should be based on established concepts of crisis intervention, because cancer is a major life crisis. Counseling should be designed to support adaptive behaviors and feelings that reduce the psychological stress, restore and consolidate the patient's self-image, and normalize sexual functioning as quickly as possible.

The Suicidal Patient

The World Health Organization (WHO) reports that suicide rates have increased 60% worldwide in the last 45 years, with 870,000 annual deaths. Approximately 30,000 people commit suicide each year in the United States. Cooper, Rosa, and Daniel studied over 6,000 individuals and found that hopelessness ranked the highest of all symptoms associated with suicidal ideation in psychiatric patients and adolescents.

A surgeon probably will not know if a patient is contemplating suicide unless the patient admits to thinking about ending her life or unless a family member voices concern. Subtle warning signs include a chronic state of depression, lethargy, an inability to relate to others, weight loss or gain, lack of interest in life in general or the surgical procedure in question, a change in personal appearance, abnormal sleep patterns, or any strange behavior uncharacteristic of the particular patient. Many of these symptoms are normal for the presurgical and postsurgical patient, so it is easy to see how suicidal tendencies could hide within the maze.

To determine a patient's suicide potential, ask: Have you been troubled with thoughts of hurting yourself? Barbee advises physicians to ask directly: Have you ever thought of taking your own life? Do you feel like taking your life now? If the patient answers yes, the physician should find out if the patient has a simple, straightforward suicide plan that is likely to succeed.

A patient with low to moderate suicide potential is noticeably depressed but can identify some support system. There may be suicidal thoughts but no specific plan.

A patient with a high suicide potential feels profoundly helpless. Little or no support system seems to exist. Thoughts of suicide are frequent, and a plan exists that is likely to succeed.

The surgeon may be the first person to realize the patient is in emotional trouble, and he or she might be the only support system available if the patient has significantly withdrawn from others. Crisis therapy for the suicidal patient begins when the patient requests help or when someone recognizes her potential for self-destruction. By showing interest in her feelings and concern for her welfare, the surgeon initiates crisis intervention.

Rare Causes for Concern

Pelvic Injury from Traumatic Accident

In a review of high-impact pelvic fractures, Harvey-Kelly et al. found that 35.9% of men and 39.6% of women experience sexual dysfunction, and they believe the numbers may be underreported. Patient age, urogenital injuries in particular, and specific fracture types B with accompanying rotational instability, but vertical stability, and type C with double instability were the highest risk factors. In conclusion, they advised that sexual function in both sexes should be assessed no sooner than 1 year, and no more than 3 years after the injury using the International Index of Erectile Function and the Female Sexual Function Index.

Disorders of Sexual Development

The terminology of Disorders of Sexual Development (DSD) has changed in an effort to reflect a more accurate description of the pathophysiology (Table 3.4).

TABLE 3.4 Terminology of Disorders of Sexual Development	
PREVIOUS	**REVISED**
Female pseudohermaphrodite	46,XX DSD
Male pseudohermaphrodite	46,XY DSD
True hermaphrodite	Ovotesticular DSD
XX Male	46,XX testicular DSD
XY Sex reversal	46,XY complete gonadal dysgenesis

Hutchinson et al. say that once children are diagnosed with ambiguous genitalia or other manifestations of DSD (ideally from birth), a team of specialists is required to counsel the parents and teach them how to deal with their specific set of circumstances. Interestingly, clinical and basic science research now shows gender identity development *begins* in utero.

Ocal lists four issues causing the current intense debates about how to manage intersexual patients:

• Etiologic diagnosis
• Assignment of gender
• Genital surgery indication and timing
• Disclosure of medical information to patient and parents

A government publication emphasizes that the psychologist chosen must have knowledge of sexual development, gender identity development, factors that influence sex role behavior, and sexuality; he or she must understand the trajectory of a DSD across the individual's life. Thus, the role of the psychologist as part of the individual's holistic team is routine, preemptive, and reactive as time passes and important issues arrive.

These children offer all of humanity a glimpse into how we came to be female or male. The contributions they make are without bounds.

Premature Ovarian Insufficiency

In Premature Ovarian Insufficiency (POI), a woman's ovaries cease to function properly before her 40th birthday. Symptoms are irregular or absent menstrual periods, hot flashes, night sweats, vaginal dryness, and decreased sexual desire. Infertility is common, though 5% to 10% of women with POI are able to conceive without medical intervention.

Because there are fewer than 200,000 cases in the United States, POI is classed as a "rare" disease, and 90% of the causes remain unknown, mysteries yet to be solved. Some guesses are genetic history, a woman's ovaries attacked by her own immune system, infection, chemotherapy and radiation cancer treatments, or something environmental.

DEALING WITH DEATH

Death is a taboo subject for most physicians. Many doctors go to great lengths to avoid discussing the eventuality, and most are uncomfortable dealing with the emotional consequences of the death of a patient. To many physicians, death is viewed as a personal failure. Regardless of any internal attitudes he or she may have, the surgeon is responsible for communicating the facts of the death to the family and for being the first person to help them cope with the loss of their loved one.

When a patient dies, explain to the family, to the best of your ability, exactly what happened. Assure them that everything medically possible was done. Ufema suggests the following guidelines to make the death experience as bearable as possible for all concerned.

• Ask about donations for transplantation.
• Provide an area where the family members can say goodbye.
• If it is true, tell the family members how the patient affected you personally.
• Transfer your protective feelings for the patient to the family members.
• Begin the grief process by saying, "Jane's body is ready for the morgue now. Would you like to say a final goodbye?"
• If family members want a lock of hair, allow them to take it.
• Give family members the patient's belongings.
• Provide an escort for any family member who is alone.
• Help the hospital staff cope with the loss.

Remember that it is permissible for the physician to show emotion with the family if the emotion is genuine. Someone is gone and will never see tomorrow.

FUTURE TRENDS

The new millennium was heralded with great joy and celebration. Its predominant theme was one of hope, and nowhere is this more evident than in the field of medicine, especially women's health issues. The hand that rocks the cradle now rules important aspects of the research world. During the next 20 years, 45 million women will enter menopause and live one-third to one-half of their lives postmenopausally. Research into improving the quality of their lives and subsequently all those they touch has never been more important or timely.

Guidelines for Practice

Pelvic exams are a source of dread for most gynecologic patients. Many women will applaud new guidelines from the American College of Obstetrics and Gynecology that state no pelvic exam is necessary on healthy asymptomatic women under 21 years of age or over 21 years of age if they, too, are asymptomatic and have had the uterus removed, fallopian tubes removed for benign conditions, no history of cancer, and some forms of precancerous neoplasia; are neither HIV positive nor immunocompromised; and were not exposed to diethylstilbestrol in utero.

Common sense and patient wishes should dictate whether a pelvic exam is done on asymptomatic low-risk women, because no evidence supports or refutes benefits from the annual pelvic exam or speculum and biannual exam for this group of patients.

Some women, because of age and other health issues, choose not to seek treatment for conditions detected during the pelvic exam. Physicians may honor their wish to end the pelvic examinations.

As a multitude of women move through the life stages of maiden, mother, and crone, the health care they receive during one stage will be reflected in all those that follow. Baby boomer women, born between 1946 and 1964, will continue their legacy of reform by participating in medical clinical studies concerning endocrinology, gynecology, neurology, oncology, genetics, and finally, geriatrics. The daughters and sons they presented to the world will advance reproductive technology in all its genetic and social ramifications.

Robotics

Robotic gynecologic surgery, a recent gift of the technologic world, is being performed routinely now. It is envisaged that most surgery in the future can and will be performed robotically. The systems currently in use are not intended to act independently from surgeons or to replace them. They provide a means for the skilled surgeon to complete complex and advanced procedures with increased precision and with a minimally invasive approach. Medical students will soon be able to perfect their surgical techniques using cyber scalpels, simulated lifelike patient bodies, three-dimensional models, and long-distance mentors. The space industry has also yielded a smart surgical probe that will be used for breast biopsies. The small disposable needle with multiple sensors will be able to distinguish normal tissue from tumor tissue and greatly reduce the 18,000 breast biopsies per week now performed on women with suspicious lesions. Originally conceived as a robotic tool to aid astronaut/physicians during long-duration space flights, it has already found a medical application in neurosurgery.

In 2005, the FDA approved the use of a robotic system (da Vinci built by Intuitive Inc.) for use in gynecology. While most advanced gynecologic surgeries are still performed through an abdominal incision (teaching hospitals 82%, nonteaching hospitals 77%), laparoscopic surgeries have less blood loss, fewer complications, shorter hospital stays, and quicker recoveries than do abdominal or vaginal procedures. The da Vinci Robotic System allows less experienced laparoscopic surgeons to perform complex procedures.

Weinberg, Rao, and Escobar found that although there is widespread adoption of the robotic platform, there have been *no* randomized trials comparing its efficacy and safety with traditional surgical approaches. Their comprehensive work updates previous published reviews and focuses only on actual comparative observational studies. In conclusion, they believe, given the caveats of appropriate patient selection and proper physician training, robotic surgery could be advantageous, but they cautioned that until larger, well-designed observational studies or randomized control trials are completed with long-term outcomes, the superiority of robotic surgery over other methods cannot be determined.

Wright, like the former researchers, cautions against over-exuberant use and rapid adoption of robotic-assisted surgery, also citing the absence of randomized trial evidence validating its use. In addition, higher costs are noted compared to conventional surgery for many of the procedures. There is marked concern that the sole manufacturer of the FDA-approved devices controls the market by regulating the product's cost, buying up the competition, and using unsubstantiated advertising claims.

Makary et al. at Johns Hopkins had similar concerns when they analyzed 400 randomly selected websites for US hospitals that had 200 beds or more. They found that 89% of them touted the clinical superiority of robotic surgery over conventional surgeries but failed to provide substantiation or to disclose any associated risks. Again, no randomized controlled studies to date show that patients benefit from robotic surgeries over any others. It is known that robotic surgeries take more time, keep patients under anesthesia longer, and cost more.

Makary believes hospitals are perceived as trusted advisers by the public and should have no conflicts of interest when recommending one service or product over the other. Hospital website use of manufacturer provided text and images was blatant.

Johns Hopkins forbids the use of industry-provided content on its websites.

The Old is the New New

Old sciences and contemporary science hold that optimal therapeutic results are obtained when the patient actively participates in the healing process. The use of traditional or alternative therapies is not only popular among some patients but can also be effective.

Schiff, Gurgevich, and Caspi advocate for scientific studies to determine if hypnosis and acupuncture used concomitantly would work better than either works alone. Acupuncture is based on the principle that channels of energy in the body become blocked and result in disease or discomfort. Theta waves produced during hypnosis result in a heightened state of relaxation *or* a state of laser-focused attention.

During acupuncture, the patient lies still for 20 to 30 minutes. Listening to hypnotic suggestions (of the patient's choosing) during this time might double-prime the individual to expect and receive positive health results.

The possibilities for relief of chronic pain, chemotherapy-induced nausea, childbirth, and success making those vital lifestyle changes are just a few of the possibilities of combining the two modalities into what might be called hypnopuncture.

Psychosomatic Medicine

Psychosomatic medicine is a system of medicine that aims at discovering the exact nature of the relationship between the emotions and bodily function, affirming the principle that the mind and body are one.

Psychosomatic medicine is an idea whose time has come. The discipline is particularly useful for those mysterious symptoms that are experienced by 30% to 40% of all medical patients. Chronic illnesses account for the expenditure of 80% of health care dollars. These patients will never be cured, but the quality of their lives can be dramatically improved if areas other than the illness itself are explored.

Psychosomaticism tries to determine the character of the relationship between the body and the mind and what's going on between them to make or keep the patient ill. Is it an unresolved problem from the past? Is it recent trauma? Is it an unhealthy lifestyle? If hard, cold, biologic, diagnostic tests can't confirm or deny a causal agent, what is the culprit?

Fava et al.'s comprehensive review of psychosomatic literature elucidates the progress already made when an interdisciplinary approach of investigation is applied, with patient, physician, psychotherapists, nurses, other clinicians, and family members all working together in the best interest of the patient. Allostasis is the goal.

Allostasis means the ability of an organism to achieve stability through change. Productive positive change can only occur if the individual has the necessary coping mechanisms to deal with the destabilizing circumstances affecting the illness or the patient's quality of life.

Infertility

Wurn and Wurn et al. conducted original research to determine if noninvasive physical therapy could open completely blocked fallopian tubes in infertile women. Not only is this a major cause of infertility, both natural and in vitro, but of abdominopelvic pain and pain during intercourse.

For inclusion, the patients had to have a history indicative of abdominopelvic adhesions, with:

- Documented complete bilateral or unilateral (if one tube had already been surgically removed) tubal occlusion
- A history of meeting the US requirement for infertility by failing to achieve a natural intrauterine pregnancy after a minimum of 1 year of unprotected intercourse
- Documented radiologic, surgical, or pregnancy reports after treatment

All therapists had been specifically trained to treat pelvic adhesions. Fallopian tubes were accessed via external, internal, and bimanual manipulation of neighboring soft tissue structures. Truly occluded fallopian tubes are not known to spontaneously open. Confirmed patency or natural intrauterine pregnancy within a 2-year follow-up was considered success.

Within that time frame, 9 (53%) of the 17 patients with confirmed patency reported a natural or intrauterine insemination.

Researchers concluded that, though the study was small, a noninvasive manual soft tissue physical therapy approach to reopen blocked fallopian tubes absolutely exists and is pregnant with possibility.

Depression

Jackson et al. ask the critical question of whether successful treatment of depression, a profound source of human suffering, can prevent the occurrence of other disease processes. Thus far, clinical trials have not shown this to be true, so there could be an unknown, yet-to-be-discovered factor that causes both depression and comorbid disease.

Scrutiny of body–mind interactions may soon spawn radical new approaches to the practice of Western medicine and spell the end of traditional separation of the two entities.

Those Stimulating Seniors

The next time you see senior citizens, you might want to thank them for your job.

The Census Bureau records that 10,000 baby boomers retire every day, and one American turns 65 every 13 seconds. By 2030, 70 million people will be seniors. Directly or indirectly, they will influence the creation of 20 million jobs, many in health care and others in the financial industry, real estate, the legal profession, and technology.

The Congressional Budget Office estimates that $135 billion is spent every year just on long-term care for seniors. Of the most rapidly growing businesses in the United States, 10 out of 20 are in health care.

Jonathan Tilly told attendees at the North American Menopause Society 22nd Annual Meeting that a woman's ticking biologic clock may not be inevitable. Maybe the ovaries don't "fail"; maybe they just go into a state of suspended animation.

His study took half the ovary tissue from a mouse he had forced into menopause and grafted it into a young wild mouse. The dormant premeiotic germline stem cells became active again when exposed to the young mouse's ovaries. They produced oocytes.

Human oogonial stem cells will spontaneously generate what appear to be immature oocytes in vitro. To determine if this is possible in vivo, the researchers transplanted cells from a menopausal woman into immunodeficient mice. There was clear evidence of positive oocytes in the grafted tissue.

Tilly believes ovarian replacement therapy could improve the life course of women, and not just women who wish to reproduce. Will women be able to function better if the biologic clock is turned back?

Tilly and team compared a menopausal mouse to her non-menopausal sisters. The sisters did not suffer the ravages of time such as loss of hair, wrinkly skin, or cancer, whereas the menopausal sister looked "ratty."

As surgeons, it will be your duty and privilege to witness, record, and practice the new knowledge and incorporate it with what is already known so that you can make a positive difference in the lives of women now living as well as those yet to be born.

CONCLUSION

Advanced technology cannot change the fact that women are emotional creatures by nature. Few experiences give women more satisfaction than do sexuality and conception. Surgery on or near her reproductive tract is potentially fraught with emotional sequelae. The gynecologic surgeon's responsibility transcends a stunning technical performance in the surgical arena. The accomplished surgeon must considerably manage the patient's return to physical and psychological health. The most important thing a doctor will ever do is learn to listen, even in these, what will someday be known as, the halcyon days of technology.

BIBLIOGRAPHY

Abel G. How to avoid being accused of sexual harassment. The American Association of Sex Educators, Counselors, and Therapists (AASECT), 2000 Annual Conference, May 10–14, 2000.

Advincula AP, Falcone T. Laparoscopic robotic gynecologic surgery. *Obstet Gynecol Clin North Am.* 2004;31:599, ix.

Agency for Health Care Policy and Research. *Health services research on hysterectomy and alternatives*. Fact sheet. AHCPR Publication No. 97-R021. Rockville, MD: Agency for Health Care Policy and Research. http://www.ahrq.gov/research/hysterec.htm

American Society of Colon and Rectal Surgeons. *Bowel incontinence (patient brochure)*. Arlington Heights, IL: American Society of Colon and Rectal Surgeons (ASCRS).

Andersen BL, Hacker NF. Psychosexual adjustment following pelvic exenteration. *Obstet Gynecol* 1983a;61:331.

Andersen BL, Hacker NF. Psychosexual adjustment of gynecologic oncology patients: a proposed model for future investigation. *Gynecol Oncol* 1983b;15:214.

Andrews J. Urinary Incontinence—New Hope. *Research Activities*, Updated July, 2012.

Angelos P. When the evidence isn't there: seeking informed consent for new procedures. *Virtual Mentor*. Updated January, 2011. http://virtualmentor.ama-assn.org

Barbee MA. Recognizing suicide. *Nursing* 1993;23:32N.

Barber CA, Margolis K, Luepker RV, et al. The impact of the Women's Health Initiative Study on discontinuation of postmenopausal hormone therapy: the Minnesota Heart Survey (2000-2002). *J Women's Health (Larchmt)* 2004;13:975.

Barnes AB, Tinkham CG. Surgical gynecology. In: Notman MT, Nadelson CC, eds. *The woman patient: medical and psychological interfaces*. New York: Plenum Press, 1978.

Benjamin-Pratt AR, Howard FM. Management of chronic pelvic pain. *Minerva Ginecol* 2010;62:447.

Blair TMH, Warner CG. Sexual assault. *Top Emerg Med* 1992;(Dec):58.

Bloch R. Disclosing cancer diagnosis to a patient. *J Natl Cancer Inst* 1994;86:38.

Bluestein D, Starling E. Helping pregnant teenagers. *West J Med* 1994;161:140.

Brain CE, Creighton SM, Mushtaq I, et al.; US Gov Pub. Holistic Management of DSD. *Best Pract Res Clin Endocrinol Metab* 2010;24:335–354.

Brown J, Seeley D, et al. Correspondence re: Urinary incontinence after hysterectomy. *Lancet* 2000;356:2012.

Bruns D. *Matters of life and death*. Greeley, CO: Health Psychology Associates, 1997.

Butler RN, Hoffman E, Whitehead DE, et al. Love and sex after sixty: how physical changes affect intimate expression. *Geriatrics* 1994;49:20.

Colditz GA. Estrogen, plus progestin therapy, and risk of breast cancer. *Clin Cancer Res* 2005;11(2 Pt 2):909S. ISSN:1078-0432.

Daly MJ, Sadock BJ, Kaplan HI, et al. Psychological impact of surgical procedures on women. In: Sadock BJ, Kaplan HI, Freedman AM, eds. *The sexual experience*. Baltimore, MD: Williams & Wilkins, 1976:308.

Davey DA. HRT: some unresolved clinical issues in breast cancer, endometrial cancer and premature ovarian insufficiency. *Womens Health* 2013;9:59.

Davis H, Johnston M. The effects of communication/counselling in medical practice: an evaluation. *J R Soc Med* 1994;87:429.

Dennerstein AO, Franz CP. Conference report: Third annual female sexual function forum: new perspectives in the management of female sexual dysfunction. U.S. National Health and Social Life Survey and Kinsey Institute for Research on Sex, Gender, and Reproduction, Indiana University, October 26–29, 2000. Boston, MA.

Derogatis LR. Breast and gynecologic cancers: their unique impact on body image and sexual identity in women. In: Vaeth JM, Blomberg RC, Adler L, eds. *Body image, self-esteem, and sexuality in cancer patients*. New York: Karger, 1980.

Diaz-Arrastia C, Jurnalov C, Gomez G, et al. Laparoscopic hysterectomy using a computer-enhanced surgical robot. *Surg Endosc* 2002;16.

Diaz-Gilbert M. Culturally diverse patients. *Nursing* 1993;23:44.

Eunice Kennedy Shriver National Institute of Child Health and Human Development. Primary Ovarian Insufficiency (POI) overview. http://www.nichd.nih.gov/health/topics/poi. US Gov Pub

Fava GA, Sonino N. Psychosomatic medicine. *Int J Clin Pract* 2010;64:1155.

Feldhaus-Dahir M. Female sexual dysfunction: barriers to treatment. *Urol Nurs* 2009;29:81.

Female Sexual Function Forum. U.S. National Health and Social Life Survey, October 26–29, 2000, Boston, MA.

Freeman MG. Introduction to the sexual history. In: Walker HK, Hall WD, Hurst JW, eds. *Clinical methods*, 2nd ed. Boston, MA: Butterworth, 1980.

Galovotti C, Richter DL. Talking about hysterectomy: the experiences of women from four cultural groups. *J Womens Health Gend Based Med* 2000;9(suppl 2):S63.

Gross J. Our bodies, but my hysterectomy. *The New York Times.* June 1994.

Hammond CB. Management of the menopausal woman. *Am J Manag Care* 11:541.

Hammond CB. The Women's Health Initiative Study: perspectives and implications for clinical practice. *Rev Endocr Metab Disord* 2005;6:93.

Hammond C, Love S. Controversies in hormone replacement therapy. ACOG 46th Annual Clinical Meeting, 4th Scientific Session, May 9–13, 1998. New Orleans, LA.

Hammond CB, Rackley CE, Fiorica J, et al. Consequences of estrogen deprivation and the rationale for hormone replacement therapy. *Am J Manag Care* 2000;6(14 suppl):S746.

Harvey-Kelly KF, Kanakaris NK, Eardley I, et al. Little known about sexual dysfunction after pelvic trauma. *J Urol* 2011;185. Medscape. May 05, 2011.

Hensley S. Morphine may block PTSD after serious injury. National Public Radio. January 4, 2013. 8:58 AM. http://www.npr.org/blogs/health/2010/01/morphine_ptsd.html

Hufnagel V, Golant S. *No more hysterectomies.* New American Library, 1989.

Jackson JL, DeZee K, Berbano E. Can treating depression improve disease outcomes? *Ann Intern Med* 2004;140:1054.

Kaplan HI, Sadock BJ. *Comprehensive textbook of psychiatry*, 5th ed. Baltimore, MD: Williams & Wilkins, 1989:1563.

Kelley WE Jr. Robotic surgery: the promise and early development. *Laparoscopy and SLS Report* 2002;1:6.

Kritz-Silverstein D, Wingard DL, Barrett-Conner E, et al. Hysterectomy, oophorectomy, and depression in older women. *J Wom Health* 1994;3:255.

Kronos Longevity Research Institute (KLRI).

Kuzmarov IW, Bain J. Sexuality in the aging couple, Part I: the aging woman. *Geriatrics and Aging* 2008;11:589.

Lebrun CE, van der Schouw YT, de Jong FH, et al. Endogenous oestrogens are related to cognition in healthy elderly women. *Clin Endocrinol (Oxf)* 2005;63:50.

Lewis CE, Groff JY, Herman GJ, et al. Overview of women's decision making regarding elective hysterectomy, oophorectomy and hormone replacement therapy. *J Womens Health Gend Based Med* 2000:9 (Suppl 2):S5.

Love S, Lindsey K. *Dr. Susan Love's hormone book.* New York: Random House, 1997.

Love S, Lindsey K, Williams M. *Dr. Susan Love's breast book.* Reading, MA: Addison Wesley Longman, 1990.

Makary M, Jin Linda X, Ibrahim AA, et al. Johns Hopkins research shows hospital websites use industry-provided content and overstate claims of robotic success. http://www.hopkinsmedicine.org. Updated May 18, 2011. Johns Hopkins Medicine.

Margossian H, Falcone T. Robotically assisted laparoscopic hysterectomy and adnexal surgery. *J Laparoedosc Adv Surg Tech A* 2001;11:161.

Maslow A. A theory of human motivation. *Psychol Rev* 1984; 50:370.

Massler DJ, Devansan MM. Sexual consequences of gynecologic operations. In: Comfort A, ed. *Sexual consequences of disability.* Philadelphia, PA: George F. Stickley, 1978.

McCully KS, Jackson S. Hormone replacement therapy and the bladder. *J Br Menopause Soc* 2004;10:30.

Meador C. The unheard heart: a metaphor for medicine in the digital age. In Health beat by Maggie Mahar. Commentary on health care, the economy, politics, and public health. http://www.healthbeat-blog.org/

Medscape. Pelvic exams: new guidelines for asymptomatic women. http://www.medscape.com. Updated Jul 24, 2012. 999.

Mericli M, Nadasy GL, Szekeres M, et al. Estrogen replacement therapy reverses changes in intramural coronary resistance arteries caused by female hormone depletion. *Cardiovasc Res* 2004;61:317.

Miller MM, Monjan AA, Buckholtz NS. Estrogen replacement therapy for the potential treatment or prevention of Alzheimer's Disease. *Ann N Y Acad Sci* 2001;949:223.

Mull DJ. Cross-cultural communication in the physician's office. *West J Med* 1993;159:609.

NASA Ames Research Center. Smart surgical probe licensed to fight breast cancer. Moffett Field, CA: Computational Sciences Division, 2000. Press release, December 22, 2000.

Novack DH, Plumer R, Smith RL, et al. Changes in physician's attitude toward telling the cancer patient. *JAMA* 1979;241:897.

Ocal G. Current concepts in disorders of sexual development. *J Clin Res Pediatr Endocrinol* 2011;3:105.

Paget L, Nedza S, Kurtz P, et al. *Patient-clinician communication: basic principles and expectations.* Washington, DC: Institute of Medicine of the National Academies, Updated June 2011. http://www.iom.edu/Global/Perspectives/2012/PatientClinician.aspx?page=1. Accessed June 1, 2012.

Parker WH, Broder MS, Liu Z, et al. Ovarian conservation at the time of hysterectomy for benign disease. *Obstet Gynecol* 2005;106:219.

Pelvic Pain Support Network. Talking about pelvic pain. http://www.pelvicpain.org.uk/index

Peters AAW, Trimbos-Kemper GCM, Admiraal C, et al. A randomized clinical trial on the benefit of adhesiolysis in patients with intra-peritoneal adhesions and chronic pelvic pain. *Br J Obstet Gynaecol* 1992;99:59.

Pines A. What is the actual lesson from the WHI study upon its completion? *Harefuah* 2004;143:722, 766.

Plourde EL. *The ultimate rape: what every woman should know about hysterectomies and ovarian removal.* Irvine, CA: New Voice, 1998.

Prentice RL, Langer R, Stefanick ML, et al. Combined postmenopausal hormone therapy and cardiovascular disease: toward resolving the discrepancy between observational studies and the Women's Health Initiative clinical trial. *Am J Epidemiol* 2005;162:404.

Richter DL, Kenzig MJ, Greaney ML, et al. Physician-patient interaction and hysterectomy decision making: the ENDOW study. Ethnicity, needs, and decisions of women. *Am J Health Behav* 2002;26:431.

Roeske NCA. Hysterectomy and other gynecologic surgeries: a psychological view. In: Notman MT, Nadelson CC, eds. *The woman patient: medical and psychological interfaces.* New York: Plenum, 1978.

Roovers JPWR, van der Vaart CH, et al. Correspondence re: urinary incontinence after hysterectomy. *Lancet* 2000;356(9246):2012.

Rosen C. New devices and truly informed consent. *Virtual Mentor* 2010;12:73.

Sardonis J. Moon Pendant. http://www.sardonis.com

Schain WS. Sexual functioning, self-esteem and cancer care. In: Vaeth JM, Blomberg RC, Adler L, eds. *Body image, self-esteem, and sexuality in cancer patients.* New York: Karger, 1980.

Schiff E, Gurgevich S, Caspi O. Potential synergism between hypnosis and acupuncture—is the whole more than the sum of its parts? *Evid Based Complement Alternat Med* 2007;4:233.

Schwartz SA, Williams DE. Psychological aspects of gynecologic surgery. *CME J Gynecol Oncol* 2002;7:268.

Shelton AJ, Groff JY. Hysterectomy: beliefs and attitudes expressed by African-American women. *Ethn Dis* 2001;11:732.

Sherwin BB. Estrogen and cognitive functioning in women. *Proc Soc Exp Biol Med* 1998;217:17.

Shute N. Menopause is no disease. Interview 3/24/97 with Susan Love. U.S. News & World Report. http://www.usnews.com

Simon JA. Problems of sexual function in menopausal women. *Menopausal Medicine* 2012;20.

Singh M, Rivlin ME, et al. Chronic pelvic pain in women: treatment and management. Updated December 4, 2012. http://emedicine.medscape.com/article/258334-treatment

Snyder H, Sickmund M. *Juvenile offenders and victims: 1999 national report.* Washington, DC: Office of Juvenile Justice and Delinquency Prevention. http://www.buildingblocksforyouth.org/justiceforsome/conclusion.html

Sternberg E. *The balance within: the science connecting health and emotions.* New York: W.H. Freeman and Co., 2001.

Takahashi K, Tanaka E, Murakami M, et al. Long-term hormone replacement therapy delays the age related progression of carotid intima-media thickness in healthy postmenopausal women. *Maturitas* 2004;49:170.

Tjaden P, Thoennes N. *Full report of the prevalence, incidence, and consequences of violence against women: findings from the National Violence Against Women survey*. Washington, DC: US Department of Justice, Office of Justice Programs, National Institute of Justice, 2000.

U.S. Cancer Statistics Working Group. *United States Cancer Statistics: 1999-2009 incidence and mortality web-based report*. Atlanta, GA: Department of Health and Human Services, Centers for Disease Control and Prevention, and National Cancer Institute, 2013. (http://apps.nccd.cdc.gov/uscs/). Available at http://www.cdc.gov/uscs. http://apps.nccd.cdc.gov/uscs/

Ufema J. Helping loved ones say goodbye. *Nursing* 1991;21:42.

Ustecka Z. Psychological intervention improves health of breast cancer patients. http://www.medscape.com Updated February 1, 2008.

Wagner JR, Russo P. Urologic complications of major pelvic surgery. *Surg Oncol* 2000;18:216.

Warga C. *Menopause and the mind: the complete guide to coping with memory loss, foggy thinking, verbal confusion, and other cognitive effects of perimenopause and menopause*. New York: Simon & Schuster, 1999.

Warren MP; Halpert S. Hormone replacement therapy: controversies, pros and cons. *Best Prac Res Clin Endocrino Metab* 2004; 18:317.

Weinberg L, Rao S, Escobar PF. Robotic surgery in gynecology: an updated systematic review. *Obstetrics and Gynecology International* 2011;2011:852061.

Woodis BC, McLendon AN, Muzyk AJ. Testosterone supplementation for hypoactive sexual desire disorder in women. *Pharmacotherapy* 2012;32:38. doi: 10.1002/PHAR.1004.

Wright K. Essay: Why isn't everyone excited about robotic assisted surgery?. http://www.kevinmd.com. minimally invasive gynecologic surgery fellow. Cost of Care 2011 healthcare essay contest.

Wu K, Jennifer M, Hundley A, et al. Predicting the number of women who will undergo incontinence and prolapse surgery, 2010-2050. *Am J Obstet Gynecol* 2011;205:230.e1.

Wurn BF, Wurn LJ, King R, et al. Treating fallopian tube occlusion with a manual pelvic physical therapy. *Altern Ther Health Med* 2008;14:18.

Yates J, Barrett-Connor E, Barlas S, et al. Rapid loss of hip fracture protection after estrogen cessation: evidence from the national osteoporosis risk assessment. *Obstet Gynecol* 2004;103:440.

Youngs DD, Ehrhardt AA, Wise TN. Psychological sequelae of elective gynecologic surgery. In: *Psychosomatic obstetrics and gynecology*. New York: Appleton-Century-Crofts, 1980:255.

Yin S. Mice can avoid menopause, but can women? http://www.medscape.com. Updated Sep 27, 2011.

CHAPTER 4
Risk Prevention, Risk Management, and Professional Liability

Gerald B. Hickson and Ilene N. Moore

DEFINITIONS

Adverse event (AE)—Undesired occurrence resulting from complication and/or error.

Adverse outcome (AO)—Undesired clinical outcome without implying cause. AOs may be due to: (a) the underlying pathologic disease process, (b) complication of treatment, (c) medical error, or (d) perception of a disappointing result.

Complication—A known risk of a specified procedure, operation, medication, therapy, or treatment plan.

Medical error—Failure of a planned action to be completed as intended or the use of a wrong plan to achieve an aim.

Near miss—Event or deviation from best practice that did not cause harm but may signal risk for other patients.

This chapter addresses the myths and realities surrounding "risk management." The goals of the chapter are for the gynecologic surgeon to better understand:

- Health care's increasing focus on safety (**Introduction**)
- Incidence of AEs, which patients sue, why they sue, and whom they sue (**Section I: The Genesis of Malpractice Claims**)
- Best practices for professional self- and group-regulation and learning from near-misses and AEs in order to promote patient safety and reduce claims risk (**Section II: Professionalism and Risk Prevention**)
- Best practices for managing the aftermath of risk events (**Section III: Managing Risk Events**)
- Medical malpractice law, discovery, trial, settlement, alternative dispute resolution (ADR), and tort reform (**Section IV: Litigation**)

We begin with a case:

Ms. AJ is a 46-year-old G3P3Ab0 female with a 5-year history of uterine fibroids. She notes increasing menorrhagia and pelvic pressure over the past 2 years with an increase in uterine size to 20 weeks. Dr. GYN has treated her conservatively but now recommends a hysterectomy. He engages Ms. AJ in an informed consent discussion, covering treatment options and their potential risks and benefits. Ms. AJ agrees to a total abdominal hysterectomy (TAH), and surgery is scheduled.

On the day of the procedure, her husband waits in the surgical waiting room for word that his wife is out of the operating room. He inquires several times at the reception desk, always told, "Someone will come out to talk with you." No one does before his wife is transported to her inpatient room.

On arrival to his wife's room, Mr. J meets the advanced practice nurse on Dr. GYN's team, Ms. NP. In response to Mr. J's questions, Ms. NP states, "You will have to ask Dr. GYN."

Dr. GYN does not round on Ms. AJ until the following morning. Ms. AJ mentions that she expected to see him after surgery. Dr. GYN states, "I'm here now, so what do you want to know?" and proceeds to discuss in general terms that the surgery took a little longer than anticipated but overall the procedure went well. He checks her dressing, turns, and leaves the room.

On postoperative day (POD) 3, Ms. AJ tells Ms. NP that she is having low abdominal pain. Ms. NP states that pain is normal postoperatively, and she will prescribe some pills to take at home. She discharges Ms. AJ and instructs her to keep her post-op follow-up appointment with Dr. GYN, scheduled for 3 weeks hence.

INTRODUCTION

Health care delivery in the United States is evolving. Press coverage related to the Institute of Medicine (IOM)'s landmark studies, *To Err Is Human* and *Crossing the Quality Chasm*, accelerated public and industry recognition of patient harm caused by medical care. Most distressing was the IOM's estimate that 98,000 people die annually in the United States as a result of medical error, with countless more injured. Unfortunately, progress aimed at making health care safer has been slow despite more than a decade of increased awareness and investment in research and safety initiatives. A study of 10

North Carolina hospitals by Landrigan et al. illustrates this point. The hospitals' overall harm rate did not change between 2002 and 2007. Furthermore, two thirds of the harms were judged preventable. Despite the overall finding, a closer look at the data revealed a range of results among the study sites, suggesting that some appeared to have tackled risk issues more successfully than did others.

The fact is, safety and quality vary among, and even within, practices, hospitals, and health care systems. Some patients experience well-coordinated, timely, efficient, and effective service, while others receive fragmented, delayed, redundant, or inadequate care. As society becomes less tolerant of unsafe conditions and avoidable AEs, the focus on claims management must shift to an emphasis on risk prevention.

Utilizing evidence-based best practices, professionals must move patients out of harm's way through risk surveillance, apply analytic methodologies to identify factors that contribute to AEs, fix defective systems, and hold professionals accountable. Furthermore, professionals must treat patients, their families, and each other with respect. Private and public payors are leveraging their market power to encourage practices that promote safety, improve outcomes, and manage costs. The Centers for Medicare and Medicaid Services (CMS), for example, uses a payment withholding and reward system to incentivize professionals and hospitals to achieve lower hospital-acquired infections rates, reduced need for hospital readmissions, and integration of patient perceptions of care into quality standards. Payors also deny reimbursement for the extra care needed to treat outcomes they deem avoidable or place liens for reimbursement against patient-claimants' jury awards and settlements.

SECTION I: THE GENESIS OF MALPRACTICE CLAIMS

KEY POINTS: GENESIS OF CLAIMS

- Many patients with valid potential claims do not sue.

- Noneconomic factors play a significant role in patients' and families' decisions to sue.

- Claims are nonrandomly distributed.

- 3% to 8% of physicians by specialty account for over half of all risk management expenses.

- Risk status appears constant over time.

- Unsolicited patient complaints are related to malpractice claims risk.

- Intervention with high-complaint physicians can lower claims risk.

Incidence of AEs

Responding to the malpractice insurance crisis of the 1970s, the California Hospital Association organized a study in which 21,000 medical charts from all 1974 hospitalizations at 23 California hospitals were reviewed. Mills reported that the study found almost 5% of inpatients (7% if over 65) experienced AEs. Nearly one fifth of the AEs were further classified as injuries for which the professional staff and/or hospital would likely be liable, that is, due in whole or in part to medical negligence.

The Harvard Medical Practice Study I (HMPS I) reported similar findings from a review of 30,000 New York State hospital records from the year 1984. The overall AE rate was 3.7%; for those over 65, the AE rate was 5%. Twenty-eight percent of the AEs involved negligence (Fig. 4.1). Replicating the study in Colorado and Utah, the researchers found essentially the same results.

Other studies, including some from the international community, also confirm that the majority of AEs do not involve negligence.

Who Sues?

Or, to rephrase, who are the claimants in medical malpractice cases?

Danzon reported that in the 1970s no more than one out of 10 patients injured by care filed suit. In the HMPS III, Localio and colleagues found an even lower claims rate among injured patients. HMPS III matched 47 malpractice cases to the 30,000 1984 HMPS I hospitalizations. In only eight of the 47 cases did medical record review demonstrate evidence of negligence. However, these eight cases represented only two percent of the patients with AEs attributable to medical negligence. The majority of claims were instead filed by patients whose AE did not result from negligence; for every suit with an AE attributed to negligence, five to six suits lacked such evidence. The results were consistent with Mills' earlier observation that "most patients who file lawsuits for medically caused disabilities do so without real knowledge about presence or absence of legal fault as the cause of their disability". HPMS III remains an important study for its insight into the fact that much of the legal activity involving allegations of medical malpractice represents circumstances where care was appropriate, but the patient or family do not appear to understand or accept.

A later study of 1,452 medical malpractice cases conducted by Studdert et al. found that, in comparison to HMPS III, three out of five claims are legally justifiable. What might account for the higher proportion of cases deemed valid? We suggest

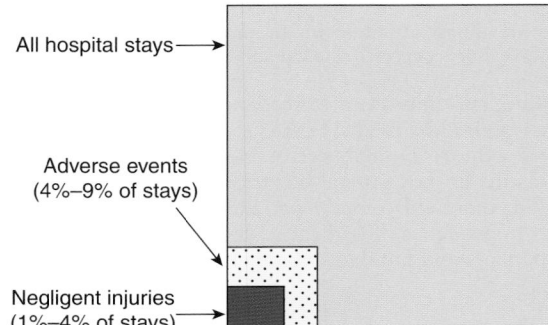

FIGURE 4.1 Adverse events versus negligent injuries. Adapted from Bovbjerg RR. *Medical malpractice: problems & reforms—a policy-maker's guide to issues and information*. Washington, DC: The Intergovernmental Health Policy Project, George Washington University, 1995; Mills DH. Whither malpractice regulation? *West J Med* 1988;149:611; deVries EN, Ramrattan MA, Smorenburg SM, et al. The incidence and nature of in-hospital adverse events: a systematic review. *Qual Saf Health Care* 2008;17:216; Brennan TA, Leape LL, Laird NM, et al. Incidence of adverse events and negligence in hospitalized patients: results of the Harvard Medical Practice Study I. *N Engl J Med* 1991;324:371.

four potential factors: (a) study methodology, (b) threshold for finding preventable harm, (c) evolving error disclosure practices, and (d) case selection.

The study methodologies differed in that HMPS III reviewed patients' medical records for evidence of AEs and negligence, while Studdert reviewed insurers' closed claims. Documentation in medical records can be incomplete or absent. In contrast, insurers' files contain deposition transcripts and/or witness interviews that may reveal evidence of negligent events not found in medical records.

Second, because of our evolving understanding of how faulty systems and human factors intersect to cause error, some of the "no negligence" AEs in HMPS III might be characterized today as avoidable error-based AEs. The IOM definition of error ("the failure of a planned action to be completed as intended or the use of wrong plan to achieve an aim") captures the notion that occurrence of an unintended outcome itself signals likelihood that faulty systems and/or human decision-making contributed. Reassignment of some of the 47 HMPS III cases would likely have brought HMPS III's valid:invalid ratio closer to Studdert's.

The third potential reason for Studdert finding a higher percentage of justifiable claims may relate to increasing error disclosure. Some patients who might otherwise never realize medical error caused them harm may sue once this information is disclosed. However, the data so far suggest that disclosure does not lead to more suits nor an increase in overall liability costs; rather, disclosure may reduce suit and claims rates, time to resolution, average payouts, and legal costs.

A fourth factor is that plaintiff's attorneys today are likely more selective about which cases they accept. Attorneys take malpractice cases on a contingency (rather than hourly pay) basis and are not paid if they lose. Thus, accepted cases must potentially yield a recovery large enough to cover attorney fees and upfront costs, including experts' travel expenses and billings for time spent reviewing cases, executing certificates of merit (in states where required), and testifying.

> Rice reports: "Experienced malpractice attorneys say they tend to be very judicious about what they pursue."
>
> Shepherd reports that "Over 75 percent of the attorneys… survey[ed] indicate[d] that they reject more than 90 percent of the cases that they screen…over half…responded that, even for a case they are almost certain to win on the merits, they will not accept the case unless expected damages are at least $250,000."

In sum, it is important to recognize that there are patients who are injured by medical care, and a significant proportion of injury is due to avoidable error. However, most patients with valid claims do not pursue litigation. Although many claims are valid, there still remain patients who file claims despite little or no evidence of bad care. We now examine what motivates patients and families to contact an attorney.

Why Do Patients Sue?

Some professionals assert it is all about "ambulance-chasing lawyers" and plaintiffs' desire for money; however, the evidence suggests that decisions to sue are more complex. In one study where families were asked why they had sued their obstetrician, many offered more than one reason. Money was mentioned as a reason for contacting an attorney by a quarter of the families, but most identified a host of noneconomic reasons: wanting to "make sure this doesn't happen to anyone else" (19%), needing information (20%), feeling their loved one would have no future (20%), believing there was a cover-up (24%), and advice from an "influential other" (33%). Only one respondent

indicated that she had been solicited by an attorney. In the United Kingdom, Vincent et al. also found noneconomic factors more prominent in patients' decisions to sue than the need for financial compensation.

While some factors are outside a professional's control, how and what information a professional provides to the patient is not. As gynecologic surgeons reflect about their personal risk prevention strategies, it is beneficial to examine the types of informational issues families cited as reasons for filing: no one would tell them what was wrong, their physician would not answer questions, and no one warned them that the problems might be permanent. The need to understand is normal. Patients want answers if only to help dispel fears that somehow something they did contributed to the AO.

If patients do not raise questions, do not assume they have none. Make clear through your verbal and nonverbal communications that you want to address their questions. If you are asked questions, say what you know but be careful about speculation. If you do not know the answer, say so. Specify when you expect to be able to follow up with more answers, and make certain that you *do* follow up.

Patients and families may claim they did not receive clear explanations of what happened even when the professional tried. When you provide answers, seek to confirm that they understood utilizing "teach-back" methods; do not equate a head nod with comprehension.

Ineffective communication may also lead to allegations of cover-up or incompetence, especially if other professionals provide conflicting information or "joust" (criticize the treating professional, practice, or health care institution). For the one third of families in the study who decided to file suit based on the "advice" of an "influential other," most often it was a health care professional who told them the bad outcome was a result of poor care and/or that they should sue. The following represent examples of reported communications:

> "The nurse practitioner told me, "They gave you the wrong medication when they discharged you. That's why you're having this problem."
>
> "After talking to the anesthesiologist, I realized it clearly was the surgeon's fault. I had no idea that the bad outcome was related to Dr. XX's care until he suggested…."

"Influential others" fill gaps when patients have unanswered questions, residual concerns, lack of trust in the professional, or worries about the future. Healthcare professionals should remain alert to the possibility of error by others. However, by jousting and offering gratuitous negative comments, they bear some responsibility for inflaming and undermining colleagues' relationships with their patients, which can contribute to unnecessary litigation. Thus, professionals should ask themselves a set of questions before commenting about care delivered by others:

- Do I have all the data?
- Am I certain the history provided by the patient is accurate?
- Do I have the expertise, or am I making a judgment about someone who practices in another field?

Whenever possible, professionals should seek direct clarification of the facts of the case from colleagues who provided care to the patient. If direct contact is not possible, reviewing the medical records may shed light.

If needed information is not available or what is learned does not reassure, then reporting through appropriate channels is professional. In the group setting, the reporter can make practice leaders aware. In the hospital setting, one should utilize an online reporting system (if available) and/or directly contact designated personnel such as risk managers and/or safety and quality officers. In other words, commitment to safety means that colleagues and team members raise questions with the involved parties, route concerns for objective review, and if information emerges that impacts the patient, share it with him/her in a professional manner. Arguing at the patient's bedside or rushing to tell a patient or to comment in the medical record that a previously treating professional "messed up" is not consistent with principles of professional disclosure.

Inflammation and communication failures can trigger unnecessary claims. Examples of such circumstances include the following: (a) The AO is not due to medical mishap, but the patient believes it is; (b) a medical error did not result in harm, but the patient believes it to be the cause of his/her outcome; and (c) medical error caused harm, but failed opportunities to address the patient's and family's needs spurred their decision to pursue legal action and/or to make unreasonable demands. Understanding the reasons families sue can help professionals reflect and act in ways to prevent claims that might be avoided.

Who Gets Sued?

Many physicians assert there is little they can do to prevent malpractice claims, citing as "fact" that "everyone in my specialty gets sued." It is true that overall claims rates vary by specialty. Jena et al. and Kane found neurosurgeons and cardiothoracic surgeons to share claims rates of 19% per annum; general surgeons, 15%; and obstetrician–gynecologists, 12%. (Obstetrician–gynecologists also account for the highest number of indemnity payments of over one million dollars.) In comparison, psychiatrists, family physicians, and pediatricians experience overall rates of 3% to 5%.

Such aggregate statistics suggest that claims are common and likely inevitable over the course of a career. They do not tell the whole story, however, for claims rates do not address the distribution of claims among physicians. In fact, claims are nonrandomly distributed, and a small subset of physicians within any specialty accounts for a disproportionate share of claims and payouts. Studying physicians in Florida, Sloan and colleagues reported that, depending on the specialty, 3% to 8% of physicians account for 75% to 85% of all indemnity payouts within their specialty: 8% of surgical subspecialists, 6% of obstetrician–gynecologists, and 3% of medical specialists.

Other studies have confirmed nonrandom distribution of claims and payouts within multi-specialty groups. Furthermore, the propensity to attract claims persists over time; physicians with high numbers of past claims appear to continue this pattern into the future.

Is there something different about physicians who experience multiple claims compared with peers who are seldom or never sued, or are they just unlucky? Four likely hypotheses are that high suit physicians: (a) care for a more litigious population, (b) care for the sickest patients, (c) are less technically or clinically competent than low-suit colleagues, and/or (d) do not "connect" as well with patients.

Well-educated, higher income patients are more likely to sue than are those who are elderly, poor, or uninsured. However, Entman and colleagues found no difference in practice demographics for obstetrician-gynecologists with a history of multiple claims when compared with peers in their community with few or no claims.

Review of patient medical charts from the practices of high versus low claims obstetrician–gynecologists also revealed no significant differences in patient mix, acuity, documentation practices, or evidence of marginal care. The area in which high claims physicians did differ, however, was in how they were perceived by patients. The researchers asked open-ended questions of the patients (none of whom had filed suit against their physician) whether any aspects of care failed to meet or exceed their expectations. Their responses could be sorted into concerns about their physician's communication skills, care and treatment, access and availability, and "humaneness" during labor and delivery. The following are sample patient comments from the interviews:

> "He did a very poor job of communicating... discounted everything that we said."
> "Dr. X offered no information. I felt he was hiding information."
> "...never gives me more than 5 minutes."
> "He was terrible with this pregnancy and was even worse with the next one, but the HMO said I had to stay with him. I kept hoping to get his partner, but never lucked out. I'm not getting pregnant anymore because of him."

Patients whose obstetricians had a history of multiple lawsuits voiced three times more complaints about their care than did patients of low-suit physicians. In other words, the same small group of physicians responsible for high numbers of malpractice cases was also associated with higher numbers of patient complaints and dissatisfaction.

Identifying Professionals at High Risk of Claims

If physicians with high numbers of malpractice cases have significantly higher complaint rates than do their peers with few or no claims, is the converse also true? Do patient complaints identify physicians at high risk for claims? If they do, perhaps it is possible to identify high-risk physicians by a method other than waiting for lawsuits.

Unsolicited "patient complaints" are the stories patients and families share with practice and hospital representatives about their care experiences:

> "The GYN... didn't listen... just cut me off... made me worry about the treatment plan."
> "[Patient] described the exam as torture... Dr. XX was yanking and shoving the speculum... it hurt worse than her surgery."
> "They left me sitting in the stirrups... then Dr. XX made a very inappropriate remark and left the room... I felt humiliated."

Capturing patient complaints allows opportunities for "service recovery," that is to say, helping to "make right" what patients and families perceive as wrong. Hickson and colleagues hypothesized that coding and aggregating unsolicited patient complaints over time would reveal risk patterns. Studying unsolicited patient complaints at an academic medical center Hickson et al. and Moore et al. found:

- Most physicians were associated with few or no unsolicited patient complaints over a 6-year audit period. Five percent of physicians were associated with nearly one third of all patient complaints (Fig. 4.2).
- Risk management activity was associated with three characteristics of physician practice: unsolicited complaint numbers, specialty, and productivity as measured by relative value units (RVUs) by discipline. Logistic regression analysis revealed, however, that of the three predictors of risk,

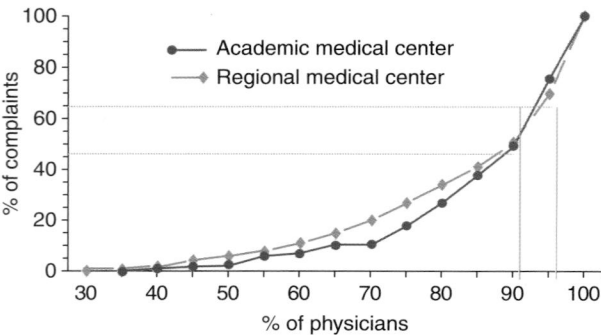

FIGURE 4.2 Distribution of patient complaints. Adapted from Hickson GB, Pichert JW. Identifying and intervening with high-malpractice-risk physicians to reduce claims. *Physician Insurer* 2007: 29. Adapted with permission from the Fourth Quarter 2007 issue of Physician Insurer Magazine, Physician Insurers Association of America. Copyright © 2007.

unsolicited complaints and risk management activity were most closely linked.

- Association of physician productivity with lawsuit risk was minor when compared with patient complaints and disappeared for physicians with multiple lawsuits. In other words, the unique ability of a physician and his/her practice to create dissatisfaction among patients overwhelmed productivity as a predictor of high claims experience.
- Nine percent of physicians, as a group, were associated with the highest numbers of unsolicited complaints and 50% of all risk management expenditures and payouts.

A follow-up study at a regional medical center affirmed the results (Fig. 4.2).

Stelfox et al., Fullam et al., Cydulka et al., and Levtzion-Korach et al. have confirmed the relationship between patient complaints and claims experience. Furthermore, any relationship between patient satisfaction survey data and risk management activity disappears once patient complaints are entered into the model. Complaint distribution patterns similar to those from the multispecialty group studies are also seen for single physician specialty groups including trauma, urology, and cardiothoracic surgeons and can support targeted interventions to help reduce unnecessary risk.

In sum, the empirical data demonstrate that professionals' own behaviors and practices are primarily responsible for inspiring claims rather than external factors. Malpractice claims should not be viewed as just an expected "cost of doing business." Rather, AOs are more likely to lead to claims when patients are dissatisfied with their physician's practice and/or interpersonal behaviors. Unless high-risk professionals are willing and able to address sources of patient dissatisfaction, their malpractice costs will continue to exceed those of their low-risk colleagues.

SECTION II: PROFESSIONALISM AND RISK PREVENTION

Traditional risk management programs focus primarily on managing claims. Skillful management of potential claims is, of course, important to gynecologic surgeons when their patients are unhappy about outcomes of care. Modern risk prevention programs, however, also proactively identify sources of risk through surveillance and monitoring, utilize

methodologies that elucidate "sharp end" (obvious) and "blunt end" (less obvious) contributors to AEs, and take corrective action to fix defective systems and remedy deficient human performance and behavior. Both risk mitigation and proactive management of potential claims (Section III) reduce medicolegal costs.

Organizations with a knowledgeable risk prevention/management department and stakeholders with aligned interests can help reduce risk of patient harm and individual professionals' risk for claims. One way to lessen your own risk is to practice in a setting with a good, integrated, aligned risk prevention program.

KEY POINTS: BEST PRACTICES FOR RISK PREVENTION

- Promoting professional behaviors to support teamwork
- Early reporting and timely review of unexpected AOs, suspected errors, and near misses
- Event analysis methodologies to understand "how and why" the risk event occurred and a process for fixing system defects
- Remediation of human performance and behaviors that threaten patient safety and increase risk of medical malpractice claims

---

Professionalism

Professionalism is the fundamental human force behind the goal of making medicine safer and kinder. Professionalism requires more than clinical knowledge. Beyond the need for cognitive and technical competence are the essential behavioral dimensions: modeling respect, communicating effectively, being available, and demonstrating willingness to give and receive feedback. The Joint Commission's requirement for Ongoing Professional Practice Evaluations reflects growing recognition that the ability to deliver safe, high-quality patient care requires competency in this complex skill set.

Professionalism promotes teamwork; unprofessional behavior creates team dysfunction. Rosenstein and O'Daniel's survey of perioperative personnel found disruptive behaviors to be common. Study participants linked unprofessional behaviors with communication failures as well as distractions leading to momentary lapse of attention, well documented by others as contributors to errors and AEs. Sample comments from study participants included:

> "Some surgeons seem to believe that they have the right to be rude...and disrespectful to non-physicians. It makes it very difficult to perform at a high level when one is constantly in fear of being screamed at."
> "We have some... team-oriented surgeons... but the ones who are disruptive make it so intensely difficult that it is overwhelming. Unfortunately, as good as the good ones are, they can't outweigh how bad the bad ones are."

Professionals are committed to self-assessment of their performance and continually seek ways to improve. Professionals are also committed to group regulation. Risk prevention, therefore, includes methodologies to identify and address unprofessional interpersonal and practice behaviors that threaten safety. Professionals' commitment to group regulation is evidenced by their participation in related activities, including peer review. Professionals further assume personal responsibility for identifying faulty systems within the environment, work to "fix" systems thus identified, and disseminate information about best practices.

Reporting and Timely Review

How do professionals learn about threats to safety within their practice, group, or health care institution? Active reporting is a critical component of a risk prevention program. Professionals, support staff, patients, and families are all observers, and by lowering barriers to reporting, they help identify threats to safety and quality. Information on how to report should be disseminated so that all potential reporters, including patients, know how to report within the practice or health system (e.g., by phone, written contact, face-to-face, and/or electronic reporting) and to whom they should report (e.g., patient relations personnel, practice leaders, or a risk manager).

Practices, health care organizations, and malpractice insurance carriers should make clear in their policies what types of events health care professionals and personnel are to report. These should include sentinel events, errors or suspected errors with consequences (e.g., lengthened hospital stay, temporary or permanent disability, death), near misses, coworker concerns about performance or conduct, information about unsafe conditions or faulty equipment, and patient/family complaints of which they are aware.

Early reporting of suspected risk events, near misses, or patient injury to the professional's risk manager or malpractice carrier is always good. Reporting permits timely review and optimal management of a potential claim. Designated personnel must promptly address each report, review the asserted issues, and assemble a response and action plan. Reports should also be entered into a database for tracking, trending, and identifying patterns.

Early reporting also allows an opportunity to quickly address patient and family concerns and rebuild trust. In particular, when avoidable error with harm is identified, disclosure with apology may reduce inflammation and therefore risk of a lawsuit. Emerging evidence suggests that honesty and proactive risk prevention strategies help avert litigation and reduce claims costs.

Despite its critical importance, professionals sometimes hesitate to report. Possible reasons include lack of clarity about the mechanism for reporting and loyalty to the professionals involved in the incident. Because of concerns that even anonymous reporting will invite retribution from those who are the subject of the report, explicit nonretaliation language should be a part of the reporting policy to protect reporters and must be enforced.

Ultimately, failure to report is not consistent with being a professional. Reporting is part of one's commitment to self- and group-regulation. Success of surveillance relies on team members recognizing the value of reporting safety risks, understanding it is an expectation and part of their professionalism, and making it psychologically safe for all to speak up when they observe practices that appear unsafe.

Event Analysis Methodologies

If harm or the potential for harm is suggested by a report, professionals try to understand what happened and why. Event analysis methodologies represent best practices in seeking to understand how errors occur and how to prevent them. Practices, health care organizations, and medical malpractice insurance carriers should endorse utilization of event analysis in order to identify and address faulty systems and individuals.

Common event analysis techniques include: (a) risk management file review (b) root cause analysis (RCA), also termed event analysis, or multicausal analysis and (c) multidisciplinary morbidity, mortality, and improvement (MMM&I) conference. The tools support a balanced focus on systems and individual accountability, and the information uncovered by the analyses is what drives risk prevention efforts.

Protecting event analysis activities from discovery may vary by state, and you will want to seek legal advice to set up these processes. Even in states where legal protection of such activities is untested, professionals' commitment to continual learning and improvement can help them work through how best to achieve what is right for patients and their care.

Risk Management File Review

Risk management file review is the foundation for evaluating all claims and potential claims, whether the insurer is a carrier or a self-insured entity. The case is assessed for potential liability by reviewing, for example, medical records, witness interviews, and consultant/expert reports. Reviewers seek to identify strengths and weaknesses in individual cases, including medical conditions likely to have led to the same outcome in the absence of medical or nursing error, and patient actions that may have contributed.

The risk prevention lens, in contrast, views cases as opportunities to learn about modifiable contributory factors that can prevent future occurrences. For example, a traditional risk manager may focus on poor documentation that represents a weakness in a case and suggest better documentation in the future to make cases more defensible. A risk prevention lens would disseminate the notion that poor documentation impairs team communication and therefore the ability of the team to achieve intended outcomes. Exhorting improved documentation practices through the latter lens serves to increase patient safety in a broader sense.

Although the traditional risk management model cautions against sharing results of a review for fear the opposing litigant could gain access to that information during discovery, modern risk prevention recognizes that waiting years for a case to close before disseminating lessons learned inhibits professionals' ability to improve care. Coded and aggregated medicolegal data can be used to identify recurring safety themes and individual and group patterns, and when consolidated with claims files data within larger consortia (e.g., the Harvard-based CRICO/RMF), allow identification of common areas of risk. Larger databases can help prioritize areas in which best practice standards should be developed, disseminated and implemented. For example, the American Society of Anesthesiologists (ASA)'s review of over 5,000 closed claims dating from the 1970s through 1994 transformed a medical discipline's safety record. Practice changes such as use of end-tidal CO_2 monitoring and intraoperative pulse oximetry, virtually eliminated claims for undetected esophageal intubation and inadequate ventilation.

Root Cause Analysis

RCA is a tool for drilling down and understanding what caused an AE. RCAs are designed to explore AEs for factors that represent variation in performance by systematically teasing out both sharp and blunt end contributors to AEs. RCAs attempt to answer three questions: What happened? Why did it occur? ("Ask five times.") What can be done to prevent recurrence? Follow-up should occur and the action plan assessed for effectiveness.

In smaller practices, a designated group can develop expertise in RCAs. In larger settings, participants in RCAs generally include a trained facilitator, team members, managers of involved service areas, risk managers, and quality and safety officers. Causative factors are coded, action plans developed, and professionals and staff educated. Percarpio and Watt's recent study of Veterans Affairs medical centers suggests that committing resources to RCAs results in safety improvements such as lower postoperative complication rates.

Multidisciplinary Morbidity, Mortality, and Improvement Conference

The MMM&I conference is an educational forum, open to a broader range of individuals than attend an RCA. MMM&I attendees include professional, clinical, administrative, and clerical staff. In the hospital setting, attendees likely also include pharmacists and learners. The conference is designed to help attendees feel comfortable speaking up about circumstances and behaviors that contributed to an AE (psychological safety) and to lessen the inhibitory effect of the hierarchy. In addition, by reminding everyone that errors occur, the MMM&I can help start the healing process for professionals involved in the case.

In contrast to traditional M&M (morbidity and mortality) conferences, which tend to focus on individual performance (sometimes perceived as "shame and blame"), MMM&I conferences review a case within a framework of factors known as common contributors to failures or errors resulting in AEs. In one model, six domains (policies, environment, equipment, communication, procedures, and people) are set up as a "fishbone" or cause-and-effect Ishikawa diagram to identify all factors that contributed to failures. The "I" (Improvement) of the MMM&I results when a work group prioritizes identified issues and develops a follow-up action plan and assigned team members complete tasks and provide feedback.

Aggregating analyses from MMM&I conferences can identify recurring factors that underlie failures and help focus efforts on highest-yield projects. For example, one department of obstetrics-gynecology aggregated analyses of inpatient women's health cases and identified contributory factors such as jousting, ineffective communications, lost and overlooked documents, inadequate supervision, failure to follow policies, and equipment issues. Patterns suggested that improved systems for alerting key professionals for emergencies and facilitating intercaregiver communication would help remedy these issues. As a result, the department established a team to identify best practices and trained all clinical personnel.

Remediating Human Performance and Behavior

Unsolicited patient complaints support risk prevention efforts. Complaints help identify opportunities for service recovery, learning about threats to safety, and supporting interventions for professionals at high risk for claims.

Only a fraction of the patients who are unhappy with their care complain. For each patient who voices a complaint, many dissatisfied patients do not (estimated ratios range from one out of three to fewer than one in fifty). Patients who do not share their concerns with you or your group may instead tell family, friends, neighbors, and, increasingly, the general public via social media. Professionals should therefore make every effort to narrow the gap between voiced and unvoiced dissatisfaction by making it easy for patients to file complaints and responding professionally to those complaints by providing service recovery.

Patients and families also serve as the "canary in the mine." Murff found, for example, that admissions with surgical complications generate more complaints than surgical admissions without complications. Unsolicited complaints at times are the first (and sometimes only) notice of errors and sentinel events:

> "I had a cystocele and a rectocele... After surgery I went for my checkup and she explained that it was my rectocele falling and now I had an enterocoele... she never repaired the rectocele during my first surgery... because she thought if she pulled everything up tight, it would take care of it... I am now faced with a third surgery for same problem."

Additionally and as previously discussed, patient complaints may be used to identify and address professionals with a disproportionate share of complaints and at high malpractice claims risk. Vanderbilt's Patient Advocacy Reporting System is a risk prevention tool that utilizes a reliable process to collect and code complaints and aggregate and analyze the data. The tool supports a risk prevention program in which professionals are made aware of their high numbers of complaints and associated high-risk status through a committee organized in accordance with the requirements of their state's peer-review statutes.

Volunteer peer "messengers" are trained to conduct nondirective, nonjudgmental interventions with identified professionals and share individualized and local and national comparative data. The messenger asks his/her colleague to reflect on why he or she appears to stand out. The majority of professionals respond to peer-based intervention by reducing complaint numbers and claims risk.

Follow-up data are provided at intervals to help professionals evaluate the effectiveness of self-directed changes in their practice or interactive style. As illustrated by the Promoting Professionalism Pyramid model (Fig. 4.3), if complaints continue after peer-based interventions, the professional is escalated to the next tier. An appropriate "authority figure" then develops a specific accountability action plan designed to assist the professional. The plan may include coaching, relevant continuing education, a practice review and redesign, and/or medical evaluation to rule out conditions that require further attention, such as substance abuse, psychiatric disorder, or cognitive impairment.

The Role of the Insurance Carrier and Risk Manager

As a gynecologic surgeon, reflect on your relationship with your malpractice carrier (or self-insured health system), risk manager, and any personal experience you may have had with claims. Identifying patterns and threats to safety helps professionals focus on education and resources where they can most favorably impact patient care and risk prevention.

Do your carrier and risk manager:

- Encourage and make early reporting accessible?
- Support risk management file review, RCAs, and MMM&Is?
- Promote patient complaint collection, analysis, and intervention with high-risk individuals?

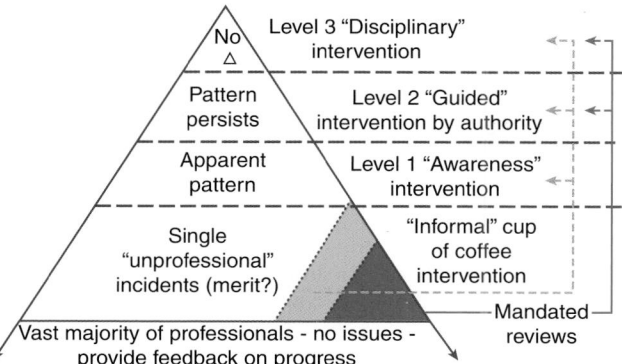

FIGURE 4.3 Promoting Professionalism Pyramid. Adapted from Hickson GB, Pichert JW, Webb LE, et al. A complementary approach to promoting professionalism: identifying, measuring, and addressing unprofessional behaviors. *Acad Med* 2007;82:1040. Copyright © 2007 Association of American Medical Colleges.

- Offer on-site practice review to identify risk issues?
- Incentivize you to adopt risk prevention procedures and participate in safety initiatives?

SECTION III: MANAGING A RISK EVENT

In spite of the best risk prevention strategies, some confluence of the human condition and systems failures interact in ways to create a risk event. Even so, it may be possible to identify early and respond in a way to avert the level of anger that can make managing risk more challenging.

The genesis of a potential lawsuit may begin before an AE occurs or is recognized. From the time a patient first calls a physician's office for an appointment, or tries to find a parking space, the practice is either building credit or is creating debt with the patient:

In Ms. AJ's case, Dr. GYN seemed professional at their first meeting, providing an explanation of her procedure and answering questions. Her postoperative experience created concern. Postdischarge, Ms. AJ's frustration mounted.

At home (POD 4), Ms. AJ continues to have low abdominal discomfort. She feels her abdomen is swollen and experiences persistent back pain. Ms. AJ calls Dr. GYN's office and asks to speak with him. Ms. NP returns the call. Ms. NP states she doubts symptoms are related to surgery. She promises to get back to Ms. AJ as soon as she has a chance to talk with Dr. GYN. Ms. AJ does not receive a callback that day. The next morning (POD 5), Ms. AJ leaves a voice mail as prompted by the office messaging system, asking if she can be checked by Dr. GYN because she is feeling "really bad."

Ms. AJ does not hear back. That afternoon, Ms. AJ calls her primary care physician who suggests she go to the emergency department for evaluation. Dr. ED orders an abdominal CT scan with contrast. The study reveals extravasation of dye into the abdominopelvic region. An intravenous pyelogram (IVP) confirms leaking dye from the left ureter. Dr. ED calls Dr. GYN's answering service. Dr. GYN's partner calls back and asks Dr. ED to call a urologist to admit Ms. AJ because Dr. GYN is out of town and the patient will need a urologic procedure.

Ms. AJ is admitted. Dr. GYN is informed the next morning.

Once a professional realizes that his/her patient has experienced an AE, some thoughts may come to mind:

- This is a recognized complication, right? (It was covered in the informed consent process....)
- What do I say to my patient?

- Should I report this to my practice leaders, risk manager, or malpractice carrier?
- Do I have liability exposure? Will I be sued?
- I wonder what Dr. ED and Dr. Urology are saying to my patient....
- Could the "complication" have been identified sooner?

Knowing that the practice and/or health care organization is principled, "aims to do right" by patients and families, has the right tools to manage the situation, and offers guidance to team members, can help make an uncomfortable situation more tolerable for professionals. If your carrier or hospital does not offer information about a comprehensive approach to risk management after an event, you should ask what they do.

Dr. GYN goes to see Ms. AJ. She appears upset. Ms. AJ tells Dr. GYN that no one in his office listened when she reported continued discomfort, and she feels she should not have had to contact her primary care physician to get help; Dr. GYN did the surgery so he should have responded. She fears that the delay has led to a more serious problem. Ms. AJ also mentions that the urologist kept shaking his head when she told him how no one in Dr. GYN's office seemed to take her seriously.

At the time an AE is recognized, the cause—*complication? error? combination?*—is often not clear. In some cases, objective review never fully elucidates the answer. Even if a professional is confident that what the patient is experiencing is a complication that happens under even the best of circumstances, patients and their families may still wonder if extra care might not have prevented the event. So, too, should the involved professional.

KEY POINTS: BEST PRACTICES FOR RISK MANAGEMENT AFTER AN AE

- Coordinate care for the patient's medical and emotional needs

- Support emotional needs of involved team members

- Notify your carrier or group or hospital risk manager if an error is identified, suspected, or unclear

- If appropriate, dispatch trained individuals within the practice, group, or hospital to meet with the patient and family to assist with service recovery

- Engage in a process of disclosure with the patient and offer an apology if error is identified. "Patient" includes family members or other parties authorized by the patient or legal guardians

- Consider reimbursement of out-of-pocket expenses and early settlement offers. (This is done by risk management professionals.)

Coordinating Care for the Patient's Medical Needs

After an AE, a professional should not delay care for his/her patient but does need to ask, "Do I need help in caring for the patient?" "Do I have the expertise to address the adverse outcome?" Do not be tempted to deliver care outside your usual scope of practice; arrange appropriate consultations from other professionals.

Furthermore, irrespective of whether you or another specialist manages the patient's current medical needs, it is important that you do not abandon your patient. Continue to visit and follow the patient. If patients do not see their physician, especially after an AE with error, patients may believe you are avoiding them for one of two reasons: either you don't care or you feel guilty.

After an event, physicians and nursing professionals set the tone for the patient and family's ongoing relationship with the health care team and the ability to move forward. Because the patient and family are likely experiencing feelings of loss, guilt, anger, and fear (whether or not expressed), professionals should engage without defensiveness.

Supporting the Emotional Needs of Involved Team Members

Situational stress poses risk. Professionals should be cautioned when error is suspected or confirmed that they may experience intense emotions of fear, guilt, or anger (often about other team members' performance) and/or disorientation due to an altered sense of one's abilities. Such feelings cloud judgment. When appropriate, team members should be encouraged to obtain professional help for themselves during a crisis.

Notifying Risk Management or Insurer

Risk managers and insurers want to hear about AEs as soon as possible. Make them aware of any outcome that has the potential to result in a claim, *even* if you believe you have no liability and *even* if you believe you have such a great relationship that "she would never sue me." Treat each potential risk event the same way.

Risk managers who learn about risk events can facilitate timely review, help team members prepare for disclosure to the patient and family, and sequester defective equipment (e.g., an IV pump that dispensed heparin 10 times faster than programmed) in accordance with federal regulatory requirements. Furthermore, evidence demonstrates that professional and prompt engagement with the patient decreases overall malpractice costs.

Engaging in Service Recovery

Trained patient relations personnel in a practice, group, or hospital setting are a valuable resource in managing the aftermath of an AE by focusing on the needs of the patient. Service recovery aims to facilitate communication among the patient, family, and health care professionals and to identify ways to assist the patient and family. They can also help defuse situations in which professionals come under verbal assault from angry family members.

Commencing Disclosure

> Dr. GYN is aware of the results of the imaging studies that show a ureteral transection, almost certainly related to Ms. AJ's TAH. Dr. GYN is confident that the laceration did not result from carelessness but rather the challenges of the procedure. Before surgery, Dr. GYN discussed possible complications with Ms. AJ. He recognizes he needs to talk with Ms. AJ.
>
> Dr. GYN promptly notifies his insurer and risk manager about the AE and discusses a disclosure plan. They agree that Dr. GYN proceed with speaking with Ms. AJ and her husband, but not speculate on the cause of the injury until the review is completed.

The move toward disclosure of AOs and errors is fairly recent. Not that long ago, some malpractice carriers recommended against disclosing to patients and families the fact that a poor outcome was due to problems with care, or policy language prohibited admissions of liability.

Such policies appear counterproductive. Prohibiting direct admission of error or fault can create ethical dilemmas for professionals who believe they should be honest with their patients, consistent with principles long embedded within professional codes of ethics. Such policies also create risk; patients may find other professionals who reinforce their concerns, leading to the belief that litigation is the only option to compel truthful answers.

Insurers or risk managers who encourage nondisclosure may do so because they believe that admission of fault increases likelihood of lawsuits or makes cases harder to defend. A growing body of evidence suggests, however, that a more transparent model lessens the risk of suits and moderates payouts. In such a model, specific information about AEs is shared with the affected patient and sincere and specific apology offered for error that caused or contributed to the outcome. Progressive risk prevention/management programs now encourage training in disclosure for professionals so they know how and when to share information related to AEs with patients and families. Training reinforces that respect for the patient is paramount.

Specific skills sets are required for effective communication; disclosure is no different. Disclosure, if done appropriately, can promote understanding and builds trust. Done poorly, it increases anxiety and destroys trust. Gynecologic surgeons would be prudent to ask their insurance carrier and any health care institution in which they care for patients about their disclosure policy and relevant training programs.

Training helps professionals prepare for the skills needed to manage four key disclosure scenarios:

1. AO is recognized, but the "why" (disease process? complication? error?) is uncertain at the moment.
2. Obvious error has occurred with obvious consequences.
3. The professional suspects error by another professional.
4. The patient believes that error caused the AO despite a review that finds no supporting evidence.

Disclosure is a process that takes place over time. The team leader for the patient's care, usually the physician, has primary responsibility for communicating with the patient after an event and managing disclosure. The professional needs to recognize what he or she knows (really) about the event and when. Share with the patient and family the known *facts*, if only to say, "I do not yet know the cause, but these are our observations so far...." Speculating or saying nothing may be equally destructive and increase probability of misunderstanding with the patient (especially if he or she asks others what they think).

If medical error is identified and confirmed to have caused harm or potential future consequences for the patient's care, professionals should disclose and offer an apology. Disclosure training should prepare professionals to anticipate questions patients might ask and to deal with a range of reactions from the family, such as shock, hostility, rage, or emotional breakdown.

How might one categorize the type of disclosure scenario Dr. GYN initially faces? At the time Dr. GYN first engages with Ms. AJ after identification of the ureteral leak, what he knows is that there is a tear in the ureter and that the patient's ultimate outcome is unclear at this time. He believes he conducted the procedure correctly, but may wonder whether he or others within his practice might have identified Ms. AJ's "complication" sooner. Dr. GYN decides that this case contains uncertainty.

Disclosure: Uncertainty as to the Cause of the AO

When a patient suffers an AO, it is important that professionals not jump to the conclusion that someone did something wrong nor summarily dismiss the possibility. Professionals should refrain from becoming confessional or defensive. In an "uncertainty" scenario, the team must quickly discern the facts that are known and what information is not yet clear. Professionals should not speculate, even when asked by patients or family, but instead affirm their commitment to the review process.

Conversation in the face of an AE should always contain an expression of human concern. An expression of human concern should not be confused with apology. Apology is offered when the injury resulted from error.

> Dr. GYN meets with his patient. "Ms. AJ, as you recall, because of your symptomatic fibroids, we discussed treatment options and then scheduled you for a total abdominal hysterectomy. I know you've not felt well since leaving the hospital. Because of your symptoms, the emergency medicine physician ordered a CT scan and IVP, and as you are aware, the tests confirmed a leak from your left ureter, and fluid is collecting in your pelvis and abdomen. I am sorry that you have experienced a ureteral tear. You are in good hands with Dr. URO."
>
> Ms. AJ asks Dr. GYN why this happened. He tells her that he requested a review of the case; there are several potential causes, and he does not want to speculate. He promises Ms. AJ he will share what is learned. Dr. GYN states he realizes it must be hard for her to go through additional surgery and the hospitalization. He offers to continue to follow her progress, if she will permit, as the urology team provides care.

Disclosure: Obvious Error, Obvious Consequences

"Obvious–obvious" refers to those circumstances where error has occurred with clear clinical consequences. If certain that an error occurred—for example, retained foreign body, wrong procedure, wrong patient, wrong plan, failure to follow up on an abnormal test, or failure to get the patient in sooner—the professional with primary responsibility for the patient shares the information with the patient. The professional should:

- Review "how we got here." Summarize the medical condition for which the patient was treated, the treatment provided, and the patient's current clinical status.
- Specify what happened: what the error was, when and where it occurred, and its cause (if known).
- Offer an apology.
- Describe actions taken so far to reduce the gravity of the harm, and additional actions needed.
- Convey who will manage ongoing care (you or someone else? what is the patient's preference?).
- Provide contact information for ongoing communications.
- Assess the need for counseling or other support, and if indicated, make an appropriate referral.

When offering an apology for error with harm, acknowledge the specific nature of the error and the resulting impact on the patient. The apology must be sincere in both words and body language. Remember that patients may conditionally accept an apology; they will wait and see if you follow through on promises they heard during disclosure or reserve judgment until they see how you care for them subsequently.

If the patient believes you promised something, be sure you do it. Failure to follow up may inflame.

If review reveals that the care, including follow-up, was appropriate and the AE was due to an unavoidable complication, apology is neither necessary nor appropriate. Nonetheless, we hope that professionals would still regret that their patient experienced a complication.

A review of Ms. AJ's case determines that Dr. GYN made reasonable efforts to identify the ureter at the time of surgery, but despite these efforts, ureteral injury occurred, likely due to complex anatomy. There was no evidence Dr. GYN's intraoperative technique deviated from best practices. Notwithstanding this conclusion, a team is assigned to review the literature to see if postoperative cystoscopy with indigo carmine flush is emerging as a best practice. If so, it can be considered for future patients.

The review also finds that Ms. AJ was placed at increased risk by the challenges seeking care after discharge. The reviewers agree that Ms. AJ's best chance for restoration of ureteral function would have been recognition of the transection at the time of the TAH. However, once discharged, the additional 2 days' delay in making the diagnosis did not otherwise affect her prognosis for success of the repair procedure.

Dr. GYN returns to speak with Ms. AJ. He expresses his regret that Ms. AJ experienced the complication and apologizes for the failure of his office to afford her access to be seen more timely. In fact, he is distressed that Ms. AJ had difficulty being seen, voice messages were not checked, and his partner did not call him but instead asked the emergency department to have Urology admit his patient. Dr. GYN, however, does not feel an apology is appropriate for the ureteral injury, as he does not believe he was negligent. Dr. GYN shares with Ms. AJ:

> "The results of the review confirm that the initial surgery was performed appropriately, and your ureteral injury was a recognized complication. The intent is never to cut the ureter. I am sorry you have had this complication and that you needed a second hospitalization and surgery.
>
> The review also concluded that we did not get you back into our office quickly enough when you tried to let us know things were not going well. I apologize to you about the problems you experienced gaining access to my office and the resulting delay in making the diagnosis. I know you spent extra days in pain and were worried about what was going on."

It is important to recognize that a sincerely felt and expressed apology is good, but some apologies are not offered or not received well. Remember that an apology is delivered within an existing relationship and that related and previous events may increase or decrease the probability it is accepted. If previous interactions have created trust, this is helpful. If events unfold in a way that create doubt, then the apology is less likely to be accepted. Patients and families also are impacted by nonverbal communication: How do you look? Do you appear distracted? Are you sitting or standing? Does your communication device go off?

Be aware also of the apology that inflames:

- The nonapology apology: "I'm sorry you feel that way."
- Blaming the victim: "I'm sorry it happened, but you should have been more insistent when you called."
- Blaming colleagues: "I'm sorry for my [sorry] APN who clearly should have made sure I saw you right away."
- Narcissistic: "I am so sorry but this has never happened to *me* before... affects my reputation in the community."

> Dr. GYN continues:
> Because of your case, our office manager and I have reviewed our policies and procedures for postoperative patients. We have made some changes to make sure future patients have a different experience.

Ms. AJ thanks Dr. GYN for the information and tells him she appreciates his candor. Then she states, "There are going to be costs, and I'm going to miss more work than anticipated. Who is going to pay the bill for the second surgery, antibiotics, and hospitalization? And who is going to compensate me for my lost income? I'm not going to be able to teach my fall course now; that is going to impose a big loss."

Many professionals may want to reassure a patient asking "Who is going to pay?" and tell them, "Don't worry, it will be taken care of." But what does that mean, really? In most cases, treating professionals do not have the authority to make promises to waive bills (except perhaps their own) or to provide compensation. Practices and organizations should have a designated group and process for conducting a review and determining what should be done about associated costs. Professionals should also keep in mind that CMS and, increasingly, other payors are denying coverage for "never" events and outcomes deemed avoidable.

Expenses Reimbursement and Early Settlement

Humane gestures can create goodwill and reduce risk of litigation. Some risk managers and insurers are finding ways to help support families of patients with AEs through hospitalization and beyond. For instance, COPIC, a Colorado insurer, offers a program to reimburse out-of-pocket medical and recovery time expenses without requiring a determination of negligence or waiver of the right to sue. Over a 10-year period, 2,000 patients received an average payment of $5,000. Only 3.4% of these patients sued; 0.6% received indemnity payment through the tort system.

Other options include offering patients a pre-suit mediation process and/or early settlement in appropriate cases. Early settlement can help the patient and family move forward emotionally and provides them with money when they have the most need for it. Note, however, that once the patient hires an attorney, the opportunity to directly engage with the patient is foreclosed; all communication related to the case thereafter must be handled attorney to attorney.

Unfortunately, not all carriers and health systems know the literature or support disclosure and early offer. Those that do understand these principles, however, realize that the goal is to do the right and professional thing for the patient.

Special Cautionary Circumstances

- If you are asked by a patient for permission to record a conversation, or suddenly realizes a conversation is being recorded, you should remain calm and ask the patient (without anger or defensiveness) why. If the reason does not seem to have a legitimate clinical basis or the purpose appears adversarial, explain that recording is potentially counterproductive to the relationship. Politely ask the patient to stop recording. If the patient refuses, then you should end the visit and offer to reschedule if the patient will agree to a visit without recording devices. You should also contact your insurer (or risk manager) to inform them of the encounter.
- If you receive a call or written query from a plaintiff's attorney regarding a patient you have treated (and even if the attorney assures you that the patient has no intention of suing you but just has questions about care received from others), respond by referring the attorney to your medical malpractice insurance carrier or risk manager.

- If you receive a request for records from a plaintiff's attorney, contact your insurer or risk manager, confirm that the request is accompanied by a valid release from the patient or legal representative (e.g., court-appointed conservator or parent for minor patient) authorizing release to that attorney, and release only those records specifically authorized by the patient or representative. Collect reasonable charges for duplication and preparation of records.

SECTION IV: LITIGATION

Sometimes, in spite of efforts to avoid or defuse potential claims, patients file suit. When the health care professional is sued, he or she enters a different world filled with unfamiliar rules, strange standards of proof, and, at times, confusing outcomes. Furthermore, the plaintiff's attorney represents an opponent whose methods of inquiry may feel manipulative or accusatory. Health care professionals should recognize the differences between the health care and legal worlds and respect them.

This section discusses common concepts of the legal process and provides a simplified overview of how medical malpractice cases progress. It will not make you an expert. If you are sued or need legal advice, consult a licensed and experienced attorney.

KEY POINTS: WHAT TO REMEMBER IF YOU ARE SUED

- Errors occur, and some patients are injured by negligent care.
- Patients have a right in our society to dispute.
- Notify and consult your malpractice insurance carrier and hospital risk manager.
- Discuss what you know about the case with your attorney; do not discuss details of the case with others except in venues your attorney deems protected from discovery under state law.
- Do not alter health care records or destroy equipment related to the suit.
- Being sued can threaten one's sense of well-being. If stressed or depressed, seek professional help.

The Start of Litigation

Eleven months after Ms. AJ's ureteral repair surgery, she files a medical malpractice lawsuit against Dr. GYN. The summons is delivered to Dr. GYN in the office in the middle of a busy day. He immediately contacts his carrier.

Law is traditionally divided into two major categories, civil and criminal. Medical malpractice actions belong to that branch of civil law called tort (as opposed to contract). A tort is a breach of an existing legal duty that impairs a person's legal right or causes damage to his person or property; tort law seeks to redress these violations of conduct (Prosser, 1971).

Medical malpractice is a subtype of tort law called negligence. Negligence can be defined as failing to take the appropriate level of care. The difference between medical malpractice and simple negligence is that the legal duties health care professionals owe to their patients are established by norms of the profession. To prove a case of medical negligence to a lay jury requires expert testimony to describe the applicable norms in the case at hand, demonstrate how the defendant failed to meet those norms, and show linkage between that failure and the claimant's injury (Prosser, 1971).

The plaintiff initiates a lawsuit by filing a "complaint" alleging the medical malpractice cause of action. A cause of action is a claim on which a court can grant relief. The complaint must be filed before the statute of limitations expires or the plaintiff will be barred from filing. In most jurisdictions, the limitation is 1 to 2 years and begins to run when a plaintiff knows, or should have known, that his/her injuries may have been caused by negligent medical care. In some states, the limitation period is longer for minors. Some states require plaintiffs to give "notice of intent to file" to defendants prior to filing a suit. Other jurisdictions require plaintiffs to obtain a certificate or affidavit of merit, or to present the proposed medical malpractice case to a panel for a determination of merit.

After the suit is filed, a defendant is served with a "summons," a notification that he or she is being sued. Defendants have a limited period in which to "answer," either admitting or denying the allegations (Garner, 2009). If you receive a summons, do not let it sit on your desk. Notify your carrier or risk manager immediately; an attorney will need to file the answer on your behalf. Failure to respond within the required timeframe may result in a default judgment against you; in other words, you may lose without a chance to defend (Garner, 2009).

Discovery

Once the answer is filed, the case moves on to "discovery." The purpose of discovery is to obtain information that may lead to admissible evidence. Each party is able to subpoena (compel) production of records, written answers to interrogatories (a set of questions), and witness deposition (the taking of testimony under oath outside of court) (Garner, 2009). Today, parties also commonly subpoena each other to produce any e-mail communications, images on smartphones, text messages, or social media pages that could lead to admissible evidence Fed. R. Civ. P. 26(a)(1)(A). Either party may file a "motion to quash" (ask the court to deny or nullify) a discovery request, which the court will then adjudicate; the presumption, however, is strongly in favor of discovery Fed. R. Civ. P. 45(a)(3).

Deposition is an important part of discovery. During deposition, each side has an opportunity to learn what evidence might be presented to the jury by the other side and, therefore, learn the strength of the other's case. Further, each side has an opportunity to observe the demeanor and "likeability" of their own and the opposing side's witnesses. Deposition transcripts also serve an important role at trial; parties attempt to impeach witnesses' credibility by showing the jury discrepancies between their recorded deposition and testimony in court.

Health care professionals should never go to a deposition without their lawyer. Equally important is that defense counsel must adequately prepare clients for deposition in advance. The deponent (person being deposed) should guard against volunteering information beyond what is asked for by opposing counsel; saying more than necessary is disadvantageous in a litigation context, for plaintiff's attorneys can use the defendant's words against him/her at trial or in settlement negotiations. Deponents should listen carefully to each question, wait to see if his/her attorney objects, then provide a succinct and narrow response. If one does not understand the question, or the question has several parts, ask for it to be rephrased. If the

deponent does not have an actual recollection or is not certain, he or she should state so.

A defendant deponent's role at deposition is as a witness, not an expert. Experts can offer opinions, but defendants should only state the facts as they know them. Thus, if a defendant is asked his/her opinion about a hypothetical case, he or she might reply, "I am not here as an expert witness. I have no opinion." If asked about something that happened in the patient-plaintiff's case, they should refer to the relevant note in the medical record.

Defendants are allowed to testify during deposition (and trial) as to their "habit and custom" if information is not documented in the chart and they do not have a specific recollection (Garner, 2009). As an example, if the medical record contains a notation that an informed consent discussion took place but no further detail is documented, the health care professional would likely not have a *specific* recollection of having informed *this* patient about a particular risk such as a transected ureter. However, he or she could testify (of course *only if true*) that "it would be my habit and custom to include that risk in any informed consent discussion for this procedure." It is far better to have the documentation of what was discussed.

> Ms. AJ's attorney deposes Dr. GYN. Dr. GYN does well explaining the indications for the procedure, the findings at surgery, and the procedure itself. He states he was unaware that Ms. AJ had called the office and spoken with Ms. NP.
> Ms. NP is also deposed. She states that she mentioned to Dr. GYN that Ms. AJ had called and told him about their conversation. Upon being pressed by Ms. AJ's attorney, Ms. NP states that Dr. GYN was busy when she spoke with him; he nodded but did not suggest anything else. Ms. NP states she called Ms. AJ back. When asked how she knows she called, Ms. NP asks to look at the medical record and states, "I didn't write it down, but it would have been my habit to call; I am good about calling patients back."

Trial

The Standard of Proof

The "trier of fact" in malpractice cases may be a jury, single arbitrator, arbitration panel, or judge ("bench trial"). Their role is to hear and evaluate the evidence to determine if the plaintiff satisfied his "burden of proof" (Prosser, 1971). The evidence presented must demonstrate that each of the four elements of the medical malpractice case is "more likely than not" to be true or, in other words, to have a greater than a 50% (a "feather's weight") likelihood of being true. These elements are:

1. The defendant owed a duty of care to the plaintiff.
2. There occurred a breach in the standard of care, that is to say, the defendant failed to exercise "that degree of care and skill which is expected of a reasonably competent practitioner in the same class to which (s)he belongs, acting in the same or similar circumstances".
3. Damages were proximately caused by a breach of the standard of care (in other words, without the defendant's acts, the damages would not have occurred).
4. Actual damages resulted.

Prior to trial or arbitration, parties may "stipulate" agreement as to certain facts or elements of the case; these facts or elements are then no longer in dispute. There usually is no controversy over whether the defendant owed a duty of care to the plaintiff except in those rare cases where the parties litigate as a threshold issue whether a physician–patient relationship existed. Sometimes, defendants agree pretrial to stipulate to liability, that is, admit that the standard of care was breached and caused the plaintiff injury, because the real issue is the disagreement over amount of damages; in this circumstance, the damages dispute becomes the sole issue at trial or arbitration.

The Defendant

During the trial, plaintiffs and defendants call witnesses and usually testify themselves. As in your deposition, remember that your role as a defendant is to state the facts within your personal knowledge and to not opine; your experts will do that on your behalf. The plaintiff's attorney may use any of your court testimony that differs from your deposition to attempt to impeach your credibility. If your recall of any fact now differs from what you testified to on deposition, discuss with your attorney who will then advise. You must do your best to remain calm and professional. You do not want to alienate a jury.

"Likeability," in particular, is important for defendants. If the jury interprets the professional's demeanor as arrogant or "clueless," they may infer that this is how he or she acted at the time of the event in question. Attorneys are generally able to assess in advance if one of their clients will not make a good witness, an observation that may enter into a recommendation to settle pretrial (Peters, 2007b). If a client or other party witness does not do a good job when testifying at trial, the attorney may attempt to settle the case before the case goes to the jury.

Missing records or evidence of an improper attempt to alter a medical record entry can hurt a defendant's credibility. Paper records can be analyzed for discrepancy between asserted timing of a written entry and actual entry. Entries are all timed in electronic medical records, so timeline discrepancies can be fatal to cases.

Expert Witnesses

As noted, medical malpractice cases depend heavily on expert testimony when jury members are laypersons without medical training. In a typical case, both sides will present experts to testify as to the standard of care under the facts of the case and whether the defendant met that standard, whether the plaintiff's damages were caused by a breach of that standard, and the quantum of damages that resulted from the events in question.

One of the reasons why going before a jury can be risky is illustrated by the fact that after review of the same records, experts often reach different conclusions about the standard of care and whether the care provided caused the plaintiff's outcome. In other words, the legal system uses indistinct borders to separate AEs with negligence from those without negligence. A more skeptical view is the consideration that because experts are not court appointed but instead hired by the plaintiff or defense attorney, their opinion may be influenced by that affiliation, whether intentional or not.

If a party asks you to review and consult on a case of possible medical malpractice, keep in mind that if your opinion supports their position, they may also ask you to testify as an expert witness. Before and during the review, ask yourself the following questions:

1. Do I (really) have the expertise related to the medical practice in question?
2. Am I current? After all, medical practice evolves quickly.
3. Am I biased in a way that will impact my review, for example, am I against all plaintiffs or against doctors who don't practice the way I do?
4. Is the money the party is paying me affecting my opinion? (Dollars influence in very subtle ways.)
5. *Can I serve a professional role?*

The Jury: Verdict and Damages Awards

The judge provides "jury instructions" that explain applicable law and instructs the jury to apply the law to the facts presented to decide the case. The jury determines if the defendant is liable and, if so, what the damages award for the plaintiff should be.

One of the goals of medical malpractice law is to compensate those negligently injured by care and make them "whole" for their loss. Damages are intended to make up for the difference between how the person was prior to the injury—including what they would have been projected to earn and the type of life they would likely have had if not for the injury—and their "new normal" (Restatement of Torts, 1979). Two types of damages are awarded in malpractice cases: special damages and general damages.

"Special" or "economic" damages refer to the plaintiff's monetary losses and expense burdens resulting from the injury. Special damages include replacement of lost past and future earnings as well the cost of care necessary to restore or optimize the injured party's physical and emotional health over the length of time care will be needed. With serious, permanent injury, the care plan may be lifelong.

"General" or "noneconomic" damages (also referred to as "pain and suffering") are awarded to compensate for intangible losses related to mental anguish, pain, loss of enjoyment of life, loss of consortium (i.e., loss of normal marital relations and companionship), and disfigurement. Juries place dollar values on pain and suffering. The valuation often represents a significant percentage of the total damages award and may exceed the amount granted for special damages.

"Punitive" damages, intended to "teach the defendant a lesson," are rare in medical malpractice cases. Some states prohibit punitive damages or allow only for fraud, malice, or gross negligence. Plaintiffs who successfully prove battery (an intentional tort) may also receive punitive damages.

It is often asserted that juries are predisposed to find liability for a "sympathetic plaintiff." Vidmar found jurors to be careful listeners, alert to plaintiffs who contribute to their poor outcome, and disinclined to punish doctors for imperfect human decision making. Furthermore, juries do not grant large awards because they view physicians or corporate defendants as able to pay. Rather, juries award substantial damages when they believe there is negligent care and award higher damages to more severely injured plaintiffs.

Even when jurors keep an open mind and listen carefully to the evidence, in the end, they are human; a host of factors may impinge on their deliberations. These factors influence the jury's view of each witness' credibility, acceptance of one expert's theory over another, or their evaluation of an appropriate award.

Settlement and Alternative Dispute Resolution

At the start of a lawsuit, a defendant may believe he or she "did nothing wrong" and the plaintiff may feel that no amount could sufficiently compensate their suffering and loss. External review and discovery can impact some of this confidence. Settlement allows parties to weigh the relative risks and costs of going to trial against allowing some monetary transfer from defendant to plaintiff. Settlement remains an option at every stage of litigation. For example, a party that becomes aware of a significant weakness in its case will try to settle before spending more money. On the other end, parties may settle on the eve of trial, during jury deliberation, or after a verdict if the losing party makes clear it will appeal.

> Dr. GYN has refused to settle and wants his carrier to defend the case. His attorney explains his concerns about aspects of the case that might not sit well with a jury and could lead to a generous award. Counsel reminds Dr. GYN that his office's telephone records confirm that the patient called several times. There is, however, no documentation that Dr. GYN called her back. Counsel agrees that it was not unreasonable for Ms. NP to field the request; unfortunately, however, Ms. NP gave the patient advice that proved to be inadequate, and the evidence suggests she did not follow up with the patient as promised.
>   Dr. GYN's attorney further shares that plaintiff's expert will testify that the standard of care required cystoscopy with intravenous indigo carmine dye contrast to look for ureteral injury at the end of the procedure. The defense attorney assures Dr. GYN that their own expert will dispute this assertion; it will be up to the jury to weigh the two testimonies.
>   Dr. GYN's defense attorney makes a recommendation to Dr. GYN to settle the case.

Throughout a lawsuit, plaintiff and defense attorneys assess their strategy for achieving an optimal result for their client (and themselves). Attorneys weigh the facts of the case that emerge from record review, interviews with witnesses and experts, and discovery. They observe performance at deposition to anticipate how witnesses and experts will do at trial. Trial attorneys also remain sensitive to the fact that cases can turn on a single weakness. For example, a key defense witness who no longer works for the practice or organization may not wish to cooperate, or a medical chart entry by a team member appears to criticize the patient's care.

Client motivations, too, play a role in settlement decisions. A defendant may wish to avoid publicity or have concern that a jury will not fully understand a subtle defense. (Imagine a case with a serious error, a patient with a bad outcome, but no likely causal connection between the two.) A plaintiff may fear exposure of embarrassing information at trial or, in need of cash, decide to accept less than to wait years for trial without guarantee of a larger jury award.

Ultimately, the decision to settle is a microeconomic assessment. Each side calculates the damages at stake discounted by the probability that the plaintiff will win in comparison to the cost of continued litigation. If the two sides' valuations are similar, they are likely to settle. Parties have trouble settling when both perceive their own case as strong, the plaintiff overestimates the chance that it will win and the defendant underestimates, or they are unable to assign a realistic valuation because previous jury awards for similar injuries vary widely (especially for pain and suffering awards).

Mediation, a form of alternative dispute resolution (ADR), can help the settlement process. The mediators' role is to facilitate information sharing, finding areas of agreement, and negotiating based on mutual benefit. Mediation is particularly helpful when parties enter with a realistic idea of the settlement value of their case.

Arbitration, another ADR format, differs from mediation in that a third party makes a decision on the merits of the case. In other words, arbitration declares a winner and a loser. Arbitrators tend to have experience in the field (e.g., practice as a medical malpractice litigator), and so can assess each side's position on the basis of previous cases within the jurisdiction.

With nonbinding arbitration, parties are free to reject the arbitration decision and proceed to trial. Binding arbitration, on the other hand, is based on an existing contract in which the patient-plaintiff agrees to waive the right to go to court to adjudicate disputes and accepts binding arbitration as his/her sole venue for recourse. Courts generally uphold binding arbitration agreements as long as the agreements conform to state statutory requirements.

> Ms. AJ and Dr. GYN agree to mediate. At mediation, Ms. AJ's attorney puts forth a demand far in excess of a million dollars. Dr. GYN's team counters with a significantly smaller offer, explaining the ureteral injury was not the result of negligence but a known complication, mentioned in the informed consent discussion and consent form (which Ms. AJ signed). The defense acknowledges that it took longer than it might for the diagnosis to be made, but this did not affect Ms. AJ's outcome.
>   The mediator urges the parties to make a realistic assessment of their cases and provide numbers that are closer to what they would be willing to settle for.
>   Dr. GYN tells his attorney that he still believes he did not do anything wrong and is unhappy with the idea of settling the case. However, the suit has created enormous stress, and he just wants the case to "go away."
>   Over the course of the next 6 hours, with some back and forth, the parties agree to a settlement amount. The parties agree that the amount will be kept confidential.

In sum, parties to a medical malpractice case must recognize that whether the care was negligent is not necessarily dispositive of the case. Other factors influence the outcome and the decision to settle. While settlement or verdict decisions may not seem fair to health care professionals accustomed to rigorous standards of proof, attorneys and medical malpractice insurance carriers understand the risks and advise settlement or defense strategies accordingly.

Does the Medical Malpractice Legal System Achieve its Goals?

Although variation among cases and wide ranges of awards for similar categories of injuries create an impression of randomness, data suggest that the US legal system does a reasonable job sorting filed claims. Compared with meritorious suits, nonvalid suits result in more case withdrawals, trial loss, or lower settlement payments. Sixty to sixty-five percent (60–65%) of claims are dropped or dismissed without payment, and about one fourth to one third of cases settle. Five to fifteen percent of cases proceed to trial. In 80–90% of trials, there is a verdict for the defense (physician).

Unfortunately, a gynecologic surgeon who believes the legal outcome in his/her particular case was wrong probably does not feel any better if told the system usually gets it right. As someone trained to understand scientific probabilities, awarding a plaintiff a lot of money on only a 51% level of certainty feels different from the 95% probability medical professionals demand before they are persuaded the effect is real and not due to chance. Furthermore, awareness that weaker claims are sometimes paid because trial costs will likely exceed the settlement amount also may seem unfair. In any event, even legal vindication at trial does not erase incurred defense costs or the emotional burden of a suit.

Despite outcomes that are not perfect in all cases, it is reasonable to consider if, overall, medical malpractice tort law achieves its goals. These goals are: (a) compensation of injured patients, (b) vindication of the injured plaintiff's sense of justice, (c) deterrence of undesirable (negligent) behavior, and (d) structural improvement of the medical care system to reduce risk of patient harm in the future.

Compensation

Some injured patients are made whole by the system, but overall only a fraction of injured patients are ever compensated. As discussed earlier, only a small percentage of patients harmed by negligent care actually sue. Some patients forgive. Others resign themselves to the outcome. Also, as we have seen, patients are commonly thwarted in their efforts to sue by lawyers' selectivity of cases. Attorneys' selectivity of cases also means many injured patients are unable to receive compensation. Finally, in the absence of express disclosure, it is likely that a large group of patients never learn that the harm they suffered was avoidable.

For patients who win their cases, the award may not sufficiently cover their financial needs once attorney fees and costs are deducted. Tort reform such as caps on noneconomic damages (see below) also contributes to undercompensation, especially in cases of severe injury. Furthermore, lags of up to four years to resolve litigated cases mean that many patients lack current funds to pay for needed medical care or support for their families.

Some states are attempting to shift resources to serve more people. Lower-cost arbitration in some states is linked to increased claims frequency, suggesting that more claimants are gaining access to compensation. In addition, some states have enacted no-fault administrative systems for certain conditions, such as birth-related injury, in order to remove the unpredictability of the tort system, lower its cost, and accelerate payment.

Vindication

Litigation affords the ability to, according to Bovbjerg, "command more attention from providers", which can help achieve closure for many plaintiffs, especially in cases where they sued to find out what happened. The need for accountability is one of the deficits of a no-fault compensation system for medical injury.

Public exposure of a health care professional's claims also can provide a sense of vindication for plaintiffs. Information about filed lawsuits and named physicians are increasingly available on public databases in many jurisdictions. One can identify physicians who are sued (and those sued repeatedly). However, not all states and counties provide claims information, and others require a "per query" payment.

The Healthcare Quality Improvement Act of 1986 established the National Practitioner Data Bank (NPDB) as a federal repository for information regarding health care professionals' malpractice payments and disciplinary actions. Individual consumers cannot query the database. However, Public Citizen Congress Watch, a consumer watch group, reports that 16 years of cumulative NPDB data show 6% of physicians responsible for 58% of all malpractice payments, 2% account for 33% of all payments, and 1% for 20% of payments. The nonrandom distribution of medical malpractice payouts in the NPDB database is consistent with Sloan's conclusions of twenty-plus years ago that lawsuits are nonrandomly distributed.

Deterrence

Medical malpractice tort law aims to deter future conduct of the type that led to the patient's injury. Litigation achieves this goal when health care professionals understand that different actions likely would have prevented injury, and then act with greater caution in the future.

The tort system leads to other incentives for change. For example, medical malpractice actions may deter if they raise medical malpractice insurance costs. With enough claims, carriers may drop insureds from coverage. The risk that one will be uninsurable or shifted into a high-risk pool with very high premiums may motivate some individuals to take extra precautions to avoid patient injury. Others find the experience of being deposed and cross-examined, perceived or real reputational effects, and the anxiety associated with being involved in a lawsuit incentive enough to change behaviors and practices in ways that lower risk.

Unfortunately, litigation may not deter when physicians sued repeatedly continue to see claims as random events, a cost of doing business, and a nuisance that one simply cannot do anything to prevent. Fatalistic "acceptance" of claims suggests lack of awareness that suits are nonrandomly distributed. Thus, other means of professional regulation besides tort law, such as identifying and intervening with high risk physicians as discussed in Section II, are needed to change behavior.

The malpractice tort system has also led to "overdeterrence" or the practice of "defensive medicine." Defensive medicine is a self-focused reaction to the malpractice tort system in which unnecessary tests and imaging studies are ordered in an effort to protect from suits. Refusing to see patients with complex problems or terminating "difficult" patients in the name of lowering risk increases patient risk in other ways.

Structural Change

Another goal of medical malpractice tort law is to induce movement toward structural change in the health care system in order to protect future patients. Certain liability rules such as joint and several liability and enterprise liability for malpractice can encourage such movement.

Joint and several liability makes full compensation for injured plaintiffs a higher priority than limiting codefendants' liability for damages to their proportional contribution to the injury. Specifically, defendants who co-contribute to injury are liable not only for their own apportioned share of the damages but also for the share of any co-defendant who does not pay (Wright, 1988). Such cross-subsidization should incentivize "deep pocket" defendants to therefore more carefully choose and monitor those with whom they share patients.

The doctrine of enterprise liability for malpractice holds health care organizations responsible for medical liability in place of, or in addition to, individuals. Enterprise liability encourages integration of professionals, systems, services, and practices into a system that can exert more uniform control and supervision over processes, behavior, and performance. Emerging data suggest that such integration results in lower defense costs than in less integrated settings.

Despite the tort system's partial ability to increase structural accountability, it alone cannot achieve safer care for reasons that include its retrospective nature, high transaction costs, and failure to draw on our increasing knowledge of risk prevention best practices. The retrospective quality of litigation allows injuries to keep occurring, for it focuses primarily on compensation rather than prevention. Going forward, defendants may fix systems and remediate individuals, but they are always playing catch-up.

The system's excessively high transaction costs represent wasted resources that could be used to compensate more patients who suffer harm from care. Fifty-four cents of every dollar spent goes toward administrative, attorney, and expert costs. Defensive medicine, too, adds to the unnecessary costs stimulated by the litigation system, wasting billions of national health care dollars.

In sum, the medical malpractice tort system cannot act as a primary corrective agent. Rather, in order to prevent patient injury, we must use risk prevention best practices to reliably and promptly identify risk (monitoring and reporting), review for contributors to AEs (risk management file reviews, RCAs, MMM&Is), and address behaviors and systems that undermine safety and performance.

Tort Reform

Over the past four decades, varying medical malpractice tort reforms have been implemented throughout the United States. The earliest enactments were spurred by escalating liability costs that threatened the ongoing availability of medical malpractice insurance. Medical malpractice insurance costs have since stabilized, but the tort reform debate continues. Although a lengthy discussion on tort reform is outside the scope of this chapter, we present a brief overview of some common types of tort reform.

Some reforms primarily affect the litigation process. These include (a) screening cases for legitimacy prior to filing suit (e.g., mandatory panel review, medical reviewer affidavits or certificates of merit), (b) imposing a shorter statute of limitations (e.g., reducing the statute of limitations to 1 year), and (c) placing stricter criteria for expert witness eligibility (e.g., requiring that an expert is in active practice within the same specialty as the defendant).

Reforms that impact damage awards include (a) collateral source rule modifications in which any compensation plaintiff receives from another ("collateral") source such as auto or worker's compensation insurance is subtracted from the damages award ("offset"), (b) caps that place an upper limit on the plaintiff's noneconomic damages award, and (c) tiered contingency fee rates that direct more of the award toward the seriously injured plaintiff than would result from standard contingency fee agreements. California's Medical Injury Compensation Reform Act of 1975 or MICRA is a well-known example of tort reform. The statute provides for various reforms that include collateral source rule modification, a $250,000 cap on noneconomic damages, and limits on attorney fees to 40% of the first $50,000 awarded, 33% of the next $50,000, 25% of the next $500,000, and 15% of any amount over $600,000.

Of the tort reform features discussed, only noneconomic damages caps are consistently shown to lower the payout per claim and numbers of paid claims.

CONCLUSION

Health care professionals want to deliver exemplary care and reduce risk of patient injury. To achieve these goals, they must be willing to regulate their own and group members' performance and behavior. Professionalism is essential for effective teamwork and achieving intended outcomes.

Professionals should utilize risk prevention tools to identify and address variation from best practices. When errors negatively impact clinical outcomes, professionals share information with the patient and remain engaged.

Understanding why patients sue and best practices for managing potential claims can help professionals avoid claims. Still, patients sometimes sue. Therefore, health professionals should gain familiarity with the medical malpractice tort law process and rely on trusted legal professionals for guidance.

ACKNOWLEDGMENTS

The authors wish to acknowledge and thank Ruth Schimmel for her research assistance and helpful suggestions and comments. Thanks also to Peggy Westlake for her research and technical support and Nancy Yelton and Anna C. Hayden for their research assistance.

BIBLIOGRAPHY

Allsop J, Mulcahy L. *Adverse events, complaints, and clinical negligence claims: what do we know?* London, UK: UK Department of Health, 2002:14.

AMA Council on Ethical and Judicial Affairs. *Principles of medical ethics.* Chicago, IL: American Medical Association, 2001.

Andrews L. Studying medical error in situ: implications for malpractice law and policy. *DePaul Law Rev* 2005;54:357–392.

Annandale E, Hunt K. Accounts of disagreements with doctors. *Soc Sci Med* 1998;46:119.

Avraham R. An empirical study of the impact of tort reforms on medical malpractice settlement payments. *J Legal Stud* 2007;36(S2):S183.

Bagian JP, Gosbee J, Lee CZ, et al. The Veterans Affairs root cause analysis system in action. *Jt Comm J Qual Improv* 2002;28:531.

Beckman HB, Markakis KM, Suchman AL, et al. The doctor–patient relationship and malpractice: lessons from plaintiff deposition. *Arch Intern Med* 1994;154:1365.

Benjet B. A review of state law modifying the Collateral Source Rule: seeking greater fairness in economic damages awards. *Def Couns J* 2009;76:210.

Bismark M, Dauer E, Paterson R, et al. Accountability sought by patients following adverse events from medical care: the New Zealand experience. *CMAJ* 2006;175:889.

Black B, Silver C, Hyman DA, et al. Stability, not crisis: medical malpractice claim outcomes in Texas, 1988–2002. *J Empir Leg Stud* 2005;2:207.

Boothman RC, Blackwell AC, Campbell DA, et al. A better approach to medical malpractice claims? The University of Michigan experience. *J Health Life Sci Law* 2009;2:125.

Bovbjerg RR. *Medical malpractice: problems & reforms—a policymaker's guide to issues and information.* Washington, DC: The Intergovernmental Health Policy Project, George Washington University, 1995.

Bovbjerg RR, Petronis KR. The relationship between physicians' malpractice claims history and later claims. Does the past predict the future? *JAMA* 1994;272:1421.

Bovbjerg RR. Medical malpractice on trial: quality of care is the important standard. *Law Contemp Probl* 1986;49:321.

Bovbjerg RR, Sloan FA, Blumstein JF. Public policy: valuing life and limb in tort: scheduling "pain and suffering." *Nw U L Rev* 1989;83:908.

Brennan TA, Leape LL, Laird NM, et al. Incidence of adverse events and negligence in hospitalized patients: results of the Harvard Medical Practice Study I. *N Engl J Med* 1991;324:371.

Burstin HR, Johnson WG, Lipsitz SR, et al. Do the poor sue more? *JAMA* 1993;270:1697.

Cal. Bus. & Prof. Code § 6146(a) (West 2014).

Cal. Civ. Code § 3333.1-3333.2 (West 2014).

Cheney FW. The American Society of Anesthesiologists Closed Claims Project: what have we learned, how has it affected practice, and how will it affect practice in the future? *Anesthesiology* 1999;91:552.

Christensen JF. The heat of darkness: the impact of perceived mistakes on physicians. *J Gen Intern Med* 1992;7:424.

Classen EC, Resar R, Griffin F, et al. 'Global Trigger Tool' shows that adverse events in hospitals may be ten times greater than previously measured. *Health Aff (Millwood)* 2011;30:581.

Clayton EW, Hickson GA, Githens PB, et al. Doctor–patient relationship. In: Sloan FA, Githens PB, Clayton EW, et al., eds. *Suing for medical malpractice.* Chicago, IL: University of Chicago Press, 1993:65.

Cohen JR. Advising clients to apologize. *S Calif Law Rev* 1999;72:1009.

COPIC. https://www.callcopic.com/copic-services/safety-and-risk/Pages/3rs.aspx. Accessed on May 13, 2013.

CRICO/RMF. http://www.rmf.harvard.edu/

Cunningham L. *The quality connection in health care.* San Francisco, CA/Oxford, UK: Jossey-Bass, 1991:94.

Custin RE, Tehrani S. The golden standard? California as a model for national medical malpractice tort reform. *J Bus Ethics* 2012;18:91.

Cydulka RK, Tamayo-Sarver J, Gage A. Association of patient satisfaction with complaints and risk management among emergency physicians. *J Emerg Med* 2011;41:405.

Daniels S, Martin J. Plaintiffs' lawyers, specialization, and medical malpractice. *Vand Law Rev* 2006;59:1051.

Danzon PM. The frequency and severity of medical malpractice claims: new evidence. *Law Contemp Probl* 1986;49:57.

Danzon P, Lillard L. The resolution of medical malpractice claims: research results and policy implications. The Rand Corp. Report No. R-2793-ICJ. 1982. http://www.rand.org/content/dam/rand/pubs/reports/2007/R2793.pdf. Accessed on December 4, 2014.

Danzon PM, Lillard LA. Settlement out of court: the disposition of medical malpractice claims. *J Legal Stud* 1983;12:345.

Deis JN, Smith KM, Warren MD, et al. Transforming the morbidity and mortality conference into an instrument for system-wide improvement. In: Henricksen K, et al., eds. *Advances in patient safety: new directions and alternative approaches*, Vol. 2: Culture and Redesign. Rockville, MD: Agency for Healthcare Quality and Research, 2008.

deVries EN, Ramrattan MA, Smorenburg SM, et al. The incidence and nature of in-hospital adverse events: a systematic review. *Qual Saf Health Care* 2008;17:216.

Donn SM. Medical liability, risk management, and the quality of health care. *Semin Fetal Neonatal Med* 2005;10:3.

Duclos CW, Eichler M, Taylor L. Patient perspectives of patient–provider communication after adverse events. *Int J Qual Health Care* 2005;17:479.

Engalla v. Permanente Medical Group, Inc. 15 Cal. 4th 951, 938 P.2d 903(1997).

Entman SS, Glass CA, Hickson GB, et al. The relationship between malpractice claims history and subsequent obstetric care. *JAMA* 1994;272:1588.

Fed. R. Civ. P. 12(b)(6).

Fed. R. Civ. P. 26.

Fed. R. Civ. P. 45.

Felps W, Mitchell TR, Bylington E. How, when, and why bad apples spoil the barrel: negative group members and dysfunctional groups. *Res Organ Behav* 2006;27:175.

Fullam F, Garman AN, Johnson TJ, et al. The use of patient satisfaction surveys and alternative coding procedures to predict malpractice risk. *Med Care* 2009;47:553.

Furrow BR. The patient injury epidemic: medical malpractice litigation as a curative tool. *Drexel Law Rev* 2011;4:41.

Furrow BR. Adverse events and patient injury: coupling detection, disclosure, and compensation. *N Engl Law Rev* 2012;46:437.

Galanter M. Reading the landscape of disputes: what we know and don't know (and think we know) about our allegedly contentious and litigious society. *UCLA Law Rev* 1983;31:4.

Gallagher TH, Studdert D. Disclosing harmful medical errors to patients. *N Engl J Med* 2007;356:2713.

Gallagher TH, Bell SK, Smith KM, et al. Disclosing harmful medical errors to patients: tackling three tough cases. *Chest* 2009;136:897.

Garner, BA, ed. *Black's law dictionary*, 9th ed. St. Paul, MN: West, 2009.

Gawande A. *Complications: a surgeon's notes on an imperfect science.* New York City: Metropolitan Books, Henry Holt and Co., 2002.

Gluck PA. Medical error theory. *Obstet Gynecol Clin N Am* 2008;35:11.

Golann D. Dropped medical malpractice claims: their surprising frequency, apparent causes, and potential remedies. *Health Aff (Millwood)* 2011;30:1343.

Gordon LA. Can Cedars-Sinai's "M+M Matrix" save surgical education? *Bull Am Coll Surg* 2004;89:16.

Grossberg B. Uniformity, federalism, and tort reform: the Erie implications of medical malpractice certificate of merit statutes. *Univ Penn Law Rev* 2010;159:217.

Hain PD, Pichert JW, Hickson GB, et al. Using risk management files to identify and address causative factors associated with adverse events in pediatrics. *Ther Clin Risk Manag* 2007;3:625.

Haskins interview. http://sph.umn.edu/mha-executive-interview-paul-haskins/. Accessed on December 4, 2014.

Hayden AC, Pichert JW, Fawcett J, et al. Best practices for basic and advanced skills in health care service recovery: a case study of a re-admitted patient. *Jt Comm J Qual Patient Saf* 2010;36:310.

Health Insurance Portability and Accountability Act of 1996 (HIPAA). Pub. L. 104–191 (1996); 45 CFR §§ 164.502, 164.508.

Healthcare Quality Improvement Act (HCQIA) 42 U.S.C. §§ 11131 et seq (2006).

Hickson GB, Altemeir WA, Perrin JM. Physician reimbursement by salary or fee-for-service: effect on physician practice behavior in a randomized prospective study. *Pediatrics* 1987;80:344.

Hickson GB, Clayton EW, Entman SS, et al. Obstetricians' prior malpractice experience and patients' satisfaction with care. *JAMA* 1994;272:1583.

Hickson GB, Clayton EW, Githens PB, et al. Factors that prompted families to file medical malpractice claims following perinatal injuries. *JAMA* 1992;267:1359.

Hickson GB, Entman SS. Physician practice behavior and litigation risk: evidence and opportunity. *Clin Obstet Gynecol* 2008; 51:688.

Hickson GB, Entman SS. Physicians influence and the malpractice problem. *Obstet Gynecol* 2010;115:682.

Hickson GB, Federspiel CF, Blackford JU, et al. Patient complaints and malpractice risk in a regional healthcare center. *South Med J* 2007a;100:791.

Hickson GB, Federspiel CF, Pichert JW, et al. Patient complaints and malpractice risk. *JAMA* 2002;287:2951.

Hickson GB, Gentile DA, Githens PB, et al. Liability. In: Sloan FA, Githens PB, Clayton EW, et al., eds. *Suing for medical malpractice.* Chicago, IL: The University of Chicago Press, 1993:65.

Hickson GB, Jenkins AD. Identifying and addressing communication failures as a means of reducing unnecessary malpractice claims. *N C Med J* 2007b;68:362.

Hickson GB, Moore IN, Pichert JW, et al. Balancing systems and individual accountability in a safety culture. In: Berman S, ed. *From front office to front line.* 2nd ed. Oakbrook Terrace, IL: Joint Commission Resources, 2012:1.

Hickson GB, Pichert JW. Identifying and intervening with high-malpractice-risk physicians to reduce claims. *Physician Insurer* 2007d:29.

Hickson GB, Pichert JW. Identifying and addressing physicians at high risk for medical malpractice claims. In: Youngberg B, ed. *Patient safety handbook*, 2nd ed. Sudbury, MA: Jones and Bartlett, 2013:360.

Hickson GB, Pichert JW, Federspiel CF, et al. Development of an early identification and response model of malpractice prevention. *Law Contemp Probl* 1997;60:7.

Hickson GB, Pichert JW, Webb LE, et al. A complementary approach to promoting professionalism: identifying, measuring, and addressing unprofessional behaviors. *Acad Med* 2007c;82:1040.

Holman M, Vidmar N, Lee P. Most claims settle: implications for alternative dispute resolution from a profile of medical-malpractice claims in Florida. *Law Contemp Probl* 2011;74:103.

Hsiao WC, Braun P, Becker ER, et al. *A national study of resource-based relative value scales for physician services: phase III final report to the health care financing administration.* Boston, MA: Harvard School of Public Health, 1992:179, 215. HCFA Contract No. 18-C-98795/1–03.

Hyman CS, Liebman CB, Schechter CB, et al. Interest-based mediation of medical malpractice lawsuits: a route to improved patient safety? *J Health Polit Policy Law* 2012;35;797.

Hyman DA, Black B, Silver C, et al. Estimating the effect of damages caps in medical malpractice cases: evidence from Texas. *J Legal Anal* 2009;1:355.

Hyman DA, Silver C. Five myths of medical malpractice. *Chest* 2013;143:222.

Hyman DA, Silver C. Medical malpractice litigation and tort reform: it's the incentives, stupid. *Vand Law Rev* 2006;59:1085.

Imershein AW, Brents AH. The impact of large medical malpractice awards on malpractice awardees. *J Leg Med* 1992;13:33.

Institute of Medicine. *Crossing the quality chasm: a new health system for the 21st century.* Washington, DC: National Academy Press, 2001.

Ishikawa K. *Guide to quality control*, 2nd ed. revised. Tokyo: Asian Productivity Organization, 1986:226.

Issacharoff S, Silver C, Syverud KD. *Bargaining impediments and settlement behavior.* http://www.utexas.edu/law/faculty/csilver/class/DisputeResolution.htm. Accessed on May 9, 2013.

James BC, Savitz, LA. How Intermountain trimmed health care costs through robust quality improvement efforts. *Health Aff (Millwood)* 2011;6:1185.

Jena AB, Chandra A, Lakdawalla D, et al. Outcomes of medical malpractice litigation against US physicians. *Arch Intern Med* 2012;172:892.

Jena AB, Seabury S, Lakdawalla D, et al. Malpractice risk according to physician specialty. *N Engl J Med* 2011;365:629.

Kachalia A, Kaufman SR, Boothman R, et al. Liability claims and costs before and after implementation of a medical error disclosure program. *Ann Intern Med* 2010;153:213.

Kachalia A, Mello MM. New directions in medical liability reform. *N Engl J Med* 2011;364:1564.

Kachalia A, Shojania KG, Hofer TP, et al. Does full disclosure of medical errors affect malpractice liability? The jury is out. *Jt Comm J Qual Saf* 2003;29:503.

Kachalia A, Gandhi TK, Puopolo AL, et al. Missed and delayed diagnoses in the emergency department: a study of closed malpractice claims from 4 liability insurers. *Ann Emerg Med* 2007;49:196.

Kane CK. Medical liability claim frequency: a 2007–2008 snapshot of physicians. *Policy Research Perspectives No. 2010-1*. Chicago, IL: American Medical Association, 2010, http://www.ama-assn.org/resources/doc/health-policy/prp-201001-claim-freq.pdf

Kaplan HS, Fastman BR. Organization of event reporting data for sense making and system improvement. *Qual Saf Health Care* 2003;12:ii68.

Kauffmann RM, Landman MP, Shelton J, et al. The use of a multidisciplinary morbidity and mortality conference to incorporate ACGME general competencies. *J Surg Educ* 2011;68:303.

Kesselheim AS, November MT, Lifford KL, et al. Using malpractice claims to identify risk factors for neurological impairment among infants following non-reassuring fetal heart rate patterns during labour. *J Eval Clin Pract* 2010;16:476.

Kohn L, Corrigan J, Donaldson M, eds. *To err is human: building a safer health system. Report of the Institute of Medicine.* Washington, DC: National Academy Press, 1999.

Kraman SS, Cranfill L, Hamm G, et al. Advocacy: the Lexington Veterans Affairs Medical Center. *Jt Comm J Qual Improv* 2002:646.

Kramen SS, Hamm G. Risk management: extreme honesty may be the best policy. *Ann Intern Med* 1999;131:963.

Krauss MI. A medical liability toolkit, including ADR. *J Law* 2012;2:349.

Kripalani S, Weiss BD. Teaching about health literacy and clear communication. *J Gen Intern Med* 2006;21:888.

Landrigan CP, Parry GJ, Bones CB, et al. Temporal trends in rates of patient harm resulting from medical care. *N Engl J Med* 2010;363:2124.

Lavery JP. The physician's reaction to a malpractice suit. *Obstet Gynecol* 1988;71:138.

Leape LL, Berwick DM. Five years after To Err Is Human: what have we learned? *JAMA* 2005;293:2384.

Leape LL, Shore MF, Dienstag JL, et al. A culture of respect. Part 1. The nature and causes of disrespectful behavior by physicians. *Acad Med* 2012;87:845.

Leape LL, Shore MF, Dienstag JL, et al. A culture of respect, Part 2: the nature and causes of disrespectful behavior by physicians. *Acad Med* 2012;87:853.

Lee JD, Lindahl BA. *Modern tort law: liability and litigation.* West Group, 1990.

Lembitz A. *Litigation alternative: COPIC's 3Rs program.* http://www.aaos.org/news/aaosnow/sep10/managing7.asp. Accessed on December 4, 2014.

Levtzion-Korach O, Frankel A, Alcalai H, et al. Integrating incident data from five reporting systems to assess patient safety: making sense of the elephant. *Jt Comm J Qual Patient Saf* 2010; 36:402.

Livanovitch v. Livanovitch, 99 Vt. 327, 328, 131 A. 799, 800 (1926).

Localio AR, Lawthers AG, Brennan TA, et al. Relation between malpractice claims and adverse events due to negligence. Results of the Harvard Medical Practice Study III. *N Engl J Med* 1991; 325:245.

Long AL, Horvath MM, Jansen J, et al. The Leapfrog CPOE Evaluation Tool: one academic medical center's experience. *Patient Saf Qual Healthcare* 2010:48.

Madison KM. The evolution of reporting as a quality improvement tool. *J Leg Med* 2012;33:63.

McClellan FM, White AA, Jimenez RL, et al. Do poor people sue doctor more frequently? Confronting unconscious bias and the role of cultural competency. *Clin Orthop Relat Res* 2012;470:1393.

McDonald, TB, Helmchen LA, Smith KM, et al. Responding to patient safety incidents: the "seven pillars". *Qual Saf Health Care* 2010;19:1.

Medical Injury Compensation Reform Act of 1975 (MICRA). http://mittelmanlawfirm.com/medical-injury-compensation-reform-act-of-1975-micra/. Accessed on December 4, 2014.

Mello MM. Of swords and shields: the role of clinical practice guidelines in medical malpractice litigation. *Univ Penn Law Rev* 2001;149:645.

Mello MM. Medical malpractice: impact of the crisis and effect of state tort reform. *The Synthesis Project* 2006;10:1. http://www.rwjf.org/content/dam/supplementary-assets/2006/05/15168.medmalpracticeimpact.report.pdf. Accessed on December 4, 2014.

Mello MM, Chandra A, Gawande AA, et al. National costs of the medical liability system. *Health Aff (Millwood)* 2010;29:1574.

Metzloff TB. Resolving malpractice disputes: imaging the jury's shadow. *Law Contemp Probl* 1991;54:43.

Metzloff TB. Alternative dispute resolution strategies in medical malpractice. *Alaska Law Rev* 1992;9:429.

Meyers AR. Lumping it: the hidden denominator of the medical malpractice crisis. *Am J Public Health* 1987;77:1544.

Miller A. Hospital reporting and "never" events. *Medicare Patent Manag* 2009;4:20.

Mills DH, ed. *Report on the medical insurance feasibility study/sponsored jointly by California Medical Association and California Hospital Association.* San Francisco, CA: Sutter Publications, Inc., 1977.

Mills DH. Medical insurance feasibility study. A technical summary. *West J Med* 1978;128:360.

Mills DH. Whither malpractice regulation? *West J Med* 1988; 149:611.

Moore IN, Pichert JW, Hickson GB, et al. Rethinking peer review: detecting and addressing medical malpractice claims risk. *Vand Law Rev* 2006;59:1175.

Morris JA, Carrillo YM, Jenkins JM, et al. Surgical adverse events, risk management and malpractice outcome: morbidity and mortality review is not enough. *Ann Surg* 2003;237:844.

Morse RB, Pollak MM. Root cause analyses performed in a children's hospital: events, action plan strength, and implementation rates. *J Healthcare Qual* 2012;34:55.

Mukherjee K, Pichert JW, Cornett MB, et al. All trauma surgeons are not created equal: asymmetric distribution of malpractice claims risk. *J Trauma* 2010 Sep;69:549.

Mulcahy L, Tritter JQ. Pathways, pyramids and icebergs? Mapping the links between dissatisfaction and complaints. *Sociol Health Illn* 1998;20:825.

Murff HJ, France DJ, Blackford J, et al. Relationship between patient complaints and surgical complications. *Qual Saf Health Care* 2006;15:13.

National Health Policy Forum. The basics: relative value units (RVUs), 2009. http://www.nhpf.org/library/the-basics/Basics_RVUs_02-12-09.pdf. Accessed on December 4, 2014.

O'Neil AC, Petersen LA, Cook EF, et al. Physician reporting compared with medical-record review to identify adverse medical events. *Ann Intern Med* 1993;119:370.

Patient Protection and Affordable Care Act (PPACA). PL 111-148 §3023 and §3025, 2010.

Patient Safety Network. Medicare says it won't cover hospital errors, 2007. http://psnet.ahrq.gov/resource.aspx?resourceID=5818. Published on August 19, 2007. Accessed on December 4, 2014.

Patient Safety Network. Never events, 2012 http://psnet.ahrq.gov/primer.aspx?primerID=3. Published October 2012. Accessed on December 4, 2014.

Percarpio KB, Watts BV. A cross-sectional study on the relationship between utilization of root cause analysis and patient safety at 139 Department of Veterans Affairs medical centers. *Jt Comm J Qual Patient Saf* 2013;39:32.

Percarpio KB, Watts BV, Weeks WB. The effectiveness of root cause analysis: what does the literature tell us? *Jt Comm J Qual Patient Saf* 2008;34:391.

Peters PG. What we know about malpractice settlements. *Iowa Law Rev* 2007a;92:1783.

Peters PG. Doctors and juries. *Mich Law Rev* 2007b;105:1453.

Peterson KF. Medical negligence: statute of limitations—tolling events. In: Conlin RB, Cusimano GS, eds. *Litigating tort cases.* Eagan, MN:AAJ Press, 2012:§61:20.

Pichert JW, Hickson GB, Bledsoe S, et al. Understanding the etiology of serious medical events involving children: implications for pediatricians and their risk managers. *Pediatr Ann* 1997;26:160.

Pichert JW, Moore IN, Karrass J, et al. An Intervention Model That Promotes Accountability: Peer Messengers and Patient/Family Complaints. *Jt Comm J Qual Patient Saf* 2013;39:435.

Pichert JW, Hickson GB, Moore IN. Using patient complaints to promote patient safety: the Patient Advocacy Reporting System (PARS). In: Henriksen K, Battles JB, Keyes MA, Grady ML, eds. *Advances in patient safety: new directions and alternative approaches.* Bethesda, MD: Agency for Healthcare Research and Quality (AHRQ), 2008;2:421.

Pichert JW, Hickson GB, Pinto A, et al. Communicating about unexpected outcomes, and adverse events, and errors. In: Carayon P, ed. *Human factors and ergonomics in health care and patient safety,* 2nd ed. Boca Raton: CRC Press, 2012:401.

Pichert JW, Johns JA, Hickson GB. Professionalism in support of pediatric cardio-thoracic surgery: a case of a bright young surgeon. *Prog Pediatr Cardiol* 2011;32:89.

Priest GL, Klein B. The selection of disputes for litigation. *J Legal Stud* 1984;13:1.

Prince JM, Vallabhaneni R, Zenati MS, et al. Increased interactive format for morbidity & mortality conference improves educational value and enhances confidence. *J Surg Educ* 2007;64:266.

Prosser WL. *Handbook of the law of torts.* St. Paul, MN: West Publishing Co., 1971.

Public Citizen Congress Watch. *The great medical malpractice hoax; NPDB data continue to show medical liability system produces rational outcomes. 1991–2005,* 2007:12, http://www.citizen.org/documents/NPDB%20Report_Final.pdf. Accessed on December 14, 2014.

Rand Corporation. *Analysis of medical malpractice.* http://www.rand.org/pubs/technical_reports/TR562z17/analysis-of-medical-malpractice.html. Accessed on December 4, 2014.

Raper SE. No role for apology: remedial work and the problem of medical injury. *Yale J Health Policy Law Ethics* 2011;11:296.

Reason J. Human error: models and management. *Br Med J* 2000;320:768.

Reason JT. *Managing the risks of organizational accidents.* Aldershot, UK: Ashgate Publishing, 1997.

Reiter CE, Hickson GB, Pichert JW. Addressing behavior and performance issues that threaten quality and patient safety: what your attorneys want you to know. *Prog Pediatr Cardiol* 2012;33:37.

Report on Medicare Compliance. *CMS targets readmission through payment, audits; 'coaching' model reduces rate.* 2008;17.

Restatement (Second) of Torts. Philadelphia, PA: American Law Institute, 1979: § 901.

Rex JH, Turnbull JE, Allen SJ, et al. Systematic root cause analysis of adverse drug events in a tertiary referral hospital. *Jt Comm J Qual Improv* 2000;26:563.

Rhodes R, Strain JJ. Whistleblowing in academic medicine. *J Med Ethics* 2004;30:35.

Rice S. Harmed in the hospital? Should you sue?, 2011. http://www.cnn.com/2011/HEALTH/03/24/ep.malpractice.sue.or.not/index.html. Accessed on February 26, 2013.

Rosenstein AH, O'Daniel M. Disruptive behavior and clinical outcomes: perceptions of nurses and physicians. *Am J Nurs* 2005;105:54.

Rosenstein AH, O'Daniel M. Impact and implications of disruptive behavior in the perioperative arena. *J Am Coll Surg* 2006;203:96.

Sage WM. Enterprise liability and the emerging managed health care system. *Law Contemp Probl* 1997;60:159.

Sage WM. The forgotten third: liability insurance and the medical malpractice crisis. *Health Aff (Millwood)* 2004;23:10.

Sage WM, Hastings KE, Berenson RA. Enterprise liability for medical malpractice and health care quality improvement. *Am J Law Med* 1994;20:1.

Sage WM, Zivin JG, Chase NB. Bridging the relational-regulatory gap: a pragmatic information policy for patient safety and medical malpractice. *Vand Law Rev* 2006;59:1263.

Samuel FE. Safe Medical Devices Act of 1990. *Health Aff (Millwood)* 1991;10:192.

Schaffner W, Way WA, Federspiel CF, et al. Improving antibiotic prescribing in office practice. *JAMA* 1983;250:1728.

Schlesinger M, Mitchell S, Elbel B. Voices unheard: barriers to expressing dissatisfaction to health plans. *Milbank Q* 2002;80:709.

Schwappach DLB, Boluarte TA. The emotional impact of medical error involvement on physicians: a call for leadership and organisational accountability. *Swiss Med Wkly* 2008;138.

Shannon SW. How a captive insurer uses data and incentives to advance patient safety. *Pat Saf Qual Healthcare* 2009;18, http://www.rmf.harvard.edu/~/media/Files/_Global/KC/News/Shannon.pdf. Accessed on December 4, 2014.

Shapiro RS, Simpson DE, Lawrence SL, et al. A survey of sued and nonsued physicians and suing patients. *Arch Intern Med* 1989;149:2190.

Shepherd J. Uncovering the silent victims of the American Medical Liability System. *Vanderbilt Law Rev* 2014;67:151.

Shilkret V. Annapolis Emergency Hospital Assn. 276 Md. 187, 349 A.2d 245, 1975.

Skaggs L. Hospital risk management programs in the age of health care reform. *Kansas J Law Publ Policy* 1995;4:89.

Sloan FA, Githens PB, Hickson GB. The dispute resolution process. In: Sloan FA, Githens PB, Clayton EW, Hickson GB, Gentile DA, David PF, eds. *Suing for medical malpractice.* Chicago, IL: University of Chicago Press, 1993a:155.

Sloan FA, Githens PB, Hickson FB, et al. Compensation. In: Sloan FA, Githens PB, Clayton EW, Hickson GB, Gentile DA, David PF, eds. *Suing for medical malpractice.* Chicago, IL: University of Chicago Press, 1993b:188.

Sloan FA, Mergenhagen PM, Bovbjerg RR. Effects of tort reform on the value of closed medical malpractice claims: a microanalysis. *J Health Polit Policy Law* 1989;14:663.

Sloan FA, Mergenhagen PM, Burfield WB, et al. Medical malpractice experience of physicians. Predictable or haphazard? *JAMA* 1989;262:3291.

Stein A. Toward a theory of medical malpractice. *Iowa Law Rev* 2012;97:1201.

Stelfox HT, Gandhi TK, Orav EJ, et al. The relation of patient satisfaction with complaints against physicians and malpractice lawsuits. *Am J Med* 2005;118:1126.

Stimson CJ, Pichert JW, Moore IN, et al. Medical malpractice claims risk in urology: an empirical analysis of patient complaint data. *J Urol* 2010;183:1971.

Struve CT. Expertise in medical malpractice litigation: special courts, screening panels, and other options. *Pew Project Med Liabil* 2003:1.

Studdert DM, Mello MM, Brennan TA. Medical malpractice. *N Engl J Med* 2004a;350:283.

Studdert DM, Mello MM, Gawande AA, et al. Disclosure of medical injury to patients: an improbable risk management strategy. *Health Aff (Millwood)* 2007;26:215.

Studdert DM, Mello MM, Gawande AA, et al. Claims, errors, and compensation payments in medical malpractice litigation. *N Engl J Med* 2006;354:2024.

Studdert DM, Mello MM, Sage WM, et al. Defensive medicine among high-risk specialist physicians in a volatile malpractice environment. *JAMA* 2005;293:2609.

Studdert DM, Yang YT, Mello MM. Are damages caps regressive? A study of malpractice jury verdicts in California *Health Aff (Millwood)* 2004b;23:54.

Szekendi MK, et al. Using patient safety morbidity and mortality conferences to promote transparency and a culture of safety. *Jt Comm J Qual Patient Saf* 2010;36:3.

The Joint Commission. Ongoing Professional Practice Evaluation (OPPE), 2014. http://www.jointcommission.org/mobile/standards_information/jcfaqdetails.aspx?StandardsFAQId=470&StandardsFAQChapterId=74. Revised on March 6, 2013. Accessed on December 4, 2014.

The Joint Commission. Sentinel event, 2014. http://www.jointcommission.org/sentinel_event.aspx. Accessed on November 30, 2014.

The Joint Commission. Sentinel Event Alert #40 (July 2008), Behaviors that undermine a culture of safety, 2008. http://www.jointcommission.org/assets/1/18/SEA_40.PDF. Accessed on November 30, 2014.

Thomas EJ, Studdert DM, Burstin HR, et al. Incidence and types of adverse events and negligent care in Utah and Colorado. *Med Care* 2000;38:261.

U.S. Department of Veterans Affairs National Center for Patient Safety: Root Cause Analysis. http://www.patientsafety.va.gov/professionals/onthejob/rca.asp. Accessed on December 4, 2014.

Vidmar N. Medical malpractice lawsuits: an essay on patient interests, the contingency fee system, juries, and social policy. *Loy L A Law Rev* 2005;38:1217.

Vidmar N, Gross F, Rose M. Jury awards for medical malpractice and post-verdict adjustments of those awards. *DePaul Law Rev* 1998;48:265.

Vincent C, Neale G, Woloshynowych M. Adverse events in British hospitals: preliminary retrospective record review. *Br Med J* 2001;322:517.

Vincent C, Phillips A, Young M. Why do people sue doctors? A study of patients and relatives taking legal action. *Lancet* 1994;343:1609.

Viscusi WK, Born PH. Damages caps, insurability, and the performance of medical malpractice insurance. *J Risk Insur* 2005;72:23.

Wachter RM. The end of the beginning: patient safety five years after "To Err Is Human." *Health Aff (Millwood)* 2004;23:534.

Wachter RM, Shojania KG. *Internal bleeding: the truth behind America's terrifying epidemic of medical mistakes.* New York: Rugged Land, LLC, 2004.

Walsh KE, Landrigan CP, Adams WG, et al. Effect of computer order entry on prevention of serious medication errors in hospitalized children. *Pediatrics* 2008;121:e421.

Waterman AD, Garbutt J, Hazel E, et al. The emotional impact of medical errors on practicing physicians in the United States and Canada. *Jt Comm J Qual Patient Saf* 2007;3:467.

Waters RM, Budetti PP, Claxton G, et al. Impact of state tort reforms on physician malpractice payments. *Health Aff (Millwood)* 2007;26:500.

Weingart SN, Saadeh MG, Simchowitz B, et al. Process of care failures in breast cancer diagnosis. *J Gen Intern Med* 2009;24:702.

Weycker DA, Jensen GA. Medical malpractice among physicians: who will be sued and who will pay? *Health Care Manag Sci* 2000;269.

Whetten-Goldstein K, Kulas E, Sloan F, et al. Compensation for birth-related injury. *Arch Pediatr Adolesc Med* 1999;153:41.

White AA, Pichert JW, Bledsoe SH, et al. Cause-and-effect analysis of closed claims in obstetrics and gynecology. *Obstet Gynecol* 2005;105:1031.

White AA, Wright S, Blanco R, et al. Cause-and-effect analysis of risk management files to assess patient care in the emergency department. *Acad Emerg Med* 2004;11:1035.

Williams AG. The cure for what ails: a realistic remedy for the medical malpractice "crisis". *Stanford Law Policy Rev* 2012;23:101.

Williams PM. Techniques for root cause analysis. *BUMC Proc* 2001;14:154.

Wright RW. Allocating liability among multiple responsible causes: a principled defense of joint and several liability for actual harm and risk exposure. *Univ Calif Davis Law Rev* 1988;21:1141.

Wu AW. Medical error: the second victim: the doctor who makes the mistake needs help too. *Br Med J* 2000;320:726.

Wu AW, Lipshutz AK, Pronovost PJ. Effectiveness and efficiency of root cause analysis in medicine. *JAMA* 2008;299:685.

Wynn WP. In re medical review panel for the claim of Maria Moses: the Supreme Court parts a red sea of questions—the doctrine of continued tort applied to medical malpractice claims. *Loy Law Rev* 2001;47:1605.

Yee F. Mandatory mediation: the extra dose needed to cure the medical malpractice crisis. *Cardozo J Confl Resol* 2006;7:393.

Zablotsky P. From a whimper to a bang: the trend toward finding occurrence based statutes of limitations governing misdiagnosis of diseases with long latency periods. *Dick Law Rev* 1999;103:455.

CHAPTER 5
The Changing Environment in Which We Practice Gynecologic Surgery

Eric J. Bieber

DEFINITIONS

Accountable Care Organization (ACO)—An organization of health care providers (hospitals, providers, and others) that agrees to be accountable for the quality, cost, and overall care of the beneficiaries.

Hospitalist/laborist—Physician/providers who dedicate all or part of their practices to providing care specifically to patients within the hospital.

Institute for Healthcare Improvement (IHI)—A not-for-profit organization founded in 1991 and dedicated to improving health care throughout the globe. Initiated the 100,000 lives campaign (www.ihi.com).

Institute of Medicine (IOM)—Not-for-profit organization chartered in 1970 as part of the National Academy of Sciences to provide unbiased, evidence-based guidance to improve health in the United States (www.iom.com).

Patient Protection and Affordable Care Act (PPACA)—A federal statute approved in 2010 by President Obama and upheld by the Supreme Court in June 2012. The act aims to increase the health insurance coverage for Americans via mandates, subsidies, and tax credits.

Pay for performance (P4P)—A broad construct that attempts to pay providers or health care organizations for achieving predetermined quality thresholds.

Value-based purchasing—Authorized by PPACA, this is a payment method for rewarding quality of care through financial incentives.

As gynecologic surgeons and care providers of women, we have witnessed major changes in our practices over the years. When we think back to our days as medical students and residents, even the youngest of us is able to appreciate the palpable differences that exist today: from how we manage our offices to how we approach diagnostic testing and treatment. Most recently, the passage of the PPACA, the advent of Accountable Care Organizations, and the focus on value and value-based purchasing have begun to rapidly change our external environment.

The cornerstone of the modern practice of medicine continues to be the resounding theme of evidence-based medicine. Quality initiatives from the IHI recommendations, National Committee for Quality Assurance (NCQA), and more recently the efforts of many organizations with the Partnership for Patients as well as many other initiatives have made attempts to promote the safest, most effective care of our patients. Pay for performance and adherence to quality metrics and benchmarks are becoming commonplace. Hospitals have their patient satisfaction scores transparently available for patients to evaluate, and we expect doctor scores to similarly be available in the coming years. We are also being challenged to move from a time when surgical and other treatments were the mainstay of our practice to a new time of screening, prevention, wellness, and the ultimate promise of genomics.

Few of us appreciated how profound a role the computer would play in our daily practice or how this tool might empower us to provide the best possible care in each encounter. The electronic health record (EHR), its implementation and daily use, and its significant benefits and pitfalls will be reviewed in part. We also review the changes that are occurring in medical education from residency to postgraduate training.

We discuss one of the latest trends: a move for at least some physicians, including obstetrician–gynecologists, to choose to function as hospital-based providers or hospitalists. Finally, we review the importance of evaluating evidence-based methodologies for rating our literature.

HEALTH CARE REFORM

The PPACA has profoundly changed the landscape of medicine in the United States. Signed into law in 2010 and upheld by the Supreme Court in 2012, this large body of legislation will continue to impact all care providers for decades to come. Undoubtedly, there will be alteration to the original, but the main tenets of the law are likely to be enacted over the next few years.

Accountable Care Organizations or ACOs had been proposed and piloted in the late 2000s. They are called out specifically within the PPACA, and by law, pilots had to be started. The Centers for Medicare & Medicaid Services (CMS) is the responsible party for overseeing the Medicare Shared Savings Program (MSSP). The Center for Medicare & Medicaid Innovation (CMMI) launched the initial Pioneer ACO program composed of 32 initial ACOs. Since this time, there has been a proliferation of both Medicare ACOs and more recently of commercial ACOs. The main tenet of an ACO is patient-centered care with a view to optimizing care over the continuum including wellness and preventative care. Don Berwick's triple aims of improving the health of the population, enhancing patient experience, and decreasing cost or improving efficiency are core to ACOs mission. In addition, the MSSP calls out 33 key quality metrics that must be met to share in savings. These metrics are in the four core areas of patient/caregiver experience, care coordination/patient safety, preventative health, and care of at-risk populations. A different variation on patient-centric care is the advent of the patient-centered medical home (PCMH). NCQA has defined the PCMH as a "health care setting that facilitates partnerships between individual patients, and their personal physicians, and when appropriate, the patient's family. Care is facilitated by registries, information technology, health information exchange (HIE), and other means to assure that patients get the indicated care when and where they need and want it in a culturally and linguistically appropriate manner."

Additional changes brought about through PPACA include the introduction of "value-based purchasing" where providers are either rewarded or penalized for their efforts relative to quality and efficiency. Discussed in more detail later, this is a true pay-for-performance program. Bundled payment demonstrations are also called out in the legislation and aim to better align providers, hospitals, and others to work together to optimize care over the continuum by providing a single payment for an entire episode of care. The issue of readmissions has also been brought to the forefront with penalties now beginning for many hospitals. Also, key to the PPACA is the expansion

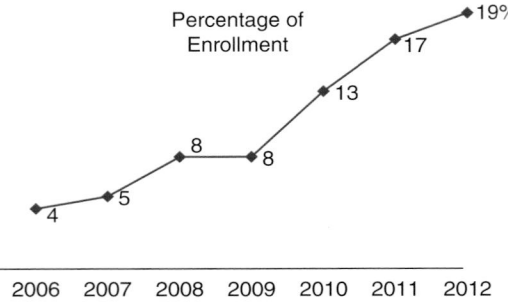

Studies: High Deductible Plans can Reduce Utilization up to 25%

FIGURE 5.1 Increasing enrollment in high-deductible health plans. Data from Towers Watson. *2012 health care changes ahead survey report.* http://www.towerswatson.com/DownloadMedia. aspx?media={24F68B2F-90F6-48C9-ADF3-CA61A378300A}. Published on October 2012.

of Medicaid by many states and the formation of health care exchanges with the goal of providing health care coverage to the majority of the citizens of the United States. The details of many of these issues remain to be worked out as of the time of this writing and are outside the scope of this chapter. Indeed, many states have chosen to opt out of Medicaid expansion in 2015, and health exchanges have largely only been attempted in Utah and Massachusetts. The true impact on health care at an individual level as well as a population level remains to be seen. Other issues such as the physician and nursing workforce required to care for the additional millions of individuals who will now have health care coverage continue to be hotly debated topics.

Another evolving area is the increase in high-deductible or consumer-driven health plans (**Fig. 5.1** and **Table 5.1**). Because of the ever-increasing cost of health care premiums, many

TABLE 5.1 High-Deductible Health Plan: National Enrollment

2012 DATA BY STATE	TOTAL ENROLLMENT IN HIGH-DEDUCTIBLE HEALTH PLANS
California	1,002,000
Texas	755,000
Illinois	717,000
Ohio	**663,000**
Florida	540,000
New York	495,000
Minnesota	487,000
Pennsylvania	406,000

Source: Buck K. *Health savings accounts and account-based health plans: research highlights.* America's Health Insurance Plans (AHIP) Center for Policy and Research. http://www.ahip.org/HSAHighlightsReport072012/. Published on July 2012.

companies and employees have chosen to accept the potential of greater out-of-pocket expense for the concomitant reduction in health insurance premiums. The outcome of patients having to pay these "first dollar amounts" to providers is more and more patients asking about the cost of visits, surgeries, and radiologic studies. Given the complexities of charges and billings, this may be challenging for many organizations. This advent of consumerism in health care is consistent with the government's desire to increase transparency of both quality and pricing in an effort to increase the value for patients. With the significant increase in the number of these plans across the country, the issues of cost, access, and transparency of information are likely to become of even greater interest for patients.

QUALITY INITIATIVES

In 2010, Daniel Levinson of the Office of the Inspector General of the Department of Health and Human Services released a report on safety issues for Medicare beneficiaries. After evaluation of numerous patient records, including review by multiple physicians, the report concluded that 13.5% of hospitalized Medicare patients experience at least one adverse event during a hospitalization. An additional 13.5% of all patients experienced an event that led to temporary harm. In the subsequent review by physicians, they noted that 44% of these events were preventable. The total yearly cost estimate appeared to be close to $4.4 billion.

Few clinicians would argue that quality is the most important parameter in health care today. Yet, it is becoming ever more evident that many patients do not receive state-of-the-art health care. In a landmark article published in 2006, Asch et al. from the Rand Health group evaluated 30 chronic and acute conditions and used 439 indicators of quality to access if patients had received appropriate care. Unfortunately, overall, only 54.9% of patients received what would be considered recommended care. Some sociodemographic differences existed: Women received 56.6% of care versus men at 52.3%, and those with annual household income greater than $50,000 received 56.6% versus those less than $15,000 at 53.1%. However, what is striking is the low level of achieving recommended care for all the groups studied regardless of the sociodemographic differences.

In 1999, the IOM released a report suggesting that 98,000 patients per year die secondary to inadequate care being rendered. Many subsequent debates ensued regarding the methodologies used to attain these numbers. However, this report created a call to arms, challenging those individuals and organizations who provide care to improve the quality of care delivered to all patients. Furthermore, it has caused a number of initiatives from a broad base of organizations. In December 2004, the IHI, at its 16th Annual National Forum on Quality Improvement in Health Care, announced a goal to save 100,000 lives by June 2006. The campaign invited all US hospitals to join in implementing six broad initiatives that have demonstrated efficacy in well-performed clinical trials. These include

1. Prevention of surgical site infections
2. Prevention of ventilator-associated pneumonia
3. Prevention of central line infections
4. Prevention of adverse drug events (ADEs) through medication reconciliation
5. Deployment of rapid response teams
6. Delivery of evidence-based care for acute myocardial infarction

What is particularly impressive about the IHI campaign is the extent of support across a broad range of disparate federal, state, political, and private organizations, including—but not limited to—the CMS, Veterans Health Administration, American Medical Association, American Nurses Association, Centers for Disease Control and Prevention, Joint Commission on Accreditation of Healthcare Organizations, the Leapfrog Group, and multiple others.

Ultimately, the IHI released information suggesting that these initiatives were able to save 122,300 patients. This was good news and suggested that progress was indeed being made. Unfortunately, a more recent publication reviewed hospital admissions from 2002 to 2007 in North Carolina hospitals. The authors found a rate of 25.1 harms per 100 admissions with no statistical change over the 5 years of the study. The challenge to implement the IHI recommendations as well as multiple other quality initiatives has caused a number of hospitals and large organizations to create chief quality officer positions that are largely responsible for implementing and monitoring compliance to these programs. In essence, this may be the confluence of patient safety, performance improvement, utilization review, and other previous orphan committees.

Consistent with the IHI initiatives, other initiatives have come from CMS, including recommendations for optimization of diabetic patients. These include bundles of care much like the IHI central line bundle, in which appropriate care consists of all elements being appropriately performed or delivered within the correct time frame. Unfortunately, as the bundles become more complicated, it becomes more and more difficult for the provider to remember what has or has not been done. This may be yet another opportunity for the EHR to allow both the clinician and the patient to know what tests or interventions need to be performed, thus optimizing the encounter. The Joint Commission has also continued to evolve its recommendations, including core measure sets for venous thromboembolism, the surgical care improvement project, and most recently a core measure set for perinatal care. In addition, there continue to be updates and new releases of National Patient Safety Goals (Table 5.2). We expect that with increasing evidence-based knowledge, many additional quality-driven initiatives will come forward.

Another key safety initiative is the Partnership for Patients, a public–private partnership that aims to improve quality, safety, and affordability. An amazing 3,700 hospitals have signed on to portions of this program whose two primary goals are the reduction of hospital-acquired infections by 40% by the end of 2013 (as compared to 2010) and reducing complications using care transitions to effect a 20% reduction in hospital readmissions. Twenty-six hospital engagement networks were awarded $218 million to lead these efforts. The patient safety areas of focus include (but are not limited to) the following (many of which an obstetrician–gynecologist may encounter):

1. Adverse drug events
2. Catheter-associated urinary tract infections
3. Central line–associated bloodstream infections
4. Injuries from falls and immobility
5. Obstetrical adverse events
6. Pressure ulcers
7. Surgical site infections
8. Venous thromboembolism
9. Ventilator-associated pneumonia
10. Readmissions

TABLE 5.2 2013 Hospital National Patient Safety Goals

Identify patients correctly	
NPSG.01.01.01	Use at least two ways to identify patients. For example, use the patient's name and date of birth. This is done to make sure that each patient gets the correct medicine and treatment.
NPSG.01.03.01	Make sure that the correct patient gets the correct blood when they get a blood transfusion.
Improve staff communication	
NPSG.02.03.01	Get important test results to the right staff person on time.
Use medicines safely	
NPSG.03.04.01	Before a procedure, label medicines that are not labeled, for example, medicines in syringes, cups, and basins. Do this in the area where medicines and supplies are set up.
NPSG.03.05.01	Take extra care with patients who take medicines to thin their blood.
NPSG.03.06.01	Record and pass along correct information about a patient's medicines. Find out what medicines the patient is taking. Compare those medicines to new medicines given to the patient. Make sure the patient knows which medicines to take when they are at home. Tell the patient it is important to bring their up-to-date list of medicines every time they visit a doctor.
Prevent infection	
NPSG.07.01.01	Use the hand cleaning guidelines from the Centers for Disease Control and Prevention or the World Health Organization. Set goals for improving hand cleaning. Use the goals to improve hand cleaning.
NPSG.07.03.01	Use proven guidelines to prevent infections that are difficult to treat.
NPSG.07.04.01	Use proven guidelines to prevent infection of the blood from central lines.
NPSG.07.05.01	Use proven guidelines to prevent infection after surgery.
NPSG.07.06.01	Use proven guidelines to prevent infections of the urinary tract that are caused by catheters.
Identify patient safety risks	
NPSG.15.01.01	Find out which patients are most likely to try to commit suicide.
Prevent mistakes in surgery	
UP.01.01.01	Make sure that the correct surgery is done on the correct patient and at the correct place on the patient's body.
UP.01.02.01	Mark the correct place on the patient's body where the surgery is to be done.
UP.01.03.01	Pause before the surgery to make sure that a mistake is not being made.

The purpose of the National Patient Safety Goals is to improve patient safety. The goals focus on problems in health care safety and how to solve them.
This is an easy-to-read document. It has been created for the public. The exact language of the goals can be found at www.jointcommission.org. Copyright © The Joint Commission, 2013. Reprinted with permission.

Because of the breadth of the Partnership for Patients effort and the collaborative nature of the learning, there is real hope that sustainable change may be able to be accomplished.

It was previously believed that organizations with higher caseloads of a particular disease might be better positioned to deliver recommended care. Lindenauer et al. studied this tenet as it relates to pneumonia in the acute care setting. Surprisingly, they found both hospitals and physicians who had a higher caseload of pneumonia patients actually had reduced adherence to recommended guidelines—such as influenza and pneumococcal vaccine administration or early antibiotic administration—and had no better outcomes.

Quality initiatives are currently being led by a number of organizations, including some physician groups. For example, in Washington State, a physician-led group has brought all hospitals to the table to evaluate discrete performance measures regarding cardiac revascularization. Similarly, the California Perinatal Quality Care Collaborative in 1998 targeted improving antenatal steroid use as an initiative. They accumulated baseline data, developed educational materials, and broadly disseminated this information. They concluded that regional collaboration allowed an improvement from a baseline rate of administration of 76% to 86% post implementation. Callcut and Breslin discuss how private groups, such as the Leapfrog Group, are playing an important role in moving the private regulatory movement forward and suggest that surgeons need to become more active participants in this process of reshaping and redefining our future.

How to best implement quality improvement programs in a given setting is also continuing to be investigated. A recent evaluation of hospital quality improvement implementation and subsequent impact on discrete patient-safety metrics suggested that involvement by multiple units within a hospital might have a negative impact on results. Alternatively, having a higher percentage of physicians involved was associated with better scores on at least two of the four safety indicators. Interestingly, having a higher percentage of hospital staff or senior management involved had no impact on any of the indicators.

TABLE 5.3 Key Steps for Initiating, Improving, Evaluating, and Sustaining a Quality Improvement Program

Initiating or improving a quality improvement program

1. Do background work: Identify motivation, support teamwork, and develop strong leadership.
2. Prioritize potential projects and choose the projects to begin.
3. Prepare for the project by operationalizing the measures, building support for the project, and developing a business plan.
4. Do an environmental scan to understand the current situation (structure, process, or outcome), the potential barriers, opportunities, and resources for the project.
5. Create a data collection system to provide accurate baseline data and document improvement.
6. Create a data reporting system that will allow clinicians and other stakeholders to see and understand the problem and the improvement.
7. Introduce strategies to change clinician behavior and create the change that will produce improvement.

Evaluating and sustaining a quality improvement program

1. Determine whether the target is changing with ongoing observation, periodic data collection, and interpretation.
2. Modify behavior change strategies to improve, regain, or sustain improvements.
3. Focus on sustaining interdisciplinary leadership and collaboration for the quality improvement program.
4. Develop and sustain support from the hospital leadership.

From Curtis JR, Cook DJ, Wall RJ, et al. Intensive care unit quality improvement: a "how-to" guide for the interdisciplinary team. *Crit Care Med* 2006;34:211, with permission. Copyright © 2006 by the Society of Critical Care Medicine and Lippincott Williams.

TABLE 5.4 Amount Available Each Year Controlled by Statute

2013	1.00% of base-operating DRG payments
2014	1.25%
2015	1.50%
2016	1.75%
2017	2.00%

Most clinicians have not been trained in how to develop and implement quality improvement programs. Curtis et al. have published a how-to paper that came out of an outcomes task force of the Society of Critical Care Medicine but has wide applicability to many areas of medicine (Table 5.3). The generalized lack of education and training in quality may explain some of the lethargy that Leape and Berwick allude to in their article "Five Years after *To Err Is Human:* What Have We Learned?." They suggest that extraordinary quality improvements have been achieved by implementing discrete strategies in specific environments. If each of our organizations could fractionally achieve similar success, the impact on patient care might be quite remarkable.

PAY FOR PERFORMANCE

In many settings, multiple quality measures are being subjected to pay for performance, with groups achieving higher levels of patient compliance being awarded higher levels of reimbursement. This is a marked change from being paid for delivery of units of health care or procedures in which disease states are being managed. As of 2013, 100s of pay-for-performance initiatives have been started by a wide variety of sponsors, ranging from employers to the federal government. The most important current pay-for-performance effort is the value-based purchasing program sponsored by CMS. In this program, up to 2.0% of a hospital's base-operating diagnosis related group (DRG) payments will be at risk (Table 5.4). CMS calculates the incentive adjustment based on a total performance score achieved by the hospital. The program is structured to allow a continual evolution with measures and weighting changing each year. Because almost $1 billion dollars is at risk, many organizations have highly focused efforts around the measures. As can be seen, CMS is moving from a time when surrogate measures, such as core measures, were the key drivers to outcomes and efficiency metrics (Fig. 5.2 and Table 5.5). The PPACA also required a Hospital-Acquired Condition (HAC) Reduction Program with another potential 1% payment reduction if performance thresholds are not met. Currently, there are eight measures in two domains, but these will likely increase over time (Table 5.6). In addition, many of these measures have applicability for obstetrician–gynecologists. The final major pay-for-performance program is aimed at reducing readmissions. In this program, payments are again reduced (1% in 2013, 2% in 2013, and 3% in 2015 and beyond) if readmission rates exceed the expected level. While the initial disease states being evaluated are acute myocardial infarction, pneumonia, and heart failure, all Medicare discharges are penalized. Reviewing Figure 5.3 demonstrates the significant potential for hospital revenue reductions as all of these programs are phased in.

In an early article on the subject of paying for high-quality care, Epstein et al. called for several significant changes to facilitate adoption of pay-for-performance initiatives. These recommendations included an expansion in the scope of the efforts, as well as the amount of incentive available to the clinician or group; the importance of large groups such as CMS becoming involved; an expansion from the current small cadre of clinical indicators; an improvement in our ability to establish reliable metrics for evaluation of quality; and, finally, a call for investment in electronic infrastructure to facilitate all of the above.

A Cochrane systematic review of the subject of targeted payments to affect outcomes in primary care was unable to reach a conclusion because of limitations in prior study quality and power. Kouides et al. evaluated the use of financial incentives to increase rates of influenza vaccine administration and found that modest incentive increased an already high baseline administration rate. In another study on immunizations, Fairbrother et al. evaluated use of cash bonus, enhanced fee for service, and feedback for improving baseline vaccination rates. They found only the bonus group statistically improved (increased by 25.3%), although they believed much of this effect was due to better documentation versus actual increased administration of vaccine. Roski et al. noted that in incentivized groups, documentation of tobacco use was markedly increased, as was accession to counseling programs.

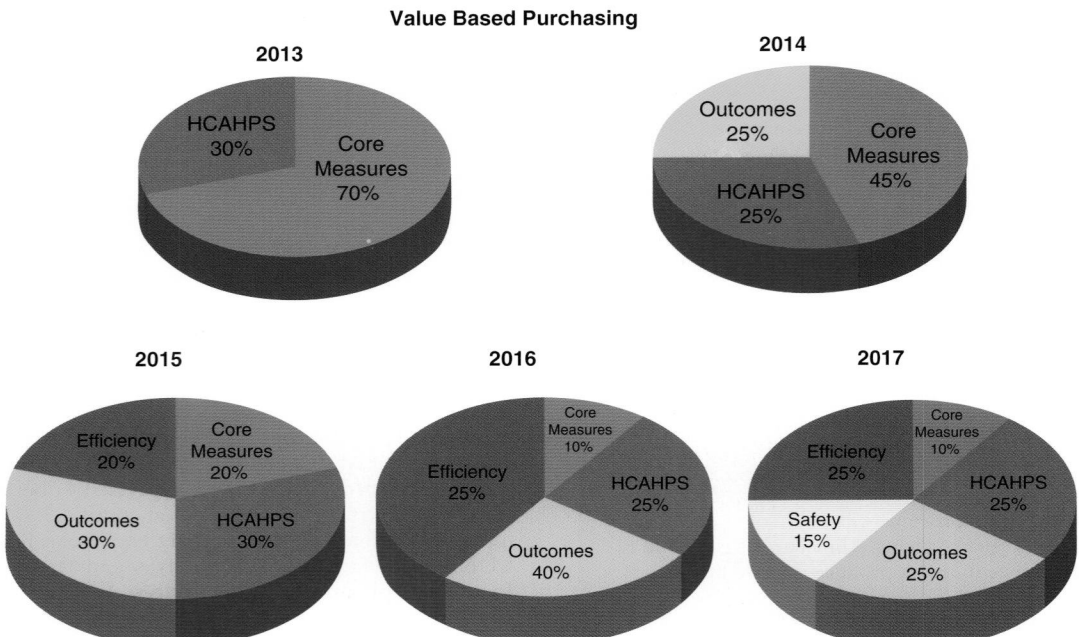

FIGURE 5.2 Evolution of value based purchasing from 2013 to 2017.

Unfortunately, other important clinical end points showed no difference.

A more recent investigation evaluated a pay-for-performance initiative by PacifiCare Health Systems. Three quality measures were evaluated: cervical cancer screening, mammography, and HgbA1c. Unfortunately, only in the cervical cancer screening group was there an improvement after the intervention, and in spite of $3.4 million paid in pay-for-performance incentives, only nominal gains were made. Also, physicians with the highest initial baseline performance had the least improvement but were the recipients of the greatest portion of the paid bonus. This trial demonstrates the potential limitation of identifying discrete end points to reward heterogeneous groups of providers, all of whom start from different baseline levels of efficacy. Dudley has suggested that how an incentive is offered (i.e., reward or penalty) and factors such as what percentage of patients in a provider's panel incentives are applicable to may affect the success of these programs. Rosenthal et al., in evaluating multiple trials and multiple industries in which pay for performance has applicability, found little evidence that paying for quality is effective. They noted that even in other industries, results are inconsistent. They raise the concern that incentives may be too low, with limited penetrance within a given provider's or group's practice panel. An additional concern is making the target for incentive so much higher than baseline that the providers feel it is unachievable and therefore do not try. This is consistent with data from Beckman et al., who interviewed providers in a pay-for-performance program. Interestingly, providers reviewed their personal profiles but did not always change their functional behaviors in response to the data.

Bundled payments are a variation on pay for performance where all the providers are paid for the entire care episode and certain outcomes are achieved. In January 2013, CMS announced that a number of organizations had been selected to become part of the Bundled Payments for Care Improvement Initiative. In the program, organizations and providers enter into payment programs that generally include financial and quality performance metrics. For the CMS program, participants could pick from a menu of 48 different episodes of care to bundle. The hope is that by aligning all providers across the continuum that coordination of care and thus quality and cost will be improved. These types of programs may have had the greatest initial application in the area of cardiovascular surgery, for which outcome metrics of individual surgeons and hospitals have been reported for several years. In addition, there are well-defined clinical algorithms regarding "best practice." This may have driven the American Heart Association's Reimbursement, Coverage, and Access Policy Development Workgroup to publish a statement on pay for performance. More recently,

TABLE 5.5 Outcome Measures			
MEASURE DESCRIPTION	**2014**	**2015**	**2016 (PROPOSED)**
Acute myocardial infarction mortality rate	X	X	X
Heart failure mortality rate	X	X	X
Composite patient safety indicators		X	X
Central line–associated bloodstream infection (CLABSI)		X	X
Catheter-associated urinary tract infection			X
Surgical site infections			X

TABLE 5.6 Proposed Measures for the HAC Reduction Program			
MEASURE DESCRIPTION	**FY 2015**	**FY 2016**	**FY 2017**
Domain 1: AHRQ patient safety indicators			
Pressure ulcer rate	X	X	X
Foreign object left in the body	X	X	X
Iatrogenic pneumothorax rate	X	X	X
Postoperative physiologic and metabolic derangement rate	X	X	X
Postoperative pulmonary embolus (PE)/deep vein thrombosis (DVT) rate	X	X	X
Surgery patients with recommended venous thromboembolism prophylaxis ordered	X	X	X
Accidental puncture and laceration rate	X	X	X
Domain 2: CDC Hospital acquired infection (HAI) measures			
Central line–associated bloodstream infection (CLABSI)	X	X	X
Catheter-associated urinary tract infection	X	X	X
Surgical site infection (SSI): SSI following colon surgery SSI following abdominal hysterectomy		X	X
Methicillin-resistant Staphylococcus aureus (MRSA)			X
Clostridium difficile			X

the American Hospital Association has evaluated bundled payments and asked the following eight questions:

1. To which conditions should bundled payments be applied?
2. What providers and services should be included in the bundled payment?
3. How can provider accountability be determined?
4. What should be the time frame of a bundled payment?
5. What capabilities are needed for organizations to administer a bundled payment?
6. How should payments be set?
7. How should the bundled payment be risk adjusted?
8. What data are needed to support bundled payment?

It is believed that the results from the demo project will provide clarity around many of these issues, although one

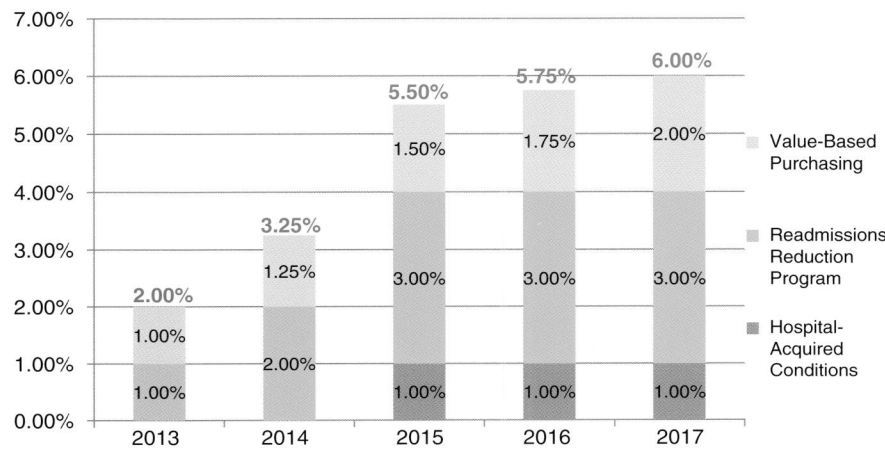

FIGURE 5.3 Total hospital revenue at risk from major Medicare quality programs.

could argue that obstetrician–gynecologists have been doing bundled payments for obstetric care for many years.

In addition to the previously noted problems with pay-for-performance programs, another limitation is that most programs to date have focused on single disease states or outcomes (such as immunization or Pap test or mammogram compliance). In reality, many patients aged 65 or older have multiple medical problems and treating single disease states in isolation may not lead to overall improved outcomes and enhanced quality. It is not surprising that 89% of Medicare's annual budget is consumed by patients with three or more chronic conditions. Boyd et al. evaluated current clinical practice guidelines (CPGs), which are often used in pay-for-performance programs, but which also focus on single disease states. In a hypothetical 79-year-old female patient with the common comorbidities of chronic obstructive pulmonary disease, diabetes, osteoporosis, hypertension, and osteoarthritis, they found that following each CPG would lead to 12 prescribed medications and a potential outlay of $406 per month. There were also significant issues with the potential for drug–drug interactions if this "optimal" regimen was followed. They concluded that pay for performance based on CPGs for single disease states may create "perverse incentives" and actually decrease quality of care and that significant effort should be placed on effectively treating the multiple chronic conditions that many of our patients have.

While these initiatives are only still beginning, there will likely be future pressures both at the state and federal level to achieve an ever-higher level of quality. In addition, pay for performance needs to evolve to incorporate these early findings into rationale paradigms for physicians, which align the needs of our patients, payers, and providers. It may also become quite difficult for groups and practices that do not have access to electronic data to be able to participate in such projects.

ELECTRONIC HEALTH RECORD

The advent of the EHR has changed forever how medicine will be practiced. Many of us were trained in a time where orders and notes were handwritten and charts were sent to a large repository (i.e., medical records). Many notes written by our colleagues were difficult to read or were unable to be located. Certainly, these were not often available in real time, across specialties or from home. Authentication of results was performed by hand and had to be reassociated with the correct chart, wasting significant time and resources that might be better directed. Prescriptions were written and handed to

patients who then delivered them to a pharmacy. In a best-case scenario, writing was legible, charts were placed in their appropriate position within the repository, and the pharmacist could read the prescription. Unfortunately, often this was not the case.

In many areas of the United States, much of this has changed. Numerous opportunities exist with the EHR to overcome many of the technical issues associated with handwriting, but the opportunities go well beyond legibility. In addition, groups like the American Medical Informatics Association's College of Medical Informatics has called for integration of the EHR and personal health records (PHR) to provide the greatest value for our patients. Much of the current focus on EMR implementation is being driven by the billions of dollars available to providers who can attest to "meaningful use." The American Recovery and Reinvestment Act (ARRA), which was enacted in 2009, includes the Health Information Technology for Economic and Clinical Health (HITECH) Act, wherein meaningful use in three separate stages is called out (Fig. 5.4). Incentive payments range from $44,000 over 5 years or $63,750 over 6 years to providers attesting to Medicare or Medicaid, respectively (Fig. 5.5). Importantly, if providers fail to attest by the designated time, not only do they lose the meaningful use dollars, there will also be a negative adjustment to their Medicare/Medicaid fees.

Multiple studies have suggested the potential positive consequences of an EHR implementation. The Kaiser group reported that with an implementation of an EHR in the northwest United States, age-adjusted outpatient visits dropped by 9%, with only a slight increase in phone calls from patients but no change or a slight improvement in quality metrics. Embi et al. found that by using EHR data to define patient eligibility into a clinical trial and then causing an electronic prompt to let the provider know of patient eligibility, they were able to double study enrollment as well as improve physician referrals to their study. In an obstetric EMR study, Klatt and Hopp demonstrated that through the use of best practice alerts in the EMR, they were able to significantly improve influenza documentation rates in pregnant women. The alert fired at each prenatal visit if the patient was either unvaccinated or didn't have documentation regarding refusal. Such alerts can be configured for a number of different clinical issues. However, a key to success is not creating "alert" fatigue and limiting the number of hard stops requiring active clinician input. The EMR is also only as good the data within it. We are aware that patients with gestational diabetes (GDM) are at increased risk for type 2 diabetes. Stuebe evaluated documentation of GDM in the EMR of a large health system. They found that only

- CMS established 3 stages of meaningful use
- Stage 1 and 2 requirements final
- Stage 3 to follow

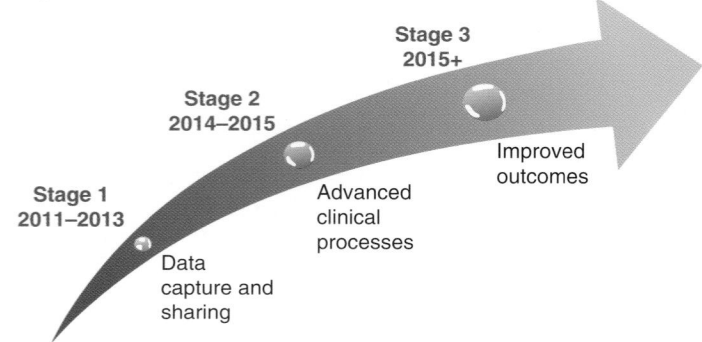

FIGURE 5.4 Meaningful use roadmap.

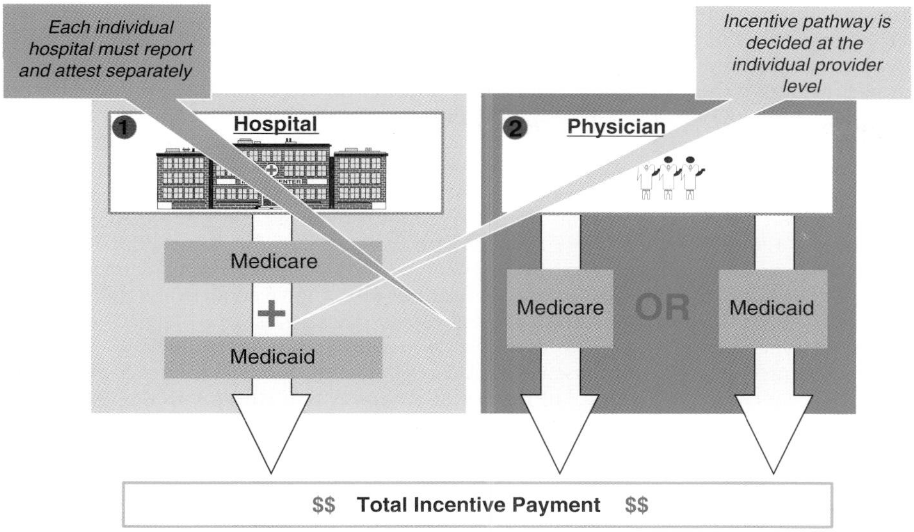

FIGURE 5.5 Meaningful use incentive roadmap.

45.8% of patients had the GDM history documented in the electronic problem list. This lack of documentation could lead to poor communication to the patient's primary care physician and the potential risk that the patient will not be screened when not pregnant.

There are multiple factors that have made the adoption of the EHR difficult for some providers and groups. Likely highest among these is the cost to implement as well as maintain the EHR. Multiple third-party vendors exist that have various EHR platforms. These range from simple documentation and chart programs to software and hardware that integrate patient care across both inpatient and ambulatory platforms and the PHR. There are currently efforts to standardize EHR language, but many of these efforts are in their infancy. It will become critical as we evolve to an all digital-based health record that these systems are able to communicate with one another, allowing patients to have their records available anywhere and anytime. Ford et al. evaluated EHR adoption rates in small physician groups of 10 or fewer partners. Using models, they projected the potential for broad adoption of EHR into the future. They suggest that it may take until 2024 for small groups to fully implement EHRs, which is much longer than is currently being called for by agencies interested in quality initiatives and cost containment. Unfortunately, the health digital information superhighway continues to have a long way to go to be completed.

Baron et al. detail their personal experience as a small group of internists (four members) with implementing an EHR. They described alterations in work flow and the initial deterioration in their office environment for staff, patients, and physicians alike. However, they also state that in spite of the various limitations, "...none of us would go back to paper health records." They identified five key issues that are likely relevant for both small and large groups involved with implementing an EHR:

1. Financing of the EHR
2. Interoperability, standardization, and connectivity
3. Work-flow redesign issues
4. Technical support
5. Issues of change management

More recently, there have been questions regarding whether the EHR is really the panacea for moving medicine to Six-Sigma quality. Computerized physician order entry (CPOE) has been suggested as a key element in decreasing errors and improving quality. Several papers have recently addressed this issue with different conclusions. Upperman et al. evaluated the rates of ADEs pre- and post-CPOE implementation. They noted an improvement in verbal order regulatory compliance, as well as an elimination of transcription errors after implementation. They also noted a statistical decrease in harmful ADEs and suggested that this improvement would result in one less harmful ADE for every 64 patient days. Han et al. noted a different experience when implementing a CPOE system in an academic tertiary care children's hospital. Surprisingly, they noted that the mortality rate increased from 2.8% before CPOE implementation to 6.57% after, an increase that remained significant even after multivariate analysis. It is noteworthy that in this paper, the authors document that the CPOE training was given 3 months before implementation. They also note that the implementation itself occurred over a period of only 6 days for the entire pediatric hospital. This may be too long an interval from training and too short a period for implementation. It is interesting that two papers, both published from the same institution, could have such different conclusions.

Ash et al. have suggested that the mere implementation of an EHR is not in and of itself enough to insure that unexpected errors won't occur. They suggest that these errors fall into two broad categories: "those in the process of entering and retrieving information and those in the communication and coordination process that the patient care information system is supposed to support." The key for powering the CPOE and the EHR is likely through well-thought-out algorithms that allow us to take advantage of the computer's ability to maintain data while attempting to best understand what a particular patient needs and while limiting changes in underlying clinical functionality, unless that change actually improves functionality.

There has also been a push to allow patients to have access to their records. This may enhance patient engagement and activation by facilitating the patients' ability to participate in their own care in a way not previously thought possible. Patients are able to view data within the EHR for accuracy, reviewing current or prior medications, allergies, etc. They could also be made aware of when lab test or studies are due or overdue, helping to improve compliance and screening. An even more novel concept that has been introduced by several groups is the ability of the patient to communicate with her care providers through Web-based messaging. Initially, providers were concerned regarding the potential for overuse, but little evidence demonstrates this type of abuse. Indeed, in a time when it may be quite difficult to locate your patient during the course of a business day, dyssynchronous communication may be a preferable manner to communicate nonemergent information with patients. In addition, these data may be appropriately security encrypted at 128 bits and easily made part of the health record.

HIE are currently being pursued by a number of organizations and states. The hope would be true interconnectivity so that patient data could be viewed regardless of the point of presentation. Numerous technologic barriers exist to limit this functionality at present, but the hope of multidirectional data flow with immediate access to this vital information promises improved care for our patients.

CHANGES IN EDUCATION

One of the most significant changes in medical education has been the limitation of resident duty hours. Such regulation of work hours has been common in industries such as aviation, in which pilots and other crew are limited both in the number of hours worked and requirements for time off between work episodes. Although many gynecologists were trained in a time of every second- or third-night call, this is no longer acceptable or allowable. New York led the way in creating legal mandates, but the Accreditation Council for Graduate Medical Education (ACGME) and the various specialty resident review committees have quickly followed. In July 2003, the ACGME put into effect new requirements and regulations (www.acgme.org). These regulations limited total duty hours to 80 hours per week when averaged over 4 weeks, limited in-house call to no more than every third night with 1 day off in 7, and limited continuous patient care hours to 30, with the last 6 hours to patient handoffs and educational activities, such as grand rounds. In addition, there had to be 10 hours between shifts worked. In 2009, the IOM opined that based on fatigue-related errors noted in other industries, residents should have a period of protected sleep of no less than 5 hours during any shift of more than 16 hours. In July of 2011, the ACGME further revised the standards mandating that duty hours for interns not exceed 16 hours. Second-year residents and above may work up to 24 hours of continuous duty, but there is a recommendation for "strategic napping." These changes represent a paradigm shift that is a dramatic departure from times past. While recent data have suggested that decision-making as well as technical skills may suffer with sleep deprivation, it is much less clear how these changes have affected patient care, safety and quality, as well as overall resident experience.

Hutter in 2006 evaluated the impact of changing to the 80-hour workweek on surgical residents in Boston. They noted that after implementation of the 80-hour workweek, residents had lower burnout scores and less emotional exhaustion, whereas sleep and motivation to work were improved. Objective quantitative measurement demonstrated no differences in the quality of patient care. In contrast, another pre– and post–duty-hour implementation study from the surgery department of University of California, Irvine, did not show changes in measures of burnout. They did note a decrease in weekly work hours from 100.7 to 82.6 after implementation and found a significant decrease in formal educational time. Of interest, time in the operating room, on clinical rounds, and in the clinic was not significantly different.

In contrast to previous publications, a report from University of California, San Francisco, internal medicine residency did not demonstrate improvement in educational satisfaction with the onset of the new duty-hour regulations. Similarly, another obstetric and gynecologic survey pre- and postimplementation of duty hours at the University of Colorado demonstrated no differences in overall satisfaction with the residency. However, some key elements were found to be statistically elevated after implementation, including reading, reviewing literature, doing research, and some clinical aspects of training.

More recently, Volpp reported on protected sleep for interns. Their prospective trial suggested that implementation of a "protected sleep period" did have a significant impact on the amount of sleep but also improved alertness the following morning as assessed by a sleepiness scale.

Two pivotal papers were published in 2013 on a number of these issues. Desai et al. from Johns Hopkins compared the effects of the 2003 duty-hour regulation with the changes the ACGME put in place in 2011. Using a crossover study design, they randomly assigned interns to a model that was compliant to the 2003 regulations or to two different models compliant with the 2011 recommendations. Both 2011-compliant models increased sleep duration while on call; however, handoffs were more than doubled, educational time was decreased, and there was a perception by residents and nurses that quality was negatively impacted. In the same journal, Sen et al. reported on results from the Intern Health Study, a prospective longitudinal cohort. They evaluated interns from before the 2011 change (2009 and 2010) and after the change with 51 residencies at 14 academic and community training programs represented. In studying the 2,300 interns, they noted a decrease in duty hours (67.0 to 64.3) with no significant impact on total sleep hours, depressive symptoms, or sense of well-being. Of concern, the number of interns self-reporting an error that caused harm to a patient increased from 19.9% prior to the rule change in 2011 to 23.3% after.

Obstetric residencies have responded to these directives and made significant changes in underlying residency structure. Nuthalapaty et al., in querying obstetric residency programs, found that 98% reported changing their programs in response to the new regulations, 94% changed their on-call structure, 85% changed distribution of responsibility, and 80% modified how residents participate in rendering care to patients.

Outside this country, even more stringent regulations exist. For example, in Brazil, the Brazilian National Committee on Medical Residency created requirements in 1981 that limit maximum weekly work hours to 60, with 30 consecutive days of vacation each year and 10% of total hours mandated to be dedicated to education. Importantly, Brazil is not the most aggressive country to implement these changes; multiple countries around the globe have decreased duty hours to 48 to 56 hours per week. It is reasonable to ask the question: Have we seen the full evolution of these changes in the United States?

It has also been noted that in some cases, residents may work fewer hours than what might be seen in a private setting, in which every-other-night call may be commonplace. One article that questioned residents in internal medicine noted that at least half of residents believed sleep deprivation was a necessary foundation in residency training. A question for the future is whether regulations such as those that have been put in place for residents may also come to exist for all physicians. Certainly, given the potential for significant manpower limitations in some specialties, as well as a trend away from rural- and toward hospitalist-type practices, this would be especially problematic and require significant redistribution of resources. There are additional issues with the duty-hour limitations, including the need to transition patient care from the previous on-call residents and the likelihood that some cases that are seen during the resident's call (especially from the emergency room) may come under the care of a different resident and result in a loss of continuity for both the resident and the patient. Whether such handoffs and the decrease in continuity are responsible for some of the results noted earlier is still in question. Although such changes have caused us to rethink classic patient flow in training programs, there is a need to learn how to appropriately transition care from one service to another. This will be critical as residents become attending physicians. One methodology for training teams to work together and communicate better is called TeamSTEPPS (team strategies and tools to enhance performance and patient safety). The tool has been developed by the Department of Defense and the Agency for Healthcare Research and Quality (http://teamstepps.ahrq.gov/index.htm). Regardless of the tool used, optimized communication and team function remain critical as there will continue to be pressure to decrease worked hours and concomitant increases in handoffs among care providers.

In recent residency matches, both general surgical and obstetric and gynecology slots have been filled at much higher percentages than in the years immediately prior to the institution of work hour limitations. Whether this is consistent with senior medical students sensing a change after the decrease in duty hours, thus creating a new perception of these "difficult" specialties, remains to be seen.

Less investigation has been performed on the impact of the duty-hour changes to medical students and how this might affect their learning. Brasher et al. used completed end-of-rotation evaluations pre- and postimplementation and found more negative comments after implementation, including decreased scores of residents as supervisors and teachers, and in teaching activities. What is less clear is this: As programs and residents have acclimated to these new standards, will there be adaptation as we get farther out from the change?

There remains limited information regarding real change in the quality of care rendered in this new paradigm. Indeed, the proponents for change would suggest the opposite: that a fresh team will deliver better care.

POSTGRADUATE TRAINING

Questions continue regarding how best to train clinicians in the postgraduate environment. Most find learning easy while in residency, with time often dedicated to didactic lectures. Few practicing physicians are afforded similar luxury, and yet, significant technologic and medical advances continue throughout our careers. Given the limitations that state-by-state licensure imposes, as well as malpractice constraints, it is also difficult for physicians to cross state boundaries to learn novel surgical procedures and be tutored. Fortunately, there have also been advances in our ability to educate with Web-based or computer technology. The classic forum of the in-person lecture remains the gold standard for education. However, some institutions have moved to Web-based programs to allow transmission of grand rounds or other educational forums in real time. This allows attendees to log on and participate regardless of their location, be it at home, in the office, or in the hospital. It also allows for lecturers to limit their time away from work as they may deliver their lecture from afar with remote transmission to multiple sites. In a time of shrinking grand-round budgets and limited external support for lectures, this may be one methodology for continuing to deliver state-of-the-art education to a diverse, ever-changing audience.

As we continue our transition from open surgery to minimal invasive surgery and now to robotic surgery, there continue to be questions regarding how to best credential surgeons on new technology. The issues discussed previously regarding limitations in postgraduate opportunities to mentor and train are the origin of some of these problems. How many preceptor cases are adequate for an individual surgeon to be able to demonstrate mastery? Unfortunately, most of us as educators realize there are profound differences between cases and surgeons. What one surgeon is able to master in 20 cases, another may be able to conquer in five or fewer. At the writing of this chapter, most residents will garner adequate experience with minimal invasive techniques during their training, but less will master robotics during this time.

Previously, many gynecologic services existed in a silo, consulting other services only when specific situations existed. In the new practice of medicine, we are being faced with many multidisciplinary procedures requiring seamless transition between multiple providers and specialties to assure the best outcome. Uterine artery embolization would be one such example. Generally, gynecologists see the patient with symptomatic myomata, but on occasion, patients will self-refer to an interventional radiologist. In most cases, the interventionalist performs the procedure, but often, this individual does not have admitting privileges. If the patient requires admission for pain management, the gynecologic service may be asked to admit and manage the patient. In addition, appropriate preoperative evaluation will need to be performed to decrease the risk of a failed or inappropriate procedure. Generally, all of the above are best accomplished in a setting where excellent communication exists between the services, and the patient seamlessly transitions through the treatment and is not held hostage to political or other logistic issues that often exist in the complicated systems we work within. This requires physicians and surgeons from multiple specialties to decide in advance how such programs should work and what each individual team member is responsible for providing. This often requires identification of specific team leaders (physician and nursing) from each discipline, as well as a specific leader who will have proximate authority to resolve issues that will predictably arise in such complex interactions. When services work in this manner, functioning at a high level, patient care is optimized. Because of the need to act across disciplines and in a team-like manner, resident and even medical student curriculums have begun to emphasize the need to work as teams—a concept adopted long ago in the business world but adopted much more slowly in the world of independent thinking and functioning within medicine. In fact, team-building retreats are becoming departmental norms in many training programs around the country.

HOSPITALISTS/LABORISTS

In the last decade, there has been a move toward some practitioners working solely within the hospital setting to care for inpatients, a practice common outside the United States for decades. This started when data suggested that in some cases, patient care might be optimized and length of stay (LOS) reduced by having a single individual responsible for overseeing a patient's stay in the hospital. Emergency department physicians have performed shift work for decades, but the change was most dramatic for hospitalists who are generally internists or family practitioners—fields that were more typically associated with primary care. With the advent of the resident 80-hour workweek, some services have been unable to be covered by residents, and again, the utility of a hospitalist coverage arrangement began to make sense.

Wachter and Goldman reviewed published studies and abstracts regarding hospitalist services and noted only 2 of 19 studies didn't demonstrate decreased LOS. The range of LOS reductions was 7% to 27%, which even on the lower end often translate into significant savings to health care organizations. Several variations on the hospitalist model exist, including use of combinations of private staff, academic staff, and house staff. One study evaluated differences between community physicians, a private hospitalist service, and an academic hospitalist group within the same tertiary care hospital and found a 20% LOS and 10% cost reduction on the academic service versus 8% and 6% reductions for the private hospitalists and the community physicians, respectively. They did not note differences in mortality rates (either inpatient or 30-day) or readmission rates between the three groups. Another variation is to use the hospitalist to cover patients typically covered by surgical services. One trial evaluated use of a hospitalist in managing elderly hip fracture patients along with orthopedic surgeons. They noted decreased time to get patients to surgery, decreased length of hospitalization after surgery, and overall decreased LOS with no adverse impact on mortality or readmission. Another area of question has been how a hospitalist service might affect teaching and education for students and residents. Hauer et al. analyzed 1,587 house staff and student evaluations on internal medicine rotations during a 2-year period. They scored the hospitalist group (vs. traditional attending physicians) higher in teaching effectiveness, knowledge, and feedback. More recently, the hospitalist trend in internal medicine and family practice has carried over to pediatric hospitals that have now created pediatric hospitalist services. Dwight et al. describe that with manpower reductions and limitations in house staff, among other issues, some Canadian hospitals have begun to successfully use a non–house staff–based model effectively. Landrigan et al. performed a systematic review of the pediatric hospitalist literature, and consistent with nonpediatric hospitalist studies, these programs had an average LOS and cost decrease of 10%. They do note that many of the programs themselves do not generate adequate revenue to not lose money. An interesting article on keys to success for creating a pediatric hospitalist program suggests six key principles that may have broad applicability to establishment of similar programs in obstetrics and gynecology (Table 5.7).

Over the last 10 years, this trend has carried over into obstetrics and gynecology. Weinstein first introduced the concept of the laborist in 2003. Since that time, a number of hospitals have moved forward with establishing programs.

In a time when clinicians have become highly interested in balancing lifestyle and workplace activities, it is understandable why this concept may become more prevalent. Funk

TABLE 5.7 Six Principles to Establish a Successful Pediatric Hospitalist Practice

1. Voluntary referrals
2. Local design
3. Minimum physician-training requirements
4. Arrangement for appropriate follow-up
5. Communication among primary care physicians, subspecialists, and hospitalists
6. Data collection and outcome measures

Adapted from Percelay JM, Strong GB. American Academy of Pediatrics Section on Hospital Medicine. Guiding principles for pediatric hospitalist programs. *Pediatrics* 2005;115:1101. Reproduced with permission. Copyright © 2005 American Academy of Pediatrics.

TABLE 5.8 Classification of References and Recommendations According to the U.S. Preventive Services Task Force

REFERENCES	
Level I	Evidence obtained from at least one properly conducted randomized clinical trial
Level II-1	Evidence obtained from well-designed controlled study without randomization
Level II-2	Evidence from well-designed cohort or case–control studies, preferably from more than one center or research group
Level II-3	Evidence obtained from multiple time series with or without intervention
Level III	Opinions of respected authorities, based on clinical experience, descriptive studies, or reports of expert committees
Meta-analysis	A systematic structured process that is more than a literature review
Decision analysis	Use of mathematical models of sequences of several strategies to determine which is optimal
Cost-efficient analysis	Comparison of health care practice or techniques in terms of the relative economic efficiencies in providing health benefits
RECOMMENDATIONS	
Level A	Based on good and consistent scientific evidence
Level B	Based on limited or inconsistent scientific evidence
Level C	Based primarily on consensus and expert opinion
Level D	Fair evidence against the recommendation
Level E	Evidence against the recommendation

Adapted from American College of Obstetricians and Gynecologists. *Reading the medical literature: applying evidence to practice.* Washington, DC: American College of Obstetricians and Gynecologists, 1998.

TABLE 5.9 New U.S. Preventive Services Task Force Grade Definitions After July 2012

GRADE	DEFINITION	SUGGESTIONS FOR PRACTICE
A	The USPSTF recommends the service. There is high certainty that the net benefit is substantial.	Offer or provide this service.
B	The USPSTF recommends the service. There is high certainty that the net benefit is moderate, or there is moderate certainty that the net benefit is moderate to substantial.	Offer or provide this service.
C	The USPSTF recommends selectively offering or providing this service to individual patients based on professional judgment and patient preferences. There is at least moderate certainty that the net benefit is small.	Offer or provide this service for selected patients depending on individual circumstances.
D	The USPSTF recommends against the service. There is moderate or high certainty that the service has no net benefit or that the harms outweigh the benefits.	Discourage the use of this service.
I statement	The USPSTF concludes that the current evidence is insufficient to assess the balance of benefits and harms of the service. Evidence is lacking, of poor quality, or conflicting, and the balance of benefits and harms cannot be determined.	Read the clinical considerations section of USPSTF Recommendation Statement. If the service is offered, patients should understand the uncertainty about the balance of benefits and harms.

surveyed obstetrician–gynecologists and noted that laborists were slightly younger and had a high rate of career satisfaction. More recently, the American Congress of Obstetricians and Gynecology has released a committee opinion supporting the concept.

Srinivas reported that 40% of National Perinatal Information Center/Quality Analytic Services member hospitals were using laborists in 2010. They noted an association with delivery volume but not geography or presence of residents. Unfortunately, while the laborist movement is growing quickly, there are presently few data regarding improved maternal or neonatal outcomes, enhanced patient experience, or the impact on resident education. Undoubtedly, we will begin to see some of this data in the literature, similar to that published and previously mentioned in medicine and pediatrics.

RATING SCIENTIFIC EVIDENCE

It has become increasingly important for physicians to evaluate the adequacy of data to which we are constantly exposed. There has been a transition in articles published in the peer-reviewed literature over the last 10 to 15 years with a significant effort toward asking and answering questions in the most rigorous manner possible. Numerous methodologies exist for evaluating these trials, which place differing values on the quality, quantity, and consistency domains expressed within each report. Given the subtleties of these differing methodologies, a paper may be deemed to be stronger or weaker. The Agency for Healthcare Research and Quality (AHRQ) has reported on an evaluation of these various systems and describes the differences relative to the type of trial being evaluated (e.g., randomized control trial vs. observational).

The most commonly used systems are seen in Tables 5.8 and 5.9 as described by the U.S. Preventive Services Task Force (USPSTF). These methods describe the type of trial and give a recommendation regarding the strength of the conclusion. It is relevant for us as practicing surgeons to be able to differentiate between data and reports that are merely interesting and those that should cause us to reevaluate our practice patterns. It is also important to understand not only what the grading system means but how the conclusions are reached for each of these unique systems. Because there are presently a number of systems and no one is universally used in journals or textbooks, this is an even greater challenge.

In a review of 55 American Congress of Obstetricians and Gynecologists practice bulletins, Chauhan et al. found that only 29% of 438 recommendations were level A (good and consistent evidence), whereas 33% of recommendations were level B (limited or inconsistent evidence) and 38% were level C (consensus and expert opinion). This is the quandary in medicine today: Evidence-based medicine is how all of us would like to practice, but unfortunately, all questions have not been answered to the extent needed. Because of this, panels of experts may by necessity have to revert to the best available data, which may be less than optimal. However, even in the field of medical ethics, there is an effort toward moving to formal tools for evaluating the validity of discussions and data. If the last 10 years is any indication to what will happen in the future, there will be an increasing number of randomized controlled trials that are well thought out and executed to aid us in determining how to best counsel our patients.

CONCLUSION

The examples illustrated in this chapter are but a small sampling of the numerous ongoing changes occurring daily. Many of these changes will likely affect our lives and practices—some more than others—but all are a radical departure from times not too distant. It will be interesting to evaluate how these changes evolve over editions of this textbook. Changes underscore the importance of lifelong education, not only in the functional practice of medicine but also in the art of the practice of medicine. It certainly makes our profession an exciting place to be—stay tuned!

BEST SURGICAL PRACTICES

- Resident education has been transformed to being less service oriented and more competency based. The 80-hour workweek has effected revolutionary changes in the mindsets of today's trainees and the people who train them.
- Quality has always been important to physicians in theory, but new initiatives, such as the Partnership for Patients program, are making evidence-based practice a reality.
- The EHR continues to evolve. This modality will alter every aspect of care delivered by physicians and effect communication between providers and their patients.
- By being dedicated providers for inpatients, hospitalists will render more efficient and timely care and therefore more effectively manage patients, with an eye to improving quality and decreasing error.
- Pay for performance is being used by both governmental and third-party payors as a means to reward providers and health care organizations for optimizing predefined outcomes and quality metrics.

BIBLIOGRAPHY

Accreditation Council Graduate Medical Education common program requirements. http://www.acgme.org/dh_dutyhourscommonPR.pdf. Accessed on August 26, 2006.

American College of Obstetricians and Gynecologists. The obstetric-gynecologic hospitalist. *Obstet Gynecol* 2010;116:237.

American College of Obstetricians and Gynecologists. Reading the medical literature: applying evidence to practice. Washington, DC: American College of Obstetricians and Gynecologists, 1998.

American Hospital Association 2010 Committee on Research. AHA research synthesis report bundled payment. Chicago. American Hospital Association. 2010.

ARHQ. Systems to rate the strength of scientific evidence. Prepared for ARHQ. http://www.ncbi.nlm.nih.gov/books/bv.fcgi?rid=hstat1.chapter.70996. Accessed August 26, 2006.

Asch SM, Kerr EA, Keesey J, et al. Who is at greatest risk for receiving poor-quality health care? *N Engl J Med* 2006;354:1147.

Ash JS, Berg M, Coiera E. Some unintended consequences of information technology in health care: the nature of patient care information system-related errors. *J Am Med Inform Assoc* 2004;11:104.

Baker G, Carter B. *Provider pay-for-performance incentive programs: 2004 national study results.* San Francisco, CA: Med-Vantage, 2005.

Baron RJ, Fabens EL, Schiffman M, et al. Electronic health records: just around the corner? Or over the cliff? *Ann Intern Med* 2005;143:222.

Beckman H, Suchman AL, Curtin K, et al. Physician reactions to quantitative individual performance reports. *Am J Med Qual* 2006;21:192.

Boyd CM, Darer J, Boult C, et al. Clinical practice guidelines and quality of care for older patients with multiple comorbid diseases: implications for pay for performance. *JAMA* 2005;294:716.

Brasher AE, Chowdhry S, Hauge LS, et al. Medical students' perceptions of resident teaching: have duty hours regulations had an impact? *Ann Surg* 2005;242:548.

Buck K. Health savings accounts and account-based health plans: research highlights. America's Health Insurance Plans (AHIP) Center for Policy and Research. http://www.ahip.org/HSAHighlightsReport072012/. Published on July 2012.

Bufalino V, Peterson ED, Burke GL, et al. American Heart Association's reimbursement, coverage, and access policy development workgroup. Payment for quality: guiding principles and recommendations: principles and recommendations from the American Heart Association's reimbursement, coverage, and access policy development workgroup. *Circulation* 2006;113:1151.

Callcut RA, Breslin TM. Shaping the future of surgery: the role of private regulation in determining quality standards. *Ann Surg* 2006;243:304.

Chauhan SP, Berghella V, Sanderson M, et al. American College of Obstetricians and Gynecologists practice bulletins: an overview. *Am J Obstet Gynecol* 2006;194:1564.

Curtis JR, Cook DJ, Wall RJ, et al. Intensive care unit quality improvement: a "how-to" guide for the interdisciplinary team. *Crit Care Med* 2006;34:211.

de Oliveira Filho GR, Sturm EJ, Sartorato AE. Compliance with common program requirements in Brazil: its effects on resident's perceptions about quality of life and the educational environment. *Acad Med* 2005;80:98.

Desai SV, Feldman L, Brown L, et al. Effect of the 2011 vs. 2003 duty hour regulation—complaint models on sleep duration, trainee education, and continuity of patient care among internal medicine house staff. *JAMA Intern Med* 2013;173:649.

Dudley RA. Pay-for-performance research: how to learn what clinicians and policy makers need to know. *JAMA* 2005;294:1821.

Dwight P, MacArthur C, Friedman JN, et al. Evaluation of a staff-only hospitalist system in a tertiary care, academic children's hospital. *Pediatrics* 2004;114:1545.

Embi PJ, Jain A, Clark J, et al. Effect of a clinical trial alert system on physician participation in trial recruitment. *Arch Intern Med* 2005;165:2272.

Epstein AM, Lee TH, Hamel MB. Paying physicians for high-quality care. *N Engl J Med* 2004;350:406.

Fairbrother G, Hanson KL, Friedman S, et al. The impact of physician bonuses, enhanced fees, and feedback on childhood immunization coverage rates. *Am J Public Health* 1999;89:171.

Ford EW, Menachemi N, Phillips MT. Predicting the adoption of electronic health records by physicians: when will health care be paperless? *J Am Med Inform Assoc* 2006;13:106.

Funk C, Anderson BL, Schulkin J, et al. Survey of obstetric and gynecologic hospitalist and laborists. *Am J Obstet Gynecol* 2010;203:177.e1.

Garrido T, Jamieson L, Zhou Y, et al. Effect of electronic health records in ambulatory care: retrospective, serial, cross sectional study. *BMJ* 2005;330:581.

Gelfand DV, Podnos YD, Carmichael JC, et al. Effect of the 80-hour workweek on resident burnout. *Arch Surg* 2004;139:933.

Giuffrida A, Gosden T, Forland F, et al. Target payments in primary care: effects on professional practice and health care outcomes. *Cochrane Database Syst Rev* 2000;CD000531.

Goldfield N, Burford R, Averill R, et al. Pay for performance: an excellent idea that simply needs implementation. *Qual Manag Health Care* 2005;14:31.

Goss JR, Maynard C, Aldea GS, et al. Clinical outcomes assessment program. Effects of a statewide physician-led quality-improvement program on the quality of cardiac care. *Am Heart J* 2006;151:1033.

Halasyamani LK, Valenstein PN, Friedlander MP, et al. A comparison of two hospitalist models with traditional care in a community teaching hospital. *Am J Med* 2005;118:536.

Han YY, Carcillo JA, Venkataraman ST, et al. Unexpected increased mortality after implementation of a commercially sold computerized physician order entry system. *Pediatrics* 2005;116:1506.

Harris RP, Helfand M, Woolf SH, et al.; Methods Work Group, Third U.S. Preventive Services Task Force. Current methods of the U.S. Preventive Services Task Force: a review of the process. *Am J Prev Med* 2001;20:21.

Hauer KE, Wachter RM, McCulloch CE, et al. Effects of hospitalist attending physicians on trainee satisfaction with teaching and with internal medicine rotations. *Arch Intern Med* 2004;164:1866.

Hutter MM, Kellogg KC, Ferguson CM, et al. The impact of the 80-hour resident workweek on surgical residents and attending surgeons. *Ann Surg* 2006;243:864.

Klatt TE, Hopp E. Effect of a best-practice alert on the rate of influenza vaccination of pregnant women. *Obstet Gynecol* 2012;119:301.

Koch EG. Springtime for obstetrics and gynecology: will the specialty continue to blossom? *Obstet Gynecol* 2004;103:198.

Kohn KT, Corrigan JM, Donaldson MS. *To err is human: building a safer health system.* Washington, DC: National Academy Press, 1999.

Kouides RW, Bennett NM, Lewis B, et al. Performance-based physician reimbursement and influenza immunization rates in the elderly. The primary-care physicians of Monroe county. *Am J Prev Med* 1998;14:89.

Landrigan CP, Rothschild JM, Cronin JW, et al. Effect of reducing interns' work hours on serious medical errors in intensive care units. *N Engl J Med* 2004;351:1838.

Landrigan CP, Conway PH, Edwards S, et al. Pediatric hospitalists: a systematic review of the literature. *Pediatrics* 2006;117:1736.

Landrigan CP, Parry GJ, Bones CM, et al. Temporal trends in rates of patient harm resulting from medical care. *N Engl J Med* 2010; 363:2124.

Leach DC. Resident duty hours: the ACGME perspective. *Neurology* 2004;62:E1.

Leape LL, Berwick DM. Five years after *To Err Is Human:* what have we learned? *JAMA* 2005;293:2384.

Lindenauer PK, Behal R, Murray CK, et al. Volume, quality of care, and outcome in pneumonia. *Ann Intern Med* 2006;144:262.

Lund KJ, Teal SB, Alvero R. Resident job satisfaction: one year of duty hours. *Am J Obstet Gynecol* 2005;193:1823.

McCullough LB, Coverdale JH, Chervenak FA. Argument-based medical ethics: a formal tool for critically appraising the normative medical ethics literature. *Am J Obstet Gynecol* 2004;191:1097.

Nuthalapaty FS, Carver AR, Nuthalapaty ES, et al. The scope of duty hour-associated residency structure modifications. *Am J Obstet Gynecol* 2006;194:282.

Percelay JM, Strong GB. American Academy of Pediatrics Section on Hospital Medicine. Guiding principles for pediatric hospitalist programs. *Pediatrics* 2005;115:1101.

Phy MP, Vanness DJ, Melton LJ III, et al. Effects of a hospitalist model on elderly patients with hip fracture. *Arch Intern Med* 2005;165:796.

Rosen IM, Bellini LM, Shea JA. Sleep behaviors and attitudes among internal medicine housestaff in a U.S. university-based residency program. *Acad Med* 2004;79:407.

Rosenthal MB, Frank RG. What is the empirical basis for paying for quality in health care? *Med Care Res Rev* 2006;63:135.

Rosenthal MB, Frank RG, Li Z, et al. Early experience with pay-for-performance: from concept to practice. *JAMA* 2005;294:1788.

Roski J, Jeddeloh R, An L, et al. The impact of financial incentives and a patient registry on preventive care quality: increasing provider adherence to evidence-based smoking cessation practice guidelines. *Prev Med* 2003;36:291.

Sen S, Kranzler HR, Didwania AK, et al. Effects of the 2011 duty hour reforms on interns and their patients. *JAMA Intern Med* 2013;173:657.

Srinivas SK, Lorch S. The laborist model of obstetric care: we need more evidence. *Am J Obstet Gynecol* 2012;207:30.

Srinivas SK, Shocksnider J, Caldwell D, et al. Laborist model of care: who is using it? *J Matern Fetal Neonatal Med* 2012;25:257.

Stuebe A, Ecker J, Bates DW, et al. Barriers to follow-up for women with a history of gestational diabetes. *Am J Perinatol* 2010;27:705.

Tang PC, Ash JS, Bates DW, et al. Personal health records: definitions, benefits, and strategies for overcoming barriers to adoption. *J Am Med Inform Assoc* 2006;13:121.

Towers Watson. 2012 health care changes ahead survey report. http:// www.towerswatson.com/DownloadMedia.aspx?media={24F68B2F-90F6-48C9-ADF3-CA61A378300A}. Published on October 2012.

Upperman JS, Staley P, Friend K, et al. The impact of hospital-wide computerized physician order entry on medical errors in a pediatric hospital. *J Pediatr Surg* 2005;40:57.

Vidyarthi AR, Katz PP, Wall SD, et al. Impact of reduced duty hours on residents' educational satisfaction at the University of California, San Francisco. *Acad Med* 2006;81:76.

Volpp KG, Shea JA, Small DS, et al. Effect of a protected sleep period on hours slept during extended overnight in-hospital duty hours among medical interns. *JAMA* 2012;308:2208.

Wachter RM, Goldman L. The emerging role of "hospitalists" in the American health care system. *N Engl J Med* 1996;335:514.

Wachter RM, Goldman L. The hospitalist movement 5 years later. *JAMA* 2002;287:487.

Weiner BJ, Alexander JA, Baker LC, et al. Quality improvement implementation and hospital performance on patient safety indicators. *Med Care Res Rev* 2006;63:29.

Weinstein L. The laborist: a new focus of practice for the obstetrician. *Am J Obstet Gynecol* 2003;188:310.

Wirtschafter DD, Danielsen BH, Main EK, et al.; California Perinatal Quality Care Collaborative. Promoting antenatal steroid use for fetal maturation: results from the California Perinatal Quality Care Collaborative. *J Pediatr* 2006;148:606.

Levinson DR. Adverse events in hospitals: national incidence among Medicare beneficiaries. https://oig.hhs.gov/oei/reports/oei-06-09-00090.pdf

CHAPTER 6
Training the Gynecologic Surgeon: Maintaining and Improving Surgical Skills

Tola B. Fashokun and Victoria L. Handa

DEFINITIONS

Assessment—The process of measuring a trainee's knowledge skills, judgment, or professional behavior against defined standards.

Deliberate practice—A highly structured form of training that consists of focused, repetitive practice in which the subject continuously monitors his or her performance and subsequently corrects, experiments, and reacts to immediate and constant feedback, with the aim of steady and consistent improvement.

Global Rating Index for Technical Skills (GRITS)—A validated assessment tool used for evaluation of intraoperative performance.

Learning style—The process by which a person understands and retains information, thereby gaining knowledge or skill.

Learning theories—Conceptual frameworks and principles that attempt to explain the learning process.

Mental imagery (mental practice)—The cognitive rehearsal of a task with or without physical movement. It can be used to enhance the acquisition of new technical skills.

Objective Structured Assessment of Technical Skills (OSATS)—A valid and reliable examination in which subjects perform standardized surgical procedures while being evaluated by an expert surgeon.

Simulation—The act of reproducing or imitating a real-life event, process, or procedure. It can be utilized both as an effective training technique and assessment tool.

Vaginal Surgical Skills Index (VSSI)—A validated procedure-specific assessment tool used for intraoperative evaluation of vaginal surgical skills.

---

*"It would take me one year to teach a trainee **how** to do an operation, five years to teach them **when** to do the operation, but a lifetime to teach them **when not** to do an operation."*

Lord Smith, past President of The Royal College of Surgeons of England

HISTORY OF SURGICAL EDUCATION

For more than a century, the surgical teaching model introduced to Johns Hopkins Hospital in 1889 by Dr. William Halsted has been the standard approach for training surgeons. Under this apprenticeship model, the surgeon trainee experiences "...the orderly exposure to graduated clinical experience in the operating room during several years of residency under the close tutelage of dedicated senior attending surgeons...." This widely accepted and historically successful model traditional paradigm "to see one, do one, teach one" led to the declaration that "the operating room is the surgeon's classroom."

However, there are limitations to this surgical education model. Variability in the number and type of surgical cases and duration of apprenticeship will impact training. Second, this model does not provide for remediation. Even Dr. Halsted recognized this limitation. Halsted observed, "experience can mean doing the same thing wrong over and over again." Finally, this traditional method of training may not be practical given the current pressures of residency work hour restrictions, increasing numbers and complexity of surgical procedures, and financial and ethical constraints of teaching surgical skills in the operating room.

EDUCATIONAL THEORIES: HOW DO ADULTS LEARN?

A contemporary approach to surgical training requires consideration of not only *what* the trainee is learning but *how* they learn. Advances in educational research have identified principles of adult learning, and accumulating evidence suggests that surgical trainees have specific learning styles. The three basic types of learning styles are visual, auditory, and tactile. To learn, we depend on our senses to process the information around us. Most people tend to use one of their senses more than the others; however, it is not unusual to use a different style to learn a particular skill. For example, some novice surgeons may find it difficult to hear and then duplicate instruction on how to correctly apply a clamp; they may learn best by first observing and then performing the illustrated task. The latter method might have a direct impact on the efficiency of intraoperative teaching. This does not imply that one style is better than the other, but one style may be more preferable given the learning environment, and the trainee may need to make adjustments to minimize any obstacles to effective learning.

A better understanding of the factors that impact the process of learning new surgical skills will hopefully lead to a more effective and efficient educational model for surgical educators and novice surgeons. Dr. Reznick et al. have suggested that "adult learning is enhanced by an approach that is self-directed and centers on the learner rather than the teacher. Adult learning is facilitated by focusing on a problem or task. Abstract, subject-centered learning is less effective as a motivator. Adults also come to an educational activity, such as learning operative skills, with a vast amount of past experience that must be recognized and utilized." Because the development of surgical skills is an active learning process, a surgeon's optimal surgical education should be based on learning theory.

One learning model relates to the psychological states involved in the process of progressing from incompetence to

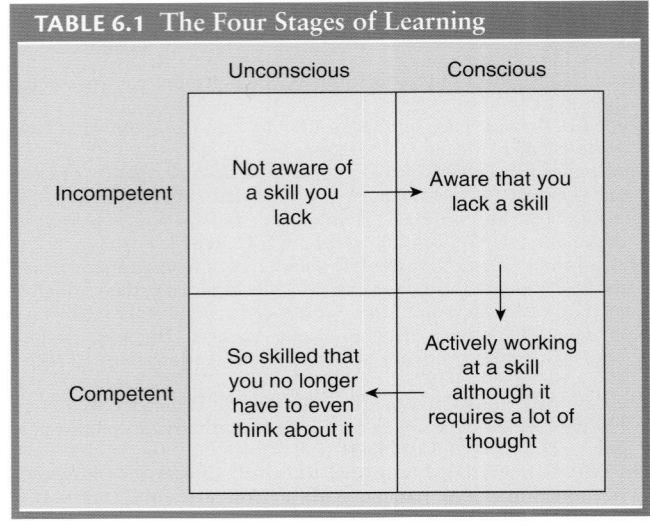

TABLE 6.1 The Four Stages of Learning

	Unconscious	Conscious
Incompetent	Not aware of a skill you lack	Aware that you lack a skill
Competent	So skilled that you no longer have to even think about it	Actively working at a skill although it requires a lot of thought

competence in a skill (Table 6.1). This theory outlines four stages. The first stage is "Unconscious Incompetence": You don't know that you don't know something. The second stage is "Conscious Incompetence": You are now aware that you are incompetent at something. Next is stage 3, "Conscious Competence": You develop a skill in that area but have to think about it. In the final stage is "Unconscious Competence": You are now so good at it, and it now comes naturally. Obviously, most surgeons would agree that their goal is to achieve the final stage when a particular surgical skill becomes "second nature"; however, this may have a direct impact on one's ability to teach this skill or procedure. Surgical educators are most effective when they are able to "break down" a complex procedure to its basic elements, which can be challenging if they are not "conscious" about the process.

Modern research in surgical education has also examined the specific steps involved in attaining motor skills. Fitts and Posner's three-stage theory of motor skill acquisition (Fig. 6.1) is widely accepted in both the motor skills and surgical literature. In the first, cognitive stage, the learner is still in the process of obtaining information about how to correctly perform the skill, through reading or direct observation. In this stage, performance is relatively slow, abrupt, inefficient, and inconsistent. The learner must concentrate on the task, and attentional demands are high. In the second associative stage, through deliberate practice and feedback, the movement becomes more fluid with fewer interruptions and attentional demands decrease. After extensive practice, the performer reaches the final, autonomous stage, which is characterized by fluent and

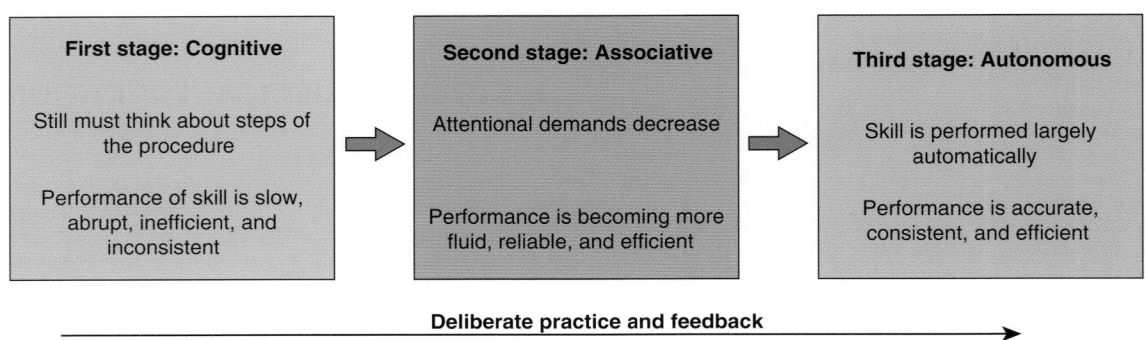

First stage: Cognitive

Still must think about steps of the procedure

Performance of skill is slow, abrupt, inefficient, and inconsistent

Second stage: Associative

Attentional demands decrease

Performance is becoming more fluid, reliable, and efficient

Third stage: Autonomous

Skill is performed largely automatically

Performance is accurate, consistent, and efficient

Deliberate practice and feedback

FIGURE 6.1 Fitts and Posner's three-stage theory of motor skill acquisition.

seemingly effortless motions. Movements are accurate, consistent, and efficient. The skill is performed largely automatically at this stage, and movement execution requires little or no attention. The understanding of skill acquisition has important implications in surgical training and is best illustrated by an example given by Reznick and MacRae, "....with a surgical skill as simple as tying a knot, in the cognitive stage the learner must understand the mechanics of the skill—how to hold the tie, how to place the throws, and how to move the hands. With practice and feedback, the learner reaches the associative stage, in which knowledge is translated into appropriate motor behavior. The learner is still thinking about how to move the hands and hold the tie, but is able to execute the task more fluidly, with fewer interruptions. In the autonomous stage, practice gradually results in smooth performance. The learner no longer needs to think about how to execute this particular task and can concentrate on other aspects of the procedure...."

Surgical trainees must have a firm understanding of basic skills first before they can progress to more complex and elaborate tasks, and the quality of performance requires assessment at every stage. Therefore, the earlier stages of teaching fundamental technical skills should take place outside the operating room; practice with constructive feedback is the rule until automaticity in basic skills is achieved. The mastery of basic skills allows trainees to focus on more complex tasks in the operating room.

OUT OF OPERATING ROOM LEARNING EXPERIENCES

Simulation

The advent of surgical simulation has resulted in significant and dynamic changes to surgical education. The use of simulation has been adopted from other disciplines, most notably the aviation industry. An obvious advantage of simulation training

is that core skills can be learned prior to application in the operating room, theoretically improving safety and efficiency. Also, with a simulation curriculum, training opportunities are not constrained by the available clinical experience. Simulation offers the opportunity for repeated practice in a safe and controlled environment, focusing on trainees and tailored to their needs. Most surgical educators would agree that fundamental surgical principles and technical skills should be taught outside the operating room. Although some training programs include surgical training models in their surgical curricula, no simulation model has gained sufficient acceptance to be considered a gold standard. Simulation practices vary widely across and within residency programs. Several research studies have confirmed the positive impact on surgical skill of practice outside the operating room using surgical simulators. Trainees whose initial learning occurs in a simulated environment make fewer errors and complete the "real" operation faster than those without such training. In essence, better skills translate into better surgery.

There are a variety of types of surgical training models, including bench models, virtual reality trainers (computer-generated models), surgical simulation in live animal models, and surgical simulation in human cadavers (Table 6.2). These various simulators have advantages and disadvantages. All are believed to result in improved trainee performance that is transferable to the operating room.

However, it is unclear which type of trainer is superior. A number of studies have reached differing conclusions. For example, a Cochrane Database Systematic Review of the effectiveness of virtual reality training compared with physical reality simulators concluded that these two training methods result in similar laparoscopic skill acquisition, but that the virtual reality trainers may result in better transferability of skills into the operating room (especially for more complex tasks). In contrast, Denadai et al. demonstrated that the acquisition of suture skills was similar on a low- and high-fidelity bench model. Practice on either model was shown to improve

TABLE 6.2 Simulation Methods			
SIMULATION	**DESCRIPTION/COST**	**PROS**	**CONS**
Bench models	Suture boards and foam models Low to mid cost	Inexpensive, safe, generally reusable; can perform basic tasks	Decreased realism; not able to perform more complex tasks
Mannequin	May be entire anatomy or pelvis Mid to high costs	Multiple use; can perform basic or more complex procedures, patient specific Team training	Limited realism, not "exact" anatomy, limited applications
Computer/virtual reality surgical simulators	Virtual software, computer visual-haptics Can practice basic laparoscopic skills High cost	Multiple use, data capture, minimal setup time; provide performance feedback, can make patient-specific	Cost, maintenance, and down time; realism varies
Live animals	Primate, sheep, pig, rabbits High cost	Closer to human anatomy; can perform entire operation or complex procedures	Expensive, differences in anatomy, single use; requires special facilities and personnel, tissue compliance, infection risks, ethical concerns
Cadavers	Entire anatomy, best used for continuing medical education High cost	Accurate anatomy; can perform the entire operation	Expensive limited availability, single use, compliance of tissue, infection risks, and ethical concerns

performance compared to training with only didactic materials. However, another systematic review (performed by Sutherland et al.) of 30 randomized controlled trials concluded that simulation training was superior to no training but was not consistently superior to traditional training methods. Most investigators would agree that the effective use of surgical training models requires standardization of instruction, feedback, and evaluation.

Ultimately, the role of simulation in teaching surgical skills is to facilitate practice of technical skills. Ericsson et al. showed that becoming an expert takes about 10,000 hours of *deliberate* and *distributed* practice, regardless of whether the goal is to become a competent surgeon, a chess master, or a professional musician. Deliberate practice is defined as a "highly structured activity, the explicit goal of which is to improve performance." In other words, time spent practicing a new surgical skill is most useful if the learner reflects on or receives feedback on performance (either self-evaluation or through formal assessment) and has numerous sessions distributed over time (e.g., throughout residency or fellowship), rather than the same number of hours compressed into a single training session. This confirms what other educators have suggested that "practice does not make perfect; perfect practice makes perfect."

Simulation may also facilitate the evaluation of surgical skills. However, for simulation to provide a robust and valid assessment tool, the simulation exercise must be highly standardized, widely available, and focused on the critical aspects of performance. It is important that simulation is incorporated as part of a standard surgical curriculum, with well-defined learning goals and objectives that should be completed at specific time intervals.

MENTAL IMAGERY (MENTAL PRACTICE)

Mental imagery, also called visualization and mental imagery rehearsal, is "the cognitive rehearsal of a task with or without physical movement." It can be used to enhance the acquisition of new technical skills and increase emotional preparedness to perform in stressful situation, both qualities applicable to the training of novice surgeons.

Educational researchers have examined whether the experience of mental imagery affects the degree of learning. For example, imagining playing a 5-finger piano exercise (mental practice) resulted in a significant improvement in performance over no mental practice—though not as great an improvement as that produced by physical practice. Mental practice alone seems to be sufficient to promote the modulation of neural circuits involved in the early stages of motor skill learning.

So how does this translate to the use of mental practice to teach surgical skills? Several studies support the use of this training tool to teach surgical skills. In a multicenter randomized controlled trial, gynecology residents who had performed three of fewer cystoscopies were randomized to preoperative mental imagery sessions or reading a book chapter describing cystoscopy. The imagery group's surgical performance assessment was 15.9% significantly higher than controls ($p = 0.03$). In addition, residents considered mental imagery to be a more useful preoperative preparation. Two additional studies using mental imagery to teach medical students demonstrated similar results. Medical students who used mental imagery techniques had at least equivalent and sometimes superior results when compared to traditional methods of learning new skills.

Despite evidence to support its usefulness, the exact role of mental imagery in surgical training has yet to be clearly defined, and there is no ideal way to use this technique. Based on prior research, mental practice is most effective when the

leaner is familiar with the task and the actual performance immediately follows the imagery session. Novice surgeons could use this technique in preparation for an "actual" surgery by reviewing details of an entire surgical procedure with the appropriate hand movements for the operation. Thus, this approach may offer a less expensive, efficient, and ethical way for a surgeon to acquire a new skill before operating on a "live" patient.

WEB-BASED LEARNING

In recent years, Web-based learning has become an emerging technology for learning and teaching surgical skills. This online learning environment includes access to videos as well as live surgeries viewed remotely. These resources support the learner-centered teaching approach, facilitating interactions with experts and with other learners. The availability of online surgical videos provides a useful resource that complements the more traditional options, including textbooks and case observation. However, the quality of materials available on the Internet is variable, and the materials available are typically not subject to peer review. Despite these limitations, Web-based learning may be a valuable resource for more seasoned surgeons interested in obtaining knowledge about a newer procedure or technique. In fact, most webcasts are created for surgeons already familiar with certain aspects of a surgical procedure or basic technical skills; surgical webinars provide an opportunity for these surgeons to interact live with an expert surgeon and may be the catalyst for a surgeon to seek more formal training.

TEACHING IN THE OPERATING ROOM

Simulation training and other surgical educational opportunities only complement traditional surgical educational experience (in operating room learning) but cannot replace it. The operating room is obviously a unique educational setting for several key reasons; first it can be a very high-stress environment for surgical educators and learners alike given the concern for providing an optimal surgical outcome in a safe, controlled, and efficient manner. In addition, it provides the teacher and learner with uninterrupted time together, and this time can and should be used for clinical teaching and learning. Operating room teaching should be similar to other structured learning activities in which key learning objectives and goals for the learner are reviewed prior to case. It is not acceptable or ethical for novice surgeon to learn a "new" technical skill without supervision. Dr. Roberts et al. emphasized the importance of deliberate and guided instruction in the operating room. The authors refer to this teaching method as "briefing, intraoperative teaching, and debriefing" or BID. The educational framework for this teaching begins with the "briefing" component before the surgery at the scrub sink; with a short interaction between the surgical educator and the learner assessing the needs of the learner and identifying mutual learning objectives. It is important that the learner is active in this process because it encourages the learner to reflect on areas that may need improvement (from previous surgeries) and formulate needs to be addressed in the current surgery. The "intraoperative teaching" should involve coaching and guiding the learner through the surgery, but the didactics or "teaching script" used during the operation should focus on the preestablished learning objectives. This more tailored approach is to avoid overloading the learner with too much information, which then becomes difficult to apply to future practice. The "debriefing" should occur at the end of the procedure and concentrate on four areas of discussion: reflection, rules, reinforcement, and correction. Details about this process are discussed later in the chapter.

Surgical educational researchers have consistently identified certain principles of effective intraoperative teaching: They include explaining reasons behind decisions, providing clear answers to questions, involving learners (letting them "actually operate") with direct supervision, and providing feedback without belittling.

SURGICAL SKILLS ASSESSMENTS

Assessment is the process of measuring a trainee's knowledge, skills, judgment, or professional behavior against defined standards. Ideally, the assessment tool should be objective, reliable, and reproducible. Assessment can have different and multiple purposes, including aiding learning through constructive feedback, measuring progress over time, and/or determining a level of competence.

There are distinct differences between constructive feedback and evaluation of surgical skills. Ideally, in order for feedback to be most effective, it should be performed in a timely fashion; however, this can be a challenge for "in operating room" learning experiences. If time permits, the feedback should be given immediately after the surgical case or at the conclusion of the surgery day through a "debriefing process." This is a systematic process of providing constructive feedback with the focus on changing or reinforcing surgical techniques, motivating the learner, and encouraging self-assessment. The feedback is direct and specific and gives the learner direction for improvement. Some of the initial questions asked of the learner such as "How do you think you did performing the vaginal hysterectomy?" "What part of the case went well?" and "What part of the case could have gone better?" can help facilitate the discussion. More specific questions about certain steps of a procedure, for example, "How do you think you did entering the posterior cul-de-sac?," may help the learner identify a particular deficiency and methods to improve their skills. It is through this process that novice surgeons become more comfortable with self-assessment. Self-evaluation can be difficult because it requires surgeons to admit to knowledge or skill deficits. However, an objective critique of one's own surgical performance is beneficial to both novice and experienced surgeons and is the first key step in learning from past mistakes to advance as a surgeon.

When providing constructive feedback, "how" something is said is often just as important as "what" is said; Fenner encourages surgical educators to adhere to some basic rules when giving feedback. Some of the dos and don'ts that we follow at our institution are listed in Table 6.3.

TABLE 6.3 The "Dos" and "Don'ts" of Feedback

DOS	DON'TS
Be descriptive, rather than elusive	Embarrass the learner
Be specific, rather than general	Give too much feedback at one time
Focus on behavior, rather than personality	Create a negative environment
Focus on modifiable issues	
Time the interaction	
Listen to the learner	
Follow up	

It should be the goal of both surgical educators and learners to foster an environment of constructive feedback, which means that giving feedback should be routinely performed and unsolicited. However, if it is not routine practice for the surgical educator to provide this constructive assessment, then it becomes the responsibility of the learner to seek this feedback.

Traditionally, formal evaluation of surgical skills is performed in the operating room with direct observation of a trainee's surgical performance by the supervising attending. Although this has been the standard evaluation process, studies have shown that an unstructured assessment using direct observation has limited reliability as an assessment method. In fact, one of the major issues with this approach is that the observation itself is not wholly successful and may be based on indirect observation or incomplete direct observation. In addition, this strategy is subjective and may be biased by factors such as the evaluator's prior knowledge of the trainee and the outcome of the surgery. Recognition of these limitations has led to a search for more valid methods of evaluating surgical skills.

The Objective Structured Assessment of Technical Skills (OSATS) is an examination in which subjects perform standardized surgical procedures while being evaluated by an expert surgeon. The assessment is based on a task-specific checklist in which all important steps of a procedure are identified and a mark is assigned for every step the candidate completes correctly. Using a 10-point scale, it grades the trainee on seven important elements of any operation, concerning a combination of skill-based, rule-based, and knowledge-based behaviors: (a) respect for tissue, (b) time and motion, (c) instrument handling, (d) knowledge of instruments, (e) use of assistants, (f) flow of operation, and (g) knowledge of the procedure. Studies have repeatedly demonstrated the reliability and validity of this assessment tool. Through the use of specialty-specific OSATS in an obstetrics and gynecology residency program, researchers have also determined that evaluators could assess their own residents as reliably as an evaluator who did not know the resident. An OSATS can also be used to evaluate a specific curriculum.

An alternative to the evaluation of the explicit steps of the procedure is the rating of general technical skill. The Global Rating Index for Technical Skills (GRITS) (Table 6.4) is a valid and reliable assessment tool, created to provide a defensible and practical evaluation of resident's surgical skills. The GRITS was based on Global Rating Scales (GRS) previously validated in the setting of OSATS and the Global Operative Assessment of Laparoscopic Skills. The GRITS consists of 9 items, each scored from 1 to 5. These items were selected to be general markers of technical skill, rather than procedure-specific steps. Therefore, the GRITS tool could be applied to a wide variety of procedures without modification. Two items applied only to laparoscopic cases.

More recently, procedure-specific assessment tools have been created for gynecology. For example, the Vaginal Surgical Skills Index (VSSI) (Table 6.5) is a reliable and valid instrument to assess vaginal surgical skills. In a study conducted at two academic medical centers, trainees were directly assessed in the operating room by supervising surgeons while performing a vaginal hysterectomy. Assessment tools for this research included the VSSI, a GRS, and a visual analogue scale used to measure the trainees' overall surgical performance. Trainees were assessed again by the same surgeons 4 weeks after the live surgery and by a blinded outside reviewer using a videotape of the case. The researchers determined that VSSI scores correlated with global rating score and visual analogue scale scores. A higher VSSI score indicates better performance, and

TABLE 6.4 Modified Global Rating Index for Technical Skills

	1	2	3	4	5
1. Respect for tissue:	(Novice) Frequently used unnecessary force on tissue or caused damage by inappropriate use of instruments		(Competent) Careful handling of tissue but occasionally caused inadvertent damage		(Fully independent) Consistently handled tissues appropriately with minimal damage
2. Time and motion:	Many unnecessary moves		Efficient time/motion but some unnecessary moves		Clear economy of movement and maximum efficiency
3. Instrument handling:	Repeatedly makes tentative or awkward moves with instruments by inappropriate use of instruments		Competent use of instruments but occasionally appeared stiff or awkward		Fluid moves with instruments and no awkwardness
4. Knowledge of instrument:	Frequently asked for wrong instrument or used inappropriate instrument		Knew names of most instruments and used appropriate instrument		Obviously familiar with the instruments and their names
5. Flow of operation:	Frequently stopped operating and seemed unsure of next move		Demonstrated some forward planning with reasonable progression of procedure		Obviously planned course of operating with effortless flow from one move to the next
6. Use of assistants:	Consistently placed assistants poorly or failed to use assistants		Appropriate use of assistants most of the time		Strategically used assistants to the best advantage at all times
7. Knowledge of specific procedure:	Deficient knowledge. Needed specific instructions at most steps		Knew all important steps of operation		Demonstrated familiarity with all aspects of operation
8. Depth perception	Constantly overshoot, swings wide, slow correction		Some overshooting but quick to correct		Accurately directs instruments in correct plane
9. Bimanual dexterity	Uses only one hand, poor coordination between hands		Uses both hands but does not optimize their interaction		Expertly uses both hands to provide optimal exposure
10. Does the trainee demonstrate competency to perform this procedure independently? (circle one)	Yes No				
11. Overall, how prepared do you think you were for this procedure? (circle one):	Not at all prepared	Somewhat prepared	Adequately prepared	Very well prepared	Extremely prepared

TABLE 6.5 Vaginal Surgical Skills Index

Trainee's Name:

Date of Operation:

Procedure(s) the trainee performed:

Proportion of the procedure(s) that the trainee performed:

1. _____ ≤50 % or 50%
2. _____ ≤50 % or 50%
3. _____ ≤50 % or 50%

Please evaluate each trainee according to the criteria below and check the box that most corresponds to his or her performance.

	0	1	2	3	4	
1. Initial inspection (*check one*)	Incomplete and unsystematic inspection of relevant pelvic and vaginal structures	Partially complete and unsystematic inspection of relevant pelvic and vaginal structures	Complete but unsystematic inspection of relevant pelvic and vaginal structures	Complete and somewhat systematic inspection of relevant pelvic and vaginal structures	Systematic and complete assessment of relevant pelvic and vaginal structures	Not observed
2. Incision (*check one*)	Does not perform appropriate incision(s) safely and does not use incision(s) effectively ensuring optimal exposure	Incompletely performs appropriate incision(s) safely and does not use incision(s) effectively ensuring optimal exposure	Performs appropriate incision(s) safely but does not use incision(s) effectively ensuring optimal exposure	Performs appropriate incision(s) safely and partially uses incision(s) effectively ensuring optimal exposure	Performs appropriate incision(s) safely and uses incision(s) effectively ensuring optimal exposure	Not observed
3. Maintenance of visibility (*check one*)	Almost never or never obtains appropriate exposure	A few times (less than half the time) obtains appropriate exposure	Sometimes (about half the time) obtains appropriate exposure	Most time (more than half the time) obtains appropriate exposure	Almost always or always obtains appropriate exposure	Not observed
4. Use of assistants (check one)	Almost never or never strategically used assistant(s) to the best advantage	A few times (less than half the time) strategically uses assistant(s) to the best advantage	Sometimes (about half the time) strategically uses assistant(s) to the best advantage	Most time (more than half the time) strategically uses assistant(s) to the best advantage	Almost always or always strategically uses assistant(s) to the best advantage at all times	Not observed
5. Knowledge of instruments (check one)	Almost never or never uses and is familiar with correct instruments	A few times (less than half the time) uses and is familiar with correct instruments	Sometimes (about half the time) uses and is familiar with correct instruments	Most time (more than half the time) uses and is familiar with correct instruments	Almost always or always uses and is familiar with correct instruments	Not observed

(Continued)

TABLE 6.5 Vaginal Surgical Skills Index (Continued)

	0	1	2	3	4	
6. Tissue and instrument handling (*check one*)	Almost never or never appropriately handles tissue and instruments	A few times (less than half the time) appropriately handles tissue and instruments	Sometimes (about half the time) handles tissue and instruments appropriately	Most time (more than half the time) handles tissue and instruments appropriately	Almost always or always handles tissue and instruments appropriately	Not observed
7. Electrosurgery (check one)	Almost never or never uses electrosurgery safely and efficiently	A few times (less than half the time) uses electrosurgery safely and efficiently	Sometimes (about half the time) uses electrosurgery safely and efficiently	Most time (more than half the time) uses electrosurgery safely and efficiently	Almost always or always uses electrosurgery safely and efficiently	Not observed
8. Knot tying/ligation (*check one*)	Almost never or never quickly and correctly performs suture ligation and knot tying	A few times (less than half the time) quickly and correctly performs suture ligation and knot tying	Sometimes (about half the time) quickly and correctly performs suture ligation and knot tying	Most time (more than half the time) quickly and correctly performs suture ligation and knot tying	Almost always or always quickly and correctly performs suture ligation and knot tying	Not observed
9. Hemostasis (*check one*)	Almost never or never exposes bleeders and uses correct technique to obtain hemostasis safely and effectively	A few times (less than half the time) exposes bleeders and uses correct technique to obtain hemostasis safely and effectively	Sometimes (about half the time) exposes bleeders and uses correct technique to obtain hemostasis safely and effectively	Most time (more than half the time) exposes bleeders and uses correct technique to obtain hemostasis safely and effectively	Almost always or always exposes bleeders and uses correct technique to obtain hemostasis safely and effectively	Not observed
10. Procedure completion (*check one*)	Almost never or never completely removes fluid and debris and thoroughly inspects for bleeding	A few times (less than half the time) completely removes fluid and debris and thoroughly inspects for bleeding	Sometimes (about half the time) completely removes fluid and debris and thoroughly inspects for bleeding	Most times (more than half the time) completely removes fluid and debris and thoroughly inspects for bleeding	Almost always or always completely removes fluid and debris and thoroughly inspects for bleeding	Not observed
11. Time and motion (*check one*)	Almost never or never efficiently performs movements with no awkward or unnecessary moves	A few times (less than half the time) efficiently performs movements with no awkward or unnecessary moves	Sometimes (about half the time) efficiently performs movements with no awkward or unnecessary moves	Most time (more than half the time) efficiently performs movements with no awkward or unnecessary moves	Almost always or always efficiently performs movements with no awkward or unnecessary moves	Not observed

	0	1	2	3	4	
12. Flow of operation and forward planning (*check one*)	Almost never or never demonstrates forward planning allowing for proper flow of the procedure	A few times (less than half the time) demonstrates forward planning allowing for proper flow of the procedure	Sometimes (about half the time) demonstrates forward planning allowing for proper flow of the procedure	Most time (more than half the time) demonstrates forward planning allowing for proper flow of procedure	Almost always or always demonstrates forward planning allowing for proper flow of the procedure	Not observed
13. Knowledge of specific procedure (*check one*)	Almost never or never demonstrates familiarity with all aspects of the operation	A few times (less than half the time) demonstrated familiarity with all aspects of the operation	Sometimes (about half the time) demonstrates familiarity with all aspects of the operation	Most time (more than half the time) demonstrates familiarity with all aspects of the operation	Almost always or always demonstrates familiarity with all aspects of the operation	Not observed

Comments:

increasing VSSI scores significantly correlated with year of training and surgical volume (with an estimated increase in score of 0.3 per hysterectomy performed).

Simulation of surgical skills seems to offer an opportunity for a structured assessment of technical proficiency. Simulation exercises could potentially complement knowledge assessments, such as professional board examinations. However, the value of simulation-based assessment has not yet gained wide acceptance. An exception is in the board certification process for general surgeons. Since 2008, candidates for the American Board of Surgeons certification process have been required to complete the Fundamentals of Laparoscopic Surgery course, including a simulation exercise. Surgeons are not eligible for board certification until they have successfully completed this curriculum. This provides a potential model for the incorporation of surgical simulation exercises into the credentialing process.

In the future, credentialing bodies may require surgeons to demonstrate technical proficiency in a simulation environment. However, for such an assessment to be used in the assessment of surgeon quality, it would be necessary to demonstrate its construct validity, as well as the ability of raters to provide reproducible and consistent assessments of performance. In addition, members of the profession would have to agree that the tasks included in such an assessment are critical to surgical performance and representative of critical tasks in clinical practice. Nevertheless, this type of assessment seems desirable and potentially could play a role in a more comprehensive evaluation of surgeon proficiency.

At the present time, there is not a standard evaluation process for assessing surgeons as they progress through training, and the number of evaluations needed to determine competency in surgery has yet to be determined. Training programs are given guidance from the Accreditation Council for Graduate Medical Education (ACGME) with regard to the type of surgical cases residents should perform, and recently, the Residency Review Committee for Obstetrics and Gynecology has established minimal thresholds for surgical procedures at the residency level. However, ACGME notes that the achievement of the minimum numbers of listed procedures does not signify achievement of an individual resident's competence in a particular listed procedure. Therefore, each program is charged with the task of determining how, what, when, and how often residents need to have their surgical skills evaluated. The ACGME provides Reznick's GRS as an assessment instrument for evaluating surgical skills. Some surgical training programs have chosen to use a combination of structured simulation assessments, as well as global and procedure-specific evaluation tools. When and how often a learner is assessed is also variable; while some institutions require formal evaluation after every procedure, other programs only evaluate when a resident or fellow believes that he/she has achieved "competency" for a certain procedure and requests an assessment or at the end of a rotation. Also, it is not known how many surgeries are required before a surgeon becomes "competent" and can perform that particular surgery independently. Thus, residency requirements for surgical volume are not evidence based; there is limited evidence in the literature about the optimal number of cases needed to achieve or maintain competence. A study performed to establish minimum cutoff scores for intraoperative assessments using both the GRS and VSSI determined on average, trainees met cutoffs for competency after performing 21 and 27 vaginal hysterectomies, respectively. Obviously, more studies are needed to determine if an "ideal number" exists, given the variation of learning styles and that some surgical trainees acquire technical skills faster than others.

CHALLENGES IN SURGICAL EDUCATION

The challenges in resident surgical education include shrinking resources for the training of residents as well as an expanding variety of surgeries in the gynecologic armamentarium. Residents must master an increasing number of surgeries within a 4-year curriculum. For example, as the number of hysterectomies performed in the United States continues to decrease, the variety of approaches to hysterectomy has increased. Traditionally, gynecologists performed abdominal and vaginal hysterectomies. However, current practice also includes laparoscopic-assisted vaginal hysterectomy, total (and subtotal) laparoscopic hysterectomy, and robotic hysterectomy. The skills required for one of these approaches may not translate into proficiency with the alternative approaches. Thus, it is a challenge for a gynecologic resident to acquire adequate experience in all of these techniques during a 4-year residency.

Our profession also faces a challenge in the development of training options for practicing gynecologists who wish to expand their areas of expertise or to master a new surgical technique. Currently, there are limited opportunities for the acquisition of new surgical skills after residency. New techniques may be discussed at a postgraduate course, sometimes with an opportunity to practice on an inanimate model or in a cadaver laboratory. However, it is not obvious that this type of training translates into the effective mastery of a new skill or the successful incorporation of new skills into technical practice. Hospitals face the challenge of determining when an established surgeon should be considered sufficiently proficient as to allow surgical privileges. In addition, there are limited avenues for retraining surgeons who have been out of the profession for a period of time and for those who require remediation. Outside of a traditional residency training environment, such surgical "retraining" and proctoring raise a number of very complicated ethical, legal, and economic issues. Nevertheless, to insure that all women have access to expert surgical care, our profession must develop strategies for evaluating and monitoring surgical proficiency after the completion of residency training.

FUTURE DIRECTIONS

Apprenticeship Model to Structured Curriculum

Due in part to the increasing evidence that the traditional model of surgical education is not sufficient and due also to increasing concerns about the impact of work hour restrictions on surgical experience, more teaching intuitions are augmenting operating room experience with a formal surgical curricula. More than a decade ago, only 29% of US obstetrics and gynecology residency programs provided a formal surgical curriculum. In contrast, a more recent survey of obstetrician–gynecologist residencies indicated that more than two thirds had created some type of formal surgical curriculum. Of those, 62% had developed a curriculum specifically for laparoscopic skills. In addition, an increasing number of residency programs were using validated assessment tools for evaluating surgical skills.

Developing a formal surgical curriculum across residency programs would require a consensus about several key issues, including how and when skills are taught, which tasks are the most critical, and how to accurately assess competency. To avoid the inconsistencies inherently associated with training surgeons using the traditional apprenticeship model, a surgical curriculum cannot rely solely on "in operating room" surgical experiences. The ideal curriculum would augment operating room learning opportunities with a combination of lectures and simulation activities (possibly including bench models, animal laboratory, and/or computer simulation). Surgical simulation should have a strong focus on the acquisition, refinement, and formal assessment of fundamental surgical skills. Incorporating simulation models into residency and fellowship training will provide a safe, low-stress environment in which students can gain surgical skills and receive constructive feedback.

CONCLUSION

Surgical education continues to evolve through the standardization of surgical training, competency-based assessments, and evidence-based educational research. The historical teaching adage of "see one, do one, teach one" will soon be replaced with the new surgical teaching adage of "read about and see several," "do many first in a simulated environment with assessment" before operating room experience, and "teach using effective and constructive feedback." However, it is important to note that the mastery of surgical technical skills, which has been the focus of this chapter, is just one component of surgical competence. Training the gynecologic surgeon requires that we not only focus on the acquisition of clinical and technical skills but the development of surgeons with sound decision-making abilities, communication, leadership, and surgical skills capable of educating the next generation of surgeons.

BEST SURGICAL PRACTICES

- Although the regulatory agencies have created some guidelines for education in the surgical specialties, there is considerable latitude for optimization of the educational experience.
- Training the gynecologic surgeon should be based on evidence-based educational research and a structured curriculum to assure acquisition, refinement, and formal assessment of fundamental surgical skills.

BIBLIOGRAPHY

Accreditation Council for Graduate Medical Education. *Milestones.* ACGME, 2012.

Batholon S, Dorion D, Darveau S, et al. Cognitive skills analysis, kinesiology, and mental imagery in the acquisition of surgical skills. *J Otolaryngol* 2005;34:328.

Beard JD, Marriot J, Purdie H, et al. Assessing the surgical skills of trainees in the operating theatre: a prospective observational study of the methodology. *Health Technol Assess* 2011;15:i,1.

Bell RH Jr. Why Johnny cannot operate. *Surgery* 2009;146:533.

Bridges M, Diamond DL. The financial impact of teaching surgical residents in the operating room. *Am J Surg* 1999;177:28.

Buyske J. The role of simulation in certification. *Surg Clin North Am* 2010;90:619.

Carter BN. The fruition of Halsted's concept of surgical training. *Surgery* 1952;32:518.

Chen CC, Korn A, Klingele C, et al. Objective assessment of vaginal surgical skills. *Am J Obstet Gynecol* 2010;203:79.e1.

Chipman JG, Schmitz CC. Using objective structured assessment of technical skills to evaluate a basic skills simulation curriculum for first-year surgical residents. *J Am Coll Surg* 2009;209:364.

Chou B, Handa VL. Simulators and virtual reality in surgical education. *Obstet Gynecol Clin North Am* 2006;33:283.

Cohen SL, Chen CCG, Satin A. Use of simulators in gynecology. *Contemporary OB/GYN* 2010;55:30.

Denadai R, Oshiiwa M, Saad-Hossne R. Does bench model fidelity interfere in the acquisition of suture skills by novice medical students? *Rev Assoc Med Bras* 2012;58:600.

Doyle JD, Webber EM, Sidhu RS. A universal global rating scale for the evaluation of technical skills in the operating room. *Am J Surg* 2007;193:551; discussion 555.

Ericsson KA, Krampe RT, Tesch-Romer C. The role of deliberate practice in the acquisition of expert performance. *Psychol Rev* 1993;100:363.

Fenner D. Avoiding pitfalls: lessons in surgical teaching. *Obstet Gynecol Clin North Am* 2006;33:333.

Fitts PM, Posner MI. *Human performance.* Belmont, CA: Brooks/Cole Publishing, 1967.

Gurusamy KS, Aggarwal R, Palanivelu L, et al. Virtual reality training for surgical trainees in laparoscopic surgery. *Cochrane Database Syst Rev* 2009;(1):CD006575.

Halsted WS. The training of the surgeon. *Bull Johns Hopkins Hosp* 1904;15:267.

Komesu Y, Urwitz-Lane R, Ozel B, et al. Does mental imagery prior to cystoscopy make a difference? A randomized controlled trial. *Am J Obstet Gynecol* 2009;201:218.e1.

Lee JY, Mucksavage P, Sundaram CP, et al. Best practices for robotic surgery training and credentialing. *J Urol* 2011;185:1191.

Moulton CE, McRae H, Graham B, et al. Teaching surgical skills: what kind of practice makes perfect? A randomized, controlled trial. *Ann Surg* 2006;244:400.

Nasca TJ, Philbert I, Brigham T, et al. The next GME accreditation system—rationale and benefits. *N Engl J Med* 2012;366:1051. doi: 10.1056/NEJMsr1200117.

Pugh CM, DaRosa DA, Glenn D, et al. A comparison of faculty and resident perception of resident learning needs in the operating room. *J Surg Educ* 2007;64:250.

Reznick RK, MacRae H. Teaching surgical skills-changes in the wind. *N Engl J Med* 2006;355:2664.

Reznick R, Regehr G, MacRae H, et al. Testing technical skill via an innovative "bench station" examination. *Am J Surg* 1997;173:226.

Roberts NK, Williams RG, Kim MJ, et al. The briefing, intraoperative teaching, debriefing model for teaching in the operating room. *J Am Coll Surg* 2009;208:299.

Roberts NK, Brenner MJ, Williams RG, et al. Capturing the teachable moment: a grounded theory study of verbal teaching interactions in the operating room. *Surgery* 2012;151:643.

Rogers RG. Mental practice and acquisition of motor skills: examples from sports training and surgical education. *Obstet Gynecol Clin North Am* 2006;33:297.

Sanders CW, Sadoski M, Bramson R, et al. Comparing the effects of physical practice and mental imagery rehearsal on learning basic surgical skills by medical students. *Am J Obstet Gynecol* 2004;191:1811.

Smith CD. Teaching surgical techniques and procedures using advanced educational tools and concepts. *Asian J Surg* 2005;28:159.

Sullivan G, Simpson D, Cooney T, et al. A Milestone in the Milestones Movement: the JGME Milestones Supplement. *J of Graduate Med Ed* 2013;5:1.

Sutherland LM, Middleton PF, Anthony A, et al. Surgical simulation: a systematic review. *Ann Surg* 2006;243:291.

Van Sickle KR, Ritter EM, Smith CD. The pretrained novice: using simulation-based training to improve learning in the operating room. *Surg Innov* 2006;13:198.

PRINCIPLES OF ANATOMY AND PERIOPERATIVE CONSIDERATIONS

CHAPTER 7
Surgical Anatomy of the Female Pelvis

John O. L. DeLancey

DEFINITIONS

Endopelvic fascia—The endopelvic fascias are those tissues outside of the muscularis of the pelvic organs that attach these organs to the pelvic sidewall. There is also some extension of loose areolar tissue over the surfaces of the organ. The surgical fascia used by gynecologists during pelvic reconstructive surgery, however, is primarily composed of the muscularis of the vaginal wall.

Pelvic diaphragm—The term *pelvic diaphragm* refers to the levator ani muscle and its covering fasciae, both the superior fascia and the inferior fascia. The term *pelvic floor* refers to all of the supportive structures that are involved with pelvic organ support. Sometimes the term *pelvic floor* and *pelvic diaphragm* can be used interchangeably, especially in the British literature.

Pelvic spaces—The space between the bladder and the anterior portion of the pelvic walls is the perivesical space or space of Retzius. The space between the lower urinary tract and the genital tract is the vesicovaginal or vesicocervical space. This is bounded laterally by the "bladder pillars," which is the region in which the tissues that go to the vagina separate from those that go to the bladder base. The rectovaginal space lies between the posterior vaginal wall and the anterior surface of the rectum, and lies primarily above the top of the perineal body.

Urethra and vesicle neck—The urethra is that portion of the lower urinary tract outside of the bladder that the urethral lumen traverses. That portion of the urethra lumen that is surrounded by the bladder vasculature is referred to as the vesicle neck.

Urinary trigone—The urinary trigone is a triangular visible area in the bladder, the apices of which are the ureteral orifices and the internal urinary meatus. This is a layer of smooth muscle connecting the ureters and the urethra, the edges of which are visible cystoscopically and when the bladder is open.

VULVA AND ERECTILE STRUCTURES

The bony pelvic outlet is bordered by the ischiopubic rami anteriorly and the coccyx and sacrotuberous ligaments posteriorly. It can be divided into anterior and posterior triangles, which share a common base along a line between the ischial tuberosities. The tissues filling the anterior triangle have a layered structure similar to that of the abdominal wall (Table 7.1). There is a skin and adipose layer (vulva) overlying a fascial layer (perineal membrane) that lies superficial to a muscular layer (levator ani muscles).

Subcutaneous Tissues of the Vulva

The structures of the vulva lie on the pubic bones and extend caudally under the pubic arch (Fig. 7.1). They consist of the mons, labia, clitoris, vestibule, and associated erectile structures and their muscles. The mons consists of hair-bearing skin over a cushion of adipose tissue that lies on the pubic bones. Extending posteriorly from the mons, the labia majora are composed of similar hair-bearing skin and adipose tissue, which contain the termination of the round ligaments of the uterus and the obliterated processus vaginalis (canal of Nuck). The round ligament can give rise to leiomyomas in this region, and the obliterated processus vaginalis can be a dilated embryonic remnant in the adult.

The labia minora, vestibule, and glans clitoris can be seen between the two labia majora. The labia minora are hairless skin folds, each of which splits anteriorly to run over, and under, the glans of the clitoris. The more anterior folds unite to form the hood-shaped prepuce of the clitoris, whereas the posterior folds insert into the underside of the glans as the frenulum.

Unlike the skin of the labia majora, the cutaneous structures of the labia minora and vestibule do not lie on an adipose layer but on a connective tissue stratum that is loosely organized and permits mobility of the skin during intercourse. This loose attachment of the skin to underlying tissues allows the skin to be easily dissected off the underlying fascia during skinning vulvectomy in the area of the labia minora and vestibule.

In the posterior lateral aspect of the vestibule, the duct of the major vestibular gland can be seen 3 to 4 mm outside

TABLE 7.1 Layers of the Anterior Triangle of the Perineum

Skin
Subcutaneous tissue
    Camper fascia
    Colles fascia
Superficial space
    Clitoris and its crura
    Ischiocavernous muscle
    Vestibular bulb
    Bulbocavernous muscle
    Greater vestibular gland
    Superficial transverse perineal muscle
Deep space-perineal membrane
    Compressor urethrae
    Urethrovaginal sphincter

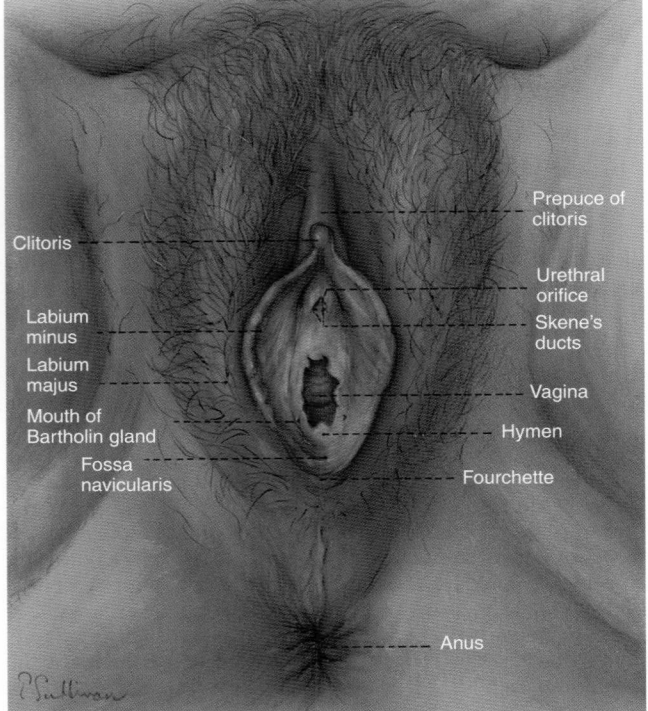

FIGURE 7.1 External genitalia.

the hymenal ring. The minor vestibular gland openings are found along a line extending anteriorly from this point, parallel to the hymenal ring and extending toward the urethral orifice. The urethra bulges slightly around the surrounding vestibular skin anterior to the vagina and posterior to the clitoris. Its orifice is flanked on either side by two small labia. Skene ducts open into the inner aspect of these labia and can be seen as small, punctate openings when the urethral labia are separated.

Within the skin of the vulva are specialized glands that can become enlarged and thereby require surgical removal. The holocrine sebaceous glands in the labia majora are associated with hair shafts, and in the labia minora, they are freestanding. They lie close to the surface, which explains their easy recognition with minimal enlargement. In addition, lateral to the introitus and anus, there are numerous apocrine sweat glands, along with the normal eccrine sweat glands. The former structures undergo change with the menstrual cycle, having increased secretory activity in the premenstrual period. They can become chronically infected, as in hidradenitis suppurativa, or neoplastically enlarged, as in hidradenomas, both of which may require surgical therapy. The eccrine sweat glands in the vulvar skin rarely present abnormalities, but on occasion form palpable masses as syringomas.

The subcutaneous tissue of the labia majora is similar in composition to that of the abdominal wall. It consists of lobules of fat interlaced with connective tissue septa. Although there are no well-defined layers in the subcutaneous tissue, regional variations in the relative quantity of fat and fibrous tissue exist. The superficial region of this tissue, where fat predominates, has been called Camper fascia, as it is on the abdomen. In this region, there is a continuation of fat from the anterior abdominal wall, called the digital process of fat.

In the deeper layers of the vulva, there is less fat, and the interlacing fibrous connective tissue septa are much more

evident than those in Camper fascia. This more fibrous layer is called Colles fascia and is similar to Scarpa fascia on the abdomen. Its interlacing fibrous septa of the subcutaneous tissue attach laterally to the ischiopubic rami and fuse posteriorly with the posterior edge of the perineal membrane (i.e., urogenital diaphragm). Anteriorly, however, there is no connection to the pubic rami, and this permits communication between the area deep to this layer and the abdominal wall. These fibrous attachments to the ischiopubic rami and the posterior aspect of the perineal membrane limit the spread of hematomas or infection in this compartment posterolaterally but allow spread into the abdomen. This clinical observation has led to the consideration of Colles fascia as a separate entity from the superficial Camper fascia, which lacks these connections.

Superficial Compartment

The space between the subcutaneous tissues and perineal membrane, which contains the clitoris, crura, vestibular bulbs, and ischiocavernous and bulbocavernosus muscles, is called the superficial compartment of the perineum (Fig. 7.2). The deep compartment is the region just above the perineal membrane; it is discussed later.

The erectile bodies and their associated muscles within the superficial compartment lie on the caudal surface of the perineal membrane. The clitoris is composed of a midline shaft (body) capped with the glans. This shaft lies on, and is suspended from, the pubic bones by a subcutaneous suspensory ligament. The paired crura of the clitoris bend downward from the shaft and are firmly attached to the pubic bones, continuing dorsally to lie on the inferior aspects of the pubic rami. The ischiocavernous muscles originate at the ischial tuberosities and the free surfaces of the crura to insert on the upper crura and body of the clitoris. A few muscle fibers, called the superficial transverse perineal muscles, originate in common with the ischiocavernous muscle from the ischial tuberosity and lie medial to the perineal body.

The paired vestibular bulbs lie immediately under the vestibular skin and are composed of erectile tissue. They are covered by the bulbocavernosus muscles, which originate in the perineal body and lie over their lateral surfaces. These muscles, along with the ischiocavernous muscles, insert into the body of the clitoris and act to pull it downward.

The Bartholin greater vestibular gland is found at the tail end of the bulb of the vestibule and is connected to the vestibular mucosa by a duct lined with squamous epithelium. The gland lies on the perineal membrane and beneath the bulbocavernosus muscle. The intimate relation between the enormously vascular erectile tissue of the vestibular bulb and the Bartholin gland is responsible for the hemorrhage associated with removal of this latter structure.

The perineal membrane and perineal body are important to the support of the pelvic organs. They are discussed in the section on the pelvic floor.

Pudendal Nerve and Vessels

The pudendal nerve is the sensory and motor nerve of the perineum. Its course and distribution in the perineum parallel the pudendal artery and veins that connect with the internal iliac vessels (Fig. 7.3). The course and division of the nerve are described with the understanding that the vascular channels parallel them.

The pudendal nerve arises from the sacral plexus (S2–S4), and the vessels originate from the anterior division of the internal iliac artery. They leave the pelvis through the greater sciatic foramen by hooking around the ischial spine and

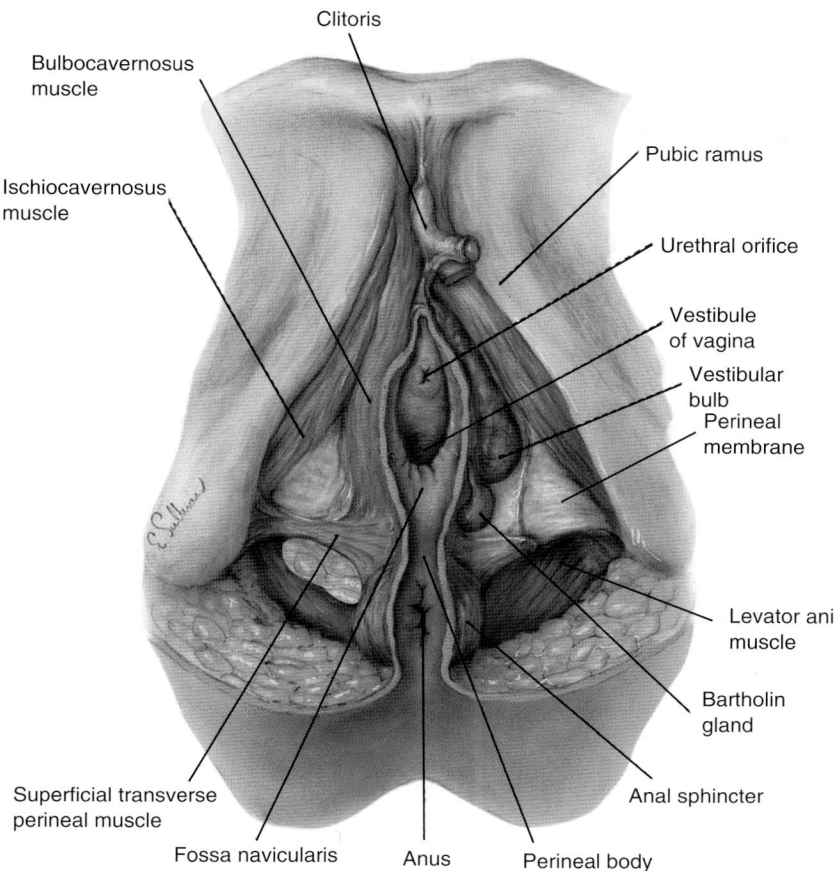

FIGURE 7.2 Superficial compartment and perineal membrane.

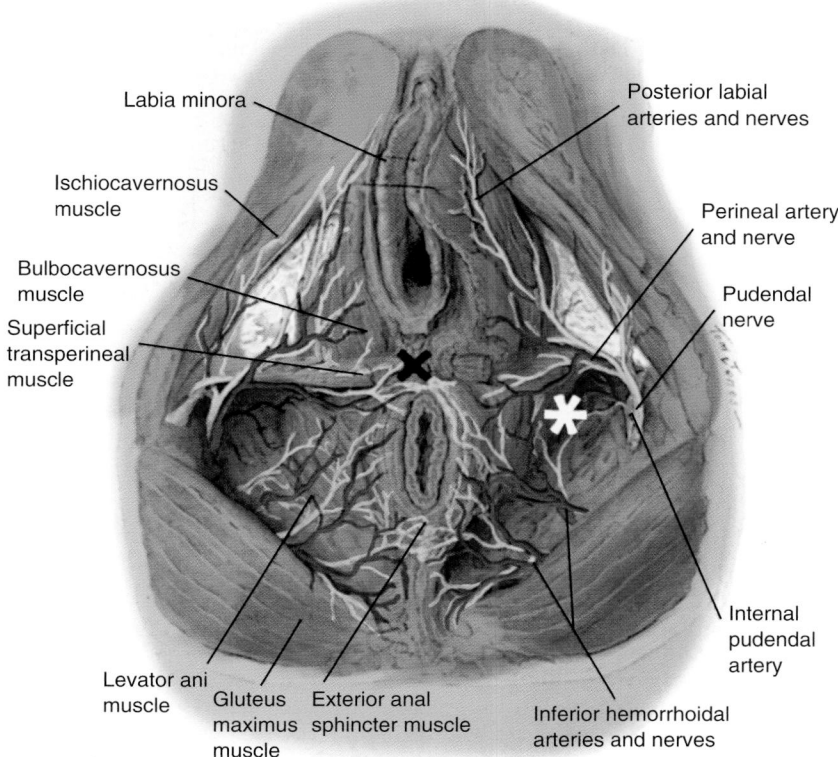

FIGURE 7.3 Pudendal nerve and vessels, with the position of the ischiorectal fossa (*asterisk*) and the perineal body (×) indicated. (From Anson BJ. *An atlas of human anatomy*. Philadelphia, PA: WB Saunders, 1950, with permission.)

sacrospinous ligament to enter the pudendal (Alcock) canal through the lesser sciatic foramen.

The nerve and vessels have three branches: the clitoral, perineal, and inferior hemorrhoidal. The clitoral branch lies on the perineal membrane along its path to supply the clitoris. The perineal branch (the largest of the three branches) enters the subcutaneous tissues of the vulva behind the perineal membrane. Here, it supplies the bulbocavernosus, ischiocavernous, and transverse perineal muscles. It also supplies the skin of the inner portions of the labia majora, labia minora, and vestibule. The inferior hemorrhoidal branch goes to the external anal sphincter and perianal skin.

Lymphatic Drainage

The pattern of the vulvar lymphatic vessels and drainage into the superficial inguinal group of lymph nodes has been established by both injection studies and clinical observation. It is important to the treatment of vulvar malignancies; an overview of this system is provided here. This area is described and illustrated in more detail in Chapter 33.

Tissues external to the hymenal ring are supplied by an anastomotic series of vessels in the superficial tissues that coalesce to a few trunks lateral to the clitoris and proceed laterally to the superficial inguinal nodes (Fig. 7.4). The vessels draining the labia majora also run in an anterior direction, lateral to those of the labia minora and vestibule. These lymphatic channels lie medial to the labiocrural fold, establishing it as the lateral border of surgical resection.

Injection studies of the urethral lymphatics have shown that lymphatic drainage of this region terminates in either the right or left inguinal nodes. The clitoris has been said to have some direct drainage to deep pelvic lymph nodes, bypassing the usual superficial nodes, but the clinical significance of this appears to be minimal.

The inguinal lymph nodes are divided into two groups—the superficial and the deep nodes. There are 12 to 20 superficial nodes, and they lie in a T-shaped distribution parallel to and 1 cm below the inguinal ligament, with the stem extending down along the saphenous vein. The nodes are often divided into four quadrants, with the center of the division at the saphenous opening. The vulvar drainage goes primarily to the medial nodes of the upper quadrant. These nodes lie deep in the adipose layer of the subcutaneous tissues, in the membranous layer, just superficial to the fascia lata.

The large saphenous vein joins the femoral vein through the saphenous opening. Within 2 cm of the inguinal ligament, several superficial blood vessels branch from the saphenous vein and femoral artery. They include the superficial epigastric vessels that supply the subcutaneous tissues of the lower abdomen; the superficial circumflex iliac vessels that course laterally to the region of the iliac crest; and the superficial external pudendal vessels that supply the mons, labia majora, and clitoral hood.

Lymphatics from the superficial nodes enter the fossa ovalis and drain into one to three deep inguinal nodes, which lie in the femoral canal of the femoral triangle. They pass through the fossa ovalis (saphenous opening) in the fascia lata, which lies approximately 3 cm below the inguinal ligament, lateral to the pubic tubercle, along with the saphenous vein on its way to the femoral vein. The membranous layer of the subcutaneous tissues spans this opening as a trabeculate layer called a fascia cribrosa, pierced by lymphatics. The deep nodes are found under this fascia in the femoral triangle.

The femoral triangle is the subfascial space of the upper one third of the thigh. It is bounded by the inguinal ligament, sartorius muscle, and adductor longus muscle. Its floor is formed by the pectineal, adductor longus, and iliopsoas muscles. The femoral artery bisects it vertically between the anterosuperior iliac spine and pubic tubercle. The femoral vein lies medial to the artery; the femoral nerve is lateral to it.

As these vessels pass under the inguinal ligament, they carry with them an extension of the transversalis fascia, which is the extraperitoneal connective tissue deep to the rectus abdominis muscle called the femoral sheath. These sheaths extend about 2 to 3 cm below the inguinal ligament before fusing with the vascular adventitia. Besides the two parts of the femoral sheath that accompany these vessels, a third portion—the femoral canal—can be found in the space medial to the vein. The abdominal opening of this is the femoral ring. The femoral canal contains the deep inguinal lymph nodes. Lymph channels from these nodes pierce the membrane, filling the femoral ring to communicate with the external iliac nodes. Also within this region, the femoral vessels give rise to the deep external pudendal vessels. The external pudendal vessels run deep to the femoral vein over the pectineal muscle to pierce the fascia lata. Here, they become subcutaneous and form anastomoses

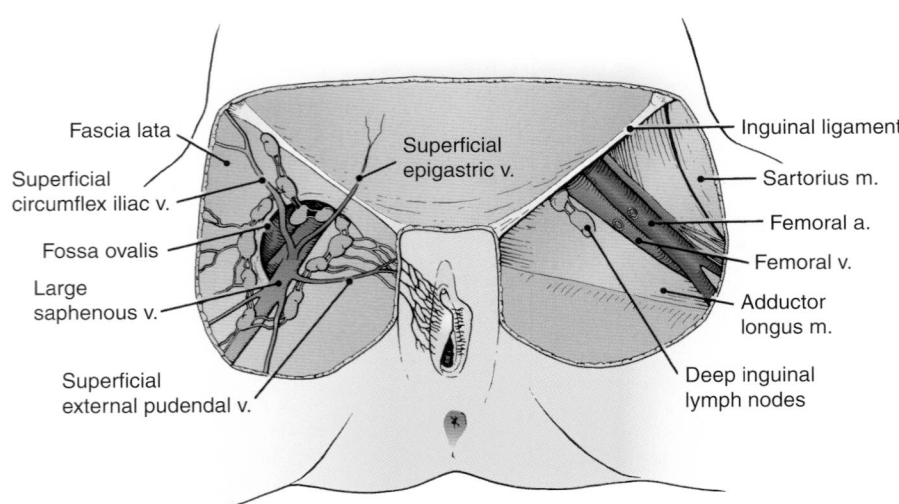

Fascia lata
Superficial circumflex iliac v.
Fossa ovalis
Large saphenous v.
Superficial external pudendal v.
Superficial epigastric v.
Inguinal ligament
Sartorius m.
Femoral a.
Femoral v.
Adductor longus m.
Deep inguinal lymph nodes

FIGURE 7.4 Lymphatic drainage of the vulva and femoral triangle. Superficial inguinal nodes are shown in the right thigh, and deep inguinal nodes are shown in the left thigh. Fascia lata has been removed on the left.

with branches of the internal pudendal vessels as well as the deep femoral and lateral circumflex femoral arteries.

THE PELVIC FLOOR

When humans assumed the upright posture, the opening in the bony pelvis came to lie at the bottom of the abdominopelvic cavity. This required the evolution of a supportive system to prevent the pelvic organs from being pushed downward through this opening. In the woman, this system must withstand these downward forces but allow for the passage of the large and cranially dominant human fetus. The supportive system that has evolved to meet these needs consists of a fibromuscular floor that forms a shelf spanning the pelvic outlet and that contains a cleft for the birth canal and excretory drainage. A series of visceral ligaments and fasciae tethers the organs and maintains their position over the closed portions of the floor. The floor consists of the levator ani muscles and perineal membrane. The openings in these structures for parturition and elimination have required the development of ancillary fibrous elements that are concentrated over open areas in the muscular floor to support the viscera in these weak areas. This section discusses the structures of the pelvic floor; the fibrous supportive system is described in the section on the pelvic viscera and cleavage planes and fascia.

Perineal Membrane (Urogenital Diaphragm)

The perineal membrane forms the inferior portion of the anterior pelvic floor. It is a triangular sheet of dense, fibromuscular tissue that spans the anterior half of the pelvic outlet (Fig. 7.2). It was previously called the urogenital diaphragm, and this change in name reflects the appreciation that it is not a two-layered structure with muscle in between, as was previously thought. It lies just caudal to the skeletal muscle of the striated urogenital sphincter (formerly the deep transverse perineal muscle). Because of the presence of the vagina, the perineal membrane cannot form a continuous sheet to close off the anterior pelvis in the woman, as it does in the man. It does provide support for the posterior vaginal wall by attaching the perineal body and vagina and perineal body to the ischiopubic rami, thereby limiting their downward descent. This layer of

the floor arises from the inner aspect of the inferior ischiopubic rami above the ischiocavernous muscles and the crura of the clitoris. The medial attachments of the perineal membrane are to the urethra, walls of the vagina, and perineal body.

Just cephalad to the perineal membrane lie two arch-shaped muscles that begin posteriorly to arch over the urethra (Fig. 7.5). These are the compressor urethral and the urethrovaginal sphincters. They are a part of the striated urogenital sphincter muscle in the woman and are continuous with the sphincter urethrae muscle. They act to compress the distal urethra. Posteriorly, intermingled within the membrane are skeletal muscle fibers of the transverse vaginal muscle and some smooth muscle fibers. The dorsal and deep nerve and vessels of the clitoris are also found within this membrane and are described later.

The primary function of the perineal membrane is related to its attachment to the vagina and perineal body. By attaching these structures to the bony pelvic outlet, the perineal membrane supports the pelvic floor against the effects of increases in intra-abdominal pressure and against the effects of gravity. The pubococcygeal and puborectal portions of the levator ani muscles lie just at the upper margin of the perineal membrane contacting its cranial surface. Contraction of these muscles elevates the medial margin of the perineal membrane along with the vagina and relaxation allows for its caudal movement. The amount of downward descent that is permitted by the connections of the perineal membrane to the midline structures can be assessed during an examination under anesthesia by placing a finger in the rectum, hooking it forward, and gently pulling the perineal body downward. If the perineal membrane has been torn during parturition, then an abnormal amount of descent is detectable, and the pelvic floor sags and the introitus gapes.

Perineal Body

Within the area bounded by the lower vagina, perineal skin, and anus is a mass of connective tissue called the perineal body (Fig. 7.3). The term *central tendon of the perineum* has also been applied to this structure and is descriptive, suggesting its role as a central point into which many muscles insert.

The perineal body is attached to the inferior pubic rami and ischial tuberosities through the perineal membrane and

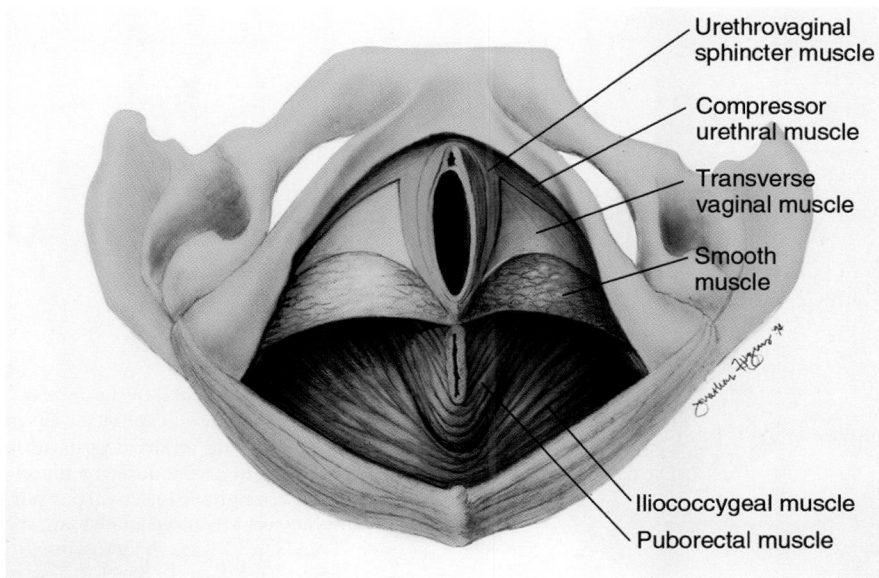

FIGURE 7.5 Structures visible after removal of the perineal membrane and superficial perineal muscles. (Copyright 1995 John O. L. DeLancey, with permission.)

Urethrovaginal sphincter muscle

Compressor urethral muscle

Transverse vaginal muscle

Smooth muscle

Iliococcygeal muscle

Puborectal muscle

superficial transverse perineal muscles. Anterolaterally, it receives the insertion of the bulbocavernosus muscles. On its lateral margins, the upper portions of the perineal body are connected with some fibers of the pelvic diaphragm. Posteriorly, the perineal body is indirectly attached to the coccyx by the external anal sphincter that is embedded in the perineal body, and it is attached at its other end to the coccyx. These connections anchor the perineal body and its surrounding structures to the bony pelvis and help to keep it in place.

Posterior Triangle: Ischiorectal Fossa

In the posterior triangle of the pelvis, the ischiorectal fossa lies between the pelvic walls and the levator ani muscles (**Fig. 7.3**). It has an anterior recess that lies above the perineal membrane. It is bounded medially by the levator ani muscles and anterolaterally by the obturator internus muscle. The main portion of the fossa is lateral to the levator ani and external anal sphincter, and it has a posterior portion that extends above the gluteus maximus. Traversing this region is the pudendal neurovascular trunk.

Anal Sphincters

The external sphincter lies in the posterior triangle of the perineum (**Fig. 7.6**). It is a single mass of muscle that has traditionally been divided into superficial and deep portions. The subcutaneous portion lies attached to the perianal skin and forms an encircling ring around the anal canal. It is responsible for the characteristic radially oriented folds in the perianal skin. The superficial part attaches to the coccyx posteriorly and sends a few fibers into the perineal body anteriorly and forms the bulk of the anal sphincter seen separated in third-degree midline obstetric tears. The fibers of the deep part generally encircle the rectum and blend indistinguishably with the puborectalis, which forms a loop under the dorsal surface of the anorectum and which is attached anteriorly to the pubic bone (**Fig. 7.6**).

The internal anal sphincter is a thickening in the circular smooth muscle of the anal wall. It lies just inside the external anal sphincter and is separated from it by a visible intersphincteric groove. It extends downward inside the external anal sphincter to within a few millimeters of the external sphincter's caudal extent. The internal sphincter can be identified

just beneath the anal submucosa in repair of a chronic fourth-degree laceration of the perineum as a rubbery white layer that is often erroneously been referred to as fascia during obstetrical repair of fourth-degree laceration. The longitudinal smooth muscle layer of the bowel, along with some fibers of the levator ani, separates the external and internal sphincters as they descend in the intersphincteric groove.

Levator Ani and Pelvic Wall

The typical depiction of the levator ani muscles in anatomy textbooks is unfortunately distorted by the extreme abdominal pressures generated during embalming that forces them downward. Many of these illustrations therefore fail to give a true picture of the horizontal nature of this strong supportive shelf of muscle. Examination of the normal standing patient is the best way to appreciate the nature of this closure mechanism, because the lithotomy position causes some relaxation of the musculature. During routine pelvic examination of the nullipara, the effectiveness of this closure can be appreciated, because it is often difficult to insert a speculum if the muscles are contracted and not relaxed.

The pelvic canal is spanned by the muscles of the pelvic diaphragm. This diaphragm consists of two components: (a) a thin horizontal shelf-like layer formed by the iliococcygeal muscle and (b) a thicker "U"-shaped sling of muscles that surround the levator hiatus that include the medial pubococcygeal and lateral puborectal muscles (**Fig. 7.7**). The open area within the U through which the urethra, vagina, and rectum pass is called the levator hiatus, and the portion of the hiatus anterior to the perineal body is called the urogenital hiatus.

The pubococcygeal muscle arises from a thin aponeurotic attachment to the inner surface of the pubic bone and inserts to the distal lateral vagina, perineal body, and anus. Some fibers also attach to the superior surface of the coccyx; hence the name pubococcygeus. Because the majority of the attachments, however, are to the vagina and anus, the term pubovisceral muscle is replacing this older term. The puborectal muscle is distinct from the pubococcygeal muscle and lies lateral to it. Its fibers originate from the lower pubis and some from the top of the perineal membrane. The muscle fibers pass beside the rectum forming a sling behind the anorectal junction.

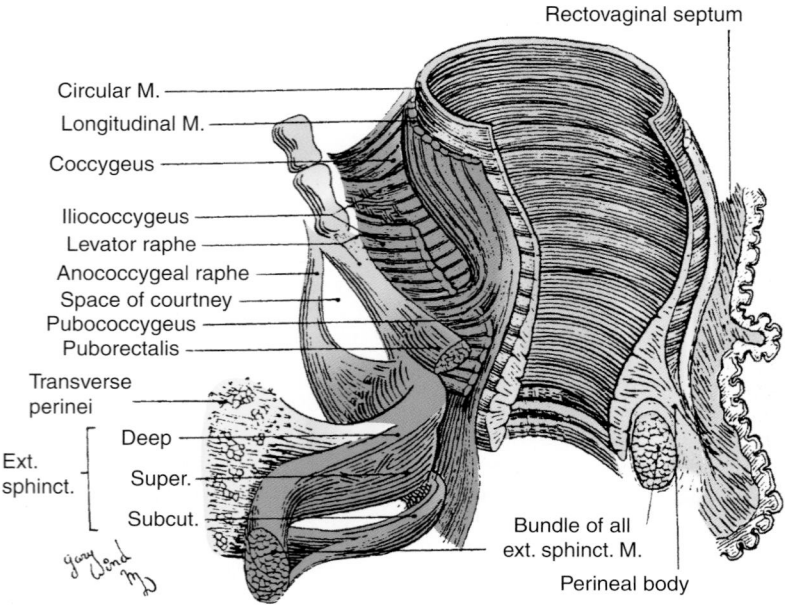

Labels on figure:
- Rectovaginal septum
- Circular M.
- Longitudinal M.
- Coccygeus
- Iliococcygeus
- Levator raphe
- Anococcygeal raphe
- Space of courtney
- Pubococcygeus
- Puborectalis
- Transverse perinei
- Ext. sphinct.
- Deep
- Super.
- Subcut.
- Bundle of all ext. sphinct. M.
- Perineal body

FIGURE 7.6 Semidiagrammatic dissection of the anorectal region in the woman with the external sphincter cut in the anterior midsagittal plane and reflected posteriorly (mucosa removed). The origin of the anterior muscle bundle is clarified, and the remaining anterolateral portions of the external sphincters are interdigitated into the transverse perinei. (From Oh C, Kark AE. Anatomy of the external anal sphincter. *Br J Surg* 1972;59:717, with permission.)

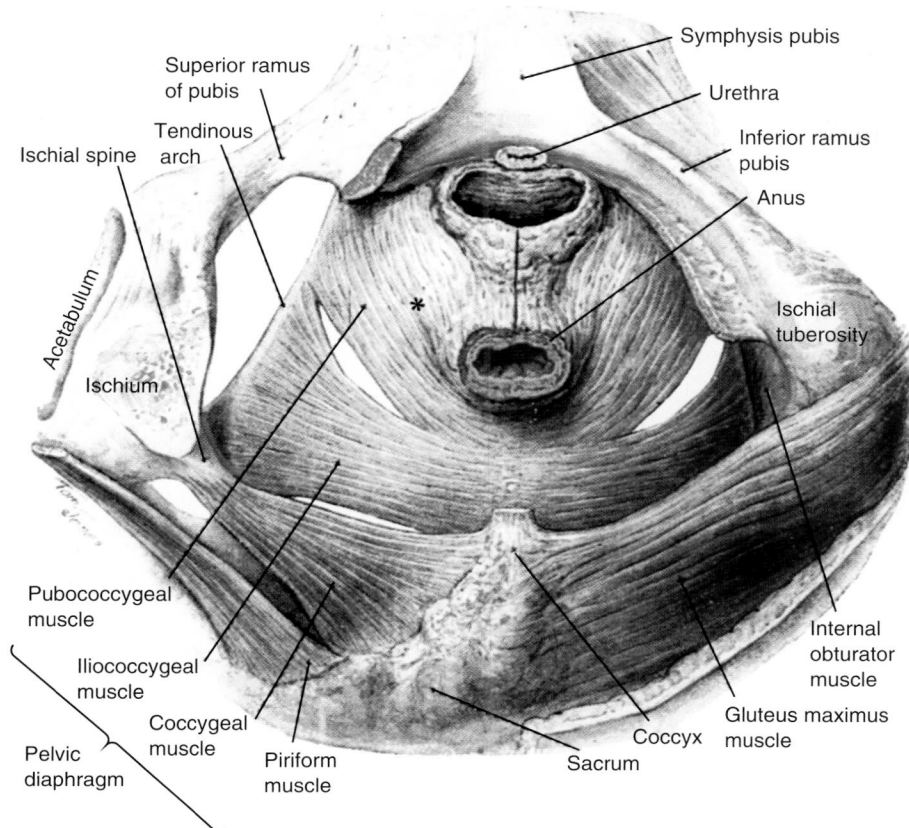

Symphysis pubis

Urethra

Inferior ramus
pubis

Anus

Ischial
tuberosity

Superior ramus
of pubis

Tendinous
arch

Ischial spine

Acetabulum

Ischium

Pubococcygeal
muscle

Iliococcygeal
muscle

Coccygeal
muscle

Pelvic
diaphragm

Piriform
muscle

Sacrum

Coccyx

Gluteus maximus
muscle

Internal
obturator
muscle

FIGURE 7.7 Anatomy of the pelvic floor. The *asterisk* indicates the puborectalis portion of the levator ani muscle. (From Anson BJ. *An atlas of human anatomy.* Philadelphia, PA: WB Saunders, 1950, with permission.)

The iliococcygeal muscle arises from a fibrous band overlying the obturator internus called the arcus tendineus levatoris ani. From these broad origins, the fibers of the iliococcygeal muscle pass behind the rectum and insert into the midline anococcygeal raphe and the coccyx. The coccygeal muscle arises from the ischial spine and sacrospinous ligament to insert into the borders of the coccyx and the lowest segment of the sacrum.

These muscles are covered on their superior and inferior surfaces by superior and inferior fasciae. When the levator ani muscles and their fasciae are considered together, they are called the pelvic diaphragm, not to be confused with the urogenital diaphragm (perineal membrane).

The normal tone of the muscles of the pelvic diaphragm keep the base of the U pressed against the backs of the pubic bones, keeping the vagina and rectum closed. The region of the levator ani between the anus and coccyx formed by the anococcygeal raphe (see previous discussion) is clinically called the levator plate. It forms a supportive shelf on which the rectum, upper vagina, and uterus can rest. The relatively horizontal position of this shelf is determined by the anterior traction on the fibrous levator plane by the pubococcygeal and puborectal muscles and is important to vaginal and uterine support.

The levator ani muscles receive their innervation from an anterior branch of the ventral ramus of the third and fourth sacral nerves called, appropriately, the nerve to the levator ani. Some aspects of the puborectal muscle may also receive a small contribution to the inferior hemorrhoidal branch of the pudendal nerve.

This section on the pelvic viscera discusses the structure of the individual pelvic organs and considers specific aspects of their interrelations (Fig. 7.8). Those aspects of blood supply, innervation, and lymphatic drainage that are idiosyncratic to the specific pelvic viscera are covered here. However, the

section on the retroperitoneum, where the overall description of these systems is given, provides the general consideration of these latter three topics.

Genital Structures

Vagina

The vagina is a pliable hollow viscus with a shape that is determined by the structures surrounding it and by its attachments to the pelvic wall. These attachments are to the lateral margins of the vagina, so that its lumen is a transverse slit, with the anterior and posterior walls in contact with one another. The lower portion of the vagina is constricted as it passes through the urogenital hiatus in the levator ani. The upper part is much more capacious. The vagina is bent at an angle of 120 degrees by the anterior traction of the levator ani muscles at the junction of the lower one third and upper two thirds of the vagina (Fig. 7.9). The cervix typically lies within the anterior vaginal wall, making it shorter than the posterior wall by about 3 cm. The former is about 7 to 9 cm in length, although there is great variability in this dimension.

When the lumen of the vagina is inspected through the introitus, many landmarks can be seen. The anterior and posterior walls have a midline ridge, called the anterior and posterior columns, respectively. These are caused by the impression of the urethra and bladder and the rectum on the vaginal lumen. The caudal portion of the anterior column is distinct and is called the urethral carina. The recesses in front of and behind the cervix are commonly called the anterior and posterior fornices of the vagina, and the creases along the side of the vagina, where the anterior and posterior walls meet, are called the lateral vaginal sulci.

The vagina's relations to other parts of the body can be understood by dividing it into thirds. In the lower third, the

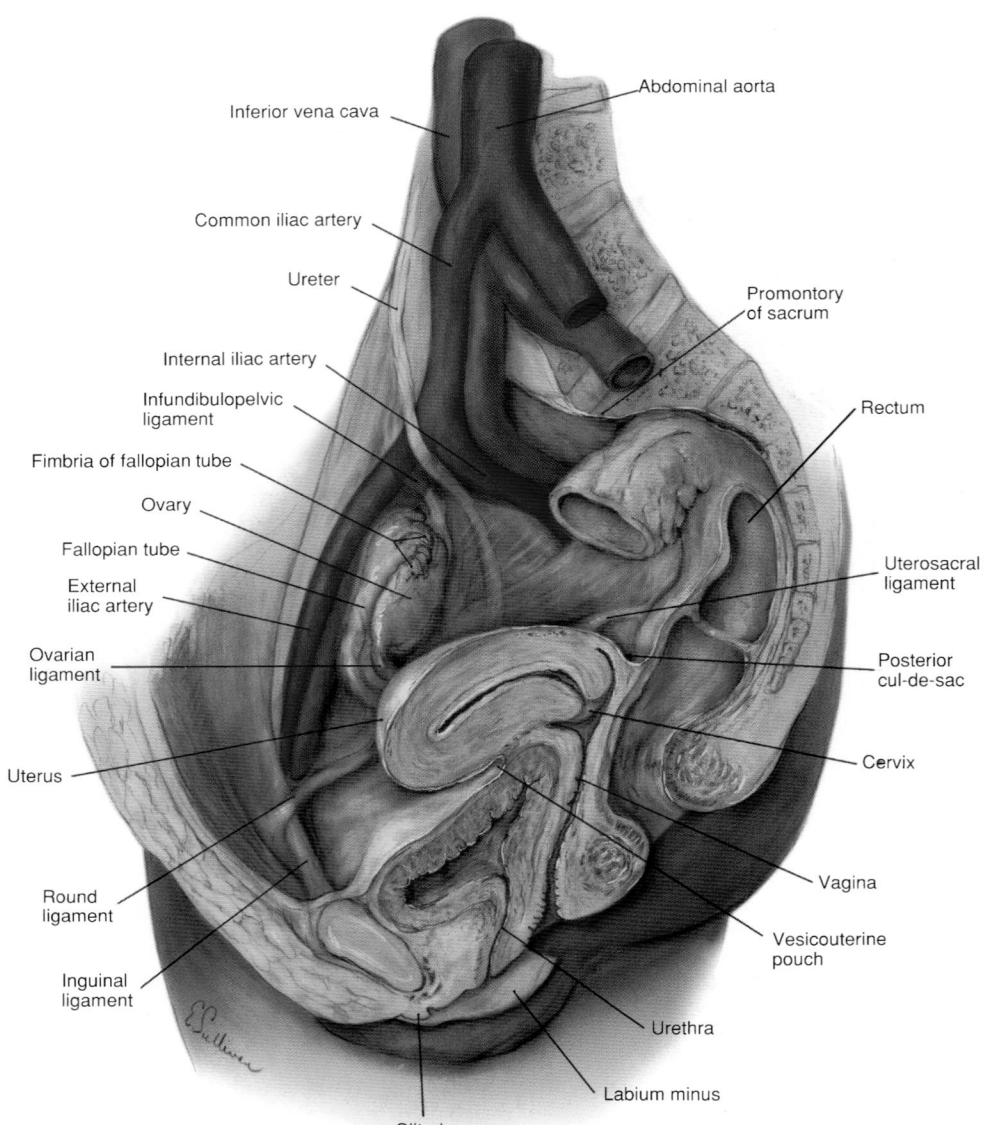

Inferior vena cava

Common iliac artery

Ureter

Internal iliac artery

Infundibulopelvic ligament

Fimbria of fallopian tube

Ovary

Fallopian tube

External iliac artery

Ovarian ligament

Uterus

Round ligament

Inguinal ligament

Clitoris

Labium minus

Urethra

Vesicouterine pouch

Vagina

Cervix

Posterior cul-de-sac

Uterosacral ligament

Rectum

Promontory of sacrum

Abdominal aorta

FIGURE 7.8 The pelvic viscera.

vagina is fused anteriorly with the urethra, posteriorly with the perineal body, and laterally to each levator ani by the "fibers of Luschka." In the middle third are the vesical neck and trigone anteriorly, the rectum posteriorly, and the levators laterally. In the upper third, the anterior vagina is adjacent to the bladder and ureters (which allow these latter structures to be palpated on pelvic examination), posterior to the cul-de-sac, and lateral to the cardinal ligaments of the vagina.

The vaginal wall contains the same layers as all hollow viscera (i.e., mucosa, submucosa, muscularis, and adventitia). Except for the area covered by the cul-de-sac, it has no serosal covering. The mucosa is of the nonkeratinized stratified squamous type and lies on a dense, dermislike submucosa. The similarity of these layers to dermis and epidermis has resulted in their being called the "vaginal skin."

The vaginal muscularis is fused with the submucosa, and the pattern of the muscularis is a bihelical arrangement. Outside the muscularis, there is an adventitia that has varying degrees of development in different areas of the vagina. This layer is a portion of the connective tissue in the pelvis called the endopelvic fascia and has been given a separate name because of its unusual

development. When it is dissected in the operating room, the muscularis is usually adherent to it, and this combination of specialized adventitia and muscularis is the surgeon's "fascia," which might better be called the fibromuscular layer of the vagina, as Nichols and Randall suggested in *Vaginal Surgery*.

Uterus

The uterus is a fibromuscular organ with shape, weight, and dimensions that vary considerably, depending on both estrogenic stimulation and previous parturition. It has two portions: an upper muscular corpus and a lower fibrous cervix. In a woman of reproductive age, the corpus is considerably larger than the cervix, but before menarche, and after the menopause, their sizes are similar. Within the corpus, there is a triangularly shaped endometrial cavity surrounded by a thick muscular wall. That portion of the corpus that extends above the top of the endometrial cavity (i.e., above the insertions of the fallopian tubes) is called the fundus.

The muscle fibers that make up most of the uterine corpus are not arranged in a simple layered manner, as is true

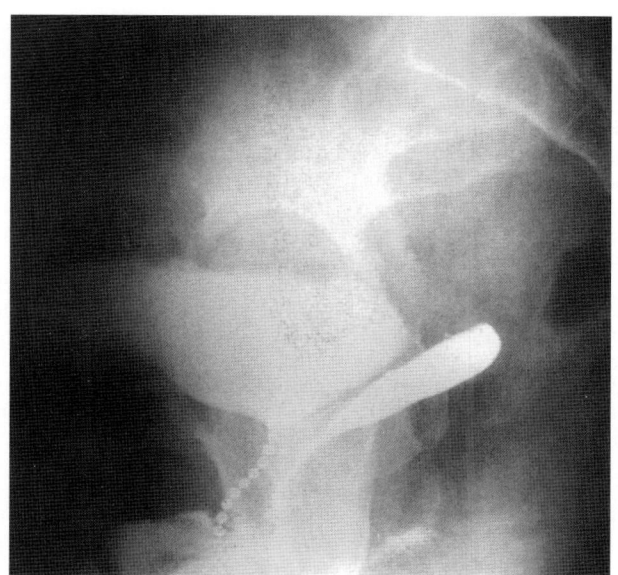

FIGURE 7.9 Bead chain cystourethrogram with barium in the vagina showing normal vaginal axis in a patient in the standing position.

in the gastrointestinal tract, but are arranged in a more complex pattern. This pattern reflects the origin of the uterus from paired paramesonephric primordia, with the fibers from each half crisscrossing diagonally with those of the opposite side.

The uterus is lined by a unique mucosa, the endometrium. It has both a columnar epithelium that forms glands and a specialized stroma. The superficial portion of this layer undergoes cyclic change with the menstrual cycle. Spasm of hormonally sensitive spiral arterioles that lie within the endometrium causes shedding of this layer after each cycle, but a deeper basal layer of the endometrium remains to regenerate a new lining. Separate arteries supply the basal endometrium, explaining its preservation at the time of menses.

The cervix is divided into two portions: the portio vaginalis, which is that part protruding into the vagina; and the portio supravaginalis, which lies above the vagina and below the corpus.

The substance of the cervical wall is made up of dense fibrous connective tissue with only a small (about 10%) amount of smooth muscle. What smooth muscle is there lies on the periphery of the cervix, connecting the myometrium with the muscle of the vaginal wall. This smooth muscle and accompanying fibrous tissue are easily dissected off the fibrous cervix and form the layer reflected during intrafascial hysterectomy. It is circularly arranged around the fibrous cervix and is the tissue into which the cardinal and uterosacral ligaments and pubocervical fascia insert.

The portio vaginalis is covered by nonkeratinizing squamous epithelium. Its canal is lined by a columnar mucus-secreting epithelium that is thrown into a series of V-shaped folds that appear like the leaves of a palm and are therefore called plicae palmatae. These form compound clefts in the endocervical canal, not tubular racemose glands, as formerly thought.

The upper border of the cervical canal is marked by the internal os, where the narrow cervical canal widens out into the endometrial cavity. The lower border of the canal, the external os, contains the transition from squamous epithelium of the portio vaginalis to the columnar epithelium of the endocervical canal. This occurs at a variable level relative to the os and changes with hormonal variations that occur during a woman's life. It is in this active area of cellular transition that the cervix is most susceptible to malignant transformation.

There is little adventitia in the uterus, with the peritoneal serosa being directly attached to most of the corpus. The anterior portion of the uterine cervix is covered by the bladder; therefore, it has no serosa. Similarly, as discussed in the following, the broad ligament envelops the lateral aspects of the cervix and corpus; therefore, it has no serosal covering there. The posterior cervix does have a serosal covering.

Adnexal Structures and Broad Ligament

The fallopian tubes are paired tubular structures 7 to 12 cm in length (Fig. 7.10). Each has four recognizable portions. At the uterus, the tube passes through the cornu as an interstitial

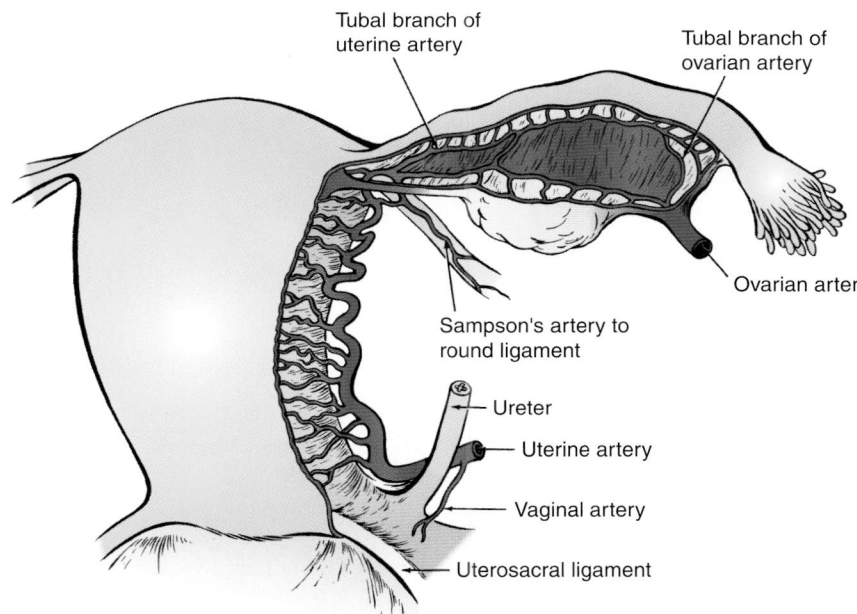

Tubal branch of uterine artery

Tubal branch of ovarian artery

Ovarian artery

Sampson's artery to round ligament

Ureter

Uterine artery

Vaginal artery

Uterosacral ligament

FIGURE 7.10 Uterine adnexa and collateral circulation of uterine and ovarian arteries. The uterine artery crosses over the ureter in the cardinal ligament and gives off cervical and vaginal branches before ascending adjacent to the wall of the uterus and anastomosing with the medial end of the ovarian artery. Note the small branch of the uterine or ovarian artery that nourishes the round ligament (Sampson's artery).

portion. On emerging from the corpus, a narrow isthmic portion begins with a narrow lumen and thick muscular wall. Proceeding toward the abdominal end, next is the ampulla, which has an expanding lumen and more convoluted mucosa. The fimbriated end of the tube has many frondlike projections to provide a wide surface for ovum pickup. The distal end of the fallopian tube is attached to the ovary by the fimbria ovarica, which is a smooth muscle band responsible for bringing the fimbria and ovary close to one another at the time of ovulation. The outer layer of the tube's muscularis is composed of longitudinal fibers; the inner layer has a circular orientation.

The lateral pole of the ovary is attached to the pelvic wall by the infundibulopelvic ligament and the ovarian artery and vein contained therein. Medially, it is connected to the uterus through the utero-ovarian ligament. During reproductive life, it measures about 2.5 to 5 cm long, 1.5 to 3 cm thick, and 0.7 to 1.5 cm wide, varying with its state of activity or suppression, as with oral contraceptive medications. Its surface is mostly free but has an attachment to the broad ligament through the mesovarium, as discussed in the following.

The ovary has a cuboidal to columnar covering and consists of a cortex and medulla. The medullary portion is primarily fibromuscular, with many blood vessels and much connective tissue. The cortex is composed of a more specialized stroma, punctuated with follicles, corpora lutea, and corpora albicantia.

The round ligaments are extensions of the uterine musculature and represent the homolog of the gubernaculum testis. They begin as broad bands that arise on each lateral aspect of the anterior corpus. They assume a more rounded shape before they enter the retroperitoneal tissue, where they pass lateral to the deep inferior epigastric vessels and enter each internal inguinal ring. After traversing the inguinal canal, they exit the external ring and enter the subcutaneous tissue of the labia majora. They have little to do with uterine support.

The ovaries and tubes constitute the uterine adnexa. They are covered by a specialized series of peritoneal folds called the broad ligament. During embryonic development, the paired müllerian ducts and ovaries arise from the lateral abdominopelvic walls. As they migrate toward the midline, a mesentery of peritoneum is pulled out from the pelvic wall from the cervix on up. This leaves the midline uterus connected on either side to the pelvic wall by a double layer of peritoneum.

Within the upper layers of these two folds, called the broad ligament, lie the fallopian tubes, round ligaments, and ovaries (Fig. 7.11). The cardinal and uterosacral ligaments are at the lower margin of the broad ligament. These structures are visceral ligaments; therefore, they are composed of varying amounts of smooth muscle, vessels, connective tissue, and other structures. They are not the pure ligaments associated with joints in the skeleton.

The ovary, tube, and round ligament each have their own separate mesentery, called the mesovarium, mesosalpinx,

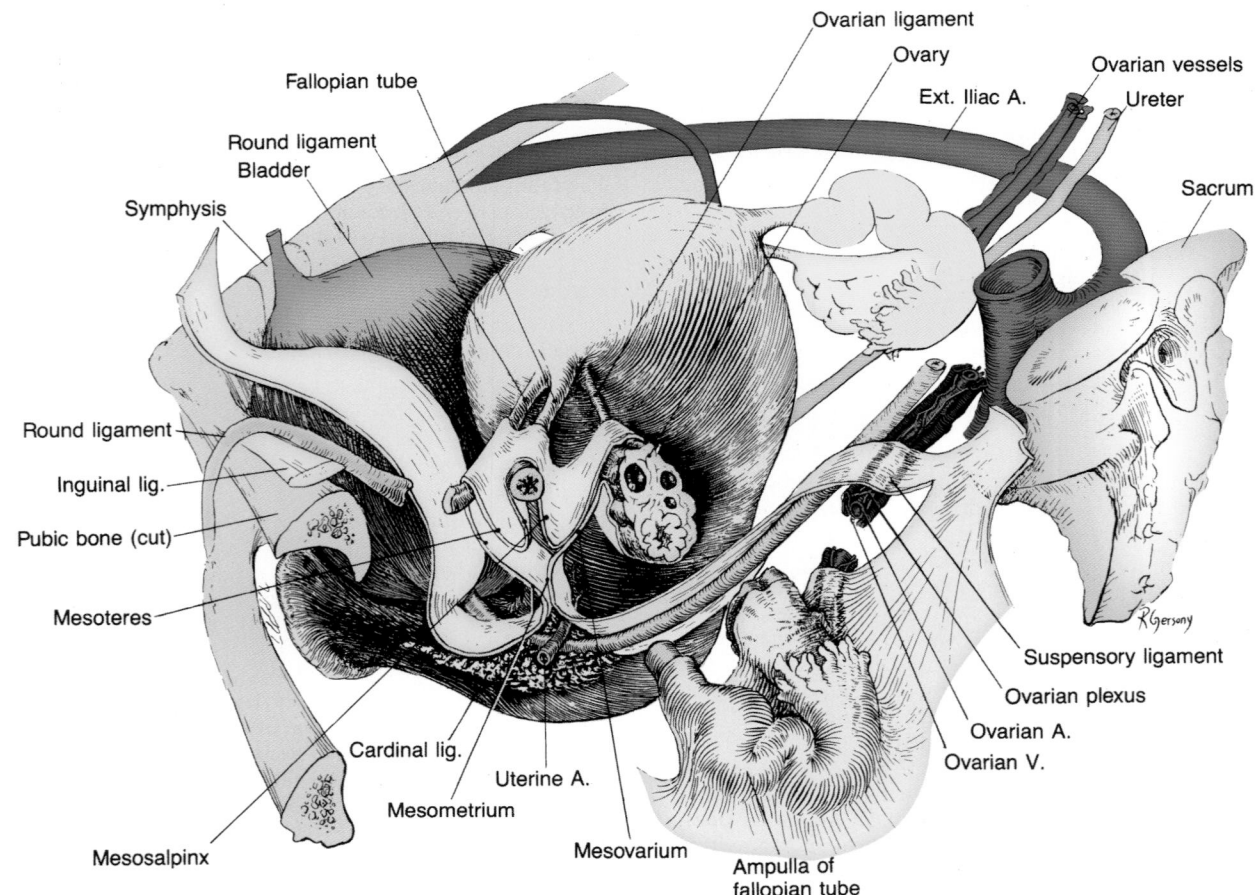

FIGURE 7.11 Composition of the broad ligament.

and mesoteres, respectively. These are arranged in a constant pattern, with the round ligament placed ventrally, where it exits the pelvis through the inguinal ligament, and the ovary placed dorsally. The tube is in the middle and is the most cephalic of the three structures. At the lateral end of the fallopian tube and ovary, the broad ligament ends where the infundibulopelvic ligament blends with the pelvic wall. The cardinal ligaments lie at the base of the broad ligament and are described under the section on supportive tissues and cleavage planes.

Blood Supply and Lymphatics of the Genital Tract

The blood supply to the genital organs comes from the ovarian arteries and uterine and vaginal branches of the internal iliac arteries. A continuous arterial arcade connects these vessels on the lateral border of the adnexa, uterus, and vagina (Fig. 7.10).

The blood supply of the upper adnexal structures comes from the ovarian arteries that arise from the anterior surface of the aorta just below the level of the renal arteries. The accompanying plexus of veins drains into the vena cava on the right and the renal vein on the left. The arteries and veins follow a long, retroperitoneal course before reaching the cephalic end of the ovary. They pass along the mesenteric surface of the ovary to connect with the upper end of the marginal artery of the uterus. Because the ovarian artery runs along the hilum of the ovary, it not only supplies the gonad but also sends many small vessels through the mesosalpinx to supply the fallopian tube, including a prominent fimbrial branch at the lateral end of the tube.

The uterine artery originates from the internal iliac artery. It usually arises independently from this source but can have a common origin with either the internal pudendal or vaginal artery. It joins the uterus near the junction of the corpus and cervix, but this position varies considerably, both with the individual and the amount of upward or downward traction placed on the uterus. Accompanying each uterine artery are several large uterine veins that drain the corpus and cervix.

On arriving at the lateral border of the uterus (after passing over the ureter and giving off a small branch to this structure), the uterine artery flows into the side of the marginal artery that runs along the side of the uterus. Through this connection, it sends blood both upward toward the corpus and downward to the cervix. Because the marginal artery continues along the lateral aspect of the cervix, it eventually crosses over the cervicovaginal junction and lies on the side of the vagina.

The vagina receives its blood supply from a downward extension of the uterine artery along the lateral sulci of the vagina and from a vaginal branch of the internal iliac artery. These form an anastomotic arcade along the lateral aspect of the vagina at the 3- and 9-o'clock positions. Branches from these vessels also merge along the anterior and posterior vaginal walls. The distal vagina also receives a supply from the pudendal vessels, and the posterior wall has a contribution from the middle and inferior hemorrhoidal vessels.

Lymphatic drainage of the upper two thirds of the vagina and uterus is primarily to the obturator and internal and external iliac nodes, and the distal-most vagina drains with the vulvar lymphatics to the inguinal nodes. In addition, some lymphatic channels from the uterine corpus extend along the round ligament to the superficial inguinal nodes, and some nodes extend posteriorly along the uterosacral ligaments to the lateral sacral nodes. These routes of drainage are discussed more fully in the discussion of the retroperitoneal space.

The lymphatic drainage of the ovary follows the ovarian vessels to the region of the lower abdominal aorta, where they drain into the lumbar chain of nodes (paraaortic nodes).

The uterus receives its nerve supply from the uterovaginal plexus (Frankenhäuser ganglion) that lies in the connective tissue of the cardinal ligament. Details of the organization of the pelvic innervation are contained in the section on retroperitoneal structures.

Lower Urinary Tract

Ureter

The ureter is a tubular viscus about 25 cm long, divided into abdominal and pelvic portions of equal length. Its small lumen is surrounded by an inner longitudinal and outer circular muscle layer. In the abdomen, it lies in the extraperitoneal connective tissue on the posterior abdominal wall, crossed anteriorly by the left and right colic vessels. Its course and blood supply are described in the section on the retroperitoneum.

Bladder

The bladder can be divided into two portions: the dome and base (Fig. 7.12). The musculature of the spherical bladder does not lie in simple layers, as do the muscular walls of tubular viscera, such as the gut and ureter. It is best described as a meshwork of intertwining muscle bundles. The musculature of the dome is relatively thin when the bladder is distended. The base of the bladder, which is thicker and varies less with distention of the dome, consists of the urinary trigone and a thickening of the detrusor, called the detrusor loop. This is a U-shaped band of musculature, open posteriorly, that forms the bladder base anterior to the intramural portion of the ureter. The trigone is made of smooth muscle that arises from the ureters that occupy two of its three corners. It continues as the muscle of the vesical neck and urethra. There it rests on the upper vagina. The shape of the bladder depends on its state of filling. When empty, it is a somewhat flattened disk, slightly concave upward. As it fills, the dome rises off the base, eventually assuming a more spherical shape.

The distinction between the base and dome has functional importance, because they have differing innervations. The bladder base has α-adrenergic receptors that contract when stimulated and thereby favor continence. The dome is responsive to β or cholinergic stimulation, with contraction that causes bladder emptying.

Anteriorly, the bladder lies against the lower abdominal wall. It lies against the pubic bones laterally and inferiorly and abuts the obturator internus and levator ani. Posteriorly, it rests against the vagina and cervix. These relations are discussed further in consideration of the pelvic planes and spaces.

The blood supply of the bladder comes from the superior vesical artery, which comes off the obliterated umbilical artery and inferior vesical artery, which is either an independent branch of the internal pudendal artery or arises from the vaginal artery.

Urethra

The urethral lumen begins at the internal urinary meatus and has a series of regional differences in its structure. It passes through the bladder base in an intramural portion for a little less than a centimeter. This region of the bladder, where the urethral lumen traverses the bladder base, is called the vesical neck.

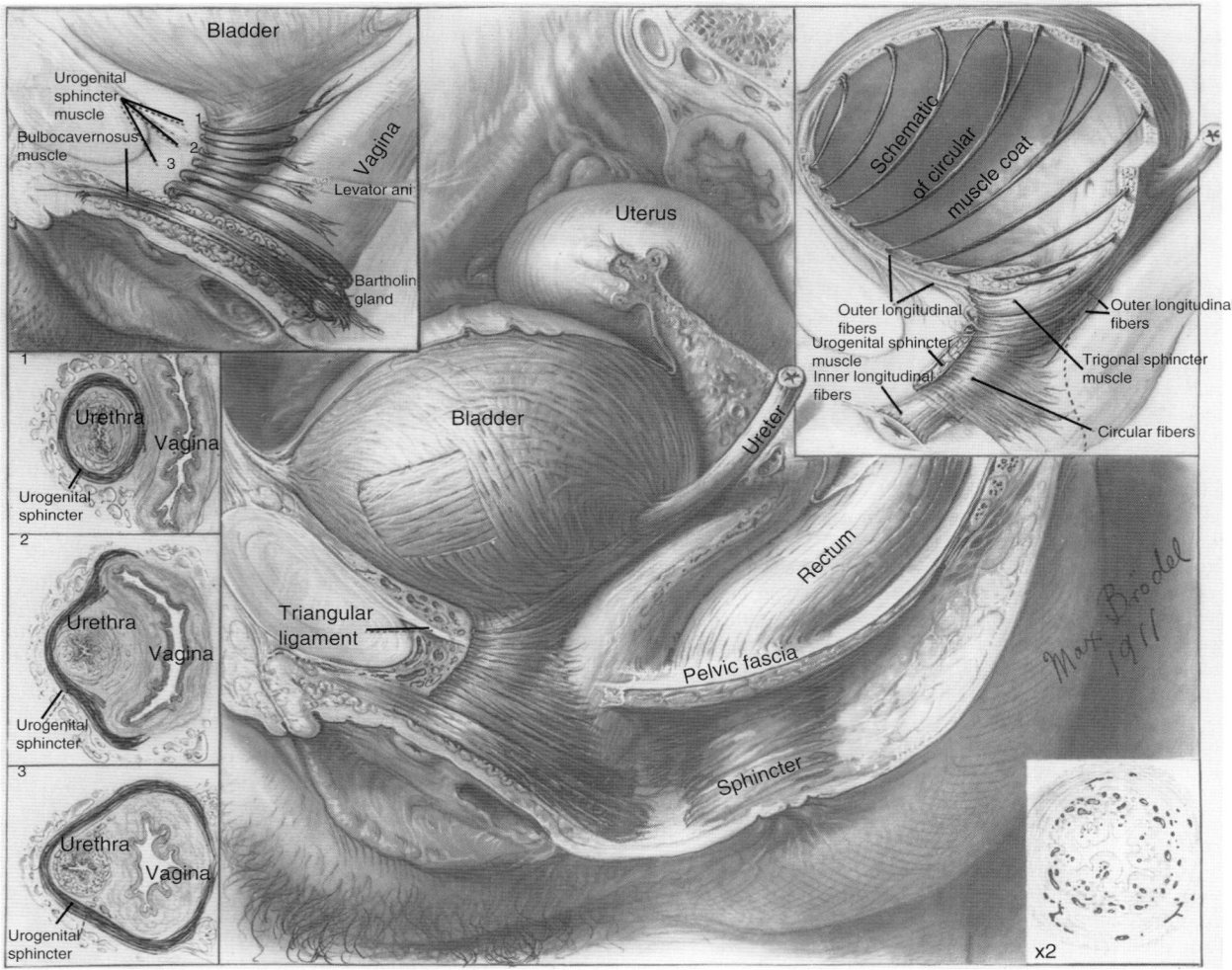

FIGURE 7.12 Lateral view of the pelvic organs showing the urethra and bladder. **Inset 3:** Two portions of the striated urogenital sphincter muscle, namely, the urethrovaginal sphincter and the urethral sphincter. The compressor urethra is not seen. (The original illustration is in the Max Brödel Archives in the Department of Art as Applied to Medicine, The Johns Hopkins University School of Medicine, Baltimore, MD, USA, with permission.)

The urethra itself begins outside the bladder wall. In its distal two thirds, it is fused with the vagina (**Fig. 7.12**), with which it shares a common embryologic derivation. From the vesical neck to the perineal membrane, which starts at the junction of the middle and distal thirds of the bladder, the urethra has several layers. An outer, circularly oriented skeletal muscle layer (urogenital sphincter) mingles with some circularly oriented smooth muscle fibers. Inside this layer is a longitudinal layer of smooth muscle that surrounds a remarkably vascular submucosa and nonkeratinized squamous epithelium that responds to estrogenic stimulation.

Within the submucosa is a group of tubular glands that lie on the vaginal surface of the urethra. These paraurethral (or Skene's) glands empty into the lumen at several points on the dorsal surface of the urethra, but two prominent openings on the inner aspects of the external urethral orifice can be seen when the orifice is opened. Chronic infection of these glands can lead to urethral diverticula, and obstruction of their terminal duct can result in cyst formation. Their location on the dorsal surface of the urethra reflects the distribution of the structures from which they arise.

At the level of the perineal membrane, the distal portion of the urogenital sphincter begins. Here the skeletal muscle of

the urethra leaves the urethral wall to form the urethrovaginal sphincter (**Fig. 7.5**) and compressor urethrae (formerly called the deep transverse perineal muscle). Distal to this portion, the urethral wall is fibrous and forms a nozzle for aiming the urinary stream. The mechanical support of the vesical neck and urethra, which are so important to urinary continence, is discussed in the section of this chapter devoted to the supportive tissues of the urogenital system.

The urethra receives its blood supply both from an inferior extension of the vesical vessels and from the pudendal vessels.

Sigmoid Colon and Rectum

The sigmoid colon begins its S-shaped curve at the pelvic brim. It has the characteristic structure of the colon, with three tenia coli lying over a circular smooth muscle layer. Unlike much of the colon, which is retroperitoneal, the sigmoid has a definite mesentery in its midportion. The length of the mesentery and the pattern of the sigmoid's curvature vary considerably. It receives its blood supply from the lowermost portion of the inferior mesenteric artery: the branches called the sigmoid arteries.

As it enters the pelvis, the colon straightens its course and becomes the rectum. This portion extends from the pelvic brim

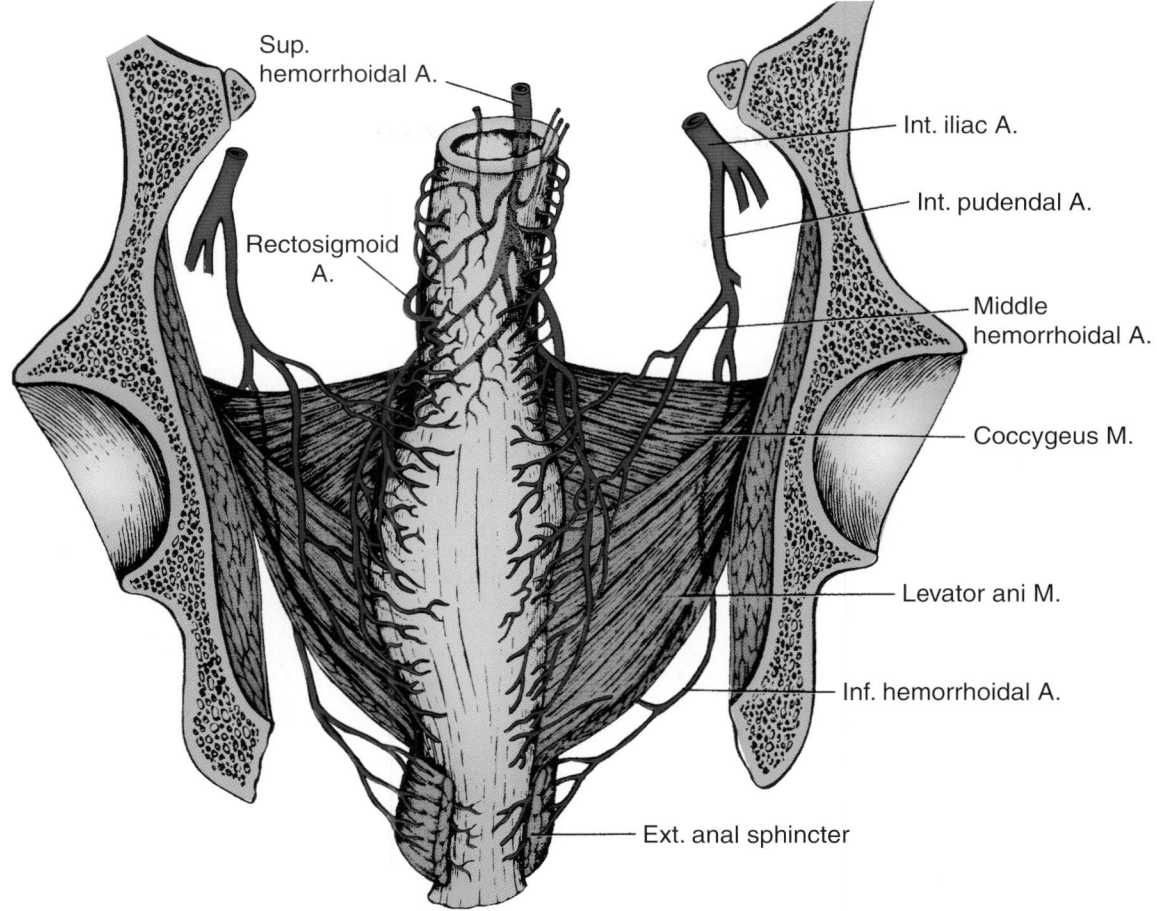

FIGURE 7.13 Rectosigmoid colon and anal canal showing collateral arterial circulation from superior hemorrhoidal (inferior mesenteric), middle hemorrhoidal (hypogastric or internal iliac), and inferior hemorrhoidal (internal pudendal) arteries.

until it loses its final anterior peritoneal investment below the cul-de-sac. It has two bands of smooth muscle (anterior and posterior). Its lumen has three transverse rectal folds that contain the mucosa, submucosa, and circular layers of the bowel wall. The most prominent fold, the middle one, lies anteriorly on the right about 8 cm above the anus, and it must be negotiated during high rectal examination or sigmoidoscopy.

As the rectum passes posterior to the vagina, it expands into the rectal ampulla. This portion of the bowel begins under the cul-de-sac peritoneum and fills the posterior pelvis from the side. At the distal end of the rectum, the anorectal junction is bent at an angle of 90 degrees where it is pulled ventrally by the puborectalis fibers' attachment to the pubes and posteriorly by the external anal sphincter's dorsal attachment to the coccyx.

Below this level, the gut is called the anus. It has many distinguishing features. There is a thickening of the circular involuntary muscle called the internal sphincter. The canal has a series of anal valves to assist in closure, and at their lower border, the mucosa of the colon gives way to a transitional layer of non–hair-bearing squamous epithelium before becoming the hair-bearing perineal skin.

The relations of the rectum and anus can be inferred from their course. They lie against the sacrum and levator plate posteriorly and against the vagina anteriorly. Inferiorly, each half of the levator ani abuts its lateral wall and sends fibers to mingle with the longitudinal involuntary fibers between the internal and external sphincters. Its distal terminus is surrounded by the external anal sphincter.

The anorectum receives its blood supply from a number of sources (**Fig. 7.13**). From above, the superior rectal (hemorrhoidal) branch of the inferior mesenteric artery lies within the layers of the sigmoid mesocolon. As it reaches the beginning of the rectum, it divides into two branches and ends in the wall of the gut. A direct branch from the internal iliac artery arises from the pelvic wall on either side and supplies the rectum and ampulla above the pelvic floor. The anus and external sphincter receive their blood supply from the inferior rectal (hemorrhoidal) branch of the internal pudendal artery, which reaches the terminus of the gastrointestinal tract through the ischiorectal fossa.

PELVIC CONNECTIVE TISSUE AND CLEAVAGE PLANES

The pelvic viscera are connected to the lateral pelvic wall by their adventitial layers and thickenings of the connective tissue that lie over the pelvic wall muscles (**Fig. 7.14**). These attachments, as well as the attachments of one organ to another, separate the different surgical cleavage planes from one another. These condensations of the adventitial layers of the pelvic organs have assumed supportive roles, connecting the viscera to the pelvic walls, in addition to their role in transmitting

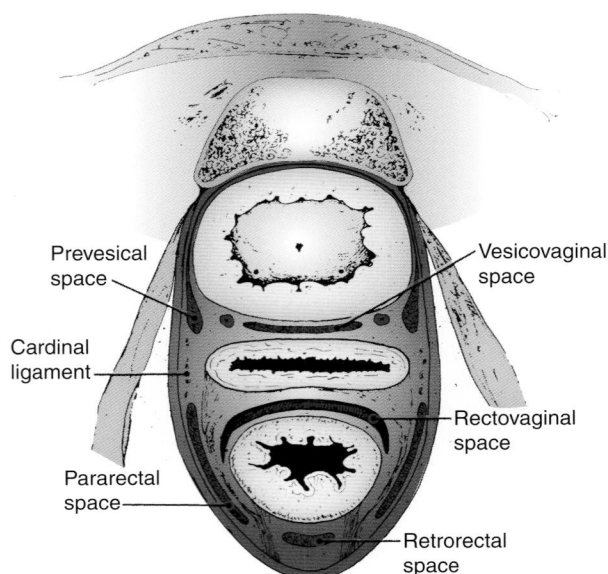

FIGURE 7.14 Cross section of the pelvis showing cleavage planes.

the organs' neurovascular supply from the pelvic wall. They are somewhat like a mesentery that connects the bowel, for example, to the body wall. They have a supportive function as well as a role in carrying vessels and nerves to the organ. An understanding of their disposition is important to both vaginal and abdominal surgery.

The tissue that connects the organs to the pelvic wall has been given the special designation of *endopelvic fascia*. It is not a layer similar to the layer encountered during abdominal incisions (rectus abdominis "fascia"). It is composed of blood vessels and nerves, interspersed with a supportive meshwork of irregular connective tissue containing collagen and elastin. These structures connect the muscularis of the visceral organs to pelvic wall muscles. In some areas, there is considerable smooth muscle within this tissue, as is true in the area of the uterosacral ligaments. Although surgical texts often speak of this fascia as a specific structure separate from the viscera, this is not strictly true. These layers can be separated from the viscera, just as the superficial layers of the bowel wall can be artificially separated from the deeper layers, but they are not themselves separate structures.

Pelvic Connective Tissue

The term *ligament* is most familiar when it describes a dense connective tissue band that links two bones, but it also describes ridges in the peritoneum or thickenings of the endopelvic fascia. The ligaments of the genital tract are diverse. Although they share a common designation (i.e., ligament), they are composed of many types of tissue and have many different functions.

Uterine Ligaments

The broad ligament comprises peritoneal folds that extend laterally from the uterus and cover the adnexal structures. They have no supportive function and were discussed in the section on the pelvic viscera.

At the base of the broad ligament, beginning just caudal to the uterine arteries, there is a thickening in the endopelvic fascia that attaches the cervix and upper vagina to the pelvic side walls (**Fig. 7.15**), consisting of the cardinal and uterosacral

ligaments (parametrium). Use of the term *ligament* has caused confusion over the years because it implies a separate structure that connects two structures. In fact, they are mesenteries that transmit vessels and nerves to the genital tract.

The term *uterosacral ligament* refers to that portion of this tissue that forms the medial margin of the parametrium and that borders the cul-de-sac of Douglas. The term *cardinal ligament* is used to refer to that portion that attaches the lateral margins of the cervix and vagina to the pelvic walls. The course of the ureter as it forms a tunnel between the cardinal and uterosacral ligament forms a point of division between these two structures. The term *parametrium* refers to all of the tissue that attaches to the uterus (both cardinal and uterosacral ligaments), and the term *paracolpium* refers to the portion that attaches to the vagina (cardinal ligament of the vagina).

The uterosacral ligament portion of the parametrium is composed predominantly of smooth muscle, the autonomic nerves of the pelvic organs, and some intermixed connective tissue and blood vessels, whereas the cardinal ligament portion consists primarily of perivascular connective tissue and the pelvic vessels. Although they are often described as extending laterally from the cervix to the pelvic wall, in the standing position, they are almost vertical as one would expect for a suspensory tissue. Near the cervix, they are discrete, but they fan out in the retroperitoneal layer to have a broad, if somewhat ill-defined, area of attachment over the second, third, and fourth segments of the sacrum. These ligaments hold the cervix posteriorly in the pelvis over the levator plate of the pelvic diaphragm.

The cardinal ligaments lie at the lower edge of the broad ligament, between their peritoneal leaves, beginning just caudal to the uterine arteries. They attach to the cervix below the isthmus and fan out to attach to the pelvic walls over the piriformis muscle in the area of the greater sciatic foramen. Although when placed under tension they feel like ligamentous bands, they are composed simply of perivascular connective tissue and nerves that surround the uterine artery and veins. Nevertheless, these structures have considerable strength, and the lack of a separate "ligamentous band" in this area does not detract from their supportive role. They provide support not only to the cervix and uterus but also to the upper portion of the vagina (paracolpium) to keep these structures positioned posteriorly over the levator plate of the pelvic diaphragm and away from the urogenital hiatus.

Vaginal Fasciae and Attachments

The attachments of the vagina to the pelvic walls are important in maintaining the pelvic organs in their normal positions. Failure of these attachments, along with damage to the levator ani muscles, result in the clinical conditions of uterine prolapse, cystocele, rectocele, and enterocele.

The term fascia has many meanings. The layer that is dissected during anterior or posterior colporrhaphy and referred to as the vaginal fascia is the muscularis of the vagina. Histologically, it has an abundance of connective tissue interspersed between the smooth muscle. It is not a layer that is separate from the vagina. Laterally, the mesenteric structures of the cardinal and uterosacral ligaments connect the vagina and uterus to the muscles and connective tissues that cover the lateral walls of the pelvis. They suspended these structures within the pelvis by the downward extension on the lateral margins of the genital track (Fig. 7.15). Between the vagina and bladder is the vesicovaginal space; posterior to it is the cul-de-sac and rectovaginal space. In the midvagina, the vagina is attached laterally to the arcus tendineus fasciae pelvis. The arcus tendineus fasciae pelvis is a fibrous band that extends from its ventral attachment at the pubic bone to its dorsal attachment to the ischial spine. These

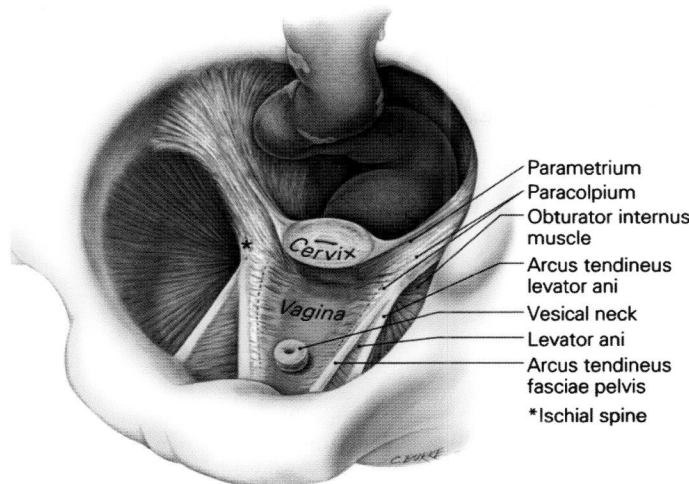

Parametrium
Paracolpium
Obturator internus muscle
Arcus tendineus levator ani
Vesical neck
Levator ani
Arcus tendineus fasciae pelvis
*Ischial spine

A

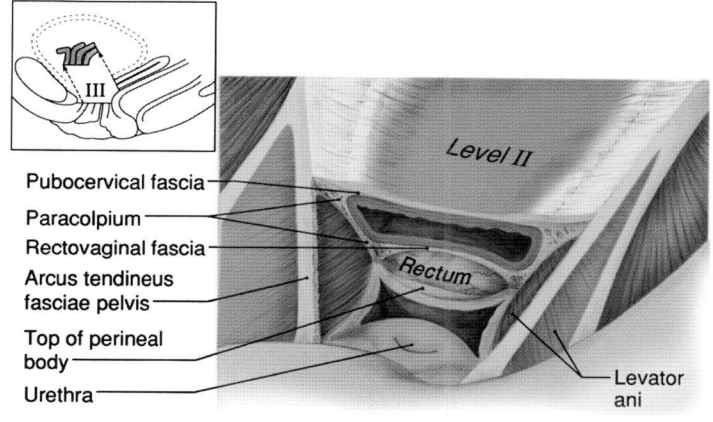

Pubocervical fascia
Paracolpium
Rectovaginal fascia
Arcus tendineus fasciae pelvis
Top of perineal body
Urethra

Level II

Rectum

Levator ani

B

FIGURE 7.15 A: Suspensory ligaments of the female genital tract seen with the bladder removed. **B:** Close-up of the lower portion of the middle vagina (level II) shows how the lateral attachments of the vagina result in an anterior layer under the bladder (pubocervical fascia) and a posterior layer in front of the rectum (rectovaginal fascia). The cephalic surfaces of the transected distal urethra and vagina (level III) are shown. (From DeLancey JOL. Anatomic aspects of vaginal eversion after hysterectomy. *Am J Obstet Gynecol* 1992;166:1717, with permission. Copyright © 1992, Elsevier.)

lateral attachments suspend the anterior vaginal wall across the pelvis and prevent its downward descent with increases in abdominal pressure. The structural layer formed by the vaginal wall and its lateral attachments to the arcus tendineus is clinically referred to as the pubocervical fascia.

Support of the posterior vaginal wall prevents the rectum from bulging forward in the clinical condition known as rectocele. This support varies in different levels of the vagina. In the distal 2 or 3 cm of the posterior vaginal wall, attachments of the perineal body to the ischiopubic rami hold the perineal body in place and prevent protrusion of the distal rectum (Fig. 7.16). In the midvagina above this, the vagina is attached laterally to the fascia covering the inside of the levator ani muscles (Fig. 7.17). This connection prevents the middle of the posterior vaginal wall from moving forward and downward during increases in abdominal pressure. The adventitial tissues between the vaginal wall and rectum contain a thickened layer called the *fascia of Denonvilliers* that extends from the bottom of the cul-de-sac of Douglas to the top of the perineal body. It is relatively thin and whether or not it provides significant support is a matter of controversy.

Urethral Supports

The support of the proximal urethra plays a role in the maintenance of urinary continence during times of increased abdominal pressure. Although it is now known that stress incontinence is primarily caused by a weak urethral sphincter mechanism (low urethral closure pressure), urethral support does play an important, if secondary, role. Therefore, considering the normal mechanisms of urethral support is appropriate.

The distal portion of the urethra is inseparable from the vagina because of their common embryologic derivation from the urogenital sinus. These tissues are fixed firmly in position by connections of the periurethral tissues and vagina to the pubic bones through the perineal membrane (Fig. 7.18). Cranial to this, beginning in the mid-urethra, a hammocklike layer composed of the endopelvic fascia, and anterior vaginal wall provides the support of the proximal urethra. This layer is stabilized by its lateral attachments both to the arcus tendineus fasciae pelvis and the medial margin of the levator ani muscles. The arcus tendineus fasciae pelvis is a fibrous band stretched from a ventral attachment at the lower portion of the pubic bones about 1 cm above the lower margin of the pubic bones and 1 cm from the midline to the ischial spine. The muscular attachment of the endopelvic fascia allows contraction and relaxation of the levator ani muscles to elevate the urethra and to let it descend.

It had previously been thought that the status of the urethral support system was the primary factor determining whether a woman had stress incontinence of urine. Recent studies have, however, shown that the strength of the urethral

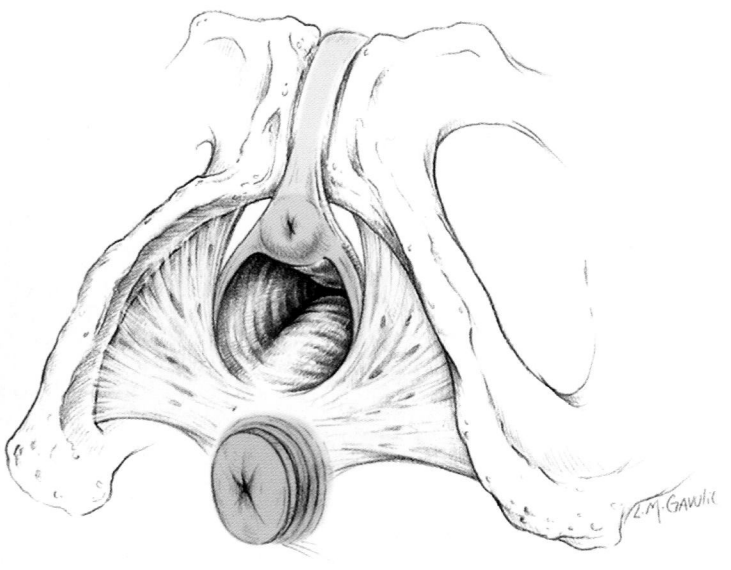

FIGURE 7.16 The peripheral attachments of the perineal membrane to the ischiopubic rami and direction of tension on fibers uniting through the perineal body. (From DeLancey JOL. Structural anatomy of the posterior compartment as it relates to rectocele. *Am J Obstet Gynecol* 1999;180:815, with permission. Copyright © 1999, Elsevier.)

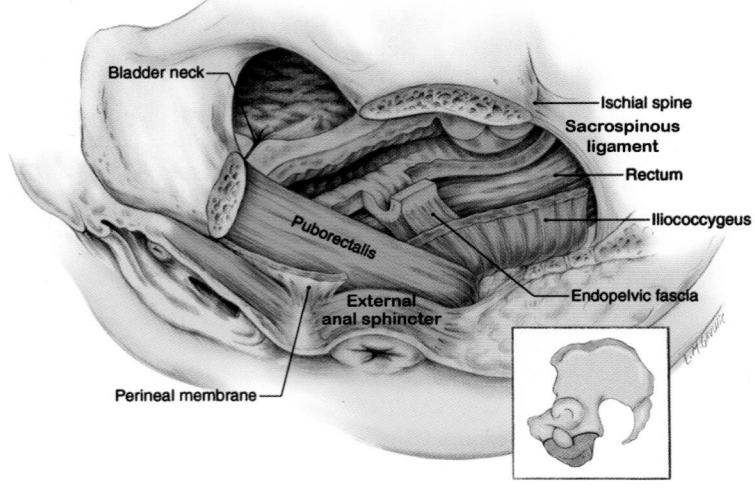

FIGURE 7.17 Lateral view of the pelvic organs after removal of the left ischial bone and ischial tuberosity. The bladder, vagina, and cervix have been cut in the sagittal plane to reveal their lumens. The rectum has been left intact. A strip of the posterior/lateral vaginal wall with its attached endopelvic fascia are shown, indicating their position relative to the levator ani muscle and this fascia's course and attachment. The two portions of the levator ani muscle (puborectalis and iliococcygeus) are visible. The ischial spine and the intact sacrospinous ligament are above the level of the removed ischial tuberosity. The left half of the perineal membrane (urogenital diaphragm) is shown just caudal to the puborectalis portion of the levator ani muscle after its detachment from the inferior pubic ramus that has been removed. (From DeLancey JOL. Structural anatomy of the posterior compartment as it relates to rectocele. *Am J Obstet Gynecol* 1999;180:815, with permission. Copyright © 1999, Elsevier.)

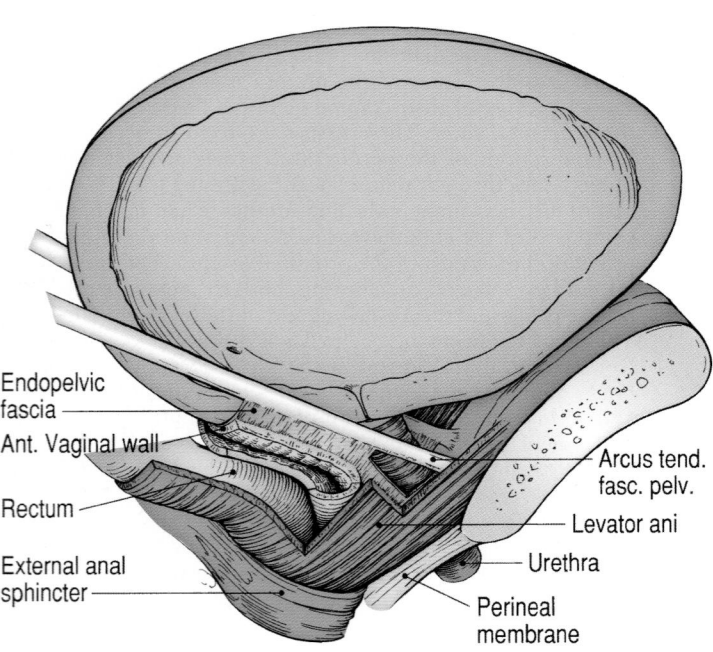

FIGURE 7.18 Lateral view of the urethral supportive mechanism transected just lateral to the midline. The lateral wall of the vagina and a portion of the endopelvic fascia have been removed so that one can see the deeper structures. (Redrawn from DeLancey JOL. Structural support of the urethra as it relates to stress urinary incontinence: the hammock hypothesis. *Am J Obstet Gynecol* 1994;170:1713, with permission. Copyright © 1994, Elsevier.)

sphincter is the primary determining factor with urethral support playing a secondary role. The way in which urethral support plays a role in continence can be understood as follows. During increases in abdominal pressure, the downward force caused by increased abdominal pressure on the ventral surface of the urethra compresses the urethra closed against the hammocklike supportive layer, thereby closing the urethral lumen against the increases in intravesical pressure. The stability of the fascial layer determines the effectiveness of this closure mechanism. If the layer is unyielding, it forms a firm backstop against which the urethra can be compressed closed; however, if it is unstable, the effectiveness of this closure is compromised. Therefore, the integrity of the attachment to the arcus tendineus and the levator ani is critical to the stress continence mechanism.

The muscular attachment is responsible for the voluntary control of vesical neck position visible during vaginal examination or fluoroscopy when the pelvic muscles are contracted and relaxed. Relaxation of these muscles with descent of the vesical neck is associated with the initiation of urination and contraction with arrest of the urinary stream. The limit of downward vesical neck motion is determined by the connective tissue elasticity in the attachments to the arcus tendineus fasciae pelvis.

Cul-de-sacs, Cleavage Planes, and Spaces

Each of the pelvic viscera can expand somewhat independently of its neighboring organs. The ability to do this comes from their relatively loose attachment to one another, which permits the bladder, for example, to expand without equally elongating the adjacent cervix. This allows the viscera to be easily separated from one another along these lines of cleavage. These surgical cleavage planes are called spaces, although they are not empty but rather are filled with fatty or areolar connective tissue. The pelvic spaces are separated from one another by the connections of the viscera to one another and to the pelvic walls.

Anterior and Posterior Cul-de-sacs

Properly termed the *vesicouterine and rectouterine pouches*, the anterior and posterior cul-de-sac separate the uterus from the bladder and rectum.

The anterior cul-de-sac is a recess between the dome of the bladder and the anterior surface of the uterus (Fig. 7.19). The peritoneum is loosely applied in the region of the anterior cul-de-sac, unlike its dense attachment to the upper portions of the uterine corpus. This allows the bladder to expand without stretching its overlying peritoneum. This loose peritoneum forms the vesicouterine fold, which can easily be lifted and incised to create a bladder flap during abdominal hysterectomy or cesarean section. It is the point at which the vesicocervical space is normally accessed during abdominal surgery.

The posterior cul-de-sac is bordered ventrally by the vagina anteriorly, the rectosigmoid posteriorly, and the uterosacral ligaments laterally. Its peritoneum extends for approximately 4 cm along the posterior vaginal wall below the posterior vaginal fornix where the vaginal wall attaches to the cervix. This allows direct entry into the peritoneum from the vagina when performing a vaginal hysterectomy, culdocentesis, or colpotomy. The anatomy here contrasts with the anterior cul-de-sac. Anteriorly, the peritoneum lies several centimeters above the vagina whereas posteriorly, the peritoneum covers the vagina. Keeping this anatomic difference in mind facilitates entering both the anterior and the posterior cul-de-sacs during vaginal hysterectomy.

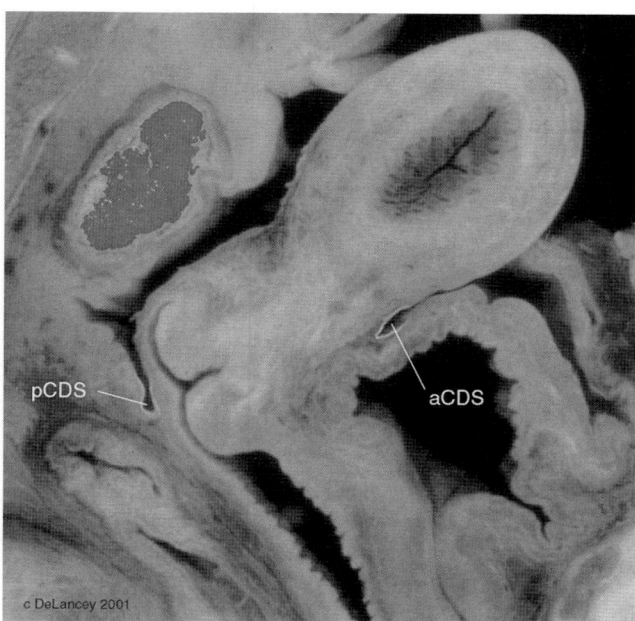

FIGURE 7.19 Sagittal section from the cadaver of a 28-year-old woman showing the anterior cul-de-sac (aCDS) and the posterior cul-de-sac (pCDS). Note how the posterior cul-de-sac peritoneum lies on the vaginal wall, whereas the anterior cul-de-sac lies several centimeters from the depth of the peritoneum in this area. (Peritoneum digitally enhanced in photograph to aid visibility.) (Copyright 2001 John O. L. DeLancey, with permission.)

Prevesical Space

The prevesical space of Retzius (Fig. 7.14) is separated from the undersurface of the rectus abdominis muscles by the transversalis fascia and can be entered by perforating this layer. Ventrolaterally, it is bounded by the bony pelvis and the muscles of the pelvic wall; cranially, it is bounded by the abdominal wall. The proximal urethra and bladder lie in a dorsal position. The dorsolateral limit to this space is the attachment of the bladder to the cardinal ligament and the attachment of the pubocervical fascia to the arcus tendineus fasciae pelvis. These separate this space from the vesicovaginocervical space. This lateral attachment is to the arcus tendineus fasciae pelvis, which lies on the inner surface of the obturator internus and pubococcygeal and puborectal muscles.

Important structures lying within this space include the dorsal clitoral vessels under the symphysis at its lower border and the obturator nerve and vessels as they enter the obturator canal. A branch to the obturator canal often comes off the external iliac artery and lies on the pubic bone; therefore, dissection in this area should be performed with care (Fig. 7.20). Lateral to the bladder and vesical neck is a dense plexus of vessels that lie at the border of the lower urinary tract. They are deep to the pubovesical muscle, and although they bleed when sutures are placed here, this venous ooze usually stops when the sutures are tied. Also within this tissue, lateral to the bladder and urethra, lie the nerves of the lower urinary tract. The upper border of the pubic bones that form the anterior surface of this region has a ridgelike fold of periosteum called the iliopectineal line. This is sometimes used to anchor sutures during urethral suspension operations.

Vesicovaginal and Vesicocervical Space

The space between the lower urinary tract and the genital tract is separated into the vesicovaginal and vesicocervical spaces

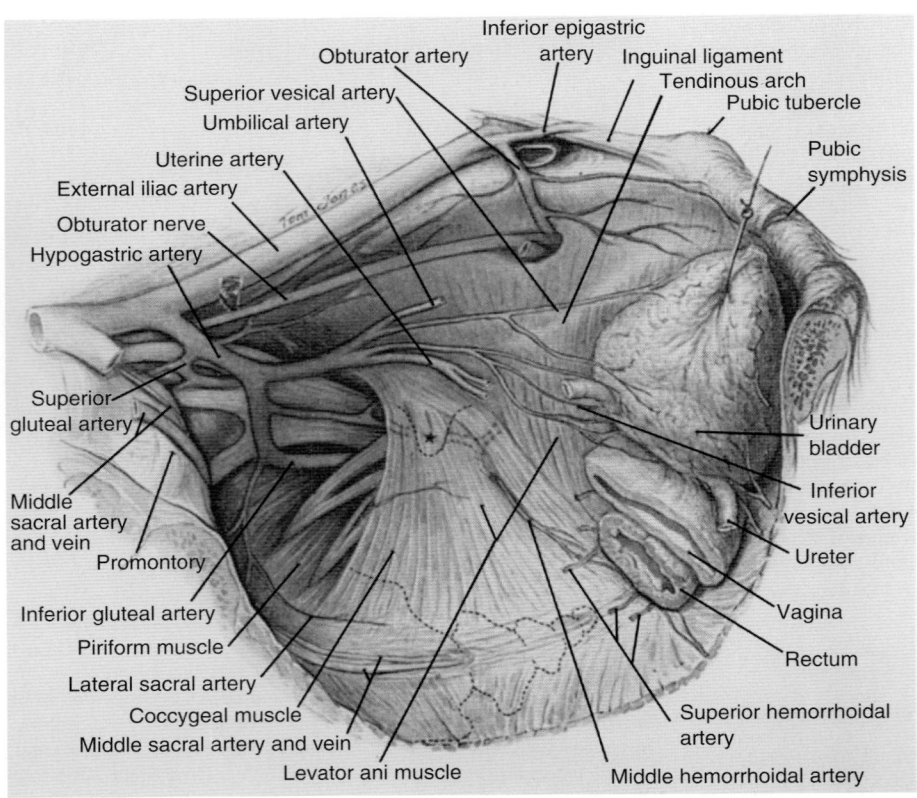

FIGURE 7.20 Structures of the pelvic wall. (From Anson BJ. *An atlas of human anatomy*. Philadelphia, PA: WB Saunders, 1950, with permission.)

(**Fig. 7.14**). The lower extent of the space is the junction of the proximal one third and distal two thirds of the urethra, where it fuses with the vagina, and it extends to lie under the peritoneum at the vesicocervical peritoneal reflection. It extends laterally to the pelvic side walls, separating the vesical and genital aspects of the cardinal ligaments.

Rectovaginal Space

On the dorsal surface of the vagina lies the rectovaginal space (**Fig. 7.14**). It begins at the apex of the perineal body, about 2 to 3 cm above the hymenal ring. It extends upward to the cul-de-sac and laterally around the sides of the rectum to the attachment of the rectovaginal septum to the parietal endopelvic fascia. It contains loose areolar tissue and is easily opened with finger dissection.

At the level of the cervix, some fibers of the cardinal-uterosacral ligament complex extend downward behind the vagina, connecting it to the lateral walls of the rectum and then to the sacrum. These are called the rectal pillars. They separate the midline rectovaginal space in this region from the lateral pararectal spaces. These pararectal spaces allow access to the sacrospinous ligament (mentioned later). They also form the lateral boundaries of the retrorectal space between the rectum and sacrum.

Region of the Sacrospinous Ligament

The area around the sacrospinous ligament is another region that has become more important to the gynecologist operating for problems of vaginal support. The sacrospinous ligament lies on the dorsal aspect of the coccygeal muscle (**Fig. 7.20**). The rectal pillar separates it from the rectovaginal space.

As its name implies, the sacrospinous ligament courses from the lateral aspect of the sacrum to the ischial spine.

In its medial portion, it fuses with the sacrotuberous ligament and is a distinct structure only laterally. It can be reached from the rectovaginal space by perforation of the rectal pillar to enter the pararectal space or by dissection directly under the enterocele peritoneum. This area is covered in more detail in Chapter 35.

Many structures are near the sacrospinous ligament, and their location must be remembered during surgery in this region. The sacral plexus lies immediately to the ligament on the inner surface of the piriformis muscle. Just before its exit through the greater sciatic foramen, the plexus gives off the pudendal nerve, which, with its accompanying vessels, passes lateral to the sacrospinous ligament at its attachment to the ischial spine. The nerve to the levator ani muscles lies on the inner surface of the coccygeal muscle in its midportion. In developing this space, the tissues that are reflected medially and cranially to gain access contain the pelvic venous plexus of the internal iliac vein, as well as the middle rectal vessels. If they are mobilized too vigorously, they can cause considerable hemorrhage.

RETROPERITONEAL SPACES AND LATERAL PELVIC WALL

The retroperitoneal space of the posterior abdomen, presacral space, and pelvic retroperitoneum contain the major neural, vascular, and lymphatic supply to the pelvic viscera. These areas are explored during operations to identify the ureter, interrupt the pelvic nerve supply, arrest serious pelvic hemorrhage, and remove potentially malignant lymph nodes. Because this area is free of the adhesions from serious pelvic infection or endometriosis, it can be used as a plane of dissection when the peritoneal cavity has become obliterated.

The structures found in these spaces are discussed in a regional context, because that is the way they are usually approached in the operating room.

Retroperitoneal Structures of the Lower Abdomen

The aorta lies on the lumbar spine slightly to the left of the vena cava, which it overlies. The portion of this vessel below the renal vessels is encountered during retroperitoneal dissection to identify the paraaortic lymph nodes (Fig. 7.21). The renal blood vessels arise at the second lumbar vertebra. The ovarian vessels also arise from the anterior surface of the aorta in this region. In general, the branches of the vena cava follow those of the aorta, except for the vessels of the intestine, which flow into the portal vein, and the left ovarian vein, which empties into the renal vein on that side.

Below the level of the renal vessels and just below the third portion of the duodenum, the inferior mesenteric artery arises from the anterior aorta. It gives off ascending branches of the left colic artery and continues caudally to supply the sigmoid through the three or four sigmoid arteries that lie in the sigmoid mesentery. These vessels follow the bowel as it is pulled from side to side, so that their position can vary, depending on retraction.

Inferiorly, a continuation of the inferior mesenteric artery forms the superior rectal artery. This vessel crosses over the external iliac vessels to lie on the dorsum of the lower sigmoid. It supplies the rectum, as described in the section concerning that viscus.

The aorta and vena cava have segmental branches that arise at each lumbar level and are called the lumbar arteries and veins. They are situated somewhat posteriorly to the aorta and vena cava and are not visible from the front. When the vessels are mobilized, as is done in excising the lymphatic tissue in this area, they come into view.

At the level of the fourth lumbar vertebra (just below the umbilicus), the aorta bifurcates into the left and right common iliac arteries. After about 5 cm, the common iliac arteries (and the medially placed veins) give off the internal iliac vessels from their medial side and continue toward the inguinal ligament as the external iliac arteries. These internal iliac vessels lie within the pelvic retroperitoneal region and are discussed later.

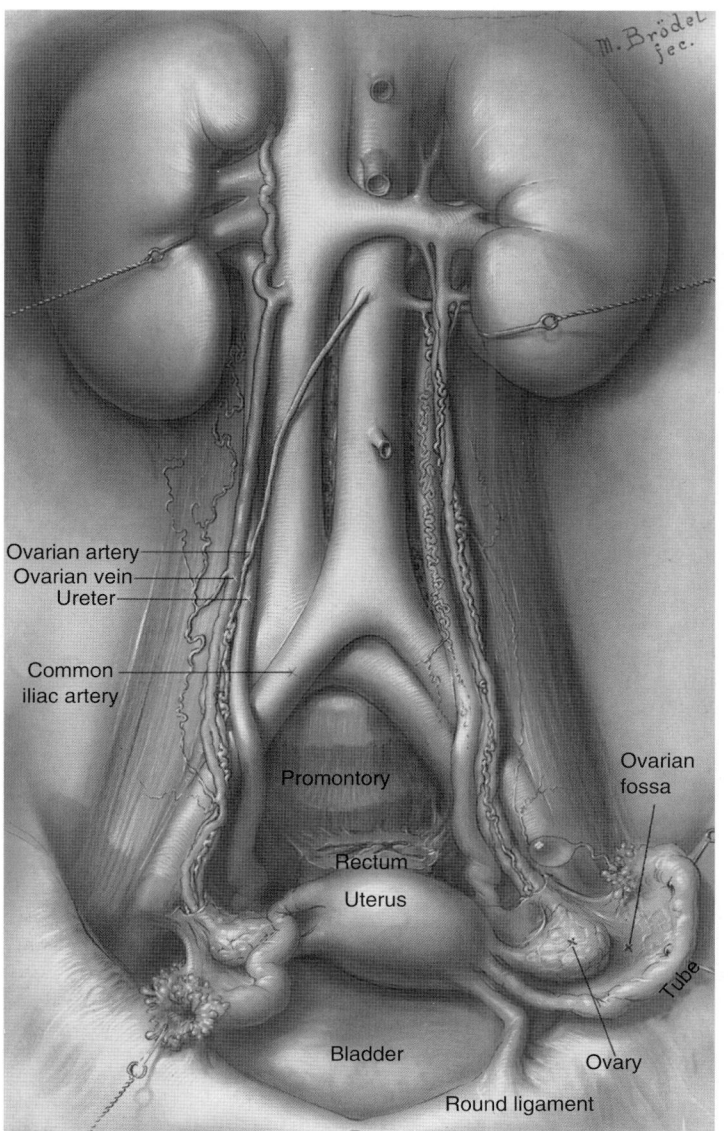

FIGURE 7.21 Structures of the retroperitoneum. Note the anomalous origin of the left ovarian artery from the left renal artery rather than from the aorta. (The original illustration is in the Max Brödel Archives in the Department of Art as Applied to Medicine, The Johns Hopkins University School of Medicine, Baltimore, MD, USA, with permission.)

The aorta and vena cava in this region are surrounded by lymph nodes on all sides. Surgeons usually refer to this lumbar chain of nodes as the paraaortic nodes, reflecting their position. They receive the drainage from the common iliac nodes and are the final drainage of the pelvic viscera. In addition, they collect the lymphatic drainage from the ovaries that follows the ovarian vessels and does not pass through the iliac nodes. The nodes of the lumbar chain extend from the right side of the vena cava to the left of the aorta and can be found both anterior and posterior to the vessels.

The ureters are attached loosely to the posterior abdominal wall in this region, and when the overlying colon is mobilized, they remain on the body wall. They are crossed anteriorly by the ovarian vessels, which contribute a branch to supply the ureter. Additional blood supply to the abdominal portion comes from the renal vessels at the kidney and the common iliac artery.

This region can be exposed either by a midline peritoneal incision to the left of the small bowel mesentery or, retroperitoneally, by reflection of the colon. During embryonic development, the colon and its mesentery fuse with the abdominal wall. A cleavage plane exists here that allows the colon and its vessels to be elevated to expose the structures of the posterior abdominal wall. Because the ureter and ovarian vessels originally arise in this area, they are not elevated with the colon.

Presacral Space

The presacral space begins below the bifurcation of the aorta and is bounded laterally by the internal iliac arteries (Figs. 7.22 and 7.23). Lying directly on the sacrum are the middle sacral artery and vein, which originate from the dorsal aspect of the aorta and vena cava (and not from the point of bifurcation, as sometimes shown). Caudal and lateral to this are the lateral sacral vessels. The venous plexus of these vessels can be extensive, and bleeding from it can be considerable.

Within this area lies the most familiar part of the pelvic autonomic nervous system, the presacral nerve (superior hypogastric plexus). The autonomic nerves of the pelvic viscera can be divided into a sympathetic (thoracolumbar) and parasympathetic (craniosacral) system. The former is also called the adrenergic system, and the latter is called the cholinergic system, according to their neurotransmitters. α-Adrenergic stimulation causes increased urethral and vesical neck tone, and cholinergic stimulation increases contractility of the detrusor muscle. Similarly, adrenergic stimulation in the colon and rectum favors storage, and cholinergic stimulation favors evacuation. β-Adrenergic agonists, which are used for tocolysis, suggest that these influence contractility of the uterus. As is true in the man, damage to the autonomic nerves during

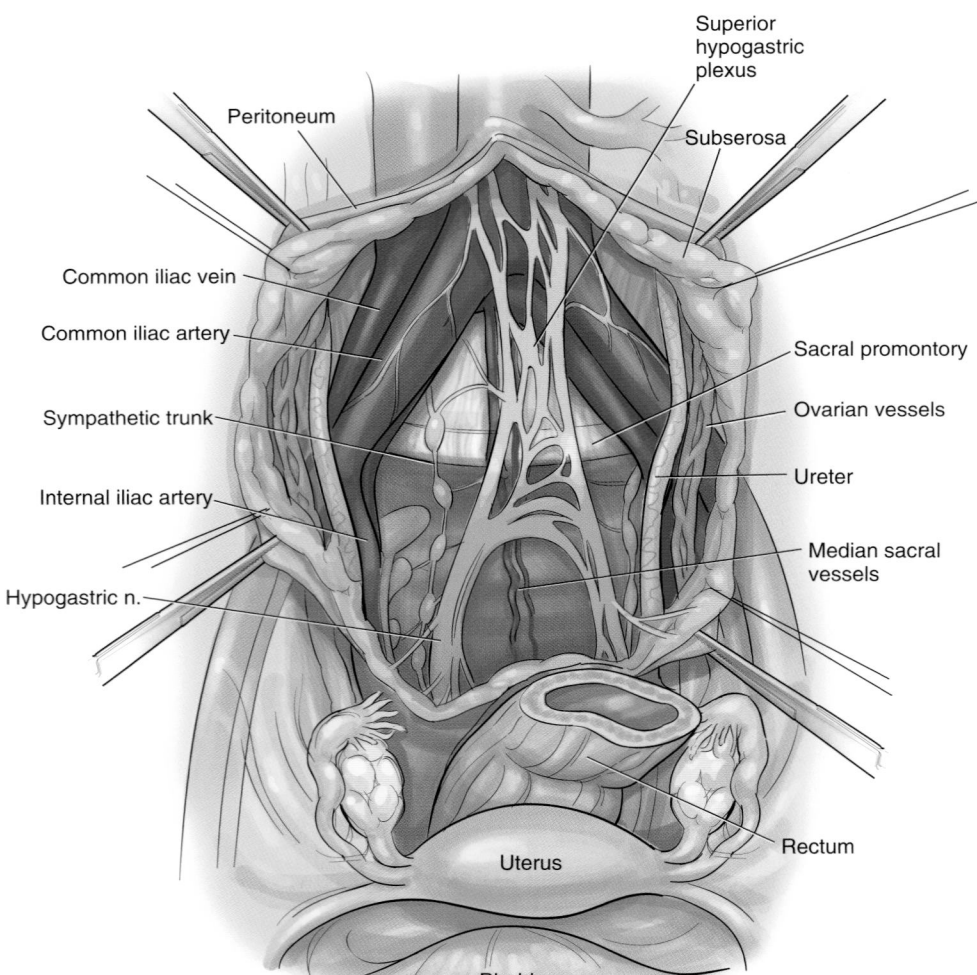

FIGURE 7.22 Presacral nerve plexus, showing passage of sympathetic trunk over bifurcation of aorta. Observe the division of the trunk into left and right presacral nerves. (Redrawn from Curtis AH, Anson BJ, Ashley FL, et al. The anatomy of the pelvic autonomic nerves in relation to gynecology. *Surg Gynecol Obstet* 1942;75:743, with permission.)

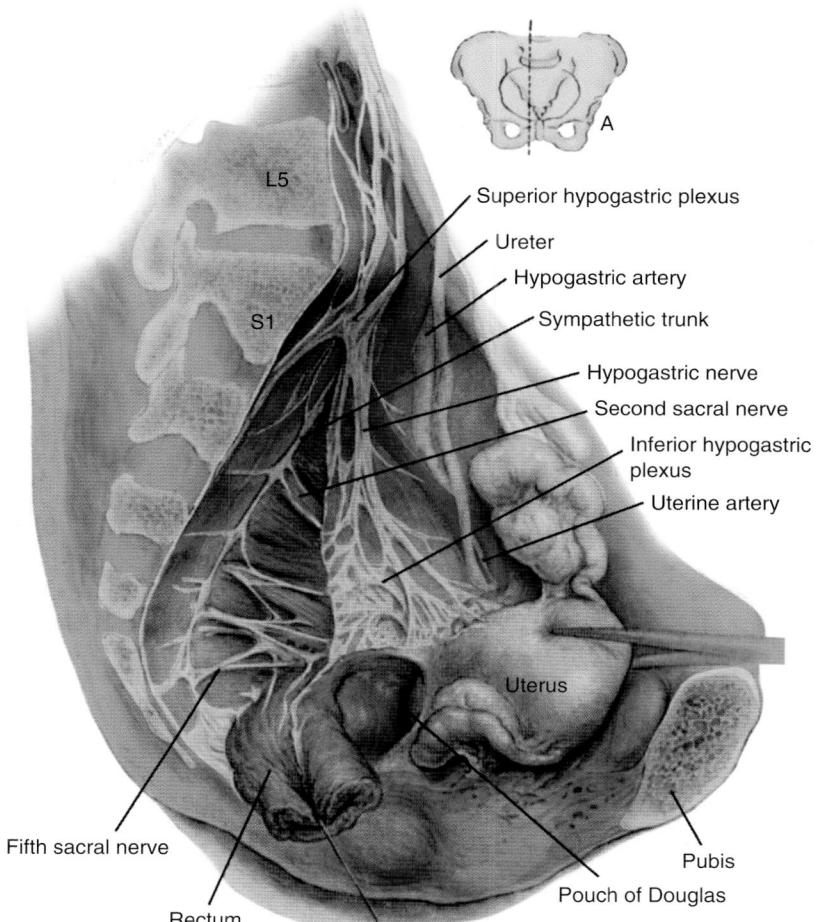

Superior hypogastric plexus
Ureter
Hypogastric artery
Sympathetic trunk
Hypogastric nerve
Second sacral nerve
Inferior hypogastric plexus
Uterine artery
L5
S1
A
Uterus
Fifth sacral nerve
Pubis
Pouch of Douglas
Rectum

FIGURE 7.23 Nerves of the female pelvis. (From Anson BJ. *An atlas of human anatomy*. Philadelphia, PA: WB Saunders, 1950, with permission.)

pelvic lymphadenectomy can have a significant influence on orgasmic function in the woman.

How these autonomic nerves reach the organs that they innervate has surgical importance. The terminology of this area is somewhat confusing, because many authors use idiosyncratic terms. However, the structure is simple: It consists of a single ganglionic midline plexus overlying the lower aorta (superior hypogastric plexus) that splits into two trunks without ganglia (hypogastric nerves), each of which connects with a plexus of nerves and ganglia lateral to the pelvic viscera (inferior hypogastric plexus).

The superior hypogastric plexus lies in the retroperitoneal connective tissue on the ventral surface of the lower aorta and receives input from the sympathetic chain ganglia through the thoracic and lumbar splanchnic nerves. It also contains important afferent pain fibers from the pelvic viscera, which makes its transection effective in primary dysmenorrhea. It passes over the bifurcation of the aorta and extends over the proximal sacrum before splitting into two hypogastric nerves that descend into the pelvis in the region of the internal iliac vessels. The hypogastric nerves end in the inferior hypogastric plexus. The hypogastric plexuses are broad expansions of the hypogastric nerves. Their sympathetic fibers come from the downward extensions of the superior hypogastric plexus and pelvic splanchnic nerves from the continuation of the sympathetic chain into the pelvis. Parasympathetic fibers come from sacral segments two through four by way of the pelvic

splanchnic nerves (nervi erigentes) to join these ganglia. They lie in the pelvic connective tissue of the lateral pelvic wall, lateral to the uterus and vagina.

The inferior hypogastric plexus (sometimes called the pelvic plexus) is divided into three portions: the vesical plexus anteriorly, uterovaginal plexus (Frankenhäuser ganglion), and the middle rectal plexus. The uterovaginal plexus contains fibers that derive from two sources. It receives sympathetic and sensory fibers from the tenth thoracic through the first lumbar spinal cord segments. The second input comes from the second, third, and fourth sacral segments and consists primarily of parasympathetic nerves that reach the inferior hypogastric plexus through the pelvic splanchnic nerves. The uterovaginal plexus lies on the dorsal (medial) surface of the uterine vessels, lateral to the sacrouterine ligaments' insertion into the uterus. It has continuations cranially along the uterus and caudally along the vagina. This latter extension contains the fibers that innervate the vestibular bulbs and clitoris. These nerves lie in the tissue just lateral to the area where the uterine artery, cardinal ligament, and uterosacral ligament pedicles are made during a hysterectomy for benign disease, and within the tissue removed during a radical hysterectomy.

The location of the sensory fibers from the uterine corpus in the superior hypogastric nerve (the presacral nerve) allows the surgeon to alleviate visceral pain from the corpus by transecting this structure. It does not provide sensory innervation to the adnexal structures or to the peritoneum and is therefore not useful for alleviating pain in those sites. Another important way in which the autonomic nervous system is involved is through damage to the inferior hypogastric plexus during radical hysterectomy. The extension of the surgical field lateral to the viscera interrupts the connection of the bladder and sometimes the rectum to their central attachments.

The ovary and uterine tube receive their neural supply from the plexus of nerves that accompany the ovarian vessels and that originate in the renal plexus. These fibers originate from the tenth thoracic segment, and the parasympathetic fibers come from extensions of the vagus.

As the lumbar and sacral nerves exit from the intervertebral and sacral foramina, they form the lumbar and sacral plexuses. The lumbar nerves and plexus lie deep within the psoas muscle on either side of the spine. The sacral plexus lies on the piriformis muscle, and its major branch, the sciatic nerve, leaves the pelvis through the lower part of the greater sciatic foramen. The sacral plexus supplies nerves to the muscles of the hip, pelvic diaphragm, and perineum, as well as to the lower leg (through the sciatic nerve). The femoral nerve from the lumbar plexus is primarily involved in supplying the muscles of the thigh.

Pelvic Retroperitoneal Space

Division of the internal and external iliac vessels occurs in the area of the sacroiliac joint. Just before passing under the inguinal ligament to become the femoral vessels, the external iliac vessels contribute the deep inferior epigastric and deep circumflex iliac arteries. There are no other major branches of the external iliac artery in this region.

Internal Iliac Vessels

Unlike the external iliac artery, which is constant and relatively simple in its morphology, the branching pattern of the internal iliac arteries and veins is extremely variable (**Figs. 7.24** and **7.25**). A description of a common variant is included here. The internal iliac artery supplies the viscera of the pelvis and

many muscles of the pelvic wall and gluteal region. It usually divides into an anterior and posterior division about 3 to 4 cm after leaving the common iliac artery (Table 7.2). The vessels of the posterior division (the iliolumbar, lateral sacral, and superior gluteal) leave the internal iliac artery from its lateral surface to provide some of the blood supply to the pelvic wall and gluteal muscles. Trauma to these hidden vessels should be avoided during internal iliac artery ligation as the suture is passed around behind vessels.

The anterior division has both parietal and visceral branches. The obturator, internal pudendal, and inferior gluteal vessels primarily supply muscles, whereas the uterine, superior vesical, vaginal (inferior vesical), and middle rectal vessels supply the pelvic organs. The internal iliac veins begin lateral and posterior to the arteries. These veins form a large and complex plexus within the pelvis, rather than having single branches, as do the arteries. They tend to be deeper in this area than the arteries, and their pattern is highly variable.

Ligation of the internal iliac artery has proved helpful in the management of postpartum hemorrhage. Burchell's arteriographic studies showed that physiologically active anastomoses between the systemic and pelvic arterial supplies were immediately patent after ligation of the internal iliac artery (**Fig. 7.25**). These anastomoses, shown in Table 7.2, connected the arteries of the internal iliac system with systemic blood vessels either directly from the aorta, as is true for the lumbar and middle sacral artery, or indirectly through the inferior mesenteric artery, as with the superior hemorrhoidal vessels. These in vivo pathways were quite different from the anastomoses that had previously been hypothesized on purely anatomic grounds.

Pelvic Ureter

The course of the ureter within the pelvis is important to gynecologic surgeons and is fully considered in Chapter 37. A few of the important anatomic landmarks are considered here (**Fig. 7.24**). After passing over the bifurcation of the

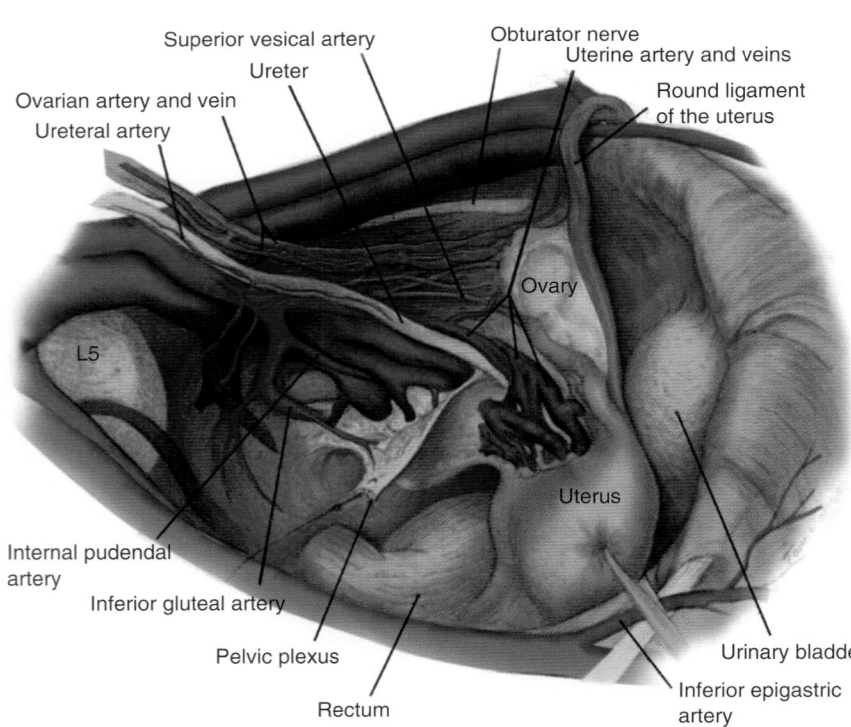

FIGURE 7.24 Arteries and veins of the pelvis. (From Anson BJ. *An atlas of human anatomy.* Philadelphia, PA: WB Saunders, 1950, with permission.)

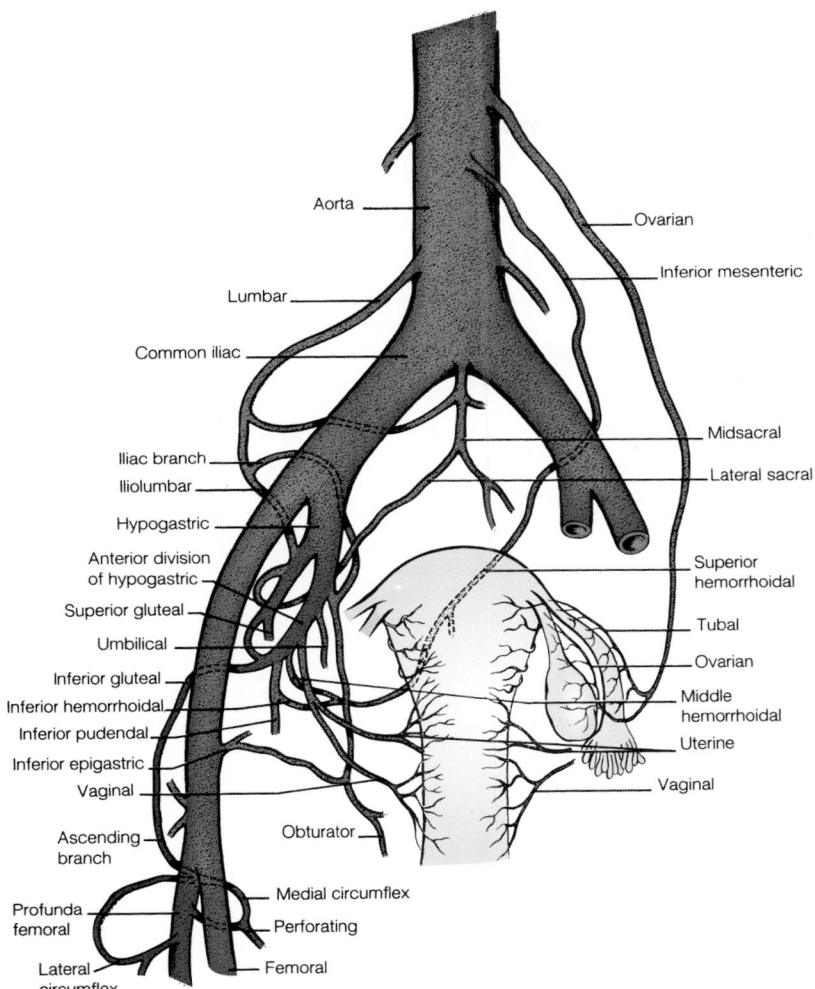

FIGURE 7.25 Collateral circulation of the pelvis.

internal and external iliac arteries, just medial to the ovarian vessels, the ureter descends within the pelvis. Here, it lies in a special connective tissue sheath that is attached to the peritoneum of the lateral pelvic wall and medial leaf of the broad ligament. This explains why the ureter still adheres to the peritoneum and does not remain laterally with the vessels when the peritoneal space is entered.

The ureter crosses under the uterine artery ("water flows under the bridge") in its course through the cardinal ligament. There is a loose areolar plane around it to allow for its peristalsis here. At this point, it lies along the anterolateral surface of the cervix, usually about 1 cm from it. From there, it comes

to lie on the anterior vaginal wall and then proceeds for a distance of about 1.5 cm through the wall of the bladder.

During its pelvic course, the ureter receives blood from the vessels that it passes, specifically the common iliac, internal iliac, uterine, and vesical arteries. Within the wall of the ureter, these vessels are connected to one another by a convoluted vessel that can be seen running longitudinally along its outer surface.

Lymphatics

The lymph nodes and lymphatic vessels that drain the pelvic viscera vary in their number and distribution, but they can be organized into coherent groups. Because of the extensive interconnection of the lymph nodes, spread of lymph flow, and thus malignancy, is somewhat unpredictable. Therefore, some important generalizations about the distribution and drainage of these tissues are still helpful. Distribution of the pelvic lymph nodes is discussed further in Chapter 46 on invasive carcinoma of the cervix. Figures 46.22 through 46.25 show this anatomy.

The nodes of the pelvis can be divided into the external iliac, internal iliac, common iliac, medial sacral, and pararectal nodes. The medial sacral nodes are few and follow the middle sacral artery. The pararectal nodes drain the part of the rectosigmoid above the peritoneal reflection that is supplied by

TABLE 7.2 Collateral Circulation after Internal Iliac Artery Ligation
INTERNAL ILIAC SYSTEMIC
Iliolumbar
Lateral sacral
Middle hemorrhoidal
Lumbar
Middle sacral
Superior hemorrhoidal

the superior hemorrhoidal artery. The medial and pararectal nodes are seldom involved in gynecologic disease.

The internal and external iliac nodes lie next to their respective blood vessels, and both end in the common iliac chain of nodes, which then drain into the nodes along the aorta. The external iliac nodes receive the drainage from the leg through the inguinal nodes. Nodes in the external iliac group can be found lateral to the artery, between the artery and vein, and on the medial aspect of the vein. These groups are called the anterosuperior, intermediate, and posteromedial groups, respectively. They can be separated from the underlying muscular fascia and periosteum of the pelvic wall along with the vessels, thereby defining their lateral extent. Some nodes at the distal end of this chain lie in direct relation to the deep inferior epigastric vessels and are named according to these adjacent vessels. Similarly, nodes that lie at the point where the obturator nerve and vessels enter the obturator canal are called obturator nodes.

The internal iliac nodes drain the pelvic viscera and receive some drainage from the gluteal region along the posterior division of the internal iliac vessels as well. These nodes lie within the adipose tissue that is interspersed among the many branches of the vessels. The largest and most numerous nodes lie on the lateral pelvic wall, but many smaller nodes lie next to the viscera themselves. These nodes are named for the organ by which they are found (e.g., parauterine).

Not only is it difficult in the operating room to make some of the fine distinctions mentioned in this anatomic discussion, but also there is little clinical importance in doing so. Surgeons generally refer to those nodes that are adjacent to the external iliac artery as the external iliac group of nodes and to those next to the internal iliac artery as the internal iliac nodes. This leaves those nodes that lie between the external iliac vein and internal artery, which are called interiliac nodes.

The direction of lymph flow from the uterus tends to follow its attachments, draining along the cardinal, uterosacral, and even round ligaments. This latter connection can lead to metastasis from the uterus to the superficial inguinal nodes, whereas the former connections are to the internal iliac nodes, with free communication to the external iliac nodes and sometimes to the lateral sacral nodes. The anastomotic connection of the uterine and ovarian vessels makes lymphatic connections between these two drainage systems likely and metastasis in this direction possible.

The vagina and lower urinary tract have a divided drainage. Superiorly (upper two thirds of the vagina and the bladder), drainage occurs along with the uterine lymphatics to the internal iliac nodes, whereas the lower one third of the vagina and distal urethra drain to the inguinal nodes. However, this demarcation is far from precise.

The common iliac nodes can be found from the medial to the lateral border of the vessels of the same name. They continue above the pelvic vessels and occur around the aorta and the vena cava. These nodes can lie anterior, lateral, or posterior to the vessels.

THE ABDOMINAL WALL

Knowledge of the layered structure of the abdominal wall allows the surgeon to enter the abdominal cavity with maximum efficiency and safety. A general summary of these layers is provided in Table 7.3. The abdomen's superior border is the lower edge of the rib cage (ribs 7 through 12). Inferiorly, it ends at the iliac crests, inguinal ligaments, and pubic bones. It ends posterolaterally at the lumbar spine and its adjacent muscles.

TABLE 7.3 Table of Abdominal Wall Layers
Skin
Subcutaneous layer
Camper fascia
Scarpa fascia
Musculoaponeurotic layer
Rectus sheath—formed by conjoined aponeuroses of the external oblique muscle
Internal oblique muscle: fused in lower abdomen
Transverse abdominal muscle
Transversalis fascia
Peritoneum

Skin and Subcutaneous Tissue

The fibers in the dermal layer of the abdominal skin are oriented in a predominantly transverse direction following a gently curving concave upward line. This predominance of transversely oriented fibers results in more tension on the skin of a vertical incision and in a wider scar.

Between the skin and musculoaponeurotic layer of the abdominal wall lie the subcutaneous tissues. It is made of globules of fat held in place and supported by a series of branching fibrous septa. In the more superficial portion of the subcutaneous layer, called Camper fascia, the fat predominates, and the fibrous tissue is less apparent. Closer to the rectus sheath, the fibrous tissue predominates relative to the fat in the region known as Scarpa fascia. Camper and Scarpa fasciae are not discrete or well-defined layers but represent regions of the subcutaneum. Scarpa fascia is best developed laterally and is not seen as a well-defined layer during vertical incisions.

Musculoaponeurotic Layer

Deep to the subcutaneous tissue is a layer of muscle and fibrous tissue that holds the abdominal viscera in place and controls movement of the lower torso (Figs. 7.26 and 7.27). Within this area are two groups of muscles: vertical muscles in the anterior abdominal wall and oblique flank muscles. The rectus abdominis muscle is found on either side of the midline, and the pyramidalis muscle is located just above the pubes. Lateral to these are the flank muscles: the external oblique, internal oblique, and transverse abdominal. The broad, sheet-like tendons of these muscles form aponeuroses that unite with their corresponding member of the other side, forming a dense white covering of the rectus abdominis muscle properly called the rectus sheath (rectus "fascia").

Rectus Abdominis and Pyramidal Muscles

Each paired rectus abdominis muscle originates from the sternum and cartilages of ribs 5 through 7 and inserts into the anterior surface of the pubic bone. Each muscle has three tendinous inscriptions. These are fibrous interruptions within the muscle that firmly attach it to the rectus abdominis sheath. In general, they are confined to the region above the umbilicus, but they can be found below it. When this happens, the rectus sheath is attached to the rectus muscle there, and these two structures become difficult to separate during a Pfannenstiel incision.

The pyramidal muscles arise from the pubic bones and insert into the linea alba in an area several centimeters above the symphysis. Their development varies considerably among individuals. Their strong attachment to the midline makes separation of their attachment here difficult by blunt dissection.

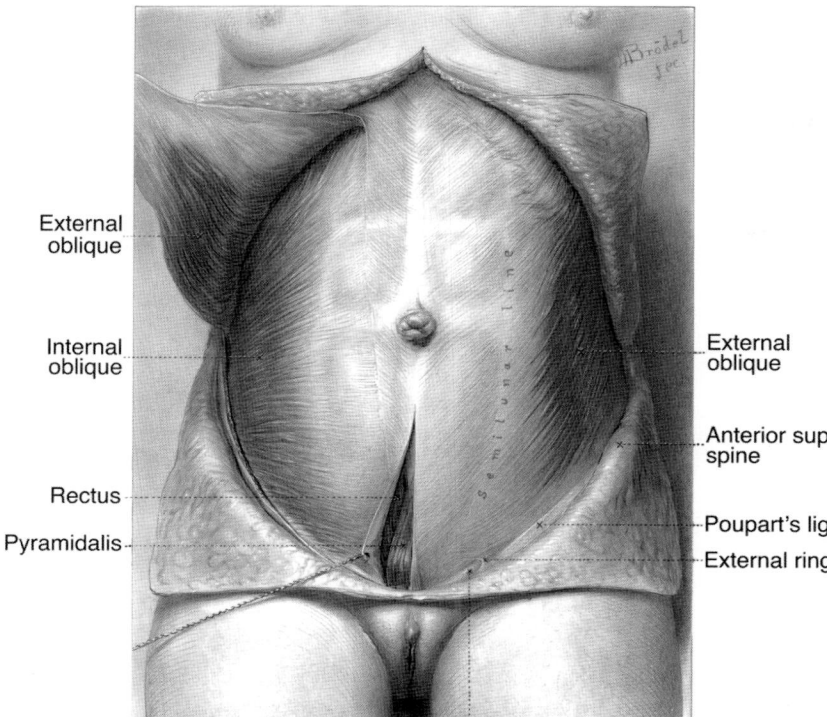

FIGURE 7.26 External oblique, internal oblique, and pyramidal muscles. (The original illustration is in the Max Brödel Archives in the Department of Art as Applied to Medicine, The Johns Hopkins University School of Medicine, Baltimore, MD, USA, with permission.)

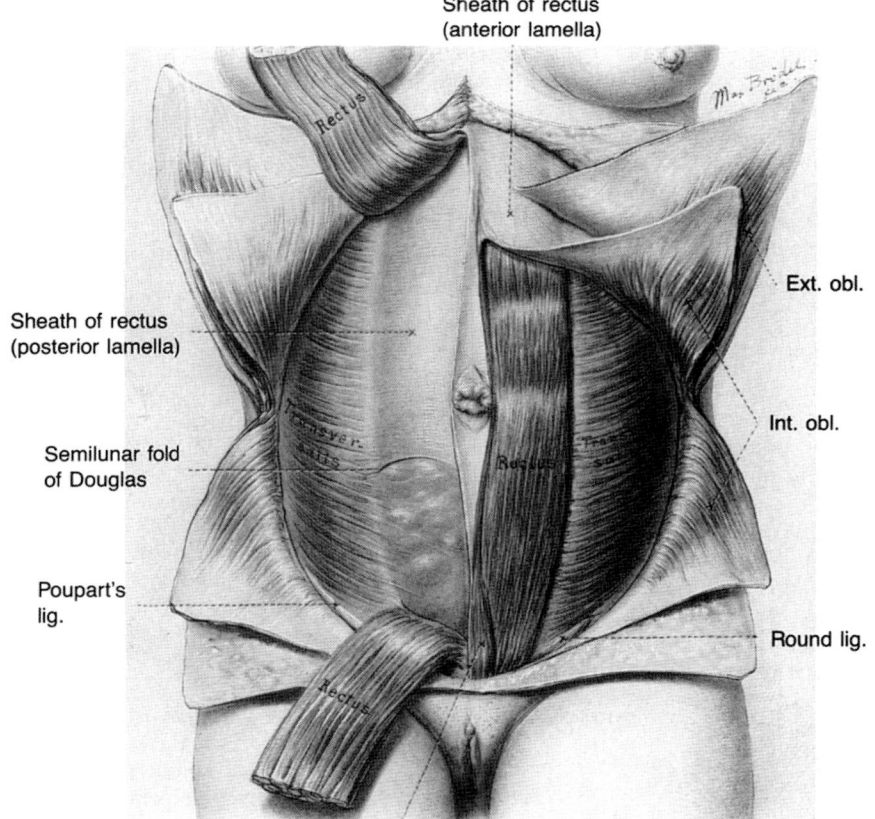

FIGURE 7.27 Transverse abdominal and rectoabdominal muscles. (The original illustration is in the Max Brödel Archives in the Department of Art as Applied to Medicine, The Johns Hopkins University School of Medicine, Baltimore, MD, USA, with permission.)

Flank Muscles

Lateral to the rectus abdominis muscles lie the broad, flat muscles of the flank. The aponeurotic insertions of these muscles join to form the conjoined tendon, or rectus sheath, which covers the rectus abdominis. Because of its importance, the rectus sheath is further discussed below.

The most superficial of these muscles is the external oblique. Its fibers run obliquely anteriorly and inferiorly from their origin on the lower eight ribs and iliac crest. Unlike the external oblique muscle's fibers, which run obliquely downward, the fibers of the internal oblique muscle fan out from their origin in the anterior two thirds of the iliac crest, the lateral part of the inguinal ligament, and the thoracolumbar fascia in the lower posterior flank. In most areas, they are perpendicular to the fibers of the external oblique muscle, but in the lower abdomen, their fibers arch somewhat more caudally and run in a direction similar to those of the external oblique muscle.

As the name *transversus abdominis* implies, the fibers of the deepest of the three layers have a primarily transverse orientation. They arise from the lower six costal cartilages, the thoracolumbar fascia, the anterior three fourths of the iliac crest, and the lateral inguinal ligament. The caudal portion of the transverse abdominal muscle is fused with the internal oblique muscle. This explains why, during transverse incisions of the lower abdomen, only two layers are discernible at the lateral portion of the incision.

Although the fibers of the flank muscles are not strictly parallel to one another, their primarily transverse orientation and the transverse pull of their attached muscular fibers place vertical suture lines in the rectus sheath under more tension than transverse ones. For this reason, vertical incisions are more prone to dehiscence.

Rectus Sheath (Conjoined Tendon)

The line of demarcation between the muscular and aponeurotic portions of the external oblique muscle in the lower abdomen occurs along a vertical line through the anterosuperior iliac spine (Fig. 7.28). The internal oblique and transverse abdominal muscles extend farther toward the midline, coming closest at their inferior margin, at the pubic tubercle. Because of

this, fibers of the internal oblique muscle are found underneath the aponeurotic portion of the external oblique muscle during a transverse incision. In addition, it is between the internal oblique and transverse abdominal muscles that the nerves and blood vessels of the flank are found and their injury avoided.

In forming the rectus sheath, the conjoined aponeuroses of the flank are separable lateral to the rectus muscles but fuse near the midline. As they reach the midline, these layers lose their separate directions and fuse. Many specialized aspects of the rectus sheath are important to the surgeon. In its lower one fourth, the sheath lies entirely anterior to the rectus muscle. Above that point, it splits to lie both ventral and dorsal to it. The transition between these two arrangements occurs midway between the umbilicus and the pubes and is called the arcuate line. Cranial to this line, the midline ridge of the rectus sheath, the linea alba, unites these two layers. Sharp dissection is usually required to separate these layers during a Pfannenstiel incision. A vertical peritoneal incision cuts the posterior sheath.

The lateral border of the rectus muscle is marked by the semilunar line of the rectus sheath. Above the arcuate line, this is the level at which the anterior and posterior layers of the sheath split. Below it the transversalis fascia fuses with the sheath. The semilunar line is not always where the three layers of flank muscles join. During a transverse lower abdominal incision, the external and internal oblique aponeuroses are often separable near the midline.

The inguinal canal lies at the lower edge of the musculofascial layer of the abdominal wall. Through the inguinal canal, in the woman, the round ligament extends to its termination in the labium majus. In addition, the ilioinguinal nerve and the genital branch of the genitofemoral nerve pass through the canal.

Transversalis Fascia, Peritoneum, and Bladder Reflection

Inside the muscular layers, and outside the peritoneum, lies the transversalis fascia, a layer of fibrous tissue that lines the abdominopelvic cavity. It is visible during abdominal incisions as the layer just underneath the rectus abdominis muscles suprapubically. It is separated from the peritoneum by a variable layer of adipose tissue. It is frequently incised or bluntly dissected off the bladder to take the tissues in this region "down by layers."

The peritoneum is a single layer of serosa. It is thrown into five vertical folds by underlying ligaments or vessels that converge toward the umbilicus. The single median umbilical fold is caused by the presence of the urachus (median umbilical ligament). Lateral to this are paired medial umbilical folds that are raised by the obliterated umbilical arteries that connected the internal iliac vessels to the umbilical cord in fetal life, and the corresponding lateral umbilical folds caused by the inferior epigastric arteries and veins.

The reflection of the bladder onto the abdominal wall is triangular in shape, with its apex blending into the medial umbilical ligament. Because the apex is highest in the midline, incision in the peritoneum lateral to the midline is less likely to result in bladder injury.

Neurovascular Supply of the Abdominal Wall

Vessels of the Abdominal Wall

Knowing the location and course of the abdominal wall blood vessels helps the surgeon anticipate their location during abdominal incisions and during the insertion of laparoscopic

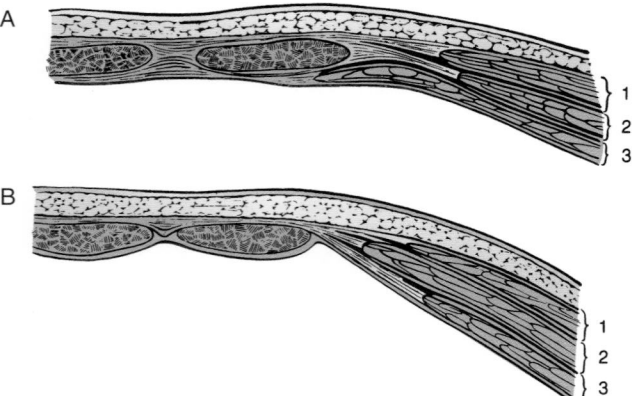

FIGURE 7.28 Cross section of lower abdominal wall. **A:** The anterior fascial sheath of the rectus muscle from external oblique (*1*) and split aponeurosis of internal oblique (*2*) muscles. The posterior sheath is formed by aponeurosis of the transverse abdominal muscle (*3*) and split aponeurosis of the internal oblique muscle. **B:** Lower portion of the abdominal wall below arcuate line (linea semicircularis) with absence of a posterior fascial sheath of the rectus muscle and all of the fascial aponeuroses (*1,2,3*) forming the anterior rectus muscle sheath.

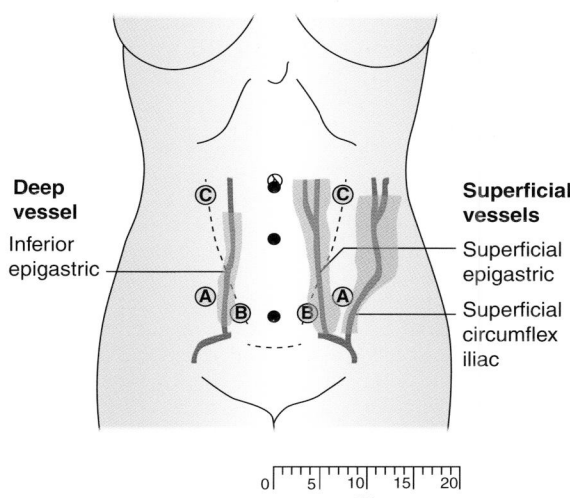

Deep vessel

Inferior epigastric

Superficial vessels

Superficial epigastric

Superficial circumflex iliac

FIGURE 7.29 Normal variation in epigastric vessels. *A, B,* and *C* designate safe spots for laparoscopic trocar insertion. *Dotted lines* indicate lateral border of rectus muscle. (From Hurd WW, Bude RO, DeLancey JOL, et al. The location of abdominal wall blood vessels in relationship to abdominal landmarks apparent at laparoscopy. *Am J Obstet Gynecol* 1994;171:642, with permission. Copyright © 1994, Elsevier.)

trocars (**Fig. 7.29**). The blood vessels that supply the abdominal wall can be separated into those that supply the skin and subcutaneous tissues and those that supply the musculofascial layer. Although there is only one set of epigastric vessels in the subcutaneous tissues (superficial epigastric), there are both superior and inferior epigastric vessels in the musculofascial layer, so care must be taken in using these terms to avoid confusion.

The superficial epigastric vessels run a diagonal course in the subcutaneum from the femoral vessels toward the umbilicus, beginning as a single artery that branches extensively as it nears the umbilicus. Its position can be anticipated midway between the skin and musculofascial layer, in a line between the palpable femoral pulse and the umbilicus. The external pudendal artery runs a diagonal course from the femoral artery medially to supply the region of the mons pubis. It has many midline branches, and bleeding in its territory of distribution is heavier than that from the abdominal subcutaneous tissues. The superficial circumflex iliac vessels proceed laterally from the femoral vessels toward the flank.

The blood supply to the lower abdominal wall's musculofascial layer parallels the subcutaneous vessels. The branches of the external iliac, the inferior epigastric, and the deep circumflex iliac arteries parallel their superficial counterparts (**Fig. 7.29**). The circumflex iliac artery lies between the internal oblique and transverse abdominal muscle. The inferior epigastric artery and its two veins originate lateral to the rectus muscle. They run diagonally toward the umbilicus and intersect the muscle's lateral border midway between the pubis and umbilicus. Below the point at which the vessels pass under the rectus, they are found lateral to the muscle deep to the transversalis fascia. After crossing the lateral border of the muscle, they lie on the muscle's dorsal surface, between it and the posterior rectus sheath. As the vessels enter the rectus sheath, they branch extensively, so that they no longer represent a single trunk. The angle between the vessel and the border of the rectus muscle forms the apex of the Hesselbach triangle (inguinal triangle), the base of which is the inguinal ligament.

Lateral laparoscopic trocars are placed in a region of the lower abdomen where injury to the inferior epigastric and superficial epigastric vessels can occur easily. The inferior epigastric arteries and the superficial epigastric arteries run similar courses toward the umbilicus. Knowing the average location of these blood vessels helps in choosing insertion sites that will minimize their injury and the potential hemorrhage and hematomas that this injury can cause. Just above the pubic symphysis, the vessels lie approximately 5.5 cm from the midline, whereas at the level of the umbilicus, they are 4.5 cm from the midline (**Fig. 7.30**). Therefore, placement either lateral or medial to the line connecting these points minimizes potential vascular injury. In addition, the location of the inferior epigastric vessel can often be seen (**Fig. 7.31**) by following the round ligament to its point of entry into the inguinal ring, recognizing that the vessel lies just lateral to this point.

Nerves of the Abdominal Wall

The innervation of the abdominal wall (**Fig. 7.30**) comes from the abdominal extension of intercostal nerves 7 through 11, subcostal nerve (T12), and iliohypogastric and ilioinguinal nerves (both L1). Dermatome T10 lies at the umbilicus.

After giving off a lateral cutaneous branch, each intercostal nerve pierces the lateral border of the rectus sheath. There it provides a lateral branch that ends in the rectus muscle. The anterior branch then passes through the muscle and perforates the rectus sheath to supply the subcutaneous tissues and skin as the anterior cutaneous branches. Incisions along the lateral border of the rectus lead to denervation of the muscle, which can render it atrophic and weaken the abdominal wall. Elevation of the rectus sheath off the muscle during the Pfannenstiel incision stretches the perforating nerve, which is sometimes ligated to provide hemostasis from the accompanying artery. This may leave an area of cutaneous anesthesia.

The iliohypogastric and ilioinguinal nerves pass medial to the anterosuperior iliac spine in the abdominal wall. The former supplies the skin of the suprapubic area. The latter supplies the lower abdominal wall, and by sending a branch through the inguinal canal, it supplies the upper portions of the labia majora and medial portions of the thigh. These nerves can be entrapped in the lateral closure of a transverse incision and may lead to chronic pain syndromes.

The genitofemoral (L1 and L2) and femorocutaneous (L2 and L3) nerves can be injured during gynecologic surgery. The genitofemoral nerve lies on the psoas muscle (**Fig. 7.31**), where pressure from a retractor can damage it and lead to anesthesia in the medial thigh and lateral labia. The femoral cutaneous nerve can be compressed either by a retractor blade lateral to the psoas or by too much flexion of the hip in the lithotomy position, causing anesthesia over the anterior thigh.

BEST SURGICAL PRACTICES

- Important anatomic relationships of the ureter include the following:
  - The ureter lies medial to the ovarian vessels at the bifurcation of the internal and external iliac arteries entering the pelvic brim.
  - The ureter courses under the uterine artery approximately at 1.5 cm lateral to the cervix.
  - The ureter lies directly on the anterior vaginal wall very near the place where the vagina is detached from the cervix during the hysterectomy.
- Branches of the ilioinguinal and iliohypogastric nerves run in the region of the abdominal wall involved in lower

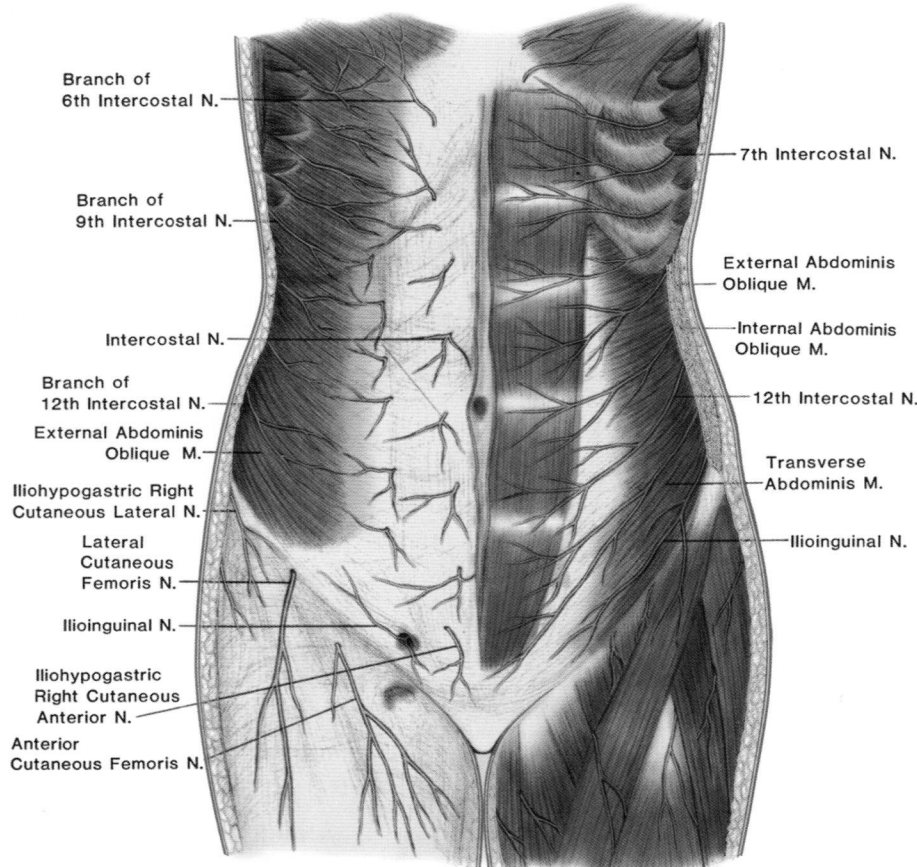

FIGURE 7.30 Nerve supply to the abdomen. **Right:** Deep innervation of T6BT12 to the transverse abdominal, internal oblique, and rectal muscles. **Left:** Superficial distribution, including cutaneous nerves, after penetration and innervation of the external oblique muscle and fascia. Innervation of the groin and thigh also is shown.

Labels (left illustration):
- Branch of 6th Intercostal N.
- Branch of 9th Intercostal N.
- Intercostal N.
- Branch of 12th Intercostal N.
- External Abdominis Oblique M.
- Iliohypogastric Right Cutaneous Lateral N.
- Lateral Cutaneous Femoris N.
- Ilioinguinal N.
- Iliohypogastric Right Cutaneous Anterior N.
- Anterior Cutaneous Femoris N.

Labels (right illustration):
- 7th Intercostal N.
- External Abdominis Oblique M.
- Internal Abdominis Oblique M.
- 12th Intercostal N.
- Transverse Abdominis M.
- Ilioinguinal N.

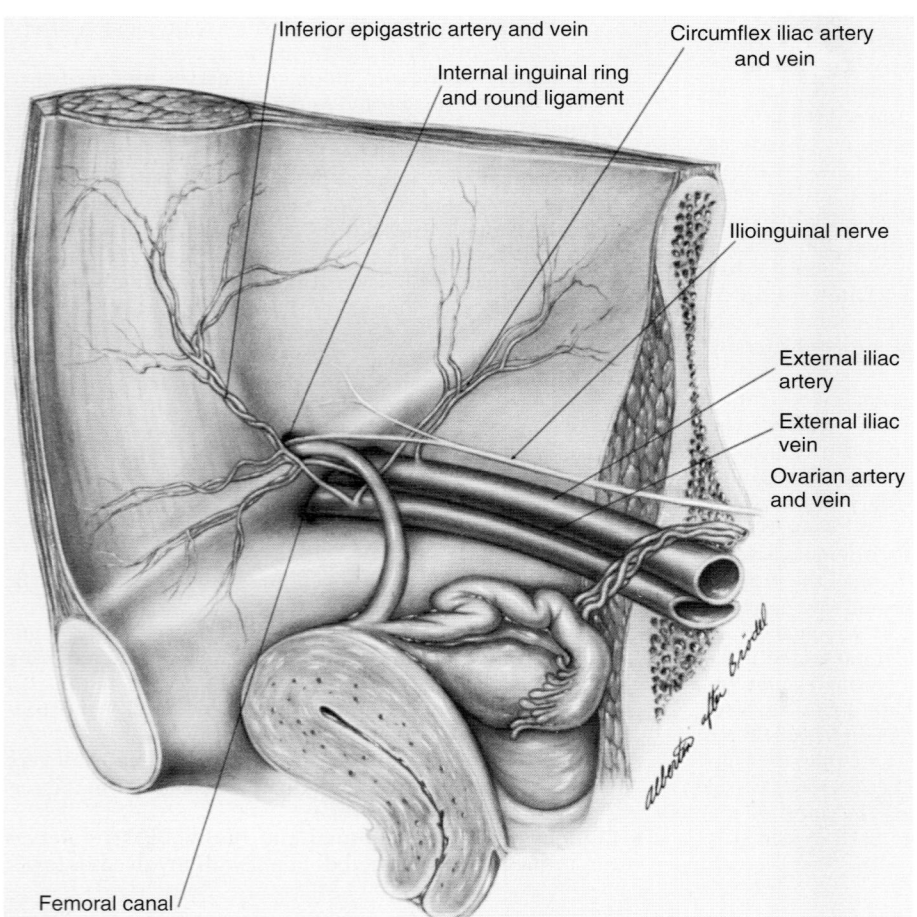

Labels:
- Inferior epigastric artery and vein
- Internal inguinal ring and round ligament
- Circumflex iliac artery and vein
- Ilioinguinal nerve
- External iliac artery
- External iliac vein
- Ovarian artery and vein
- Femoral canal

FIGURE 7.31 Sagittal view of female pelvis, showing inguinal and femoral anatomy. (The original illustration is in the Max Brödel Archives in the Department of Art as Applied to Medicine, The Johns Hopkins University School of Medicine, Baltimore, MD, USA, with permission.)

abdominal transverse incision and can be involved with nerve entrapment syndromes after these incisions.

- Support of the pelvic organs comes from the combined action of the levator ani muscles that close the genital hiatus and provide a supportive layer on which the organs can rest and by the attachment of the vagina and uterus to the pelvic sidewalls.
- The internal iliac vessels supply the pelvic organs and pelvic wall and gluteal regions. The complexity of these multiple branches varies from individual to individual, but the key feature is the multiple areas of collateral circulation that come into play immediately after internal iliac artery ligation so that blood supply to the pelvic organs has diminished pulse pressure but continues to have flow even after the ligation.
- The blood supply to the female genital tract is an arcade that begins at the top with input from the ovarian vessels, lateral supply by the uterine vessels, and distal supply by the vaginal artery. There is an anastigmatic artery that runs along the entire length of the genital tract. For this reason, ligation of any single one of these arteries does not diminish flow to the uterus itself.

BIBLIOGRAPHY

Anson BJ. *An atlas of human anatomy*. Philadelphia, PA: WB Saunders, 1950:241.

Burchell RC. Arterial physiology of the human female pelvis. *Obstet Gynecol* 1968;31:855.

Campbell RM. The anatomy and histology of the sacrouterine ligaments. *Am J Obstet Gynecol* 1950;59:1.

Cox HT. The cleavage lines of the skin. *Br J Surg* 1941;29:234.

Curry SL, Wharton JT, Rutledge F. Positive lymph nodes in vulvar squamous carcinoma. *Gynecol Oncol* 1980;9:63.

Dalley AF. The riddle of the sphincters. *Am Surg* 1987;53:298.

Daseler EH, Anson BJ, Reimann AF. Radical excision of the inguinal and iliac lymph glands. *Surg Gynecol Obstet* 1948;87:679.

DeLancey JOL. Anatomic aspects of vaginal eversion after hysterectomy. *Am J Obstet Gynecol* 1992;166:1717.

DeLancey JOL. Correlative study of paraurethral anatomy. *Obstet Gynecol* 1986;68:91.

DeLancey JOL. Structural anatomy of the posterior compartment as it relates to rectocele. *Am J Obstet Gynecol* 1999;180:815.

DeLancey JOL. Structural aspects of the extrinsic continence mechanism. *Obstet Gynecol* 1988;72:296.

DeLancey JOL. Structural support of the urethra as it relates to stress urinary incontinence: the hammock hypothesis. *Am J Obstet Gynecol* 1994;170:1713.

DeLancey JOL, Toglia MR, Perucchini D. Internal and external anal sphincter anatomy as it relates to midline obstetric lacerations. *Obstet Gynecol* 1997;90:924.

Fernstrom I. Arteriography of the uterine artery. *Acta Radiol* 1955;122(suppl):21.

Fluhmann CF, Dickmann Z. The basic pattern of the glandular structures of the cervix uteri. *Obstet Gynecol* 1958;11:543.

Forster DS. A note on Scarpa's fascia. *J Anat* 1937;72:130.

Funt MI, Thompson JD, Birch H. Normal vaginal axis. *South Med J* 1978;71:1534.

Goerttler K. Die architektur der muskelwand des menschlichen uterus und ihre funktionelle bedeutung. *Morph Jarb* 1930;65:45.

Goff BH. The surgical anatomy of cystocele and urethrocele with special reference to the pubocervical fascia. *Surg Gynecol Obstet* 1948;87:725.

Hudson CN. Lymphatics of the pelvis. In: Philipp EE, Barnes J, Newton M, eds. *Scientific foundations of obstetrics and gynecology*, 3rd ed. London, UK: Heinemann, 1986:1.

Huffman J. Detailed anatomy of the paraurethral ducts in the adult human female. *Am J Obstet Gynecol* 1948;55:86.

Hughesdon PE. The fibromuscular structure of the cervix and its changes during pregnancy and labour. *J Obstet Gynaecol Br Emp* 1952;59:763.

Huisman AB. Aspects on the anatomy of the female urethra with special relation to urinary continence. *Contrib Gynecol Obstet* 1983;10:1.

Hurd WW, Bude RO, DeLancey JOL, et al. The location of abdominal wall blood vessels in relationship to abdominal landmarks apparent at laparoscopy. *Am J Obstet Gynecol* 1994;171:642.

Hutch JA. *Anatomy and physiology of the bladder, trigone and urethra*. New York: Appleton-Century-Crofts, 1972.

Klink EW. Perineal nerve block: an anatomic and clinical study in the female. *Obstet Gynecol* 1953;1:137.

Krantz KE. The anatomy of the urethra and anterior vaginal wall. *Am J Obstet Gynecol* 1951;62:374.

Krantz KE. Innervation of the human uterus. *Ann N Y Acad Sci* 1959;75:770.

Kuhn RJ, Hollyock VE. Observations on the anatomy of the rectovaginal pouch and septum. *Obstet Gynecol* 1982;59:445.

Lawson JON. Pelvic anatomy. I. Pelvic floor muscles. *Ann R Coll Surg Engl* 1974;54:244.

Lawson JON. Pelvic anatomy. II. Anal canal and associated sphincters. *Ann R Coll Surg Engl* 1974;54:288.

Milley PS, Nichols DH. The relationship between the pubo-urethral ligaments and the urogenital diaphragm in the human female. *Anat Rec* 1971;170:281.

Milloy FJ, Anson BJ, McAfee DK. The rectus abdominis muscle and the epigastric arteries. *Surg Gynecol Obstet* 1960;110:293.

Morley GW, DeLancey JOL. Sacrospinous ligament fixation for eversion of the vagina. *Am J Obstet Gynecol* 1988;158:872.

Muellner SR. Physiology of micturition. *J Urol* 1951;65:805.

Nesselrod JP. An anatomic restudy of the pelvic lymphatics. *Ann Surg* 1936;104:905.

Nichols DH. Sacrospinous fixation for massive eversion of the vagina. *Am J Obstet Gynecol* 1982;142:901.

Nichols DH, Milley PS, Randall CL. Significance of restoration of normal vaginal depth and axis. *Obstet Gynecol* 1970;36:251.

Nichols DH, Randall CL. *Vaginal surgery*, 3rd ed. Baltimore, MD: Williams & Wilkins, 1989.

O'Connell HE, Hutson JM, Anderson CR, et al. Anatomical relationship between urethra and clitoris. *J Urol* 1998;159:1892.

Oelrich TM. The striated urogenital sphincter muscle in the female. *Anat Rec* 1983;205:223.

Oh C, Kark AE. Anatomy of the external anal sphincter. *Br J Surg* 1972;59:717.

Oh C, Kark AE. Anatomy of the perineal body. *Dis Colon Rectum* 1973;16:444.

Parry-Jones E. Lymphatics of the vulva. *J Obstet Gynaecol Br Emp* 1963;70:751.

Plentl AA, Friedman EA. *Lymphatic system of the female genitalia*. Philadelphia, PA: WB Saunders, 1971.

Ramanah R, Berger MB, Parratte BM, et al. Anatomy and histology of apical support: a literature review concerning cardinal and uterosacral ligaments. *Int Urogynecol J* 2012;23:1483.

Ramsey EM. Vascular anatomy. In: Wynn RM, ed. *Biology of the uterus*. New York: Plenum Press, 1977:60.

Range RL, Woodburne RT. The gross and microscopic anatomy of the transverse cervical ligaments. *Am J Obstet Gynecol* 1964;90:460.

Reiffenstuhl G. The clinical significance of the connective tissue planes and spaces. *Clin Obstet Gynecol* 1982;25:811.

Ricci JV, Lisa JR, Thom CH, et al. The relationship of the vagina to adjacent organs in reconstructive surgery. *Am J Surg* 1947;74:387.

Ricci JV, Thom CH. The myth of a surgically useful fascia in vaginal plastic reconstructions. *Q Rev Surg Obstet Gynecol* 1954;2:253.

Richardson AC, Edmonds PB, Williams NL. Treatment of stress urinary incontinence due to paravaginal fascial defect. *Obstet Gynecol* 1981;57:357.

Roberts WH, Habenicht J, Krishingner G. The pelvic and perineal fasciae and their neural and vascular relationships. *Anat Rec* 1964;149:707.

Roberts WH, Harrison CW, Mitchell DA, et al. The levator ani muscle and the nerve supply of its puborectalis component. *Clin Anat* 1988;1:256.

Roberts WH, Krishingner GL. Comparative study of human internal iliac artery based on Adachi classification. *Anat Rec* 1967;158:191.

Sampson JA. Ureteral fistulae as sequelae of pelvic operations. *Surg Gynecol Obstet* 1909;8:479.

Sato K. A morphological analysis of the nerve supply of the sphincter ani externus, levator ani and coccygeus. *Acta Anat Nippon* 1980;44:187.

Schreiber H. Konstruktionsmorphologische Betrachtungen uber den Wandungsbau der menschlichen Vagina. *Arkiv fur Gynaekologie* 1942;174(B43):222.

Skandalakis JE, Gray SW, Rowe JS. *Anatomical complications in general surgery.* New York: McGraw-Hill, 1983:297.

Stein TA, DeLancey JO. Structure of the perineal membrane in females: gross and microscopic anatomy. *Obstet Gynecol* 2008;111:686.

Stulz P, Pfeiffer KM. Peripheral nerve injuries resulting from common surgical procedures in the lower portion of the abdomen. *Arch Surg* 1982;117:324.

Tobin CE, Benjamin JA. Anatomic and clinical re-evaluation of Camper's, Scarpa's and Colles' fasciae. *Surg Gynecol Obstet* 1949;88:545.

Uhlenhuth E, Nolley GW. Vaginal fascia, a myth? *Obstet Gynecol* 1957;10:349.

Zacharin RF. The anatomic supports of the female urethra. *Obstet Gynecol* 1968;32:754.

CHAPTER 8
Preoperative Care of the Gynecologic Patient

Victoria L. Handa

Preoperative care is a critical factor in achieving successful outcomes of both emergent and scheduled gynecologic surgical procedures. This chapter is designed to address the essential features of preoperative care from the preoperative examination in the office, or emergency room, to the time of surgery. Included are suggestions relating to appropriate preoperative testing and evaluation. Foremost, it is essential to keep in mind that each woman must be considered individually, based on her medical findings and needs, and that no suggestions can be completely adapted to all women preparing for gynecologic surgery.

The goals of the preoperative evaluation are to answer the following three questions, as outlined by Roizen:

1. Is the patient in optimal health?
2. Can, or should, the patient's physical or mental condition be improved before surgery?
3. Does the patient have health problems or use any medications that could unexpectedly influence perioperative events?

PREOPERATIVE COUNSELING

It is most important to dedicate a portion of the preoperative care time to a discussion with the patient of options for management of her gynecologic problem, including both short- and long-term potential complications. All patients must be given sufficient medical information to allow them to make an educated decision about whether to proceed with the planned surgery. Not only is the discussion time useful in fostering a good physician–patient relationship, but it becomes extremely important if outcomes of surgery are less than expected, particularly if the discussion was documented in the patient's record. The informed consent process should include patient education regarding the goals of the planned surgery, the alternatives, and the possible hazards. The preoperative discussion is also an opportunity to discuss expectations for the recovery period, including the expected duration of hospitalization and recommended activity restrictions for the postoperative period. This is also an opportunity to review the patient's wishes regarding advanced directives.

SCREENING FOR PERIOPERATIVE RISK

Once a decision has been made to proceed with surgery, it is the responsibility of the surgeon to assess the patient for medical and surgical conditions that could increase her risk of complications. The most important part of the evaluation is the history. A screening questionnaire may also be of value (Table 8.1). The goal is to detect preexisting conditions shown to be associated with perioperative adverse events. Women with these risk factors should be further evaluated. Depending on the complexity of the situation, the surgeon may partner with the patient's primary physician or with consultants to provide additional evaluation and management.

The risks of perioperative morbidity and mortality are strongly associated with the type of surgery planned. For example, the risk of cardiac death or myocardial infarction is 1% to 5% after major intraperitoneal surgery but less than 1% for ambulatory surgeries. Thus, the extent of the planned surgery, the nature of the pathologic condition indicating surgery, and the impact of any planned adjuvant treatments should be considered.

Risk factors for major cardiac complications (including myocardial infarction, pulmonary edema, ventricular fibrillation, cardiac arrest, and complete heart block) are well established. These risk factors include history of prior myocardial infarction, heart failure, cerebrovascular disease, insulin-dependent

TABLE 8.1 Preanesthetic Screening Questionnaire
1. Do you usually get chest pain or breathlessness when you climb up two flights of stairs at normal speed?
2. Do you have kidney disease?
3. Has anyone in your family (blood relatives) had a problem following an anesthetic?
4. Have you ever had a heart attack?
5. Have you ever been diagnosed with an irregular heartbeat?
6. Have you ever had a stroke?
7. If you have been put to sleep for an operation, were there any anesthetic problems?
8. Do you suffer from epilepsy or seizures?
9. Do you have any problems with pain, stiffness, or arthritis in your neck or jaw?
10. Do you have thyroid disease?
11. Do you suffer from angina?
12. Do you have liver disease?
13. Have you ever been diagnosed with heart failure?
14. Do you suffer from asthma?
15. Do you have diabetes that requires insulin?
16. Do you have diabetes that requires tablets only?
17. Do you suffer from bronchitis?

Reprinted with permission from Asbury AJ, Hilditch WG, Jack E, et al. Validation of a pre-anaesthetic screening questionnaire. *Anaesthesia* 2003;58:874, with permission. Copyright © 2003, John Wiley and Sons.

TABLE 8.2 Classification of Physical Status, Established by the American Society of Anesthesiologists

CLASS	DESCRIPTION
P1	A normal healthy patient
P2	A patient with mild systemic disease
P3	A patient with severe systemic disease
P4	A patient with severe systemic disease that is a constant threat to life
P5	A moribund patient who is not expected to survive without the operation
P6	A declared brain-dead patient whose organs are being removed for donor purposes

Excerpted from ASA Manual for Anesthesia Department Organization and Management, American Society of Anesthesiologists, Park Ridge, IL, 2003–2004. A copy of the full text can be obtained from ASA, 520 N. Northwest Highway, Park Ridge, IL 60068-2573.

diabetes, and serum creatinine >2.0 mg/dL. Among gynecologic surgery patients with none of these risk factors, the risk of a major cardiac complication is less than 1%. Other important factors include the age of the patient, dependent functional status (defined as unable to perform activities of daily living without assistance), and American Society of Anesthesiologists' class (Table 8.2). The patient's exercise tolerance can be used as a guide: Poor exercise tolerance is defined as inability to walk four blocks or to climb two flights of stairs as a part of normal daily activities. A more diligent preoperative evaluation is appropriate for women at high risk, possibly including exercise stress test and referral for cardiology evaluation.

Diabetes mellitus is a potential risk factor for cardiovascular morbidity and perioperative infections. The risk of surgical site infection is higher among women with preoperative serum glucose >200 mg/dL. The risk of infection is also significantly increased by postoperative hyperglycemia. In addition, an assessment for end-organ failure (such as renal or cardiac disease) is appropriate for women with long-standing diabetes, and especially those with a history of poor control and those with other sequelae from their diabetes.

Clinically significant pulmonary complications occur in 5% to 10% of surgeries. In a systematic review, Smetana and colleagues found that risk factors for pulmonary complications include age over 50 years, functional dependence (requiring assistance to perform activities of daily living), obstructive sleep apnea, surgery lasting greater than 3 hours, and cigarette smoking. Smoking duration is also a risk factor for perioperative complications. Well-controlled asthma is not a risk factor for perioperative pulmonary complications.

VALUE OF SCREENING LABORATORY STUDIES AND OTHER TESTING

The practice of a routine battery of preoperative laboratory tests is no longer recommended. Using data from National Surgical Quality Improvement Program, Benarroch-Gampel and colleagues demonstrated that the patient's medical history, age, and the type of surgery planned are better predictors of surgical complications than are the results of laboratory tests. Similar findings were obtained by Fritsch and colleagues. The indiscriminate use of "routine" preoperative tests not only fails to identify high-risk patients but also leads to unnecessary costs. Also, false-positive results can lead to unnecessary surgical delays and interventions. Thus, preoperative tests should not be ordered routinely but should be based on the characteristics of the patient and the planned surgery.

Preoperative testing recommendations at Johns Hopkins Bayview Medical Center are summarized in Table 8.3. Testing recommendations for gynecologic surgery are based on the patient's risk factors, which are derived from the history and physical examination. Coagulation studies are rarely recommended prior to gynecologic surgery but may be considered for those with menorrhagia, if clinically indicated. Chest x-ray is indicated only if the patient has experienced a recent acute episode of respiratory distress or flare of chronic pulmonary disease. A urine pregnancy test is obtained on the day of surgery for women who, by history, may be pregnant. Tests that have been performed recently (within 6 months) should not be repeated if the patient's condition has not changed. This is because the result is unlikely to be different; Macpherson and colleagues found a less than 1% probability of an abnormal laboratory test result in an adult with a normal value within the past year.

Preoperative hematocrit (or complete blood count) is probably the most commonly used preoperative laboratory study. Baseline hemoglobin can be useful in the interpretation of postoperative anemia and the management of patients with acute surgical blood loss. Therefore, a preoperative hematocrit should be ordered if the planned surgery is likely to result in substantial blood loss or if the patient's history suggests a high risk for preoperative anemia.

Serum electrolytes should not be ordered routinely but may be useful in women on diuretics or with a history that suggests an electrolyte imbalance is likely. A routine BUN and creatinine are appropriate for women with diabetes or hypertension. Routine BUN and creatinine may also be useful in older patients. Serum glucose is recommended for women on chronic corticosteroids.

A preoperative electrocardiogram should be considered in women with known cardiovascular disease, peripheral artery disease, or cerebrovascular disease. This is because a baseline electrocardiogram can be useful in the management of acute perioperative cardiovascular events. However, an electrocardiogram is a poor screening test and is unlikely to alter management in the asymptomatic patient. Routine preoperative electrocardiogram should be considered in women over age 50.

A cardiac stress test should be considered if the patient reports poor exercise tolerance or if cardiac symptoms are present. Other indications for a preoperative cardiac evaluation include a history of prior myocardial infarction, known or suspected heart failure, cerebrovascular disease, insulin-dependent diabetes, and serum creatinine >2.0 mg/dL.

Preoperative chest x-ray and pulmonary function tests do not predict postoperative pulmonary complications and therefore should not be routinely ordered before surgery. A thorough clinical assessment will detect most high-risk conditions. Women with dyspnea, poor exercise tolerance, or unexplained cough should be considered for further evaluation.

Cervical cytology should be obtained before hysterectomy for benign disease. The goal is to identify women with cervical cancer, for whom a simple hysterectomy is not appropriate. If the patient is up to date on screening cytology and the last study was normal, cytology should not be repeated.

TABLE 8.3 Johns Hopkins Bayview Medical Center Preoperative Evaluation Center Preadmission Screening Guidelines

MEDICAL CONDITION	CBC	SERUM ELECTROLYTES	PT/PTT	LIVER FUNCTION TESTS	EKG
Age >50					X
Hypertension		X			X
Cardiac disease or arrhythmia	X	X			X
Diabetes		X			X
Renal disease		X			X
Diuretic/ACE inhibitor/chemotherapy		X			X
Hematologic or liver disease	X		X	X	
Hysterectomy	X				
Hysteroscopy		X			
Highly invasive procedures: Radical surgery Preoperative bowel prep Anticipate >500 mL blood loss	X	X	X		X

These are screening guidelines only; further testing based on the patient's medical history, surgeon's evaluation, or primary care physician's discretion.
Data from Johns Hopkins Bayview Medical Center Preoperative Evaluation Center pre-admission guidelines.

To minimize infectious complications of surgery, active infections (such as urinary tract infection) should be identified and treated completely before surgery unless surgery is urgent. In addition, American College of Obstetricians and Gynecologists recommends screening for and treating bacterial vaginosis before hysterectomy to minimize the risk of cuff infection. However, an alternative is the routine use of preoperative metronidazole. This option may be cost-effective at the time of hysterectomy if the prevalence of bacterial vaginosis is at least 1%.

PERIOPERATIVE MANAGEMENT OF MEDICATIONS TAKEN CHRONICALLY

The management of chronic medications varies by institution, and there is little evidence to guide best practices. However, most medications taken chronically are safely continued in the perioperative period. Cessation should not be recommended for beta-blockers (especially if used to control arrhythmia or angina), statins, alpha 2 agonists, H2 blockers, proton pump inhibitors, and inhaled asthma medications (including steroids, beta-agonists, and anticholinergics).

There is considerable controversy about whether to stop oral contraceptives in the perioperative period. The rationale for stopping hormonal contraception is to minimize phlebitis risk. However, concerns regarding unwanted pregnancy are also valid. Therefore, the most practical option is probably to continue oral contraception.

Medications that should be stopped before surgery include herbal preparations, including Ephedra, Garlic, Ginkgo, Ginseng, Kava, and St. John's Wort.

Typically, warfarin is stopped before elective surgery to minimize the risks of significant bleeding or hematoma formation. However, the risk of thrombosis is increased by cessation of warfarin before surgery. Thus, patients at high risk of thrombosis should be managed by transitioning from warfarin to enoxaparin (Lovenox) 1 mg/kg subcutaneously twice a day in the preoperative period, usually beginning 5 days before elective surgery. Once the international normalized ratio is less than 1.5, the risk of bleeding is further minimized if enoxaparin can be held for 24 hours before surgery. An inferior vena cava filter is an alternative to perioperative enoxaparin. Warfarin can be continued if the planned procedure is such that the risk of surgical bleeding is minimal.

Traditionally, patients have been asked to refrain from using aspirin before elective surgery. The rationale to stop aspirin is the increased risk of hematoma and bleeding complications. However, among women who are on maintenance therapy with aspirin for cardiovascular prevention, aspirin cessation may lead to an increase in thrombosis. Aspirin withdrawal leads to an increase in perioperative risk of cardiac and thromboembolic complications among women who use aspirin for cardiovascular prevention. Therefore, current recommendations are to continue maintenance aspirin therapy for women who use this for cardiovascular prevention. However, casual use of aspirin in the perioperative period should be avoided.

PREOPERATIVE MANAGEMENT OF RISK FACTORS

Women at highest risk for perioperative cardiac events should be considered for treatment with a beta-blocker. A number of large clinical trials have investigated the benefit of perioperative beta-blockers to reduce cardiac events. Based on evidence of benefit, especially for women undergoing cardiac surgery, the American Heart Association has recommended that high-risk patients receive perioperative beta-blockers, beginning at least 1 week before surgery (preferably 30 days). Those felt to benefit from this intervention included women with ischemic heart disease, those with heart failure, women with a history of cerebrovascular disease, women with diabetes mellitus, and those with renal insufficiency (serum creatinine >2 mg/dL).

However, the 2008 PeriOperative ISchemic Evaluation (POISE) trial suggested that perioperative beta-blockade was associated with an increased risk of stroke. As a result, enthusiasm for prophylaxis has waned. The current recommendations for perioperative beta-blockade are focus on high-risk groups, with initiation of therapy well before the planned surgery in order to titrate dosage to control heart rate while avoiding bradycardia and hypotension. Beta-blockers should not be initiated on the day of surgery. As previously noted, withdrawal of beta-blockers should be avoided in patients receiving this therapy chronically.

Revascularization, including angioplasty and coronary stents, may be employed as a strategy to reduce risk in women with ischemic heart disease. However, the risk of myocardial infarctions or death is increased in the first few weeks after angioplasty or stenting. Therefore, if possible, elective gynecologic surgery should not be performed in the first 6 weeks after angioplasty or stenting. For women who have received a drug-eluting stent, elective surgery should be avoided for 1 year.

Optimal control of diabetes should be obtained before elective surgery to reduce surgical complications, especially surgical site infections. The risk of surgical infection is higher in diabetics with poor glucose control before surgery and in the immediate postoperative period. More specifically, among 55,000 diabetics undergoing surgery, King and colleagues found that infection risk was marginally increased for postoperative serum glucose 150 to 250 mg/dL but increased 50% for women with serum glucose greater than 250 mg/dL. Thus, the goal of perioperative management of diabetes is to maintain a serum glucose <200 mg/dL in the perioperative period. Women with diabetes should be assessed preoperatively for renal impairment.

Perioperative adrenal insufficiency can occur among women receiving glucocorticoids. Women who have received more than 20 mg/day of prednisone (or equivalent) for at least 3 weeks over the 6 months preceding surgery should be treated with "stress steroids." A typical regimen for "stress steroids" would include preoperative administration of 50 mg IV hydrocortisone and postoperative administration of 25 mg IV hydrocortisone every 8 hours for 24 hours.

Women who smoke cigarettes should be encouraged to quit prior to elective surgery. Smoking cessation should be attempted as far in advance of surgery as possible. Risks related to smoking are dramatically reduced by at least 2 months of smoking cessation prior to surgery.

Controversy surrounds the practice of perioperative mechanical bowel preparation. A 2005 meta-analysis demonstrated no benefit to preoperative mechanical bowel preparation. Some surgeons continue the practice for vaginal or laparoscopic surgery with the goal of decompressing the bowel.

RISK REDUCTION ON THE DAY OF SURGERY

Most gynecologic surgeons are familiar with strategies for prevention of deep venous phlebitis. The risk of perioperative phlebitis is influenced by both patient and surgical characteristics. Most women undergoing gynecologic surgery will be classified as moderate or high risk, depending on the duration of the procedure (<30 or >30 minutes) and the age of the patient (<60 or >60 years). For both groups, recommended prophylactic options include heparin (5,000 u SQ q12h), enoxaparin

(Lovenox) 40 mg daily, or intermittent pneumatic compression stockings. Prophylaxis should be initiated before surgery and continued at least through hospital discharge. It is not clear whether these measures are beneficial if they are initiated after surgery.

Surgical site infection is defined by the Centers for Disease Control and Prevention (CDC) as infections at or near the surgical incision occurring within 30 days of an operative procedure or within 1 year if an implant is left in place. Surgical site infections can be minimized by preoperative preparation, such as optimal glucose control among diabetics and identification and preoperative treatment of infection. Prevention of surgical site infection includes skin preparation. Hair removal does not reduce surgical site infections. If hair removal at the surgical site is necessary or preferred by the surgeon, the hair should be clipped rather than shaved. Specifically, the risk for surgical site infection is more than doubled by shaving versus clipping.

Traditionally, skin preparation with povidone–iodine has been used to minimize surgical site infection. However, a randomized study by Darouiche and colleagues suggested that chlorhexidine–alcohol is superior to povidone–iodine preparation. Thus, chlorhexidine–alcohol should be preferred for preparation of abdominal skin.

Povidone–iodine remains the standard for vaginal skin preparation. The optimal vaginal preparation for women with iodine allergy is not established. Chlorhexidine has been suggested as an alternative, but the current labeling of chlorhexidine warns of use in genital area, and therefore many surgeons are hesitant to consider the use of this agent in the vagina. Moreover, the value of chlorhexidine preparation was questioned by a recent retrospective cohort study of greater than 7,000 abdominal hysterectomies in Sweden. Kjølhede and colleagues found no difference between vaginal cleansing with chlorhexidine solution versus no vaginal preparation. In contrast, other studies have suggested a benefit from chlorhexidine vaginal preparation. In summary, povidone–iodine remains the preferred preparation, with some surgeons opting to use chlorhexidine in women who report allergy to iodine.

Preoperative intravenous antibiotics can further reduce surgical site infections in clean-contaminated surgeries, such as hysterectomy. The American College of Obstetricians and Gynecologists recommends antibiotic prophylaxis prior to hysterectomy and urogynecology procedures (including those involving mesh). Cephazolin is recommended, although alternatives include cefotetan, cefoxitin, cefuroxime, or ampicillin–sulbactam. In case of penicillin allergy, clindamycin plus gentamicin is the recommended alternative. Prophylactic antibiotics should be administered within 60 minutes prior to the start of surgery. The goals are to insure serum levels of the drug at the time of incision and to minimize the risk of a severe allergic reaction at the time of induction of anesthesia.

Recommendations have changed for perioperative antibiotics for prevention of endocarditis. The American Heart Association and other international organizations no longer recommend endocarditis prophylaxis for any gynecologic procedures, including hysterectomy.

In contrast, the use of prophylactic antibiotics for women with prosthetic joints undergoing invasive procedures remains controversial. In the past, intravenous antibiotics were recommended to reduce bacteremia at the time of genital tract surgery, in an effort to reduce hematogenous infection of prosthesis. However, in December 2012, The American Academy of Orthopedic Surgeons and the American Dental Association issued a statement recommending against the practice of routinely prescribing prophylactic antibiotics for patients with hip and knee prosthetic joint implants undergoing dental procedures. This was after an evidence-based review failed to demonstrate any benefit from antibiotics in this setting. However, it is not clear whether those recommendations represent the best practices for women undergoing gynecologic surgery. For women at highest risk, the gynecologic surgeon might consider administering a single dose of cefazolin, cefoxitin, or ampicillin–sulbactam. Risk factors have been defined as immunosuppression, history of inflammatory arthropathies (e.g., rheumatoid arthritis, systemic lupus erythematosus), history of joint infection, and insulin-dependent (Type 1) diabetes. The value of antibiotic prophylaxis in these groups is unclear.

BIBLIOGRAPHY

ACOG Committee on Practice Bulletins—Gynecology. ACOG Practice Bulletin No. 104: Antibiotic prophylaxis for gynecologic procedures. *Obstet Gynecol* 2009;113:1180.

Ang-Lee MK, Moss J, Yuan CS. Herbal medicines and perioperative care. *JAMA* 2001;286:208.

Asbury AJ, Hilditch WG, Jack E, et al. Validation of a pre-anaesthetic screening questionnaire. *Anaesthesia* 2003;58:874.

Barrera R, Shi W, Amar D, et al. Smoking and timing of cessation: impact on pulmonary complications after thoracotomy. *Chest* 2005;127:1977.

Benarroch-Gampel J, Sheffield KM, Duncan CB, et al. Preoperative laboratory testing in patients undergoing elective, low-risk ambulatory surgery. *Ann Surg* 2012;256:518.

Centre for Clinical Practice at NICE (UK). Prophylaxis against Infective Endocarditis: Antimicrobial Prophylaxis Against Infective Endocarditis in Adults and Children Undergoing Interventional Procedures [Internet]. London, UK: National Institute for Health and Clinical Excellence (UK), 2008. (NICE Clinical Guidelines, No. 64.) Available from: http://www.ncbi.nlm.nih.gov/books/NBK51789/

Cohen MM, Duncan PG, Tate RB. Does anesthesia contribute to operative mortality? *JAMA* 1988;260:2859.

Committee on Practice Bulletins—Gynecology, American College of Obstetrician and Gynecologists. ACOG Practice Bulletin No 84: Prevention of deep vein thrombosis and pulmonary embolism. *Obstet Gynecol* 2007;110:429.

Committee on Standards and Practice Parameters, Apfelbaum JL, Connis RT, Nickinovich DG, et al. Practice advisory for preanesthesia evaluation: an updated report by the American Society of Anesthesiologists Task Force on Preanesthesia Evaluation. *Anesthesiology* 2012;116:522.

Culligan PJ, Kubik K, Murphy M, et al. A randomized trial that compared povidone iodine and chlorhexidine as antiseptics for vaginal hysterectomy. *Am J Obstet Gynecol* 2005;192:422.

Darouiche RO, Wall MJ Jr, Itani KM, et al. Chlorhexidine-alcohol versus povidone-iodine for surgical-site antisepsis. *N Engl J Med* 2010;362:18.

Devereaux PJ, Goldman L, Cook DJ, et al. Perioperative cardiac events in patients undergoing noncardiac surgery: a review of the magnitude of the problem, the pathophysiology of the events and methods to estimate and communicate risk. *CMAJ* 2005;173:627.

Douketis JD, Spyropoulos AC, Spencer FA, et al. Perioperative management of antithrombotic therapy: antithrombotic therapy and prevention of thrombosis, 9th ed: American College of Chest Physicians Evidence-Based Clinical Practice Guidelines. *Chest* 2012;141:e326S.

Douketis JD, Woods K, Foster GA, et al. Bridging anticoagulation with low-molecular-weight heparin after interruption of warfarin therapy is associated with a residual anticoagulant effect prior to surgery. *Thromb Haemost* 2005;94:528.

Dunkelgrun M, Boersma E, Schouten O, et al. Bisoprolol and fluvastatin for the reduction of perioperative cardiac mortality and myocardial infarction in intermediate-risk patients undergoing noncardiovascular surgery: a randomized controlled trial (DECREASE-IV). *Ann Surg* 2009;249:921.

Fleisher LA, Beckman JA, Brown KA, et al. 2009 ACCF/AHA focused update on perioperative beta blockade incorporated into the ACC/AHA 2007 guidelines on perioperative cardiovascular evaluation and care for noncardiac surgery: a report of the American college of cardiology foundation/American heart association task force on practice guidelines. *Circulation* 2009;120:e169.

Fritsch G, Flamm M, Hepner DL, et al. Abnormal pre-operative tests, pathologic findings of medical history, and their predictive value for perioperative complications. *Acta Anaesthesiol Scand* 2012;56:339.

Gerstein NS, Schulman PM, Gerstein WH, et al. Should more patients continue aspirin therapy perioperatively?: clinical impact of aspirin withdrawal syndrome. *Ann Surg* 2012;255:811.

Girish M, Trayner E Jr, Dammann O, et al. Symptom-limited stair climbing as a predictor of postoperative cardiopulmonary complications after high-risk surgery. *Chest* 2001;120:1147.

Gupta PK, Gupta H, Sundaram A, et al. Development and validation of a risk calculator for prediction of cardiac risk after surgery. *Circulation* 2011;124:381.

Hawn MT, Houston TK, Campagna EJ, et al. The attributable risk of smoking on surgical complications. *Ann Surg* 2011;254:914.

Karachalios GN, Charalabopoulos A, Papalimneou V, et al. Withdrawal syndrome following cessation of antihypertensive drug therapy. *Int J Clin Pract* 2005;59:562.

King JT Jr, Goulet JL, Perkal MF, et al. Glycemic control and infections in patients with diabetes undergoing noncardiac surgery. *Ann Surg* 2011;253:158.

Kjølhede P, Halili S, Löfgren M. Vaginal cleansing and postoperative infectious morbidity in vaginal hysterectomy. A register study from the Swedish National Register for Gynecological Surgery. *Acta Obstet Gynecol Scand* 2011;90:63.

Lee TH, Marcantonio ER, Mangione CM, et al. Derivation and prospective validation of a simple index for prediction of cardiac risk of major noncardiac surgery. *Circulation* 1999;100:1043.

Little JW, Jacobson JJ, Lockhart PB, et al. The dental treatment of patients with joint replacements: a position paper from the American Academy of Oral Medicine. *J Am Dent Assoc* 2010;141:667.

Macpherson DS, Snow R, Lofgren RP, et al. Preoperative screening: value of previous tests. *Ann Intern Med* 1990;113:969.

Malone DL, Genuit T, Tracy JK, et al. Surgical site infections: reanalysis of risk factors. *J Surg Res* 2002;103:89.

McElligott KA, Havrilesky LJ, Myers ER, et al. Preoperative screening strategies for bacterial vaginosis prior to elective hysterectomy: a cost comparison study. *Am J Obstet Gynecol* 2011;205:500.e1.

Mills E, Eyawo O, Lockhart I, et al. Smoking cessation reduces postoperative complications: a systematic review and meta-analysis. *Am J Med* 2011;124:144.e8.

Moller AM, Maaloe R, Pedersen T. Postoperative intensive care admittance: the role of tobacco smoking. *Acta Anaesthesiol Scand* 2001;45:345.

POISE Study Group; Devereaux PJ, Yang H, Yusef F, et al. Effects of extended-release metoprolol succinate in patients undergoing noncardiac surgery (POISE trial): a randomised controlled trial. *Lancet* 2008;371:1839.

Qaseem A, Snow V, Fitterman N, et al. Risk assessment for and strategies to reduce perioperative pulmonary complications for patients undergoing noncardiothoracic surgery: a guideline from the American College of Physicians. *Ann Intern Med* 2006;144:575.

Reilly DF, McNeely MJ, Doerner D, et al. Self-reported exercise tolerance and the risk of serious perioperative complications. *Arch Intern Med* 1999;159:2185.

Roizen MF, Foss JF, Fischer SP. Preoperative evaluation. In: Miller RD, ed. *Anesthesia*, 5th ed. Philadelphia, PA: Churchill Livingstone, 2000:824.

Roizen MF. Anesthetic implications of concurrent diseases. In: Miller RD, ed. Anesthesia, 5th ed. Philadelphia, PA: Churchill Livingstone, 2000:903.

Roizen MF. More preoperative assessment by physicians and less by laboratory test [editorial comment]. The value of routine preoperative medical testing before cataract surgery. *N Engl J Med* 2000;342:168.

Shammash JB, Trost JC, Gold JM, et al. Perioperative beta-blocker withdrawal and mortality in vascular surgical patients. *Am Heart J* 2001;141:148.

Smetana GW, Lawrence VA, Cornell JE, et al. Preoperative pulmonary risk stratification for noncardiothoracic surgery: systematic review for the American College of Physicians. *Ann Intern Med* 2006;144:581.

Tanner J, Norrie P, Melen K. Preoperative hair removal to reduce surgical site infection. *Cochrane Database Syst Rev* 2011;(11):CD004122.

Wallace AW, Au S, Cason BA. Association of the pattern of use of perioperative β-blockade and postoperative mortality. *Anesthesiology* 2010;113:794.

Wille-Jørgensen P, Guenaga KF, Matos D, et al. Pre-operative mechanical bowel cleansing or not? An updated meta-analysis. *Colorectal Dis* 2005;7:304.

Wilson SH, Fasseas P, Orford JL, et al. Clinical outcome of patients undergoing non-cardiac surgery in the two months following coronary stenting. *J Am Coll Cardiol* 2003;42:234.

Wilson W, Taubert KA, Gewitz M, et al. Prevention of infective endocarditis: guidelines from the American Heart Association: a guideline from the American Heart Association Rheumatic Fever, Endocarditis, and Kawasaki Disease Committee, Council on Cardiovascular Disease in the Young, and the Council on Clinical Cardiology, Council on Cardiovascular Surgery and Anesthesia, and the Quality of Care and Outcomes Research Interdisciplinary Working Group. *Circulation* 2007;116:1736.

CHAPTER 9
Postanesthesia and Postoperative Care

Alexander Duncan, Jonathan E. Sevransky, and Ira R. Horowitz

DEFINITIONS

Hospital-acquired pneumonia (HAP)—Pneumonia that develops 48 hours or more after hospital admission because of organisms that were not incubating at the time of admission.

Hypoxic pulmonary vasoconstriction—Local reflex in the lung that diverts blood away from poorly oxygenated regions.

Low molecular weight heparin (LMWH)—Product that acts by inhibiting factor Xa.

Tissue plasminogen activator (t-PA)—Compound used for nonsurgical thrombolysis.

Venous thrombotic event—A venous thromboembolism that includes vascular clotting, such as deep vein thrombosis, and pulmonary embolism.

Virchow triad—Factors that increase the risk of vascular thromboembolism, for example, hypercoagulability, stasis, trauma to vessels.

V/Q abnormalities—Ventilation/perfusion abnormalities, which can lead to mismatching of pulmonary blood flow and ventilation.

Postoperative complications are the most important factors in defining the outcome of the first 72 hours following a patient's surgical procedure. It is critical to monitor basic physiologic parameters—such as renal, cardiovascular, and respiratory functions—and laboratory tests to optimize and sustain recovery from surgery and anesthesia.

Postoperative morbidity can be minimized by an appropriate preoperative assessment of the surgical patient. This should include emphasis on identifying the patient at risk for venous thromboembolic complications and administering prophylactic anticoagulation. Optimized nutritional status and support has also been shown to improve wound healing and decrease the postoperative recovery time and length of hospital stay.

POSTOPERATIVE VASCULAR COMPLICATIONS

About 3 million venous thrombotic events, or venous thromboembolisms (VTEs), occur in the United States each year. About 2,000,000 plus of these events are deep vein thrombosis (DVT) in the hospital, and as many as 600,000 are pulmonary embolisms (PEs). Twenty-five percent of PEs are fatal, and VTE has been recognized as the biggest preventable cause of morbidity and mortality in United States hospitals. Ten percent of hospital deaths in the US are due to PE, and some patient groups, especially gynecologic malignancy patients, have a higher-than-usual risk for VTE, with a general incidence of about 15% to 20%. The risk of fatal postoperative PE among these patients is closer to 40% with no prophylaxis. More than 90% of PE patients have a lower or upper extremity DVT concomitantly.

PE has few defining characteristics, but the onset of respiratory distress compounded by hypotension, chest pain, and cardiac arrhythmias can be harbingers of impending death and are complications that convert an otherwise successful surgery into a postoperative fatality. Only 70% of patients who die of a PE have it considered in their differential diagnosis.

Modern diagnostic studies have provided more accurate information about the frequency of vascular complications and can identify those patients at risk of an embolic event. Pre- and postoperative prophylaxis with heparin or low molecular weight heparins (LMWHs) and concomitant use of embolic stockings and intermittent pneumatic compression (IPC) devices have significantly reduced the risk of VTE in the moderate- and high-risk patients. Clarke-Pearson and colleagues, using univariate and regression analysis, designed a prognostic model to evaluate the risk of postoperative VTE for an individual patient. In a group of 411 gynecology patients, the prognostic factors they identified included type of surgery, age, leg edema, non-Caucasian ethnicity, severity of varicose veins, previous radiotherapy, and a prior history of DVT.

More than 130 years ago, Rudolph Virchow conceptualized the factors leading to postoperative thrombosis. These included venous stasis, changes in the blood constituents, and impaired function of the vessel wall. The blood clotting process is complicated (Fig. 9.1), but it is initiated by the actions of tissue factor (TF) on factor VIIa after injury to vessels exposes the subendothelium and promotes platelet adhesion and aggregation to form a primary platelet plug. The process is completed by the actions of multiple components and factors in the blood that generate thrombin, the potent rate-regulating enzyme, which then interacts with fibrinogen and factor XIII to form an insoluble clot (Fig. 9.2). Much recent evidence has focused on the role of cell-derived circulating microparticles (MPs) as potent etiologic agents for enhanced risk of VTE. This is because these MPs carry TF and other procoagulant phospholipids on their surfaces that potentiate activation of the coagulation pathways and may promote angiogenesis.

When patients have cancer or sustain venous damage from the surgical procedure, such as occurs with skeletonization of the pelvic vasculature, the up-regulation of thrombin generation has more profound effects. TF, fibrin, and thrombin

II

Coagulation Mechanism

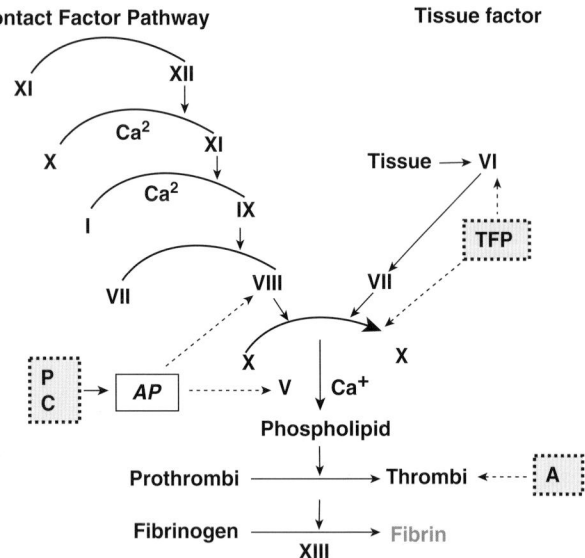

FIGURE 9.1 Formation of venous thrombus following various surgical procedures with the activation of clotting factors and aggregation of platelets. AP, activated protein, PC, protein C, TFP, tissue factor peptide.

all have angiogenic properties that can interfere with tissue structural properties by degrading matrix metalloproteinases, promoting cell migration, and enhancing metastasis. Tumors also up-regulate the production of TF and its inclusion into MPs as well as plasminogen activator inhibitor-1 (PAI-1), thus promoting the generation of procoagulant activity. This multifactorial derived activity helps to explain the high incidence of VTE in the gynecologic cancer patient.

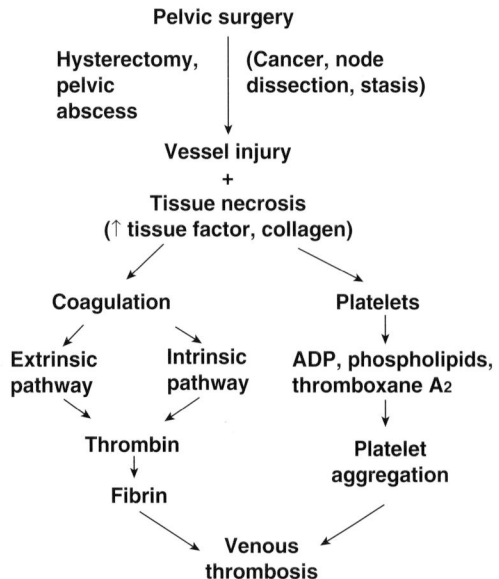

FIGURE 9.2 Schematic representation of the cascade clotting mechanism, illustrating the role of extrinsic and intrinsic factors. Increases in tissue thromboplastin-like substance and collagen-activated factor XII initiate the formation of fibrin through the extrinsic and intrinsic pathways, principally by the activation of factor X. ADP, adenosine diphosphate.

These tumorigenic effects on coagulation occur in addition to the typical acute postsurgical reactions seen in many hemostasis proteins. These include increases in fibrinogen, factor V, factor VIII, and von Willebrand factor, which promotes platelet adhesion and function. There is usually an increase in platelet number in the postoperative period, and the normal fibrinolytic response is blunted by the increase in PAI-1 and thrombin-activatable fibrinolysis inhibitor. Essentially, the fibrinolytic system is nonfunctional for several days following surgery, which down-regulates the ability of plasmin to impede wound healing by preventing degradation of fibrin and other matrix proteins.

Venous stasis is thought to be the cornerstone of postoperative thrombosis. Venous stasis in the pelvis and lower extremities results in platelet activation, promoting the adhesion of platelets to the endothelial cells lining the vessel, which are already stressed in a procoagulant mode. This results in conditions that encourage the development of a thrombus. These physiologic changes in venous hemodynamics occur in the pre-, peri-, and postoperative periods. Doran has shown that venous return from the lower extremities is decreased by half during surgical procedures because of the impact of muscle relaxation from anesthetic agents. Scanning using I^{125} fibrinogen has demonstrated that venous thrombosis is initiated during the surgery in 50% of patients who subsequently manifest a DVT. Lower extremity blood flow has been shown to decrease to about 75% of the normal drainage flow in the immediate postoperative period. This is an important reflection of Virchow triad on the role of adequate vessel flow. This reduction in flow persists for about 14 days after surgery because of the loss of muscle-pumping function in the legs. The major site of thrombus formation is the soleal venous sinuses of the calf, a portion of the venous arcade that joins the posterior tibial and peroneal veins draining the soleal muscle. Thrombi from these sinuses often occur posterior to valves located at the junction where these sinuses drain into the collecting veins. Thrombi often occur in these sinuses and in valve cusps in bedridden patients.

Another contributing factor to venous stasis during prolonged surgery is the use of tight packing of the intestines in the upper abdomen with obstruction of the underlying vena cava. The type and length of operation are directly related to the incidence of postoperative VTE, as outlined in Table 9.1.

Diagnosis of Venous Thromboembolism

The traditional clinical methods used to diagnose venous thrombosis of the lower extremities are of limited value, with error rates approaching 50% for both false-negative and false-positive rates. Most of the diagnostics problems occur because of the insidious nature of venous thrombosis in the lower extremity, which takes place in the soleal veins. Modern imaging methods have evolved considerably in recent years, ranging from I^{125} fibrinogen scanning to venography to Doppler duplex ultrasound, impedance plethysmography (IPG), and magnetic resonance imaging (MRI) technique studies. Although for DVT venography remains the gold standard, modern compression ultrasonography is now the dominant technique, having a good negative predictive value (98%) for proximal DVT and slightly lower (96%) for calf DVT. However, it is still inferior to venography, which remains the reference source (Table 9.2).

Venography

The venogram has had the most extensive and rigorous use in clinical practice of all imaging techniques. However, it is no longer routinely used because it is invasive, uses contrast dye, has limitations, and provides an increased risk in many

TABLE 9.1 Levels of Thromboembolism Risk in Surgical Patients without Prophylaxis

LEVEL OF RISK EXAMPLES	CALF DVT, %	PROXIMAL DVT, %	CLINICAL PE, %	FATAL PE, %	SUCCESSFUL PREVENTION STRATEGIES
Low risk Minor surgery in patients <40 y with no additional risk factors	2	0.4	0.2	0.002	No specific measures Aggressive mobilization
Moderate risk Minor surgery in patients with additional risk factors; nonmajor surgery in patients aged 40–60 y with no additional risk factors; major surgery in patients <40 y with no additional risk factors	10–20	2–4	1–2	0.1–0.4	LDUH q12h, LMWH, ES, or IPC
High risk Nonmajor surgery in patients >60 y or with additional risk factors; major surgery in patients >40 y or with additional risk factors	20–40	4–8	2–4	0.4–1.0	LDUH q8h, LMWH, or IPC
Highest risk Major surgery in patients >40 y plus prior VTE, cancer, or molecular hypercoagulable state; hip or knee arthroplasty, hip fracture surgery; major trauma; spinal cord injury	40–80	10–20	4–10	0.2–5	LMWH, oral anticoagulants, IPC/ES + LDUH/LMWH, or ADH

Modified from Gallus et al. and International Consensus Statement. Reprinted with permission from Geerts WH, Heit JA, Clagett GP, et al. Prevention of venous thromboembolism (Sixth ACCP Consensus Conference on Antithrombotic Therapy) *Chest* 2001;119(suppl 1): 132S. Copyright © 2008, American College of Chest Physicians.

patients who have renal compromise. However, the use of computed tomography (CT) venography in conjunction with CT angiography had proven to increase the sensitivity of DVT diagnosis from 83% to 90% in the PIOPED-II study.

I^{125}-Labeled Fibrinogen Scanning

This technique first developed in the 1960s was used widely for many years. It involves the intravenous injection of isotope-labeled fibrinogen, which is expected to be incorporated into the evolving thrombus and can be imaged by a scintillation scanner. Because of the use of isotopes, it is technically cumbersome and rarely used, despite many large studies validating its use in the 1970s and 1980s and its high correlation with venography.

Impedance Plethysmography

Impedance plethysmography is based on the principal of electrical resistance in specific areas of the body. When there is resistance to blood flow that is due to a thrombus, there is marked reduction in the electrical resistance over that vessel. IPG is most useful in proximal venous thrombosis but is relatively poor in visualizing thrombi below the knee because of the small caliber and slow flow rates through the soleal sinuses. The technique is only about 50% accurate compared with venography in detecting DVT below the popliteal vessels.

Huisman and colleagues evaluated 471 outpatients clinically suspected of acute-onset DVT. Four sequential IPGs were obtained on days 1, 2, 5, and 10 of the study. Of the 137 patients with abnormal results, 117 (85%) had abnormal results on day 1, with the other 20 patients becoming positive by day 10. When compared with venography, serial IPG had a specificity of 92% and a sensitivity of 100%. The use of serial testing clearly improved the ability to diagnose DVT. Another similar study by Vaccaro and associates involving 252 patients using single-test IPG gave a sensitivity of 84% and a specificity of 78%, confirming the superiority of the serial testing protocol. Given the short length of hospital stays now, it is unlikely that serial IPG would be possible despite its proven high correlation with venography.

Doppler Ultrasound

The use of Doppler ultrasound, often with computer color enhancement, has become the most widely used imaging technique for diagnosis of DVT. Its major physiologic use is in the measurement of flow velocity in larger blood vessels. In this technique, a reflected sound signal is converted to both an audible form and visual image on a computer screen. In the presence of a thrombosis, there is a decrease in the reflected signal that can be heard or, more likely, can be visualized. Most modern ultrasound machines use color enhancement to identify arteries (red) and veins (blue). This technique is again very useful to identify DVTs in the iliac, femoral, or popliteal veins, but its sensitivity falls off markedly when applied to the small vessels in the calf, usually to less than 60%.

Real-Time Ultrasound

Real-time ultrasound has been compared with venography, and in a study by Aitken and Godden, it demonstrated a sensitivity of 94% and a specificity of 100% in a small study of

TABLE 9.2 Diagnosis of Deep Venous Thrombosis

METHOD	SENSITIVITY AND SPECIFICITY	INDICATION AND COMMENTS
Clinical history and physical examination		Classic symptoms often absent in proven DVT <60% with suggestive symptoms proven to have DVT Absence of symptoms does not exclude PE
D-dimer ELISA (plasma)	Sensitivity 97% Specificity: poor	Useful to exclude the diagnosis if D-dimer ELISA is <500 µg/mL Many conditions increase D-dimer levels (false-positive results)
B-mode compression ultrasonography ± Doppler	Symptomatic proximal DVT: Sensitivity 93%–97% Specificity 98% Asymptomatic DVT: Sensitivity 38%–59% Specificity: high	Noninvasive test First-line modality for confirming diagnosis in symptomatic patients Not useful for screening of asymptomatic patients Compression component best for thigh DVT
IPG	Symptomatic DVT: Sensitivity 90% Specificity 95% Asymptomatic DVT: Sensitivity 22% Specificity 98%	Noninvasive test Limited to *serial* examination in symptomatic patients with proximal DVT Insensitive to calf-vein thrombi and nonocclusive thrombi
MR venography	Proximal DVT: Sensitivity 100% Specificity 96% Calf-vein DVT: Sensitivity 87% Specificity 97%	Noninvasive but expensive Ability to screen for DVT in asymptomatic patients Can also image lungs for PE in same setting
Contrast-enhanced CT venography	Distal and proximal DVT: Sensitivity 100% Specificity 96%	Noninvasive test Superior to venography in evaluating the great vessels Expensive Less contrast than conventional venography Can image lungs for PE in same setting
Ascending contrast venography phlebography	Reference standard	Invasive test Reference standard but expensive Risk for contrast nephropathy and allergic reactions Risk for thrombogenicity (usually superficial veins) Negative test does not exclude PE Equivocal results in recurrent DVT

Reprinted with permission from De Wet CJ, Pearl RG. Venous thromboembolism: deep-vein thrombosis and pulmonary embolism. *Anesthesiol Clin North Am Clin* 1999;17:895. Copyright © 1999, Elsevier.

46 patients. In a slightly larger study of 121 patients by Appelman and colleagues, the sensitivity was found to be 96%, and specificity was 97%.

Compression Ultrasound

This technique has been used in some large DVT trials, such as the PREVENT trial, but there have been few studies directly comparing it with venography. In a recent small study by Tomkowski and colleagues involving 160 medically ill patients, 12 patients had venographically proven DVT. Compression ultrasound technique had a sensitivity of 28% and a specificity of 98%, but despite the small numbers of venographically confirmed patients, the method performed poorly, having both false-positive and false-negative findings.

Duplex Doppler Ultrasound

This is a combination technique using real-time and Doppler methods in a procedure known as B mode or duplex Doppler imaging. It allows a radiologist to visualize the vessel and identify any thrombus in it. In a study by Langsfeld and colleagues, 431 patients were examined; 86 patients had a DVT. This gave a sensitivity of 100%, but two false positives dropped the specificity to 78%. Technical issues may have given one incorrect result, the second patient was pregnant, and the study was considered falsely positive because of aortocaval compression from the pregnant uterus.

In a study by Kristo and associates comparing duplex Doppler, venography, and single bilateral IPG, the respective sensitivities and specificities were as follows: ultrasound, 92% and 100%; venography, 100% and 75%; and IPG, 50% and 83%.

For many reasons, duplex B mode imaging has become the noninvasive imaging method of choice, essentially replacing venography as the "practical" gold standard.

Light Reflection Rheography

Light reflection rheography (LRR) uses infrared light directed at the skin. The backscattered rays are quantitated, which allow an estimation of blood volume. A decreased venous emptying rate of 0.35 is considered positive for DVT. In a study in patients with gastrointestinal problems in which 69 limbs were tested by venography and LRR, the sensitivity for LRR was 96%, the specificity was 83%, the positive predictive value was 79%, and the negative predictive value was 97%.

Light reflection rheography could prove to be a low-cost, sensitive tool for DVT detection. Further studies are needed to determine if the technique fulfills its early promise. However, in one study of 411 asymptomatic pregnant women in the second and third trimesters who did not have DVT, the use of LRR denoted a significant false-positive rate of 25% and an inadequate study rate of 19%. This gave an overall specificity of only 45%, indicating that LRR is not for use in DVT diagnosis in pregnant women.

Radioisotope Imaging

Various imaging methods have been tried using radioisotopes to try to detect thrombi in both arteries and veins by labeling components of the clotting system, such as platelets or fibrinogen. These labeled components became incorporated into the developing thrombus, and the focused radioactivity would then allow "visualization" by a detector. Radioactive-tagged antibodies to both platelets and factors have also been used for DVT diagnosis.

Indium[111]-labeled platelets have demonstrated good success with high sensitivity and specificity. The same is true for fibrinogen[125]- and technetium[99m]-labeled platelets.

Although all of these radioisotope-labeled methods have some proponents, the advances in computer software technology and imaging methods will probably outweigh significant development of radioisotopic methods for routine clinical VTE diagnosis.

Indirect Computed Tomography Venography

The new and evolving technique of indirect CT venography, using intravenous contrast medium injection followed by CT scanning of the limbs or chest, has a high potential for detecting DVT or PE. Some early studies have indicated detection of thrombi at least to calf level and perhaps lower. There are few studies comparing CT venography and CT pulmonary angiography. A recent study by Nchimi evaluated 1,408 patients with both techniques for PE detection and included lower-extremity DVT as a secondary finding. They found that in 48% of patients with DVT, the upper end of the thrombus was between the ankle and the knee. Comparing the two techniques, CT venography detected 17% more VTE than did CT pulmonary angiography.

Magnetic Resonance Imaging/Magnetic Resonance Imaging Venography

The use of MRI techniques with or without contrast media is another new approach to VTE detection. There are several different technologies using MRI, but all basically use the differences in signal intensities to distinguish flowing blood from stagnant blood (i.e., clot). Although there have been few large-scale studies published, the major advantage of MRI is that no contrast medium is required, allowing the technique to be used in pregnant women. One study by Carpenter and colleagues indicated no statistical differences between contrast venography and MRI in DVT diagnosis. Magnetic resonance imaging techniques for routine VTE and arterial thromboses diagnosis will likely continue, as improvements in computer software will provide for the advancement of MRI-based method as tools for vascular diagnostics.

Evolving Imaging Techniques

Because of progress in instruments and computer software in conjunction with ongoing concerns about radiation exposure to patients, several new technical modifications are being evaluated, especially for PE diagnosis. These include multidetector computed tomography angiography (MDCTA), electrocardiogram (ECG)-gated CT angiography, and dual-energy/dual-source CT angiography. Early studies suggest that these methods, especially the dual-source CT angiography, may have significantly enhanced accuracy using the very latest detection technology to minimize the radiation required to provide good diagnostic images.

Nonimaging Methods

The use of laboratory tests as a means of exclusion of VTE has gained momentum in the last decade. The use of the *automated quantitative* D-*dimer assays* has gained widespread acceptance, especially in emergency rooms, to exclude VTE. In a study by Wells and associates comparing IPG and D-dimer with contrast venography, the combination of IPG and a negative (normal) D-dimer test gave a negative predictive value of 97%. In this same study, the combination of positive IPG and positive D-dimer had a positive predictive value of 93% for any DVT and 90% for proximal DVT.

The use of an appropriate D-dimer assay in isolation has been shown to have about 98% negative predictive value for exclusion of DVT. Despite numerous studies, there is still no proven consistent correlation between a positive D-dimer assay and the presence of venous thrombosis.

The utility and power of D-dimer assays for exclusion of PE and DVT have been enhanced by the use of pretest probability scores. Several of these exist, namely, the Wells model criteria for DVT and PE diagnosis as well as the Geneva score or other modifications such as the Pisa score. All of these scoring systems are simple and applicable to most emergent VTE diagnostic situations. In conjunction with D-dimer assays, they all enhance the negative predictive value for VTE exclusion and hence the need for unnecessary imaging studies.

Because the diagnosis of PE can be difficult in many older patients, especially those with heart failure or other cardiovascular complications, some preliminary studies have been done using combinations of D-dimer, B-type natriuretic peptide, and cardiac troponins to determine if a better distinction can be made between a PE and an underlying cardiac complication. These studies are likely to be the forerunners for other combinations of biomarker lab tests to identify more specific negative or even positive predictive markers for VTE. This is especially important since many older patients with VTEs have some degree of renal impairment, and the use of contrast dyes in imaging can be problematic.

Risk Factors for Vascular Complications

Several clinical factors are known to identify the patient with an increased risk for VTE (Table 9.3). The most prevalent and important include age >40 years, obesity >20% above ideal weight, prolonged surgery, and immobility in the pre-, peri-, and postoperative periods. Pelvic malignancy, prior VTE, known thrombophilia risk, severe diabetes, heart failure, prior radiation therapy, and chronic obstructive pulmonary disease all increase the VTE risk.

TABLE 9.3 Profile of Patient at High Risk for Venous Thrombosis

FACTOR	CONDITION
Age	<40 Major surgery
Age	>60 Nonmajor surgery
Obesity	
Moderate	75–90 kg or >20% above ideal weight
Morbid	115 kg or >30% above ideal weight with reduced fibrinolysin and immobility
Immobility	
Preoperative	Prolonged hospitalization; venous stasis
Intraoperative	Prolonged operative time; loss of pump action of calf muscles; compression of vena cava
Postoperative	Prolonged bed confinement; venous stasis
Trauma	Damage of wall of pelvic veins
Radical pelvic surgery	
Malignancy	Release of tissue thromboplastin[a]
Activation of factor X; reduced fibrinolysin	
Radiation	Prior radiation therapy
Medical diseases	Diabetes mellitus
Cardiac disease; heart failure	
Severe varicose veins	
Previous venous thrombosis with or without embolization[a]	
Chronic pulmonary disease	
Molecular hypercoagulable state	

[a]Highest risk.

changes promote sludging of red cells and activation of platelets, setting the stage for VTE during the operative period. This is one of the main risk factors described by Virchow for the etiology of thrombosis.

Studies done using I^{125} fibrinogen scanning presurgery and immediately postsurgery have indicated that in 50% of patients who subsequently developed VTE, the initiation of clot formation occurred during the surgical procedure. This is amplified during prolonged anesthesia, with generalized muscle relaxation further promoting venous stasis in the lower extremities, which compounds the thromboembolic risk. For this risk, the judicious use of prophylactic anticoagulation in the high-risk patient should include the operative phase and continue at a minimum until the patient is fully ambulatory.

Postoperative immobility also promotes VTE risk by continuing venous stasis, and studies have shown that 66% of patients who develop a DVT do so in the first 48 hours after surgery. Other compounding issues include sitting with legs crossed or dangling over the bed or the exaggerated Fowler position. These positions all produce impairment of lower extremity venous return. Postoperative patients should be ambulated early and aggressively; if ambulation is not possible, they should have their legs elevated to 15 degrees above the horizontal.

Other Factors

Other factors include previous VTE, varicose veins, severe diabetes, cardiac failure, chronic obstructive pulmonary disease, and underlying thrombophilia. Given the high incidence of factor V Leiden (5%) and the G20210A prothrombin gene mutations (3%) in the Caucasian populations, which are well-recognized risk factors for venous thrombosis (Table 9.4), these genetic risk factors are common enough to make a major contribution to preoperative thrombosis, even in the patient with no prior VTE history.

Underlying malignancy is a huge contributor to risk, most likely because of the significant up-regulation of TF that is known to occur with many malignancies. Up-regulation of TF increases thrombin generation by several mechanisms, promotes platelet activation, and enhances the generation of MPs and angiogenesis, as discussed earlier.

A review of these risk factors clearly identifies the high-risk VTE patient, and it is essential that these surgical risk variables are identified and understood in designing appropriate thromboprophylaxis and monitoring parameters to prevent venous thrombosis. Many countries including the United States have produced national consensus documents from their clinical

Age

An autopsy study by Sevitt and Gallagher demonstrated that DVT was most prevalent in patients older than 60 years. Several studies have shown a linear risk of fatal PE with increasing age. Approximately 10% of hospitalized patients' deaths are due to PE, and only about 35% of these are diagnosed ante mortem. Contributing factors include degenerative changes in the vascular tree, increases that occur in the concentration of many coagulation factors, and, possibly, increased platelet adhesiveness.

Immobility

Prolonged inactivity in the preoperative patient promotes an impairment of venous flow in the lower extremities. Many diagnostic techniques also produce a decrease in muscle tone with a secondary decrease in venous flow. These hemodynamic

TABLE 9.4 Risk of Thromboembolism

Deficiency/dysfunction
  Antithrombin
  Protein C
  Protein S
  Heparin cofactor II
Factor V Leiden
Prothrombin variant 20210A
Antiphospholipid antibodies
  Lupus anticoagulant
  Anticardiolipin
Hyperhomocystinuria
Dysfibrinogenemia
Decreased levels of plasminogen
Decreased levels of plasminogen activators
Heparin-induced thrombocytopenia

oncology societies for both treatment and prophylaxis for VTE in cancer patients.

Prophylaxis

Prevention remains the most effective tool in the treatment of VTE. Between 5% and 45% of gynecologic surgery patients develop DVT in their legs; of these, 20% have popliteal or femoral involvement; and of these, 40% will progress to PE with its high mortality. It is imperative that methods for prophylaxis are planned and implemented before surgery (Table 9.5).

In the Sixth American College of Chest Physicians (ACCP) Consensus Conference, Geerts and colleagues—in a review of PE in 7,000 gynecologic surgery patients in prospective clinical trials—reported a reduction in the rate of fatal PE of 75% using thromboprophylaxis (Table 9.6). The current 2012 Chest (ACCP) guidelines recommend the routine use of LMWH or unfractionated heparin (UFH) and mechanical compression stockings given the high risk in this population. They do not recommend the use of inferior vena cava (IVC) filters.

TABLE 9.5 Agents Used in Venous Thromboembolism		
AGENT	**MECHANISM OF ACTION**	**COMMENTS**
Heparin	Combines with AT-III and neutralizes activated factors: IIa (thrombin activity) Xa (responsible for thrombin generation) XIIa, XIa, IXa	Prevention and treatment of VTE Risk of heparin-induced thrombocytopenia Requires monitoring (APTT) when used for treatment

LMWH
  Ardeparin
  Dalteparin
  Enoxaparin
	Combines with AT-III and prevents thrombin generation through its anti-factor Xa effect	Prevention and treatment of VTE
		Risk of heparin-induced thrombocytopenia
		
		No anti-IIa activity (if molecular weight <5.6 kDa)
		APTT does not reflect anticoagulation state
		More predictable pharmacokinetic profile
		Renal failure and dehydration increase effective plasma concentration

Heparinoid Danaparoid	Same as LMWH High anti-Xa/IIa ratio	Prevention and treatment of VTE Similar to LMWH but may be used for anticoagulation when heparin-induced thrombocytopenia is present
Direct thrombin inhibitors and hirudin	Directly inhibits thrombin activity	Prevention and treatment of VTE May be used for heparin-induced thrombocytopenia

Plasminogen activators:
Nonselective
  Streptokinase
  Urokinase
	Activates plasminogen, which leads to the formation of plasmin, which dissolves fibrin clot (no effect on polymerized fibrin clot)
	Also degrades fibrinogen, which leads to fibrinogen degradation products and decreases in plasma fibrinogen
		Treatment of life-threatening DVT or PE
		High risk of bleeding
		Many contraindications such as recent surgery or trauma

Thrombus-selective tissue plasminogen activator	Activates fibrin-bound plasminogen Degrades fibrinogen (to a lesser extent)	
Warfarin	Inhibits correct synthesis of vitamin K–dependent coagulation factors (II, VII, IX, X) These factors cannot bind calcium and therefore remain inactive Inhibits protein C (vitamin K dependent)	Long-term treatment and prevention of VTE Contraindicated in pregnancy (teratogenic) High risk of bleeding Requires anticoagulation monitoring Numerous drug interactions
Inferior vena caval filters	Trap larger emboli	Used as prevention of PE when anticoagulation fails or is contraindicated Used prior to pulmonary embolectomy or pulmonary endarterectomy
External pneumatic leg compression	Prevents venous stasis Stimulates fibrinolytic system	Used as prophylaxis for DVT Possibly contraindicated in peripheral arterial disease

Reprinted with permission from DeWet CJ, Pearl RG. Venous thromboembolism: deep-vein thrombosis and pulmonary embolism. *Anesthesiol Clin North Am* 1999;17:895. Copyright © 1999, Elsevier.

TABLE 9.6 Prevention of Deep Venous Thrombosis after Gynecologic Surgery[a]

REGIMEN	NO. OF TRIALS	NO. OF PATIENTS	INCIDENCE OF DVT, %	95% CI	RELATIVE % REDUCTION
Untreated control subjects	12	945	16	14–19	—
Oral anticoagulants	5	183	13	8–18	22
IPC	3	253	9	6–13	44
LDUH	11	1092	7	6–9	56
ES	1	104	0	0–3	"99"

[a]Pooled data from randomized trials that used routine I[125] fibrinogen-uptake test (FUT) as the primary outcome.
Reprinted with permission from Geerts WH, Heit JA, Clagett GP, et al. Prevention of venous thromboembolism (Sixth ACCP Consensus Conference on Antithrombotic Therapy) *Chest* 2001;119(1 suppl):132S. Copyright © 2008, American College of Chest Physicians.

Low-Dose Unfractionated Heparin

Low-dose UFH has been the mainstay of prophylactic treatment for many years, with numerous prospective randomized clinical trials validating a risk reduction in DVT incidence from 35% to 45% to about 7% in the high-risk patient. In one large study by Kakkar and colleagues (Table 9.7) incorporating 4,000 patients at multiple centers, patients were randomized to 5,000 U USP calcium heparin subcutaneously starting 2 hours before surgery and subsequently every 8 hours thereafter for the next 7 days. The reduction in VTE between the control group (25%) and the treatment group (8%) was highly significant. The most important finding was the decrease in fatal PE from 16 patients in the control group to 2 in the treatment group confirmed by autopsy.

Because there is no change in the activated partial thromboplastin time (APTT) because of the low level of subcutaneous heparin, there was no increase in postoperative bleeding. This is because the main impact of the low-dose heparin is exerted via antithrombin through factor Xa, as well as directly on thrombin. There is also a secondary effect in which heparin releases tissue factor pathway inhibitor (TFPI), which also helps to down-regulate factor Xa by forming a complex involving TF:F Xa:F VIIa:TFPI.

TABLE 9.7 Pulmonary Embolism and Deep Venous Thrombosis in Patients on Low-Dose Heparin and in Controls

	LOW-DOSE HEPARIN	CONTROL
Number of patients	2045	2076
Number of deaths from all causes	80	100
Deaths caused by PE (verified at autopsy)	2	16
Deep venous thrombosis	8%	25%

Reprinted with permission from Kakkar W, Corrigan TP, Fossard DP. Prevention of postoperative pulmonary embolism by low dose heparin. *Lancet* 1975;2:45. Copyright © 1975, Elsevier.

These studies, as well as those shown in Table 9.8, clearly validate the efficacy of low-dose UFH in reducing VTE in surgical patients using an initial dose of 5,000 U 2 hours before surgery and then 5,000 U every 12 hours for the next 5 days. For the truly high-risk patient, such as those with a prior VTE or multiple risk factors, 5,000 U every 8 hours should be used. In current clinical practice, the use of UFH has been superseded by the use of LMWHs.

Low-Dose Unfractionated Heparin/Dihydroergotamine

The combination of low-dose UFH and dihydroergotamine (DHE) treatment was shown to work well by adding the known effect of DHE as a selective venous vasoconstricting agent to the anticoagulant properties of UFH.

Dextran 70/Dextran 40

In 1972, Bonnar and Walsh described the use of dextran 70 to prevent thrombosis after pelvic surgery. A subsequent study by Bernstein and colleagues involving radical hysterectomy patients using dextran 70 as prophylaxis showed a decrease in DVT incidence from 33% to 5%. Dextran works by interfering with platelet function, interacts with factor V and VIII, and inhibits fibrinolysis. Despite some comparable studies between dextran and low-dose UFH, the Sixth ACCP Consensus Conference in 2001 recommended against using dextran products in VTE prophylaxis.

Low Molecular Weight Heparins

Low molecular weight heparins (LMWHs) act by primarily inhibiting factor Xa with a small component of activity against thrombin. They have become mainstay of anticoagulant prophylaxis and treatment and continue to replace all other forms of drug therapy. The drugs have a longer half-life than does UFH and are much more biopredictable. If LMWH levels are measured in patients using an anti-Xa assay, there is a remarkable homogeneity of response. This has led the U.S. Food and Drug Administration to recommend against the need to monitor when LMWHs are used for VTE prophylaxis. There are currently four LMWH drugs available in the United States (Fragmin, Lovenox, Innohep, and Arixtra). They are subtly different in molecular weights and in manufacturing processes but in essence are almost identical in clinical efficacy. They are not, however, dosed in the same way, some using milligrams and other units, or even units per kilogram. Pharmacists can provide accurate dosage information about any of the products available.

TABLE 9.8 Results of Prophylactic Treatment of Venous Thrombosis after Gynecologic Surgery[a]

INVESTIGATORS	YEAR	TYPE OF SURGERY	NUMBER OF PATIENTS	VENOUS THROMBOSIS (%)					
				CONTROL	HEPARIN	LMWH	DEXTRAN	AC	PNEUMATIC CALF COMPRESSION
Bonnar et al.	1973	Simple hysterectomy	260	15.0	—	—	0.1	—	—
		Radical malignant	62	33.0	—	—	5.0	—	—
Ballard et al.	1973	Major gynecologic, age 40	110	29.0	3.6	—	—	—	—
McCarthy et al.	1974	Major gynecologic	130	—	10.9	—	16.2	—	—
Baertschi et al.	1975	Major gynecologic	458	—	2.3	—	—	4.7	—
Gjonnaess and Abildgaard	1976	Major gynecologic, age 50	95	8.0	2.0	—	—	—	—
Adolf et al.	1978	Major gynecologic	454	29.3	7.0	—	—	—	—
Taberner et al.	1978	Major gynecologic	146	23.0	6.0	—	—	6.0	—
Clarke-Pearson et al.	1983a	Gynecologic malignant	185	12.4	14.8	—	—	—	—
Clarke-Pearson et al.	1984	Gynecologic malignant	107	34.6	—	—	—	—	12.7
Borstad et al.	1992	Major gynecologic malignant	141	—	0.00	0.00[b]	—	—	—

[a]Detected by ^{125}I-labeled fibrinogen scan.
[b]One patient had PE 3 days after discontinuation of LMWH.
AC, anticoagulants; LMWH, low-molecular-weight heparin.

Multiple studies reported in the literature essentially show equivalence or better for the LMWHs compared with UFH and/or Coumadin in the prevention of VTE, but almost all of these show a much lower bleeding risk for the LMWH treatment groups, even with hard data for bleeding risk being quantitated by transfusion requirements. LMWHs have also been compared with dextran and used in combination with DHE with good outcomes, but the reality is that *in normal clinical practice, LMWHs by themselves provide adequate protections with minimal complications.* One other advantage of the LMWH preparations is their much lower incidence of heparin-induced thrombocytopenia (HIT) when used as de novo therapy. However, if a patient has had HIT in the past, these preparations should not be used because there is a 90% cross-reactivity between UFH and LMWH for the antibody causing HIT. The one exception to this is Arixtra, the synthetic factor Xa inhibitor, which has been shown to cause clinical HIT in two to three cases to date.

It is highly likely, given the once-per-day dosage requirement and the lack of HIT risk, that LMWHs will continue to dominate for thromboprophylaxis therapy in VTE.

Newer Oral Anticoagulants

In the past 18 months, three new oral anticoagulants have been approved for use in various medical conditions. One of these drugs, dabigatran (Pradaxa), is an anti-IIa (thrombin) inhibitor approved for atrial fibrillation similar to a new oral anti-Xa inhibitor apixaban (Eliquis). However, the third new drug, an oral anti-Xa inhibitor, rivaroxaban (Xarelto), has been approved for treatment and prophylaxis of VTE although not specifically tried in cancer-related VTE.

The fact that Xarelto is oral, does not require any monitoring, and has few side effects is likely to promote increased use especially from the patient compliance perspective where the need for subcutaneous injections remains a problem.

Compression Modalities

As long ago as 1944, Stanton et al. used static compression to decrease venous stasis by decreasing the luminal diameter of the veins, thereby increasing blood flow velocity. In the mid-1970s, Sigel and colleagues showed an increase in blood velocity of 20% using graduated compression stockings but a 200% increase in velocity using intermittent sequential compression.

Mittelman and colleagues showed that uniform intermittent calf compression was not as effective as intermittent sequential compression at increasing thigh blood flow. This is another example of a component of Virchow triangle, namely, stasis being involved in the VTE protection mechanism.

It is possible that another component of the triad—the coagulation system—is also influenced by IPC because several groups have shown that it stimulates fibrinolysis, perhaps by increasing prostacyclin production. Prostacyclin is a potent natural vasodilator and antiplatelet agent released from endothelial cells. Guyton and colleagues found increased quantities of 6-keto prostaglandin $F_{1\alpha}$ in patients undergoing IPC compared with controls. The 6-keto prostaglandin $F_{1\alpha}$ is a specific breakdown product of prostacyclin. Frango and associates have shown a 16-fold increase in prostacyclin production in cultured endothelial cells submitted to pulsatile shear stress compared with a twofold increase with contact shear stress.

Graduated Compression Stockings Initial studies evaluating antiembolic stockings proved inconclusive and relied on several different methods to diagnose VTE, which compounded the uncertainty. Sigel and colleagues designed a compression thromboembolism deterrent (TED) hose with graduated pressures of 18, 14, 12, 10, and 8 mm Hg from the ankle to the upper thigh. Scurr and associates evaluated TED hose in a study of 70 patients older than 40 years undergoing major abdominal surgery in which only one leg had TED hose applied. Using I^{125} fibrinogen scanning as the diagnostic tool, 19 patients had DVTs in the control leg, and only 1 had a DVT in the TED hose leg. A subsequent similar study by Inada and colleagues found a DVT frequency of 14.5% in the control leg and only 3.6% in the TED leg. Malignancy is a powerful predisposition to VTE secondary to stasis and tissue factor production by the tumor. In a study by Allan and associates assessing the efficacy of TED stocking in patients undergoing abdominal surgery for malignant and benign diseases, the incidence of DVT in the benign disease group was 24.5% in the control limb and 6.1% in the TED limb. However, in the malignant disease group, the incidence of DVT was only slightly increased in the control limb at 27.9%, but the incidence of DVT in the TED limb was significantly higher at 11.5%, clearly amplifying the impact of the tumor on the DVT risk. The Sixth ACCP Consensus Conference suggested that TED hose with early ambulation was an acceptable and effective means of VTE prophylaxis in the low-risk gynecology surgery patient.

External Intermittent Pneumatic Compression These techniques also promote increased blood flow in the lower extremities that is due to decreased stasis and improved fibrinolysis. Nicolaides and colleagues compared intermittent sequential pneumatic compression, nonsequential (one chamber) pneumatic compression, and UFH in the prevention of VTE. Using pressures of 35, 30, and 20 mm Hg sequentially for 12 seconds at the ankle, calf, and thigh, respectively, they observed a 240% increase in peak blood velocity. In contrast, using the single-chamber device at 35 mm Hg, the increase was only 180%. The intermittent sequential device was more effective than was the single-chamber device and was as effective as 5,000 U of UFH every 12 hours in preventing DVT. In addition, the intermittent sequential device increased the time interval for clot formation proximal to the calf compared with UFH. In another study, the same authors compared electrical calf stimulus, low-dose UFH, intermittent sequential compression, and TED hose in 150 patients older than 30 years undergoing major abdominal surgery. The incidence of proven DVT was 18%, 9%, and 4%, respectively.

In a similar study in patients undergoing surgery for gynecologic malignancy comparing no thromboprophylaxis to nonsequential external compression, the control group had a VTE frequency of 34.6%. In the compression treatment group, the VTE incidence was reduced to 12.7%. Diagnostic tools for VTE were IPG and I^{131}.

Treatment of Venous Thrombosis

The initial treatment of VTE in most hospitals still involves the use of intravenous UFH, although LMWHs are approved for treatment of VTE. Given the potential variability of the hypercoagulable state in these patients, constant intravenous infusion UFH still remains the easiest drug to use. Most patients are now treated using a weight-based heparin nomogram and are given a loading dose of 80 U/kg to a maximum of 10,000 U. They are maintained on a constant infusion of 18 U/kg, and the first APTT or factor Xa assay should be done at 4 to 6 hours after the initiation of therapy. Because of the large thrombus burden these patients may have, they can clear or use UFH at an accelerated rate; thus, they are often undertreated. Patients with gynecologic malignancies will typically require higher-than-average doses until the cancer has been surgically removed or treated. Care must be taken to reduce the infusion, or these patients are susceptible to bleeding that is due to heparin overdose. There is little place for intermittent bolus treatment with UFH in modern anticoagulation practice.

If the APTT is used to monitor efficacy of UFH therapy, it should be used in conjunction with the laboratory heparin monitoring nomogram. Because APTT reagents can vary widely between institutions, the old concept of using a ratio of 1.5 to 2 times some poorly defined control APTT value is completely outmoded and can lead to erroneous and inadequate anticoagulation therapy. Any modern coagulation lab should have a heparin treatment weight-based nomogram specific for their reagent and APTT instrument combination.

Standard clinical practices—such as leg elevation to minimize or treat leg edema after a DVT—are still appropriate. Patients should probably not be aggressively mobilized as long as they have significant leg edema. Most patients will require 5 to 7 days of UFH or LMWH treatment, and the modern trend is to rapidly introduce oral anticoagulation, usually within 24 to 48 hours after initiation of heparin therapy. This will not always be possible in this population, but any UFH or LMWH treatment should be continued until the international normalized ratio is in the therapeutic range of 2 to 3 for several days. The new oral anticoagulants (Xarelto) can be initiated in place of Coumadin anticoagulation immediately after surgery and do not require any time to become therapeutic. Similar to Coumadin, they need to be continued for 3 to 6 months or longer, depending on the circumstances and any other complicating factors (i.e., prior VTE or congenital thrombophilia).

The patient who is found to have an asymptomatic DVT of the lower extremity poses a dilemma for some physicians. Some feel that this is not a significant risk and should not be treated, but the risk of thrombus extension into the proximal and popliteal veins remains high and is a possibility. Although this is still a small risk for most patients, the longer-term complications of postphlebitic syndrome from the damaged valves in those veins can produce significant morbidity for such patients, leading to chronic leg edema and venous stasis ulceration. For that reason, most practitioners would elect to anticoagulate women with asymptomatic DVT. With the onset of widespread DVT prophylaxis in many hospitals, the problem of whether to treat asymptomatic DVT is becoming moot.

POSTOPERATIVE PULMONARY COMPLICATIONS

Postoperative pulmonary complications (PPCs) after abdominal surgery remain an important cause of increased morbidity, mortality, and resource use. Atelectasis, pneumonia, and pulmonary thromboembolic disease following abdominal surgery continue to occur frequently despite continuing advances in anesthetic, surgical, and postoperative treatment. The incidence of PPCs has surpassed that of postoperative cardiac complications, and PPCs have a greater impact on postoperative outcomes. Gynecologic surgery is increasingly performed in patients with advanced age, multiple comorbid conditions, and increased risk for the development of PPCs. Risk factors

TABLE 9.9 Risk Factors for Postoperative Pulmonary Complications in Gynecologic Surgery Patients

Age >60 y
Cancer
Congestive heart failure
Smoking within 8 wk of surgery
Upper abdominal incision
Vertical incision
Incision length >20 cm

for PPCs in patients undergoing a gynecologic surgery procedure vary among studies but are consistent with other patient groups undergoing abdominal surgical procedures (Table 9.9). The most important PPCs in terms of incidence, morbidity, mortality, and resource use are atelectasis, pneumonia, respiratory failure, and pulmonary thromboembolic disease.

An understanding of the physiology that predisposes to PPCs, the risk factors for their development, and the preventive and therapeutic measures to minimize and treat them are of critical importance to gynecologic surgeons.

Perioperative Respiratory Physiology

Effects of Anesthesia

General anesthesia results in important alterations in respiratory physiology (Table 9.10). Anesthetic agents influence not only the ventilatory response to oxygen and carbon dioxide but also the pattern of respiration. Inhalational agents and intravenous agents both result in a reduction of the ventilatory response but differ in their effects on respiratory pattern. The classic breathing pattern produced by inhalational anesthetics is a rhythmic, rapid, and shallow pattern of respiration with no intermittent sighs (large breaths), whereas intravenous anesthesia is associated with slow, deep respirations. Little metabolism of inhalational anesthetics occurs during surgery, with most of the anesthetic agents stored in the tissues, such as muscle and fat.

At the conclusion of anesthesia, most of the stored anesthetic agent is eliminated via the lungs. As a result of tissue stores, significant concentrations of the anesthetic agent may be present well into the recovery phase, particularly after high anesthetic doses, long anesthetic times, or the presence of cardiopulmonary disease. This prolonged anesthetic effect can lead to clinically significant respiratory depression in the postoperative period.

The number of functional alveolar units participating actively in gas exchange is directly related to the functional residual capacity (FRC). General anesthesia is associated with a reduction in FRC by approximately 16%, irrespective of the

anesthetic techniques used. The cause of the reduction in FRC is multifactorial and includes cranial movement of the diaphragm, chest wall relaxation with reduction in thoracic volume, reduction in respiratory compliance, and shift of central blood volume from the thorax into the abdomen. Reduction in FRC can have marked adverse effects on perioperative gas exchange, especially the development of hypoxemia.

Atelectasis is defined as the absence of gas from a part or the whole of the lungs that is due to the failure of expansion or resorption of gas from the alveoli. It occurs in the dependent areas of the lungs within 5 minutes of anesthetic induction in a patient with healthy lungs and leads to shunt physiology. Atelectasis may be caused by compression, gas resorption, or surfactant impairment. Compression occurs when the distending pressure in the alveolus is reduced to a level that causes the alveolus to collapse. In the setting of general anesthesia, compression occurs mainly as result of impairments in diaphragmatic position and function. In addition to the cephalad movement of the diaphragm that is due to relaxation from anesthesia as described above, increased intra-abdominal pressure from bowel edema, peritoneal fluid, and hematoma forces the diaphragm cephalad and contributes substantially to compressive atelectasis. The contractile function of the diaphragm is not altered as a result of an effect of anesthesia itself because diaphragmatic dysfunction, which almost always presents after upper abdominal surgery, does not arise after lower abdominal surgery.

Other factors contributing to postanesthesia pulmonary complications include reabsorption hypoxic pulmonary vasoconstriction and ventilation/perfusion abnormalities.

Although most gynecologic surgery is done in the pelvis, upper abdominal operations are sometimes done by gynecologic oncologists, and extension of the surgical incision and operative procedure into the upper abdomen produce increased respiratory effects. Respiratory muscle dysfunction is the major effect of upper abdominal surgery on respiratory physiology (Table 9.11). Tidal breathing depends on inspiratory muscle function, especially the function of the diaphragm. Other accessory muscles of respiration are recruited when work of breathing increases, such as when diaphragmatic dysfunction is present, during states of increased oxygen consumption, and in the presence of cardiopulmonary disease. In addition to breathing, respiratory muscles play an integral role in the generation of cough and act as stabilizers of the thorax and abdomen. Upper abdominal surgery may affect each of these respiratory muscle functions by several different mechanisms.

An important change following upper abdominal surgery is a shift in respiratory pump function from the diaphragm to accessory inspiratory and expiratory muscles of respiration. This results in a rapid shallow breathing pattern of respiration. The contractile function of the diaphragm is impaired by inhibition of phrenic nerve output by stimulation of visceral and somatic nerve pathways during manipulation of the abdominal

TABLE 9.10 Effects of Anesthesia on Respiratory Physiology

Reduced ventilatory response to oxygen and carbon dioxide
Rhythmic rapid shallow breathing pattern
Reduced functional residual capacity
Diaphragmatic dysfunction
Atelectasis
Ventilation–perfusion mismatching
Blunting of hypoxic pulmonary vasoconstriction
Impairment in mucociliary clearance

TABLE 9.11 Effects of Upper Abdominal Surgery on Respiratory Physiology

Reduction in lung volumes: residual volume, total lung capacity, functional residual capacity and vital capacity
Reflex inhibition of phrenic nerve activity resulting in decreased diaphragmatic function
Increased neck and intercostal inspiratory accessory muscle use
Tonic and phasic contraction of abdominal expiratory muscles

viscera and the peritoneum. The less efficient accessory muscles of inspiration, such as the intercostals and neck muscles, assume an increased share of the respiratory effort. Tonic and phasic contraction of the expiratory abdominal muscles also occurs. The net effect on respiratory mechanics is a reduction in lung volumes, including the FRC (which leads to atelectasis), V/Q abnormalities, and hypoxemia. These changes may be aggravated by hypoventilation that is due to the residua of general anesthesia, postoperative sedative–hypnotic therapy, and pain. In addition to a submaximal voluntary activation of inspiratory muscles, pain may also have a direct effect, through unknown mechanisms, on inspiratory muscle function.

Atelectasis

Clinically significant atelectasis occurs in 15% to 20% of patients undergoing abdominal surgery. The pathophysiologic effects of atelectasis include decreased respiratory compliance, increased pulmonary vascular resistance, predisposition to acute lung injury, and hypoxemia. Atelectasis may also be a precursor to more serious PPCs, such as postoperative pneumonia. The definition of atelectasis is not uniform across clinical studies, with most investigations incorporating a global definition of a PPC that includes atelectasis. However, generally accepted criteria for the diagnosis of atelectasis include impaired oxygenation in a clinical setting where atelectasis is likely, unexplained temperature of greater than 38°C, and chest radiographic evidence of volume loss or new airspace opacity. Risk factors implicated in the development of atelectasis after abdominal surgery include advanced age, obesity, intraperitoneal sepsis, prolonged anesthesia time, nasogastric tube placement, and smoking.

The risk of atelectasis may be reduced by a number of interventions (Table 9.12). Preoperative smoking cessation is effective if it is started well in advance of surgery (6 to 8 weeks before operation). If smoking cessation is attempted in close proximity to a planned surgical procedure, the improvement in mucociliary clearance in combination with reduced cough may lead to a secretion burden that paradoxically increases the risk of PPCs. Atelectasis is effectively prevented and treated by deep breathing exercises and mobilization. Voluntary lung inflation exercises enable redistribution of gas into areas of low compliance. Mechanical aids, such as incentive spirometry, have not been shown to be superior to properly performed deep breathing maneuvers. Effective deep breathing exercises require the patient to be conscious and cooperative. Chest physiotherapy is extremely labor intensive and has potential disadvantages in that it may exhaust the patient, cause pain, induce bronchospasm, and cause transient hypoxemia. Because chest physiotherapy has never been shown to be superior to deep breathing exercises in preventing or treating atelectasis, it is not recommended after abdominal surgery. Continuous positive airway pressure reduces the incidence of significant postoperative hypoxemia and may reduce rates of pneumonia and intubation. However, the cost, complexity, and potential complications of continuous positive airway pressure limit the practicality of routine application of this technique to patients undergoing abdominal surgery.

Although evidence suggests that effective postoperative pain control reduces PPC, there is inconclusive evidence as to whether postoperative epidural analgesia is superior to patient-controlled analgesia. Both modalities, however, appear to be superior to on-demand narcotic analgesia in reducing PPCs. Laparoscopic procedures reduce postoperative pain scores, as well as have less adverse effect on postoperative respiratory muscle function. Through these mechanisms, atelectasis is reduced with a laparoscopic as opposed to open abdominal surgical procedure. Irrespective of the procedure used, postoperative gastric decompression should be used selectively rather than routinely for postoperative nausea, symptomatic abdominal distention, or inability to tolerate oral intake. Routine nasogastric tube use significantly increases rates of atelectasis without reducing risk of aspiration in comparison with selective decompression.

Postoperative Pneumonia

Hospital-acquired pneumonia (HAP) is defined as pneumonia that develops 48 hours or more after hospital admission because of an organism that was not incubating at the time of hospitalization. Hospital-acquired pneumonia after abdominal surgery has a high attributable mortality, increases hospital length of stay and cost, and has lasting effects on patient-centered outcomes, including increased hospital length of stay of approximately 11 days and increased hospital charges by 75%. Hospital-acquired pneumonia is also associated with a fourfold increase in risk of discharge to a skilled nursing facility. Women have a risk of developing HAP after abdominal surgery that is twice that of men.

Hospital-acquired pneumonia is caused by a wide spectrum of bacterial pathogens and is occasionally due to viral or fungal pathogens in immunocompetent patients (Table 9.13). Common pathogens include the aerobic gram-negative bacilli and *Staphylococcus aureus* species. Early-onset HAP, defined as occurring within the first 4 days of hospitalization, is usually associated with a better prognosis and is more likely to be caused by antibiotic-susceptible pathogens. Late-onset HAP (occurring on or after 5 days of hospitalization) is more likely to be caused by multidrug-resistant (MDR) pathogens, which are associated with increased morbidity and mortality. The risk of HAP from MDR pathogens is related to characteristics of the patient, the health care environment, and the prescribed medical treatment (Table 9.14).

TABLE 9.12 Prevention and Treatment of Atelectasis

Smoking cessation 8 wk before elective surgery
Laparoscopic procedure
Deep breathing exercises
Mobilization
Adequate analgesia (epidural or patient-controlled analgesia preferred)
Selective gastric decompression

TABLE 9.13 Common Pathogens Causing Hospital-Acquired Pneumonia

Early onset (≤4 d)
Streptococcus pneumoniae
Methicillin-sensitive *Staphylococcus aureus*
Methicillin-resistant *S. aureus*
Haemophilus influenzae
Escherichia coli
Klebsiella pneumoniae
Enterobacter species
Proteus species
Serratia marcescens
Late onset (≥5 d)
All of the above plus:
Pseudomonas aeruginosa
Multidrug-resistant *Klebsiella pneumoniae*
Acinetobacter species

TABLE 9.14 Risk Factors for Multidrug-Resistant Pathogens Causing Hospital-Acquired Pneumonia

Immunosuppressive disease or therapy
Home infusion therapy
Chronic dialysis
Home wound care
Residence in a nursing home or extended care facility
Antimicrobial therapy in the preceding 90 d
Current hospitalization of 5 d or more
Hospitalization for 2 d or more in the preceding 90 d
High frequency of antibiotic resistance in the community,
    hospital, or patient care unit

TABLE 9.15 Interventions to Decrease Risk for Hospital-Acquired Pneumonia

Strict adherence to infection control procedures
Early removal of invasive devices
Semirecumbent positioning of the patient
Early mobilization of the patient
Restriction of acid suppression therapy
Restrictive red blood cell transfusion strategy
Strict control of hyperglycemia

Bacterial colonization of the lower respiratory tract under conditions that promote bacterial invasion is necessary for HAP to develop. Sources of colonization include air, water, equipment, fomites, and direct transfer from health care providers. Among conditions that promote invasion are severity of underlying illness, comorbid conditions, prior exposure to antimicrobials, and exposure to invasive devices, such as nasogastric and endotracheal tubes. Risk of colonization may be modified by several means (Table 9.15). Infection control procedures, including guidelines for alcohol-based hand disinfection and appropriate barrier precautions, should strictly be observed. Early removal of invasive devices, in particular nasogastric tubes, and avoidance of endotracheal intubation when noninvasive ventilation is feasible, will reduce the risk of HAP. As one of the mechanisms for initial colonization of the lower respiratory tract includes microaspiration of gastrically residing bacteria, measures to minimize aspiration and to reduce gastric bacterial overgrowth are important preventive measures. All patients should be maintained in at least a semirecumbent position with the head elevated to 30 to 45 degrees. Restriction of the use of stress ulcer prophylaxis to patients who meet criteria (i.e., receiving mechanical ventilation or coagulopathy/therapeutic anticoagulation) is critical in controlling a possible risk factor for HAP. Implementation of a restrictive red blood cell transfusion strategy in patients without evidence of active bleeding is proven to reduce infectious complications of all kinds, including HAP. Adherence to

such a strategy not only reduces infectious complications but reduces overall in-hospital mortality and may reduce recurrence of malignancy. In most patients, a hemoglobin target of 7.0 should be adopted, with a hemoglobin target of 9.0 reserved for patients with active cardiac ischemia or hemodynamic instability. Strict control of hyperglycemia has been widely adopted as a means of reducing morbidity and mortality, including the risk of infection. Although the optimal glucose target and the means of achieving that target remain controversial, an attempt to limit capillary blood glucose to less than 150 mg/dL in both diabetic and nondiabetic patients appears warranted.

The clinical definition of HAP includes a new opacity on chest radiograph (posterior–anterior and lateral views preferred) plus two of the following: fever greater than 38°C, leukocytosis or leukopenia, and purulent respiratory secretions. The diagnosis of HAP should be supported by sampling of lower respiratory tract secretions, with either an endotracheal aspirate or a bronchoscopic specimen, before the initiation of empiric antibiotic therapy. Importantly, antibiotics should not be excessively delayed while awaiting obtaining these samples in patients who are critically ill. The initial step in choosing antibiotic therapy for suspected HAP is determination of the patient's risk of infection with an MDR pathogen (Fig. 9.3). Knowledge of local microbiologic data including pathogens and sensitivity will assist with proper selection of antimicrobials. One of the consequences of increasing antimicrobial resistance is an increased probability of inappropriate initial empiric treatment. Inappropriate or delayed empiric treatment results in a substantial excessive attributable mortality

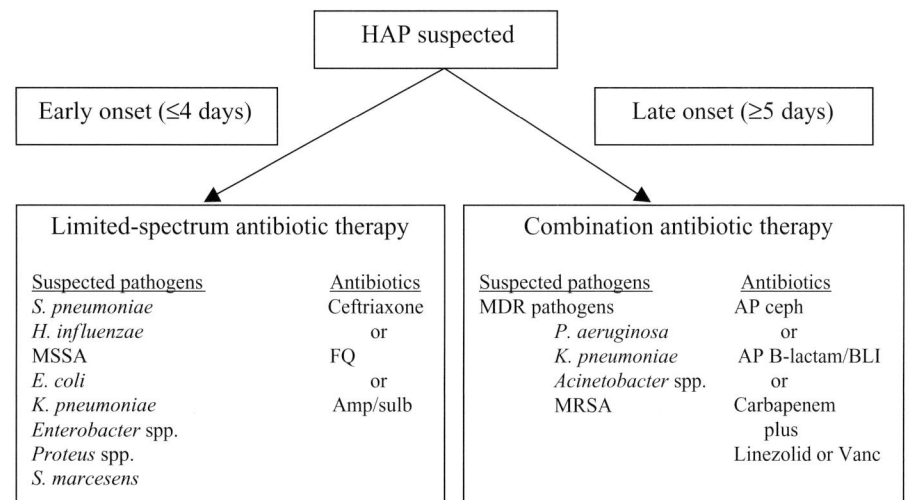

MSSA, methicillin-sensitive *S. aureus*; FQ, fluoroquinolone; Amp/sulb, ampicillin/sulbactam; MDR, multidrug-resistant; MRSA, methicillin-resistant *S. aureus*; AP ceph, antipseudomonal cephalosporin; AP B-lactam/BLI, antipseudomonal B-lactam/B-lactamase inhibitor; Vanc, vancomycin.

FIGURE 9.3 Algorithm for initiating empiric antibiotic therapy for hospital-acquired pneumonia (HAP).

and hospital length of stay. Prompt institution of appropriate empiric therapy based on risk stratification for the presence of a possible MDR pathogen is crucial to improving patient outcome in HAP.

Initial therapy should be administered intravenously, with a switch to the enteral route of administration in selected patients with a good clinical response and a functional gastrointestinal tract. Combination therapy should be used initially if patients are at high risk of being infected with an MDR pathogen. Monotherapy is appropriate for those patients deemed to be low risk. Duration of therapy should be based on clinical response and may often be safely terminated after 8 days, provided the etiologic pathogen is not *Pseudomonas aeruginosa*, which requires a longer course of 15 days. Clinical improvement usually takes 48 to 72 hours, and therapy should not be changed during this time unless there is a rapid clinical decline. The responding patient should have therapy tailored to the most focused regimen possible on the basis of microbiologic studies. The nonresponding patient should be evaluated for drug-resistant organisms, complications of pneumonia (e.g., parapneumonic effusion or empyema), extrapulmonary sites of infection, or noninfectious causes of symptoms and signs of pneumonia (e.g., drug fever with drug-induced lung injury).

Respiratory Failure

Respiratory failure denotes either the inability to maintain normal tissue oxygen transport or the normal excretion of carbon dioxide. Clinically, respiratory failure is usually diagnosed by levels of arterial PO_2 and PCO_2, although the levels that constitute the threshold for respiratory failure are arbitrary. An arterial PO_2 of less than 60 mm Hg or an arterial PCO_2 of greater than 45 mm Hg generally indicates significant respiratory compromise in patients without preexisting lung disease. The diagnostic and therapeutic approach to the patient with respiratory failure is dictated by the underlying mechanism of abnormal gas exchange (Table 9.16).

Five basic pathophysiologic mechanisms cause acute hypoxemic respiratory failure. These include hypoventilation, V/Q abnormalities, shunt, diffusion limitation, and low inspired fraction of oxygen. All of these causes of hypoxemia are responsive to supplemental oxygen except shunt. Hypoventilation is usually due to depression of respiratory drive at the level of the central nervous system as a result of drug therapy or the residua of anesthesia as described above. V/Q abnormalities are common causes of hypoxemic respiratory failure and result from

such conditions as airflow obstruction from asthma and chronic obstructive pulmonary disease and pulmonary thromboembolic disease. Shunt is frequently caused by pneumonia and atelectasis. Diffusion limitation and low inspired fraction of oxygen are uncommon causes of hypoxemia in the absence of chronic lung disease and high altitude, respectively.

The spectrum of causes of hypoxemia often can be narrowed according to the appearance of the chest radiograph. A simplified approach to chest radiographic interpretation for other than the pulmonary or critical care medicine specialist involves classifying the pulmonary parenchyma as generally white or black (normal). The causes of a white chest radiograph include atelectasis, pneumonia, pulmonary edema, and acute lung injury. Further characterization of a white chest radiograph includes the description of the radiographic opacities as diffuse or localized. Diffuse infiltrates are commonly associated with hydrostatic pulmonary edema that is due to cardiac pump failure, nonhydrostatic pulmonary edema that is due to lung injury from a variety of causes (e.g., aspiration or pancreatitis), or atypical pneumonias that are rarely hospital acquired (e.g., influenza, *Mycoplasma*, or *Chlamydia pneumoniae*). Focal infiltrates are suggestive of atelectasis or pneumonia. The causes of a black or a normal chest radiograph include pulmonary thromboembolic disease, microatelectasis, exacerbation of underlying obstructive lung disease, intracardiac or pulmonary arteriovenous right-to-left shunt, and a low cardiac output state. In the case of a black or white chest radiograph, information obtained from the history and physical examination may be crucial for determining the nature of further diagnostic testing to pinpoint the etiology of respiratory failure.

Ventilatory failure, the inability to maintain an appropriate arterial PCO_2, is caused by three major mechanisms: insufficient respiratory drive, excessive respiratory workload including increased dead space, or respiratory pump dysfunction. Insufficient ventilatory drive is usually due to drug therapy or the residua of anesthesia as stated above but may also be due to a primary central nervous system disorder (such as stroke, intracranial hemorrhage, and obesity–hypoventilation syndrome) or due to toxic–metabolic encephalopathy as a result of a wide variety of underlying conditions. Increased ventilatory workload may result from increased CO_2 production, increased dead space, altered respiratory mechanics (increased airway resistance or decreased pulmonary compliance), or compensation for metabolic acidosis.

Increased CO_2 production is a by-product of overall increases in metabolism. Fever, delirium with marked agitation, severe sepsis, overfeeding, and hyperthyroidism are examples of clinical states associated with increased CO_2 production. Increased dead space is a hallmark of severe chronic obstructive pulmonary disease; in patients with normal lung function, increased dead space is usually due to either pulmonary thromboembolic disease or a change in respiratory pattern. Rapid shallow breathing as a result of the physiologic changes is induced by anesthesia, and upper abdominal surgery produces an increase in the proportion of ventilation to the anatomic dead space and a decrease in effective alveolar ventilation. In addition to anesthesia and upper abdominal surgery as causes of respiratory pump dysfunction in the postoperative patient, any other cause of respiratory muscle weakness may result in ventilatory failure. Endocrine disorders, such as myasthenia gravis or hypothyroidism, as well as electrolyte abnormalities, such as hypophosphatemia, are examples of conditions that could significantly contribute to respiratory muscle weakness and pump dysfunction.

Treatment of acute respiratory failure depends on the underlying cause and is best accomplished in an appropriately

---

TABLE 9.16 Pathophysiologic Mechanisms of Hypoxemic Respiratory Failure and Ventilatory Failure

HYPOXEMIC RESPIRATORY FAILURE	VENTILATORY FAILURE
Hypoventilation	Insufficient respiratory drive
V/Q abnormalities (shunt, dead space)	Excessive respiratory workload
Venous admixture	Respiratory pump dysfunction
Diffusion limitation	
Low inspired fraction of oxygen	

monitored environment, such as the intensive care unit with the aid of a specialist in critical care medicine, as mechanical support of ventilation—via either conventional invasive mechanical ventilation through an endotracheal tube or noninvasively through a tight fitting nasal or facial mask—may be necessary (Fig. 9.4). Management of mechanical ventilation and its consequences has acquired a level of complexity that mandates subspecialist care and is beyond the scope of this chapter.

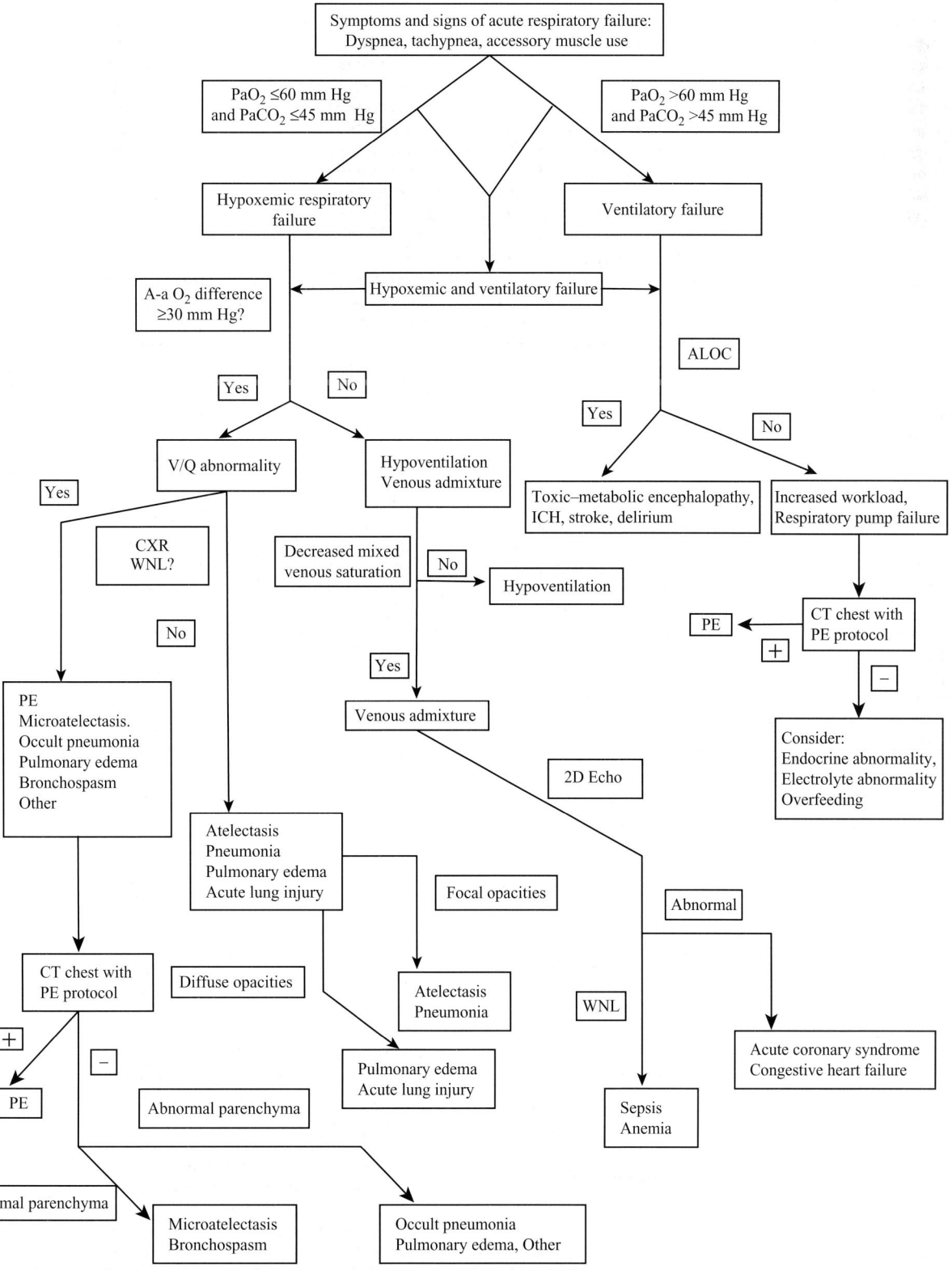

FIGURE 9.4 Algorithm for the evaluation of respiratory failure. ALOC, altered level of consciousness; CT, computed tomography; CXR, chest x-ray; ICH, intracranial hemorrhage; PE, pulmonary embolism; WNL, within normal limits.

POSTOPERATIVE CARE OF THE URINARY BLADDER

The most common postoperative problem in the female bladder is atony caused by overdistention and the reluctance of the patient to initiate the voluntary phase of voiding. After abdominal/pelvic surgery, the patient is often unwilling to contract the abdominal muscles to produce sufficient intra-abdominal pressure against the dome of the bladder to initiate the voiding reflex. After anterior colporrhaphy, spasm, edema, and tenderness of the pubococcygeal muscles may obstruct the process of voiding. The operative trauma from plication of the pubovesicocervical fascia causes edema of the urethral wall and submucosa, especially at the urethrovesical junction, thus contributing to the urinary obstruction.

For spontaneous voiding to occur, the parasympathetic function of the bladder detrusor must be coordinated with the voluntary motor function of the abdominal wall and the levator muscles. In the past, it was customary to insert an indwelling urethral catheter for 5 or more days after vaginal plastic surgery. Although this technique is still used in many clinics, a suprapubic catheter has proved to be an effective alternative. The suprapubic technique was developed and introduced to the gynecologic literature in 1964. When inserted at the time of surgery, the suprapubic Silastic tube eliminates the necessity for repeated bladder catheterization until spontaneous voiding occurs. Although used preferentially after anterior vaginal colporrhaphy, suprapubic bladder catheterization also is useful when the need for prolonged bladder drainage is anticipated, such as after radical Wertheim hysterectomy. A suprapubic catheter also can be inserted when a Marshall-Marchetti-Krantz urethral suspension is performed.

The procedure for suprapubic bladder drainage is performed either before or after the operative procedure. Catheter placement consists of insertion of a 12F Silastic (silicone) catheter into the bladder through a needle trocar (Fig. 9.5). A 12F pigtail (Bonanno) Teflon catheter and other modifications also have been used by many surgeons. The bladder is filled with 300 mL of sterile water, and the needle trocar is inserted through the surgically cleaned anterior abdominal wall about 2 cm above the symphysis pubis. When the stylet is removed from the trocar, clear fluid should pass from the bladder under pressure. About 10 cm of the suprapubic catheter is threaded through the trocar, after which the trocar is removed by sliding it over the indwelling tube. The opposite end of the Silastic catheter is connected to a sterile 1-L drainage bottle or to a sterile closed drainage urinometer bag. The tubing should be filled with fluid at all times and should be anchored to the skin with silicone paste or sutured to the skin to avoid accidental removal. A two-way stopcock is inserted between the catheter and drainage tubing for easy opening and closing of the system. The system is not irrigated unless there is plugging of the bladder catheter and failure of drainage.

Alternatively, at the Emory University Hospital, a Foley catheter is placed through the abdominal wall. After placing a Kelly clamp through the urethra and elevating the dome of the bladder, an incision is made in the abdominal wall superior to the Kelly clamp. A 14F Foley catheter is then pulled into the bladder and connected to gravity drainage. If a suprapubic urethropexy is performed, a 2- to 3-cm opening is made in the dome of the bladder, and the bladder is inspected to ensure that no sutures penetrated the mucosa. The Foley catheter is placed in the bladder and sutured in place with a no. 2.0 absorbable purse-string suture. Using the preceding techniques for insertion of a suprapubic Foley catheter, we have decreased the frequency of catheter obstruction. Seven to ten days postoperatively, the suprapubic catheters are clamped and postvoid residuals are evaluated. Patients with more than 100 mL of residual urine after spontaneous voiding require an extended period of catheterization. If the urinary residual is less than

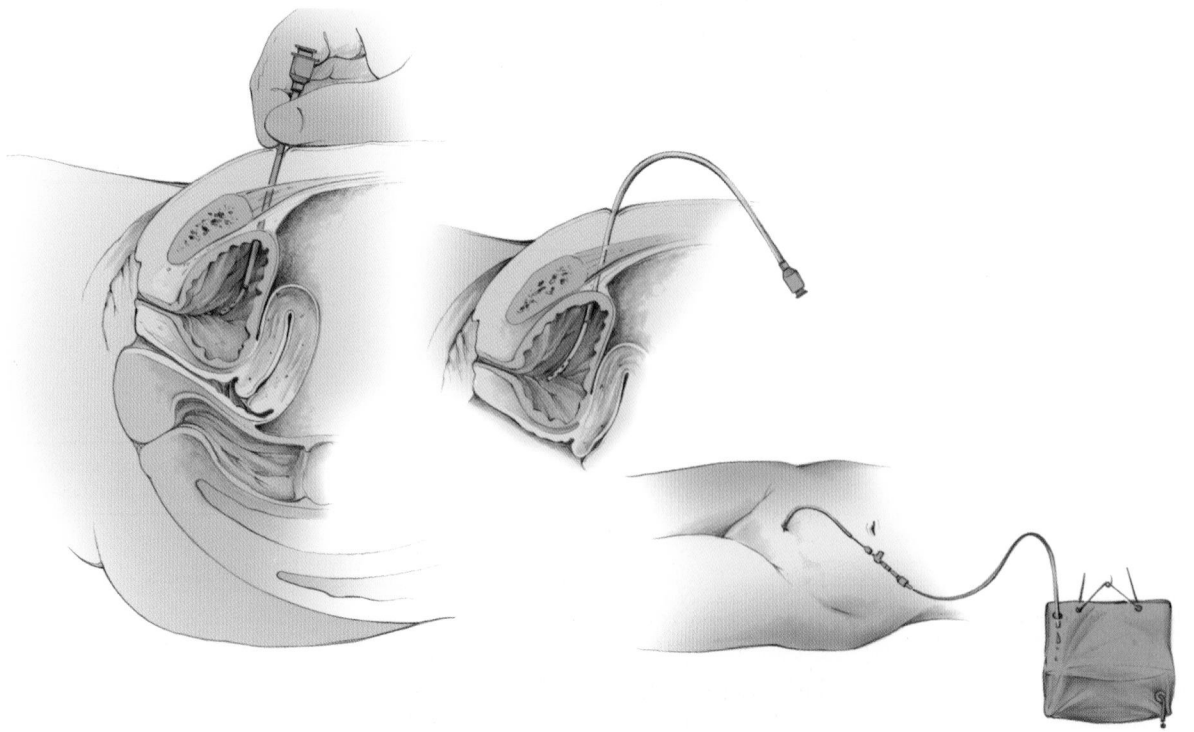

FIGURE 9.5 Method of inserting a suprapubic tube into the bladder through a needle, with resultant drainage into a bottle. Suprapubic catheterization avoids the trauma to the urethra caused by repeated catheterization of an indwelling catheter.

100 mL on two successive voidings of more than 200 mL each, the suprapubic catheter can be removed. In many patients who require prolonged catheterization following radical hysterectomy or pelvic support surgery, intermittent self-catheterization using a clean but not sterile technique has become favored by many gynecologists. We believe, as do other authors, that prophylactic antibiotics given during the use of an indwelling bladder catheter are ineffective in preventing urinary tract infection. Although urinary tract symptoms may be delayed with the use of prophylactic antibiotics, it is our experience that the incidence of infection is unchanged and that a subsequent urinary tract infection may result from resistant organisms that are more difficult to treat later. Therefore, we prefer to treat only patients who have significant bacteriuria and pyuria, which includes about 10% to 15% of the patients with suprapubic drainage.

POSTOPERATIVE GASTROINTESTINAL TRACT MANAGEMENT

Dysfunction of the gastrointestinal tract remains a challenge in postoperative management. Each patient should be treated as an individual and not placed on a standard protocol for advancing diets. Patients who have had uncomplicated surgery may be given a regular diet on the first postoperative day if bowel sounds are present, if abdominal examination reveals no distention, and if the patient is no longer nauseated from her anesthesia. Seriously ill or malnourished patients or patients requiring extensive bowel surgery may benefit from preoperative and postoperative parenteral nutrition.

It is important to differentiate between postoperative ileus and postoperative obstruction (Table 9.17) if proper therapy is to be initiated promptly with beneficial results. The distinction may be difficult. This is because partial bowel obstruction is often accompanied by a secondary ileus as part of the clinical picture. Only by close clinical monitoring of the bowel sounds, serial abdominal radiographic studies, and frequent white blood cell counts can one clearly separate these two postoperative complications. Adynamic ileus is the more common clinical entity, a fact that may mislead the surgeon into a

false sense of security unless he or she remains acutely aware of the distinguishing features of intestinal obstruction. Serial monitoring of the white blood cell count and differential count is an important method for differentiating between bowel obstruction and paralytic ileus. A key feature of advancing bowel obstruction is necrosis of the bowel wall, which causes progressive leukocytosis, along with distention and peritonitis. The most common gynecologic disease process associated with both ileus and intestinal obstruction is severe pelvic inflammatory disease (PID). Notoriously acute exacerbation of PID or rupture of a pelvic abscess is associated with prolonged ileus. Occasionally, fibrous adhesions form, and secondary bowel obstruction occurs. Postoperative pelvic peritonitis from any cause, including cellulitis resulting from hematoma formation and secondary infection of the vaginal cuff, is often associated with ileus, whereas intestinal obstruction only rarely results from such a complication.

Total Parenteral Nutrition

Nutritional support has proved efficacious in patients undergoing major surgery and in patients with impaired bowel function, inadequate oral intake, or cancer. A few patients require total parenteral nutrition (TPN) for prolonged periods secondary to their inability to obtain adequate calories orally. Parenteral nutrition may be administered through a peripheral or central access, depending on the patient's initial nutritional status and the time required on TPN.

Hospitalized patients may require TPN for disease processes such as gastrointestinal tract obstruction, prolonged ileus, short-bowel syndrome, radiation enteritis, intra-abdominal abscess, pancreatitis, regional enteritis, and enterocutaneous fistula. A patient with any condition that prevents oral intake of adequate amounts of food for more than 7 to 10 days probably requires central parenteral nutrition. Because it is much easier to maintain an adequate nutritional state than to improve a poor one, the decision to use TPN should not be delayed.

TPN is not without complications. Many of these pertain to the need for central venous access. Catheter tip infection is one of the more frequently encountered problems. Meticulous aseptic technique when placing the central venous catheter and adherence

TABLE 9.17 Differential Diagnosis Between Postoperative Ileus and Postoperative Obstruction		
CLINICAL FEATURE	**POSTOPERATIVE ILEUS**	**POSTOPERATIVE OBSTRUCTION**
Abdominal pain	Discomfort from distention but not cramping pains	Cramping progressively severe
Relation to previous surgery	Usually within 48–72 h of surgery	Usually delayed, may be 5–7 d for remote onset
Nausea and vomiting	Present	Present
Distention	Present	Present
Bowel sounds	Absent or hypoactive	Borborygmi with peristaltic rushes and high-pitched tinkles
Fever	Only if related to associated peritonitis	Rarely present unless bowel becomes gangrenous
Abdominal radiographs	Distended loops of small and large bowels; gas usually present in the colon	Single or multiple loops of distended bowel (usually small bowel) with air–fluid levels
Treatment	Conservative with nasogastric suction, enemas, cholinergic stimulation	Conservative management with nasogastric decompression Surgical exploration

to aseptic technique when using the catheter minimizes the risk of infection. Antibiotic-coated central venous catheters have been around for more than a decade and are coming more into favor as compelling data surface suggesting decreased infection rates with their use. At the Emory University Hospital, central venous catheters coated with chlorhexidine and silver sulfasalazine are being used. Other potential problems with central venous catheters include catheter or air embolism and pneumothorax or hemothorax. Total parenteral nutrition itself can cause fluid overload, electrolyte abnormalities, or metabolic disturbances.

Patient Evaluation

A complete medical history and physical examination must be obtained before parenteral nutrition is initiated. Particular attention should be paid to identifying patients with cardiovascular or renal disease, hyperlipidemia, diabetes, and thyroid disease. Total parenteral nutrition modification can include decreasing or eliminating fat emulsion in patients with severe cardiovascular disease or hyperlipidemia, administering low-nitrogen TPN to patients with renal failure, and increasing the insulin dosage in patients with diabetes mellitus.

The patient's degree of malnutrition should be assessed by taking measurements of several physical indicators, such as actual body weight (ABW) and ideal body weight (IBW), usual body weight (UBW; preillness), creatinine-to-height index, triceps skin fold thickness (TSFT), and arm circumference (AC). The arm muscle circumference (AMC) is calculated and used as an index of nutritional status.

$$AMC = AC - (TSFT \times 3.14)$$

Fat stores are reflected in the triceps skin fold measurement, whereas somatic proteins are evaluated by measuring muscle mass, such as the AMC. The Frisancho standards (1984) are used to interpret body weight (kilograms), triceps (millimeters), and bone-free arm muscle area (square centimeters). Patients found to be in the 5th to 10th percentiles are severely malnourished and require an anabolic environment. Weight loss is considered significant when the (UBW – ABW)/ UBW × 100 is >10%. Weight loss during starvation occurs at a rate of 0.4 kg/d. Survival also is compromised when the ABW falls below the 70th percentile of the IBW. In addition to the preceding physical measurements, a thorough evaluation of chemical indicators is required (Table 9.18) before initiating TPN. Extensive monitoring is required while the patient is receiving TPN (Table 9.19).

TABLE 9.18 Pretreatment Screening

LABORATORY EVALUATION
Complete blood count with differential
Prothrombin time/partial thromboplastin time
Electrolytic panel
Chemistry panel
Albumin
Transferrin
Total lymphocyte count
Triglycerides
Magnesium
Phosphorus
Copper
Zinc
Selenium

TABLE 9.19 Treatment Monitoring

TEST	FREQUENCY
Electrolyte panel	Twice weekly
Chemistry panel	Weekly
Magnesium	Weekly
Transferrin	Weekly
Triglycerides	Monthly, or as needed
Zinc	Monthly, or as needed
Copper	Monthly, or as needed
Selenium	Monthly, or as needed

The physical and chemical measurements of malnutrition are subject to many influences during illness and should be treated as confounding variables. For example, albumin values less than 3.2 g/dL are frequently used to indicate malnutrition. Starker and colleagues observed that in hospitalized patients, albumin and body weight measurements in conjunction provided better indications of sodium balance and extracellular fluid volume. In addition, albumin serum levels are required for maintenance of the intravascular colloid oncotic pressure and as a carrier protein.

The half-life of albumin is 20 days and thus reflects a depletion of visceral proteins of at least 3 weeks' duration. Transferrin, with a half-life of 8 to 9 days, provides the clinician with a measurement of recent protein status changes. Because transferrin is required to bind Fe^{2++}, its level is affected by intravascular iron status and can increase during pregnancy, in patients with hepatitis, and in patients receiving estrogen supplementation. Serum protein content can be reduced in protein-losing enteropathy, nephropathy, chronic infections, uremia, and during catabolism. Transferrin reflects recent losses and remains a better indicator of protein status and change than is albumin. Total lymphocyte counts of less than 1,500 mL are indicative of an immunocompromised patient. Immunologic skin testing for recall antigens and total lymphocyte counts has been correlated with both nutritional status and morbidity and mortality. Its usefulness in the assessment of nutritional status is limited to confounding variables such as cancer, side effects of cancer treatment protocols, stress of trauma or surgery, and infection. Phosphorus and the trace elements are thoroughly evaluated before initiating TPN and during TPN because they are often depleted with many disease states and are required when alimenting (Tables 9.7, 9.8, and 9.18 to 9.21).

Nutritional Requirements

Total parenteral nutrition consists of six components: carbohydrates, fat, protein, electrolytes, vitamins, and trace elements. The Harris-Benedict basal energy expenditure (BEE) accounts for two thirds of the total daily energy requirements, with the remaining one third obtained from protein. Daily requirements for protein are between 1.5 and 2.5 g/kg/d. Patients receiving TPN who are severely malnourished and stressed require larger amounts of protein daily.

The BEE is calculated as follows:

$$BEE(kcal/d) = 655 + 9.56(wt) + 1.85(ht) - 4.68(age)$$

TABLE 9.20 Design of Parenteral Nutrition Programs: Examples

Nonobese patient weighing 60 kg; assume basal Harris-Benedict equation estimate of daily caloric requirements of 1,250 kcal/d

Patient characteristics
1. Euvolemic, normal urine output, and no unusual gastrointestinal losses; therefore, appropriate initial estimate of daily fluid requirement is 30 mL/kg body weight
2. Moderately stressed with normal renal and hepatic function; therefore, appropriate to provide 1.2 g protein per kg body weight
3. Nonobese; therefore, appropriate to provide Harris-Benedict estimate plus 20% for calories, i.e., 1,250 kcal plus 20% = 1,500 kcal

Program design
1. Fluid requirement: 30 mL × body weight; 30 × 60 = 1,800 mL
2. Caloric requirement: Harris-Benedict estimate plus 20%; 1250 kcal + 250 kcal = 1,500 kcal
3. Protein requirement for moderately stressed patient: 1.2 g/kg body weight; 60 × 1.2 = ~70 g protein. 70 g protein × 4 kcal/g protein = 280 kcal
4. Fat requirement: 30% of total calories; 30% × 1,500 kcal = 450 kcal
5. Carbohydrate requirement: caloric requirement minus the sum of protein and fat calories; 1,500 − (280 + 450 kcal) = 770 kcal. 770 kcal carbohydrate − kcal/g carbohydrate (3.4) = ~225 g carbohydrate
6. Therefore, consider the following parenteral nutrition formula: 1.5 L amino acids, 5% dextrose, 15%; plus 250 mL of 20% fat emulsion, which provides 1,750 mL, 1565 kcal, 75 g protein, 225 g carbohydrate, and 500 fat calories. Note that 5% amino acids equals 50 g protein per liter
7. If institution uses three-in-one admixture (amino acids plus dextrose plus fat in one container) and stock solutions of 10% amino acids, 70% dextrose, and 20% lipid, a comparable parenteral nutrition program would be 1.5 L amino acids, 5%; dextrose, 15%; fat, 3.5%

Similar patient characteristics except patients volume-expanded
1. Consider the following fluid-restricted parenteral nutrition formula: 1 L of amino acids, 7%; dextrose, 20%; plus 250 mL 20% fat emulsion, which provides 1,250 mL, 1,460 calories, 70 g protein, 200 g carbohydrate, and 500 fat calories

Reprinted with permission from McMahon MM. Parenteral nutrition. In: Goldman L, Ausiello D, eds. *Cecil textbook of medicine*, 22nd ed. Philadelphia, PA: WB Saunders Company, 2004. Copyright © 2004, Elsevier.

Height is in centimeters; weight is in kilograms.

Once the patient has reached the estimated daily calorie goal, a 24-hour nitrogen balance study is performed by obtaining a 24-hour urine collection and an AM electrolyte panel. If a large quantity of fluid from the nasogastric tube, ileostomy, fistula, or wound is present, this also should be collected and sent for nitrogen measurements.

$$N_2 (g) \, \text{balance} = N_2 (g) \, \text{in} - N_2 (g) \, \text{out}$$

Adding 4 to the N_2 out value accounts for nitrogenous losses in the stool and skin. This does not include an estimate of the losses from the gastrointestinal tract and wound, as previously described.

$$N_2 (g) \, \text{balance} = N_2 (g) \, \text{in} \times \left[N_2 (g) \, \text{out} + 4 \right]$$
$$N_2 (g) \, \text{out} = \text{urine volume} \, (mL) \times \text{urine urea} \, N_2 \, (mg/dL)$$
$$N_2 (g) \, \text{in} = \text{amino acids per day} / 6.24$$
$$6.24 = g \, \text{protein} / g \, \text{nitrogen}$$

Patients with normal renal and liver function are started on standard total hyperalimentation solution (THAS) (Table 9.18). Each liter provides a total of 1,020 kcal, including 41 g of amino acids and 250 g of dextrose. The osmolality of this solution is 1,850 mOsm, which therefore necessitates a central venous access. The calories-to-nitrogen ratio of this solution is 157:1 and is optimal in nonstressed patients. The addition of lipids also is effective in promoting a positive nitrogen balance.

The total daily sodium concentration should be equivalent to that of normal saline (150 mEq/L). This can be altered to accommodate patients who require sodium restriction or loading. Table 9.22 outlines the recommendation for daily electrolyte requirements. It should be noted that acetate serves as a precursor to bicarbonate, because the latter is not compatible in the THAS solution. Multivitamins are added daily to 1 L of THAS, whereas trace elements are divided equally in the volume to be infused during a 24-hour period. The recommended daily allowances for both fat- and water-soluble vitamins are outlined in Table 9.23.

Blood glucose levels in patients receiving TPN should be between 100 and 200 mg/dL. A minimum of 10 IU should be added to each liter when required. This permits about 50% to adhere to the plastic tubing. This can be supplemented with subcutaneous doses of regular insulin to obtain the desired blood glucose level. About one half to two thirds of the previous day's requirements are added in divided doses to the THAS solutions.

Intravenous lipids provide a nonprotein source of energy and serve as a source of essential fatty acids. Ten percent fat emulsions (550 kcal/500 mL) and 20% fat emulsions (1,000 kcal/500 mL) are commercially available. In patients receiving standard TPN, 500 mL of 10% fat emulsion are infused twice weekly at a rate of 42 mL/h. However, when fat emulsion is used with peripheral THAS, the patient requires 2 L of peripheral THAS and 1 L of 10% fat emulsion daily. Twenty percent fat emulsions also can be used for calories in patients with glucose intolerance or patients who require a decreased protein–calorie percentage.

TABLE 9.21 Trace Minerals

MINERALS AND LEVELS	DEFICIENCY		TOXICITY	
	SYMPTOMS	ETIOLOGY	SYMPTOMS	ETIOLOGY
Zinc, 55–150 mg/dL	Diarrhea, mental depression, alopecia, night blindness, dermatosis, impaired taste, hypogonadism, impaired wound healing	Gastrointestinal (failure of ingestion, absorption, retention) Large wounds Protein–energy malnutrition Cancer	Vomiting Diarrhea Neurologic damage ("zinc shakes")	Increased ingestion from galvanized containers Metal fume fever
Selenium, 90–150 µg/dL (synergism with vitamin E)	Myositis with muscle weakness Cardiomyopathy with arrhythmias and congestive heart failure	Unsupplemented TPN	Liver cirrhosis Alopecia Pathologic loss of nails Dermatitis	Increased ingestion (rare)
Chromium, 50–200 µg/d	Neuropathy Encephalopathy New insulin–dependent diabetes mellitus	Unsupplemented TPN Increased renal loss secondary to injury Gastrointestinal losses	Respiratory Lung cancer	Workers manufacturing products containing hexavalent chromium
Phosphorus, 3.0–4.5 mg/dL	Nausea, vomiting, anorexia, dysarthria, paresthesia, hemolytic anemia, peripheral neuropathy, respiratory depression, congestive heart failure, renal glycosuria	Gastrointestinal (failure of ingestion, absorption, retention) Cellular anabolism Respiratory or metabolic alkalosis Al(OH)$_3$ antacids Alcoholism	Neurotoxicity secondary to compensatory hypocalcemia	Renal failure Hypoparathyroidism
Magnesium, 136–145 mEq/L	Nausea, vomiting, muscle weakness, lethargy, tetany, muscle tremor, personality changes	Gastrointestinal (failure of ingestion, absorption, retention) Cellular catabolism, acidosis, K$^+$ depletion Glomerular dysfunction	Hyporeflexia, lethargy, respiratory depression, cardiac arrest	Magnesium supplementation in patients with renal compromise
Copper, 70–155 µg/dL	Hypochromic anemia not responsive to iron, neutropenia	THAS without copper or high amino acids Gastrointestinal (failure of ingestion, absorption, retention) Pregnancy, lactation (increased requirements) Renal losses	Jaundice–hepatic necrosis Intravascular hemolysis Gastric hemorrhage Tremors, choreoathetoid movements, dementia, rigidity, dysarthria	Iatrogenic Wilson disease Absorption of copper nitrate salves in burn patients

THAS, total hyperalimentation solution; TPN, total parenteral nutrition.

Patients deficient in fatty acids present with dermatitis, hemolytic anemia, thrombocytopenia, elevated liver enzymes, and poor wound healing.

To improve glucose tolerance, the first liter should be started at a rate of 42 mL/h. On the second day, the solution can be increased to 84 mL/h; on day three, it can be increased to 124 mL/h. If the patient is unable to tolerate this schedule, increments can be decreased to 21 mL/h each day. Treatment monitoring is outlined in Table 9.19. Total nitrogen balance should be recalculated if there is a marked change in the patient's condition or in the parenteral nutrition administered.

Recent data in the surgical literature suggest that supplementing TPN with glutamine dipeptides improves nitrogen balance, preserves intestinal permeability and absorption, and improves recovery of lymphocytes. These authors also demonstrated a shorter hospital stay in postoperative patients receiving glutamine dipeptide–enriched TPN compared with controls receiving TPN alone.

Initiating Total Parenteral Nutrition

Safe venous access is required for initiating TPN. A reliable intravenous catheter should be placed into a large central vein with the catheter tip located so that blood flow dilutes the highly concentrated nutritional fluids. The insertion site also should allow easy fixation of the catheter at the entrance site, minimum catheter movement during body

TABLE 9.22 Daily Electrolyte Requirements for Parenteral Nutrition	
ELECTROLYTE	**DOSAGE (mEq/d)**
Sodium	60–150
Potassium	60–240
Phosphate	30–45
Calcium	10–15
Magnesium	8–26
Acetate	80–120
Chloride	60–150

movements, and easy dressing changes. A subclavian vein approach satisfies the requirements for safe catheter placement, but neither internal jugular vein nor antecubital fossa placement is optimal. The internal jugular vein should be used only if the subclavian approach has failed. Movement of the head and neck results in an increased incidence of occluding venous access when the internal jugular vein has been cannulated.

Anatomy of Infraclavicular Subclavian Vein

In 1952, Aubaniac, a French physician, was among the first to advocate use of the subclavian vein for intravenous infusions. Wilson and colleagues cannulated the superior vena cava through a percutaneous puncture of the subclavian vein. They reported a high percentage of successful cannulations and a low incidence of complications.

As **Figure 9.6** shows, the subclavian vein is located within the costoclavicular–scalene triangle, which is bounded anteriorly by the medial end of the clavicle, posteriorly by the upper surface of the first rib, and laterally by the anterior scalene muscle. The anterior scalene muscle separates the subclavian vein from the subclavian artery, which lies beneath and along the lateral aspect of the muscle. The subclavian vein is covered by 5 cm of the clavicle medially and joins the internal jugular vein near the medial border of the anterior scalene muscle to form the innominate vein. The innominate vein descends behind the sternum and joins with the opposite innominate vein to form the superior vena cava. The subclavian vein, which is about 3 or 4 cm long, continues as the axillary vein below the clavicle en route to the axilla. Several other significant structures occupy this region. The phrenic nerve courses across the anterior surface of the anterior scalene muscle near its attachment to the first rib and courses medially to lie posterior to the subclavian vein. It can be injured if the posterior wall of the vessel is penetrated. The internal thoracic nerve and apical pleura are in contact with the posterior surface of the subclavian vein at its junction with the internal jugular vein. The roots of the brachial plexus formed by the fifth, sixth, seventh, and eighth cervical and first thoracic nerves lie lateral to the anterior scalene muscle on the lateral side of the subclavian artery. If a cannulating needle is directed too far laterally, the brachial nerve plexus could be injured or the subclavian artery could be punctured. The thoracic duct on the left side and the lymphatic duct on the right cross the anterior scalene muscle on either side of the thorax to enter the superior aspect of each subclavian vein near its junction with the internal jugular vein. These lymphatic vessels are rarely encroached on during subclavian catheterization.

Subclavian Catheter Placement

As illustrated in **Figure 9.7A**, the subclavian catheter is inserted with the patient in the supine position, with the foot of the bed elevated 6 to 12 inches to increase the pressure in the subclavian vein and produce venous distention. After meticulous

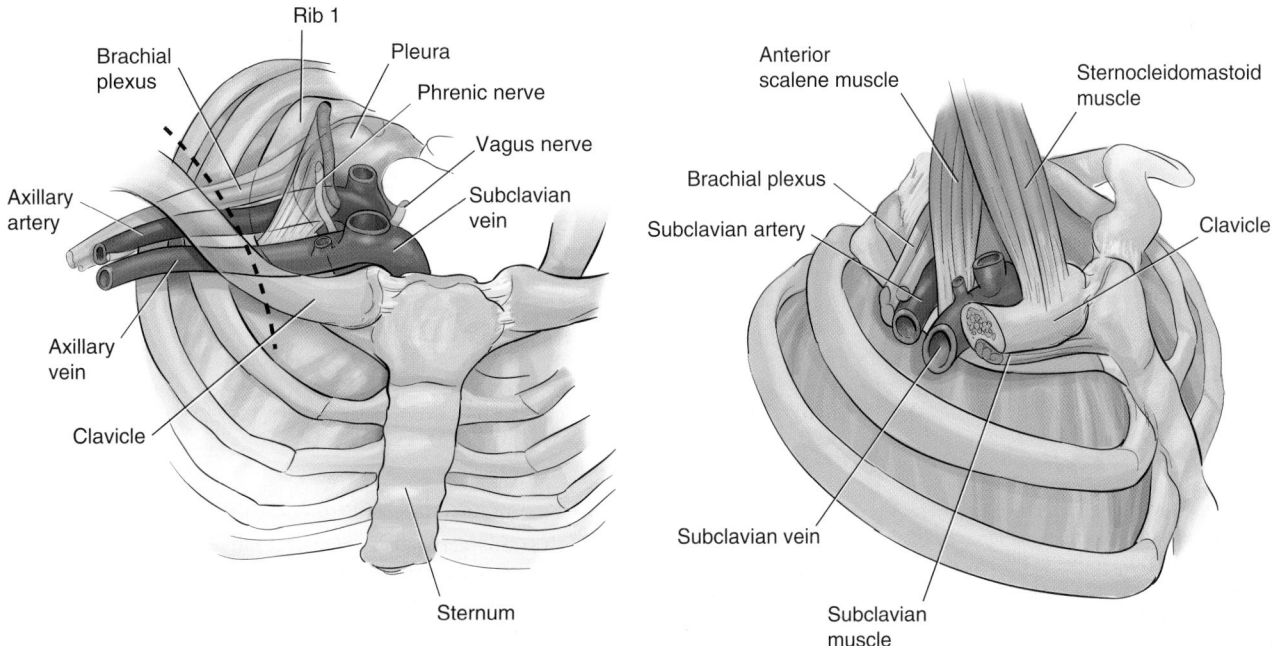

FIGURE 9.6 Anatomic relations of the subclavian vein. The broken line represents the location of the transverse section for lateral view.

TABLE 9.23 Recommended Dietary Allowances[a]

PATIENT PARAMETERS					FAT-SOLUBLE VITAMINS							
	WEIGHT[b]		HEIGHT[b]		PROTEIN,	VITAMIN	VITAMIN	VITAMIN	VITAMIN	ASCORBIC	THIAMINE	RIBOFLAVIN
AGE (Y)	(KG)	(LB)	(CM)	(IN)	G	A, >MG RE[c]	D, IU[d]	E, IU[e]	K, >MG	ACID (C), MG	(B₁), MG	(B₂), MG
Females 11–14	46	101	157	62								
15–18	55	120	163	64	44	800	400	12	55	60	1.1	1.3
19–24	58	128	164	65	46	800	400	12	60	60	1.1	1.3
25–50	63	138	163	64	50	800	200	12	65	60	1.1	1.3
51+	65	143	160	63	50	800	200	12	65	60	1.0	1.2

[a]The allowances, expressed as average daily intakes over time, are intended to provide for individual variations among most normal persons as they live in the United States under usual environmental stresses. Diets should be based on a variety of common foods in order to provide other nutrients for which human requirements have been less well defined.
[b]Weights and heights of reference adults are actual medians for the U.S. population of the designated age, as reported by National Health and Nutrition Examination Survey II (NHANES II). The median weights and heights of those under 19 years of age were taken from Hamill PV et al. *Am J Clin Nutr* 1979;32:607. The use of these figures does not imply that the height-to-weight ratios are ideal.

aseptic preparation of the skin with povidone–iodine (Betadine), the skin and subcutaneous tissues are infiltrated with a 1% solution of lidocaine (Xylocaine) if the patient is awake. The point of needle insertion is about 1 cm below the junction of the inner and middle third of the clavicle. Most central venous catheter units include an external introducer catheter (Teflon) and an internal (silicone) infusion catheter. The outer Teflon sheath accommodates a no. 12 needle, which fits snugly into and protrudes beyond the end of the Teflon catheter. The needle and sheath are introduced into the skin with the shaft of the needle held almost parallel with the anterior chest wall (Fig. 9.7A). The needle is directed medially and advanced along the undersurface of the clavicle. It is not necessary to scrape the posterior surface of the clavicle to ensure that the pleura is protected from puncture. By applying suction constantly, the needle passes beneath the skin and immediately aspirates dark red blood, which confirms entry into the vein. If the vein is not entered, the needle is withdrawn

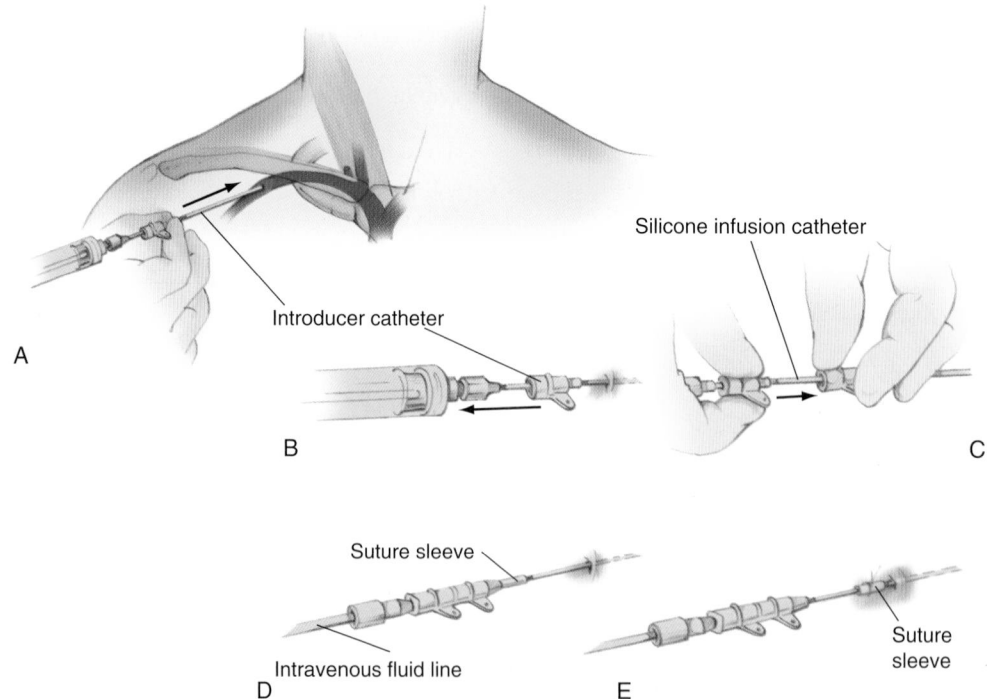

FIGURE 9.7 Insertion of subclavian catheter for monitoring central venous pressure. **A:** After locally anesthetizing the puncture site, the needle with overlying introducer catheter is directed medially between the first rib and the clavicle at the junction of the middle and inner third of the clavicle. The needle is held parallel to the anterior chest wall and advanced along the undersurface of the clavicle. Entry into the vein is evident with aspiration of blood in the attached syringe. **B:** The needle and syringe are removed from the Teflon sheath, and a finger is held over the end of the open catheter to prevent entry of air. **C:** The silicone infusion catheter is inserted through the introducer catheter until the two connectors meet and lock firmly. **D:** The intravenous fluid line is connected to the silicone infusion catheter. **E:** The suture sleeve is advanced to the skin surface, where the catheter is sutured II firmly to the skin.

WATER-SOLUBLE VITAMINS				MINERALS						
NIACIN (B₃), MG	PYRIDOXINE (B₆), MG	FOLATE, >MG	CYANOCOBALAMIN (B₁₂), >MG	CALCIUM, MG	PHOSPHORUS, MG	MAGNESIUM, MG	IRON, MG	ZINC, >MG	IODINE, >MG	SELENIUM, MG
15	1.5	180	2	1200	1200	300	15	12	150	50
15	1.6	180	2	1200	1200	280	15	12	150	55
15	1.6	180	2	800	800	280	15	12	150	55
13	1.6	180	2	800	800	280	10	12	150	55

^{c}Retinol equivalents. 1 retinol equivalent = 1 mg retinol or 6 mg β-carotene.
^{d}As cholecalciferol. 10 mg cholecalciferol = 400 IU of vitamin D.
$^e\alpha$-Tocopherol equivalents. 1 mg D-α-tocopherol = α-TE = 1.49 IU.
Reprinted with permission from the: National Academy of Sciences. *Recommended Dietary Allowances*, 10th ed. Washington, DC: National Academy Press, 1989. Copyright © 1989, National Academy of Sciences.

and readvanced in a similar manner but in a slightly more cranial or caudal direction. Use of real-time sonography has been shown to increase the likelihood of successful subclavian catheter placement. As soon as a free flow of blood is obtained, the introduced Teflon sheath is advanced far enough to be certain that it is securely placed within the vein. The sheath is held in place by the connector, the finger is placed over the end of the needle to prevent air embolism, and the internal needle is replaced (Fig. 9.7B) by the silicone infusion catheter that accompanies the central venous pressure kit (Fig. 9.7C). A thin wire stylet inside the infusion catheter allows the catheter to be advanced easily; occasionally, the stylet must be withdrawn slightly to advance the catheter as far as possible into the innominate vein and superior vena cava. The silicone infusion catheter is advanced until the attached connector can be securely wedged into the connector of the Teflon sheath (Fig. 9.7C). After the infusion catheter is connected to an intravenous fluid line, the Teflon sheath is carefully withdrawn from the vein, remaining partially in the subcutaneous tissue while leaving an ample length of the infusion catheter in the vena cava (Fig. 9.7D). A suture sleeve on the introducer sheath is slid down to the puncture site and sutured to the skin (Fig. 9.7E). The tip of the catheter is preferably positioned in the superior vena cava and should not be advanced into the right atrium or ventricle, where it could cause accidental trauma to the heart wall or cardiac arrhythmias. To ensure its continued sterility and proper function, the subclavian vein catheter should not be used to replace fluids or withdraw blood for laboratory studies, if it is at all possible to avoid these uses. A central venous line for hyperalimentation is an exception to this rule. The dressing should be changed daily and the catheterization site cleaned with povidone–iodine or a similar antimicrobial solution.

Cardiac and Respiratory Insufficiency

Patients with congestive heart failure require decreased sodium and decreased total fluid volume. The best solution can be prepared from the most concentrated solutions of glucose, amino acid, and fat available. Fluid-restricted solutions also may be beneficial for patients with respiratory failure, who should receive less total glucose in favor of more fat because the respiratory quotient (CO_2/O_2) of glucose (1.00) is greater than that of fat (0.70) and because excess glucose will increase the load of CO_2 the lungs must excrete. Excessive

total caloric intake resulting in fat synthesis from glucose substrate may severely compromise respiratory function because large amounts of CO_2 are released (respiratory quotient 8.0).

Discontinuing Total Parenteral Nutrition

Before discontinuing TPN, the patient should tolerate an enteral diet that provides adequate calories. It is permissible to aliment patients with an enteral diet before decreasing the THAS solution. An abrupt discontinuation of central parenteral nutrition results in rebound hypoglycemia. Our recommendation is to decrease the THAS stepwise to 42 mL/h before discontinuation. Some institutions recommend that the patient receive 10% dextrose for an additional 12 hours once central parenteral nutrition has been discontinued.

Team Approach to Total Parenteral Nutrition

Total parenteral nutrition can now be safely administered to patients in many hospitals because of the existence of a team of physicians, nurses, and health care professionals. Although the composition and exact function of the team members vary between hospitals, most teams consist of a physician, nurse, pharmacist, and nutritionist. The role of the team varies in each institution from consultation to complete management of the patient's nutritional needs. The team approach by either method is highly beneficial because it provides a high concentration of personnel with knowledge, expertise, and interdisciplinary communication at the patient's bedside. Team members can provide continuing education on nutrition therapy, continuously audit and collect quality control data, and investigate ways to improve the safety and efficacy of TPN as a treatment modality. Most teams operate with a standardized protocol that covers patient assessment, catheter insertion techniques, solutions used, and monitoring functions performed.

Enteral Nutrition

Enteral nutrition is preferable to TPN. The old adage "if the gut works, use it," applies for several reasons. Ease of administration, economic considerations, and decreased number of complications are all advantages of enteral feeding over parenteral nutrition. Several studies have shown TPN and

TABLE 9.24 Protocol for Enteral Tube Feeding

Nasogastric route: Use small-bore, flexible tube (8F preferred); obtain radiograph after placement to confirm position.

Elevate the head of the bed at least 30 degrees.

Use feeding pump for continuous feeding.

Begin with full-strength formula at 25–30 mL/h and, if tolerated, increase by 25–30 mL/h at 12-h intervals until desired total volume is reached.[a]

Check gastric residuals every 4 h; if >100 mL, hold feeding, and repeat at hourly intervals until residuals are <100 mL before resuming feeding.

Irrigate with 30–50 mL of water after each residual check or after any medications are given. (If the patient requires additional free water, use greater volumes of water for irrigation.)

If the patient experiences diarrhea or intestinal cramping, slow rate of feeding or decrease concentration of formula.

[a]When using hypertonic formulas or feeding into the jejunum with a nasojejunal or jejunostomy tube, diluting the formula to one-half or three-quarter strength may improve tolerance initially. The concentration then can be increased after the desired volume is reached.

enteral nutrition equally efficacious in achieving nitrogen balance. Patients with good bowel function should receive enteral feedings. Relative contraindications to enteral feeding include gastrointestinal bleeding, diarrhea, and intestinal obstruction. Small-bore nasal feeding tubes are placed in the stomach, duodenum, or jejunum. An abdominal radiograph should be obtained to confirm placement. Failure to obtain appropriate studies may result in tube placement in the trachea. Alternatively, a gastrostomy or jejunostomy tube could be placed for long-term enteral nutrition (Table 9.24). Several products are commercially available (Table 9.25). Enteral tube feedings are routinely administered by pump, with either bolus feeds to the stomach or continuous feeds to the small bowel, and should be administered by pump at 25 to 30 mL/h with gastric residuals evaluated every 4 hours. Table 9.26 shows the essential and nonessential amino acids.

ROUTINE ORDERS

When the patient has fully recovered from the anesthetic and is ready for return to the nursing floor and routine postoperative care, we have found the basic postoperative orders shown in Figure 9.8 to be useful. They are only a general outline. This list should be expanded to include the special needs of each postoperative patient.

It is imperative that each patient be evaluated before being transferred from the recovery room. If the patient is not ready for transfer, additional efforts are made to stabilize the patient or transfer her to an intensive care bed. On transferring, the frequency of physicians' rounds should be based on the severity of the patient's condition. All patients should be evaluated on the evening of surgery and appropriate documentation made in the chart. A thorough evaluation of the vital signs, catheter drainage (nasogastric, peritoneal, and Foley), and pulmonary status is required, and abdominal examination is performed. Each physician has a desired protocol for postoperative management. The routine orders outlined in this chapter provide

TABLE 9.25 Commonly Used Adult Commercial Enteral Feeding Formulas[a]

CATEGORY FORMULATION				
POLYMERIC BALANCED	**1.0 KCAL/ML**	**1.2 KCAL/ML**	**1.5 KCAL/ML**	**2.0 KCAL/ML**
≤16% protein	Ensure, Resource, Isocal, Osmolite, Nutren 1.0		Nutren 1.5, Ensure Plus, Resource Plus, Boost Plus, Comply	Nutren 2.0, Deliver, Magnacal
17%–20% protein	Osmolite HN, Isocal HN, Ensure HN, Ultracel, Jevity		Ensure Plus HN	TwoCal HN
≥20% protein	Sustacal, Replete, Promote, Protein XL (22%), Isosource VHN (25%)		TraumaCal	
Modified conventional				
≤16% protein	Peptamen, Reabilan, Vivonex Plus, Criticare HN			
17%–20% protein	Vital HN, Reabilan HN, Alitra Q			
Peptide based	Peptamen (16%), Reabilan (12.5%), Criticare HN (14%), Peptamen VMP (25%), Reabilan HN (17.5%), Alitra Q (21%), Vital HN (16%), SandaSource Peptical (20%)		Crucial (25%)	
Elemental	Tolerex (8%), Vivonex T.E.N. (15%), Vivonex Plus (18%)			

TABLE 9.25 Commonly Used Adult Commercial Enteral Feeding Formulas[a]   (*Continued*)

CATEGORY FORMULATION				
POLYMERIC BALANCED	**1.0 KCAL/ML**	**1.2 KCAL/ML**	**1.5 KCAL/ML**	**2.0 KCAL/ML**
Modified-disease specific (% protein)[b]				
Critical care	Immun-Aid (32%), Impact (22%), Impact/Fiber (22%)	Perative (20%)		
Glucose intolerance	Glytrol (18%), Choice dM (17%), Glucema (16.7%), Diabetasource (20%)			
Hepatic	Travasorb Hepatic (11%), Hepatic-Aid (15%)	Hepatic-Aid II (15%)	NutriHep (11%)	
Malabsorption renal			Lipisorb (17%), Travasorb Renal (7%)	Renal Cal (6%–9%), Amin-Aid (4%)
Pulmonary			Nutrivent (18%), Respalor (20%), Pulmocare (16.7%)	
Modular supplements				
Protein	Casec, ProMod			
Carbohydrate fat	Modical, Polycose Microlipid, MCT oil			

[a]This table includes only a partial listing of commercial products.
[b]Manufacturers market these products as disease specific. The author's use of this designation is intended neither to endorse the manufacturer's claims of special efficacy in the diseases specified nor to deny that the polymeric-balanced or modified-conventional formulas might be appropriate or even superior in these conditions.
MCT, medium-chain triglyceride.
Reprinted with permission from Rombeau JL. Enteral nutrition. In: Goldman L, Ausiello D, eds. *Cecil textbook of medicine*, 22nd ed. Philadelphia, PA: WB Saunders Company, 2004. Copyright © 2004, Elsevier.

the clinician with a framework to design patient care plans that address the individual patient's requirements. Laboratory and radiographic evaluation of the postoperative patient also is tailored to the individual patient. Unfortunately, many physicians are predominantly concerned with quantitative test values. However, it is just as important to develop a close rapport with the patient, the patient's family, and the nursing staff. Only through good communication can the gynecologic surgeon deliver optimum medical care.

BEST SURGICAL PRACTICES

- Approximately 500,000 hospitalized patients develop DVT and approximately 200,000 PE.
- Ten percent of hospital deaths in the United States are secondary to a PE.
- Tumors up-regulate the production of TF and PAI-1, which promotes coagulation and VTE.
- Anti–factor Xa assay can be used to monitor patients who are anticoagulated with LMWHs.
- General anesthesia is associated with a reduction of FRC by approximately 16%.
- Atelectasis occurs in 15% to 20% of patients undergoing abdominal surgery.
- An arterial PO_2 of less than 60 mm Hg or an arterial PCO_2 of greater than 45 mm Hg indicates significant respiratory compromise in patients without preexisting lung disease.
- Increased CO_2 production is a by-product of increased metabolism (i.e., fever, marked agitation, severe sepsis, overfeeding, and hypothyroidism).
- During stress, urinary nitrogen levels may increase greater than or equal to 20 g in 24 hours, corresponding to a loss of 600 g of hydrated body protein.

TABLE 9.26 Amino Acids

ESSENTIAL	NONESSENTIAL
Arginine	Alanine
Histidine	Asparagine
Isoleucine	Aspartic acid
Leucine	Cysteine
Lysine	Glutamic acid
Methionine	Glutamine
Phenylalanine	Glycine
Threonine	Proline
Tryptophan	Serine
Valine	Tyrosine

BASIC POSTOPERATIVE ORDERS

Patient's Name: _____.

1. Admit to Unit #____
2. Diagnosis:
3. Allergies:
4. Condition:
5a. Vital signs:
    ____ q 15 minutes until stable
    ____ q 2 hours for 24 hours
    ____ q 8 hours, if stable
5b. Notify House Officer (H.O.) if
    BP < 90/60, > 160/100
    Pulse <60, >120
    Temp >38.0°C
6. Activity:
    ____ Bed rest
    ____ Ambulate
    ____ Other (specify)
7. Diet:
    ____ NPO
    ____ Other (specify)
8. Intravenous fluids:
9. Incentive inspirometer q 2 hours while awake
10. Encourage deep breathing
11. Drains:

Type	Location	Drainage
____ Nasogastric	____ Stomach	____ Low/intermittent suction
____ Peritoneal	____ Pelvis	____ Bulb suction
____ Foley catheter	____ Bladder	____ Gravity

12a. Fluid intake and output chart.
12b. Notify H.O. if urine output <30 cc/h.
13. Pain medication: Specify
    (a) route of administration
    (b) dosage
14. Antiemetic medication: Specify
    (a) route of administration
    (b) dosage
15. Antibiotics
16. Venous thrombosis prophylaxis
17. Other medications
18. Catheterize q 6 hours, or sooner, if bladder is full and patient unable to void.

FIGURE 9.8 Sample of basic postoperative orders.

BIBLIOGRAPHY

Adolf J, Buttermann G, Weidenbach A, et al. Optimization of postoperative prophylaxis of thrombosis in gynecology. *Geburtshilfe Frauenheilkd* 1978;38:98.

Aitken AGF, Godden OJ. Real-time ultrasound diagnosis of deep vein thrombosis: a comparison with venography. *Clin Radiol* 1987;38:309.

Allan A, Williams JT, Bolton JP, et al. The use of graduated compression stockings in the prevention of postoperative deep vein thrombosis. *Br J Surg* 1983;70:172.

Almond DJ, Guillou PJ, McMahon MJ. Effect of i.v. fat emulsion on natural killer cellular function and antibody-dependent cell cytotoxicity. *Hum Nutr Clin Nutr* 1985;39:227.

American Thoracic Society. Guidelines for the management of adults with hospital-acquired, ventilator-associated, and healthcare-associated pneumonia. *Am J Respir Crit Care Med* 2005;171:388.

Apelgren KN. Triple lumen catheters: technological advance or setback? *Am Surg* 1987;53:113.

Appelman PT, DeJong TE, Lampmann LE. Deep venous thrombosis of the leg: US findings. *Radiology* 1987;163:743.

Askanazi J, Carpentier YA, Elwyn DH, et al. Influence of total parenteral nutrition on fuel utilization in injury and sepsis. *Ann Surg* 1980;191:40.

Askanazi J, Elwyn DH, Silverberg PA, et al. Respiratory distress secondary to a high carbohydrate load. *Surgery* 1980;87:596.

Aubaniac R. L'injection intraveineuse sous claviculaire: avantages et technique. *Presse Med* 1952;60:1456.

Auler JO Jr, Miyoshi E, Fernandez CR, et al. The effects of abdominal opening on respiratory mechanics during general anesthesia in normal and morbidly obese patients: a comparative study. *Anesth Analg* 2002;94:741.

Baertschi U, Schaer A, Bader P, et al. A comparison of low dose heparin and oral anticoagulants in the prevention of thrombo-phlebitis following gynaecological operations (author's translation). [German] *Geburtshilfe Frauenheilkd* 1975;35:754.

Baker JP, Detsky AS, Wesson DE, et al. Nutritional assessment: a comparison of clinical judgment and objective measurements. *N Engl J Med* 1982;306:969.

Ballantyne JC, Carr DB, deFerranti S, et al. The comparative effects of postoperative analgesic therapies on pulmonary outcome: cumulative meta-analyses of randomized, controlled trials. *Anesth Analg* 1998;86:598.

Ballantyne JC, Carr DB, Chalmers TC, et al. Postoperative patient-controlled analgesia: meta-analyses of initial randomized control trials. *J Clin Anesth* 1993;5:18.

Ballard RM, Bradley-Watson PJ, Johnstone FD, et al. Low doses of subcutaneous heparin in the prevention of deep vein thrombosis after gynaecological surgery. *J Obstet Gynaecol Br Commonw* 1973;80:469.

Barbul A, Fishel RS, Shimazu S, et al. Intravenous hyperalimentation with high arginine levels improves wound healing and immune function. *J Surg Res* 1985;38:328.

Bearman GM, Munro C, Sessler CN, et al. Infection control and the prevention of nosocomial infections in the intensive care unit. *Semin Respir Crit Care Med* 2006;27:310.

Bernstein K, Ulmsten U, Astedt B, et al. Incidence of thrombosis after gynecologic surgery evaluated by an improved 125I-fibrinogen uptake test. *Angiology* 1980;31:606

Bistrian BR, Blackburn GL, Hallowell E, et al. Protein status of general surgical patients. *JAMA* 1974;230:858.

Bjornson HS, Colle R, Bower RH, et al. Association between microorganism growth at the catheter site and colonization of the catheter in patients receiving total parenteral nutrition. *Surgery* 1982;92:20.

Blackburn GL, Bistrian BR, Maini BS, et al. Nutritional and metabolic assessment of the hospitalized patient. *J Parenter Enteral Nutr* 1977;1:11.

Blackburn GL, Etter G, Mackenzie T. Criteria for choosing amino acid therapy in acute renal failure. *Am J Clin Nutr* 1978;31:1841.

Bluman LG, Mosca L, Newman N, et al. Preoperative smoking habits and postoperative pulmonary complications. *Chest* 1998;113:883.

Bohner H, Kindgen-Milles D, Grust A, et al. Prophylactic nasal continuous positive airway pressure after major vascular surgery: results of a prospective randomized trial. *Langenbecks Arch Surg* 2002;387:21.

Bonnar J. Venous thromboembolism and gynecologic surgery. *Clin Obstet Gynecol* 1985;28:432.

Bonnar J, Walsh J. Prevention of thrombosis after pelvic surgery by British dextran 70. *Lancet* 1972;1:614.

Bonnar J, Walsh J, Haddon M, et al. Coagulation system changes induced by pelvic surgery and the effect of dextran 70. *Bibl Anat* 1973;12:351.

Borstad E, Urdal K, Handeland G, et al. Comparison of low molecular weight heparin vs. unfractionated heparin in gynecological surgery: II. Reduced dose of low molecular weight heparin. *Acta Obstet Gynecol Scand* 1992;71:471.

Bower RH, Talamini MA, Sax HC, et al. Postoperative enteral versus parenteral nutrition: a randomized controlled trial. *Arch Surg* 1986;121:1040.

Brenner DA. Total parenteral nutrition at home. *Outpatient Ther Med* 1987;2:1.

Brooks-Brunn JA. Postoperative atelectasis and pneumonia: risk factors. *Am J Crit Care* 1995;4:340.

Brooks-Brunn JA. Risk factors associated with postoperative pulmonary complications following total abdominal hysterectomy. *Clin Nurs Res* 2000;9:27.

Brun-Buisson C, Brochard L. Corticosteroid therapy in acute respiratory distress syndrome: better late than never? *JAMA* 1998;280:182.

Bullock TK, Waltrip TJ, Price SA, et al. A retrospective study of nosocomial pneumonia in postoperative patients shows a higher mortality rate in patients receiving nasogastric tube feeding. *Am Surg* 2004;70:822.

Carpenter JP, Holand GA, Baum RA, et al. Magnetic resonance venography for the detection of deep venous thrombosis: comparison with contrast venography and duplex Doppler ultrasonography. *J Vasc Surg* 1993;18:734.

Carrier M, Le Gal G, Cho R, et al. Dose escalation of LMW heparin to manage recurrent VTE events despite systemic anticoagulation in cancer patients. *J Thromb Haemost* 2009;7:760.

Celli BR, Rodriguez KS, Snider GL. A controlled trial of intermittent positive pressure breathing, incentive spirometry, and deep breathing exercises in preventing pulmonary complications after abdominal surgery. *Am Rev Respir Dis* 1984;130:12.

Chastre J, Fagon JY, Bornet-Lecso M, et al. Evaluation of bronchoscopic techniques for the diagnosis of nosocomial pneumonia. *Am J Respir Crit Care Med* 1995;152:231.

Chory ET, Mullen JL. Nutritional support of the cancer patient: delivery systems and formulations. *Surg Clin North Am* 1986;66:1105.

Christenson M, Hitt JA, Abbott G, et al. Improving patient safety: resource availability and application for reducing the incidence of healthcare-associated infection. *Infect Control Hosp Epidemiol* 2006;27:245.

Chumillas S, Ponce JL, Delgado F, et al. Prevention of postoperative pulmonary complications through respiratory rehabilitation: a controlled clinical study. *Arch Phys Med Rehabil* 1998;79:5.

Clarke-Pearson DL, Coleman RE, Siegel R, et al. Indium 111 platelet imaging for the detection of deep venous thrombosis and pulmonary embolism in patients without symptoms after surgery. *Surgery* 1985;98:98.

Clarke-Pearson DL, Coleman RE, Synan IS, et al. Venous thromboembolism prophylaxis in gynecologic oncology: a prospective controlled trial of low-dose heparin. *Am J Obstet Gynecol* 1983;145:606.

Clarke-Pearson DL, Synan IS, Hinshaw WM, et al. Prevention of postoperative venous thromboembolism by external pneumatic calf compression in patients with gynecologic malignancy. *Obstet Gynecol* 1984;63:92.

Clinical Nutrition Cases. Is chromium essential for humans? *Nutr Rev* 1988;46:17.

Cook D, Guyatt G, Marshall J, et al. A comparison of sucralfate and ranitidine for the prevention of upper gastrointestinal bleeding in patients requiring mechanical ventilation. Canadian Critical Care Trials Group. *N Engl J Med* 1998;338:791.

Delafosse B, Bouffard Y, Viale JP, et al. Respiratory changes induced by parenteral nutrition in postoperative patients undergoing inspiratory pressure support ventilation. *Anesthesiology* 1987;66:393.

DeWet CJ, Pearl RG. Venous thromboembolism: deep-vein thrombosis and pulmonary embolism. *Anesthesiol Clin North Am* 1999;17:895.

Dinsmore RE, Wedeen V, Rosen B, et al. Phase-offset technique to distinguish slow blood flow and thrombus on MR images. *AJR Am J Roentgenol* 1987;148:634.

Dodek P, Keenan S, Cook D, et al. Evidence-based clinical practice guideline for the prevention of ventilator-associated pneumonia. *Ann Intern Med* 2004;141:305.

Doran FSA. Prevention of deep vein thrombosis. *Br J Hosp Med* 1971;6:773.

Duggan M, Kavanagh BP. Pulmonary atelectasis: a pathogenic perioperative entity. *Anesthesiology* 2005;102:838.

Fabregas N, Ewig S, Torres A, et al. Clinical diagnosis of ventilator associated pneumonia revisited: comparative validation using immediate post-mortem lung biopsies. *Thorax* 1999;54(10):867.

Fagevik Olsen M, Wennberg E, Johnsson E, et al. Randomized clinical study of the prevention of pulmonary complications after thoracoabdominal resection by two different breathing techniques. *Br J Surg* 2002;89:1228.

Falanga A, Marchetti M, Vignoli A. Coagulation in cancer: biological and clinical aspects. *J Thromb Haemost* 2013;11:223.

Falanga A, Tartari CJ, Marchetti M. Microparticles in tumour progression. *Thromb Res* 2012;129(suppl 1):S132.

Flanders SA, Collard HR, Saint S. Nosocomial pneumonia: state of the science. *Am J Infect Control* 2006;34:84.

Ford GT, Rosenal TW, Clergue F, et al. Respiratory physiology in upper abdominal surgery. *Clin Chest Med* 1993;14:237.

Frango JA, Eskin SG, McIntire LV. Flow effects on prostacyclin production by cultured human endothelial cells. *Science* 1985;227:1477.

Fragou M, Gravvanis A, Dimitriou V, et al. Real-time ultrasound-guided subclavian vein cannulation versus the landmark method in critical care patients: a prospective randomized study. *Crit Care Med* 2011;39:1607.

Gazzaniga AB, Day AT, Sankary H. The efficacy of a 20 per cent fat emulsion as a peripherally administered substrate. *Surg Obstet Gynecol* 1985;160:387.

Geerts WH, Heit JA, Clagett GP, et al. Prevention of venous thromboembolism (Sixth ACCP Consensus Conference on Antithrombotic Therapy). *Chest* 2001;119(1 suppl):132S.

Gjonnaess H, Abildgaard U. Bleeding in gynecological surgery: influence of low dose heparin. *Int J Gynaecol Obstet* 1976;14:9.

Gould M, Garcia J, Wien SM, et al. Prevention of VTE in the nonorthopedic surgical population (Ninth ACCP Consensus Conference) on antithrombotic therapy. *Chest* 2012;141:S145.

Greene KE, Peters JI. Pathophysiology of acute respiratory failure. *Clin Chest Med* 1994;15:1.

Groeben H. Epidural anesthesia and pulmonary function. *J Anesth* 2006;20:290.

Guyton DP, Khayat A, Schreiber H, et al. Endogenous plasminogen activator and venous flow: therapeutic implications. *Crit Care Med* 1987;15:122.

Guyton DP, Khayat A, Schreiber H. Pneumatic compression stockings and prostaglandin synthesis: a pathway to fibrinolysis? *Crit Care Med* 1985;13:266.

Hall JC, Tarala R, Harris T, et al. Incentive spirometry versus routine chest physiotherapy for prevention of pulmonary complications after abdominal surgery. *Lancet* 1991;337:953.

Hall JC, Tarala R, Tapper J, et al. Prevention of respiratory complications after abdominal surgery: a randomised clinical trial. *BMJ* 1996;312:148.

Hall JC, Tarala RA, Hall JL. A case-control study of postoperative pulmonary complications after laparoscopic and open cholecystectomy. *J Laparoendosc Surg* 1996;6:87.

Hamill PV, Drizd TA, Johnson CL, et al. Physical growth: National Center for Health Statistics percentiles. *Am J Clin Nutr* 1979;32:607.

Hauser CJ, Shoemaker WC, Turpin I, et al. Oxygen transport responses to colloids and crystalloids in critically ill surgical patients. *Surg Gynecol Obstet* 1980;150:881.

Haydock DA, Hill GL. Improved wound healing response in surgical patients receiving i.v. nutrition. *Br J Surg* 1987;74:320.

Hebert PC, Wells G, Blajchman MA, et al. A multicenter, randomized, controlled clinical trial of transfusion requirements in critical care. Transfusion Requirements in Critical Care Investigators, Canadian Critical Care Trials Group. *N Engl J Med* 1999;340(6):409.

Hedenstierna G, Rothen HU. Atelectasis formation during anesthesia: causes and measures to prevent it. *J Clin Monit Comput* 2000;16:329.

Heird WC, Grundy SM, Hubbard VS. Structured lipids and their use in clinical nutrition. *Am J Clin Nutr* 1986;43:320.

Hilgard P. Experimental vitamin K deficiency and spontaneous metastases. *Br J Cancer* 1975;35:391.

Hodgkinson CP, Hodari AA. Trocar suprapubic cystostomy for postoperative bladder drainage in the female. *Am J Obstet Gynecol* 1966;96:773.

Hoover JC, Ryan JP, Anderson EJ, et al. Nutritional benefits of immediate postoperative jejunal feeding of an elemental diet. *Am J Surg* 1980;139:153.

Huisman MV, Buller HR, Ten Cate JW, et al. Serial impedance plethysmography for suspected deep venous thrombosis in outpatients. The Amsterdam General Practitioner Study. *N Engl J Med* 1986;314:823.

Inada K, Koike S, Shirai N, et al. Effects of intermittent pneumatic leg compression for prevention of postoperative deep venous thrombosis with special reference to fibrinolytic activity. *Am J Surg* 1988;155:602.

Ireton-Jones CS, Turner WW Jr. The use of respiratory quotient to determine the efficacy of nutrition support regimens. *J Am Diet Assoc* 1987;87:180.

Jourdain B. Role of quantitative cultures of endotracheal aspirates in the diagnosis of nosocomial pneumonia. *Am J Respir Crit Care Med* 1995;152:241.

Kakkar W, Corrigan TP, Fossard DP. Prevention of postoperative pulmonary embolism by low dose heparin. *Lancet* 1975;2:45.

Khorana AA, Connolly GC. Assessing risk of VTE in patient with cancer. *J Clin Oncol* 2009;27:4839.

Knill RL. Control of breathing: effects of analgesic, anaesthetic and neuromuscular blocking drugs. *Can J Anaesth* 1988;35(3[Pt 2]):S4.

Kollef MH. Inadequate antimicrobial treatment: an important determinant of outcome for hospitalized patients. *Clin Infect Dis* 2000;31(suppl 4):S131.

Konrad F, Schreiber T, Grunert A, et al. Measurement of mucociliary transport velocity in ventilated patients: short-term effect of general anesthesia on mucociliary transport. *Chest* 1992;102:1377.

Kristo DA, Perry ME, Kollef MH. Comparison of venography, duplex imaging and bilateral impedance plethysmography for diagnosis of lower extremity deep vein thrombosis. *South Med J* 1994;87:55.

Laghi F, Tobin MJ. Disorders of the respiratory muscles. *Am J Respir Crit Care Med* 2003;168:10.

Langsfeld M, Hershey FB, Thorpe L, et al. Duplex B-mode imaging for the diagnosis of deep venous thrombosis. *Arch Surg* 1987;122:587.

Lawrence VA, Hilsenbeck SG, Mulrow CD, et al. Incidence and hospital stay for cardiac and pulmonary complications after abdominal surgery. *J Gen Intern Med* 1995;10:671.

Lawrence VA, Dhanda R, Hilsenbeck SG, et al. Risk of pulmonary complications after elective abdominal surgery. *Chest* 1996;110:744.

Lawrence VA, Cornell JE, Smetana GW. Strategies to reduce postoperative pulmonary complications after noncardiothoracic surgery: systematic review for the American College of Physicians. *Ann Intern Med* 2006;144:596.

Lazo-Langner A, Goss GD, Spaans JN, et al. The effect of low-molecular weight heparin on cancer survival: a systematic review and meta-analysis of randomized trials. *J Thromb Haemost* 2007;5:729.

Leiter LA, Marliss EB. Survival during fasting may depend on fat as well as protein stores. *JAMA* 1982;248:2306.

Lyman GH, Khorana AA, Falanga A, et al. American Society of Clinical Oncology guideline: recommendations for VTE prophylaxis and treatment in patients with cancer. *J Clin Oncol* 2007;25:5495.

Magnusson L, Spahn DR. New concepts of atelectasis during general anaesthesia. *Br J Anaesth* 2003;91:61.

Malhotra A. Intensive insulin in intensive care. *N Engl J Med* 2006;354:516.

McAlister FA, Bertsch K, Man J, et al. Incidence of and risk factors for pulmonary complications after nonthoracic surgery. *Am J Respir Crit Care Med* 2005;171:514.

McCarthy TG, McQueen J, Johnstone FD, et al. A comparison of low dose subcutaneous heparin and intravenous dextran 70 in the prophylaxis of deep venous thrombosis after gynaecological surgery. *J Obstet Gynaecol Br Commonw* 1974;81:486.

McMahon MM. Parenteral nutrition. In: Goldman L, Ausiello D, eds. *Cecil textbook of medicine*, 22nd ed. Philadelphia, PA: WB Saunders Company, 2004.

Mirtallo JM, Schneider PT, Mauko K, et al. A comparison of essential and general amino acid infusions in the nutritional support of patients with compromised renal function. *J Parenter Enteral Nutr* 1982;6:109.

Mittelman JS, Edwards WS, McDonald JB. Effectiveness of leg compression in preventing venous stasis. *Am J Surg* 1982;144:611.

Moller AM, Vilebro N, Pedersen T, et al. Effect of preoperative smoking intervention on postoperative complications: a randomised clinical trial. *Lancet* 2002;359:114.

Moore FD. Energy and the maintenance of the body cell mass. *J Parenter Enteral Nutr* 1980;4:228.

Moosman DA. The anatomy of infraclavicular subclavian vein catheterization and its complications. *Surg Gynecol Obstet* 1973;136:71.

Morgan G, Mikhail M, Murray M. *Clinical anesthesiology*, 4th ed. New York: McGraw-Hill, 2006:127.

Morlion BJ, Stehle P, Wachtler P, et al. Total parenteral nutrition with glutamine dipeptide after major abdominal surgery: a randomized, double-blind, controlled study. *Ann Surg* 1998;227:302.

Moudgil R, Michelakis ED, Archer SL. Hypoxic pulmonary vasoconstriction. *J Appl Physiol* 2005;98:390.

Nagendran J, Stewart K, Hoskinson M, et al. An anesthesiologist's guide to hypoxic pulmonary vasoconstriction: implications for managing single-lung anesthesia and atelectasis. *Curr Opin Anaesthesiol* 2006;19:34.

National Academy of Sciences. *Recommended Dietary Allowances*, 10th ed. Washington DC: National Academy Press, 1989.

Nchimi A. Incidence and distribution of lower extremity deep venous thrombosis at indirect computed tomography venography in patients suspected of pulmonary embolism. *Thromb Haemost* 2007;97:566.

Nelson R, Edwards S, Tse B. Prophylactic nasogastric decompression after abdominal surgery. *Cochrane Database Syst Rev* 2005; (1):CD004929.

Nicolaides AN, Fernandes IF, Pollock AV. Intermittent sequential compression of the legs in the prevention of venous stasis and postoperative deep venous thrombosis. *Surgery* 1980;87:69.

Nourdine K, Combes P, Carton MJ, et al. Does noninvasive ventilation reduce the ICU nosocomial infection risk? A prospective clinical survey. *Intensive Care Med* 1999;25:567.

Padberg FT, Ruggiero J, Blackburn GL, et al. Central venous catheterization for parenteral nutrition. *Ann Surg* 1981;193:264.

Pappachen S, Smith PR, Shah S, et al. Postoperative pulmonary complications after gynecologic surgery. *Int J Gynaecol Obstet* 2006;93:74.

Platell C, Hall JC. Atelectasis after abdominal surgery. *J Am Coll Surg* 1997;185:584.

Rayburn W, Wolk R, Mercer N, et al. Parenteral nutrition in obstetrics and gynecology. *Obstet Gynecol* 1986;41:200.

Reilly JJ, Gerhardt AL. Modern surgical nutrition. *Curr Probl Surg* 1985;22:1.

Richards MJ, Edwards JR, Culver DH, et al. Nosocomial infections in medical intensive care units in the United States. National Nosocomial Infections Surveillance System. *Crit Care Med* 1999;27:87.

Rombeau JL. Enteral nutrition. In: Goldman L, Ausiello D, eds. *Cecil textbook of medicine*, 22nd ed. Philadelphia, PA: WB Saunders Company, 2004.

Rose D, Yarborough MF, Canizaro PC, et al. One hundred and fourteen fistulas of the gastrointestinal tract treated with total parenteral nutrition. *Surg Gynecol Obstet* 1986;163:345.

Rucquoi M. Respiratory dead space and anesthesia. *Acta Anaesthesiol Belg* 1988;39(3 suppl 2):29.

Sadigh G, Kelly AM, Cronin P. Challenges, controversies and hot topics in PE Imaging. *Am J Roentgenol* 2011;196:497.

Sanders RA, Sheldon GF. Septic complications of total parenteral nutrition: a five year experience. *Am J Surg* 1976;132:214.

Sandstedt S, Lennmarken C, Symreng T, et al. The effect of preoperative total parenteral nutrition on energy-rich phosphates, electrolytes and free amino acids in skeletal muscle of malnourished patients with gastric carcinoma. *Br J Surg* 1985;72:920.

Sevitt S, Gallagher NG. Venous thrombosis and pulmonary embolism: a clinical pathological study in injured and burned patients. *Br J Surg* 1961;48:475.

Shils ME, Young VR, eds. *Modern nutrition in health and disease*, 7th ed. Philadelphia, PA: Lea & Febiger, 1988.

Shulman SM, Chuter T, Weissman C. Dynamic respiratory patterns after laparoscopic cholecystectomy. *Chest* 1993;103:1173.

Siafakas NM, Mitrouska I, Bouros D, et al. Surgery and the respiratory muscles. *Thorax* 1999;54:458.

Sigel B, Edelstein AL, Savitch L, et al. Type of compression for reducing venous stasis. A study of lower extremities during inactive recumbency. *Arch Surg* 1975;110:171.

Smeeta GW. Preoperative pulmonary evaluation. *N Engl J Med* 1999;340:937.

Stanton JR, Freis ED, Wilkins RW. Acceleration of linear flow in deep veins with local compression. *J Clin Invest* 1944;28:553.

Starker PM, Gump FE, Askanazi J, et al. Serum albumin levels as an index of nutritional support. *Surgery* 1982;91:194.

Starker PM, LaSala PA, Askanazi J, et al. The influence of preoperative total parenteral nutrition on morbidity and mortality. *Surg Gynecol Obstet* 1986;162:569.

Stella MH, Knuth SL, Bartlett D Jr. Respiratory response to mechanical stimulation of the gallbladder. *Respir Physiol Neurobiol* 2002;130:285.

Taberner DA, Poller L, Burslem RW, et al. Oral anticoagulants controlled by the British: comparative thromboplastin versus low-dose heparin in prophylaxis of deep vein thrombosis. *Br Med J* 1978;1:272.

Tablan OC, Anderson LJ, Besser R, et al. Guidelines for preventing health-care–associated pneumonia, 2003: recommendations of CDC and the Healthcare Infection Control Practices Advisory Committee. *MMWR Recomm Rep* 2004;53(RR-3):1.

The Multicenter Trial Committee. Dihydroergotamine-heparin prophylaxis of postoperative deep vein thrombosis: a multicenter trial. *JAMA* 1984;251:2960.

Thompson DA, Makary MA, Dorman T, et al. Clinical and economic outcomes of hospital acquired pneumonia in intra-abdominal surgery patients. *Ann Surg* 2006;243:547.

Tobin WR, Kaiser HE, Groeger AM, et al. The effects of volatile anesthetic agents on pulmonary surfactant function. *In Vivo* 2000;14:157.

Tomkowski WZ, Davidson BL, Wisniewska J, et al. Accuracy of compression ultrasound in screening for deep venous thrombosis in acutely ill medical patients. *Thromb Haemost* 2007;97:191.

Torosian MH, Daly JM. Nutritional support in the cancer-bearing host: effects on host and tumor. *Cancer* 1986;58(suppl 8):1915.

Tracey KJ, Legaspi A, Albert JD, et al. Protein and substrate metabolism during starvation and parenteral refeeding. *Clin Sci* 1988;74:123.

Trousseau A. *Phlegmasia alba dolens: clinique medicale de l'Hotel Dieu de Paris*, vol. 3. London, UK: New Sydenham Society, 1868:695.

Vaccaro P, Van Aman M, Miller S, et al. Shortcomings of physical examination and impedance plethysmography in the diagnosis of lower extremity deep venous thrombosis. *Angiology* 1987;38:232.

van den Berghe G, Wouters P, Weekers F, et al. Intensive insulin therapy in the critically ill patients. *N Engl J Med* 2001;345:1359.

Vamvakas EC, Blajchman MA. Deleterious clinical effects of transfusion-associated immunomodulation: fact or fiction? *Blood* 2001;97:1180.

Vassilakopoulos T, Mastora Z, Katsaounou P, et al. Contribution of pain to inspiratory muscle dysfunction after upper abdominal surgery: a randomized controlled trial. *Am J Respir Crit Care Med* 2000;61(4[Pt 1]):1372.

Vernet O, Christin L, Schutz Y, et al. Enteral versus parenteral nutrition: comparison of energy metabolism in lean and moderately obese women. *Am J Clin Nutr* 1986;43:194.

Villanueva C, Colomo A, Bosch A, et al. Transfusion strategies for acute upper gastrointestinal bleeding. *N Engl J Med* 2013;368:11.

Vinton NE, Laidlaw SA, Ament ME, et al. Taurine concentrations in plasma and blood cells of patients undergoing long-term parenteral nutrition. *Am J Clin Nutr* 1986;44:398.

Virchow R. *Handbuch der speciellen Pathologie und Therapie*, vol. II. Erlangen and Stuttgart, Germany: F Enke, 1854.

Walder B, Schafer M, Henzi I, et al. Efficacy and safety of patient-controlled opioid analgesia for acute postoperative pain: a quantitative systematic review. *Acta Anaesthesiol Scand* 2001;45(7):795.

Wells PS, Brill-Edwards P, Stevens P, et al. A novel and rapid whole-blood assay for D-dimer in patients with clinically suspected deep vein thrombosis. *Circulation* 1995;91:2184.

Wells PS, Anderson DR, Rogers M, et al. Derivation of a simple clinical model to categorize patient probability of PE with D dimer assay. *Thromb Haemost* 2000;83:416.

Wilson JT, Rogers FB, Wald SL, et al. Prophylactic vena cava filter insertion in patients with traumatic spinal cord injury: preliminary results. *Neurosurgery* 1994;35:234.

Young GP, Thomas RJ, Bourne DW, et al. Parenteral nutrition. *Med J Aust* 1985;143:597.

CHAPTER 10
Water, Electrolyte, and Acid–Base Metabolism

Jack B. Basil and Devin D. Namaky

DEFINITIONS

Anion gap—The anion gap is the difference between the measured cations and anions in serum, plasma, or urine. For serum, it is estimated by subtracting the sum of the chloride and bicarbonate anions from the sodium cations and is usually expressed in mmol/L or mEq/L:

$$\left[Na^+\right] - \left(\left[Cl^-\right] + \left[HCO_3^-\right]\right)$$

Bowman space—This is the capsular-shaped space that surrounds the glomerulus at the beginning of the tubular nephron in the kidney. It receives the initial glomerular filtrate.

Effective intravascular volume—This is the proportion of the intravascular volume that is effective in determining the filling pressure of the ventricles and is usually directly related to the central venous pressure. This may not always correlate with the *actual* intravascular volume.

Extracellular fluid—The body fluid that exists outside of cells. It contains approximately one third of the volume of total body water.

Fractional excretion of sodium—This is the amount of sodium excreted in the urine, expressed as a percentage of the sodium that is filtered by the kidney:

$$\%E/F_{Na} = 100 \left\{ \left(\left[Na^+\right]_{Urine} \left[Cr\right]_{Serum}\right) / \left(\left[Na^+\right]_{Serum} \left[Cr\right]_{Urine}\right) \right\}$$

where $[Na^+]_{Urine}$ is the concentration of sodium in the urine. $[Na^+]_{Serum}$ is the concentration of sodium in the serum, $[Cr]_{Serum}$ is the concentration of creatinine in the serum, and $[Cr]_{Urine}$ is the concentration of creatinine in the urine.

Henderson-Hasselbalch—An equation for calculating the pH of an acid or buffered solution. A modification of this equation may be used to calculate the pH of blood as follows:

$$pH = pK_{a\,H_2CO_3} + \log\left\{\left[HCO_3^-\right]/\left[k_{HCO_2}\left(PCO_2\right)\right]\right\}$$

where $pK_{a\,H_2CO_3} = 6.1$, $\left[HCO_3^-\right]$ = concentration of bicarbonate in the blood, $k_{H\,CO_2} = 0.03$ mmol/mm Hg.

Intracellular fluid—The body fluid that exists inside of cells. It contains approximately two thirds of the volume of total body water.

Intravascular volume—This is the same as blood volume and includes intravascular water, as well as plasma, plasma proteins, and other blood products such as red cells.

Metabolic acidosis—Acidosis resulting from increase in acids other than carbonic acid or resulting from the inability of the body to form bicarbonate in the kidney.

Metabolic alkalosis—Alkalosis in which plasma bicarbonate is increased directly, or indirectly as a result of decreased hydrogen ion concentration.

Oncotic pressure—The osmotic pressure exerted by proteins in solution, usually pulling water into the intravascular space. This is also commonly called the *colloid osmotic pressure*.

Orthostatic hypotension—A decrease in perfusion that is caused by a change from a supine to a standing position. This is generally diagnosed by a decrease in systolic blood pressure of more than 20 mm Hg, or a decrease in diastolic blood pressure of more than 10 mm Hg, and is further suggested by a pulse increase of more than 30 bpm.

Osmotic pressure—The pressure that is needed to prevent water flow between two solutions of different concentrations that are separated by a semipermeable membrane.

Plasma osmolality—The measure of solute per kilogram of plasma. For the purposes of this chapter, this is used interchangeably with plasma *osmolarity*, which is the measure of solute per *liter* of plasma. This can be estimated for normal plasma:

$$P_{OSM} = 2\left[Na^+\right] + \left[glucose\right] + \left[urea\right]$$

Respiratory acidosis—Acidosis secondary to decreased ventilation, usually with a proportionate increase in plasma carbon dioxide.

Respiratory alkalosis—Alkalosis secondary to increased ventilation, usually with a proportionate decrease in plasma carbon dioxide.

Specific gravity—This is the ratio of the density of a substance to the density of water. Under most conditions encountered, this is equal to the *apparent* specific gravity, which is the ratio of the weight of a substance to the weight of an equal volume of water.

Proper management of fluids and electrolytes in the gynecologic surgical patient is of extreme importance. Gynecologic surgical patients can differ in age, baseline nutritional status, and in the complexity of medical problems that they possess. The stresses of surgery and the bodies' complex responses to that stress need to be understood to best care for these patients. The tendency to standardize postoperative care for all patients should be avoided.

This chapter focuses on the clinical aspects of water and electrolyte balance, and an understanding of basic renal physiology is a prerequisite.

CLINICAL ASSESSMENT OF DISORDERS OF WATER AND ELECTROLYTE METABOLISM

Disorders of extracellular fluid (ECF) electrolyte composition may be detected by measurement of the serum electrolyte concentrations. Identification of the process (or processes) behind the disturbance of electrolyte composition and the planning of subsequent therapy are critically dependent on the clinician's ability to accurately assess whether the disturbance in ECF electrolyte composition is associated with volume expansion, volume contraction, or a normal volume.

In the evaluation of a patient's ECF volume status, it must be kept clearly in mind that the critical volume that is effective in determining cardiac output is the effective intravascular volume (IVV). The most effective IVV is that which maintains an optimal cardiac output and thus maximizes tissue perfusion. Although the actual IVV and the effective IVV are the same in many clinical situations and can be expected to change in direct proportion, in a number of important clinical states, the actual IVV is different from the effective IVV. For example, in acute metabolic acidosis, increased venoconstriction can develop, resulting in an abnormal increase in central venous pressure (CVP) and cardiac output. Under this circumstance, the actual IVV could be less than normal, whereas the effective IVV is greater than normal. Because of the increase in venous tone, an IVV that is lower than normal can maintain a normal effective IVV.

Acute changes in venous tone induced by drugs (e.g., morphine, furosemide, norepinephrine), changes in acid–base status, and the presence of bacterial endotoxin also can disrupt the normal relation between the actual IVV and the effective IVV.

The most reliable clinical means for assessing the status of the effective IVV is the pulmonary capillary wedge pressure. This measurement is an estimate of the pulmonary capillary pressure, which is a measure of the filling pressure of the left ventricle. Factors that increase pulmonary capillary wedge pressure tend to increase cardiac output by increasing capillary outflux. When effective IVV is considered within these constraints, it becomes clear that under virtually any physiologic or pathophysiologic circumstance, an optimal effective IVV is one that results in a pulmonary capillary wedge pressure that is high enough to promote optimal cardiac output but low enough to prevent pulmonary edema.

Fortunately, in most clinical situations, it is not necessary to resort to measuring pulmonary wedge pressure to assess whether a disturbance of ECF composition is associated with an effective IVV that is abnormally high, abnormally low, or normal. Instead, an accurate assessment of the effective IVV usually can be made by a careful clinical assessment using the criteria listed in Table 10.1. This table lists the bedside and laboratory means to assess volume status according to whether the findings are consistent with an effective IVV that is less than normal or an effective IVV that is nearly normal or expanded.

Also shown in Table 10.1 are the conditions under which the given means for evaluating the IVV must be qualified (i.e., the conditions that may render the meaning of the finding indeterminate with respect to the evaluation of IVV). For example, the relation between an increase in weight and a change in IVV is rendered indeterminate if, at the same time, the patient has developed a third space, as in bowel obstruction. In this instance, the entire weight gain could be caused by the accumulation of fluid outside the IVV. Thus, the finding of weight gain in this setting cannot be used as evidence of an increase in effective IVV. Whenever a finding can be significantly qualified,

TABLE 10.1 Assessment of Effective Intravascular Volume

SUGGESTIVE EVIDENCE	QUALIFYING CONDITIONS[a]
Significantly decreased effective IVV	
History of fluid and electrolyte deprivation or loss (e.g., vomiting, diarrhea)	Difficulty in establishing by history whether the magnitude of loss or deprivation is sufficient to result in negative balance of water and electrolytes
Decrease in body weight below normal not explained by inadequate caloric intake	None
Blood pressure less than usual for the patient with orthostatic hypotension	1. The patient receiving methyldopa (Aldomet), prazosin (Minipress), minoxidil (Loniten), or other drugs that interfere with vascular α-receptors 2. Autonomic insufficiency as in diabetics, quadriplegics, and after prolonged bed rest
Elevated serum creatinine associated with concentrated urine ($U_{osm}/P_{osm} > 1.5$) and Na^+ conservation: ($U_{Na} < 20$ mEq/L) or $\%E/F_{Na} < 1\%$	Decreased renal perfusion owing to (a) severe hepatic failure (hepatorenal syndrome) and (b) severe cardiac failure. Acute, high-grade urinary tract obstruction (see text)
Low CVP or pulmonary capillary wedge pressure	See text
Decreased tissue turgor	See text
Hematocrit above normal	Presence of conditions that may cause erythrocytosis
Nearly normal or expanded effective IVV (i.e., absence of significant intravascular volume depletion)	
Hypertension with the patient in sitting or standing position and no orthostatic fall in blood pressure	None
Presence of cardiac failure: left ventricular failure: audible third heart sound or pulmonary edema	Patients with markedly reduced cardiac output and very large left ventricles may have decreased effective IVV despite an audible third heart sound
Right ventricular failure: peripheral edema with increased venous pressure (neck vein distention, increased intravenous pressure)	Right ventricular failure but normal left ventricular function (see text)
Increase in weight above normal not explained by increased caloric intake	1. Significant hypoalbuminemia 2. Development of third spaces (e.g., ascites, bowel obstruction)
Increased CVP	See text
Increased pulmonary capillary wedge pressure	See text
Edema, ascites, or pleural effusion	See text
Hematocrit less than normal	Presence of conditions that can cause loss, destruction, or decreased production of red blood cells

[a]Qualifying conditions are circumstances that can render the meaning of the finding indeterminate with respect to the evaluation of the effective IVV.
$\%E/F_{Na}$, percentage of excretion of filtered sodium (see text).

it should not be used in the assessment of the effective IVV. As many independent means as practical should be used to assess the effective IVV to minimize the effect of possible error on the final decision. The greater the number of independent, unqualified findings that agree in favor of a given clinical decision, the more likely it is that the decision is correct. If such a systematic approach to clinical decision making is used, it should be possible to arrive at an accurate evaluation of volume status in most circumstances.

DATABASE FOR ASSESSMENT OF EFFECTIVE INTRAVASCULAR VOLUME

Body Weight

All patients should be weighed on admission to the hospital and then periodically during their hospital stay. In patients undergoing surgery, or in whom problems in fluid and electrolyte balance are anticipated, weight must be measured daily.

Alterations in body weight are the result of changes in body water content plus solid tissue content (fat, protein, bone). Gains or losses of solid tissue are almost always related to changes in caloric intake and seldom exceed 0.25 kg/24 hours. For example, a patient who takes no calories for 24 hours is forced to consume her endogenous stores of fat and protein to meet the energy requirements for continued life. The complete oxidation of fat yields 9 cal/g, and protein yields 4 cal/g. It can be readily calculated that the complete oxidation of 0.25 kg of solid tissue (in starvation, a mixture of about 87% fat, 13% protein) yields enough calories to meet basal daily energy needs. Thus, changes in weight exceeding 0.25 kg/24 hours are almost always attributable to changes in water balance. Although the relation between body weight and effective IVV can be variable, usually the relation between changes in body weight and IVV can be correctly assessed by the application of the guidelines. The first is that a decrease in body weight below normal (for the patient), and not explained on the basis of inadequate caloric intake, can be assumed to be accompanied by a decrease in IVV. The second is that an increase in body weight above normal not explained by increased nutrition can be assumed to be accompanied by an increase in IVV except when the weight gain develops in association with the following conditions:

- Significant hypoalbuminemia: serum albumin less than 2.5 g/dL
- Venous obstruction or congestion
- Development of third spaces (e.g., obstructed or ischemic bowel)

Under these three general conditions, an increase in body weight may not reflect an increase in the effective IVV.

Renal Function

Creatinine, a by-product of muscle energy metabolism, is produced at a constant rate that is related to muscle mass. Nearly all of the creatinine produced is excreted by glomerular filtration. Therefore, changes in the concentration of serum creatinine reflect changes in the glomerular filtration rate (GFR), and the clearance of creatinine is an index of the GFR.

Normally, as muscle mass increases, the GFR increases proportionally less. Therefore, on the average, children have lower serum creatinine values than do adults, and large adults have higher serum creatinine levels than do small adults. Because of these considerations, a single range of serum creatinine values cannot be applied to everyone.

The following guidelines are suggested for the evaluation of the IVV in light of the state of renal function. Azotemia can be assumed to result from decreased renal perfusion if the serum creatinine level is elevated, the urine is concentrated (specific gravity higher than 1.015), and renal sodium conservation is present (urine sodium level <20 mEq/L) on a random and untimed urine sample. If the fractional excretion of sodium is below 1%, azotemia can be attributed to decreased IVV, unless the patient has severe liver or cardiac disease causing end-organ hypoperfusion. If severe cardiac failure and severe liver failure (hepatorenal syndrome) can be excluded, the decreased renal perfusion can be assumed to be caused by a decreased effective IVV.

Edema, Ascites, and Pleural Effusion

Effective IVV is increased when edema, pleural effusion, or ascites occurs in the setting of congestive heart failure (CHF). Increased effective IVV cannot be assumed in the presence of edema, ascites, or pleural effusion if there is significant hypoalbuminemia or venous obstruction or if the accumulation of fluid is in a relatively small area of capillary injury (e.g., pleural effusion caused by pulmonary infarction).

Tissue Turgor

Tissue turgor is a function of the elasticity of the solid components of tissue and the degree of distention of the tissues by interstitial fluid. If tissue is depleted of interstitial fluid, it becomes less elastic (i.e., it less readily returns to its original shape after being deformed). Skin turgor is best assessed on the forehead and anterior chest. In patients less than 50 years of age, the turgor of the dorsum of the hand also can be used. In older patients, the elasticity of the solid components of tissue is decreased, and the turgor of the skin becomes unreliable in interpreting changes in interstitial volume.

Central Venous Pressure

The measurement of CVP is a relatively simple but useful means for monitoring cardiac function and cardiovascular status. For the valid measurement of CVP, the catheter must be placed in the large intrathoracic veins near the right atrium (as assessed by chest radiograph), and the catheter must be patent (as assessed by the cyclic variation of CVP with ventilatory movements: decreased CVP during inspiration, increased CVP during expiration).

In normal adults, CVP is about 5 to 12 cm H_2O. CVPs below 3 cm H_2O are commonly seen in children and young adults who have no evidence of a decreased effective IVV. In older adults and elderly persons, CVP of less than 3 cm H_2O can be assumed to reflect a significant decrease in effective IVV.

Central venous pressure is an index of the filling pressure of the right atrium, which, in turn, is an index of the filling pressure of the right ventricle. In uncomplicated circumstances, expansion of the IVV results in increased CVP, whereas contraction of the IVV results in decreased CVP. Central venous pressure cannot be used to assess the adequacy of left ventricular function in patients in whom left ventricular function may be impaired relative to right ventricular function. Central venous pressure also is unreliable when lung disease is present, because it is commonly falsely elevated. In such patients, left ventricular function can be monitored by observing for signs and symptoms of left ventricular failure (dyspnea, development of an audible third heart sound, or pulmonary edema), or by direct measurement of pulmonary capillary wedge pressure. Under normal circumstances, the pulmonary capillary wedge pressure is about equal to the CVP plus 6 mm Hg.

Pulmonary Capillary Wedge Pressure

Technical refinements of the Swan-Ganz catheter make it possible to measure pulmonary artery systolic and diastolic pressure, CVP, pulmonary wedge pressure, and cardiac output using the thermodilution technique with the same catheter. This permits a definitive assessment of the volume status of the patient, because it can be determined whether the cardiac output is appropriate for a given pulmonary wedge pressure. Specific guidelines for the interpretation of the relation between pulmonary wedge pressure and cardiac output are discussed in the following sections.

Patients with Normal Volume Status

Pulmonary wedge pressure can be expected to be between 8 and 12 mm Hg in a patient with a normal cardiopulmonary system and a normal effective IVV. Cardiac output is normal. Pulmonary wedge pressure can be less than 8 mm Hg without indicating volume contraction; in this circumstance, the cardiac output is normal despite the unusually low pulmonary wedge pressure.

Patients Who Are Volume Contracted

Patients who have a normal cardiopulmonary system but who are significantly volume depleted usually have a pulmonary wedge pressure below 8 mm Hg and their cardiac output is less than normal. In patients with chronic pulmonary hypertension (e.g., those with chronic left ventricular failure), a higher than normal pulmonary wedge pressure is needed to drive a satisfactory cardiac output. Thus, in such patients, pulmonary wedge pressure can be above the normal range but be inappropriately low for the patient. This situation can be identified by showing that: (a) cardiac output is less than normal, despite the elevated pulmonary wedge pressure; (b) volume infusion causes an increase in cardiac output toward a more favorable range; and (c) despite further increase in pulmonary wedge pressure with volume expansion, pulmonary function does not deteriorate. (PaO_2 does not decrease, $PaCO_2$ does not increase, and pulmonary compliance does not worsen.)

Patients Who Are Volume Expanded

In patients with a normal cardiopulmonary system, pulmonary wedge pressure usually is above 18 mm Hg when volume expansion is substantial. Cardiac output is above normal. If cardiac function is impaired, cardiac output will be inappropriately low for the level of pulmonary wedge pressure.

When a given pulmonary wedge pressure is being interpreted, the serum albumin level also should be taken into consideration, because this opposes the effect of capillary hydrostatic pressure to cause migration of fluid from the capillary lumen to the interstitial space. Thus, at any given elevated pulmonary wedge pressure, pulmonary edema develops more rapidly in a patient who is hypoalbuminemic than in one who has a normal serum albumin concentration. In some patients, it is not possible to obtain a reliable pulmonary wedge pressure. In most of these patients, the pulmonary artery diastolic pressure is a good estimate of the pulmonary wedge pressure. If pulmonary hypertension is present, then pulmonary vascular resistance is increased; thus, pulmonary artery diastolic pressure may not be a good index of the pulmonary wedge pressure. In such patients, it is important to be able to obtain a wedge pressure. Finally, in patients who are being ventilated with high levels of positive end-expiratory pressure, pulmonary wedge pressure may become an unreliable index of left atrial filling pressure because the high intrapulmonary pressures may cause obstruction of the catheter orifice. Patients must be briefly taken off the ventilator for accurate measurements. Other circumstances in which pulmonary artery wedge pressure measurements may be inaccurate include the presence of mitral stenosis or pulmonary venous obstruction.

Blood Pressure

The following guidelines are suggested for the evaluation of the effective IVV from measurement of blood pressure.

1. A nearly normal or expanded effective IVV can be assumed in patients with hypertension that is demonstrated in the sitting or standing position.
2. Effective IVV may be decreased in patients who previously were hypertensive but who have become normotensive.
3. Effective IVV may be decreased in patients who develop orthostatic hypotension (a drop in systolic pressure greater than 10 mm Hg in changing from the supine to the sitting or standing position).

Orthostatic hypotension also can be present, in the absence of volume contraction, as a result of prolonged bed rest, during the use of such antihypertensive agents as methyldopa (Aldomet) or of vasodilators (prazosin, minoxidil). If the pulse rate does not rise as blood pressure falls when a patient stands, autonomic neuropathy should be considered as a cause of postural hypotension.

Systemic Vascular Resistance

Normal values are 50 to 150 dyne-s/cm for pulmonary vascular resistance and 800 to 1,200 dyne-s/cm for systemic vascular resistance. Pulmonary vascular resistance is elevated in hypovolemic shock, cardiogenic shock, pulmonary embolism, or airway obstruction; it is diminished in septic shock. Systemic vascular resistance is elevated in hypovolemic shock, cardiogenic shock, pulmonary embolism, and sometimes in right ventricular infarct and cardiac tamponade; it is decreased in end-stage liver disease and septic shock.

CLINICAL ASSESSMENT OF DISORDERS OF EXTRACELLULAR FLUID COMPOSITION

Hyponatremia

The schema for the evaluation of a hyponatremic patient depends on the assessment of volume status. That is, it must first be determined whether the patient's hyponatremia is associated with an effective IVV that is decreased, normal, or increased. Once this is decided on the basis of the assessment of IVV, a further separation, based only on the state of renal sodium and water excretion, is made. Each of the final categories contains relatively few diagnostic possibilities, and the presence or absence of each of these conditions in a given patient usually can be readily determined. The scheme for the evaluation of a hypernatremic patient is analogous, except that it depends on the assessment of the state of renal water excretion.

Clinical Assessment

In the discussion that follows, only patients with true hyponatremia are considered (i.e., hyponatremia in which serum osmolality is decreased in proportion to the reduction in serum sodium concentration, after appropriate correction for any elevation in the plasma urea nitrogen). By making this distinction, hyponatremia caused by accumulation of ECF solutes such as glucose or mannitol can be excluded. In this type of hyponatremia, the decreased concentration of ECF sodium is the result of the shift of water from cells to the ECF in response to the osmotic gradient caused by the accumulation of the solute. As a consequence, the hyponatremia is associated with an increased plasma osmolality. These patients also can be readily identified either by the presence of hyperglycemia sufficient to explain the decrease in serum sodium concentration or by a history of administration of large amounts of mannitol (0.100 g in adults), usually in the presence of a decreased capacity to excrete mannitol (decreased GFR).

Also to be excluded are patients with spurious hyponatremia that results from the abnormal accumulation of plasma lipids or proteins. In such circumstances, the concentration of sodium in plasma water is normal; however, the concentration of sodium expressed per liter of whole plasma is reduced because an abnormally large volume of whole plasma is occupied by the lipids or proteins, which do not contain plasma water and electrolytes. Thus, when aliquots of hyperlipemic or hyperproteinemic plasma are analyzed, a lower amount of sodium is determined to be present in a given volume of whole plasma. Plasma osmolality, however, is normal because lipids and proteins do not contribute importantly to plasma osmolality (see section on osmotic forces). Patients with spurious hyponatremia can be readily identified by the presence of markedly elevated total serum protein levels (e.g., multiple myeloma) or grossly lipemic serum. The distinction can be readily made if lipemic serum is subjected to centrifugation and the lipoprotein layer is removed before evaluation, if flame photometry is being used for measurement of serum Na^+. Spurious hyponatremia is no longer a consideration in most laboratories, because serum Na^+ concentration is determined by ion-specific electrodes, and increased levels are not affected by lipemic serum. Symptoms of hyponatremia include increased tendon reflexes, lethargy, mental confusion, and muscle twitching, which are followed by convulsions, coma, and possibly death if levels fall below 115 mEq/L.

Hyponatremia and Volume Depletion Associated with Renal Sodium Wasting

The normal renal response to volume depletion and hyponatremia is the virtual elimination of sodium from the urine

(Fig. 10.1; see section on sodium balance). Thus, the presence of an excessive amount of urinary sodium under these conditions indicates that renal sodium loss is the cause or a major contributing factor to the state of sodium depletion. A spot urine sodium concentration greater than 40 mEq/L, a %E/F^{Na} above 1%, or a urinary sodium excretion rate greater than intake indicates such renal sodium wasting. The conditions discussed in the following sections are associated with hyponatremia, IVV depletion, and renal sodium wasting.

Chronic Renal Disease All types of renal disease can be associated with renal salt wasting. In adults with such a disorder, the serum creatinine level is virtually always above 2 mg and usually much higher before a significant salt leak develops. These azotemic patients usually require 85 to 170 mEq of sodium daily (5 to 10 g of sodium chloride) to maintain salt balance at a normal effective IVV. Thus, if sodium intake is decreased in azotemic patients by anorexia or vomiting, or if additional sodium losses occur (e.g., diarrhea or diuretic therapy), the inability of the diseased kidneys to conserve sodium and water normally may rapidly lead to the development of significant sodium and water deficits. Water intake usually continues; therefore, sodium balance is more adversely affected than is water balance. As a consequence, the patient becomes volume contracted with hyponatremia. With the onset of CHF or the nephrotic syndrome, the salt leak of chronic renal failure usually disappears, and salt intake must be restricted.

Diuretic Therapy The diuretics include thiazide agents or loop diuretics, such as furosemide, bumetanide, and ethacrynic acid. Diuretics induce a renal salt–wasting state, and if the urinary output of sodium exceeds intake, sodium depletion ensues. Rarely, diuretics cause hyponatremia without evidence of volume depletion if severe potassium depletion has resulted from their use (Fig. 10.1).

Adrenal Insufficiency (Addison Disease) Destruction of the adrenal gland or sudden withdrawal of chronic, daily glucocorticoid therapy results in inadequate adrenal function. The lack of mineralocorticoid causes wasting of renal salt but retention of renal potassium and leads to sodium depletion. The lack of glucocorticoid results in a decreased capacity to excrete a water load and leads to hyponatremia but not to volume depletion or hyperkalemia.

Hyponatremia and Volume Depletion Associated with Renal Sodium Conservation

A spot urine sodium concentration of less than 20 mEq/L or a %E/F$_{Na}$ below 1% in a hyponatremic, volume-contracted patient is evidence of normal renal sodium conservation and indicates that the cause of the sodium depletion is nonrenal in origin or that it occurred during previous diuretic therapy. The fact that the serum sodium concentration is lower than normal indicates that water balance is less negative than is sodium

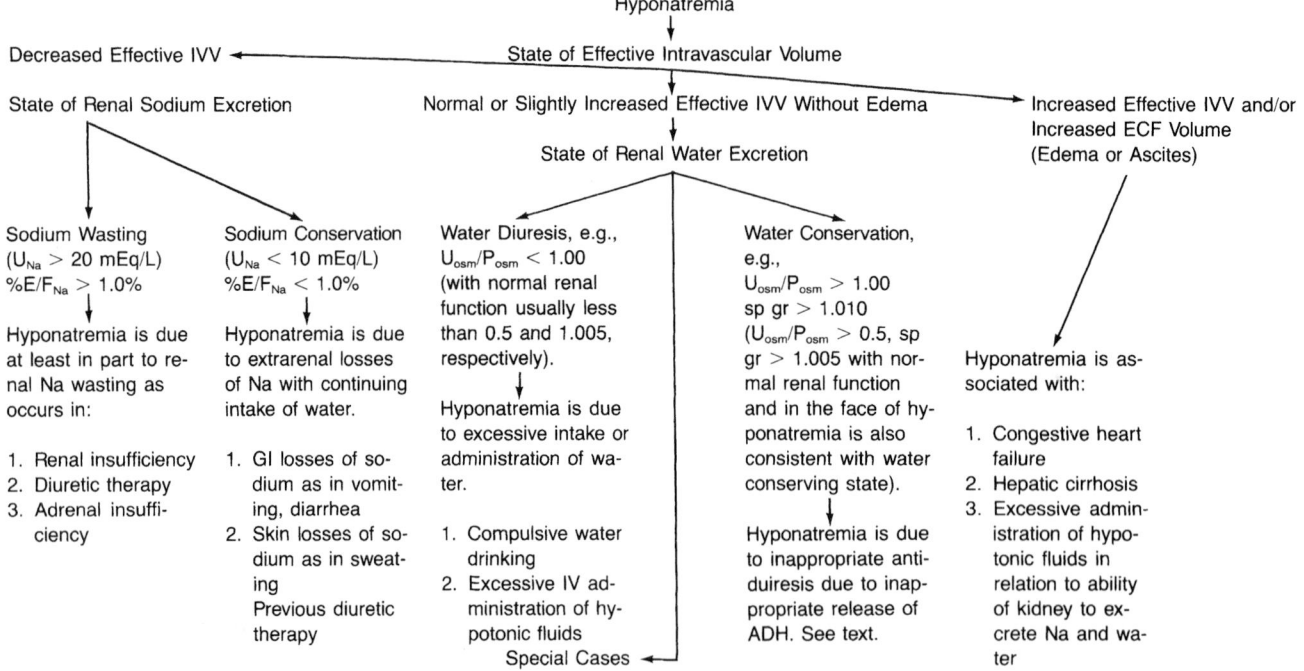

(Hyponatremia with essentially normal effective IVV but water diuresis occurs with water loading, and water conservation occurs with water restriction.)

1. Severe K$^+$ depletion associated with diuretic therapy. Identifying features: history of diuretic administration, presence of hypokalemic metabolic alkalosis.
2. Resetting of "osmostat." Probably a rare complication of chronic disease. See text.
3. Polydipsic vomiting. Identifying features: protracted vomiting but continued large oral intake of water, metabolic alkalosis.

FIGURE 10.1 Approach to the assessment of a hyponatremic patient. This approach considers only patients with true hyponatremia (i.e., in nonazotemic patients, serum osmolality is reduced in proportion to the decrease in serum sodium). Thus, patients are excluded who have lowered concentrations of serum sodium because of hyperlipidemia, hyperproteinemia, or the abnormal accumulations of solutes in the extracellular fluid (ECF), such as glucose or mannitol. ADH, antidiuretic hormone; ECT, extracellular fluid; %E/F$_{Na}$, fractional excretion of sodium; GI, gastrointestinal; IVV, intravascular volume.

balance. The conditions discussed in the following sections can result in volume depletion and hyponatremia as a result of extrarenal losses of sodium.

Gastrointestinal Losses If losses of fluid from the upper gastrointestinal tract (e.g., vomiting, gastric aspiration) cause the hyponatremia, and if the gastric juice is normally acid, metabolic alkalosis is present. If diarrheal losses cause the hyponatremia, metabolic acidosis may be present. In patients with gastric achlorhydria, upper gastrointestinal losses also can lead to metabolic acidosis.

Losses of Sodium from the Skin Sweat contains about 50 mEq/L of sodium and is a hypotonic fluid. If sweat losses are not replaced, then hypernatremia can develop. In most situations, the water losses from the skin are replaced more adequately than are the sodium losses. Thus, most patients with significant sodium losses that are due to sweating become hyponatremic. Skin losses of fluid and electrolytes also can occur after burns or other skin injuries. These are isotonic losses of sodium and lead to hyponatremia if the water losses are more adequately replaced than are the sodium losses.

Losses of Sodium from Prior Diuretic Therapy The natriuretic action of most diuretics lasts less than 24 hours. Hyponatremia is made worse if water intake is excessive.

Hyponatremia and Normal Volume Status Associated with Water Diuresis

In a patient with normal renal function who has become hyponatremic as a result of the administration or ingestion of excessive amounts of water, intravascular and ECF volume are normal to slightly expanded, and high rates of urine flow in association with maximally, or nearly maximally, dilute urine can be expected. In a patient with preexisting renal functional impairment, water loading also increases urine flow rate and dilution of the urine; however, maximally dilute urine cannot be formed. Hyponatremia secondary to water loading may occur in compulsive water drinkers, who usually are severely neurotic or psychotic, or after excessive IV administration of hypotonic fluids. Many of these patients also have high levels of antidiuretic hormone (ADH) for various reasons (e.g., drugs, psychosis). Without this elevation of ADH, presuming normal renal function, consumption of 20 L of water a day would be necessary for development of frank hyponatremia.

Hyponatremia and Normal to Slightly Elevated Volume Status Associated with Water Conservation

As discussed, it is appropriate to observe a brisk water diuresis in a patient with normal renal function who is hyponatremic and has evidence of normal or slightly elevated IVV without edema. When high flow rates of hypotonic urine are not observed, the patient is exhibiting an inappropriate antidiuresis. This may result from the inappropriate release of ADH, although other mechanisms also can be involved (e.g., decreased renal blood flow, certain drugs). Another characteristic of such patients is that administered sodium is promptly excreted in the urine, perhaps because of the effect of atrial natriuretic factors. On the other hand, when sodium intake is curtailed, renal sodium conservation is observed. These patients also exhibit normal adrenal and renal function and are not edematous. The syndrome of inappropriate antidiuresis has been associated with various clinical states, including malignant tumors (e.g., in the lung or pancreas), central nervous system (CNS) disorders (e.g., head trauma, meningitis),

infections (e.g., tuberculosis, bacterial pneumonias), the postoperative state, hypopituitarism, and myxedema, as well as with many drugs (Table 10.2). Infusion of oxytocin to induce uterine contraction also can cause hyponatremia because of the antidiuretic effects of oxytocin.

Within the category of hyponatremia associated with normal IVV are three special categories. The feature that sets these apart is that patients may exhibit evidence of water conservation when water is withdrawn or an appropriate or nearly appropriate water diuresis when water is administered. That is, it appears that osmoregulation has been reset to "defend" a lowered plasma osmolality. The first special category includes patients who have an unusual response to diuretic therapy, characterized by hyponatremia, severe potassium depletion, and metabolic alkalosis. Despite the hyponatremia and normal IVV, exchangeable sodium is nearly normal, suggesting intracellular movement of sodium. Magnesium levels should be assessed, and potassium replacement must be accomplished before specific treatment of hyponatremia. The second category involves patients with an unusual manifestation of a chronic illness, such as pulmonary tuberculosis, that resets the osmostat. The third category includes patients with sodium depletion resulting from any cause in whom the decrease in effective IVV is minimized by excessive water intake and retention. This effect of excessive water intake can occur in any of the causes of sodium depletion.

Hyponatremia Associated with Increased Effective Intravascular Volume or Increased Extracellular Fluid Volume (Edema or Ascites)

Congestive Heart Failure When hyponatremia develops spontaneously in the course of chronic CHF (i.e., is not the result of excessive water administration or diuretic therapy), it usually is indicative of severe cardiac insufficiency and has a poor prognosis. The cause of the hyponatremia in such patients has been ascribed to a decreased capacity to increase renal free water clearance perhaps because of (a) increased fractional reabsorption of glomerular filtrate proximal to the renal diluting sites of the distal nephron and (b) an elevated ADH level.

Cirrhosis of the Liver Patients with cirrhosis and ascites have a decreased capacity to excrete a water load, possibly because of the same mechanisms at work in patients with CHF.

Excessive Administration of Hypotonic Fluids This usually is an iatrogenic situation and must be especially guarded against

---

TABLE 10.2 Antidiuretic Drugs

Sulfonylureas (chlorpropamide, tolbutamide)
Cytotoxic agents (vincristine, cyclophosphamide)
Nicotine
Morphine
Barbiturates
Carbamazepine
Psychotropics (tricyclics)
Clofibrate
Isoproterenol
Nonsteroidals
Salicylates
Acetaminophen
Vasopressin
Oxytocin

in postoperative patients whose ADH levels are elevated because of stress, pain, hypovolemia, or drugs, as well as in elderly patients who are unable to maximally dilute their urine.

Hypernatremia

All patients with hypernatremia are volume contracted, except those in whom the disorder develops as a result of excessive administration of hypertonic saline or sodium bicarbonate and the rare patients with essential hypernatremia (Fig. 10.2). The following discussion considers only the first group of patients; the latter section on treatment discusses all forms of hypernatremia. Patients with hypernatremia usually have CNS deficits, and they may also have confusion and neuroseizures. Autopsy findings often reveal hemorrhages or thromboses of brain tissue.

Hypernatremia Associated with Formation of Concentrated Urine

The normal renal response to decreased intake of water or increased extrarenal losses of water is the formation of maximally concentrated urine. In most clinical situations in which hypernatremia is the result of water depletion, the expected renal response is a $U_{osm}:P_{osm}$ ratio greater than 1.5 and a specific gravity above 1.015. Thus, the finding of hypernatremia with evidence of renal conservation of water indicates that the hypernatremia is caused by excessive nonrenal losses of water or solute diuresis.

Excessive Nonrenal Water Loss Hypernatremia typically develops in patients with accelerated rates of nonrenal water loss owing to a hot environment, fever, or hyperventilation, and in whom water losses are not replaced because the patient cannot perceive or communicate thirst. Despite the hypernatremia, sodium deficits usually are present because initially, as water deficits develop, renal sodium excretion increases to maintain normal plasma osmolality and serum sodium concentration.

When more than about 15% of ECF volume is lost, renal conservation of sodium occurs; if the water losses continue, hypernatremia develops. The presence of volume deficits is indicated by the signs of IVV depletion, as previously described. Urine flow rate usually is less than 35 mL/h.

Solute Diuresis The amount of water that must accompany the excretion of a given amount of solute in the urine is determined by the osmolality of the renal medullary interstitial fluid (with which the collecting duct fluid must equilibrate) and the plasma level of ADH activity (which determines the permeability of the collecting duct to water and, therefore, the rate at which water moves from the collecting duct to medullary interstitial fluid to achieve osmotic equilibrium). Hypernatremia results if water intake does not keep pace with renal water losses, because although renal sodium excretion also is increased in solute diuresis, renal sodium reabsorption is affected proportionally less than is water reabsorption. Large amounts of mannitol infused intravenously or high-protein mixtures fed by nasogastric tube (each gram of protein yields 8 mOsm as urea, phosphate, and potassium) can cause a solute diuresis sufficient to cause hypernatremia if water intake is inadequate. In solute diuresis, urine volume usually is greater than 35 mL/h.

Hypernatremia Associated with Formation of Dilute Urine

The finding of hypernatremia in combination with isotonic or hypotonic urine indicates that, at least in part, the hypernatremia results from failure of normal renal conservation of water. Failure to concentrate the urine under these conditions may result from the lack of ADH (hypothalamic–pituitary diabetes insipidus) or impaired renal tubular function that interferes with the development of a hypertonic medullary interstitium (renal tubular damage).

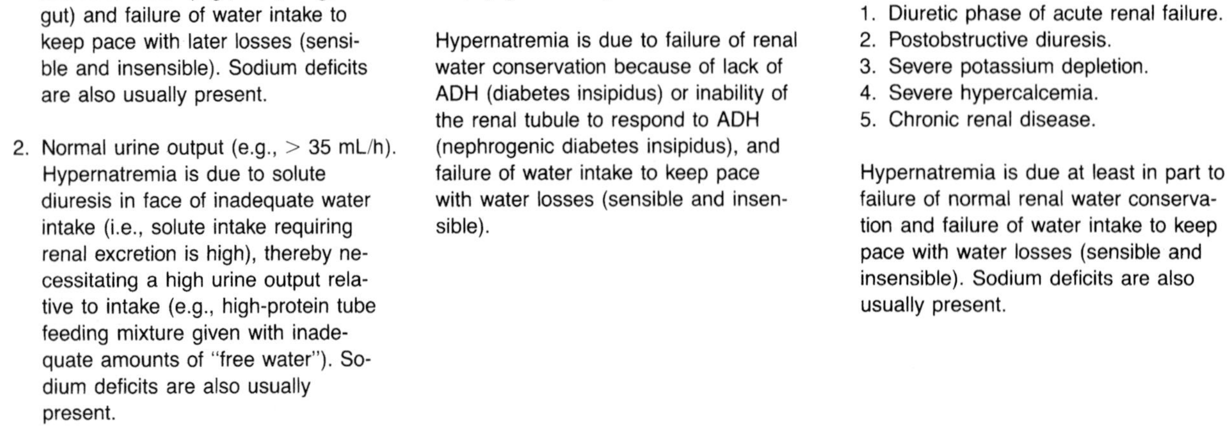

Hypernatremia

State of Renal Water Excretion

Concentrated Urine
($U_{osm}/P_{osm} > 1.5$, sp gr > 1.015):

1. Low urine output (e.g., < 35 mL/h). Hypernatremia is due to nonrenal losses of water (e.g., skin, lung, gut) and failure of water intake to keep pace with later losses (sensible and insensible). Sodium deficits are also usually present.

2. Normal urine output (e.g., > 35 mL/h). Hypernatremia is due to solute diuresis in face of inadequate water intake (i.e., solute intake requiring renal excretion is high), thereby necessitating a high urine output relative to intake (e.g., high-protein tube feeding mixture given with inadequate amounts of "free water"). Sodium deficits are also usually present.

Diabetes insipidus or nephrogenic diabetes insipidus (usually $U_{osm}/P_{osm} < 0.5$, sp gr < 1.005):

Hypernatremia is due to failure of renal water conservation because of lack of ADH (diabetes insipidus) or inability of the renal tubule to respond to ADH (nephrogenic diabetes insipidus), and failure of water intake to keep pace with water losses (sensible and insensible).

Dilute Urine
($U_{osm}/P_{osm} < 1.00$, sp gr < 1.010):

Renal tubular damage
(usually $U_{osm}/P_{osm} \sim 1.0$, sp gr ~ 1.010):

1. Diuretic phase of acute renal failure.
2. Postobstructive diuresis.
3. Severe potassium depletion.
4. Severe hypercalcemia.
5. Chronic renal disease.

Hypernatremia is due at least in part to failure of normal renal water conservation and failure of water intake to keep pace with water losses (sensible and insensible). Sodium deficits are also usually present.

FIGURE 10.2 Approach to the assessment of a hypernatremic patient. This approach does not consider patients with hypernatremia secondary to excessive administration of hypertonic saline. ADH, antidiuretic hormone.

Central diabetes insipidus or nephrogenic diabetes insipidus should be suspected immediately in a patient with hypernatremia when the urine is very dilute (a $U_{osm}:P_{osm}$ ratio <0.5, or specific gravity <1.005).

In patients with renal tubular damage, the ability to concentrate and dilute the urine is decreased. As a result, under all conditions, the urine is isotonic or nearly isotonic with plasma. Hypernatremia can supervene when water losses exceed sodium losses and water intake does not keep pace with water losses. Despite the hypernatremia, significant sodium deficits usually are present because renal sodium wasting also usually is a feature of these disorders. The following sections are examples of clinical situations in which renal tubular damage can be associated with hypernatremia.

Diuretic Phase of Acute Renal Failure Occasionally, in a patient recovering from acute renal injury, tubular function is more severely affected than is glomerular function. Thus, an inordinately large fraction of the glomerular filtrate escapes reabsorption, resulting in high urine flow rates. The period of inappropriate diuresis can persist for a few days to several weeks.

Postobstructive Diuresis The sudden release of chronic urinary tract obstruction often is followed by several days or weeks in which urine flow rates are abnormally high. Short-lived nephrogenic diabetes insipidus develops in some patients.

MANAGEMENT OF WATER AND ELECTROLYTE BALANCE

Water requirements should be carefully monitored, especially in hospitalized patients. Patients with known fluid deficits or excesses should be approached as demonstrated in Tables 10.3

TABLE 10.3 General Guidelines for Planning Fluid and Electrolyte Therapy in Complicated Cases

Volume-contracted patients (from water and electrolyte loss)

Deficit Replacement
Moderate volume contraction (e.g., decreased effective IVV causing azotemia but not hypotension). Plan to replace deficits in about 24 h (e.g., 0.9% saline at 200–250 mL/h). If the patient is hypernatremic, 0.9% and 0.45% saline can be alternated.
Severe volume contraction (e.g., decreased effective IVV causing hypotension). Give 0.9% saline as rapidly as practicable until the hypotension is corrected.
Estimate maintenance needs, and add this amount to the fluids used to correct the preexisting water and electrolyte deficits.

For patients with normal renal function and no abnormal losses:

Maintenance	*Equivalent Intravenous Fluid Orders*
Water: 2,500–3,000 mL/24 h	Alternate:
Sodium: 150 mEq/24 h	5% dextrose in 0.45% saline with
Potassium: 40 mEq/24 h	5% dextrose in 0.25% saline
	Each day add:
	Multivitamins to first liter
	Potassium chloride 20 mEq to first and second liters
	Infuse at 100–125 mL/h

Nutrition (Short Term)
At least 400 carbohydrate calories/24 h

For patients with acute renal failure with no urine output and no abnormal losses:

Maintenance	*Equivalent Intravenous Fluid Orders*
Water: 600 mL/24 h	600 mL 20% glucose in water and multivitamins per 24 h
Sodium: 0	
Potassium: 0	

Nutrition (Long Term)
At least 400 carbohydrate calories/24 h
Monitor the patient frequently:
Weigh daily.
Measure serum creatinine and electrolyte levels daily or more frequently if necessary.
Measure CVP or pulmonary wedge pressure in complicated cases. If the patient has normal cardiopulmonary function, CVP is sufficient. If cardiac disease or pulmonary hypertension is suspected, pulmonary wedge pressure measurement is preferred.
Evaluate water and electrolyte needs daily or more frequently in patients with high rates of abnormal losses.

Volume-expanded patients (increased effective IVV)

Correct volume excess:
Mild (e.g., simple edema): Decrease NaCl intake.
Moderate (e.g., mild pulmonary vascular congestion): Induce diuresis with diuretic and allow the sodium and water losses to go unreplaced.
Severe volume excess (e.g., severe pulmonary edema): Steps 1 and 2 and phlebotomy or ultrafiltration (if the patient is anemic) and/or digitalis, vasodilators, if heart disease is present.
Estimate ongoing losses (as above) and begin replacing when volume excesses have been corrected.
Monitor the patient frequently.

CVP, central venous pressure; IVV, intravascular volume.

TABLE 10.4 Major Sources, Loss Rates, and Replacement Fluids in Abnormal Water and Electrolyte Loss

SOURCES	RATE OF LOSS	REPLACEMENT FLUID
Fever	Insensible water losses (normally 450 mL/24 h from the skin and 450 mL/24 h from the lung) increase by about 10% per degree Fahrenheit or 20% per degree Celsius for each degree of temperature above normal.	Replace with 5% dextrose in water
Hyperventilation	Doubling alveolar ventilation (i.e., 50% reduction in $Paco_2$) increases insensible water losses from the lung by 50%. Thus, the increase in alveolar ventilation required to reduce $Paco_2$ from 40 to 20 mm Hg increases insensible loss from the lung from 450 to 675 mL/24 h.	Replace with 5% dextrose in water
Gastric fluid	Rates of loss from nasogastric suction usually are 1–2 L/24 h but can be much greater. Normal composition of gastric juice is about H^+, 100 mEq/L; sodium, 40 mEq/L; potassium, 10 mEq/L; and chloride, 150 mEq/L.	Replace with 0.45 normal saline and potassium chloride (usually 20–40 mEq/L) as needed[a]
Diarrheal fluid	Losses can vary from trivial to several liters daily. In adults, diarrheal fluid usually resembles ECF except that the bicarbonate concentration is higher (about 30–50 mEq/L) and chloride concentration is lower (about 80 mEq/L). Potassium concentration is variable (10–40 mEq/L)	Replace with 0.45 normal saline and 50 mEq of sodium bicarbonate/liter and potassium chloride (usually 20 mEq/L), as needed[a]
Urine in acute renal failure	Because of tubular injury, urine sodium concentration usually is between 40 and 80 mEq/L and is largely independent of urine flow rate.	Replace with 0.45 normal saline and potassium chloride, as needed[a]

[a]The rate of potassium replacement usually is determined by the serum potassium concentration rather than the rates of potassium loss. For example, even though a patient in acute renal failure may be losing 30 mEq/24 h potassium in the urine, it may not be necessary to replace this amount, since potassium may be entering the extracellular fluid (ECF) at an even faster rate because of catabolism of cellular proteins. On the other hand, the potassium losses in gastric fluid may amount to only 10–20 mEq/24 h, yet far greater amounts of potassium may have to be administered to maintain a normal serum potassium level, since gastric aspiration may lead to metabolic alkalosis, causing renal potassium wasting and extensive diffusion of potassium into intracellular fluid.

and 10.4. *Minimum* maintenance requirements can be calculated from two simple formulas.

The first is the 4-2-1 rule (Table 10.5). A more simplified method of calculation using this formula in adults would be to administer 60 mL/h of fluid for the first 20 kg of body weight. Subtract 20 from the patient's weight (in kilograms) and add this difference to calculate the hourly rate. For example, a patient who weighs 65 kg has a maintenance requirement of 105 mL/h. The 4-2-1 method was originally established in children, and characteristically overestimates fluid needs for adults since adults have lower body surface area per unit of weight and, as a result, less insensible losses.

The second method is to calculate the body surface area and multiply by 1,000. A patient with a body surface area of 1.5 m² would require 1,500 mL of fluid daily.

Intraoperative Fluid Administration

The guidelines for fluid replacement during the perioperative period are dictated by (maintenance) basal requirements, deficits, intraoperative losses, and third space losses. The basal requirement has been discussed. Deficits include actions of general or spinal anesthesia on effective blood volume, intestinal losses (bowel obstruction or diarrhea), perspiration, and blood loss. In some cases, a CVP or Swan-Ganz catheter may be needed to assess IVV.

Intraoperative losses of fluid occur through several routes. Evaporation from peritoneal surfaces occurs, but quantifying

it is difficult. The most obvious source of fluid loss, blood loss, is first assessed by looking into the suction canister. Fluid from irrigation should be subtracted. A soaked lap pad contains about 50 mL of blood, and a 4 × 4 pad contains about 5 mL. These are crude approximations. For instance, a moistened lap pad absorbs less than a dry one. Most researchers recommend a replacement rate of 3 to 1 for blood loss using crystalloid suspension and 1 to 1 using colloid suspension. While anesthetized, patients experience third space loss. This phenomenon is the movement of isotonic fluid from the intravascular space to the interstitial space. A replacement of 2 to

TABLE 10.5 Maintenance Requirements by 4-2-1 Rule[a]

BODY WEIGHT CATEGORY	FLUID RATE (ML/KG)	WEIGHT CATEGORY (KG)	FLUID (ML/H)
0–10	4	10	40
11–20	2	10	20
21+	1	40	40

[a]Patient weighs 60 kg. Fluid requirement would be 100 mL/h.

TABLE 10.6 Composition of Parenteral Fluids[a]

SOLUTIONS	CATIONS				ANIONS		
	Na	K	Ca	Mg	Cl	HCO₃	OSMOLALITY (mOsm)
Extracellular fluid	142	4	5	3	103	27	280–310
Lactated Ringer solution	130	4	3	—	109	28[b]	273
0.9% sodium chloride	154	—	—	—	154	—	308
D₅ 45% sodium chloride	77	—	—	—	77	—	407
D₅W	—	—	—	—	—	—	253
3% sodium chloride	513	—	—	—	513	—	1,026

[a]Electrolyte count in mEq/L.
[b]Present in solution as lactate that is converted to bicarbonate.

4 mL/kg/h is usually adequate to accommodate third space losses. Actual total intraoperative losses may be difficult or impossible to monitor during long and difficult surgical procedures. Monitoring of vital signs and urine output (optimal, 0.5 mL/kg/h) is extremely important. Sometimes invasive monitoring can be used to guide the clinician.

Crystalloid solutions contain only sugars and electrolytes (Table 10.6). Lactated Ringer solution is usually used because its composition more closely resembles the extracellular component than does normal saline. Generally, solutions that contain less sodium than lactated Ringer solution does should not be used in the perioperative setting. Although D₅W solutions have an osmolality greater than 250, they are unsuitable as routine perioperative replacement because the sugar is metabolized. Normal saline is another popular crystalloid solution. It is preferred over lactated Ringer solutions in the perioperative period when the patient is hyponatremic or if brain injury is present. Hypertonic saline is rarely used in the perioperative setting. Because water tends to follow sodium, its theoretic advantage is that water is drawn into the intravascular space from the interstitial space; hence, smaller volumes of hypertonic solution than isotonic solution are needed to provide the same intravascular expansion. Crystalloid solutions are preferentially used over colloid solutions for perioperative fluid replacement.

Colloid solutions include albumin, hetastarch, and dextran. Blood is also a colloid but is discussed in another chapter. Colloids are used primarily when patients have a low colloid oncotic pressure or when large amounts of crystalloids have been infused. For example, if a patient has suffered a significant protein loss from ascites secondary to pelvic malignancy, colloids should be used early in the fluid replacement process. If a patient's blood pressure becomes difficult to maintain after infusion of sufficient crystalloid, colloids should be used.

Albumin, hetastarch, and dextran are three commonly used colloid solutions. Albumin is the most popular of the colloid solutions. It is a blood product but has the advantage of complete absence of infectious agents. In addition, it is treated with heat, eliminating the possibility of transmission of hepatitis or human immunodeficiency virus (HIV). It comes in 5% and 25% concentrations. In a prior Cochrane review, perioperative use of albumin in critically ill patients was shown to be associated with an increased risk of death. However, several subsequent studies in various populations, including septic and critically ill patients, have shown that albumin is safe and may reduce morbidity and mortality. Albumin may be especially useful when large volumes of fluid may be needed or if

other blood products are limited or not available. Hetastarch consists of large polymer molecules and comes in a solution of saline. It is synthetic; therefore, its use does not affect the blood supply. There is no risk for viral transmission. Hetastarch is metabolized by the kidney and so must be used judiciously in those who have renal disease. Other disadvantages include potential volume overload, dilution hypoproteinemia, and decreased coagulation. The half-life of hetastarch can be as long as 13 days. More recently, serious safety concerns have arisen regarding the use of hetastarch. Hetastarch has been associated with an increased risk of mortality and kidney injury in critically ill and septic patients. In addition, several trials utilizing hetastarch have been retracted because of scientific misconduct. Given the associated risks, with questionable benefit, further use of hetastarch compounds should be limited to clinical trials. Dextran is similar to hetastarch in mode of action. Additional problems with this substance are interference with cross matching and histamine release.

In summary, crystalloids should be used primarily for perioperative volume replacement. Colloid solutions may be considered under the following conditions:

1. Large amounts of crystalloid are needed to maintain normal hemodynamics.
2. Assessment of circulatory status is difficult.
3. The patient has an elevated pulmonary capillary wedge pressure.
4. The colloid pressure is below 12 mm Hg.

Colloid oncotic pressure may be difficult to ascertain in a routine clinical setting; therefore, total protein or albumin levels can be used to give a rough approximation of colloid pressure. If blood loss is more than 25% of total blood volume, transfusion of red cells may be considered. Hemoglobin concentrations can be useful. Experience has shown that hemoglobin levels between 7 and 8 g/dL are generally well tolerated in healthy adults. If the patient has significant comorbidities, then transfusion may be considered to achieve a higher hemoglobin level, especially prior to surgery.

Correction of Volume Deficits

Estimating the Magnitude of Sodium or Water Deficits

If the patient has been weighed daily, the magnitude of the water deficit owing to external losses of water can be estimated from the decrease in body weight. The coexisting sodium deficits can be estimated by examining the weight deficits in light of the serum sodium concentration. For example, if the patient has acutely lost 3 kg and the serum sodium concentration is within 10% either way of normal serum sodium concentration (i.e., 126 to 154 mEq/L), little error is incurred by assuming that the patient has lost 3 L of ECF (i.e., isotonic saline); therefore, replacement therapy should be about 3 L of 0.9% saline (155 mEq/L). Using an equivalent amount of lactated Ringer solution offers no advantage, because the kidneys adjust electrolyte excretion to make up for small differences between the composition of the ECF and the isotonic saline.

In patients in whom sodium and water deficits cannot be documented by changes in body weight, or in whom the losses are from the IVV into internal third spaces, approximate but useful guidelines are available to estimate the magnitude of the IVV deficit. These guidelines are as follows:

1. A loss equivalent to 15% of ECF volume (about 2 to 3 L in the average adult) results in a decrease in tissue turgor, but blood pressure and renal function, as judged by serum creatinine level, usually are normal.
2. Losses of sodium and water in excess of 15% of ECF volume usually are accompanied by decreased tissue turgor, orthostatic or frank hypotension, and significant elevation of serum creatinine level.

Correction Rates and Criteria for Assessment

Sodium and water losses great enough to result in hypotension represent a medical emergency, and rapid IV administration of isotonic saline is indicated until the hypotension is reversed. Thereafter, the rate of IV therapy is guided by the adequacy of the IVV as assessed by other criteria, particularly the measurement of blood pressure and pulse in the supine and sitting positions, urine flow rate, and CVP. In patients with less severe degrees of volume depletion, salt and water deficits often can be corrected by increasing oral intake. Salt can be added to food (the salt packets commonly present on hospital trays provide slightly more than 1 g of sodium chloride), or plain sodium chloride tablets can be given, with unrestricted water allowance, letting the patient's thirst mechanism dictate water intake. As a guide to the amount of sodium chloride that should be added to the diet to restore the deficits, 1 L of ECF contains 140 mEq of sodium, or about 9 g of sodium chloride. The adequacy of replacement therapy can be assessed over the ensuing days by measurement of change in body weight and blood pressure and by the decrease in serum creatinine level.

Correction of Volume Excess

Expansion of effective IVV sufficient to precipitate pulmonary edema is a medical emergency and requires the usual treatment of pulmonary edema, including placement of the patient in the sitting position or elevation of the head of the bed and administration of oxygen, vasodilators—such as nitrates, hydralazine, or angiotensin-converting enzyme inhibitors (e.g., captopril, enalapril, lisinopril)—digitalis, and loop diuretics, as needed. If the pulmonary edema does not improve, then phlebotomy may be required to relieve the vascular congestion. If the volume excess is less severe (e.g., simple edema), the problem usually can be controlled by decreasing salt intake, adding a diuretic drug, or both. The effectiveness of treatment can be guided by the decrease in body weight and periodic measurement of serum electrolyte and creatinine levels.

Correction of Hyponatremia

The approach to the correction of hyponatremia depends on (a) whether the patient has significant CNS symptoms as a result of the hyponatremia (coma or seizures) and (b) the cause of the hyponatremia. If the patient has coma or seizures as a result of hyponatremia, the serum sodium level is commonly below 125 mEq/L and the reduction usually has occurred rapidly, over a few hours to days. In these situations, regardless of the cause of the hyponatremia, the serum sodium level should be rapidly raised toward normal by the IV administration of 3% saline. The serum sodium level should be raised to 125 mEq/L at a rate of 1 to 2 mEq/h. The rate of replacement can be slowed once the serum sodium level reaches 125 mEq/L, because neurologic symptoms are rare above this concentration. Rapid elevation of the serum sodium concentration to normal or hypernatremic levels must be avoided, because it may cause central pontine myelinolysis. The correction using 3% saline (513 mEq/L) can be calculated as follows:

$$\text{volume TBW} = 0.6 \text{ H total body weight in kg}$$

$$\text{volume TBW} \times \left(\text{desired}\left[Na^+\right] - \text{actual}\left[Na^+\right]\right) = \text{total } Na^+ (mEq)$$

where:
$[Na^+]$ is expressed in mEq/L; and TBW = total body water.

The total amount of sodium required can then be replaced at a rate of 2 mEq/h using hypertonic saline. For example, if a 71-kg woman with neurologic symptoms has a serum sodium level of 113 mEq/L, correction to a serum sodium level of 125 mEq/L can be achieved as follows:

$$\text{volume TBW} = 0.6 \times 71 = 42.6$$
$$42.6 \times (125 - 113) = 511 \text{ mEq } Na^+$$

Therefore, since 1 L of 3% saline contains 513 mEq of sodium, this patient requires 1 L of 3% saline to raise her serum sodium level by 12 mEq. The liter of hypertonic saline is administered over 6 to 12 hours. Serum electrolyte levels should be checked every few hours and rates of replacement readjusted as necessary. The infusion of hypertonic saline results in diffusion of water from ICF to ECF until isosmotic conditions are restored. This results in reduction of cell volume and an increase of ICF osmolality toward normal as well as in an expansion of ECF volume. The expansion of the ECF by the hypertonic saline may precipitate or worsen CHF. Therefore, patients who receive hypertonic saline should be carefully observed for signs of pulmonary edema and, if such signs are present, vigorously treated with a loop diuretic.

Hyponatremia Associated with Volume Depletion

The administration of isotonic saline in amounts sufficient to replace existing sodium deficits usually results in complete correction of the hyponatremia, as discussed, in connection with the treatment of volume depletion, because restoration of effective IVV toward normal allows a water diuresis. If specific disease states, such as adrenal insufficiency or diarrhea, are associated with the development of the hyponatremia and volume depletion, these also require treatment.

Hyponatremia Associated with Normal Intravascular Volume

If the hyponatremia is associated with excessive intake of water, restricting water intake to normal corrects the problem.

If the hyponatremia is owing to an inappropriate antidiuresis, water intake must be restricted below normal—for example, to about 800 mL of measured liquid intake daily in an average-sized adult. This usually results in negative water balance, a decrease in body weight, and an increase in serum sodium concentration toward normal. If a specific cause for the inappropriate antidiuresis can be identified, it should be eliminated.

Hyponatremia Associated with Expanded Intravascular Volume and Extracellular Fluid

The spontaneous development of hyponatremia in the course of severe CHF or liver failure is an ominous sign. The hyponatremia usually does not cause any clinical symptoms, and although it can be successfully treated by water restriction, clinical improvement usually does not follow. Furthermore, during such treatment, patients complain bitterly of thirst. Thus, water restriction sufficient to raise the serum sodium concentration to normal is not indicated. Water intake should be restricted, however, to prevent the serum sodium concentration from decreasing to less than 120 mEq/L in an effort to prevent possible CNS symptoms of hyponatremia.

Correction of Hypernatremia

Hypernatremia Secondary to Water Depletion

The amount of water needed to correct the serum sodium concentration toward normal should be determined based on the clinical volume status of the patient. Hypotonic solutions can be used to correct hypernatremia over a period of 24 to 48 hours. Serial sodium levels should be used to avoid overcorrection and hyponatremia. Furosemide should not be used to correct hypernatremia or decreased urine output in a patient with decreased IVV.

Hypernatremia Secondary to Excessive Administration of Hypertonic Saline

In the rare instance of hypernatremia secondary to excessive administration of hypertonic saline, which occurs when intra-amniotic infusion of hypertonic saline is used to induce abortion, hypernatremia is owing solely to positive sodium chloride balance. Therefore, treatment involves simply inducing a state of negative sodium chloride balance while maintaining a slightly positive water balance. If the hypernatremia is associated with impairment of CNS function (Na^+ usually exceeds 160 mEq/L), 2 to 3 L of 5% solution of glucose in water should rapidly be given IV, along with sufficient furosemide to induce a urine flow rate of about 10 to 20 mL/min. About 100 mg of IV furosemide is an appropriate initial dose. This results in the excretion of urine containing about 140 mEq/L of sodium and chloride and 10 mEq/L of potassium. If, at the same time, only the water and potassium are replaced (e.g., replacement of each 1,000 mL of urine with 1,000 mL of 5% solution of glucose in water plus 10 to 20 mEq of potassium chloride, given IV), the patient is selectively depleted of sodium chloride, and plasma electrolytes can be restored to normal within several hours. During this period of correction, serum and urine electrolyte levels must be monitored frequently to assess the adequacy of IV replacement therapy, particularly the rate of potassium administration.

POTASSIUM METABOLISM

Disorders of potassium metabolism frequently coexist with disorders of sodium and water balance. For example, sodium and potassium losses often accompany gastrointestinal losses of water and electrolytes. The recognition and management of potassium depletion under these circumstances were discussed earlier in connection with the management of disorders of sodium and water balance. Even small movements of potassium into and out of cells can cause significant changes in the serum potassium since more than 90% of potassium resides intracellularly. It also is important to recognize disorders in which disturbances of potassium balance are the primary abnormality or the major feature of the electrolyte disturbances.

Hyperkalemia

Hyperkalemia is defined as a serum potassium level greater than 5 mEq/L. Serum potassium levels between 5 and 6 mEq/L usually cause little or no functional abnormality, but such levels indicate that an abnormality of potassium regulation is present. This sign should be heeded and its cause investigated, because further small elevations in serum potassium concentration can seriously impair cardiac and skeletal muscle function. At a serum potassium level of 6 or 7 mEq/L, the electrocardiogram (ECG) begins to show tall, peaked T waves, and skeletal muscle weakness may be present. At a serum potassium level greater than 7 mEq/L, severe ECG abnormalities may be present, including complete suppression of atrial activity and an idioventricular rhythm that can then lead to ventricular tachycardia and fibrillation. Profound skeletal muscle weakness leading to respiratory arrest also may develop. If serious hyperkalemia is suspected, an ECG should be obtained immediately along with a blood specimen for potassium measurement. The ECG findings establish whether life-threatening hyperkalemia is present. Table 10.7 lists the principal clinical conditions associated with hyperkalemia.

Pseudohyperkalemia can result from hemolysis of red blood cells as a result of the mechanical trauma of venipuncture. Such pseudohyperkalemia should be readily recognized, because both potassium and hemoglobin are released by the damaged cells. If the serum potassium level has been significantly raised by in vitro hemolysis, the serum is visibly pink because of the presence of free hemoglobin. Patients with extraordinarily high white blood cell counts or platelet counts also can exhibit pseudohyperkalemia as the result of excessive traumatic in vitro lysis of these cells. Pseudohyperkalemia can be avoided by drawing venous blood samples under low pressure into a heparinized syringe.

Management

Life-Threatening Hyperkalemia Electrocardiogram shows sine waves or loss of atrial activity and a broad QRS complex. Serum potassium level usually is higher than 7 mEq/L.

1. Infuse 10 mL of 10% calcium gluconate intravenously over a few minutes with ECG monitoring to observe for reversal of ECG changes toward normal. The same infusion of 10 mL of 10% calcium gluconate can be repeated once. Calcium ion directly antagonizes the effects of potassium on myocardial metabolism. The onset of action is a few minutes. If the patient is taking digitalis, consider not giving the calcium and proceed on to the next step.
2. Infuse 50 g of glucose, 10 U of regular insulin, and 50 mEq of sodium bicarbonate. The onset of action is about 15 minutes. Additionally, an IV infusion of glucose, insulin, and sodium bicarbonate (e.g., 500 mL of 10% dextrose in water plus 15 units of regular insulin plus 50 mEq of sodium bicarbonate) may be started. Infuse over several hours. This maneuver causes potassium to

TABLE 10.7 Causes of Hyperkalemia

CAUSE	EFFECT
Excessive intake of potassium Transfusion of blood stored for prolonged periods	Shortened life span of stored RBCs after transfusion leads to excessive release of RBC potassium to ECF. Plasma potassium of stored blood also is increased (30 mEq/L) after 14 days of storage.
Excessive oral or intravenous intake of potassium	Acute ingestion of 500 mEq potassium chloride can cause fatal hyperkalemia with normal renal function. If renal function is impaired, even normal potassium intake can cause severe hyperkalemia.

Excessive release of intracellular stores of potassium
  Chemotherapy of malignancies
  Catabolism of hematomas
  Rhabdomyolysis
  Succinylcholine action on muscle
  Sepsis with excessive catabolism of muscle protein
  Acute digitalis poisoning
  Familial hyperkalemic periodic paralysis
  Intravenous hypertonic glucose or mannitol
  Intravenous arginine
  Metabolic acidosis
	The potential for any of these conditions to cause serious hyperkalemia is greatly increased when they coexist with impaired renal function.
	
	H^+ displaces K^+ from intracellular sites, causing increased diffusion of K^+ into ECF.

Impaired renal capacity to excrete potassium Grossly reduced GFR	Almost all of filtered potassium is reabsorbed. Excreted potassium represents almost exclusively potassium secreted by the tubules. Nevertheless, grossly reduced GFR is associated with grossly reduced tubular function and hence the tendency to hyperkalemia.
Impaired tubular function Hyperkalemic renal tubular acidosis	Some patients with normal or mildly reduced GFR can have substantial impairment of potassium secretion (e.g., lupus patients with interstitial nephritis, mild obstructive uropathy).

Decreased aldosterone secretion
  Addison disease
  Primary hypoaldosteronism
  Hyporeninemic hypoaldosteronism
	Aldosterone is necessary for normal potassium and H^+ secretion and normal Na^+ absorption in the distal renal tubule.
	
	Common in patients with diabetes mellitus or obstructive uropathy.

Drugs that suppress angiotensin formation
  β-Blocking agents (e.g., propranolol)
  Prostaglandin synthetase inhibitors (e.g., indomethacin, ibuprofen)
  Angiotensin-converting enzyme inhibitors (e.g., captopril, enalapril, lisinopril)
	Angiotensin II causes aldosterone secretion; β-blockers and nonsteroidal anti-inflammatory drugs directly suppress angiotensin formation by suppressing renin production. Captopril prevents angiotensin II formation by blocking conversion of angiotensin I.

Drugs that interfere with renal potassium secretion	Spironolactone competitively inhibits the action of aldosterone. Triamterene and amiloride block potassium secretion even in the absence of aldosterone.
Ureteral implantation into jejunal loop	Increased reabsorption of potassium from jejunum causes predisposition to hyperkalemia.

ECF, extracellular fluid; GFR, glomerular filtration rate; RBCs, red blood cells.

move intracellularly. The amount of glucose infused must be altered or omitted in hyperglycemic diabetic patients.
3. Nebulized albuterol at a dose of 10 to 20 mg is recommended. The peak action is approximately 90 minutes.
4. As soon as practical, give sodium polystyrene sulfonate (Kayexalate) by mouth, nasogastric tube, or retention enema (e.g., 20 to 50 g of Kayexalate every 2 to 4 hours). An equal number of grams of sorbitol should be given if the Kayexalate is administered into the upper gastrointestinal tract. Sorbitol, a sugar that is poorly absorbed from the intestine, causes an osmotic diarrhea and prevents concretions of Kayexalate from forming within the gut. Kayexalate is an ion-exchange resin that removes potassium by binding potassium and releasing sodium into body fluids.
5. Hemodialysis may be required in patients in whom these measures fail.

TABLE 10.8 Causes of Hypokalemia

CAUSE	COMMENTS ON PATHOGENESIS
Decreased potassium intake	With 0 mEq potassium intake, stool potassium is about 10 mEq/2 h, urinary potassium is <30 mEq/24 h or is <20 mEq/L.
Excessive renal losses of potassium	Urinary potassium usually >30 mEq/24 h or 20 mEq/L.
Diuretic therapy	All diuretics except for spironolactone, triamterene, and amiloride cause renal potassium wasting. *Mechanism:* Diuretics cause increased sodium delivery to distal tubular sites where sodium is reabsorbed in exchange for potassium or hydrogen ion.
Diuretic phase of acute tubular necrosis and other causes of osmotic diuresis	*Mechanism:* Same as above.
Metabolic alkalosis	*Mechanism:* renal tubular cell potassium concentration increased resulting in enhanced potassium secretion.
Gentamicin or amphotericin B nephrotoxicity	Renal tubular damage presumably causes increased back flux of potassium into renal tubules in the case of amphotericin.
Increased renal mineralocorticoid effects	Increased activity of distal tubular site, which reabsorbs sodium in exchange for potassium or H^+.
Mineralocorticoid therapy (deoxycorticosterone acetate, 9 α-fludrocortisone)	
Primary aldosteronism	
Secondary aldosteronism (e.g., cirrhosis of the liver, renal artery stenosis, malignant hypertension)	
Cushing syndrome	
Excessive licorice or chewing tobacco (glycyrrhizic acid)	
Bartter syndrome	
Renal tubular acidosis	*Mechanism:*
	Distal: Possibly increased renal potassium secretion in exchange for sodium at the distal tubular site because of decreased availability of H^+ for secretion
	Proximal: Increased bicarbonate excretion leads to increased renal potassium excretion.
Excessive gastrointestinal losses of potassium	
Vomiting, gastric drainage, diarrhea, laxative abuse	Renal potassium excretion also increased in the case of vomiting or gastric drainage.
Villous adenoma of the rectum	Loss of potassium-rich mucus per rectum
Shift of potassium from the extracellular to the intracellular fluid	
Correction of metabolic acidosis	H^+ leaves cells, K^+ enters cells during correction of metabolic acidosis.
Correction of hyperglycemia	K^+ enters cells with glucose to provide cation to balance anion that forms during metabolism of glucose
Hypokalemic periodic paralysis	Unexplained familial disorder
Miscellaneous	
Ureterosigmoidostomy	Colonic secretion of HCO_3^- and K^+ with absorption of Na^+ and Cl^- results in hypokalemic metabolic acidosis.

Moderate Hyperkalemia Electorocardiogram shows only peaked T waves; serum potassium level usually is below 7 mEq/L.

1. Reduce potassium intake (normal potassium intake is 60 to 100 mEq/24 h). Reducing dietary potassium to 50 to 60 mEq/24 h usually is sufficient to correct mild hyperkalemia.
2. Kayexalate may be needed periodically to control the serum potassium level.
3. Correct metabolic acidosis if present.
4. Stop administration of medications that can contribute to hyperkalemia, such as angiotensin-converting enzyme inhibitors, nonsteroidal anti-inflammatory drugs, and potassium-sparing diuretics.

Hypokalemia

Hypokalemia is defined as a serum potassium level below 3.5 mEq/L (Table 10.8). Significant symptoms usually do not result from hypokalemia unless the serum potassium level is less than 3 mEq/L. An important exception is in patients who are receiving digitalis preparations. In such patients, hypokalemia, or even low-normal serum potassium levels, can increase myocardial irritability and lead to serious arrhythmias. In addition to increasing myocardial irritability, hypokalemia can cause profound muscle weakness and ileus. Chronic severe hypokalemia also can cause metabolic alkalosis and decreased capacity to concentrate the urine. The ECG in hypokalemia often shows U waves, although this finding is not diagnostic of hypokalemia.

Management

Mild Asymptomatic Hypokalemia This usually can be corrected simply by eliminating the cause of the potassium wasting or by increasing potassium intake. If the hypokalemia is caused by diuretic therapy, potassium depletion usually can be avoided by administering spironolactone or triamterene. Potassium supplementation also can be used, but if the patient is on a low sodium chloride intake, the potassium supplement must be given as potassium chloride. The use of other, more palatable potassium salts (e.g., gluconate, citrate, acetate) and all forms of potassium in food is much less effective in correcting hypokalemia, and this treatment is used primarily in patients on a normal sodium chloride intake.

Severe or Symptomatic Hypokalemia This usually requires IV administration of potassium chloride. In general, the use of IV solutions that contain more than 40 mEq/L of potassium should be avoided, because infusing high concentrations of potassium can cause hyperkalemia or cardiac disturbance. In correcting even severe potassium deficits, it is seldom necessary to infuse more than 120 to 160 mEq/24 hours of potassium chloride. When higher rates are used, frequent monitoring of the patient's ECG and serum potassium level is essential. Intravenous replacement of potassium should never run at a rate of greater than 10 mEq/h. The oral route of potassium replacement should be used whenever possible.

Calcium

Approximately 99% of body calcium is contained in bone. Up to 40% of the extracellular calcium that circulates in the bloodstream is bound to plasma proteins. However, the unbound or ionized form of calcium is the form that exerts physiologic activity. Total calcium is a measure of both the bound and unbound or ionized form. Serum albumin levels affect the total serum calcium, as albumin is the plasma protein to which the majority of calcium is bound.

$$\text{corrected calcium in mg / dL}$$
$$= \text{measured calcium} + \left[(4 - \text{albumin in g / dL}) \times 0.8\right]$$

Ionized or unbound calcium can be measured if specifically requested. Its concentration is affected by the serum pH. With alkalosis when the pH is increased, a decrease in ionized calcium results from the increased protein binding of calcium. Conversely, with acidosis, a decrease in protein binding causes an increase in ionized calcium.

The homeostasis of calcium is quite complex, and calcium serves many important functions. Calcium plays a role in regulation of muscle contraction and nerve conduction. Additionally, it functions in the coagulation cascade. The majority of calcium is stored in bone; however, calcium is under the control of several other organ systems, including the integument, endocrine, and renal. Parathyroid hormone (PTH) appears to be the major hormone effecting calcium homeostasis. Vitamin D must be present, however, for it to exert its maximal effect. PTH causes the following.

- Mobilization of calcium and phosphorus from bone
- Increased renal tubular reabsorption of calcium
- Increased intestinal absorption of calcium
- Decreased renal tubular reabsorption of phosphorus

Hypocalcemia

Clinical manifestations of hypocalcemia (defined as a calcium level below 8 to 8.5 mg/dL) are characterized by neuromuscular irritability. Symptoms can include numbness, muscle cramping, paresthesias, Chvostek (twitching of facial muscles) and Trousseau (carpal spasm) signs, tetany, and seizures. Patients can also experience psychosis and memory loss. On physical examination, patients may have hyperactive deep tendon reflexes. ECG findings of hypocalcemia include a prolonged QT interval, which can lead to heart block or ventricular fibrillation. Causes of hypocalcemia are shown in Table 10.9.

Treatment of hypocalcemia should be directed at its underlying cause. A low total calcium level with a normal ionized calcium level signifies a low level of plasma proteins. These patients usually are asymptomatic, and calcium replacement in this setting usually is not necessary.

For patients with acute symptomatic hypocalcemia, calcium gluconate or chloride should be given intravenously. These may cause a local cellulitis or tissue necrosis if infiltration occurs. If infiltration occurs, especially with the chloride solution in emergent situations, 10 mL of 10% calcium gluconate can be administered intravenously over 15 minutes. In addition, 10 to 20 mL of calcium gluconate can be placed in 1 L of D_5W and administered over 24 hours. If the serum albumin level is below 2 mg/dL, then it may be prudent to replace albumin, especially if the urine output is low. Because albumin is heat treated, there is no risk of hepatitis or HIV exposure. In cases of symptomatic hypocalcemia, magnesium levels must be checked and corrected if necessary. In those patients with metabolic acidosis and hypocalcemia, the hypocalcemia should be treated initially followed by the correction of the acidosis.

Long-term treatment of hypocalcemia involves adequate nutritional supplementation of calcium, vitamin D, or both. If the serum phosphorus level is high, hypoparathyroid disease must be suspected and the patient treated accordingly. If the serum phosphorus is normal or low, then primary bone disease (hungry bone) must be considered. It is imperative that magnesium levels be checked because replenishment of calcium cannot be accomplished in a patient who is hypomagnesemic.

Hypercalcemia

The clinical manifestations of hypercalcemia usually are seen when the total serum calcium is greater than 12 mg/dL. Common presenting symptoms include weakness, fatigue, nausea, vomiting, constipation, polyuria, polydipsia, lethargy, and confusion. Psychiatric disturbances and coma can be seen in severe cases of hypercalcemia. Electrocardiogram changes include prolongation of PR and QRS intervals with a shortening of the QT interval. Complete heart block and cardiac arrest can occur in profound hypercalcemia. Additional laboratory

TABLE 10.9 Causes of Hypocalcemia

Deficiency or absence of PTH
Vitamin D deficiency—decreased intestinal absorption
Septic shock—suppression of PTH products
Renal failure—decreased 1:25 dihydroxycholecalciferol
Hypomagnesemia—decreased PTH release and decreased organ response to calcium
Hyperphosphatemia

abnormalities can include elevations in serum amylase and creatinine levels. The phosphorus level is critical in establishing the cause of hypercalcemia. A phosphorus level below 3.5 mg/dL suggests hyperparathyroidism, whereas an elevated phosphorus level suggests an underlying malignancy.

Hypercalcemia, unlike many other electrolyte disturbances, is rarely iatrogenically induced. There are several causes of hypercalcemia. The majority of hospitalized patients with hypercalcemia have an underlying malignancy, whereas the most common etiology of hypercalcemia in the ambulatory setting is hyperparathyroidism. Additional causes of hypercalcemia include thiazide diuretics, lithium, vitamin D intoxication, hyperthyroidism, and sarcoidosis. In the setting of gynecology, hypercalcemia is most often seen with malignancy. In patients with cancer, hypercalcemia results from increased bone resorption and decreased renal excretion. Metastasis to the bony skeleton causes an increase in osteoclastic activity that increases bone resorption. Some gynecologic tumors, however, may cause hypercalcemia by production of a substance similar to PTH, causing bone resorption without evidence of bony metastasis.

Volume expansion is crucial in the treatment of acute hypercalcemia. Replacement with normal saline solution decreases calcium reabsorption in the proximal renal tubule, thus improving renal function. Initial IV fluid therapy should be aggressive, with rates of 250 to 500 mL/h, as most patients are volume contracted. Addition of loop diuretics such as furosemide may aid in increasing urinary calcium excretion, but caution must be used because these drugs may result in volume contraction and hypokalemia. After initial volume is restored, 3 to 6 L/d of normal saline solution should be given. Close monitoring of daily patient weights, intake and output, and frequent monitoring of serum electrolytes is necessary in patients with hypercalcemia.

Bisphosphonates are commonly used for the treatment of hypercalcemia. This class of drugs inhibits osteoclast precursors and induces osteoclast cytotoxicity, thereby decreasing serum calcium levels. Etidronate disodium (Didronel) is given at a dose of 7.5 mg/kg IV over 2 hours daily for 3 to 7 days. Alternatively, pamidronate (Aredia) is given as a single dose of 60 to 90 mg IV over 4 to 24 hours. Peak onset of action with these medications is usually seen in 48 to 96 hours and may last 2 to 3 weeks. The single dose of 90 mg IV of pamidronate is recommended for severe cases of hypercalcemia because of its effectiveness.

Zoledronic acid (Zometa) is a new-generation, nitrogen-containing bisphosphonate that has been shown to be superior to pamidronate at inhibiting the induction of hypercalcemia of malignancy. Zometa can be given over 5 minutes in a 4-mg dose for the initial treatment of hypercalcemia and an 8-mg dose for relapsed or refractory hypercalcemia. The duration of response with zoledronic acid is approximately 32 days with a 4-mg dose and 43 days with an 8-mg dose compared with 18 days with a 90-mg dose of pamidronate.

Calcitonin increases renal excretion of calcium and inhibits osteoclastic activity. In patients with hypercalcemia, calcitonin can be given at a dose of 4 to 8 IU/kg intramuscularly or subcutaneously every 6 to 12 hours. Commercial calcitonin preparations are generally from salmon. It has a rapid onset of action, and serum calcium levels may decrease within several hours. Its effect usually subsides after several days but may be potentiated by concomitant glucocorticoid administration. Calcitonin has minimal side effects. Tachyphylaxis is seen with calcitonin, limiting its repeated usage and causing it to be less consistently effective compared with other available hypercalcemic treatments.

Glucocorticoids decrease the intestinal absorption of calcium, promote urinary excretion of calcium, and may lower calcium levels by a direct cytolytic effect on some tumor cells.

Lowering of serum calcium levels with glucocorticoids may take 5 to 10 days. Dosages may vary from 20 to 100 mg of oral prednisone or its IV equivalent per day. Side effects limit the long-term use of glucocorticoids for hypercalcemia.

Another potent inhibitor of bone resorption is gallium nitrate. Its onset of action is usually seen in 1 to 2 days, with a peak at 5 to 10 days after administration. Gallium nitrate is administered in a dose of 100 to 200 mg/kg/d for 5 days in a continuous drip. It is important to maintain a saline diuresis of at least 2 L/d during this therapy. Side effects are relatively uncommon, but renal toxicity may be seen. Gallium nitrate in early studies was significantly more effective than was calcitonin with or without the addition of corticosteroids. Its obvious disadvantage over the biphosphonates is that it requires continuous IV infusion over 4 or 5 days.

Oral and IV phosphorus has been used successfully to treat hypercalcemia. It has fallen out of favor, however, because it causes decreased excretion of calcium from the kidneys. Intravenous phosphorus can also lead to soft tissue deposition of calcium compounds and renal failure. It was used in patients with serum phosphorus levels less than 3 mg/dL and normal renal function. For patients with extremely high calcium levels and severe symptoms (e.g., coma, arrhythmia), renal dialysis may be necessary for rapid correction of hypercalcemia.

Plicamycin (mithramycin) is an antibiotic that blocks bone resorption, thus lowering serum calcium. The recommended dose of plicamycin in the treatment of hypercalcemia is 25 mg/kg IV over 4 to 6 hours and may be repeated every 24 to 48 hours. Its onset of action is relatively quick, and peak action is usually noted in 2 to 3 days. Side effects can be severe and include nausea, vomiting, bleeding, thrombocytopenia, renal failure, and hepatotoxicity. These side effects are more common with repeated doses of plicamycin. Because of these side effects, plicamycin usually is reserved for hypercalcemia of malignancy or hypercalcemia refractory to other therapies.

Magnesium

Magnesium has several functions in the human body. Its primary role is in neuromuscular function, but it also serves as an enzyme cofactor in protein and carbohydrate metabolism. The majority (60%) of magnesium in the body is contained within the bone. Most of the remainder is found intracellularly, with only about 1% found in the ECF. Normal serum magnesium levels are between 1.2 and 2.2 mEq/L. Magnesium metabolism depends on potassium and calcium levels. The kidney serves as the organ primarily responsible for magnesium homeostasis. Magnesium is filtered at the glomerulus and reabsorbed in the ascending loop of Henle and to a lesser degree in the proximal and distal tubules.

Hypomagnesemia

Hypomagnesemia is more common than hypermagnesemia. Hypomagnesemia results from decreased gastrointestinal absorption with conditions such as chronic diarrhea, malabsorption syndromes, and nasogastric suction. Increased renal and gastrointestinal losses from osmotic diuresis, hypercalcemia, and medications such as cisplatin, diuretics, and aminoglycosides also can cause hypomagnesemia. Hypomagnesemia can result from decreased intake in malnutrition. For example, 10% to 15% of hospitalized patients and more than half of patients in intensive care units exhibit low magnesium levels. Patients with heavy alcohol use may have hypomagnesemia.

Symptoms and signs of hypomagnesemia are usually nonspecific but may manifest by neuromuscular excitability. Hypomagnesemia is often seen in combination with hypokalemia, hypocalcemia, and metabolic alkalosis. Neurologic abnormalities include weakness, dizziness, lethargy, confusion, tremors, fasciculations, and seizures. Typical ECG findings are prolonged PR and QT intervals; however, atrial and ventricular arrhythmias can result.

The treatment of hypomagnesemia involves the replacement of magnesium. Mild or chronic cases may be treated with oral magnesium supplements. Oral repletion is also preferred in asymptomatic patients. This is accomplished by giving 240 mg of elemental magnesium one to four times a day. Diarrhea is the most common side effect. For severe or acute cases, IV magnesium is indicated. Obstetricians and gynecologists are familiar with the 4-g magnesium load mixed with 50 mL of D_5W infused over 30 minutes. Deep tendon reflexes should be evaluated frequently because hyperreflexia suggests hypermagnesemia. Long-term oral therapy can be provided with magnesium oxide 300 mg/d. Patients should receive proper nutritional counseling and be warned to avoid alcohol. Any underlying medical disorder that may contribute to magnesium losses should be treated. Hydration status should be evaluated because overhydration can lead to mild forms of hypomagnesemia. Gastrointestinal tract losses and alcohol consumption also should be addressed in the evaluation of this disease process.

Hypermagnesemia

Hypermagnesemia is rare and usually iatrogenic. Causes of hypermagnesemia include therapy with magnesium-containing antacids or laxatives or secondary to administration of parenteral hyperalimentation. Often hypermagnesemia is seen in patients with some degree of renal insufficiency and in preeclamptic or preterm labor patients treated with IV magnesium.

Mild to moderate hypermagnesemia usually is asymptomatic, but patients with severe cases may present with several symptoms. Clinical manifestations are normally seen if magnesium levels are greater than 4 mEq/L. Signs and symptoms include nausea, vomiting, weakness, lethargy, and somnolence. A prolonged PR interval, widening of the QRS complex, and increased T-wave amplitude can be seen with levels greater than 5 mEq/L. Areflexia occurs at levels above 6 to 7 mEq/L. Respiratory arrest, bradycardia, and hypotension can be seen when levels are higher than 10 to 11 mEq/L. Finally, cardiac arrest can occur when serum magnesium is above 14 mEq/L.

Discontinuation of magnesium intake is the primary therapy for symptomatic hypermagnesemia. Patients with severe cases should be given 10% calcium gluconate, 10 to 20 mL IV over 10 minutes. The calcium therapy antagonizes the effects of magnesium and is cardioprotective. Supportive therapy and mechanical ventilation may be necessary in those with respiratory failure. Hemodialysis may be required in patients with hypermagnesemia and renal insufficiency.

Phosphorus

As with magnesium, the majority of phosphorus is contained in the bony skeleton and the intracellular space, and only 1% is found in the ECF. As a result, serum phosphate levels may not accurately reflect total body phosphate stores. A normal range for serum phosphorus is 3 to 4.5 mg/dL. Phosphorus serves as an important energy source by means of high-energy phosphates. It is a key component to protein and lipid structure and is a vital component for carbohydrate metabolism.

Hypophosphatemia

Causes of hypophosphatemia defined as a serum phosphate below 2.5 mg/dL include a redistribution of phosphate into the cells, a decrease in intestinal absorption, or an increase in

TABLE 10.10 Causes of Moderate to Severe Hypophosphatemia (<1.5 mg/dL)
Respiratory alkalosis
Malabsorption
Vitamin D deficiency
Hyperalimentation
Treatment of diabetic ketoacidosis
Hyperparathyroidism
Excessive alcohol use

renal excretion. Several causes of hypophosphatemia are listed in Table 10.10. Most patients with mild hypophosphatemia are asymptomatic. Moderate to severe hypophosphatemia causes neuromuscular abnormalities, including weakness, rhabdomyolysis, paresthesias, confusion, seizures, and coma. Erythrocyte, leukocyte, and platelet dysfunction also can be seen because of a depletion of cellular adenosine triphosphate and 2,3-diphosphoglycerate.

Most patients with serum phosphate levels between 1 and 2.5 mg/dL usually are asymptomatic. Treatment is aimed at correcting the underlying cause. In cases of chronic hypophosphatemia, oral repletion can be instituted at a dose of 500 to 1,000 mg of elemental phosphorus two to three times per day, and the most common side effect is diarrhea. This can be given in the form of sodium/potassium phosphate tablets called Neutra-Phos or Neutra-Phos K (each contains 250 mg of elemental phosphorus). Parenteral administration of phosphorus is indicated when serum phosphorus levels are below 1 mg/dL. Infusion at a dose of 2.5 to 5 mg elemental phosphorus/kg given every 6 hours is recommended. When the serum levels are greater than 1.5 to 2 mg/dL, patients may be switched to oral supplements. Care must be taken to avoid hyperphosphatemia. Also, concomitant calcium supplementation often is needed to prevent hypocalcemia. Serum magnesium, calcium, and potassium levels should be monitored closely.

Hyperphosphatemia

Hyperphosphatemia is relatively rare and is seen either with an increased endogenous or exogenous phosphorus load or with a decrease in renal clearance of phosphorus. Renal failure is the most common cause of hyperphosphatemia. Elevated phosphorus levels also may be seen secondary to rhabdomyolysis, tumor lysis syndrome, hypoparathyroidism, and respiratory or metabolic acidosis. Clinical manifestations include numbness, tingling, muscle cramps, paresthesias, and tetany and are caused by hypocalcemia. Hyperphosphatemia causes hypocalcemia by decreasing calcium absorption from the gastrointestinal tract.

Addressing the underlying cause is the cornerstone of management for hyperphosphatemia. In acute cases, saline diuresis can be used in patients with normal renal function. Additionally, administration of glucose and insulin causes a shift in phosphorus from ECF to the intracellular space. Dialysis may be required if renal failure is present. Oral phosphate binders such as calcium carbonate can be used in patients with chronic hyperphosphatemia.

ACID–BASE METABOLISM

Chemicals that are able to provide a hydrogen ion (H+), such as HCl and H_2CO_2, are defined as acids. Bases are defined as chemicals with the ability to accept a H+ and include OH− and HCO_3^-. The acidity of a solution is governed by the concentration of hydrogen ions it contains. The pH of a system is defined as the negative logarithm of hydrogen ions within that system expressed in moles per liter. The normal pH of human ECF ranges from 7.35 to 7.45.

Buffer Systems

In order for optimal cellular function to occur within the body, the pH must remain in this range. Humans have the ability to absorb excess acids or alkali in circumstances of abnormal pH. The lungs correct for acid–base disorders in an acute setting until the kidneys can compensate. In acidotic states, patients will hyperventilate to decrease CO_2 levels in the blood. Conversely, in alkalotic states, patients will hypoventilate, driving up the level of CO_2 in the blood. Renal function will gradually compensate by retaining or releasing bicarbonate and hydrogen ions. The most important human buffer system is the bicarbonate system. It is the principal extracellular buffer. Organic phosphates and peptides are the other major intracellular buffers.

Table 10.11 shows the directional changes in acid–base parameters for the primary acid–base disorders. If the kidney detects a respiratory acidotic state, CO_2 and H_2O in renal tubule cells are converted by carbonic anhydrase to carbonic acid (H_2CO_3). This dissociates into H_2CO_3, which is secreted back into ECF, and H+, which is exchanged for sodium from the renal tubule. This in effect causes excretion of the hydrogen ion into the urine, where it is buffered with ammonium and phosphate ions or acted on by carbonic anhydrase (in the tubule) to ultimately form CO_2 and H_2O. The CO_2 is absorbed back into the cell, where more bicarbonate can be generated to buffer ECF acidosis. If a patient has a respiratory alkalosis, available levels of CO_2 are low, causing a decrease in hydrogen excretion.

Primary Acid–Base Disorders

Metabolic Acidosis

Metabolic acidosis begins as a reduction in plasma HCO_3 and a rise in H+. In response to these changes, alveolar ventilation is increased, resulting in a decrease in $PaCO_2$ and restoration of H+ toward normal. Metabolic acidosis can be divided into normal anion gap and increased anion gap acidosis. Table 10.12 shows the major causes of metabolic acidosis.

Increased Anion Gap Renal failure, either acute or chronic, can result in an increased anion gap metabolic acidosis resulting from the kidneys' inability to excrete inorganic acids, such as phosphate and sulfate. Organic acid accumulation also results in an increased anion gap metabolic acidosis. In the case of lactic acidosis, cellular respiration is disturbed. This occurs as a result of anaerobic glycolysis in muscle, red blood cells, and other tissues. Conditions such as shock, hypoxemia, and septicemia can produce lactic acidosis by causing inadequate oxygen delivery to tissues. Conditions such as diabetic ketoacidosis, alcoholic ketoacidosis, and starvation cause an accelerated rate of organic acid production by lipolysis and ketogenesis. Ingestion of substances such as salicylates, methanol, ethylene glycol, and paraldehyde can result in an increased anion gap metabolic acidosis.

Normal Anion Gap Normal anion gap metabolic acidosis occurs with abnormal increases in net bicarbonate losses. This can occur when the kidney fails to reabsorb bicarbonate in proximal renal tubular acidosis. The administration of carbonic anhydrase inhibitors can also cause normal anion gap metabolic acidosis. Excessive diarrhea or small bowel/pancreatic drainage can cause bicarbonate losses from the gastrointestinal tract. Hyperchloremic acidosis occurs when the kidney fails to regenerate bicarbonate in conditions such as distal renal tubular acidosis and hyporeninemic hypoaldosteronism. Administration of acid salts can result in chloremic acidosis.

MANAGEMENT

The treatment for metabolic acidosis depends on the severity of acidosis and the underlying cause. A clinical manifestation of metabolic acidosis is hyperventilation. In the surgical patient, metabolic acidosis is commonly due to hypoxia secondary to inadequate tissue perfusion and subsequent accumulation of lactic acid. Volume resuscitation, including blood transfusion, will correct many of these cases of metabolic acidosis. Volume resuscitation and insulin are recommended to correct diabetic ketoacidosis. Patients with this form of metabolic acidosis will often require 4 to 5 L of intravenous fluid on diagnosis. Regular insulin can be given with a loading dose of 15 to 20 IU, followed by a continuous insulin infusion at 5 to 10 IU/h. In cases of renal tubular acidosis, bicarbonate therapy, thiazide diuretics, and a low-salt diet are used for correction.

In cases of acute, severe acidosis (pH <7.1, bicarbonate <10), patients will become dyspneic with depressed cardiac function and mental status changes. It may be necessary to administer intravenous bicarbonate to these patients. In general, the serum bicarbonate concentration should not be acutely raised to levels greater than 15 to 18 mEq/L. Too-rapid correction requires infusion of large amounts of sodium bicarbonate, which can cause overexpansion of the ECF and CHF. Finally,

TABLE 10.11 Primary Disorders of Acid–Base Regulation

ACID–BASE DISTURBANCE	PRIMARY (INITIATING) EVENT	SECONDARY (COMPENSATORY) EVENT	RESULTANT CHANGE IN BLOOD H+ AND PH
Metabolic acidosis	↓ HCO_3^-	↓ PCO_2^-	H+ ↑, pH ↓
Metabolic alkalosis	↑ HCO_3^-	↑ PCO_2 (minimal and only with severe increase in HCO_3^-)	H+ ↓, pH ↑
Respiratory acidosis Acute (24 h)	↑ $PaCO_2$	Negligible ↑ HCO_3^-	H+ ↑, pH ↓
Chronic (3–7 days or longer)	↑ $PaCO_2$	Important ↑ HCO_3^-	
Respiratory alkalosis	↓ $PaCO_2$	↓ HCO_3^-	H+ ↓, pH ↑

TABLE 10.12 Major Causes of Metabolic Acidosis
Increased anion gap
Accumulation of acids
Alcoholic ketoacidosis
Diabetic ketoacidosis
Lactic acidosis
Starvation
Salicylate ingestion
Methanol ingestion
Ethylene glycol ingestion
Paraldehyde ingestion
Reduced excretion of acids
Renal failure
Normal anion gap
Excessive bicarbonate loss
Diarrhea
Ureterosigmoidostomy
Proximal renal tubular acidosis
Small bowel or pancreatic drainage
Carbonic anhydrase inhibitors
Excessive acid production
Ammonium chloride
Arginine HCl
Lysine HCl
Hyperalimentation-containing acids
Decreased renal bicarbonate production
Distal renal tubular acidosis
Hyporeninemic hypoaldosteronism

rapidly restoring the plasma bicarbonate level to normal may produce alkalosis because of persistence of a low $Paco_2$. That is, if plasma bicarbonate is rapidly restored to normal or above in the treatment of metabolic acidosis, alveolar ventilation frequently persists at elevated levels for an additional 24 to 48 hours. Thus, the low Pco_2 with normal plasma bicarbonate level can result in severe alkalosis, which, in turn, can cause cardiac arrhythmias, tetany, and seizures.

METABOLIC ALKALOSIS

Metabolic alkalosis occurs when extracellular bicarbonate concentration is increased and renal excretion of this excess bicarbonate is decreased. This cascade may begin with the loss of a hydrogen ion. The major causes of metabolic alkalosis are listed in Table 10.13.

One of the most common causes of metabolic alkalosis is vomiting or gastric suction. Volume contraction ensues, and bicarbonate is saved in the kidney. Profound potassium depletion can also increase renal reabsorption of bicarbonate and cause a metabolic alkalosis. Diuretics cause a metabolic alkalosis by inducing a sodium chloride excretion without bicarbonate, excretion of potassium, and secondary aldosteronism.

Gastric acid secretion normally has no net effect on acid–base regulation. If the gastric HCl is lost from the body and is not replaced, metabolic alkalosis will ensue (Fig. 10.3).

Mineralocorticoid excess in conditions such as hyperaldosteronism, Bartter syndrome, Liddle syndrome, and Cushing

TABLE 10.13 Major Causes of Metabolic Alkalosis
Extracellular volume depletion
Mineralocorticoid excess
Increased renal acid excretion
Massive alkali administration

syndrome can cause metabolic alkalosis. The mechanism for alkalosis in these conditions is an increase in bicarbonate via the kidneys. Hypercalcemia can result in an increase in proximal tubular reabsorption of bicarbonate leading to metabolic alkalosis. Massive alkali administration in the form of massive blood and/or platelet transfusion or $NaHCO_3$ ingestion can lead to metabolic alkalosis.

Management

Metabolic alkalosis can have serious consequences, such as tetany, major motor seizures, production of hypokalemia and cardiac arrhythmias (particularly in patients receiving digitalis), suppression of alveolar ventilation, and decrease in cerebral blood flow. Furthermore, the presence of metabolic alkalosis often is a sign that the patient is significantly volume contracted. For these reasons, it is important to treat metabolic alkalosis and its underlying causes. Effective treatment consists of replacing sodium, potassium, and chloride deficits as they occur, as discussed. Rarely, it is necessary to treat metabolic alkalosis with IV infusion of hydrochloric acid, ammonium chloride, arginine hydrochloride, or a carbonic anhydrase inhibitor (acetazolamide). This form of treatment is necessary in patients who cannot undergo the sodium bicarbonate diuresis necessary to correct the metabolic alkalosis. This inability usually is the result of severely impaired renal or cardiac function.

Respiratory Acidosis

Inadequate alveolar ventilation leads to respiratory acidosis. Acutely, this can occur with depression of the medullary respiratory center by sedating drugs or narcotics, by impaired respiratory excursion of the thorax by paralysis or trauma, and by airway obstruction. Chronic respiratory acidosis can be seen in conditions such as emphysema, severe kyphoscoliosis, and extreme obesity with Pickwickian syndrome.

Management

The treatment for respiratory acidosis is to increase alveolar ventilation (by endotracheal intubation, mechanical ventilation, or bronchodilation). Within minutes, severe respiratory acidosis can be reversed with adequate ventilation. In patients with chronic respiratory acidosis, severe posthypercapnic alkalosis develops if the $Paco_2$ is rapidly restored to normal and the patient is unable to initiate and sustain a bicarbonate diuresis. This inability usually results from sodium chloride or potassium chloride deficits. If sodium chloride or potassium chloride is provided to correct volume contraction and intracellular potassium deficits, a bicarbonate diuresis ensues, and correction of metabolic alkalosis is achieved.

Respiratory Alkalosis

Respiratory alkalosis occurs when hyperventilation decreases Pco_2, resulting in an increase in pH. Hyperventilation may be secondary to conditions such as pulmonary embolism and CHF, which can cause hypoxia. Fever, sepsis, salicylate toxicity, and hepatic failure all can increase alveolar ventilation and cause respiratory alkalosis. This condition can also be iatrogenically induced by mechanical ventilation. Chronic hyperventilation can be seen in pregnancy, exposure to high altitudes, and underlying pulmonary disease.

Management

The symptoms of acute respiratory alkalosis (e.g., paresthesia, lightheadedness, tetany) can be rapidly controlled by raising $Paco_2$ to normal (e.g., by rebreathing into a paper bag). If the patient is being supported on a ventilator, the dead space can be increased, or tidal volume and respiratory rate can be decreased

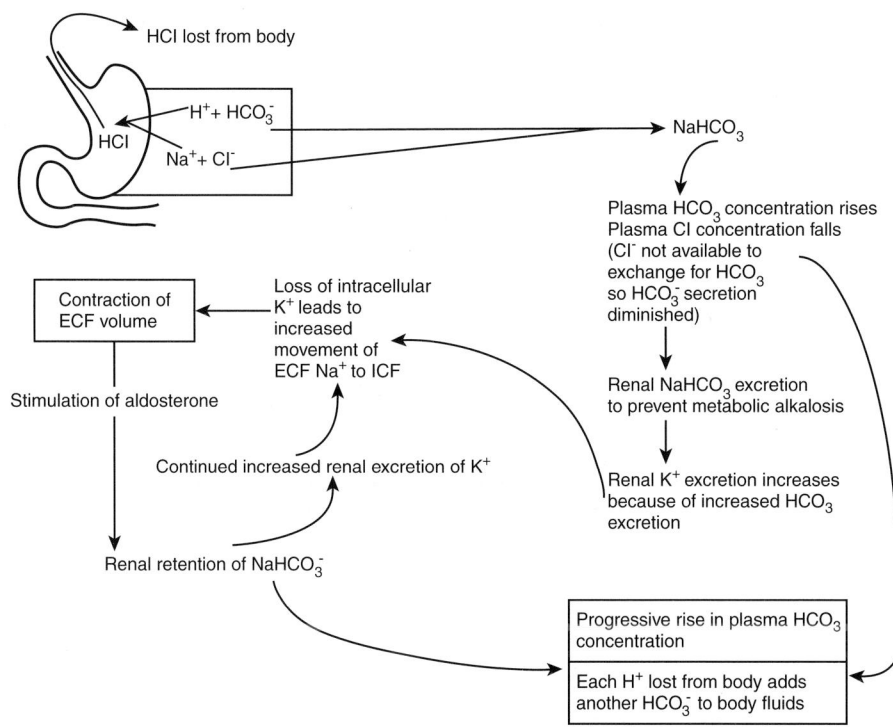

FIGURE 10.3 Pathogenesis of metabolic alkalosis from loss of gastric hydrochloric acid.

while oxygenation is maintained. Definite treatment consists of removing the cause of hyperventilation. Respiratory alkalosis also can cause tetany and seizures and predispose to cardiac arrhythmias (by causing an intracellular shift of potassium), particularly in patients receiving digitalis. If the patient is septic, aggressive measures should be taken to alleviate this. She should be treated with appropriate antibiotics and adequate volume replacement. Surgery may be necessary if the patient has an abscess.

Mixed acid–base disturbances can commonly be seen in severely ill patients. Anion gap measurements and careful evaluation of compensatory changes in the pH, HCO_3^-, and PCO_2 are necessary in the workup and management of these patients. The treatment of mixed acid–base disturbances is aimed at the underlying disease process.

BEST SURGICAL PRACTICES

- An accurate assessment of the effective IVV usually can be made based on a careful clinical assessment of the patient.
- Maintenance fluids in a hospitalized patient should be calculated by taking the body surface area and multiplying by 1,000 to come up with the daily fluid requirement in mL.
- The syndrome of inappropriate antidiuresis has been associated with malignant tumors, CNS disorders, infections, the postoperative state, hypopituitarism, and myxedema, as well as with many drugs. Infusion of oxytocin to induce uterine contraction also can cause hyponatremia because of the antidiuretic effects of oxytocin.
- Symptoms of hyponatremia include increased tendon reflexes, lethargy, mental confusion, and muscle twitching, which are followed by convulsions, coma, and possibly death if levels fall below 115 mEq/L.
- The initial step in correcting either hyponatremia or hypernatremia is an accurate assessment of the patient's volume status.
- Furosemide should not be used to correct hypernatremia or decreased urine output in a patient with decreased IVV.
- Intravenous replacement of potassium should never run at a rate of greater than 10 mEq/h. The oral route of potassium replacement should be used whenever possible.

- In severe life-threatening hyperkalemia (ECG showing sine waves and broad QRS complexes), patients should first receive 10 mL of calcium gluconate IV for cardioprotective purposes. These patients should receive an amp of D50, 10 U of regular insulin, and 50 mEq of sodium bicarbonate. Subsequently, these patients should then receive 20 to 50 g of Kayexalate every 2 to 4 hours and infusions of glucose and insulin.
- Magnesium metabolism is closely related to potassium and calcium levels. In cases of hyponatremia or hypocalcemia, magnesium and potassium must be checked and corrected accordingly.
- If the patient has significant comorbidities, then transfusion may be considered to achieve a higher hemoglobin level, especially prior to surgery.
- For any acid–base disturbance, it is important to elucidate the underlying cause for both the diagnosis and the treatment to be effective and successful.

BIBLIOGRAPHY

Agus Z. Hypomagnesemia. *J Am Soc Nephrol* 1999;10:1616.
Altura BT, Brust M, Bloom S, et al. Magnesium dietary intake modulates blood lipid levels and atherogenesis. *Proc Natl Acad Sci U S A* 1990;87:1840.
American Diabetes Association. Magnesium supplementation in the treatment of diabetes. *Diabetes Care* 1992;14:1065.
Antonelli M, Sandroni C. Hydroxyethyl starch for intravenous volume replacement: more harm than benefit. *JAMA* 2013;309:723.
Aono T, Kurachi K, Miyata M, et al. Influence of surgical stress under general anesthesia on serum gonadotropin levels. *J Clin Endocrinol Metab* 1976;42:144.
Arbus GS. An in vivo acid–base nomogram for clinical use. *Can Med Assoc J* 1973;109:291.
Arieff AI. Hyponatremia, convulsions, respiratory arrest, and permanent brain damage after elective surgery in healthy women. *N Engl J Med* 1986;314:1529.
Arieff AI, deFronzo RA. *Fluid, electrolyte and acid–base disorders.* New York, NY: Churchill Livingstone, 1985.
Ayus JC, Krothapalli RK, Arieff AI. Treatment of symptomatic hyponatremia and its relation to brain damage: a prospective study. *N Engl J Med* 1987;317:1190.
Beutler B, Cerami A. Cachectin and tumor necrosis factor as two sides of the same biological coin. *Nature* 1986;320:584.

Bilezikian JP. Management of acute hypercalcemia. *N Engl J Med* 1992;326:1196.

Breen P. Arterial blood gas and pH analysis: clinical approach and interpretation. *Anesthesiol Clin North Am* 2001;19:885.

Brown JM, Grosso MA, et al. Cytokines, sepsis and the surgeon. *Surg Gynecol Obstet* 1989;169:568.

Claes Y, Van Hemelrijck J, Van Gerven M, et al. Influence of hydroxyethyl starch on coagulation in patients during the perioperative period. *Anesth Analg* 1992;75:24.

Claybaugh JR, Share L. Vasopressin, renin, and cardiovascular responses to continuous slow hemorrhage. *Am J Physiol* 1973;224:519.

Cochrane Injuries Group Albumin Reviewers. Human albumin administration in critically ill patients: systematic review of randomized controlled trials. *BMJ* 1997;317:235.

Cockcroft DW, Gault MH. Prediction of creatinine clearance from serum creatinine. *Nephron* 1976;16:31.

Cohen JJ, Kassirer JP. *Acid base.* Boston, MA: Little, Brown, 1982.

Dacey M. Endocrine and metabolic dysfunction syndromes in the critically ill: hypomagnesemic disorders. *Crit Care Clin* 2001;17:155.

Delaney AP, Dan A, McCaffrey J, et al. The role of albumin as a resuscitation fluid for patients with sepsis: a systematic review and meta-analysis. *Crit Care Med* 2011;39:386.

Epstein FH. Signs and symptoms of electrolyte disorders. In: Maxwell MH, Kleeman CR, eds. *Clinical disorders of fluid and electrolyte metabolism.* New York, NY: McGraw-Hill, 1980.

Fisken RA, Heath DA, Somers S, et al. Hypercalcemia in hospital patients: clinical and diagnostic aspects. *Lancet* 1981;1:202.

Fuss M, Cogan E, Gillet C, et al. Magnesium administration reverses the hypocalcaemia secondary to hypomagnesemia despite low circulating levels of 25-hydroxyvitamin D and 1,25-dihydroxyvitamin D. *Endocrinology* 1985;22:807.

Golzarian J, Scott WH. Hypermagnesemia induced paralytic ileus. *Dig Dis Sci* 1994;39:1138.

Haase N, et al. Hydroxyethyl starch 130/0.38-0.45 versus crystalloid or albumin in patients with sepsis: systematic review with meta-analysis and trial sequential analysis. *BMJ* 2013;346:f839.

Harrington JL. Metabolic alkalosis. *Kidney Int* 1984;26:88.

Heinsimer JA, Lefkowitz RJ. Adrenergic receptors: biochemistry, regulation, molecular mechanisms and clinical indications. *J Lab Clin Med* 1982;100:641.

Kapoor M, Chan G. Fluid and electrolyte abnormalities. *Crit Care Clin* 2001;17:503.

Kendler KS, Weitzman RE, Fisher DA. The effect of pain on plasma arginine vasopressin concentrations in man. *Clin Endocrinol* 1978;8:89.

Klahr S. *The kidney and body fluids in health and disease.* New York, NY: Plenum, 1984.

Klee GG, Kao PC, Heath H III. Hypercalcemia. *Endocrinol Metab Clin North Am* 1988;573:600.

Knochel JP. Neuromuscular manifestation of electrolyte disorder. *Am J Med* 1982;72:521.

Lennon EJ, Lemann J Jr. Fluid and electrolyte balance. In: Te Linde RW, Mattingly RF, eds. *Operative gynecology,* 6th ed. Philadelphia, PA: JB Lippincott, 1985.

Leone BJ, Spahn DR. Anemia, hemodilution, and oxygen delivery. *Anesth Analg* 1992;75:651.

Levi M, Cronin RE, Knochel JP. Disorders of phosphate and magnesium metabolism. In: Coe FC, Favus MJ, eds. *Disorders of bone and mineral metabolism.* New York, NY: Raven, 1992:587.

Major P, Lortholary A, Hon J, et al. Zoledronic acid is superior to pamidronate in the treatment of hypercalcemia of malignancy: a pooled analysis of two randomized, controlled clinical trials. *J Clin Oncol* 2001;19:558.

Martinez F, Lash R. Intensive care unit complications: endocrinologic and metabolic complications in the intensive care unit. *Clin Chest Med* 1999;20:401.

Matthay MA. Invasive hemodynamic monitoring in critically ill patients. *Clin Chest Med* 1983;4:233.

Maxwell MH, Kleeman CR, Narins RG. *Clinical disorders of fluid and electrolyte metabolism,* 4th ed. New York, NY: McGraw-Hill, 1987.

Narins RG. Therapy of hyponatremia: does haste make waste? *N Engl J Med* 1986;314:1573.

Narins RG, Emmett M. Simple and mixed acid–base disorders: a practical approach. *Medicine* 1980;59:161.

Ponce SP, Jennings AE, Madias NE, et al. Drug-induced hyperkalemia. *Medicine* 1985;64:357.

Riggs JE. Neurologic manifestations of electrolyte disturbances. *Neurol Clin* 2002;20:227.

Roacha E, Silva M, Velasco IT, et al. Hypertonic saline resuscitation: saturated salt-dextran solutions are equally effective, but induce hemolysis in dogs. *Crit Care Med* 1990;18:203.

Robertson G, Aycinesa P, Zerbe R. Neurogenic disorders of osmoregulation. *Am J Med* 1986;2:339.

Schrier RW. Pathogenesis of sodium and water retention in high-output and low-output cardiac failure, nephrotic syndrome, cirrhosis and pregnancy. *N Engl J Med* 1988;319:1065.

Schrier RW, ed. *Renal and electrolyte disorders,* 2nd ed. Boston, MA: Little, Brown, 1980.

Skillman JJ, Lauler DP, Hickler RB, et al. Hemorrhage in normal man: effect of renin, cortisol, aldosterone, and urine composition. *Ann Surg* 1967;166:865.

Slotman GJ, Burchard KW, Gann DS. Thromboxane and prostacyclin in clinical acute respiratory failure. *J Surg Res* 1985;39:1.

Spiegel A. The parathyroid glands: hypercalcemia and hypocalcemia. In: Goldman L, ed. *Cecil textbook of medicine,* 21st ed. Philadelphia, PA: WB Saunders, 2000:1399.

Steiner RW. Interpreting the fractional excretion of sodium. *Am J Med* 1984;77:699.

Vincent JL, Navickis RJ, Wilkes MM. Morbidity in hospitalized patients receiving human albumin: a meta-analysis of randomized, controlled trials. *Crit Care Med* 2004;32:2029.

Waters J, Miller L. Cause of metabolic acidosis in prolonged surgery. *Crit Care Med* 1999;27:2142.

Wilkes MM, Navickis RJ. Patient survival after human albumin administration: a meta-analysis of randomized, controlled trials. *Ann Intern Med* 2001;135:149.

Williams SE. Hydrogen ion infusion for treating severe metabolic alkalosis. *BMJ* 1976;2:1189.

Zarychanski R, Abou-Setta AM, Turgeon AF, et al. Association of hydroxyethyl starch administration with mortality and acute kidney injury in critically ill patients requiring volume resuscitation: a systematic review and meta-analysis. *JAMA* 2013;309:678.

Ziegler, R. Hypercalcemic crisis. *J Am Soc Nephrol* 2001;12 (17 suppl):S3.

CHAPTER 11
Postoperative Infections: Prevention and Management

W. David Hager and Mark J. Dougherty

DEFINITIONS

Bacteremia—Infection of the bloodstream can complicate any pelvic infection, but is seen most frequently in association with abscesses, peritonitis, and necrotizing fasciitis.

Cuff cellulitis—A soft tissue infection of the surgical margin in the upper vagina where the uterus was removed.

Drug fever—Elevated temperature that is due to an adverse reaction to medications.

Febrile morbidity—A temperature of 38°C (100.4°F) or greater recorded on two occasions, at least 6 hours apart, more than 24 hours after the surgical procedure.

Necrotizing fasciitis—A severe synergistic bacterial infection of the fascia, subcutaneous tissue, and skin that is often caused by group A beta-hemolytic streptococci, often in combination with other bacteria including methacillin-resistant *Staphylococcus aureus* (MRSA), anaerobes, and aerobic, gram-negative bacilli.

Surgical Site Infections (SSI)—Recent CDC criteria for SSI's have been developed using National Health Safety Network (NHSN) criteria; NHSN data provide regularly updated risk stratified rates of SSI for comparison between individual surgeons and between hospitals. (Edwards and colleagues, 2009).

Urinary tract infection—The criterion for defining a urinary tract infection (UTI) is more than 100,000 colonies/mL of a single pathogen from a clean-catch urine and more than 10,000 colonies/mL from a catheterized specimen.

Vaginal cuff hematoma/cuff abscess—A walled-off collection of blood originating from an oozing vascular pedicle or along the vaginal cuff. If the collection becomes infected, it creates an abscess.

Wound cellulitis—Soft tissue infection localized to the skin and adipose tissue above the fascia that is characterized by erythema, warmth, swelling, and tenderness.

Wound seroma—A collection of serous fluid beneath the skin surface.

Infection complicating surgical procedures has been the consternation of gynecologists since the first operations were performed. Multiple interventions have proven value in reduction of SSI, including appropriate perioperative antimicrobial prophylaxis, avoidance of shaving, appropriate skin preparation (such as with chlorhexidine/alcohol), and monitoring of surgeon-specific infection rates.

It is imperative that the gynecologic surgeon understand basic infectious disease concepts in order to treat infected patients appropriately. Diagnosis and treatment are not guesswork but depend on understanding basic principles.

An understanding of bacteria that are a part of the normal vaginal flora enables the gynecologist to recognize the pathogenic bacteria that contribute to postoperative infection. Certain risk factors play a role in increasing postoperative infection rates. Knowledge of these factors can enable the surgeon to take action to alter those risks, and/or be alert for those who are at increased risk. There are various types of postoperative infection, each with its own unique time of onset and usual bacterial etiology. Knowledge about likely causes of a disorder can facilitate decision making when an antibiotic is empirically selected to treat the patient.

Appropriate patient evaluation, including proper culturing techniques, is critical to this diagnostic process. Steps to prevent infection must become routine with every surgeon on every case. These steps are necessary not only for the operator but also for all personnel participating in the surgical and medical management of the patient. These steps are described later in this chapter.

FEBRILE MORBIDITY

In the evaluation of patients who have an elevated temperature in the postoperative period, it is important to recognize that all febrile morbidity is not infectious morbidity. Treating a fever without a definite cause of infection will often do more harm than good.

Several different definitions of febrile morbidity have been used, and this may create confusion for the surgeon. The most frequent definition is a temperature of 38°C (100.4°F) or greater recorded on two occasions, at least 6 hours apart, more than 24 hours after the surgical procedure. This excludes a fever during the first 24 hours. Operative site infections during this time are unusual unless there is preexisting infection at the operative site or gross contamination of the site. Some

investigators have used a definition of a single temperature elevation of 39°C (102°F) or greater recorded on any occasion in the postoperative period as indicative of febrile morbidity. We prefer the former definition.

Regardless of the choice of definition of febrile morbidity, it is important to treat infection and not fever. Fever may trigger sensitivity to the possibility of infection, but complete assessment of the patient including assessment for UTI, pneumonia, pelvic infection, DVT, intravascular catheter infection, and drug fever should be performed before antibiotic treatment is initiated.

INCIDENCE

New NHSN definitions for SSI have been created and data collected so that hospitals and surgeons can be compared through public reporting. Many states now legally require public reporting of health care associated events, including SSI. The Centers for Medicare and Medicaid Services has initiated "Pay-for-performance" programs that include financial penalties/rewards based on provider performance with SSI rates used as part of the formula. National Health Safety Network data provide risk-stratified percentile rates so that, for instance, median abdominal hysterectomy rates for risk class 0, 1, and 2/3 in 2008 were 0.32, 1.61, and 3.41, respectively. Hospitals in the top 25th percentile had zero infections. The U.S. Department of Health and Human Services has set a national 5-year target to reduce SSI by 25% starting in 2012. In order to achieve this goal, risk factors for infection will need to be reduced.

VAGINAL FLORA

The most frequent source of bacteria that cause postoperative pelvic infection among women is the vagina. The vagina is colonized by large numbers of a variety of bacteria that normally exist in a symbiotic relationship. Several factors influence the vaginal flora, including age, sexual activity, stage of the menstrual cycle, use of antibiotic or immunosuppressive agents, and any invasive procedure.

Mean bacterial counts in vaginal secretions are 10^8 to 10^9 bacteria/mL, with three to six different species present. The most frequent aerobic bacteria are *Lactobacilli* sp., *Gardnerella vaginalis*, coagulase-negative *Staphylococcus*, *Corynebacterium* sp., *Enterococcus faecalis* species of *Streptococcus*, and *Enterobacteriaceae*. Anaerobes outnumber aerobes and include *Peptostreptococcus* sp., *Peptococcus* sp., *Prevotella bivia*, *Prevotella disiens*, and members of the *Bacteroides fragilis* group (Table 11.1). These same bacteria are frequently isolated from sites of pelvic infection among women who have undergone gynecologic surgery. This indicates, as Schottmueller proposed at the turn of the century, that pelvic infections are principally a result of endogenous sources of bacteria. The concepts of antibiotic prophylaxis and antiseptic douching before surgery or preoperative placement of antiseptic gel are related to reducing these large numbers of bacteria. Although investigators have found that colonization rates change in relation to the stage of the menstrual cycle, no data have supported the concept that timing of gynecologic surgery in relation to menses alters infection rates.

Surgery itself alters the numbers and types of bacteria in the vagina and cervix. After vaginal and abdominal hysterectomy, the number of lactobacilli decreases, and the number of facultative gram-negative rods, *B. fragilis* group species, and enterococci increases. Preoperative hospitalization before surgery on a gynecologic ward also alters the vaginal flora in a direction toward more virulent organisms.

TABLE 11.1 Bacteria Composing Normal Vaginal Flora

AEROBES	ANAEROBES
Staphylococcus aureus	*Peptostreptococcus* sp.
Coagulase-negative Staphylococcus	*Peptococcus* sp.
Group B streptococcus	*Bacteroides* sp.
Streptococcus sp.	*Fusobacterium* sp.
Enterococcus faecalis	*Prevotella bivia*
Lactobacilli	*Prevotella disiens*
Corynebacterium sp. *Escherichia coli* *Klebsiella* sp. *Gardnerella vaginalis*	*Bacteroides fragilis* group

RISK FACTORS FOR INFECTION

Several factors alter the infectious risk morbidity of postoperative patients (Table 11.2). Many of these risk factors may be modified by the surgeon. Appropriate use of perioperative antibiotic prophylaxis, including administration within 1 hour of incision, significantly reduces infection risk. Blood glucose control in diabetes and reduction of immunosuppressive medications may decrease risk. Avoidance of hair removal at the surgical site, especially shaving, by the patient or operative team may significantly reduce risk. Skin preparation with chlorhexidine/alcohol or other appropriate antiseptic also reduces postoperative infection rate. Strict adherence to hand hygiene by health care personnel in the preoperative, perioperative, and postoperative period may also play a significant role in SSI risk.

When a hysterectomy is performed through an infected operative site, there is an increased risk of postoperative infection. Likewise, contamination of the operative field by break

TABLE 11.2 Risk Factors for Postoperative Infection

Altered immunocompetence
Premenopausal age
Obesity
Radical surgery
Bacterial vaginosis
Prolonged preoperative hospitalization
Excessive intraoperative blood loss
Hematoma or serous fluid collection
Operator inexperience/surgical skill
Lower socioeconomic status
Prolonged operative time
Poor nutrition
Excessive devitalized (necrotic) tissue
Foreign bodies
Diabetes mellitus
Systemic disease
Failure to use prophylactic antibiotics correctly
Shaving of the operative site
Inadequate skin preparation
Surgery in an infected operative site

in sterile technique or injury to the bowel promotes infection. Duration of surgery is considered to be a risk for infection in most studies, but this actually may reflect experience of the operating surgeon, complexity of the case, or inadequate hemostasis. Lack of adequate hemostasis increases the risk of undrained collections of blood and creates an ideal culture medium for contaminating bacteria. Low hemoglobin and hematocrit levels, preoperatively or postoperatively, have been mentioned as factors in increased rates of postoperative infection, especially of abdominal incisions. No data, however, have indicated that raising the volume of red blood cells decreases the rate of infection. Leaving an excessive amount of devitalized tissue (e.g., large, ligated pedicles) and failure to close dead spaces can predispose to a greater risk of infection. Pedicles should be trim and dry, dead space should be closed, and hemostasis obtained. Lysis of adhesions may increase the risk of infection if a bowel injury occurs.

The use of a vaginal cuff drain has been shown to have a significant beneficial effect on decreasing morbidity but has fallen out of favor because of the simplicity and effectiveness of antibiotic prophylaxis.

Bacterial vaginosis, characterized by increased vaginal concentrations of certain anaerobic and facultative bacteria, has been shown to increase the relative risk of postoperative infection in gynecologic procedures. The presence of increased concentrations of pathogenic bacteria adjacent to the site of incision in the vagina allows for ascending spread of these organisms in a susceptible host. Although treatment of bacterial vaginosis in pregnant women may decrease their risk of preterm delivery and preterm, premature rupture of membranes, no studies have shown a decreased rate of postoperative infection in bacterial vaginosis–positive women treated before gynecologic surgery.

ETIOLOGY

All women have bacteria colonizing the vagina in greater or lesser numbers. Women without symptoms have a mean of 4.2 species present. It is these same bacteria normally existing in a symbiotic relationship that ultimately can invade tissue altered by surgery, leading to clinical infection. The virulence of the bacteria and the volume inoculated are countered by the host's immune defense mechanisms and may be aided by prophylactic antibiotics to combat the occurrence of infection.

The bacteria listed in Table 11.3, which are responsible for postoperative infection after gynecologic surgery, are the same organisms that can be recovered from vaginal cultures of women before hysterectomy, according to Hemsell. The volume of bacteria present and their proximity to the operative site promote a polymicrobial infection in women who experience posthysterectomy infectious morbidity. Aerobic bacteria may initiate the infectious process; as tissue is devitalized and the oxidation reduction potential is altered, anaerobes proliferate and add to the tissue damage. Large, necrotic tissue pedicles and undrained collections of blood are ideal sites for infection to occur. Once the infection has begun, the body's host immune defense mechanisms initiate an inflammatory response, and attempt to wall off and localize the infection. Infected hematomas and abscesses can result when this occurs.

CATEGORIES OF INFECTION

Not all women who have temperature elevation after gynecologic surgery are infected, and not all of those who are infected have the same clinical syndrome. It is important to categorize the infectious process because treatment can vary accordingly.

TABLE 11.3 Pathogens Responsible for Infections After Gynecologic Surgery

Aerobic gram-positive cocci
Staphylococcus aureus
Coagulase-negative Staphylococcus
Streptococcus viridans group
Group B streptococci
Streptococcus faecalis

Aerobic gram-negative bacilli
Escherichia coli
Proteus mirabilis
Klebsiella sp.
Gardnerella vaginalis

Anaerobes
Peptostreptococcus sp.
Peptococcus sp.
Prevotella bivia
Prevotella disiens
Bacteroides melaninogenicus
Bacteroides capillosus
Bacteroides fragilis group
 B. fragilis
 B. ovatus
 B. thetaiotaomicron
 B. distasonis
 B. vulgatus
Clostridium perfringens
Fusobacterium sp.

Cuff Cellulitis

Cuff cellulitis is an infection of the surgical margin in the upper vagina where the uterus was removed. Symptoms and signs of infection usually begin late in the hospital course or even after discharge from the hospital. These patients' immediate postoperative course may have been completely benign. There is always an element of induration, erythema, and edema in the vaginal cuff immediately after hysterectomy. If the patient becomes infected, she will often have initial symptoms of lower abdominal pain, pelvic pain, back pain, fever, and abnormal vaginal discharge. Examination may reveal persistent hyperemia, induration, and tenderness of the vaginal cuff, and possibly purulent discharge along with fever. The parametrial and adnexal areas are nontender. The white blood cell count usually is mildly to moderately elevated.

Gram-positive aerobes, facultative gram-negative aerobes, and obligate anaerobes can all contribute to the cause of cuff cellulitis. Single- or multiple-agent broad-spectrum antibiotic coverage is effective in treating this infection, although single agents usually are preferred to reduce costs and the likelihood of an allergic reaction.

Infected Vaginal Cuff Hematoma or Cuff Abscess

Hysterectomy can result in small amounts of oozing from vascular pedicles or along the vaginal cuff. This bleeding may result in a walled-off collection of blood called a hematoma. If this localized mass above the vaginal cuff becomes infected, an abscess may result. Bacteria, especially anaerobes, flourish in this environment.

Women with a vaginal cuff abscess present with fever that is usually early in the postoperative period. Other symptoms include chills, pelvic pain, and rectal pressure. Clinical findings include temperature elevation; lower abdominal and vaginal cuff tenderness; the presence of a tender, fluctuant mass near the cuff; and, occasionally, purulent drainage from the cuff. The pain and tenderness is often more predominant on one side.

An infected cuff hematoma actually can present later in the postoperative course than an abscess and usually is associated with a drop in the hemoglobin and hematocrit levels. The hematoma may not be readily palpable but can be delineated on pelvic ultrasound or computed tomographic (CT) scan.

Postoperative Ovarian Abscess

The patient who develops fever and abdominal and pelvic pain late in the postoperative hospital course or after hospital discharge may have a pelvic abscess, possibly of ovarian origin. If there is a sudden increase in abdominal or pelvic pain, a rupture may have occurred. A ruptured abscess should be managed as a surgical emergency, proceeding to a laparoscopy or a laparotomy with excision or drainage of the infected mass. The inciting site for an ovarian abscess is a place of recent follicle expulsion or a site of surgical trauma to an ovary in a premenopausal woman. Ovaries should not be aspirated or probed at the time of hysterectomy for fear that bacteria from the vagina may penetrate the ovary and initiate infection. Once again, anaerobes are the predominant bacteria in an ovarian abscess.

If an ovarian abscess is suspected, then a CT scan should be ordered. The CT scan not only identifies the size and location of the abscess but also allows for visualization and evaluation of the ureters, bladder, and colon. A pelvic ultrasound also may be useful to localize the abscess but does not provide the ancillary information. Many abscesses respond to broad-spectrum antibiotic therapy; but if a tender, fluctuant mass persists, drainage is necessary. A radiologic interventionist may be able to accomplish percutaneous drainage with a needle or catheter using CT or ultrasound guidance, or colpotomy drainage may be possible. For colpotomy drainage to be accomplished safely, the abscess must be fluctuant, fixed in the cul-de-sac, and dissecting the upper third of the rectovaginal septum. With either approach, a closed suction drain should be placed to ensure complete and continued evacuation during the next 2 to 3 days. Some abscesses are amenable to a laparoscopic approach with incision and drainage. Copious irrigation and suctioning are critical if this approach is chosen.

Septic Pelvic Thrombophlebitis

Septic pelvic thrombophlebitis (SPT) complicates gynecologic surgery in 0.1% to 0.5% of procedures. It is usually a diagnosis of exclusion, made when a postoperative patient with febrile morbidity does not respond to appropriate parenteral antibiotic therapy in the absence of an undrained abscess or infected hematoma. The development of SPT is enhanced by venous stasis (e.g., obesity, diabetes), vascular injury, or bacterial contamination of pelvic vessels.

Two forms of SPT have been described. The classic form is seen in association with abdominal surgery. This form occurs 2 to 4 days after surgery and is characterized by fever, tachycardia, gastrointestinal distress, unilateral abdominal pain, and, in 50% to 67% of cases, a palpable abdominal cord resulting from acute thrombus formation. The enigmatic form complicates parturition or pelvic surgery and is characterized by spiking temperatures despite clinical improvement on antibiotics; tachycardia during the temperature spikes; and small, diffusely scattered thrombi in small pelvic vessels. Pelvic findings are minimal in both forms. The diagnosis often may be confirmed by CT scan or magnetic resonance imaging (MRI).

The traditional mainstay of treatment for SPT is anticoagulation with heparin for 7 to 10 days. Some experts recommend changing antibiotics or extending coverage before heparin is considered. All patients should be treated with antibiotics effective against heparinase-producing *Bacteroides* sp. Long-term anticoagulation is not required unless septic pulmonary emboli have occurred. Lysis of fever may occur 24 to 48 hours after starting heparin, yet other cases may require much longer for complete resolution. Treatment should be continued until the patient is afebrile for 48 hours and clinically well.

Osteitis Pubis

Osteitis pubis rarely complicates gynecologic procedures adjacent to the symphysis pubis, such as retropubic urethral suspension, radical vulvectomy, or pelvic exenteration. Direct or contiguous seeding of the periosteum from pelvic bacteria results in a delayed-onset infection 6 to 8 weeks after the original procedure. Patients report pain and tenderness along the symphysis pubis, especially with ambulation. Low-grade fever, an elevated erythrocyte sedimentation rate, and a moderate leukocytosis have been reported, as well as positive cultures from blood or the bone itself. Aggressive antibiotic therapy covering *Staphylococcus aureus* and facultative gram-negative bacilli is essential for adequate recovery. If the response is not adequate, surgical debridement of the pubis is necessary.

Wound Infection

Surgical wound infection is possible with any transabdominal gynecologic procedure, but especially with those that are contaminated. Extensive study of the epidemiology of wound infections resulted in a classification of operative wounds in relation to contamination and increasing risk of infection (Table 11.4). Because the vagina is entered during hysterectomy, even an uninfected hysterectomy is classified as a clean-contaminated operation. Fortunately, prophylactic antibiotics and minimally invasive, laparoscopic procedures have greatly reduced the risk of severe, surgical wound infections.

The Centers for Disease Control and Prevention (CDC) definitions of surgical wound infection were modified by Horan et al. This system divides infections into two major categories: (a) an organ/space surgical site infection (SSI) and (b) superficial and deep incision infection. An SSI may be in any anatomic area that was opened or manipulated during a surgical procedure other than the incision itself. This would include most of the infections that develop after hysterectomy. It must develop within 30 days of the procedure and be accompanied by one of the following: diagnosis by a surgeon or attending physician; an abscess or other evidence of infection identified during reoperation or by radiologic or histopathologic examination; aseptically obtained organ/space fluid or tissue, the culture of which resulted in bacterial isolates; or purulent drainage from a drain placed through a stab wound into the organ/space.

Wound Cellulitis

Abdominal wound infections are categorized by their location and severity. The least severe are localized to the skin and adipose tissue above the fascia. Wound cellulitis is characterized by erythema, warmth, swelling, and tenderness. If there is no purulent drainage, antibiotic therapy alone with a cephalosporin or augmented penicillin often is effective. *S. aureus*, coagulase-negative staphylococci, and streptococci cause most of these infections. If wound cellulitis fails to improve, the possibility of resistant organism infection, such as MRSA, or occult abscess should be considered.

TABLE 11.4 Classification of Operative Wounds in Relation to Contamination and Increasing Risk of Infection

Clean
  Elective, primarily closed and undrained
  Nontraumatic, uninfected
  No inflammation encountered
  No break in aseptic technique
  Respiratory, alimentary, genitourinary tracts not entered

Clean-Contaminated
  Alimentary, respiratory, or genitourinary tract entered under controlled conditions and without unusual contamination
  Appendectomy
  Vagina entered
  Genitourinary tract entered in absence of culture-positive urine
  Minor break in technique
  Mechanical drainage

Contaminated
  Open, fresh traumatic wounds
  Gross spillage from gastrointestinal tract
  Entrance of genitourinary tract in presence of infected urine
  Major break in technique
  Incisions in which acute nonpurulent inflammation is present

Dirty or Infected
  Traumatic wound with retained devitalized tissue, foreign bodies, fecal contamination, or delayed treatment, or wounds from a dirty source
  Perforated viscus encountered
  Acute bacterial inflammation with pus encountered during operation

Source: Altemeier WA, Burke JF, Pruitt BA, et al. *Manual on control of infection in surgical patients*, 2nd ed. Philadelphia: JB Lippincott, 1984:28, with permission.

Wound Seroma

A collection of serous fluid beneath the skin surface is a seroma. A small amount of serous drainage may be managed with limited opening of the incision, drainage, and cleansing. Larger collections may require more extensive incision and drainage. Antibiotic therapy is not necessary with an uninfected seroma. If a seroma intermittently or continuously leaks, it may become infected and require antibiotic therapy.

Deep Wound Infection

When purulent drainage is noted, the wound should be opened widely to allow drainage and removal of necrotic tissue. The incision should be probed gently to evaluate fascial integrity. If the fascia is intact, healing is hastened by mechanical debridement followed by loose, wet-to-dry packing with gauze moistened with saline; dilute hydrogen peroxide (1:1 mixture with saline) or Dakin's solution, 0.5%. Povidone–iodine is to be discouraged because it does not promote the development of granulation tissue. An antibiotic effective against anaerobes such as piperacillin–tazobactam, metronidazole, or a carbapenem must be used.

Evisceration of bowel may occur if the infection involves the fascia. This is a surgical emergency requiring identification of the defect, freshening of the fascial edges, placement of intra-abdominal and subcutaneous closed suction drains, and reinforced closure of the fascia. Some surgeons leave the skin open for delayed closure; others close it primarily.

Necrotizing Fasciitis

This severe complication results from synergistic bacterial infection of the fascia, subcutaneous tissue, and skin. This rapidly progressive infection is initially characterized by pain and toxicity out of proportion to physical findings with subsequent development with cutaneous necrosis and hemorrhagic bullae. Perineal necrotizing fasciitis is commonly caused by group A, beta-hemolytic streptococci, but may be a polymicrobial, synergistic infection with anaerobic bacteria or *Clostridium perfringens*. Methicillin-resistant Staphylococcus aureus has been increasingly identified as a causative agent, and empiric IV antibiotics may be needed to cover this organism, pending culture data. Diabetes, alcoholism, and immunocompromise all represent significant risk factors for development of necrotizing fasciitis. Patients usually present with severe pain in the area of involvement; clinical signs of sepsis; and a viscous, cloudy, malodorous drainage. The wound edges may be purple or even necrotic. If gangrene occurs in the area of fasciitis, bullae of the skin and crepitus in the subcutaneous tissue may occur. Necrotizing fasciitis carries a high mortality potential and may be initially difficult to recognize. Therefore, a high index of suspicion must be maintained. Although C/T and MRI scans may be of benefit in the diagnosis of necrotizing fasciitis, aggressive surgical intervention/exploration and antibiotic therapy with activity against beta-hemolytic streptococci, anaerobes, enteric gram-negative bacilli, and MRSA should be initiated.

Urinary Tract Infection

Infection of the lower urinary tract is a frequent complication of gynecologic surgery. The patient may have low-grade fever, dysuria, frequency, and urgency, but in many situations has no symptoms. The criterion for defining a UTI is more than 100,000 colonies/mL of a single pathogen from clean-catch urine and more than 10,000 colonies/mL from a catheterized specimen. Appropriate sterile technique for insertion and management of indwelling catheters is important in preventing UTI. In general, urethral catheters should be removed as soon as possible after surgery unless the surgery has involved the bladder itself. Attachment of the urethral catheter to the leg with a locking device lowers UTI risk by preventing pistoning that leads to secondary urethral trauma. Treatment of a documented UTI should be with an appropriate oral or parenteral antibiotic. Although quinolone antibiotic previously provided antibiotic activity against most urinary pathogens, increasing quinolone resistance has limited quinolone efficacy. Alternate antibiotic choices include trimethoprim/sulfamethoxazole, amoxicillin/clavulanic acid, and cefpodoxime. Some *Escherichia coli* strains with quinolone, trimethoprim–sulfamethoxazole, and amoxicillin/clavulanic acid resistance are still sensitive to cefpodoxime. Some *E. coli* strains are now so highly resistant that only carbapenem therapy is effective.

Bacteremia

Infection of the bloodstream can complicate any pelvic infection but is seen more frequently in association with abscesses, peritonitis, and SPT. Antibiotics effective against the isolated organism should be used. Duration of therapy for gram-negative bacteremia

should be 7 to 14 days. Parenteral antibiotics should be used initially but may be converted to oral if improvement has occurred and the patient has been afebrile for 24 to 48 hours. Antibiotic duration for *S. aureus* bacteremia should be 2 to 6 weeks of parenteral antibiotics due to the frequency of metastatic infection with serious sequelae, including endocarditis. Infectious disease consultation should be considered for *S. aureus* bacteremia or fungemia due to the high risk of serious secondary complications. Therapeutic intervention for bacteremia/fungemia includes identification and eradication of the source.

Drug Fever

This diagnosis should be considered when appropriate parenteral antibiotics have been used, and there are no localizing signs of infection, normal or low WBC, eosinophilia, rash, elevated liver enzymes, no undrained fluid collection, and no evidence of SPT. Fevers associated with medications may be unusually high, in some cases greater than 105°F. Medications that are more common causes of drug fever, such as antibiotics, metoclopramide, anti-convulsants, antipsychotics, and allopurinol, should be discontinued.

EVALUATION OF THE PATIENT WITH SUSPECTED INFECTION

Fever is the most common sign of postoperative infection, but it is important to remember that fever is not always caused by infection in the postoperative patient (Table 11.5). In a large study of 537 women who underwent major gynecologic surgery, Fanning et al. found that 39% developed postoperative fever, but only 17 patients (8%) actually had a documented infection. Other signs and symptoms of postoperative infection can include erythema, induration, and/or tenderness around the incision, drain, or intravenous infusion site; leg pain; tenderness or swelling; costovertebral angle (CVA) tenderness; cough; or dysuria. When any of these or other signs or symptoms alerts the surgeon to the possibility of a postoperative

---

TABLE 11.5 Fever Evaluation in Gynecologic Patients

History
  Time of onset
  Surgical procedure
  Risk factors
  Antibiotic prophylaxis
  Symptoms
  Ancillary illnesses

Physical Examination
  Upper respiratory
  Lower respiratory
  Gastrointestinal
  Urinary tract
  Wound
  Pelvis

Laboratory
  Complete blood cell count with differential
  Catheterized urinalysis
  Chemistry panel
    Cultures
    Urine
    Blood
    Surgical site

infection, an appropriate workup is indicated. A diagnosis of infection should be made or at least a high probability of infection should be present before antibiotics are started.

History

Careful history taking often can be the source of helpful clues to the cause of postoperative infection. The time of onset of the complicating infection is important. Ledger emphasized that the interval between surgery and the onset of fever is helpful in determining the cause of infection. For example, Garibaldi and colleagues suggested that most cases of early postoperative fever are not infectious in origin. Possible noninfectious causes include pulmonary atelectasis, hypersensitivity reactions to antibiotics or anesthetics, pyrogenic reactions to tissue trauma, or hematoma formation. Infectious causes of early postoperative fever include aspiration pneumonia, group A α-hemolytic streptococcal wound infection, or surgery in a previously infected site (e.g., pelvic inflammatory disease or recent D&C or cone biopsy). Other important aspects of history include the surgical procedures performed (e.g., abdominal versus vaginal approach, whether ovaries were invaded), risk factors encountered (pelvic abscess, bowel injury), use of antibiotic prophylaxis, symptoms, and whether the patient had any ancillary illnesses (smoking history, history of cardiac valvular disease, immunosuppression).

Physical Examination

Gynecologic surgeons tend to focus on the pelvis as the source of all postoperative infections. Instead, a comprehensive evaluation of the entire patient should be carried out. The upper respiratory tract should be examined to rule out otitis, pharyngitis, and bronchitis and the lower respiratory tract to rule out pneumonia. The gastrointestinal tract should be checked to evaluate bowel function, distention, and tenderness. Breast examination is usually only important in postpartum patients. The urinary tract should be evaluated, and the possibility of pyelonephritis must be considered. Intravenous access, especially central lines or other indwelling foreign bodies, should be carefully inspected and palpated for evidence of infection. The surgical wound must be examined carefully, and if the site of infection has not been identified or symptoms suggest a pelvic infection, a pelvic examination should be carried out. The pelvic examination should evaluate the vaginal cuff for discharge, erythema, and induration. Palpation for tenderness and for masses should be done and cultures obtained if pus is identified.

Laboratory and Imaging Evaluation

In recent years, it has become clear that a routine postoperative "fever workup"—including a variety of studies, such as a complete blood count, urine analysis, chest x-ray, and multiple cultures—is largely unrewarding in identifying the site of postoperative infections. A careful history and physical examination are the best guides to which laboratory tests, if any, are indicated. In a retrospective review of 257 patients who underwent major gynecologic surgery, Lyon et al. found that a urine culture was positive in only 9% of the patients who were cultured and less than 2% of all febrile patients. Fewer chest x-rays were ordered, and they were almost always negative, with only 1.5% of all febrile patients having a significant finding. Similar results were described by Fanning et al., who also noted that none of the 77 blood cultures in their series of 211 febrile postoperative patients was positive.

In a follow-up study, Schwandt et al. outlined a protocol for evaluating postoperative gynecologic patients as follows: (a) record temperatures every 4 hours; (b) for temperatures greater than 38°C (100.4°F), evaluate the patient by history and physical examination; (c) when no significant signs or symptoms are identified, order no tests, and observe the patient. Antibiotics are not started at this point. The authors felt that this protocol of selectively ordering lab tests to evaluate a postoperative fever did not compromise patient care and saved considerable resources. Similar findings also have been reported in a retrospective review by McNally et al.

Although current practice discourages the use of "routine" testing to evaluate a postoperative fever, the clinician must be sensitive to special circumstances, unusual signs or symptoms, or persistent fever or other warning signs. Special circumstances could include a patient who was at high risk for infection because of immunosuppression, gross bacterial contamination at surgery, infection already present before surgery, or a patient in such a frail or unstable condition that any postoperative infection could be fatal. Unusual signs or symptoms, which include evidence of necrotizing fasciitis or gas-forming organisms and, most common of all, persistence of fever or other signs or symptoms of infection, definitely warrant a more exhaustive evaluation and, in most cases, prompt aggressive therapy.

A complete blood count with differential usually is indicated, and electrolytes, renal function tests, and liver-associated tests may be useful if sepsis is anticipated, prior damage to these organs exists, and/or antibiotics excreted or metabolized by these organs may be used. Acute pancreatitis can be ruled out by a normal serum amylase and lipase.

Blood cultures are not always indicated. In patients who will receive parenteral antibiotics, those with high fever, with persistent fever despite antibiotics, or who are immunocompromised, they should be drawn. This is particularly true when patients have indwelling central lines for longer than a few days, especially if these lines have been used for several functions (blood transfusions, antibiotics, electrolytes, etc.), and/or the patient had bacteremia that could seed the tip of the line. In these cases, at least one culture should be taken through the central line catheter. Other cultures of pus from an abdominal incision, the vaginal cuff, an undrained collection, or a drainage tube occasionally may be helpful in a patient who is not responding to antibiotics or in whom an unusual infection (*Actinomyces*) is suspected. A sputum Gram stain and culture is rarely useful but should be considered in a symptomatic, immunosuppressed patient who could have tuberculosis, coccidioidomycosis, or some other atypical pneumonia.

A number of different imaging techniques may be useful in special circumstances. A CT scan of the abdomen/pelvis should identify an abscess; allow evaluation of ureteral and bowel function; and provide information about pulmonary status. In many cases, CT-guided percutaneous catheter drainage in combination with intravenous antibiotics is the treatment of choice. Renal function always should be satisfactory before administering intravenous contrast for a CT or intravenous pyelogram. Ultrasound can be used to scan the abdominal incision and pelvis for an abscess or hematoma. Ultrasound of the heart can diagnose valvular vegetations associated with bacterial endocarditis. It also is useful for evaluation of the leg veins for venous thrombosis. Pelvic or abdominal vein thrombosis can be diagnosed easily in most cases using CT scanning. Radioactive-tagged white blood cell scans can be useful for localizing occult infections, but these have largely been replaced by CT scans.

TREATMENT

The following factors must be considered when making antibiotic choices for the treatment of postoperative infections.

1. Pelvic infections are polymicrobial in etiology.
2. The most frequent causative organisms are aerobic, gram-positive cocci (*Streptococci* and *S. aureus*), facultative gram-negative rods (*E. coli*, *Klebsiella* sp., *Enterobacter* sp.), anaerobic cocci (peptostreptococci), and anaerobic rods (*Prevotella* sp., *Bacteroides* sp., *B. fragilis*).
3. Enterococci may occasionally cause sepsis or be a sole isolate but usually accompany other bacteria and are not principal pathogens.
4. The choice of an antibiotic is made empirically before culture results are available.
5. The timing of onset of the infection may be an indicator of a pathogen group.
6. Resistance to frequently used antibiotics is developing.
7. Single agents may be as effective as multiple agents in treating postoperative infections.

The polymicrobial nature of postoperative pelvic infections results in about 20% aerobic gram-positive cocci, 20% gram-negative rods, and 60% anaerobes. Infections that occur in the first 24 hours after surgery usually are caused by gram-positive cocci or occasionally by facultative gram-negative rods. Infections that occur after the first 48 hours more frequently have an anaerobic component often in association with facultative, gram negatives. The effect of timing should be considered in making the initial choice of an antibiotic because an extended-spectrum penicillin or cephalosporin may be the best choice in early-onset infections (Table 11.6).

The gold standard for treating gynecologic postoperative infections has been gentamicin, 2 mg/kg loading dose, followed by 1.5 mg/kg maintenance dose for patients with normal renal function, plus clindamycin, 900 mg, both administered parenterally every 8 hours. Unfortunately, increasing resistance among anaerobes to clindamycin along with increasing *E. coli* resistance to gentamicin is altering the effectiveness of this regimen. Gentamicin carries potential for nephrotoxicity and ototoxicity, although these are both rare when used for short-term therapy in young, healthy women. Aminoglycoside serum levels should be obtained if the treatment is expected to last more than 72 hours. The addition of ampicillin to the previous combination extends the spectrum of coverage to include many, but not all, enterococci.

Metronidazole has excellent activity against anaerobic bacilli but has minimal activity against anaerobic gram-positive cocci. Metronidazole in combination with levofloxacin has been frequently used as combination therapy; however, gram-negative resistance to quinolones makes this a less attractive option. The oral absorption of metronidazole is superb, resulting in blood levels that are equivalent to parenteral administration. Metronidazole is only effective against anaerobes and has minimal to no aerobic spectrum.

Investigators have studied various extended-spectrum penicillins and cephalosporins as single agents for the treatment of mild to moderately severe postoperative pelvic infections. These agents have an extended spectrum of in vitro antibacterial activity and β-lactamase stability. Single agents—such as cefoxitin, cefotetan, cefuroxime, ampicillin/sulbactam, and piperacillin/tazobactam—avoid the problems of admixture with multiple agents and the potential for aminoglycoside toxicity. If resistant gram-negative organisms are expected due to prolonged hospitalization or prior antibiotic therapy, a carbapenem antibiotic such as, meropenem, would be a reasonable empiric choice pending culture data. The increasing incidence of resistant organisms elevates the importance of obtaining a deep wound or abscess culture prior to starting antibiotics.

TABLE 11.6 Treatment Choices for Gynecologic Infection

POSTOPERATIVE INFECTION	RECOMMENDED REGIMEN	FAILURES	PENICILLIN ALLERGY
Mild to moderate	Extended-spectrum penicillin or cephalosporin (e.g., piperacillin/tazobactam, 4.5 g/6 h; [this dose goes with pip/tazo] ticarcillin/clavulanic acid, 3.1 g/4–6 h; metronidazole 500 mg/6 h and levofloxacin 500 mg/d ceftriaxone, 2 g followed by 1 g/24 h; cefoxitin, 2 g/6 h; cefotetan 2 g/12 h; cefotaxime, 1 g/8 h [IV doses]).	Clindamycin/gentamicin or metronidazole/gentamicin	Clindamycin/gentamicin
Severe	Metronidazole/gentamicin or clindamycin/gentamicin (e.g., metronidazole, 500 mg/6 h or clindamycin, 900 mg/8 h plus gentamicin, 2 mg/kg followed by 1.5 mg/kg/8 h or a single daily dose of 5 mg/kg [ampicillin, penicillin, or vancomycin may be added to cover enterococci]).	Add ampicillin to clindamycin/gentamicin; imipenem or meropenem	Clindamycin/gentamicin
Pelvic abscess	Meropenem 500 mg–1 g/IV q8h; clindamycin/gentamicin; metronidazole/gentamicin	Evaluate need for surgical drainage	NA
Septic pelvic thrombophlebitis	Meropenem 500 mg–1 g/IV q8h; or metronidazole plus heparin		NA

NA, not applicable.

If a superficial wound abscess is identified on exam by palpation of fluctuance, a simple incision and drainage should be performed. In patients who have larger abscesses on CT scan (>3 to 4 cm), either surgical drainage or CT scan guided drainage should be considered. Parenteral antibiotics should be continued until the patient is afebrile and otherwise clinically improved for 24 to 48 hours. At that point, antibiotics may be converted to oral, and the patient may be discharged.

If there is not a good response to appropriate antibiotic therapy within 72 hours, the patient should be completely reevaluated. After another review of the history and physical examination, imaging studies should be considered. Perhaps a chest x-ray may indicate new consolidation or an abdominal and pelvic CT scan may identify a fluid collection or abscess, a retained foreign body, or even septic thrombophlebitis. If a fever persists, antibiotics may be discontinued, and the patient recultured/reevaluated before new antibiotics are started. SPT and necrotizing fasciitis should be considered.

PREVENTION OF INFECTION

Tremendous potential morbidity and economic burden are imposed by perioperative infections. In a 5-year study of wound infections after abdominal hysterectomy, Kandula and Wenzel found that women with infections were hospitalized an average of 3.55 days longer, resulting in a significant financial impact. It is important to implement specific strategies aimed at preventing postoperative infection and to use these unfailingly with every patient. In doing so, a significant number of infections can be prevented. Identifying risk factors is important preoperatively and intraoperatively. Major risks are obesity, bacterial vaginosis, prior history of wound infection, radical surgery, uncontrolled diabetes, and excessive blood loss (>1,000 mL).

Some guidelines for infection prevention apply to all situations, and some are specific to certain types of infection. Meticulous hand washing before and after any patient contact is particularly important, but unfortunately has poor general compliance. Multiple prior studies have revealed only 40% to 50% physician compliance with hand washing. In our institution, hand hygiene compliance has dramatically improved over the course of the past 5 years through improved access to alcohol hand gels, intensive educational efforts, and use of anonymous observers with feedback to noncompliant medical personnel. Concurrent with an increase in hand hygiene compliance to over 90%, a significant decline in transmission of hospital-associated organisms (MRSA, vancomycin-resistant enterococci, and resistant gram-negative rods) has been documented.

The skin is colonized with bacteria, some of which are transient and reside on the integument for only a short time, and some of which are resident and are present continuously. One can effectively remove the transient microflora with routine hand washing with soap. Alcohol-based hand gels have a more protracted effect in reducing transient microflora, often up to 2 hours. The resident organisms require antimicrobial products for their inhibition of growth or elimination. Hand washing is a cornerstone for preventing the spread of infection (Table 11.7).

Prevention of Postoperative Pneumonia

All patients who undergo general endotracheal anesthesia are at risk for retention of pulmonary secretions, alveolar collapse, and, in turn, atelectasis and possibly pneumonia. Atelectasis is frequently a cause of immediate postoperative fever. To help prevent this complication, all patients undergoing surgery, and especially those with chronic obstructive airway disease, should be encouraged to discontinue or decrease smoking and have any upper respiratory infections assessed before operation.

TABLE 11.7 Recommendations for Hand Washing

In the absence of a true emergency, personnel should always wash their hands:

- Before performing invasive procedures (chlorhexidine gluconate 1% solution and ethyl alcohol 61% have been used to replace water-aided hand scrubs with soap in many institutions. We recommend that the initial scrub of the day be with traditional washing for 5 min).
- Uniformly when entering and exiting all patient rooms
- After situations during which microbial contamination of hands is likely to occur, particularly those involving contact with mucous membranes, blood, body fluids, secretions, or excretions. Gloves should be worn in this situation.
- After touching inanimate sources that are likely to be contaminated with virulent or epidemiologically important microorganisms
- After taking care of an infected patient or one who is likely to be colonized with microorganisms of special clinical or epidemiologic significance, such as multiple drug–resistant bacteria. Gloving should be uniformly worn in this situation with hand cleansing prior to placement of gloves and after removing gloves.

Sources: Garner JS, Favero MS. Guideline for hand washing and hospital environmental control, 1985. In: *Guidelines for the prevention and control of nosocomial infections.* Washington, DC: US Department of Health and Human Services, PB82–9234401, 1985:7; Boyce et al. Guidelines for hand hygiene in the health care setting. *MMWR Recomm Rep* 2002;51(RR-16):1.

Postoperatively, coughing, deep breathing, and devices to encourage alveolar expansions should be used. Adequate analgesia to control pain that interferes with respiratory effort should be administered. Early ambulation should be encouraged.

Prevention of Urinary Tract Infection

Urinary tract infections can complicate gynecologic surgery because of the proximity of the urethra to the operative site in the vagina. This effect is augmented by the placement of an indwelling urinary catheter. To limit UTIs, appropriate placement and management of catheters is essential. Personnel should be instructed in the proper sterile placement of catheters, maintained as a closed drainage system without traction on the device. Bladder catheters should be placed only when absolutely necessary, should be removed as soon as feasible, and should be maintained with correct fixation to the leg in order to avoid a pistoning effect resulting in urethral trauma. Many of the minimally invasive procedures, including hysterectomy, in our institution have their catheters removed in the postoperative recovery room.

Prevention of Operative Site and Wound Infections

Other Considerations

Multiple studies have demonstrated that antibiotic prophylaxis significantly reduces infectious morbidity following both vaginal and abdominal hysterectomy. These results do not mean that the important surgical principles that have been shown to reduce morbidity can be ignored, but the use of prophylactic antibiotics in many gynecologic surgical procedures has reduced the incidence of postoperative surgical site infections from 30% to 50% to about 15% in most series.

Theory of Antibiotic Prophylaxis

At the time of hysterectomy, vaginal or cervical bacteria are inoculated into the surgical site, and it is hypothesized that antibiotics in these tissues at this time augment host defense mechanisms to reduce the incidence of clinical infections. For antibiotic prophylaxis to work effectively, several important criteria must be fulfilled. First, the operative procedure must have a significant risk of bacterial contamination and, in the absence of prophylactic antibiotics, an appreciable incidence of operative site infection. Hysterectomy or other gynecologic procedures involving the cervix, vagina, or vulva all meet this criterion. Second, the prophylactic antibiotic administered should be effective against expected pathogens and have a low rate of side effects. Third, the antibiotic should not be one that would be routinely used therapeutically. Although many antibiotic regimens have proven effective in prospective, randomized trials for gynecologic surgery, the first- and second-generation cephalosporins have emerged as the generally recommended antibiotics because of their effectiveness, low incidence of side effects, and low cost. Finally, for effective antibiotics prophylaxis, the tissue levels of the chosen antibiotic need to be optimal at the time bacterial contamination of the surgical site occurs. This means that the antibiotic needs to be administered shortly before the start of surgery, usually at the time the patient is brought into the operating room and anesthesia is induced.

Choice of Antibiotics for Prophylaxis

As noted, the antibiotic selected for a given procedure should be effective, have few side effects, be administered in a way that results in a minimal risk of antibiotic-resistant infections, and be inexpensive. In a meta-analysis of 25 prospective, randomized trials of prophylactic antibiotics for abdominal hysterectomy, Mittendorf et al. reported a reduction of serious postoperative infections from 21.1% to 9%. The most commonly used antibiotic for hysterectomy is cefazolin, because it meets the preceding criteria and has a relatively long half-life of 1.8 hours. Recommended prophylactic antibiotic regimens for various gynecologic procedures are listed in Table 11.8.

Cephalosporins generally should not be given to patients with a history of penicillin anaphylaxis but may be given to patients with milder penicillin allergies. Metronidazole and clindamycin have been particularly effective when anaerobic contamination is anticipated in B-lactam-allergic patients.

In women with damaged or artificial heart valves or others at increased risk for bacterial endocarditis, combination antibiotics such as ampicillin (2 g) and gentamicin (1.5 mg/m^2) are recommended. If the patient is allergic to penicillin, vancomycin (1 g over 1 to 2 hours) is substituted for ampicillin. Unlike prophylactic antibiotics given for operative site infections when only a single dose is administered, it is recommended that a second dose be given 6 hours later.

Adverse Reactions

Although reactions to cephalosporins may occur in 1% to 10% of patients, severe side effects such as anaphylaxis have been reported in only about 0.02% of patients. The majority of reactions are skin rashes and urticaria, which usually are resolved by the time the patient has recovered from anesthesia postoperatively. *Clostridium difficile*–related colitis was previously associated

---

TABLE 11.8 Antimicrobial Prophylactic Regimens by Procedure

PROCEDURE	ANTIBIOTIC	DOSE
Vaginal/abdominal	Cefazolin	1 or 2 g single dose IV
Hysterectomy[a]	Cefoxitin	1 or 2 g single dose IV
	Cefotetan	1 or 2 g single dose IV
	*For B lactam allergic clindamycin/gentamicin	900 mg/1.5 mg/kg single dose IV
Laparoscopy	None	—
Laparotomy	None	—
Hysteroscopy	None	—
Hysterosalpingogram[b]	Doxycycline	100 mg twice daily/5 d orally
IUD insertion	None	—
Endometrial biopsy	None	—
Induced abortion/D&C	Doxycycline	100 mg orally 1 h before procedure and 200 mg orally after the procedure
	Metronidazole	500 mg twice daily orally for 5 d
Urodynamics	None	—

[a]A convenient time to administer antibiotic prophylaxis is in the operating suite, just before induction of anesthesia.
[b]If hysterosalpingogram demonstrated dilated tubes. No prophylaxis indicated for a normal study.
D&C, dilation and curettage; IV, intravenously; IUD, intrauterine device.
Source: ACOG Practice Bulletin 2001;23:269, with permission. Copyright © 2006 The American College of Obstetricians and Gynecologists.

with primarily beta-lactam antibiotics and clindamycin but is now being increasingly induced by quinolone antibiotics, particularly levofloxacin. A new, more potent strain of *C. difficile*, NAP-1, carries a significant morbidity and mortality potential.

Miller et al. identified *Clostridium difficile* as the most common hospital-associated infection, superseding MRSA. Although the induction of bacterial resistance to commonly used antibiotics has been a theoretical concern, this has not been a clinical problem when prophylactic antibiotic use is limited to one to three doses of early-generation cephalosporins. More potent broad-spectrum antibiotics should be reserved for specific indications and not used in a prophylactic setting to avoid induction of resistant organisms.

Surveillance for nosocomial infections must be carried out by the hospital infection control program so that surgeons are aware of their individual rates of postoperative infection. Several studies have shown that surgeon-specific wound infection rates can be reduced effectively by such reporting mechanisms.

The classic work of Cruse and Foord helped to delineate specific factors that influence wound infection rates. Others have added to this work so that preoperative and intraoperative management routines can be recommended even though they have not all been confirmed in controlled trials. Preoperative hospitalization should be limited as much as possible. Same-day admission is not just cost-effective for third-party payors; it makes good sense from an infection control perspective. Hair removal should be avoided unless there is an abundance of hair at the operative site. Using a depilatory or clipping the hair is suggested if removal is necessary. Patients should be discouraged from shaving themselves at home before admission, since this results in microtrauma to the skin with a secondary increase in bacterial colonization and infection risk.

Because bowel entry is a major cause of contamination and subsequent wound or surgical site infection, great care should be given to a thorough inspection of the bowel intraoperatively whenever there has been a risk of injury. The use of a povidone–iodine douche or insertion of gel has been recommended for the night before admission or the day of surgery. Although this practice has been recommended for many years, and povidone–iodine solution and gel have been demonstrated to decrease vaginal bacterial counts to undetectable levels 10 minutes after application, the bacterial flora gradually return to approximately one half pretreatment levels in 2 hours. Appropriate preparation of the patient's skin in the operating room is essential to decreasing skin contaminants prior to an incision being made. The benefit of vaginal cleansing with an anti-infective agent the night before, or even immediately before surgery, has not been evaluated in a prospective, randomized trial.

Bacterial vaginosis has been found to be a risk factor for postoperative infection when present before surgery in women undergoing hysterectomy. In a prospective study of 175 women who underwent major gynecologic surgery, Lin et al. found a 36% incidence of postoperative febrile morbidity in patients who had bacterial vaginosis preoperatively and only a 20% incidence of fever among the women who had a lactobacillus-predominant vaginal flora ($P = 0.045$). Although some data support the benefit of treating pregnant women with bacterial vaginosis to decrease the rates of preterm labor, premature rupture of the membranes, and intra-amniotic infection, no data have shown a beneficial effect of preoperative treatment of hysterectomy patients. In light of the obstetric data, some gynecologists recommend screening hysterectomy patients preoperatively and treating those who are infected with metronidazole because anaerobes play such a significant role in postoperative gynecologic infections.

All gynecologists should employ careful hand-washing techniques or Avagard use preoperatively and when seeing patients. Appropriate gowns and eye coverings should be worn. Wearing double gloves is an effective way to decrease the chances of percutaneous injury. Careful surgical technique is essential to minimize postoperative infections. In cases where extensive adhesiolysis is carried out, careful inspection of the bowel should be done. Adequate hemostasis should be obtained whenever possible. The amount of dead space should be limited. Large areas of necrotic tissue should be excised, and vascular pedicles should be short. Closing the subcutaneous space has no benefit, and using suture there can actually increase the rate of superficial wound infection. If the case is dirty, consideration should be given to delayed wound closure. If drains are used, they should be closed suction drains, not gravity drains. Draining the subcutaneous space often is helpful in large patients to eliminate serous and bloody fluid.

UNIVERSAL PRECAUTIONS

The epidemics of acquired immunodeficiency syndrome and hepatitis B viral infection have brought to light the risks of lethal infection of the surgeon or other members of the operative team by blood or tissue fluids in association with surgery. Believing that all at-risk situations can be identified by history, physical examination, or laboratory data is naive and dangerous. To overcome this prevalent thought, universal blood and body fluid precautions were developed. This concept treats all patients' blood and certain other body fluids capable of transmitting blood-borne pathogens as potentially infectious. Universal precautions include the following requirements: (a) the use of gloves when touching blood and body fluids, mucous membranes, or broken skin, or when handling items or surfaces soiled with blood or body fluids; (b) the use of masks and eye protection during procedures that can generate splashing or droplets in the air; (c) the use of a gown or plastic apron if splashing of blood is anticipated; (d) careful hand washing if hands are contaminated with blood or body fluids; (e) extraordinary care in handling needles or other sharp objects, and proper disposal of sharp objects in puncture-resistant containers; (f) the availability of emergency resuscitation devices to minimize the need for emergency mouth-to-mouth resuscitation; and (g) the exclusion from patient care of personnel with exudative lesions or weeping dermatitis until these conditions are resolved.

Assuming that every patient is potentially infected, using specific protocols for the safe use of invasive procedures and taking steps to avoid any and all risk-taking behavior by medical personnel can help to prevent nosocomial infections.

Multiple studies have shown that double gloving significantly reduces the risk of blood contamination to the surgeon and other members of the operative team. In a large study from Finland, Laine and Aarnio reported a 7.4% glove perforation rate for single gloves in 1,020 surgeon uses. When double gloves were used, the inner glove was perforated in only 0.52% of 1,148 uses. Overall, someone in the surgical team had a glove perforation during 18.9% of the operative procedures, and the literature quotes rates of up to 61% in orthopedics and trauma surgery. The most common site of perforation is the index finger of the left hand of the surgeon; but all members of the team are at risk, and gloves can be torn in clamps or retractors as well as punctured by needlestick injuries. Manufacturing defects in the gloves themselves are uncommon but do occur and may go unnoticed until blood is seen on the finger or hand. Although double gloving does reduce dexterity and tactile sensation, it also reduces the potential for blood contamination almost 10-fold. It is a good general practice and always should be used in high-risk situations.

BEST SURGICAL PRACTICE

- Major risk factors for postoperative infection include immunocompromise, obesity, bacterial vaginosis, prolonged surgery, radical surgery, and excessive blood loss (>1,000 mL).
- Prophylactic antibiotics have been shown to reduce infectious morbidity for most major gynecologic surgery, including hysterectomy. For antibiotic prophylaxis to work effectively, several important criteria must be fulfilled: (a) the operative procedure must have a significant risk of bacterial contamination; (b) the prophylactic antibiotic administered should be effective against expected pathogens and have a low rate of side effects; (c) the antibiotic should not be one that would be routinely used therapeutically; and (d) the tissue levels of the antibiotic need to be optimal at the time surgery occurs.
- Infections that occur in the first 24 hours after surgery usually are caused by gram-positive cocci or occasionally by facultative gram-negative rods. Infections that occur after the first 48 hours more frequently have an anaerobic component. Pelvic infections are polymicrobial in etiology: 20% aerobic gram-positive cocci, 20% gram-negative rods, and 60% anaerobes.
- Rather than routine "fever workup" for postoperative fever evaluation, a careful history and physical examination are the best guides to which laboratory tests, if any, are indicated. Possible noninfectious causes of early postoperative fever include pulmonary atelectasis, hypersensitivity reactions to antibiotics or anesthetics, pyrogenic reactions to tissue trauma, or hematoma formation.
- In order to manage deep wound infection, the incision should be probed gently to evaluate fascial integrity. If the fascia is intact, healing is hastened by mechanical debridement followed by loose, wet-to-dry packing with gauze moistened with saline; dilute hydrogen peroxide (1:1 mixture with saline) or Dakin solution, 0.5%. Povidone–iodine is to be discouraged because it does not promote the development of granulation tissue.
- Careful hand-washing technique is critical to reduction in postoperative infections.
- Evisceration of bowel may occur if a postoperative wound infection involves the fascia. This is a surgical emergency requiring identification of the defect, freshening of the fascial edges, placement of intra-abdominal and subcutaneous closed suction drains, and reinforced closure of the fascia. Some surgeons leave the skin open for delayed closure; others close it primarily.
- The use of universal precautions to minimize the risk of the surgeon, surgical team, or health care worker acquiring a potentially fatal human immunodeficiency or hepatitis B viral infection from the patient is strongly encouraged. Although high-risk patients may be identified, all patients pose a potential risk to the surgeon.

BIBLIOGRAPHY

American College of Obstetricians and Gynecologists. Bulletin-74 ACOG, 2006. *Antibiotic prophylaxis for gynecologic procedures.* Washington, DC: ACOG, 2006:1216.

Barton J, Sibai B. Severe sepsis and septic shock in pregnancy. *Obstet Gynecol* 2012;120:689.

Boyce JM, Pittet D; Healthcare Infection Control Practices Advisory Committee; HICPAC/SHEA/APIC/IDSA Hand Hygiene Task Force. Guideline for hand hygiene in health-care settings. Recommendations of the Healthcare Infection Control Practices Advisory Committee and the HICPAC/SHEA/APIC/IDSA Hand Hygiene Task Force. Society for Healthcare Epidemiology of America/Association for Professionals in Infection Control/Infectious Diseases Society of America. *MMWR Recomm Rep* 2002;51(RR-16):1.

Brill A, Ghosh K, Gunnarsson C, et al. The effects of laparoscopic cholecystectomy, hysterectomy, and appendectomy on nosocomial infection risks. *Surg Endosc* 2008;22:112.

Brough SJ, Hunt TM, Barrie WW. Surgical glove perforations. *Br J Surg* 1988;75:317.

Brown CEL, Lowe TW, Cunningham FG, et al. Puerperal pelvic thrombophlebitis: impact on diagnosis and treatment using x-ray computed tomography and magnetic resonance imaging. *Obstet Gynecol* 1986;68:789.

Centers for Disease Control and Prevention. CDC Surgical Site Infection Events. January 2013.

Centers for Disease Control and Prevention. Public Health Service guidelines for the management of health-care worker exposure to HIV and recommendations for postexposure prophylaxis. *MMWR Morb Mortal Wkly Rep* 1998;47(RR-7):1.

Centers for Disease Control and Prevention. The 2002 USPHS/IDSA guidelines for preventing opportunistic infections among HIV-infected persons. *MMWR Morb Mortal Wkly Rep* 2002;51(RR-8):xx.

Classen DC, Evan RS, Pestotnik SL, et al. The timing of prophylactic administration of antibiotics and the risk of surgical-wound infection. *N Engl J Med* 1992;326:281.

Condon RE, Schulte WJ, Malongoni MA, et al. Effectiveness of a surgical wound surveillance program. *Arch Surg* 1983;118:303.

Cruse PJE, Foord R. The epidemiology of wound infection: a 10 year prospective study of 62,939 wounds. *Surg Clin North Am* 1980;60:27.

Cuchural GJ, Tally FP, Jacobus NV, et al. Susceptibility of the *Bacteroides fragilis* group in the United States: analysis by site of isolation. *Antimicrob Agents Chemother* 1988;32:717.

Culver DH, Horan TC, Gaynes RF. Surgical wound infection rates by wound class: operative procedure and patient risk index. *Am J Med* 1991;91:152S.

Dellinger EP, Gross PA, Barrett TL, et al. Quality standard for antimicrobial prophylaxis in surgical procedures. Infectious Disease Society of America [review]. *Clin Infect Dis* 1994;18:422.

DeSouza MV. New fluoroquinolones: a class of potent antibiotics. *Mini Rev Med Chem* 2005;5:1009.

Dinsmoor MJ. Imipenem-cilastatin. *Obstet Gynecol Clin North Am* 1992;19:475.

Donowitz GR, Mandell GL. Beta lactam antibiotics. *N Engl J Med* 1988;318:490.

Duff P. The aminoglycosides. *Obstet Gynecol Clin North Am* 1992;19:511.

Duff P. Prophylactic antibiotics for hysterectomy. In: Mead PB, Hager WD, Faro S, eds. *Protocols for infectious diseases in obstetrics and gynecology*, 2nd ed. Malden, MA: Blackwell Scientific, 2000:476.

Eason E, Wells G, Garber G, et al. Antisepsis for abdominal hysterectomy: a randomized controlled trial of povidone-iodine gel. *BJOG* 2004;111:695.

Edwards JR, Peterson KD, Yi Mu, et al. National Healthcare Safety Network (NHSN) report: data summary for 2006 through 2008, issued December 2009. *Am J Infect Control* 2009;37:783.

Evaldson GR, Frederici H, Jullig C, et al. Hospital-associated infections in obstetrics and gynecology: effects of surveillance. *Acta Obstet Gynecol Scand* 1992;71:54.

Fanning J, Neuhoff RA, Brewer JE, et al. Frequency and yield of postoperative fever evaluation. *Infect Dis Obstet Gynecol* 1998;6:252.

Fille M, Mango M, Lechner M, et al. *Bacteroides fragilis* group: trends in resistance. *Curr Microbiol* 2006;52:153.

Gallup DC, Gallup DG, Nolan TE, et al. Use of a subcutaneous closed drainage system and antibiotics in obese gynecologic patients. *Am J Obstet Gynecol* 1996;175:358.

Garibaldi RA, Brodine S, Mutsumiya S, et al. Evidence for the non-infectious etiology of early postoperative fever. *Infect Control* 1985;6:273.

Garner JS, Favero MS. Guideline for hand washing and hospital environmental control, 1985. *Guidelines for the prevention and control of nosocomial infections*. Washington, DC: US Department of Health and Human Services, 1985:7.

Grossman JH, Adams RL. Vaginal flora in women undergoing hysterectomy with antibiotic prophylaxis. *Obstet Gynecol* 1979;53:23.

Hager WD, Pascuzzi M, Vernon M. Efficacy of oral antibiotics following parenteral antibiotics for serious infections in obstetrics and gynecology. *Obstet Gynecol* 1989;73:326.

II

Hager WD, Rapp RP. Metronidazole. *Obstet Gynecol Clin North Am* 1992;19:475.

Haley RW, Culver DH, White JW, et al. The efficiency of infection surveillance and control programs in preventing nosocomial infections in US hospitals. *Am J Epidemiol* 1985;121:182.

Harris WJ. Early complications of abdominal and vaginal hysterectomy. *Obstet Gynecol Surv* 1995;50:795.

Hemsell DL. Gynecologic postoperative infections in obstetric and gynecologic infectious disease. In: Pastorek JG, ed. *Obstetric and gynecologic infectious disease*. New York, NY: Raven Press, 1994:141.

Hemsell DL, Bowden RE, Hemsell PG, et al. Single-dose cephalosporin for prevention of major pelvic infection after vaginal hysterectomy: cefazolin vs cefoxitin vs cefotaxime. *Am J Obstet Gynecol* 1987;156:1201.

Hemsell DL, Johnson ER, Bowden RE, et al. Ceftriaxone and cefazolin prophylaxis for hysterectomy. *Surg Gynecol Obstet* 1985;161:197.

Hemsell DL, Johnson ER, Heard MC, et al. Single-dose piperacillin vs triple-dose cefoxitin prophylaxis at vaginal and abdominal hysterectomy. *South Med J* 1984;82:438.

Hemsell DL, Nobles B, Heard MC. Recognition and treatment of posthysterectomy pelvic infections. *Infect Surg* 1988;7:47.

Horan TC, Gaynes RP, Martone WJ, et al. CDC definitions of nosocomial surgical site infections, 1992: a modification of CDC definitions of surgical wound infections. *Am J Infect Control* 1992;20:271.

Hoyme UB, Tamimi HK, Eschenbach DA, et al. Osteomyelitis pubis after radical gynecologic operations. *Obstet Gynecol* 1984;63:475.

Hunter J, Quarterman C, Waseem M, et al. Diagnosis and management of necrotizing fasciitis. *Br J Hosp Med (Lond)* 2011;72:7.

Jaffe TA, Nelson RC, DeLong DM, et al. Practice patterns in percutaneous image-guided intraabdominal abscess drainage: survey of academic and private practice centers. *Radiology* 2004;233:750.

Jenson SL, Kristensen B, Fabrin K. Double gloving as self protection in abdominal surgery. *Eur J Surg* 1997;163:163.

John JF. What price success? The continuing saga of the toxic therapeutic ratio in the use of aminoglycoside antibiotics. *J Infect Dis* 1988;158:1.

Kamat AA, Brancazio L, Gibson M. Wound infection in gynecologic surgery. *Infect Dis Obstet Gynecol* 2000;8:230.

Kandula PV, Wenzel RP. Postoperative wound infection after total abdominal hysterectomy: a controlled study of the increased duration of hospital stay and trends in postoperative wound infection. *Am J Infect Control* 1993;21:201.

Kaye KS. Infection prevention and control in the hospital. *Infect Dis Clin North Am* 2011;25:140.

Kim K, Kim K, Lee J, et al. Can necrotizing fasciitis be differentiated from non-necrotizing infectious fasciitis with MR imaging? *Radiology* 2011;259:816.

Korn AP, Gullon K, Hessol N, et al. Does vaginal cuff closure decrease the infectious morbidity associated with abdominal hysterectomy? *J Am Coll Surg* 1997;185:404.

Laine T, Aarnio P. How often does glove perforation occur in surgery? Comparison between single gloves and a double-gloving system. *Am J Surg* 2001;181:564.

Lars P, Naver S, Gottrup F. Incidence of glove perforations in gastrointestinal surgery and the protective effect of double gloves: a prospective, randomised, controlled study. *Eur J Surg* 2000;166:293.

Larsen JW, Hager WD, Livengood CH, et al. Guidelines for the diagnosis, treatment and prevention of postoperative infections. *Infect Dis Obstet Gynecol* 2003;11:65.

Leaper D, Ayliffe GA, Gilchrist B. Postoperative wound infection. *J Wound Care* 1996;5:330.

Ledger W. Diagnosis and treatment of salpingitis. *J Reprod Med* 1983;28(10 Suppl):709.

Lin L, Song J, Kimber N, et al. The role of bacterial vaginosis in infection after major gynecologic surgery. *Infect Dis Obstet Gynecol* 1999;7:169.

Lyon DS, Jones JL, Sanchez A. Postoperative febrile morbidity in the benign gynecologic patient. *J Reprod Med* 2000;45:305.

Mage G, Masson FN, Canis M. Laparoscopic hysterectomy. *Curr Opin Obstet Gynecol* 1995;7:283.

McNally CG, Krivak TC, Alagoz T. Conservative management of isolated post hysterectomy fever. *J Reprod Med* 2000;45:572.

Mead PB, Hager WD, Faro S. *Protocols for infectious diseases in obstetrics and gynecology*, 2nd ed. Malden, MA: Blackwell Scientific, 2000.

Miller BA, Chen LF, Sexton DJ. Hospital associated infections. *Infect Control Hosp Epidemiol* 2011;32:387.

Mittendorf R, Aronson MP, Berry RE, et al. Avoiding serious infections associated with abdominal hysterectomy: a meta-analysis of antibiotic prophylaxis. *Am J Obstet Gynecol* 1993;169:1119.

Morgan MS. Diagnosis and management of necrotizing fasciitis. *J Hosp Infect* 2010;75:249.

Ong CT, Kuti JL, Nicolau DP. Pharmacodynamic modeling of imipenem-cilastatin, meropenem and piperacillin-tazobactam for empiric therapy of skin and soft tissue infections: a report from the OPYAMA program. *Surg Infect* 2005;6:419.

Persson E, Bergstrom M, Larsson PG, et al. Infections after hysterectomy: a prospective, nation-wide Swedish study. *Acta Obstet Gynecol Scand* 1996;75:757.

Peters WA. Bartholinitis after vulvovaginal surgery. *Am J Obstet Gynecol* 1998;178:1143.

Rhomberg PR, Fritsche TR, Sader HS, et al. Clonal occurrences of multidrug-resistant Gram-negative bacilli: a report from the meropenem yearly susceptibility test information collection program in the United States (2004). *Diagn Microbiol Infect Dis* 2006;54:249.

Sawyer RG, Pruett TL. Wound infections. *Surg Clin North Am* 1994;74:519.

Schwandt A, Andrews SJ, Fanning J. Prospective analysis of a fever evaluation algorithm after major gynecologic surgery. *Am J Obstet Gynecol* 2001;184:1066.

Shapiro M, Munoz A, Tager IB, et al. Risk factors for infection at the operative site after abdominal or vaginal hysterectomy. *N Engl J Med* 1982;307:1661.

Solomkin J, Teppler H, Graham DR, et al. Treatment of polymicrobial infections: *post hoc* analysis of three trials comparing ertapenem and piperacillin-tazobactam. *J Antimicrob Chemother* 2004;53(suppl S2):51.

Soper DE. Bacterial vaginosis and postoperative infections. *Am J Obstet Gynecol* 1993;169:467.

Thomason JL, Gelbart SM, Scaylione NJ. Bacteria vaginosis: current review with indications for asymptomatic therapy. *Am J Obstet Gynecol* 1991;165:1210.

CHAPTER 12
Shock in the Gynecologic Patient

Addison K. May

DEFINITIONS

Categories of the etiologies of shock—
- Hypovolemic
  - Blood loss, dehydration, and diarrhea
- Distributive
  - Sepsis, endocrine, spinal, and anaphylaxis
- Obstructive
  - PE, tamponade, pericarditis, and pulmonary hypertension
- Cardiogenic
  - MI, myopathy, and valvular lesions

Classification of the severity of hemorrhagic shock—
- Class I—up to 15% of blood volume

  Compensation maintains normal cardiac output and blood pressure

– Class II—15% to 30% of blood volume

Compensation cannot maintain normal cardiac output, but systolic blood pressure is maintained; pulse pressure is narrowed (compensated shock)

– Class III—30% to 40% of blood volume

Cardiac output and blood pressure are decreased; significant tachycardia (uncompensated shock)

– Class IV—greater than 40% blood loss

Cardiac output and blood pressure are profoundly decreased; very significant tachycardia

Compensated shock—A state of global, inadequate organ perfusion, and oxygen delivery with normal blood pressure.

Cytopathic hypoxia—A state of mitochondrial injury and dysfunction resulting from hypoxia and oxidative stress where oxidative phosphorylation is interrupted, thus mandating ATP generation through lactate generation.

Sepsis—The presence of SIRS due to an infectious etiology.

Septic shock—Sepsis advanced to the point of distributive shock.

Severe sepsis—When sepsis has progressed to a severity to manifest organ dysfunction such as delirium, acute lung injury, or acute kidney injury.

Severe SIRS—When SIRS has progressed to a severity to manifest organ dysfunction such as delirium, acute lung injury, or acute kidney injury.

Severe SIRS with shock—SIRS advanced to the point of distributive shock.

Shock—A state of global inadequate organ perfusion and oxygen delivery.

Systemic inflammatory response syndrome (SIRS)—Global activation of the inflammatory cascade, by a variety of stimuli, manifest by two or more of the following:

– Hyper- or hypothermia (>38°C or <036°C)

– Tachycardia (heart rate >90)

– Increased minute ventilation (respiratory rate >20)

– Leukocytosis or leukopenia (WBC > 12,000 or <4,000, or >10% bands)

Shock is defined as a state of global inadequate organ perfusion and may arise from a variety of diverse etiologies. Regardless of the etiology, the shock state will contribute to oxidative stress, cellular injury, and systemic activation of the inflammatory cascade (SIRS) and potentiate or lead to multisystem organ dysfunction syndrome (MODS). Both uncompensated and compensated shock will contribute to cellular changes that potentiate the severity of shock itself. An understanding of the physiologic derangements introduced by shock as well as the therapeutic interventions to mitigate the various etiologies of shock is required to optimally manage patients with this condition. In the chapter to follow, the etiologies, the physiologic cellular and organ derangements caused by the shock state, the interaction with the inflammation and organ injury, and the therapeutic interventions to target each are discussed.

DEFINITION AND ETIOLOGIES OF SHOCK

Shock is defined as a state of systemic or global inadequate organ perfusion and may be caused by a variety of insults. Most commonly, shock is recognized by hypotension, defining *uncompensated shock*. However, inadequate organ perfusion can occur with relatively normal vital signs, as occurs in *compensated shock*. Recognition that shock may exist without significant alterations in hemodynamics is critical to minimizing cellular and organ injury that may be introduced by occult hypoperfusion.

The various etiologies of shock are most frequently classified into four different categories based upon the underlying pathophysiologic alteration: hypovolemic, cardiogenic, obstructive, and distributive. Common causes of *hypovolemic shock* include hemorrhage, dehydration, and diarrheal diseases. *Cardiogenic shock* may be caused by an acute myocardial infarction, valvular lesions, and myopathies induced by ischemia, viral diseases, and inflammatory conditions. Causes of *obstructive shock* include tension pneumothorax, cardiac tamponade, constrictive pericarditis, acute pulmonary embolism, and severe pulmonary hypertension. The various causes of *distributive shock* include sepsis, spinal cord injury with neurogenic shock, adrenal insufficiency, vasopressin deficiency, anaphylaxis, and ischemia/reperfusion. Distributive shock physiologically differs from the other three classifications of shock in that a decline in cardiac output is not universally present. In fact, due to the decrease in systemic vascular resistance, cardiac output is frequently increased unless an underlying cardiac dysfunction also exists.

Appropriate therapeutic interventions for the treatment of shock should be directed toward the underlying pathophysiologic defect, which varies between and within classifications. While shock may be induced by a single etiology, recognizing that multiple etiologies may coexist and that one type of shock may cause or exacerbate a second is crucial to decisions regarding appropriate therapy. Changes induced by shock and the interdependence that may exist are outlined below.

PHYSIOLOGIC RESPONSE

Response to Decreased Cardiac Output

The predominant response to decreased cardiac output is to preserve perfusion to the heart and brain. This acute physiologic response is best characterized and understood in the context of hemorrhagic shock. Additionally, compensated shock is most easily understood in acute hemorrhagic shock, although inadequate organ perfusion with normal hemodynamics clearly exists in other forms of shock.

Acute hemorrhagic shock may be classified into four classes (Table 12.1). In *class I* shock, less than 15% of blood volume (approximately 750 mL in a 70 kg individual) has been lost. At this degree of blood loss, an increase in cardiac contractility and heart rate can maintain cardiac output and thus organ perfusion. In *class II* hemorrhagic shock, 15% to 30% of blood volume (approximately up to 1,500 mL in a 70-kg individual) has been lost. At this magnitude of blood loss, the acute compensatory mechanisms of increased heart rate and contractility can no longer maintain cardiac output. To maintain perfusion pressure, vasoconstriction of peripheral and mesenteric vascular beds increases resistance to blood flow, maintaining systolic blood pressure and increasing diastolic pressure (narrowed pulse pressure). While systolic blood pressure is preserved, cardiac output and delivery are decreased. This is the state of *compensated shock*. *Class III* hemorrhagic shock is defined as blood loss at 30% to 40% (approximately >1,500 mL in a 70-kg individual) of total body blood volume. At this degree of blood loss, cardiac output is severely altered and vasoconstriction can no longer maintain systolic pressure. Thus, perfusion pressure of the brain and heart are both now altered. Mental status changes and obvious signs of shock ensue. *Class IV* hemorrhagic shock is defined as greater than 40% of blood volume. At this degree of shock, profound hypotension, tachycardia, and severely depressed level of consciousness are manifested.

TABLE 12.1 Hemorrhagic Shock: Estimated Blood Loss[a] Based on Patient's Initial Presentation

	CLASS I	CLASS II	CLASS III	CLASS IV
Blood loss (mL)	<750	750–1,500	1,500–2,000	>2,000
Blood loss (% blood volume)	≤15%	15%–30%	30%–40%	≥40%
Pulse rate	<100	100–120	120–140	>140
Blood pressure	Normal	Normal	Decreased	Decreased
Pulse pressure (mm Hg)	Normal or increased	Decreased	Decreased	Decreased
Capillary refill	Normal	Delayed	Delayed	Delayed
Respiratory rate	14–20	20–30	30–40	>35
Urine output (mL/h)	>30	20–30	5–15	Negligible
CNS/mental status	Slightly anxious	Mildly anxious	Anxious, confused	Confused, lethargic
Fluid replacement	Crystalloid	Crystalloid	Crystalloid and blood	Crystalloid and blood

[a]Estimate based upon a 70-kg male.

It is important to recognize that greater than roughly 1,500 mL of blood in a 70-kg individual must be lost before compensatory mechanisms are overwhelmed and hypotension develops. Significant blood loss with associated hypoperfusion of vital organs may exist prior to the development of hypotension. Inadequate organ perfusion induces cellular insult, as outlined below, regardless of blood pressure and must be recognized and treated.

Cellular Biochemical Changes

Shock, or inadequate perfusion, creates hypoxia of the cells involved, which results in anaerobic rather than aerobic metabolism for cellular functions. This period of anaerobic metabolism produces "hypoxic priming" within the affected cells, characterized by a marked reduction in adenosine triphosphate (ATP) generation by the cell, an increase in oxidative stress, loss of antioxidant potential, and a buildup of acidic by-products, including lactic acid. The decrease in ATP production within hypoxic cells leads to a cascade of events including decreased ion exchange by the sodium–potassium adenosine triphosphatase pumps (Na^+/K^+-ATPase), calcium (Ca^{2+}), cellular swelling, Ca^{2+} activation of phospholipases with activation of the arachidonic acid cascade, and generation of fatty acid reactive oxidant species. Additionally, cellular hypoxia leads to the ischemic generation of *xanthine oxidase* by irreversible proteolytic cleavage of xanthine dehydrogenase, the enzyme that normally catalyzes the metabolism of hypoxanthine (product of ATP utilization) to xanthine and subsequently uric acid via the generation of NADH from NAD^+.

Reperfusion of cells following a period of hypoxic priming induces further oxidant injury and activation of the inflammatory cascade through several mechanisms. The xanthine oxidase enzyme, generated during hypoxia, catalyzes the conversion of hypoxanthine and oxygen to xanthine and subsequently uric acid and generating the oxidative species, superoxide (O_2^-). Additionally, hypoxia followed by reperfusion induces increased activity of nitric oxide synthetase and enhanced production of nitric oxide (NO), another oxidative

species. NO and O_2^- interact to form yet another oxidative species, peroxynitrite (ONOO). These oxidative species generated by hypoxia and reperfusion directly injure mitochondria, proteins, chromosomes, and membrane structures. In severe shock states, oxidative stress can be greatly potentiated by cellular mitochondrial injury, a condition known as *cytopathic hypoxia*. Oxidative species, such as ONOO, can oxidize the components of the electron transport chain and open pores in the mitochondrial membrane, both contributing to mitochondrial dysfunction and loss of aerobic metabolism by the affected cells. The loss of mitochondrial function mandates anaerobic metabolic pathways by the affected cells, an ongoing reduction of ATP generation, thus further potentiating oxidative stress. The oxidative cellular injury introduced by shock potentiates oxidative injury produced by tissue trauma, infection, and sepsis as shown in Figure 12.1.

Global hypoxia and reperfusion directly activates the proinflammatory nuclear transcription factor NF-κB with increased production of cytokines (TNF, IL-1, IL-6, IL-8), chemokines, coagulation factors, adhesion molecules, and activation of tissue macrophages and neutrophils. The shock state also directly activates the innate immune system through the release of a variety of substances (referred to as "damage-associated molecular patterns" or DAMPs) that are recognized by toll-like receptors (particularly TLR4) expressed on endothelial cells, neutrophils, and tissue macrophages. Systemic activation of macrophages and neutrophils results in direct tissue damage and still further cellular oxidant injury. As in the case oxidant generation, activation of the proinflammatory state and the innate immune system by shock potentiates the activation of the inflammatory cascade caused by other insults such as tissue trauma, infection, and sepsis.

Shock and SIRS

The persistence of the shock state creates a nonlinear increase in oxidative injury and activation of the inflammatory cascade and innate immune system. Increasing severity and persistence of shock will produce systemic inflammatory response syndrome (SIRS) and organ dysfunction, culminating in MODS.

Simplified Model of Oxidant Stress in Sepsis, Shock, and Trauma

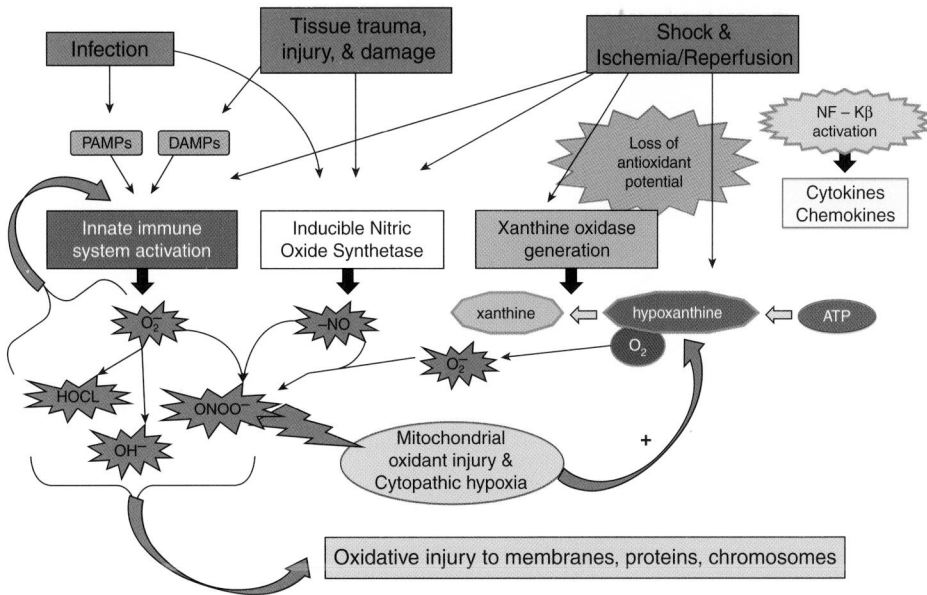

FIGURE 12.1 This simplified model of oxidant stress in sepsis, shock, and trauma demonstrates the overlapping nature of oxidant generation from these insults. Infection, tissue injury, and ischemia/reperfusion injury all activate the innate immune system via the molecular patterns recognized by toll-like receptors on immune cells which in turn produce several oxidative species. Additionally, nitric oxide production is up-regulated. Shock and ischemia/reperfusion injury may also irreversibly cleave xanthine dehydrogenase to xanthine oxidase, increasing the production of oxidant stress. Finally, significant cellular oxidative stress can induce mitochondrial injury and cytopathic hypoxia. PAMPs, pathogen-associated molecular patterns, DAMPs, damage-associated molecular patterns. Oxidative species: HOCL, hypochlorous acid; O_2^-, superoxide; NO, nitric oxide; OH^-, hydroxide; $ONOO^-$, peroxynitrite.

Additionally, shock also creates and enhances vasodilation resulting in distributive shock. SIRS can result from or be exacerbated by shock. Activation of the inflammatory cascade and the subsequent proinflammatory state outlined above produces physiologic changes in temperature (hyperthermia, temperature > 38°C or less commonly hypothermia, temperature < 36°C), heart rate (tachycardia HR > 90), minute ventilation (respiratory rate > 20), and changes in white blood cell count (leukocytosis WBC > 12,000, bandemia > 10% bands, or less commonly leukopenia WBC < 4,000), with two or more of these changes defining *SIRS*. As the severity of this process progresses, organ dysfunction will be manifest, thus defining *severe SIRS*. The presence of SIRS and severe SIRS in which the etiology is infectious defines *sepsis* and *severe sepsis*, respectively. In critically ill patients, SIRS and sepsis are very common, occurring in roughly 75% to 80% of this population. However, SIRS is significantly more common than is sepsis, a fact that should be considered when making decisions regarding empiric antibiotics in response to fever and leukocytosis.

Vasodilation

During shock, vascular smooth muscle function is altered leading to vasodilation. Vascular smooth muscle function is directly altered by a loss of ATP production, decreased cytoplasmic calcium and decreased phosphorylation of myosin, decreasing smooth muscle contraction. The resulting vasodilation is propagated by the up-regulation of nitric oxide synthetase and subsequently increased nitric oxide production, resulting in even greater vascular smooth muscle relaxation. As a result, systemic vascular resistance falls and distributive (or vasodilatory) shock develops. Thus, a distributive shock state may develop secondary to other forms of shock. The vasodilated state may persist for days and may require

prolonged vasoconstrictive agents to ensure adequate mean arterial pressure (MAP) to ensure tissue perfusion. Increasing severity and length of hypoperfusion increases the magnitude of this series of events. Thus, hypovolemic, obstructive, and cardiogenic shock may all initiate a state of distributive or vasodilatory shock following resuscitation. After correction of the original underlying physiologic defect (e.g., hemorrhagic shock), subsequent therapy may be required to correct the vasodilatory component rather than continuing pure volume replacement.

Additionally, tissue hypoxia and sepsis both may lead to defects in the production of *vasopressin* by the hypothalamus and *cortisol* by the adrenal glands. Additionally, the use of etomidate as an induction agent for endotracheal intubation is commonly associated with a period of adrenal insufficiency. Deficiencies of either vasopressin or cortisol will produce vasodilation and distributive shock that is refractory to inotropic support. These deficiencies will coexist with the distributive shock resulting from nitric oxide–induced vasodilation and may complicate management of other forms of shock.

Coagulopathy

While large volumes of blood loss may be sustained without the development of coagulopathy if normotension is maintained, coagulopathy develops at much a much smaller volume of blood loss if shock is present. Tissue hypoxia directly potentiates coagulopathy, and on-going shock will worsen derangements that are introduced by blood loss, hypothermia, and infection. Significant overlap of the coagulation system, the anticoagulant and fibrinolytic pathways, and the inflammatory system exists, and hypoperfusion and tissue hypoxia will potentiate alteration in both pro- and anticoagulation arms of the coagulation system via multiple mechanisms. Hypoxia may directly alter the release of tissue factor, tissue plasminogen activator, and activation of protein C. These changes overlap and exacerbate those introduced by hemorrhage, hypothermia, and sepsis. Thus, during resuscitation and treatment of patients in shock, recognition that coagulopathy may develop during and be exacerbated by the shock state is important to minimize the chance of potentiation of bleeding and complications related to the derangements in the coagulation system.

Cardiac and Renal Dysfunction

In general, the physiologic response to decreasing perfusion or perfusion pressure is to preserve blood flow and pressure to the brain and the heart. As delivery becomes inadequate, organs that require consistently high levels of ATP production to maintain normal function become altered, specifically the heart and kidney. The alteration in cardiac and renal function following shock complicates the resuscitation of patients with shock, particularly if shock has been prolonged or severe.

Cardiac dysfunction following shock may be quite significant but unrecognized after resuscitation. Cardiac dysfunction may occur even in previously young, healthy individuals and is typically severe in patients who are elderly or have underlying cardiac disease. At rest, the heart has the highest oxygen extraction ratio of all the organs. The increased heart rate that occurs as a consequence of shock greatly increases oxygen demand by the heart, while decreasing the diastolic perfusion time. In shock states, decreasing perfusion pressure and increasing demands coupled with increasing heart rate quickly create hypoxic conditions, necessitating anaerobic metabolism and a loss of ATP production. Sodium/potassium (Na/K) and sodium/calcium (Na/Ca) ATPase pumps become dysfunctional. Thus, cellular swelling, a loss of contractility, and a decrease in compliance of the heart develop. To achieve adequate filling of the ventricles postshock, higher central venous pressures (CVP) are required, and to achieve adequate contractility, inotropic agents may be necessary. Assessing adequacy of delivery by specific measures of perfusion such as trends in serum lactate, mixed venous or central venous oxygen saturation, and cardiac index or oxygen delivery may be necessary.

Renal function and renal concentrating ability may be significantly altered during periods of either compensated or uncompensated shock. To maintain normal function, the kidneys also require consistent ATP generation. The kidneys concentrate urine by maintaining concentration gradients within the renal medulla; under normal conditions, the renal medulla is relatively hypoxic. During limited perfusion, ATPase pumps cannot maintain adequate concentration gradients; upon reperfusion, urine output may be excessive and dilute. Thus, urine output by the kidney may be a measure of adequate perfusion following periods of shock.

Assessment of Organ Perfusion

The goal of therapeutic interventions for shock, regardless of etiology, is to restore adequate tissue perfusion in order to limit cellular and organ injury because sustained tissue hypoxia is one of the most important cofactors in the development of multiple organ injury. Tissue perfusion is dependent upon forward flow of oxygenated blood and adequate perfusion pressure. As noted in sections above, assessment of adequate organ perfusion during and after resuscitation may be complicated by (a) the presence of compensated shock,

(b) changes in cardiac compliance and function, (c) alteration in renal function, and (d) the distributive shock that develops secondary to tissue hypoxia. Unfortunately, no single measure is adequately sensitive or specific in all settings to document adequacy of organ perfusion. Thus, an array of techniques may be required. A brief overview of commonly employed measures is provided below, outlining settings in which measures are adequate and inadequate.

The most commonly used measures of organ perfusion are the assessment hemodynamic parameters and organ function. Significant tachycardia, hypotension, low urine output, cool extremities to physical exam, and alteration in mental status all indicate inadequate perfusion absent conditions that specifically alter each individual measure. However, as noted above, significant limitations to organ perfusion may exist despite all of these being normal. In young, otherwise healthy patients without a period of significant shock, these parameters are most likely adequate, if normal. However, if a period of significant shock is suspected, these measures lose their value. Additionally, in geriatric patients suffering significant stress or insult, these measures are frequently inadequate.

One approach to assessing adequacy of perfusion is to assess the accumulation of by-products of inadequate perfusion through the assessment of either *serum lactate* or *base deficit* (BD). Cells with inadequate perfusion must undergo anaerobic metabolism to continue ATP production. By-products of anaerobic metabolism include the generation of lactic acid as well as the buildup of other acids generated by ATP metabolism and accumulation of acids used in the mitochondrial respiratory process that contribute to BD. While these two measures are similar, they have different characteristics and limitations. Additionally, while these measures may indicate inadequate perfusion, they do not indicate the physiologic defect or defects contributing to the tissue hypoxia such as hypovolemia, cardiac dysfunction, or distributive shock. Thus, they typically must be used in the context of additional information that provides assessment of the underlying defect.

BD can be a sensitive measure of hypoperfusion but, unfortunately, lacks specificity. BD is calculated by the formula $BD = -[(HCO_3) - 24.8 + (16.2 \times (pH - 7.4))]$ and reflects the buildup of acids within the circulation. In the setting of inadequate tissue perfusion and hypoxia, numerous acids accumulate including lactic acid, by-products of ATP metabolism, and products used by the mitochondria. BD tends to change more rapidly than does serum lactate and may reflect hypoperfusion even when lactate is within normal limits. During pregnancy, recognition that maternal circulation is preserved over fetal circulation and that elevated BD or a decline in serum bicarbonate is important to ensure fetal perfusion. However, numerous therapeutic interventions may alter BD independent of adequacy of perfusion, including the choice of fluid provided to the patient (lactated ringers versus normal saline). Elevated BD predicts poor outcome in acutely injured patients, even in the setting of normal lactate. Thus, this measure can alert the practitioner to occult hypoperfusion but must be interpreted with caution, particularly after resuscitation has been initiated.

Serum lactate is a more specific measure of the adequacy of organ perfusion than is BD but does have significant limitations. Lactate is generated under conditions of anaerobic metabolism to allow ongoing glycolysis and generation of 2 ATP through the conversion of pyruvate by the lactate dehydrogenase enzyme and the generation of NAD from NADH. Serum lactate elevation and its persistence in sepsis and trauma strongly correlate with organ dysfunction and death.

Studies suggest that resuscitation efforts directed to normalize serum lactate improve outcome, but this remains inadequately studied. Lactate is effectively metabolized and cleared from the serum by the liver; thus, it only rises if hepatic clearance is exceeded and may rise relatively slowly. Metabolic processes that convert NAD to NADH, such as alcohol metabolism, limit the mitochondrial oxidative phosphorylation by consuming NAD and limiting pyruvates conversion to acetyl-CoA and entry into the tricarboxylic acid cycle (TCA or Krebs cycle). Additionally, epinephrine can directly elevate lactate. Other processes that confound the use of lactate as a marker of adequacy of perfusion include hepatic insufficiency and cytopathic hypoxia. In both cases, lactate may be elevated despite normal organ perfusion. In cytopathic hypoxia, the inability of the mitochondria to utilize oxygen mandates ongoing glycolysis and lactate generation.

Venous Oxygen Saturation

Another measure of adequacy of delivery and resuscitation is the use of venous oxygen saturation as a surrogate for the balance between systemic oxygen delivery (D_{O2}), global oxygen consumption (V_{O2}), and the fraction of delivered oxygen that is consumed (extraction ratio—ER_{O2}) in critically ill patients. As oxygen consumption increases relative to delivery, the extraction ratio increases and is reflected as a decline in venous saturation. The most precise measurement of global venous saturation is the mixed venous oxygen saturation (SvO_2), reflecting venous blood from all portions of the body, including the coronary sinus. However, its measurement requires the placement of a pulmonary artery catheter. An alternative is the use of central venous oxygen saturation ($ScvO_2$) via a central line positioned in the superior vena cava or right atria. The two differ slightly, and some data suggest that they may not be interchangeable. The $ScvO_2$ may be up to 6% higher than SvO_2, but trends in either appear to adequately reflect resuscitation. Generally, values of less than 70% for both measures reflect increased, compensatory extraction. Changes in SvO_2 and $ScvO_2$ occur rapidly; thus, venous saturation can be used as a real-time assessment of resuscitative efforts. The use of venous saturation as a guide to resuscitation in sepsis and other forms of shock has been shown to improve targeted resuscitation and outcomes and may outperform lactate in certain settings.

Limitations to venous saturation include its requiring invasive procedures for placement of either a pulmonary catheter or central line. Additionally, in patients with true shunts (e.g., patients with liver failure) and in patients who have developed cytopathic hypoxia, extraction oxygen extraction will be diminished and venous saturation may be supranormal.

Assessments of Cardiac Filling and Function

Assessments of cardiac filling and cardiac output are both frequently used to guide resuscitation. To maintain adequate oxygen delivery to tissues, the heart must maintain adequate cardiac output. Output by the heart is determined by heart rate and stroke volume, and stroke volume is determined by filling and contractility. CVP, pulmonary artery pressure, and pulmonary wedge pressure, pulse pressure variation and pulse contour analysis, and ultrasound and echocardiography may all be used to estimate filling. The first three measures all provide an assessment of pressure and one must recognize that pressures do not directly assess volume. With changes in the compliance of the heart, as occurs during shock and resuscitation, the volume for a given pressure changes as well. This is

very significant limitation of these values when used to assess adequacy of filling. Ultrasound and echocardiography may be used to provide an estimate of filling but may be technically difficult in many settings of critical illness.

Assessment of cardiac output and function may be determined by pulmonary artery catheter, pulse pressure variation and pulse contour analysis, and transesophageal echocardiography. However, each method has settings in which accuracy of these values may be limited. Additionally, knowledge of the cardiac output does not necessarily equate to adequate oxygen delivery. Tissue perfusion is dependent upon both delivery and perfusion pressure. Oxygen demand by tissues also is not static, and no specific cardiac output is indicative of adequate perfusion in all settings.

Other Assessments of Oxygen Delivery

Research to identify noninvasive measures that can detect occult tissue hypoxia and assure adequacy of resuscitation continues. Additional tools that have been or continue to be investigated include regional capnometry, near-infrared spectroscopy, and sidestream dark-field video microscopy. However, none have achieved widespread acceptance or use.

TREATMENT OF SHOCK

The treatment of shock should be directed toward correcting the underlying physiologic defect or defects that are contributing to inadequate organ perfusion, such as (a) hypovolemia, (b) vasodilatation, or (c) cardiac dysfunction. Both compensated (or occult) and uncompensated shock should be corrected expeditiously to prevent exacerbation of organ dysfunction and propagation of the derangements outlined above. Additionally, during pregnancy, care must be taken to ensure adequate fetal perfusion. While a single underlying insult, such as hemorrhage or infection, most frequently initiates the development of shock, understanding that the physiologic derangements introduced by severe shock frequently include more than one type of shock (i.e., hypovolemic, distributive, and cardiogenic components) is paramount to achieving the best outcome. These secondary components of shock develop as a result of tissue hypoxia; thus, aggressive correction of the underlying primary cause of the shock may fail to improve or even aggravate the other components of shock in the complex patient. The magnitude of each of the various components changes during the course of the illness and recognition of the dynamic nature of the process is important.

While the appropriate treatment of the underlying defect will improve the shock state, incorrectly treating the combination of physiologic defects may worsen hypoperfusion or contribute to other secondary problems such as abdominal compartment syndrome or acute volume overload. For example, treatment of patients with hypotension due to low cardiac output with vasoconstrictive agents will increase systemic vascular resistance, raising blood pressure, but actually decrease cardiac output and delivery. This circumstance may occur when either hemorrhagic shock or cardiogenic failure is treated with high-dose Levophed rather than appropriately treating with either blood products or medications to specifically improve inotropy.

Hemorrhagic Shock

The most common cause of shock in the obstetric and gynecologic patient is hemorrhage. In 2005, hemorrhagic shock was the third leading cause of maternal death due to obstetric factors in the United States. Significant advances in our understanding of resuscitation of patients with severe hemorrhagic shock have been made in the past decade, predominately through the trauma literature. The expected signs and symptoms for the degree of shock is provided in Table 12.1, as put forth in the ATLS guidelines. While patients with limited blood loss, class I and class II hemorrhagic shock, may respond to crystalloid resuscitation, patients with larger volume of hemorrhage will require blood and blood component therapy. Goals during the resuscitation of patients in hemorrhagic shock are to achieve replacement of adequate circulating volume while avoiding coagulopathy, hypothermia, progressive acidosis, and excessive crystalloid administration.

Patients with significant hemorrhagic shock may have alterations in their level of consciousness, and an assessment of the safety of their airway and ability to maintain oxygenation should be undertaken and an airway established as required. Two large bore IVs (18 gauge or larger) should be established to ensure the ability to provide crystalloid and blood products without limitation of flow and cell lysis by the catheter. Efforts should be made to maintain patient normothermia. These may include (a) warm fluids, (b) fluid warming devices, (c) heated ventilator circuits with temperature turned to 38°C to 40°C, (d) forced air warming devices, and (e) ambient room temperature set at 26.5°C to 29°C. While beyond the scope of this chapter, prompt intervention to control the source of hemorrhage is required while resuscitative efforts are continued.

As noted in Table 12.1, patients with hemorrhage of up to 30% of their blood volume may be treated with crystalloid resuscitation without necessarily requiring blood products, assuming on-going hemorrhage has been controlled and pre-existing ischemic cardiac disease is not present. Patients with blood loss greater than 30% will require blood and blood product administration. The approach to transfusion in a patient with hemorrhagic shock with ongoing blood loss should be different than in those patients with large volume blood loss without shock. Traditionally, resuscitation for hemorrhage has been centered on replacing circulating volume with crystalloid and packed red blood cells (PRBCs). In situations in which blood loss has been matched by fluid and blood replacement without limitations in blood flow (isovolemic blood loss), large volumes of blood may be administered without the development of coagulopathy, and administration of other blood products like fresh frozen plasma (FFP), cryoprecipitate, and platelets should be based upon abnormal laboratory analysis. However, as outlined above, the presence of shock and tissue hypoxia contributes to coagulopathy, and empiric treatment with other components may be indicated. Data predominately from civilian and military trauma literature support an approach in patients with massive hemorrhage which limits crystalloid resuscitation and provides replacement of blood products approximating a 1:1:1 ratio of PRBCs, FFP, and platelets. To achieve this, most centers have developed massive transfusion protocols (MTPs) to provide the correct ratios of products, once activated. An example of the MTP implemented at Vanderbilt University Medical Center is provided in Figure 12.2. Absolute activation points are difficult to establish for all patients. The use of MTPs should be considered in patients with ongoing hemorrhage (or risk of ongoing hemorrhage) and hypotension (systolic blood pressure <90 mm Hg) after initial 2 U of PRBCs. The use of MTPs should be considered in a bleeding patient with severe acidosis, existing coagulopathy, thrombocytopenia, or hypothermia[444]. The use and timing of other products such as cryoprecipitate or recombinant factor VII remains controversial and variable in practice.

Distributive Shock

The most common cause of distributive shock in obstetric and gynecologic patients is sepsis although other etiologies should also be considered such as severe SIRS following ischemia/reperfusion, adrenal insufficiency, vasopressin deficiency, and anaphylaxis. In all cases of distributive shock, the underlying problem is predominantly vasodilation with inadequate perfusion pressure. Thus, therapy should be directed predominantly to increasing vascular vasomotor tone. The therapeutic agents and approach to achieve appropriate vasoconstriction vary depending on the cause and are discussed below.

Sepsis and Septic Shock

Sepsis is a common problem and is one of the most common causes of critical illness in both obstetric and gynecologic surgery patient populations. The diagnosis of sepsis may be difficult to establish in critically ill patients with insults that may initiate the SIRS. Diagnostic criteria for sepsis, severe sepsis, and septic shock are outlined in Tables 12.2 and 12.3. The treatment of *septic shock* involves three critical components: (a) source control, (b) appropriate empiric antibiotic therapy, and (c) restoration of cellular perfusion. While beyond the scope of this chapter, the importance of adequate *source control* cannot be overemphasized. Elimination of necrotic or infected tissues, elimination of infected fluid collections, elimination or control of enteric connections, and reduction of bacterial load are all components of adequate source control. A specific anatomical diagnosis for the source of infection should be sought, either establishing or excluding potential sources within the differential as soon as possible and interventions to establish control within 12 hours after the diagnosis of sepsis as possible. Critically ill patients with previous efforts to establish source control and with an appropriate course of antibiotic therapy who are not responding appropriately should be evaluated for failure of primary source control, typically with diagnostic imaging such as computed tomography.

Empiric Antibiotic Therapy

Timely and appropriate *empiric antibiotic therapy* is also critical in patients with septic shock. Significant observational data demonstrate that inadequate empiric antibiotic coverage (not active against all pathogens) significantly increases mortality, despite altering therapy when sensitivities return. Thus, broad empiric antibiotic coverage targeted to cover all likely pathogens should be initiated and then de-escalated once culture and sensitivity data are available. Additionally, antibiotics should be initiated as soon as sepsis and septic shock is suspected, ideally within 1 hour. In one large observational study of critically ill patients with septic shock, each 1 hour delay in antibiotic therapy from the onset of shock was associated with a 12% increase in mortality. Appropriate culture data should be obtained to allow de-escalation of therapy and the antibiotic regimen narrowed to the least number of agents required to appropriate treat the pathogens involved. As noted above, patients not responding to therapy in an appropriate manner should be evaluated for inadequate source control rather than simply extending antibiotic courses beyond 7 days.

Background: Protocolized transfusion has been shown to improve clinical outcomes as well as transfusion efficiency in patients who require massive transfusion (>10 U in 24 hours). This document provides guidelines for utilization of the massive transfusion protocol (MTP).

1. Patient selection
   a. Patients with current, ongoing, or impending massive blood loss should be considered for activation of MTP.
   b. Activation of massive transfusion protocol should be considered for patients who received greater than 2 u of blood in the emergency department (1).
2. Activation
   a. MTP may be activated by the attending surgeon, intensivist or designated surrogate. If surrogate activates MTP, attending surgeon of record must be provided to blood bank (BB).
   b. MTP may be activated by trauma/surgical cc faculty, fellows and instructors; anesthesiology faculty; and selected surgical faculty ONLY.
   c. Upon suspicion of MTP activation, type and screen must be sent to BB as soon as possible.
   d. To activate MTP, call BB at _____ and provide the following information
      i. "This is Dr. _____ activating the MTP....."
      ii. Patient name
      iii. Patient MRN. This will be repeated by BB personnel for verification purposes.
      iv. Patient age
      v. Patient gender
      vi. Current or intended location
3. Product breakdown
   a. Each round of MTP provides 6U PRBC, 4U FFP, 1 dose pack of platelets Repeat rounds of MTP contain identical product "doses"
4. Administration
   a. Products are delivered, and BB calls patient location to verify continuation of MTP. Default is to continue MTP until verbally discontinued by faculty physician.
   b. MTP boxes are intended to be given in their entirety until completed. If not all products are desired, strong consideration should be given to MTP discontinuation.
5. Endpoints/termination
   a. When appropriate endpoints are reached, the MTP must be discontinued to limit resource utilization.
   b. Most reliable transfusion endpoint is a collaborative decision based on operative field examination, laboratory results, and clinical parameters.
   c. Premature discontinuation of MTP should be avoided to minimize catch-up reactive transfusion.
6. Pitfalls, common errors
   a. Failure to send type and screen.
      i. T&S must be sent upon suspicion of MTP requirement.
   b. Returning platelets on ice.
      i. Cold temperature destroys platelets. Must be returned in cooler side pouch.
   c. Failure to identify significant hemorrhage, delayed MTP activation.
      i. Result in delayed activation, over activation is anticipated
   d. Premature termination.
      i. Consider continuing MTP until patient stabilizes in the ICU.
   e. Failure to provide entire box/dose.
      i. If not all products are required, d/c MTP and transfuse PRN.
      ii. Collaborate with intensivist/anesthesiologist regarding transfusion plan.
   f. Reliability on laboratory tests alone for transfusion indication.
      i. Laboratory tests are unreliable in the hyperacute setting.
   g. Inappropriate personnel activating MTP.
      i. BB personnel are empowered to refuse MTP to callers who are not authorized to activate protocol.

References:
1. Nunez, TC, Voskresensky, IV, Dossett, LA, et al. Early prediction of massive transfusion in trauma: simple as ABC (assessment of blood consumption)? *The Journal of Trauma* 2009;66:346–352.
2. Vanderbilt University Medical Center Trauma and Surgical Critical Care, Nashville, TN.

FIGURE 12.2 Massive Transfusion Protocol.

TABLE 12.2 Diagnostic Criteria for Sepsis

Infection, documented or suspected, and some of the
  following:
General variables
  Fever (>38.3°C)
  Hypothermia (core temperature < 36°C)
  Heart rate > 90/min⁻¹ or more than two SD above the
    normal value for age
  Tachypnea
  Altered mental status
  Significant edema or positive fluid balance (>20 mL/kg
    over 24 h)
  Hyperglycemia (plasma glucose > 140 mg/dL or
    7.7 mmol/L) in the absence of diabetes

Inflammatory variables
  Leukocytosis (WBC count > 12,000 µL⁻¹)
  Leukopenia (WBC count < 4,000 µL⁻¹)
  Normal WBC count with >10% immature forms
  Plasma C-reactive protein more than two SD above the
    normal value
  Plasma procalcitonin more than two SD above the
    normal value

Hemodynamic variables
  Arterial hypotension (SBP < 90 mm Hg, MAP < 70 mm
    Hg, or an SBP decrease > 40 mm Hg in adults or <2
    SD below normal for age)

Organ dysfunction variables
  Arterial hypoxemia (PaO₂/FIO₂ < 300)
  Acute oliguria (urine output < 0.5 mL/kg/h for at least 2 h
    despite adequate fluid resuscitation)
  Creatinine increase > 0.5 mg/dL or 44.2 µmol/L
  Coagulation abnormalities (INR > 1.5 or aPTT > 60 s)
  Ileus (absent bowel sounds)
  Thrombocytopenia (platelet count < 100,000 µL⁻¹)
  Hyperbilirubinemia (plasma total bilirubin > 4 mg/dL or
    70 µmol/L)

Tissue perfusion variables
  Hyperlactatemia (>1 mmol/L)
  Decreased capillary refill or mottling

WBC, white blood cell; SBP, systolic blood pressure; MAP, mean
arterial pressure; INR, international normalized ratio; aPTT,
activated partial thromboplastin time.
Adapted from Dellinger RP, et al. Surviving sepsis campaign:
international guidelines for management of severe sepsis and
septic shock: 2012. *Crit Care Med* 2013;41:580–637. Copyright
© 2013 by the Society of Critical Care Medicine and Lippincott
Williams & Wilkins.

TABLE 12.3 Severe Sepsis and Septic Shock

Severe sepsis definition = sepsis-induced tissue
  hypoperfusion or organ dysfunction (any of the following
  thought to be due to the infection)
  Urine output < 0.5 mL/kg/h for >2 h despite adequate
    fluid resuscitation
  Acute lung injury with PaO₂/FIO₂ < 250 in the absence of
    pneumonia as infection source
  Acute lung injury with PaO₂/FIO₂ < 200 in the presence
    of pneumonia as infection source
  Creatinine > 2.0 mg/dL (176.8 µmol/L)
  Bilirubin > 2 mg/dL (34.2 µmol/L)
  Platelet count < 100,000 µL
  Coagulopathy (international normalized ratio > 1.5)
  Lactate above upper limits laboratory normal (tissue
    hypoperfusion)
  Sepsis-induced hypotension (septic shock)

Adapted from Dellinger RP, et al. Surviving sepsis campaign:
international guidelines for management of severe sepsis and
septic shock: 2012. *Crit Care Med* 2013;41:580–637. Copyright
© 2013 by the Society of Critical Care Medicine and Lippincott
Williams & Wilkins.

organ perfusion should be constantly monitored to access the effectiveness of the resuscitation and provide indicators to adjust therapy. General recommended goals of resuscitation include the following:

a. CVP of 8 to 12 mm Hg
b. MAP of ≥65 mm Hg
c. Urine output ≥0.5 mL/kg/h
d. Normal assessment of tissue oxygenation
   – Central venous (superior vena cava) or mixed venous
     oxygen saturation of 70% or 65%, respectively
   – Normalization of serum lactate

Recognition that preexisting comorbidity or other clinical conditions may require an alteration of these end points is important to appropriately target resuscitation. For instance, during the third trimester of pregnancy, the normal values for the end points cited above are altered: CVP 4 to 10 mm Hg, MAP 84 to 96 mm Hg, mixed venous saturation >80%.

An example of an algorithm to direct resuscitation in patients with severe sepsis and septic shock is provided in **Figure 12.3**. Initial therapy is directed at replacing the volume deficits with crystalloid fluid resuscitation in a volume of up to 30 mL/kg. Additional crystalloid may be required based upon the analysis of volume status. Additional fluid resuscitation should be based upon ongoing assessments of volume responsiveness; excessive crystalloid administration may worsen acute lung injury, edema, and increase the risk of abdominal compartment syndrome. Patients with large fluid requirements may benefit from provision of albumen. Patients with hypotension or hypoperfusion after adequate fluid resuscitation should have vasopressor therapy added. Norepinephrine is the first-line vasopressor of choice, demonstrating better return of splanchnic perfusion than do other agents. Patients with depressed cardiac function may require the addition of an inotropic agent to achieve adequate cardiac output. Epinephrine may be required in addition to or instead of norepinephrine. Alternative inotropic agents may be considered in combination with norepinephrine such as dobutamine or milrinone.

Restoration of Cellular Perfusion

The third critical component of the treatment of patients with septic shock is the *restoration of cellular perfusion.* Septic patients typically have both volume depletion and vasodilatory components to their shock. Additionally, some patients may also have altered cardiac function. Thus, a quantitative resuscitation managed by a specific protocol should be undertaken. As resuscitation precedes, an evaluation of volume status, blood pressure, organ function, and

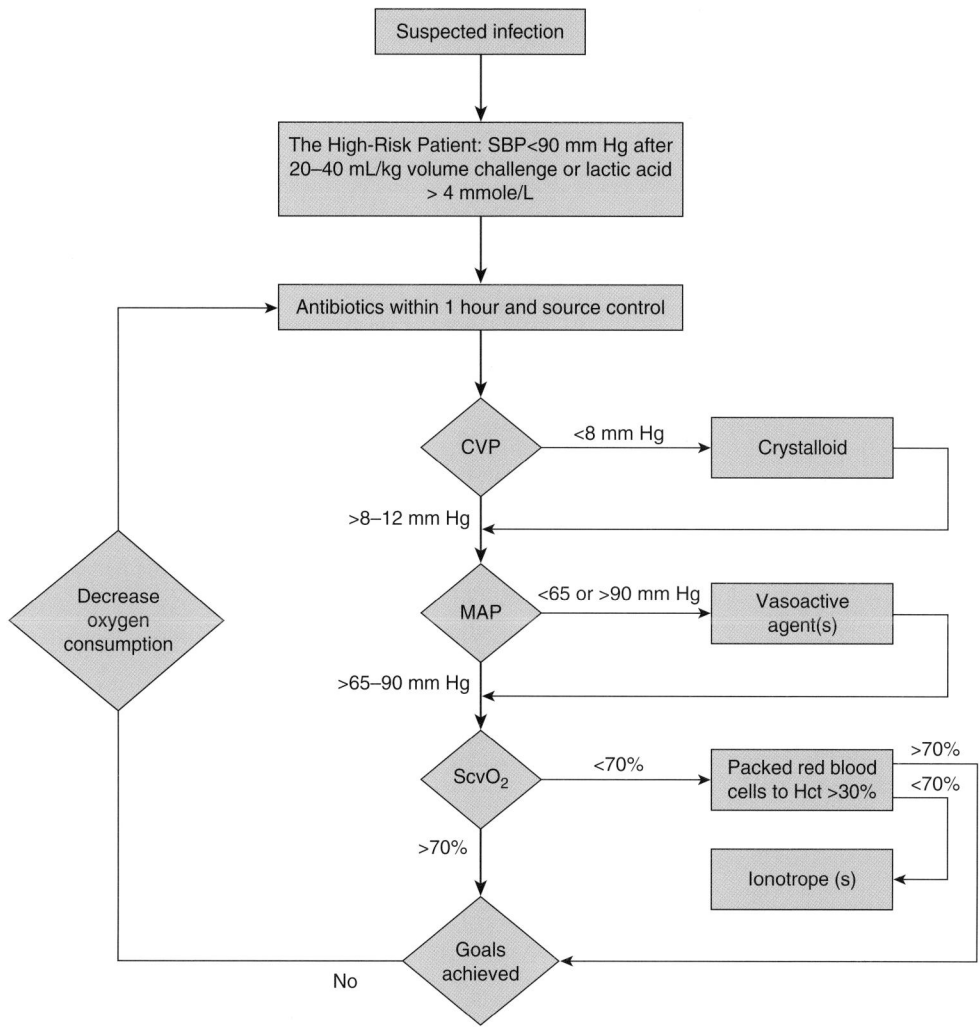

FIGURE 12.3 Algorithm for the goal-directed resuscitation of patients with severe sepsis and septic shock.

Vasopressin and Adrenal Insufficiency

Patients with severe sepsis and septic shock may develop distributive shock related to either vasopressin deficiency or adrenal insufficiency. Patients in whom blood pressure is poorly responsive to or requires high doses of norepinephrine may be *vasopressin deficient*. The addition of a vasopressin infusion at 0.03 to 0.04 units/min may be initiated with responsiveness determined by a decline in norepinephrine requirements. Due to the pronounced vasoconstrictive effects of vasopressin, this agent should not be used as a first-line agent and the use of doses above the recommended range should only be used as salvage therapy. *Adrenal insufficiency* may also develop as a result of sepsis and be a cause of inadequate response to vasopressor therapy. An absolute value of serum hydrocortisone that indicates either adequate or inadequate production is not currently assessable. Thus, presumptive therapy of adrenal insufficiency is currently recommended in patients who appear unresponsive to vasopressor support. Recommended treatment is with hydrocortisone (50 mg every 6 hours) and tapered when vasoactive support is no longer needed and blood pressure is normal.

Other conditions may lead to either vasopressin or adrenal insufficiency. Tissue hypoxia and severe shock may contribute to both. Assessment of serum cortisol levels in these settings remains controversial as an absolute level of serum cortisol for a given state is difficult to establish.

SUMMARY

An understanding that compensated and uncompensated shock create a nonlinear increase in cellular and organ dysfunction is important for the practicing obstetrician and gynecologist. Persistent shock is a self-replicating process, and prompt, targeted therapy directed toward the appropriate contributing components is paramount. Early correction of cellular perfusion limits organ dysfunction and improves outcomes.

BIBLIOGRAPHY

Abraham E, Singer M. Mechanisms of sepsis-induced organ dysfunction. *Crit Care Med* 2007;35:2408.

American College of Surgeons Committee on Trauma. Shock. In: *Advanced trauma life support for doctors: ATLS student course manual.* Chicago, IL: American College of Surgeons, 2008:61.

Annane D, Bellissant E, Bollaert PE, et al. Corticosteroids in the treatment of severe sepsis and septic shock in adults: a systematic review. *JAMA* 2009;301:2362.

Barie PS, Hydo LJ, Shou J, et al. Influence of antibiotic therapy on mortality of critical surgical illness caused or complicated by infection. *Surg Infect (Larchmt)* 2005;6:41.

Bone RC, Balk RA, Cerra FB, et al. Definitions for sepsis and organ failure and guidelines for the use of innovative therapies in sepsis. The ACCP/SCCM Consensus Conference Committee American College of Chest Physicians/Society of Critical Care Medicine. *Chest* 1992;101:1644.

Bradburn E, Rogers FB, Krasne M, et al. High-risk geriatric protocol: improving mortality in the elderly. *J Trauma Acute Care Surg* 2012;73:435.

Cairns CB, Moore FA, Haenel JB, et al. Evidence for early supply independent mitochondrial dysfunction in patients developing multiple organ failure after trauma. *J Trauma* 1997;42:532.

Callaway DW, Shapiro NI, Donnino MW, et al. Serum lactate and base deficit as predictors of mortality in normotensive elderly blunt trauma patients. *J Trauma* 2009;66:1040.

Claridge JA, Crabtree TD, Pelletier SJ, et al. Persistent occult hypoperfusion is associated with a significant increase in infection rate and mortality in major trauma patients. *J Trauma* 2000;48:8.

Cohen MJ. Towards hemostatic resuscitation: the changing understanding of acute traumatic biology, massive bleeding, and damage-control resuscitation. *Surg Clin North Am* 2012;92:877.

Cohen WR. Hemorrhagic shock in obstetrics. *J Perinat Med* 2006;34:263.

Cotton BA, Guillamondegui OD, Fleming SB, et al. Increased risk of adrenal insufficiency following etomidate exposure in critically injured patients. *Arch Surg* 2008;143:62.

Cotton BA, Reddy N, Hatch QM, et al. Damage control resuscitation is associated with a reduction in resuscitation volumes and improvement in survival in 390 damage control laparotomy patients. *Ann Surg* 2011;254:598.

Crouser ED. Mitochondrial dysfunction in septic shock and multiple organ dysfunction syndrome. *Mitochondrion* 2004;4:729.

Crowl AC, Young JS, Kahler DM, et al. Occult hypoperfusion is associated with increased morbidity in patients undergoing early femur fracture fixation. *J Trauma* 2000;48:260.

Davies MG, Hagen PO. Systemic inflammatory response syndrome. *Br J Surg* 1997;84:920.

De Backer D, Aldecoa C, Njimi H, et al. Dopamine versus norepinephrine in the treatment of septic shock: a meta-analysis*. *Crit Care Med* 2012;40:725.

De Backer D, Creteur J, Silva E, et al. Effects of dopamine, norepinephrine, and epinephrine on the splanchnic circulation in septic shock: which is best? *Crit Care Med* 2003;31:1659.

Dellinger RP, Levy MM, Rhodes A, et al. Surviving sepsis campaign: international guidelines for management of severe sepsis and septic shock: 2012. *Crit Care Med* 2013;41:580.

Duchesne JC, McSwain NE, Jr, Cotton BA, et al. Damage control resuscitation: the new face of damage control. *J Trauma* 2010;69:976.

Dunham CM, Siegel JH, Weireter L, et al. Oxygen debt and metabolic acidemia as quantitative predictors of mortality and the severity of the ischemic insult in hemorrhagic shock. *Crit Care Med* 1991;19:231.

Dunham CM, Watson LA, Cooper C. Base deficit level indicating major injury is increased with ethanol. *J Emerg Med* 2000;18:165.

Dunne JR, Tracy JK, Scalea TM, et al. Lactate and base deficit in trauma: does alcohol or drug use impair their predictive accuracy? *J Trauma* 2005;58:959.

Dutton RP. Resuscitative strategies to maintain homeostasis during damage control surgery. *Br J Surg* 2012;99(suppl 1):21.

Englehart MS, Schreiber MA. Measurement of acid–base resuscitation endpoints: lactate, base deficit, bicarbonate or what? *Curr Opin Crit Care* 2006;12:569.

Fink MP. Bench-to-bedside review: cytopathic hypoxia. *Crit Care* 2002;6:491.

Guinn DA, Abel DE, Tomlinson MW. Early goal directed therapy for sepsis during pregnancy. *Obstet Gynecol Clin North Am* 2007;34:459.

Gurgel ST, do Nascimento PC, Jr. Maintaining tissue perfusion in high-risk surgical patients: a systematic review of randomized clinical trials. *Anesth Analg* 2011;112:1384.

Holley A, Lukin W, Paratz J, et al. Review article: part two: goal-directed resuscitation—which goals? Perfusion targets. *Emerg Med Australas* 2012;24:127.

Holmes CL, Patel BM, Russell JA, et al. Physiology of vasopressin relevant to management of septic shock. *Chest* 2001;120:989.

Ibrahim EH, Sherman G, Ward S, et al. The influence of inadequate antimicrobial treatment of bloodstream infections on patient outcomes in the ICU setting. *Chest* 2000;118:146.

James JH, Luchette FA, McCarter FD, et al. Lactate is an unreliable indicator of tissue hypoxia in injury or sepsis. *Lancet* 1999;354:505.

Jansen TC, van BJ, Schoonderbeek FJ, et al. Early lactate-guided therapy in intensive care unit patients: a multicenter, open-label, randomized controlled trial. *Am J Respir Crit Care Med* 2010;182:752.

Keel M, Trentz O. Pathophysiology of polytrauma. *Injury* 2005;36:691.

Kollef MH, Sherman G, Ward S, et al. Inadequate antimicrobial treatment of infections: a risk factor for hospital mortality among critically ill patients. *Chest* 1999;115:462.

Kumar A, Roberts D, Wood KE, et al. Duration of hypotension before initiation of effective antimicrobial therapy is the critical determinant of survival in human septic shock. *Crit Care Med* 2006;34:1589.

Levy RJ. Mitochondrial dysfunction, bioenergetic impairment, and metabolic down-regulation in sepsis. *Shock* 2007;28:24.

Luna CM, Vujacich P, Niederman MS, et al. Impact of BAL data on the therapy and outcome of ventilator-associated pneumonia. *Chest* 1997;111:676.

Marshall JC. Inflammation, coagulopathy, and the pathogenesis of multiple organ dysfunction syndrome. *Crit Care Med* 2001;29:S99.

Martel MJ, MacKinnon KJ, Arsenault MY, et al. Hemorrhagic shock. *J Obstet Gynaecol Can* 2002;24:504.

Marx G, Reinhart K. Venous oximetry. *Curr Opin Crit Care* 2006;12:263.

Montravers P, Gauzit R, Muller C, et al. Emergence of antibiotic-resistant bacteria in cases of peritonitis after intraabdominal surgery affects the efficacy of empirical antimicrobial therapy. *Clin Infect Dis* 1996;23:486.

Mosdell DM, Morris DM, Voltura A, et al. Antibiotic treatment for surgical peritonitis. *Ann Surg* 1991;214:543.

Nduka OO, Parrillo JE. The pathophysiology of septic shock. *Crit Care Clin* 2009;25:677.

Pacheco LD, Saade GR, Costantine MM, et al. The role of massive transfusion protocols in obstetrics. *Am J Perinatol* 2013;30:1.

Pacheco LD, Saade GR, Gei AF, et al. Cutting-edge advances in the medical management of obstetrical hemorrhage. *Am J Obstet Gynecol* 2011;205:526.

Rios FG, Risso-Vazquez A, Alvarez J, et al. Clinical characteristics and outcomes of obstetric patients admitted to the intensive care unit. *Int J Gynaecol Obstet* 2012;119:136.

Rivers EP, Ahrens T. Improving outcomes for severe sepsis and septic shock: tools for early identification of at-risk patients and treatment protocol implementation. *Crit Care Clin* 2008;24:S1.

Rivers EP, Coba V, Visbal A, et al. Management of sepsis: early resuscitation. *Clin Chest Med* 2008;29:689.

Rivers EP, Coba V, Whitmill M. Early goal-directed therapy in severe sepsis and septic shock: a contemporary review of the literature. *Curr Opin Anaesthesiol* 2008;21:128.

Rivers EP, Elkin R, Cannon CM. Counterpoint: should lactate clearance be substituted for central venous oxygen saturation as goals of early severe sepsis and septic shock therapy? No. *Chest* 2011;140:1408.

Rushing GD, Britt LD. Reperfusion injury after hemorrhage: a collective review. *Ann Surg* 2008;247:929.

Scalea TM, Simon HM, Duncan AO et al. Geriatric blunt multiple trauma: improved survival with early invasive monitoring. *J Trauma* 1990;30:129.

Schulman AM, Claridge JA, Carr G, et al. Predictors of patients who will develop prolonged occult hypoperfusion following blunt trauma. *J Trauma* 2004;57:795.

Seal JB, Gewertz BL. Vascular dysfunction in ischemia-reperfusion injury. *Ann Vasc Surg* 2005;19:572.

Walley KR. Use of central venous oxygen saturation to guide therapy. *Am J Respir Crit Care Med* 2011;184:514.

CHAPTER 13
Wound Healing, Suture Material, and Surgical Instrumentation

Gary H. Lipscomb

DEFINITIONS

Absorbable sutures—Sutures that lose the majority of their tensile strength before 60 days when implanted in body tissues.

Healing by primary intention—Wound healing that occurs if the wound layers are reapproximated following injury.

Healing by secondary intention—Wound healing that occurs if wounds are left open after injury and allowed to close spontaneously from the formation of granulation tissue.

Healing by third intention—Wound healing that occurs when the wound is closed after an initial period of delay of several days also referred to as *delayed primary closure.*

Knot-pull tensile strength—Breaking strength of a suture when tied around a plastic tube using a surgeon's flat knot and stressed from either end.

Nonabsorbable sutures—Sutures that maintain the majority of their tensile strength before 60 days when implanted in body tissues.

WOUND HEALING

Ideally, organic tissue lost by destruction or injury would be replaced with tissue identical in form and function. This process is known as *regeneration*. Although tissue regeneration does occur in lower animals (e.g., salamanders), humans have lost this ability for the most part. With the exception of the epidermis of the skin, mucosa of the intestinal tract, and liver, damaged human tissue heals by the laying down of collagen, a repair process better known as *scarring*. This process is responsible for emergently sealing the wound and ultimately providing long-term structural support for the injured organ but is unable to reproduce other functions of the replaced tissue. As a result, the healing process also leads to disease if an organ becomes unable to function properly owing to extensive replacement of functioning tissue by nonfunctioning scar. Heart failure following a massive myocardial infarction is an example. In other cases, the healing process itself directly produces disease (e.g., postoperative adhesion formation following surgical procedures or tubal occlusion after pelvic inflammatory disease).

Physiology of Wound Healing

The healing of a wound involves several distinct biologic processes: (a) inflammation, (b) epithelialization, (c) fibroplasia, (d) wound contraction, and (e) scar maturation. Although considered distinct, these processes do not occur in a strict sequence but often occur simultaneously with each other. These repair mechanisms are also nonspecific. They are activated whether a wound is made with a surgical scalpel and sutured closed or by trauma and then allowed to heal without surgical closure. However, the nature of the wound influences the degree to which each individual process is involved, and this in turn can affect the ultimate success of the repair.

Inflammation

The inflammatory phase of healing is the initial response to any injury involving more than an epithelial surface. This phase can be divided into two separate but simultaneously occurring responses: a vascular and a cellular response. Both are initiated by amines, most notably histamine, as well as the kinins and proteolytic enzymes released by the injured tissue. Immediately after injury, a transient vasoconstriction of the local vasculature lasts for 5 to 10 minutes. Vasoconstriction is followed by vasodilatation and an increase in vascular permeability. Edema caused by the escape of plasma through altered vessel walls becomes clinically apparent at this point.

The cellular response is characterized by the migration of leukocytes into the injured area. Although the agents responsible for this active migration of leukocytes remain unclear, chemotactic factors are thought to play a major role. Initially, the polymorphonuclear leukocytes and monocytes in the wound are present in the same concentration as in the systemic circulation. As a result, polymorphonuclear leukocytes predominate for the first 3 days. Because polymorphonuclear leukocytes are relatively short-lived compared with monocytes, the latter stages of the inflammatory phase are characterized by a predominance of monocytes that transform into macrophages. These leukocytes actively phagocytize bacteria, foreign proteins, and necrotic debris. As polymorphonuclear leukocytes die, their intracellular enzymes and debris are released into the wound and become part of the wound exudate. These released enzymes also facilitate the breakdown of material not phagocytized by the leukocytes. This accumulated exudate or pus develops even in the absence of bacteria. Even when this exudate is sterile, the presence of proteolytic enzymes, including collagenase, can interfere with epithelialization and fibroplasia and, thus, interfere with continued wound healing. Poor wound healing, however, is more common in wounds contaminated with bacteria and foreign material. In these cases, the inflammatory response may persist for long periods of time.

Epithelialization

By virtue of their exposed location, the epithelial surfaces of the gastrointestinal, urogenital, and respiratory tract as well as the skin itself are continually subjected to the physical and chemical trauma associated with the activities of daily living. As a result, these surfaces are constantly replacing damaged or destroyed cells through a process known as *epithelialization*. Epithelialization occurs by migration and subsequent maturation of immature epithelial cells from the deeper basal layers of surrounding areas. If the cellular damage is confined entirely to the epithelium, the healing response is merely an exaggerated form of the basic normal replacement process.

If an injury involves the supporting connective tissue beneath the epithelium, however, the other components of the healing processes, in addition to epithelialization, become involved. If the injury severs blood vessels, the vessels retract, and the process of hemostasis is initiated. If bleeding is not too severe, a blood clot soon forms. This clot subsequently contracts, dehydrates, and becomes a scab. Within 12 hours, basal cells from the surrounding epithelial surfaces begin migrating onto the injured surface. Epithelial cells move beneath the scab, detaching it from the wound and sealing the surface. In incised and sutured wounds, epithelialization generally produces a watertight seal within 24 hours of injury. This new layer of epithelial cells is initially thin and poorly attached to the underlying surface, rendering it susceptible to injury from even minor trauma. Final epithelial healing is accomplished by differentiation and maturation of the migrated cells and by scar formation through fibroplasia.

Fibroplasia

The process by which wounds regain strength is termed *fibroplasia*. Fibroplasia results in the production of the collagen necessary to form a fibrous scar and ultimately determines the final strength of the healed wound. This process begins with the differentiation of mesenchymal cells into fibroblasts. Fibroblasts then migrate into the wound, apparently along fibrin strands produced during clot formation. Once at the injury site, fibroblasts proliferate and manufacture the glycoproteins and mucopolysaccharides that make up the ground substance of connective tissue. Ground substance is an amorphous matrix that is believed to induce aggregation of collagen subunits and influences the final orientation of the fibers.

Once the ground substance is produced, fibroblasts begin to synthesize the basic building block of collagen–tropocollagen. Tropocollagen is a stiff elongated macromolecule of three helically intertwined chains of amino acids consisting of two identical $\alpha1$ chains and one $\alpha2$ chain. Within the ground substance and at the proper pH, osmolality, and temperature, tropocollagen molecules polymerize into collagen fibrils by forming covalent bonds with their neighbor. These fibrils bond with other fibrils to form collagen bundles. It is not until 4 to 5 days after injury that the wound produces enough collagen to result in a measurable increase in wound tensile strength. Before this time, the wound is held together only by fibrous adhesion. This time frame between wounding and an increase in tensile strength originally was referred to by Howes and Harvey as the "lag period" of wound healing.

Wound Contraction

The manner in which tissue heals is dependent on whether tissue integrity is simply interrupted (as in a surgical incision) or tissue is removed (as in an avulsion injury). In both types of injury, tissue seals itself, begins to reepithelialize, and synthesizes collagen for structural support. However, when large amounts of tissue are missing, the edges of the wound must be brought closer together so that the previously noted tissue responses can repair the defect. This process is known as *contraction*. Contraction of wound margins begins about 5 days after injury and corresponds with the fibroplasia phase of healing. Because this process can be inhibited by cytochrome poisons, such as potassium cyanide, and by smooth muscle relaxants, older theories attributing wound contraction to passive collagen changes have been discarded. Instead, wound contraction appears to be an active process produced by contractile proteins within the fibroblasts. If the area is too large for contraction to bring the edges together, the wound remains covered with granulation tissue, or if small enough, it is covered with epithelium only. Epithelialization of such a wound prevents weeping, but without the normal underlying supporting stroma, it remains too fragile to provide lasting protection. Pathologic progression of skin contraction ultimately may result in restriction of joint or limb mobility. This deformity is termed *contracture* and should not be confused with contraction.

Scar Maturation

The bulky scar formed during the fibroplasia phase consists of randomly oriented soluble collagen fibers. This scar has little tensile strength. During scar maturation, the disordered fibers are replaced with fibers arranged in a more orderly fashion, producing a denser and stronger scar. Collagen fibers also continue to form covalent bonds within fibrils as well as between adjacent fibrils and fibers, resulting in a continued increase in wound tensile strength over time. This maturation process may continue for years.

During scar maturation and remolding, the breakdown of old disordered collagen slightly exceeds production of new organized collagen fibers. The resulting new scar is softer and less bulky than is the original scar but also is stronger because of its more organized and extensively cross-linked nature. However, if collagen production exceeds breakdown, then a keloid or hypertrophied scar results.

Surgical Wound Healing

Depending on the manner of wound closure, three types of surgical wound healing are recognized: primary, secondary, and third intention. Figure 13.1 illustrates these types of wound healing.

Primary intention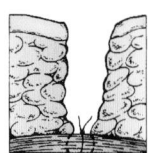

Secondary intention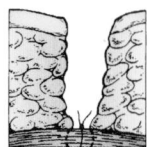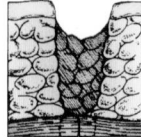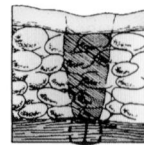

Third intention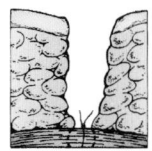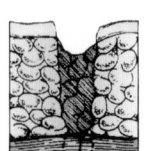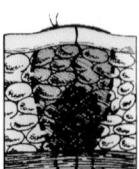

FIGURE 13.1 Types of wound healing.

Primary Intention

Healing occurs by primary intention if the wound layers are reapproximated following injury. This apposition of tissue layers allows healing to occur in a minimum of time, with no separation of wound edges and with minimum scar formation. This is the desired mode of healing for surgical incisions.

Secondary Intention

It has been known for centuries that a wound has a higher resistance to infection when left open rather than closed. This was demonstrated experimentally in dogs by Bilroth, who applied dressings soaked in liquid feces and pus to wounds. Wounds left open remained healthy in appearance, whereas those that were subsequently closed became infected. As a result, contaminated or infected surgical wounds often are left unapproximated and allowed to close spontaneously. This type of wound healing is referred to as healing by secondary intention. This healing process obviously is more complicated and prolonged than that of primary intention. The wound eventually heals by a combination of contraction and the formation of granulation tissue with the wound gradually filling in from the raw surfaces. This type of healing is slow and frequently characterized by formation of excessive scar tissue. Granulation tissue from the healing wound also may protrude above the wound margin during this process. This can prevent final epithelialization of the surface and require further treatment for complete healing.

Third Intention

Wound healing by third intention, also known as *delayed primary closure*, refers to the technique of wound closure after a period of delay. This method often is used after postoperative wound breakdown or as an alternative to healing by secondary intention of wounds that should not be closed primarily, such as grossly contaminated or infected wounds. The timing of closure is important. After delays of 7 to 8 days, the wound edges become increasingly difficult to approximate because of the increasing collagen content. Edlich and colleagues have suggested that closure on or after the 4th day appears to be ideal. This concept also is supported by Lowery and Curtis, who showed that wounds closed after a delay of between 3 and 6 days have the lowest infection rates. Furthermore, studies by Fogdestam revealed that wounds closed during this time frame also have greater wound strength at 20 days than do wounds closed primarily.

Methods of Wound Closure

Wound dehiscence with evisceration is a serious complication of abdominal surgery. This complication is associated with prolonged morbidity and high mortality. Published mortality figures range from 18% to 35%, with a mean of 20%. Wound dehiscence occurs in 0.5% to 5% of all abdominal surgeries but is less frequent (0.1% to 0.7%) with gynecologic abdominal procedures. Potential reasons for the decreased rate of dehiscence associated with gynecologic surgery include the use of transverse incisions, healthier patients, lower infection rates, and a lower rate of bowel enterotomies.

Traditionally, gynecologic surgeons have been taught that vertical incisions are associated with a greater likelihood of dehiscence than are transverse incisions. Critical review of the earlier data supporting this conclusion reveals that significant confounding variables often were ignored. In general, vertical incisions often were performed emergently on sicker patients or those who had other risk factors for dehiscence, such as

cancer. Transverse incisions typically were performed on relatively healthy patients undergoing elective surgery. At least two randomized studies by Greenall and colleagues and Stone and associates have shown no difference in hernia formation or dehiscence between vertical and transverse incisions.

Proper suture selection is critical in preventing wound dehiscence. The wound may break down if the suture has too little initial tensile strength or if the suture is absorbed too quickly before the wound regains enough strength to resist normal stress. The suture also is only as strong as the knots placed in it. If the knot is tied using an improper technique or too few knots are placed, the knot can slip and the suture line fail. The issues involved with proper suture selection and knot security are discussed in detail later in this chapter. Proper surgical technique is one of the most critical factors in preventing wound dehiscence. Several studies have indicated that the most common cause of wound dehiscence is intact sutures pulling through fascia. Animal studies have confirmed that incisions closed with wide loose fascial bites have greater tensile strength than do those closed using smaller fascial bites. Sanders and DiClementi also have shown that tightly tied fascial sutures result in fascial necrosis beneath the sutures. Thus, the old adage that one should "approximate and not strangulate fascia" is well taken.

Although the use of loose, wide fascial bites appears to reduce the likelihood of suture pull-through, the optimum distance sutures should be placed from the fascial edge is unknown. However, data obtained by Campbell and colleagues can provide some guidelines. When the pullout force and pullout energy of sutures placed in cadaver fascia were plotted against bite size, bites of 0.9 cm yielded the maximum pullout force, but maximum pullout energy was obtained with bite sizes of 1.2 to 1.5 cm. Unfortunately, it is unknown whether pullout energy or pullout force is more clinically relevant.

Tera and Aberg, working with human cadavers, have shown that the strength of a sutured midline incision is approximately doubled if sutures are placed lateral enough to include the edge of rectus muscle. Normally a bite of approximately 1.5 to 2 cm is required to include rectus muscle in a midline closure. From these studies, it appears that fascia sutures should be placed at least 1.0 cm from the fascia edge and that bites of 1.5 cm or larger are probably preferable.

The use of large tissue bites may be responsible, in part, for the success of mass closure techniques, such as retention sutures, or the Smead-Jones closure, in which wide sutures are passed through fascia, muscle, and peritoneum. The Smead-Jones mass closure consists of a combination "far" mass closure bite at least 2.5 cm from the fascial edge on each side of the incision with a second "near" bite through the fascial edge. This far–far/near–near technique is considered the gold standard for vertical closure because it has been shown consistently to be more secure than simple layered closure.

Unfortunately, the Smead-Jones technique is time consuming and requires a large number of sutures. One solution to this problem has been the use of a continuous running mass closure. In gynecologic surgery, abdominal incisions traditionally have been closed in layers with interrupted sutures. The belief that interrupted sutures provide greater wound security than does a continuous suture is not well documented, and there are several well-performed studies using both general surgery and gynecologic oncology patient populations showing continuous closure to be comparable to Smead-Jones closure provided that adequate tissue bites are taken. A recent meta-analysis of available randomized trials suggests that a continuous technique also is associated with decrease in subsequent ventral hernia formation. The continuous technique not only is the most rapid of all the mass closure methods but also

TABLE 13.1 U.S. Pharmacopeia–Required Knot-Pull Tensile Strength (LB)

	ABSORBABLE SUTURES		NONABSORBABLE SUTURES		
SIZE	NATURAL	SYNTHETIC	CLASS I	CLASS II	CLASS III
4-0	1.7	2.4	1.3	1.0	1.8
3-0	2.7	3.9	2.1	1.5	3.0
2-0	4.4	6.2	3.2	2.3	4.0
1-0	6.1	8.8	4.8	3.2	7.5
1	8.4	11.6	6.0	4.0	10.5

is more rapid than are traditional interrupted layer techniques. One theoretical advantage of a continuous suture line is that any stress on the incision is distributed along the entire suture line and not confined to one loop of suture, thereby potentially decreasing the likelihood of suture pullout.

Mass closure techniques classically have used a nonabsorbable permanent suture. The use of nonabsorbable sutures occasionally produces painful palpable knots or results in the formation of suture sinuses. The development of slowly absorbed synthetic sutures has allowed the use of these sutures for running continuous closures, thus avoiding the potential complications of nonabsorbable sutures. Several studies are now available showing excellent results using a continuous absorbable suture line for fascial closure even in high-risk patients. Although the use of continuous polyglycolic acid and polyglactin 910 sutures to close vertical midline incisions has been discouraged by some surgeons, others have obtained good results in patients at low risk for dehiscence. Since these initial studies, other synthetic absorbable sutures (polydioxanone and polyglyconate) that retain their tensile strength much longer than polyglycolic acid and polyglactin 910 have become available. Because of this delayed loss of tension strength compared with other absorbable suture material, polydioxanone and polyglyconate sutures are especially well suited for continuous fascial closure and should be considered the absorbable sutures of choice for mass closure of patients at high risk for dehiscence.

The manner in which the incision is made also may influence the dehiscence rate. Although no good data are available, it has been suggested that the shearing produced when scissors are used to incise the fascia results in increased fascia necrosis and an increased breakdown rate when compared with incisions produced by a scalpel. Likewise, the use of electrosurgery to incise the fascia has been implicated by some data to result in an increase in the dehiscence rate. These factors are magnified if the fascia then is closed improperly. Because such fascia necrosis generally occurs only at the cut edge of the fascia, the use of generous fascia bites during fascial closure probably is more important in preventing fascial dehiscence than is the manner of opening the fascia.

SUTURE MATERIAL

It is unknown when humankind first learned to use strings or animal sinews to ligate bleeding vessels or approximate tissue. Any material used for this purpose is commonly referred to as *suture*, whereas the act of reapproximating tissue with suture is known as *suturing*. The first recorded use of suture and suturing dates to the 16th century BC in the Edwin Smith papyrus, the oldest record of a surgical procedure. Over the

centuries, many different materials have been used as sutures. These materials include metals (gold, silver, and tantalum wire), plant material (linen and cotton), and animal products (horsehair, tendons, intestinal tissue, and silk).

The United States Pharmacopeia (USP) is the official compendium that defines the various classes of suture as well as sets standards for dimensions and minimum tensile strength for each class of suture marketed in the United States. Most sutures today significantly exceed the minimum tensile strength required by the USP (Table 13.1).

Sutures are divided into size categories based on diameter as defined by the USP. Sutures progressively larger than 0 are numbered in increasing numerical order; that is, 1, 2, etc. Sizes progressively smaller than 0 are indicated by an increasing number of zeros; that is, 0, 00, 000. The smaller the suture, the more zeros. For simplicity, the smaller numbers often are written numerically as 1-0, 2-0, etc., where the first numeral refers to the number of zeros.

The USP characterizes sutures based on their rate of absorption by bodily tissues. Sutures initially are classed as either absorbable or nonabsorbable. Absorbable sutures lose the majority of their tensile strength before 60 days when implanted in body tissues. Absorbable sutures are further subdivided by the USP into natural and synthetic sutures. Figure 13.2 illustrates the percentages of tensile strength remaining for common absorbable sutures at various postoperative time intervals.

Nonabsorbable sutures are defined as sutures that maintain the majority of their tensile strength for more than 60 days in body tissue. These sutures are further subdivided by the USP into three classes: class I is composed of silk or synthetic fibers; class II is composed of cotton or linen fibers or coated natural or synthetic fibers, with the coating forming a casting of significant thickness but not contributing appreciably to strength (these coatings typically are added to improve handling characteristics or resist degradation); and class III sutures are composed of monofilament or multifilament metal wire.

Natural Absorbable Sutures

Plain and Chromic Catgut

One of the oldest suture materials is plain catgut. Catgut consists of highly purified strands of collagen obtained from the submucosa of animals. Despite its name, catgut normally is obtained from sheep or cattle intestines. The name is believed to have originated from the Arabic term *kitgut*, which referred to the strings of a musical instrument known as a kit. Kitgut was made from sheep intestines and probably served as a readily available source of suture material. Over the years, the term has evolved into *catgut*.

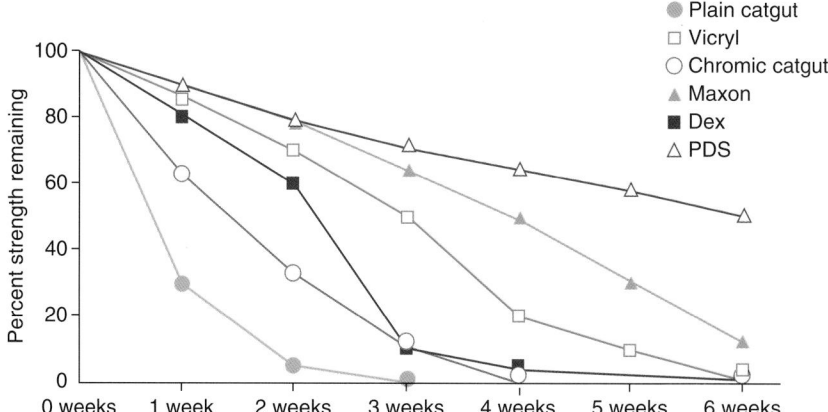

FIGURE 13.2 Percentage of in vivo tensile strength of absorbable sutures remaining at various postoperative times.

Because plain catgut is a foreign protein, it elicits a marked inflammatory response in tissue. It is rapidly degraded by proteolytic enzymes released by white blood cells. This suture loses more than 70% of its tensile strength in 7 days and is totally digested by 70 days. Plain gut is used in tissue in which strength is needed for very short periods of time. It is ideal for Pomeroy tubal ligations because it dissolves rapidly and thus allows the severed ends to fall apart. Less rapidly absorbed sutures, particularly permanent suture, are associated with higher failure rates, probably because of fistula formation.

Chromic catgut is treated with chromic acid salts that bind to the antigen sites in the collagen. The resulting suture elicits less inflammatory response and subsequently is more resistant to degradation. Chromic catgut maintains more than half of its tensile strength at 7 to 10 days, with some measurable strength up to day 21. It is suitable for tissue in which long-term strength is not needed. Examples of such tissue include serosal, visceral, and vaginal tissues. This suture should not be used in skin because the inflammatory response can cause scarring, and the suture often serves as a nidus for infection. Because natural absorbable sutures are degraded by the proteolytic enzymes released by inflammatory cells, these sutures lose strength more rapidly in infected tissue. Because catgut is derived from animal intestines, primarily cow and sheep, there has been increasing concerns over the possibility of theoretical infection with transmissible spongiform encephalopathies (TSE), such as "mad cow." Intestines are currently classified as tissues of medium infectivity with regard to TSE. Furthermore, because all inactivation processes for TSE cause severe changes to catgut, it is not possible to apply these methods to these sutures to eliminate infectious agents. Risk management is only possible by restricting sources to TSE-free herds. Because of these concerns, catgut sutures have been taken off the market in many countries of Europe as well as Japan. Where available, catgut has become progressively more expensive. Because the primary advantage of catgut over many of the synthetics has been cost, many believe use of catgut sutures will soon become obsolete.

Synthetic Absorbable Sutures

Polyglycolic Acid, Polyglactin 910, Lactomer 9-1, and Glycomer 631

During the 1970s, two synthetic absorbable sutures (polyglycolic acid and polyglactin 910) became available in the United States. These sutures were designed to be stronger, longer lasting, and less reactive than catgut. Both sutures are composed of braided filaments of a synthetic polymer. Polyglycolic acid (Dexon: Sherwood/Davis & Geck, St. Louis, MO) is a copolymer of glycolic acid, whereas polyglactin 910 (Vicryl: Ethicon, Somerville, NJ) is a copolymer of lactic and glycolic acid. The two sutures have very similar biologic properties. Breakdown is by hydrolysis rather than digestion by proteolytic enzymes. The result is minimal inflammatory reaction and a constant absorption rate. There essentially is no loss in tensile strength in the first 7 to 10 days after implantation. Approximately 50% to 60% of tensile strength remains after 14 days, 20% to 30% after 21 days, and almost no tensile strength at 28 days. The initial tensile strength of both these sutures is significantly greater than catgut suture of equal size. In fact, the tensile strength of the synthetic absorbable sutures is almost equal to the tensile strength of a catgut suture one size larger.

Glycomer 631 (Biosyn: Covidien, Mansfield, MA) introduced in 1995 is a triblock polymer of glycolide, dioxanone, and trimethylene carbonate. Advances in polymer chemistry allowed production of a monofilament suture equivalent to polyglactin 910 and polyglycolic acid. Glycomer 631 maintains its tension strength longer than the two sutures in this class with 75% of the tension strength remaining at 2 weeks and 40% remaining at 3 weeks.

Lactomer 9-1 (Polysorb: Covidien, Mansfield, MA) is a braided absorbable suture composed of glycolide and lactide in a 9:1 ratio. The surfaces of Polysorb have been coated with an absorbable mixture of caprolactone/glycolide copolymer and calcium stearoyl lactylate to decrease their coefficient friction. At 2 weeks, nearly 80% of the tensile strength remains, and approximately 30% of the tensile strength is retained at 21 days. Absorption is essentially complete by days 56 to 70.

One disadvantage of the synthetic absorbable sutures is that they do not handle as well as catgut suture. To counter this difficulty, manufacturers have attempted to enhance the handling qualities of their products by offering versions with various surface coatings or variations with finer and more tightly woven filaments. Although these refinements improve handling characteristics, they increase the tendency of knots to slip. As a result, additional throws may be needed when using these suture versions.

These sutures can be used in most situations in which chromic catgut would be used and have replaced catgut almost entirely for many surgeons. Because they retain tensile strength longer than do natural absorbable sutures, they are acceptable for fascial closure in patients at low risk for fascial dehiscence.

Polyglyconate and Polydioxanone

Sutures of polyglycolic acid and polyglactin are by necessity composed of braided filaments because the inherent rigidity of the polymers produces a monofilament suture too stiff for general surgical use. A newer class of polymers, first available in the 1980s, allowed the production of pliable monofilament sutures. This type of suture is represented by polyglyconate (Maxon) and polydioxanone (PDS). Although subtle differences exist between the two sutures, they are similar enough to consider them together when discussing the biologic properties of this suture class.

The initial tensile strength of these monofilament sutures is comparable to that of the multifilament absorbable sutures. However, this class of suture undergoes absorption at a much slower rate than do other absorbable sutures. As a result, tensile strength is maintained for a longer period of time. More than 90% of initial tensile strength is maintained by the end of the first postoperative week, 80% at 2 weeks, 50% at 4 weeks, and 25% at 6 weeks. As with the other synthetic sutures, inflammatory response is minimal. An additional advantage is that these monofilament sutures lack interstices that could serve as a nidus for bacterial infection. As a result, chronic inflammation is rarely seen with this class of monofilament sutures. In comparison, infected absorbable braided sutures have been shown experimentally by Buckall to contain bacteria even after 70 days of implantation.

Because of their delayed absorption profile, both polyglyconate and polydioxanone are excellent choices for fascial closure. Because these sutures are composed of only one fiber, care must be taken to insure that the strand is not inadvertently damaged by instruments, needles, or other sharp-edged material. Such damage may not be easily recognized in the operating room but can seriously weaken a monofilament suture and may result in suture line disruption postoperatively. This precaution is even more critical when a continuous suture line is used. Additionally, the use of the commonly used loop-to-strand closure to end a suture line produces a very weak knot when monofilament suture is used. The use of two sutures, with each starting at one end of the incision and then tied strand to strand, is recommended when monofilament sutures are used in high load–bearing situations such as fascial closure. A more detailed discussion is provided later in this chapter in the discussion of surgical knots.

Poliglecaprone 25, Polyglactin 910 (Rapide), and Polyglytone 6211

With further advances in polymer chemistry, it is now possible to manufacture the synthetic equivalent of surgical gut. First introduced in 1993, poliglecaprone 25 (Monocryl) has the absorption similar to chromic catgut. Unlike natural collagens, poliglecaprone 25 produces highly uniform and predictable absorption patterns. Like the other synthetic sutures, poliglecaprone 25 is absorbed by hydrolysis and thus does not induce the inflammatory response of catgut. This monofilament suture retains approximately 50% to 60% of its original tensile strength at 7 days postoperatively, 20% to 30% at 14 days, and by 21 days has lost essentially all tensile strength. This particular suture has the advantages of chromic catgut suture but without many of the disadvantages (i.e., intense inflammatory response and somewhat unpredictable absorption rate). Although it is similar to chromic catgut in tensile strength and actually maintains its tensile strength longer than does chromic catgut, it is not recommended by the manufacturer for use for fascial closure or in any tissue in which approximation under stress is required.

Polyglactin 910 Rapide (Vicryl Rapide) released in 1995 is identical in chemical structure to polyglactin 910 but is of lower molecular weight. It has been treated with gamma rays to speed absorption. The result is a braided suture with performance characteristics similar to plain catgut. Absorption is rapid, with 70% of tensile strength lost in the first 7 days. After 10 to 14 days, essentially no strength remains. It is intended for use in the superficial soft tissue where only short-term support is needed. It can be used for skin closure because of its rapid absorption and minimal inflammatory response. The sutures typically begin to fall off at 7 to 10 days. Because sutures remaining in skin longer than 7 days may cause scarring, any suture remaining at this time can be wiped off with sterile gauze or, if necessary, cut. Although this suture does not meet USP strength requirements for synthetic absorbable sutures, its tensile strength exceeds the tensile strength specifications for similar size natural collagen suture.

Polyglytone 6211 (Caprosyn: Covidien, Mansfield, MA) released in 2002 is composed of glycolide, caprolactone, trimethylene carbonate, and lactide. The absorption profile is similar to that of polyglactin 910 Rapide. However, in contrast to polyglactin 910 Rapide, polyglytone 6211 is a monofilament suture.

These sutures are an excellent choice for first- and second-degree episiotomy and vaginal laceration closure. Because of the intense inflammatory response produced, gut sutures are associated with more significantly postepisiotomy pain than are synthetic sutures, whereas long-delayed absorbable synthetic sutures are associated with the presence of unabsorbed suture and knots after the postpartum period.

Nonabsorbable Sutures

By definition, nonabsorbable sutures are suitably resistant to the action of living mammalian tissue. These sutures, however, are not completely resistant to absorption. Over time, these sutures also lose tensile strength, and in the case of natural fiber, sutures eventually are completely absorbed or digested. Despite beliefs to the contrary, the initial tensile strength of many nonabsorbable sutures is less than that of comparable-size absorbable suture (Table 13.1). Nonabsorbable sutures, however, have the advantage of maintaining tensile strength for long periods of time. Disadvantages of nonabsorbable sutures include the potential suture-related pain, palpable sutures, and occasionally the formation of suture sinuses.

Natural Nonabsorbable Sutures

Modern nonabsorbable natural fiber sutures are composed of either surgical silk or cotton. Silk suture is one of the best handling sutures. The handling and knot-tying characteristics of silk suture remain the standard against which other sutures are judged. This suture has little "memory"; that is, it does not tend to return to its original form after being bent or twisted. As a result, it handles well, ties easily, and possesses excellent knot security. Silk suture loses more than half of its tensile strength after 1 year of implantation and frequently cannot be found after 2 years. In this respect, it can be viewed as a delayed absorbable suture. Because silk is a foreign animal protein, it initiates the greatest inflammatory response of the nonabsorbable sutures. The multifilament nature and the capillary action of this suture make it unsuitable in contaminated tissue or in tissues in which the potential for infection is high.

Cotton is the other nonabsorbable natural suture material still available today. It is rarely used in modern surgical practice. Cotton is the weakest of the nonabsorbable sutures. Cotton loses 50% of its original tensile strength within 6 months of implantation but still has 30% to 40% remaining at the end of 2 years. Unlike silk, which loses tensile strength when exposed to moisture, wet cotton is 10% stronger than dry cotton. Because wet cotton also is easier to handle, it is commonly moistened before use.

Synthetic Nonabsorbable Sutures

A wide variety of nonabsorbable synthetic sutures exist. Nylon is a synthetic polyamide polymer derived from coal, air, and water. It is available both as a braided polyfilament suture (Nurolon, Surgilon) and as a monofilament suture (Dermalon, Ethilon). Monofilament nylon has slightly greater tensile strength than braided nylon, but braided nylon handles better and has better knot security than the monofilament nylon suture. Monofilament nylon suture incites less inflammatory reaction and is less prone to infection than the braided nylon sutures. However, because nylon is relatively inert, all types of nylon suture produce minimal tissue reaction. Nylon undergoes slow hydrolysis in tissue over extended periods of time. It loses approximately 15% to 20% of tensile strength each year.

Polyester sutures are produced only in braided forms. Most differences in the properties of these sutures are determined by whether they are coated and by the type of coating. The uncoated forms (Mersilene, Dacron) generally offer the best knot security. As with synthetic absorbable suture, coatings can improve the handling characteristics of the polyester sutures. Knot security of coated polyester sutures is generally poorer than that of uncoated sutures. Coatings currently used include polytetrafluoroethylene, also known as Teflon (Polydek, Ethiflex, and Tevdek), polybutilate (Ethibond), and silicone (Ti-Cron).

Polypropylene (Prolene, Surgilon) is a monofilament suture composed of a linear hydrocarbon polymer. It has the least tissue reactivity of all nonabsorbable sutures. Although polypropylene has a high memory, it also exhibits a small degree of plasticity. If it is tied carefully and the knots set firmly, a flattening occurs where the strands cross. This flattening helps lock the knot and thus provides somewhat greater knot security than is possible with many other monofilament nonabsorbable sutures. As with the absorbable monofilament sutures, the same precautions to prevent damage to the suture must be observed with the monofilament nonabsorbable sutures.

Metal Sutures

Although silver wire was used by Sims for closure of vesicovaginal fistulas, metal sutures are rarely used in gynecologic surgery today. Historically, metal sutures have been used in infected sites or for repair of wound dehiscence and evisceration. Stainless steel once was used routinely by the military for closure of battle wounds of the abdomen. Metal sutures have the highest tensile strength of all suture material. They are also particularly nonreactive. Metal sutures, however, are difficult to handle, require the use of special instruments, and tend to puncture gloves and tissue. With the availability of other nonabsorbable suture materials that also offer high tensile strength and low reactivity but are easier to handle, little reason exists to use these sutures in gynecologic surgery today.

Barbed Suture

The barbed suture is a recent development in sutures. The use of barbed suture has particular advantages in laparoscopy and in dermal closure. Since knots are eliminated and an equal level of tissue approximation is applied throughout tissue closure, these sutures may have advantages over smooth suture in many other surgical applications.

In 2004, the Quill bidirectional barbed suture (Angiotech, Vancouver, British Columbia, Canada) became the first barbed suture to be approved by the FDA. In 2009, the FDA approved the V-Loc barbed suture (Covidien, Mansfield, MA). The Quill system is a bidirectional suture with needles swaged to each end of the suture, while the V-Loc system is unidirectional with only one needle with the other end being a closed loop to avoid the need for a knot to initially anchor the suture. Both sutures are available in a variety of both absorbable and nonabsorbable sutures. The Quill system is available with sutures composed of poliglecaprone 25, polydioxanone, nylon, and polypropylene. The V-Loc system is available as the V-Loc 90 composed of glycomer 631, the V-Loc 180 with polyglyconate, and V-Loc PBT composed of polybutester. The numerical designation of the V-Loc 90 and 180 indicates the time to complete suture absorption.

Because effective diameter of the suture is decreased during the manufacturing process, bidirectional suture is rated one USP size smaller than its equivalent smooth suture, that is, a 2-0 smooth suture and a 3-0 bidirectional suture are actually the same diameter. Unidirectional suture is rated equal to its USP smooth suture equivalent.

Choice of Suture for Fascial Closure

Tensile strength is critical, although many factors are important in choosing a suture for fascial closure. As noted, the most common cause of dehiscence is sutures pulling through fascia. Because a fascial closure can only be as strong as the weakest component, suture for fascial closure should maintain a tensile strength greater than that of the fascia through the critical healing period. Because the incidence of wound infection is related to the amount of suture material placed in the wound, it would also seem reasonable to use the smallest suture able to provide this necessary tensile strength.

All sutures marketed in the United States must meet minimum tensile strength requirements as defined by the USP. The tensile strength measurement required by USP is knot-pull tensile strength. In measuring knot-pull tensile strength, the suture is tied around a plastic tube using a flat surgeon's knot with one end held in place and the opposite end attached to a tensilometer. Although these data are easily obtained from the various suture manufacturers and are frequently used in suture advertisements, knot-pull tensile strength is not particularly applicable to actual surgical situations. A more useful measurement of strength is obtained using the knotted loop model as suggested by Herman. In this model, a loop is formed by tying a suture around a glass rod using sufficient square knots to prevent slippage. The rod is removed and the loop placed over two right angle rods gripped in the jaws of a tensilometer. The jaws are then separated at a constant rate until breakage occurs. This model stresses the material and the knot more comparably to actual in vivo situations and also allows estimation of knot security. Assuming no slippage at the knot, tensile strength calculated using the knotted-loop model is approximately twice the knot-pull tensile strength.

The force required to pull a loop of suture through intact fascia (pullout force) is frequently cited as 8.3 pounds. This figure is derived from work on the fascia of dogs by Howes and Harvey in 1929 and does not necessarily apply to humans. Fortunately, several studies are now available that have measured the strength of human fascia (Campbell et al., Tera and Aberg, and Boerema). Two of these studies, by Campbell and colleagues and Tera and Alberg, were performed using human cadavers. The third study by Boerema measured the pullout force of fascia at the time of surgery on living patients. All three produced data that indicated the pullout force for human fascia was approximately 15.2 to 24.2 pounds.

Fascial incisions regain their strength slowly, achieving approximately 10%, 25%, 30%, and 40% of original strength by postoperative weeks 1, 2, 3, and 4, respectively. The point at which fascia has regained enough strength to resist the stress of daily activities is unknown. Some

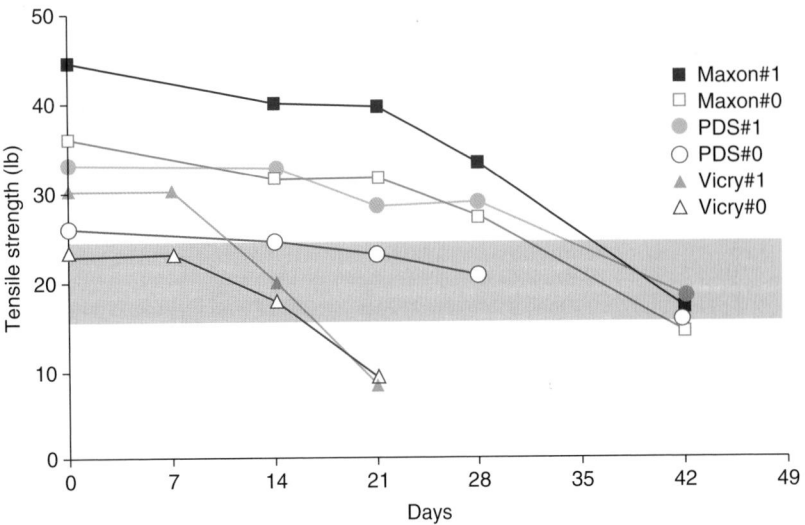

FIGURE 13.3 The tensile strength of various implanted suture materials over time and the point at which tensile strength is less than fascial pullout strength (14.5 to 24.2 pounds).

estimation of this time frame can be obtained from available data on fascial dehiscence. The majority of fascial dehiscence occurs between 2 and 12 days postoperatively, with a mean occurring around days 7 to 8. Dehiscence rarely occurs after postoperative day 12 but has been reported up to day 18. This suggests that in most patients, fascia has regained enough strength by 2 weeks after surgery to resist reasonable stresses but that in a limited number of patients, fascia may not regain sufficient strength to prevent dehiscence until 3 weeks postoperatively.

Using the fascia pullout data, tensile strength as measured by the knotted-loop model following various lengths of implantation in animals, and dehiscence data, the appropriate size absorbable suture for fascial closure can now be estimated. As can be seen in **Figure 13.3**, both 1 and 0 polydioxanone and polyglyconate retain tensile strength greater than the fascial pullout force for 4 to 6 weeks, but polyglycolic acid sutures of the same size maintain adequate tensile strength only for 7 to 14 days. Based on this model, a 1 or 0 polydioxanone or polyglyconate suture appears to be the most appropriate absorbable suture for fascial closure. Unfortunately, although these types of data are theoretically appealing, there are little clinical data to support these conclusions. It must be realized that in most healthy patients, fascial dehiscence does not occur, even when rapidly absorbed sutures are used. Before the development of the synthetic absorbable sutures, 1 and 0 chromic catgut sutures were frequently used for fascial closure. In fact, based on a survey of ob/gyn residency programs, chromic catgut still was being used for fascial closure in 16.1% of vertical fascial incisions and 23.4% of transverse fascial incisions as of 1979. Although fascial dehiscence in healthy patients remained uncommon after fascial closure with chromic catgut, dehiscence rates of up to 11% were reported for other patient populations. Likewise, polyglycolic acid and polyglactin 910 sutures have been used for fascial closure with good success, even in patients at risk for dehiscence.

Surgical Needles

Needles are necessary to carry suture material through tissue. The specific needle required for a procedure is determined by the tissue type, its location and accessibility, and the surgeon's personal preference. All surgical needles have three basic components: the eye, the body, and the point.

The eye of the needle is the point of attachment for suture. Eyes may be classed as closed, French, or swaged. Closed eyes are similar to those on household sewing needles, whereas French eye needles have a slit with ridges inside the slit to catch and hold the suture. Swaged or eyeless needles have the suture mechanically attached to the end of the needle to form a continuous unit. Eyed needles have several disadvantages over swaged needles, including difficulties with threading and the need to pull a double loop of suture through the tissue. Swaged needles are available with either the suture permanently attached or attached in such a manner that it can be removed from the needle by a slight straight tug on the suture. These controlled-release needles, also known as "pop-off" needles, increase the speed at which interrupted sutures can be placed.

The shape of the body or shaft of a needle determines how easily the needle performs in different applications (Fig. 13.4). The longitudinal shape of the body may be straight, half-curved, curved, or compound. Straight needles are used commonly when tissue is easily accessible. This type of needle is rarely used by gynecologists except for skin closure. Half-curved, or ski, needles may be used to close skin but have primarily been used in gynecology to facilitate laparoscopic suturing. Curved needles require less space for maneuvering than do other needles, and thus are ideally suited for most surgical procedures. Curved needles are commonly named based on the percentage of a circle they complete; that is, a ½ circle needle is one half of a full circle. Curved needles are available in various curvatures, with the ⅜ circle the most commonly used. The less of an arc the needle completed, the more shallow a bite the needle takes. For example, a ⅝ needle is useful in deep wounds in which a deep, narrow bite is required. Compound curve needles were originally developed for anterior segment ophthalmic surgery and are not used in gynecologic surgery.

The point of the needle begins at the widest part of the needle body and extends to the extreme tip. The two types of needle points are the cutting point and the tapered point (Fig. 13.4). Tapered points are used in easily penetrated tissue, such as bowel or peritoneum. A variation of the taper point is the blunt point, which has a rounded blunt tip at the end of a tapered shaft. This needle tip was designed for use in friable tissue but has been advocated by some surgeons for use with other tissues because of its reduced likelihood to penetrate the surgeon's gloves or skin. Cutting needles are used in

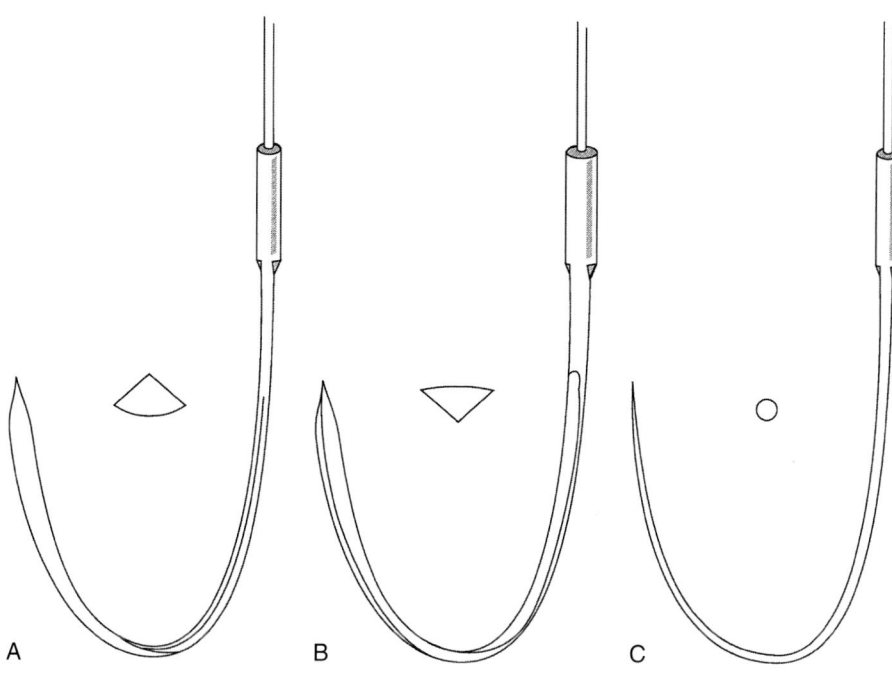

FIGURE 13.4 Common points and body shapes for curved needles.

tough tissue, such as skin. The most common cutting needle is the reverse cutting needle. Its sharp edge is on the outside of the outer curvature of the needle. Conventional cutting points have the sharp edge on the inside of the curvature. Variations of the cutting point include spatula and lancet points and are used for specialized applications such as ophthalmology.

Needle Holders

Straight needles can be held and pushed through tissue with the fingers. Straight needles can be used only to sew in a straight line, and only then when the tissue is easily accessible. When straight needles are used, sewing is done in a direction away from the operator.

In the depths of a wound, curved needles are needed. A needle holder is required when curved needles are used. All needle holders have a broad head with a variety of surfaces to prevent the needle from slipping or rotating. Needle holders may be large and heavy, or small and delicate, depending on the size needle to be used. Many needle holders have ring finger grips and locking mechanisms. Two common types of basic needle holders used in gynecology are Wagensteen (straight) or Heaney (angled) (**Fig. 13.5**). Curved needle holders are especially useful in vaginal surgery, for which the angled head allows easier needle placement. The needle is loaded so that the angled tip is pointed toward the needle eye and not the tip. Sewing using needle drivers is performed toward the operator.

Surgical Knots

The surgical knot has been described as the weakest link in any knotted suture, regardless of the knot configuration and the type of suture used. If tied improperly, a surgical knot will fail before the tensile strength of the suture is reached. Even when performed perfectly, the mere placement of a knot in suture reduces its overall tensile strength by 30% to 35%. Therefore, some knowledge of surgical knots is imperative for all surgeons.

All surgical knots can be divided into two basic groups: flat knots (square, surgeon's, and granny) and sliding knots

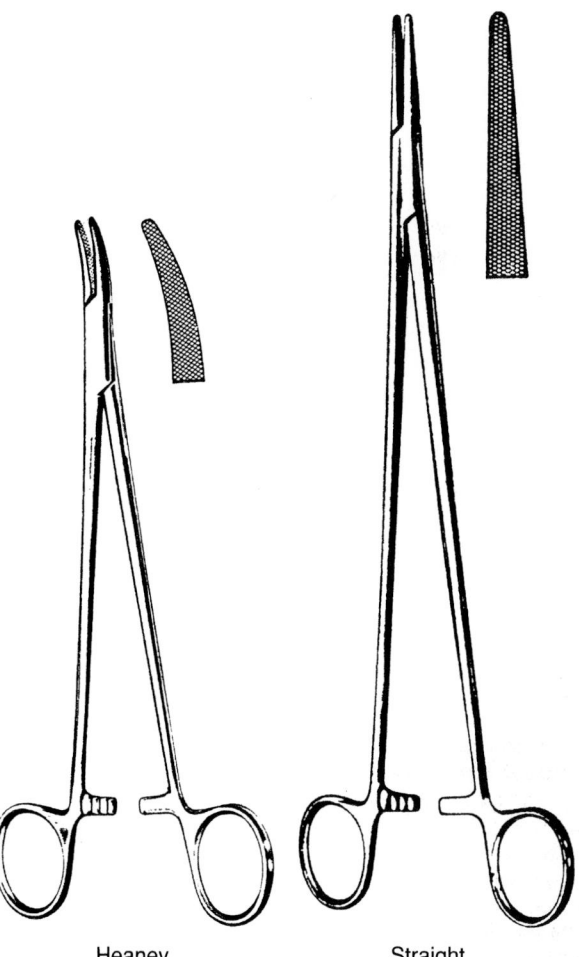

Heaney   Straight

FIGURE 13.5 Needle holders. (Courtesy of Zinnanti Surgical Instruments, Inc., Chatsworth, CA.)

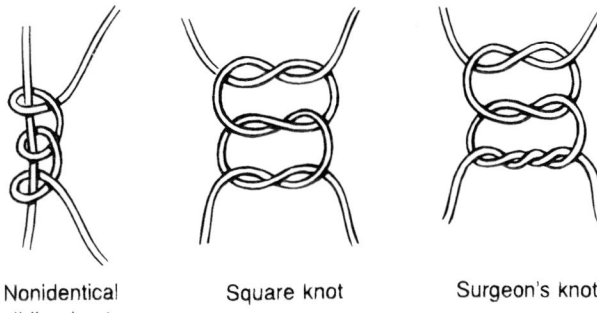

Nonidentical Square knot Surgeon's knot
sliding knot

FIGURE 13.6 Flat and sliding knots.

(identical and nonidentical) (**Fig. 13.6**). Flat knots are formed with half hitches tied with equal tension on the ends of the suture. Surgeon's knots are formed by adding an additional loop to the first throw of the half hitch. Sliding knots are two half hitches either nonidentical (square knot) or identical (granny knot), tied with greater tension on one segment than the other.

The term *sliding knot* suggests the tendency of the knot to slip compared with the flat, but this is not completely true. Simple sliding knots of two or three throws do slip often and should not be used as surgical knots. Brouwers and colleagues have shown, however, that flat knots with only two throws also tend to slip rather than break.

The flat square knot is the most secure of all the surgical knots and theoretically the most desirable knot for tying suture. However, according to a study by Trimbos, sliding knots are used more commonly by gynecologists than are square knots. It has been shown also that many surgeons actually tie sliding knots despite being convinced they tie flat knots. Sliding knots frequently are used in actual surgical practice for two reasons. The crossing of the surgeon's hands needed to tie square knots unavoidably releases tension on the knot, and this can lead to knot slippage. The tying of deep ligatures is most easily performed by keeping constant tension on one suture. Thus, sliding knots may be preferable to square knots in certain situations. Whichever knot is used, the operator should be aware of the knot being used and the number of throws needed to obtain maximum knot capacity.

The number of throws required for knot security is frequently debated. Too few throws and the knot is weaker than the suture; additional throws above that needed to equal the sutures tensile strength adds unneeded suture to the wound and may increase the infection rate. When flat square knots are used, Brown has shown that maximum knot-holding capacity was achieved with four throws in all non-coated suture tested. In fact, three throws were sufficient to achieve maximum knot-holding capacity except for sutures composed of nylon (both monofilament and braided). The addition of coating to improve handling characteristics also decreases knot security. In a 1983 study, Rodeheaver and colleagues showed that coated suture required two additional flat throws to equal the maximum knot-holding capacity of uncoated suture. In a similar study by Van Rijssel and colleagues, the knot-holding capacity of a sliding knot with one extra throw equaled that of square knots in smaller gauge (3-0) suture. In larger sutures (0), square knots remained stronger than sliding knots with an extra throw, but sliding knots with more than five throws were not tested. From these studies, it appears that a surgical knot of four to six throws is adequate for most sutures. The exact number of throws required, of course, depends on the type of suture and whether a flat or sliding knot is formed.

It is common practice for some surgeons to leave suture tails long to prevent knot disruption should the knot slip. As might be expected, the usefulness of this practice is dependent on the type of suture involved. It has been shown that any knot slippage in nylon, polydioxanone, and polypropylene sutures results in total knot disruption. In other sutures (polyglyconate and polyglactin), initial knot slippage is followed by knot recomposition. The reconstituted knot remains intact until greater force is applied. A long suture tail is only helpful in preventing knot disruption in this latter class of suture.

Knot security is of utmost importance when using a continuous suture line. This is of critical importance if a monofilament suture is used in a strength critical suture line. It is common practice for many surgeons to form the terminal knot in a continuous suture line by tying the ending single strand to the last loop of suture. This "loop-to-strand" knot is a potentially weak configuration. Unlike multifilament sutures that lock in place with each throw, monofilament sutures do not lock and are prone to slippage. Unless multiple square knots are used, the single strand may slip from the knot when placed under tension. As a result, the entire suture line disrupts. At reoperation, the strand may appear broken, but, in fact, one of the three terminal knot ends has slipped through what appears to be an intact knot (**Fig. 13.7**). A safer method for tying continuous suture is to run two sutures to the midpoint of the incision and tie the two single strands to each other, thus avoiding the "loop-to-strand" knot. Alternatively, polydioxanone is available in a looped version that eliminates the initial knot and permits ending the suture line in a strand-to-strand configuration. The disadvantage is the large increase in the mass of suture placed into the wound.

SURGICAL INSTRUMENTATION

A multitude of surgical instruments are designed to perform one unique function or slightly improve on the performance of another instrument. This section is not intended to be a comprehensive list of all instruments available but a review of the basic surgical instrumentation needed for most common gynecologic procedures.

Scalpel

The scalpel is the first instrument used in most surgeries and remains the best instrument for dividing tissue with minimal trauma to surrounding tissue. Scalpel blades come in various sizes and shapes to allow performance of different tasks (**Fig. 13.8**). The basic scalpel blade has a straight ribbed back and an oval cutting surface. This basic blade is commonly available in sizes 10, 15, 20, and 22. The 10 scalpel blade is the most versatile and the most commonly used size. The smaller blades are used for fine dissection and when precise turns are required in making the incision—that is, plastic surgery—although the larger blades are used to rapidly perform an incision. Blades such as the 11 and 12 are designed for specific purposes. The 11 blade is bayonet-shaped and used to perform stab incisions for drains and in draining abscesses. The 12 blade is hook-shaped and was originally used for myringotomies. It is infrequently used by gynecologists.

Scissors

The scissors are the second most commonly used instrument to divide tissue. In addition to cutting, scissors also can be

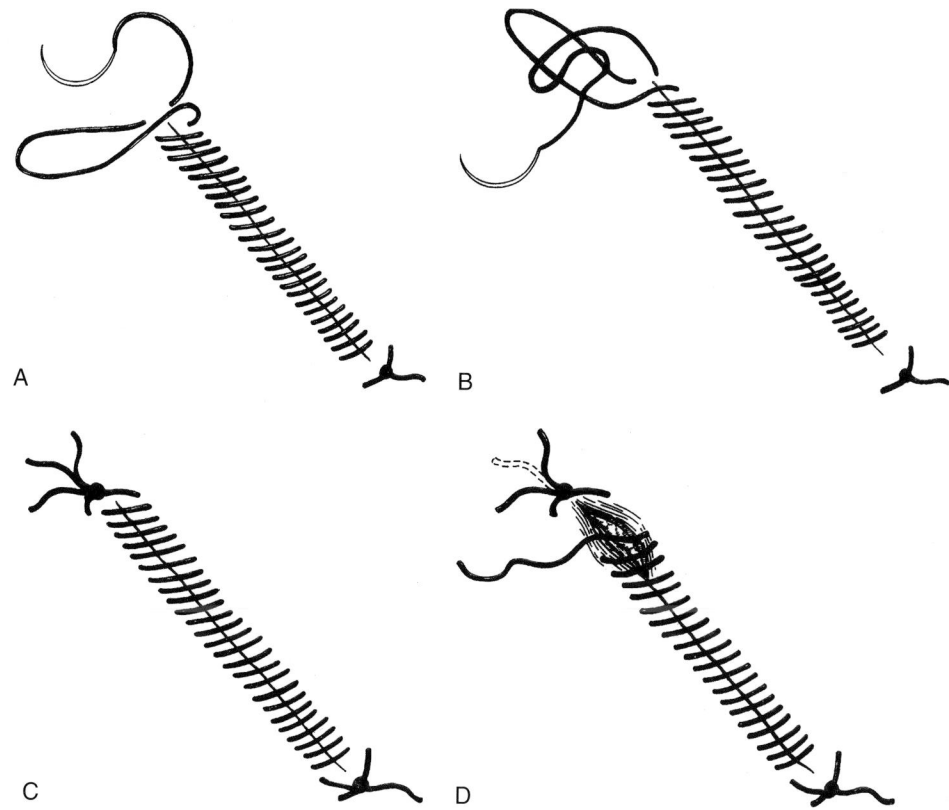

FIGURE 13.7 Development of suture line.

used for blunt dissection by opening the scissors after the tips have been inserted into a tissue plane. The basic scissors designs used in gynecology surgery are the Mayo, Metzenbaum, and Iris scissors. All come in both straight and curved versions (Fig. 13.9). Curved scissors allow horizontal cutting deep in a wound and thus improve visibility. Curved scissors also are used to cut tissue in a smooth curve, such as for incising the vaginal cuff in an abdominal hysterectomy.

Mayo scissors are used when dividing tough tissue, such as the rectus fascia, parametrial tissue, or vaginal cuff. Metzenbaum scissors are more delicate than are the heavier Mayo scissors and are used for cutting thinner tissue, such as peritoneum

and adhesions. Metzenbaum scissors are frequently use for retroperitoneal dissection or for developing tissue planes in adhered or distorted tissue.

Iris scissors are small scissors used for delicate dissection. Originally designed for ophthalmic surgery, they are used in gynecology for precise vulvar and vaginal surgery, such as fistula repair or colporrhaphy.

Suture scissors are used only to cut suture and never tissue. Suture scissors are general-purpose scissors with blunt ends to avoid the possibility that the tips will injure structures distal to the suture.

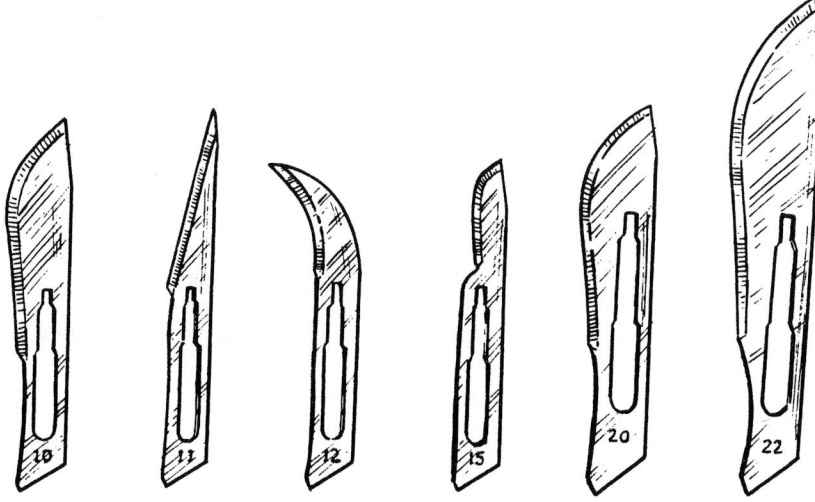

FIGURE 13.8 Surgical scalpel blades.

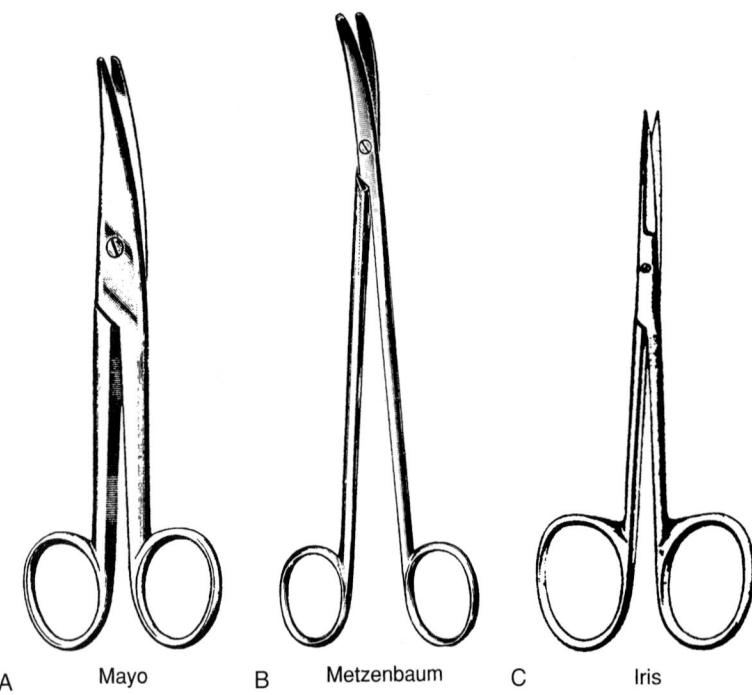

FIGURE 13.9 Surgical scissors. (Courtesy of Zinnanti Surgical Instruments, Inc., Chatsworth, CA.)

A   Mayo   B   Metzenbaum   C   Iris

Tissue Forceps

Tissue or thumb forceps consist of two strips of metal joined at one end (Fig. 13.10). The opposable ends of the forceps are used to grasp and hold tissue during dissection, suturing, or cutting. These ends are of varying shapes and configuration, depending on the purpose for which the forceps are intended. The most common alteration to the ends is the addition of teeth. Smooth forceps without teeth are used when handling friable or delicate tissue. DeBakey forceps have long fine smooth tips that provide precise control of small or delicate tissue deep in the wound. They are commonly used in vascular surgery or retroperitoneal node dissection. Toothed forceps bite into tissue, providing a firm grip with minimal pressure. The teeth can vary from one to many and be fine or large. Adson forceps are equipped with fine teeth and are commonly used to approximate skin for staple or suture placement. Ring-tipped and Russian forceps increase the grasping force without using teeth by increasing the surface area of the grasping tips. These forceps are used when a secure hold is needed on structures that would be traumatized by toothed forceps. Bonney tissue forceps are heavy-toothed forceps with serrations along the shaft for maximum gripping power. They are used when sewing fascia.

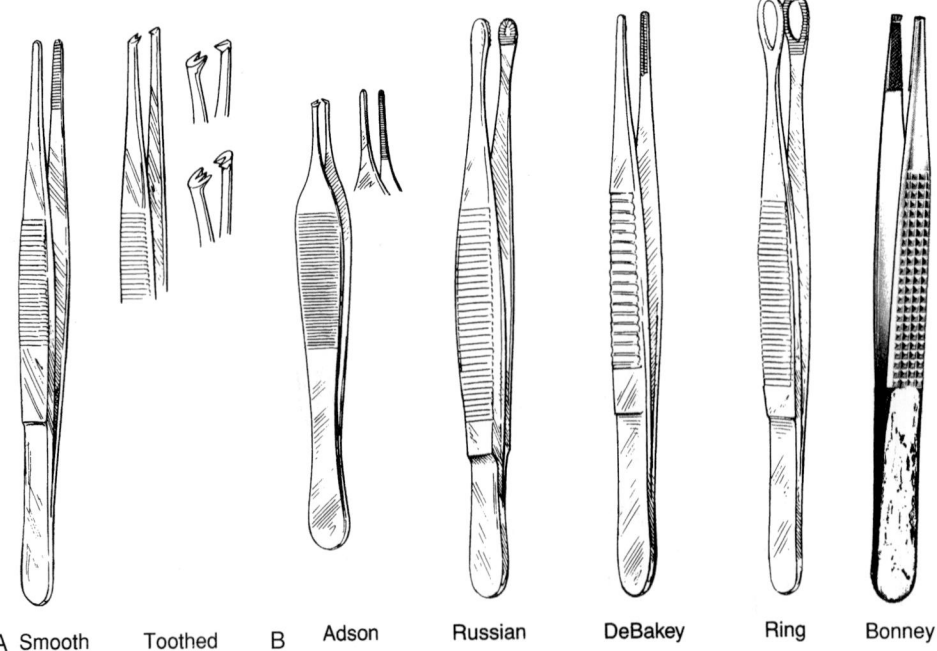

A Smooth   Toothed   B   Adson   Russian   DeBakey   Ring   Bonney

FIGURE 13.10 Tissue (thumb) forceps. (Courtesy of Zinnanti Surgical Instruments, Inc., Chatsworth, CA.)

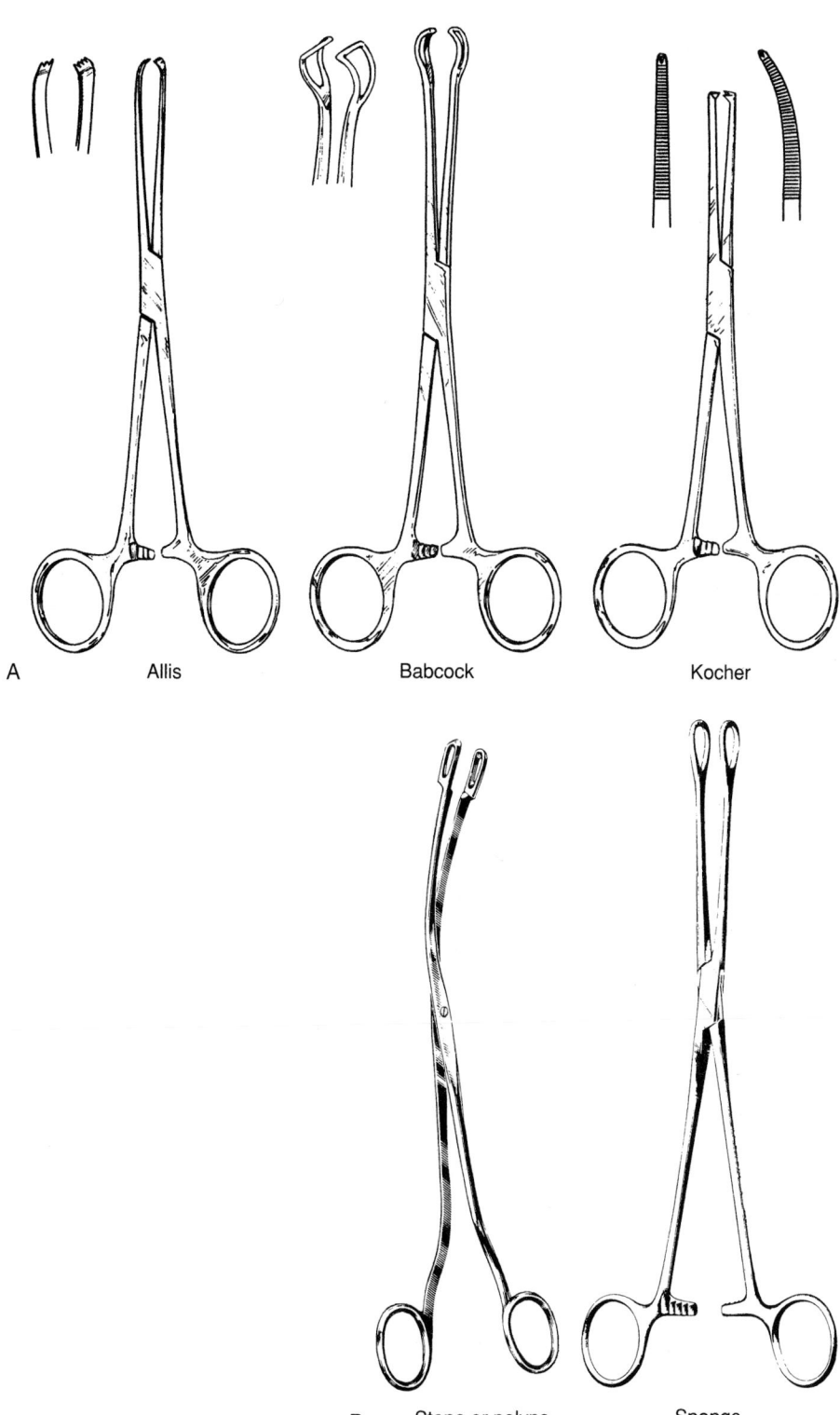

A   Allis   Babcock   Kocher

B   Stone or polyps   Sponge

FIGURE 13.11 Tissue clamps. (Courtesy of Zinnanti Surgical Instruments, Inc., Chatsworth, CA.)

Clamps

Grasping forceps, commonly referred to as clamps, are designed to grasp and apply traction to tissues (Fig. 13.11). All have finger rings and a locking mechanism. Babcock clamps have no teeth and are atraumatic. These clamps can grasp and hold delicate tissues such as fallopian tube or bowel without causing damage. Allis clamps have serrated edges with short teeth. This clamp has much more grasping power than does the Babcock clamp. Kocher/Ochsner clamps have transverse ridges along the shaft and interlocking teeth at the tip. Because of their design, tissue within the clamp is unlikely to slip. These clamps are frequently used to grasp heavy tissue such as fascia and occasionally are used as hysterectomy clamps. Ring forceps can be used like ring-tipped

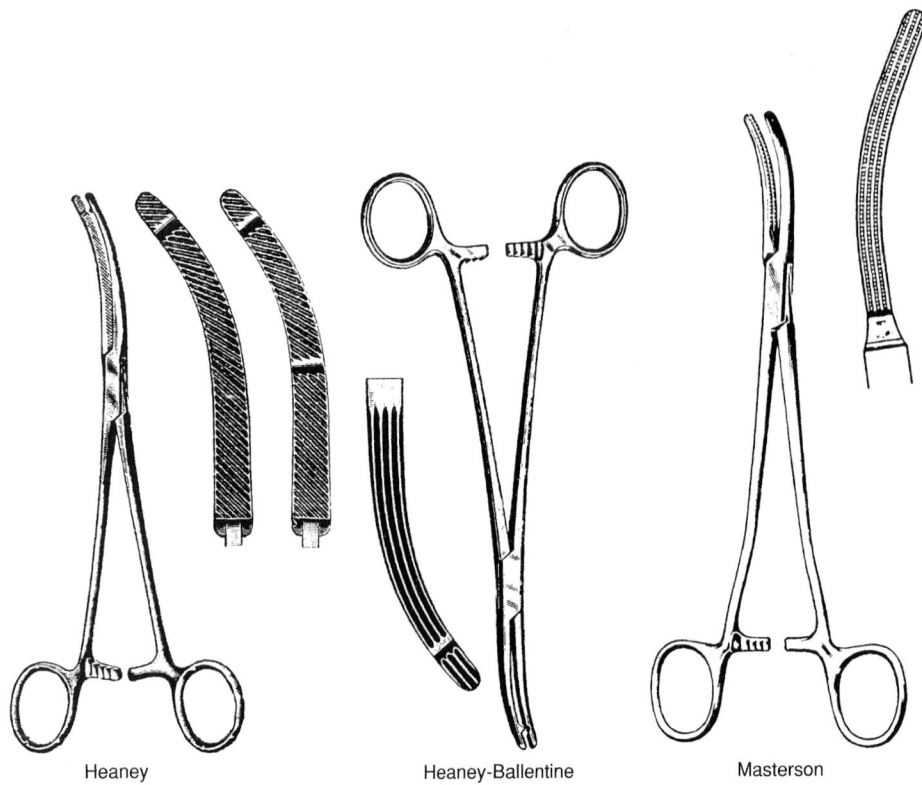

Heaney   Heaney-Ballentine   Masterson

FIGURE 13.12 Hysterectomy clamps. (Courtesy of Zinnanti Surgical Instruments, Inc., Chatsworth, CA.)

tissue forceps but more commonly are used to hold folded sponges. In this fashion, they can be used to retract tissue, sponge fluid or blood, or apply solutions to the skin in preparation for surgery. Renal stone forceps were designed to remove stones from the renal pelvis but are commonly used by the gynecologic surgeon to explore the uterine cavity for polyps or retained tissue. When used in this capacity, they are inserted, opened, rotated 180 degrees, closed, and withdrawn.

Heaney, Heaney-Ballentine, and Masterson clamps are the commonly used clamps for clamping the parametrial and paracervical tissue during hysterectomy (**Fig. 13.12**). Hysterectomy clamps are heavy crushing clamps with ridged shafts. The classic clamps (Heaney, Heaney-Ballentine) also have toothed tips. The more recent Masterson clamp lacks a toothed tip and was designed to generate the least amount of crushing force.

Retractors

Retractors are used to hold tissue out of the operative field to improve exposure during surgical procedures (**Fig. 13.13**). Retractors are either held by an assistant (manual retractors) or use counterpressure from other tissue (self-retaining retractors) to hold themselves in place.

Self-retaining retractors frequently are used to hold the sides of the incision apart during gynecologic surgery. Gynecologists seem to favor the O'Conner-O'Sullivan retractor when performing pelvic surgery. General surgeons, on the other hand, prefer the Balfour retractor. The O'Conner-O'Sullivan is a circular retractor with four blades, two permanently attached lateral retractors to retract the sidewalls, and a removable upper and lower blade to retract the bowel and bladder, respectively. This retractor is available with large or small lateral blades, whereas the removable blades

come in several sizes. The Balfour retractor also has two lateral blades but only one additional retractor blade. This blade normally is employed as an upper blade with a manual retractor used for bladder retraction if needed. However, if the bowel is carefully packed away with laparotomy packs, the third blade can be used as a bladder retractor. All blades of the Balfour retractor are removable and available in different sizes.

The Bookwalter retractor is the most versatile of retractors, providing excellent exposure to the operative field. It consists of a circular metal ring to which a wide variety of retractors can be attached at any point. Its best use is during radical pelvic surgery or when operating on massively obese patients. In extremely obese patients, it may be necessary to attach the Bookwalter retractor to the operating table.

Manual retractors allow maximum flexibility in providing exposure (**Fig. 13.14**). They can be used alone or as a supplement to self-retaining retractors. Common manual retractors include the Heaney, Deaver, and Richardson retractors. Specialized retractors include the Briesky-Navratil (used during sacrospinous vault suspension), Army-Navy, and Parker retractors (used for skin and subcutaneous tissue).

Dilators

Dilators are metal or plastic cylinders used to dilate the cervical os to sufficient size to admit other surgical instruments (**Fig. 13.15**). Dilators may have tapered (Hank and Pratt) or rounded (Hegar) tips. Dilators with tapered tips require less force to perform dilatation than do dilators with rounded tips. The sizes are measured either by diameter or by circumference. The unit of measurement for diameter is millimeters, whereas the unit of measurement for circumference is in French calibration. The relationship of the two measurements can be calculated by the formula for the circumference of a circle where

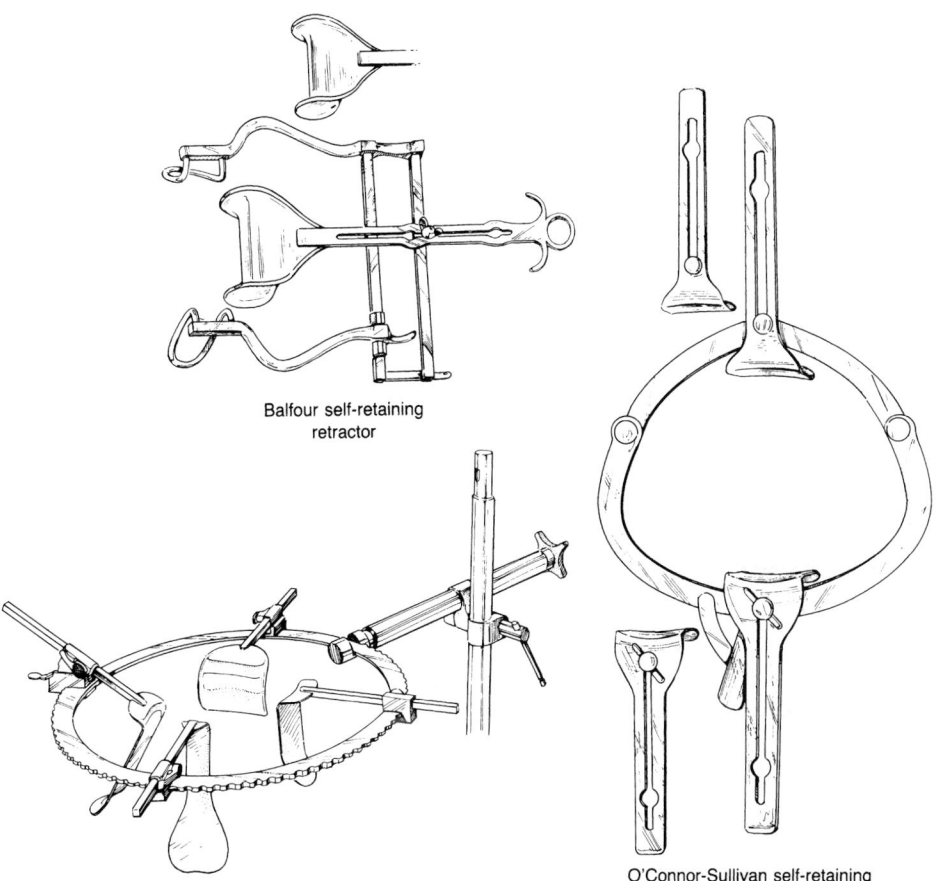

Balfour self-retaining retractor

Bookwalter retractor

O'Connor-Sullivan self-retaining retractor

FIGURE 13.13 Retractors. (Courtesy of Zinnanti Surgical Instruments, Inc., Chatsworth, CA.)

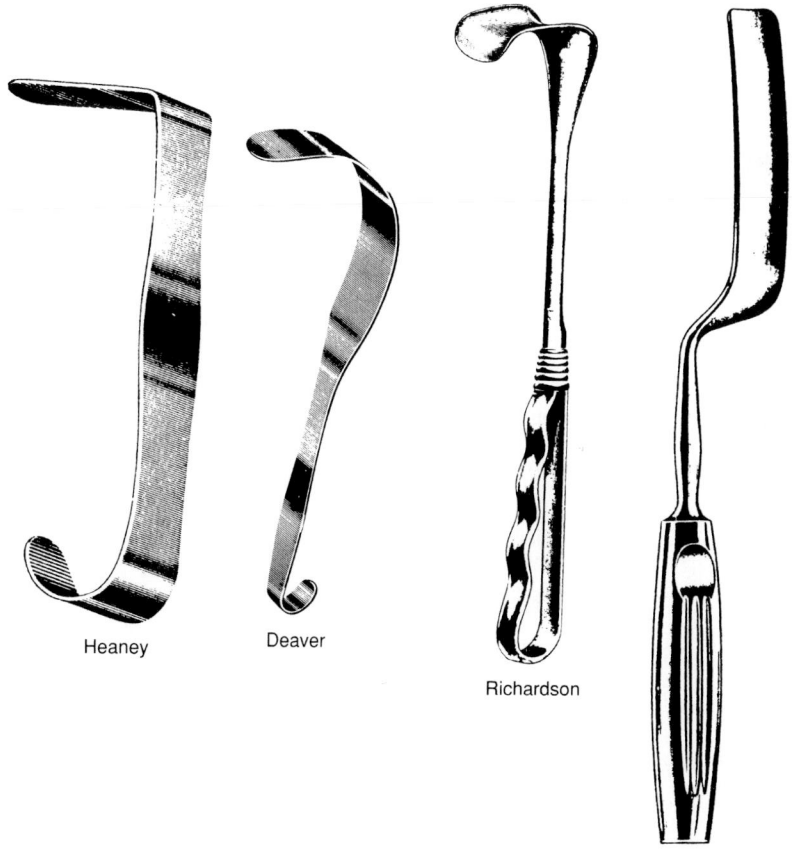

Heaney

Deaver

Richardson

Breisky

FIGURE 13.14 Manual retractors. (Courtesy of Zinnanti Surgical Instruments, Inc., Chatsworth, CA.)

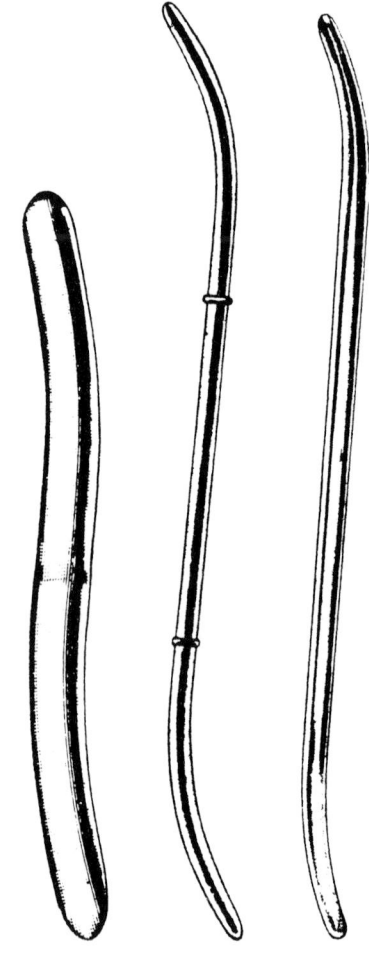

Hegar   Hank   Pratt

FIGURE 13.15 Common cervical dilators. (Courtesy of Zinnanti Surgical Instruments, Inc., Chatsworth, CA.)

the diameter times pi (3.14) equals the circumference. For comparison purposes, approximately 3 French equals 1 mm of diameter.

CONCLUSION

This chapter has attempted to present an introduction to the mechanisms of wound healing, wound closure, suture material, and instrumentation. It is hoped that this chapter will be a useful resource not only for those embarking on a surgical career but also for experienced surgeons as well.

BEST SURGICAL PRACTICES

- Secondary wound closure should ideally be performed on day 4.
- Proper surgical technique is one of the most critical factors in preventing wound dehiscence.
- Abdominal wall fascia should be loosely closed with suture bites of 1 to 1.5 cm.
- The use of mass closure techniques using long-delayed or permanent suture to close fascia is recommended to reduce fascial dehiscence.

- The use of catgut sutures has been limited in many countries because of increasing concerns over the possibility of theoretical infection with TSE, such as "mad cow" disease.
- Suture knots produced by tying a loop of suture to a single strand are less secure than are those tied using a strand to strand. This is particularly critical when using monofilament suture.

BIBLIOGRAPHY

Alexander HC, Prudden JF. The causes of abdominal wound disruption. *Surg Gynecol Obstet* 1966;124:1223.

Archie JP, Feltman RW. Primary abdominal wound closure with permanent, continuous running monofilament sutures. *Surg Gynecol Obstet* 1981;153:721.

Bilroth T. Beobachtungs-studien über wundfieber und accidentelle wundkrankheiten. *Arch Klin Chir* 1866;6:443.

Boerema I. Cause and repair of large incisional hernias. *Surgery* 1971;69:111.

Bourne RB, Bitar H, Andreae PR, et al. In-vitro comparison of four absorbable sutures: Vicryl, Dexon Plus, Maxon and PDS. *Can J Surg* 1988;31:43.

Brouwers JE, Oosting H, Haas D, et al. Dynamic loading of surgical knots. *Surg Gynecol Obstet* 1991;173:443.

Brown RP. Knotting material and suture. *Br J Surg* 1992;79:399.

Bryant WM. Wound healing. In: Bekiesz B, ed. *Ciba clinical symposia*. Ciba-Geigy 1977;29:2.

Buckall TE. Abdominal wound closure: choice of suture. *J R Soc Med* 1981;74:580.

Campbell JA, Temple WJ, Frank CR, et al. A biomechanical study of suture pullout in linea alba. *Surgery* 1989;106:888.

Corman ML, Veidenheimer MC, Coller JA. Controlled clinical trial of three suture materials for abdominal wall closure after bowel operations. *Am J Surg* 1981;141:510.

Douglas DM. The healing of aponeurotic incisions. *Br J Surg* 1952;40:79.

Edlich RF, Rogers W, Kasper G, et al. Studies on the management of the contaminated wound. I. Optimal time for closure of contaminated open wounds. *Am J Surg* 1969;117:323.

Ethicon. *Wound closure manual*. Somerville, NJ: Ethicon Inc., 1985.

Ethicon. *Wound closure manual*. Somerville, NJ: Ethicon Inc., 1994.

Fagniez PL, Hay JM, Lacaine F, et al. Abdominal midline incision closure. *Arch Surg* 1985;120:1351.

Fogdestam I. A biomechanical study of healing rat skin incisions after delayed primary closure. *Surg Obstet Gynecol* 1981;153:191.

Gallup DG, Talledo EO, King LA. Primary mass closure of midline incisions with a continuous running monofilament suture in gynecologic patients. *Obstet Gynecol* 1989;73:675.

Greenall MJ, Evans M, Pollack AV. Midline or transverse laparotomy? A random controlled clinical trial. *Br J Surg* 1980;67:180.

Greenburg AG, Salk RS, Peskin GW. Wound dehiscence: pathology and prevention. *Arch Surg* 1979;114:143.

Hartko WJ, Ghanekar G, Kemmann E. Suture materials currently used in obstetric-gynecologic surgery in the United States: a questionnaire survey. *Obstet Gynecol* 1982;59:241.

Herman JB. Tensile strength and knot security of surgical suture materials. *Am Surg* 1971;37:209.

Higgins GA, Antkowiak JG, Esterkyn SH. A clinical and laboratory study of abdominal wound closure and dehiscence. *Arch Surg* 1969;98:421.

Hodgson NC, Malthaner RA, Ostbye T. The search for an ideal method of abdominal fascial closure: a meta-analysis. *Ann Surg* 2000;231:436.

Hoffman MS, Villa A, Roberts WS, et al. Mass closure of the abdominal wound with delayed absorbable suture in surgery for gynecologic cancer. *J Reprod Med* 1991;36:356.

Howes EL, Harvey SC. The strength of the healing wound in relation to the holding strength of the chromic catgut suture. *N Engl J Med* 1929;200:1285.

Hunter J. *Treatise on blood, inflammation and gunshot wounds*. London, UK: Nichol, 1794:216.

Katz AR, Mukherjee DB, Kagnanov AL, et al. A new synthetic mono-filament absorbable suture made from polytrimethylene carbonate. *Surg Gynecol Obstet* 1983;161:213.

Kim YB, DuBeshter B, Nilaoff JM. Continuous single-layer closure of midline abdominal incisions in high-risk gynecologic patients. *J Gynecol Surg* 1992;8:15.

Knight CD, Griffen FD. Abdominal wound closure with continuous monofilament polypropylene suture. Experience with 1000 cases. *Arch Surg* 1983;118:1305.

Lichtenstein IL, Herzoikoff S, Shore JM, et al. The dynamics of wound healing. *Surg Gynecol Obstet* 1970;130:685.

Lowery KF, Curtis GM. Delayed suture in the management of wounds: analysis of 721 traumatic wounds illustrating the influence of time interval in wound repair. *Am J Surg* 1950;80:280.

Orr JW, Orr P, Barrett JM, et al. Continuous or interrupted fascial closure: a prospective evaluation of No. 1 Maxon in 402 gynecologic procedures. *Am J Obstet Gynecol* 1990;163:1485.

Paterson-Brown S, Dudley HAF. Knotting in continuous mass closure of the abdomen. *Br J Surg* 1986;73:679.

Peacock EE. Wound healing. In: Schwartz SI, Shires GT, Spenser FC, et al., eds. *Principles of surgery*, 3rd ed. New York: McGraw-Hill, 1979:303.

Ray JA, Doddi N, Regula D, et al. Polydioxanone (PDS), a novel monofilament synthetic absorbable suture. *Surg Gynecol Obstet* 1981;151:497.

Reul GJ. The role of sutures in the complications in vascular surgery and their relationship to pseudoaneurysm formation. In: Bernham VM, Town JB, eds. *Complications in vascular surgery*. New York: Grune & Stratton, 1981:615.

Rodeheaver GT, Tacker JG, Edlich RF. Mechanical performance of polyglycolic acid and polyglactin-910 synthetic absorbable suture. *Surg Gynecol Obstet* 1981;153:835.

Rodeheaver GT, Tacker JG, Edlich RF, et al. Knotting and handling characteristics of coated synthetic sutures. *J Surg Res* 1983;35:525.

Sanders RJ, DiClementi D. Principles of abdominal wound closure: II. Prevention of dehiscence. *Arch Surg* 1977;112:1188.

Sanders RJ, DiClementi D, Ireland K. Principles of abdominal wound closure: I. Animal studies. *Arch Surg* 1977;112:1184.

Sanz LE. Sutures: a primer on structure and function. *Contemp Obstet Gynecol* 1990;33:99.

Sanz LE. Wound management: technique and suture material. In: Sanz LE, ed. *Gynecologic surgery*. Oradell, NJ: Medical Economics, 1988:21.

Sanz LE, Patterson JA, Kamath R, et al. Comparison of Maxon suture with Vicryl, chromic catgut, and PDS sutures in fascial closure in rats. *Obstet Gynecol* 1988;71:418.

Sloop RD. Running synthetic absorbable suture in abdominal closure. *Am J Surg* 1981;141:572.

Stone HH, Hoefling SJ, Strom PR, et al. Abdominal incisions: transverse vs vertical placement and continuous vs interrupted closure. *South Med J* 1983;76:1106.

Stone IK, von Fraunhofer JA, Masterson BJ. The biomechanical effects of tight suture closure upon fascia. *Surg Obstet Gynecol* 1986;163:448.

Tera H, Aberg C. Tissue strength of structures involved in musculo-aponeurotic layer sutures in laparotomy incisions. *Acta Chir Scand* 1976;142:349.

Trimbos JB. Security of various knots commonly used in surgical practice. *Obstet Gynecol* 1984;64:274.

Trimbos JB, Van Rijssel EJC, Klopper PJ. Performance of sliding knots in monofilament and multifilament suture material. *Obstet Gynecol* 1986;68:425.

The United States Pharmacopeia, 23th rev. Taunton, MA: Rand McNally, 1994.

Van Rijssel EJC, Trimbos JB, Booster MH. Mechanical performance of square knots and sliding knots in surgery: a comparative study. *Am J Obstet Gynecol* 1990;162:93.

Wasiljew BK, Winchester DP. Experience with continuous absorbable suture in the closure of abdominal incisions. *Surg Obstet Gynecol* 1982;154:375.

Wilhelm DL. Inflammation and healing. In: Anderson WA, Kissane JM, eds. *Pathology*, 7th ed. St. Louis, MO: CV Mosby, 25.

CHAPTER 14
Incisions for Gynecologic Surgery

James J. Burke II

DEFINITIONS

Arcuate line—The demarcation above which the posterior lamella of the internal oblique aponeurosis fuses with the aponeurosis of the transversalis muscle and passes posterior to the rectus muscles. Below this line, the aponeurosis of the internal oblique passes anterior to the rectus muscles.

Cherney incision—A transverse abdominal incision in which the rectus muscles are transected at their insertion on the pubic symphysis. The fascia may or may not be dissected free from the rectus muscles. Entry into the peritoneum may be vertical or transverse.

Dehiscence—Disruption of a surgical wound, either superficial or deep. Superficial dehiscence is separation of the skin and subcutaneous tissue because of seroma, hematoma, or abscess formation. Fascial dehiscence describes the separation of the fascia without extrusion of the bowel.

Evisceration—Disruption of the fascia with extrusion of the bowel through the wound.

Gridiron incision—A muscle-splitting, oblique incision, useful for a transperitoneal or extraperitoneal approach to pelvic organs; similar to a McBurney incision.

Hernia—A late complication of wound disruption. A fascial disruption occurs with protrusion of the peritoneum, bowel, and omentum. The skin and subcutaneous tissue are intact.

Langer lines—The natural, anatomic tissue lines on the abdominal skin.

Linea alba—Where the aponeurosis of the internal and external oblique muscles insert, anterior to the rectus musculature.

Maylard incision—A transverse abdominal incision in which the rectus muscles are transected after ligation of the inferior epigastric vessels. The fascia is not dissected free of the rectus muscles. The peritoneum is usually entered in a transverse fashion.

Panniculectomy—Surgical removal of the pannus, excess skin, and subcutaneous fat, which hangs like an apron from the abdomen. Removal facilitates gynecologic surgery.

Pfannenstiel incision—A commonly used transverse abdominal incision in which the rectus muscles are not cut and the fascia is dissected superiorly and inferiorly along the rectus muscles. The peritoneum is usually entered vertically.

Schuchardt incision—An incision made in the vagina, along the sulcus of the vagina from the lateral fornix to the introitus and through the perineum. This incision can increase room in the vagina so as to aid in difficult vaginal surgeries.

Smead-Jones closure—An interrupted closure of the anterior abdominal wall using a far–far, near–near approach. The closure includes all of the abdominal wall structures on the far–far portion and only the fascia on the near–near portion.

Although the buzz in gynecologic surgery is a minimally invasive approach, certain benign and malignant gynecologic disease states still require a laparotomy to treat. One of the lasting marks of any abdominal surgery, and most noticeable to the patient, is the scar made by the incision. In selecting an incision, the gynecologist must take into consideration the underlying pathology prompting the surgery, the suspicion of malignancy, the absence or presence of upper abdominal disease, and the underlying comorbid state of the patient. Although there are many types of incisions for gynecologic surgery, selection of any incision must be highly individualized. However, selection of an incision should not be dictated by patient choice to preserve cosmesis if it may compromise the surgical approach. Conversely, unduly large or poorly positioned incisions may increase the likelihood of infection, herniation, or dehiscence, as well as unsightly cosmesis. During the surgical consenting process, the patient should be counseled on the location of the incision, the rationale for the particular incision, and any possible complication that may arise from the planned incision. This chapter presents the classic incisions used by gynecologists to perform most gynecologic surgery. Finally, discussion about the prevention and management of common complications associated with abdominal incisions is presented.

ANATOMY OF THE ANTERIOR ABDOMINAL WALL

To avoid injury to vessels and nerves and to close any incision with minimal chance of dehiscence, abdominal wall anatomy should be thoroughly understood. The abdominal wall protects the visceral organs and vasculature within the abdominal cavity. Cephalad, the anterior abdominal wall extends to the costal margins and the xiphoid process. The costal cartilages of the seventh, eighth, ninth, and tenth ribs form a portion of the cephalad boundary. Lateral boundaries include the iliac crests; inferiorly, the abdominal wall is delineated by the inguinal ligaments, the pubic crests, and the superior border of the symphysis pubis. The principal anatomic structures of the abdominal wall include the overlying skin, subcutaneous tissue, muscles, fascia, and the neurovascular supply to these structures. Many factors—such as age, muscle mass and tone, obesity, intra-abdominal pathology, previous pregnancies, and posture—can result in variation in the contour of the abdominal wall. These variations can affect abdominal wall topography and may present impediments to the correct choice and placement of laparotomy incisions.

Skin and Lymphatics

The skin contains small vessels, lymphatics, and nerves. A minimal loss of skin sensation can result from any abdominal incision. Numbness below a transverse incision frequently occurs. As stated in the discussion on nerve supply (below), laterally extended transverse abdominal incisions can result in numbness of the skin on the anterior thigh.

The lymphatic drainage of the upper abdominal wall passes directly to the axillary lymph nodes. The lymphatic drainage of the lower abdomen passes to the inguinal nodes and then to the iliac chain. Some lymphatics around the umbilicus drain toward the liver through the falciform ligament. When an incision is placed transversely in the lower abdomen, lymphatic drainage of the abdominal wall above the incision site is disrupted. Some tissue swelling may develop temporarily until collateral lymphatic drainage can be established. Patients should be counseled about this possible swelling before undergoing surgery.

In 1861, Austrian anatomist Karl Langer described cleavage lines of the skin while working with cadavers. Langer punctured numerous holes at short distances from each other into the skin of a cadaver with a tool that had a circular-shaped tip, similar to an ice pick. He noticed that the resultant punctures in the skin had ellipsoidal shapes. From this testing, he observed patterns and was able to determine "line directions" by the longer axes of the ellipsoidal holes and lines. These have become known as Langer lines (Fig. 14.1). Across the abdomen, these lines usually run horizontally, and when making vertical incisions in the skin of the abdomen, cuts perpendicular to Langer lines are made, whereas transverse incisions cut parallel to these. Thus, transverse incisions heal with a relatively fine scar, and vertical incisions can heal with a broad scar, particularly in the lower abdomen.

Muscles and Fascia

The abdominal muscles assist in respiration, defecation, urination, coughing, and childbirth by increasing intra-abdominal pressure. They work synergistically with the muscles of the back to flex, extend, and rotate the trunk and pelvis. There are two groups of muscles that form the musculature of the anterior abdominal wall. The flat muscles include the external oblique, the internal oblique, and the transversalis. These muscle fibers run diagonally or transversely. The second group, composed of the recti muscles and the paired pyramidalis muscles, have fibers that run vertically (Fig. 14.2). The recti, with their thin investing fascia, are muscles of locomotion and posture. The paired pyramidalis muscles arise from the crest of the pubic symphysis and insert into the lower linea alba. Preservation of the pyramidalis muscles is not essential when making incisions. The integrity of the anterior abdominal wall is not associated with this second group of muscles.

A cross section of the lower abdominal wall shows that the fascia of the abdominal muscles envelops the anterior and posterior surfaces of the rectus muscles and anchors the external oblique, internal oblique, and transversalis muscles to the vertical (rectus) muscles (Fig. 14.3). There is excellent fascial support anteriorly and posteriorly to the rectus muscles above the arcuate (semicircular) line. In this location, the fascial aponeurosis of the external oblique and the split fascial aponeurosis of the internal oblique fuse together anterior to the rectus muscle and insert in the midline (linea alba). Above the arcuate line, the posterior lamella of the internal oblique aponeurosis

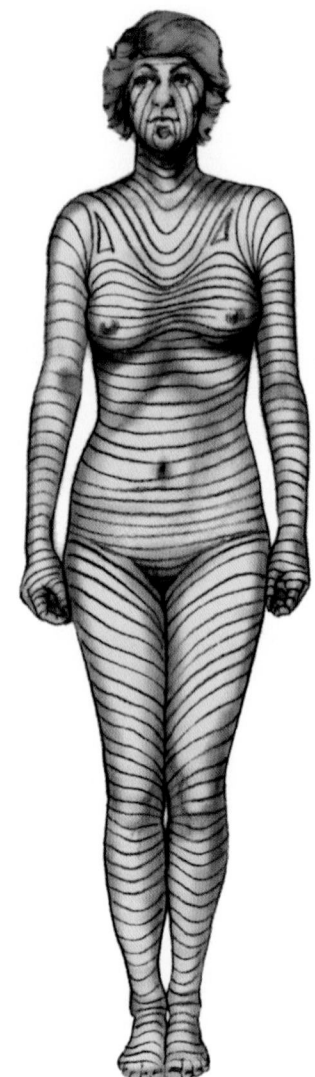

FIGURE 14.1 Langer lines run horizontally across the lower abdomen. A transverse incision cuts parallel to the Langer lines and usually heals with a fine scar.

fuses with the aponeurosis of the transversalis muscle, passing posterior to the rectus muscle and inserting in the midline. The lower half of the lower abdominal wall is weakened below the arcuate line, at a level about horizontal to the anterior superior iliac spines, where the posterior division of the rectus sheath disappears. In this location, the divided lamella of the internal oblique muscle combines and passes anterior to the rectus muscle. From this lower portion of the lower abdominal wall to the pubic rami, only the attenuated transversalis fascia and the peritoneum lie adjacent to the posterior surface of the muscle. It is in this weakened section of the lower abdomen that most incisional hernias occur after open pelvic surgery through lower midline incisions. In the lower abdomen, the force required to approximate edges of a vertical incision is 30 times greater than the force required to approximate edges of a transverse incision.

The external oblique muscle and its aponeurosis form the most anterior layer of the flat muscles. The external oblique muscle originates from the lower eight ribs. Superiorly, the fibers of this muscle run transversely; inferiorly, they assume an oblique downward course. A portion of the muscle gives rise

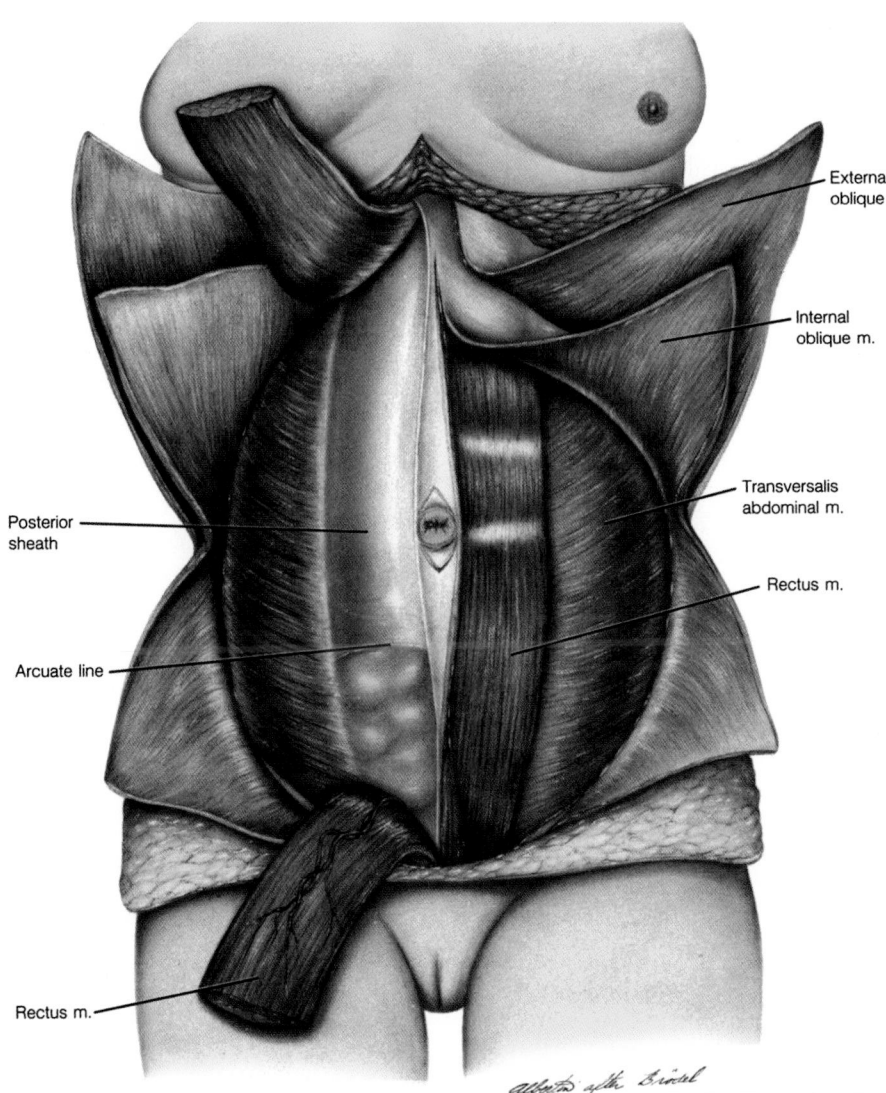

Posterior sheath

Arcuate line

Rectus m.

External oblique m.

Internal oblique m.

Transversalis abdominal m.

Rectus m.

albatar after Brödel

FIGURE 14.2 Musculature of the abdominal wall (**left**), showing reflection of external and internal oblique muscles along with the anterior division of the rectus sheath, which exposes the transversalis and rectus muscles. Tendinous inscriptions in the rectus sheath are visible above the umbilicus. The rectus muscle has been reflected (**right**) to demonstrate the posterior rectus sheath and the abrupt cessation of the posterior lamella of the internal oblique at the linea semicircularis (*arcuate line*). Below the *arcuate line*, the intestines are separated from the abdominal wall by the peritoneum and the attenuated fascia of the transversalis muscle.

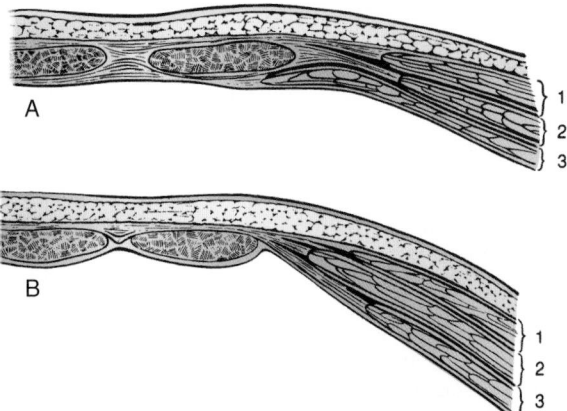

FIGURE 14.3 Cross section of lower abdominal wall. **A:** The anterior fascial sheath of the rectus muscle from external oblique muscle (*1*) and split aponeurosis of internal oblique muscle (*2*). The posterior sheath is formed by aponeurosis of transversalis muscle (*3*) and split aponeurosis of internal oblique muscle. **B:** Lower portion of abdominal wall below arcuate line (linea semicircularis) with absence of a posterior fascial sheath of the rectus muscle and all of the facial aponeuroses (*1–3*) forming the anterior rectus sheath.

to a broad fibrous aponeurosis, which courses medially, anterior to the rectus muscle. The next posterior fanlike muscle is the internal oblique, which originates primarily from the iliac crest, the thoracolumbar fascia, and the inguinal ligament. The midportion of this muscle runs an upward oblique course and gives rise to the aponeurosis of the internal oblique. As noted, at the lateral border of the rectus musculature, the aponeurosis splits and forms a sheath around the rectus muscle, rejoining medial to the rectus to help form the linea alba. The third flat muscle, the transversus abdominis, arises from the lower six costal cartilages, thoracolumbar fascia, and the internal lip of the iliac crest. This muscle has a truly transverse course. Above the midway point between the umbilicus and pubis, the aponeurosis of this muscle passes behind the rectus muscle and contributes to the posterior rectus sheath. Below this point, the aponeurosis passes anterior to the rectus muscle, contributing to the anterior rectus sheath. Medial to the rectus muscle, the fasciae of all three flat muscles insert to form the linea alba.

The major functions of the flat muscles are to assist with respirations and to assist in increasing intra-abdominal pressure. Each time these muscles contract, they pull at the linea alba. Because the linea alba represents the insertion of six major abdominal muscles (three on each side), cutting it, as with lower midline incisions, actually interrupts the major portion of the insertion of these six muscles. Thus, contractions of these muscles in the postoperative period can result in considerable tension on a suture line in the linea alba and can cause considerable discomfort.

The rectus abdominis muscle arises from the pubic crest and courses superiorly, inserting into the xiphoid process with the upper attachments being three times as broad as its pubic insertion. It has three or four fibrous insertions. One is at the level of the umbilicus; two are usually halfway between the umbilicus and the insertions, superiorly and inferiorly, respectively. Of note, the fibrous insertions are tightly adherent to the anterior rectus sheath. These limit the retraction of the muscle when it is cut. Thus, when performing a transverse-muscle–cutting incision, it is not necessary to reapproximate the rectus muscle. The pyramidalis, a triangular muscle, usually lies anterior to the rectus and arises from the anterior portion of the pubic symphysis, inserting into the inferior portion of the linea alba. The midportion of this muscle usually has an avascular raphe, which can easily be incised to adequately expose the space of Retzius.

Blood Supply

The abundant blood supply to the anterior abdominal wall comes from several sources. The main arterial supply consists of the superior epigastric, musculophrenic, deep circumflex iliac, and inferior epigastric vessels. The medial abdominal wall receives blood from the epigastric arteries, whereas the lateral wall is supplied by the musculophrenic and deep circumflex iliac arteries. The lateral wall is also supplied by the lower intercostal and lumbar arteries (T8 to T12 and L1). This freely anastomosing vascular system provides one continuous arterial and venous channel on both sides of the anterior abdominal wall, extending from the subclavian artery and vein (cephalad) to the external iliac vessels (caudad) (Fig. 14.4). Because of the rich anastomosis, vascular deficiency is usually not a complication of abdominal wall surgery. The linea alba is relatively bloodless. The limited vascular supply in this area of fascial fusion can impair wound healing when lower midline incisions are used. Thus, a secure closure is mandatory to avoid dehiscences, eviscerations, or incisional hernias.

Conversely, the epigastric vessels are subject to injury, particularly when a muscle-splitting incision is used. Also, the deep circumflex or musculophrenic vessels can be injured when an extraperitoneal approach is chosen.

The superior epigastric artery is a continuation of the internal thoracic (mammary) artery. This vessel enters the sheath of the rectus from behind the seventh costal cartilage and descends posterior to the rectus muscle. It has multiple branches in the substance of the rectus muscle and anastomosis to the inferior epigastric artery. In the upper abdomen, cephalad to the umbilicus, the main branch of the artery tends to lie posterior to the midportion of the rectus muscle (Fig. 14.5). The inferior epigastric artery arises from the external iliac artery near the midinguinal point. It continues in a cephalad course along the posterolateral portion of the rectus muscle and has an anastomosis with the superior epigastric arteries. The lower a transverse incision is made, the more laterally the inferior epigastric arteries are encountered. Bleeding from branches of the inferior epigastric vessels beneath the rectus muscle can dissect cephalad or caudad along the entire length of the posterior sheath. Below the arcuate line, bleeding can dissect laterally and inferiorly along the retroperitoneal planes and spaces, resulting in extensive hematomas of the abdominal wall and

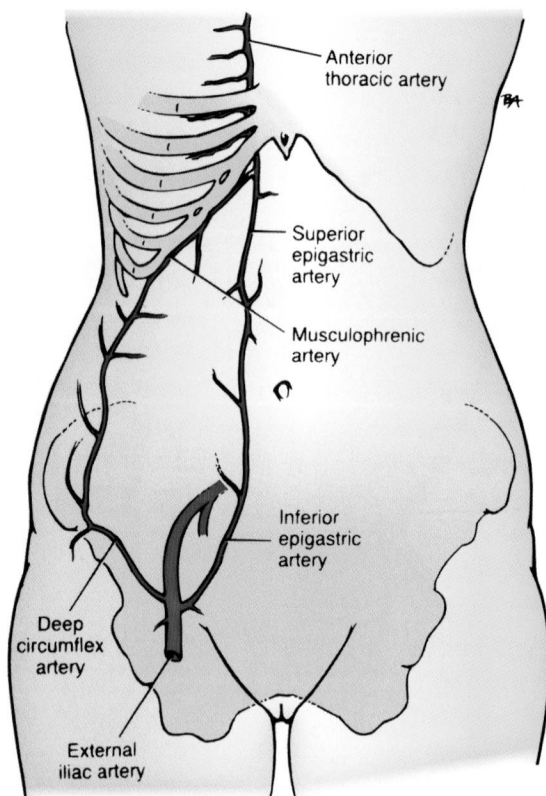

FIGURE 14.4 The major arterial blood supply of the anterior abdominal wall consists of four major vessels. Two lateral and two medial contribute to the rich anastomosis. (Reprinted from Gallup DG. Opening and closing the abdomen and wound healing. In: Gershenson D, Curry S, DeCherney A, eds. *Operative gynecology*, 1st ed. Philadelphia, PA: WB Saunders, 1993:127, with permission. Copyright 1993 Elsevier.)

pelvis. Such bleeding can produce confusing acute abdominal signs in the postoperative patient, with large quantities of blood being lost in these loose tissues and spaces.

The musculophrenic artery, arising from the internal (mammary) thoracic artery, courses along the costal margin posterior to the cartilages. It has an anastomosis with the deep circumflex artery, which originates from the external iliac at about the same level as the inferior epigastric artery. The deep circumflex courses behind the inguinal ligament and along the iliac crest, eventually piercing the transversalis muscle and digitating between that muscle and the internal oblique. Before its anastomosis with the musculophrenic, this vessel can be relatively large. Care must be taken not to injure this vessel when these muscles are incised laterally.

The venous drainage of the abdominal wall accompanies the arterial supply. The veins of the abdominal wall may be dilated in patients with obstruction of blood flow through the liver and porta hepatis.

Innervation

The nerve supply to the anterior abdominal wall is easily damaged by some incisions. The anterior abdominal wall is supplied by the thoracoabdominal nerves, the iliohypogastric nerves, and the ilioinguinal nerves. The thoracoabdominal

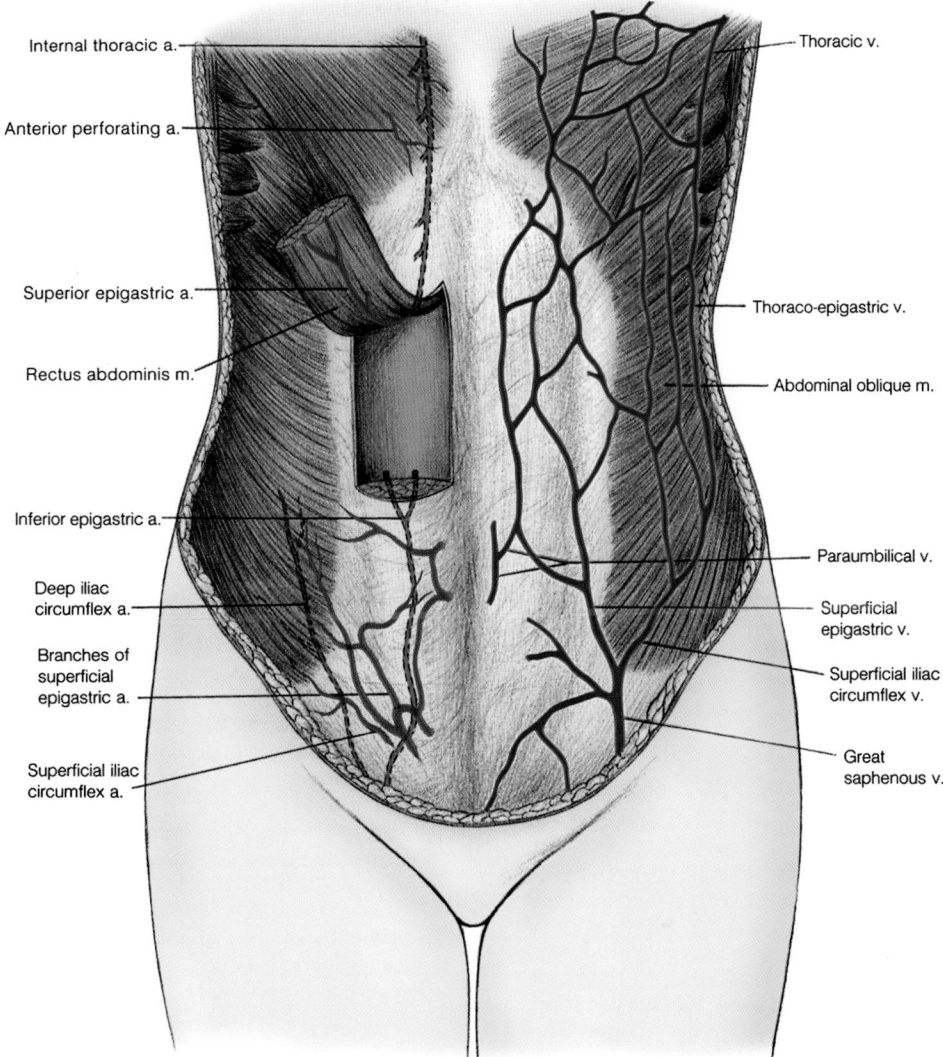

FIGURE 14.5 Arterial and venous circulation of abdominal wall. The superior and inferior epigastric arteries provide a rich arcade for the rectus muscles, arising superiorly from the internal thoracic artery and inferiorly from the external iliac artery. The venous system has a similar origin, with the exception that the superficial inferior epigastric vein communicates with the saphenous vein of the leg.

nerves, which are the 7th to 11th intercostal nerves, leave the intercostal spaces and travel caudad and anterior between the transversalis and internal oblique muscles. These nerves innervate these muscles as well as the external oblique. These nerves enter the sheath of the rectus muscle, and their branches innervate the rectus muscle and the overlying skin. Nerve roots from several vertebrae supply most of the nerves of the abdominal wall, whereby any one nerve will contain fibers from at least two or three intercostal nerves. When incisions are made lateral to the midline, a transverse type is the least likely to cause neural injury. In the upper abdomen, an obliquely caudad and laterally directed incision is least likely to cause significant nerve injury. In the lower part of the abdomen, an obliquely directed cephalad and laterally directed incision is relatively nerve sparing.

A vertical incision that passes lateral to the rectus muscle or through the muscle itself can denervate medially lying tissue. Depending on the length of the incision, atony or atrophy of the muscle can then occur. A midline incision in the linea alba or a transverse incision (even through the rectus muscle),

however, does not interfere with motor innervation of the abdominal musculature.

A minimal loss of skin sensation can result from abdominal incisions and is unavoidable in most cases. The iliohypogastric and ilioinguinal nerves, which are chiefly derived from the first lumbar nerve root, are sensory in function (Fig. 14.6). Injury to the former, when wide transverse incisions are used, can result in sensation changes in the skin over the mons, whereas injury to the latter can result in sensation changes to the labia majora. A widely placed transverse incision can also result in numbness of the skin over the upper anterior thigh. Although they lie for a distance between the internal oblique and the transversalis muscles, they do not enter the rectus sheath. They do not innervate the external oblique or the rectus muscle. Both nerves supply the lower fibers of the internal oblique and transversalis muscles. If damage occurs to these nerves at the level of the anterosuperior iliac spine, these muscle fibers will be denervated, resulting in weakening of the normal inguinal canal–controlling mechanism and predisposing the patient to an inguinal hernia.

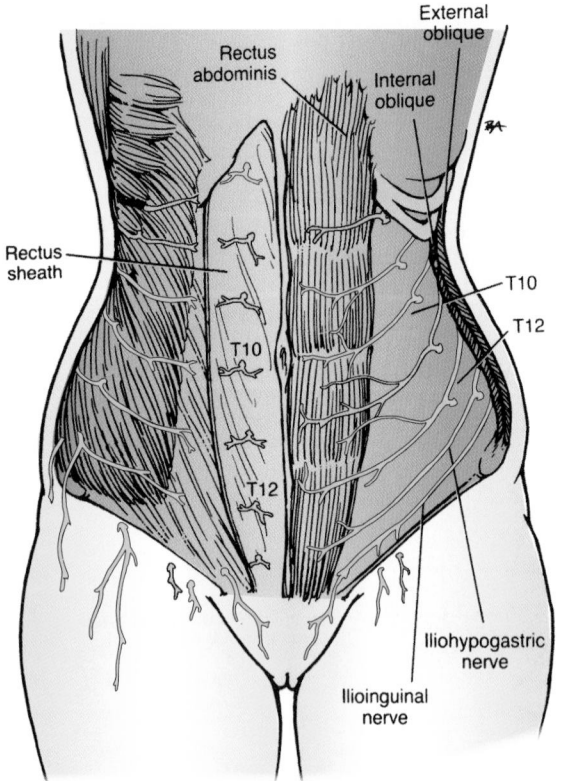

FIGURE 14.6 Major innervation of the anterior abdominal wall. The iliohypogastric nerves and ilioinguinal nerves supply the sensory innervation of the lower abdominal wall. (Reprinted from Gallup DG. Opening and closing the abdomen and wound healing. In: Gershenson D, Curry S, DeCherney A, eds. *Operative gynecology*, 1st ed. Philadelphia, PA: WB Saunders, 1993:127, with permission. Copyright 1993 Elsevier.)

PHYSIOLOGY OF WOUND HEALING

When making a surgical incision, tissue integrity is violated in order to gain access to diseased organs for treatment. These acute wounds heal in a progressive, systematic, and balanced repair process, consisting of four phases: hemostasis, inflammation, proliferation, and remodeling (Fig. 14.7).

The hemostatic phase is initiated immediately upon injury, whereby the intrinsic and extrinsic clotting cascades are activated. When an injury occurs, collagen, von Willebrand factor, and tissue factor are exposed from the subendothelium to the bloodstream, acting as the inciting catalyst for the systemic repair process. A platelet plug forms, composed of platelets and fibrin. Platelets release granules containing multiple growth factors, which act as chemoattractants, and thromboxane A2, which acts as a potent vasoconstrictor. Transforming growth factor beta (TGF-β) is the key growth factor released, playing a central role in wound healing.

The inflammatory phase occurs from days 1 to 10 and is characterized by an inflammatory cell wound infiltration and initiation of epithelialization occurring at 1 to 2 mm from the wound edges. The ordered cellular influx begins with neutrophils that act as scavengers, cleaning cellular debris through phagocytosis and killing bacteria through oxidative burst. Neutrophils secrete elastase and matrix metalloproteinases (MMPs) to degrade the extracellular matrix, facilitating cellular migration. Monocytes from the blood convert to macrophages arriving at 48 hours, which are the key coordinating cells for transitioning to the proliferative phase by releasing additional growth factors, mediating angiogenesis and fibroplasia, and synthesizing nitric oxide.

The proliferative phase starts when fibroblasts arrive at the wound, usually around day 5. At this time, type III collagen is deposited with neovascularization and initiation of granulation tissue formation. Granulation tissue is perfused connective tissue, which forms the framework for further epithelialization. Fibroblasts in the wound convert to myofibroblasts to allow wound contraction, a key component for healing via secondary intention. Cellular signaling for this conversion is mediated by macrophages through TGF-β. Fibroblasts also secrete MMP, which aids cellular migration.

From day 8 through year 1, wound remodeling and maturation occur. Initial deposition of collagen is disordered, and over time, remodeling of collagen at areas of increased stress allows for increased tensile strength. By the 3rd week, type III collagen has been replaced for type I collagen, which is the most common type of collagen in the human body and provides 30% of its final strength. The maximal tensile strength of the tissue is reached approximately 8 weeks after injury and at a level which is 80% of its original strength.

When this ordered repair process fails, an acute wound is converted into a chronic wound. Factors negatively affecting proper

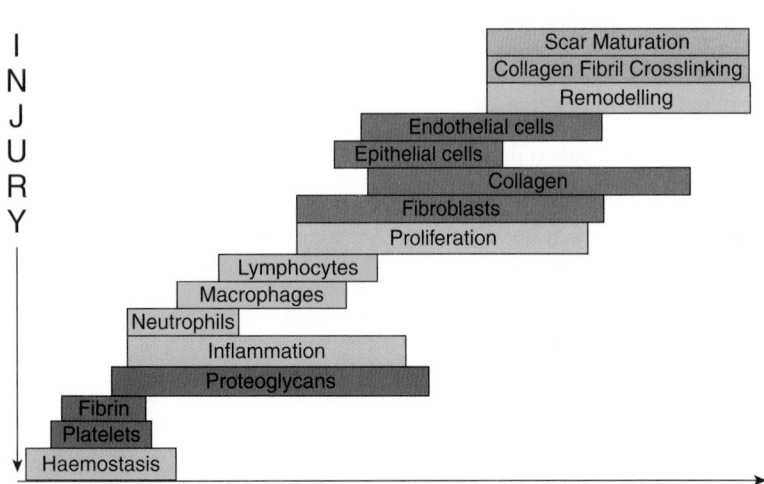

FIGURE 14.7 Orderly steps in wound healing.

TABLE 14.1 Wound Classification

CLASS	CATEGORY	DEFINITION	WOUND INFECTION RATE (%)
I	Clean	Wounds are made under ideal operating room conditions. The procedures are usually elective, and no entry is made into the oropharyngeal cavity or lumen of the respiratory, alimentary, or genitourinary tract. Inflammation is not encountered, and no break in technique occurs. The wounds are always primarily closed and seldom drained. Almost 75% of all operations are included in this group.	1–5
II	Clean-contaminated	Wounds occur from entry into the oropharyngeal cavity, respiratory, alimentary, or genitourinary tract without significant spillage. Clean wounds are included in this category when there is a minor break in surgical technique. These procedures include about 16% of all operations.	3–11
III	Contaminated	This category includes open, fresh, and traumatic wounds, operations with a major break in sterile technique, and incisions encountering acute, nonpurulent inflammation, such as in cholecystitis or cystitis.	4–17
IV	Dirty	Old (>4 h) traumatic wounds, perforated viscera, or operations involving clinically evident infections are included in this category. Wounds containing foreign bodies or devitalized tissue are also considered dirty.	5–27

From Ortega G, Rhee DS, Papandria DJ, et al. An evaluation of surgical site infections by wound classification system using the ACS-NSQIP. *J Surg Res* 2012;174:33; Cruse PJE, Foord R. The epidemiology of wound infection: a 10-year prospective study of 62,939 wounds. *Surg Clin North Am* 1980;60:27; and Culver DH, Horan TC, Gaynes RP, et al. Surgical wound infection rates by wound class, operative procedure and patient risk index. National Nosocomial Infections Surveillance System. *Am J Med* 1991;91:152S.

wound healing include age; comorbid conditions such as cardiac disease, connective tissue disorders, diabetes, and liver diseases; lifestyle factors such as nutritional status, obesity, smoking, and illicit drug usage; and therapeutic modalities such as prior irradiation, chemotherapy, steroid usage, and NSAID usage. In addition to these factors, bacterial burden can impact wound healing and interrupt the progressive, ordered repair process. Bacteria colonize a wound within 48 hours. Most bacteria have low virulence and do not invade the tissue. The wound relationship with bacteria consists of a continuum from contamination to wound septicemia. Contamination within a wound is defined by non-replicating bacteria, whereas colonization is defined as replicating bacteria adherent to the wound without tissue damage, both of which do not delay wound healing. However, critical colonization may delay wound healing. In acute wounds, bacteria exist as free-floating planktonic organisms and must be rapidly controlled to prevent tissue destruction and wound sepsis (see below skin preparation for surgery). Bacteria in chronic wounds do not exist as planktonic organisms but rather as biofilms able to resist the host inflammatory cascade and antibiotic therapy.

The risks of wound infections are directly related to the classification of wounds (Table 14.1). Most of the abdominal procedures performed by gynecologists include a hysterectomy, and whenever the vagina is entered, the procedure is classified as a clean-contaminated procedure. Prevention of surgical site infections (SSIs) is critical to improve quality surgical care and reduce health care costs associated with such infections (see Prevention of Surgical Site Infections).

SUTURES

Many types of sutures have been used throughout the years for closure of wounds, to relieve healing tissues of the disruptive forces. Some of these materials include linen; cotton; silk; wires of gold, silver, iron, and steel; dried gut; animal hair; tree bark; and other plant fibers. In recent years, with advancements in polymer technology, a wide range of synthetic compounds have emerged as suture material. To date, however, no study, or surgeon, has definitively shown there to be a perfect suture for all situations.

The ideal suture material should have the following characteristics: knot security, inertness, adequate tensile strength, flexibility, ease in handling, smooth passage through tissue, nonallergenicity, resistance to infection, and absorbability at a predictable rate. Despite these ideal attributes, the presence of suture material (foreign bodies) in wounds induces an excessive tissue inflammatory response that lowers the body's defense mechanism against infection and interferes with the proliferative phase of wound healing (see above), ultimately leading to inferior wound strength due to excessive scar tissue formation.

Currently available suture material can be classified in many ways: suture size, tensile strength, absorbable versus nonabsorbable, multifilament versus monofilament, stiffness and flexibility, and, finally, smooth versus barbed. Table 14.2 lists the common sutures that are utilized in obstetrical and gynecologic surgical procedures, the relative tensile strength, the type of degradation (if any), and the handling characteristics.

There are two standards to describe the size of suture material: the US Pharmacopeia (USP) and the European Pharmacopoeia (EP). The USP is the more commonly used standard, which was established in 1937 for standardization and comparison of suture materials, corresponding to metric measures. This standardization sets out limits on the average diameter, and the minimum knot pull tensile strengths of the three classes of sutures are collagen, synthetic absorbable, and nonabsorbable. Size refers to the diameter of the suture strand and is denoted as zeroes. The more zeroes characterizing a suture size, the smaller the resultant strand diameter (e.g., 4-0 is larger than 5-0). Intuitively, the smaller the strand size, the less knot pull tensile strength of the suture. However, the tensile strength also is dependent upon the makeup of the suture.

TABLE 14.2   Available Absorbable and Nonabsorbable Sutures and Characteristics

SUTURE	TENSILE STRENGTH/ABSORPTION					HANDLING CHARACTERISTICS	
ABSORBABLE MULTIFILAMENT	TIME TO LOSS OF 50% TENSILE (D)	TIME TO LOSS 100% TENSILE (D)	TIME TO COMPLETE ABSORPTION (D)	ABSORPTION RATE	TISSUE REACTION/ DEGRADATION	HANDLING	MEMORY
Plain gut (twisted)	3–5	14–21	70	Unpredictable	High/proteolysis	Fair	Low
Chromic gut (twisted)	7–10	14–21	90–120	Unpredictable	High/proteolysis	Fair	Low
Fast-absorbing coated polyglactin 910 (Braided) (Vicryl Rapide)	5	14	42	Predictable	Low/hydrolytic	Best	Low
Coated polyglactin 910 (Braided) (Vicryl)	21	28	56–70	Predictable	Low/hydrolytic	Best	Low
Coated polyglycolide (Dexon II) (Monofilament)	14–21	28	60–90	Predictable Predictable	Low/hydrolytic	Best	Low
Polyglytone 6211 (Caprosyn)	5–7	21	56	Predictable	Low/hydrolytic	Good	Low
Poliglecaprone 25 (Monocryl)	7	21	91–119	Predictable	Low/hydrolytic	Good	Low
Glycomer 631 (Biosyn)	14–21	28	90–110	Predictable	Low/hydrolytic	Good	Low
Polyglyconate (Maxon)	28–35	56	180	Predictable	Low/hydrolytic	Fair	High
Polydioxanone (PDS II) (Barbed)	28–42	90	183–238	Predictable	Low/hydrolytic	Fair	High
Poliglecaprone 25 (Monoderm)	7–10	21	90–120	Predictable	Low/hydrolytic	Good	Low

Polydioxanone (PDO) (Nonabsorbable multifilament)	28–42	90	180	Predictable	Low/hydrolytic	Fair	High
Silk (Braided)	180	365	730	Unpredictable	High/proteolysis	Best	Low
Cotton (twisted)	180	>730	n/a	Unpredictable	High/proteolysis	Best	Low
Polyester (Braided)	n/a	n/a	n/a	n/a	Low/none	Good	Medium
Nylon (Braided) (Nurolon, Surgilon) (Monofilament)	n/a year 1, 89%; year 2, 72%; year 11, 66%	n/a	n/a	Unpredictable	Low/hydrolytic	Good	High
Polypropylene (Prolene, Surgilene)	n/a	n/a	n/a	n/a	Low to none/none	Poor	High
Nylon (Ethilon, Dermalon, Monomid)	See above	See above	See above	Unpredictable	Low/hydrolytic	Poor	High
Polybutester (Novafil)	n/a	n/a	n/a	n/a	Low/none	Good	Low
Stainless steel	n/a	n/a	n/a	n/a	Low to none/none	Fair	High

Adapted from Greenberg JA, Clark RM. Advances in suture material for obstetrics and gynecologic surgery. *Rev Obstet Gynecol* 2009;2:146, with permission. Reviews in Obstetrics and Gynecology is a copyrighted publication of MedReviews, LLC. All rights reserved.

The tensile strength of a suture will depend upon the diameter of the suture and the material that makes up the suture and is simply the force (measured in weight [pounds or kilograms]) necessary to cause the suture to rupture. This measurement is typically presented in two forms: straight pull and knot pull. A straight pull tensile measurement is the tension that causes rupture of the suture when that force is applied to either end of the suture, where a knot pull measurement is the force necessary to rupture the suture after a knot has been tied in the middle of the suture.

Suture materials are classified as being absorbable or nonabsorbable based upon whether they lose their entire tensile strength within 2 to 3 months or retain their strength for longer than 2 to 3 months. The degradation of suture material depends whether the material is a natural material (such as surgical gut–collagen sutures made from sheep or cow intestines) or synthetic materials (such as polyglactin 910 or polydioxanone), where the former is degraded by proteolysis and the later by hydrolysis. Although both degradative processes cause intense inflammatory responses in tissue, the response to synthetic materials is much less than the response to natural protein analogues.

If a suture is manufactured with more than one fiber, it is deemed a multifilament suture. In regard to wound healing, there are no advantages of a multifilament suture over a monofilament suture or vice versa. However, multifilament sutures inflect more microtrauma to tissue, induce a more intense inflammatory response, demonstrate enhanced capillarity (more crevices and spaces) with an increase in spread of microorganisms, and contribute to a larger knot size than do monofilaments of equal sizes. But the improved handling characteristics and flexibility of multifilament suture material may be more advantageous and outweigh any wound healing detriments as compared to the handling of monofilament sutures.

Suture stiffness and flexibility can be as important, as strength and absorption when it comes to classifying sutures as these traits determine the materials' handling or feel. Stiffness describes whether a suture is soft or hard, gives it memory or recoil, and determines the ease with which knots can be tied. Furthermore, stiffness is associated with the presence or absence of mechanical irritation of the suture due to its ability, or inability, to comply with the topology of the surrounding tissues.

Considering all of the characteristics mentioned above, knot tying of sutures is almost as integral to the surgery as the suture itself. A knot is needed as an anchor to the tissue to avoid suture slippage and acute and chronic wound complications (dehiscence and hernia formation). However, there may be unequal distribution of tension on the knots rather than on the length of the suture line, which may subtly interfere with uniform wound healing and remodeling. Irrespective of the knot configuration and material, the weakest spot along the suture is the knot, and the second weakest point is the portion immediately adjacent to the knot with reductions in tensile strength being reported from 35% to 95% depending upon the study and suture material used. It is these weak areas that generally represent the site of failure of a suture. Finally, knot security will depend on suture size and the tissue needing approximation. Although sliding knots, also known as *nonidentical sliding knots*, can be safely used for pelvic viscera, sutures used to close abdominal wall fascia should be tied with square knots, and the number of throws will depend upon the suture material. Sometimes it is convenient to tie a loop-to-strand knot as a way of terminating a continuous suture rather than tying a single-strand to single-strand knot. Hurt and colleagues eloquently conducted a safety evaluation of tying a loop-to-strand knot with a monofilament suture, poliglecaprone (Monocryl). In these experiments, the authors used 0-0- and 2-0-gauge suture, randomly comparing single-strand with single-strand square knots, loop-to-strand square knots,

and loop-to-single-strand, nonidentical sliding knots. A total of 40 knots were tied in each group and evaluated by tensiometry. The major outcome studied was the proportion of knots becoming untied in each group. The authors found that when monofilament sutures were tied loop-to-single strand with nonidentical sliding knots, 85% of the 0-0-guage suture and 55% 2-0-gauge sutures untied. None of the single-strand to single-strand square knots untied, and only 15% of the 0-0 and 5% of the 2-0-gauge sutures, when tied loop-to-single strand with square knots, untied. Although these conditions were carefully controlled and conducted ex vivo, care must be taken to lay down square knots (six throws) while tying monofilament suture in a loop-to-single-strand fashion. Van Rissel and colleagues observed poor knot performance when a surgeon's knot plus two square knots was made with monofilament sutures.

In addition to understanding the physical properties and characteristics of the variety of suture material available, the surgeon must consider the tissue and physiologic milieu in which the suture will be placed, before choosing said material. However, since all materials induce some degree of unwanted inflammatory reaction, choosing a balance between strength and inflammation is key to selecting a particular suture for a particular tissue closure. For example, due to the high disruptive forces on rectus fascia, repair of these wounds needs suture material that has relatively longer tensile strength than suture materials used in other areas of gynecology. A recent meta-analysis by Hodgson et al. reviewed absorbable versus nonabsorbable sutures for the closure of rectus fascia and found a statistically significant increase in hernia formation with polyglycolic acid sutures, but no difference in risk with polydioxanone when compared with nonabsorbable nylon and polypropylene. However, there was a statistically significant increase in both suture sinuses and wound pain with nonabsorbable suture compared to absorbable suture. In typical conditions, the reasoned suture selection for closing abdominal fascia for gynecologic operations would seem to be one of the delayed absorption monofilament sutures, such as polydioxanone or polyglyconate, although polyglycolic acid–based sutures are not unreasonable (especially for closure of transverse fascial incisions) given their long safety history in obstetrics and gynecology.

Drains

Sometimes, drainage of the abdominal cavity is appropriate after an operation for a tuboovarian abscess or some other type of pelvic infection. In addition, intraperitoneal drainage may be helpful for oozing peritoneal surfaces after complicated hysterectomies or other pelvic surgery. Although used in the past for prevention of lymphoceles or ureteral fistulae, retroperitoneal drains are not routinely used after radical pelvic surgery.

The use of prophylactic drains in the subcutaneous space to reduce the formation of hematoma and seroma or to reduce abscess and infection remains controversial. Recently, a large meta-analysis of the subject was reported, showing that subcutaneous drains could be omitted after cesarean section, breast reduction surgeries, abdominal surgeries (clean-contaminated wounds), femoral wounds, and hip and knee joint replacement. Furthermore, the authors suggested that drains should not be placed prophylactically secondary to a patient being obese. Farnell and associates, in a prospective study, analyzed 3,282 incisions of the wound varieties listed in Table 14.1. When patients with clean-contaminated or contaminated wounds received subcutaneous closed drainage systems, alone or with antibiotics or saline irrigation, no significant advantage was noted compared with primary closure without

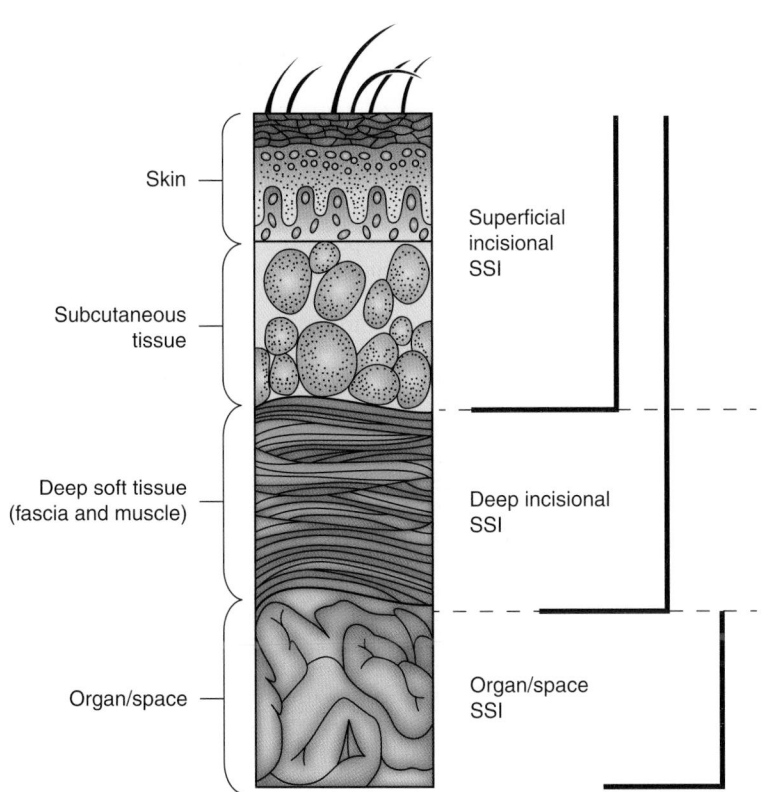

Skin

Superficial incisional SSI

Subcutaneous tissue

Deep soft tissue (fascia and muscle)

Deep incisional SSI

Organ/space

Organ/space SSI

FIGURE 14.8 Cross section of abdominal wall depicting CDC classifications of surgical site infection. (Reprinted from Horan TC, Gaynes RP, Martone WJ, et al. CDC definitions of nosocomial surgical site infections, 1992: a modification of the CDC definitions of surgical wound infections. *Infect Control Hosp Epidemiol* 1992; 13:606, with permission. Copyright 1992, The Society for Hospital Epidemiology of America, Inc. and SLACK Incorporated.)

III

drainage. However, a trend favoring subcutaneous drainage and antibiotic irrigation was seen in patients with contaminated wounds.

Drains can be classified into two categories: passive and active. The passive drain functions primarily as an overflow "valve" being assisted by gravity, while the latter drain is connected to some type of suction device. If a drain is used at all, the preferred system is a closed drainage system such as a Jackson-Pratt or a Blake. Both have small reservoirs (100 mL) that are relatively easy for paramedical personnel to manage on the ward and at home. The Blake drain, with its longitudinal ridges, offers less chance of obstruction from small tissue fragments or clots than does the Jackson-Pratt drain. However, no large prospective, randomized trials comparing these two systems have been done to substantiate that claim. To avoid clot formation and subsequent obstruction, the drain is placed on suction early, usually while completing closure of the incision. In addition, the nursing staff (and other caregivers) should be instructed to "strip" the drain catheter each shift (or several times throughout the day) while the drain is in place. Drains in the subfascial or subcutaneous spaces should be removed and not advanced as has been done in the past. Once the drainage is less than 50 mL per 24 hours, usually by postoperative day 2 or 3, it can be safely removed.

PREVENTION OF SURGICAL SITE INFECTIONS

Surgical site infection (SSI) is defined as an infection that occurs at or near a surgical incision within 30 days of a procedure or within 1 year if an implant is left in place. The Centers for Disease Control further categorize SSIs as being incisional or organ/space. Incisional SSIs are further divided into those that involve only the skin and subcutaneous tissues (superficial incisional SSI) and those involving deeper soft tissues

of the incision (deep incisional SSI) (Fig. 14.8). The CDC estimates that approximately 500,000 SSIs occur annually in the United States and account for 38% of all nosocomial infection. Two thirds of these SSIs are confined to the incision and one third involves organs or spaces accessed during the operation. These infections reduce patients' quality of life and account for 3.7 million excess hospital days and more than $1.6 billion in excess costs annually. Surgical wound classification was introduced in 1964 by the National Academy of Sciences (Table 14.1) and lists estimates of SSI for each class of wound. The rate of SSI with gynecologic operations is typically 8% to 10% and is related to many factors, including surgeon experience, the indication for the procedure, the procedure performed, and the comorbid condition of the patient.

In preparation for surgery, there are several patient-centered and operative characteristics that must be considered and completed to reduce the rate of SSI. The CDC recommendations to reduce SSI have been published, and the reader is directed to this reference for the full recommendations. However, a brief synopsis is presented here.

Patient Issues

Several patient characteristics have been associated with increased risk of SSI and include coincident remote site infections or colonization, prolonged preoperative hospital stay, diabetes, tobacco usage, steroid use, obesity (body mass index [BMI] ≥ 30 kg/m^2), extremes of ages, poor nutritional status, and perioperative transfusion of blood products.

Preoperative Issues

Although multiple studies have shown that preoperative showers or baths the night before surgery with chlorhexidine gluconate did a better job of reducing bacterial colony counts as compared to povidone–iodine or triclocarban-medicated soap, no study has definitively shown that such a practice reduces postoperative SSI rates. A recent, fourth, meta-analysis update on the topic by Webster and Osborne demonstrated (in seven trials included in the analysis, with over 10,000 patients) no conclusive evidence exists that preoperative showering with chlorhexidine over other wash products (iodine or regular soap) reduced SSI. At this time, this issue is still unresolved, and for our patients, we do not recommend the practice.

Traditionally, patients undergoing surgery have hair removed from the site of incision in order to reduce the chance of SSI. Some studies have shown that if hair removal is accomplished by shaving, 24 hours or more, before an operation, microscopic cuts in the skin serve as foci for bacterial multiplication. A recent, large meta-analysis of this practice was completed by Tanner et al. and showed that although hair can be removed by several different methods (shaving, clipping, the use of depilatories to dissolve hair) and at several different time points prior to an operation (the day before surgery versus immediately preoperatively), existing research studies are too small and methodologically flawed to make strong recommendations for or against hair removal or for which technique of hair removal is superior to affect postoperative SSIs. However, the authors' recommendation is that if hair must be removed to facilitate the surgery or application of adhesive dressings, clipping rather than shaving, immediately before surgery, appears to result in fewer SSIs.

There are several antiseptic agents for preoperative preparation of the abdominal skin and vaginal area for gynecologic surgery (Table 14.3). The iodophors, alcohol-containing products, and chlorhexidine gluconate are the most commonly used agents and require various amounts of time to apply and to dry depending upon the agent and the presence of hair on the skin. Darouiche et al. performed a multicenter, prospective randomized trial comparing povidone–iodine to chlorhexidine–alcohol skin preparation for 849 adults undergoing clean-contaminated surgery. These investigators showed that the chlorhexidine–alcohol patient cohort had a significantly lower SSI rate versus the povidone–iodine group (9.5% versus 16.1%, $p = 0.004$). In addition, the chlorhexidine group had fewer superficial infections (4.2 versus 8.6, $p = 0.008$) and deep incisional infections (1% versus 3%, $p = 0.05$). There was no difference in the organ/space infection rate between the two groups. A meta-analysis by Lee et al. included nine randomized controlled trials (inclusive of the study above and a total of 3,614 patients) comparing chlorhexidine preparations to iodine preparations for reduction of SSI. The authors found that chlorhexidine antisepsis significantly reduced the rate of SSIs by 36% (risk ratio 0.64, 95% confidence interval 0.51 to 0.80) across a wide variety of surgical procedures versus iodine antisepsis. It is important to note that when using the chlorhexidine–alcohol (2% chlorhexidine gluconate and 70% isopropyl alcohol, ChloraPrep) preparation of the abdominal skin, the skin must be scrubbed with the preloaded applicator and allowed to dry prior to draping. For preparation of the vagina, currently, no study of sufficient power has been completed that would lead to a strong recommendation for or against chlorhexidine or povidone–iodine cleansing of the vagina to reduce SSI. In our institution, the vagina is cleansed with the povidone–iodine prep routine or chlorhexidine (4% Hibiclens) prep if the patient is iodine sensitive.

The surgical scrub is the process that each member of the surgical team performs by washing the hands and forearms

TABLE 14.3 Antiseptic Solutions for Operative Preparation of Abdominal Skin

ANTISEPTIC	MECHANISM OF ACTION	ANTIMICROBIAL COVERAGE	ONSET	DURATION	APPLICATION	EXAMPLES
Aqueous–iodophor	Free iodine causes protein and DNA damage.	Excellent for gram+ bacteria; good for gram–, fungi, virus, Mtb	Intermediate	2 h	Two-step scrub and paint	Betadine Scrub Care
Aqueous–CHG	Disrupts cell membranes	Excellent for gram+; good for gram– and virus; fair for fungi; poor for Mtb	Intermediate	6 h	Two-step scrub and dry; repeat X1	Hibiclens
Alcohol–iodophor	Ethyl alcohol/ethanol (ETOH) denatures protein. Free iodine causes protein and DNA damage.	Same as aqueous iodophor, but improved gram and Mtb activity	Rapid	48 h (DuraPrep) 96 h (Prevail-Fx)	One-step paint *Dry time*—3 min on hairless surface	DuraPrep solution Prevail-Fx
Alcohol–CHG	ETOH denatures protein. CHG disrupts cell membranes.	Same as aqueous–CHG, but improved gram, fungal, and Mtb activity	Rapid	48 h	1-step scrub for dry site—30 s 1-step scrub for moist site—2 min *Dry time*—3 min on hairless surface	ChloraPrep

Mtb, *Mycobacterium tuberculosis*; CHG, chlorhexidine gluconate; Betadine, Purdue Products, LP (Stamford, CT); Scrub Care and Prevail-FX, Cardinal Health (Dublin, OH); Hibiclens Mölnlycke Health Care US, LLC (Norcross, GA); 3 M DuraPrep Surgical Solution, 3 M Health Care (St. Paul, MN); ChloraPrep, CareFusion, Inc. (Leawood, KS)
Adapted from Hemani ML, Lepor H. Skin preparation for the prevention of surgical site infection: Which agent is best? *Rev Urol* 2009;11:190, with permission. *Reviews in Urology* is a copyrighted publication of MedReviews, LLC. All rights reserved.

prior to donning surgical gowns and approaching the operative sterile field. Recent studies have shown that scrubbing for at least 2 minutes is as effective as the time-honored 10-minute scrub in reducing bacterial colony counts. In addition, the first scrub of the day should include a thorough cleaning under the fingernails (usually with a "pick" and brush). Limited data exist concerning reusable versus disposable surgical attire and different drapes used for different surgeries and the risk of SSI for patients. However, the Occupational Safety and Health Administration does require these "barriers" be present to protect personnel of the surgical team from exposure to body fluids and recommends that surgical attire be changed if visibly soiled.

Most incisions will be closed primarily after the surgical procedure, and a dressing for the incision is applied. Generally, this cover is left in place for 24 to 48 hours prior to being removed. If the incision is left open to be closed at a later time (delayed primary closure) or to heal by secondary intention, then it is packed with sterile dressing. Sometimes, a wound vacuum is placed to aid healing by negative pressure (see below). In general, delayed closure should be used for contaminated or dirty wounds. Alternatively, intermittent staples can be placed in the skin with intervening saline-moistened "wicks" into the subcutaneous spaces. When a bacteria-containing organ is opened (the unprepped bowel or abscessed gynecologic organs) and delayed closure is not used, copious saline irrigation of all layers for closure should be instituted. In addition, a monofilament nonabsorbable or slowly absorbable suture should be used in the fascia closure to further reduce bacterial loads.

Prophylactic antibiotic administration has been shown to decrease SSI in patients undergoing abdominal or vaginal hysterectomy and is aimed at reducing colonization from endogenous bacteria from the skin or ascending, endogenous, pathogenic bacteria from the vagina, opened at the time of hysterectomy. Unfortunately, these antibiotics either are not given or are given at inappropriate times prior to the surgical incision. The theory is that an antibiotic present in tissue will aid the host immune defense mechanism in killing bacteria that are inoculated into the wound (i.e., when a skin incision is made or the vagina opened).

The ideal antibiotic should be of low toxicity, have an established safety record, not be routinely used for the treatment of serious infections, have a spectrum of activity that includes the microorganisms most likely to cause infection, reach useful concentration in relevant tissue during the procedure, be administered for a short duration, and be administered in a fashion that will ensure it is present at the site of surgery, at the time of incision. The American Congress of Obstetricians and Gynecologists has published a practice bulletin covering the topic of antibiotic prophylaxis, and the reader is directed to this publication for a more thorough discussion.

Although more than 30 prospective, randomized clinical trials and two meta-analyses support the use of prophylactic antibiotics to substantially reduce postoperative infectious morbidity and decrease length of stay in women undergoing hysterectomy, no antibiotic regimen is superior to all others. Table 14.4 shows the acceptable prophylactic antibiotic regimens to be dosed within 1 hour of incision for hysterectomy. First- and second-generation cephalosporins are typically used in patients not sensitive to β-lactam agents. Most patients need only one dose of prophylactic antibiotic; however, for procedures lasting longer than the half-life of the antibiotic, redosing is appropriate (3 to 4 hours for most first-generation cephalosporins). Similarly, if there is a large loss of blood (>1,500 mL), then a second dose of the antibiotic is appropriate. All prophylactic antibiotics need to be stopped within 24 hours of completion of the surgery.

In 2002, the CDC and the Centers for Medicare and Medicaid Services (CMS) collaborated on the Surgical Infection Prevention (SIP) project to develop quality improvement measures, which included the timeliness, appropriate selection and duration of perioperative prophylactic antibiotics, normothermia for colorectal procedures, euglycemia, and appropriate hair removal, in 55 participating hospitals. Investigators found that in the 44 hospitals that reported results, the rate of SSI decreased 27%, from 2.3% in the first 3 months of participation to 1.7% in the last 3 months. In 2006, the SIP evolved into the current Surgical Care Improvement Project with the goal of reducing the rate of surgical complications, and CMS has now tied payment to the hospital based upon participation and reduction of these complications. There are 20 measures covering various discrete elements of patient care; nine of these measures are publicly reported and seven measures focus on SSI reduction, of which five pertain to hysterectomy.

TABLE 14.4 Recommended Prophylactic Antibiotics for Hysterectomy and Urogynecology Procedures

PROCEDURE	ANTIBIOTIC	DOSE (SINGLE DOSE)
Hysterectomy	Cefazolin[a]	1 g or 2 g IV[b]
Urogynecology procedures, including those with mesh	Clindamycin plus gentamicin[c] OR	600 mg IV/1.5 mg/kg IV
	Quinolone[d] OR	400 mg IV
	Aztreonam	1 g IV
	Metronidazole plus gentamicin OR	500 mg IV/1.5 mg/kg IV
	Quinolone	400 mg IV

[a]Acceptable alternatives include cefotetan, cefoxitin, cefuroxime, or ampicillin–sulbactam.
[b]A 2 gm dose I recommended in women with a body mass index (BMI) >35 kg/m² or weight >100 kg or 220 pounds
[c]Antimicrobial choice in women with a history of immediate hypersensitivity to penicillin.
[d]Ciprofloxacin or levofloxacin or moxifloxacin.
IV, intravenously.
Adapted from ACOG Committee on Practice Bulletins-Gynecology. Antibiotic prophylaxis for gynecologic procedures. ACOG Practice Bulletin No. 104 American Congress of Obstetricians and Gynecologists. *Obstet Gynecol* 2009;113:180, with permission. Copyright 2009. The American Congress of Obstetricians and Gynecologists.

BEST PRACTICE

- Prophylactic antibiotic administration within 1 hour of surgical incision (within 2 hours if the patient is receiving vancomycin or fluoroquinolones).
- Appropriate prophylactic antibiotic for the specific procedure (Table 14.4).
- Prophylactic antibiotic must be discontinued 24 hours after surgery end time.
- Surgical site hair removal (clipping or depilation versus no hair removal) if hair interferes with the incision/surgery.
- Urinary catheter removal on postoperative day 1.
- Colorectal surgery patients with perioperative temperature management.
- For cardiac surgery patients, a controlled 6 AM postoperative blood glucose (<200 mg/dL).

Because of concerns about wound complications, a prior dictum was that incisions of the abdominal skin should not be made with electrosurgery. A recent meta-analysis looking at wound complication rates between incisions made with a scalpel or electrosurgery found no difference in wound complications regardless of method of incision creation. The review included nine randomized controlled trials (1,901 participants) and found no significant difference in overall wound complication rates (risk ratio 0.9, 95% confidence interval 0.68 to 1.18) or rates of wound dehiscence (risk ratio 1.04, 95% confidence interval 0.36 to 2.98). No statement could be conclusively made concerning blood loss, pain, or incision time. The authors concluded that current evidence suggests that making an abdominal incision with electrosurgery may be as safe as using a scalpel.

Discarding the skin knife, which continues as an archaic practice to date, has not been shown to reduce wound infection rates but instead leaves an extra "sharp" on the operative field, which may injure members of the health care team. In a randomized prospective study, the rate of postoperative wound infections was not different after the use of one or two scalpels for the incision. The same scalpel used on the skin can be safely used for subcutaneous and deep incisions.

ABDOMINAL INCISIONS

In general, abdominal incisions used for most gynecologic procedures can be divided into transverse or vertical incisions. For extraperitoneal incisions and access to organs not associated with the female genital tract, modifications of oblique incisions are sometimes used. Because of the ease and rapid entry, the abdomen was originally routinely opened by a midline incision in the linea alba. One of the first successful abdominal operations was performed by McDowell in 1809. In the early days of abdominal surgery, transverse incisions were generally avoided because they were more time consuming. Also, an unfounded fear was that transection of the rectus muscle would leave a defect because of retraction of the muscle. As previously stated in the section on anatomy, the adherence of the recti musculature to its anterior fascia by several transverse inscriptions prevents retraction. In the late 1800s and early 1900s, several transverse incisions were developed, such as the Küstner, Pfannenstiel, Maylard, and Cherney incisions. Most of the transverse incisions used for pelvic surgery are identified by the name of the surgeon who first described them, whereas the few vertical abdominal incisions have no such eponyms.

Transverse Incisions

Transverse incisions for pelvic surgery are attractive because they produce the best cosmetic results. Additionally, low transverse incisions are as much as 30 times stronger than midline incisions, are less painful, and result in less interference with postoperative respirations. Wound dehiscence is allegedly more common with vertical incisions. The older literature suggests that wound evisceration was three to five times more common and hernia formation was two to three times more common when vertical incisions were used compared with transverse incisions. Many earlier studies reported an increased incidence of eviscerations with midline incisions that could be associated with inappropriate closures. More recent studies, however, have shown no difference in the risk of wound dehiscence or even a slight advantage for midline incisions. A large study, completed at Hutzel Hospital in Detroit by Hendrix and colleagues, found that there was no difference in fascial dehiscence between transverse (Pfannenstiel) and vertical incisions.

Transverse incisions have certain associated disadvantages. They are relatively more time consuming and relatively more hemorrhagic. Occasionally, nerves are divided, and division of multiple layers of fascia and muscle can result in formation of potential spaces with subsequent hematoma or seroma formation. Ability to explore the upper abdominal cavity adequately is compromised with most low transverse incisions.

Pfannenstiel Incision

Most surgeons would agree that the Pfannenstiel incision provides the best wound security of all gynecologic incisions. The cosmetic results are excellent, but exposure is limited (especially to the upper abdomen). This type of incision should be used in select patients with certain gynecologic malignancies. It should not be used (or should be used in very select patients) when pelvic exposure is needed in certain nonmalignant conditions, such as severe endometriosis, and large leiomyomata with distortion of the lower uterine segment, or when reoperating on a patient for postoperative hemorrhage.

The original, true Pfannenstiel incision is described as a transverse incision that is slightly curved (concavity upward) and may be made at any level suitable to the surgeon (Fig. 14.9A). It is usually 10 to 15 cm long and extends through the skin and subcutaneous fat to the level of the rectus fascia. The rectus fascia is incised transversely on either side of the linea alba, which is cut separately, joining the two lateral incisions but leaving the rectus fascia intact across the midline (Fig. 14.9B). The rectus sheath is separated from the underlying muscle by inserting the fingers on either side of the cut edge of the sheath and pulling the fascia in opposite directions, with one hand toward the head and the other hand toward the feet (or alternatively, cutting the attachments in the midline). This maneuver frees the fascia from the anterior surface of the rectus muscle as far as desired between the symphysis and the umbilicus (Fig. 14.9C). The rectus muscles are then separated in the midline, and the peritoneum is opened vertically (Fig. 14.9D). This procedure avoids the necessity of dissecting the subcutaneous fat away from the anterior rectus fascia, as is done in the Küstner incision. It separates the perforating nerves and small blood vessels, which enter the fascia from the underlying muscles to supply the fascia, although it possibly weakens the incision.

If the Pfannenstiel incision is extended laterally beyond the edge of the rectus muscles and into the substance of the external and internal oblique muscles, injury to the iliohypogastric or ilioinguinal nerves can occur, with resulting neuroma formation. In addition, closure of this extended fascial incision can entrap these nerves in either the closing suture or surrounding scar tissue. To avoid these nerve injuries in laterally extended incisions, including a Cherney or Maylard incision, the lateral extensions should have sutures placed only in the external oblique fascia.

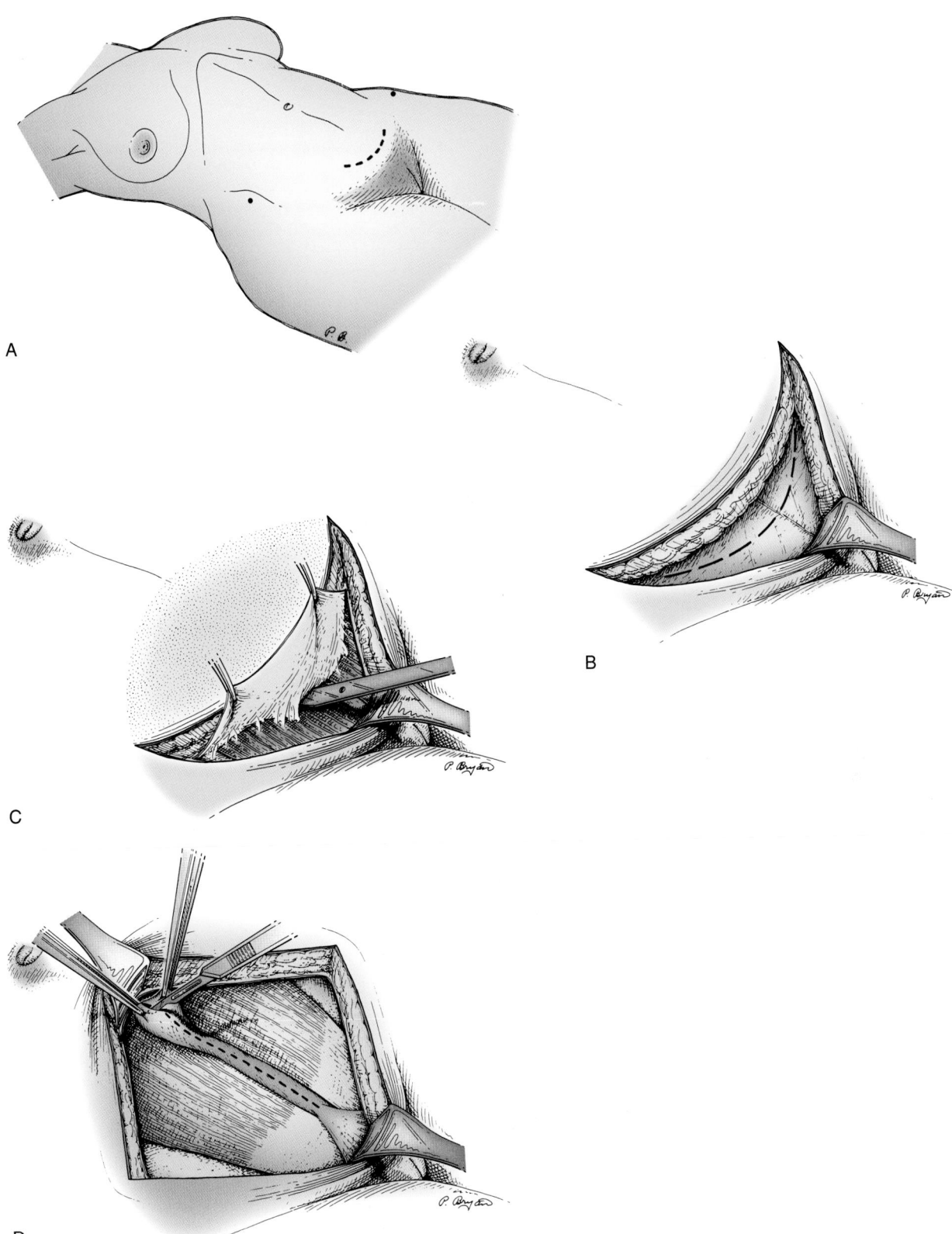

FIGURE 14.9 A: The skin incision for a Pfannenstiel incision is elliptical just above the symphysis pubis. **B:** The skin, subcutaneous fat, and fascia of the abdominal wall are incised transversely. **C:** The fascia is separated from the rectus muscle superiorly, inferiorly, and laterally. Small perforating vessels require ligation or coagulation. **D:** The rectus muscles are separated, and the peritoneum is incised in the midline.

The fascia can be closed with a running technique in patients with clean wounds or clean-contaminated wounds. Polyglycolic acid, polyglactin 910, or one of the delayed absorbable sutures can be used. Subcutaneous sutures are usually unnecessary, and the skin is closed with a subcuticular suture (preferably monofilament), reinforced surgical tape (e.g., Steri-Strips), skin glue, or staples.

Küstner Incision

Some surgeons advocate a Küstner incision, incorrectly referred to as a modified Pfannenstiel incision. The slightly curved transverse skin incision begins below the level of the anterior superior iliac spine and extends just below the pubic hairline, through subcutaneous fat, down to the aponeurosis of the external oblique muscle and the anterior sheath of the recti musculature, in the same manner as all other transverse incisions (**Fig. 14.10A**). The superficial branches of the inferior epigastric artery and vein may be encountered in the subcutaneous fat at the lateral margin of the incision. When encountered, they can be ligated or sealed with electrocautery. The fascia is cleaned superiorly and inferiorly until a sufficient area is exposed from the region of the umbilicus to the symphysis to permit an adequate vertical incision in the linea alba. Excessive separation of the fat from the fascia in the

lateral margins of the incision is unnecessary and can provide sites for small postoperative hematomas. Separation of the rectus muscles and entrance into the peritoneum are performed in the same manner in the ordinary midline incision (**Fig. 14.10B**). Because of the importance of obtaining adequate hemostasis in the subcutaneous fat of the skin flaps, this incision is definitely more time consuming than the low midline incision or the Pfannenstiel incision. It offers little or no tensile strength advantage, and its extensibility is severely limited. If this incision is used, strong consideration of subcutaneous, closed suction drainage should be given, due to the large amount of "dead space" created.

Cherney Incision

The Cherney differs from the muscle-dividing Maylard incision by the location of transection of the rectus muscles. In both incisions, the skin and fascia are divided transversely as with a Pfannenstiel incision, but Cherney advocated freeing the rectus muscles at their tendinous insertion into the symphysis pubis. The rectus muscles are then retracted cephalad to improve exposure. The transverse Cherney incision is about 25% longer than a midline incision measured from the umbilicus to the symphysis.

The Cherney incision provides excellent access to the space of Retzius and excellent exposure of the pelvic side wall.

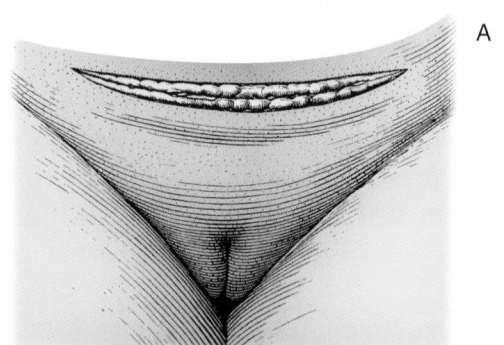

A

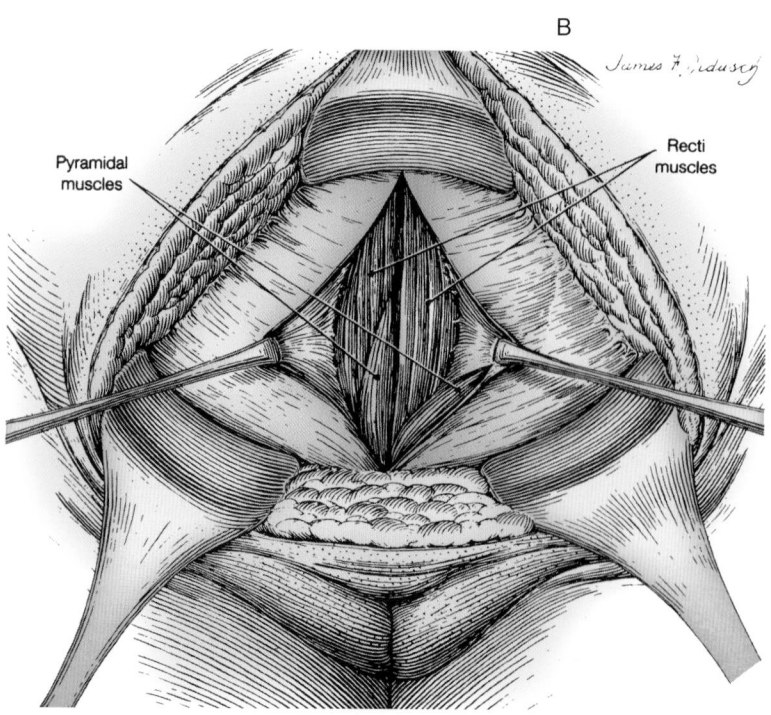

B

Pyramidal muscles

Recti muscles

FIGURE 14.10 Küstner incision. **A:** Skin incision just below the hairline. **B:** Midline incision through fascia, exposing rectus and pyramidalis muscles. The rectus muscles are retracted laterally, and the peritoneum is incised in the midline.

Occasionally, the surgeon who uses a Pfannenstiel incision finds that incision inadequate for exposure for hemostasis or not large enough to expose areas of associated abnormal conditions deep in the pelvis. Under these circumstances, the safe approach is not to transect the rectus muscles halfway, but to perform a Cherney incision. Partial incision of the rectus muscle can lead to injury of the inferior epigastric vessels on the lateral border of the rectus muscles. Also, if conversion to a Maylard is attempted after a previous Pfannenstiel incision, the anterior rectus sheath will have already been widely separated from the rectus muscles. In this case, the ends of the muscle are likely to retract and will not reunite when the edges of the fascia are later reapproximated. In this situation, it may be necessary to reapproximate the rectus muscle ends with horizontal mattress sutures (which may be difficult due to the retraction).

Even if the peritoneum is opened, the space of Retzius can be bluntly dissected (Fig. 14.11). The inferior epigastric vessels, which course more laterally on the rectus muscles, are identified. The pyramidal muscles are sharply dissected. The fibrous tendinous rectus muscles are then dissected sharply from their insertion into the symphysis pubis (Fig. 14.12). Bleeding is negligible in this area, and the inferior epigastric vessels do not need to be ligated. The peritoneal incision can be extended laterally about 2 cm cephalad to the bladder while the vessels are visualized.

As stated earlier, transverse incisions, particularly the Cherney and the later-described Maylard, can result in nerve injury. The femoral nerve is particularly at risk when a self-retaining retractor with deep lateral blades is used in these widely extended incisions. If a self-retaining retractor is used with either of these incisions, the lateral blades should only be deep enough to fit under the edges of the incision and not rest on the psoas muscles.

In closing a Cherney incision, the ends of the rectus tendons are united to the inferior portion of the lower flap of the rectus sheath with five or six interrupted delayed absorbable or permanent sutures in horizontal mattress configuration (Fig. 14.13). To avoid osteomyelitis, the rectus muscles should not be sutured to the periosteum of the symphysis pubis. Fascial closure is then accomplished with a running continuous suture of No. 0 or No. 1 delayed absorbable material, as in the Pfannenstiel. Although the lines of tension favor transverse incisions as opposed to vertical incisions, running sutures should be

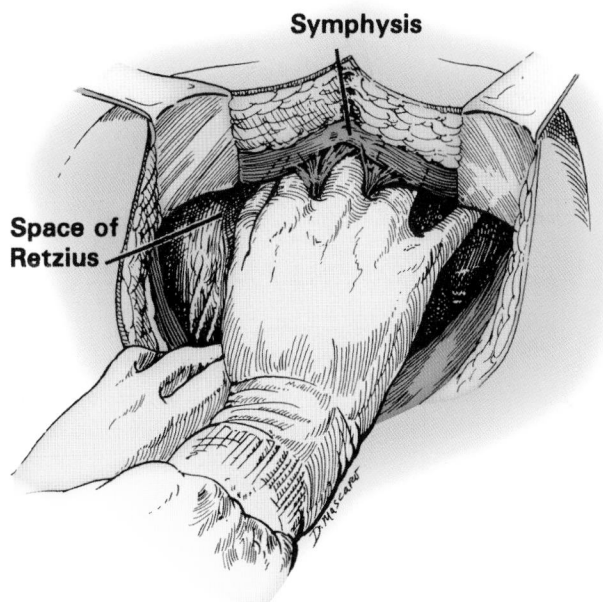

FIGURE 14.11 Developing the space of Retzius. The weight of the hand of the operator easily separates the bladder from the overlying symphysis in the relatively bloodless midline. (Reprinted from Gallup DG. Opening and closing the abdomen. In: Phelan JP, Clark SL, eds. *Cesarean delivery*. New York: Chapman & Hall, 1988:449, with permission; from Taylor and Francis Group LLC, with permission.)

placed at least 1.5 cm from the fascial edge and 1.0 cm from one another. The remainder of the closure is similar to the Pfannenstiel closure, depending on the surgeon's preference.

Maylard Incision

The Maylard incision is a true transverse-muscle–cutting incision in which all layers of the lower abdominal wall are incised transversely. This incision was originally described by Ernest Maylard in 1907. The incision provides excellent pelvic exposure and is used by many surgeons for radical pelvic surgery,

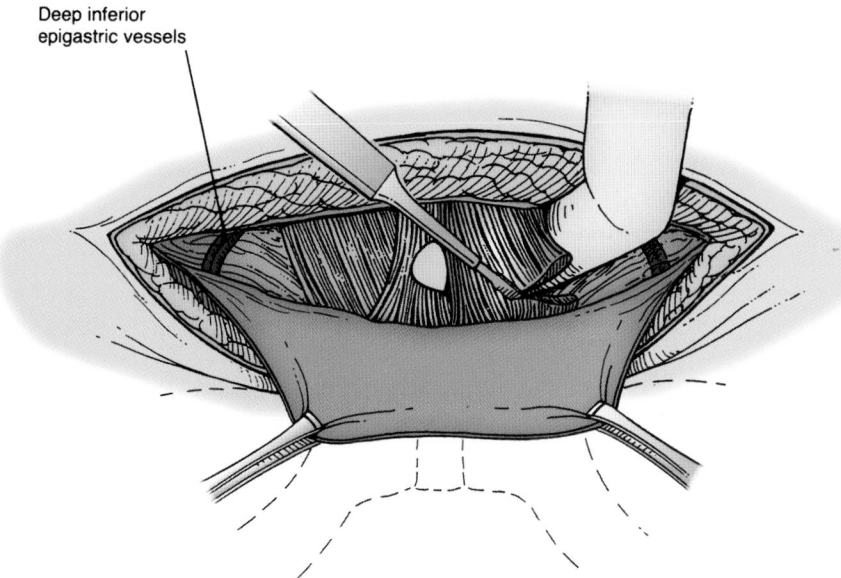

FIGURE 14.12 The finger of the operator is placed posterior to the rectus muscle, and with gentle traction, the muscle is pulled cephalad. The rectus muscle can then be dissected from its insertion at the symphysis by the Bovie device. The peritoneal incision can then be extended laterally, avoiding the inferior epigastric vessels, which are positioned laterally. (Reprinted from Gallup DG. Abdominal incisions and closures. In: Gallup DG, Talledo OE, eds. *Surgical atlas of gynecologic oncology*. Philadelphia, PA: WB Saunders, 1994:43, with permission. Copyright © 1995, Elsevier.)

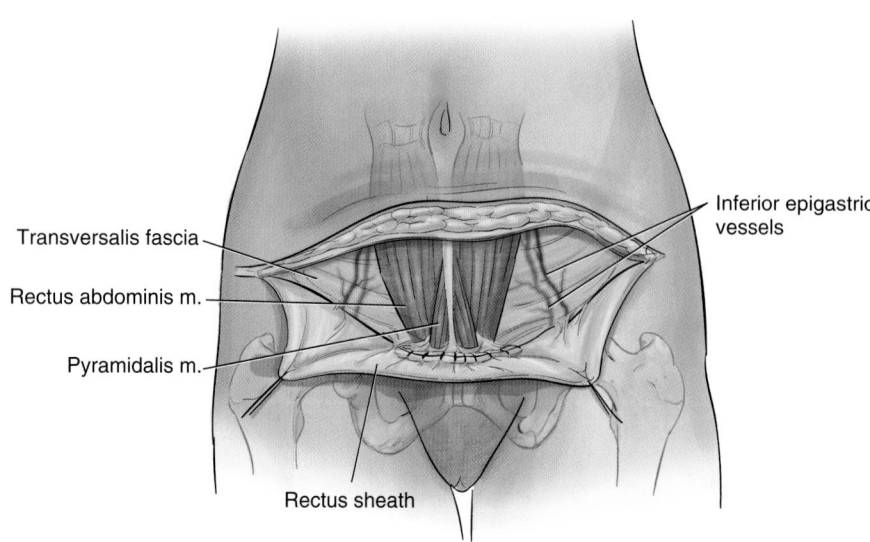

Transversalis fascia

Rectus abdominis m.

Pyramidalis m.

Rectus sheath

Inferior epigastric vessels

FIGURE 14.13 Reuniting of the rectus tendons to the inferior portion of the lower flaps. The deep inferior epigastric vessels are positioned laterally in the caudad portion of the abdomen. (Reprinted from Gallup DG. Opening and closing the abdomen. In: Phelan JP, Clark SL, eds. *Cesarean delivery.* New York: Chapman & Hall, 1988:449, with permission; from Taylor and Francis Group LLC, with permission.)

including radical hysterectomy with pelvic lymph node dissection and pelvic exenteration. Although midline incisions are preferable for patients with suspicious adnexal masses, patients with adnexal masses, which are questionable for malignancy by radiographic and serologic studies, may be candidates for this more cosmetic incision. Patients must be informed that if malignancy is found, the transverse incision will take the form of a "hockey stick" or "J" incision (Fig. 14.14), or a separate upper abdominal incision will be used to evaluate the upper abdominal cavity and retroperitoneal paraaortic nodes.

The Maylard-Bardenheuer incision has been modified in several aspects since its original description. Before the skin incision is made, a series of three to four perpendicular markings with a sterile marking pen are made across the planned line of the incision. These markings help later to reapproximate the skin edges. The transverse skin incision is made about 3 to 8 cm above the pubic symphysis, depending on the indications for surgery and patient age and weight. The skin incision should never be made in a deep skin crease or beneath a large panniculus, because of the anaerobic environment

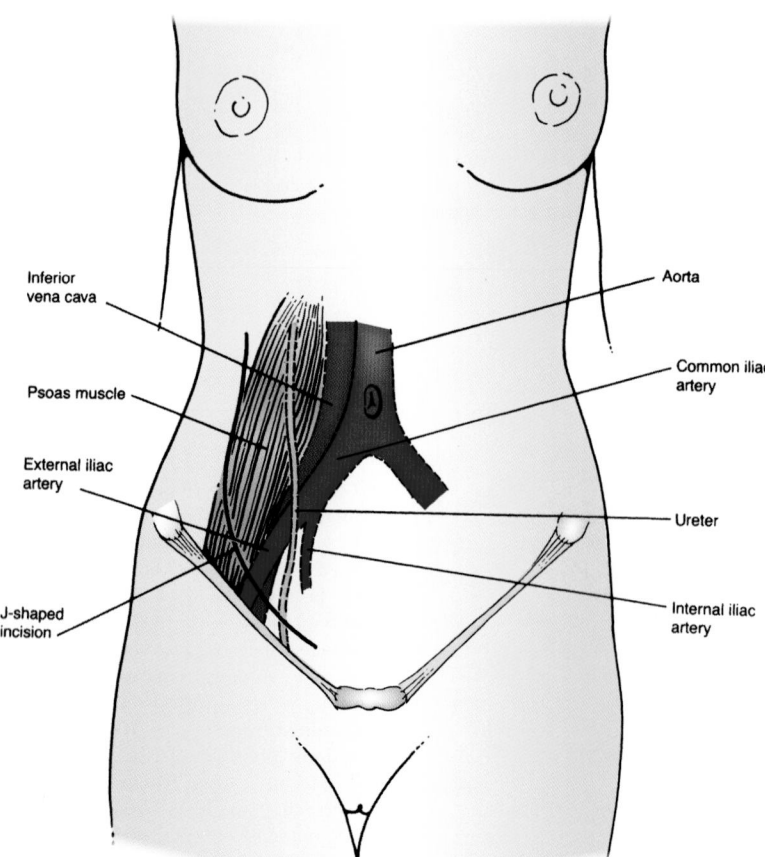

Inferior vena cava

Psoas muscle

External iliac artery

J-shaped incision

Aorta

Common iliac artery

Ureter

Internal iliac artery

FIGURE 14.14 J-shaped incision on the right is shown in relation to deeper structures, the ureter, iliac vessels, and great vessels. It is initiated about 3 cm cephalad to the umbilicus and is carried inferiorly parallel to the round ligament. (Reprinted from Gallup DG. Abdominal incisions and closures. In: Gallup DG, Talledo OE, eds. *Surgical atlas of gynecologic oncology.* Philadelphia, PA: WB Saunders, 1994:43, with permission. Copyright 1995, Elsevier.)

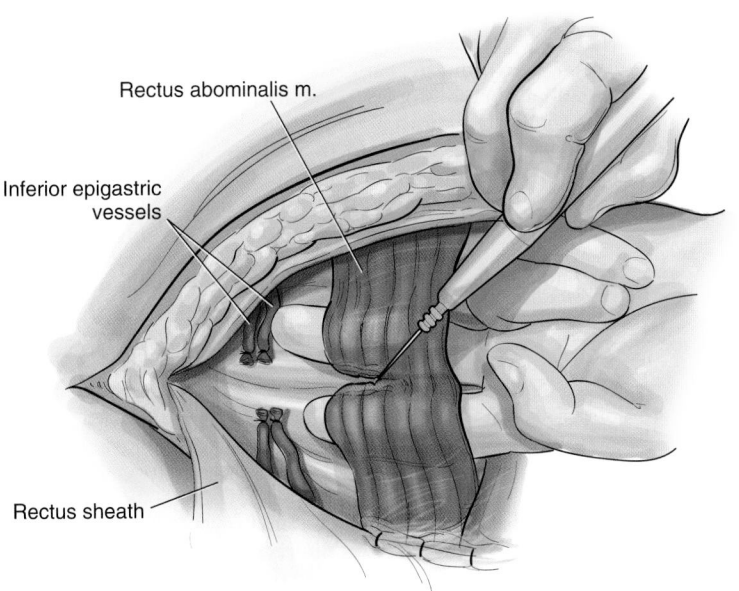

Rectus abominalis m.

Inferior epigastric vessels

Rectus sheath

FIGURE 14.15 Maylard incision. The rectus muscles are incised with a knife or a Bovie device. The hand of the surgeon is withdrawn as the muscle is cut. The inferior epigastric vessels were previously isolated, sectioned, and ligated. (Reprinted from Gallup DG. Opening and closing the abdomen. In: Phelan JP, Clark SL, eds. *Cesarean delivery.* New York: Chapman & Hall, 1988:449, with permission; from Taylor and Francis Group LLC, with permission.)

in this location and increased risk of wound complications. The fascia is incised transversely, and the aponeurosis is not detached from the underlying muscle.

Once the transverse fascia incision has been carried lateral to the borders of the rectus muscles, the inferior epigastric vessels, lying on the posterolateral border of each muscle, are identified. (Some surgeons suggest preservation of these vessels even when the rectus muscles are transected.) The vessels are "teased" away from their attachments by using blunt dissection with an instrument or gentle finger dissection. The vessels are ligated before incising the rectus muscles to avoid tearing of the vessels, vessel retraction, and hematoma formation (Fig. 14.15). The fingers of the surgeon tease the overlying rectus muscle from the peritoneum, and the muscles are sectioned between the fingers by using an electrocautery.

For better approximation of the muscles during closure, suture the underlying muscle to the overlying fascia before entering the peritoneum. A 2-0 delayed absorbable "U" suture is used, and the knots are placed anterior to the fascia. The peritoneum is incised transversely.

Closure of the fascia is similar to the running technique for other transverse incisions. The muscles do not need to be reapproximated with individual sutures (exception noted above), although some surgeons prefer to close the parietal peritoneum with a running polyglycolic suture. Drainage of the subfascial space is the surgeon's prerogative (Fig. 14.16).

Caution should be exercised in using the Maylard incision in patients with impaired circulation to the leg secondary to obstruction of the common iliac arteries or terminal aorta. In this situation, blood flow from the inferior epigastric artery may provide the only additional collateral circulation to the lower extremity. Ligation of this artery could result in lower extremity ischemia and a real vascular surgical emergency. In the gynecologic patient with clinical evidence of impaired circulation in the lower extremity, a midline incision should be used.

Vertical Incisions

Generally, vertical incisions afford excellent exposure, can be easily extended, and provide rapid entry to the abdominal cavity. Whether the incision is made midline or paramedian, the resulting scar may be wide.

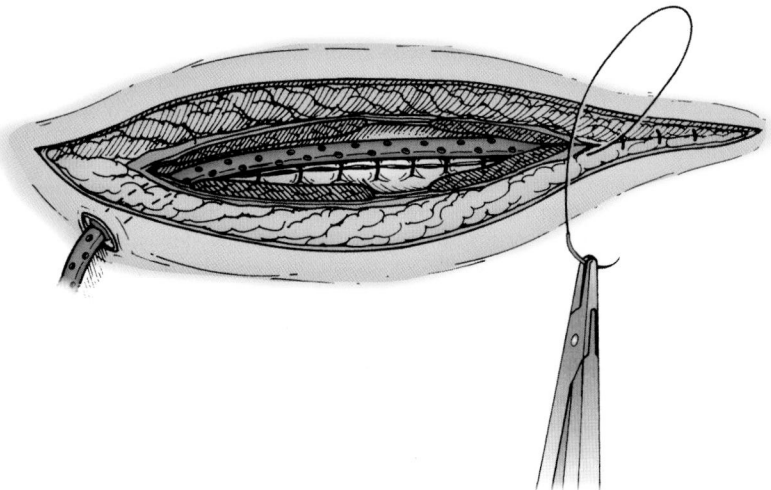

FIGURE 14.16 The peritoneum has been closed with 2-0 polyglycolic acid sutures. A closed drainage system is used if hemostasis is not absolute. A running delayed absorbable suture is used, placing the bites about 1.5 cm from the fascial edge. (Reprinted from Gallup DG. Abdominal incisions and closures. In: Gallup DG, Talledo OE, eds. *Surgical atlas of gynecologic oncology.* Philadelphia, PA: WB Saunders, 1994:43, with permission. Copyright 1995, Elsevier.)

Midline (Median) Incision

As stated in the section on anatomy, the midline incision is the least hemorrhagic incision, as well as the incision that affords rapid entry into the abdominal/pelvic cavity. Exposure is excellent, and minimal nerve damage occurs. However, dehiscence and hernias are said to be more common. Abdominal wound disruption is one of the most serious postoperative problems associated with gynecologic surgery. The "burst abdomen," or evisceration, seen more frequently in general surgery patients, occurs with a frequency of 0.3% to 0.7% in gynecologic patients and is associated with a mortality of 10% to 35%. The type of incision is only one factor associated with evisceration. Mechanical factors—such as wound hematomas, paroxysmal coughing associated with chronic lung disease, and gastrointestinal problems (retching, vomiting, ileus)—can lead to evisceration. However, better perioperative care, newer suture material, and better closure techniques have been shown to lower the rates of wound infection, dehiscence, and hernia formation.

The midline incision is the most easily mastered gynecologic incision because the fascial area is relatively bloodless and the rectus muscles are usually separated in parous women. If the patient has a prior midline incision, the surgeon should incise the skin and peritoneum more cephalad to the earlier incision to avoid injury to possibly adherent bowel. In nulliparous women, the midline separation between the rectus muscles may not be obvious. In these cases, the pyramidalis muscles are useful landmarks in directing the surgeon to the midline separation of the rectus muscles, inferiorly. Because this incision can be extended easily, the midline incision is the most versatile of all incisions used by gynecologists.

Hemostasis of the anterior layers of the abdomen should always be complete before the peritoneum is entered (Fig. 14.17). Once the abdomen is explored (in a systematic fashion), the bowel is carefully packed out of the pelvis. Seldom are more than two or three moist laparotomy packs needed to accomplish exposure of the pelvis. If more packs are required or there is a struggle to pack the upper abdominal contents, anesthesia may be inadequate, or in patients with prior abdominal surgery, adhesive disease may be obstructing movement. The more packs used, the more likely small-bowel terminal nerve endings will be damaged, resulting in postoperative adynamic ileus. Use of more modern table-fixed retractors, such as the Bookwalter retractor, not only improves exposure in vertical and transverse incisions but also limits the use of excessive packs.

Paramedian Incision

The true paramedian incision is placed lateral to the midline and splits the rectus muscle longitudinally. Like the midline or median incision, the paramedian incision has excellent extensibility and exposure, particularly on the side of the pelvis where the incision is made. However, because it splits the rectus muscle, the risk of bleeding and nerve injury is increased, relative to the median incision. A modified paramedian incision retracts the rectus muscle laterally before incising the posterior rectus sheath and peritoneum. This approach avoids the potential risks associated with splitting the rectus muscle. Paramedian incisions have been advocated over midline incisions because of alleged greater strength. A recent meta-analysis, comparing outcomes of midline incisions with transverse and paramedian incisions, showed that midline incisions had higher hernia rates as compared to transverse incisions (risk ratio 1.77, 95% confidence interval 1.09 to 2.87) and paramedian incisions (risk ratio 3.41, 95% confidence interval 1.02 to 11.45).

Fascial Closure of Vertical Incisions

Although midline incisions allow quick entry into the abdomen and provide excellent exposure to abdominal and pelvic anatomy, the relatively avascular nature of the anatomy, as well as the lateral pulling forces, make these types of incisions weaker and prone to early (see SSIs above and evisceration below) and late postoperative complications. Incisional hernia is a frequent complication of midline abdominal surgery with a reported incidence of 3% to 13% and typically results in some future surgical intervention, increasing patient morbidity and decreasing patient quality of life. Most incisional hernias seem to develop during the early postoperative period and are related to early separation of the fascial edges. Because the regenerative capability of fascia is limited, the ability of the closing suture line to hold these edges together during the early postoperative period is paramount. The fascia heals quite slowly and needs to have support from the suture utilized for at least 6 weeks to reduce the risk of incisional hernia formation. The surgeon can control several variables (e.g., reducing SSIs [as discussed above], choosing an appropriate suture for closure, employing proper suturing technique) to reduce the rate of hernia formation.

Selecting a suture to close midline abdominal incisions is the prerogative of the surgeon; although a myriad of options exist, no consensus on the choice of suture material (or even technique of closure) exists. Over the last two decades, multiple prospective randomized clinical trials have been completed comparing one suture to another and evaluating for wound complications, such as evisceration, hernia formation, wound infection, suture sinus formation, and wound pain. Although some classes of suture outperformed others, to date, no single suture has emerged as the sole superior choice for closure of midline incisions. However, several types of nonabsorbable and slowing absorbable suture material have come to the forefront for closure of midline incisions with resulting reduction of hernia formation versus closure with quickly absorbing suture material. As mentioned above, one of the most important factors of closure of the midline incision is that the fascial edges need to be approximated for at least 6 weeks to reduce hernia formation. Nonabsorbable monofilament and slowly absorbable (e.g., PDS; see Table 14.2) suture material produce low rates of incisional hernia, as compared to fast-absorbing suture, which support the fascia for less than 6 weeks. In addition, the rate of SSI is lower with monofilament suture compared to multifilament material, owing to the interstitial spaces where bacteria can evade phagocytosis. Diener et al. recently performed a meta-analysis of midline laparotomy closure, reviewing the literature, including five systematic reviews (dating from 1998) and 14 trials (published between 1981 and 2009), and including 7,711 patients (6,752 midline incisions). The authors reported that the five systematic reviews contained significant heterogeneity and did not meet their criteria for analysis. However, the 14 trials included in their review demonstrated no statistical heterogeneity for patients undergoing elective midline laparotomy closure. Their findings showed that hernia rates were significantly lower with absorbable suture versus nonabsorbable suture (odds ratio 0.41, 95% confidence interval 0.43 to 0.82, $P = 0.001$) and slowly absorbable versus quickly absorbable sutures (odds ratio 0.65, 95% confidence interval 0.19 to 0.88, $P = 0.02$). No statistical differences were noted among the secondary end points of wound dehiscence, suture sinus formation, wound infection, and wound pain, whether wounds were closed with nonabsorbable versus slowly absorbable or slowly absorbable versus quickly absorbable suture material. The authors concluded that for elective primary or secondary laparotomy through midline incisions, the abdominal fascia should be closed with slowly absorbable (monofilament) suture material in a continuous fashion. The authors had no recommendation for closure of the abdominal fascia in emergency setting.

Suturing technique goes hand in hand with the suture material used for midline laparotomy closures. Several meta-analyses have been performed assessing outcome after

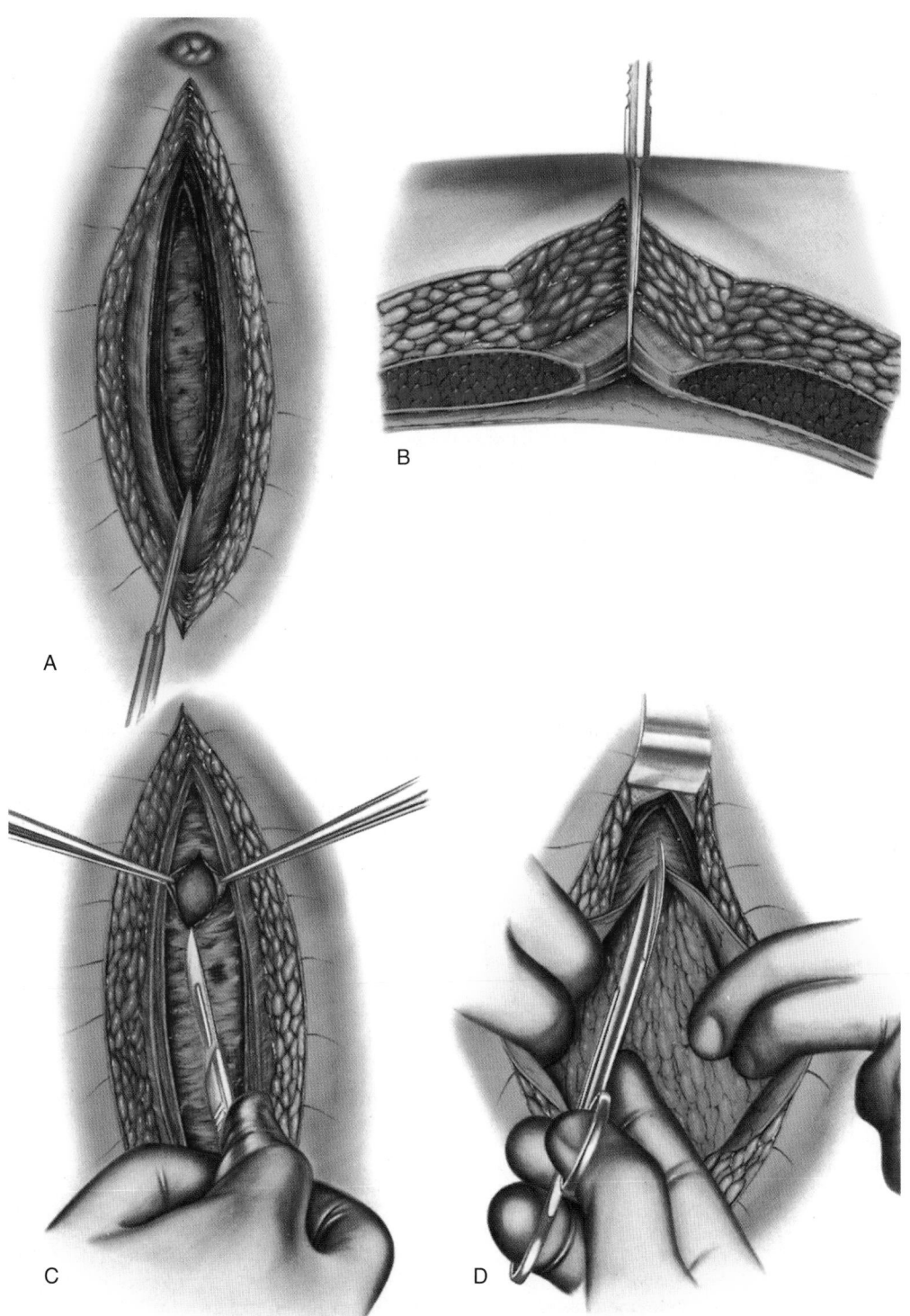

FIGURE 14.17 A: Cutting of linea alba in low midline incision with scalpel. **B:** Cross section of abdominal wall showing skin, subcutaneous fat, anterior and posterior rectus sheaths, and underlying peritoneum. **C:** Opening of peritoneum with knife, and demonstration of small bowel protruding into peritoneal opening. **D:** Enlargement of peritoneal opening to the region of the umbilicus with Mayo scissors.

continuous closure (with varying types of suture material) versus interrupted closures (with various types of suture material). In general, these reviews showed that incisional hernias, wound dehiscence, suture sinus formation, wound infection, and wound pain were less for continuous closure as compared to interrupted closure. In addition, the continuous closure technique is significantly easier and faster than interrupted

closure (Fig. 14.18) Further, closing the wound in one single layer has produced lower dehiscence rates than closure with several layers, and including the peritoneum in the suture line does not contribute to the tensile strength of the wound.

Standardizing the tension applied on sutures in the clinical setting during closure of the abdomen is difficult. However, higher tension is correlated with higher rates of SSI than with

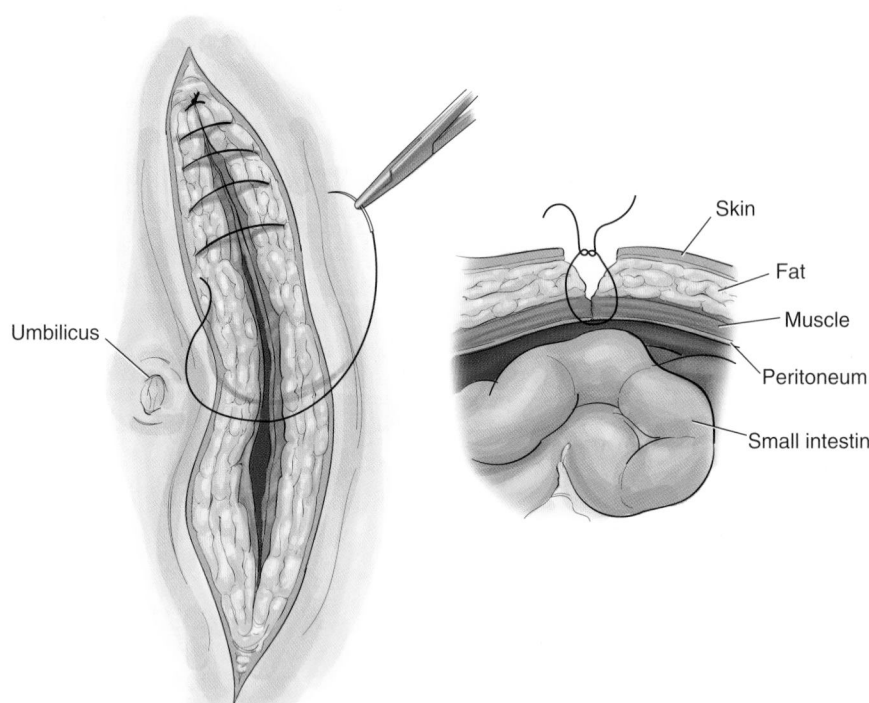

FIGURE 14.18 Closure of a midline incision using a No. 2 polypropylene, running mass closure. The anterior fascia, muscle, posterior fascia, and peritoneum are included in the bites (**inset**), which are taken 1.5 to 2 cm from the fascial edge and about 1 cm apart. With permanent polypropylene suture, a hemoclip can be used on the short end to avoid suture unraveling.

lower tension. This may be due to soft tissue that is included in the stitch, which gets compressed and devitalized, leading to tissue necrosis and increasing the rate of SSI. For continuous closure, the *suture length to wound length* (SL-to-WL) ratio is directly correlated with incisional hernia formation (fewer hernias with SL-to-WL ratio of 4 or higher) but depends upon the number of stitches, the size of the stitches, the tension on the suture line, and the length of the wound.

$$\text{Calculation of SL-to-WL ratio} : \left(A - [B + C]\right) / D$$

A = length of suture used
B = length of suture remnants at the starting knot
C = length of suture remnants at the finishing knot
D = length of skin incision

High SL-to-WL ratio can be accomplished with large stitches or with small stitches placed at closer intervals. For several decades, it had been recommended to place large stitches at least 1 to 1.5 cm from the wound edge and 1 cm apart. This surgical dictum was purely based upon experimental data. However, recent experimental data from Cengiz et al., and taking into account SL-to-WL ratio, showed that smaller stitches, placed 5 to 8 mm from the wound edge and at close intervals of 4 to 5 mm, resulted in a stronger wound 4 days after closure compared to wounds closed with larger stitches, placed 10 mm from the edge and 10 to 15 mm apart. More recently, Millbourn et al. showed that keeping the SL-to-WL ratio at 4 or greater, but using smaller stitch sizes as described above, resulted in an incisional hernia rate significantly lower than if large stitches were used to maintain the same SL-to-WL ratio (5.6% versus 18.0%, $P = 0.001$). In addition, SSI rates were less with small stitch size versus larger stitches (5.2% versus 10.2%, $P = 0.02$).

Although interesting from a historical perspective, the interrupted Smead-Jones closure technique (**Fig. 14.19**) has not been shown to be superior to a continuous closure technique in patients at high risk for wound disruption.

However, this technique is a far–far, near–near, interrupted, mass closure technique. The first (far–far) bite includes both the fascia and peritoneum on each side, and only the anterior fascia is included in the near–near bite. The widely spaced initial pass takes the tension off the healing incision, while the carefully placed near–near bites approximate the fascial edges. A nonabsorbable or slowly absorbable suture is used, with the key to the success of this closure being widely spaced far–far bites (at least 1.5 to 2 cm from the fascial edges).

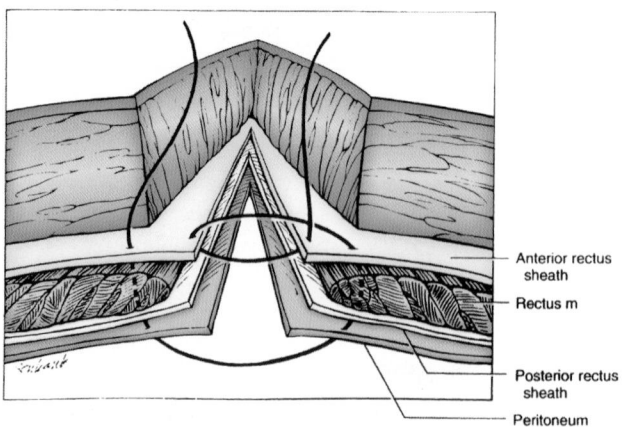

FIGURE 14.19 Smead-Jones layered closure. This is a far–far, near–near suturing technique, with the anterior fascia being included in the near–near bite. A No. 1 nylon or No. 1 polypropylene suture (or some other delayed absorbable suture) is used, with the key to the success of this closure being widely spaced far–far bites (at least 1.5 to 2 cm from the fascial edges). This closure technique may be performed in an interrupted fashion or as running suture. (Reprinted from Morrow CP, Curtin JP. Incisions and wound healing. In: *Gynecologic cancer surgery.* Churchill Livingstone, 1996:152, with permission: from Elsevier Health Science Books, with permission.)

BEST PRACTICE

- Use a monofilament suture material, slowly absorbable or nonabsorbable.
- Use a continuous suture technique.
- Close the wound in one layer.
- Avoid high tension on the suture—adapt but do not compress the fascia edges.
- Place the stitches in the fascia only, 5 to 8 mm from the wound edge and at close intervals 4 to 5 mm apart.
- The SL-to-WL ratio should be 4 or greater.

Oblique Incisions

Oblique incisions can be used for a transperitoneal or an extraperitoneal approach.

Gridiron (Muscle-Splitting) Incision of McBurney

The McBurney incision is an excellent choice for an uncomplicated appendectomy and can be used for the extraperitoneal drainage of an abscess from pelvic inflammatory disease. In pelvic inflammatory disease, when drainage becomes necessary for an indolent broad ligament abscess that does not respond to antibiotics and does not point into the cul-de-sac for drainage, drainage through a gridiron incision is most effective. The incision is constructed as for an appendectomy, except that it is made a little lower, and the peritoneal cavity is not entered. Similarly, if drainage of the pelvis is required during a pelvic laparotomy, the drain should not exit through the midline incision but rather through a small gridiron (stab wound) incision in the lower abdomen. In treating a large tuboovarian abscess that extends out of the pelvis and does not respond to antibiotic therapy, extraperitoneal drainage through a McBurney incision is also possible by approaching the abscess laterally. This permits entrance into the site of infection without soiling the peritoneal cavity.

The gridiron incision is made obliquely downward and inward over the McBurney point (Fig. 14.20A). The location can be varied when the incision is performed for appendectomy during pregnancy or when it is used for abscess drainage, as mentioned above. The incision in the skin can be made at a lower

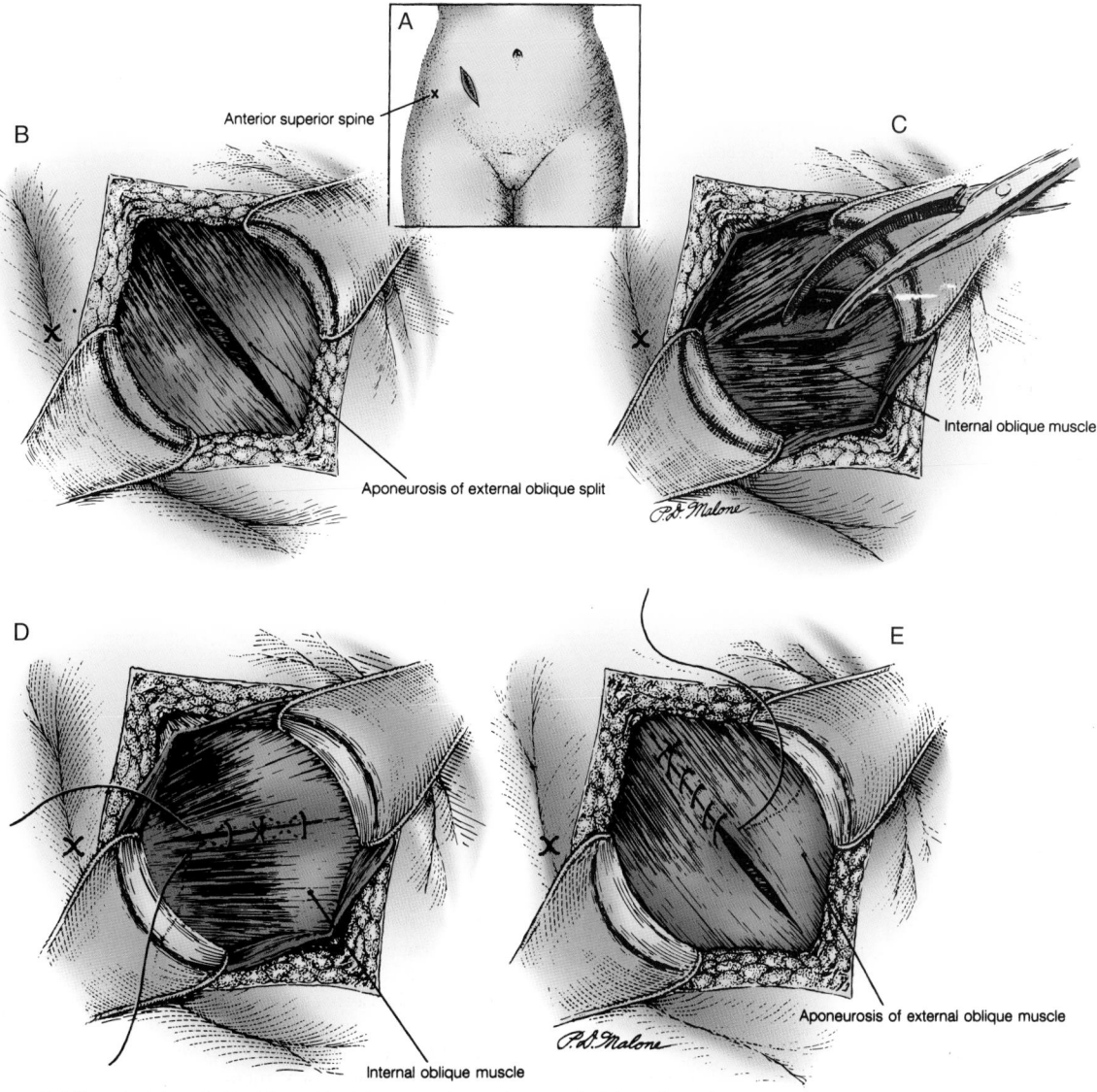

FIGURE 14.20 Gridiron incision. **A:** Position of incision. **B:** Fibers of external oblique have been split. **C:** Internal oblique muscle being split with a Kelly clamp. **D:** In closing, internal oblique fibers are approximated with figure-of-eight No. 0 delayed absorbable sutures. **E:** Aponeurosis of external oblique is closed with continuous or interrupted No. 0 delayed absorbable sutures.

level to preserve the cosmetic appearance of the abdominal wall. The incision is carried through the skin and subcutaneous fat to the external oblique muscle. The fibers of the muscle are separated in the direction in which they run (**Fig. 14.20B**). The internal oblique and the transverse abdominis are separated in the line of their fibers (**Fig. 14.20C**). At this point, the internal oblique and the transversus abdominis course in the same direction and are closely fused. Retractors are avoided, if possible. Instead, the peritoneum should be gently reflected away from the abdominal wall inferiorly and the abscess entered beneath the round ligament for extraperitoneal drainage. Thickened indurated tissue may make this step difficult. If the parietal peritoneum is adherent to the peritoneal surface of the abscess, drainage still may be possible without transversing free space in the peritoneal cavity. The surgeon should avoid contaminating the peritoneal cavity with pus, if possible.

The gridiron incision can be used in the left lower quadrant to drain an abscess on the left side of the pelvis as well as to perform sigmoid colostomy. Closure is depicted in **Figure 14.20D, E** and is best made with a monofilament slowly absorbable suture.

Rockey-Davis Incision

An alternative to the McBurney incision is the Rockey-Davis (or Elliot) incision. It is a transverse incision placed at the junction of the middle and lower thirds of a line extending from the anterosuperior iliac spine to the umbilicus. Medially, the incision extends to the border of the rectus muscle. The aponeurosis of the external oblique muscle is split in the line of its fibers. The internal oblique and transversus muscle fibers can be separated by blunt finger dissection. The peritoneum is incised transversely. This incision has provided satisfactory exposure to pathology in either lower abdominal quadrant. A similar incision made lower on the abdomen preserves the cosmetic appearance of the abdominal wall.

Incisions for Obese Patients

The prevalence of obesity is increasing in the United States, with 30% of adults being classified as being obese BMI ≥ 30 kg/m²) and 20% as being classified as extremely obese (BMI ≥ 40 kg/m²). Obesity is a recognized risk factor for postoperative wound infections, and thus, placement of an

abdominal incision can be challenging in these patients. Pitkin first observed increased operative and postoperative risks when abdominal hysterectomy is performed on obese patients. He noted significantly more postoperative fever in the obese patients versus nonobese (59% versus 36%) and a significant difference in wound complications for obese patients over nonobese (29% wound complication rate versus 4%). Krebs and Helmkamp reported a wound infection rate of 24% in massively obese patients when a periumbilical transverse incision was used. Because muscle cutting is needed for this transverse incision, entry time can be lengthy and relatively hemorrhagic. If any transverse incision is chosen for obese patients, it should be far removed from the anaerobic moist environment of the subpannicular fold (**Fig. 14.21**).

In 1977, Morrow and colleagues suggested modifications of preoperative care, intraoperative techniques, and postoperative care in obese gynecologic patients and observed only a 13% wound infection rate. Gallup subsequently modified Morrow's techniques. He reported his experience in a group of 97 obese patients, comparing them to obese patients not operated on by the modified protocol. Obese patients who were managed with the modified protocol had a wound infection rate of 3% versus 42% in those patients not operated on by protocol.

In the obese patient, the umbilicus is deviated caudally on a vertical axis in the supine and dorsal lithotomy positions. When relating the position of the umbilicus to the pubic symphysis, it can sometimes be at or below the level of the pubic symphysis, depending upon the size of the panniculus. Any incision should not be performed in the suprapubic fold after lifting the fat pad because of the poorly vascularized skin, which is typically thin and submitted to intense maceration due to the moist warm anaerobic environment that promotes the proliferation of numerous organisms (**Fig. 14.21**).

Several options for incisions on the obese abdomen exist. Querleu described a transverse incision, similar to the Maylard incision described above. But the midline incision seems to be the incision of choice for most surgeons. This incision is made by first retracting the panniculus caudad, below the inferior margins of the symphysis (**Fig. 14.21**). The skin incision is a periumbilical incision because it is usually extended around the umbilicus and more cephalad due to the caudally deviated position of the umbilicus. The fascial incision is always extended to the symphysis. A supraumbilical longitudinal

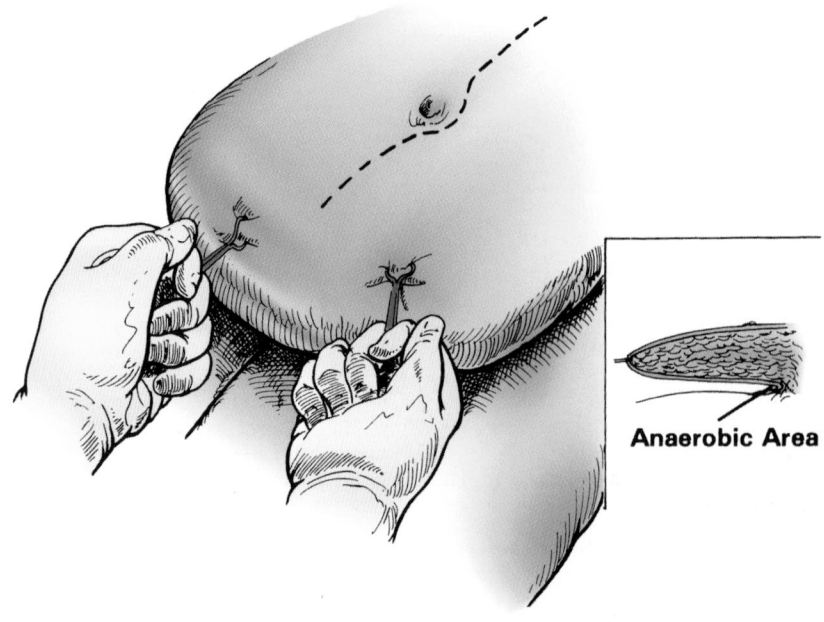

Anaerobic Area

FIGURE 14.21 Midline incision in an obese patient. The panniculus is retracted inferiorly, and the incision avoids the moist anaerobic environment (**inset**) beneath the subpannicular fold. (Reprinted from Gallup DG. Opening and closing the abdomen. In: Phelan JP, Clark SL, eds. *Cesarean delivery*. New York: Chapman & Hall, 1988:449, with permission; from Taylor and Francis Group LLC, with permission.)

incision, as described by Greer and Gal, is a variation, where the entire incision is above the umbilicus, in the flat area of the abdomen above the panniculus.

After the operation is completed, the abdominal fascia is closed with a monofilament slowly absorbing (or occasionally monofilament nonabsorbable) suture in a continuous closure. Subcutaneous sutures and or drains are not used. The skin is closed with staples, which are left in place for 2 weeks.

Panniculectomy and Abdominoplasty

An alternate surgical approach in the massively obese patient is to remove the large panniculus before the intended pelvic surgery. As observed by Kelly in 1910, wound complications can be avoided and cosmesis can be achieved by this procedure. Exposure to the pelvic organs is certainly improved. In 1978, Pratt and Irons reported on 126 panniculectomies, and 85 of these were performed to facilitate exposure to the surgical field. The average hospital stay was only 14 days, but 34.5% of the patients had some degree of morbidity. In the series by Voss and colleagues, 5 of 76 (6.6%) patients undergoing panniculectomy and hysterectomy developed pulmonary embolism. In another series, investigators encountered excessive blood loss and acknowledged the need for transfusion in combined surgery. More recently, several series have noted the relative safety of combining abdominoplasty with other surgical procedures. Hopkins and colleagues performed a retrospective review of patients who underwent panniculectomy at the time of gynecologic surgery. They identified 78 patients (average weight 278 pounds) on whom the procedure was performed. Their infection rate was a laudable 2.6%, with an equally impressive average blood loss of 71 mL. Four of the patients had minimal incisional separations.

As more sophisticated monitoring, better antibiotics, better suture material and techniques, and a safer blood supply have become more available, selective use of combined gynecologic procedures and plastic surgical removal of the panniculus is increasing. Extended antibiotic prophylaxis to prevent SSI in morbidly obese patients who do have the combined hysterectomy and medically indicated panniculectomy may be indicated. In a cohort study conducted at the Mayo Clinic, investigators showed that morbidly obese women who received standard prophylactic antibiotics and continued oral ciprofloxacin until drains were removed, had fewer SSIs compared to morbidly obese women who received only standard prophylactic antibiotic treatment (5.9% for extended antibiotics versus 27.9% in the standard treatment group). In a study of patients who had a mean weight of 261 pounds, Morrow et al. found no operative mortality and a mean hospital stay of 8.2 days. Only 11% of the patients required transfusion. The investigators in this series emphasized that the panniculectomy should be performed first to improve exposure.

Although removal of a large panniculus results in better exposure, patient selection for this potentially morbid procedure should be carefully considered. Also, the patient must be counseled and must be strongly motivated to lose weight and change her nutritional habits. If the patient is not committed to these lifestyle changes, it seems impractical to perform an extensive abdominoplastic procedure and incur the associated morbidity. If the surgical procedure is not urgent, an alternative would be to defer the procedure until the patient has achieved 40% to 50% of the planned weight loss.

Of the various operative techniques available for panniculectomy and abdominoplasty, the elliptical transverse incision, originally described by Kelly, has proven to be the procedure of choice. Two modifications of the transverse panniculectomy can be useful. The most common procedure includes an elliptical "watermelon" incision (**Fig. 14.22A**), extending from the lateral aspect of the lumbar regions to

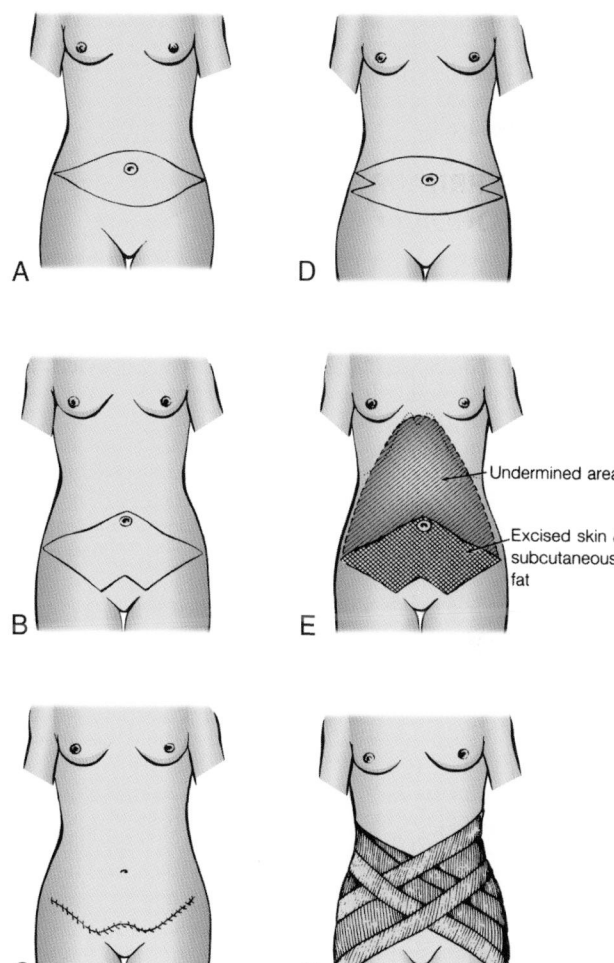

FIGURE 14.22 Panniculectomy incisions. **A:** Elliptical transverse incision extending from the region of iliac crest passes above and below the umbilicus. **B:** V-shaped incision in lateral angles eliminates folds of skin in abdominal wall. **C:** W-shaped incision over the mons pubis extends along the inguinal ligament to the iliac crest. **D:** The upper incision passes above the umbilicus. Wide mobilization of the upper skin flap is carried to the sternum and rib margins. **E:** After removal of panniculus and skin, the upper skin flap is sutured without tension to the lower skin margin. **F:** A firm elastic dressing is crisscrossed over the abdominal wall for abdominal support and prevention of seroma formation.

about 3 to 4 cm above the umbilicus. If the patient requests the preservation of the umbilicus, it can be excised and transplanted to the upper pedicle of skin. However, as shown by Cosin and colleagues, this transplantation can lead to increased wound complications. Inferiorly, the transverse incision follows the concave skin fold that separates the overhanging panniculus from the suprapubic skin. The underlying fat is excised deeply in a slightly wedged manner, with the deep portion of the fat extending outward and slightly beyond the skin margin to avoid ischemia of the skin edge. Meticulous attention must be given to absolute hemostasis (a time-consuming procedure) to avoid postoperative hematoma formation and infection. The excessive use of cautery, which produces a favorable environment for bacterial growth in devitalized tissue, should be avoided. The lateral angles of the incision may require separate "V" incisions to avoid the unsightly folds of redundant fat (**Fig. 14.22B**). When these V-shaped wedges are closed, the angle of the incision is converted into a

Y-shaped configuration, which eliminates the excessive skin in the lateral aspects of the abdominal wall. After the removal of the large panniculus, the abdomen can be opened either transversely or vertically. A vertical incision has been advocated to improve exposure.

DELAYED PRIMARY CLOSURE AND SECONDARY CLOSURE

The value of delayed primary wound closure in managing possible contaminated wounds has been recognized by military surgeons for many years. In 1968, Grosfeld and Solit reported that patients with perforating appendicitis had a reduction in wound infection rates from 34.1% to 2.3% when delayed closure was used. Similarly, in a high-risk group of patients—which included patients with obesity, cancer, possible contamination from above-and-below procedures, infection, and bowel content contamination—Brown and colleagues found a marked reduction in wound infection rates when delayed primary closure was used compared with immediate closure in matched patients. The infection rate for the former group was 2.1%; for the latter, 23.3%. Possible candidates for such a closure include patients with ruptured appendicitis, ruptured tuboovarian abscess, extensive bowel injury, or diverticulitis with contamination.

After closure of the fascia, the wound is irrigated with copious amounts of saline and then packed with 0.1% Dakin solution (sodium hypochlorite). The wound dressing sponges are changed two to three times a day with a wet-to-dry technique, using sterile saline or 0.1% Dakin solution. Once the signs of infection are gone, the Dakin solution should be stopped, as it can impede epithelialization. In 4 to 5 days, depending on the appearance of granulation tissue in the subcutaneous tissues, the previously placed sutures are tied to approximate the skin edges. Tincture of benzoin is placed at the lateral edges of the closed incision, and Steri-Strips are used to approximate uneven skin edges.

Alternatively, the skin edges of the incision can be closed with widely spaced staples, "wicking" the intervening spaces with saline-soaked (Dakin solution in the face of infection) gauze (e.g., Nu Gauze or Kerlix strips). Once adequate granulation tissue is present, the skin edges can be reapproximated with nonabsorbable monofilament sutures and local lidocaine at the patient's bedside before discharge from the hospital.

Superficial separation of layers anterior to the fascia is usually associated with wound infections, seromas, or hematomas. Many centers suggest opening the wound, usually the entire length, obtaining appropriate cultures for antibiotic choice, and allowing healing by second intention, with once- or twice-daily wound dressing changes. Although most cleansing in a second-intention scenario is accomplished by home health care personnel, patients are inconvenienced by this method. A trend in many centers and practices has been to perform delayed closure after a period of 2 to 5 days. In 1988, in a prospective randomized study, Hermann and associates found that secondary closure, performed 2 days after wound drainage had ceased, resulted in a significant reduction in healing time when compared with healing by second intention.

In a larger series of patients on an obstetrics and gynecology service, Walters and colleagues found a similar advantage in delayed closure of wounds. In 35 patients who underwent reclosure, 85.7% had their wounds successfully closed. Patients in this study had abdominal incisions that had been opened owing to infection, hematoma, or seroma. The fascia was intact in all patients, and all patients had wound debridement and cleansing for a minimum period of 4 days. All patients in this series had reclosure performed in the operating room and received three doses of cefazolin. The closure was done by an en bloc technique, using No. 2 monofilament nylon sutures. In a series from the University of Mississippi (Dodson et al.), patients with superficial wound dehiscence were randomized to en bloc closure with No. 1 polypropylene versus a superficial closure through the skin using No. 2 polypropylene vertical mattress sutures. There was no statistical difference in the number of days needed to complete wound healing. However, the en bloc group required longer time for closure, and these patients experienced more pain. Of note, none of these patients received prophylactic antibiotics, and all wounds were reclosed under local anesthesia in the patient care area 2 to 6 days after reopening the wound.

Our technique for reclosing wounds is similar to that reported by Dodson and associates. After reopening the wound in patients with superficial wound dehiscence, the subcutaneous tissues are debrided daily, and wet-to-dry dressings using sterile saline are placed in the wound two to three times daily. Antibiotics are generally not used unless the patient has a concomitant infection (e.g., cellulitis or cuff infection). The wound is closed when a healing bed of granulation tissue without exudate or necrotic debris is present. Many wounds require sharp debridement, but most can still be closed within 5 days of reopening.

Wounds are closed in the treatment room on the ward or in the office with local 1% lidocaine anesthesia after premedication with anxiolytics and narcotic pain medication. The skin is then prepped with a povidone–iodine solution, and the sutures are placed 1 cm from the skin edges and 2 cm apart. The suture of choice is a No. 0 polypropylene suture or a similar permanent or delayed absorbable suture. We leave the sutures in for 2 weeks.

An alternative to secondary closure with suture is negative pressure wound therapy (NWPT). Since the first reports of this type of therapy for chronic wounds in 1997, NWPT has overwhelmed the wound healing world, including treatment of postoperative wound complications. This method utilizes a pump to produce subatmospheric pressures (50 to 125 mm Hg), a polyurethane foam (which is black in color) with pore sizes ranging from 400 to 600 μm or polyvinyl alcohol foam (which is white) (both of which can be cut to conform to the wound), tubing to connect the foam to the pump and to the fluid reservoir, and occlusive material to create a seal to maintain negative pressure. The mode of the pump is either intermittent or continuous. The mechanism of action is that the foam occludes the wound, allowing for quicker epithelialization, and drains away any exudates. In addition, the subatmospheric pressure creates tissue strain, stimulating cellular proliferation, angiogenesis, and growth factor elaboration. Further, inflammation and edema is reduced, with all the associated mediators, and the bacterial load in the wound is reduced. The black foam, which has the larger pores, is considered most effective at stimulating wound contraction and formation of granulation tissue. The white foam has a smaller pore size and is utilized to restrict granulation tissue growth. Contraindications to NWPT include exposed vessels, anastomotic sites, organs, nerves, malignancy, untreated osteomyelitis, nonenteric and unexplored fistulae, and necrotic tissue. The presence of necrotic tissue requires aggressive debridement prior to NWPT. It is important to note that no randomized clinical trial comparing NWPT to delayed closure has been done despite a robust use of this technology for disrupted, postoperative wounds.

COMPLETE WOUND DEHISCENCE AND EVISCERATION

Technically, wound dehiscence means separation of all layers of the abdominal incision, but wound dehiscence has been subdivided based on the layers of tissue that have separated. Incomplete or partial dehiscence (superficial dehiscence) means separation of the skin and all tissue layers posterior to the skin, sometimes including the fascia. However, if the disruption includes the peritoneum, the disruption is called a complete dehiscence. Should the intestine protrude through the wound, the term *evisceration* (also a burst abdomen) is used. The frequency of fascial dehiscence ranges between 0.3% and 3% of all cases of pelvic surgery.

Evisceration is one of the most feared and dangerous postoperative complications, with a reported incidence of 0.4% to 3.5%, rates that have remained constant over the last several decades despite advances in perioperative care, surgical techniques, and materials. The mortality rate associated with evisceration has been reported to be as high as 35% and is usually associated with other complications, such as sepsis. However, Helmkamp's 10-year study noted a mortality rate of only 2.9% in 70 cases, which may reflect improved supportive care available for these patients in recent years. Evisceration is less likely to occur in gynecology patients than in general surgery patients.

Older studies reported that the type and location of the incision and the type of suture used were major causative factors in evisceration. However, many of the predisposing factors for complete wound disruption or evisceration are metabolic and include malnutrition, poorly controlled diabetes, corticosteroid use, and older age. Mechanical factors associated with dehiscence and evisceration include obesity, intra-abdominal distention (including rapid postoperative reaccumulation of ascites), infection, retching, and coughing. In addition, any process that can impair wound healing, such as radiotherapy or chemotherapy, can contribute to an increased risk for wound disruption.

Complete wound dehiscence and evisceration are usually problems associated with tissue failure and not suture failure, with the main mechanism being suture cutting through the suture holding tissues. If the suture holding tissues disintegrate due to a necrotizing infection, this usually occurs 7 to 10 days after wound closure, as it takes time for an infection to develop. However, rates of severe SSI causing dehiscence of evisceration are quite low (0.1%). The most common cause for wound dehiscence is most likely the quality of the suture technique (see above). Maintenance of a SL-to-WL ratio over 4 and utilizing a continuous closure versus interrupted are both associated with low rates of dehiscence and evisceration.

Rollins and associates noted that about half of their patients with serious wound complications had prior abdominal or pelvic surgery. In the series reported by Jurkiewicz and Morales, 88% of eviscerated wounds had tearing of suture through the fascia, with knots and suture intact. Thus, large loose sutures with secure knots are always preferable to tight strangulating sutures that cause ischemia of the incision margin.

Eviscerations usually occur from day 5 to 14 after operation, with a mean of about 8 days. One of the early signs of complete dehiscence and impending evisceration is the seepage of serosanguineous pink discharge from an apparently intact wound. It can be present for several days before evisceration occurs and occurs in 23% to 84% of cases. Although occult hematomas are usually the cause of such discharge, these wounds need to be examined carefully by probing with a cotton-tipped swab to assess the integrity of the fascial closure. Frequently, the patient is conscious of something giving way, "tearing," or "popping" immediately before the burst abdomen becomes clinically apparent.

With few exceptions, complete dehiscence or eviscerations should be closed as soon as they are recognized. In case of evisceration, when a delay of several hours is anticipated because of a recent meal, the bowel can be replaced by using sterile gloves, gently packing it in place with lap pads soaked in saline, and securing it with an abdominal binder. Broad-spectrum antibiotics should be initiated, and baseline blood counts and serum electrolyte studies should be obtained.

Closing an evisceration should be performed in the operating room (never on the floor) and always under general anesthesia so that the extent of the dehiscence may be determined. Necrotic tissue clots and suture material should be removed, and aerobic and anaerobic cultures should be obtained. The bowel and omentum should be inspected and thoroughly cleansed with several liters of warm normal saline. If the fascial margins can be located and are not ragged, a continuous, mass closure technique with a slowly absorbable monofilament suture, achieving an SL-to-WL ratio of 4 or more, is advised. When completing the closure, it is unknown whether small or large stitch size is better, but the SL-to-WL ratio can be maintained with either. The subcutaneous tissue and skin are packed open for later delayed closure or NWPT placement.

If the wound edges are ragged or the patient's condition is poor, a through-and-through retention suture of No. 2 nylon or polypropylene is used. The sutures are placed at least 2.5 to 3 cm from the skin edges and are passed through all layers. To allow for edema, they are placed 2 cm apart (**Fig. 14.23**).

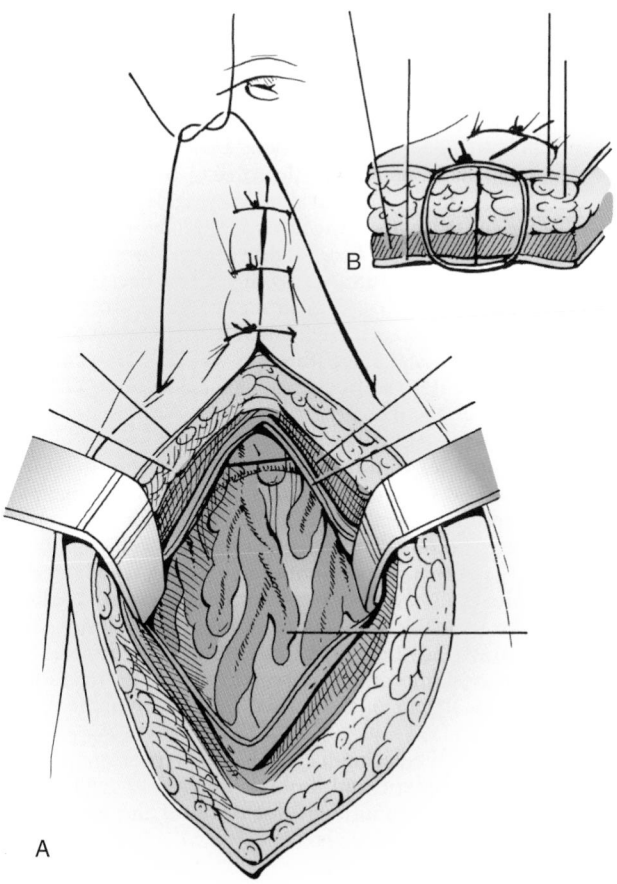

FIGURE 14.23 A: Secondary closure of an evisceration with retention sutures (usually No. 1 polypropylene sutures—rubber dams can be included) and preferably No. 2 polypropylene sutures. **B:** All layers are incorporated.

To prevent inclusion of the underlying intestine in a suture, all sutures are held up before the first one is tied. Skin edges unopposed between the through-and-through sutures can be approximated with interrupted 3-0 polypropylene. The through-and-through sutures should be left in place for 3 weeks. A nasogastric tube should be used in the immediate postoperative period to avoid abdominal distention, and broad-spectrum antibiotics should be continued and modified according to culture results.

INCISIONAL HERNIA

Incisional hernia is a frequent complication after midline incisions (and less frequently in transverse incisions) of the abdominal wall. In this situation, the peritoneum remains intact, and the fascial margins and adjacent muscles separate, leaving a defect beneath the subcutaneous tissue into which the bowel and omentum may herniate.

Causes of herniation are similar to those of evisceration; however, the skin, subcutaneous tissue, and peritoneum remain intact. Most cases of ventral hernia follow an incisional infection, weakening the supporting tissues. Increased intra-abdominal pressure from coughing and vomiting, along with necrosis of the fascial margins, permits the sutures to pull through the edge of the fascia. These changes result in separation of the wound edges and failure of fibroblastic bridging of the fascia. This complication occurs more frequently in lower abdominal incisions because of the anatomic deficit of the posterior fascial sheath beneath the rectus in the area inferior to the semicircular line. Ventral hernias occur after low midline incisions in about 0.5% to 1% of all gynecologic operations, with the incidence rising to about 10% after a wound infection. Similarly, reclosure after dehiscence increases the chance of hernia formation to about 25%.

Although the initial fascial defect may be small, the size of the resultant hernia can assume varying proportions and involve the entire length of the lower abdominal wall. The size of the hernia depends on the mobility of the bowel and omentum and the final aperture size of the ventral defect. A large amount of small bowel and omentum can escape from a small fascial defect into an easily expandable subcutaneous space. The smaller the fascial defect through which small bowel can herniate, the greater the frequency of incarceration, obstruction, and infarction.

Patients with ventral hernias often report lower abdominal discomfort, and with large ventral hernias, the abdominal wall is distended to varying degrees. Patients with large hernias may note bowel peristalsis beneath the skin and report that the bulge becomes smaller when they are in a recumbent position. The hernia is more noticeable during coughing and straining and can increase in size over time because of enlargement of the hernial ring or incorporation of additional segments of bowel into the hernial sac. Rarely, a ventral hernia produces acute symptoms of visceral torsion, incarceration, and infarction. Repair of the hernia is preferably done on an elective basis.

Advances in the technique of hernia repair as well as the materials (synthetic and biologic meshes) to repair such hernias have made a thorough discussion of the topic here, beyond the scope of this chapter.

PERINEOTOMY INCISIONS

Adequate exposure is just as important with vaginal surgery as it is with abdominal surgery. When exposure is not adequate with abdominal operations, the incision is extended, or some other measure is used to improve exposure. Certain measures also can improve exposure with vaginal operations. A tight vaginal introitus may restrict exposure of the upper vagina but can be enlarged at the beginning of the operation by making a midline or mediolateral episiotomy incision. A mediolateral incision can be made on one or both sides of the vaginal introitus. If a midline episiotomy is made and closed transversely, the vaginal introitus can be made larger than before, if that is deemed advisable. These incisions can be closed with 2-0 or 3-0 delayed absorbable suture.

Sometimes, the entire vagina is small in caliber because of virginity or nulliparity, atrophic shrunken vaginal mucosa, previous colporrhaphy, or previous irradiation or disease. The vaginal vault may be fixed in a relatively high position, with relatively little descensus. Because adequate exposure through the vagina may be impossible, some operations may require an abdominal approach. On the other hand, required exposure may be obtained by making a Schuchardt incision. The entire vagina can be enlarged with this incision, achieving remarkable improvement in exposure of the upper vagina. Therefore, a patient whose problem might otherwise have necessitated an abdominal approach can have the advantage of a perfectly satisfactory vaginal operation if a Schuchardt incision is made.

According to Speert (1958), Langenbeck made a deep relaxing incision into the perineal body in attempting vaginal hysterectomy for uterine cancer in 1828. Similar incisions were used by Olshausen in 1881 and Duhrssen in 1891. Karl Schuchardt described his incision in 1893:

> to make more accessible from below a uterus whose mobility is limited.... With the patient in the lithotomy position and her buttocks elevated, a large, essentially sagittal incision is made, somewhat convex externally, beginning between the middle and posterior third of the labium majus, ...extending posterior toward the sacrum, and stopping two fingerbreaths [*sic*] from the anus. The wound is deepened only in the fatty tissue of the ischiorectal fossa, leaving the funnel of the levator ani muscle, the rectum behind it, and the sacral ligaments intact. Internally, the sidewall of the vagina is opened into the ischiorectal fossa and the vagina divided in its lateral aspect by a long incision extending up to the cervix. There thus results a surprisingly free view of all the structures under consideration.

The incision is ordinarily made on the patient's left side by a right-handed operator (Fig. 14.24). A left-handed operator may find it technically easier to make the incision on the patient's right side. Bilateral incisions have been advocated in extreme cases. The side on which the incision is made may be dictated by the location of the pathology to be removed. Injection of the tissues to be incised with sterile saline solution can be helpful, especially beneath the vaginal mucosa in the line of the incision. The assistant pulls upward to the left with the index finger placed as deep as possible in the vagina just to the left of the urethra. The operator makes countertraction by placing two fingers in the vagina and pulling downward to the right. This pull and counterpull in opposite directions stretches the left vaginal wall. The incision is made with the electrosurgical unit beginning at the 4 o'clock position at the introitus and extending downward in the skin of the buttock to the level of the anus. The incision is then carried upward through the vaginal mucosa into the upper third of the vagina. As the incision is deepened, the fingers of the operator's left hand are used to displace the rectum medially to protect it from injury. The ischiorectal fossa fat is visible

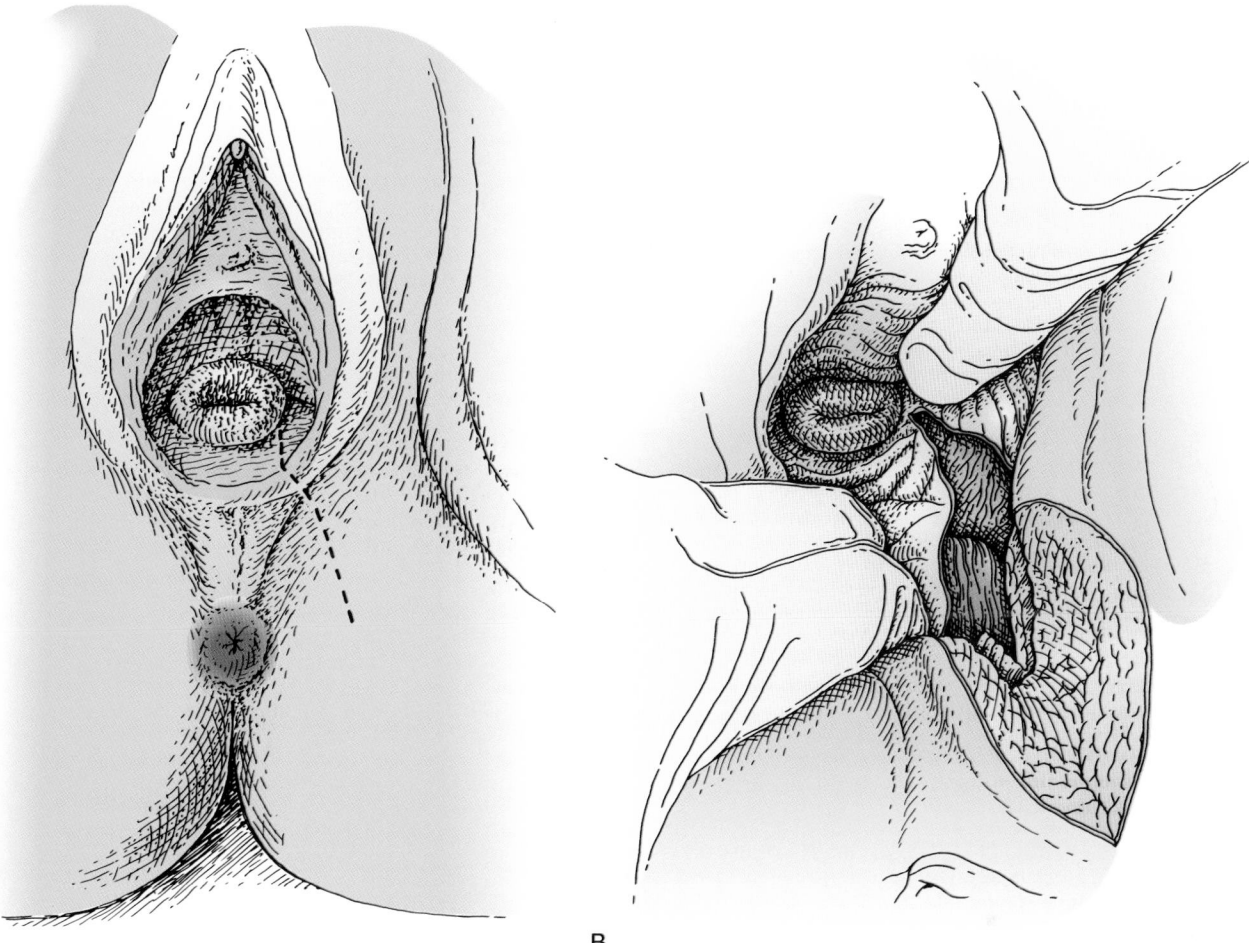

A   B

FIGURE 14.24 A: The Schuchardt incision begins at the 4-o'clock position in the vaginal introitus and extends into the buttock and up the posterolateral wall of the vagina to the cervix. **B:** The ischiorectal fossa fat is exposed. The puborectalis muscle is divided. The left paravesical and pararectal spaces can be exposed through the incision.

below the puborectalis muscle, which is incised with the electrosurgical knife (**Fig. 14.24**). If necessary, the left paravesical space can be developed. For the best possible exposure, the apex of the vaginal incision should intersect any incision made around the cervix, achieving hemostasis by coagulation or ligation.

At the end of the operation, the Schuchardt incision is closed with 2-0 and 3-0 delayed absorbable sutures, attempting to reapproximate the puborectalis muscle edges and to obliterate the dead space in the ischiorectal fossa. Drainage of these incisions is usually not necessary.

The Schuchardt incision most often is used for extensive vaginal hysterectomy for early invasive cervical cancer. We also have used it when performing extensive dissections to remove endometriosis in the vaginal vault, to gain better exposure for difficult vaginal hysterectomy or vesicovaginal fistula repair, to repair injuries to the lower ureter, to remove organized hematomas just above the puborectalis muscle, to drain lymphocysts vaginally, or to remove benign cystic teratomas in the lower presacral area behind the rectum. It can convert a technically difficult, complicated, and dangerous vaginal operation into one that is simple, easy, and safe. It is difficult to understand why perineotomy incisions are so

quickly performed for obstetric operations and so reluctantly for gynecologic operations.

BEST SURGICAL PRACTICES

- During counseling for surgery, location of the incision, rationale, and any potential complications must be presented to the patient.
- Fascial closures (of midline and some transverse incisions) should be accomplished with delayed absorbable monofilament suture (see above). Plain catgut or chromic catgut should *never* be used for fascial closures.
- Closed drainage systems (i.e., Jackson-Pratt or Blake) should be used when drains are considered. Passive drains, such as Penrose drains, should not be used.
- Monofilament sutures should be tied with either three square knots (six throws) or one surgeon's knot and two square knots (four throws).
- For superficial dehiscence, consider delayed closure or NPWT over secondary-intention closure with wet-to-dry dressing changes for improved patient healing. Delayed closure in the office may be less expensive and more convenient for the patient compared to NPWT.

BIBLIOGRAPHY

Alexander HC, Prudden JF. The causes of abdominal wound disruption. *Surg Gynecol Obstet* 1966;122:1223.

Alexander JW, Aerni S, Plettner JP. Development of a safe and effective one-minute preoperative skin preparation. *Arch Surg* 1985;120:1367.

Altman AD, Nelson G, Nation J, et al. Vacuum assisted wound closures in gynecologic surgery. *J Obstet Gynaecol Can* 2011;33:1031.

ACOG Committee on Practice Bulletins-Gynecology. Antibiotic prophylaxis for gynecologic procedures. ACOG Practice Bulletin No. 104. American Congress of Obstetricians and Gynecologists. *Obstet Gynecol* 2009;113:1180.

Archie JP, Feldman RW. Primary wound closure with permanent continuous running monofilament sutures. *Surg Gynecol Obstet* 1981;153:721.

Balthazar ER, Colt JD, Nicols RL. Preoperative hair removal: a random prospective study of shaving versus clipping. *South Med J* 1982;75:799.

Beale EW, Hoxworth RE, Livingston EH, et al. The role of biological mesh in abdominal wall reconstruction: a systematic review of the current literature. *Am J Surg* 2012;204:510.

Bickenbach KA, Karanicolas PJ, Ammori JB, et al. Up and down or side to side? A systematic review and meta-analysis examining the impact of incision on outcomes after abdominal surgery. *Am J Surg* 2013;206:400. pii: S0002-9610(13)00154-2. doi: 10.1016/j.amjsurg.2012.11.008

Bourne RB, Bitar H, Andrese PR, et al. In-vivo comparison of four absorbable sutures: Vicryl, Dexon Plus, Maxon and PDS. *Can J Surg* 1988;31:43.

Bratzler DW, Hunt DR. The surgical infection prevention and surgical care improvement project: national initiatives to improve outcomes for patients having surgery. *Clin Infect Dis* 2006;43:322.

Broughton G II, Janis JE, Attinger CE. Wound healing: an overview. *Plast Reconstr Surg* 2006;117:1e-S.

Brown SE, Allen HH, Robins RN. The use of delayed primary wound closure in preventing wound infections. *Am J Obstet Gynecol* 1977;127:213.

Bucknall TE, Cox PJ, Ellis H. Burst abdomen and incisional hernia: a prospective study of 1129 major laparotomies. *Br Med J* 1982;284:931.

Bucknall TE. Factors influencing wound complications: a clinical and experimental study. *Ann R Coll Surg Engl* 1983;65:71.

Burger JW, Lange JF, Halm JA, et al. Incisional hernia: early complications of abdominal surgery. *World J Surg* 2005;29:1608. doi: 10.1007/s00268-005-7929-3

Campbell JA, Temple WJ, Frank CB, et al. A biomechanical study of suture pullout in linea alba. *Surgery* 1989;106:888.

Cengiz Y, Blomquist P, Israelsson LA. Small tissue bites and wound strength: an experimental study. *Arch Surg* 2001;136:272.

Charoenkwan K, Chotirosniramit N, Rerkasem K. Scalpel versus electrosurgery for abdominal incisions. *Cochrane Database Syst Rev* 2012;6:CD005987. doi: 10.1002/14651858.CD005987.pub2

Cherney LS. A modified transverse incision for low abdominal operations. *Surg Gynecol Obstet* 1941;72:92.

Chu CC. Classifications and general characteristics of suture materials. In: Chu CC, von Fraunhofer JA, Greisler HP, eds. *Wound closure biomaterials and devices*. Boca Roton, FL: CRC Press, 1997:39.69.

Clancy CM. SCIP: making complications of surgery the exception rather than the rule. *AORN J* 2008;87:621.

Cosin JA, Powell JL, Donovan JT, et al. The safety and efficacy of extensive abdominal panniculectomy at the time of pelvic surgery. *Gynecol Oncol* 1994;55:36.

Cox PJ, Ausobsky JR, Ellis H, et al. Towards no incisional hernias: lateral paramedian versus midline incisions. *J R Soc Med* 1986;79:711.

Cruse PJE, Foord R. A five-year prospective study of 23,649 surgical wounds. *Arch Surg* 1973;107:206.

Cruse PJE, Foord R. The epidemiology of wound infection: a 10-year prospective study of 62,939 wounds. *Surg Clin North Am* 1980;60:27.

Cruse PJE. Infection surveillance: identifying the problem and the high-risk patient. *South Med J* 1977;70(suppl 1):40.

Culver DH, Horan TC, Gaynes RP, et al. Surgical wound infection rates by wound class, operative procedure and patient risk index. National Nosocomial Infections Surveillance System. *Am J Med* 1991;91:152S.

Darouiche RO, Wall MJ Jr, Itani KMF, et al. Chlorhexidine-alcohol versus povidone iodine for surgical site antisepsis. *N Engl J Med* 2010;362:18.

Daversa B, Landers D. Physiologic advantages of the transverse incision in gynecology. *Obstet Gynecol* 1961;17:305.

Dellinger EP, Hausmann SM, Bratzler DW, et al. Hospitals collaborate to decrease surgical site infections. *Am J Surg* 2005;190.

Desai KK, Hahn E, Pulikkotill B, et al. Negative pressure wound therapy: an algorithm. *Clin Plast Surg* 2012;39:311.

Diener MK, Voss S, Jensen K, et al. Elective midline laparotomy closure: the INLINE systemic review and meta-anaylsis. *Ann Surg* 2010;251:843.

Dineen P. A critical study of 100 conservative wound infections. *Surg Gynecol Obstet* 1961;113:91.

Dodson MK, Magann EF, Sullivan DL, et al. Extrafascial wound dehiscence: deep en bloc closure versus superficial skin closure. *Obstet Gynecol* 1994;83:142.

Dougherty SH, Simmons RL. The biology of surgical drains. *Curr Probl Surg* 1992;9:648.

Edlich RF, Panek RH, Rodeheaver GT, et al. Physical and chemical configuration of suture in the development of surgical infection. *Ann Surg* 1973;177:679.

Edwards R, Harding KG. Bacteria and wound healing. *Curr Opin Infect Dis* 2004;17:91.

Ellenhorn JDI, Smith DD, Schwarz RE, et al. Paint-only is equivalent to scrub-and-paint in preoperative preparation of abdominal surgery sites. *J Am Coll Surg* 2005;201:737.

Ellis H, Heddle R. Does the peritoneum need to be closed at laparotomy? *Br J Surg* 1977;64:733.

El-Nashar SA, Diehl CL, Swanson CL, et al. Extended antibiotic prophylaxis for prevention of surgical site infections in morbidly obese women who undergo combined hysterectomy and medically indicated panniculectomy: a cohort study. *Am J Obstet Gynecol* 2010;202:e1.

Farnell MB, Worthington-Self S, Mucha P Jr, et al. Closure of abdominal incisions with subcutaneous catheters. *Arch Surg* 1986;126:641.

Flegal KM, Carroll MD, Kit BK, et al. Prevalence of obesity and trends in the distribution of body mass index among US adults, 1999–2010. *JAMA* 2012;307:491.

Fletcher HS, Joseph WL. Bleeding into the rectus abdominis muscle. *Int Surg* 1973;58:97.

Gal D. A supraumbilical incision for gynecologic neoplasm in the morbidly obese patients. *J Am Coll Surg* 1994;179:18.

Galle PC, Homesley HD, Rhyne AL. Reassessment of the surgical scrub. *Surg Gynecol Obstet* 1978;147:214.

Gallup DG. Abdominal incisions and closures. In: Gallup DG, Talledo OE, eds. Surgical atlas of gynecologic oncology. Philadelphia, PA: WB Saunders, 1994:43.

Gallup DG. Opening and closing the abdomen. In: Phelan JP, Clark SL, eds. *Cesarean delivery*. New York: Chapman & Hall, 1988:449.

Gallup DG. Opening and closing the abdomen and wound healing. In: Gershenson D, Curry S, DeCherney A, eds. *Operative gynecology*, 1st ed. Philadelphia, PA: WB Saunders, 1993

Gallup DG, Nolan TE, Smith RP. Primary mass closure of midline incisions with a continuous polyglyconate monofilament absorbable suture. *Obstet Gynecol* 1990;76:872.

Gallup DG, Talledo OE, King LA. Primary mass closure of midline incisions with a continuous running monofilament suture in gynecologic patients. *Obstet Gynecol* 1989;73:67.

Gallup DG. Modification of celiotomy techniques to decrease morbidity in obese gynecologic patients. *Am J Obstet Gynecol* 1984;150:171.

Goldberg SR, Diegelmann RF. Wound healing primer. *Surg Clin North Am* 2010;90:1133.

Greenberg JA, Clark RM. Advances in suture material for obstetric and gynecologic surgery. *Rev Obstet Gynecol* 2009;2:146.

Greenburg G, Salk RP, Peskin GW. Wound dehiscence: pathophysiology and prevention. *Arch Surg* 1979;114:143.

Greer BE, Cain JM, Figge DC, et al. Supraumbilical upper abdominal midline incision for pelvic surgery in the morbidly obese patient. *Obstet Gynecol* 1990;76:71.

Grosfeld JL, Solit RW. Prevention of wound infection in perforated appendicitis: experience with delayed primary wound closure. *Ann Surg* 1968;168:891.

Guillou PJ, Hall TJ, Donaldson DR, et al. Vertical abdominal incisions: a choice? *Br J Surg* 1980;67:359.

Gutwein LG, Panigrahi M, Schultz GS, et al. Microbial barriers. *Clin Plast Surg* 2012;39:229.

Hamilton HW, Hamilton KR, Lone FJ. Preoperative hair removal. *Can J Surg* 1977;20:269.

Hasselgren AO, Harbery E, Malmer H, et al. One instead of two knifes for surgical incision. *Arch Surg* 1984;118:917.

Helmkamp BF, Krebs HB, Amstey MS. Correct use of surgical drains. *Contemp Ob Gyn* 1984;23:123.

Helmkamp BF. Abdominal wound dehiscence. *Am J Obstet Gynecol* 1977;128:803.

Hemani ML, Lepor H. Skin preparation for the prevention of surgical site infection: Which agent is best?. *Rev Urol* 2009;11:190.

Hendrix SL, Schimp V, Martin J, et al. The legendary superior strength of Pfannenstiel incision: a myth? *Am J Obstet Gynecol* 2000;182:1446.

Hermann GG, Bagi P, Christofferson I. Early secondary suture versus healing by second intention of incisional abscesses. *Surg Gynecol Obstet* 1988;167:16.

Higson RH, Kettlewell MGW. Parietal wound drainage in abdominal surgery. *Br J Surg* 1978;65:326.

Hodgson NC, Malthaner RA, Ostbye T. The search for an ideal method of abdominal fascial closure: a meta-analysis. *Ann Surg* 2000;231:436.

Hoer J, Lawong G, Klinge U. Factors influencing the development of incisional hernia: a retrospective study of 2983 laparotomy patients over a period of 10 years. *Chirurg* 2002;73:474.

Hopkins MP, Shriner AM, Parker MG, et al. Panniculectomy at the time of gynecologic surgery in morbidly obese patients. *Am J Obstet Gynecol* 2000;182:1502.

Horan TC, Gaynes RP, Martone WJ, et al. CDC definitions of nosocomial surgical site infections, 1992: a modification of the CDC definitions of surgical wound infections. *Infect Control Hosp Epidemiol* 1992;13:606.

Hugh TB, Nakivel C, Meagher AP, et al. Is closure of the peritoneal layer necessary in the repair of midline surgical abdominal wounds? *World J Surg* 1990;14:2231.

Hurt J, Unger JB, Ivy JJ et al. Tying a loop-to-strand suture: is it safe? *Am J Obstet Gynecol* 2005;192:1094.

Israelsson LA, Millbourn D. Closing midline abdominal incisions. *Langenbecks Arch Surg* 2012;397:1201.

Ivy JJ, Unger JB, Hurt J, et al. The effect of number of throws on knot security with non-identical sliding knots. *Am J Obstet Gynecol* 2004;191:1618.

Jenkins TPN. The burst abdominal wound: a mechanical approach. *Br J Surg* 1976;63:873.

Jurkiewicz MJ, Morales L. Wound healing, operative incisions, and skin grafts. In: Hardy JD, ed. *Hardy's textbook of surgery*. Philadelphia, PA: JB Lippincott Co, 1983:108.

Keill RH, Keitzer WF, Henzel J, et al. Abdominal wound dehiscence. *Arch Surg* 1973;106:573.

Kelly HA. Excision of the fat of the abdominal wall: lipectomy. *Surg Gynecol Obstet* 1910;10:229.

Kim JC, Lee YK, Lim BS, et al. Comparison of tensile and knot security properties of surgical sutures. *J Mater Sci Mater Med* 2007;18:2363.

Knight CD, Griffen FD. Abdominal wound closure with a continuous monofilament polypropylene suture. *Arch Surg* 1983; 118:1305.

Kosins AM, Scholz T, Cetinkaya M, et al. Evidence-based value of subcutaneous surgical wound drainage: the largest systematic review and meta-analysis. *Plast Reconstr Surg* 2013;132:443.

Kowalsky MS, Dellenbaugh SG, Erlichman DB, et al. Evaluation of suture abrasion against rotator cuff tendon and proximal humerus bone. *Arthroscopy* 2008;24:329.

Krasner DL, Rodeheaver GT, Sibbald RG. *Chronic wound care: a clinical source book for healthcare professionals.* Malvern, PA: HMP Communications, 2007.

Krebs HB, Helmkamp F. Transverse periumbilical incision in the massively obese patient. *Obstet Gynecol* 1984;63:241.

Krupski WC, Sumchai A, Effeney DJ, et al. The importance of abdominal wall collateral blood vessels. *Arch Surg* 1984;119:854.

Küstner O. Der suprasymphysare kreuzschnitt, eine methode der coeliotomie bei wenig umfanglichen affektioen der weiblichen beckenorgane. *Monatsschr Geburtsh Gynakol* 1896;4:197.

Landis SJ. Chronic wound infection and antimicrobial use. *Adv Skin Wound Care* 2008;21:531.

Langer K. Cleavage of the cutis (the anatomy and physiology of the skin): presented at the Meeting of the Royal Academy of Sciences, April 25, 1861. *Clin Orthop* 1973;91:3.

Lee I, Agarwal RK, Lee BY, et al. Systematic review and cost analysis comparing use of chlorhexidine with the use of iodine for preoperative skin antisepsis to prevent surgical site infection. *Infect Control Hosp Epidemiol* 2010;31:1219.

Lilienfeld DE, Valhov D, Tenney JH, et al. Obesity and diabetes as risk factors for postoperative wound infections after cardiac surgery. *Am J Infect Control* 1988;16:3.

Lineweaver W, Howard R, Soucy D, et al. Topical antimicrobial toxicity. *Arch Surg* 1985;120:1985.

Macht SC, Krizek TJ. Sutures and suturing: current concepts. *J Oral Surg* 1978;36:240.

Mangrum AJ, Horan TC, Pearson ML, et al. Guideline for prevention of surgical site infection, 1999. Hospital Infection Control Practices Advisory Committee. *Infect Control Hosp Epidemiol* 1999;20:250.

Martone WJ, Nichols RL. Recognition, prevention, surveillance and management of surgical site infections: introduction to the problem and symposium overview. *Clin Infect Dis* 2001;33(suppl 2):S67.

Mayer AD, Ausobsky JR, Evans M, et al. Compression suture of the abdominal wall: a controlled trial in 302 major laparotomies. *Br J Surg* 1981;68:632.

Mayland AE. Direction of abdominal incision. *Br Med J* 1907;2:895.

McBurney C. The incision made in the abdominal wall in cases of appendicitis, with a description of a new method of operating. *Ann Surg* 1894;20:38.

McDowell E. Three cases of extirpation of diseased ovaria: 1817. *Am J Obstet Gynecol* 1995;172:1632.

McMinn RMH, Hutchings RJ, Logan BM. *Color atlas of applied anatomy*. Chicago, IL: Mosby Year Book, 1984:110.

Mead PB. Managing infected abdominal wounds. *Contemp Ob Gyn* 1979;14:69.

Mendenez MA. The contaminated wound. In: O'Leary JP, Waltering EA, eds. *Techniques for surgeons*. New York: John Wiley and Sons, 1985:36.

Menke MN, Menke NB, Boardman CH, et al. Biological therapeutics and molecular profiling to optimize wound healing. *Gynecol Oncol* 2008;111:S87.

Metz SA, Chegini N, Masterson BJ. In vivo tissue reactivity and degradation of suture materials: a comparison of Maxon and PDS. *J Gynecol Surg* 1989;5:37.

Millbourn D, Cengiz Y, Israelsson LA. Effect of stitch length on wound complications after closure of midline incisions: a randomized controlled trial. *Arch Surg* 2009;144:1056.

Mishriki SF, Law DJ, Jeffery PJ. Factors affecting the incidence of post-operative wound infections. *J Hosp Infect* 1990;16:223.

Molokova OA, Kecherukov AI, Aliev FSh, et al. Tissue reactions to modern suturing material in colorectal surgery. *Bull Exp Biol Med* 2007;143:767.

Montz FJ, Creasman WT, Eddy G, et al. Running mass closure of abdominal wounds using an absorbable looped suture. *J Gynecol Surg* 1991;7:107.

Morris DM. Preoperative management of patients with evisceration. *Dis Colon Rectum* 1982;25:249.

Morrow CP, Hernandez WL, Townsend DE, et al. Pelvic celiotomy in the obese patient. *Am J Obstet Gynecol* 1977;127:335.

Moylan JA, Kennedy B. The importance of gown and drape barriers in the prevention of wound infection. *Surg Gynecol Obstet* 1980;151:465.

O'Shaughnessy M, O'Malley VP, Corbett G, et al. Optimum duration of surgical scrub time. *Br J Surg* 1991;78:685.

Olson M, O'Connor MO, Schwartz ML. A 5-year prospective study of 20,193 wounds at Minneapolis VA Medical Center. *Ann Surg* 1984;199:253.

Ortega G, Rhee DS, Papandria DJ, et al. An evaluation of surgical site infections by wound classification system using the ACS-NSQIP. *J Surg Res* 2012;174:33.

Oster PJ, Gjode P, Mortensen BB, et al. Randomized comparison of polyglycolic acid and polyglyconate sutures for abdominal fascial

III

closure after laparotomy in patients with suspected impaired wound healing. *Br J Surg* 1995;82:1080.

Osterberg B. Enclosure of bacteria within capillary multifilament sutures as protection against leukocytes. *Acta Chir Scand* 1983;149:663.

Papadia A, Ragni N, Salom EM. The impact of obesity on surgery in gynecological oncology: a review. *Int J Gynecol Cancer* 2006;16:944.

Parsons L, Ulfelder H. *Atlas of pelvic surgery*, 2nd ed. Philadelphia, PA: WB Saunders, 1968:156.

Pearl ML, Rayburn WF. Choosing abdominal incision and closure techniques. *J Reprod Med* 2004;49:662.

Peipert JF, Weitzen S, Cruickshank C, et al. Risk factors for febrile morbidity after hysterectomy. *Obstet Gynecol* 2004;103:86.

Perencevich EN, Sands KE, Cosgrove SE, et al. Health and economic impact of surgical site infections diagnosed after hospital discharge. *Emerg Infect Dis* 2003;9:196.

Peterson AF, Rosenberg A, Alatary SO. Comparative evaluation of surgical scrub preparation. *Surg Gynecol Obstet* 1978;146:63.

Pfannenstiel JH. Uber die vortheile des suprasymphysaren fascienguerschnitt fur die gynaekologischen koeliotomien. *Samml Klin Vortr Gynaekol (Leipzig) Nr 268* 1900;97:1735.

Pharmacopoeia. Pharmacopoeia Web site. http://www.pharmacopoeia.com.cn.html. Accessed April 14, 2013.

Pitkin RM. Abdominal hysterectomy in obese women. *Surg Gynecol Obstet* 1976;142:532.

Poussier M, Denève E, Blanc P, et al. A review of available prosthetic material for abdominal wall repair. *J Visc Surg* 2013;150:52. http://dx.doi.org/10.1016/j.jviscsurg.2012.10.002

Pratt JH, Irons B. Panniculectomy and abdominoplasty. *Am J Obstet Gynecol* 1978;132:165.

Pratt JH. Wound healing: evisceration. *Clin Obstet Gynecol* 1973;16:126.

Querleu D. Voies d'abord. *Techniques chirurgicales en Gynècologies*. Paris, France: Masson Ed., 1995;14.

Rahbari NN, Knefel P, Diener MK, et al. Current practice of abdominal wall closure in elective surgery-is there any consensus? *BMC Surg* 2009;9:8. doi: 10.1186/1471-2482-9-8

Rees VL, Coller FA. Anatomic and clinical study of the transverse abdominal incision. *Arch Surg* 1943;47:136.

Richards PC, Balch CM, Aldrete JS. Abdominal wound closure. *Ann Surg* 1983;197:238.

Salkind AR, Rao, KC. Antibiotic prophylaxis to prevent surgical site infections. *Am Fam Physician* 2011;83:585.

Sanz LE, Patterson JA, Kamath R, et al. Comparison of Maxon suture with Vicryl, chromic catgut, and PDS sutures in fascial closure in rats. *Obstet Gynecol* 1988;71:918.

Sanz LE, Smith S. Mechanism of wound healing, suture material, and wound closure. In: Buchsbaum HJ, Walton LA, eds. *Strategies in gynecologic surgery*. New York: Springer Verlag, 1986:53.

Savage RC. Abdominoplasty combined with other surgical procedures. *Plast Reconstr Surg* 1982;70:437.

Schimp VL, Worley C, Brunello S, et al. Vacuum-assisted closure in the treatment of gynecologic oncology wound failures. *Gynecol Oncol* 2004;92:586.

Schuchardt K. Eine neue Methode der Gebarmutterexstirpation. *Sentralbl Chir* 1893;20:1121.

Seiler CM, Bruckner T, Diener MK, et al. Interrupted or continuous slowly absorbable sutures for closure of primary elective midline abdominal incisions: a multicenter randomized trial (INSECT). *Ann Surg* 2009;249:576.

Seropian R, Reynolds BM. Wound infections after preoperative depilatory versus razor preparation. *Am J Surg* 1971;121:251.

Shepherd JH, Cavanagh D, Riggs D, et al. Abdominal wound closure using a nonabsorbable single-layer technique. *Obstet Gynecol* 1983;61:248.

Shull BL, Verheyden CN. Combined plastic and gynecologic procedures. *Ann Plast Surg* 1988;20:252.

Simchen E, Rozin R, Wax Y. The Israeli study of surgical infection of drains and the risk of wound infection in operations for hernia. *Surg Gynecol Obstet* 1990;170:331.

Stone HH, Holfling SJ, Strom PR, et al. Abdominal incisions, transverse vs. vertical placement and continuous vs. interrupted closure. *South Med J* 1983;76:1106.

Sutton G, Morgan S. Abdominal wound closure using a running, looped monofilament polybutester suture: comparison to Smead-Jones closure in historical controls. *Obstet Gynecol* 1992;80:650.

Tanner J, Norrie P, Melen K. Preoperative hair removal to reduce surgical site infection. *Cochrane Database Syst Rev* 2011;(11): CD004122. doi: 10.1002/14651858.CD004122.pub4

Tera H, Aberg C. Strength of knots in surgery in relation to type of knot, type of suture material and dimension of suture thread. *Acta Chir Scand* 1977;143:75.

Tera H, Aberg C. Tissue strength of structures involved in musculoaponeurotic layer sutures in laparotomy incisions. *Acta Chir Scand* 1976;142:349.

Tera J, Aberg C. Tensile strengths of twelve types of knot employed in surgery, using different suture materials. *Acta Chir Scand* 1976;142:1.

Thompson JB, Maclean KF, Collier FA. Role of the transverse abdominal incision and early ambulation in the reduction of postoperative complications. *Arch Surg* 1949;59:1267.

Thorek P. *Anatomy in surgery*, 3rd ed. New York: Springer-Verlag, 1985:368.

Tollefson DG, Russell KP. The transverse incision in pelvic surgery. *Am J Obstet Gynecol* 1954;68:410.

Trimbos JB, Brohim R, van Rijssel EJ. Factors relating to the volume of surgical knots. *Int J Gynaecol Obstet* 1989;30:355.

Valentine RJ, Weigelt JA, Dryer D, et al. Effect of remote infections on clean wound infection rates. *Am J Infect Control* 1986; 14:64.

van Ramshorst GH, Eker HH, Harlaar JJ, et al. Therapeutic alternatives for burst abdomen. *Surg Technol Int* 2010;19:111.

van Rissel EJC, Trimbos BJ, Booster MH. Mechanical performance of square knots and sliding knots in surgery: a comparative study. *Am J Obstet Gynecol* 1990;162:93.

van't Riet M, Steyerberg EW, Nellensteyn J, et al. Meta-analysis of techniques for closure of midline abdominal incisions. *Br J Surg* 2002;89:1350.

Velasco E, Thuler LC, Martins CA, et al. Risk factors for infectious complications after abdominal surgery for malignant disease. *Am J Infect Control* 1996;24:1.

Venturi ML, Attinger CE, Mesbahi AN, et al. Mechanisms and clinical applications of the vacuum-assisted closure (VAC) device: a review. *Am J Clin Dermatol* 2005;6:185.

Von Fraunhofer JA, Chu CC. Mechanical properties. In: Chu CC, von Fraunhofer JA, Greisler HP, eds. *Wound closure biomaterials and devices*. Boca Roton, FL: CRC Press, 1997:111.

Voss SC, Sharp HC, Scott JP. Abdominoplasty combined with gynecologic surgical procedures. *Obstet Gynecol* 1986;67:181.

Vowden K, Voweden P. Wound bed preparation. Retrieved from: http://www.worldwidewounds.com/2002/april/Vowden/WoundBed-Preparation.html#Fig8. March 2002.

Wallace D, Hernandez W, Schlaerth JB, et al. Prevention of abdominal wound disruption utilizing the Smead-Jones closure technique. *Obstet Gynecol* 1980;56:226.

Walsh C, Scaife C, Hopf H. Prevention and management of surgical site infections in morbidly obese women. *Obstet Gynecol* 2009:113:411.

Walters MD, Dombroski RA, Davidson SA, et al. Reclosure of disrupted abdominal incisions. *Obstet Gynecol* 1990;76:597.

Webster J, Osborne S. Preoperative bathing or showering with skin antiseptics to prevent surgical site infections. *Cochrane Database Syst Rev* 2012;(9):CD004985. doi: 10.1002/14651858.CD004985. pub4

Wechter ME, Pearlman MD, Hartman KE. Reclosure of the disrupted laparotomy wound: a systematic review. *Obstet Gynecol* 2005;106:376.

Weiland DE, Bay RC, Del Sordi S. Choosing the best abdominal closure by meta-analysis. *Am J Surg* 1998;176:666.

Witte MB, Barbul A. Role of nitric oxide in wound repair. *Am J Surg* 2002;183:406.

CHAPTER 15
Principles of Electrosurgery and Laser Energy Applied to Gynecologic Surgery

Ted L. Anderson and May S. Thomassee

DEFINITIONS

Active electrode—The electrode in monopolar circuits that carries the radiofrequency energy to the patient operative site.

Active electrode monitoring—A system with a sleeve placed around the active electrode to detect stray energy and to carry the induced energy to ground. Stray energy generally occurs from breaks in insulation or capacitive coupling.

Alternating current (AC)—Sinusoidal energy waveform (60 Hz) used in household electrical appliances and in electrosurgery.

Ammeter—Device that measures the amount of current flowing through a conductor at a specific moment.

Ampere—Quantity of electrons that move through a conductor over time (coulombs per second).

Bipolar—Closed circuit system where the active and passive electrodes are located within the energy device. This system does not use the patient as part of the circuit.

BLEND—Variation of electrical "on" and "off" time, where the current is interrupted at a variation of time, other than the standard CUT and COAG settings. (The current is "on" usually between 25% and 50% and varies with each BLEND setting.)

Capacitance—The buildup of electrical charge surrounding the active blade or even insulator of an electrosurgical device.

Capacitive coupling—Occurs when two conductors are separated by an insulator. Is always present, but not always dangerous. Becomes dangerous when the discharge of electrical energy occurs outside of the surgeon's field of view or when it is not recognized as conducting energy to nearby tissue through electromagnetic current.

Circuit—An electrical network that has a closed loop giving a delivery and return path for electrical current, accomplishing work by routing electrons.

COAG—Function on electrosurgical unit to describe interrupted, modulated, or damped current. The voltage of this waveform is always, higher than it is with CUT waveforms, given the same power output.

Coulomb—Measure of a quantity of electrons.

Current (power) density—Total amount of energy output per unit area of tissue. Affected by size of active electrode, shape, and power output (settings) of electrosurgical generator. Measured in watts (W). The smaller the spot of contact, the greater the density (current concentrated at the surface area of an electrode in contact with tissue during electrical flow) and the greater the heat effect for the same amount of time. Related to the square root of the area of contact.

Current (amperes)—Flow rate of a quantity (coulombs) of electrons.

CUT—Function on electrosurgical unit to describe uninterrupted, unmodulated, or undamped current in a continuous sinusoidal waveform. At the same power settings, the voltage of the waveform is always lower than it is with COAG or BLEND waveforms.

Desiccation—A form of coagulation achieved by "drying out" tissue through making contact with the active electrode. Either CUT or COAG waveforms may be used, but CUT waveform is preferable to reduce depth of penetration. Intracellular temperature stays below 100°C, which leads to cell shrinkage and dehydration.

Direct coupling—Occurs when two conductive materials in the same circuit touch during electrical activation or are close enough that arcing can occur. This can be intentional or unintentional. A break in the insulation of an active electrode that allows sparking to tissue is an example of unintended direct coupling.

Dwell time—Length of time an activated electrosurgical device is held at a specific tissue location.

Edge density—Affinity of electrons to concentrate at the edges of flat or irregularly shaped electrodes as they exit the electrode. This feature enhances the cutting ability of blade-shaped electrodes.

Electricity—Movement of electrons between two oppositely charged poles, positive and negative.

Electrocautery—Use of electricity to heat an object with subsequent direct transfer of energy by heat, such as a hot iron. Electrons do not move into the affected tissue; only heat is transferred.

Electrosurgery—Concentrated transfer kinetic energy (via electrons) from an active electrode to tissue creating a passive transfer of heat, using an electrosurgical generator.

Energy (joules)—Quantity of work produced over time. Energy (joules) equals work (watts) multiplied by time (seconds).

Faradic effect—Stimulation of tetanic muscle contractions, including cardiac muscle, when using electrical current with radiofrequency less than 100,000 cycles per second.

Fulguration—A form of coagulation achieved by arcing or spraying of "sparks" to tissue surface using high-voltage, damped, or interrupted (COAG) function with active electrode not touching tissue. Immediately causes charring and carbonization of the superficial tissue. Used to coagulate bleeding vessel or for treatment of endometriosis.

Heat (thermal energy)—Produced as electrons move from the low resistance of an electrosurgical probe to the high resistance of tissue. This energy may boil (vaporize) or denature (coagulate) tissue, depending on the extent and rapidity with which heat is generated.

Hertz (Hz)—Unit of measurement of electromagnetic sine wave. 1 Hz = 1 cycle per second.

Hybrid laparoscopic trocar sleeve—Conductive trocar sleeve used in laparoscopy that is covered by an outer nonconductive locking sleeve. Not used often anymore.

Impedance (ohms)—Resistance to flow of electrons through a conductor. Although resistance refers to direct current through a uniform wire, such as copper, it is generally substituted for impedance. Impedance is correctly applied with changes in voltage (alternating or fluctuating), frequency (modulating or demodulating), or tissue type (lipid membranes, soft tissue, fibrous tissue, fat, muscle, bone, or artificial appliances). It can measure the combination of tissue resistance and capacitance. Impedance in human tissue is generally 100 to 1,000 V; in the fallopian tube, it is 400 to 500 V.

Isolation ground circuitry—Safety feature that uses transformers not in contact with the parent generator so that the induced flow "floats" its own separate circuit. If a break in the floating circuit occurs, all energy within that circuit stops and does not seek ground.

Kilohertz (kHz)—Equal to 1,000 cycles of electromagnetic radio waves per second.

Kinetic energy—The energy that an object possesses due to its motion.

Monopolar—Type of electrode or electrical system in which the active electrode is small (high current density) and the passive electrode is large (low current density), and they are located remotely from each other. Most monopolar generators are calibrated against a 500-V load of resistance.

Open circuit (open "activation")—State when the electrosurgical instrument is activated prior to touching the tissue. A charge density can build up at the tip of the electrode and spark or stray to an unintended site if activated for a prolonged period of time remote from the site of intended effect. Open circuitry is used to start fulguration.

Return electrode (passive or dispersive electrode)—Large conductive pad (low current density) placed on the patient to complete an electrosurgical pathway and return electrosurgical energy to the generator.

Return electrode monitoring—A system of modern electrosurgical generators whereby the return electrode consists of a dual pad system with internal monitoring capabilities to sound an alarm on the generator if not placed properly.

Radiofrequency—High-frequency electrical current in the range of 3 kilohertz (kHz) to 300 gigahertz (GHz), or 3,000 to 3 billion cycles per second.

Sparking (arcing)—Transmission of electrical energy through gas (air, argon). Used in a noncontact technique with COAG interrupted waveform for tissue fulguration.

Vaporization—Raising the cellular temperature rapidly above 100°C, which causes cell wall rupture, releasing steam. CUT mode is preferred for this with a noncontact technique.

Voltage (volts)—Electromotive force (pressure) that drives current.

Watts (work)—Amount of work produced by electron flow (current). Work (watts) equals force (volts) multiplied by current rate (amperes).

Waveform—The pattern of sinusoidal oscillation of an alternating electrical current from positive to negative.

Waveform frequency—Number of oscillations of an alternating electrical current, usually between 350,000 and 4 million cycles per second in electrosurgery.

INTRODUCTION

The practice of medicine and surgery has increasingly relied on applications of energy since the late 1800s. Indeed, the majority of gynecologic surgical procedures performed today incorporate some form of applied energy. However, the underlying physical principles that govern the desired biologic effects remain marginally understood by most surgeons. The typical resident graduating from an obstetrics and gynecology program has received limited formal training concerning the principles and application of electrosurgery, as was often the case for his or her faculty mentors. Importantly, these limitations in a surgeon's knowledge of electrosurgical principles can permit delivery of unintended energy, resulting in immediate or delayed complications.

Over the past decade, electrosurgical instruments and generators have evolved into complex systems that can interact with biophysical properties of tissues to modulate, limit, and even discontinue energy delivery in response to measured parameters. In some cases, multiple energy modalities can be delivered by the same instrument. Thus, it is imperative that the contemporary gynecologic surgeon has a comfortable

working knowledge of energy generation, delivery, and tissue effects in order to use these devices and systems effectively and safely.

Our goal in this chapter is to provide the basic fundamental principles of electrosurgery and laser technology. More specifically, we wish to provide a very practical approach that illustrates how these are applied within the field of gynecologic surgery to promote safe use of the available instruments.

HISTORY AND THE DEVELOPMENT OF ELECTROSURGERY

As early as the 4th century BC, the Egyptians described the treatment of wounds using a device called a "fire drill," which turned rapidly to produce heat along its shaft. In the early writings of the Hippocratic Corpus (approximately 400 BC), followers of Hippocrates described the treatment of various tumors, as well as hemorrhoids, through direct application of heat. During this period, the use of heat was frequently accomplished through specific heating of a metal device and placing it directly on the wound, essentially inflicting third-degree burns without the ability to modulate tissue effect. Accordingly, the word "cautery" arose from the Greek term *kauterion*, meaning "hot iron." Around 1600, the English physician and scientist William Gilbert introduced the term *electricus* meaning "like amber" as he discovered attraction of objects to each other after rubbing them against an amber rod. Once electricity was widely available, this concept was further expanded to "electrocautery." *Electrocautery* is the use of electricity to heat the metal tip of a device and subsequently apply direct heat to the tissue. Thus, up until this point, all applications of heat to medicine were in the form of cautery or electrocautery.

It was actually Benjamin Franklin's eighteenth century experiments with electricity that led to the idea that direct application of electrical current to tissue might be used to advantage in medicine. While John Wesley (England), Johann Kruger (Germany), and Jean-Antoine Nollet (France) experimented with paralytic conditions, Franklin and his Dutch colleague Jan Ingenhousz described a "highly elated state" after several unintended nonlethal shocks to the head and proposed this as therapy for melancholy.

Two significant discoveries paved the way for modern application of electricity in medicine. First was the recognition of electromagnetic induction by Michael Faraday and Robert Todd, leading to the ability to harness and store electrical energy reliably. This gave rise to a pathway for development of electrosurgical generators. The second was an extension of the work of Luigi Galvani, who demonstrated that electricity applied to frog legs induced muscle contraction, when William Morton and Arsenne D'Arsonval recognized application of electricity at a frequency of greater than 100 kHz allowed electricity to pass through the body without inducing pain or burn and without inducing muscle (including cardiac) spasm, the so-called faradic effect. D'Arsonval further noted that the current directly influenced body temperature, oxygen absorption, and carbon dioxide elimination, increasing each as the current passed through the body. Of note, the temperature was determined to increase proportionally to the square of the "current density."

The French surgeon Joseph Rivière in the early 1900s was perhaps the first to use electricity clinically, in the form of an electrical shock to treat a hand ulcer. However, in the 1920s, it was Grant Ward who demonstrated that a continuous sinusoidal electrical waveform was superior for cutting tissue, and an interrupted electrical sinusoidal waveform resulted in more effective coagulation. This led to the now infamous collaboration between Harvey Cushing and physicist William Bovie to produce an electrosurgical unit (ESU) (generator) designed to achieve intraoperative hemostasis during neurosurgical procedures. They published the results of a case series of intracranial tumor excisions in 1928, with an excerpt by Dr. Bovie describing the principles of superficial dehydration (desiccation), cutting, and coagulation as they applied to the tissue. These landmark events led to the era of modern applications of electricity in medicine.

BASIC PRINCIPLES OF ELECTROSURGERY

Electrocautery and electrosurgery are not synonymous. We distinguish between the two terms electrocautery and electrosurgery based on many differences as described in this chapter. *Electrocautery* refers to the application of electric current to an instrument of high resistance, resulting in heating, and then applying this hot instrument for direct transfer of heat to destroy tissue, without the ability to modify the depth of tissue penetration or tissue effect. For example, as described earlier, this would be like burning the skin with a hot iron. Conversely, *electrosurgery* is the employment of kinetic energy in the form of alternating current (AC) radiofrequency to transfer energy to tissue, raising intracellular temperature, which can be modulated to achieve desired tissue effects.

In order to achieve electrosurgery, there are three specific elements we must have. First, there must be a generator or ESU to accept electricity delivered from the electrical outlet on the wall of the operating room, modulate it to a higher frequency, and deliver it in the required conformation. Second, there must be an active electrode to deliver electricity to the tissue of interest in the form required. Third, there must be a return electrode to deliver the electricity away from the tissue to complete the electrical circuit.

The flow of electricity from an ESU through tissue follows the basic principles of physics. Particles of energy (*electrons*) are forced through tissue in a maximal direction from a positively charged pole to a negatively charged pole, in a sinusoidal waveform. The term circuit is used to describe the path the electrons take. In electric circuits, electricity is typically carried through conductors such as wire. However, electricity can also be carried through ion-containing substances like living tissue. Electron flow through cells creates changes in polarity of the cellular electrolytes (Na^+, Ca^{++}, K^+, Cl^-, etc.). Electromagnetic energy causes the anions to migrate toward the positive electrode and cations toward the negative, which is referred to as the galvanic effect. Importantly, the high-frequency flow of electrons in the radiofrequency spectrum surpasses that required for cellular membrane depolarization and does not affect the opening of sodium or calcium channels. Rather, the frictional forces of these charged intracellular ions create kinetic excitation and subsequent intracellular thermal heating as a result of thermodynamic changes.

The flow of electrons through a conductor is called *current,* which is governed by two opposing forces, namely *voltage* (the force pushing electrons along a circuit) and *resistance* (opposition to the free flow of electrons). This relationship is defined by Ohm law, which is depicted in **Figure 15.1**. You can see from this relationship that in order to increase electron flow (current), you must either increase the electromotive force (voltage) or decrease the impedance to free flow (resistance).

$$\text{Current (I)} \atop \text{(amps)} = \frac{\text{Voltage (V) (volts)}}{\text{Resistance (R) (ohms)}}$$

FIGURE 15.1 Ohm law describes the flow of electrons through a circuit.

It may help to think of this in terms of water flowing through a hose in your garden. If you kink the hose (increase resistance), your water flow (current) is going to decrease. The only way to accommodate for this is to increase the water pressure (voltage) proportionally.

We can further explore the relationship between resistance and voltage by examining the concept of *power*, defined as the instantaneous energy required per unit time to perform a function, measured in watts. Specifically, power is defined by the electromotive force (voltage) times the flow of electrons (current), or $W = V \times I$. With mathematical substitution of Ohm law ($I = V/R$), we can derive that power (watts) is related to the voltage squared divided by resistance, or $W = V^2/R$. In practical terms, this means that as resistance increases, in order to maintain the power required to perform a function, the electromotive force (voltage) must increase exponentially. As we shall see, it is the voltage that we must harness and control to accomplish electrosurgical tasks effectively and safely. If we go back to our hose analogy, this means that if you increase resistance (kink the hose), in order to maintain the watts or instantaneous energy required per unit time to perform a function of work (to water the garden), the voltage (water pressure) must increase. Therein, we have the basic mathematical and physical basis for applied electrosurgery.

ELECTROSURGICAL GENERATORS

Generators of ESUs deliver AC the surgical field carried by an electrosurgical instrument (active electrode). More specifically, the ESU must take the electrical current supplied from the wall outlet and change it to direct current. Then, through the use of oscillators, it must be modulated back to AC with higher frequency and the appropriate characteristics needed to produce the desired effects on tissues. The frequency delivered is between 500,000 and 5 million cycles per second and is sufficiently rapid to avoid stimulation of muscle contraction by surpassing the threshold for calcium and sodium channel depolarization. Because this frequency is in the range of AM radio waves, it is often referred to as radiofrequency (RF) current. Frequencies below 100,000 cycles per second are capable of causing tetanic muscle contraction, which is referred to as the *faradic effect*. On occasion, harmonic demodulation can occur, which produces small amounts of RF at less than 100,000 Hz presumably by alteration of current through interactions with the biophysical environment, which produces minor muscle twitches or nerve stimulation. Conversely, usual household appliances, such as hair dryers or blenders, use 60 cycles per second (or 60 Hertz, Hz) and are at much lower frequency than that of electrosurgical instrumentation (Fig. 15.2).

Most modern solid-state ESUs are capable of producing over 8,000 V, which is capable of pushing electrons up to 3 mm in room air under standard atmospheric conditions. However, more common outputs in typical use are in the 1,000 to 3,000 V range with a frequency upward of 350,000 Hz. Further, most generators today are calibrated to power output, with the power set reflecting the power available at the start of the electrosurgical application. As tissue impedance increases with heating in response to applied energy, we know from our prior calculations that power decreases. Additionally, many modern ESUs are best described as adaptive generators. Often designed to work in concert with specific instruments, they have the ability to adjust computer-controlled output in real time. They measure tissue impedance at the operative site and modulate output accordingly. Additionally, there are features for limiting maximum voltage, thereby reducing unintended effects of "stray energy."

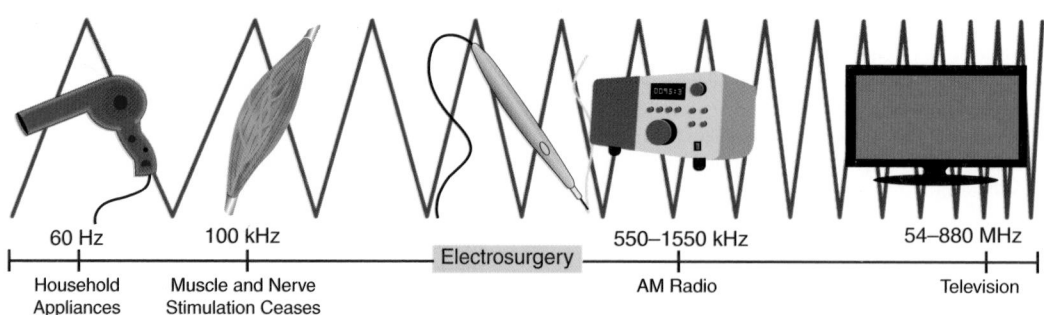

60 Hz	100 kHz	Electrosurgery	550–1550 kHz	54–880 MHz
Household Appliances	Muscle and Nerve Stimulation Ceases		AM Radio	Television

FIGURE 15.2 Radiofrequency spectrum. The frequency produced by electrosurgical generators overlaps with the range of AM radio waves and is thus referred to as "radiofrequency" (RF).

Three fundamental principles that have guided the evolution of the modern ESU are "electricity must complete a circuit or it will not flow," "electricity goes to ground," and "electricity follows the path of least resistance." Older generator models were ground referenced, which means that a "grounding pad" was required to return the electrical current delivered to the patient (complete the electrical circuit). However, given the other principles just mentioned, currents often traveled through alternative grounding pathways, including EKG clips, creating unintended patient thermal injury. Isolated ESUs were introduced in the late 1960s, whereby current delivered by the ESU was returned to the ESU, not to ground, to complete the circuit. Further, the current delivered to the patient was generated in transformers insulated from the ESU frame. Thus, when the electrical circuit is interrupted, the electrons do not seek ground; no current flows. This introduced the concept of "return electrode" rather than "grounding pad," although the two terms are often (incorrectly) used interchangeably. This advancement dramatically reduced thermal injury hazards associated with earlier grounded systems. However, if return electrodes were not properly or completely placed, or if they began to peel off intraoperatively, burns could occur at these sites due to electrical arching and increased charge density.

Return electrode monitoring was introduced in the 1980s. In this system, still used today, return electrodes consist of two side-by-side conductive pads. Built-in monitors measure integrity of pad contact with skin and balance of contact between the two pads through a low-impedance feedback with the ESU. If there is an imbalance, poor contact, or a breach in contact, an alarm sounds and generator output is automatically discontinued. It should be noted that for these return electrodes to function effectively, both pads should be equal distance from the operative field with the largest edge facing the site.

MONOPOLAR AND BIPOLAR

All modern ESUs offer the ability to modulate electrical current output. The radiofrequency output can be delivered in *monopolar* or *bipolar* circuits (see Figs. 15.3 and 15.5 below). Further, radiofrequency can be delivered by providing a continuous or interrupted pattern RF energy. By convention, we typically refer to these two patterns as *CUT* and *COAG* (respectively) in homage to the description of tissue effects by Ward and Bovie in the 1920s.

Of course, *monopolar* current is a misnomer, as all electrical circuits must be bipolar. The more appropriate distinction would be the location of the active and return electrodes with respect to each other. With monopolar circuits, the active electrode (instrument delivering RF energy) and the return electrode (sometimes called dispersive or passive electrode) are located remotely from each other. Thus, the RF energy enters the body (conductor) through the active electrode and is dispersed through a myriad of pathways following the path of least resistance to the return electrode to complete the electrical circuit (Fig. 15.3). The concentration

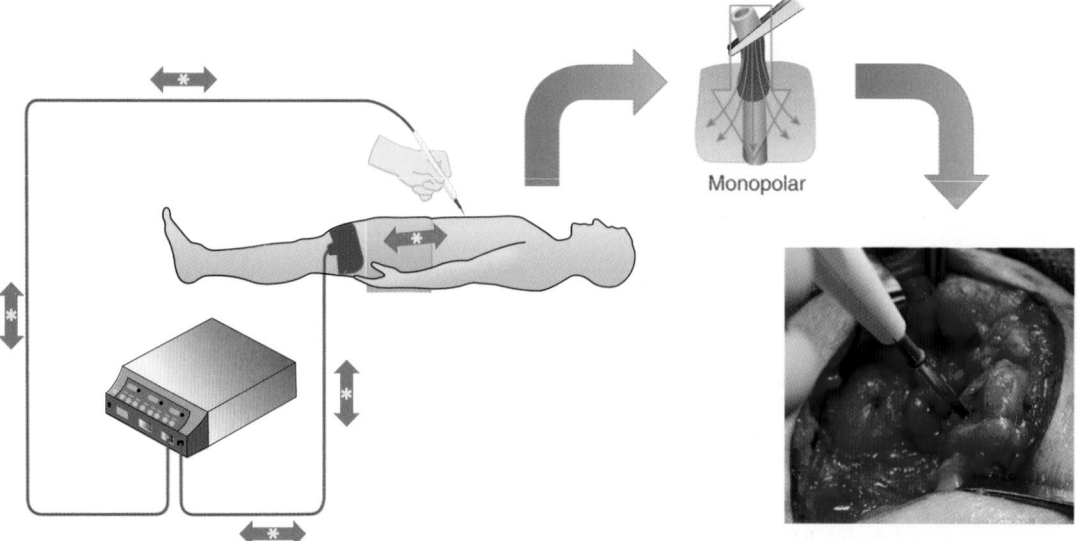

Monopolar

FIGURE 15.3 Monopolar electrical circuit. RF is delivered from the ESU through an active electrode to the patient, is dispersed through the patient, and is returned to the ESU via a remotely placed return electrode to complete the circuit.

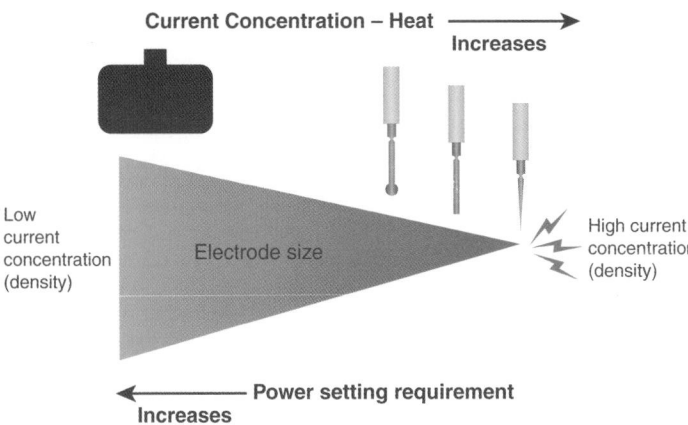

Current Concentration – Heat ⟶ **Increases**

Low current concentration (density)

Electrode size

High current concentration (density)

⟵ **Power setting requirement** **Increases**

FIGURE 15.4 Current density. The higher concentration of RF energy at the active electrode is responsible for the tissue effect achieved at that site. Increasing the electrode size decreases charge density and lessens the local effect. Further, as electrical current radiates away from the active electrode, the tissue effect is dramatically decreased.

III

of RF energy at the active electrode is responsible for local tissue effect (e.g., burn) at that site. Conversely, the dispersed nature of RF energy through the body and at the site of the return electrode explains why there is minimal, if any, recognizable effect. This concept is known as "current density." You may notice this concept readily when comparing the tissue effect using a standard electrosurgical spatula electrode with the edge versus the wide face of the blade facing the tissue. This is further illustrated by the increased tissue effect when using a needle tip electrode without decreasing the ESU output (Fig. 15.4).

In bipolar circuits, the active and return electrodes are components of the same instrument. The charge density is basically identical at both electrodes. The only part of the patient involved in the circuit is that tissue directly located between the electrodes (Fig. 15.5).

In monopolar circuits, RF energy may be delivered either in a continuous waveform or in interrupted pulses electrical current, referred to as *CUT* or *COAG*, respectively, in deference to tissue effect described by Grant Ward in the 1920s. In CUT mode, there is delivery of a continuous uninterrupted sinusoidal waveform through the active electrode (continuous

duty cycle). Alternatively, in COAG mode, the RF energy is delivered in pulses whereby over a given time RF energy is only delivered approximately 4% of the time (interrupted duty cycle). During the "off time," desiccated, cooled, and coagulated tissue with denatured proteins increases resistance and thus increases voltage required for energy delivery. Most ESUs offer a "BLEND" mode in which the duty cycle is increased to 40%, but off 60% of the time, allowing for a mixture of cutting and coagulation properties (Fig. 15.6).

In bipolar circuits, RF energy is delivered by the ESU in CUT setting, which is a continuous sinusoidal waveform with low voltage. Modern instruments available to use in the bipolar mode also employ use of compressive force to reduce vascular pulse pressure and subsequently blood flow through the intervening tissue. This further helps the energy to remain concentrated between the electrodes in order to achieve maximal desired tissue effect. Further, there is often the incorporation of feedback mechanisms to determine when the intervening tissue is sufficiently desiccated. This feedback allows an adaptive ESU to recognize increased tissue resistance and discontinue energy delivery when complete tissue effect has been achieved.

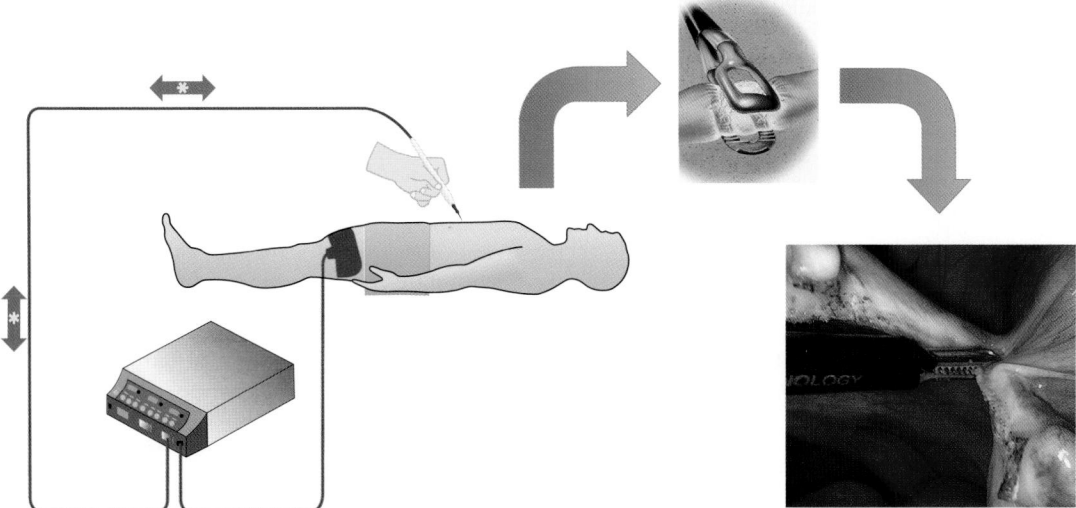

FIGURE 15.5 Bipolar electrical circuit. RF is delivered from the ESU through an active electrode to the patient and is returned to the ESU via return electrode located in the same instrument to complete the circuit. Only the tissue located between the electrodes is involved in the circuit.

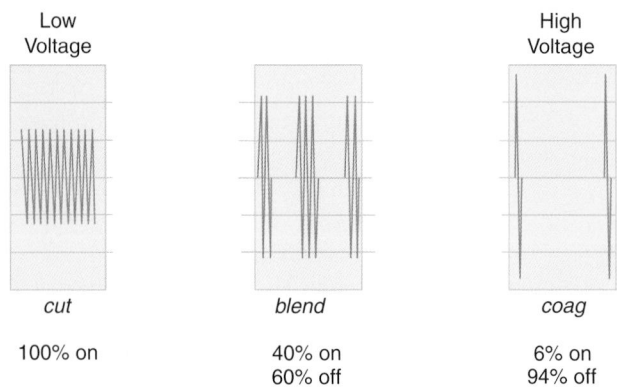

FIGURE 15.6 Continuous (CUT) versus interrupted (COAG) duty cycles differ in the duration that RF energy is delivered over time and by the voltage required to deliver that energy. Most generators offer a BLEND mode that offers some features of both extremes by varying the duration of the duty cycle.

TISSUE EFFECTS

Although the terms "CUT" and "COAG" have become ingrained in our electrosurgical lexicon, it is more useful to think of waveform and technique with respect to the tissue effect achieved. RF energy may be used to cut through tissue via rapid increase in temperature in a noncontact mode (vaporize) or coagulate tissue through slow deep dehydration and denaturation of proteins (desiccate) or by the superficial spray of electrons (fulgurate), often resulting in tissue carbonization (Table 15.1). Temperature changes have been identified with each of these effects. Normal resting human physiologic temperature is 37°C. Irreversible damage in tissue occurs at ≥50°C by intracellular protein denaturation and coagulation. Cellular dehydration (evaporation of water) occurs when tissue is heated to ≥90°C, which is referred to as *desiccation*. Rapid temperature rise to ≥100°C will cause cell walls to rupture as liquid water changes to steam by a process known as *vaporization*. At temperatures ≥250°C, tissues begin to char and carbonize leading to a *fulguration* effect.

As mentioned earlier, the CUT mode delivers a continuous sinusoidal waveform alternating from positive to negative at the frequency output of the ESU. This RF, delivered through a small active electrode (high current density), generates rapid and intense intracellular heat, which vaporizes the surrounding cells. The steam vapor occupies a space much greater than the water of the cell, creating two effects. First, it literally explodes the cells. Second, and equally importantly, it dissipates the heat generated to reduce thermal damage to adjacent tissue. Consequently, there is little or no coagulation effect. This mode is used to maximal advantage if the RF energy is engaged immediately before touching the tissue. If the active electrode is moved too slowly, or allowed to dwell in one spot too long, the tissue becomes dehydrated, resistance is increased, and tissue is more slowly dehydrated (desiccated). Therefore, for efficient and effective cutting of tissue, the surgeon should use a continuous waveform (CUT) with a small or thin active electrode that is activated just prior to tissue contact. With a peak voltage of about 200 V, the ionized air facilitates a layer of steam as the electrode glides by exploding cells with minimal surrounding heat or tissue coagulation.

In the COAG mode with a frequency of 500 kHz, bursts of RF energy occur over 31,000 times per second. However, this accounts for less than 5% of the time in pure COAG mode. It is during the "off" intervals that tissue is cooled and denatured (coagulated), which increases resistance. If the COAG waveform had the same peak voltage as the CUT waveform, the average power delivered per unit time would be less because the RF energy is off the majority of the time. In order to deliver the same power, the COAG waveform must deliver the same average voltage as the CUT waveform. To do so, there must be large peak voltages during the percentage of time that the RF energy is being delivered (Fig. 15.7). The high-voltage sparks created are more widely dispersed, and, due to the intermittent heating effect, cellular temperature does not increase rapidly or sufficiently to vaporize. Consequently, cells are more slowly dehydrated and do not explode to create an incision in tissue, but greater tissue resistance is the result. Because of the higher peak voltage (greater electromotive force), COAG waveforms can drive current through higher resistances, which permit fulguration (superficial), even after dehydration has occurred, and deeper desiccation of tissue. Fulguration and desiccation are both forms of tissue coagulation. With desiccation, concentration of current is related to the area of tissue contact with the active electrode. This creates deep penetration of heat and minimal charring of the tissue surface. On the other hand, fulguration occurs when (noncontact) superficial sparking occurs. Due to the high peak voltage at high current density, the sparks are sprayed in a random fashion in repeated intermittent cycles, resulting in tissue necrosis and charring. Given equal current density, noncontact fulguration is more efficient at creating surface necrosis and charring. However, contact desiccation yields a greater depth of tissue dehydration.

Coaptive coagulation is a term that refers to grasping of a bleeding vessel with a conductive metal instrument using sufficient pressure to stop blood flow. Subsequently, the active electrode is used to transfer energy through the instrument, causing coagulation and protein denaturation of the tissue. The surface of the tissue is coagulated first, with subsequent desiccation of the deeper tissue. The CUT waveform should always be used during coaptive coagulation since it has lower voltage and will reduce the chance of desiccation of the surrounding tissue.

Desired tissue effects can vary based on multiple factors and are not as simple as using CUT current when "cutting" is needed and COAG current when "coagulation" is needed. In 1928, Bovie described three distinct tissue effects of electrosurgery: *superficial dehydration*, *cutting*, and *tissue coagulation*. Superficial dehydration involves using the active electrode at a very short distance above the tissue, not in contact with, and causing electron "spraying" across the surface for dehydration of a thin layer of tissue. The cutting mechanism involves using current to separate the tissues ahead of the active electrode without using the electrode as a manual cutting device. This technique relies on an arc of electrons ahead of the electrode tip, prior to contacting the tissue. This method can be altered to perform coagulation by "damping" or interrupting the waveform to produce a coagulation effect in highly vascular tissue, while current remains the same. Lastly, he described tissue coagulation ("electrocoagulation") in which an electrode cannot perform the same effects as that of cutting. This type of tissue manipulation is based on two factors, the current density at the electrode tip and the dwell time of the activated instrument. The larger the area of tissue to be

TABLE 15.1 Tissue Effect Can Be Altered by Altering the Waveform and using the Active Electrode with a Contact or Noncontact Technique

	NO CONTACT	CONTACT
CUT (continuous)	Vaporization	Desiccation
COAG (interrupted)	Fulguration	Desiccation

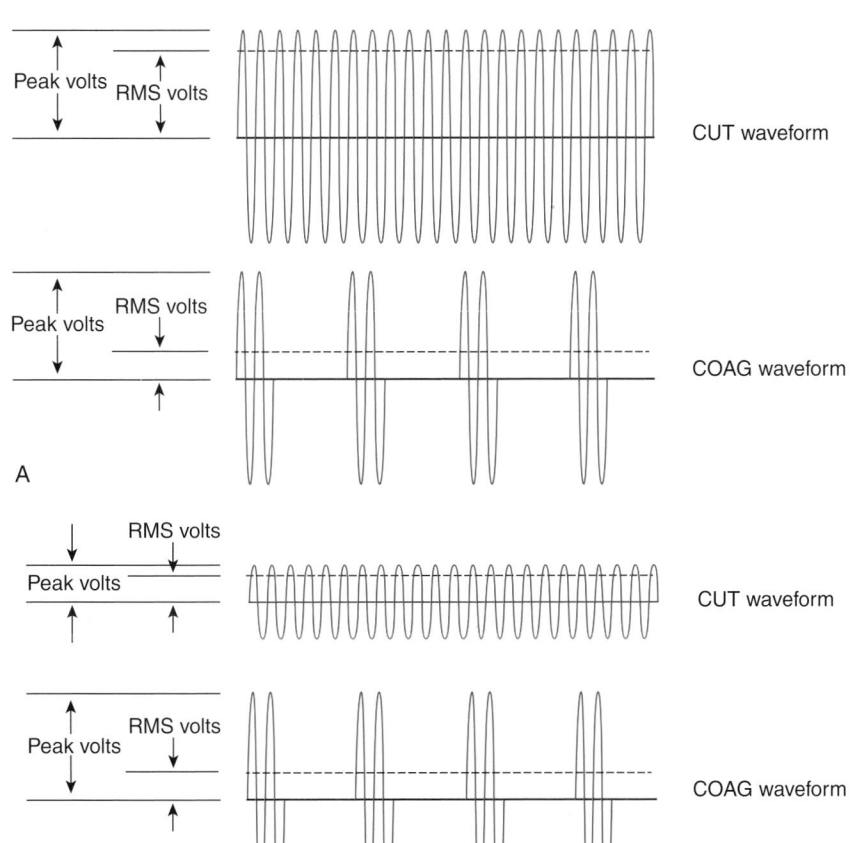

FIGURE 15.7 When the voltage is the same between pure CUT and pure COAG current, the amount of power delivered in COAG is only one third that of CUT. Conversely, when the power is the same between pure CUT and pure COAG current, the peak voltage of COAG is about three times greater than that of CUT. (RMS, root mean square.)

coagulated, the weaker the current needed with a longer dwell time. If a stronger current is used, the superficial tissue becomes quickly dehydrated or carbonized, causing cessation of flow to the surrounding tissue. If the dwell time is activated for longer than necessary to achieve the desired effect, there is possibility of unintended stray current to nearby tissues.

To achieve numerous desired tissue effects, the surgeon can use a combination of waveforms, current waveforms, active electrode characteristics, and surgical technique (Fig. 15.8). We have already discussed the effects achieved by electrode contact versus noncontact (Table 15.1) and different waveforms (Figs. 15.6 and 15.7). Additional manipulation of tissue effects may be accomplished by altering the size of the electrode, which controls current density. A needle tip electrode will yield greater current density than the broad surface of an electrosurgical bladed electrode. Therefore, at a given power using a continuous waveform, the needle tip electrode will produce quicker higher temperatures favoring vaporization (cutting), whereas

the broad blade will result in a lower current density and slower and lower rise in temperature, favoring tissue desiccation. The speed with which the active electrode is moved can also contribute significantly to tissue effect. Recall that at an ideal speed, the active electrode glides through a path of vaporizing cells to cut tissue with minimal collateral effects. On the other hand, moving the electrode too slowly (increased dwell time) will generate increased heat in surrounding tissues resulting in a proportional degree of tissue coagulation. Once the superficial tissue is fulgurated, it acts as its own insulator. Dwelling over the same tissue longer than is required for the fulguration effect has potential to cause deeper tissue injury with potential for stray paths of electron flow. Similarly, moving the active electrode too fast will result in a continuous waveform contact mode (desiccation) as it overshoots the microenvironment of ionized air that creates a layer of steam from vaporized cells.

Finally, in order to achieve a desired tissue effect, the surgeon must take into consideration the constitution of the target tissue.

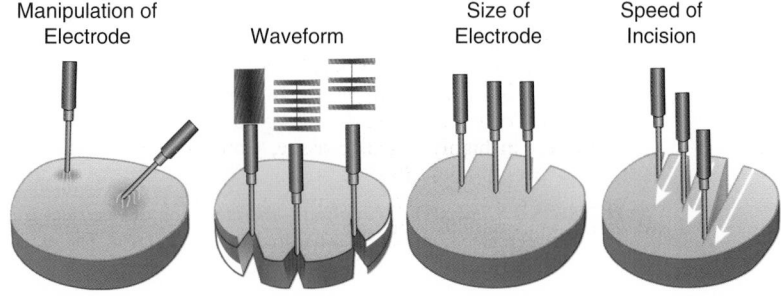

FIGURE 15.8 Variables that moderate tissue effects include electrode manipulation (contact versus noncontact), waveform (CUT versus COAG or BLEND), size of electrode (current density), and speed of active electrode movement.

Tissue impedance (resistance), which primarily depends on water content, will also affect the electrosurgical outcome. Impedance is high in desiccated tissues, moderate in adipose tissues, and very low in vascular tissues with higher water content. The impedance of tissue is dynamic during electrosurgery. Moreover, the power needed to accomplish a particular electrosurgical effect may vary from one patient to another. Lean, muscular patients are better overall conductors of electricity. Obese or emaciated patients may provide more tissue impedance to the electrical current and so may require more applied power to achieve the same effect. Power requirements to achieve a given electrosurgical effect will be higher whenever an electrode is applied to an area of higher impedance. With higher resistance, there is increased possibility of stray current seeking alternative sites of action. For example, as water evaporates and tissue coagulates, impedance rises—at times to the point that current is inhibited from flowing through the tissue. If the surgeon reflexively increases the power setting and consequently the output voltage, the current is more likely to overcome the tissue resistance and seek an alternative pathway of least resistance to the ground, which may lead to unintended thermal injury. Therefore, it is always advisable to use the lowest power setting to achieve the desired tissue effect.

ELECTROSURGERY AND PATIENT SAFETY

As we have seen, the principles of Ohm law along with the rules "electricity must complete a circuit or it will not flow," "electricity goes to ground," and "electricity follows the path of least resistance" provide the basis of predictable use of RF energy in surgical applications. However, these same principles illustrate the potential dangers of unintended energy paths. Complications arise when electrosurgical principles are not thoroughly understood and devices are not properly used. Injuries from electrosurgical devices have been reported anywhere from 2.2 to 5/1,000. Of note, these are recognized injuries at the time of surgery. Electrosurgical injuries do not always present at the time of surgery and can frequently present complications between 3 and 7 days postoperatively. It is believed that there are a larger number of unrecognized injuries, some of which do not become substantial and are thus underreported. Unintended thermal injury to tissue can be related to many factors, including direct and indirect application of energy. We discuss here examples of the most common sources of unintended energy application, potentially leading to patient injury.

Open Activation

Intentionally activating the active electrode prior to contact with tissue (open activation), the surgeon can create a fulguration effect (discussed earlier). Perhaps the best example of this is the use of a ball electrode to fulgurate the bed of a cervical loop electrosurgical excision procedure (LEEP). However, this becomes a potential hazard when the active electrode is at a sufficient distance away from the target tissue (e.g., activating the RF energy in a laparotomy incision when the active electrode is a few inches away from the target). The energy charge builds up at the tip of the electrode as it encounters the very high resistance of air. With sufficient power, the electromotive force (voltage) can cause the RF energy to discharge the energy across the resistance of the insulator to the nearest (often unintended) site, much like a lightning bolt discharge.

Direct Coupling

Direct coupling occurs when an active electrode comes into contact with a conductive instrument that channels RF energy

to another site (tissue) with which it is in contact. An intentional use of this principle would be passing current from an active electrode through a pair of forceps that is grasping a vessel at the operative site. A common example of untended direct coupling in laparoscopy occurs when activated monopolar scissors touch adjacent bowel graspers, causing direct transfer of RF energy to the unintended site (bowel). Alternatively, this may occur when the active electrode touches the laparoscope, which is in contact with bowel.

Insulation Failure

This type of "stray energy" perhaps occurs more frequently in laparoscopy than in laparotomy. It is frequently unrecognized, owing to the fact that less than 15% of the operative field is typically seen when using a video camera and laparoscope. Laparoscopic instruments are covered by an insulator to direct current to the active electrode at the tip of the instrument. When there is a break in the insulated shaft of an instrument, which can occur through a variety of mechanisms such as moving the instrument repeatedly through a trocar or when cleaning and processing for reuse, RF energy can discharge through these breaks with effects like that described in open activation. The bowel is a frequently affected target of stray RF energy form insulation failure. Usually, blanching of sigmoid wall (or other tissue) occurs, and the surgeon should assume that tissue destruction is deeper than is visible. This type of tissue injury (pale, blanching) has a higher likelihood of breaking down in the future. However, this may be more indirect if, for example, the RF discharge were to the laparoscope, which is in turn in contact with bowel. Should such injury to the bowel occur, the correct method of action for the bowel is excision or resection and reanastomosis.

Capacitive Coupling

Capacitance refers to the ability of an object to store an electrical charge. Capacitance coupling may occur when two conductors in proximity to one another are separated by an insulator. It is best described as a mechanism whereby electrical current in the active electrode induces a current in another nearby conductor (unintended) despite otherwise intact insulation. For example, when using an operative laparoscope, the insulated active electrode (scissors, for example) is passed through a channel within the operative scope. This produces the ideal situation for capacitive coupling of the laparoscope by the active electrode (**Fig. 15.9**).

Some degree of capacitive coupling occurs with all standard monopolar electrosurgical instruments, but it is not always

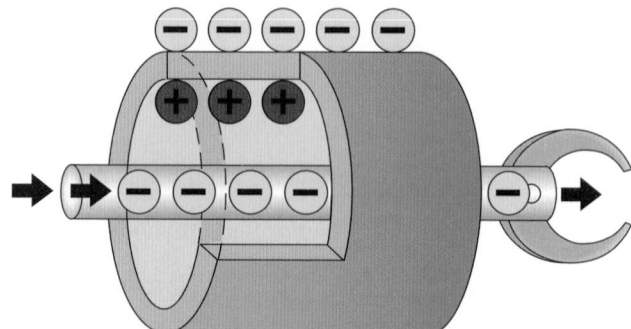

FIGURE 15.9 Capacitance coupling is the induction of electrical current between two conductors separated by an insulator. The active electrode carries active current and induces a separate current in the nearby conductor.

a hazard. Whether the "stray energy" of capacitive coupling causes clinical injury depends on (a) the total amount of current transferred, (b) the ability to prevent arcing discharge of the built-up energy to an unintended tissue target, and (c) concentration of the current (i.e., the current density) as it makes its way back to the patient return electrode. Higher voltages increase capacitive coupling. The low-voltage CUT mode exhibits less capacitive coupling than COAG does. Thin insulation decreases the effective separation of the electrode from the surrounding conductor and will increase the amount of induced current.

Common conditions exist where capacitive coupling can cause sufficient current to cause an injury. When a metal trocar is used, it can be capacitively coupled to the active electrode. Additionally, when a conventionally insulated electrode is passed through a metal suction–irrigator, approximately 70% of the current may be induced in the suction–irrigator. The same situation can occur when an active electrode is passed through the operating channel of a laparoscope. An all-metal cannula through the abdominal wall will "bleed off" stray current through the abdominal wall as the RF energy is discharged over a larger surface area on its way to the return electrode with minimal or no effect. However, if the metal trocar is anchored by a plastic sleeve in the first example, or if a plastic trocar is used, then RF energy can build up until it overcomes the impedance of surrounding air to discharge through the path of least resistance to an often unintended tissue target. Another common and rarely recognized example occurs when the wire of a monopolar electrosurgical instrument is wrapped around a hemostat attached to a surgical drape for stabilization. With prolonged use of the electrosurgical instrument, the hemostat may become charged through capacitive coupling and that electrical energy may discharge seeking ground through the path of least resistance causing a drape fire or a burn to the patient (**Fig. 15.10**).

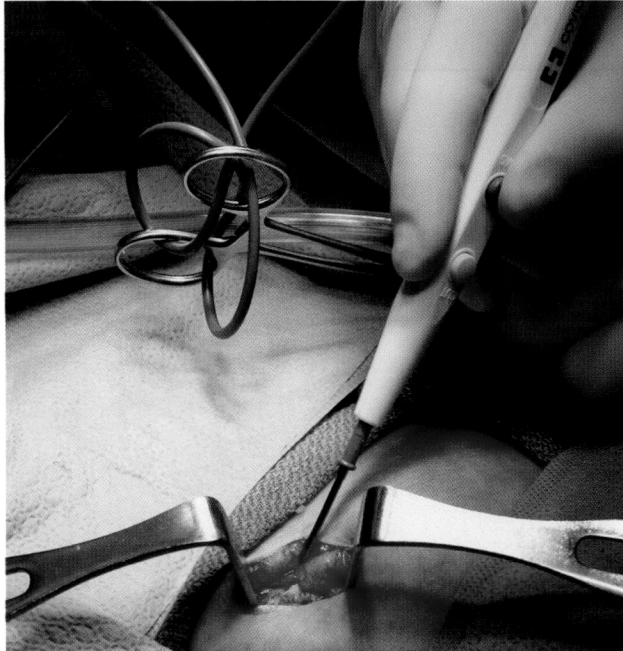

FIGURE 15.10 Securing the wire of an electrosurgical instrument to the drape with a hemostat provides an opportunity for capacitive coupling and discharge of built-up energy to create a drape fire or a patient burn.

Bipolar Instruments

Bipolar electrosurgical instruments became popular in the mid-1970s as an alternative to monopolar instruments with hopes to avoid complications of stray current as described above. Although bipolar electrosurgical instruments are safer than monopolar instruments with respect to stray RF injury, they are not without possibility of complication. It is important to remember that the zone of thermal damage may extend beyond that of the electrodes at the instrument tip. Once the tissue is sufficiently desiccated, further application of electricity can propagate heated water and subsequent steam to adjacent tissue, causing a thermal spreading effect. In order to reduce this potential, the surgeon should cease desiccation once vapor is no longer visualized and when the tissue becomes white in color.

Excessive desiccation can cause stickiness of the tissue as a result of carbonization, often referred to as an "amalgam." Additionally, the active electrode can become adherent to the tissue, due to molecular breakdown of the cellular contents into sugars if the COAG function is used improperly or for a prolonged period of time. When deep tissue desiccation is required, the CUT function should be used to ensure deep penetration of tissue. If the COAG function is used instead, in tubal sterilization for example, it can cause immediate surface char and cessation of the flow of electrons while increasing tissue impedance, increasing lateral thermal spread, and preserving patency of the underlying tubal lumen. Use of the CUT mode allows a more precise and controlled spread of energy within the tissue due to its continuous, low-voltage waveform.

When using bipolar instruments, the use of an "in-line ammeter" is recommended to help monitor the increase in tissue resistance indicating complete tissue desiccation.

ADVANCED MONOPOLAR AND BIPOLAR DEVICES

Unique instruments are now widely available that dramatically reduce the potential for injury though unintended RF energy discharge in monopolar instruments. Further, with the advent of bipolar electrosurgical devices in the mid-1970s, there came a recognized need for more versatile instruments, including the ability to offer both tissue desiccation and cutting abilities in the same instrument. Having these functions within one instrument provides more efficiency to the surgeon and avoids the need to change out surgical instruments for various tissue effects. There was a simultaneous desire to reduce the thermal spread, tissue carbonization resulting in instrument sticking, and increased "plume" formation of conventional bipolar instruments. Several instruments are now available that can be used to grasp, dissect, seal vessels up to 7 mm in diameter, and transect tissue. These tissue-sealing devices all employ the three components of pressure, temperature, and time to coapt tissue; denature and mobilize collagen and other proteins within the tissue at elevated temperatures; and fix or reorganize the collagen fibers to form a tissue seal. Then, some mechanism is used to transect the sealed tissue.

Active Electrode Monitoring

The potential for injury from capacitive coupled currents can be reduced with an understanding of the biophysics but can be eliminated by active electrode monitoring systems that "collect" stray current and confine capacitive coupling to the surgical instrument. Such a device is commercially available that eliminates the risk of capacitance regardless of the type of trocar sleeve used (Encision, Inc., Boulder, CO). This device

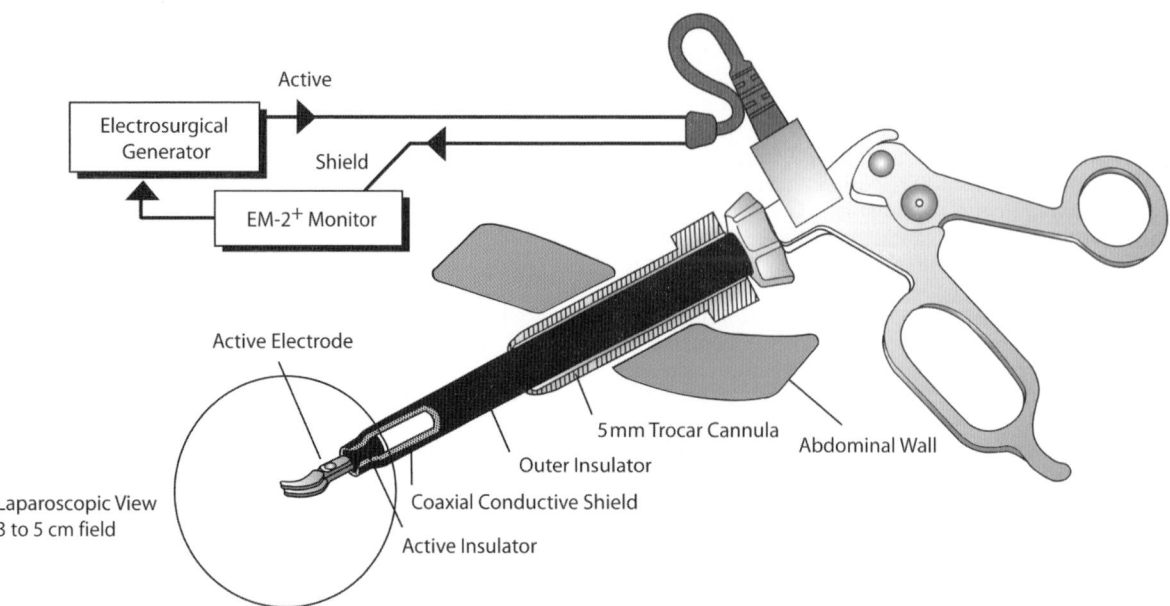

FIGURE 15.11 The Encision (formerly Electroshield) system eliminates the threat of unintentional capacitance injury when using monopolar instruments during laparoscopy by returning capacitance-induced current back to the generator. If an insulation breakdown occurs, the surgeon is alerted.

consists of a shroud over the active electrode shaft that shunts all capacitance-coupled current back through a return electrode to the electrosurgical unit, which avoids unintentional RF energy discharge. Additionally, if there is any breech in the insulation of the active electrode that could promote direct coupling to other metal instruments or adjacent tissue, the surgeon is alerted with an audible alarm (Fig. 15.11).

Argon Beam Coagulator

The argon beam coagulator is a monopolar active electrode housed inside an insulated cannula through which argon gas is dispelled at up to 12 L per minute (laparotomy) or 4 L per minute (laparoscopy). This instrument is superior for controlled noncontact superficial fulguration of tissue, owing to two unique properties of argon gas. First, electrons prefer to follow a stream of argon gas rather than pass through room air or carbon dioxide (CO_2), as each of the latter has a higher resistance to electron flow. Accordingly, because electrons choose to flow the path of least resistance, they stay collimated (parallel alignment) in the flow of argon, so sparks can be directed with efficiency. Second, the ionization properties of argon gas flowing over the active electrode enhance the distance the spark can travel to complete the circuit to the tissue surface. These properties create a bright bluish hue to the sparks, which makes them easy to see and aim at the bleeding surface (Fig. 15.12). The gas, expelled under pressure, blows the pooled blood away from the surface bleeders, making coagulation more discrete and efficient. To create the planned fulguration effect, the wand must move like a paintbrush to prevent deep tissue damage.

Plasma Kinetic Technology

The PlasmaKinetic platform (Olympus America, Center Valley, PA) employs an advanced solid-state adaptive generator with software to deliver pulsed RF energy with continuous tissue impedance. This vapor pulse coagulation generates less

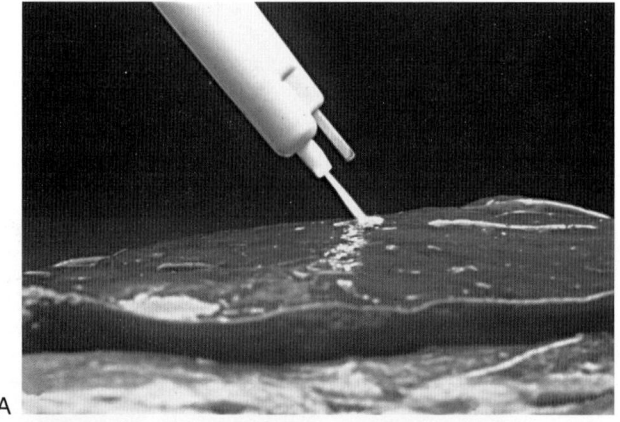

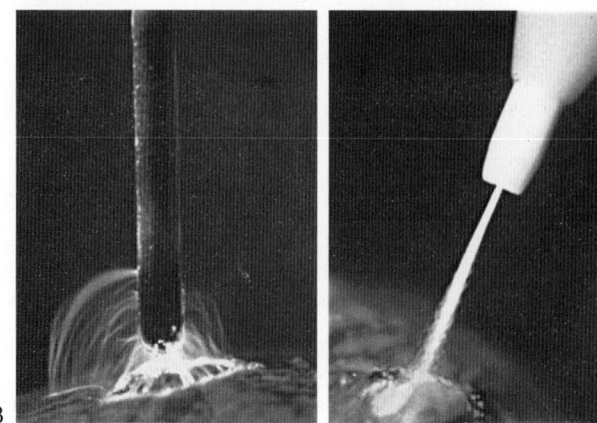

FIGURE 15.12 Argon beam coagulator. The ionized gas has its own unique blue hue that makes the sparks easily visible for accurate fulguration. **A:** The argon beam coagulator at work. **B:** Sparking effect of standard electrode (**left**) compared with argon beam coagulator (**right**).

heat overall but ensures reaching temperature for effective collagen denaturation without rapid desiccation. As the generator delivers a pulse of RF energy, tissue impedance is measured and voltage is altered (decreased) to match the impedance. In between pulses, the tissue cools, allowing for renaturation (fixing) of the collagen. This cycle continues until complete tissue sealing and desiccation has been accomplished. Instruments for use with laparoscopy, laparotomy, and vaginal surgery are available with this technology. Several related devices are available using this platform. The HALO device (Olympus America, Center Valley, PA) includes a knife blade that can be advanced after desiccation to cut the tissue. The newest device in this line (ThunderBeat) offers the option of advanced bipolar technology or a combination of advanced bipolar together with ultrasonic technology for simultaneous sealing and cutting of tissue.

LigaSure

The LigaSure device (Covidien, Boulder, CO) achieves true tissue fusion using a combination of pressure and pulsed energy to denature collagen and elastin in tissue bundles, vessel walls, and lymphatics to reform into a permanent plastic-like seal that resists deformation with tensile strength up to three times the normal systolic pressure. The tissue to be sealed is grasped in the jaws of the instrument, and a calibrated force is applied to the tissue during energy delivery. Using proprietary adaptive generator technology and software, the type of tissue held in the forceps is recognized and tissue impedance is monitored while delivering the appropriate amount of RF energy required to seal the tissue. During the process, elastin and collagen are denatured, creating a permanent seal that resists deformation. A cutting blade is then deployed to cut the sealed tissue. Instruments for use with laparoscopy, laparotomy, and vaginal surgery are available with this technology.

EnSeal

The EnSeal Laparoscopic Vessel Fusion System (Ethicon Endo-Surgery, Cincinnati, Ohio) uses a set of high-compression plastic jaws embedded with nanometer-sized spheres of nickel through which the temperature of the tissue pedicle is predetermined by local conductivity. A patented positive temperature coefficient system utilizes a carbon crystalline matrix to limit tissue temperature along the seal line. This creates a conductive polymer chain at temperatures less than 100°C that dissociates at temperatures greater than 100°C, thus limiting energy delivery and lateral thermal spread. The device has a central mechanical blade used to compress the tissue to force water out of the cells and reduce lateral thermal spread by reducing excess steam within the tissue being desiccated. This feature also serves as the cutting function of the tool.

ULTRASONICS

Ultrasonic devices generate tissue effects similar to advanced bipolar devices. However, the source of thermal energy generation is ultrasonic vibration of the active shaft of the device at greater than 20,000 vibrations per second. An ultrasonic generator delivers AC to the handpiece to achieve excitation in pizoelectrodes interspersed between metal cylinders. This process results in mechanical energy by vibrating the cylinders at frequencies between 23 and 55 kHz. The shaft of the instrument, which is the active element or nonarticulating jaw, is in contact with the cylinders and oscillates linearly at the same frequency.

Different tissue effects can be achieved by variation in the oscillation distance of the shaft. The higher setting (100 μ) is better for rapid tissue transection while minimizing lateral thermal spread, but the effectiveness in coagulation of tissue and vessels is decreased. Alternatively, a shorter oscillation (50 μ) is superior for tissue and vessel sealing, yet results in greater potential for lateral thermal spread and cavitation. Cavitation occurs when steam released from vaporized cells expands tissue planes. Although this does occur to some extent with monopolar vaporization, it occurs at lower temperatures with ultrasonic energy due to the oscillating tip. Thus, ultrasonic devices are similar to advanced bipolar devices in that they both sequentially convert electrical energy to mechanical energy to thermal energy to facilitate tissue effects. However, with bipolar devices, the source of friction is intracellular (molecular), whereas ultrasonic devices create extracellular friction from the oscillating shaft followed by intracellular heating without the passage of electrical current through the tissue.

There are multiple ultrasonic devices currently available, including the Harmonic Scalpel and Harmonic ACE (Ethicon Endo-Surgery, Cincinnati, OH), Autosonix and Sonicision (Covidien, Boulder, CO), and SonoSurg (Olympus America, Center Valley, PA). A recently available device by Olympus, ThunderBeat, combines both advanced bipolar and ultrasonic technology in the same device in a manner, allowing the surgeon to use the different energy sources independently or sequentially.

SPECIAL SURGICAL SITUATIONS

Pregnancy

No data indicate that using electrosurgical techniques in a pregnant patient has any untoward effect on the fetus at any stage of development. Owing to the dispersion effect, the fetus, bathed in electrolyte-rich amniotic fluid, is protected from any concentration of electrical current. Just as the output frequency of all electrosurgical generators is above the faradic effect (the level that stimulates muscle contraction) for adult electrosurgery, the same is true for the fetus.

During a cesarean section, the only concern is the accidental touching of an activated electrode to the fetus, which causes tissue heating. This does not mean that the usual technique of making an incision in the uterus would preclude using an electrosurgical incision, but rather that a "backstop" under the incision line, between the amniotic membrane and the muscle wall, should be in place. Although using a nonconductive material, such as a plastic suction tip, may seem wise, a metal ribbon retractor also can be used because it has a large surface area serving to diffuse the current density. Caution should be exercised when using the gloved finger of the surgeon as a backstop because if open activation is used, the increased voltage may create a hole in the glove.

Body Piercing and Prosthetic Implants

There have been no documented electrosurgical injuries reported in the literature in relation to body piercing. Nonetheless, faulty instrument insulation can theoretically transmit current from the surgical active electrode to the metal object, causing a skin burn. Therefore, conventional wisdom indicates that removal of umbilical and labial piercings prior to a surgical procedure is prudent when possible. It is not necessary to remove piercings or other metal jewelry distant from the operative site. These objects are too far away from the active electrode to receive substantial electrical current. If removal of rings and/or piercings is not desired or possible, then taping the metal object down to the skin to create the greatest surface area contact will decrease current density and minimize any potential risk.

The same principles apply to metal-implanted prosthetic devices. The large surface area would minimize the potential of patient burn, and there have been no reported adverse patient events related to prosthetic devices and electrosurgery. It is noteworthy that the overlying scar has more potential for affecting the electrical circuit through increased resistance, and that is minimal as well.

Implantable Devices

Any implanted cardiac pacemaker, implantable cardioverter–defibrillator, resynchronization device, or ventricular assist device is referred to as a cardiac implantable electronic device (CIED). The nature of any device type and patient reliance on that device must be investigated preoperatively. Failure to do so can lead to adverse outcomes. The potential for electromagnetic interference with CIEDs depends upon the distance from the active and return electrodes, the RF frequency used, and the current pathway. Attention must be paid to place the return electrode in a location so that the path between the active and return electrodes does not travel near the CIED generator or leads. If so, then the risk of interference is low, although there is at least some potential for interference as the RF circuit does not travel linearly between the active and return electrode.

Possible adverse effects of CIEDs with electrosurgery include permanent damage to the device, inability of the device to function properly, resetting of the device, or inappropriate delivery of implantable cardiac defibrillator (ICD) therapy leading to patient effects of hypotension, tachyarrhythmia or bradyarrhythmia, myocardial tissue damage, and myocardial ischemia or infarction. When planning a surgical procedure in a patient who is heavily dependent on the CIED, alternative monopolar instruments should be replaced whenever possible with bipolar instruments where current is limited to tissue between the tips of the forceps and stray RF energy is rare.

Preoperative management of the CIED may include reprogramming or disabling algorithms and suspending antitachyarrhythmia functions. Clinical magnets positioned over the CIED can change pacing to an asynchronous mode in pacemakers and suspend tachycardia therapies in implantable cardiac defibrillators. However, magnets should not be routinely used over an ICD. Temporary pacing and defibrillation equipment should be immediately available before, during, and after the procedure.

Although continuous monitoring by EKG is critical, that signal can also be subject to electromagnetic interference, which can complicate detection of CIED malfunction. Thus, peripheral perfusion by pulse oximetry or invasive arterial waveform should also be monitored.

There are noncardiac devices using electric current that could potentially be affected by RF energy during electrosurgery. These include neural stimulators and gastric neurostimulators used to treat gastroparesis. Minimizing interference with these devices is desirable. However, the consequences of malfunction are not immediately life threatening, as with CIEDs.

ELECTROSURGICAL APPLICATIONS IN OPERATIVE HYSTEROSCOPY

The same electrosurgical principles that have been discussed previously in this chapter apply to hysteroscopy as well, with one notable exception, that is, the need to create distension of the uterine cavity and provide an electrically insulated environment (replacing the insulation of air during laparotomy or CO_2

gas during laparoscopy). This is accomplished through the use of nonionic fluids such as glycine, mannitol, or sorbitol. These media are absorbed to varying degrees, depending on factors such as operative time, intracavitary pressure, and vascular nature of the resected tissue. With excessive absorption come the hazards of fluid and electrolyte imbalances and complications from metabolism of the medium itself (e.g., glycine is metabolized to water and ammonia). However interesting and important, these issues are beyond the focus of this chapter.

Some surgeons employ endometrial loop resection, some use ball ablation, and some employ both techniques sequentially. Further variability is noted in watts used, speed of the electrode, and even pressure applied by the rollerball to the uterine lining (more pressure results in greater active electrode contact and decreased current density). Some surgeons use only COAG waveform, while others use CUT or even some sequential or spatial combination of the two. However, we do know that by using the CUT waveform, there is less bubble generation and accumulation on the anterior surface of the cavity. At the end of the ablation procedure, some surgeons switch to a COAG waveform at 75 W. With the increased peak voltage of this waveform, electrons driven by higher electromotive force "seek out" undertreated areas of lower impedance, ensuring complete tissue coagulation.

There are three common, if not unique, electrosurgical complications associated with operative hysteroscopy, aside from the fluid management issue described briefly above. The first is due to uterine perforation by an active electrode during RF energy application. This can be minimized by (a) never advancing the hysteroscope with the active electrode extended and (b) only energizing the active electrode while retracting the active electrode toward the hysteroscope. If this type of complications does occur, then laparoscopy or laparotomy (depending on skill level) must be undertaken to evaluate possible pelvic or abdominal organ injury. The second is accidental burns to the vagina or perineum through capacitive coupling of the outer sheath of the resectoscopic hysteroscope. Because the inner and outer sheaths of the resectoscope (conductors) are separated by air (insulator), capacitive coupling can occur. Relatively high current density in the outer sheath touching small areas of genital tissue can create a burn injury. Finally, injuries can also occur from defects in electrode insulation, especially when interrupted COAG current is used and the cervix is overdilated and is in contact with less than 2 cm of the outer sheath. The high electromotive force created by prolonged activation along already desiccated tissue (increased resistance) and subsequent current diversion is responsible for this type of injury.

BIPOLAR HYSTEROSCOPIC SURGERY

A family of instrumentation is available for hysteroscopy that uses bipolar technology to attain the desired electrosurgical effect. Two advantages of bipolar electrosurgery include the ability to use in a saline environment, mitigating the potential hazards of nonionic fluid absorption. Additionally, isolation of the electrical circuit occurs between a set of closely separated electrodes separated by a ceramic insulator. Performance is similar to its monopolar counterpoint, providing tissue vaporization and desiccation while retaining all of the inherent safety features of bipolar electrosurgery.

The VERSAPOINT system (Ethicon Women's Health and Urology, Somerville, NJ) consists of a dedicated bipolar electrosurgical generator and a variety of specialized hysteroscopic bipolar electrodes for different tissue effects. A key feature of the system is its ability to adjust automatically to an optimal power setting depending on the type of electrode.

The VERSAPOINT adaptive generator varies the output power in response to local impedance changes at the active electrode. A high-impedance vapor pocket is created that surrounds and insulates the active electrode from completing the circuit through the normal saline until tissue contact is made. Once contact occurs, current flows through the tissue and, by seeking the path of least resistance, returns through the saline to the proximal return electrode and finally back to the generator. Similar bipolar resectoscopic systems are also available through Karl Storz Endoscopy America (El Segundo, CA) and Richard Wolf Medical Instruments (Vernon Hills, IL).

BIPOLAR ENDOMETRIAL ABLATION

Nonresectoscopic bipolar endometrial ablation is possible using the NovaSure Global Endometrial Ablation System (Hologic, Marlborough, MA). This system includes a single-use, three-dimensional bipolar device and adaptive RF generator that produces a controlled destruction of the endometrium in an average of 90 seconds. After inserting the device transcervically into the uterine cavity, it is seated by retracting a protective sheath to deploy a fan-shaped bipolar electrode that conforms to the uterine cavity. During deployment, the measured endometrial cavity length and width are entered into the generator, which calculates the power output required to ensure ablation of the uterine cavity. During activation, a vacuum is used to ensure good electrode tissue contact, as well as to remove blood, endometrial debris, and steam, eliminating any uncontrollable steam ablation effect. The term "global" refers to the fact that the entire cavity is treated simultaneously (Fig. 15.13).

Using a constant power output generator, the maximum power delivered is 180 W. The depth of ablation is controlled by monitoring tissue impedance during the procedure. A

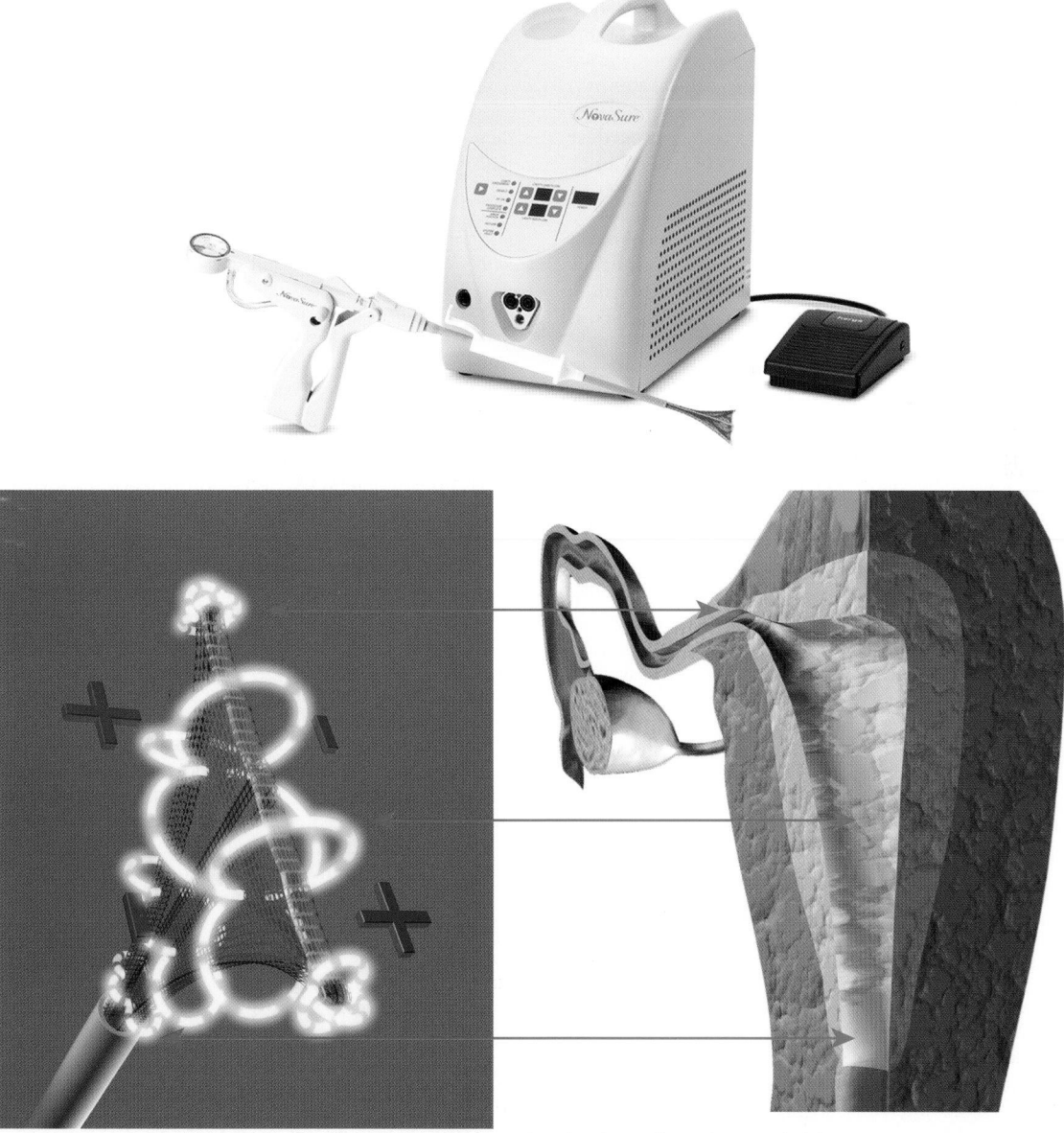

FIGURE 15.13 The NovaSure Global Endometrial Ablation System is a bipolar device for endometrial ablation using a metalized mesh electrode, vacuum for firm tissue contact, and an impedance-controlled generator designed to create a shallower depth of desiccation at the cornual area and lower uterine segment, with a deeper ablation in the uterine midbody. (Courtesy of HOLOGIC, Inc. and affiliates.)

shorter center-to-center distance between electrodes provides a more shallow depth of desiccation at the areas and lower uterine segment. A wider center-to-center distance between electrodes provides for a deeper ablation in the uterine corpus. The endometrium does not require pretreatment or thinning prior to treatment. RF energy delivery continues until monitored tissue impedance reaches 50 ohms (representing a distinction between the lower resistance of the endometrium and the higher resistance of the myometrium) or after 2 minutes, at which time the NovaSure System discontinues energy delivery.

LASER TECHNOLOGY

Historical Perspective and Background

Although the basis of laser technology was first described by Albert Einstein in 1917, working lasers did not appear until 1960 and were not applied to medicine until about 5 years later. LASER is actually an acronym for "light amplification by stimulated emission of radiation." Energy from lasers is derived by the ability to generate light emissions that are both highly collimated (parallel rays) and coherent (in phase, noninterfering wavelengths) and that can be delivered to the surgical site by a series of mirrors or fibers without measurable degeneration of these properties. In doing so, virtually any surgical procedure requiring vaporization, cutting, or coagulation of tissue can be performed using lasers. Laser energy can destroy tissue layer by layer, without touching it, with minimal thermal damage.

Lasers generate light energy through the release of photons from excited atoms in a medium contained within an optically resonant chamber. The nature of the active lasing medium, a collection of atoms usually in the form of crystals or gas, is how the type of laser derives its name. When the medium is stimulated by an external source (e.g., electricity), the atoms circulating the nucleus of the medium are stimulated into a higher-energy orbit. As the electrons decay to resting levels, light energy in the form of a photon is released. This process is known as spontaneous emission. Not only can electrons be stimulated by an external energy source, they can be bombarded by photons, which causes decay and emission of a photon that is identical in phase (coherent), in wavelength, and in color (monochromatic) and travels in the same direction without divergence (collimated). This process is called stimulated emission.

The optical cavity in which the electrons reside, and where the photons are produced, is lined by mirrors. All of the mirrors are completely reflective, except for a semitransparent mirror at one end of the linear axis of the optical cavity. The direction in which photons are emitted is totally random. They are focused by the mirrors so that most resonate back and forth along the axis of the optical chamber. Photons that are aligned with the optical axis of the chamber are released when the laser is "fired," emerge through the semitransparent mirror, and are emitted from the laser as the monochromatic parallel coherent laser beam.

Laser generators have focusing attachments for delivery of the light energy for superficial use (e.g., colposcopy or lower genital tract), for laparotomy, and for laparoscopy. Historically, all lasers have been able to transmit energy via a flexible quartz fiber except for the CO_2 laser, which was transmitted along rigid tubes reflected by mirrors. However, a hollow-core flexible fiber delivery system recently has been developed for delivery of CO_2 laser energy (OmniGuide, Cambridge, MA) with adapters for external, laparoscopy, and robotic use.

Laser Tissue Interactions

Just as the surgeon can manipulate the active electrode to modify the effects of RF energy at the surgical site, there are three parameters that impact the amount of laser energy delivered. The first variable is wattage. For most applications, energy in the order to 5 to 10 W is sufficient; it is rarely necessary to exceed 20 W.

The second parameter is time. Simply put, the longer the laser remains focused on one spot, the more energy is applied to that area. This can be modified either by moving a continuous wave beam around within the desired treatment area or by delivering the laser energy in pulses. In pulsed modes, laser energy can be delivered as a single pulse or a series of pulses. Generally, a single pulse is less than 0.25 second. Timed pulses of short duration can be useful in controlling delivery.

The third parameter that can be controlled is the spot size of the beam. This is analogous to altering the current density of RF energy at the tip of the active electrode to alter tissue effects. Power density, expressed in watts/cm², is inversely proportional to the area of the spot size, such that doubling the beam diameter reduces power density to one fourth. Conversely, decreasing spot size in half results in a fourfold increase in power density.

As previously mentioned, laser energy emerges from the generator in a coherent and parallel fashion. This could hypothetically travel in this form to infinitely. However, the laser light is focused to a fixed focal length, depending on the application of the device (external, laparotomy, or laparoscopy use). The surgeon can further alter the focus with additional lenses or mechanical devices. By focusing or defocusing the laser energy, it is used as a cutting or coagulating tool.

Applications of Lasers

The first gynecologic application of laser technology was reported in 1973 when Kaplan and colleagues used CO_2 laser to treat cervical lesions. Potassium titanyl phosphate (KTP) and neodymium:YAG (Nd:YAG) lasers became increasingly popular for laparoscopic applications, especially related to treatment of endometriosis and infertility patients, partially because of their specific properties but equally because a flexible fiber delivery system was comparatively easier to use than the rigid mirrored system of the CO_2 laser. However, because of increasing cost consciousness and availability of superior advanced RF-based devices in the late 1990s, laser technology for all but external lower genital tract disease dramatically decreased.

There are three zones of laser tissue damage: (a) the area vaporized, (b) the area of tissue death that results from the heated tissue short of vaporization, and (c) the area of tissue damage caused by conduction of the heat away from the lased site. Because it removes tissue with vaporization and evacuation, the suctioned plume allows the tissue base to heal without a devitalized tissue covering. Postoperative pain is reduced because nerve endings are sealed by the beam.

In gynecologic surgery, the most commonly used lasers are CO_2, argon, KTP, and Nd:YAG (Table 15.2). The argon and KTP lasers produce light waves of a specific wavelength, giving a characteristic color. The Nd:YAG and CO_2 lasers have wavelengths in the nonvisible spectrum. Accordingly, a helium–neon laser (632 nm, red) is typically coupled with them to use as a beam aiming guide and to aid in focus.

CO_2 Laser

The CO_2 laser is the most versatile and most widely used laser. Laser energy is absorbed, scattered, or affected by the thermal conductivity and local circulation of the tissue. Soft tissue is about 80% water by volume, which absorbs CO_2 laser energy readily, limiting penetration. Indeed, it has a shallow depth of penetration (up to 0.5 mm), and minimal lateral thermal damage is limited to about 0.5 mm. The CO_2 laser is therefore relatively safe and can be used in critical areas where RF energy application would be more dangerous, such as near

TABLE 15.2 Laser Characteristics

TYPE	LASING MEDIUM	WAVELENGTH (NM)	COLOR	DEPTH OF PENETRATION
Argon	Argon gas	488–512	Blue–green	0.5 mm
KTP	Potassium titanyl phosphate	532	Green	1–2 mm
Nd:YAG	Neodymium-doped yttrium aluminum garnet	1,064	Near infrared	3–4 mm
CO_2	CO_2 gas	10,600	Infrared	0.1 mm

the bladder, on the lateral side wall near the ureter, and on the bowel serosa. A sharply focused laser beam produces narrow tissue vaporization comparable to an incision made by a scalpel. However, defocusing the beam enlarges the spot, and using the same settings, power density is reduced to treat a thin surface rapidly. The CO_2 laser provides excellent vaporization and cutting by increasing the power density and excellent coagulation with slight defocusing of the beam. The amount of damage caused by heat conduction is directly proportional to the amount of time spent in lasing.

Disadvantages of the CO_2 laser include focusing of the helium–neon beam as well as production of smoke referred to as "plume," which needs frequent evacuation to allow adequate visualization of the target.

Nd:YAG Laser

Similar to CO_2 lasers, Nd:YAG lasers emit an invisible beam requiring a helium–neon spot for guidance. However, this energy penetrates tissue to greater depths of 3 to 4 mm, and, because the Nd:YAG energy scatters in tissue, its thermal damage is greater than that of CO_2. Poorly absorbed by water, it is not as good for vaporization, but it has much better coagulation properties. Because of its depth of penetration and its performance in a liquid environment, it was used to advantage in the early days of hysteroscopic procedures, including endometrial ablation. Although this laser fiber is typically used in a noncontact technique, adding a sapphire tip to the end of the fiber, the laser energy can be focused and converted into heat and used in a contact mode. This improves its vaporization abilities, but the tips need to be cooled with gas or liquid through the fiber.

KPT and Argon Lasers

The KTP and argon lasers have similar wavelengths in the visible light spectrum and are delivered via a fiberoptic fiber. The advantages of these lasers over the CO_2 laser include selective absorption by hemoglobin and other pigmented tissues and less plume production. These lasers produce a moderate scatter, 100 times that of the CO_2 laser, resulting in significantly reduced cutting ability but substantially increased coagulation effectiveness.

The main disadvantage is the need to wear special glasses that distort the view of the pelvis and make it difficult to visualize small implants of endometriosis.

LASER SAFETY

Lasers have been used in gynecologic surgery for nearly 40 years. Although there has generally been good safety record, there is great potential for injury. It is recommended that surgeons wishing to use laser technology undergo both didactic and practical training in laser use. There are also a few guidelines that should be kept in mind related to use of laser technology:

- Place an appropriate warning sign on the door of the operating room indicating when lasers are being used.
- All operating room personnel should wear protective safety glasses, matched for the wavelength of the laser used.
- When the laser is not actively being fired, it should be placed in standby mode.
- Drapes near the operative field should be flame resistant and kept wet if possible.
- Adequate suction should be available to collect all plume produced by laser use. Understand their specific tissue interactions of the laser being used. It is much easier to cause damage to a vessel or ureter when using deep penetrating energy such as that produced by the Nd:YAG laser than when using the CO_2 laser energy.
- Fibers used to transmit laser energy are delicate and can break, deliver laser energy at the break point, and potentially injure the patient and/or operating room personnel.

SUMMARY

When electricity is used in surgical applications, it follows Ohm law and three general rules: (a) Electricity must complete a circuit or it will not flow, (b) electricity goes to ground, and (c) electricity follows the path of least resistance. An understanding of these concepts, continuous and interrupted waveforms produced by electrosurgical generators and electrical circuits, and the tissue effects produced by active electrode characteristics and manipulation, the surgeon can use radiofrequency energy to advantage in the operating room. Conversely, a lack of understanding by the surgeon can result in poor surgical outcome and unnecessary complications. Just as physicians are expected to understand and prescribe drugs in a precise and logical manner, so should they have a working knowledge of the energy sources they choose to use in surgery.

BEST SURGICAL PRACTICES

Fundamental Principles of Electrosurgery

- Ohm law describes the underlying electrical principle of electrosurgery. Current (flow of electrons) is directly related to voltage (electromotive force) and inversely related to impedance (resistance to flow of electrons).
- Three rules explain the flow of electrons in tissue: (a) Electricity must complete a circuit or it will not flow; (b) electricity goes to ground; and (c) electricity follows the path of least resistance.

- An electrosurgical generator produces sinusoidal waveforms, variants of current, and voltage as a continuous (undamped) output current called CUT, a highly interrupted (damped) output called COAG, or a moderately interrupted (damped) output called BLEND.
- Electrosurgery creates a desired tissue effect by delivering high-frequency AC with active electrodes that manipulate electrons to sufficient concentration (current density) in living tissue.
- In most circumstances, the CUT waveform should be used to cut and desiccate tissue, reserving the COAG waveform for surface fulguration to control small open bleeders and for superficial coagulation.
- Specific tissue effects can be achieved by using specific waveforms, using contact or noncontact techniques, altering the size and shape of the active electrode, and altering the movement speed of the active electrode (dwell time). The educated surgeon can integrate these variables to achieve the desired result.
- The lower-voltage CUT waveform should be used to incise tissue and for coaptive sealing of larger blood vessels. The higher voltage of the COAG current produces rapid tissue desiccation and carbonation, resulting in increased tissue resistance limiting coagulation to superficial small vessels. The BLEND current may provide a satisfactory combination for cutting through fatty tissues, such as the subcutaneous tissue or omentum.
- Coaptive sealing of the uterine and ovarian vessels using any type of monopolar current may be ineffective if the blood flow remains uninterrupted. Unless a vessel is sufficiently squeezed before electricity is applied, current density is dramatically reduced by conduction in blood, as any heat is dissipated by convection. Bipolar cautery is recommended for these larger pedicles.

Fundamental Principles to Reduce Risk during Electrosurgery

- Place electrode pencils in their safety holster when not in use. This will avoid accidental activation delivering unintended RF energy.
- Inspect each instrument's insulation before use.
- Any alcohol preparation near the field of surgery should be completely dried before initiation of an electrosurgical device to avoid fire.
- With monopolar systems, use a monitored return electrode system (frequently referred to as a REM system). Place return electrodes close to the operative site on a clean, dry, shaved area, avoiding bony prominence and scar tissue. The longest edge should face the operative site, and REM pads should never be cut.
- Cords to electrosurgical devices should be secured using a nonconductor (or plastic) clamp. The cord should never be wrapped around a metal clamp, as this has potential for direct coupling with high output of power or if there is an insulation failure in the device cord.
- Activate CUT for all desiccation–coagulation procedures; use COAG for fulguration procedures.
- Activate the electrode in short bursts (about 3 seconds) to minimize capacitive coupling. Use the manufacturer's recommended connection cables. Inspect instrument insulation before each use. If the usual power settings seem inadequate, do not increase the power until the circuit is checked, especially the return electrode.
- Select the lowest voltage that will create the desired effect. For any given power setting, CUT current produces a lower peak voltage than COAG current.

- If open activation occurs at a site remote from the intended area, the charge has potential to build at the tip of the instrument and discharge via arcing to an alternate site. Moreover, this can cause unrecognized injury out of the operative field of view if performed during laparoscopic procedures. If the surgeon desires true fulguration or vaporization of tissue, the instrument should be activated as near to the tissue as possible without actually touching it.
- Consider using bipolar methods. Bipolar systems deliver current as an uninterrupted CUT waveform calibrated against a lower resistance than monopolar systems. As such, it is wise to use a current flow meter to confirm complete desiccation of tissue, especially during tubal sterilization. In some tissues, the thermal effect will be limited such that monopolar application will be preferable.
- Consider using bipolar energy for patients with pacemakers and other implanted cardiac devices. If monopolar must be used, follow safety advice from the implant manufacturer.
- The degree of thermal necrosis on tissue that is electrically incised is dependent on the velocity of passage as well as electrode size and shape and the electrosurgical waveform.
- As one electrode is changed to another, the surgeon should keep charge density, waveform, and electrode characteristics in mind and adjust the generator output to match the task at hand.
- The most common complication during electrosurgery is return electrode burns, owing to improper application of the electrode. Prophylactic measures include proper skin preparation and site application. Alternate site burns, such as to cardiac leads, usually result from improper grounding, use of too much power, and high-voltage application.

Fundamental Principles of Electrosurgery Techniques

- Before taking any electrosurgical action, determine the source of bleeding and its proximity to vital anatomy using mechanical tamponade with active hydrolavage. If the bowel, bladder, or ureter is in close proximity to the bleeder, mobilize that structure sufficiently before applying energy.
- Because the output voltage of COAG current is very high, contact coagulation is generally limited to superficial layers. That is because of the accelerated buildup of tissue resistance from rapid desiccation and superficial carbonization. Conversely, electrode contact using the lower-voltage CUT current heats tissue more gradually, leading to deeper and more reliable penetration.
- Preferentially use BLEND or COAG current for a wider zone of hemostasis during incision of vascular tissues and to facilitate dissection of tissues with greater impedance, such as fatty or desiccated pedicles and adhesions. On the other hand, it is more prudent to use the lower-voltage CUT current via the edge of an electrode whenever lateral thermal spread may pose extra liability to adjacent tissues.
- If bleeding in the vicinity of the bowel, bladder, or ureter cannot be controlled with pressure alone, carefully direct short bursts of noncontact COAG current with a broad-surface electrode to attain hemostasis with the least possible amount of electrosurgical penetration. Still, visceral bleeding is best controlled by mechanical means, using the patience of pressure or suture ligation.
- Although the flow of current is restricted to the tissue between the poles during bipolar electrosurgery, this does not eliminate the risk of thermal injury to tissue that is distant from the site of directed hemostasis. As current is applied between the poles, the intervening tissue gradually desiccates until it becomes thoroughly dehydrated.

- Unwanted thermal damage can be minimized by terminating the flow of current at the end of the visible vapor phase, applying current in a pulsatile fashion to permit tissue cooling, and securing pedicles by a stepwise process that alternates between partial desiccation and incremental cutting.
- Because the rate of temperature generation is a direct function of the volume of tissue being desiccated, thermal spread can also be reduced by using the sides or tips of a slightly open forceps to press or lift, rather than coapt for hemostasis.
- As with contact monopolar coagulation, tissue between the electrodes of a bipolar instrument may become adherent during desiccation. Repeated attempts to shake the tissue free may lead to traumatic avulsion of a key vascular pedicle. A stuck vascular pedicle can usually be unglued by energizing the opened device while immersed in a conductive irrigant, such as saline.

BIBLIOGRAPHY

Bellina JH. Gynecology and the laser. *Contemp Obstet Gynecol* 1974;4:24.

Bellina JH, Fick AC, Jackson JD. Application of the CO_2 laser to infertility surgery. *Surg Clin North Am* 1984;64:899.

Brill AI. Energy systems for operative laparoscopy. *J Am Assoc Gynecol Laparosc* 1998;5:333.

Brill AI. Bipolar electrosurgery: convention and innovation. *Clin Obstet Gynecol* 2008;51:153.

Cushing H, Bovie W. Electrosurgery as an aid to the removal of intracranial tumors. *Surg Gynecol Obstet* 1928;47:751.

D'Arsonval M. Action physiologique des courants alternatifs a grande frequence. *Arch Physiol Pathol* 1893;5:401.

Ewing J. *A treatise on tumors*, 2nd ed. Philadelphia, PA: WB Saunders, 1922:17.

Kelly HA, Ward GE. *Electrosurgery*. Philadelphia, PA: WB Saunders, 1932.

Licht SH. *The history of therapeutic heat*, 2nd ed. New Haven, CT: Elizabeth Licht Publications, 1965.

Loffer FD, Pent D. Indications, contraindications and complications of laparoscopy. *Obstet Gynecol Surv* 1975;30:407.

Luciano A, Soderstrom R, Martin D. Essential principles of electrosurgery in operative laparoscopy. *J Am Assoc Gynecol Laparosc* 1994;1:189.

Major RH. *History of medicine*. Volumes I and II. Springfield, MA: Charles C. Thomas, 1954.

Massarweh NN, Cosgriff N, Slakey DP. Electrosurgery: history, principles, and current and future uses. *J Am Coll Surg* 2006; 202:520.

Feldman LS, Brunt LM, Fuchshuber P, et al. Rationale for the fundamental use of surgical energy (FUSE) curriculum assessment: focus on safety. *Surg Endosc* 2013;27:4054.

Nduka CC, Super PA, Monson JRT, et al. Cause and prevention of electrosurgical injuries in laparoscopy. *J Am Coll Surg* 1994;179:161.

Odell RC. Pearls, pitfalls, and advancement in the delivery of electrosurgical energy during laparoscopy. In: Amaral JF, ed. *Problems in general surgery*. Philadelphia, PA: Lippincott Williams & Wilkins, 2002:5.

Reidenbach HD. Fundamentals of bipolar high-frequency surgery. *Endosc Surg Allied Technol* 1993;1:85.

Soderstrom RM. Electrosurgical injuries during laparoscopy: prevention and management. *Curr Opin Obstet Gynecol* 1994;6:248.

Sutton C, Abbott J. History of power sources in endoscopic surgery. *J Minim Invasive Gynecol* 2013;20:271.

Vaincaillie TG. Electrosurgery at laparoscopy: guidelines to avoid complication. *Gynaecol Endosc* 1994;3:143.

Vilos GA, Rajakumar C. Electrosurgical generators and monopolar and bipolar electrosurgery. *J Minim Invasiv Gynecol* 2013; 20:279.

CHAPTER 16
Diagnostic and Operative Laparoscopy

Howard T. Sharp and Marisa R. Adelman

DEFINITIONS

Aqua dissection—The use of fluid, most often sterile water or saline, under force, to separate one anatomical plane from another. Laparoscopic suction–irrigators are an excellent tool for performing aqua dissection.

Chromopertubation—A procedure in which a colored dye is passed through the fallopian tubes to confirm patency.

Colpotomy—A surgical incision in the vagina. The -*tomy* part of the word is from the Greek word *tome*, meaning cutting.

High definition—A term initially introduced in the 1930s to define the then-new technology that replaced the experimental systems ranging from 15 lines to about 220 lines of resolution. High-definition television is now defined as resolution 1,080 or 720 lines. HD is broadcast digitally and consequently produces a more vivid and realistic picture.

Morcellate—To divide into small portions.

Reposable—A trocar/sleeve kit in which disposable trocars are used with reusable sleeves in an effort to reduce the cost of disposable products while ensuring sharp, undamaged instruments more commonly found in the disposable kits.

Veres needle—A spring-loaded needle designed to allow entry into body cavities without trauma to underlying organs during laparoscopy.

Laparoscopic surgical advances have accelerated remarkably over the past decades. What was initially a primitive tool for diagnostic purposes and simple procedures such as tubal sterilization has evolved into a more coordinated system for the repair or removal of diseased abdominal and pelvic organs. As operative laparoscopy has become more complex and technology has continued to advance, new challenges and complications have been recognized. The proper use of equipment and techniques can greatly add to patient safety and satisfaction. To this end, the purpose of the chapter is to review contemporary equipment, commonly used surgical techniques, and strategies to avoid and manage complications associated with laparoscopic surgery.

HISTORY

The first description of endoscopy is attributed to Phillip Bozzini in 1805, as he attempted to view the urethral mucosa with a simple tube and candlelight. Hysteroscopy was the first gynecologic endoscopic procedure performed when Pantaleoni used a cystoscope to identify uterine polyps in 1869. Laparoscopy was first performed by Jacobaeus of Sweden in 1910, wherein a Nitze cystoscope, composed of a candle and a hollow tube, was used to illuminate the peritoneal cavity. Kalk of Germany was instrumental in developing laparoscopy into a diagnostic and surgical procedure in the early 1930s. By the end of the 1930s, laparoscopy was being used in the diagnosis of ectopic pregnancy and the performance of tubal sterilization. Raoul Palmer of France reported the use of gaseous distention with lithotomy–Trendelenburg positioning in 1947. The use of "cold light" and fiberoptics were landmark innovations credited to Fourestier, Gladu, Valmiere, and Kampany and Hopkins, respectively. Monopolar electrosurgery for tubal sterilization was popularized in the 1960s. Semm of Germany reported advanced operative laparoscopic procedures such as salpingectomy, myomectomy, oophorectomy, ovarian cystectomy, and salpingostomy in the 1970s. These pioneers of endoscopic surgery and many others have laid the crucial groundwork that has enabled modern gynecologic surgeons to perform advanced operative laparoscopy on a routine basis, with a variety of energy systems under increasingly ergonomic and efficient conditions.

INDICATIONS FOR LAPAROSCOPY

Diagnostic Laparoscopy

Laparoscopy can provide valuable clinical information in a number of circumstances. It can aid in the evaluation of patients with acute pelvic and abdominal pain, including ovarian torsion, ovarian cyst rupture, ectopic pregnancy, appendicitis, and pelvic inflammatory disease. In the evaluation of less emergent conditions, such as chronic pelvic pain and infertility, it is useful to identify pelvic adhesions, endometriosis, hernias, uterine fibroids, and adnexal masses. Before performing diagnostic laparoscopy, a thorough history, detailed physical examination, and appropriate imaging studies should be completed.

Operative Laparoscopy

Most surgeries traditionally performed by the abdominal or vaginal approach can now be performed laparoscopically. Studies are still needed to better define which advanced procedures are most appropriate to perform laparoscopically from an economic and safety vantage point. Operator experience is a critical factor that must be considered. Commonly performed laparoscopic procedures include adhesiolysis, treatment of endometriosis, tubal sterilization, ovarian cystectomy, oophorectomy, salpingectomy, salpingostomy, and hysterectomy. More advanced procedures include repair of pelvic organ prolapse, tubal reanastomosis, myomectomy, radical hysterectomy, and lymphadenectomy.

EQUIPMENT

Contemporary laparoscopy equipment consists of an imaging system comprising a telescope (laparoscope) and video camera system, an insufflation or abdominal wall lift system, and specialized surgical instruments. Digitization and robotics are areas that continue to evolve.

Imaging Systems

Imaging systems consist of a laparoscope, light source, fiberoptic cord, camera unit, and monitors. High-definition digital cameras are compatible with the increased resolution capabilities of high-definition flat screen monitors. Most imaging systems are also equipped with a printer, video recorder, or DVD recorder for documentation.

The laparoscope in its basic form is a telescope. Laparoscopes range from 1.8 to 12 mm in diameter, with a distal end (objective) available in varying viewing angles (Fig. 16.1). The 0-degree deflection-angle telescope is most commonly used and provides a straightforward view, whereas a 30-degree foroblique lens allows for visualization in a large frontal view but must be continuously directed to maintain field orientation.

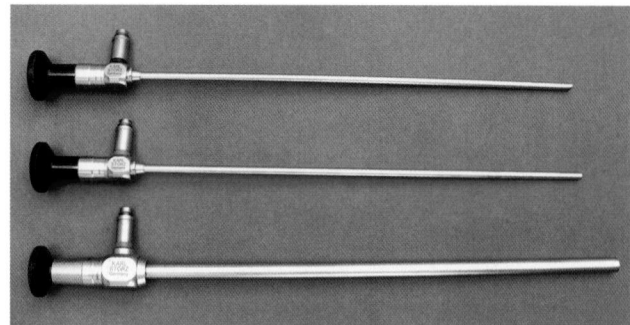

FIGURE 16.1 Telescopes used in laparoscopy. **Top:** 5-mm, 45-degree viewing angle laparoscope. **Middle:** 5-mm, 0-degree viewing angle laparoscope. **Bottom:** 10-mm, 0-degree viewing angle laparoscope.

Operative laparoscopes are equipped with a central channel that allows laser, electrosurgical, or mechanical instruments to be introduced into the abdomen. Light is introduced through the laparoscope with a fiberoptic cable powered by a light source. It is important that the light source has sufficient power to deliver adequate light through the fiberoptic cable. Ideally, high-intensity light sources that use xenon or halogen are used. Though a significant amount of original light is lost from the original hot light source, the fiberoptic cable is able to transmit enough heat to burn paper drapes as well as patient's skin; therefore, caution should be used to avoid inadvertent contact with drapes or the patient.

The camera unit consists of a camera head, cable, and camera control. The camera head attaches to the eyepiece of the laparoscope and captures images transmitted by the laparoscope. Camera/laparoscopes are now available as combined, fused units that are fully autoclavable, with push-button zoom and autofocus features. The basis of laparoscopic cameras is the solid-state silicon computer chip or charge-coupled device (CCD). This is composed of silicon elements, which emit an electric charge when exposed to light. Each silicon element contributes one pixel unit to the image produced. The image resolution is dependent on the number of pixels on the chip. CCDs are housed within the camera head of rigid scopes, in comparison to complementary metal oxide semiconductors, which are located at the tip of flexible scopes. Most laparoscopic cameras have 250,000 to 2,073,600 pixels. Three-chip CCDs provide better image quality but are more expensive, as they have a separate chip for each primary color, as opposed to the single-chip CCD. High-definition displays, with 1,080 lines, are needed to provide optimal visualization. Newer developments include the use of wireless systems, designed to provide central control over operating room devices, using either a microphone or a movable touch-pad screen.

Abdominal Lifting Systems

Insufflation systems allow gas to fill the abdominopelvic cavity to optimize visualization. Insufflators are designed to deliver gas at low rates during initial Veres needle insertion, but are also able to provide high flow rates when gas is lost to maintain a relatively constant, set intra-abdominal pressure during surgery. Insufflation may be achieved with a Veres needle or the Hassan trocar, filtered tubing, an insufflator, and gas tanks. Insufflation tubing with a 0.3-micron filter is recommended to prevent intraperitoneal contamination with bacteria, microparticles, and debris from the insufflator and gas tank. A Veres needle is often used to create a pneumoperitoneum, although other methods, such as direct trocar insertion and open laparoscopy, will be discussed. The Veres needle is available in reusable or disposable

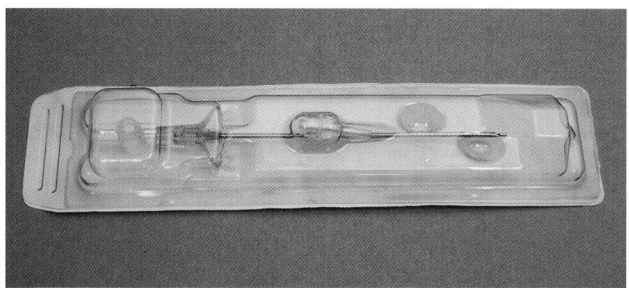

FIGURE 16.2 Disposable Veres needle.

models containing a spring-loaded tip that retracts as it pierces the abdominal wall, allowing a blunt tip to engage on entry to the peritoneal cavity (Fig. 16.2). This is designed to avoid damaging the bowel or other intra-abdominal organs. Though filtered room air has been used, carbon dioxide is most commonly used today. Carbon dioxide has the advantage of being rapidly absorbed by blood. However, it is converted to carbonic acid on moist peritoneal surfaces, which can cause pain. For this reason, nitrous oxide or helium is preferred by some, especially in cases using local anesthesia or conscious sedation. Some have advocated the use of heated or hydrated gas to prevent hypothermia during laparoscopy. A Cochrane review concluded that during laparoscopic abdominal surgery, heated gas insufflation, with or without humidification, had minimal benefit on patient outcomes. Specifically, there was no effect on postoperative pain, changes in core temperature, or length of hospitalization observed. This is partly because insufflators that contain a heating unit will ultimately have little or no effect on temperature by the time the gas has traveled 50 to 100 cm in tubing. In longer surgeries, prevention of hypothermia is better achieved by using a heated body surface blanket or a device that delivers heated and hydrated gas. Gasless laparoscopy can also be performed with the use of a mechanical lifting arm that attaches to a fanlike retractor along the peritoneal surface of the abdominal wall, obviating the need for gas distension. Some favor this approach in patients with cardiopulmonary risk factors.

Surgical Instrumentation

Trocars and sleeves are used to pierce the abdominal wall for placement of the laparoscope and surgical instruments (Fig. 16.3). Trocar sleeves range from 3 to 15 mm

in diameter and are available as reusable, disposable, and reposable systems. Disposable systems consist of completely disposable trocars and sleeves. They offer the advantage of consistent sharpness but are more expensive. Reusable trocars offer the advantage of being the most cost effective, but they must be maintained for sharpness. Reposable systems are composed of a disposable bladed or nonbladed trocar with a reusable sleeve. All are acceptable for use. Most sleeves contain a Luer-Lok port that attaches to insufflation tubing. Trocar tips may be pyramidal, conical (reusable), bladed, or blunt tipped or have optical access (disposable). Conical and blunt-tipped trocars have the advantage of making smaller fascial defects but require greater force to place. Optical access trocars enable the surgeon to visualize the layers of the abdominal wall during placement. Expandable trocar sheaths are available that are initially placed through the abdominal wall with a Veres needle and then expand to accept a 5- to 12-mm port. These offer the advantage of creating smaller abdominal wall defects and thereby reducing the risk of hernia formation and injury to the inferior epigastric vessels.

Ancillary instruments may be placed through secondary trocar sleeves to aid in diagnostic and operative laparoscopy (Figs. 16.4 and 16.5A, B). These include blunt probes; a variety of graspers, including toothed and atraumatic graspers; scissors; needle drivers; knot pushers; biopsy forceps; suction–irrigators; energy delivery tools; specimen retrieval bags; and tissue morcellators. A uterine manipulator may be used to improve access to the uterus, fallopian tubes, ovaries, and the posterior and anterior cul-de-sacs. These are available in reusable and disposable models (Fig. 16.6A–C). Some manipulators are inserted in a fixed position and allow limited uterine mobility, whereas others are hinged and allow the uterus to be moved anteriorly, posteriorly, and laterally. Many of these also offer the ability to perform chromotubation for evaluation of fallopian tube patency. Colpotomizer cups are included, or can be attached to most uterine manipulators, and engulf the cervix, allowing the surgeon to cut against it when resecting the uterus and cervix from the vagina during laparoscopic hysterectomy. The colpotomizer delineates the vaginal fornices, allowing for maximal preservation of vaginal length, and optimizes separation of the ureters from the uterine arteries, in order to avoid injury. At least one of the current cups on the market utilizes light, in order to better identify the cervicovaginal junction. The same device may also include a balloon that is inflated to prevent the pneumoperitoneum from escaping through the

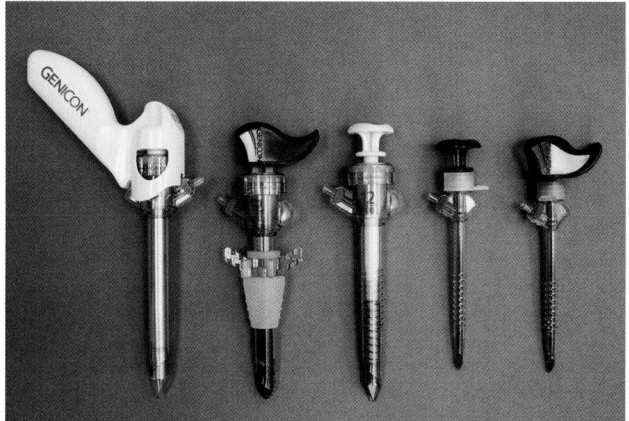

FIGURE 16.3 Trocars and sleeves. Shown from left to right: 12-mm blunt optical tip, 12-mm Hasson blunt tip, 12-mm shielded tip, 5-mm pyramidal tip, and 5-mm bladeless tip. (Courtesy of Genicon.)

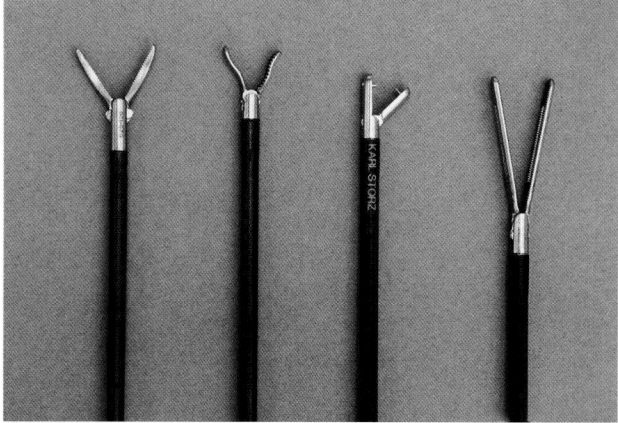

FIGURE 16.4 Ancillary instruments for laparoscopic surgery. Shown from *left* to *right*: Maryland dissector, atraumatic forceps, biopsy forceps, and bowel grasper.

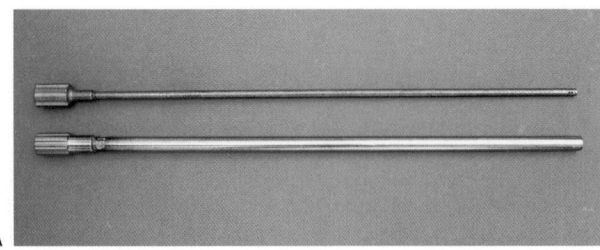

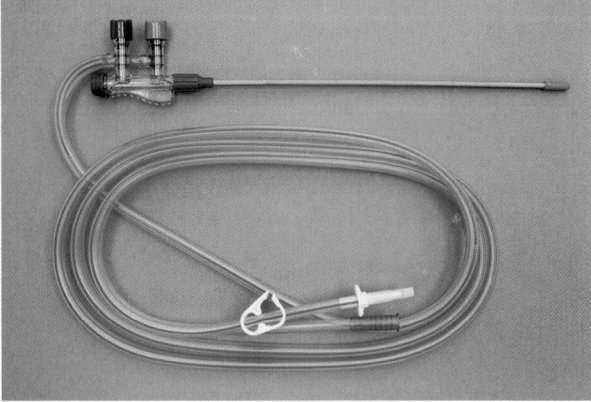

FIGURE 16.5 A: Reusable suction tips. **B:** Disposable suction irrigator. (Courtesy of Genicon.)

vagina (pneumooccluder) once the colpotomy has been made. Though these instruments can significantly facilitate the hysterectomy, they are more expensive than other manipulators, and the time required to insert them can potentially contribute

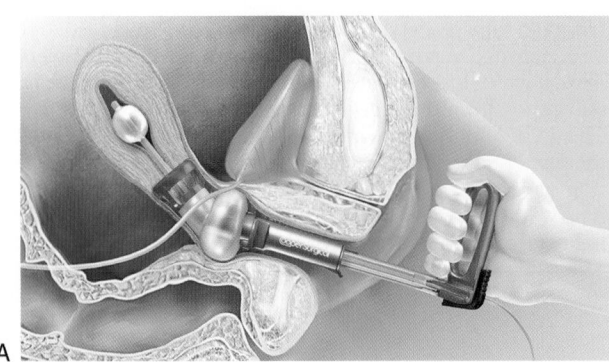

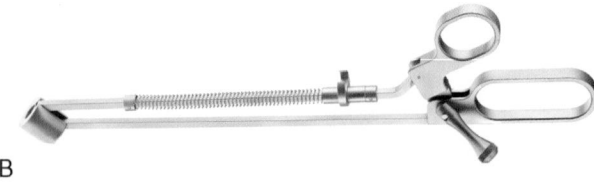

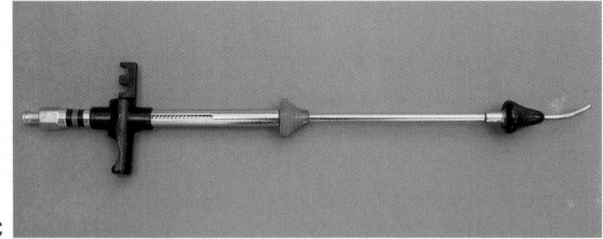

FIGURE 16.6 Uterine manipulators. **A:** Rumi. (CooperSurgical.) **B:** Pelosi. (CooperSurgical.) **C:** Acorn.

to the overall anesthesia time. An alternative to a colpotomizing cup is a sponge-stick or EEA sizer.

Energy and Hemostasis

The application of energy systems to laparoscopy has expanded laparoscopic surgeons' ability to perform complex surgeries with the capability to rapidly divide tissues and maintain hemostasis. This technology has also introduced a new set of complications, such as unrecognized bowel burns from inadvertent direct and capacitive coupling. In an effort to reduce risks associated with monopolar electrosurgical devices, several options are available. One is the use of endomechanical energy; a second is the use of bipolar electrosurgery, laser, or ultrasonic energy; and a third is the gaining of a better understanding of electrosurgical principles. Though our understanding of laparoscopically applied electrophysics has improved, gynecologic surgeons often have no formal electrosurgical training or credentialing, in contrast to the once-common laser safety courses.

Endomechanical Energy

Endomechanical energy can be used for tissue division and hemostasis in a number of ways, including suturing, stapling, and the application of vascular clips.

Suture The simplest laparoscopic ligature to apply is the pre-tied loop, available as a slip knot on a push rod that is used to push a suture loop around a tissue pedicle for hemostasis. The Roeder loop, which was modified by Kurt Semm for laparoscopic use, can also be tied in the operating room using standard suture. Laparoscopic suturing can be performed using stock suture, ideally 36 to 48 inches in length (Fig. 16.7). Needle drivers are used to drive needles through tissue, and knots may be tied outside the laparoscopic port (extracorporeal knot) or within the body (intracorporeal knot). Extracorporeal knots are usually performed as sliding square knots, pushed through the trocar sleeve to the tissue by multiple passes of a knot pusher, which serves as the surgeon's finger (Fig. 16.8). Intracorporeal knots are tied within the abdomen by looping the suture material around the laparoscopic needle holders using the same technique as an "instrument tie" (Fig. 16.9). Laparoscopic suturing requires considerable practice to confidently load the needle into the needle driver and place sutures accurately. To this end, the Endo Stitch (Covidien) was developed, wherein the needle is preloaded and the suture is passed through tissue up to 2 cm thick by closing a handle and a toggle switch. Interrupted or continuous suturing can be accomplished. The Endo Stitch is a 10-mm disposable instrument, which uses device-specific suture cartridges. There are several other automatic suturing devices, both disposable and reusable, some of which are able to articulate. Both absorbable clips and titanium knots are available to secure the ends of suture, obviating the need for knots. In an effort to accommodate surgeons desiring to use the laparoscopic needle driver and suture, self-righting needle drivers were designed, which automatically fix the needle at a perpendicular or oblique position to the needle driver. Such devices can facilitate suturing laparoscopically.

Staplers The Endo GIA, originally designed for gastrointestinal anastomosis, can be used in gynecologic laparoscopy as a stapling device for securing and dividing tissue. After placing and firing the preloaded device, six staggered rows of staples, 3 cm in length and 1 cm in width, are left behind. A knife blade simultaneously divides the tissue, leaving three rows of staples on each side of the incision.

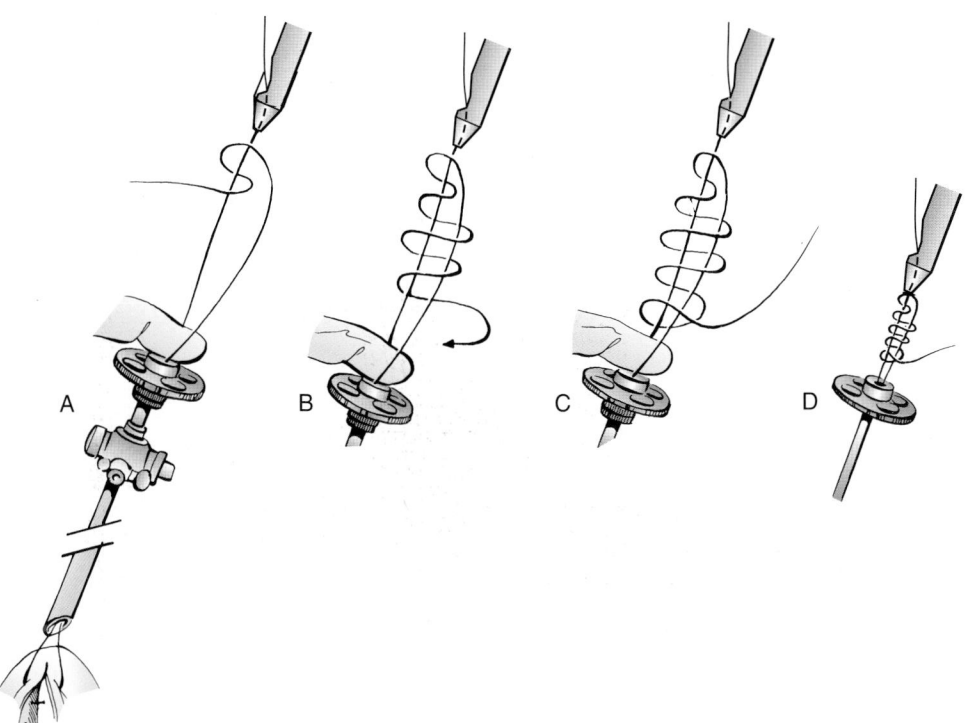

FIGURE 16.7 Extracorporeal knot tying with slip knot. **A:** With both suture ends outside the body, the suture is cut below the needle. A single throw is made. **B:** With the free end of the suture, three revolutions are made around both suture strands. **C:** The tail of the suture is inserted through the lowest loop. **D:** The tail is pulled to tighten the knot, the suture is cut above the knot, and the slip knot is pushed with a closed-nose knot pusher to the desired position. (Modified from Murphy AA. Operative laparoscopy. *Fertil Steril* 1987;47:1, with permission. Copyright © 1987 Elsevier.)

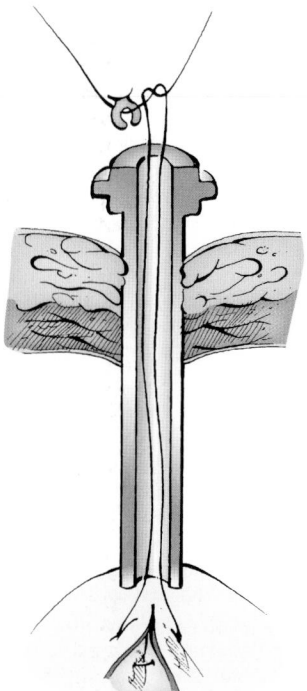

FIGURE 16.8 Extracorporeal knot tying with the Clarke knot pusher. (Modified from Hulka JF, Reich H. *Textbook of laparoscopy*, 2nd ed. Philadelphia, PA: WB Saunders, 1994:202, with permission. Copyright © 1987 Elsevier.)

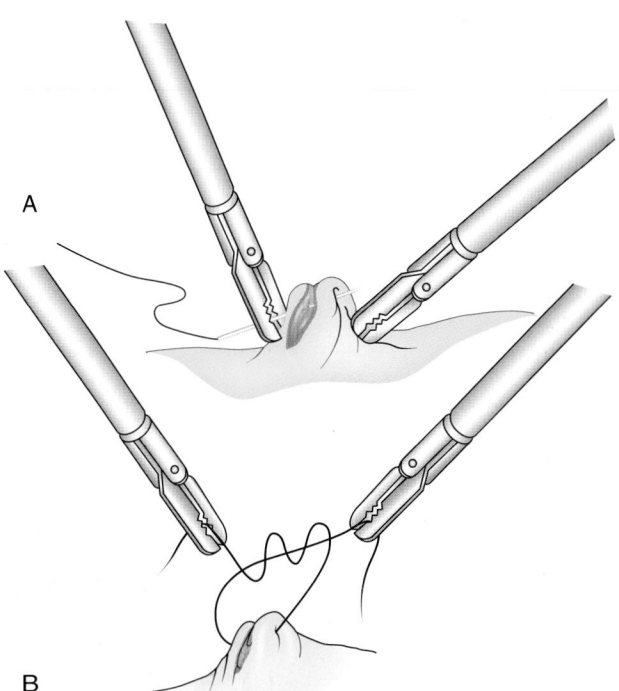

FIGURE 16.9 Intracorporeal knot tying. **A:** The needle is passed through the tissue. **B:** A surgeon's knot is made with the instruments and pulled tight.

Vascular Clips Endoscopic vascular clips may be used to achieve hemostasis for bleeding vessels or pedicles. These offer the advantage of being used near vital structures, where the use of other forms of energy may otherwise result in lateral thermal damage.

Laser Energy

The term *laser* is an acronym for *l*ight *a*mplification by *s*pontaneous *e*mission of *r*adiation. Surgical lasers available for gynecologic use include CO_2, argon, potassium titanyl phosphate, and neodymium:yttrium–aluminum–garnet. These have the ability to vaporize, cut, and, to varying degrees, coagulate tissue (see Chapter 15).

Ultrasonic Energy

The HARMONIC ACE Scalpel (Ethicon) uses vibration at a rate of 55,000 cycles per second, as an energy source to break hydrogen bonds in tissue, resulting in cutting or coaptation of vessels. The Harmonic devices are available for use in vaginal, abdominal, and laparoscopic procedures. The laparoscopic device, termed the Harmonic Ace (Fig. 16.10), is approved for sealing vessels up to 5 mm in diameter. It can be used to grasp, seal, and incise structures, or the active blade can be used alone for dissection and transection of tissue. This modality results in minimal lateral thermal spread of energy, and there is no risk of electrical injury.

Electrosurgery

Monopolar and bipolar electrosurgical instruments are frequently used to perform tubal sterilization and to obtain hemostasis. Monopolar instruments use current that flows from an active electrode through a patient's tissue, and exits by way of a return electrode plate (usually placed on the patient's thigh), to the electrosurgical unit (ESU). Needlepoint electrodes, L-hooks, and most endoscopic scissors are examples of monopolar electrosurgical instruments. Bipolar instruments, such as the Kleppinger forceps and the newer impedance-controlled bipolar systems, use current that flows from an active electrode through tissue and returns back to the ESU through a return electrode within the same instrument. With bipolar energy, a return electrode plate is not necessary. Both monopolar and bipolar electrosurgery can be used for cutting or coagulating (see Chapter 15).

Electrosurgical instruments conduct high-frequency alternating current (AC), which forces electrons through the tissue and accomplishes resistive heating. With AC, electrons flow back and forth between positive and negative poles, as compared with direct current, in which electrons only flow in one direction. Household electrical outlets conduct low-frequency AC, at 60 cycles per second (Hz). Electrosurgical generators convert low-frequency AC to high-frequency AC, in the range of radiofrequency (300 to 600 kHz). The waveform of radiofrequency current is continuous and sinusoidal. The waveform can thus be interrupted to produce different effects (Fig. 16.11).

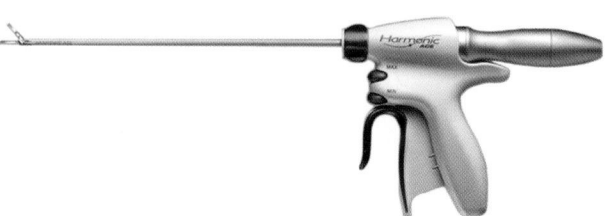

FIGURE 16.10 HARMONIC ACE. (Courtesy of Ethicon.)

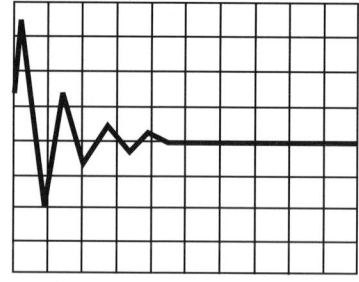

Coagulating Wave Form

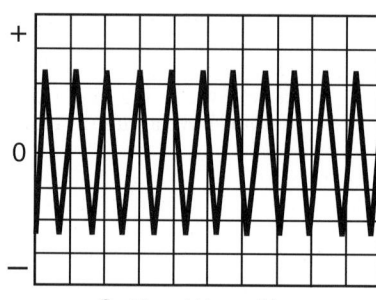

Cutting Wave Form

FIGURE 16.11 Coagulating and cutting waveforms.

Cutting mode utilizes continuous uninterrupted low-voltage energy, inducing resistive heating and causing cells to vaporize at their boiling point of 100°C. There is very little elevation in surrounding tissue temperature, therefore minimizing the amount of lateral thermal damage. Modifications in the waveform refer to blend 1 (80% on, 20% off), blend 2 (60% on, 40% off), blend 3 (50% on, 50% off), and coagulation (6% on, 94% off). Electrosurgical generators will maintain a constant power output; therefore, when the highly interrupted waveform of *coagulation mode* is utilized, and current is reduced, a higher output voltage will be generated (watts = voltage × current). These "bursts" of high voltage increase the temperature of surrounding tissues, resulting in denaturation and charring, giving the effect of coagulation and hemostasis, rather than cutting. Understanding the concepts of cutting and coagulation is clinically relevant when bleeding is encountered. For example, when there is surface oozing, fulguration is used to achieve enough superficial lateral thermal spread to cause hemostasis. Fulguration is superficial coagulation, which uses the coagulation mode to achieve high-voltage sparking. The highly interrupted, high-voltage current causes random sparks to arc between the electrode and tissue, rapidly elevating superficial tissue temperatures, in order to achieve hemostasis. Vessels up to 2 mm in diameter can be controlled in this manner, although it is ineffective in wet surgical fields, as the current is conducted and the energy is widely disbursed. Conversely, in the case of a larger bleeding vessel or pedicle, it is best to desiccate the tissue by applying pressure (coaptation) and cutting current. This causes fibrous bonding of the dehydrated cells of the endothelium without significant lateral thermal spread. It also decreases the risk of thermal bowel injury from capacitive coupling (see Chapter 15), as lower voltage is used. Conversely, when the coagulation waveform is used in this scenario, instead of causing bonding inside the vessel, superficial lateral thermal spread is more likely to occur along the tissue surface, resulting in eschar formation and subsequent bleeding.

Current density refers to the amount of current flow per cross-sectional area, described in amps per meters squared.

This concept has several direct applications to the use of electrosurgical energy in laparoscopy and is used to safely return current from the patient to the ESU. Because current density is described in terms of current per meter squared, applying energy to a small area of bleeding or to a bleeding tissue pedicle will result in an intended thermal effect, inversely related to the electrode size. For example, the use of a needlepoint electrode will have high-current density, compared with a much larger spatula tip, resulting in greater energy applied to a small surface in the former. The current density principle is used to allow current to exit the body without causing injury, as it exits through a relatively large surface area of the return electrode, usually placed on the patient's thigh. This does not cause an exit site burn because of low current density. Exit site burns have typically occurred when part of the return electrode has peeled away from the patient, resulting in a smaller area of surface contact, thus creating high current density at the exit site. Newer systems have a built-in fault, whereby the active electrode will not deliver current if the pad is no longer in complete contact with the patient.

Bipolar instruments have undergone significant transformation in recent years. Simple bipolar systems, such as the ESU with a Kleppinger forceps, have evolved to devices that provide bipolar energy that senses tissue impedance to perform controlled energy delivery. The LigaSure Vessel Sealing Device (Covidien) (Fig. 16.12A) applies high coaptive pressure at temperatures below 100°C, to denature and reform hydrogen cross-links, forming a vascular seal. Tissue fusion and vessel sealing use the body's own collagen and elastin to create a permanent fusion zone. Hemostasis is achieved by reforming the collagen and elastin in vessel walls to form an autologous seal. Tissue impedance is monitored 3,333 times a second, in order to provide real-time adjustment of energy output. The EnSeal Laparoscopic Vessel Fusion System (Ethicon) (Fig. 16.12B) is also able to produce high-coaptive pressures and does so uniformly across the length of the jaw, as a mechanical blade is advanced. The plastic jaws are thermoelastic and contain conductive carbon spheres. When the temperature exceeds 100°C, the polymer of the jaws expands, and the spheres are separated such that they cannot conduct current. Tight temperature regulation is thus maintained, avoiding elevation in temperature of surrounding tissue. Additionally, the offset electrode configuration, whereby the positive electrode is located within the nonhinged lower jaw and all jaw components serve as the negative electrode, is designed to minimize thermal spread. The combination of coaptive pressure and heat results in a tissue seal. PlasmaKinetic technology (Gyrus ACMI, a division of Olympus) makes two laparoscopic instruments, both of which deliver pulsed, ultra–low-voltage, high-current radiofrequency energy and utilize continuous impedance feedback. The HALO PKS Cutting Forceps (Fig. 16.12C) uses a mechanical blade, while the PKS Omni delivers both bipolar coagulation and cutting. The newest device on the market, the ThunderBeat (Olympus) (Fig. 16.12D), combines bipolar and ultrasonic energy. Sealing can be achieved alone by applying bipolar energy, or sealing and cutting can occur simultaneously with a combination of bipolar and ultrasonic energy. Bipolar energy is applied laterally, while ultrasonic energy is applied centrally. All of these devices are approved to seal vessels up to 7 mm in diameter.

In several comparative studies between the HARMONIC ACE, LigaSure, and EnSeal, failure rates and mean burst pressure tended to increase for all instruments with increasing vessel diameter, but the lowest burst pressures measured were still three times higher than that of normal systolic pressure. EnSeal and LigaSure had less radial adventitial collagen denaturation than the Harmonic ACE. Representative histologic samples were found to have less than 3 mm of coagulative necrosis for all instruments; therefore, 5 mm is likely a safe margin of distance from an instrument, in order to avoid histologic damage. When change in temperature was measured at varying distances, no changes were recorded at distances greater than 1 cm from the tips of monopolar, bipolar, Harmonic, and LigaSure devices in a porcine model. It is worth noting that the maximum temperature during and after activation is approximately 200°C for ThunderBeat and Harmonic, and that those devices require almost twice the time to cool to less than 60°C, as compared to LigaSure. The maximum temperature during and after activation therefore requires some caution, in order to avoid inadvertent thermal damage to surrounding structures.

Energy systems are commonly used for making the colpotomy, although there are reports of introducing a scalpel laparoscopically. Monopolar hooks, bipolar hooks, spatulas, lasers, and the active ultrasonic blades of the Harmonic and ThunderBeat devices run the gamut of what is available

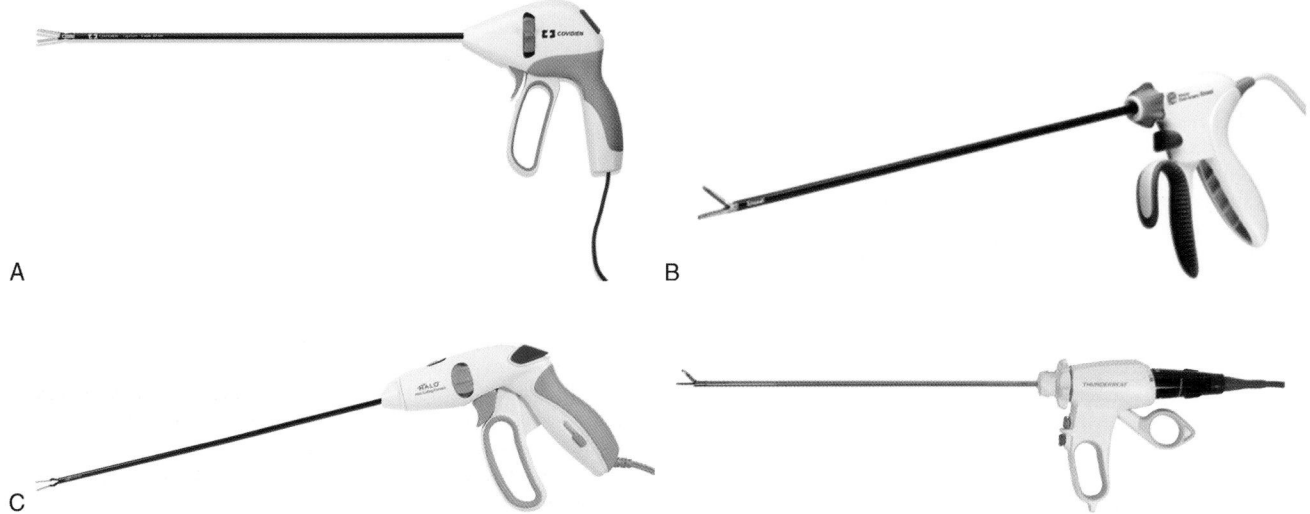

A B C

FIGURE 16.12 Bipolar energy devices. **A:** LigaSure. (Copyright © 2012 Covidien. All rights reserved. Used with permission of Covidien.) **B:** EnSeal. (Courtesy of Ethicon.) **C:** HALO PKS Cutting Forceps. (Courtesy of Gyrus.) **D:** ThunderBeat. (Courtesy of Olympus.)

and typically used. Several companies manufacture monopolar loops for assisting in performance of supracervical hysterectomy. They typically operate at high wattages (100 to 130 watts), using moderately interrupted current (20% coagulation, 80% cut), and can transect the uterine corpus from the cervix in approximately 5 seconds. The loops may also assist in transection of broad-based pedunculated myomas, especially when visualization of the stalk is obscured. It is important when using a monopolar loop, however, to ensure that no viscera are entrapped prior to activation. Many other monopolar, bipolar, and ultrasonic devices can accomplish the same tasks, but not with the same degree of efficiency. The time saved in the operating room must be balanced by the cost of additional instrumentation.

Robotics

In 1994, the first U.S. Food and Drug Administration–approved robotic surgical device called AESOP (Automated Endoscopic System for Optimal Positioning, Computer Motion, Inc.) was introduced. With this system, the surgeon could control the orientation of the laparoscope through voice commands. The da Vinci Robotic Surgical System (Intuitive Surgical) and Zeus Robotic Surgical System (Computer Motion) allow the surgeon to operate from a remote station with hand controls that can provide increased dexterity and minimize fatigue, tremors, or incidental hand movement (see Chapter 17).

POSITIONING THE PATIENT FOR LAPAROSCOPIC SURGERY

The patient should be placed on the operating table in the low lithotomy position with the buttocks at or slightly over the table's edge to allow placement and use of an intrauterine manipulator and to have access to the perineum if needed during surgery. The patient's thighs should be in the same plane as the abdomen to allow freedom of motion for laparoscopic instrumentation. When the knees are bent and elevated above the plane of the abdominal wall, it is difficult to gain access to the upper abdomen and pelvic brim without bumping into the legs because of the fulcrum effect of instruments placed into lower ports. Stirrups should have ample padding to support the lower leg without creating pressure points. Particular attention should be given to preventing injury to the peroneal nerve, which is especially vulnerable to compression injury. It is preferable to use a stirrup that can be elevated without undraping the patient so that a high lithotomy position can be used for easier vaginal access if needed. To avoid stretch injury to the femoral, sciatic, or obturator nerves, the thigh should be flexed no more than 90 degrees, and the hips should be abducted no more than 45 degrees. External rotation should be avoided.

Systems to prevent slippage while in steep Trendelenburg include nonslip pads, beanbags, and shoulder braces. Nearly all of these setups require that the arms be tucked to the side. Caution should be exercised when using shoulder braces, as brachial plexus injuries can result when placed too medially.

Surgical Suite

Efficient orientation of the surgical suite is critical for efficient laparoscopic surgery. In general, a right-handed surgeon stands on the patient's left side with the surgical assistant on the patient's right; however, some surgeons prefer the patient's right side. The monitor is usually placed between the patient's

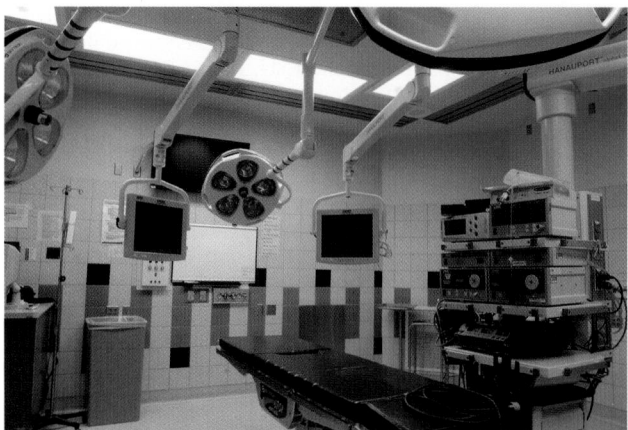

FIGURE 16.13 Ergonomic surgical suite with ceiling-mounted, movable flat screens.

legs if only one is available. In the case of two monitors, these are usually placed near the patient's lower legs in the direct line of vision of the surgeons. Newer surgical suites have done away with towers and have ceiling-mounted, movable flat screens, which are highly ergonomic (Fig. 16.13). The insufflation monitor is usually placed across from the surgeon so intra-abdominal pressure can be viewed. Insufflation tubing, light cords, electrosurgical cords, and suction–irrigation tubing should be out of the surgeon's path if perineal access is necessary. Knowledgeable operating room personnel are likewise critical to the laparoscopic mission. The scrub technician usually stands caudad to the surgical assistant. A circulating technician assists in troubleshooting equipment and obtaining supplies and equipment.

ENTERING THE ABDOMINAL CAVITY

The abdominal cavity may be initially entered at the umbilicus or alternative sites by Veres needle, open laparoscopy, or direct trocar insertion.

Umbilical Site Veres Needle Technique

When the umbilical site and Veres needle technique is used, the Veres needle is first placed into the abdominal cavity to establish a pneumoperitoneum, and a trocar is subsequently placed into the pneumoperitoneum. A meta-analysis of methods used to establish pneumoperitoneum compared open access (Hasson type) with closed access (needle/trocar) and two types of closed access techniques (direct trocar versus needle/trocar). It was noted that deaths were only reported in the needle/trocar group. However, because of the rarity of death as an outcome, the statistical risk could not be compared meaningfully. The meta-analysis was underpowered to adequately compare the two closed techniques. Therefore, the question of which technique for initial port placement is safest has not been definitively answered to date.

A scalpel is used to make a small skin incision in accordance with the size of the trocar to be placed at the umbilicus or in the left upper quadrant (discussed later in Alternatives to Umbilical Entry). The skin should be elevated in the case of umbilical entry, and the scalpel should be held parallel to the long axis of the patient, to avoid incidentally lacerating the great vessels, which lie in close proximity to the umbilicus. Having the anesthesiologist decompress the stomach with a nasogastric tube will decrease the risk of inserting the Veres

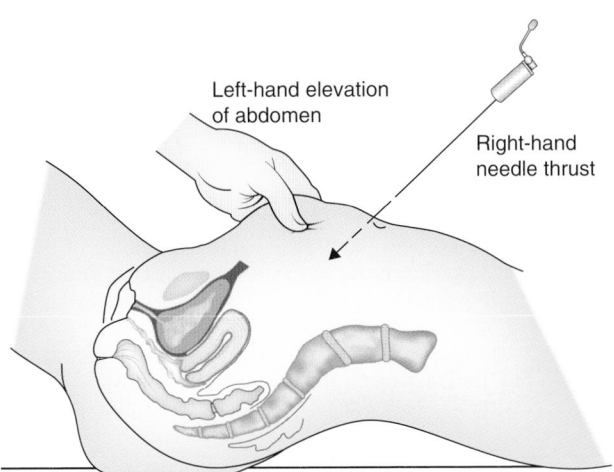

Left-hand elevation
of abdomen

Right-hand
needle thrust

FIGURE 16.14 Insertion of the Veres needle.

needle or trocar into an overdistended stomach, especially in the case of a left upper quadrant entry. The patient's abdomen should be relaxed by neuromuscular blockade if general anesthesia is being used to allow adequate elevation for Veres needle and trocar insertion. The patient should be lying in a flat or neutral position on the operating table, because the use of Trendelenburg positioning may cause the trajectory of the Veres needle or trocar to be closer to the great vessels rather than the pelvic cavity. In the thin patient, the Veres needle or trocar should be directed toward the hollow of the sacrum to avoid the great vessels (Fig. 16.14). In the obese patient, the aorta is typically above the level of the umbilicus; therefore, the Veres needle or trocar may be inserted vertically (90 degrees to the long axis of the patient), as long as the abdominal wall has been elevated adequately (Fig. 16.15). Placing the Veres needle close to the base of the umbilicus takes advantage of the thin natural confluence of tissue planes at the umbilicus. Separate clicks can be heard or felt as the needle traverses the fused fascia of the rectus muscles and then peritoneum.

Correct placement of the Veres needle into the abdominal cavity can be assessed by several techniques. The hanging drop technique is used by placing a small amount of sterile saline in the top of the Veres needle to verify a negative intra-abdominal pressure as it descends into the abdominal cavity. Alternatively, the syringe barrel test can be performed by watching the column of saline descend the barrel of a syringe attached to the Veres needle. Aspiration of a syringe attached to the Veres needle can test for blood or gastrointestinal

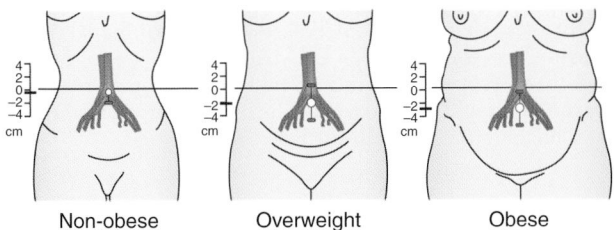

Non-obese   Overweight   Obese

FIGURE 16.15 The location of the umbilicus in relationship to the major vessels in nonobese, overweight, and obese patients. (Modified from Hurd WW, Bude RO, DeLancey JO, et al. The relationship of the umbilicus to the aortic bifurcation: implications for laparoscopic technique. *Obstet Gynecol* 1992;80:48, with permission. Copyright © 1992, The American Congress of Obstetricians and Gynecologists.)

contents. Low-flow insufflation should be performed at a flow rate of approximately 1 L/min, until further signs of intra-abdominal needle placement are confirmed, such as low intra-abdominal pressure (<10 mm Hg) or loss of dullness to percussion over the right upper quadrant. If the "intra-abdominal" pressure reading is higher than 10 mm Hg, the probability of extraperitoneal insufflation is high, and the approach should be reassessed. A prospective, observational study of four tests to ascertain Veres needle placement compared the double click test, the hanging drop test, the aspiration test, and the initial five insufflation pressures in 345 women. High insufflation pressures were the most sensitive for preperitoneal insufflation. Occasionally, high insufflation pressures may be encountered with correct intra-abdominal entry, such as in the case of morbid obesity or when the omentum is in close proximity. Often, the abdominal wall can be lifted, allowing the omentum to dislodge from the Veres, and an appropriate opening pressure will be observed. If elevating the abdomen does not result in a more appropriate pressure within several seconds, it must be assumed that the Veres needle is in the incorrect space and must be reinserted. High-flow insufflation may occasionally be used in the presence of reassuring signs of correct needle placement. During insufflation, intra-abdominal pressures should not exceed 20 to 25 mm Hg to avoid interfering with diaphragmatic excursion and central venous return from caval compression. After an adequate pneumoperitoneum has been established, ranging from 1 to 5 L depending on body habitus, a trocar is inserted at the umbilicus, paying attention to the angle of insertion based on body habitus, as discussed. Once the trocar is placed, the bladed or central portion is removed, and the laparoscope is placed through the trocar sleeve to ensure correct placement before attaching the insufflation tubing to the trocar sleeve.

Alternates to Umbilical Entry

When Veres needle insufflation is not successful, or in patients who are at risk for adhesions near the umbilicus, placing the Veres needle at a site other than the umbilicus is usually successful. Two commonly used sites are Palmer point and the left ninth intercostal space. Palmer point is located 3 cm from the midline and 3 cm below the left rib cage. The needle is directed 15 degrees cephalad after the skin has been stretched caudally. This will help direct the Veres needle at a 90-degree angle to the peritoneum, facilitating entry. If the ninth intercostal space is used, the Veres needle should be placed between the ninth and tenth rib, grazing the top of the tenth rib. This grazing minimizes the risk of damaging the intercostal neurovascular bundle. The rib cage provides a natural elevation of a space devoid of bowel regardless of patient weight. There is a remote chance of pneumothorax with this technique. Before performing either of these techniques, palpation for splenomegaly should be performed. After Veres needle placement, a 5-mm trocar is usually placed at Palmer point.

Open Laparoscopy

Hasson described the technique of open laparoscopy in 1971 as a way of avoiding blind trocar placement. A small incision is made at the umbilicus. Allis clamps are used to grasp the fascia, which is incised, and the peritoneum is entered directly. A Hasson-type cannula is used that can be anchored to sutures in the rectus fascia. In a review of more than 5,000 cases over nearly three decades, this technique has been shown to be associated with a low complication rate.

III

Direct Trocar Insertion

Direct trocar placement has also been described by placing the trocar through the umbilicus initially, rather than using the Veres needle.

SECONDARY TROCAR PLACEMENT

One or two secondary ports are usually adequate for most laparoscopic procedures. More complicated surgeries may require up to five. These may be placed lateral to the inferior epigastric artery or in the midline above the bladder. The size and number of trocars will depend on the procedure and equipment to be used. A 3- to 5-mm trocar may be used for diagnostic laparoscopy to maneuver pelvic organs for adequate visualization. Most instruments for tissue manipulation will fit through a 5-mm port. Some energy delivery systems and tissue retrieval systems require the use of larger ports (8 to 15 mm). Anticipating the need for larger ports can lead to significant cost savings when disposable trocars are used.

The placement of lateral trocars can be associated with injury to the inferior epigastric vessels. Before lateral trocar placement, these vessels can usually be seen along the anterior abdominal wall, as they branch off the external iliac vessels. They can also be found in the anterior abdominal wall triangle, delineated medially by the medial umbilical ligament and laterally by the insertion of the round ligament (**Fig. 16.16**). Laparoscopic visualization of the inferior epigastric vessels has been shown to be successful in 88% of normal weight women, decreasing to 63% in obese women. The ability to visualize the superficial epigastric vessels with transillumination, however, is much more dependent upon weight, with 84% identified in normal weight women and only 23% identified in obese women. Insertion of a spinal needle through the anterior abdominal wall at the intended site of trocar insertion can help find a safe trajectory away from the inferior epigastric vessels. If the vessels cannot be seen, a safe location can usually be found by measuring 5 cm superior to the pubic symphysis and 8 cm lateral. In a study in which ultrasonography was used to measure the distance between the inferior epigastric artery and the umbilicus, a median of 4.75 cm was observed. Additionally, the distance from the midline

at the levels of the umbilicus and the ASIS never exceeded 6 cm. Six centimeters should therefore be considered the minimum safe distance from the midline. Secondary trocars should be inserted in a controlled fashion, under direct vision. Placement of suprapubic secondary trocars should be placed well above the bladder. Two fingerbreadths measured above the pubic symphysis has been standard terminology for midline trocar placement. Because of the significant differences in finger widths among surgeons and considering the increased risk of bladder injury using the suprapubic location, it is also worth placing a spinal needle through the anterior abdominal wall in the midline to ensure that the port is well above the bladder. If the patient has had a prior laparotomy, the bladder may be tented superiorly, and it may be necessary to place the trocar higher.

TISSUE REMOVAL

Small tissue fragments, such as peritoneal biopsy specimens, may be removed through 5-mm trocar sleeves. Large, dense specimens, such as leiomyoma fragments, require larger ports (10 to 15 mm). Fluid-filled specimens, such as ovarian cysts, may be placed in a plastic specimen removal bag (**Fig. 16.17**) and drained while in the bag to avoid spillage. A posterior colpotomy can also be performed for specimen removal. Colpotomy may be performed vaginally, as one would when performing vaginal hysterectomy, or laparoscopically. Laparoscopic colpotomy is performed by first inserting a lubricated sponge stick into the posterior vaginal fornix for cul-de-sac elevation. An incision is then made between the uterosacral ligaments into the posterior vaginal fornix, using the sponge stick as a backstop. Laser, unipolar scissors, or the Harmonic Scalpel may be used as an energy source. An endoscopic specimen bag may be removed through the colpotomy incision. A wet lap pad may be placed vaginally to allow optimal pneumoperitoneum for laparoscopic closure of the colpotomy, or the colpotomy may be closed vaginally. Alternatively, morcellation may be performed with an electromechanical or bipolar morcellator (**Fig. 16.18A–D**). There are several electromechanical morcellators, both disposable and reusable, which either are battery powered or utilize a generator. They range 12 to 15 mm in diameter, although the disposable units are typically only available in a 15-mm diameter. The blades are single use and can be retracted during specimen retrieval, when the morcellator function is not needed. A bladeless morcellator is now available, which uses bipolar energy, and a product line–specific generator. For safety reasons, it is important that the tip of the morcellator be in view at all times. Keeping the cutting tip elevated and parallel with the abdominal wall adds to visualization and decreases the risk of inadvertently injuring bowel and other vital structures, as severe injuries have been reported, including injury to the pancreas. The specimen should be drawn up into the morcellator rather than pushing the morcellator into the specimen.

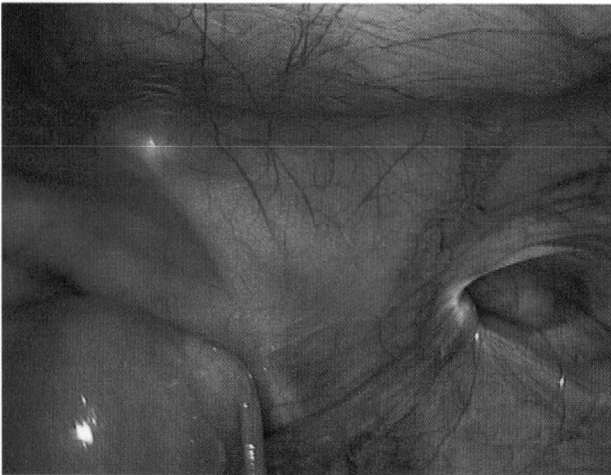

FIGURE 16.16 Note the relationship of the inferior epigastric vessels to the medial umbilical ligament and the insertion of the round ligament.

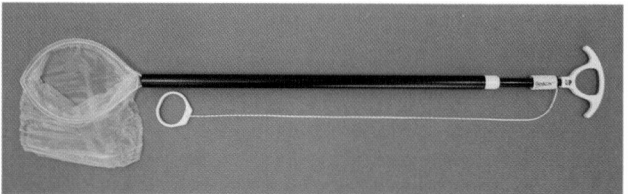

FIGURE 16.17 Specimen retrieval bag. (Courtesy of Genicon.)

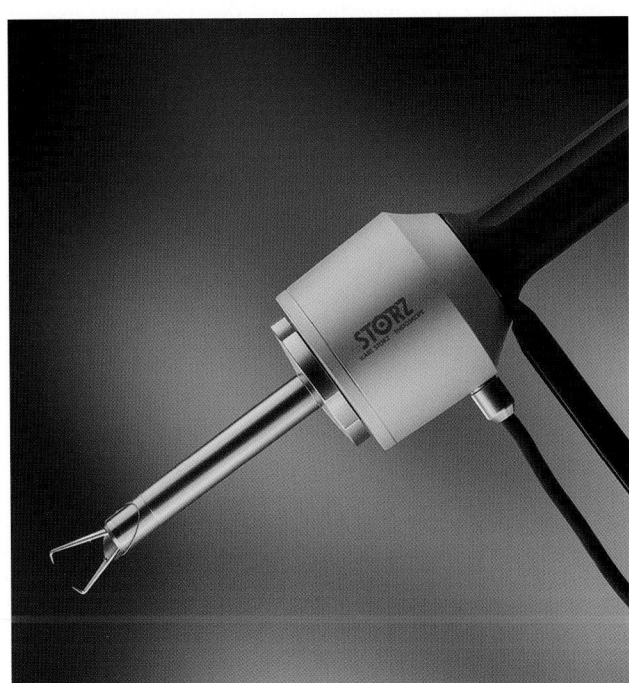

A

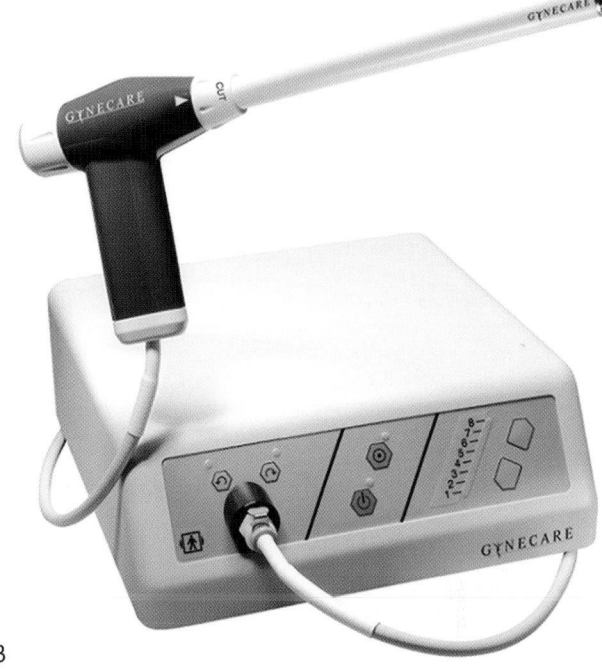

B

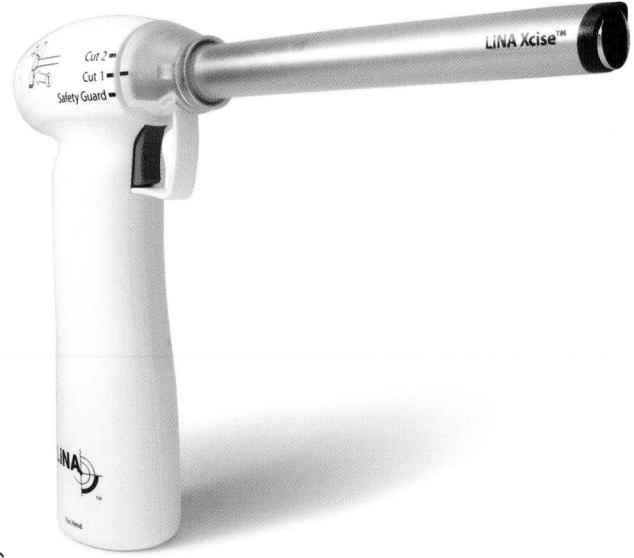

C

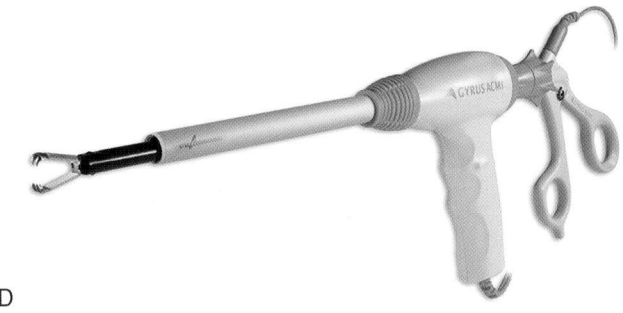

D

III

FIGURE 16.18 Tissue morcellators. **A:** Rotocut. (© 2013 Photo Courtesy of KARL STORZ Endoscopy-America, Inc.) **B:** Morcellex. (Courtesy of Gynecare.) **C:** LiNA Xcise. (Courtesy of LiNA Medical.) **D:** PKS PlasmaSORD. (Courtesy of Olympus.)

FASCIAL CLOSURE

Fascial defects should be closed when measuring 10 mm or greater. This can be done directly, by visualizing the fascia, and securing it in an interrupted or figure-of-eight fashion, utilizing a UR6 needle. Alternatively, a fascial closure device can be used and is especially helpful in patients with a thick anterior abdominal wall, when the fascia is difficult to visualize (Fig. 16.19A–D). These closure devices are used under direct laparoscopic visualization. Some designs require the retrieval of a suture loop, while others are designed to autoretrieve the end of the suture. Additionally, certain designs will allow for any width of fascial closure, while others secure a predetermined width of fascia. Whether performed abdominally or laparoscopically, it is important to secure an appropriate width of fascia to avoid tearing and subsequent herniation.

DIAGNOSTIC LAPAROSCOPY

A systematic approach to diagnostic laparoscopy, like checklists for pilots, can help ensure thoroughness in what is regarded as a routine surgery. After insertion of the laparoscope, the abdomen should be carefully examined, particularly the area in the trajectory of the Veres needle or trocar, to ensure that inadvertent bowel or vascular damage was not caused. Trendelenburg positioning should then be used to view the pelvic cavity and organs.

With the assistance of a uterine manipulator, the uterus can be anteverted to visualize the posterior aspect of the uterus, from the fundus to the posterior cul-de-sac. This should begin with a panoramic view and proceed with a close-up magnification view to detect subtle findings, such as atypical manifestations of endometriosis. The presence of peritoneal windows or defects in the posterior cul-de-sac should be noted if present.

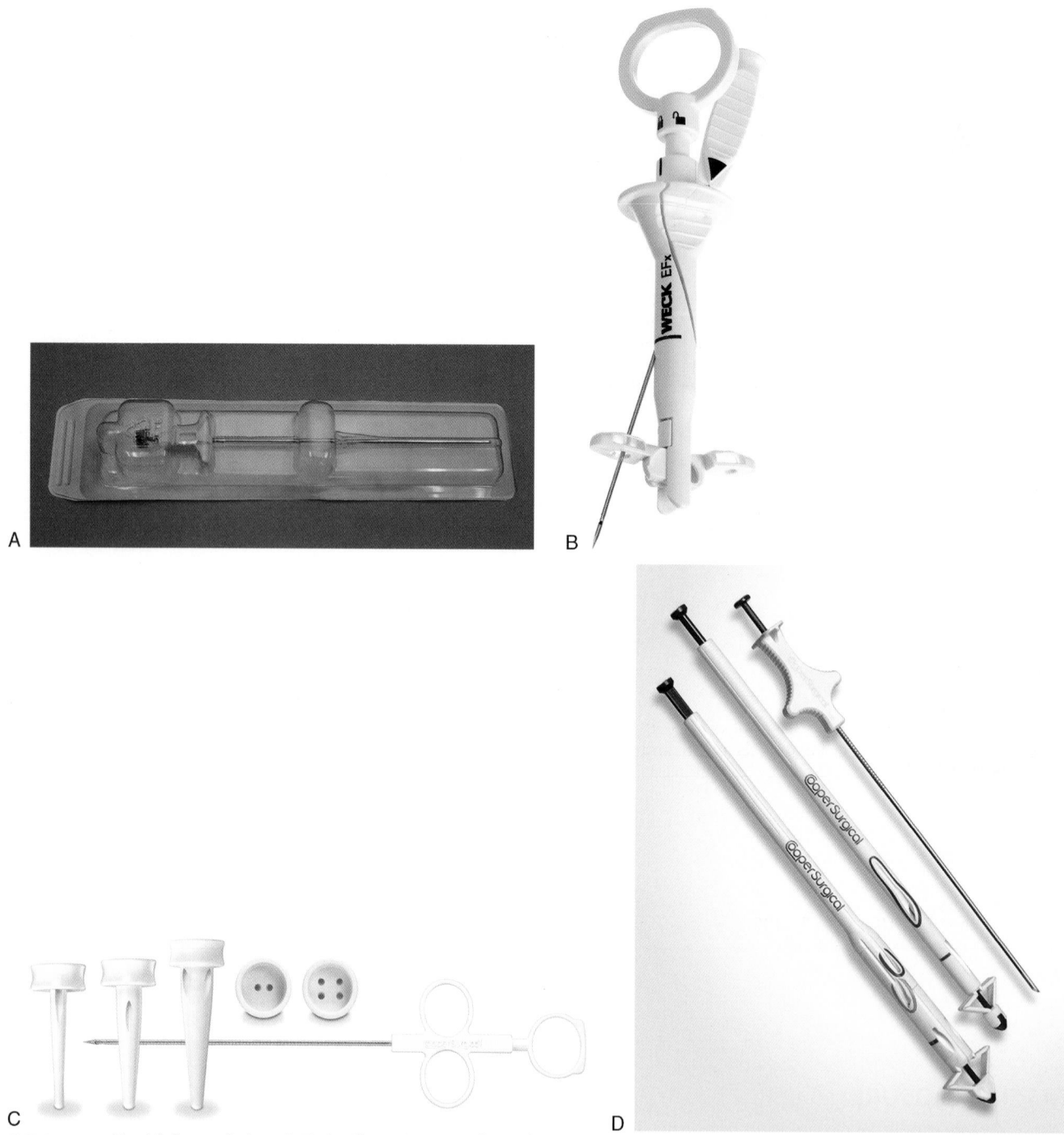

FIGURE 16.19 Fascial closure devices. **A:** Endo Close. (Courtesy of Covidien.) **B:** Weck EFx. (Courtesy of Teleflex.) **C:** Carter-Thomason. (Courtesy of CooperSurgical.) **D:** Carter-Thomason II. (courtesy of CooperSurgical.)

The posterior cul-de-sac should also be probed with an instrument such as a blunt probe or atraumatic grasper to palpate any hidden endometriotic nodules that may be imbedded within the rectovaginal septum. Anytime a shallow posterior cul-de-sac is noted, this should be considered, as an obliterated endometriotic posterior cul-de-sac can have a deceivingly normal-appearing peritoneal surface. The uterosacral ligaments should have the appearance of a "V" with the apex at the cervix. If peritoneal fluid is obscuring the posterior cul-de-sac, the fluid should be removed by suction. The broad ligaments should be inspected for the presence of endometriosis, adhesions, or fibroids.

The ovaries should be viewed globally. This can be accomplished by simply flipping the ovary superiorly with a probe or other blunt instrument, or the utero-ovarian ligament can be grasped with an atraumatic grasper from the contralateral port and rotated by twisting the grasper clockwise for the left ovary and counterclockwise for the right ovary. This provides an excellent view of the undersurface of the ovary that can be easily held in place for inspection of the ovarian fossa and pelvic sidewall. With the ovary lifted up away from the sidewall, the transperitoneal course of the ureter can usually be seen. The ureter is optimally visualized by looking for peristalsis as it crosses the common iliac artery at the pelvic brim. One advantage of identifying the ureter early during surgery is that the peritoneal surface can become edematous as the case proceeds, likely from prolonged carbon dioxide exposure and manipulative contact. The fallopian tube should be handled with care. Fallopian tube forceps are available that allow the tube to be grasped at the mesosalpinx while surrounding the tube. The proximal portion of the tube should be examined for nodules, which may be indicative of salpingitis isthmica nodosa. The fimbria should be examined delicately, looking for any sign of phimosis. Anterior to the fallopian tubes, the round ligaments should be viewed and traced laterally to identify the presence of hernia. The anterior cul-de-sac is best seen by using the uterine manipulator to place the uterus in a retroverted position. In this position, the anterior surface of the uterus and the bladder parietal peritoneum can be seen well. The anterior abdominal wall should be viewed for the presence of endometriosis or hernia.

The appendix should be viewed for any sign of inflammation, endometriosis, or fecalith. This is best performed by using an atraumatic bowel grasper. The upper abdomen should also be inspected, taking note of the liver, gallbladder, and diaphragmatic surfaces. If needed, the large and small intestine can also be inspected by "running" the bowel with two atraumatic bowel graspers. A panoramic, 360-degree evaluation is helpful to ensure that no upper abdominal adhesions have been missed that may have caused the intestine to be adherent to the anterior abdominal wall. It is possible in the presence of such adhesions to place a trocar through and through the intestine unknowingly. This condition can be ruled out by placing the laparoscope through one of the lower ports for visualization of the umbilical port. Chromopertubation may be performed by instilling a diluted indigo carmine solution through the uterine manipulator. Lack of spill may be due to obstruction, tubal spasm, or leakage from the cervix. It is therefore important to have a tight uterine cannula seal at the cervix.

OPERATIVE LAPAROSCOPIC PROCEDURES

Adhesiolysis

Pelvic adhesions have been associated with infertility and chronic pelvic pain. It should be recognized that chronic pelvic pain is often a complex condition, and in the absence of gastrointestinal obstructive symptoms, adhesiolysis is usually often not curative of pain. To better understand the nature of symptomatic adhesion, pain mapping under conscious sedation may be a useful technique. In performing adhesiolysis, optimal results depend on the use of microsurgical technique, gentle tissue handling, and meticulous hemostasis with minimal tissue fulguration. Adhesiolysis can be performed by a number of techniques, including blunt and sharp dissection, electrodissection, aquadissection, and laser dissection.

Blunt dissection is the most rudimentary form of adhesiolysis. Although not recommended, this technique is usually used in treating thin, avascular adhesions. Virtually any type of laparoscopic instrument can be used to place traction on an adhesion to cause separation. If bleeding or significant resistance is encountered, this technique should be abandoned.

Sharp dissection is the preferred method for dealing with all adhesions, especially thick avascular adhesions. The advantage of sharp dissection over electrodissection is the decreased risk of inadvertent electrosurgical injury. This is performed in a similar fashion to laparotomy. The adhesion is held on tension with an atraumatic grasper, and scissors are used to lyse the adhesive band. It is important to turn the tip of the scissors toward the optical viewing angle to avoid vascular or bowel injury.

Aqua dissection can be used to free adhesions from the pelvic sidewall to avoid injury to ureter or the great vessels. It is also a useful technique in removing endometriotic nodules. With this technique, the peritoneum is grasped, and an incision is made large enough to place the tip of a powered suction–irrigation device. Irrigation is used to force fluid under the peritoneum, causing it to balloon out from deeper tissues. The adhesion or peritoneum can then be dissected free.

Monopolar energy and *bipolar energy* are frequently used to lyse thicker vascular adhesions. When using electrosurgery, care must be used to avoid injury to bowel. It is always best to start from known to unknown. As known areas are freed from adhesions, unknown areas become recognizable. Monopolar instruments, like scissors and needlepoint electrodes, are ideal for these adhesions. Bipolar instruments, such as Kleppinger forceps, bipolar scissors, or newer tissue-controlled bipolar energy instruments that seal vessels, can be used.

Laser dissection has been used in laparoscopy with great success as a result of minimal lateral thermal spread, as compared with most forms of electrosurgery. However, it should be noted that this form of energy is indeed still an energy source and obtains hemostasis through lateral thermal spread. The small spot size of laser makes this a useful tool for precision adhesiolysis. The CO_2 laser has a depth of penetration of 0.1 mm and is excellent for cutting. With the adhesion on tension, the CO_2 laser is introduced through the operating channel of the laparoscope or through a secondary port.

The Harmonic Scalpel is used with a technique similar to both bipolar and monopolar dissection, depending whether tissue is grasped or the active blade is used alone. This technique does not use electrosurgery. Ultrasonic energy has the advantage of limited lateral thermal spread, similar to the newer bipolar electrosurgical instruments.

Sidewall and Retroperitoneal Space Dissection

It is often necessary to identify the course of ureter and iliac vessel in cases of pelvic sidewall adhesions or endometriosis. If the ureter is able to be identified at the pelvic brim but then is obscured by adhesions, endometriosis, or an ovarian mass along its caudad course, the peritoneum overlying the sidewall can be grasped and opened with scissors (Fig. 16.20). A Maryland dissector can be used to gently

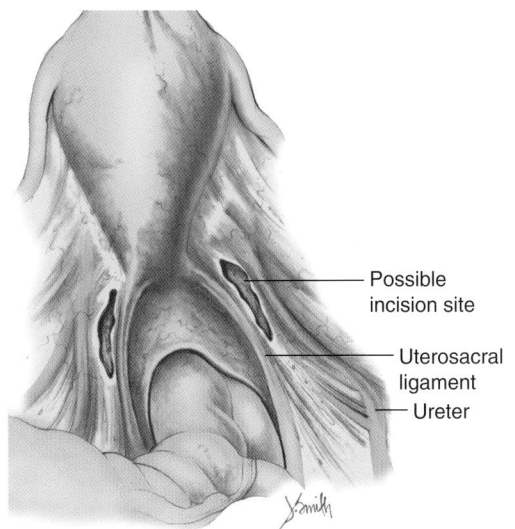

Possible incision site

Uterosacral ligament

Ureter

FIGURE 16.20 Pelvic sidewall dissection. The peritoneum has been incised so that the retroperitoneal structures can be visualized.

spread the peritoneum to view the ureter. If the anatomy is distorted, it may be necessary to start the dissection at the pelvic brim or by opening the round ligament. If the round ligament is to be opened, it should be divided with an energy source as lateral as possible, and a blunt grasper can be used to dissect the retroperitoneal space, watching for the ureter on the medial leaf of the broad ligament and avoiding the iliac vessels. Developing the pararectal space can help to define anatomic landmarks to avoid inadvertent vascular or ureteral injury. Once the ureter and uterine artery are located, adhesions can be lysed with an energy system of the surgeon's choice.

Posterior Cul-De-Sac Dissection

When endometriosis or pelvic adhesions partially or completely obliterate the posterior cul-de-sac and are associated with pelvic pain or infertility, a surgical approach is usually indicated. Cul-de-sac obliteration secondary to endometriosis often involves deep fibrotic endometriosis that may involve the rectum, rectovaginal septum, or uterosacral ligaments. Dissection of the posterior cul-de-sac may be necessary and can be performed laparoscopically by skilled surgeons. The goal is to lyse adhesions, excise large or deep endometriotic lesions, and resect or vaporize small superficial lesions.

The patient should undergo a bowel prep before surgery. A uterine manipulator is used to antevert the uterus, and a rectal probe is placed in the rectum to delineate and retract the rectum posteriorly. A sponge stick placed in the vagina can further delineate the rectum from the vagina (**Fig. 16.21**). The anterior rectum is carefully dissected from the posterior aspect of the uterus or vagina with scissors, laser, Harmonic Scalpel, or tissue-controlled bipolar energy system. The use of monopolar and traditional bipolar energy can result in significant thermal injury to the rectum. Aquadissection may also be useful. Dissection should continue until the loose areolar tissue of the rectovaginal space is reached. If a ureter is near the site of dissection, the position of the ureter should be confirmed before any dissection takes place. The fibrotic endometriosis can then be excised from the posterior vagina or uterosacral ligaments. If endometriosis extends to the vaginal mucosa, this is excised, and the posterior vagina is closed vaginally or laparoscopically. Palpation of the endometriotic nodule before and after removal is helpful to ensure complete excision.

Oophorectomy and Salpingo-Oophorectomy

STEPS IN THE PROCEDURE

Salpingo-Oophorectomy

- Ensure that the tube and ovary are free of all adhesions.

- Identify the ureter. If it is not possible to visualize the ureter through the peritoneum, incise the peritoneum, and identify the ureter by dissecting the pararectal space.

- The infundibulopelvic ligament is isolated and sealed with either bipolar or ultrasonic energy and transected. The utero-ovarian ligament is sealed and transected.

- The intervening mesosalpinx is incised parallel to the round ligament.

- All pedicles are inspected for hemostasis.

Several techniques for laparoscopic oophorectomy or salpingo-oophorectomy have been described. One procedure involves the placement of three loop ligatures around the ovary and adnexa. Before placement of the loops, the structures must be free of adhesions. Incisions in the mesosalpinx are sometimes necessary to facilitate placement. The ovary or adnexa is cut distal to the three loops. Small bleeding points can be coagulated on the stump, but care must be taken not to coagulate the suture.

Alternatively, the peritoneum is opened, and the ureter is identified by dissecting the pararectal space (**Fig. 16.22A, B**). Lactated Ringer solution or saline can be injected into the retroperitoneal space to push the ureter away from the site of coagulation and increase the margin of safety. The utero-ovarian ligament is coagulated or sealed with bipolar energy or ultrasonic energy and transected, and the infundibulopelvic ligament is then coagulated or sealed and transected. If the fallopian tube is to be removed with the ovary, the proximal fallopian tube and utero-ovarian ligament are coagulated or sealed before transection (**Fig. 16.23A–C**). The intervening mesosalpinx is similarly transected. Pedicles are examined for hemostasis, and the ovary is removed by one of the described methods of tissue removal. Laparoscopic stapling devices can also be used on the pedicles, but care must be used to avoid the ureter.

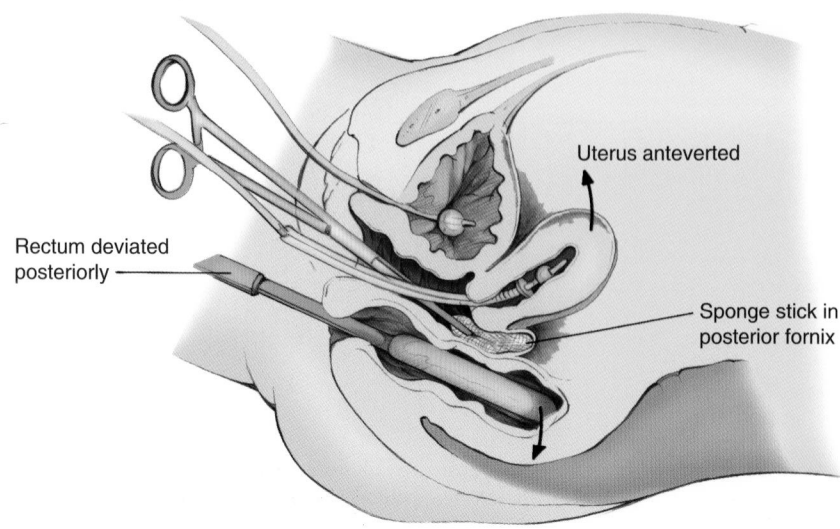

Rectum deviated posteriorly

Uterus anteverted

Sponge stick in posterior fornix

FIGURE 16.21 Dissection of the posterior cul-de-sac. Instruments in the uterus, posterior fornix of the vagina, and rectum help define the anatomy.

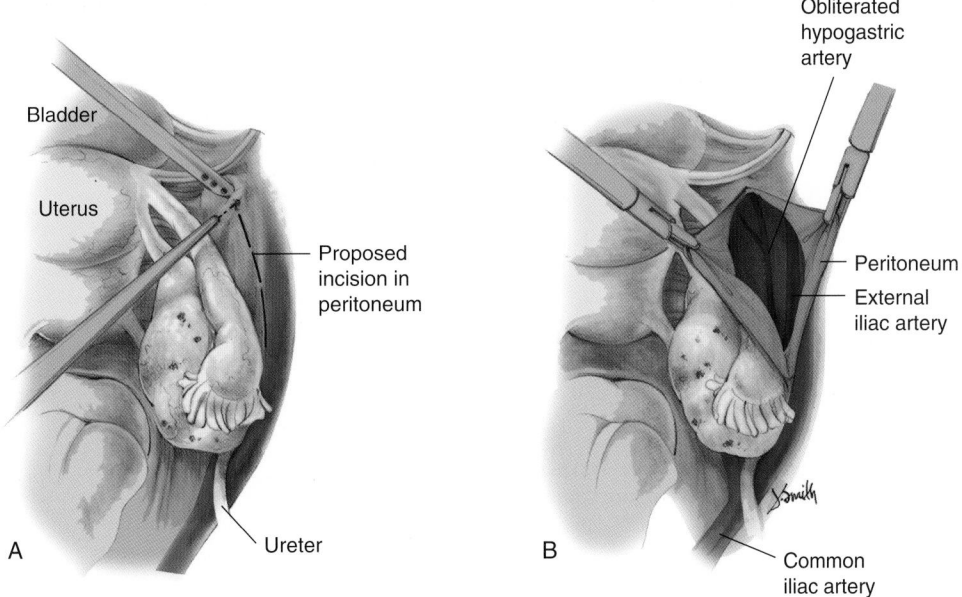

FIGURE 16.22 Dissecting the retroperitoneal space. **A:** The peritoneum overlying the pelvic sidewall is incised. **B:** The peritoneum is opened, and the ureter and vessels are identified.

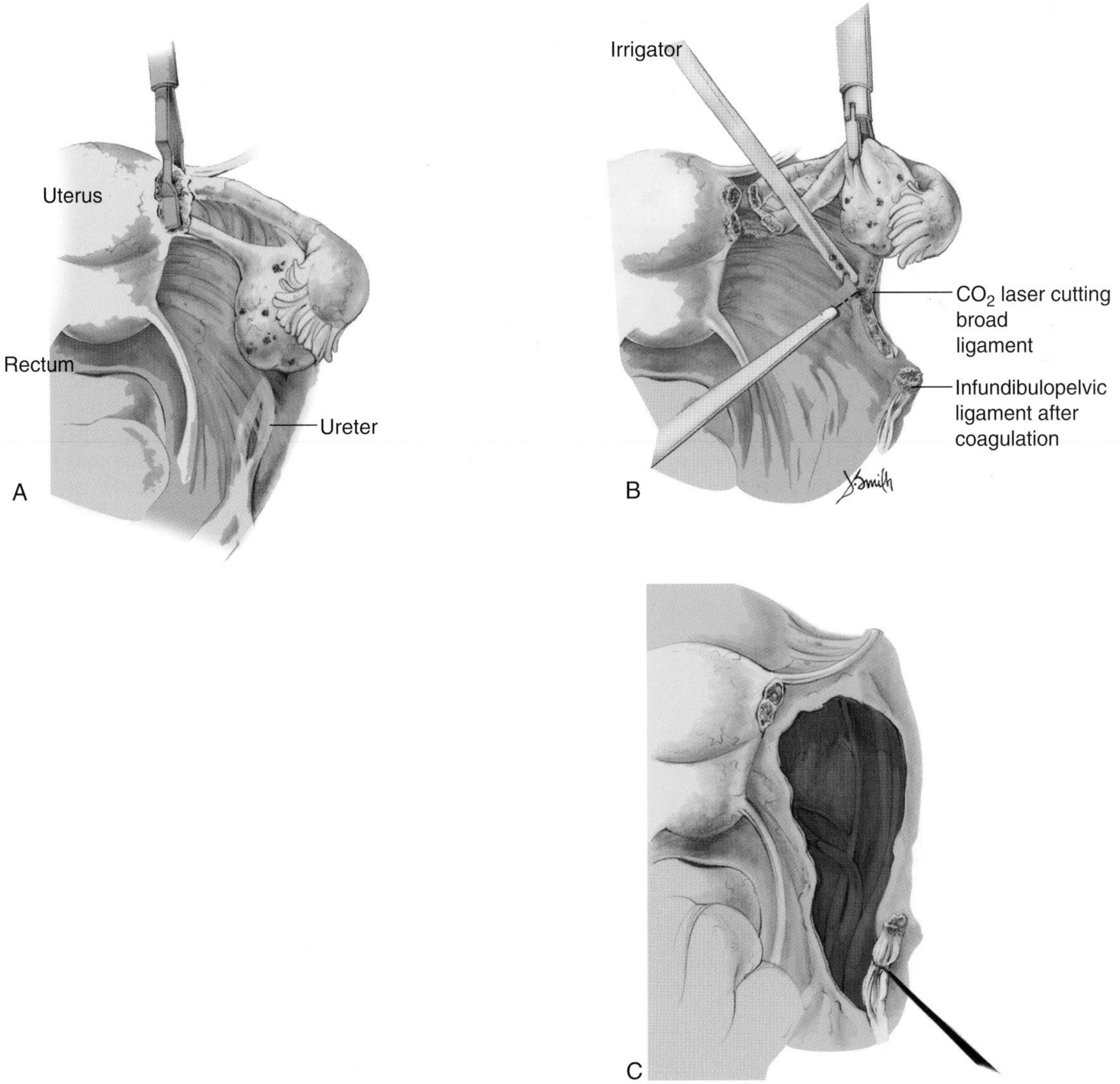

FIGURE 16.23 Oophorectomy with the use of bipolar coagulation. **A:** The utero-ovarian ligament is coagulated and then transected. **B:** The infundibulopelvic ligament is coagulated with bipolar forceps and then cut. **C:** An Endoloop may be placed on the infundibulopelvic ligament after transaction for added hemostasis.

LAPAROSCOPIC MYOMECTOMY

STEPS IN THE PROCEDURE

Myomectomy

- A hemostatic agent, such as dilute vasopressin, is injected into the myometrium, either through a port or transabdominally.

- The uterine serosa is incised with a laser, needle electrode, or ultrasonic energy.

- A myoma screw is introduced into the fibroid, or a tenaculum is used to grasp the fibroid.

- The fibroid is enucleated with a combination of traction and countertraction, as well as electrosurgery where indicated.

- The defect is closed in two to three layers.

Laparoscopic myomectomy is a heterogeneous procedure that can range from a simple procedure to one of the more difficult laparoscopic surgeries requiring expert laparoscopic suturing skills. For example, large pedunculated fibroids (8 to 10 cm) can be detached in a few minutes. Large intramural fibroids may take several hours to remove and repair in the hands of expert laparoscopic surgeons. Two case–control studies comparing open with laparoscopic myomectomy have both demonstrated significantly longer mean operating room time and shorter hospital stays with the laparoscopic group. The use of a preoperative gonadotropin-releasing hormone (GnRH) agonist may be considered in patients who are anemic. A prospective randomized study using leuprolide acetate in patients undergoing laparoscopic myomectomy also demonstrated significantly lower blood loss and operative times in the treatment group. The authors of this study noted increased operative time in the subset of markedly hypoechoic fibroids because of increased fibroid softness. Other studies have shown longer operative times and a higher conversion to laparotomy rate associated with the use of GnRH agonists in laparoscopic myomectomy because of difficult cleavage planes.

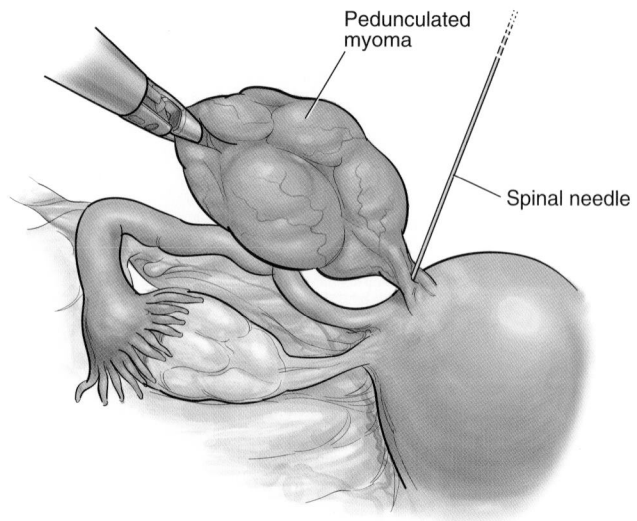

FIGURE 16.24 Excision of a pedunculated myoma. The base is thoroughly coagulated and cut.

Pedunculated myomas can be resected by coagulating and transecting the base, and the defect does not typically require suturing (**Fig. 16.24**). Intramural and subserosal fibroids require an incision to be made with scissors, laser, needle electrode, or Harmonic Scalpel. Before incising the uterine serosa, it is advisable to inject hemostatic agents into the serosa and myoma. A dilute vasopressin solution or bupivacaine plus epinephrine may be injected transabdominally into the myometrium through a spinal needle. A randomized placebo-controlled trial demonstrated significantly lower blood loss, total operative and enucleation time, and degree of surgical difficulty associated with bupivacaine plus epinephrine compared with saline. When the whorled white appearance of the myoma is seen, the edges of the uterine serosa are held open with atraumatic graspers, and a corkscrew retractor is screwed into the myoma. Using upward traction with the corkscrew retractor, the myoma is peeled away from the uterine corpus (**Fig. 16.25**). Hemostasis is

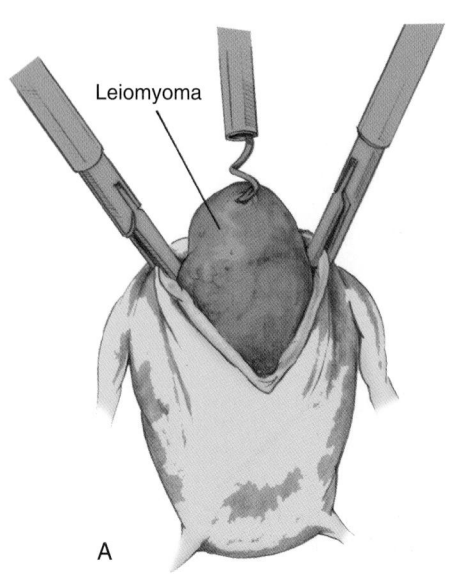

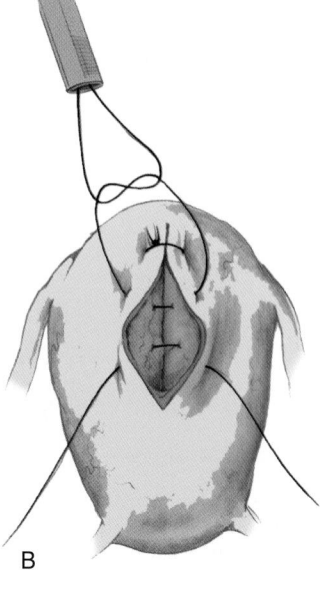

FIGURE 16.25 Myomectomy. **A:** The leiomyoma is grasped with forceps or a corkscrew and is dissected from the myometrium with careful blunt and sharp dissection. **B:** The defect, if large, is closed with sutures in two layers.

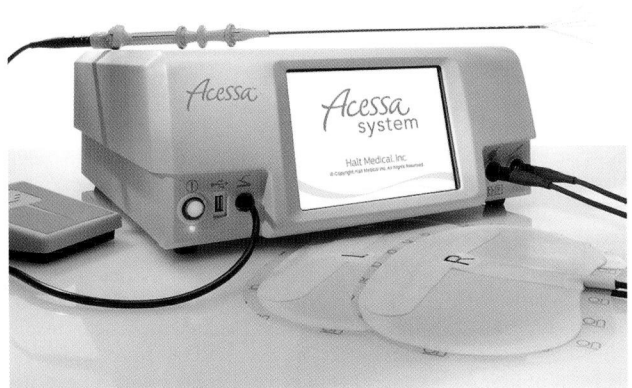

FIGURE 16.26 Acessa System. (Courtesy of Halt Medical.)

achieved with electrosurgery or Harmonic Scalpel. The defect is sutured closed in two or three layers, depending on the depth of the defect, using a delayed absorbable suture as described previously. In order to close a defect under tension, an intracorporeal cinch knot, an extracorporeal sliding knot, or a barbed suture can be used. Another option is to perform uterine closure through a minilaparotomy if the fundus or area to be sutured can be delivered through a small incision. Morcellation can be performed, or smaller specimens can be delivered through a posterior colpotomy. It is best to avoid losing myoma pieces that become detached, as there have been reports of specimens becoming infected, parasitic, or continuing to grow at the trocar incision site. Loss of tissue, however, is not necessarily an indication for laparotomy, as a case series of 12 retained specimens, three of which were myomas, resulted in no sequelae with 2-year follow-up. Uterine rupture has been reported in patients undergoing laparoscopic myomectomy, and pregnancy should be monitored with the same caution given to patients who have undergone abdominal myomectomy. It is not known whether laparoscopic repairs are equivalent to repair by laparotomy, although healing time is certainly improved.

A radiofrequency ablation system, which utilizes an electrode array to accommodate fibroids of varying size, can now be delivered laparoscopically. The Acessa System (Halt Medical) (Fig. 16.26) uses monopolar radiofrequency, with real-time temperature feedback control, to achieve a target temperature of 100°C. The electrosurgical probe contains a needle electrode array, consisting of seven straight electrodes, which is inserted percutaneously through a 2-mm skin incision. The procedure is performed in conjunction with real-time laparoscopic ultrasound. In a 12-month prospective follow-up study, mean uterine volume decreased by 25.1%, mean fibroid volume decreased by 44.3%, and a clinically significant reduction in menstrual bleeding was observed in 68.8% of subjects. A median of 5 days was missed from work, return to normal activities occurred at a mean of 9 days, and 95% of patients reported being satisfied with the treatment at 12 months. A total of 674 fibroids were treated, with a mean of five fibroids per patient. There were four device-related adverse events and one surgical reintervention.

LAPAROSCOPY USING LOCAL ANESTHESIA OR CONSCIOUS SEDATION

Laparoscopy can be performed under conscious sedation in the operating room or in a nonhospital environment, such as physician's office. Microlaparoscopy is often used with 2- or 3-mm instrumentation. Local anesthesia and conscious

sedation has long been used to perform tubal ligation. The use of microlaparoscopic instrumentation has assisted in performing laparoscopy under conscious sedation in the office setting for pain mapping in chronic pelvic pain patients. Pain mapping may be useful in patients with chronic pelvic pain of uncertain etiology, as this enables the patient to participate in the evaluation of the pelvis, and to decipher between incidental versus painful adhesions and endometriosis. If conscious sedation is to be performed in the office without the presence of an anesthesiologist, it is important to follow state guidelines. The American College of Surgeons has developed guidelines that have been endorsed by the American Congress of Obstetricians and Gynecologists, which detail requirements for an optimally safe environment and resuscitation.

Laparoscopy under conscious sedation is usually performed by combining local anesthesia with intravenous sedation. Proper patient selection is important, as patients must be able to withstand lifting the abdomen at the umbilicus for trocar insertion and tolerate local infiltration at the umbilicus. The umbilicus is infiltrated at the skin and then down through the fascia with a 25-gauge needle, using approximately 10 mL of 1% lidocaine or 0.25% bupivacaine. If conscious sedation is used, short-acting narcotics, such as remifentanil, are ideal if pain mapping is to be performed, so that the patient is able to respond to intraperitoneal stimuli. If tubal sterilization is to be performed, an anxiolytic drug such as midazolam is useful.

COMPLICATIONS

Nerve Injury

Most nerve injuries occurring during laparoscopic surgery are neurapraxia or nerve contusion and will usually resolve within 6 weeks. Neurotmesis, or complete division of the nerve, is the most severe form of nerve injury, often resulting in permanent disability. Proper preoperative and intraoperative patient positioning—as well as knowledge of known risk factors associated with mononeuropathies—is an important part of providing a safe environment for laparoscopic surgery. Femoral neuropathy occurring during laparoscopy can be associated with excessive hip flexion or abduction or long operating times. When the lithotomy position is used in patients undergoing vaginal or laparoscopic surgery, the thigh should be flexed no greater than 90 degrees and abducted no greater than 45 degrees. If a patient's position is changed intraoperatively from low lithotomy to high lithotomy, these relationships should be maintained. Obturator neuropathy is most commonly associated with direct injury during radical pelvic surgery or lymphadenectomy, but can also occur as a result of excessive hip flexion. As the obturator nerve leaves the obturator foramen, it lies directly against bone and can become acutely angulated and deformed if the hips are excessively flexed, particularly during prolonged surgery. The obturator neurovascular bundle is also vulnerable during laparoscopic retropubic dissection, particularly during the paravaginal repair of lateral defects of the anterior vaginal wall. Surgeons who operate in these spaces should be well versed in the anatomy of the obturator nerve.

The iliohypogastric and ilioinguinal nerves can be injured from lateral trocars with subsequent suture ligature and fibrotic entrapment. Care should be taken to avoid extreme lateral trocar placement; however, there is considerable anatomic variation in the course of these nerves, and injury cannot always be avoided. Mapping of nerves in fresh frozen cadavers revealed that the ilioinguinal nerve enters the abdominal wall with an average of 3.1 cm medial and 3.7 cm inferior to the ASIS and that the iliohypogastric nerve enters the abdominal wall with an average of 2.1 cm medial and 0.9 cm inferior to the ASIS. Placement of trocar sites 2 cm above the level of the ASIS, at any point medially, would avoid almost all of the ilioinguinal and iliohypogastric nerves identified in the study, although such placement may not always be practical.

Sciatic neuropathy during laparoscopic surgery can be a result of nerve stretching. Injury to the sciatic nerve has been reported in procedures lasting as short as 35 minutes in free-hanging stirrups. The peroneal division of the sciatic nerve is under the least amount of tension when the knee and hip are flexed, as the nerve is fixed at the sciatic notch and the fibular head. Tension along the nerve is increased with hip flexion when the knee joint becomes straightened or externally rotated. Patients at increased risk of sustaining sciatic nerve injury are long legged, obese, or short in stature. In hanging-type stirrups, long-legged or obese patients have a tendency for external hip rotation, and shorter patients have less flexion at the knee. In such cases, stirrups that support the ankle and calf may be more appropriate.

In a large retrospective study, at a single institution, a total of 19,461 cases were reviewed, encompassing 56 surgical procedures performed in the lithotomy position. Fifty-five patients were found to have persistent neuropathy of the lower extremity, defined as a motor deficit if at least 3 months' duration. The majority were neuropathies of the common peroneal nerve, of which there were 43. The remaining neuropathies included eight sciatic and four femoral. At 12 months, approximately 50% of patients with common peroneal and femoral neuropathies had regained complete motor function, while none of the patients with sciatic neuropathies had regained complete motor function. The most important risk factor, found to have a relative risk of 100, was each hour spent in lithotomy. Decreasing the amount of time spent in the lithotomy position should therefore be the primary preventative strategy.

The incidence of brachial plexus injuries is 0.16% and can be particularly devastating, especially when bilateral. The brachial plexus arises from the anterior nerve roots of C5–T1; passes behind the clavicle, over the first rib; and is partially fixed to the fascia of the upper arm. The upper roots can be stretched when a patient is positioned in steep Trendelenburg, and the body slides relative to outstretched arms, or when shoulder braces are positioned too medially. This results in weakness of the upper arm and a constellation of sequelae termed Erb palsy. The lower roots can be compressed between the clavicle and first rib when the arms are abducted greater than 90 degrees. This results in weakness of the distal forearm and hand and a constellation of sequelae termed Klumpke paralysis.

Vascular Injuries

Of all the injuries associated with laparoscopy, vascular injuries are the most acutely life threatening, particularly in the case of injury to the aorta, vena cava, or iliac vessels. Injury can occur during Veres needle placement, during trocar insertion, or during tissue dissection. Injury to the great vessels requires immediate laparotomy, manual compression, repair, and usually transfusion. Injury to smaller vessels can usually be rendered hemostatic with the use of bipolar electrosurgery, hemostatic clips, or laparoscopic suturing techniques. Injury to the inferior epigastric vessels can occur during placement of the lateral trocar. The inferior epigastric artery can usually be seen as it branches off the external iliac artery running cephalad along the abdominal wall peritoneum. If it is injured, a bipolar forceps can be placed through the contralateral port

in an attempt to coagulate. Alternatively, endoscopic fascial closure devices can be used to place suture on either side of the vessel for vascular occlusion. Hemostasis can usually be immediately achieved by placing a 30-mL Foley catheter through the trocar site and inflating the balloon for tamponade. The Foley catheter can then be secured with an 8-inch clamp. This injury can also be managed by enlarging the trocar site to visualize, clamp, and ligate the bleeding vessel.

Gastrointestinal Injury

Gastrointestinal injury is the most lethal injury associated with laparoscopy, with a mortality rate reported as high as 3.6%. Injury may occur from Veres needle placement, trocar insertion, adhesiolysis, tissue dissection, devascularization injury, or thermal injury. As a general rule, Veres needle injuries need no repair as long as the puncture is not associated with bleeding or a subsequent rent from additional tissue manipulation. In the case of colonic puncture without tearing, nonoperative management with antibiotics, copious irrigation, and suction has been suggested. There has been little evidence-based literature published about stomach injury during laparoscopy, but it is estimated that gastric perforation occurs in approximately 1 in 3,000 cases. Risk factors for stomach injury include a history of upper abdominal surgery and difficult induction of anesthesia, as a gas-distended stomach can distend to below the level of the umbilicus. Orogastric or nasogastric suction before Veres needle or trocar placement can help lower this risk. Trocar injury to the stomach requires repair by laparoscopy or laparotomy. The defect may be oversewn with a delayed absorbable suture in layers, and the abdominal cavity should be irrigated and suctioned, being sure to remove any food particles as well as gastric juices. Nasogastric suction is usually maintained postoperatively until normal bowel peristalsis occurs.

Veres needle and trocar injury to the small intestine may not be obvious because of small-bowel redundancy and a tendency for small bowel to fall out of view. Furthermore, a through-and-through trocar injury may be hidden from laparoscopic view. Potential injury should be investigated when multiple anterior abdominal wall adhesions are present. A lower quadrant secondary port can be used to view the umbilical port site. If there are no abdominal wall adhesions but a bowel injury is suspected, the bowel should be run with laparoscopic bowel graspers, or manually by standard laparotomy, until an injury is satisfactorily ruled out. A full-thickness injury to the small bowel of 5 mm or greater should be repaired in two layers with an interrupted layer of 3-0 delayed absorbable suture to approximate the mucosa and muscularis and a serosal layer of 3-0 interrupted silk suture placed perpendicular to the long axis of the intestine to avoid stricture formation. This is usually performed by laparotomy or by minilaparotomy at the umbilical site, where the injured bowel loop is pulled through to the skin surface and repaired. Laparoscopic repair has also been reported as effective by surgeons with advanced gastrointestinal surgical skills. If the laceration to the small bowel exceeds one half of the luminal diameter, segmental resection is recommended.

Trocar injury to the colon is reported to occur with a frequency of approximately 1 per 1,000 cases. Undetected injury to the large intestine can be associated with significant morbidity, compared with injury to the small intestine and stomach, because of the high concentration of coliform bacteria. Therefore, if injury to the colon is suspected, the area should be inspected carefully, using atraumatic bowel graspers, or laparotomy may be performed. The management of large intestinal injuries depends on size, site, and length of time from injury to diagnosis. In general, once the diagnosis of colonic injury is made, broad-spectrum antibiotics should be administered, and consultation should be sought with a surgeon who has experience with bowel injury. In the case of a small rent with minimal soilage, the defect can be closed in two layers with copious irrigation. When a larger injury has occurred and the bowel has not been prepared with a mechanical or antibiotic regimen, or when the injury involves the intestinal mesentery, a diverting colostomy is usually necessary. In the case of delayed (postoperative) diagnosis, a diverting colostomy should be performed. If injury to the rectosigmoid colon is suspected, filling the posterior cul-de-sac with normal saline, injecting air into the rectum through a catheter-tipped bulb syringe, and looking laparoscopically for bubbles may aid in detection (flat tire test). Alternatively, proctosigmoidoscopy may be performed or used to inject air into the rectum.

Thermal injuries are histologically different from traumatic injuries and therefore must be treated differently. Thermal bowel injuries can be differentiated histologically from traumatic injury by the presence of coagulation necrosis and the absence of capillary ingrowth and white cell infiltrate in the former. Because of this coagulation necrosis, thermal injuries require wide resection, even though the bowel may still have a normal appearance adjacent to the injury, as it may take days for the extent of the injury to become apparent.

Trocar Site Hernia

In a retrospective review of more than 3,500 laparoscopies in 1993, the frequency of incisional hernias was reported to be 0.17%. The fascia should be closed in trocar sites that are 10 mm and larger. Although there are case reports of hernia occurring at 5-mm trocar sites, closing 5-mm trocar sites usually requires enlarging the skin incision, or using laparoscopic fascial closure devices, which may not be warranted in this rare possibility. Closing the fascia may not entirely prevent hernia formation. A survey of more than 3,200 gynecologists noted that 18% of hernias occurred despite fascial closure and appeared to be related to the number of laparoscopies performed, rather than the length of the surgeon's career. Trocar site hernias can present as occult or incarcerated hernias. A defect is usually palpable over the trocar site incision with Valsalva, or a mass can be seen. If the patient presents with signs of bowel obstruction, the bowel must be inspected carefully, and if there is evidence of necrosis or vascular compromise, the bowel should be resected.

Urinary Tract Injury

Bladder injury during laparoscopy is estimated to occur 1 in 300 cases. Higher injury rates have been reported with laparoscopic hysterectomy and bladder neck suspension. Risk factors for bladder injury include a distended bladder during suprapubic trocar insertion; previous surgery with distortion of bladder anatomy, causing it to be pulled cephalad with the parietal peritoneum; and endometriosis obliterating the anterior cul-de-sac. Inserting a Foley catheter into the bladder before trocar placement, and using lateral trocar sites, will lessen the risk of bladder injury. In cases when a midline, suprapubic trocar is used, and the superior aspect of the bladder cannot be deciphered, filling the bladder with 300 mL of water or saline will define the bladder margins. Intraoperative signs of bladder injury include clear fluid in the operative field, visible bladder laceration, and gas distention of the Foley bag. To adequately make the diagnosis, the bladder wall can be inspected directly, or methylene blue or indigo carmine, diluted with 200 to 300 mL of sterile normal saline, may be instilled retrograde through the Foley catheter. Intentional cystotomy or cystoscopy may be performed to inspect the extent of the injury and to ensure that there is no ureteric involvement.

Recommendations for repair of bladder injuries have been reviewed in a consensus statement of the International Society of Urology (Société Internationale d'Urologie). In the acute setting, bladder injuries can be treated with catheter drainage alone if the injury is small, uncomplicated, and isolated. A cystogram should be performed on the 10th day of drainage, when more than 85% of bladder injuries will be healed. A surgical repair should be performed if the Foley catheter is unable to provide adequate drainage because of blood clots or persistent extravasation or if there is concomitant injury to the urethra or ureter. Cystotomy closure should be performed using a watertight, multilayered repair, with absorbable suture. Laparoscopic repair may be performed in the case of a small injury with adequate exposure and surgical expertise, as long as the ureters and bladder neck are not compromised.

According to a nationwide Finnish record linkage study, although the overall complication rates for laparoscopy are decreasing, the rate of ureteral injury has remained steady at 1%, with the greatest risk associated with laparoscopic hysterectomy. A review of the world literature through 2003 concluded that laparoscopically assisted vaginal hysterectomy was the most frequently performed surgery associated with ureteral injury. The usual time to diagnosis in postoperative patients with ureteral injury is typically between 2 and 7 days, but has been reported as late as 33 days after surgery. Patients often present with symptoms of abdominal pain, fever, hematuria, flank pain, or peritonitis. Leukocytosis is a common finding. Management of ureteral injury should be undertaken in collaboration with a surgeon trained in ureteral injury repair. In the majority of cases, percutaneous or cystoscopic stenting techniques can be used. Laparotomy is usually performed for end-to-end anastomosis or reimplantation of the ureter into the bladder, but in experienced hands, repair may be performed laparoscopically. The literature is growing in favor of intraoperative diagnostic cystoscopy after complex vaginal, laparoscopic, and abdominal pelvic surgery, in an effort to avoid delayed diagnosis of injuries to the urinary tract. It appears that cases in which the diagnosis is delayed are most likely to result in the greatest morbidity and legal repercussions.

CONCLUSION

Laparoscopy has become a mainstay of gynecologic surgery. Laparoscopic technology continues to evolve, requiring continual education and research. The main benefits of laparoscopic surgery have been shorter hospitalization, improved cosmesis, and, in some cases, improved safety and cost. Evidence-based surgical studies are difficult to perform but will be required to fully understand the role of each laparoscopic procedure in terms of long-term outcomes and cost.

BEST SURGICAL PRACTICES

- A good laparoscopic surgeon should know his or her limitations and not hesitate to call for help.
- Conversion to laparotomy is not considered failure.
- Careful selection of patients is the first key to success in any surgery.
- Preparation is essential in laparoscopic surgery and may include a "pilot's checklist" and/or "dress rehearsal" to avoid being caught with too few inappropriately sized trocars.
- "Shortcuts," which modify a surgical procedure, "change" the procedure. Once the surgical technique has been

changed, success rates obtained from literature or prior experience cannot be attributed to the new procedure.

- Careful positioning of the patient can help avoid nerve injuries, as can minimizing operative time.
- Traction–countertraction and exposure are important in both open and laparoscopic surgeries. To maximize these, an additional trocar port is often helpful.
- Consider intraoperative cystoscopy with indigo carmine in complex pelvic surgery.
- Understand your energy source.

BIBLIOGRAPHY

Batres F, Barclay DL. Sciatic nerve injury during gynecologic procedures using the lithotomy position. *Obstet Gynecol* 1983;62:92S.

Birch DW, Manouchehri N, Shi X, et al. Heated CO_2 with or without humidification for minimally invasive abdominal surgery. *Cochrane Database Syst Rev* 2011;(1):CD007821. doi: 10.1002/14651858. CD007821.pub2

Brill AI. Electrosurgery: principles and practice to reduce risk and maximize efficacy. *Obstet Gynecol Clin North Am* 2011;38:687.

Chudnoff SG, Levine DJ, Galen DI, et al. Prospective 12-Month Follow Up of Quality-of-Life Improvement Following 135 Consecutive Cases of Laparoscopic and Ultrasound-Guided Radiofrequency Ablation of Fibroids. Data presented at the 41st Global Congress of Minimally Invasive Gynecology.

Gomez RG, Ceballos L, Coburn M, et al. Consensus statement on bladder injuries. *BJU Int* 2004;94:27.

Grainger AH, Soderstrom RM, Schiff SF, et al. Ureteral injuries at laparoscopy: insights into diagnosis, management and prevention. *Obstet Gynecol* 1990;75:839.

Guido RS, Levine DJ, Galen DI, et al. Reduction in Uterine and Fibroid Volumes in 135 Consecutive Subjects following Laparoscopic and Ultrasound-Guided Radiofrequency Ablation of Fibroids: 12-Month Follow-Up. Data presented at the 41st Global Congress of Minimally Invasive Gynecology.

Harkki-Siren P, Sjoberg J, Kurki T. Major complications of laparoscopy: a follow-up Finnish study. *Obstet Gynecol* 1999;94:94.

Hershlag A, Loy RA, Lavy G, et al. Femoral neuropathy after laparoscopy: a case report. *J Reprod Med* 1990;35:575.

Hulka JF, Reich H. Textbook of laparoscopy, 2nd ed. Philadelphia, PA: WB Saunders, 1994:202.

Hurd WW, Bude RO, DeLancey JO, et al. The relationship of the umbilicus to the aortic bifurcation: implications for laparoscopic technique. Obstet Gynecol 1992;80:48.

Hurd WW, Amesse LS, Gruber JS, et al. Visualization of the epigastric vessels and bladder before laparoscopic trocar placement. *Fertil Steril* 2003;80:209.

Irvin W, Andersen W, Taylor P, et al. Minimizing the risk of neurologic injury in gynecologic surgery. *Obstet Gynecol* 2004;103:374.

Kadar N, Reich H, Liu CY, et al. Incisional hernias after major laparoscopic gynecologic procedures. *Am J Obstet Gynecol* 1993;168:1493.

Krebs HB. Intestinal injury in gynecologic surgery: a ten-year experience. *Am J Obstet Gynecol* 1986;155:509.

Leal JG, Leon IH, Saenz LC, et al. Laparoscopic ultrasound-guided radiofrequency volumetric thermal ablation of symptomatic uterine leiomyomas: feasibility study using the halt 2000 ablation system. *J Minim Invasive Gynecol* 2011;18:364.

Levy BS, Soderstrom RM, Dail DH. Bowel injuries during laparoscopy. *J Reprod Med* 1985;30:660.

Loffer F, Pent D. Indications, contraindications and complications of laparoscopy. *Obstet Gynecol Surv* 1975;30:407.

Montz FJ, Holschneider CH, Munro MG. Incisional hernia following laparoscopy: a survey of the American Association of Gynecologic Laparoscopists. *Obstet Gynecol* 1994;84:881.

Murphy AA. Operative laparoscopy. *Fertil Steril* 1987;47:1.

Newcomb WL, Hope WW, Schmelzer TM, et al. Comparison of blood vessel sealing among new electrosurgical and ultrasonic devices. *Surg Endosc* 2009;23:90.

Nezhat C, Nezhat F, Ambrose W, et al. Laparoscopic repair of small bowel and colon: a report of 26 cases. *Surg Endosc* 1993;7:88.

Nezhat C, Seidman D, Nezhat F, et al. The role of intraoperative proctosigmoidoscopy in laparoscopic pelvic surgery. *J Am Assoc Gynecol Laparosc* 2004;11:47.

Nezhat CH, Seidman DS, Nezhat F, et al. Laparoscopic management of intentional and unintentional cystotomy. *J Urol* 1996;156:1400.

Oh BR, Kwon DD, Park KS, et al. Late presentation of ureteral injury after laparoscopic surgery. *Obstet Gynecol* 2000;95:337.

Ostrzenski A, Radolinski B, Ostrzenska KM. A review of laparoscopic ureteral injury in pelvic surgery. *Obstet Gynecol Surv* 2003;58:794.

Palter SF, Olive DL. Office microlaparoscopy under local anesthesia for chronic pelvic pain. *J Am Assoc Gynecol Laparosc* 1996;3:359.

Pellegrino MJ, Johnson EW. Bilateral obturator nerve injuries during urologic surgery. *Arch Phys Med Rehabil* 1988;69:46.

Person B, Vivas DA, Ruiz D, et al. Comparison of four energy-based sealing and cutting instruments: a porcine model. *Surg Endosc* 2008;22:534.

Seehofer D, Mogl M, Boas-Koop S, et al. Safety and efficacy of new integrated bipolar and ultrasonic scissors compared to conventional laparoscopic 5-mm sealing and cutting instruments. *Surg Endosc* 2012;26:2541.

Spinelli P, Di Felice G, Pizzetti P, et al. Laparoscopic repair of full-thickness stomach injury. *Surg Endosc* 1991;5:156.

Siprasad S, Yu DF, Muir GH, et al. Positional anatomy of vessels that may be damaged at laparoscopy: new access criteria based on CT and ultrasonography to avoid vascular injury. *J Endourol* 2006;20:498.

Sutton PA, Awad S, Perkins AC, et al. Comparison of lateral thermal spread using monopolar and bipolar diathermy, the Harmonic Scalpel and the Ligasure. *Br J Surg* 2010;97:428.

Taylor R, Weakley FL, Sullivan BH. Non-operative management of colonic perforation with pneumoperitoneum. *Gastrointest Endosc* 1978;24:124.

Tulikangas PK, Gill IS, Falcone T. Laparoscopic repair of ureteral injuries. *J Am Assoc Gynecol Laparosc* 2001;8:259.

Van Der Voort M, Heijnsdijk EA, Gouma DJ. Bowel injury as a complication of laparoscopy. *Br J Surg* 2004;91:1253.

Wang PH, Lee WL, Yuan CC, et al. Major complications of operative and diagnostic laparoscopy for gynecologic disease. *J Am Assoc Gynecol Laparosc* 2001;8:68.

Warner MA, Martin JT, Schroeder DR, et al. Lower-extremity motor neuropathy associated with surgery performed on patients in a lithotomy position. *Anesthesiology* 1994;81.

Whiteside JJ, Barber MD, Walters MD, et al. Anatomy of ilioinguinal and iliohypogastric nerves in relation to trocar placement and low transverse incisions. *Am J Obstet Gynecol* 2003;189:1574.

Wu MP, Lin YS, Chou CY. Major complications of operative gynecologic laparoscopy in southern Taiwan. *J Am Assoc Gynecol Laparosc* 2001;8:61.

CHAPTER 17
Robotic Surgery

Jed Delmore and Kevin E. Miller

DEFINITIONS

Learning curve—Defined as the length of time or number of cases to reach a predictable operating time, the fewest complications, or lowest blood loss.

Patient-side cart—A mobile cart composed of a camera arm and three operating arms that attach to the laparoscopic ports.

Robot—A machine capable of carrying out a complex series of actions automatically, especially one programmable by a computer.

Surgeon console—A mobile cart composed of a stereoscopic viewer, master controllers, and a series of foot pedals.

Uterine manipulator—One of several instruments inserted in the uterus with an attached colpotomy ring to facilitate movement of the uterus and visualization of the vaginal fornix.

Vision cart—A mobile cart containing the vision system for image processing, light source, carbon dioxide insufflator and energy sources, and usually a video monitor.

INTRODUCTION

History

The technologic advances in minimally invasive surgery, specifically gynecologic surgery, over the past 50 years are staggering. Using monocular laparoscopes with continuous carbon dioxide insufflation of the peritoneal cavity, most gynecologists in the United States in the early 1970s were performing diagnostic laparoscopy and tubal sterilizations. Within a short period of time, video laparoscopy allowed a rapid expansion in procedures performed by the minimally invasive approach. Salpingectomy, oophorectomy, myomectomy, resection and ablation of endometriosis, hysterectomy, and a long list of other procedures, are now commonly performed. Until recently, most technologic advances in laparoscopy have involved video equipment, instrumentation, and newer energy sources. A combination of astounding technologic advances has resulted in the introduction of robotic or robotically assisted surgery in gynecology, and astute, aggressive marketing to physicians and the public has resulted in the rapid assimilation of robotic surgery into today's surgical practices. However, controlling the application of robotic technology and teaching the procedures seem to lag behind the marketing.

According to the Oxford Dictionary, "robot" is derived from the Czech word *robota* meaning "forced labor." The term was introduced in Karel Čapek's play "*Rossum's Universal Robots*" in 1920. A robot is defined as a machine capable of carrying out a complex series of actions automatically, especially one programmable by a computer. The history of robotic surgery is best described as a convergence of research performed in multiple locations in the 1980s. Expanding on the technique of stereotactic brain biopsies, Kwoh and colleagues modified an industrial robot, the Unimation PUMA (Programmable Universal Machine for Assembly) 200, for the biopsy of brain tumors in 1988. In 1991, Davies et al., at the Imperial College of Science, Technology, and Medicine in London reported the use of a modified PUMA 560 robot, which later became PROBOT, for transurethral resection of prostatic tumors. During the 1980s and early 1990s, researchers at the National Aeronautics and Space Administration Ames Research Center were working on virtual environments while researchers at the Stanford Research Institute were working on robotics and a telemanipulator system for hand surgery. As described in a review by Satava, the Department of Defense and the Defense Advanced Research Projects Agency funded research directed toward the concept of telepresence surgery for combat casualty care. This culminated in the demonstration of a telepresence vascular anastomosis in the swine model in 1996 by Bowersox and telesurgical laparoscopic cholecystectomy in 1998 by Himpens. In 1993, Yulun Wang, PhD, formed Computer Motion, which developed a robotic camera holder for laparoscopy called Automated Endoscopic System for Optimal Positioning (AESOP) and ultimately created an integrated robotic system that attached to the operating table called ZEUS. In

1995, Frederic Moll, MD, acquired the license for the telepresence surgical system and created Intuitive Surgical. In 2003, Computer Motion and Intuitive Surgical merged into a single entity, Intuitive Surgical. Presently, da Vinci is the only robotic surgical system approved by the U.S. Food and Drug Administration (FDA) (Intuitive Surgical, Sunnyvale, CA). As a result, any reference to robotic surgery or robotic platform in the remainder of this chapter pertains to the Intuitive, da Vinci system. This is not meant to be an endorsement of this or any other product; it simply reflects the fact that there are no other commercially available robotic platforms at present.

Advantages and Disadvantages

The November 2009 American Congress of Obstetricians and Gynecologists Committee Opinion concerning types of hysterectomy concluded that vaginal hysterectomy is the approach of choice whenever feasible, on the basis of its well-documented advantages and lower complication rates. Laparoscopic hysterectomy is an alternative to abdominal hysterectomy for those patients in whom vaginal hysterectomy is not indicated or feasible. "The experience with robot-assisted hysterectomy is limited at this time; more data are necessary to determine its role in the performance of hysterectomy." The advantages of robotic surgery include those experienced by the patient, the hospital, and by the surgeon. The advantages to the patient include smaller incisions compared to laparotomy, shorter hospital stay, less blood loss, and a more rapid return to normal activity. Laparoscopic surgery provides the same benefits; but because of technical considerations noted below, the range of surgical procedures is greater with robotic surgery. The advantages to a surgeon include enhanced visibility with a three-dimensional (3D) view, enhanced image magnification, and stable camera platform devoid of first-assistant fatigue that can result in an unstable field of view with camera motion. The instruments utilized by the surgeon are wristed to allow a full range of motion and angles similar to an open procedure. In distinction to conventional laparoscopy, which relies on a fulcrum effect and requires movement of the handle of the instrument in the opposite direction to the desired movement of the tip, robotic surgery allows hand and instrument movement in the same direction. Surgeon hand tremor is minimized, and the ratio of hand motion to robotic instrument motion can be adjusted. Sarlos reported that fatigue and back discomfort may be reduced by a more ergonomically correct position at the surgeon console. This benefit may be the greatest during longer cases. Robotic suturing may be considerably easier for most surgeons compared to laparoscopic suturing in studies reported by Andenberg and Chandra. For instructing resident physicians and fellows-in-training, the video monitor on the vision cart allows the educator to draw on the monitor that can be seen by the trainee at the console. Sonographic or computed tomographic images from preoperative studies can be projected onto the surgeon console screen for viewing during surgery. The newest da Vinci Si model allows surgeons at two separate consoles to operate simultaneously on the same patient, or it allows a mentor to intervene during a trainee's procedure. The potential advantage to the hospital or institution is a shorter patient hospital stay for procedures that historically resulted in a longer stay if performed by laparotomy. Potential disadvantages to the patient include a longer operative time and facial edema from protracted Trendelenburg position.

The major disadvantage to all parties is the cost of the robot, associated instruments, drapes, and maintenance contracts. The cost of a da Vinci robotic system varies between $1,000,000 and $2,300,000. Wristed robotic instruments, which have a limit of 10 uses, cost approximately $1,300.

For point of reference, the 2011 purchase price paid by one of our community hospitals for typical laparoscopic instruments utilizing different energy sources ranges from $350 to $450. Annual maintenance costs for the robotic system are estimated at $150,000 (Intuitive Surgical, Second Quarter Investor Presentation, http://phx.corporate-ir.net/phoenix.zhtml?c=122359&p=irol-IRHome).

Because of the size of the entire robotic system, larger operating rooms (ORs) are required for optimal efficiency and may add expense to the institution. Size and position of the robotic arms when docked may cause difficulty for the bedside assistant when passing sutures, retracting tissues, or manipulating the uterus with a vaginal manipulator.

From the surgeon's standpoint, the major disadvantage is the lack of haptic or tactile sense with the instruments. Those surgeons accustomed to blunt dissection of tissues will be required to enhance their sharp dissection skills and rely on anatomic landmarks. Those in residency training may suffer from diminished experience with traditional open procedures and operative technologies as more and more gynecologic surgical procedures are done using minimally invasive and robotic techniques.

ROBOTIC TRAINING

In 2007, Javier Magrina explained that robotic surgery "… is nothing more than an enhancement along the continuum of laparoscopic technologic advances and represents only the beginning of numerous more forthcoming advances."

Obstacles and Challenges to Teaching and Learning

Currently, there is no standardized training model or validated method to teach robotic surgery. Two notable obstacles to teaching the application of this new technology result from the unique features of robotics. Until recently, a single surgeon controlled the robotic operation without the use of a second set of independent controls for the assistant or trainee. The teacher/instructor had no ability for immediate hands-on correction as he or she would have had with traditional teaching. Thus, potential patient safety issues become a concern with implementation of robotics. The situation is likened to a student pilot on final approach without the flight instructor being able to take control of the airplane's pitch and power controls to avoid a potentially dangerous landing. The robotics instructor must correct the trainee with prompt, understandable, and verbal commands. However, dual consoles are now available, although they are expensive and not widely available. These dual consoles allow cosurgeons to work on the same patient with three moving instruments controlled by the cosurgeons in contrast to two moving instruments with a single console. Additionally, a mentor and a trainee can operate on the same patient simultaneously. The single-surgeon console in use at most facilities is a "resident-unfriendly" platform. The resident initially functions as a table-side assistant or observer, which is quite different from the usual hands-on learning experience. Hanly suggested that wider availability of mentoring consoles will likely improve resident and nonresident learning experiences and enhance patient safety. The telestration feature enables the teacher/mentor to point, draw, or illustrate directly on the video touch screen monitor as the surgeon sees this on the surgeon console screen in real time.

Another obstacle to learning robotic surgery is the lack of tactile sensation and feedback to the surgeon. Palpation of the tissues is not translated to the surgeon in the same way as one "feels" the tissues with open procedures or conventional laparoscopy. This lack of tactile sensation or haptics presents an initial challenge to learning until one is conditioned to develop a "sensation of feel" on the basis of the visual cues as proposed by Hagen and colleagues. This may be likened to an experienced pilot transitioning to flying a remote-controlled drone aircraft from a virtual cockpit far from the area of flight. Despite these obstacles, Dharia and Falcone, Stefanidis et al., and Suh et al. suggest that the robotic features of instrument motion comparable to open procedures, tremor reduction, 3D high-definition image, wristed instrument articulation, and downscaling movements have made more difficult advanced laparoscopic surgical cases with steep learning curves easier to learn and apply to patient care.

Training Methods

Initially, most robotic training regimens were developed and sponsored by Intuitive Surgical, Inc., the maker of da Vinci Surgical System. The manufacturer has been active in developing training methods and recommendations to introduce the techniques of robotic surgery to potential customers. However, with increased experience of surgeons and institutions, locally developed training protocols have placed less emphasis on the manufacturer to provide training. Initial training protocols incorporated a combination of "on-site" (hospital) training, "off-site" (laboratory) hands-on courses, as well as Internet-based modules and surgical videos. All OR team members require basic training on mechanical and technical aspects of robotic system functions (*system training*). This specifically includes learning the components of the system, how to dock, set up, and insert instruments, implement safety features, and troubleshoot malfunctions. The second aspect of training deals with acquiring the technical skills to perform surgery (*procedure training*). Training modules and videos may be accessed at http://www.davincisurgerycommunity.com.

Since there is only one commercially available robotic surgical system available in the United States today, the technical system training is still largely provided by the manufacturer. This system training can be completed with the Internet-based Intuitive Surgical curriculum including system overview, setup/docking, surgeon console functions, and safety features. The setup module instructs on port placement, camera arm positioning, instrument arm positioning, docking, endoscope insertion and removal, and instrument insertion and removal. The surgeon console module instructs on system setup and vision, ergonomic, and instrument control. The safety features module teaches how to troubleshoot fault messages, emergency switch location and use, energy source control, and procedure conversion to open or standard laparoscopy.

Procedure training is surgeon and procedure specific and directed at acquiring the needed technical skills. For the gynecologist/pelvic surgeon, a sample of the procedures performed robotically include hysterectomy, adnexal surgery, lymphadenectomy, radical hysterectomy, myomectomy, sacrocolpopexy, Burch retropubic urethropexy, endometriosis resection, and ureteral and fistula repairs. Commercially produced and Web-based surgical videos provided by surgeons are available. Inanimate simulator training, live animal models (pig lab), and case observation have been required of surgeons learning robotic techniques before being proctored by an experienced surgeon. After certification of completion of both system and procedure training, experienced gynecologic surgeons desiring to obtain robotic surgical privileges are commonly proctored at their home institution with a minimum of two to five cases before independent-use privileging is granted. Because of the high expense of animal laboratory courses ($3,000 per one to five trainees), these may not be feasible for some residency/fellowship training programs. Hoekstra and Geller have reported on nonstandardized methods developed to achieve didactic and procedural training within their institution. Completion of a procedure training program described by Geller and associates at the University of North Carolina is required before residents or fellows performing robotic surgery. This "System Skills Practicum" includes developing proficiency in four surgical skills: (a) "manipulation drill" that requires transfer of rubber rings from tower to tower to learn wristed instrument movements and camera manipulation (clutching), (b) "dissection drill" that requires dissection of a vessel encased in gelatin using scissors and grasping instruments, (c and d) "suturing drills." The "suturing drills" are timed and involve reapproximating linear and jagged lacerations on an inanimate model to teach needle-driver use and intracorporeal knot tying with camera and instrument clutching. These suturing drills are the most difficult to master. Surgical training programs such as residency and fellowship also typically require involvement in a minimum number of case observations in addition to working as first assistant with progressive hands-on experience.

The simulation training module connecting to the da Vinci Si model functions the same as a flight simulator or video game box. The surgeon works directly at the console on a series of exercises to learn and maintain proficiency skills in manipulation of the robotic controls. The simulation unit scores and records each exercise to allow quantification of progress. Manipulation skills of the wristed instruments, camera control, clutching, dissection, energy control, and needle driving are performed in various combinations. Surgical facilities responsible for credentialing may be able to utilize this module to assess surgeon skill retention and possibly to maintain privileges.

Does Previous Experience with Operative Laparoscopy Matter?

Several studies have evaluated experienced surgeons and inexperienced/novice surgeons with regard to skill development when learning simple and complex robotic techniques. Stefanidis and Suh found that previous experience as an assistant surgeon on robotic surgical cases shortens the learning curve, and all trainees have lessened physical demands and decreased workload with improved accuracy and precision in comparison to standard laparoscopic techniques. They also reported that surgical novices seem to learn difficult tasks such as robotic suturing more easily than experienced surgeons. Interestingly, other high-intensity hand–eye coordination activities, such as prior high-volume video game experience, were found to have a negative impact on learning robotic suturing in a study by Harper. Overall, it appears that lack of previous laparoscopic experience does not seem to be a major obstacle in learning the technical aspects of the robotic platform.

Experience with Various Energy Sources

As with standard operative laparoscopy, the surgeon performing robotic surgery should be familiar with the various energy sources, as the power settings and depth of thermal spread may be new or different from what they are accustomed to with standard laparotomy, vaginal, or laparoscopic procedures. Energy sources used with the da Vinci system include bipolar cautery, monopolar cautery (scissors), PlasmaKinetic (PK), and harmonic energy sources. If bedside assistants will be operating conventional laparoscopic energy sources, adequate education and experience are required.

What Is the Learning Curve for Robotic Surgery?

Operating time may represent an indirect measure of the learning curve for a specific surgical procedure. An efficient OR team should lead to decreased operating times. Because of the significant technical training robotic surgery requires of the entire surgical team, safety and efficiency in robotic surgery require a well-trained, experienced team, which is used to working together. The importance of the same team working together frequently with the same surgical procedures cannot be overemphasized. Several components contributing to operating times include OR personnel, surgeon, and patient factors. First, efficiency is dependent upon the OR personnel for room turnover, equipment processing and setup, and assisting the surgeon in positioning and draping the patient. Second, surgeon factors depend on his/her learning curve or experience performing the particular operation. As with any other surgical method, operating times decrease and technical proficiency increases as the frequency and volume of cases increase to a certain number. Third, patient-dependent factors that increase the difficulty of the surgery, such as morbid obesity, previous surgeries, and presence of extensive adhesions, are to be considered. The patient factors should be considered especially when selecting initial cases and will depend on the surgeon's experience and skill level. A study by Hoekstra and colleagues found a learning curve of 5 to 10 cases to demonstrate proficiency in simple hysterectomy, cuff closure, and pelvic lymph node dissection for gynecologic oncology fellows. Useful methods of teaching were verbal feedback, telestration teaching, and demonstration of a portion of the procedure after a first attempt by the fellow. Looking at hysterectomy performed in a community-based practice, Lenihan and associates found that surgical time stabilized at a total time of 95 minutes after 50 cases.

In a recent study of gynecologic surgeons learning robotic surgery skills, Woelk et al. concluded that "surgical proficiency" with the new techniques required performing many more robotic procedures than previously thought. A total of 325 robotic hysterectomies were done by eight different gynecologic surgeons over a 3-year period at the Mayo Clinic. Operative time and intraoperative and postoperative complications were recorded for each surgeon, and results were analyzed in 6-month blocks of time. Operative time and postoperative length of hospital stay declined significantly over the 3-year study, but complications did not change significantly, although there was a trend toward fewer complications as surgical experience accumulated.

The risk of complications and length of surgery continued to decline and did not level off for any of the surgeons over the 6 to 36 months of evaluation, which included up to 150 hysterectomies for one of the surgeons. None of the surgeons monitored had a complication rate of greater than double the local benchmark rate for abdominal hysterectomy (11.4%), but only one surgeon, the most experienced, was able to achieve a complication rate of less than the abdominal hysterectomy benchmark (5.7%)—and this was finally achieved after 91 robotic hysterectomies. This was the only surgeon who actually did over 90 robotically assisted hysterectomies during the course of the study.

Credentialing Requirements

Credentialing and granting hospital privileging vary throughout the United States. Individual institutions may rely on recommendations from local or national experts for guidelines regarding robotic surgical privileges. The robotic platform is a complex surgical tool, and surgeons should be expected to be specifically credentialed to perform each operation, for example, hysterectomy, using robotic techniques. Credentialing in basic operative laparoscopic skills makes sense, as robotics is an adaptation of laparoscopy. However, advanced laparoscopic skills are not necessarily required or helpful for the robotic surgeon. For experienced surgeons, two to five proctored robotic surgical procedures are usually required before independent robotic privileges are granted. Residents and fellows will likely have a more protracted exposure to robotics and may require performance or significant involvement in more cases before showing proficiency.

In our institution, credentialing criteria for robotic surgery include core privileges in the specialty (gynecology, urology, general surgery, etc.) with documented attendance at a basic certified course in robotics and observation of a minimum of two full robotic cases before being granted temporary privileges. Documentation of robotic training during residency or fellowship may satisfy the above requirements. Before performing proctored procedures, the surgeon must perform a minimum of two documented simulated runs with OR staff and the robotic instrument specialist. After this, two proctored cases are observed by a physician with robotic privileges. Surgeons are then able to operate independently and must perform a minimum of eight procedures within the next year to maintain robotic privileges. The Department of Obstetrics and Gynecology places the surgeon in a period of focused review for ongoing evaluation of outcomes and patient safety.

How Will Resident Training Be Altered with the Advent of the Robotic Platform?

As the technologic advances in minimally invasive surgical procedures increase, the demands placed on resident training are in constant flux. During the late 1980s, vaginal, simple laparoscopic, and open surgery progressed to incorporate more advanced hysteroscopic and laparoscopic techniques. Eventually, this led to the more common use of total and subtotal laparoscopic hysterectomy. Twenty years later, in an era of robotic surgery, the gynecologic surgeon in training has a wider spectrum of procedures to master in the same 4-year time frame. Will resident physicians graduate with an adequate number of each type of hysterectomy to be proficient? Will it become rare to perform the traditional open abdominal hysterectomy? Will the vaginal hysterectomy be utilized less frequently? How do we teach patient selection for robotic surgery? While robotic surgery may replace abdominal hysterectomy for many indications, vaginal hysterectomy is associated with low morbidity, short operating time, rapid postoperative recovery, and low cost, so it should remain the technique of choice when technically possible.

With regard to resident training in hysterectomy, in the United States, obstetrics and gynecology residents perform an average of 120 hysterectomies during their training. This is an overall decrease in the total number of hysterectomies compared to years past, with a notable decrease in the number of vaginal hysterectomies as reported by Pulliam. Now, with robotic training, there is the potential for a significant decrease in the number of abdominal hysterectomies performed by the average gynecologic surgeon as well as the resident-in-training. In our community, we found that abdominal hysterectomies decreased significantly after robotic surgery became available, but no decrease in vaginal and/or laparoscopic-assisted vaginal hysterectomy was detected.

ROBOT COMPONENTS AND INSTRUMENTATION

Although the da Vinci robotic system is currently the only FDA-approved robotic system for surgery, there are three models currently in use: the original standard unit, the S model, and the Si model. The models vary in instrument length, camera capability, presence of a third operating arm, and the availability of high-definition video capability. Each system consists of the patient-side cart, the surgeon console, and the vision cart/console.

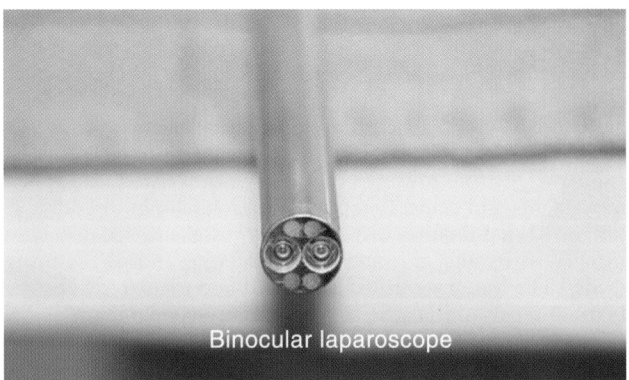

FIGURE 17.1 Binocular, 3D laparoscope.

Vision Cart

A 12-mm endoscope (Fig. 17.1) that is passed through the camera port in the patient is internally composed of two 5-mm lenses attached to the camera head, all of which are on the sterile field. The camera cables are passed off the field and attached to the vision system, which processes the images from the two 5-mm lenses and produces the 3D stereoscopic view. In addition to the vision system, the vision cart/console also contains the light source, heated carbon dioxide insufflator, and cautery unit or another energy source (Fig. 17.2).

The vision console is usually equipped with a video monitor that provides a 2D view of the operative field and allows telestration. The touch screen monitor allows the table-side assistant, educator, or colleague to draw on the monitor, which projects over the field visualized by the surgeon at the surgeon console. This allows for education of the surgeon, trainee, or members of the surgical team (Fig. 17.3). The vision cart is mobile and pulled adjacent to the operating table once the surgical procedure has begun.

Patient-Side Cart

The patient-side cart (Fig. 17.4) is placed immediately next to the operating table by either straight docking between the patient's legs or side docking at the level of the right or left hip. The standard system was designed with a camera arm and two operating arms. The S and Si systems have three operating arms and a camera arm. Positioning of the camera arm and operating arms varies with the procedure to be performed. The arms are attached to laparoscopic ports through which the wristed instruments or camera is placed. Without a second surgeon console, only two of the robotic operating arms are

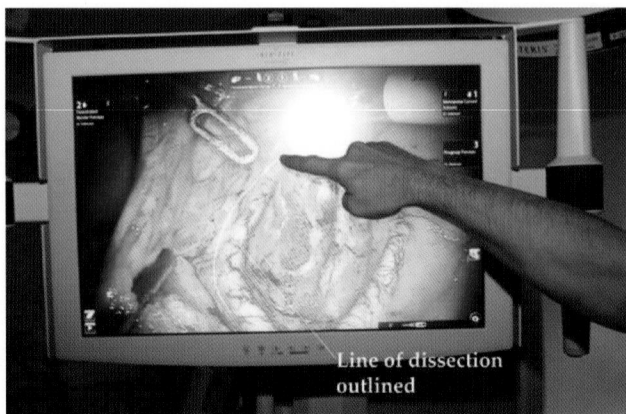

FIGURE 17.2 Vision cart.

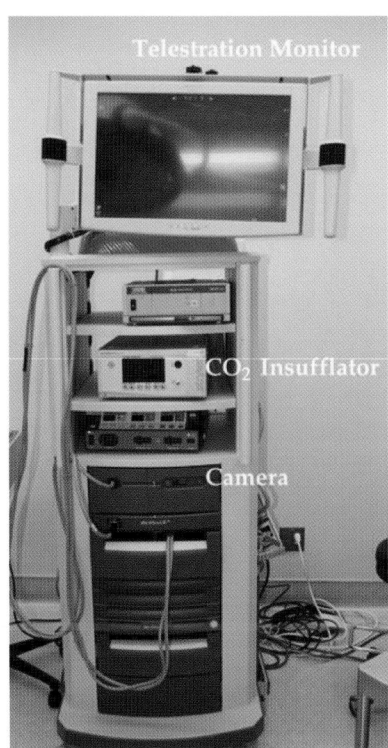

FIGURE 17.3 Telestration monitor.

capable of movement at any point in time. If the third arm is docked, one of the arms can serve as a retractor while the surgeon utilizes the other two arms for surgery. The surgeon may alternate or toggle between the available robotic operating arms. Instruments are interchangeable between all three operating arms. Most surgeons will use monopolar scissors for

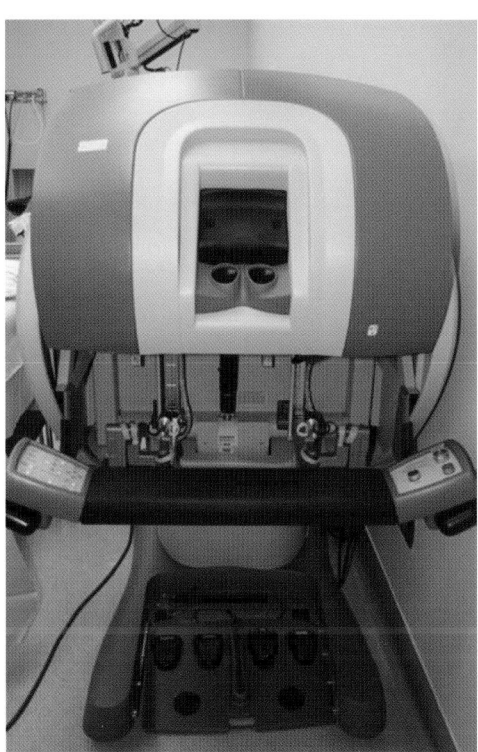

FIGURE 17.5 S model surgeon console.

dissection in one arm and a grasper utilizing bipolar cautery, PK, or harmonic shears for hemostasis in the opposite hand.

Surgeon Console

The surgeon console (Fig. 17.5) is composed of a stereoscopic viewer through which the surgeon views the surgical field: two master controllers used to manipulate instruments and move, rotate, and focus the camera and a series of foot pedals. Foot pedals on the right side are used to activate the energy sources for the two operating instruments. A camera pedal on the left side allows movement of the camera. The S system has a pedal to focus the camera and a separate pedal on the left side to switch between two operating arms (Fig. 17.6). The Si system does not have a foot pedal to focus the camera, as that function is accomplished with the master controllers. A toggle switch is built into the side of the Si unit that is foot-activated to alternate operating instruments (Fig. 17.7). As mentioned earlier, the Si system allows a second surgeon at a separate console to

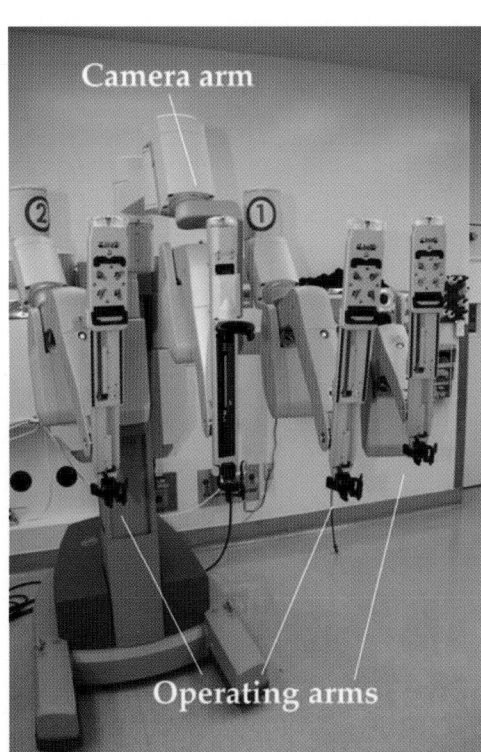

FIGURE 17.4 Patient-side cart.

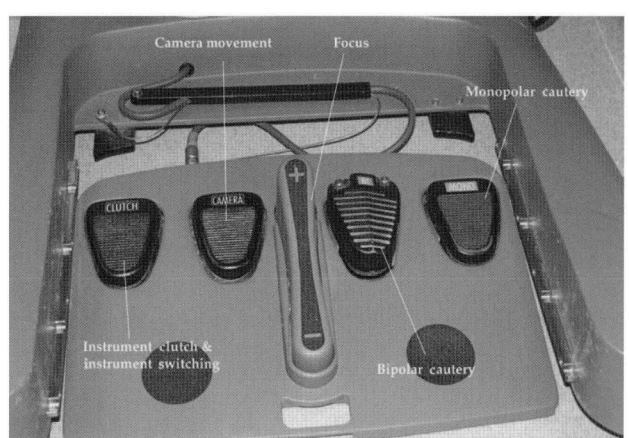

FIGURE 17.6 S model foot pedals.

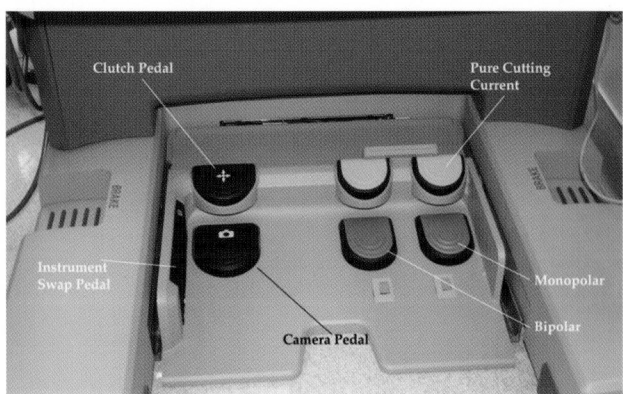

FIGURE 17.7 Si model foot pedals.

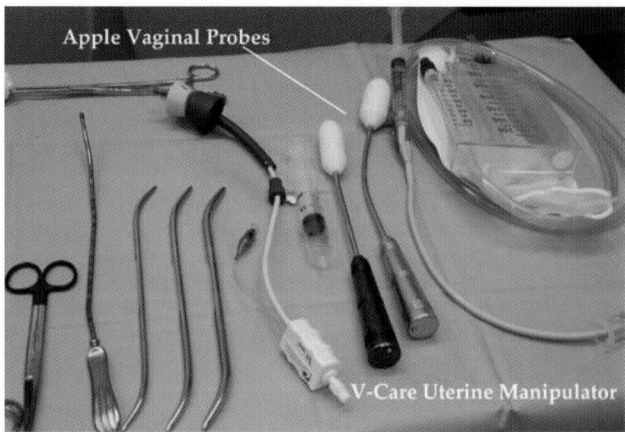

FIGURE 17.9 Uterine and vaginal manipulators.

operate in parallel with the primary surgeon by controlling the third operating arm. In addition, the Si system allows visualization of radiographic images by the surgeon in the surgeon console display. While the surgeon sees intraoperative images in high definition and three dimensions, the OR staff sees conventional images on the accessory monitors. The Si unit also allows for a teaching/simulation unit to be attached and operated from the surgeon console.

Instruments

A variety of interchangeable instruments (Fig. 17.8) specific to robotic surgery are available for use. As mentioned previously, most surgeons will utilize scissors with monopolar cautery in one operating arm and a grasper with attached energy source for hemostasis in the opposite arm. A fenestrated grasper is available for the third arm. Additional instruments include vascular forceps, a single-tooth tenaculum, a monopolar spatula, and several types of needle drivers. Each da Vinci–specific instrument may be reused up to 10 times. The table-side assistant may use a laparoscopic atraumatic grasper, irrigator/aspirator, energy source, and needle driver through the right or left upper quadrant assistant port. If a hysterectomy is performed for reasons other than cervical cancer, most surgeons will utilize a uterine manipulator. Two popular manipulators are the RUMI system (CooperSurgical, Trumbull, CT) with Koh ring or a VCare Manipulator (ConMed EndoSurgery, Utica, NY). If manipulating the cervix is contraindicated, the Apple vaginal probe (Apple Medical Corp, Marlborough, MA) is helpful (Fig. 17.9).

Energy Sources

The use of an energy source for tissue dissection and cutting will usually involve monopolar electrocautery with a da Vinci scissor or spatula. Bipolar cautery may be applied with a fenestrated forceps or Maryland dissector. Additional energy sources used with robotic instruments include Harmonic ACE (ultrasonic shears) (Ethicon Endo-Surgery, Cincinnati, OH) and the Gyrus PK dissecting forceps (advanced bipolar) (Gyrus ACMI, Maple Grove, MN).

OR AND TABLE SETUP

If possible, the largest available OR should be assigned as home for the robotic system. Sufficient room must be allowed for the operating table to be positioned for a variety of cases involving the pelvis, upper abdomen, thorax, and head and neck region. The patient-side cart and vision cart are mobile and parked away from the operating table until needed. Once needed, they are positioned adjacent to the operating table for surgery. Gynecology cases will involve two operating table setups: one for placing vaginal instruments and one larger table for the abdominal portion of the procedure (Figs. 17.10 and 17.11). Most operating tables currently in use will allow for patient weight in excess of 600 pounds and 30 degrees of Trendelenburg position. To avoid movement of the patient in steep Trendelenburg position, the table should be equipped with a warmed gel pad allowing for friction with the patient's bare skin or a beanbag device, which molds to the patient (Figs. 17.12 and 17.13). Another option is an inverted egg

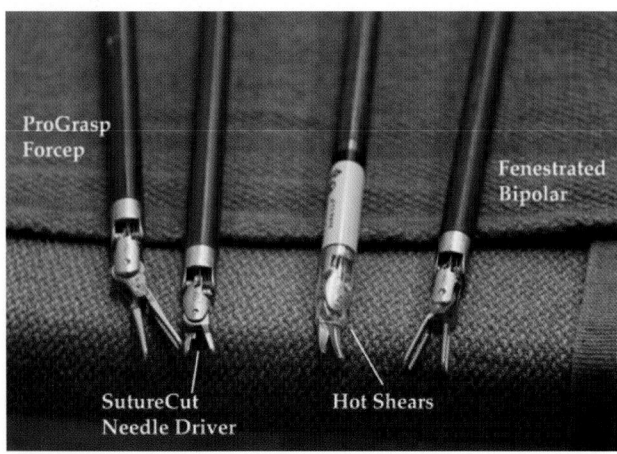

FIGURE 17.8 Commonly used robotic instruments.

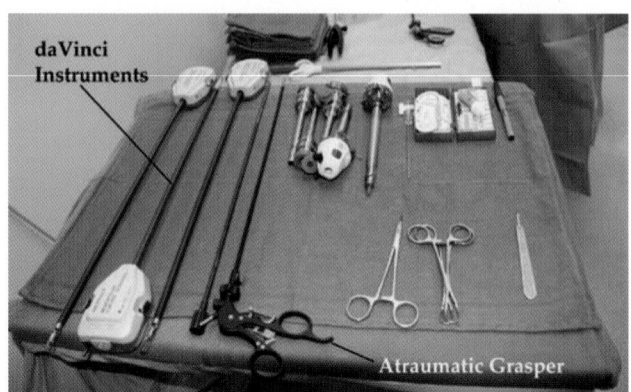

FIGURE 17.10 Mayo stand setup.

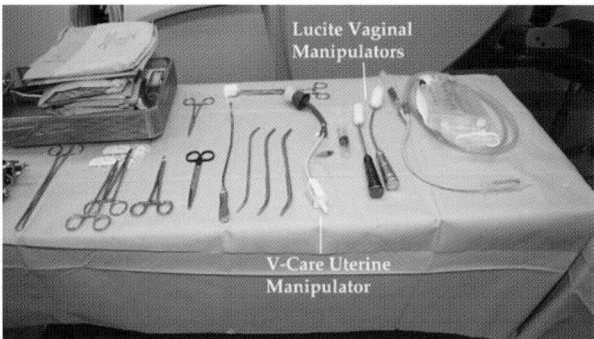

FIGURE 17.11 Vaginal table setup.

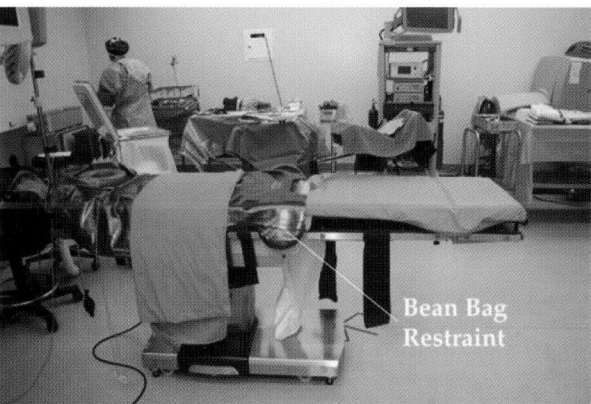

FIGURE 17.12 Beanbag restraint.

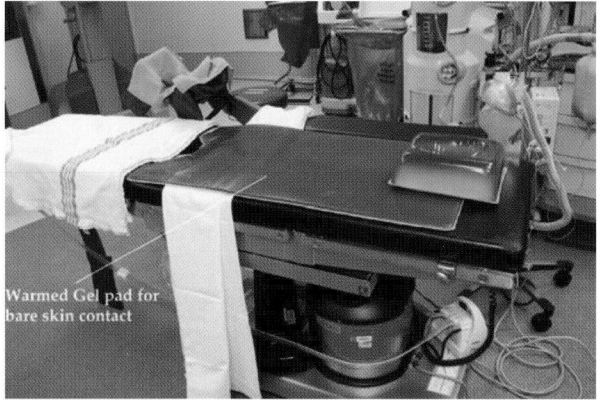

FIGURE 17.13 Gel pad restraint.

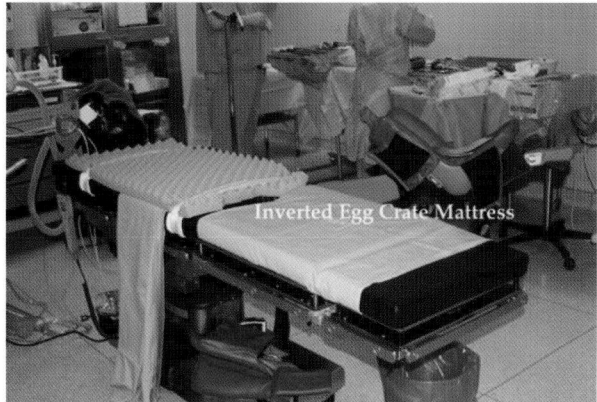

FIGURE 17.14 Inverted egg crate mattress restraint.

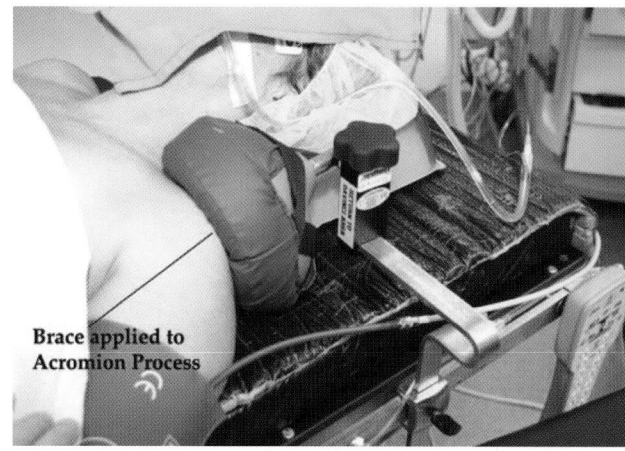

FIGURE 17.15 Shoulder brace.

mattress taped to the bed for bare skin contact (Fig. 17.14). The patient's arms are padded with foam, tucked to her side, and secured with bedsheets. Shoulder braces may be used with care to prevent movement of the patient (Fig. 17.15). If not positioned carefully, the shoulder braces may put the patient at risk for nerve injury. Adjustable stirrups in standard and bariatric sizes are needed to allow placement of vaginal instruments. With motion of the camera arm, there is risk of contact with the patient's face, resulting in injury. Padding of the patient's face will be addressed in the anesthesia section.

Anesthetic Considerations

Anesthetic concerns regarding OR procedures for robotic surgeries include the use of steep Trendelenburg, tucking and padding both arms, covering both legs, and padding and covering the patient's face. Airway pressures may be elevated due to increasing patient size and steep Trendelenburg positioning. Intra-abdominal pressures created by carbon dioxide insufflation and intestines resting on the diaphragm can create an anesthetic challenge. Over time, surgeons and anesthesiologists have become more comfortable with these challenges. When our program started, all patients had two large bore intravenous (IV) sites, and in many cases, an arterial line was placed. Currently, invasive monitoring is seldom needed, and in most cases, a single IV site is utilized. We have made an effort to assess all patients in the preanesthesia clinic several days prior to surgery, therefore providing the safest possible surgery and anesthetic experience. Many gynecologic procedures will involve placing a laparoscopic port in the left upper quadrant of the abdomen for use by the first assistant. We routinely place an orogastric tube to decompress the stomach and avoid gastric trauma from port placement. An important anesthetic consideration is knowing that gastric secretions may track along the orogastric tube to fill the mouth or stain the patient's face. As mentioned earlier, the camera arm of the robot is in constant motion and may come in contact with the patient's face, especially when the camera port is placed well above the umbilicus or a 30-degree, downward lens is used. To prevent trauma, eye shields are placed on the patient; followed by foam padding; and then a face shield allows egress of the endotracheal tube, esophageal stethoscope, and orogastric tube (Fig. 17.16). In cases of lymphadenectomy, the IV fluid rates are kept at a minimum by anesthesia to avoid venous distention.

The Dedicated OR Team

As the surgeon is sitting at the surgeon console without patient contact, he or she relies exclusively on the dedicated OR team to be the hands and eyes at the table. Dedicated

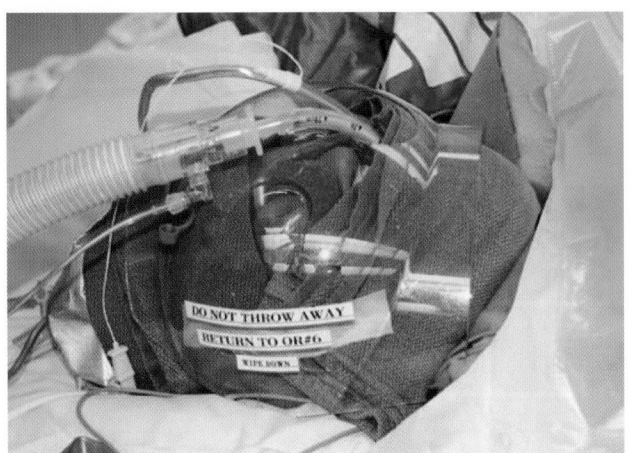

FIGURE 17.16 Eye protection and facial padding.

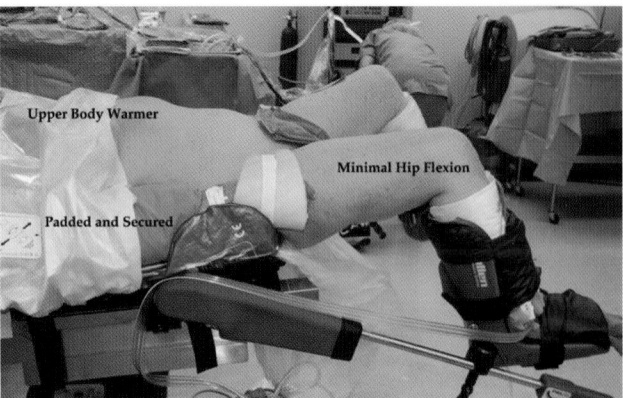

FIGURE 17.18 Patient positioned and padded.

implies two definitions: team members who are personally committed to the most efficient and safe robotic procedures possible, and OR management that will assign the same skilled staff for all cases rather than rotating multiple OR staff. Members of our team include a circulating registered nurse familiar with the variety of robotic procedures, driving the patient-side cart and troubleshooting any problems with console error messages and instrument needs. In addition, we utilize two table-side assistants, one of whom will provide retraction, pass instruments or suture, irrigate the field when needed, and address any conflicts between robotic arms. The second table-side assistant is responsible for uterine manipulation and specimen retrieval (Fig. 17.17). Both assistants drape the upper abdomen while the surgeon places the uterine manipulator. The two bedside assistants may be surgical scrub technicians, certified surgical first assistants, physician assistants, nurse practitioners, or resident physicians. The most efficient operations will be associated with the most experienced table-side assistants.

The Surgeon

In addition to operating the instruments, the surgeon has several other important perioperative responsibilities. The surgeon is responsible for assuring a reasonable period of time for the initial learning curve, appropriate patient selection, preoperative preparation of the patient, and calm leadership of the rest of the team. There are several possible definitions of the "learning curve" for robotic surgery. It may be defined

as the length of time or number of cases to reach a predictable operating time, the fewest complications, or lowest blood loss. It is not in the patient or surgeon's best interest to start with the most complicated procedures. Dealing with a morbidly obese patient, multiple previous abdominal procedures, large fibroid tumors of the uterus, or severe pelvic endometriosis while still learning to effectively manipulate the robotic instruments will result in more complications, unnecessarily long surgical times, and surgeon frustration. Accommodating to the use of different surgical instruments and the lack of haptic sensation is best dealt with by scheduling less complicated cases at the onset of training. Once appropriate patient selection has been completed, the surgeon should explain the aspects of surgery and provide detailed postoperative instructions in advance of the surgery. We have been emphatic about the need to avoid straining or Valsalva maneuvers in the first 2 weeks postoperatively and avoiding any vaginal sexual intercourse for 6 weeks following surgery. On the basis of the type of procedure planned, the surgeon will decide on placement of the camera port, first-assistant port, and two or three operating ports. The operating table will be positioned to allow either side docking or docking between the patient's legs. The surgeon will place the uterine manipulator and, in many cases, place sutures in the cervix if a hysterectomy is planned. The surgeon will tell the table-side assistant which instruments and energy sources will be needed. Once the patient is in Trendelenburg position and ports are in place (Figs. 17.18 and 17.19), the robot is docked and instruments are placed.

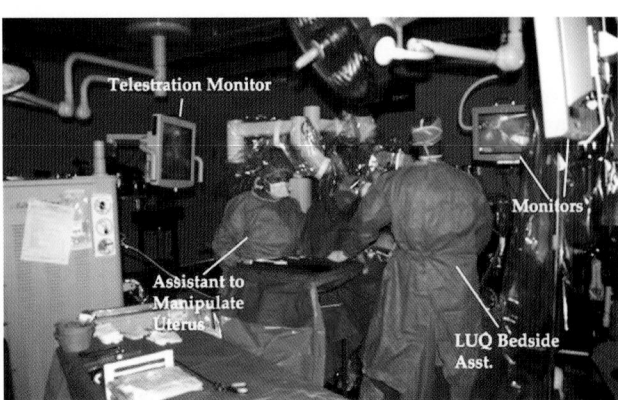

FIGURE 17.17 Surgical assistants' positioning.

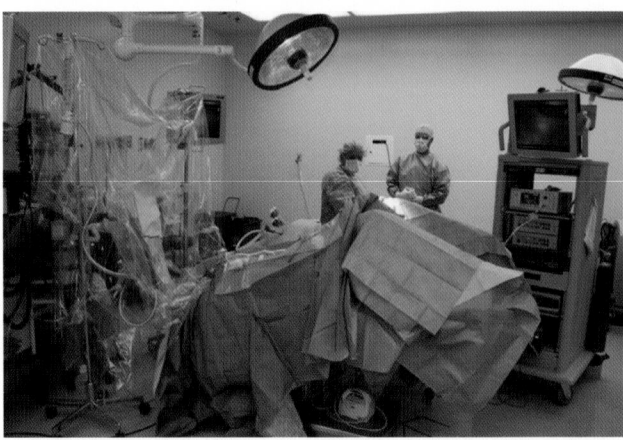

FIGURE 17.19 Ports in place and 30 degrees of Trendelenburg.

At that point, the surgeon assumes control of the surgeon console and initiates the internal portion of the procedure. Once the procedure is complete, the robot is undocked, the abdomen is deflated, and port site skin incisions are closed. Using noncutting trocars, for the 8-mm and 12-mm ports, we have not routinely closed the fascial incisions. All incisions are injected with local anesthetic.

Postoperative Care

One of the greatest advantages of minimally invasive surgical procedures, whether laparoscopic or robotic assisted, is the early mobility and dismissal of patients. At the completion of the procedure, if renal function is normal and the patient is well hydrated, IV ketorolac is given before leaving the OR. A 1- to 2-L bolus of intravenous fluids is given in the recovery room, and the Foley catheter is removed prior to discharge from the recovery room. Regular diet, oral analgesics, and IV ondansetron are part of the routine postoperative orders. Patients are discharged home once they are able to tolerate a liquid diet, demonstrate adequate pain control, and void without difficulty. More than 50% of patients can be dismissed the day of surgery and more than 95% dismissed in less than 24 hours after the surgery is complete.

GYNECOLOGIC PROCEDURES PERFORMED ROBOTICALLY

Although many types of gynecologic procedures have been performed, we will focus on the five most common: robotic hysterectomy, robotic hysterectomy and staging lymphadenectomy, robotic radical hysterectomy, robotic myomectomy (RM), and robotic sacrocolpopexy (RSCP). The first report of uterine horn reanastomosis in an animal model was reported by Margossian in 1998, followed by a pilot study by Falcone and colleagues applying robotic surgery for tubal reanastomosis in humans in 2000. In 2002, Diaz-Arrastia and colleagues at the University of Texas Medical Branch in Galveston reported 11 patients undergoing robotic hysterectomy and bilateral salpingo-oophorectomy. Blood loss ranged from 50 to 1,500 mL, and operative times ranged from 4.5 to 10 hours. By 2006, Reynolds and Advincula reported their experience with 16 patients: 12 undergoing robotic-assisted laparoscopic hysterectomy and 4 treated with supracervical hysterectomy. Blood loss ranged from 50 to 300 mL, and operative times ranged from 170 to 432 minutes. Following these initial publications, multiple institutions and investigators have reported their experience with robotic hysterectomy or comparisons among robotic hysterectomy, laparoscopic hysterectomy, and abdominal hysterectomy. These experiences will be listed in detail later. To date, no randomized trials have compared these techniques, although a multi-institutional, international trial to compare abdominal radical hysterectomy to laparoscopic or robotic radical hysterectomy for early-stage cervical cancer has been proposed by Obermair.

Hysterectomy for Benign Indications

Following the initial feasibility studies noted previously, a 2007 study by Kho and associates reported the initial experience with 91 patients undergoing robotic-assisted hysterectomy with or without removal of adnexa, appendix, and lysis of adhesions. Estimated blood loss was 78 mL, mean operating time was 127 minutes, average length of stay was

1.35 days, and a complication rate of 8% was reported. A study by Matthews and another by Landeen compared robotic hysterectomy to laparoscopic hysterectomy and open hysterectomy. Reports by Payne, Shashoua, Nezhat, and Giep have compared robotic hysterectomy to laparoscopic hysterectomy. Table 17.1 summarizes several published reports of robotic hysterectomy for benign indications. In general, robotic hysterectomy was associated with a longer operating time, lower blood loss, similar to shorter length of stay, and similar complication rates when compared to laparoscopic hysterectomy. When compared to abdominal hysterectomy, surgery times were longer, blood loss was lower, length of stay was shorter, and complication rates were lower for patients treated with robotic hysterectomy. It should be noted that all of these studies were retrospective in design. Open hysterectomy and laparoscopic hysterectomy used for comparison were performed prior to the introduction of robotic hysterectomy.

In a study of 256 patients undergoing robotic hysterectomy with uteri weighing 250 to 3,020 g, with the median weight at 453 g, Payne et al. reported median operating times of 167 minutes for women with uteri weighing 500 g or greater, compared to 126 minutes for women with uteri weighing less than 500 g. Blood loss increased as uterine size increased, hospital length of stay was 1 day, and a major complication rate of 2% was reported.

Surgical Technique of Robotic Hysterectomy

STEPS IN THE PROCEDURE

Robotic Hysterectomy with or without Bilateral Salpingo-oophorectomy

- Preoperative assessment including history and physical examination with review of indications for surgery. Assessment in the preanesthesia clinic if indicated. Equally important is the assessment for the robotic approach, including patient size; associated medical conditions, which may impact the ability to tolerate steep Trendelenburg positioning; and ventilation.

- Following induction of anesthesia, placing a temporary Foley catheter, cervical sutures, and uterine manipulator if planned for use will complete the vaginal portion.

- Camera port positioning well above (25 cm) the fundus of the uterus to allow an unobstructed field of view is essential. Operating ports and first-assistant ports are placed after insufflation with CO_2 to assure there is no external conflict/contact between arms.

- The patient is placed in the maximum Trendelenburg position required for the procedure, and the patient-side cart is docked.

- The retroperitoneum is developed on each side to allow optimal visualization of the ureters. If salpingo-oophorectomy is planned, the ovarian vasculature is coagulated/sealed and divided. If the adnexa are to be preserved, the utero-ovarian ligaments are coagulated and divided.

- The uterus is placed under traction to one side, and the peritoneum of the anterior and posterior broad ligament is incised to skeletonize the uterine vasculature adjacent to the cervix.

- The anterior peritoneum and bladder are dissected away from the cervix and bladder to allow visualization of the impression of the colpotomy ring of the uterine manipulator distending the anterior vaginal fornix.

- The uterine vessels are coagulated/sealed at the level of the colpotomy ring with the bladder gently displaced distally.

- An anterior colpotomy is created on top of the colpotomy ring and extended circumferentially around the vaginal fornix allowing the uterus and cervix to be detached from the vagina and delivered through the colpotomy.

- A damp laparotomy sponge is placed in the vagina to prevent loss of CO_2, and the field is assessed for hemostasis.

- The vaginal angles are secured, and the vaginal cuff is closed with running or interrupted absorbable suture placed 1 cm back from the edge of the vagina to minimize cuff dehiscence.

- After the abdominal incisions are closed, the vaginal pack is removed and the vagina is inspected for evidence of any lacerations or bleeding.

- Orders are placed to remove the Foley catheter in the recovery room and start the patient on oral analgesics, regular diet, and most will be dismissed the same day.

- Patients are instructed to avoid vaginal intercourse for seven weeks postoperatively.

On the day prior to surgery, we have requested patients limit themselves to a full liquid diet and take one bottle of magnesium citrate at noon.

Prior to induction of general anesthesia, the patient is positioned on the operating table utilizing a gel pad, inverted egg crate mattress, or beanbag positioner. Depending on the patient's size, shoulder braces may be needed but used with caution. Once the patient is anesthetized, prepped, and draped, an indwelling catheter is placed in the bladder and sutures of size 0 polyglactin are placed at the 3 o'clock and 9 o'clock positions in the cervix. The cervix is dilated,

TABLE 17.1 Robotic Hysterectomy Compared to Laparoscopic and Abdominal Routes

AUTHORS	NO. OF SUBJECTS	EBL MEAN (RANGE)	OPERATIVE TIME MINUTES MEAN (RANGE)	LOS	COMPLICATION RATE (%)
Diaz-Arrastia et al. (2002)	11	50–1,500 mL	4.5–10 h		
Reynolds and Advincula (2006)	16	96 (50–300)	242 (170–432)		
Kho et al. (2007)	91	78	127	1.35 ± 0.69	8
Payne et al. (2008)	100	61 ± 60	119 ± 59	1 ± 0.7	
Shashoua et al. (2009)	26	113 (50–300)	142 (90–218)	1.0 (0–2)	
Boggess et al. (2009)	152	79 ± 132	122 ± 48	1.05 ± 0.69	3.50
Nezhat et al. (2009)	26	250 (100–1,000)	276 (150–440)	1.0 (1–1)	
Giep et al. (2010)	237	59 ± 75	89 ± 37.5	1.0 ± 0.1	3.80
Matthews et al. (2010)	65	82 ± 106	NL	1.5 ± 0.7	4.20
Payne et al. (2010)	256	98 ± 106	151 ± 57	1.1 ± 0.7	3.50
Feuer et al. (2011)	55	63.5 ± 3.76	80.9 ± 3.4	1.3 ± 0.15	1.80
Landeen et al. (2011)	569	109 ± 143	117 ± 59	1.3 ± 0.6	8.40
Laparoscopic Hysterectomy					
Payne et al. (2008)	100	113 ± 85	92 ± 29	1.6 ± 1.4	
Shashoua et al. (2009)	44	98 (50–450)	122 (60–245)	1.4 (0–5)	
Nezhat et al. (2009)	50	300 (110–750)	206 (110–420)	1.05 (1–3)	
Giep et al. (2010)	265	167 ± 146	124 ± 48	1.2 ± 0.7	1.90
Matthews et al. (2010)	21	353 ± 303	NL	1.8 ± 0.8	6.80
Feuer et al. (2011)					
Landeen et al. (2011)	227	182 ± 185	118 ± 45	1.8 ± 1.5	8.80
Abdominal Hysterectomy					
Matthews et al. (2010)	113	430 ± 417		3.5 ± 3.2	23.40
Feuer et al. (2011)					
Landeen et al. (2011)	274	269 ± 385	83 ± 33	2.7 ± 1.4	14

EBL, estimated blood loss; LOS, length of stay.

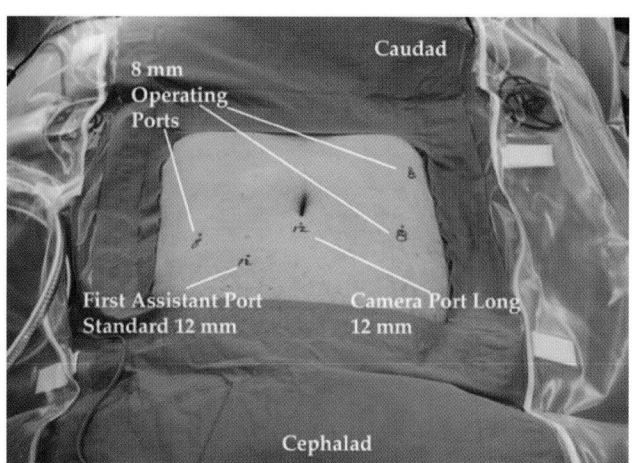

FIGURE 17.20 Port site marking.

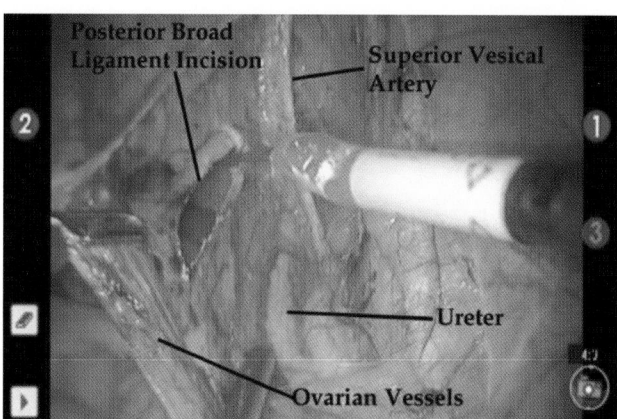

FIGURE 17.22 Incising the posterior broad ligament.

III

and a uterine manipulator is placed. We prefer to use the VCare Manipulator (ConMed EndoSurgery, Utica, NY). The sutures are brought through the colpotomy ring for traction to allow removal of the uterus later. The abdomen is then approached, and a decision regarding camera port placement is made. In virtually all cases, the camera port is above the umbilicus; however, the distance from the umbilicus depends on the uterine size. A distance of 20 to 24 cm above the uterine fundus is ideal. Once the abdomen is insufflated, sites are marked for the additional ports. Eight-millimeter ports for the operating arms are usually placed 10 cm lateral to the midline at or just below the level of the umbilicus. A 12-mm port is placed for the first assistant in the left upper quadrant, and an additional 8-mm port for the third operating arm of the robot is placed in the right lower quadrant (Figs. 17.20 and 17.21). The patient is placed in 30 degrees of Trendelenburg, and the bowel is displaced from the pelvis. Conventional laparoscopic instruments may be needed for dissection of omental and bowel adhesions to enhance port positioning and visualization. The robotic arms are then docked to the ports, and instruments are placed. We usually use a fenestrated bipolar grasper in one operating port and monopolar scissors in the opposite port. A Prograsp forceps is frequently placed in the third operating port. The first assistant uses an atraumatic grasper, bariatric needle driver,

and irrigator/aspirator through the 12-mm port in the left upper quadrant.

The technical steps in a hysterectomy follow those of a standard abdominal hysterectomy except for entry into the vagina. The uterus is grasped at the cornua and displaced to one side with the Prograsp forceps that runs parallel to the anterior abdominal wall. Once the ureter is identified in the retroperitoneum (Fig. 17.22), the round ligament is coagulated and divided. If salpingo-oophorectomy is planned, the ovarian vasculature is coagulated and divided at this time (Fig. 17.23). The anterior and posterior broad ligaments are incised, and uterine vasculature is then skeletonized and coagulated (Fig. 17.24). The uterine artery can be coagulated at the level of the hypogastric artery to minimize bleeding if extended dissection of the uterus due to leiomyoma or endometriosis is anticipated (Fig. 17.25). Once the above procedures have been completed on both sides, the bladder is dissected clear of the uterus and cervix, allowing identification of the colpotomy ring distending the anterior vaginal fornix (Fig. 17.26). With the bladder well dissected and displaced inferiorly, the anterior colpotomy is made and carried circumferentially around the vaginal fornix on top of the colpotomy ring (Fig. 17.27). When completely detached, the uterus and cervix (and adnexa if included) are delivered through the vagina. At this point, the bedside assistant will place a dry laparotomy sponge within a sterile surgical glove to occlude the vagina, thus preventing

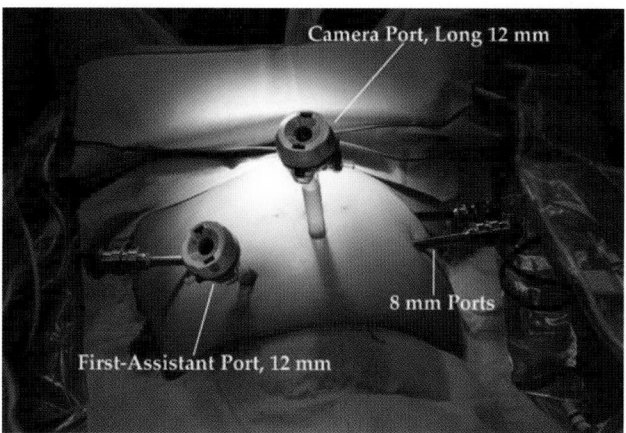

FIGURE 17.21 Ports in place.

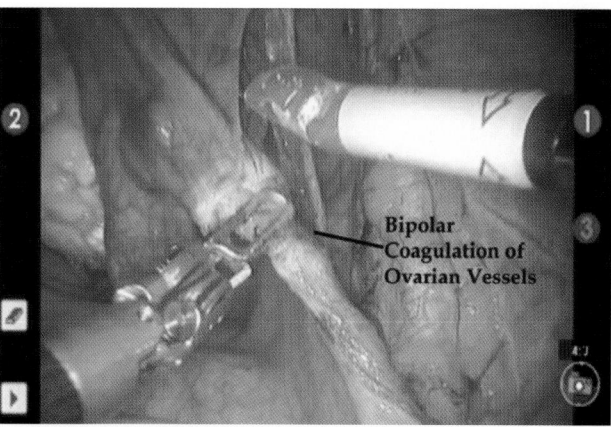

FIGURE 17.23 Coagulation of ovarian vessels.

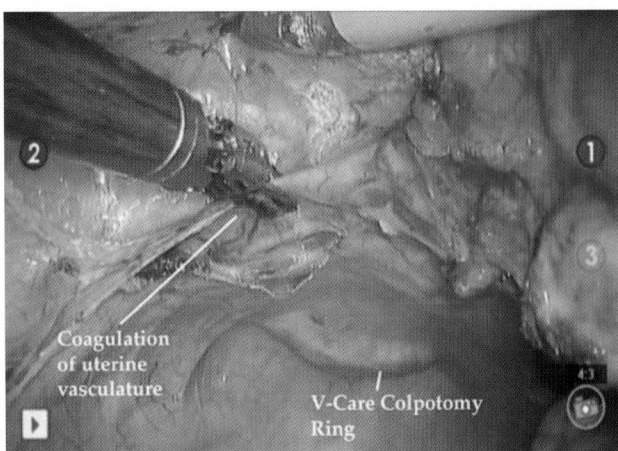

FIGURE 17.24 Coagulation of uterine vessels.

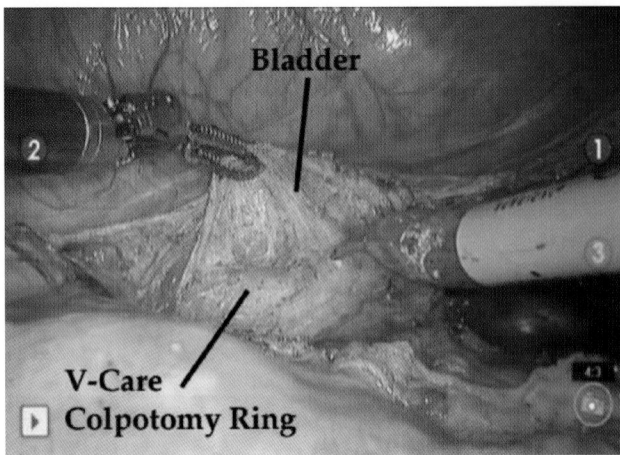

FIGURE 17.26 Bladder dissection.

loss of carbon dioxide (Fig. 17.28). Monopolar scissors are replaced with a needle driver, and the vaginal cuff is closed. A 0 polyglactin suture in either an interrupted figure-of-eight placement or running from each angle to the midline is used to close the vaginal apex (Fig. 17.29). Support is provided by incorporation of the cardinal and uterosacral ligaments into the angle closure. In the case of uterine leiomyomata, which prevents delivery of the uterus through the vagina, we secure the uterus with the third operating arm while bivalving or quartering the uterus with monopolar cautery. Once all vascular pedicles are inspected, the instruments are removed, the robot undocked, the abdomen deflated, and ports removed. As we use only noncutting trocars, none of the fascial incisions are closed. All incisions are injected with 0.25% bupivacaine with epinephrine following subcutaneous closure and before applying a liquid skin adhesive. In the absence of contraindications, we will give 15 to 30 mg of ketorolac intravenously at the end of the case and 1 to 2 L of IV fluid in the recovery room. Oral analgesics are prescribed once dismissed from the recovery room. Most patients will be discharged home within 24 hours with instructions to ambulate frequently, avoid straining for 2 to 3 weeks, and avoid sexual intercourse for 6 weeks.

Robotic Hysterectomy and Lymphadenectomy for Endometrial Cancer

Perhaps, the area of gynecologic surgery most enthusiastically adopting robotic techniques is in treatment of endometrial cancer. Because of age, health issues, and size, this group of women represents the highest risk for surgical complications. Table 17.2 represents most of the available literature regarding the application of robotic surgery for treatment of uterine cancer. Studies by Boggess, Bell, and Lim compare hysterectomy and staging lymphadenectomy performed robotically, laparoscopically, or as an open procedure. In general, blood loss and length of postoperative hospitalization were the lowest in the robotic group. Operating times were shortest in the open group and comparable in the robotic and laparoscopic groups. Complications were lowest in the robotic group. Lymph node counts were similar across all three groups. Studies by Seamon, Holz, and Cardenas-Goicoechea compare hysterectomy and staging lymphadenectomy performed robotically with those performed laparoscopically. Surgical time was shorter, and length of stay for robotic surgeries was shorter in two of the three studies. Estimated blood loss was lower for robotic surgery in all three studies. Node counts were higher in the robotic group in one study and comparable in the other two studies. Conversion to an open procedure was less likely in the robotic group compared to the laparoscopy group. Studies by Veljovich and DeNardis comparing robotic hysterectomy and staging lymphadenectomy to an open procedure confirm that operating times are longer, blood loss is less, and length of stay is shorter in the robotic group. Node counts are comparable in both groups.

Because of the association between obesity and endometrial cancer, the role of robotic surgery in that patient group is

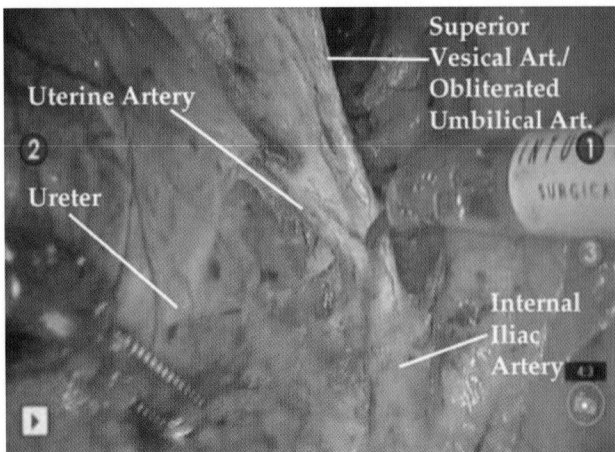

FIGURE 17.25 Visualization of uterine artery.

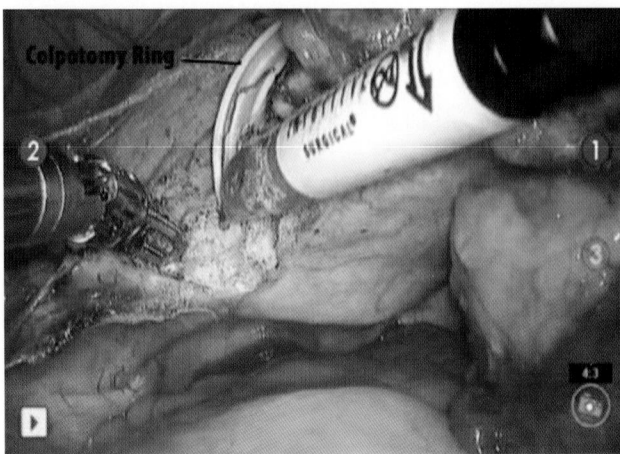

FIGURE 17.27 Colpotomy.

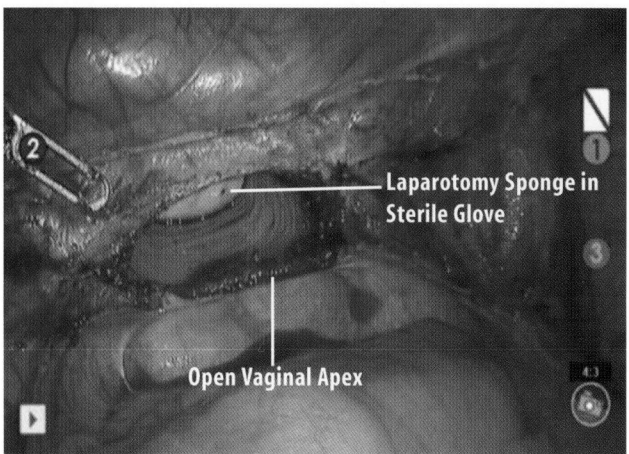

FIGURE 17.28 Open vaginal cuff.

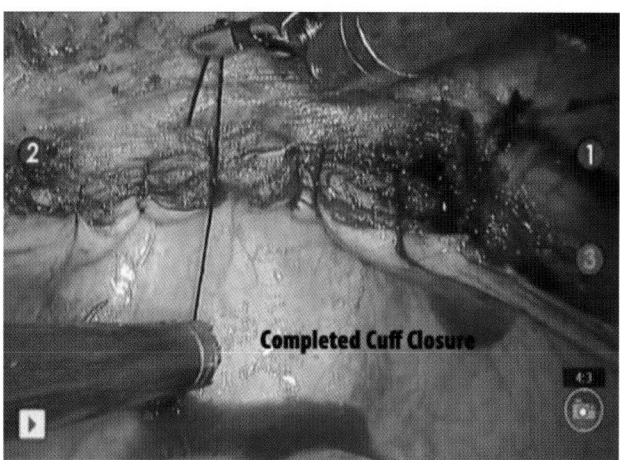

FIGURE 17.29 Vaginal cuff closure.

III

TABLE 17.2 Hysterectomy and Staging Lymphadenectomy

			ROBOTIC TECHNIQUE			
AUTHORS	NO. OF SUBJECTS	EBL MEAN ± SD OR (RANGE)	OPERATIVE TIME MINUTES MEAN (RANGE)	NO. OF NODES	LOS	COMPLICATION RATE (%)
Boggess et al. (2008)	103	74 ± 101	191 ± 36	32 ± 26	1 ± 0.2 d	
Veljovich et al. (2008)	25	66 (10–300)	283 (171–4,430)	17 (2–32)	40 h (17–215)	
DeNardis et al. (2008)	56	105 ± 77	177 ± 55	18.6 ± 12	1.0 ± 0.5 d	
Bell et al. (2008)	40	166 ± 225	184 ± 41	17 ± 7.8	2.3 ± 1.3	7.50
Gehrig et al. (2008)	49 (obese)	50 (25–300)	189 (111–263)	31 (6–73)	1.02 (1–2)	
Lowe et al. (2009)	405	87 ± 97	170 ± 68	15.5 ± 9.6	1.8 ± 2.8	
Holloway et al. (2009)	100	103 ± 80	171 ± 50	18.7 ± 11	1.2 ± 0.93	
Seamon et al. (2009)	105	88 (20–500)	242 ± 53	31 ± 7.6	1 (1–46)	13
Seamon et al. (2009)	92 (obese)	109	228 ± 43	24.7 ± 13.2	1 (1–2)	11
Lim et al. (2010)	56	89 ± 45	162 ± 53	26 ± 12	1.6 ± 0.7	12
Cardenas-Goicoechea et al. (2010)	102	109 ± 83	237 ± 57	22 ± 10	1.88 ± 1.167	7.80
Holz et al. (2010)	13	84.6 ± 32	192 ± 38	13 ± 4.5	1.7 ± 0.6	15
Lim et al., 2011	122	81 ± 45	147 ± 48	25 ± 12.7	1.5 ± 0.9	10.50
Laparoscopic Technique						
Boggess et al. (2008)	81	145 ± 105	213 ± 34	23 ± 11	1.2 ± 0.5 d	
Bell et al. (2008)	30	253 ± 427	171 ± 36	17 ± 7.1	2.0 ± 1.2	20
Gehrig et al. (2008)	32 (obese)	150 (50–700)	215 (156–324)	24 (3–59)	1.27 (1–4)	
Seamon et al. (2009)	76	200 (50–650)	287 ± 55	33 ± 8.4	2 (1–9)	14
Lim et al. (2010)	56	209 ± 91	192 ± 55	45 ± 20	2.6 ± 0.9	23
Cardenas-Goicoechea et al. (2010)	173	187 ± 187	178 ± 58	23 ± 12		7.50
Holz et al. (2010)	20	150 ± 111	156 ± 49	8.5 ± 5.4		15
Lim et al. (2011)	122	207 ± 109	186 ± 59	43 ± 17	3.2 ± 2.3	19.60
Abdominal Technique						
Boggess et al. (2008)	138	266 ± 184	146 ± 48	14.9 ± 11	4.4 ± 2.0 d	
Veljovich et al. (2008)	131	197 (25–900)	139 (69–294)	13 (1–42)	127 h (13–576)	
DeNardis et al. (2008)	106	241 ± 115	79 ± 17	18 ± 9.6	3.2 ± 1.2	
Bell et al. (2008)	40	316 ± 282	108 ± 41	15 ± 4.8	4.0 ± 1.5	27.50
Seamon et al. (2009)	162 (obese)	394	142 ± 47	23.9 ± 11.8	3 (3–4)	27
Lim et al. (2010)	36	266 ± 145	136 ± 32	55 ± 23	4.9 ± 1.9	25

EBL, estimated blood loss; LOS, length of stay.

of great interest. Gehrig and colleagues reported on 49 obese patients with endometrial cancer treated robotically compared to 32 matched patients treated laparoscopically. Robotic surgery was associated with a lower estimated blood loss, shorter operating times, shorter hospital stay, and increased node counts. When comparing robotic surgery for endometrial cancer in the obese patient to an open procedure, Seamon and colleagues demonstrated lower blood loss, fewer complications, shorter length of stay, and comparable node counts with robotic surgeries. However, longer operating times were also reported for the patients treated robotically. To date, there are no prospective studies comparing robotic hysterectomy and staging lymphadenectomy to laparoscopic or open approaches.

Surgical Technique for Lymphadenectomy

We prefer to perform the pelvic lymphadenectomy prior to the hysterectomy and the aortic node sampling after the hysterectomy. By developing the retroperitoneum, including the paravesical and pararectal spaces, the medial leaf of the broad ligament serves as a barrier between the node-bearing tissues and the rectosigmoid. The extent of the lymph node dissection in the pelvis includes the distal common iliac nodes, the nodes surrounding the external iliac artery and vein, and the obturator lymph nodes (Fig. 17.30). At the completion of the pelvic lymphadenectomy, all nodal tissues from both sides are placed in a sterile plastic pouch to be delivered through the vagina at the completion of the hysterectomy. The hysterectomy is performed as described previously. Once the vaginal cuff is closed, the monopolar scissors replace the needle driver and the right-sided aortic node sampling is performed. The peritoneum overlying the right common iliac artery is incised to the level of the lower aorta and inferior mesenteric artery. The nodal tissue overlying the lower aorta and distal vena cava is dissected clear of those vessels while retracting the right ureter laterally (Fig. 17.31). The right-sided aortic nodes are placed in the thumb of a sterile glove and brought out through the first-assistant port. The left aortic lymphadenectomy is similar but less difficult because there is no vena cava on the left side. The left ureter should be identified and carefully avoided.

Since less IV fluid is given intraoperatively to minimize venous filling, extra fluid is given in the recovery room prior to transfer. As with the patients undergoing robotic hysterectomy for benign conditions, many patients can be dismissed on the day of surgery and more than 90% of patients are dismissed in less than 24 hours of surgery.

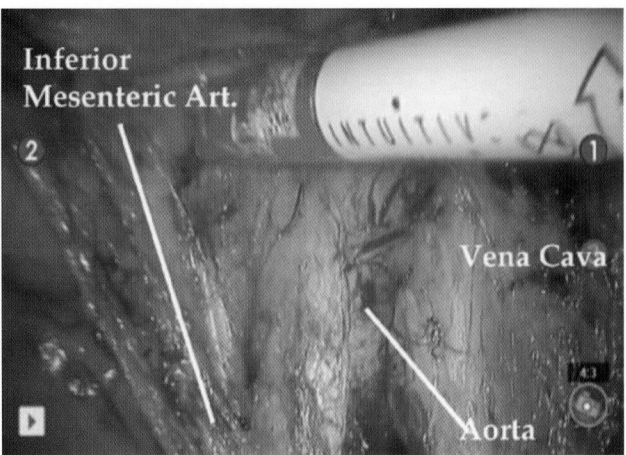

FIGURE 17.31 Aortic node sampling.

Robotic Radical Hysterectomy and Pelvic Lymphadenectomy

Table 17.3 lists 13 studies published since 2008 with a total of 432 patients treated by robotic radical hysterectomy and pelvic lymphadenectomy. Studies by Fanning, Kim, Persson, and Lowe describe the experience of the authors performing the robotic procedure. Five studies by Boggess, Ko, Maggioni, Geisler, and Cantrell compare robotic radical hysterectomy to abdominal radical hysterectomy. Nezhat and Tinelli compared robotic radical hysterectomy to laparoscopic radical hysterectomy. Finally, studies by Magrina and Estape compare robotic radical hysterectomy to laparoscopic radical hysterectomy and abdominal radical hysterectomy. In the study by Magrina, robotic surgery resulted in a decreased length of stay compared to open procedures and comparable length of stay compared to laparoscopic procedures. Operating times for robotic surgery were similar to open procedures but shorter than the laparoscopic approach. Blood loss was greatest in the open group when compared to robotic and laparoscopic techniques. There was no difference in lymph node counts or complications between the three groups. The results reported by Estape differ somewhat in that robotic surgery was longer than open procedures but comparable in length to the laparoscopic approach. Robotic surgery resulted in a higher lymph node count when compared to open and laparoscopic approaches. When looking at the comparative studies of robotic radical hysterectomy to open procedures by Geisler, Maggioni, Cantrell, and Ko, estimated blood loss and length of stay are shorter, operating times in general are longer, and lymph node counts and complications are comparable. There are no prospective studies comparing robotic radical hysterectomy to laparoscopic or open procedures, although an international phase III randomized trial comparing the three approaches has been proposed by Obermair.

Robotic Radical Hysterectomy Technique

Patient positioning for robotic radical hysterectomy is the same as described earlier in the chapter. Uterine manipulators are usually replaced with a Lucite vaginal probe to facilitate dissection of the bladder and to assess the length of the vaginal cuff. Depending on the patient preference, age, and gross appearance, the ovaries may be preserved or removed. Paravesical and pararectal spaces are developed, and the uterine artery is coagulated and divided at its origin from the hypogastric artery. The ureter is then dissected from the medial broad ligament, and the ureteral tunnel is exposed. The anterior vesicle ligament is cauterized and divided, thus unroofing the ureter from the cardinal

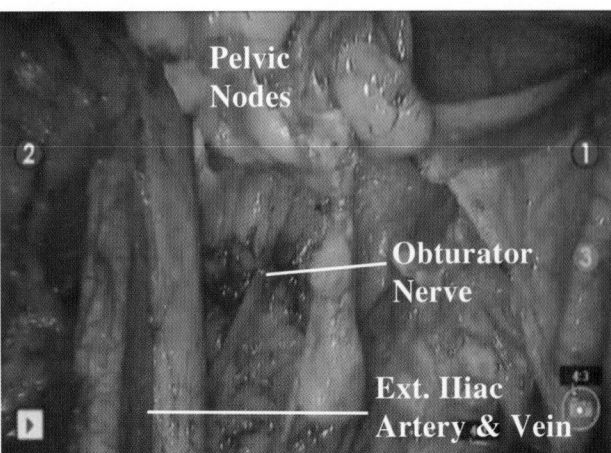

FIGURE 17.30 Pelvic lymphadenectomy.

TABLE 17.3 Radical Hysterectomy Comparison

AUTHORS	NO. OF SUBJECTS	EBL MEAN (RANGE)	OPERATIVE TIME MINUTES MEAN (RANGE)	NO. OF NODES	LOS	COMPLICATION RATE (%)
ROBOTIC TECHNIQUE						
Boggess et al. (2008b)	51	96 ± 85	210 ± 45	33 ± 14	1	7.80
Magrina et al. (2008)	27	133 ± 108	189 ± 43	26 ± 6.3	1.7 (0.9)	7
Fanning et al. (2008)	20	300 (100–475)	390 (210–510)	18 (15–35)	1 d	10
Kim et al. (2008)	10	355 (200–450)	207 (120–240)	27.6 (12–52)	7.9 (5–17) d	10
Ko et al. (2008)	16	81.9 (20–400)	290 (199–364)	15.6 (4–34)	1.7 (1–4)	18
Nezhat et al. (2008)	13	157 (50–400)	323 (232–453)	24.7 (11–51)	2.7 (1–6) d	30
Persson et al. (2009)	80	150 (25–1,300)	262 (132–475)			
Estape et al. (2009)	32	130 ± 119	144 ± 48	32 ± 10	2.6 ± 2.1	18.80
Maggioni et al. (2009)	40	78 ± 94	272 ± 42	20.4 ± 6.9	3.7 ± 1.2	5.00
Lowe et al. (2009b)	42	50 (25–150)	215 (120–606)	25 (12–60)	1	16.80
Geisler et al. (2010)	15	165	154	25	1.4 d	
Cantrell et al. (2010)	63	50 (20–400)	213 (73–290)	29 (13–99)	1 (1–3)	4
Tinelli et al. (2011)	23	157 ± 7	323 ± 30	24.7 ± 5	3 ± 1	
Laparoscopic Technique						
Magrina et al. (2008)	31	208 ± 105	220 ± 37	25.9 (7.8)	2.4 (1.5)	6
Nezhat et al. (2008)	30	200 (100–500)	318 (200–464)	31 (10–61)	3.8 (2–11)	205
Estape et al. (2009)	17	209 ± 169	132 ± 42	18.6 ± 5.3	2.3 ± 1.4	23.50
Tinelli et al. (2011)	76	95 ± 5	255 ± 25	27 ± 4.7	4 ± 2	
Abdominal Technique						
Boggess et al. (2008)	49	416 ± 188	247 ± 48	23.3 ± 12.7	3.2	16.30
Magrina et al. (2008)	35	443 ± 253	166 ± 33	27.7 (6.6)	3.6 (1.2)	9
Ko et al. (2008)	32	665 (200–3,500)	219 (113–308)	17.1 (4–38)	4.9 (3–8)	12
Estape et al. (2009)	14	621 ± 194	114 ± 26	25.7 ± 11.5	4.0 ± 1.7	28.60
Maggioni et al. (2009)	40	221.8 ± 132	199.6 ± 65.6	26.2 ± 11.7	5.0 ± 2.4	12.00
Geisler et al. (2010)	30	323	166	26	2.8 d	
Cantrell et al. (2010)	64	400 (100–1,200)	240 (181–420)	24 (4–72)	4 (3–8)	6

EBL, estimated blood loss; LOS, length of stay.

ligament all the way to its entry into the bladder. Once this has been accomplished on both sides, the bladder is dissected away from the upper third of the vagina, and the posterior vaginal wall and uterosacral ligaments are exposed. The uterosacral ligaments are divided at the level of the anterior rectum. At this point, an upper vaginotomy is performed, and adequate vaginal margin is determined on the basis of the size of the cervical cancer. The specimen is removed through the vagina, and a dry laparotomy sponge in a sterile glove is placed in the vagina to maintain the pneumoperitoneum. Bilateral total pelvic lymphadenectomy is then performed. Common iliac nodes are removed through the first-assistant port and labeled separately. The pelvic nodes are placed in a sterile pouch and brought out through the vagina. The vaginal cuff is closed with interrupted or running 0 polyglactin sutures. Patients are usually dismissed the following morning with an indwelling catheter with plans for a voiding trial in 1 week.

Robotic Use in Reconstructive Pelvic Surgery

Robotic Sacrocolpopexy

The primary application of robotics in reconstructive pelvic surgery has been sacrocolpopexy. Sacrocolpopexy has been the most important operation in the abdominal approach for repair of enterocele and vaginal vault prolapse. It may also be utilized for apical support with concurrent hysterectomy. The procedure is reported by Nygaard as a durable repair with approximately a 90% long-term success rate. Permanent synthetic graft material, usually type I macroporous polypropylene mesh, is used most commonly. In the mid-1990s, the laparoscopic approach to perform this operation was reported by Nezhat and colleagues. However, this was a technically difficult operation to learn with a steep learning curve. Laparoscopic sacrocolpopexy offers similar success rates as open abdominal surgery with the benefits of minimally invasive surgery, such as shorter hospital stay, more rapid recovery, and possibly less morbidity. However, those benefits are associated with longer operating times. Because of the technical difficulties associated with the learning curve and maintaining proficiency as well as the benefits of the vaginal reparative approach, this technique has not been widely adopted. The availability of robotics is changing the trend from the open and laparoscopic approaches.

Several retrospective reports on RSCP or sacrohysteropexy are presented in Table 17.4. Akl and associates evaluated 80 patients treated with RSCP and followed them for 1 to 24 months. Five percent of patients required conversion to an open procedure, and a 6% graft exposure rate was reported. Operative time decreased by 25% after the first 10 cases. In three separate studies, Daneshgari, Göçmen, and Kramer describe case series of 12 to 21 patients with overall low blood loss, comparable operative times, and short hospital stays. Kramer described 21 patients who underwent RSCP, with 12 patients requiring additional repairs at a later date.

TABLE 17.4 Robotic Sacrocolpopexy

AUTHORS	NO. OF SUBJECTS		FOLLOW-UP DURATION	EBL (ML)	OPERATIVE TIME	LOS (DAYS)	OUTCOME
Geller (2008)	73	RSCP	6 wk	103 ± 96	328 ± 55 min	1.3 ± 0.8	Comparable point C improvement
	105	ASCP		255 ± 155	225 ± 61 min	2.7 ± 1.4	
Elliot (2006)	30	RSCP	24 mo (12–36)	3.1 h (2.15–4.75)	1.03 (1–2)		
Akl (2009)	80	RSCP	4.8 mo (1–24)		198 min		Operative time decreased 25% after the first 10 cases
Daneshgari (2007)	12	RSCP	6 mo	81 (50–150)		2.4 (1–7)	
Göçmen (2011)	12	RSCP	12 mo	12.5 (10–20)	150.5 (114–189) min		
Geller (2011a)	28	RSCP	14.8 mo				Pelvic floor function improved
Kramer (2009)	21	RSCP			3 h 14 min	1	

RSCP, robotic sacrocolpopexy; ASCP, abdominal sacrocolpopexy; EBL, estimated blood loss; LOS, length of stay.

Reported complications include small bowel obstruction, ileus, pelvic abscess, bladder injury, ureteral injury, and conversion to an abdominal approach. The overall complication rate appears to be no higher than abdominal sacrocolpopexy (ASCP). Geller and colleagues in 2008 reported the largest series but only compared RSCP to ASCP. Geller and colleagues found a significantly longer operating time, shorter length of hospital stay, and lower blood loss for RSCP compared to ASCP. At 6-week follow-up, they reported similar pelvic organ prolapse quantification point C improvement in both groups. Geller and associates treated 28 patients with RSCP at a mean follow-up of 14.8 months. They found improved pelvic floor function with stable support and sexual function. Two patients with graft exposures and two recurrent prolapse were reported. Acknowledging the small volume of published reports, these initial data and unpublished experiences seem to indicate safe and reliable use of the robotic platform for sacrocolpopexy.

Surgical Technique The initial technical aspects are similar to preparation for hysterectomy as described above. Either a straight or side dock technique is utilized. Port placement for the camera is usually above the umbilicus approximately halfway or higher between the pubic symphysis and xiphoid process (12-mm dilating trocar). Two 8-mm da Vinci dilating trocars are placed approximately 10 cm or greater, lateral to midline at a level usually between the anterior superior iliac spines and umbilicus (below the level of the camera port). The assistant 12-mm port is placed in either the left or right upper quadrant. The third da Vinci robotic arm is not usually required but is prepared for possible additional retraction on more challenging cases. The upper pelvis and abdominal wall are cleared of omental and bowel adhesions with laparoscopy before docking, at which point further adhesions deeper in the pelvis are cleared with the monopolar shears. If the sigmoid colon is excessively redundant or unruly due to poor bowel preparation, it may be retracted to the left anterior abdominal wall with a traction suture to be released at completion of the case. Usually, the assistant is required to retract the sigmoid colon to the left. The vagina is distended with a Lucite probe or large stainless steel bowel sizer (or two as needed) for vaginal manipulation. The rectum also may be stented with a probe to aid in the deep posterior dissection. Other instruments such as Breisky-Navratil retractors may be placed vaginally as needed to improve visualization of dissection planes and suture placement. We will frequently place an Allis clamp in the midline vagina anteriorly and posteriorly where we anticipate placing the most distal aspect of the mesh arms. Placement of the Allis clamps is dependent upon the patient's anatomic defects. Placement of the Allis clamps also helps in identifying how far to extend the dissection in the vesicovaginal and rectovaginal spaces. The upper pelvic structures including the aortic bifurcation, right common iliac artery, right ureter, and sacral promontory are identified. Care is taken to identify the left common iliac vein as it crosses the field. The peritoneum over the first sacral joint (S1) is opened, and the areolar, fatty, and lymphatic tissues are carefully cleared to expose the anterior longitudinal ligament and middle sacral vessels while keeping clear of the left common iliac vein (Fig. 17.32).

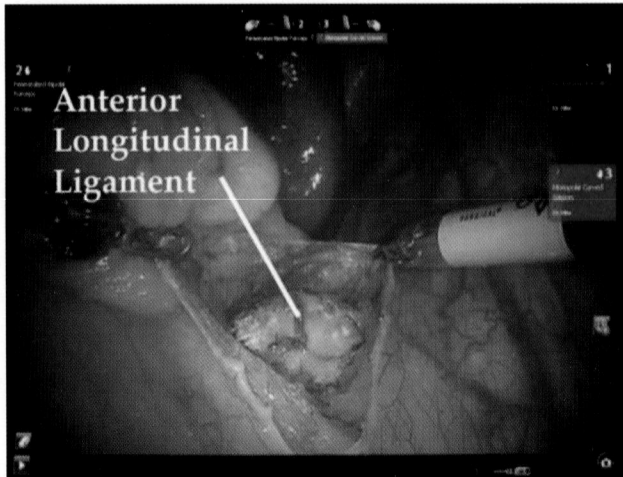

FIGURE 17.32 Exposing anterior longitudinal ligament.

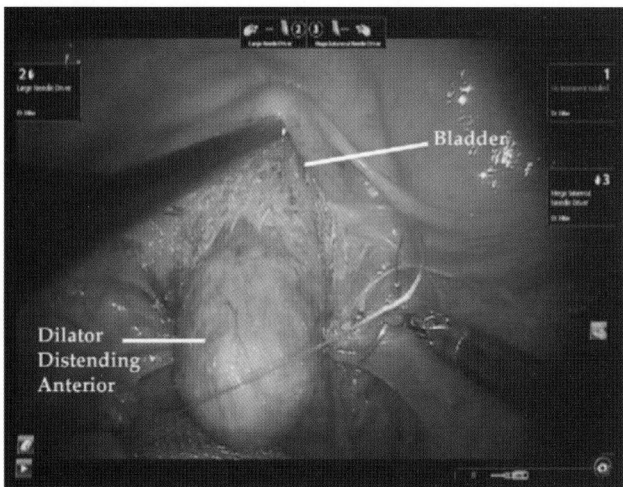

FIGURE 17.33 Exposing anterior vagina.

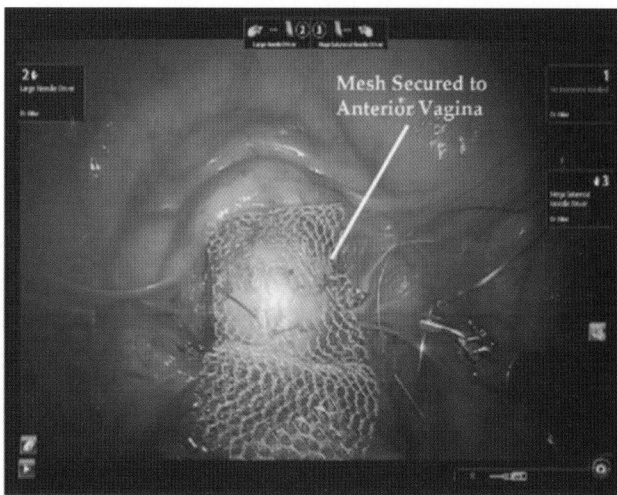

FIGURE 17.35 Mesh secured to anterior vagina.

The middle sacral vessels may be coagulated once skeletonized. A 30-degree downward-directed scope may be helpful for this dissection in some patients. The line of dissection is then carried over the peritoneum and the underlying fatty tissue to the right of the sigmoid colon and medial to the ureter to the pelvic floor and vaginal apex. Care is taken to avoid trauma to the presacral, lateral sacral, and hypogastric veins. Next, the peritoneum over the vagina is opened to develop the rectovaginal and vesicovaginal spaces (Figs. 17.33 and 17.34). The table-side assistant is instructed to manipulate the vaginal stent to assist the dissection. Once these spaces are opened and the bladder and rectum are mobilized, an assessment is made of length for the mesh arms. A self-constructed or prefabricated type I macroporous, polypropylene Y-shaped mesh with two arms and a width of 4.5 to 5 cm is cut to the desired length (usually 4 to 8 cm) with a tail for attachment to the sacrum. The mesh is applied over a wide surface area with multiple placements of permanent suture through the full thickness of the vaginal wall. The mesh is attached to the anterior vagina and then the posterior vagina (Figs. 17.35 and 17.36). The 30-degree upward-directed scope may be useful for placement of the low posterior sutures. The vagina is then elevated toward S1, is taken off of tension, and marked for attachment to the anterior longitudinal ligament with a permanent suture placed transversely, usually under the middle sacral vessels. The tail is secured with two or three sutures (Fig. 17.37). The peritoneum is then closed over the mesh with a delayed absorbable suture to cover the bridge of mesh between vaginal apex and sacrum in an attempt to

decrease the risk of adhesions and bowel obstruction. We close the peritoneum from distal to proximal, taking care not to kink or damage the ureter during the closure. A vaginal pack may be used to keep the vagina distended against the mesh. Antibiotic irrigation may also be used to irrigate the mesh.

Robotic Burch Retropubic Urethropexy

There are currently no studies looking specifically at the use of robotic retropubic urethropexy, although three patients undergoing the procedure are mentioned in reports by Partin and Daneshgari. This surgical procedure is primarily utilized in conjunction with RSCP for the treatment of overt or occult stress incontinence especially with urethrovesical junction hypermobility or urethrocele. The major obstacle to overcome is the lack of tactile sensation for placing the periurethral sutures. The advantages of laparoscopic retropubic urethropexy (LRPU) and robotic Burch retropubic urethropexy are improved hemostasis, visualization, and accurate, symmetric suture placement and tensioning. Paravaginal repair for additional lateral midvaginal support may also be placed.

Surgical Technique The technique is initially the same as performing an LRPU (Marshall-Marchetti-Krantz procedure or Burch procedure). With a Foley catheter in the bladder, the peritoneum is incised in an inverted U incision over the bladder dome following the pelvic arch from the intersection of the pubic ramus and obliterated umbilical vessels to the same spot on the contralateral side. The pubic bone is exposed,

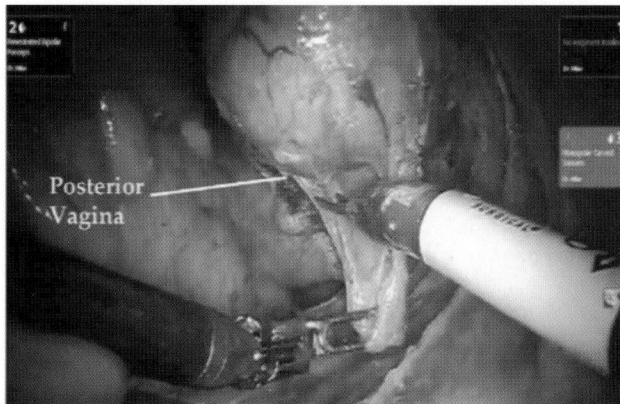

FIGURE 17.34 Exposing posterior vagina.

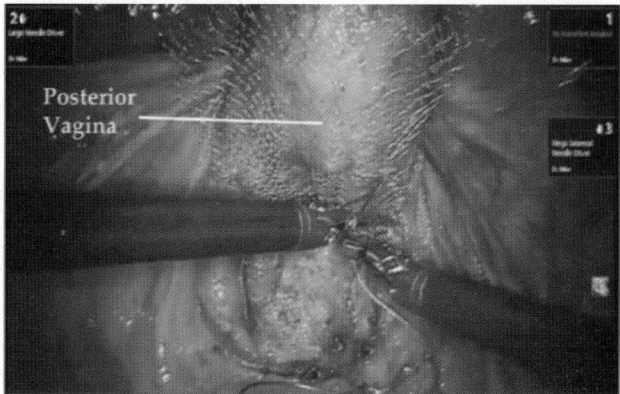

FIGURE 17.36 Mesh secured to posterior vagina.

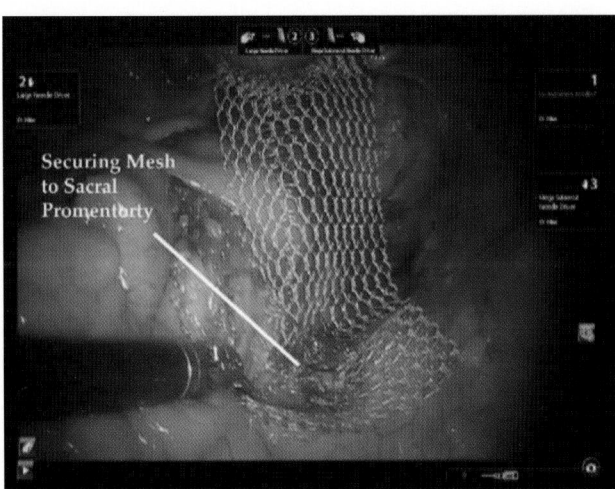

FIGURE 17.37 Mesh secured to sacral promontory.

and the avascular retropubic space of Retzius is entered to mobilize the bladder and open the space widely, taking care to avoid the obturator neurovascular structures laterally and identify the bladder neck, obturator internus muscle, arcus tendineus fasciae pelvis, and pearly white fibromuscular anterior vaginal wall (pubocervical fascia). One of the table-side assistants places a large cervical dilator in the vagina adjacent to the urethra and bladder neck in the same way one would place fingers for an open or laparoscopic dissection while the second table-side assistant retracts the fatty tissue and bladder medially. Venous bleeders are coagulated with the fenestrated bipolar, and monopolar shears are used for the dissection. A double purchase of 0-Dacron suture on a CT-2 needle is placed 2 cm lateral to the mid- to proximal urethra over the elevated vaginal dilator and is secured to the cartilaginous periosteum of the pubic bone median raphe (Marshall-Marchetti-Krantz stitch). This is repeated on the opposite side, and the next suture is placed cephalad and lateral to the MMK stitch 2 cm lateral to the urethra–vesicle junction with double purchase and secured to Cooper ligament (Burch stitch). The knots for these sutures are tied using a sliding knot for tensioning to leave a 2- to 3-cm suture bridge (Fig. 17.38). Due to the lack of tactile sense, it is easy to fracture the sutures if not tensioned carefully using visual clues. Reperitonealization is optional. IV indigo carmine dye is administered, and cystoscopy is performed with

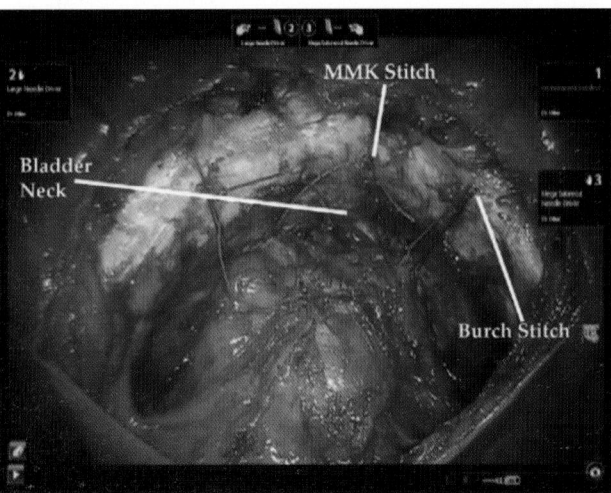

FIGURE 17.38 Placement of Burch and MMK stitches for urethropexy.

a 70- or 110-degree telescope to confirm that no sutures were placed in the bladder and for assessment of ureteral patency.

Robotic Myomectomy

As with sacrocolpopexy and lymph node dissection, myomectomy is another procedure traditionally performed by laparotomy. Although successfully performed laparoscopically, it is technically challenging with a steep learning curve. The robotic platform has been adapted for this operation.

Table 17.5 lists the five retrospective, observational studies that have evaluated RM compared to open abdominal myomectomy (AM) or laparoscopic myomectomy (LM). Advincula and Nash each compared RM to AM. Both studies found that RM group took considerably longer, especially as the volume of the myomas increased. The RMs resulted in shorter hospital length of stay, but hospital charges were significantly higher, although AM had higher nursing costs. The weight of myomas removed was similar in the study by Advincula, but was lower for RM versus AM in the Nash study. Bedient and Nezhat compared RM to LM. Uterine size, myoma size, and number of myomas in the LM group were greater compared to the RM in the Bedient study but not in the Nezhat study. Barakat and colleagues evaluated RM, LM, and AM. They identified larger myoma weights in the RM group compared to LM, but they detected slightly smaller weights than those removed in the AM group. Overall, these studies seem to indicate that at least in the early stages of RM, operating times are longer with less blood loss and shorter length of stay. Complications and conversion to laparotomy do not appear to be increased. There are no long-term pregnancy data, and cost for RM is higher.

Surgical Technique The initial technical aspects are similar to preparation for hysterectomy as described previously. Either a straight or side dock technique is utilized. Depending on uterine volume and size, the 8-mm port sites should be placed higher and more lateral if possible for larger myomatous uteri. The surgical principles are the same as for open AM and LM. As described by Frick and Falcone, an intrauterine catheter may be placed to instill indigo carmine dye to detect if there is entry into the endometrial cavity during dissection. Vasopressin is injected either directly through the abdominal wall or via an accessory port into the myometrium for initial vasoconstriction and hemostasis. A monopolar hook or shears are used to make the incision. It is preferable to utilize one uterine incision for multiple myomas if possible. The table-side assistant provides countertraction on the myoma with a grasper or a single-tooth tenaculum. For this operation, the third robotic operating arm is useful for providing countertraction, stabilization, and retraction during the dissection. Bipolar or Gyrus PK may be required to seal larger vessels. If multiple myomas are removed, they should be counted to ensure they are not lost into the upper abdomen. Once the myomas are enucleated, the myometrium is closed in the usual way with layered reapproximation using either interrupted or running delayed absorbable suture (Vicryl, PDS, or V-Loc barbed suture) to close dead space and minimize hematoma formation. Usually, myomas are reduced and removed by a commercial morcellator.

Additional Robotic Procedures in Gynecology

Magrina and colleagues reported on 85 patients undergoing robotic adnexectomy compared to 91 patients undergoing the same procedure laparoscopically. Blood loss, operating time, length of stay, and complications were similar in both groups

TABLE 17.5 Robotic Myomectomy

AUTHORS	SUBJECTS	PROCEDURE	MAX. MYOMA DIAMETER (CM)	WEIGHT OF MYOMAS REMOVED (G)	NO. OF MYOMAS REMOVED	OPERATION TIME (MIN)	EBL (ML)	LOS (DAYS)	CONVERSION TO LAPAROTOMY
Advincula (2007)	29	RM		227.86		231 ± 85	196	1.48	2
	29	AM		223.76		154 ± 43	365	3.62	
Nezhat (2009b)	15	RM	5.1 (4–8.5)	116 (25–350)	3 (1–7)	234 (144–445)	370	1	0
	35	LM	6.4 (3–12)	156 (15–420)	4 (1–21)	203 (95–330)	420	1.05 (1–3)	0
Bedient (2009)	40	RM	4.7 (0.2–14.4)	210 (7–1,076)	2.7 (1–9)	141 (50–277)	100	5	0
	41	LM	7.0 (1.3–13.5)	350 (10–1,316)	6.5 (1–26)	166 (68–315)	250	9 (>2 d LOS)	2
Nash (2011)	27	RM		20–102		184–280	150	0.5–1.2	
	106	AM		57–208		106–158	150	2.3–2.65	
Barakat (2011)	89	RM	7.7	223		181	150	1	
	93	LM	6.7	96.65		155	100	1	
	393	AM	7.5	263		126	200	3	

RM, robotic myomectomy; LM, laparoscopic myomectomy; AM, abdominal myomectomy; EBL, estimated blood loss; LOS, length of stay.

with no clear advantage to the robotic approach. Additional gynecologic procedures performed robotically and reported by Magrina, Ramirez, Burnett, and Sundaram include radical trachelectomy, staging for early ovarian cancer, and vesicovaginal fistula repair. Nam and colleagues reported the use of robotic technology applied to single-incision laparoscopic surgery. Without question, the robotic platform will be applied to an increasing number of gynecologic procedures.

COST ANALYSIS

While robotic surgery may reduce blood loss and length of stay, shorten recovery time compared to laparotomy, and show comparable results to laparoscopic surgery, cost remains the most significant drawback. Table 17.6 lists results of studies by Holz, Barnett, Bell, Landeen, Jonsdottir, and Sarlos comparing costs among robotic hysterectomy, conventional abdominal hysterectomy, laparoscopic hysterectomy, and vaginal hysterectomy. Three of the studies make comparisons between procedures performed for benign reasons, while the remaining three studies address cost comparisons in the treatment of endometrial cancer. Cost analyses are difficult to interpret on the basis of a high number of variables and variation in how hospital systems attribute expenses and depreciate equipment. Most studies are retrospective and do not collect real-time expenses, which should vary over time. In addition to hospital expenses, estimates of societal expenses such as recovery time and time off work vary greatly. Bell and colleagues compared actual costs and estimated societal costs of robotic hysterectomy, laparoscopic hysterectomy, abdominal hysterectomy, and staging lymphadenectomy in endometrial cancer patients. Robotic surgery costs were significantly less than abdominal hysterectomy and comparable to laparoscopic surgery. When comparing actual costs for robotic surgery to laparoscopic surgery for endometrial cancer, Holz and colleagues found hospital costs to be significantly higher for

robotic surgery. The higher costs are mostly attributable to the price of disposable instruments. Societal costs were not included in the calculations.

In a well-publicized review of the billing data of almost 10,000 hysterectomies done at many different hospitals in the United States, Wright et al. reported that the median total cost for robotic hysterectomy was $2,200 more than the cost of a laparoscopic hysterectomy. This study showed that cost did not decrease significantly with increasing surgeon experience. The median total cost (not charges) for a laparoscopic hysterectomy in the United States in 2010 was $6,679, while the cost for a robotic hysterectomy was $8,868. These costs were direct costs for the operative procedure and did not reflect capital costs to purchase the instrumentation or societal costs of patient loss of functionality during recovery.

Using decision modeling to compare costs among robotic, laparoscopic, and open procedures for treatment of endometrial cancer, Barnett and colleagues included societal costs as a component of the calculations. They found laparoscopic surgery to be the least expensive, with robotic surgery less costly than abdominal hysterectomy. The differences in cost would be minimized if disposable equipment costs decreased. When comparing abdominal, laparoscopic, vaginal, and robotic hysterectomy for benign conditions, Jonsdottir and colleagues found vaginal hysterectomy to have the lowest operative cost and robotic surgery to have the highest operative cost. However, when total hospital cost for all four procedures was compared, little difference was noted. As a general summary of cost-effectiveness, the initial purchase and maintenance of robotic equipment cannot be understated. If an increasing number of procedures that previously would have been performed by laparotomy are performed by the minimally invasive robotic approach, shorter hospital stays, fewer complications, and a shorter recovery times would benefit the patient and society. That said, there

TABLE 17.6 Robotic Cost Comparison		ROBOTIC SURGERY	LAPAROSCOPIC SURGERY	STANDARD LAPAROTOMY	VAGINAL
	SOURCE OF COSTS	**HOSPITAL COST**	**HOSPITAL COST**	**HOSPITAL COST**	**HOSPITAL COST**
Holz et al. (2010)	Actual costs	5,084 (median)	3,615 (median)		
Barnett et al. (2010)	Decision modeling				
	Societal perspective	11,476	10,128	12,847	
	Hospital perspective and purchase of robot	8,770	6,581	7,009	
	Hospital perspective with existing robot	7,478	6,581	7,009	
Bell et al. (2008)	Actual costs	8,212 (average)	7,569 (average)	12,943 (average)	
Jonsdottir et al. (2011), benign	Actual total costs	11,004 (mean)	12,329 (mean)	12,678 (mean)	11,820 (mean)
	Actual operative costs	10,528 (mean)	7,710 (mean)	6,215 (mean)	4,210 (mean)
Landeen et al. (2011), benign (indirect and direct cost with depreciation)	Actual costs	8,135 (average)	6,900 (average)	7,005 (average)	5,505 (average)
Sarlos et al. (2010), benign	Actual costs	4,067 (average) Euros	2,151 (average) Euros		

is currently little proof to support this assumption. Ideally, a large randomized trial comparing surgery performed by laparotomy, laparoscopy, or robotics would give a more precise conclusion. Given the current level of surgeon and patient bias, it is unlikely that being randomized to laparotomy would be acceptable.

IMPLEMENTING A ROBOTIC SURGERY PROGRAM

The decision to start a program in robotic surgery is complex and costly. In some circumstances, the decision is forced, as in the case of communities unable to recruit urologists out of training due to lack of availability of a robot for radical prostatectomy. In other cases, the decision is elective and designed to enhance an existing surgical program. At times, the robotic program is for marketing purposes to attract more patient referrals for the hospital and surgeons: the "build it, and they will come" theory. Regardless of the original reason to start a robotic surgical program, commitment is the essential requirement. Commitment must come from four unified sectors: the hospital or clinic making the financial outlay, a dedicated group of surgeons, the anesthesia department, and the nursing department. Weak or missing commitment from any of the above members will almost guarantee failure. From an institutional standpoint, commitment to the initial purchase, ongoing maintenance, designation of a sufficiently large OR, and willingness to assign designated, competent staff is required. Anesthesiologists and anesthetists are faced with caring for a patient in 30 degrees of Trendelenburg position, without access to patient extremities, and minimal access to a fully padded face. Ventilatory requirements become more challenging as patient size increases and more complex cases are scheduled. Dedicated bedside assistants and circulating nurses are a critical component to assembling an outstanding robotic surgical team because they are committed to perform a sufficient number and variety of robotic cases to acquire skills needed to become increasingly more efficient. Finally, the surgeons must commit to a protracted learning curve, selecting appropriate patients, and to constantly making fine adjustments to enhance the program. The ultimate goal is shifting complex laparotomy cases to minimally invasive robotic cases with improved outcomes, lower complication rates, shorter recovery times, and improved quality of life for the patients.

BEST SURGICAL PRACTICES

- The surgeon considering adding robotic techniques to his or her practice should be committed to a sufficient number and frequency of cases to maintain the newly acquired skills.
- For surgeons unaccustomed to utilizing different energy sources during open or laparoscopic procedures, the robotic platform will be more challenging and potentially associated with a greater risk of injury until adequate experience is acquired.
- Sharp dissection and attention to normal tissue planes rather than blunt dissection will result in better visibility and reduced bleeding and trauma.
- Patient selection, optimal positioning of the patient on the operating table, and correct positioning of the uterine manipulator will minimize surgeon frustration.
- Vaginal cuff dehiscence can be minimized by extending the bladder dissection off the anterior vagina, avoiding excessive thermal damage to the vaginal incision, placing sutures well back from the vaginal incision, minimizing tension on the vaginal cuff closure, and stressing to the patient the importance of avoiding sexual intercourse for at least 6 weeks following surgery.
- Set the expectations for early dismissal and rapid return to normal activity when robotic surgery is proposed.
- Insist on developing an efficient, competent, and committed surgical team.

BIBLIOGRAPHY

Advincula AP, Xu X, Goudeau S IV, et al. Robot-assisted laparoscopic myomectomy versus abdominal myomectomy: a comparison of short-term surgical outcomes and immediate costs. *J Minim Invasive Gynecol* 2007;14:698.

Akl MN, Long JB, Giles DL, et al. Robotic-assisted sacrocolpopexy: technique and learning curve. *Surg Endosc* 2009; 23:2390.

Barakat EE, Bedaiwy MA, Zimberg S, et al. Robotic-assisted, laparoscopic, and abdominal myomectomy: a comparison of surgical outcomes. *Obstet Gynecol* 2011;117(2, Pt 1):256.

Barnett JC, Judd JP, Wu JM, et al. Cost comparison among robotic, laparoscopic, and open hysterectomy for endometrial cancer. *Obstet Gynecol* 2010;116:685.

Bedient CE, Magrina JF, Noble BN, et al. Comparison of robotic and laparoscopic myomectomy. *Am J Obstet Gynecol* 2009;201: 566.e1.

Bell MC, Torgerson J, Seshadri-Kreaden U, et al. Comparison of outcomes and cost for endometrial cancer staging via traditional laparotomy, standard laparoscopy and robotic techniques. *Gynecol Oncol* 2008;111:407.

Boggess JF, Gehrig PA, Cantrell L, et al. A comparative study of 3 surgical methods for hysterectomy with staging for endometrial cancer: robotic assistance, laparoscopy, laparotomy. *Am J Obstet Gynecol* 2008;199:360.e1.

Boggess JF, Gehrig PA, Cantrell L, et al. A case-control study of robot-assisted type III radical hysterectomy with pelvic lymph node dissection compared with open radical hysterectomy. *Am J Obstet Gynecol* 2008;199:357.e1.

Boggess JF, Gehrig PA, Cantrell L, et al. Perioperative outcomes of robotically assisted hysterectomy for benign cases with complex pathology. *Obstet Gynecol* 2009;114:585.

Bowersox JC, Shah A, Jensen J, et al. Vascular applications of telepresence surgery: initial feasibility studies in swine. *J Vasc Surg* 1996;23:281.

Burnett AF, Stone PJ, Duckworth LA, et al. Robotic radical trachelectomy for preservation of fertility in early cervical cancer: Case series and description of technique. *J Minim Invasive Gynecol* 2009;16:569.

Cantrell LA, Mendivil A, Gehrig PA, et al. Survival outcomes for women undergoing type III robotic radical hysterectomy for cervical cancer: a 3-year experience. *Gynecol Oncol* 2010; 117:260.

Cardenas-Goicoechea J, Adams S, Bhat SB, et al. Surgical outcomes of robotic-assisted surgical staging for endometrial cancer are equivalent to traditional laparoscopic staging at a minimally invasive surgical center. *Gynecol Oncol* 2010;117:224.

Chandra V, Nehra D, Parent R, et al. A comparison of laparoscopic and robotic assisted suturing performance by experts and novices. *Surgery* 2010;147:830.

Daneshgari F, Kefer JC, Moore C, et al. Robotic abdominal sacrocolpopexy/sacrouteropexy repair of advanced female pelvic organ prolapse (POP): utilizing POP-quantification-based staging and outcomes. *BJU Int* 2007;100:875.

Davies BL, Hibberd RD, Ng WS, et al. The development of a surgeon robot for prostatectomies. *Proc Inst Mech Eng H* 1991; 205:35.

DeNardis SA, Holloway RW, Bigsby GE IV, et al. Robotically assisted laparoscopic hysterectomy versus total abdominal hysterectomy and lymphadenectomy for endometrial cancer. *Gynecol Oncol* 2008;111:412.

Diaz-Arrastia C, Jurnalov C, Gomez G, et al. Laparoscopic hysterectomy using a computer-enhanced surgical robot. *Surg Endosc* 2002;16:1271.

Dharia SP, Falcone T. Robotics in reproductive medicine. *Fertil Steril* 2005;84:1.

Elliott DS, Krambeck AE, Chow GK. Long-term results of robotic assisted laparoscopic sacrocolpopexy for the treatment of high grade vaginal vault prolapse. *J Urol* 2006;176:655.

Estape R, Lambrou N, Diaz R, et al. A case matched analysis of robotic radical hysterectomy with lymphadenectomy compared with laparoscopy and laparotomy. *Gynecol Oncol* 2009; 113:357.

Falcone T, Goldberg JM, Margossian H, et al. Robotic-assisted laparoscopic microsurgical tubal anastomosis: a human pilot study. *Fertil Steril* 2000;73:1040.

Fanning J, Fenton B, Purohit M. Robotic radical hysterectomy. *Am J Obstet Gynecol* 2008;198:649.e1–e4.

Feuer G, Hernandez P, Barker J. Surgical technique enhances the efficiency of robotic hysterectomy. *Int J Med Robot* 2011;7:1.

Frick AC, Falcone T. Robotics in gynecologic surgery. *Minerva Ginecol* 2009;61:187.

Gehrig PA, Cantrell LA, Shafer A, et al. What is the optimal minimally invasive surgical procedure for endometrial cancer staging in the obese and morbidly obese woman? *Gynecol Oncol* 2008;111:41.

Geisler JP, Orr CJ, Khurshid N, et al. Robotically assisted laparoscopic radical hysterectomy compared with open radical hysterectomy. *Int J Gynecol Cancer* 2010;20:438.

Geller EJ, Siddiqui NY, Wu JM, et al. Short-term outcomes of robotic sacrocolpopexy compared with abdominal sacrocolpopexy. *Obstet Gynecol* 2008;112:1201.

Geller EJ, Parnell BA, Dunivan GC. Pelvic floor function before and after robotic sacrocolpopexy: one-year outcomes. *J Minim Invasive Gynecol* 2011a;18:322.

Geller EJ, Schuler KM, Boggess JF. Robotic surgical training program in gynecology: how to train residents and fellows. *J Minim Invasive Gynecol* 2011b;18:224.

Giep BN, Giep HN, Hubert HB. Comparison of minimally invasive surgical approaches for hysterectomy at a community hospital: robotic-assisted laparoscopic hysterectomy, laparoscopic-assisted vaginal hysterectomy and laparoscopic supracervical hysterectomy. *J Robot Surg* 2010;4:167.

Göçmen A, Sanlkan F, Uçar MG. Robotic-assisted sacrocolpopexy/ sacrocervicopexy repair of pelvic organ prolapse: initial experience. *Arch Gynecol Obstet* 2012;285:683.

Hagen ME, Meehan JJ, Inan I, et al. Visual clues act as a substitute for haptic feedback in robotic surgery. *Surg Endosc* 2008; 22:1505.

Hanly EJ, Miller BE, Kumar R, et al. Mentoring console improves collaboration and teaching in surgical robotics. *J Laparoendosc Adv Surg Tech A* 2006;16:445.

Harper JD, Kaiser S, Ebrahimi K, et al. Prior video game exposure does not enhance robotic surgical performance. *J Endourol* 2007;21:1207.

Himpens J, Leman G, Cadiere GB. Telesurgical laparoscopic cholecystectomy. *Surg Endosc* 1998;12:1091.

Hoekstra AV, Morgan JM, Lurain JR, et al. Robotic surgery in gynecologic oncology: impact on fellowship training. *Gynecol Oncol* 2009;114:168.

Holloway RW, Ahmad S, DeNardis SA, et al. Robotic-assisted laparoscopic hysterectomy and lymphadenectomy for endometrial cancer: analysis of surgical performance. *Gynecol Oncol* 2009;115:447.

Holz DO, Miroshnichenko G, Finnegan MO, et al. Endometrial cancer surgery costs: robot vs laparoscopy. *J Minim Invasive Gynecol* 2010;17:500.

Jonsdottir GM, Jorgensen S, Cohen SL, et al. Increasing minimally invasive hysterectomy: effect on cost and complications. *Obstet Gynecol* 2011;117:1142.

Kho RM, Hilger WS, Hentz JG, et al. Robotic hysterectomy: technique and initial outcomes. *Am J Obstet Gynecol* 2007;197: 113.e1. Erratum in *Am J Obstet Gynecol* 2007;197:332.

Kim YT, Kim SW, Hyung WJ, et al. Robotic radical hysterectomy with pelvic lymphadenectomy for cervical carcinoma: a pilot study. *Gynecol Oncol* 2008;108:312.

Ko EM, Muto MG, Berkowitz RS, et al. Robotic versus open radical hysterectomy: a comparative study at a single institution. *Gynecol Oncol* 2008;111:425.

Kramer BA, Whelan CM, Powell TM, et al. Robot-assisted laparoscopic sacrocolpopexy as management for pelvic organ prolapse. *J Endourol* 2009;23:655.

Kwoh YS, Hou J, Jonckheere EA, et al. A robot with improved absolute positioning accuracy for CT guided stereotactic brain surgery. *IEEE Trans Biomed Eng* 1988;35:153.

Landeen LB, Bell MC, Hubert HB, et al. Clinical and cost comparisons for hysterectomy via abdominal, standard laparoscopic, vaginal and robot-assisted approaches. *S D Med* 2011;64:197.

Lenihan JP Jr, Kovanda C, Seshadri-Kreaden U. What is the learning curve for robotic assisted gynecologic surgery? *J Minim Invasive Gynecol* 2008;15:589.

Lim PC, Kang E, Park do H. Learning curve and surgical outcome for robotic-assisted hysterectomy with lymphadenectomy: case-matched controlled comparison with laparoscopy and laparotomy for treatment of endometrial cancer. *J Minim Invasive Gynecol* 2010;17:739.

Lim PC, Kang E, Park do H. A comparative detail analysis of the learning curve and surgical outcome for robotic hysterectomy with lymphadenectomy versus laparoscopic hysterectomy with lymphadenectomy in treatment of endometrial cancer: a case-matched controlled study of the first one hundred twenty two patients. *Gynecol Oncol* 2011;120:413.

Lowe MP, Johnson PR, Kamelle SA, et al. A multiinstitutional experience with robotic-assisted hysterectomy with staging for endometrial cancer. *Obstet Gynecol* 2009;114(2, Pt 1):236.

Lowe MP, Chamberlain DH, Kamelle SA, et al. A multi-institutional experience with robotic-assisted radical hysterectomy for early stage cervical cancer. *Gynecol Oncol.* 2009;113:191.

Maggioni A, Minig L, Zanagnolo V, et al. Robotic approach for cervical cancer: comparison with laparotomy: a case control study. *Gynecol Oncol* 2009;115:60.

Magrina JF. Robotic surgery in gynecology. *Eur J Gynaecol Oncol* 2007;28:77.

Magrina JF, Kho RM, Weaver AL, et al. Robotic radical hysterectomy: comparison with laparoscopy and laparotomy. *Gynecol Oncol* 2008;109:86.

Magrina JF, Espada M, Munoz R, et al. Robotic adnexectomy compared with laparoscopy for adnexal mass. *Obstet Gynecol* 2009;114:581.

Magrina JF, Zanagnolo V, Noble BN, et al. Robotic approach for ovarian cancer: perioperative and survival results and comparison with laparoscopy and laparotomy. *Gynecol Oncol* 2011; 121:100.

Margossian H, Garcia-Ruiz A, Falcone T, et al. Robotically assisted laparoscopic microsurgical uterine horn anastomosis. *Fertil Steril* 1998;70:530.

Matthews CA, Reid N, Ramakrishnan V, et al. Evaluation of the introduction of robotic technology on route of hysterectomy and complications in the first year of use. *Am J Obstet Gynecol* 2010;203:499.e1.

Nam EJ, Kim SW, Lee M, et al. Robotic single-port transumbilical total hysterectomy: a pilot study. *J Gynecol Oncol* 2011; 22:120.

Nash K, Feinglass J, Zei C, et al. Robotic-assisted laparoscopic myomectomy versus abdominal myomectomy: a comparative analysis of surgical outcomes and costs. *Arch Gynecol Obstet.* 2012;285:435.

Nezhat CH, Nezhat F, Nezhat C. Laparoscopic sacral colpopexy for vaginal vault prolapse. *Obstet Gynecol* 1994;84:885.

Nezhat FR, Datta MS, Liu C, et al. Robotic radical hysterectomy versus total laparoscopic radical hysterectomy with pelvic lymphadenectomy for treatment of early cervical cancer. *JSLS* 2008; 12:227.

Nezhat C, Lavie O, Lemyre M, et al. Laparoscopic hysterectomy with and without a robot: Stanford experience. *JSLS* 2009a;13:125.

Nezhat C, Lavie O, Hsu S, et al. Robotic-assisted laparoscopic myomectomy compared with standard laparoscopic myomectomy—A retrospective matched control study. *Fertil Steril* 2009b; 91:556.

Ng WS, Davies BL, Timoney AG, et al. The use of ultrasound in automated prostatectomy. *Med Biol Eng Comput* 1993;31:349.

Nygaard IE, McCreery R, Brubaker L, et al. Abdominal sacrocolpopexy: a comprehensive review. *Obstet Gynecol* 2004; 104:805.

Obermair A, Gebski V, Frumovitz M, et al. A phase III randomized clinical trial comparing laparoscopic or robotic radical hysterectomy with abdominal radical hysterectomy in patients with early stage cervical cancer. *J Minim Invasive Gynecol* 2008; 15:584.

ACOG Committee Opinion No. 444: Choosing the route of hysterectomy for benign disease. *Obstet Gynecol* 2009;114:1156.

Partin AW, Adams JB, Moore RG, et al. Complete robot-assisted laparoscopic urologic surgery: a preliminary report. *J Am Coll Surg* 1995;181:552.

Payne TN, Dauterive FR. A comparison of total laparoscopic hysterectomy to robotically assisted hysterectomy: surgical outcomes in a community practice. *J Minim Invasive Gynecol* 2008; 15:286.

Payne TN, Dauterive FR, Pitter MC, et al. Robotically assisted hysterectomy in patients with large uteri: Outcomes in five community practices. *Obstet Gynecol* 2010;115:535.

Persson J, Reynisson P, Borgfeldt C, et al. Robot assisted laparoscopic radical hysterectomy and pelvic lymphadenectomy with short and long term morbidity data. *Gynecol Oncol* 2009; 113:185.

Pulliam SJ, Berkowitz LR. Smaller pieces of the hysterectomy pie: current challenges in resident surgical education. *Obstet Gynecol* 2009;113(2, Pt 1): 395.

Ramirez PT, Schmeler KM, Malpica A, et al. Safety and feasibility of robotic radical trachelectomy in patients with early-stage cervical cancer. *Gynecol Oncol* 2010;116:512.

Reynolds RK, Advincula AP. Robot-assisted laparoscopic hysterectomy: technique and initial experience. *Am J Surg* 2006; 191:555.

Sarlos D, Kots L, Stevanovic N, et al. Robotic hysterectomy versus conventional laparoscopic hysterectomy: outcome and cost analyses of a matched case-control study. *Eur J Obstet Gynecol Reprod Biol* 2010;150:92.

Satava RM. Robotic surgery: from past to future—a personal journey. *Surg Clin North Am* 2003;83:1491, xii.

Seamon LG, Cohn DE, Henretta MS, et al. Minimally invasive comprehensive surgical staging for endometrial cancer: robotics or laparoscopy? *Gynecol Oncol* 2009;113:36.

Shashoua AR, Gill D, Locher SR. Robotic-assisted total laparoscopic hysterectomy versus conventional total laparoscopic hysterectomy. *JSLS* 2009;13:364.

Stefanidis D, Wang F, Korndorffer JR Jr, et al. Robotic assistance improves intracorporeal suturing performance and safety in the operating room while decreasing operator workload. *Surg Endosc* 2010;24:377.

Stefanidis D, Hope WW, Scott DJ. Robotic suturing on the FLS model possesses construct validity, is less physically demanding, and is favored by more surgeons compared with laparoscopy. *Surg Endosc* 2011;25:2141.

Suh I, Mukherjee M, Oleynikov D, et al. Training program for fundamental surgical skill in robotic laparoscopic surgery. *Int J Med Robot* 2011;7:327.

Sundaram BM, Kalidasan G, Hemal AK. Robotic repair of vesicovaginal fistula: case series of five patients. *Urology* 2006;67:970.

Tinelli R, Malzoni M, Cosentino F, et al. Robotics versus laparoscopic radical hysterectomy with lymphadenectomy in patients with early cervical cancer: a multicenter study. *Ann Surg Oncol* 2011;18:2622.

Veljovich DS, Paley PJ, Drescher CW, et al. Robotic surgery in gynecologic oncology: program initiation and outcomes after the first year with comparison with laparotomy for endometrial cancer staging. *Am J Obstet Gynecol* 2008;198:679.e1; discussion 679.e9.

Woelk JL, Casiano ER, Weaver AL, et al. The learning curve of robotic hysterectomy. *Obstet Gynecol* 2013;121:87.

Wright JD, Ananth CV, Lewis SN, et al. Robotically assisted vs laparoscopic hysterectomy among women with benign gynecologic disease. *JAMA* 2013;309:689.

CHAPTER 18
Operative Hysteroscopy

Mindy S. Christianson, Kyle J. Tobler, and Howard A. Zacur

DEFINITIONS

Hysteroscopy—Direct visual inspection of the cervical canal and uterine cavity through a rigid or flexible hysteroscope.

Index of refraction—The bending of light caused by the ratio of its velocity in room air to its velocity within an optical fiber.

Resectoscope—A specialized electrosurgical endoscope that consists of an inner and outer sheath equipped with a 30-degree telescope. The inner sheath has a common channel for the telescope fluid medium and electrode.

Uterine synechiae—Adhesions that form between the anterior and posterior walls of the uterus as a result of trauma or infection in a milieu of estrogen deprivation.

INTRODUCTION

Hysteroscopy is a term derived from the Greek words *hystera*, which means uterus, and *skopeo*, which means "to view." In 1869, Pantaleoni successfully performed this procedure in a living human subject. He used a tube with an external light source to detect "vegetations within the uterine cavity." No attempt was made at this time to distend the uterine cavity. During the past 145 years, developments in optics, fiberoptics, instruments, and distending media have resulted in new equipment and techniques that allow the gynecologic surgeon to diagnose and treat many intrauterine cavity disorders. Hysteroscopy is a standard part of the gynecologic surgeon's armamentarium and the preferred minimally invasive choice for treatment of intrauterine pathology.

Abnormal vaginal bleeding may occur as the result of many different intrauterine cavity disorders. Dilating the endocervical canal and then blindly probing or curetting the uterine cavity to diagnose and treat these disorders would seem far less effective than performing a diagnostic and/or operative hysteroscopy. Critics have cautioned, however, about the risk of disseminating endometrial cells into the peritoneal cavity from the pressure of either gaseous or liquid distending medium during hysteroscopy. In 2000, reports by Zerbe and colleagues and Obermair and colleagues demonstrated that endometrial cancer cells could be found in peritoneal fluid following hysteroscopy with saline as distending medium in women with endometrial cancer. Whether to use hysteroscopy in evaluating abnormal bleeding in women at risk for endometrial cancer was questioned by the authors of these reports. A retrospective cohort analysis by Soucie and associates in 2012 linked a registry of women diagnosed with endometrial cancer with performance of hysteroscopy, staging of endometrial cancer, and death rates. This study concluded that hysteroscopy in women with endometrial cancer was not associated with causing a higher stage of disease. The authors concluded that hysteroscopy should continue to be used as a safe diagnostic tool for abnormal uterine bleeding.

With the emergence of minimally invasive gynecology surgery as a recognized advantage to patients, operative hysteroscopy has earned a special niche in this area. The advantages of hysteroscopy as an accurate diagnostic technique are that it not only allows direct visual observation and accurate localization of pathology but also provides a means to sample the site most likely to yield positive results. Hysteroscopy generally is a low-risk technique that uses the endocervical canal, the natural passageway of the body, to gain entry into the intrauterine environment. Commonly performed procedures utilizing hysteroscopy include diagnostic hysteroscopy, tubal sterilization, polypectomy, myomectomy, and excision of uterine septa. Nonhysteroscopic techniques to treat intrauterine septa and adhesions are obsolete. Ablation or resection of the endometrium is considered an acceptable alternative to hysterectomy for the management of abnormal uterine bleeding. Submucous myomas no longer require hysterectomy because they can be satisfactorily managed conservatively by operative hysteroscopy. Cornual obstruction and interstitial tubal obstruction also are now managed hysteroscopically. Teaching operative hysteroscopy techniques is a key aspect of residency training curriculums and postgraduate seminars. However, as operative hysteroscopy case numbers have increased, the number of complications has also risen. Most of these complications are caused by operator error and inexperience.

Learning how to perform an adequate hysteroscopy and then becoming competent to do hysteroscopic surgery are practice, skill-related techniques. Older methods of acquiring endoscopic skills focused on course attendance, preceptorship, and practice. During the late 1990s and continuing to the present, simulators have been developed to facilitate hand–eye coordination exercises. Several of the computer-based models with advanced interactive graphics provide sophisticated models for the student to shave myomas, ablate endometrium, and pass cannulas into tubal ostia (Fig. 18.1A, B).

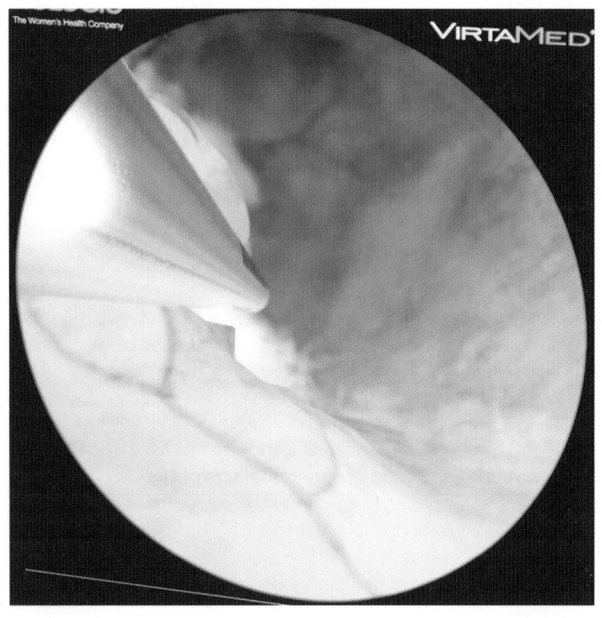

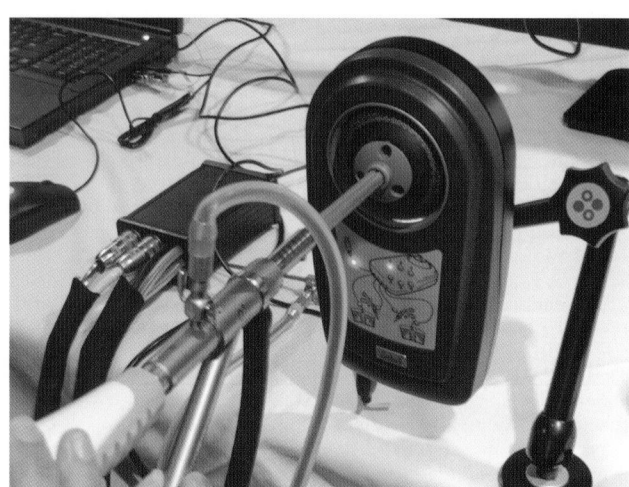

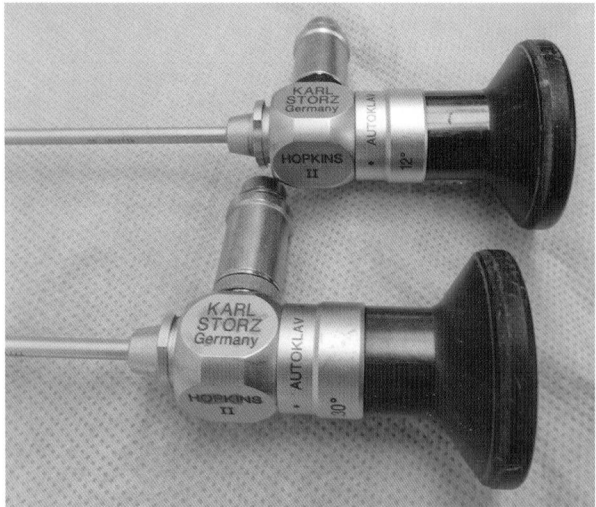

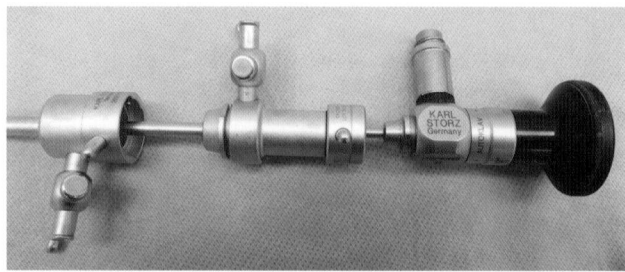

FIGURE 18.1 A: Computerized simulation permits the gynecologist to interact by manipulating a hysteroscopic morcellator and resecting a virtual submucosal myoma or polyp. **B:** The simulator uses equipment that is balanced similar to actual hysteroscopes. **C:** Two common 4-mm telescopes are shown here. *Top* is a 12-degree, and the *bottom* is a 30-degree telescope. **D:** Telescopes must couple to a 5-mm sheath to be practically functional. The distention liquid or gaseous medium gains access to the uterine cavity via the inner sheath, and fluid exits the uterus via the outer sheath.

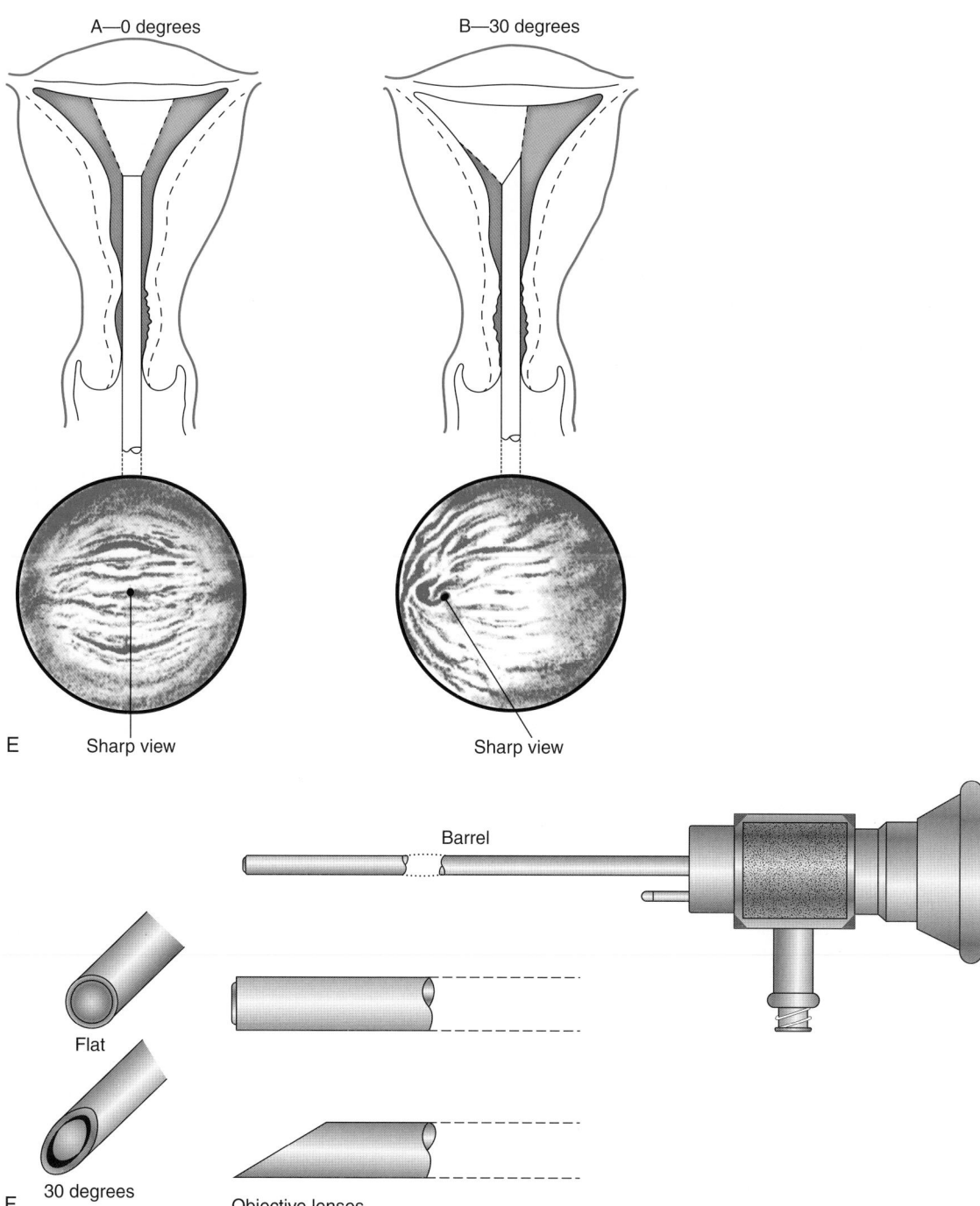

FIGURE 18.1 (*Continued*) **E:** Telescopes are available with either straight-on (0 degrees) or foreoblique (30 degrees) viewing objective lenses. **F:** A telescope can be conveniently subdivided into three parts: eyepiece, barrel, and objective lens. (Parts A and E reprinted from Baggish MS, Valle RF, Guedj H. *Hysteroscopy: visual perspectives of uterine anatomy, physiology and pathology*, 3rd ed. Philadelphia, PA: Lippincott Williams & Wilkins, 2007, with permission. Copyright © 2007, Lippincott Williams.)

However, the most basic skill levels a hysteroscopist must attain are the ability to insert the scope safely into the uterine cavity followed by satisfactory distension of the cavity to obtain clear visualization of that cavity. The preceding is not taught by simulation and must be learned in vivo. Without this skill set, hysteroscopy cannot be successfully performed.

INSTRUMENTATION

Hysteroscopes may be classified as rigid or flexible and possessing fixed or variable focus and be designated for either diagnostic or operative use. Scope diameter, lens offset, sheath diameter, ability to be used with a variety of distending media,

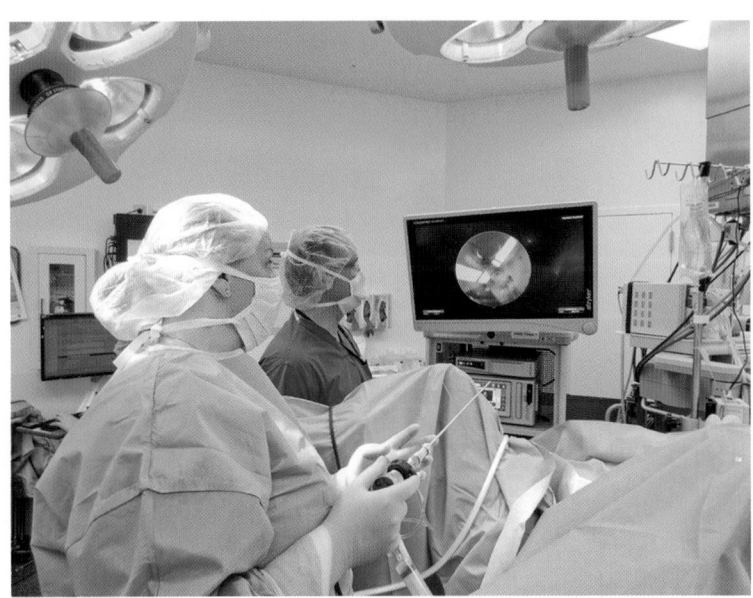

FIGURE 18.2 Contemporary operative hysteroscopy is performed with a digital camera attached to the eyepiece of the telescope. The operator and assistants all view the field by way of a high-resolution video monitor.

and ability to use either bipolar or monopolar cautery are key characteristics of the instrumentation.

Viewing through the hysteroscopic telescope may still be done by using the naked eye, but is now almost always done by using a camera and video screen. As might be expected, the images obtained by the hysteroscope may vary depending upon the type of camera and video screen used with high-definition systems providing the sharpest images (Fig. 18.2).

Telescopes

The telescope has three parts: the eyepiece, the barrel, and the objective lens (Fig. 18.1F). The 4-mm telescope (lens) gives the sharpest, clearest image in addition to a small outside diameter (Fig. 18.1C). The most desirable optics provide a large field that subtends an angle of approximately 105 degrees. However, 3-mm diameter telescopes, which have greatly improved optics, provide comparable views. These contemporary 3-mm diameter telescopes coupled to endoscopic video systems with zoom lenses are highly satisfactory for office hysteroscopy as well as for operative hysteroscopy. Telescopes are available in a variety of viewing angles with the 0-degree straight-on or a 30-degree fore-oblique view being the most common (Fig. 18.1E). Other viewing angles available include 12 degrees, 15 degrees, and 70 degrees. The major advantage of the 0-degree lens is that it allows the operator to see operative devices as a relatively distant panorama, whereas this view is lost when 30-degree lens is used. Surrounding the optics are numerous small-diameter incoherent fiberoptic bundles that provide intense cold illumination to the operative field.

Light Generators

The quality and power of light delivered to the telescope depend on the wattage and characteristics of the remote light generator and the type and structural integrity of the connecting fiberoptic light cable. Three general types of light generators are available: tungsten, metal halide, and xenon. The xenon white light is a powerful generator that provides high-quality color and intensity and is the most commonly used today.

Fiberoptic light cables must be intact to convey the optimal light from the generator to the telescope. Broken fibers can be easily identified by viewing the stretched-out cable against a dark background and looking for light emitting through the sides of the cable. The liquid cable conducts light effectively and provides superior light when combined with a xenon generator.

Diagnostic and Operative Sheaths

A diagnostic sheath is required to deliver the distending medium into the uterine cavity. The telescope fits into the sheath and is secured by means of a watertight seal that locks into place. The sheath is 4 to 5 mm in diameter, depending on the outer diameter of the telescope, with a 1-mm clearance between the inner wall and the telescope, through which either carbon dioxide (CO_2) or liquid distending medium is transmitted (Fig. 18.1D). Medium instillation into the sheath is controlled by means of an external stopcock. Even the 5-mm instrument allows easy access through the narrow endocervical canal past the point of maximal constriction, the internal os. Therefore, diagnostic hysteroscopy usually can be performed without cervical canal dilatation. If the hysteroscope is inserted into the canal under direct vision, and if the axis of the cervical and uterine canal is carefully followed until the corpus is reached, there should be no risk of creating a false passage or perforation. Imprecise or loose coupling between the telescope and sheath will result in leakage of the medium at that interface.

Operative sheaths have a larger diameter than do diagnostic sheaths, ranging in size from 7 to 10 mm and average 8 mm in diameter (Fig. 18.3). The operative sheath allows space for instillation of the medium, for the 3- to 4-mm telescope, and for the insertion of operating devices. The operating channel is sealed with a rubber nipple or gasket to prevent leakage of the distending medium (Fig. 18.3C). The standard operating sheath consists of a single common cavity shared by the medium, telescope, and operating tools. Disadvantages of this type of sheath are inability to flush the uterine cavity with the distending medium and difficulty manipulating the operative tools within the cavity. Hysteroscopes with isolated channels overcome the problems inherent to the common cavity sheath (Fig. 18.4). The dual operating channels permit flushing of the cavity and precise placement of operating

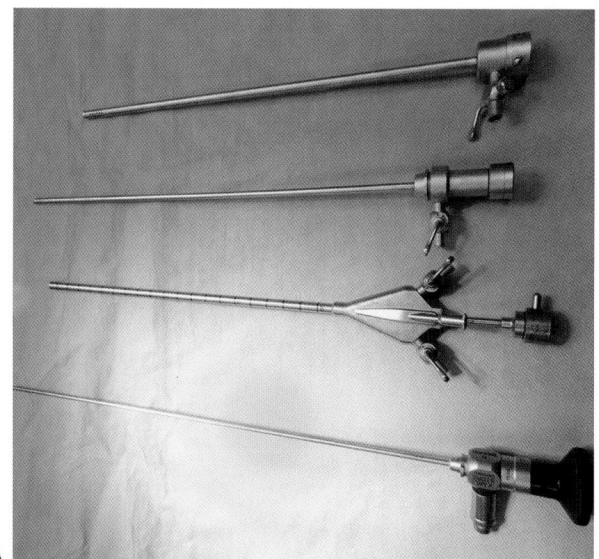

A

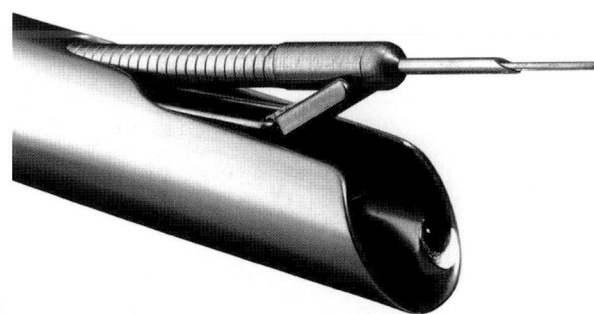

B

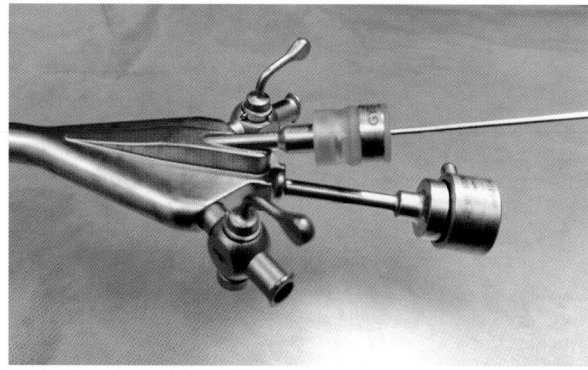

C

FIGURE 18.3 A: Instrumentation for hysteroscopic procedures. From top down: outer sheath of the diagnostic scope; the inner sheath of the diagnostic scope (not coupled together); operative sheath that includes inflow, outflow, and an instrument port; 4-mm telescope capable of insertion into either the operative sheath or diagnostic sheath. **B:** The terminal bridge reflects the cannula to angulate and facilitate its entry into the tubal ostium. (Reprinted from Baggish MS, Valle RF, Guedj H. *Hysteroscopy: Visual perspectives of uterine anatomy, physiology and pathology*, 3rd ed. Philadelphia, PA: Lippincott Williams & Wilkins, 2007, with permission. Copyright © 2007, Lippincott Williams.) **C:** An operating sheath with input and output channels as well as flushing capability. The operating channel is sealed with a rubber nipple and has a 7-F instrument inserted.

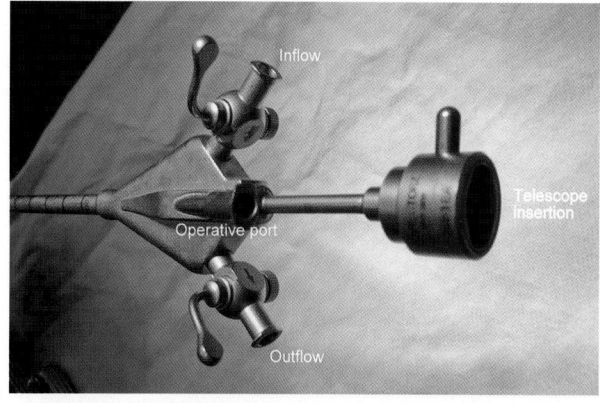

A

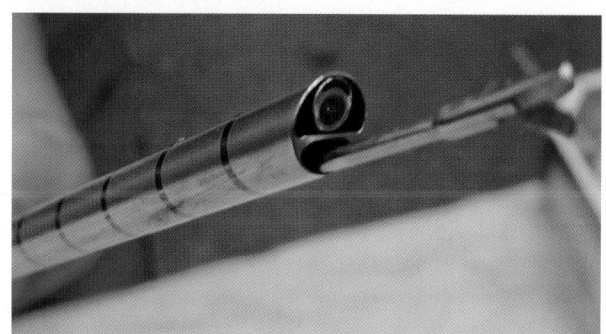

B

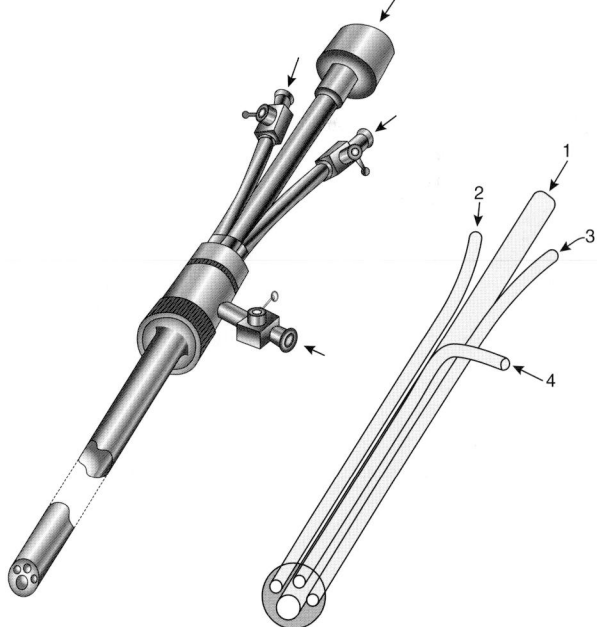

C

FIGURE 18.4 A: A single-channel operating sheath consists of a single cavity that the telescope, distending medium, and operating instruments share. **B:** Terminal portion of the operative sheath with scissors extended through. The top channel allows placement of the telescope, inflow, and outflow. The lower port allows passage of the operative instrument. **C:** A dual-channel operating sheath is constructed with (*1*) isolated channels for a telescope, (*2 and 3*) two operating devices, and (*4*) distending medium.

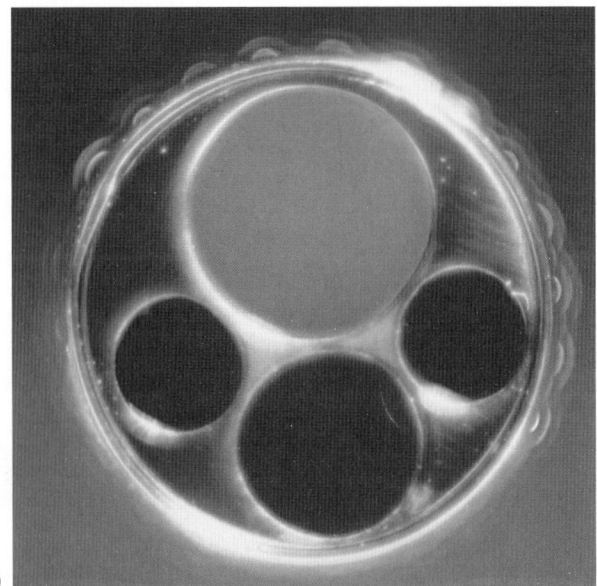

D

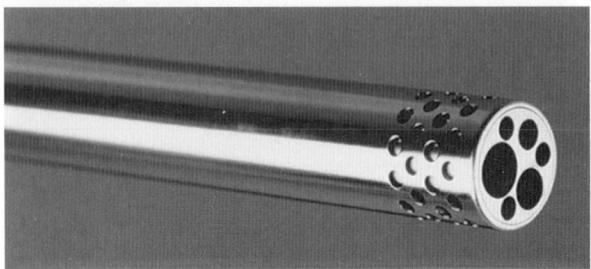

E

FIGURE 18.4 (*Continued*) **D:** The terminal portion of the second-generation isolated-channel hysteroscope shows the channel for the 4-mm optic (**top**) and a 3-mm operating channel for a variety of large accessory instruments (**bottom**). The two channels at either side are the fluid intake channels. **E:** The double sheath mechanism of the isolated-channel hysteroscope. The perforations in the outer sheath are for fluid return. The uterus is continuously flushed.

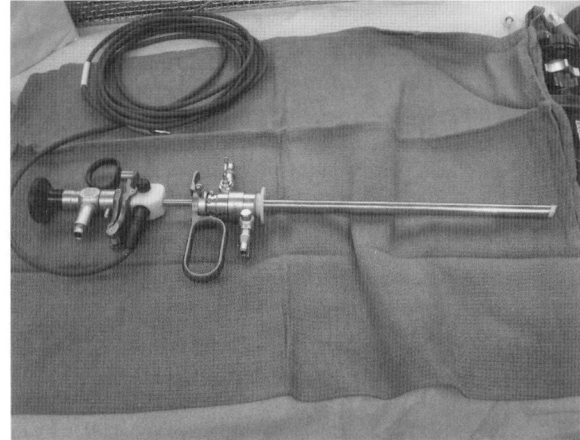

A

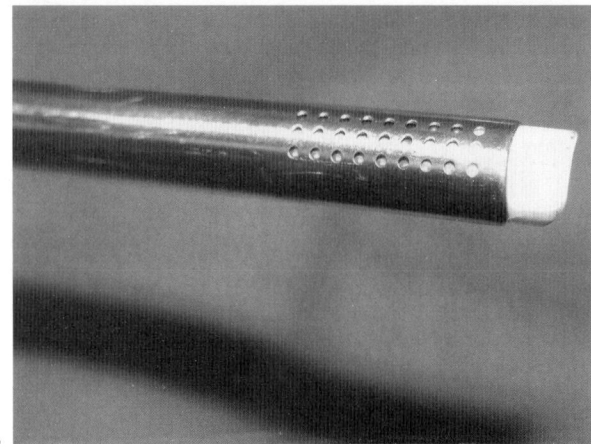

B

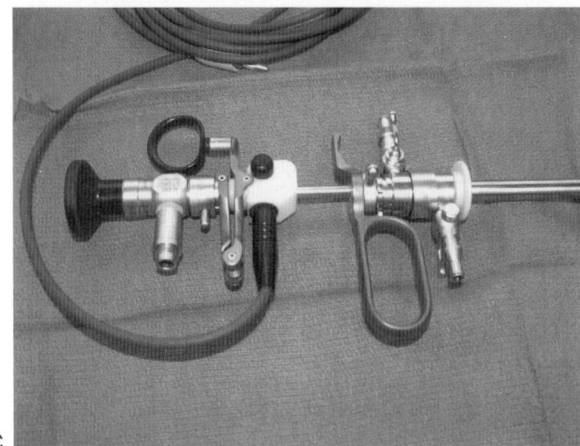

C

FIGURE 18.5 A: The resectoscope shown here is equipped with fluid entry and exit ports. A flushing sheath as the trigger mechanism is pulled back the electrode extends out from the terminal portion of the sheath. **B:** The terminal portion of the sheath shows the output external sheath. Fluid enters through the inner sheath (terminus white). **C:** A 30-degree telescope couples to the sheath. The electric cord carries current, which is transmitted to the electrode.

accessories. A popular model today is the isolated-channel sheath consisting of a double-flushing sheath (**Fig. 18.4D, E**) that permits media instillation by way of the inner sheath and media return by way of the perforated outer sheath. The constant flow of the fluid medium in and out of the cavity creates a very clear operative field. The single isolated operating channel has a diameter sufficiently large (3 mm) to permit an entirely new generation of larger, sturdier operating tools to be used (**Fig. 18.4**). The new sheath combines the advantages of the resectoscope with the facility of the operating hysteroscope.

The resectoscope is a specialized electrosurgical (monopolar or bipolar) endoscope that consists of an inner sheath and outer sheath (**Fig. 18.5A**). The outer sheath is for fluid return as described above. The inner sheath has a common channel for the telescope, fluid medium, and electrode (**Fig. 18.5B**). The double-armed electrode is fitted to a trigger device that pushes the electrode out beyond the sheath and then pulls it back within the sheath (**Fig. 18.5C**). The operating tools consist of four basic electrodes: a cutting loop, ball, button, and angulated needle (**Fig. 18.5D–G**). Most resectoscopes are equipped with a 30-degree telescope. The lens is angled toward the electrode to permit a clear view of the near operative field. Vision of the

electrode is lost when the electrode is fully extended outward. Most operating sheaths measure 8 mm or more in outer diameter, so dilatation is usually required for insertion. Contemporary small-diameter resectoscopes use a 3-mm telescope and a 7- to 7.5-mm sheath.

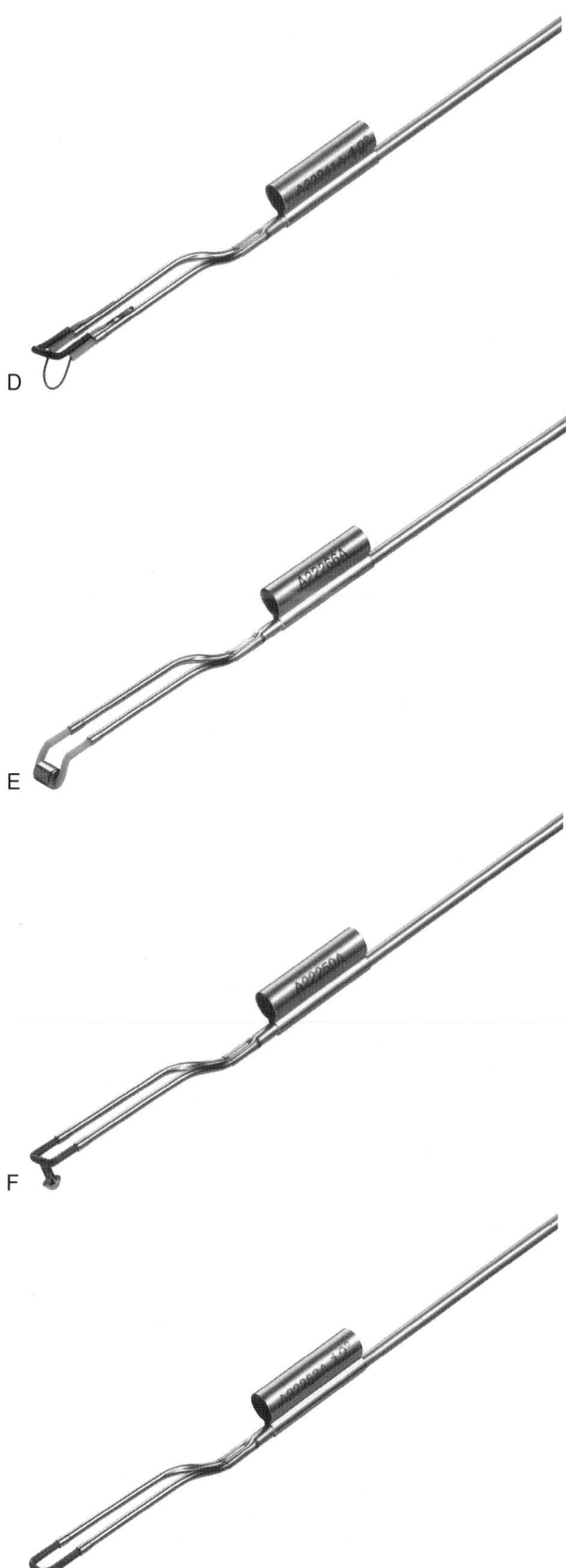

III

FIGURE 18.5 (*Continued*) **D:** The cutting loop electrode is the instrument for shaving submucous myomas. **E:** The ball or barrel electrode is the instrument most utilized for endometrial ablation. **F:** The button electrode is specifically employed to point coagulation. **G:** The angulated needle electrode is favored for fine cutting, for example, adhesions or pedunculated myomas.

CAMERA

In most cases today, hysteroscopy employs the endoscopic microchip camera coupled directly to the telescope, with digital cameras and digital recorders. Endoscopic video camera lenses range in focal length from 25 to 38 mm. A 28- to 30-mm lens provides satisfactory magnification. The view with the coupled camera provides magnification comparable to that obtained during microsurgery. If a video recorder is available, a permanent record of the procedure can be recorded. A xenon light generator provides the best illumination for video techniques, although less expensive light sources may be satisfactory when coupled to newer cameras, which are highly light sensitive.

ACCESSORY INSTRUMENTS

The standard accessories are the 7-F (i.e., 2.3-mm) alligator grasping forceps, biopsy forceps, and scissors. The small size of these semirigid instruments makes them particularly fragile, as excessive torque at the junction of the shaft and handle frequently leads to breakage. Flexible devices are less likely to fracture and are equally as facile compared with the semirigid variety. Development of the large isolated-channel sheath has made the use of totally flexible 3-mm operating instruments feasible. The scissors and graspers are substantially heavier and much less prone to breakage (**Fig. 18.6A–D**).

A variety of monopolar and bipolar electrodes are also now available for operative hysteroscopy. Monopolar balls, needles, shaving loops (3 mm), and ridged (vaporizing) loops can be inserted through the large operating channel. Bipolar needles for myolysis, as well as bipolar ball and cutting loop electrodes, have been manufactured (**Fig. 18.7**), together with bipolar scissors and needles. The hysteroscopic sheath has an advantage over the resectoscopic sheath, allowing insertion of an aspirating cannula (2.3 or 3 mm), which permits the operator to selectively clear the field of bubbles and debris that cannot be removed by the way of the return second sheath. Nevertheless, the resectoscope is generally easier to use for the average gynecologist.

A complete bipolar system marketed under the trade name of Versapoint (Gynecare, Ethicon, Somerville, NJ) permits cutting and ablation via operative hysteroscopes or via a dedicated bipolar resectoscope. The mechanism for the bipolar current flow through the electrode is illustrated in **Figure 18.8A**. The electrodes measure 5-F diameter (i.e., 2 mm) and therefore can be accommodated by standard and isolated hysteroscopic channels (**Fig. 18.8B**). The biggest advantage of this bipolar technology is that saline may be used as the distending medium for the operative hysteroscopy. This obviates the risk of hyponatremia (see sections on media and complications). Hysteroscopic morcellators have also been developed as an alternative to the resectoscope in removing uterine submucosal myomas. Two such systems are TRUCLEAR hysteroscopic morcellator (Smith & Nephew, Andover, MA) and the MyoSure tissue removal system (Hologic, Bedford, MA) (**Fig. 18.9A, B**). Both systems use suction-based, mechanical energy, rotating tubular cutter systems rather than the high-frequency electrical energy used by resectoscopes. The benefits of these systems include the ability to use isotonic distension media such as normal saline and an improved visual field as resected "fibroid chips" are removed.

The Flexible Hysteroscope

The 4.8-mm-diameter fiberoptic hysteroscope consists of three sections: a soft flexible front section, a rigid rotating middle section, and a semirigid rear section. In 1990, Lin

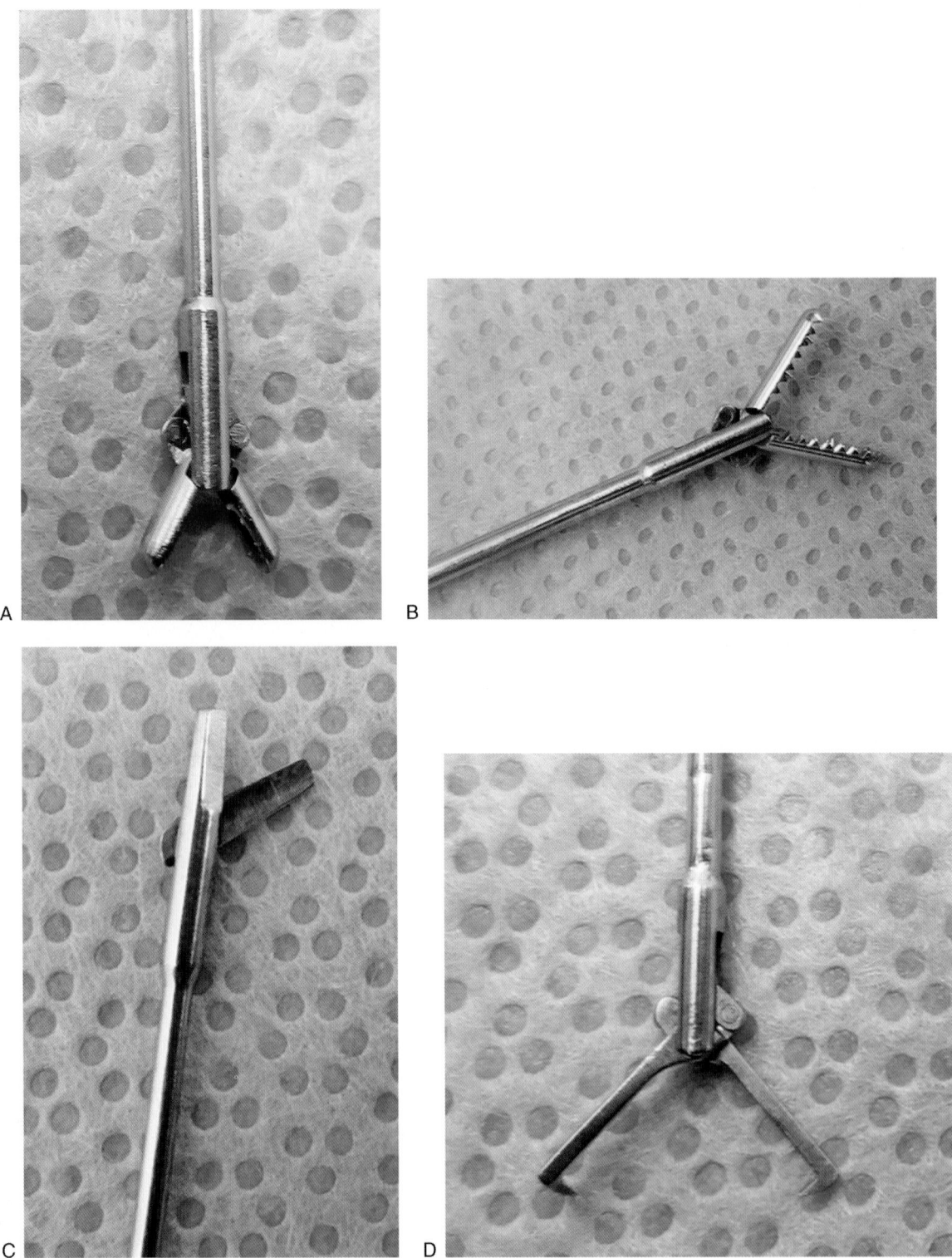

FIGURE 18.6 A: Direct vision intrauterine biopsies may be performed utilizing the biopsy forceps. **B:** Crocodile-jawed forceps are ideal for grabbing and retaining devices or tissue within the uterine cavity. **C:** Scissors have a variety of intrauterine applications, including cutting adhesions and uterine septa. **D:** Tenaculum allows a puncturing grasp that is more secure than that of the crocodile-jawed forceps.

and colleagues reported their experiences with this instrument in 153 procedures, including transcervical tubocornual recanalization, chorionic villus sampling, and retrieval of lost intrauterine devices (IUDs). The flexible hysteroscope has particular advantage in its ease of aligning the catheter for tubal canalization. Several manufacturers now produce fiberoptic (flexible hysteroscopes) (Fig. 18.10). Contemporary fiberoptic hysteroscopes are available with single-use, sterile sheaths that eliminate need to sterilize equipment between cases.

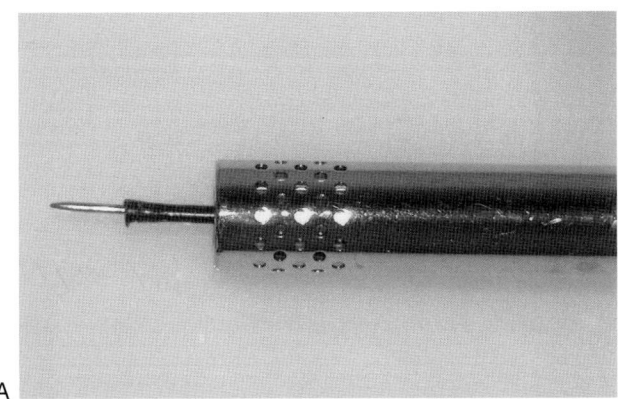

A

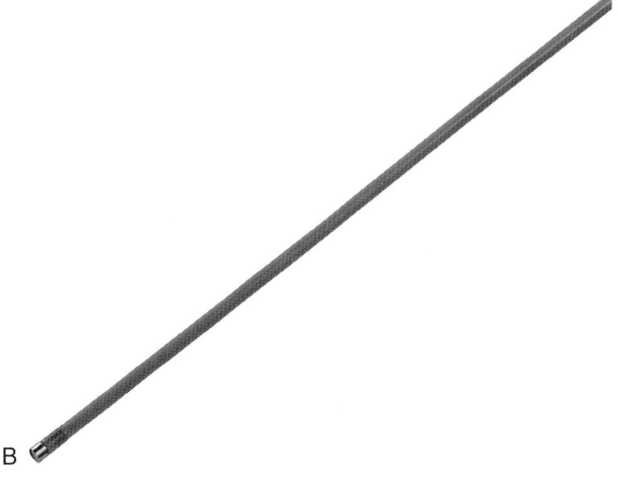

B

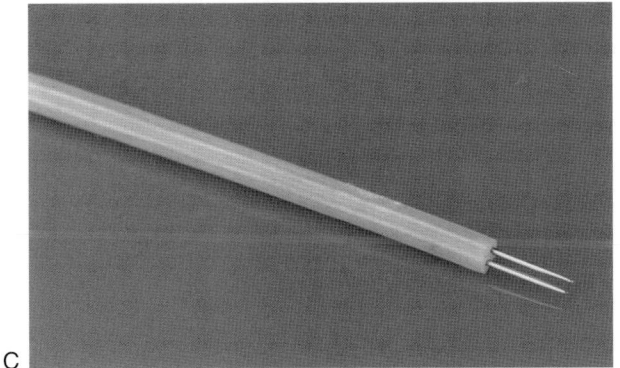

C

III

FIGURE 18.7 A: This straight cutting needle (insulated with Teflon) protrudes from the terminal portion of the sheath of a flushing operating hysteroscopy. This device can cut septa, adhesions, myomas, and polyps. **B:** The button electrode may be inserted through the operating channel and used for coagulation indications but never for cutting. **C:** A 3-mm bipolar needle that can be inserted into a submucous myoma for myolysis.

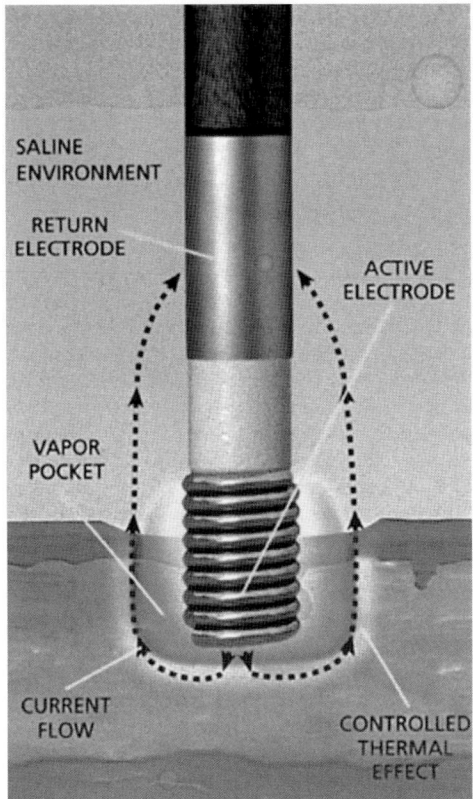

A

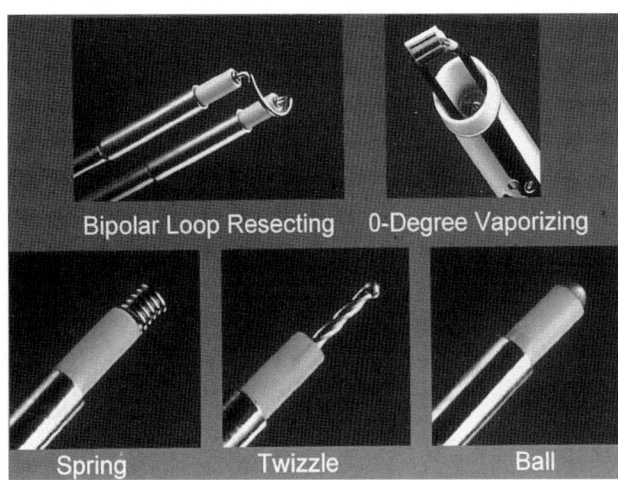

B

FIGURE 18.8 A: The mechanism of action for the Versapoint bipolar electrode is illustrated. The coiled bottom portion is the active electrode, and the upper (separately illustrated) metal portion serves as the return electrode. The saline medium facilitates the conduction of current between the two poles. **B:** Several bipolar electrodes are shown. The major advantage of bipolar devices is the ability to use normal saline as the distending fluid medium.

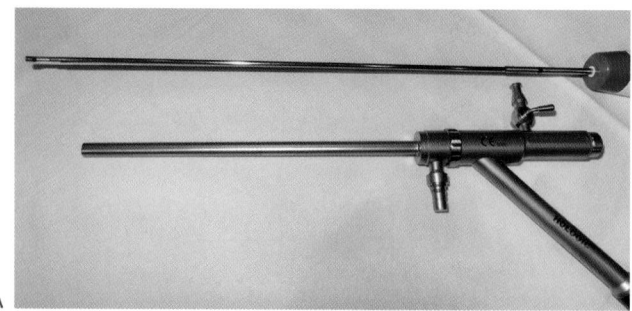

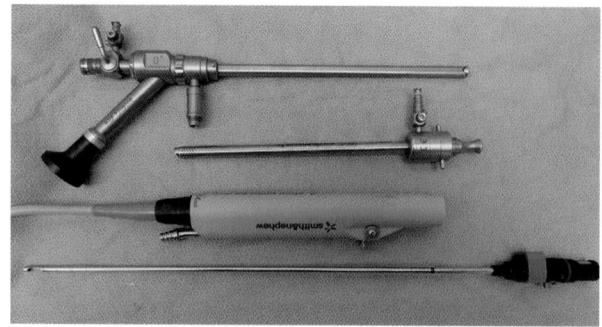

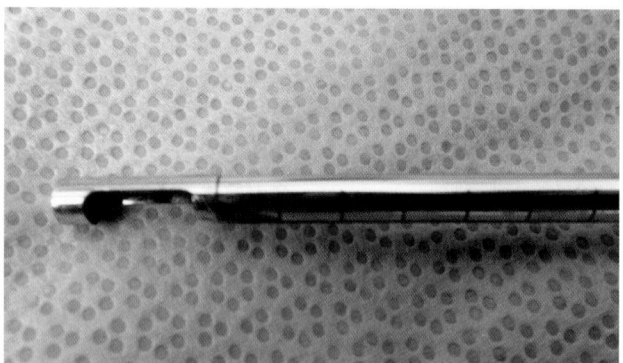

FIGURE 18.9 A: Hysteroscopic morcellator setup by Hologic. Note the angled telescopic portion, which allows the camera to be attached. Disposable device is inserted down an operative channel. **B:** Hysteroscopic morcellator setup by MyoSure. From top down is the angled telescope with an operative channel and media inflow port. The outer sheath includes an articulated obturator that allows for a blind entry if preferred by the surgeon. The motor attaches to suction and the below disposable morcellating piece. **C:** The working/cutting end of the morcellator. Note the blunt end with a protected rotating blade located inside the curvature, which oscillates cutting tissue and pulling cut portions inside the lumen of the instrument for removal. Cutting can only occur along the lateral open edge.

DISTENDING MEDIA

Under normal circumstances, the uterine cavity is a potential space, with the anterior and posterior walls in close apposition. To achieve a panoramic view within the uterus, the walls must be separated. The thick muscle of the uterine wall requires a minimum pressure of 40 mm Hg to distend the cavity sufficiently to see with a hysteroscope. Because the endometrium is richly endowed with blood vessels, touching it with the sheath of the hysteroscope often produces bleeding. Although a variety of distending media can be used to attain the desired degree of distention, it usually requires pressures approximating 70 mm Hg, which at the same time propels the medium through the oviducts into the peritoneal cavity. Over-dilatation of the cervix with a loosely applied hysteroscopic

sheath results in leakage of the medium, suboptimal pressure, and poor expansion of the uterine cavity. In contrast, a tight application of the sheath maintains the medium within the cavity, keeps intrauterine pressure above mean arterial pressure, and maintains a clear operative field.

Media can be conveniently divided into gaseous or liquid. The latter may be further subdivided into high-viscosity and low-viscosity fluids.

GASEOUS MEDIA

Carbon Dioxide

CO_2 is a colorless gas that is highly soluble when mixed with blood. It can be used to safely distend the uterus when instilled with a proper insufflation apparatus. CO_2 is ideal for diagnostic hysteroscopy. The hysteroscopic insufflator (Fig. 18.11) delivers CO_2 into the uterus at a flow rate measured in cubic centimeters per minute, in contrast to the laparoscopic insufflator, which allows CO_2 to flow in at a rate of liters per minute. The laparoscopic insufflator is both unsuitable and unsafe for hysteroscopic insufflation. The rate of flow of CO_2 into the uterus should never exceed 100 mL per minute, and pressure should be adjusted below 150 mm Hg. Before CO_2 is infused, the hysteroscopic tubing and the hysteroscope must be purged of air. Additionally, the Trendelenburg position should be avoided.

When CO_2 flow is excessive, bubbles appear and obscure the field. CO_2 tends to flatten the endometrium, and this artifact can obscure pathology. When CO_2 is improperly instilled, emboli form and can produce severe derangements in cardiovascular physiology. Advantages of CO_2 as a distention medium include its neatness. It does not foul instruments, it does not mess up the office or operating room, and it allows entry evaluation of the endocervical canal. CO_2 is therefore an excellent diagnostic medium. The disadvantage of CO_2 is that it cannot be used for operative hysteroscopy due to risk of CO_2 embolism.

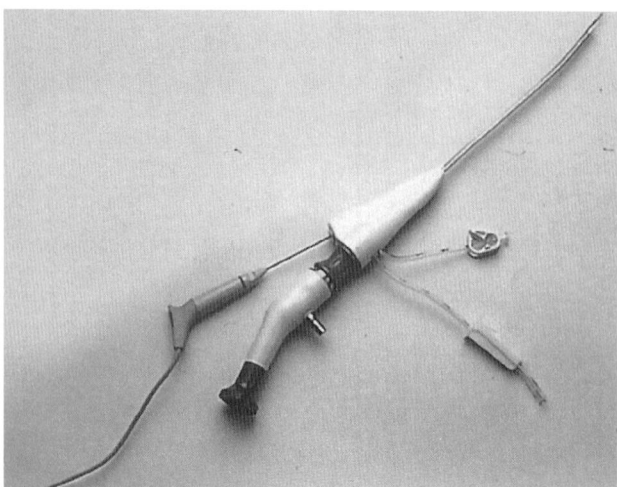

FIGURE 18.10 Flexible fiberoptic hysteroscopes can be manipulated to turn at virtually any angle.

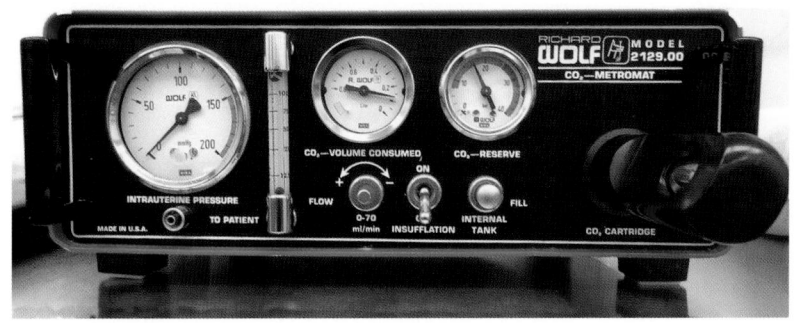

FIGURE 18.11 CO_2 is infused using a specific hysteroscopic insufflator that measures the flow rate (100 mL per minute) and uterine pressure (not to exceed 150 mm Hg). Laparoscopic CO_2 insufflation devices cannot be used for hysteroscopy due to a much higher flow rate designed to expand the abdominal cavity.

LIQUID MEDIA

High Viscosity

Hyskon (32% dextran 70 in dextrose) is a colorless, viscid solution that is rarely used today for diagnostic and operative hysteroscopy. An advantage of Hyskon is its immiscibility with blood, which permits excellent visualization, even during active bleeding. A disadvantage of Hyskon is that dried residue tends to harden and clog hysteroscopic sheath channels. Two types of severe patient reactions unique to Hyskon have been reported: a syncratic anaphylactoid reaction and a bleeding diathesis. The hematologic reaction is caused by excessive vascular uptake of dextran, which allows a more general manifestation of its physiologic actions, including fibrinoplastic action, stearic exclusion, alteration of platelet adhesiveness, and interference with von Willebrand factor (factor VIIIR). Hyskon also places a patient at risk for fluid overload. The osmotic activity of dextran is such that for each gram of Hyskon instilled into the vascular space, 20 mL of interstitial water will be pulled into the circulation; 100 mL of Hyskon (32% dextran) will expand the plasma volume by 32 g × 20 mL, or a total of 640 mL. As the volume of intravascular Hyskon increases, a critical level is reached, and pulmonary edema occurs. Finally, dextran 70 (Hyskon) is a mixture of macromolecules ranging from 25 to 125 kd. Although the lower-weight molecules are rapidly excreted, the larger molecules can interfere with glomerular filtration and will remain in the bloodstream for 4 to 6 weeks.

Low Viscosity

Low-viscosity fluids must be continuously flushed through the uterine cavity if a clear view is to be obtained. Delivered fluid must be continuously circulated out of the cavity and clean fluid constantly added to make up for the deficit and maintain uterine distension. A standard diagnostic sheath does *not* allow for flushing. Therefore, if a low-viscosity fluid is used for distension, the view may be suboptimal because blood can mix with the distending fluid, creating a colored fluid through which the operator will see the field. The safest distending medium will be isoosmolar—that is, the electrolyte content will amount to 300 mOsm. Additionally, the sodium content of the fluid should approximate 140 mEq/L. The ideal low-viscosity fluid medium is 0.9% sodium chloride.

Regardless of the type of medium infused, the surgeon is responsible for monitoring the infused volume and reconciling that volume with the collected volume. Positive infusion differences require that the procedure be stopped when deficits range from 500 mL (for hypoosmolar fluids) to 1,000 mL (isoosmolar fluids). The surgeon and anesthesiologist must communicate, because fluid overload scenarios will usually necessitate the anesthesiologist helping to manage the ensuing pathophysiology. Additionally, intravenous fluids infused by the anesthesia team will add to the increased circulatory volume. Finally, any fluid including physiologic salt solutions can produce pulmonary edema when excessive volumes are administered via the hysteroscope, because the pressure gradient to maintain uterine distension is 60 to 70 mm Hg and subendometrial venous pressure is 4 mm Hg. Inevitably, fluids will diffuse into the venous circulation.

Low-viscosity distention media may be delivered by hanging a 2- to 3-L bag or bottle of fluid 6 to 8 feet above the operating table, permitting the fluid to infuse by gravity feed (Fig. 18.12A). An alternative is instilling low-viscosity fluid by rotary pump (Fig. 18.12B). The newest pumps weigh the fluid in real time and give the surgeon a constant readout of flow rate and total volume of fluid infused (Fig. 18.12C, D). Use of an automated fluid pump and monitoring system is advocated by both the American Congress of Obstetricians and Gynecologists and the American Association of Gynecologic Laparoscopists to most accurately monitor inflow and outflow and prevent complications associated with fluid overload.

Normal Saline, Ringer Lactate

Normal (physiologic) saline (0.9% sodium chloride) is perhaps the safest of any hysteroscopic media. Complications of excessive vascular absorption include fluid overload and pulmonary edema, which are managed by diuresis and support. The medium is readily available in 3-L sterile bags that can be mounted on an intravenous pole or given via an infusion pump. Garry and colleagues (1992) reported excellent safety results and precise maintenance of uterine pressure by using a pump delivery system, which was combined with one of the operating channels of the dual-channel operating sheath to provide an outflow tract and thus a constant flow rate through the uterine cavity.

Unfortunately, because saline is an efficient conductor of electrons, it does not permit a current density that is high enough for tissue action when using a monopolar system. Saline is therefore not suitable for monopolar electrosurgery, although it is effective when the Nd:YAG laser, the KTP/532 laser, bipolar electrode, and mechanical devices such as scissors are the hysteroscopic accessories of choice.

The optimal drape for the operating room is the urologic pouch (tucked under the buttocks) with a plastic reservoir pocket into which the outflow fluid may be collected and quantified to determine the fluid deficit (the difference between instilled fluid and returned fluid). The surgeon should be given a running account by a nurse or surgical assistant of the volume of fluid instilled, which is calculated as the liters of fluid hung minus volume of return fluid. Whenever any significant fluid deficit is calculated, usually considered 2.5 L for isotonic saline, the procedure should be discontinued and scheduled for completion at a later date.

Glycine 1.5% and Sorbitol 3%

Glycine (1.5%) and sorbitol (3%) solutions were first used in urologic surgery, principally for male patients. They were adopted later by gynecologists for use with monopolar

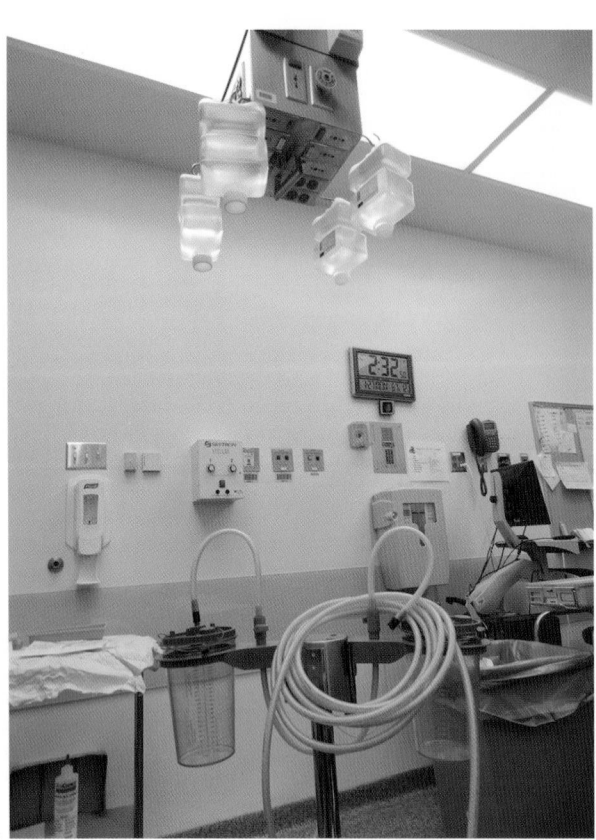

A

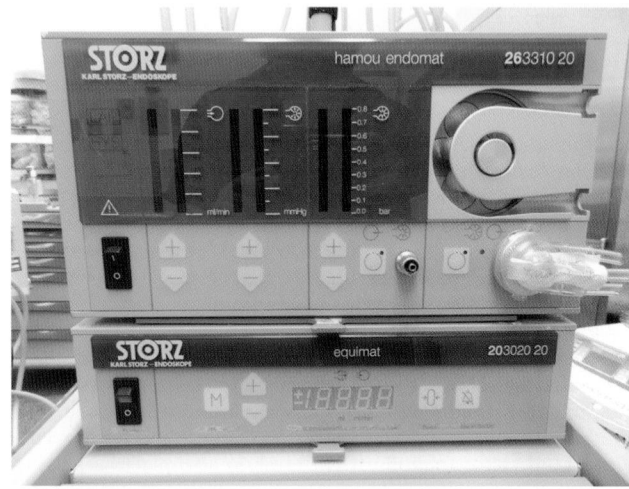

B

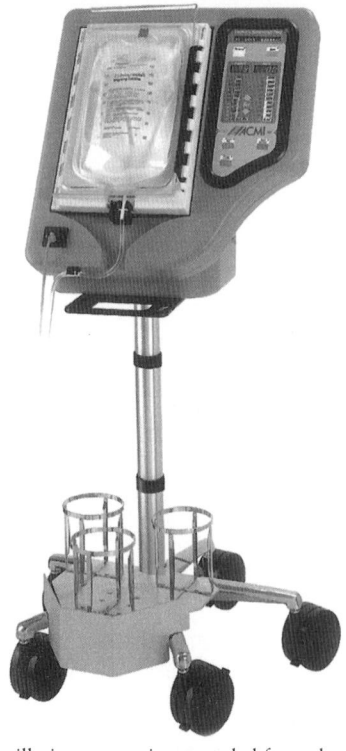

C

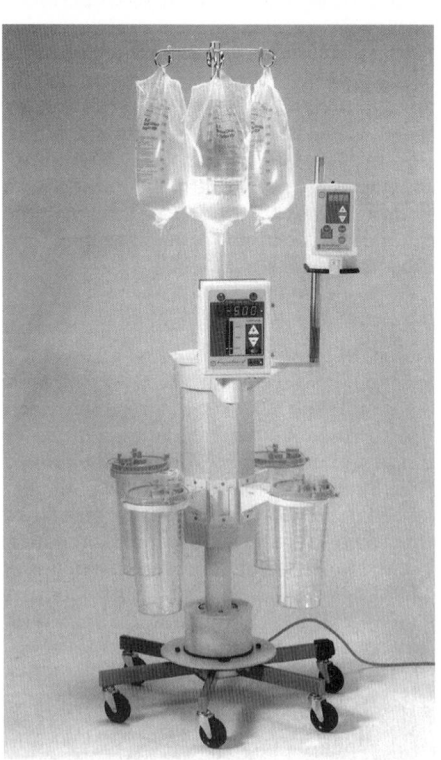

D

FIGURE 18.12 A: This fluid instillation system is suspended from the ceiling and is equipped to handle four 3-L bottles or bags. The height is easily adjusted to provide a head of pressure to infuse into the uterus. **B:** The advantage of this pump relates to its ability to provide a constant flow of low-viscosity fluid and to maintain sufficient pressure to keep the uterine walls distended. **C:** This pump delivery system not only delivers fluid but also weighs each bag and continuously calculates fluid volume infused and volume collected. **D:** This apparatus is very similar to the technology shown in part (**C**), but permits the usage of multiple bags of fluid.

electrosurgical devices such as the resectoscope. Both glycine and sorbitol are used for hysteroscopic distension, but both have disadvantages inherent to their composition. Since these solutions are hypoosmolar (sorbitol, 178 mOsm/L; glycine, 200 mOsm/L), the principal hazard relates to their vascular absorption and the creation of an acute hyponatremic, hypoosmolar state. A fluid deficit equal to or greater than 750 mL should alert the surgeon to a likelihood of hyponatremia and hypoosmolality. Two reports have presented data concerning significant complications secondary to hyponatremia. In one series of four women, two died (50% mortality); in the other, one of four women died (25% mortality). Absorption of hypoosmolar solutions produces a gradient between the circulating blood and the brain cells. The brain cells respond by pumping cation out to diminish the positive infusion of water into the brain. Unfortunately, the cation pumping mechanism of the brain is deficient in women, secondary probably to the actions of progesterone, and women are at significantly greater risk for the development of life-threatening cerebral edema when a hypoosmolar state exists. At a minimum, intraoperative and 4-hour postoperative serum sodium levels should be requested on a stat basis if concern for a fluid deficit using a hypoosmolar medium exists. A unique disadvantage of glycine is that it can be metabolized to ammonia and cause neurologic damage.

5% Mannitol and 2.2% Glycine

Mannitol (5%) and glycine (2.2%) may be used with electrosurgical devices and are approximately isoosmolar. Mannitol has an osmolality of 285 mOsm and is an osmotic diuretic. Its optical characteristics are equivalent to glycine and sorbitol; however, it is a safer medium. In a study of 181 hysteroscopic examinations using isotonic 2.2% glycine, although there was a mean decrease in sodium of 9 mmol/L in patients absorbing 1,000 mL, the serum osmolality remained normal with no significant adverse sequelae.

DIAGNOSTIC HYSTEROSCOPY TECHNIQUES

Diagnostic hysteroscopy can be performed in an office setting under local anesthesia. The injection of lidocaine 1%, 10 to 15 mL, directly into the cervix produces adequate anesthesia. Discomfort for the patient can be further diminished by ibuprofen (Motrin), 600 to 800 mg, administered 30 minutes before the procedure. Patients who require cardiac prophylaxis (e.g., artificial heart valves) should be covered by appropriate antibiotics. Informed consent clearly reviewing the risks, benefits, and alternatives should be obtained.

Accurate knowledge of the position of the uterus is critical to safely facilitate the procedure. The optimal view of the uterus is obtained during the proliferative phase of the menstrual cycle. After placing the patient in the dorsal lithotomy position, the perineum and vagina are gently swabbed with Betadine or another suitable antiseptic solution. A Sims retractor or breakaway speculum is inserted to allow visualization of the cervix (Fig. 18.13). The edge of the cervix at the 12 o'clock position is grasped with a single-toothed tenaculum. A suitable

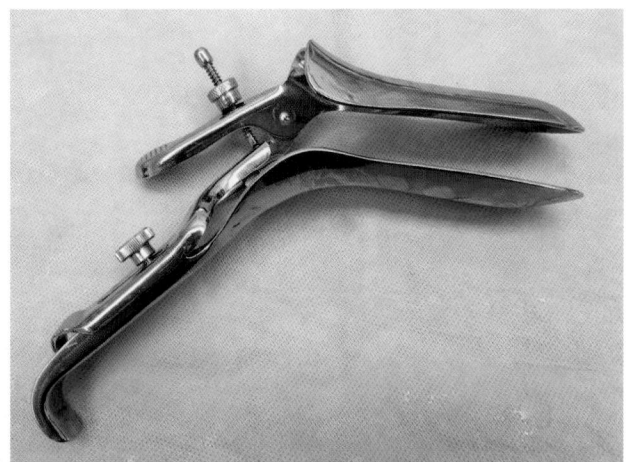

A   B

FIGURE 18.13 A: The Sims retractor is excellent for retracting the posterior vaginal wall and is easily removed following placement of the hysteroscope. **B:** Bivalve speculum can be used with similar results as the Sims retractor and is ideal for use in the absence of an assistant. The speculum or Sims retractor should be removed once the hysteroscope is positioned in the external cervical os to allow full mobility with a direct entry technique.

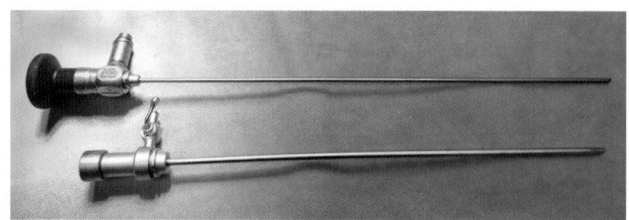
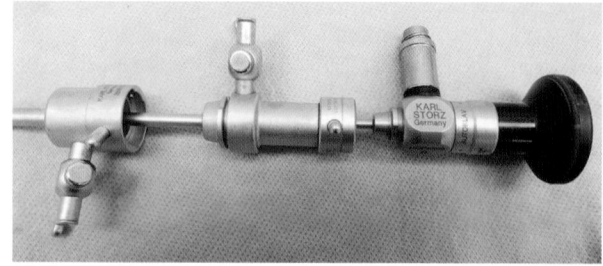

A   B

FIGURE 18.14 A: The diagnostic lens (telescope) and its 5-mm inner diagnostic sheath are excellent instruments for office or surgicenter outpatient hysteroscopy. **B:** Close-up showing 4-mm telescope engaging into both the inner and outer diagnostic sheaths (note: the locking pins are still in the open position).

telescope is selected and checked by the operator for clarity of the eyepiece and objective lens. If necessary, the lens is cleansed with a soft saline-soaked or water-soaked sponge. The light generator is switched on, and the fiberoptic cable is attached to the telescope. The telescope is inserted into the diagnostic sheath, and the selected medium is flushed through the sheath to expel any air within the sheath (Fig. 18.14A, B).

If CO_2 is the selected medium, the flow rate is adjusted to deliver 30 mL per minute. The hysteroscope is engaged into the external cervical os. As the endoscope is advanced, the gas separates the walls of the endocervix, allowing an excellent view of the endocervical folds and crypts. The internal os is seen above as the endoscope is manipulated along the axis of the canal and through the os under direct vision (Fig. 18.15A, B). Flow is adjusted to a rate 60 mL per minute when the isthmus is entered.

Routine dilatation of the cervix should be avoided, because even gentle insertion of cervical dilators can traumatize the endocervix and endometrium. Typically, the endocervical canal shows longitudinal folds, papillae, and clefts. The internal os appears as a narrow constriction at the top of the endocervical canal. The isthmus is a cylindrical extension above the os. The corpus is a capacious cavity above the isthmus. The central point of müllerian duct fusion is seen projecting down from the fundus. The cornua occupy either

side of this fused area. The tubal ostia are visible at the upper extremities of the fundal cornua and show great variation in their appearance and angle of entry into the uterine cavity. The uterine endometrium is smooth and pink-white in color during the proliferative phase. The gland openings appear as white-ringed elevations surrounded with netlike vessels. During the secretory phase of the cycle, the endometrium is lush and velvety; it protrudes into the cavity irregularly and can be easily mistaken for small polyps. The hue of secretory endometrium is magenta. When CO_2 is the distending medium, the endometrium is artificially flattened. Although the cornua are easily recognized, the tubal ostia may not be seen during the latter phase of the menstrual cycle.

OPERATIVE HYSTEROSCOPY TECHNIQUES

To begin, the telescope is inserted into the operative or resectoscope sheath. If the operative sheath is used, a proper nipple is selected and attached to the opening of the operating channel (Fig. 18.16A, B). The sheath is flushed with the distending medium, and the light cable is attached. Careful dilatation with Pratt dilators should be performed until the operative sheath negotiates a tight passage through the cervix. With the medium flowing, the hysteroscope can be inserted into

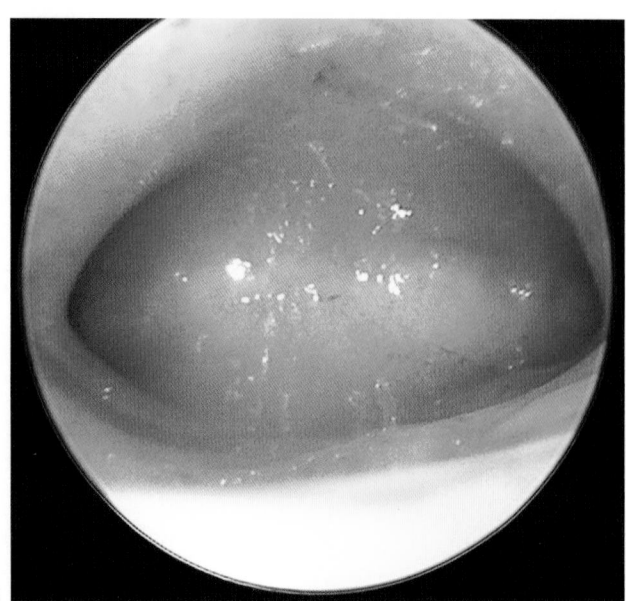
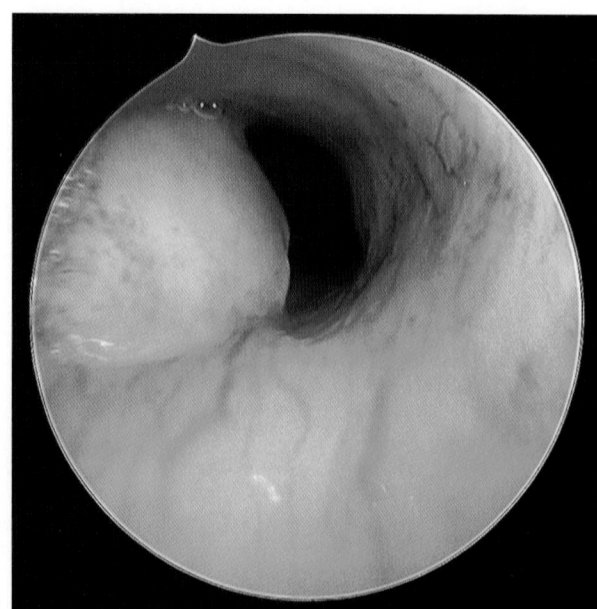

A   B

FIGURE 18.15 A: Hysteroscopic image using CO_2 to distend the intrauterine cavity. The hysteroscope's objective lens is just above the internal os allowing a panoramic view of the cavity. The recesses to the right and left are the cornu. **B:** This view is taken within the distended cervix looking upward into the dark corpus. Note a paracervical polyp along the lateral edge.

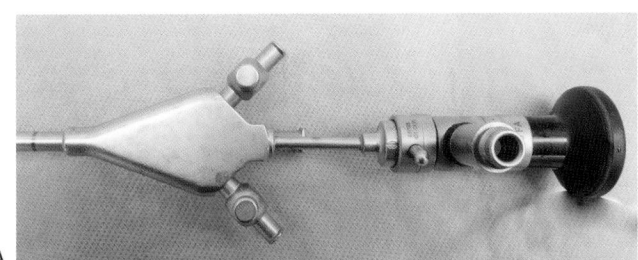
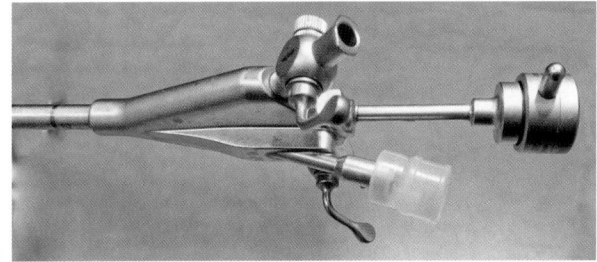

A   B

FIGURE 18.16 A: The telescope is secured by means of a watertight pin and screw mechanism. **B:** Close-up of operating sheath. A pink-colored nipple cover is attached to the operating channel, which allows passage of the instrument without backflow of distention media. The two stopcocks are for infusion of the distending medium and return and jettison of circulating fluid. Note all stopcocks are opened.

the uterine cavity under visualization. The uterine cavity is scanned, and the operator mentally notes landmarks (e.g., the tubal ostia, depth of the cornua, the location and attachments of the lesion, the proximity of the internal cervical os). The flow of the debris with the liquid medium will also help the operator locate the tubal ostia. If there is difficulty viewing the cavity clearly, the hysteroscope has probably been inserted too deeply, and the telescope has come in contact with the uterine wall. When the view is blocked, the most prudent first maneuver is to pull the instrument back with the medium flowing into the uterus.

After a clear view is obtained, the operating device (e.g., electrode or scissors) is inserted into the cavity and advanced to make contact with the endometrium for relative calibration and spatial orientation within the cavity. The cavity can also be further distended with a constant flow sheath by closing off the return valve stopcock. The valve is then opened, and the cavity is flushed clear.

In certain cases, it is advantageous to perform a simultaneous laparoscopy to permit an assistant to view the serosal surface of the uterus to provide some additional insurance against inadvertent perforation. Clinical scenarios in which simultaneous laparoscopy may be beneficial include excision of a septum, lysis of uterine adhesions, and excisions of large submucous myomas.

ELECTROSURGICAL DEVICES AND LASERS

Electrosurgical devices and lasers both exert their tissue actions in a similar fashion. Light energy from lasers is transformed to thermal energy by electron flow. Lasers and electrosurgical devices both produce coagulation at 60 to 70°C and vaporization at 100°C (Table 18.1), and both require sufficient power density to exert the desired action. Similar tissue actions can be produced by raising the power density or by keeping the power constant and increasing the tissue exposure time. A 1-mm laser fiber delivering 30 watts (W) of power to tissue will create a power density of 3,000 W/cm². A 3-mm ball electrode will need to generate 300 W of power to create a similar power density. The Nd:YAG laser, which works by thermal energy, is the preferred laser for hysteroscopic surgery. The Nd:YAG laser beam can be transmitted equally well with any distending medium, whereas monopolar electrosurgical devices operate most effectively in an electrolyte-free medium.

The surgeon must be familiar with the physics governing the actions of electrosurgical tools and lasers and with the tissue actions exerted by these energized devices. A knowledgeable surgeon would not use a ball device to cut or a loop electrode

to coagulate tissue. Proper selection of wattage depends on disease pathology and location. High power applied for a long period of time is risky and puts the patent at risk for tissue injury.

Regardless of whether a resectoscope, handheld electrode, or laser is used, depth of tissue action is extremely important. Transmural injury is possible at high-power densities or with prolonged exposure. One must keep in mind that the thickness of the distended uterine wall (0.5 to 1 cm) is considerably less than that of the nondistended uterine wall (1.5 to 2 cm) (Fig. 18.17A, B). Uterine perforation by either a laser fiber or an electrode is much more serious than perforation by scissors or another mechanical device, because the thermal energy can inflict great damage to surrounding structures (e.g., bowel or bladder). The injury may not attain its maximum damage until 2 or 3 days after surgery. Therefore, either laparoscopy or laparotomy is indicated in such cases to determine the extent of injury.

TABLE 18.1 Gross Effects of Thermal Injury as Caused by Both Laser and Electrosurgery Apparatus

APPROXIMATE DEGREE OF HEAT	THERMAL DAMAGE CAUSED
<40°C	No significant cell damage.
>40°C	Reversible cell damage, depending on the duration of exposure.[a]
>49°C	Irreversible cell damage (denaturation).[a]
>70°C	Coagulation (Latin: coagulation 5 clotting). Collagens are converted to glucose.
>100°C	Phase transition from liquid to vapor of the intracellular and extracellular water. Tissue rapidly dries out (desiccation) (Latin: ex sico 5 dehydration). Glucose has an adhesive effect after dehydration.
>200°C	Carbonization (Latin: *carbo* 5 coal). Medical pathologic burns of the fourth degree.

[a]According to Bender and Schramm (1968).

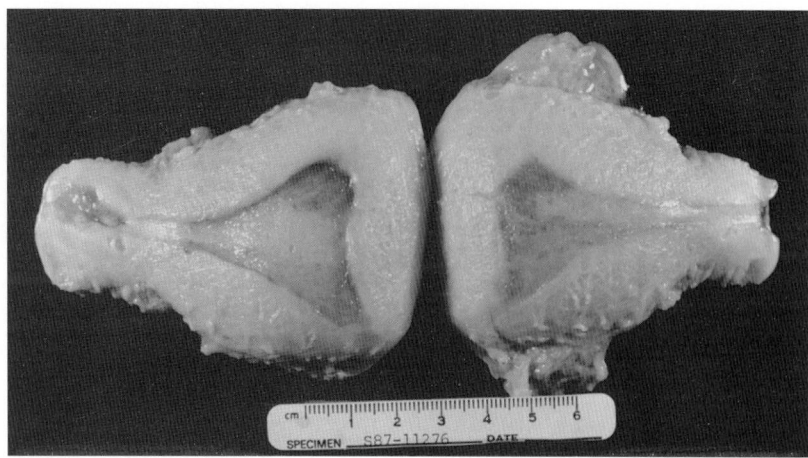
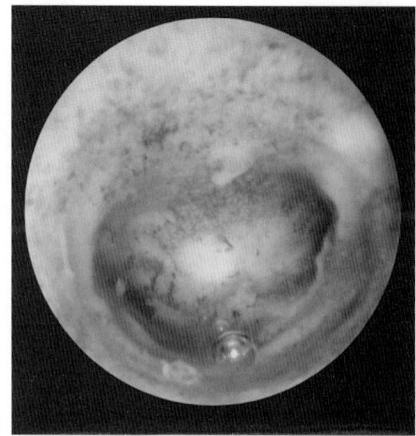

FIGURE 18.17 A: A uterus that is removed at hysterectomy shows the thick walls of the myometrium. These walls average approximately 1.5 cm in thickness, with the exception of the cornu, where the myometrium is thinner. **B:** The uterus is distended with the liquid medium. The walls of the uterus are now much thinner, averaging 0.5 to 1 cm in thickness.

SPECIFIC PROCEDURES IN HYSTEROSCOPIC SURGERY

Septate Uterus

Modern hysteroscopy has rendered the correction of the septate uterus relatively simple and straightforward by the transcervical route. Uterine septae are a treatable factor contributing to pregnancy wastage usually secondary to spontaneous abortion. The diagnosis of a uterine septum is usually made after a hysterosalpingogram or during a diagnostic hysteroscopy. Unfortunately, neither of the studies mentioned above differentiates between septate and bicornuate uteri. Historically, a diagnostic laparoscopy has been most helpful for an accurate differential diagnosis. A laparoscopic view of a septate uterus will reveal a wide but otherwise normal fundus, whereas the bicornuate uterus typically appears heart shaped. More recently, MRI of the pelvic has emerged as an imaging modality that in most cases can differentiate between a septate and bicornuate uterus. A bicornuate uterus, if pregnancy wastage is demonstrated, should be treated by a Jones or Strassman procedure. A septate uterus should be treated hysteroscopically. The standard technique, first reported in 1978 by March and colleagues, is to cut the septum with scissors under direct hysteroscopic view.

Cararach and colleagues compared hysteroscopic incision of septate uteri during a 5-year period (81 women) using a scissors or resectoscope approach and found only marginal benefit in favor of the former. Choe and Baggish used the Nd:YAG laser fiber to transect septa in 14 women. Of 13 patients who conceived, 10 delivered a live-born, term infant (87%), compared with a preoperative term pregnancy rate of 11%. Laser, resectoscope, or needle electrodes are more appropriate for the broad and usually vascular septum. Four recent studies by Litta et al., Pabuccu and Gomel, Saygili-Yilmaz, and Patton and Novy evaluated reproductive outcomes following hysteroscopic metroplasty. The percentage of pregnancies reaching term following metroplasty ranged from 50% to 83%.

Uterine rupture during pregnancy and more specifically in labor has been reported after hysteroscopic metroplasty with or without uterine perforation. It would therefore be prudent to inform the patient who will undergo metroplasty of the subsequent risk, so that she is knowledgeable and can inform her obstetrician should she become pregnant.

Hysteroscopic Technique

The uterine septum is viewed from the level of the internal cervical os. The endoscope is moved into each chamber of the divided uterine cavity, and the locations of the tubal ostia are noted. The hysteroscope is again withdrawn to a level just above the internal os. The appropriate operating instrument is inserted through the sheath, and the septum is divided in its midportion (**Figs. 18.18** and **18.19**). There is usually no need to remove tissue, as the septal tissue retracts after it is incised. In many cases, it is beneficial to perform simultaneous laparoscopy. As the fundus is approached, the operator depends on a signal from the assistant performing the laparoscopy to indicate when the quality of the hysteroscope light demonstrates transmission through the intact uterine wall. A dialog between the hysteroscopist and laparoscopist prevents perforation. A newer technique permits the operator to scan the uterus ultrasonographically to

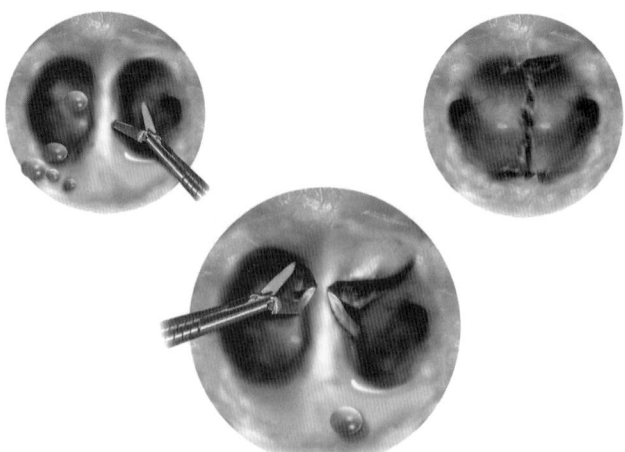

FIGURE 18.18 *Upper left:* Hysteroscopic view of a septate uterus immediately before cutting the septum. *Center:* The septum is cut approximately at midpoint, taking care not to drift too far posteriorly. Thicker septa are cut from periphery inward to the center. *Upper right:* The septum has been completely incised. (Reprinted with permission from Baggish MS, Valle RF, Guedj H. *Hysteroscopy: visual perspectives of uterine anatomy, physiology and pathology*, 3rd ed. Philadelphia, PA: Lippincott Williams & Wilkins, 2007, with permission.)

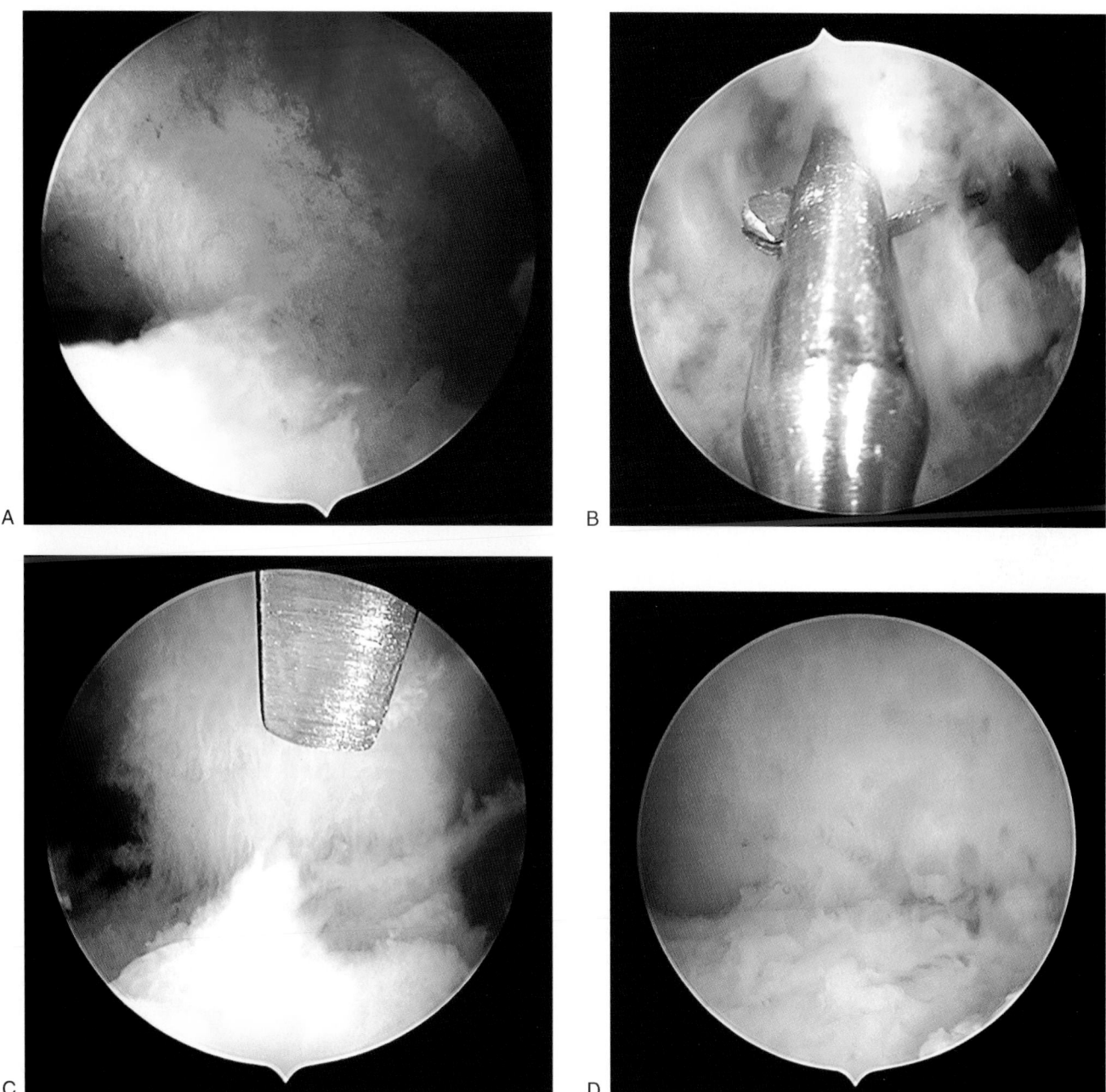

FIGURE 18.19 A: Hysteroscopic view of a septate uterus taken immediately before incising the septum. **B:** The septum is cut at its midpoint via hysteroscopic scissors. **C:** The central portion of the septum with the initial incision. **D:** Complete resection of the septum. Note the avascular and fibrous appearance of the septum, just lateral to the resection both cornea are congruent with the resection. (Photographs courtesy of Dr. Lauren Schwartz.)

determine whether the myometrium has been entered and to monitor the amount of space existing between the operating device and the serosal surface of the uterus. The surgeon should be aware of the common tendency of the cutting instrument to drift posteriorly and should clip the septum squarely in the middle. When the drift goes unnoticed, the operating instrument can cut into the myometrium and cause pulsatile bleeding. Similarly, correcting the septum too perfectly at the level of the fundus will result in deep penetration into the myometrium and subsequent hemorrhage. If a multichannel hysteroscope is used, a 3-mm ball electrode may be used to coagulate the bleeding

vessel. The double-needle bipolar electrode is a safe alternative method for electrocoagulation.

If bleeding does ensue, a Foley catheter with a 10-mL balloon can be inserted into the endometrial cavity at the end of the procedure and inflated to 5 to 6 mL. The pressure exerted by the bag on the uterine walls is sufficient to control the bleeding promptly. The bag is deflated 6 to 12 hours postoperatively and is removed if no further bleeding ensues. Patients are usually advised to take conjugated estrogen daily following surgery. Antibiotics are not routinely administered.

Uterine Synechiae

Adhesions form between the anterior and posterior walls of the uterus as a result of trauma or infection in a milieu of estrogen deprivation. This condition is often referred to as Asherman syndrome. Classically, this problem follows an abortion or postpartum hemorrhage, for which a vigorous curettage has been performed to control the bleeding. Friedler and associates reported the incidence of adhesions after one abortion to be 16.3%. This figure rose to 32% after three or more abortions. The severity of adhesions also typically rises as the number of abortions increases. In most cases, the patient does not resume menstruation; however, a minority of patients continues to menstruate normally. Because the patient is subsequently infertile or amenorrheic, a hysterogram is performed. The radiograph reveals filling defects that vary from minimal to severe (i.e., virtually obliterating the endometrial cavity). Previous treatment of uterine synechiae consisted of blind curettage, and the results were predictably poor. With the advent of operative panoramic hysteroscopy, treatment progressed to identification of adhesions and sharp incision of the adhesions with scissors (Fig. 18.20).

Adhesiolysis surgery is probably the most difficult of hysteroscopic operations. Because numerous vascular channels are opened, the risk of intravascular absorption of the medium is high. Rock and colleagues reported a technique of laparoscopically injecting the uterus with leucomethylene blue dye to help identify the junction at which the anterior and posterior walls were adhered. Capella-Allouc and associates reported 31 cases of severe adhesions that underwent hysteroscopic lysis ranging over one to four operations. The number of subsequent pregnancies after treatment was 43%, and the live birth rate was 32%. A 2004 report from Belgium of 46 women with Asherman syndrome, of whom one third had severe adhesions, described live births as greater than 40%.

Hysteroscopic Technique

A thorough diagnostic hysteroscopy is performed to assess the degree of adhesion formation and deformity of the cavity. Small openings in the curtain of adhesions in which there are flow patterns of tiny blood fragments and tissue debris are helpful and should be sought out, as are any normal anatomic landmarks. Photographs, videotapes, and detailed drawings are helpful reminders in planning the strategy for cutting these adhesions.

Simultaneous laparoscopy is often prudent to prevent and immediately recognize perforation of the uterus. Flexible or semirigid scissors, the resectoscope, Versapoint, or the Nd:YAG laser are the operating instruments of choice, although some operators use the monopolar needle electrode at 40 to 50 W of cutting power, BLEND 1 or 2. The laser is initially set to deliver 30 to 50 W of power. The medium is instilled into the cavity by way of an operating sheath. Filmy and central adhesions should be cut first, always following the fluid flow. Marginal and dense adhesions should be tackled last, always cutting from below and moving upward. A second key to success is to maintain the hysteroscope in mid-channel relative to the uterine walls. The cavity can usually be restored to reasonably normal architecture. Bleeding is not uncommon during this operation, particularly when cutting marginal adhesions, because the border between adhesion and myometrium is blurred.

The patient should be placed on conjugated estrogens during postoperative recovery. Placement of an IUD or uterine stent (Cook OB/GYN) (Fig. 18.21) within the cavity to keep the walls from adhering is a standard postoperative measure.

Cannulation of Fallopian Tube

Novy and associates described a technique for passing a special catheter into the tubal ostium and through the obstructed interstitial portion of the tube. The procedure was successful in 92% of the cases. Dumesic and Dhillon reported a tubal cannulation procedure in which they used a flexible guiding insert to facilitate passage of the cornual cannulation catheter. These techniques are useful for treating interstitial obstruction secondary to cellular debris and tubal spasm. The obvious advantage of this cannulation technique is its usefulness in treating cases that might otherwise require tubocornual anastomosis. Pregnancy rates range from 25% to 54% in 6 months.

Hysteroscopic Technique

A 5.5-F Teflon cannula with a metal obturator (Cook OB/GYN) is introduced through the operating channel of the hysteroscopic sheath. The obturator is removed. A 3-F catheter with a guide cannula wire is introduced into the 5.5-F cannula by

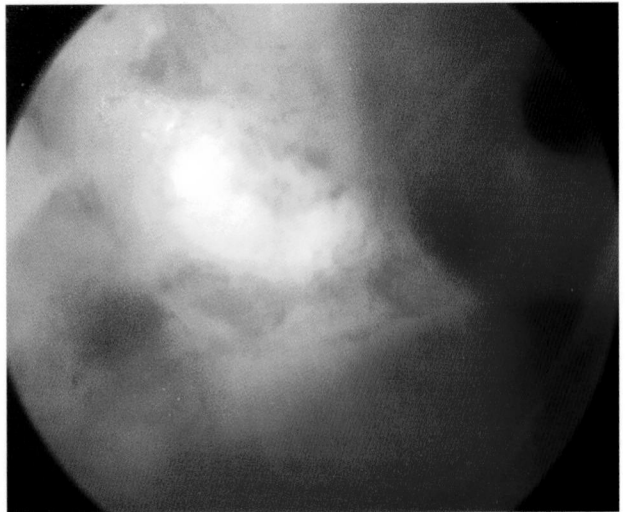

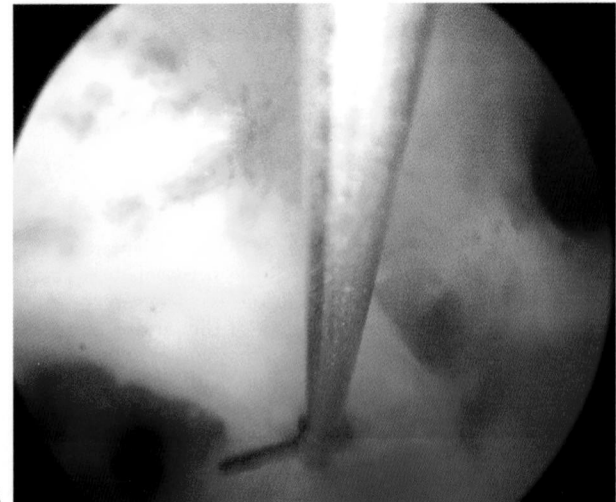

A B

FIGURE 18.20 A: A thin transverse adhesion spanning the intrauterine cavity between the lateral and anterior–posterior walls. **B:** Hysteroscopic Mayo scissors used to incise the adhesion. Note: due to high risk for uterine perforation, no electrocautery is used.

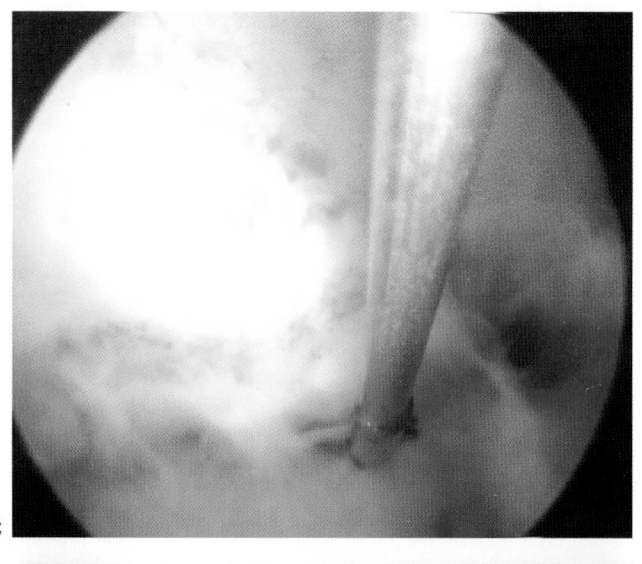

C

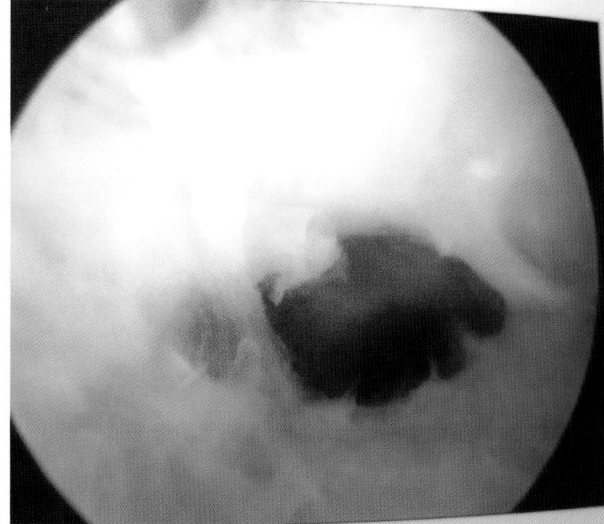

D

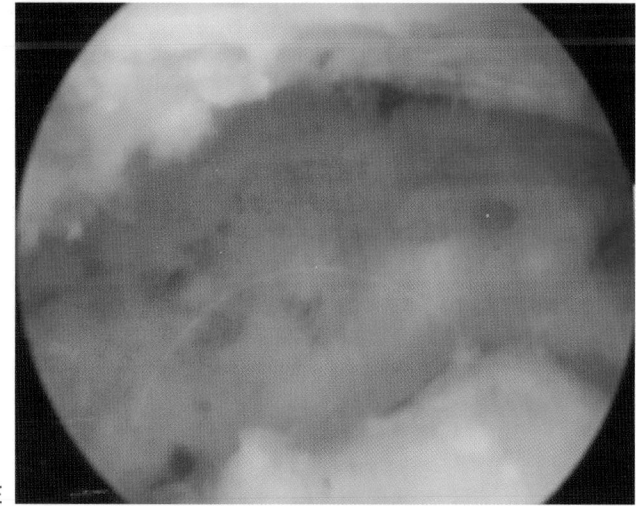

E

III

FIGURE 18.20 (*Continued*) **C:** Incision moving laterally. **D:** Opening into the upper/superior portion of the uterine cavity now visualized. **E:** Complete visualization of the newly opened intrauterine cavity.

way of a Y-adapter on the end of the cannula, engaged into the tubal ostium, and gently advanced into the tube. When the cornual portion of the tube is negotiated or when resistance is encountered, the guide wire is withdrawn and indigo carmine dye injected through the 3-F catheter. Simultaneous laparoscopy allows one to see the dye exit the fimbriated end of the tube and confirm patency. Alternatively, one can place a radiologic plate beneath the patient and inject opaque dye (Fig. 18.22).

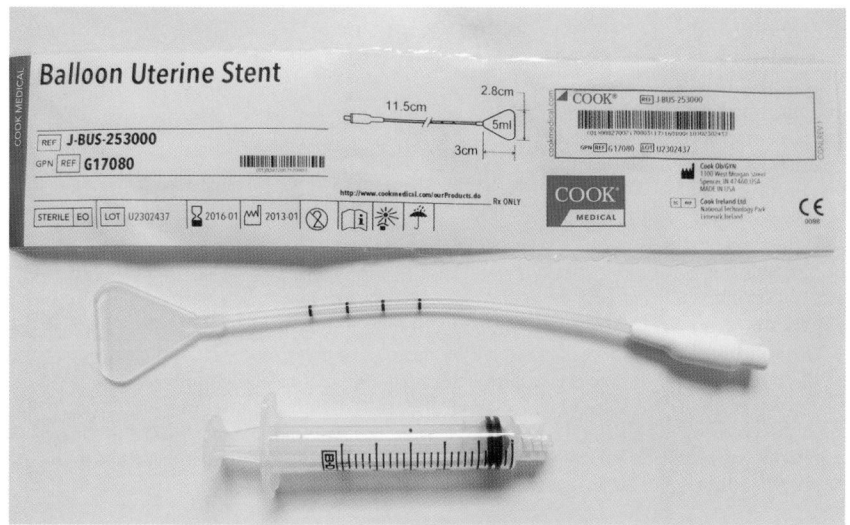

FIGURE 18.21 This specially designed balloon may be placed within the uterine cavity. Uninflated, it can be used to prevent formation of adhesions following hysteroscopic lysis of adhesions. When inflated, it can be used to tamponade bleeding from the uterine wall. The intrauterine pressure will usually control bleeding. A 10-mL Foley catheter (balloon inflated to 5 mL) may be used for this same purpose.

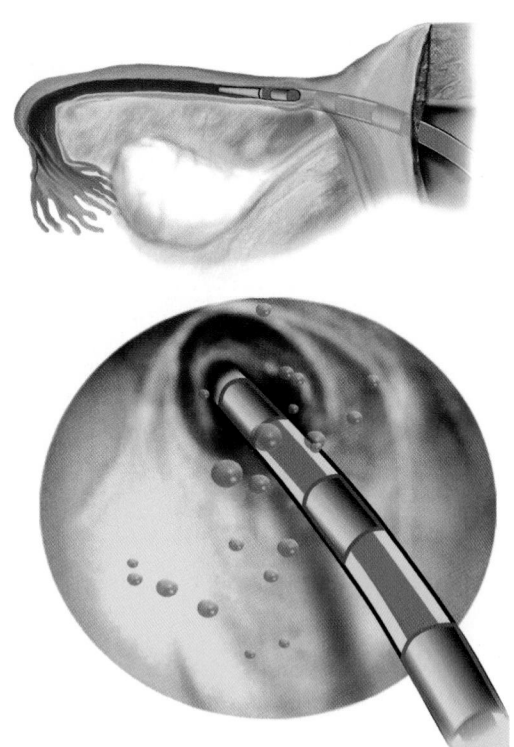

FIGURE 18.22 An inner guide wire is inserted via direct hysteroscopic view into the tubal ostium and advanced. An outer cannula is then advanced over the guide wire. Indigo carmine may be injected to demonstrate tube patency to an assistant viewing from above via laparoscopy. (Reprinted from Baggish MS, Valle RF, Guedj H. *Hysteroscopy: Visual perspectives of uterine anatomy, physiology and pathology*, 3rd ed. Philadelphia, PA: Lippincott Williams & Wilkins, 2007, with permission.) Copyright © 2007, Lippincott Williams & Wilkins.)

Uterine Polyps

Functional and nonfunctional polyps are a common cause of abnormal uterine bleeding. Functional polyps tend to be smaller than nonfunctional polyps. If a hysterogram is performed, a focal filling defect will be seen. Diagnosis is directly and readily made by hysteroscopy. Polyps protrude into the endometrial cavity. A functioning polyp has a lining identical to the surrounding endometrium. The nonfunctioning polyp presents as a white protuberance covered with branching surface vessels. Thick-walled vessels are usually seen within the depths of the polyps. Polyps are relatively easy to diagnose and treat. Gebauer and colleagues compared blind removal of uterine polyps (curettage and polyp forceps) with hysteroscopy. Polyps were diagnosed in 43% of cases by curettage. Out of 45 cases in which polyp forceps removed the polyp, remnants of or complete polyps remained in 31 cases. The authors concluded that hysteroscopically controlled polyp extraction was superior to blind techniques.

Endometrial polyps secondary to tamoxifen therapy in women undergoing treatment for breast cancer is a problem for which hysteroscopy may prove to be indispensable. Taponeco and colleagues reported on 414 breast cancer patients who underwent hysteroscopy (334 treated with tamoxifen and 80 controls). Significant differences were found in malignant (7.8%) and atypical (9%) hyperplastic polyps between the treated group versus controls (0 cases). The authors recommended that hysteroscopy and biopsy should be performed on any woman receiving tamoxifen who reports uterine bleeding.

Garuti and colleagues compared the accuracy of blind sampling of the endometrium versus hysteroscopically directed biopsies in postmenopausal women receiving tamoxifen for breast cancer. The authors reported a sensitivity and negative predictive value of 100% with each technique. However, the specificity (80% versus 68%) and positive predictive value (69% versus 43%) were better for hysteroscopic versus blind sampling.

Hysteroscopic Technique

A multichannel operating hysteroscope is inserted into the uterine cavity, and a retractable electric snare loop is inserted through the 3-mm channel of the operating sheath. The polyp is encircled by the loop such that the loop encompasses the polyp base as it is tightened. The polyp is cut off at the base with 30 to 40 W of power for cutting current. The snare is then removed, and an alligator jaw forceps is inserted. The polyp is grabbed by the forceps. The hysteroscope is withdrawn, removing with it the freed polyp, which is sent to the pathology laboratory for histologic evaluation. The site of removal is inspected again and the procedure terminated. If any bleeding is observed, a 3-mm ball electrode is applied to the site for coagulation (40 to 50 W). Alternatively, a polyp may be cut at its base with a needle electrode or laser fiber. The polyp may also be shaved by means of the resectoscope (**Fig. 18.23**).

Myoma Uteri

Submucous myomas characteristically appear as white spherical masses covered with a network of fragile thin-walled vessels when viewed by hysteroscopy. Myomas typically are sessile or pedunculated. A hysterogram shows a filling defect that is not dissimilar to that produced by a polyp. Unfortunately, blind dilation and curettage is a grossly inaccurate method of diagnosing this disorder. Although subserous and intramural myomas rarely produce alarming symptoms, even when they attain

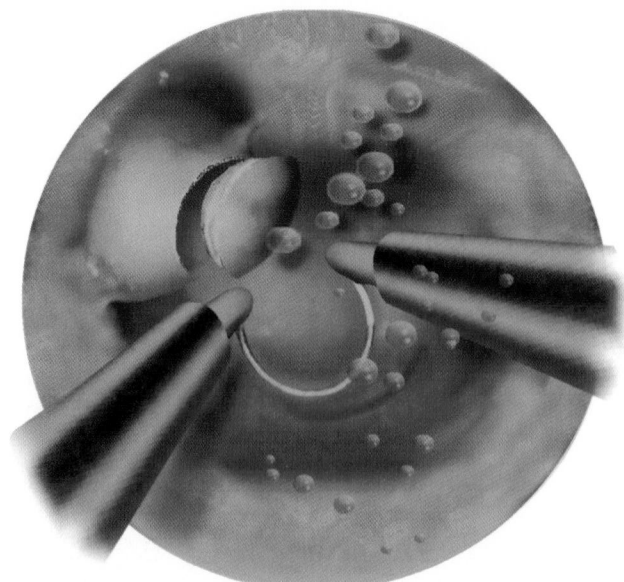

FIGURE 18.23 A functioning polyp on the right corpal wall of the uterus is resected by means of a resectoscopic loop electrode. Note that the technique is the same as the one employed for shaving a submucous myoma. (Reprinted with permission from Baggish MS, Valle RF, Guedj H. *Hysteroscopy: visual perspectives of uterine anatomy, physiology and pathology*, 3rd ed. Philadelphia, PA: Lippincott Williams & Wilkins, 2007, with permission.)

relatively large size, smaller lesions in the submucous location invariably cause considerable bleeding.

In the past, a diagnosis of submucous myoma was usually followed by a recommendation for hysterectomy. Today, hysteroscopic surgery offers a therapeutic alternative to that radical approach. Gonadotropin-releasing hormone (GnRH) analogues such as leuprolide acetate (Lupron) or goserelin acetate (Zoladex) have been recommended as supplementary preoperative medical therapy. The general plan is to treat symptomatic patients for 2 to 3 months preoperatively to reduce the size and vascularity of the lesion during surgery. All patients should be given detailed information concerning the need for typing and holding of blood and the possibility of hysterectomy if intractable bleeding occurs.

Valle in 1990 reported data on 59 cases of abnormal bleeding, dysmenorrhea, and infertility that were diagnosed as submucous myomas. Hysteroscopy eliminated or markedly decreased bleeding in 52 of these cases. In 1989, Baggish and Sze treated 71 patients with symptomatic myomas and four patients with incidental submucous myomas. The treatment methods used with the multichannel hysteroscope were Nd:YAG laser ($n = 41$), monopolar loop ($n = 6$), monopolar needle ($n = 6$), bipolar needles ($n = 10$), and electrosurgery or scissors and laser ($n = 12$). As with Valle's series, results were excellent; 65 of 75 (87%) returned to normal menses postoperatively.

Emanuel and colleagues reported 285 women who underwent hysteroscopic resection of submucous myomas. The median follow-up was approximately 4 years (1 to 104 months), and 85.5% of the operated patients required no further surgery. Clark and associates treated 37 women using the bipolar Versapoint electrode via ablation or excision. Improvement of bleeding symptoms was reported in 78% of the patients, and 92% were satisfied with the treatment. No significant complications were reported.

Hysteroscopic Technique

Several variations of hysteroscopic procedures are now available to manage submucous myomas. Resectoscopic instrumentation has vastly improved in recent years compared with earlier instruments. Self-flushing sheaths, straight and offset cutting loops, and diminished-diameter, low-profile scopes are among these recent improvements. In addition, electrosurgical generators have been modernized and are safer devices than instruments from the 1970s and 1980s. Under video control, the resectoscopic technique consists of progressive shaving of the myoma and harvesting pieces of tissue for subsequent histologic evaluation. For fundal myomas, the straight electrode is the most effective device, whereas the angulated electrode is preferred for lesions located on the anterior or posterior walls (Fig. 18.24A). The electrode should be activated only while returning toward the hysteroscope, never while advancing outward away from the lens. The greatest disadvantage to this technique centers on the need to repeatedly remove the shaved nuggets of tissue (Fig. 18.24).

Other electrosurgical techniques may be employed in conjunction with the large isolated-channel, flushing hysteroscope. Three-mm needles, shaving loops, and bipolar electrodes may be used to perform all of the optional operations described above for the resectoscope (Fig. 18.25). The fine-needle electrode can be substituted for laser fiber to excise pedunculated or section sessile myomas. The 3-mm retractable cutting loop can perform shaving procedures in a fashion similar to that of the resectoscope loop. The bipolar needles can be plunged many times into the substance of the submucous myoma of any size to coagulate the interior of the myoma (myolysis).

If postoperative bleeding occurs, a 10-mL Foley balloon is placed in the cavity and blown up to 5 mL for 6 to 12 hours. If the cavity is large, a 30-mL balloon inflated with 10 to 15 mL of water can be used. Some gynecologic surgeons prefer to do

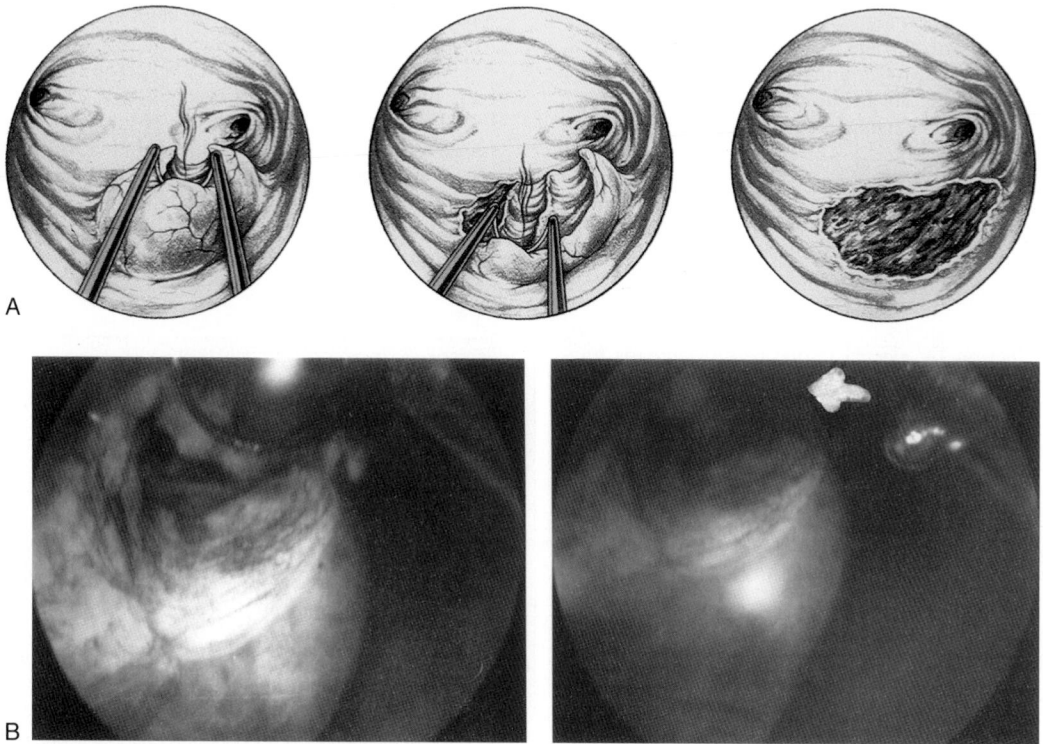

FIGURE 18.24 A: The shaving technique for the elimination of a submucous myoma is shown using an angulated loop electrode via the resectoscope. (Reprinted from Baggish MS, Barbot J, Valle RF. *Diagnostic and operative hysteroscopy*, 2nd ed. St. Louis, MO: Mosby-Year Book, 1999, with permission. Lippincott Williams & Wilkins, 2007.) **B:** A chunk of tissue has been cut out of this myoma. The resectoscopic loop is seen above (**left**). The picture to the right shows the loop extended farther into the cavity (*arrow*).

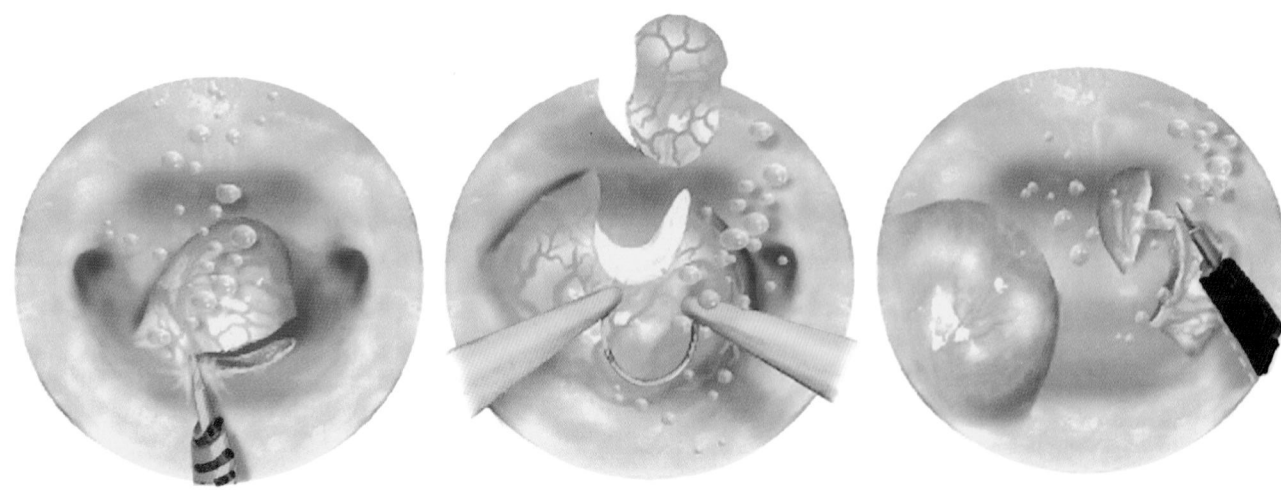

A. Laser fiber   B. Bipolar electrode   C. Electrosurgical needle

FIGURE 18.25 A–C: Several techniques and instruments may be used to deal with submucous myomas. **A:** shows a laser fiber within an irrigation cannula cutting a myoma at its base. **B:** shows an electrode shaving a myoma. **C:** shows an electrosurgical needle cleaving a piece of a submucous myoma. (Reprinted from Baggish MS, Valle RF, Guedj H. *Hysteroscopy: visual perspectives of uterine anatomy, physiology and pathology*, 3rd ed. Philadelphia, PA: Lippincott Williams & Wilkins, 2007, with permission.)

a simultaneous laparoscopy when large myomas (3 to 5 cm) are resected and extracted. Regardless of myoma size, a simultaneous laparoscopy should be performed whenever concern for perforation exists. The central fundal myoma is associated with the greatest risk of uterine perforation.

Reports caution that uterine rupture can occur during pregnancy after hysteroscopic myomectomy. This is particularly the case when the operator attempts to resect the intramural portion of the submucous myoma. As such, patients should inform their obstetricians of a history of a hysteroscopic myomectomy in the event they become pregnant. Regarding risk of malignancy from submucosal fibroids, the risk of leiomyosarcoma is less than 1%. Nevertheless, any myoma or part of a myoma that is excised should be sent to the pathology laboratory for evaluation. This, of course, includes resectoscopic fragments.

Sterilization

Surgical methods of performing female sterilization from tubal ligation to total salpingectomy are discussed in other chapters of this book. These methods are well established and in widespread use with low failure rates. Attempts to perform female sterilization hysteroscopically using plugs or causing proximal obstruction by electrical or chemical means have been attempted in the past. High complication and failure rates resulted in cessation of their use. In November 2002, the Food and Drug administration (FDA) approved the use of the Essure microinsert, which is inserted hysteroscopically. Essure is widely used today. A detailed description of the Essure microinserts and the technique for placing them via hysteroscopy can be found in Chapter 27 of this text.

Endometrial Ablation

Since the first practical method of hysteroscopic ablation was described in 1981, several thousand cases have been performed by a variety of techniques, including the Nd:YAG laser, the resectoscopic roller ball or loop, and, most recently, the long hysteroscopic ball electrodes. Garry and associates in 1995 reported 600 endometrial laser ablations performed on 524 women. No major operative morbidity was reported. The success rate (mean age, 43 years) was 83.4%. Baggish and Sze have performed 568 ablations; 401 of these were performed

with the Nd:YAG laser and 167 by electrosurgery. Excellent results were obtained in 89% of the women treated, and amenorrhea was achieved in 58%. Again, no major operative complications were observed. Magos and coworkers reported 250 cases of endometrial resection with a 92% improvement in abnormal bleeding. However, data obtained from the Royal College of Obstetricians and Gynaecologists' MISTLETOE (Minimally Invasive Surgical Technique—Laser, Endothermal, or Endoresection) Study in 1997 revealed a 6.4% rate of significant complications associated with endometrial resection alone and a rate of 11.4/1,000 with emergency hysterectomy. This compares with complication rates of 2.7% and 2.1% for laser and rollerball, respectively. The latter two techniques had emergency hysterectomy rates of 1.3/1,000 (i.e., 11 times less than endometrial resection). Nonhysteroscopic minimally invasive techniques for endometrial ablation have emerged in recent years and replaced hysteroscopic endometrial ablation in most settings. These techniques, which include thermal balloon ablation, microwave endometrial ablation, and radiofrequency electromagnetic energy, are reviewed in detail in Chapter 26.

Hysteroscopic Technique

STEPS IN THE PROCEDURE

Operative Hysteroscopy

- Patient in lithotomy position.
- Bimanual examination: uterus anteverted or retroverted.
- Position fluid collection bag under the buttocks.
- Prior to starting, verify the following: hysteroscope assembly and outflow inflow tubes correctly connected, light cord and camera attached to telescope, and white balance.
- Verify correct distention media.
- Verify pressure, flow, and fluid deficit alarm settings on automated pump delivery system.
- Cervix visualized with bivalve speculum or Sims retractor.

- Tenaculum applied to the anterior lip of the cervix.

- Dilation of cervix, if required (dilation not required for diagnostic scope); do not overdilate.

- Place hysteroscope in external os, with distention media flowing; insert under direct visualization; countertraction applied using tenaculum (verify that inflow valve is open and outflow valve is closed).

- Once inside uterine cavity, remove speculum or Sims retractor with the hysteroscope in place; verify/orient position by identifying the tubal ostia.

- Insert operative instruments (must have rubber stopper over port prior to opening instrument port valve); maintain the distal end of the hysteroscope in constant visualization while inserting the instrument.

- Operative portion: If visualization is cloudy, open outflow valve to clear, then reclose; may leave slightly open for fluid circulation if necessary.

- Attempt to only touch intrauterine walls when necessary to avoid bleeding, which will cloud the field.

- Check fluid deficit: Approximately every 5 minutes, halt procedure at a deficit of 1000–1500 mL (hypoosmolar) or 2,500 mL (isoosmolar) depending on distention media used.

- Termination of procedure: fluid deficit calculated and recorded in operative notes/dictation.

All patients who might be candidates for endometrial ablation should have been managed first by hormonal treatment in an attempt to control the abnormal uterine bleeding. If this strategy fails, and if the woman does not desire to bear children, then she is a candidate for endometrial ablation. A preoperative diagnostic hysteroscopy, endometrial sampling, or both should be performed to exclude endometrial carcinoma or atypical hyperplasia, and all pertinent hematologic studies and consultations should be performed. All patients are pretreated to atrophy the endometrium with medication such as a GnRH agonist.

A simultaneous laparoscopy is not performed during endometrial ablation unless a perforation or other transmural injury is suspected. Depending on the technique selected, either 5% mannitol or 0.9% saline is used as the distending medium. The operating hysteroscope or resectoscope is inserted into the uterine cavity. One method to treat the fundus is by dragging the laser fiber or the ball electrode from side to side (cornu to cornu) (Fig. 18.26A). The anterior and lateral walls are ablated next, before the posterior wall. Ablation should not be extended below the internal os into the cervix (Fig. 18.26B). Power settings for the electrosurgical generator range from 50 to 150 W, depending on the size of the ball, barrel, or loop electrode (Figs. 18.27 and 18.28). Laser power is set at 40 to 60 W. The goal of the ablation operation is to destroy the visible endometrium, including the cornual endometrium, to a depth of 1 to 2 mm. The conduction heat will actually spread deeper, usually to 3 to 5 mm, depending on how long the device remains on the tissue. This penetration translates into extensive superficial myometrial destruction and coagulation of the radial branches of the uterine cavity

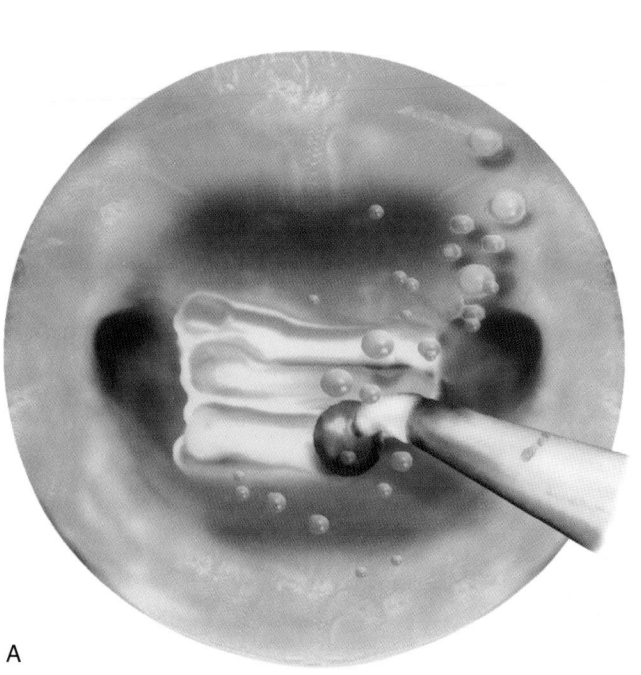

A

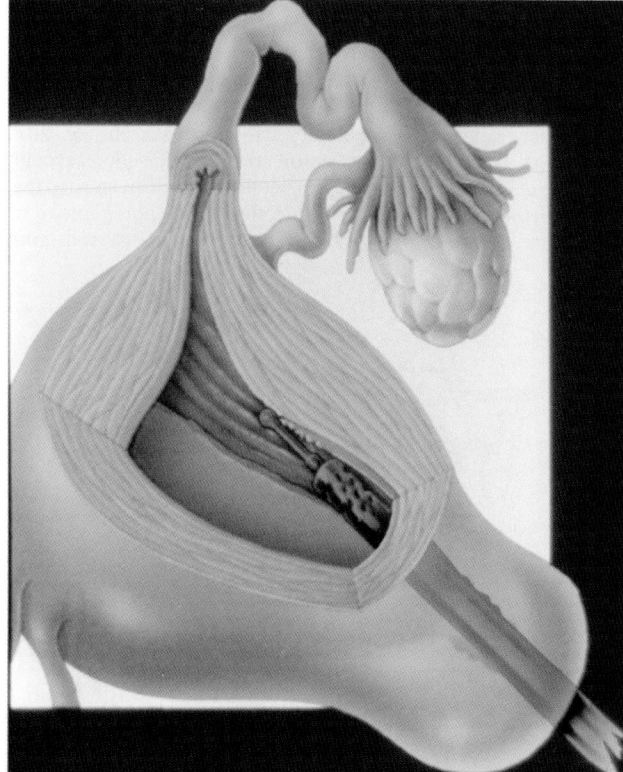

B

FIGURE 18.26 A: The ball electrode is dragged from side to side via moving the entire hysteroscope, thereby ablating the uterine fundus. **B:** The anterior and posterior walls are ablated by dragging the energized ball electrode from above downward. This creates 2- to 3-mm furrows in the endometrium. Conduction heat damage can extend another 1 to 2 mm. (Reprinted from Baggish MS, Valle RF, Guedj H. *Hysteroscopy: visual perspectives of uterine anatomy, physiology and pathology*, 3rd ed. Philadelphia, PA: Lippincott Williams & Wilkins, 2007, with permission.)

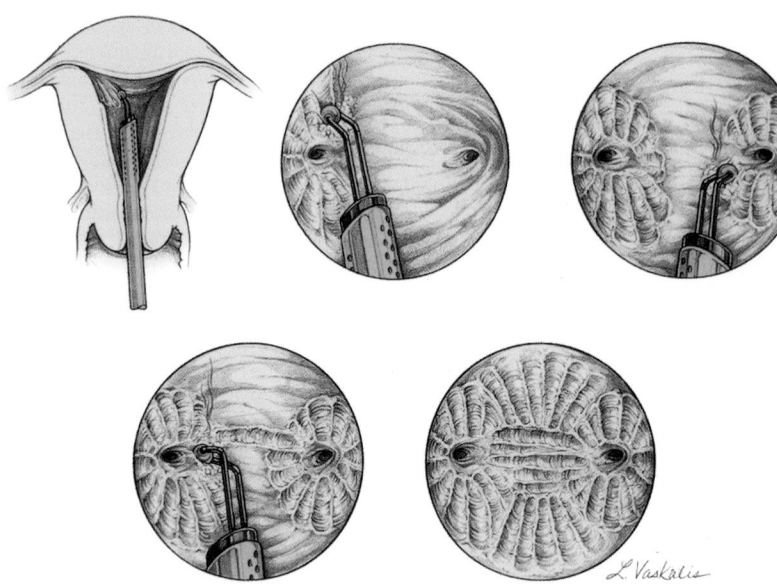

FIGURE 18.27 The resectoscope with ball electrode attached is inserted into the uterine cavity. Initially, the cornu and fundus are carefully ablated, taking care to keep dwell time low to reduce the risk of deep heat conduction injury. Next, the anterior wall is ablated, followed by the posterior wall. (Reprinted from Baggish MS, Valle RF, Guedj H. *Hysteroscopy: Visual perspectives of uterine anatomy, physiology and pathology*, 3rd ed. Philadelphia, PA: Lippincott Williams & Wilkins, 2007, with permission.)

(Fig. 18.29). When the endometrium sloughs, regeneration is prevented because basal and spiral arterioles do not survive the 100°C heat exposure. Over a period of 6 to 8 weeks, the uterine walls scar and shrink. Subsequent sampling or hysteroscopy is possible after endometrial ablation (Fig. 18.30). The mean duration of the operation is about 30 minutes. Patients usually are sent home on the day of surgery. The operation is usually completed with little or no blood loss.

Miscellaneous Procedures

Intrauterine Device Removal

The gynecologist is occasionally called to search for and remove an IUD with an indicator string that is not seen in the cervix. In such circumstances, the operating hysteroscope is a vital tool with which to locate the device and remove it under direct visualization. The hysteroscope is inserted, and

the device is viewed. If a string is seen, an alligator jaw forceps is inserted, and the string is grasped. The hysteroscope is withdrawn, pulling the device through the uterine cavity and the cervix to the exterior. If the IUD is embedded, then a rigid grasping forceps is required. The IUD is located, and the large jaws of the rigid instrument grab the extruded portion of the IUD itself. Strong pressure is exerted on the jaws as the sheath of the hysteroscope is slowly withdrawn from the uterus, into the cervix, and out of the vagina.

Biopsy of Intrauterine Lesions

When a tumor is suspected, the operative hysteroscope is inserted into the cavity, a 9-F biopsy forceps is directed to the tumor site, and multiple biopsy specimens are obtained in a fashion analogous to that used with colposcopic biopsies. A 9-F plastic cannula is inserted by way of the operating channel, and strong suction is applied to the mouth of the cannula

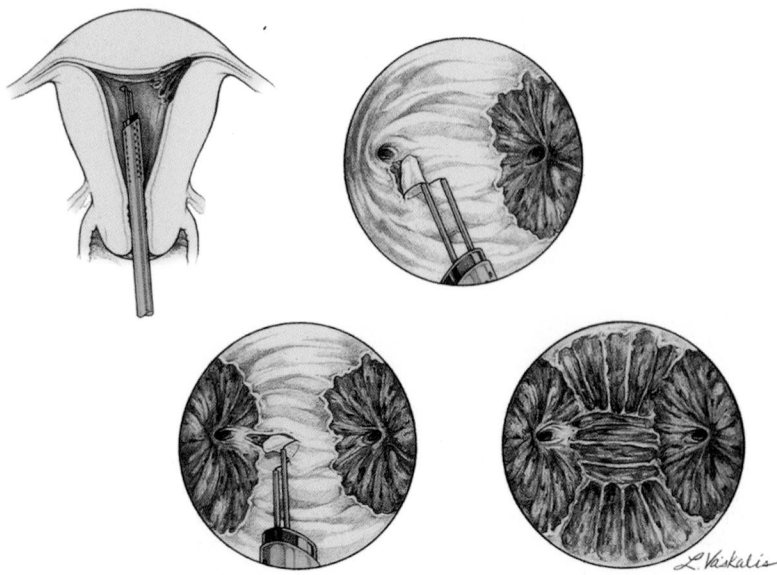

FIGURE 18.28 Endometrial resection is performed in a manner similar to ablation; however, instead of a ball electrode, a cutting loop is substituted. This is clearly a riskier procedure compared with ablation by either laser or ball electrode, particularly relative to deep myometrial resection with the accompanying risks of hemorrhage and/or perforation. (Reprinted from Baggish MS, Valle RF, Guedj H. *Hysteroscopy: visual perspectives of uterine anatomy, physiology and pathology*, 3rd ed. Philadelphia, PA: Lippincott Williams & Wilkins, 2007, with permission.)

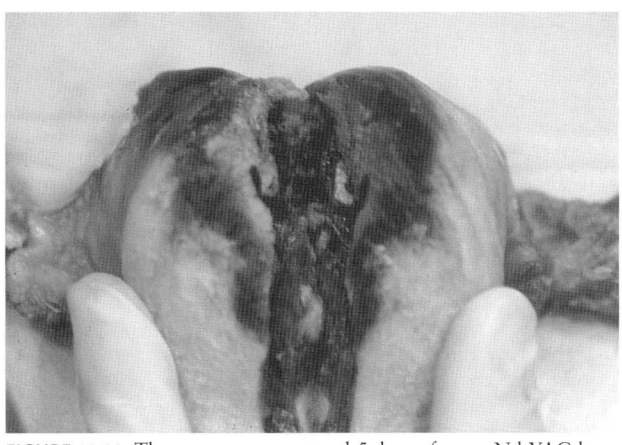

FIGURE 18.29 The uterus was removed 5 days after an Nd:YAG laser ablation. Note the extensive laser injury involving about half the thickness of the myometrium. Laser penetration depends not only on power but also on the length of time the laser beam remains in contact with the tissue.

by means of a 30-mL syringe. The cannula is removed, and the contents are flushed out with saline into a bottle of fixative. Similarly, a 9-F curette can be inserted under direct vision. Alternatively, a diagnostic hysteroscope can be inserted into the uterus. The site of pathology is noted. The endoscope is withdrawn, a Novak curette is inserted into the cavity, and biopsy specimens are taken at the previously located site. Finally, the hysteroscope is pulled back to the level of the internal cervical os, a small Novak curette is inserted alongside the hysteroscope, and a directed biopsy specimen is obtained.

COMPLICATIONS

Unfortunately, accurate data concerning complications are hard to obtain. As greater numbers of gynecologists have begun to perform operative hysteroscopy, the rate of complications has increased. Complications include bleeding, uterine perforation, creation of false passages, and excess fluid absorption and subsequent pathologic responses. Propst and colleagues reviewed data on 925 women who had hysteroscopies. Operative complications occurred in 2.7% of patients.

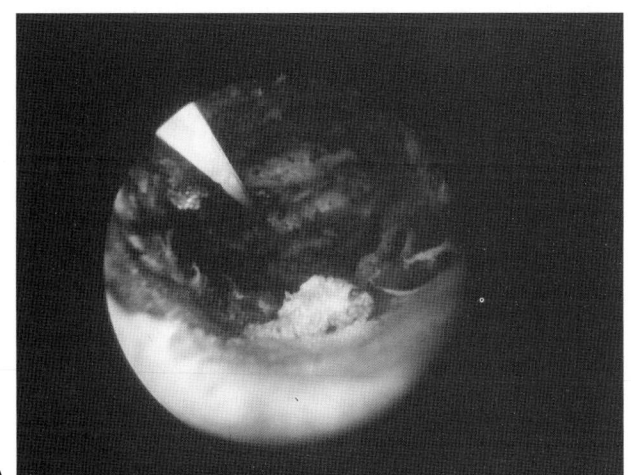

A

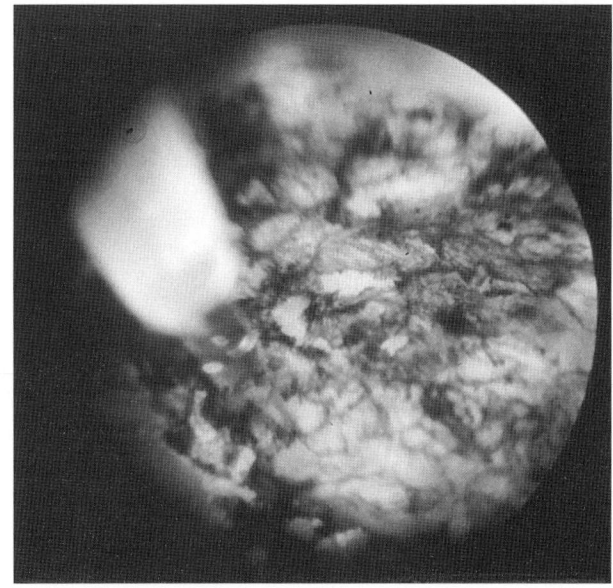

B

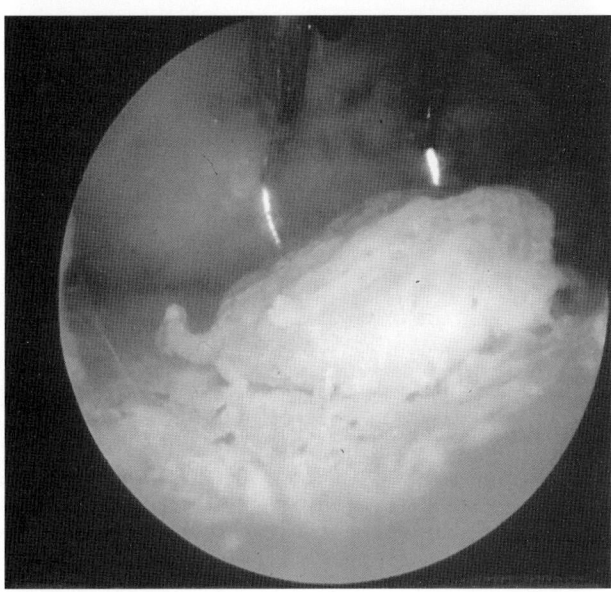

C

FIGURE 18.30 A: Complete destruction of the endometrium has been afflicted by means of Nd:YAG laser ablation. The fiber is seen at the 11 o'clock position. **B:** Close-up view of ablated endometrium shown in part A. Note the laser fiber to the left. **C:** Endometrial resection is performed via a shaving technique utilizing the resectoscope.

Excessive fluid absorption was the most common complication. Myomectomy and resection of uterine septum had greatest odds for complication (odds ratio [OR] 7.4).

Intraoperative and Postoperative Bleeding

The most common complications inherent to hysteroscopic surgical procedures are intraoperative and postoperative bleeding. Intraoperative bleeding can be managed by aspirating the blood and by increasing the pressure of the distending medium so that it exceeds arterial pressure and compresses the walls of the uterus sufficiently to stop bleeding. The bleeding vessel may then be coagulated with a 3-mm ball electrode and the use of forced coagulation at 30 to 40 W of power or by multiple jabs with bipolar needles at 20 to 30 W of power with the generator set for automatic bipolar. If the counterpressure of the medium is relaxed (at the termination of the procedure) and bleeding continues, then control is best obtained by inserting an intrauterine balloon initially inflated to 2 to 5 mL. If this pressure does not promptly stop the bleeding, then a larger balloon can be distended to 10 mL until the bleeding has stopped (Fig. 18.21). More distension may be required for larger uteri. Care must be taken because overinflation of an intrauterine balloon can itself rupture the uterus. The balloon remains in place for 6 to 8 hours, is partially deflated for 6 hours, and, finally, is totally deflated before removal. When the bleeding is pulsatile, the source is arterial rather than venous. If this type of bleeding is not immediately controlled by balloon compression, then emergent hysterectomy or uterine artery embolization will usually be required. Delayed postoperative bleeding is most commonly associated with endometrial slough (after ablation), chronic endometritis, or spontaneous extrusion and expulsion of the intramyometrial portion of a previously resected submucous myoma. Bleeding–clotting studies should be obtained in cases of late postoperative bleeding, particularly if these studies were not performed preoperatively in women with a diagnosis of abnormal uterine bleeding (preoperative endometrial ablation or myomectomy).

A French group in 2003 prospectively studied a decade of operative hysteroscopies (2,116 cases). Thirteen cases of major bleeding were reported, with six requiring intrauterine catheter placements. The highest-risk procedure for associated hemorrhage was hysteroscopic adhesiolysis.

Uterine Perforation

Uterine perforation can occur during any operative hysteroscopy procedure but is most common during septum resection, myomectomy, and lysis of adhesions. The best insurance against this complication is simultaneous laparoscopy. Among novice operators, perforation can occur even during insertion of the hysteroscope. With appropriate care, this sort of perforation should not happen, because the cervix and internal os should be negotiated under direct visualization, and the cavity should likewise be entered under direct visualization. Examination under anesthesia is also simple and lets the operator know the direction of the uterine axis.

As we noted above, the most dangerous perforations are those associated with lasers and electrosurgical devices. The risk of this type of injury can be reduced by not activating the energy device during a thrusting or forward movement. The foot pedal is activated only during the return phase of the laser fiber or electrosurgical electrode. If a perforation does happen with an energy device, then laparotomy or laparoscopy is required to ensure that no injury has been inflicted on the intestine, bladder, or ureter (Fig. 18.31).

A risk of perforation is associated with the septum transection in its final phase at the level of the uterine fundus because the operator may have some difficulty determining

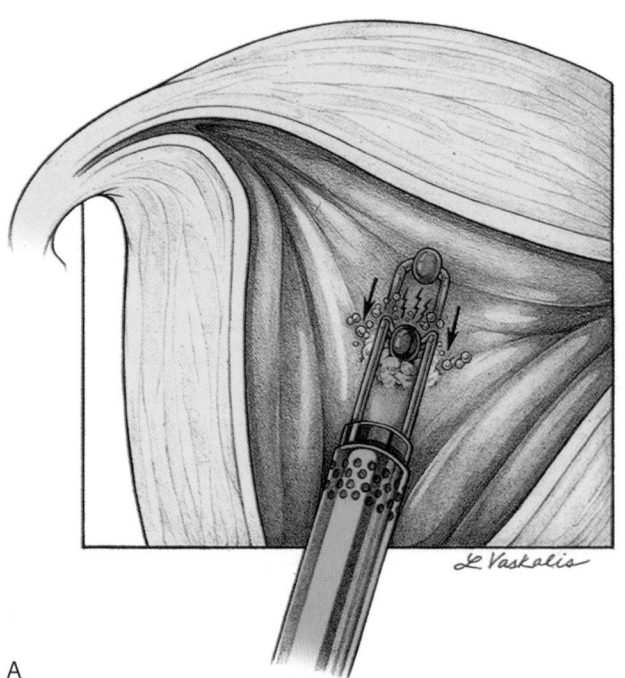

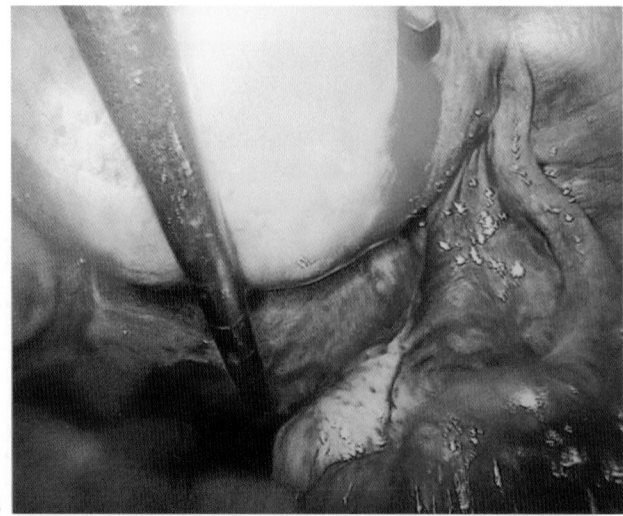

FIGURE 18.31 A: The operator should never apply power to an energy device while advancing the electrode. The power can safely be applied as the electrode returns toward the sheath. (Reprinted from Baggish MS, Valle RF, Guedj H. *Hysteroscopy: Visual perspectives of uterine anatomy, physiology and pathology*, 3rd ed. Philadelphia, PA: Lippincott Williams & Wilkins, 2007, with permission.) **B:** Laparoscopic image of a uterine perforation that occurred while using the hysteroscopic resection loop.

where the septum ends and the myometrium begins. This risk is constant regardless of the cutting instrument used. The operator rapidly becomes aware that uterine perforation has occurred because distention becomes difficult to maintain and the flow of the distending medium exits at the perforation site (Fig. 18.32). An alert assistant viewing by laparoscope should warn the hysteroscopist of impending perforation the moment an increasing intensity of light transmission through the thinning uterine wall is observed. If perforation is unnoticed and if simultaneous laparoscopy is not performed, a serious complication is even possible with a nonenergy instrument, but this is far less common than those occurring with lasers or electrodes. Nevertheless, if a perforation is suspected, that patient should be carefully observed in the hospital. Injuries to the iliac vessels can occur as the result of uterine perforation. An unexplained falling blood pressure, together with medium leakage, should alert the surgeon to this possibility. Perforation of the uterus during hysteroscopy can place a woman at an increased risk for uterine rupture during a future pregnancy.

As uterine perforation often occurs during the dilation prior to actually placing the hysteroscope, there has been much interest in optimizing the dilatation process to avoid perforation and other complications such as creating a false passage and cervical laceration. Use of misoprostol, a synthetic prostaglandin E_1, has been studied extensively as a cervical dilator prior to hysteroscopy to prevent complications associated with dilatation. A 2011 systemic review by Selk and Kroft did not rule out a beneficial effect of misoprostol on cervical dilation or surgical complications in operative hysteroscopy, but the authors were unable to conclude that evidence currently supports the routine use of misoprostol prior to hysteroscopy.

Management of Fluid Overload

Fluid overload associated with hysteroscopy is rare, with 1 study of 21,676 patients reporting the complication in 0.02% of cases. However, the pathophysiologic ramifications for the patient can be severe and life-threatening. Therefore, the gynecologic surgeon must be vigilant in preventing this important complication. The risk of complications varies with the distention medium.

Methods to prevent fluid overload include the following: (a) Use isotonic fluids such as normal saline whenever possible, (b) monitor the fluid deficit closely, (c) maintain intrauterine fluid pressure at 70 to 80 mm Hg, and (d) limit surgical operating time to 1 hour or less. Serious complications due to hyponatremia have been reported from use of hypoosmolar fluids such as sorbitol and glycine. For instance, absorption of 1,000 mL of glycine distension medium during hysteroscopy is associated with a reduction in serum sodium of approximately 10 mEq/L. The American Congress of Obstetricians and Gynecologists' Committee on Gynecologic Practice recommends termination of a case with a deficit of 750 mL with hypoosmolar fluids when patient is elderly or has comorbid conditions. The case should be terminated for a deficit of 1,000 to 1,500 mL for all other patients. When an isotonic distension medium is used, the case should be terminated when the deficit reaches 2,500 mL. With this finding, in addition to terminating the case, a stat sodium level should be sent and patient should be administered a loop diuretic such as furosemide. Severe hyponatremia should be managed in cooperation with an intensive care specialist; the patient should be very closely monitored and may require hypertonic saline.

Poor Visibility in the Operative Field

Inability to see the operative field is a common problem. The usual cause of this problem is deep insertion of the hysteroscope so that the telescope lies directly in contact with the endometrium. The surgeon will see nothing but a red blur. The natural tendency is to push the hysteroscope deeper in. This strategic mistake invariably leads to perforation. Another cause of visibility problems is blood within the uterine cavity secondary to dilatation. The fastest way to deal with a bloody cavity is rapid flushing with the hysteroscopic medium combined with aspiration using a cannula placed into the cavity via the operating channel.

Overdilatation of the cervix is an equally common mistake that results in excessive leakage of distending medium and an inability to maintain distension, with the resultant inability to perform the operative hysteroscopy. Blood and debris can cloud the field to such a degree that accurate operative endoscopy is impossible. If the operator cannot clearly see the field, it is better to discontinue the procedure rather than press on

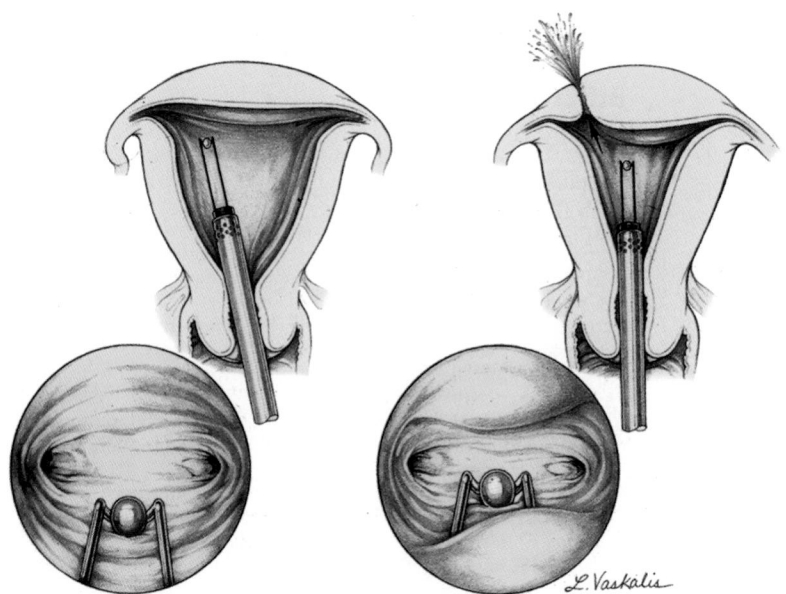

FIGURE 18.32 Perforation should be immediately suspected when the endometrial cavity depressurizes and collapses around the hysteroscope, creating a compromised view of the cavity. (Baggish MS, Valle RF, Guedj H. *Hysteroscopy: visual perspectives of uterine anatomy, physiology and pathology*, 3rd ed. Philadelphia, PA: Lippincott Williams & Wilkins, 2007, with permission.)

and risk a catastrophic error. It is easy to become disoriented in the uterine cavity if normal anatomic landmarks cannot be recognized.

Gas Embolus

Gas embolism is a well-documented complication of operative hysteroscopy using CO_2 as the distending medium, with a 0.51% incidence of subclinical events and a 0.03% incidence of symptomatic events in a review of 3,932 cases by Brandner et al. As previously mentioned, a fatal CO_2 gas embolism is especially likely to occur if a laparoscopic CO_2 insufflator is connected to the diagnostic hysteroscope.

Air embolism may also occur commonly during operative hysteroscopy when fluid distending media are used, with an incidence from 10% to 50% having been reported. Differences in incidence rates are most likely due to differences in methods used to detect embolization. Methods include noticing a decrease in end-tidal CO_2, which is not very specific, and detecting a mill-wheel murmur. Transesophageal echocardiography appears to be the most sensitive and specific monitoring method. Introduction of ambient air into the uterine cavity by repeated passes of the hysteroscope or by creation of vapors by use of electrosurgery is thought to be responsible for causing air emboli. Air then passes into venous sinuses of the uterus either passively or actively from the pressure of the liquid media. If a gas embolism is suspected, the procedure should be stopped immediately. Avoiding the Trendelenburg position during operative hysteroscopy has been suggested to decrease the risk of gas embolism.

Infection

Infection is an unlikely complication associated with hysteroscopy. Hysteroscopy should be avoided in the presence of gross cervical infection, uterine infection, or salpingitis. Infection is otherwise uncommon after even extensive intrauterine surgery (e.g., adhesiotomy or myomectomy). Prophylactic antibiotics should be administered only when indications exist such as a history of rheumatic carditis, congenital heart defect, or prolapsed mitral valve or in cases of suspected chronic endometritis (submucous myoma or imbedded IUD). Baggish and colleagues in 1999 observed only 13 infections out of 5,000 cases that could be casually related to the hysteroscopic operation. Salat-Baroux and associates reported 7 mild infections out of 4,000 hysteroscopic examinations. On the other hand, McCausland and coworkers reported three cases of tuboovarian abscess after operative hysteroscopy. Agostini and colleagues reported 30 infections associated with 2,116 operative hysteroscopies. Eighteen of these infections were cases of endometritis.

Operator Technique

The most serious complications happen because of operator error. Most often, these are the result of inexperience and are avoidable. Difficult cases beyond the capabilities of the primary care gynecologist should be referred to the expert hysteroscopist. Skill in one area of endoscopy (e.g., operative laparoscopy) does not confer similar expertise in operative hysteroscopy. Indeed, the opposite may be truer.

During the postoperative period, operative complications should be the initial exclusion diagnosis for any patient who is not recovering according to the usual pattern. Worsening postoperative pain, fever, nausea, distension, and free intraperitoneal air are the signals of bowel injury. Diminished urinary output, fever, and distension suggest bladder or ureteral trauma. Falling blood pressure and rapid thready pulse, with or without distension, should raise concerns of a vascular problem and third-space hemorrhage.

Most negligence cases adjudicated in favor of the plaintiff have involved delayed initiation of appropriate treatment for an operative complication. Cases involving injury recognized at the time of surgery and correctly managed in a timely fashion do not usually become medicolegal problems.

Equipment Failure

As previously reviewed in this chapter, diagnostic and operative hysteroscopic procedures utilize complex equipment requiring attention for correct instrument assembly, connection to electrical or laser energy sources as well as connections to video cameras and monitors for proper administration of distending media. In a recent prospective observation study by Courdier, equipment failures were divided into four categories: imaging, transmission of fluids and light, the electric circuit, and surgical instruments. During 51 operative hysteroscopies, 37.3% (19) were complicated by equipment failures. Most common problems included nonavailable or damaged hysteroscopic connections and fittings, faulty connections, or an incorrect setting of the suction system. Surgeon error and staff error contributed to many of the documented errors. Surgeons performing diagnostic and operative hysteroscopy should be able to assemble and disassemble the hysteroscopic instruments, be able to connect and activate the video monitoring systems, and be capable of operating the hysteroscopic fluid monitoring systems. Creation of checklists for surgeons and assistants to review prior to performing the hysteroscopic procedure may be of value.

BEST SURGICAL PRACTICES

- Abnormal uterine bleeding is most comprehensively evaluated by hysteroscopy and sampling as opposed to blind curettage.
- A gynecologist or gynecologist-in-training can best learn hysteroscopy by performing 25 to 50 diagnostic hysteroscopies before initiating operative procedures.
- Infusion of liquid, low-viscosity media during operative hysteroscopy must be accurately measured and recorded, especially hypoosmolar media such as glycine or sorbitol.
- Perforation during operative hysteroscopy with an energy device requires laparotomy to inspect intraabdominal structures for thermal injury.
- A clear, unobstructed view of the intrauterine milieu is necessary before the initiation of any endouterine surgery.

BIBLIOGRAPHY

AAGL Advancing Minimally Invasive Gynecology Worldwide; Munro MG, Storz K, Abbott JA, et al. AAGL Practice Report: Practice Guidelines for the Management of Hysteroscopic Distending Media. *J Minim Invasive Gynecol* 2013;20:137.

Aberdeen Endometrial Ablation Trials Group. A randomized trial of endometrial ablation versus hysterectomy for the treatment of dysfunctional uterine bleeding: outcome at four years. *Br J Obstet Gynaecol* 1999;106:360.

Agostini A, Cravello L, Desbriere R, et al. Hemorrhage risk during operative laparoscopy. *Acta Obstet Gynecol Scand* 2002;81:878.

Agostini A, Cravello L, Shojai R, et al. Postoperative infection and surgical hysteroscopy. *Fertil Steril* 2002;77:766.

Alborzi S, Dehbashi S, Parsanezhad ME. Differential diagnosis of septate and bicornuate uterus by sonohysterography eliminates the need for laparoscopy. *Fertil Steril* 2002;78:176.

Aydeniz B, Gruber IV, Schauf B, et al. A multicenter survey of complications associated with 21,676 operative hysteroscopies. *Eur J Obstet Gynecol Reprod Biol* 2002;104:160.

Baggish MS, Barbot J, Valle RF. *Diagnostic and operative hysteroscopy: a text and atlas.* Chicago, IL: Mosby-Year Book, 1989.

Baggish MS, Barbot J, Valle RF. *Diagnostic and operative hysteroscopy*, 2nd ed. St. Louis, MO: Mosby-Year Book, 1999, Lippincott Williams & Wilkins, 2007.

Baggish MS, Brill AI, Rosenzweig B, et al. Fatal acute glycine and sorbitol toxicity during operative hysteroscopy. *J Gynecol Surg* 1993;9:137.

Baggish MS, Sze EHM. Experience with 568 endometrial ablation procedures. *J Gynecol Surg* 1996;174:908.

Baggish MS, Sze EHM, Morgan G. Hysteroscopic treatment of symptomatic submucous myomata uteri with the Nd-YAG laser. *J Gynecol Surg* 1989;5:127.

Baggish MS, Valle RF, Guedj H. *Hysteroscopy: visual perspectives of uterine anatomy, physiology and pathology*, 3rd ed. Philadelphia, PA: Lippincott Williams & Wilkins, 2007.

Brink DM, DeJong P, Fawcus S, et al. Carbon dioxide embolism following diagnostic hysteroscopy. *Br J Obstet Gynaecol* 1994;101:717.

Brandner P, Neis KJ, Ehmer C. The etiology, frequency, and prevention of gas embolism during CO(2) hysteroscopy. *J Am Assoc Gynecol Laparosc* 1999;6:421.

Brundin J, Thomasson K. Cardiac gas embolism during carbon dioxide hysteroscopy: risk and management. *Eur J Obstet Gynecol Reprod Biol* 1989;33:241.

Cameron IM, Mollison J, Pinion SB, et al. A cost comparison of hysterectomy and hysteroscopic surgery for the treatment of menorrhagia. *Eur J Obstet Gynecol Reprod Biol* 1996;70:87.

Capella-Allouc S, Morsad F, Rongieres-Bertrand C, et al. Hysteroscopic treatment of severe Asherman's syndrome and subsequent fertility. *Human Reprod* 1999;14:1230.

Cararach M, Penella J, Ubeda A, et al. Hysteroscopic incision of the septate uterus: scissors versus resectoscope. *Hum Reprod* 1994;9:87.

Ceci O, Bettocchi S, Marello F, et al. Hysteroscopic evaluation of the endometrium in postmenopausal women taking tamoxifen. *J Am Assoc Gynecol Laparosc* 2000;7:185.

Christianson MS, Barker MA, Lindheim SR. Overcoming the challenging cervix: techniques to access the uterine cavity. *J Low Genit Tract Dis* 2008;12:24.

Clark TJ, Mahajan D, Sunder P, et al. Hysteroscopic treatment of symptomatic submucous fibroids using a bipolar intrauterine system: a feasibility study. *Eur J Obstet Gyn Reprod Biol* 2002;100:237.

Corson SL, Brooks PG, Soderstrom RM. Gynecologic endoscopic gas embolism. *Fertil Steril* 1996;65:529.

Courdier S, Garbin O, Hummel M, et al. Equipment failure: causes and consequences in endoscopic gynecologic surgery. *J Minim Invasive Gynecol* 2009;16:28.

Creinin M, Chen M. Uterine defect in a twin pregnancy with a history of hysteroscopic fundal perforation. *Obstet Gynecol* 1992;79:879.

Dumesic DA, Dhillon SS. A new approach to hysteroscopic cannulation of the fallopian tube. *J Gynecol Surg* 1991;7:7.

Dwyer N, Hutton J, Stirkat GM. Randomized controlled trial comparing endometrial resection with abdominal hysterectomy for surgical treatment of menorrhagia. *Br J Obstet Gynaecol* 1993;100:237.

Emanuel MH, Wamsteker K, Hart AA, et al. Long-term results of hysteroscopic myomectomy for abnormal uterine bleeding. *Obstet Gynecol* 1999;93:743.

Fisher JC. Principles of safety in laser surgery and therapy. In: Baggish MS, ed. *Basic and advanced laser surgery in gynecology*. Norwalk, CT: Appleton-Century-Crofts, 1985:85.

Friedler S, Margalioth EJ, Kafka I, et al. Incidence of post-abortion intrauterine adhesions evaluated by hysteroscopy: a prospective study. *Hum Reprod* 1993;8:442.

Gabriele A, Zanetta G, Pasta F, et al. Uterine rupture after hysteroscopic metroplasty and labor induction. *J Reprod Med* 1999;44:642.

Garry R, Hasham F, Kokri MS, et al. The effect of pressure of fluid absorption during endometrial ablation. *J Gynecol Surg* 1992;8:1.

Garry R, Shelley-Jones D, Mooney P, et al. Six hundred endometrial laser ablations. *Obstet Gynecol* 1995;85:24.

Garuti G, Cellani F, Colonnelli M, et al. Hysteroscopically targeted biopsies compared with blind samplings in endometrial assessment of menopausal women taking tamoxifen for breast cancer. *J Am Assoc Gynecol Laparosc* 2004;11:62.

Gebauer G, Hafner A, Siebzehnrubl E, et al. Role of hysteroscopy in detection and extraction of endometrial polyps: results of a prospective study. *Am J Obstet Gynecol* 2002;186:1104.

Goldenberg M, Zolti M, Seidman DS, et al. Transient blood oxygen desaturation, hypercapnia and coagulopathy after operative hysteroscopy with glycine used as the distending medium. *Am J Obstet Gynecol* 1994;170:25.

Goldrath MH. Vaginal removal of the pedunculated submucous myoma: the use of laminaria. *Obstet Gynecol* 1987;70:670.

Goldrath MH, Fuller T, Segal S. Laser photovaporization of endometrium for the treatment of menorrhagia. *Am J Obstet Gynecol* 1981;140:14.

Gonzales R, Brensilver JM, Rovinsky JJ. Post-hysteroscopic hyponatremia. *Am J Kidney Dis* 1994;23:735.

Groenman FA, Peters LW, Rademaker BM, et al. Embolism of air and gas in hysteroscopic procedures: pathophysiology and implication for daily practice. *J Minim Invasive Gynecol* 2008;15:241.

Halverson LM, Aserkoff RD, Oskowitz SP. Spontaneous uterine rupture after hysteroscopic metroplasty with uterine perforation. *J Reprod Med* 1993;38:236.

Hidlebaugh DA, Orr RK. Long-term economic evaluation of resectoscopic endometrial ablation versus hysterectomy for the treatment of menorrhagia. *J Am Assoc Gynecol Laparosc* 1998;5:351.

Howe RS. Third trimester uterine rupture following hysteroscopic uterine perforation. *Obstet Gynecol* 1993;81:827.

American Congress of Obstetricians and Gynecologists. Technology Assessment in Obstetrics and Gynecology No. 7: hysteroscopy. *Obstet Gynecol* 2011;117:1486.

Istre O, Skajaa K, Schjoensby AP, et al. Changes in serum electrolytes after transcervical resection of endometrium and submucous fibroids with use of glycine 1.5% for uterine irrigation. *Obstet Gynecol* 1992;80:218.

Jansen FW, Vredevoogd CB, van Ulzen K, et al. Complications of hysteroscopy: a prospective, multicenter study. *Obstet Gynecol* 2000;96:266.

Jones HW, Seegar-Jones G. Double uterus as an etiological factor in repeated abortion: indications for surgical repair. *Am J Obstet Gynecol* 1953;65:325.

Kivnick S, Kanter MH. Bowel injury from rollerball ablation of the endometrium. *Obstet Gynecol* 1992;79:833.

Lefler HT Jr. Long-term follow-up of endometrial ablation by modified loop resection. *J Am Assoc Gynecol Laparosc* 2003;10:517.

Lin BL, Iwata Y, Liu KH, Valle RF. Clinical applications of a new Fujinon operating fiberoptic hysteroscope. *J Gynecol Surg* 1990;6:81.

Litta P, Pozzan C, Merlin F, et al. Hysteroscopic metroplasty under laparoscopic guidance in infertile women with septate uteri: follow-up of reproductive outcome. *J Reprod Med* 2004;49:274.

Lobaugh ML, Bammel BM, Duke D, et al. Uterine rupture during pregnancy in a patient with a history of hysteroscopic metroplasty. *Obstet Gynecol* 1994;83:838.

MacLean-Fraser E, Penava D, Vilos GA. Perioperative complication rates of primary and repeat hysteroscopic endometrial ablations. *J Am Assoc Gynecol Laparosc* 2002;9:175.

Magos AL, Baumann R, Lockwood GM, et al. Experience with the first 250 endometrial resections for menorrhagia. *Lancet* 1991;337:1074.

March CM. Hysteroscopy for infertility in diagnostic and operative hysteroscopy. In: Baggish MS, Barbot J, Valle RF, eds. *Diagnostic and operative hysteroscopy: a text and atlas*. Chicago, IL: Mosby-Year Book, 1989:136.

March CM, Israel R. Gestational outcome following hysteroscopic lysis of adhesions. *Fertil Steril* 1981;36:455.

March CM, Israel R. Hysteroscopic management of recurrent abortion caused by septate uterus. *Am J Obstet Gynecol* 1987;156:834.

March CM, Israel R, March AD. Hysteroscopic management of intrauterine adhesions. *Am J Obstet Gynecol* 1978;130:65.

Mints M, Radestad A, Rylander E. Follow up of hysteroscopic surgery for menorrhagia. *Acta Obstet Gynecol Scand* 1998;77:435.

Neuwirth RS. Hysteroscopic management of symptomatic submucous fibroids. *Obstet Gynecol* 1983;62:509.

Neuwirth RS. Hysteroscopic resection of submucous leiomyoma. *Contemp Obstet Gynecol* 1985;25:103.

III

Neuwirth RS. A new technique for and additional experience with hysteroscopic resection of submucous fibroids. *Am J Obstet Gynecol* 1978;131:91.

Neuwirth RS, Amin HK. Excision of submucous fibroids with hysteroscopic control. *Am J Obstet Gynecol* 1976;126:95.

Novy MJ, Thurmond AS, Patton P, et al. Diagnosis of cannula obstruction by transcervical fallopian tube cannulation. *Fertil Steril* 1988;50:434.

Obermair A, Geramou M, Gucer F, et al. Does hysteroscopy facilitate tumor cell dissemination? Incidence of peritoneal cytology from patients with early stage endometrial carcinoma following dilatation and curettage (D & C) versus hysteroscopy and D & C. *Cancer* 2000;88:139.

Overton C, Hargreaves J, Maresh M. A national survey of complications of endometrial destruction for menstrual disorders: the Mistletoe study. *Br J Obstet Gynaecol* 1997;104:1351.

Pabuccu R, Gomel V. Reproductive outcome after hysteroscopic metroplasty in women with septate uterus and otherwise unexplained infertility. *Fertil Steril* 2004;81:1675.

Pantaleoni D. On endoscopic examination of the cavity of the womb. *Med Press Circ* 1869;8:26.

Patton PE, Novy MJ. The diagnosis and reproductive outcome after surgical treatment of the complete septate uterus, duplicated cervix and vagina septum. *Am J Obstet Gynecol* 2004;190:1669.

Perlitz Y, Rahav D, Ben-Ami M. Endometrial ablation using hysteroscopic instillation of hot saline solution into the uterus. *Eur J Obstet Gynecol Reprod Biol* 2001;99:90.

Perry CP, Daniell JF, Gimpelson RJ. Bowel injury from Nd-YAG endometrial ablation. *J Gynecol Surg* 1990;6:199.

Perry PM, Baughman VL. A complication of hysteroscopy: air embolism. *Anesthesiology* 1990;73:546.

Propst AM, Liberman RF, Harlow BL, et al. Complications of hysteroscopic surgery: predicting patients at risk. *Obstet Gynecol* 2000;96:517.

Quinones RG. Hysteroscopy with a new fluid technique. In: Siegler AM, Lindemann HJ, eds. *Hysteroscopy: principles and practice.* Philadelphia, PA: JB Lippincott Co., 1984:41.

Reed TP, Erb RA. Hysteroscopic tubal occlusion with silicone rubber. *Obstet Gynecol* 1983;61:388.

Roberts S, Long L, Jonasson O. The isolation of cancer cells from the bloodstream during uterine curettage. *Surg Gynecol Obstet* 1960;111:3.

Rock JA, Singh M, Murphy A. A modification of technique for hysteroscopic lysis of severe uterine adhesions. *J Obstet Gynecol* 1993;9:191.

Rogerson L, Gannon MJ, Donovan PJ. Outcome of pregnancy following endometrial ablation. *J Gynecol Surg* 1997;13:155.

Romer T. Benefit of GnRH analogue pretreatment for hysteroscopic surgery in patients with bleeding disorders. *Gynecol Obstet Invest* 1998;45(suppl 1):12.

Ruiz JM, Neuwirth RS. The incidence of complications associated with the use of Hyskon during hysteroscopy: experience in 1793 consecutive patients. *J Gynecol Surg* 1992;8:219.

Salat-Baroux J, Hamou JE, Maillard G, et al. Complications from micro-hysteroscopy. In: Siegler A, Lindemann H, eds. *Hysteroscopy.* Philadelphia, PA: JB Lippincott Co., 1984.

Saygili-Yilmaz E, Yildiz S, Erman-Akar M, et al. Reproductive outcome of septate uterus after hysteroscopic metroplasty. *Arch Gynecol Obstet* 2003;268:289.

Schmitz MJ, Nahhas WA. Hysteroscopy may transport malignant cells into the peritoneal cavity: case report. *Eur J Gynaecol Oncol* 1994;15:121.

Selk A, Kroft J. Misoprostol in operative hysteroscopy: a systematic review and meta-analysis. *Obstet Gynecol* 2011;118:941.

Siegler AM, Kemmann EK. Hysteroscopic removal of occult intrauterine contraceptive device. *Obstet Gynecol* 1975;46:604.

Siegler AM, Kemmann EK. Hysteroscopy: a review. *Obstet Gynecol Surg* 1975;30:567.

Smith DC, Donohue LR, Waszak SJ. A hospital review of advanced gynecologic endoscopic procedures. *Am J Obstet Gynecol* 1994;170:1635.

Soucie JE, Chu PA, Ross S, et al. The risk of diagnostic hysteroscopy in women with endometrial cancer. *Am J Obstet Gynecol* 2012;207:71.e1.

Sowter MC, Singla AA, Lethaby A. Pre-operative endometrial thinning agents before hysteroscopic surgery for heavy menstrual bleeding. *Update in Cochrane Database Syst Rev* 2002;(3):CD001 124;PMID:12137619

Strassman EO. Plastic unification of double uterus. *Am J Obstet Gynecol* 1952;64:25.

Sullivan B, Kenney P, Seibel M. Hysteroscopic resection of fibroid with thermal injury to sigmoid. *Obstet Gynecol* 1992;80:546.

Taponeco F, Curcio C, Fasciani A, et al. Indication of hysteroscopy in tamoxifen treated breast cancer. *J Exp Clin Cancer Res* 2002;21:37.

Tapper AM, Heinonen PK. Experience with isotonic 2.2% glycine as distension medium for hysteroscopic endomyometrial resection. *Gynecol Obstet Invest* 1999;47:263.

Valle RF. Hysteroscopic evaluation of patients with abnormal uterine bleeding. *Surg Gynecol Obstet* 1981;153:521.

Valle RF. Hysteroscopic removal of submucous leiomyomas. *J Gynecol Surg* 1990;6:89.

Valle RF. Hysteroscopy for gynecologic diagnosis. *Clin Obstet Gynecol* 1983;26:253.

Valle RF, Sciarra JJ. Hysteroscopy: a useful diagnostic adjunct in gynecology. *Am J Obstet Gynecol* 1975;122:230.

Valle RF, Sciarra JJ, Freeman DW. Hysteroscopic removal of intrauterine devices with missing filaments. *Obstet Gynecol* 1977;49:55.

Vilos GA. Intrauterine surgery using a new coaxial bipolar electrode in normal saline solution (Versapoint): a pilot study. *Fertil Steril* 1999;4:740.

Yaron Y, Shenhav M, Jaffa AJ, et al. Uterine rupture at 33 weeks' gestation subsequent to hysteroscopic uterine perforation. *Am J Obstet Gynecol* 1994;170:786.

Zerbe MJ, Zhang J, Bristow RE, et al. Retrograde seeding of malignant cells during hysteroscopy in presumed early endometrial cancer. *Gynecol Oncol* 2000;79:55.

Zikopoulos KA, Kolibianakis EM, et al. Live delivery rates in subfertile women with Asherman's syndrome after hysteroscopic adhesiolysis using the resectoscope or the Versapoint system. *Reprod Biomed Online* 2004;8:720.

CHAPTER 19
Control of Pelvic Hemorrhage

Lindsay M. Kuroki and David G. Mutch

DEFINITIONS

Argon beam—Ionizing energy transmitted through argon gas stream that achieves hemostasis by creating eschar, tissue destruction, and formation of necrotic tissue with less depth of penetration than conventional electrocoagulation.

Autologous blood transfusion—Transfusion performed with the patient's own blood. This may benefit patients with a rare blood type and antibodies and may even be an acceptable alternative to Jehovah's Witness patients. However, these are the exceptions, and in general, autologous blood donation is not routinely recommended due to evidence that shows that autologous blood donors are more likely to undergo any transfusion (autologous and/or allogeneic blood) due to lower baseline preoperative hematocrit and a more liberal transfusion policy when using autologous blood.

Bogota bag—Sterile plastic bag used for temporary abdominal closure in setting of damage control protocol, suspected intra-abdominal compartment syndrome, or as a temporizing abdominal closure in the face of severe hemorrhage requiring packing and future evaluation with delayed closure.

Hemostatic clips—Small V-shaped clips of stainless steel, titanium, or plastic that can be applied on small vessels or tissue for hemostasis.

Homologous blood transfusion—Transfusion of blood or blood products from another human being.

Parachute pack—Sometimes called an umbrella pack. A towel or large sheet is inserted through the vagina into the pelvis, and it is then filled from below with gauze packing. The edges are twisted together, and the pack is pulled down against the pelvic floor to control deep pelvic bleeding after pelvic surgery, most commonly exenteration.

Peanut dissector—A long clamp with a small cotton bud placed in the tip of the jaws. It is a useful tool for blunt pressure dissection of small spaces.

Total blood volume—About 8% of total body weight or between 4.5 and 5.0 L in the average woman. Acute blood loss of 25% of total blood volume (about 1,500 mL) produces symptoms of tachycardia, hypotension, and decreased urine output. Transfusion should be considered when operative blood loss exceeds 15% of total blood volume. This can be roughly calculated by multiplying the patient's weight in kilograms by 10 (750 mL for a 75-kg woman).

The prevention and control of bleeding are fundamental to the success of any operation. Preoperative, intraoperative, and postoperative hemorrhage are potential complications in every patient undergoing gynecologic surgery. Preoperative hemorrhage is encountered in a variety of circumstances, such as intraperitoneal bleeding from a ruptured ectopic pregnancy or in patients on anticoagulation who have intraperitoneal hemorrhage associated with ovulation. Intraoperative hemorrhage can result from vascular injury, and postoperative bleeding is often due to unrecognized bleeding at the time of surgery that was obscured by reflex vasoconstriction or hypotension.

Surgical techniques and operations are designed to control bleeding and avoid hemorrhage, but inevitably, every surgeon will be confronted with uncontrolled bleeding. The surgeon who anticipates the next procedural step has the fund of knowledge to troubleshoot and the surgical skill set to act quickly will exhibit the leadership necessary to direct the operative team so that control of bleeding can be accomplished promptly and effectively.

Many benign gynecologic conditions are associated with abnormal uterine bleeding (AUB). Daily dietary intake of iron usually is sufficient to replace the iron lost with normal menstruation but may be inadequate to compensate for acute blood loss anemia. Outpatient preoperative evaluation of such patients should include a pregnancy test; complete blood count (CBC), including mean corpuscle volume (MCV); measurement of thyroid-stimulating hormone (TSH); and a Pap smear. Based on the history elicited, testing for *Chlamydia trachomatis* should be considered in patients who are at high risk for infection; coagulation studies in those who have a strong personal or family history of bleeding disorders; and an endometrial biopsy in patients suspected of hyperplasia or malignancy. Transfusion before elective gynecologic surgery may be indicated; however, other alternatives such as hormonal therapy and iron supplementation may also help optimize the patient's hemoglobin and iron stores. The preoperative use of epoetin alfa (recombinant erythropoietin) for correction of preoperative anemia has been used successfully in orthopedics. However, its application in gynecologic surgery remains unclear and is probably most applicable in gynecologic patients with chronic renal failure, nonmyeloid

(hematopoietic) leukemia, or human immunodeficiency virus (HIV). Occasionally, a patient's personal or religious beliefs (e.g., Jehovah's Witnesses) may not be compatible with receiving blood products and therefore require more extensive preoperative counseling and/or treatment planning before elective surgery. Some of these patients may also benefit from recombinant erythropoietin.

FUNDAMENTAL CONCEPTS OF NORMAL COAGULATION

Every surgeon should understand the basic mechanisms of normal hemostasis that can be applied when surgical injury to tissue is inflicted. Bleeding during gynecologic surgery usually results from cutting or injuring a vessel, but occasionally, it may result from a preexisting condition or defect in the clotting mechanism. The surgeon should be able to quickly recognize when normal hemostasis is interdicted and operate efficiently to correct vascular injuries and coagulopathies and minimize blood loss.

The following is a discussion of the principles and concepts of normal hemostasis, abnormal hemostasis (congenital and acquired), and management techniques. Coagulation is the working interrelation of five aspects of a complex biochemical and vascular system that causes the formation and dissolution of the fibrin platelet plug. These five components are (a) vasculature, (b) platelets, (c) plasma clotting proteins, (d) fibrinolysis and clot inhibition, and (e) the hypercoagulable response. How these five components interrelate in the normal setting must be understood before one can appreciate how they relate to bleeding or abnormal clotting in disease states. For the purposes of this chapter, we will focus on the first three factors.

Vasculature

The vasculature presents an endothelial-lined flexible conduit through which red cells, white cells, platelets, and all of the plasma proteins flow. At the interface between the flowing blood and vessel wall are several inhibitory biochemical systems that prevent the generation of the platelet–thrombin clot. The antiplatelet substance prostacyclin, produced in the vessel wall, inhibits platelet adhesion to the site of injury. The surface antithrombin III–heparin sulfate complex inhibits deposition of thrombin and fibrin.

A tear in the vessel wall removes the endothelial cell layer, exposing the basement membrane, smooth muscle, collagen, and supporting adventitia. These substances are biochemical activators of platelets and have their own thromboplastic activity. This activity initiates fibrin generation and deposition. A disease or medication that interferes with or intensifies this process can cause bleeding or inappropriate clotting, respectively. The vessel wall is diagrammed in **Figure 19.1**.

Congenital diseases associated with inadequate connective tissue and vascular dysfunction associated with bleeding are rare. The more frequently seen conditions are hereditary hemorrhagic telangiectasia, Ehlers-Danlos syndrome, and Marfan syndrome, which are characterized by defects in collagen, leading to poor clot formation and platelet activation at the injured site.

Acquired diseases associated with bleeding include deficiencies in vitamin C; Cushing syndrome; acute and chronic inflammatory diseases, such as infectious vasculitis and immune vasculitis; pyrogenic purpura; embolic purpura; and anaphylactoid reactions from drugs. Myeloproliferative disorders, such as multiple myeloma and Waldenström macroglobulinemia,

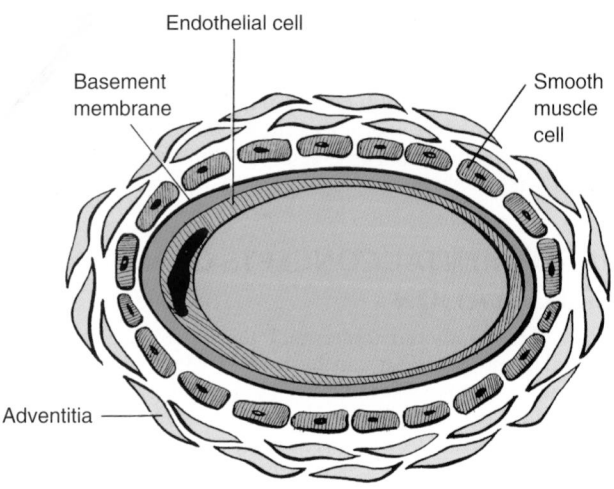

FIGURE 19.1 Vessel cross-section.

TABLE 19.1 More Commonly Seen Rare Congenital Clotting Disorders		
NAME	**INCIDENCE (PER MILLION)**	**TREATMENT**
Factor VIII (classic hemophilia A, sex-linked)	60–80	FVIII concentrate
Factor IX (classic hemophilia B, sex-linked)	15–20	FIX concentrate
von Willebrand disease (dominant, autosomal)	5–10	Cryoprecipitate (DDAVP), factor VIII concentrate with von Willebrand factor

DDAVP, deamino-D-arginine vasopressin.
The remainder of the known congenital clotting factors are very rare and occur with such low frequency that their discussion, diagnosis, and management can be found elsewhere (see Harker LA. *Hemostasis manual*, 2nd ed. Philadelphia, PA: FA Davis, 1974; Corriveau DM, Fritsma GA. *Hemostasis and thrombosis.* Philadelphia, PA: JB Lippincott Co., 1988; Triplett DA, ed. *Laboratory evaluation of coagulation.* Chicago, IL: ASCP Press, 1982).

produce abnormal proteins that interfere with vascular function and therefore permit bleeding.

Platelet Function

Platelets are disk-shaped fragments of the large multinucleated megakaryocytes released from the bone marrow on a daily basis (normal count is 150×10^3/mL to 400×10^3/mL), with a lifespan between 8 and 10 days (Fig. 19.2). The surface activation of the receptor sites on the platelet results in a biochemical chain reaction, generating thromboxane A_2, which in turn causes contraction of the protein thrombosthenin. This triggers platelet release of dense granules with nonmetabolic adenosine diphosphate (ADP). ADP is a potent platelet-aggregating agent that stimulates more platelets and eventually generates a platelet plug.

The congenital diseases associated with poor platelet function are divided into four types of dysfunction: (a) adhesion to collagen, (b) adhesion to subendothelium, (c) release reaction defects, and (d) ADP aggregation defects. Von Willebrand disease (vWD) (Table 19.1) is the most common hereditary coagulation abnormality, although acquired forms have

been described. Excessive bleeding results from the absence, decreased production, or abnormal function of von Willebrand factor, a large multimeric protein synthesized by megakaryocytes and vascular endothelium. This protein is responsible for the proper binding of platelets to the exposed collagen surface at the site of vascular injury. Its absence, therefore, prevents formation of the platelet plug necessary for hemostasis. Clinical manifestations of vWD vary in severity and often go unrecognized until some form of vascular trauma occurs or surgery is performed. In addition, such patients are particularly sensitive

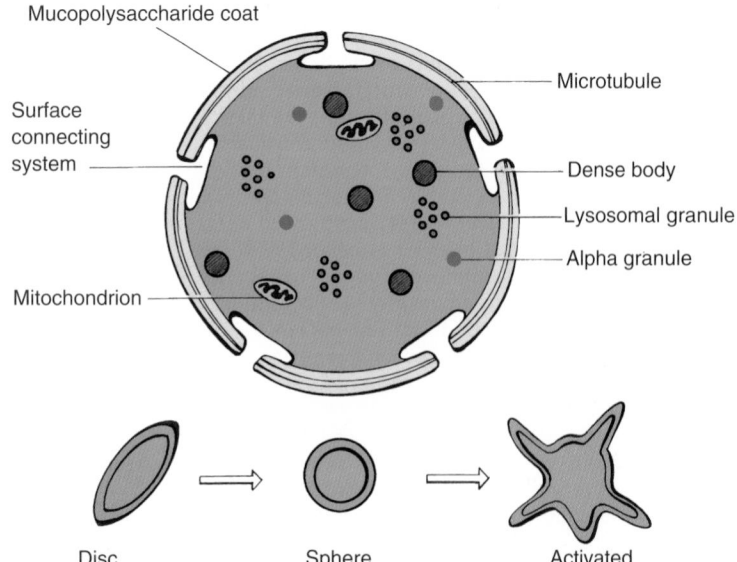

FIGURE 19.2 Platelet cross-section.

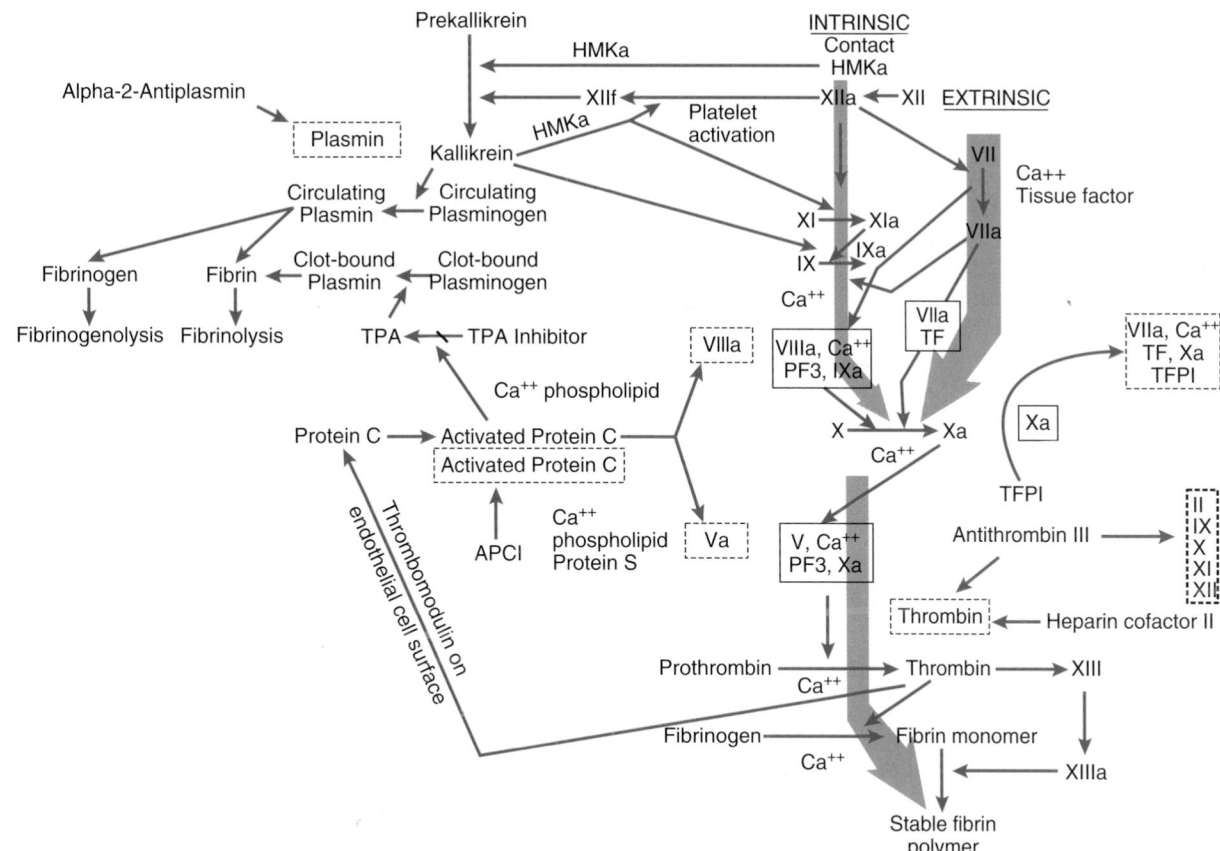

FIGURE 19.3 Coagulation system. *Dashed boxes* indicate destruction of factors. (APC1, activated protein C1; HMKa, high molecular weight kininogen; PF3, platelet factor 3; TPA, tissue plasminogen activator; TF, tissue factor; TFPI, tissue factor pathway inhibitor.)

to aspirin or other antiplatelet medications, increasing their tendency to bleed more at the time of surgery.

Acquired defects in platelet function are much more common and can be classified into two groups: (a) those due to an underlying condition, such as renal failure, myeloproliferative disorders (polycythemia vera, chronic myelogenous leukemia), and increased fibrin split products in consumptive coagulopathies, and (b) those that are iatrogenic, such as defects caused by medications (aspirin, nonsteroidal anti-inflammatory drugs, antibiotics, antihistamines, tricyclic antidepressants, dextran) and cardiopulmonary bypass surgery.

The laboratory assessment of platelet function has been extrapolated from the research laboratory and is now more readily available. The routine analysis of platelet function should begin with a platelet count and platelet function analyzer (PFA-100). However, in special cases, evaluation of platelet adhesion and aggregation and/or biochemical markers for measuring platelet turnover (e.g., platelet factor 4 and β-thromboglobulin assays) may be useful, although not predictive of surgical bleeding.

Plasma Clotting Proteins

Plasma clotting proteins are a group of serine proteases and cofactors that interact in a synergistic system to generate fibrin. The activation of the clotting system can be initiated in two ways: either by contact activation with factor XII or through thromboplastin activation of factor VII. The clotting cascade is diagrammed in **Figure 19.3**. The most common congenital factor deficiencies associated with bleeding are hemophilia A (factor VIII deficiency) and hemophilia B (factor IX deficiency). Both are seen in males and rarely in female disorders with sex-linked inheritance patterns. The majority of other congenital bleeding disorders have an autosomal recessive inheritance pattern or a dominant pattern with variable penetrance, making them extremely rare and less pertinent to this discussion.

However, acquired factor deficiencies are common. For example, critically ill patients on antibiotics that kill vitamin K–producing bacteria in the intestine and those who are diet restricted to nothing by mouth are at high risk for a coagulopathy due to loss of vitamin K–dependent factors II, VII, IX, and X. Other commonly acquired multifactor deficiencies are seen in acute and chronic liver disease such as viral hepatitis and alcoholic cirrhosis; consumptive coagulopathies, as in sepsis and placenta abruption; washout coagulopathies, seen in patients who require multiple transfusions after severe blood loss anemia; and major trauma.

The laboratory assessment of the plasma clotting factors has traditionally begun with prothrombin time (PT; factors V, VII, and X, prothrombin, and fibrinogen) and activated partial thromboplastin time (APTT; factors VIII, IX, XI, and XII). Specific factor assays also can identify the exact deficiencies. One must remember that a factor deficiency as low as 30% can generate a normal PT and APTT. This relation is important in investigating minimal prolongations of the PT or APTT that appear insignificant but nonetheless could be obscuring a deficiency. The tissue factor pathway inhibitor modulates activated factors X and VIII but is not apparently clinically significant.

TABLE 19.2 Pertinent Medical History to Screen for Coagulation Problems

History of spontaneous bruising or bleeding
History of unusual bruising or excessive bleeding after surgery
Family history of bruising or bleeding after surgery
Medication associated with bruising or bleeding
Current medication within past week
Previous coagulation testing
Current coagulation testing

PREOPERATIVE COAGULATION ASSESSMENT FOR SURGICAL PATIENTS

Preoperative evaluation of any patient may be divided into two general categories: elective versus emergency surgery.

Elective Surgery

The elective gynecologic surgical patient must be evaluated by general medical history and specific nature of the surgery. Table 19.2 highlights the most important positive and negative findings. Preoperative coagulation screening (Table 19.3) should supplement the history and physical and be individualized according to risk factors elicited (e.g., a prior emergency surgical procedure; positive personal or family history of spontaneous bleeding or easy bruising; use of medications that can affect coagulation, such as antiplatelet medication; acquired vitamin K deficiency; and fibrinolytic therapy).

The risks of blood-borne infections and adverse reactions are always present, but the documented need for blood transfusion(s) as a lifesaving measure will validate the decision so long as it is congruent with the patient's religious and personal beliefs. Standard preoperative orders for blood require knowledge of the specific needs of the patient and the indicated surgery. For the routine gynecologic procedure, such as simple hysterectomy in an otherwise healthy woman, a type and screen is appropriate. If an unexpected antibody is identified, the blood bank should notify the ordering physician and set aside 2 units of antigen-negative, crossmatched, compatible blood. In an emergency, the blood bank can always release universal donor type O–negative blood immediately.

In more complex procedures such as pelvic exenteration for cancer, where there usually is significant blood loss, a type and crossmatch for the average number of units used are appropriate and encouraged. With extremely difficult procedures or other complicating medical conditions, additional blood, fresh frozen plasma, and platelets may be required during the procedure and should be requested preoperatively.

Emergency Surgery

As an emergency procedure proceeds, decisions regarding blood replacement must be made. A direct approach to blood replacement therapy and the complications of such therapy depends on a clear understanding of the following concepts.

1. Transfusion with packed red cells may help compensate for the volume of the estimated blood loss but iatrogenically may cause a bleeding disorder (e.g., thrombocytopenic hemophilia). Therefore, platelets and fresh frozen plasma may also be indicated.
2. The patient's bleeding potential is dynamic and will change rapidly and frequently with the loss of blood and replacement therapy.
3. Direct monitoring before, during, and after surgery offers the best chance to diagnose and manage bleeding problems. It also allows formulation of plans and adjustment of the replacement therapy.

COMPONENT THERAPY FOR REPLACEMENT BEFORE SURGERY

With surgery planned, the preoperative data can be evaluated. Assuming the patient does not have hemophilia, vWD, severe liver disease, or liver failure, a prolonged PT and APTT may suggest a less common acquired or congenital bleeding disorder. Assistance from a clinical pathologist or hematologist should be requested if an intrinsic bleeding disorder is suspected.

TABLE 19.3 Tests to Indicate Coagulation Status

TEST	REFERENCE RANGE[a]	LEVEL OF ALARM	SIGNIFICANCE
Hematocrit (%)	37–47	25	Tissue anoxia
White cell count (mL)	4×10^3 to 12×10^3	3×10^3 to 25×10^3	Susceptibility to infection, leukemia
Platelet count (mL)	140×10^3 to 400×10^3	100×10^3 to 700×10^3	Bleeding, myeloproliferative disorder
Fibrinogen (mg/dL)	150–400	100	Bleeding, liver disease, intravascular consumption
Prothrombin time (s)	10–13	14	Bleeding factor deficiency
Activated partial thromboplastin time (s)	28–38	40	Bleeding factor deficiency, inhibitor
PFA-100	Collagen–epinephrine	Prolonged closure time	Screen for medication effect
Bleeding time (will not predict surgical bleeding)			

[a]Reference ranges may vary in each laboratory, reflecting method, instrumentation, and reagents.

COMPONENT THERAPY FOR REPLACEMENT DURING SURGERY

According to Schifman and Steinbronn, when intraoperative blood loss exceeds 15% of the patient's estimated blood volume, the surgeon should consider red blood cell transfusion to replace the acute blood loss. As a general rule, 15% of an adult's blood volume (in milliliters) equals the patient's weight (in kilograms) times 10. For example, for a 75-kg woman (165 pounds), 15% of blood volume is (75 × 10) 750 mL. When considering the risks and benefits of transfusing blood, the following should be considered: the patient's estimated blood volume and hemoglobin/hematocrit prior to surgery, the estimated intraoperative blood loss, the anticipated additional blood loss, and the risk of hypoxic and metabolic complications.

When massive blood replacement therapy is under way, intraoperative monitoring of coagulation at 2-hour intervals or after every 10 units of blood transfused is usually sufficient. It is important to remember that a patient bleeding during a surgical procedure has a higher demand for clotting factors and platelets than does a patient at bed rest. The use of blood and blood components in the management of massive bleeding that is due to a major vessel rupture has the following objectives:

1. To maintain sufficient blood volume and circulating red cells to carry enough oxygen to sustain life.
2. To replace blood sufficiently to achieve adequate coagulation and hemostasis, assuming there was extensive loss of plasma clotting factors and platelets.
3. To avoid falling so far behind in replacement that consumptive coagulopathy leads to exacerbated bleeding at the microvascular level due to insufficient clotting factors and platelets.

These objectives require repeated assessment of the patient throughout the surgical procedure and clear communication with anesthesia and the operating room staff.

The following guidelines are recommended for component therapy in clinical situations requiring massive blood replacement to maintain normal hemostasis.

Correction of the deficit in blood volume with crystalloid volume expanders will generally maintain hemodynamic stability, while transfusion of packed red blood cells is used to improve and maintain tissue oxygenation. Each unit of packed cells contains approximately 250 mL of red cells and, in an adult, will raise the hematocrit by roughly 3% unless there is continued bleeding (Table 19.4). Development of massive transfusion protocols has resulted in improved outcomes and decreased mortality. Most protocols focus on delivering a minimum ratio of 2 units (500 mL) of fresh frozen plasma for every 3 units of packed red blood cells and 1 unit of platelets (300 mL) for every 5 units of packed red blood cells. The size and age of the patient affect blood replacement. Posttransfusion labs should include CBC, PT, and APTT.

Platelets should be given when the platelet count falls below 100,000/mL in massive hemorrhage (measurement error of a platelet count can be as high as 62,000/mL in a bleeding patient). When a long surgical procedure is anticipated, or when more than 6 units of blood are given, 6 units of platelets in a volume of 300 mL should be given toward

TABLE 19.4 Blood Products

BLOOD PRODUCT	VOLUME (ML)	ADDITIONAL FACTORS	EXPECTED RESPONSE	COMMON INDICATIONS
PRBC 1 unit	200–250	Fibrinogen: 10–75 mg	Increase: 1 mg/dL Hgb 3% Hct	ABLA MTP Surgical blood loss
Platelets SDA RDP[a]	300–500 50 per unit	Fibrinogen: 2–4 mg/mL (360–900 mg) Clotting factors: Equivalent of 200–250 mL of plasma "6 pack" of pooled RDP similar to SDP	Increase: 30–60 K/mm³	Plt count <10 K MTP Bleeding with known qualitative plt defect
FFP[b] 1 unit	180–300	Fibrinogen: 400 mg Clotting factors: 1 mL contains 1 active unit of each factor	Decrease: PT/INR PTT	Coagulopathy Warfarin overdose DIC
Cryo 10 pack		Fibrinogen: 1,200–1,500 Clotting factors: VIII, vWF, XII	Decrease: PT/INR PTT Increase: Fibrinogen	vWD DIC Hemophilia A

[a]4–10 RDP units are pooled prior to transfusion.
[b]Duration of FFP effect is approximately 6 h.
Reprinted from Klingensmith ME, Abdulhameed A, Bharat A, et al., eds. *The Washington manual of surgery*, 6th ed. Lippincott Williams & Wilkins, 2012:133, with permission. Copyright © 2011, Lippincott Williams & Wilkins/Wolters Kluwer Health.
ABLA, acute blood loss anemia; Cryo, cryoprecipitate; DIC, disseminated intravascular coagulation; FFP, fresh frozen plasma; Hct, hematocrit; Hgb, hemoglobin; MTP, massive transfusion protocol; plt, platelets; PRBC, packed red blood cells; RDP, random donor platelets; SDP, single-donor platelets; vWD, von Willebrand disease, vWF, von Willebrand factor.

the end of the surgical procedure or when surgical hemostasis is achieved. This amount should be administered once to provide a maximum bolus effect. Because platelets are often difficult to obtain, their use should be reserved until near the end of the procedure. Pooling and transporting the platelets can take up to an hour, so the blood bank should be given sufficient notice to have them readily available in surgery when needed. In assessing the patient's coagulation status, it should be remembered that clotting factors are constantly changing.

When the PT and APTT are prolonged (more than 14 and 40 seconds, respectively) after replacement therapy, intrinsic disease must be considered initially, if only to be ruled out later. A borderline hemophiliac or patient with liver disease may manifest excessive bleeding after stress, trauma, or blood replacement because of the increased coagulation needs. Therefore, administration of fresh frozen plasma in 2 units (500-mL) doses should begin to correct the deficiencies caused by massive red blood cell replacement. If oozing continues despite the rapid transfusion of 6 units of fresh frozen plasma, a clotting problem or other ongoing bleeding disorders should be suspected and additional support sought.

When the fibrinogen level falls below 100 mg/dL, transfusion of 20 units of cryoprecipitate will provide about 150 mg/dL fibrinogen in a 70-kg person. A low fibrinogen level is rare because fibrinogen is stable and present in fresh frozen plasma. Liver disease or intravascular consumption must be suspected if the fibrinogen level is initially less than 100 mg/dL and remains low throughout surgery and recovery. Twenty units of cryoprecipitate will achieve therapeutic levels quickly and permit monitoring over several hours.

The goals of intraoperative monitoring are as follows:

- To assess changes in the coagulation mechanism resulting from blood loss and replacement therapy.
- To identify the coagulation components affected and determine the correct components to initiate therapy and achieve the following values: PT less than 14 seconds, APTT less than 40 seconds, fibrinogen more than 100 mg/dL, and platelets more than 80×10^3/mL. Posttransfusion laboratory monitoring should be drawn after 1 to 2 hours to determine the success of replacement.
- To assess the efficacy of replacement component therapy in an extensive operative procedure.

COMPONENT THERAPY FOR POSTOPERATIVE REPLACEMENT

The presurgical and intraoperative threshold levels for hematocrit, platelet count, PT, APTT, fibrinogen, and clot retraction also apply postoperatively, and a comparison of these values provides an accurate assessment of the bleeding patient. When laboratory values are abnormal, however, further surgery can be delayed until an attempt at aggressive specific component therapy is made. When abnormal coagulation studies exist, the following causes predominate, in order of frequency (most frequent first):

1. Low platelet count owing to transfusion of only packed red cells or fresh frozen plasma.
2. Prolonged PT and APTT due to transfusion of packed red cells without fresh frozen plasma. Careful monitoring of venous and arterial pressure, as well as cardiac output, should be considered in blood component therapy. Often, a slower rate of administration can achieve hemostasis without cardiovascular overload. If nearly normal coagulation values are achieved, but bleeding continues, surgical causes for bleeding should be considered.
3. Low fibrinogen level owing to dilution with plasma expanders or concurrent development of a disseminated intravascular coagulation (DIC).

The goals of postoperative monitoring are as follows:

- To assess for a coagulopathy and determine possible etiologies, including blood replacement.
- To determine the effectiveness of specific component therapy and identify the need for additional components.
- To enable the surgeon to distinguish surgical from nonsurgical bleeding.

Close postoperative monitoring, whether the patient is bleeding or not, will achieve these objectives with the ultimate goal of recognizing and resolving bleeding disorders in a timely manner.

RISKS OF BLOOD TRANSFUSION

Transfusions of whole blood were given sporadically before 1900, usually to treat specific diseases rather than to replace lost blood volume. It was not until the work of Cannon and Bayliss in 1919, and of Blalock in 1930, that it was proven that the important factors in shock were the loss of circulating blood volume and the decreased return of venous blood to the right heart. Eventually, banking and storage of donated blood became possible with refrigeration and the addition of sugar and later sodium citrate as an anticoagulant.

Homologous blood must be collected from carefully selected volunteer donors and properly matched to the potential recipient. The risks of red blood cell transfusion were reviewed by a National Institutes of Health and Food and Drug Administration Consensus Development Conference on Perioperative Red Cell Transfusion and published in 1988. The following excerpt is taken directly from their report.

In deciding whether to use red blood cell transfusion in the perioperative period, the need for possibly improved oxygenation must be weighed against the risks of adverse consequences, both short term and long term. The disadvantages are of two general types (Table 19.5): transmission of infection and adverse effects attributable to immune mechanisms. In addition, massive transfusion, defined as the replacement by transfusion of more than 50% of a patient's blood volume in 12 to 24 hours, may be associated with a number of hemostatic and metabolic complications (e.g., ionized calcium, potassium, and acid–base disturbances).

In modern blood banking practice, bacterial contamination of red blood cell units is rare. For practical purposes, the transmissible agents of greatest concern are viruses.

- Cytomegalovirus infection occurs with moderate frequency among those recipients without prior infection. Most of these infections are asymptomatic, except among immunocompromised people. The use of the newer leukocyte reduction filters ($<5 \times 10^6$) is under extensive clinical study and application as an alternative to cytomegalovirus-negative blood.
- Human T-cell lymphotropic viruses occur with low but not negligible frequency among donor populations in the United States. It is not known whether transfusion-transmitted infection with these viruses results in T-cell leukemia/lymphoma and/or neurologic disease several to many years later.
- On rare occasions, other microbial agents—including parvoviruses, malaria, *Toxoplasma*, Epstein-Barr virus, and *Babesia*—cause infection and disease.

TABLE 19.5 Blood Transfusion Risks

DISEASE OR SITUATION	RISK
Viral infection	
HIV	1:1.9 million
HTLV	1:250,000–1:2.0 million
Hepatitis B	1:180,000
Hepatitis C	1:1.6 million
Bacterial contamination	
Platelet packs (stored at room temperature)	1:12,000
Packed or whole red blood cells	1:5 million
Fatal red cell hemolytic reaction	1:250,000–1:1.1 million
Delayed red cell hemolytic reaction	1:1,000–1:1,500
TRALI	1:5,000
Febrile red cell nonhemolytic reaction	1:100
Allergic (urticarial reaction)	1:100
Anaphylactic reaction	1:150,000

HIV, human immunodeficiency virus; HTLV, human T-cell lymphotropic virus; TRALI, transfusion-related acute lung injury.
From Zoon KC. Ten years after: what has been achieved by Consent Decrees: the FDA view. *Paper presented at: Fifth Annual FDA and the Changing Paradigm for Blood Regulation*; January 16–18, 2002; New Orleans, LA, 2002; Schreiber GB, Busch MP, Kleinman SH, et al. The risk of transfusion-transmitted viral infections: the retrovirus epidemiology donor study. *N Engl J Med* 1996;334:1685; Dziecxkowski JS, Anderson KC. Transfusion biology and therapy. In: Fauci AS, Martin JB, Braunwald E, et al., eds. *Harrison's principles of internal medicine*. 14th ed. New York, NY: McGraw-Hill, 1998:718; Goodnough LT, Breacher ME, Kanter MH, et al. Transfusion medicine: first of two parts—blood transfusion. *N Engl J Med* 1999;340:438.

It is known that the incidence of hepatitis transmission increases with the number of donor exposures. This relationship is probably true for other transfusion-transmitted infections. HIV presently poses only a remote hazard because of strict donor selection and laboratory screening procedures. The consequences of HIV infection are rarely seen until 2 or many more years have elapsed, but ultimately, morbidity and mortality are extremely high.

Immunologic consequences also complicate homologous red blood cell transfusion. Hemolytic and nonhemolytic reactions are largely caused by alloimmunization to red blood cell and leukocyte antigens. Compatibility testing virtually has eliminated immediate hemolytic transfusion reactions; however, if they occur, they are largely due to human error. Nonhemolytic febrile reactions occur in 1% to 2% of recipients due to sensitization to leukocyte antigens but may be reduced by the use of leukocyte reduction filters ($<5 \times 10^6$).

It is important for gynecologic surgeons to discuss with their patients the possible need for transfusion of blood products and review the risks, benefits, and alternatives of such treatment. The most common transfusion-related viral infection, however, is non-A, non-B hepatitis, which accounts for 90% to 95% of cases of previous transfusion-acquired hepatitis and possibly as many as 3,000 deaths per year in the United States. When mortality or significant morbidity occurs with blood transfusion, the gynecologic surgeon must be able to show that the transfusion was indicated.

There are alternatives to blood and blood component transfusion that may be considered in critically ill patients such as those with sepsis and DIC. The drug-activated protein C, drotrecogin alfa (Xigris), is recombinant human-activated protein C (drotrecogin alfa, activated). It is used in replacement therapy in sepsis and holds a great promise in the management and survival in sepsis. By replacing this essential naturally occurring anticoagulant, there is reversal of the bleeding and thrombosis seen with sepsis. Its specific application in septic gynecologic surgical patients has not been reported in any large study.

Recombinant-activated factor VII (FVII) (NovoSeven) has been clinically demonstrated to successfully manage patients with FVIII and FIX inhibitors. It has also been used in the management of bleeding in cardiovascular surgery, liver failure, Coumadin overdose, and DIC. It has significantly reduced the use of blood components in these disorders, and although expensive, it has the potential to greatly improve patient outcomes.

By reducing the need for blood and blood components with the use of activated protein C (drotrecogin alfa), and recombinant-activated FVII, one can reduce the infectious disease exposure of blood as well as the generation of allogeneic antibodies.

AUTOLOGOUS BLOOD TRANSFUSION

Blood collected from a patient for retransfusion at a later time into the same patient is called autologous blood. Autologous blood transfusions account for over 5% of blood donated in the United States, with the majority obtained by preoperative donation, and have been endorsed by the Council on Scientific Affairs of the American Medical Association and by the Committee on Hospital Transfusion Practice of the American Association of Blood Banks.

The American Association of Blood Banks' standards for elective preoperative autologous blood donation include the following guidelines:

- A hemoglobin of no less than 11 g/dL or a packed cell volume of no less than 34%.
- Phlebotomy no more frequently than every 3 days and not within 72 hours of surgery.

Preoperative autologous donation is generally discouraged in patients over the age of 80 and absolutely contraindicated in patients with an active infection, and any of the following conditions would also preclude a patient from undergoing preoperative autologous donation: unstable angina or angina at rest, a myocardial infarction within the last 3 months, heart failure, aortic stenosis, ventricular arrhythmias, transient ischemic attacks, or marked hypertension.

If established screening and administration guidelines are followed, autologous blood has potential to be the safest type of blood for transfusion. It minimizes the risks of immunologically mediated hemolytic, febrile, or allergic reactions as well as viral transmissions such as hepatitis, malaria, cytomegalovirus, and HIV. In patients with rare blood types who have antibodies to common blood antigens, it may be the only blood available for transfusion. Autologous blood transfusion may be acceptable to Jehovah's Witnesses and should be offered preoperatively if a patient meets criteria for donation and based on the indicated procedure.

Despite these benefits, several aspects of the provision of preoperative blood donation remain controversial, including extent of testing, release of infectious units, participation of known infectious donors, transfusion of autologous blood to other recipients, the use of erythropoietin, and cost-effectiveness. Furthermore, improper handling, storage, or labeling of saved units has potential to cause several complications including hemolysis, bacterial infection/sepsis, and pulmonary edema due to volume overload, respectively. A meta-analysis by Forgie et al. found that patients who underwent preoperative autologous donations were more likely to undergo any transfusion with autologous and/or allogeneic blood (odds ratio 3.0) due to both a lower preoperative hematocrit (average of 3.5 units lower in patients who donated autologous blood compared to controls) and a more liberal transfusion policy when using autologous blood. Another drawback of autologous blood donation is the high cost that accounts for the extra time, enhanced clerical requirements, storage, and early delivery to the hospital. This expense is only exacerbated by the fact that approximately 50% of donated blood is generally wasted, rather than transfused to other patients. Depending on the age of the patient and likelihood of transfusion, the cost-effectiveness of autologous transfusion ranges from $235,000 to $23 million per quality adjusted year of life saved. Given these disadvantages, and considering that only about 2% of patients undergoing elective hysterectomy require blood transfusion(s), routine preoperative autologous donation cannot be recommended.

Intraoperative Autologous Transfusion

The frequency of intraoperative autologous transfusion has increased appreciably in the past decade, especially for cardiovascular operations. Keeling and colleagues reported on the use of the Haemonetics Cell Saver for autologous intraoperative transfusion in 725 consecutive general hospital patients. Seventy-five percent were cardiovascular patients, but a variety of other patients, including gynecology and obstetric patients, were represented. At least until additional data are available to the contrary, intraoperative autologous transfusion is contraindicated in patients with malignant disease and in patients with bacterial contamination of blood in the operative field. A series of 25 myomectomy operations by Shapiro and Toledo demonstrated that intraoperative autologous transfusion is convenient to use and does not interfere with the performance of the procedure.

The Haemonetics Cell Saver operates by retrieving blood from the operative site by suctioning it into a double-lumen catheter, in which it is immediately anticoagulated with heparin. It is then collected in a cardiotomy reservoir, where a filter removes gross debris. The blood is then pumped to a spinning centrifuge bowl, where the red blood cells are separated, washed with normal saline solution, and then concentrated to a hematocrit of about 50%. The supernatant waste that is subsequently collected contains saline, anticoagulant, activated coagulation factors, platelets, leukocytes, free hemoglobin, and other small debris. The washed, packed red blood cells are pumped into a reinfusion bag. The blood is then directly transfused to the patient through a filter. It takes approximately 8 to 10 minutes to process about 250 mL of packed cells. The machine is maintained and operated by a trained technician.

BASIC SURGICAL PRINCIPLES TO AVOID EXCESSIVE BLEEDING IN PELVIC SURGERY

Knowledge of basic anatomy and precise surgical technique are the basis for avoiding hemorrhage. Good exposure, appropriate instruments and correct placement of clamps, skillful dissection technique, and careful suture placement may help minimize blood loss. The surgeon who knows the patient, the disease entity being treated, the technical details of the planned surgical procedure, and his or her own technical abilities can confidently make judgments that minimize risks and complications, allowing for the best possible surgical outcome.

Among the many contributions to surgery made by William S. Halsted, first chief of surgery at Johns Hopkins Hospital, was a surgical technique that emphasized meticulous dissection, gentleness in the handling of tissues, accuracy in hemostasis, precision in wound approximation, and asepsis. It is impossible to place too much emphasis on the need for optimal exposure to limit blood loss. During vaginal operations, a contracted pelvic outlet will limit access and visibility, and often, a leiomyomatous uterus may require morcellation to allow sufficient exposure for safe vaginal removal. A Schuchardt incision may be required to improve exposure during vaginal operations. If exposure is inadequate, bleeding from vessels in the upper broad ligament may not be controllable from below, and an abdominal incision may be necessary to achieve final hemostasis. When hemorrhage is a problem during vaginal or laparoscopic surgery, the question always arises, "When should the operation be converted to an open abdominal procedure so that improved exposure and better access can be used to control the bleeding?" The answer to this question will vary depending on a variety of circumstances, but good exposure will go a long way. Once the decision is made to convert to an exploratory laparotomy, the exposure achieved will depend on the choice of incision, the method of retracting, the placement and intensity of the lights, and presence of assistants. Suction should be available and is preferred over sponges for two reasons. First, sponges can cause damage to delicate serosal surfaces. Second, a determination of the amount of blood lost can be more accurate if the largest percentage has actually been suctioned into a calibrated bottle and measured. One can then add to this exact amount an estimate of the amount of blood lost on the drapes, sponges, and lap packs. Good lighting of the surgical field is important. In addition to the standard surgical room lights, a headlight worn by the surgeon and/or the assistants is very useful in providing focused lighting deep in the pelvis. There are also lighted retractors and disposable, fiberoptic, and lighted suction irrigators, which may be helpful in vaginal surgery.

For pelvic laparotomy, the patient usually is placed in Trendelenburg position and the bowel is packed with moist laparotomy sponges to allow better exposure into the pelvis. Depending on the incision type, a Bookwalter or Balfour retractor with a C-arm may be useful.

It usually is possible and always desirable to keep the number of clamps in the operative field to an absolute minimum so as not to obscure the source of bleeding. The length of the instruments may vary depending on the thickness of the abdominal wall and depth of the pelvis. The handles of the instruments should come all the way out and above the level of the incision so as not to interfere with the operator's view of the pelvis. The surgeon must stand high enough to see down into the pelvis, and the patient's abdominal wall should be at about the level of the operator's umbilicus.

Cushing, a neurosurgeon, introduced the hemostatic silver metal clip in 1911, to occlude cranial vessels inaccessible to ligation. More recently, clips have been made of stainless steel, tantalum, and the new synthetic absorbable nonopaque polydioxanone polymer. The latter has the advantage of not causing the streaked artifact of metal clips when subsequent computed tomography (CT) of the pelvis is performed. Clips cause little tissue reaction, are available in different sizes, are easily applied, and provide secure control of bleeding vessels in relatively inaccessible places in the pelvis where ligation would be more difficult. A small vessel can be quickly occluded with a clip even before the vessel is cut, thus keeping the field dry. Clips are especially useful in retroperitoneal dissections. Disposable applicators loaded with multiple clips are available, obviating the need for reloading and facilitating rapid use. If appropriately used, clips can reduce blood loss, facilitate dissection, and reduce operating time.

Working with Bovie, Cushing also pioneered the use of electrosurgery for hemostasis. Modern electrosurgical units are radiofrequency generators that supply 500,000 to 2 million Hz of alternating current to the tip of the electrode. An electrosurgical instrument can be used to coagulate small vessels or to cut through fat or muscle. If a "blend" cut is used, small vessels will be coagulated as the instrument divides the tissue.

The needlepoint electrode can be used for precise incisions with minimal tissue injury from collateral thermal effect. Superficial coagulation of small vessels can be achieved by holding the electrode close to the tissue, pressing the "coagulation" button, and allowing the sparks to jump to the tissue surface. It is important to not let blood pool, as dry surfaces are much more effectively coagulated with the electrosurgical instrument. If bleeding is brisk, the vessel is grasped with a fine-pointed clamp or forceps, and hemostasis can be achieved by touching the metal clamp with the tip of the electrosurgical instrument and applying current. Bipolar electrodes built into tissue forceps are also very effective for coagulating smaller vessels during tedious dissections. Experience in the use of electrosurgery will result in maximum efficiency with minimum tissue damage.

Argon beam coagulation is another technique to achieve hemostasis that uses a unipolar current of inert argon gas. Since its introduction in the late 1980s, the argon beam coagulator has found wide utility in gynecology but is most commonly utilized in complete cytoreduction of advanced ovarian carcinoma, especially if the liver and diaphragm are involved. It provides a more homogenous, adherent eschar with less depth of necrosis compared with standard electrosurgical coagulation. The flow of argon gas clears and controls the bleeding, and the ionizing energy is transmitted through the argon gas stream. The maximum temperature reached is 110°C, compared with the 205°C of traditional electrosurgical generators, thereby minimizing tissue destruction, charring, and formation of necrosis. With a thorough knowledge of pelvic anatomy, the surgeon should emphasize the development of pelvic planes and spaces. This will avoid unnecessary bleeding and allow more accurate placement of clamps on vessels. Certain parts of the dissection can be delayed until later, especially if blood loss is likely to be increased. For example, during an abdominal hysterectomy, dissection of the bladder away from the cervix and vagina may be associated with blood loss and should not be performed at the beginning of the case. Furthermore, exposure of the anterior lower uterine segment and cervix is not required until the uterine vessels and broad ligament need to be clamped.

In the early days of abdominal pelvic surgery, postoperative hemorrhage was common because an effective technique of hemostasis was not known. The usual method of performing abdominal hysterectomy involved use of a ligature en masse around the lower uterus. It was not until 1889 that Stimson published a technique for secure individual ligation of the uterine and ovarian vessels that significantly reduced

the incidence of postoperative hemorrhage. Kelly published a similar technique with illustrations in 1891. In abdominal operations today, all major vascular pedicles should be individually ligated, twice if technically feasible. Delayed-absorbable sutures should be used and square knots firmly tied. Vascular pedicles should be small and the vessels skeletonized as much as possible so that a secure ligature with little extraneous tissue can be accomplished. A vascular pedicle where the tip of the clamp is free, such as the infundibulopelvic ligament, should always be ligated first with a free tie to occlude the vessels. The pedicle is then secured with a transfixion suture ligature placed between the previous free tie and the clamp. This technique avoids hematoma formation and the rare occurrence of a traumatic arteriovenous fistula. If a suture ligature is to be held long for traction or later identification, there is a danger that it will become loosened or be pulled off, with a resulting hematoma or bleeding. Sutures used to ligate vessels should usually be cut and rarely held for traction for that reason. Specifically during a vaginal hysterectomy, the upper broad ligament containing the utero-ovarian ligament and the fallopian tube should be doubly clamped. The lateral-most clamp is replaced by a free tie completely around the pedicle. Tied tightly, this ligature compresses the vessels in the pedicle so that the most medial clamp (the one closest to the uterus) can then be replaced with a suture ligature placed through the pedicle, passed around the tip of the clamp both ways, and tied tightly around the pedicle. This second transfixion ligature is one vascular ligature that is usually held long for identification purposes.

The newer delayed-absorbable sutures and smaller-gauge sutures are strong enough to ligate vessels. However, it is dangerous to use fine suture to ligate large pedicles. The suture may break or cut through the tissue if there is too much tension on the pedicle. Fine needles with small sutures are useful for controlling localized venous or arterial bleeding, but larger suture with bigger bites is less likely to pull through infected or malignant tissue. Proper suture selection for the specific technique is an important part of obtaining hemostasis.

INTRAOPERATIVE MEASURES TO CONTROL PELVIC HEMORRHAGE

Despite adequate technical skills and careful dissection, serious hemorrhage can suddenly complicate any operative procedure. Excessive bleeding in an area of dissection stains tissues, obscures visibility, restricts technical freedom, and gradually adds up to a significant amount of blood loss that may require replacement. The outcome of such situations is dependent on the surgeon's quick reaction time, knowledge base, technical ability, and leadership to produce a good outcome. The first task is to control the hemorrhage. A finger should immediately be placed on the bleeding point for prompt, atraumatic control. When the blood has been suctioned out and the fingertip exposed, it may be gently rolled off the bleeding point while a fine-tipped clamp or forceps is poised to compress the bleeding vessel and suction is ready to provide exposure. Depending on the location of the bleed and adjacent structures, the Bovie may be used safely by touching the metal clamp with the tip of the electrosurgical instrument and applying current. In most instances, this will adequately control the hemorrhage, although it is often necessary to place another clamp, clip, or suture adjacent to the first in order to control the other side of the lacerated vessel or other nearby bleeders. It is most important to avoid placing too many clamps in the area because this will obscure the bleeding site and cause additional trauma to the vessels. Multiple sutures and/or clips may also cause more bleeding and can injure adjacent structures, such as the ureter, bladder, pelvic vessels, and nerves. Electrocautery should not be used to attempt to control significant bleeding. It will only cause increased bleeding and more tissue injury.

If an immediate attempt to control the hemorrhage by simple means is unsuccessful, the bleeding should be controlled again with pressure, with a fingertip, with a sponge forceps, or occasionally by packing. The surgeon should step back, take a deep breath, and carefully consider the situation. The anesthesiologist should be made aware of the hemorrhage and consulted about the patient's stability, blood loss up to this point, availability of blood for transfusion, and intravenous access. The anesthesiologist will play an important role in fluid and blood replacement, monitoring coagulation factors and ensuring perfusion of vital organs. Therefore, it is important that he or she be fully aware of the situation and an active participant in such decisions as how long to safely proceed with surgery. The anticipated difficulty in controlling the hemorrhage must be continually reassessed and clearly communicated among the surgical team. The surgeon should request appropriate help to alleviate the situation, which may include additional suction, specific instruments, more scrub and/or circulating nurses, and even more experienced assistants or intraoperative consults (e.g., gynecologic oncologist, urologist, colorectal surgeon, general surgeon, vascular surgeon). It is prudent to anticipate these things and account for the time it will take for help to arrive. If the patient is stable and any necessary equipment has been readied, it is reasonable to reconsider the anatomy, obtain good exposure, and have another try at controlling the bleeding. Often, the 10 minutes or so that the hemorrhage has been controlled by pressure will result in a substantial reduction in the bleeding. Perhaps the vessel or bleeding site can be more clearly seen and controlled with a clamp, stitch, or clip. Arterial bleeding in the pelvis is usually readily identified due to blood spurting and easier to control because the vessels have thick walls and are not as easily torn further. If the artery can be clamped, it usually can be ligated, a clip can be applied, or both. If an artery has mostly retracted from view with only one small edge still visible, that edge may be grasped with a clamp and gently twisted, thus decreasing the amount of bleeding sufficiently to allow clipping or ligation. Venous hemorrhage in the pelvis may be a much more difficult problem. Such bleeding can vary in magnitude from a trivial ooze to life-threatening hemorrhage. Pelvic veins can be fragile, tortuous, hidden from view, and distended. Blood returning through the lacerated vein can come from multiple deeper sources that are unavailable for ligation. Placing clamps and sutures blindly is dangerous, can inadvertently injure surrounding structures, and can even cause more bleeding. Avoid electrocoagulation of a laceration in a large vein as it will inevitably create a larger hole, making it even more difficult to secure.

Sometimes, the best procedure is to hold a finger or a pack against the bleeding site for a minimum of 5 minutes, after which the bleeding may stop or decrease so that the bleeding vessel can be identified and controlled with a clip or a suture. Digital pressure to control venous bleeding takes advantage of the fact that the pressure in pelvic veins is very low, and atraumatic compression is less likely to cause further tearing injury to the vein. Sometimes, careful dissection is required to free the vessel above and below the source of bleeding to allow more precise ligation or clipping. If the vessel can be sufficiently liberated, another instrument is gently slipped beneath the first one so that its point is free. Then, a fine ligature is placed around the clamp. If necessary, clips can also be placed on each side of the tie.

If the bleeding has still not been controlled at this point or if bleeding cannot be controlled by pressure on the bleeding site, consultation should be requested for additional help and expertise. By this time, the surgeon may feel frustrated, and it is important to maintain control of the operation and the surgical team. Blood and clotting factors should be replaced as discussed earlier in this chapter, the patient kept warm, and the whole situation reevaluated with input from all members of the team. One should appreciate the importance of avoiding acidosis and hypothermia, as both have potential to interfere with normal functioning of the coagulation system (e.g., assembly of coagulation factor complexes involving calcium and negatively charged phospholipids and enzymatic activity of plasma coagulation proteins, respectively). The surgeon must maintain focus and exert good judgment and leadership. This includes using the skills and ideas of each member of the surgical team and knowing which ideas to use, when to use them, and when to ask for help.

Special Techniques

Diffuse venous oozing, which may be associated with malignancy, inflammation, or extensive lysis of adhesions, can usually be controlled by electrocautery or packing for 5 to 15 minutes. When these techniques are not effective, various hemostatic agents may be considered. However, it is important to remember that the patient must have normal clotting factors for these products to be most effective. Most of these agents have been studied in animal models, with very little literature comparing these agents head to head in human subjects.

Older agents such as oxidized, regenerated cellulose (ORC) come in a thin, pliable, woven sheet (Surgicel NuKnit, Johnson & Johnson, USA) or a soft, multiple-layered, fuzzy pad that can be separated into thin sheets or used as a pliable pad (Surgicel Fibrillar, Johnson & Johnson, USA). Additionally, it has bactericidal activity against gram-positive and gram-negative organisms and takes approximately 14 days to be fully absorbed. Absorbable, gelatin foam pads (Gelfoam, Pharmacia and Upjohn, USA) are also available in several sizes and can be cut to fit. These stiff sponges are about 4 mm thick and can be applied dry or moistened with saline to make them pliable. Both of these sheets or pads can be applied to an oozing surface and covered with a pressure pack for 5 minutes or so, during which time clot formation will form on the cellulose or gelatin matrix.

Microfibrillar collagen "flour" (Avitene, Davol, USA or InStat, Johnson & Johnson, USA) is a soft, granular material that can be placed on a semidry surface or into a small crevice for hemostasis. This bovine collagen material acts as a fibrin nidus to accelerate thrombus formation on the surface of the vessel. It will only control bleeding from a small arteriole or venule. Caution must be exercised when using this material because it can produce secondary fibrosis in the pelvis and even a persistent palpable mass. There have been reports of retroperitoneal fibrosis and ureteral obstruction secondary to the use of this hemostatic agent.

Other attempts to control severe bleeding from deep pelvic veins include a combination preparation such as Floseal (thrombin/gelatin) or a combined approach with Gelfoam and Avitene, stacked one on top of the other. If coagulation factors have been depleted because of multiple transfusions, the Gelfoam can be soaked in thrombin. When the material is applied, the field should be as dry as possible. Constant pressure can be applied by placing sutures that can be tied on top of the sandwiches. There is a new commercial product made of absorbable collagen sponge coated with human coagulation factor and thrombin that sounds very good, but it is not yet U.S. Food and Drug Administration (FDA) approved for use in the United States (TachoSil, Nycomed, Denmark).

Malviya and Deppe have reported the successful use of fibrin glue, a biodegradable tissue adhesive sealant and topical hemostatic agent, to control life-threatening hemorrhage in one obstetric and two gynecologic patients. The fibrin glue (Tisseal, Baxter Pharma, USA or Crosseal, Ethicon, USA) is prepared from equal amounts of cryoprecipitate (highly concentrated human fibrinogen) and bovine thrombin. It imitates the last stages of physiologic coagulation at the local site. It is available as a spray applicator or in a dual syringe set. This technique has been used successfully in microvascular, cardiovascular, and thoracic surgical procedures and has recently been reported in controlling hemorrhage in liver transplantation. Schwartz and colleagues compared spray-on fibrin sealant to standard techniques for hemostasis in 121 patients undergoing liver resection. Time to achieve hemostasis and postoperative complications was significantly less in the patients randomized to fibrin sealant. This technique should be helpful in extensive pelvic dissections for gynecologic cancer, especially to control low-pressure pelvic vein bleeding that is not controllable by other standard measures.

Gynecologic surgeons usually do not have the luxury of using tourniquets to control bleeding. There are, however, two special procedures in which tourniquets may be useful—myomectomy and uterine unification operations. The tourniquet is fashioned in the manner used by vascular, thoracic, and trauma surgeons to occlude major vessels. A vessiloop or a small Silastic pediatric catheter can be used for this purpose. A tourniquet loop can be placed around the uterine isthmus through a small hole made in the broad ligament just lateral to the uterine vessels. Loops also can be placed around both infundibulopelvic ligaments through the same hole in the broad ligament. When these are snugged down tightly and held with a Kelly clamp, the entire circulation to the uterus can be occluded. This technique can reduce blood loss to a minimum in these two procedures.

Similarly, vessel loops or vascular clips can be used above and below the defect when repairing a sizable hole in the wall of a large vein or artery that cannot be sacrificed.

For completeness of discussion, hypotensive anesthesia has been used for radical pelvic surgery in the past, but it is rarely used and not recommended for routine gynecologic surgery. Reducing the circulation to the operative field by deliberate induction of hypotension has the potential to be a safe and effective anesthetic technique in carefully selected patients.

Hypogastric Artery Ligation

One of the methods of controlling severe pelvic hemorrhage is ligation of both hypogastric arteries. In 1893, at the Johns Hopkins Hospital, Howard Kelly performed bilateral hypogastric artery ligation to control hemorrhage during a hysterectomy for uterine cancer. Hypogastric artery ligation was later reintroduced by Mengert and colleagues and then extensively investigated by Burchell, who demonstrated that the arterial pulse pressure just distal to the point of ligation was decreased significantly (77%) on the same side. If both hypogastric arteries are ligated, the pulse pressure is decreased by 85%, presumably allowing blood clots to form at the site of bleeding from damaged vessels. Blood flow in vessels distal to the point of ligation is decreased by only 48%.

Because it is important to preserve some of the collateral circulation to the pelvis—including the lumbar, iliolumbar, middle sacral, lateral sacral, superior and middle hemorrhoidal, and gluteal arteries—it is important to ligate the anterior division of the hypogastric artery distal to the origin of the posterior parietal branch, as demonstrated in **Figure 19.4**. In ligating the hypogastric artery, the peritoneum is opened over the external iliac artery from the round ligament to the infundibulopelvic ligament, and the hypogastric artery is identified and

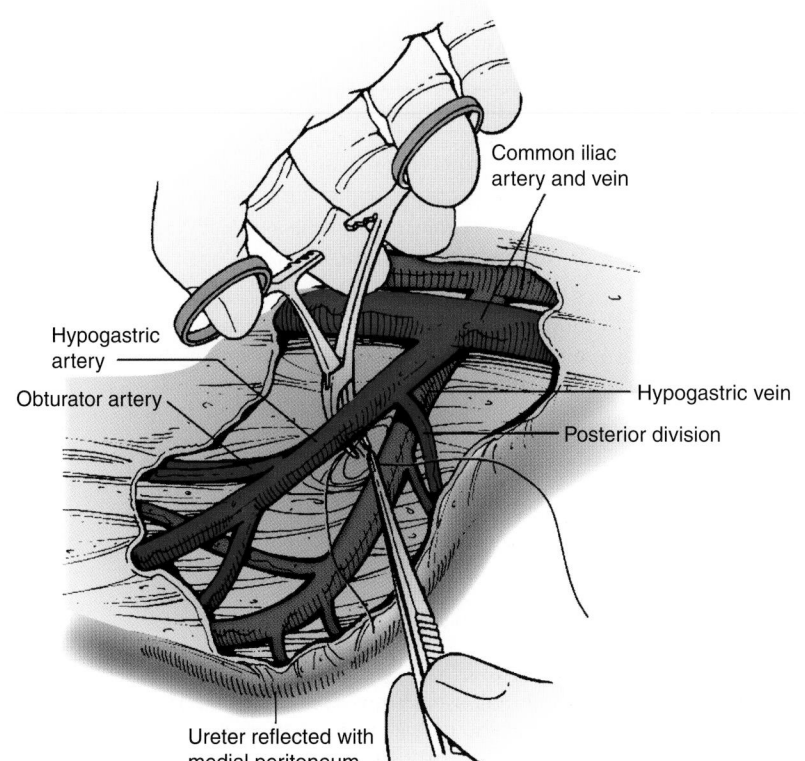

Common iliac artery and vein

Hypogastric artery

Obturator artery

Hypogastric vein

Posterior division

Ureter reflected with medial peritoneum

FIGURE 19.4 Ligation of the right hypogastric artery. The clamp is passed laterally to medial, and the ligature is placed around the anterior division of the hypogastric artery. Note the ureter is attached to the peritoneum, which is reflected medially.

gently skeletonized. The ureter is left attached to the medial peritoneal reflection to avoid disturbing its blood supply. The hypogastric vein is also identified on the pelvic sidewall, if possible; but as long as the artery is well visualized and dissected from the sidewall, it is not necessary to risk more bleeding by isolating the hypogastric vein. The posterior branch of the hypogastric artery must be clearly identified before double ligation of the anterior division is performed. Nonabsorbable suture is passed around the artery with a right-angle clamp and tied. A second free-tie suture is placed distal to the initial ligature to avoid recanalization. Transfixion or division of the vessel is not recommended in this procedure. The hypogastric arteries should be ligated bilaterally, if possible, to obtain the best results. In addition, we believe that the arterial branch closest to the bleeding point should be ligated if this can be done without increasing bleeding or risk to other pelvic structures. For example, because the uterine artery is the first visceral branch of the hypogastric artery, it may be feasible to identify this artery and ligate it separately if the bleeding is from the uterus. This may be a somewhat more difficult than ligating the entire anterior division of the hypogastric artery and should not be attempted in the face of massive pelvic bleeding, distorted pelvic anatomy, or shock.

When massive bleeding is present but there is no indication to remove the uterus (e.g., certain obstetric operations), it is important to ligate both ovarian arteries in addition to bilateral hypogastric artery ligation. This procedure is easily accomplished by extending the lateral peritoneal incision up and parallel to the infundibulopelvic ligaments. It is imperative to first identify the ureter. The ovarian artery should be ligated with a single, permanent ligature, but the artery should not be cut. This avoids the need for multiple ligatures and the risk of retraction and retroperitoneal bleeding of the vessel. A single hemoclip also can be placed on each ovarian artery as a quicker and easier method of occlusion. Care should be taken to avoid injury to the ovarian vein. If there is difficulty in distinguishing the artery from the ovarian vein, ligation of both the ovarian artery and vein within the infundibulopelvic ligament is acceptable. Even though ligating both the arterial and venous circulation to the ovary leads to a high incidence of postoperative cystic enlargement of the ovary, this complication is preferable to the risk of recurrent pelvic bleeding when the ovarian arteries are not ligated. Pregnancy after hypogastric artery ligation has been studied, and many reports of full-term deliveries after bilateral hypogastric artery ligation with and without bilateral ovarian artery ligation have been described. Such testimony provides compelling evidence of the abundant collateral blood supply to the uterus that can develop over time. According to Burchell, the blood flow to the pelvis is reduced by as much as 50%; however, ischemic necrosis of pelvic tissues does not occur unless additional collateral pathways are destroyed.

Ovarian Artery and Uterine Artery Ligation

As an alternative to ligating the ovarian artery in the infundibulopelvic ligament, Cruikshank and Stoelk have described a technique of ligating this artery at the point of its anastomosis with the uterine artery in the medial mesosalpinx. This point of ligation allows maintenance of the blood flow to the tube and ovary but occludes the ovarian artery blood flow to the uterus (Fig. 19.5). Because this technique allows uninterrupted blood supply to the ovaries, it is probably preferable.

For post–cesarean delivery hemorrhage, Fehrman has recommended bilateral ligation of the uterine arteries as primary treatment. First, the uterus should be elevated upward and angled away from the targeted uterine artery. The artery should be identified by palpation, and a 0 absorbable suture is passed into and through the myometrium about 2 cm medial to and below the uterine vessels. The needle is brought out through an avascular area in the broad ligament, cephalad and lateral to the uterine vessels. The suture is tied and the procedure is repeated on the other side. When this method was used in 66 patients, only 6 required hysterectomy to achieve hemostasis. If bilateral uterine ligation is not effective in controlling the uterine bleeding, supplementary ligation of the round and the ovarian ligaments at their junction with the uterine corpus is recommended.

The vaginal artery can originate as a separate branch from the hypogastric artery. Uncontrollable bleeding from the vagina may not be stopped by hysterectomy or by ligation of the uterine arteries and therefore requires hypogastric artery ligation.

The collateral circulation of the female pelvis is extensive and provides a variety of intercommunicating sources of arterial blood from various sites. These collateral vessels anastomose with the hypogastric artery and the blood supply to the uterus through a number of circuitous arterial pathways in the pelvis. During a difficult hysterectomy, the collateral circulation can create problems in achieving adequate hemostasis. Therefore, it is important to have a clear understanding of the various extrapelvic arteries that communicate with the pelvic circulation. If bleeding occurs postoperatively, one can consider embolization utilizing interventional radiology.

STEPS IN THE PROCEDURE

Surgical Control of Pelvic Hemorrhage

Hypogastric Artery Ligation
- Open the peritoneum over the external iliac artery from the round ligament to the infundibulopelvic ligament.
- Identify hypogastric artery at its origin from the common iliac artery or at the medial margin of the psoas muscle, and follow it up to the common iliac artery bifurcation.

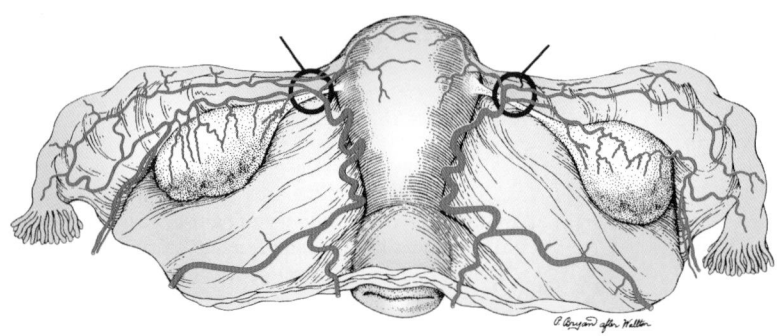

FIGURE 19.5 In addition to ligation of the anterior division of the hypogastric artery, the blood flow to the uterus through the ovarian artery can be ligated in the medial mesosalpinx without interfering with the blood flow to the tube and ovary.

- Leave the ureter attached to the medial peritoneal reflection.

- Identify the hypogastric vein more laterally on the pelvic sidewall.

- If possible, identify the anterior and posterior branches of the hypogastric artery.

- About 2 cm distal to the origin of the hypogastric artery, using a right-angle clamp, pass a nonabsorbable suture around the artery.

- Place a second free-tie suture distal to the initial ligature to avoid recanalization.

- Transfixion or division of the vessel is not recommended.

Ovarian Vessel Ligation

- Extend the lateral peritoneal incision up and parallel to the infundibulopelvic ligaments.

- Identify the ureter.

- Ligate the ovarian vessel with a single, permanent ligature, avoiding the ovarian vein.

- A single clip also can be placed on each ovarian artery as a quicker and easier method of occlusion.

Uterine Artery Ligation

- The uterus should be elevated upward and angled away from the targeted uterine artery.

- Identify the uterine artery by visualization or palpation.

- A 0 absorbable suture is passed into and through the myometrium about 2 cm medial to and below the uterine vessels. The needle is brought out through an avascular area in the broad ligament, cephalad and lateral to the uterine vessels. The suture is securely tied.

Packing Techniques

In rare cases, standard techniques of pressure, clipping, ligation, or application of hemostatic agents is unsuccessful for controlling bleeding. Several techniques may be considered in these cases. Trauma surgeons will occasionally pack persistent venous bleeding and close the abdomen when the procedure has been prolonged and/or the patient is unstable. The patient is then reoperated on in 24 to 48 hours when coagulation factors and blood volume have been repleted. In some cases, the packing can be brought out through a large, hollow, soft rubber drain placed in a separate incision in the abdominal walls. The packing can then be removed through the drain in 48 hours under a light general anesthesia without opening the abdomen. If bleeding persists, it can sometimes be controlled by vascular embolization by interventional radiology.

Some surgeons have found the parachute pack, or umbrella pack, to be useful as a last resort to control persistent venous bleeding from the pelvic floor muscles after pelvic exenteration. This area is very deep in the pelvis, and exposure may be unsatisfactory from either above or below. This technique involves the formation of a large pack of loose gauze within an outstretched, opened piece of gauze or plastic sheet. The center of the sheet is inserted through the vagina and positioned in the pelvic cavity from above. The pack is then stuffed from below with multiple gauze packing rolls (**Fig. 19.6A**). When an adequate volume has been obtained, the corners of the sheet are twisted together, and the stuffed packing is pulled down against the pelvic floor, compressing the vessels of the pelvic floor muscles and paravaginal tissues (**Fig. 19.6B**). Downward traction is maintained by clamping the twisted sheet at the vaginal introitus with several sturdy clamps. These are padded with gauze or foam rubber as they rest tightly against the perineum. The handles should be taped shut but may be reclamped from time to time to maintain pressure on the towel as it stretches. Place a Jackson-Pratt or Blake drain(s) in the pelvis to monitor for continued bleeding and an indwelling urinary catheter (if the bladder is still present) to avoid outflow obstruction and monitor urine output. The pack can be left in place with perineal traction for 24 to 48 hours until the bleeding has diminished and coagulation factors and other parameters have normalized. The pack is removed vaginally by first withdrawing the internal gauze and then the outside bags, sheet, or towel.

Temporary abdominal closure techniques are commonly practiced due to concern for abdominal compartment syndrome but should also be part of the surgeon's repertoire when enforcing damage control due to excessive pelvic hemorrhage. Because a second operative procedure is required for definitive repair, the abdomen is intentionally left open to facilitate reexploration, and the patient is closely monitored in an intensive care unit to correct for hypovolemic shock, hypothermia, metabolic abnormalities, and any coagulopathy. Several techniques for temporary abdominal closure include the Bogota bag, absorbable mesh, negative pressure systems (towel- and sponge-based), pack dressings, and the Wittmann patch or Velcro burr. Regardless of the technique used, they are characterized by a tension-free closure.

The Bogota bag, first described in 1984 by Oswaldo Borráez in Bogotá, Colombia, is a sterile plastic bag (typically a 3-L urinary irrigation bag), which is placed over the abdominal defect and sutured to the skin or fascia of the anterior abdominal wall. It serves as a hermetic barrier to minimize fluid loss, avoid evisceration, and prevent musculoaponeurotic necrosis and has the additional benefit of allowing direct visualization of abdominal contents should ischemic bowel be a concern.

Different types of mesh closures using porous material have been used. For example, an Esmarch rubberized dressing can be sutured to the skin or fascia. Alternatively, a fenestrated plastic dressing can be used to drape over the abdominal contents and securely tucked into the paracolic gutters. Jackson-Pratt drains are placed superiorly and inferiorly, and a sterile operating room pack is positioned over the drape. Then, an Ioban dressing is used to effectively close the wound.

Velcro dressings are another useful addition to abdominal closures that are sutured to the fascia and then advanced every 4 to 6 hours, bringing the fascia closer together. This technique has a lower risk of abdominal compartment syndrome since the Velcro will unfasten as the intra-abdominal pressure increases. It also has the advantage of easy access/reentry into the abdomen, by simply unfastening the Velcro at the midline.

In addition to abdominal packing, other potential etiologies of abdominal compartment syndrome that are pertinent to gynecologic patient include blunt or penetrating abdominal trauma, intra-abdominal or retroperitoneal bleeding, patients with massive ascites, bowel wall edema, and those postsurgical patients who may be third spacing due to shock. It is imperative to have a high level of suspicion and recognize an early triad of abdominal compartment syndrome—oliguria, elevated peak airway pressures, and elevated intra-abdominal pressure.

III

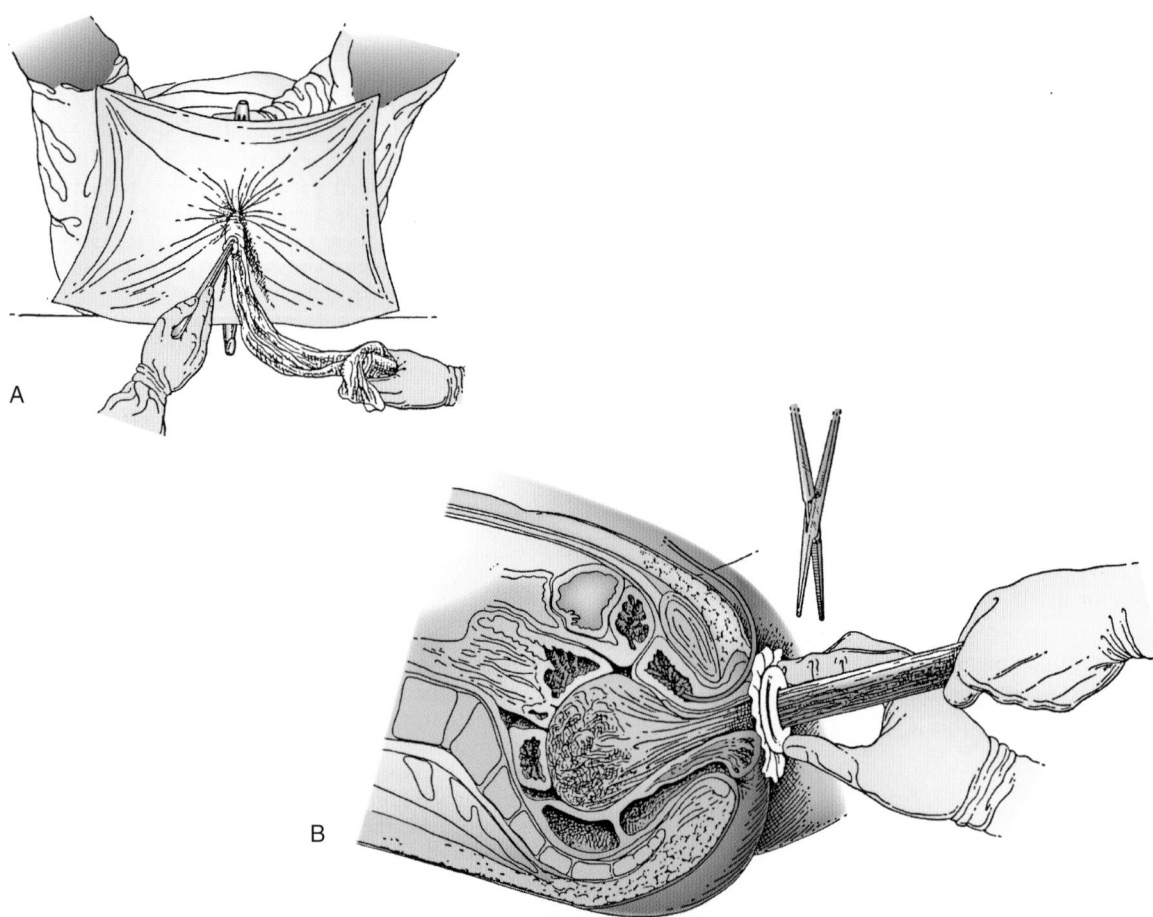

FIGURE 19.6 A and B: The parachute pack can be used to control bleeding from the deep pelvic veins after pelvic exenteration. A plastic sheet or towel is packed with gauze rolls through the vaginal or perineal opening. The ball of gauze packing is then pulled down to exert pressure against the vessels of the pelvic floor.

One of the first opportunities to assess for elevated intra-abdominal pressure is in the operating room, during abdominal closure. If the peak inspiratory pressure on the ventilator rises by 15 to 20 mm Hg, it is likely that the abdominal viscera are compressing the diaphragms. If the retroperitoneal pressure exceeds that within the inferior vena cava (IVC), venous return is compromised, leading to diminished cardiac output hypotension. Measurement of intravesical pressure (>25 mm Hg) is the standard method to screen intra-abdominal hypertension and abdominal compartment syndrome.

Potentially Troublesome Anatomic Locations

Iliac Vessels

One of the most dangerous places in the pelvis to dissect is in the region of the bifurcation of the common iliac artery and vein. This landmark is the superior border for pelvic lymphadenectomy in many gynecologic oncology staging procedures. The hypogastric vein and its branches are at risk of injury when dissecting between the distal common iliac artery and the psoas muscle, as well as deeper in the area of lumbosacral nerve trunks. When the surgeon places gentle traction on surrounding areolar tissue, a relatively loose and thin-walled vein may inadvertently be torn or pulled into the dissecting scissors. One should proceed cautiously, being cognizant of important adjacent structures, especially since the vein wall may not be distinct. Severe hemorrhage threatening exsanguination can result from

laceration of either the external iliac vein or the hypogastric vein where they join together, or from laceration of their major branches. On the medial side of these veins, the lateral sacral veins disappear into the sacral foramina. Fatal hemorrhage can result from laceration of these vessels as well, especially if they are torn where they enter the foramina, preventing adequate exposure of the cut end and inability to clamp, ligate, or clip the vessel. Instead, they are kept open by their attachment to the walls of the foramina, and extreme measures may be required to control such bleeding. One can try to pack the foramen with bone wax, but this usually is not successful. Alternatively, multiple layers (sandwiches) of absorbable gelatin sponge (Gelfoam) and microfibrillar collagen (Avitene) can be held in place with a strong pressure pack for 20 minutes and, perhaps, ultimately the packing can be fixed with sutures. This area deserves its reputation as the "corona mortis" of the pelvis.

Obturator Fossa

Numerous variations in the branches of the hypogastric artery and vein are encountered in dissecting the obturator fossa, especially in the floor of the fossa. The "web" of paracervical tissue separating the paravesical and pararectal spaces contains branches of the hypogastric artery and vein. These vessels must be carefully ligated with clips or sutures during a radical hysterectomy. The dissection can be carried down between the paravesical and pararectal space by carefully ligating or clipping each vessel encountered, thus uniting those two spaces.

The obturator artery and vein are usually found just below the obturator nerve. If injured, they may be ligated or clipped. Should these vessels retract through the obturator foramen into the upper thigh without being ligated, bleeding into the thigh may be a significant problem.

Pararectal Space

Development of the pararectal space between the ureter and the hypogastric artery must be done carefully because of the danger of injuring the internal iliac veins against the pelvic sidewall. The dissection is directed posteriorly at first, but soon changes to a more caudal direction. Failure to make this directional change can result in laceration and bleeding from veins in the bottom of the space. If development of the pararectal space is difficult, such as after pelvic radiation therapy, the paravesical space should be opened first, allowing the cardinal ligament to be identified and taken down in a serial fashion starting with the uterine vessels at their origin. The pararectal space should gradually be opened inferiorly, with the ureter identified medially and the iliac veins visualized laterally. The pararectal space can be expanded with sharp dissection or with pressure a from a peanut dissector, and with care to avoid excessive force.

Aortic Area

The removal of lymph nodes around the aorta and vena cava can result in serious hemorrhage from either vessel if not done carefully and with adequate exposure. An abdominal incision that provides sufficient exposure for a routine pelvic operation is not ordinarily sufficient for dissection around the aorta and vena cava unless the incision is extended. Although the vena cava usually can be ligated without serious problems, a laceration in the vena cava should be repaired. Bleeding is controlled by placing a finger over the site of injury and gaining the necessary exposure by retraction and suctioning. A running stitch using 5-0 Prolene suture on a small vascular needle is used to close the laceration from side to side as the finger is slowly withdrawn. The same technique can be used to repair lacerations in other large veins, such as the common and external iliac veins. Often, there are no untoward results, but repair of the laceration is often preferable. A patch graft of Gore-Tex or other materials can be sewn over the hole. Since veins are of low pressure, this is often successful and maintains the function of the vein. In contrast, lacerations of the common and external iliac arteries must always be repaired. These vessels cannot be ligated without serious consequences, and if the injury is not repairable, the artery should be replaced.

Presacral Space

In the presacral region, bleeding usually can be avoided by choosing a plane of dissection that is superficial to the anterior sacral artery and vein. The retrorectal space can easily be entered using blunt dissection staying in the correct plane superficial to the presacral fascia and the vessels that overlie the periosteum of the sacrum. If done properly, this plane can be developed inferiorly to the tip and lateral margins of the sacrum without appreciable bleeding. Timmons and colleagues and Khan and associates have recommended using metal thumbtacks to control presacral hemorrhage when the usual methods fail. Sterilized metal thumbtacks are placed directly over the bleeding point in the presacral fascia and pushed all the way into the sacrum with the thumb. Others have used a combination of bone wax, thumbtacks, packs, and hemostatic agents with success. Careful attention should be taken when using clips, ligatures, or cautery, as bleeding from the veins can be aggravated by imprecise use of these techniques.

POSTOPERATIVE BLEEDING

With normal hemostasis and proper surgical technique, postoperative hemorrhage is a rare occurrence. Every patient, however, should be carefully monitored postoperatively for signs of occult bleeding. The intensity and duration of the monitoring will depend on the type of surgery, any complications, and the medical condition of the patient. In addition to measuring vital signs and strict urine output, the abdominal incision and/or the perineum, and any intraperitoneal/subcutaneous drains, should be inspected for bleeding. Any sign of restlessness in the patient may be an indication of blood loss. Maintain a low threshold to check a CBC if there is a suspicion of postoperative bleeding or acute blood loss anemia. Because the risk of postoperative hemorrhage is low in routine, uncomplicated gynecologic surgery, many experts do not recommend routinely checking the hematocrit or hemoglobin postoperative. But in more extensive or complex surgery, a follow-up hematocrit or hemoglobin 4 to 12 hours after surgery may be helpful to guide postoperative management.

Occult intraperitoneal bleeding is one of the most serious postoperative complications after abdominal or vaginal surgery. Early warning signs may be insidious and not recognized until 12 to 18 hours after surgery was completed. However, the patient may suddenly develop severe hypotension, tachycardia, tachypnea, restlessness, and abdominal distention, prompting expedited intervention(s). In most cases, a small vessel has been slowly bleeding. Only after a significant blood loss has occurred do changes in the vital signs or symptoms of abdominal distention alert the clinician to a problem. In retrospect, subtle signs of hypovolemia, including tachycardia and decreased urine output, usually have been present.

Nonetheless, diagnosis of intraperitoneal bleeding in the postoperative patient can be difficult. Peritoneal signs are subtle and can be masked by incisional pain and analgesic medications. Unfortunately, the initial examination of the abdomen may be quite benign, as the peritoneal cavity has a large capacity for occult blood loss without appreciable abdominal distention. As much as 3,000 mL of blood (about 65% of the total blood volume of a 70-kg person) can be hidden in the peritoneal cavity, with only a 1-cm increase in the radius of the abdomen. Abdominal ultrasound is a rapid, noninvasive, readily available method of confirming the diagnosis of intraperitoneal bleeding. Alternatively, if a patient has experienced an unexpected drop in hematocrit postoperatively but is stable, an abdominal and pelvic CT scan is another good way to identify (or rule out) intra-abdominal hemorrhage or a hematoma (**Fig. 19.7**).

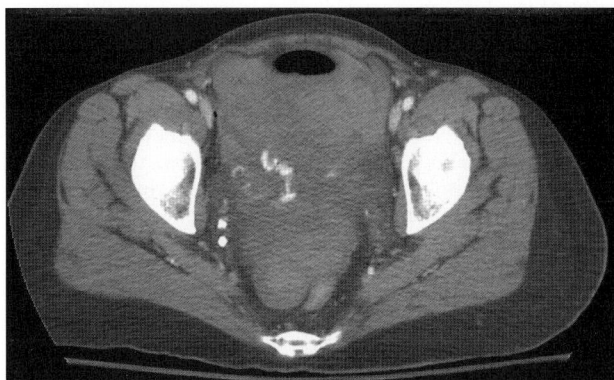

FIGURE 19.7 Axial CT image of the pelvis in a 52-year-old woman who is 5 hours post-op from a vaginal hysterectomy. Note the extravasation of contrast from an arterial injection into the right internal iliac artery.

Sometimes, it is difficult for the surgeon who performed the original operation to convince himself or herself that bleeding is persistent and intervention is urgently needed. Consultation with a colleague is often helpful in these situations. A routine coagulation profile, ordered at the first suspicion, or even simple observation of clot formation in a tube of blood at the bedside is helpful. However, the experienced surgeon knows that the most common reason for intraperitoneal blood and postoperative shock is loss of surgical hemostasis—a vessel has become disligated. The question now becomes: Should the patient be immediately taken back to the operating room to identify and control the bleeding or taken to the radiology suite in an attempt to control the bleeding by embolization? Both techniques are highly effective, and most often, the decision is dictated by the stability of the patient as well as the suspected source of bleeding. For instance, if the patient is unstable with a rapid pulse, falling blood pressure, and/or low urine output, or if the interval since surgery is short, suggesting fairly rapid hemorrhage, it is recommended to quickly return to the operating room where a team of anesthesiologists and direct one-to-one monitoring of the patient can allow prompt replacement of blood products and treatment of hemorrhagic shock. On the other hand, if the patient is reasonably stable and bleeding does not appear to be brisk, then it is reasonable to try to identify the bleeding artery and embolize it by transcatheter interventional radiologic techniques. A CT angiogram is useful in distinguishing if there is bleeding that can be embolized.

Whichever plan is selected, one or more large-bore intravenous lines should be started, and fluid replacement should begin with packed red blood cells ordered and started as indicated and available. A Foley catheter should be in place to allow close monitoring of urine output, and broad-spectrum antibiotics should be started. If the patient is not in the recovery room, she should be transferred there or to a monitored bed with easy access to the operating room. Preprocedure labs should be obtained, including coagulation studies, and the operating room and anesthesia service should be notified, as well as the interventional radiology team if appropriate.

Arterial Embolization

In 1969, Nusbaum and colleagues described arterial embolization to control bleeding from esophageal varices by selectively cannulating the superior mesenteric artery and infusing small doses of vasopressin into terminal vessels. The subsequent use of particulate matter to achieve hemostasis within bleeding viscera developed rapidly. Selective angiographic arterial embolization has been used to control hemorrhage after abdominal and vaginal hysterectomy and other gynecologic operations, hemorrhage from cervical cancer and gestational trophoblastic disease, postpartum hemorrhage, hemorrhage from abdominal pregnancy, and retroperitoneal hemorrhage. Experience has shown that selective pelvic artery embolization is a comparatively simple and safe procedure. Dramatic results can be seen. Clinical success rates of more than 90% are routinely reported when embolization is used for postsurgical and posttraumatic hemorrhage. Therefore, embolization rather than surgical ligation is appropriately selected as the primary procedure to control bleeding in patients who are stable or who cannot tolerate another operation.

Intravascular embolization requires the expertise of a skilled interventional radiologist. Percutaneous catheterization of the femoral artery under local anesthesia provides direct access in a retrograde manner to the hypogastric artery (Fig. 19.8).

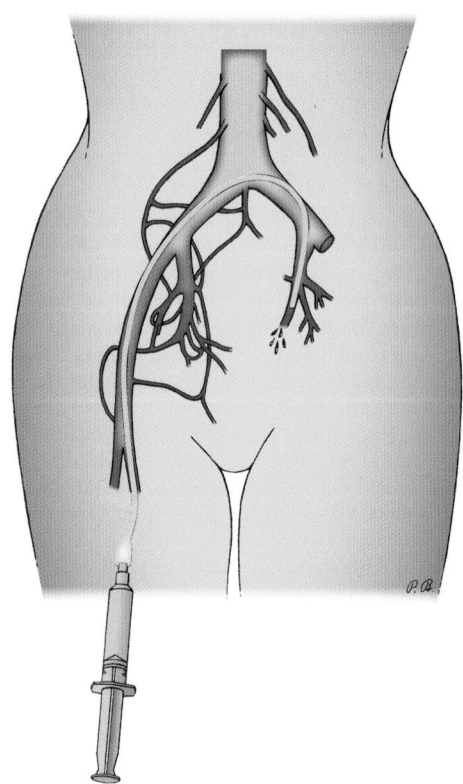

FIGURE 19.8 The femoral artery can be catheterized under local anesthesia to provide access to the hypogastric artery and its branches.

The brachial artery can also be used for access to the vascular system. If prior hypogastric artery ligation has obstructed this pathway, arteriography of the pelvic vasculature through one of the collateral arteries usually localizes the specific bleeding vessel or vessels, although with greater difficulty. The site of bleeding can be accurately identified with angiography and fluoroscopy if the rate of bleeding is 2 to 3 mL per minute or more. The hypogastric artery or the specific collateral vessel is cannulated for injection (Fig. 19.9A–C). A variety of materials can be used for embolization, including small pieces of Gelfoam, metal coils, small Silastic spheres, autologous clot, subcutaneous tissue, and other hemostatic materials. Gelfoam is one of the most practical and easily injected materials. It is sterile and nonantigenic, remains in the vessel for 20 to 50 days, and forms a fibrin mesh framework on which blood clots can develop. Its immediate effect is to obstruct the distal artery or arteriole and reduce pulse pressure in the bleeding vessel, thereby permitting clot formation and cessation of bleeding. Material is injected under angiographic observation. When it becomes evident by repeat angiography that the bleeding vessel has been occluded, the catheter is removed and the patient is carefully monitored for evidence of further bleeding.

After embolization, patients usually have no complications or evidence of the effects of local ischemia. Those who have not had a hysterectomy will resume normal menstruation. Some patients will exhibit evidence of a mild postembolization syndrome, including pain, fever, leukocytosis resulting from vascular thrombosis, and tissue necrosis. A few isolated cases of more serious problems have been reported, including bladder necrosis, vesicovaginal fistula, neuropathies, and renal toxicity from the contrast medium. The overall complication rate is estimated to be less than 10%.

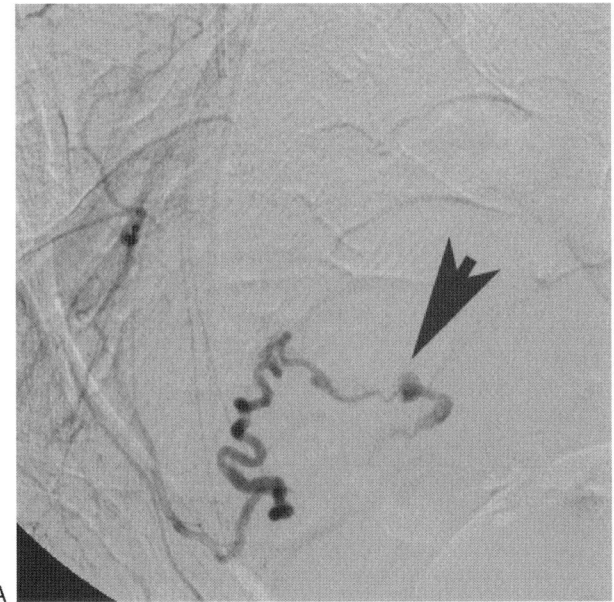

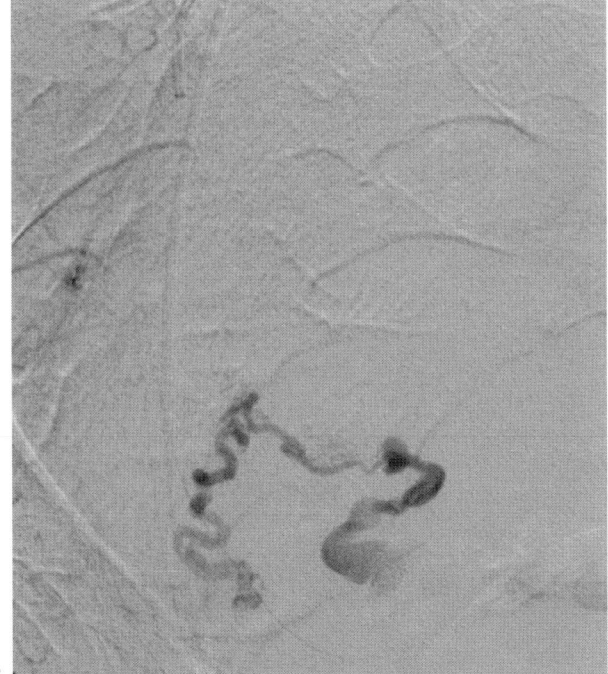

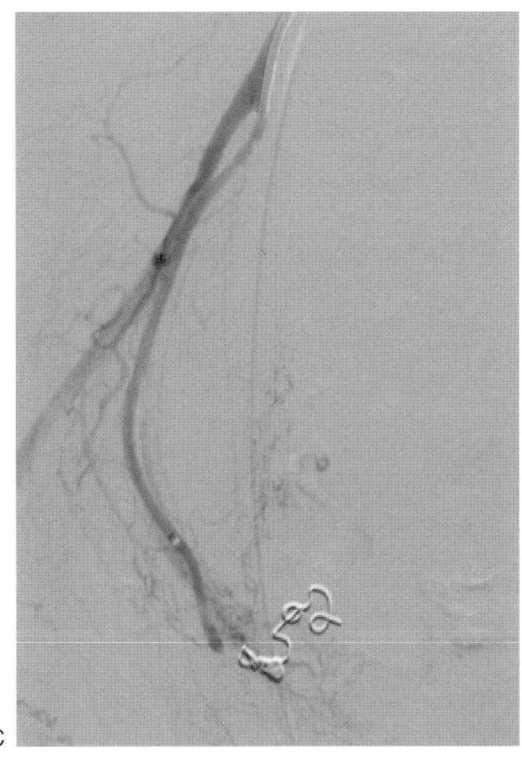

III

FIGURE 19.9 Selective angiogram with the catheter tip positioned in the right internal iliac artery (same patient as shown in **Fig. 19.8**). **A:** The tortuous right uterine artery is filled and some wispy extravasation is seen (**arrow**). **B:** A delayed image shows more extensive extravasation. **C:** After five microcoils have been injected, the bleeding has been controlled. No extravasation is seen with an injection of contrast in the common iliac artery. (Courtesy of Dr. Leann Stokes, Vanderbilt University.)

Reoperation

If reoperation is selected, the patient should be as stable as possible, with blood actively being transfused or at least available in the room. Two suctions should be ready and an adequate staff with sufficient number of assistants involved. If the patient has previously had an abdominal operation, the incision should be reopened. A preoperative ultrasound or CT scan should have identified the bleeding as intraperitoneal or retroperitoneal. The previous procedure should be mentally reviewed to identify any possible ligatures that were tentative or any troublesome bleeding sites that may have continued to bleed. When the abdomen is opened, the clots should be evacuated and a search instituted for the bleeding sites, starting with

the most likely locations. Care should be taken when removing clots from the pelvic area.

Bleeding sites should be carefully ligated, sutured, or clipped. It is not unusual to reopen the abdomen and find no active bleeding sites. This is somewhat disconcerting because of the concern that the problem will repeat itself after the abdomen is again closed. Every attempt should be made to identify the source of bleeding, including irrigation with warm, sterile water to allow better visualization.

During reoperation, patients are at increased risk of ureteral injury. In addition to exercising care in clamping and ligating bloodstained tissue with distorted anatomy, it may be wise to prove ureteral integrity at the end of the operation. This can be done by injecting 5 mL of indigo carmine dye intravenously and observing efflux of dye from each ureteral orifice through the cystoscope or by direct visualization if the bladder dome is already opened. After reoperation, patients are also at increased risk of developing postoperative complications such as pulmonary atelectasis, ileus, postoperative infection, incisional complications, and coagulation disorders from multiple transfusions. The anticipation of these complications allows the adoption of measures to prevent or manage them correctly should they occur.

Postoperative hemorrhage from the vaginal vault usually comes from the vaginal artery in the lateral vaginal fornix or from one of its branches. Most often, the lateral vaginal angle, including the vaginal artery, is not properly secured or slips off the pedicle. To prevent such bleeding, this stitch should be anchored to more lateral tissue so that the angle cannot slip out of the ligature. This stitch should not be held because traction will loosen it. Excessive vaginal bleeding may be noted in the recovery room or after the patient has returned to her room. Every attempt should be made to establish an objective measurement of the amount of blood lost and to follow vital signs and serial hematocrit values. One must realize that the vagina is a distensible organ. If a clot occludes the vaginal introitus, a large amount of blood—sometimes several hundred milliliters—can distend the vagina behind it and not be evident on a perineal pad. When significant vaginal bleeding is present, the patient should be examined in dorsal lithotomy position. This may be possible in the recovery room with analgesia, but a return to the operating room for an examination under anesthesia should be used if necessary. The vaginal apex should be inspected. If the source of bleeding is visualized, it should be clamped and ligated from below. Figure-of-eight using 0 delayed-absorbable transfixion sutures should be placed to include the vaginal mucosa and underlying paravaginal tissue. Care must be taken to avoid the inadvertent placement of a suture into the musculature of the bladder wall, the ureter, or the underlying rectum. If bleeding is not controlled by this technique, it is unwise to continue to add suture on top of suture in a frantic effort to control the vaginal bleeding. In such cases, it is probable that the bleeding vessels have retracted well above the vaginal apex and cannot be reached by this approach.

If surgical hemostasis cannot be achieved transvaginally, laparotomy may be necessary. A vaginal pack will not control significant bleeding from the vaginal vault that has already required a return to the operating room, although a temporary pack may slow the blood loss while the patient is prepared for laparotomy. A Foley catheter should already be in place. In some patients, the hemorrhage will be delayed until 10 to 14 days after surgery, when the sutures lose their tensile strength. Furthermore, posthysterectomy disruption of the vaginal vault with hemorrhage also can result from coitus.

Bleeding from anterior and posterior colporrhaphy usually is from veins that have not been secured. In this situation, a fairly tight vaginal pack effectively compresses these vessels and controls the bleeding. It seldom is necessary to reexplore an anterior or posterior colporrhaphy to locate and ligate a specific bleeding vessel. Again, a Foley catheter is necessary while the pack is in place to bypass urethral obstruction.

A postoperative pelvic hematoma can cause serious morbidity, especially if it is large and becomes infected. Hematomas can develop above the vaginal vault, along the pelvic sidewall, in the retroperitoneum extending up to the kidneys, in the paravesical space, in the abdominal wall, and in the ischiorectal fossa and vulva. A hematoma in the ischiorectal fossa and on the vulva may be obvious on examination when the patient reports discomfort in the area. If it is below the puborectalis

muscle attachment to the vagina, it will not dissect into the pelvis but rather be limited to the perineum and buttocks. A pelvic hematoma may be recognized in a patient whose postoperative discomfort and anemia exceed what is normally expected, whose temperature is progressively increasing, and whose postoperative abdominal distention is slow to resolve. A definitive diagnosis can be made by ultrasound or CT scan, which is helpful in delineating its exact size and location. An extended, postoperative course may be alleviated if a large hematoma can be evacuated and drained via a small closed suction drain placed by interventional radiology. However, in specific cases, drain placement may be difficult to perform or even contraindicated, in which case it may be preferable to allow the hematoma to gradually resolve over a few months. Unfortunately, sometimes a hematoma will not resolve completely, and residual fibrosis will persist and continue to be symptomatic. Hemorrhage after uterine curettage is extremely rare, even when complicated by perforation. Under most circumstances, the curettage should be stopped and the patient's vital signs checked for several hours. Most patients have an uncomplicated postoperative recovery and are stable to be discharged home the same day. However, if the perforation was caused by a wide, blunt instrument (such as a curette or a suction device), if the uterus is pregnant or contains cancer, or if fatty tissue appears in the curettage specimen, then overnight observation should be considered and the patient closely observed for intraperitoneal bleeding or a broad ligament hematoma. Diagnostic laparoscopy should be performed immediately after perforation if significant injury is suspected to assess for damage to surrounding organs, especially bowel, and determine if a hematoma or active bleeding is present. Alternatively, if the perforation is midline and no trauma is suspected, careful observation is a reasonable option. A misdirected curette can lacerate the uterine artery and vein, with subsequent intraperitoneal bleeding or broad ligament hematoma formation. In such cases, laparotomy may be necessary to fully evaluate and control the bleeding. As a last resort, hysterectomy may not be indicated if there is severe damage to the uterus or to control bleeding.

Hemorrhage from cervical conization can occur in the first 24 hours or 7 to 14 days later when cervical sutures lose their tensile strength. Patients may also bleed heavily after a loop electrosurgical procedure (LEEP) due to inadequate electrocautery, possible vaginal laceration, or delayed relaxation of small vessels that were initially vasoconstricted at the completion of the procedure. If the patient is bleeding heavily at any time after conization or LEEP, a speculum exam should be performed and the cervix and vaginal walls should be thoroughly inspected. Measures to control the bleeding include resuturing, electrocautery, and Monsel solution. If bleeding is not profuse, Monsel solution, Gelfoam, and/or a small vaginal pack can be tried. In taking the conization specimen, one must be certain that the apex of the cone intersects the endocervical canal. If the cervical incision is misdirected to one side or the other, the uterine vessels are in danger of laceration and cause serious hemorrhage or broad ligament hematoma. To prevent this problem, the cervix should first be sounded to ascertain the direction of the endocervical canal and the incision planned accordingly.

SUMMARY

Careful preoperative evaluation of the patient and thoughtful preoperative planning on the part of the surgeon and surgical team will help prevent or minimize significant operative blood loss. However, intraoperative or postoperative hemorrhage does occur from time to time and represents a significant challenge to the technical skill and the emotional control of the surgeon. He or she must take charge of the situation, organize a plan to control the bleeding, clearly communicate with other members of the surgical team, and, finally, execute the technical steps necessary to obtain hemostasis. Each part of this approach is important. We hope that the ideas and techniques discussed in this chapter will make the reader more prepared to meet this challenge.

BEST SURGICAL PRACTICES

- Preparation to prevent and control operative bleeding starts before the surgical procedure. The patient should be thoroughly evaluated for risk factors that may increase the possibility of hemorrhage. Congenital and acquired coagulation disorders need to be diagnosed by a careful and thorough history and appropriate lab tests. The surgical approach should be individualized to the patient's condition, goals of treatment, and the abilities of the surgical team. Preoperative consultations with other specialists should be sought if indicated. All medical conditions of the patient should be optimized prior to elective surgery.
- The possibility and risks of blood transfusion should always be discussed with the patient as part of informed consent before surgery. The risk of a febrile reaction to transfusion is approximately 1%. Transmission of hepatitis B via transfusion occurs about 1 in every 180,000 transfusions, whereas the risk of HIV transmission with modern blood banking procedures is approximately 1 in 1.9 million.
- During the operative procedure, good exposure, keen awareness of the anatomy, and careful dissection, clamping, and suturing are all important technical skills that will reduce the risk of uncontrolled hemorrhage. Ultimately, excellent surgical judgment and leadership must be used to achieve the best possible outcome for the patient.
- When life-threatening intraoperative hemorrhage occurs, the surgeon should identify the source of the bleeding, apply pressure, and orchestrate the operative team to help achieve hemostasis. This is one of the most challenging of all emergencies and requires leadership; sound judgment; knowledge; precise, efficient technical skills; and clear communication lines.
- When intraoperative blood loss exceeds 15% of the patient's blood volume (about 500 to 1,000 mL), transfusion should be considered. The patient's medical history, vital signs, the probability of additional blood loss, and anticipated course of management should dictate how urgent to initiate transfusion of specific blood products (e.g., packed red blood cells, platelets, cryoprecipitate).
- Hematocrit and coagulation factors—as well as serum calcium, electrolytes, and glucose—should be followed at least every 120 minutes or after 10 units of transfusion. Although it is best to use actual serum levels of coagulation factors, as a rough guide, after every 6 to 8 units of packed red cells, 2 units of fresh frozen plasma should be given. If fibrinogen levels fall below 100 mg/dL, 20 units of cryoprecipitate should be given. A bolus of 6 units of platelets should be given if the platelet count falls below 100,000 and the patient is actively bleeding.
- The gynecologic surgeon should be able to use special techniques such as packing, thrombotic agents, and hypogastric artery ligation and know their indications for the control of pelvic hemorrhage.
- Postoperative bleeding may be difficult to diagnose, but a high level of suspicion due to intraoperative complications and attention to clinical detail (vital signs, strict ins and outs especially output from the Foley catheter and any pelvic drains, incisional or vaginal bleeding, etc.) will facilitate prompt recognition and appropriate management. Abdominal and pelvic ultrasound and CT imaging are also very helpful in making the diagnosis of postoperative bleeding and localizing the site of bleeding.
- Embolization of arterial bleeders by interventional radiology and reoperation are both effective techniques to manage postoperative hemorrhage. When the patient is relatively stable and an experienced interventional radiology team is available, embolization is generally preferred because it is associated with less morbidity.

BIBLIOGRAPHY

Abbas FM, Currie JL, Mitchell S, et al. Selective vascular embolization in benign gynecologic conditions. *J Reprod Med* 1994;39:492.

Albala DM, Lawson JH. Recent clinical and investigational applications of fibrin sealant in selected surgical specialties. *J Am Coll Surg* 2006;202:685.

Alvarez M, Lockwood CJ, Ghidini A, et al. Prophylactic and emergent arterial catheterization for selective embolization in obstetric hemorrhage. *Am J Perinatol* 1992;9:441.

Amrein PC, Ellman L, Harris WH. Aspirin-induced prolongation of bleeding time and perioperative blood loss. *JAMA* 1981;245:1825.

Arepally GM, Ortel TL. Clinical practice: heparin-induced thrombocytopenia. *N Engl J Med* 2006;355:809.

Baggaley RF, Boily MC, White RG, et al. Risk of HIV-1 transmission for parenteral exposure and blood transfusion: a systematic review and meta-analysis. *AIDS* 2006;20:805.

Barrett NA, Kam PC. Transfusion-related acute lung injury: a literature review. *Anaesthesia* 2006;61:777.

Behnam K, Jarmolowski CR. Vesicovaginal fistula following hypogastric embolization for control of intractable pelvic hemorrhage. *J Reprod Med* 1982;27:304.

Berkowitz RL, Bussel JB, McFarland JG. Alloimmune thrombocytopenia: state of the art 2006. *Am J Obstet Gynecol* 2006;195:907.

Bernard GR, Vincent JL, Laterre PF, et al. Efficacy and safety of recombinant human activated protein C for severe sepsis. *N Engl J Med* 2001;344:699.

Bertina RM, Koeleman BPC, Koster T, et al. Mutation in blood coagulation factor V associated with resistance to activated protein C. *Nature* 1994;369:64.

Bickell WH, Wall MJ, Pepe PE, et al. Immediate versus delayed fluid resuscitation for hypotensive patients with penetrating torso injuries. *N Engl J Med* 1994;331:1105.

Blajchman MA. The clinical benefits of the leukoreduction of blood products. *J Trauma* 2006;60:S83.

Burchell RC. The umbrella pack to control pelvic hemorrhage. *Conn Med* 1968;32:734.

Carless PA, Henry DA. Systematic review and meta-analysis of the use of fibrin sealant to prevent seroma formation after breast cancer surgery. *Br J Surg* 2006;93:810.

Chung AF, Menon J, Dillon TF. Acute postoperative retroperitoneal fibrosis and ureteral obstruction secondary to the use of Avitene. *Am J Obstet Gynecol* 1978;132:908.

Ciavarella S, Reed RL, Counts RB, et al. Clotting factor levels and the risk of diffuse microvascular bleeding in the massively transfused patient. *Br J Haematol* 1987;67:365.

Clark SL, Phelan JP, Yeh SY, et al. Hypogastric artery ligation for obstetric hemorrhage. *Obstet Gynecol* 1985;66:353.

Collins JA. Problems associated with the massive transfusion of stored blood. *Surgery* 1974;75:274.

Corriveau DM, Fritsma GA. *Hemostasis and thrombosis.* Philadelphia, PA: JB Lippincott Co., 1988.

Cruikshank SH, Stoclk EM. Surgical control of pelvic hemorrhage: bilateral hypogastric artery ligation and method of ovarian artery ligation. *South Med J* 1985;78:539.

Cushing H. The control of bleeding in operations for brain tumors: with description of silver "clips" for occlusion of vessels inaccessible to the ligature. *Ann Surg* 1911;54:1.

Dagi RF. The management of postoperative bleeding. *Surg Clin North Am* 2005;85:1191.

Dahlback B, Carlsson M, Svensson PH. Familial thrombophilia due to a previously unrecognized mechanism characterized by poor anti-coagulant response to activated protein C: prediction of a cofactor to activated protein C. *Proc Natl Acad Sci U S A* 1993;90:1004.

DeBernardo RL Jr, Perkins RB, Littell RD, et al. Low-molecular-weight heparin (dalteparin) in women with gynecologic malignancy. *Obstet Gynecol* 2005;105:1006.

Dehaeck CMC. Transcatheter embolization of pelvic vessels to stop intractable hemorrhage. *Gynecol Oncol* 1986;24:9.

Dodd RY. The risk of transfusion transmitted infections. *N Engl J Med* 1992;327:419.

Dubay ML, Holshausen CA, Burchell RC. Internal iliac artery ligation for postpartum hemorrhage: recanalization of vessels. *Am J Obstet Gynecol* 1980;136:689.

Dziecxkowski JS, Anderson KC. Transfusion biology and therapy. In: Fauci AS, Martin JB, Braunwald E, et al., eds. *Harrison's principles of internal medicine*. 14th ed. New York, NY: McGraw-Hill, 1998:718.

Edmunds LH, Addonizio VP. Massive transfusion. In: Colman RW, Hirsh J, Marder VJ, et al., eds. *Hemostasis and thrombosis: basic principles and clinical practice*, 2nd ed. Philadelphia, PA: JB Lippincott Co., 1987:913.

Ereth MH, Oliver WC, Santrach PJ. Perioperative interventions to decrease transfusion of allogeneic blood products. *Mayo Clin Proc* 1994;69:575.

Esmon NL, Owen W, Esmon C. Isolation of a membrane-bound cofactor for thrombin-catalyzed activation of protein C. *J Biol Chem* 1982;257:859.

Etchason J, Petz L, Keeler E, et al. The cost effectiveness of pre-operative autologous blood donations. *N Engl J Med* 1995;332:719.

Evans S, McShane P. The efficacy of internal iliac artery ligation in obstetric hemorrhage. *Surg Gynecol Obstet* 1985;160:250.

Fehrman H. Surgical management of life-threatening obstetric and gynecologic hemorrhage. *Acta Obstet Gynecol Scand* 1988;67:125.

Ferraris VA, Swanson E. Aspirin usage and perioperative blood loss in patients undergoing unexpected operations. *Surg Gynecol Obstet* 1983;156:439.

Forgie MA, Wells PS, Laupacis A, et al. Preoperative autologous donation decreases allogeneic transfusion but increases exposure to all red blood cell transfusion: results of a meta-analysis. International Study of Perioperative Transfusion (ISPOT) Investigators. *Arch Intern Med* 1998;158:610.

Gewirtz AS, Miller ML, Keys TF. The clinical usefulness of the preoperative bleeding time. *Arch Pathol Lab Med* 1996;120:353.

Given FT, Gates HS, Morgan BE. Pregnancy following bilateral ligation of the internal iliac (hypogastric) arteries. *Am J Obstet Gynecol* 1964;89:1078.

Goodnough LT, Breacher ME, Kanter MH, et al. Transfusion medicine: first of two parts—blood transfusion. *N Engl J Med* 1999;340:438.

Gunter O, Au B, Isbell J, et al. Optimizing outcomes in damage control resuscitation: identifying blood product ratios associated with improved survival. *J Trauma* 2008;65:527.

Haas S. The use of a surgical patch coated with human coagulation factors in surgical routing: a multicenter postauthorization surveillance. *Clin Appl Thromb Hemost* 2006;12:445.

Harima Y, Shiraishi T, Harima K, et al. Transcatheter arterial embolization therapy in cases of recurrent and advanced gynecologic cancer. *Cancer* 1989;63:2077.

Harker LA. *Hemostasis manual*, 2nd ed. Philadelphia, PA: FA Davis Co., 1974.

Hillyer CD, Emmens RK, Zago-Novaretti M, et al. Methods for the reduction of transfusion-transmitted cytomegalovirus infection: filtration versus the use of seronegative donor units. *Transfusion* 1994;34:929.

Hong YM, Loughlin KR. The use of hemostatic agents and sealants in urology. *J Urol* 2006;176:2367.

Johnson H, Knee-Ioli S, Butler TA, et al. Are routine preoperative laboratory screening tests necessary to evaluate ambulatory surgical patients? *Surgery* 1988;104:639.

Judd WB. Pretransfusion testing in clinical laboratory medicine. In: McClatchey KD, ed. *Clinical Laboratory Medicine*. Baltimore, MD: Williams & Wilkins, 1994:1733.

Kanji S, Devlin J, Piekos K, et al. Recombinant human activated protein C, drotrecogin alfa (activated): a novel therapy for severe sepsis. *Pharmacotherapy* 2001;21:1389.

Kaplan EB, Sheiner LB, Boeckmann AJ, et al. The usefulness of preoperative laboratory screening. *JAMA* 1985;253:3576.

Keeling MM, Gray LA Jr, Brink MA, et al. Intraoperative autotransfusion. Experience in 725 consecutive cases. *Ann Surg* 1983;197:536.

Kelly HA. Ligation of both internal iliac arteries for hemorrhage in hysterectomy for carcinoma uteri. *Bull Johns Hopkins Hosp* 1894;5:53.

Kelly HA. Ligature of the trunks of the uterine and ovarian arteries as a means of checking hemorrhage from the uterus and broad ligaments in abdominal operations. *Johns Hopkins Hosp Rep* 1891;2:220.

Kermode JC, Zheng Q, Milner EP. Marked temperature dependence of the platelet calcium signal induced by human von Willebrand factor. *Blood* 1999;94:199.

Ketchum L, Hess JR, Hiippala S. Indications for early fresh frozen plasma, cryoprecipitate, and platelet transfusion in trauma. *J Trauma* 2006;60:S51.

Khan FA, Fang DT, Nivatvongs S. Management of presacral bleeding during rectal resection. *Surg Gynecol Obstet* 1987;165:275.

Klingensmith ME, Abdulhameed A, Bharat A, et al., eds. *The Washington manual of surgery*, 6th ed. Lippincott Williams & Wilkins, 2012:133.

Lattouf JB, Beri A, Klinger CH, et al. Practical hints for hemostasis in laparoscopic surgery. *Minim Invasive Ther Allied Technol* 2007;16:45.

Lee VS, Tarassenko L, Bellhouse BJ. Platelet transfusion therapy: platelet concentrate preparation and storage. *J Lab Clin Med* 1988;111:371.

Leonard F, Lecuru F, Rizk E, et al. Perioperative morbidity of gynecological laparoscopy: a retrospective monocenter observational study. *Acta Obstet Gynecol Scand* 2000;79:129.

Levy GG, Nichols WC, Lian EC, et al. Mutations in a number of the ADAMTS gene family cause thrombotic thrombocytopenic purpura. *Nature* 2001;413:488.

Lier H, Krep H, Schroeder S, et al. Preconditions of hemostasis in trauma: a review. The influence of acidosis, hypocalcemia, anemia, and hypothermia on functional hemostasis in trauma. *J Trauma* 2008;65:951.

Lovisetto F, Zonta S, Rota E, et al. Use of human fibrin glue (Tissucol) versus staples for mesh fixation in laparoscopic transabdominal preperitoneal hernioplasty: a prospective, randomized study. *Ann Surg* 2007;245:222.

MacLennan S, Williams LM. Risks of fresh frozen plasma and platelets. *J Trauma* 2006;60:S46.

Madjdpour C, Heindl V, Spahn DR. Risks, benefits, alternatives and indications of allogeneic blood transfusions. *Minerva Anestesiol* 2006;72:283.

Madjdpour C, Spahn DR, Weiskopf RB. Anemia and perioperative red blood cell transfusion: a matter of tolerance. *Crit Care Med* 2006;34:S102.

Malviya VK, Deppe G. Control of intraoperative hemorrhage in gynecology with the use of fibrin glue. *Obstet Gynecol* 1989;73:284.

Mannucci PM. Hemostatic drugs. *N Engl J Med* 1998;339:245.

Mannucci PM. Desmopressin (DDAVP) in the treatment of bleeding disorders: the first 20 years. *Blood* 1997;90:2515.

Mannucci PM, Tenconi PM, Gastaman G, et al. Comparison of four virus-inactivated plasma concentrates for treatment of severe von Willebrand disease; a cross-over randomized trial. *Blood* 1992;79:3130.

Mannucci PM, Tripodi A. Laboratory screening of inherited thrombotic syndromes. *Thromb Haemost* 1987;57:247.

Mengert WF, Burchell RC, Blumstein RW, et al. Pregnancy after bilateral ligation of the internal iliac and ovarian arteries. *Obstet Gynecol* 1969;34:664.

Mintz PD, Henry JB, Boral LI. The type and antibody screen: symposium on blood banking and hemotherapy. *Clin Lab Med* 1982;2:169.

Mitty HA, Sterling KM, Alavarez M, et al. Obstetric hemorrhage: prophylactic and emergency arterial catheterization and embolotherapy. *Radiology* 1993;188:183.

Morgan CH, Penner JA. Bleeding complications during surgery: part I. Defects of primary hemostasis and congenital coagulation. *Lab Med* 1986;17:207.

Morgan CH, Penner JA. Bleeding complications during surgery: part II. Acquired hemorrhagic disorders. *Lab Med* 1986;17:262.

Moscardo F, Perez F, de la Rubia J, et al. Successful treatment of severe intra-abdominal bleeding associated with disseminated intravascular coagulation using recombinant activated FVII. *Br J Haematol* 2001;114:174.

Nordestgaard AG, Bodily KC, Osborne RW, et al. Major vascular injury during laparoscopic procedures. *Am J Surg* 1995;169:543.

Nusbaum M, Baum S, Blakemore WS. Clinical experience with the diagnosis and management of gastrointestinal hemorrhage by selective mesenteric catheterization. *Ann Surg* 1969;170:506.

Ozier Y, Schulmberger S. Pharmacological approaches to reducing blood loss and transfusions in the surgical patient. *Can J Anaesth* 2006;53:S21.

Papp Z, Toth-Pal E, Papp C, et al. Hypogastric artery ligation for intractable pelvic hemorrhage. *Int J Gynaecol Obstet* 2006;92:27.

Pearl ML, Braga CA. Percutaneous transcatheter embolization for control of life-threatening pelvic hemorrhage from gestational trophoblastic disease. *Obstet Gynecol* 1992;80:571.

Perioperative red cell transfusion. *NIH Consens Dev Conf Consens Statement* 1988;7:1.

Poon MC. Use of recombinate FVIIa in hereditary bleeding disorders. *Curr Opin Hematol* 2001;8:312.

Prati D. Transmission of hepatitis C virus by blood transfusions and other medical procedures: a global review. *J Hepatol* 2006;45:607.

Repine TB, Perkins JG, Kauvar DS, et al. The use of fresh whole blood in massive transfusion. *J Trauma* 2006;60:S78.

Rock WA Jr, Meeks GR. Managing anemia and blood loss in elective gynecologic surgery patients. *J Reprod Med* 2001;46:507.

Rodgers RP, Levin J, ed. A critical reappraisal of the bleeding time. *Semin Thromb Hemost* 1990;16:1.

Rohrer MJ, Michelotti MC, Nahrwold DL. A prospective evaluation of the efficacy of preoperative coagulation testing. *Ann Surg* 1988;208:554.

Rosen NR, Bates LH, Herod G. Transfusion therapy: improved patient care and resource utilization. *Transfusion* 1993;33:341.

Rutherford EJ, Skeete DA, Brasel KJ. Management of the patient with an open abdomen: techniques in temporary and definitive closure. *Curr Probl Surg* 2004;41:815.

Santoso JT, Saunders BA, Grosshart K. Massive blood loss and transfusion in obstetrics and gynecology. *Obstet Gynecol Surv* 2005;60:827.

Santoso JT, Lin DW, Miller DS. Transfusion medicine in obstetrics and gynecology. *Obstet Gynecol Surv* 1995;50:470.

Schafer M, Lauper M, Krahenbuhl L. Trocar and Veress needle injuries during laparoscopy. *Surg Endosc* 2000;15:275.

Schreiber GB, Busch MP, Kleinman SH, et al. The risk of transfusion transmitted viral infections: the retrovirus epidemiology donor study. *N Engl J Med* 1996;334:1685.

Schwartz M, Madariago J, Hirose R, et al. Comparison of a new fibrin sealant with standard topical hemostatic agents. *Arch Surg* 2004;139:1148.

Shah HN, Hegde S, Shah JN, et al. A prospective, randomized trial evaluating the safety and efficacy of fibrin sealant in tubeless percutaneous nephrolithotomy. *J Urol* 2006;176:2488.

Shinagawa S, Nomura Y, Kudoh S. Full-term deliveries after ligation of bilateral internal iliac arteries and infundibulopelvic ligaments. *Acta Obstet Gynecol Scand* 1981;60:439.

Sieber PR. Bladder necrosis secondary to pelvic artery embolization: case report and literature review. *J Urol* 1994;151:422.

Simon PH, Conner C, Delcour C, et al. Selective uterine artery embolization in the treatment of cervical pregnancy: two case reports. *Eur J Obstet Gynecol Reprod Biol* 1991;40:159.

Sitges-Serra A, Insenser JJ, Membrilla E. Blood transfusions and postoperative infections in patients undergoing elective surgery. *Surg Infect (Larchmt)* 2006;7(suppl 2):S33.

So-Osman C, Nelissen RG, Eikenboom HC, et al. Efficacy, safety and user-friendliness of two devices for postoperative autologous shed red blood cell re-infusion in elective orthopaedic surgery patients: a randomized pilot study. *Tranfus Med* 2006;16:321.

Sproule MW, Bendomir AM, Grant KA, et al. Embolisation of massive bleeding following hysterectomy, despite internal iliac artery ligation. *Br J Obstet Gynaecol* 1994;101:908.

Stehling L. Fluid replacement in massive transfusion. *Massive Transfus AABB* 1994;1.

Stimson LA. On some modifications in the technique of abdominal surgery, limiting the use of the ligature en masse. *Trans Am Surg Assoc* 1889;7:65.

Strumper-Groves D. Perioperative blood transfusion and outcome. *Curr Opin Anaesthesiol* 2006;19:198.

Svensson PJ, Dahlback B. Resistance to activated protein C as a basis for venous thrombosis. *N Engl J Med* 1994;330:517.

Swanson K, Dwyre DM, Krochmal J, et al. Transfusion-related acute lung injury (TRALI): current clinical and pathophysiologic considerations. *Lung* 2006;184:177.

Thompson JD. Anemia due to gynecologic disease: its correction by the use of iron orally. *South Med J* 1957;50:679.

Timmons MC, Kohler MF, Addison WA. Thumbtack use for control of presacral bleeding, with description of an instrument for thumbtack application. *Obstet Gynecol* 1991;78:313.

Traver MA, Assimos DG. New generation tissue sealants and hemostatic agents: innovative urologic applications. *Rev Urol* 2006;8:104.

Triplett DA, ed. *Laboratory evaluation of coagulation*. Chicago, IL: ASCP Press, 1982.

Vanderlinde ES, Heal JM, Blumberg N. Autologous transfusion. *Br Med J* 2002;324:772.

Werner EJ, Broxson EH, Tucker EL, et al. Prevalence of von Willebrand disease in children: a multiethnic study. *J Pediatr* 1993;1123:893.

Yamashita Y, Harada M, Yamamoto H, et al. Transcatheter arterial embolization of obstetric and gynaecological bleeding: efficacy and clinical outcome. *Br J Radiol* 1994;67:530.

Yugi H, Mizui M, Tanaka J, et al. Hepatitis B virus (HBV) screening strategy to ensure the safety of blood for transfusion through a combination of immunological testing and nucleic acid amplification testing—Japanese experience. *J Clin Virol* 2006;36 (suppl 1):S56.

Zoon KC. Ten years after: what has been achieved by Consent Decrees: the FDA view. *Paper presented at: Fifth Annual FDA and the Changing Paradigm for Blood Regulation*; January 16–18, 2002. New Orleans, LA, 2002.

III

CHAPTER 20
The Impact of Assisted Reproductive Technology on Gynecologic Surgery

Hey-Joo Kang and Zev Rosenwaks

DEFINITIONS

Controlled ovarian hyperstimulation—Administration of exogenous gonadotropins to induce growth of multiple ovarian follicles within a single menstrual cycle.

Developmental states—*Morula*—The stage between 72 and 96 hours after insemination, from the 16-cell stage to formation of the blastocyst. *Blastocyst*—The stage consisting of an inner cell mass from which the fetus develops and a trophectoderm from which the placenta develops. It is distinguished from the morula by the presence of a fluid-filled cavity.

Embryo transfer—The delivery of viable embryos to the uterine fundus for implantation. This is traditionally done transcervically or less commonly by laparoscopic cannulation of the fallopian tubes.

Intracytoplasmic sperm injection (ICSI)—Procedure by which a single sperm is injected directly into a mature oocyte assisted fertilization.

Mature oocyte—An oocyte at metaphase II of meiosis. Fertilization may occur at this stage of development.

Noncommunicating hydrosalpinx—Accumulation of distal tubal fluid that is unable to pass into the peritoneal cavity.

Oocyte—The immature female gamete.

Oocyte retrieval—The removal of oocytes after controlled ovarian hyperstimulation by ultrasound-guided needle aspiration. In rare instances, laparoscopic retrieval may be necessary.

Ovarian hyperstimulation syndrome (OHSS)—A complication of assisted reproductive technology that occurs almost exclusively with the use of gonadotropin stimulation. It is a condition of vascular hyperpermeability secondary to the release of vasoactive substances (vascular endothelial growth factor, tumor necrosis factor-alpha, interleukins) from the overstimulated ovaries. The transudation of protein-rich fluid from the intravascular to the extravascular compartment can lead to ascites, hemoconcentration, electrolyte imbalance, or hepatic and renal dysfunction. Severe OHSS can lead to vascular collapse, acute respiratory distress syndrome (ARDS) and even death.

Prezygote—The stage of pronuclear formation after penetration of the mature (MII) oocyte by spermatozoon. At this stage, male and female pronuclei are evident as well as the second polar body. This is the stage immediately preceding syngamy, the fusion of two nuclei to form a single nucleus of the zygote.

Zona pellucida—The glycoprotein membrane surrounding the plasma membrane of an oocyte.

Zygote—Single cell stage after pronuclear breakdown (syngamy) but before first cleavage.

ASSISTED REPRODUCTIVE TECHNOLOGY

Assisted reproductive technology (ART) is inclusive of any procedure involving fertilization of the oocyte outside the body. The first live birth from ART was reported in 1978 by Patrick Steptoe and Robert Edwards following laparoscopic retrieval of a single oocyte from a naturally stimulated ovary. The most frequently practiced ART procedure is in vitro fertilization (IVF). It involves a sequence of events beginning with controlled ovarian hyperstimulation, harvesting of oocytes, fertilization with spermatozoa, culturing of embryos, and replacement into the uterine cavity. Also under the umbrella of ART are laparoscopic tubal transfer of gametes (gamete intrafallopian transfer; GIFT), zygotes (zygote intrafallopian transfer; ZIFT), and embryos (tubal embryo transfer; TET). These techniques have largely been supplanted by IVF in light of their requirement for laparoscopy and considerable technical advances in both IVF and embryo culture conditions.

Assisted Reproductive Technology and the Expectations of Pregnancy

Consideration should first be made to the success rates of ART without surgical intervention. If this is deemed reasonable, it may be prudent to forgo surgery—and the inherent risks therein—and proceed directly to IVF. The decision to proceed with surgical intervention also requires detailed knowledge of its impact on subsequent pregnancy rates and should only be entertained if pregnancy rates could be significantly improved or the need for ART eliminated altogether.

Data on ART outcomes are collected every year to provide information to prospective patients as well as clinicians. The 2010 data from the Society for Assisted Reproductive Technology (SART) report pregnancy rates for fresh and frozen nondonor oocytes per cycle of IVF (Table 20.1). Success rates are clinic specific, and this information is available through http://sart.org.

Female age is the single most important predictor of IVF success rate due to the direct relationship between advancing female age and genetic instability of the oocyte. Over 90% of maternally derived aneuploidy stems from meiosis I chromosomal segregation errors. Two main mechanisms for oocyte aneuploidy have been described by Fragouli and colleagues. The first occurs exclusively during meiosis I with premature division of a chromosome into its two sister chromatids, followed by their random segregation. The second error is nondisjunction of entire chromosomes during meiosis I and meiosis II leading to hyperhaploid ($n = 24$) and hypohaploid ($n = 22$) gametes. As a result, advancing age of the female partner is inextricably

TABLE 20.1 2010 Success Rates of IVF Cycles[a] Using Fresh Embryos from Nondonor Oocytes

	AGE RANGES				
	<35	**35–37**	**38–40**	**41–42**	**>42**
Number of cycles	39,473	20,250	20,706	9,650	5,546
Percentage of cycles resulting in pregnancies	47.7	38.8	29.9	20.1	8.9
Percentage of cycles resulting in live births	41.7	31.9	22.1	12.5	4.1
Reliability range	(41.2–42.1)	(31.3–32.6)	(21.5–22.7)	(11.8–13.1)	(3.6–4.7)
Percentage of retrievals resulting in live births	44.6	35.5	25.4	14.9	5.3
Percentage of transfers resulting in live births	47.8	38.4	28.1	16.8	6.3
Percentage of cycles with elective single embryo transfer	9.6	5.3	1.7	0.6	0.5
Percentage of cancellations	6.6	10.0	12.9	16.5	22.0
Implantation rate	36.9	27.0	17.7	9.6	3.7
Average number of embryos transferred	2.0	2.2	2.6	3.0	3.1
Percentage of live births with twins	32.4	27.2	22.1	16.9	9.6
Percentage of live births with triplets or more	1.5	1.5	1.1	1.1	0.9

[a]Data collected from Society for Assisted Reproductive Technology (SART) member clinics.
Reprinted with permission from SART Clinic Summary Report (2010). https://www.sartcorsonline.com/rptCSR_PublicMultYear.aspx?ClinicPKID=0. Copyright 2013 SART, All Rights Reserved.

coupled with a decline in pregnancy and live birth rates. Coincidental with age, ovarian reserve also plays a major role in a woman's reproductive potential. Thus, any discussion of prognosis should be made in the context of ovarian reserve assessment.

ASSISTED REPRODUCTIVE TECHNOLOGY AND ENDOMETRIOSIS

Endometriosis is endometrial tissue found outside the uterus. This ectopic tissue responds to the hormonal changes of a menstrual cycle and can be a significant cause of morbidity. The precise pathophysiology of endometriosis and its impact on fertility depend upon the degree of endometriosis present in the ovaries and pelvis. Proposed mechanisms include distortion of pelvic anatomy and abnormal peritoneal environment characterized by increased inflammatory cytokines and oxidative stress, which may interfere with follicular development, ovum pickup, fertilization, and embryo development.

For patients who are infertile and have no other cause for infertility, it can be tempting to explore the pelvis via laparoscopy to diagnose and ultimately ablate lesions from endometriosis. There are two randomized prospective trials evaluating the efficacy of laparoscopic ablation of mild-to-moderate endometriosis and postoperative natural fecundity. The Canadian Collaborative Group on Endometriosis (ENDOCAN) randomized 341 patients with unexplained infertility for 2 years or more to diagnostic laparoscopy versus ablation and followed patients for 36 months. They found a modest increase in fecundity rates in those whose endometriosis was ablated, from 2.4% to 4.7%. Ultimately, eight women required surgery to achieve one additional pregnancy. The second, an Italian study led by Parazzini,

randomized 96 women to diagnostic laparoscopy versus ablation followed for 1 year and found no increase in spontaneous conception rates. However, when adjuvant GnRH agonist was used postoperatively over a brief time interval, spontaneous conception was increased from 18% to 39%.

In the context of ART, pregnancy rates in patients with mild-to-moderate endometriosis who forgo surgery are comparable to patients with unexplained infertility. The conception rates after ART are significantly higher compared to those who are managed expectantly for up to 24 months following ablative surgery. In a study by Suzuki et al., even patients with more advanced endometriosis experienced monthly fecundity rates of 22% to 25%, questioning the need for laparoscopic intervention prior to ART. Thus, surgery can marginally improve spontaneous conception rates in individuals with infertility and stage I–II endometriosis but does not approach success rates achieved with ART.

There are several considerations to be made in women with asymptomatic severe endometriosis and fertility. If there is significant anatomic distortion, surgery vis-à-vis fimbrioplasty or lysis of adhesion, in instances where adnexa are adherent to surrounding structures, can improve fertility. Reports on postoperative natural pregnancy rates are sparse and in the range of 7% to 15% over 12 months.

Garcia-velasco and Arici demonstrated that with respect to ovarian endometriomas, laparoscopic cystectomy prior to IVF does not appear to improve pregnancy rates. Since endometrias can be destructive to the ovarian reserve of young women, surgical intervention may be appropriate for this patient group. Rapidly growing endometriomas may indicate an underlying malignancy or borderline tumor. Therefore, any adnexal structure with a documented increase in size over a short time interval should be investigated for pathologic diagnosis. Depending on its size and location within the ovary, endometriomas may present structural impedance at oocyte retrieval. Each scenario provides a legitimate reason to favor removal prior to IVF.

ASSISTED REPRODUCTIVE TECHNOLOGY AND TUBAL INFERTILITY

Tubal factor infertility accounts for 30% of cases of female infertility and 9% of diagnoses among couples who underwent ART treatments in the United States in 2010. Tubal health is evaluated by hysterosalpingogram (HSG). In this procedure, contrast is placed into the uterine cavity and the fallopian tubes are visualized using fluoroscopy. The luminal diameter should be less than 1 mm at the isthmic portion of the fallopian tube and typically increases to 2 to 3 mm at the ampullary end. Free spill of contrast should be visualized to confirm tubal patency. Assisted reproductive technology was originally devised as a method to overcome tubal factor infertility. Statistically, current success rates after IVF exceed that of surgical repair. However, IVF can be financially and emotionally burdensome, and there are some instances when surgical correction can restore normal reproductive anatomy and should be considered before proceeding to IVF.

The optimal candidate for tubal reconstruction is young (<30) with a history of voluntary surgical sterilization without coexistent infertility factors. She should be counseled regarding postrepair conception rates, which range from 18% to 45% over a 12-month period, as well as ectopic pregnancy rates of 7% to 25%, as reported by Collins. Postoperative fecundity rates are subject to patient selection, technical skill of the surgeon, as well as the final length of the repaired fallopian tube.

Proximal Obstruction

The final diagnosis of proximal tubal disease by HSG should be reserved until confirmed with further testing. Tubal spasm or failure to produce adequate anterograde pressure of dye can be misinterpreted as proximal occlusion. Procedural options permitting simultaneous diagnosis and correction of proximal obstruction are fluoroscopic cannulation, laparoscopic chromotubation, and hysteroscopic catheterization. Each of these is sufficient to assign a final diagnosis of proximal tubal obstruction. If proximal obstruction is confirmed and efforts to establish patency are unsuccessful, IVF is the treatment of choice for these patients.

Hysteroscopic Catheterization—This procedure begins with appropriate distention media. A hypoosmotic media like glycine is ideal because it is immiscible with blood, ensuring clear visualization of the tubal ostia. First, standard chromopertubation of the fallopian tubes is done to confirm the diagnosis of proximal obstruction. The hysteroscope is then introduced through the cervical os, and tubal ostia are visualized. A soft flexible catheter with a metal introducer is directed through the obstructed side to a depth of 1 to 2 cm, and the inner metal introducer is removed while the outer sheath is advanced further into the isthmic portion of the fallopian tube. Indigo carmine is introduced through the operator's end of the catheter. A concurrent laparoscopy confirms spill of dye through the fimbriated end, and the catheter is removed. Laparoscopy also ensures prompt recognition of bleeding or tubal perforation.

Distal Obstruction/Hydrosalpinges

Surgical correction of mild tubal disease may be appropriate for young women. Correction may involve lysis of peritubal adhesions or fimbrioplasty. In fimbrioplasty, every effort should be made to use a laparoscopic approach to reduce the risk of adhesion formation. If tubal caliber is normal and the fimbriated end agglutinated, the closed tip of a pair of fine forceps

is introduced through the distal end and gently separated. The procedure should be repeated to reduce the rate of reocclusion. Care should be taken to avoid bleeding, as this increases the risk of scarring the delicate fimbria. Peritubal adhesions should be filmy and clear and separated without the use of cautery. Patton reported fecundity rates of parous women after this procedure in the range of 63% over 24 months, with a 5% ectopic pregnancy rate. However, women with severe distal disease and those over 37, who have diminished of ovarian reserve and increased aneuploidy rates, should forego surgery and proceed directly to IVF.

The study of ART outcomes has altered our management of hydrosalpinx. Patients with dilated, fluid-filled fallopian tubes may experience decreased pregnancy rates with IVF. The theories behind such observations include embryo toxicity and alterations in endometrial receptivity markers from exposure to tubal fluid. An interruption in embryo–endometrial cross talk could result from retrograde flow of tubal fluid. In fact, a recent survey of reproductive endocrinologists conducted by Omurtag and colleagues reported increased consideration of salpingectomy for hydrosalpinx without evidence of spill into the peritoneal cavity by HSG, presuming a greater degree of retrograde flow. In general, when the decision has been made to intervene surgically prior to ART, proximal tubal occlusion with bipolar cautery or surgical clips has comparable benefit to salpingectomy in patients with challenging access to adnexa.

Most studies support removal of ultrasound-visible hydrosalpinges prior to IVF; however, individual consideration should be made in women who are poor surgical candidates secondary to adhesive disease. Some of these patients may benefit from hysteroscopic placement of coiled tubes passed anterograde into the tubal ostia. In this procedure, flexible inserts containing polyethylene terephthalate fibers are guided by the hysteroscope and passed directly into the fallopian tubes. The inserts induce a fibrotic reaction that will permanently occlude the tube and thereby prevent retrograde flow of fluid into the uterine cavity. A follow-up HSG 3 months after insertion will confirm complete occlusion.

Because the current success rate of IVF in women with tubal disease exceeds that of surgical repair, it remains the treatment of choice. However, American Society for Reproductive Medicine (ASRM) practice guidelines state that tubal reconstructive surgery is a reasonable treatment option for young women with mild tubal disease and for those with ethical, religious, or financial restrictions that preclude IVF.

ASSISTED REPRODUCTIVE TECHNOLOGY AND SURGICAL MANAGEMENT OF UTERINE MYOMAS

Advising the infertile female on the management of an asymptomatic fibroid is a frequent clinical dilemma. It is unclear whether the presence of fibroids without cavitary involvement can be considered the sole cause for infertility. Theories behind adverse sequelae of myomas include mechanical obstruction of tubal ostia, chronic intracavitary inflammation, and increased uterine contractility.

There exist very few randomized trials to guide the gynecologic surgeon on the reproductive benefit of surgery in this situation. Metwally and colleagues identified that only three randomized clinical trials exist evaluating the effect of surgical intervention on subfertility, and a vast number of retrospective and observational studies make up the remaining body of literature. Two of the RCTs compare laparoscopic versus abdominal myomectomy and find they appear to have similar outcomes in miscarriage, pregnancy, and live birth rates.

Only one RCT evaluates surgical intervention versus no intervention and subsequent fertility. Casini et al. randomized 181 young women with myomas less than 4 cm and unexplained infertility to surgical intervention or expectant management for 1 year. Women with submucous myomas benefited from intervention with an increase in pregnancy rate of 27% in the expectantly managed group to 43% in the operative group ($P < 0.05$). Improvement after surgery in women with intramural myomas without cavitary involvement ($n = 76$) did not reach significance but trended higher in the operative group.

It is generally accepted that subserous myomas do not adversely affect pregnancy or live birth rates, thus removal is rarely warranted. Pritts' review showed agreement among studies on the topic: submucous myomas decrease pregnancy rates and increase the incidence of miscarriage. For the majority of patients with submucous myomas, surgical resection restores pregnancy rates to match those with a normal uterine cavity.

The management of intramural myomas not distorting the uterine cavity has become the focus of much debate in the ART world. Large intramural myomas appear to diminish pregnancy and live birth rates in infertile women; however, there is no conclusive evidence that surgical removal restores these rates. Therefore, the decision must weigh risks versus potential benefit of myomectomy. Risks for morbidity include bleeding necessitating hysterectomy or transfusion; postoperative adhesions, especially involving the fallopian tubes; and infection. When the potential obstetric complication of uterine rupture and an increased likelihood of cesarean section are considered, it is clear that there is reason for caution about recommending myomectomy for unproven benefit.

ASSISTED REPRODUCTIVE TECHNOLOGY AND THE INDICATION FOR HYSTERECTOMY

Prior to ART, it was standard practice to remove the uterus and bilateral adnexa in cases of pelvic pain from endometriosis or adnexal mass. The uterus was considered a vestigial organ without the accompanying adnexa and a source for carcinoma of the cervix or endometrium later in life. Now, patients with these conditions achieve pregnancies through the use of donor oocytes. The uterus should also be conserved for premenopausal women who have the opportunity and desire to cryopreserve oocytes/embryos prior to surgery.

ASSISTED REPRODUCTIVE TECHNOLOGY AND THE PRESERVATION OF FERTILITY AFTER SURGICAL MENOPAUSE

Improved survival rates for women with cancer have led to the pursuit of fertility preservation. As such, recent years have witnessed the development of methods for gamete, embryo, and ovarian tissue cryopreservation from the prepubertal girl to the adult woman. Although it is beyond the scope of this chapter to describe the technical aspects of cryopreservation, the fundamental principles of cryopreservation and success rates upon thaw will be reviewed. The purpose of this section is to provide the gynecologic surgeon with appropriate options that should be offered to the patient about to undergo bilateral oophorectomy or gonadotoxic therapy.

Ovarian Tissue Cryopreservation

This method offers the ability to cryopreserve thousands of primordial follicles without a delay in cancer treatment. In the majority of diagnosed cancers, chemotherapy is initiated soon after diagnosis. Because gonadotropin stimulation and oocyte retrieval usually require 2 to 3 weeks, it may be time-prohibitive to freeze embryos for potential future use. Breast cancer patients may have a brief window between surgery and chemotherapy, but supraphysiologic estrogen levels seen with IVF—especially in those with ER/PR+ tumors—risk stimulation of the primary tumor.

Strips of ovarian cortical tissue are surgically removed by laparoscopy or laparotomy and immediately frozen through slow cooling or vitrification. The tissue can later be thawed and the primordial follicles matured in vitro or can be autotransplanted back into the patient. Returning the tissue at or near the original location is referred to as orthotopic transplantation, while placing the tissue in a separate site such as the forearm or abdominal wall is heterotopic transplantation. With a forearm graft, the ovarian tissue is grafted into the subcutaneous space located above the brachioradialis fascia. The patients then must undergo gonadotropin stimulation, harvest, and uterine embryo transfer to conceive.

There have been approximately 20 reports of human live births using ovarian cortical tissue cryopreservation with autotransplantation, the first one reported in 2004. Thus, this technique should be considered experimental. Of note, this is the only treatment option for prepubertal girls. The potential drawbacks to be discussed are potential reseeding of tumor cells, especially in systemic cancers such as in leukemia, and in cases of high tumor potential as in BRCA gene carriers.

Oocyte Cryopreservation

Candidates for oocyte cryopreservation include premenopausal women scheduled for prophylactic oophorectomy for BRCA gene mutation, severe pelvic pain for endometriosis, or oncologic patients requiring gonadotoxic therapy. Oocyte cryopreservation necessitates a minimum delay in treatment for the primary disease of 2 to 3 weeks, and toleration of a transient rise in estrogen levels up to 4,000 pg/mL. In breast cancer patients with ER/PR+ tumors, some medical oncologists allow for one cycle of oocyte cryopreservation in the brief window between surgery and chemotherapy. It is prudent in these patients to use an aromatase inhibitor in conjunction with gonadotropin stimulation to maintain a low estradiol level.

Since the first pregnancy from frozen oocytes was described by Chen in 1986, there has been intense interest in the potential of oocyte cryopreservation. Since embryo cryopreservation using the slow-cooling method was an established technique with reasonable thaw survival and pregnancy rates, the application of slow cooling was extended to oocyte freezing. However, the oocyte has much higher water content compared to the embryo, and initial success was hampered by formation of ice crystals during cooling, causing a disruption in the meiotic spindle. In mature oocytes, metaphase chromosomes are lined up along the equatorial plate by the meiotic spindle, and this delicate spindle is easily damaged by ice crystal formation. Ultimately, changes to the sucrose and sodium concentrations were able to improve outcomes with the slow-freeze technique.

Vitrification is the solidification of a solution without formation of ice crystals. Oocytes are exposed to high concentrations of cryoprotectant followed by immersion into liquid nitrogen, creating a glass-like state. Its advantage over slow freeze is the avoidance of ice crystal formation and thus any consequent damage to the meiotic spindle. Hardening of the zona pellucida after thaw can create a challenge to successful fertilization, but is overcome by the use of intracytoplasmic sperm injection (ICSI). The majority of studies on thaw survival rates and pregnancy rates favor vitrification over the slow-freeze technique.

The ASRM reports number of live births following oocyte cryopreservation remains small but is rapidly rising. Thaw survival rates are approaching 98%, and pregnancy rate per thawed oocyte is 4.2%. Although pregnancy rates are slowly improving with more experience, some published data touting success rates approaching that of fresh embryo transfers should be interpreted with caution given these data are derived from donor oocytes from young women without a history of infertility. Both chromosomal and congenital aneuploidy rates in thawed oocytes and live births are comparable to rates following natural conception.

Oocyte freezing can be offered to any patient from adolescence to adulthood about to undergo bilateral oophorectomy or gonadotoxic therapy if the diagnosis will allow for the required time and hormonal stimulation necessary for oocyte harvest. Success rates as well as potential risks (OHSS,

postoperative intraabdominal bleeding, and infection following oocyte retrieval) can now be reasonably quantified to allow for informed decision making.

Embryo Cryopreservation

If the patient has a stable partner at the time of diagnosis, embryo cryopreservation is the treatment of choice. This is a routine procedure in ART laboratories with reliable success rates performed through aforementioned techniques of slow freeze or vitrification. Embryos can be cryopreserved at any developmental stage, from prezygote, zygote, preembryo, morula, or blastocyst stage (Fig. 20.1). Decisions on the optimal

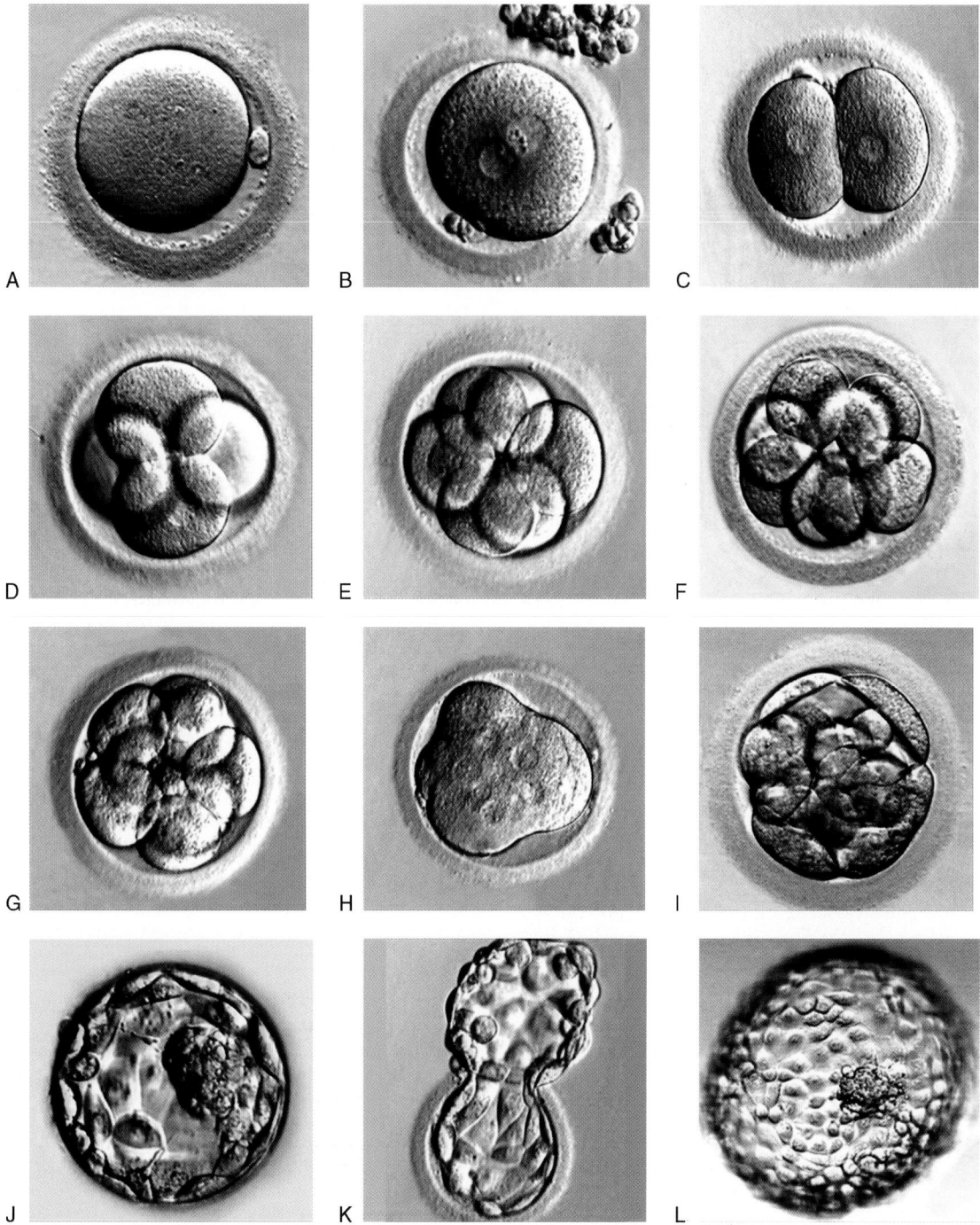

FIGURE 20.1 Embryos can be cryopreserved at any developmental stage (A–L).

stage to freeze depend upon the experience of individual clinics. Although success rates vary by many factors—clinic experience, female age at the time of cryopreservation, and number and quality of embryos banked—a pregnancy rate of up to 60% can be reasonably achieved.

CONCLUSION

The natural inclination of a gynecologic surgeon is to intervene in the setting of visible pathology. With regard to endometriosis, the benefit of surgical intervention varies based on degree of disease and intended fertility treatment. In cases of tubal occlusion, access to ART dictates whether surgical intervention is necessary. Each case is unique and must be considered individually. Therefore, the true challenge in treating the infertile couple in the age of ART is to understand whether surgical intervention is beneficial or an unnecessary delay to achieving pregnancy.

BEST SURGICAL PRACTICES

- The success rates of ART without surgical intervention should be considered before a recommendation for surgery is made.
- Success rates of ART are largely dependent on female age.
- Oocyte aneuploidy rates rise with advancing female age.
- For mild-to-moderate endometriosis, surgery can marginally improve spontaneous conception rates but does not approach success rates with ART.
- Patients with severe endometriosis may benefit from surgery prior to ART if lysis of adhesions is performed to restore female anatomy, thus reducing potential complications of oocyte retrieval.
- Pathologic diagnosis should be made for any rapidly expanding ovarian cyst to exclude malignancy prior to ART.
- Evidence does not support prophylactic removal of an asymptomatic endometrioma prior to ART with a goal of increasing pregnancy rates. However, removal should be considered in patients where size and location may obstruct oocyte harvest.
- Only young women (<35) with reasonable remaining tubal length and no coexistent risk factor for infertility should be considered for tubal reanastomosis. In the majority of patients with bilateral tubal disease or history of voluntary sterilization, ART should be recommended.
- Surgery for severe tubal disease should be reserved for young women who have ethical, religious, or financial restrictions that preclude IVF.
- Hydrosalpinges visible on transvaginal ultrasound should be removed prior to ART.
- Women with noncommunicating hydrosalpinges not visible on ultrasound could benefit from salpingectomy prior to ART. It is also reasonable to proceed directly to ART and reconsider salpingectomy if an initial attempt is unsuccessful.
- Subserous myomas do not adversely affect pregnancy or live birth rates, thus removal is rarely warranted.
- Submucous myomas decrease pregnancy rates and increase risk of miscarriage. Removal of submucous myomas should be advocated.
- Intramural myomas that do not distort the cavity may still reduce pregnancy rates and increase miscarriage rates. It is unclear if removal restores pregnancy rates to match rates

achieved by women with unexplained infertility without myomas. Decisions made should be specific to the size, location, and coexistent conditions of the patient.
- Ovarian tissue cryopreservation can be performed without significant delay, does not require ovarian stimulation, and is the only fertility preservation option for prepubertal girls. It is currently considered experimental with a limited number of live births to date.
- Oocyte cryopreservation can be offered to adolescent and single adult women where controlled ovarian hyperstimulation and a delay in gonadotoxic treatment would not adversely affect the patient's outcome.
- Embryo cryopreservation remains the treatment of choice in fertility preservation for adult women with stable partners.

BIBLIOGRAPHY

Casini ML, Rossi F, Agostini R, et al. Effects of the position of fibroids on fertility. *Gynecol Endocrinol* 2006;22:106.

Centers for Disease Control and Prevention. 2010 Assisted Reproductive Technology National Summary Report: National Summary and Fertility Clinic Success Rate Reports. Available from: www.cdc.gov/ART/ART2010

Chen C. Pregnancy after human oocyte cryopreservation. *Lancet* 1986;1(8486):884.

Collins JA, Van steirteghem A. Overall prognosis with current treatment of infertility. *Hum Reprod Update* 2004;10:309.

Donnez J, Dolmans MM, Demylle D, et al. Livebirth after orthotopic transplantation of cryopreserved ovarian tissue. *Lancet* 2004;364:1405.

Fragouli E, Wells D, Delhanty JD. Chromosome abnormalities in the human oocyte. *Cytogenet Genome Res* 2011;133:107.

Garcia-velasco JA, Arici A. Surgery for the removal of endometriomas before in vitro fertilization does not increase implantation and pregnancy rates. *Fertil Steril* 2004;81:1206.

Marcoux S, Maheux R, Bérubé S. Laparoscopic surgery in infertile women with minimal or mild endometriosis. Canadian Collaborative Group on Endometriosis. *N Engl J Med* 1997;337:217.

Martínez-burgos M, Herrero L, Megías D, et al. Vitrification versus slow freezing of oocytes: effects on morphologic appearance, meiotic spindle configuration, and DNA damage. *Fertil Steril* 2011;95:374.

Metwally M, Cheong YC, Horne AW. Surgical treatment of fibroids for subfertility. *Cochrane Database Syst Rev* 2012;11:CD003857.

Omurtag K, Grindler NM, Roehl KA, et al. How members of the Society for Reproductive Endocrinology and Infertility and Society of Reproductive Surgeons evaluate, define, and manage hydrosalpinges. *Fertil Steril* 2012;97:1095.

Parazzini F. Ablation of lesions or no treatment in minimal-mild endometriosis in infertile women: a randomized trial. [Gruppo Italiano per lo Studio dell'Endometriosi]. *Hum Reprod* 1999;14:1332.

Patton GW. Pregnancy outcome following microsurgical fimbrioplasty. *Fertil Steril* 1982;37:150.

Practice Committee of American Society for Reproductive Medicine. Essential elements of informed consent for elective oocyte cryopreservation: a Practice Committee opinion. *Fertil Steril* 2007;88:1495.

Practice Committee of American Society for Reproductive Medicine. The role of tubal reconstructive surgery in the era of assisted reproductive technologies. *Fertil Steril* 2008;90(5, suppl 1):S250.

Pritts EA, Parker WH, Olive DL. Fibroids and infertility: an updated systematic review of the evidence. *Fertil Steril* 2009;91:1215.

Steptoe PC, Edwards RG. Birth after the reimplantation of a human embryo. *Lancet* 1978;2:366.

Suzuki T, Izumi S, Matsubayashi H, et al. Impact of ovarian endometrioma on oocytes and pregnancy outcome in in vitro fertilization. *Fertil Steril* 2005;83:908.

CHAPTER 21
Reconstructive Tubal Surgery

Victor Gomel

DEFINITIONS

Falloposcopy—A transvaginal endoscopic procedure to examine the fallopian tubes, especially the intramural and isthmic segments.

Fimbrial phimosis—Agglutination of the fimbriae.

Fimbrioplasty—The reconstruction of the fimbriae or tubal infundibulum.

Hydrosalpinx—A distally occluded tube, usually secondary to infection, which distends with accumulation of serous fluid.

Hysterosalpingography (HSG)—An x-ray–based contrast test to assess the uterine cavity and the fallopian tubes.

Pelvic inflammatory disease (PID)—An inflammatory disorder of the uterus, fallopian tubes, and adjacent pelvic structures usually secondary to a sexually transmitted infection.

Salpingo-ovariolysis—The division and/or excision of periadnexal adhesions with the aim of restoring normal anatomy.

Salpingoscopy—An endoscopic examination of the ampullary portion of the tubal lumen.

Salpingostomy—The creation of a new stoma in a tube with a completely occluded distal end.

Tubal cannulation—The passage of a flexible guide wire and narrow-gauge cannula through the proximal tubal ostia along the length of the tube.

Tubotubal anastomosis—The surgical approximation of tubal segments after tubal sterilization or excision of an occluded or diseased portion of tube.

The fallopian tube is a very important organ for the survival of our species. Human life normally originates in the proximal ampulla of the fallopian tube where the oocyte and sperm meet and where fertilization takes place. The physiologic functions of the human oviduct include pro-ovarian sperm transport to the site of fertilization, ovum pickup and prouterine transport of the ovum, ampullary retention of the fertilized oocyte (approximately 72 hours), provision of a suitable environment for fertilization to occur and for the zygote to survive, and, eventually, transport of the zygote from the ampulla to the uterine cavity. Alterations in any of these functions (caused by either damage to the ciliated epithelium or tubal distortion or occlusion) can result in tubal implantation (owing to the lack of transport of the zygote to the uterus) or infertility (owing to the prevention of sperm meeting the oocyte).

In vitro fertilization (IVF) techniques, which have experienced significant improvement in the past three decades, in effect replicate most of the functions of the fallopian tube, except for transport of the preembryo into the uterine cavity. This last step (embryo replacement) is performed using a cannula into which the embryo(s) is aspirated; the cannula then is introduced into the uterus through the cervical canal, and the embryo(s) is deposited in the uterine cavity.

TUBAL FACTOR INFERTILITY

Much of the increase in the incidence of both infertility and tubal pregnancy in the past four decades has been the result of tubal damage after sexually transmitted pelvic infections.

The commonly isolated organisms are *Chlamydia trachomatis*, *Neisseria gonorrhoeae*, and *Mycoplasma hominis*, of which *Chlamydia* is the most common. These organisms appear to account for most primary invasions; however, in 15% to 60% of cases of acute pelvic inflammatory disease (PID), aerobic or anaerobic bacteria, or both, can also be identified. The clinical picture can vary from an almost asymptomatic condition to a life-threatening event. As demonstrated by Westrom and colleagues, and by Paavonen and Egert-Kruuse, patients with a more severe clinical appearance often have both aerobic and anaerobic infections.

The classic clinical picture of PID, which includes pain, fever, and lower genital tract infection, occurs in less than 50% of affected patients. Gomel reported that more than half of the patients who were investigated for infertility and were found to have a hydrosalpinx gave no previous history of acute PID. This observation has since been confirmed. Indeed, the wide variation in the clinical presentation makes the diagnosis problematic.

It has been estimated that acute PID occurs at a rate of 10 cases per 1,000 women per year in the age group 15 to 39 years and at a rate of 20 cases per 1,000 women per year in the age group 15 to 24 years. Just as there is difficulty in diagnosing PID, there is difficulty in ascertaining the trend in its incidence. Westrom and colleagues reported that in PID cases, the rate of isolating *Chlamydia* per population of 100,000 has increased annually since 1984.

Data from Westrom and colleagues, and from Paavonen and Egert-Kruuse, indicate the infertility rate after a single episode of PID correlates with the degree of residue of tubal damage. Tubal infertility also increases with recurrent episodes of PID. Infertility occurred in 8% of patients with one episode, 20% with two episodes, and 40% in those with three or more episodes of PID. Further, up to two thirds of cases of tubal factor infertility and one third of cases of ectopic pregnancy may be attributable to *C. trachomatis* infection.

INVESTIGATION

The investigation of the infertile couple should be concluded rapidly, accurately, and inexpensively, with as little invasion as possible. In addition, the emotional needs of the couple must be recognized and addressed. Investigation must commence with a thorough clinical assessment of the couple. A detailed history followed by a thorough physical examination permits the selection of the necessary tests to undertake. A positive history of PID or the finding of *Chlamydia* antibodies has a predictive value for tubal pathology of odds ratio (OR) 3.7 (1.7 to 8.4) and that of ruptured appendicitis of OR 4.4 (2.5 to 7.6). This chapter discusses only investigations specific to tubal and peritoneal factors of infertility.

Tubal Insufflation

Tubal insufflation is a tubal patency test, first described by Rubin, which is now rarely performed. The procedure uses an endocervical cannula connected, by rubber tubing, to a mercury manometer and a source of carbon dioxide (CO_2). The rate of gas flow through the system is gradually increased to approximately 30 to 60 mL per minute. Tubal patency is determined by one or more of the following: a written record of the rise and rapid fall of the gas pressure, auscultation of the lower abdomen for the gas passing through the tubes into the peritoneal cavity, or direct visualization of the pressure changes on a mercury manometer.

This historic tubal patency test has been replaced by hysterosalpingography (HSG) and/or salpingosonography. Both of these tests should be performed before ovulation, about the tenth day of the cycle. Administration of one of the nonsteroidal anti-inflammatory medications is helpful to the patient as it reduces her discomfort due to uterine cramping and thus diminishes diagnostic errors.

Hysterosalpingography

Hysterosalpingography is a contrast study of the uterine cavity and fallopian tubes. It is a simple, inexpensive, safe, and rapid diagnostic procedure that, when performed properly, provides valuable information about the uterine cavity and tubal patency and architecture.

Contraindications to HSG include pregnancy, uterine bleeding, lower genital tract infection, PID, and allergy to the contrast material. In women with a history of recurrent PID, or with any suggestion of a recent exacerbation, there is a significant risk of reactivation of quiescent PID. This occurs in approximately 3% of such patients. To combat this risk, some centers prophylactically administer antibiotics. During the preliminary history and physical examination, the physician must search for possible contraindications and screen for and treat any lower genital tract infections, before performing an HSG. Prophylactic antibiotics prior to HSG are indicated in selected cases, particularly if hydrosalpinx is suspected.

Technique

Hysterosalpingography must be timed to occur between the complete cessation of menstruation and ovulation. This will avoid the risk of disturbing a luteal phase pregnancy. Such timing also avoids radiation exposure to the oocyte that will resume meiosis after the luteinizing hormone surge. Administration of a nonsteroidal anti-inflammatory medication before the procedure reduces the patient's discomfort and diminishes errors associated with HSG. The latter is especially applicable to errors regarding cornual occlusion. This has been clearly demonstrated in a study by Lang and Dunaway.

An oil-soluble or water-soluble contrast medium can be used. A recent Cochrane meta-analysis by Luttjeboer et al. concluded that use of an oil-soluble media increases subsequent pregnancy rates when compared with *no* intervention (OR 3.30; 95% confidence interval [CI] 2.00 to 5.43); however, there was no significant difference in the odds of pregnancy with oil-soluble versus water-soluble media (OR 1.49; 95% CI 0.95 to 1.54). Water-soluble media are most widely used; they are better tolerated by the patient; further, water-soluble media coat the surfaces without sticking to them, producing sharp and finely shaded images and greater visual detail of the lesions. These characteristics enable better assessment of the intraluminal architecture (Fig. 21.1). The contrast material is eliminated within 30 minutes.

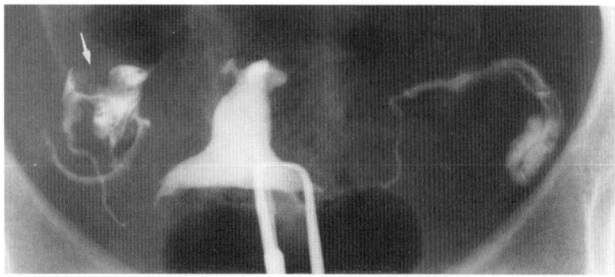

FIGURE 21.1 Hysterosalpingogram. Early film demonstrates a normal uterus and a left hydrosalpinx. On the right, there is an ampullary defect (*arrow*) at the site of a previous tubal pregnancy, which was treated with parenteral methotrexate administration.

After the patient has emptied her bladder, she is placed on the radiographic table. A bivalve speculum is inserted into the vagina, and the cervix and upper vagina are washed with an antiseptic solution. The appropriate cannula, which is filled with contrast material and emptied of any air, is attached to the cervix in such a way as to ensure a tight seal. The speculum is removed before the injection of contrast material. Removal of the speculum is important (especially if the metal variety is used), not only to decrease the patient's discomfort but also to avoid obscuring the cervical canal and vaginal fornices on the x-ray films.

Hysterosalpingography must be performed under fluoroscopic control with the use of an image intensifier. With the syringe attached to the cannula, the contrast material is injected very slowly to avoid discomfort, contraction of the uterus, spasm of the uterotubal junction, and obscuring of the lesions with a large quantity of contrast material. Films are taken to record salient features as they appear on the monitor. An average of three to five films are taken. Preliminary films are of limited value; they can be used to identify misplaced intrauterine contraceptive devices or areas of pelvic calcification. Such information can also be gained by examining the first film.

As the contrast material is injected slowly and intermittently, the endocervical canal, isthmus, and uterine cavity are visualized. To straighten the uterus, firm traction is maintained on the cervix. A film is taken at this point. It is essential to obtain films early during the procedure to record any intrauterine lesions and details of the intratubal architecture. Such details are obscured by larger amounts of contrast material in the uterus, tubes, and peritoneal cavity. Another film is taken when the contrast material starts to escape into the peritoneal cavity (Fig. 21.1). Injection of medium is continued slowly until tubal patency is unquestionably established. Manipulation of the uterus with the cannula may be necessary to display specific tubal segments. A film is obtained when abnormal findings are encountered. In certain cases, a true lateral film may provide useful information. When taking this exposure, the traction on the cervix is temporarily released to obtain information regarding the position of the uterus, the location of intrauterine lesions, and the course and configuration of the tubes.

The last phase of the procedure includes a delayed fluoroscopic examination and a film taken 10 to 20 minutes (when water-soluble contrast material is used) after removal of the cannula. This examination and film may yield information about the external contour of the internal genitalia, the shape of the ovarian fossa, and the presence of periadnexal adhesions.

With adherence to proper technique, complications are rare. Major complications include PID, uterine perforation, bleeding from the tenaculum site, and intolerance to iodine, especially if intravasation of contrast occurs. Oil-soluble media may cause granulomas in the pelvis and serious complications if intravasation occurs; a case of cerebral embolization has been reported by Dan et al.

Hysterosalpingography performed using water-soluble media provides precise information about the uterus and oviducts that can assist in patient management. Abnormal uterine findings include fusion anomalies, T-shaped uterus, submucous fibroids and endometrial polyps, intrauterine synechiae (Fig. 21.2), and other less commonly identified lesions, such as adenomyosis. Tubal abnormalities that can be observed are listed in Table 21.1 and shown in figures from Gomel and colleagues (Figs. 21.3 to 21.6).

It must be noted that HSG has limitations: (a) it often does not indicate the exact nature of intrauterine lesions; (b) it is associated with false-positive results with regard to cornual occlusion, which may necessitate a selective salpingography and/or tubal cannulation; and (c) it has a low positive

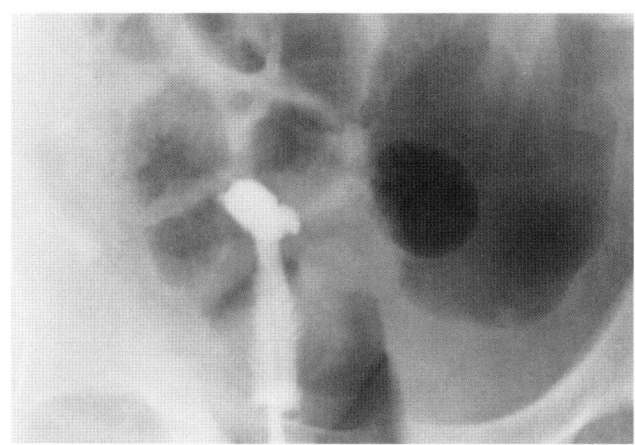

FIGURE 21.2 Hysterosalpingogram in a patient with Asherman syndrome. Contrast material outlines the cervical canal and a part of the lower uterine cavity, the remainder of which is obliterated by synechiae. (From Gomel V, Taylor PJ. *Diagnostic and operative gynecologic laparoscopy*. St Louis, MO: Mosby, 1995:106, with permission.)

predictive value in the diagnosis of periadnexal adhesions and endometriosis. For these reasons, laparoscopy and, when necessary, hysteroscopy are undertaken to elucidate the diagnosis. Indeed, HSG and laparoscopy are complementary, not competitive, procedures in the investigation of infertility associated with tubal and peritoneal factors.

In many instances, HSG demonstrates the presence of severe tubal damage or conditions deemed inoperable. Severe intratubal adhesions, and distal tubal occlusion in association with cornual lesions, such as salpingitis isthmica nodosa, are examples of contraindications of reconstructive surgery. In such instances, the couple may be advised of the significance of the findings, and IVF may be recommended as primary treatment, without recourse to laparoscopy.

We have been viewing and continue to view a well-performed HSG as a good, inexpensive, initial test to assess the uterine cavity and the fallopian tubes and are pleased to note concurrence in the American Society for Reproductive Medicine's (ASRM's) committee opinion in this regard: *"There is good evidence to support HSG as the standard first line test to asses tubal patency, but it is limited by false positive diagnoses of proximal tubal blockage."* It further states: *"The evidence is fair to recommend tubal cannulation for proximal tubal obstruction in young women with no other significant infertility factors."*

IV

TABLE 21.1 Abnormalities of the Oviduct

ABNORMALITIES OF THE OVIDUCT		
ABNORMALITY	**SIGNS**	**COMMENTS**
TUBOCORNUAL REGION		
Failure of contrast to enter tube	Simple obstruction	May be owing to tubal spasm; may be unilateral or bilateral
Salpingitis isthmica nodosa (SIN)	Appears as a simple obstruction or as spicules of contrast radiating from tubal lumen	May be unilateral or bilateral
Endometriosis	Similar to SIN, usually with more pronounced punctate pattern	May be unilateral or bilateral
Polyps	Small globular or elongated vacuoles surrounded by contrast medium	
ISTHMUS		
Occlusion	Contrast outlines portion of the isthmic segment.	Most commonly owing to prior surgical sterilization or tubal pregnancy, less commonly to SIN, and uncommonly to tuberculosis and endometriosis
AMPULLA		
Intraluminal adhesions	Patchy filling defects	Caused by endosalpingeal infection
Tubal pregnancy	Obstruction, stenosis, round defect, occasionally calcification	
INFUNDIBULUM		
Hydrosalpinx	Obstruction usually bilateral	Most common type of occlusion
Phimosis of distal tubal ostium	Intraluminal retention of contrast medium and slow intraperitoneal spill from stenosed tube	Both conditions are usually sequelae of PID
INTRAPERITONEAL SPREAD		
Adhesions	Localized pooling and loculation of contrast medium around distal end of oviducts	

Modified from Gomel V, Taylor PJ. *Diagnostic and operative gynecologic laparoscopy*. St Louis, MO: Mosby, 1995:105.

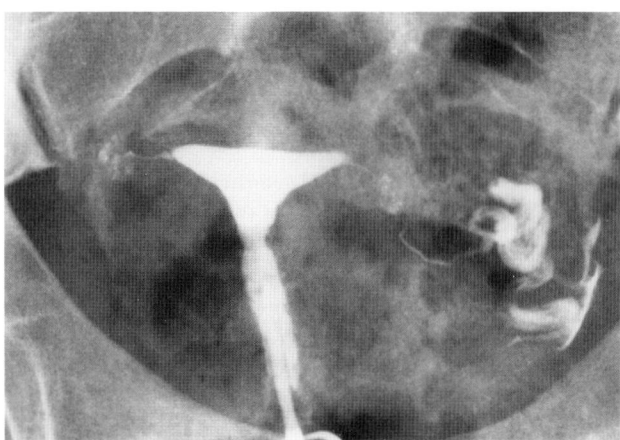

FIGURE 21.3 Hysterosalpingogram showing bilateral proximal isthmic lesions typical of salpingitis isthmica nodosa. The right tube is occluded, whereas the left is still patent. (From Gomel V, Taylor PJ. *Diagnostic and operative gynecologic laparoscopy*. St Louis, MO: Mosby, 1995, with permission.)

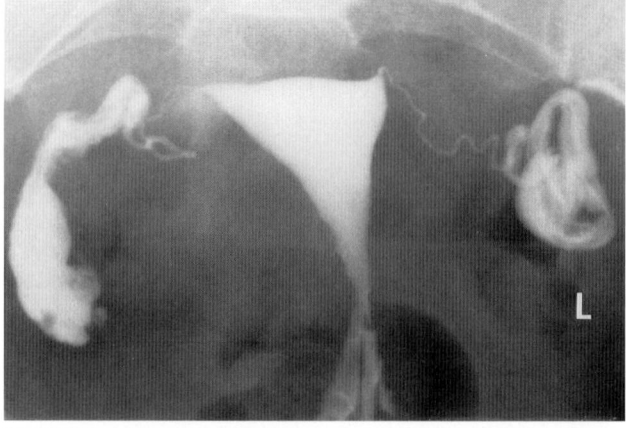

FIGURE 21.5 Hysterosalpingogram showing bilateral hydrosalpinx. The longitudinal epithelial folds are preserved in the left tube. (From Gomel V, Taylor PJ. *Diagnostic and operative gynecologic laparoscopy*. St Louis, MO: Mosby, 1995:106, with permission.)

Selective Salpingography and Tubal Cannulation

Selective salpingography is the injection of a contrast medium directly into the uterine tubal ostium with the use of a special radiopaque cannula inserted through the cervix. The increased pressure generated by the direct injection helps to overcome obstructions associated with mucous plugs or minor synechiae. Data from Thurmond, Novy et al, and Papaioannou et al. indicate selective salpingography is technically possible in approximately 90% of available tubes.

Cannulation of the tube requires the use of a special flexible guide wire and narrow-gauge cannula. This cannulation system is introduced through the larger cannula, which is used for selective salpingography.

If HSG demonstrates a cornual or proximal tubal obstruction (Fig. 21.7), selective salpingography with or without tubal cannulation (Fig. 21.8) should be the next step; this is ideally performed in the same setting. These techniques are useful in differentiating true from false cornual occlusion. The benefits of this approach have been shown for apparent cornual spasm, obstructions caused by amorphous material (tubal plugs), and tubal synechiae. Indeed, half of the tubes that were proximally blocked at selective salpingography were found to be normal after tubal catheterization in the largest series reported to date. It is doubtful that these techniques have a real therapeutic effect on pathologic occlusions that are due to obliterative fibrosis, chronic follicular salpingitis, salpingitis isthmica nodosa, or endometriosis.

Salpingosonography

Salpingosonography is a sonographic technique to assess the uterine cavity and tubal patency. After the insertion of a Foley catheter into the cervix, transvaginal sonography is carried out to assess the pelvic structures. Then, a 20-mL syringe is filled with 10 mL of saline solution followed by 10 mL of air. Air is injected first slowly, and passage is followed through the tube; saline is then injected to cause the air bubbles to flow more visibly through the tube. Air-filled albumin microspheres have also been used for this purpose. Several authors (Chenia et al., Inki et al., Strandell et al.) found salpingosonography to have a concordance with laparoscopy of

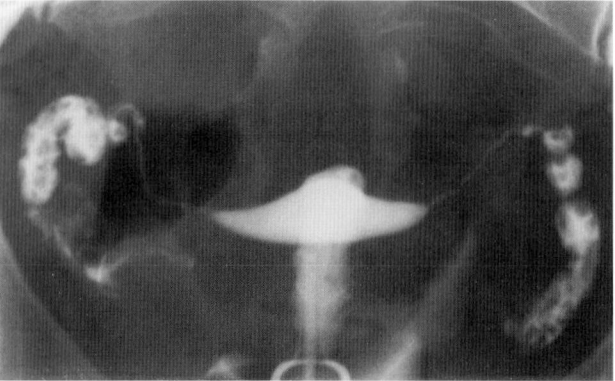

FIGURE 21.4 Hysterosalpingogram. Both tubes exhibit extensive intratubal adhesions. (From Gomel V, Taylor PJ. *Diagnostic and operative gynecologic laparoscopy*. St Louis, MO: Mosby, 1995:106, with permission.)

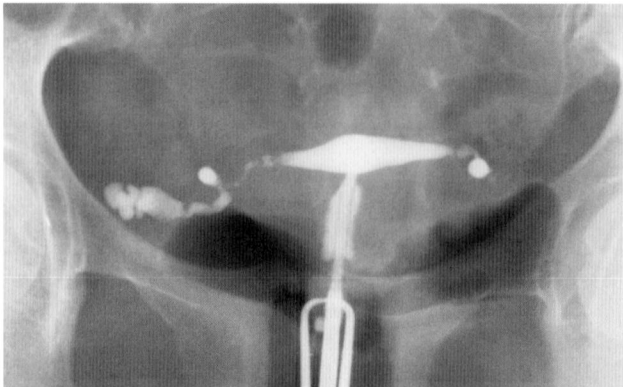

FIGURE 21.6 Hysterosalpingogram. The tubes exhibit findings typical of a prior tuberculous salpingitis. (From Gomel V, Taylor PJ. *Diagnostic and operative gynecologic laparoscopy*. St Louis, MO: Mosby, 1995:108, with permission.)

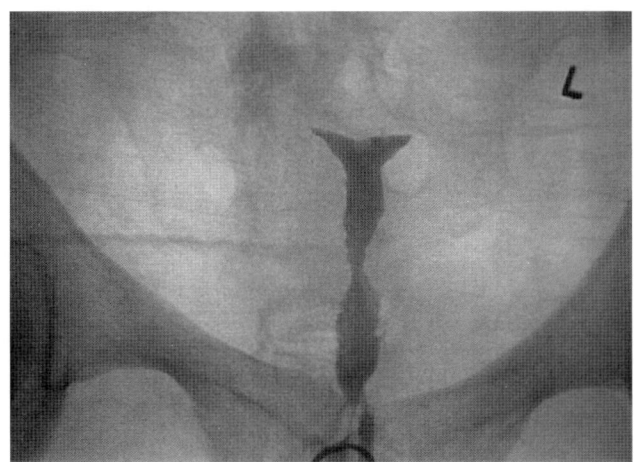

FIGURE 21.7 Hysterosalpingogram showing bilateral cornual occlusion. (From Gomel V, Taylor PJ. *Diagnostic and operative gynecologic laparoscopy.* St. Louis, MO: Mosby, 1995:109, with permission.)

approximately 80% and with HSG between 72% and 90%. Although the concordance with HSG with regard to passage of contrast into the peritoneal cavity appears high, it is important to remember that salpingosonography does not provide any information about the intratubal architecture. Yet, the pain scores associated with both of these techniques were comparable, as demonstrated in a prospective study by Cheong and Li in 2005.

Salpingoscopy

Salpingoscopy is the endoscopic examination of the ampullary portion of the tubal lumen. This can be accomplished with a small-gauge rigid or flexible endoscope during either laparoscopy or laparotomy. If the distal tube is totally occluded (hydrosalpinx), it is necessary to make a small opening at the fimbriated end to permit the introduction of the scope. The tubal lumen is visualized while distended with physiologic solution injected through the outer sheath of the rigid endoscope or the channel of the flexible scope. The distal end of the tube must be appropriately manipulated to bring it into the axis of the scope. Salpingoscopy permits direct assessment of the tubal epithelium. The findings have been classified into

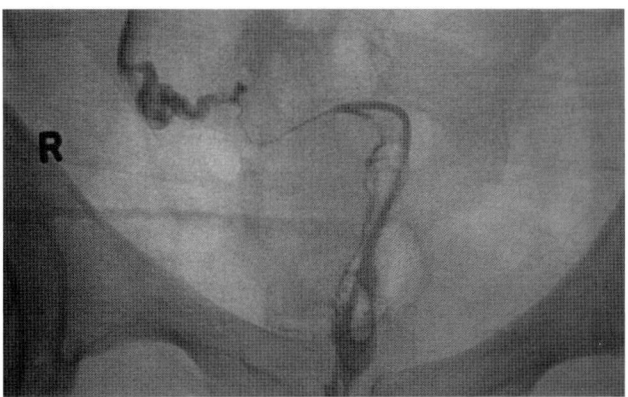

FIGURE 21.8 Tubal cannulation (same patient as in Fig. 21.7). The occlusion has been relieved, and the tube has opacified. (From Gomel V, Taylor PJ. *Diagnostic and operative gynecologic laparoscopy.* St. Louis, MO: Mosby, 1995:109, with permission.)

five grades. Grade 1 refers to normal mucosal architecture. Grade 2 refers to tubes that demonstrate variable degrees of flattening of both major and minor mucosal folds, which are largely preserved. Grade 3 refers to tubes that demonstrate focal adhesions between mucosal folds. Grade 4 refers to tubes with extensive intraluminal adhesions or disseminated flattened epithelial areas. Grade 5 refers to tubes that are rigid and hollow with a complete loss of epithelial folds. Findings at salpingoscopy appear to be predictive and prognostic of pregnancy outcome.

Microsalpingoscopy has been used to examine the integrity of the tubal mucosa more closely. Microsalpingoscopy uses an endoscope that has magnification capability enabling visualization of individual cells of the tubal epithelium. The epithelium is stained with concentrated methylene blue solution injected through the cervical cannula. It is then assessed under magnification. The level of staining of the nuclei of the tubal cells is inversely proportional to functional integrity of the mucosa. This technique is at present investigational; thus, its value remains to be determined.

Falloposcopy

Falloposcopy is a transvaginal microendoscopic technique aimed at exploring the entire length of the tube, especially the intramural and isthmic segments. A linear eversion catheter system has been used to perform falloposcopy without the need for preliminary hysteroscopy and anesthesia. The patient requires premedication to decrease the discomfort associated with the procedure.

The system includes a linear eversion catheter with an outer plastic polymer body 2.8 mm in diameter and a sliding stainless steel inner body 0.8 mm in diameter, containing a 0.48-mm fiberoptic endoscope. The tip of the outer catheter is angulated so it can be directed toward the uterotubal junction. Once the tubal ostium is identified, the tip of the catheter is held against the ostium. The pressure within the eversion catheter is increased, and the membrane of the eversion catheter is introduced into the fallopian tube for a short distance. The endoscope is pushed down the lumen to the tip of the introduced catheter. The image obtained is displayed on a high-resolution color monitor. The eversion catheter and the endoscope it houses are advanced in the described manner, slowly and gradually, with the endoscope always maintained within the inverting membrane to prevent the tip of the endoscope from piercing the tubal wall.

Falloposcopy may be used as a means of tubal catheterization and has the added benefit of permitting assessment of the lumen of the tube, especially its intramural and isthmic segments. Kerin et al. proposed a classification based on a scoring system that takes into account the degree of tubal patency, tubal dilatation, epithelial and vascular changes, intratubal adhesions, and other abnormal findings.

This technique, which requires expensive disposable equipment, did not gain clinical acceptance.

Tests Designed to Assess Tubal Function

Salpingography, salpingoscopy, and falloposcopy are designed to assess tubal patency and morphology. Many procedures designed to assess tubal function have been proposed but did not attain clinical acceptance.

Early attempts at using radioactive microspheres as oocyte surrogates to evaluate egg transport did not appear to be clinically valuable. Uher et al. have introduced biodegradable microspheres into the pouch of Douglas by either cul-de-sac puncture or laparoscopy. These microspheres, which

IV

were recognizable by fluorescence, were collected in a cervical cup 24 hours later. Microspheres were present in the cup in 66% of 69 patients with unexplained infertility and in 100% of 20 patients with male factor infertility.

Radionuclide Hysterosalpingography

Radionuclide HSG is a scintigraphic procedure designed by Brundin and colleagues to evaluate the spontaneous pro-ovarian transport of microspheres in the genital tract. A solution containing ^{99m}Tc-labeled albumin microspheres is squirted toward the external cervical os of the cervix and upper vagina. The subsequent transport of the microspheres through the cervix, uterus, and tubes is monitored by a gamma camera equipped with a pinhole collimator. The pro-ovarian transport of microspheres depends on both the anatomic patency and the functional integrity of the uterus and oviducts. This test is designed to assess primarily the sperm transport function of the uterus and tubes. This technique is still experimental, but preliminary work reported by Lundberg et al. indicates it is not predictive of fertility potential.

Laparoscopy

Laparoscopy permits direct visualization of the peritoneal cavity, pelvis, and internal reproductive organs. It can also test tubal patency with the use of concomitant chromopertubation. It is the most accurate way to identify periadnexal adhesive disease and endometriosis. Laparoscopy also provides the necessary surgical access to perform surgical procedures. Hysteroscopy and salpingoscopy, when indicated, may be performed during the same setting. Laparoscopy is an invasive procedure that usually requires a general anesthetic. It is important to be reminded that most of the major vascular and bowel injuries occur with the initiation of laparoscopy, during the introduction of the Veress needle, principal trocar, and ancillary trocars.

There are those who argue in favor of an immediate laparoscopy bypassing HSG. An analysis of 18 published series demonstrates good congruence between laparoscopic and HSG findings. These collected data indicate that the sensitivity and specificity of HSG are approximately 76% and 83%, respectively. These studies represent a selected population of patients in whom the prevalence of tubal occlusion was 38%. This prevalence figure falls to 10% in studies of large numbers of unselected patients, which reflects more accurately the general population. If the sensitivity and specificity figures reported above are applied to a hypothetical group of patients with a 10% rate of tubal occlusion, only 3% of those with a normal HSG will have an abnormal laparoscopy. Thus, the laparoscopy will be normal in approximately 97% of patients. These data support delaying endoscopy for 4 to 6 months in those with an apparently normal HSG, except in women of older reproductive age.

Based on the preceding information, a well-performed HSG should be the preliminary investigation for tubal factor infertility. This approach permits the identification of (a) uterine anomalies and lesions; (b) cornual occlusion or lesions, even in the presence of cornual patency; (c) distal tubal occlusion; and (d) assessment of intratubal architecture. This information is of paramount importance to the surgeon at the time of laparoscopy, especially if the condition is amenable to laparoscopic surgery, which should be performed in the same setting. Indeed, with the advanced imaging techniques and newer therapeutic modalities available today, laparoscopy, solely for the purpose of diagnosis, should be rarely required.

Laparoscopic Survey

A thorough laparoscopic survey will identify any adhesions, along with their extent and nature; reveal the presence of endometriosis, its extent, and other abdominal and pelvic lesions; and permit assessment of the uterus, ovaries, and tubes. The information yielded by the prior HSG and this survey enable the surgeon to undertake reconstructive laparoscopic surgery and to recommend surgery by open access or the use of assisted reproductive technologies. These will be discussed later.

A bimanual pelvic examination is performed on the anesthetized patient. The cervix is then exposed, and a uterine cannula is attached to the cervix. In addition to permitting intraoperative chromopertubation, the cannula enables manipulation of the uterus and enhances laparoscopic visualization.

Once the laparoscope is inserted, the entire peritoneal cavity is inspected. Inspection commences in the upper abdomen and includes the liver and the undersurface of the diaphragm, which are inspected in a clockwise fashion. Particular attention is then focused on the lower abdomen and pelvis. To improve access to the pelvis, the patient is placed in the Trendelenburg position. The bowel is displaced upward, initially by manipulating the uterus and thereafter by using a probe or other appropriate instrument inserted through a second puncture, usually placed suprapubically in the midline, or in one of the lower quadrants.

A general panoramic inspection of the pelvis is performed with the laparoscope at some distance from the pelvic organs. This permits a general impression to be formed. Subsequently, a systematic survey is performed. The laparoscope is advanced; appropriate manipulation of the uterus, with the cervical cannula, and of the suprapubic probe enhances visibility of specific organs. The uterus is assessed, along with its anterior surface, the vesicouterine pouch, and the dome of the bladder.

The uterus is then moved into anteversion. The fundus and the posterior surface of the uterus, the uterosacral ligaments, and the pouch of Douglas are thoroughly inspected. If fluid is present in the pouch, its nature is noted. It may be necessary to aspirate the fluid to inspect the underlying peritoneal surfaces. To aspirate the fluid, the probe is replaced by a suction cannula, which also can be used as a manipulating probe. The aspirated fluid can be sent for microbiologic or biochemical studies as deemed necessary. The cul-de-sac and the lateral peritoneal surfaces are inspected for any scarring or evidence of endometriosis. In addition, the peritoneum over the pararectal spaces and over the sacrum should be evaluated.

The extent and type of pelvic and periadnexal adhesions are noted (Fig. 21.9). Each tube and ovary and the respective pelvic sidewalls are thoroughly scrutinized. Once the anterior surface of the ovary is inspected, the ovary is elevated and flipped upward with the probe, exposing its posterior surface, the fossa ovarica, and the pelvic sidewall down to the level of the uterosacral ligament, which are assessed. The tube is inspected from the proximal to the distal end. Attention is paid for any evidence of fusiform swelling at the uterotubal junction (which is usually caused by salpingitis isthmica nodosa or endometriosis); the distal end of the tube is scrutinized for the presence of fimbrial phimosis or frank distal tubal occlusion (hydrosalpinx) (Fig. 21.10). The ovarian fimbrial relation is assessed, and the fimbriae are viewed en face. Once the other adnexa are similarly assessed, chromopertubation is performed by injection of dilute indigo carmine or methylene blue solution through the uterine cannula. The passage of the dye solution is followed through the tube, and the nature of the spill is examined by viewing the fimbriae to determine the presence of prefimbrial phimosis or fine fimbrial adhesions that may impede ovum pickup.

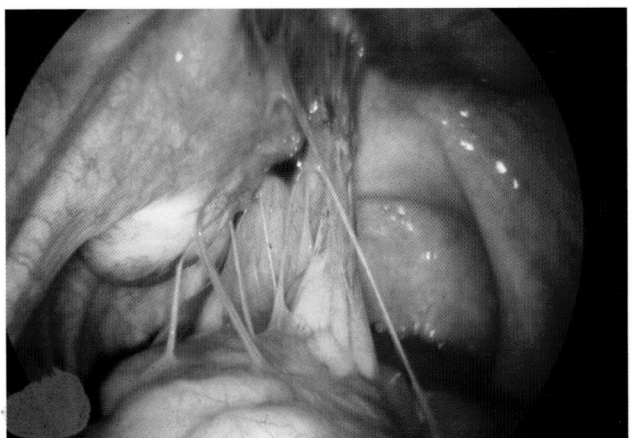

FIGURE 21.9 Laparoscopy. Periadnexal adhesions cover and fix the distal half of the fallopian tube.

Abdominal, pelvic, and periadnexal adhesions may impede laparoscopic access to the pelvis and the adnexa; this may necessitate preliminary adhesiolysis.

Hydroculdoscopy (Fertiloscopy)

Hydroculdoscopy was introduced to visualize the fallopian tubes, ovaries, and the cul-de-sac of Douglas. The technique is a modification of the traditional "culdoscopy," which has been largely abandoned. It was introduced as a diagnostic technique to replace laparoscopy in the investigation of infertile women, hence the name "fertiloscopy."

With the patient properly positioned, a bimanual examination is carried to examine the pelvic organs and confirm that the pouch of Douglas is free. The posterior fornix of the vagina is exposed, and the pouch of Douglas is entered using a Veress-type needle. Once the needle is appropriately placed, 200 to 250 mL of saline solution is introduced into the pouch of Douglas through the Veress needle. A trocar/cannula that permits the introduction of a small-caliber endoscope or a "fertiloscope" is then inserted.

The procedure permits the visualization of the pouch of Douglas, the posterior surface of the uterus, the fallopian tubes, and ovaries. Tubal patency can be ascertained by the introduction of a dilute methylene blue solution into the uterine cavity, through an appropriate cannula. If tubal damage is suspected, a salpingoscopy may be performed during the same procedure.

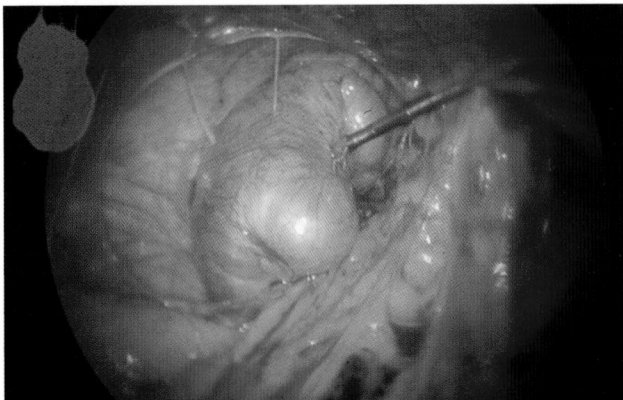

FIGURE 21.10 Laparoscopy. Thin-walled dilated hydrosalpinx with extensive pelvic and periadnexal adhesions.

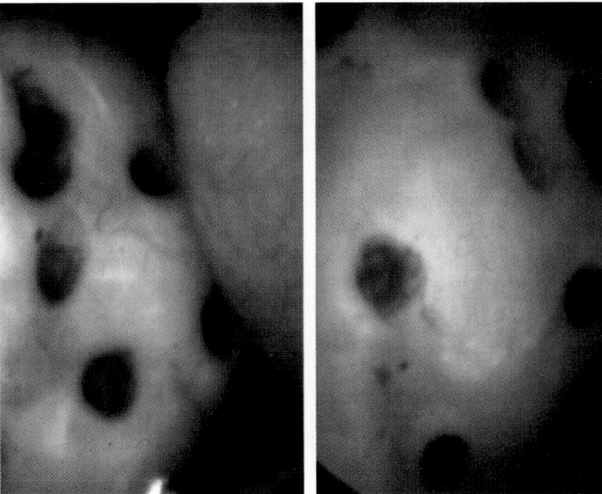

FIGURE 21.11 Fertiloscopy: views of ovarian drilling via hydroculdoscopy using a bipolar electrode.

Initially introduced as a diagnostic tool, the technique has also provided surgical access for certain therapeutic procedures including minor adhesiolysis and ablation of minor endometriotic lesions; it also permits performance of ovarian drilling.

The first ovarian drilling by hydroculdoscopy was performed in France in 1999 at the Antoine Beclère Hospital by Hervé Fernandez, introducing a bipolar Versapoint probe into the pouch of Douglas through a site lateral to that of the endoscope. The patient was markedly obese and was found to have polycystic ovaries as reported by Fernandez in 2001 (Fig. 21.11). Ovarian drilling using this access has since been performed in many centers; the reported results appear similar to those performed by laparoscopy.

It is evident that the procedure cannot be undertaken if the cul-de-sac of Douglas is occluded. The view obtained with hydroculdoscopy is localized and very different from the panoramic view obtained by laparoscopy; furthermore, it does not offer the wide surgical applications that laparoscopic surgical access offers. However, it does have a role in replacing a laparoscopy in appropriately selected patients.

TREATMENT OF TUBAL INFERTILITY

Until the mid to late 1980s, reproductive surgery was the main option of treatment for the infertile woman with damaged fallopian tubes to achieve a pregnancy. This changed dramatically due to significant progress realized in IVF in the decade of the 1990s. The Society for Assisted Reproductive Technology reports rates in the United States progressed from 12.3% of births per initiated cycle in 1990 to 25.4% in 1999, 2004. The 1990s also witnessed the introduction and acceptance of intracytoplasmic sperm injection (ICSI), which proved to be a panacea in the treatment of male infertility.

There are now two realistic treatment options for the treatment of tubal and peritoneal factor infertility: reconstructive surgery and assisted reproduction techniques (ART). Surgery also experienced significant progress and development in the last three decades. Furthermore, presence of a credible alternative with IVF permits the reproductive surgeon to operate on cases with a better prognosis, which was not the case before the end of the 1980s. We have known for a long time that one of the important factors influencing surgical outcome is the degree of tubal damage. Operating on patients with better prognosis translates in superior outcomes as has been well demonstrated. Surgery and IVF must not be regarded as competitive but rather as complementary treatments necessary to achieve the desired goal. The choice of treatment is ideally dependent on multiple considerations, both technical and nontechnical.

Technical considerations refer to proper assessment of the clinical findings of the couple. It is evident that IVF is the only treatment option for women with inoperable fallopian tubes and tubal disease coincident with another important fertility factor, such as male factor infertility. Not infrequently, a woman will require reconstructive surgery to make IVF possible or more frequently to increase the success rate with IVF. Some patients are better served with surgery.

The provision of accurate information regarding both IVF and tubal surgery is essential in the decision-making process of the couple. The couple must be given the live birth rate per cycle of IVF, the cumulative birth rate after multiple cycles of treatment, and the potential complication rates, including multiple pregnancy, abortion, and ectopic pregnancy. In addition, the effect of frozen embryo replacement on the cumulative pregnancy rate must be considered in the analysis. Similar information must also be provided regarding reconstructive tubal surgery. It is imperative that such figures reflect the experience of the center in which treatment will be performed and not those reported in international journals.

Nontechnical considerations include age, cost, and the wishes of the couple. Female fecundity is adversely affected by age. Fecundity begins to decline at approximately 31 years of age. This trend has been observed both in "normal" couples and in those with unexplained infertility. This decline becomes even more evident after 35 years of age. In women of advanced reproductive age, the marked decline of fecundity rate per cycle of IVF must be weighed against the fact that reconstructive surgery offers multiple cycles during which conception can occur. Therefore, although the younger woman may consider surgery for a given condition, those in more advanced reproductive age, 37 and over, may be advised to consider IVF first.

Health insurance coverage and the cost of the procedure, depending on the jurisdiction, and the resources of the couple play important roles in the decision-making process. Another, often underestimated potential factor is the economic impact of a multiple pregnancy, which occurs much more frequently with IVF.

The perceptions and wishes of the couple regarding treatment options depend on many influences, including their own values and ethical views. There may be disagreement between partners. The physician should provide detailed information for the couple as clearly and accurately as possible and should abstain from interfering with their decision making except to clarify misunderstandings and misinterpretations. The physician must advise against active treatment when the prognosis is poor because treatment with essentially no chance of success cannot be justified.

The significant improvement in the outcomes of ART was largely due to the simplification of techniques, both clinical and laboratory, progress made in cryopreservation, and the replacement of multiple embryos. Another important factor was the commercialization of these services, which proved lucrative. The number of IVF programs in the United States increased from 267 in 1994 to 461 in 2004, and the number of cycles performed quadrupled during the intervening 20 years from approximately 32,000 to 128,000, which represented a $1.25 billion business. During the same period, there has been a significant decline in the use and teaching of reconstructive infertility surgery. In vitro fertilization started increasingly to be offered, as primary treatment option, in most cases of tubal factor infertility. These changes have occurred despite the acceptance of laparoscopic access to perform many of the reconstructive tubal operations and the use of minilaparotomy incision for more complex anastomotic procedures, both of which have become day care procedures. Concerned with this trend, as early as 1992, we emphasized that both therapeutic options had a place, that treatment should be individualized based on the clinical findings and circumstances of the couple, and that these two options were not competitive but rather complementary. We are of the same opinion today.

Assisted reproduction has revolutionized reproductive medicine; we are in full recognition of this fact. We also believe that reproductive surgery has an important place in the treatment of tubal infertility and in assisting to improve ART outcomes in those who need preliminary surgery. We are gratified to find in ASRM's "Committee Opinion: Role of Tubal Surgery in the Era of Assisted Reproductive Technology" published in March 2012 support for many opinions we have held about the role of reproductive surgery since early 1990s, when ART results started to show significant progress. We strongly recommend the reader to obtain a copy of this document.

In Vitro Fertilization and Embryo Transfer

Reconstructive tubal surgery was the only treatment option for infertile women with damaged fallopian tubes, until the recent past. This is no longer the case due to significant improvement in outcomes and much wider availability of IVF and ART that provide such couples with a realistic therapeutic alternative.

Data collected prospectively for ART treatments during the year 2009, the last year for which there was a detailed analysis available at the time of writing, from 441 clinics in the United States provided the following outcome data, which were tabulated by the Centers for Disease Control and Prevention (CDC) in 2011. There were 146,244 cycles of ART in 2009. Of these 102,478 (70.1%) were fresh nondonor and 26,069 (17.8%) were frozen nondonor cycles; 11,038 (7.5%) were fresh donor and 6,659 (4.6%) were frozen donor cycles. The majority of the women treated (61.1%) were 35 years of age and more, and only 38.9% were under 35. The overall live birth rate per cycle started in the fresh nondonor group was 30% and in the frozen nondonor group was also 30%. The birth rate was the same in 2010. In cycles that resulted in a clinical pregnancy, 81.3% resulted in live births. Of live births, 69.5% were singleton births and 28.9% were twins and 1.6% triplets or greater multiples.

Of note, a 2013 report from the CDC indicates the number of ART cycles performed in the United States has more than doubled from 64,036 cycles in 1996 to 147,260 in 2010. More important is the improvement in the overall live birth rate per cycle started from 12.3% in 1990 to 30% in 2010.

Intracytoplasmic sperm injection represents a very important progress in ART; it has proven to be a panacea in the treatment of male infertility. As early as 2003, it was demonstrated that in male factor infertility, the use of ICSI is associated with a success rate that almost equals that of standard IVF in the absence of male factor (Table 21.2). Furthermore, since the same time there has been an increasing use of ICSI for fertilization of oocytes even in couples without a male factor. In the United States in 2010, ICSI was used in 66% of IVF cases.

The outcome of both standard IVF and ICSI is adversely affected by the age of the female partner. There is a linear decline after age 35 in both the overall live birth rates and the implantation rate of embryos as clearly evident in Table 21.3 that summarizes the US IVF results for the year 2010.

TABLE 21.2 CDC 2003 Assisted Reproductive Technology Report

LIVE BIRTHS PER OOCYTE RETRIEVAL IN ART CYCLES 2003					
	AGE (YEARS)				
	<35	35–37	38–40	41–42	>42
Male factor infertility					
IVF	42.6%	35.9%	26.2%	16.1%	6.0%
IVF with ICSI	41.8%	35.0%	24.1%	13.5%	4.2%
No male factor infertility					
IVF	42.6%	35.9%	26.2%	16.1%	6.0%
IVF with ICSI	37.8%	32.2%	21.8%	11.0%	4.2%

ART, assisted reproductive technology; IVF, in vitro fertilization; ICSI, intracytoplasmic sperm injection.

There has been an increase in the use of frozen nondonor embryos and improvement in outcomes. Frozen nondonor embryos were used in approximately 18% of all ART cycles performed in 2009, compared to 14% in 2003. The rate of thawed embryos resulting in live births is 30.3%, similar to the overall rate with fresh nondonor cycles, which is quite impressive. Although replacement of frozen thawed embryos improves the cumulative success rate for a couple, the overall net effect remains limited because not all of the cycles provide spare embryos and not all of the frozen embryos withstand the thawing process.

In vitro fertilization and embryo transfer is not risk free, especially in stimulated cycles. Although uncommon, ovarian hyperstimulation, bleeding, and infection can occur. Pregnancies resulting from IVF have an abortion rate of approximately 17%. The overall tubal pregnancy rate is approximately 1% to 2% of ART cycles. A 1991 study from our center by Zouves et al. demonstrated a tubal pregnancy rate of 2.6% (of clinical pregnancies) among IVF patients without tubal factor infertility. However, this rate was 12% in patients with prior tubal disease and tubal surgery.

Assisted reproductive technology procedures are associated with a significant increase in the rate of multiple pregnancies (relative risk [RR] >20). The Centers for Disease Control (CDC) Assisted Reproductive Technology report for 2009 indicated that of the resulting live births, only 69.5% were singletons, 28.9% twins, and 1.6% triplets or higher order. These results show a modest improvement compared to those of 2003, which were 65.8%, 31.0%, and 3.2%, respectively. The high rate of multiple pregnancies is due to the number of embryos transferred. Since transfer of more embryos improves the overall pregnancy rate, there is a temptation to do so. In Europe, where in many jurisdictions the number of embryos to be transferred is limited, both the live birth outcomes and the multiple pregnancy rates are lower (Table 21.4).

The high rate of multiple births has a tremendous personal and social impact. Perinatal morbidity and mortality are markedly increased in pregnancies complicated by multiple gestations. The cost, both emotionally and financially, of caring for premature or abnormal children is great. It was demonstrated that monofetal pregnancies also are associated with elevated risk as compared with non-ART singleton pregnancies; more than 10% of monofetal births are preterm, and the perinatal mortality rate (approximately 19 per 1,000) is higher than non-ART singleton pregnancies. This has not changed; the 2009 US outcomes for fresh nondonor ART cycles indicate preterm birth rates of 11.6% for singletons from single-fetus pregnancy, 19.0% for singletons from multiple-fetus pregnancy, 60% for twins, and 97.5% for triplets or more. The percentages of low-birth-weight infants for the same group were 8.7%, 16.7%, 56.1%, and 92.1%, respectively.

A 1994 study by Rufat et al. from France that analyzed a total of 1,637 IVF pregnancies resulting in 1,263 deliveries and 1,669 live born or stillborn children demonstrated a preterm birth rate of 22.7% of all deliveries and 12.2% of singleton deliveries compared with 5.6% among all deliveries in France, and 34.7% of babies weighed less than 2,500 g compared with 5.2% among all deliveries in France. The rates of perinatal, neonatal, and infant mortality were higher than the national

TABLE 21.3 ART Results in the United States for the Year 2000[a]

AGE	<35	35–37	38–40	41–42	42–44	>44
Implant %	36.5	26.9	17.7	9.6	4.2	1.7
Live birth %	41.5	31.9	22.1	12.4	5.0	1.0
Twins%	32.9	27.3	21.6	15.0	8.1	2.3
Triplet+%	2.6	3.1	3.7	3.0	0.6	2.3

[a]Percentage of live births per cycle; 147,260 cycles from 443 clinics. Intracytoplasmic sperm injection in 66% CDC Reproductive Health; www.cdc.gov/art/ART.2010

TABLE 21.4 ART Results in Europe for the Year 2007

DELIVERY/OPU %	IVF	ICSI	MULTIPLE PREGNANCY
Europe	21.1	20.2	22.3
France	19.2	20.5	19.3
Germany	16.0	16.1	21.8
Italy	15.2	14.3	23.4
United Kingdom	26.4	27.5	17.9

From de Mouzon J, et al. Assisted reproductive technology in Europe, 2007: results generated from European registers by ESHRE. *Hum Reprod* 2012;27:954, with permission. Copyright 2012, Oxford University Press.

average. Another important study by Bergh et al. from Sweden compared the obstetric outcomes of babies conceived with IVF ($n = 5,856$) to all babies born in the general population during a span of 13 years (1982–1995) demonstrated that children resulting from IVF conception had increased rates of low birth weight (RR = 5), major malformations (RR = 1.4), cerebral palsy (RR = 4), and death (RR = 2). Such elevated personal and societal costs must be considered when embarking on any ART procedure.

REPRODUCTIVE SURGERY

Reproductive surgery encompasses much more than procedures designed to improve fertility, as understood by some. In fact, in addition to fertility-promoting procedures, such as reconstruction of fallopian tubes and salpingo-ovariolysis, it includes all surgical procedures performed on the pelvic organs of female children, adolescents, and childbearing age women, and not only when performed in those who present with infertility. It must be noted that *"female infertility is frequently caused by misdiagnosis or delayed diagnosis and treatment of acute conditions in young and/or reproductive age women, such as PID, ectopic pregnancy, appendicitis, etc. It is also caused by surgical procedures that are unnecessary, unnecessarily extensive and/or traumatic, resulting in damage to or loss of normal reproductive organs and development of post-operative adhesions."* These observations clearly demonstrate the need to stress the importance of reproductive surgery, and to avail surgeons and especially gynecologists with training opportunities in this field.

Surgery was the only available therapeutic option for infertility caused by tubal and peritoneal factors until the mid-1980s. Traditional surgical techniques often yielded poor outcomes frequently as a result of extensive postoperative adhesions. In my textbook "Microsurgery in Female Infertility" published in January 1983, I wrote "I have vivid recollections of the frustration and disappointment I felt, when assisting as a resident at second-look laparotomies for removal of prosthetic devices such as Mulligan hoods, at finding extensive adhesions in the peritoneal cavity; with bowel, omentum, and the internal genitalia adherent to one another. Extensive adhesiolysis and separation of structures were often necessary in order to visualize the oviducts and remove the prosthetic devices left in situ during the prior reconstructive operation."

We have had important developments in the field of reproductive surgery in the past four decades. Gynecologic microsurgery was introduced in the early 1970s; simultaneously, laparoscopic surgical access was used for tubal reconstruction, especially in distal tubal disease. Used initially by open access, microsurgical tenets were also applied in procedures performed by laparoscopic access. The use of magnification and especially microsurgical principles yielded significantly improved outcomes, particularly in tubal anastomosis.

The use of laparoscopy for surgical access provided the advantages that are now well recognized: less postoperative discomfort and analgesic requirement, shorter hospital stay and postoperative recovery period, improved cosmetics, and frequently reduced costs. Many laparoscopic interventions became ambulatory procedures, the patient being able to return home the same day. It also did not take long to realize that this mode of surgical access yielded results that were not dissimilar to those obtained via laparotomy, provided of course the technique used was the same. Experience with laparoscopy permitted modification of open interventions for more complex cases, such as tubocornual anastomosis, where a small minilaparotomy incision replaced a formal laparotomy, permitting such procedures also to be performed on ambulatory basis.

The overall risks of reconstructive tubal surgery are small and include the recognized complications of anesthesia and surgery. Surgery, if successful, offers multiple cycles in which to achieve conception and the opportunity to have more than one pregnancy. The abortion rate subsequent to reconstructive tubal surgery is not increased over that of the normal population. The live birth and ectopic pregnancy rates depend on the specific nature of the tubal disease and the extent of tubal damage.

MICROSURGERY

Principles

Microsurgery has been defined as "surgery under magnification." In fact, magnification is only a single facet of microsurgery, which embraces a broad concept of tissue care designed to minimize tissue damage and the use of measures that prevent and/or decrease an acute inflammatory reaction in the peritoneal cavity. These are measures applicable to both open and laparoscopic access; they include the following:

- Use of a delicate, atraumatic technique designed to minimize tissue injury, which in addition includes judicious use of electrical or laser energy and frequent intraoperative irrigation with heparinized lactated Ringer solution to keep serosal surfaces moistened to prevent desiccation
- Prevention of foreign body contamination of the peritoneal cavity
- Obtaining meticulous pinpoint hemostasis, using a microelectrode, minimizing adjacent tissue damage.
- Complete excision of abnormal tissues
- Identifying proper cleavage planes and precisely align and approximate tissue planes with fine nonreactive sutures
- Performing a thorough pelvic lavage using heparinized lactated Ringer solution at the close of the procedure to remove from the peritoneal cavity any blood clots, foreign body, or debris that may be present.

Additional measures help to decrease acute inflammatory reaction. Specifically before the close of the procedure, we leave 300 to 500 mL of lactated Ringer solution with 500 mg of hydrocortisone succinate in the peritoneal cavity. General measures assist in this regard: use of preoperative and postoperative antiinflammatory medications, for example, Voltaren suppository, infiltration of a local anesthetic before placing the incision, and the administration of a single dose of prednisone postsurgery.

Magnification, with an operating microscope or with an endoscope, provides many advantages; it permits prompt identification of abnormal morphologic changes, recognition and avoidance of surgical injury, and application of the preceding principles with the use of fine instruments and suture materials. Microsurgery is a surgical attitude as much as a technique.

In the late 1960s, Swolin used magnification with loops—electrosurgery with a fine electrode for the reconstruction of distal tubal occlusion. In addition, he strived to reduce peritoneal trauma by keeping the operative site moistened by frequent irrigation. In Vancouver, we expanded the microsurgical techniques; using an operating microscope, we applied them in the correction of pathologic cornual and midtubal occlusions (tubocornual anastomosis and tubotubal anastomosis) and in reversal of sterilization. This approach permitted us to perform tubocornual anastomosis as opposed to a tubouterine implantation—which was the standard procedure at the time—in cases of pathologic cornual occlusion. An anastomosis in such cases preserves tubal integrity and thus is a more physiologic approach of tubal reconstruction.

Microsurgery, in fact, finds its ultimate application in tubal anastomosis. The use of magnification, microsurgical instruments, and sutures enables the recognition of subtle abnormalities—even in the presence of tubal patency, excision of abnormal tissues, and correct alignment of the tubal segments and precise apposition of each layer. Indeed, the application of microsurgery has significantly improved the outcome of such procedures. However, in the treatment of distal tubal occlusion, any improvement attributable to the use of microsurgical techniques has been relatively modest, despite the reduction in postoperative adhesions and improved tubal patency rates.

The introduction of microsurgery into gynecology has yielded benefits much greater than simple improvement in the outcome of certain fertility operations. It created a great awareness of the effects of peritoneal trauma and the resulting postoperative adhesions. It also promoted the use of conservative approaches that are now considered standard *of* care for women undergoing surgical treatment for benign gynecologic disease. These are additional and important reasons to continue to teach reconstructive infertility surgery. Thus, microsurgery is a surgical philosophy, a delicate surgical approach designed to minimize peritoneal trauma and tissue disruption and prevent postoperative adhesions while increasing the accuracy of the procedure and improving the outcome.

Microsurgical techniques are equally applicable to both open and laparoscopic access. We demonstrated the applicability of microsurgical techniques by laparoscopy for adhesiolysis, salpingo-ovariolysis, fimbrioplasty, and salpingostomy as early as the mid-1970s. Microsurgical techniques must be used in all reproductive operations, irrespective of the mode of access. This is especially important today because most such procedures are performed by laparoscopy and minilaparotomy.

The laparoscope also provides a degree of magnification. Bringing the distal end of the laparoscope close to the area of interest, one achieves excellent visibility and illumination. There are microsurgical advantages inherent to laparoscopic access. Operating within a closed peritoneal cavity eliminates the need to use packs and prevents the introduction of foreign materials such as lint and talcum powder. The pressure effect of the pneumoperitoneum diminishes venous oozing and permits spontaneous coagulation of minor vessels. It is possible to perform intraoperative irrigation to expose any bleeding vessels and keep tissues moistened. Fine electrodes can also be used to achieve precise electrosurgical hemostasis. Like microsurgery, laparoscopic procedures are performed with few instruments. The instrument manufacturers have at last recognized the need for proper microsurgical instruments for laparoscopy; they are now readily available.

We must stress, however, that the large volume of gas insufflation necessary in operative laparoscopy causes desiccation of the mesothelial cells that line the peritoneum; furthermore, it has been recognized that CO_2 is toxic to mesothelial cells. This phenomenon may enhance the development of postoperative adhesions. Hypoxia causes retraction of the mesothelial cells exposing the extracellular matrix. This causes substances and cellular elements that enhance adhesion formation or decrease repair to enter the peritoneal cavity. Both animal and more recently human work demonstrated that the noxious effects of CO_2 pneumoperitoneum may largely be avoided by modifying the gas mixture by adding small percentages of O_2 and N_2O, keeping the gas mixture fully humidified and at a temperature of 31°C.

Major Equipment and Surgical Instruments

The major equipment includes an electrosurgical generator suitable for both general and microsurgical work and, depending on the access mode used, either an operating microscope or appropriate laparoscopic equipment. Most of the good modern electrosurgical generators can be used for both general work and microsurgical work. Such generators are now standard equipment in most operating rooms.

When access to the pelvis is achieved by laparotomy or minilaparotomy, magnification is obtained by the use of an operating microscope or loops. Loops provide low levels of fixed magnification. It is difficult to work with loops that provide a magnification greater than four times. They are suitable for use only in simple short procedures and are quite helpful when used to divide adhesions or excise endometriotic lesions located deep in the pelvis. Magnification is best obtained with an operating microscope that provides magnification ranges from 2 to 40 times; coaxial illumination of a constant visual field enables precise focusing and change of levels of magnification. In gynecologic microsurgery, an objective lens with a focal distance of 250 to 300 mm allows for a suitable working distance under the lens. The microscope can be mounted on the floor or ceiling. Focusing, varying the level of magnification, and other functions of the microscope can be manual or motorized. The latter version is preferable because changes can be readily accomplished through controls on a foot pedal while the surgeon's hands remain in the operative field. Most modern operating microscopes are equipped with beam splitters, which permit the fitting of two pairs of binoculars so that both the surgeon and the assistant can simultaneously view the operative field. A miniature television camera can also be fitted to the same beam splitter, which enables the operating room personnel to follow the surgery on the monitor and allows video recordings of the procedure to be made.

When laparoscopic access is used, a good laparoscope equipped with a high-resolution mini TV camera and a high-resolution monitor is required. The laparoscope does not offer the stereoscopic vision and the excellent depth of field that the operating microscope provides. Nonetheless, first generations

IV

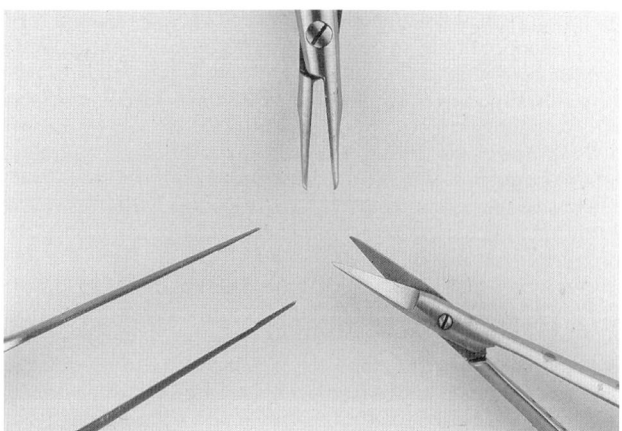

FIGURE 21.12 The working tips of the principal microsurgical instruments: plain forceps, scissors, and needle holder.

of three-dimensional laparoscopic equipment and magnification devices have been produced. Progress is under way.

Good microsurgical instruments for open access have been present since the 1970s. Microsurgical instrument for laparoscopic access became available in the last two decades. Although their shapes are obviously different, their functions are similar. The basic microsurgical instruments are few and include plain and toothed platform microforceps, microscissors, microneedle holder, and straight scissors and/or a microblade to transect the tube (**Fig. 21.12**). The forceps have rounded tips with a shaft designed so that they, like the scissors and needle holder, have good ergonomics and can be used comfortably. Teflon-coated probes with variable rounded tips are used for retraction.

Electromicrosurgery requires the use of a true insulated microelectrode of 100 or 150 μm in diameter with a free pointed conical tip. The microelectrode is connected to the handle of the electrosurgical unit with an adaptor. A rocker switch mounted on the handle allows delivery of current in cutting, coagulating, or blend modes. Irrigation can be performed with an appropriate laparoscopic irrigator. For open procedures, a device with a fingertip control (Gomel irrigator) (**Fig. 21.13**) is commercially available and enables accurate irrigation.

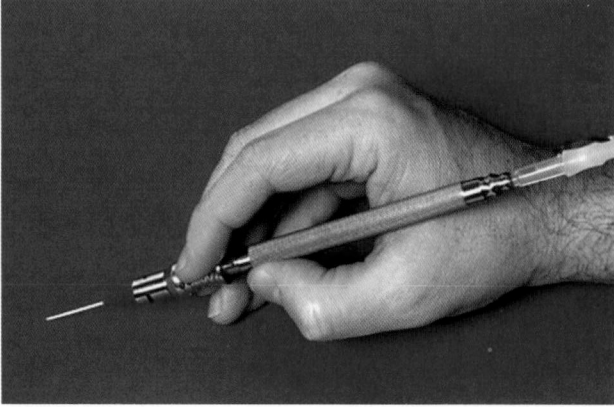

FIGURE 21.13 The Gomel microsurgical irrigator. An intravenous cannula has been attached to the tip of the irrigator. Fingertip control of the sliding valve permits one to initiate or stop irrigation.

Immediate Preoperative Preparation

Before the induction of anesthesia, the surgeon must ensure that all necessary equipment and instruments are present and in working order. After the induction of anesthesia, the patient's bladder is catheterized with a Foley catheter, which is connected to continuous drainage. If intraoperative chromopertubation is required, either a pediatric Foley catheter or an appropriate uterine cannula is introduced through the cervix and fixed in place. The catheter or cannula is connected either directly or by means of an extension tube to a syringe filled with dilute dye solution.

When open surgical access is used, anteversion and elevation of the uterus can be achieved either by selecting a suitable uterine cannula or by packing the vagina. With the latter option, a pediatric Foley catheter should first be placed in the uterine cavity if intraoperative chromopertubation is desired.

Surgical Access

As indicated earlier in the text, many reconstructive tubal operations can be performed by laparotomy, minilaparotomy, or laparoscopic access. The selection of the specific access route depends on the nature of the lesion, the type of procedure required, and the skill of the surgeon. The aim is to select the access route that will yield the best outcome for the patient.

Many reconstructive operations, especially those for distal tubal disease, can be efficiently performed by laparoscopic access. Because of the advantages inherent in undertaking such a procedure at the time of the initial diagnostic laparoscopy, it is preferable that a surgeon trained in this type of surgery perform the initial laparoscopy.

Access by Laparoscopy

Once a proper pneumoperitoneum is obtained, the principal trocar and cannula are inserted (usually intraumbilically), the trocar is removed, and the laparoscope is introduced through the cannula. The details of performing a laparoscopy will not be described in this chapter. A thorough laparoscopic survey is performed as described earlier in this text, and the nature and extent of the tubal and pelvic lesions is assessed. The information yielded by the prior complemented by the laparoscopic findings and the status of the other fertility parameters, permits the surgeon to select the therapeutic approach that is best for the patient.

The laparoscopic survey requires the establishment of a secondary portal for the introduction of a probe or other appropriate instrument. This ancillary portal is placed suprapubically in the midline or in one of the lower abdominal quadrants. The undertaking of reconstructive surgery will necessitate the establishment of additional portals of entry. These are placed, depending on the clinical findings and the procedure to be performed, at sites that permit easy access to the operative field.

Open Access: Minilaparotomy

In reconstructive tubal surgery, a transverse suprapubic incision is the type used most often. Since 1985, we have used a small, minilaparotomy, suprapubic transverse or vertical (if a midline or paramedian scar is present) incision to gain access to the pelvis. The length of this minilaparotomy incision is usually 4.5 to 6 cm. The prior pelvic findings and especially the depth of the patient's subcutaneous adipose layer determine the length of the incision. The site of the proposed incision is infiltrated with a long-acting anesthetic agent, such as

0.25% bupivacaine (Marcaine) solution. A transverse suprapubic incision is made and extended down to the fascia. The subcutaneous fat is dissected over the fascia, in the midline upward and downward. The fascia is then incised vertically in the midline. The recti muscles are separated in the midline, and the peritoneum is incised vertically, with the incision curbed laterally at the lower end to avoid the bladder. The subcutaneous tissues are reinfiltrated with the same solution before closure of the skin incision. Thereafter, a bilateral ilioinguinal nerve block is established. The small size of the incision; the lack of bowel manipulation, along with gentle handling of tissues during the procedure; and the use of local anesthesia reduce postoperative discomfort and analgesia requirements. This approach permits prompt mobilization of the patient and discharge from the hospital or surgical center usually on the same day. These patients return to normal activity almost as rapidly as those who have had their procedures performed laparoscopically.

It is essential that the surgical personnel thoroughly wash their gloves after they have been put on and again before making the peritoneal incision. Once the peritoneal cavity is entered, retraction is obtained with a disposable device that provides both wound protection and circumferential retraction with maximal exposure for the incision size. Varying sizes of such devices are available from many manufacturers and are preferable to standard retractors. Pads soaked in heparinized (5,000 U/L) lactated Ringer solution can be introduced into the pouch of Douglas to further elevate the uterus and isolate the bowel already displaced by a mild (10- to 15-degree) Trendelenburg tilt.

Once the surgical site is well exposed, the operating microscope is positioned. Although the operating microscope can be draped, we have not found this to be necessary, particularly if foot pedals control the microscope. Intraoperative irrigation is performed with heparinized lactated Ringer solution in an intravenous bag that is elevated and connected with intravenous tubing to a Gomel microsurgical irrigator (Fig. 21.12). This enables periodic irrigation of the exposed peritoneal surfaces and ovaries to prevent desiccation and to visualize individual bleeders.

Pelvic Lavage

At the close of a reconstructive procedure, irrespective of the type and the mode of access, the operative site is inspected to ensure that complete hemostasis has been achieved. Any bleeding vessels are electrodesiccated. A thorough pelvic lavage is then performed with the irrigation solution until the fluid remains clear. Pelvic lavage serves to remove from the peritoneal cavity any blood clots or other debris that may be present.

When laparoscopic access is used for the procedure, underwater examination of the operative site may be performed. When the irrigation fluid remains clear, the pneumoperitoneum pressure is reduced and the region inspected with the distal end of the laparoscope under the surface of the fluid. This permits prompt recognition of any small bleeding vessels, which can be desiccated with the use of a microelectrode or microbipolar forceps.

Once the irrigation fluid is completely suctioned out of the pelvis, some investigators leave varying amounts of physiologic solution in the peritoneal cavity to reduce postoperative adhesions. We use 300 to 500 mL of lactated Ringer solution to which 500 mg of hydrocortisone succinate is added. There are promising new products designed to prevent adhesion formation that are easy to apply by both open and laparoscopic access; these are currently undergoing clinical trials. The topic of ancillary measures for adhesion prevention is outside the purview of this chapter and will not be discussed further.

SURGICAL TECHNIQUE

In this chapter, the following procedures are discussed: salpingo-ovariolysis, fimbrioplasty, salpingostomy, tubotubal anastomosis to repair midtubal disease or to reverse a prior sterilization, tubocornual anastomosis to treat proximal tubal disease, and other procedures performed rarely in unusual circumstances. The techniques used for these procedures are essentially the same irrespective of the access route.

Whereas procedures for distal tubal disease are very amenable to laparoscopic access, anastomotic procedures are technically more difficult to accomplish by this route. Isthmic–isthmic and isthmic–ampullary anastomosis (usually used for sterilization reversal) have been performed with varying degrees of accuracy via laparoscopic access, but accomplishing other types of anastomoses (especially tubocornual) through this access route is much more challenging.

With microsurgical procedures, our aim has always been to keep the techniques as simple as possible for the outcomes to be reproducible, not only by surgical virtuosi but also by all physicians who practice in this field. Our more recent technical modifications, including access through a minilaparotomy incision and the use of a protractor, were the result of the same thought process. Although we remain enthusiastic proponents of laparoscopic access, we do not let this enthusiasm blind us to the possibility that some procedures may still be performed better by modifications and improvements in traditional methods.

Salpingo-Ovariolysis

Pelvic and periadnexal adhesions usually are the sequel of PID. These adhesions may be broad or shallow; they are usually not too vascular and extend from one structure to another. In so doing, they tend to leave a space or potential space between the involved structures, an aspect that facilitates adhesiolysis (Fig. 21.14). Dense cohesive adhesions often result from prior surgery. In this case, adjacent structures are intimately conglutinated. The adherent surface is devoid of the superficial mesothelial layer of the peritoneum. In other words, the underlying stromal layers of the two structures coalesce. The lysis of such an adhesive process is technically difficult and is associated with a very high percentage of recurrence.

Periadnexal adhesions usually coexist with other types of tubal damage. Thus, salpingo-ovariolysis is often an integral part of other reconstructive procedures. However, periadnexal adhesive disease may be the sole apparent lesion, in which case

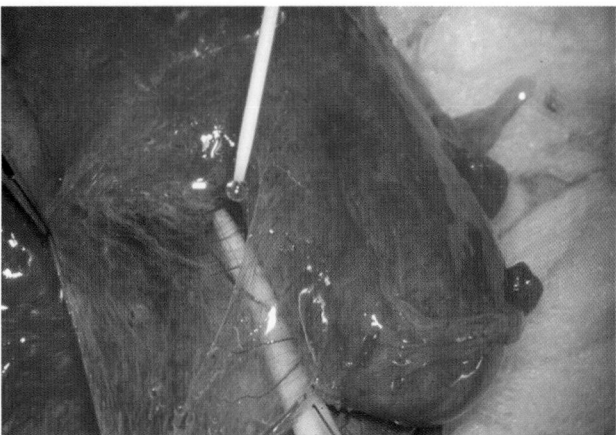

FIGURE 21.14 Salpingolysis. The space between the two involved structures facilitates division.

fertility depends on the severity and nature of the adhesions. Even in the presence of a patent tube, extensive adhesions may encapsulate the tube (especially the fimbriated end, the ovary, or both) and prevent ovum pickup (Fig. 21.9). By fixing the fimbriated end of the patent tube away from the ovary, adhesions may distort their spatial relationship and, hence, the functional proximity that exists between these two organs. For example, the fimbriated end of a patent tube may be adherent to the anterior abdominal wall or the uterine fundus, whereas the ovary is fixed in the pouch of Douglas. Periovarian adhesions may also affect follicular development, as has been demonstrated in both animal and human studies. Human studies were usually performed on patients undergoing IVF treatment.

When salpingo-ovariolysis is performed by open access, adhesiolysis is usually commenced by defining the distal margins of the adhesions. The division of adhesions at their distal attachment frees the adnexa, making it possible to elevate and bring them closer to the abdominal wall. This move facilitates the remainder of the procedure. Elevation of the adnexa is achieved by the use of inert pads soaked in the irrigation fluid. Adhesiolysis is then completed by systematically excising the adhesions from the tubal serosa or ovarian surface (Fig. 21.14). With laparoscopic access, it is usually preferable to reverse this order and commence the adhesiolysis at the level of the adnexa.

Adhesions are put on tension with a toothed forceps, and the site of incision is exposed. Division is effected electrosurgically or with appropriate microsurgical scissors. It is imperative to divide adhesions one layer at a time, slightly lateral to their attachments to the organ to avoid damaging the adjacent peritoneum. Adhesions are often composed of two layers, even though they may initially appear as a single layer. They tend to attach to an organ at two different levels. It is essential to enter between the two layers first; this permits exposure of the demarcation line between the adhesion and the mesothelium of the adjacent structure. Each layer of adhesion is then put on a stretch with toothed forceps, the demarcation line is identified, and the adhesion is transected. With open access, placement of a Teflon rod under the incision line enhances exposure. Damage to the peritoneum or ovarian surface is avoided by keeping the transection line 1 mm away from these surfaces. Prominent vessels along the transection line are individually electrodesiccated.

When a microelectrode is used for this purpose, the electrosurgical unit is put on the blend or cut setting. Pure coagulating current (coag mode) may be used to obtain hemostasis of individual bleeders, which are exposed under a jet of irrigation fluid. With open access, an elongating adaptor may be attached to the handle of the electrosurgical unit to facilitate adhesiolysis in the deeper parts of the pelvis.

All of the broad adhesions are excised and removed from the pelvis. Shallow adhesions are simply divided. In this case, a small opening is made on the adhesion, through which a fine instrument or Teflon rod is introduced. This permits separation of the adjacent structures and better visualization of the adhesion, which is incised without damaging these structures. The procedure is completed with a thorough pelvic lavage with the irrigation solution mentioned earlier in the text.

The technical principles are identical when laparoscopic access is used for the procedure. In this case, however, because there is no need to lift the adnexa close to the abdominal wall, the salpingo-ovariolysis is commenced with the tube and ovary. Once again, the performance of effective and safe salpingo-ovariolysis requires clear identification of each adhesive layer, which is grasped and retracted, permitting clear identification of the attachments to the organ of interest. The adhesions are incised parallel to the organ of interest and approximately 1 mm away to prevent damaging its mesothelial envelope (Figs. 21.15 and 21.16).

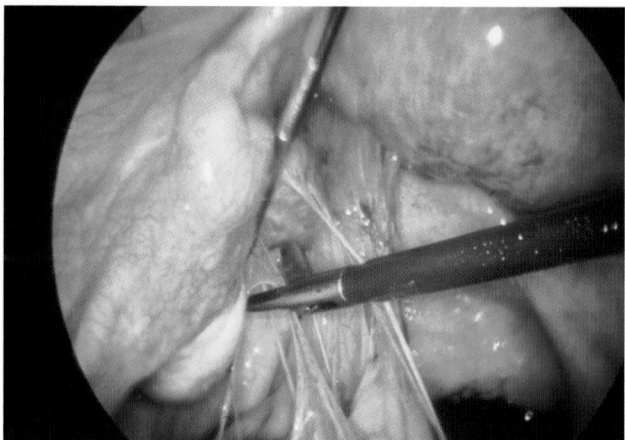

FIGURE 21.15 Salpingo-ovariolysis by laparoscopic access (same patient as in Fig. 21.9). Division of adhesions parallel to the tube.

Division is accomplished electrosurgically with a microelectrode or mechanically with fine scissors. We use scissors for laparoscopic salpingo-ovariolysis and electrodesiccation to secure obvious vessels or bleeders encountered along the incision line. As described earlier, shallow adhesions are simply divided, whereas broad adhesions are excised (by dissecting them free at all points of attachment) and removed through one of the ancillary portals (Fig. 21.16).

Cohesive adhesions require identification of the dissection plane. This is achieved by making a small incision and developing a tissue plane either by spreading the jaws of the scissors, by blunt dissection, or by hydrodissection (injecting irrigation solution into the site under pressure). It is important to abstain from using thermal energy in such cases because of the inherent danger.

It should not be necessary to use open access, excepting rare circumstances, for the purpose of salpingo-ovariolysis. Our primary approach in such cases has always been by laparoscopic access and whenever possible at the time of the diagnostic survey.

Results of Salpingo-Ovariolysis

The reported intrauterine pregnancy rates resulting from open microsurgical salpingo-ovariolysis range from 41% to 57%. The rates for live births are 37% to 57%, and the rates for ectopic pregnancies are 5% to 8% of operated patients. In one of these studies, 33 of 63 (52.4%) patients who underwent open microsurgical salpingo-ovariolysis achieved intrauterine pregnancies; in addition, 3 (4.8%) had ectopic pregnancies at 2-year follow-up. These 63 patients reported by Tulandi had been randomized to two cutting modalities: electrosurgery ($n = 33$) and CO_2 laser ($n = 30$). The results were identical in both subgroups. Indeed, there has been no demonstrable improvement in the outcome of such procedures with the use of lasers in both clinical and experimental studies.

The preexisting tubal patency and the uncontrolled nature of the salpingo-ovariolysis series reported in the literature may cast doubt on the value of this procedure. The Canadian Infertility Evaluation Study Group addressed this issue by studying treatment-dependent and treatment-independent pregnancies in patients with periadnexal disease whose fallopian tubes were not completely occluded. This was a multicenter, controlled, randomized study. The cumulative pregnancy rates reported by Tulandi and colleagues in 1989 were 59% among 69 patients in the group who underwent microsurgical salpingo-ovariolysis and only 16% among the

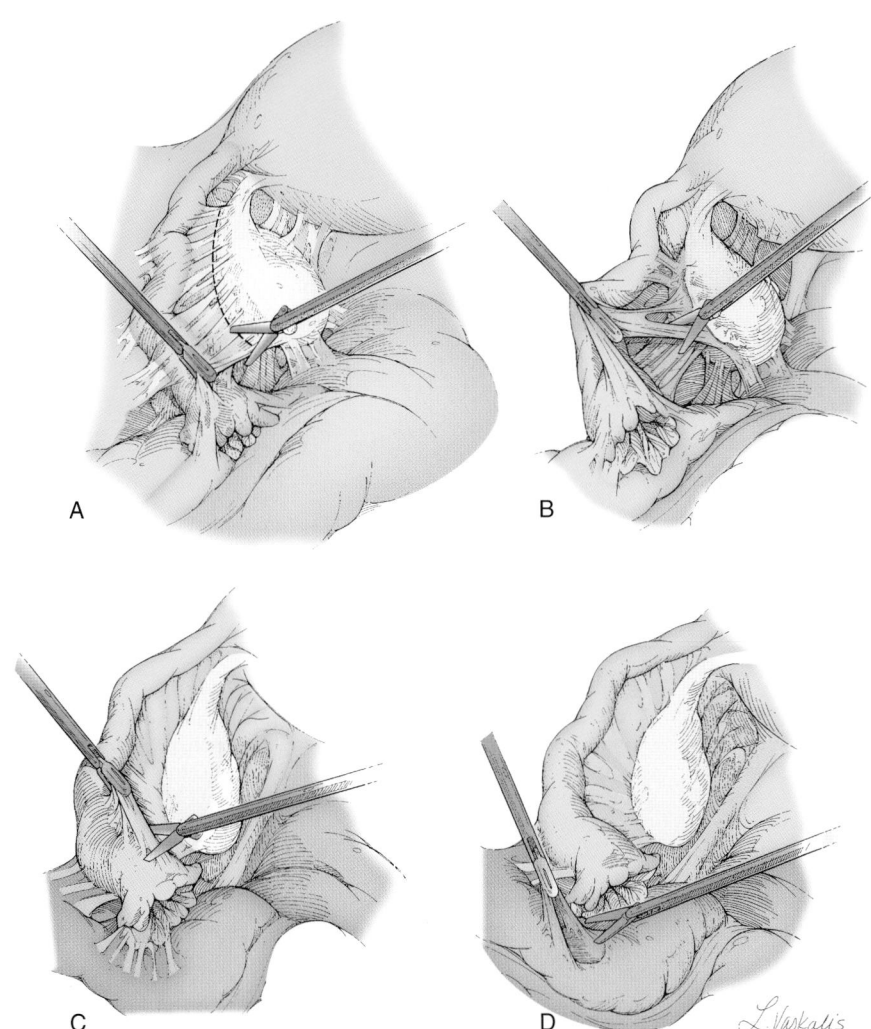

FIGURE 21.16 Salpingo-ovariolysis. **A:** Division of adhesions commences in a well-exposed area. **B:** Adhesions are stretched and are divided one layer at a time parallel to the organ of interest. **C:** Broad adhesions are freed at all points and removed from the peritoneal cavity. **D:** Salpingo-ovariolysis being completed. (From Gomel V, Taylor PJ. *Diagnostic and operative gynecologic laparoscopy.* St Louis, MO: Mosby, 1995:171, with permission.)

78 control patients who were not treated. This study confirms that pregnancies may occur in a small proportion of women with periadnexal adhesions and patent tubes and also proves the therapeutic value of salpingo-ovariolysis in such cases.

In the early stages of development of operative laparoscopy, we demonstrated that laparoscopic salpingo-ovariolysis yields results similar to those obtained by open access. We also stressed the importance of adhering to microsurgical principles in the performance of such procedures by both open and laparoscopic access. In 1983, we reported a series of 92 patients who underwent salpingo-ovariolysis by laparoscopy. The duration of involuntary infertility was longer than 20 months for all patients. Periadnexal adhesions were severe in 79 patients and moderate in 13. Moreover, the series included only those patients in whom ovum pickup by the tube on the side with lesser disease was deemed impossible or greatly hampered. At the time of the survey, the patients had been monitored postoperatively for a period of 9 months or longer. Of the 92 patients, 57 (62%) achieved at least one intrauterine pregnancy, 54 (59%) had one or more live births, and 5 (5.4%) had ectopic pregnancies. Ten of the patients who did not get pregnant had a second-look laparoscopy that demonstrated no significant residual adhesive process.

Similar results were corroborated by Bruhat et al. and Donnez et al. at other centers in Europe and by Fayez in North America. This demonstrates that the results of laparoscopic salpingo-ovariolysis, as expected, depend on the severity of the adhesions. The reported intrauterine pregnancy rates after laparoscopic salpingo-ovariolysis range from 51% to 62%, and ectopic pregnancy rates range from 5% to 8% of operated cases. Although no prospective, randomized trials exist, these results appear similar to those yielded by laparotomy.

Fimbrioplasty

Fimbrioplasty is the reconstruction of the fimbriae or infundibulum in a tube that exhibits fimbrial agglutination or prefimbrial phimosis and results in partial distal occlusion. Often, the tube and ovary are involved in adhesions, in which case salpingo-ovariolysis must precede the fimbrioplasty. The technique of fimbrioplasty, which will be described further, is the same irrespective of the access route used. Our approach is invariably by laparoscopic access.

Fimbrial phimosis results from the agglutination of the fimbriae. A small opening is usually present at the distal end of the tube unless this opening is covered by fibrous tissue. The latter usually becomes evident when the tube is distended by transcervical chromopertubation. When the opening is covered by fibrous tissue, this tissue must be incised or excised

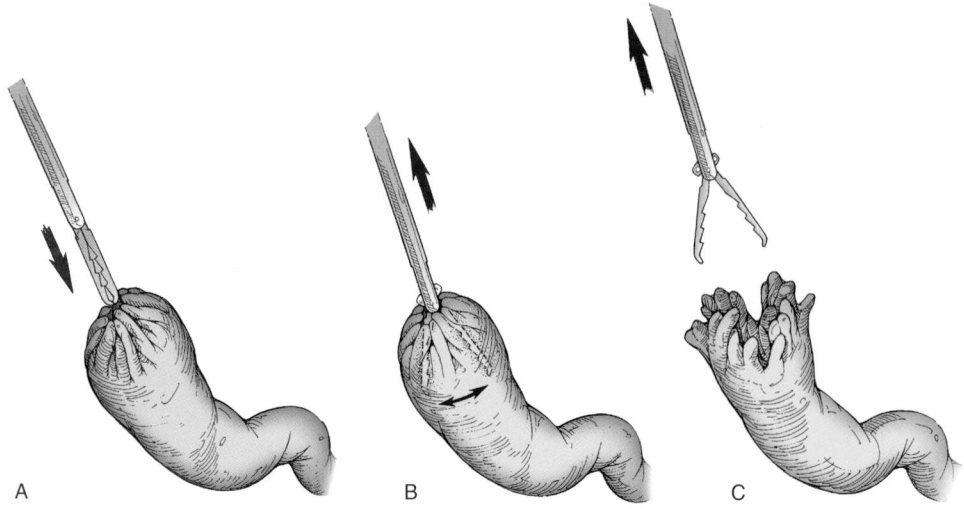

FIGURE 21.17 Fimbrioplasty: to free agglutinated fimbriae. **A:** The 3-mm alligator-jawed forceps is introduced through the stenosed opening. **B:** The jaws of the forceps are opened within the tube. **C:** The forceps is gently withdrawn while the jaws are kept open. (From Gomel V, Taylor PJ. *Diagnostic and operative gynecologic laparoscopy.* St Louis, MO: Mosby, 1995:173, with permission.)

to gain access to the fimbriae (**Fig. 21.17**). Agglutination of the fimbriae can be corrected simply by introducing a fine forceps, a 2-mm alligator forceps with jaws closed through the phimotic fimbrial opening. The jaws of the forceps are opened within the tubal lumen, and the forceps are gently withdrawn with the jaws open. Deagglutination is achieved by repeating this movement a few times, varying the direction in which the jaws of the forceps are opened (**Fig. 21.18**). When sufficient gentleness is used during this manipulation, bleeding is usually negligible and stops spontaneously.

When the stenosis is located at the level of the true abdominal tubal ostium, which is located at the apex of the infundibulum, the fimbriae may have a normal appearance. However, when chromopertubation is performed, the ampullary portion of the tube distends before any exit of dye solution. In this instance, it is necessary to place an incision on the antimesosalpingeal border of the tube, which commences at the infundibulum and continues past the stenotic area into the distal ampulla. The tube is stabilized by introducing a thin Teflon probe through the stenotic opening into the distal ampulla; the incision is made electrosurgically by using a microelectrode. This is the approach we generally use. Alternatively, the area can be injected with 1 mL of dilute vasopressin solution (1 IU in 30 mL of normal saline) and the incision made mechanically with microsurgical scissors. Bleeders are desiccated electrosurgically. The edges of the two flaps thus created are folded back either by securing them to the adjacent ampullary serosa with no. 7-0 or 8-0 polyglactin 910 (Vicryl) sutures or by electrosurgery (or a defocused CO_2 laser beam),

which desiccates the serosal aspect of the flaps, causing them to fold backward (**Fig. 21.19**).

Results of Fimbrioplasty

Very few investigators have classified fimbrioplasty as an independent procedure. Most include such patients in their salpingostomy series. French and Belgian centers include fimbrioplasty (correction of partial distal tubal occlusion) as stage 1 in their salpingostomy series.

Patton et al., in a series of microsurgical fimbrioplasty procedures in 40 patients, reported total intrauterine and ectopic pregnancy rates of 63% (25 patients) and 5% (2 patients), respectively, after 24 months of follow-up. The outcome of the intrauterine pregnancies and the live birth rates were not provided.

In 1983, we reported 40 such patients, all treated by laparoscopic access. Live births occurred in 19 (48%), and two patients (5%) had tubal gestations. In 1979, Mettler et al. reported a crude pregnancy rate of 31% among 51 women. The anatomic location and outcome of these pregnancies were not recorded. In 1990, Dubuisson et al. reported 31 such patients. After 18 months of follow-up, eight patients (25.8%) had intrauterine pregnancies, and four (12.9%) had ectopic pregnancies. In 1986 in a series of 100 patients, Donnez et al. reported a total pregnancy rate of 61%. The location and outcome of these pregnancies were not provided. A 1991 report by Canis et al. included 32 such patients with their salpingostomy patients; 16 (50%) of these achieved intrauterine pregnancies, but the outcome was not reported. Surprisingly, there were no tubal pregnancies.

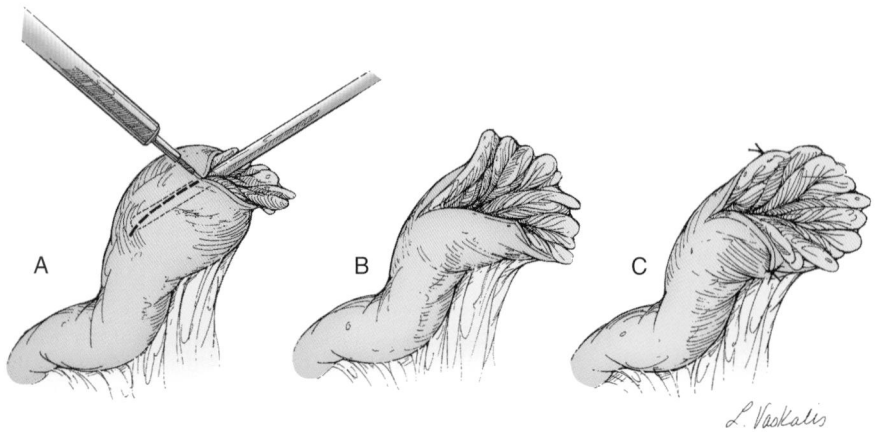

FIGURE 21.18 Fimbrioplasty: correction of prefimbrial phimosis. **A and B:** An incision is placed at the antimesosalpingeal border of the tube. **C:** Completed procedure with flaps everted. (From Gomel V, Taylor PJ. *Diagnostic and operative gynecologic laparoscopy.* St Louis, MO: Mosby, 1995:173, with permission.)

L. Vaskalis

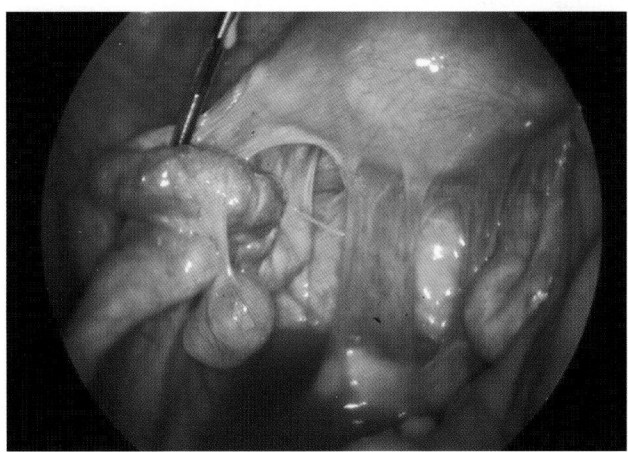

FIGURE 21.19 Bilateral hydrosalpinx with periadnexal and pelvic adhesions.

Salpingostomy (Salpingoneostomy)

Salpingostomy, or salpingoneostomy, is the creation of a new stoma in a tube with a completely occluded distal end (hydrosalpinx). Salpingostomy can be terminal, ampullary, or isthmic, depending on the anatomic location at which the new stoma is fashioned.

Isthmic and ampullary salpingostomy are of historic interest, except for the reversal of prior fimbriectomy (Kroener sterilization), in which ampullary salpingostomy may have a place. We demonstrated that success with ampullary salpingostomy in such cases is dependent on ampullary length and

suggested that reconstructive surgery should only be undertaken when more than one half of the ampulla is present. In 1980, we reported a small series of 14 patients submitted to ampullary salpingostomy for reversal of sterilization. They all met the requirement of having more than one half of the ampullary segment preserved, at least on one side. Six of these women had one or more intrauterine pregnancies (42.9%); of whom five had live births (35.7%); the other had a midtrimester abortion. There were no ectopic pregnancies. Subsequently, experiments by Halbert et al. performed on rabbits corroborated the necessity of having one half or more of the ampulla preserved. This recommendation is corroborated by a 2001 study, by Tourgeman et al. reporting on 41 women who had fimbriectomy reversal.

Distal tubal occlusion is usually associated with varying degrees of pelvic and periadnexal adhesions that must first be lysed. Thereafter, the distal end of the tube is examined to ensure that it is not adherent to the ovary or other structures. If the distal tube is adherent, it must be dissected free until the tubo-ovarian ligament is exposed. Only by freeing the tube can the surgeon ensure that the neostomy is being performed at the appropriate site.

Once the salpingo-ovariolysis is completed and the tube is totally freed, it is distended by transcervical chromopertubation. The occluded terminal end of the tube is examined under magnification, which permits recognition of the relatively avascular zones that radiate from a central punctum. The tube is entered at this central point with use of the microelectrode or microsurgical scissors, and the incision is extended toward the ovary over an avascular line (**Figs. 21.20A, B,** and **21.21A**). This incision fashions a new fimbria ovarica that maintains the tuboovarian relation. At this point in the procedure, it becomes

IV

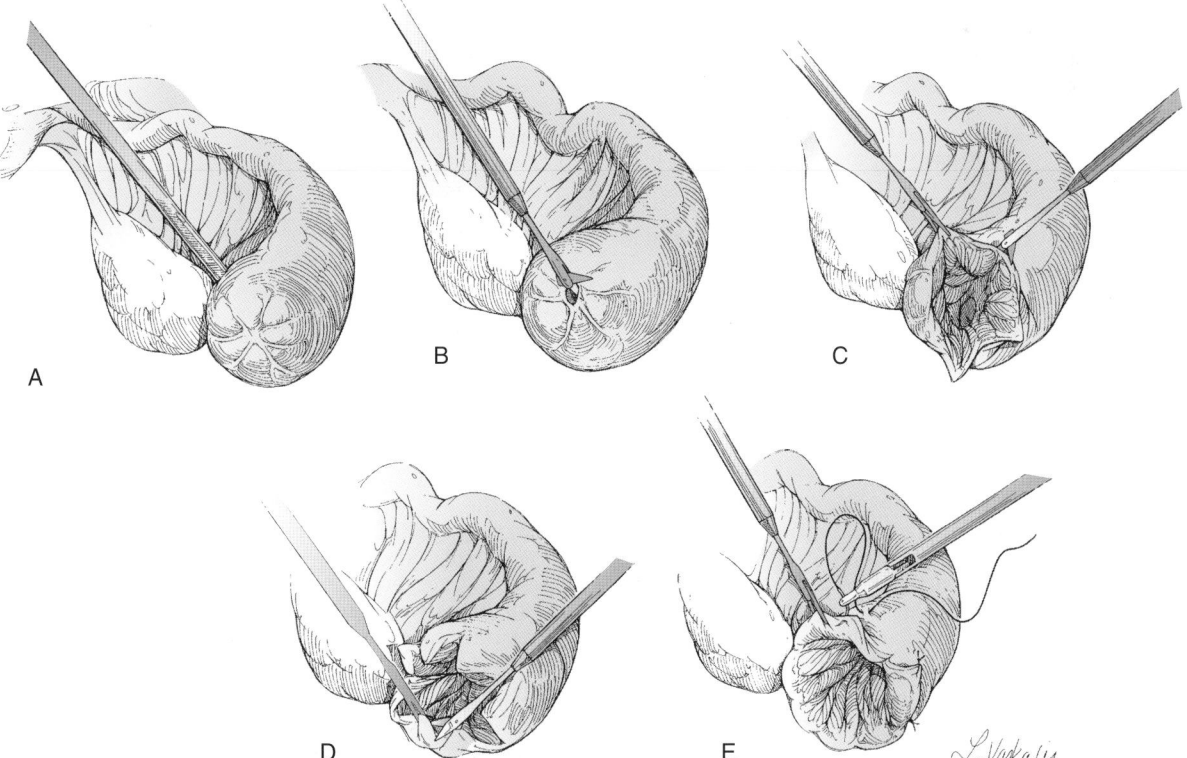

FIGURE 21.20 Salpingostomy. **A:** The occluded distal end of the tube usually has a centrally placed avascular area, from which avascular scarred lines extend in a cartwheel manner. **B:** The first incision is made along an avascular line toward the ovary. **C:** Avascular lines are incised by viewing from within the tube along the circumference of the initial opening. **D:** Cutting along the avascular lines is continued until a satisfactory stoma is fashioned. **E:** The flaps can be everted by placing two or three no. 6-0 absorbable synthetic sutures. (From Gomel V, Taylor PJ. *Diagnostic and operative gynecologic laparoscopy.* St Louis, MO: Mosby, 1995:174, with permission.)

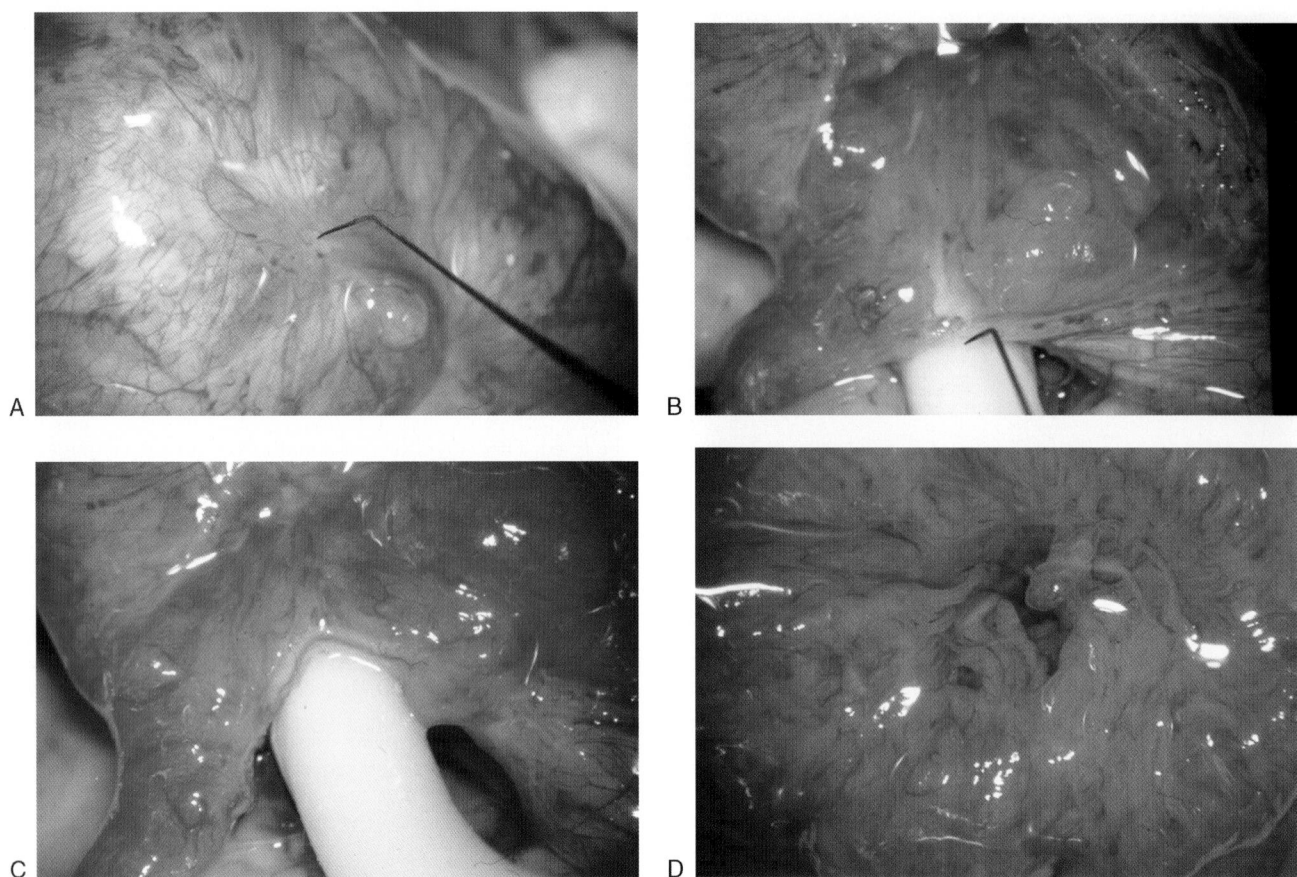

FIGURE 21.21 Microsurgical salpingostomy by open access. **A:** The terminal end of the tube is entered at an avascular central point, and the incision is extended toward the ovary. **B and C:** The tube is then viewed from within, and small incisions are placed along the circumference of the tube. **D:** Completed salpingostomy; the infundibular portion of the tube has well-preserved epithelium and folds.

possible to view the tube from within when placing additional incisions along its circumference to complete the creation of a new stoma. These additional incisions are made between endothelial folds over avascular areas. In so doing, one avoids cutting through vascular mucosal folds, which will be shaped as fimbriae, and bleeding is minimized as a result (Figs. 21.20C, D and 21.21B, C). Any bleeding points that occur are exposed under a jet of irrigation fluid and desiccated individually with a microelectrode or microbipolar forceps. Once a satisfactory stoma is achieved, the flaps created in the process are everted either by securing them without tension to the ampullary seromuscularis with interrupted no. 7-0 or 8-0 Vicryl sutures (Fig. 21.20E)—this is the approach we prefer—or by desiccating their serosal surface, which causes them to fold backward. Desiccation is achieved either electrosurgically with a small ball-shaped electrode and a low power density or with CO_2 laser using a defocused beam. The procedure is concluded with a thorough pelvic lavage, as described earlier in this chapter (Fig. 21.21D).

Considering the results of salpingostomy obtained by laparoscopy approach and those obtained by open access, and considering further the significant improvement in IVF results, an open salpingostomy should rarely be indicated.

If during the initial diagnostic laparoscopy, the surgeon decides to perform the salpingostomy, or for that matter any other reconstructive tubal procedure, by open access, and if pelvic and/or periadnexal adhesions exist, these adhesions can be lysed laparoscopically at their distal margins, thus mobilizing the adnexa. Such an undertaking permits the subsequent

salpingostomy or other procedure to be readily performed through a minilaparotomy incision.

Results of Salpingostomy

In the major published series, the live birth rate after microsurgical salpingostomy ranges from 20% to 37%, and the ectopic pregnancy rate ranges from 5% to 18% (Table 21.4). Work performed in the past 40 years has made it evident that the major determinants of the outcome of salpingostomy are the degree of preexisting tubal damage, the extent and nature of periadnexal adhesions (Figs. 21.21 and 21.22), and the surgical technique (Fig. 21.23). The following factors were quantified in a numerical scoring system to predict the prognosis of the surgical outcome: ampullary diameter, tubal wall thickness, nature of the tubal endothelium, extent of adhesions, and type of adhesions. This scoring system was approved by the American Fertility Society (current ASRM) and published in 1988. In cases deemed favorable (mild), the reported live birth rates after microsurgical salpingostomy range from 40% to 60%. This rate drops to less than 20% in cases considered unfavorable (severe).

In 1990, we reported a series of 90 patients who underwent microsurgical salpingostomy with a minilaparotomy incision. Nineteen (21.1%) were lost to follow-up and were considered failures. Twenty-seven (30%) patients achieved one or more intrauterine pregnancies, and eight (8.9%) had tubal pregnancies. Ectopic gestations occurred in two additional patients

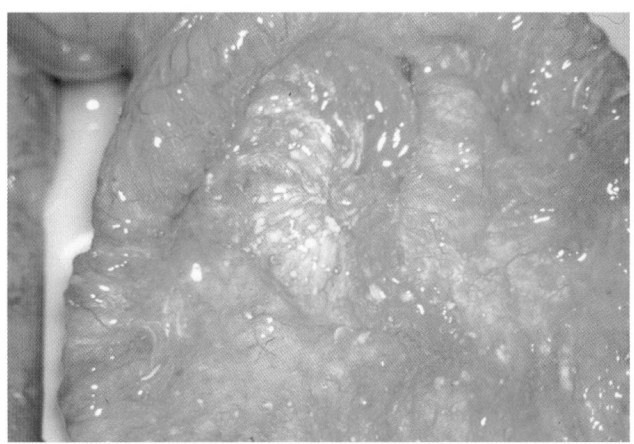

FIGURE 21.22 Microsurgical salpingostomy by open access. The tube is markedly dilated and exhibits a flat epithelium with poorly preserved folds.

who also had intrauterine pregnancies. Twenty-three (25.6%) women were successful in having one or more live births. These 90 patients were assessed with the classification approved by the American Fertility Society. On the basis of this classification, 73 patients had extensive (severe) damage, and 17 had limited (mild) damage. In the group of 73 patients, 15 (20.5%) had one or more intrauterine pregnancies, and 13 (17.8%) had one or more live births. In the "mild" group of 17 patients, 12 (70.6%) had one or more intrauterine pregnancies, and 10 (58.8%) had one or more live births ($P < 0.05$) (Table 21.5). These observations emphasize the importance of a thorough preoperative investigation and proper patient selection.

On the surface, the results yielded by laparoscopic salpingostomy appear to be somewhat inferior to those obtained by open access. However, laparoscopic salpingostomy offers distinct advantages: it can be performed during the initial diagnostic laparoscopy, avoiding a second intervention and resulting in cost savings.

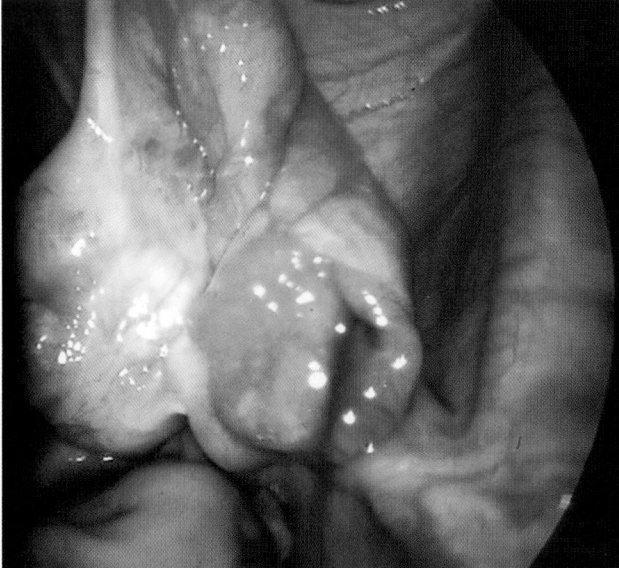

FIGURE 21.23 Second-look laparoscopy following salpingostomy demonstrating a patent tube and a paucity of adhesions (the same patient as Fig. 21.10).

The ASRM's committee opinion, in regard to fimbrioplasty and salpingotomy, is as follows: "Although IVF is preferred over salpingostomy for mild hydrosalpinges in older women and for those with male factor or other infertility factors, salpingostomy before IVF may improve the subsequent likelihood of success of IVF while still giving the patient the option to attempt spontaneous conception.... The evidence is fair to recommend laparoscopic fimbrioplasty and neo-salpingostomy for the treatment of mild hydrosalpinges in young women with no other significant infertility factors."

Hydrosalpinx and IVF

Since the work of Strandell et al. in 1994, 1999, and 2001, many more reports confirmed the deleterious effect of hydrosalpinx on the outcome of IVF treatment and corroboration on the benefit of salpingectomy before IVF, which significantly increases the rate of success. A Cochrane meta-analysis by Johnson et al. in 2004 confirms the earlier work of Strandell et al. in demonstrating that the odds of ongoing pregnancy and live birth (OR 2.13, 95% CI 1.24 to 3.65) were increased after laparoscopic salpingectomy for unilateral or bilateral hydrosalpinges, visible by ultrasonography, before IVF.

Surprisingly, there have been few reports on the effect of a salpingostomy, as opposed to a salpingectomy, on pregnancy outcomes with subsequent IVF.

Several hypotheses have been put forward to explain the detrimental effect of a hydrosalpinx on fertility and specifically IVF outcome. A "washout effect" owing to the passage of the collected tubal fluid to the uterine cavity at the time when embryos are transferred is one such—and more likely—hypothesis. This washout may also occur sometime after transfer. As evidence indicates, many embryos ascend to the tube after transfer and eventually return to the uterus when the tube assumes a prouterine transport. It is at this time that the fluid contained in the hydrosalpinx, by passing to the uterus, may wash the embryos out. Other hypotheses related to the hydrosalpinx fluid include an embryotoxic effect, bioactive factors in the fluid adversely affecting endometrial receptivity, and an inadequate glucose supply in this fluid. These latter hypotheses have not been confirmed scientifically; the washout effect remains the most likely mechanism.

The assumption that the deleterious effect of large hydrosalpinges may be owing to a washout of the transferred embryos is supported by a study of Van Voorhis et al. in 1998. They compared women with hydrosalpinges ($n = 34$) with women who had tubal disease but no hydrosalpinges ($n = 124$) undergoing IVF treatment. Women with hydrosalpinges were found to have a reduced clinical pregnancy rate (18% vs. 37%, $P = 0.053$), a reduced ongoing pregnancy rate (15% vs. 34%, $P = 0.051$), and a reduced implantation rate (7% vs. 18%, $P = 0.003$) after IVF procedures. Among women who had hydrosalpinges, 16 had their hydrosalpinges aspirated at the time of oocyte retrieval and 18 did not. Aspiration of hydrosalpinges was associated with a higher clinical pregnancy rate (31% vs. 5%, $P = 0.07$), a higher ongoing pregnancy rate (31% vs. 0%, $P = 0.015$), and a higher implantation rate (14 vs. 1%, $P = 0.015$) as reported by Van Voorhis et al. However, others have indicated that aspiration of hydrosalpinx fluid is of little value before oocyte retrieval or embryo transfer.

In a study performed in our department reported by McComb and Taylor, in 2001, 23 infertile women, with a duration of infertility of 19 to 146 months (mean 53.6 months) and who had a unilateral hydrosalpinx and a patent contralateral patent tube, were submitted to a laparoscopic salpingostomy of their terminally occluded fallopian tube. The subsequent intrauterine and ectopic pregnancy rates were

IV

TABLE 21.5 Results of Microsurgical Salpingostomy

INVESTIGATORS	YEAR	PATIENTS	INTRAUTERINE PREGNANCIES	LIVE BIRTHS	ECTOPIC PREGNANCIES
ACCESS BY LAPAROTOMY					
Swolin[a]	1975	33	9	8 (24.2%)	6
Gomel[b]	1978	41	12	11 (26.8%)	5
Gomel[b]	1980	72	22	21 (29.2%)	7
Larsson[c]	1982	54	21	17 (31.5%)	0
Verhoeven et al.[d]	1983	143	34	28 (19.6%)	3
Tulandi and Vilos[e]	1985	67	15	NS	3
Boer-Meisel et al.	1986	108	31	24 (22.2%)	19
Donnez and Casanas-Roux[a]	1986	83	26	NS	6
Kosasa and Hale	1988	93	37	34 (36.6%)	13
Schlaff et al.	1990	82	14	NS	6
Winston and Margara	1991	323	106	74 (22.9%)	32
Schippert et al.[f]	2010	153	53	32 (22.2)	12
ACCESS BY MINILAPAROTOMY					
Gomel	1990	90	27	23 (25.6%)	8
ACCESS BY LAPAROSCOPY					
Gomel[g]	1977	9	4	4	0
Daniell and Herbert[h]	1984	22	4	3 (13.6%)	1
Dubuisson et al.	1990	34	10	NS	1
Canis et al.	1991	55	13	NS	6
McComb and Paleologou	1991	22	5	5 (22.7%)	1
Dubuisson et al.	1994	90	29	26 (29.9%)	4
Oh	1996	82	29	NS	8
Millingos et al.	2000	61	14	NS	2
Taylor et al.	2001	139	44	25 (18%)	23

[a]Follow-up period more than 8 years.
[b]Follow-up period more than 1 year.
[c]Follow-up period more than 4 years.
[d]Twenty-three of these were iterative procedures; only three of these patients (13%) had live births.
[e]Thirty-seven of these procedures were performed with the carbon dioxide laser.
[f]The total number of salpingostomies was not given; 153 is the number of patients who responded to the questionnaire.
[g]Eight of the nine patients had prior salpingostomy by conventional techniques that resulted in reocclusion.
[h]Performed with the carbon dioxide laser.
NS, not stated.

43.5% and 4%, respectively. The average time to conception was 13.4 months (range 0 to 71 months). If a single patient whose surgery–pregnancy time interval was 71 months is excluded, the average surgery–pregnancy time interval of the others becomes 7 months. Both the high intrauterine pregnancy and low ectopic pregnancy rates and the short surgery–pregnancy time frame strongly suggest these conceptions occurred through the previously patent (lesser damaged) oviduct. It also suggests that salpingostomy alleviated the deleterious effect of the unilateral hydrosalpinx on embryo implantation.

The beneficial effect of salpingostomy in IVF was demonstrated in 1998 by Murray and colleagues in a small number of cases. Obviously salpingostomy, in addition, offers the woman the potential of achieving a pregnancy naturally. This and other evidence suggest that there may well be a place for laparoscopic salpingostomy, instead of salpingectomy, in selected cases.

We in Vancouver have preferred to perform a salpingostomy instead of a salpingectomy preceding IVF treatment in the absence of factors contraindicating this approach. The ASRM's committee opinion, in this regard, is as follows: "Although IVF is preferred over salpingostomy for mild hydrosalpinges in older women and for those with male factor or other infertility factors salpingostomy before IVF may improve the subsequent likelihood of success of IVF while still giving the patient the option to attempt spontaneous conception.... Patients with poor-prognosis hydrosalpinges are better served by salpingectomy followed by IVF." And further on the text: "Intuitively, it makes sense that laparoscopic neo-salpingostomy before IVF should improve the pregnancy rate, but there are still no confirmatory studies."

Tubotubal Anastomosis

The term *tubotubal anastomosis* refers to an anastomosis performed anywhere along the tube either to treat occlusions resulting from disease processes or to reverse a prior sterilization. The procedure used to repair proximal or cornual tubal disease is usually referred to as *tubocornual anastomosis*.

Microsurgery finds its ultimate application in tubotubal anastomosis. The precision afforded by this technique allows total excision of occluded or diseased portions, proper alignment, and excellent apposition of each layer of the proximal and distal tubal segments.

Depending on the tubal segments that are approximated, tubotubal anastomosis can be intramural–isthmic, intramural–ampullary, isthmic–isthmic, isthmic–ampullary, ampullary–ampullary, or ampullary–infundibular. This section first describes the fundamentals of tubotubal anastomosis and then the technical variations necessary to deal with each specific type of anastomosis.

Basic Principles of Tubotubal Anastomosis

When periadnexal adhesions are present, salpingo-ovariolysis is first completed. When access is achieved through minilaparotomy, the side to be worked on is elevated with the use of pads soaked in the irrigation solution. The contralateral adnexa are left in their natural position to prevent desiccation. When access occurs by way of laparoscopy, the mesosalpinx under the site of anastomosis may be injected with 1 to 2 mL of dilute vasopressin solution to reduce oozing and facilitate hemostasis.

The principles of tubotubal anastomosis are the same, irrespective of the mode of access used. The proximal tubal segment is distended by transcervical chromopertubation. This helps in the identification of the site of occlusion. The tube is transected, with appropriate scissors, adjacent to the site of the occlusion or, in the case of a previous tubal sterilization, near the occluded end. The occluded end or the occluded segment of the tube is grasped with a strong-toothed forceps to expose the site and facilitate the transection (Fig. 21.24A, B), which

is effected with straight scissors or a sharp microblade. It is essential to halt the incision at the mesosalpinx, in the immediate periphery of the tubal muscularis, to avoid damaging the adjacent vascular arcade. Dye solution can now escape from the transected tubal lumen (Fig. 21.24C).

The occluded tubal segment is excised from the mesosalpinx electrosurgically or with scissors, the line of incision kept close to the tube to avoid damaging the vessels mentioned earlier (Fig. 21.24D, E). The cut surface is examined under high magnification to ensure that the tube is normal. Healthy tube is devoid of scarring and exhibits normal muscular and vascular architecture together with intact mucosal folds (Fig. 21.24F). Hemostasis is obtained by precise electrodesiccation of the more significant bleeders, which are located between the serosa and muscularis. Each is exposed by irrigation and desiccated with an insulated microelectrode. If open access is used, gentle compression of the tube between thumb and forefinger facilitates this process. Desiccation of minor bleeders is unnecessary because they stop spontaneously. Desiccation of the tubal epithelium must be avoided to prevent damaging it and adversely affecting future tubal function. Major tubal vessels (such as those composing the vascular arcade) may be divided inadvertently or by necessity. These can be electrodesiccated with monopolar or bipolar current. Overzealous electrodesiccation must be avoided to prevent devitalizing the anastomosis site.

When there is no significant luminal disparity between the two segments, the distal portion is prepared in a similar manner. Before transection, the distal segment is distended by

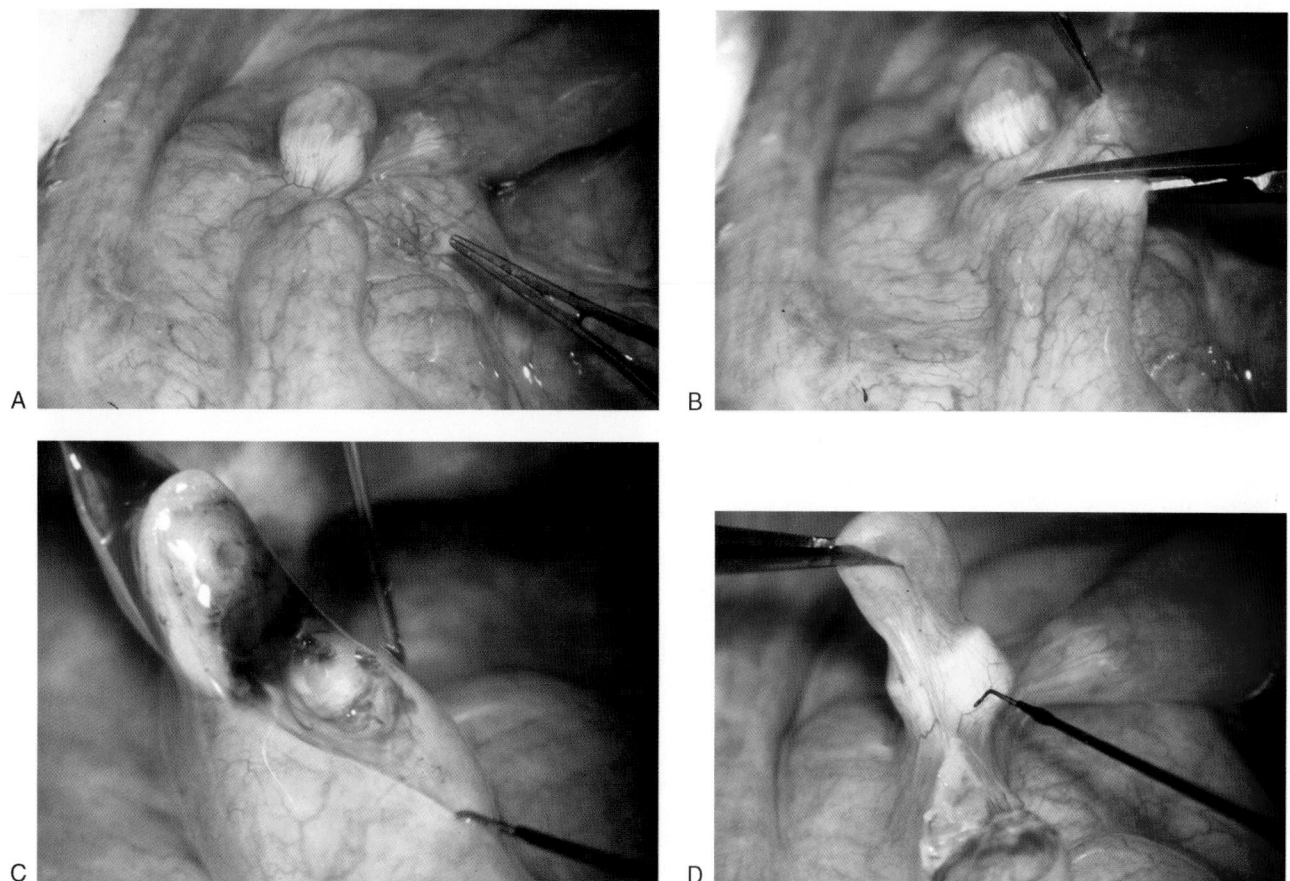

FIGURE 21.24 Microsurgical tubotubal anastomosis for reversal of Fallope-ring sterilization. **A:** Prior tubal sterilization with Fallope ring. **B:** The occluded end of the isthmus is grasped, and the tube is transected with scissors. **C:** Dye solution escapes from the lumen. **D:** The occluded tubal segment is excised from the mesosalpinx electrosurgically by the use of a microelectrode.

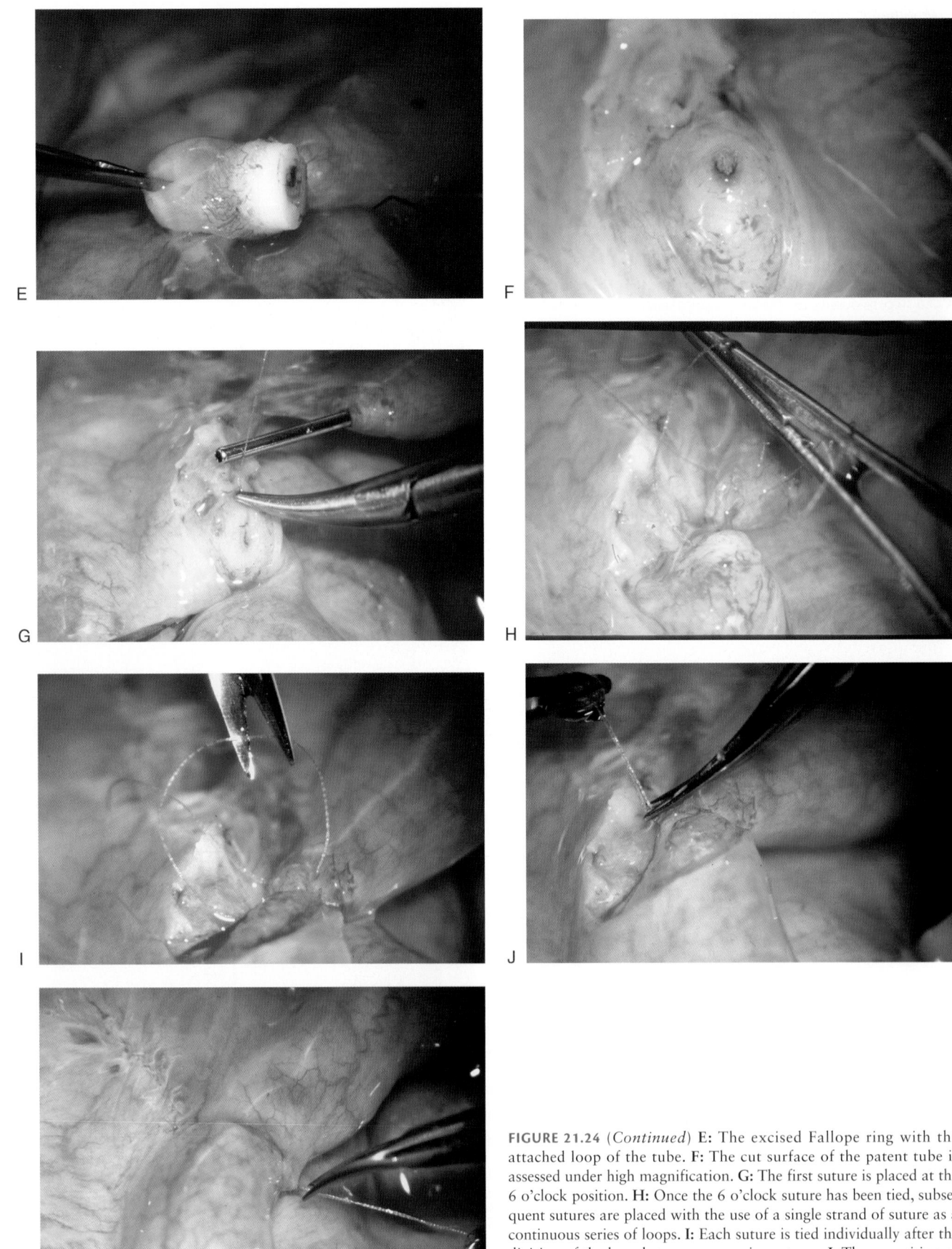

FIGURE 21.24 (*Continued*) **E:** The excised Fallope ring with the attached loop of the tube. **F:** The cut surface of the patent tube is assessed under high magnification. **G:** The first suture is placed at the 6 o'clock position. **H:** Once the 6 o'clock suture has been tied, subsequent sutures are placed with the use of a single strand of suture as a continuous series of loops. **I:** Each suture is tied individually after the division of the loop between successive sutures. **J:** The apposition of the inner musculoepithelial layer is complete. **K:** The anastomosis is completed with approximation of the serosa.

descending hydropertubation, which consists of injecting a few milliliters of irrigation fluid or dilute dye solution through the fimbriated end to identify the distal limit of the occluded portion or, in the case of a prior sterilization, to identify the real extremity of the stump. The tubal segments are approximated in two layers. The first of these joins the epithelium and muscularis, and the second joins the serosa. We generally use no. 8-0 Vicryl sutures swaged on a 130-micron shaft, 4- or 5-mm-long, taper-cut needle for tubal anastomosis. The first suture of the inner musculoepithelial layer is always placed at the mesosalpingeal border (6 o'clock position) to ensure proper alignment of the two segments of the tube (Fig. 21.24G). All of the sutures are placed in a way that positions the knots peripherally.

In exceptional circumstances when the distance between the two segments is great, the mesosalpinx adjacent to the cut ends of the two tubal segments can be approximated first, using a single interrupted no. 7-0 or 8-0 suture. This step brings the tubal segments into close proximity; thus, it facilitates placement of the sutures of the inner layer and reduces the tension that would have existed when tying these sutures.

Once the 6 o'clock suture is tied, the placement of three or more additional sutures (depending on the type of anastomosis) is required to appose the inner layer. These additional sutures can be placed by using a single strand of suture as a continuous series of loops, including the muscularis and the epithelium of the two segments (Figs. 21.24H and 21.25). The sutures are tied individually, after the division of the loop between each successive suture (Fig. 21.24I). This approach facilitates and speeds up suture placement. We advise against the use of a splint in the lumen of the tube because this does not facilitate the procedure and may traumatize the endothelium. Instead, if necessary, the cut surface may be stained with methylene blue or indigo carmine solution to accentuate the visibility of the individual layers.

After approximation of the inner layer (Fig. 21.24J), chromopertubation should demonstrate tubal patency and a watertight anastomotic site. The serosa is joined either with interrupted sutures or with two continuous sutures, one that runs anteriorly and the other posteriorly, starting at the anti-mesosalpingeal border (12 o'clock). Finally, the defect in the mesosalpinx is repaired (Fig. 21.24K).

Tubotubal Anastomosis to Repair Midtubal Disease

The most common reason to perform a tubotubal anastomosis is reversal of sterilization. Midtubal occlusions resulting from disease processes are rare. Such lesions usually affect the intramural or proximal isthmic segments and require a tubocornual-type anastomosis.

The causes of midtubal occlusion include endometriosis and tubal pregnancy, usually undiagnosed or treated by observation and rarely medically. A tubal pregnancy treated medically with methotrexate administration or surgically by linear salpingotomy may result in tubal occlusion at the gestational site (Fig. 21.26A–C). As described by Urma et al., treatment of tubal pregnancy by segmental excision will leave the tube in two segments, as with a tubal sterilization. Rare causes of occlusion include congenital absence of a midtubal segment and tuberculosis. In the latter instance, reconstruction is contraindicated.

In an intact tube, the site of occlusion may be apparent on inspection; palpation of the tube may identify an indurated segment that is the likely site of occlusion. As mentioned earlier, transcervical chromopertubation distends the proximal segment up to the site of occlusion and helps the surgeon define its proximal limit. The tube is transected either immediately proximal to the occluded segment or in the occluded zone itself. Successive transection of the tube at 1- to 2-mm intervals helps identify the normal segments proximal and distal to the occlusion site.

Irrespective of the type of anastomosis, the basic steps of the procedure are the same. The luminal diameter of the tube is not uniform and is significantly greater in the ampullary segment. The technical variations required largely depend on the disparity of the luminal calibers of the two segments to be joined.

Intramural–Isthmic Anastomosis

Anastomosis between the intramural and isthmic segments is the type of anastomosis most often required to treat cornual disease. In most cases of reversal of sterilization, a short segment of isthmus is usually present. This short segment is frequently adherent to the side of the uterus as a result of retraction of the adjacent mesosalpinx, thus giving the appearance of total absence of the proximal tube. The presence of

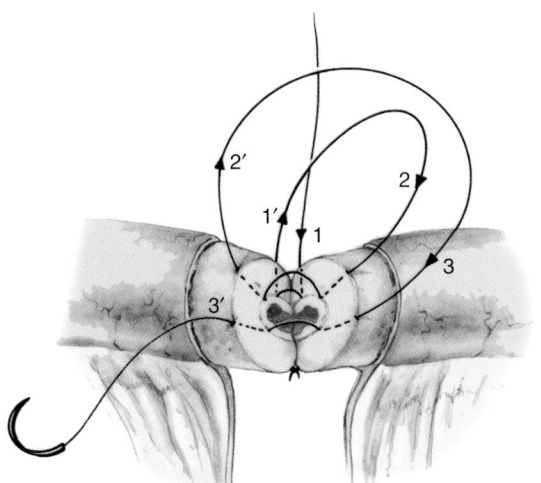
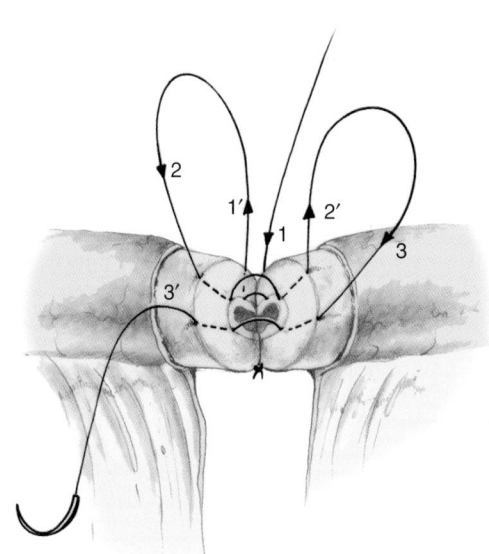

FIGURE 21.25 Microsurgical tubotubal anastomosis: after the 6 o'clock suture has been tied, placement of subsequent sutures using a single strand of suture as a continuous series of loops.

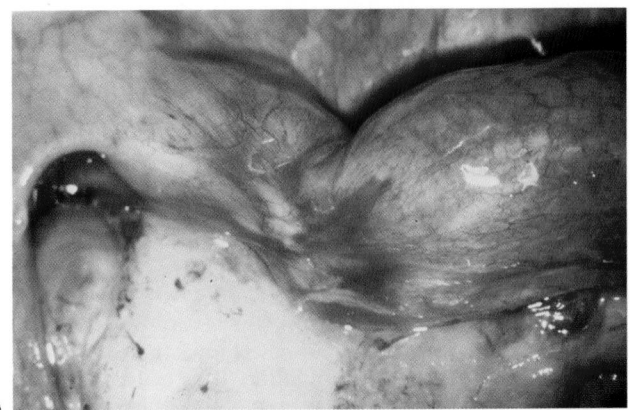

A

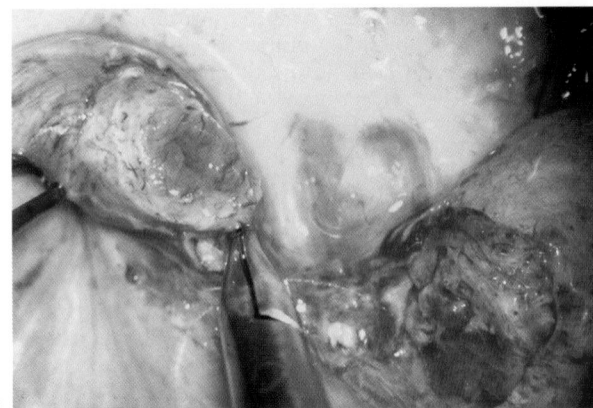

B

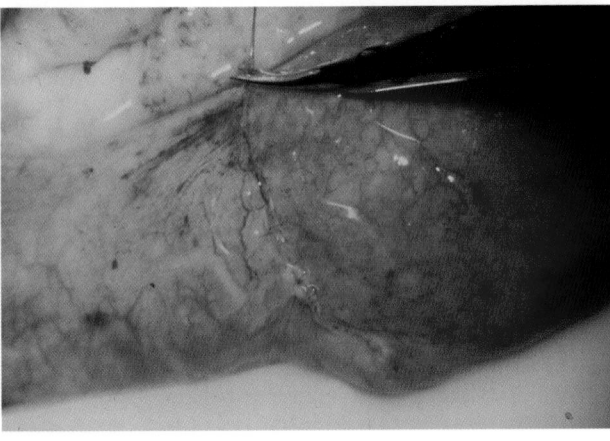

C

FIGURE 21.26 **A:** Midtubal occlusion due to prior ectopic pregnancy. **B:** The occluded portion of the tube has been excised and **(C)** two layer anastomosis performed between the two normal-appearing tubal segments.

a portion of isthmus would have been evident from HSG. Transcervical chromopertubation distends this small segment of isthmus, facilitating identification of its distal margin and its dissection from the uterus. The dissection must be effected carefully to avoid damaging the tube itself and the vessels supplying it. The conservation and appropriate preparation of this segment, even when very small, converts the anastomosis to an isthmic–isthmic type and facilitates the procedure.

In the absence of any isthmus (as may be the case subsequent to either a tubal sterilization or excision of an isthmic pregnancy), maintenance of uterine distention by chromopertubation will indicate the site where the intramural segment should be sought, between the uterine insertion points of the round and ovarian ligaments. Excision of the serosa and underlying scar tissue over the distended area may permit the dye solution to stream out of the intramural segment. In some instances, to access normal tube, it is also necessary to dissect the muscularis of this segment from the surrounding uterine muscle for 1 or 2 mm with microscissors or a microelectrode. After this, the tube is transected with microscissors. This process may have to be repeated until the patent and normal tube is reached, at which point dye solution should stream out of the lumen.

Because of extensive vascularity, dissection in the cornu usually causes significant oozing that hinders visibility. When more than superficial dissection of this region is anticipated, initial infiltration with dilute vasopressin solution (1 U of vasopressin in 30 mL of normal saline) significantly decreases capillary oozing and facilitates the procedure. With the use of a 30-gauge needle on a 3-mL syringe, the cornual region of the uterus is injected with 2 mL of this solution in a circular fashion under the serosa 1 cm medial to the uterotubal junction. The resulting vasoconstriction is recognized by serosal blanching.

In this type of anastomosis, there is no significant luminal disparity between the two segments of the tube. Hence, the isthmus is simply transected near the occluded end and prepared, as described earlier. A two-layer anastomosis is then performed. Once the inner layer has been joined, the serosa and superficial muscle of the cornual region are approximated to the serosa of the isthmus. The defect under the tube is repaired by suturing the mesosalpinx to the serosa of the lateral edge of the uterus.

Intramural–Ampullary Anastomosis

The salient feature of intramural–ampullary anastomosis is the considerable luminal disparity that exists between the intramural and ampullary segments. The key technical issue lies in the preparation of the occluded proximal end of the ampulla, where an opening into the ampullary lumen, which is not much larger than that of the intramural segment, must be fashioned.

The intramural segment is first prepared as described under intramural–isthmic anastomosis. To identify the occluded end of the ampulla, which may be buried between the leaves of the mesosalpinx, the tube is distended with a few milliliters of dye or irrigation solution introduced through the fimbriated end. Alternatively, a malleable blunt probe can be introduced through the infundibulum and gently threaded toward the occluded end. With the use of microscissors, the serosa over the tip of the ampullary stump is incised in a circular manner. The serosa and any scar tissue under it are then excised to expose the muscularis of the occluded end. The center point of the exposed muscularis is grasped with toothed microforceps, and a small incision is made into the ampullary lumen with the microscissors. This opening is enlarged to correspond in size

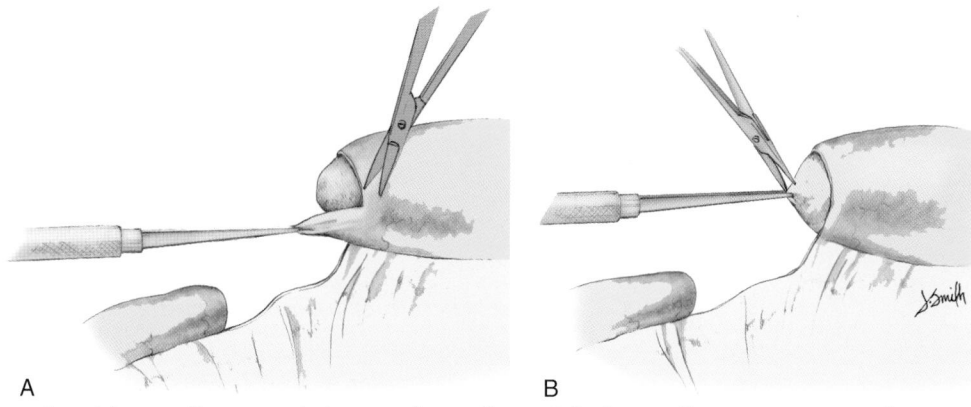

A   B

FIGURE 21.27 Preparation of the ampullary stump in intramural–ampullary or isthmic–ampullary anastomosis. **A:** The serosa over the tip of the ampullary stump is incised in a circular manner and excised. **B:** The center point of the exposed muscularis is grasped, and a small opening is made into the lumen.

to the lumen of the proximal tubal segment by excising a tiny circular portion of muscularis and epithelium (Figs. 21.27A, B and 21.28). The resulting opening is slightly larger than the intramural lumen, and because of absence of significant disparity, anastomosis of the two segments can be performed as described for isthmic–isthmic anastomosis (Fig. 21.29).

Isthmic–Isthmic Anastomosis

Isthmic–isthmic anastomosis is the simplest type of anastomosis to perform. The lumina are comparable in size. The technique is the same as that described earlier under the basic principles of tubotubal anastomosis.

Isthmic–Ampullary Anastomosis

The salient feature of this type of anastomosis is also the considerable luminal disparity that usually exists between the lumina of the isthmic and ampullary segments. The isthmic stump is prepared as described under "basic principles of tubotubal anastomosis." In most instances, the occluded end of the ampullary stump will be free, enabling a lumen of appropriate diameter (comparable in size to that of the isthmic segment) to be fashioned, as described under intramural–ampullary anastomosis (Figs. 21.27A, B and 21.28). A two-layer anastomosis is then performed as described under the basic principles of tubotubal anastomosis (Fig. 21.25). Although the muscularis of the ampulla is considerably thinner than that

of the isthmus, this poses no problem in approximating the epithelium and muscularis of the two segments.

Occasionally, circumstances will not permit the use of the technique described earlier in the preparation of the occluded ampullary end. The ampullary stump may be occluded by a permanent suture or clip, and removal of this suture or clip may lead to the creation of an opening that is much larger than the isthmic lumen and through which lush epithelial folds will prolapse. If the opening into the ampullary lumen is significantly larger than that of the isthmic segment (either inadvertently or by necessity), it will be necessary to either enlarge the isthmic lumen or narrow the ampullary lumen. To enlarge the lumen of the isthmic segment, a 2- to 3-mm slit is made with scissors at its antimesosalpingeal border. Partial excision of the corners thus created results in an enlarged oval opening (Fig. 21.30A). To approximate the inner musculoepithelial layer, the 6 o'clock suture is placed first and tied. Five additional sutures are usually required, and these are placed as described earlier. The 12 o'clock suture must incorporate the muscularis and epithelium of the ampulla and the same tissues at the apex of the isthmic slit (Fig. 21.30B). Approximation of the serosa and closure of the defect in the mesosalpinx complete the anastomosis. An alternative approach is to reduce the size of the large ampullary opening. This is achieved by plicating the muscular layer

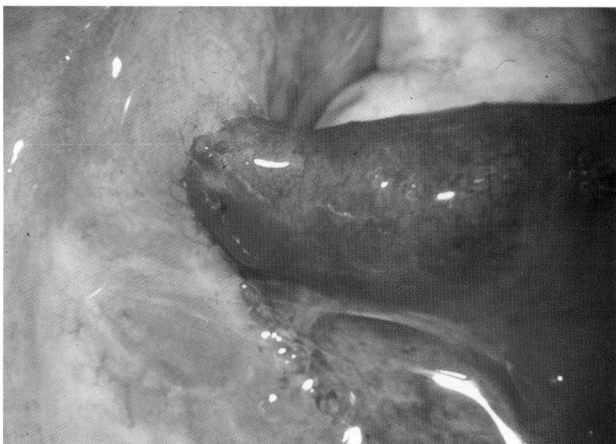

FIGURE 21.29 Tubocornual anastomosis (intramural–ampullary) completed. The anastomosis site is patent, as evident from the distention and blue discoloration of the tube as a result of chromopertubation. There is no leakage from the anastomotic site.

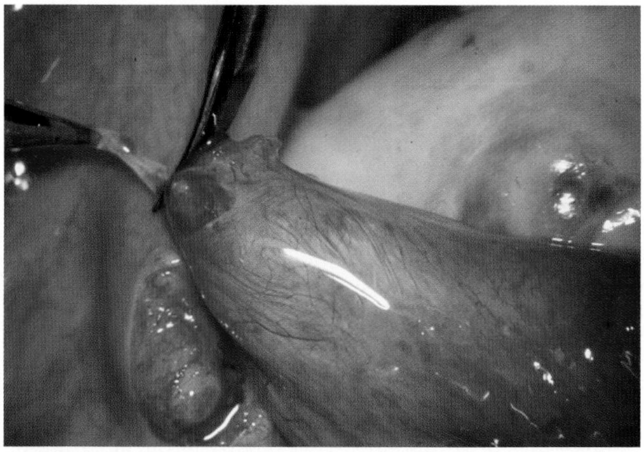

FIGURE 21.28 Preparation of the ampullary stump in intramural–ampullary or isthmic–ampullary anastomosis.

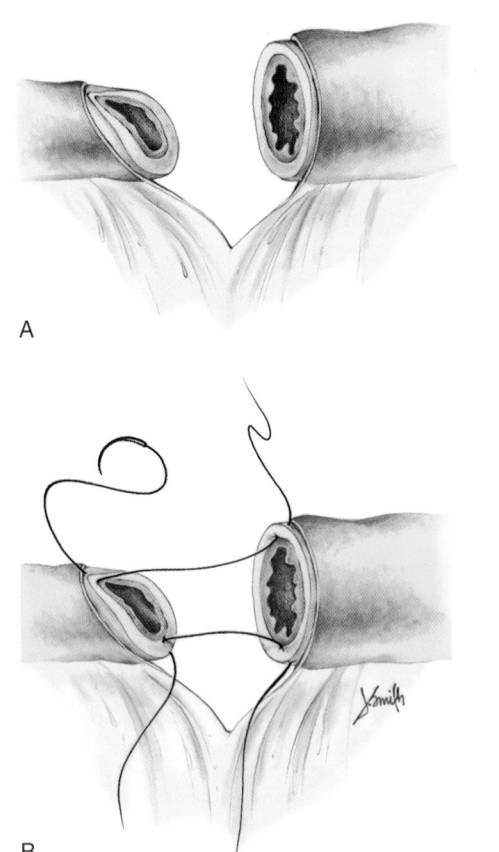

A

B

FIGURE 21.30 Isthmic–ampullary anastomosis in the presence of significant luminal disparity. **A:** Enlargement of the isthmic lumen. **B:** Placement of the 12 o'clock suture.

surrounding the opening with interrupted sutures, after which the prolapsing epithelium is invaginated.

Ampullary–Ampullary Anastomosis

The proximal ampullary segment is transected near the occluded end, which is then excised from the mesosalpinx as previously described. An opening that corresponds in size to the lumen of the proximal segment is made in the occluded end of the distal ampullary segment, as described under isthmic–ampullary anastomosis.

In this type of anastomosis, the major difficulty to be overcome is the propensity of the ampullary epithelium to prolapse through the lumen. Although investigators such as Winston have advocated excision of these epithelial fronds, we advise against this approach because it may lead to development of intratubal adhesion formation at this site. The epithelial fronds can be replaced with pressure from the irrigating solution or with the tip of the plain microforceps while the successive sutures of the inner layer are tied. One must be careful not to include these epithelial fronds within a suture or knot or between the segments that are being approximated. Because of the larger circumference of the ampulla, approximation of the two ampullary segments will require a greater number of interrupted sutures than in an isthmic–isthmic anastomosis.

Ampullary–Infundibular Anastomosis

An ampullary–infundibular anastomosis may be necessary when a distal ampullary portion of the tube has been ablated or excised either during a prior sterilization or during removal of a tubal gestation, leaving distally the infundibular segment only. The occluded ampulla is prepared as described previously. To make anastomosis of the two segments possible, it is necessary to fashion an opening in the infundibular portion. To do so, a Teflon probe with a conical tip is introduced into the infundibulum from the fimbriated end, and a circular opening is fashioned with microscissors, from the medial side, corresponding in size to the lumen of the ampullary segment. A two-layer anastomosis is then performed.

Results of Tubotubal Anastomosis for Reversal of Sterilization

The major published series report live birth rates between 40% and 80% after microsurgical tubotubal anastomosis for reversal of sterilization (Table 21.6). The ectopic gestation rates are usually low.

The factors that affect the outcome of such procedures are multiple and include the following: the type of prior sterilization, the site of anastomosis, and the length of the reconstructed tube or tubes, which are interrelated factors; the presence of single versus double reconstructed oviducts; the status of the tubes (presence or absence of disease); the extent and nature of adhesions and the presence of other pelvic disease; the status of other fertility parameters, especially that of the male partner; and significantly the age of the woman and the surgical technique used. Therefore, the outcome depends on the degree of rigor in selection criteria and the quality of the surgical technique. This is corroborated by the results of two relatively recent reports on sterilization reversal, which include two large series from Korea by Kim and colleagues in 1997 (Table 21.6). In our experience, in the absence of a male factor, the three most important parameters that predict outcome are the age of the female partner, the length of the reconstructed tube, and the surgical technique. A reconstructed tubal length of less than 4 cm adversely affects outcome; this likely reflects the loss of ampullary length and consequent loss of oviductal oocyte retention.

It is possible to perform tubotubal anastomosis by laparoscopic access to reconstruct a previous tubal sterilization. The outcomes reported in the literature are very variable, and most report results inferior to those obtained by open access. This is largely due to modification of the recognized microsurgical technique to make the laparoscopic procedure simpler to perform.

The first report on laparoscopic tubotubal anastomosis was a case report by Sedbon et al. in 1989; instead of microsurgical suturing for the apposition of the tubal segments, they used biologic glue over a stent. Pregnancy outcome was not reported. Early reports on tubotubal anastomosis were small case series, performed with simplified techniques, and despite the majority of the cases in these series were reversal of simpler types of sterilization reversal, the results were relatively poor.

Most surgeons who attempted tubotubal anastomosis by laparoscopic access using the microsurgical technique, described earlier in this text, found that operating times are prolonged. Many attempted to simplify the technique by using glue as described above or using only two sutures for the apposition of the prepared tubal segments, as first reported by Dubuisson and Swolin in 1995. In this technique, the first suture (4-0 Vicryl) approximates the mesosalpinx immediately beneath the two segments of the tube and the second (6-0 Vicryl) the tube at 12 o'clock position. The second suture incorporates the serosa and muscularis of the two segments of the tube. There are several recent reports in the literature on this type of modified technique.

TABLE 21.6 Results of Microsurgical Tubotubal Anastomosis for Reversal of Sterilization

INVESTIGATORS	YEAR	PATIENTS	INTRAUTERINE PREGNANCIES	LIVE BIRTHS	ECTOPIC PREGNANCIES
ACCESS BY LAPAROTOMY					
Gomel	1974	14	8	NS	1
Gomel	1980c	118	76	NS	1
Winston	1980	105	63	NS	3
Gomel[a]	1983b	118	96	93 (78.8%)	2
DeCherney et al.[b]	1983	124	84	72 (58.1%)	8
Schlosser et al.	1983	119	NS	44 (37%)	11
Silber and Cohen[c]	1984	48	33	31 (64.6%)	2
Henderson	1984	95	61	51 (53.7%)	5
Paterson	1985	147	93	87 (59.2%)	5
Spivak et al.[d]	1986	83	48	39 (47%)	6
Boeckx et al.	1986	63	44	NS	3
Rock et al.	1987	80	58	49 (61.3%)	10
Xue and Fa[e]	1989	117	98	95 (81.2%)	2
Putman et al.	1990	86	64	55 (64%)	NS
teVelde et al.	1990	215	156	137 (63.7%)	8
Kim JD et al.[f]	1997	387	329	295 (76.2%)[f]	6
Kim SH et al.[g]	1997	1,118	505	366 (32.7%)[g]	42
Cha et al.	2001	44	31	NS	1
Wiegerinck et al.	2005	41	26	NS	1
Gordts et al.[b]	2009	172	119	98 (60.0%)	10
Schippert et al.	2011	89	65	45 (50.6%)	6
Moon SM et al.[i]	2012	961	732	630 (71.1%)	22
ACCESS BY LAPAROSCOPY					
Dubuisson et al.[j]	1998	32	17	13 (40.6%)	NS
Bisonette et al.[j]	1999	102	64	49 (50.5%)	5
Yoon et al.[k]	1999	202	154	98 (48.5%)[l]	5
Mettler et al.[j,m]	2001	28	15	15 (53.6%)	2
Cha et al.[k]	2001	37	28	NS	1
Ribeiro et al.	2003	26	13	NS	0
Wiegerinck et al.[n]	2005	41	15	NS	1
Schepens et al.[o]	2010	134	74	NS[o]	5
ROBOTIC					
Falcone et al.	2000	10	5	NS	0
Caillet et al.[p]	2010	97	66	58 (59.8%)	NS

[a]Resurvey of 1980 series; follow-up period more than 18 months.

[b]Follow-up period more than 18 months.

[c]Follow-up period more than 4 years.

[d]Follow-up period more than 1 year.

[e]Follow-up period more than 3.5 years.

[f]Follow-up period more than 2 years. There were eight ongoing pregnancies in addition to the live births.

[g]Follow-up period more than 5 years. There were 31 ongoing pregnancies in addition to the live births.

[b]Excluded 89 patients lost to follow-up and 8 patients who did not attempt a pregnancy from their series of 172 women, limiting the evaluation to the remaining 164.

[i]They only reviewed 886 of the 961 patients. The 71.1% birth rate is the result of 630 births from the 886 cases included in the analysis.

[j]Tubal anastomosis performed with single-suture technique.

[k]Tubal anastomosis performed by using two-layer microsurgical technique.

[l]There were 31 ongoing pregnancies in addition to the live births.

[m]A screening laparoscopy was performed, and only those having a distal tubal segment of 4 cm and a proximal segment of 3 cm were included.

[n]Comparative study with cases performed with open access. Laparoscopic anastomosis performed without sutures; the technique is described in the text.

[o]Excluded 7 patients lost to follow-up, analyzing 127 of the 134 cases. The text does not give birth rates; it indicates that 51 of 120 women with bilateral anastomosis and 4 of 7 women with unilateral anastomosis had ongoing pregnancies. Therefore, 55 of the 127 women (43%) had ongoing pregnancies.

[p]They excluded 14 of the 160 cases for various reasons together with 49 lost to follow-up, and analyzed the remaining 97 patients.

NS, not stated.

There are also publications reporting on the laparoscopic use of a truly microsurgical, two-layer anastomosis technique. The largest of these series is from 1999 by Yoon et al. from Korea, which includes 202 cases. Fifteen of these were lost to follow-up, and one had no partner. The remaining 186 were monitored for a minimum of 12 months. One hundred fifty-four achieved intrauterine pregnancies, a rate of 77% if we consider, as most series do, 15 cases lost to follow-up as failures. Ninety-eight delivered healthy infants, 25 pregnancies ended in abortion, and 31 patients had ongoing pregnancies at the time of the survey. If we assume all 31 ongoing pregnancies resulted in a live birth, the live birth rate in this series would have been 64%. There were five cases of ectopic pregnancy. These results are not too dissimilar to those achieved by open access, which supports the premise of the importance of the technique used and not the mode of access. In 2001, Cha et al., also from Korea, further supported this assumption. In their study, they compare the fertility outcome in 81 women who had microsurgical reversal of sterilization, 37 by laparoscopic and 44 by open access. The outcomes include only intrauterine and tubal pregnancy rates, which were similar in both groups: 75.7% and 70.5%, respectively; there was one tubal pregnancy in each group (Table 21.6).

Attempts to develop simple techniques that would yield equivalent results by laparoscopic access continue to be made. A 2005 study by Wiegerinck et al. reports the use of the following laparoscopic technique for tubal anastomosis: *"Once the tubal ends to be anastomosed were prepared, a splint was inserted into the proximal tube through a guiding catheter inserted vaginally."* The splint was then introduced into the distal portion of the tube. The distal portion was aligned with the proximal segment over the splint. The seromuscularis of the two segments was fixed at the 3 and 9 o'clock positions using microclips of 3-mm size. Subsequently, fibrin glue was applied on the anastomotic surface. The splint was taped externally to the Foley catheter and removed 4 hours after the end of the procedure. Although they report similar results for both the laparoscopic group and a control group (selected from patients whose procedure was performed through a Pfannenstiel incision), it is surprising that the cumulative rate of ongoing pregnancy at 3 years in the control group was only 52% and in the laparoscopic group only 45%. This, despite the fact that in the latter group more than 90% of the sterilizations had been performed by clips or Silastic rings, and their average age was only 34.9 years. Schepens et al. from the same group more recently reported on 134 patients; due to the fact that the patient population includes cases from 1997 to 2008, they must have included the 41 reported earlier (Table 21.6).

Several groups have explored robotically assisted tubal anastomosis. Initial reports in 2000 of small series by Falcone and Degueldre, both of whom were proficient in microsurgery, used a technique similar to that described earlier in this text. They reported the use of the robot-facilitated suturing but increased the length of the procedure. A recent large series that included Degueldre reported a birth rate of 60% following robotic-assisted reversal of sterilization. They stressed the fact that the use of the robot was associated with prolonged operating times and increased costs. Tubotubal anastomosis is a relatively simple operation for a physician skilled in microsurgery. It is difficult at this stage to justify the use of a robot for such cases, while it use would better serve more complex surgical procedures.

Using metaanalysis, Watson et al. examined the role of microsurgery versus macrosurgery in the reversal of sterilization. The available studies were limited by the lack of randomized controlled trials and the use of historical control groups. However, as expected, the use of magnification and microsurgical approach for sterilization reversal and for adhesiolysis and salpingostomy led to higher intrauterine pregnancy and lower ectopic rates.

Microsurgical tubotubal anastomosis for reversal of sterilization produces excellent results that are principally dependent on the status and the length of the reconstructed tube. Live birth rates of 60% to 80% can be achieved, provided that the reconstructed tube is longer than 4 cm and the ampullary portion greater than 2 cm. The second most important factor is the woman's age. The tubal pregnancy rates are usually low.

The advantages of laparoscopic access are well recognized. These include a shorter hospital stay and recovery time and lower postoperative analgesic requirements. We tried laparoscopic access for sterilization reversal and decided to continue using an operation microscope through a minilaparotomy incision. Our experience demonstrates that access by a minilaparotomy incision, using the technique described earlier in this text, provides the same advantages. We perform tubal anastomosis for reversal of sterilization, tubocornual anastomosis for pathologic tubal occlusion, and other more complex reconstructive microsurgical procedures via minilaparotomy. Patients are admitted to hospital on the morning of surgery and most are discharged a few hours postoperatively. Each surgeon must balance patient factors, his or her expertise, and the resources of the center in deciding how to approach such procedures.

The ASRM's committee opinion in regard to sterilization reversal supports the position we have held for more than three decades and is as follows: *"There is good evidence to support the recommendation for microsurgical anastomosis for tubal ligation reversal… it can be accomplished by mini-laparotomy as an outpatient procedure."* Comparable results may be obtained by laparoscopy if the procedure is performed *"in an identical fashion to open microsurgical tubal anastomosis.... Operating times are prolonged.... Only surgeons who are very facile with laparoscopic suturing and who have extensive training in conventional tubal microsurgery should attempt this procedure."*

Tubocornual Anastomosis for Proximal Tubal Disease

Various disease processes can affect the proximal tube and occlude the region of the uterotubal junction. On the basis of histologic studies on resected tubal segments, these occlusive lesions in order of frequency are as follows: obliterative fibrosis, chronic inflammation, salpingitis isthmica nodosa, intratubal endometriosis, and, rarely, ectopic gestation and tuberculosis. All of the published series report a varying but usually low percentage of cases with no demonstrable lesions. This may be related to tubal spasm (at the time of HSG or laparoscopy) or to the presence of tubal plugs or synechiae. Such conditions, as opposed to occlusive disease, are amenable to treatment with selective salpingography and tubal cannulation, as was discussed earlier in this chapter.

The management strategy in proximal tubal occlusion must take into account other variables, including the condition of the distal tube, the extent and nature of pelvic adhesions, the presence of associated pelvic disease, and the status of other fertility parameters, especially male factor infertility. This strategy must also respect the following principles: simplicity, reproducibility, and cost-effectiveness.

The selection of treatment must be individualized according to the investigative findings, the wishes of the couple, the expertise of the surgeon, and the results achieved by the center in which the couple will be managed. Figure 21.31 diagrammatically summarizes a process to manage proximal tubal occlusion.

The traditional surgical treatment of occlusive proximal tubal disease was uterotubal implantation. The application of microsurgery has made it possible to perform an anastomosis instead, after removal of the affected tubal segment. Central to this approach is the complete excision of the affected portion of the tube, whether it is intramural or isthmic. In cases

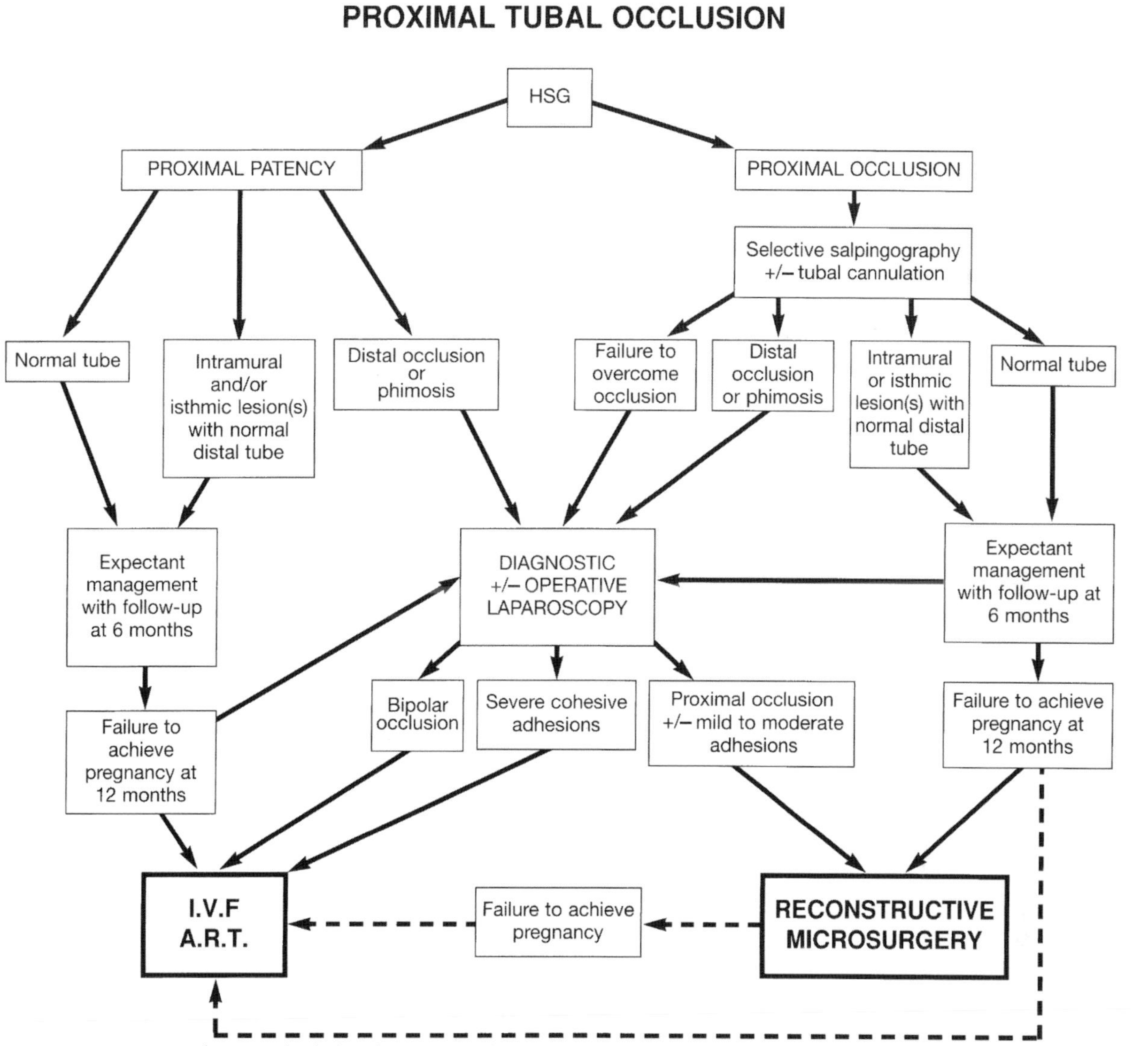

PROXIMAL TUBAL OCCLUSION

```
                                    HSG
                   ┌─────────────────┴─────────────────┐
          PROXIMAL PATENCY                      PROXIMAL OCCLUSION
                                                         │
                                              Selective salpingography
                                                +/- tubal cannulation
```

Boxes under PROXIMAL PATENCY: Normal tube | Intramural and/or isthmic lesion(s) with normal distal tube | Distal occlusion or phimosis

Boxes under Selective salpingography +/- tubal cannulation: Failure to overcome occlusion | Distal occlusion or phimosis | Intramural or isthmic lesion(s) with normal distal tube | Normal tube

Second-level boxes (left): Expectant management with follow-up at 6 months → Failure to achieve pregnancy at 12 months

Center: DIAGNOSTIC +/- OPERATIVE LAPAROSCOPY

Under DIAGNOSTIC: Bipolar occlusion | Severe cohesive adhesions | Proximal occlusion +/- mild to moderate adhesions

Right: Expectant management with follow-up at 6 months → Failure to achieve pregnancy at 12 months

Final boxes: I.V.F A.R.T. ← Failure to achieve pregnancy ← RECONSTRUCTIVE MICROSURGERY

FIGURE 21.31 Management of proximal tubal occlusion. HSG, hysterosalpingogram; IVF, in vitro fertilization; ART, artificial reproductive technology. (Modified from Gomel V, Dubuisson JB. *References en gynecologie et obstetrique.* Poulnoy, France: SPEI, 1995:251.)

of pathologic occlusion, a portion of healthy intramural tube is usually spared, permitting the conservation of sometimes all but more often a part of this segment. In other instances, the whole intramural segment is involved in the disease process and must be excised. In such cases, microsurgery permits an anastomosis to be performed between the uterine tubal ostium and the healthy portion of the isthmus. Depending on the extent of intramural tube that is excised and thus the site at which the anastomosis is performed, tubocornual anastomosis may be juxtamural, intramural, or juxtauterine (**Fig. 21.32**).

The cornual region of the uterus is infiltrated with dilute vasopressin solution. This is done by injecting 2 mL of this solution in a circular fashion under the serosa 1 cm medial to the uterotubal junction with the use of a 30-gauge needle on a 3-mL syringe. The vasoconstriction that follows is recognized by the blanching of the serosa. The tube is then incised at the uterotubal junction, with care taken not to divide the arteriovenous arcade at its mesosalpingeal margin. After transection of the tube, patency of the intramural segment is assessed by transcervical chromopertubation, and the normalcy of the cut surface is evaluated under high magnification (**Fig. 21.33A**).

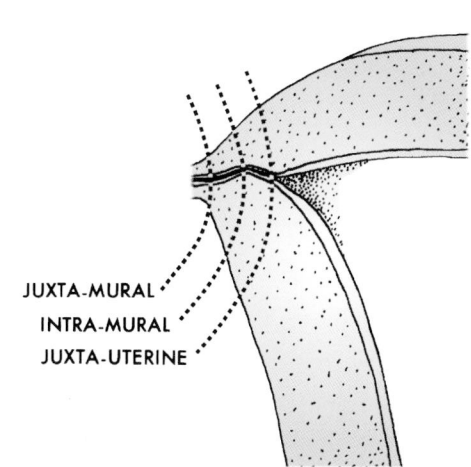

FIGURE 21.32 Types of tubocornual anastomosis.

JUXTA-MURAL
INTRA-MURAL
JUXTA-UTERINE

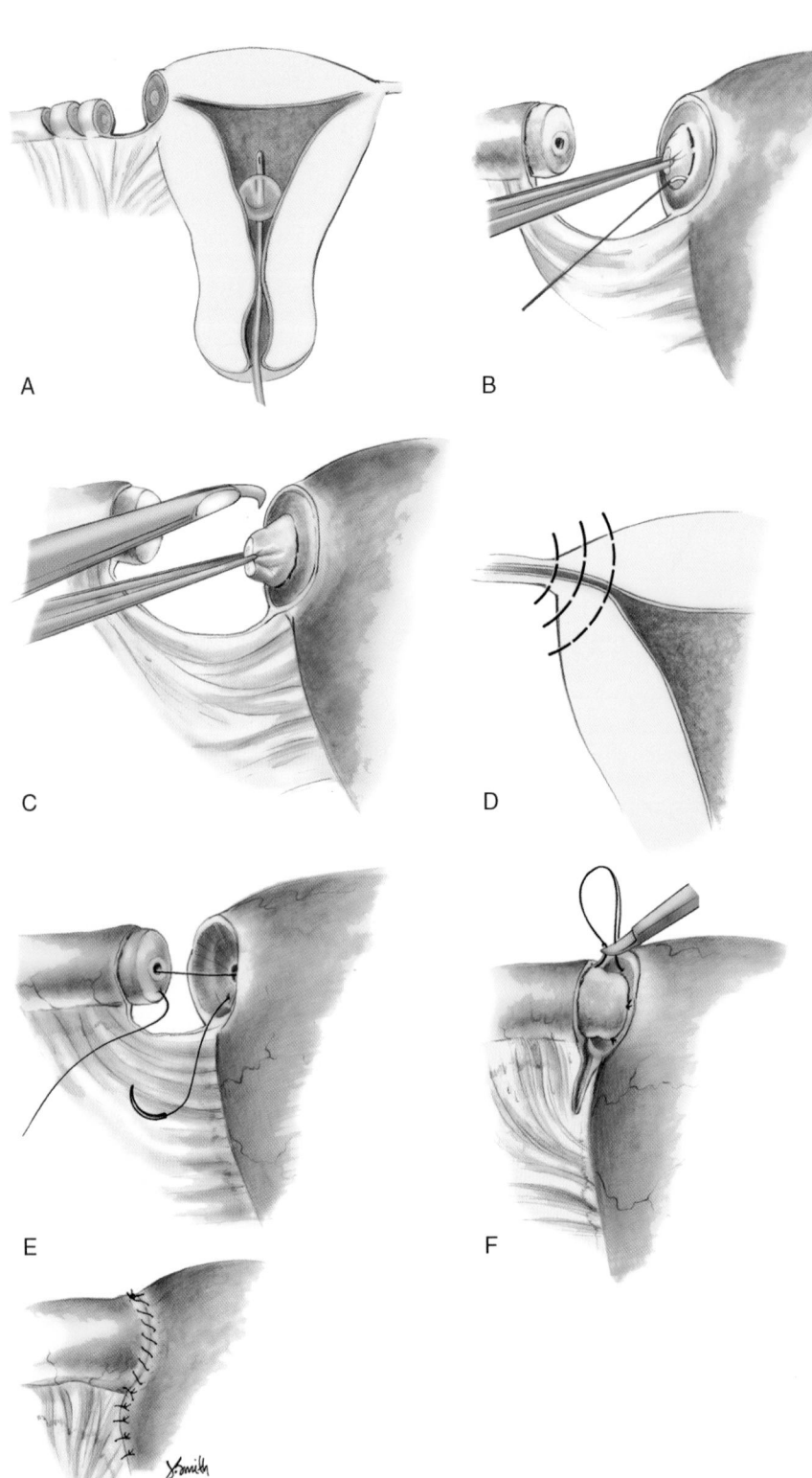

FIGURE 21.33 Microsurgical tubocornual anastomosis for proximal tubal disease. **A:** The tube is transected at the uterotubal junction (UTJ). Commencing at the UTJ, serial cuts are made on the isthmus until patent and normal tube is identified. **B:** The intramural tube is dissected electrosurgically, by using a microelectrode, from the surrounding uterine muscle, 1 to 2 mm at a time, and (**C** and **D**) transected until patent and normal tube is reached. **E:** The first anastomotic suture of the inner musculoepithelial layer is placed at the 6 o'clock position. **F:** Subsequent sutures are placed with a single strand of suture. **G:** After the apposition of the inner layer, the seromuscularis of the uterus is joined to the serosa of the tube and the mesosalpinx is joined to the lateral aspect of the uterus.

If the intramural tube is found to be occluded or abnormal at this site, its musculature is dissected further from the surrounding uterine muscle, 1 to 2 mm at a time, toward the uterine cavity (Fig. 21.33B, D). The small portion of the tube thus dissected is transected, and the cut surface is reassessed. If the intramural tube is still occluded or abnormal, the same procedure is repeated until normal patent tube is reached. Dye solution will spurt from the open lumen. It

is essential that dissection of the intramural tube from the surrounding uterine muscle be effected at the level of the immediate periphery of the tubal muscularis. The preoperative HSG usually provides information about the length of the normal intramural segment and the extent of excision required. Transection of successive portions of the intramural tube can be achieved with either curved microscissors or especially designed cornual blade (Gomel cornual blade,

Spingler-Tritt, Jestetten, Germany). By limiting the excised tissue to the intramural tube, there is little risk of creating a large defect at the cornu.

After the preparation of the cornual end, the occluded or abnormal isthmic segment is prepared by making serial cuts 1 to 2 mm apart, beginning at the initial transection site at the uterotubal junction and continuing until normal patent tube is identified (Fig. 21.33A). Patency of the distal segment is confirmed by descending hydropertubation, with injection of a few milliliters of dye or irrigation solution through the fimbriated end. Hemostasis of the cut end of the normal distal tube is obtained by precise electrocoagulation of bleeders located between the muscularis and serosa. The intervening abnormal tubal segments are excised from the mesosalpinx mechanically or electrosurgically, avoiding the vascular arcade beneath the tube.

The intramural and isthmic segments are approximated in two layers as follows: The initial suture of the first layer, which incorporates the muscularis and epithelium of the two segments, is placed at the 6 o'clock position (Fig. 21.33E). If the anastomosis is superficial (juxtamural type), the suture is tied.

With anastomoses located deep in the cornua, as in intramural or juxtauterine types, the 6 o'clock suture is held with a clip until the remaining sutures have been placed, because tying this initial suture would make placement of the subsequent sutures difficult if not impossible. In such cases, the subsequent sutures are placed with the use of a continuous strand of suture, as described earlier (Fig. 21.25). This approach facilitates suture placement and prevents the individual sutures from becoming tangled. Three additional sutures, placed at cardinal points, are usually sufficient to join the inner layer. If the cornual crater is deep and the placement of sutures is difficult, this task can be facilitated by making a small coronal incision on the uterus, above the cornual crater. The edges of this incision must be properly approximated at the end of the procedure.

If the distance between the two segments of the tube is significant or if there is undue tension, it is necessary to hold the distal tubal segment close to the intramural segment while tying the sutures. Alternatively, a single no. 7-0 Vicryl suture is passed through the mesosalpinx below the cut end of the distal segment of the tube and then through the border of the uterus immediately beneath the cornual crater. The suture is tied to bring the two segments into close proximity. The 6 o'clock suture is tied first. Then, the loop between each succeeding suture is divided and tied in turn. After approximation of the first layer, the seromuscularis of the uterus is joined to the serosa of the tube with no. 8-0 sutures. The defect under the tube is closed by approximating the mesosalpinx to the lateral edge of the uterus (Fig. 21.33F, G).

Compared with tubouterine implantation, microsurgical tubocornual anastomosis offers several advantages: It largely maintains the integrity of the uterine cornu; preserves a longer tube; obviates the need for a cesarean section, except for obstetric reasons; and yields better results (Fig. 21.34).

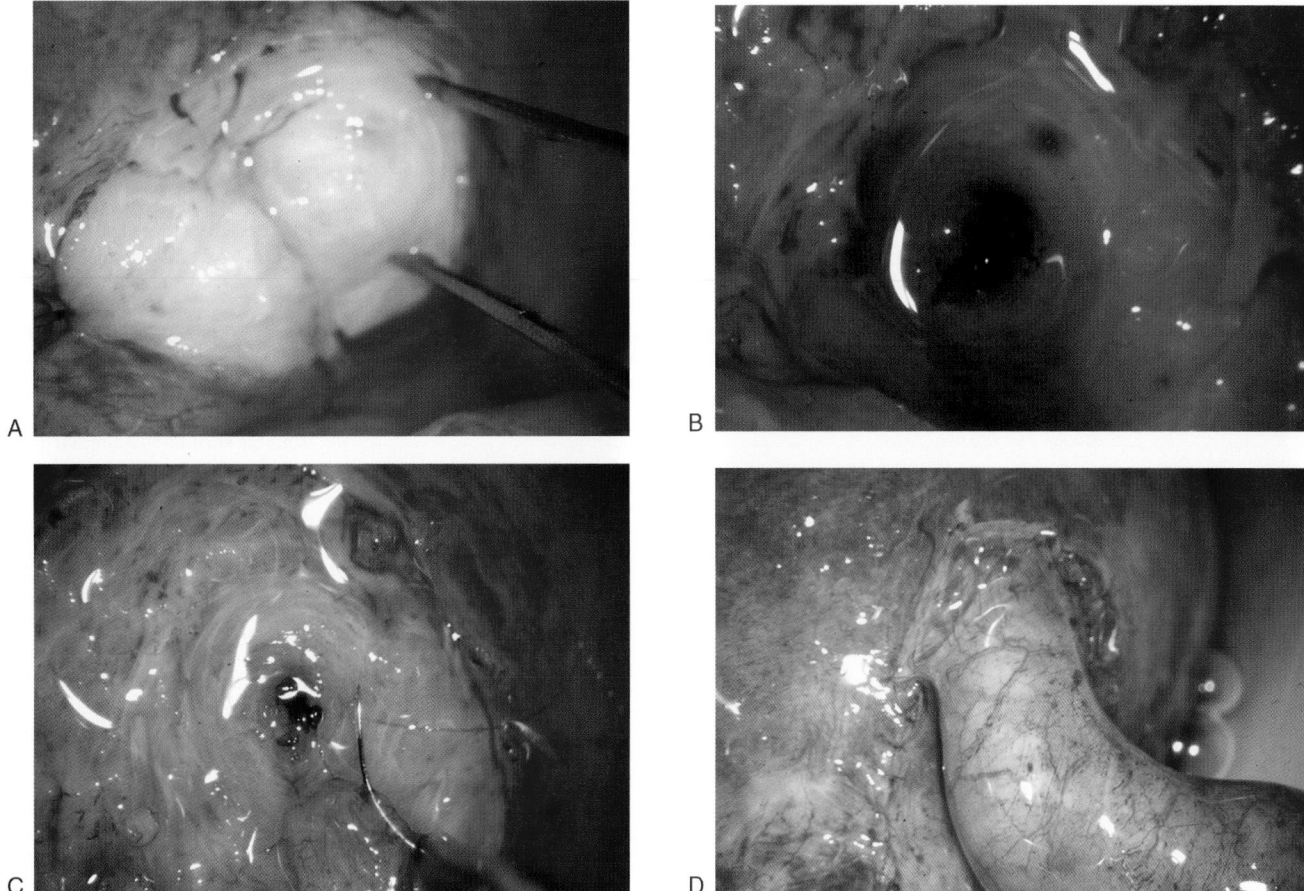

FIGURE 21.34 Microsurgical tubocornual anastomosis for proximal tubal disease. **A:** Serial cuts are made through the intramural segment to reach normal tube. **B:** Normal-appearing tube; methylene blue solution coming through. **C:** Subsequent to the 6 o'clock sutures the other sutures are in process of being placed. **D:** The procedure is completed by apposing the seromuscularis of the uterus to the serosa of the tube and the mesosalpinx to the lateral aspect of the uterus.

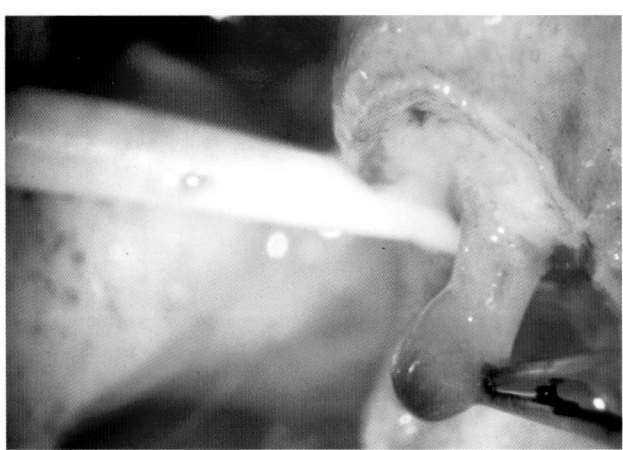

FIGURE 21.35 Cornual polyp.

Cornual polyps, when large, may cause infertility (Fig. 21.35). They can be removed placing a small coronal incision in the cornual region to access the tube at the site of the polyp. The polyp is excised, and the incision is closed in layers.

Results of Tubocornual Anastomosis

Microsurgical tubocornual anastomosis for the treatment of occlusive cornual disease yields fairly good results in centers experienced with this procedure. The published series report live birth rates between 33% and 56% and ectopic pregnancy rates between 5% and 7% (Table 21.7). This table makes it clearly evident that there has been a paucity of reports regarding this procedure for more than a decade. Tubocornual anastomosis for pathologic proximal occlusion is the most difficult type of tubal anastomosis. This procedure is performed less and less with such patients referred for IVF. We continue to perform this procedure in Vancouver and continue to obtain live birth rates of approximately

50%. It is imperative to confirm the cornual obstruction with selective salpingography and/or tubal cannulation, before recommending this procedure.

The ASRM's committee opinion states: "*Unless the proximal blockage on HSG is clearly due to SIN, selective salpingography or tubal cannulation can be attempted... Before performing this procedure, there should be confirmation of normal distal tubal anatomy.*"

"*In these cases, IVF is preferred to resection and microsurgical anastomosis... However microsurgery may be considered after failed tubal cannulation if IVF is not an option for the patient, but it should be attempted only by those with appropriate training.*"

Rare Procedures and Technically Difficult Cases

Rare circumstances may be encountered that are amenable to microsurgical correction. Some of these circumstances are discussed in this section.

The technical difficulty of a procedure must be differentiated from the prognosis that the procedure offers. Furthermore, difficulty is a relative term because what is commonplace work for some may be difficult or even impossible for others to achieve. From the patient's standpoint, what is important is the prognosis, the yield associated with the surgical procedure. Furthermore, the prognosis is not necessarily inversely proportional to the difficulty of the procedure. For example, microsurgical tubocornual anastomosis to treat occlusive cornual lesions is one of the technically more difficult reconstructive tubal operations. However, centers experienced in this procedure achieve excellent results. An even more technically difficult operation is tubo-ovarian transposition.

Tubo-Ovarian Transposition

In the case of a unicornuate uterus without an ipsilateral tube and ovary, the contralateral tube and ovary, if present, may be transposed while preserving their vascular pedicle.

TABLE 21.7 Results of Microsurgical Tubocornual Anastomosis for Occlusive Proximal Tubal Disease

INVESTIGATORS	YEAR	PATIENTS	INTRAUTERINE PREGNANCIES	LIVE BIRTHS	ECTOPIC PREGNANCIES
Gomel	1977	13	NS	7 (53.8%)	1
Gomel	1980	38	21	20 (52.6%)	2
Winston	1980	49	NS	16 (32.7%)	2
McComb	1986	26	15	14 (53.8%)	2
Donnez and Casanas-Roux	1986	82	NS	36 (43.9%)	6
Gillett and Herbison	1989	32	19	18 (56.3%)	2
Tomazevic et al.[a]	1996	59	NS	27 (45.8%)	NS
Awartani and McComb	2003	26	12	NS	3

[a]Of the 32 operated patients who did not deliver within 2 years after surgery, 21 were treated with 66 cycles of IVF, resulting in live births for 12.

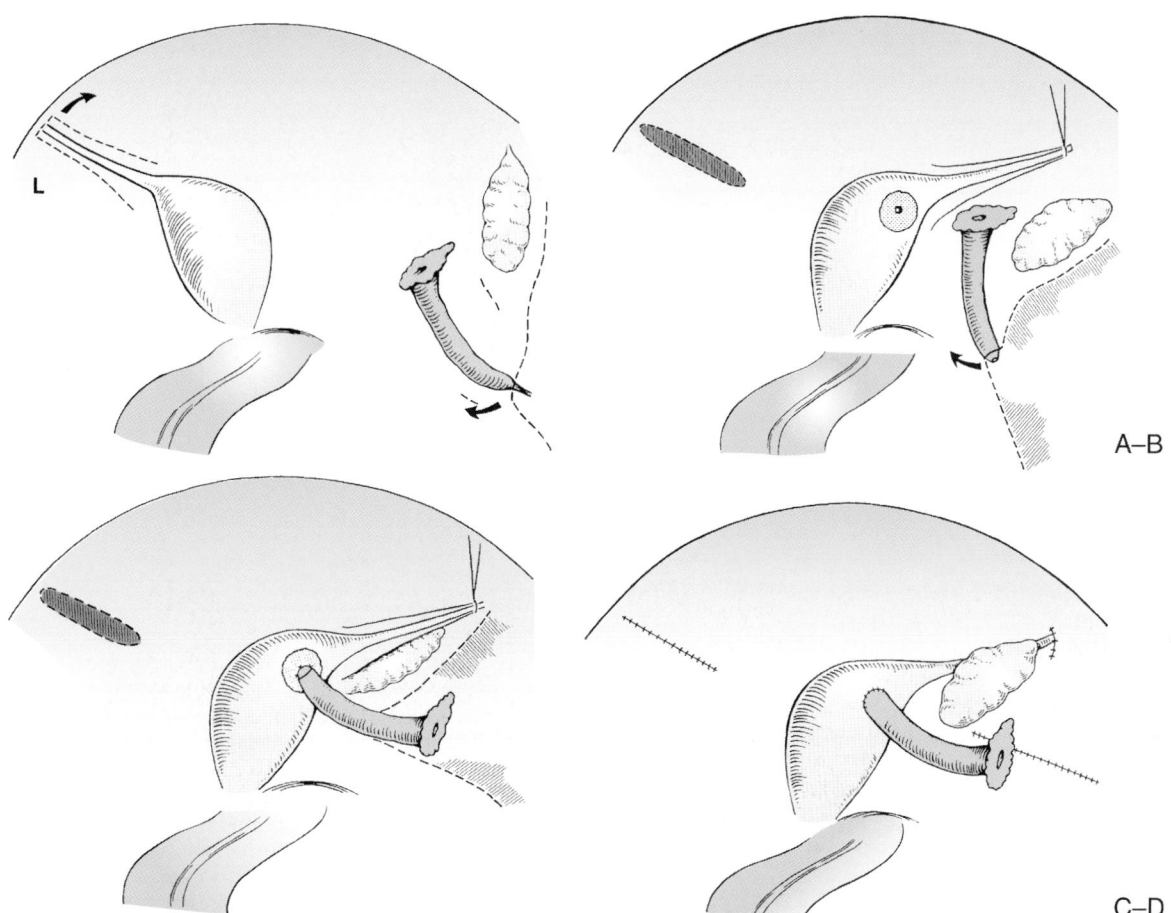

FIGURE 21.36 Microsurgical tubo-ovarian transposition. **A:** Schematic drawing of the findings. **B:** The uterus was centered by moving the left round ligament and attaching it to right inguinal fossa. The intramural segment of the left tube is identified. **C:** The right adnexa is mobilized, with its vascular pedicle intact. The right tube is rotated clockwise to bring its ampullary stump in proximity of the left intramural segment, and permit a two layer anastomosis to be performed. **D:** the anastomosis is completed by apposition of the cornual seromuscularis to the serosa of the tube. All peritoneal incisions are closed. The *dotted lines* indicate the peritoneal incisions made during the procedure. (L = left side.) (From Gomel V, McComb P. Microsurgical transposition of the human fallopian tube and ovary with subsequent pregnancy. *Fertil Steril* 1985;43:804, with permission. Copyright 1985 American Society for Reproductive Medicine. Published by Elsevier Inc. All rights reserved.)

We performed such a procedure in a woman with a single left unicornuate uterus whose ipsilateral tube and ovary were removed subsequent to a left tubal pregnancy. On the right side, placed high on the pelvic sidewall, were an ovary and a short oviduct, composed of infundibulum and ampulla only (Fig. 21.36A).

The uterus was mobilized centrally as follows: The left round ligament was divided near its inguinal insertion and dissected from the broad ligament with its vascular supply intact (Fig. 21.36A). The divided end of the round ligament was then affixed to the right inguinal region (Fig. 21.36B). Microsurgical transposition of the right ovary and tube with preservation of their vascular supply permitted anastomosis between the left intramural and right ampullary tubal segments (Fig. 21.36C). The ovary was mobilized further to achieve the proper spatial relation with the fimbrial extremity of the tube (Fig. 21.36D). In the third postoperative cycle, the patient was successful in achieving an intrauterine pregnancy, which resulted in a normal live birth. Subsequently, she had two additional pregnancies resulting in live births. Since the publication of this report in May 1985, there have been at least five case reports

of successful transposition of the fallopian tube without the ovary. These reports clearly illustrate the potential of surgery, even though technically difficult, in restoring fertility in the face of unusual pelvic anatomy.

Other Unusual Procedures

The following procedures are of historic interest and have little place—excepting very unusual circumstances—in view of the results ART presently offers.

Correction of Bipolar Tubal Disease

The results associated with surgical correction of bipolar (both proximal and distal) tubal occlusion are dismal. A report from the Mayo Clinic included 31 such patients: bipolar tubal occlusion of both tubes ($n = 13$) or their only remaining tube ($n = 5$), bilateral distal and unilateral proximal occlusion ($n = 7$), and bilateral proximal and unilateral distal occlusion ($n = 6$). Despite a mean follow-up period of more than 3 years, pregnancies occurred in only three patients. Furthermore, two of these were ectopic, and one was a spontaneous abortion.

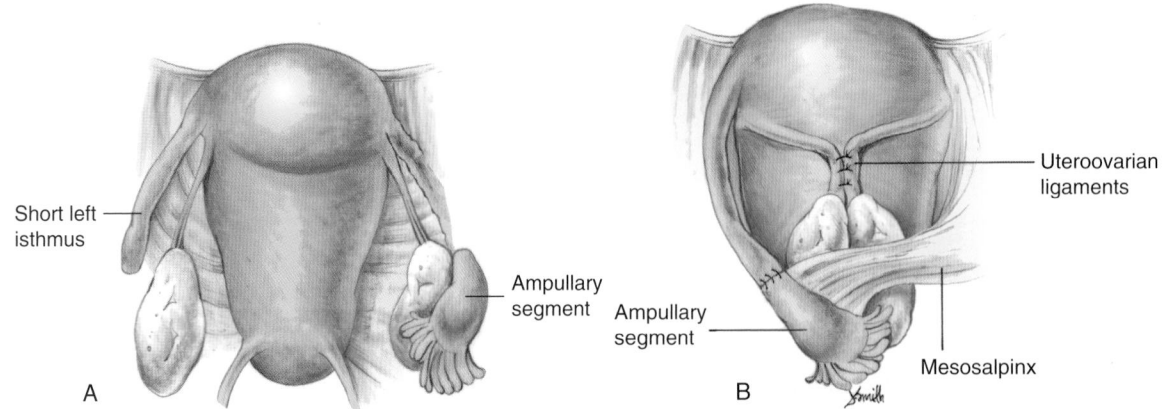

FIGURE 21.37 Microsurgical anastomosis of contralateral tubal segments. **A:** Isthmic segment of the tube on the left and ampullary–infundibular segment on the right. **B:** The uteroovarian ligaments are approximated with nonabsorbable sutures behind the uterus; the left isthmic segment of the tube is anastomosed to the right ampullary–infundibular segment.

Anastomosis of Contralateral Tubal Segments

A patient may have a healthy proximal segment of tube on one side and an ampullary–infundibular segment on the other. In such a circumstance, microsurgical reconstruction of one functional tube can be achieved by anastomosis of the contralateral tubal segments behind the uterus, maintaining the physiologic relation between the tubal infundibulum and ovary. In the presence of both ovaries, the utero-ovarian ligaments are first approximated with interrupted, nonabsorbable no. 4-0 or 5-0 Nylon sutures. This brings the ovaries together and helps reduce tension in achieving the subsequent tubal anastomosis (**Fig. 21.37**). Successful delivery after such a procedure has been reported.

Approximation of the Fimbriated End of the Oviduct to the Contralateral Ovary

When a single ovary exists on the side opposite the patient's only tube, simple approximation of the fimbriated extremity of the tube to the ovary may be possible. The ovary is mobilized, and the mesovarium is fixed to the posterior surface of the uterus with nonabsorbable sutures. The contralateral oviduct is mobilized, and its mesosalpinx is sutured to the posterior aspect of the uterus. The nonabsorbable sutures are placed on the mesosalpinx approximately 1 cm from the tube. This will effectively place the infundibulum in close proximity to the ovary. Alternatively, the ovary can be transposed to the contralateral side with its vascular pedicle kept intact.

Iterative Reconstructive Surgery

Except in rare circumstances, there are no data to support the undertaking of an iterative surgical procedure when a prior reconstructive operation has failed. Rare exceptions include cases of tubotubal anastomosis that failed for purely technical reasons, provided sufficient lengths of healthy tube are available for reconstruction. In such instances, an iterative microsurgical anastomosis may be undertaken if tubal cannulation fails to restore patency.

Tubal cannulation, performed at the time of the postoperative control HSG that demonstrates an obstruction at the anastomosis site, may prove beneficial in a small percentage of cases by breaking down synechiae or dislodging debris that may be present at this site.

Iterative surgery yields a modest success rate if the initial procedure was performed with the use of conventional techniques. However, the success rate of iterative procedures is disappointing when they are undertaken after a failed microsurgical intervention. Most of the available data on iterative surgery concern salpingostomy. Of the 119 such cases reported in the literature, 18 (15.1%) achieved live births, 5 had spontaneous abortions, and 7 (5.9%) had ectopic gestations. All of these 119 patients had their first procedure performed by conventional techniques and their second intervention performed by microsurgery.

The first report on laparoscopic salpingostomy by Gomel in 1997 included, except for one case, iterative procedures on patients who had previously undergone surgery with conventional techniques. This fact may explain the satisfactory rate of success that was obtained.

The conception rate after iterative microsurgical fertility-promoting procedures is significantly lower than that obtained with primary microsurgical interventions. Thie et al. (1986) reported a conception rate of 51% after various primary microsurgical procedures in 161 patients. This rate was only 18% at 3-year follow-up in a similar group of 21 patients who had microsurgery after a failed primary operation performed by conventional techniques.

The preceding data strongly suggest that iterative surgery may be indicated in selected, rare instances and that most of these patients may be better served with IVF.

Observations on Current Practice

The enormous progress in IVF and ART in the past 20 years has been accompanied with the commercialization of this technology and its services all over the world. In parallel fashion, there has been a significant decline in the practice and teaching of reconstructive surgery. There is a paucity of publications on this subject. In vitro fertilization is offered now, as a primary treatment option, in most cases of tubal factor infertility. These changes have occurred despite the greater acceptance of laparoscopic access to perform many of the reconstructive tubal operations and the use of minilaparotomy incision for more complex anastomotic procedures, which represents a major progress in gynecologic surgery. These changes have occurred despite the satisfactory results yielded by reconstructive surgery in appropriately selected cases and despite the fact that surgery offers the couple the opportunity to attempt a pregnancy over a long period of time and to conceive more than once. Furthermore, as already stated before, the presence of a credible alternative with IVF permits the reproductive surgeon to operate on cases with better prognosis, which translates in superior outcomes as has been well demonstrated.

In addition, training in microsurgery renders the gynecologist much more conscious of avoiding peritoneal trauma and more careful in tissue handling and tissue care. It makes him/her more conscious of conservation and overall a better surgeon. Skills that may well be lost with lack of teaching of reconstructive microsurgery.

The evidence suggests that surgery should retain its place in the treatment of tubal infertility. Preservation of the place of surgery will require a concerted effort on the part of the teaching institutions. We are pleased to note the recommendations in support of this approach in ASRM's recent "Committee Opinion: Role of Tubal Surgery in the Era of Assisted Reproductive Technology."

Surgery and ART are complementary approaches that can be used singly or in combination to improve the outlook of couples suffering from tubal infertility. This was clearly demonstrated in a study by Tomazevic published in 1996. Fifty-nine women with pathologic cornual occlusion were treated by microsurgical tubocornual anastomosis; 27 of these (45.8%) had live births. The 32 women in whom the surgery did not yield a birth were offered IVF treatment; 21 of them had a total of 66 cycles of IVF. Twelve of these had a live birth, bringing the total of women with a baby to 39 (66.1%). The reader must be reminded that the success rate with IVF in the late 1980s and early 1990s was fairly low compared to current outcomes.

In the preface of the book *Microsurgery in Female Infertility,* published in early 1983, it is stated: "This manuscript has been completed during a time of rapid change and expansion with the understanding that it represents not an end point but merely an accounting at a given point in time. Further developments are also occurring in the area of IVF and embryo transfer (IVF & ET), which will undoubtedly produce improved results. Nonetheless, I do not consider the techniques of microsurgery on the one hand and IVF & ET on the other as competitive; on the contrary, I see them as complementary, enabling us to achieve a greater success rate among those patients presenting with complex fertility problems." This statement is still valid today.

BIBLIOGRAPHY

Aitola P, Airo I, Kaukinen S, et al. Comparison of N_2O and CO_2 pneumoperitoneums during laparoscopic cholecystectomy with special reference to postoperative pain. *Surg Laparosc Endosc* 1998;8:140.

Ajonuma LC, Ng EH, Chan HC. New insights into the mechanisms underlying hydrosalpinx fluid formation and its adverse effect on IVF outcome. *Hum Reprod Update* 2002;8:255.

ASRM. Committee opinion: role of tubal surgery in the era of assisted reproductive technology. *Fertil Steril* 2012;97:539–545.

Benadiva CA, Kligman I, Davis O, et al. In vitro fertilization versus tubal surgery: Is pelvic reconstructive surgery obsolete? *Fertil Steril* 1995;64:1051.

Bergh T, Ericson A, Hillensjo T, et al. Deliveries and children born after in-vitro fertilization in Sweden 1982–95: a retrospective cohort study. *Lancet* 1999;354:1579.

Bisonette F, Lapensee L, Bouzayen R. Outpatient laparoscopic tubal anastomosis and subsequent fertility. *Fertil Steril* 1999;72:549.

Boeckx W, Gordts S, Buysse K, et al. Reversibility after female sterilization. *Br J Obstet Gynaecol* 1986;93:839.

Boer-Meisel ME, teVelde ER, Habbema JDF, et al. Predicting the pregnancy outcome in patients treated for hydrosalpinx: a prospective study. *Fertil Steril* 1986;45:23.

Bowman MC, Cooke ID. Comparison of fallopian tube intraluminal pathology as assessed by salpingoscopy with pelvic adhesions. *Fertil Steril* 1994;61:464.

Brosens IA, Puttemans PJ. Double-optic laparoscopy: salpingoscopy, ovarian cystoscopy and endo-ovarian surgery with the argon laser. *Baillieres Clin Obstet Gynaecol* 1989;3:595.

Bruhat MA, Mage G, Manhes H, et al. Laparoscopy procedures to promote fertility ovariolysis and salpingolysis: results of 93 selected cases. *Acta Eur Fertil* 1983;14:113.

Brundin A, Dahlborn M, Ahlberg-Ahre E, et al. Radionuclide hysterosalpingography for measurement of human oviduct function. *Int J Gynecol Obstet* 1989;28:53.

Canis M, Mage G, Pouly JL, et al. Laparoscopic distal tuboplasty: report of 87 cases and a 4 year experience. *Fertil Steril* 1991; 56:616.

Centers for Disease Control and Prevention. 2003 assisted reproductive technology success rates. www.cdc.gov/ART/ART2003

Centers for Disease Control and Prevention. 2009 assisted reproductive technology success rates: National Summary and Fertility Clinic Reports. 2011. www.cdc.gov/ART/ART2009

Centers for Disease Control and Prevention. 2010 assisted reproductive technology success rates. 2013. www.cdc.gov/ART/ART2010

Cha SH, Lee MH, Kim JH, et al. Fertility outcome after tubal anastomosis by laparoscopy and laparotomy. *J Am Assoc Gynecol Laparosc* 2001;8:348.

Chapron C, Querleu D, Bruhat MA, et al. Surgical complications of diagnostic and operative gynaecological laparoscopy: a series of 29,966 cases. *Hum Reprod* 1998;13:867.

Chenia F, Hofmeyr GJ, Moolla S, et al. Sonographic hydrotubation using agitated saline: a new technique for improving fallopian tube visualization. *Br J Radiol* 1997;70:833.

Cheong YC, Li TC. Evidence based management of tubal disease and infertility. *Curr Obstet Gynaecol* 2005;15:306.

Dan U, Oelsner G, Gruberg L, et al. Cerebral embolization and coma after hysterosalpingography with oil-soluble contrast medium. *Fertil Steril* 1990;53:939.

Daniell JF, Herbert CM. Laparoscopic salpingostomy using the CO_2 laser. *Fertil Steril* 1984;41:558.

DeCherney AH, Mezer HC, Naftolin F. Analysis of failure of microsurgical anastomosis after mid-segment, non-coagulation tubal ligation. *Fertil Steril* 1983;39:618.

Degueldre M, Vandromme J, Huong PT, et al. Robotically assisted laparoscopic microsurgical tubal reanastomosis: a feasibility study. *Fertil Steril* 2000;74:1020.

de Mouzon J, Goossens V, Bhattacharya S, et al. Assisted reproductive technology in Europe, 2007: results generated from European registers by ESHRE. *Hum Reprod* 2012;27:954.

Dicker D, Ashkenazi J, Feldberg D, et al. Severe abdominal complications after transvaginal ultrasonographically guided retrieval of oocytes for in vitro fertilization and embryo transfer. *Fertil Steril* 1993;59:1313.

Donnez J, Casanas-Roux F. Prognostic factors of fimbrial microsurgery. *Fertil Steril* 1986a;46:200.

Donnez J, Casanas-Roux F. Prognostic factors influencing the pregnancy rate after microsurgical cornual anastomosis. *Fertil Steril* 1986;46:1089.

Donnez J, Nisolle M, Casanas-Roux F. CO_2 laser laparoscopy in infertile women with adnexal adhesions and women with tubal occlusion. *J Gynecol Surg* 1989;5:47.

Dubuisson JB, Bouquet de Joliniere J, Aubriot FX, et al. Terminal tuboplasties by laparoscopy: 65 consecutive cases. *Fertil Steril* 1990;54:401.

Dubuisson JB, Chapron C. Single suture laparoscopic tubal re-anastomosis. *Curr Opin Obstet Gynecol* 1998;10:307.

Dubuisson JB, Chapron C, Morice P, et al. Laparoscopic salpingostomy: fertility results according to the tubal mucosal appearance. *Hum Reprod* 1994;9:334.

Falcone T, Goldberg JM, Margossian H, et al. Robotic-assisted laparoscopic microsurgical tubal anastomosis: a human pilot study. *Fertil Steril* 2000;73:1040.

Fayez JA. An assessment of the role of operative laparoscopy in tuboplasty. *Fertil Steril* 1983;39:476.

Fernandez H, Alby JD, Gervaise A, et al. Operative transvaginal hydrolaparoscopy for treatment of polycystic ovary syndrome: a new minimally invasive surgery. *Fertil Steril* 2001;75:607.

Filmar S, Gomel V, McComb P. The effectiveness of CO_2 laser and electromicrosurgery in adhesiolysis: a comparative study. *Fertil Steril* 1986;45:407.

Gillett WR, Herbison GP. Tubocornual anastomosis: surgical considerations and coexistent infertility factors in determining the prognosis. *Fertil Steril* 1989;51:241.

Gomel V. Tubal reconstruction by microsurgery. Presented at the Eighth World Congress on Fertility and Sterility (IFFS), Buenos Aires, Argentina. 1974; Abstract No. 391.

Gomel V. Laparoscopic tubal surgery in infertility. *Obstet Gynecol* 1975;46:47.

Gomel V. Tubal anastomosis by microsurgery. *Fertil Steril* 1977;28:59.

Gomel V. Reconstructive surgery of the oviduct. *J Reprod Med* 1977;18:181.

Gomel V. Salpingostomy by laparoscopy. *J Reprod Med* 1977;18:265.

Gomel V. Profile of women requesting reversal of sterilization. *Fertil Steril* 1978;30:39.

Gomel V. Salpingostomy by microsurgery. *Fertil Steril* 1978;29:380.

Gomel V. Causes of failure of reconstructive infertility microsurgery. *Clin Obstet Gynecol* 1980;23:1269.

Gomel V. Clinical results of infertility microsurgery. In: Crosignani PG, Rubin BL, eds. *Microsurgery in female infertility*. London, UK: Academic Press, 1980:77.

Gomel V. Microsurgical reversal of sterilization: a reappraisal. *Fertil Steril* 1980;33:587.

Gomel V, Swolin K. Salpingostomy: microsurgical technique and results. *Clin Obstet Gynecol* 1980;23:1243.

Gomel V. The impact of microsurgery in gynecology. *Clin Obstet Gynecol* 1980;23:1301.

Gomel V, McComb PF. Unexpected pregnancies in women afflicted by occlusive tubal disease. *Fertil Steril* 1981;36:529.

Gomel V. An odyssey through the oviduct. *Fertil Steril* 1983;39:144.

Gomel V. *Microsurgery in female infertility*. Boston, MA: Little, Brown, 1983.

Gomel V. Salpingo-ovariolysis by laparoscopy in infertility. *Fertil Steril* 1983;34:607.

Gomel V, McComb PF. Microsurgical transposition of the human fallopian tube and ovary with subsequent intrauterine pregnancy. *Fertil Steril* 1985;43:804.

Gomel V. Distal tubal occlusion. *Fertil Steril* 1988;49:946.

Gomel V. Operative laparoscopy: time for acceptance. *Fertil Steril* 1989;52:1.

Gomel V, Erenus M. The American Fertility Society, 46th Annual Meeting. Program Supplement 1990:P-097–S106(abst).

Gomel V, Taylor PJ. In vitro fertilization versus reconstructive tubal surgery. *J Assist Reprod Genet* 1992;9:306.

Gomel V. From microsurgery to laparoscopic surgery: a progress. *Fertil Steril* 1995;63:464.

Gomel V, Dubuisson JB. *References en gynecologie et obstetrique*. Poulnoy, France: SPEI, 1995:251.

Gomel V, Rowe TC. Microsurgical tubal reconstruction and reversal of sterilization. In: Wallach EE, Zacur HA, eds. *Reproductive medicine and surgery*. St Louis, MO: Mosby, 1995:1074.

Gomel V, Taylor PJ. *Diagnostic and operative gynecologic laparoscopy*. St Louis, MO: Mosby, 1995.

Gomel V. Reproductive surgery. *Minerva Ginecol* 2005;57:21.

Gomel V, McComb PF. Microsurgery for tubal infertility. *J Reprod Med* 2006;51:177.

Gordts S, Boeckx W, Vasquez G, et al. Microsurgical resection of intramural tubal polyps. *Fertil Steril* 1983;40:258.

Gordts S, Campo R, Puttemans P et al. Clinical factors determining pregnancy outcome after microsurgical tubal reanastomosis. *Fertil Steril* 2009;92:1198.

Heikkinen H, Tekay A, Volpi E, et al. Transvaginal salpingosonography for the assessment of tubal patency in infertile women: methodological and clinical experiences. *Fertil Steril* 1995;64:293.

Henderson SR. The reversibility of female sterilization with the use of microsurgery: a report on 102 patients with more than one year of follow-up. *Am J Obstet Gynecol* 1984;149:57.

Henry-Suchet J, Loffredo V, Tesquier L, et al. Endoscopy of the tube (5 tuboscopy): its prognostic value for tuboplasties. *Acta Eur Fertil* 1985;16:139.

Hunter JG, Staheli J, Oddsdottir M, et al. Nitrous oxide pneumoperitoneum revisited. Is there a risk of combustion? *Surg Endosc* 1995;9:501.

Inki P, Palo P, Anttila L. Vaginal sonosalpingography in the evaluation of tubal patency. *Acta Obstet Gynecol Scand* 1998;77:978.

James C, Gomel V. Surgical management of tubal factor infertility. *Curr Opin Obstet Gynecol* 1990;2:200.

Johnson NP, Mak W, Sowter MC. Surgical treatment for tubal disease in women due to undergo in vitro fertilisation. *Cochrane Database Syst Rev* 2004;(3):CD002125.

Jones HW Jr, Rock JA. On the reanastomosis of fallopian tubes after surgical sterilization. *Fertil Steril* 1978;29:702.

Kerin JF, Williams DB, San Roman GA, et al. Falloposcopic classification and treatment of fallopian tube lumen disease. *Fertil Steril* 1992;57:731.

Kim JD, Kim KS, Doo JK, et al. A report on 387 cases of microsurgical tubal reversals. *Fertil Steril* 1997;68:875.

Kim SH, Shin CJ, Kim JG, et al. Microsurgical reversal of tubal sterilization: a report on 1118 cases. *Fertil Steril* 1997;68:865.

Lang EK, Dunaway HH. Recanalization of obstructed fallopian tube by selective salpingography and transvaginal bougie dilatation: outcome and cost analysis. *Fertil Steril* 1996;66:210.

Larsson B. Late results of salpingostomy combined with salpingolysis and ovariolysis by electromicrosurgery in 54 women. *Fertil Steril* 1982;37:156.

Lauritsen JG, Pagel JD, Vangsted P, et al. Results of repeated tuboplasties. *Fertil Steril* 1982;37:68.

Letterie GS, Luetkehans T. Reproductive outcome after fallopian tube canalization and microsurgery for bipolar tubal occlusion. *J Gynecol Surg* 1992;8:11.

Lundberg S, Wramsby H, Bremmer S, et al. Radionuclide hysterosalpingography is not predictive in the diagnosis of infertility. *Fertil Steril* 1998;69:216.

Luttjeboer F, Harada T, Hughes E, et al. Tubal flushing for subfertility. *Cochrane Database Syst Rev* 2007;(3):CD003718.

Madelenat P, DeBrux J, Palmer R. L'etiologie des obstructions tubaires proximales et son rle dans le prognostic des implantations. *Gynecologie* 1977;28:47.

Mahadevan MM, Wiseman D, Leader A, et al. The effects of ovarian adhesive disease upon follicular development in cycles of controlled stimulation for in vitro fertilization. *Fertil Steril* 1985;44:489.

Marana R, Muscatello P, Muzii L, et al. Perlaparoscopic salpingoscopy in the evaluation of the tubal factor in infertile women. *Int J Fertil* 1990;35:211.

Marchino GL, Gigante V, Gennarelli G, et al. Salpingoscopic and laparoscopic investigations in relation to fertility outcome. *J Am Assoc Gynecol Laparosc* 2001;8:218.

Marret H, Harchaoui Y, Chapron C, et al. Trocar injuries during laparoscopic gynaecological surgery. Report from the French Society of Gynaecological Laparoscopy. *Gynaecol Endosc* 1998;7: 235.

McComb P, Gomel V. Cornual occlusion and its microsurgical reconstruction. *Clin Obstet Gynecol* 1980;23:1229.

McComb P. Microsurgical tubocornual anastomosis for occlusive cornual disease: reproducible results without the need for tubouterine implantation. *Fertil Steril* 1986;46:571.

McComb PF, Lee NH, Stephenson MD. Reproductive outcome after microsurgery for proximal and distal occlusions in the same fallopian tube. *Fertil Steril* 1991;56:134.

McComb PF, Paleologou A. The intussusception salpingostomy technique for the therapy of distal oviductal occlusion at laparoscopy. *Obstet Gynecol* 1991;78:443.

McComb PF, Taylor RC. Pregnancy outcome after unilateral salpingostomy with a contralateral patent oviduct. *Fertil Steril* 2001;76:1278.

Mettler L, Giesel H, Semm K. Treatment of female infertility due to tubal obstruction by operative laparoscopy. *Fertil Steril* 1979;32:384.

Mettler L, Ibrahim M, Lehmann-Willenbrock E, et al. Pelviscopic reversal of tubal sterilization with the one- to two-stitch technique. *J Am Assoc Gynecol Laparosc* 2001;8:353.

Millingos SD, Kallipolitis GK, Loutradis DC, et al. Laparoscopic treatment of hydrosalpinx: factors affecting pregnancy rate. *J Am Assoc Gynecol Laparosc* 2000;7:355.

Moon HS, Joo BS, Park GS et al. High pregnancy rate after microsurgical tubal reanastomosis by temporary loose parallel 4-quadrant sutures technique: a long long-term follow-up report on 961 cases. *Hum Reprod* 2012;27:1657.

Munro MG, Gomel V. Fertility-promoting laparoscopically directed procedures. *Reprod Med Rev* 1994;3:29.

Murray DL, Sagoskin AW, Widra EA, et al. The adverse effect of hydrosalpinges on in vitro fertilization pregnancy rates and the benefit of surgical correction. *Fertil Steril* 1998;69:41.

Musset R. *An atlas of hysterosalpingography.* Québec, Canada: Les Presses de l'Université Laval, 1979.

Novy MJ, Thurmond AS, Patton P, et al. Diagnosis of cornual obstruction by transcervical fallopian tube cannulation. *Fertil Steril* 1988;50:434.

Oh ST. Tubal patency and conception rates with three methods of laparoscopic terminal salpingostomy. *J Am Assoc Gynecol Laparosc* 1996;3:519.

Paavonen J, Eggert-Kruse W. *Chlamydia trachomatis*: impact on human reproduction. *Hum Reprod Update* 1999;5:433.

Pabuccu R, Ulgenalp I, Baser I, et al. Microsurgical transposition of the human fallopian tube. *Gynecol Obstet Invest* 1991;31:51.

Palermo G, Joris H, Devroey P, et al. Pregnancies after intracytoplasmic injection of single spermatozoon into an oocyte. *Lancet* 1992;340:17.

Papaioannou S, Afnan M, Girling AJ, et al. Diagnostic and therapeutic value of selective salpingography and tubal catheterization in an unselected infertile population. *Fertil Steril* 2003;79:613.

Patton PE, Williams TJ, Coulam CB. Results of microsurgical reconstruction in patients with combined proximal and distal tubal occlusion: double obstruction. *Fertil Steril* 1987;48:670.

Patterson PJ. Factors influencing the success of microsurgical tuboplasty for sterilization reversal. *Clin Reprod Fertil* 1985;3:57.

Pauerstein CJ, Turner T, Eddy CA. A technique for evaluating functional patency of the oviduct. *Fertil Steril* 1977;28:777.

Putman JM, Holden AEC, Olive DL. Pregnancy rates following tubal anastomosis: Pomeroy partial salpingectomy versus electrocautery. *J Gynecol Surg* 1990;6:173.

Ribeiro SC, Tormena RA, Giribela CG, et al. Laparoscopic tubal anastomosis. *Int J Gynaecol Obstet* 2004;84:142.

Rock JA, Guzick DS, Katz E, et al. Tubal anastomosis: pregnancy success following the reversal of Falope ring or monopolar cautery sterilization. *Fertil Steril* 1987;48:13.

Rock JA, Katayama KP, Martin EJ, et al. Factors influencing the success of salpingostomy techniques for distal fimbrial obstruction. *Obstet Gynecol* 1978;52:591.

Rogers AK, Goldberg SM, Hammel JP, et al. Tubal anastomosis by robotic compared to outpatient minilaparotomy. *Obstet Gynecol* 2007;109:1375.

Rowe TC, Gomel V, McComb P. Investigations of tuboperitoneal causes of female infertility. In: Insler V, Lunenfeld B, eds. *Infertility, male and female.* Edinburgh, UK: Churchill Livingstone, 1993:253.

Rubin IC. Non-operative determination of patency of fallopian tubes in sterility: intrauterine inflation with oxygen and production of a subphrenic pneumoperitoneum. *JAMA* 1920;74:1017.

Rubin IC. Roentgendiagnostik der uterus tumorens mit hilfe von intrauterine collargol injektionen vorlaeufige mitteilung. *Zentralbl Gynakol* 1914;38:658.

Rubin IC. Therapeutic aspects of uterotubal insufflation in sterility. *Am J Obstet Gynecol* 1945;50:621.

Rufat P, Olivennes F, deMouzon J, et al. Task force report on the outcome of pregnancies and children conceived by in vitro fertilization (France: 1987 to 1989). *Fertil Steril* 1994;61:324.

Schepens JJ, Mol BW, Wiegerinck MA, et al. Pregnancy outcomes and prognostic factors from tubal sterilization reversal by sutureless laparoscopical re-anastomosis: a retrospective cohort study. *Hum Reprod* 2011;26:354.

Schippert C, Hille U, Bassler C, et al. Organ-preserving and reconstructive microsurgery of Fallopian tubes in tubal infertility: still an alternative to in vitro fertilization (IVF). *J Reconstr Microsurg* 2010;26:317.

Schlaff WD, Hassiakos DK, Damewood MD, et al. Neosalpingostomy and distal tubal obstruction: prognostic factors and impact of surgical technique. *Fertil Steril* 1990;54:984.

Schlösser HW, Frantzen C, Mansour N, et al. Sterilisation Refertilisierung. Erfahrungen und Ergebnisse bei 119 microchirurgisch refertilisierten Frauen. *Geburtshilfe Frauenheilkd* 1983;43:213.

Sedbon E, BouquetdelaJolinieres J, Boudouris O, et al. Tubal desterilization through exclusive laparoscopy. *Hum Reprod* 1989;4:158.

Silber SJ, Cohen R. Microsurgical reversal of tubal sterilization: factors affecting pregnancy rate, with long-term follow-up. *Obstet Gynecol* 1984;64:679.

Singhal V, Li TC, Cooke ID. An analysis of factors influencing the outcome of 232 consecutive tubal microsurgery cases. *Br J Obstet Gynaecol* 1991;98:628.

Society for Assisted Reproductive Technology (SART), The American Fertility Society. In vitro fertilization-embryo transfer (IVF-ET) in the United States: 1990 results from the IVF-ET Registry. *Fertil Steril* 1992;57:15.

Society for Assisted Reproductive Technology, American Society for Reproductive Medicine. Assisted reproductive technology in the United States and Canada: 1993 results generated from the American Society for Reproductive Medicine/Society for Assisted Reproductive Technology Registry. *Fertil Steril* 1995;64:13.

Spivak MM, Librach CL, Rosenthal DM. Microsurgical reversal of sterilization: a six-year study. *Am J Obstet Gynecol* 1986;154:355.

Strandell A, Bourne T, Bergh C, et al. Sonographic hydrotubation using agitated saline: a new technique for improving fallopian tube visualization. *Ultrasound Obstet Gynecol* 1999;14:200.

Strandell A, Bourne T, Bergh C, et al. The assessment of endometrial pathology and tubal patency: a comparison between the use of ultrasonography and X-ray hysterosalpingography for the investigation of infertility patients. *Ultrasound Obstet Gynecol* 1999;14:200.

Strandell A, Lindhard A, Waldenstrom U, et al. Hydrosalpinx and IVF outcome: a prospective, randomized, multicentre trial in Scandinavia on salpingectomy before IVF. *Hum Reprod* 1999;14:2762.

Strandell A, Lindhard A, Waldenstrom U, et al. Hydrosalpinx and IVF outcome: cumulative results after salpingectomy in a randomized, controlled trial. *Hum Reprod* 2001;16:2403.

Strandell A, Waldenstrom U, Nilsson L, et al. Hydrosalpinx reduces in-vitro fertilization/embryo transfer pregnancy rates. *Hum Reprod* 1994;9:863.

Stumpf PG, March CM. Febrile morbidity following hysterosalpingography: identification of risk factors and recommendations for prophylaxis. *Fertil Steril* 1980;33:487.

Swolin K. Fertiltatsoperationen: Teil I and II. *Acta Obstet Gynecol Scand* 1967;46:204.

Swolin K. Electro microsurgery and salpingostomy: long-term results. *Am J Obstet Gynecol* 1975;121:418.

Taylor PJ, Collins JA. *Unexplained infertility.* New York: Oxford Medical Publications, 1992.

Taylor RC, Berkowitz J, McComb PF. Role of laparoscopic salpingostomy in the treatment of hydrosalpinx. *Fertil Steril* 2001;75:594.

Templeton AA, Mortimer D. The development of a clinical test of sperm migration to the site of fertilization. *Fertil Steril* 1982;37:410.

te Velde ER, Boer ME, Looman CW, et al. Factors influencing success or failure after reversal of sterilization: a multivariate approach. *Fertil Steril* 1990;54:270.

IV

Thie JL, Williams TJ, Coulam CB. Repeat tuboplasty compared with primary microsurgery for postinflammatory tubal disease. *Fertil Steril* 1986;45:784.

Thurmond AS. Selective salpingography and fallopian tube recanalization. *AJR Am J Roentgenol* 1991;156:33.

Tomazevic T, Ribic-Pucelj M, Omahen A, et al. Microsurgery and in-vitro fertilization and embryo transfer for infertility resulting from pathological proximal tubal blockage. *Hum Reprod* 1996;11:2613.

Tourgeman DE, Bhaumik M, Cooke GC, et al. Pregnancy rates following fimbriectomy reversal via neosalpingostomy: a 10 years retrospective analysis. *Fertil Steril* 2001;76:1041.

Trimbos-Kemper TCM. Reversal of sterilization of women over 40 years of age: a multicenter survey in the Netherlands. *Fertil Steril* 1990;53:575.

Tsereteli Z, Terry ML, Bowers SP, et al. Prospective randomized clinical trial comparing nitrous oxide and carbon dioxide pneumoperitoneum for laparoscopic surgery. *J Am Coll Surg* 2002;195:173.

Tulandi T. Salpingo-ovariolysis: a comparison between laser surgery and electrosurgery. *Fertil Steril* 1986;45:489.

Tulandi T, Collins JA, Burrows E, et al. Treatment-dependent and treatment-independent pregnancy among women with periadnexal adhesions. *Am J Obstet Gynecol* 1990;162:354.

Tulandi T, Vilos GA. A comparison between laser surgery and electrosurgery for bilateral hydrosalpinx: a two year followup. *Fertil Steril* 1985;44:846.

Tureck RW, Garcia C-R, Blasco L, et al. Perioperative complications arising after transvaginal oocyte retrieval. *Obstet Gynecol* 1993;81:590.

Uher J, Rypacek F, Presl J. Transport of novel ovum surrogates in the human fallopian tube: a clinical study. *Fertil Steril* 1990;54:278.

Urman B, Gomel V, McComb P, et al. Midtubal occlusion: etiology, management, and outcome. *Fertil Steril* 1992;59:747.

Urman B, Zouves C, Gomel V. Fertility outcome following tubal pregnancy. *Acta Eur Fertil* 1991;22:205.

Van Voorhis BJ, Sparks AE, Syrop CH, et al. Ultrasound guided aspiration of hydrosalpinges is associated with improved pregnancy and implantation rates after in-vitro fertilization cycles. *Hum Reprod* 1998;13:736.

Verhoeven HC, Berry H, Frantzen C, et al. Surgical treatment for distal tubal occlusion: a review of 167 cases. *J Reprod Med* 1983;28:293.

Watrelot A, Nisolle M, Chelli H, et al. International Group for Fertiloscopy Evaluation. Is laparoscopy still the gold standard in infertility assessment? A comparison of fertiloscopy versus laparoscopy in infertility. Results of an international multicentre prospective trial: the 'FLY' (Fertiloscopy-LaparoscopY) study. *Hum Reprod* 2003;18:834.

Watson A, Vandekerckhove P, Lilford R. Techniques for pelvic surgery in subfertility. *Cochrane Database Syst Rev* 2003;(3):CD000221.

Westrom L. Effect of acute pelvic inflammatory disease on fertility. *Am J Obstet Gynecol* 1975;121:707.

Westrom L. Incidence, prevalence and trends of pelvic inflammatory disease and its consequences in industrialized countries. *Am J Obstet Gynecol* 1980;138:880.

Westrom L, Joesoef MR, Reynolds GH, et al. Pelvic inflammatory disease and infertility. *Sex Transm Dis* 1992;14:185.

Wiegerinck MA, Ronkema M, Van Kessel PH, et al. Sutureless re-anastomosis by laparoscopy versus microsurgical re-anastomosis by laparotomy for sterilization reversal: a matched cohort study. *Hum Reprod* 2005;20:2355.

Winston RML. Reversal of sterilization. *Clin Obstet Gynecol* 1980;23:1261.

Winston RML, Margara RA. Microsurgical salpingostomy is not an obsolete procedure. *Br J Obstet Gynaecol* 1991;98:637.

Xue P, Fa Y-Y. Microsurgical reversal of female sterilization. *J Reprod Med* 1989;34:451.

Yoon TK, Sung HR, Kang HG, et al. Laparoscopic tubal anastomosis: fertility outcome in 202 cases. *Fertil Steril* 1999;72:1121.

Zouves C, Erenus M, Gomel V. Tubal ectopic pregnancy after in vitro fertilization and embryo transfer: a role for proximal occlusion or salpingectomy after failed distal tubal surgery? *Fertil Steril* 1991;56:691.

CHAPTER 22
Endometriosis

John S. Hesla and John A. Rock

DEFINITIONS

Adenomyoma—A manifestation of adenomyosis characterized as localized, encapsulated disease of the uterine wall, as compared with the more common diffuse pattern of extension of endometrial glands and stroma in the myometrium.

Adenomyosis—Heterotopic endometrial glands and stroma located deep within the myometrium, with glandular extension below the endometrial–myometrial interface of at least 2.5 mm.

American Society for Reproductive Medicine (ASRM) classification of endometriosis—A scoring system to quantify the location and extent of endometriosis with a scalar rather than numeric terminology. This documentation has been proposed to allow direct comparison of patient responses to medical and surgical treatments and to identify factors predictive of disease outcome.

Atypical peritoneal implants of endometriosis—Lesions of varying appearance, including vesicles, flat plaques, raised blebs, polypoid structures, areas of fibrosis and adhesion formation, and peritoneal defects. May be clear, yellow, brown, blue, or black in color, as compared with the readily recognized red or gray implants.

Cancer antigen 125 (CA-125)—A high molecular weight glycoprotein expressed on the cell surface of some derivatives of embryonic coelomic epithelium. CA-125 is often elevated in cases of mild-to-severe endometriosis, as well as other conditions, including acute pelvic inflammatory disease, adenomyosis, uterine leiomyoma, menstruation, pregnancy, epithelial ovarian cancer, pancreatitis, and chronic liver disease.

Endometrioma—A solitary, nonneoplastic mass containing endometrial tissue and blood.

Endometriosis—The presence and growth of functioning endometrial tissue containing glandular and stromal elements in places other than the uterus that often results in severe pain and infertility.

Hydrodissection—Forceful injection of physiologic irrigant through a small defect created in the surfaces to be separated, such as the peritoneum from the retroperitoneal tissue. This may aid in establishment of the plane of dissection.

Presacral neurectomy—Division of the superior hypogastric plexus; useful as an adjunctive procedure to eliminate the uterine component of dysmenorrhea that results from endometriosis.

Reflux menstruation—Reflux of menses through fallopian tube to ectopic site, especially the peritoneal cavity. Proposed by John Sampson as a mechanism for the origin of endometriosis in many women.

Uterine suspension—Surgical technique of elevation of the adnexa to reduce adhesion formation at denuded peritoneal surfaces of the posterior cul-de-sac, uterine serosa, and broad ligament.

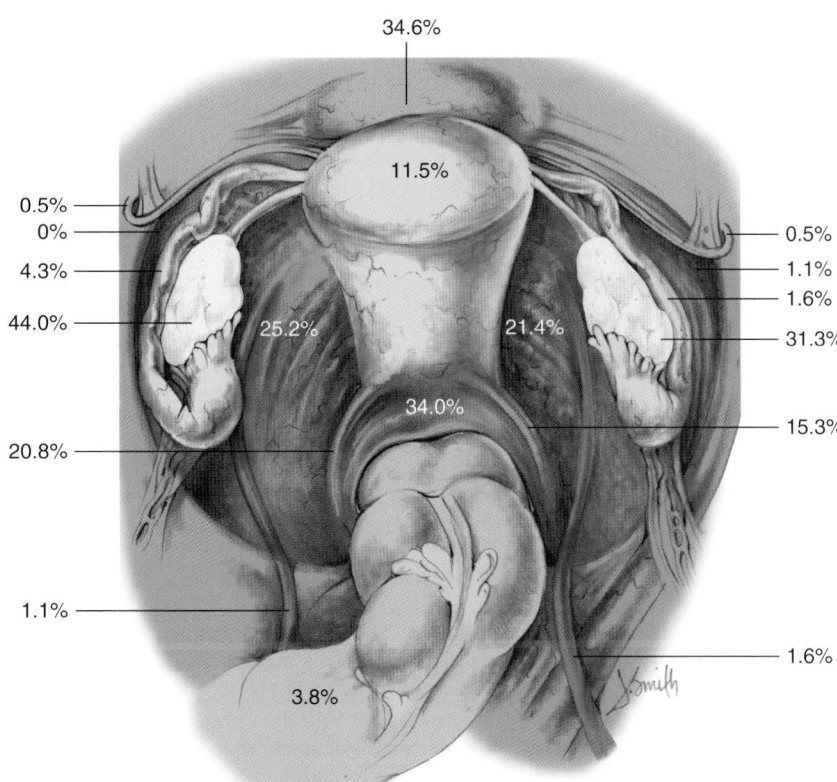

34.6%

11.5%

0.5%
0%
4.3%
44.0%
25.2%   21.4%
34.0%
20.8%

0.5%
1.1%
1.6%
31.3%

15.3%

1.1%

1.6%

3.8%

FIGURE 22.1 Anatomic locations of endometriosis implants in 182 consecutive infertility patients found to have endometriosis by laparoscopy. The rates shown indicate the percentage of all patients with implants in a given locale (Redrawn with permission from Jenkins S, Olive DL, Haney AF. Endometriosis: pathogenic implications of the anatomic distribution. *Obstet Gynecol* 1986;67:335. Copyright © 1986, The American College of Obstetricians and Gynecologists).

Endometriosis is a clinical and pathologic entity initially described by von Rokitansky in 1860 that is characterized by the presence of tissue resembling functioning endometrial glands and stroma outside the uterine cavity. These ectopic implants can be located throughout the pelvic cavity, including the ovaries, uterine ligaments, rectovaginal septum, parietal peritoneum, intestinal serosa, and appendix. Less common sites of involvement include the cervix, hernial sacs, the umbilicus, laparotomy and episiotomy scars, and the pleural and pericardial cavities (**Fig. 22.1**).

Although endometriosis has been extensively investigated over the past century, it remains an enigmatic disease process. The association between endometriosis and infertility is still undefined, and there are insufficient data to support many of the hormonal and surgical therapies that have been proposed. In addition, the often subtle and varied appearances of endometriosis can make recognition of lesions and surgical staging difficult, thereby casting doubt on the utility of the classification systems that have been developed. Nevertheless, the findings of well-designed clinical trials and recent studies that have elucidated the pathogenesis of endometriosis have enabled a more rational approach to the medical and surgical management of this disease.

PREVALENCE

The estimated prevalence of endometriosis among population groups varies depending on the presenting symptoms. Endometriosis affects 6% to 10% of reproductive-age women. Among women with pelvic pain, the prevalence of endometriosis ranges from approximately 30% to 80%. The disease has been diagnosed in 40% to 52% of women with severe dysmenorrhea and 70% of patients with chronic pelvic pain. Cramer and colleagues, in a multicenter study, diagnosed endometriosis in 17% of women with primary infertility, and

in other series, the prevalence varied from approximately 9% to 50%. Verkauf prospectively identified endometriosis in 38.5% of infertile women and 5.2% of fertile women. Other studies have confirmed the odds that infertile women are seven to 10 times more likely to have endometriosis than are their fertile counterparts. However, any postmenarchal woman is at risk, because endometriotic implants have been identified in postmenopausal women, in women with primary amenorrhea secondary to müllerian anomalies, and in 69.6% of teenagers who underwent diagnostic laparoscopy for chronic pelvic pain. Twin and family studies suggest a genetic component. Simpson and colleagues reported a 6.9% occurrence rate in first-degree female relatives, which compared with 1% for the non–blood-related control group. Genes involved in implantation of tissue, fibrinolysis, or ovarian steroidogenesis may be aberrantly expressed at a higher frequency in family members with endometriosis. Other risk factors include alcohol use, smoking, and low body mass index.

HISTOGENESIS

The mechanism by which endometriosis develops is unknown, although there has been much discussion as to its origin (**Table 22.1**). Variations in the location and presentation of implants have compromised a complete understanding of the histogenesis of the aberrant endometrial cells. Four major theories have been proposed:

1. The reflux and direct implantation theory suggests that viable endometrial cells reflux through the fallopian tubes during menstruation and implant on surrounding pelvic structures.
2. The coelomic metaplasia theory suggests that the multipotential cells of the coelomic epithelium may be stimulated to transform into endometrial-like cells.

> **TABLE 22.1** Theories for the Histogenesis of Endometriosis
>
> Transtubal regurgitation or retrograde menstruation
> Direct implantation of endometrial cells
> Metaplasia of coelomic epithelium
> Lymphatic dissemination
> Hematogenous spread
> Activation of embryonic cell rests
> Activation of wolffian rests
> Metaplasia of urothelium
> Hereditary factor
> Immunologic factor

3. The vascular dissemination theory suggests that endometrial cells enter the uterine vasculature or lymphatic system at menstruation and are transported to distant sites.
4. The autoimmune disease theory suggests that endometriosis is a disorder of immune surveillance that allows ectopic endometrial implants to grow.

Reflux and Direct Implantation Theory

John Sampson first postulated that endometriosis arose from retrograde flow of fragments of endometrial tissue through the oviducts and into the peritoneal cavity. Much evidence validates this theory. The anatomic distribution of endometriosis as noted at laparoscopy is consistent with a reflux pattern of development; the most common sites of disease in the infertile woman are the ovary and uterosacral ligament, followed by the posterior uterus, posterior cul-de-sac, and posterior broad ligament. Endometriosis developed in monkeys when the uterus was surgically inverted to cause menstruation to occur intraperitoneally. Exposure of abraded peritoneum to endometrial cells has resulted in the growth of endometriotic implants in rabbits and rats. Endometriosis has developed in laparotomy, episiotomy, and cesarean section scars after surgical entrance into the endometrial cavity, and anomalies of the müllerian tract are associated with an increased occurrence of endometriosis. Endometriosis is a common finding in women with stenosis of the external cervical os. Epidemiologic data suggest that women who menstruate more frequently, more heavily, or for a longer duration have an increased likelihood of disease development. Prolonged lactation and multiparity are protective.

Peritoneal implants of endometriosis and the presence of endometriomas are more common on the left side of the pelvis than the right. The position of the sigmoid colon creates a sequestered microenvironment around the left adnexa, which facilitates implantation of endometrial cells regurgitated through the left tube. The large intestine does not provide the right hemipelvis with this anatomical shelter, because the cecum lies more cranial in position. In addition, the retrograde menstruation theory is supported by the finding of a higher prevalence of endometriosis in the subphrenic region, since the falciform ligament may trap refluxed endometrium in the right hypochondrium.

Focal endometriosis has been identified in 16% to 63% of proximal tubal segments after cautery or Pomeroy tubal sterilization, perhaps as a consequence of recurrent bathing of the healing terminal area with menstrual products. Nevertheless, bloody peritoneal fluid has been observed in 90% of women with patent fallopian tubes undergoing laparoscopy during the perimenstrual time period, a figure much greater than the estimated 2% to 5% prevalence of symptomatic endometriosis in women of reproductive age. Additionally, peritoneal implants have been identified in women who had a prior tubal ligation procedure and were undergoing laparoscopy for the evaluation of pelvic pain. Hence, other factors evidently are present to promote the ectopic implantation.

Coelomic Metaplasia Theory

The germinal epithelia of the ovary, endometrium, and peritoneum all originate from the same totipotential coelomic epithelium. The metaplasia theory postulates that these totipotential cells are transformed by repeated exposure to hormonal or infectious stimuli. This may explain the development of endometriotic lesions in unusual locations and in the odd cases of male patients in whom endometriosis develops after prostatectomy, orchiectomy, or prolonged treatment with estrogen. Reports of endometriosis in women with primary amenorrhea and an absence of functioning uterine endometrium and of endometriosis identified in mature teratomas also lend support to the metaplasia theory.

Vascular Dissemination Theory

Endometrial cells can be transported to extrauterine sites by blood vessels or the lymphatic system or by contamination of the pelvis or abdominal wall incision if the uterine cavity is surgically entered. Retroperitoneal endometriosis is hypothesized to arise from lymph vascular spread; 29% of patients with pelvic endometriosis documented on autopsy had pelvic lymph nodes that contained endometriosis. Theories of vascular dissemination help explain how endometriosis can develop in the lung or pericardium.

Autoimmune Disease Theory

Alterations in cellular immunity can facilitate the successful implantation of translocated endometrial cells. Compared with control subjects, monkeys with spontaneous endometriosis had both a lowered cell-mediated response to autologous endometrial tissue, as determined by skin testing, and a decreased in vitro blastogenesis response. Similar studies performed in women demonstrated that lymphocytes obtained from control patients were significantly more efficient in cytolysis of isolated endometrial stromal cells than were lymphocytes obtained from patients with endometriosis. This decreased cytotoxic response to endometrial cells may be due to a defect in natural killer cell activity, such as a decreased lytic effect toward stroma that allows ectopic development of endometrial fragments. In addition, there may be an increased resistance of endometrium in women with endometriosis to natural killer cytotoxicity.

Promoting Factors

Clinical and laboratory studies support the concept that endometriosis is an estrogen-dependent condition. Estradiol concentrations greater than approximately 60 pg/mL have been identified as necessary for proliferation of endometriotic lesions. Nevertheless, estrogen and progesterone receptors are found in much lower concentrations in endometriotic tissue than in normal endometrium tissue; such endometriotic tissue also frequently fails to show cyclic variations of development in response to hormonal changes. Early data from primate studies suggested that endometriosis required no steroidal supplementation to become initially established, but later studies demonstrated that chronic exposure to ovarian steroids is necessary for the survival of these experimentally induced endometrial plaques.

Growth factors can originate from the peritoneal environment to stimulate endometrial development. Platelet-derived growth factor, a macrophage secretory product, enhance endometrial stromal cell proliferation in a dose-dependent manner. Similarly, macrophage-conditioned media promote mouse endometrial stromal cell proliferation in vitro, and this activation is enhanced with the addition of estrogen. Increased concentrations of macrophage-derived growth factors, including vascular endothelial growth factor, have been identified in the peritoneal fluid of women with endometriosis. This suggests that changes in the vascular permeability and angiogenesis play an important role in the pathophysiology of this disease.

Molecular alterations in steroidogenic enzyme function have been implicated in the pathogenesis of endometriosis. Endometrial tissue from patients with endometriosis expresses aromatase P-450, whereas endometrium from control women without identifiable endometriosis does not. The presence of aromatase within endometriosis results in higher local production of estrogen necessary to support the growth and metabolic activity of the lesion.

Menstrual effluent contains factors that induce alterations in the peritoneal mesothelium, facilitating adhesion of endometrial cells. Attachment of endometrial cells is enhanced by induction of adhesion molecules and their receptors and the overexpression of matrix metalloproteinases and plasminogen activators. These factors ensure local destruction of the extracellular matrix. Suppression of matrix metalloproteinase production by progesterone decreased ectopic implantation of endometrium in the nude mouse, implicating these proteinases in the pathogenesis of endometriosis.

In summary, no single theory explains all cases of endometriosis, although the direct implantation mechanism seems the likely cause for most disease locations. Immunologic factors, inducing substances, or other mediators may explain the development of endometriosis in more distant sites.

NATURAL HISTORY

The natural history of endometriosis is not clearly understood. The disease appears to progress in most untreated patients, although spontaneous regression can occur in as many as 58% of milder cases. Falcone and Lebovic analyzed the findings of follow-up laparoscopies performed 6 to 39 months following the initial diagnostic procedure among 162 patients in several previous endometriosis surgical trials that were randomized to the placebo control group rather than surgical excision/ablation. There was nearly equal distribution of those with progressive disease (31%), unchanged (31%), and improvement in extent of lesions (38%).

Surgical and medical therapies may promote a temporal regression but may not effectively eliminate microscopic, retroperitoneal, and hormonally resistant disease. Dmowski and Cohen described persistent disease in 15% of patients treated with danazol, and Henzl and associates noted a progression of disease during the course of treatment in 4% to 8% of patients receiving danazol or an analogue of gonadotropin-releasing hormone (GnRH). When conservative surgery was combined with danazol or GnRH agonist therapy, the overall recurrence rate at 36 months was between 13.5% and 33%.

The effect of pregnancy on the clinical course of endometriosis is uncertain. Although Sampson proposed that pregnancy induces involution of implants, other authors recently described a variable response of endometriosis to pregnancy. McArthur and Ulfelder analyzed the clinical effect of pregnancy on endometriosis in 24 patients. They found that the behavior of endometriosis during the gravid state was extremely variable and that the regression of disease appeared to be due to decreased tissue responsiveness to hormonal stimulation rather than to actual necrosis of the lesions. More patients in their series experienced disease persistence than permanent regression. Monkey studies have confirmed these findings; the response of endometrial implants to pregnancy varied from total regression to significant progression.

Approximately 2% to 4% of early postmenopausal women suffer from endometriosis. These cases are usually associated with exogenous intake of estrogens or tamoxifen. Nevertheless, there are reports of symptomatic endometriosis in women older than 60 years of age who have not received steroid replacement therapy. Such cases presumably are secondary to the responsiveness of the residual lesions to low levels of estrogens that arise from peripheral conversion of ovarian and adrenal androgens.

PATHOPHYSIOLOGY

Gross Appearance

Signs of endometriosis may be evident on physical examination. Endometriosis can form tender nodules on the uterosacral ligaments that are readily palpable on rectovaginal examination. It may infiltrate the deepest portion of the rectouterine pouch and cause pain with defecation and, rarely, cyclic rectal bleeding. Lesions of endometriosis have been identified in the umbilicus, in the vulva, and in episiotomy scars. Complete ureteral obstruction has been reported. This can be temporarily reversed with the administration of GnRH agonists, progestogens, and danazol. Diaphragmatic involvement can lead to chronic, recurrent pneumothorax at the time of menstruation. Lesions have been identified in the upper and lower extremities, the pericardium, and the lung.

The gross appearance of endometriosis is extremely variable. On entering the abdomen, the surgeon may find a small, adherent nodule on one or both sides of the pelvis, usually attached to the posterior cul-de-sac and posterior surface of the uterus. Frequently, release of ovarian adhesions to mobilize the adnexa results in an egress of chocolate-colored or dark red fluid that is highly suggestive of endometriosis. Examination of the ovary may disclose a cyst that is rarely larger than 10 cm and has a dark, hemorrhagic lining. Endometriomas develop over a time span of a few months as a result of extensive intracystic hemorrhage. Reddish blue, fibrinous areas that represent small islands of endometriosis may be present on the ovarian cortex. Peritoneal implants vary in appearance from black, puckered lesions surrounded by a variable extent of fibrosis, to red polypoid material, to clear vesicles. Other appearances include yellow-brown peritoneal discoloration, white plaques, or scarring. The strong inflammatory stimulus of superficial lesions of endometriosis may promote fibrosis and invagination of adjacent peritoneal surfaces. Red lesions are the most metabolically active and are found mainly in younger patients.

The fallopian tube is usually nonobstructed and free of gross disease, although peritubal adhesions can extend to adjacent structures, particularly in patients with extensive disease. Deeply infiltrating endometriotic nodules extend more than 5 mm beneath the peritoneum and may involve the uterosacral ligaments, bladder, ureters, or vagina. The depth of invasion has been correlated with pain symptomatology. Endometrial invasion of the rectal or sigmoidal wall can simulate malignancy or produce complete obstruction.

Microscopic Appearance

The essential diagnostic criterion is the presence of endometrial tissue, both stroma and glandular elements. This aberrant tissue resembles the uterine mucosa both histologically and physiologically. Secretory change and decidualization are seen in response to hormone influences in the luteal phase, and estrogen stimulates proliferation of the ectopic implants. Nevertheless, these functional changes are less uniform for implants than for the uterine mucosa.

The ultrastructural features of endometriosis are consistent with an incomplete response to the hormonal milieu. Endometriotic implants contain lower concentrations of progesterone receptors than do corresponding normal endometrium, so the histologic response to progesterone is less profound. Gould and colleagues reported that the nucleus of endometriotic stromal cells had a marked degree of estrogen binding throughout the menstrual cycle, whereas stromal binding sites in the uterine endometrium were present only during the proliferative phase and not the secretory phase of the cycle. The differing responses of the two tissue types to steroid hormones were reflected by the modulation of estrogen binding and changes in glandular histology. Estrogen receptors did not undergo downregulation during the luteal phase of the cycle in endometriotic foci, despite an increase in endogenous progesterone concentration. Alterations in the quantity, activation, or function of the progesterone receptor may be responsible for this lack of change in estradiol receptors, the abnormal response of the ectopic endometrium to progesterone, and the failure of hormonal therapy in some patients.

Estrogens play a primary role in the establishment and maintenance of endometriotic tissue. There is evidence of local estrogen production within endometriotic cells. Pellegrini and colleagues observed an overexpression of estrogen receptors α and β, which belong to the nuclear receptor family and act as activated transcription factors. Cyclin D1 and c-myc are estrogen-related genes implicated in cell cycle control that are overexpressed in endometriotic cells.

Because of the pressure of retained blood in the cyst cavities of endometriomas, a large concentration of endothelial leukocytes heavily laden with hemosiderin (pseudoxanthoma cells) may be found, and the glandular lining may be nearly absent and replaced by reactive connective tissue elements. Biopsy may fail to yield histologic proof of the endometrial glands and stroma in approximately one third of all cases of typical clinical endometriosis, even if many tissue sections are analyzed.

The "chocolate cyst" description of the ovary is used synonymously with endometrial cyst or endometrioma. Nevertheless, other types of ovarian cysts may have a similar fluid content, including the hemorrhagic follicle, corpus luteum, or cystadenoma. Pathologic confirmation of the diagnosis is always advised.

Approximately 0.7% to 1.0% of patients with endometriosis have lesions that undergo malignant transformation. Atypical glandular changes have been found in 3% to 6% of cases of ovarian endometriosis. Several histologic tumor types have been described (Table 22.2). Endometrioid adenocarcinomas account for 69% of reported lesions, with the ovary being the primary site in most cases. Rapidly enlarging endometriomas or those measuring greater than 10 cm should be sectioned carefully to search for malignant foci. Tumors arising in endometriosis are predominantly of low grade and confined to the site of origin. Progestogen therapy is recommended after surgical resection of these lesions.

Clinical Characteristics

The clinical features of endometriosis are varied, and the presentation depends on the site of growth and the severity of disease. The classic triad of dysmenorrhea, dyspareunia, and infertility has been described as characteristic of the disease (Table 22.3). Nevertheless, patients with extensive endometriosis may be clinically symptom-free, and women with only minimal involvement may manifest disabling pelvic pain. Dysmenorrhea is a common symptom that most likely is associated with endometriosis if it develops after age 20 years, is

TABLE 22.2 Histology of Tumors Arising in Endometriosis		
HISTOLOGY	**NUMBERS**[a]	**INCIDENCE (%)**
Endometrioid carcinoma		
Adenocarcinoma	96	46.4
Adenoacanthoma	43	20.8
Adenosquamous carcinoma	4	1.9
Clear cell carcinoma	28	13.5
Sarcoma, including mixed mesodermal tumor	24	11.6
Serous cystadenocarcinoma	6	2.9
Squamous cell carcinoma	3	1.4
Mucinous cystadenocarcinoma	2	1.0
Mixed germ cell tumor and adenocarcinoma	1	0.5
Totals	207	100

[a]Two patients had two different histologic patterns.
From Heaps JM, Nieberg RK, Berek JS. Malignant neoplasms arising in endometriosis. *Obstet Gynecol* 1990;75:1023, with permission. Copyright © 1990, The American College of Obstetricians and Gynecologists and Lippincott Williams & Wilkins.

TABLE 22.3 Symptoms Associated with Endometriosis

Pelvic
    Dysmenorrhea
    Dyspareunia
    Chronic pelvic pain
    Sciatica
    Premenstrual spotting

Gastrointestinal
    Constipation
    Diarrhea
    Dyschezia
    Tenesmus
    Hematochezia

Urinary
    Flank pain
    Back pain
    Abdominal pain
    Urgency
    Frequency
    Hematuria

Pulmonary
    Hemoptysis
    Catamenial chest pain
    Pneumothorax

Infertility

---

clearly attributed to anatomic distortion. Also, the oxidative stress associated with endometriomas may lead to follicular depletion and vascular compromise of the ovarian cortex. However, the pathophysiology of infertility in patients with less advanced disease is more controversial.

Endometriotic implants within the fallopian tube or ovary may promote a local inflammatory response that has a direct, deleterious effect on tubal function (Table 22.4). Oocyte capture by the fallopian tube may be prevented despite the normal process of oocyte maturation and ovulation. Endometriosis and especially adenomyosis are associated with impeded hyperperistaltic and dysperistaltic uterotubal transport capacity. Chronic salpingitis was detected in 29 of 87 (33%) fallopian tubes of patients undergoing laparotomy for ovarian endometriosis; tubal obstruction was demonstrated in only one of these cases, although adhesions were present in 24%. Endometriosis has been identified in the resected segments of fallopian tubes in women undergoing tubocornual anastomosis for proximal tubal obstruction when there was no evidence of implants elsewhere in the pelvis. Others have reported a correlation between tubal endometriosis and chronic salpingitis in similar cases, although this finding has not been uniform.

Altered folliculogenesis or ovulation has been described in endometriotic patients who have undergone serial sonogram studies. An abnormal follicular growth rate and total growth period may disturb the normal synchronization of oocyte maturation, uterine receptivity, and ovulation. Tummon and coworkers reported that women with minimal endometriosis had more, yet smaller, follicles and lower preovulatory estradiol levels at the time of midcycle luteinizing hormone (LH) surge.

IV

---

progressive, and is not well relieved by nonsteroidal antiinflammatory agents or oral contraceptives. Spasmodic pain beginning before the onset of menstrual bleeding is another common symptom of patients with endometriosis. When the rectovaginal septum or uterosacral region is involved, the pain is often referred to the rectum or lower sacral and coccygeal regions because of premenstrual and menstrual swelling of ectopic implants. Dyschezia and constipation may be present. Dyspareunia is common, especially in cases of uterosacral or vaginal infiltration, fixed retroversion of the uterus, or ovarian fixation by adhesions. Again, there is no absolute correlation between the amount of visible endometriosis as seen at surgery and the extent of symptoms; minor disease involvement may result in severe pain, whereas massive areas of superficial endometriosis may cause no discomfort.

Other presenting symptoms can include signs of urinary tract involvement, such as hematuria or ureteral obstruction, unusual abdominal or adnexal masses, cyclic sciatica, catamenial pneumothorax or hemoptysis, and swollen and painful scars. Premenstrual spotting can occur for 3 to 7 days before the start of menses; this is a poorly recognized but relatively consistent sign of endometriosis. An endometrioma can leak, causing considerable pain, or it can rupture and produce a clinical picture much like that seen with a ruptured ectopic pregnancy or acute appendicitis. Nearly 10% of patients with endometriosis present with acute symptoms that require exploration for diagnosis and treatment.

Approximately 20% to 40% of women with endometriosis are infertile. Vercellini and colleagues report the monthly fecundity rate for those with endometriosis is 2% to 10%, as compared to 15% to 20% in fertile couples. When extensive pelvic scarring or large endometriomas are present in the patient with endometriosis, the associated infertility can be

TABLE 22.4 Possible Mechanisms by Which Endometriosis Causes Infertility

Mechanical interference
    Pelvic adhesions
    Chronic salpingitis
    Altered tubal motility
    Distortion of tuboovarian relations
    Impaired oocyte pickup

Alterations in peritoneal fluid
    Increased concentration of prostaglandins
    Increased number of activated macrophages
    Increased production of cytokines
    Enhanced phagocytosis of sperm

Abnormal systemic immune system response
    Increased cell-mediated gamete injury
    Increased prevalence of autoantibodies
    Antiendometrial antibody production

Hormonal or ovulatory dysfunction
    Defective folliculogenesis
    Luteinized unruptured follicle syndrome
    Hyperprolactinemia
    Luteal phase deficiency

Fertilization or implantation failure
Early spontaneous abortion

From Surrey ES, Halme J. Endometriosis as a cause of infertility. *Obstet Gynecol Clin North Am* 1989;16:79, with permission. Copyright © 1989, Elsevier.

Luteinized unruptured follicle (LUF) syndrome, a condition of normal ovulatory hormone secretion and luteinization of the follicle without the expected occurrence of ovulation, has been reported to be more common in patients with endometriosis. Mio and colleagues performed transvaginal ultrasound at least every other day from cycle day 8 through the third day after human chorionic gonadotropin (hCG) administration on 47 patients with endometriosis, predominantly minimal and mild, and 28 control patients with male factor infertility. Luteinized unruptured follicle syndrome was diagnosed in 20 of 81 (24.7%) monitored cycles in endometriosis patients and in only 3 of 44 (6.8%) monitored cycles in control patients, a difference that achieved statistical significance. Schenken and associates also noted an increased rate of LUF and associated luteal phase deficiency in monkeys with surgically induced moderate-to-severe endometriosis. An absence of sonographic evidence of midcycle follicular collapse in patients with mild endometriosis has ranged from 4% to 35% in the literature.

Luteal phase function has been evaluated by endometrial biopsy and peripheral progesterone concentrations. There is insufficient evidence to conclusively link endometriosis with a deficiency of corpus luteum activity, although some studies have suggested the existence of a shortened luteal phase, delayed increase in progesterone secretion after ovulation, decreased progesterone secretion in the late luteal phase, and lowered serum estradiol levels during the early follicular phase.

The effect of endometriosis on fertilization and preimplantation development is widely debated. Peritoneal fluid from patients with endometriosis had a deleterious effect on sperm–oocyte interaction in homologous mouse and hamster fertilization assays. In vitro studies involving human zona pellucida confirmed an adverse effect of peritoneal fluid on sperm binding in this patient population, although others reported that peritoneal fluid from women with low-stage endometriosis had no detrimental effect on sperm motility characteristics. Peritoneal fluid from women with moderate and severe endometriosis caused declines in sperm motility and velocity. Exposure of two-cell mouse embryos to the peritoneal fluid or serum of patients with endometriosis has resulted in a decreased rate of cleavage and development to the blastocyst and hatching stages as compared with control nonendometriotic specimens. However, this association was not verified by similar studies of mouse embryo development and apoptosis.

Aberrant gene expression in eutopic and ectopic endometrium may be related to infertility or the establishment of the disease. Integrins are ubiquitous cell adhesion molecules that undergo dynamic alterations during the normal menstrual cycle in the human endometrium. The $\alpha v \beta 3$ vitronectin receptor integrin is normally expressed in endometrium during the periimplantation period; such expression may be lost in women with mild endometriosis, which may affect uterine receptivity. The endometrium of infertile women with endometriosis may synthesize low levels of L-selectin, a protein that coats the trophoblast on the surface of the blastocyst. This may be another mechanism for impaired implantation. Women with lower levels of expression of *HOXA*10 have lower implantation rates. This gene is involved in endometrial regeneration in each menstrual cycle.

A high frequency of spontaneous abortions in infertile women with endometriosis has been reported, although the relation was questioned because of potential control group bias. Naples and coworkers found that patients with endometriosis who refused treatment had the same abortion rate before and after diagnosis (26% and 25.5%). Studies of the last decade with appropriate control groups have demonstrated no substantial increase in the incidence of spontaneous abortion in women with endometriosis.

Mechanisms Influencing Symptoms

Because of the uncertain mechanisms causing infertility and pelvic pain in patients with minimal and mild endometriosis, many investigators have attempted to identify specific alterations in the peritoneal environment that would explain these symptoms. Significant increases or decreases in peritoneal fluid volume that are due to increased production by the ovaries, altered mesothelial permeability, or increases in the colloid osmotic pressure have been hypothesized to inhibit ovum capture by the fallopian tube or to adversely affect tubal transport. Koninckx and associates reported elevations in peritoneal fluid volume during cycle days 1 through 5 in patients with mild and moderate endometriosis. The quantity of fluid was comparable to that in control subjects during the remainder of the follicular phase. These authors described reduced volumes in the early luteal phase, which directly contrasts with findings reported by Oak and colleagues. Rock and associates evaluated patients during cycle days 8 through 12 and measured no difference in fluid vols in patients with endometriosis compared with that in control subjects. Similar findings were noted by Rezai and associates. Hence, it appears unlikely that fluid volume alone plays a role in the establishment of infertility.

Peritoneal fluid from patients with minimal and mild endometriosis has been shown to increase macrophage proliferation in vitro. In addition, several studies have described increases in total macrophage number in the peritoneal fluid of patients with endometriosis. Hill and coworkers measured significant elevations in total leukocytes, macrophages, helper T cells, lymphocytes, and natural killer cells in women with stages I and II endometriosis. Activated macrophages may affect the reproductive process by altering sperm motility, fimbrial ovum capture, sperm–oocyte interaction, and early embryonic growth. Increased sperm phagocytosis by macrophages has been demonstrated by in vivo animal and in vitro human studies. Suginami and Yano demonstrated the presence of an ovum capture inhibitor in peritoneal fluid from patients with endometriosis, which reduces fimbrial activity for ovum capture in vitro. This macromolecule may prevent contact between the fimbrial cells and cumulus oophorus.

Prostaglandins, interleukins, and other substances produced by macrophages may be harmful to reproduction. Fakih and colleagues demonstrated that interleukin-1 was present in the peritoneal fluid of almost all patients with endometriosis, but not in the fertile control group. Interleukins have been shown to adversely affect mouse embryo growth in vitro. In addition, interleukin-1 stimulated fibroblast proliferation, collagen deposition, and fibrinogen formation; hence, elevated concentrations of such lymphokines may account for the development of fibrosis and adhesions in advanced stages of endometriosis. Interleukin-6 secretion in vitro is up-regulated in ectopic and eutopic endometrial stromal cells from women with endometriosis. Nevertheless, not all studies have confirmed the existence of a difference in interleukin activity between endometriosis patients and control groups. Decreased plasminogen activator activity in endometriotic implants may also be a cause for increased adhesion formation.

Bleeding from ectopic endometrial implants may promote the formation of free oxygen radicals. The iron in hemoglobin may be the catalyst of free radical reactions. Free radicals may damage proteins, carbohydrates, nucleotides, and lipids, resulting in tissue damage and de novo adhesions.

Chronic elevations in the level of peritoneal prostaglandins have been hypothesized to interfere with ovulation, to alter tubal mobility such that the embryo may arrive in the uterus at a suboptimal time for implantation, or to diminish corpus luteum function. Drake and associates measured the metabolites of prostacyclin and thromboxane A_2 in peritoneal fluid and noted a 10-fold increase in these levels in patients with endometriosis. Ylikorkla and colleagues confirmed these observations, although the increase in prostanoid metabolites in the patients with endometriosis was less than twice that of the controls. When cycle stage was experimentally controlled, Rock and coworkers, Rezai and associates, and others failed to demonstrate a significant change in prostaglandin levels in peritoneal fluid from patients with endometriosis as compared with control groups. In addition, prostaglandin concentrations did not vary between the follicular and luteal phase in either endometriosis patients or controls. Variations in collection of samples during the menstrual cycle, selection of control groups, and collection techniques have compromised the interpretation of data regarding the relative importance of prostanoid content in peritoneal fluid in the studies that have been published on this topic.

Alterations in the systemic immune response of endometriosis patients may influence fecundity. Cellular and humoral abnormalities have been reported in the peripheral blood and peritoneal fluid of women with endometriosis. Translocated endometrial cells may implant only in patients with an inherent defect in cell-mediated immunity. Functional changes in monocytes and macrophages, natural killer cells, cytotoxic T lymphocytes, and B cells suggest decreased surveillance, recognition, and destruction of misplaced endometrial cells and possible facilitation of their implantation. The endometrial proteins of menstrual fluid may be recognized as foreign by the host and trigger an autoimmune response. This host reaction can be variable, thus explaining why some women with a weak autoimmune response and varying extent of disease can conceive with no difficulty. Other investigators have confirmed a high prevalence of autoantibodies against endometrial and ovarian tissues in the sera and cervical and vaginal secretions of women with endometriosis. Nonspecific polyclonal B-cell activation has been postulated to exist in endometriosis, but there is a lack of substantive data to demonstrate that this association contributes significantly to endometriosis-associated subfertility.

Dioxin, a pollutant that is known to decrease cell-mediated cytotoxicity by reducing the number of helper T cells, has been suggested as a causative factor in the high incidence of endometriosis in developed countries. Heilier and associates documented an increase in dioxin-like compounds in the serum of women with peritoneal endometriosis and deep endometriotic (adenomyotic) nodules. Moreover, a dose-dependent relation existed between dioxin exposure and the subsequent development and severity of endometriosis in the rhesus monkey after a latent period of more than 5 years.

Nevertheless, other studies have suggested that endometriosis may not be associated with immunologic alterations in the pelvis. In a retrospective analysis of the cell count and volume of peritoneal fluid in 135 infertile women with endometriosis, Haney and colleagues found a negative correlation between total cell numbers and extent of disease and no significant correlation between fluid volume and extent of disease. Similarly, in the rabbit model of endometriosis, there was no difference in peritoneal fluid volume, macrophage numbers, or macrophage activation in treated versus control animals.

Hence, the exact cause-and-effect relation between endometriosis and infertility in the absence of a distortion in pelvic

anatomy remains unknown. In a recent study using an adhesion-free rabbit model of endometriosis, peritoneal implants did not adversely affect the number of corpora lutea, the oocyte recovery or fertilization rates, tubal transport, embryonic development and cleavage, or nidation index. Similarly, Mahmood and Templeton were unable to detect differences in hormonal patterns of the menstrual cycle, follicular growth, preovulatory peritoneal fluid volume and sex steroid concentration, rate of LUF, oocyte maturity, fertilization rate, or cleavage rate between patients with minimal and mild endometriosis and control women.

Little is known about the mechanisms by which endometriosis induces pain symptoms. Dyspareunia may be related to stimulation of pain fibers by stretching of scarred, inelastic tissue or by direct pressure on nodules of endometriosis embedded in fibrotic tissue. Endometriosis implants may secrete inflammatory substances such as prostaglandins, cytokines, and growth factors that initiate the sequence of events that result in the development of pain. Moreover, the extravasated debris and blood from endometriotic implants may stimulate an inflammatory reaction within the peritoneal cavity with production of the aforementioned substances.

DIAGNOSIS

Symptoms

Dysmenorrhea, dyspareunia, and pelvic, back, and rectal pain—the more common symptoms of endometriosis—have been assumed to be caused by endometrial implants. However, the development of such symptoms is not diagnostic of the disease state. In one random survey of women in the general population, more than 60% reported dyspareunia at some point in their lives, and 33% had persistent discomfort. The prevalence of laparoscopically diagnosed endometriosis in patients with chronic pelvic pain has ranged from 4% to 52% in published series. Leibson et al. reported the age of peak diagnosis of endometriosis based on presenting symptom is pelvic pain, age 15 to 24 years; infertility, age 25 to 34 years; and dysfunctional uterine bleeding, age 35 to 44 years.

Some authorities have suggested that the symptoms may be dependent on the location of the implants, the presence of adhesions, distortion of ovarian anatomy by endometriosis, and involvement of other organs, such as the ureter or rectum. However, Fedele and colleagues found no significant association between the American Fertility Society (AFS; now known as the American Society for Reproductive Medicine) classification of stage and the presence and severity of dysmenorrhea, pelvic pain, and dyspareunia in a prospective study of 160 women. The pain profiles of the patients with ovarian lesions were similar to those of the patients with peritoneal or ovarian and peritoneal disease. Conversely, in a later study by the same group, ovarian endometriomas were the only lesions significantly associated with severe dysmenorrhea and pelvic pain in infertile women. In a more recent prospective study of symptoms experienced by women diagnosed with histologically proven endometriomas, Chapron et al. showed no correlation of the intensity of the pain with the size of the endometrioma. In this study, severe pelvic pain was significantly associated with the secondary finding of deeply infiltrating endometriotic lesions.

Koninckx and coworkers demonstrated that the presence of pelvic pain did not correlate with the total area of endometriosis, type of lesion, or volume of disease. The only significant discriminator proved to be the depth of infiltration; endometriotic lesions greater than 1 cm in depth were associated with

IV

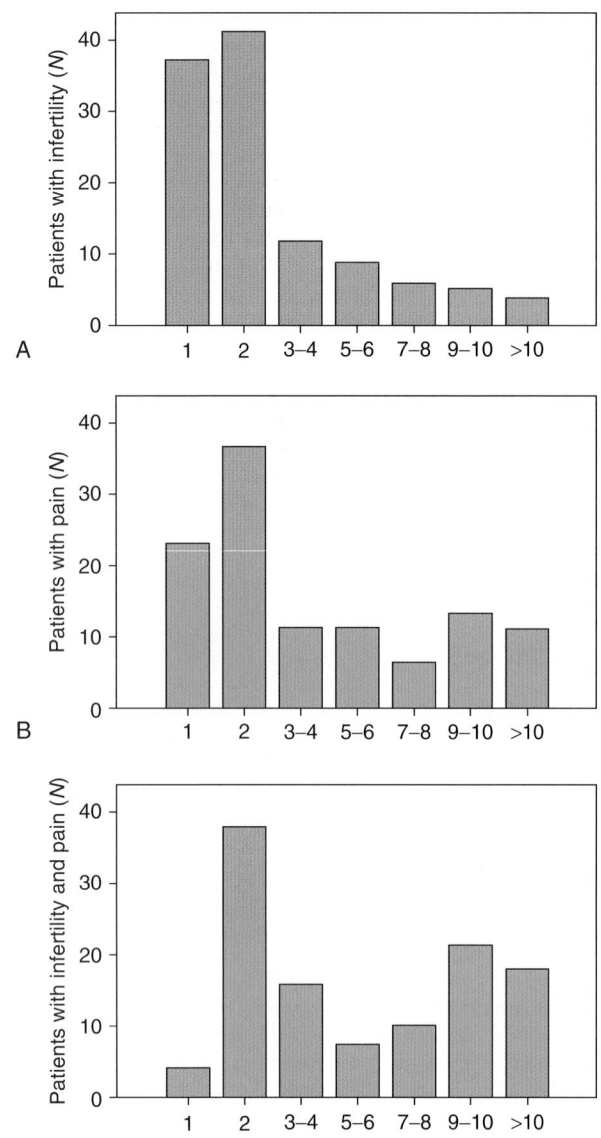

FIGURE 22.2 Frequency distributions of depth of infiltration of pelvic endometriosis in women with (**A**) infertility (N = 283), (**B**) pain (N = 119), or (**C**) infertility and pain (N = 48) (Redrawn with permission from Koninckx PR, Mueleman C, Demeyere S, et al. Suggestive evidence that pelvic endometriosis is a progressive disease, whereas deeply infiltrating endometriosis is associated with pelvic pain. *Fertil Steril* 1991;55:759. Copyright © 1991, Elsevier).

severe discomfort (Fig. 22.2). This supports earlier data that strongly linked pain with deep infiltration of the fibromuscular tissue of the pelvis. Hsu and colleagues found dysuria and midline anterior pain were the only symptoms associated with the location of superficial endometriosis lesions.

Pain symptoms generally correlate with fluctuations in steroid hormone concentrations. In response to cyclic stimulation by ovarian estradiol and progesterone, endometriotic lesions undergo epithelial and stromal proliferation, variable secretory changes, stromal pseudodecidual reaction, and periodic regression in a manner more disorganized than, yet similar to, that of normal endometrium. Surgical castration and ovarian hormonal suppressive therapy result in diminution of pain in most patients.

Physical Findings

Bimanual pelvic examination may reveal tender uterosacral ligaments, cul-de-sac nodularity, induration of the rectovaginal septum, fixed retroversion of the uterus, adnexal masses, and generalized or localized pelvic tenderness. The adherent tube and ovary may constitute a tender, irregular mass that is similar in characteristics to the mass palpated in cases of chronic salpingo-oophoritis. Uterosacral nodules occasionally reach 1 cm or more in size. Lesions implanted in the retrocervical area or rectovaginal wall are frequently more easily felt than seen and can be missed if the physical examination is omitted. A perceptible, painful swelling of the implant before and at menstruation remains a classic and reliable clinical sign of active rectovaginal or retrocervical endometriosis.

Cancer antigen 125 (CA-125), a high molecular weight glycoprotein expressed on the cell surface of some derivatives of embryonic coelomic epithelium, is often elevated toward the end of the luteal phase and during menstruation in patients with AFS stages II to IV endometriosis. Barbieri and colleagues reported that a value higher than 35 U/mL had a positive predictive value of 0.58 and a negative predictive value of 0.96 in establishing the presence of endometriosis. Many other conditions have been associated with an elevated CA-125 concentration, including acute pelvic inflammatory disease, adenomyosis, uterine leiomyoma, menstruation, pregnancy, epithelial ovarian cancer, pancreatitis, and chronic liver disease. Pittaway and colleagues reported that 80% of women with pelvic pain and endometriosis had a CA-125 titer greater than 16 U/mL, whereas only 6% of patients with pelvic pain and without endometriosis had an increased serum concentration of this cell surface antigen.

Increased concentrations of CA-125 and placental protein 14 (PP14) have been related specifically to the presence of endometriotic cysts and deep endometriosis. The results of most studies, however, suggest that CA-125 is not sufficiently sensitive to identify lesser stages of endometriosis and is therefore not reliable as a screening test.

Somigliana and colleagues report transvaginal ultrasonography has high sensitivity (84% to 100%) and specificity (90% to 100%) in identifying ovarian endometriomas as based upon characteristics of low-level, homogeneous internal echoes. Doppler sonographic evaluation of resistance indices in the vessels of adnexal masses increases the sensitivity and negative predictive values of two-dimensional sonography and CA-125, but this yields many false-positive results because of the neovascularity of benign tumors. Magnetic resonance imaging (MRI) may be helpful in assessing deep pelvic and extrapelvic endometriosis, including lesions that involve the bladder, vagina, or sigmoid (Table 22.5). Small studies have indicated that transrectal sonography or rectal endoscopic sonography is useful for detecting rectal wall involvement if performed by a skilled radiologist or gastroenterologist.

Visual Findings

The patient with unexplained lower abdominal pain or a presentation suggesting endometriosis requires laparoscopy for definitive diagnosis. Ultrasonography and other noninvasive procedures cannot provide the specific information needed to diagnose or classify the extent or severity of disease. For proper laparoscopic evaluation, a double puncture technique is essential. The ancillary probe or forceps placed through the lower abdominal sheath permits mobilization of the tubes and ovaries. A methodical regimented approach should be used to thoroughly inspect the lateral sidewalls, all ovarian surfaces, both sides of the broad ligaments, the

TABLE 22.5 Accuracy of MRI for the Diagnosis of Adenomyotic Endometriosis According to Location

LOCATION	SENSITIVITY (%)	SPECIFICITY (%)	ACCURACY (%)
Uterosacral ligaments	76	83	80
Rectovaginal	80	98	97
Rectosigmoid	88	98	95
Bladder	88	99	98
Vagina	76	95	93

From Bazot M, Darai E, Hourani R, et al. Deep pelvic endometriosis: MR imaging for diagnosis and prediction of extension of disease. *Radiology* 2004;232:379, with permission. Copyright © 2004 RSNA.

bladder and bowel serosa, and the inferior aspects of the cul-de-sac. Uterine manipulation with a cannula fixed to the cervix facilitates evaluation of the uterosacral ligaments and rectal serosa. Photography and video recording are useful for documentation of findings.

Awareness of the wide range of visual appearances of endometriosis is necessary for accurate diagnosis and appropriate surgical therapy of the disease. Although darkly pigmented lesions are readily recognizable and are considered a classic presentation of endometriosis, less discernible yet common forms of implants were described as early as the 1920s, when Sampson noted "red raspberries, purple raspberries, blueberries, blebs, and peritoneal pockets." The black or blue puckered "powder-burn" implant is a late consequence of cyclic growth and regression of the lesion, to the point that bleeding and hemosiderin staining of the tissue have occurred. Biopsy of such areas reveals inactive endometrial glands and fibrous stroma.

Distinctive morphologic variations include vesicles, flat plaques, raised lesions, polypoid structures, areas of fibrosis and adhesion formation, and peritoneal defects (Table 22.6). Yellow, brown, blue, or black coloration is proportional to the amount of hemosiderin deposition. Red polypoid lesions share the closest histologic characteristics with native endometrium and are thought to have the greatest metabolic activity, as is suggested by their high concentrations of prostaglandin metabolites. Biopsy of nonpigmented implants (i.e., implants that are the same color as adjacent peritoneum) may reveal active endometriotic glands and stroma. White lesions are predominantly fibromuscular scarring with scattered glandular

and stromal elements, and brown lesions are mainly hemosiderin deposits. Peritoneal defects and subovarian adhesions contain endometriosis in 40% to 70% of cases. Because other peritoneal lesions share morphologic features similar to those of endometriosis, the differential diagnosis is broad and includes old suture locations, epithelial malignancies, endosalpingiosis, hemangioma, inflammatory reaction to infection or oil-based hysterosalpingogram dye, and carbon deposition from laser surgery. Rectovaginal endometriotic lesions consist of smooth muscle with active glandular epithelium and scanty stroma. They share similar characteristics to adenomyomas.

Small endometriotic lesions become more visible during the premenstrual and menstrual phases of the cycle, because during this time, microfoci of peritoneal disease become congested with blood and debris. In addition, vascular dilatation, superficial hemorrhage, and ecchymosis formation cause accentuation of the more typical features of endometriosis. Performance of laparoscopy at a time when ovarian steroidogenesis is suppressed by medications such as GnRH analogues or progestogens can lead to inaccuracies in the assessment of extent of disease.

Jansen and Russell reported the presence of nonpigmented lesions in 38% of their 202 patients with biopsy-proven endometriosis; 15% had only nonpigmented implants. Most areas of pigmented endometriosis are surrounded by nonpigmented endometriosis. These subtle lesions may represent the first stage of development of peritoneal disease. Recognition of nonpigmented endometriosis may be enhanced by "painting" the peritoneum with the patient's blood or by filling the pelvis with irrigation fluid and submerging the laparoscope to appreciate the three-dimensional configuration of clear lesions. Subtle lesions are likely to originate from microscopic glands; they appear and disappear like blebs on the peritoneal surface. With progressive fibrosis, these implants become the classic pigmented, scarred lesions, and finally, when fibrosis replaces the stroma, they appear as white, inactive disease.

The ability to detect subtle lesions of endometriosis increases with the experience of the surgeon and is reinforced by histologic confirmation. Although depth perception is impaired when the monocular lens of the laparoscope is used to view the pelvic cavity, the magnification ability of this lens when closely approximated to the peritoneum may allow identification of subtle surface irregularities present in occult disease. Magnification up to 10× power can be obtained with the laparoscope, depending on the working distance. Microscopic implants of endometriosis not visible even with 10× magnification have been documented by scanning electron microscopy in peritoneal biopsies of patients with unexplained infertility who had no evidence of disease at the time of laparoscopy. A scanning electron microscopy study of samples of supposedly normal tissue from endometriosis patients has documented the presence of endometriotic foci in 25% of cases. Lesions as

TABLE 22.6 Histologic Confirmation of Lesions Categorized by Appearance

INVESTIGATORS	CONFIRMATION BY APPEARANCE (%)						
	BLACK	WHITE	RED	GLANDULAR	SUBOVARIAN ADHESIONS	YELLOW-BROWN PATCHES	POCKETS
Jansen and Russell (1986)	—	81	81	67	50	47	47
Stripling et al. (1988)	97	91	75	—	—	33	—
Martin et al. (1989)	94	80	75	66	39	22	39

small as 200 μm have been identified through this technique. Hence, surgical treatment of all visible disease is more accurately described as cytoreductive rather than ablative.

An ovarian endometrial cyst is usually formed by an inversion of the ovarian cortex. The frontal surface of the ovary in proximity to the hilus is the most common site for the invagination process to occur. Repetitive bleeding from the endometrial implants on the surface of the ovary may promote the growth of such lesions. Alternatively, invaginated epithelial inclusions may form endometriomas through coelomic metaplasia. Adhesions are common from the ovary to the fossa ovarica or to the posterior leaf of the parametrium.

Preoperative sonographic evaluation is a useful screening test for the presence of small endometrial cysts; their identification may affect the disease categorization to which the patient is assigned. Sonographic patterns may indicate purely cystic features, cystic features with few septations or minimal debris, complex combinations of cystic and solid elements, and largely solid features. More recently, fat-saturated MRI has been shown to be an acceptable tool for detecting endometriomas larger than 4 mm in diameter.

An adnexal mass in a patient with known pelvic endometriosis cannot be assumed to be an endometrial cyst of the ovary. Ovarian malignancy must remain in the differential diagnosis; the size of the mass has been correlated with malignancy. In a study of 180 women, 1% of masses smaller than 5 cm, 11% of masses between 5 and 10 cm, and 72% of masses larger than 10 cm were malignant. Most of these malignant tumors were adenocarcinoma.

The rules that apply to the management of all women in whom an adnexal mass develops also apply to patients with endometriosis with an adnexal mass. Among women of reproductive age, unilateral adnexal masses that are cystic and unilocular with regular borders on ultrasound examination are likely to be benign, whereas masses with solid areas, septa, papillations, or irregular borders have a greater likelihood of being malignant. Endometriomas vary in their appearance but usually have regular borders and slightly thickened and diffuse internal echoes unless fresh hemorrhage is present. Sensitivity and specificity of transvaginal ultrasound have been reported by Eskenazi and colleagues to be 84% to 100% and 90% to 100%, respectively.

Recognition of deep ovarian endometriosis is necessary for correct surgical staging. Small endometriomas were diagnosed in 48% of infertile women with mildly enlarged ovaries (3.5 to 5 cm in diameter) when the ovaries were punctured with a 16-gauge needle. The ovarian surfaces were without gross disease in this series of patients. Deep ovarian endometriosis is frequently associated with the presence of intestinal or more extensive pelvic disease.

Vercellini and colleagues studied the visual diagnostic parameters of ovarian endometriomas at laparotomy in 245 women with ovarian cysts. The gross characteristics that established the diagnosis included a size smaller than 12 cm in diameter; adhesions to the pelvic sidewall, to the posterior broad ligament, or to both; the presence of powder-burn lesions; superficial endometriosis with adjacent puckering on the surface of the ovary; and tarry, thick, chocolate-colored fluid content. These criteria yielded a sensitivity of 97%, a specificity of 95%, and an accuracy of 96%.

The depth of peritoneal infiltration by endometriosis cannot be evaluated by inspection alone. Deep endometriosis, which is almost exclusively localized to the posterior cul-de-sac and the uterosacral ligaments, is better detected by palpation and becomes even more apparent during excision. Deep endometriosis has been recognized to become smaller with increasing depth, although in some women, the largest volume

is hidden under an adhesion involving the bowel or is buried in the rectovaginal septum. Diagnosis is enhanced if clinical examinations are performed during menstruation in women with chronic pelvic pain, severe dysmenorrhea, or deep dyspareunia. In most cases, a nodule is more palpable at this time.

Koninckx and Martin have described three types of infiltrating endometriosis. Type I is characterized by a large pelvic area of typical or subtle lesions surrounded by white sclerotic tissue. During excision, deep disease becomes obvious and grows progressively smaller with deeper sectioning of tissue (like a cone). Type II is formed by retraction of the bowel and is recognized clinically as a small classic lesion associated with retraction. In some women, no implant is visible, but induration is associated with the retraction. Excision usually reveals the presence of a nodule. Type III is nodular endometriosis of the rectovaginal septum. This category is clinically suspected at the time of rectovaginal examination when painful nodularities are noted. Occasionally, nodular endometriosis presents as small, typical lesions at laparoscopy or as dark blue cysts at the vaginal fornix during speculum examination. Type III disease is the most severe and often spreads laterally to involve the ureter.

CLASSIFICATIONS

Many endometriosis classification systems have been introduced to allow direct comparison of patient responses to medical and surgical treatments and to identify factors predictive of disease outcome. No system has yet been devised that is entirely satisfactory. The AFS (renamed the American Society for Reproductive Medicine) organized a panel of experts in 1979 to develop a classification system that might serve as a basis for evaluating various therapies. The committee devised an innovative scheme based on the natural progression of the disease. Three anatomic areas—the peritoneum, ovary, and fallopian tube—were examined for the presence of endometriosis or adhesions, with allowances made for unilateral involvement. However, the system was not weighted for depth of infiltration of peritoneal implants. A point system instead assigned values to each area of disease involvement based on the presumption that implant area and adhesion characteristics were most often associated with disease prognosis. The stage of disease was determined by the cumulative score of the assigned points. This classification system was criticized for its arbitrary division of endometriosis into categories that did not necessarily reflect the true relative risk of disease sequelae, pain, and infertility.

The AFS classification was revised in 1985 to provide a more standard assessment of endometriosis for correlation of surgical treatment with distribution and severity of implants (Table 22.7). The point range of mild disease was expanded, and greater weight was given to deep endometriosis, dense adhesions, and cul-de-sac obliteration by adhesive disease. Although the revised staging system appropriately acknowledges the importance of adhesive disease and endometriomas, most women with extensive peritoneal disease in the absence of ovarian involvement, particularly deeply invasive implants, receive a very low score on laparoscopic inspection of the lesions.

This revised AFS classification has been widely used by investigators to categorize disease states. Nevertheless, direct comparison of treatment outcome is compromised by inconsistencies in the application of the staging criteria and by the great variations in medical and surgical therapeutic options being applied in the management of endometriosis. Evaluation of the extent of disease by laparoscopy may be limited by a lack of recognition of atypical implants, particularly if the patient is hypoestrogenic as a result of recent discontinuation of medical therapy for endometriosis. Furthermore, the divisions between stages of endometriosis remained arbitrary, the

TABLE 22.7 The American Society for Reproductive Medicine Revised Classification of Endometriosis[a]

ENDOMETRIOSIS	<1 CM	1–3 CM	>3 CM
Peritoneum			
Superficial	1	2	4
Deep	2	4	6
Ovary			
Right superficial	1	2	4
Right deep	4	16	20
Left superficial	1	2	4
Left deep	4	16	20
Posterior		Partial	Complete
Cul-de-sac			
Obliteration		4	40
Adhesions	<1/3 enclosure	1/3–2/3 enclosure	>2/3 enclosure
Ovary			
Right filmy	1	2	4
Right dense	4	8	16
Left filmy	1	2	4
Left dense	4	8	16
Tube			
Right filmy	1	2	4
Right dense	4[b]	8[b]	16
Left filmy	1	2	4
Left dense	4[b]	8[b]	16

[a]Determination of the stage or degree of endometrial involvement is based on a weighted point system. The following categories have been established: stage I (minimal disease) 1–5 points, stage II (mild disease) 6–15 points, stage III (moderate disease) 16–40 points, and stage IV (severe disease) >40 points.
[b]If the fimbriated end of the fallopian tube is completely enclosed, change the point assignment to 16.

point score for ovarian involvement was weighted too heavily, and the classification scheme did not address disease involving the fallopian tubes, intestines, or urinary tract. Also, there were no parameters to indicate the present activity and state of evolution of the disease.

The Endometriosis Classification Subcommittee of the American Society for Reproductive Medicine (ASRM) released new recommendations in 1996 for the documentation of the extent and location of disease. One concern over the reproducibility of the scoring system was directed at the variability in assessing ovarian endometriosis and cul-de-sac obliteration. The subcommittee indicated that an endometriotic cyst should be confirmed by histology or by the presence of the following features: (a) cyst diameter less than 12 cm, (b) adhesion to pelvic sidewall and/or broad ligament, (c) endometriosis on the surface of the ovary, and (d) tarry, thick, chocolate-colored fluid content. Cul-de-sac obliteration should be considered partial if some normal peritoneum is visible below the uterosacral ligaments, but adhesions or endometriosis has obliterated part of the cul-de-sac. Complete obliteration exists when no peritoneum is visible below the uterosacral ligaments. Because information is accumulating to suggest that the morphologic appearance of the endometriotic implants may correlate with biologic activity and consequently fertility, the newly revised classification scheme requests the categorization of lesions as red, white, and black. The percentage of surface involvement of each implant type is to be documented.

This revised ASRM classification system is oriented toward the infertile population. Muzii and colleagues, using a pain questionnaire administered to women before surgery, found a significant correlation between the severity of dysmenorrhea and total revised ASRM score, partial score for deep disease, and partial score for adhesions. However, they found no correlation between the pain score for dysmenorrhea and the partial score for superficial disease, number of typical and atypical implants, or the total number of implants. Limited knowledge of the specific pathophysiologic alterations by which endometriosis can cause these symptoms has so far prevented any precise categorization of disease based on response to conventional therapies for these symptoms.

The Enzian classification was developed in 2005 and subsequently revised in 2010 and 2011 to provide a means to characterize deeply infiltrating endometriosis, retroperitoneal structures, and the involvement of other organs. In 2003, Haas et al. observed a correlation was observed between the rASRM severity grade and the location of lesions in the Enzian classification, and pain and dysmenorrhea correlated strongly with the Enzian staging system score. The Enzian classification has thus far not been widely accepted and applied in clinical settings outside of Europe.

THERAPIES

Although women with endometriosis can present with a range of symptoms, therapy is usually initiated for the correction of pain, infertility, or a persistent pelvic mass. Pain and infertility can coexist in a patient; nevertheless, many women with endometriosis-associated infertility have relatively little or no discomfort. Treatment options vary depending on the clinical history and findings at the time of surgery.

Expectant Management

Treatment of mild and moderate endometriosis with hormonal preparations does not offer any advantage over expectant management in promoting conception in women with infertility. A Cochrane review of 13 randomized controlled trials that included almost 800 infertile women with endometriosis found no evidence that medications that suppressed ovulation were superior to placebo in women who wished to conceive. In studies by Seibel and colleagues, Hull and associates, and Telimaa, patients assigned to expectant management conceived earlier than the medically treated group, and the cumulative pregnancy rate was not higher for women receiving progestogens or danazol. This lack of enhancement of fecundity may be related to the lower number of estrogen, progesterone, and androgen receptors in endometriotic lesions as compared with normal endometrium. Nevertheless, patients who have pelvic pain or dysmenorrhea and minimal or mild disease do benefit from hormonal therapy.

The age of the patient and the duration of her infertility are important factors to consider in determining the appropriate therapy for the symptomatic individual. Laparoscopic laser ablation of milder stages of endometriosis appears to lessen the interval to conception, although the cumulative pregnancy rate may not be greater than that of women managed expectantly. Surgical therapy for more advanced disease results in a higher pregnancy rate than does expectant management or hormonal treatment, partly because of correction of mechanical factors that may be inhibiting ovulation or tubal function.

There is no direct evidence to support the contention that surgical treatment of minimal or mild endometriosis in the asymptomatic patient will hinder future disease progression and sequelae. The potential benefits of cytoreductive therapy must be weighed against the risk of adhesion formation through surgical devitalization of peritoneal surfaces.

Medical Treatment

Mild pain symptoms associated with endometriosis may be effectively treated with nonsteroidal anti-inflammatory agents and oral contraceptives (Fig. 22.3). Additional endocrinologic therapies include progestogens, GnRH agonists, and danazol.

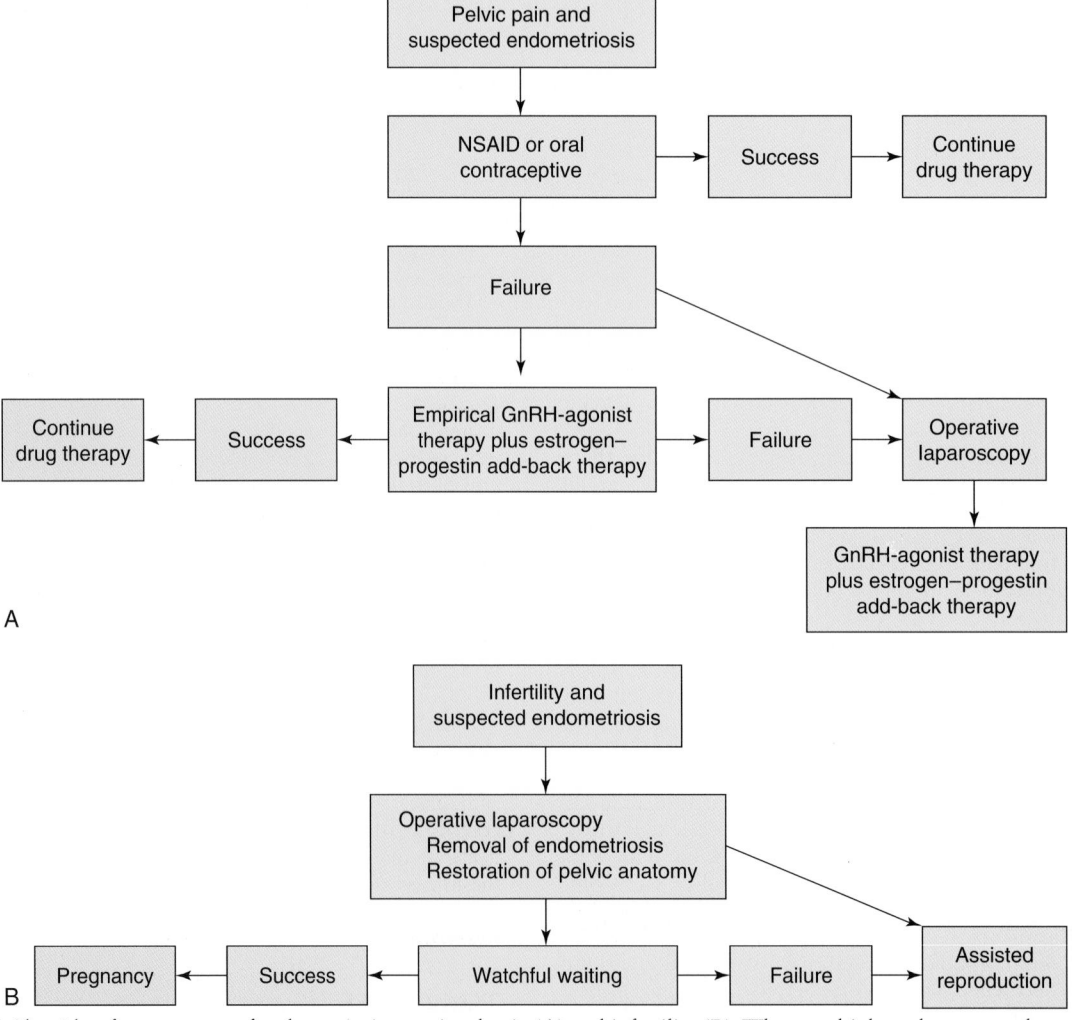

FIGURE 22.3 Algorithm for treatment of endometriosis-associated pain (**A**) and infertility (**B**). Where multiple pathways are shown, the path is guided by medical judgment and patient preference. In the infertility pathway, some practitioners dispense with the operative laparoscopy and recommend assisted reproductive technologies directly (From Olive DL, Pritts EA. Drug therapy: treatment of endometriosis. *N Engl J Med* 2001;345:267, with permission. Copyright © 2001, Massachusetts Medical Society).

These agents have similar degrees of efficacy in the relief of pain symptoms; side effects vary depending on their mechanism of action. At restoration of ovulation and of physiologic levels of estrogen, both eutopic and ectopic endometria resume metabolic activity. Therefore, medical therapy is symptomatic rather than curative, and most patients experience pain relapse at suspension of treatment.

Progestogens

By inhibiting the pituitary release of LH, progestogens suppress ovarian steroidogenesis and promote endometrial glandular atrophy, apoptosis, and extensive decidual transformation of the stroma. Progestogens oppose the growth-promoting effects of estrogens on the endometrial tissue by altering the clearance of the nuclear estrogen receptor and inducing 17β-hydroxysteroid dehydrogenase, which converts estradiol to the weaker estrone. Moreover, by eliminating cyclic bleeding and suppressing uterine contractility, progestogens prevent reflux menstruation, a potential stimulus for continued endometriosis development. Progestogens may prevent implantation and growth of regurgitated endometrium by inhibiting the expression of matrix metalloproteinase and plasminogen activators. Moreover, progestogens have anti-inflammatory properties.

Luciano and colleagues administered medroxyprogesterone acetate, 50 mg daily for 4 months, to symptomatic women with moderate-to-severe endometriosis. Improvement of pain, pelvic nodularity, and tenderness on examination occurred in 80% of patients. Twenty percent of women experienced breakthrough bleeding, and an additional 10% reported persistent cyclic bleeding. Minor weight gain, edema, and increased irritability were other described side effects, which were generally well tolerated. A lower daily dose of 30 mg may provide equivalent relief of symptoms. Bergqvist and Theorell administered this dose to patients for 6 months and found a similar improvement in quality-of-life scores as that achieved with the GnRH agonist nafarelin. Compared with the cost of GnRH agonists and danazol, which are the other commonly prescribed agents, the low cost of the medroxyprogesterone acetate is a notable advantage.

Norethindrone acetate, a 19-nortestosterone progestin, has been shown to be effective in achieving amenorrhea and controlling disease symptoms, even with rectovaginal endometriosis. When used to treat moderate or severe pelvic pain after unsuccessful conservative surgery for symptomatic rectovaginal endometriosis, a dose of 3.5 mg per day for 12 months resulted in a 73% satisfaction rate (33/45). In 2005, Vercellini and colleagues reported a substantial reduction in dysmenorrhea, deep dyspareunia, nonmenstrual pelvic pain, and dyschezia scores. Low-dose norethindrone acetate could be considered an effective, tolerable, and inexpensive first-choice medical alternative to repeat surgery in those with recurrent pain. More recently, Vercellini et al. compared the effect of conservative surgery at laparoscopy with daily oral norethindrone acetate 2.5 mg per day. The progestin group took longer to respond to therapy, but the laparoscopy group started to experience a return of symptoms before the end of the study. At 12 months, surgery and progestin therapy were equally effective in the treatment of deep dyspareunia in women with rectovaginal endometriosis, whereas medical therapy performed significantly better than excisional treatment in those without deeply infiltrating lesions (33% vs. 63%; adjusted odds ratio [OR], 0.23; 95% confidence interval [CI], 0.07 to 0.76; $P = 0.02$).

A similar response rate can be obtained with megestrol acetate. Doses of 40 mg per day for up to 24 months resulted in significant relief of dysmenorrhea, noncyclic pelvic pain, and dyspareunia in 86% of subjects.

Parenteral depot medroxyprogesterone acetate has also been used to produce long periods of amenorrhea and elicit direct progestational changes of the endometrial tissue. A regimen of 150 mg intramuscularly every 3 months for 1 year has been used to manage endometriosis patients with moderate-to-severe pelvic pain. Twenty-nine of 40 subjects (72.5%) were satisfied with their pain relief after 1 year of therapy. An alternative regimen is 104 mg subcutaneously every 3 months. Frequent breakthrough bleeding can be troublesome to correct.

The rate of recurrence of symptomatic endometriosis after progestogen therapy appears to be related to the length of follow-up. Riva and colleagues reported an 18% rate after an average of 11 months, whereas Moghissi and Boyce described a 42% recurrence rate during a 2-year interval after discontinuation of medication.

Cyclic administration of low-dose oral contraceptive pills may result in relief of pelvic pain, particularly cramping associated with menstruation. This line of therapy should be considered for the woman with mild symptoms who is not attempting to conceive. A randomized, controlled trial by Harada and colleagues showed the superiority of combined oral contraceptives over placebo in decreasing baseline pain scores for dysmenorrhea (by 45% to 52% vs. 14% to 17%) and the volume of ovarian endometriomas (by 48% vs. 32%). Long-term continuous oral contraceptive use has been proposed for women with symptomatic endometriosis and menstruation-related pain who have failed a cyclic pill regimen. With such a regimen, the endometrium remains thin on sonogram studies, and endometriotic plaques subjected to a progestin-dominant pill are less active and usually less painful and will undergo apoptosis.

Low-dose (20 to 35 mg ethinyl estradiol) combination oral contraceptives may be given daily for 6 to 9 months without break to relieve pain or more severe dysmenorrhea. The dose may be increased to two or more tablets per day for several days to alleviate episodes of breakthrough bleeding. In a study by Vercellini and colleagues in 2003, 80% (40/50) of patients were satisfied or very satisfied with continuous use of an oral contraceptive containing ethinyl estradiol (0.02 mg) and desogestrel (0.15 mg) for 2 years, and 96% experienced pain relief, although spotting and breakthrough bleeding were frequent side effects.

The levonorgestrel intrauterine device (IUD) has proven effective in relieving pelvic pain symptoms caused by peritoneal and rectovaginal endometriosis and in reducing the risk of recurrence of dysmenorrhea after conservative surgery. In a study by Lockhat and colleagues, an improvement in symptoms was observed in 96% throughout the 36 months of use, with only 11% experiencing pain symptoms at 18 months. A recent randomized study by Tanmahasamut showed that the immediate postoperative placement of a levonorgestrel-releasing IUD after conservative surgery significantly prevented recurrence of moderate-to-severe dysmenorrhea, pelvic pain, and dyspareunia and improved the quality-of-life scores of the patients in the treatment group at 1 year postlaparoscopy. The progestogen released by the IUD is rapidly absorbed by the subendometrial vascular network, which reduces menstrual flow by 70% to 90%.

Danazol

Danazol is a synthetic (2,3-isoxazole) derivative of 17α-ethinyl testosterone that was introduced into clinical practice by Greenblatt and colleagues in 1971 after good performance in uncontrolled trials. The drug gained rapid acceptance because of its effectiveness in relieving pain associated with endometriosis and in enhancing fertility. All of the progestational and

IV

the weak androgenic effects of the drug result from retention of the methyl group in the 19 position of the steroid nucleus, whereas the oral activity of danazol is ascribed to the ethinyl group at position 17.

The pharmacologic action of danazol is complex. By directly inhibiting GnRH secretion, the midcycle LH surge is ablated, although basal gonadotropin concentrations are maintained. The drug interacts with endometrial androgen and progesterone receptors, suppresses the activity of multiple enzymes necessary for ovarian and adrenal steroidogenesis, and displaces androgens from sex hormone–binding globulin, thereby augmenting androgen action on endometrial receptors. The decline in sex hormone–binding globulin induced by danazol lowers estradiol binding, increases estradiol clearance, and promotes a decline in the circulating level of this hormone. Hence, the derivative has direct androgenic and antiprogestational action on endometrial implants and creates a hypoestrogenic, hypoprogestational environment antagonistic to endometriosis. Moreover, by producing amenorrhea, danazol prevents peritoneal seeding of refluxed endometrial tissue. In addition, danazol is capable of suppressing elevated autoantibodies in several autoimmune diseases and has been shown to decrease immunoglobulin and autoantibody levels in women with endometriosis. In contrast to GnRH agonists, danazol use maintains a normal estrogenic state and increases bone mineral density over baseline.

The adverse effects of danazol reflect its anabolic, androgenic, and antiestrogenic properties and may be dose related. Weight gain, muscle cramps, decreased breast size, and vasomotor symptoms are noted in 50% or more of patients maintained on doses of 400 to 800 mg per day. In Buttram's 1985 series, 41% of patients treated with the standard dose of 800 mg per day gained more than 10 pounds during the course of therapy. The threefold increase in free testosterone can cause acne, oily skin, and deepening of the voice in a small percentage of recipients. High-density lipoprotein (HDL) cholesterol declines by 50% or more in response to the altered steroid concentrations; an 80% decrease in the HDL_2 subfraction has been reported. Most series have described a concomitant increase in low-density lipoprotein (LDL) cholesterol; the alteration in the ratio of HDL to LDL cholesterol may be an unacceptable risk to some patients. Because danazol is metabolized by the liver, modest elevations in serum glutamic oxaloacetic transaminase and serum glutamate pyruvate transaminase may arise. Reported idiopathic drug reactions include gastrointestinal disturbances, weakness, dizziness, skin rashes, headaches, and muscle cramps. Bothersome side effects occur in as many as 85% of patients, and at least 10% of women receiving danazol discontinue pharmacologic treatment because the adverse effects are intolerable. Combining danazol therapy with aerobic exercise appears to reduce the incidence of many of these androgenic side effects. Preliminary data from trials using danazol vaginal rings and insertion of daily 200 mg vaginal tablets suggest that this route of administration may result in symptomatic improvement of pain while avoiding the androgenic side effects noted with oral administration.

Because of the potential androgenic action of this hormone on the developing fetus, the patient must not be pregnant when initiating therapy. Barrier contraception has been recommended for the entire course of treatment to eliminate the possibility of conception, although high doses of danazol usually cause anovulation.

The amenorrhea induced by danazol has been found to benefit patients with dysmenorrhea, dyspareunia, and cyclic pelvic pain associated with endometriosis. Young and

Blackmore reviewed the effects of different dosages of oral danazol with respect to relief of symptoms in 452 patients. At a dose of 800 mg, 95% of patients noted relief of dysmenorrhea, and 89% reported relief of pelvic pain. At a dose of 400 mg, posttherapeutic relief was reduced by 10%. Moore and associates reported that pain associated with minimal and moderate pelvic endometriosis appeared to respond well to doses of danazol of 400 mg or less per day, whereas severe endometriosis was best treated with doses greater than 400 mg per day. A 6-year prospective study that evaluated the effectiveness of danazol at two doses (400 and 800 mg) in carefully classified patients concluded that there was no difference in side effects between the two doses and that gross resolutions of disease at second-look laparoscopy were similar. However, ovarian endometriosis greater than 1 cm did not respond as well to either dose of danazol as did peritoneal or ovarian disease less than 1 cm.

Recurrence of pain symptoms within 4 to 12 months of discontinuation of danazol therapy approached 50% in most studies. Lower daily doses of medication or courses of treatment less than 4 months in duration may result in a shorter symptom-free interval.

Clinical trials designed to assess the efficacy of medical therapy of minimal, mild, and moderate stages of disease refute the notion that danazol may enhance conception. Furthermore, conception is delayed while the patient is receiving danazol.

Gonadotropin-Releasing Hormone Agonists

Gonadotropin-releasing hormone (GnRH) agonists are available for use in the treatment of estrogen-dependent diseases such as endometriosis. Some of the more frequently studied analogues include leuprolide, nafarelin, buserelin, and goserelin. Alteration of the amino acid at position 6 and ethylamide replacement of the C-terminal amino acid of the native decapeptide hormone results in a GnRH agonist with increased resistance to lysosomal degradation. Pituitary receptor binding is enhanced, resulting in a decline in the number of receptors available for further occupancy. Continued administration of the GnRH agonist leads to a desensitization of the pituitary gonadotrope receptor and a reversible down-regulation of the pituitary–ovarian axis. Ovarian estrogen secretion may reach castrate levels.

The initial response to GnRH agonist administration is a markedly increased secretion of pituitary stores of follicle-stimulating hormone (FSH) and LH. If therapy is begun in the follicular phase of the menstrual cycle, the developing follicle may respond to the flare in circulating gonadotropin levels with a rapid increase in estradiol production. Estradiol levels may remain elevated for 3 weeks before declining. GnRH agonist administration in the luteal phase leads to a more rapid decline in estrogen secretion, although FSH and LH levels remain elevated for 1 and 4 weeks, respectively.

Gonadotropin-releasing hormone agonist treatment results in improvement or resolution of pain symptoms in all stages of disease. Lemay and colleagues reported resolution of pain in 70% and improvement in discomfort in 15% of 24 subjects after 2 to 4 months of treatment with the agonist buserelin. Dyspareunia improved in 9% and disappeared in 91% of patients studied. The depot formulation of leuprolide acetate has also been shown to significantly reduce dysmenorrhea, pelvic pain, and pelvic tenderness in patients with endometriosis.

Henzl and associates, in a double-blind, multicenter study, treated 213 patients with either danazol or nafarelin. After 6 months of treatment, more than 80% of patients in all groups experienced a significant reduction in visible implants. A 43% reduction in AFS score was noted for each treatment group; there was no difference in response among patients receiving the 0.4- and 0.8-mg daily dose of nafarelin. Most patients continued to demonstrate some visible implants at the time of follow-up laparoscopy, and, as with danazol, there was some diminution in size of endometriomas but no effect on preexisting adhesions.

The optimal interval of GnRH analogue administration has been widely debated. Six months of medication has been traditionally prescribed, although a significant reduction in implant volume occurs as early as 2 weeks after initiation of treatment in the rat model. A maximal effect was measured after 4 weeks of therapy in this animal study, suggesting that short courses of drug may be as efficacious as 6 months of continuous therapy. The regrowth of lesions after estrogen therapy has been reported years after the menopause; hence, hypoestrogenism results in inactivation rather than resolution of the disease.

Response to therapy may be dependent on route of administration. Donnez and colleagues reported that buserelin administration by a long-acting subcutaneous implant led to a greater reduction in endometriosis score, mitotic index, and endometrial cyst diameter than when given in an intranasal form. This may have been due to a greater consistency in hormonal release by the injected preparation.

As occurs with danazol and progestogen regimens, symptoms recur at variable periods after discontinuation of GnRH analogue therapy. Subjective return of pain occurred in 57% of patients within 6 months of discontinuing leuprolide, although 37% with moderate or severe pelvic pain at baseline were still improved at 1 year. Franssen and colleagues noted a lasting and significant amelioration of dysmenorrhea and dyspareunia 6 months after completion of treatment; however, scores for chronic pelvic pain had nearly reached their pretreatment level once this time had elapsed. Patients with a higher disease stage at the onset are more likely to experience recurrence and to experience it earlier than patients with minimal disease. One treatment option for such patients may be a second 3-month course of GnRH analogue. Henzl reported a significant decrease in mean pain scores and essentially no change in compact bone density in most patients when nafarelin was readministered for 3 months after a treatment-free interval of 6 months or more.

Most of the side effects associated with GnRH analogue therapy are related to hypoestrogenism. Hot flashes are common and can lead to sleep disturbances and chronic fatigue in extreme cases. Vaginal dryness, superficial dyspareunia, headaches, and depression have been reported. In general, these adverse effects are better tolerated than those experienced with danazol use. In addition, there are no undesirable changes in HDL, LDL, or total cholesterol throughout the prolonged period of hypoestrogenism induced by GnRH analogue, unlike the changes accompanying danazol intake.

A decline in trabecular bone mineral content and an increase in urinary calcium excretion to menopausal levels occur during the course of GnRH analogue therapy in approximately two thirds of patients. Quantitated computed tomographic (CT) studies consistently show significant loss of trabecular bone of the vertebrae and hip with GnRH analogue exposure. Restoration of normal estrogen production after cessation of therapy appears to at least partially reverse these bone changes. In a study of the GnRH agonist goserelin, an 8.2% decline in density of the lumbar spine was measured after completion of 6 months of treatment; this improved to a mean loss of 5.4% at 6 month after cessation. Others found no significant change from baseline after a 6-month course of GnRH analogue when bone density was assessed 6 months after treatment.

Concomitant administration of a progestogen during the course of GnRH analogue therapy has been examined to ameliorate vasomotor symptoms and retard both urinary calcium excretion and radiologic evidence of loss of bone mineral density. Cedars and coworkers reported a diminution in the side effects mentioned earlier when medroxyprogesterone acetate was administered at a dose of 20 to 30 mg per day during the 6-month course of agonist therapy; however, laparoscopic evaluation after completion of therapy failed to reveal any improvement or suppression of active endometriosis with the combination regimen, and the regimen failed to significantly reduce symptoms of pelvic pain. Conversely, Makarainen and colleagues reported that medroxyprogesterone acetate, 100 mg per day, diminished hot flashes and the urinary excretion of calcium in women treated with goserelin acetate, 3.6 mg monthly, for 6 months. Second-look laparoscopy revealed equivalent diminution in extent of endometriosis when compared with the goserelin–progestin placebo group.

Norethindrone, the 19-nortestosterone progestin, has been shown to suppress both the painful symptoms of endometriosis and the extent of disease at laparoscopy when used in daily doses of 1.4 to 10 mg during GnRH agonist therapy. A randomized, double-blind study has demonstrated that GnRH agonist therapy may be safely and effectively extended for up to 1 year in the management of endometriosis-associated pelvic pain when prescribed in conjunction with low-dose sex steroid hormones. Hornstein et al. reported that norethindrone acetate, 5 mg, alone or in combination with conjugated equine estrogens, 0.625 mg daily, from the onset of depot leuprolide acetate therapy alleviated hypoestrogenic symptoms and preserved bone density while resulting in equivalent pain relief to that achieved by the placebo estrogen–progestin patient group. Others have treated a limited number of patients with a similar regimen for up to 10 years without detecting an adverse effect on bone mineral density. For women with relapse of endometriosis-associated pain, GnRH agonist with "add-back" progestin or progestin/estrogen therapy provides patients with a better quality of life than GnRH analogue alone or oral contraceptive regimens.

The addition of calcium carbonate and alendronate or etidronate sodium, which are organic bisphosphonates, to the low-dose norethindrone acetate add-back therapy in patients with symptomatic endometriosis receiving prolonged GnRH agonist treatment may further minimize the adverse side effects of hypoestrogenism.

In a review of randomized clinical trials of the Cochrane Menstrual Disorders and Subfertility Group register, there was no difference in pain relief between GnRHas, levonorgestrel, and danazol. Additional controlled studies will better establish the optimal medical management of this condition.

Conservative Surgery

Surgery is indicated for correction of pain, infertility, or other symptoms in patients with extensive pelvic endometriosis or when hormonal manipulation fails to adequately diminish pain symptoms in women with lesser stages of disease. Surgery is successful in relieving pain in a very high percentage of cases and offers a better prognosis for pregnancy than does endocrine therapy in many cases of advanced disease.

The surgeon who has mastered the specialized techniques of operative laparoscopy can treat a wide range of pathologic findings at the time of diagnosis. Therapeutic planning depends on many factors, including the age of the patient, her desire for fertility or pain relief, the duration and intensity of her symptoms, the extent of disease, and previous treatments that have been undertaken. Preoperative rectoscopy–sigmoidoscopy and intravenous pyelography are recommended in patients with

IV

symptoms suggestive of deeply invasive endometriosis of the posterior cul-de-sac and rectovaginal septum. Magnetic resonance imaging or sonography may also be helpful in predicting the extension of disease (Table 22.5).

The decision of whether to perform surgical resection of endometriosis through the laparoscope or open abdomen is not entirely dependent on the stage of disease that is encountered. Laparoscopy can be considered for all cases unless there is difficulty in establishing the appropriate tissue planes of dissection or unless improved access is necessary for atraumatic manipulation of the involved organs. Specific endoscopic procedures include ablation of endometriotic implants, adhesiolysis, ovarian cystectomy, oophorectomy, and salpingectomy. Although the results and complications are similar, the cost savings with respect to decreased hospital expenses and loss of work time favor laparoscopy over laparotomy when other factors regarding risks and outcome are equal. Laparoscopy provides superior visualization of the posterior cul-de-sac and allows a high degree of magnification of peritoneal surfaces, which aids in the identification of subtle disease.

Conservative resection of disease by laparotomy is most valuable in cases of extensive, dense pelvic adhesions, or endometriomas greater than 5 cm in diameter. In addition, deep involvement of the rectovaginal septum with fibrotic extension into the perirectal fossa, invasion of the bowel muscularis, and endometriotic infiltration in the region of the uterine vessels and ureter is generally best approached through the open abdomen for all but advanced endoscopic surgeons. The objective of the laparotomy procedure is complete excision of all endometriosis and associated adhesive disease to restore normal functional anatomy of the reproductive tract. The usual surgical approach is through a transverse suprapubic incision. A Maylard incision provides adequate exposure for presacral neurectomy and reconstructive surgery of ovarian endometriomas of almost any size.

Principles of Microsurgery

Microsurgical technique, or the philosophy of gentle manipulation of tissue in an attempt to avoid trauma, is the major tenet of pelvic reconstruction. The inflammation, trauma, coagulation, and foreign materials associated with conventional macrosurgical technique lead to tissue ischemia and adhesion formation because of local failure of the intrinsic peritoneal fibrinolytic system. Adhesion formation can be reduced by the application of loupe magnification or use of the operating microscope; reconstruction with fine, nonreactive sutures; precise hemostasis; and frequent irrigation of tissues with warmed lactated Ringer solution. Nevertheless, there are no definitive data to suggest that use of the particularly costly ancillary laser and the operating microscope has appreciably improved the reproductive prognosis in the surgical management of endometriosis through laparotomy. The magnification provided by laparoscopy in a closed surgical field matches these microsurgical principles.

Several basic techniques are available for the endoscopic ablation of endometriosis, including excision, coagulation, and vaporization. Coagulation can be achieved by monopolar or bipolar cautery, thermocoagulation, or, in some circumstances, laser, depending on the wavelength of energy applied. The extent of tissue penetration in electrocautery is related to the power and type of current, the duration of application, and the size of the electrode. Less tissue damage is achieved with bipolar than with monopolar cautery. The carbon dioxide (CO_2) laser is more precise than the fiber lasers, although CO_2 laser energy is strongly absorbed by water molecules and is rendered ineffective in the presence of blood. Meticulous

technique that maintains serosal integrity may reduce the incidence of de novo adhesion formation.

Sites of Conservative Surgery

Peritoneum Small lesions of superficial peritoneal endometriosis less than 5 mm in diameter are easily treated with laser or bipolar coagulation while under a constant stream of irrigation. Deep lesions or more extensive peritoneal disease must be excised with a tissue margin of at least 2 to 4 mm, because, as noted previously, microscopic lesions are commonly present in tissue adjacent to visible implants (Fig. 22.4). Ablation of deep disease by monopolar microdiathermy or CO_2 laser vaporization rather than excision of the disease may result in inadequate resection and a greater amount of ischemic damage to the tissue, heightening the propensity toward adhesion formation. Immobilizing adhesions can be merely divided during the preparatory phase of the procedure; precise excision is more easily accomplished after the involved organs are freed. Before dissection of the pelvic sidewall, the ureter must be identified and isolated; it frequently is displaced from its normal location by endometriotic adhesive disease. A Lucite, Teflon, or laparoscopic titanium probe can be used to isolate adhesions and protect adjacent structures during separation of the tissue planes. Suture placement can lead to foreign body reaction, tissue anoxia, and fibrosis and should therefore be avoided. Covering hemostatic, deperitonealized surfaces with an absorbable, oxidized, regenerated cellulose barrier (Interceed) significantly reduces the incidence, extent, and severity of postsurgical pelvic adhesions, even in patients with severe endometriosis. Alternatively, application of the Gore-Tex surgical membrane has been shown to result in a statistical reduction in adhesion score; this barrier can be removed at the time of a second-look laparoscopic procedure if its presence would impair tuboovarian function.

Estimations of the depth of endometrial implants at the time of laparoscopic resection relate well with histologic measurements. Superficial implants can be destroyed by bipolar cauterization; however, 25% of patients have lesions greater than 5 mm in depth. Deep (<5 mm) and very deep (<10 mm) lesions represent an active form of the disease and occur almost exclusively in patients who report pain. The superficial action of nonvaporizing modalities such as bipolar or thermal coagulation is not sufficient for deep disease. The diagnosis of retroperitoneal endometriosis is suggested by preoperative digital rectovaginal palpation and laparoscopic blunt probe palpation. The depth of infiltration of deep lesions appears to correlate poorly with the visible surface area of involvement. The laparoscopic treatment of deep disease is often complicated by the proximity of implants to vital structures such as the ureter, bladder, and vessels (Table 22.8).

Laparoscopic forceps are used to elevate and isolate the tissue to be excised. Instruments should be placed with care, because surgical manipulation of tissue that will not be resected may result in de novo adhesion formation. The diseased peritoneum may also be separated from underlying tissue by the technique of hydrodissection, which forcefully injects physiologic irrigant retroperitoneally through a small defect created in the peritoneum (Fig. 22.5). This retroperitoneal placement of fluid acts to dissipate CO_2 laser energy and, in so doing, promotes safer dissection or vaporization of the peritoneal surface. Coagulation or vaporization of disease in the ovarian fossa or near the uterosacral ligament should be undertaken only after clear identification of the ureter. Uterine manipulation with a Valtchev retractor or other uterine manipulator may be used while treating lesions of the posterior cul-de-sac.

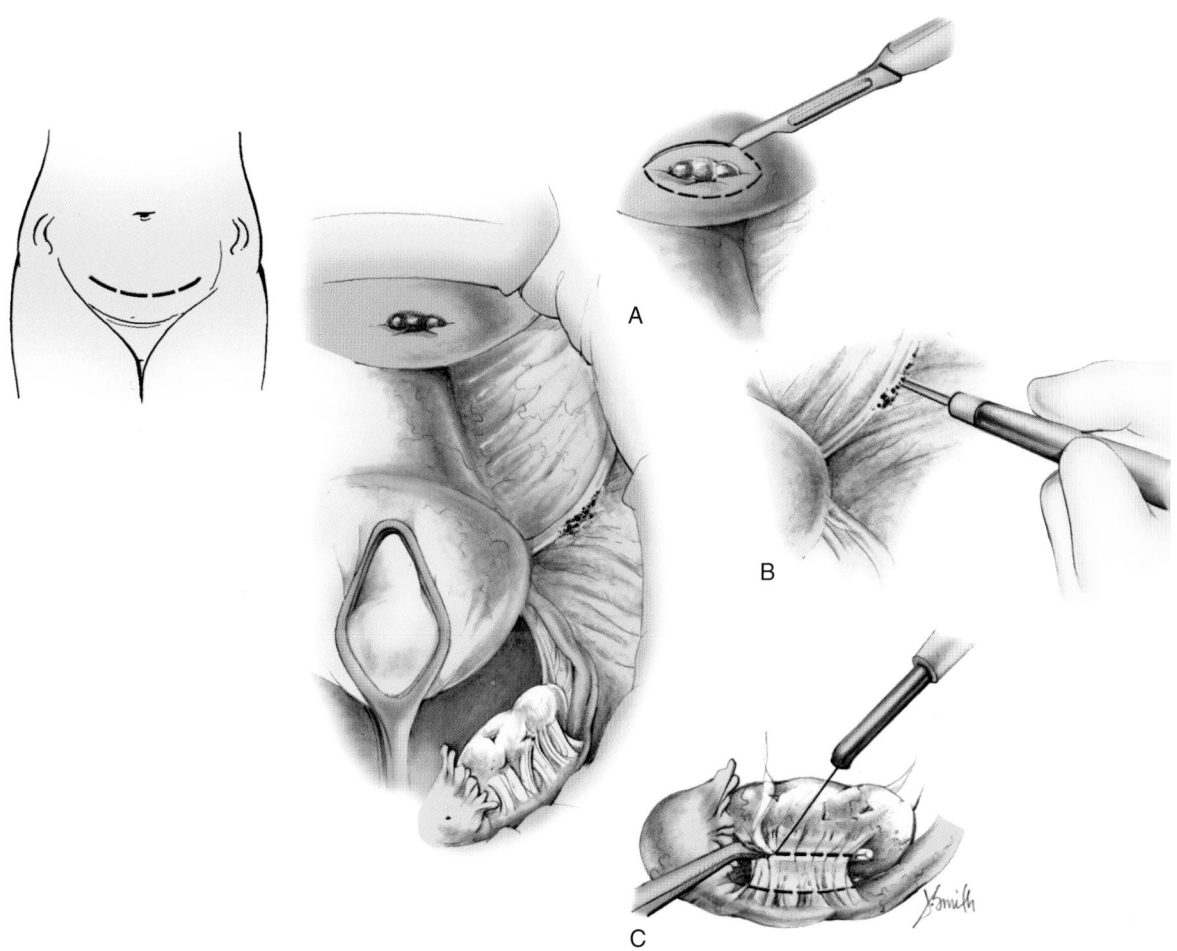

FIGURE 22.4 Excision or CO_2 laser vaporization of peritoneal implants. **A:** Superficial implants are vaporized by use of power densities between 1,000 and 3,000 W/cm², with a spot size of 0.8 to 1 mm, or they are cauterized with microbipolar forceps. More extensive peritoneal disease is excised. Very large defects can be closed with 5-0 or 6-0 polyglactin or polydioxanone sutures. Adhesion barriers can be placed. **B:** Endometriosis can be associated with extensive adnexal adhesions. **C:** Wide adhesion bands can be retracted with a glass rod or similar nonconductive probe and completely excised with a monopolar microelectrode.

TABLE 22.8 Suggested Surgical Procedure According to Classification of Deeply Infiltrating Endometriosis (DIE)

DIE CLASSIFICATION	OPERATIVE PROCEDURE
A: Anterior DIE	
Al: Bladder	Laparoscopic partial cystectomy
P: Posterior DIE	
P1: Uterosacral ligament	Laparoscopic resection of USL
P2: Vagina	Laparoscopically assisted vaginal resection of DIE infiltrating the posterior fornix
P3: Intestine	
Solely intestinal location	
Without vaginal infiltration (V–)	Intestinal resection by laparoscopy or by laparotomy
With vaginal infiltration (V+)	Laparoscopically assisted vaginal intestinal resection or exeresis by laparotomy
Multiple intestinal location	Intestinal resection by laparotomy

USL, uterosacral ligament.
From Chapron C, Fauconnier A, Vieira M, et al. Anatomical distribution of deeply infiltrating endometriosis: surgical implications and proposition for a classification. *Hum Reprod* 2003;18:157, with permission. Copyright © 2003, Oxford University Press.

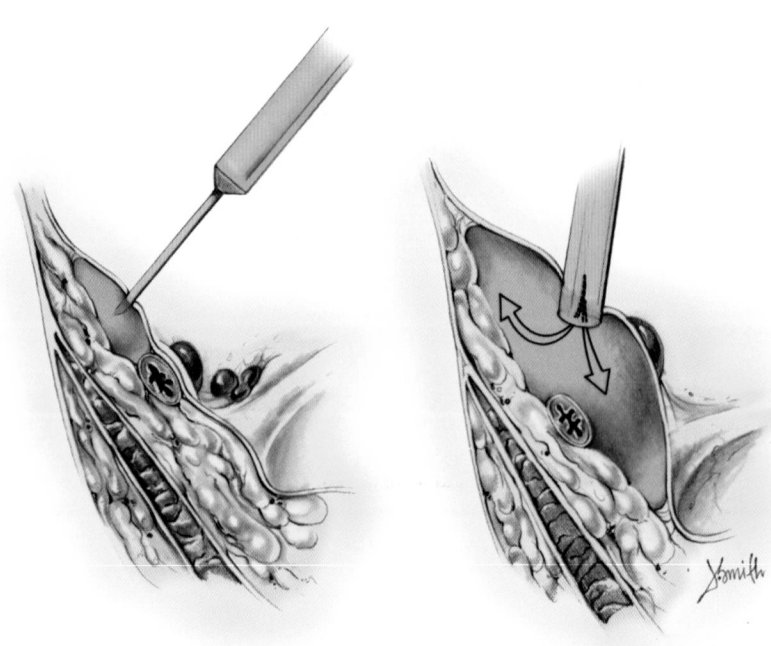

FIGURE 22.5 Hydrodissection.

It is difficult to evaluate the depth of tissue damage with electrocauterization; however, laser vaporization allows visualization of the three-dimensional boundaries of every lesion. The laser beam should be applied until the bubbling of retroperitoneal areolar tissue is noted. The zone of thermal necrosis is minimal with the CO_2 laser, particularly when applied in the superpulse mode. In the region of the ureter, urinary bladder, colon, or large blood vessels, a single or repeat pulse mode of 0.05 to 0.1 second allows a depth of penetration of 100 to 200 μm. Irrigation of the pelvis washes off debris and carbon deposition and better exposes the base of the site of laser impact. A 2- to 4-mm clear margin is desired around each lesion treated. Excision of the involved peritoneum is superior to vaporization of implants when the extent of tissue penetration cannot be recognized.

Dissection of retroperitoneal disease can be facilitated by placing a bougie probe in the rectum and a sponge forceps in the vagina (Fig. 22.6). Traction in either direction opens the rectovaginal and perirectal spaces. Initial dissection of the anterior rectum provides a landmark of the rectovaginal space and permits posterior mobilization of the nodule. Subsequent lateral dissection is performed, followed by anterior dissection, which permits retrieval of the involved tissue.

Resection of deep posterior cul-de-sac nodules requires great endoscopic expertise. A combined laparoscopic–vaginal approach may be necessary to effectively remove these implants (Fig. 22.7). It is often helpful to have an assistant place his or her fingers deep in the vaginal fornices or a bougie probe in the rectum to indicate the sites of the nodules to ensure their complete removal. The direct palpation made possible through laparotomy may be required to recognize all indurated, deep lesions. A complete bowel preparation is mandatory in all cases of suspected deep endometriosis.

Electrosurgery should be avoided when extensive dissection is performed because it may be associated with widespread thermal damage and difficulty in recognizing tissue planes. Superficial invasion of the muscularis of bowel or bladder can be treated with laser vaporization or endocoagulation because of the precision and lack of penetration of these energy sources. Anterior cul-de-sac treatment should be accompanied by continuous bladder drainage.

Tubal endometriosis may distort the normal anatomic relationship of the distal tube to the ovary and in severe cases may cause complete fimbrial obstruction. Short pulses of CO_2 laser may be used to vaporize lesions while minimizing thermal damage. Endoscopic adhesiolysis of the distal tube may be accomplished with fine scissors or careful application of laser. Unipolar electrocautery should not be used on this tissue.

Defects in the parietal peritoneal surface are frequently associated with endometriosis and are most commonly found in the posterior cul-de-sac region. These defects should be explored and ablated even if they appear grossly normal because of the frequency of microscopic disease.

Ovary Superficial endometriosis of the ovary usually presents as small, dark, punctate lesions located on and immediately beneath the cortical surface. This disease can be readily treated with laser or bipolar forceps under constant irrigation. Occasionally, however, the small, visible lesion may be merely the tip of a large endometrial cyst. If there is any doubt, the implant should be excised and the ovary explored to determine the extent of disease. Care should be taken to minimize thermal injury to surrounding ovarian tissue. This is particularly important near the fimbria ovarica, because postoperative adhesion formation could compromise distal tubal function. Inability to elevate the ovary is usually a sign of adhesions and endometriotic implants of the inferolateral surface of the ovary and the peritoneum of the ovarian fossa. Excising the fibrotic pelvic sidewall and/or uterosacral ligament lesions to which the ovary was attached will reduce disease recurrence.

RECONSTRUCTION BY LAPAROTOMY Extensive ovarian endometriosis is often associated with periovarian and peritubal adhesions. These adhesions may become apparent while manipulating the ovary to visualize the lateral surface adjacent to the broad ligament. Filmy adhesions are elevated with delicate tissue forceps and can be resected with fine-needle cautery, a scalpel, or the laser. Care must be taken to maintain the integrity of the ovarian capsule. After the appropriate adhesiolysis is accomplished, the posterior cul-de-sac is packed with moist, lint-free packs, and a silicone surgical platform can be placed to stabilize the adnexa. The ovary should be carefully

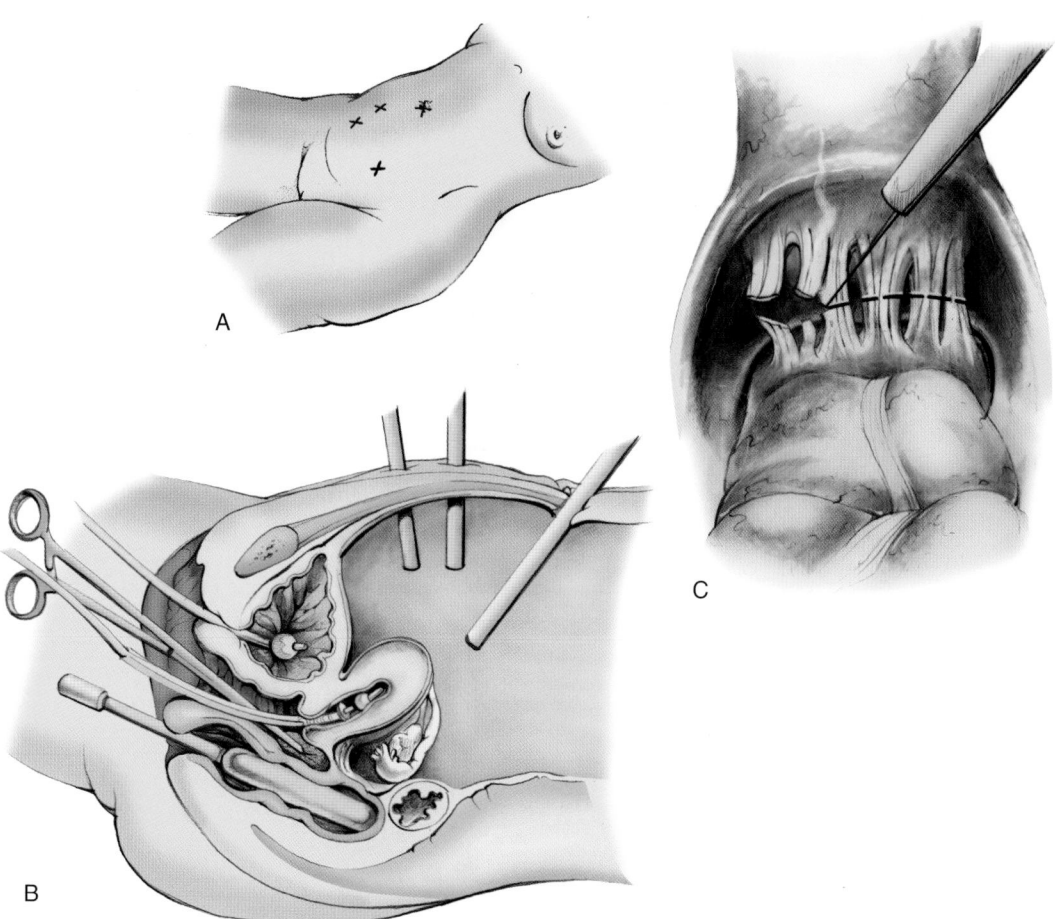

FIGURE 22.6 Laparoscopic therapy for endometriosis. **A:** Dorsal lithotomy positioning for surgery, with multiple puncture sites marked for placement of ancillary instruments. **B:** Traction on bougie in rectum and sponge forceps in vagina mobilize rectovaginal and perirectal spaces. Uterine manipulation cannula, bladder drainage, and multiple transabdominal instruments facilitate safe dissection. **C:** CO_2 laser division of endometriosis-associated adhesions extending from lower uterus to rectal serosa.

examined for extent of disease involvement before creation of the initial incision. Peritoneal spillage of the contents of the endometrioma can be avoided by placement of a lint-free pack around the platform.

The cortical incision should be made in a way that will preserve the normal anatomic relations of the ovary with the uteroovarian ligament and fimbria ovarica (**Fig. 22.8**). This is best accomplished by making a shallow longitudinal incision over the endometrioma with the monopolar microneedle, scalpel, or laser. The surgeon should attempt to remove the endometrioma in an intact state; however, if the cyst cavity is inadvertently entered, an elliptical incision around the site of rupture is useful for exposure. The intact endometrioma can be transfixed with a traction suture of 2-0 nylon to facilitate creation of a cleavage plane between the cyst and normal ovarian tissue. Blunt, curved scissors or a flat probe or knife handle is used for dissection. Particular care must be taken when dissecting the hilar region to maintain hemostasis and preserve primordial follicles. An attempt should be made to preserve as much of the normal ovarian cortex as possible; pregnancies have been achieved with only a small fraction of remaining ovary.

The ovary is reconstructed by placing one or two purse-string sutures of 4-0 or 5-0 polyglactin, polyglycolic acid, or polydioxanone to eliminate the dead space and maximize hemostasis. This may be followed by placement of a running subcortical 5-0 suture of the same delayed absorbable material (**Fig. 22.8**),

if necessary. In some circumstances, less tissue distortion can be achieved by placing a deep layer of interrupted mattress sutures followed by additional layers of running sutures (**Fig. 22.8**). Suture on or extruding through the surface should be strictly avoided because of its adhesiogenic properties.

After the ovary has been carefully approximated, the posterior surfaces of the uterus and broad ligament are inspected for hemostasis wherever the ovary was previously adhered. Microbipolar cauterization may be necessary. Placement of an adhesion barrier is useful in separating raw peritoneal surfaces during the healing process.

ENDOSCOPIC THERAPY OF OVARIAN ENDOMETRIOSIS Surgical treatment of endometriosis less than 4 to 5 cm in diameter can be accomplished with relative ease. However, endoscopic resection of larger lesions may be compromised by the presence of dense, cohesive adhesions and by difficulties removing the entire cyst wall because of the inability to find the plane of attachment of the fibrotic endometrioma to the ovarian cortex. When performing a cystectomy, the experience and skill of the surgeon influence the extent to which healthy ovarian tissue is removed and the ovary is devascularized. A recent histologic study of endometriomas by Romualdi et al. indicated that more follicles are involuntarily removed when smaller cysts are excised, particularly when the capsule is less defined due to fibrosis.

IV

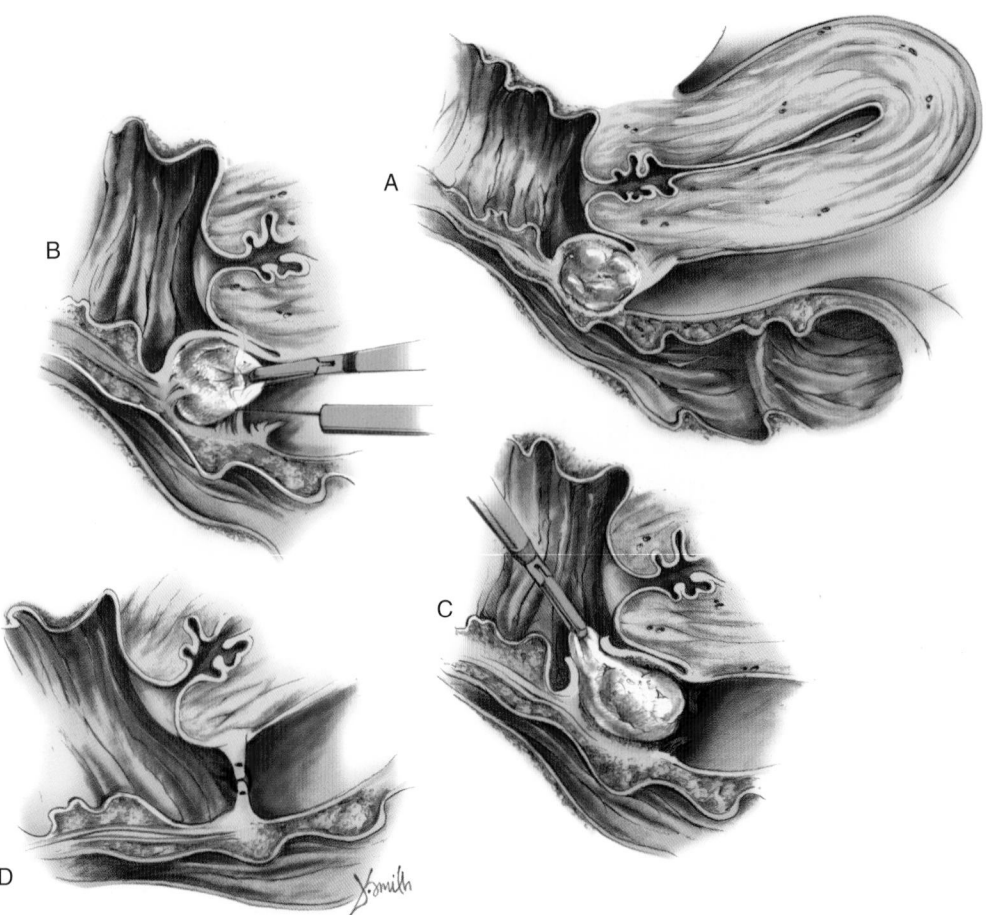

FIGURE 22.7 **A:** Deep laparoscopic dissection of the rectovaginal space, in combination with colpotomy, for the excision of a large endometriotic nodule of the rectovaginal septum. **B:** Initial laparoscopic dissection of nodule. **C:** Completion of dissection by way of colpotomy incision. **D:** Vaginal suture placement to reapproximate the rectovaginal septal defect.

The endometrioma can be excised in an intact or ruptured state during the laparoscopic procedure. In either case, the technique is initiated by longitudinally incising the cortex overlying the cyst after achieving full mobilization of the ovary by adhesiolysis. The incision is generally made along the inferior pole on the opposite side to the hilus in such a manner as to preserve the apposition of healthy ovarian tissue to the fimbria. Laser, scissors, or a unipolar needle electrode may be used for this purpose. Hydrodissection may be used to separate the cyst wall from the ovarian stroma. If the cyst is entered, its contents are immediately drained with the suction cannula, and the cavity is irrigated and inspected for papillary structures or other suspicious features. Often, the cyst ruptures during dissection of adhesions that bind the ovary to the pelvic sidewall. Under this circumstance, the plane of dissection between the cyst wall and the ovarian cortex can be established after identifying the site of rupture. The endometriosis tissue typically penetrates the cyst wall less than 2 mm. The opening can be extended with the use of the needle electrode or laser.

With larger endometriomas, the normal ovarian cortex is stabilized with atraumatic forceps, and the cyst wall is grasped with a second pair of 5-mm forceps and stripped from the bed of normal ovarian tissue (Fig. 22.9). As demonstrated by Muzii et al., dissection may be facilitated by removing a small circular rim of tissue around the adhesion site to begin the stripping procedure in a clearer field, where the endometrioma

wall is less adhered to healthy ovarian tissue. Judicious use of the needle electrode or hydrodissection may facilitate separation of the tissue planes. Remaining fragments of the cyst wall near the hilum should be vaporized with CO_2 laser, if possible, rather than electrocautery to destroy the mucosal lining and reduce the extent of thermal damage to the vasculature. If necessary, hemostasis may be achieved with minimized application of bipolar cautery. The key to successful surgery is to avoid bleeding, since the application of energy to control bleeding results in loss of functional ovarian tissue.

An alternative technique involves sharp and blunt dissection to remove the cyst in an intact state. Hydrodissection is particularly useful with this approach. The cyst contents are carefully drained in a plastic laparoscopy pouch to facilitate clean removal from the peritoneal cavity.

Very small endometriomas less than 1 to 2 cm in size may be effectively treated by electrocoagulation of the mucosal lining. Because CO_2 laser is absorbed by fluid, complete ablation of the cyst wall with this energy source may be compromised in an environment rich in blood and hemosiderin, although laser ablation may be less harmful to healthy ovarian tissue than electrocoagulation.

The ovarian defect is usually left to heal spontaneously. Ischemia associated with suture placement can provoke adhesion formation after laparoscopic ovarian reconstruction. Low-power continuous CO_2 laser or bipolar coagulation can be applied to the inside wall of the redundant ovarian capsule

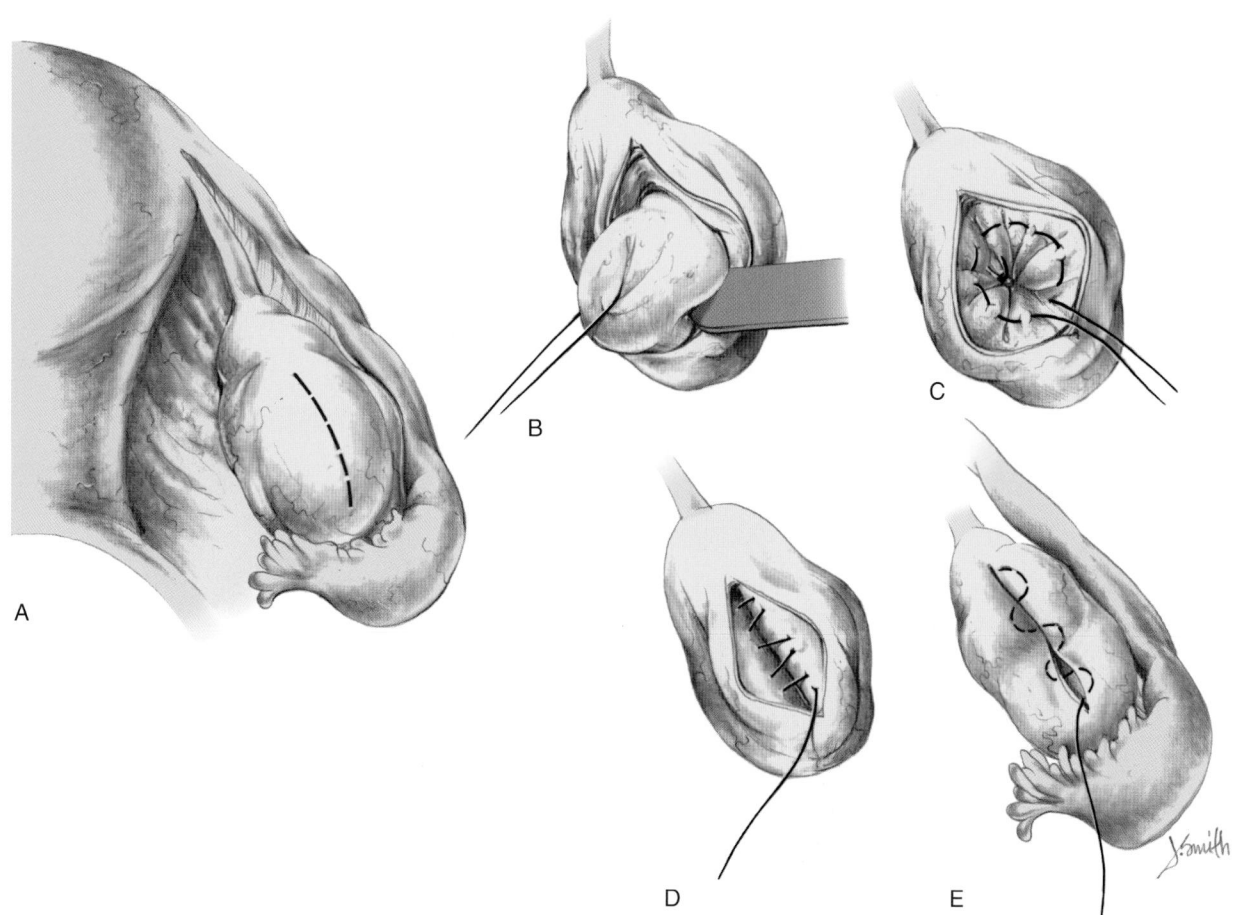

FIGURE 22.8 Excision of ovarian endometrioma through laparotomy. **A:** The ovarian cortex is gently incised so that the endometrial cyst is not entered. The incision is made along the longitudinal axis of the ovary. **B:** The endometrioma is then peeled out with the blunt knife handle. **C and D:** The ovarian defect is closed with two layers of purse-string sutures of 4-0 or 5-0 absorbable, nonreactive material. **E:** In the case of a deep defect, a more superficial running suture may be necessary before the cortical edges are approximated with 5-0 nonreactive, delayed absorbable sutures.

to cause an inversion of the incised cortex. Most authors have reported excellent results with this no-suture technique.

Under the rare circumstances of persistent bleeding or poor apposition of ovarian tissue, the cortex may be reapproximated with sutures. If fine absorbable suture is used, the knot should be placed internally to minimize the possibility of it becoming a nidus for adhesion formation. The high incidence of adhesion formation after surgery for endometriosis, particularly at the site of the ovary or where dense adhesions were divided, underscores the importance of optimizing surgical techniques to potentially reduce adhesion formation.

Extensive cauterization of ovarian tissue can lead to a rise in FSH levels postoperatively and should be avoided. Goksever Celik et al. demonstrated that laparoscopic removal of endometriomas by the stripping technique causes a decrease in ovarian follicular reserve at 6 months after surgery as measured by serum antimüllerian hormone levels. This change in serum markers of ovarian reserve was not different whether laparoscopic suturing or bipolar coagulation was used to achieve hemostasis in a recent randomized trial by Ferrero et al. Postsurgical ovarian failure after laparoscopic excision of bilateral endometriomas is a rare but possible complication. There were three cases of premature ovarian failure among 126 patients who underwent laparoscopic excision of bilateral endometriomas in a recent series by Busaccca and colleagues, corresponding to a rate of 2.4%. This may be caused by irreversible

trauma to ovarian vasculature by electrocoagulation, excessive removal of ovarian tissue, and an autoimmune reaction caused by a severe, local inflammatory process. Coccia et al. found the mean age of menopause is lower in patients who have undergone surgery for bilateral endometriomas.

Fayez and Vogel prospectively evaluated four laparoscopic methods for the treatment of endometriomas. Patients were treated postoperatively with danazol and underwent a second-look laparoscopy 8 weeks after their initial surgery. Complete excision with scissors successfully eliminated recurrence of the cysts, but adnexal adhesions had developed postoperatively in all cases. Mere incision and drainage of the cyst contents, followed by stripping or CO_2 laser vaporization of the lining, resulted in adhesion formation in only 25% to 37% of cases, but endometrioma cysts recurred in 21% to 22%. Other authors have used the potassium titanyl phosphate laser to photocoagulate or remove the cyst lining of large endometriomas and have reported a very low rate of recurrence at 6 months after the procedure.

In a prospective study by Beretta and colleagues, patients were randomly allocated at the time of laparoscopy to undergo either cystectomy or drainage of the endometrioma and bipolar coagulation of the inner lining. No preoperative or postoperative adjunctive medical therapies were administered. The excision technique resulted in a lower 24-month cumulative recurrence rate of dysmenorrhea, deep dyspareunia, and

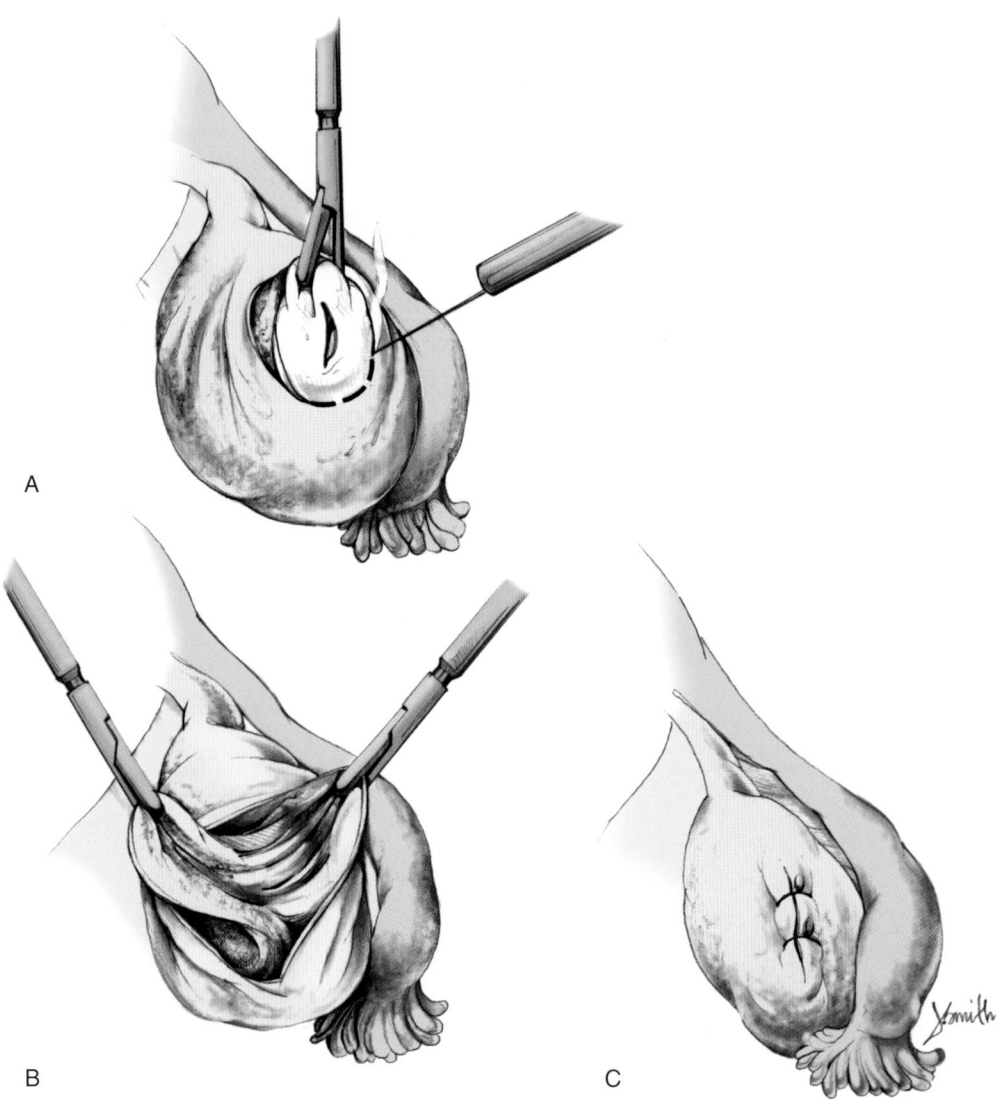

FIGURE 22.9 Laparoscopic ovarian cystectomy after fenestration of the cyst. **A:** The cut edges of the ovarian cortex and cyst wall are held and teased apart. **B:** The cyst wall can be stripped off by twisting it around the grasping forceps. Hydrodissection may be helpful. **C:** Large defects can be closed with laparoscopic suturing. Most incisions are left to heal by second intention.

nonmenstrual pelvic pain. The median interval between the operation and the recurrence of moderate-to-severe pelvic pain was longer in the cystectomy group (19 months) versus the drainage and coagulation group (9.5 months). In addition, the 24-month cumulative pregnancy rate was statistically significantly higher in the former group than in the latter group (66.7% vs. 23.5%, respectively).

In a 2004 prospective, randomized clinical trial by Alborzi and associates, the rate of recurrence of pelvic pain and dysmenorrhea over a 2-year postoperative period was significantly less for those who underwent cystectomy (15.8%) as compared with those undergoing fenestration and coagulation (56.7%). Moreover, the rate of reoperation was 5.8% in the former group and 22.9% in the latter group. The cumulative pregnancy rate was significantly higher in the cystectomy group (59.4%) than in fenestration/coagulation group (23.3%) at 1-year follow-up.

If there is evidence of functional destruction of the ovary or if the patient has chronic, incapacitating pelvic pain secondary to ovarian endometriosis and does not plan to become pregnant in the future, appropriate therapy may consist of oophorectomy. The infundibulopelvic and utero-ovarian ligaments can be ligated with an Endoloop ligature, bipolar coagulation, the harmonic scalpel, or surgical staples before excision of the structure. The ovary is retrieved by morcellation, minilaparotomy, or posterior colpotomy. This type of surgery must be performed carefully when adnexal adhesions are present to avoid ovarian remnant syndrome.

Intestines Intestinal involvement has been estimated to occur in 3% to 15% of women with endometriosis and in up to 50% of patients with severe disease. The most common areas of intestinal involvement are the rectum and rectosigmoid colon, followed by the sigmoid colon, cecum, terminal ileum, proximal colon, and appendix. The incidence of appendiceal endometriosis has been estimated at approximately 0.8% of all appendectomies; 3% to 5% of patients with endometriosis have appendiceal involvement.

Symptoms that should arouse suspicion of colorectal involvement include constipation alternating with diarrhea, rectal pain, tenesmus, dyspareunia, and dysmenorrhea. Cyclic rectal bleeding is seen in as many as one third of women with rectosigmoid involvement, but the mucosa is rarely invaded. Small intestine disease accounts for up to 16% of gastrointestinal endometriosis and most often involves the terminal ileum. The most common symptom associated with disease in this location is midabdominal cramping pain. Ten percent of small bowel involvement presents with obstruction requiring surgery. The more common large bowel disease results in clinical obstruction in only 1% of cases.

The differential diagnosis of intestinal endometriosis includes primary carcinoma, metastatic carcinoma, diverticulitis, inflammatory bowel disease, irritable bowel syndrome, pelvic inflammatory disease, radiation colitis, and ischemic stricture. Endometrial adenocarcinomas have been reported in the colon and rectum but are exceedingly rare in comparison with the relatively large numbers of patients with colorectal endometriosis.

Preoperative or intraoperative rigid sigmoidoscopy may be helpful in ruling out primary colorectal malignancy. An intact mucosa effectively rules out primary colorectal malignancy. The greatest chance of diagnosing colorectal endometriosis occurs when the examination is performed at the time of menstruation. Although endometriosis rarely invades the intestinal mucosa, mucosal distortion is possible secondary to infiltration of the submucosa.

Pelvic and rectal pain is the major symptom that leads to colorectal resection in patients with advanced endometriosis. Bowel resection should be undertaken in the symptomatic patient or when there is a suspicion of malignancy; however, the frequency of such indications is small. In a series authored by Prystowsky and colleagues of 1,573 consecutive patients with endometriosis, only 11 women (0.7%) required bowel resection. Bowel resection is usually undertaken for lesions producing partial obstruction because most of these lesions are fibrotic and unresponsive to hormonal manipulation. This would include those with bowel occlusion of greater than 50% of the circumference, lesions of greater than 2 to 3 cm in size, or when muscularis involvement of disease is greater than 7 to 8 cm. Recommended approaches for less extensive lesions include CO_2 laser vaporization of superficial serosal disease of the rectum or large intestine, excision without entering the mucosa, and oophorectomy or hormonal suppression. A harmonic scalpel may be used laparoscopically to shave an endometriotic nodule in the prerectal fascia. As demonstrated by Koninckx et al., most recurrences occur at the posterior fornix of the vagina, and complete excision is important in this area, particularly since the vaginal cuff heals well following resection of deep endometriosis in this area. The use of electrocautery or fiber lasers should be avoided because of their greater risk of causing transmural thermal damage.

A full mechanical and antibiotic bowel preparation is carried out preoperatively. A technically difficult and prolonged surgery is expected when the nodule is greater than 3 cm in diameter, firmly attached to the ischial spine, and localized in the sigmoid or when adhesions are present because of previous incomplete surgery or past in vitro fertilization (IVF) procedures that resulted in perforation of the nodule with the aspiration needle. When the nodule of deep endometriosis is attached to the ischial spine or ischiosacral ligament, dissection should be performed carefully because of the risk of extensive bleeding that may be difficult to control.

Lesions less than 2 cm in size or less than one third of the rectal circumference can be excised in a full-thickness manner either transabdominally or laparoscopically. In cases of large lesions that encroach on the mucosa, full-thickness excision of involved bowel can be undertaken either by disk excision

of small, isolated lesions or by segmental resection for larger lesions, particularly those invading the bowel lumen. During the dissection of the nodule from the bowel, a layer of fibrosis may be left in situ to avoid entering the mucosa. The anastomosis can be hand sewn with a continuous single layer of absorbable monofilament suture or created with surgical staples; however, patients with cul-de-sac disease must be in the lithotomy position to allow transanal placement of the stapler. A circular end-to-end stapler has limitations to the amount of rectal wall that can be resected. The risks of rectovaginal fistula may be reduced by the interposition of a pedicled omentoplasty between the two suture lines and performance of a defunctioning stoma and pelvic drainage.

Excision of a sigmoid nodule is difficult without sigmoid resection, since the nodule is often localized mesenterically, thus impairing blood flow after excision, and the mobility of the sigmoid makes discoid resection and suture repair technically challenging. These procedures have been performed by or with the assistance of general surgeons.

A one-time dose of antibiotic is administered intraoperatively if the vagina is entered; a course of 4 to 7 days is recommended for muscularis defect with single-layer suturing or full-thickness resection and double-layer suture repair, respectively.

The short-term complications associated with bowel resection for endometriosis include leak at the anastomosis site, pelvic abscess and fistula, and bowel and bladder dysfunction. The lower the anastomosis, the higher the probability of postoperative leakage and rectovaginal fistula formation. Bowel perforation is usually identified within the week after surgery and may be treated with suturing and lavage if laparoscopy is performed within 24 hours after perforation. Later diagnoses associated with peritonitis necessitate colostomy. For those who have undergone low rectal resections, 15% or more experience leaks. Urinary retention usually resolves within a few weeks. Local excision with transmural discoid excision is associated with a lower risk of short- and long-term complications than rectal resection and has acceptable clinical outcomes for most patients.

Appendectomy should be considered when there is physical evidence of peritonitis, when implants are large and active, when associated adhesive disease to adjacent bowel may result in partial or complete angulation and obstruction, or when the benign nature of the lesion is in doubt. Spontaneous perforation of the appendix that is due to endometriotic involvement is very rare. The technique of incidental endoscopic appendectomy is similar to that performed through laparotomy, although the stump need not be buried in the cecum. The tip of the appendix is grasped and elevated. The appendiceal vessels are bipolar cauterized or occluded with surgical clips near the base of the appendix before being excised. Two loop ligatures are placed immediately next to each other at the base, and a third Endoloop is then secured approximately 5 mm distal to the first two. The appendix may then be transected between the second and third ligature and placed in a surgical pouch for safe retrieval from the abdominal cavity. Judicious application of bipolar cautery at the stump sterilizes the raw surface of the pedicle without causing damage to the adjacent cecum.

Coronado and colleagues reported a complete relief of pelvic symptoms in 49% and an improvement in 39% of patients who underwent full-thickness resection of the colon; 39% of patients in the series achieved a term pregnancy. In a later series by the same colorectal surgeons of 130 patients who underwent aggressive, conservative surgical management for advanced disease, the operative procedures performed included low anterior resection with anastomosis to the extraperitoneal rectum ($n = 109$), sigmoid resection ($n = 10$), disk excision of the rectum ($n = 7$), ileocecal resection ($n = 2$), and small bowel resection ($n = 2$). Twenty-four of forty nine patients (49%) who attempted to conceive delivered a viable child.

Ferrero and colleagues compared open-bowel resection to laparoscopic resection in women with rectosigmoid endometriosis. They showed improved pregnancy rates when the procedure was performed laparoscopically. However, Vercellini et al., in a nonrandomized study in 2006, showed no higher rate of conception following resection of deeply infiltrating rectovaginal endometriosis via laparotomy over that achieved with expectant management among 105 women who were followed over a 2-year period. The cumulative 24-month probability of becoming pregnant was 44.9% in the surgery arm and 46.9% in the expectant management arm.

The sequelae of intestinal endometriosis may not appear until the patient is postmenopausal. Although the endometriosis can become inactive, the resulting cicatrization can lead to a decrease in the bowel lumen and to symptoms of obstruction.

Urinary Tract Endometriosis involving the urinary tract is relatively rare. The spectrum of disease severity varies from incidental findings at laparoscopy, laparotomy, or cystoscopy to more significantly associated hematuria, flank pain, hypertension, and ureteral obstruction. Bladder and ureteral involvement represent 85% and 15% of cases, respectively. Cystoscopy and intravenous pyelography are helpful studies in documenting the extent of disease. Magnetic resonance imaging may further delineate the extent of involvement. Vesical endometriosis can be treated by hormonal suppressive therapy or partial cystectomy. These nodular lesions develop within the muscularis and are typically seen with partial or complete obliteration of the anterior cul-de-sac. Fedele et al. deomonstrated conservative surgical treatment of bladder endometriosis is effective in ensuring long-term relief in most cases of endometriosis affecting the vesical dome, whereas success rates for deeper lesions involving the vesical base and the vesicouterine septum are lower, depending on the degree of surgical radicalness. The bladder wall is sutured in two layers, and a bladder catheter is left in place for 7 to 10 days postoperatively.

Extrinsic ureteral compression by endometriosis presents four times more frequently than intrinsic involvement and is most likely to occur in the distal third near the region of the ovarian fossa. The left ureter is more commonly affected. Patients with paracervical and extensive uterosacral ligament disease are also at risk. In patients with deep endometriosis, hydronephrosis should be excluded before surgery because it requires preoperative placement of a ureteral stent. The preferred treatment for ureteral obstruction is ureterolysis or resection of the involved segment followed by ureteroneocystostomy or ureteroureterostomy. When hydronephrosis is present, the stricture can be removed over the stent with resection of a defined lesion in greater than 80% of patients.

Involvement of peritoneum overlying the ureter is amenable to resection by laparotomy or laparoscopy. An incision is made in normal peritoneum adjacent to the involved area. The inferior margin of the incision is grasped and deviated medially, and the ureter is separated from the peritoneum bluntly or by hydrodissection. The peritoneal lesion can be excised or vaporized. Periureteral vessels must remain intact to prevent ischemia and resultant fistula formation. If the peritoneum is adhered and the lesion cannot be dissected, the ureter is likely involved in the disease process. Ureteroneocystostomy should be considered.

Incisional Scars Surgical scars are occasionally the sites of endometriotic implantation. Perineal, vaginal, and vulvar scars, particularly episiotomies, colporrhaphies, and Bartholin gland excisions, are likely areas for involvement by endometriosis. There is often a history of delayed wound healing of the incisional scar infiltrated with endometriosis. These implants typically appear as either deep-lying or subcutaneous nodules infiltrating the fascia and muscle. Bleeding into the tissues at the time of menstruation can cause cyclic local pain, tenderness, and discoloration; however, the nodule may lie too deep for detection of any color change through the skin. If the nodule is superficial, cyclic bleeding or ulceration may be apparent.

In most instances, incisional endometriomas have followed surgical procedures that violated the uterine cavity and allowed the endometrium to be transplanted. Wespi and Kletzhändler suggested that the frequency might approach 5% among patients having cesarean section or hysterectomy. Metroplasty and myomectomy also increase the risk of incisional endometriosis. Indeed, endometriosis has been reported along the needle tracts after amniocentesis or saline injection for abortion. Careful flushing and irrigation of the abdomen and of the incision during closure should minimize the chance of contamination when incision into the uterine cavity is required.

Episiotomy scars and cervical and vaginal lacerations also serve as implantation sites after delivery. The chance is significantly increased when postpartum curettage is performed. Paull and Tedeschi reported 15 instances in 2,208 deliveries when curettage was carried out and no instances in 13,800 deliveries without curettage.

Management, usually best accomplished by local excision, is both diagnostic and curative. Various hormonal regimens may be appropriate if it is imperative to avoid surgery. However, malignancy can occur in each area of ectopic endometriosis, and histologic confirmation of the tentative diagnosis is recommended.

Thorax Thoracic endometriosis is an uncommon disease with varying clinical presentations. The diagnosis is almost always established on clinical grounds. In a report of 65 cases of thoracic endometriosis by Foster et al., pleural and lung parenchymal disease presented with different clinical features. Ninety-three percent of women with pleural disease developed pain with right-sided pneumothorax or pleural effusion. Because numerous right diaphragmatic defects were noted in patients with pleural involvement, pleural implants are believed to be secondary to tubal regurgitation and transport of endometrial tissue through the diaphragmatic defects. Other symptoms may include upper quadrant abdominal pain or referred pain to the shoulder. Disease involving the lung parenchyma produced hemoptysis rather than the pleuritic symptoms. Previous pelvic surgery was more common among women who had parenchymal endometriosis; however, pelvic endometriosis was found more often in those with pleural disease.

Catamenial pneumothorax or hemoptysis should alert the physician to the possibility of thoracic endometriosis. The chest roentgenogram is usually of little value in diagnosing this disease; however, cytology, aspiration biopsy, and pleuroscopy may be useful. Chest CT scan may reveal pulmonary or pleural nodules, particularly if performed during menses. Massive effusion and bleeding can occur, but this presentation is more commonly associated with a malignancy. GnRH agonist or surgical treatment may be effective in the symptomatic patient. Chemical pleurodesis or surgical pleural abrasion may be superior to hormonal treatment in the long-term management of pneumothorax.

Sciatic Nerve Endometriosis may compress the sciatic nerve within the pelvis, at the sciatic notch, in the gluteal region distal to the notch, or within the sheath of the sciatic nerve. The lesion may be identified with magnetic resonance neurography. Patients present with pain in the hip and the buttock radiating down the back of the leg to the foot. The discomfort begins a few days before menstruation and becomes progressively more severe before subsiding 2 or 3 days to 2 weeks after cessation of menstruation. Over time, the sciatica may be constantly present, with excruciating exacerbation during menses. Neuropathic injury and muscle denervation may lead to progressive weakness of the leg. Two thirds of patients with sciatic nerve endometriosis have right-sided lesions. CT-guided biopsy is possible to confirm the diagnosis. Surgical exploration of the sciatic nerve is not necessary in most cases. Patients may experience remission of symptoms with GnRH agonist administration or during pregnancy.

Adjunctive Procedures of Conservative Surgery

Uterine Suspension
Uterine suspension techniques have been devised to reduce adhesion formation at denuded peritoneal surfaces of the posterior cul-de-sac, uterine serosa, and broad ligament. Elevation of the adnexa may prevent adhesion reformation of the ovary or fallopian tube at a site where existing adhesions have been excised. This procedure may be particularly useful in the case of a posterior or retroflexed uterus. It is indicated in selected cases of dyspareunia after resection of posterior cul-de-sac endometriosis. There is no evidence to suggest that uterine suspension is detrimental to subsequent pregnancies, although it is of unproven efficacy in enhancing fertility or as an adjunct in the treatment of endometriosis-associated pelvic pain. The modified Gilliam procedure offers certain advantages over other uterine suspensions because of its maintenance of normal anatomic relations. Shortening the round ligament through the internal inguinal ring eliminates the opening that is made lateral to the point of the ligament's attachment to the abdominal wall in the Olshausen suspension procedure.

When a modified Gilliam suspension is performed via laparotomy, the uterus is elevated, and a 2-0 absorbable suture is placed around each round ligament approximately 3 to 4 cm from its insertion into the uterus (**Fig. 22.10**). The edge of the rectus fascia is grasped by a Kocher clamp at the level of the anterosuperior spine of the ileum. The adjacent peritoneal edge is grasped with a Kelly clamp. The rectus fascia is separated from the underlying musculature with blunt dissection. A long Kelly clamp is inserted between the fascia and muscle to the level of the inguinal ring while displacing the peritoneum superiorly. This clamp is inserted through the ring and along the round ligament by gently opening and closing the instrument. The insertion is facilitated by placing traction on the suture to stabilize the round ligament. The peritoneum overlying the ligament is then incised at a point adjacent to the suture, and the suture is grasped by the Kelly clamp. By withdrawing the clamp, the round ligament is brought through the internal ring and outside of the peritoneal cavity; it can then be sutured to the rectus sheath with 2-0 interrupted delayed absorbable sutures. These sutures must be placed through the round ligament without encircling the ligament and thus occluding its blood supply. This procedure is repeated on the opposite side.

At the end of the suspension, the surgeon's hands should be introduced into the abdomen to ascertain whether there is a loop of round ligament lateral to the point where the ligament has been withdrawn from the peritoneal cavity. If so, this should be corrected to prevent strangulation of the involved segment lying between the ligament and abdominal wall. In addition, the fallopian tube should be inspected to ensure that its course has not been disturbed. This can occur if the traction suture has been placed through a segment of round ligament too close to the uterus.

Laparoscopic suspension is possible after placement of a trocar and sheath approximately 5 cm lateral to the midline and 3 cm above the inguinal ligament. The anterior rectus fascia in this site is tagged with suture. The round ligament is grasped at the usual site with laparoscopic forceps to elevate the ligament to the tagged anterior fascia, where it is sutured in place with nonabsorbable suture. The desired positioning of the uterus is confirmed laparoscopically.

Presacral Neurectomy
Presacral neurectomy, or division of the superior hypogastric plexus, is useful as an adjunctive procedure to eliminate the uterine component of dysmenorrhea that results from endometriosis. Sixty to eighty-five percent of patients with secondary dysmenorrhea experience complete relief of symptoms. There is no evidence that presacral neurectomy enhances fertility.

A significantly greater relief of midline pelvic pain is achieved when endometriosis resection is combined with presacral neurectomy as compared with conservative resection alone. In a series by Tjaden and colleagues, all 17 patients undergoing presacral neurectomy noted a complete resolution of midline pelvic pain, and only two of these had a recurrence of pain within the 42-month follow-up period. Endometriosis rarely provokes exclusively midline pelvic pain, however, and lateralizing adnexal pain and deep dyspareunia are not affected by this procedure. Careful patient selection is necessary if the desired outcome is to be achieved.

The hypogastric plexus consists of fine strands of nerves embedded in a delicate areolar tissue. The plexus is formed as a continuation of the aortic and inferior mesenteric plexuses and passes over the bifurcation of the aorta. It then continues below the promontory of the sacrum before dividing into the right and left inferior hypogastric nerves. The presacral neurectomy procedure can be performed through a transverse Maylard incision or longitudinal incision that adequately exposes the region of the bifurcation of the aorta (**Fig. 22.11**). At the time of laparotomy, the descending colon is packed superiorly and to the left to expose the left margin of the hypogastric plexus. The posterior peritoneum overlying the sacrum is elevated and incised with the scalpel. The incision is extended caudally with scissors for approximately 5 cm to the third or fourth sacral vertebra and cranially to just below the bifurcation of the aorta. The margin of the posterior peritoneum can be drawn upward and outward by a stay suture or an Allis clamp. A Kittner sponge is then used to dissect the areolar tissue and associated nerve fibers off the posterior aspect of the peritoneal flap. The right ureter is readily visible and can be retracted laterally, and the areolar tissue is dissected from it without disturbing its blood supply. The common iliac artery, which lies just below the ureter, is freed superiorly from the adjacent tissue. A right angle clamp or probe can be introduced medially next to the promontory to elevate the sheath and allow blunt dissection underneath it. Care must be taken to avoid the middle sacral vessels that may be left intact on the surface of the promontory. Injury to the middle sacral vein can result in significant blood loss. Hemorrhage is controlled with cautery, suture ligation, hot packs, hypogastric vessel ligation, use of an absorbable gelatin sponge (Gelfoam) or microfibrillar collagen (Avitene), or packing with bone wax.

The areolar tissue is taken off the left flap of peritoneum until the superior hemorrhoidal vessels are exposed. These vessels should remain on the peritoneum but are bluntly freed from the overlying tissue. By elevating the sheath, several vessels that feed into the left common iliac vein can be identified. These branches are isolated, clamped, and tied as they are visualized. When the plexus has been isolated, a Babcock clamp

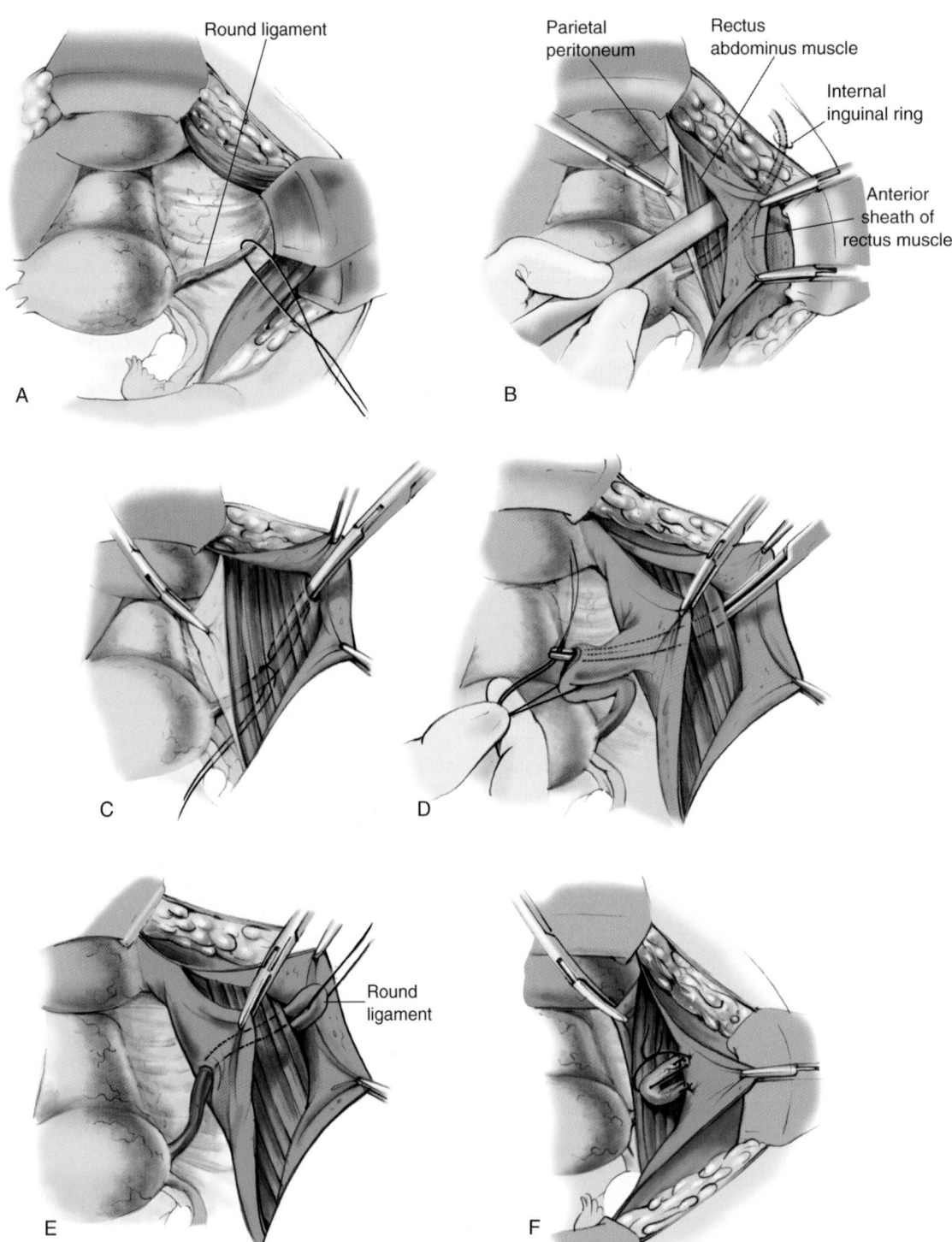

FIGURE 22.10 Modified Gilliam suspension. **A:** A chromic suture is placed around the round ligament approximately 3 to 4 cm from the uterine cornu. **B:** The rectus fascia is grasped with Kocher clamps and separated from the belly of the rectus muscle bluntly with the index finger or knife handle. **C:** The parietal peritoneum is grasped with Kelly forceps. A long Kelly forceps is introduced through the internal inguinal ring as it passes over the belly of the rectus. **D:** The Kelly clamp is brought through the internal inguinal ring and along the round ligament to a point adjacent to the chromic stay suture. A knife is used to open the peritoneum. The ends of the chromic suture are grasped by the Kelly clamp. **E:** As traction is applied to the suture, a knuckle of the round ligament passes through the internal ring. **F:** Three sutures of 2-0 delayed absorbable or silk suture are placed, fixing the ligament to the rectus fascia in a manner that will not interrupt the blood supply.

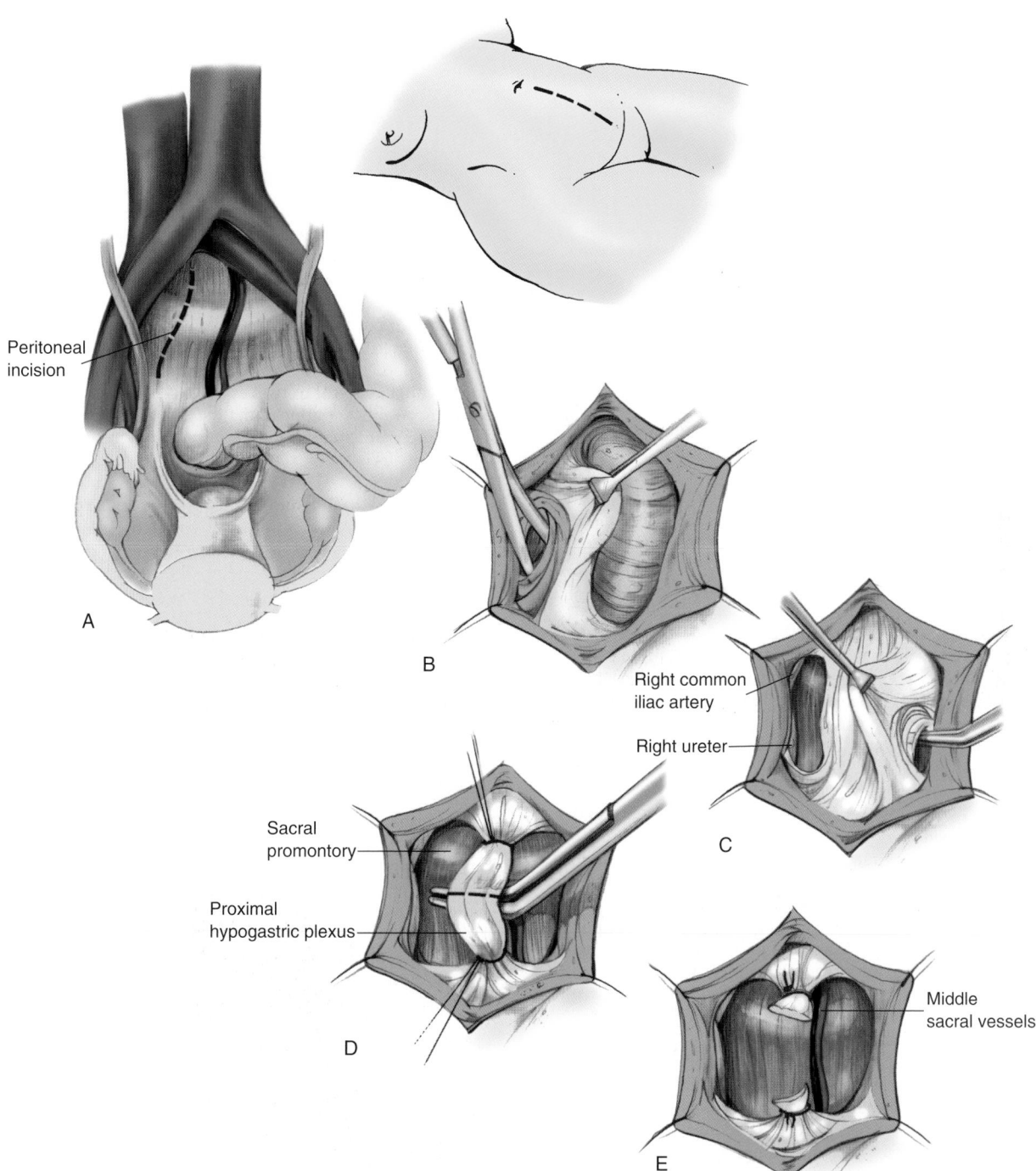

FIGURE 22.11 Presacral neurectomy. **A:** Location of incision in relation to anatomic landmarks. A Maylard incision can also be used in some cases. The descending colon is displaced superiorly and to the left for good exposure of the left margin of the hypogastric plexus. **B:** A Kittner sponge is used to dissect the areolar tissue medially and off the posterior aspect of the peritoneal flap. The right ureter can be identified easily. **C:** The areolar nerve-bearing tissue is dissected from the peritoneum on the left side, exposing the left internal iliac vessels and superior hemorrhoidal vessels. **D:** The plexus is isolated and elevated off the sacral promontory. A segment of plexus approximately 5 cm in length is isolated with 2-0 silk sutures. **E:** The plexus is excised. Note the relation between pedicles of the nerve bundle and adjacent structures.

can be used to elevate the sheath. Two 2-0 absorbable or silk sutures are placed around the proximal and distal aspects of a 5-cm segment of the plexus and are loosely tied. The tonsil clamp is applied to each end of the nerve bundle. As the clamps are removed, the sutures are slipped down over the crushed areas and tied securely. The intervening portion of the plexus is

then excised. The peritoneum may then be approximated with absorbable suture.

In less than 10% of cases, the pelvic mesocolon is inserted in front of the interiliac trigone and the nerve bundle cannot be reached by simple incision of the peritoneum. In these cases, the chief branches of the inferior mesenteric artery must be moved to the left to expose the triangular space between the two common iliac arteries. Unless there is adequate exposure and meticulous dissection, incomplete resection of the superior hypogastric plexus can occur, resulting in suboptimal denervation.

A laparoscopic approach to presacral neurectomy has also been described. This technique involves insertion of a 10-mm trocar sheath 3 cm above the symphysis pubis and placement of two accessory ports in each iliac fossa. Steep Trendelenburg position with a left lateral tilt is required to allow displacement of the intestines cephalad to expose the bifurcation of the aorta and sacral promontory. After retraction of the sigmoid colon and vasopressin infiltration of the sacral promontory area, the parietal peritoneum is grasped and elevated, and a transverse incision is performed from the major vessels or ureter on the right to the mesentery of the sigmoid on the left. The presacral nerve is isolated by developing the avascular space between the nerve and right internal iliac artery down to the periosteum via blunt dissection. Segments of the superior hypogastric plexus are removed by sharp dissection after thorough diathermy. The entire length of removed nerve plexus should not exceed 3 to 4 cm. Venous bleeding is controlled with bipolar cautery. Meticulous hemostasis must be ensured at the completion of the operation. This technique should only be performed by experienced laparoscopic surgeons because the vascular complications can be serious. In a review of 655 laparoscopic presacral neurectomy procedures, Chen and Soong reported a 0.6% rate of major complications, including one case of injury of the right internal iliac artery and three cases of chylous ascites.

Polan and DeCherney reported that the combination of presacral neurectomy and conservative surgery in women with chronic pelvic pain, endometriosis, and pelvic inflammatory disease increased total postoperative pain relief from 26% to 75%, although only a small number of patients were included in this laparotomy series. Lee and coworkers performed presacral neurectomy via laparotomy in 50 women with chronic pelvic pain. Dysmenorrhea resolved in 73% of the cases, dyspareunia lessened in 77%, and acyclic pain improved in 63%. The uterosacral ligaments were resected in half of the subjects in this study, but this did not seem to affect the overall rate of pain relief. In a randomized clinical trial of women with moderate-to-severe endometriosis and pelvic pain undergoing conservative surgical therapy, Candiani and colleagues reported a recurrence of midline menstrual pain in 23% of women who underwent presacral neurectomy versus a 42% recurrence in those who did not. This difference reached the limit of statistical significance ($P = 0.06$).

In an uncontrolled laparoscopic study by Nezhat and associates of 100 women subjected to vaporization of endometriosis and presacral neurectomy, the symptoms of pelvic pain, dysmenorrhea, and dyspareunia were reduced by more than 50% in 74, 61, and 55 patients, respectively, over the 1-year follow-up period. The stage of endometriosis did not correlate with the degree of pain improvement achieved. More recently, in a prospective, randomized, double-blind, controlled trial, Zullo and colleagues reported that the performance of laparoscopic presacral neurectomy improved the cure rate in women treated with conservative laparoscopic surgery for severe dysmenorrhea caused by endometriosis as compared with those who underwent mere ablation of endometriosis (85.7% vs. 57.1% at 12 months, $P < 0.05$). A significant improvement in the quality of life was observed after surgery in both groups.

Two common side effects of the presacral neurectomy procedure have been observed. Constipation may require laxatives or stool softeners for a period of 3 to 4 months. The vaginal dryness that develops in as many as 10% to 15% of patients is transient and usually resolves within 6 months.

Difficulty with micturition is an infrequent complication that rarely lasts for more than 1 or 2 months. A painless first stage of labor has been reported in women who have undergone presacral neurectomy.

Uterine Nerve Ablation The technique of uterosacral neurectomy was initially described by Ruggi in 1899. Later popularized by Doyle, it has since been adapted for performance during laparoscopic procedures for the alleviation of dysmenorrhea. Sympathetic fibers T10 to L1 are contained within the inferior hypogastric plexus and course along the inferior vena cava and sacrum to enter the uterus through the nerves of the uterosacral ligaments and accompanying uterine arteries. The parasympathetic components of the paracervical nerves originate from S1 through S3 or S4, travel within the nervi erigentes, and emerge in the lateral pelvis to form the Frankenhäuser ganglia lateral to the cervix. Division of the uterosacral ligaments at a point approximately 1.5 cm distal to the cervix should interrupt many sensory nerve fibers of the cervix and uterine corpus.

Lichten and Bombard published a small randomized, prospective, double-blind study of laparoscopic uterosacral nerve ablation for the treatment of severe or incapacitating dysmenorrhea unresponsive to oral contraceptives and nonsteroidal anti-inflammatory agents. None of the control patients noted improvement, whereas 9 of 11 in the treated group had almost complete relief at 3 months, and 5 of 11 described complete relief from dysmenorrhea 1 year after surgery. Patients with endometriosis were not included in this small series.

Surgical resection of pelvic endometrial implants may be all that is necessary to alleviate discomfort in most endometriosis patients. In a double-blind, randomized controlled laparoscopic trial, Johnson and colleagues found that uterine nerve ablation was effective in reducing dysmenorrhea in the absence of endometriosis, but the addition of this procedure to the surgical treatment of endometriosis was not associated with a significant difference in any pain outcomes. Similarly, Vercellini and colleagues could not demonstrate the efficacy of this procedure.

Uterine nerve ablation by laparotomy fell from favor before it was revived as an endoscopic technique. The potential neurologic, intestinal, orthopedic, and psychological components of pain should be considered before subjecting the patient to a procedure that, although now performed endoscopically, carries some surgical risk and whose effectiveness has been questioned because of the small number of cases evaluated. Complications associated with transection of the uterosacral ligaments include ureteral damage, bowel damage, and postoperative hemorrhage, which, if undetected, may result in death. Uterine prolapse has been described as a potential long-term side effect of the procedure.

Second-Look Laparoscopy

Second-look laparoscopy has been suggested as an appropriate procedure for additional lysis of pelvic adhesions in patients who have undergone a laparotomy or a laparoscopy for the resection of endometriosis. If scheduled 8 days to 6 weeks after the initial dissection, second-look laparoscopy allows separation of de novo adhesions that are still relatively filmy in consistency. In addition, laparoscopy after pelvic reconstructive surgery provides an opportunity to assess future prognosis for fertility.

Early second-look laparoscopy after endoscopic treatment of endometriomas has revealed a recurrence rate of endometriomas of 15% to 20%. Equally significant are the nearly 20% incidence of de novo adhesion formation and the 40% to

82% recurrence rate of dense adhesions. Second-look laparoscopy allows treatment of these findings; however, there is little direct evidence that this secondary surgical procedure will increase the cumulative pregnancy rate.

Some surgeons have proposed a three-step protocol to both surgically and medically treat large endometriomas more than 5 to 6 cm in size. During the initial diagnostic laparoscopy, the endometrioma is opened, drained, and biopsied. The patient is then treated with GnRH agonists for 12 weeks, and the second-look laparoscopy is performed. The endometrioma is opened, and the interior wall of the cyst is laser vaporized. The epithelial lining of the cyst is atrophic and thinned, and the use of the CO_2 laser results in minimal thermal damage to the normal ovarian tissue. This three-step approach may result in less compromise to ovarian follicular reserve than stripping of the cyst wall.

Surgical Outcomes

No classification schedule for endometriosis provides an accurate correlation between extent of disease and pregnancy rate. Nevertheless, point categorization through the revised ASRM classification does provide a framework in which to report outcomes of therapy.

Fertility In a review of the surgical outcome expected through laparoscopic therapy for minimal and mild endometriosis, Cook and Rock found the crude pregnancy rate following cautery or laser ablation of implants was 54% to 58%. Life table analysis showed similar conception rates following laparoscopy and laparotomy to excise minimal or mild stages of endometriosis. Hence, the performance of a laparotomy is not warranted for lesser stages of disease.

Treatment of mild endometriosis via laparoscopic excision or electrocoagulation resulted in similar reproductive outcomes in a retrospective study by Tulandi and Al-Took. The total pregnancy rate was 53.5% in the excision group and 57.1% in the electrosurgery group. The mean interval between surgery and conception was 10.7 months in the electrosurgery group and 13.3 months in the excision group. Excision of tissue may result in more complete removal of infiltrating endometriosis, which should be of particular benefit to patients with deep nodules.

The stage of disease as categorized by the modified ASRM classification of endometriosis did not predict subsequent reproductive performance in a 2006 study by Vercellini and colleagues. Five hundred and thirty-seven infertile women with endometriosis undergoing first-line conservative laparoscopic surgery were followed for a mean of 32 months postoperatively. The cumulative probability of pregnancy at 3 years following laparoscopy was 47% (51% at stage I, 45% at stage II, 46% at stage III, and 44% at stage IV; log-rank test, [chi]^2 = 1.50, P = 0.68).

Expectant management of mild-to-moderate endometriosis after diagnosis by laparoscopy yields a crude pregnancy rate of approximately 50%, which has brought into question whether surgical therapy of lesser stages of disease actually enhances fertility. In a retrospective study comparing the efficacy of electrosurgical treatment of endometriosis with the efficacy of expectant management in minimal and mild endometriosis-associated infertility, Tulandi and Mouchawar reported that the cumulative probability of conception was significantly higher among patients treated surgically. Moreover, meta-analysis of the two randomized prospective trials showed that laparoscopic electrosurgery or laser to resect or ablate stages I–II endometriosis implants and

adhesions resulted in a significantly higher fecundity rate as compared with the control group undergoing diagnostic laparoscopy only. The largest trial, conducted by Marcoux et al. in 1997, clearly supported this outcome, with an increased chance of pregnancy (OR 2.03, 95% CI 1.28 to 3.24) and ongoing pregnancy rate after 20 weeks (OR 1.95, 95% CI 1.18 to 3.22) (**Fig. 22.12**), but the smaller trial, by Parazzini in 1999, did not show benefit (pregnancy OR 0.76, 95% CI 0.31 to 1.88; live birth OR 0.85, 95% CI 0.32 to 2.28). When the ongoing pregnancy and live birth rates from these two studies were combined, Jacobson et al. found a statistically significant increase with surgery (OR 1.64, 95% CI 1.05 to 2.57). The findings suggest that for every 12 patients having stage I or II endometriosis diagnosed at laparoscopy, there will be one additional successful pregnancy if ablation or resection of visible endometriosis is performed, compared with no treatment. This number needed to treat applies only to those patients who are found to have endometriosis. Approximately 70% of patients with otherwise unexplained infertility and no signs or symptoms to suggest endometriosis would be found to not have endometriosis during diagnostic laparoscopy.

Operative treatment of moderate or severe disease does offer a greater likelihood of conception than expectant management, in part because of correction of mechanical factors such as adhesions. The overall crude pregnancy rate reported by various studies of conservative laparotomy for endometriosis that stratified reproductive results by disease severity was 38%, with a monthly fecundity rate averaging 1.4% to 1.5%. Laparoscopic treatment of endometriosis offered a mean crude pregnancy rate of 47.6% in a small compilation of series. Hence, expert laparoscopists have reported results that appear to be as good as those obtained through the open abdomen, although there are inadequate data for direct comparison of outcomes of the two surgical modalities, and the correct identification and classification of disease may vary between laparotomy and laparoscopy groups. A 2012 Cochrane review of two randomized control trials concluded that excision of ovarian endometriomas was superior to ablative therapy of endometriomas in improving the chance of spontaneous pregnancy, with an odds ratio of 5.21. Life table analysis demonstrated that pregnancy is most likely to occur during the first 36 months after surgery. Furthermore, the duration of

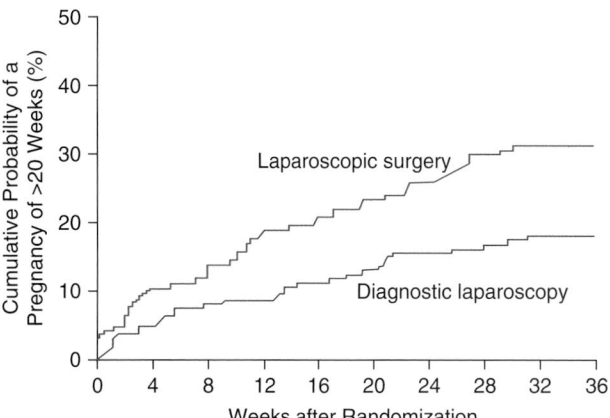

FIGURE 22.12 Cumulative probability of a pregnancy carried beyond 20 weeks in the 36 weeks after laparoscopy in women with endometriosis, according to study group (From Marcoux S, Maheux R, Béribé S. Laparoscopic surgery in infertile women with minimal or mild endometriosis. *N Engl J Med* 1997;337:217. Copyright © 1997, Massachusetts Medical Society).

IV

infertility and, perhaps, patient age may have a greater impact on cumulative pregnancy rates than the actual stage (revised ASRM stages I through IV) of the disease.

Rectovaginal endometriosis is usually associated with pain symptoms, but the effect of disease in this location on fertility is uncertain. According to the results of 11 selected studies reviewed by Vercellini et al. in 2012, the mean postoperative conception rate in all women desiring pregnancy was 39% (223/571), irrespective of the preoperative fertility status and whether the patient pursued IVF after surgery. This rate dropped to 24% (123/510) in infertile patients who attempted to conceive spontaneously after surgery.

Pain In a prospective, randomized, double-blind, controlled trial of laser laparoscopy in the treatment of pelvic pain associated with minimal-to-moderate endometriosis, Sutton and associates found that 62.5% of the laser-treated women reported symptom improvement at 6 months as compared with 22.6% of those treated expectantly. Symptom relief continued at 1 year in 90% of those who initially responded. Moreover, in a more recent randomized, blinded, crossover study by Abbott et al., 80% percent of patients who underwent excisional surgery had symptomatic improvement as compared with 30% of the placebo group. A 2010 Cochrane analysis concluded that laparoscopic surgery for pelvic pain associated with endometriosis was superior to diagnostic laparoscopy alone, with an odds ratio of 7.72.

The technique of surgically treating lesser stages of endometriosis may not significantly influence pain relief, as long as the surgeon is aware of the depth of extension of the lesions. In a recent randomized study by Wright and colleagues, both excision and ablation of mild endometriosis produced good symptomatic relief and reduction of pelvic tenderness (67%).

Long-term improvement in quality of life can be achieved with laparoscopic excision of endometriosis. In a prospective, observational cohort study of 176 women with chronic pelvic pain with surgically diagnosed endometriosis, pain scores were highly significantly reduced at 2 to 5 years following resection in the categories of dysmenorrhea, dyspareunia, nonmenstrual pain, and dyschezia. The chance of requiring further surgery was 36%. Of note, almost one third who had further surgery had no evidence of endometriosis, either macroscopically or histologically, at the time of reoperation.

Aggressive and complete or near-complete excision of deep endometriosis is justified. Resection of deep endometriosis relieved dyspareunia in 40% and dysmenorrhea in 60% of cases. Nezhat and associates noted moderate-to-complete relief of pain in 162 of 175 women; however, some patients in this series had several surgical interventions. Preliminary analysis of the surgical results in 250 women in whom deep endometriosis had been excised with CO_2 laser showed a cure rate of pelvic pain in 70% and a recurrence rate of less than 5% over a 5-year follow-up period. Vercellini and colleagues reported that conservative surgery for rectovaginal endometriosis in infertile women did increase the pain-free survival time, although it did not modify the reproductive prognosis over expectant management. Recurrence of symptoms after surgery requiring reoperation may be dependent on surgeon experience and the use of postoperative suppressive therapy. It is progressive with time and is reported to by Falcone and Lebovic be approximately 15% at 1 year, 36% at 5 years, and 50% at 7 years. After bowel resection in patients with extensive endometriosis, pain symptoms have been improved by at least 70%, with recurrence in 0% to 34% in published trials. Women under 30 years of age at the time of initial operation are more likely to undergo a second surgical procedure to treat recurrent pain.

Endometriosis is often not identified in patients with chronic pelvic pain who undergo reoperation following their initial surgery for endometriosis. Persistence of dysmenorrhea and nonmenstrual pain after optimal endometriosis surgery may indicate adenomyosis. In a recent study by Parker and colleagues, chronic pelvic pain was significantly more likely to persist with uterine junctional zone thickness greater than 11 mm on preoperative MRI.

Recurrent Surgery

Rock and colleagues have shown that 13.5% of patients initially treated with conservative surgery required subsequent operative procedures. Wheeler and Malinak noted a cumulative recurrence rate at 3 and 5 years after conservative surgery of 13.5% and 40.3%, respectively. Neither the initial staging nor the ability to conceive after the initial surgery greatly affected the recurrence rates. Repeat conservative surgery for pelvic pain associated with recurrent endometriosis has similar efficacy and limitations as primary surgery, with long-term cumulative recurrence rates ranging from 20% to 40% as reported by Belanda et al.

Laparoscopic excision of ovarian endometriomas by the stripping technique is associated with a lower reoperation rate than that of fenestration. In a study of patients who underwent laparoscopic cystectomy of ovarian endometriomas of greater than 3 cm in diameter, Busacca and colleagues reported a cumulative rate of ultrasonographic recurrence of 11.7% over 48 months. Two studies that evaluated patients up to 49 and 60 months following surgery for endometriomas noted recurrent rates of up to 57%.

A second cytoreductive procedure may benefit some infertile women who have undergone surgery in the past if they do not pursue assisted reproductive technologies. A cumulative pregnancy rate of 32.4% at 35.4 months was achieved by Fedele and colleagues in 2006 after a second conservative laparoscopic stripping procedure for recurrent endometriomas. The recurrence of pain (17.4%) was similar to that experienced after the primary laparoscopic stripping procedure. However, if the initial surgery fails to restore fertility in patients with stage III or stage IV endometriosis, IVF may be more beneficial than reoperation for those who are otherwise asymptomatic. Pagidas and colleagues compared the outcome of a second operation for stage III or IV endometriosis-related infertility versus proceeding directly to IVF. The cumulative pregnancy rate 9 months after surgery was 24.4%, compared with a pregnancy rate of 33.4% after one trial of IVF and a cumulative pregnancy rate of 69.6% after two trials of IVF.

Combination Medical and Surgical Treatment

Preoperative and postoperative medical therapies have been proposed as treatment adjuncts to conservative resection of endometriosis to enhance fertility. Preoperative suppression of disease with hormonal agents may facilitate the surgical procedure by reducing tissue vascularity, and the greater ease in tissue dissection may decrease adhesion formation during the postoperative period. The preoperative hormonal agents also eliminate the corpus luteum that might otherwise be mistaken for an endometrioma. However, they may also reduce the size of endometriosis implants, making them less recognizable after short-term drug therapy. In a controlled clinical trial by Muzii et al., a 3-month course of GnRH agonist treatment before laparoscopy for endometrioma excision failed to result in a reduction in operative time or recurrence rate of disease during a 1-year follow-up period. There are no substantive data to justify hormonal treatments before surgery to improve the success of surgery.

Initiation of postoperative medical therapy may inhibit the activity of any residual disease, suppress ovulation, and decrease the possibility of adverse effects of peritoneal spillage of disease at the time of resection. However, postoperative medical therapy has a serious drawback; the patient is unable to attempt conception for several months. Andrews and Larsen have noted that the best chance for postsurgical conception occurs during the first 6 months after conservative surgery by laparotomy. Thus, suppressing ovulation during that critical period may be counterproductive. Treatment with a GnRH agonist after surgery does not improve fertility as compared with expectant management.

Contemporary management of women with endometriosis-associated pelvic pain involves both surgical and long-term medical therapy. When cytoreductive laparoscopy is followed by a 6-month course of GnRH analogue, there is a significant delay in the return of endometriosis symptoms requiring further treatment. In a randomized, prospective study, Hornstein and colleagues found that this interval was more than 24 months in those receiving nafarelin versus 11.7 months in the placebo group. A shorter duration of hormonal therapy during the postoperative period may be inadequate in reducing recurrence risk. A 3-month course of nafarelin following surgical therapy of stages III and IV endometriosis was ineffective in reducing pain scores as compared with placebo. Postoperative administration of low-dose, cyclic oral contraceptives for 6 months delayed the recurrence of pain symptoms and endometriomas at 12 months, but no significant differences were detected at 24 months or 36 months following laparoscopic excision. A 2012 systematic review and meta-analysis by Vercellini et al in 2012 indicated that a more prolonged course of postoperative oral contraceptive use (≥12 months) dramatically decreased the risk of endometrial cyst recurrence and pain symptoms. Because of these data, patients should be advised of the potential benefit of regular contraceptive use following surgery until such time as pregnancy is desired.

Hysterectomy

The number and rate of hysterectomies performed for endometriosis increased steadily from the 1960s to the 1980s, more so than for other diagnoses. The reported rate for 1982 to 1984 was more than double the rate for 1965 to 1967, although the exact reasons for the increase remain uncertain. Although statistically significant increases for hysterectomy rates were observed from 1994 through 1998, the increase was limited, and the curve remained nearly flat. Endometriosis was the primary indication for 20.8% of white women and 9.7% of black women undergoing hysterectomy in the United States from 1994 to 1999. Because of concern over the risk of recurrence even after definitive surgical therapy, bilateral oophorectomy was performed at the time of hysterectomy in 52% of women 44 years of age or younger and in 81% of women 45 years of age or older.

Definitive surgery offers prompt, complete, and long-term relief of pain from endometriosis more often than do the various available medical regimens. Most hysterectomies for endometriosis are performed by the abdominal route; in selected cases, laparoscopy may allow lysis of complicating adhesions or large implants, thus allowing safe vaginal hysterectomy. When the posterior cul-de-sac is obliterated and extensive fibrosis is present deep in the pelvis, subtotal hysterectomy may be indicated.

The recurrence of cyclic pain associated with endometriosis after hysterectomy with preservation of normal ovaries has been estimated at 3% to 7%. Nevertheless, in a study of 138 women who underwent hysterectomy with the diagnosis of endometriosis at the Johns Hopkins Hospital, ovarian conservation was associated with a 6.1 times greater risk of development of recurrent pain and an 8.1 times greater risk of reoperation as compared with oophorectomy at the time of hysterectomy. Recent data from a 7-year follow-up study by Shabika et al. showed that in women undergoing hysterectomy, the reoperation-free rates at 2, 5, and 7 years for those with ovarian preservation were 95%, 86%, and 77%, respectively, as compared with 96%, 91%, and 91% for those patients without ovarian preservation. Hysterectomy does not improve symptoms in 25% of cases of chronic pelvic pain when the uterus is believed to be the source of the pain.

Minute, hormonally active ovarian fragments may be detected in women with symptomatic endometriosis, even after total abdominal hysterectomy and bilateral salpingo-oophorectomy. Laparoscopic resection of invasive peritoneal and intestinal disease that persists after castration may result in an improvement in pain symptoms. Ovarian remnant syndrome is the result of incomplete excision of cortical tissue at the time of extirpative surgery for endometriosis or pelvic inflammatory disease. Most ovarian remnants are retroperitoneal in location, and they are often densely adhered to pelvic sidewall structures, including the ureter, hypogastric vessels, and bladder base. Complete surgical removal may be difficult.

Estrogen replacement therapy after total hysterectomy and bilateral oophorectomy is associated with less than a 10% rate of recurrence of endometriosis. A cause-and-effect relation between estrogen replacement and malignancy in endometriosis has not been established, suggesting that progestational agents need not be prescribed together with estrogens after hysterectomy for a diagnosis of endometriosis. However, administering both progestin and estrogen may be theoretically beneficial if the disease was incompletely resected or deeply invasive, contained atypical epithelial changes, or is recurrent. A study by Matorras et al. showed an endometriosis recurrence rate of 3.5% in women treated with cyclic estrogen and progestogen replacement during a mean 46 months of follow-up as compared to 0% recurrence rate in untreated controls. Women who begin estrogen replacement therapy immediately after total abdominal hysterectomy and bilateral salpingo-oophorectomy are at no greater risk of recurrent pain than those who delay estrogen therapy for more than 6 weeks postoperatively.

Women with endometriosis were shown by Modugno and colleagues to be at increased risk of developing ovarian cancer (OR 1.32; 95% CI 1.06 to 1.65). An analysis by Melin et al. of data from the National Swedish Cancer Register showed that complete surgical removal of endometriosis lesions, even when the ovaries are unaffected, as well as removing the affected ovary in case of ovarian endometriosis, may significantly decrease the risk of ovarian cancer. In addition, hysterectomy and the use of oral contraceptives for greater than 10 years substantially reduce this risk.

ENDOMETRIOSIS AND ASSISTED REPRODUCTIVE TECHNOLOGIES

If spontaneous conception is not achieved within 3 years of surgical resection of endometriosis or within 1 year of repair of tubal obstruction associated with endometriosis, the odds are poor that it ever will occur. Techniques in assisted reproduction have been widely used during the past three decades. IVF removes gametes and zygotes from a potentially harmful environment and may bypass pelvic adhesions associated with endometriosis. Endometriosis is the sole identifiable cause of infertility in 25% to 35% of women undergoing IVF/embryo transfer.

IV

The impact of endometriosis on the outcome of IVF has been controversial. Several studies have noted that the responses to gonadotropic stimulation, the numbers of pre-ovulatory oocytes, the fertilization and cleavage rates, and the clinical pregnancy rates associated with stage I and stage II endometriosis have been equivalent to rates associated with tubal disease and unexplained infertility. Kuivasaari et al. reported that there was a significantly lower pregnancy rate and embryo implantation rate per fresh embryo transfer after pooled cycles (1 to 4) among women with stage III/IV endometriosis (22.6%) compared with stage I/II (40%) or tubal infertility (36.6%). However, when adjusted for confounding variables, Barnhart and colleagues in 2002 found that there was a significantly negative association between endometriosis of all stages and IVF outcome. This meta-analysis pooled data from 22 nonrandomized studies regarding IVF success rates in patients with endometriosis versus control patients without endometriosis and with tubal infertility. Most of these series included small numbers of subjects. The authors concluded that there was a 54% reduction in pregnancy rate after IVF in patients with endometriosis and that the success rate was even lower when the staging of endometriosis was higher. Subsequent studies have disputed these findings.

Poor IVF outcome in severe endometriosis may be related to oocyte or embryo factors rather than decreased uterine receptivity. Diaz and colleagues found that a history of severe endometriosis in recipients of donor oocytes had no effect on embryo implantation rates or clinical pregnancy rates as compared with recipients who did not have a history of endometriosis. Oocytes originating from women with endometriotic ovaries and donated to disease-free women led to reduced implantation rates.

In general, women with endometriosis have a lower ovarian response to gonadotropin stimulation. One reason for this response may be previous ovarian resection. Studies recruiting women with a history of surgical excision of a unilateral endometrioma and comparing subsequent ovarian responsiveness to gonadotropin stimulation in the affected and contralateral intact gonad indicate that excision of endometriomas is associated with quantitative damage to ovarian follicular reserve. However, this lower oocyte yield following surgery has not necessarily led to decreased pregnancy rates.

Recent retrospective studies have suggested that routine laparoscopic cystectomy for endometriomas before commencing an IVF cycle does not improve IVF outcomes. Aside from a lower peak estradiol level on the day of hCG administration and a higher total gonadotropin dose administered to women previously operated on for an endometrioma, no significant differences were found between the resected endometrioma group and the intact endometrioma group among the different variables analyzed by Garcia-Velasco et al. Pre-IVF excision of ovarian endometriomas in symptomatic women did not impair nor enhance IVF or intracytoplasmic sperm injection success rates.

A 2005 retrospective study by Suzuki et al. indicated that women with a history of past or current endometriomas had fewer oocytes retrieved during IVF than tubal factor controls, but the fertilization rate, embryo quality, or pregnancy outcome was not affected. Conversely, Almog and colleagues found that the presence of an intact, unilateral ovarian endometrioma was not associated with a reduced number of oocytes retrieved from the affected ovary as compared to the opposite ovary or women without endometriomas.

Tinkanen and Kujansuu studied the effects of operative treatment of recurrent ovarian endometriosis on the pregnancy rate with IVF. They compared 45 patients with ultrasound-diagnosed ovarian endometriosis during IVF treatment,

36 of the cases being recurrences after previous operation, with 55 patients who had undergone past endometrioma resection and had no evidence of recurrence before IVF. Patients with endometriomas had significantly more embryos for transfer compared with women without endometriomas. The clinical pregnancy rate was 38% in the endometrioma group compared with 22% in the no-endometrioma group. The women who had surgery with no recurrent endometriosis may have had a more extensive resection as compared with those with recurrent endometriomas following initial surgery.

Hence, the hypothesis that surgical therapy of endometriosis increases IVF pregnancy rates is not clearly validated by the available evidence. Endometrioma resection may compromise or destroy adjacent normal ovarian tissue by removing part of the ovarian cortex and thus reducing ovarian reserve. On the other hand, larger endometriomas may interfere with follicular recruitment, may impose difficulties during oocyte retrieval, and may theoretically produce substances that are toxic to maturing oocytes and affect cell cleavage after fertilization. However, a systematic review by Benschop et al. concluded that surgical intervention for women with endometriomas 3 cm or larger has no benefit over expectant management on the outcome of assisted reproductive technology. The European Society of Human Reproduction and Embryology recommends laparoscopic ovarian cystectomy before IVF if the patient has an endometrioma $\geq$ 4 cm in diameter in order to confirm the diagnosis histologically and to reduce the potential risks of transvaginal aspiration of follicles in women with large cysts.

In vitro fertilization offers a high cumulative pregnancy rate in patients with colorectal endometriosis who have not undergone prior surgery for deep infiltrating endometriosis. However, the subgroup of patients with concomitant uterine adenomyosis has a low pregnancy rate. Several studies have found that adenomyosis had no adverse effects on IVF outcome in infertile women with proven endometriosis when they were pretreated with long-term GnRH agonist.

The presence of significant pelvic pain symptoms, number of previous surgical interventions for endometriosis, the size of the cyst, accessibility of ovaries for transvaginal aspiration of follicles, and the patient's age and ovarian reserve must be taken into consideration in establishing an individualized treatment plan (Fig. 22.3). Resection of large cysts before IVF may reduce the risk of inadvertent needle puncture or drainage of endometriomas at the time of oocyte retrieval for IVF, which is associated with an increased risk of infection, even if prophylactic antibiotics are administered. Further randomized clinical trials are needed to elucidate the relative effects of mild peritoneal endometriosis and advanced stages of disease associated with endometriomas and pelvic adhesions on the outcome of IVF.

The relative value of initial medical therapy before use of assisted reproductive technologies remains controversial. Dicker and associates noted that 35 women with severe endometriosis who underwent 6 months of ovarian suppression with a GnRH analogue had a higher clinical pregnancy rate per cycle and per transfer than did 32 women who received ovarian stimulation for IVF without prior GnRH treatment (per cycle, 25% vs. 3.9%; per transfer, 33% vs. 5.3%). Sallam et al., in a Cochrane review of three randomized, controlled trials involving 165 participants, ovarian steroid suppression with GnRH agonist for 3 to 6 months before IVF in women with stages II to IV endometriosis led to a fourfold increase in clinical pregnancy rates. However, the very high reported clinical pregnancy rates in the treatment arms of two of these studies suggest that more data are necessary to better understand the relative value of this suppressive therapy.

TABLE 22.9 Cycle Fecundity in Women with Stage I or II Endometriosis, According to Treatment

GROUP TREATMENT	UNEXPLAINED INFERTILITY	ENDOMETRIOSIS-ASSOCIATED INFERTILITY			
	GUZICK ET AL.	DEATON ET AL.	CHAFFKIN ET AL.	FEDELE ET AL.	KEMMANN ET AL.
No treatment or intracervical					
Insemination	0.02	0.033	—	0.045	0.028
IUI	0.05[a]	—	—	—	—
Clomiphene	—	—	—	—	0.066
Clomiphene/IUI	—	0.095[a]	—	—	—
Gonadotropins	0.04[a]	—	0.066	—	0.073[a]
Gonadotropins/IUI	0.09[a]	—	0.129[a]	0.15[a]	—
IVF	—	—	—	—	0.222[a]

[a]$P < 0.05$ for treatment versus no treatments.
IUI, intrauterine insemination; IVF, in vitro fertilization.
From the Practice Committee of the American Society for Reproductive Medicine. Endometiosis and infertility. *Fertil Steril* 2004;82 (suppl 1):S40, with permission. Copyright © 2004, Elsevier.

Controlled ovarian hyperstimulation (COH) with clomiphene citrate, letrozole, human menopausal gonadotropins, or FSH together with intrauterine insemination (IUI) has been proposed as a method to increase cycle fecundity of patients with endometriosis, although few series have been published to date (Table 22.9). By increasing the number of oocytes released at the time of ovulation and introducing a high concentration of spermatozoa into the female reproductive tract, the chance for conception is improved, merely because of the larger number of gametes available for fertilization. In addition, subtle abnormalities of folliculogenesis, corpus luteum function, tubal motility, or sperm function may be corrected with this therapy. Cycle fecundity rates associated with COH/IUI therapy in patients with endometriosis-associated infertility have ranged from 9% to 13%, although these series did not include a nontreatment control group. One recent prospective randomized study found a higher pregnancy rate with COH/IUI following at least 6 weeks of GnRH agonist suppression in patients with advanced stages of endometriosis.

Fedele and associates reported that superovulation with timed intercourse was not associated with a better cumulative, crude pregnancy rate than expectant management in infertile women with endometriosis stages I and II, although the cycle fecundity rate was improved. However, a more recent randomized, controlled trial of COH and IUI for infertility associated with stages I and II endometriosis demonstrated a live birth rate of 11% per cycle in the treatment group and 2% in the control group. Nuoja-Huttunen and colleagues reported that ovarian stimulation or induction using gonadotropins results in higher fecundity rates than no treatment, but the clinical pregnancy rate after treatment was still significantly lower in the endometriosis group (6.5%) than in women with unexplained infertility (15%). There was no surgical treatment of endometriosis before therapy with COH and IUI in these latter studies.

In a 2006 retrospective study by Webrouck and colleagues, the clinical pregnancy rate per cycle of COH and IUI in women with minimal or mild endometriosis who underwent laparoscopic excision of lesions within 7 months of onset of treatment was 21% or 18.9%, respectively, which was comparable to that achieved in patients with unexplained infertility, 20.5%. The mean age of the patients with endometriosis in this study was 31 years. The cumulative live birth rate of nearly 70% within four cycles suggests that COH and IUI may be appropriate first-line therapy in patients younger than 35 who have not become pregnant within 6 to 12 months after

surgical treatment of minimal-to-mild endometriosis and who have no other infertility risk factors. In a 2012 study by Abu Hashim et al. of women with a mean age of 31 years who had undergone laparoscopic treatment of minimal-to-mild endometriosis 6 to 12 months earlier, the clinical pregnancy rates were 15.9% and 14.5%, respectively, with letrozole–IUI and clomiphene–IUI therapy.

Temporary exposure to very high estradiol levels in women during COH for IVF or IUI is not a major risk factor for endometriosis recurrence in women treated with assisted reproductive technology.

Women with endometriosis have been shown to have adverse obstetrical outcomes as compared to those without endometriosis. Preterm birth, preeclampsia, antepartum bleeding or placental complications, and cesarean sections were more common in women diagnosed with endometriosis in a Swedish cohort study by Stephansson et al. of data from the national medical birth registry. It is uncertain whether these associations were related to endometriosis, being infertile, or the antiretroviral therapy treatment that may have been undertaken to achieve the pregnancy.

ADENOMYOSIS

Adenomyosis is defined as heterotopic endometrial glands and stroma located deep within the myometrium associated by hyperplasia of the adjacent smooth muscle. This disease can be categorized as diffuse or local in its distribution. Diffuse adenomyosis can be relatively localized but is never encapsulated (Fig. 22.13). The uterus itself is usually mildly enlarged, rarely to more than twice-normal size, and is generally symmetric. Cut sections of the myometrium reveal a coarse trabecular pattern of interlacing musculature and fibrous tissue with small islands of endometrium that are often dark and hemorrhagic. Localized, encapsulated disease of the uterine wall is termed *adenomyoma*, to distinguish this manifestation of adenomyosis from the more usual diffuse pattern. An adenomyoma is always located mainly within the wall of the uterus but may project into the uterine cavity to become further known as a *submucous adenomyoma*. This encapsulated, submucous form of adenomyosis disease resembles the leiomyoma.

The most widely accepted theory of the origin of adenomyosis is that endometrial tissue within the myometrium is of müllerian origin. Its presence in this location is the result of a direct, downward extension of the endometrium of the uterine cavity.

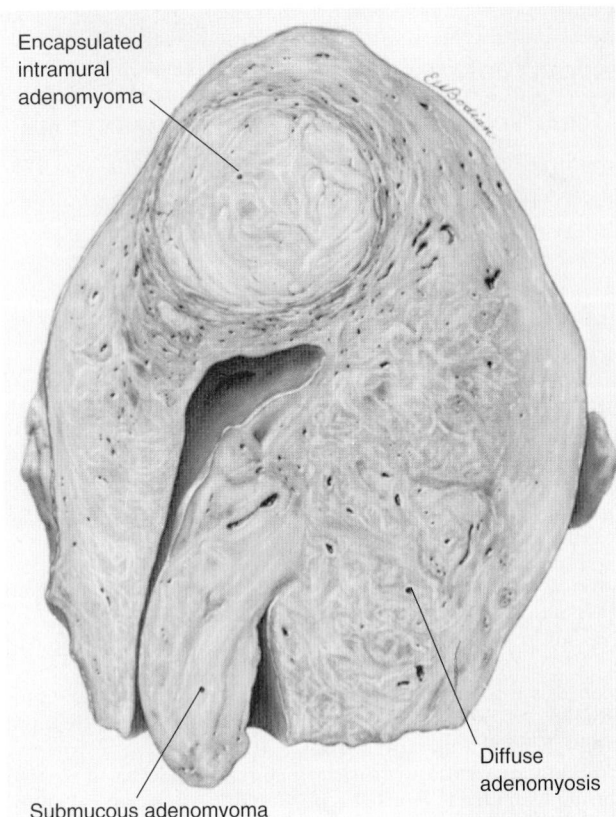

Encapsulated intramural adenomyoma

Diffuse adenomyosis

Submucous adenomyoma

FIGURE 22.13 Uterus showing three types of adenomyomatous growth: encapsulated intramural adenomyoma, submucous adenomyoma, and diffuse adenomyosis of walls.

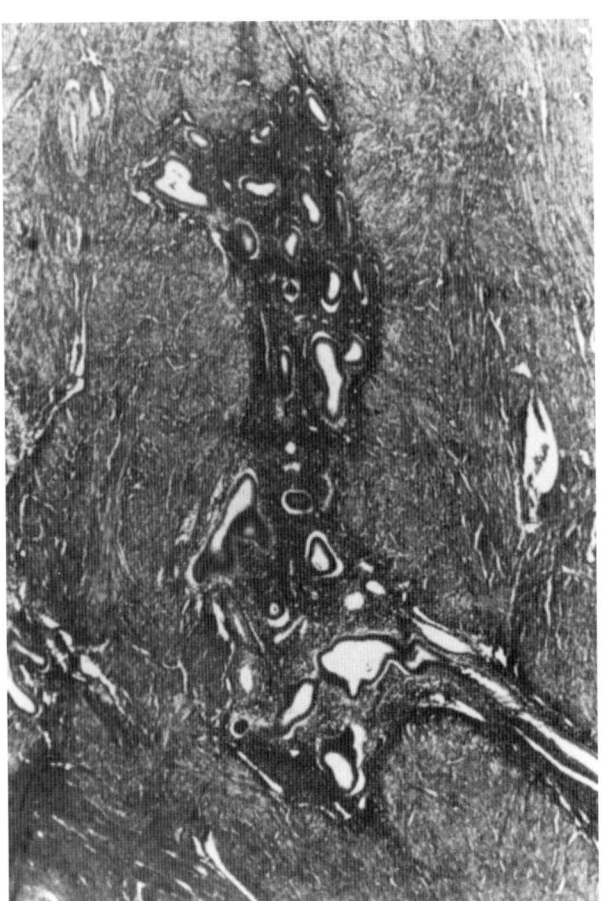

FIGURE 22.14 Area of adenomyosis. Compact stroma and proliferative, slightly hyperplastic glands surrounded by hypertrophied myometrium.

Serial sectioning of tissue has revealed a direct continuity between the basalis portion of the endometrium and the endometrial islands within the areas of adenomyosis. Endometrial extensions sometimes are present through the full thickness of the myometrium to the serosal surface of the uterus. Occasionally, only subserosal adenomyosis is seen. Subserosal adenomyosis is often associated with pelvic endometriosis and may cause the lymphatic spread of endometrial fragments.

The intramural islands generally have the same histologic appearance as the basalis of the endometrium (Fig. 22.14) and often respond to estrogen stimulation by demonstrating a proliferative or, occasionally, cystic hyperplastic pattern. Cellular atypia is rare. The effect of progestational agents on the ectopic endometrium is less predictable. Secretory changes in the glands are uncommon except in pregnancy, when a decidual reaction of the stroma is anticipated. Unlike endometriosis, adenomyotic lesions are not characterized by a pronounced hemorrhagic tendency or inflammatory response. In the absence of hormonal stimulation, adenomyosis becomes atrophic. Adenocarcinomas involving adenomyosis are characterized by a history of prior exogenous estrogen use, by low histologic grades, and by an excellent prognosis.

Adenomyosis can be definitively diagnosed only through histologic sections of myometrium. The reported incidence of the disease varies widely among from 8% to 62%, depending on the criteria used for diagnosis and on the thoroughness with which the excised uterine tissue is studied. The usual criterion for diagnosis is glandular extension below the endometrial–myometrial interface of greater than 2.5 mm, whereas adenomyosis subbasalis can be defined as minimally invasive adenomyosis extending less than 2 mm beneath the basal

endometrium. The incidence of adenomyosis begins to rise in the mid-30s and peaks in the fifth decade. Infertility is not common, although most patients are multiparous. Approximately 12% have coexisting external endometriosis. Adenomyosis is often discovered incidentally in patients undergoing surgery for uterine leiomyomata.

Symptoms

Adenomyosis is often an incidental pathologic finding, and approximately 35% of cases are asymptomatic. Dysmenorrhea is more likely to be reported when glandular invasion exceeds 80% or more of the myometrium. Pain can be severe, cramping, or knifelike and may occur up to 1 week before the onset of menstrual flow. The pattern of dysmenorrhea is likely associated with bleeding episodes within the deep-lying islands of endometrium. Menorrhagia can be a consequence of the increased surface area of the enlarged uterine cavity. In addition, extensive involvement of the myometrium can interfere with the normal contractility of the uterine musculature and can lead to excessive bleeding. Nevertheless, data collected from 1,851 hysterectomies for the prospective, multicenter Collaborative Review of Sterilization study indicate that adenomyosis occurs as often in asymptomatic uteri removed for prolapse (19%) as in uteri removed for excessive bleeding (22%) or pain symptoms (15%). Uterine adenomyosis is significantly associated with pelvic endometriosis, with a prevalence of up to 90%. By impairing uterine sperm transport, adenomyosis may be a leading factor of infertility in women with endometriosis.

Pelvic Findings

The uterus may be very firm to palpation and is usually enlarged to not more than twice its normal size. As it is classically described, the adenomyotic enlargement occurs in the anteroposterior dimension, a reflection of the more prominent involvement of the posterior uterine wall. In the more common diffuse type of adenomyosis, the uterus is a symmetrically enlarged, globular structure. Encapsulated adenomyomas may cause the uterus to be irregular or asymmetric, much as it is when leiomyomata are present. At times, particularly during menstruation, the enlarged uterus is tender on examination.

Diagnosis

Adenomyosis should always be suspected in a woman with dysmenorrhea and menorrhagia of increasing severity her fourth or fifth decade, particularly if the uterus is symmetrically enlarged, firm, and tender. An exact preoperative diagnosis is often difficult to establish because dysfunctional uterine bleeding and multiple small leiomyomata can present in a similar fashion. Gambone and colleagues reported that a presumptive diagnosis of adenomyosis was verified in only 38% of hysterectomy specimens. The diagnosis can be histologically established before hysterectomy only in the rare case in which excessive myometrium is removed during curettage or a polypoid submucous adenomyoma is excised. However, hysteroscopic myometrial biopsy of the posterior uterine wall with use of a 5-mm loop electrode has been shown to effectively establish the diagnosis in women with menorrhagia.

Hysterosalpingography of the adenomyomatous uterus with water-based media can occasionally demonstrate multiple spiculations or tuft defects leading from the uterine cavity to the myometrial wall; however, similar findings can occur in cases of vascular or lymphatic extravasation. MRI has proved to be highly accurate for distinguishing adenomyosis from leiomyomata; on T2-weighted images, adenomyosis appears as an ill-defined, relatively homogeneous, low-signal-intensity area embedded with sparse, high-intensity spots. The optimal junctional zone thickness value for establishing the diagnosis of adenomyosis is 12 mm or more. Several studies have shown that the sensitivity and specificity of MRI to diagnose adenomyosis range from 86% to 100% in a symptomatic patient population.

Recent studies have also suggested an important role for transvaginal ultrasound in distinguishing adenomyosis from leiomyomata. By using the diagnostic criterion of the presence of unencapsulated, heterogeneous, myometrial areas within round anechoic areas 1 to 3 mm in diameter, Fedele and colleagues noted a sensitivity of 80%, a specificity of 74%, a negative predictive value of 81%, and a positive predictive value of 73%. Nevertheless, when transvaginal sonography and MRI have been prospectively compared, the latter has been significantly more accurate in correctly establishing the diagnosis.

Hormone receptor studies have documented the presence of steroid receptors in adenomyotic foci. Estrogen receptors are more consistently present than are progesterone receptors, which are completely absent in 40% of cases evaluated. Progestins or cyclic estrogen–progestin combination preparations offer little aid in treatment, although recent reports indicated that adenomyosis-associated menorrhagia can be controlled with the insertion of a levonorgestrel-releasing intrauterine device or a danazol-loaded intrauterine device. GnRH agonist therapy for 6 months resulted in the disappearance of pain symptoms and a decline in uterine volume in 65% of cases of biopsy-proven adenomyosis, but the dysmenorrhea and menorrhagia recurred at the end of treatment. Nevertheless, extended intermittent use of these agonists can effectively

relieve pain symptoms while having the significant advantage of preserving fertility between treatments.

Curettage does not aid in establishing the diagnosis of adenomyosis and is ineffective as treatment, although it may be required because of abnormal bleeding. The need for surgery, therefore, is based on continued menorrhagia and dysmenorrhea rather than on an estimation of uterine size or even the known presence of adenomyosis or leiomyomata. The definitive treatment for abnormal bleeding caused by adenomyosis is hysterectomy. The vaginal route is preferred if the size of the uterus is appropriate and no other pelvic abnormalities are present. Under certain circumstances, as with a younger patient who wishes to retain her reproductive capability, excision of an encapsulated adenomyoma should be considered instead of hysterectomy. Such situations arise infrequently because adenomyosis is generally diffuse and usually occurs in multiparous women who are no longer interested in childbearing. The precise efficacy of hysteroscopic endometrial resection, laparoscopic myometrial reduction, and myometrial excision as conservative surgical procedures for adenomyosis has yet to be proved. Endometrial ablation is ineffective as treatment for deep, subserosal adenomyosis that penetrates more than 2 mm. Attempting to resect deeper myometrial tissue carries the risk of increased bleeding. Thermal balloon and radiofrequency ablation has been used recently to treat excessive bleeding in women with adenomyosis. Ectopic, deeper endometrial glands not resected may persist under the scar and eventually proliferate through the area of ablation or resection to cause symptoms such as dysmenorrhea.

Excisional surgery of adenomyosis is best performed by laparotomy because of the value of palpating the uterus to assess the extent of disease and the greater ease in achieving hemostasis. Fujishita and colleagues described a modified approach called the transverse H technique, where one vertical and two crossing horizontal incisions are made. This allows easier removal of a more limited volume of adenomyotic tissue than classical reduction and resulted in a greater improvement in symptoms.

The use of GnRH analogues postoperatively may reduce the recurrence of symptoms in patients who undergo cytoreductive surgery. Wang et al. followed 165 women treated with surgery alone or surgery followed by a 6-month course of ovarian suppressive therapy with GnRH analogues. They found that the symptom-relapse rates in the surgical–medical group were significantly lower than those in the surgery-alone group (28.1% vs. 49.0%, respectively). There was no significant difference in the clinical pregnancy rates (79.5% vs. 74.1%, respectively) or the delivery rates (72.7% vs. 63.0%) among the 44 women in the surgical–medical group and the 27 patients in the surgery-alone group who tried to conceive upon completion of the course of treatment for adenomyosis.

In a recent series of 104 patients, Osada and colleagues described a technique of radical resection of adenomyomatous tissue along with a triple-flap method for reconstructing the uterine wall. All of the patients in the report had adenomyosis involving more than 80% of the anterior and posterior uterine walls with more than 6 cm of wall thickness as verified by MRI and ultrasound. A supracervical tourniquet was applied, and the uterus was bisected at the midline along the sagittal plane until the uterine cavity was opened. Adenomyotic tissues were excised from surrounding myometrium, leaving a myometrial thickness of 1 cm from serosa to endometrium. The endometrium was reapproximated with suture, and the myometrium was repaired with a triple-flap reconstruction. The serosal surface of the underlying flaps was stripped to ensure that only myometrial tissues apposed each other. Only four cases (3.8%) had recurrence of symptoms after 2 years. Sixteen pregnancies were reported out of twenty six women who wished to conceive (61%) and three-fourths of these were achieved through IVF. The deliveries occurred through cesarean section.

There have been several reports of uterine rupture in the second and third trimester of women who have undergone cytoreductive surgery, so careful patient counseling and close obstetrical management are necessary if conservative surgery is being contemplated, especially if it entails significant resection of a portion of the myometrium.

Interventional radiologic techniques have been described to selectively embolize the uterine vessels in women with adenomyosis. Although short-term results from Pelage et al. of uterine artery embolization to treat adenomyosis appeared encouraging, midterm results were disappointing, with only 55% of treated patients showing clinical improvement after 2 years. In a review by Popovic et al. of 15 studies in which uterine artery embolization was performed to treat symptomatic adenomyosis in 208 women, 64.9% reported long-term satisfaction. Preliminary trials have suggested that magnetic resonance–guided focused ultrasound surgery may be used in the future to destroy focal adenomyosis.

Hysterectomy should be considered in the severely symptomatic patient when ultrasonography, MRI, or myometrial biopsy demonstrates deep adenomyosis. The surgical procedure may be performed abdominally, vaginally, or laparoscopically. Subtotal hysterectomy should be avoided, as adenomyosis may recur in the cervical stump or the rectovaginal septum.

BEST SURGICAL PRACTICES

- Surgery is indicated for correction of pain, infertility, or other symptoms in patients with extensive pelvic endometriosis or when hormonal manipulation fails to adequately diminish pain symptoms in women with lesser stages of disease. Surgical management of endometriomas has no significant effect on IVF pregnancy rates as compared to no treatment. Resection of large endometriomas (>5 cm in size) allows a histologic confirmation of the etiology of the cyst and may reduce the risk of bacterial seeding of the endometrial cyst during transvaginal aspiration of follicles for IVF.
- Preoperative rectoscopy–sigmoidoscopy and intravenous pyelography are recommended in patients with symptoms suggestive of deeply invasive endometriosis of the posterior cul-de-sac and rectovaginal septum. Preoperative ultrasound and MRI may help to categorize the extent of ovarian involvement and location of deeply infiltrating disease. A bowel prep before surgery may facilitate optimal performance and safety of the surgical procedure, particularly when deep disease is anticipated.
- Laparoscopy can be considered for all cases unless there is difficulty in establishing the appropriate tissue planes of dissection or unless improved access is necessary for atraumatic manipulation of the involved organs. Conservative resection of disease by laparotomy is most valuable in cases of extensive, dense pelvic adhesions or endometriomas greater than 5 cm in diameter. In addition, deep involvement of the rectovaginal septum with fibrotic extension into the perirectal fossa, invasion of the bowel muscularis, and endometriotic infiltration in the region of the uterine vessels and ureter are generally best approached through the open abdomen for all but advanced endoscopic surgeons.
- The philosophy of gentle manipulation of tissue in an attempt to avoid trauma is the major tenet of pelvic reconstruction. Adhesion formation can be reduced by magnification of the surgical site, avoidance of suture unless clearly indicated, reconstruction with fine nonreactive suture, precise hemostasis, and frequent irrigation of tissues with warmed solution.
- Less tissue damage is achieved with bipolar than with monopolar cautery. Ablation of deep disease by monopolar microdiathermy or CO_2 laser vaporization rather than excision of the disease may result in inadequate resection and a greater amount of ischemic damage to the tissue, heightening the propensity toward adhesion formation. Deep lesions or more extensive peritoneal disease must be excised with a tissue margin of at least 2 to 4 mm, because microscopic lesions are commonly present in tissue adjacent to visible implants. Twenty-five percent of patients have lesions greater than 5 mm in depth.
- Coagulation or vaporization of disease in the ovarian fossa or near the uterosacral ligament should be undertaken only after clear identification of the ureter. Resection of deep posterior cul-de-sac nodules requires great endoscopic expertise. A combined laparoscopic–vaginal approach may be necessary.
- Inability to elevate the ovary is usually a sign of adhesions and endometriotic implants of the inferolateral surface of the ovary and the peritoneum of the ovarian fossa. When removing an endometrioma, the cortical incision should be made in a way that will preserve the normal anatomic relations of the ovary with the uteroovarian ligament and fimbria ovarica. Suture on or extruding through the surface should be avoided when possible because of its adhesiogenic properties. With larger endometriomas, the normal ovarian cortex is stabilized with atraumatic forceps, and the cyst wall is grasped with biopsy forceps and stripped from the bed of normal ovarian tissue. The dissection may be facilitated by removing a small circular rim of tissue around the adhesion site to begin the stripping procedure in a clearer field, where the endometrioma wall is less adhered to healthy ovarian tissue. The rate of recurrence of pelvic pain and dysmenorrhea over a 2-year postoperative period is significantly less for those patients who are managed by cystectomy as compared with those undergoing fenestration and coagulation. Moreover, the rate of reoperation is less and the cumulative pregnancy rate is higher in the cystectomy group. Extensive cauterization or resection of ovarian tissue can lead to a decline in follicle number and a rise in FSH levels postoperatively and should be avoided.
- Aggressive and complete excision of deep endometriosis is justified. The recurrence rate of clinically detectable endometriosis is higher when the depth of infiltration is greater than 5 mm at the time of initial surgery, no matter the site of the lesion. A second cytoreductive procedure may benefit some infertile women who have undergone surgery in the past, although assisted reproductive technologies would lead to a higher chance of conceiving for most patients who failed primary surgery. The hypothesis that surgical therapy of endometriosis increases IVF pregnancy rates is not clearly validated by the available evidence.
- Uterine suspension is of unproven efficacy in enhancing fertility or as an adjunct in the treatment of endometriosis-associated pelvic pain.
- Presacral neurectomy, or division of the superior hypogastric plexus, is useful as an adjunctive procedure to eliminate the uterine component of dysmenorrhea that results from endometriosis. Uterine nerve ablation may be effective in reducing dysmenorrhea in the absence of endometriosis, but the addition of this procedure to the surgical treatment of endometriosis has not been associated with a significant difference in any pain outcomes.

BIBLIOGRAPHY

Abbott JA, Howe J, Clayton RD, et al. The effects and effectiveness of laparoscopic excision of endometriosis: a prospective study with 2–5 year follow-up. *Hum Reprod* 2003;18:1922.

Abbott J, Howe J, Hunter D, et al. Laparoscopic excision of endometriosis: a randomized, placebo-controlled trial. *Fertil Steril* 2004;82:878.

Aboulghar MA, Mansour RT, Serour G, et al. The outcome of *in vitro* fertilization in advanced endometriosis with previous surgery: a case-controlled study. *Am J Obstet Gynecol* 2003;188:371.

Abu Hashim A, El Rakhawy M, Abd Elaal I. Randomized comparison of superovulation with letrozole vs. clomiphene citrate in an IUI program for women with recently surgically treated minimal to mild endometriosis. *Acta Obstet Gynecol Scand* 2012; 91:338.

Adamson GD, Subak LL, Pasta DJ, et al. Comparison of CO_2 laser laparoscopy with laparotomy for the treatment of endometriomata. *Fertil Steril* 1992;57:965.

Adamson GD, Hurd SJ, Pasta DJ, et al. Laparoscopic endometriosis treatment: is it better? *Fertil Steril* 1993;59:35.

Albourzi S, Momtahan M, Parsanezhad M, et al. A prospective, randomized study comparing laparoscopic ovarian cystectomy versus fenestration and coagulation in patients with endometriomas. *Fertil Steril* 2004;82:1633.

Almog B, Shehata F, Sheizaf B, et al. Effects of ovarian endometrioma on the number of oocytes retrieved for in vitro fertilization. *Fertil Steril* 2011;95:525.

American Fertility Society. The classification of endometriosis. *Fertil Steril* 1979;32:633.

American Fertility Society. Revised American Fertility Society classification of endometriosis: 1985. *Fertil Steril* 1985;43:351.

American Society for Reproductive Medicine. Revised American Society for Reproductive Medicine classification of endometriosis: 1996. *Fertil Steril* 1997;67:817.

Andrews WE, Larsen GD. Endometriosis: treatment with hormonal pseudopregnancy and/or operation. *Am J Obstet Gynecol* 1974;118:643.

Ascher SM, Arnold LL, Patt RH, et al. Adenomyosis: prospective comparison of MR imaging and transvaginal sonography. *Radiology* 1994;190:803.

Awadalla SG, Friedman CI, Haq AU, et al. Local peritoneal factors: their role in infertility associated with endometriosis. *Am J Obstet Gynecol* 1987;157:1207.

Ayers JW, Birenbaum DL, Menon KM. Luteal phase dysfunction in endometriosis: elevated progesterone levels in peripheral and ovarian veins during the follicular phase. *Fertil Steril* 1987;47:925.

Badawy SZA, Cuenca V, Kaufman L, et al. The regulation of immunoglobulin production by B cells in patients with endometriosis. *Fertil Steril* 1989;51:770.

Bailey HR, Ott MT, Hartendorp P. Aggressive surgical management for advanced colorectal endometriosis. *Dis Colon Rectum* 1994;37:747.

Ballester M, Mathieu d'Argent E, Morcel K, et al. Cumulative pregnancy rate after ICSI-IVF in patients with colorectal endometriosis: results of a multicentre study. *Hum Reprod* 2012;27:1043.

Barbieri RL. Etiology and epidemiology of endometriosis. *Am J Obstet Gynecol* 1990;162:565.

Barbieri RL. Hormone treatment of endometriosis: the estrogen threshold hypothesis. *Am J Obstet Gynecol* 1992;166:740.

Barbieri RL. Stenosis of the external os: an association with endometriosis in women with chronic pelvic pain. *Fertil Steril* 1998; 70:571.

Barbieri RL, Ryan KJ. Danazol: endocrine pharmacology and therapeutic applications. *Am J Obstet Gynecol* 1981;141:453.

Barbieri RL, Niloff JM, Bast RC Jr, et al. Elevated serum concentrations of CA-125 in patients with advanced endometriosis. *Fertil Steril* 1986;45:630.

Barnhart K, Dunsmoor-Su R, Coutifaris C. Effect of endometriosis on *in vitro* fertilization. *Fertil Steril* 2002;77:1148.

Benschop L, Farquhar C, van der Poel N, et al. Interventions for women with endometrioma prior to assisted reproductive technology. *Cochrane Database Syst Rev* 2010;(11):CD008571. doi: 10.1002/14651858.CD008571.pub2

Beretta P, Franchi M, Ghezzi F, et al. Randomized clinical trial of two laparoscopic treatments of endometriomas: cystectomy versus drainage and coagulation. *Fertil Steril* 1998;70:1176.

Bergqvist A, Theorell T. Changes in quality of life after hormonal treatment of endometriosis. *Acta Obstet Gynecol Scand* 2001;80:628.

Berlanda N, Vercellini P, Fedele L. The outcomes of repeat surgery for recurrent symptomatic endometriosis. *Curr Opin Obstet Gynecol* 2010;22:320.

Biberoglu KO, Behrman SJ. Dosage aspects of danazol therapy in endometriosis: short term and long term effectiveness. *Am J Obstet Gynecol* 1981;138:645.

Bridoux V, Roman H, Kianifard B, et al. Combined transanal and laparoscopic approach for the treatment of deep endometriosis infiltrating the rectum. *Hum Reprod* 2012;27:418.

Brosens IA, Koninckx PR, Corvelyn PA. A study of plasma progesterone, oestradiol-17β, prolactin and LH levels and of the luteal phase appearance of the ovaries in patients with endometriosis and infertility. *Br J Obstet Gynaecol* 1978;85:246.

Brosens I, Vasquez G, Gordts S. Scanning electron microscopy study of the pelvic peritoneum in unexplained infertility and endometriosis. *Fertil Steril* 1984;41:215.

Bruner KL, Mastrisian LM, Rodgers WH, et al. Suppression of matrix metalloproteinases inhibits establishment of ectopic lesions by human endometrium in nude mice. *J Clin Invest* 1997;99:2851.

Busacca M, Marana R, Caruana P, et al. Recurrence of ovarian endometriomas after laparoscopic excision. *Am J Obstet Gynecol* 1999;180:519.

Busacca M, Riparini J, Somigliana E, et al. Postsurgical ovarian failure after laparoscopic excision of bilateral endometriomas. *Am J Obstet Gynecol* 2006;195:421.

Buttram VC Jr, Reiter RC, Ward S. Treatment of endometriosis with danazol: report of a 6 year prospective study. *Fertil Steril* 1985;43:353.

Cakmak H, Taylor HS. Molecular mechanisms of treatment resistance in endometriosis: the role of progesterone-hox gene interactions. *Semin Reprod Med* 2010;28:69.

Candiani GB, Vercellini P, Fedele L. Laparoscopic ovarian puncture for correct staging of endometriosis. *Fertil Steril* 1990;53:994.

Candiani GB, Fedele L, Vercellini P, et al. Repetitive conservative surgery for recurrence of endometriosis. *Obstet Gynecol* 1991;77:421.

Candiani GB, Vercellini P, Fedele L, et al. Conservative surgical treatment for severe endometriosis in infertile women: are we making progress? *Obstet Gynecol Surv* 1991;48(suppl 7):490.

Candiani GB, Fedele L, Vercellini P, et al. Presacral neurectomy for the treatment of pelvic pain associated with endometriosis: a controlled study. *Am J Obstet Gynecol* 1992;167:100.

Candiani GB, Vercellini P, Fedele L, et al. Conservative surgical treatment of rectovaginal septum endometriosis. *J Gynecol Surg* 1992;8:177.

Canis M, Mage G, Wattiex A, et al. Second-look laparoscopy after laparoscopic cystectomy of large ovarian endometriomas. *Fertil Steril* 1992;58:617.

Carpenter SE, Markham SM, Rock JA. Exercise may reduce side effects of danazol. *Infertility* 1988;2:259.

Cedars MI, Lu JK, Meldrum DR, et al. Treatment of endometriosis with a long-acting gonadotropin releasing hormone agonist plus medroxyprogesterone acetate. *Obstet Gynecol* 1990;75:641.

Chaffkin LM, Nulsen JC, Luciano AA, et al. A comparative analysis of the cycle fecundity rates associated with combined human menopausal gonadotropin (hMG) and intrauterine insemination (IUI) versus either hMG or IUI alone. *Fertil Steril* 1991;55:252.

Chapron C, Santulli P, de Ziegler D, et al. Ovarian endometrioma: severe pelvic pain is associated with deeply infiltrating endometriosis. *Hum Reprod* 2012;27:702.

Cheesman KL, Ben-Nun I, Chatterton RT Jr, et al. Relationship of luteinizing hormone, pregnanediol-3-glucuronide and estriol-16-glucuronide in urine of infertile women with endometriosis. *Fertil Steril* 1982;38:542.

Cheesman KL, Cheesman SD, Chatterton RT, et al. Alterations in progesterone metabolism and luteal function in infertile women with endometriosis. *Fertil Steril* 1983;40:590.

Chen FP, Soong YK. The efficacy and complications of laparoscopic presacral neurectomy in pelvic pain. *Obstet Gynecol* 1997; 90:974.

IV

Chong AP, Luciano AA, O'Shaughnessy AM. Laser laparoscopy versus laparotomy in the treatment of infertility patients with severe endometriosis. *J Gynecol Surg* 1990;6:179.

Coccia ME, Rizzello F, Mariani G, et al. Ovarian surgery for bilateral endometriomas influences age at menopause. *Hum Reprod* 2011;26:3000.

Coddington CC, Oehninger S, Cunningham DS, et al. Peritoneal fluid from patients with endometriosis decreases sperm binding to the zona pellucida in the hemizona assay: a preliminary report. *Fertil Steril* 1992;57:783.

Confino E, Harlow L, Gleicher N. Peritoneal fluid and serum autoantibody levels in patients with endometriosis. *Fertil Steril* 1990;53:242.

Cook AS, Rock JA. The role of laparoscopy in the treatment of endometriosis. *Fertil Steril* 1991;55:663.

Cornillie FJ, Oosterlynck D, Lauweryns JM, et al. Deeply infiltrating pelvic endometriosis: histology and clinical significance. *Fertil Steril* 1989;53:978.

Coronado C, Franklin RR, Lotze EC, et al. Surgical treatment of symptomatic colorectal endometriosis. *Fertil Steril* 1990;53:411.

Cramer DW, Missmer SA. The epidemiology of endometriosis. *Ann N Y Acad Sci* 2002;955:11.

Cramer DW, Wilson E, Stillman RJ, et al. The relation of endometriosis to menstrual characteristics, smoking, and exercise. *JAMA* 1986;255:1904.

Cullen TS. The distribution of adenomyomata containing uterine mucosa. *Arch Surg* 1919;80:130.

Czernobilsky B, Morris W. A histologic study of ovarian endometriosis with emphasis on hyperplastic and atypical changes. *Obstet Gynecol* 1979;53:318.

Czernobilsky B, Silverstein A. Salpingitis in ovarian endometriosis. *Fertil Steril* 1978;30:45.

Damewood MD, Hesla JS, Schlaff WD, et al. Effect of serum from patients with minimal to mild endometriosis on mouse embryo development in vitro. *Fertil Steril* 1990;54:917.

Daniell JF. Fiberoptic laser laparoscopy. *Baillieres Clin Obstet Gynaecol* 1989;3:545.

Davis GD, Brooks RA. Excision of pelvic endometriosis with the carbon dioxide laser laparoscope. *Obstet Gynecol* 1988;72:816.

Dawood MY. Impact of medical treatment of endometriosis on bone mass. *Am J Obstet Gynecol* 1993;168:674.

Dawood MY, Kahn-Dawood FS, Wilson L Jr. Peritoneal fluid prostaglandins and prostanoids in women with endometriosis, chronic pelvic inflammatory disease, and pelvic pain. *Am J Obstet Gynecol* 1984;148:391.

De Cicco C, Corona R, Schonman R, et al. Bowel resection for deep endometriosis: a systematic review. *Br J Obstet Gynaecol* 2011;118:285.

DeLeon FD, Vijayakumar R, Brown M, et al. Peritoneal fluid volume, estrogen, progesterone, prostaglandin, and epidermal growth factor concentrations in patients with and without endometriosis. *Obstet Gynecol* 1986;68:189.

Diaz I, Navarro J, Blasco L, et al. Impact of stage III–IV endometriosis on recipients of sibling oocytes: matched case–control study. *Fertil Steril* 2000;74:31.

Dicker D, Feldberg D, Goldman JA, et al. The impact of long-term gonadotropin-releasing hormone analogue treatment on preclinical abortions in patients with severe endometriosis undergoing in vitro fertilization-embryo transfer. *Fertil Steril* 1992;57:597.

Dickey RP, Olar TT, Taylor SN, et al. Relationship of follicle number, serum estradiol, and other factors to birth rate and multiparity in human menopausal gonadotropin-induced intrauterine insemination cycles. *Fertil Steril* 1991;56:89.

diZerega G, Hodgen G. Endometriosis: role of ovarian steroids in initiation, maintenance, and suppression. *Fertil Steril* 1980;33:649.

Dlugi AM, Miller JD, Knittle J, et al. Lupron depot (leuprolide acetate for depot suspension) in the treatment of endometriosis: a randomized, placebo-controlled, double-blind study. *Fertil Steril* 1990;54:419.

Dmowski WP, Cohen MR. Treatment of endometriosis with an antigonadotropin, danazol: a laparoscopic and histologic evaluation. *Obstet Gynecol* 1975;46:147.

Dmowski WP, Steele RW, Baker GF. Deficient cellular immunity in endometriosis. *Am J Obstet Gynecol* 1981;141:377.

Dmowski WP, Radwanska E, Binor Z, et al. Mild endometriosis and ovulatory dysfunction: effect of danazol treatment on success of ovulation induction. *Fertil Steril* 1986;46:784.

Döberl A, Berquist A, Jeppson S, et al. Regression of endometriosis following the shorter treatment with, or lower dose of, danazol. *Acta Obstet Gynecol Scand Suppl* 1984;123:51.

Dodin S, Lemay A, Maheux R, et al. Bone mass in endometriosis patients treated with GnRH agonist implant or danazol. *Obstet Gynecol* 1991;77:410.

Dodson WC, Haney AF. Controlled ovarian hyperstimulation and intrauterine insemination for treatment of infertility. *Fertil Steril* 1991;55:457.

Donnez J, Casanas-Roux F, Ferin J, et al. Tubal polyps, epithelial inclusions, and endometriosis after tubal sterilization. *Fertil Steril* 1984;41:56.

Donnez J, Nisolle-Pochet M, Clerckx-Braun F, et al. Administration of nasal buserelin as compared with subcutaneous buserelin implant for endometriosis. *Fertil Steril* 1989;52:25.

Doyle JB. Paracervical uterine denervation by transection of the cervical plexus for the relief of dysmenorrhea. *Am J Obstet Gynecol* 1955;70:11.

Drake TS, O'Brien WF, Ramwell PW, et al. Peritoneal fluid thromboxane B_2 6-keto-prostaglandin F_{1a} in endometriosis. *Am J Obstet Gynecol* 1981;140:401.

Dunselman GA, Dumoulin JC, Land JA, et al. Lack of effect of peritoneal endometriosis on fertility in the rabbit model. *Fertil Steril* 1991;56:340.

Eskenazi B, Warner M, Bonsignore L, et al. Validation study of nonsurgical diagnosis of endometriosis. *Fertil Steril* 2001;76:929.

Evers JL. The second look laparoscopy for evaluation of the results of medical treatment of endometriosis should not be performed during ovarian suppression. *Fertil Steril* 1987;47:502.

Fahaeus L, Larsson-Cohn U, Ljungberg S, et al. Profound alterations of the lipoprotein metabolism during danazol treatment in premenopausal women. *Fertil Steril* 1984;42:52.

Fakih HN, Tamura R, Kesselman A, et al. Endometriosis after tubal ligation. *J Reprod Med* 1985;30:939.

Fakih H, Baggett B, Holtz G, et al. Interleukin-1: a possible role in the infertility associated with endometriosis. *Fertil Steril* 1987;47:218.

Falcone T, Lebovic DI. Clinical management of endometriosis. *Am J Obstet Gynecol* 2011;118:691.

Fayez JA, Collazo LM. Comparison between laparotomy and operative laparoscopy in the treatment of moderate and severe endometriosis. *Int J Fertil* 1990;35:252.

Fayez JA, Vogel MF. Comparison of different treatment methods of endometriomas by laparoscopy. *Obstet Gynecol* 1991;78:660.

Fedele L, Parazzini F, Bianchi S, et al. Stage and localization of pelvic endometriosis and pain. *Fertil Steril* 1990;53:155.

Fedele L, Bianchi S, Bocciolone L, et al. Pain symptoms associated with endometriosis. *Obstet Gynecol* 1992;79:767.

Fedele L, Bianchi S, Dorta M, et al. Transvaginal ultrasonography in the differential diagnosis of adenomyoma versus leiomyoma. *Am J Obstet Gynecol* 1992;167:603.

Fedele L, Bianchi S, Marchini M, et al. Superovulation with human menopausal gonadotropins in the treatment of infertility associated with minimal or mild endometriosis: a controlled randomized study. *Fertil Steril* 1992;58:28.

Fedele L, Bianchi S, Zanconato G, et al. Long-term follow-up after conservative surgery for bladder endometriosis. *Fertil Steril* 2005;83:1729.

Fedele L, Bianchi S, Zanconato G, et al. Laparoscopic excision of recurrent endometriomas: long-term outcome and comparison with primary surgery. *Fertil Steril* 2006;85:694.

Ferrero S, Anserini P, Abbamonte LH, et al. Fertility after bowel resection for endometriosis. *Fertil Steril* 2009;92:41.

Ferrero S, Venturini PL, Gillott DJ, et al. Hemostasis by bipolar coagulation versus suture after surgical stripping of bilateral ovarian endometriomas: a randomized controlled trial. *J Minim Invasive Gynecol* 2012;19:722.

Foster DC, Stern JL, Buscema J, et al. Pleural and parenchymal pulmonary endometriosis. *Obstet Gynecol* 1981;58:552.

Franssen AM, Kaver FM, Chadha DR, et al. Endometriosis: treatment with gonadotropin-releasing hormone agonist buserelin. *Fertil Steril* 1989;51:401.

Fujishita A, Masuzaki H, Khan KN, et al. Modified reduction surgery for adenomyosis. A preliminary report of the transverse H incision technique. *Gynecol Obstet Invest* 2004;57:132.

Gambone JC, Reiter RC, Lerich JB, et al. The impact of a quality assurance process in the frequency and confirmation rate of hysterectomy. *Am J Obstet Gynecol* 1990;163:545.

Gant NF. Infertility and endometriosis: comparison of pregnancy outcomes with laparotomy versus laparoscopic techniques. *Am J Obstet Gynecol* 1992;166:1072.

Garcia-Velasco JA, Mahutte NG, Corona J, et al. Removal of endometriomas before in vitro fertilization does not improve fertility outcomes: a matched, case–control study. *Fertil Steril* 2004;81:1194.

Glatt AE, Zinner SH, McCormack WM. The prevalence of dyspareunia. *Obstet Gynecol* 1990;75:433.

Goksever Celik H, Dogan E, Okyay E, et al. Effect of laparoscopic excision of endometriomas on ovarian reserve: serial changes in the serum antimullerian hormone levels. *Fertil Steril* 2012;97:1472.

Gould SF, Shannon JM, Cunha GR. Nuclear estrogen binding sites in human endometriosis. *Fertil Steril* 1983;39:520.

Granberg S, Wikland M, Jansson I. Macroscopic characterization of ovarian tumors and the relation to the histologic diagnosis: criteria to be used for ultrasound evaluation. *Gynecol Oncol* 1989;35:139.

Greenblatt RB, Dmowski WP, Mahesh VB, et al. Clinical studies with an antigonadotropin danazol. *Fertil Steril* 1971;22:102.

Grow DR, Filer RB. Treatment of adenomyosis with long-term GnRH analogues: a case report. *Obstet Gynecol* 1991;78:538.

Gruenwald P. Origin of endometriosis from the mesenchyme of the coelomic walls. *Am J Obstet Gynecol* 1942;44:470.

Guzick DS. Clinical epidemiology of endometriosis and infertility. *Obstet Gynecol Clin North Am* 1989;16:43.

Haas D, Oppelt P, Shebl O, et al. Enzian classification: does it correlate with clinical symptoms and the rASRM score? *Acta Obstet Gynecol Scand* 2013;92:962.

Habuchi T, Okagaki T, Miyakawa M. Endometriosis of bladder after menopause. *J Urol* 1991;145:361.

Halme J, Hammond MG, Hulka JK, et al. Retrograde menstruation in healthy women and in patients with endometriosis. *Obstet Gynecol* 1984;64:151.

Halme J, White C, Kauma S, et al. Peritoneal macrophages from patients with endometriosis release growth factor activity in vitro. *J Clin Endocrinol Metab* 1988;66:1044.

Haney AF, Jenkins S, Weinberg JB. The stimulus responsible for the peritoneal fluid inflammation observed in infertile women with endometriosis. *Fertil Steril* 1991;56:408.

Harada T, Momoeda M, Taketani Y, et al. Low-dose oral contraceptive pill for dysmenorrhea associated with endometriosis: a placebo-controlled, double-blind, randomized trial. *Fertil Steril* 2008;90:1583.

Hart RJ, Hickey M, Maouris P, et al. Excisional surgery versus ablative surgery for ovarian endometriomata. *Cochrane Database System Rev* 2011(5):CD004992. doi: 10.1002/14651858. CD004992.pub3

Heaps JM, Nieberg RK, Berek JS. Malignant neoplasms arising in endometriosis. *Obstet Gynecol* 1990;75:1023.

Heilier JF, Nackers F, Verougstraete V, et al. Increased dioxin-like compounds in the serum of women with peritoneal endometriosis and deep endometriotic (adenomyotic) nodules. *Fertil Steril* 2005;84:305.

Henzl MR. Gonadotropin-releasing hormone analogs: update on new findings. *Am J Obstet Gynecol* 1992;166:757.

Henzl MR, Corson SL, Moghissi K, et al. Administration of nasal nafarelin as compared with oral danazol for endometriosis. *N Engl J Med* 1988;318:485.

Hickman TN, Namnoum AB, Hinton EL, et al. Timing of estrogen replacement therapy following hysterectomy with oophorectomy for endometriosis. *Obstet Gynecol* 1998;91:673.

Hill JA, Faris HM, Schiff I, et al. Characterization of leukocyte subpopulations in the peritoneal fluid of women with endometriosis. *Fertil Steril* 1988;50:216.

Hornstein MD, Hemmings R, Yuzpe AA, et al. Use of nafarelin versus placebo after reductive laparoscopic surgery for endometriosis. *Fertil Steril* 1997;68:860.

Hornstein MD, Surrey ES, Weisberg GW, et al. Leuprolide acetate depot and hormonal add-back in endometriosis: a 12-month study. *Obstet Gynecol* 1998;91:16.

Houston DE, Noller RL, Melton LJ III, et al. Incidence of pelvic endometriosis in Rochester, Minnesota 1970–1979. *Am J Epidemiol* 1987;125:959.

Hsu AL, Sinaii N, Segars J, et al. Relating pelvic pain location to surgical findings of endometriosis. *Obstet Gynecol* 2011;188:223.

Hughes E, Brown J, Collins JJ, et al. Ovulation suppression for endometriosis. *Cochrane Database Syst Rev* 2007;18:CD000155.

Hull ME, Moghissi KS, Magyar DF, et al. Comparison of different treatment modalities of endometriosis in infertile women. *Fertil Steril* 1987;47:40.

Igarashi M, Abe Y, Fukuda M, et al. Novel conservative medical therapy for uterine adenomyosis with a danazol-loaded intrauterine device. *Fertil Steril* 2000;74:412.

Ishimaru T, Masuzaki H. Peritoneal endometriosis: endometrial tissue implantation as its primary etiologic mechanism. *Am J Obstet Gynecol* 1991;165:210.

Jacobson TZ, Duffy JM, Barlow D, et al. Laparoscopic surgery for subfertility associated with endometriosis. *Cochrane Database Syst Rev* 2009;4:CD001398.doi: 10.1002/14651858.CD001398.pub2

Jacobson TZ, Duffy JM, Barlow D, et al. Laparoscopic surgery for pelvic pain associated with endometriosis. *Cochrane Database Syst Rev* 2010;(11):CD001300.

Jadoul P, Kitajima M, Donnez O, et al. Surgical treatment of ovarian endometriomas: state of the art? *Fertil Steril* 2012;98:556.

Jänne O, Kauppila A, Kukko E, et al. Estrogen and progestin receptors in endometriosis lesions: comparison with endometrial tissue. *Am J Obstet Gynecol* 1981;141:562.

Jansen RP, Russell P. Nonpigmented endometriosis: clinical, laparoscopic, and pathologic definition. *Am J Obstet Gynecol* 1986;155:1154.

Javert CT. Pathogenesis of endometriosis based on endometrial homeoplasia direct extension, exfoliation and implantation, lymphatic and hematogenous metastasis. *Cancer* 1949;2:399.

Jenkins S, Olive DL, Haney AF. Endometriosis: pathogenetic implications of the anatomic distribution. *Obstet Gynecol* 1986;67:335.

Johnson JV, Roxek MM, Moreno AC, et al. Surgically induced endometriosis does not alter peritoneal factors in the rabbit model. *Fertil Steril* 1991;56:343.

Johnson NP, Farquhar CM, Crossley S, et al. A double-blinded randomized controlled trial of laparoscopic uterine nerve ablation for women with chronic pelvic pain. *Br J Obstet Gynaecol* 2004;111:950.

Killick S, Elstein M. Pharmacologic production of luteinized unruptured follicles by prostaglandin synthetase inhibitors. *Fertil Steril* 1987;47:773.

Kim CH, Cho YK, Mok JE. Simplified ultralong protocol of gonadotrophin-releasing hormone agonist for ovulation induction with intrauterine insemination in patients with endometriosis. *Hum Reprod* 1996;11:398.

Koninckx PR, Martin DC. Deep endometriosis: a consequence of infiltration or retraction or possibly adenomyosis externa? *Fertil Steril* 1992;58:924.

Koninckx P, Ide P, Vandenbroucke W, et al. New aspects of the pathophysiology of endometriosis and associated infertility. *J Reprod Med* 1980;24:257.

Koninckx PR, Mueleman C, Demeyere S, et al. Suggestive evidence that pelvic endometriosis is a progressive disease, whereas deeply infiltrating endometriosis is associated with pelvic pain. *Fertil Steril* 1991;55:759.

Koninckx PR, Rittinen L, Seppälä M, et al. CA-125 and placental protein 14 concentrations in plasma and peritoneal fluid of women with deeply infiltrating pelvic endometriosis. *Fertil Steril* 1992;57:523.

Koninckx PR, Braet P, Kennedy SH, et al. Dioxin pollution and endometriosis in Belgium. *Hum Reprod* 1994;9:1001.

Koninckx PR, Ussia A, Adamyan L, et al. Deep endometriosis: definition, diagnosis, and treatment. *Fertil Steril* 2012;98:564.

Kuivasaari P, Hippeläinen M, Anttila M, et al. Effect of endometriosis on IVF/ICSI outcome: stage III/IV endometriosis worsens cumulative pregnancy and live-born rates. *Hum Reprod* 2005;20:3130.

Lamb K, Hoffman RG, Nichols TR. Family trait analysis: a case–control study of 43 women with endometriosis and their best friends. *Am J Obstet Gynecol* 1986;154:596.

Laufer MR. Identification of clear vesicular lesions of atypical endometriosis: a new technique. *Fertil Steril* 1997;68:739.

IV

Laufer MR, Goitein L, Bush M, et al. Prevalence of endometriosis in adolescent girls with chronic pelvic pain not responding to conventional therapy. *J Pediatr Adolesc Gynecol* 1997;10:199.

Leach RE, Arneson BW, Ball GD, et al. Absence of antisperm antibodies and factors influencing sperm motility in the cul-del-sac fluid of women with endometriosis. *Fertil Steril* 1990;53:351.

Lee NC, Dicker RC, Rubin GL, et al. Confirmation of the preoperative diagnoses for hysterectomy. *Am J Obstet Gynecol* 1984;150:283.

Lee RB, Stone K, Magelssen D, et al. Presacral neurectomy for chronic pelvic pain. *Obstet Gynecol* 1986;69:517.

Leibson CL, Good AE, Hass SL, et al. Incidence and characterization of diagnosed endometriosis in a geographically defined population. *Fertil Steril* 2004;82:314.

Lemay A, Maheux R, Faure N, et al. Reversible hypogonadism induced by a luteinizing hormone-releasing hormone (LH-RH) agonist (buserelin) as a new therapeutic approach for endometriosis. *Fertil Steril* 1984;41:863.

Lessey BA, Castelbaum AJ, Sawin SW, et al. Aberrant integrin expression in the endometrium of women with endometriosis. *J Clin Endocrinol Metab* 1994;79:643.

Lichten EM, Bombard J. Surgical treatment of primary dysmenorrhea with laparoscopic uterine nerve ablation. *J Reprod Med* 1987;32:37.

Lockhat FB, Emembolu JO, Konje JC. The efficacy, side-effects and continuation rates in women with symptomatic endometriosis undergoing treatment with an intra-uterine administered progestogen (levonorgestrel): a 3 year follow-up. *Hum Reprod* 2005;20:789.

Loh FH, Tan AT, Kumar J, et al. Ovarian response after laparoscopic ovarian cystectomy for endometriotic cysts in 132 monitored cycles. *Fertil Steril* 1999;72:316.

Luciano AA, Hauser KS, Chapler FK, et al. Effects of danazol on plasma lipids and lipoprotein levels in healthy woman and in women with endometriosis. *Am J Obstet Gynecol* 1983;145:422.

Luciano AA, Turksoy RN, Carleo J. Evaluation of oral medroxyprogesterone acetate in the treatment of endometriosis. *Obstet Gynecol* 1988;72:323.

Mahmood TA, Templeton A. Pathophysiology of mild endometriosis: review of literature. *Hum Reprod* 1990;5:765.

Mahmood TA, Templeton A. Folliculogenesis and ovulation in infertile women with mild endometriosis. *Hum Reprod* 1991;6:225.

Mahmood TA, Templeton A. Peritoneal fluid volume and sex steroids in the preovulatory period in mild endometriosis. *Br J Obstet Gynaecol* 1991;98:179.

Mahmood TA, Arumugam K, Templeton AA. Oocyte and follicular fluid characteristics in women with mild endometriosis. *Br J Obstet Gynaecol* 1991;98:573.

Makarainen L, Ronnberg L, Kauppila A. Medroxyprogesterone acetate supplementation diminishes the hypoestrogenic side effects of gonadotropin-releasing hormone agonist without changing its efficacy in endometriosis. *Fertil Steril* 1996;65:29.

Marcoux S, Maheux R, Bérubé S, et al. Laparoscopic surgery in infertile women with minimal or mild endometriosis. *N Engl J Med* 1997;337:217.

Marrs RP. The use of potassium-titanyl-phosphate laser for laparoscopic removal of ovarian endometriomas. *Am J Obstet Gynecol* 1991;164:1622.

Martin D. Laparoscopic treatment of ovarian endometriomas. *Clin Obstet Gynecol* 1991;34:452.

Martin DC, Hubert GD, Levy BS. Depth of infiltration of endometriosis. *J Gynecol Surg* 1989;5:55.

Martin DC, Hubert GD, Vander Zwaag R, et al. Laparoscopic appearances of peritoneal endometriosis. *Fertil Steril* 1989;51:63.

Matorras R, Elorriaga MA, Pijoan JI, et al. Recurrence of endometriosis in women with bilateral adnexectomy (with or without total hysterectomy) who received hormone replacement therapy. *Fertil Steril* 2002;77:303.

Max E, Sweeney WB, Bailey HR, et al. Results of 1,000 single-layer continuous polypropylene intestinal anastomoses. *Am J Surg* 1991;162:461.

McArthur JW, Ulfelder H. The effect of pregnancy upon endometriosis. *Obstet Gynecol Surv* 1965;20:709.

McCausland AM. Hysteroscopic myometrial biopsy: its use in diagnosing adenomyosis and its clinical application. *Am J Obstet Gynecol* 1992;166:1619.

Meldrum DR, Chang RJ, Lu J, et al. "Medical oophorectomy" using a long-acting GnRH agonist: a possible new approach to the treatment of endometriosis. *J Clin Endocrinol Metab* 1982;54:1081.

Melin AS, Lundholm C, Malki N, et al. Hormonal and surgical treatments for endometriosis and risk of epithelial ovarian cancer. *Acta Obstet Gynecol Scand* 2013;92:546.

Meresman GF, Auge L, Baranao RI, et al. Oral contraceptives suppress cell proliferation and enhance apoptosis of eutopic endometrial tissue from patients with endometriosis. *Fertil Steril* 2002;77:1141.

Metzger DA, Olive DL, Stohs GF, et al. Association of endometriosis and spontaneous abortion: effect of control group selection. *Fertil Steril* 1986;45:18.

Meyer R. Über Stand der Frage der Adenomyositis und Adenomyome im Allgemeinen und ins Besondere über Adenomyositis seroepithelialis und Adenomyometritis sarcomatosa. *Zentralbl Gynakol* 1919;36:745.

Mio Y, Toda T, Harada T, et al. Pathophysiology of infertility associated with endometriosis: luteinized unruptured follicle in the early stages of endometriosis as a cause of unexplained infertility. *Am J Obstet Gynecol* 1992;167:251.

Missmer SA, Hankinson SE, Spiegelman D, et al. Reproductive history and endometriosis among premenopausal women. *Obstet Gynecol* 2004;104:965.

Missmer SA, Hankinson SE, Speigelman D, et al. Incidence of laparoscopically confirmed endometriosis by demographic, anthropometric, and lifestyle factors. *Am J Epidemiol* 2004;160:784.

Mittal KR, Barwick KW. Endometrial adenocarcinoma involving adenomyosis without true myometrial invasion is characterized by frequent preceding estrogen therapy, low histologic grades, and excellent prognosis. *Gynecol Oncol* 1993;49:197.

Modugno F, Ness RB, Allen GO, et al. Oral contraceptive use, reproductive history, and risk of epithelial ovarian cancer in women with and without endometriosis. *Am J Obstet Gynecol* 2004;191:733.

Moen M, Bratlie A, Moen T. Distribution of HLA antigens among patients with endometriosis. *Acta Obstet Gynecol Scand Suppl* 1984;123:25.

Moghissi KS, Boyce CR. Management of endometriosis with oral medroxyprogesterone acetate. *Obstet Gynecol* 1976;47:265.

Moore JG, Hibbard LT, Growdon WA, et al. Urinary tract endometriosis: enigmas in diagnosis and management. *Am J Obstet Gynecol* 1979;134:162.

Moore EE, Harger JH, Rock JA, et al. Management of pelvic endometriosis with low-dose danazol. *Fertil Steril* 1981;36:15.

Moore JG, Binstock MA, Growdon WA. The clinical implications of retroperitoneal endometriosis. *Am J Obstet Gynecol* 1988;158:1291.

Morcos RN, Gibbons WE, Findlay WE. Effect of peritoneal fluid on in vitro cleavage of 2-cell mouse embryos: possible role in infertility associated with endometriosis. *Fertil Steril* 1985;44:678.

Murphy AA, Green WR, Bobbie D, et al. Unsuspected endometriosis documented by scanning electron microscopy in visually normal peritoneum. *Fertil Steril* 1986;46:522.

Murphy AA, Schlaff WD, Hassiakos D, et al. Laparoscopic cautery in the treatment of endometriosis-related infertility. *Fertil Steril* 1991;55:246.

Muscato JJ, Haney AF, Weinberg JB. Sperm phagocytosis by human peritoneal macrophages: a possible cause of infertility in endometriosis. *Am J Obstet Gynecol* 1982;144:503.

Muzii L, Marana R, Caruana P, et al. The impact of preoperative gonadotropin-releasing hormone agonist treatment on laparoscopic excision of ovarian endometriotic cysts. *Fertil Steril* 1996;65:1235.

Muzii L, Marana R, Pedulla S, et al. Correlation between endometriosis-associated dysmenorrhea and the presence of typical and atypical lesions. *Fertil Steril* 1997;68:19.

Muzii L, Marana R, Caruana P, et al. Postoperative administration of monophasic combined oral contraceptives after laparoscopic treatment of ovarian endometriomas: a prospective, randomized trial. *Am J Obstet Gynecol* 2000;183:588.

Muzii L, Bellati F, Palaia I, et al. Laparoscopic stripping of endometriomas: a randomized trial on different surgical techniques. Part I: clinical results. *Hum Reprod* 2005;20:1981.

Namnoum AB, Hickman TN, Goodman SB, et al. Incidence of symptom recurrence after hysterectomy for endometriosis. *Fertil Steril* 1995;64:898.

Naples JD, Batt RE, Sadigh A. Spontaneous abortion rate in patients with endometriosis. *Obstet Gynecol* 1981;57:509.

Nezhat C, Nezhat F, Pennington E. Laparoscopic treatment of infiltrative rectosigmoid colon and rectovaginal septum endometriosis by the technique of video laparoscopy and the CO_2 laser. *Br J Obstet Gynaecol* 1992;99:664.

Nezhat C, Seidman DS, Nezhat F, et al. Laparoscopic surgical management of diaphragmatic endometriosis. *Fertil Steril* 1998;69:1048.

Nezhat CH, Seidman DS, Nezhat FR, et al. Long-term outcome of laparoscopic presacral neurectomy for the treatment of central pelvic pain attributed to endometriosis. *Obstet Gynecol* 1998; 91:701.

Nishida M. Relationship between the onset of dysmenorrhea and histologic findings in adenomyosis. *Am J Obstet Gynecol* 1991;165:229.

Noble LS, Simpson ER, John A, et al. Aromatase expression in endometriosis. *J Clin Endocrinol Metab* 1996;81:174.

Nuoja-Huttunen S, Tomas C, Bloigu R, et al. Intrauterine insemination treatment in subfertility: an analysis of factors affecting outcome. *Hum Reprod* 1999;14:698.

Oak MK, Chantler EN, Williams CA, et al. Sperm survival studies in peritoneal fluid from infertile women with endometriosis and unexplained infertility. *Clin Reprod Fertil* 1985;3:297.

Olive DL, Henderson DY. Endometriosis and müllerian anomalies. *Obstet Gynecol* 1987;69:412.

Olive DL, Lee KL. Analysis of sequential treatment protocols for endometriosis-associated infertility. *Am J Obstet Gynecol* 1986;154:613.

Olive DL, Martin DC. Treatment of endometriosis-associated infertility with CO_2 laser laparoscopy: the use of one- and two-parameter exponential models. *Fertil Steril* 1987;48:18.

Olive DL, Montoya I, Riehl RM, et al. Macrophage-conditioned media enhance endometrial stromal cell proliferation in vitro. *Am J Obstet Gynecol* 1991;164:953.

Oosterlynck DJ, Cornillie FJ, Waer M, et al. Women with endometriosis show a defect in natural killer cell activity resulting in a decreased cytotoxicity to autologous endometrium. *Fertil Steril* 1991;56:45.

Osada H, Silber S, Kakinuma T, et al. Surgical procedure to conserve the uterus for future pregnancy in patients suffering from massive adenomyosis. *Reprod Biomed Online* 2011;22:94.

Pagidas K, Falcone T, Hemmings R, et al. Comparison of reoperation for moderate (stage III) and severe (stage IV) endometriosis-related infertility with in vitro fertilization-embryo transfer. *Fertil Steril* 1996;65:791.

Parazzini F. Ablation of lesions or no treatment in minimal-mild endometriosis in infertile women: a randomized trial. Gruppo Italiano per lo Studio dell'Endometriosi. *Hum Reprod* 1999;14:1332.

Parazzini F, Fedele L, Busacca M, et al. Postsurgical medical treatment of advanced endometriosis: results of a randomized clinical trial. *Am J Obstet Gynecol* 1994;171:1205.

Parker JD, Leondires M, Sinaii N. Persistence of dysmenorrhea and nonmenstrual pain after optimal endometriosis surgery may indicate adenomyosis. *Fertil Steril* 2006;86:711.

Paull T, Tedeschi LG. Perineal endometriosis at the site of episiotomy scar. *Obstet Gynecol* 1972;40:28.

Pelage JP, Jacob D, Fazel A, et al. Midterm results of uterine artery embolization for symptomatic adenomyosis: initial experience. *Radiology* 2005;234:948.

Pellegrini C, Gori I, Achtari C, et al. The expression of estrogen receptors as well as GREB1, c-MYC, and cyclin D1, estrogen-regulated genes implicated in proliferation, is increased in peritoneal endometriosis. *Fertil Steril* 2012;98:1200.

Pinkert T, Catlow C, Straus R. Endometriosis of the urinary bladder in a man with prostatic carcinoma. *Cancer* 1979;43:1562.

Pittaway DE, Douglas JW. Serum CA-125 in women with endometriosis and chronic pelvic pain. *Fertil Steril* 1989;51:68.

Pittaway DE, Daniell JF, Maxson WS. Ovarian surgery in an infertility patient as an indication for a short-interval second-look laparoscopy: a preliminary study. *Fertil Steril* 1985;44:611.

Pittaway DE, Vernon C, Fayez JA. Spontaneous abortions in women with endometriosis. *Fertil Steril* 1988;50:711.

Pokras R, Hufnagel VG. Hysterectomy in the United States, 1965–84. *Am J Public Health* 1988;78:852.

Polan ML, DeCherney A. Presacral neurectomy for pelvic pain in infertility. *Fertil Steril* 1980;34:557.

Popovic M, Puchner S, Berzaczy D, et al. Uterine artery embolization for the treatment of adenomyosis: a review. *J Vasc Interv Radiol* 2011;22:901.

Prystowsky JB, Stryker SJ, Ujiki GT, et al. Gastrointestinal endometriosis: incidence and indications for resection. *Arch Surg* 1988;123:855.

Punnonen R, Soderstrom P, Alanen A. Isthmic tubal occlusion: etiology and histology. *Acta Eur Fertil* 1984;15:39.

Ranney B. Endometriosis IV: hereditary tendency. *Obstet Gynecol* 1971;37:734.

Redwine DB. The distribution of endometriosis in the pelvis by age groups and fertility. *Fertil Steril* 1987;47:173.

Redwine DB. Peritoneal blood painting: an aid in the diagnosis of endometriosis. *Am J Obstet Gynecol* 1989;161:865.

Redwine DB. Endometriosis persisting after castration: clinical characteristics and results of surgical management. *Obstet Gynecol* 1994;83:405.

Redwine DB. Ovarian endometriosis: a marker for more extensive pelvic and intestinal disease. *Fertil Steril* 1999;72:310.

Ret Davalos ML, De Cicco C, D'Hoore A, et al. Outcome after rectum resection: a review for gynecologists. *J Minim Invasive Gynecol* 2007;12:33.

Rezai N, Ghodgaonkar RB, Zacur HA, et al. Cul-de-sac fluid in women with endometriosis: fluid volume, protein and prostanoid concentration during the periovulatory period—days 13 to 18. *Fertil Steril* 1987;48:29.

Rier SE, Martin DC, Bowman RE, et al. Endometriosis in rhesus monkeys (*Macaca mulatta*) following chronic exposure to 2,3, 7,8-tetrachloro-dibenzo-p-dioxin. *Fundam Appl Toxicol* 1993; 21:433.

Riva HL, Kawasaki DM, Messinger AJ. Further experience with norethynodrel in treatment of endometriosis. *Obstet Gynecol* 1962;19:111.

Rivlin ME, Miller JD, Krueger RP, et al. Leuprolide acetate in the management of ureteral obstruction caused by endometriosis. *Obstet Gynecol* 1990;75:532.

Rock JA, Guzick DS, Jones HW Jr. The efficacy of accessory surgical intervention in conjunction with resection and fulguration of endometriosis. *Infertility* 1981;4:193.

Rock JA, Guzick DS, Sengos C, et al. Evaluation of pregnancy success with respect to extent of disease as categorized using contemporary classification systems. *Fertil Steril* 1981;35:131.

Rock JA, Parmley TH, King TM, et al. Endometriosis and the development of tuboperitoneal fistulas after tubal ligation. *Fertil Steril* 1981;35:16.

Rock JA, Dubin NH, Ghodgaonkar RB, et al. Cul-de-sac fluid in women with endometriosis: fluid volume and prostanoid concentration during the proliferative phase of the cycle—days 8–12. *Fertil Steril* 1982;37:747.

Romualdi D, Franco Zannoni G, Lanzone A, et al. Follicular loss in endoscopic surgery for ovarian endometriosis: quantitative and qualitative observations. *Fertil Steril* 2011;96:374.

Rown J, Pan A, Hart RJ. Gonadotrophin-releasing hormone analogues for pain associated with endometriosis. *Cochrane Database Syst Rev* 2010;(12):CD008475.

Ruggi G. Della sympatectamia al collo ed ale adome. *Policlinico* 1899;1:193.

Sakamoto A. Subserosal adenomyosis: a possible variant of pelvic endometriosis. *Am J Obstet Gynecol* 1991;165:198.

Saleh A, Tulandi T. Reoperation after laparoscopic treatment of ovarian endometriomas by excision and by fenestration. *Fertil Steril* 1999;72:322.

Sallam HN, Garcia-Velasco JA, Dias S, et al. Long-term pituitary down-regulation before in vitro fertilization (IVF) for women with endometriosis. *Cochrane Database Syst Rev* 2006;(1):CD004635. doi: 10.1002/14651858.CD004635.pub2

Sampson JA. Benign and malignant endometrial implants in peritoneal cavity, and their relation to certain ovarian tumors. *Surg Gynecol Obstet* 1924;38:287.

Sampson JA. Peritoneal endometriosis due to menstrual dissemination of endometrial tissue into the peritoneal cavity. *Am J Obstet Gynecol* 1925;14:422.

IV

Sangi-Haghpeykar H, Poindexter AN. Epidemiology of endometriosis among parous women. *Obstet Gynecol* 1995;85:983.

Schenken RS, Asch RH, Williams RF, et al. Etiology of infertility in monkeys with endometriosis: luteinized unruptured follicles, luteal phase defects, pelvic adhesions and spontaneous abortions. *Fertil Steril* 1984;41:122.

Schenken RS, Williams RF, Hodgen GD. Effect of pregnancy on surgically induced endometriosis in cynomolgus monkeys. *Am J Obstet Gynecol* 1987;157:1392.

Schlaff WD, Dugoff L, Damewood MD, et al. Megestrol acetate for treatment of endometriosis. *Obstet Gynecol* 1990;75:646.

Schmidt CL. Endometriosis: a reappraisal of pathogenesis and treatment. *Fertil Steril* 1985;44:157.

Schneider VL, Schneider A, Reed KL, et al. Comparison of Doppler with two-dimensional sonography and CA-125 for prediction of malignancy of pelvic masses. *Obstet Gynecol* 1993;81:983.

Schweppe KW, Wynn RM. Ultrastructural changes in endometriotic implants during the menstrual cycle. *Obstet Gynecol* 1981;58:465.

Schweppe KW, Wynn RM, Beller FK. Ultrastructural comparison of endometriotic implants and eutopic endometrium. *Am J Obstet Gynecol* 1984;148:1024.

Seibel MM, Berger MJ, Weinstein FG, et al. The effectiveness of danazol on subsequent fertility in minimal endometriosis. *Fertil Steril* 1982;38:534.

Sekiba K, Obstetrics and Gynecology Adhesion Prevention Committee. Use of Interceed (TC7) absorbable adhesion barrier to reduce postoperative adhesion reformation in infertility and endometriosis surgery. *Obstet Gynecol* 1992;79:518.

Serta RT, Rufo S, Seibel MM. Minimal endometriosis and intrauterine insemination: does controlled ovarian hyperstimulation improve pregnancy rates? *Obstet Gynecol* 1992;80:37.

Shakiba K, Bena JF, McGill KM, et al. Surgical treatment of endometriosis: a 7-year follow up on the requirement for further surgery. *Obstet Gynecol* 2008;111:1285.

Shook TE, Nyberg LM. Endometriosis of the urinary tract. *Urology* 1988;31:1.

Simpson JL, Elias S, Malinak LR, et al. Heritable aspects of endometriosis. I. Genetic studies. *Am J Obstet Gynecol* 1980;137:325.

Simpson JL, Malinak LR, Elias S, et al. HLA associations in endometriosis. *Am J Obstet Gynecol* 1984;148:395.

Somigliana E, Vercellini P, Viganc P, et al. Should endometriomas be treated before IVF-ICSI cycles? *Hum Reprod Update* 2006;12:57.

Somigliana E, Vercellini P, Vigano P, et al. Non-invasive diagnosis of endometriosis: the goal or own goal? *Hum Reprod* 2010;25:1863.

Steele RW, Dmowski WP, Marmer DJ. Immunologic aspects of human endometriosis. *Am J Reprod Immunol* 1984;6:33.

Stephansson O, Kieler H, Granath F, et al. Endometriosis, assisted reproduction technology, and risk of adverse pregnancy outcome. *Hum Reprod* 2009;24:2341.

Stock RJ. Postsalpingectomy endometriosis: a reassessment. *Obstet Gynecol* 1982;60:560.

Stovall TG, Ling FW, Crawford DA. Hysterectomy for chronic pelvic pain of presumed uterine etiology. *Obstet Gynecol* 1990;75:676.

Strathy JH, Molgaard CA, Coulam CB, et al. Endometriosis and infertility: a laparoscopic study of endometriosis among fertile and infertile women. *Fertil Steril* 1982;38:667.

Stripling MC, Martin DC, Chatman DL, et al. Subtle appearance of pelvic endometriosis. *Fertil Steril* 1988;49:425.

Sueldo CE, Lambert H, Steinleitner A, et al. The effect of peritoneal fluid from patients with endometriosis on murine sperm–oocyte interaction. *Fertil Steril* 1987;48:697.

Suginami H, Yano K. An ovum capture inhibitor (OCI) in endometriosis peritoneal fluid: an OCI-related membrane responsible for fimbrial failure of ovum capture. *Fertil Steril* 1988;50:648.

Surgical Membrane Study Group. Prophylaxis of pelvic sidewall adhesions with Gore-Tex surgical membrane: a multicenter clinical investigation. *Fertil Steril* 1992;57:921.

Surrey ES, Halme J. Effect of platelet-derived growth factor on endometrial stromal cell proliferation in vitro: a model for endometriosis? *Fertil Steril* 1991;56:672.

Surrey ES, Gambone JC, Lu JK, et al. The effects of combining norethindrone with a gonadotropin-releasing hormone agonist in the treatment of symptomatic endometriosis. *Fertil Steril* 1990;53:620.

Surrey ES, Voigt B, Fournet N, et al. Prolonged gonadotropin-releasing hormone agonist treatment of symptomatic endometriosis: the role of cyclic sodium etidronate and low-dose norethindrone "add-back" therapy. *Fertil Steril* 1995;63:747.

Sutton CJ, Ewen SP, Whitelaw N, et al. Prospective, randomized, double-blind, controlled trial of laser laparoscopy in the treatment of pelvic pain associated with minimal, mild, and moderate endometriosis. *Fertil Steril* 1994;62:696.

Suzuki T, Ixumi S, Matsubayashi H, et al. Impact of ovarian endometrioma on oocytes and pregnancy outcome in in vitro fertilization. *Fertil Steril* 2005;83:908.

Takahashi K, Okada S, Ozaki T, et al. Diagnosis of pelvic endometriosis by "fat-saturation" technique. *Fertil Steril* 1994;62:973.

Tamaya T, Motoyama T, Ohono Y, et al. Steroid receptor levels and histology of endometriosis and adenomyosis. *Fertil Steril* 1979;31:396.

Tanmahasamut P, Rattanachaiyanont M, Angsuwathana S, et al. Postoperative levonorgestrel-releasing intrauterine system for pelvic endometriosis-related pain. *Obstet Gynecol* 2012;119:519.

Te Linde RW, Scott RB. Experimental endometriosis. *Obstet Gynecol* 1978;130:569.

Telimaa S. Danazol and medroxyprogesterone acetate inefficacious in the treatment of infertility in endometriosis. *Fertil Steril* 1988;50:872.

Thomas EJ, Lenton EA, Cooke ID. Follicle growth patterns and endocrinological abnormalities in infertile women with minor degrees of endometriosis. *Br J Obstet Gynaecol* 1986;93:852.

Tinkanen H, Kujansuu E. In vitro fertilization in patients with ovarian endometriomas. *Acta Obstet Gynecol Scand* 2000;79:119.

Tjaden B, Schlaff WD, Kimball A, et al. The efficacy of presacral neurectomy for the relief of midline dysmenorrhea. *Obstet Gynecol* 1990;76:89.

Togashi K, Ozasa H, Konishi I, et al. Enlarged uterus: differentiation between adenomyosis and leiomyoma with MR imaging. *Radiology* 1989;171:531.

Tseng JF, Ryan IP, Milam TD, et al. Interleukin-6 secretion in vitro is upregulated in ectopic and eutopic endometrial stromal cells from women with endometriosis. *J Clin Endocrinol Metab* 1996;81:1118.

Tulandi T, Al-Took S. Reproductive outcome after treatment of mild endometriosis with laparoscopic excision and electrocoagulation. *Fertil Steril* 1998;69:229.

Tulandi T, Mouchawar M. Treatment-dependent and treatment-independent pregnancy in women with minimal and mild endometriosis. *Fertil Steril* 1991;56:790.

Tummon IS, Maclin VM, Radwanska E, et al. Occult ovulatory dysfunction in women with minimal endometriosis and unexplained infertility. *Fertil Steril* 1988;50:716.

Tummon IS, Colwell KA, MacKinnoa CJ, et al. Abbreviated endometriosis-associated infertility correlates with in vitro fertilization success. *J In Vitro Fert Embryo Transf* 1991;8:149.

Tummon IS, Asher LJ, Martin JS, et al. Randomized controlled trial of superovulation and insemination for infertility associated with minimal or mild endometriosis. *Fertil Steril* 1997;68:8.

Uchima FD, Edery M, Iguchi T, et al. Growth of mouse endometrial luminal epithelial cells in vitro: functional integrity of the oestrogen receptor system and failure of oestrogen to induce proliferation. *J Endocrinol* 1991;128:115.

Uohara JK, Kovara TY. Endometriosis of the appendix: report of 12 cases and review of the literature. *Am J Obstet Gynecol* 1975;121:423.

Vaughan Williams CA, Oak MK, Elstein M. Cyclical gonadotrophin and progesterone secretion in women with minimal endometriosis. *Clin Reprod Fertil* 1986;4:259.

Vercellini P, Fedele L, Bianchi S, et al. Pelvic denervation for chronic pain associated with endometriosis: fact or fancy? *Am J Obstet Gynecol* 1991;165:745.

Vercellini P, Vendola N, Bocciolone L, et al. Reliability of visual diagnosis of ovarian endometriosis. *Fertil Steril* 1991;56:1198.

Vercellini P, De Giorgi O, Oldani S, et al. Depot medroxyprogesterone acetate versus an oral contraceptive combined with very-low-dose danazol for long-term treatment of pelvic pain associated with endometriosis. *Am J Obstet Gynecol* 1996;175:396.

Vercellini P, Chapron C, Fedele L, et al. Evidence for asymmetric distribution of sciatic nerve endometriosis. *Obstet Gynecol* 2003;102:383.

Vercellini P, Frontino G, De Giorgi O. Continuous use of an oral contraceptive for endometriosis-associated recurrent dysmenorrhea that does not respond to a cyclic pill regimen. *Fertil Steril* 2003;80:560.

Vercellini P, Chapron C, Fedele L, et al. Evidence for asymmetric distribution of lower intestinal endometriosis. *Br J Obstet Gynaecol* 2004;111:1213.

Vercellini P, Pietropaolo G, De Giorgi O, et al. Treatment of symptomatic rectovaginal endometriosis with an estrogen-progestogen combination versus low-dose norethindrone acetate. *Fertil Steril* 2005;84:1375.

Vercellini P, Fedele L, Aimi G, et al. Reproductive performance, pain recurrence and disease relapse after conservative surgical treatment for endometriosis: the predictive value of the current classification system. *Hum Reprod* 2006;21:2679.

Vercellini P, Pietropaolo G, De Giorgi O, et al. Reproductive performance in infertile women with rectovaginal endometriosis: is surgery worthwhile? *Am J Obstet Gynecol* 2006;195:1303.

Vercellini P, Abbiati A, Vigano' P, et al. Asymmetry in distribution of diaphragmatic endometriosis lesions: evidence in favour of the menstrual reflux theory. *Hum Reprod* 2007;22:2359.

Vercellini P, Barbara G, Buggio L, et al. Effect of patient selection on estimate of reproductive success after surgery for rectovaginal endometriosis: literature review. *Reprod Biomed Online* 2012;24:389.

Vercellini P, Somigliana E, Consonni D, et al. Surgical versus medical treatment for endometriosis-associated deep dyspareunia: I. Effect on pain during intercourse and patient satisfaction. *Hum Reprod* 2012;27:3450.

Vercellini P, De Matteis S, Somigliana E, et al. Long-term adjuvant therapy for the prevention of postoperative endometrioma recurrence: a systematic review and meta-analysis. *Acta Obstet Gynecol Scand* 2013;92:8.

Verkauf BS. The incidence, symptoms, and signs of endometriosis in fertile and infertile women. *J Fla Med Assoc* 1987;74:671.

Vernon MW, Beard JS, Graves K, et al. Classification of endometriotic implants by morphologic appearance and capacity to synthesize prostaglandin F. *Fertil Steril* 1986;46:801.

Vigano P, Vercellini P, Di Blasio AM, et al. Deficient antiendometrium lymphocyte-mediated cytotoxicity in patient with endometriosis. *Fertil Steril* 1991;56:894.

von Rokitansky C. Ueber Uterusdrusen-Neubildung im Uterus und Varialsarcomen. *Zkk Gesellsch d Aerzte zu Wien* 1860;37:577.

Wang PH, Liu WM, Fuh JL, et al. Comparison of surgery alone and combined surgical-medical treatment in the management of symptomatic uterine adenomyoma. *Fertil Steril* 2009;92:876.

Wardle PG, Hull MG. Is endometriosis a disease? *Baillieres Clin Obstet Gynaecol* 1993;7:673.

Weed JC, Arquembourg PC. Endometriosis: can it produce an autoimmune response resulting in infertility? *Clin Obstet Gynecol* 1980;23:885.

Wentz AC. Premenstrual spotting: its association with endometriosis but not luteal phase inadequacy. *Fertil Steril* 1980;33:605.

Werbrouck E, Spiessens C, Meuleman C, et al. No difference in cycle pregnancy rate and in cumulative live-birth rate between women with surgically treated minimal to mild endometriosis and women with unexplained infertility after controlled ovarian hyperstimulation and intrauterine insemination. *Fertil Steril* 2006;86:566.

Wespi HJ, Kletzhändler M. Uber Narbenendometriosen. *Mschr Geburtsh Gynakol* 1940;111:169.

Wheeler JM, Malinak LR. Recurrent endometriosis: incidence, management, and prognosis. *Am J Obstet Gynecol* 1983;146:247.

Wheeler JM, Johnston BM, Malinak LR. The relationship of endometriosis to spontaneous abortion. *Fertil Steril* 1983;39:656.

Wihemsson L, Lindblom B, Wiqvist N. The human uterotubal junction: contractile patterns of different smooth muscle layers and the influence of prostaglandin E_2, prostaglandin $F_{2\alpha}$ and prostaglandin I_2 in vitro. *Fertil Steril* 1979;32:303.

Wilcox LS, Koonin LM, Pokras R, et al. Hysterectomy in the United States, 1988–1990. *Obstet Gynecol* 1994;83:549.

Wood C, Maher P, Hill D. Biopsy diagnosis and conservative surgical treatment of adenomyosis. *Aust N Z J Obstet Gynaecol* 1993;33:319.

Wright J, Lotfallah H, Jones K, et al. A randomized trial of excision versus ablation for mild endometriosis. *Fertil Steril* 2005;83:1830.

Yanushpolsky EH, Best CL, Jackson KV, et al. Effects of endometriomas on oocyte quality, embryo quality, and pregnancy rates in in vitro fertilization cycles: a prospective, case-controlled study. *J Assist Reprod Genet* 1998;15:193.

Yaron Y, Peyser MR, Samuel D, et al. Infected endometriotic cysts secondary to oocyte aspiration for in-vitro fertilization. *Hum Reprod* 1994;9:1759.

Ylikorkla O, Koskimies A, Laathainen T, et al. Peritoneal fluid prostaglandins in endometriosis, tubal disorders, and unexplained infertility. *Obstet Gynecol* 1984;63:616.

Young MD, Blackmore WP. The use of danazol in the management of endometriosis. *J Int Med Res* 1977;5(suppl 3):86.

Zanagnolo VL, Beck R, Schlaff WD, et al. Time-related effects of gonadotropin-releasing hormone analog treatment in experimentally induced endometriosis in the rat. *Fertil Steril* 1991;55:411.

Zullo F, Palomba S, Zupi E, et al. Effectiveness of presacral neurectomy in women with severe dysmenorrhea caused by endometriosis who were treated with laparoscopic conservative surgery: a 1-year prospective randomized double-blind controlled trial. *Am J Obstet Gynecol* 2003;189:5.

CHAPTER 23
Surgical Conditions of the Vulva

Ira R. Horowitz, Joseph Buscema, and Bhagirath Majmudar

DEFINITIONS

Bubo—Enlarged, suppurative inguinal lymph node characteristic of chancroid.

Burow solution—A soothing aluminum sulfate solute that can be used as a soak or wet compress for inflamed or irritated skin or mucous membrane.

Cavitron ultrasonic surgical aspirator (CUSA)—An electromechanical surgical instrument that is useful in soft tissue dissection. Using focused ultrasound, superficial tissue is sheared off and aspirated through the wand tip. It has been used to treat condyloma and vulvar intraepithelial neoplasia.

Donovan body—An intracytoplasmic gram-negative, rod-shaped bacteria characteristically identified in histiocytes associated with granuloma inguinale.

Fournier gangrene—An older term for necrotizing fasciitis.

Keyes biopsy instrument—A pencil-like biopsy instrument with a sharp, hollow, cylindrical tip that is rotated while pressed against the skin. It cuts a small, cylindrical biopsy, which is then elevated with tissue forceps and cut off at the base with scissors or a knife.

Necrotizing fasciitis—A severe, rapidly progressive, life-threatening infection of the subcutaneous tissue and fascia that may involve the vulva. Synergistic bacterial infection with multiple organisms, it is associated with vascular thrombosis leading to necrosis of the skin and subcutaneous tissue of fascia. It is treated with aggressive broad-spectrum antibiotic coverage and wide surgical debridement.

Silvadene cream—A 1% silver sulfadiazine cream commonly used on the vulva following laser therapy or surgery to minimize the risk of cellulitis or wound infection and to sooth the postoperative wound site.

Vulvar intraepithelial neoplasia (VIN)—A preinvasive neoplastic condition of the vulva.

Vulvar vestibulitis—A painful condition of the vulva of uncertain etiology. It is characterized by (a) severe pain on vestibular touch or attempted vaginal entry, (b) tenderness to pressure localized within the vulvar vestibule, and (c) minimal physical findings consisting of slight erythema within the vestibule.

Word catheter—A small latex catheter with an inflatable balloon to hold it in place. It is inserted to drain a Bartholin duct abscess.

The vulva and the adjacent perianal skin are designated the anogenital area. These tissues are derived from ectoderm and are considered separately from the vagina and cervix, which are of mesodermal origin. Multifocal diseases, particularly human papillomavirus (HPV), can affect all of the aforementioned epithelia. A complete vulvar examination should, therefore, include the vulva, perineum, anal area, urethral meatus, buttocks, and thighs. It is difficult to appreciate subtle skin changes in patients with dark skin; therefore, an adequate light source is necessary.

VULVAR DERMATOSES

In 1987, the International Society for the Study of Vulvovaginal Diseases (ISSVD) revised the terminology to describe the nonneoplastic epithelial disorders of the vulva, which include psoriasis, lichen planus, lichen simplex chronicus, candidiasis, and condyloma acuminata. In their 1976 classification, the ISSVD categorized hyperplastic dystrophy with and without atypia. In the classification of 1987, squamous cell hyperplasia is without atypia, and lesions with atypia are considered vulvar intraepithelial neoplasia (VIN). In 2006, the ISVD published the Classification of Vulvar Dermatoses. The benign lesions were categorized as spongiotic, acanthotic, lichenoid, dermal homogenization/sclerosis vesiculobullous, acantholytic, granulomatous, and vasculopathic patterns. This was further simplified in 2011 when the ISSVD formulated a classification that would be easier for clinicians (Table 23.1).

TABLE 23.1 International Society for the Study of Vulvovaginal Diseases Classification of Vulvar Pain

A. Vulvar pain related to a specific disorder
- Infectious
- Inflammatory
- Neoplastic
- Neurologic

B. Vulvodynia
1. Generalized
   a. Provoked (sexual or nonsexual)
   b. Unprovoked (spontaneous)
   c. Mixed (provoked and nonprovoked)
2. Localized (i.e., vestibule, clitoris, vulva)
   Provoked (sexual or nonsexual)
   Unprovoked (spontaneous)
   Mixed (provoked and nonprovoked)

The terms *kraurosis* and *leukoplakia* have been overused in the past. In 1877, Schwimmer reported that leukoplakia on the buccal surfaces of the mouth was a premalignant lesion, and Beisky later described kraurosis as an atrophic lesion similar to lichen sclerosus. Because of these early reports, every lesion on the vulva that appeared white and constricted the vaginal outlet was called kraurosis. Moreover, conditions as varied as leukoderma and invasive cancer have been called leukoplakia. Other terms, such as *primary senile atrophy* and *atrophic leukoplakia*, have been used interchangeably. They are nonspecific and should be eliminated. The epidermis may be thickened and the skin markings accentuated (lichenification), but the extent of the epithelial proliferation cannot be assessed without biopsy. Usually a 3- or 4-mm Keyes punch biopsy is used to obtain a small biopsy in the office under local anesthesia (Fig. 23.1). The specimen is oriented with the epithelial surface up on a square of filter paper or Telfa before being placed in fixative. This allows correct orientation of the tissue so that a full-thickness, nontangential, microscopic section can be prepared. Occasionally, experienced clinicians make a tentative diagnosis based on history and physical examination. A trial of topical therapy may be used for 6 to 8 weeks to evaluate the response; if the response is less than satisfactory or if there is any suspicion of invasive cancer, a biopsy must be done.

Although some physicians have suggested that lichen sclerosus and kraurosis have different histopathologies, their microscopic appearance is similar. A safe approach would be for surgeons to describe the anatomic appearance (i.e., whether the vulva is shrunken and constricted or thickened and leathery), leaving it up to the pathologist, who is familiar with both histology and anatomy, to define the cellular and histologic abnormalities.

Hyperkeratosis

Both chronic infections and benign tumors, most commonly condylomata acuminata, appear white because keratin absorbs moisture, which reflects light back to the observer.

To avoid the ambiguous term *leukoplakia*, Jeffcoate, in 1966, introduced the term *dystrophy* into the nomenclature of benign epithelial lesions of the vulva. Predictions about the malignant potential of vulvar dystrophy vary; of all the types of dystrophy, the one most often benign is lichen sclerosus. As noted earlier, the terminology for vulvar dystrophies has been altered. Vulvar dystrophy has been classified in three categories: squamous hyperplasia, lichen sclerosus, and VIN. Typical squamous cell hyperplasia is characterized by a thickened, hyperkeratotic squamous epithelium, elongated rete pegs, and often an infiltration of the underlying tissue with chronic inflammatory cells. Typical hyperplasia is a benign form of chronic dermatitis with hyperkeratosis and acanthosis; thus, the designation "dystrophy" should be eliminated.

Depigmentation Lesions

Leukoderma and *vitiligo* are terms that are used interchangeably. Treatment is not required unless the symptoms of the commonly associated chronic dermatitis cannot be controlled by local medications. The hyperkeratotic lesions comprise a number of diverse entities that share a white to grayish white epithelial appearance in a moist environment. Biopsy is the only reliable criterion for accurate assessment.

Lichen Sclerosus

Lichen sclerosus is characterized by hyperkeratosis, thinning of the epidermis, loss of rete peg architecture, collagenization of the underlying tissue, and associated middermal inflammatory infiltrate (Fig. 23.2). In 2006, the ISSVD classified lichen

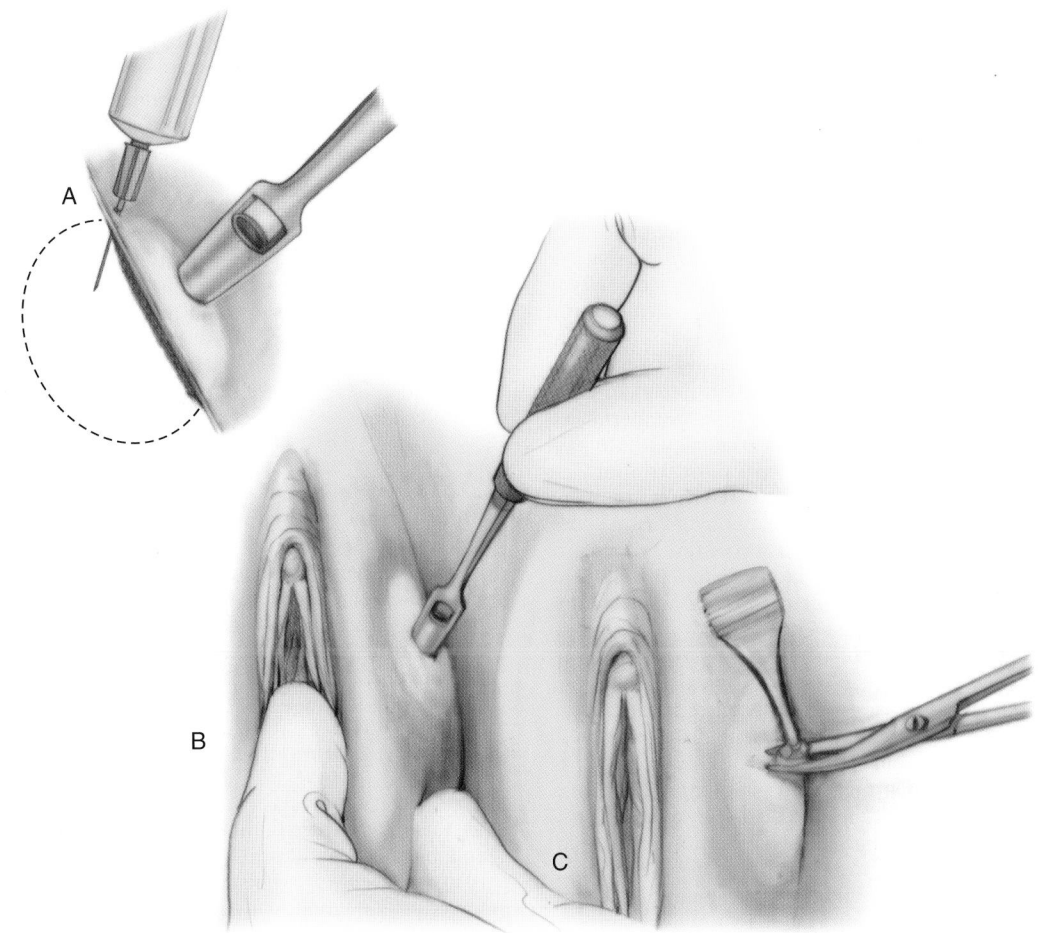

FIGURE 23.1 Biopsy of the vulva. **A:** The skin and subcutaneous tissue are infiltrated with local anesthetic using a small needle. **B:** A 3- or 4-mm Keyes punch biopsy instrument is firmly pressed against the skin to be biopsied and gently rotated. **C:** The small core of skin and subcutaneous tissue separated by the Keyes punch is elevated by small toothed tissue forceps and trimmed off at the base with curved iris scissors. Pressure is applied to the biopsy site, and the base is cauterized with silver nitrate sticks.

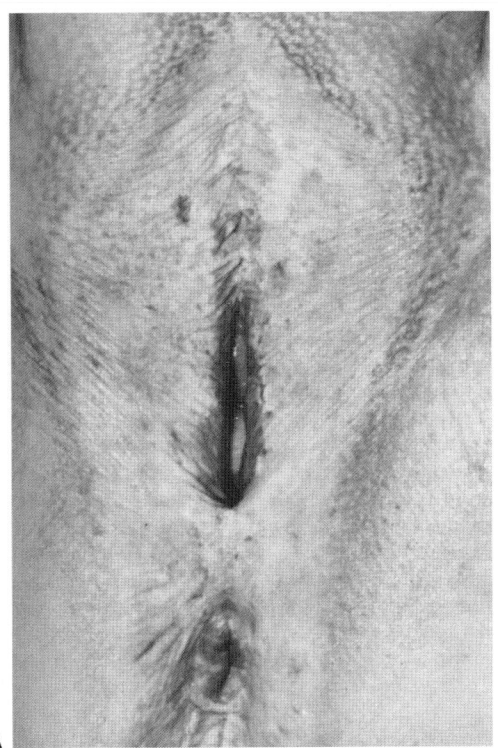

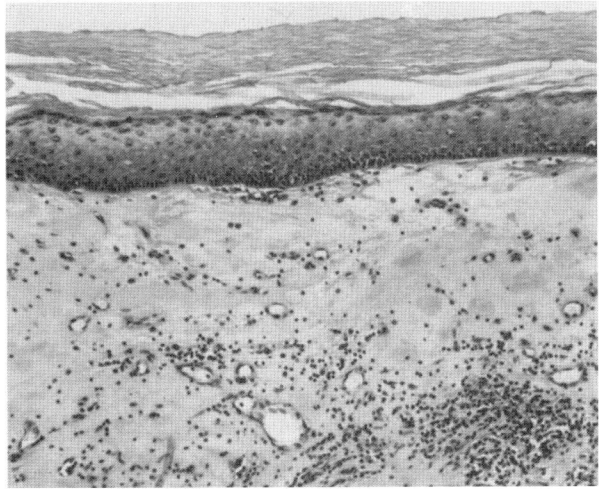

FIGURE 23.2 Vulvar dystrophy; lichen sclerosus. **A:** Distorted vulva with superficial ulcerations and extensive hyperkeratosis and loss of normal architecture. **B:** Microscopic picture of lichen sclerosus composed of epidermal diminution, subepidermal collagenization, and middermal lymphocytic infiltrate.

IV

sclerosis as lichenoid pattern. It can occur at any age. The disease has been noted in the prepubertal child, and it occurs during the menstrual years. Nevertheless, it is seen most often in the postmenopausal woman when the lesions more commonly are symptomatic, perhaps because of the additional epithelial compromise caused by atrophy. The genetic aspects of lichen sclerosus have not been clearly identified, but the finding of lesions in both mother and child has been documented.

If biopsy specimens reveal lichen sclerosus, the patient should be treated with ultrapotent corticosteroids. Many series over the past few years have shown an excellent clinical response to 0.05% clobetasol proportionate topical ointment or cream. In a series of 81 women with biopsy-proven lichen sclerosus, Lorenz and coworkers reported that 77% had complete remission of symptoms and another 18% experienced significant improvement. Patients were treated with topical application of clobetasol cream twice daily for 1 month, at bedtime for another month, and, finally, twice a week for 3 months. They continued to use the cream on an "as-needed" basis once or twice a week. Many patients continue to require occasional episodic therapy for symptomatic flareups, but the long-term effects of these ultrapotent steroids on the vulva have not been well studied. Some experts recommend maintenance therapy with lower potency corticosteroids, such as triamcinolone or 0.1% betamethasone. Topical testosterone has been recommended in the past, but Bornstein and associates compared the results of 2% testosterone propionate with 0.05% clobetasol dipropionate; at 1-year follow-up, 80% of the clobetasol-treated patients reported symptomatic improvement compared with 40% of those treated with testosterone.

Many patients with chronic vulvar dermatitis, stenosis of the outlet specifically related to lichen sclerosus, and vestibulitis have an associated constriction of the vaginal outlet with resultant dyspareunia. Local intravaginal or vulvar applications of estrogen do not improve this condition. Plastic surgery to the outlet (**Fig. 23.3**) may be helpful. By excising a triangular area of skin beneath the fourchette, the surgeon can undermine and evert the adjacent vaginal epithelium, incise the transverse perineal muscle and fascia, and cover the denuded area with a flap of vaginal mucosa. The procedure is simple, and the use of delayed absorbable suture material lessens the incidence of wound breakdown that commonly occurs when absorbable suture is used. The results of this procedure have been most satisfactory; approximately 95% of patients are greatly relieved of dyspareunia. Breech and Laufer have reported good results in a few patients by suturing a protective covering of oxidized regenerated cellulose gauze (Surgicel, Johnson & Johnson, Arlington, TX) to the raw surfaces of the inner labia and clitoris after division of intracoital adhesions to prevent recurrence.

VULVAR INTRAEPITHELIAL NEOPLASIA

The first two cases of carcinoma in situ (CIS) of the skin were described by Bowen in 1912. Bowen also stated that although stromal invasion had not developed in patients observed over periods of 12 to 16 years, curettage and cauterization did not eliminate recurrence of the lesions.

In 1958, Woodruff and Hildebrandt reported 13 cases of VIN. They suggested that because the histology varied from one area to another in the same section, the general term CIS should be used to designate the lesion. Today, the term VIN is commonly used, and vulvar intraepithelial lesions were originally subdivided into VIN I, corresponding to mild dysplasia; VIN II, similar to moderate dysplasia; and VIN III, corresponding to severe dysplasia or CIS, similar to the classification of cervical disease.

However, in 2004, the ISSVD changed the classification, eliminating the term *VIN I*. VIN I is thought to be secondary to viral changes and not a reproducible diagnosis. In addition to eliminating VIN I, they combined VIN II and VIN III as simply VIN, the expectation being that these lesions will be treated as high-grade preinvasive neoplasms. Jones and colleagues, in their review of 405 women with VIN, reported a decrease in the mean age of patients with VIN from 50 in 1980 to 39 in 2003. The increased prevalence of HPV infection as well as increased awareness by patients, clinicians, and pathologists have resulted in an increase in the diagnosis of VIN and, perhaps, a more common identification of these lesions in younger women. In an international study, de Sanjose and colleagues identified HPV 16, HPV 33, and HPV 18 in descending order.

Symptoms

Pruritus is the predominant symptom of most vulvar disease, including cancer, yet itching was the primary symptom in only 50% of patients with in situ cancer in a series reported by Buscema and associates. Other presenting symptoms were the presence of a lump, bleeding, and pain. In a small percentage of the cases, the lesion was discovered on routine examination; but in others, the diagnosis commonly was made in patients seen during follow-up of cervical neoplasia.

Diagnosis

The best technique for early diagnosis is careful inspection of the external genitalia—including perianal areas, thighs, and buttocks—under a bright light (**Fig. 23.4**). If suspicion is aroused either by history or preexisting neoplasia in the lower genital canal or by the suggestion of an abnormal configuration, magnification should be used. An experienced colposcopist can describe white lesions and areas of abnormal vasculature. As a screening procedure, however, colposcopy has not contributed to the early detection of vulvar neoplasia. The use of nuclear staining, specifically 1% toluidine blue and tetracycline fluorescence, has delineated foci of increased metabolic activity, but the false-negative and false-positive rates are high enough to make the results unpredictable.

Careful visual evaluation of the vulvar region should be directed at the focally white, hyperkeratotic areas and at the more important, slightly elevated, papillary areas of the skin. Atypical pigmentation, most significantly gray-white areas that are even minimally ulcerated or slightly elevated above the surrounding skin, should be viewed with suspicion (**Fig. 23.5**). Biopsy provides the final diagnosis.

Multifocal areas of neoplasia that involve the external genitalia, perineum, and the epithelium of the lower genital canal are common; in fact, more than half of the patients with intraepithelial disease in the lower genital tract have multifocal lesions. These lesions suggest an infectious, possibly viral, origin for the neoplasia. In contrast, patients older than 60 years of age with invasive or in situ cancer more commonly have unifocal disease. Benedet and Murphy noted an increase in unifocal and diffuse disease in patients older than 50 years of age. When the vulva is the primary site of the lesion, the cervix, vagina, and perianal areas are frequent sites for associated neoplastic alterations. The combination of vulvar and cervical cancer comprises approximately 20% of all multicentric neoplasia in the lower genital tract.

The most pressing question about multifocal disease is whether invasive disease that develops from in situ lesions will arise in many foci or in only one focus. Only two of our patients with in situ neoplasia younger than 40 years of age have developed invasive cancer, and both cases appeared as

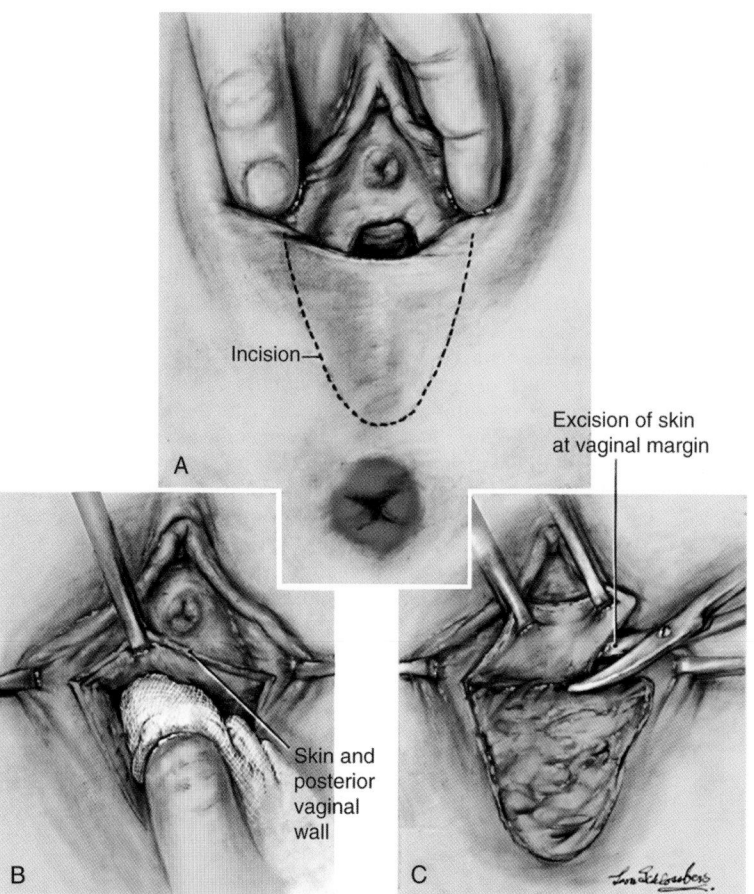

Incision

Excision of skin
at vaginal margin

Skin and
posterior
vaginal
wall

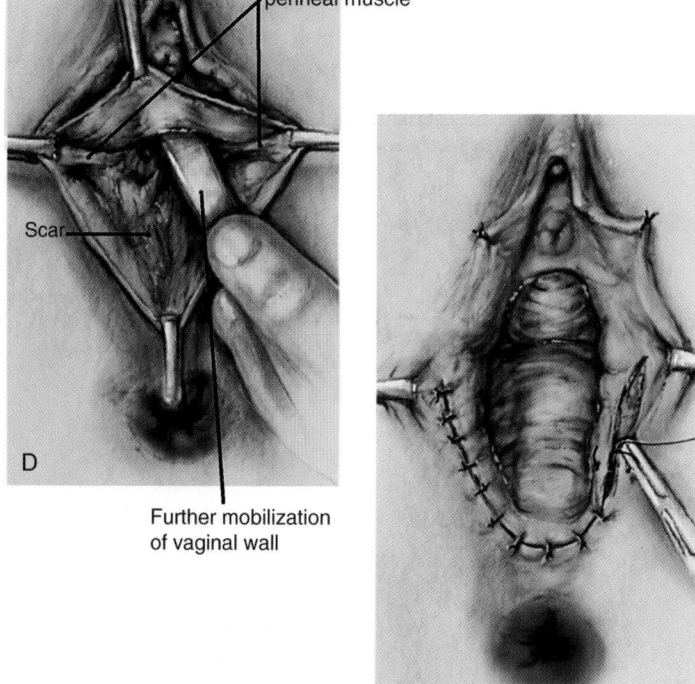

Superior transverse
perineal muscle

Scar

Further mobilization
of vaginal wall

FIGURE 23.3 Perineoplasty. **A:** The incisional line is identified. The incision must be sufficiently extensive to allow for postoperative retraction and subsequent constriction of the outlet. **B:** The vagina is undermined to allow for exteriorization without tension. **C:** The scarred skin of the fourchette is excised. The vaginal epithelium is preserved for exteriorization. The vaginal epithelium is sufficiently undermined for the margins to be approximated to the skin (**D**) without tension (**E**). Occasionally, a small incision is made into the midline of the exteriorized mucosa to allow for an adequate outlet without tension.

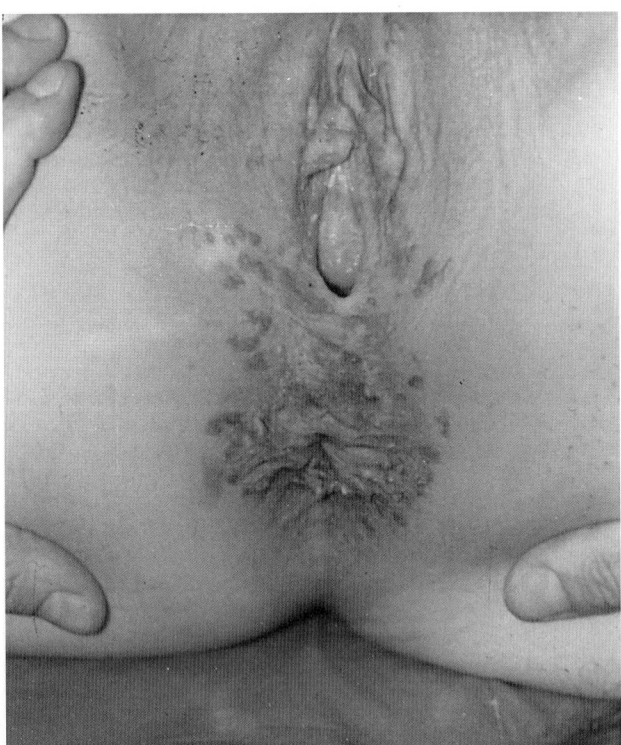

FIGURE 23.4 Multiple foci of CIS in a young patient. Note the vulvar and perianal involvement.

solitary perianal lesions. Because the vulva and the cervix are of different embryologic origins, the tendency to correlate the histopathology of one area with that of the other may be unrewarding. For example, the full-thickness changes that signal cervical intraepithelial neoplasia are not as comparable when they occur on the vulva. Keratinization at the rete tips with intraepithelial pearl formation may indicate, on the other hand, a preinvasive disease in the anogenital area anywhere.

Pathologic Diagnosis

Biopsy with a Keyes punch can be performed in the office with the use of local anesthesia. Knife biopsies often are tangential and contain only the superficial layers, which results in a less than accurate histologic interpretation. An alternative is to use a cervical biopsy forceps to obtain a small specimen that can be evaluated. Correct orientation of the tissue in the fixative is mandatory if accurate evaluation of the specimen is to be rendered. Such orientation can be obtained by placing the biopsy specimen on filter paper or Telfa with the epithelial surface exposed, so that the pathologist can embed the specimen accurately. Tangential cutting may result in the erroneous diagnosis of invasive disease. Cytology has not proved to be a satisfactory screening technique in the evaluation of the precursory cellular atypias in vulvar neoplasia.

The classic bowenoid changes vary from one microscopic section to another, but typical sections show loss of polarity, hyperchromasia, anaplasia, individual cell keratinization, corps ronds, and mitotic activity on the surface (Fig. 23.6). Abnormal mitosis may abound. Other gross variations include the erythroplastic lesion (erythroplasia of Queyrat) with immature cells extending from base to surface and lesions that appear almost normal, being marked only by intraepithelial pearl formation at the rete tips in a background of marked dysplasia. Papillary lesions showing changes of high-grade dysplasia were previously designated as *bowenoid papulosis*, a term discontinued by ISSVD.

Treatment and Results

Although *surgical excision* of VIN is favored, patients typically do not require total vulvectomy. Modesitt and colleagues found invasive cancer in 22% of patients with biopsies consistent with VIN III. Vulvectomy may be appropriate for selected patients who are elderly, particularly if they have extensive disease, or for patients with Paget disease. Wide local excision usually is successful, but an attempt should be made to

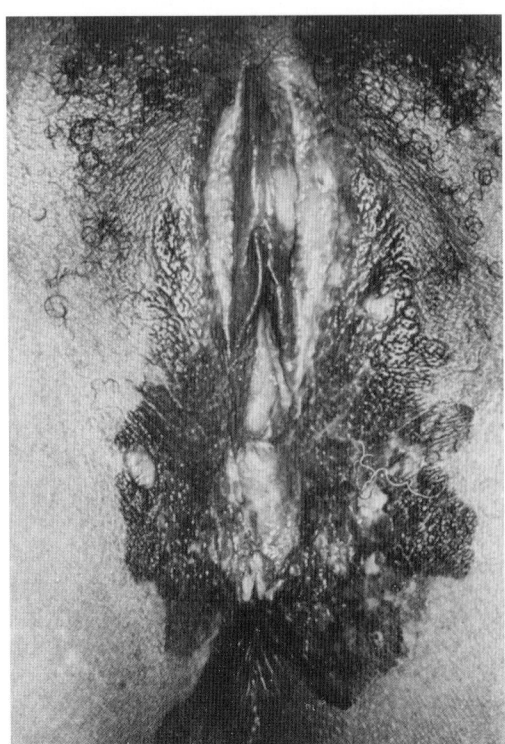

FIGURE 23.5 Carcinoma in situ of vulva showing multiple patterns, particularly atypical pigmentation.

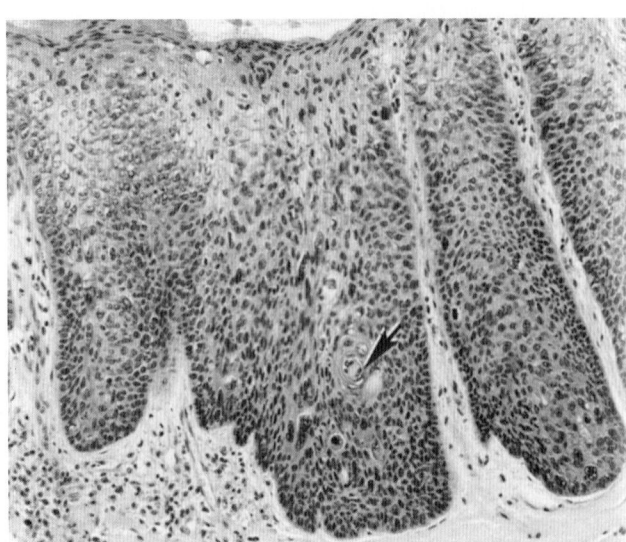

FIGURE 23.6 Carcinoma in situ of the vulva. There is full-thickness alteration in the architecture with elongation and distortion of the rete pegs. At *arrow*, there is intraepithelial pearl formation (160×).

obtain clear margins. The adjacent loose skin of the vulva provides sufficient extra skin to cover minor defects without a skin graft and without significant deformity. The incidence of recurrence is no greater with local excision than with total vulvectomy, but it still approaches 30% to 40%. Positive margins have been indicative of an increased risk of recurrence in some series. Unless invasive cancer is suspected in the area of the positive margins, immediate reexcision is usually not indicated, but careful follow-up is necessary because recurrence is common. Brown has suggested that CO_2 laser vaporization around the surgical margins will decrease the risk of recurrence.

A *skinning vulvectomy*, in which the epidermis and underlying dermis of the vulva and often the perineal area are removed and replaced by a skin graft, has been used for the treatment of extensive or multifocal vulvar in situ disease. This procedure is usually recommended in younger women with extensive lesions in an attempt to restore normal anatomy and sexual function. However, the technique requires surgery at a donor site, which produces an additional scar in a patient who usually is young. Furthermore, it imposes prolonged bed rest, near-complete immobilization of the lower extremities, and indwelling bladder catheterization for 5 to 6 days while the skin graft heals.

The *carbon dioxide laser* has been successfully used in the treatment of in situ vulvar neoplasia. This approach is of particular appeal for the younger patient with multifocal, viral proliferative disease. This subset of patients with VIN is undoubtedly at lower risk for occult invasion. Emphasis in therapy should be directed toward preservation of maximum tissue and vulvar function. Given these considerations and the reality of recurrences, laser ablation provides an effective medium. Pretreatment requirements include careful examination of the lower genital tract and the liberal use of biopsies to identify areas of possible invasion and multicentric disease. The risk of invasive cancer is greater in the older patient. The desire for cosmetic results is less, so the use of surgical excision is favored in older women.

The laser itself is directed colposcopically after examination of tissues prepared by the application of dilute acetic acid. The latter may enhance detection of minimal viral changes not readily seen with the naked eye. Although benign condylomata can be adequately treated by superficial vaporization (so-called first and second plane), laser treatment of VIN must address the extension of disease into the hair follicles (pilosebaceous ducts). This mandates deeper laser vaporization beyond the papillary dermis and into the upper reticular dermis (third plane). The colposcope permits recognition of landmarks that characterize these levels. Baggish and coworkers identified skin appendage involvement in 36% of cases of vulvar in situ carcinoma and predicted that laser vaporization to a depth of 2.5 mm would effectively treat involved appendages in 95% of cases. Shatz and associates advocated ablation of VIN to a depth of 1 to 2 mm in nonhairy and hairy skin to achieve similar success. In laser treatment of VIN, the use of appropriate power densities should be emphasized. Low-power densities lead to thermal conduction injury in adjacent and underlying normal tissue. The latter increases the risk of scarring. Power densities of greater than 750 W/cm^2 are recommended. However, the deeper extent of vaporization required for VIN III, particularly in hair-bearing areas of the vulva, results in considerably greater postoperative pain, a longer period of healing, and an increased risk of scarring and subsequent chronic pain and dyspareunia; therefore, many experts have abandoned the use of the laser in favor of surgical excision for VIN III. Bornstein and Kaufman have proposed combining laser ablation with surgical excision in the treatment of

selected patients with VIN. Laser is used particularly in areas where excision hampers preservation of anatomy, such as in the clitoral region. Laser therapy for VIN should probably be reserved for experienced laser surgeons and colposcopists.

The *ultrasonic surgical aspirator* can assist the surgeon in ablating to depths comparable to those achieved with the CO_2 laser. The advantage of this instrument is its ability to obtain additional tissue that might identify an occult cancer. Ultrasonic surgical aspirator and laser ablation also may be used to treat perianal intraepithelial neoplasia. In this setting, two concerns should be kept in mind. This location appears to be associated with a greater risk for the development of invasive squamous cancer, and the likelihood of fibrosis, scarring, and stricture is heightened. As with all treatments for VIN, the potential for recurrence and the need for further follow-up must be appreciated. With ablative approaches such as laser, diligence must be exercised to exclude invasion.

Topical agents have been used in the treatment of VIN with inconsistent results. Most notable among these topical treatments has been 5-fluorouracil (5-FU, Efudex 5%). Efudex is not recommended by the manufacturer for this use, and they specifically recommend against its use in the vagina. The mechanism of action appears to be related to the inhibition of DNA and RNA synthesis; the latter is not specific to dysplastic or HPV-infected cells. Normal epithelium is susceptible to the agent, and a component of hypersensitivity reaction appears operative in its mode of action. For cases in which treatment is effective, denudation of the epithelium is a requisite for success. This understandably leads to localized discomfort and pain, often reported as intense burning. Treatment regimens with topical 5-FU are diverse, and no standardized administration protocol has been widely adopted. One technique is topical application on an alternate-night basis for as long as 6 weeks; patient compliance problems typically lead to earlier curtailment. Among young patients with erythroplastic VIN, a 50% to 60% complete response rate has been reported. The hyperkeratotic VIN lesion has not proved to be as responsive to 5-FU.

In a 41-year review of 405 women, Jones and colleagues observed that more than 50% of women treated with laser ablation or surgical resection required an additional procedure within 14 years. Fifty percent of patients with positive surgical margins required additional treatment within 5 years. In comparison with positive margins, women with negative margins had a 15% chance of requiring additional therapy. Brown and colleagues, in a small series of 33 patients, noted a decrease in recurrence with a combination of surgical excision and laser vaporization at the margins.

TECHNIQUE OF CONSERVATIVE (SIMPLE) VULVECTOMY

Conservative (simple) vulvectomy is recommended in many patients with widespread VIN when it may be difficult to rule out invasive cancer or Paget disease of the vulva. It may also be appropriate when premalignant lesions, such as granulomatous diseases, do not respond to medical therapy or wide local excision.

An outline of the surgical margins is made with a surgical marking pen (Fig. 23.7). The initial incision should be made at the vaginal outlet so that the urethral borders can be well demarcated and the vaginal epithelium undermined for a short distance. If the incision is begun at the lateral skin margins, bleeding can mask the area, making the incision at the outlet more difficult to define. When the first incision is made at the outlet, a small pack can be placed into the vagina to control the bleeding while the elliptic incision at the outer skin margins of

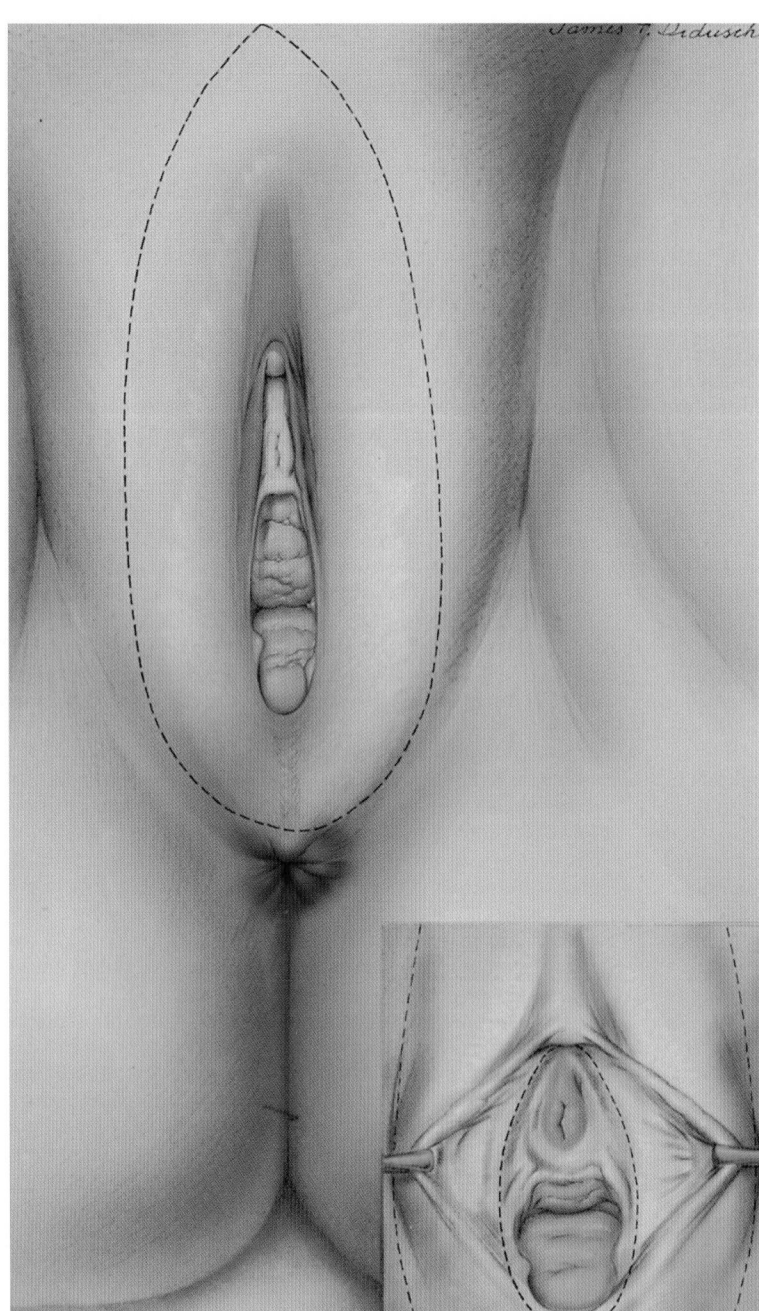

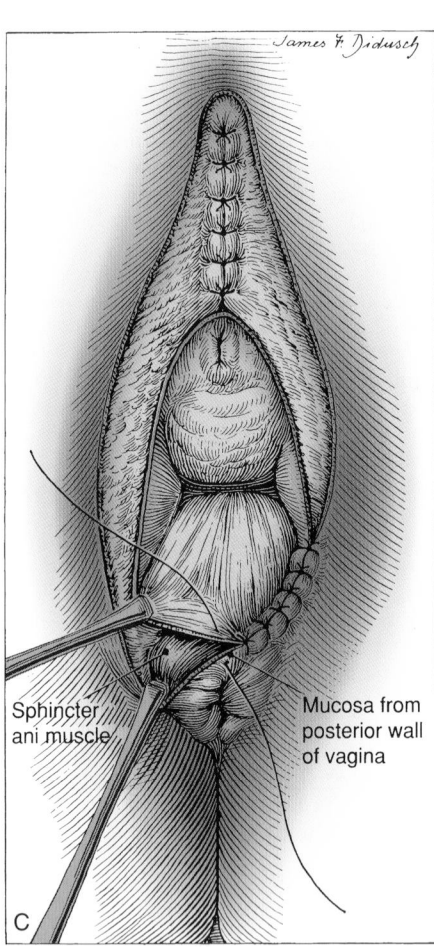

Sphincter ani muscle

Mucosa from posterior wall of vagina

FIGURE 23.7 Conservative vulvectomy for vulvar CIS.

the lesion is made. The skin incision usually encompasses most of the labia majora, depending on the extent of the lesion. The incision through the skin is made with a knife to avoid tissue necrosis that occurs at the skin margins when an electrosurgical instrument is used. Minor vessels can be coagulated.

Major bleeding concerns may arise at the clitoris, particularly from the dorsal vein. Hemostatic sutures must be used to control the bleeding. A second point of concern is the pudendal vessels, which enter at the lower one third of the vulva close to the opening of the Bartholin duct. Branches of the pudendal vessels extend down to the anus as the inferior hemorrhoidals, and bleeding may be rather profuse in this area.

Because the lesions for which conservative vulvectomy is performed are superficial, dissection does not need to extend

down to the deep fascia or to the muscles of the urogenital diaphragm. Although it is unnecessary to remove the bulbocavernous and ischiocavernous muscles, they may be difficult to avoid when the vulva is quite atrophic. Removal of some of the adipose tissue, particularly in the obese patient, allows for better approximation of the skin edges to the vaginal mucosa. The incision can be carried almost to the anal orifice; careful dissection here is important so that the external anal sphincter is not damaged. If the disease extends onto the anal mucosa or the protruding hemorrhoidal tissue, the mucosa should first be carefully dissected from the underlying external sphincter, excised with the tumor-free margins, and sutured to the perianal skin with 3-0 delayed absorbable material. In the remaining vulva, the underlying tissues are approximated in layers with absorbable sutures, and the skin edges are approximated with interrupted absorbable sutures (Fig. 23.7). If bleeding is a problem, a small suction drain can be placed at the lower end of the incision, but it is much better to achieve meticulous hemostasis and use a firm pack against the area for 24 hours.

During closure of the perineal defect above the anal orifice and posterior vaginal introitus, the surgeon should evert the vaginal epithelium over the perineum in approximation to the anal orifice rather than suture the lateral skin edges snugly across the perineum and fourchette. Everting the vaginal mucosa allows for satisfactory coitus, whereas tightly approximated skin across the posterior fourchette may constrict the vaginal introitus and predispose to pain, dyspareunia, and fissuring.

When the firm packing has been removed after 24 hours, the entire area should be exposed. Initial application of ice packs to the operative site for 24 to 48 hours seems to provide more comfort to the patient than heat. Later, warm air blown across the perineum is both comforting and therapeutic because it helps to keep the operative site dry and stimulates blood flow, enhancing the healing process. An indwelling urethral catheter or a suprapubic catheter is used while the suture line undergoes initial healing of the skin edges. The suprapubic catheter can be maintained for 4 to 5 days, if desired. A single dose of a cephalosporin such as Cefazolin (1 g) intravenously is recommended immediately before surgery. Infrequently, a local cellulitis may develop, necessitating antibiotic therapy; extended-spectrum cephalosporins and semisynthetic penicillins have proved effective.

VULVAR RECONSTRUCTION

Procedures performed for extensive VIN III or Paget disease include total or partial vulvectomy, skinning vulvectomy, and multiple wide excisions. These may occasionally result in large denuded areas, creating challenges for reconstruction. With the advent of laser ablation and the ultrasonic surgical aspirator, fewer procedures such as skinning vulvectomy are performed for VIN.

Reconstructive efforts for superficial excisions typically require split-thickness grafts. Such grafts are ill suited for reconstruction after radical excision because the depth of tissue defect is too great, and poor cosmetic and functional results ensue. A buttock donor site is preferred. Perioperative antibiotics are used. Bowel preparation and slow postoperative feeding minimize contamination of the graft site.

Split-thickness skin grafts can be procured with an air-driven dermatome. The size of the vulvar defect helps to determine donor site excision. Meticulous hemostasis should be sought before application of the graft. Fine absorbable sutures are used to secure the skin edges of the graft. The donor site should be covered with an occlusive dressing, such as Op-Site or Tegaderm, until significant healing occurs. A soft pressure dressing is tied over the graft site and kept in place for 5 days, accompanied by an indwelling catheter for urinary drainage.

VULVAR PRURITUS

The most common symptom associated with vulvar dermatoses and many other vulvar conditions is pruritus. In most cases, pruritus is a symptom of an underlying disease process, and although treatment of this annoying symptom is important, the clinician should attempt to diagnose and treat the disease that causes the symptom of pruritus.

Before any therapy for vulvar lesions caused by chronic irritation is begun, an accurate tissue diagnosis must be established. All patients should be given detailed instructions to eliminate local irritants. A history of urinary incontinence may suggest a source of chronic vulvar irritation. Associated vaginitis should be treated vigorously. Topical medications for control of the symptoms must be given a satisfactory trial. Vulvectomy should not be performed for chronic dermatitis or for the benign dystrophies, including lichen sclerosus, before careful histologic evaluation is done. Systemic etiologies such as diabetes, anxiety, Sjögren syndrome, hepatic or renal diseases, or drug reactions may exist. Cutaneous etiologies, such as candidiasis, vaginitis, and contact or atopic dermatitis, can also occur.

Topical Agents

Topical agents have been effective in treating vulvar pruritus and should be tried initially. When they are ineffective, often, it is secondary to their inability to penetrate the thickened hyperkeratotic surface. Initially, treatment for a specific disease should be instituted. For example, topical steroids should be used for psoriasis, antifungals for candidiasis, and appropriate ablative therapy for molluscum contagiosum and condylomata acuminata. Vulvar dermatoses such as lichen sclerosus, lichen simplex chronicus, lichen planus, seborrheic dermatitis, and plasma cell vulvitis can be effectively treated with high-potency topical steroids such as betamethasone. Many of these patients also present with vulvar dysesthesia (vulvar burning) and can be treated with tricyclic medications such as amitriptyline and nortriptyline.

For historic purposes, no chapter on vulvar pruritus would be complete without mentioning alcohol injection and the Mering procedure. Before treatment with amitriptyline became popular, patients with recalcitrant pruritus and vulvar dysesthesia were treated with local alcohol injection. The anogenital area was prepped and draped in a sterile manner after the induction of general or regional anesthesia. The region was then divided into 1-cm squares with a marking pen of brilliant green. Absolute alcohol, 0.2 mL, was then injected subcutaneously at the intersection of these lines (Fig. 23.8). Postoperatively, the patients were treated with cold packs and cool sitz baths for 1 week.

Mering Procedure

Because of the effectiveness of topical high-potency steroid creams, the Mering procedure is rarely used to treat vulvar pruritus in the United States today. It requires hospitalization and careful surgical technique (Fig. 23.9). The skin is shaved and thoroughly cleaned, and the incision is outlined with a marking pencil. The incision is made on the outer surface of the labium majus. It extends to the fascia of the urogenital diaphragm from the level of the clitoris to slightly beyond the fourchette and may continue inferiorly to the level of the anal orifice, depending on the extent of the pruritus. The nerves in the adjacent tissue are severed with a finger placed on each side, moving from the lateral aspect of the clitoris toward the midline, over the clitoris, where the fingers meet. The procedure interrupts branches of the ilioinguinal and genitofemoral nerves (Fig. 23.10). Blunt dissection extends posteriorly to the lateral side of the rectum, outside the external anal sphincter. If the perianal area is involved, blunt dissection may extend to the posterior limit of the anal orifice, where the two fingers meet behind the anus in the midline breaking up the branches of the pudendal nerve.

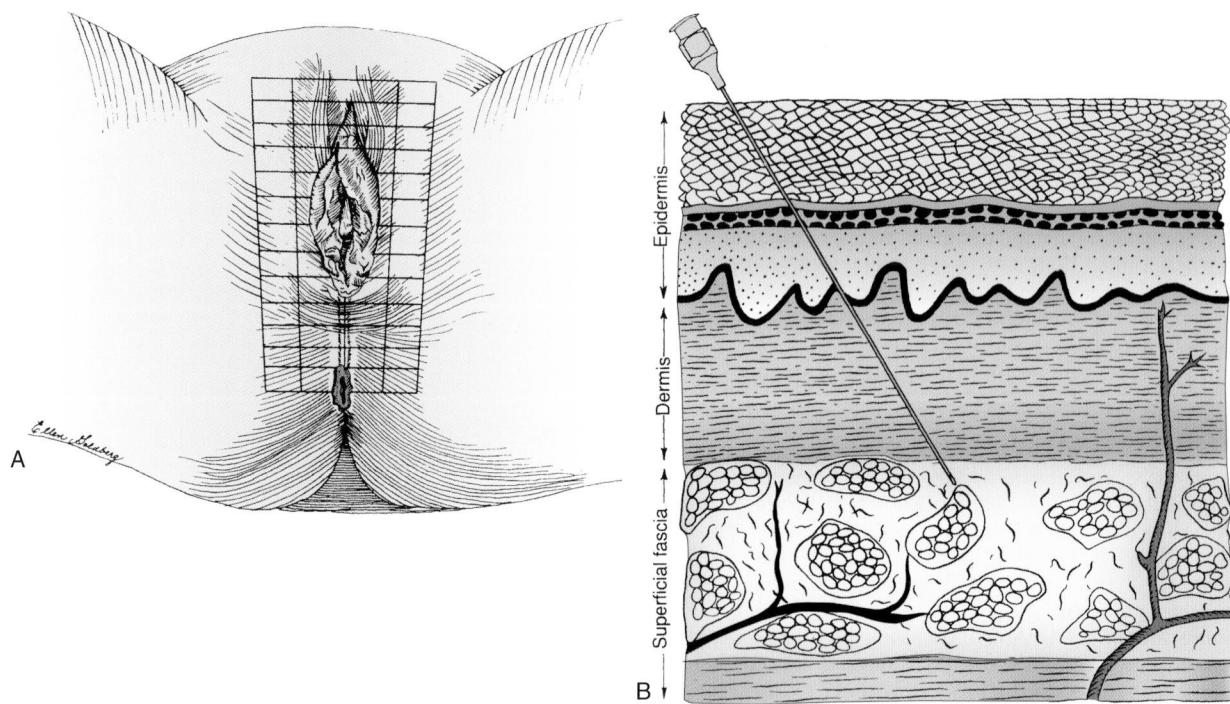

FIGURE 23.8 A: Marking of external genitalia into 1-cm squares in preparation for alcohol injection. **B:** Depth of penetration of 25-gauge needle into the subcutaneous tissue. (From Woodruff JD, Thompson B. Local alcohol injection in the treatment of vulvar pruritus. *Obstet Gynecol* 1972;40:18, with permission. Copyright © 1972 The American College of Obstetricians and Gynecologists.)

It is important that hemostasis be meticulously maintained. A small, flat Jackson-Pratt drain should be placed under the flap on each side. The subcutaneous tissue is approximated with absorbable sutures, and the skin is sutured with polyglycolic acid or polyglactin 910 material. The area must be packed tightly for 24 hours, and the patient should use ice packs or cool tub baths. Domeboro sitz baths (Burow solution) may help to relieve edema.

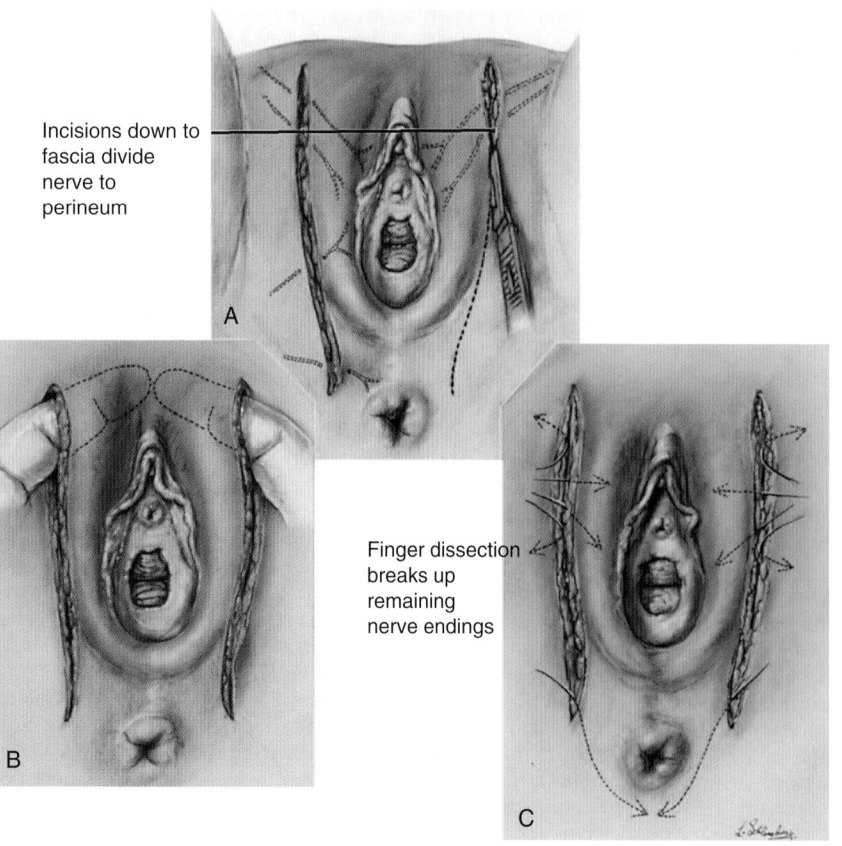

Incisions down to fascia divide nerve to perineum

Finger dissection breaks up remaining nerve endings

FIGURE 23.9 The Mering procedure. **A:** The incisions are made at the lateral margins of the labia majora, extending to the level of the clitoris superiorly and the anal orifice inferiorly. The depth of dissection is the deep fascia, to incise the adipose tissue and the nerves. **B:** The finger dissects the underlying tissue, breaking up the fibers of the pudendal, ilioinguinal, and genitofemoral nerves. **C:** The underlying tissues are carefully approximated to attain good hemostasis. A small drain should be inserted at the most dependent aspect of the incision to avoid the accumulation of blood in the operative sites.

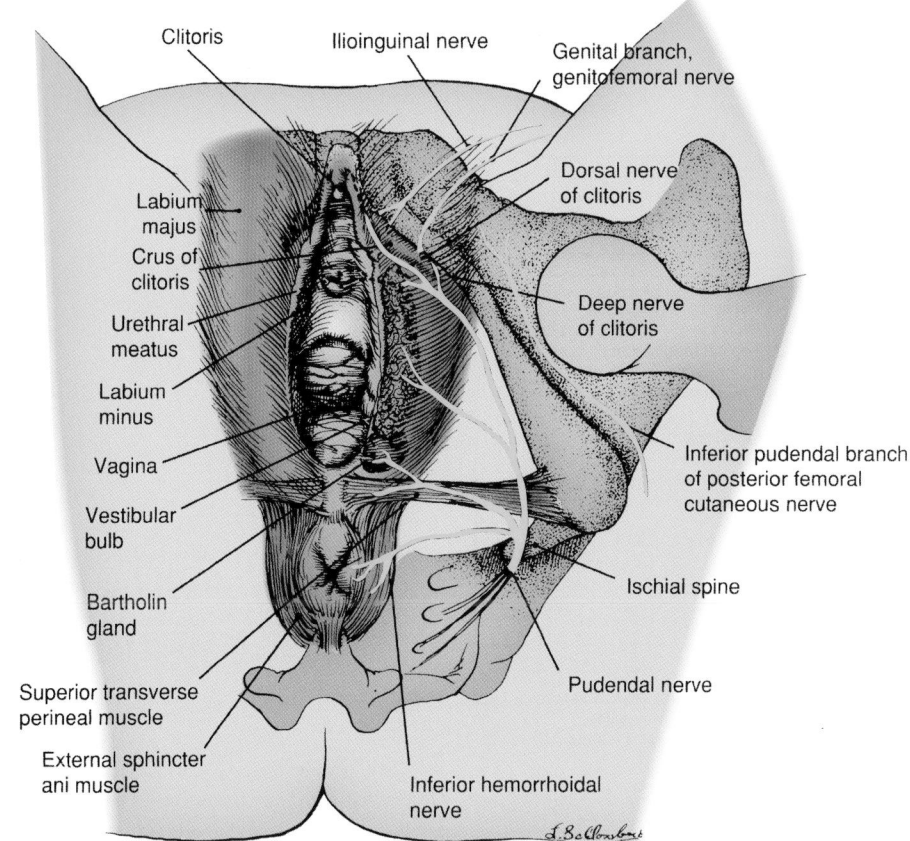

FIGURE 23.10 Nerve supply to anogenital region. (From Woodruff JD, Julian CG. In: Ridley JH, ed. *Gynecologic surgery: errors, safeguards and salvage.* Baltimore: Williams & Wilkins, 1974, with permission. Copyright © 1974 Williams & Wilkins.)

IV

VULVAR PAIN AND VULVODYNIA

Vulvar pain is another common symptom of vulvar disease. It may be produced by a wide variety of vulvar conditions, or, occasionally, primary vulvodynia without any identifiable underlying diagnosis may be encountered. The ISSVD has defined vulvodynia as "vulvar discomfort, most often described as burning pain, occurring in the absence of relevant visible findings or a specific, clinically identifiable, neurologic disorder." The classification of vulvar pain is presented in Table 23.1.

There are many types of vulvar conditions that cause vulvar pain, including infections (candidiasis, herpes, etc.), inflammatory conditions (contact dermatitis), neoplasia (VIN, Paget disease, etc.), and neurologic conditions (herpetic neuralgia, neuroma, etc.). A careful diagnostic evaluation, usually including a biopsy of the vulva, is indicated to identify any of these lesions so that the correct therapy can be instituted. However, despite a careful and thorough workup, some patients will have vulvar pain for which an underlying diagnosis cannot be found. These patients are thus diagnosed with vulvodynia as defined above. The syndrome may be either localized to one area of the vulva or generalized, and the pain may be present all the time (unprovoked) or only when the vulva is touched or pressed (provoked). Vulvodynia involving the vulvar vestibule has been called *vulvar vestibulitis* or *vestibulodynia*. It is a clinical syndrome consisting of the following characteristics: (a) severe pain on vestibular touch or attempted vaginal entry, (b) tenderness to pressure localized within the vulvar vestibule, and/or (c) physical findings confined to vestibular erythema of varying degrees. This syndrome is chronic and multifactorial. Etiologies include chronic or recurrent candidiasis, HPV infections, recurrent bacterial vaginosis, trauma, chemical and surgical destructive techniques, alterations of vaginal pH, irritants (soaps, detergents, douches, deodorants), and idiopathic causes. **Figure 23.11** summarizes the evaluation and management of vulvodynia.

Medical Treatment

A careful diagnostic evaluation is essential because of the apparent multifactorial etiology of vestibulodynia. If an infectious etiology is present, it is imperative to treat it. Recombinant alpha-interferon is efficacious in treating vulvodynia with a history of condylomata acuminata or subclinical HPV. Triamcinolone acetonide 0.1% and bupivacaine can also be injected monthly. An alternative combination is methylprednisolone and lidocaine submucosal.

Chronic recurrent candidiasis is treated with prolonged oral administration of ketoconazole or fluconazole. Topical anticandidal regimens should be prescribed when oral antifungal medications are discontinued.

In addition to being treated for the infectious etiology, all patients should be started on a course of topical steroids. Horowitz treats all patients with vulvodynia with hydrocortisone acetate 1% or 2.5% with 1% pramoxine hydrochloride ointment (Pramosone) for 2 to 3 months. After 3 months of this therapy, the patients are placed on desoximetasone 0.25% ointment (Topicort). Only after failing topical steroids are the patients considered for surgical treatment. Oral amitriptyline is also an important part of the therapeutic regimen. Doses of 25 to 75 mg taken 3 hours before bedtime are prescribed. Patients with vulva dysesthesia or interstitial cystitis benefit most from medical therapy with amitriptyline. Oral gabapentin is also helpful in some patients. It should be started with a gradual dose escalation and tapered off when discontinued.

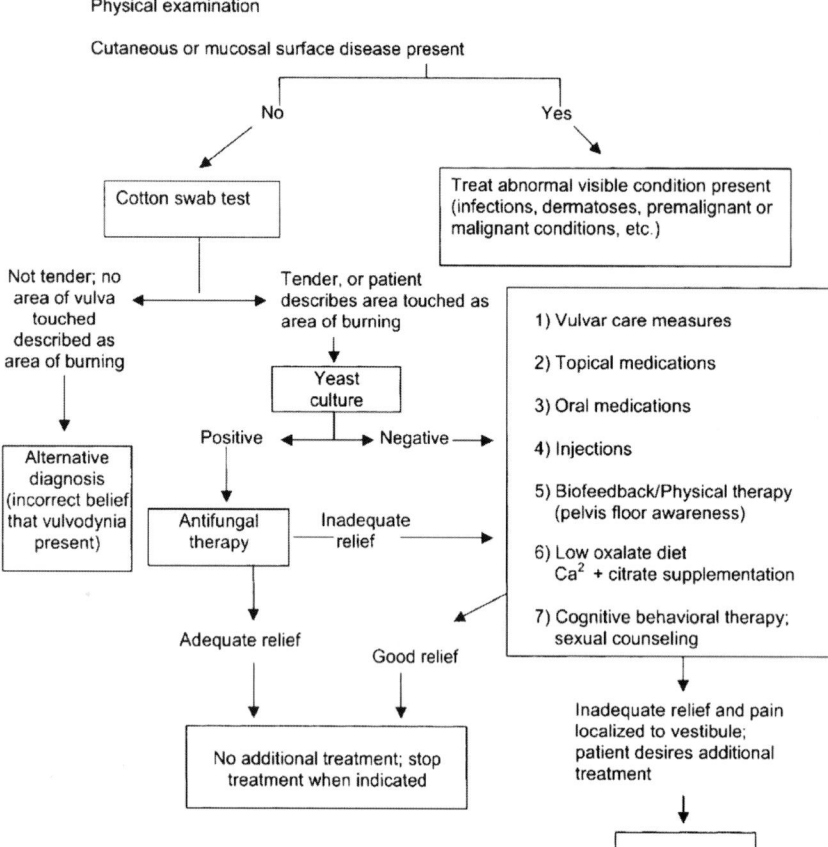

FIGURE 23.11 Vulvodynia algorithm. (Reprinted with permission from Haefner HK, Collins ME, Davis GD, et al. The vulvodynia guideline. *J Low Genit Tract Dis* 2005;9:42. Copyright © 2005, The American Society for Colposcopy and Cervical Pathology.)

Surgical Treatment

Carbon dioxide laser ablation of the vestibular glands has not been shown to be optimal and has resulted in scarring and increased dyspareunia in some patients. In 1995, Reid and associates reported long-term results with the flashlamp-excited dye laser in nonresponders to medical therapy. Those with poor responses to laser vaporization were then treated with gland resection. Overall response rates were 62% to 80%, depending on the distribution of tenderness. However, long-term follow-up has been disappointing, and this approach remains controversial.

Primary surgical therapy has produced relief of symptoms in 75% to 90% of patients. This technique was initially described by Woodruff and associates in 1981 and Friedrich in 1987 and was modified by Marinoff and Turner in 1991 to include the periurethral Skene gland openings. The outer incision extends circumferentially from the periurethral glands along Hart line to the contralateral glands. The proximal vaginal margin is just inside the hymenal ring. This horseshoe-shaped epithelium is superficially excised and sent for histologic diagnosis. In almost all cases, the histology consists of nonspecific periglandular chronic inflammation, much less impressive than might be expected based on the severe symptoms reported. As in a perineoplasty, the vaginal mucosa is undermined and the vagina advanced to approximate edges. The wound is closed in two interrupted layers of 3-0 polyglactin 910 (Vicryl) or polyglycolic acid (Dexon) sutures (Fig. 23.12). Postoperative treatment is the same as for perineoplasty. Coitus should be avoided for 2 to 3 months after surgery.

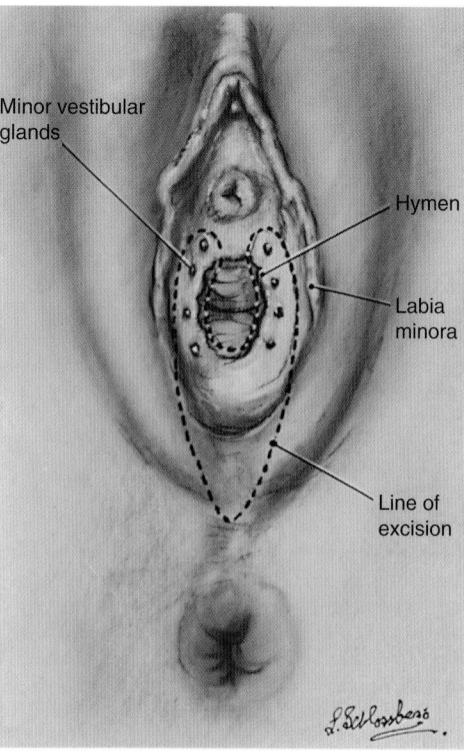

FIGURE 23.12 The minor vestibular glands exit lateral to the hymenal ring. They are very superficial and thus seldom produce definable "nodules," even when chronically infected.

TABLE 23.2 CDC-Recommended Treatment of Sexually Transmitted Diseases

DISEASE	PRIMARY TREATMENT	ALTERNATE TREATMENT
Herpes		
First episode	Acyclovir 400 mg PO TID × 7–10 d	Acyclovir 200 mg PO 5 × day × 7–10 d
	Famciclovir 250 mg PO TID 7–10 d	
	Valacyclovir 1 g PO BID 7–10 d	
Suppressive	Acyclovir 400 mg PO BID	Famciclovir 250 mg PO BID
	Valacyclovir 500 mg PO daily	
	Valacyclovir 1 g PO daily	
Episodic	Acyclovir 400 mg PO TID × 5 d	Acyclovir 800 mg PO BID × 5 d
	Acyclovir 800 mg PO BID × 2 d	
	Famciclovir 125 mg PO BID × 5 d	
	Famciclovir 1,000 mg PO BID × 1 d	
	Famciclovir 500 mg once, followed by 250 mg BID × 2 d	
	Valacyclovir 500 mg PO BID × 3 d	
	Valacyclovir 1.0 g daily × 5 d	

BID, twice a day; PO, by mouth; TID, three times a day.
Available at http://www.cdc.gov/STD/treatment/2010/STD-Treatment-2010-RR5912.pdf

IV

Several of Horowitz's patients (unpublished report) had severe levator spasm secondary to anticipation of activities associated with vulvar pain. This learned response has been treated successfully with biofeedback in several patients. Glazer and colleagues were the first to report the treatment of vulvar vestibulitis syndrome with electromyographic biofeedback of pelvic floor musculature. Seventy-eight percent (22 of 28) resumed coitus by the end of the treatment period.

VULVAR INFECTIONS

Although infections involving the vulva are treated with antibiotics rather than surgery, their appearance may resemble CIS or even invasive cancer of the vulva. An accurate diagnosis may require cultures, viral testing, or even biopsy. Appropriate therapy is based on a correct diagnosis. Treatment of vulvitis secondary to an infectious process varies depending on the infection present. Viral infections such as HPV are strongly associated with intraepithelial neoplasia and carcinoma. These lesions are discussed later in this chapter.

TABLE 23.3 Types of Genital Herpes Simplex Infection

- Primary infection: Initial infection with either HSV-1 or HSV-2 without evidence of prior exposure to either (i.e., antibodies)
- Nonprimary first episode: Initial clinical episode with HSV-1 or HSV-2 in patient with prior exposure to the other viral serotypes
- Recurrent infection: Reactivation of latent virus

HSV, herpes simplex virus.
From Sweet RL. Sexually transmitted diseases. In: Bieber EJ, Sanfilippo JS, Horowitz IR, eds. *Clinical Gynecology*. Philadelphia: Churchill Livingstone Elsevier, 2006:249. Copyright © 2006, Elsevier.

Molluscum contagiosum, a member of the pox family, requires accurate identification and resection of the umbilicated lesions with a dermal curette. These lesions are usually circular and umbilicated. *Molluscum contagiosum* in an adult may be an indicator of underlying human immunodeficiency virus (HIV) infection. Therefore, the patient's background should be appropriately discussed.

Herpes genitalis is caused by the herpes simplex virus (HSV). Between 500,000 and 1 million new cases are diagnosed annually in the United States, a ninefold increase between 1966 and 1997. More than 25% of women are seropositive for HSV type 2. The patients with primary herpes present with high fevers, malaise, myalgias, painful vulvovaginal lesions, and inguinal adenopathy. The ulcers are small but coalesce into larger ulcers. The primary treatment of these sexually transmitted diseases is presented in Table 23.2. The three categories of HSV infection are outlined in Table 23.3.

Granuloma inguinale (donovanosis) is caused by *Klebsiella granulomatis* and presents as painless papular nodules or ulcerations. These lesions can occur in the genital, perianal, oral, and inguinal regions. Fewer than 100 new cases are reported annually in the United States. When large and destructive, *Granuloma inguinale* can simulate malignancy. Cytology and biopsy accompanied with Warthin Starry stains may establish the true diagnosis. The condition should be considered in all cases in which clinically malignant lesions are repetitively negative by biopsies. No U.S. Food and Drug Administration (FDA)-approved polymerase chain reaction (PCR) tests are available to date. The 2010 Centers for Disease Control and Prevention (CDC)-recommended treatment regimen is doxycycline 100 mg orally twice daily for 3 weeks or until lesions have completely healed. Alternative treatment regimens include the following:

Azithromycin 1 g orally once per week for at least 3 weeks and until all lesions have completely healed

OR

Ciprofloxacin 750 mg orally twice a day for at least 3 weeks and until all lesions have completely healed

OR

Erythromycin base 500 mg orally four times a day for at least 3 weeks and until all lesions have completely healed

OR

Trimethoprim–sulfamethoxazole one double-strength (160/800 mg) tablet orally twice a day for at least 3 weeks and until all lesions have completely healed

Lymphogranuloma venereum (LGV) is caused by *Chlamydia trachomatis* types L1, L2, and L3. *Lymphogranuloma venereum* presents with papular or vesicular lesions on the vulva that can also ulcerate. Lesions are usually painless and heal spontaneously. As with herpes, these patients present with headaches, myalgias, arthralgias, and inguinal adenopathy. The 2010 CDC treatment guidelines recommend doxycycline 100 mg orally twice daily for 21 days. Alternatively, the patient can be treated with erythromycin base 500 mg orally four times daily for 21 days.

Chancroid is caused by *Haemophilus ducreyi*. The chancroid lesions present as multiple papules that become pustular and ulcerate. These lesions are very tender and have a ragged edge sitting on an erythematous base (halo). More than 50% of these patients present with large inguinal lymph nodes called buboes. These lymph nodes may become suppurative. Lymph nodes and soft tissue in the inguinal area can also be involved secondary to LGV and granuloma inguinale. The 2010 CDC treatment guidelines include the following recommended regimens:

Azithromycin 1 g orally in a single dose

OR

Ceftriaxone 250 mg intramuscularly in a single dose

OR

Ciprofloxacin 500 mg orally twice a day for 3 days (ciprofloxacin is contraindicated for pregnant and lactating women)

OR

Erythromycin base 500 mg orally three times a day for 7 days

Syphilis is caused by the spirochete *Treponema pallidum*. The primary lesions usually have a painless, coin-shaped ulcer with a raised border and an indurated base. They can present 10 to 90 days after exposure and resolve in 2 to 6 weeks. Untreated syphilis results in a secondary phase characterized by skin rash, generalized adenopathy, and moist, papular anogenital lesions called condyloma latum. This is followed by a latent phase leading to tertiary syphilis. The latter can involve the cardiovascular, musculoskeletal, or central nervous system. *Treponema pallidum* can also cross the placenta and result in syphilis in the newborn infant. More than one sexually transmitted disease can be seen in the same patient and can combine with acquired immunodeficiency syndrome. See Table 23.4 for CDC 2010 guidelines.

Necrotizing Fasciitis

Necrotizing fasciitis of the vulva is a very serious destructive infection characterized by rapid progression and a high mortality rate ranging from 12% to 60%. It represents a surgical emergency. Multiple bacterial pathogens are implicated, including staphylococci, *A. streptococci*, *Escherichia coli*, *Peptostreptococcus*, *Prevotella* and *Porphyromonas* spp., *Bacteroides fragilis*, and *Clostridium* spp. Associated vascular thrombosis leads to skin and subcutaneous tissue necrosis. Fisher criteria have been emphasized in the diagnosis and help to exclude clostridial infections. Brook and Frazier isolated mixed aerobic–anaerobic flora in 68% of specimens, 10% facultative or aerobic bacteria, and 22% exclusively anaerobic organisms. Diabetes mellitus is the most common predisposing condition, although other factors, such as radiation, have been identified. The most common clinical findings are necrosis, fever tachycardia, leukocytes, edema, and foul odor.

Devascularization of the skin proceeds with sparing of underlying muscle and bone. Early skin changes include hemorrhagic bullous formation. Typically, the underlying fascial necrosis exceeds the boundaries of visible skin involvement. Inflammatory alterations and edema usually are present. Most patients present with fever, tachycardia, and signs of systemic toxic reaction. Crepitus is present in 37% to 50% of patients. Prompt diagnosis is important because this disorder progresses rapidly.

Treatment combines expeditious surgery, antibiotics, and maintenance of circulation and tissue oxygenation. Surgical treatment should include aggressive excision of nonviable skin, subcutaneous tissue, and avascular fascia. Extensive debridement down to and including the fascia must be performed until viable, well-vascularized tissue margins are identified. Wounds are packed, not primarily closed. High-dose broad-spectrum antibiotic coverage is administered, and associated medical conditions such as dictates are managed aggressively. These patients are frequently very sick, and renal failure and acute adult respiratory distress syndrome commonly complicate their management. The operation for additional debridement or subsequent skin grafting is also common. *Fournier gangrene* presents in a manner similar to that of necrotizing fasciitis and nonclostridial myonecrosis. Infections develop in the labia and spread to the perineum, buttocks, and abdominal wall. Treatment consists of a combination of surgery, broad-spectrum antibiotics, and hyperbaric oxygen (Table 23.5).

Hidradenitis Suppurativa

An infectious process commonly demanding extensive local surgery is hidradenitis suppurativa. Hidradenitis suppurativa was initially described by Aristide Verneuil in 1854. This pustular disease begins as an infection in the apocrine sweat glands. The early manifestations often are cyclic, because the secretory activity of the apocrine glands corresponds to the progestational phase of the menstrual cycle. Consequently, in the early stages of the disease or in the chronic pruritic phase (Fox-Fordyce disease), the use of hormonal therapy, such as oral contraceptives, may help to modify the secretory activity of the glands. Once the disease extensively involves the deeper tissues, local and systemic agents usually are ineffective. Isotretinoin (Accutane) has been effective in some cases, but care must be taken in prescribing this agent because it is a powerful teratogen. Antiandrogens such as cyproterone acetate have been successful in some patients. Dapsone and anti-TNF alpha drugs have also proven efficacious. Culturing exudates and treating with appropriate antibiotics may provide palliation and further delay surgery. The pustules often infect the entire area, so that pressure at one point may produce exudation of purulent material from sinus tracts (Fig. 23.13A). Multiple bacteria have been isolated from

TABLE 23.4 CDC-Recommended Treatment of Syphilis in Adults, 2010

Primary and secondary syphilis
Recommended regimen
Benzathine penicillin G, 2.4 million units IM in a single dose
Penicillin allergy (nonpregnant)
Doxycycline 100 mg orally twice a day for 14 d
OR
Tetracycline 500 mg orally four times a day for 14 d

Latent syphilis
Early latent syphilis (<1 y)—recommended regimens
Benzathine penicillin G, 2.4 million units IM in a single dose
Late latent syphilis (>1 y)—recommended regimens
Benzathine penicillin G, 7.2 million units total, administered as three doses of 2.4 million units
    IM each, at 1-week intervals
Penicillin allergy (nonpregnant)
Doxycycline 100 mg orally twice a day
OR
Tetracycline 500 mg orally four times a day
Both drugs administered for 14 d if duration of infection known to have been <1 y; otherwise,
    administer for 28 d

Tertiary syphilis
Recommended regimen
Benzathine penicillin G, 7.2 million units total, administered as three doses of 2.4 million units
    IM, at 1-week intervals
Penicillin allergy (nonpregnant)—Infectious Disease Consultation
Doxycycline 100 mg orally twice a day

Neurosyphilis
Recommended regimen
Aqueous crystalline penicillin G 18 million to 24 million units per day, administered in 3 million
    to 4 million units IV every 4 hours, for 10–14 d
Alternative regimen (if compliance assured)
Procaine penicillin 2.4 million units IM daily
PLUS
Probenecid 500 mg orally four times a day, both for 10–14 d
Penicillin allergy (nonpregnant)
Ceftriaxone 2 g daily either IM or IV for 10–14 d (Consider Infectious Disease Consultation)

Syphilis during pregnancy
Recommended regimens
Penicillin regimen appropriate for the pregnant woman's stage of syphilis. Some experts
    recommend additional therapy (e.g., a second dose of benzathine penicillin 2.4 million units
    IM) 1 wk after the initial dose, particularly for women in the third trimester and for those who
    have secondary syphilis during pregnancy.
Penicillin allergy—Infectious Disease Consultation

IM, intramuscularly; IV, intravenously.
Available at http://www.cdc.gov/STD/treatment/2010/STD-Treatment-2010-RR5912.pdf

patients with hidradenitis suppurativa (Table 23.6). Because the entire anogenital area is honeycombed by the underlying infection, simple incision into a few of the pustules is useless. Extensive debridement must be performed to allow healing from the base.

The incision extends into the underlying fat, and the involved skin is removed in segments, leaving bridges of normal skin between the excised pustules. Loose approximation of the skin edges can be performed with polyglycolic acid or polyglactin 910 suture material; more commonly, the entire area is left open and treated locally to promote granulation (Fig. 23.13B). Results of therapy are rewarding in most cases, and skin grafting usually is unnecessary. The patient must be treated with antibiotics based on cultures obtained from the draining sinuses both before and after surgery. Radical vulvectomy is occasionally indicated for extensive disease of the vulvar, inguinal, and perineal areas, but generally, simple vulvectomy is usually effective. It is imperative that a thorough histologic evaluation be performed by the pathologist. Squamous cell carcinoma has been reported to arise in diffuse perineal hidradenitis suppurativa. Myocutaneous flaps or split-thickness skin grafts can be placed in a two-stage procedure. This will allow the infections to clear before the raw vulvar surface is grafted. Wet to dry dressings are used 48 hours to 2 weeks before grafting.

Harrison and colleagues have reported a 37% recurrence rate in patients with inguinal or perineal lesions. In their series of 106 patients, Rompel and Petres experienced 17.8% complication rate with surgery and only a 2.5% recurrence in the operative field.

TABLE 23.5 Antibiotic Regimens for Treatment of NSTI

ANTIBIOTIC	BACTERIAL COVERAGE AND DOSE
Piperacillin/tazobactam	Gram-negative and gram-positive facultative 3.375–4.5 g, q6 h
Ticarcillin/clavulanic acid	Facultative and obligate anaerobes 3.1 g, q6 h
Ampicillin/sulbactam	3 g, q6 h
Gentamicin	Effective against gram-negative facultative anaerobes, acts synergistically with penicillin against enterococci 5 mg/kg of body weight q24 h, or 2 mg/kg of body weight as a loading dose followed by 1.5 mg/kg of body weight q8 h
Clindamycin	Effective against obligate anaerobes Effective against 80% of *Streptococcus agalactiae* and MRSA 900 mg q8 h
Metronidazole	Effective against obligate anaerobes 500 mg q8 h

NSTI indicates necrotizing soft tissue infections.
Adapted with permission from Faro S, Faro J. Necrotizing soft-tissue infections in obstetric and gynecologic patients. *Clin Obstet Gyncol* 2012;55:875. Copyright © 2012, Lippincott Williams.

TABLE 23.6 Bacteria Involved in Hidradenitis Suppurativa

GRAM-POSITIVE ORGANISMS	GRAM-NEGATIVE ORGANISMS
Staphylococcus aureus	*Acinetobacter*
Staphylococcus epidermidis	*Pseudomonas aeruginosa*
Staphylococcus hominis	*Bacteroides*
Streptococcus milleri	*Fusobacterium*
Streptococcus pyogenes	*Prevotella*
Propionibacterium acnes	
Peptostreptococcus	
Corynebacterium	
Lactobacillus	

From Faro S. Vulvovaginal infections. In: Bieber EJ, Sanfilippo JS, Horowitz IR, eds. *Clinical Gynecology.* Philadelphia: Churchill Livingstone Elsevier, 2006;249–258. Copyright © 2006, Elsevier.

CROHN DISEASE

Crohn disease, a chronic granulomatous inflammatory disease of the bowel, affects the vulva and perianal area in about 25% to 30% of the cases in which there is classic intestinal involvement. The draining sinuses often communicate with the vagina or the rectum, thus resulting in the formation of fistulous tracts (Fig. 23.14A). On rare occasions, the vulva may be primarily involved, even though the small and large bowel apparently are not affected or affected subsequently. Crohn disease can also present as unilateral labial hypertrophy.

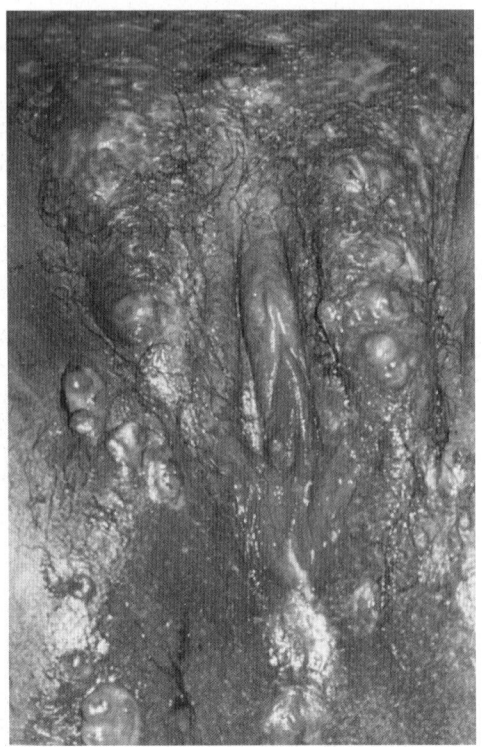
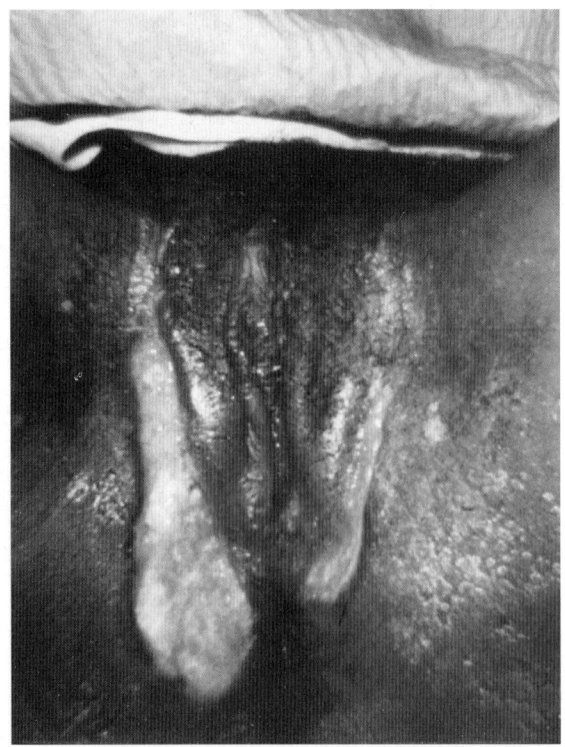

FIGURE 23.13 A: Extensive hidradenitis suppurativa with numerous communicating sinuses. **B:** Same vulva 4 weeks after debridement with exuberant granulations (complete healing in 2 months).

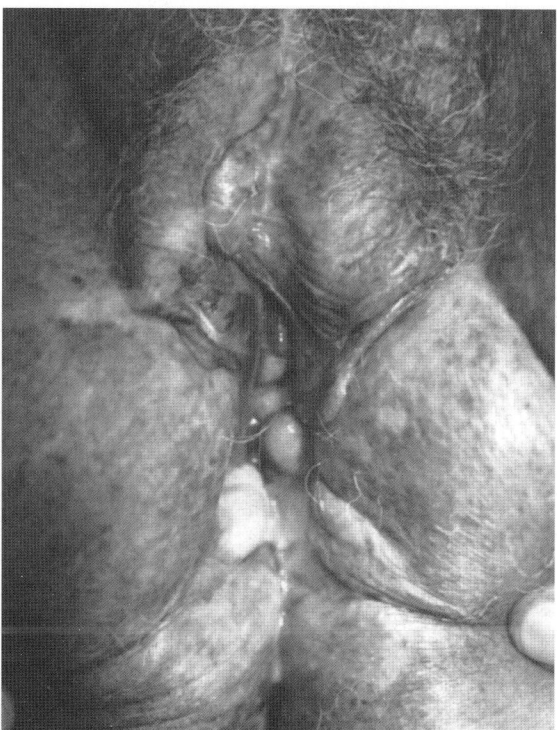
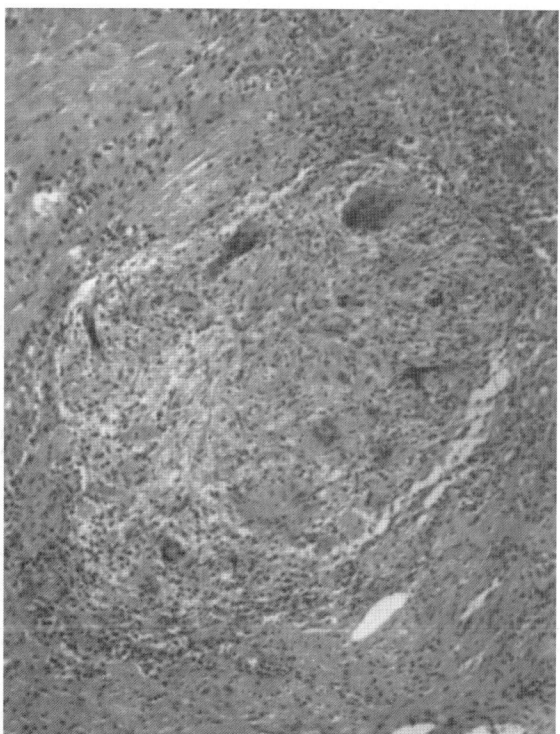

FIGURE 23.14 Crohn disease. **A:** Vulva showing multiple fistulae and fibrosis causing tissue contraction and distortion. **B:** Microscopic section to show noncaseating granuloma. No microorganisms were seen by special stains.

Before any surgical therapy is begun, the diagnosis can be confirmed by studying the bowel or by obtaining a biopsy specimen of the affected tissues in the perineum. The presence of noncaseating granuloma without demonstrable organisms is characteristic of Crohn disease (**Fig. 23.14B**). Further deterioration of the tissue may result from attempts to excise a draining sinus produced by Crohn disease. Rectal incontinence can result from destruction of the anal sphincter or the development of a rectovaginal fistula. Approximately 9% of rectovaginal fistulas are secondary to Crohn disease.

Immunocytochemistry of Crohn lesions has documented *E. coli* and streptococcal antigens. In addition to short-term metronidazole, patients have responded to prolonged treatment (3 to 6 months) with broad-spectrum antibiotics such as ciprofloxacin. Methotrexate therapy is effective in reducing the requirement for prednisone in patients with chronically active Crohn disease. Other drugs used in the medical management of Crohn disease include 5-aminosalicylic acid, cyclosporine, azathioprine, 6-mercaptopurine, mesalamine, and infliximab (Remicade).

In addition to pharmacotherapy, a submucosal anal pull-through procedure may bring relief. Layered surgical repair of a fistula caused by Crohn disease usually is unsuccessful, particularly without appropriate medical management. However, after appropriate medical therapy, surgical excision of the tract is usually effective (see Chapter 39). Results are difficult to predict because multiple areas of the terminal colon and small intestine may be affected, and any affected area may involve the vagina or perineum. Medical therapy should always be given during this type of surgical procedure and should be continued postoperatively for at least 2 months.

TRAUMA

Major trauma to the vulva most often occurs when young girls experience injuries as a result of sledding or bicycling accidents.

Hematomas and occasionally lacerations can develop when the vaginal area forcefully comes in contact with the crossbar of a bicycle (as during a fall from a bicycle seat) or when the girl is thrown from a sled against an obstacle such as a tree or fence. Trauma also can result from sexual assault, and the gynecologist must be sensitive to this possibility even when the initial history suggests another etiology. Women or girls who are victims of sexual assault should receive testing for pregnancy and sexually transmitted diseases. These patients should be referred to counseling and encouraged to report the abuse to state officials. All minors should be reported to the state by the examining physician.

Most traumatic injuries do not require surgical attention. An examination under anesthesia may be useful to adequately evaluate the extent of the injury. If surgical repair is not required, patients should be treated conservatively with activity restriction and with the immediate and continued use of Burow solution (aluminum sulfate, calcium acetate; available as Domeboro tablets or powder) added to the sitz bath to reduce edema. Antibiotics may be used as prophylaxis against superinfection in damaged tissues. If a hematoma increases in size and extends well into the perineum or over the lower abdominal wall, incising the vulvar skin, evacuating the hematoma, and ligating the bleeding vessels may reduce the period of convalescence. An alternative would be to use selective arterial embolization. Goldman and coworkers reported 30% of patients with genital trauma not associated with parturition have a urologic injury. When a hematoma produces urethral obstruction, evacuation may reduce the time an indwelling urethral catheter is needed. If the hematoma is not expanding, it should be followed conservatively. Most vulvar hematomas resolve spontaneously; surgical intervention, on the other hand, can result in significant morbidity, including infection. Frequently, a distinct bleeding site is not identified. If, however, the clot becomes secondarily infected, it requires prompt evacuation and drainage. Lacerations into the rectum or urethra should be repaired expeditiously.

CYSTS OF THE VULVA

Bartholin Duct Cysts

Obstruction of the Bartholin duct, usually near the orifice, is common. Although such obstructions can result from gonococcal infection, other infections and trauma more commonly explain the occlusion. During a mediolateral episiotomy or a posterior colporrhaphy, for example, sutures can easily injure or even ligate the duct. The lining of the main cyst is transitional epithelium. The mucus-secreting glands are not affected by the obstruction but may be distorted by the infectious process. During the acute infection, which may precede the actual cyst formation, an abscess often develops with symptoms of tenderness, swelling, and erythema. Depending on the cause, secretion from the cyst may be mucoid or cloudy.

Incision and drainage bring almost immediate relief to the patient and can be accomplished under local anesthesia. A small wick can be left in the cavity to maintain adequate drainage. A small incision (2 cm) is made in the cyst wall in the area of the normal duct orifice, and a culture is obtained for *Neisseria gonorrhoeae*, *Chlamydia*, and aerobic and anaerobic bacteria. A Word catheter (**Fig. 23.15**) is inserted and the catheter bulb inflated with 2 to 3 mL of saline. If the catheter remains in place for 3 to 4 weeks, the tract becomes epithelialized, and the catheter can be removed. Broad-spectrum antibiotics are given before surgery.

Marsupialization seldom can be accomplished during the acute stage, but the procedure is useful for chronic or recurrent abscesses. Injection of an antibiotic into the abscess has been tried as treatment for the acute infection but has proved to be less effective than systemic antibiotic therapy.

Most Bartholin duct cysts are uninfected and asymptomatic. They are usually found during routine pelvic examinations. Patients may even be unaware of large cysts. When symptoms do occur, most patients report discomfort during coitus or pain while sitting or walking. These require marsupialization only if they are symptomatic. Table 23.7 differentiates between a Bartholin cyst and abscess.

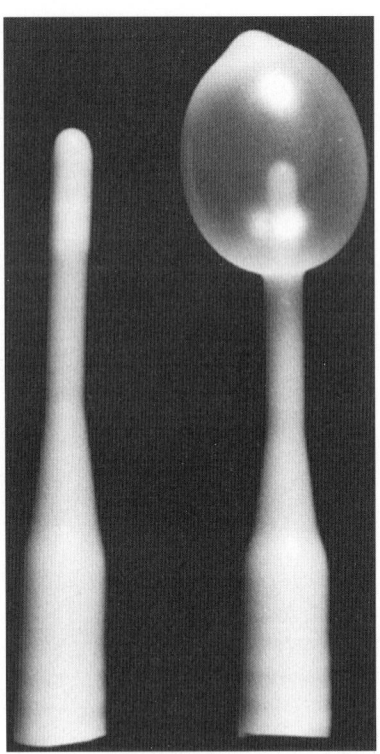

FIGURE 23.15 The Word catheter (*left*) is inserted into the Bartholin duct cyst through a vaginal incision. The bulb is inflated with saline solution (*right*), and the end of the catheter is placed in the vagina.

Technique of Marsupialization

Drainage of a Bartholin duct cyst by marsupialization is not as technically involved as excision and eliminates many complications. The procedure makes it possible to avoid excising the gland with the cyst and to preserve the secretory function of the gland for lubrication.

Marsupialization has had limited use since the Word catheter was introduced. The catheter accomplishes the same result as surgery with minimal or no trauma. The nipple of the catheter can be inserted into the vagina. There is essentially no

TABLE 23.7 Differentiation between Bartholin Abscess and Bartholin Cyst	
BARTHOLIN ABSCESS	**BARTHOLIN CYST**
Enlarged gland	Enlarged gland
Erythema present in skin overlying and surrounding the gland	Erythema absent
Skin overlying the gland typically warm to the touch	No increase in temperature
Fever present, especially with tachycardia	Fever absent
Advancing cellulitis can be present.	Cellulitis absent
WBC count elevated	WBC count not elevated
Bacteria and WBCs are present in fluid (pus) contained within gland.	No bacteria or WBCs present in (serous) fluid contained within the cyst

WBC, white blood cell.
From Faro S. Vulvovaginal infections. In: Bieber EJ, Sanfilippo JS, Horowitz IR, eds. *Clinical Gynecology*. Philadelphia: Churchill Livingstone Elsevier, 2006;249. Copyright © 2006, Elsevier.

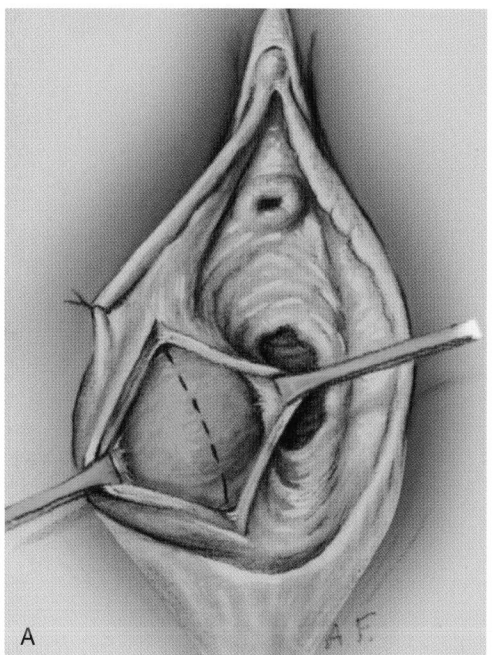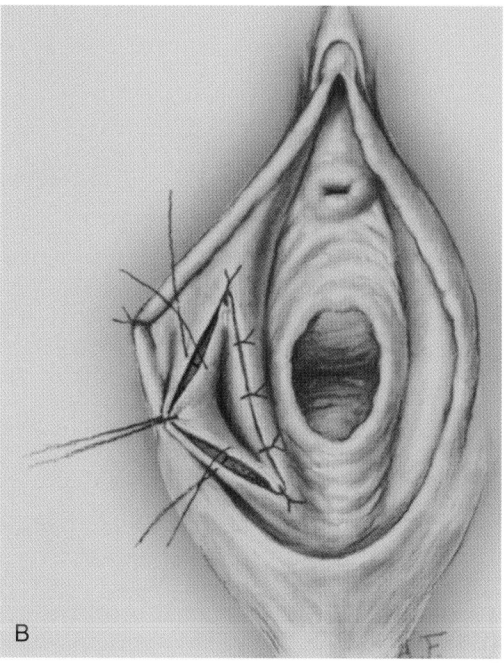

FIGURE 23.16 **A:** Incision for marsupialization. **B:** Marsupialization. (From Tancer ML, Rosenberg M, Fernandez D. Cysts of the vulvovaginal [Bartholin's] gland. *Obstet Gynecol* 1956;7:609. Copyright © 1956, The American College of Obstetricians and Gynecologists.)

discomfort with the procedure, and coitus can be resumed normally. Because this procedure can be performed with local analgesia in the office setting and yields results comparable to those of marsupialization, its use should be encouraged.

The marsupialization can be performed under local, regional, or general anesthesia. A wedged-shaped, vertical incision is made in the vaginal mucosa over the center of the cyst, just outside the hymenal ring, with a no. 15 blade (**Fig. 23.16A**). The incision should be as wide as possible to enhance the postoperative patency of the stoma. After the cyst wall is opened and the cyst is drained of its contents, the lining of the cyst is everted and approximated to the vaginal mucosa with interrupted sutures of 3-0 delayed absorbable material (**Fig. 23.16B**). Drains and packs are not necessary, but the patient's postoperative care should include daily sitz baths beginning on the third or fourth postoperative day.

As a result of closure and secondary fibrosis of the orifice after marsupialization, 10% to 15% of cysts recur. Abscess formation is another occasional sequela of marsupialization.

Technique of Excision

It is seldom necessary to excise a Bartholin duct cyst, particularly in the younger patient, unless there is induration at the base. The latter may signify deep-seated infection that is inaccessible by marsupialization. Conversely, this may represent neoplasm in the base of the gland, an issue of greater concern in the patient older than 40 years of age or in patients with coexisting Paget disease. An elliptical incision in the vaginal mucosa is made as close as possible to the site of the gland orifice with a no. 15 blade (**Fig. 23.17**). An incision on the mucosal side is preferable because an incision through the vulvar skin makes it difficult to dissect the cyst wall from the skin without incising or tearing the skin. If an opening is accidentally made through the skin, a permanent fenestration may result. Difficulty is not usually encountered during dissection of the cyst from the inner surface of the vulvar skin when the incision is made on the mucosal side. Excising a small ellipse of mucosa with the cyst allows the surgeon to

have a site for traction and reduces the risk of rupturing the cyst. Because cyst formation usually is preceded by inflammation, the wall is adherent and cannot be easily enucleated with blunt dissection only. The blunt-pointed Mayo scissors serve admirably for sharp dissection of the cyst from its bed (**Fig. 23.17C**). The cyst can be mobilized further with the handle of the scalpel. A large cyst may develop posteriorly and may approximate the rectum. The rectal wall can easily be distinguished from the cyst by inserting a finger into the rectum during dissection.

Complete removal of the gland tissue adherent to the cyst wall is essential because residual glandular tissue may result in the formation of a tender nodule or recurrent cyst. If the margins of the cyst have become obscured, the cyst can be opened and the wall dissected from the surrounding tissue.

Directly beneath the Bartholin duct is the vestibular bulb, which is composed of anastomosing venous channels. In the dissection of the gland from the vestibular bulb, additional care must be taken to avoid troublesome bleeding. To ensure permanent hemostasis, the entire cavity must be obliterated by approximating the walls with fine delayed absorbable suture material after excision of the cyst.

Approximation of the vaginal mucosa is best accomplished with a continuous or interrupted mucosal suture of 3-0 delayed absorbable material. Persistent bleeding from the labia or vestibular bulb may cause a postoperative hematoma of the labia, which can progress to include the mons pubis and the abdominal wall beneath the Scarpa fascia. Bed rest, ice packs, and a pressure dressing on the vulva are the methods of treatment for a hematoma; attempts to ligate the venous bleeding points are futile. Although the blood usually reabsorbs with time, sometimes, evacuation and drainage are necessary. If the bleeding deep in the bed of the gland seems uncontrollable, deep mattress sutures can be placed from the skin through the bleeding bed into the vagina. The sutures should not be tied too tightly because necrosis may result, with fenestration of the vaginal outlet. A small drain should be stitched into the bed with fine absorbable sutures to avoid the accumulation of blood and serous fluid.

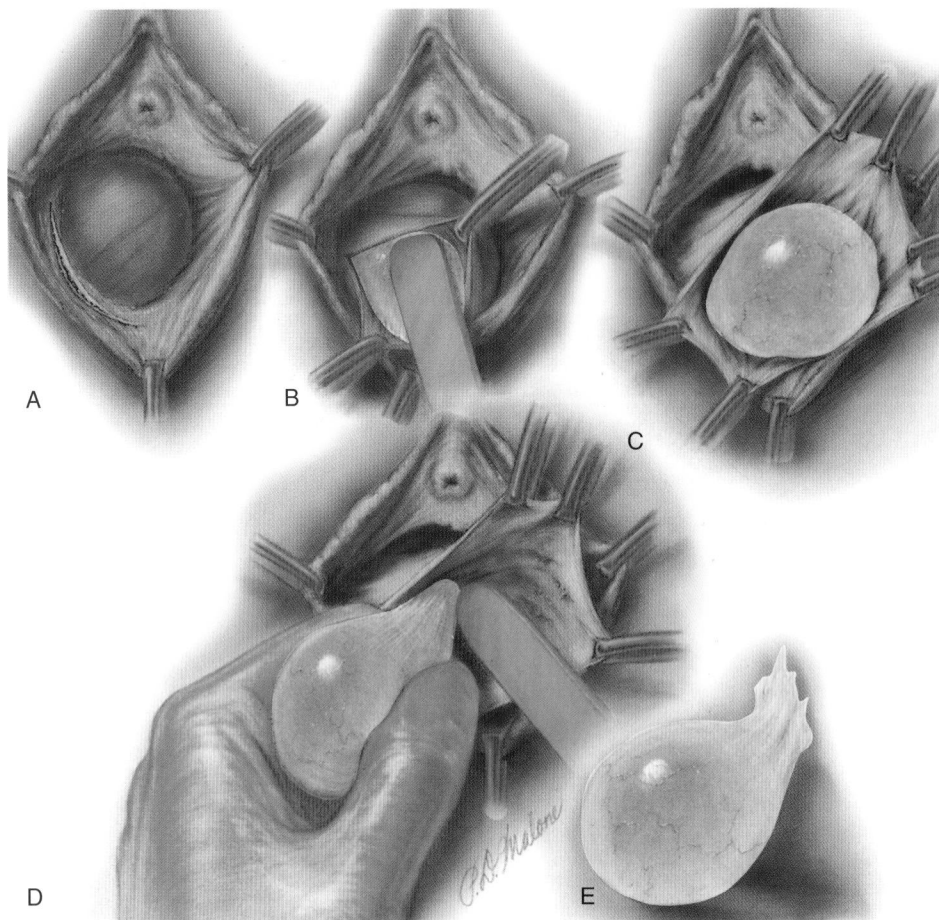

FIGURE 23.17 Excision of a Bartholin gland cyst. **A:** An incision is made in the mucosa over the cyst. **B:** Dissection is begun, using the handle of the scalpel. **C:** Dissection has been continued by sharp and blunt dissection. **D:** Dissection is almost complete. **E:** Intact cyst after removal.

Hydrocele or Cyst of the Canal of Nuck

Hydrocele is an uncommon vulvar cyst. The cyst appears as a dilatation in the labium majus and adjacent labium minus and must be differentiated from a Bartholin duct cyst. **Figure 23.18** shows a hydrocele. The patient underwent two procedures for drainage of a Bartholin duct cyst, but the mass recurred after each procedure.

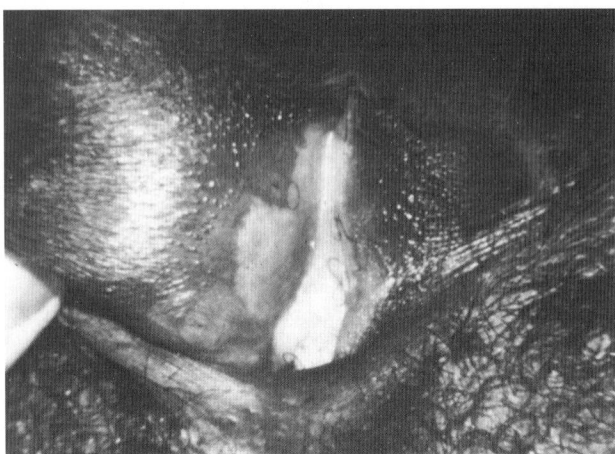

FIGURE 23.18 A hydrocele is caused by the extension of a peritoneal sac with the round ligament from the inguinal canal into the vulva.

A hydrocele is a cystic, fluid-filled hernia of the peritoneum that accompanies the round ligament and extends from the inguinal canal into the vulva. When this sac extends into the inguinal canal, it is known as a cyst of the canal of Nuck. On rare occasions, a loop of intestine may follow the pathway of the round ligament, forming a hernia in the vulva. When a hydrocele is treated as a Bartholin duct cyst by incision and drainage, peritoneal fluid may reaccumulate above the drainage site, and the hydrocele recurs.

Surgical treatment for a hydrocele begins with an incision into the cystic mass. The external inguinal ring is identified by inserting a finger in the cyst anteriorly to the inguinal canal. The peritoneal lining is excised from the cavity, and the external inguinal ring is closed along with the subjacent tissue in the anterior vulva. If a hernia is present, inguinal herniorrhaphy should be performed along with excision of the peritoneal covering of the round ligament.

SOLID TUMORS OF THE VULVA

The incidence of solid, benign tumors in the vulva is low, but a variety of benign tumors, including fibromas, fibromyomas, lipomas, hemangiomas, neurofibromas, and endometriomas, have been reported. These tumors can originate from any of the three germinal layers that constitute the anogenital area. One occasionally sees a solid vulvar tumor composed of benign breast tissue or a benign fibroadenoma (**Fig. 23.19**). Lactational changes can be seen in this tissue. Such an event is

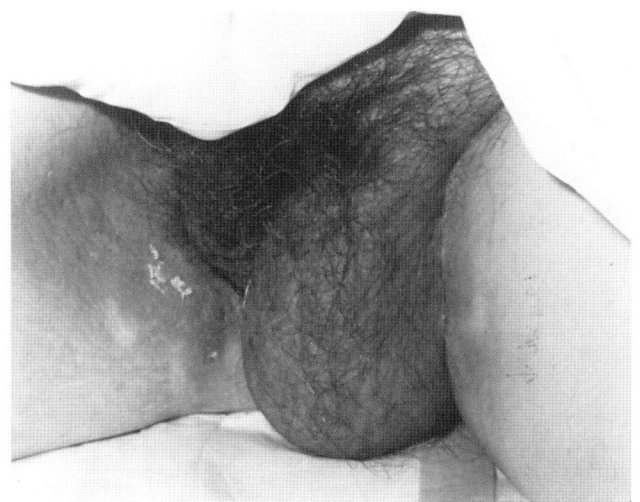

FIGURE 23.19 Fibroadenoma of the vulva arising from the embryonic breast tissue, the caudal end of the milk line.

accounted for by the embryologic milk line caudally ending in the vulvar area. Degenerative changes and necrosis often occur in the larger tumors and should not be confused with malignancy. Lipomas often are mistaken for cystic lesions because of their consistency, whereas hernias and hydroceles of the canal of Nuck must be differentiated from neoplastic growths because they require different surgical approaches.

Most solid tumors should be excised, both to ascertain the diagnosis and to relieve the patient's discomfort. Small, pedunculated tumors can be removed by simple ligation of the stalk; the deeply situated lesions require more extensive local dissection. All nevi showing hemorrhage, sudden enlargement, and pruritus should be suspected to be melanomas and excised widely.

The boundaries of such mesodermal tumors are difficult to delineate, but most of the tumors are benign. Even recurrence does not signify malignant alteration; a fibromyoma may recur if incompletely excised, even when the original specimen had no histologic evidence of malignancy. Although a sarcoma rarely arises in the vulva, histologic studies must be carefully made because degenerating atypical multinucleated cells of a benign or reactive tissue can be mistakenly diagnosed as malignant.

As in any vulvar surgery, hemostasis is important because compression is difficult to obtain in these soft tissues. Extravasation of blood can dissect the fascial planes well out to the vulva, thigh, flanks, and abdominal wall. Closed suction drains should be used in the wounds if hemostasis is not complete.

Condyloma Acuminatum

Condyloma acuminatum is one morphologic manifestation of HPV infection in the lower genital tract. These polypoid lesions have an incubation period ranging from several weeks to 8 months; however, clinical infection usually is apparent 6 to 8 weeks after exposure. Transmission of the virus is attributed to coitus, and the process is efficient, because most sexual partners are affected subclinically if not clinically. The disease process continues increasing in prevalence. Interestingly, clinically apparent condyloma constitutes only a fraction of HPV infections. Most are undetected in asymptomatic patients with no clinical findings.

Numerous HPV subtypes have been identified. Human papillomavirus subtypes 6, 11, 16, 18, 31, 33, 35, 39, 45, 51, 52, 56, 58, 59, 68, and 69 account for most genital tract infections. Careful histopathologic and virologic study of vulvar lesions has demonstrated an association of HPV 6 and HPV 11 with approximately 90% of exophytic vulvar condylomata

as well as flat cervical condylomas and some low-grade cervical dysplasias. The quadrivalent vaccine provides protection against HPV subtypes 6, 11, 16, and 18. It is not effective for the treatment of already existing condyloma or HPV infections. This vaccine is further discussed in Chapter 46.

Condylomata acuminata that manifest on the vulva are frequently associated with cervical, vaginal, and anal HPV infection. Careful clinical evaluation mandates vaginal/cervical cytology and colposcopy in patients who present with vulvar warts. This is appropriate not only to exclude cervical and vaginal dysplasia but also to define the extent of condylomatous involvement and permit appropriate tailoring of regional therapy.

Condylomata acuminata are small and usually multifocal lesions. They may be accompanied by pruritic discomfort or irritation. Warts initially may be reddish brown because of parakeratosis; however, with time and exposure to local trauma, they become gray or white. The latter appears to be associated with hyperkeratosis and the generalized keratin disturbance associated with viral infection (**Fig. 23.20**). Unless they are traumatized, bleeding is not a typical feature. In pregnancy, however, because of marked vascular alterations, condyloma of the vagina and perineum can be a source of abundant bleeding if laceration occurs. Massive vulvar and perianal condylomata may occur in certain circumstances, preventing identification of the introitus and anal orifice; conditions that foster this growth potential include immunosuppression and, less frequently, pregnancy (**Fig. 23.21**). Those lesions that were previously called *giant condyloma* are now regarded as *verrucous carcinoma*. In the spectrum of condylomatous growths, the dividing line between condyloma and verrucous carcinoma is indistinct because of the structural benignancy of both.

Various treatment approaches are available and are characterized by their inability to eliminate the offending agent: the virus. Interferon offers a nonspecific antiviral therapy. Flu-like effects should be anticipated for at least several weeks. Efficacy has been demonstrated with this technique, although treatment is cumbersome, can be costly, and remains investigational. Its primary role has not been defined.

Topical Therapy

At the present time, only a variety of ablative approaches are available for the management of condyloma. These should be individualized with consideration of prior treatment, volume and location of disease, the presence or absence of associated dysplasia, and other idiosyncratic patient factors. The most common approach to vulvar condylomata is the local application of 25% podophyllum resin, often prepared in benzoin. This method, although reasonably well tolerated in the office setting, often requires numerous applications. Burning discomfort ensues after sustained contact, which is necessary for efficacy. Most recommend that the agent be left in place for 6 hours before tub baths, so compliance may be problematic. Podophyllum appears to be more effective on exophytic, rather than flat, condylomata. Use is restricted to the vulva in nonpregnant patients; vaginal application may lead to undesirable absorption and neurotoxicity. An alternative is halogenated acetic acid, either bichloracetic or trichloroacetic acid (TCA). Our preference is 90% TCA. This agent quickly interacts with cellular proteins, inducing a coagulative effect, and rapidly turns lesions a brilliant white. Advantages include its ability to sustain a prompt chemical effect on the condyloma, its availability for intravaginal use and use during pregnancy, and the fact that it can be rapidly neutralized with sodium bicarbonate, which may be dissolved in water and applied as a cooling paste. The patient may apply the following to treat external vulvar warts: Podofilox 0.5% solution or gel, Imiquimod 5% cream, and sinecatechins 15% ointment.

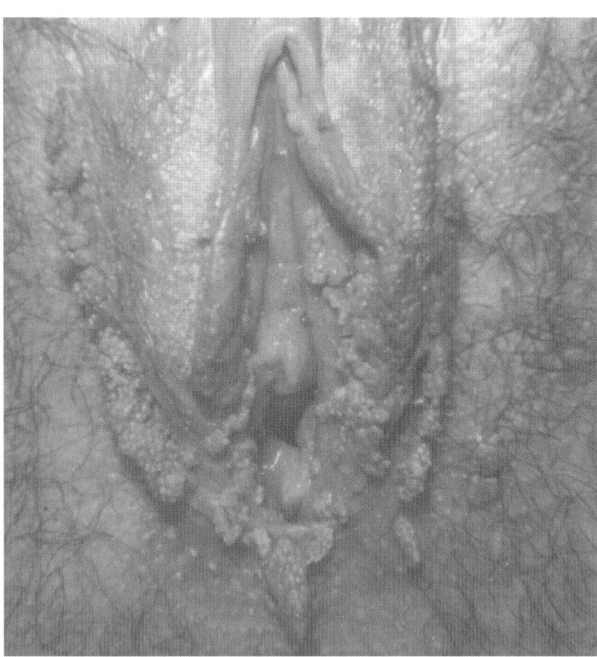

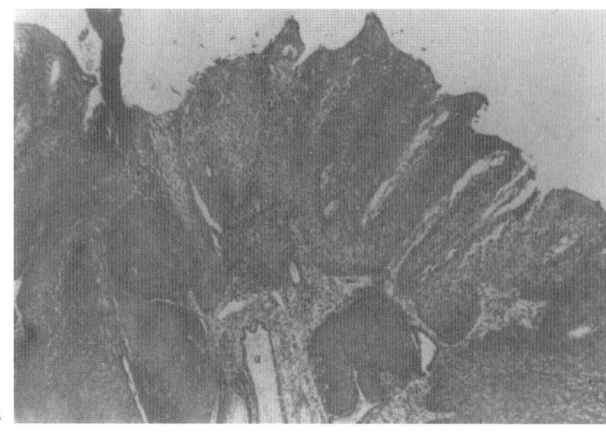

FIGURE 23.20 A: Condylomata acuminata, gross. Condylomata acuminata involving labia majora and minora. Note exophytic quality and lack of pigmentation. **B:** Condylomata acuminata, microscopic. Epidermal hyperplasia featuring acanthosis and elongated, distorted rete pegs is evident. Keratin disturbances are present.

Excision or Ablation

Surgical excision, electrosurgical, destruction, and laser ablation are reserved for certain patients.

Criteria for selection may include the following:

- Extensive volume of condylomata exceeding what may be resolved with chemical agents

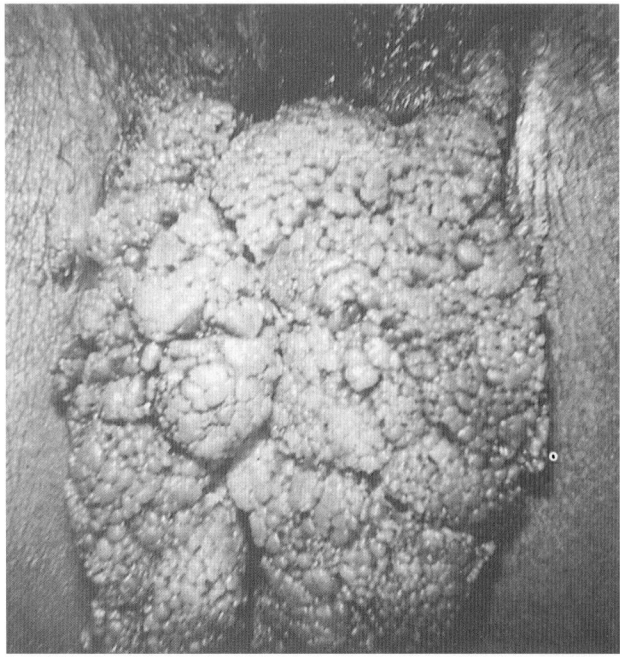

FIGURE 23.21 Massive condylomata acuminata now considered as verrucous carcinoma. Note abundant exophytic lesions producing confluent, cauliflower-like growth. Lesion is present on perineum and totally obscures anal orifice. Patient is 23 years old and is maintained on prednisone because of neurosarcoidosis.

- Multicentric HPV infections, particularly with involvement of the vagina, urethra, or anus
- Failure of concerted office therapy with topical chemical agents
- Additional presence of significant intraepithelial neoplasia
- Immunocompromised state in some hosts

One should certainly use biopsy liberally to evaluate presumed condylomata that are refractory to topical treatment or that have an atypical appearance. This helps prevent sustained, ineffective chemical treatment of high-grade VIN, often presenting as a flat and pigmented verrucous lesion in the younger patient, and helps exclude a frank cancer with warty features. Large, sessile condylomata or those that grow rapidly, bleed abnormally, or become necrotic or invasive should arouse the suspicion of malignancy.

Cryotherapy has been used on the vulva to eradicate warts. The freezing induces localized tissue necrosis. Although healing usually is satisfactory, and numbing effects induce analgesia, application is limited by delivery systems and probe-tip sizes. Larger condylomatous masses are more difficult to treat, as are vaginal lesions. Depth of apparent tissue destruction can be difficult to assess.

Electrocautery with a loop has been used effectively, particularly with massive lesions. Analgesic needs are definitely a factor in this approach. Smaller lesions may be fulgurated. Buildup of charred tissue can be removed by abrasion to identify residual warty tissue. The precision and depth of tissue injury can be problematic.

Colposcopically directed laser ablation performed by trained personnel in appropriately selected cases may afford effective treatment. Condylomatous lesions may be vaporized; starting at the center of the lesion causes the wart to collapse inward toward the beam. The level of the adjacent normal skin should be selected as a landmark. In treating condylomata, there is no need for deep laser vaporization into the dermis, exceeding the so-called first laser surgical plane. Issues of appropriate power density may be debated; however, the inexperienced laser surgeon should use lower-power densities (larger spot size or lower laser output) to protect against unnecessarily deep laser injury. In experienced hands, higher laser output may be feasible, which speeds the procedure. Power densities of 500 to 800 W/cm^2 normally are used for vaporization. Lower-power densities are associated with undesirable thermal injury to adjacent tissues. Sites of laser vaporization should be wiped with moistened gauze sponges to remove carbon and thermally coagulated tissue and to permit accurate assessment of depth and remaining disease. Large lesions can be dealt with by laser excision followed by vaporization at the base (see Chapter 15). Clinicians are advised to use protective eyewear during vaporization to prevent possible conjunctival condyloma.

Brush laser vaporization of the normal epithelium surrounding warty lesions is commonly done to destroy subclinical HPV and reduce the risk of clinical recurrence. This technique uses lower-power densities (200 to 300 W/cm^2) to superficially denude 1 to 2 cm of adjacent epidermis. The rationale for this approach is the presence of HPV in tissue proximal to the condyloma, as demonstrated by Ferenczy and colleagues. Brush vaporization and laser treatment of so-called subclinical HPV infection that may be appreciated with the colposcope have been proposed to lessen the viral reservoir and reduce recurrence rates.

Even with vaporization of grossly normal tissue surrounding the visible lesions, recurrences must be anticipated in 25% to 50% of patients with extensive disease treated with the laser, particularly if the patient is immunocompromised. These patients require further treatment with either laser or chemical approaches, such as 5-FU topically. If disease is minimal, they can be observed.

Patients subjected to extensive laser treatment require considerable local care while healing proceeds. Cool tub or sitz baths with Burow solution followed by the application of silver sulfadiazine (Silvadene) cream and 5% lidocaine (Xylocaine) ointment often afford relief and protect against bacterial superinfection. Narcotics for pain management are appropriate short-term drugs. Prophylactic systemic antibiotics do not appear to be indicated. Weekly office follow-up is advised for 2 to 3 weeks to assess tissue healing, prevent undesirable areas of tissue agglutination, and allow potential early identification of recurrences, which can be managed with chemical ablation. Patients should be followed up carefully for several months after treatment to monitor for recurrences.

The Cavitron ultrasonic surgical aspirator (CUSA) has also been efficacious in treating condyloma. Tissue cell damage is 25 to 30 mm, which is similar to that caused by a cold scalpel. This contrasts with electrocautery at 75 to 100 mm. The tip vibrates at 23,000 cycles per second. Tissue is fragmented and aspirated, providing a specimen for histologic evaluation. Regardless of the selected approach to therapy, all patients should be advised to have their consorts examined to lessen the risk of reexposure to lesions with a large viral burden. This theoretically helps diminish treatment failures. Patients with HIV or other types of immunosuppression need to be more closely followed up.

Hidradenoma (Sweat Gland Tumor) of the Vulva

A rare benign tumor of the vulva, hidradenoma, was first described by Schickele in 1902. The tumor is characterized by its intricate papillary adenomatous pattern, which may be readily mistaken for cancer.

Clinically, a hidradenoma is small, rarely more than 1 cm in diameter (Fig. 23.22A). Its consistency can range from firm to as soft as a sebaceous cyst, with which it is often confused. Most of these lesions are found in the interlabial folds, in the labia majora, or in the perineum. Because these tumors are apocrine in origin, the labia minora location is unusual. The occasional occurrence of reddish brown pulpy material on the surface results when the tumor is evulsed through the duct of the sweat gland.

These lesions have been carefully studied in numerous laboratories, and the complex microscopic patterns have been repeatedly stressed (Fig. 23.22B). The superficial papillary adenomatous pattern appears aggressive, but careful inspection shows that the glandular structures are lined by a single layer of well-organized cuboidal cells. In some parts of the tumor, the pink-staining secretory elements can be identified superficial to the basal layer. Beneath the epithelium is an indefinite layer of flattened myoepithelial cells. When the clear cell variant of the

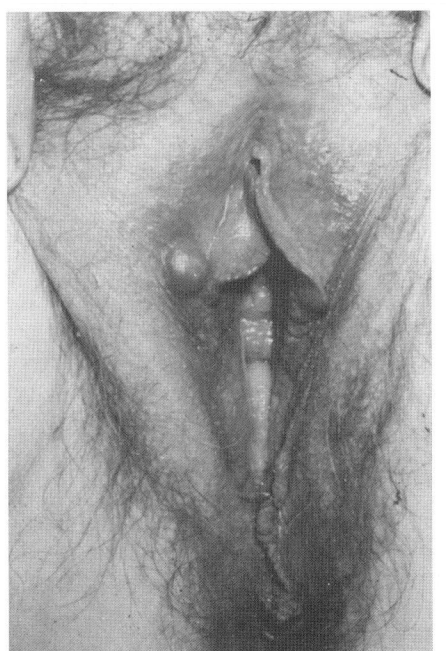

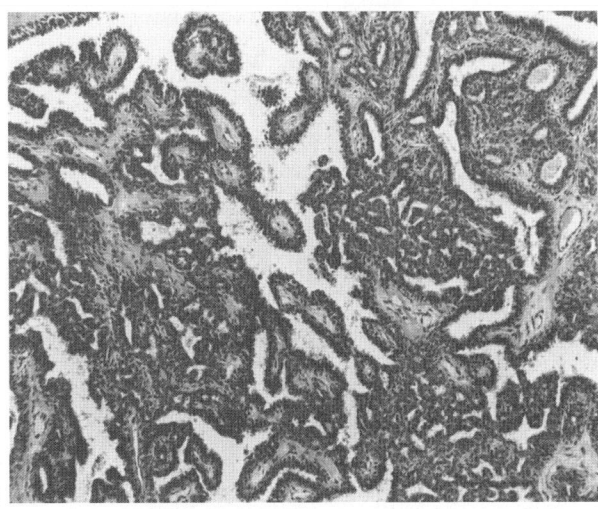

FIGURE 23.22 A: Hidradenoma of the vulva. **B:** Low-power magnification section of hidradenoma of the vulva. (A: From Novak E, Woodruff JD. *Obstetric and gynecologic pathology.* 7th ed. Philadelphia, PA: WB Saunders, 1974. Copyright © 1974 Elsevier.)

myoepithelium proliferates, an ominous picture is created, yet this clear cell hidradenoma also behaves in a benign manner. Although hidradenocarcinoma occasionally does occur, a finding of distinct adenocarcinoma in the vulva should initiate a search to rule out a metastatic lesion from another primary site.

Hidradenomas are classically asymptomatic, and most lesions are discovered during a routine pelvic examination. Curative treatment consists of local excision; recurrences result only from incomplete excision.

Granular Cell Tumors

Granular cell tumors (GCTs) were first described by Weber in 1854. It was not until 1926 that Abrikossoff coined the term *myoblastoma*. Later, the tumor was termed *granular cell schwannoma*. The current nomenclature recognizes the term *granular cell tumor*. Although frequently benign, GCTs can present as a malignant form that is multicentric and metastatic in vital organs. Horowitz and associates reported on 20 patients presenting with GCTs of the vulva over a 31-year period at the Emory University Teaching Hospitals. Seventy percent of the patients were African American, and the mean age was 50 years. Ninety percent of the lesions were on the labia majora, with lesion size ranging from 0.4 cm × 0.4 cm to 7 cm × 8 cm × 12 cm. Nineteen of twenty patients were treated with a wide local excision. The twentieth patient required radical excision because of the size of the lesion. This patient eventually died of pulmonary metastasis. Only two patients presented with multiple lesions. Twelve lesions were stained for S100. All were positive, which suggests a neural Schwann cell origin.

Sometimes, the overlying pseudoepitheliomatous changes are misinterpreted as invasive cancer (Fig. 23.23). Identification is possible with recognition of the granular cells dispersed within the underlying stroma or within the tumor. In a few patients, GCT has behaved in a malignant fashion, but an

appearance of a second lesion at a site outside the vulva usually indicates multiple primary lesions rather than metastasis.

Hemangioma

Hemangiomas are common vulvar lesions that usually do not require treatment. The lesions normally are small, are often multiple, and may bleed with trauma. On occasion, keratinization causes the superficial surface to appear white or gray-white (angiokeratoma). Hemangiomas should be differentiated from small varicosities, which commonly are seen in the postmenopausal patient.

An accurate diagnosis is imperative because a malignant melanoma can be misinterpreted as a hemangioma. The abrupt appearance of any pigmented lesion demands biopsy. In 2 of 11 melanomas seen in our clinic, the lesions were diagnosed as hematoma or angioma, and a correct diagnosis was provided only by histologic study. Angiokeratoma, a benign tumor, is a distinct clinicopathologic entity. Aggressive angiomyxoma, although structurally benign, is known for its large size and local recurrences. Some tumors, although benign, can be massive in size and thereby pose operative problems (Fig. 23.24).

The best treatment for congenital hemangioma is careful observation. The lesions regress spontaneously in almost all cases, and attempts at excision may be mutilating. If bleeding is a problem, the troublesome vascular channels can be treated by surgical ligation or embolization.

Varicocele and Varices

Varices are common on the vulva, and the larger lesions are almost routinely unilateral. As with most varicosities, treatment depends on size and symptoms. Whereas varicoceles in the scrotum arise from dilatation of the veins in the pampiniform plexus of the inguinal canal, the lesions on the vulva arise from the pudendal veins (Fig. 23.25). Careful evaluation usually demonstrates more extensive involvement of the tributaries of the hypogastric vein with varicosities of the gluteal vessels over the buttock.

If the patient experiences discomfort from the engorgement that follows exercise or standing for long periods, ligation is indicated with excision of the segment of vulvar skin that contains the varices. Knowledge of the intricate vascular system that supplies the external genitalia is necessary to ensure that surgery will result in long-term success and will prevent recurrences. Horowitz has treated several patients using selective embolization with success.

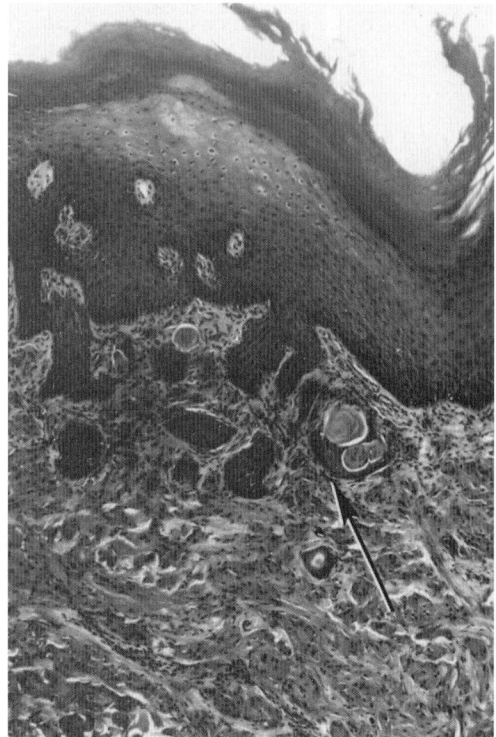

FIGURE 23.23 Granular cell tumor. Note the pseudoepitheliomatous hyperplasia, nests of large, pale "granular cells" beneath the epithelium (*arrow*).

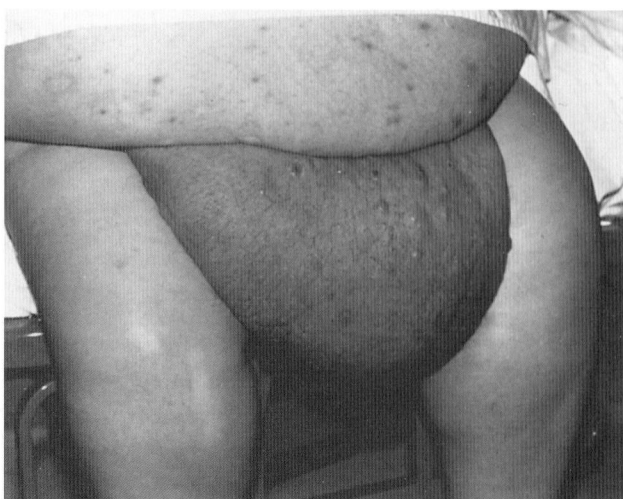

FIGURE 23.24 A benign angiolipoma noted for its massive size.

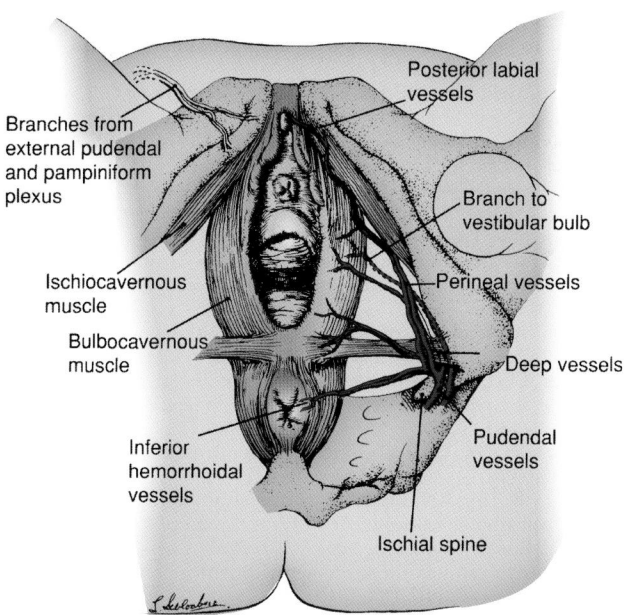

FIGURE 23.25 Vascular supply of the vulva.

Labels on figure:
Branches from external pudendal and pampiniform plexus
Ischiocavernous muscle
Bulbocavernous muscle
Inferior hemorrhoidal vessels
Posterior labial vessels
Branch to vestibular bulb
Perineal vessels
Deep vessels
Pudendal vessels
Ischial spine

BEST SURGICAL PRACTICES

- Vulvar diseases are multiple and may be difficult to diagnose. Many inflammatory conditions clinically resemble cancer.
- Bartholin gland abscesses are usually treated with antibiotics and insertion of a Word catheter. Marsupialization or excision is rarely used today. The possibility of cancer of Bartholin gland should be considered in the postmenopausal women with a new mass involving the Bartholin gland.
- Vulvodynia can be caused by infectious, inflammatory, neurologic, or neoplastic conditions of the vulva. When no underlying cause of vulvar pain can be demonstrated, oral amitriptyline and gabapentin as well as topical steroid creams should be tried. Local injection with triamcinolone and bupivacaine can also be used. If vulvar vestibulodynia is diagnosed, an extended perineoplasty has been effective in many patients.
- Vulvar condyloma are caused by some types of HPV (90% are due to types 6 and 11). These lesions may be self-limiting and resolve spontaneously. They do not undergo malignant transformation. If numerous, large, or symptomatic, they can be successfully treated with topical podophyllin, podofilox, or TCA. These lesions may also be destroyed or removed with electrosurgical desiccation, CUSA, CO_2 laser, or simple excision. These lesions may be difficult or impossible to eradicate in immunocompromised patients.
- Vulvar intraepithelial neoplasia should be diagnosed by biopsy. It may be caused by certain types of HPV, especially in younger women. If untreated, it may progress to invasive cancer. It can be treated by laser ablation, but surgical excision is usually recommended. A variety of techniques have been used, depending on the size and location of the lesion or lesions.

ACKNOWLEDGMENTS

The authors want to recognize the late Dr. J. Donald Woodruff, who has been a coauthor of this chapter for several editions and who has served as a mentor to the current authors.

BIBLIOGRAPHY

Abdel-Mesih A, Daya D, Omuma K, et al. Interobserver agreement for assessing invasion in stage 1A vulvar squamous cell carcinoma. *Am J Surg Pathol* 2013;37:1336.

Abramov Y, Elchalal U, Abramov D, et al. Surgical treatment of vulvar lichen sclerosus: a review. CME review article. *Obstet Gynecol* 1996;51:3.

Abrikossoff AI. Über myome, ausgehend von der guer gestriften willkürlichen muskulatur. *Virchows Archiv für pathologische Anatomie and Physiologie and für Klinische Medizin* 1926;260:215.

Adelson MD. Ultrasonic surgical aspiration in the treatment of vulvar disease [Letter, Comment]. *Obstet Gynecol* 1991;78(3 Pt 1):477.

Anderson T. Green SD, Childers BJ. Massive soft tissue injury: diagnosis and management of necrotizing fasciitis. *Plast Reconstr Surg* 2006;14:127.

Aranda FI, Laforga JB. Nodular fasciitis of the vulva: report of a case with immunohistochemical study. *Pathol Res Pract* 1998;194:805.

Ault KA, Giuliano AR, Edwards RP, et al. A phase I study to evaluate a human papillomavirus (HPV) type 18 L1 VLP vaccine. *Vaccine* 2004;22:3004.

Bachmann GA, Raymond R, Arnold LD, et al. Chronic vulvar and other gynecologic pain: prevalence and characteristics in a self-reported survey. *J Reprod Med* 2006;1:3.

Baggish MS, Miklos JR. Vulva pain syndrome: a review. *Obstet Gynecol Surv* 1995;50:618.

Baggish MS, Sze EH, Adelson MD, et al. Quantitative evaluation of the skin and accessory appendages in vulvar carcinoma in situ. *Obstet Gynecol* 1989;74:169.

Barbero M, Micheletti L, Preti M, et al. Biologic behavior of vulvar intraepithelial neoplasia: source, logic and clinical parameters. *J Reprod Med* 1993;38:108.

Beisky A. Über Kraurosis Vulvae. *Z Heik (Prague)* 1885;6:69.

Benedet JL, Murphy KJ. Squamous carcinoma in situ of the vulva. *Gynecol Oncol* 1982;14:213.

Bloss JD. The use of electrosurgical techniques in the management of premalignant diseases of the vulva, vagina, and cervix: an excisional rather than an ablative approach. *Am J Obstet Gynecol* 1993;169:1081.

Bronstein J, Abramovici H. Combination of subtotal perineoplasty and interferon for the treatment of vulvar vestibulitis. *Gynecol Obstet Invest* 1997;44:53.

Bronstein J, Heifetz S, Kellner Y, et al. Clobetasol dipropionate 0.05% versus testosterone propionate 2% topical application for severe vulvar lichen sclerosus. *Am J Obstet Gynecol* 1998;178:80.

Bornstein J, Kaufman RH. Combination of surgical excision and carbon dioxide laser vaporization for multifocal vulvar intraepithelial neoplasia. *Am J Obstet Gynecol* 1988;158:459.

Bornstein J, Lahat N, Sharon A, et al. Telomerase activity in HPV-associated vulvar vestibulitis. *J Reprod Med* 2000;45:643.

Bornstein J, Pascal B, Abramovici H. Intramuscular beta-interferon treatment for severe vulvar vestibulitis. *J Reprod Med* 1993;38:117.

Bornstein J, Sova Y, Atad J, et al. Development of vaginal adenosis following combined 5-fluorouracil and carbon dioxide laser treatments for diffuse vaginal condylomatosis. *Obstet Gynecol* 1993;81:896.

Bornstein J, Zarfati D, Fruchter O, et al. A repetitive DNA sequence that characterizes human papillomavirus integration site into the human genome is present in vulvar vestibulitis. *Eur J Obstet Gynaecol Reprod Biol* 2000;89:173.

Bouchard S, Yazbech S, Lallier M. Perineal hemangioma, anorectal malformation, and genital anomaly: a new association? *J Pediatr Surg* 1999;34:1133.

Bowen JD. Precancerous dermatoses. *J Cutan Dis* 1912;30:241.

Breech LL, Laufer MR. Surgicel in the management of labial and clitoral hood adhesions in adolescents with lichen sclerosus. *J Pediatr Adolesc Gynecol* 2000;13:21.

Bresci G, Parisi G, Banti S. Long term therapy with 5-aminosalicylic acid in Crohn's disease: is it useful? Our four years' experience *Int J Clin Pharmacol Res* 1994;14:133.

Brook I, Frazier EH. Clinical and microbiological features of necrotizing fasciitis. *J Clin Microbiol* 1995;33:2382.

IV

Brown JV III, Goldstein BH, Rettenmaier MA, et al. Laser ablation of surgical margins after excisional partial vulvectomy for VIN: effect on recurrence. *J Reprod Med* 2005;50:345.

Buscema J, Naghashfar Z, Sawada E, et al. The predominance of human papillomavirus type 16 in vulvar neoplasia. *Obstet Gynecol* 1988;71:601.

Buscema J, Stern J, Woodruff JD. The significance of histologic alterations adjacent to invasive vulvar carcinoma. *Am J Obstet Gynecol* 1980;137:902.

Buscema J, Woodruff JD, Parmley TH, et al. Carcinoma in situ of the vulva. *Obstet Gynecol* 1980;55:225.

Calvillo O, Skaribas IM, Rockett C. Computed tomography-guided pudendal nerve block: a new diagnostic approach to long-term anoperineal pain: a report of two cases. *Reg Anesth Pain Med* 2000;25:420.

Centers for Disease Control and Prevention. National Disease and Therapeutic Index (IMS American Ltd.). Available at www.cdc.gov

Collins CG, Hansen LH, Theriot EA. Clinical stain for use in selecting biopsy sites in patients with vulvar disease. *Obstet Gynecol* 1966;28:158.

Coppelson M. Colposcopic features of papillomaviral infection and premalignancy in the female lower genital tract. *Dermatol Clin* 1991;9:251.

Crum CP, McLachlin CM, Tate JE, et al. Pathobiology of vulvar squamous neoplasia. *Curr Opin Obstet Gynecol* 1997;9:63.

Dalziel KL, Millard R, Wojnarowska F. The treatment of vulval lichen-sclerosus with a very potent topical steroid (clobetasol propionate 0.05%) cream. *Br J Dermatol* 1991;124:461.

Davis BL, Robinson DG. Diverticula of the female urethra: assay of 120 cases. *J Urol* 1970;104:850.

de Sanjosé S, Alemany L, Ordi J, et al. Worldwide human papillomavirus genotype attribution in over 200 cases of intraepithelial and invasion lesions of the vulva. *Eur J Cancer* 2013;49:3450.

DeSimone CP, Crisp MP, Ueland FR. Concordance of gross surgical and final fixed margins in vulvar intraepithelial neoplasia 3 and vulvar cancer. *J Reprod Med* 2006;6:1285.

DiBonito L, Falconieri G, Bonifacio-Gori D. Multicentric papillomavirus infection of the female genital tract: a study of morphologic pattern, possible risk and viral prevalence. *Pathol Res Pract* 1993;189:1023.

DiPaola GR, Gomez-Rueda N, Arrighi L. Relevance of microinvasion in carcinoma of the vulva. *Obstet Gynecol* 1975;45:647.

Edwards L. New concepts in vulvodynia. *Am J Obstet Gynecol* 2003;189(suppl):S24.

Ersan Y, Ozgultelxin R, Cetinkale O, et al. Fournier-gangran. *Langenbecks Arch Chir* 1995;380:139.

Farley DE, Katz VL, Dotters DT. Toxic shock syndrome associated with vulvar necrotizing fasciitis. *Obstet Gynecol* 1993;82:660.

Faro S, Faro J. Necrotizing Soft-tissue Infections in Obstetric and Gynecologic Patients. *Clin Obstet Gynecol* 2012;55:875.

Farrell AM, Randall VA, Vafaee T, Dawber RP. Finasteride as a therapy for hidradenitis suppurativa. *Br J Dermatol* 1999;141:1138.

Feagan BG, Rochon J, Fedorak RN, et al. Methotrexate for the treatment of Crohn's disease: the North American Crohn's Study Group Investigators. *N Engl J Med* 1995;332:292.

Feller ER, Ribaudo S, Jackson ND. Gynecologic aspects of Crohn's disease. *Am Fam Physician* 2001;64:1725.

Ferenczy A, Mitao M, Nagai N, et al. Latent papillomavirus and recurring genital warts. *N Engl J Med* 1985;313:784.

Fischer GO. The commonest causes of symptomatic vulvar disease: a dermatologist's perspectives. *Australas J Dermatol* 1996;1:12.

Fisher JR, Conway MJ, Takeshita RT, et al. Necrotizing fasciitis: importance of roentgenographic studies for soft-tissue gas. *JAMA* 1979;241:803.

Fleming DT, McQuillian GM, Johnson RE, et al. Herpes simplex virus type 2 in the United States, 1976 to 1994. *N Engl J Med* 1997;337:1105.

Foster DC. Vulvar disease. *Obstet Gynecol* 2002;100:145.

Frega A, di Renzi F, Stentella P, et al. Management of human papillomavirus vulvoperineal infection with systemic *b*-interferon and thymostimulin in HIV-positive patients. *Int J Gynaecol Obstet* 1994;44:255.

Friedman-Kien AE, Eron LJ, Conaut M, et al. Natural interferon alpha for treatment of condylomata acuminata. *JAMA* 1988;259:533.

Friedrich EG Jr. International Society for the Study of Vulvovaginal Disease. New nomenclature for vulvar disease: report of the Committee on Terminology. *Obstet Gynecol* 1976;47:122.

Friedrich EG Jr. Topical testosterone for benign vulvar dystrophy. *Obstet Gynecol* 1971;37:677.

Friedrich EG Jr. *Vulvar disease: diagnosis and management.* 2nd ed. Philadelphia, PA: WB Saunders, 1983:488.

Friedrich EG Jr, Kalra PS. Serum levels of sex hormones in vulvar lichen sclerosus and the effect of topical testosterone. *N Engl J Med* 1984;310:488.

Friedrich EG Jr, Wilkinson EJ. Mucous cyst of the vulvar vestibule. *Obstet Gynecol* 1973;42:407.

Friedrich EG, Wilkinson EJ, Steingraeber PH, et al. Paget's disease of the vulva and carcinoma of the breast. *Obstet Gynecol* 1975;46:130.

Friedrich EG Jr. Vulvar vestibulitis syndrome. *J Reprod Med* 1987;32:110.

Furlonge CB, Thin RN, Evans BE, et al. Vulvar vestibulitis syndrome: a clinicopathological study. *Br J Obstet Gynaecol* 1991;98:703.

Gerber S, Bongiovanni AM, Ledger WJ, et al. A deficiency in interferon-alpha production in women with vulvar vestibulitis. *Am J Obstet Gynecol* 2002;186:361.

Glazer HI, Radke G, Swencionis C, et al. Treatment of vulvar vestibulitis syndrome with electromyographic biofeedback of pelvic floor musculature. *J Reprod Med* 1995;40:283.

Goldman HB, Idom CB, Dmochowski RR. Traumatic injuries of the female external genitalia and their association with urological injuries. *J Urol* 1998;159:956.

Haefner HK. Critique of new gynecologic surgical procedures: surgery for vulvar vestibulitis. *Clin Obstet Gynecol* 2000;43:689.

Haefner HK, Collins ME, Davis GD, et al. The vulvodynia guideline. *J Low Genit Tract Dis* 2005;9:40.

Haefner HK, Tate JE, McLachlin CM, et al. Vulvar intraepithelial neoplasia: age, morphological phenotype, papillomavirus DNA, and coexisting invasive carcinoma. *Hum Pathol* 1995;26:147.

Haley JC, Mirowski GW, Hood AF. Benign vulvar tumors. *Semin Cutan Med Surg* 1998;17:196.

Harrison BJ, Mudge M, Hughes LE. Recurrence after surgical treatment of hidradenitis suppurativa. *BMJ* 1987;294:487.

Haslund P, Lee RA, Jemec GB. Treatment of hidradenitis suppurativa with tumor necrosis factor-alpha inhibitors. *Acta Derm Venereal* 2009;89:595.

Hatch K. Colposcopy of vaginal and vulvar human papillomavirus and adjacent sites. *Obstet Gynecol Clin North Am* 1993;20:203.

Hatch KD. Vulvovaginal human papillomavirus infections: clinical implications and management. *Am J Obstet Gynecol* 1991;165:1183.

Herzog TJ, Rader JS. The Ultrasonic Surgical Aspirator in the gynecologic oncology patient. *Adv Obstet Gynecol* 1994;1:325.

Hoffman MS, Pinelli DM, Finan M, et al. Laser vaporization for vulvar intraepithelial neoplasia III. *J Reprod Med* 1992;37:135.

Hoffman MS, Roberts WS, LaPolla JP, et al. Laser vaporization of grade 3 vaginal intraepithelial neoplasia. *Am J Obstet Gynecol* 1991;165:1342.

Horowitz BJ. Interferon therapy for condylomatous vulvitis. *Obstet Gynecol* 1989;73:446.

Horowitz IR, Copas P, Majmudar B. Granular cell tumors of the vulva. *Am J Obstet Gynecol* 1995;173:1710.

Horowitz IR, Gomella LG, eds. *Obstetrics and gynecology on call*, 1st ed. East Norwalk, CT: Appleton & Lange, 1992:167.

International Society for the Study of Vulvar Disease, Committee on Terminology. New nomenclature for vulvar disease. *Obstet Gynecol* 1989;160:769.

Japaze H, Dinh T, Woodruff JD. Verrucous carcinoma of the vulva: study of 24 cases. *Obstet Gynecol* 1982;60:462.

Jeffcoate TNA. Chronic vulvar dystrophies. *Am J Obstet Gynecol* 1966;95:61.

Jeffries DJ. Acyclovir update. *BMJ* 1986;293:1523.

Jemal A, Simard EP, Dorell C, et al. Annual report to the Nation on the Status of Cancer, 1975–2009, featuring the burden and trends in human papillomavirus (HPV)-associated cancers and HPV vaccination coverage levels. *J Natl Cancer Inst* 2013;105:175.

Jones RW, Rowan DM, Stewart AW. Vulvar intraepithelial neoplasia: aspects of the natural history and outcome of 405 women. *Obstet Gynecol* 2005;106:1319.

Joseph MA, Jayaseelan E, Ganapathi B. et al. Hidradenitis suppurativa treated with finasteride. *J Dermatolog Treat* 2005;16:75.

Julian CG, Callison J, Woodruff JD. Plastic management of extensive vulvar defects. *Obstet Gynecol* 1971;38:193.

Kaur MR, Lewis HM. Hidradenitis suppurativa treated with dapsone: a case series of five patients. *J Dermatol Treat* 2006;17:211.

Kehoe S, Luesley D. Pathology and management of vulval pain and pruritus. *Curr Opin Obstet Gynecol* 1995;1:16.

Kent HL, Wisniewski PM. Interferon for vulvar vestibulitis. *J Reprod Med* 1990;35:1138.

Kizer JR, Bellah RD, Schnaufer L, et al. Meconium hydrocele in a female newborn: an unusual case of a labial mass. *J Urol* 1995;153:188.

Kornbluth A, Marion JF, Solomon P, et al. How effective is current medical therapy for severe ulcerative and Crohn's colitis? An analytic review of selected trials *J Clin Gastroenterol* 1995;20:280.

Koutsky LA, Ault KA, Wheeler CM. A controlled trial of a human papillomavirus type 16 vaccine. *N Engl J Med* 2002;347:1645.

Larsen J, Peters K, Petersen CS, et al. Interferon alpha-2b treatment of symptomatic chronic vulvodynia associated with koilocytosis. *Acta Derm Venereol* 1993;73:385.

Le T, Hicks W, Menard C, et al. Preliminary results of 5% imiquimod cream in the primary treatment of vulva intraepithelial neoplasia grade 2/3. *Am J Obstet Gynecol* 2006;194:377.

Lijnen RL, Blindeman LA. VIN III (bowenoid type) and HPV infection. *Br J Dermatol* 1994;131:728.

Lorenz B, Kaufman RH, Kutzner S. Lichen sclerosus–therapy with clobetasol propionate. *J Reprod Med* 1998;43:790.

Lynch PJ, Moyal-Barracco, M, Scurry J, et al. 2011 ISSVD Terminology and classification of vulvar dermatological disorders: an approach to clinical diagnosis. *J Low Genit Tract Dis* 2012;16:339.

Lynch PJ, Moyal-Barrocco M, Bogliatto F, et al. 2006 ISSVD classification of vulvar dermatoses pathologic subsets and their clinical correlates. *J Reprod Med* 2007;52:3.

Majmudar B. Tumors of the vulva, Section 15. In: *Conn's current therapy 2000*. Philadelphia, PA: WB Saunders, 2000.

Majmudar B, Castellano PZ, Wilson RW, et al. Granular cell tumors of the vulva. *J Reprod Med* 1990;35:1008.

Mann MS, Kaufman RH, Brown D Jr, et al. Vulvar vestibulitis: significant clinical variables and treatment outcome. *Obstet Gynecol* 1992;79:122.

Mao C, Koutsky LA, Ault KA, et al. Efficacy of human papillomavirus-16 vaccine to prevent cervical intraepithelial neoplasia: a randomized controlled trial. *Obstet Gynecol* 2006;107:18.

Marinoff SC, Turner ML. Vulvar vestibulitis syndrome: an overview. *Am J Obstet Gynecol* 1991;165:1228.

Marinoff SC, Turner ML, Hirsch RP, et al. Intralesional alpha interferon: cost-effective therapy for vulvar vestibulitis syndrome. *J Reprod Med* 1993;38:19.

Massad LS. Applying the new ISSVD terminology on precursors of vulvar squamous cell carcinoma to management. *J Low Genit Tract Dis* 2006;10:135.

Matthews D. Marsupialization in the treatment of Bartholin's cyst and abscesses. *Obstet Gynaecol Br Commonw* 1966;73:1010.

McKay M. Dysesthetic (essential) vulvodynia treatment with amitriptyline. *J Reprod Med* 1993;38:9.

McKay M. Subsets of vulvodynia. *J Reprod Med* 1988;3308:695.

McKay M. Vulvodynia: diagnostic patterns. *Dermatol Clin* 1992;10:423.

McKay M, Frankman O, Horowitz BJ, et al. Vulvar vestibulitis and vestibular papillomatosis: report of the ISSVD Committee on Vulvodynia. *J Reprod Med* 1991;36:413.

Mering JH. A surgical approach to intractable pruritus vulvae. *Am J Obstet Gynecol* 1952;64:619.

Modesitt SC, Waters AB, Walton L, et al. Vulvar intraepithelial neoplasia III: occult cancer and the impact of margin status on recurrence. *Obstet Gynecol* 1998;92:962.

Morin C, Bouchard C, Brisson J, et al. Human papilloma-viruses and vulvar vestibulitis. *Obstet Gynecol* 2000;95:683.

Moscicki A, Palefsky JM, Gonzales J, et al. Colposcopic and histologic findings and human papillomavirus (HPV) DNA test variability in young women positive for HPV DNA. *J Infect Dis* 1992;166:951.

Moyal-Barracco M, Lynch P. 2003 ISSVD terminology and classification of vulvodynia. *J Reprod Med* 2004;49:772.

Murina F, Tassan P, Roberti P, et al. Treatment of vulvar vestibulitis with submucous infiltrations of methylprednisolone and lidocaine: an alternative approach. *J Reprod Med* 2001;46:713.

Novak ER, Woodruff JD. *Gynecologic and obstetric pathology*, 8th ed. Philadelphia, PA: WB Saunders, 1979.

O'Connell JX, Young RH, Nielsen GP, et al. Nodular fasciitis of the vulva: a study of six cases and literature review. *Int J Gynecol Pathol* 1997;16:117.

O'Farrell N. Donovanosis. In: Holmes KK, Sparling PF, Mardh P-A, et al. (Eds.). *Sexually transmitted diseases*. New York: McGraw-Hill, 1999:525.

Paavonen J. Vulvodynia: a complex syndrome of vulvar pain. *Acta Obstet Gynecol Scand* 1995;74:2343.

Parks JS, Jones RW, McLean MR, et al. Possible etiologic heterogeneity of vulvar intraepithelial neoplasia: a correlation of pathologic characteristics with human papillomavirus detection by in situ hybridization and polymerase chain reaction. *Cancer* 1991;67:1599.

Patsner B. Treatment of vaginal dysplasia with loop excision: report of five cases. *Am J Obstet Gynecol* 1993;169:179.

Pincus SH. Vulvar dermatoses and pruritus vulvae. *Dermatol Clin* 1992;10:297.

Price LM, Mendolsohn SS, Youngs GR, et al. Unilateral vulvar hypertrophy and Crohn's disease. *Int J STD AIDS* 1995;6:146.

Rader JS, Leake JF, Dillon MB, et al. Ultrasonic surgical aspiration in the treatment of vulvar disease. *Obstet Gynecol* 1991;77:573.

Raley JC, Followwill KA, Zimet GD, et al. Gynecologists' attitudes regarding human papilloma virus vaccination: a survey of Fellows of American College of Obstetricians and Gynecologists. *Infect Dis Obstet Gynecol* 2004;12:127.

Reed BD, Caron AM, Gorenflo DW, et al. Treatment of vulvodynia with tricyclic antidepressants: efficacy and associated factors. *J Low Genit Tract Dis* 2006;4:245.

Reid R, Greenberg M, Jenson AB, et al. Sexually transmitted papillomaviral infections. I. The anatomic distribution and pathologic grade of neoplastic lesions associated with different viral types. *Am J Obstet Gynecol* 1987;156:212.

Reid R, Greenberg MD, Lorincz AT, et al. Superficial laser vulvectomy. IV. Extended laser vaporization and adjunctive 5-fluorouracil therapy of human papillomavirus–associated vulvar disease. *Obstet Gynecol* 1990;76:439.

Reid R, Greenberg MD, Pizzuti DJ, et al. Superficial laser vulvectomy. *Am J Obstet Gynecol* 1992;166:815.

Reid R, Omoto KH, Precop SL, et al. Flashlamp-excited dye laser therapy of idiopathic vulvodynia is safe and efficacious. *Am J Obstet Gynecol* 1995;172:1684.

Revuz J. Hidradenitis suppurativa. *Presse Med* 2010;39:1254–1264.

Rompel R, Petres J. Long-term results of wide surgical excision in 106 patients with hidradenitis suppurativa. *Dermatol Surg* 2000;26:638.

Santos JV, Baudet JA, Lasellas FJ, et al. Intravenous cyclosporine for steroid-refractory attacks of Crohn's disease: short and long term results. *J Clin Gastroenterol* 1995;20:207.

Schickele G. Weitere Beiträge zur Lehre der mesonephris chen Tumoren. Hegars Beitr. zur Geburtshilfe und gynäkologic, Bd. 6, H.3, 1902.

Schover L, Youngs DD, Cannata NW. Psychosexual aspects of the evaluation and management of vulvar vestibulitis. *Am J Obstet Gynecol* 1992;167:630.

Schwimmer E. Die idiopathischen Schleimhautplaugues der mundhohle (Leukoplakia buccalis). *Arch Dermat Syph* 1877;9:611.

Scurry J, Campion M, Scurry B, et al. Pathologic audit of 164 consecutive cases of vulvar intraepithelial neoplasia. *Int J Gynecol Pathol* 2006;25:176.

IV

Scurry J, Wilkinson EJ. Review of terminology of precursors of vulvar squamous cell carcinoma. *J Low Genit Tract Dis* 2006;10:161.

Shakla VK, Hughes LE. A case of squamous cell carcinoma complicating hidradenitis suppurativa. *Eur J Surg Oncol* 1995;21:106.

Shatz P, Bergeron C, Wilkinson EJ, et al. Vulvar intraepithelial neoplasia and skin appendage involvement. *Obstet Gynecol* 1989;74:769.

Sherman KJ, Daling JR, Chu J, et al. Genital warts, other sexually transmitted diseases, and vulvar cancer. *Epidemiology* 1991;2:257.

Sideri M, Jones RW, Wilkinson EJ, et al. Squamous vulvar intraepithelial neoplasia: 2004 modified terminology. ISSVD Vulvar Oncology Subcommittee. *J Reprod Med* 2005;50:807.

Sobel JD. Management of recurrent vulvovaginal candidiasis with intermittent ketoconazole prophylaxis. *Obstet Gynecol* 1985;65:435.

Sonnendecker EW, Sonnendecker HE, Wright CA, et al. Recalcitrant vulvodynia: a clinicopathological study. *S Afr Med J* 1993;83:730.

Taussig FJ. *Diseases of the vulva*. New York: Appleton Century-Crofts, 1931.

Theusen B, Andreasson B, Bock JE. Sexual function and somatopsychic reactions after local excision of vulvar intra-epithelial neoplasia. *Acta Obstet Gynecol Scand* 1992;71:126.

Turner ML, Marinoff SC. General principles in the diagnosis and treatment of vulvar diseases. *Dermatol Clin* 1992;10:275.

Umpierre SA, Kaufman RH, Adam E, et al. Human papillomavirus DNA in tissue biopsy specimens of vulvar vestibulitis patients treated with interferon. *Obstet Gynecol* 1991;78:693.

van Beurden M, ten Kale FJ, Smits HL, et al. Multifocal vulvar intraepithelial neoplasia grade III and multicentric lower genital tract neoplasia associated with transcriptionally active human papillomavirus. *Cancer* 1995;75:2879.

Villa LL, Costa RLR, Petta CA, et al. Prophylactic quadrivalent human papillomavirus (types 6, 11, 16, and 18) L1 virus-like particle vaccine in young women: a randomised double-blind placebo-controlled multicentre phase II efficacy trial. *Lancet Oncol* 2005;6:271.

Vuopala S, Pollanen R, Kaappila A, et al. Detection and typing of human papillomavirus infection affecting the cervix, vagina, and vulva: comparison of DNA hybridization with cytological, colposcopic and histological examination. *Arch Gynecol Obstet* 1993;253:75.

Weber CO. Anatomische Untersuchang einer hypertropphischen Zunge nebst Bemrkungen uber die nenbildung guergestreifter muskel fasern. *Virchows Arch A Pathol Anat Histopathol*, 1854;7:115.

Welsh DA, Powers JS. Elevated parathyroid hormone-related protein and hypercalcemia in a patient with cutaneous squamous cell carcinoma complicating hidradenitis suppurativa. *South Med J* 1993;86:1403.

Wharton LR Jr, Everett HS. Primary malignant Bartholin gland tumors. *Obstet Gynecol Surv* 1951;6:1.

Wilkinson EJ, Guerrero E, Daniel R, et al. Vulvar vestibulitis is rarely associated with human papillomavirus infection types 6, 11, 16, or 18. *Int J Gynecol Pathol* 1993;12:344.

Woodruff JD, Genadry R, Poliakoff S. Treatment of dyspareunia and vaginal outlet distortions by perineoplasty. *Obstet Gynecol* 1981;57:750.

Woodruff JD, Hildebrandt EE. Carcinoma in situ of the vulva. *Obstet Gynecol* 1958;12:414.

Woodruff JD, Julian C, Paray T, et al. The contemporary challenge of carcinoma in situ of the vulva. *Am J Obstet Gynecol* 1973;115:677.

Woodruff JD, Richardson EH Jr. Malignant vulvar Paget's disease. *Obstet Gynecol* 1957;10:10.

Woodruff JD, Sussman J, Shakfeh S. Vulvitis circumscripta plasmacellularis. *J Reprod Med* 1989;34:369.

Woodruff JD, Thompson B. Local alcohol injection in the treatment of vulvar pruritus. *Obstet Gynecol* 1972;40:18.

Woodruff JD, Genadry R, Poliakoff S. Treatment of dyspareunia and vaginal outlet distortions by perineoplasty. *Obstet Gynecol* 1981;57:750.

Wu AY, Sherman ME, Rosenshein NB, et al. Pathologic evaluation of gynecologic specimens obtained with the Cavitron ultrasonic surgical aspirator (CUSA). *Gynecol Oncol* 1992;44:28.

Wysoki RS, Majmudar B, Willis D. Granuloma inguinale (donovanosis) in women. *J Reprod Med* 1988;33:709.

CHAPTER 24
Surgical Conditions of the Vagina and Urethra

Y. Hernandez Suarez, John A. Rock, and Ira R. Horowitz

DEFINITIONS

Genitoplasty—Surgical reconstruction of the external genitals.

Hematocolpos—A condition in which menstrual blood accumulates inside the vagina and distends it, most commonly associated with obstructing vaginal anomalies.

Hermaphroditism—A condition in which there is a combination of disparate or contradictory elements most commonly used to describe an individual who has both male and female sexual characteristics and organs (synonyms: intersex, androgyne).

Imperforate hymen—The hymen usually is perforated during embryonic life to establish a connection between the lumen of the vaginal canal and the vaginal vestibule, and it usually is torn early in the prepubertal years. If canalization fails and there are no perforations, the hymen is called imperforate.

Pseudohermaphroditism—A condition in which the gonads are of one sex (genetically XX or XY), but in which the physical/phenotypical appearance is of the opposite sex. Genetically female individuals (chromosomes XX, thus with female gonads/ovaries) presenting with significant male secondary sex characteristics and genetically male individuals (chromosome XY, thus with male gonads/testes) presenting with significant female secondary sex characteristics.

OBSTRUCTIVE LESIONS OF THE VAGINA

Imperforate Hymen

Imperforate hymen is the most common obstructive congenital lesion of the female genital tract. The hymen, the junction of the sinovaginal bulbs with the urogenital sinus (UGS), is a thin mucous membrane, sometimes cribriform in appearance, composed of endoderm from the UGS epithelium. The müllerian ducts meet the sinovaginal bulbs at the most cephalad tip of the invaginating UGS. The vaginal plate elongates and canalizes to form the vagina. If the vaginal plate does not canalize, a transverse vaginal septum is the result. Canalization of the most caudal portion of the vaginal plate at the UGS establishes a patent hymen. The hymen usually is perforated during embryonic life to establish a connection between the lumen of the vaginal canal and the vaginal vestibule, and it usually is torn early in the prepubertal years. If canalization fails and there are no perforations, the hymen is called *imperforate*. It is usually an isolated finding with no associated anatomic anomalies.

Although variations in hymen development occur, complete blockage by the hymen of the vaginal orifice is rare, occurring in approximately 0.05% to 0.1% of newborn girls. In 1986, Mor and colleagues described the types of hymeneal shape in the newborn infant from examination performed within the first 24 hours of life. In 53.5%, a smooth hymen with a central orifice was observed; a folded hymen with a central orifice was seen in 27%; a folded hymen with an eccentric orifice occurred in 4.5%; an anterior opening of the hymen was found in 10.8%; a posterior opening was found in 0.6%. The researchers found that 3% had hymeneal bands and 0.3% of the newborns had imperforate hymens.

Stelling and colleagues have evaluated the genetic transmission of imperforate hymen and reported that the occurrence of imperforate hymen in two consecutive generations of a family is consistent with a dominant mode of transmission, either sex linked or autosomal. Examination of newborns with a family history of imperforate hymen is of particular importance.

Symptoms

Cases that are recognized at birth present with a thin bulging membrane between the labia, which represents a mucocolpos. When the hymen is incised, the vagina is found to contain mucoid fluid that is the result of accumulated cervical secretion. This is caused by the stimulation of the infant's cervical mucous glands by maternal estrogen in the presence of an intact hymen. Prenatal diagnosis of imperforate hymen and mucocolpos has been described with second-trimester antenatal sonography demonstrating a thin membrane that distended the vagina and spread the labia majora.

Although by performing a careful inspection of the external genitalia, an imperforate hymen may be diagnosed at any age, most commonly imperforate hymen is not detected until puberty, with girls presenting at age 13 to 15 years when symptoms begin to appear with no external evidence of menstruation. In 2005, Posner and Spandorfer reported a bimodal distribution of age at diagnosis with 43% (*n* = 10) of girls diagnosed younger than age 8 and 57% (*n* = 13) at or older than age 8. Among older girls, 100% were symptomatic with abdominal pain and/or urinary symptoms. They found that in the young girls, in 90% of cases the diagnosis was incidental. On review of the older girls' medical records,

they found that the majority lacked description of breast and pubic hair development, and almost half did not have menstrual history documented. The older group was more likely to present symptomatically and to undergo ancillary testing. They conclude that incorporating an examination of the external genitalia into routine practice of clinicians caring for children can prevent the significant delays in diagnosis of imperforate hymen, misdiagnosis, and potential morbidity associated with the latter group.

The symptoms of imperforate hymen after the onset of puberty are due to the accumulation of menstrual blood within the vaginal outlet tract. The blood of the first few cycles is collected in the vagina, which can hold a large volume of blood without undue stretching. This accumulated menstrual blood in the vagina is called *hematocolpos*. The patient may feel slight fatigue and have cramping discomfort suggesting menstruation, but she has no history of any passage of menstrual blood through the vaginal outlet. **Figure 24.1A** shows bulging of the imperforate hymen, which may be dark in color because of occult blood showing through the stretched mucous membrane; **Figure 24.1B** shows extrusion of accumulated blood after the hymen is incised.

With continuing menstruation, the vagina distends, the cervical canal dilates, and hematometra (the filling of the endometrial cavity with blood) occurs. When the intrauterine pressure reaches a certain point, retrograde passage of blood into the tubes causes hematosalpinx. Rarely, blood passes freely into the peritoneal cavity (**Fig. 24.2**) causing all the symptoms and signs of peritonitis.

The most common symptoms of vaginal overdistention are lower abdominal pain, discomfort in the pelvis, and pain in the lower back. A tender mass may be palpable suprapubically, the result of uterine enlargement and upward displacement, bladder distention, or both. Hematocolpos should be included in the differential diagnosis of amenorrheic girls presenting with persistent lower back pain. Irritation of the sacral plexus is believed to be the etiology of this referred pain pattern. The lower abdominal discomfort often is aggravated on defecation, and if extensive blood accumulation occurs in the vagina,

IV

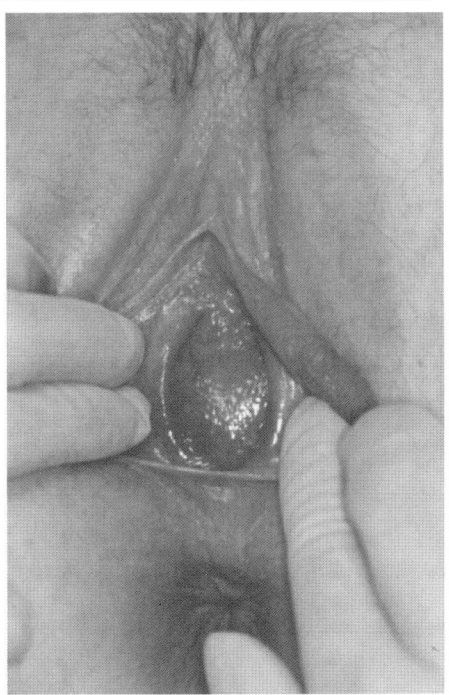

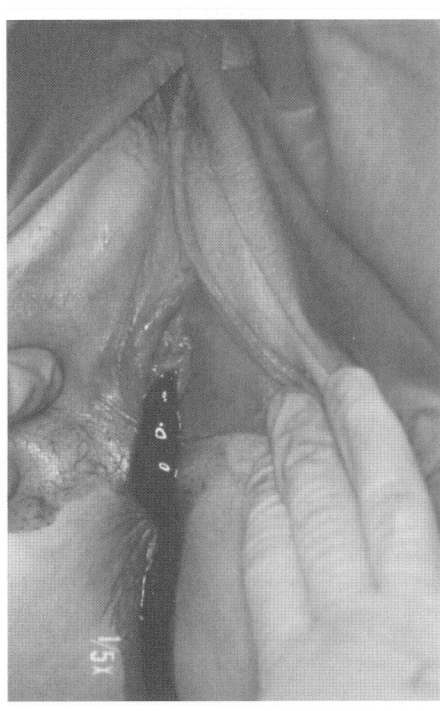

A   B

FIGURE 24.1 A: An imperforate hymen, membrane protrusion with a dark-tinged posterior representing a hematocolpos. **B:** Extrusion of accumulated blood at the time of incision into the membrane.

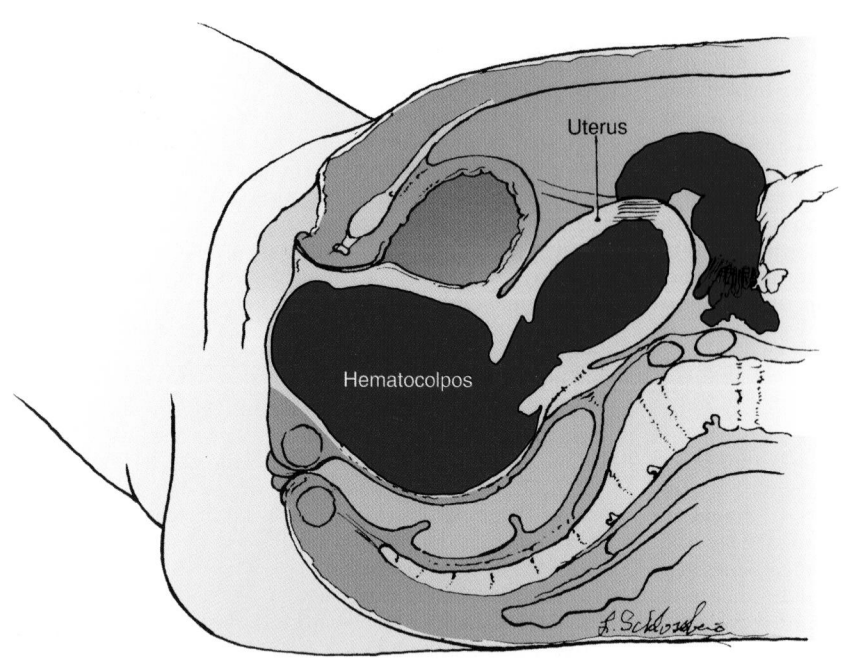

FIGURE 24.2 Hematocolpos, hematometra, hematosalpinx, and hemoperitoneum consequent to an imperforate hymen.

constipation may result from pressure and obstruction of the underlying rectum. Urination can be difficult as a result of pressure of the distended vagina, which can compress the urethra and prevent emptying of the bladder; urinary obstruction can ensue. Bladder symptoms can present as cramplike pains in the suprapubic region, along with symptoms of dysuria, frequency, and urgency; overflow incontinence may eventually develop, and hydronephrosis is a rare complication. Girls presenting with severe dysmenorrhea and duplicate vagina and didelphic uterus should be evaluated for unilateral imperforate hymen.

Pelvic ultrasound should be performed in the evaluation of imperforate hymen particularly prior to surgical intervention. Concomitant diagnostic laparoscopy in patients with imperforate hymen has not demonstrated an association with pelvic endometriosis, and laparoscopy should not be included in the standard evaluation of imperforate hymen.

Treatment

Approach to the surgical management of imperforate hymen requires cultural sensitivity. The importance of hymeneal integrity varies among cultures and religions. Options should be carefully explained to patients and their families, and the choice of surgical approach should be reached through shared decision making. In the patient diagnosed in infancy, surgery may be delayed until adolescence to ensure optimum long-term vaginal functionality and reduce the small risk of repeat surgery. The goals of surgical management of imperforate hymen are both long and short term. In the short term, the obstruction of the vagina is alleviated. In the long term, satisfactory cosmesis, sexual function, and fertility are preserved.

In the standard approach, the hymenal membrane is incised in a stellate fashion, preferably at the 2-, 4-, 8-, and 10-o'clock positions. The quadrants of the hymen are then excised, and the mucosal margins are approximated with fine delayed absorbable suture (**Fig. 24.3**). To prevent scarring and stenosis, the hymenal tissue should not be excised too close to the vaginal mucosa. The vagina should be carefully drained with a suction probe. In patients in whom hematometra is present, all intrauterine instrumentation should be avoided (**Fig. 24.2**), as there is significant risk of perforating the thin, overstretched uterine wall. Patients should be followed for 2 to 3 weeks to ensure adequate resolution of the hematometra. Rarely, secondary dilatation of the cervix may be needed.

For patients in whom the perception of hymeneal "integrity" is important, the procedure may be modified to exclude the excision of the hymen. A simple vertical incision of the hymeneal membrane is performed with oblique suturing of the hymen to form an annular opening. Sutures may be avoided with the placement of a Foley catheter and topical estrogen cream for 2 weeks postoperatively. These approaches have anecdotally resulted in satisfactory cosmesis and defloration.

Rock and colleagues followed pregnancy success subsequent to the surgical correction of imperforate hymen between 1945 and 1981 at the Johns Hopkins Hospital. Twenty-two patients of mean age 14.7 years were admitted for surgical correction of imperforate hymens. Associated anomalies, including urinary tract anomalies, were rare. Thirteen patients subsequently conceived, and 10 patients were observed to have living children. Liang and colleagues in 2003 reported on the long-term postoperative evaluation of 15 patients with imperforate hymen. They conducted questionnaires and telephone interviews regarding sexuality, fertility, menstrual problems, micturition, and defecation. The mean postoperative follow-up was 8.5 years, with the mean age at diagnosis being 13.2 years. The women reported being markedly relieved of their presenting symptoms after hymenectomy. There were some who reported having irregular menstruation, and 6/15 reported dysmenorrhea. The authors reported that most patients fared well in terms of fertility and sexual function. It is important to counsel patients and their families about the favorable prognosis of fertility and pregnancy in women with correction of imperforate hymen.

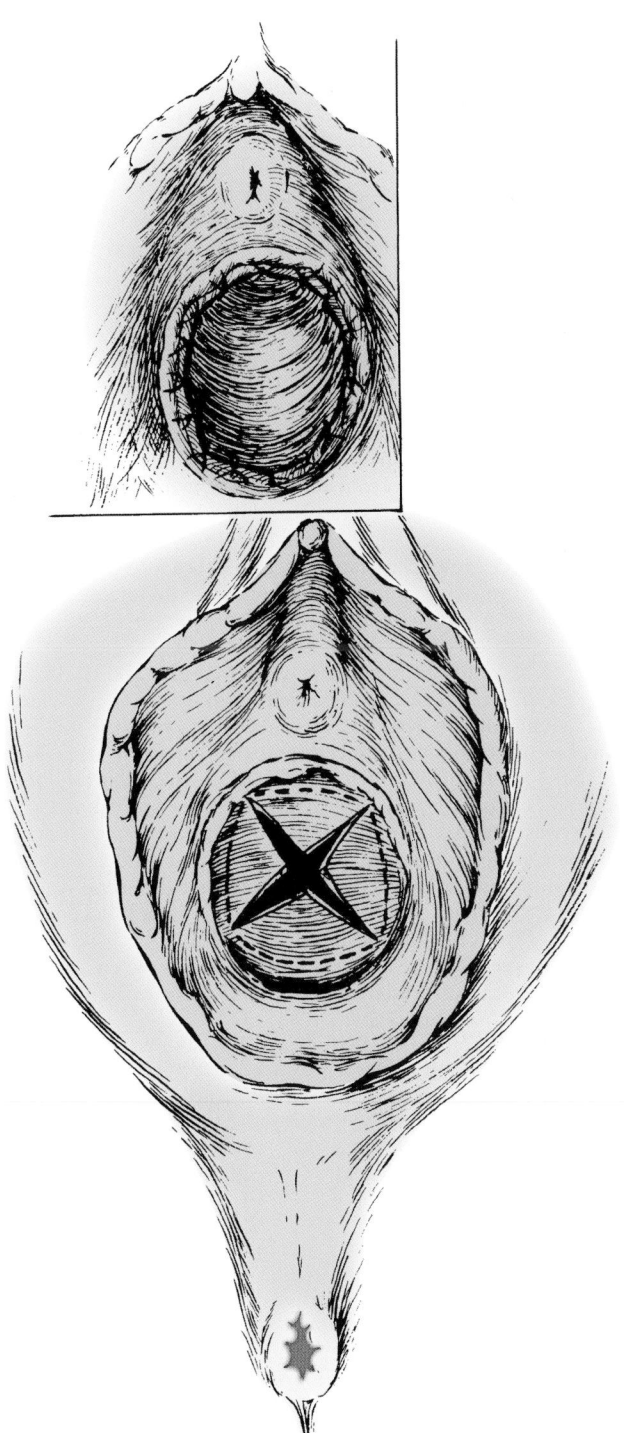

FIGURE 24.3 Excision of imperforate hymen. Stellate incisions are made through the hymenal membrane at the 2-, 4-, 8-, and 10-o'clock positions. The individual quadrants are excised along the lateral wall of the vagina, avoiding excision of the vagina (**inset**). Margins of vaginal mucosa are approximated with fine delayed absorbable suture.

Transverse Vaginal Septum

Transverse vaginal septum is a rare cause of congenital vaginal obstruction. Presenting symptoms are identical to imperforate hymen, but diagnosis is frequently delayed in the setting of a normal vulvovaginal exam. Transverse vaginal septum is diagnosed on pelvic ultrasound with hematocolpos identified cephalad to the septum. Concomitant uterine and renal malformations have been described. Magnetic resonance imaging (MRI) may be helpful in identifying the anatomy. Joki-Erkkila and Heinonen in 2003 identified 26 women with obstructive vaginal malformations. Thirteen underwent incision of an imperforate hymen and 3 excision of a complete transverse vaginal septum, with a mean follow-up period of 13 years. The remaining 10 had obstructive hemivagina and incision of a "longitudinal" vaginal septum with a mean follow-up period of 16 years. The women with transverse obstruction (imperforate hymen or transverse vaginal septum) were diagnosed within a month from their primary symptoms compared with 27 months for those with longitudinal obstruction. None with imperforate hymen required reoperation, but 2/3 with transverse vaginal septum did for vaginal constriction, and 3/10 with longitudinal vaginal septum had reexcision of their septum. All of the 10 women with longitudinal obstruction had uterine and renal malformations, whereas in those with a transverse vaginal obstruction, only 6 underwent renal evaluation, and of these, 2 had double ureters. Dysfunctional uterine bleeding was reported by 19% of those in the transverse group and 40% of those in the longitudinal obstruction group, dyspareunia was reported in 30% of the transverse and none in the longitudinal, and dysmenorrhea was reported in 19% of transverse and 20% of longitudinal. No endometriosis was found in women who subsequently had a laparotomy or laparoscopy (18/26). In the 14 who were attempting to conceive, difficulty with fertility was not diagnosed. Twenty-five (89%) out of twenty eight pregnancies ended in delivery, the live birth rate of the longitudinal group being 82%, and 94% in those with transverse obstruction. The authors concluded that accurate diagnosis, along with adequate treatment, can reduce the need for reoperations and that no specific long-term clinical gynecologic symptoms were identified in these women with obstructing vaginal anomalies.

Sequelae of Female Genital Mutilation

Female genital mutilation (FGM) is defined by the World Health Organization as "all procedures that involve partial or total removal of the external female genitalia, or other injury to the female genital organs for non-medical reasons." The WHO estimates that more than 100 million worldwide have undergone some type of FGM. It is estimated that approximately 250,000 girls and women with FGM are currently living in the United States. Female genital mutilation is practiced in Africa, Southeast Asia, and the Middle East, and is most commonly performed in puberty. Late complications of FGM include strictures, obstruction, and fistula formation. Complete obstruction of the vagina resulting in hematocolpos and hematometra has been reported. Women with FGM may seek gynecologic consultation to alleviate dyspareunia or dysmenorrhea or in preparation for childbirth. Defibulation is a vertical incision made to open scarring and reconstruct external genitalia. In a study by Nour et al. at the African Women's Health Center at the Brigham and Women's Hospital, 40 women were identified as having undergone defibulation between 1995 and 2003. Indications for defibulation were pregnancy (30%), dysmenorrhea (30%), apareunia (20%), and dyspareunia (20%). Almost 50% were found to have an intact clitoris underneath the scar. More than 90% of women stated they would highly recommend the procedure to others. 100% were satisfied with appearance and sexual function. The American Congress of

IV

Obstetricians and Gynecologists has prepared a toolkit for clinicians caring for patients with FGM that includes photographs and detailed instructions.

Anomalies of the External Genitalia and Vagina

Sexually Ambiguous External Genitalia

Sexually ambiguous external genitalia defects of the UGS are remarkably constant in appearance, regardless of the etiology of the anomaly. Such genitalia differ only in their degree of malformation and occupy a range of positions somewhere intermediate to the genitalia of a normal female and that of a normal male. These anomalies can be anatomically identical to each other, whether their etiologic factor is congenital adrenal hyperplasia (CAH), male hermaphroditism, true hermaphroditism, or some other intersex syndrome. External genitalia proceeds along the female lines except in the presence of some virilizing influence acting on the developing embryo (i.e., androgens). The conversion of testosterone to dihydrotestosterone by 5α-reductase activity occurs in the skin of the external genitalia and UGS in early gestation. Masculinization of the external genitalia ensues in the presence of functional androgens regardless of genetic sex. In the case of female pseudohermaphroditism—XX chromosomes in the presence of a virilizing influence—the fusion of the scrotolabial folds may be sufficient to obscure or conceal the vagina from the outside or even to entirely suppress its formation. The urethra can be formed for varying distances or along the entire length of the phallus. Therefore, the operative procedure for reconstruction of ambiguous genitalia into feminine genitalia does not vary in its essential elements, regardless of the cause of the intersexuality. The common goals for the female reconstruction of ambiguous genitalia include reduction of clitoral size, creation of labia minora, and exteriorization of the vagina.

Any reconstruction of the external genitalia with the objective of producing normal female appearance and function requires a full understanding of the surgical anatomy. It is essential to accurately identify the site of communication of the vagina with the UGS. In their classic paper in 1969, Hendren and Crawford recognized the variability of the communication of the vaginal insertion into the UGS. **Figure 24.4** illustrates the spectrum of vaginal communication with the urethra, with **Figure 24.4A** representative of a low distal communication (infrasphincteric) and **Figure 24.4B** representative of a high proximal communication (suprasphincteric). In 95% of cases, the vaginal communication

is in relation to the caudal UGS derivatives (infrasphincteric) with the vagina communicating with that portion of the UGS that in a man gives rise to the membranous portion of the male urethra and that in the woman becomes the vaginal vestibule. If this usual relation is confirmed at surgery, the persistent, anomalous UGS may be incised to the vaginal communication without fear of disturbing the urinary sphincter. In less than 5% of cases, the vagina communicates high, with the portion of the UGS that becomes the prostatic urethra in the man or the entire urethra in the woman (suprasphincteric). Knowledge of the possible variants in communication of the vagina with the UGS is critical before entertaining surgical correction. Preoperatively, genitography showing the relationship of the UGS, urethra, vagina, and bladder may be helpful. Contrast is injected retrogradely through the perineal meatus of the UGS. Delineation of this anatomy can be elucidated at the time of surgery with the use of endoscopy to evaluate where the vagina communicates with the UGS. In 1989, Bargy and colleagues described the anatomic lesions in the intersexual states based on clinical and anatomic observations.

One objective of the reconstruction procedure for external genitalia is to delay the procedure until the anomalous structures are of a size to permit easy identification of all structures. As observed by Azziz and coworkers, vaginal repair may be delayed until menarche, when maturity and the desire for sexual activity are usually well established. There is present debate in the need for early reconstruction for the sole purpose of cosmesis to prevent embarrassment or anxiety to the patient's family. Crouch and Creighton revisited the long-standing dictum of early surgical correction of ambiguous genitalia for intersex conditions. They report that some advocate the "one-stage" procedure in infancy, but that others advocate deferral of vaginal surgery until after puberty, especially given that many patients require further surgery at adolescence. It has been believed that the intersex child may be psychologically damaged by the "appearance" of uncorrected external genitalia if not performed at infancy, but unfortunately to date little research on this exists.

Most hermaphrodites reared as girls have a vagina or vaginal pouch, although in some instances, it is rudimentary. Only rarely is there no vagina, despite ambiguity of the external genitalia. The choice of operative procedure must conform to the observed anatomy. Thus, these choices are considered in the context of several categories based on anatomic structure of the anomaly.

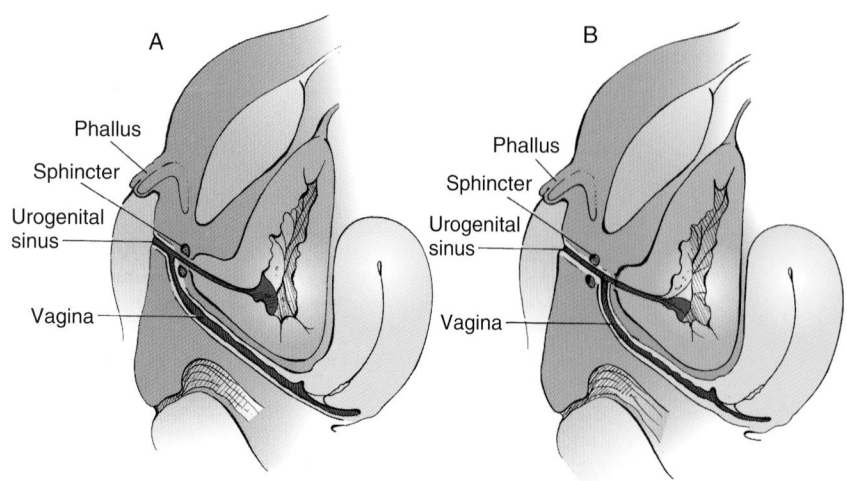

FIGURE 24.4 Illustration of the spectrum of vaginal communication with the urethra. **A:** Representative of a low distal communication (infrasphincteric). **B:** Representative of a high proximal communication (suprasphincteric).

When the Vagina Is Present and the Vaginosinus Communication Is Low The basic operation is, in essence, a modification of one described at length by Young that was previously performed successfully by various surgeons, notably in Europe. Patients with adrenal hyperplasia usually require only reconstruction of the external genitalia. However, when exploratory laparotomy is necessary to remove contradictory sex structures in other types of intersexuality or to establish the diagnosis, reconstruction of the genitalia may be considered at the same operation.

If an operation is deemed necessary at a very young age, the structures can be so small that it is impossible to introduce a finger into the UGS, and all tissues must be grasped throughout the operation with fine delicate tissue forceps. Operating loupes (2.5 to 3) are of great benefit to the surgeon. Small bipolar forceps and microscissors are also useful. Fine 5-0 or 6-0 synthetic absorbable sutures on an atraumatic needle are used throughout the procedure.

In cases of simple labial fusion, a cutback vaginoplasty (Fig. 24.5) would be sufficient to restore "normal" female genital anatomy. In cases of low vaginal confluence with the UGS (Fig. 24.4A), reconstruction may be done either by freeing the posterior vaginal wall and suturing up to the perineal external opening (Fig. 24.6) or—if a patient has copious subcutaneous fat and difficulty exists in approximating the vagina to the perineal skin—by use of a posterior flap technique, as used by Fortunoff and coworkers (Fig. 24.7).

Initially, the UGS may be thoroughly investigated with a small McCarthy panendoscope to determine accurately the position and size of the vaginal communication. If a sound or catheter can be easily introduced into the meatus of the UGS and into the vagina, use of the endoscope may be omitted. Special care is needed not to introduce the sound into the urethra.

A sound accidentally introduced into the urethra poses the danger of incising the distal urethral meatus. After the UGS is incised (to within 2 or 3 cm of the anus), the urethral orifice may be identified (Fig. 24.6A, B). A small Foley catheter may then be introduced through the urinary meatus for purposes of identification throughout the remainder of the operation. To attach the edges of the vagina to the skin, it is usually necessary to free the vagina posteriorly and laterally to secure sufficient mobilization so that these structures meet with no tension. It is unnecessary to free the vagina anteriorly, because this requires its separation from the urethra. Sufficient mobilization can ordinarily be obtained by lateral and posterior dissection. When sufficient freedom has been attained, the edges of the vagina may be secured to the skin with interrupted 5-0 sutures on an atraumatic reverse cutting needle. In the infant, four or five sutures around the edge of the vagina are usually sufficient. The edges of the incised sinus membrane may then be sutured to the skin anteriorly (Fig. 24.6D–G). A small sponge impregnated with petroleum jelly may be introduced into the vagina to maintain its patency during the healing process. The indwelling catheter may be left in place for a few days until edema of the surrounding structures has subsided. An indwelling catheter is particularly useful in children with metabolic disorders that require accurate urine collection. A pressure dressing for 24 hours reduces the incidence of incisional hematoma.

Figure 24.7 illustrates vaginoplasty with a posterior flap as advocated by Fortunoff and is useful in cases with anticipated difficulty in bringing the vaginal orifice to the outside. Briefly, a posterior-based U-flap is drawn, with corners on either side of the perineal body near the rectum (Fig. 24.7A–C). This flap must be wide enough for tension-free anastomosis. This posterior flap is dissected in the midline and is carried out between the rectum and UGS.

Sutures are individually placed through the posterior-based flap and into the split posterior vagina. Sutures are tied after all have been placed. Because the anterior wall is not disturbed, no anterior flap is required. Finally, the phallic skin is divided in the midline and moved inferiorly to create the labia minora.

Surgical reconstruction of an enlarged clitoris has undergone significant evolution. Traditionally, the clitoris was simply amputated, and a nonfunctioning cosmetic clitoris was fashioned. Although several children so treated now have normal adult sexual function, the literature is lacking in follow-up data on large patient groups. Surgical efforts now focus on concealment, plication, resection, and reduction, with an attempt to provide a normal cosmesis without sacrificing sensation or vascularity of the glans.

The clitoral flap technique has provided a somewhat better cosmetic result than simple amputation. This procedure attempts to preserve a shell of the glans on a pedicle flap. The shaft of the clitoris is subtotally resected, and the stumps are reanastomosed (Fig. 24.8). The nerve supply to the glans is severed during this procedure, with the result that sensation in the glans is diminished. Sexual function, however, seems to be satisfactory.

Rajfer and colleagues have suggested a dorsal approach to the subtotal resection of the corpora (Fig. 24.9), which has the advantage of preserving the ventral nerve supply and which should preserve sensation in the glans. This approach is theoretically desirable and can be recommended for suitable cases. As mentioned earlier, however, lack of clitoral sensation does not seem to significantly affect the later sexual behavior of patients treated by procedures that sever the dorsal nerves to the glans.

In 1999, Baskin and colleagues described the anatomic studies of the human clitoris. As in the human penis, the nerves in the clitoris form an extensive network surrounding the tunica

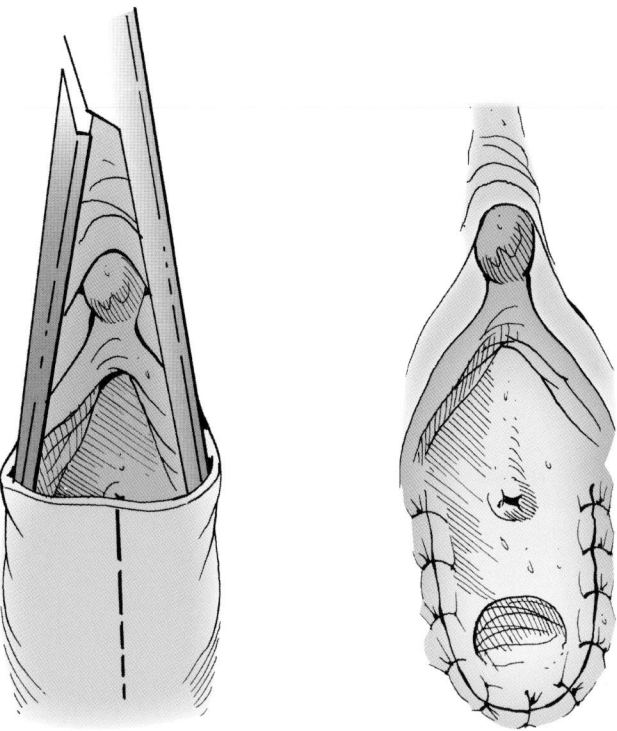

FIGURE 24.5 In cases of simple labial fusion, a cutback vaginoplasty is sufficient to restore "normal" female genital anatomy.

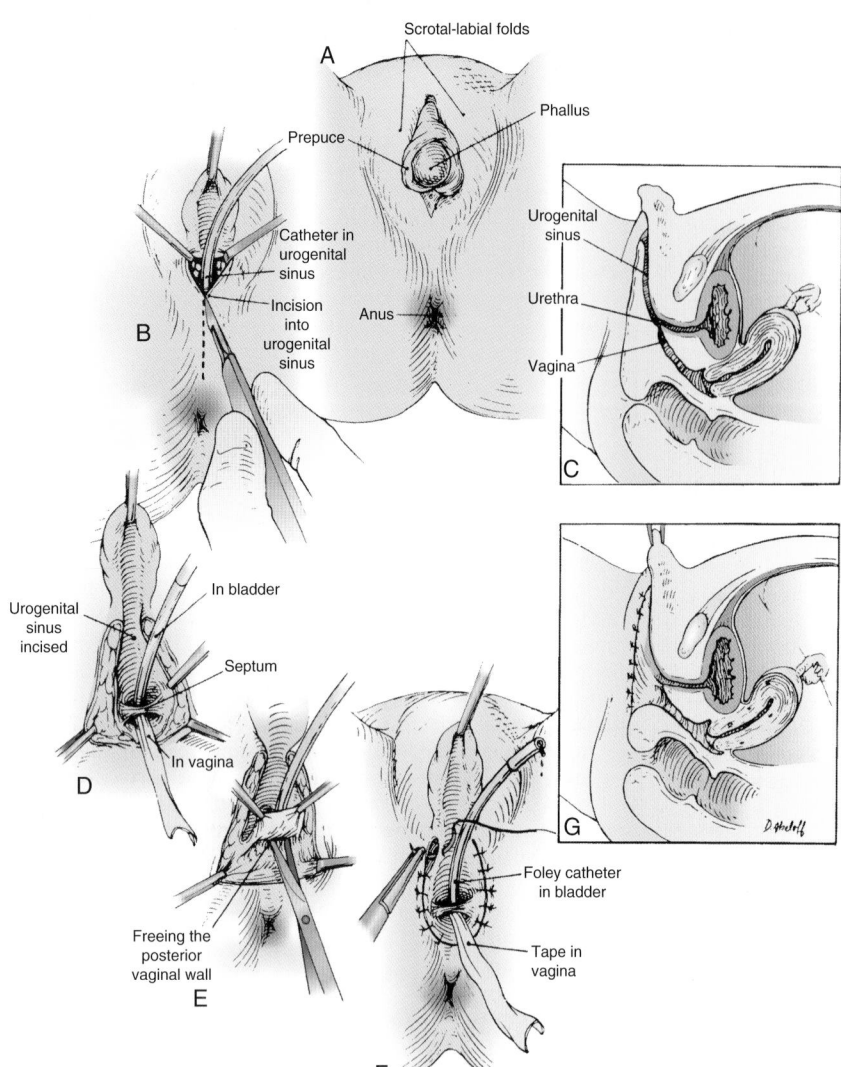

FIGURE 24.6 A: The external genitalia of an 18-month-old girl with CAH. The operation is the same, regardless of the etiology of the "virilizing" deformity. B: Beginning of the operation. Incision into the UGS. If the external meatus is large enough and the UGS will accommodate it, it is sometimes possible to introduce a catheter into the bladder through the urethra and introduce a sound into the vagina beside this. When the structures are large enough, this maneuver greatly facilitates the operative procedure by ensuring their identification. C: Lateral view showing the relations among the various structures. D: Situation after incision of the UGS. E: With the glass catheter in the bladder, the posterior vaginal wall is freed to make it possible to bring it to the skin edge without undue tension. F: The operative situation after the edges of the vagina are sutured to the skin and after the edges of the mucous membrane of the UGS are also sutured to the skin along the line of incision. G: Lateral view at the completion of the operation.

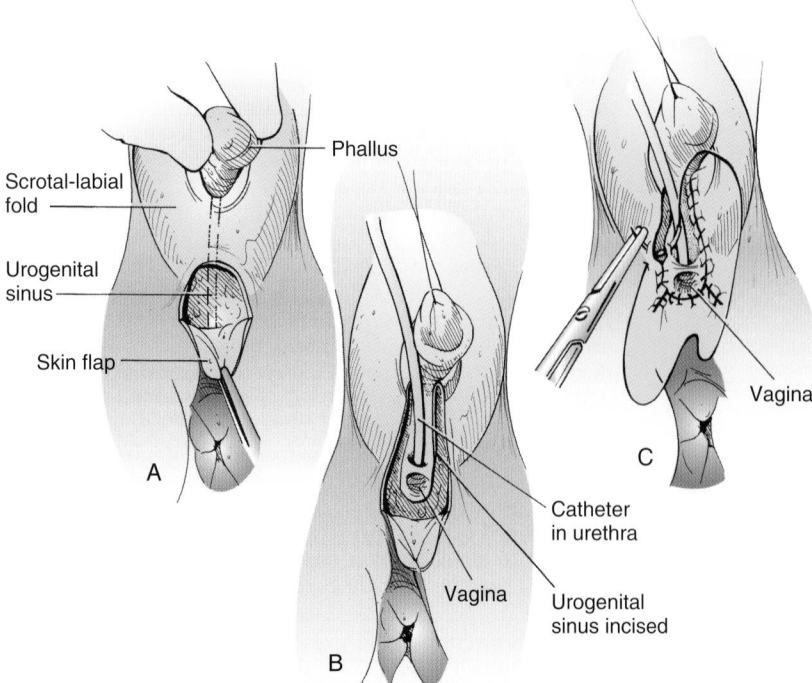

FIGURE 24.7 A posterior flap technique for when there is difficulty bringing the vaginal orifice to the outside.

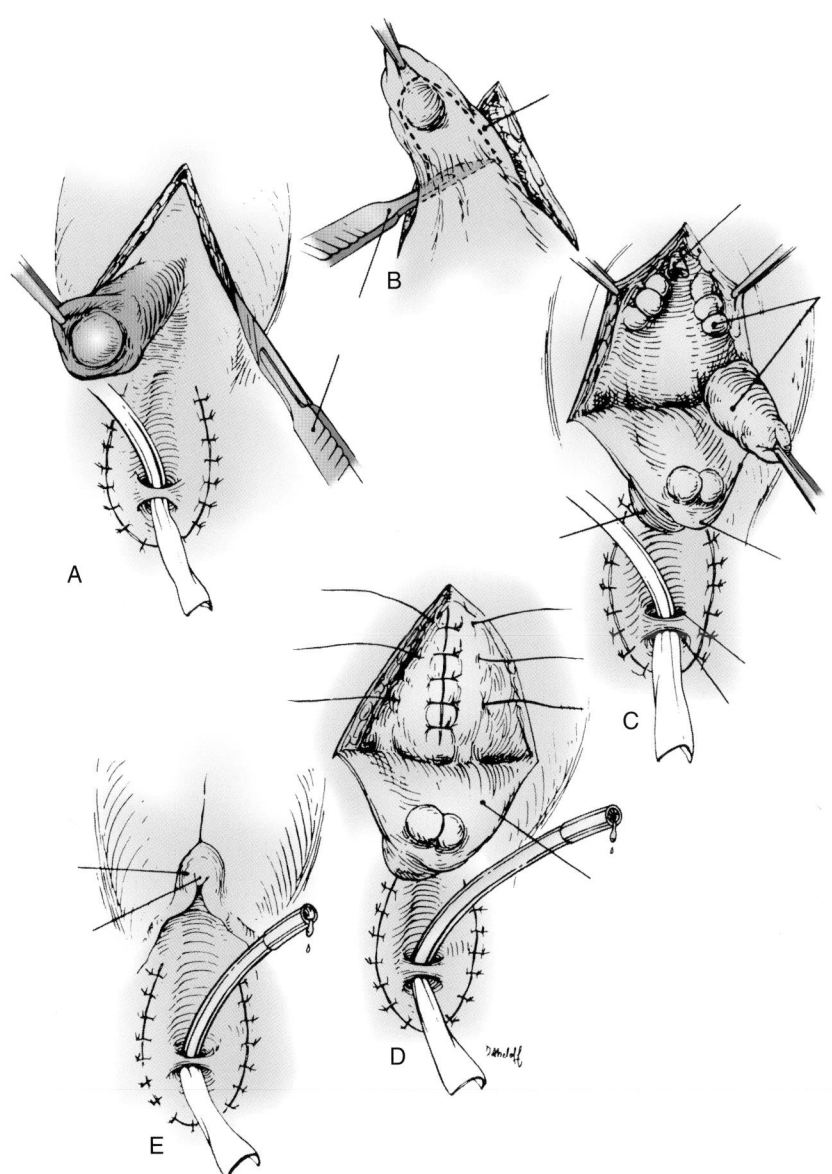

FIGURE 24.8 Clitoral reduction via the clitoral flap technique. **A:** The initial incision. **B:** The flap must be as wide as possible at the base to preserve the circulation for the glans. The glans cannot be preserved completely because the blood supply will be insufficient to maintain it. It must be as thin a shell of the glans as possible. **C:** The shaft of the phallus has been removed. **D:** There has been some closure of the space from which the corpora were removed. **E:** The flap has been sutured into place.

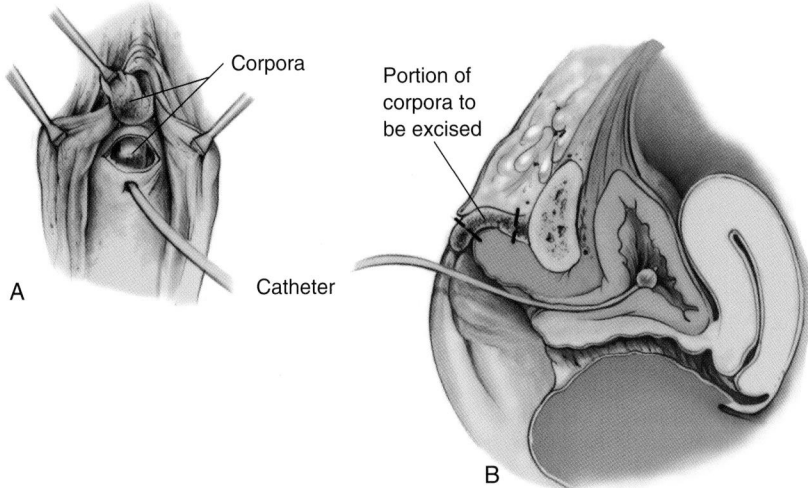

FIGURE 24.9 Clitoral reduction with the corpora exposed through a dorsal incision (operation of Rajfer et al.). **A–C:** Corpora are approached and removed through a posterior incision in the phallus.

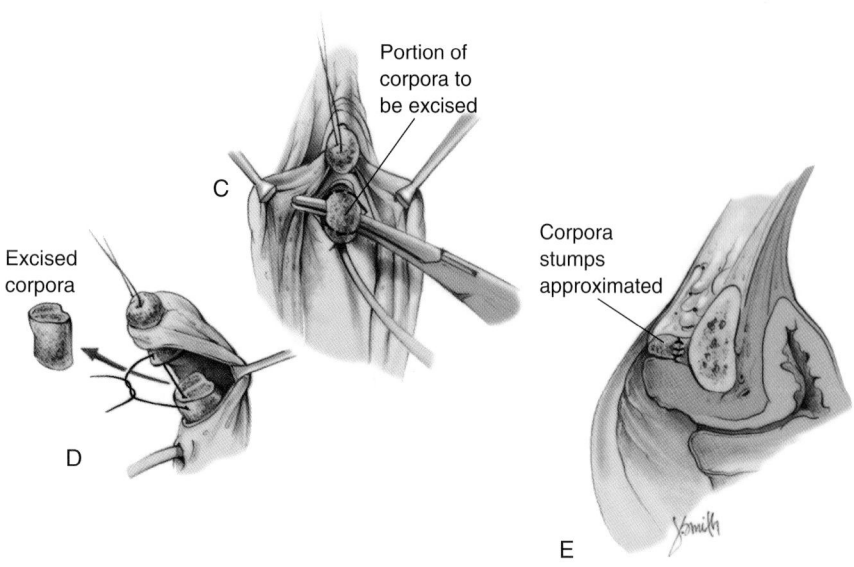

FIGURE 24.9 (*Continued*) **D:** Diagram of the excised portion of the corpora. **E:** The corpora are removed and stumps approximated.

of the corporeal body with a nerve-free zone at the 12-o'clock position. The normal clitoris has corporeal bodies that are smaller but analogous to those of the penis. The surgeon should be mindful of their function if extensive resection is considered with care to preserve the dorsal aspect of the glans.

Rink and Adams in 1998 reviewed feminizing genitoplasty. They advocated clitoral reduction without sacrificing sensation or vascularity of the glans, recommending a subtunical reduction of erectile tissue as described by Kogan and colleagues in the 1980s. The glans is preserved with its neurovascular supply intact along Buck fascia and the dorsal tunic of the corpora, yet the cavernous erectile tissue is excised. **Figure 24.10** illustrates this surgical management; additionally, the phallus is degloved, and this skin is used to create the labia minora. An incision is made around the corona of the phallus and continued inferiorly around the urethral meatus. Preservation of this meatal plate improves cosmesis and increases blood supply to the glans. The neurovascular bundle is identified, with lateral incisions into the tunica of the corpora along the phallus from the glans backward proximal to the corporal bifurcation. The cavernous erectile tissue is dissected from the inferior aspect

of the dorsal tunic and excised, and the proximal and dorsal corpora are suture ligated. The glans is secured to the inferior aspect of the pubis or to the corporal stumps.

In a pilot study of six women in 2003, Crouch and colleagues reported on genital sensation after feminizing genitoplasty for women with CAH. These women were assessed for thermal, vibratory, and light touch sensory thresholds in the clitoris and vagina using a genitosensory analyzer and Von Frey filaments. Highly abnormal results for sensation in the clitoris were found in the six women studied. In three who had an introitus capable of admitting a vaginal probe, the vaginal sensory data was considered normal. Given an abnormal clitoral sensation and normal vaginal sensation, the authors hypothesize that the abnormal clitoral findings may result from the surgical reconstruction rather than an effect of CAH. A self-administered sexual function assessment revealed that these women had sexual difficulties, particularly in the areas of infrequency of intercourse and anorgasmia. The authors voiced their concerns with the stated superiority of modern surgery. They stated that the vascularity of the glans remains vulnerable and that the risk of damage to the neurovascular bundles is inherent in any technique that

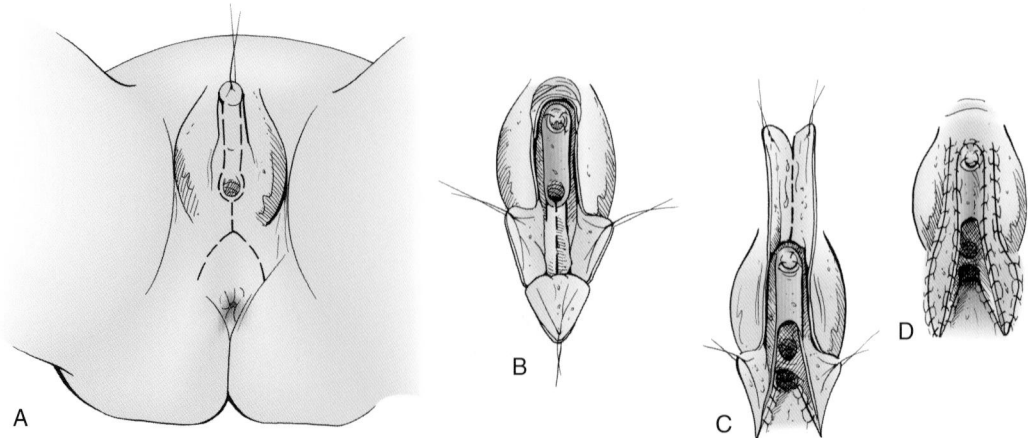

FIGURE 24.10 Surgical management of the clitoris with creation of labia minora and a posterior flap technique for vaginoplasty. **A:** Incision around the corona of the phallus continued inferiorly around the urethral meatus. **B:** Proposed incision into the posterior wall of the UGS. **C:** Degloving of the phallus. Sutures are individually placed through the posterior-based flap and into the split posterior vagina. **D:** The phallic skin is divided in the midline and moved inferiorly to create the labia minora. (From Rink RC, Adams MC. Feminizing genitoplasty: state of the art. *World J Urol* 1998;16:212. Copyright © 1998, Springer-Verlag Berlin Heidelberg. With kind permission from Springer Science and Business Media.)

entails their separation from the corporal tissue. They concluded that even after seemingly successful clitoral reduction, the sensory function is significantly impaired, and this should be taken into consideration during counseling. Larger studies are presently under way to further evaluate these findings.

When the Vaginal Orifice Is Obscured   As mentioned previously, preoperative identification and catheterization or sounding of the vaginal orifice is key to the performance of a successful, one-stage procedure. When the vagina cannot be located by sounding, it sometimes can be seen by endoscopy. When sounding and vision both fail, an attempt before surgery to introduce a small (no. 4 or 5) ureteral catheter into the vagina by blindly probing through the endoscope along the posterior wall of the UGS may assist in the identification of the vagina. Sometimes, this catheter finds the orifice. If so, it may be left within the vagina as a guide during surgical exposure of the area (**Fig. 24.11**). If the vaginal orifice cannot be located, a planned two-stage operation is indicated. The objective of the first stage is to obtain cosmetically satisfactory female genitalia by reducing the clitoris and partially excising

the UGS without exteriorizing the vagina. During the planned second stage, exteriorization of the vagina can be performed. The second stage should be postponed until identification of the vaginal orifice by sounding becomes possible. This may require waiting for puberty for estrogenization of the area. If dilators are needed for patency postoperatively, this surgery should be delayed until the girl is sufficiently mature for their appropriate use. This will maximize the success of the reoperation.

When the Vaginosinus Communication Is Blocked   Rarely does the vagina not communicate with the UGS. The vagina with the UGS is homologous with the hymenal area, and the hymen rarely is imperforate in an otherwise normal woman. For such a circumstance, we have found it helpful to pass a uterine sound downward through the fundus via hysterotomy into the vagina, thus forming a protrusion on the perineum. With such a guide, the edges of the vaginal epithelium can be located and sutured to the skin (**Fig. 24.12**). Until the uterus enlarges somewhat from its infantile state, the cavity is not large enough to accommodate even a uterine sound. Therefore,

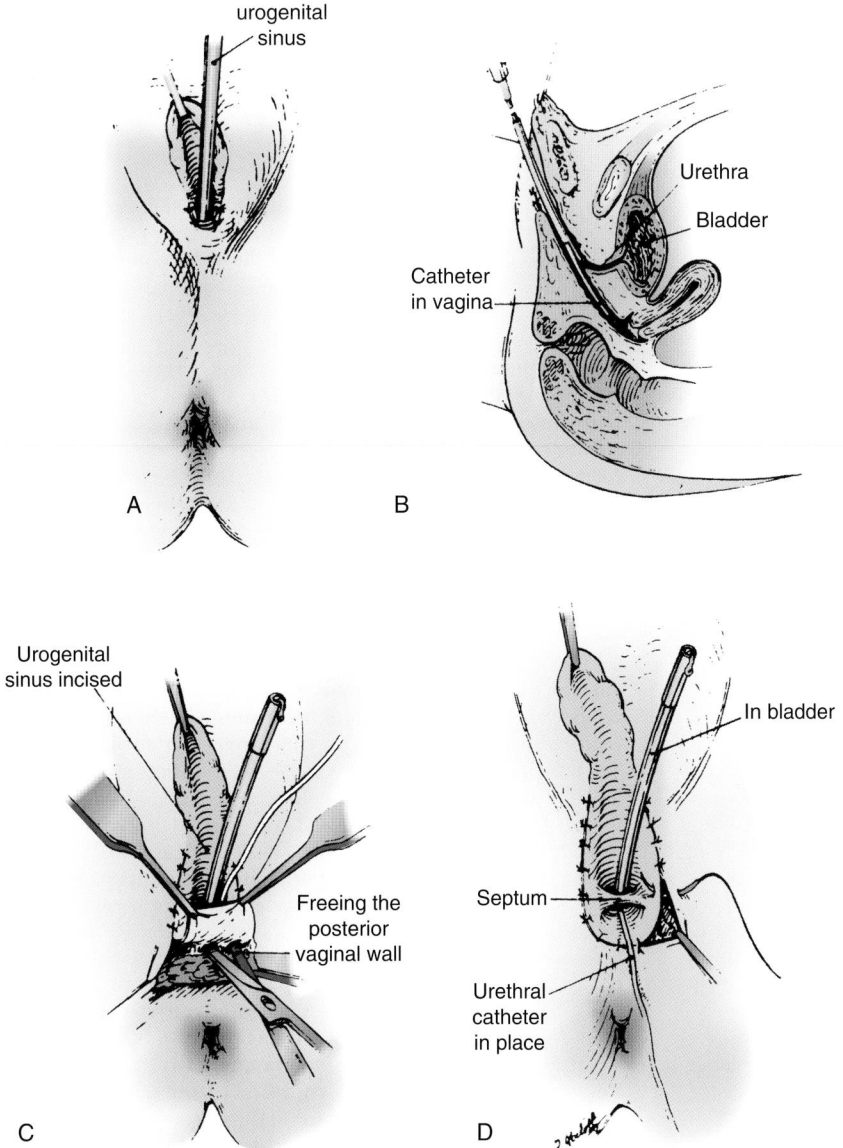

FIGURE 24.11 Operative procedure when it is difficult to locate vaginal orifice by sounding. An operative endoscope can be used to probe with a small ureteral catheter. **A:** The orifice is enlarged to accommodate the endoscope. **B:** The tip of the catheter has found the vaginal opening and entered the vagina. **C:** Freeing the posterior vaginal wall with the ureteral catheter in the vagina and a stiff catheter in the urethra. **D:** The vaginal portion of the operation is complete.

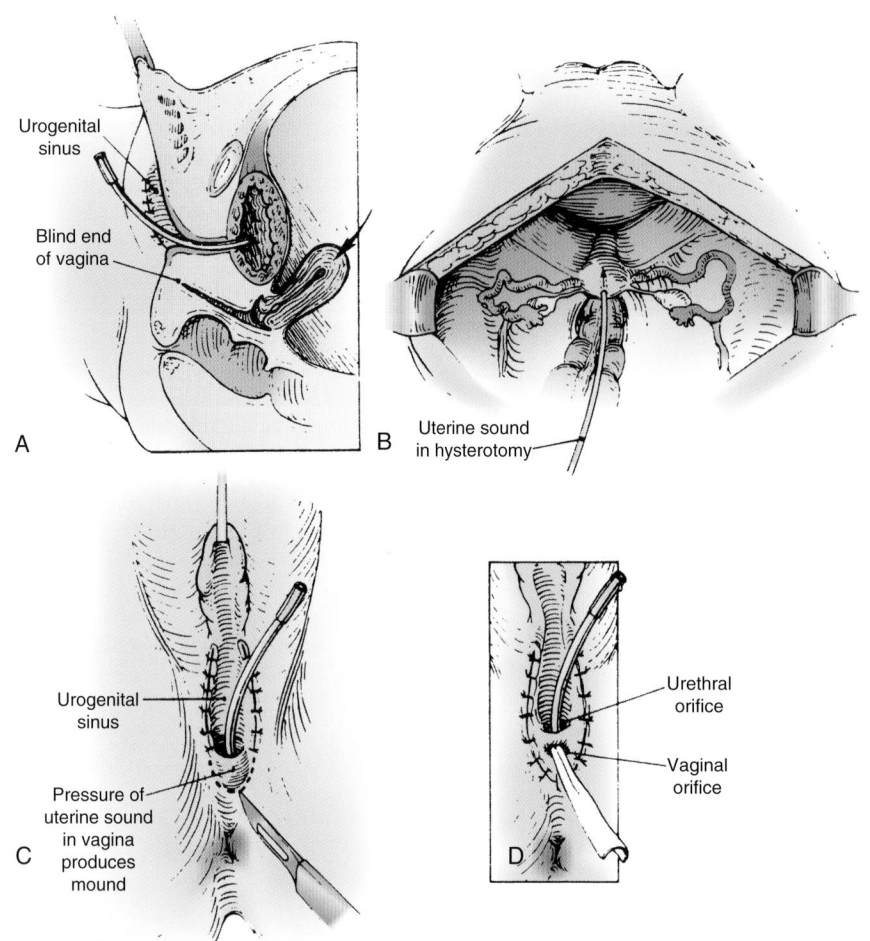

FIGURE 24.12 A: A situation in which the vaginal orifice is imperforate. **B:** A uterine sound has been passed through the fundus into the vagina. **C:** The tip of the sound can be palpated in the perineum. **D:** The completed procedure.

if such an operation is contemplated, it should not be done until there is a palpable enlargement of the uterus at the onset of puberty. Evaluation of uterine volume sonographically as a predictor of uterine size adequacy may be helpful.

When the Vaginosinus Communication Is High Hendren has been especially interested in patients whose vaginosinus communication involves the proximal urethra (suprasphincteric). He has advocated an operation that disconnects the vagina from the urethra and repositions the vaginal orifice in the perineum, the "pull-through" vaginoplasty. In his hands, this procedure seems to have been satisfactory for some patients. The procedure requires positioning the new vaginal orifice in the perineum (**Fig. 24.13**). The vast majority of patients with ambiguous external genitalia and a vagina have a vaginosinus communication well distal to the proximal urethra (infrasphincteric), and consideration of the procedure advocated by Hendren is not necessary. In patients in whom the vagina enters the UGS proximal to the external sphincter, the pull-through vaginoplasty of Hendren and Crawford or the method described by Passerini-Glazel can be used to prevent incontinence. Hendren and Crawford's vaginal pull-through remains the basis for reconstruction today. Modification to this procedure has evolved in an attempt to decrease the complexity and decrease the tendency of an isolated vagina toward stenosis. Rink and coworkers have favored a one-stage procedure using a perineal prone approach with no division of the rectum.

Results of Revision of External Genitalia Among 28 patients with adrenogenital syndrome and good follow-up treated at the Johns Hopkins Hospital, 22 (87.6%) needed further vaginal reconstructive surgery to achieve an adequate vaginal size to allow comfortable intercourse. Of the 22 patients, 5 had undergone more than 1 surgical attempt at reconstruction. The mean age of patients undergoing repeat procedures was 7.1 years. The mean age at first surgery for the whole group was 23.6 months. Vaginal reconstructive surgery was performed on 18 of these patients and was successful in 13 (72%) of the procedures. It generally is recommended that exteriorization of the vagina be postponed until near puberty, when feminization occurs and the young woman is sufficiently mature to comply with a postoperative dilatation program. The results of exteriorization performed during infancy must be followed up carefully for evidence of narrowing. In 1997, Costa and colleagues evaluated the vaginal size and sexual activity after different techniques of feminization of external genitalia in patients with pseudohermaphroditism. In their series of patients, all who underwent clitoroplasty reported orgasms, and 29% of the patients who had clitoridectomy reported no orgasms. Fifty percent of the patients who submitted to neovaginoplasty reported pain or bleeding during sexual intercourse. Satisfactory sexual intercourse was reported by 87% after vaginal dilation with acrylic molds.

In 2000, Krege and colleagues reported on the long-term follow-up of female patients with CAH from 21-hydroxylase deficiency, with special emphasis on the results of vaginoplasty.

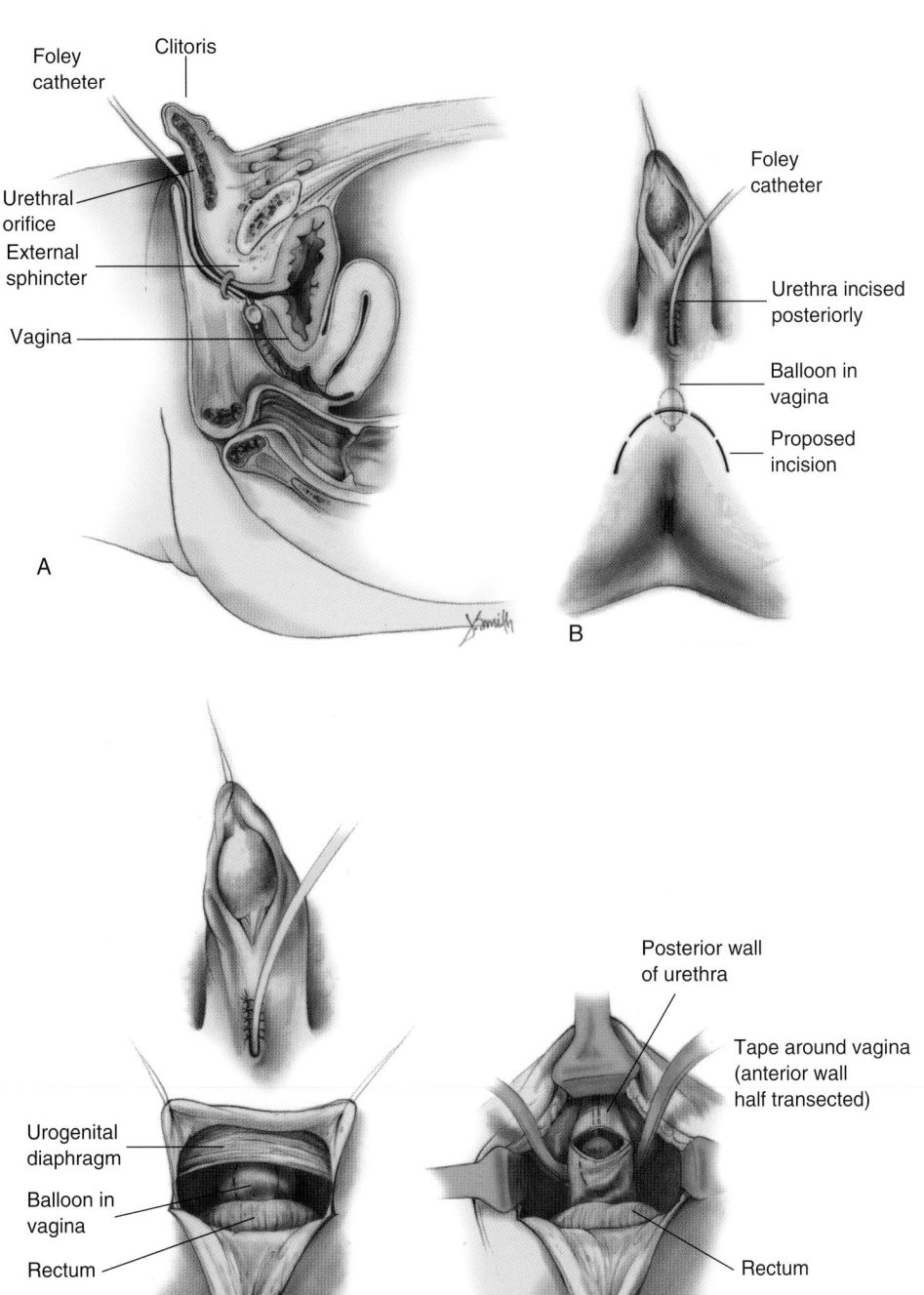

FIGURE 24.13 A perineal pull-through vaginoplasty according to Hendren. **A:** Sagittal view in diagram of high suprasphincteric vaginal communication to the UGS. A small Foley catheter is placed in the vagina to aid in its manipulation and localization. **B:** The location of the initial incision in relation to the balloon in the vagina. **C:** The flap is retracted posteriorly, and the dissection is carried along the anterior wall of the rectum until the vagina (as identified by the balloon) is approached. **D:** The vagina is identified by the Foley balloon catheter. The vagina is open. Care should be taken to pull a flap of vagina distal so that there will be no problem in closing the urethra.

They reported that the main problem during the long-term follow-up was intravaginal stenosis, with all those affected—9 of 25 (36%)—having undergone a single-stage procedure early in life to correct ambiguous genitalia (mean age, 4.7 years; range, 2 to 9 years). The authors suggested that vaginoplasty should be undertaken at the beginning of puberty, because higher estrogen levels may prevent stenosis and dilatation may be performed. In addition, 16 patients answered questionnaires that included psychological profile, and the researchers found that 14 had problems with their overall body image. Patients with correction of vaginal stenosis were particularly anxious

about sexual intercourse and had problems with orgasm. Creighton and colleagues in 2001 retrospectively evaluated the cosmetic and anatomical outcomes of 44 adolescent patients who had undergone feminizing surgery for ambiguous genitalia during their childhood. The authors reported that cosmetic results were judged as poor in 18 (41%) and that 43/44 (98%) required further treatment to the genitalia for cosmesis, tampon use, or intercourse. Of the genitoplasties planned as one-stage procedures, 23/26 (89%) required further major surgery.

Davies and colleagues in 2005 reported on urinary symptoms in adult women with CAH. The authors reported on

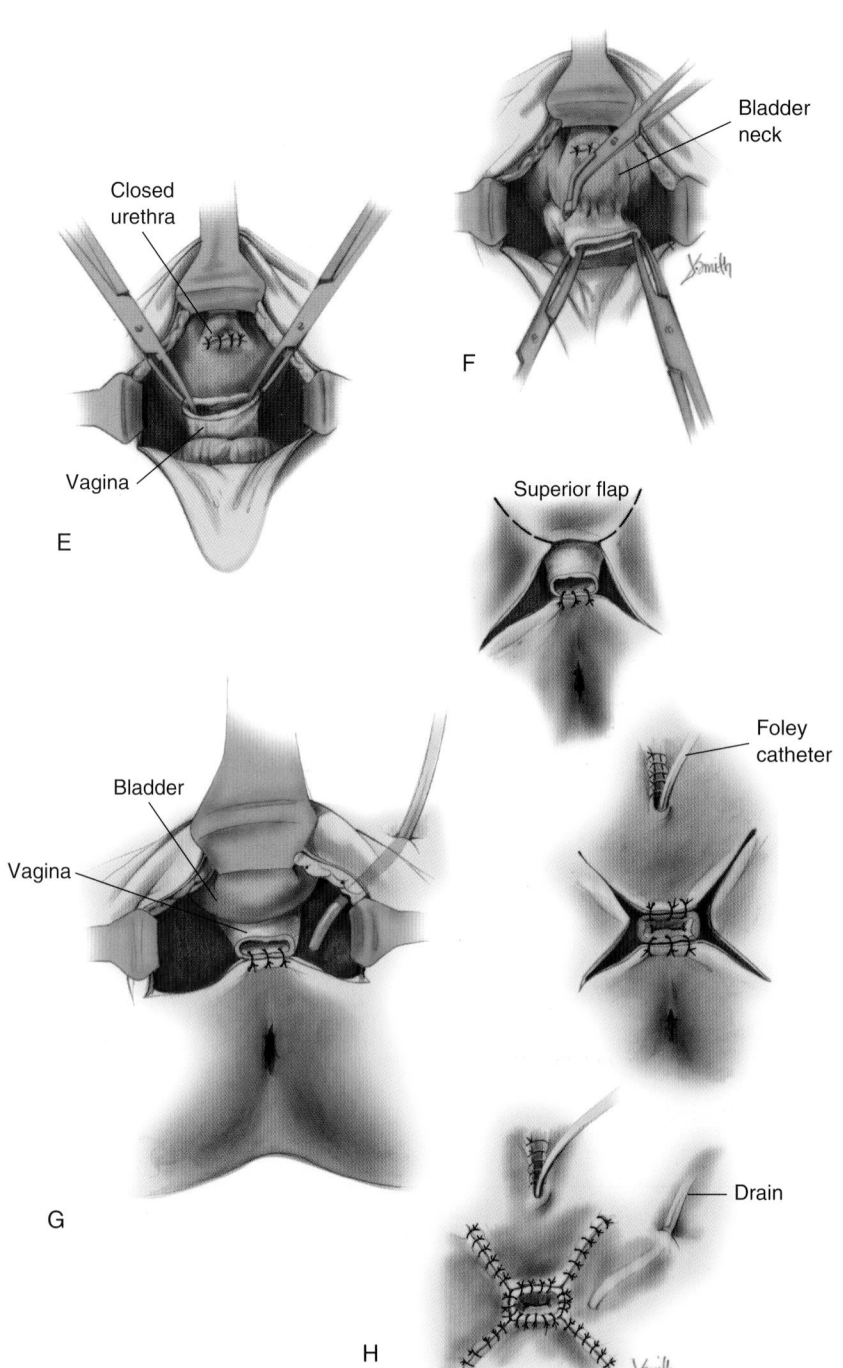

FIGURE 24.13 (*Continued*) **E:** The urethra is closed. Clips are placed on the vagina to bring it down to the perineum. **F:** The vagina is further mobilized. **G:** The edge of the vagina is attached to the original flap of perineal skin. **H:** Anterior and lateral flaps are attached. Note the use of a drain in the perivaginal space. (From Hendren WH. Reconstructive problems of the vagina and the female urethra. *Clin Plast Surg* 1980;7:207, with permission.)

19 women with CAH, of whom 16 had childhood feminizing genital surgery, and compared them with age-matched women without CAH. The Bristol Female Lower Urinary Tract Symptoms (BFLUTS) questionnaire was given to all of the women. Sixty-eight percent of the women with CAH reported urge incontinence compared with 16% of controls ($P = 0.003$). Stress incontinence was present in 47% of CAH and 26% of the controls. Nine of the CAH women reported that their urinary symptoms had an adverse effect on their lives, whereas only one of the controls did ($P = 0.008$). The authors concluded that women with CAH are more likely to have urinary symptoms than controls. It is important to emphasize that it is

not known whether these results are associated with the surgical procedures that the women underwent or an effect of CAH itself. For counseling purposes, this information is important because in two thirds of these CAH women, urinary symptoms persisted.

Historically, it has been assumed that psychosexual development of infants with intersex disorders is mostly due to rearing rather than being intrinsic. Over the past decade, the role of testosterone imprinting of the fetal brain has been studied to evaluate the role of this hormone in determining male sexual orientation. Studies in the 1990s of girls with CAH have confirmed that such children engage in more rough-and-tumble play than their affected peers and that difficulties with adjustment to their assigned sex may exist. Nonetheless, few studies have been conducted to address the social, psychological, and sexual outcomes for affected adolescents and adults, although it appears that most function in the normal range and are well adjusted. The majority of girls appear not to overtly demonstrate sexual identity problems.

Ozbey and coauthors reported on the experience of sex (re)assignment in genotypic female (46XX) patients with CAH when complicated by delayed presentation and inadvertent assignment. They reported on 70 patients with CAH who between 1983 and 2002 were counseled for sex assignment. They evaluated age at diagnosis and operation, the degree of virilization, parental consanguinity, and the sex preference of the families as factors determining sex (re)assignment decision-making. Forty-one of 70 (59%) presented after the neonatal period, and in these cases, all of the parents had assumed or were advised of a sex based on external genitalia appearance. Forty-nine of 70 were reared as girls, and 21 were reared as "boys." Of these 21 "boys," only 9 could be reassigned as girls (mean age, 7.9 months), and the other 12, with mean age at presentation of 55.8 months, were reared as "boys" in compliance with the parents' and the study group's decision. These "boys" underwent appropriate masculinizing reconstructive surgery. They concluded that age of presentation was critical for the ability to correctly assign the sex of patients with CAH.

Secondary Operations A secondary operation on the vaginal outlet may be required. This is generally the case if the basic operation is deliberately accomplished in two stages, whatever the reason. A secondary operation may be indicated, for example, when an infant's vaginal orifice is not readily identifiable, yet it seems desirable to construct cosmetically acceptable female genitalia at a very early age. Care should be taken when considering the appropriate age for performing a clitoroplasty. Some have recommended that this can be done in the newborn and that the vagina may be exteriorized at puberty as a second operation. Alizai and colleagues reported on the outcome of feminizing genitoplasty in 14 postpubertal girls (mean age, 13.1 years) with CAH. These girls were assessed under anesthesia by a pediatric urologist, plastic/reconstructive surgeon, and gynecologist. Thirteen of fourteen had previously undergone feminizing genitoplasty in early childhood. The authors reported that the outcome of clitoral surgery was unsatisfactory (clitoral atrophy or prominent glans) in six of the girls. Additional vaginal surgery was necessary for normal comfortable intercourse in 13 of the girls. In the girls with a history of vaginal reconstruction in infancy, fibrosis and scarring were prominent. The authors concluded that these results were disappointing, even in the girls who had their surgery performed by specialist surgeons. The authors highlighted the importance of late follow-up and the challenges in the prevailing assumption that total correction can be achieved with a single-stage operation in infancy. When the complete operation is attempted at an early age, the vagina is sometimes not satisfactorily exteriorized. Vaginal stenosis may require reconstruction at the time of puberty (**Fig. 24.14**). In this circumstance, there usually has been a failure to carry the midline incision far enough posteriorly, and a second procedure is required to complete the first one by continuing the midline incision far enough posteriorly.

In other cases, contraction at the vaginal outlet may occur even if the operation is adequately performed. A minor revision of the vaginal orifice is required to enlarge the vaginal orifice by making an incision in the midline and closing it at

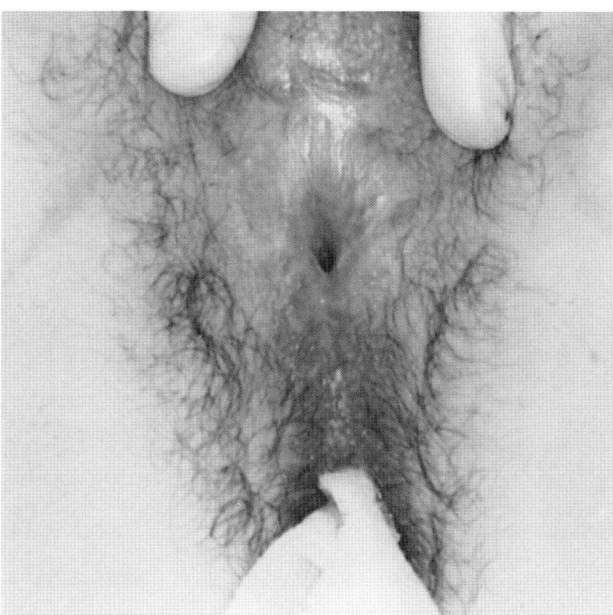

FIGURE 24.14 External genitalia of a 15-year-old patient with vaginal stenosis. Revision of the external genitalia, including an exteriorization of the vagina, had been performed in infancy.

90 degrees to the original axis of the incision (**Fig. 24.15**). In some instances, it may be necessary to create flaps to enlarge the vaginal orifice (**Fig. 24.16**).

It should be emphasized that simple exteriorization of the lower vaginal tract can be combined with cosmetic correction of virilized external genitalia in infancy, but in most cases, it is best to defer definitive reconstruction of the intermediate or high vagina until after puberty.

Exstrophy–Epispadias Complex

Exstrophy–epispadias complex (ECC) is a rare congenital anomaly occurring in live births in a 1:25,000 to 1:40,000 ratio. There is a male predominance over females in a ratio of about 2:1. Classic ECC is characterized by (a) absence of the lower anterior abdominal wall, (b) absence of the anterior wall of the posterior bladder so that the posterior bladder wall and the ureteric orifices are exposed, (c) a poorly defined bladder neck and urethra, and (d) wide separation of the pubic symphysis. A genital abnormality typically present in girls with bladder exstrophy is anterior displacement and narrowing of the vagina (**Fig. 24.17**) and separation of the clitoris into two distinct bodies (**Fig. 24.18**).

Bladder exstrophy, cloacal exstrophy, and epispadias are variants of the ECC. These defects have been attributed to failure of the normal process of ingrowth of mesoderm and the consequent lack of reinforcement of the cloacal membrane. The normal cloacal membrane is bilaminar and occupies the caudal end of the germinal disc. An ingrowth of mesenchyme between the ectodermal and endodermal layers of the cloacal membrane forms the lower abdominal wall musculature and the pelvic bones. After mesenchymal ingrowth occurs, descent of the urorectal septum divides the cloacal membrane into the bladder anteriorly and the rectum posteriorly. The urorectal septum eventually meets with the posterior remnant of the cloacal membrane, which perforates to form the anal and UGS openings. The paired genital tubercles migrate medially and fuse in the midline anterior to the

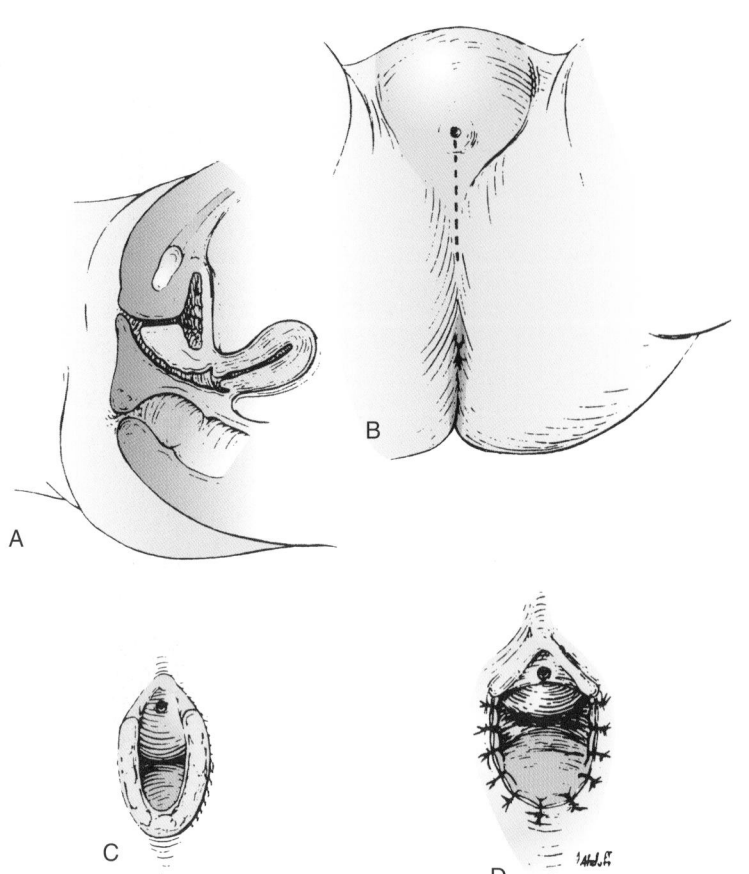

FIGURE 24.15 **A:** Repeated operation on the vaginal outlet when the operation was not completed at the first procedure. **B:** The posterior incision. **C:** The vagina is exposed. **D:** The closure.

cloacal membrane before perforation. Without its normal support from mesenchymal derivatives, the cloacal membrane is subject to premature rupture. Depending on the extent of the infraumbilical defect and the stage of development when rupture occurs, bladder exstrophy, cloacal exstrophy, or epispadias develops (**Fig. 24.19**). Jones reviewed the records of all female patients diagnosed with bladder exstrophy at Johns Hopkins Hospital over a 20-year time span. Of 18 patients with adequately described external genitalia, 13 had small,

anteriorly displaced vaginal orifices, and the remaining five patients had vaginal orifices of normal size and location. In this series, only a third of patients with ECC demonstrated the defect of narrowing of the vagina.

Exstrophy–epispadias complex may be associated with a wide range of both genital and extragenital abnormalities. Stanton reviewed 70 patients with bladder exstrophy and observed an increased incidence of various müllerian anomalies. Eleven patients were observed to have associated rectal

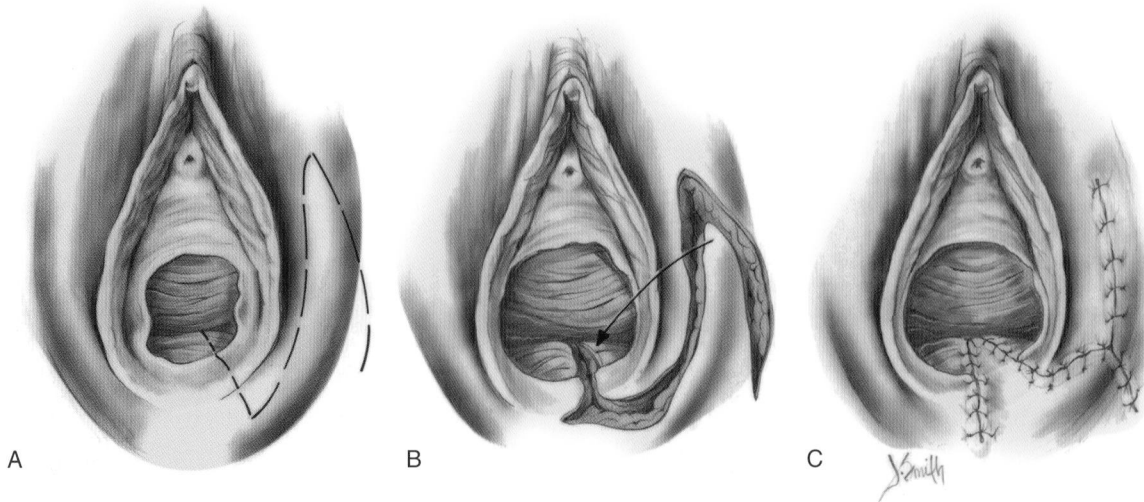

FIGURE 24.16 Labial cutaneous flap. **A:** An incision is made through the labia skin and subcutaneous fat. **B:** The flap is rotated into the perineotomy incision. **C:** The flap is sutured in place by interrupted 3-0 delayed absorbable sutures. This may be repeated on the other side if required.

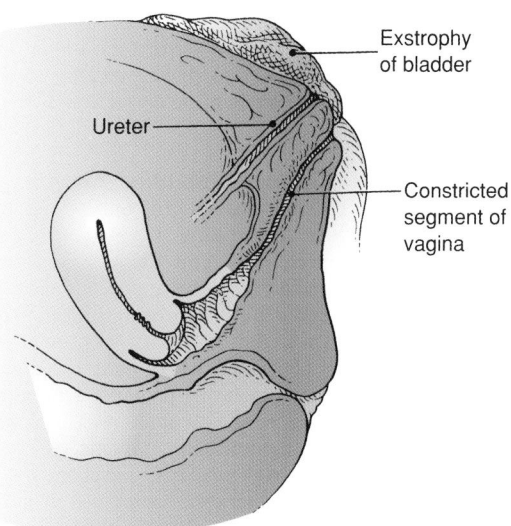

FIGURE 24.17 Common gynecologic anomaly seen in women with bladder exstrophy. The vagina is rotated anteriorly and constricted over its distal portion.

prolapse. Blakely and Mills observed various extragenital abnormalities in their series, including rectal prolapse, imperforate anus, exophthalmos, renal agenesis, and spina bifida.

Treatment Our understanding of appropriate urologic management of bladder exstrophy has evolved greatly over the past few decades; improved management has markedly increased the life expectancy and quality of life of these patients. Historical methods of treatment involved bladder excision and a urinary diversion procedure such as ureterosigmoidostomy. These techniques were complicated by serious sequelae, including pyelonephritis, hyperchloremic acidosis, rectal incontinence, ureteral obstruction, and later development of malignancy. Modern care of the patient with complex pelvic congenital disorders mandates a multidisciplinary approach that includes gynecologic surgeons, urologists, neurologists, endocrinologists, pediatricians, and allied health professionals.

Urologic management of bladder exstrophy relies on a staged approach to functional bladder closure. The initial

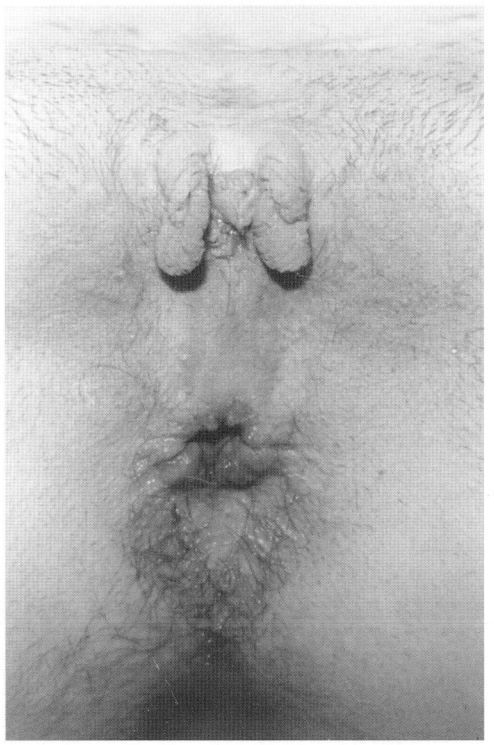

FIGURE 24.18 Preoperative photograph of a patient undergoing reconstruction of the external genitalia. Note the bifid clitoris and small anterior vaginal orifice.

procedure consists of primary bladder closure with or without iliac osteotomies to aid closure of the pelvic ring and growth and improvement of bladder capacity. The second-stage procedures usually involve bladder neck reconstruction to improve continence and bilateral ureteral reimplantations to prevent reflux. Both failures and primary reconstruction have also been performed using continence urostomies, such as the Mainz II pouch. Mingin and coworkers and Gerharz and colleagues have reported their success using this technique.

Genital anomalies in ECC can usually be sufficiently corrected to allow for sexual activity and pregnancy. The adjunctive gynecologic procedures in ECC attempt to correct the

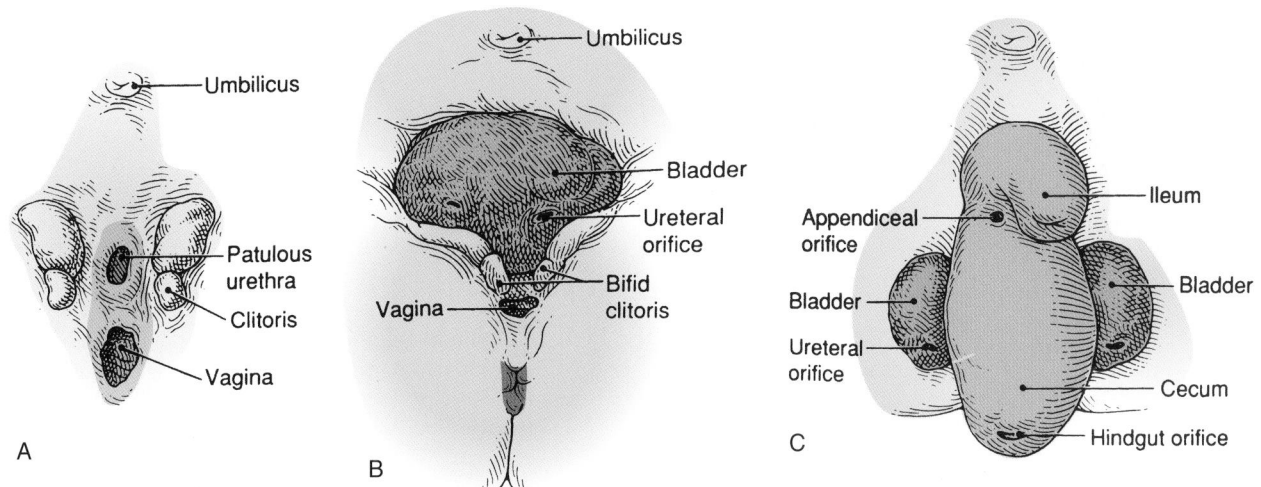

FIGURE 24.19 Anatomic features of (**A**) epispadias, (**B**) classic bladder exstrophy, and (**C**) cloacal exstrophy in females.

anterior displacement and narrowing of the vagina and the bifid separation of the clitoris.

The surgical approach to the external genitalia in patients with ECC has evolved from that first described by Howard Jones Jr. in 1973. Particular emphasis is placed on attainment of an adequate vaginal diameter without further predisposing to subsequent prolapse. The first step is vertical incision into the posterior raphe of what resembles fused scrotolabial folds; next, Allis clamps are placed laterally for traction. Fine-needle point electrocautery is then used to further open the incision, with special care taken not to take this incision too far posteriorly. The lateral portions of the incision are secured with 3-0 nonreactive absorbable sutures for further traction. The posterior vaginal edges are undermined to allow their mobilization to the exterior. The vaginal mucosa is then approximated to the perineal surface with interrupted and figure-of-eight sutures, incorporating the superficial perineal muscles into the closure. In the more posterior portion of the closure, 2-0 nonreactive absorbable suture is used, because this is the area of greatest tension. At completion, there is a significant increase in the diameter of the vagina, and the vaginal orifice usually accommodates two fingers.

Experience with management of ambiguous genitalia has shown a decrease in the incidence of postoperative vaginal stenosis if dilatation therapy is employed during the constrictive phase (the first 6 weeks) of healing. For this reason, following reconstruction of the external genitalia and exteriorization of the vagina, appropriately sized Lucite dilators are used once or twice a day for this 6-week period or until healing is complete. Patients who undergo surgical correction in early infancy are at risk for vaginal stenosis as they age. In a series by Cerveillone, one third of patients corrected in infancy underwent vaginoplasty by age 15.

Reapproximation of the bifid clitoris (**Fig. 24.20**) is primarily cosmetic and may disrupt erogenous sensitivity. The technique involves excising a diamond-shaped area of skin and subcutaneous tissue between the clitoral bodies. The medial aspect of each side of the clitoris is then denuded and undermined to allow a central reapproximation with a side-to-side closure.

Other surgical approaches have been described to optimize cosmesis. Stanton performed perineotomy in six patients with bladder exstrophy in which the labia and clitoris were reapproximated by a Z-plasty technique. Still others have described extraordinary efforts to restore the mons pubis and female escutcheon with skin flaps of hair-bearing areas. These latter reports, however, fail to mention correction of the vaginal anomaly.

Pregnancy and Exstrophy–Epispadias Complex Several series have reviewed subsequent pregnancy outcomes in patients with bladder exstrophy. Clemetson extensively reviewed the literature in 1958 and found 45 patients who underwent 64 pregnancies. A very high incidence of uterine prolapse was observed both before and after pregnancy. In addition, there was a higher incidence of premature labor and malpresentations (24%). Krisiloff and colleagues also reported a high incidence of uterine prolapse related to pregnancy, which occurred in 6 of 7 women. Burbige and coworkers reported on 14 pregnancies in patients with a history of bladder exstrophy. Uterine prolapse occurred in 7 of 11 patients, all of whom had undergone a previous urinary diversion procedure.

The mode of delivery in patients with prior urinary diversion procedures has primarily been spontaneous vaginal delivery. The increased incidence of premature labor and malpresentation, however, has warranted an increased rate of cesarean sections for obstetric indications. In patients with a prior bladder reconstruction, most surgeons advocate an elective cesarean section to eliminate stress on the pelvic floor and to avoid trauma to the delicate urinary sphincter mechanism.

Pelvic Prolapse and Exstrophy–Epispadias Complex Several mechanisms have been proposed to explain the high incidence of uterine prolapse in patients with bladder exstrophy. These mechanisms include (a) a deficiency of the pelvic floor that is due to the wide separation of the pubic symphysis, (b) an inherent deficiency of the cardinal ligament complex, and (c) the abnormal axis and short length of the vagina.

Because wide separation of the pubic symphysis results in an enlarged genital hiatus and deficiency of the pelvic floor, it is possible that iliac osteotomy may be helpful in deterring pelvic organ prolapse by closer approximation of the levator ani and puborectal muscles. Although Gearhart and Jeffs suggest

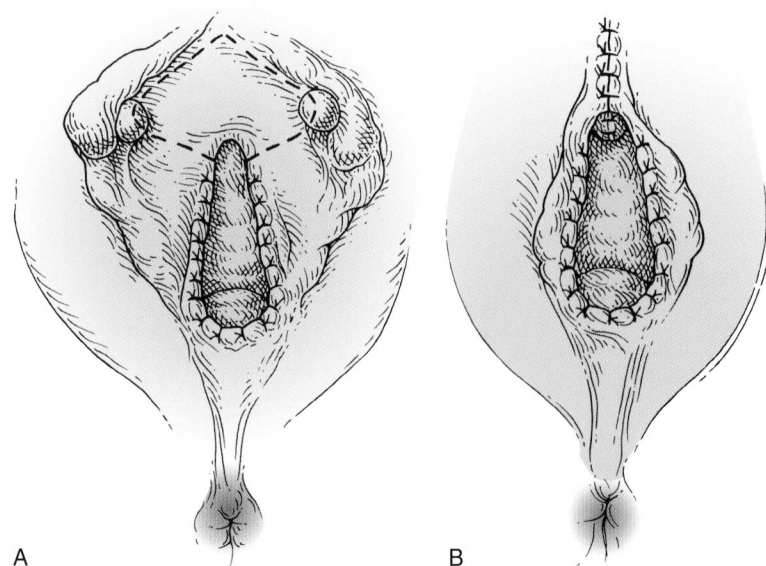

A   B

FIGURE 24.20 Schematic depiction of procedure to reapproximate the clitoris. A vulvovaginoplasty has already been performed to exteriorize the vagina. **A:** A diamond-shaped piece of skin and subcutaneous tissue between the clitoral bodies is excised. **B:** The clitoral bodies are then undermined and mobilized to the center for a side-to-side reapproximation.

that iliac osteotomies may not be necessary if primary bladder closure is performed in the first 72 hours of life, perhaps the procedure should be given increased consideration in female patients who present such a high risk for uterine prolapse later in life.

It appears important not to extend the midline perineal incision too far posteriorly in revision of the genitalia in these patients. As the incision proceeds posteriorly, the midline septum thickens to approximately 2 cm. At this point, the levator ani muscles may be severed, further enlarging the genital hiatus. It is prudent, therefore, to be more conservative; postoperative dilator therapy may aid in achieving further vaginal diameter if needed. A case referred to us illustrates this point. A 16-year-old nulliparous patient with bladder exstrophy and a history of staged bladder reconstruction underwent revision of the external genitalia. A large posterior incision into the perineal body had left a gaping introitus, and uterine prolapse had occurred several months after this procedure. Our initial approach was to reconstruct the perineal body to help contain the uterus and improve support to the pelvic floor. This reconstruction has been successful, without further prolapse 5 years after the procedure. Blakely and Mills, who observed uterine prolapse occurring very soon after enlargement of the vaginal introitus, reported a similar case.

Management of uterine prolapse associated with bladder exstrophy is particularly difficult when the patient desires preservation of childbearing. Sacrospinous fixation of the cervix may be considered, although an abnormally short vagina may produce difficulty in obtaining the suspension without significant suture bridges. An abdominal sacrocervicopexy may also be considered. Dewhurst and coworkers described this approach in 1980. They suspended the uterus to the sacrum using Ivalon sponge in a patient with procidentia following repair of bladder exstrophy.

Of note, the multiple operative and cystoscopic procedures performed on this group of patients have resulted in latex sensitization rates similar to that seen in health care workers. Ricci and coworkers evaluated 17 patients (15 children, 2 young adults) with bladder exstrophy for latex allergy. Twelve had latex sensitization, with five demonstrating serious symptoms.

Cosmetic Gynecologic Surgery

Women may seek surgical procedures to address the appearance of their external genitalia. It is the obligation of gynecologic surgeons to educate women on the wide range of normalcy of the female genitalia. Medical indications for labioplasty may include labial hypertrophy or asymmetrical labial growth. This procedure may be performed via simple linear removal, wedge resection, or Z-plasty. Some women may seek surgical procedures to enhance sexual function. There are few long-term safety or efficacy studies to support these interventions, which include reduction of the clitoral hood, perineoplasty, vaginoplasty, and hymenoplasty, and are often bundled under the lay term "vaginal rejuvenation." These procedures are not sanctioned by the American Congress of Obstetricians and Gynecologists and, like all vulvovaginal surgery, carry the risk of infection, dyspareunia, scarring, and unsatisfactory cosmesis.

Vaginal Trauma Post Sexual Assault

The National Violence Against Women Survey estimates that more than 300,000 women are the victims of sexual assault every year. Of these, about half are under the age of 18. Although the risk of surgical injury to the vagina is low in most cases of sexual assault, the risk increases under certain circumstances. These include when the perpetrator utilizes a weapon in the assault and/or is under the influence of drugs or alcohol at the time of the assault. Careful history and a judicious examination are needed to rule out acute genital trauma. In most urban settings, rape is initially evaluated in hospital-based programs. Gynecologists who are called to evaluate the victims of sexual assault should be familiar with the forensic and legal implications of the examination.

THE URETHRA

The female urethra develops from the caudal end of the UGS after it separates from the vaginal canal between the eighth and twelfth week of embryologic life. Because the vagina and urethra are so closely integrated, the urethra shares many common disease processes and anatomic defects with the vagina. Bacteria in the lower genital tract frequently colonize in the outer urethra, harbor in the paraurethral glands, and enter the bladder to produce acute infections. A bacterial infection in the lower genital tract may not become clinically manifest for several years, until a Skene duct cyst or a urethral diverticulum develops. Estrogen deficiency causes atrophic changes of the vaginal mucosa and can have a similar effect on the urethral mucosa. Thinning of the epithelium and irritation of the sensory nerve fibers can cause urinary frequency and dysuria. Prolapse at the external meatus also may result from atrophic changes of the urethra.

Diverticulum of the Urethra

Urethral diverticulum is characterized by urethral mucosa herniating into surrounding tissues. The condition probably occurs more frequently than it is diagnosed; whenever an article reporting on urethral diverticulum appears in the literature, there is a coincident upsurge in the number of cases diagnosed. According to the National Hospital Discharge Survey (1979 to 1998), 27,000 inpatient procedures were performed for the repair of urethral diverticula in the United States over a 19-year period.

Etiology

In 1941, Parmenter suggested several congenital factors that could develop into a urethral diverticulum, including Gartner duct, a faulty union of primal folds, cell nets, and wolffian ducts or vaginal cysts that rupture into the urethra. Additional possible causes include trauma at childbirth, surgical trauma, urethral stone, urethral stricture, and infection of the urethral glands. Malignancy has been reported in a small percentage of cases.

The most probable etiology of urethral diverticulum is chronic infection of the suburethral tissue by vaginal flora. Huffman's experiments support the notion that a suburethral infection can develop into an abscess that becomes lined with epithelium. Huffman demonstrated periurethral openings by constructing wax models of infected urethras. The usual organisms cultured are *Escherichia coli*, *Aerobacter aerogenes*, and other gram-negative bacilli; *Staphylococcus aureus*; and *Streptococcus faecalis*.

Symptoms

Dysuria, urgency, frequency, and hematuria occurred together in 85% to 90% of 32 cases reviewed by Peters and Vaughn. Other frequently occurring symptoms are a lump in the vagina caused by protrusion of the diverticulum sac into the vagina, dyspareunia (intermittent discharge from the urethra), and pain on walking. Pyuria and cystitis also occur, depending on the location of the diverticular orifice. If the opening is sufficiently close to the outer end of the urethra, there may be no leakage of purulent exudate back into the bladder, which may explain the absence of symptoms of cystitis in 5% of cases. If the diverticulum is located in the posterior urethra near the urethrovesical junction, stress urinary incontinence may be a significant symptom. In a review of 70 cases from the Johns Hopkins Hospital, Ginsberg and Genadry found that 17% of the diverticula were located in the proximal (outer) urethra, 43% in the midurethra, and 31% in the distal (posterior) urethra; in the remaining cases, the site was not specifically identified. Urethral diverticulum should be considered in all cases of refractory urinary tract infection in women.

Diagnosis

Urethral diverticula usually are small, varying from 3 mm to 3 cm in diameter. Some of the larger sacs cover the entire length of the urethra. They are almost exclusively present on the distal two thirds of the posterior wall of the urethra. On palpation of a suburethral mass, tenderness commonly is found. Pressure on the mass may cause the escape of urine or exudate from the urethral meatus.

An examination of the floor of the urethra through the water cystoscope while suburethral pressure is being applied reveals an opening in 50% to 70% of cases. The pressure may force contents of the diverticulum into the urethra while it is being viewed. Some of the openings are extremely small and may be missed. Inflammatory swelling can result in edema of the orifice, which makes visualization difficult or impossible.

The diagnosis of urethral diverticulum is firmly established by means of positive-pressure urethrography (PPUG). A special catheter is used to block the urethra at both ends and to fill it and the diverticulum under pressure with water-soluble contrast medium (**Figs. 24.21** to **24.23**). If the urethral orifice to the diverticulum is quite large, a voiding cystourethrogram together with a positive pelvic film may demonstrate the diverticulum. Although not as sensitive as PPUG, voiding cystourethrography (VCUG) may assist in identifying a urethral diverticulum. Wang and Wang compared VCUG and PPUG in evaluating 120 women. Twenty of 120 women demonstrated diverticulum. Thirteen were positive on PPUG and 10 with VCUG. If the surgeon's suspicion is high for urethral diverticulum, MRI should be considered if both the PPUG and VCUG studies are negative.

Gerrard and colleagues have shown that transvaginal ultrasound is effective for evaluating patients with suspected urethral diverticulum. The technique is accurate, low cost, readily available, and should be considered as an initial screening technique for women when one suspects a urethral diverticulum. Computerized tomography and MRI have better defined diverticular anatomy. Neitlich and colleagues have suggested MRI to be more sensitive than double balloon urethrography. These techniques should be considered after other conventional methods have not defined the diverticulum.

Occasionally, a diverticulum occurs with no clinical evidence of inflammation. If the diverticulum is diagnosed during a careful pelvic examination, and if the patient is completely asymptomatic except for a previous history of urinary tract problems, surgery is not necessary. With a complication rate of 15% to 20%, diverticulectomy should not be considered a quick and easy procedure. Removal of an asymptomatic urethral diverticulum may create more problems than it prevents, particularly if the sac is small

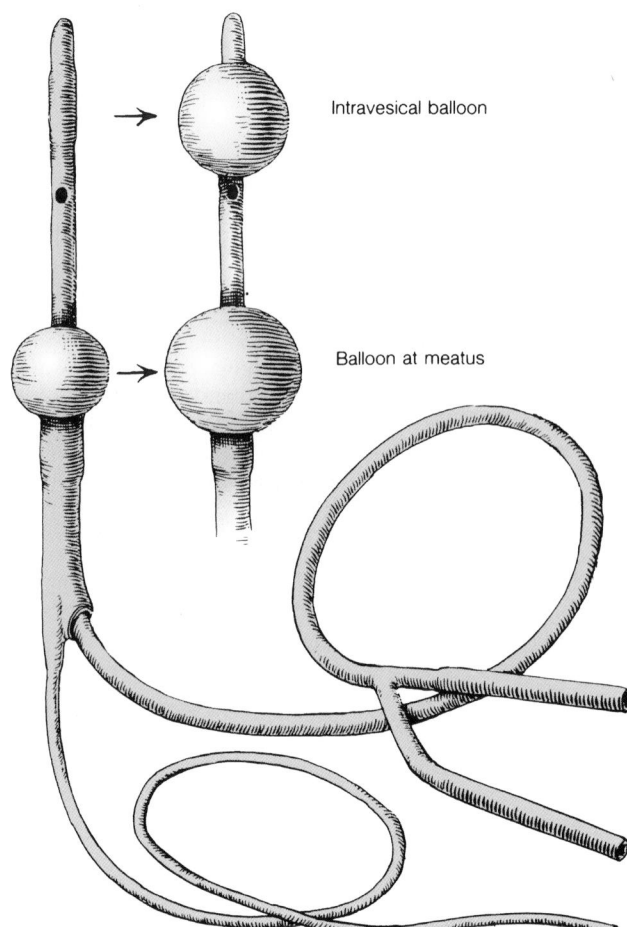

FIGURE 24.21 Double-ballooned catheter for PPUG. (From Davis HJ, Cian LG. Positive pressure urethrography: a new diagnostic method. *J Urol* 1958;80:34, with permission.)

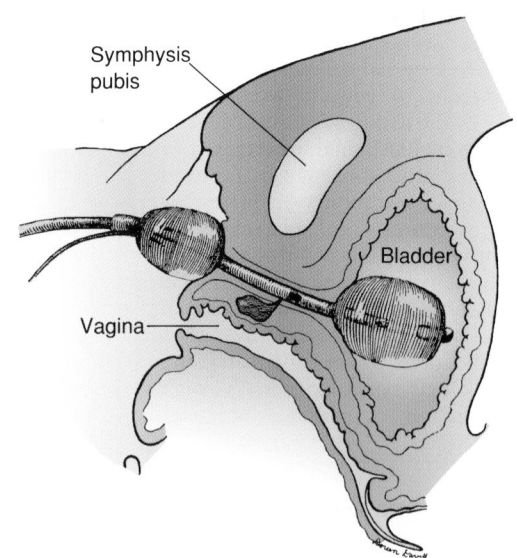

FIGURE 24.22 Double-ballooned catheter inserted for PPUG. (From Davis HJ, Cian LG. Positive pressure urethrography: a new diagnostic method. *J Urol* 1958;80:34, with permission.)

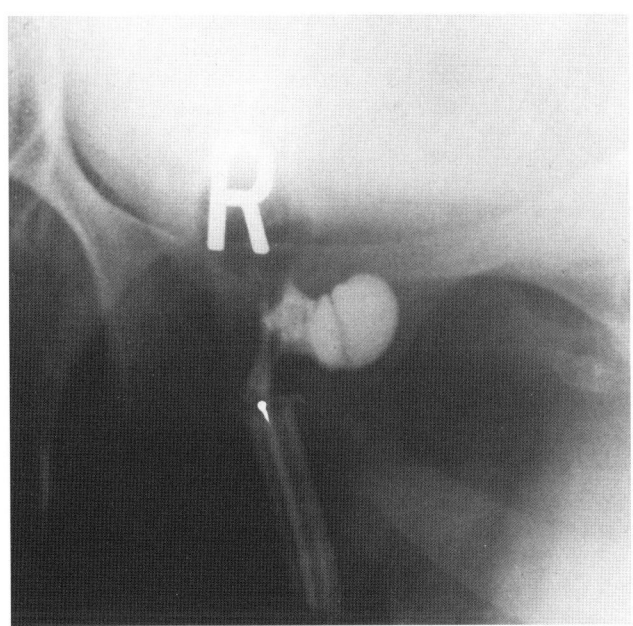

FIGURE 24.23 A large urethral diverticulum filled with contrast medium.

or located in the floor of the posterior urethra. Only if a patient experiences acute or recurrent symptoms should urethral surgery be performed. Leng and McGuire classify urethral diverticulum as true versus pseudodiverticulum (Table 24.1).

Treatment

A diverticulum that requires treatment must be completely excised before the defect in the urethra can be closed. Failure to remove the entire diverticulum results only in recurrence of the problem. Many techniques have been used to identify the anatomic boundaries of the diverticulum. One popular method is to pass a sound into the diverticulum through the urethral orifice. Another method is to distend the diverticulum by injecting it with fibrinogen and thrombin mixed in a syringe to form a firm fibrin clot. However, direct anatomic dissection

TABLE 24.1 Urethral Diverticulum	
TRUE DIVERTICULUM	**PSEUDODIVERTICULUM**
No prior urethral surgery	History of urethral surgery
Chronic recurring symptoms of urgency, dysuria, dyspareunia, dribbling	Relatively few voiding symptoms
Chronic lower urinary tract infections	Cystoscopy demonstrates broad-mouthed ostium to diverticulum
Narrow-necked ostium not readily apparent on radiography or cystoscopy	More likely to have stress incontinence
Reprinted from Leng WW, McGuire EJ. Management of female urethral diverticula: a new classification. *J Urol* 1998;160:1297. Copyright © 1998, Elsevier.	

of the diverticulum from the paraurethral fascia and vaginal wall without visual enhancement of the anatomic boundaries offers a better success rate. The smooth covering of a diverticulum protruding into the vagina can be easily distinguished from the rugal folds of the vaginal mucosa.

If the wall of the diverticulum is left unopened until the dissection has reached the base of the diverticulum sac, its neck can be visualized directly while it is removed. Inadvertent removal of a portion of the urethral floor along the base of the diverticulum is too common an error; if the mucosa is closed with too much tension, a urethral stricture or a postoperative fistula may result.

Excision and Layered Closure A midline incision is made through the vaginal mucosa, which is then separated from the wall of the diverticulum (**Fig. 24.24A**). The wall of the diverticulum also is dissected from the paraurethral fascia in as wide a circumference as can be developed.

The diverticulum is opened, and the interior of the cavity is inspected. If the orifice of the diverticulum is large, the opening of the urethra can easily be seen, especially if a catheter has been placed in the urethra and bladder (**Fig. 24.24B**). The rest of the thin, friable mucosa of the diverticulum is separated from the vaginal mucosa and fascia before the neck of the diverticulum is trimmed near the urethral orifice. The lining of the diverticulum is friable because of inflammatory changes and the thin layer fragments during the dissection. Meticulous sharp dissection is required to separate the lining completely from the vagina and from the floor of the urethra. We repeat, in caution, that the neck of the diverticulum should be carefully resected to avoid eversion and to prevent the removal of mucosa from the urethral floor.

The urethral defect is closed with 3-0 delayed absorbable sutures interrupted so that the edges can be inverted (**Fig. 24.24C**). After the interrupted sutures are tied, the paraurethral fascia is closed in a double-layer "vest-over-pants" technique in which the layer of fascia from one side of the urethra is sutured beneath the opposite and overlapping fascia and fastened to the urethral wall on that opposite side. The top layer of fascia is then sutured at its edge to the underlying fascial layer. The fascial margins are sutured by more durable 2-0 delayed absorbable sutures (**Fig. 24.24D, E**), and the vaginal mucosa finally is trimmed and closed, also with interrupted 2-0 delayed absorbable sutures. Faerber as well as Leng and McGuire have advocated diverticulectomy and placement of pubovaginal slings. Faerber uses the sling for intrinsic sphincter deficiency, whereas Leng and McGuire have recommended fascial slings to close the defect if it is too large for reinforcement.

The bladder is filled with 300 mL of distilled water, and a suprapubic Silastic catheter is inserted and left in place until the morning of the fifth postoperative day. A suprapubic catheter is used in preference to a urethral catheter for three major reasons: to avoid trauma to the operative site, to avoid the necessity for transurethral catheterization during attempts to initiate voiding, and to avoid the discomfort of a urethral catheter. On the fifth day after surgery, the patient should attempt to void with the three-way stopcock of the suprapubic catheter closed to allow the bladder to fill.

Urethrotomy Urethrotomy has been used by Edwards and Beebe and by Kropp to treat diverticula. Splitting the floor of the urethra from the meatus down its full length to the site of the orifice of the diverticulum allows the sac to be well visualized during excision. As a rule, however, cases of urethral

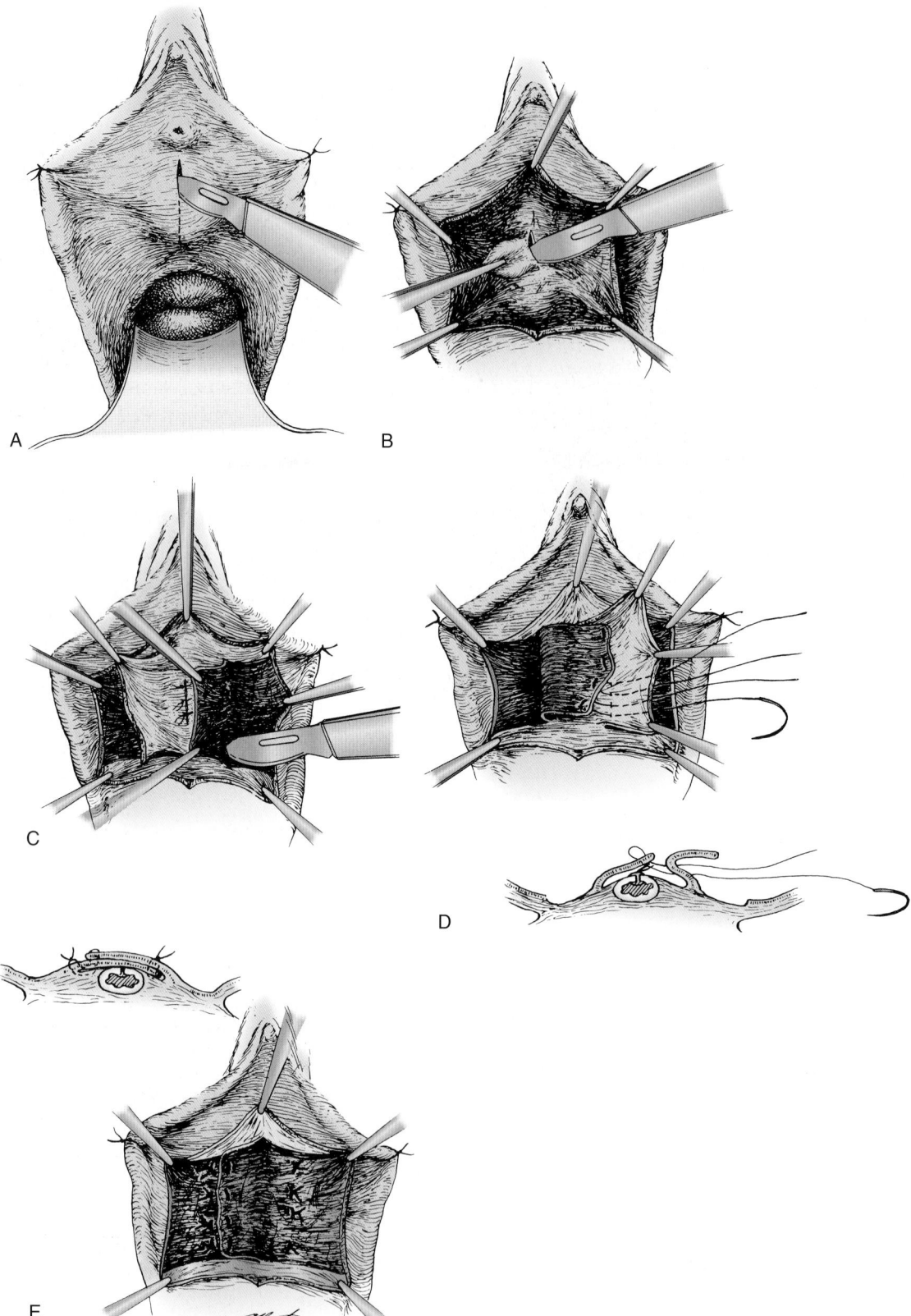

FIGURE 24.24 Suburethral diverticulum. **A:** A midline vaginal incision is made over the diverticulum. **B:** The diverticulum is dissected from the vaginal mucosa and surrounding fascia. Freed diverticulum is excised from the floor of the urethra, avoiding removal of an excessive amount of the urethral wall. **C:** The urethra is closed with interrupted 3-0 delayed absorbable sutures placed through the muscularis and mucosa to ensure mucosa-to-mucosa approximation. The paraurethral fascia is mobilized with sharp dissection from the vaginal mucosa. **D:** The paraurethral fascia is plicated beneath the urethral incision, using the vest-over-pants technique. The inner layer of fascia is sutured to the undersurface of the outer layer using horizontal mattress sutures of 2-0 delayed absorbable material. The inset is a cross-sectional view of suture placement. **E:** Completion of vest-over-pants plication of paraurethral fascia over the floor of the urethra. The free margin of the outer fascia is sutured to the inner fascial layer. The inset is a cross-sectional view of suture placement.

diverticula can be successfully repaired without such an extensive incision that requires the floor of the urethra to heal along its entire length. Healing is particularly a problem if there has been recent infection in the diverticulum.

Marsupialization In 1970, Spence and Duckett recommended marsupialization of the diverticulum to prevent recurrence, to minimize operating time, and to reduce blood loss. This procedure has been endorsed by Lichtman and Robertson and by Ginsberg and Genadry. Stress urinary incontinence has not been reported as a complication, but only, we suspect, because marsupialization is not used to treat lesions in the posterior urethra near the bladder base. Marsupialization is a useful procedure when diverticula occur in the outer third of the urethra, where a permanent opening in the outer floor of the urethra would not adversely influence intraurethral pressure.

Complications of Diverticulectomy

Complications arise in about 20% of cases treated for diverticula of the urethra. Urethral stricture can occur when too much urethral mucosa is removed, but strictures usually can be resolved by urethral dilatations. Urethral fistula, a serious and troublesome complication of diverticulectomy, occurs in about 5% of treated patients.

Postoperative fistulas frequently develop when acute or subacute infection in the walls of the diverticulum causes the urethral mucosa to become friable; the urinary incontinence that develops from urethral fistulas is far more troublesome than the initial symptoms of the diverticulum.

Closure of a urethral fistula is difficult because the blood supply to the floor of the urethra is delicate, and scarring and infection often develop with repeated efforts to close the urethra. A fistula in the outer part of the urethra may be asymptomatic and may not need to be repaired, but there normally are reports with an outer fistula of spraying of urine when voiding.

Urethral Prolapse

Although there have been few recent reports of urethral prolapse, nearly 400 cases have been published in the English literature since 1732. More than half of these cases occurred in infants and children; the remainder occurred in elderly patients.

Urethral prolapse is characterized by a sliding outward of the urethral mucosa around the entire urethral meatus. The urethra may become cyanotic, edematous, and infarcted (Fig. 24.25). Symptoms vary greatly. Prolapse may cause no discomfort, in which case it is detected only by bloody discharge of congested tissues that are breaking down, but more often there are reports of severe and continuous pain, urinary

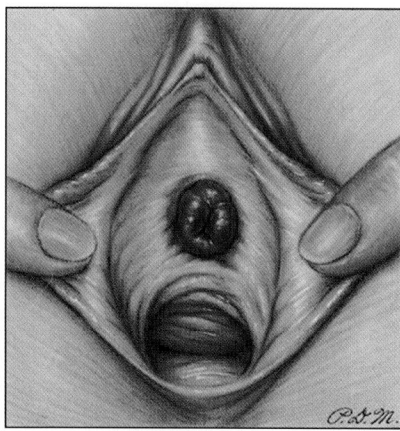

FIGURE 24.25 Prolapsed urethra.

frequency, and tenesmus. Occasionally, in a small child, tissue reaction and edema of the outer urethra produces urinary retention rather than the more usual urinary frequency.

Urethral prolapse is thought to be the result of poor development of or atrophic changes in the collagen and elastic tissues of the submucosa. In infants, prolapse usually follows a severe coughing or crying spell. In some older patients, too, prolapse has followed paroxysms of coughing. In older patients, diminished tone and elasticity of tissue alone may be sufficient to cause some cases of urethral prolapse.

Treatment of urethral prolapse may be palliative or surgical. Hot, moist compresses provide temporary comfort. A small mass of tissue can be reduced, but recurrence is common.

Surgical Techniques

Several surgical procedures have been suggested, including the one advocated by Kelly and Burnam, in which the prolapsed mucosa is excised by a circular incision (Fig. 24.26A). The cut edges are then sutured with 3-0 delayed absorbable suture material, avoiding an excessive number of stitches, which can result in stricture of the urethral meatus (Fig. 24.26B). In most cases, this circumcision technique has proved to be the preferred method of correction.

Cryosurgery also has been used to treat urethral prolapse. The method is extremely effective in producing complete annular necrosis and healing of the prolapsed tissue (Fig. 24.27). The cryosurgery procedure can be performed without anesthesia, although for a young child, a local anesthetic is advisable. A suprapubic Silastic catheter is inserted and is left in postoperatively to permit bladder drainage until complete, spontaneous

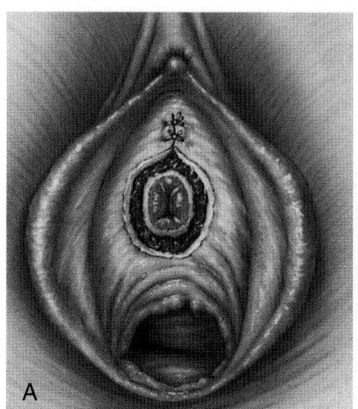
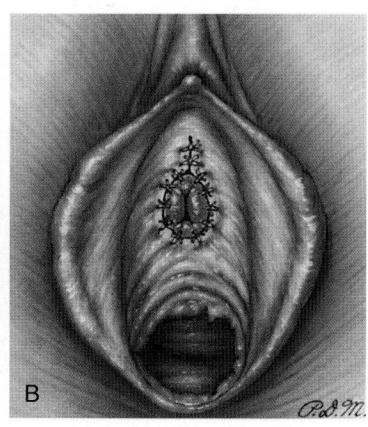

FIGURE 24.26 Operation for urethral prolapse. **A:** The prolapsed mucosa has been excised. **B:** Completed operation. Cut edges of urethral and vaginal mucosa are sutured with 3-0 delayed absorbable sutures.

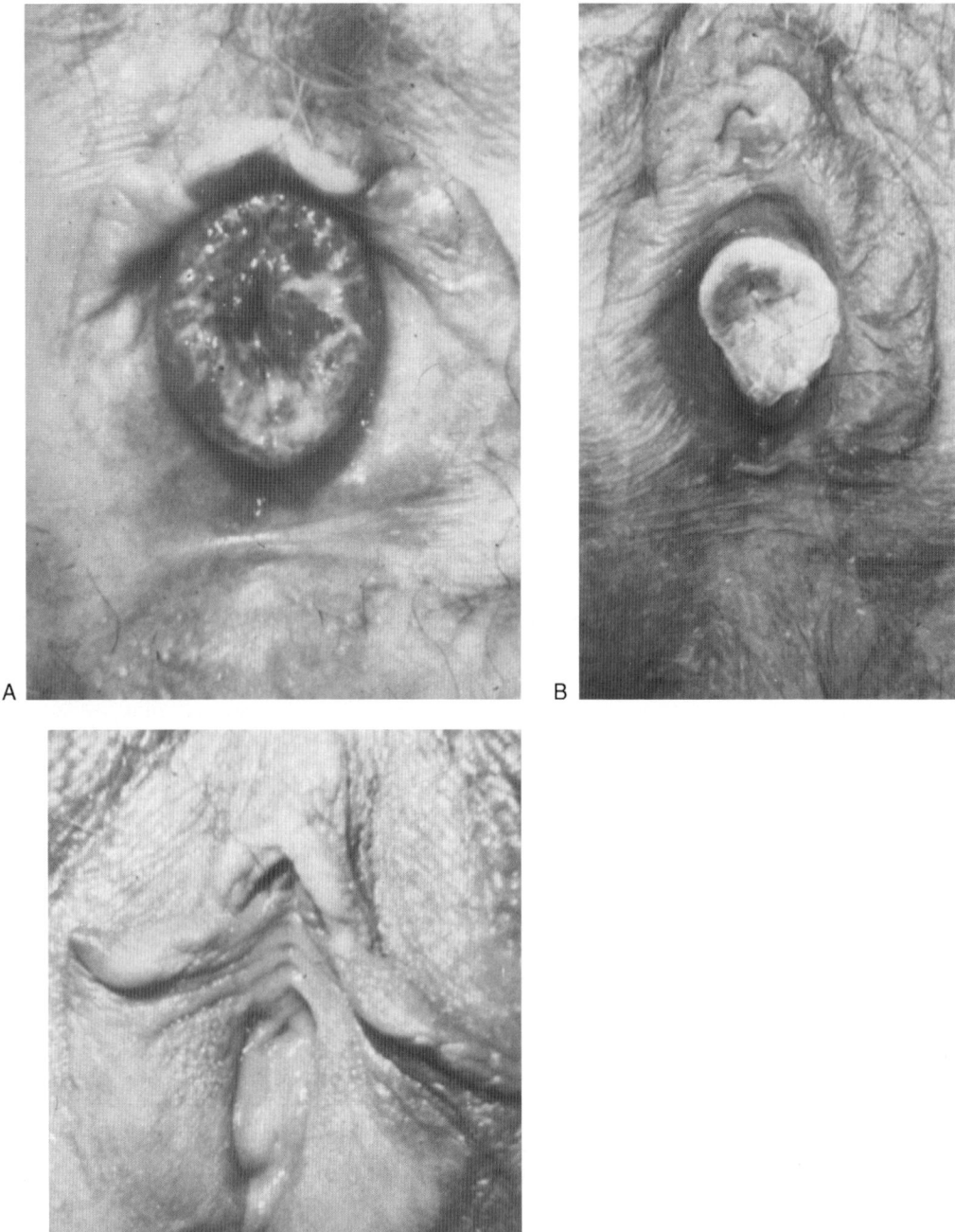

FIGURE 24.27 Cryosurgery in the treatment of urethral prolapse. **A:** Urethral prolapse in an elderly woman. **B:** Regression of urethral prolapse after cryosurgery. **C:** Repeated cryosurgery of urethral prolapse resulted in complete regression and healing of the urethral meatus within 8 weeks.

voiding can occur. The catheter also helps to prevent postoperative trauma at the suture line around the meatus.

Carcinoma of the Vagina

Carcinoma of the vagina is uncommon, occurring in less than 2% of patients with gynecologic malignancies. The average age at presentation is 60 years. Vaginal carcinoma is most frequently secondary to metastases from tumors of the cervix and vulva rather than originating in the vagina. Lesions that encroach on the outer vagina from the vulva must be separated from lesions that originate in the vaginal canal to be considered a vaginal primary.

The International Federation of Obstetrics and Gynecology (FIGO) has agreed on the following exclusionary criteria for the classification of vaginal cancer:

1. A vaginal growth extending to the portion of the cervix and reaching the area of the external os should always be considered a carcinoma of the cervix.
2. A vulvar growth that has extended to the vagina should be classified as carcinoma of the vulva.
3. A vaginal growth that is limited to the urethra should be classified separately as carcinoma of the urethra.

Clinicians now satisfy the staging criteria for the diagnosis of primary carcinoma of the vagina by showing a histologically negative cervix, urethra, vulva, and endometrium.

The criteria for the definition of primary carcinoma of the vagina were established after many clinicians reported the recurrence of vaginal lesions after treatment of carcinoma in situ of the cervix. Tumors recurred in 1% to 6% of cases. Today, extension of carcinoma in situ and invasive carcinoma of the cervix to the vaginal fornices or upper vagina can be easily identified with the use of colposcopy.

The clinical stages of carcinoma of the vagina agreed on by FIGO are listed in Table 24.2. In 1973, Perez and coworkers proposed that stage II be divided into stages IIa and IIb to provide a more accurate definition of the extent of the lesion. In the proposed modified FIGO classification, stage IIa includes subvaginal infiltration not extending into the parametrial regions, whereas stage IIb includes parametrial or paravaginal infiltration not extending to the pelvic wall. This classification has not been accepted by FIGO. Creasman and colleagues queried the National Cancer Data Base (NCDB), a central registry of hospital case data, from 1985 through 1994. Of the 4,885 cases, 75% were invasive and 90% epithelial. Survival at 5 years was as follows: stage 0, 96%; stage I, 73%; stage II, 58%; and stage III to IV, 36%. The overall 5-year survival rate with melanoma was 14%.

Symptoms

The diagnosis of vaginal tumors frequently is delayed because of the lack of early symptoms. Progressive vaginal discharge and postmenopausal bleeding are the most frequent symptoms. Postcoital bleeding can also herald the presence of a vaginal or cervical carcinoma. More than 10% of patients are asymptomatic at the time of diagnosis.

Women with a history of vaginal, vulvar, and cervical intraepithelial neoplasia have an increased risk of vaginal carcinoma.

These patients should receive annual Papanicolaou smears even if they have undergone a hysterectomy. Having a hysterectomy for other than preneoplastic or neoplastic conditions does not increase the risk for developing vaginal carcinoma.

The symptoms of vaginal carcinoma resemble those of cervical carcinoma, except that obvious bleeding occurs later than with neoplasms on the cervix. The overt bleeding eventually forces the patient to see her physician for diagnosis. The type of pelvic pain is frequently indicative of lesion location. The posterior vagina, the most common location of vaginal carcinomas, presents with tenesmus and other bowel symptoms. Anterior tumors, on the other hand, result in urethral and bladder symptoms.

Histopathology

The most common histologic type of primary vaginal tumor is squamous carcinoma, which accounts for 84% to 90% of all vaginal cancers (Table 24.3). Adenocarcinoma, including diethylstilbestrol (DES)-related cases, represents approximately 4% to 9% of vaginal cancers. Sarcomas, including leiomyosarcoma and sarcoma botryoides, account for 2% to 3% of vaginal lesions, and melanomas account for 1% to 2% of malignant neoplasms of the vagina. Rare tumors, such as endodermal sinus tumors or neoplasms originating in embryologic cloacal remnants, may form a transitional cell neoplasm that involves the vagina.

Squamous carcinoma of the vagina is discovered in 10% to 15% of cases after the finding of squamous cancer in other parts of the lower genital tract, such as the vulva or cervix. This has led to the theory of multicentric origin of squamous cancer in the lower genital tract. Woodruff and Parmley and others emphasize this correlation and have recommended that patients with squamous cancer in one area be categorized as high risk for the development of squamous carcinoma in other sites of the lower genital tract. A viral etiology, such as the human papillomavirus, is most likely responsible for these findings.

Carcinoma may arise in the neovagina lined with a split-thickness skin graft from the buttock or lateral thigh. Carcinoma of the neovagina is a rare cancer; only nine cases have been reported. The primary carcinoma seems to be related to the transplanted tissue. In three cases, adenocarcinoma was associated with the use of a large or small bowel intestinal graft for vaginal reconstruction. Five cases of squamous cell cancer arising from the graft have been documented. The transplanted epithelium in the vagina may be exposed to an unidentified carcinogen or mutagen, as has been documented with the vulva, and can undergo malignant transformation in

IV

TABLE 24.2 International Federation of Obstetrics and Gynecology Classification of Vaginal Carcinoma

Preinvasive Carcinoma	
Stage 0	Carcinoma in situ, intraepithelial carcinoma
Invasive Carcinoma	
Stage I	Carcinoma limited to the vaginal wall
Stage II	Carcinoma involving the subvaginal tissue, but not extending onto the pelvic wall
Stage III	Carcinoma extending onto the pelvic wall
Stage IV	Carcinoma extending beyond the true pelvis or involving the mucosa of the bladder or rectum. Bullous edema that does not permit a case to be allotted to stage IV
Stage IVa	Spread of the growth to adjacent organs
Stage IVb	Spread to distant organs

From Pettersson F, ed. *Annual report on the results of treatment in gynecologic cancer.* Stockholm, Sweden: FIGO, 1988:174

TABLE 24.3 Histologic Types of Vaginal Cancer and Frequency of Occurrence

TYPE	FREQUENCY (%)
Squamous carcinoma	85–90
Adenocarcinoma (including DES related)	4–9
Sarcoma	2–3
Melanoma	2–3
Other	1–2
DES, diethylstilbestrol.	

this environment. These observations underscore the need for regular pelvic examinations after operative vaginoplasty with either a bowel graft or a split-thickness skin graft.

Diethylstilbestrol, a nonsteroidal estrogenic hormone thought to enhance embryo implantation and placental development, was introduced into clinical obstetrics in 1944 in Boston and became popular and widely used during the next two decades. Women with a history of previous spontaneous abortions or other risk factors for early pregnancy loss of multiple gestations were given DES. It is known now that DES use during the first trimester of pregnancy may cause vaginal neoplasia. It was not until the late 1960s, however—when a cluster of cases of adenocarcinoma appeared in young women younger than age 25 years (all offspring of DES-treated women)—that Herbst and colleagues connected the result with the unusual cause.

From 1944 to 1970, approximately 1.5 to 2 million female offspring were exposed to DES. Fortunately, the incidence of vaginal adenocarcinoma in these young women has been quite low, ranging from 0.14 to 1.4 in 1,000 exposed women. More than 500 documented cases have been reported to the DES registry to date.

Observations of the development of vaginal adenosis and adenocarcinoma in teenage girls whose mothers were given DES before the eighteenth week of pregnancy brought new insights to the study of squamous tumor cells in the lower genital tract and greatly increased our understanding of the embryologic development of the vagina. The effect of the DES drug provided an indisputable histologic foundation for the development of an uncommon vaginal adenocarcinoma in women younger than 29 years of age. Twenty-five percent of women exposed in utero have anatomic cervical, vaginal, and urinary tract abnormalities.

The DES-associated adenocarcinoma originally was thought to arise from mesonephric remnants in the vagina, and the disease consequently was mislabeled as a clear cell carcinoma. However, electron microscopic analysis of the ultrastructure of both the adenocarcinoma and the vaginal adenosis allowed Fenoglio and colleagues to clearly define these lesions as composed of columnar epithelium, similar in all respects to endocervical epithelium, and of paramesonephric (müllerian) origin. The colposcopic studies of Stafl and Mattingly and of others confirm these observations.

Vaginal adenosis has been found by colposcopic examination to occur in 34% to 90% of exposed offspring and vaginal adenocarcinoma in 50%. Although the hypothesis is still unproven, there is a strong possibility that the benign vaginal lesion is the cell of origin for vaginal adenocarcinoma. The risk of development of clear cell adenocarcinoma in an exposed woman between birth and age 34 is 1 in 1,000.

Etiology

During embryologic development, the vagina is formed from the columnar epithelium of the müllerian ducts and UGS. The tissue then transforms into squamous epithelium, so that the vaginal and cervical epithelium have a common embryologic origin. Squamous metaplasia within the vaginal adenosis has been observed with a colposcope, and transformation of the metaplastic tissue also has been demonstrated in the development of intraepithelial neoplasia. Although many agents have been postulated as carcinogenic factors, none have been positively demonstrated. It is quite possible that squamous carcinoma arises from the effects of an oncogenic agent on the transformation zone within the foci of vaginal adenosis. The studies now being done on the effects of DES may find some interesting causative factors that influence vaginal carcinoma.

Carcinoma of the vagina also may share a common causative denominator with cervical carcinoma. Because slightly more than 50% of the cases occur in the posterior wall of the upper third of the vagina, which is the end point of vaginal coitus, vaginal carcinoma could be venereally induced. As with cervical carcinoma, primary carcinoma of the vagina usually occurs in sexually active women. Except for the cases of adenocarcinoma in young women exposed to DES, squamous carcinoma of the vagina is unquestionably associated with sexual activity. As with cervical intraepithelial neoplasia and carcinoma, the human papillomavirus is probably responsible for the majority of vaginal carcinomas.

Site of Lesion

Plentl and Friedman found that 51% of vaginal carcinoma lesions occur in the upper third of the vagina, 30% in the lower third, and 19% in the middle third. In the lower third, lesions most often occur in the anterior wall, whereas in the upper third, lesions most often appear in the posterior vaginal wall. Although the location is observed on diagnosis, the precise site of origin is difficult to pinpoint because the tumors usually have spread to various parts of the vagina by that time.

Pathways of Spread

The lymphatic drainage of the vagina takes place through different pathways. The upper third drains by way of the cervical lymphatics, the lower third passes by way of the vulvar lymphatics, and the middle third communicates with both the upper and the lower lymphatic channels. The vaginal vault and the anterior wall of the upper vagina drain to the inter-iliac pelvic lymph nodes, where they communicate with the external iliac, the hypogastric, and the common iliac nodes. The lymphatic drainage of the posterior vagina communicates directly with the deep pelvic nodes, including the inferior gluteal, sacral, and rectal nodes.

Because the major pathways of lymphatic drainage are to the superior and inferior gluteal muscles and the common iliac lymph nodes, the potential for extrapelvic spread of vaginal carcinoma is great. When extrapelvic spread occurs, prognosis usually is poor. The primary site of origin of the tumor is an important indicator of lymph node metastases, whether the tumor will metastasize to the inguinal–femoral chain or to the deep pelvic lymph nodes. When the disease involves the lower third of the vagina, 6% to 7% of patients have metastases to the inguinal–femoral lymph nodes.

Diagnosis

In general, invasive carcinoma of the vagina appears as either a raised exophytic lesion or an ulcerative, depressed lesion in the vaginal wall. Biopsy can be performed on both types of lesions easily, and diagnosis can be established without difficulty. Vaginal cytology usually is positive if an adequate cell sample is obtained from the exfoliated lesion, although, as often happens with cervical carcinoma, many cases of false-negative cytology occur even when an invasive lesion is present. Colposcopy, Lugol solution, or both can be used to demarcate the areas for biopsy, although iodine staining usually is unnecessary if the lesion is clearly visible.

Identifying vaginal carcinoma at an early stage can be a major problem because the first lesions appear within the epithelial cells, frequently indistinguishable from the remainder of the vaginal epithelium. Only by colposcopic examination or with iodine staining can alterations in the surface epithelium of the vagina be identified. Ng and associates have achieved an accuracy of 88% to 90% in detecting dysplastic lesions in DES-exposed patients with adenosis, but their technique requires separate, four-quadrant vaginal smears from the walls of the vagina to increase the sensitivity of the Papanicolaou smear. Herbst and coworkers emphasize the advantage of iodine staining of the vagina to reveal occult lesions that may be associated with adenosis. Stafl and Mattingly reported an accuracy of 96% in detecting abnormal epithelial lesions of the vagina in DES-exposed women by careful examination and colposcopy.

Because the vaginal speculum can obscure surface lesions and delay early diagnosis, the instrument should be rotated during the examination so that the entire canal can be inspected. With iodine staining, the clinician can detect multifocal lesions, but the entire vagina also should be cytologically tested. A thorough colposcopic examination can be used to detect vaginal carcinoma if the clinician has that expertise.

Treatment

Primary vaginal carcinoma is treated either with surgery or with radiotherapy. The choice of treatment depends on three factors: the size of the lesion, the location of the tumor in the vagina, and the clinical stage of the disease.

Stage 1 Lesions Easiest to treat by far is vaginal intraepithelial neoplasia III (VAIN III), and it offers the most hopeful prognosis. Either surgery or radiotherapy can be used, depending on the location of the lesion. If the disease is located in the upper vagina and the margins of the disease are distinct, a partial vaginectomy, with or without hysterectomy, is a practical and successful method of treatment.

The carbon dioxide laser has proved to be a simple, effective means of treating noninvasive vaginal carcinoma. Laser therapy offers conservative treatment for both focal and multicentric lesions without impairment of normal coital function. Because there is a risk of residual disease in 10% of laser-treated patients, careful colposcopic and cytologic follow-up are critical. Histologic study is difficult after the carbon dioxide laser vaporizes the treated lesions. An alternative ablative technique is the ultrasonic surgical aspirator, the tip of which vibrates 23,000 times per second, fragmenting and aspirating the tissue in contact with it. This technique permits histologic evaluation of the collected tissue fragments. The operative site also heals faster secondary to decreased thermal damage. Robinson and colleagues reported their experience in treating 46 patients with VAIN. Sixty-six percent (29) of those initially treated with ultrasonic surgical aspiration did not have recurrence. Fifty-two percent of patients treated for recurrent disease (17) did not experience a recurrence. The mean duration of follow-up was 21 months.

Nonsurgical methods such as administration of 5-fluorouracil vaginal cream have also proved efficacious in treating VAIN.

Radiation therapy is rarely used to treat VAIN. However, radiation is an excellent modality for suspected invasion when the medical risk for further evaluation by surgery is too great.

A vaginal cylinder, such as the Bloedorn applicator, can be used for radiotherapeutic treatment to deliver 70 Gy to the vaginal surface over a period of approximately 72 hours. If the lesion is confined to the vaginal fornices, vaginal colpostats can be used to deliver a similar dosage. Lesions in the lower third of the vagina may be treated by partial vaginectomy or by intravaginal irradiation using a variety of brachytherapy techniques.

Surgery, radiation, or both are the primary modalities for treating vaginal carcinomas. Lesions in the vaginal fornix can be treated with a radical Wertheim hysterectomy, partial vaginectomy, and bilateral pelvic lymphadenectomy. Treatment for this lesion is similar to that for stage Ib cervical carcinoma. If pelvic lymph nodes are histologically positive or if paraaortic lymph nodes look suspicious, a paraaortic lymphadenectomy should be performed. If the lymph nodes are histologically positive for carcinoma, pelvic radiation with or without paraaortic radiation should be administered. As with cervical carcinoma, the size of the lesion is prognostic of our ability to adequately treat these patients with primary surgery. Large lesions not permitting clear surgical margins (e.g., proximity to the bladder or rectum) should be treated with primary radiation therapy. Radical surgery also may require the replacement of the upper vagina with a split-thickness skin graft to reestablish normal vaginal length for a sexually active woman. Irradiation therapy is an alternative treatment for this stage of disease.

The radical Wertheim hysterectomy has been quite successful in treating stage I adenocarcinoma in young women who were exposed to DES in utero. More than 75% of patients are cured. Magrina and associates treated a patient with stage I disease at their institution with laparoscopic radical parametrectomy and pelvic and aortic lymphadenectomy. The role of laparoscopy in the treatment of vaginal carcinoma will continue to expand. Although its role in parametrectomy may be debated, laparoscopy to excise the pelvic and periaortic nodes before radiation may be beneficial to patients with advanced disease.

Sentinel Node Detection Sentinel node detection in vaginal carcinoma has not gained universal acceptance. Gynecologic tumor—such as cervical and vulvar—have been much more amicable to sentinel node detection and biopsy. Van Dam and colleagues used ^{99m}TC-labeled nanocolloids in primary and recurrent vaginal carcinomas. Nodes were identified laparoscopically and resected. Three of four patients had nodes identified through sentinel node detection. Frumovitz and colleagues evaluated fourteen patients with pretreatment lymphoscintigraphy. Eleven patients had at least one sentinel node identified: five (45%) inguinal, four (36%) pelvic, and two (18%) inguinal and pelvic. Contrary to present beliefs, the location of positive sentinel nodes did not correlate to the location of the lesion.

Radiation therapy is the preferable treatment for large proximal lesions or middle or distal vaginal tumors. A combination of teletherapy (external beam) and interstitial or intracavity therapy is used.

Stage II and Stage III Lesions More extensive lesions of the vagina pose an extremely difficult therapeutic problem for the gynecologist. Because the levator ani muscles of the pelvic diaphragm surround the vagina, penetration of the lateral wall of the vagina by the invasive tumor frequently is associated with fixation of the disease to the adjacent pelvic musculature. Even radical surgery cannot effectively control the disease when it extends beyond the confines of the vagina into the paravaginal tissues. Instead, the major method of treatment for stage II and stage III lesions is radiotherapy.

When stage II lesions involve the anterior or posterior wall of the vaginal septum, an anterior or posterior exenteration with pelvic node dissection may be required. When the disease includes the lower third of the vagina, a groin dissection also is necessary. Because surgery must be so extensive, its usefulness is limited when the disease affects the paravaginal region (stage IIb) or the lateral vaginal wall (stage III).

IV

Stage IV Lesions When advanced lesions involve only the bladder or the rectum, exenteration may be required to control the disease effectively. Unfortunately, pelvic exenteration, either anterior or posterior, can be used only when there is no other extension of the disease, and it is rare for the bladder and rectum to be involved without involvement of the adjacent paravaginal tissues. If the patient is not an acceptable surgical risk for exenteration, external beam megavoltage irradiation therapy followed by intravaginal or interstitial irradiation can be used to control the local disease and to offer palliation. If the tumor does not respond after 5,000 cGY of irradiation treatment to the whole pelvis, an exenteration may be required to control the disease in properly selected patients. Exenteration is also recommended for central recurrences without lymph node metastasis.

Advanced/Recurrent Disease Pelvic exenteration is the best treatment for patients who have failed primary irradiation therapy of vaginal carcinoma. As with cervical carcinoma, it is imperative that the recurrences be central and nodes radiographically negative. Before performing the exenteration, pelvic and periaortic nodes are sent for frozen section. Depending on the age of the patient, continent urinary diversions, neovaginal, and primary end-to-end colon anastomosis are performed when possible. Berek and colleagues reported on their 45-year pelvic exoneration experience at UCLA. Survival for cervical/vaginal cancers was 73% at 1 year, 57% at 3 years, and 54% at 5 years (Fig. 24.28). Positive margins had a deleterious effect on survival (Fig. 24.29).

Irradiation Therapy

Irradiation treatment of vaginal carcinoma is easily divided between lesions in the upper and middle thirds and the lower third of the vagina.

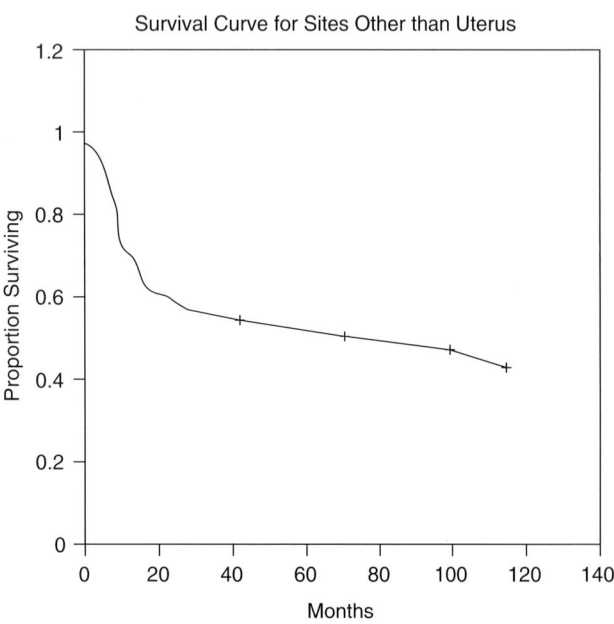

FIGURE 24.28 Survival of patients with recurrent cervical and vaginal cancers following pelvic exenteration. (Reprinted with permission from Berek JS, Howe C, Legasse LD, et al. Pelvic exenteration for recurrent gynecologic malignancy: survival and morbidity analysis of the 45-year experience at UCLA. *Gynecol Oncol* 2005;99:157. Copyright © 2005 Elsevier Inc.)

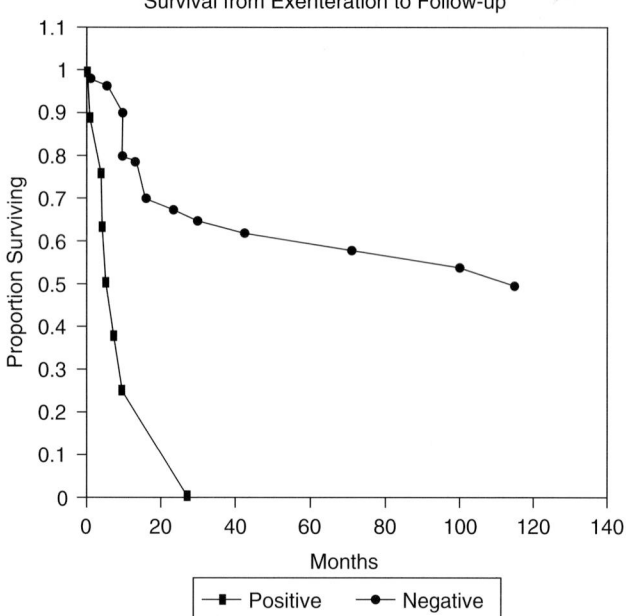

FIGURE 24.29 Survival based on status of surgical margins. (Reprinted with permission from Berek JS, Howe C, Legasse LD, et al. Pelvic exenteration for recurrent gynecologic malignancy: survival and morbidity analysis of the 45-year experience at UCLA. *Gynecol Oncol* 2005;99:158. Copyright © 2005 Elsevier Inc.)

Upper and Middle Thirds of the Vagina Because the lymphatic drainage of the upper and middle vagina extends through the hypogastric and pelvic nodes, full pelvic irradiation is necessary. Treatment usually includes a combination of techniques.

External beam megavoltage therapy using 4,500 to 5,000 cGY focused on the midplane of the pelvis is used to treat the full pelvis and to encompass the vagina. A vaginal implant of radium, cesium, or iridium follows, delivering an additional 3,000 to 4,000 cGY to a depth of 0.5 to 1.0 cm or more, depending on the thickness of the lesion.

At the MD Anderson Hospital, Brown and coworkers demonstrated the efficacy of using a radium needle implant for localized lesions. When the implant is used, high doses of radiation to the entire vagina, bladder, and rectum are avoided. Interstitial needles and iridium wires have been used as a primary treatment for localized vaginal lesions, and they can be used for persistent disease.

Lower Third of the Vagina Lesions in the lower third of the vagina frequently metastasize to the inguinal–femoral lymphatics and must be treated with full external and intravaginal irradiation followed by external beam irradiation treatment to the inguinal–femoral lymph nodes. The inguinal–femoral regions require either a surgical groin dissection or the application of 5,000 to 6,000 cGY of electron beam teletherapy in addition to full pelvic irradiation. When vaginal lesions have metastasized to the groin lymph nodes, the cure rate is equally poor for both methods. In general, the presence of tumor in the groin nodes is a poor prognostic sign, suggesting that the deep pelvic nodes also may be involved in approximately 6% to 7% of cases. Because the incidence of vaginal cancer is so low, the exact frequency with which the deep pelvic nodes are involved has not been documented.

Chemoradiation for large bulky lesions may play a role in vaginal carcinoma, just as it does in cervical or vulvar lesions. Agents such as cisplatin, 5-fluorouracil, and hydroxyurea have been successfully used.

The number of patients with vaginal carcinoma reported to the FIGO registry by international clinics between 1979 and 1981 totals 547. Seventy-eight percent of these patients were treated by radiation. Only 38.6% of these patients were alive at 5 years. Results from other institutions that primarily have followed radiation therapy show that only stage I lesions have an adequate 5-year survival rate (Table 24.4).

In a retrospective analysis of 134 patients with carcinoma of the vagina treated at Washington University, Perez and Camel report an actuarial disease-free, 5-year survival rate of 85% for stage I lesions, 51% for stage IIa lesions, 33% for stage IIb lesions, 33% for stage III lesions, and 19% for stage IV lesions. The actuarial study demonstrated that beyond stage I of the disease, control is poor. For stage IIa lesions, local control of the disease was achieved in only 65% of cases at the University of Maryland because external irradiation was not used in all cases. Pelvic control was achieved in 48% of stage IIb and stage III lesions, but in none of the seven patients (0%) with stage IV disease.

Overall survival rates for stages I through IV from published reports are outlined in Table 24.5. The highest survival rates are observed in stage I disease, whereas few patients survive for 5 years after the diagnosis of stage IV disease. Shah and colleagues reviewed the Surveillance, Epidemiology and End Results program (SEER) data on 2,149 women from 1990 to 2004. The average age at diagnosis was 65.7. The 5-year survivals were stage I (84%), stage II (75%), and stage III/IV (57%). Mortality decreased by 17% after the year 2000.

BEST SURGICAL PRACTICES

- Incorporating an exam of the external genitalia into routine practice of clinicians caring for children can prevent delays in diagnosing imperforate hymen, misdiagnosis, and potential morbidity. To prevent scarring, stenosis, and subsequent dyspareunia in women with imperforate hymen, the hymenal tissue should not be excised too close to the vaginal mucosa.
- Sexually ambiguous external genitalia defects of the UGS are remarkably constant in appearance regardless of the etiology and differ only in degree of malformation, ranging somewhere intermediate to that of a normal girl and that of a normal boy. Thus, operative procedure for reconstruction of ambiguous genitalia into feminine genitalia does not vary in its essential elements.
- The common goals for the female reconstruction of ambiguous genitalia include reduction of clitoral size, creation of labia minora, and exteriorization of the vagina. Any reconstruction of the external genitalia with the objective of producing normal female appearance and function requires a full understanding of the surgical anatomy.
- It is essential to accurately identify the site of communication of the vagina with the UGS in female reconstruction of ambiguous genitalia. Knowledge of the possible variants in communication of the vagina with the UGS is critical before entertaining surgical correction.
- One objective of the reconstruction procedure for external genitalia is to delay the procedure until the anomalous structures are of a size to permit easy identification of all structures. Repair may be delayed until menarche, when maturity and the desire for sexual activity are usually well established.
- Surgical efforts of clitoral reduction focus on concealment, plication, resection, and reduction, with an attempt to provide

TABLE 24.4 Absolute 5-Year Survival after Irradiation Therapy for Carcinoma of the Vagina

	PROPORTION SURVIVING					
FIGO STAGE	MD ANDERSON HOSPITAL[a] 1948–1967	UNIVERSITY OF MARYLAND[b] 1970–2000	WASHINGTON UNIVERSITY[c] 1957–1970	VIENNA UNIVERSITY[d] 1950–1977	1950–1977	INDIANA UNIVERSITY[f] 1987–2007
I	/16 (69%)	/50 (85%)	/6 (83%)	/39 (85%)	/60 (75%)	92%
II	/19 (68%)	/97 (78%)	/31 (64%)	/60 (47%)	/95 (45%)	82%
IIa		/20 (65%)	/39 (51%)			
IIb		/11 (63%)	/21 (33%)			
III	/15 (27%)	/39 (58%)	/20 (40%)	/12 (33%)	/145 (30%)	} 20%
IV	/11 (0%)	/7	/7 (0%)	/8 (19%)	/62 (19%)	
I–IV	/61 (46%)		/64 (52%)	/119[e] (53%)	/362 (40%)	

[a]Data from Hilgers RD. Squamous cell carcinoma of the vagina. *Surg Clin North Am* 1978;58:25.
[b]Data from Pecorelli S, ed. FIGO annual report on the results of treatment in gynecological cancer. *Int J Gynecol Obstet* 2003;83:27
[c]Data from Perez CA, Camel HM. Long-term follow-up in radiation therapy of carcinoma of the vagina. *Cancer* 1982;49:1308.
[d]Data from Kucera H, Langer M, Smekal G, et al. Radiotherapy of primary carcinoma of the vagina: management and results of different therapy schemes. *Gynecik Ibcik* 1985;21:87.
[e]Not included in the figure 119 are 15 patients of the total patient group of 134 who were stage 0.
[f]Data from Sinha B, Stehman F, Schilder J, et al. Indiana University experience in the management of vaginal cancer. *Int J Gynecol Cancer* 2009;19(4):686–693.

TABLE 24.5 Carcinoma of the Vagina: Comparison of Survival (%)

INVESTIGATORS	YEARS STUDIED	STAGE				TOTAL
		I	II	III	IV	
Puthawala et al. (1983)[a]	1976–1979	100	75	22	0	56
Gallup et al. (1987)[a]	1971–1984	100	50	0	25	43
Brown et al. (1971)[a]	1948–1967	69	68	27	0	46
Nori et al. (1983)[a]	1950–1974	71	61	33	0	42
Perez (1981)[a]	1965–1981	81	42	30	9	50
Prempree (1982)[a]	1957–1975	78	57	39	0	48
Benedet et al. (1983)[a]	1950–1980	71	50	15	0	45
Manetta et al. (1988)[a]	1976–1986	71	47	33	33	48
Eddy et al. (1991)[b]	1970–1989	84	70	45	35	28
Stock et al. (1995)[b]	1962–1992	100	67	53	0	15
Creasman et al. (1998)[b]	1985–1994	792	73	58	58	58
Frank et al. (2003)[b]	1970–2000	165	78	56	37	46
Viswanathan et al. (2003)[b]		58	70	64	32	0
Tabata et al. (2002)[b]	1957–1995	51	82	70	0	0
Mock et al. (2003)[b]		86	41	43	37	0
Otton et al. (2004)[b]	1982–1998	70	71	48		

[a]Adapted from Manetta A, Perito JL, Larson JE, et al. Primary invasive carcinoma of the vagina. *Obstet Gynecol* 1988;72:77.
[b]Adapted from Creasman WT. Vaginal cancers. *Curr Opin Obstet Gynecol* 2005;17:71.

a normal cosmesis without sacrificing sensation or vascularity of the glans. Even after seemingly successful clitoral reduction, the sensory function is significantly impaired, and this should be taken into consideration during counseling.

- Preoperative identification and catheterization or sounding of the vaginal orifice is key to the performance of a successful, one-stage procedure.
- It generally is recommended that exteriorization of the vagina be postponed until near puberty because higher estrogen levels may prevent stenosis, and sufficiently, maturity in the patient is needed to comply with a postoperative dilatation program.
- When the complete operation is attempted at an early age, the vagina is sometimes not satisfactorily exteriorized. It should be emphasized that simple exteriorization of the lower vaginal tract can be combined with cosmetic correction of virilized external genitalia in infancy, but in most cases, it is best to defer definitive reconstruction of the intermediate or high vagina until after puberty.
- Preinvasive lesions of the vagina can be treated with excision or ablative techniques.
- Early stage I carcinoma of the vulva can be treated with radiation therapy and/or surgical excision. Radical vaginectomy and pelvic lymph node dissection has few complications and excellent 5-year survival. In more advanced-stage vaginal cancers, radiation therapy is superior.

BIBLIOGRAPHY

Abramova L, Parekh J, Irvin WP, et al. Sentinel node biopsy in vulvar and vaginal melanoma; presentation of six cases and literature review. *Ann Surg Oncol* 2002;9:840.

Agrawal PP, Singhal SS, Neema JP, et al. The role of interstitial brachytherapy using template in locally advanced gynecological malignancies. *Gynecol Oncol* 2005;99:169.

Al-Kurdi M, Monaghan JM. Thirty two years experience in management of primary tumors of the vagina. *Br J Obstet Gynaecol* 1981;88:1145.

Alizai NK, Thomas DFM, Lilford RJ, et al. Feminizing genitoplasty for congenital adrenal hyperplasia: what happens at puberty? *J Urol* 1999;161:1588.

Anderson MJ. The incidence of diverticula of the female urethra. *J Urol* 1967;98:96.

Ansari DO, Horowitz IR, Katzenstein HM, et al. Successful treatment of an adolescent with locally advanced cervicovaginal clear cell adenocarcinoma using definitive chemotherapy and radiotherapy. *J Pediatr Hematol Oncol* 2012;34:e174.

Azziz R, Mulaikal RM, Migeon CJ, et al. Congenital adrenal hyperplasia: long-term results following vaginal reconstruction. *Fertil Steril* 1986;46:1011.

Bailez MM, Gearhart JP, Migeon C, et al. Vaginal reconstruction after initial construction of the external genitalia in girls with salt-wasting adrenal hyperplasia. *J Urol* 1992;148:680.

Ball HG, Berman ML. Management of primary vaginal carcinoma. *Gynecol Oncol* 1982;14:154.

Bargy F, Laude F, Barbet JP, et al. The anatomy of intersexuality. *Surg Radiol Anat* 1989;11:103.

Baskin LS, Erol A, Li YW, et al. Anatomical studies of the human clitoris. *J Urol* 1999;162:1015.

Benedet JL, Murphy KJ, Fairey RN, et al. Primary invasive carcinoma of the vagina. *Obstet Gynecol* 1983;62:715.

Benjamin J, Elliott L, Cooper JF, et al. Urethral diverticulum in the adult female: clinical aspects, operative procedure, and pathology. *Urology* 1974;3:1.

Berek JS, Howe C, Legasse LD, et al. Pelvic exenteration for recurrent gynecologic malignancy: survival and morbidity analysis of the 45-year experience at UCLA. *Gynecol Oncol* 2005;99:153.

Blaikley JB, Dewhurst CJ, Ferreira HP, et al. Vaginal adenosis: clinical and pathological features with special reference to malignant change. *J Obstet Gynaecol Br Commonw* 1971;78:1115.

Blakely CR, Mills WG. The obstetric and gynaecological complications of bladder exstrophy and epispadias. *Br J Obstet Gynaecol* 1981;88:167.

Breslow A. Thickness, cross-sectional areas, and depths of invasion in the prognosis of cutaneous melanoma. *Ann Surg* 1970;172:902.

Brown GR, Fletcher GH, Rutledge FN. Irradiation of in situ and invasive squamous cell carcinoma of the vagina. *Cancer* 1971;28:1278.

Burbige KA, Hensle TW, Chambers WJ, et al. Pregnancy and sexual function in women with bladder exstrophy. *Urology* 1986;28:120.

Burrows LJ. Surgical procedures for urethral diverticula in women in the United States, 1979–97. *Int Urogynecol J Pelvic Floor Dysfunct* 2005;16:158.

Cervellione RM, Phillips T, Baradaran N, et al. Vaginoplasty in the female exstrophy population: Outcomes and complications. *J Pediatr Urol* 2010;6:595

Choo YC, Anderson DG. Neoplasms of the vagina following cervical carcinoma. *Gynecol Oncol* 1982;14:125.

Chou CP, Huang JS, Yu CC, et al. Urethral diverticulum: diagnosis with virtual CT urethroscopy. *AJR Am J Roentgenol* 2005;184(6):1889.

Chung AF, Casey MJ, Flanner JT, et al. Malignant melanoma of the vagina: report of 19 cases. *Obstet Gynecol* 1980;55:720.

Clemetson CA. Ectopia vesicae and split pelvis: an account of pregnancy in a woman with treated ectopia vesicae and split pelvis, including a review of the literature. *J Obstet Gynaecol Br Emp* 1958;65:973.

Committee on Genetics, 1999–2000; Kaye CI, Cunniff C, et al. Evaluation of the newborn with developmental anomalies of the external genitalia. *Pediatrics* 2000;106:138.

Costa EM, Mendonca BB, Inacio M, et al. Management of ambiguous genitalia in pseudohermaphrodites: new perspectives on vaginal dilation. *Fertil Steril* 1997;67:229.

Creasman WT. Vaginal cancers. *Curr Opin Obstet Gynecol* 2005;17:71.

Creasman WT, Phillips JL, Menck HR. The National Cancer Data Base report on cancer of the vagina. *Cancer* 1998;83:1033.

Creighton SM, Minto CL, Steele SJ. Objective cosmetic and anatomical outcomes at adolescence of feminizing surgery for ambiguous genitalia done in childhood. *Lancet* 2001;358:124.

Crouch NS, Creighton SM. Minimal surgical intervention in the management of intersex conditions. *J Pediatr Endocrinol* 2004;17:1591.

Crouch NS, Minto CL, Laio KLM, et al. Genital sensation after feminizing genitoplasty for congenital adrenal hyperplasia: a pilot study. *BJU Int* 2003;91:5.

Curra QJ, Rendtorff RC, Chandler RW, et al. Female gonorrhea: its relationship to abnormal uterine bleeding, urinary tract symptoms and cervicitis. *Obstet Gynecol* 1975;45:195.

Dalrymple JL, Russell AH, Lee SW, et al. Chemoradiation for primary invasive squamous carcinoma of the vagina. *Int J Gynecol Cancer* 2004;14:110.

Damario MA, Carpenter SE, Jones HW Jr, et al. Reconstruction of the external genitalia in females with bladder exstrophy. *Int J Gynaecol Obstet* 1994;44:245.

Davies MC, Crouch NS, Woodhouse CR, et al. Congenital adrenal hyperplasia and lower urinary tract symptoms. *BJU Int* 2005;95:1263.

Davis BL, Robinson DG. Diverticula of the female urethra: assay of 120 cases. *J Urol* 1970;104:850.

Davis HJ, Cian LG. Positive pressure urethrography: a new diagnostic method. *J Urol* 1958;80:34.

Davis HJ, Te Linde RW. Urethral diverticula: an assay of 121 cases. *J Urol* 1956;75:753.

Dewhurst J, Topliss PH, Shepherd JH. Ivalon sponge hysterosacropexy for genital prolapse in patients with bladder exstrophy. *Br J Obstet Gynaecol* 1980;87:67.

DiSaia PJ, Morrow CP, Townsend DE. *Synopsis of gynecologic oncology*. New York, NY: John Wiley & Sons, 1975.

Eddy GL, Marks RD, Miler MC III, et al. Primary invasive vaginal carcinoma. *Am J Obstet Gynecol* 1991;165:282.

Edwards E, Beebe RA. Diverticula of female urethra. Review: new procedure for treatment: report of 5 cases. *Obstet Gynecol* 1955;5:729.

Faerber GJ. Urethral diverticulectomy and pubovaginal sling for simultaneous treatment of urethral diverticulum and intrinsic sphincter deficiency. *Tech Urol* 1998;4:192.

Fenoglio C, Ferenczy A, Richard RM, et al. Scanning and transmission electron microscopic studies of vaginal adenosis and the cervical transformation zone in progeny exposed in utero to diethyl-stilbestrol. *Am J Obstet Gynecol* 1976;126:170.

Fortunoff FS, Latimer JK, Edson M. Vaginoplasty technique for female pseudohermaphrodites. *Surg Gynecol Obstet* 1964;118:545.

Frank SJ, Jhingran A, Levenback C, et al. Definitive radiation therapy for squamous cell carcinoma of the vagina. *Int J Radiat Oncol Biol Phys* 2005;62:138.

Frank SJ, Jhingran A, Levenback C, et al. Definitive treatment of vaginal cancer with radiation therapy [Abstract 116]. *Int J Radiat Oncol Biol Phys* 2003;57(suppl):S194.

Frick HC. Primary carcinoma of the vagina. *Am J Obstet Gynecol* 1968;101:695.

Frick HC, Jacox HW, Taylor HC. Primary carcinoma of the vagina. *Am J Obstet Gynecol* 1968;101:695.

Frumovitz M. Gayed IW, Jhingran A, et al. Lymphatic mapping and sentinel lymph node detection in women with vaginal cancer. *Gynecol Oncol* 2008;108:478.

Gallup DG, Morley GW. Carcinoma in situ of the vagina: a study and review. *Obstet Gynecol* 1975;46:334.

Gallup DG, Talledo OE, Shah KJ, et al. Invasive squamous cell carcinoma of the vagina: a 14-year-old study. *Obstet Gynecol* 1987;69:782.

Gearhart JP, Jeffs RD. State-of-the-art reconstructive surgery for bladder exstrophy at the Johns Hopkins Hospital. *Am J Dis Child* 1989;143:1475.

Gerharz EW, Hohl UN, Weingartner K, et al. Experience with the Mainz modification of ureterosigmoidostomy. *Br J Surg* 1998;86:427.

Gerrard ER Jr, Lloyd LK, Kubricht WS, et al. Transvaginal ultrasound for the diagnosis of urethral diverticulum. *J Urol* 2003;169:1395.

Ginsberg DS, Genadry R. Suburethral diverticulum: classification and therapeutic considerations. *Obstet Gynecol* 1983;61:685.

Gurumurthy M, Cruickshank ME. Management of vaginal intraepithelial neoplasia. *J Low Genit Tract Dis* 2012;306.

Hacker NF, Eifel PJ, van der Velden J, et al. Cancer of the vagina. *Int J Gynaecol Obstet* 2002;119(suppl 2);S97.

Hamilton W, Boyd JD, Mossman HW. *Human embryology*, 3rd ed. Cambridge: W Heffer & Sons, 1962.

Hellman K, Silversward C, Nilsson B, et al. Primary carcinoma of the vagina: factors influencing the age at diagnosis. The Radiumhemmet series 1956–96. *Int J Gynecol Cancer* 2004;14:491.

Hendren WH. Reconstructive problems of the vagina and the female urethra. *Clin Plast Surg* 1980;7:207.

Hendren WH. Surgical management of urogenital sinus abnormalities. *J Pediatr Surg* 1977;12:339.

Hendren WH, Crawford JD. Adrenogenital syndrome: the anatomy of the anomaly and its repair. *J Pediatr Surg* 1969;4:49.

Herbst AL, Cole P, Norusis MJ, et al. Epidemiologic aspects and factors related to survival in 384 registry cases of clear cell adenocarcinoma of the vagina and cervix. *Am J Obstet Gynecol* 1979;153:876.

Herbst AL, Scully RE, Robbo SJ. The significance of adenosis and clear-cell adenocarcinoma of the genital tract in young females. *J Reprod Med* 1975;14:5.

Herbst AL, Ulfelder H, Poskanzer EC. Adenocarcinoma of the vagina: association of maternal stilbestrol therapy with tumor appearing in young women. *N Engl J Med* 1971;284:878.

Herman JM, Homesley HD, Dignan MB. Is hysterectomy a risk factor for vaginal cancer? *JAMA* 1986;256:601.

Herzog TJ, Rader JS. The ultrasonic surgical aspirator in the gynecologic oncology patient. In: Rock JA, Faro S, Gant NF Jr, et al., eds. *Advances in obstetrics and gynecology*, Vol. 1. St Louis, MO: Mosby-Year Book, 1994:325.

Hilgers RD. Pelvic exenteration for vaginal embryonal rhabdomyosarcoma: a review. *Obstet Gynecol* 1975;45:175.

Hilgers RD. Squamous cell carcinoma of the vagina. *Surg Clin North Am* 1978;58:25.

Hines M. Abnormal sexual development and psychosexual issues. *Baillieres Clin Endocrinol Metab* 1998;12:173.

Hines M, Kaufman FR. Androgen and the development of human sex-typical behavior: rough-and-tumble play and sex preferred playmates in children with congenital adrenal hyperplasia (CAH). *Child Dev* 1994;65:1042.

Hoffman MJ, Adams WE. Recognition and repair of urethral diverticula. *Am J Obstet Gynecol* 1965;92:106.

Honig A, Rieger L, Kristen P, et al. A case review of metastasizing invasive hydatidiform mole. Is less-less good? Review of the literature with regard to adequate treatment. *Eur J Gynaecol Oncol* 2005;26:158.

Hopkins MP, Morley GW. Squamous cell carcinoma of the neovagina. *Obstet Gynecol* 1987;69:525.

Houghton CRS, Iversen T. Squamous cell carcinoma of the vagina: a clinical study of the location of the tumor. *Gynecol Oncol* 1982;13:365.

Huffman JW. The detailed anatomy of the paraurethral ducts in the adult human female. *Am J Obstet Gynecol* 1948;55:86.

Hutch JA. *Anatomy and physiology of the bladder, trigone and urethra.* New York, NY: Appleton-Century-Crofts, 1972.

International Federation of Obstetrics and Gynecology. *Annual report on the results of treatment of carcinoma of the uterus, vagina and ovary*, Vol. 18. Stockholm, Sweden: Norestedt, 1982.

Jung, W, Wu HG, Ha SW, et al. Definitive radiotherapy for treatment of primary vaginal cancer effectiveness and prognostic factors. *Int J Gynecol Cancer* 2012;22:521.

Jahnke A, Domke R, Makovitzky J, et al. Vaginal metastasis of lung cancer: a case report. *Anticancer Res* 2005;25:1645.

Joki-Erkkila MM, Heinonen PK. Presenting and long-term clinical implications and fecundity in females with obstructing vaginal malformations. *J Pediatr Adolesc Gynecol* 2003;16:307.

Jones HW Jr. An anomaly of the external genitalia in female patients with exstrophy of the bladder. *Am J Obstet Gynecol* 1973;117:748.

Jones HW Jr, Verkauf BS. Surgical treatment in congenital adrenal hyperplasia: age at operation and other prognostic factors. *Obstet Gynecol* 1970;36:1.

Kamat MH, DelGaiso A, Seebode D. Urethral prolapse in female children. *Am J Dis Child* 1969;118:691.

Kanbour AE, Klionsky BK, Murphy AL. Carcinoma of the vagina following cervical cancer. *Cancer* 1974;34:1838.

Kelly HA, Burnam CF. Malfunctions of the urethra. In: Kelly HA, ed. *Diseases of the kidneys, ureters, and bladder.* New York: D Appleton, 1922:564.

Klaus H, Stein RT. Urethral prolapse in young girls. *Pediatrics* 1973;52:645.

Klobe JM. *Pathologische Anatomie der weiblichen Sexualorgane.* Wien, 1864.

Kogan SJ, Smey P, Levitt SB. Subtunical total reduction clitoroplasty: a safe modification of existing techniques. *J Urol* 1983;130:746.

Krege S, Walz KH, Hauffa BP, et al. Long-term follow-up of female patients with congenital adrenal hyperplasia from 21-hydroxylase deficiency, with special emphasis on the results of vaginoplasty. *BJU Int* 2000;86:253.

Krisiloff M, Puchner PJ, Tretter W, et al. Pregnancy in women with bladder exstrophy. *J Urol* 1978;119:478.

Kropp KA. The female urethra. In: Glenn JF, ed. *Urologic surgery.* Hagerstown, MD: Harper & Row, 1975.

Kucera H, Langer M, Smekal G, et al. Radiotherapy of primary carcinoma of the vagina: management and results of different therapy schemes. *Gynecik Ibcik* 1985;21:87.

Lamoreaux WT, Grigsby PW, Dehdashti F. FDG-PET evaluation of vaginal carcinoma. *Int J Radiat Oncol Biol Phys* 2005;62:733.

Latourette HB. End results of treatment of cancer of vagina. *Ann N Y Acad Sci* 1964;114:1020.

Lee RA. Diverticulum of the urethra: clinical presentation, diagnosis and management. *Clin Obstet Gynecol* 1984;27:490.

Lee RA, Symmonds RE. Recurrent carcinoma in situ of the vagina in patients previously treated for in situ carcinoma of the cervix. *Obstet Gynecol* 1976;48:61.

Leng WW, McGuire EJ. Management of female urethral diverticula: a new classification. *J Urol* 1998;160:1297.

Lialios G, Plantaniotis G, Kallitsaris A, et al. Vaginal metastasis from renal adenocarcinoma. *Gynecol Oncol* 2005;98:172.

Liang C-C, Chang S-D, Soong Y-K. Long-term follow-up of women who underwent surgical correction for imperforate hymen. *Arch Gynecol Obstet* 2003;269:5.

Lichtman A, Robertson J. Suburethral diverticula treated by marsupialization. *Obstet Gynecol* 1976;47:203.

Lintgen C, Herbert P. Clinical-pathological study of 100 female urethras. *J Urol* 1946;55:298.

Livermore GR. Treatment of prolapse of the urethra. *Surg Gynecol Obstet* 1921;32:557.

Magrina JF, Walter AJ, Schild SE. Laparoscopic radical parametrectomy and pelvic and aortic lymphadenectomy for vaginal carcinoma: a case report. *Gynecol Oncol* 1999;75:514.

Manetta A, Gutrecht EL, Berman ML, et al. Primary invasive carcinoma of the vagina. *Obstet Gynecol* 1990;76:639.

Manetta A, Perito JL, Larson JE, et al. Primary invasive carcinoma of the vagina. *Obstet Gynecol* 1988;72:77.

Marcus R Jr, Million RR, Daly JW. Carcinoma of the vagina. *Cancer* 1978;42:2507.

Marcus SL. Multiple squamous cell carcinoma involving the cervix, vagina and vulva: the theory of multicentric origin. *Am J Obstet Gynecol* 1960;80:802.

Melneck S, Cole P, Anderson D, et al. Rates and risks of DES-related clear cell adenocarcinoma of the vagina and cervix. *N Engl J Med* 1987;316:514.

Merino MJ. Vaginal cancer: the role of infectious and environmental factors [Review]. *Am J Obstet Gynecol* 1991;165:1255.

Mingin GC, Stock JA, Hanna MK. The Mainz II pouch: experience in 5 patients with bladder exstrophy. *J Urol* 1999;162:846.

Mock U, Kucera H, Fellner C, et al. High dose-rate (HDR) brachytherapy with or without external beam radiotherapy in the treatment of primary vaginal carcinoma: long-term results and side effects. *Int J Radiat Oncol Biol Phys* 2003;56:950.

Mor N, Merlob P, Reisner SH. Types of hymen in the newborn infant. *Eur J Obstet Gynecol Reprod Biol* 1986;22:225.

Murad TM, Durant JR, Maddox WA, et al. The pathologic behavior of primary vaginal carcinoma and its relationship to cervical cancer. *Cancer* 1975;35:787.

Nakagawa S, Koga K, Kuga K, et al. The evaluation of the sentinel node successfully conducted in a case of malignant melanoma of the vagina. *Gynecol Oncol* 2002;86:387.

Neitlich JD, Foster HE Jr, Glickman MG, et al. Detection of urethral diverticula in women: comparison of a high-resolution fast spin echo technique with double balloon urethrography. *J Urol* 1998;159:408.

Ng AB, Reagan JW, Hawliczek S, et al. Cellular detection of vaginal adenosis. *Obstet Gynecol* 1975;46:323.

Nomura Y, Yamakado K, Tanaka H, et al. Letters to the editor: radiofrequency ablation for the treatment of hemorrhagic vaginal cancer. *J Vasc Interv Radiol* 2005:1557.

Nori D, Hilaris BS, Shu F. Radiation therapy of primary vaginal carcinoma. *Int J Radiat Oncol Biol Phys* 1981;70:20.

Nori D, Hilaris B, Stanimir G, et al. Radiation therapy of primary vaginal carcinoma. *Int J Radiat Oncol Biol Phys* 1983;8:1471.

Nour NM, Michels KB, Bryant AE. Defibulation to treat female genital cutting: effect on symptoms and sexual function. *Obstet Gynecol* 2006;108:55.

Orr JW, Dosoretz DD, Mahoney D. Surgically (laparotomy/laparoscopy) guided placement of high dose rate interstitial irradiation catheters (LG-HDRT): technique and outcoe. *Gynecol Oncol* 2006;100:145.

Otton GR, Nicklin IL, Dickie GJ, et al. Early stage vaginal carcinoma – an analysis of 70 patients. *Int J Gynecol Cancer* 2004;14:304.

Oudoux A, Rousseau T, Bridji B. Interest of F-18 fluorodeoxyglucose positron emission tomography in the evaluation of vaginal malignant melanoma. *Gynecol Oncol* 2004;95:765.

Ozbey H, Darendeliler F, Kayserili H, et al. Gender assignment in female congenital adrenal hyperplasia: a difficult experience. *BJU Int* 2004;94:388.

Parmenter FJ. Diverticulum of the urethra. *J Urol* 1941;45:749.

Passerini-Glazel G. A new 1-stage procedure for clitorovaginoplasty in severely masculinized female pseudohermaphrodites. *J Urol* 1989;142:565.

Pathak UN, House MJ. Diverticulum of the female urethra. *Obstet Gynecol* 1970;36:789.

Perez CA. Definitive radiotherapy for carcinoma of the vagina. *Int J Radiat Oncol Biol Phys* 1981;7:20.

Perez CA, Arneson AN, Dehner LP, et al. Radiation therapy in carcinoma of the vagina. *Obstet Gynecol* 1974;44:862.

Perez CA, Arneson AN, Galakatos A, et al. Malignant tumors of the vagina. *Cancer* 1973;31:36.

Perez CA, Camel HM. Long-term follow-up in radiation therapy of carcinoma of the vagina. *Cancer* 1982;49:1308.

Peters WA III, Kumar NB, Morley GW. Carcinoma of the vagina. *Cancer* 1985;55:892.

Peters WA, Vaughn EJ Jr. Urethral diverticula in the female: etiologic factors and postoperative results. *Obstet Gynecol* 1976;47:549.

Pettersson F. *Annual report on the results of treatment in gynecological cancer.* Stockholm: FIGO, 1988:174.

Pirtoli L, Santoni R. Radiation therapy of the primary vaginal carcinoma. *Acta Radiol Oncol Radiat Phys Biol* 1980;19:353.

Plentl AA, Friedman EA. *Lymphatic system of the female genital tract.* Philadelphia, PA: WB Saunders, 1971.

Pokorny SF, Kozinetz CA. Configuration and other anatomic details of the prepubertal hymen. *Adolesc Pediatr Gynecol* 1988;1:97.

Posner JC, Spandorfer PR. Early detection of imperforate hymen prevents morbidity from delays in diagnosis. *Pediatrics* 2005; 115:1008.

Prempree T. Role of radiation therapy in the management of primary carcinoma of the vagina. *Acta Radiol [Oncol]* 1982;21:195.

Prempree T, Vlravathana T, Slawson RG, et al. Radiation management of primary carcinoma of the vagina. *Cancer* 1977;40:101.

Pride GL, Bucher DA. Carcinoma of vagina 10 or more years following pelvic irradiation therapy. *Am J Obstet Gynecol* 1977; 127:513.

Pride GL, Schultz AE, Chuprevich TW, et al. Primary invasive carcinoma of the vagina. *Obstet Gynecol* 1979;53:218.

Puthawala A, Sved AM, Nalick R, et al. Integrated external and interstitial radiation therapy for primary carcinoma of the vagina. *Obstet Gynecol* 1983;62:367.

Rajfer J, Ehrlich RM, Goodwin WE. Reduction clitoroplasty via ventral approach. *J Urol* 1982;128:341.

Rastogi BL, Bergman B, Angawall L. Primary leiomyosarcoma of the vagina: a study of five cases. *Gynecol Oncol* 1984;18:77.

Reddy S, Lee MS, Graham JE, et al. Radiation therapy in primary carcinoma of the vagina. *Gynecol Oncol* 1987;26:19.

Reid GC, Schmidt RW, Roberts JA, et al. Primary melanoma of the vagina: a clinicopathologic analysis. *Obstet Gynecol* 1989;764:190.

Reiner WG. Sex assignment in the neonate with intersex or inadequate genitalia. *Arch Pediatr Adolesc Med* 1997;151:1044.

Reuben SC, Young J, Mikuta JJ. Squamous carcinoma of the vagina: treatment, complications, and long-term follow-up. *Gynecol Oncol* 1985;20:346.

Ricci G, Gentili A, Di Lorenzo F, et al. Latex allergy in subjects who had undergone multiple surgical procedures for bladder exstrophy: relationship with clinical intervention and atopic diseases. *BJU Int* 1999;84:1058.

Ries J, Ludwig H. Zur therapie des primaren karzinoms der vagina. *Strahlentherapie* 1962;119:92.

Rink RC, Adams MC. Feminizing genitoplasty: state of the art. *World J Urol* 1998;16:212.

Rink RC, Pope JC, Kropp BP, et al. Reconstruction of the high urogenital sinus: early perineal prone approach without division of the rectum. *J Urol* 1997;158:1293.

Robinson JB, Sun CC, Bodurka-Bevers D, et al. Cavitational ultrasonic surgical aspiration for the treatment of vaginal intraepithelial neoplasia. *Gynecol Oncol* 2000;78:235.

Rock JA, Katz E. Ambiguous genitalia. *Semin Reprod Endocrinol* 1987;5:327.

Rock JA, Schlaff WD. Congenital adrenal hyperplasia: the surgical treatment of vaginal stenosis. *Int J Gynaecol Obstet* 1986; 24:417.

Rock JA, Zacur HA, Dlugi AM, et al. Pregnancy success following the surgical correction of imperforate hymen as compared to the complete transverse vaginal septum. *Obstet Gynecol* 1982;59:448.

Rubin SC, Young J, Mikuta JJ. Squamous carcinoma of the vagina: treatment, complications, and long-term follow-up. *Gynecol Oncol* 1985;20:346.

Rutledge FN. Cancer of the vagina. *Am J Obstet Gynecol* 1967;97:635.

Rutledge FN, Boronow RC, Wharton JT. *Gynecologic oncology.* New York: John Wiley & Sons, 1976.

Samant R, Tam T, Dahrouge S, et al. Radiotherapy for the treatment of primary vaginal cancer. *Radiother Oncol* 2005;77:133.

Sander R, Nuss RC, Rhadgan RM. DES-associated vaginal adenosis followed by clear-cell adenocarcinoma. *Int J Gynecol Pathol* 1986;5:362.

Schubert G. Uber scheidenbildung bei angeborenem vaginaldefekt. *Zbl Gynak* 1911;45:1017.

Shah CA, Goff BA, Lowe K, et al. Factors affecting risk of mortality in women with vaginal cancer. *Obstet Gynecol* 2009;113:1038.

Sholem SL, Wechsler M, Roberts M. Management of the urethral diverticulum in women: a modified operative technique. *J Urol* 1974;112:485.

Sinha B, Stehman F, Schilder J, et al. Indiana University experience in the management of vaginal cancer. *Int J Gyencol Cancer* 2009;19:686.

Smith FR. Clinical management of cancer of the vagina. *Ann N Y Acad Sci* 1964;114:1012.

Smith WG. Invasive carcinoma of the vagina. *Clin Obstet Gynecol* 1981;24:503.

Spence H, Duckett J. Diverticulum of the female urethra: clinical aspects and presentation of simple operative technique for cure. *J Urol* 1970;104:432.

Spirtos IM, Doshi BP, Kapp DS, et al. Radiation therapy for primary squamous cell carcinoma of the vagina: the Stanford University experience. *Gynecol Oncol* 1989;35:20.

Stafl A, Mattingly RF. Vaginal adenosis: a precancerous lesion? *Am J Obstet Gynecol* 1974;120:666.

Stanton SL. Gynecologic complications of epispadias and bladder exstrophy. *Am J Obstet Gynecol* 1974;119:749.

Stelling JR, Gray MR, Davis AJ, et al. Dominant transmission of imperforate hymen. *Fertil Steril* 2000;74:1241.

Stern A, Patel S. Diverticulum of the female urethra: value of the postvoid bladder film during excretory urography. *Radiology* 1976;121:22.

Stock RG, Chen AS, Seski J. A 30-year experience in the management of primary carcinoma of the vagina: analysis of prognostic factors and treatment modalities. *Gynecol Oncol* 1995;56:45.

Stuart GC, Allen HH, Anderson RJ. Squamous cell carcinoma of the vagina following hysterectomy. *Am J Obstet Gynecol* 1981;139:311.

Tabata T, Taheshirma N, Nishida H, et al. Treatment failure in vaginal cancer. *Gynecol Oncol* 2002;84:309.

Tait L. Saccular dilatation of the urethra: removal, cure. *Lancet* 1875;2:625.

Thigpen JT, Blessing JA, Homesley HD, et al. A phase II trial of cisplatin in advanced recurrent cancer of the vagina: a GOG study. *Gynecol Oncol* 1986;23:101.

Underwood PB, Smith RT. Carcinoma of the vagina. *JAMA* 1971;217:46.

Usherwood MM. Management of vaginal carcinoma after hysterectomy. *Am J Obstet Gynecol* 1975;122:352.

van Dam P, Sonnemans H, van Dam P-J, et al. Sentinel node detection in patients with vaginal carcinoma. *Gynecol Oncol* 2004;92:89.

Viswanathan A, Bishop K, Lee H, et al. The impact of brachytherapy dose in vaginal cancer [Abstract 1135]. *Int J Radiat Oncol Biol Phys* 2003;57(suppl):343.

Wang AC, Wang CR. Radiologic diagnosis and surgical treatment of urethral diverticulum in women: a reappraisal of voiding cystourethrography and positive pressure urethrography. *J Reprod Med* 2000;45:377.

Weed JC, Lozier C, Daniel SJ. Human papilloma virus in multifocal, invasive female tract malignancy. *Obstet Gynecol* 1983;62:832.

Wharton JT. Carcinoma of the vagina. In: Rutledge F, Boronow RC, Wharton JT, eds. *Gynecologic oncology.* New York: John Wiley & Sons, 1976:259.

IV

Wharton JT. Carcinoma of the vagina and urethra. In: Rovinsky D, ed. *Obstetrics and gynecology*. Hagerstown, MD: Harper & Row, 1972.

Wharton JT, Kearns W. Diverticulum of the female urethra. *J Urol* 1950;63:1063.

Wheeless CR Jr, McGibbon B, Dorsey JH, et al. Gracilis myocutaneous flap in reconstruction of the vulva and female perineum. *Obstet Gynecol* 1979;54:97.

Whelton JA, Kottmeier HL. Primary carcinoma of the vagina. *Acta Obstet Gynecol Scand* 1962;41:22.

Winderl LM, Silverman RK. Prenatal diagnosis of congenital imperforate hymen. *Obstet Gynecol* 1995;85(5 pt 2):857.

Woodruff JD, Parmley TH. Epidermoid carcinoma of the vagina. In: Hafez EC, Evans TN, eds. *The human vagina*. New York, NY: Elsevier North Holland, 1979.

Young HH. *Genital abnormalities, hermaphroditism and related adrenal diseases*. Baltimore, MD: Williams & Wilkins, 1937.

Young RH, Scully RE. Endodermal sinus tumor of the vagina: a report of nine cases and review of the literature. *Gynecol Oncol* 1984;18:380.

Zambo K, Koppan M, Paal A. Sentinel lymph nodes in gynaecological malignancies: frontline between TNM and clinical staging systems? *Eur J Nucl Med Mol Imaging* 2003;30:1684.

IV

CHAPTER 25
Surgery for Anomalies of the Müllerian Ducts

Lesley L. Breech and John A. Rock

DEFINITIONS

Hematometra—The distention of the uterus with blood or menstrual fluid.

Hematometrocolpos—The distention of the uterus and vagina with blood or menstrual fluid; because the vaginal wall is more distensible, the vagina will preferentially fill before the uterus.

Hydrocolpos—The distention of the vagina with fluid; often seen in infants with complex reproductive anomalies.

Metroplasty—Uterine reconstructive procedure.

Uterine anlagen—An underdeveloped uterine structure that is a remnant of a single embryologic müllerian duct.

Maldevelopment of the müllerian ducts occurs in a variety of forms, and each anomaly is distinctive. Nevertheless, some generalizations can be made. Classifications of vaginal anomalies based on certain anatomic findings are useful in organizing the type of malformation, but there usually are exceptions to each rule. Thus, what appears, after a preliminary diagnostic evaluation, to be an apparently isolated vaginal malformation may be found later to be associated with a uterine or renal anomaly. A comprehensive preoperative evaluation of patients with suspected malformations of the müllerian ducts is essential, but a clear understanding of the particular anomaly may not be established until the time of surgical correction. Reproductive surgeons must therefore be equally skilled in both uterine and vaginal reconstructions.

The patient with a uterovaginal anomaly often relies entirely on her physician to clarify the reproductive consequences associated with her diagnosis. The physician can help to allay her anxieties by making a prompt evaluation and giving a full and accurate description of the reproductive implications or the obstetric consequences of her particular uterovaginal anomaly.

CLASSIFICATION OF UTEROVAGINAL ANOMALIES

Classifications of uterovaginal anomalies originally were organized on the basis of clinical findings. Our improved understanding of the embryologic development of most uterovaginal anomalies has enabled categorization on this basis. The 1988 American Fertility Society (AFS) classification of müllerian anomalies (Table 25.1) offers an alternative based on the degree of failure of normal uterine development. Anomalies are grouped according to similarities of clinical manifestations, treatment, and prognosis for fetal salvage. The AFS classification system is weighted primarily toward disorders of lateral fusion and does not include associated vaginal anomalies, although the scheme does allow the user to describe anomalies involving the vagina, tubes, and urinary tract as associated malformations.

No classification of müllerian maldevelopment can focus entirely on the uterus; the vagina is often involved, and sometimes the tubes are involved as well. This discussion follows a suggested modification of the AFS classification of uterovaginal anomalies (Table 25.2) that comprises four groups based on embryologic considerations.

TABLE 25.1 American Fertility Society Classification of Müllerian Anomalies[a]

Class I. Segmental, müllerian agenesis–hypoplasia
  A. Vaginal
  B. Cervical
  C. Fundal
  D. Tubal
  E. Combined anomalies

Class II. Unicornuate
  A. Communicating
  B. Noncommunicating
  C. No cavity
  D. No horn

Class III. Didelphys

Class IV. Bicornuate
  A. Complete (division down to internal os)
  B. Partial

Class V. Septate
  A. Complete (septum to internal os)
  B. Partial

Class VI. Arcuate

Class VII. Diethylstilbestrol related

[a]This classification allows the user to indicate the malformation type and provides additional findings to describe associated variations involving the vagina, cervix, tubes (right, left), and kidneys (right, left).
Adapted from the American Fertility Society. The American Fertility Society classifications of adnexal adhesions, distal tubal occlusion, tubal occlusion secondary to tubal ligation, tubal pregnancies, müllerian anomalies and intrauterine adhesions. *Fertil Steril* 1988;49:944, with permission. Copyright © 1988, Elsevier.

TABLE 25.2 American Fertility Society Classification of Uterovaginal Anomalies

Class I. Dysgenesis of the müllerian ducts

Class II. Disorders of vertical fusion of the müllerian ducts
  A. Transverse vaginal septum
    1. Obstructed
    2. Unobstructed
  B. Cervical agenesis or dysgenesis

Class III. Disorders of lateral fusion of the müllerian ducts
  A. Asymmetric–obstructed disorder of uterus or vagina usually associated with ipsilateral renal agenesis
    1. Unicornuate uterus with a noncommunicating rudimentary anlage or horn
    2. Unilateral obstruction of a cavity of a double uterus
    3. Unilateral vaginal obstruction associated with double uterus
  B. Symmetric–unobstructed
    1. Didelphic uterus
      a. Complete longitudinal vaginal septum
      b. Partial longitudinal vaginal septum
      c. No longitudinal vaginal septum
    2. Septate uterus
      a. Complete
        1) Complete longitudinal vaginal septum
        2) Partial longitudinal vaginal septum
        3) No longitudinal vaginal septum
      b. Partial
        1) Complete longitudinal vaginal septum
        2) Partial longitudinal vaginal septum
        3) No longitudinal vaginal septum
    3. Bicornuate uterus
      a. Complete
        1) Complete longitudinal vaginal septum
        2) Partial longitudinal vaginal septum
        3) No longitudinal vaginal septum
      b. Partial
        1) Complete longitudinal vaginal septum
        2) Partial longitudinal vaginal septum
        3) No longitudinal vaginal septum
    4. T-shaped uterine cavity (diethylstilbestrol related)
    5. Unicornuate uterus
      a. With a rudimentary horn
        1) With endometrial cavity
          a) Communicating
          b) Noncommunicating
        2) Without endometrial cavity
      b. Without a rudimentary horn

Class IV. Unusual configurations of vertical–lateral fusion defects

Modified from the American Fertility Society. The American Fertility Society classifications of adnexal adhesions, distal tubal occlusion, tubal occlusion secondary to tubal ligation, tubal pregnancies, müllerian anomalies and intrauterine adhesions. *Fertil Steril* 1988;49:944.

Class I: Dysgenesis of the Müllerian Ducts

Dysgenesis of the müllerian ducts, which includes agenesis of the uterus and vagina (the Mayer-Rokitansky-Küster-Hauser [MRKH] syndrome), is an impairment of the reproductive system characterized by no reproductive potential other than that achieved by in vitro fertilization in a host uterus.

Class II: Disorders of Vertical Fusion of the Müllerian Ducts

Disorders of vertical fusion can be considered to represent faults in the junction between the downgrowing müllerian ducts (müllerian tubercle) and the upgrowing derivative of the urogenital sinus. Typically, these disorders are characterized by an atretic portion of the vagina that can be quite thick, extending through more than half the distance of the vagina, or it can be quite thin and limited to a small obstructing membrane.

Regardless of the length of the septum, a disorder of vertical fusion should be regarded as a transverse vaginal septum and classified as either obstructed or unobstructed. The so-called partial vaginal agenesis with uterus and cervix present is probably a misnomer for a large segment of atretic vagina. Cervical agenesis or dysgenesis is also included in the group of disorders of vertical fusion.

Class III: Disorders of Lateral Fusion of the Müllerian Ducts

Disorders of lateral fusion of the two müllerian ducts can be symmetric–unobstructed, as with the double vagina, or asymmetric–obstructed, as with unilateral vaginal obstruction. Obstructions associated with disorders of lateral fusion are particularly noteworthy in that they are observed clinically only as unilateral obstructions that almost invariably are associated with absence of the ipsilateral kidney. Bilateral obstruction is thought to be associated with bilateral kidney agenesis and subsequent nonviability of the developing embryo.

The three varieties of asymmetric obstruction with ipsilateral renal agenesis are:

1. Unicornuate uterus with a noncommunicating horn that contains menstruating endometrium
2. Unilateral obstruction of a cavity of a double uterus
3. Unilateral vaginal obstruction

The five groups of symmetric–unobstructed disorders of lateral fusion are:

1. The didelphic uterus
2. The septate uterus
3. The bicornuate uterus
4. The T-shaped uterine cavity, which may be hypoplastic and irregular and which is associated with diethylstilbestrol (DES) exposure in utero
5. The unicornuate uterus with or without a rudimentary horn

The first three groups are types of double uteri; differentiation between a septate uterus (second group) and a bicornuate uterus (third group) requires visualization of the fundus. The septum within the septate uterus is complete or partial. When the septum is complete, that inevitably involves the cervical region with a longitudinal vaginal septum that can extend to the introitus or partially down the vagina. The bicornuate uterus also can have a partial or almost complete separation of the uterine cavities. The term *arcuate uterus* is used primarily by radiologists to refer to a slight septum in the uterine fundus that forms no clear separation of the uterine cavities. This type of uterus is usually included in the category of partial septate uterus.

The unicornuate uterus may have an attached horn with a cavity that communicates with the unicornuate uterus, or there may be no uterine horn or a uterine horn with no cavity.

Some debate has focused on whether the unicornuate uterus with a communicating horn can represent a hypoplastic side of a bicornuate uterus.

Class IV: Unusual Configurations of Vertical–Lateral Fusion Defects

This final category includes combinations of uterovaginal anomalies and other disorders. Unusual uterovaginal configurations have been described that do not fit a particular category, and vertical and lateral fusion disorders can coexist.

Unusual configurations of vertical–lateral fusion defects can be seen with abnormalities of the lower urinary tract. Singh and coworkers have described a patient who was noted to have a persistent hymen and a longitudinal vaginal septum with a didelphic uterus. The patient was noted also to have a double urethra and bladder and left renal agenesis.

Obstructive lesions require immediate attention to relieve retrograde flow of trapped mucus and menstrual blood and increasing pressure on surrounding organs and structures. When no obstruction is present, attention may not be required immediately, but it will always be required eventually to establish or improve reproductive or coital function.

EMBRYOLOGY

The reproductive organs in the female (and in the male) consist of external genitalia, gonads, and an internal duct system between the two. These three components originate embryologically from different primordia and in close association with the urinary system and hindgut. Thus, the developmental history is complex (Figs. 25.1 and 25.2). Even in the 3.5- to 4-mm embryo, it is possible to recognize the bilateral thickenings of the coelomic epithelium known as the gonadal ridges medial to the mesonephros (primitive kidney) in the dorsum of the coelomic cavity. At approximately the 6th week of gestation, in the 17- to 20-mm embryo, the gonad can be distinguished as either a testis or an ovary.

In the female, the labia minora and majora develop from the labioscrotal folds, which are ectodermal in origin. The phallic portion of the urogenital sinus gives rise to the urethra. The müllerian (paramesonephric) duct system is stimulated to develop preferentially over the wolffian (mesonephric) duct system, which regresses in early female fetal life. The cranial parts of the wolffian ducts can persist as the epoöphoron of the ovarian hilum; the caudal parts can persist as Gartner ducts. The müllerian ducts persist and attain complete development to form the fallopian tubes, the uterine corpus and cervix, and a portion of the vagina.

Origin of the Müllerian Ducts

Approximately 37 days after fertilization, the müllerian ducts first appear lateral to each wolffian duct as invaginations of the dorsal coelomic epithelium. The site of origin of the invaginations remains open and ultimately forms the fimbriated ends of the fallopian tubes. At their point of origin, each of the müllerian ducts forms a solid bud. Each bud penetrates the mesenchyme lateral and parallel to each wolffian duct. As the solid buds elongate, a lumen appears in the cranial part, beginning at each coelomic opening. The lumina extend gradually to the caudal growing tips of the ducts.

Eventually, the caudal end of each müllerian duct crosses the ventral aspect of the wolffian duct. The paired müllerian ducts continue to grow in a medial and caudal direction until they eventually meet in the midline and become fused together

in the urogenital septum. A septum between the two müllerian ducts gradually disappears, leaving a single uterovaginal canal lined with cuboidal epithelium. Failure of reabsorption of this septum can result in a septate uterus. The most cranial parts of the müllerian ducts remain separate and form the fallopian tubes. The caudal segments of the müllerian ducts fuse to form the uterus and part of the vagina. The cranial point of fusion is the site of the future fundus of the uterus. Variations in this site of fusion can result in an arcuate or bicornuate uterus. Complete failure of fusion can result in a didelphic uterus.

Isolated case reports continue to challenge established embryologic mechanisms of müllerian development. Dunn and Hantes reported a case of a double cervix and vagina with a blind cervical pouch challenging the theory of unidirectional fusion. Engmann and colleagues reported a unicornuate uterus with normal external uterine morphology, with bilateral fallopian tubes; however, only the right fallopian tube communicated with the uterine cavity. The patient suffered from pain because of the obstruction egress of the stimulated endometrial tissue. The patient was treated with removal of the obstructed cavity. The authors propose that this may represent failure of canalization of one of the müllerian ducts. Additional reports are necessary to fully evaluate potential variations in embryologic development.

Development of the Vagina

The vagina is formed from the lower end of the uterovaginal canal, which developed from the müllerian ducts and the urogenital sinus (Fig. 25.2). The point of contact between the two is the müllerian tubercle. A solid vaginal cord results from proliferation of the cells at the caudal tip of the fused müllerian ducts. The cord gradually elongates to meet the bilateral endodermal evaginations (sinovaginal bulbs) from the posterior aspect of the urogenital sinus below. These sinovaginal bulbs extend cranially to fuse with the caudal end of the vaginal cord, forming the vaginal plate. Subsequent canalization of the vaginal cord occurs, followed by epithelialization with cells derived mostly from endoderm of the urogenital sinus. Recent proposals hold that only the upper one third of the vagina is formed from the müllerian ducts and that the lower vagina develops from the vaginal plate of the urogenital sinus. Recent studies also suggest that the vaginal canal is actually open and connected to a patent uterus and tubes, even in early embryonic life, and that the vagina does not form and later become canalized from an epithelial cord of squamous cells growing upward from the urogenital sinus. Most investigators now suggest that the vagina develops under the influence of the müllerian ducts and estrogenic stimulation. There is general agreement that the vagina is a composite formed partly from the müllerian ducts and partly from the urogenital sinus.

At approximately the 20th week, the cervix takes form as a result of condensation of stromal cells at a specific site around the fused müllerian ducts. The mesenchyme surrounding the müllerian ducts becomes condensed early in embryonic development and eventually forms the musculature of the female genital tract. The hymen is the embryologic septum between the sinovaginal bulbs above and the urogenital sinus proper below. It is lined by an internal layer of vaginal epithelium and an external layer of epithelium derived from the urogenital sinus (both of endodermal origin), with mesoderm between the two. It is not derived from the müllerian ducts.

Anomalies in Organogenesis of the Vagina

Anomalies in the organogenesis of the vagina are easily understood. If there is failure in the development of the müllerian

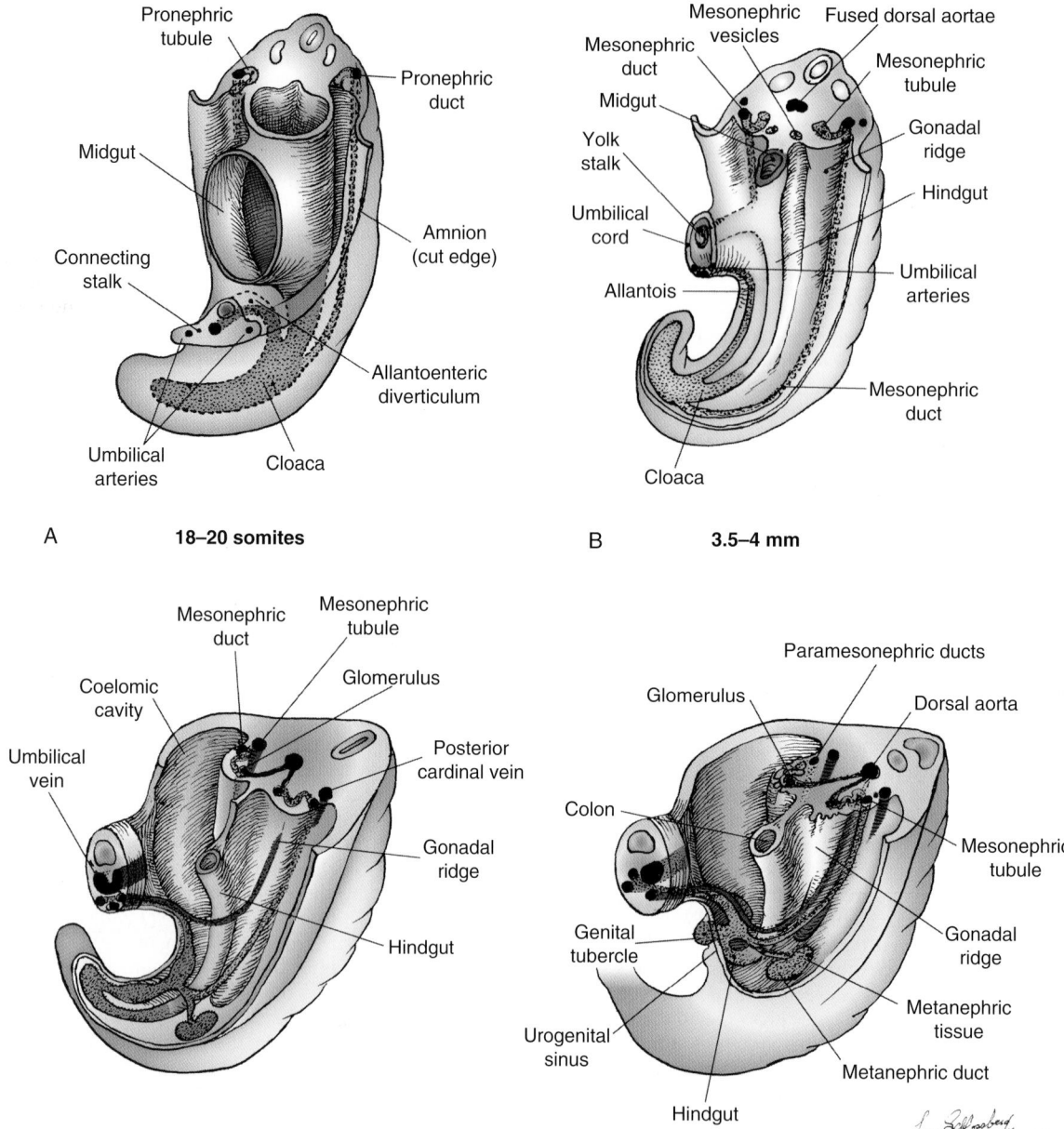

FIGURE 25.1 Diagrammatic representation of the development of the female reproductive organs and structures in early embryogenesis. **A:** At the 18- to 20-somite stage (4th week), the gonadal ridges have not yet begun to form. **B:** In the 3.5- to 4-mm embryo (5th week), the gonadal ridges can be recognized as thickenings of the coelomic cavity just medial to the mesonephric tubules. (Gonadal differentiation into either testis or ovary does not occur until the 6th week of development.) The allantoenteric diverticulum is joined caudally to the dilated cloaca. **C and D:** The genital tubercle and labial folds form in the region just anterior to the cloaca. The cloaca later divides into the ventral urogenital sinus and the dorsal rectum. The development of the urinary system closely parallels that of the reproductive system. The nonfunctioning pronephric tubules shown in (**A**) develop to form the mesonephric ducts shown in (**B**) and (**C**). The permanent kidneys eventually develop from the metanephric tissue, and the urinary collecting system develops from the metanephric ducts. The paramesonephric (müllerian) ducts are apparent by the 12- to 14-mm stage (**D**). (Their subsequent development is illustrated in **Figure 25.2.**)

ducts at any time between their origin from the coelomic epithelium at 5 weeks of embryonic age and their fusion with the urogenital sinus at 8 weeks, the sinovaginal bulbs will fail to proliferate from the urogenital sinus, and the uterus and vagina will fail to develop. Congenital absence of the uterus and the vagina, known as the MRKH syndrome, is the most common clinical example of this anomaly.

Transverse Vaginal Septum

A transverse vaginal septum can develop at any location in the vagina but is more common in the upper vagina at the point of junction between the vaginal plate and the caudal end of the fused müllerian ducts. This defect presumably is caused by failure of absorption of the tissue that separates the two or by

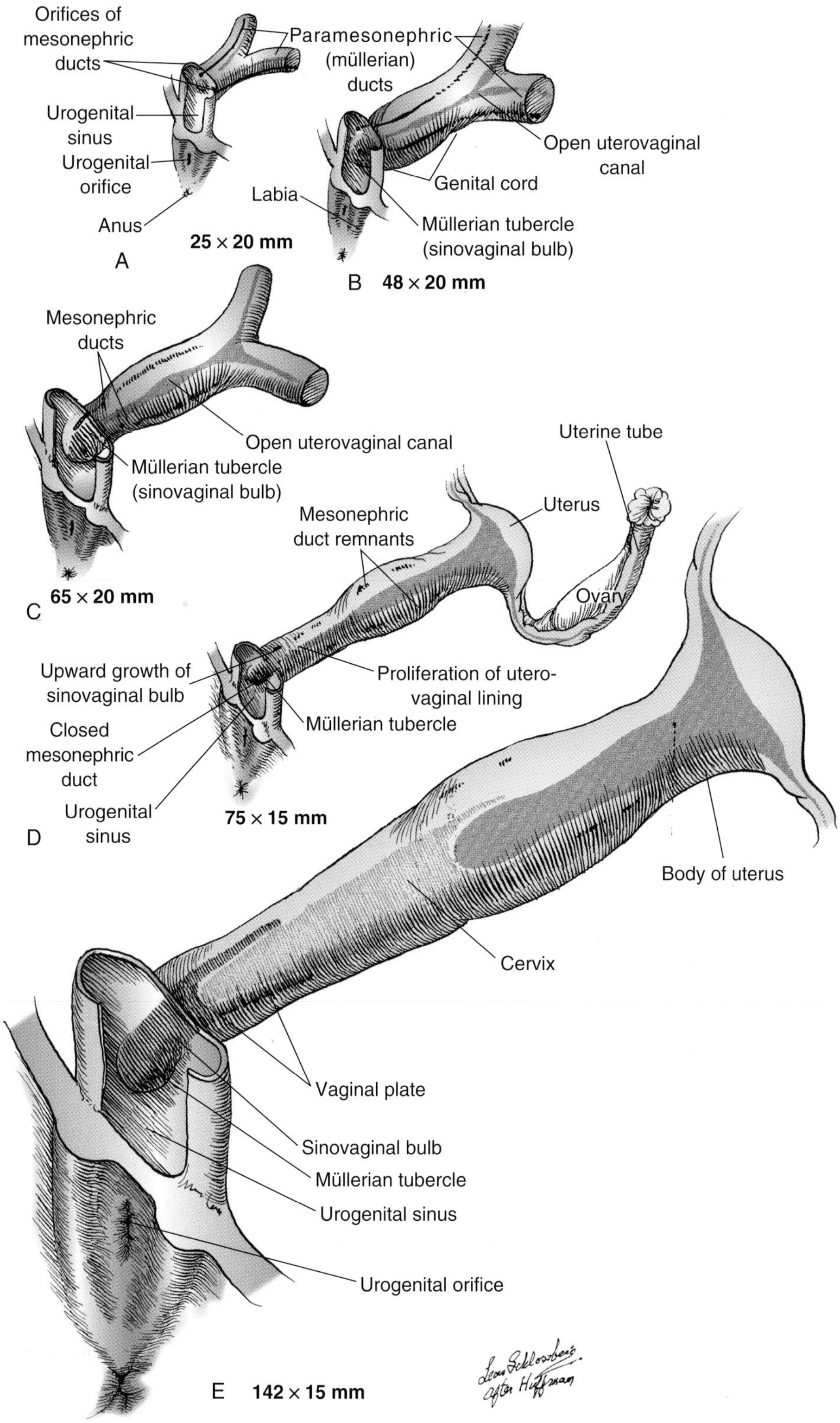

FIGURE 25.2 Further development of the paramesonephric (müllerian) ducts and the urogenital sinus. **A:** Early development of the paramesonephric ducts. The cranial ends of the paramesonephric ducts develop first. These ends remain open to form the fimbriated ends of the fallopian tubes. The paramesonephric ducts grow caudally and cross the mesonephric ducts ventrally. **B:** Eventually, they fuse together to form the uterovaginal canal. **C:** Further caudal development brings this structure into contact with the wall of the urogenital sinus, producing the müllerian tubercle. The caudal ends of the fused paramesonephric ducts form the uterine corpus and cervix. Together with the urogenital sinus, they also form the vagina. The cranial point of fusion of the paramesonephric ducts marks the location of the future uterine fundus. The fallopian tubes form from the unfused cranial parts of the paramesonephric (müllerian) ducts. The proliferation of the lining of the uterovaginal canal above the upward growth of the sinovaginal bulb from below (**D**) forms the vaginal plate (**E**), which later becomes canalized to leave an open vaginal canal. Thus, the vagina is of composite origin. The mesonephric ducts in the female degenerate but can persist into adult life as Gartner ducts.

failure of complete fusion of the two embryologic components of the vagina. A large segment of vagina can be atretic. In past reviews, this has been termed *partial vaginal agenesis with a uterus present*. Elucidation of the cause of a high transverse vaginal septum is more difficult. A local abnormality of the vaginal mesoderm or failure of canalization of the epithelial vaginal plate can provide the answer, but why the abnormality should occur at this particular site is not evident. The proportion of the vagina originating from the urogenital sinus can at times be considerably more than one fifth, and a high transverse vaginal septum thus may represent the junction of an abnormally long urogenital sinus contribution and a short müllerian portion.

Alternatively, the high transverse septum could be the sequela of a local infection of the septum at the end of the vagina. Septa in other areas of the vagina are unexplained by this theory, which has not gained widespread acceptance.

Disorders of Ineffective Suppression of Müllerian Ducts

When abnormal gonadal development is caused by ineffective suppression of the müllerian ducts, ambiguous external genitalia frequently are accompanied by a small rudimentary uterus or a partially developed vagina. Additionally, when there is a genetic loss of cytoplasmic receptor proteins within androgenic target cells, such as occurs in the androgen insensitivity syndrome (formerly called testicular feminization syndrome), the vagina is incompletely developed because the existing male gonads suppress the development of the müllerian ducts. Because these genetically XY patients have phenotypic female genital anatomy without a completely formed vagina, it is important that a vagina be nonsurgically (dilatation) or surgically created to ensure a satisfactory sexual experience.

Congenital anorectal malformations (imperforate anus with rectoperineal or rectovestibular fistula or more complex anomalies like cloaca or cloacal exstrophy) have been reported to occur with reproductive anomalies. These anomalies can be associated with maldevelopment of the müllerian and mesonephric duct derivatives.

Müllerian Duct Abnormalities

Abnormalities in the formation or fusion of the müllerian ducts can result in a variety of anomalies of the uterus and vagina: single, multiple, combined, or separate. Just as the entirely separate origin of the ovaries from the gonadal ridges accounts for the infrequent association of uterovaginal anomalies with ovarian anomalies (see this chapter), so do the close developmental relationships of the müllerian and wolffian ducts explain the frequency with which anomalies of the female genital system and urinary tract are associated. Failure of development of a müllerian duct is likewise associated with failure of development of a ureteric bud from the caudal end of the wolffian duct. Thus, the entire kidney can be absent on the side ipsilateral to the agenesis of a müllerian duct.

Depending on the timing of the teratogenic influence, renal units can be absent, fused, or in unusual locations in the pelvis. Ureters can be duplicated or can open in unusual places, such as the vagina or uterus. Jones and Rock have noted that failure of lateral fusion of the müllerian ducts with unilateral obstruction is associated consistently with absence of the kidney on the side with obstruction. Bilateral obstruction has not been observed clinically, presumably because it would be associated with bilateral renal agenesis, a condition that would not allow the embryo to develop. According to Thompson and Lynn, 40% of female patients with congenital absence of the kidney are found to have associated genital anomalies.

Much investigation has been undertaken to determine a genetic relationship in the development of disorders of the müllerian ducts. Familial aggregates of the most common disorders of the müllerian differentiation are best explained on the basis of polygenic or multifactorial inheritance. No information exists on the number and chromosomal location of responsible genes. Single mutant genes are responsible for the McKusick-Kaufman syndrome and the hand–foot–genital syndrome. Hand–foot–genital syndrome is a rare, dominantly inherited condition that affects both the distal limbs and the genitourinary tract. A nonsense mutation of the HOXA13 gene has been identified in several families. HOX

gene mutations have been reported in several families with multiple müllerian abnormalities. Genital malformations may also be associated with heterozygous DNA sequence variations of the HOXA10, HOXA11, and HOXA13 genes. To date, involvement of the Y chromosome in the pathogenesis of müllerian anomalies has not been considered. The 2004 report by Plevraki and colleagues suggests the possible role of testis-specific protein 1-Y gene in patients with uni- or bilateral gonadal agenesis and uterovaginal dysgenesis. Timmreck and colleagues narrowed the genetic considerations by noting that in an evaluation of 40 women with developmental abnormalities of the uterus and vagina and 12 normal controls, no mutations of the WNT7A gene—a gene associated with murine Müllerian duct development—were found. Reproductive abnormalities involving the uterus and vagina may also be associated with other more complex malformation syndromes in which the molecular basis of many of the syndromes remains unknown.

CONGENITAL ABSENCE OF THE MÜLLERIAN DUCTS

The disorders of müllerian agenesis include congenital absence of the vagina and uterus. Often referred to in the literature simply as congenital absence of the vagina (vaginal agenesis), this condition is more accurately labeled aplasia (or dysplasia) of the müllerian ducts because the lower vagina generally is normal, but the middle and upper two thirds are missing. Despite the absence of the uterus, rudimentary uterine primordia are found that are comparable to each other in size and appearance. Tubes and ovaries in patients with congenital absence of the müllerian ducts generally are normal. The syndrome, usually referred to as the MRKH syndrome, is associated with a heterogeneous group of disorders that have a variety of genetic, endocrine, and metabolic manifestations and associated anomalies of other body systems.

Characteristics of Women with Müllerian Agenesis

- Congenital absence of the uterus and vagina (small rudimentary uterine bulbs are usually present with rudimentary fallopian tubes)
- Normal ovarian function, including ovulation
- Sex of rearing: female
- Phenotypic sex: female (normal development of breasts, body proportions, hair distribution, and external genitalia)
- Genetic sex: female (46,XX karyotype)
- Frequent association of other congenital anomalies (skeletal, urologic, and especially renal)

Partial agenesis of the vagina with the uterus present and a transverse vaginal septum both are categorized as disorders of vertical fusion. These two disorders have a low incidence of associated urinary tract anomalies, another circumstance that sets them apart from the MRKH syndrome.

Realdus Columbus first described congenital absence of the vagina in 1559. In 1829, Mayer described congenital absence of the vagina as one of the abnormalities found in stillborn infants with multiple birth defects. Rokitansky in 1838 and Küster in 1910 described an entity in which the vagina was absent, a small bipartite uterus was present, the ovaries were normal, and anomalies of other organ systems (renal and skeletal) were frequently observed. Hauser and associates emphasized the spectrum of associated anomalies. Pinsky suggested that congenital absence of the vagina is part of a symptom

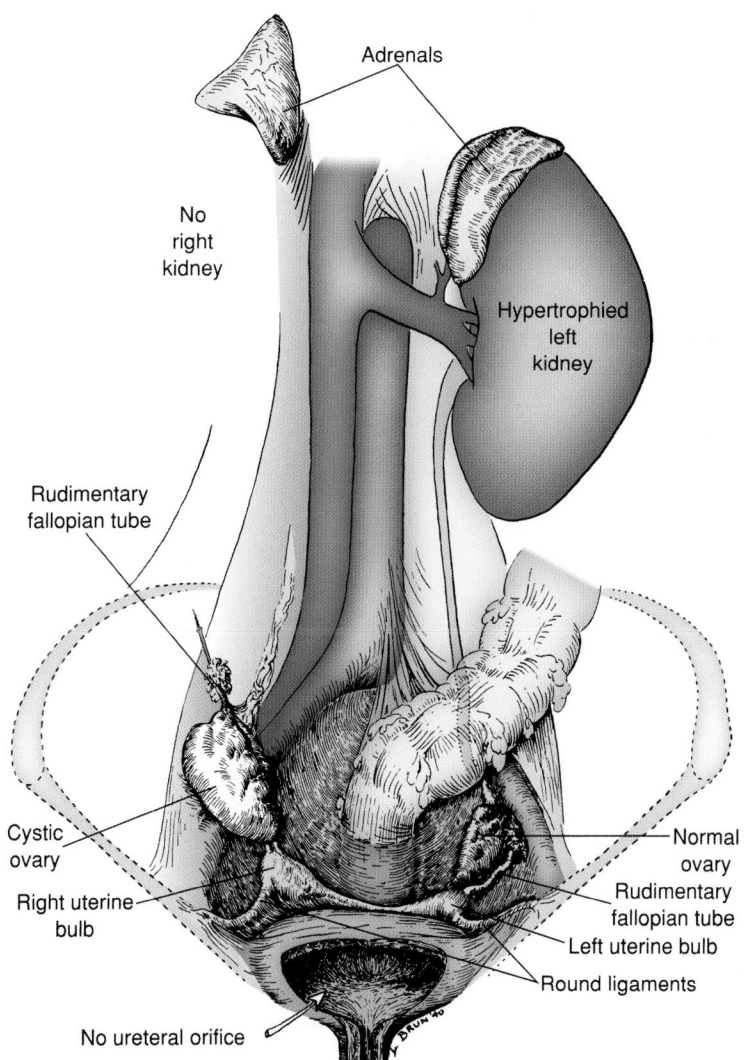

Adrenals

No
right
kidney

Hypertrophied
left
kidney

Rudimentary
fallopian tube

Cystic
ovary

Right uterine
bulb

No ureteral orifice

Normal
ovary
Rudimentary
fallopian tube
Left uterine bulb
Round ligaments

FIGURE 25.3 Typical findings in a patient with MRKH syndrome. Note the absence of the right kidney and right ureteral orifice. The uterus is represented by bilateral rudimentary uterine bulbs joined by a band behind the bladder. The ovaries appear normal although there is malposition of the right ovary.

complex and not a true syndrome. Over the years, the disorder has come to be known as the MRKH syndrome, the Rokitansky-Küster-Hauser syndrome, or simply the Rokitansky syndrome (Fig. 25.3). Counseller found that the condition occurred once in 4,000 female admissions to the Mayo Clinic. Evans estimated that vaginal agenesis occurred once in 10,588 female births in Michigan from 1953 to 1957.

Individuals with an absent vagina and the classic MRKH syndrome usually are first seen by a gynecologist at age 14 to 15 years, when the absence of menses causes concern. Such young women have a normal complement of chromosomes (46,XX) and usually have normal ovaries and secondary sex characteristics, including external genitalia. Menstruation does not appear at the usual age because the uterus is absent, but ovulation occurs regularly. There are some exceptions to the rule of normal ovaries. For example, polycystic ovaries and gonadal dysgenesis have been reported in patients with congenital absence of the vagina. Plevraki and colleagues reinforced the importance of consideration of such conditions, as one of the six women with MRKH evaluated over a 12-month period demonstrated hypergonadotropic hypogonadism that was due to the bilateral absence of gonadal tissue. Additionally, nested polymerase chain reaction demonstrated the presence of testis-specific protein 1-Y-linked (TSPY) gene in two women.

Etiologic Factors

An exclusively genetic etiology cannot be ascribed to vaginal agenesis because almost all patients have a normal karyotype (46,XX) and because the discordance of vaginal agenesis in three sets of monozygotic twins has been reported. The occurrence of complete vaginal agenesis in sisters with a 46,XX karyotype suggests an autosomal mode of inheritance for these patients. Shokeir investigated the families of 13 unrelated females with aplasia of müllerian duct derivatives. Similarly affected females were found in 10 families. Usually, there was an affected female paternal relative, suggesting female-limited autosomal dominant inheritance of a mutant gene transmitted by male relatives.

Other investigators point to the variety of associated anomalies as support for the etiologic concept of variable expression of a genetic defect possibly precipitated by teratogenic exposure between the 37th and the 41st gestational day, the time during which the vagina is formed. Knab has suggested five possible etiologic factors of the MRKH syndrome:

1. Inappropriate production of müllerian regressive factor in the female embryonic gonad
2. Regional absence or deficiency of estrogen receptors limited to the lower müllerian duct

3. Arrest of müllerian duct development by a teratogenic agent
4. Mesenchymal inductive defect
5. Sporadic gene mutation

Knab believes that the teratogenic and the mutant gene etiologies are the most probable.

Anomalies Associated with Müllerian Agenesis

Many patients with müllerian agenesis have associated anomalies of the upper müllerian duct system together with associated anomalies of other organ systems. By gentle rectal examination, the physician can feel an absence of the midline müllerian structure that should represent the uterus. The physician instead feels a smooth band (possibly a remnant of the uterosacral ligaments) that extends from one side of the pelvis to the other. In MRKH syndrome, the uterus is represented by bilateral rudimentary uterine bulbs that vary in size, are not usually palpable, are connected to small fallopian tubes, and are located on the lateral pelvic side wall adjacent to normal ovaries. Depending on their size, these rudimentary uterine bulbs may or may not contain a cavity lined by endometrial tissue (**Fig. 25.4**). If present, the endometrial tissue can appear immature or, rarely, can show evidence of cyclic response to ovarian hormones. The endometrial cavity does not communicate often with the peritoneal cavity because the tube may not be patent at the point of junction between the tube and the rudimentary uterine bulb. In rare instances, however, active endometrium can exist within the uterine anlagen and the endometrial cavity, enabling communication with the peritoneal cavity through patent fallopian tubes. Reports have described several patients with functioning endometrial tissue in one or both rudimentary uterine bulbs (**Fig. 25.4B**). The patient can develop hematometra because of cyclic accumulation of trapped blood. Cyclic abdominal pain is relieved by excision of the active uterine anlagen. A patient with MRKH syndrome was reported who had a 4-cm endometrioma removed from the left ovary by laparotomy at the time of operation to create a vagina. Myomas have been reported to form in the muscular wall of inactive uterine anlagen, and dysmenorrhea has been attributed to their presence. A small myoma has been found, in addition to the tube and ovary, in the inguinal canal and in the inguinal hernia sac. Due to the rarity of the condition,

interaction with the radiologist about the patient's history is important to make an accurate diagnosis.

Chakravarty and colleagues and Singh and Devi have demonstrated that the rudimentary bulbs have the potential for function. These authors used these rudimentary uterine bulbs to reconstruct a midline uterus. The reconstructed uterus was then connected to a newly constructed vagina. A surprising number of patients who have undergone this procedure have experienced cyclic menstruation, although recurrent stenosis and obstruction of the rudimentary horns are the most common results of such efforts. The authors of this chapter have had no experience with this technique and question its usefulness. In the majority of cases, these rudimentary uterine bulbs usually are insignificant structures that cause no problems.

Associated Urologic and Renal Anomalies

Fore and associates reported that 47% of patients in whom evaluation of the urinary tract was performed had associated urologic anomalies. In other studies, approximately one third of patients with complete vaginal agenesis were found to have significant urinary anomalies, including unilateral renal agenesis, unilateral or bilateral pelvic kidney, horseshoe kidney, hydronephrosis, hydroureter, and a variety of patterns of ureteral duplication. A significant number of patients with partial vaginal agenesis also have associated urinary tract anomalies.

Associated Skeletal and Other Anomalies

Associated skeletal anomalies have been recognized since congenital absence of the vagina was first described. In a review of 574 reported cases, Griffin and associates found a 12% incidence of skeletal abnormalities. Most of these abnormalities involve the spine (wedge vertebrae, fusions, rudimentary vertebral bodies, and supernumerary vertebrae), but the limbs and ribs also can be involved. Other anomalies include syndactyly, absence of a digit, congenital heart disease, and inguinal hernias, although the latter are more often present in patients with androgen insensitivity syndrome than in patients with MRKH syndrome (**Fig. 25.3**). Consideration of cardiac anomalies is also important, as Pittock and colleagues reported a substantial incidence of cardiac defects (16%) when reviewing a group of 25 patients with MRKH at the Mayo Clinic.

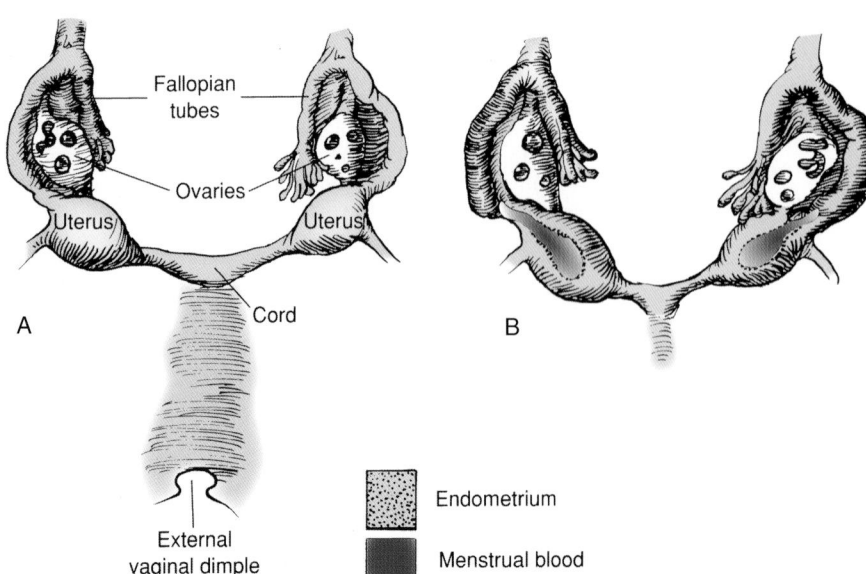

FIGURE 25.4 Patients with congenital absence of the vagina can show variation in the development of the upper müllerian ducts. **A:** Bilateral rudimentary uterine bulbs without endometrium. **B:** Bilateral rudimentary uterine bulbs containing a cavity lined with functioning endometrial tissue. Cross-sectional view shows presence of menstrual blood.

The recognized association of absent vagina with imperforate anus and rectovestibular fistula will likely be diagnosed in infants and treated by the pediatric surgeon at the time of the rectal pull through (most commonly with sigmoid neovaginoplasty). However, the condition may not be noted or treatment may be deferred to young adulthood. Knowledge of this association can be important at the time of treatment as creation of an adequate neovagina with dilation may be impaired by scarring at the previous fistula site in the vestibule. Assessment of vaginal adequacy as a young adult is important as the neovagina created in childhood may need revision or augmentation.

Treatment for Disorders of Müllerian Agenesis

Pretreatment Considerations

If functioning endometrial tissue is present with the anlagen, then symptoms from cryptomenorrhea will begin shortly after female secondary sex characteristics develop. Prompt removal of the active uterine bulbs affords complete relief of symptoms.

Occasionally, older patients with the classic MRKH syndrome consult a gynecologist because of difficult or painful intercourse. The indication for operation in these patients is obvious. Of all patients, they are the most satisfied with the operative results.

Most commonly, patients aged 14 to 16 years are seen by a gynecologist because of primary amenorrhea. An examination may not have been performed by a previous physician because the patient was "too young," but various hormonal medications may have been given with the hope that menstruation would begin. An inaccurate examination may have led to the mistaken diagnosis of imperforate hymen. Futile attempts to incise the hymen may have resulted in scarring of the apex of the vaginal dimple before a correct diagnosis of congenital absence of the vagina was finally made. In the past, it was customary to advise delaying surgery to create a vagina for these young patients until just before their marriage. More recently, it has become usual to perform the procedure when patients are 17 to 20 years old and are emotionally mature and intellectually ready to manage the potential postoperative requirements for care, including manipulation of the vaginal form or the use of dilators.

Psychological Concerns

Insufficient attention has been given to the psychological aspects of this problem. The patient with congenital absence of the vagina cannot be made into a whole person simply by creating a perineal pouch for intercourse. Establishment of sexual function is only one concern and may be the easiest problem to correct. Evans reported that 15% of his patients have real psychiatric difficulty. He and David and associates suggest that psychiatric help should be initiated before the treatment to create a neovagina. Weijenborg and ter Kuile described the effect of a group program on women with Rokitansky syndrome. The authors held group sessions conducted by a gynecologist, a female social worker, and a woman with Rokitansky syndrome. Seventeen patients participated. Three women had elected not to create a vagina, six women created a vagina by dilatation or sexual activity, and eight women had undergone a vaginoplasty. Indices of psychological distress were measured before the program, at initiation of the program, and at the last group session. The results demonstrated that women with Rokitansky syndrome felt less anxious, less depressed, and less sensitive to interpersonal contact after participation in the semistructured program. These data support the value of group interaction in patients with Rokitansky syndrome.

Learning about this anomaly, especially at a young age, is a shock and is accompanied by diminished self-esteem.

Such patients can be encouraged by having their gynecologist offer appropriate psychological and medical therapy with an experienced multidisciplinary team. The gynecologist can also point out that the patient will functionally be like other young women who have had a hysterectomy because of serious pelvic disease and who have satisfied their desire to be a parent through adoption or gestational surrogacy. When receiving this diagnosis, patients and families are looking for reassurance about the future. Liao and colleagues reported on women with Rokitansky (treated with dilation, no treatment, or surgery) who completed four questionnaires assessing health-related quality of life, emotional distress, and sexual function and underwent a vaginal examination. Of the 87 eligible participants, 56 (64%) took part in the study. Thirty-six women had used dilators in the past, and 7 (who were sexually active) had undergone vaginal surgery (laparoscopic Vecchietti 4, McIndoe 1, bowel 1, skin flap vaginoplasty 1). The range of time from surgery to participation in the study was 5 to 16 years. Twelve patients had no intervention to create a neovagina. The participants reported overall better physical health and poorer overall mental health compared with normative data. Anxiety levels were higher, especially for women who had treatment to create a neovagina (dilation or surgical treatment). Vaginal length had a positive correlation with overall sexual satisfaction but was not related to overall quality of life. Kimberley and colleagues in Australia reported on quality of life and sexual experience of patients with vaginal atresia or agenesis. Seventy patients were identified, but nine were excluded who were younger than 17 years, newly diagnosed, or developmentally delayed. Thirty-four women responded with 28 actual participants in the study. Of the 20 patients who completed the sexual satisfaction questionnaire, only four were treated surgically (Sheare procedure 3, McIndoe 1) and the remaining 16 created a neovagina with dilation. The quality-of-life outcomes as measured by the World Health Organization Quality of Life (WHOQOL-BREF) questionnaire showed overall quality of life to be comparable to that of the average Australian population. In addition to quality-of-life evaluation, psychosocial assessment is important as well. There was a strong correlation between the quality-of-life scores and sexual satisfaction, highlighting the importance of psychological and psychosocial supports in the management of young women affected by the condition. Time since diagnosis had a positive influence on overall sexual satisfaction, with 92% of women who received a diagnosis more than 5 years ago demonstrating satisfactory sexual function scores. Callens and her colleagues in the Belgian-Dutch Study Group on Disorder of Sex Development (DSD) attempted to evaluate the psychosexual and anatomical outcomes of patients after dilation or surgery to create a neovagina; however, only 7 of the 35 participants were noted to have a diagnosis of MRKH (all treated with skin graft neovaginoplasty). Of those patients, only two were examined to correlate the anatomic findings with the psychosexual responses. All of the patients completed at least some part of the Female Sexual Function Index (FSFI), a validated measure in the vaginal reconstruction population, with the mean score of 25.0, which falls below the 26.55 cutoff, implying that they are at risk for developing sexual dysfunction. The authors acknowledged that their population was not randomized for treatment, was recruited exclusively from a clinical sample, and may have been biased by including patients who created a sufficient vagina by coitus alone with those that followed a dilation program. Regardless, their results support that any treatment for vaginal hypoplasia may be of limited utility without psychological expertise to address other aspects of self-perception. More work in the area of overall quality of life, well-being, and emotional/sexual wellness is needed in this population.

When counseling patients, gestational surrogacy should definitely be included in the discussion. Until recently, the literature had provided only sparse evidence regarding the use of this modality in this population. Beski and colleagues confirmed the use of gestational surrogacy in a small population. The treatment cycles resulted in six clinical pregnancies (42.9% pregnancy rate per embryo transfer and 54.5% per oocyte retrieval) and three live births (21.4% per embryo transfer, 27.3% per retrieval, and 50% per patient). Several authors have reported on the genetic offspring of patients with vaginal agenesis. Petrozza and colleagues reported a retrospective study in 1997, describing a large number of treatment cycles for patients with Rokitansky syndrome. The authors attempted to determine an inheritance pattern of the syndrome through a questionnaire sent to all centers performing surrogacy treatment in the United States. A total of 162 in vitro fertilization/surrogacy treatment cycles were reviewed for 58 patients with congenital agenesis of the uterus and vagina. The treatment resulted in 34 live births (17 girls, 17 boys). One child had a nonspecific middle ear defect and hearing loss. The authors concluded that congenital absence of the uterus and vagina was not commonly inherited in a dominant fashion. These findings suggest that inheritance of this disorder in children of affected mothers is likely via a polygenic mechanism. In this population, none of the 17 female infants born to affected mothers exhibited Rokitansky syndrome. Ovulation induction is similar to other patients; however, oocyte retrieval may be more challenging. Typically, oocytes are retrieved transvaginally; yet, after creation of a neovagina, the ovaries may not be as easily accessible. In addition, ovaries may be ectopically located, higher in the abdomen. Barton and colleagues reported success with a transabdominal approach without decrease in safety or efficacy. Five of the sixty-nine women who underwent abdominal follicular aspiration were noted to have congenital reproductive anomalies.

Patient Cooperation

Regardless of which operative technique is chosen, the patient must cooperate if the operation is to be successful. In many of the available vaginal reconstruction techniques, dilation or use of a vaginal mold will be necessary. For example, when a McIndoe operation is performed, patients must understand the need to wear a form continuously for several months and intermittently for several years until the vagina is no longer subject to constriction and until regular intercourse is taking place. No surgery should be performed until preoperative evaluation determines that the patient understands her essential role in its success. This is especially important when the patient is a younger teenager. The single most important factor in determining the success of vaginoplasty is the psychosocial adjustment of the patient to her congenital vaginal anomaly.

Laboratory and Diagnostic Testing

A complete chromosomal analysis should be considered in all patients. If there is a suspicion of ovarian dysgenesis, androgen insensitivity syndrome, or some aberration of the classic MRKH syndrome, then a consideration of additional SRY analysis should be entertained to assess the possible presence of any Y chromosome. A contrast study such as a magnetic resonance (MR) urogram or an intravenous pyelogram should be done preoperatively. This also provides an adequate survey for anomalies of the spine. If a pelvic mass is present, then additional special studies may be indicated to differentiate

between hematometra, hematocolpos, endometrial and other ovarian cysts, and pelvic kidney. The MR urogram may facilitate the evaluation of the reproductive, urologic, and skeletal systems with one radiographic study.

Evaluation of Cyclic Pain

Some patients without a pelvic mass report cyclic pain. This pain can be ovulatory or possibly a result of dysmenorrhea originating in well-developed rudimentary uterine bulbs. The physician can differentiate between the two by asking the patient to keep a pain diary and reviewing the diagnostic imaging with an experienced reconstructive gynecologic surgeon or radiologist to ensure that an obstructed anlagen is not present. Occasionally, there is a question about whether a patient has congenital absence of the vagina or an imperforate hymen with cryptomenorrhea. The diagnosis is clarified before operative intervention by using radiographic imaging. Pelvic ultrasonography can often detect hematocolpos or an obstructed uterine anlagen distended with menstrual blood. Magnetic resonance imaging (MRI) can differentiate the two diagnoses, if necessary.

METHODS OF CREATING A VAGINA

There is no unanimity of opinion regarding the correct approach to the problem of vaginal agenesis (Table 25.3). With the development of the Ingram method for vaginal dilatation, fewer patients require surgical vaginoplasty. The American Congress of Obstetricians and Gynecologists has supported nonsurgical creation of a neovagina as first-line therapy since 2006. Increased utilization of additional surgical techniques has broadened the discussion of surgical treatment of vaginal agenesis. The role of tissue expanders in vaginoplasty has been reviewed by Patil and Hixon. Labial expansion with an expander having a capacity of 250 mL provides a flap

---

TABLE 25.3 Classification of Methods to Form a New Vagina

Nonsurgical (intermittent pressure on the perineum)
  Active dilatation
  Passive dilatation

Surgical
  Without the use of abdominal contents
    Without cavity dissection
      Vulvovaginoplasty
      Constant pressure (Vecchietti)
    No attempt to line cavity (now unacceptable)
    Lining cavity with grafts
      Split-thickness skin grafts (McIndoe operation)
      Dermis grafts
      Amnion homografts
    Lining cavity with flaps
      Musculocutaneous flaps
      Fasciocutaneous flaps
      Subcutaneous pedicled skin flaps
      Labial skin flaps (can be created with tissue expander)
      Penoplasty (transsexualism)

With use of abdominal contents (cavity lining with)
  Peritoneum
  Free intestinal graft
  Pedicled intestine

10 cm long and 8 cm wide with a 4-cm projection. Thus, well-vascularized flaps can be available to provide an outlet for stenosis-free vaginoplasty. This approach has been suggested to maximize the success of surgical vaginoplasty. A review of the methods devised for the formation of a vagina follows. The editors of this book have found the modified McIndoe technique to give the most consistently satisfactory results.

Nonsurgical Methods

In 1938, Frank described a method of creating an artificial vagina without operation. In 1940, he reported remarkably satisfactory results in eight patients treated with this method. His follow-up study showed that a vagina formed in this manner remained permanent in depth and caliber, even in patients who neglected dilatation for more than 1 year. It has been emphasized that the pelvic floor itself is embryologically deficient in some patients. Indeed, the ease with which some patients are able to create a vagina with intercourse alone or with other intermittent pressure techniques can be explained on this basis. Five patients were reported to have developed enteroceles, one after coitus alone, three after a Williams vulvovaginoplasty, and three after a McIndoe operation. This complication can develop when the vaginal mucosa is brought in close proximity to the pelvic peritoneum, but a relative embryologic weakness or an absence of endopelvic fascia can also contribute to this complication. Rock, Reeves, and associates at the Johns Hopkins Hospital reported that an initial trial of vaginal dilatation was successful in 9 of 21 patients.

Prompted by the rewarding results of Broadbent and Woolf, Ingram has described a passive dilatation technique of creating a new vagina. Instructing his patients in the insertion of dilators (Fig. 25.5) specially designed for use with a bicycle seat stool, Ingram was able to produce satisfactory vaginal depth

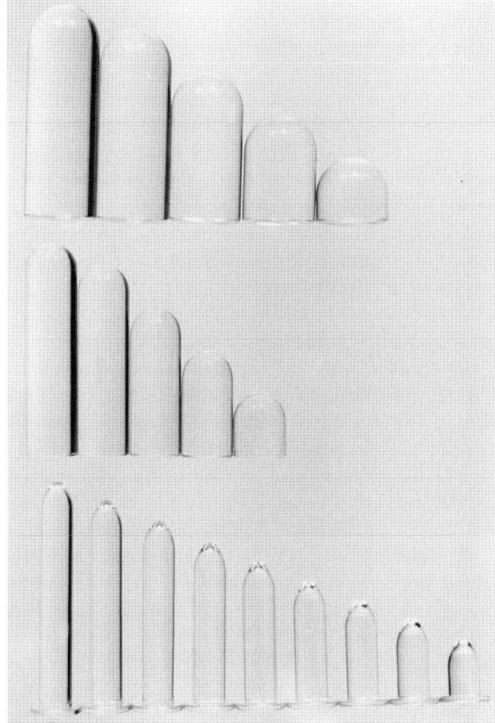

FIGURE 25.5 Vaginal dilators for use in Ingram passive dilatation technique to create a new vagina. The set from Faulkner Plastics consists of 19 dilators of increasing length and width.

and coital function in 10 of 12 cases of vaginal agenesis and 32 of 40 cases of various types of stenosis.

The Ingram technique for passive dilatation has several advantages. The patient is not required to press the dilator against the vaginal pouch. A series of graduated Lucite dilators slowly and evenly dilate the neovaginal space. The patient should be carefully instructed in the use of dilators, as recommended by Ingram, beginning with the smallest dilator. The patient is shown and instructed with the use of a mirror how to place a dilator against the introital dimple. The dilator may be held in place with a supportive undergarment and regular clothing worn over this.

The patient is shown how to sit on a racing-type bicycle seat that is placed on a stool 24 inches above the floor. She is instructed to sit leaning slightly forward with the dilator in place for at least 2 hours/day at intervals of 15 to 30 minutes. Follow-up is usually at monthly intervals, and the patient can expect to graduate to the next size larger dilator approximately every month. An attempt at sexual intercourse may be suggested after the use of the largest dilator for 1 or 2 months. Continued dilatation is recommended if intercourse is infrequent. In our experience, functional success rates are outstanding. Roberts, Haber, and Rock previously reported the largest series of vaginal agenesis patients who used the Ingram method of dilatation to create a neovagina. The records of 51 patients with müllerian agenesis were reviewed: 37 patients attempted vaginal dilatation, and 14 young women underwent a surgical intervention. Functional success was defined as satisfactorily achieving intercourse or accepting the largest dilator without discomfort in the clinic visit. All patients were followed up for at least 2 years and for an average of 9.25 years. Functional success was achieved in 91.9% of those who attempted dilatation (Table 25.4). Thus, passive dilatation should be suggested as an initial therapy for vaginal creation. If dilatation is unsuccessful, operative vaginoplasty is indicated.

Edmonds and colleagues reported on their experience with managing 360 patients with MRKH from 1998 to 2010. Two hundred forty-five patients requested vaginal dilation for treatment. The mean age of dilating patients was 18.6 years (16 to 22 years). Success was defined as achieving sexual satisfaction and functional vaginal length (6 cm) and was achieved in 232 of 245 patients (94.7%). The mean time to complete therapy was 5.5 months (2 to 19 months). Despite having large number of patients in the study, the applicability outside of the United Kingdom could be questioned. The UK program consists of an intensive program in which patients have an identified clinical nurse specialist for teaching and support, one or two specific providers, and an inpatient admission (an average of 3 days) to teach dilation technique. Also, sexual satisfaction was not measured in a structured way for all patients; a subset of 60 patients were assessed using a sexual function questionnaire with the answers compared to a normal population. In the United States,

TABLE 25.4 Outcomes of Patients with Vaginal Agenesis Who Attempted Dilatation

PATIENTS	TOTALS	PERCENT
Successful dilatation	34/37	91.9%[a]
Failed dilatation	3/37	8.1%

[a]$P < 0.001$.
Modified from Roberts CP, Haber MJ, Rock JA. Vaginal creation for müllerian agenesis. *Am J Obstet Gynecol* 2001;185:1349, with permission. Copyright © 2001, Elsevier.

V

Gargollo and colleagues described their 12-year experience treating patients with vaginal agenesis. Rokitansky syndrome was the primary diagnosis in 64 of the 69 patients included in the retrospective review. The mean age at start of vaginal dilation was 17.5 years (14 to 35 years), and mean follow-up time was 19 months (0 to 100). Progressive perineal dilation was the treatment of choice. The total success rate was 88% achieving functional success (ability to achieve satisfactory vaginal intercourse, vaginal acceptance of the largest dilator, or vaginal length of at least 7 cm), during a mean of 18.7 months of therapy. Their work not only described an outpatient regimen that could be applicable in the United States but also highlighted the integral role that the multidisciplinary team plays in patient success. They also reinforced that dilating can be successful even in patients with a small vaginal dimple; thus, validating an attempt would be reasonable in almost all patients with vaginal agenesis.

Surgical Methods

During the past three decades, experience has proved the Abbe-Wharton-McIndoe procedure (more popularly called the McIndoe operation) for dealing with complete absence of a vagina to be generally superior to others in most cases. In special circumstances, alternative methods of creation of a neovagina may be indicated.

Historical Development of Surgical Procedures

In 1907, Baldwin used a double loop of ileum to line a space dissected between the rectum and bladder, leaving the mesentery connected to the bowel. The continuity of the intestinal tract was reestablished by an end-to-end anastomosis. He reported that the new vagina was absolutely normal in every way. In 1910, Popaw constructed a vagina using a portion of the rectum that was moved anteriorly. This operation was modified by Schubert in 1911. The rectum was severed above the anal sphincter and moved anteriorly to serve as the vagina. The sigmoid was sutured to the anus to reestablish the continuity of the intestinal tract. Both operations had soberingly high morbidity and mortality rates, and their popularity declined. Today, segments of sigmoid are used most often to create a vaginal pouch or extend vaginal length in patients who have lost vaginal function as a result of extensive surgery or irradiation for pelvic malignancy. Some patients who are treated for multiple genitourinary or gastrointestinal abnormalities may be treated with a bowel vaginoplasty during a combined procedure.

Less formidable procedures involving dissection of a space between the bladder and rectum and lining of this space with flaps of skin from the labia or inner thighs also were tried. Marked scarring resulted, and hair usually grew in the vagina. Extensive plastic procedures to construct a vagina are no longer necessary or desirable and have been discarded in favor of safer procedures unless there is the problem of maintaining a vaginal canal after an extensive exenterative operation for pelvic malignancy. In this case, the physician may want to consider using the gracilis myocutaneous flap technique described by McCraw and associates in 1976.

The Abbe-Wharton-McIndoe Operation

This operation for creating a new vagina began with simple surgical attempts to create a space between the bladder and the rectum. These early attempts were often made in patients with cryptomenorrhea. However, such a space usually would constrict because the surgeon would fail to recognize the importance of prolonged continuous dilatation until the constrictive phase of healing was complete.

At the Johns Hopkins Hospital in 1938, Wharton combined an adequate dissection of the vaginal space with continuous

dilatation by a balsa form that was covered with a thin rubber sheath and was left in the space. He did not use a split-thickness skin graft. Instead, he based his operation on the principle that the vaginal epithelium has remarkable powers of proliferation and in a relatively short time will cover the raw surface. Recalling that a similar process occurs in the fetus when the epithelium of the sinovaginal bulbs and the urogenital sinus form the vaginal canal, Wharton merely applied this same principle in the adult. This simple procedure is entirely satisfactory as long as the space is kept dilated long enough to allow the epithelium to grow in. Occasionally, however, even after several years, the vault of the vagina remains without epithelial covering. Coital bleeding and leukorrhea result from the persistent granulation tissue, and there is a tendency for vaginas constructed by this method to be constricted by scarring in the upper portion. In Counseller's 1948 report from the Mayo Clinic of 100 operations to construct a new vagina, 14 were performed by the Wharton method, with excellent results in all 14 patients. It was stated that the disadvantages of persistent granulation tissue with bleeding and leukorrhea were of no consequence. This has not been the experience of the editors of this book.

When inlay skin grafts were first used to construct a new vagina, the results were poor because the necessity for dilatation of the new vagina again was not recognized. Severe contraction, uncontrolled by continuous or intermittent dilatation, almost invariably spoiled the results. Although Abbe and others preceded him by many years in using a skin-covered prosthesis in neovaginal construction, it was Sir Archibald McIndoe, at the Queen Victoria Hospital in England, who popularized the method and gave it substantial clinical trial. He emphasized the three important principles used today in successful operations for vaginal agenesis:

1. Dissection of an adequate space between the rectum and the bladder
2. Inlay split-thickness skin grafting
3. The cardinal principle of continuous and prolonged dilatation during the contractile phase of healing

Other tissues such as amnion and peritoneum have been used to line the new vaginal space, but they have not had substantial success. However, Tancer and associates reported good results with human amnion. Karjalainen and associates stated that a more physiologic result was achieved with an amnion graft than with a skin graft. Nevertheless, concerns about the transmission of human immunodeficiency virus with human amnion now limit this option.

Technique of Abbe-Wharton-McIndoe Operation

TAKING THE GRAFT After a careful pelvic examination is performed under anesthesia to verify previous findings, the patient is positioned for taking a skin graft from the buttocks. For cosmetic reasons, the graft should not be taken from the thigh or hip unless for some reason it cannot be obtained from the buttocks. Patients may be asked to sunbathe in a bathing suit before coming to the hospital so that its outline can be seen; an attempt should be made to take the graft from both buttocks within these borders. The quality of the graft determines to a great extent the success of the operation. We have found the Padgett electrodermatome to be the most satisfactory instrument for taking the graft. With relatively little experience and practice, the gynecologic surgeon can successfully cut a graft of controlled width and thickness (Fig. 25.6). The instrument is set and checked for taking a graft approximately 0.018 inch thick and 8 to 9 cm wide. The total graft length should be 16 to 20 cm. If the entire graft cannot be taken from one buttock, then a graft 8 to 10 cm long is needed from each buttock.

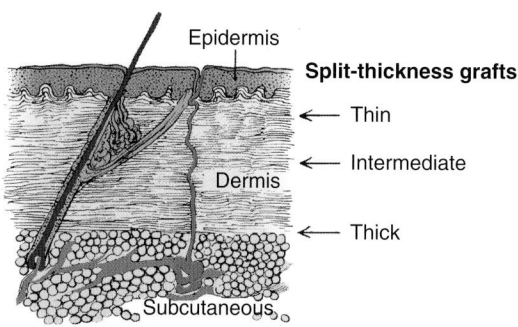

Split-thickness grafts

Epidermis

← Thin

← Intermediate

Dermis

← Thick

Subcutaneous

FIGURE 25.6 Section of split-thickness skin grafts. Grafts should be uniform in thickness. The Padgett electrodermatome is set to take a graft approximately 0.018 inch thick. A graft that is slightly thick is better than a thin graft.

The skin of the donor site is prepared with an antiseptic solution (povidone–iodine), which is then thoroughly washed away. The skin is then lubricated with mineral oil as assistants steady and stretch the skin tight. Considerable pressure should be applied uniformly across the dermatome blade. The thickness of the graft must have minimal variation. A graft that is a little too thick is better than one that is a little too thin. There should be no breaks in the continuity of the graft. The graft is placed between two layers of moist gauze, and the donor sites are dressed. The donor site is soaked with a dilute solution of epinephrine for hemostasis, and a sterile dressing is applied. A pressure dressing is then placed over the site; this dressing can be removed on the seventh postoperative day. The sterile dressing dries in place over the donor site and ultimately will fall off by itself. Moistened areas on the dressing can be dried with cool air. If there is separation and evidence of some superficial infection, then merbromin can be applied to these areas.

CREATING THE NEOVAGINAL SPACE The patient is placed in the lithotomy position, and a transverse incision is made through the mucosa of the vaginal vestibule (**Fig. 25.7A**). The space between the urethra and bladder anteriorly and the rectum posteriorly is dissected until the undersurface of the peritoneum is reached.

Median raphe

Creating space between urethra and rectum

A

B

C

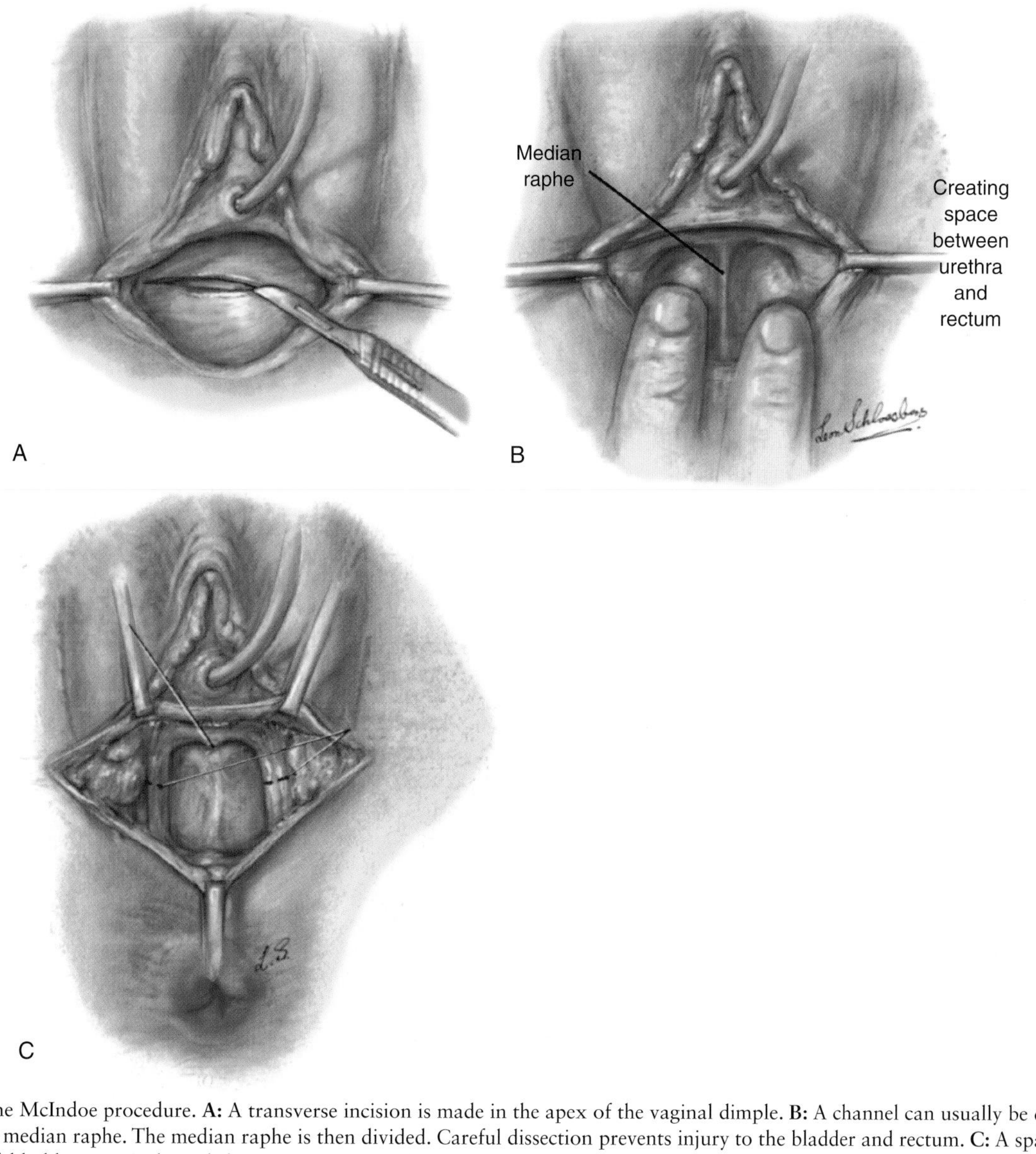

FIGURE 25.7 The McIndoe procedure. **A:** A transverse incision is made in the apex of the vaginal dimple. **B:** A channel can usually be dissected on each side of the median raphe. The median raphe is then divided. Careful dissection prevents injury to the bladder and rectum. **C:** A space between the urethra and bladder anteriorly and the rectum posteriorly is dissected until the undersurface of the peritoneum is reached. Incision of the medial margin of the puborectalis muscles will enlarge the vagina laterally.

This step may be safer with a catheter in the urethra and sometimes a finger in the rectum to guide the dissection in the proper plane. After incising the mucosa of the vaginal vestibule transversely, the physician often is able to create a channel on each side of a median raphe (Fig. 25.7B), starting with blunt dissection and then dilating each channel with Hegar dilators or with finger dissection. In some instances, it may be necessary to develop the neovaginal space by dissecting laterally and bringing the fingers toward the midline. The median raphe is then divided, thus joining the two channels. This maneuver is helpful in dissecting an adequate space without causing injury to surrounding structures.

To avoid subsequent narrowing of the vagina at the level of the urogenital diaphragm, it may be helpful to incise the margin of the puborectalis muscles bilaterally along the midportion of the medial margin (Fig. 25.7C). Although useful in all circumstances, incision of the puborectalis muscle is more important in cases of androgen insensitivity syndrome with android pelvis, in which the levator muscles are more taut against the pelvic diaphragm, than in cases of gynecoid pelvis. Incision of the puborectalis muscle causes no difficulty with fecal incontinence, significantly improves the ease with which the vaginal form can be inserted into the canal in the postoperative period, and has eliminated the problem of contracture of the upper vagina caused by a poorly applied form. The dissection should be carried as high as possible without entering the peritoneal cavity and without cleaning away all tissue beneath the peritoneum. A split-thickness skin graft will not take well when applied against a base of thin peritoneum. All bleeders should be ligated by clamping and tying them with very fine sutures. It is essential that the vaginal cavity be dry to prevent bleeding beneath the graft. Bleeding causes the graft to separate from its bed, resulting in the inevitable failure of the graft to implant in that area and in local graft necrosis.

PREPARING THE VAGINAL FORM Early skin grafts were formed over balsa, which has the advantages of being an inexpensive, easily available, light wood that can be sterilized without difficulty. It also can be whittled easily in the operating room to a proper shape to fit the new vaginal space. However, uneven pressure from the form can cause a skin graft to slough in places, and pressure spots are associated with an increased risk of fistula formation. The Counseller-Flor modification of the McIndoe technique (Fig. 25.8) uses, instead of the rigid balsa form, a foam rubber mold shaped for the vaginal cavity from a foam rubber block and covered with a condom. The foam rubber is gas sterilized in blocks measuring approximately 10 × 10 × 20 cm. The block is shaped with scissors to approximately twice the desired size, compressed into a condom, and placed into the neovagina (Fig. 25.8A–C). The form is left in place for 20 to 30 seconds with the condom open to allow the foam rubber to expand and conform to the neovaginal space (Fig. 25.8D). The condom is then closed, and the form is withdrawn. The external end is tied with 2-0 silk, and an additional condom is placed over the form and tied securely (Fig. 25.8E, F).

SEWING THE GRAFT OVER THE VAGINAL FORM The skin graft is then placed over the form and its undersurface exteriorized and sewn over the form with interrupted vertical mattress 5-0 nonreactive sutures (Fig. 25.8G, H). Where the graft is approximated, the undersurfaces of the sutured edges are also exteriorized.

The graft should not be "meshed" to make it stretch farther, and the edges of the graft should be approximated meticulously around the form without gaps. Granulation tissue develops at any place where the form is not covered with skin. Contraction usually occurs where granulation tissue forms. After the form has been placed in the neovaginal space, the edges of the graft are sutured to the skin edge with 5-0 nonreactive absorbable sutures, with sufficient space left between sutures for drainage to occur. The physician must be careful not to have the form so large that it causes undue pressure on the urethra or rectum. A balsa form should have a groove to accommodate the urethra. With a foam rubber form, this is unnecessary. A suprapubic silicone catheter is placed in the bladder for drainage. If the labia are of sufficient length, then the form can be held in place by suturing the labia together with two or three nonreactive sutures.

REPLACING WITH A NEW FORM After 7 to 10 days, the form is removed and the vaginal cavity is irrigated with warm saline solution and inspected. This is usually performed with mild sedation and without an anesthetic. The cavity should be inspected carefully to determine whether the graft has taken satisfactorily in all areas of the new vagina. Any undue pressure by the form should be noted and corrected. It is especially important that there not be too much pressure superiorly against the peritoneum of the cul-de-sac. Such a constant upward pressure could result in weakness with subsequent enterocele formation. The new vaginal cavity must be inspected frequently to detect and to prevent pressure necrosis of the skin graft.

The patient is given instructions on daily removal and reinsertion of the form and is taught how to administer a low-pressure douche of clear warm water. She is advised to remove the form at the time of urination and defecation, but otherwise to wear it continuously for 6 weeks. A neoprene form, which is much easier to remove and keep clean than a foam rubber form, is substituted for the original form in 6 weeks. A new form is molded with a sterile sheath cover (condom) to fit the size of the vaginal canal. The patient is instructed to use the form during the night for the following 12 months. If there has been no change in the caliber of the vagina by that time, then it is unlikely to occur later, and insertion of the form at night can be done intermittently until coitus is a frequent occurrence. However, if there is the slightest difficulty in inserting the form, then the patient should be advised to use the form continuously again. Most patients are able to maintain the form in place simply by wearing tighter underclothes and a perineal pad. Douches are advisable during residual vaginal healing and discharge.

RESULTS AND COMPLICATIONS Results with the McIndoe operation have improved over the years. Recently, reported percentages of satisfactory results have ranged from 80% to 100%. The serious complications formerly associated with the McIndoe operation have been significantly reduced by improvements in technique and greater experience. Serious complications do still occur, however, including a 4% postoperative fistula rate (urethrovaginal, vesicovaginal, and rectovaginal), postoperative infection, and intraoperative and postoperative hemorrhage. Failure of graft take is also still reported as an occasional complication. Failure of graft take often leads to the development of granulation tissue, which might require reoperation, curettage of the granulation tissue down to a healthy base, and even regrafting. Minor granulation can be treated with silver nitrate application. The functional result is more important than the anatomic result in evaluating the success of this operation. Although a vagina of only 4 cm is adequate for some couples, in most instances, a vagina smaller than 4 cm causes major problems.

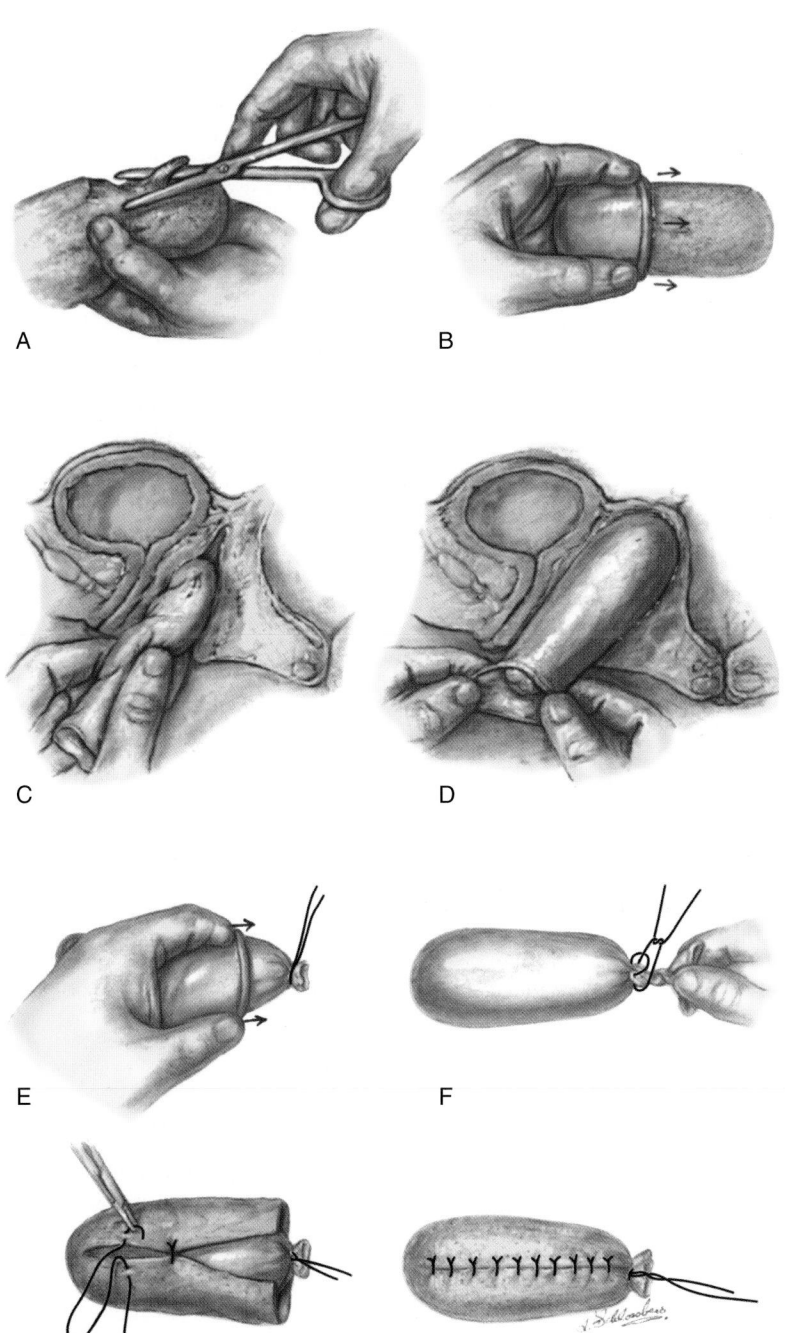

FIGURE 25.8 Counseller-Flor modification of the McIndoe technique. **A:** A form is cut from a foam rubber block. **B:** A condom is placed over the form. **C:** The form is compressed and placed into the vagina. **D:** Air is allowed to expand the foam rubber, which accommodates to the neovaginal space. The condom is closed and the form removed. A second condom is placed over the form (**E**) and tied securely (**F**). **G:** The graft is then sewn over the form with interrupted 5-0 nonreactive sutures. **H:** The undersurfaces of the sutured edges of the graft are exteriorized. The vaginal form is ready for insertion into the neovagina.

The postoperative results have improved significantly since the balsa vaginal form was replaced by the foam rubber form. Between 1950 and 1989, the McIndoe operation was performed on 94 patients at the Johns Hopkins Hospital. During these 39 years, 83% of the 94 patients had a 100% take of the graft; in only three cases was there a significant area over which the graft failed.

Urethrovaginal fistula has become even more infrequent since the introduction of the suprapubic catheter and the foam rubber form. The catheter is removed when the patient is voiding well and has no residual urine. In general, the patient is able to void without difficulty within the first few days of the procedure. Prophylactic broad-spectrum antibiotics started

within 12 hours of surgery and continued for 7 days are of definite value in reducing the incidence of graft failures from infection in the operative site.

Because of the excellent results obtained after a modified McIndoe vaginoplasty, this operation is recommended as the procedure of choice for women unable or unwilling to obtain a neovagina with dilatation methods. Women with a flat perineum with no dimple or pouch have no alternative other than the McIndoe vaginoplasty to obtain a neovagina for comfortable sexual relations.

Desirability of the modified McIndoe procedure may be increased by the use of alternative graft harvest sites to conceal possible aesthetic concerns of the buttock site, as proposed by

Höckel and colleagues. The authors proposed the use of split skin harvesting from the scalp because thin (0.25-mm) split skin grafts do not seem to hamper hair growth at the donor site nor lead to hair growth at the recipient site. Because alopecia has been reported as a complication associated with technical errors, more experience is necessary before advocating the scalp as a potential graft harvest site.

It is important that a McIndoe operation be performed correctly the first time. If the vagina becomes constricted because of granulation tissue formation, injury to adjacent structures, or failure to use the form properly, then subsequent attempts to create a satisfactory vagina are more difficult. The first operation has the best chance of success.

Ozek, like many other surgeons, modified the McIndoe procedure by describing an X-type perineal incision and the use of a perforated vaginal mold during the postoperative period. He postulated that this incision minimized stricture at the vaginal introitus and provided greater ease of dissection of the vaginal cavity. He reinforced that the overall procedure is simple with a generally uneventful postoperative course. Complications included infection, failure of skin graft take, stress urinary incontinence, partial graft loss, and vaginal stricture. All were treated satisfactorily except the patient with stress urinary incontinence.

Despite any minor modifications of the McIndoe vaginoplasty, the essential components of dissection of an adequate space, split-thickness skin grafting, and continuous dilatation during the contractile phase of healing remain unchanged. Recent reviews continue to support the safety and efficacy of the procedure. Hojsgaard and Villadsen reported 26 patients who underwent vaginoplasty, 18 of whom had Rokitansky syndrome. All patients were recorded as having a satisfactory result with complete graft take, adequate vaginal dimensions, and no strictures or fistulas giving symptoms. Complete take was achieved in 33% of patients within a week postoperatively, and after one further grafting procedure, an additional 38% had complete take. The intraoperative and early postoperative complications were perforation of the rectum in one patient (3.8%) and postoperative bleeding in three patients (11.5%). The late complications were vaginal stricture in three patients (11.5%), urethrovaginal fistula in two patients (7.7%), and rectovaginal fistula in one patient (3.8%). Alessandrescu and colleagues described the surgical management of 201 cases of Rokitansky syndrome. The surgeon substituted a modified transverse perineal incision and a perforated, rigid plastic mold. Intraoperative and postoperative complications consisted of two rectal perforations (1%), eight graft infections (4%), and 11 infections of graft site origin (5.5%). Sexual satisfaction was investigated with both objective and subjective criteria. Among the 201 cases, 83.6% had anatomic results evaluated as "good," 10% as "satisfactory," and 6.5% as "unsatisfactory." More than 71% of patients rated their sexual life as "good" or "satisfactory" and reported that they had been able to experience orgasms related to vaginal intercourse. Twenty-three percent reported the ability to have sexual intercourse but had no ability to achieve orgasm, and only 5% expressed dissatisfaction with their sexual performance. Strickland and colleagues reported on the coital satisfaction, perception of vaginal competence, and impact on lifestyle of adult women undergoing vaginoplasty as adolescents. Ten of twenty-two women responded to a questionnaire at a median of 18 years (range 5 to 13 years) following surgical intervention with a McIndoe vaginoplasty. All of the women had sexual experience, and 80% were sexually active at the time of evaluation. The most frequent difficulty reported was vaginal dryness and lack of lubrication with sexual intercourse. Ninety percent of the subjects expressed satisfaction that sexual ability was acceptable. This experience also supports the role of the McIndoe vaginoplasty in providing young women with vaginal agenesis long-term coital ability and minimal disabilities.

DEVELOPMENT OF COMPLICATIONS Several case reports exist of malignant disease developing in a vagina created by various techniques; these reports were reviewed by Gallup and colleagues, as well as others. The authors reported a patient who was initially treated for intraepithelial malignancy by total vaginectomy combined with a split-thickness skin graft vaginoplasty to reconstruct a functional vagina. The authors noted a lesion in her vaginal apex 7 years later. These findings suggest that epithelium transplanted to the vagina can assume the oncogenic potential of the lower reproductive tract. The evidence supports a risk of neoplastic change in both skin and bowel grafts, with a reported average interval from vaginoplasty to diagnosis on the order of 19 years or greater. Epithelium transplanted to the vagina will assume the oncogenic potential of the lower reproductive tract. With less than 25 cases of primary carcinoma of the neovagina reported, it is presently unclear if transplantation of bowel or other graft tissue alone changes the malignancy risk. Consideration of a plan for surveillance and counseling regarding transmission risk for virally related dysplastic change in the lower genital tract is also extremely important for any patients undergoing neovaginoplasty. Neovaginal vault prolapse has also been reported in patients managed both medically and surgically. Without apical or lateral suspension by endopelvic fascial attachments, subsequent prolapse may develop with any type of neovagina. Prolapse in neovaginal segments created by dilation, McIndoe technique, skin flaps, and bowel segments is reported. Abdominal suspension via sacrocolpopexy, abdominal suspension to the Cooper ligament, vaginal resection of redundant prolapsed bowel neovagina, and sacrospinous ligament suspension have all been described as treatment. Kondo and colleagues report a recurrence rate after surgical treatment of 25%.

The Williams Vulvovaginoplasty

Construction of a perineal bridge to help contain the vaginal mold was a routine part of the operation described by McIndoe, but it was not adopted subsequently by others. However, Williams described a similar vulvovaginoplasty procedure in 1964 and advised that it could be used to create a vaginal canal (**Fig. 25.9**). In 1976, he reported that the procedure was unsuccessful in only 1 of 52 patients. Feroze and coworkers reported that the anatomic results were good in 22 of 26 patients. According to these authors, the advantages of the Williams operation are its technical simplicity, its absence of serious local complications even when performed as a repeat procedure, the ease of postoperative care, the absence of postoperative pain, the speed of recovery, the possible elimination of dilators and consequent applicability to patients who do not intend to have regular intercourse in the near future, and the higher success rates of primary and repeat procedures. The technique is not applicable to patients with poorly developed labia. It does result in an unusual angle of the vaginal canal, which is reported to straighten to a more normal direction with intercourse. If a very high perineum is created, urine can momentarily collect in the pouch after urination, giving the impression of postvoid incontinence. Failure of the suture line to heal by primary intention results in a large area of granulation tissue and most likely an unsatisfactory result.

Williams believes that if the urethral meatus is patulous, a vulvovaginoplasty should not be performed because the urethra might be stretched further by coitus. He suggests that varying deficiencies in muscular and fascial tissue can explain

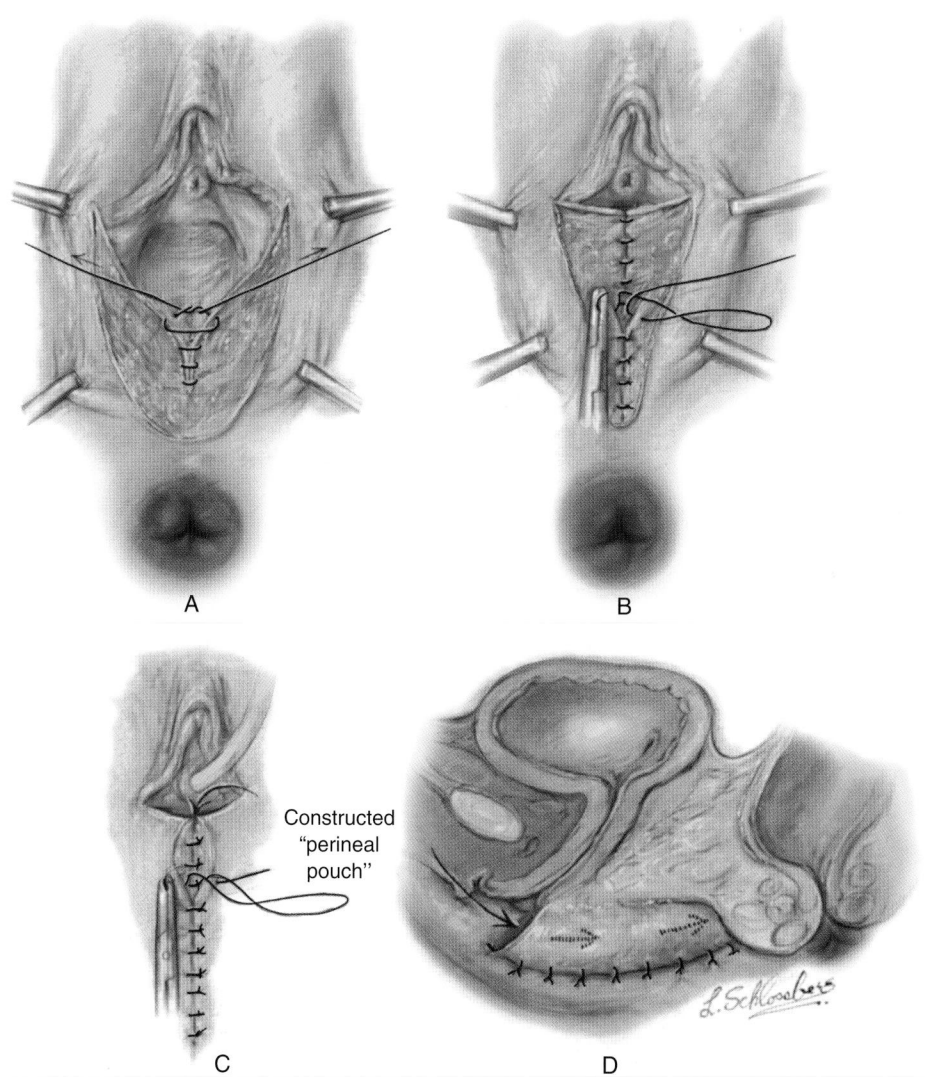

A

B

Constructed "perineal pouch"

C

D

L. Schlossberg

FIGURE 25.9 The Williams vulvovaginoplasty. **A–C:** No. 3-0 polyglycolic acid sutures can be used throughout to close both inner and outer skin margins and the tissue between. **D:** The entrance to the pouch should not cover the external urethral meatus.

why some patients with uterovaginal agenesis are able to develop a satisfactory vaginal canal with simple intermittent pressure with coitus, whereas others are prone to develop enteroceles.

The Williams vulvovaginoplasty is a useful operation and should certainly be considered the operation of choice for patients needing a follow-up to an unsatisfactory primary operation to create a neovagina or a supplement to a small vagina resulting from extensive surgery or radiation therapy, when options are limited. It remains an option for the rare patient with a solitary kidney low in the pelvis who does not have room for dissection of an adequate vaginal space.

Alternative Techniques

Schätz and colleagues reported three patients who underwent the George modification of the Wharton-Sheares neovaginoplasty technique. Wharton combined an adequate dissection of the vaginal space with continuous dilatation by a balsa form that was covered with a thin rubber sheath and was left in the space. His operation was based on the principle that the vaginal epithelium will proliferate and, in a relatively short time, will cover the raw surface. This modification of an already simple procedure may provide an alternative in areas where multidisciplinary, reconstructive pelvic surgery teams are not

available. Because the procedure includes the mere dilatation of the bilateral müllerian ducts and lining of the superior aspect with peritoneum, it eliminates some of the more complex aspects of the other surgical options. However, with a mean follow-up period reported as only 12 months (range of 2 to 23 months), reported long-term complications associated with the Wharton method (persistent granulation tissue, coital bleeding, leukorrhea, and scarring of the upper portion) cannot be fully evaluated. Longer follow-up and a larger patient experience are both necessary to consider this procedure as a primary option for patients with MRKH. Walch and colleagues from Austria reported the outcome of 10 patients with MRKH treated with the George modification of the Wharton-Sheares approach. Mean follow-up from surgery was 33.5 ± 22.4 months (range 3 to 77 months). Data collected on follow-up included cytologic smears of the neovagina, swabs, culture, and hybrid capture for human papillomavirus (HPV). The mean vaginal length was 8.3 cm (range 7 to 10 cm). Of the 8 patients from whom a biopsy was able to be obtained, all showed nonkeratinizing stratified squamous epithelium. The sexual function scores obtained by the Rosen FSFI questionnaire were comparable to previously published control patients. The authors propose that an important drawback of this technique may be the lifelong routine need for the use of vaginal dilators (Table 25.5).

TABLE 25.5 Comparison of Female Sexual Function Index Values for Different Types of Neovaginoplasty

	WHARTON-SHEARES-GEORGE SURGERY (n = 7)	SIGMOID VAGINOPLASTY (n = 11)	DAVYDOV LAPAROSCOPIC VAGINOPLASTY (n = 25)	LAPAROSCOPIC DAVYDOV TECHNIQUE (n = 40)	LAPAROSCOPIC DAVYDOV TECHNIQUE (n = 6)	LAPAROSCOPIC MODIFIED VECCHIETTI TECHNIQUE (n = 27)	LAPAROSCOPIC VECCHIETTI TECHNIQUE (n = 40)	HEALTHY WOMEN (n = 131)
Desire	4.3 ± 1.3	4.7 ± 0.9	4.4 ± 0.9	4.3 ± 0.7	3.9 ± 1.2	4.4 ± 0.8	4.2 ± 0.9	4.1 ± 1.1
Arousability	5.4 ± 0.5	4.9 ± 0.6	4.4 ± 1.1	4.7 ± 0.8	4.0 ± 1.1	4.8 ± 0.8	4.6 ± 1.0	5.0 ± 1.0
Lubrication	5.1 ± 1.5	5.0 ± 0.9	4.5 ± 1.4	5.1 ± 0.6	4.4 ± 1.0	5.0 ± 0.8	4.5 ± 1.0	5.5 ± 0.9
Orgasm	4.9 ± 1.0	5.3 ± 0.8	4.1 ± 1.3	5.0 ± 0.6	3.3 ± 1.6	4.6 ± 1.0	4.4 ± 0.9	5.0 ± 1.2
Satisfaction	5.1 ± 1.5	4.7 ± 1.6	4.6 ± 1.1	4.8 ± 1.5	4.0 ± 1.8	5.4 ± 0.6	5.2 ± 1.2	5.1 ± 1.2
Pain	5.1 ± 1.1	3.5 ± 2.4	4.4 ± 1.4	4.7 ± 1.0	1.9 ± 1.9	5.0 ± 0.9	5.2 ± 1.0	5.5 ± 1.0
Total score	29.9 ± 4.3	28.0 ± 5.0	26.5 ± 5.6	31.8 ± 0.8	21.4 ± 5.3	29.0 ± 3.2	30.2 ± 1.0	30.2 ± 6.1
Reference	Communal P H et al.		Giannes A et al.	Bianchi S et al.	Allen LM et al.	Fedele L et al.	Bianchi S et al.	Rosen R et al.

Note: Values are given as means ± SD. Patients without sexual activity within the past month were not included in this FSFI evaluation. Total FSFI score ranges from 0 to 36.
Modified from Walch. Long-term outcomes after Wharton-Sheares-George surgery. *Fertil Steril* 2011;96:492, with permission. Copyright © 2011, Elsevier.

Since the initial report of the use of oxidized cellulose material instead of a skin graft to line the neovaginal space, more than 30 cases have been reported using several different commercial products. No operative or postoperative complications have been reported and epithelialization was noted between 1 and 12 months after the procedure. Limited long-term data are available regarding this technique. Dornelas and colleagues in Brazil recently reported on 11 patients treated with this modality, eight of which had MRKH. The mean follow-up for the entire group was 14 months (6 to 24 months). Patients who were sexually active at the 6-month assessment were administered the FSFI, translated into Portuguese, with all the results in the "very good" range. The authors reinforced that if sexual intercourse is suspended for prolonged periods, vaginal dilation may be required to preserve vaginal length. The proposed advantages include the shorter operative times and easily available material that does not require additional surgical expertise. Several authors, including Adamyan, Soong et al., and Templeman and colleagues, have described the laparoscopic use of the peritoneum to create a neovagina in patients with vaginal agenesis. Adamyan and Soong et al. reported a group of 45 patients without significant postoperative complications. The most common postoperative problem involved the formation of granulation tissue at the vaginal vault. Templeman and colleagues described the laparoscopic mobilization of peritoneum for the creation of a neovagina in only one patient. The peritoneum was grasped through a perineal dissection and sutured to the introitus. A purse-string closure was placed at the apex. Stenting of the neovagina was continued for 3 months postoperatively followed by rigid dilator use. At 9-month follow-up evaluation, an 8- by 2-cm vagina was described, with squamous epithelialization present. Both groups describe the technique as safe and efficient, producing a neovagina with apical granulation tissue as the only complication. Bianchi and colleagues reported on eighty patients with Rokitansky syndrome. Forty patients underwent a Davydov procedure. The team highlighted that the Davydov procedure is a better choice in patients with female hypospadias but may have more risk in patients with a pelvic kidney or patients with previous pelvic surgery and adhesions. They also argued that the Davydov approach immediately achieves good functional results and there is less need for vaginal dilation than other methods to maintain the end result. They found a mean vaginal length of 7.25 + 2.1 cm at discharge and 8.5 + 1.6 cm at 12 months postprocedure. At 12 months postprocedure, the FSFI was completed by all the patients in the study with globally optimal results. No important complications occurred, although one patient experienced introital stenosis, which did not require surgery. However, they also again reinforced the risk of significant complications including rectal and bladder perforation. Lastly, they commented on potential limitation of the Davydov in the situation of postoperative failure. They suggest that this procedure yields poor chance of surgical correction due to the difficulty of recanalization of the urethrovesicorectal space. Giannesi and colleagues reported an assessment of sexuality via a self-report questionnaire after the laparoscopic Davydov procedure. The FSFI was also administered to both 28 women who underwent a laparoscopic Davydov procedure and 28 age-matched controls. The anatomical result was judged to be satisfactory (>6 cm) in 26 of 28 patients with a mean vaginal length of 7.2 ± 1.5 cm. No statistical difference was found between the subjects and the controls in all six domains of the FSFI; however, the authors note that 6 of the 25 (24%) operative subjects who completed the entire FSFI had a poor FSFI result. Of note, the areas of greatest concern were in the areas of lubrication and pain. Liao and colleagues reported on 31 patients with MRKH who underwent surgery with a laparoscopic Davydov procedure. Seven patients were lost to follow up, so only 24 patients completed the surgery and requested follow-up. The FSFI was administered to evaluate function of patients who became sexually active and compared them with 50 randomly selected, age-matched healthy women. There was no significant difference in the frequency of sexual intercourse between the control group and the 20 cases who were sexually active. There was no statistical difference in scores of all six domains of the FSFI between the cases and the control subjects. The data from both groups suggest positive functional results.

The Vecchietti operation was first described in 1965 by Giuseppe Vecchietti. He subsequently reported his cumulative 14-year experience in 1979 and 1980. Veronikus and colleagues reviewed the use of the technique and described a laparoscopic modification that uses cystoscopy to confirm bladder integrity. The Vecchietti procedure is a surgical technique for the treatment of vaginal agenesis that constructs a dilatation-type neovagina in 7 to 9 days. The procedure uses specialized equipment including a traction device, a ligature carrier, and an acrylic-shaped olive. The process is in two steps, with essential operative and postoperative components. The operative phase involves positioning the olive at the perineum and the traction sutures extraperitoneally. Classically performed through a Pfannenstiel incision, the ligature carrier introduces the suture into a newly dissected vesicorectal space. The olive is threaded with suture at the perineum, and the suture is reintroduced at the abdomen. The suture is then guided lateral to the rectus muscles bilaterally in a subperitoneal fashion and advanced along the sidewall. The traction device, which provides constant traction on the olive, is positioned on the abdomen. During the postoperative invagination phase, the neovagina is created by applying constant traction to the olive. The process reportedly occurs at a rate of 1.0 to 1.5 cm per day, developing a 10- to 12-cm vagina in 7 to 9 days. Prior to being discharged, patients are instructed on how to use a vaginal obturator on an outpatient basis. Borruto reported on Vecchietti's personal series of vaginal agenesis patients, comprising 522 consecutive patients. The surgical complications included one bladder and one rectal puncture with the ligature carrier and three cases of vaginal vault bleeding. At 100% follow-up at 1 month, dyspareunia was initially reported to be 12%, but resolved in all cases by 3 months. There were no reported failures of the neovaginal construction with 1- and 2-year follow-up of 70% and 30%, respectively.

Modifications of the Vecchietti approach include the use of laparoscopy and elimination of the dissection of the vesicorectal space. The first description of a laparoscopic modification was published by Gauwerky and colleagues. The vesicorectal space was dissected laparoscopically. The threads of the olive device were positioned using a probe introduced into the abdomen through the perineum. Six small abdominal incisions were used for laparoscopic instruments and the traction springs of the specialized device. In 1995, Laffarque and others described a laparoscopic intervention, creating a neovagina in three patients without dissection of the vesicorectal space. At completion of the procedure, cystoscopy was used to confirm bladder integrity. Some experts believe the theoretical risk of bladder or rectal perforation without the dissection of the vesicorectal space is unacceptably high. Brucker and colleagues in Tübingen, Germany, reported on their experience with the Vecchietti procedure in 101 patients with 93 treated for vaginal agenesis. They stratified their patients to three groups: Group 1 with conventional instruments and tunneling in the vesicorectal space, Group 2 included conventional instruments and no dissection in the vesicorectal space, and Group 3 combined both specialized instruments and no vesicorectal dissection. Group 3 had the longest mean vaginal length immediately postprocedure (9.6 cm compared to 8.9 cm in Group 1 and 7.8 in Group 2) and shortest traction time (4.8 days compared to 11.7 days in Group 1 and 7.5 days in Group 2). Mean follow-up for Group 2 was 37.7 months compared to 15.5 months in Group 3. Without tunneling and the new specialized instruments, the mean operative time was decreased from 113.0 to 47.5 minutes with a significant reduction in complication rate for bladder lesions and no bowel lesions. Bianchi and colleagues also described their experience with 80 patients who underwent laparoscopic creation of neovagina. Forty of these patients underwent a laparoscopic Vecchietti procedure. Mean operating room time was 30 ± 9.6 minutes. Their group did not perform a Vecchietti procedure for patients with female hypospadias due to risks to the urethra with introital pressure. Preferentially, they performed a laparoscopic Vecchietti for patients with a pelvic kidney, in lieu of other laparoscopic options. They noted that the Vecchietti is easier as a laparoscopic procedure since the perineal approach is not necessary with the absence of dissection in the vesicorectal space. When comparing the outcomes to the laparoscopic Davydov procedure, they reported initially longer vaginal length with the Davydov approach (6.3 ± 0.7 cm for Vecchietti, 7.25 ± 2.1 cm for Davydov), which persists at 12 months; however, both remain within the clinically normal range (7.5 ± 1.1 cm for Vecchietti, 8.5 ± 1.6 cm for Davydov). Additionally, there were no important differences in sexual quality of life, as demonstrated by FSFI scores. Fedele and colleagues modified the approach to use a combined laparoscopic–ultrasonographic technique. The ultrasound assists in identifying the space of connective tissue between the bladder and rectum. The operating time for this modified procedure was only 40 minutes. After 10 days, the patient engaged in sexual intercourse. One-month evaluation confirmed a 12-cm vaginal length. Long-term follow-up outcomes are not available. This technique may even be considered in patients who have been treated for imperforate anus with vaginal agenesis who were not treated in childhood. Sexuality after the laparoscopic Vecchietti procedure requires more data to fully assess. Fedele and colleagues provided the initial report, describing 50 of 52 cases (96%) with a vaginal length greater than 7 cm. All patients succeeded in having vaginal intercourse, 49 (82.6%) had a stable sexual relationship, and 49 (94.2%) were globally satisfied with their sexual life. Since then, the FSFI was introduced and validated as a tool to assess the sexual function in patients undergoing reconstruction. In 2008, Fedele reviewed the entire population, which at that time included 110 patients, including the 27 patients who completed the FSFI at 12 months after surgery. No significant difference was found between the patients and the controls in the domains regarding desire, arousal, and satisfaction. The scores for the domains on lubrication, orgasm, and comfort, as well as in the total score, resulted in a statistically significant difference, with slightly lower scores for patients with Rokitansky. The lowest scores were in patients who had low scores for desire and arousal, with the authors suggesting that this may actually reflect a more pervasive psychological aspect affecting the total score.

Urologic surgeons involved in urogenital reconstruction are familiar with the role of buccal mucosa in the reconstruction of the urethra and mucosally lined genital surfaces. More recently, gynecologic surgeons have reported the use of buccal mucosal grafts in surgical creation of a complete neovagina. Reports have described using buccal mucosa that was fenestrated prior to grafting to increase the size of the graft. Patients were initially hospitalized with the graft in place and then discharged to continue mold use at home for several weeks. Authors reported

vaginal lengths greater than 8 cm; however, limited patient numbers and abbreviated follow-up have been reported. Perhaps, the most advantageous role for buccal neovaginal grafting may be in augmentation vaginoplasty for patients who have had prior suboptimal attempts at vaginal reconstruction or those with more complex reconstructive needs, such as DSD conditions or cloacal anomalies. Benefits of this procedure include the tissue similarities compared to native vagina, an easily accessible source with excellent healing and no visible scar. More data are necessary to weigh the possible disadvantages of numbness of the lip/cheek and difficulty opening the mouth due to scarring or contracture at the graft donation site.

Bowel vaginoplasty is a well-known alternative for creation of a neovagina. The Ruge procedure and others are characterized by the formation of a neovagina using sigmoid colon grafts. Advocates propose that scar formation and vaginal stenosis occur less often than with other procedures; however, the disadvantage is the necessity of an abdominal laparotomy. Ota and colleagues reported a laparoscopic-assisted Ruge procedure. Mesenteric dissection and sigmoid resection were performed laparoscopically. A 3.5-cm incision was used for appropriate bowel suturing. The segment of sigmoid colon was mobilized and brought to the introitus. The serosal layer of the pediculate end was stabilized to pelvic peritoneum. The patient remained hospitalized for 14 days. The benefit of this modification is certainly the accomplishment of a difficult surgical procedure endoscopically. Other advantages include the functional, ample vaginal length (12 cm) without postoperative dilatation. Disadvantages include the extended postoperative hospitalization period and the small number of patients evaluated.

Reported surgical outcomes by authors such as Hensle and colleagues and Communal and associates support the role of sigmoid neovaginoplasty, especially in patients with MRKH. Until recently, long-term data regarding sexual function had not been available. Parsons and colleagues retrospectively reviewed 28 cases at a mean of 6.2 years after sigmoid vaginoplasty. Seventy-nine percent of patients were reportedly "very satisfied" with sexual function, and 21% were "comfortable" with the outcome. Communal and colleagues administered the FSFI to 11 patients after creation of a sigmoid neovagina. The mean score of the 8 women who were attempting intercourse was reported to be equivalent to that of "normal" patients without vaginal agenesis. Carrard et al. reported on 59 patients with MRKH, 11 treated with the Frank method and 48 who underwent sigmoid vaginoplasty. The mean time after surgery was 6 years (10 months to 17.8 years). Forty patients (68%) answered the questionnaire, 35/48 (73%) who had surgery and 5/11 (45%) who were treated with dilation. The mean total FSFI score was 28 in the operated group: 21 patients of the 30 currently sexually active respondents (70%) had a score above the cutoff for sexual dysfunction. Women with MRKH syndrome treated with sigmoid vaginoplasty could be considered "normal" in terms of desire, arousability, lubrication, orgasm, and global sexual satisfaction. However, discomfort scores were higher in these patients. The only significant between-group difference was in terms of vaginal discharge discomfort. In comparison, in the group treated by the Frank method, the mean total FSFI score was 30 and each domain score was similar to "normal" women's score. Three patients (75%) had a score above the 26.55 cutoff. Hensle and colleagues provided additional information by reporting the sexual function of 57 patients who underwent creation of a bowel neovagina. Forty-two of the patients were reported to have MRKH. Eight patients underwent ileovaginoplasty; two patients were then subsequently treated with a colonic neovagina. The follow-up period varied from 18 months to 24 years with a mean of 8.8 years. Outcomes were evaluated both by a retrospective chart review and the female sexual dysfunction questionnaire described as an Institutional Review Board–approved, validated instrument. Of the 36 patients who responded, 31 were sexually active. Seventy-eight percent of the entire group of patients, including additional diagnoses precipitating neovaginoplasty, reported sexual desire, 33% sexual arousal, 33% sexual confidence, and 78% sexual satisfaction. Also, 56% reported frequent orgasms, 22% occasional orgasms, and 22% no orgasms. Thirty-two patients (89%) reported adequate lubrication for sexual activity; 34 patients used home douching, and 20 required pads for mucus production. Djordjevic and colleagues reported on the use of the rectosigmoid in neovaginal replacement. They reported on 86 patients, of whom 54 had vaginal agenesis. The mean follow-up was 47 months (range 8 to 114 months). The mean vaginal length was 13 cm in patients with vaginal agenesis. Mucous production was reported in 19/54 (35%) in the first 6 months; however, after 6 months, only 2 (3.7%) patients noted the complaint. Introital stenosis and vaginal prolapse were each only reported in 2 cases (3.7%). Sexual outcome was evaluated with the FSFI with sexual function described as satisfactory in 46/54 patients (85.18%).

One of the long-term risks with colonic neovaginal replacement is the possible involvement of the neovagina in systemic inflammatory bowel disease. Only a handful of cases have been reported; however, involvement of the neovagina has been reported as significant, requiring reoperation and repeat vaginal replacement. Endoscopic surveillance with biopsy should be considered essential in patients with symptoms of unexplained discharge and pain.

Makinoda and colleagues reported a nongrafting method of vaginal creation. This group reported 18 women who underwent a two-step protocol. The initial step used noninvasive dilatation using a vaginal mold based on the technique of Frank. The second step was a surgical procedure via a perineal approach. The apex of the dilated vaginal space was incised, and further dissection between the bladder and rectum was carried to the peritoneal cavity. After peritoneal perforation, the uterine structures, when present, were pulled down and sutured to the newly created vaginal space. A firm vaginal mold was inserted and recommended for use for 6 months postoperatively. The authors propose a benefit of avoidance of grafting. The time course for success with the initial dilatation step may be unacceptably long in many patients (mean = 10.90 ± 9.8 months). No significant surgical complications were reported despite the theoretical risk of ureteral contortion and kinking when pulling the rudimentary uterine structures inferiorly. During the follow-up period, shrinkage of the vaginal length and diameter was noted in some patients who had been noncompliant with the mold or without coitus. The authors noted a minimal vaginal length of 5 cm in a patient who was noncompliant with the mold and not sexually active. The authors dispute the necessity of any lining of the neovaginal space. In their experience, significant narrowing or contraction of the margins did not occur. They maintain that the vaginal space is maintained by suturing the muscular buds of the uterus to the pressure-created neovaginal space.

A spatial W-plasty technique using a full-thickness unilateral groin graft has been described in a limited number of patients by Chen and others. The authors advocate an earlier intervention with the premise that a full-thickness graft may grow as the patient grows. This is recommended to eliminate psychological issues in patients who would be treated during the late teens, when sexual identity may be forming.

An exciting innovation is the use of autologous in vitro grown vaginal tissue. Panici and colleagues in Rome reported a two-step procedure. The first step involved acquiring a full-thickness biopsy of the vestibule. The tissue was processed and incubated. The time interval between the biopsy and the fully differentiated mucosal tissue for grafting was 2 weeks. When the tissue was ready for grafting, the vaginal canal was prepared in the Abbe-McIndoe technique and gauze was placed with the cell stratum facing the newly created vaginal canal walls. Surgical time was reported as 18 minutes for the second step, and estimated blood loss was less than 100 mL. The gauze was kept in place with a mold for 5 days; the mold was then removed, and the vagina was irrigated. Estimated success was 90%. Although this technique is in its infancy, the benefit of having the neovagina lined with physiologic vaginal tissue is significant both for function and psychological implications. Challenges include the logistics of the two-step procedure and the need for capabilities for tissue culture. Additional experience with this type of orthotopic vaginal grafting may lead to groundbreaking changes in the treatment of this condition.

Acquired Vaginal Insufficiency

Unusual types of infection and atrophy can rarely cause closure of part of the vagina, but acquired vaginal inadequacy most often is the result of treatment of various gynecologic malignancies with surgery or radiation, or a combination of both. Restoration and maintenance of vaginal function are important elements of the treatment plan for such malignancies, especially when the patient is young and otherwise healthy. The unique surgical challenges associated with creation of a neovagina in patients treated with radiation therapy require the experience and expertise of surgeons familiar with this population. The techniques of vaginal reconstruction in gynecologic oncology have been reviewed by Magrina and Masterson, by Pratt, and by McCraw and associates.

DISORDERS OF VERTICAL FUSION

The problems associated with vertical fusion include transverse vaginal septum with or without obstruction. Although imperforate hymen is a vertical fusion problem, the hymen is not a derivative of the müllerian ducts; therefore, this condition is discussed elsewhere (see Chapter 24).

Transverse Vaginal Septum

No reliable epidemiologic data exist regarding the incidence of transverse vaginal septum. Reported incidences vary from 1 in 2,100 to 1 in 72,000. It is probably less common than congenital absence of the vagina and uterus. It has been diagnosed in newborns, infants, and older adolescent girls. Its etiology is unknown, although McKusick has suggested that some and perhaps most cases are the result of a female sex-limited autosomal recessive transmission. There is a developmental defect in vaginal embryogenesis that leads to an incomplete fusion between the müllerian duct component and the urogenital sinus component of the vagina. The incomplete vertical fusion results in a transverse vaginal septum (AFS class IIA) that varies in thickness and can be located at almost any level in the vagina (Fig. 25.10). Lodi has reported that 46% occur in the upper vagina, 40% in the midvagina, and 14% in the lower vagina. Rock, Zacur, and associates have noted septa in the upper, middle, and lower thirds of the vagina in 46%, 35%, and 19% of patients, respectively. In general, the thicker septum is noted to be more common closer to the uterine cervix. In contrast to congenital absence of the müllerian ducts, the transverse vaginal septum is associated with few urologic or other anomalies. Imperforate anus and bicornuate uterus can be found, as

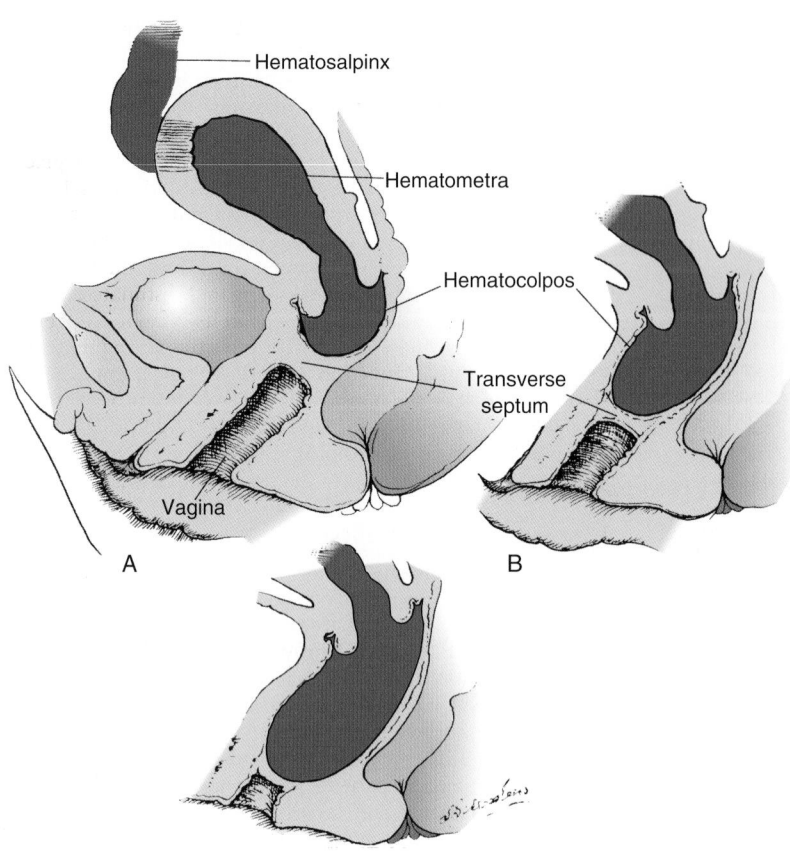

Hematosalpinx

Hematometra

Hematocolpos

Transverse
septum

Vagina

A

B

C

FIGURE 25.10 Positions of septum responsible for complete vaginal obstruction. High (**A**), mid- (**B**), and low (**C**) transverse vaginal septa. Note the position of the hematocolpos. Lower vaginal septa allow more blood to accumulate in the upper vagina. The vaginal mass shown in (**C**) is more accessible through rectovaginal examination.

reported by Mandell and colleagues. The lower surface of the transverse septum is always covered by squamous epithelium. The upper surface can be covered by glandular epithelium, which is likely to be transformed into squamous epithelium by a metaplastic process after correction of the obstruction.

In neonates and young infants, imperforate transverse vaginal septum with obstruction can lead to serious and life-threatening problems caused by the compression of surrounding organs by fluid that has collected above the septum. The fluid undoubtedly comes from endocervical glands and müllerian glandular epithelium in the upper vagina that have been stimulated by the placental transfer of maternal estrogen. Continued fluid collection in infants, even after the 1st year, has been reported; thus, the possibility of a fistula between the upper vagina and the urinary tract should be considered. The distended upper vagina creates a large pelvic and lower abdominal mass that can displace the bladder anteriorly, displace the ureters laterally with hydroureters and hydronephrosis, compress the rectum with associated obstipation and even intestinal obstruction, and limit diaphragmatic excursion to indirectly compress the vena cava and produce cardiorespiratory failure. Fatalities have been reported. The hydrocolpos develops along the axis of the upper vagina and therefore may not necessarily cause the outlet or perineum to bulge when there is compression of the mass from above. After careful preoperative radiologic and endoscopic investigations of the infant, the septum should be removed through a perineal approach. Bilateral Schuchardt incisions may be required to ensure that the septum has been removed. Because of the subsequent tendency for vaginal stenosis and reaccumulation of the fluid in the upper vagina, follow-up studies to assess

the recurrence of urinary obstruction are important. Vaginal reconstruction may be required in later years to allow satisfactory menstruation and coitus.

A hematocolpos may not develop until puberty. Symptoms include cyclic lower abdominal pain, no visible menstrual discharge, and gradual development of a central lower abdominal and pelvic mass. Sometimes, a small tract opens in the septum, some menstrual blood escapes periodically, and symptoms are variable. A septum large enough to allow pregnancy to occur can still cause dystocia during labor. Cyclic hematuria may be present if a communication between the bladder and upper vagina exists. The pelvic organs of a woman with a transverse vaginal septum are shown in **Figure 25.11**. The woman developed severe cyclic pain at the time of onset of menstruation, but there was no external bleeding until menstrual blood finally began to flow through the small sinus. Pelvic examination per rectum revealed a cervix and a normal-sized corpus. The ovaries were palpable but adherent, probably because of organized blood from hematosalpinx and hematoperitoneum. Remarkably, the woman had little dysmenorrhea after beginning to menstruate externally. Coitus was fairly satisfactory before surgical correction, but the shortness of the vagina was something of a handicap. The obstructing membrane was excised, and an anastomosis of the upper and lower vagina was performed.

The findings of 26 patients with complete transverse vaginal septum reported from the Johns Hopkins Hospital by Rock, Zacur, and colleagues have shown that associated congenital anomalies include urinary tract anomalies, coarctation of the aorta, atrial septal defect, and malformations of the lumbar spine. Vaginal patency and coital function were successfully established in all patients, and 7 of 19 patients

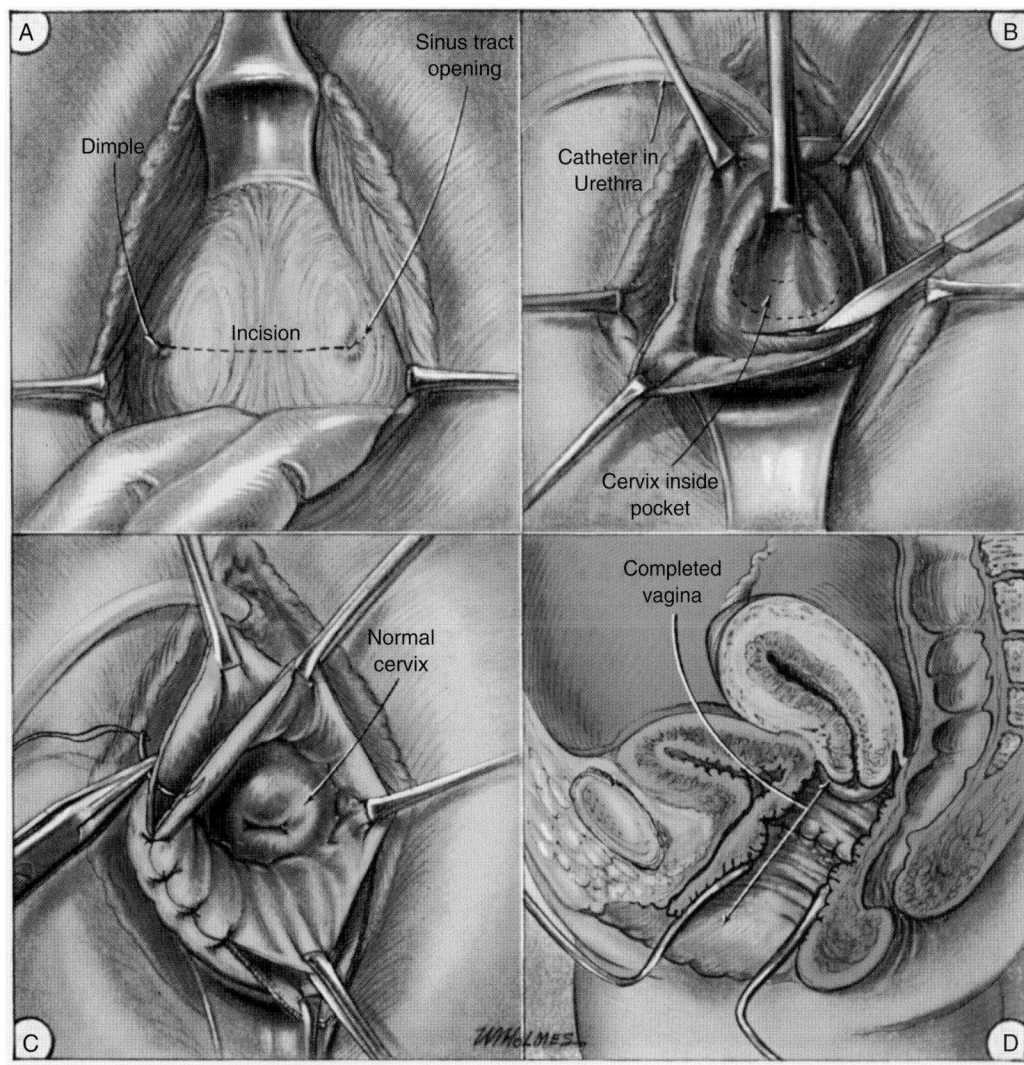

FIGURE 25.11 Surgical correction of transverse vaginal septum. **A:** The upper end of a short vagina. The small sinus tract opening, through which the patient menstruated, is shown. The line of incision is drawn through the mucous membrane between the vaginal dimple and the sinus. **B:** Areolar tissue is dissected through to the pocket of mucosa that covered the cervix. The mucosa is incised. **C:** An anastomosis is made between the lower vagina and the upper vagina. **D:** Completed vagina. It is slightly shorter than normal but of normal caliber.

attempting pregnancy eventually had children. The incidence of endometriosis and spontaneous abortion was high. A lower pregnancy rate and more extensive endometriosis were present when the transverse septum was located high in the vagina, suggesting that retrograde flow through the uterus and fallopian tubes occurs earlier in these patients. More extensive dissection between the bladder and rectum was required to identify the upper vagina when the septum was thick and high. Exploratory laparotomy was necessary in five patients to guide a probe through the uterine fundus and cervix and to assist in locating a high hematocolpos.

Surgical Technique for a Transverse Vaginal Septum

A transverse incision is made through the vault of the short vagina (**Fig. 25.11A**). A probe is introduced through the septum after a portion of the barrier has been separated by sharp and blunt dissection. The physician usually finds some areolar tissue in dissecting the space between the vagina and the rectum. Palpation of a urethral catheter anteriorly and insertion of a double-gloved finger along the anterior wall of the rectum posteriorly

provide the proper surgical guidelines so that the bladder and rectum can be avoided during this blind procedure. After the dissection is continued for a short distance, the cervix can usually be palpated, and continuity can be established with the upper segment of the vagina (**Fig. 25.11B, C**). The lateral margins of the excised septum are extended widely by sharp knife dissection to avoid postoperative stricture formation. The edges of the upper and the lower vaginal mucosa are undermined and mobilized enough to permit anastomosis with the use of interrupted delayed absorbable sutures (**Fig. 25.11C**). **Figure 25.11D** shows the completed anastomosis with a vagina that is of normal caliber but has a length slightly shorter than average. A soft foam rubber vaginal form covered with a sterile latex sheath can be placed in the vagina and removed in 10 days for evaluation of the healing process. The form can be worn for 4 to 6 weeks until complete healing has occurred. After this, coitus is permitted. If the patient is not sexually active, then vaginal dilatation may be necessary to maintain established patency. Alternatively, a silicone elastomer (Silastic) vaginal form can be inserted at night until the constrictive phase of healing is complete. A combination of a perineal (transvaginal) and

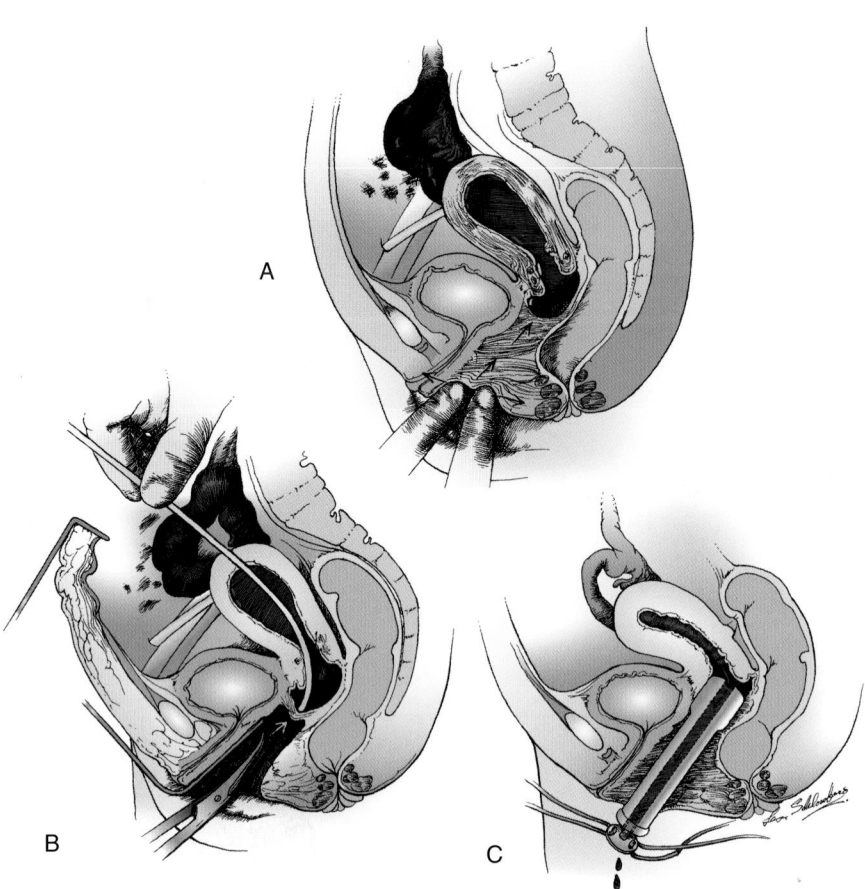

FIGURE 25.12 Correction of an atretic vagina. **A:** A large portion of atretic vagina is palpated with two fingers. Once the vaginal space is developed, it may be necessary to open the abdomen via laparotomy and pass a probe through to the uterine fundus (**B**) to tent out the septum, which may then be safely excised. **C:** An acrylic resin (Lucite) form is then placed into the vagina and secured with rubber straps.

laparoscopic approach may also be useful. Laparoscopy can provide assistance with mobilization of the upper vagina, using dissection both anteriorly at the bladder and in the posterior cul-de-sac. This technique can decrease tension on the anastomosis of upper and lower vagina and minimize the risk of stricture.

High Transverse Vaginal Septum   If the length of the obstructing transverse vaginal septum is such that reanastomosis of the upper and lower vagina is impossible, as is the case with a high transverse vaginal septum, in which a significant portion of the vagina is atretic, then a space is created between the rectum and bladder to permit identification of the obstructed vagina (**Fig. 25.12**). The mass that has resulted from accumulated menstrual blood must be distinguished from the bladder anteriorly and the rectum posteriorly, a process that is facilitated by the mass itself. When differentiation is impossible, however, exploratory laparotomy can be performed. During this procedure, a probe is passed through the fundus of the uterus to tent out the vaginal septum and enable the surgeon to excise it from below and resect it safely.

In most surgical procedures to remove the high transverse vaginal septum, the obstructing membrane can be readily identified (**Fig. 25.13**), after which the operator can probe the mass with an aspirating needle to identify old menstrual blood. The upper vagina is then opened and the septum excised. Because the distance between the septum and the upper vagina is too great to permit an anastomosis, an indwelling acrylic resin (Lucite) form, consisting of a bulbous end and a channel through which menstrual blood can drain, is placed into the vagina and anchored with a retaining harness. The bulbous end of the form, in most instances, is retained in the upper

vagina and should be left in place for 4 to 6 months while epithelialization is accomplished. After its removal, vaginal dilatation should be practiced on a daily basis for 2 to 4 months to prevent contracture of the space. It is essential to the success of the operation that the new space not become constricted; to avoid constriction, the form must be worn for many months during the constrictive phase of healing. As an alternative to the Lucite form, the physician can consider using a split-thickness graft to bridge the gap. The graft is usually sutured in situ in the vagina rather than sutured to a form. An ingenious but rather complicated Z-plasty method of bridging the gap has been described by Garcia and by Musset. A simpler flap method was described by Brenner and associates.

A transverse vaginal septum diagnosed after the onset of puberty presents numerous problems. Often, a large segment of the vagina is absent, making anastomosis of the upper and lower segments difficult. Furthermore, postoperative vaginal dilatation is necessary to prevent stenosis at the anastomosis site. Poor compliance with dilatation in a poorly motivated pubertal patient is always a concern. However, rarely is the surgeon able to delay vaginoplasty until the patient is more mature because of increasingly severe cyclic abdominal pain caused by the hematocolpos. Thus, a difficult vaginoplasty can have less than optimal results.

Hurst and Rock have described an alternative approach to maximize surgical resection and anastomosis in women with a high transverse vaginal septum. Aspiration of the hematocolpos under ultrasound guidance was necessary to relieve the acute pain and delay surgery. Continuous oral contraceptives were used to delay recurrence of hematocolpos. Most important, vaginal dilatation was used to lengthen the lower vaginal

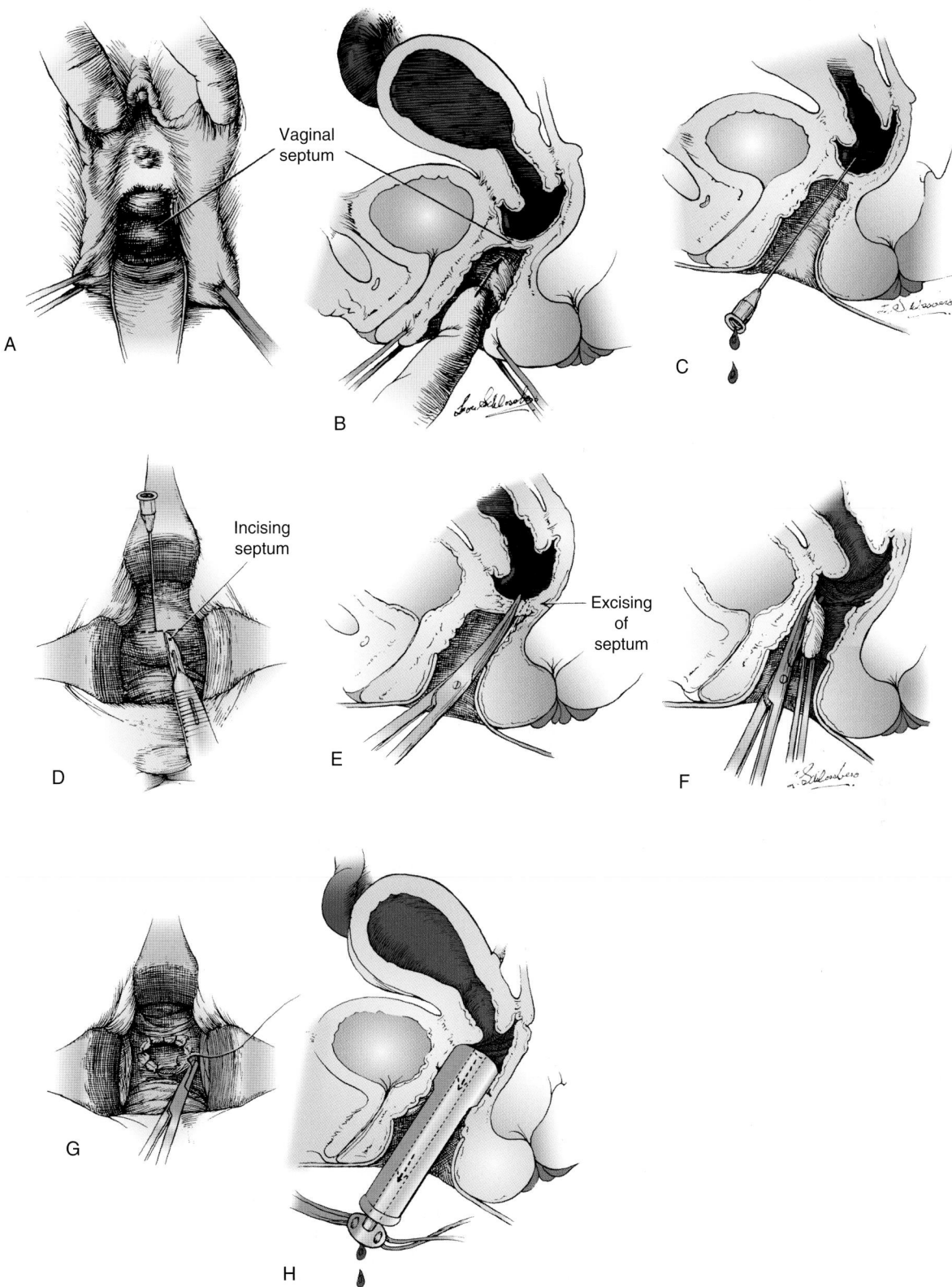

FIGURE 25.13 A high transverse vaginal septum. **A:** The neovaginal space is dissected, revealing a high obstructing vaginal membrane. **B:** This can be palpated with the middle finger. **C:** A needle is then placed into the mass. **D:** The incision is made with a sharp knife, and considerable bleeding can occur. **E:** The septum is excised. **F:** The septum is removed. **G:** After the septum is removed, the wall of the septum is oversewn with interrupted sutures of 2-0 chromic catgut. **H:** Because the distance between the septum and the upper vagina is too great to allow anastomosis, an acrylic resin (Lucite) form is placed in the vagina so that epithelialization can occur over the form while vaginal patency is maintained. The form, in place, is fitted with a plastic retainer. Rubber straps can be placed through the retainer and attached to a waist belt to allow constant upper pressure so that the form is retained in the upper vagina. Modification of this method includes a small adapter to allow drainage through the acrylic resin (Lucite) form, preventing the accumulation of old blood and mucus in the upper vagina.

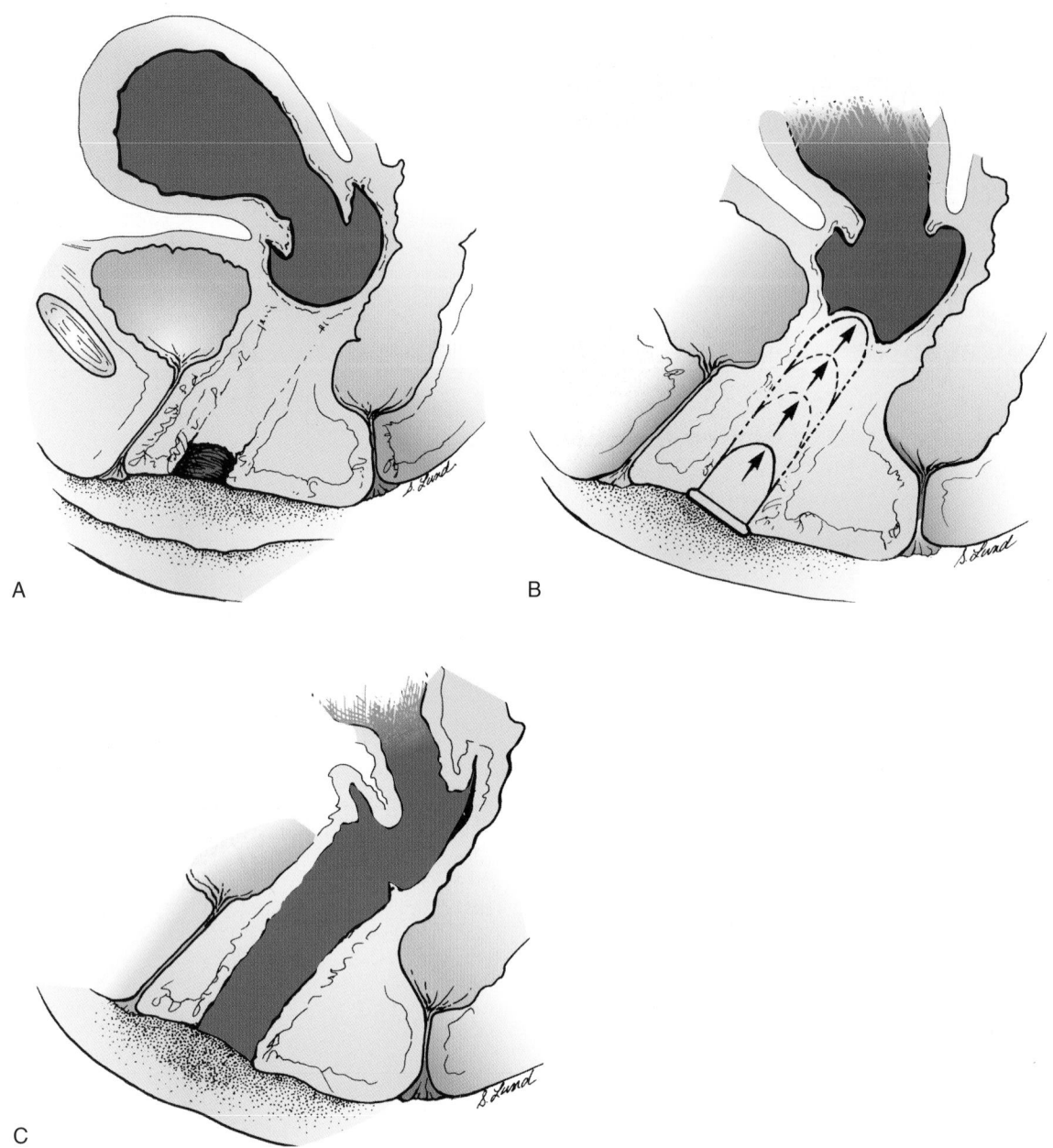

FIGURE 25.14 **A:** High transverse vaginal septum demonstrating a small hematocolpos and hematometra. Upper to lower vaginal anastomosis at this stage can result in stenosis at the anastomosed site. **B:** Vaginal depth is increased with passive dilatation using progressively larger dilators. **C:** A primary upper to lower vaginal anastomosis can be performed easily after dilatation.

segment to facilitate resection and reanastomosis (Fig. 25.14). In all three patients, the approach was successful.

Congenital Absence or Dysgenesis of the Cervix

Agenesis or atresia of the cervix (AFS class IIB) is a relatively infrequent müllerian anomaly. When this anomaly does occur, it is often in association with absence of a portion or all of the vagina. In many cases of cervical agenesis or atresia, retention of menstrual blood initiates symptoms of cyclic lower abdominal pain without menstrual flow, causing the patient to seek gynecologic evaluation and care. In past times, diagnosis was suspected on the basis of a history and physical findings but was not proved until the time of surgery. Today, diagnosis of cervical agenesis or atresia is still usually difficult before operation, but the possibility of making a correct diagnosis before surgery does exist, with the help of modern diagnostic tools.

Early diagnosis offers significant advantages in patient care, the most important of which is effective presurgical planning and preparation.

Diagnosis of Cervical Dysgenesis

Patients with congenital absence of the cervix present a diagnostic challenge. Patients with cervical aplasia with a functioning midline uterine corpus have aplasia of the lower two thirds of the vagina with an upper vaginal pouch. Similarly, some patients have a considerable atretic segment of vagina and an upper vaginal pouch with a properly developed uterine cervix and corpus above. Differentiation of these two müllerian anomalies is essential. Ultrasonography may be helpful. Valdes and associates have reported the use of preoperative ultrasonography in the evaluation of two patients with atresia of the vagina and cervix. Magnetic resonance imaging has been found to be

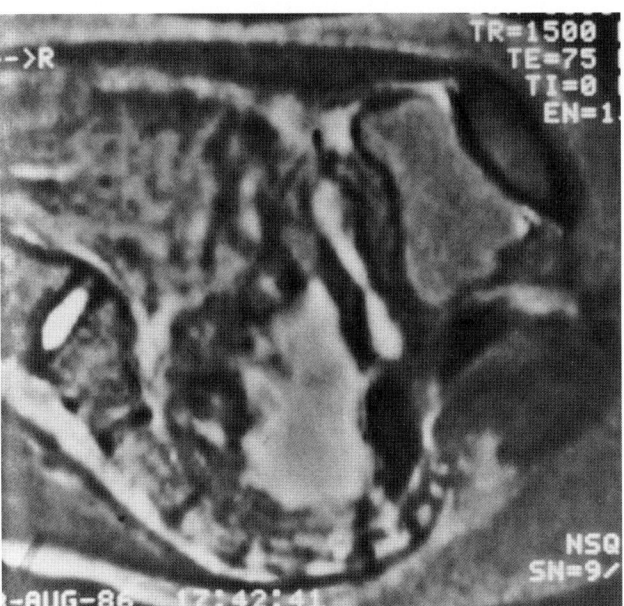

FIGURE 25.15 Magnetic resonance T1-weighted image showing atretic segment of distal cervix. The tip of an atretic cervix is shown. No vagina is noted.

helpful in confirming this diagnosis, as reported by Markham and associates. The lower uterine segment and cervical tissue can be carefully examined (**Fig. 25.15**). With cervical dysgenesis, there is no vaginal dilatation with the accumulation of blood, as seen with a high transverse vaginal septum. Both ultrasonography and MRI are most helpful when they are correlated with the findings of a careful pelvic examination under anesthesia.

Anatomic Variations of Congenital Cervical Anomalies

Two basic categories of cervical anomalies have been observed in several configurations. Patients exhibiting the first type, cervical aplasia, lack a uterine cervix (**Fig. 25.16A**), and the lower uterine segment narrows to terminate in a peritoneal sleeve at a point well above the normal communication with the vaginal apex. Omurtag and colleagues' report of uterine torsion and acute pain in a 13-year-old with hematometra reminds the reconstructive gynecologic surgeon of the consideration of uterine torsion in the absence of a well-formed cervix. The uterus can be susceptible to rotation on its horizontal axis, particularly with the mass effect of hematometra. The second type, cervical dysgenesis, can be described in four subtypes:

1. Cervical body consisting of a fibrous band of variable length and diameter (endocervical glands may be noted on pathologic examination) (**Fig. 25.16B**)
2. Intact cervical body with obstruction of the cervical os (the cervix is usually well formed, but a portion of the endocervical lumen is obliterated) (**Fig. 25.16C**)
3. Stricture of the midportion of the cervix (which is hypoplastic with a bulbous tip and no identifiable cervical lumen) (**Fig. 25.16D**)
4. Fragmentation of the cervix (with portions that can be palpated below the fundus and that are not connected to the lower uterine segment) (**Fig. 25.16E**)

Associated anomalies of the urinary tract are rare, but they do occur. Variable portions of the vagina can be atretic. Cervical obstruction is most often associated with a vagina of normal length.

Treatment

When both the vagina and cervix are absent and a functioning uterine corpus is present, it is difficult to obtain a satisfactory fistulous tract through which menstruation can occur. Many methods have been tried, most of them involving creation of a passage through the dense fibrous tissue between the uterine cavity and the vagina and placement of a stent to keep the tract open. Occasional successes in maintaining an open passageway and normal cyclic menstruation have been reported, but endocervical glands do not develop, and there is no way to compensate for the absence of the cervical mucus, which plays an important role in sperm transport. Even though cyclic ovulatory periods can be achieved in a few patients, pregnancy is unlikely. Eventually, the uterovaginal tract closes from constriction by fibrous tissue. Endometriosis can develop along the tract. Endometriosis also can develop in ovaries and other pelvic sites because of retrograde menstruation. Recurrent and severe pelvic infection is a common problem and may require total hysterectomy and removal of both ovaries. As in vitro fertilization procedures began to offer the possibility for a host uterus to carry a pregnancy to term, procedures to establish a fistulous tract were abandoned. Nevertheless, Cukier and associates in 1986 reported treating a patient with congenital absence of the cervix by construction of a splint that extended into the neocervical canal such that a split-thickness skin graft could actually be placed within the endocervical canal. This patient has continued to menstruate without difficulty, although pregnancy has not been accomplished.

Many authors have recommended hysterectomy as an initial procedure for a patient with a functioning uterine corpus and congenital absence of the cervix and vagina. A hysterectomy eliminates much needless suffering from associated problems such as cryptomenorrhea, sepsis, endometriosis, and multiple operations. If the hysterectomy is performed soon enough, before the problems become great, it may be possible to conserve the ovaries and their useful functions. The reconstructive surgeon should be prepared to perform a vaginoplasty if hysterectomy is performed, particularly if there has been a vaginal dissection. If the neovaginal space is allowed to close and scar, then future operations to develop an adequate neovagina are associated with increased risks of graft failure and fistula formation.

Despite the overall poor results from reconstruction for congenital absence of both the cervix and the vagina, clinical experience suggests that cannulization procedures can be worthwhile in a few carefully selected cases with adequate stroma to allow a cervicovaginal anastomosis. If a long segment of cervix is fibrous cord, a cervical grafting technique may be required. If a fragmented cervix is noted, then hysterectomy is usually warranted. The few patients who have achieved a pregnancy after cervical reconstruction have had a well-formed cervical body. Anecdotal reports of resection of the dysgenetic cervix and reconstruction with uterovaginal anastomosis may be promising. The isthmus of the uterus is anastomosed directly to the vagina as in patients with cervical malignancy who undergo trachelectomy. Successful pregnancies have been reported. More experience with this type of reconstruction is necessary to fully understand the unique challenges that may occur in this population compared to patients who experience disease in an otherwise normally developed cervix.

Anecdotal case reports occasionally appear in the literature confirming the necessity of palpable cervical tissue. Letterie described the development of a cervicovaginal tract in an adolescent patient with a core of cervical tissue. The tract remained patent for menstrual flow for 2 years; however, pregnancy had not yet been attempted. Data published by the

V

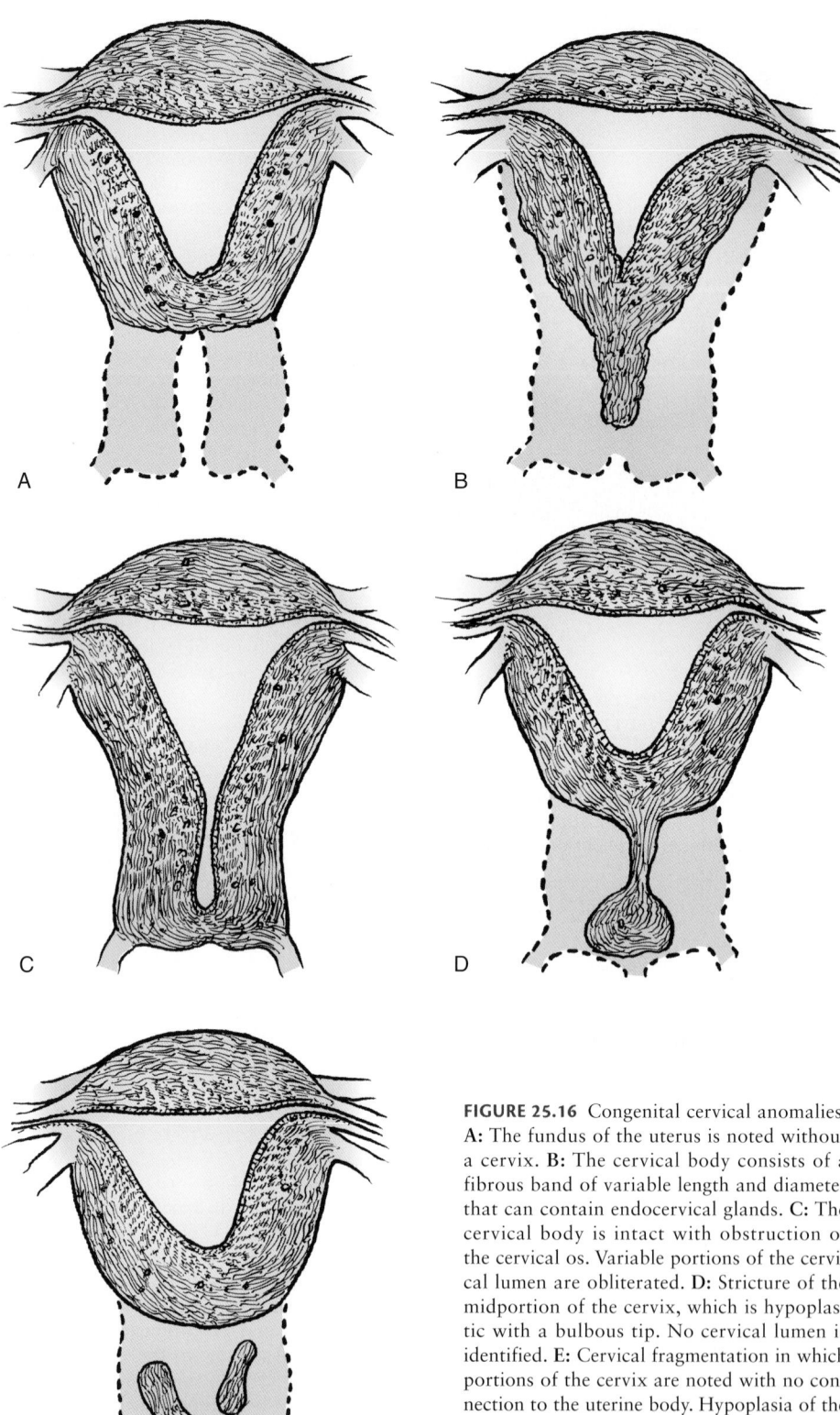

FIGURE 25.16 Congenital cervical anomalies. **A:** The fundus of the uterus is noted without a cervix. **B:** The cervical body consists of a fibrous band of variable length and diameter that can contain endocervical glands. **C:** The cervical body is intact with obstruction of the cervical os. Variable portions of the cervical lumen are obliterated. **D:** Stricture of the midportion of the cervix, which is hypoplastic with a bulbous tip. No cervical lumen is identified. **E:** Cervical fragmentation in which portions of the cervix are noted with no connection to the uterine body. Hypoplasia of the uterine cavity can be associated with cervical cord fragmentation.

senior author regarding the long-term follow-up of 21 patients with abnormal cervical development support the success of cannulization in only selected patients with sufficient rudimentary cervical tissue. All of the patients with fragmentation of the cervix (*n* = 4) eventually underwent hysterectomy. Only those patients with a well-formed cervical body, with at least a palpable cord or only distal obstruction, achieved successful surgical outcomes (4/7 patients). Only one patient with distal obstruction treated with cannulization using a full-thickness skin graft achieved pregnancy.

Others have reported the anastomosis of a well-developed distal vagina to a substantial midline uterine body. Creighton and colleagues described the use of the laparoscope for this procedure; however, Deffarges and associates examined the outcomes of 18 patients after open uterovaginal anastomosis. Twenty-two percent of patients required additional surgery. Eighty-three percent of the cases were associated with upper genital tract complications. Six spontaneous pregnancies also were reported in four of the patients. Despite the small potential for pregnancy, it is imperative to realize the potential for complications, including sepsis and even death as a result of ascending infection. Fedele and colleagues reported successful management of cervical atresia in twelve patients with vaginal aplasia with laparoscopy. All women experienced regular menstrual cycles. The mean vaginal length at 6-month follow-up was 6 cm. At the time of publication, none of the patients had attempted pregnancy. Kriplani and colleagues described 14 consecutive patients with congenital absence of the uterine cervix (Table 25.6). Laparoscopic-assisted uterovaginal anastomosis with placement of a silicone stent was performed. McIndoe vaginoplasty was performed concomitantly in patients with vaginal agenesis. Cervical dysgenesis was present in 5 (35.7%) and

cervical agenesis in 9 (64.2%). Mean follow-up after surgery was 3.8 + 1.2 years. Postoperatively, all but one patient experienced regular menses and relief of cyclic pain. One patient underwent hysterectomy because of genital infection and restenosis. The authors reported that five patients were sexually active and reported it to be satisfactory. Pregnancy occurred in 3/5 patients. Reoperation and subsequent hysterectomy have been reported in as much as half of patients undergoing cervical reconstruction as the primary procedure. Kriplani attributes the use of the silicone stent in the neocervix until the resolution of inflammation as one of the reasons the incidence of restenosis was decreased in their population. Only one patient (7.4%) required hysterectomy for recurrent infection and stenosis.

The surgical approach for the rare opportunity for cervical cannulation remains a challenge. Several additional factors may also influence the surgical outcome: the size of the created channel, the duration of stenting of the channel, the presence of rudimentary endocervical glands in the region of the created channel, the presence of a native vagina adjacent to the created channel, or the number of menses allowed to flow through the stented channel. Because the surgical approach for cervical cannulation is based only on several case reports, limited

SOURCE, YEAR	NO. OF PATIENTS	AGE, YEAR	LAPAROSCOPIC-ASSISTED PROCEDURE	CERVICAL REMNANT	VAGINA	VAGINAL LENGTH AFTER SURGERY, MEAN, CM	SEXUALLY ACTIVE/ PREGNANT
Lee et al., 1999	1	12	Reconstruction of cervix and vagina using skin graft	Absent	Absent	7	NA
Creighton et al., 2006	1	16	Uterovaginal anastomosis	Absent	Proximaplasia	NA	1/0
Fedele et al., 2008	12	12–17	Uterovestibular anastomosis	Present (n = 2)	NA	6 ± 1.6	6/NA
Raudrant et al., 2008	1	13	Uterovaginal anastomosis	Absent	Absent	Small	NA
El Saman, 2009	4	14/18	Laparoscopic canalization and combined retropubic balloon vaginoplasty	Absent	Absent	9–11	NA
Daraï et al., 2009	1	16	Uterovaginal anastomosis	Absent	Absent	6	NA
El Saman, 2010	5	13–16	Endoscopically monitored canalization	Absent	Absent in 2	NA	2/0
Nguyen et al., 2011	1	21	Laparoscopically assisted reconstruction of PTFE graft lining neocervix	Absent	Present	NA	1/0

TABLE 25.6 Published Reports of Laparoscopic-Assisted Management of Cervical Agenesis and Vaginal Aplasia

NA, data not available or not applicable; PTFE, polytetrafluoroethylene.
Modified from Kriplani A, Kachhawa G, Awasthi D, et al. Laparoscopic-assisted uterovaginal anastomosis in congenital atresia of uterine cervix: follow-up study. *J Minim Invasive Gynecol* 2012;19:477, with permission. Copyright © 2012 AAGL. Published by Elsevier Inc. All rights reserved.

data regarding safety and efficacy are available to share with patients and families. A frank discussion with both the patient and her family regarding the potential risks and morbidity is imperative. Even reportedly successful attempts have involved multiple surgical interventions, such as a reported cervicoplasty with bladder mucosa described by Bugamann and colleagues; the 12-year-old patient had to undergo at least one previously failed attempt at reconstruction before the reported successful procedure. Very young adolescents may be subjected to multiple surgical procedures without good evidence of success. These more aggressive, fertility-sparing procedures may be best suited for patients who have had good menstrual suppression and are more mature at the time of the discussion of risks and benefits and decision for surgery.

DISORDERS OF LATERAL FUSION

Failures of lateral fusion of the two müllerian ducts cause vaginal anomalies that are grouped as obstructed or unobstructed.

The Unobstructed Double Uterus (Bicornuate, Septate, or Didelphic Uterus)

Complete failure of medial fusion of the two müllerian ducts can result in complete duplication of the vagina, cervix, and uterus. Partial failure of fusion can result in a single vagina with a single or duplicate cervix and complete or partial duplication of the uterine corpus. A failure of absorption of the uterine septum between the two fused müllerian ducts causes the septum to persist inside the uterus to a variable extent while the external appearance remains that of a single uterus. The septum can be so complete that it divides both the uterine cavity and endocervical canal into two equal or unequal components. More often, incomplete disappearance of the septum leaves only the upper uterine cavities divided. Each of these and a variety of other forms of double uteri have their own individual features of clinical significance. When no obstruction is present, surgical reconstruction is performed primarily because of difficulties with reproduction.

Some aspects of lateral fusion disorders remain controversial because information is still inaccurate or incomplete. Many reports are based on small samples of selected patients, patients who have been diagnosed as having one anomaly or another based on incomplete data, and patients who have received unification operations without preliminary studies to rule out other causes of reproductive difficulty. A comparison of results from one series to the next is difficult because authors have used different classifications based on a variety of embryologic, anatomic, physiologic, functional, and radiologic considerations. Unknown numbers of uterine anomalies may have escaped detection because reproductive performance is generally acceptable and gynecologic difficulties do not necessarily occur.

The müllerian ducts undergo multiple steps in development, including caudal, medial growth followed by fusion and later resorption of the remaining septum. Apoptosis has been proposed as a mechanism by which the septum regresses. Bcl-2, a protein involved in regulating apoptosis, was found to be absent from the septa of several uteri. The absence of this critical protein may play a pivotal role in the persistence of the septum and lateral fusion disorders.

Historical Development of Surgical Procedures

Ruge, in 1882, first reported excision of a uterine septum in a woman who had suffered two pregnancy losses. The woman subsequently carried a pregnancy to term. Paul Strassmann of Berlin and later Erwin Strassmann, his son, were strong advocates of uterine unification operations. The studies of Jones and Jones have contributed greatly to modern understanding of the management of uterine anomalies. Their studies began with a report in 1953 of a series that was started in 1936. Updates have been published from time to time. Wheeless, Rock, Andrews, and others have joined in these reports.

Diagnosis of Uterine Anomalies

If a uterine anomaly is associated with obstruction of menstrual flow, then it causes symptoms that will come to the attention of the gynecologist shortly after menarche. Unobstructed uterine anomalies are diagnosed later in a variety of circumstances. Young girls may notice difficulty in using tampons or later difficulty with coitus if a longitudinal vaginal septum is present. This can lead to the diagnosis of an associated uterine anomaly. A patient with an anomalous upper urinary tract on intravenous pyelogram may be found to have a uterine anomaly on gynecologic evaluation. A uterine anomaly is occasionally found when a patient reports dysmenorrhea or menorrhagia or when a dilatation and curettage (D&C) is performed. A palpable mass may be a uterine anomaly but should be confirmed as such by ultrasonography, MRI, hysterography, or laparoscopy. Woelfer and colleagues described the use of three-dimensional ultrasonography in screening for congenital uterine anomalies. During an investigation of the correlation of uterine anomalies with obstetric complications, the authors assessed the potential value of three-dimensional ultrasound for screening. More than 100 women with uterine anomalies were identified. Seventy-two arcuate uteri, twenty nine septate, and five bicornuate uteri were described. The authors emphasized how the three-dimensional ultrasound may overcome the limitations of conventional two-dimensional ultrasonography in providing a coronal view of the uterus, thus differentiating between arcuate, bicornuate, and subseptate uteri. This technique remains investigational. Semmens has pointed out that the diagnosis of a uterine anomaly can also be made from astute observation of an abnormal uterine contour during pregnancy, either in the antepartum period or at the time of abdominal or vaginal delivery. The abnormal contour is caused by a combination of fetal malpresentation and an anomalous uterus. An anomalous uterus can also be diagnosed when a pregnancy occurs despite the presence of an intrauterine contraceptive device. Persistent postmenopausal bleeding despite recent D&C can lead to a diagnosis of an anomalous uterus. Sometimes the diagnosis is made as an incidental finding at laparotomy. Historically, most uterine anomalies were diagnosed after hysterosalpingography to evaluate infertility or reproductive loss, usually from repeated spontaneous abortion, but increasingly, uterine anomalies are detected on MRI performed for other indications.

Uterine Anomalies and Reproductive History

Although some uterine anomalies can cause infertility, most patients with uterine anomalies are able to conceive without difficulty. There is no question that uterine anomalies can be associated with perfectly normal reproductive performance. Overall, however, the incidences of spontaneous abortion, premature birth, fetal loss, malpresentation, and cesarean section are clearly increased when a uterine anomaly is present. It is impossible to predict which patients with uterine anomalies will have these problems.

Etiology of Reproductive Failure

The etiology of reproductive failure in patients with uterine anomalies remains unclear. Mahgoub believes that the presence of a uterine septum can lead to spontaneous pregnancy loss because of diminished intrauterine space for fetal growth or because of implantation of the placenta on a poorly vascularized septum. Mizuno and associates have attached importance to the inadequacy of vascularization of the uterine septum. Associated cervical incompetence, luteal phase insufficiency, and distortion of the uterine milieu have all been implicated in the etiology of increased reproductive loss. However, it is as yet unexplained why some patients with a uterine anomaly have normal reproductive function, whereas others abort early in pregnancy. Interestingly, it has been reported that the chance for a liveborn child increases with each pregnancy loss. It is unknown whether this apparent "conditioning" of the uterus is due to better vascularization, better myometrial stretching and accommodation, or some other factor.

A medical history of three or more episodes of spontaneous abortion or premature labor merits evaluation of the uterine cavity to determine whether structural abnormalities of the uterus are present. An abnormality is found in approximately 10% of such cases. Among chronic early second-trimester aborters, the incidence may be higher. The etiology of spontaneous abortion is complex, and a complete workup should be done even when an anomalous uterus has been found. A careful history should include a detailed discussion of each previous pregnancy loss and inquiry into DES exposure or other drug or chemical toxicity, specific medical illnesses, and exposure to contagious diseases. A family history should emphasize reproductive failures among family members of both the patient and her partner. Specific medical diseases such as thyroid disease, diabetes mellitus, renal disease, and systemic lupus erythematosus should be ruled out. The possibility of infection by such agents as *Neisseria gonorrhoeae*, *Chlamydia*, *Mycoplasma*, *Toxoplasma*, and *Listeria* should be considered. Chromosome analyses should be done. Abnormalities in aborted tissue are found in more than 50% of spontaneous abortions, and abnormalities appear in up to one fourth of couples with a history of habitual abortion. Identifying such couples makes it possible to offer genetic counseling for subsequent pregnancies. Uterine leiomyomas, especially lower uterine segment and submucous leiomyomas, can cause spontaneous abortion. Basal body temperature charts, serum progesterone determinations, and endometrial biopsies timed in the luteal phase help determine the presence of luteal phase deficiency. The cervix should be studied for incompetence.

Couples with multiple etiologies for reproductive loss should have all other problems corrected before metroplasty is considered. Indeed, correcting other factors first may correct the problem of reproductive loss without metroplasty. In 1977, Rock and Jones reported on seven patients who had anomalous uterine development and extrauterine factors in the etiology of their reproductive loss. These patients had already had 16 pregnancies, 5 (29%) of which resulted in a liveborn child. After therapy to correct the extrauterine factor, the success rate increased to 71%. Stoot and Mastboom reported an impressive increase in reproductive performance among uterine anomaly patients by simple improvement of abnormal carbohydrate metabolism.

Hysterographic Studies

Proper technique during the performance of hysterosalpingography to diagnose uterine anomalies is important. The hysterogram must be taken at right angles to the axis of the uterus for a true assessment of the deformity to be made. The study is best done under fluoroscopy. A septate uterus cannot be distinguished from a bicornuate uterus by hysterogram alone (**Fig. 25.17**). The external uterine configuration also cannot usually be determined by pelvic examination alone, but some idea of the configuration can be obtained by ultrasonography.

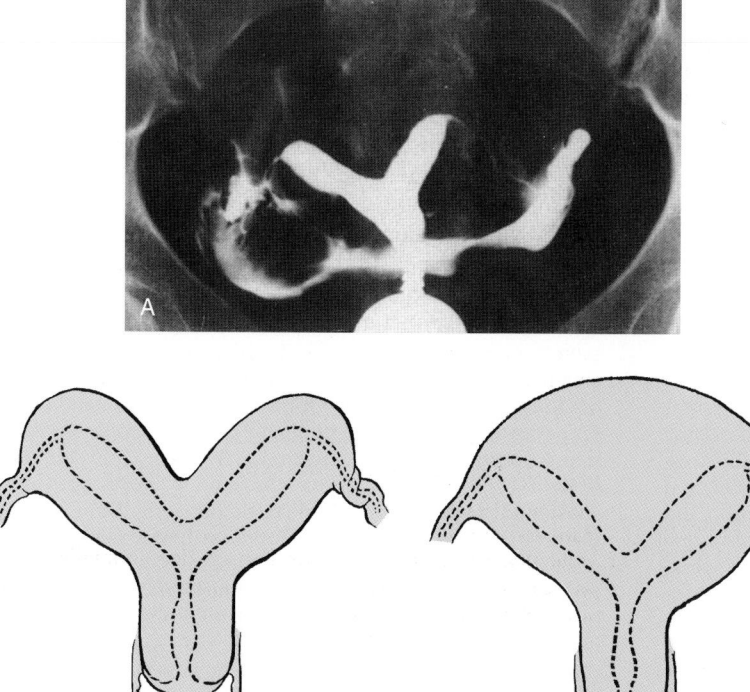

FIGURE 25.17 A: A hysterogram of a double uterus. A bicornuate uterus (**B**) and a septate uterus (**C**) are types of double uteri. Visualization of the fundus is required to determine the type of uterus.

McDonough and Tho have suggested the use of double-contour pelvic pneumoperitoneum–hysterographic studies for precise identification of müllerian malformations. Of course, laparoscopy is even more certain. If the uterine corpus has not been previously visualized, the physician must be prepared to correct either anomaly (i.e., obstructed or unobstructed), depending on the findings at surgery.

Additional Testing

A complete investigation should also include an assessment of tubal patency and an MRI urogram or an intravenous pyelogram. A variety of upper urinary tract anomalies are seen, including absence of one kidney, horseshoe kidney, pelvic kidney, duplication of the collecting system, and ectopically located ureteral orifices. The lower urinary tract (bladder and urethra) is much less often anomalous.

The Double Uterus and Obstetric Outcome

The percentage of full-term pregnancies with various types of double uteri in an unselected series of women who have not been operated on is unknown. For all types combined, it is probably approximately 25%. In patients selected for operation, it probably increases from approximately 5% to 10% to approximately 80% to 90%. Because patients with uterine anomalies who have relatively normal obstetric histories cannot be identified, there is confusion in the literature about which anomalies are more often associated with obstetric difficulties and which are relatively benign in their effect. Special diagnostic procedures to detect uterine anomalies are not usually performed before reproductive performance is tested. A didelphic uterus is the exception. This anomaly can be diagnosed easily on routine pelvic examination by identification of two complete cervices and perhaps also a longitudinal vaginal septum. A study by Heinonen in Finland of 182 women with uterine anomalies indicated that pregnancies in the septate uterus had a better fetal survival rate (86%) than they did in the complete bicornuate uterus (50%) or in the unicornuate uterus (40%). These findings differ from prevailing opinions that the septate uterus is associated with the highest reproductive loss, as proposed by Jones and Jones. A 2011 report by Woefler and associates supports Jones and Jones's opinions by noting that women with a septate uterus had a significantly higher proportion of first-trimester loss than did women with a normal uterus.

In 1968, Capraro and colleagues reported on 85 patients with uterine anomalies seen between 1962 and 1966. One uterine anomaly was seen for every 645 admissions (0.145%). Metroplasty was considered necessary in only 14 (16%) of these 85 cases. According to Jones and Jones, only one third of patients with a double uterus have important reproductive problems. In most instances, the presence of a double uterus is not in itself an indication for metroplasty.

In 1980, Jewelewicz and coworkers estimated the spontaneous abortion rate to be 33.8% in women with a bicornuate uterus, 22.2% in those with a septate uterus, and 34.6% in those with a unicornuate uterus. More recently, Ludmir and associates reported that high-risk obstetric intervention did not significantly increase the fetal survival rate for uncorrected uterine anomalies. Capraro and associates found a preoperative fetal salvage rate of 33.3% for the septate uterus, 10% for the bicornuate uterus, and 0% for the didelphic uterus. Postoperatively, the fetal salvage rate was 100% for the bicornuate uterus, 80% for the septate uterus, and 66% for the didelphic uterus. The report gives the improved salvage figures, compared with several previous studies, after abdominal metroplasty.

Ravasia and colleagues described the incidence of uterine rupture in a cohort of women with müllerian duct anomalies who attempted vaginal birth after cesarean delivery (VBAC). Of the 1,813 patients who attempted VBAC between 1992 and 1997, only 25 patients with known müllerian duct anomalies attempted a trial of labor. This included 14 patients with a bicornuate uterus, five with a septate uterus, four with a unicornuate uterus, and two with uterine didelphys. Uterine rupture was diagnosed in two patients with müllerian anomalies. The authors proposed several mechanisms for the higher incidence of uterine rupture in this population: abnormal development of the lower uterine segment, previous scar similar to a vertical or classic incision, and the possibility of abnormal traction on the uterine scar during labor.

The Didelphic Uterus A didelphic uterus with two hemicorpora is easily diagnosed because all patients have two hemicervices visible on speculum examination and most, if not all, have a longitudinal sagittal vaginal septum. In the series reported by Heinonen and associates, all 21 patients with a didelphic uterus had a vaginal septum. Conversely, a patient with a longitudinal vaginal septum usually has a didelphic uterus. The indication for uterine unification is related to the role of this anomaly as an etiologic factor in reproductive loss. Of all the uterine anomalies (except arcuate uterus), the didelphic uterus is associated with the best possibility of a successful pregnancy. However, there is still some increase in perinatal mortality, premature birth, breech presentation, and cesarean section for delivery. Heinonen and associates reported a fetal survival rate of 64% without metroplasty. Musich and Behrman stated that the didelphic uterus offers the best chance for a successful pregnancy (57%) and should not be considered an appropriate indication for metroplasty. However, W. S. Jones considered the didelphic uterus to give the worst obstetric outcome. In the opinion of the editors of this book, a unification operation for a didelphic uterus is not often indicated, and the results may be disappointing, especially when an attempt is made to unify the cervix. Not only is this procedure technically difficult in a complete didelphic anomaly, but it can also result in cervical incompetence or cervical stenosis.

The Septate Uterus Most patients who are evaluated for repeated pregnancy loss and who are found to have a uterine anomaly have a septate uterus. A few have other anomalies, mostly the bicornuate uterus. Proctor and Haney's review of women with recurrent first-trimester pregnancy loss reinforces the role of the septate uterus in repeated pregnancy loss. Of 35 women reviewed with a divided uterine cavity on hysterosalpingogram, all women were found through diagnostic hysteroscopy and laparoscopy to have a septate uterus. In our experience, fetal survival rates are higher after septate uterus repair than after other repairs. In 1977, Rock and Jones reported on 43 patients with septate uteri selected for Jones metroplasty at the Johns Hopkins Hospital. Of these 43 patients, 95% became pregnant postoperatively, 73% carried to term, and 77% delivered a liveborn child. Similarly, hysteroscopic metroplasty for the septate uterus provides a substantial improvement in obstetric outcome. Data obtained from retrospective studies suggest that hysteroscopic metroplasty is associated with favorable outcomes, with a pregnancy rate of approximately 80% and a miscarriage rate of only approximately 15%. Recent prospective observational studies reported similar findings. Pabuccu and Gomel reported the reproductive outcome of 61 patients; however, the patients had unexplained infertility, and nearly 15% were also treated with cervical cerclage. Litta and colleagues also reported an 83.3%

term delivery rate in their population of women with a septate uterus who underwent hysteroscopic metroplasty. Patton and colleagues described 16 women with a complete uterine septum. The preoperative pregnancy loss rate was 81%. Eleven of the fourteen septa treated with a hysteroscopic approach were successfully removed. The remaining three unsuccessful hysteroscopic procedures and two additional patients were treated using the Tompkins metroplasty. Postoperatively, 9 women conceived after hysteroscopic surgery, and term live births occurred in 9 of 12 (75%) conceptions. The most controversial area remains the resection of the cervical portion of the septum. Parsanezhad and colleagues reported a multicenter, randomized controlled trial regarding the management of the cervical septum. Surgical issues, complications, and pregnancy outcomes were compared. Operating times, distending media deficits, and perioperative complications were all substantially better in the cervical septum resection group. The reproductive outcomes were similar; however, the cesarean section rate was higher in the group in which the cervical septum was spared. The histologic features of the septum in this abnormal uterus have been described. Dabirashrafi and colleagues noted less connective tissue in uterine septa. Poor decidualization and placentation were suggested as a cause.

Finally, the AFS class Va uterus (a double cervix and uterine cavity with a single fundus) can result from a rotation abnormality during the descent of the müllerian ducts. Among the reported cases of the septate uterus, the incidence of the complete septum involving the cervix varies from 4% to 29%. If the dextrorotating müllerian ducts overrotate, the senior author theorizes that the septum fails to absorb after fusion of the ducts (J. A. Rock, *personal observations*, 1991). In virtually every patient with a complete septate uterus, the left cervix is higher than the right. In one patient, one cervix has been noted above the other (Fig. 25.18). This rotation abnormality may be a factor associated with lack of absorption of the uterine septum in these patients.

Uterine Anomalies and Menstrual Difficulties

Dysmenorrhea and abnormal and heavy menstrual bleeding have been reported to occur more frequently with any form

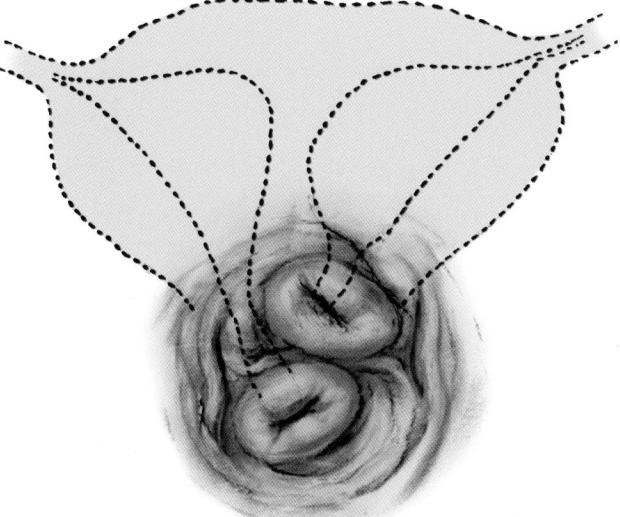

FIGURE 25.18 A double uterus with two cervices and a single fundus (class V). Note that the left cervix is positioned over the right cervix. This rotation abnormality may be a factor associated with a lack of absorption of the uterine septum.

of double uterus and to be relieved after unification operations. Capraro and associates reported several cases in which dysmenorrhea was cured by metroplasty. Erwin Strassmann also believed that all cases of dysmenorrhea and menorrhagia associated with uterine anomalies were relieved by unification of the two uterine cavities. Generally, however, dysmenorrhea and menorrhagia are inappropriate indications for uterine unification, and the operation should not be performed solely for these reasons. Grynberg and colleagues reported on women who experienced infertility, pregnancy losses, dyspareunia, or dysmenorrhea. In their series, 22 patients underwent hysteroscopic resection of complete uterine septum and resection of longitudinal vaginal septum. The data suggested that hysteroscopic incision of the septum did not improve reproductive outcomes (miscarriage rate increased from 25% to 43%, cervical cerclage rate was not significantly changed). In their series, the advantage of surgery was limited because the miscarriage and the preterm delivery rates were not improved after metroplasty. This publication reminds reconstructive gynecologists that careful consideration of indications for surgery is imperative before surgery. Until more data are available, systematic surgical intervention for young women diagnosed with complete uterine septum without evidence of pregnancy loss should be discouraged.

Uterine Anomalies and Infertility

Opinions differ considerably in terms of whether infertility is a proper indication for metroplasty. Erwin Strassmann stated that primary infertility could be cured in 60% of patients with uterine anomaly if all other causes of infertility were excluded. Strassmann reported eight metroplasties for primary sterility that yielded nine pregnancies and seven liveborn children, although the number of patients who conceived was not given. Similar reports of small numbers of patients can be found throughout the literature. Heinonen and Pystynen indicated that uterine anomalies are rarely the reason for infertility. Nonuterine causes of infertility must be ruled out before metroplasty, as a last resort, is considered.

Certainly, a full infertility investigation to rule out other causes should be completed before the anomalous uterus is blamed. Even when no other cause for infertility is found, if the uterus is septate or bicornuate, then there may not be any proper indication for metroplasty. This question of when to perform metroplasty simply has not yet been answered. The decision is difficult and becomes even more difficult when the opportunity for metroplasty presents itself because a septate or bicornuate uterus requires laparotomy for some other reason, such as endometriosis or tubal occlusion.

Surgical Technique for Uterine Unification

Historically, the septate uterus has been unified with either the Jones or the Tompkins procedure. Clinical reports by Chervenak and Neuwirth; by Daly, Walters, and colleagues; by DeCherney and associates; and Israel and March have favorably compared hysteroscopic (resectoscopic incision of a uterine septum) with the more traditional transabdominal approach. Term pregnancy rates after these procedures have approached 80% to 85%. Several attempts may be necessary to incise a wide septum, although the septum usually can be incised completely at the first operation.

Transcervical Lysis of the Uterine Septum Abdominal metroplasty for transfundal incision or for excision of the septum associated with the septate uterus generally has been abandoned. With hysteroscopic scissors, the procedure can be tedious, especially with a large, broad septum. Although

the hysteroscope and scissors are still used for cutting the septum, the resectoscope has been found to be comparable. The optics are excellent, and the septum can be electrosurgically incised with little difficulty. Laser-assisted procedures have also been described.

Before transcervical lysis of a uterine septum, a gonadotropin-releasing hormone agonist may be given for 2 months to reduce the amount of endometrium that can obscure the surgeon's view during the procedure. Many authors do not consider routine preoperative preparation of the endometrium essential and may only use medications in procedures involving exceptionally wide septa or complete septa that involve the lower one third of the uterine cavity or the cervical canal. If medical preparation is not used, surgical intervention should be scheduled during the early proliferative phase of the cycle to avoid bleeding and impaired visualization from a vascular endometrium associated with the secretory phase. Transcervical lysis is usually performed in conjunction with laparoscopy under general endotracheal anesthesia. The uterine cavity is distended with dextran 70 (Hyskon) by way of the resectoscope, which is inserted into the cervix. The septum is then electrosurgically incised by advancing the cutting loupe, using the trigger mechanism of the resectoscope. The uterine septum is incised until the tubal ostia are visualized and there is no appreciable evidence of the septum. The procedure is performed under simultaneous laparoscopy to limit the risks of uterine perforation. The laparoscopic light can be turned off so that the light from the hysteroscope can be clearly visualized through the fundus. Most patients can be discharged within 4 hours of the procedure. There is no role for placement of a postoperative intrauterine device. The benefit of routine procedure-related antibiotic therapy has not been well supported with evidence; however, it is recommended to administer antibiotics before the procedure and to continue for 5 days after surgery to limit the risks of infection. If excessive bleeding occurs after the procedure, a Foley catheter should be placed in

the uterine cavity for tamponade and removed in 4 to 6 hours. Hormonal therapy is the most commonly used postoperative treatment regimen. The aim of the treatment is the promotion of rapid epithelialization. Dabirashrafi and colleagues reported that estrogen therapy did not appear to demonstrate a benefit. Further evidence is necessary before dismissing the current trend of postoperative estrogen therapy.

Transcervical lysis also can be performed to repair a complete septate uterus (i.e., a single fundus with two cavities and two cervices). In this instance, a no. 8 Foley catheter is inserted into one cervix and indigo carmine is injected into the cavity. The other cavity is distended with dextran 70 (Hyskon) by way of the resectoscope. The septum is electrosurgically incised at a point above the internal cervical os until the Foley catheter is visualized. The septum is then incised in a superior direction until the tubal ostium is visualized and there is no appreciable septum (**Fig. 25.19**).

After transcervical lysis of a uterine septum, a 2-month delay before attempting pregnancy is suggested to allow complete resorption of the septum. Delivery may be vaginal. The Jones procedure is used to repair a septate uterus when a particularly broad septum cannot be easily incised with the resectoscope. The Strassmann procedure is used for unification of a bicornuate uterus. The safety and efficacy of hysteroscopic resection of the uterine septum in patients with a class Va septate uterus has been demonstrated by the senior author. Historically, case reports, such as that of Hundley and colleagues, were the only source of information about this interesting variant; however, one of the largest populations of patients with a complete septum was reported in 1999 by Rock, Roberts, and Hesla. The patients underwent hysteroscopic metroplasty with preservation of the cervical portion of the septum. With the exception of one case of pulmonary edema, no significant intraoperative or postoperative complications were reported. Postoperative hysteroscopy revealed only minor fundal septal remnants without clinical significance.

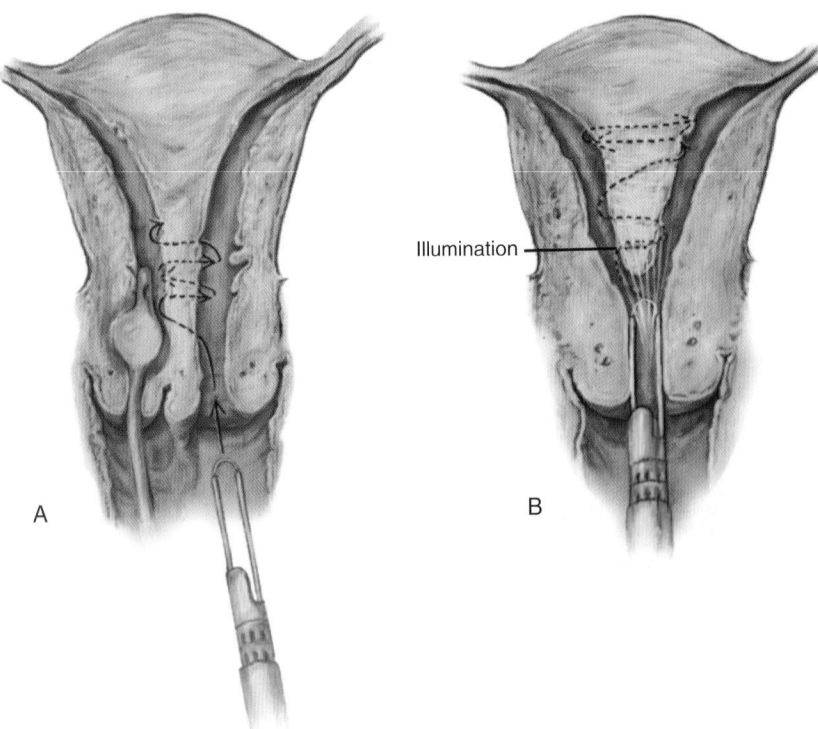

Illumination

A   B

FIGURE 25.19 Resectoscopic metroplasty. **A:** A Foley catheter is placed in one cavity of a complete septate uterus (American Fertility Society class Va uterus). The resectoscope is inserted in the opposite cavity, and the septum is incised until the Foley is visualized. The septum can be easily incised with the resectoscope until both internal os are visible. **B:** A septate uterus with a single cervix. The septum can be incised with the straight loupe of the resectoscope.

The Modified Jones Metroplasty In the modified Jones unification operation (**Fig. 25.20**), the abdomen is generally opened through a transverse incision. If only the unification operation is planned, then a Pfannenstiel incision is permissible. The pelvic viscera are inspected. The septate uterus may demonstrate a median raphe across the fundus, but it is surprising how often the corpus looks normal. To facilitate manipulation, a traction suture of heavy silk is placed through the top of the septum. This suture is removed from the site when the septum is excised.

No attempt is made to stain the uterine cavity with methylene blue. Normal unstained endometrial tissue can be easily differentiated from the myometrium.

There are essentially two methods to control bleeding during this procedure. In the first, a tourniquet is applied at the junction of the lower uterine segment and cervix by inserting a 0.5-inch Penrose drain through an avascular space in the broad ligaments just lateral to the uterine vessels on each side. The tourniquet is placed around the lower uterine segment and is tied anterior to the uterus. Because the uterine corpus receives a significant blood supply through the ovarian arteries, tourniquets should also be tied around the infundibulopelvic ligaments on each side, using the same hole in the broad ligament. All tourniquets must be tied tightly enough to occlude both the arterial supply to and the venous drainage from the uterus. If only the venous drainage is occluded, then the corpus becomes engorged and congested, and bleeding is increased. If the arterial supply is occluded, then the uterus blanches, and the bleeding is minimal. A sterile Doptone can be used to establish disappearance of uterine artery pulsations. Hypotensive anesthetic techniques used in conjunction with the tourniquets allow a uterine unification operation to be accomplished with negligible blood loss.

The alternative method for hemostasis uses up to 20 units of vasopressin that is diluted in 20 mL of saline and injected into the anterior and posterior walls of the uterus before the incision is made.

The uterine septum should be surgically excised as a wedge (**Fig. 25.20D**). The incisions begin at the fundus of the uterus. The approach to the endometrial cavity should be handled

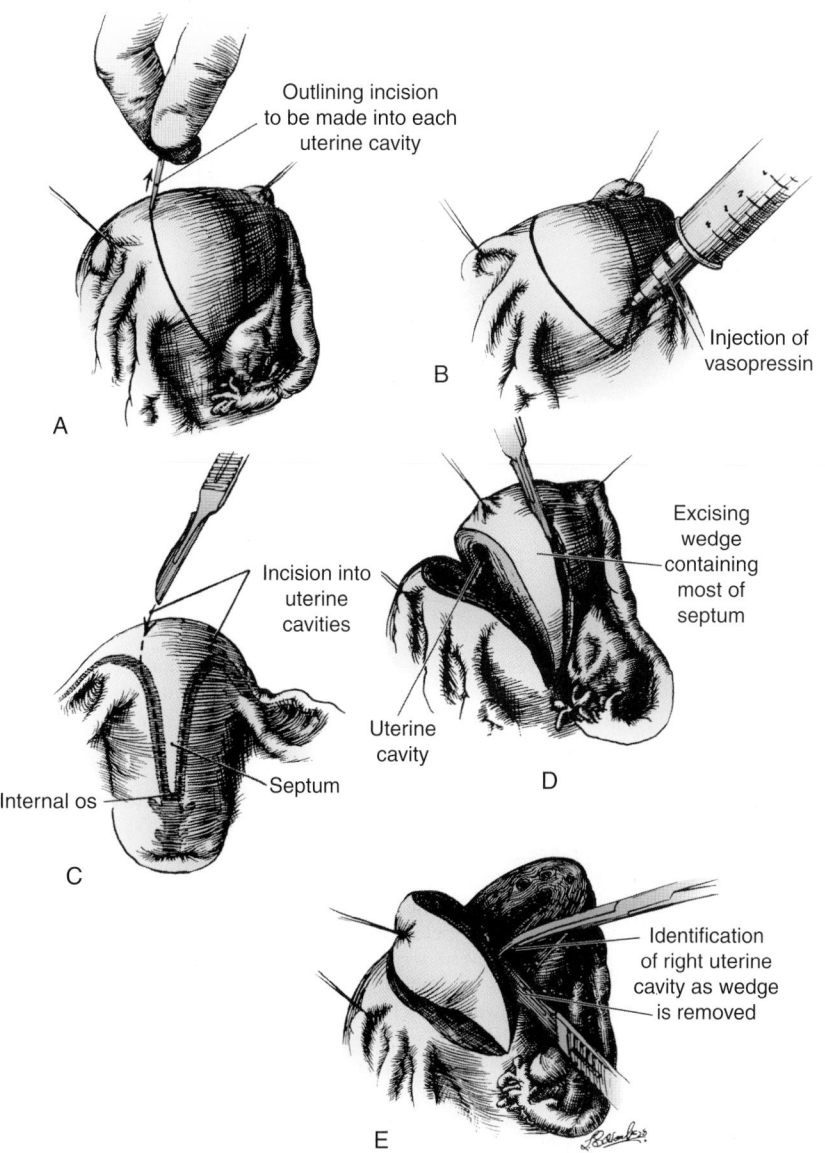

Outlining incision to be made into each uterine cavity

Injection of vasopressin

A

B

Incision into uterine cavities

Excising wedge containing most of septum

Uterine cavity

Internal os

Septum

C

D

Identification of right uterine cavity as wedge is removed

E

FIGURE 25.20 The modified Jones metroplasty. See the text for a full description of the various steps in the operative repair of a septate uterus by excision of a wedge.

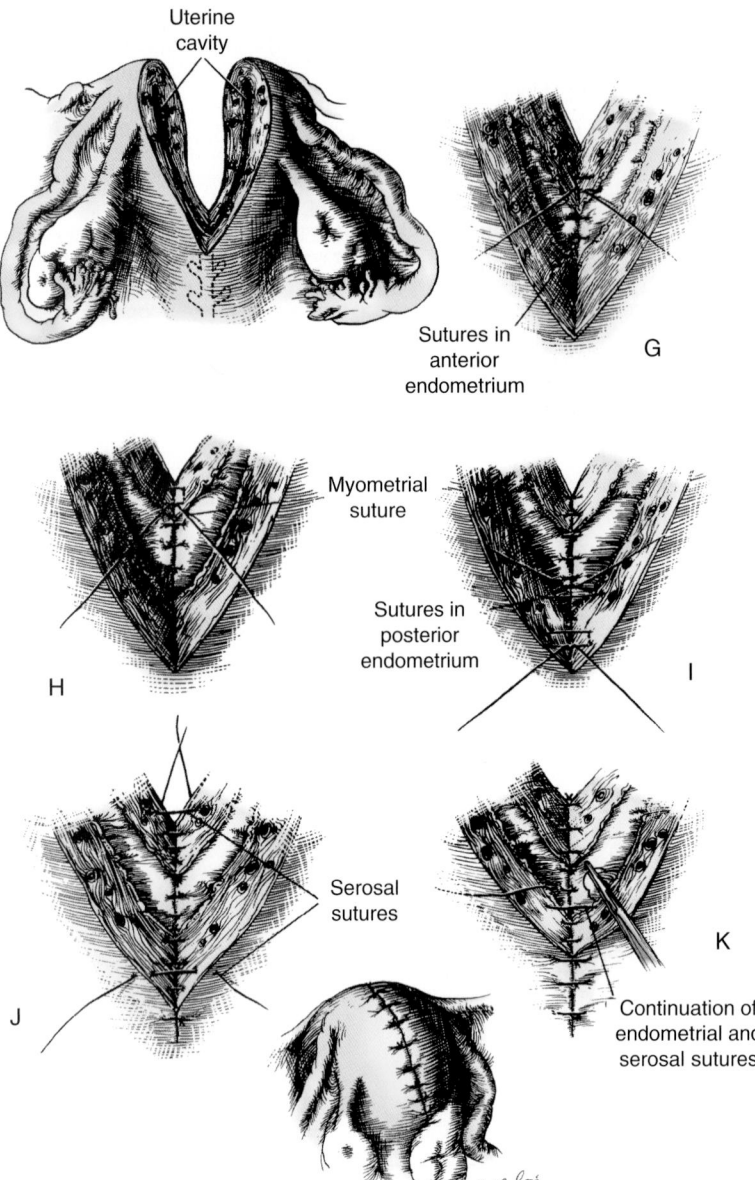

Uterine
cavity

F

Sutures in
anterior
endometrium

G

Myometrial
suture

H

Sutures in
posterior
endometrium

I

Serosal
sutures

J

K

Continuation of
endometrial and
serosal sutures

L

FIGURE 25.20 (*Continued*)

carefully so that it is not transected (Fig. 25.20E). The original incisions at the top of the fundus are usually within 1 cm—and sometimes even less—of the insertion of the fallopian tubes. If the incision is directed toward the apex of the wedge, however, there seems to be little danger of transecting the tube across its interstitial transit in the myometrium.

After the wedge has been removed, the uterus is closed in three layers with interrupted stitches; 2-0 nonreactive suture on an atraumatic tapered needle is convenient. Two sizes of needles are needed: a half-inch needle for the inner and intermediate layers and a large needle (three fourths half round) for the outer muscular layer. The inner layer of stitches must include approximately one third of the thickness of the myometrium, because the endometrium alone is too delicate to hold a suture and will be cut through. The inner sutures should be placed through the endometrium and the myometrium in such a way that the knot is tied within the endometrial cavity (Fig. 25.20G, H). While the suture is being tied, the two lateral halves of the uterus should be pressed together both manually and with the

guy sutures to relieve tension on the suture line and to reduce the possibility of cutting through. These sutures are placed alternately, first anterior and then posterior. After the first few stitches are placed and before the first layer is completed, the second layer can be started to reduce tension.

As the operation proceeds, the third layer of stitches is begun in the serosa both anteriorly and posteriorly (Fig. 25.20I–K). Finer, nonreactive suture material can be used to approximate the serosal edges of the uterus more precisely to prevent adhesion formation to the suture line (Fig. 25.20K, L). By the conclusion of the operation, the uterus appears near normal in configuration. The striking feature is usually the proximity of the insertions of the fallopian tubes. Special care must be exercised not to obstruct the interstitial portions of the fallopian tubes while placing the fundal myometrial and serosal sutures.

The final size of the uterine cavity seems to be relatively unimportant to reproductive capability; uterine symmetry appears to be a more important factor. Often, the constructed cavity is quite small compared with the normal uterus.

Whether the surgeon removes the septum with the Jones procedure or lyses the septum transcervically, postoperative hysterogram films often show small dog-ears that are leftover tags from the original bifid condition of the uterus. Such dog-ears do not seem to interfere with function, although a postoperative roentgenogram cannot be considered normal in the sense that it does not have the appearance of a normal endometrial cavity after such an operation. If a double cervix is present, the physician should not attempt to unify the cervix because an incompetent cervical os will result. To allow the uterine incision the best possible opportunity to heal, a delay of 4 to 6 months in attempting pregnancy is advised after abdominal metroplasty.

The Jones Metroplasty versus the Tompkins Procedure The technique of modified Jones metroplasty is a compromise between the classic Jones metroplasty and the Tompkins metroplasty. In the Jones operation, the entire septum is removed. In the Tompkins operation, a single median incision divides the uterine corpus and septum in half. The incision is carried inferiorly until the endometrial cavity is reached. Each lateral septal half is then incised to within 1 cm of the tubes. No septal tissue is removed. The myometrium is reapproximated, taking care not to place sutures too close to the interstitial portion of the tubes. Proponents of the Tompkins technique suggest that it is simpler than the classic Jones procedure, that it conserves all myometrial tissue and leaves the uterotubal junction in a more normal and lateral position, and that it provides better results than the Jones metroplasty. Good results with the Tompkins technique have been reported by McShane and colleagues.

The Wedge Metroplasty versus Transcervical Lysis There are obvious advantages to a transcervical incision of a uterine septum for patients with a septate uterus. Morbidity is decreased after the procedure, and delivery can be vaginal. Term pregnancy rates are comparable with those after abdominal metroplasty for repeated pregnancy wastage.

Most of the septa associated with a septate uterus can be cut through the cervix by way of the hysteroscope or the resectoscope. Nevertheless, cases of broad uterine septum can benefit from the wedge metroplasty, and reconstructive surgeons should be knowledgeable in its performance.

The Strassmann Metroplasty The Strassmann procedure is not easily adapted to the septate uterus, but it is the procedure of choice for unification of the two endometrial cavities of an externally divided uterus, both bicornuate and didelphic (Fig. 25.21). A bicornuate uterus cannot be repaired through transcervical lysis because perforation will result. When there has been failure of fusion of the two müllerian ducts, inspection of the pelvic cavity often reveals a broad peritoneal band that lies in the middle between the two lateral hemicorpora. This rectovesical ligament is attached anteriorly to the bladder, folds over and is attached between the uterine cornua, continues posteriorly in the cul-de-sac, and ends with its attachment to the anterior wall of the sigmoid and rectum. It is not invariably present, but when it is, its potential significance in the etiology of the anomaly, possibly by preventing the two müllerian ducts from joining, must be considered. This rectovesical ligament must be removed before a unification procedure can be performed (Fig. 25.21A).

For hemostasis, tourniquets are used in a manner similar to that described for the modified Jones procedure. The two uterine cornua are incised on their median sides in their longitudinal axes, deeply enough to expose the uterine cavities (Fig. 25.21B). Superiorly, the incision must not be too close to the interstitial portion of the fallopian tubes. Inferiorly, the incision is carried far enough to join the two sides into a single endocervical canal. If it appears that a deeper incision will compromise the competence of the cervix, then a double cervical canal can be left. If the cervix is already duplex, then it should not be joined. As the incision in the myometrium releases the internal stresses in the walls of the hemicorpora, each one everts and is perfectly positioned for apposition, almost as if the original intention in embryologic development is finally to be realized. The suture technique for joining the two sides (Fig. 25.21C–E) is exactly the same as for the modified Jones procedure. The suture line in the uterine corpus should be observed for several minutes to determine the adequacy of hemostasis. Occasionally, it is necessary to place one or two extra sutures to control bleeding.

A uterine suspension can be performed as necessary. However, in the event of pregnancy, the shortened round ligaments can produce symptoms from an enlarging uterus. Presacral neurectomy in association with uterine unification should be considered only in patients with severe midline dysmenorrhea.

The cervix should be dilated to ensure proper drainage from the uterine cavity. This can be accomplished transvaginally after the abdominal procedure or from above by inserting a dilator through the cervical canal into the vagina to be removed later.

The operative technique should always be consistent with the goal of maintaining or enhancing fertility and possibly achieving a successful pregnancy. Tissue surfaces should be kept moist throughout the procedure, and instruments should be selected and used in such a way that tissue damage is minimized. Abdominal packs should be placed in plastic bags to avoid adhesions, or no-lint laparotomy pads can be used. Talc should be carefully washed from gloves, and meticulous aseptic technique should be used. The appendix should not be removed. Lactated Ringer solution containing heparin and corticosteroid can be used for peritoneal lavage throughout the procedure.

Cervical Incompetence Associated with a Double Uterus

When a patient with an anomalous uterus, with or without unification, becomes pregnant, she must be watched closely for evidence of cervical incompetence, especially if a history of previous reproductive loss suggests cervical incompetence. Heinonen and associates improved fetal survival rate from 57% to 92% by cervical cerclage. Cerclage was used mostly in patients with a partial bicornuate uterus. In these patients, the fetal salvage rate was improved from 53% before cerclage to 100% afterward. Prematurity also was decreased, from 53% to 3%. The authors stress that cervical incompetence, not the uterine anomaly, is the proper indication for cerclage in these patients. However, the frequency with which these problems are found together suggests the importance of doing a careful evaluation for both problems. Some reproductive losses from a uterine anomaly might be prevented by cerclage of an incompetent cervix during metroplasty. However, routine cerclage at the time of metroplasty is not recommended.

Attempts to unify a double cervix or a septate cervix also are not recommended because of the possibility of causing cervical incompetence. However, a double or septate cervix can adversely affect the outcome of delivery if vaginal delivery is attempted, and delivery should be by cesarean section if it appears that the cervix will cause dystocia.

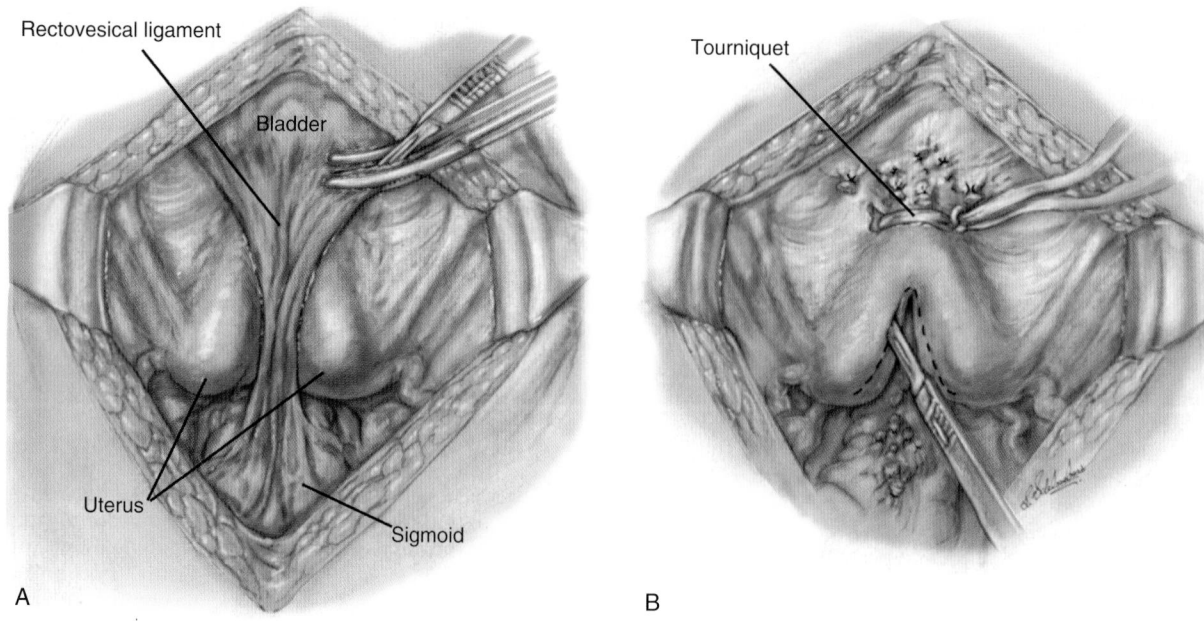

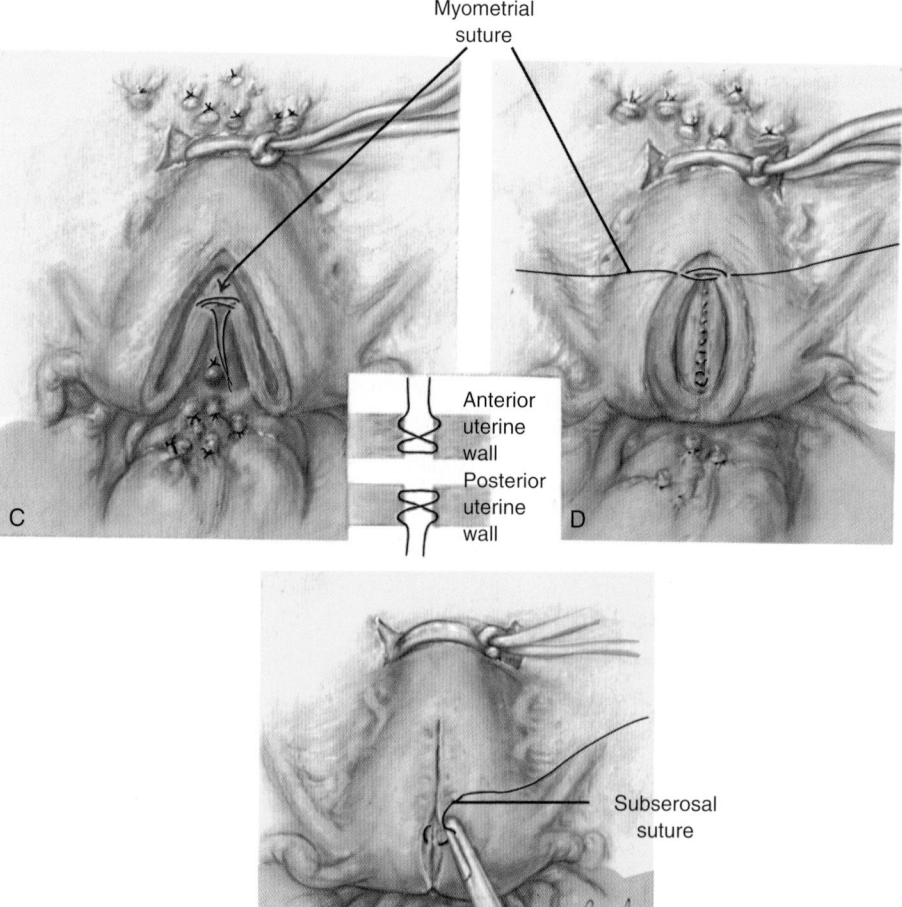

FIGURE 25.21 The Strassmann metroplasty with modification. **A:** If a rectovesical ligament is found, it should be removed. **B:** An incision is made on the medial side of each hemicorpus and carried deep enough to enter the uterine cavity. The edges of the myometrium will evert to face the opposite side. **C and D:** The myometrium is approximated by the use of interrupted vertical figure-of-eight 3-0 polyglycolic acid sutures. One should avoid placing sutures too close to the interstitial portion of the fallopian tubes. **E:** A continuous 5-0 polyglycolic acid subserosal suture is used as a final layer. Tourniquets are removed, and defects in the broad ligament are closed.

Mode of Delivery after Metroplasty

The scar formed in the myometrium after unification is as strong as, if not stronger than, the scar formed after cesarean section. The biologic conditions under which healing occurs are entirely different in these two situations. Endomyometritis is a common complication after cesarean section but is not a complication of uterine unification. Of 71 known pregnancies in Strassmann's collected series reported in 1952, 61 were delivered vaginally. There were no cases of uterine rupture during pregnancy or delivery. Lolis and colleagues reported the reproductive outcome of 22 women who underwent the Strassmann metroplasty for a bicornuate uterus; 88% achieved pregnancies that ended with the delivery of a viable infant. All were delivered by cesarean section without evidence of scar rupture. Despite evidence that the uterine scar heals securely after unification operations, our policy is to recommend delivery by elective cesarean section in all patients who have undergone abdominal metroplasty. Patients can deliver vaginally after a metroplasty by hysteroscope or resectoscope.

Diethylstilbestrol-Related Uterine Anomalies

Exposure of the female fetus to DES can cause significant anomalous development of the uterus, as reported by Kaufman and associates and by Haney and colleagues. The T-shaped uterus is the variant most commonly seen. It is associated with an increased rate of spontaneous abortions, preterm deliveries, and ectopic pregnancies.

Nagel and Malo determined the feasibility of correcting the uterine malformations seen in DES-exposed women by incising constriction rings and septa. Their goal was to incise the irregular uterine walls until the cavity assumed a smooth, straight line from the lower uterine cavity to the uterine tubal ostium. Their results suggested that metroplasty can decrease pregnancy loss but does not enhance fertility. The editors of this book suggest that the rare patient can benefit from a uterine reconstructive procedure, but that most will not. Surgeons may never develop a large series to document surgical efficacy of surgical outcomes because patients with this anomaly are close to aging out of the natural reproductive years (last dispensed in 1971 in the United States). DES-exposed patients must be monitored closely for evidence of dilatation and effacement of the cervix early in pregnancy. Cervical cerclage may be indicated in some patients.

Unicornuate Uterus

A unicornuate uterus can be present alone or with a rudimentary horn or bulb on the opposite side. In a series reported by Heinonen and associates, 11 of 13 patients with a unicornuate uterus had a rudimentary horn, and two did not. The rudimentary anlagen (uterine muscle bundle or bulb) can communicate directly with the unicornuate uterus. In some instances, there is no cavity within the anlagen, or there is no rudimentary horn. Most rudimentary horns are noncommunicating (90% according to O'Leary and O'Leary). The two sides may be connected by a fibromuscular band, or there may be no connection and no communication between the two uterine cavities. Fedele and associates have found sonography useful in determining the presence of not only a rudimentary horn but also a cavity within.

Associated Anomalies

Urinary tract anomalies are often associated with a unicornuate uterus. On the side opposite the unicornuate uterus, there may be a horseshoe or a pelvic kidney, or the kidney may be hypoplastic or absent. This is especially true if there is associated müllerian duct obstruction. When all müllerian duct derivatives and the kidney are absent on one side, this implies failure of development of the entire urogenital ridge, including the genital ridge where the ovary forms. In addition, the ovary may be malpositioned (Fig. 25.22). Rock, Parmley, and associates reported a unilateral ovary located above the pelvic brim in four cases of uterine anomalies. The orifice of the müllerian duct develops at approximately the level of the fourth thoracic vertebra (T4) in the embryo. The tip subsequently migrates along the course of the müllerian duct into the pelvis. The orifice of the duct or the fimbriated end of the tube comes to lie in the pelvis as a result of differential growth of the fetus. The subsequent differential growth is retarded so that the portion of the urogenital ridge that gives rise to both the gonad and tube does not displace into the pelvis. Malpositions of the ovary and tube are the result.

Reproductive Performance

According to Heinonen and associates, the unicornuate uterus carries the poorest fetal survival rate (40%) of all uterine anomalies. In 1957, Jones reported similar findings. The abnormal shape, the insufficient muscular mass of the uterus, and the reduced uterine volume and inability to expand may explain the poor obstetric outcome.

Moutos and colleagues compared the reproductive performance of the unicornuate uterus with that of the didelphic uterus. Twenty of the 29 women with a unicornuate uterus produced a total of 40 pregnancies, whereas 13 women with a didelphic uterus produced a total of 28 pregnancies. The percentages of pregnancies resulting in preterm delivery, term delivery, and living children were similar in both groups. The authors concluded that reproductive performance of the unicornuate uterus was not different from that of the didelphic uterus, that it is uncommon for either malformation to be a primary cause of infertility, and that there is insufficient information to support recommendation of placement of a cervical cerclage in the absence of cervical incompetence. Reichman, Laufer, and Robinson reviewed 20 published reviews on patients with a unicornuate uterus. They examined 290 total women who were reported in the literature; 175 patients conceived with 468 pregnancies reported. They reported 2.7% ectopic pregnancy, 24.3% first-trimester loss, 9.7% second-trimester abortion, 20.1% preterm delivery, and 10.5% intrauterine fetal demise. They reported a 49.9% livebirth rate. The authors also suggested that the current data available about the benefit of cervical cerclage (nonrandomized and lacking control subjects) seem inadequate to support a role for cervical incompetence for recurrent losses in patients with a unicornuate uterus.

Because most cases of unicornuate uterus have a noncommunicating rudimentary uterine horn on the opposite side, there is danger of pregnancy in the rudimentary horn from transperitoneal migration of sperm or ovum from the opposite side. According to Holden and Hart, approximately 350 cases of pregnancy in a rudimentary horn have been reported since the original case report by Mauriceau in 1669. O'Leary and O'Leary found the corpus luteum on the side contralateral to the rudimentary horn containing a pregnancy in 8% of cases. Signs and symptoms of an ectopic pregnancy develop with eventual rupture of the horn if the pregnancy is not detected early. Rupture through the wall of the vascular rudimentary horn is associated with sudden and severe intraperitoneal hemorrhage and shock. Death can occur in a few minutes. It is surprising that the current mortality rate has decreased to 5%.

Very little, if anything, can be done to improve the reproductive performance of patients with a unicornuate uterus. The physician should observe closely for signs and symptoms of preterm labor. Cervical incompetence is likely less common than previously suggested, yet if present, cerclage should be

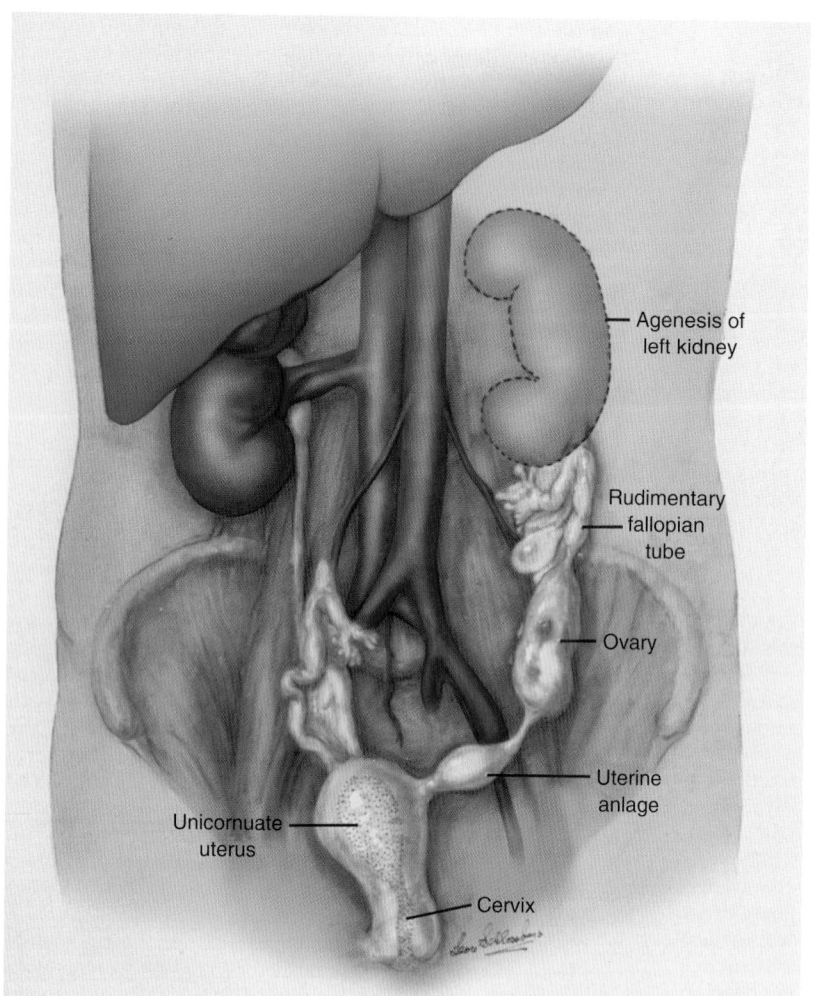

FIGURE 25.22 A unicornuate uterus associated with ovarian malposition on the left. Note that the ovary and the tube are slightly above the pelvic brim. In this instance, the ovary measured 6 inches long.

considered as indicated. Andrews and Jones have suggested that removal of the rudimentary uterine horn may improve the chances of a successful pregnancy, eliminating the risk of ectopic pregnancy in the rudimentary horn as well as the risk of possible retrograde menstruation and the development of endometriosis. Typically, the procedure is a straightforward laparoscopic procedure with the potential for substantial benefit. Cases of asymmetric development of the unicornuate uterus with an opposing rudimentary uterine horn are not amenable to unification.

Longitudinal Vaginal Septum

Failure of fusion of the lower müllerian ducts that form the vagina can result in a vagina with a longitudinal septum. The septum can be partial or complete. Young patients have difficulty using tampons. In cases of didelphic uterus with a longitudinal vaginal septum, one uterine hemicorpus is usually better developed than the other. If intercourse consistently occurs on the vaginal side connected to the uterine hemicorpus that is less well developed, then infertility or repeated pregnancy loss could result. For these reasons, the septum should be removed (when the patient is not pregnant) unless there is a contraindication. This can usually be accomplished easily with reasonable precautions against injury to the urethra, bladder, and rectum.

Haddad and colleagues reported their experience over a 24-year period with management of the longitudinal vaginal septum. The retrospective review of 202 patient charts

described a complete septum (extending from cervix to introitus) in 45.6% of patients, high partial in 36.1%, and a medium or low partial, involving only the distal vagina, in 18.3%. Uterine malformations were noted in 87.8% of cases. The frequency of uterine malformations was 99.4% in cases of complete or partial high septum and 30.3% in cases of partial medium or low septum. The most common malformation was class Va complete septate uterus in 59.5% of malformations, followed by class III uterus didelphys (24.3%), and class Vb partial septate uterus (15%). Section or resection was performed in 201 cases. Bladder injury in one patient was the only reported complication. As highlighted by the high prevalence of associated uterine malformations in this review, management should always include an assessment of uterine anatomy.

Asymmetric Obstruction of the Uterus or Vagina

Unicornuate Uterus and Noncommunicating Uterine Anlagen Containing Functional Endometrium

If one müllerian duct develops normally while the opposite müllerian duct fails to develop or develops incompletely, then a relatively normal unicornuate uterus is found on one side and the cervix, musculature, uterine cavity, endometrium, fallopian tube, blood supply, and ligamentous attachments are absent or hypoplastic to a varying degree on the other side.

Obstruction to menstruation can also occur to varying degrees on the improperly developed side. For example, if a rudimentary uterine horn does not communicate externally but does have an endometrium-lined uterine cavity, then clear symptoms of obstructed menstruation may begin soon after menarche, and severe dysmenorrhea will be present. Cryptomenorrhea can be overlooked as the diagnosis because there is cyclic menstruation from the opposite side. It is important to make the

diagnosis as soon as possible, because if the lumen of the tube communicates with the endometrial cavity of the rudimentary uterus, then retrograde menstruation and pelvic endometriosis will develop, and reproductive potential can be damaged. During the operation illustrated in Figure 25.23, which was performed to remove an obstructed rudimentary uterine horn, the fallopian tube was obstructed, and retrograde menstruation was impossible. Occasionally, the fallopian tube connected

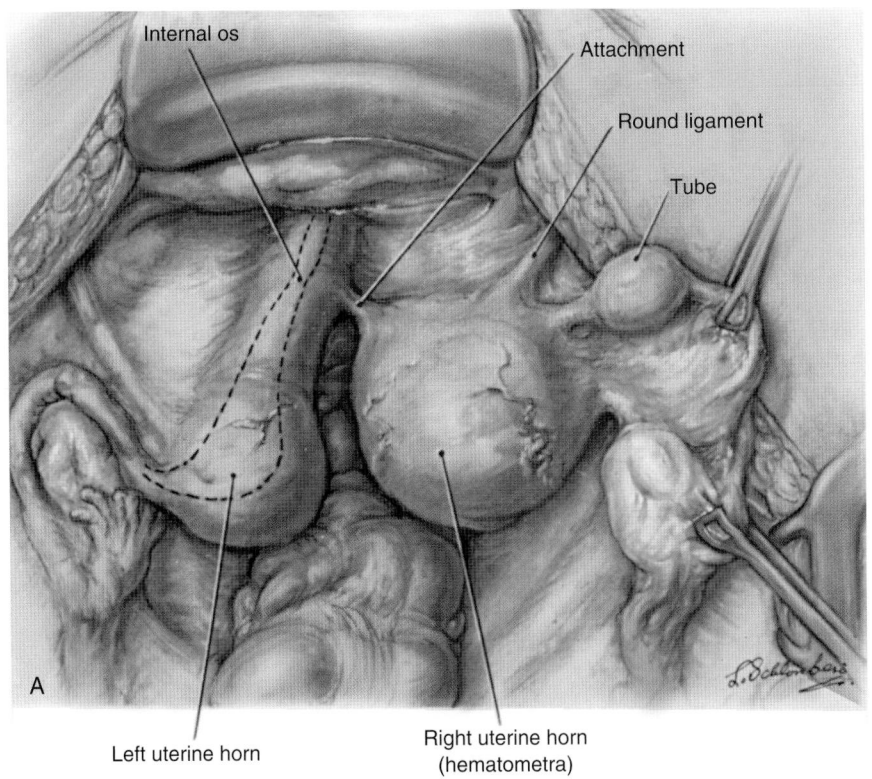

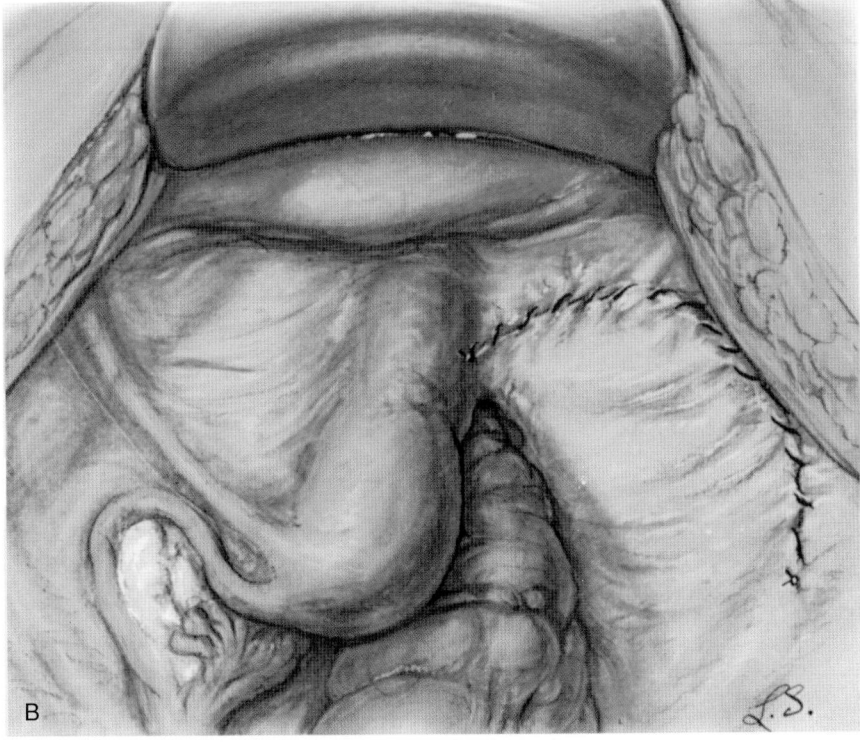

FIGURE 25.23 A: A noncommunicating rudimentary horn with functional endometrium that contains menstrual blood under pressure. Note the congenital abnormality of the fallopian tube, which prevented retrograde menstruation. B: The same patient after excision of the rudimentary horn.

to the rudimentary uterine horn may not be patent because of incomplete development. Multiple case reports regarding the laparoscopic resection of obstructed uterine anlagen have supported the use of multiple techniques (stapling, bipolar or monopolar cautery, and the harmonic scalpel). Fedele and colleagues reported a series of 10 patients who have done well; however, the follow-up was only reported out to 6 months postprocedure. The authors strongly recommend the removal of the associated fallopian tube to minimize the risk of an ectopic pregnancy.

Unilateral Obstruction of a Cavity of a Double Uterus

Another example of a rare obstructed lateral fusion problem is the complete septum between two uterine cavities illustrated in **Figure 25.24**. One cavity communicated with a cervix, and the other did not. This could represent an example of unilateral failure of cervical development. The patient reported incapacitating dysmenorrhea that appeared shortly after the menarche and lasted 5 days. A tense, cystic mass was palpable in the right half of the pelvis. The operation, described originally by Jones in the second edition of this book, consisted of making an incision through the anterior wall of the cystic right portion of the uterus. It was found to contain old menstrual blood. The entire septum was excised, and the uterus was reconstructed by anastomosis of the two cavities. A continuous lockstitch was reinforced by interrupted myometrial sutures, and the

plastic reconstruction of the uterus was completed by a third layer of interrupted sutures uniting myometrium and serosa. Steinkampf and colleagues reported a similar case in a 17-year-old girl with progressive pelvic pain. The authors described an accessory noncommunicating uterine cavity, which they treated by excision at laparotomy.

Sanders and colleagues described several cases in which the role of interventional radiology was crucial in the management of obstructive anomalies. The report described the drainage of a noncommunicating right uterine cavity distended with blood in a unicornuate uterus in a 14-year-old patient. Adequate access was established by using ultrasound-guided needle aspiration followed by a hysteroscopic excision. The assistance of interventional radiologic procedures, including percutaneous drainage and dilatation of small maldeveloped areas, may allow access to areas otherwise inaccessible by conventional mechanisms and assist in preserving reproductive function.

Double Uterus with Obstructed Hemivagina and Ipsilateral Renal Agenesis

The unique clinical syndrome consisting of a double uterus, obstruction of the vagina (unilateral, partial, or complete), and ipsilateral renal agenesis is rare. The renal agenesis (mesonephric involution) on the side of the obstructed vagina associated with a double uterus and double cervix is suggestive of an embryologic arrest at 8 weeks of pregnancy that simultaneously affects the müllerian and metanephric ducts. The exact cause is unknown.

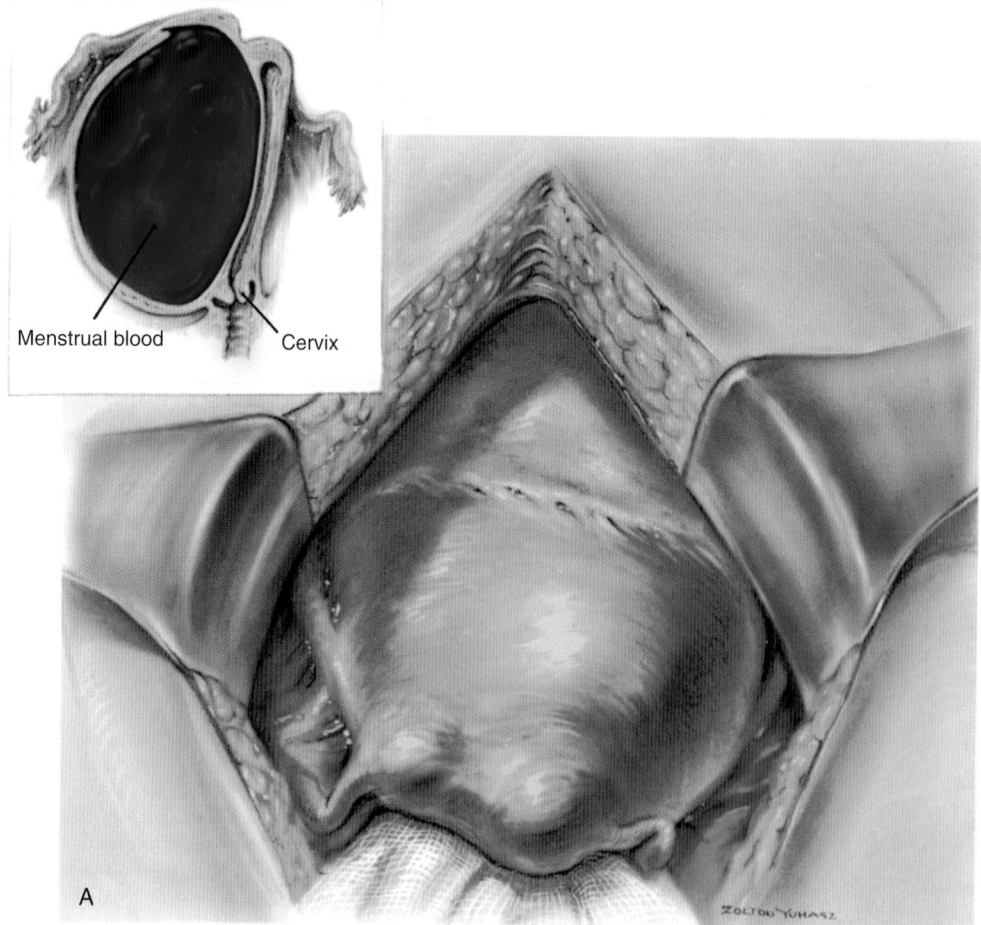

FIGURE 25.24 A: A double uterus seen at operation. Hematometra in the right uterine cavity (**inset**), which does not communicate with the other cavity or the cervical canal.

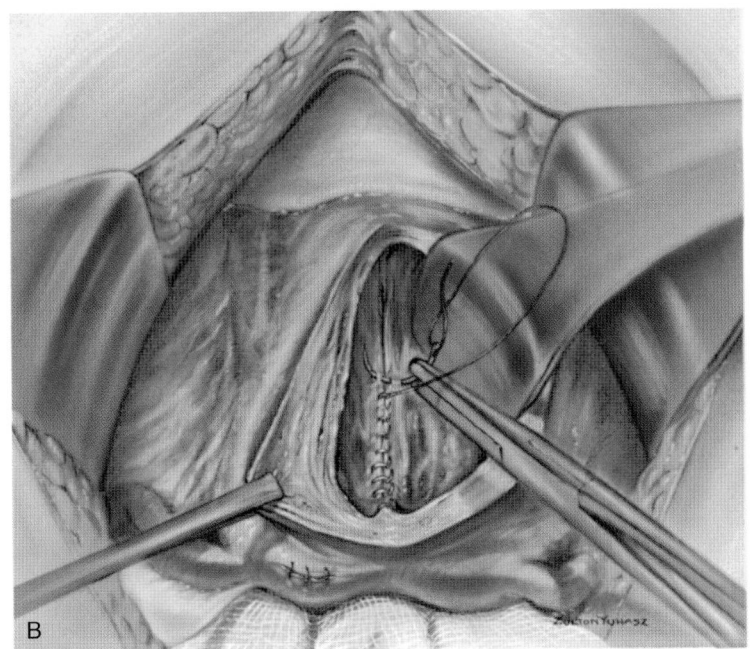

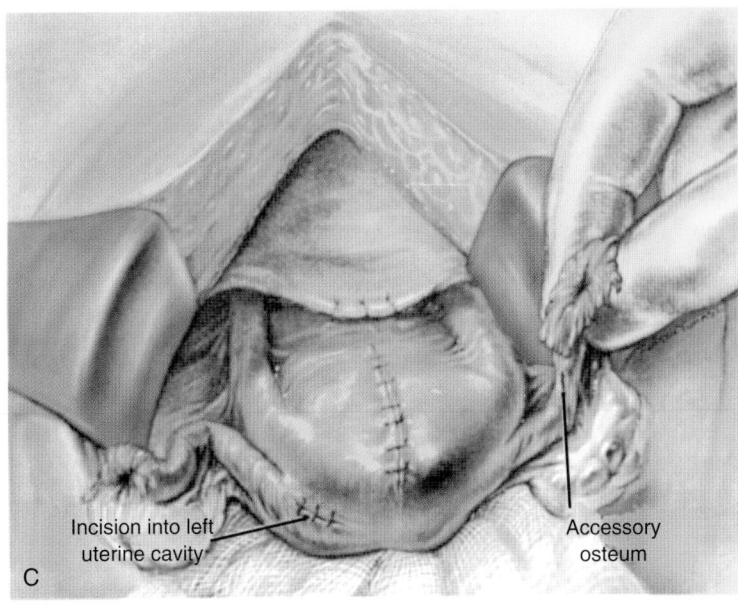

Incision into left
uterine cavity

Accessory
osteum

FIGURE 25.24 (*Continued*) **B:** The septum of the double uterus has been excised, and anastomosis is performed to unite the two cavities. **C:** Anastomosis is completed. The small incision in the left uterine cavity was made before the septum was removed for the purpose of orientation.

Diagnostic Groups

Clinical symptoms vary depending on the uterovaginal relations in individual cases, but the syndrome can be described generally in three groups. Group 1 patients have complete unilateral vaginal obstruction without uterine communication, resulting in a paravaginal mass and symptoms of severe dysmenorrhea and lower abdominal pain. Menses are regular. Group 2 patients have an incomplete unilateral vaginal obstruction without uterine communication. The presenting symptoms are lower abdominal pain, severe dysmenorrhea, excessive foul mucopurulent discharge, and, in some instances, intermenstrual bleeding. Group 3 patients have complete vaginal obstruction with a laterally communicating double uterus. They have a paravaginal mass, lower abdominal pain, and dysmenorrhea. Menses are regular. A 10-year review of patients with this anomaly was published by Phupong and colleagues. Most patients presented with dysmenorrhea (73%) or a pelvic

or paravaginal mass (71%). The right uterus and vagina were affected in 63.5% of patients.

Because menses in patients with this syndrome are rarely irregular, the possibility of this syndrome as a diagnosis can easily be overlooked. A careful pelvic examination is necessary to make the correct diagnosis. Magnetic resonance imaging can identify the obstructed vagina, double uterus, and absence of a kidney on the side of the obstruction (**Fig. 25.25**), but it may not be helpful if there is incomplete vaginal obstruction or a uterine communication. With the onset of more universal prenatal imaging, the diagnosis of unilateral renal agenesis in a female fetus should prompt the obstetric team to interact with pediatric providers about the possible association with müllerian anomalies, particularly obstructing hemivagina with double uterus. The obstructed vagina may even prolapse through the introitus in newborns with mucocolpos of the obstructed vagina. A postdelivery pelvic ultrasound, combined with renal/bladder

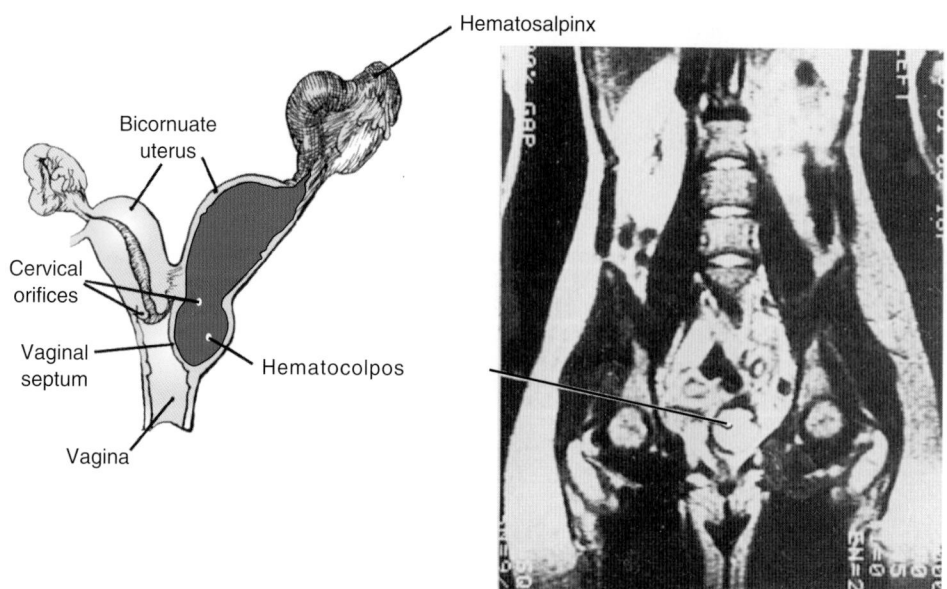

FIGURE 25.25 A double uterus with unilateral complete vaginal obstruction and ipsilateral renal agenesis. Magnetic resonance imaging reveals the left hematocolpos, both uteri, and absence of the left kidney on the side of the vaginal obstruction.

sonogram, can provide data on the uterovaginal anatomy as well as rule out hydroureter and hydronephrosis.

Complete unilateral vaginal obstruction (Group 1) can go unrecognized for a number of years after the onset of menses unless the obstructed vagina is significantly smaller causing hematometra to develop more quickly. The vagina is quite distensible and can accommodate a large amount of accumulated blood in the obstructed side. There is sufficient absorption of menstrual blood between periods so that each subsequent flow can add to the increments of accumulated blood without pain. Nevertheless, once retrograde menstruation occurs, endometriosis invariably is the result.

Surgical Treatment

Careful excision of the vaginal septum is the treatment of choice for a unilateral vaginal obstruction. Prophylactic antibiotics should be administered before surgery. After opening the vaginal pouch, the surgeon should use suction and lavage to remove the pooled blood and mucus. Phupong and colleagues' review also confirms the successful use of this primary therapy in 84.3% of patients. Haddad and colleagues reported a similar experience in a report describing patient management over a 27-year period. Excision of the vaginal septum was successful in 88% of patients, with complete excision in one procedure in 92% of those patients. In cases of pyocolpos or hematocolpos, distention and stretching of the septal tissue may increase the risk of inadequate resection and possible postoperative stenosis; the authors found the use of a two-step graduated resection advantageous to ensure adequate resection. A limited resection (3 cm) was performed to allow adequate drainage, followed by a return to the operating room in approximately 1 month to remove any remaining septum.

Because the obstructing septum is usually thick, removal can be difficult. Cooper and Merritt proposed the novel use of a tracheobronchial stent to maintain patency after excision of the obstructing vaginal septum. The stent allows maintenance of patency while epithelialization of the vaginal walls occurs. This technique can be particularly useful in high obstructing septa or in very young patients when access for reapproximation of vaginal mucosa is virtually impossible. In most cases, clamps should be used to isolate a generous vaginal pedicle

while the suture is being tied in place to prevent slippage of tissue. Such pedicles generally retract during healing, and formation of a vaginal stenosis is avoided. In most instances, surgery is restricted to excision of the septum. A handheld harmonic scalpel can be advantageous for negotiating an appropriate pedicle and providing excellent hemostasis. Abdominal exploration is usually unnecessary; however, in cases with a high vaginal obstruction, an abdominal approach may provide the best surgical access to unify the vaginas. Uterine reconstruction is not indicated for cases of lateral communication of the uterine horns. Some authors have reported the use of hemihysterectomy in patients with a high, thick-walled obstruction, massive ovarian involvement, endometriosis, or adenomyosis; however, this is generally not recommended in young patients.

Reproductive Performance

Reproductive performance for patients with this disorder is usually consistent with that of patients with a double uterus unless the delay in diagnosis and resection of the obstructing septum has been sufficient to destroy tubal function or to cause the development of endometriosis. Haddad and colleagues' review was notable for a predominance of pregnancies (80%) in the contralateral endometrial cavity.

UNUSUAL CONFIGURATIONS OF VERTICAL-LATERAL FUSION DEFECTS

Unusual configurations of both vertical and lateral fusion defects may occur simultaneously. Figure 25.26 depicts the radiographic evaluation (MRI) of a young woman in whom cryptomenorrhea developed above a transverse vaginal septum. The MRI study depicting the hematocolpos also suggests the longitudinal vaginal septum. Incision, drainage, and resection of the transverse vaginal septum allowed appropriate evaluation of the more proximal müllerian anatomy. The artist's depiction in Figure 25.26A demonstrates the unusual constellation of a uterus didelphys with an intrauterine communication of the cavities and a longitudinal vaginal septum. This type of atypical combination occurs frequently enough to emphasize the importance of proper delineation of individual anatomy preoperatively for proper surgical preparation.

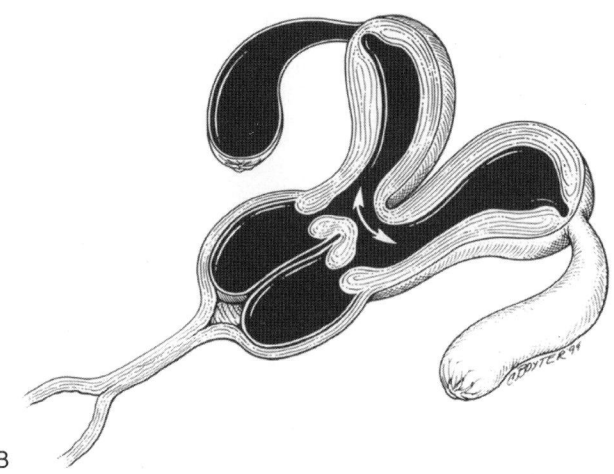

B

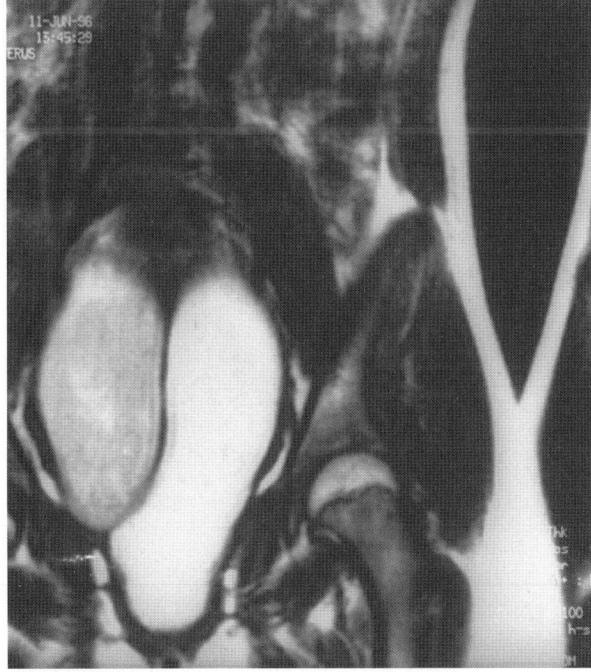

B

FIGURE 25.26 An unusual combination of both vertical and lateral fusion defects. **A:** A uterus didelphys with an intrauterine communication and a longitudinal vaginal septum are present proximal to a transverse vaginal septum. **B:** The magnetic resonance image demonstrates the presence of both septa.

Müllerian duct anomalies can occur in association with a variety of other problems. For example, Stanton reported that in a series of 70 patients with bladder exstrophy, 30 (43%) had reproductive tract abnormalities. He suggested that the true figures were actually higher. Müllerian abnormalities included absence of the vagina; septate vagina; unicornuate, bicornuate, and didelphic uterus; and absent uterus. Fewer müllerian anomalies are seen with epispadias. Jones investigated anomalies of the external genitalia and vagina in 30 patients with bladder exstrophy seen at the Johns Hopkins Hospital and suggested operative techniques for correction of these anomalies. Techniques for the management of other gynecologic and obstetric problems (especially uterine prolapse) also have been discussed by Weed and McKee and by Blakeley and Mills. A number of other rare combinations of congenital malformations of the vagina and perineum have been found in association with uterine anomalies. Their surgical correction, especially in children, is reported by Hendren and Donahoe and by others. Several authors have considered the uterovaginal anomalies that occur in association with multiple other gastrointestinal and genitourinary abnormalities. Goh and colleagues described an infant girl with complete duplication of the bladder, urethra, uterus, and vagina associated with a urogenital sinus and an anterior ectopic anus. Gastol and colleagues and Magalhaes and associates also described children with complete duplication of the bladder, urethra, vagina, and uterus. These complex anomalies include significantly more defects than lateral fusion concerns in the müllerian ducts. These cases emphasize the variable anatomy in this rare group of anomalies and that a substantial effort should be placed on defining anatomy before surgical exploration and management. Sheldon and colleagues reviewed 13 consecutive cases of vaginal reconstruction in pediatric patients with multisystem anomalies. The review emphasized several important principles involved in the surgical management: (a) all anticipated perineal reconstruction should be performed in a single stage, (b) urethral catheterization has an important role, (c) urinary reconstruction is often intimately involved in the vaginal reconstruction, (d) avoidance of overlapping suture lines is essential for optimal healing, (e) maximum growth potential of the neovagina should be considered, and (f) meticulous follow-up of proper routine dilatation of the neovagina should be expected. Coordinated reconstruction of all organ systems is especially important in these complex cases.

Müllerian duct anomalies are seen with the McKusick-Kaufman syndrome, an autosomal recessive disorder. Other clinical findings reported with this syndrome include hydrometrocolpos, postaxial polydactyly, syndactyly, congenital heart disease, intravaginal displacement of the urethral meatus, and anorectal anomalies. In 1982, Jabs and colleagues added an unusual case to the few cases previously reported in the literature.

Müllerian duct anomalies may also affect the development of the fallopian tube. Although extremely rare, episodes of unilateral or bilateral absence of the fallopian tube have been reported. Of the less than 10 cases in the literature, Eustace reported two of the described cases. He hypothesized that compromise of the local blood supply to the caudal aspect of the müllerian duct was a more likely cause than a fusion disorder. This situation could affect fallopian tube development to a variable extent with even some effect on ovarian development.

BEST SURGICAL PRACTICES

- Vaginal dilatation should be the first line of treatment for creation of a neovagina in patients with müllerian agenesis.
- The gynecologic literature supports the historical role of the McIndoe vaginoplasty as a safe and effective procedure for surgical creation of a neovagina, when necessary. The surgical tenants of the McIndoe procedure are the basis for innovative techniques in surgical creation of the neovagina.
- Appropriate preoperative evaluation of reproductive and pelvic anatomy remains a critical step before a patient is taken to the operating room for treatment of any müllerian anomaly.
- In patients with müllerian agenesis, removal of uterine anlagen that contain endometrium and have the potential to cause obstruction and subsequent pelvic pain should be strongly considered.
- Hysteroscopic metroplasty is a successful, minimally invasive technique for removal of a uterine septum.
- Resection of a uterine septum has been shown to improve pregnancy success in patients with a history of recurrent pregnancy loss.
- Strassmann metroplasty should be considered in select women with a bicornuate uterus who have experienced recurrent pregnancy loss or preterm delivery.

V

BIBLIOGRAPHY

Abbe R. New method of creating a vagina in a case of congenital absence. *Med Rec* 1898;54:836.

Adamyan LV. Laparoscopic management of vaginal aplasia with or without functional noncommunicating rudimentary uterus. In: Arrequi ME, Fitzgibbons RJ, Katkhouda N, et al., eds. *Principles of laparoscopic surgery*. New York: Springer-Verlag, 1995:646.

Adamyan LV, Maurvatov KD, Sorour YA, et al. Medicogenetic features and surgical treatment of patients with congenital malformations of the uterus and vagina. *Int J Fertil* 1996;41:293.

Alessandrescu D, Peltecu GC, Buhimschi CS, et al. Neocolpopoiesis with split-thickness skin graft as a surgical treatment of vaginal agenesis: retrospective review of 201 cases. *Am J Obstet Gynecol* 1996;175:131.

Allen LM, Lucco KL, Brown CM, et al. Psychosexual and functional outcomes after creation of a neovagina with laparoscopic Davydov in patients with vaginal agenesis. *Fertil Steril* 2010;94:2272.

American Congress of Obstetricians and Gynecologists. Müllerian agenesis: diagnosis, management, and treatment. Committee Opinion No. 562. *Obstet Gynecol* 2013;121:1134.

American Fertility Society. The American Fertility Society classifications of adnexal adhesions, distal tubal occlusion, tubal occlusion secondary to tubal ligation, tubal pregnancies, müllerian anomalies and intrauterine adhesions. *Fertil Steril* 1988;49:944.

Andrews MC, Jones HW. Impaired reproductive performance of the unicornuate uterus: intrauterine growth retardation, infertility, and recurrent abortion in five cases. *Am J Obstet Gynecol* 1982;144:173.

Bach F, Glanville JM, Balen AH. An observational study of women with mullerian agenesis and their need for vaginal dilator therapy. *Fertil Steril* 2011;96:483.

Baldwin A. Formation of an artificial vagina by intestinal transplantation. *Am J Obstet Gynecol* 1907;56:636.

Baldwin JF. The formation of an artificial vagina by intestinal transplantation. *Ann Surg* 1984;40:398.

Barton SE, Politch JA, Benson CB, et al. Transabdominal follicular aspiration for oocyte retrieval in patients with ovaries inaccessible by transvaginal ultrasound. *Fertil Steril* 2011;95:1773.

Beski S, Gorgy A, Venkat G, et al. Gestational surrogacy: a feasible option for patients with Rokitansky syndrome. *Hum Reprod* 2000;15:2326.

Blakeley CR, Mills WG. The obstetric and gynaecological complications of bladder exstrophy and epispadias. *Br J Obstet Gynaecol* 1981;88:167.

Bianchi S, Frontino G, Ciappina N, et al. Creation of a neovagina in Rokitansky syndrome: comparison between two laparoscopic techniques. *Fertil Steril* 2011;95:1098.

Borruto F. Mayer-Rokitansky-Küster syndrome: Vecchietti's personal series. *Clin Exp Obstet Gynecol* 1992;19:273.

Brenner P, Sedlis A, Cooperman H. Complete imperforate transverse vaginal septum. *Obstet Gynecol* 1965;25:135.

Broadbent TR, Woolf RM. Congenital absence of the vagina: reconstruction without operation. *Br J Plast Surg* 1977;30:118.

Brucker SY, Gegusch M, Zubke W, et al. Neovagina creation in vaginal agenesis: development of a new laparoscopic Vecchietti-based procedure and optimized instruments in a prospective comparative interventional study in 101 patients. *Fertil Steril* 2008;90:1940.

Bugamann P, Amaudruz M, Hanquinet S, et al. Uterocervicoplasty with a bladder mucosa layer for treatment of complete cervical agenesis. *Fertil Steril* 2002;77:831.

Busacca M, Perino A, Venezia R. Laparoscopic-ultrasonographic combined technique for the creation of a neovagina in Mayer-Rokitansky-Küster-Hauser syndrome. *Fertil Steril* 1996;66:1039.

Buttram VC Jr. Müllerian anomalies and their management. *Fertil Steril* 1983;40:159.

Buttram VC Jr, Gibbons WE. Müllerian anomalies: a proposed classification (an analysis of 144 cases). *Fertil Steril* 1979;32:40.

Calcagno M, Pastore M, Bellati F, et al. Early prolapse of a neovagina created with self-dilatation and treated with sacrospinous ligament suspension in a patient with Mayer-Rokitansky-Kuster-Hauser syndrome: a case report. *Fertil Steril* 2010;93:267.

Callens N, De Cuypere G, Wolffenbuttel KP, et al. Long-term psychosexual and anatomical outcome after vaginal dilation or vaginoplasty: a comparative study. *J Sex Med* 2012;9:1842.

Capraro VJ, Chuang JT, Randall CL. Improved fetal salvage after metroplasty. *Obstet Gynecol* 1968;29:97.

Carrard C, Chevret-Measson M, Lunel A, et al. Sexuality after sigmoid vaginoplasty in patients with Mayer-Rokitansky-Kuster-Hauser syndrome. *Fertil Steril* 2012;97:691.

Carvalho R, Dilworth P, Docimo S, et al. Crohn disease of the neovagina and augmented bladder in a child born with cloacal exstrophy. *J Pediatr Gastroenterol Nutr* 2009;48:106.

Chakravarty BN. Congenital absence of the vagina and uterus—simultaneous vaginoplasty and hysteroplasty. *J Obstet Gynecol India* 1977;27:627.

Chakravarty BN, Gun KM, Sarkar K. Congenital absence of vagina: anatomico-physiological consideration. *J Obstet Gynecol India* 1977;27:621.

Chen YT, Cheng T, Lin H, et al. Spatial W-plasty full thickness skin graft for neovaginal reconstruction. *Plast Reconstr Surg* 1994;94:727.

Chervenak FA, Neuwirth RS. Hysteroscopic resection of the uterine septum. *Am J Obstet Gynecol* 1981;141:351.

Communal PH, Chevret-Measson M, Golfier F, et al. Sexuality after sigmoid colpopoiesis in patients with Mayer-Rokitansky-Kuster-Hauser syndrome. *Fertil Steril* 2003;80:600.

Cooper AR, Merritt DF. Novel use of a tracheobronchial stent in a patient with uterine didelphys and obstructed hemivagina. *Fertil Steril* 2010;93:900.

Counseller VS. Congenital absence of the vagina. *JAMA* 1948;136:861.

Counseller VS, Davis CE. Atresia of the vagina. *Obstet Gynecol* 1968;32:528.

Counseller VS, Flor FS. Congenital absence of the vagina. *Surg Clin North Am* 1957;37:1107.

Creighton SM, Davies MC, Cutner A. Laparoscopic management of cervical agenesis. *Fertil Steril* 2006;85:1510.

Cukier J, Batzofin JH, Conners JS, et al. Genital tract reconstruction in a patient with congenital absence of a vagina and hypoplasia of the cervix. *Obstet Gynecol* 1986;68:325.

Dabirashrafi H, Bahadori M, Mohammad K, et al. Septate uterus: new idea on the histologic features of the septum in the abnormal uterus. *Am J Obstet Gynecol* 1995;172:105.

Daly DC, Tohan N, Walters C, et al. Hysteroscopic resection of the uterine septum in the presence of a septate cervix. *Fertil Steril* 1983;39:560.

Daly DC, Walters CA, Soto-Albors CE, et al. Hysteroscopic metroplasty: surgical technique and obstetrical outcome. *Fertil Steril* 1983;39:623.

Daraï E, Ballester M, Bazot M, et al. Laparoscopic-assisted uterovaginal anastomosis for uterine cervix atresia with partial vaginal aplasia. *J Minim Invasive Gynecol* 2009;16:92.

David A, Carvil D, Bar-David E, et al. Congenital absence of the vagina: clinical and psychological aspects. *Obstet Gynecol* 1975;46:407.

Davydov SN. Colpopoiesis from the peritoneum of the uterorectal space. In: *Proceedings of the Ninth World Congress of Obstetrics and Gynecology, Tokyo, 1979*. Amsterdam, The Netherlands: Excerpta Medica, 1980:793.

DeCherney A, Polan ML. Hysteroscopic management of intra-uterine lesions and intractable uterine bleeding. *Obstet Gynecol* 1983;61:392.

DeCherney AH, Russell JB, Graebe RA, et al. Resectoscopic management of müllerian fusion defects. *Fertil Steril* 1986;45:726.

Deffarges JV, Haddad B, Musset R, et al. Utero-vaginal anastomosis in women with uterine cervix atresia: long term follow-up and reproductive performance. A study of 18 cases. *Hum Reprod* 2001;16:1722.

Dietrich JE, Young AE, Young RL. Resection of a non-communicating uterine horn with the use of the harmonic scalpel. *J Pediatr Adolesc Gynecol* 2004;17:407.

Dillon WP, Mudaliar NA, Wingate NB. Congenital atresia of the cervix. *Obstet Gynecol* 1979;54:126.

Djordjevic ML, Stanojevic DS, Bizic MR. Rectosigmoid vaginoplasty: clinical experience and outcomes in 86 cases. *J Sex Med* 2011;8:3487.

Dornelas J, Jarmy-Di Bella ZI, Heinke T, et al. Vaginoplasty with oxidized cellulose: anatomical, functional and histological evaluation. *Eur J Obstet Gynecol Reprod Biol* 2012;163:204.

Dunn R, Hantes J. Double cervix and vagina with a normal uterus and blind cervical pouch: a rare mullerian anomaly. *Fertil Steril* 2004;82:458.

Edmonds DK, Rose GL, Lipton MG, et al. Mayer-Rokitansky-Kuster-Hauser syndrome: a review of 245 consecutive cases managed by a multidisciplinary approach with vaginal dilators. *Fertil Steril* 2012;97:686.

Ekici AB, Strissel PL, Oppelt PG, et al. HOXA10 and HOXA13 sequence variations in human female genital malformations including congenital absence of the uterus and vagina. *Gene* 2013;518:267.

El Saman AM. Combined retropubic balloon vaginoplasty and laparoscopic canalization: a novel blend of techniques provides a minimally invasive treatment for cervicovaginal aplasia. *Am J Obstet Gynecol* 2009;201:333.

El Saman AM. Endoscopically monitored canalization for treatment of congenital cervical atresia: the least invasive approach. *Fertil Steril* 2010;94:313.

Engmann L, Schmidt D, Nulsen J, et al. An usual anatomic variation of a unicornuate uterus with normal external uterine morphology. *Fertil Steril* 2004;82:950.

Eustace DL. Congenital absence of fallopian tube and ovary. *Eur J Obstet Gynecol Reprod Biol* 1992;46:157.

Evans TN. The artificial vagina. *Am J Obstet Gynecol* 1967;99:944.

Evans TN, Poland ML, Boving RL. Vaginal malformations. *Am J Obstet Gynecol* 1981;141:910.

Farber M, Marchant DJ. Reconstructive surgery for congenital atresia of the uterine cervix. *Fertil Steril* 1976;27:1277.

Farber M, Mitchell GW. Bicornuate uterus and partial atresia of the fallopian tube. *Am J Obstet Gynecol* 1979;134:881.

Farber M, Mitchell GW. Surgery for congenital anomalies of müllerian ducts. *Contemp Obstet Gynecol* 1977;9:63.

Farber M, Mitchell GW. Surgery for congenital absence of the vagina. *Obstet Gynecol* 1978;51:364.

Fayez JA. Comparison between abdominal and hysteroscopic metroplasty. *Obstet Gynecol* 1986;68:399.

Fedele L, Bianchi S, Frontino G, et al. Laparoscopically assisted uterovestibular anastomosis in patients with uterine cervix atresia and vaginal aplasia. *Fertil Steril* 2008;89:212.

Fedele L, Bianchi S, Frontino G, et al. The laparoscopic Vecchietti's modified technique in Rokitansky syndrome: anatomic, functional, and sexual long-term results. *Am J Obstet Gynecol* 2008;198:377.

Fedele L, Bianchi S, Zanconato G, et al. Laparoscopic creation of a neovagina in patients with Rokitansky syndrome: analysis of 52 cases. *Fertil Steril* 2000;74:384.

Fedele L, Bianchi S, Zanconato G, et al. Laparoscopic removal of the cavitated noncommunicating rudimentary uterine horn: surgical aspects in 10 cases. *Fertil Steril* 2005;83:432.

Fedele L, Borruto F, Bianchi S, et al. A new laparoscopic procedure for creation of a neovagina in Mayer-Rokitansky-Küster-Hauser syndrome. *Fertil Steril* 1996;66:854.

Fedele L, Doeta M, Vercellini P, et al. Ultrasound in the diagnosis of subclasses of unicornuate uterus. *Obstet Gynecol* 1988;71:274.

Feroze RM, Dewhurst CJ, Welply G. Vaginoplasty at the Chelsea hospital for women: a comparison of two techniques. *Br J Obstet Gynaecol* 1975;82:536.

Fore SR, Hammond CB, Parker RT, et al. Urologic and genital anomalies in patients with congenital absence of the vagina. *Obstet Gynecol* 1975;46:410.

Frank RT. The formation of an artificial vagina without operation. *Am J Obstet Gynecol* 1938;35:1053.

Frank RT. The formation of an artificial vagina without operation. *N Y State J Med* 1940;40:1669.

Frank RT, Geist SH. The formation of an artificial vagina by a new plastic technic. *Am J Obstet Gynecol* 1927;14:712.

Gabarain G, Garcia-Naveiro R, Ponsky TA, et al. Ulcerative colitis of the neovagina as a postsurgical complication of persistent cloaca. *J Pediatr Surg* 2012;47:e19.

Gallup DG, Castle CA, Stock RJ. Recurrent carcinoma in situ of the vagina following split thickness skin graft vaginoplasty. *Gynecol Oncol* 1987;26:98.

Garcia J, Jones HW. The split thickness graft technic for vaginal agenesis. *Obstet Gynecol* 1977;49:328.

Garcia RF. Z-plasty for correction of congenital transverse vaginal septum. *Am J Obstet Gynecol* 1967;99:1164.

Gargollo PC, Cannon GM Jr, Diamond DA, et al. Should progressive perineal dilation be considered first line therapy for vaginal agenesis? *J Urol* 2009;182:1882.

Gastol P, Baka-Jakubiak L, Skobejko-Wlodarska L, et al. Complete duplication of the bladder, urethra, vagina, and uterus in girls. *Urology* 2000;55:578.

Gauwerky JFH, Wallwiener D, Bastert G. An endoscopically assisted technique for reconstruction of a neovagina. *Arch Gynecol Obstet* 1992;252:59.

Geary WL, Weed JC. Congenital atresia of the uterine cervix. *Obstet Gynecol* 1973;42:213.

Genest D, Farber M, Mitchell GW, et al. Partial vaginal agenesis with a urinary-vaginal fistula. *Obstet Gynecol* 1981;58:130.

Giannesi A, Marchiole P, Benchaib M, et al. Sexuality after laparoscopic Davydov in patients affected by congenital vaginal agenesis associated with uterine agenesis or hypoplasia. *Hum Reprod* 2005;20:2954.

Goh DW, Davey RB, Dewan PA. Bladder, urethral, and vaginal duplication. *J Pediatr Surg* 1995;30:125.

Goodman FR, Bacchelli C, Brady AF, et al. Novel HOXA13 mutations and the phenotypic spectrum of hand-foot-genital syndrome. *Am J Hum Genet* 2000;67:197.

Goodman FR, Scambler PJ. Human HOX gene mutations. *Clin Genet* 2001;59:1.

Graves WP. Method of constructing an artificial vagina. *Surg Clin North Am* 1921;1:611.

Griffin JE, Edwards C, Madden JD, et al. Congenital absence of the vagina. *Ann Intern Med* 1976;85:224.

Grynberg M, Gervaise A, Faivre E, et al. Treatment of twenty-two patients with complete uterine and vaginal septum. *J Minim Invasive Gynecol* 2012;19:34.

Haddad B, Barranger E, Paniel BJ. Blind hemivagina: long-term follow-up and reproductive performance in 42 cases. *Hum Reprod* 1999;14:1962.

Haddad B, Louis-Sylvestre C, Poitout P, et al. Longitudinal vaginal septum: a retrospective study of 202 cases. *Eur J Obstet Gynecol Reprod Biol* 1997;74:197.

Haney AF, Hammond CB, Soules MR, et al. Diethylstilbestrol-induced upper genital tract abnormalities. *Fertil Steril* 1979;29:142.

Hauser GA, Keller M, Koller T. Das Rokitansky-Küster Syndrom. Uterus bipartitus solidus rudimentarius cum vagina solida. *Gynecologia* 1961;151:111.

Hauser GA, Schreiner WE. Das Mayer-Rokitansky-Küster Syndrom. *Schweiz Med Wochenschr* 1961;91:381.

Heinonen PK. Longitudinal vaginal septum. *Eur J Obstet Gynecol Reprod Biol* 1982;13:253.

Heinonen PK, Pystynen PP. Primary infertility and uterine anomalies. *Fertil Steril* 1983;40:291.

Heinonen PK, Saarikoski S, Pystynen P. Reproductive performance of women with uterine anomalies. *Acta Obstet Gynecol Scand* 1982;61:157.

Hendren WH, Donahoe PK. Correction of congenital abnormalities of the vagina and perineum. *J Pediatr Surg* 1980;15:751.

Hensle TW, Shabsigh A, Shabsigh R, et al. Sexual function following bowel vaginoplasty. *J Urol* 2006;175:2283.

Hickok LR. Hysteroscopic treatment of the uterine septum: a clinician's experience. *Am J Obstet Gynecol* 2000;182:1414.

Höckel M, Menke H, Germann G. Vaginolasty with split skin grafts from the scalp: optimization of the surgical treatment for vaginal agenesis. *Am J Obstet Gynecol* 2003;188:1100.

Hojsgaard A, Villadsen I. McIndoe procedure for congenital vaginal agenesis: complications and results. *Br J Plast Surg* 1995;48:97.

Holden R, Hart P. First-trimester rudimentary horn pregnancy: prerupture ultrasound diagnosis. *Obstet Gynecol* 1983;61(suppl):56.

Homer HA, Li T, Cooke ID. The septate uterus: a review of management and reproductive outcome. *Fertil Steril* 2000;73:1.

Hucke J, Pelzer V, Bruyne FD, et al. Laparoscopic modification of the Vecchietti-operation for creation of a neovagina. *J Pelvic Surg* 1995;1:191.

Hundley AF, Fielding JR, Hoyte L. Double cervix and vagina with septate uterus: an uncommon müllerian malformation. *Obstet Gynecol* 2001;98:982.

Hurst BS, Rock JA. Preoperative dilatation to facilitate repair of high transverse vaginal septum. *Fertil Steril* 1992;57:1351.

Ingram JM. The bicycle seat stool in the treatment of vaginal agenesis and stenosis: a preliminary report. *Am J Obstet Gynecol* 1981;140:867.

Israel R, March CM. Hysteroscopic incision of the septate uterus. *Am J Obstet Gynecol* 1984;149:66.

Jabs EW, Leonard CO, Phillips JA. New features of the McKusick-Kaufman syndrome. *Birth Defects Orig Artic Ser* 1982;18:161.

Jacob JH, Griffin WT. Surgical reconstruction of congenital atresia of the cervix. *Am J Obstet Gynecol* 1961;82:923.

Jacobsen LJ, DeCherney A. Shall we operate on Müllerian defects? Results of conventional and hysteroscopic surgery. *Fertil Steril* 2000;73:1376.

Jeffcoate TNA. Advancement of the upper vagina in the treatment of haematocolpos and haematometra caused by vaginal aplasia: pregnancy following the construction of an artificial vagina. *J Obstet Gynaecol Br Common* 1969;76:961.

Jewelewicz R, Husami N, Wallach EE. When uterine factors cause infertility. *Contemp Obstet Gynecol* 1980;16:95.

Jones HW. An anomaly of the external genitalia in female patients with exstrophy of the bladder. *Am J Obstet Gynecol* 1973;117:748.

Jones HW. Reproductive impairment and the malformed uterus. *Fertil Steril* 1981;36:137.

Jones HW, Delfs E, Jones GE. Reproductive difficulties in double uterus: the place of plastic reconstruction. *Am J Obstet Gynecol* 1956;72:865.

Jones HW, Jones GE. Double uterus as an etiological factor in repeated abortion: indications for surgical repair. *Am J Obstet Gynecol* 1953;65:325.

Jones HW, Mermut S. Familial occurrence of congenital absence of the vagina. *Am J Obstet Gynecol* 1972;114:1100.

Jones HW, Rock JA. *Reparative and constructive surgery of the female generative tract*. Baltimore, MD: Williams & Wilkins, 1983.

Jones HW, Wheeless CR. Salvage of the reproductive potential of women with anomalous development of the müllerian ducts: 1868–1968–2068. *Am J Obstet Gynecol* 1969;104:348.

Jones TB, Fleischer AC, Daniell JF, et al. Sonographic characteristics of congenital uterine abnormalities and associated pregnancy. *J Clin Ultrasound* 1980;8:435.

Jones WS. Obstetric significance of female genital anomalies. *Obstet Gynecol* 1957;10:113.

Karjalainen O, Myllynenl O, Kajanoja P, et al. Management of vaginal agenesis. *Ann Chir Gynaecol* 1980;69:37.

Kaufman RH, Binder GL, Gray PM, et al. Upper genital tract changes associated with exposure in utero to diethylstilbestrol. *Am J Obstet Gynecol* 1977;128:51.

Kimberley N, Hutson JM, Southwell BR, et al. Well-being and sexual function outcomes in women with vaginal agenesis. *Fertil Steril* 2011;95:238.

Knab DR. *Müllerian agenesis: a review*. Bethesda, MD: Department of Gynecology/Obstetrics, Uniformed Services University School of Medicine and Naval Hospital, 1983.

Kokcu A, Tosun M, Alper T, et al. Primary carcinoma of the neovagina: a case report. *Eur J Gynaecol Oncol* 2011;32:588.

Kondo W, Ribeiro R, Tsumanuma FK, et al. Laparoscopic promontofixation for the treatment of recurrent sigmoid neovaginal prolapse: case report and systematic review of the literature. *J Minim Invasive Gynecol* 2012;19:176.

Kriplani A, Kachhawa G, Awasthi D, et al. Laparoscopic-assisted uterovaginal anastomosis in congenital atresia of uterine cervix: follow-up study. *J Minim Invasive Gynecol* 2012;19:477.

Kuster H. Uterus bipartitus solidus rudimentarius cum vagina solida. *Z Geb Gyn* 1910;67:692.

Kusuda M. Infertility and metroplasty. *Acta Obstet Gynecol Scand* 1982;61:407.

Laffarque F, Giacalone PL, Boulot P, et al. A laparoscopic procedure for the treatment of vaginal aplasia. *Br J Obstet Gynaecol* 1995;102:565.

Lawrence A. Vaginal neoplasia in a male-to-female transsexual: case report, review of the literature, and recommendations for cytological screening. *Int J Transgenderism* 2001:1721.

Lee CL, Wang CJ, Liu YH, et al. Laparoscopically assisted full thickness skin graft for reconstruction in congenital agenesis of vagina and uterine cervix. *Hum Reprod* 1999;14:928.

Lees DH, Singer A. Vaginal surgery for congenital abnormalities and acquired constructions. *Clin Obstet Gynecol* 1982;25:883.

Letterie GS. Combined congenital absence of the vagina and cervix. *Gynecol Obstet Invest* 1998;46:65.

Liao LM, Conway GS, Ismail-Pratt I, et al. Emotional and sexual wellness and quality of life in women with Rokitansky syndrome. *Am J Obstet Gynecol* 2011;205:117.

Lin WC, Chang CY, Shen YY, et al. Use of autologous buccal mucosa for vaginoplSasty: a study of eight cases. *Hum Reprod* 2003;18:604.

Litta P, Pozzan C, Merlin F, et al. Hysteroscopic metroplasty under laparoscopic guidance in infertile women with septate uteri. *J Reprod Med* 2004;49:274.

Liu X, Liu M, Hua K, et al. Sexuality after laparoscopic peritoneal vaginoplasty in women with Mayer-Rokitansky-Kuster-Hauser syndrome. *J Minim Invasive Gynecol* 2009;16:720.

Lodi A. Contributo clinico statistico sulle malformazion della vagina osservate nella clinica Obstetrica e Ginecologica di Milano dal 1906 al 1950. *Ann Ostet Ginecol Med Perinat* 1951;73:1246.

Lolis DE, Paschopoulos M, Makrydimas G, et al. Reproductive outcome after Strassman metroplasty in women with a bicornuate uterus. *J Reprod Med* 2005;50:297.

Ludmir J, Samuels P, Brooks S, et al. Pregnancy outcome of patients with uncorrected uterine anomalies managed in a high risk obstetric setting. *Obstet Gynecol* 1990;75:907.

Maciulla GJ, Heine MW, Christian CD. Functional endometrial tissue with vaginal agenesis. *J Reprod Med* 1978;21:373.

Magalhaes ML, Campos LA, Souza LC, et al. A case of association of duplication of the urogenital and intestinal tracts. *J Pediatr Adolesc Gynecol* 1999;12:165.

Magrina JF, Masterson BJ. Vaginal reconstruction in gynecological oncology: a review of techniques. *Obstet Gynecol Surv* 1981;36:1.

Mahgoub SE. Unification of a septate uterus: Mahgoub's operation. *Int J Gynecol Obstet* 1978;15:400.

Makinoda S, Nishiya M, Sogame M, et al. Non-grafting method of vaginal construction for patients of vaginal agenesis without functioning uterus (Mayer-Rokitansky-Küster Syndrome). *Int Surg* 1996;81:385.

Mandell J, Stevens PS, Lucey DT. Diagnosis and management of hydrometrocolpos in infancy. *J Urol* 1978;120:262.

Markham SM, Parmley TH, Murphy AA, et al. Cervical agenesis combined with vaginal agenesis diagnosed by magnetic resonance imaging. *Fertil Steril* 1987;48:143.

Matsui H, Seki K, Sekiya S. Prolapse of the neovagina in Mayer-Rokitansky-Küster-Hauser syndrome. *J Reprod Med* 1999;44:548.

McCraw JB, Massey FM, Shanklin KD, et al. Vaginal reconstruction with gracilis myocutaneous flaps. *Plast Reconstr Surg* 1976;58:176.

McDonough PG, Tho PT. Use of pelvic pneumoperitoneum: a critical assessment of 12 years experience. *South Med J* 1974;67:517.

McIndoe AH. The treatment of congenital absence and obliterative conditions of the vagina. *Br J Plast Surg* 1950;2:254.

McIndoe AH, Banister JB. An operation for the cure of congenital absence of the vagina. *J Obstet Gynaecol Br Emp* 1938;45:490.

McKusick VA. Transverse vaginal septum (hydrometrocolpos). *Birth Defects Orig Artic Ser* 1971;7:326.

McKusick VA, Bauer RL, Koop CE, et al. Hydrometrocolpos as a simply inherited malformation. *JAMA* 1964;189:119.

McKusick VA, Weilbaccher RG, Gragg GW. Recessive inheritance of a congenital malformation syndrome. *JAMA* 1968;204:111.

McShane PM, Reilly RJ, Schiff I. Pregnancy outcomes following Tompkins metroplasty. *Fertil Steril* 1983;40:190.

Miller PB, Forstein DA. Creation of a neovagina by the Vecchietti procedure in a patient with corrected high imperforate anus. *JSLS* 2009;13:221–223.

Mizuno K, Koike K, Ando K, et al. Significance of Jones-Jones operation on double uterus: vascularity and dating of endometrium in uterine septum. *Jpn J Fertil Steril* 1978;23:9.

Motoyama S, Laoag-Fernandez JB, Mochizuki S, et al. Vaginoplasty with Interceed absorbable adhesion barrier for complete squamous epithelialization in vaginal agenesis. *Am J Obstet Gynecol* 2003;188:1260.

Moutos DM, Damewood MD, Schlaff WD, et al. A comparison of the reproductive outcome between women with a unicornuate uterus and women with a didelphic uterus. *Fertil Steril* 1992;58:88.

Murphy AA, Krall A, Rock JA. Bilateral functioning uterine anlagen with the Rokitansky-Mayer-Küster-Hauser syndrome. *Int J Fertil* 1987;32:296.

Musich JR, Behrman SJ. Obstetric outcome before and after metroplasty in women with uterine anomalies. *Obstet Gynecol* 1978;52:63.

Musset R. Traitement chirurgical des cloisans transversales due vagin d'origine congenitale par la plastie en "Z" a l'Hopital Lariboisiere. *Gynecol Obstet* 1956;55:382.

Nagel TC, Malo JW. Hysteroscopic metroplasty in diethylstilbestrol-exposed uterus and similar fusion anomalies. *Fertil Steril* 1993; 59:502.

Nguyen DH, Lee CL, Wu KY, et al. A novel approach to cervical reconstruction using vaginal mucosa-lined polytetrafluoroethylene graft in congenital agenesis of the cervix. *Fertil Steril* 2011;95:2433.

Niver DH, Barrette G, Jewelewicz R. Congenital atresia of the uterine cervix and vagina: three cases. *Fertil Steril* 1980;33:25.

Nunley WC, Kitchin JD. Congenital atresia of the uterine cervix with pelvic endometriosis. *Arch Surg* 1980;115:757.

O'Leary JL, O'Leary JA. Rudimentary horn pregnancy. *Obstet Gynecol* 1963;22:371.

Omurtag K, Session D, Brahma P, et al. Horizontal uterine torsion in the setting of complete cervical and partial vaginal agenesis: a case report. *Fertil Steril* 2009;91:1957.

Ota H, Tanaka J, Murakami M, et al. Laparoscopy-assisted Ruge procedure for the creation of a neovagina in a patient with Mayer-Rokitansky-Küster-Hauser syndrome. *Fertil Steril* 2000;73:641.

Ozek C, Gurler T, Alper M, et al. Modified McIndoe procedure for vaginal agenesis. *Ann Plast Surg* 1999;43:393.

Pabuccu R, Gomel V. Reproductive outcome after hysteroscopic metroplasty in women with septate uterus and otherwise unexplained infertility. *Fertil Steril* 2004;28:1675.

Panici PB, Ruscito I, Gasparri ML, et al. Vaginal reconstruction with the Abbe-McIndoe technique: from dermal grafts to autologous in vitro cultured vaginal tissue transplant. *Semin Reprod Med* 2011;29:45.

Parsanezhad ME, Alborzi S, Zarei A, et al. Hysteroscopic metroplasty of the complete uterine septum, duplicate cervix, and vaginal septum. *Fertil Steril* 2006;85:1473.

Parsons JK, Gearhart SL, Gearhart JP. Vaginal reconstruction utilizing sigmoid colon: complications and long term results. *J Pediatr Surg* 2002;37:629.

Patton PE, Novy MJ, Lee DM, et al. The diagnosis and reproductive outcome after surgical treatment of the complete septate uterus, duplicated cervix, and vaginal septum. *Am J Obstet Gynecol* 2004;190:1669.

Patil V, Hixon FP. The role of tissue expanders in vaginoplasty for congenital malformations of the vagina. *Br J Urol* 1992;70:554.

Petrozza JC, Gray MR, Davis AJ, et al. Congenital absence of the uterus and vagina is not commonly transmitted as a dominant genetic trait: outcomes of surrogate pregnancies. *Fertil Steril* 1997; 67:387.

Phupong V, Pruksananonda K, Taneepanichskul S, et al. Double uterus with unilaterally obstructed hemivagina and ipsilateral renal agenesis: a variety presentation and a ten-year review of the literature. *J Med Assoc Thai* 2000;83:569.

Pinsky L. A community of human malformation syndromes involving the müllerian ducts, distal extremities, urinary tract, and ears. *Teratology* 1974;9:65.

Pittock ST, Babovic-Vuksanovic D, Lteif A. Mayer-Rokitansky-Kuster-Hauser anomaly and its associated malformations. *Am J Med Genet* 2005;135A:314.

Plevraki E, Kita M, Goulis DG, et al. Bilateral ovarian agenesis and the presence of the testis specific protein 1-Y-linked gene: two new features of Mayer-Rokitansky-Küster-Hauser syndrome. *Fertil Steril* 2004;81:689.

Popaw DD. Utilization of the rectum in construction of a functional vagina. *Russk Virach St Peter* 1910;43:1512.

Pratt JH. Vaginal atresia corrected by use of small and large bowel. *Clin Obstet Gynecol* 1972;15:639.

Proctor JA, Haney AF. Recurrent first trimester pregnancy loss is associated with uterine septum but not with bicornuate uterus. *Fertil Steril* 2003;80:1212.

Prorocic M, Vasiljevic M, Tasic L, et al. Successful pregnancy after uterovaginal anastomosis in patients with congenital atresia of cervix uteri. *Clin Exp Obstet Gynecol* 2012;39:544.

Raudrant D, Chalouhi G, Dubuisson J, et al. Laparoscopic uterovaginal anastomosis in Mayer-Rokitansky-Küster-Hauser syndrome with functioning horn. *Fertil Steril* 2008;90:2416.

Ravasia DJ, Brain PH, Pollard JK. Incidence of uterine rupture among women with mullerian duct anomalies who attempt vaginal birth after cesarean delivery. *Am J Obstet Gynecol* 1999;181:877.

Reichman D, Laufer MR, Robinson BK. Pregnancy outcomes in unicornuate uteri: a review. *Fertil Steril* 2009;91:1886.

Reichman DE, Laufer MR. Mayer-Rokitansky-Kuster-Hauser syndrome: fertility counseling and treatment. *Fertil Steril* 2010;94:1941.

Roberts CP, Haber MJ, Rock JA. Vaginal creation for müllerian agenesis. *Am J Obstet Gynecol* 2001;185:1349.

Rock JA, Baramki TA, Parmley TH, et al. A unilateral functioning uterine anlage with müllerian duct agenesis. *Int J Gynecol Obstet* 1980;18:99.

Rock JA, Carpenter SE, Wheeless CR, et al. The clinical management of maldevelopment of the uterine cervix. *J Pelvic Surg* 1995;1:129.

Rock JA, Jones HW. The clinical management of the double uterus. *Fertil Steril* 1977;28:798.

Rock JA, Jones HW. The double uterus associated with an obstructed hemivagina and ipsilateral renal agenesis. *Am J Obstet Gynecol* 1980;138:339.

Rock JA, Jones HW Jr. Vaginal forms for dilatation and/or to maintain vaginal patency. *Fertil Steril* 1984;42:187.

Rock JA, Parmley T, Murphy AA, et al. Malposition of the ovary associated with uterine anomalies. *Fertil Steril* 1986;45:561.

Rock JA, Reeves LA, Retto H, et al. Success following vaginal creation for müllerian agenesis. *Fertil Steril* 1983;39:809.

Rock JA, Roberts CP, Hesla JS. Hysteroscopic metroplasty of the class Va uterus with preservation of the cervical septum. *Fertil Steril* 1999;72:942.

Rock JA, Roberts CP, Jones HW, Jr. Congenital anomalies of the uterine cervix: lessons from 30 cases managed clinically by a common protocol. *Fertil Steril* 2010;94:1858.

Rock JA, Schlaff WD. The obstetrical consequences of uterovaginal anomalies. *Fertil Steril* 1985;43:681.

Rock JA, Schlaff WD, Zacur HA, et al. The clinical management of congenital absence of the uterine cervix. *Int J Gynecol Obstet* 1984;22:229.

Rock JA, Zacur HA. The clinical management of repeated early pregnancy wastage. *Fertil Steril* 1983;39:123.

Rock JA, Zacur HA, Dlugi AM, et al. Pregnancy success following surgical correction of imperforate hymen and complete transverse vaginal septum. *Obstet Gynecol* 1982;59:448.

Rosen R, Brown C, Heiman J, et al. The Female Sexual Function Index (FSFI): a multidimensional self-report instrument for the assessment of female sexual function. *J Sex Marital Ther* 2000;26:191.

Rotmensch J, Rosensheim N, Dillon M, et al. Carcinoma arising in the neovagina: case report and review of the literature. *Obstet Gynecol* 1983;61:534.

Ruge E. Ersatz der durch die flexur mittels laparotomie. *Dtsch Med Wochenschr* 1914;40:120.

Sanders BH, Machan LS, Gomel V. Complex uterine surgery: a cooperative role for interventional radiology with hysteroscopic surgery. *Fertil Steril* 1998;70:952.

Schätz T, Huber J, Wenzl R. Creation of a neovagina according to Wharton-Sheares-George in patients with Mayer-Rokitansky-Küster-Hauser syndrome. *Fertil Steril* 2005;83:437.

Schubert G. Uber Scheidenbildung bei angeborenem Vaginaldefekt. *Zentralbl Gynaekol* 1911;45:1017.

Semmens JP. Abdominal contour in the third trimester: an aid to diagnosis of uterine anomalies. *Obstet Gynecol* 1965;25:779.

Sheldon CA, Gilbert A, Lewis AG. Vaginal reconstruction: critical technical principles. *J Urol* 1994;152:190.

Shokeir MHK. Aplasia of the müllerian system: evidence for probably sex-limited autosomal dominant inheritance. *Birth Defects Orig Artic Ser* 1978;14:147.

Simpson JL. Genetics of the female reproductive ducts. *Am J Med Genet* 1999;89:224.

Singh KJ, Devi L. Hysteroplasty and vaginoplasty for reconstruction of the uterus. *Int J Gynaecol Obstet* 1980;17:457.

Singh M, Gearheart JP, Rock JA. Double urethra, double bladder, left renal agenesis, persistent hymen, double vagina and uterus didelphys. *J Pediatr Adolesc Gynecol* 1993;6:99.

Soong YK, Chang FH, Lai YM, et al. Results of modified laparoscopically assisted neovaginoplasty in 18 patients with congenital absence of the vagina. *Hum Reprod* 1996;11:200.

Stanton SL. Gynecologic complications of epispadias and bladder exstrophy. *Am J Obstet Gynecol* 1974;119:749.

Steinkampf MP, Manning MT, Dharia S, et al. An accessory uterine cavity as a cause of pelvic pain. *Obstet Gynecol* 2004;103:1058.

Stoot JE, Mastboom JL. Restriction on the indications for metroplasty. *Acta Eur Fertil* 1977;8:79.

Strassmann EO. Operations for double uterus and endometrial atresia. *Clin Obstet Gynecol* 1961;4:240.

Strassmann EO. Plastic unification of double uterus. *Am J Obstet Gynecol* 1952;64:25.

Strassmann P. Die operative vereinigung eines doppelten uterus. *Zentralbl Gynakol* 1907;29:1322.

Strickland JL, Cameron WJ, Krantz KE. Long-term satisfaction of adults undergoing McIndoe vaginoplasty as adolescents. *Adolesc Pediatr Gynecol* 1993;6:135.

Tancer ML, Katz M, Veridiano NP. Vaginal epithelialization with human amnion. *Obstet Gynecol* 1979;54:345.

Templeman CL, Hertweck SP, Levine RL, et al. Use of laparoscopically mobilized peritoneum in the creation of a neovagina. *Fertil Steril* 2000;74:589.

Thompson DP, Lynn HB. Genital anomalies associated with solitary kidney. *Mayo Clin Proc* 1966;41:538.

Thompson JD, Wharton LR, Te Linde RW. Congenital absence of the vagina. *Am J Obstet Gynecol* 1957;74:397.

Timmreck LS, Pan HA, Reindollar RH, et al. WNT7A mutations in patients with müllerian duct abnormalities. *J Pediatr Adolesc Gynecol* 2003;16:217.

Tompkins P. Comments on the bicornuate uterus and twinning. *Surg Clin North Am* 1962;42:1049.

Ulfelder H, Robboy SJ. The embryologic development of the human vagina. *Am J Obstet Gynecol* 1976;126:769.

Valdes C, Malini S, Malinak L. Sonography in the surgical management of vaginal and cervical atresia. *Fertil Steril* 1983;40:263.

Vecchietti G. Neovagina nella sindrome di Rokitansky-Küster-Hauser. *Attual Ostet Ginecol* 1965;11:129.

Vecchietti G. Le neo-vagin dans le syndrome de Rokitansky-Küster-Hauser. *Rev Med Suisse Romane* 1979;99:593.

Vecchietti G. Die neovagina beim Rokitansky-Küster-Hauser-Syndrom. *Gynakologe* 1980;13:112.

Vecchietti G, Ardillo L. *La sindrome di Rokitansky-Küster-Hauser: fisiopatologia e clinica dell aplasia vaginale con corni uterini rudimentali.* Roma: Societa Editrice Universo, 1970.

Veronikus DK, McClure GB, Nichols DH. The Vecchietti operation for constructing a neovagina: indications, instrumentation, and techniques. *Obstet Gynecol* 1997;90:301.

von Rokitansky KE. Ober die sogenannten Verdoppelungen des uterus. *Med JB Obst Staat* 1938;76:39.

Walch K, Kowarik E, Leithner K, et al. Functional and anatomic results after creation of a neovagina according to Wharton-Sheares-George in patients with Mayer-Rokitansky-Kuster-Hauser syndrome-long-term follow-up. *Fertil Steril* 2011;96:492.

Weed JC, McKee DM. Vulvoplasty in cases of exstrophy of the bladder. *Obstet Gynecol* 1974;43:512.

Weijenborg PT, ter Kuile MM. The effect of a group programme on women with the Mayer-Rokitansky-Küster-Hauser-syndrome. *Br J Obstet Gynaecol* 2000;107:365.

Wester T, Tovar JA, Rintala RJ. Vaginal agenesis or distal vaginal atresia associated with anorectal malformations. *J Pediatr Surg* 2012;47:571.

Wharton LR. Congenital malformations associated with developmental defects of the female reproductive organs. *Am J Obstet Gynecol* 1947;53:37.

Wharton LR. Further experiences in construction of the vagina. *Ann Surg* 1940;111:1010.

Wharton LR. A simple method of constructing a vagina. *Ann Surg* 1938;107:842.

Williams EA. Congenital absence of the vagina, a simple operation for its relief. *J Obstet Gynaecol Br Commonw* 1964;71:511.

Williams EA. Uterovaginal agenesis. *Ann R Coll Surg Engl* 1976;58:266.

Williams EA. Vulvo-vaginoplasty. *Proc R Soc Med* 1970;63:40.

Woelfer B, Salim R, Banerjee S. Reproductive outcomes in women with congenital uterine anomalies detected by three-dimensional ultrasound screening. *Obstet Gynecol* 2001;98:1099.

Wu TH, Wu TT, Ng YY, et al. Herlyn-Werner-Wunderlich syndrome consisting of uterine didelphys, obstructed hemivagina and ipsilateral renal agenesis in a newborn. *Pediatr Neonatol* 2012;53:68.

CHAPTER 26
Normal and Abnormal Uterine Bleeding

Diana Broomfield, Alicia Armstrong, David Carnovale, and William J. Butler

DEFINITIONS

Amenorrhea—The absence of menstrual bleeding for more than 6 months.

Breakthrough bleeding—Intermenstrual bleeding that occurs despite the use of exogenous hormones.

Dysmenorrhea—Painful menstruation.

Interval bleeding—Bleeding between menstrual cycles.

Menorrhagia—Prolonged menstrual bleeding that is excessive in amount, duration, or both that occurs at regular intervals.

Metrorrhagia—Bleeding between periods.

Oligomenorrhea—Bleeding that occurs less frequently than every 35 days.

Polymenorrhea—Bleeding that occurs more often than every 21 days.

Postmenopausal bleeding—Uterine bleeding occurring more than 12 months after the last menstrual period of a menopausal woman.

PALM-COEIN—Polyp; adenomyosis; leiomyoma; malignancy and hyperplasia; coagulopathy; ovulatory dysfunction; endometrial; iatrogenic; and not yet classified. The term *dysfunctional uterine bleeding (DUB)* is discouraged since the implementation of this classification system.

INTRODUCTION

Abnormal uterine bleeding (AUB) is an extremely common gynecologic complaint. It is estimated that 30% of women experience menorrhagia annually. This debilitating condition is clinically important; Mahoney and colleagues report it is the indication for two thirds of hysterectomies and nearly 25% of gynecologic operations. Thus, the impact of this condition on the public health and health care costs is significant. Because medical therapies for AUB have significant failure rates or side effects, surgical treatment by hysterectomy remains a major therapeutic option for chronically symptomatic women. This chapter reviews normal menstruation, the pathophysiology underlying AUB, the evaluation of AUB, and current treatment modalities.

Reproductive capability in a young woman begins at the point of menarche, which is the beginning of cyclic uterine bleeding in the anatomically and physiologically normal female. Menarche marks the beginning of an important stage in a young woman's physical reproductive maturation and development. Attitudes toward menstruation, what is considered "normal," and the decision to seek medical evaluation are impacted by a variety of factors. In one cross-sectional US study of nearly 2,000 women, the authors concluded that Western cultures tend to "medicalize" menstruation, as evidenced by the media information that depicts menstruation as something that should be managed and remedied. This investigation also suggested that positive attitudes toward menstruation are more prevalent among women with higher educational levels and higher incomes. Positive attitudes were more common among women who exercised frequently and older women who were approaching menopause. Race and ethnicity also played a role in attitudes toward menstruation with non–European Americans having a more positive attitude toward menstruation. Common wisdom would suggest, and studies support, the assumption that women who do not have an understanding of normal menstrual physiology are more likely to become alarmed about any disruption in what is perceived to be normal menstruation. As health care providers, it is our responsibility to educate our patients about what is normal and what symptoms would require medical evaluation. Current medical therapies are quite effective in the management of most of the disturbances of menstrual function that occur in the absence of infection, gestation, or uterine tumor. The success of these therapies depends on a complete understanding of normal menstrual physiology and of the effects of the various agents available for treatment. In addition, new surgical diagnostic and therapeutic technologies are becoming available to aid in the management of patients who fail to respond to conventional endocrine manipulation by medical therapies.

The normal interval between menstrual cycles is 21 to 35 days, and the normal duration is generally 5 days. Although heavy bleeding has been traditionally described as a blood loss exceeding 80 mL, a more practical approach is to rely upon the patient's perception. The term *menorrhagia* has been used to define heavy bleeding, while *metorrhagia* is used to define bleeding between periods. *Oligomenorrhea* is used to describe bleeding that occurs less frequently than every 35 days, and *polymenorrhea* is used to define bleeding that occurs more often than every 21 days.

In 2011, in an effort to standardize the nomenclature used to describe uterine bleeding abnormalities, a new classification system was introduced by the International Federation of Gynecology and Obstetrics (FIGO). The classification system known by the acronym PALM-*COEIN* (polyp; adenomyosis; leiomyoma; malignancy and hyperplasia; coagulopathy; ovulatory dysfunction; endometrial; iatrogenic; and not yet classified) is also supported by the American Congress of Obstetricians and Gynecologists.

The PALM-COEIN system differs from the previously used nomenclature in that it categorizes uterine bleeding by etiology as well as bleeding pattern. Under the new classification system, terms such as menorrhagia would be replaced by heavy menstrual bleeding. The PALM-COEIN system also uses letter qualifiers to identify the etiology (**Fig. 26.1**). Prior to the implementation of the PALM-COEIN classification system, the term dysfunctional uterine bleeding (DUB) was often used interchangeably with AUB; DUB was used to indicate AUB for which there was no systemic or structural etiology. The use of the term DUB is not part of the PALM-COEIN system, and its use is discouraged by the FIGO Working Group in 2011.

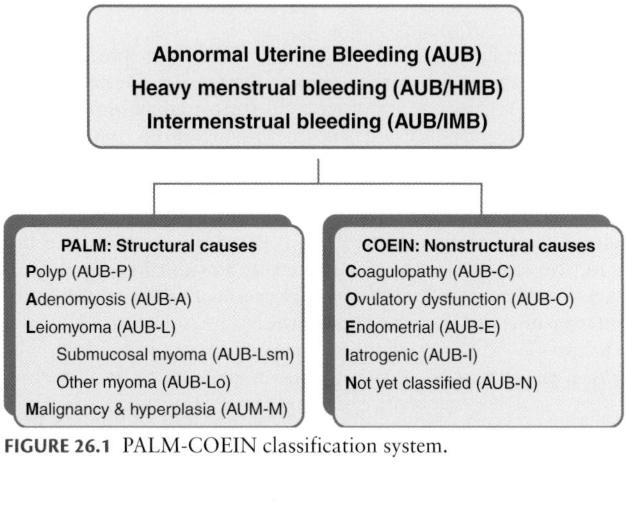

MENSTRUAL PHYSIOLOGY

Menstruation is the physiologic shedding of the endometrium associated with uterine bleeding that occurs at monthly intervals from menarche to menopause. In the years between these two physiologic landmarks, menstruation will occur 400 to 500 times in the average woman. According to the classical theory of the physiology of menstruation, it is the superficial functional layer of the endometrium that is shed during menstruation, and regeneration proceeds from the remaining intact basalis.

Recent work in humans has confirmed the presence of endometrial stem cells, which most likely are located in niches within the basalis layer. Additionally, it appears that these progenitor cells are hormonally independent. The proliferative potential of these cells is maintained in the noncycling state as demonstrated by their ability to regenerate endometrium in postmenopausal women given hormone replacement therapy.

The regenerating properties of the endometrium and its ability to support and nourish a fertilized ovum are an extremely complex system that appears to involve numerous endocrine, paracrine, and autocrine interactions. At the endometrial level, all three inhibin subunits are expressed in the human. It is believed that these dimeric glycoproteins may be involved in endometrial maturation, such as angiogenesis, decidualization, and tissue remodeling. Epidermal growth factors (EGFs) are extremely important in human embryogenesis, development, and proliferation differentiation. Human endometrial cells have been shown to express all four EGF receptors and two ligands amphiregulin and transforming growth factor alpha. Other substances with known angiogenic properties, such as leptin and erythropoietin, have also been shown to be expressed along with their receptors by human endometrium.

This process of monthly shedding and regeneration can occur as often as it does without producing permanent tissue damage possibly because most of the functional endometrium is conserved during menses and because the metamorphosis from proliferative to secretory endometria is controlled not only by processes of cell desquamation and reproliferation but also by dynamic and interactive processes of the endocrinologic and reproductive systems involving many organs. Any interruption of these normal but quite complex cyclic processes can lead to irregularities in endometrial breakdown and to AUB; the categorization of type of AUB is determined by the PALM-COEIN classification system (**Fig. 26.1**).

ENDOCRINOLOGY

The endometrium is an endocrine organ that responds to circulating blood levels of estrogen and progesterone. These two steroids alone are sufficient to induce growth and maturation of an endometrium that can support blastocyst implantation, as has been demonstrated by their sequential administration to patients with ovarian failure to prepare for the transfer of donated embryos. Estradiol (E_2) production by the developing follicle stimulates metabolic activity in the endometrium. E_2 has multiple effects that are mediated through binding to estrogen receptors. There are two estrogen receptors: alpha and beta. The estrogen receptors are members of a hormone receptor family that includes not only the other steroid receptors but

Abnormal Uterine Bleeding (AUB)
Heavy menstrual bleeding (AUB/HMB)
Intermenstrual bleeding (AUB/IMB)

PALM: Structural causes
Polyp (AUB-P)
Adenomyosis (AUB-A)
Leiomyoma (AUB-L)
  Submucosal myoma (AUB-Lsm)
  Other myoma (AUB-Lo)
Malignancy & hyperplasia (AUM-M)

COEIN: Nonstructural causes
Coagulopathy (AUB-C)
Ovulatory dysfunction (AUB-O)
Endometrial (AUB-E)
Iatrogenic (AUB-I)
Not yet classified (AUB-N)

FIGURE 26.1 PALM-COEIN classification system.

also receptors for vitamin D and thyroid hormone. All receptors in this family have three domains. The regulatory domain at the amino acid terminal binds regulatory protein factors. The hormone-binding domain on the carboxy terminal, with its contiguous hinge region, undergoes conformational changes when a steroid hormone binds to it, allowing DNA binding. The DNA-binding domain binds to the hormone-responsive elements in the target gene. The conformation of the DNA-binding domain consists of the highly conserved zinc finger structures that interact with complementary patterns in the DNA.

Steroid hormones have relatively low molecular weights and are rapidly transported into cells by passive diffusion. Binding of a steroid hormone to the intranuclear receptors transforms and activates the hormone receptor complex to allow DNA binding to specific hormone response elements and initiates subsequent transcription. Both estrogen and progesterone receptors bind to their response elements as dimers. After gene activation, the hormone receptor complex undergoes processing with dissociation and loss of activity.

Transcription of target genes with mRNA synthesis leads to translation with synthesis of proteins on ribosomes in the cytoplasm. The biologic effects of E_2 are mediated through this protein synthesis.

Estrogen and Progesterone Receptor Induction

One important function of estrogen is the induction of synthesis of its own and other steroid hormone receptors, called replenishment. Estrogen receptors reach a maximum concentration in the middle-to-late proliferative phase of the menstrual cycle. Progesterone receptors are also induced, and their concentration peaks in the late proliferative phase. Progesterone then blocks the estrogen replenishment mechanism, possibly by accelerating receptor turnover and inhibiting E_2-induced gene transcription. Enough progesterone receptors persist throughout the luteal phase, however, to maintain endometrial responsiveness and induction of deciduation.

Estrogen and Progesterone Target Genes

Target genes of the E_2 receptor complex code for the synthesis of numerous proteins, including structural proteins, enzymes, and growth factors. The relative roles played by the alpha and beta estrogen receptors in the endometrium have yet to be completely elucidated. The net effect of estrogenic stimulation is to induce DNA synthesis and mitotic activity with proliferation of the endometrial glands and stroma. The results are cessation of menstrual flow and an increase in the thickness of the endometrium.

Progesterone also has multiple biologic effects mediated through its receptors. It actively inhibits synthesis of both its own receptors and estrogen receptors, although sufficient progesterone receptors remain throughout the luteal phase of the cycle to mediate maturation and secretory differentiation of the endometrium. The net effect is to antagonize estrogenic metabolic activity with suppression of DNA synthesis in endometrial cells, which results in dynamic inhibition of cell mitosis. Progesterone is also responsible for the active induction of synthesis of various cytoplasmic enzymes, the secretion of proteins such as prolactin-dependent and progesterone-dependent endometrial peptide from decidualized stromal cells, and the stabilization of lysosomes, all of which may play an important role in the onset of menstruation.

Histology and Physiology

The postmenstrual endometrium that remains after collapse and partial shedding during menstruation consists of a thin but stable layer of basalis cells and the dense irregular remnants of the stromal cell–derived stratum spongiosum. The glands are narrow and lined by low cuboidal epithelial cells with few mitoses. The glandular stromal cells are small and spindle shaped with little cytoplasm or mitotic activity. Protein synthesis and secretory activity are minimal. It is on this substrate of basal and stromal cells that estrogen induces a proliferative response.

Early Proliferative Phase

Mitotic activity results in growth and pseudostratification of the glandular epithelial cells. With development and elongation of the glands, the epithelial cells assume a more columnar shape, with secretory granules in the cytoplasm, and glycogen begins to collect in the basal vacuoles. Arteriolar vessels grow up into the endometrium as part of the general proliferative response. The stromal cells also proliferate and expand from a dense compact state to an expanded matrix by transient edema. The combined effects of proliferation and expansion cause the endometrium to grow in this phase to a thickness of 3 to 5 mm.

The increased mitotic activity that results in proliferation is mediated by way of estrogen induction of various peptide growth factors. Epidermal growth factors and insulinlike growth factor I (IGF-I) are two potent mitogens with synthesis that is stimulated by estrogen in endometrial epithelial and stromal cells. Endothelin-1 is a vasoactive peptide with mitogenic activity; its synthesis is induced by both estrogen and growth factors, and its metabolism is enhanced by progesterone. Endothelin-1 may play a role in proliferation and in menstruation. The various peptides that are secreted from stromal and epithelial cells to form the extracellular matrix of the endometrium can be either induced or suppressed by both estrogen and progesterone. Fibronectin, for example, is suppressed by progesterone, whereas several integrin subtypes are stimulated by progesterone. These peptides may have a functional role in proliferation, differentiation, and embryo implantation.

Angiogenesis both allows repair of the endometrium after menstruation and supports cellular proliferation for regrowth during the follicular phase. It is supported and promoted by multiple growth factors. An important role is played by vascular endothelial growth factor (VEGF). Torry and Torry found VEGF mRNA expression is induced by E_2 and increases from the early proliferative phase through the secretory phase. Vascular endothelial growth factor is produced by the glandular epithelial cells, although some stromal expression is evident in the secretory phase. The increased expression throughout the cycle supports a possible role of VEGF in expansion and coiling of the spiral arterials. Kooy et al. detected changes in VEGF in women with AUB, supporting a possible role in the pathogenesis of menorrhagia.

E_2 induces several enzymes (alkaline phosphatase, 5α-reductase, and possibly phospholipase A_2). Phospholipase A_2, which releases arachidonic acid from phospholipid esters, controls the rate-limiting step in prostaglandin synthesis. E_2 also stimulates cyclooxygenase synthesis of prostaglandin $F_2\alpha$ (PGF$_2\alpha$) and prostaglandin E_2 (PGE$_2$), both of which have a role in menstrual function. PGF$_2\alpha$ has vasoconstrictive and muscle contraction effects. PGE$_2$ is generally a vasodilator but can also cause contractions in uterine smooth muscle. Alterations in the relative levels of PGF$_2\alpha$ and PGE$_2$ are known to change menstrual bleeding patterns.

Late Proliferative Phase

Ovulation with corpus luteum formation and significant progesterone secretion leads to secretory transformation in the late proliferative phase endometrium. Progesterone inhibits both estrogen and progesterone receptor synthesis and inhibits DNA synthesis and mitosis. This inhibition process is accompanied by the development of RNA-filled channels between the nucleoli and nuclear membranes that are responsible for the progesterone-induced active synthesis of cytoplasmic enzymes during the secretory phase of the cycle.

The Secretory Phase

The cytoplasmic enzymes 17β- and 20α-hydroxysteroid dehydrogenase (HSD) are induced by progesterone and modulate steroid activity. The enzyme 17β-HSD catalyzes the conversion of E_2 to the relatively weaker estrogen estrone, which, when sulfated by estrogen sulfotransferase, can no longer bind to estrogen receptors. The enzyme 20α-HSD alters progesterone receptor binding and activity. Cytoplasmic lytic enzymes such as acid phosphatase are also induced by progesterone but are kept inactive within Golgi-derived lysosomes, the membranes of which are stabilized by progesterone. Insulin-like growth factor II is synthesized locally by middle-to-late secretory phase endometrium and appears to be involved in the differentiation response of the endometrium to progesterone. Insulin-like growth factor-binding protein I also appears at this time and is regulated by the IGFs and by relaxin. Other autocrine or paracrine agents secreted locally by decidual cells are relaxin, progesterone-dependent endometrial peptide, and prolactin.

Progesterone has also been shown to induce the activity of metalloendopeptidase, which degrades the endothelin-1 peptide. Withdrawal of progesterone can lead to increased endothelin-1 activity with vasospasm and initiation of menstrual bleeding. Several investigators have described increased levels of protease inhibitors, such as α_1-antitrypsin and antithrombin III, in secretory phase uterine fluid, which may also be involved in the mechanism of menstrual bleeding.

The Luteal Phase

Morphologically, secretory transformation of the endometrium results in coiling of the spiral arterioles and endometrial glands. The endometrium reaches its maximum thickness of 5 to 6 mm and maintains this thickness throughout the luteal phase. The subnuclear intracytoplasmic glycogen vacuoles in the basal glandular cells transpose to the apex and are expelled into the glandular lumen. The stromal cells subsequently flatten into a low cuboidal form. Stromal cell differentiation from reticular spindle-shaped cells into plump predecidual cells and phagocytic granulated cells defines two layers in the functional endometrium known as the superficial compactum and the deeper spongiosum. The spongiosum has a loose edematous matrix that is the consequence of increased capillary permeability, mediated possibly by prostaglandins. The predecidual, late secretory phase stromal cells produce several metabolically active substances, as previously described, and are infiltrated by migratory leukocytes. The release of lysosomal enzymes from endometrial cells and possibly also from leukocytes may be involved in the initiation of menstruation.

Menstruation

Menstruation is controlled by many complex, interrelated, and incompletely understood factors. Normal menstruation results from progesterone withdrawal from the estrogen-primed endometrium. Changes that occur in the endometrium during menstruation were described by Markee by observation of endometrial tissue transplanted to the anterior chamber of the eyes of rhesus monkeys. Markee described cyclic changes in endometrial vascularity and the development of coiled vessels supplying the superficial two thirds of the endometrium. The estrogen-primed endometrium of the follicular phase is compact, with relatively underdeveloped vasculature. Progesterone converts this endometrium into a thick, edematous, secretory lining that is glycogen enriched and prepares the metabolically active stroma and glands with an increased vasculature to receive and nourish a fertilized ovum. If implantation does not occur, estrogen and progesterone levels fall, prostaglandin synthesis occurs, and lysosomal membranes rupture, causing constriction of the spiral arterioles, ischemic necrosis, and sloughing of the endometrium superficial to the basalis layer.

Lysosomal release and ischemic necrosis has been believed to be the main mechanism for normal menstrual bleeding for many years. However, the difficulty in detecting cell necrosis during menstruation and viability of menstrual fragments has raised a number of questions about this theory. Current data support the "metalloproteinase theory" as the mechanism leading to menstrual tissue breakdown and shedding. Matrix metalloproteinases (MMPs), lytic enzymes in conjunction with activated endometrial stromal granulocytes, macrophages, and mast cells together are now thought by most investigators to cause menstruation. It is believed that tissue inhibitors of metalloproteinases (TIMPs) remain constant throughout the menstrual cycle. Before menstruation, production and activation of MMPs increases in an environment of stable amounts of TIMPs, leading to an altered MMPs/TIMPS ratio, resulting in tissue breakdown. Estrogen and progesterone, along with cytokines, appear to play a significant role in the regulation and expressions of the MMPs. High levels of progesterone are believed to inhibit MMP production and activity. This would explain endometrial tissue breakdown that occurs coincident with decreasing progesterone levels from an involuting corpus luteum.

In the second part of the menstrual phase, mitotic activity resumes and epithelial regeneration begins. This process occurs even while menstrual bleeding continues. Horizontal growth from the stem cells of the glands present in niches within the basalis layer continues the regenerative process. New blood capillaries are formed by the stimulating effect of VEGF and thymidine phosphorylase (TP) secreted by both epithelial and stromal cells. Continuous proliferation of stem cells is ensured by high telomerase activity.

This process begins in the premenstrual phase of the cycle with cessation of synthesis and inspissation of ground substance and supporting tissues by lytic enzymes released from lysosomes, which causes loss of fluids and compression of the endometrium, tonic contractions of spiral arterioles with reduction of blood flow to the tissues, loss of stromal edema, and kinking of the coiled spiral arterioles caused by the reduction in endometrial thickness.

A generalized state of ischemia develops in the superficial layers of endometrium, and bleeding into the stroma begins. Acid phosphatase and prostaglandin substances released from autolyzed cells, together with increased endothelin-1 activity, cause more intense vasoconstriction of spiral arterioles, and devitalized tissues finally slough as small hemorrhages in the stroma coalesce. According to Beller, coagulation factors are decreased in normal menstrual discharge. Fibrinogen is absent, plasminogen is converted to plasmin by released peptidases, and the amount of plasmin inhibitor is decreased. Menstrual blood generally does not clot, but it can form red blood cell aggregates with mucoid substances, mucoproteins, and glycogen as it collects in the vagina. These red cell aggregates may appear to be blood clots, but they contain no fibrin. In the presence of very heavy flow, however, clotting can occur.

According to classical theory, during menstruation the superficial compacta and the intermediate stratum spongiosum layers of the endometrium are shed, leaving only the basalis layer intact. New endometrium is regenerated from the basalis. Regeneration of new capillaries from the basalis has been observed by Markee, and restoration of the endometrial circulation has been correlated with the cessation of menstrual bleeding. Blood loss from the process of normal menstruation is limited by recovery of tone in the myometrium and endometrial vasculature, cessation of cellular autolysis, eventual clotting over the endometrial surface, and eventual active regeneration of glands, stroma, and vessels in the basalis layer in response to rising estrogen levels in the new cycle. The retained basalis endometrium is protected from destruction by lysosomal enzymes by a mucinous carbohydrate coat that covers the free surfaces of endometrial cells. This mechanism for retention of some endometrium during menstruation may explain the lack of permanent damage during the years of menstruation.

Endometrial regression during menstruation is described by classical theory as the result of four processes: autophagia, heterophagia, extrusion of secretory products, and elimination of fluids with some, but not complete, shedding of tissue. Autophagia and heterophagia are the kindred processes of intracellular lytic digestion of debris in vacuoles and of extracellular lytic digestion of debris taken up by phagosomes. Both processes eliminate damaged tissue to allow regeneration of normal endometrial cells. With fluid loss and secretion, the functionalis (the remaining functional basalis) regresses to a resting state, ready to regenerate in the next cycle. These two processes can only partially explain the observation that initial endometrial regeneration occurs in the absence of estrogen. This initial lack of estrogen dependence can also be secondary to the lesser proliferative response required after regression, compared with complete endometrial shedding. Much work remains to be done to define the complex processes involved in menstruation.

ABNORMALITIES OF THE MENSTRUAL CYCLE

STEPS IN THE PROCEDURE

Evaluation of Abnormal Uterine Bleeding

- Rule out pregnancy
- Document ovulation
- Screen for medical disorders
- Endometrial biopsy if at risk for hyperplasia
- Treat underlying medical disorders
- Correct anatomic abnormalities
- Medical therapy in anovulatory women

Given the complexities and varieties of possible alterations of the systems that control menstruation, it is not surprising that AUB should occur even in the absence of obvious disease. Prolonged estrogen stimulation can result in endometrium that outgrows its blood supply and has asynchronous development of endometrial glands, stroma, and blood vessels. Any failure of progesterone production can also profoundly affect endometrial glands, stroma, and blood vessels. Abnormal synthesis of acid mucopolysaccharides can result in the release of excessive amounts of hydrolytic enzymes into the stroma. Lysosome release from endometrial glands, influenced by plasma progesterone levels, can affect menstrual flow. The endometrium and myometrium of patients with menorrhagia produce altered types of prostaglandins. Smith and associates have shown that the amount of menstrual flow is influenced by a change in the endometrial conversion of prostaglandin endoperoxide from PGF_2 to PGE_2 and that women with menorrhagia synthesize mainly the vasodilator PGE_2 in the endometrium.

Menstruation has three clinical characteristics: the menstrual interval or cycle length, the duration of flow, and the amount of flow. The mean cycle length is 28 to 29 days, although a menstrual interval of 21 to 35 days can be considered normal. A menstrual interval shorter than 21 days and a menstrual interval longer than 35 days are considered abnormal. Amenorrhea is the absence of menses for 6 months or longer. The menstrual interval can vary from month to month by several days. Regularity of the menstrual cycle is more important than exact approximation to the 28-day mean menstrual interval. Variation in the length of the menstrual interval in regular ovulatory cycles usually occurs in the preovulatory (proliferative) phase of the cycle and is more frequent among postmenarchal teenagers and in women approaching menopause.

A duration of flow of 7 days or less is considered normal. A patient bleeding beyond 7 days enters the intermenstrual phase of the cycle, which was previously defined as metrorrhagia and is now categorized by the American Congress of Obstetricians and Gynecologists (ACOG) as intermenstrual AUB. Regardless of the length of the menstrual flow, 70% of the blood loss usually occurs by the 2nd day and 90% by the 3rd day. The mean menstrual blood loss for a normal period is approximately 40 mL. A total blood loss of 20 to 80 mL, representing 10- to 35-mg iron, has long been accepted as within the normal range. Menstrual blood loss of 80 mL or less was established as the upper limit of normal, as this is the 95th percentile in healthy women with normal iron stores measured in a population of Swedish women in the 1960s. The clinical utility of these measures is very limited. Additionally, it has recently been shown that the 80-mL value has neither the sensitivity nor specificity for disease, compromised iron status, or adverse impact of periods. The determination of the normalcy of menstrual bleeding amount is better addressed in a clinical context. Concerns about anemia in a particular patient should be investigated with appropriate laboratory tests for iron stores. A thorough menstrual history should establish the patient's perception of the heaviness of her flow, impact on her life, difficulty with containment of flow, and associated symptoms. Quantitation of menses is difficult, and a perfect measurement tool does not exist. There have been multiple survey questionnaires that have attempted to objectively measure menstrual bleeding. These measures include surveys such as the validated Menorrhagia Impact Questionnaire (MIQ) and menstrual calendars described by Bushnell and colleagues. Although the Uterine Fibroid Quality of Life questionnaire developed and validated by Spies et al. is designed for fibroid patients, there are a number of questions within the survey that assess bleeding.

We believe that development and routine use of a convenient, standardized, objective method for measuring menstrual blood loss would significantly improve the clinical practice of gynecology. Iron deficiency anemia is a late manifestation of excessive menstruation. Serum iron (ferritin) levels are more sensitive than hematocrit and hemoglobin levels for detection of iron depletion before anemia develops, as shown by Guillebaud and colleagues. The method of Hallberg and Nilsson for quantification of iron and blood loss is based on the simultaneous use of tampons and pads for the collection of menstrual blood. Menstrual blood is extracted with 5% sodium hydroxide, which converts hemoglobin to alkaline hematin. The concentration is then determined spectrophotometrically. The method is simple and gives accurate results but is not widely used outside of clinical investigations.

Acute Abnormal Uterine Bleeding

STEPS IN THE PROCEDURE

Acute Abnormal Uterine Bleeding

- Determine patient acuity (hemodynamically unstable or hypovolemic patients require immediate intravenous access)
- Determine etiology using the PALM-COEIN classification system
- Select appropriate medical or surgical treatment

Patients who have an episode of bleeding that is sufficient to require immediate intervention should be approached in three stages. First, the patient should be rapidly assed to determine acuity. Patients who are hemodynamically unstable should have one or two large-bore intravenous lines started in the event transfusion, or clotting factor replacements are necessary. Second, the etiology of the bleeding should be determined. The determination of etiology should be guided by the PALM-COEIN classification system, which separates causes into the two broad categories of "related to structural abnormalities" and "unrelated to structural abnormalities" (Fig. 26.1). Finally, an appropriate treatment should be chosen.

Similar to nonacute abnormal bleeding, described in the following sections, the treatment of acute bleeding is medical or surgical. Hormonal management using intravenous (IV) conjugated equine estrogens can stop bleeding within 8 hours in 72% of patients compared to placebo. Oral contraceptives or progestins can be used to manage bleeding chronically. Mechanical and surgical methods to manage acute bleeding include the use of intrauterine tamponade with a 26-F Foley catheter inflated with 30 mL of saline, dilatation and curettage, and in rare cases hysterectomy. Case reports have shown that both uterine artery embolization and endometrial ablation can successfully control acute AUB according to the American Congress of Obstetricians and Gynecologists Committee Opinion on the management of acute AUB.

Abnormal Uterine Bleeding Ovulatory Dysfunction

The state of chronic anovulation is the result of unopposed estrogen stimulation of the endometrium with consequent irregular breakdown and bleeding. Chronic anovulation syndrome is a "wastebasket" diagnosis for multiple endocrine etiologies. Hyperthyroidism and hypothyroidism, hyperprolactinemia, hormone-producing ovarian tumors, and Cushing disease are all endocrine syndromes that can induce anovulation, but the primary etiology of abnormal uterine bleeding ovulatory dysfunction (AUB-O) is chronic anovulation syndrome, often commonly described as the polycystic ovary or Stein-Leventhal syndrome. Any imbalance in hypothalamic pulsatile release of gonadotropin-releasing hormone (GnRH), in pituitary synthesis or release of follicle-stimulating hormone

(FSH) or luteinizing hormone (LH), or in ovarian follicular production of E_2, androgens, or progesterone can upset the delicate balances that induce cyclic ovulation and normal menstrual function. Exogenous androgen production in the adrenal glands and estrone production in adipose tissue produce identical clinical pictures.

Anovulation is also more common at the extremes of reproductive life. Perimenarchal and perimenopausal women require evaluations modified to include diagnoses that are less common in the mid reproductive years, such as coagulopathies in the perimenarchal patient and endometrial hyperplasia in the perimenopausal patient.

Menorrhagia has been described as an early symptom in patients with subclinical hypothyroidism before diagnosis of overt disease. Thyroid replacement in a normal physiologic dosage should resolve the abnormal bleeding. Because this is one of the less common causes of AUB, there is some controversy about whether thyroid testing should be part of the initial screening of patients with AUB.

Although anovulation is a frequent cause of AUB, histologic studies consistently show that 15% to 20% of AUB patients have secretory endometrium, indicative of at least intermittent, if not regular, ovulation. Livingstone and Fraser provide evidence to suggest that ovulatory AUB is more common than AUB that is associated with ovulatory dysfunction. The differential diagnosis of abnormal bleeding with ovulation differs from that of anovulation. Ovulatory patients with abnormal bleeding are more likely to have an underlying organic pathology and are not; therefore, true AUB-O patients by strict definition.

Aksel and Jones studied endometria of patients with AUB and found hyperplasia in 63% of cases; secretory endometrium was observed in 17%, and no secretory endometrium of the interval, postmenstrual, or atrophic type made up the remaining 20%. Thus, at least 17% of patients in this series had normal cyclic hormonal function and ovulation before the endometrium was examined, and it is possible that many patients with the postmenstrual type of endometria would have shown secretory changes if curettage had been performed somewhat later. In addition to histologic confirmation of ovulation by the presence of secretory endometrium, ovulation can be documented by basal body temperature charting, urinary LH surge detection, or prospective hormonal evaluation. In some cases, the prospective hormonal studies using daily serum estrogen and progesterone levels are more accurate for defining ovulatory status than are the historically accepted studies of endometrial histology, which can be misleading because of previous hormonal therapy. Although serum progesterone concentration exceeding 3 ng/mL in the luteal phase of the cycle indicates ovulation, a single measure will only identify the presence of ovulation in that cycle. Serial measures may be necessary to identify the patient that is anovulatory on an intermittent basis.

Abnormal Uterine Bleeding Coagulopathy

Proper evaluation of abnormal bleeding in the ovulatory patient demands assessment for other less common causes of bleeding. According to Claessens and Cowell, bleeding dyscrasias are particularly common in perimenarchal patients, up to 19% of whom have a primary coagulation disorder, such as idiopathic thrombocytopenic purpura or von Willebrand disease. An ad hoc consensus conference that met in May 2004 concluded that underlying hemostatic disorders were a more common cause of menorrhagia in adult women than has been currently recognized. The most common of these coagulopathies is von Willebrand disease. The incidence of von Willebrand disease in the general population has been estimated at 0.8% to 1.3%. The consensus conference calculated, by review of the literature, an incidence of 13.2% (range 11.2% to 15.5%) in healthy women with menorrhagia. Conversely, women with von Willebrand disease report menorrhagia in 78% to 93% of patients. If von Willebrand disease is excluded, the inherited disorders of hemostasis are relatively rare. Disorders of platelet number and function have variable effects on menstrual bleeding, depending on their severity. Treatment of AUB secondary to coagulopathy may involve medical management with tranexamic acid, desmopressin acetate (DDAVP), hormonal therapy, or a progestin-containing intrauterine device (IUD). Endometrial ablation is also appropriate in these patients.

Abnormal Uterine Bleeding Iatrogenic

Hemorrhagic diatheses can occur with leukemia, with chemotherapy treatment, or secondary to oral anticoagulant therapy or ingestion of foods or drugs that inhibit platelet aggregation. Women taking anticoagulants are at risk for iatrogenic AUB. Hormonal interventions such as oral contraceptives can also result in abnormal bleeding patterns rather than improvement of symptoms. The lowest doses of oral contraceptives are more likely to be associated with spotting than formulations containing 35 μg of ethinyl estradiol. Kaunitz et al. report a higher likelihood of unscheduled bleeding with continuous and extended-cycle regimens such as Seasonale, Seasonique, and Lybrel than with the traditional 28-day schedule.

Abnormal Uterine Bleeding Not yet Classified

Although infection is considered to be a cause of AUB, infection is not one of the categories identified under the PALM-COEIN classification system. This category would therefore be classified as not yet classified. Mobiluncus species identified in cases of abnormal bleeding respond to oral metronidazole therapy. Chlamydia has been implicated in abnormal bleeding, particularly with concurrent use of oral contraceptives.

Arteriovenous malformation is a very rare cause of ovulatory bleeding. In a report by Fleming and colleagues, only two cases were diagnosed before definitive surgery; the diagnosis was by pelvic angiography.

The reported association between tubal ligation and new onset of AUB should also be noted. Although numerous anecdotal reports exist, no underlying pathologic changes in anatomy or hormone production have ever been documented. Long-term follow-up studies do not confirm an increased incidence of abnormal bleeding in these patients, but do implicate biased patient perception. Patients who discontinue oral contraceptive use after tubal ligation have heavier and more painful bleeding, whereas patients who have intrauterine devices removed after sterilization have improved menstrual symptomatology.

Pathophysiology

As stated earlier, the most common etiology for AUB is estrogen withdrawal or estrogen breakthrough bleeding in an anovulatory patient. In the absence of progesterone exposure to cause inhibition of DNA synthesis and mitosis, the estrogenic proliferative response causes stromal cell growth to exceed the structural integrity of its stromal matrix, and the endometrium breaks down with irregular bleeding. Unopposed estrogen results in vascular endometrial tissue with relatively scant stroma, giving glands a back-to-back appearance. The endometrium is fragile and undergoes repetitive spontaneous breakdown. In the absence of normal control mechanisms to limit menstrual blood loss, bleeding can be prolonged and excessive.

Other contributing factors are the lack of coordinated vasoconstriction and the release of lytic enzymes, which occurs in a normal progesterone-stimulated endometrium. The absence of progesterone stimulation of metalloendopeptidase increases endothelin-1 activity, which contributes to vasospasm. Lysosomal enzymes inappropriately released in the absence of progesterone stabilization of the lysosomal membrane further contribute to structural breakdown. The same lytic enzymes, MMPs, and their inhibitors involved in normal menstrual bleeding have been found to have aberrant locally restricted expression, activation, and uncontrolled activity in the endometrial tissue biopsy specimens from women with metrorrhagia.

Many questions still remain about the mechanisms responsible for all cases of AUB. Although the mechanisms described above can explain some cases of AUB, it does not explain clinical scenarios such as bleeding unresponsive to hormonal manipulation after structural lesions have been ruled out. Hemostasis in a bleeding endometrium depends both on coagulation, with thrombus formation forming plugs in superficial blood vessels, and on vasoconstriction of spiral arterioles; generalized endometrial collapse with compression of bleeding vessels can also contribute. The lack of coordinated vasoconstriction and the irregular structural collapse lead to irregular and often heavy bleeding. The amount of bleeding correlates directly with the level of estrogen stimulation. The chronic high estrogen milieus seen in cases of obesity and chronic anovulation, and in perimenarchal and perimenopausal patients, cause the greatest amount of AUB blood loss.

Unopposed estrogen stimulation can, over time, induce a hyperplastic response in the proliferating endometrium (Fig. 26.2). Such hyperplasia can eventually develop the cytologic changes associated with neoplasia: atypical adenomatous hyperplasia or even low-grade adenocarcinoma. Such cellular transformation takes time, as much as 10 to 20 years; a young patient with AUB has a low risk of hyperplasia or neoplasia and generally does not require endometrial sampling. Patients with a long history of chronic anovulation are at greater risk of hyperplasia and undergo histologic evaluation earlier. The perimenopausal patient has a substantially higher risk, however, and sampling is mandated.

Diagnostic Imaging Techniques

Diagnostic vaginal ultrasound can be particularly useful in cases of ovulatory AUB. A nonrandomized study of 45 otherwise unselected patients with AUB demonstrated anatomic pathology in 31% by vaginal ultrasound compared with 9% by clinical examination. Pathologic findings included leiomyoma uteri, polyps, and abnormal endometrial architecture. If these data are confirmed by later studies, the implication is that true AUB in ovulatory patients may be even more rare than the currently accepted figure of 15% to 20%. Endovaginal ultrasound is also of particular value in cases of perimenopausal and postmenopausal abnormal bleeding, which will be discussed later (Fig. 26.3).

Saline infusion sonography (SIS) is a technique to improve visualization of the endometrial cavity during transvaginal ultrasonography. Dueholm and colleagues compared the accuracy of SIS with transvaginal sonography, hysteroscopy, and magnetic resonance imaging (MRI). In 108 patients with AUB, pain, endometriosis, or myomas, SIS had an overall sensitivity comparable to the gold standard of hysteroscopy and better than either MRI or transvaginal sonography. Magnetic resonance imaging had the highest sensitivity for submucous

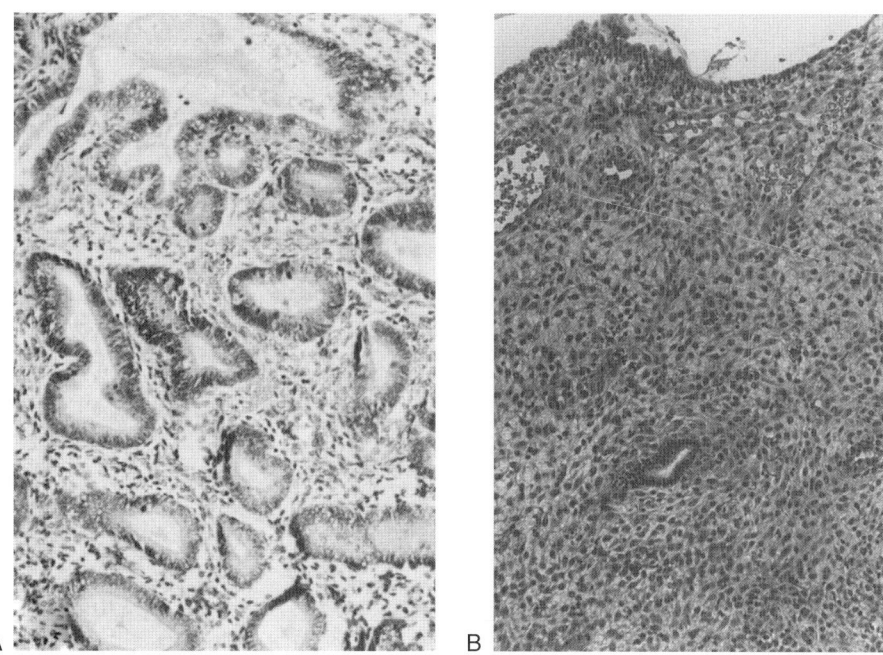

FIGURE 26.2 **A:** Endometrial hyperplasia before treatment showing hyperplastic cellular changes of glands. **B:** Hyperplastic endometrium after continuous progestin treatment.

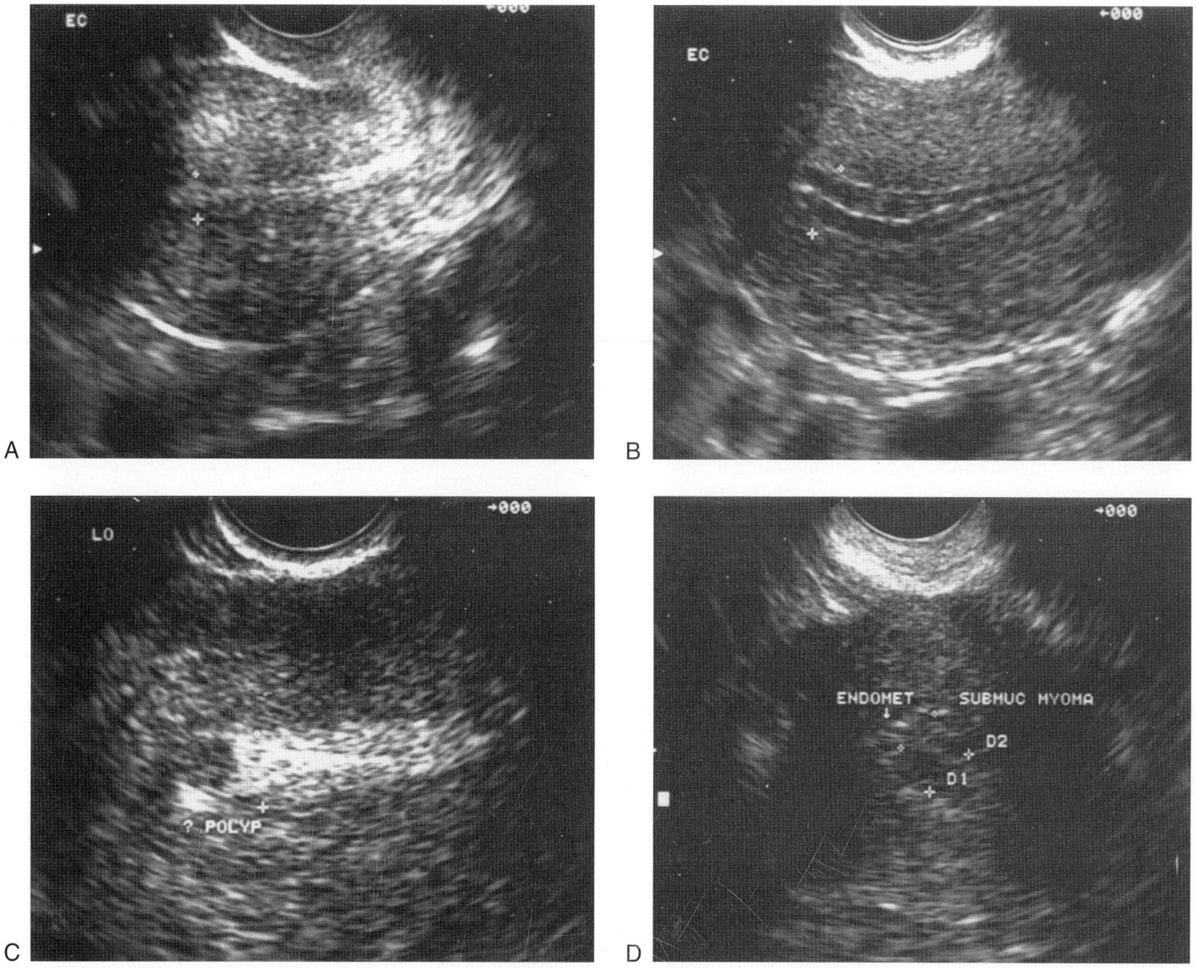

FIGURE 26.3 **A:** Single-line endometrium consistent with postmenstruation, early proliferation, and postmenopause. **B:** Three-line endometrium from estrogen stimulation, late follicular phase. **C:** Endometrial polyp in hyperechoic thickened endometrium consistent with luteal phase or hyperplasia–neoplasia. **D:** Submucous myoma with distortion of endometrial cavity marked by single-line endometrium.

myomas, but a relatively low sensitivity for other intrauterine pathology, such as polyps. As SIS is a less invasive procedure than a surgical technique, such as hysteroscopy, and is much less expensive than MRI, it should be the procedure of choice for imaging of the endometrial cavity in patients with AUB.

Differential Diagnosis of Abnormal Uterine Bleeding

Abnormal uterine bleeding occurs most frequently at the extremes of menstrual life, but it can develop at any intervening time. The characteristics of AUB are variable, from infrequent heavy flow (oligomenorrhea) to almost continuous spotting or bleeding. The age at onset and duration of irregularity can provide important clues to etiology. Anovulation is common in the perimenarchal girl. More than 50% of cycles are anovulatory in the first 2 years after menarche. Complications of pregnancy also are common in this age group and must be ruled out before initiation of treatment for AUB. New sensitive radioimmunoassays for the beta subunit of human chorionic gonadotropin are accurate for evaluating the possibility of pregnancy. Although relatively rare, endocrinologically active ovarian neoplasms do occur and should be particularly excluded in prepubertal vaginal bleeding. Other causes of irregular bleeding in the adolescent include genital trauma and coagulopathies such as idiopathic thrombocytopenic purpura and von Willebrand disease. As previously mentioned, the Claessens and Cowell review of children's hospital admissions for menorrhagia reports an overall 19% incidence of primary coagulation disorders and a 50% incidence in patients presenting at the time of menarche. Some more recent studies have disputed this high figure and cited a lower risk of 5%. Given the new data on von Willebrand disease in adult female menorrhagia, this newer figure is questionable, and coagulopathies should still be considered a significant cause of AUB in adolescents. The most common diagnosis is idiopathic thrombocytopenic purpura, but platelet disorders such as von Willebrand and Glanzmann diseases, thalassemia, and leukemia are also found.

The adult patient with AUB can have either an acute or a chronic history of menstrual irregularity. Onset at menarche and persistence into adulthood is a classic history for chronic anovulation syndrome, but nonclassical adrenal hyperplasia must be differentiated when there is coexistent androgen excess. The differential diagnosis can be made by obtaining a baseline 17α-hydroxyprogesterone level. A level less than 200 ng/dL rules out partial adrenal 21-hydroxylase enzyme deficiency. An elevated baseline 17α-hydroxyprogesterone requires a cosyntropin stimulation test to confirm the nonclassical adrenal hyperplasia diagnosis. A more acute history requires a differential diagnosis of other endocrinologic causes of anovulation, for example, thyroid and prolactin disorders, complications of pregnancy, neoplastic processes such as fibroids or hormone-producing ovarian tumors, intrauterine lesions such as polyps and synechiae, and coagulopathies. Adult patients with menorrhagia are at higher risk than previously thought to have a bleeding diathesis. Dilley and colleagues identified coagulopathies in 10.7% of 121 patients in a case–control study. The majority of cases were von Willebrand disease. Women older than the age of 30 years with a history consistent with chronic anovulation should undergo endometrial sampling because of their greater risk of hyperplasia and neoplasia. Perimenopausal women with AUB have an even higher risk of hyperplasia and neoplasia and should always undergo endometrial sampling. Several years before menopause, menstrual cycles usually shorten secondary to a decreased proliferative phase, with

resultant moderate elevation of FSH and subsequent frequent anovulatory cycles. This unopposed estrogen environment is conducive to the development of both AUB and hyperplasia. Appropriate evaluation of the premenopausal and postmenopausal patient will be discussed later in this chapter.

A diagnosis of AUB is often a diagnosis of exclusion. Problems of pregnancy such as incomplete or missed abortion, subinvolution of the placental site, placental polyp, trophoblastic disease, and extrauterine pregnancy must be ruled out. All gynecologic malignancies can cause abnormal bleeding. Common epithelial tumors of the ovary can produce estrogen and cause uterine bleeding. Submucous leiomyoma and endometrial polyps can be present in older women but are not a problem in the differential diagnosis of adolescents. Excessive anovulatory bleeding is common with polycystic ovarian disease, with functional cysts of the ovary. The patient workup for AUB should include a complete history and physical examination. Pelvic examination may disclose an adnexal mass, evidence of genital trauma or laceration, or a fibroid uterus. Laboratory studies should include thyroid function tests and the evaluation of levels of human chorionic gonadotropin, FSH, LH, prolactin, and serum androgens, if indicated. A significant increase in dehydroepiandrosterone sulfate indicates a need to screen for nonclassical adrenal hyperplasia. A serum progesterone level measurement is useful for assessment of ovulatory status. A complete blood count with platelet and coagulation studies is appropriate, and in some cases, a bleeding time may be indicated to assess platelet function. As mentioned earlier, endovaginal ultrasound and SIS are valuable adjuncts to pelvic examination. They are particularly informative for assessment of intrauterine or extrauterine pregnancies and pelvic masses detected on examination. Occasionally, they also may reveal anatomic pathology not detected by other means (Fig. 26.3). Invasive tissue-sampling procedures include endometrial sampling and sampling at the time of hysteroscopy. Diagnostic hysteroscopy can be an office procedure and has replaced blind D&C as a diagnostic test. Diagnostic hysteroscopy, with its lower false-negative rate, is preferable in the perimenopausal or postmenopausal patient. An office endometrial biopsy or diagnostic hysteroscopy is not necessary in adolescents, as patients of this age are unlikely to have structural lesions such as fibroids and polyps or endometrial hyperplasia. Hysterosalpingography and hysteroscopy will be reviewed later in this chapter.

Treatment

Because most patients with AUB have an underlying etiology of chronic anovulation with unopposed estrogen stimulation of the endometrium, medical treatment with progestational compounds is the mainstay of therapy. Precise amounts can differ depending on the patient's age, but adequate progestin stimulation will decrease DNA synthesis and cell proliferation, deplete estrogen receptors, and increase the conversion of E_2 to the less potent estrone sulfate. These effects will induce maturation of the endometrium, healing of superficial breaks, and enhancement of the stromal matrix with increased structural stability and cessation of bleeding. Withdrawal of the progestin after adequate exposure results in orderly and uniform shedding of the endometrium with a finite self-limited bleed. The progestin dosage and duration of therapy must induce a complete secretory transformation; otherwise, complete inhibition of all estrogenic effects will fail, and islands of proliferative endometrium will remain.

Although postmenopausal estrogen replacement doses are low, progesterone is needed to prevent hyperplasia. Whitehead and Frazier have shown that postmenopausal estrogen replacement mimics the unopposed estrogen environment of chronic anovulation and that 4% of patients develop endometrial hyperplasia with only 7 days of progestin exposure, 2% with 10 days of exposure, and 0% with 12 days of exposure. They recommend 12 days of progestin every month to counteract the estrogen proliferative effects. Medroxyprogesterone acetate 10 mg, or norethindrone acetate 5 mg per day, may be prescribed. After initial control of the dysfunctional bleeding, the 12-day course can be repeated at monthly intervals to prevent the development of hyperplasia. It is convenient to start each new course on the 1st day of each month. A regular withdrawal can be expected to start either during the last 2 days of progestin or within several days of the last dose. Failure to withdraw could signify pregnancy, development of a hypoestrogenic state, or, rarely, induction of ovulation by progestin stimulation of the estrogen-primed patient. In such a case of endogenous progesterone production, the menses can be delayed 2 weeks. A word of caution: This regimen is not contraceptive. It should also be noted that the numbers of women using hormonal therapy (HT) have markedly decreased since the Women's Health Initiative (WHI). In one study by MacLennan and colleagues, 64% of women using HT prior to the WHI study discontinued treatment.

An alternative method for delivery of a progestin to control dysfunctional bleeding and menorrhagia is local administration with a progestin-impregnated IUD. Numerous studies have demonstrated significant reductions in menstrual blood loss in patients using the progestin-impregnated IUD. Xiao and colleagues showed reductions of more than 80% at up to 36 months. Irvine and associates performed a randomized trial of 44 women with menorrhagia, comparing a levonorgestrel IUD with cyclic progestin therapy. The IUD group had blood loss reduced by 90%, along with higher patient satisfaction, compliance, and continuation. In a comparison of endometrial resection with the levonorgestrel IUD, Rauramo et al. showed highly significant decreases in menstrual blood loss with both treatment arms. The incidence of complications was similar in both groups, and 3-year follow-up rates were similar. Seventeen percent of the resection group required follow-up surgery. Other studies have shown a significant cost benefit to the use of the levonorgestrel IUD compared with surgical management of AUB, including hysterectomy. As noted earlier, the levonorgestrel IUD has also shown to be effective in controlling menorrhagia in patients with hemostatic disorders such as von Willebrand disease.

New research from the Los Angeles Biomedical Research Institute (LA BioMed) found a progestogen-only treatment halted bleeding in women suffering from severe menorrhagia. In a group of 48 women, Ammerman and Nelson found that injection of depo-medroxyprogesterone acetate 150 mg intramuscularly combined with 3 days of oral medroxyprogesterone acetate 20 mg every 8 hours for 9 doses had a mean time to bleeding cessation of 2.6 days, with high patient satisfaction.

Chronic unopposed estrogen can produce a very lush endometrium that can bleed heavily during progestin withdrawal. Speroff and colleagues recommend treatment using combination oral contraceptives in a step-down regimen. Two to four pills are given daily, one every 6 to 12 hours, for 5 to 7 days for acute control of bleeding. This will usually control acute bleeding within 24 to 48 hours, allowing time to complete the diagnostic evaluation. Withdrawal of medication will result in a heavy bleed. On the 5th day of this bleed, a low-dose cyclic oral contraceptive is started and repeated for three cycles to allow orderly regression of the excessive proliferative endometrium. Alternatively, the dosage of combination pills can be tapered (four times a day, then three times a day, then two

times a day) over 3 to 6 days and then continued at one pill every day. Combination oral contraceptives induce atrophy of the endometrium because the chronic estrogen–progestin exposure suppresses pituitary gonadotropins and inhibits endogenous steroidogenesis. They are useful for long-term management of AUB in patients without contraindications and have the added benefit of pregnancy prevention. Particularly in perimenarchal patients, heavy prolonged bleeding can denude the basal endometrium and make it unresponsive to progestins. Curettage for control of hemorrhage is contraindicated because of a high risk of development of intrauterine synechiae (Asherman syndrome) if the basalis is curetted. High-dose intravenous estrogen (conjugated estrogens 25 mg every 4 hours until bleeding abates) will give acute control by proliferative repair of the endometrium and by direct effects on coagulation, including increased fibrinogen and platelet aggregation. Megestrol 20 mg twice daily is also an excellent method for obtaining acute control of AUB without the side effects of intravenous estrogen treatment. It will be effective in any situation other than one in which the entire endometrium has sloughed, leaving only basalis. A progestin alone or oral conjugated estrogens in combination with a progestin can then be used to induce orderly withdrawal bleeding.

Although tranexamic acid has been available for a number of years, it has come into more widespread use. In a double-blind placebo-controlled study by Lukes et al., women who received tranexamic acid ($n = 115$) had significantly greater reduction in menstrual blood loss of –69.6 mL (40.4%) compared with –12.6 mL (8.2%) in the 72 women who received placebo ($P < 0.001$). They also had a reduction of menstrual blood loss that exceeded the prespecified amount of 50 mL. Finally, they had a reduction of menstrual blood loss that was considered meaningful to women. Compared with women receiving placebo, women treated with tranexamic acid experienced significant improvements in limitations in social or leisure and physical activities, work inside and outside the home, and self-perceived menstrual blood loss ($P < 0.01$).

Selective progesterone receptor modulators, such as ulipristal acetate (UPA), have been shown by Nieman et al. to be efficacious in the treatment of leiomyoma, and have been noted to cause amenorrhea in the vast majority of patients. Treated patients developed anovulatory amenorrhea without becoming hypoestrogenic, suggesting that decreased bleeding is mediated by a direct endometrial effect as well as inhibition of ovulation. Ulipristal acetate is currently only available as emergency contraception in the United States and for the treatment of leiomyoma in Europe, but may have potential use as a treatment of AUB.

Hysteroscopy of patients who fail to respond to hormonal therapy may reveal previously missed pathology, such as a submucous myoma or polyp. These diagnoses are particularly common in patients with ovulatory dysfunctional bleeding. If a diagnostic curettage has not been previously performed, one can be performed in conjunction with the hysteroscopy, both for diagnosis and for temporary therapy. The ACOG no longer considers D&C long-term therapy. If atypical hyperplasia has been identified and preservation of fertility is desired, more aggressive progestin therapy is recommended. Medroxyprogesterone acetate, 30 mg, or megestrol 20 to 40 mg daily for 3 months, should be prescribed, and the patient should be monitored by repeat endometrial sampling to assess the efficiency of the medical treatment (**Fig. 26.2B**). If atypical hyperplasia persists, very high-dose progestin protocols can be tried, but hysterectomy must be considered.

Menorrhagia can be reduced when PGE_2 and prostacyclin synthesis are decreased by nonsteroidal anti-inflammatory medications. These drugs inhibit the cyclooxygenase enzyme necessary for endometrial production of prostaglandin under estrogen stimulation and thus alter the relative production of the proaggregation vasoconstrictor thromboxane A_2 and the antiaggregation vasodilator prostacyclin. Pathology studies have confirmed that this improves both platelet aggregation and vasoconstriction. Fraser and colleagues demonstrated these compounds to be most effective when given in therapeutic dosages for 7 to 10 days before the expected onset of the next menstrual period in ovulatory AUB patients, but they are commonly started with the onset of menses and continued throughout the bleeding episode with good success.

For coagulation disorders, 1-desamino-8-D-arginine vasopressin (also known as desmopressin or simply DDAVP) increases coagulation factor VIII with a therapeutic effect lasting approximately 6 hours. It is best administered intravenously, 0.3 μg/kg in 50 mL saline over 15 to 30 minutes, but can be used intranasally. Antifibrinolytic agents such as ε-aminocaproic acid and tranexamic acid can decrease blood loss up to 50%, but their significant central nervous system and gastrointestinal side effects and the purported risk of intracranial arterial thrombosis have traditionally limited their applicability. New data do not support a significant thrombotic risk, and tranexamic acid is widely available in Europe for use in menorrhagia. Ergot derivatives are ineffective for treatment of menorrhagia. Local delivery of progestational agents by way of an intrauterine device has been demonstrated by Milsom and colleagues to be extremely effective, with more than a 90% reduction in bleeding in some patients. This has the potential to provide long-term therapy for patients with chronic bleeding unresponsive to other therapies.

Long-acting derivatives of GnRH agonists down-regulate pituitary synthesis of FSH and LH and induce a "medical menopause." Withdrawal of endogenous steroid stimulation will result in endometrial atrophy. Various delivery options are available, including intranasal delivery, daily subcutaneous delivery, monthly intramuscular depot, and subcutaneously implanted pellet analogue. Gonadotropin-releasing hormone agonists are not effective in acute control of abnormal bleeding. At least 2 to 4 weeks are required for adequate suppression of gonadotropin production and inhibition of steroidogenesis. Long-term therapy can effectively control blood loss with chronic AUB secondary to chronic systemic illness, thrombocytopenia, or other coagulopathies. Because of the profoundly hypoestrogenic state induced by these drugs, there is accelerated bone resorption and the risk of development of significant osteoporosis. Therefore, long-term therapy requires "add-back" treatment with an estrogen–progestin combination to prevent bone loss. Gonadotropin-releasing hormone agonists can also be used as adjuncts for endometrial preparation before endometrial ablation.

Ablation or destruction of the endometrium has been advocated for treatment of chronic abnormal bleeding unresponsive to medical management in the presence of a normal endometrial cavity and the absence of submucous leiomyomata, endometrial hyperplasia, or neoplasia. Although there has been significant disagreement regarding the appropriate indications for this procedure, it has been widely applied with varying success. The original methods included use of hysteroscopy with electrosurgical roller-ball cauterization or endomyometrial resection using a loop electrode. These hysteroscopic surgical techniques require special training. More recently, new techniques have been described to ablate the endometrial cavity without the requirement for hysteroscopy. These include thermal balloon ablation, direct instillation of heated saline, cryoablation with a cryoprobe, microwave endometrial ablation, and use of radiofrequency electromagnetic energy. Success rates reported with the various techniques have ranged from 60% to 95% of patients achieving either hypomenorrhea or amenorrhea. Brooks and Donnez et al. report pretreatment with danazol, GnRH analogues, or suction curettage to thin the endometrium appears to improve long-term success rates. Seeras and Gilliland reported resumption of menstruation in 44% of women after ablation if they had not received preoperative endometrial suppression.

A number of comparison studies have looked at success rates of the various techniques to determine relative efficacy, complication rates, and relative cost. Meyer and colleagues compared roller-ball ablation with thermal balloon ablation in a prospective, randomized trial. A greater percentage of women in the roller-ball group (27.2%) were amenorrheic at their 12-month follow-up than were women in the uterine balloon group (15.2%). The rates of hypomenorrhea plus amenorrhea were not significantly different (balloon, 80.2%; roller ball, 84.3%). Overall patient satisfaction was equivalent. The complication rate was 3.2% in the hysteroscopic roller-ball group with no significant intraoperative complications in the thermal balloon group. A comparison of thermal balloon ablation with the progestin-containing IUD showed similar results as far as overall satisfaction; however, bleeding scores were lower and amenorrhea rates higher in the IUD group (Busfield et al.). Corson, with follow-up by Goldrath, performed a prospective randomized trial of endometrial ablation using the Hydro ThermAblator (HTA; Boston Scientific Corporation, Natick, MA, USA) versus roller ball (Figs. 26.2 and 26.4). This system uses heated saline flowing free under low pressure to ablate the endometrium under hysteroscopic guidance. Success rates for both groups were comparable at 3 years with amenorrhea rates of 53% for HTA and 46% for roller ball and overall satisfaction rates of 98% and 97%, respectively. There were no significant differences in complication rates or repeat surgical procedures.

The NovaSure system (Cytyc Corporation, Palo Alto, CA, USA) uses radiofrequency current through a mesh electrode that conforms to the endometrial cavity to ablate the endometrium. Tissue desiccation is rapid compared with thermal devices and requires no pretreatment of the endometrium. The overall success rate of 88.3% and amenorrhea rate of 41% for NovaSure-treated patients were higher than 81.7% and 35% rates, respectively, for endometrial resection in a randomized

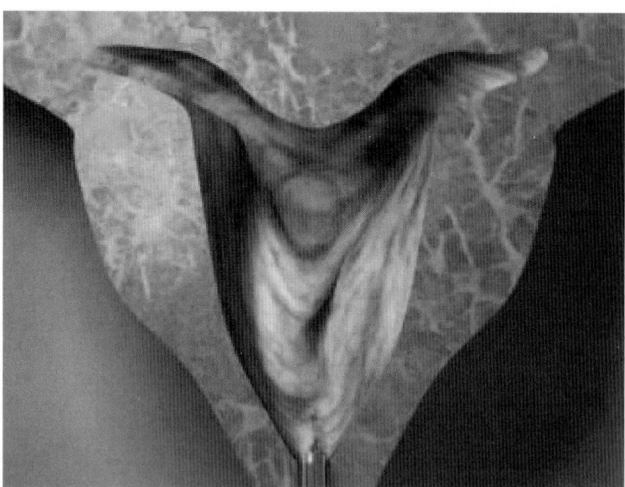

FIGURE 26.4 Hydro ThermAblator. (HTA; Boston Scientific Corporation, Natick, MA, USA.)

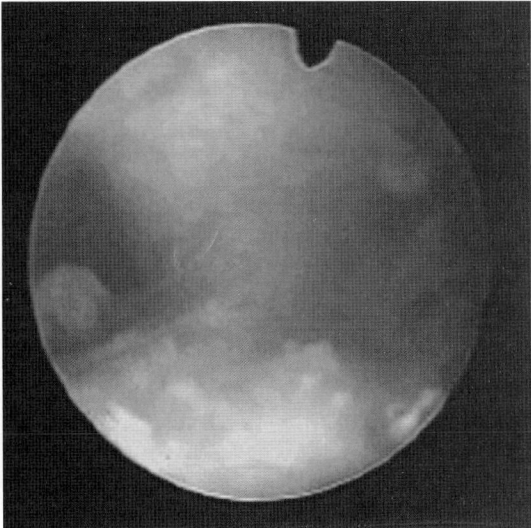

FIGURE 26.5 Endometrial cavity before and after endometrial ablation using Hydro ThermAblator.

trial by Cooper et al. A randomized trial versus hydrother-mablation (Fig. 26.5) also demonstrated higher amenorrhea rates. Microwave energy can also be used to ablate endometrium. The MEA (Microsulis Americas, Pampano Beach, FL, USA) device was tested in a prospective randomized trial by Cooper et al., comparing it with roller-ball ablation. Success rates were 87% and 83.2%, respectively, for MEA and roller ball. Amenorrhea rates were 61.3% for MEA and 51% for the roller-ball group. This trial also included patients with up to 3-cm submucous myomas. Subgroup analysis did not show any difference in the success rate in this group.

Endomyometrial resection has been reported by Kooy et al. to have higher amenorrhea rates compared with rates for other techniques. Vercellini and colleagues compared myometrial resection with endometrial ablation using a vaporizing electrode similar to a roller ball. Amenorrhea rates were 48% for the endomyometrial resection group and 36% for the ablation group, although overall patient satisfaction rates were equivalent. Difficulty of surgery and mean fluid deficit were both described as greater in the resection group. In a comparison of endometrial ablation with laser versus endomyometrial resection, Battacharya et al. showed equivalent amenorrhea rates of approximately 45%, with overall patient satisfaction rates of 90%.

Operative hysteroscopic techniques require specialized training, and complications, although relatively infrequent, can be significant. A multihospital survey by Jansen et al. in the Netherlands revealed an overall complication rate for hysteroscopy of 0.28%. Diagnostic hysteroscopy had a significantly lower complication rate than that of operative hysteroscopy (0.13% vs. 0.95%). The most frequent surgical complication was uterine perforation (0.76%). Reported complication rates for hysteroscopic ablation procedures are significantly higher. O'Connor and Magos followed 525 women for up to 5 years after endometrial resection. They reported a 6% incidence of intraoperative complications and a 3% incidence of postoperative complications. They also reported a 15% complication rate in patients who required a repeat ablative procedure. The "Mistletoe" survey led by Overton et al. from the Royal College of Obstetricians and Gynaecologists recorded endomyometrial resection complication rates of 7.2% but only 4% for roller-ball and laser ablations. A prospective trial by Meyer et al. of thermal balloon versus roller-ball ablation reported

intraoperative complications in 3.2% of the roller-ball patients but no significant intraoperative complications in the thermal balloon patients. Reported complications include uterine perforation with hemorrhage, laser or electrosurgical damage to the bowel, excessive absorption of distending medium with fluid overload, hyponatremia and pulmonary edema, and persistence of bleeding requiring repeat ablation or hysterectomy. The complication rates reported by Summitt et al. compare favorably with reported morbidity rates for women undergoing hysterectomy, which range from 7% to 15%.

There is concern regarding the potential outcome of pregnancies conceived after endometrial ablation. A literature review by Cook and Seman reports a miscarriage rate of 21.7%, a preterm rate of 26.1%, and a perinatal mortality rate of 11.8%. Of those pregnancies that continued beyond 20 weeks, 35.3% were described as having abnormal placental adherence, including placenta accreta and increta. The hysterectomy rate for this series of patients was 8.9%. These outcomes were attributed to the possible presence of intrauterine synechiae, although in most cases, no direct endometrial cavity assessment was performed.

Another concern has been possible obliteration of warning signs heralding the development of endometrial carcinoma, with subsequent delay in diagnosis. Endometrial ablation procedures usually result in a narrowed tubular uterine cavity without the obliteration seen in Asherman syndrome, but are rarely expected to result in total ablation of all endometrial tissue. Several cases of postablation endometrial carcinoma have been reported by Brooks-Carter et al. and Copperman et al.. The cost of endometrial ablation does compare favorably with that of hysterectomy, with hysterectomy reported by Vilos et al. as 58% more expensive when all costs, including lost work time, are considered.

Dilatation and curettage is most useful as a diagnostic technique when it is combined with hysteroscopy. Although D&C will acutely address AUB, it is not a long-term treatment of AUB. Removal of the structurally fragile bleeding endometrium allows restoration of normal hemostatic events, with regeneration of the integrity of the endometrium and restoration of the normal proliferative response. If the patient fails to respond to medical therapy, repeated curettage, or even endometrial ablation, then more definitive therapy, such as hysterectomy, should be considered, taking into account the age of the patient and her desire for future childbearing. It has been estimated that 2 million women in the United States are seen annually with reports of excessive uterine bleeding, and approximately 150,000 undergo hysterectomy, which accounts for 20% to 30% of all hysterectomies performed.

In general, the ovulatory type of bleeding has the poorest response to replacement hormonal therapy and the highest incidence of recurrence. Although a hysterectomy can be considered an admission of therapeutic defeat, it is frequently an expeditious method of resolving this refractory and recurrent type of AUB. When bleeding persists after repeated curettage and cyclic hormonal therapy, hysterectomy may be required. If other conditions are present that should be corrected surgically, such as a relaxed vaginal outlet, rectocele, cystocele, or uterine descensus, we recommend vaginal hysterectomy with support of the vaginal vault and repair of the vaginal wall relaxation. When hysterectomy is indicated in premenopausal women younger than 50 years of age, normal ovarian tissue is conserved. In a patient younger than 30 years of age, radical surgical treatment should be strongly avoided; one can almost always control uterine bleeding by repeated curettage or by increasing amounts of cyclic hormone therapy. Today, the availability and use of estrogen and progesterone have changed the need for hysterectomy to treat AUB. Hysterectomy is not indicated in young women but may be indicated in older women when hormonal therapy and curettage have failed. Although curettage may acutely improve bleeding, it is not a long-term therapy.

Blood transfusions are seldom required when AUB is associated with anemia, but they may be given if the anemia is so severe that symptoms are present. Oral iron therapy should be started at the first sign of heavy menstruation to prevent depletion of iron stores, and it should be given for 3 to 6 months after normal hemoglobin and hematocrit levels have been restored in patients with iron deficiency anemia.

PERIMENOPAUSAL AND POSTMENOPAUSAL BLEEDING

When uterine bleeding occurs more than 12 months after the last regular menstrual period, it is defined as postmenopausal bleeding. For a period varying from months to years before menopause, the individual patient may experience irregular patterns of bleeding. Often, the first sign is a shortening of the menstrual interval secondary to premature elevation in FSH, followed by intermittent periods of amenorrhea alternating with heavy bleeding consistent with oligoovulation or anovulation. With this clinical picture, special consideration must be given to ruling out a neoplastic process as the source of the bleeding. The first diagnostic consideration is to ensure that the bleeding originates from the uterus. In elderly women especially, bleeding from the urethra or rectum may be reported as vaginal bleeding. Vaginal or cervical lesions causing the bleeding should be diagnosed readily with careful inspection or biopsy. Cancers of the vagina or cervix or cervical polyps can also be readily diagnosed and appropriate treatment rendered.

When the source of the bleeding is determined to be the uterine cavity, sampling of the endometrium for pathology examination is usually considered to be mandatory. Although D&C at the time of hysteroscopy continues to be a commonly performed procedure for both its diagnostic and short-term therapeutic benefits, office endometrial biopsy can often expedite appropriate evaluation and therapy. Many instruments have been devised for the sampling of endometrial tissue and evaluation of the endometrial cavity. The standard instrument used for many years had been the Novak curette because of

the discomfort associated with passage of the Novak curette; newer Silastic curettes have been developed. These have a smaller diameter (3 mm), are flexible, and are often better tolerated by patients. They can be difficult to pass through a truly stenotic cervix because of their pliability. Often, there is an accompanying syringe that attaches and develops effective vacuum pressure to improve the size of the sample obtained. A four-quadrant endometrial biopsy with passes along the anterior and posterior and both lateral walls of the endometrial cavity is recommended for diagnosis of abnormal bleeding. Another potentially useful device not requiring a syringe to develop negative pressure is a disposable plastic tube with a 3.1-mm outer diameter, an aspiration port, and solid plastic obturator at its tip. The obturator fits so closely that its slow withdrawal from the uterine cavity causes sufficient suction to obtain an adequate endometrial specimen in most cases. However, the endometrial surface area sampled is small (5%) and can easily miss polyps, submucous myomas, and endometrial carcinoma that occupies only a small portion of the endometrial cavity. Because of the small aperture of this device and its almost total reliance on suction to obtain a specimen, the architecture of the obtained biopsy may be somewhat distorted.

Vacuum suction curettage has gained some popularity as an office procedure for endometrial sampling that does not require general anesthesia. A small metal or plastic cannula with an outside diameter of 3 mm that has a slightly curved tip and an opening on the concave surface for easier insertion through a small endocervical canal is connected to a plastic collection chamber, which, in newer models, is a large syringe rather than the old pumps or faucets. Several studies have compared the results of suction curettage with those of regular curettage under anesthesia in the same patient. Cohen and colleagues studied 98 patients; in 93, they found identical histologic patterns with both methods. In five patients, there was no correlation between the results of the two techniques, and none of these had cancer. At the Medical University of South Carolina, Lutz and colleagues found suction curettage to be 98% accurate in evaluating high-risk women with abnormal bleeding for endometrial malignant disease. Recent evidence from Kazandi et al. suggests that although Pipelle biopsies have equivalent diagnostic accuracy with widespread endometrial lesions they provide limited diagnostic accuracy in cases with focal pathologies.

The principal value of an endometrial biopsy is that a formal D&C under anesthesia has been avoided if the removed tissue contains adenocarcinoma. If the cause of postmenopausal bleeding is not identified in a screening endometrial biopsy and the endometrial stripe is greater than 5 mm, a hysteroscopic-directed endometrial sampling is obligatory. In office biopsies of the endometria of more than 20,000 patients of all ages, Hofmeister detected 273 cases of endometrial carcinoma, 32 of which (14.28%) were totally asymptomatic. The endometrial carcinoma detection rate was 1.76% of the total group of 23,202 patients. Hofmeister's routine office endometrial biopsies using a modification of the Novak and Randall curette provide one of the largest clinical experiences of this instrument to date. Unfortunately, only patients who had continued uterine bleeding or who demonstrated an atypical pattern in the office biopsy were subjected to a complete curettage. Therefore, the true-negative and false-negative rate for the Novak type of curette in the detection of endometrial cancer has not been determined accurately. In other studies, summarized by Cohen and colleagues, the accuracy of detection of endometrial cancer by endometrial curettage varied from 76% to 92%. However, a thorough endometrial curettage under anesthesia is also not infallible in the detection of endometrial cancer. Bettocchi and colleagues evaluated the diagnostic accuracy of endometrial curettage in 397 patients; D&C failed to detect intrauterine pathology in 62.5% of patients, including four cases of complex hyperplasia, five cases of endometrial adenocarcinoma, and many endometrial polyps and submucous myomas. The use of hysteroscopic-directed sampling may decrease that number.

Vaginal ultrasound has been investigated as a screening tool in patients with postmenopausal bleeding. The average thickness of the postmenopausal endometrial stripe has been reported as 2.3 ± 1.8 mm, with a range of 0 to 10 mm, in a series of 300 asymptomatic women. Twenty-two had endometrial stripes of 5 mm or larger, and all had benign pathology. In a series of 51 cases of postmenopausal bleeding, Nasri and colleagues reported that if the endometrial thickness was less than 5 mm, the pathology would show either inactive or no endometrial tissue. Karlsson and associates reported on 1,168 women with postmenopausal bleeding. Patients with an endometrial echo of less than 4 mm had a sensitivity of 96% and a specificity of 68% for detecting endometrial pathology. If a 5-mm cutoff was used, two endometrial carcinomas would have been missed. In another study by Gull and colleagues, 198 women screened for postmenopausal bleeding had an endometrial thickness of 5 mm or greater. Endometrial sampling diagnosed 36 primary endometrial cancers, one metastatic breast cancer, and three cases of atypical endometrial hyperplasia. Of 163 women with an endometrial stripe of 4 mm or less, only one was found to have endometrial cancer. Other series have shown that an endometrial thickness of greater than 8 mm is an indication for endometrial sampling, regardless of whether there is a report of bleeding. This will detect most, if not all, endometrial cancers. A meta-analysis by Smith-Bindman et al. reviewing the accuracy of transvaginal sonography reported that 96% of women with endometrial cancer and 92% of women with other endometrial diseases had an endometrial echo of greater than 5 mm. The false-positive rate was dependent on the use of hormone replacement therapy, with nonusers having a false-positive risk of 8%, whereas those on hormones had a 23% false-positive rate. Saline infusion sonography can be used to further evaluate patients with thickened endometrial stripes to detect structural problems such as polyps as an adjunct to endometrial sampling. Although the exact indications for patient screening and parameters for follow-up need to be more precisely defined, vaginal ultrasound appears to have promise as a noninvasive method for evaluating the postmenopausal patient.

Office hysteroscopy using new smaller-diameter flexible or rigid hysteroscopes is growing in popularity because it enables selective biopsy of the areas of visualized endometrium that appear most likely to contain a neoplastic process. A blind endometrial biopsy that reveals benign endometrial histology does not absolutely preclude the presence of a malignant process elsewhere within the endometrium. A neoplastic transformation in the endometrium is often a focal abnormality. Another major advantage of hysteroscopy is the diagnosis of endometrial polyps, submucous myomas, or other sources of bleeding that may not always be identified by endometrial biopsy or conventional curettage. In a series of 110 cases of postmenopausal bleeding, the causes of 95 were identified as endometrial polyps or submucous myomas. Only two cases of early adenocarcinoma were identified. Operative hysteroscopy, endometrial ablation, or both successfully controlled bleeding in most cases of benign disease. In cases of postmenopausal uterine bleeding, the recommended diagnostic procedures may or may not produce a tissue sample of endometrium. If the

endometrium is not atrophic, a wide range of histology can be observed. Occasionally, simple proliferative endometrium is found. The endometrium can exhibit simple hyperplasia, more marked adenomatous hyperplasia, or hyperplasia with atypical cells, resulting in a diagnosis of atypical endometrial hyperplasia. Later in the menopausal years, it is not uncommon for the endometrium to have the characteristics of cystic hyperplasia, often referred to in the older literature as "Swiss cheese hyperplasia."

Hormone-induced postmenopausal uterine bleeding can be the result of endogenous or exogenous hormonal effects. The proliferation of endometrium in a patient who is not receiving exogenous hormonal therapy is generally attributed to endogenous production of estrone. Estrone is the peripheral conversion product of the weak androgenic precursor androstenedione (85% from adrenal and 15% from ovary), and its synthesis occurs primarily in adipose tissue. In the absence of exogenous hormonal therapy, one must also exclude the possibility of an estrogen-producing ovarian tumor (granulosa cell tumor).

Management of perimenopausal bleeding in the absence of significant hyperplasia or neoplasia is essentially the same as for AUB in a younger patient. One recently accepted method that in the past was proscribed is the use of low-dose oral contraceptives. The Food and Drug Administration has approved them for patients older than 40 years of age in the absence of specific contraindications, such as hypertension, hyperlipidemia, and smoking. They provide excellent cycle control with a monthly withdrawal bleed and suppression of the endometrium. Oral contraceptives can be continued until an FSH level greater than 40 IU/L during the week of placebo pills confirms ovarian failure. Standard postmenopausal hormone replacement can then be used. A sequential program of 12 days of progestin, 5- to 10-mg medroxyprogesterone acetate, or 5-mg norethindrone acetate on a monthly basis is an alternative and is continued until failure of withdrawal bleeding occurs, indicating the need for estrogen replacement. Endometrial hyperplasia requires a more aggressive progestational regimen. Atypical adenomatous endometrial hyperplasia is considered by most to be the equivalent of an intraepithelial malignancy, and hysterectomy is often advised. Management of several types of endometrial hyperplasia other than atypical adenomatous hyperplasia can generally be accomplished by monthly administration of a progestin such as medroxyprogesterone acetate, 10 mg per day for 12 days, or norethindrone acetate, 5 mg per day for 12 days. Another endometrial biopsy should be obtained within 3 to 6 months to assess for resolution of the hyperplasia. A more aggressive hormonal regimen uses continuous high-dose progestin for 3 to 6 months (i.e., megestrol 20 to 160 mg per day).

Any of the regimens currently in use for postmenopausal hormonal replacement therapy can cause uterine bleeding. Since the WHI, the number of women using postmenopausal HT has markedly decreased, but there is still a role for this therapy in symptomatic women. A summary of the guidelines published by several major medical societies can be found in a recent publication by Dr. Pines. Unopposed estrogen is no longer recommended for postmenopausal hormone replacement in the case of an intact uterus because hyperplasia develops in 18% to 32% of cases and because unopposed estrogen has an up to sevenfold increased risk of endometrial carcinoma. Cyclic estrogen–progestin regimens significantly decrease this risk to less than 1% with 12 days of progestin. There are numerous dosage regimens for the use of conjugated estrogens 0.625 to 1.25 mg; micronized E_2 1 to 2 mg; esterified estrogens 0.625 to 1.25 mg; and E_2 patches. Although estrogen replacement therapy performs well if used for only 21 to 25 days of the month, there is no clinical reason for its discontinuance, and recent recommendations are to continue it throughout the entire cycle. The progestin regimens are those that have already been outlined. The bleeding that accompanies these commonly used continuous-estrogen and cyclic progestin regimens should occur predictably, at the conclusion of the progestin phase of the cyclic administration. Most investigators of the subject now agree that the predictable and appropriately timed withdrawal bleeding that occurs with these regimens does not require sampling for endometrial histology. As a general rule, just as intermenstrual bleeding during the regular menstruating years dictates investigation and management, so do patterns of postmenopausal bleeding not following an anticipated schedule require investigation and management.

The most important point about the significance of postmenopausal bleeding is its frequent association with gynecologic malignancy, particularly endometrial carcinoma. Although the incidence of malignancy to explain postmenopausal bleeding has decreased in recent decades, diagnostic efforts must carefully consider and rule out possible malignancy by use of appropriate diagnostic procedures, especially careful pelvic examination and uterine curettage. An endometrial biopsy is helpful for the diagnosis of suspected endometrial carcinoma only if the biopsy is positive. The definitive method for obtaining adequate histology for diagnosis is hysteroscopy and D&C.

CURETTAGE OF THE UTERUS

Indications and Contraindications

STEPS IN THE PROCEDURE
Dilatation and Curettage
• Lithotomy position, empty bladder, and sterilely drape perineum
• Thorough exam under anesthesia to evaluate uterine size and position
• Adequate exposure of the cervix with open-sided or weighted speculum
• Assess depth of uterine cavity using a uterine sound
• Curettage of the endocervix using a small box curette
• Dilatation of cervix using Hegar or Hank dilators
• Measure endometrial cavity depth using a sound
• Curettage of anterior, lateral, and posterior walls using a small or medium malleable, bluntly serrated curette

It is important that D&C be performed for the proper indications, be performed correctly to obtain the most useful information, and be performed safely. A curettage performed properly and with aseptic technique involves little risk, but if precautions are disregarded, complications and even death can result.

The chief purpose of curettage of the uterus is the removal of endometrial or endocervical tissue for histologic study of cases of AUB. Although classical curettage of the uterus continues to be a useful procedure, new practices and instrumentation permit the procurement of endometrium as a screening diagnostic test under many circumstances. Appropriate use of such procedures can reduce significantly the need for operating room curettage. Careful pelvic examination under relaxation anesthesia has been an important adjunctive diagnostic aid to conventional D&C, but the precision and availability of ultrasound and other imaging techniques have brought them to the forefront of importance in diagnosis.

Outpatient Curettage

Over the years, there have been efforts to lower the cost of D&C by making it an outpatient procedure. Today, D&C is often performed satisfactorily on an outpatient basis or in an ambulatory surgery center. Reports by Sandmire and Austin and by Martin and Rust are among many that record favorable experiences with this procedure.

As mentioned earlier, endometrial sampling today is often performed by biopsy, suction, or D&C as an office procedure. Only if they show frank adenocarcinoma can the outpatient biopsy results be considered definitive. If the histology of the office procedures is negative, a more serious condition has not been ruled out. A further note of caution is that none of the office endometrial sampling methods can ensure the removal of an endometrial polyp. Therefore, endometrial carcinoma in a polyp could be missed, as could a polyp that is a source of benign bleeding. Office sampling techniques are used only as screening procedures; if the results are negative, a more thorough evaluation using hysteroscopy is indicated. Office hysteroscopy can sometimes identify missed pathologies, such as a polyp or a submucous myoma, or to allow directed biopsy of a suspicious endometrium.

Indications for obtaining endometrial histology by one or more of the aforementioned methods include the following:

- Abnormal bleeding at any premenopausal age, especially when not corrected promptly by medical management; in women older than 35 years of age; or if a submucous myoma is suspected (include hysteroscopy or hysterosalpingography),
- Postmenopausal bleeding of any amount, regardless of a finding of atrophic vaginitis, polyp, or urethral caruncle,
- Prehysterectomy in the postmenopausal woman at risk for endocervical or endometrial carcinoma, and
- Postmenopausal vaginal surgery without hysterectomy in women at risk for endometrial pathology.

When office procedures fail to establish the diagnosis, hysteroscopy is the preferred diagnostic method. Unlike blind D&C, it allows for visualization of the uterine cavity and direct biopsies. Hysteroscopy performed under general anesthesia allows for more extensive operative procedures if indicated. Occasionally, new and important pelvic findings will be discovered. In a study of 2,666 women requiring curettage, McElin and colleagues found unanticipated adnexal masses in 30 women during pelvic examination under anesthesia before D&C. Twenty-eight masses were benign, and two were malignant. Even in women who have medical contraindications to anesthesia, office hysteroscopy can be performed with minimal anesthesia. A single curettage will not remove all of the surface endometrium completely from the uterine cavity. Repeated studies have demonstrated the inability of a thorough curettage to remove more than 50% to 60% of the endometrium when the procedure has been performed by experienced gynecologists immediately before a planned hysterectomy. Stock and Kanbour, from McGee Hospital in Pittsburgh, observed that in 60% of hysterectomy specimens studied, less than 50% of the endometrial surface had been removed by a prehysterectomy curettage. They also found 26 cases of endometrial carcinoma that had been classified as clinically normal-appearing tissue on prehysterectomy curettage; six of these carcinomas were reported as benign on frozen section. These facts and other similar experiences indicate that it is difficult to be certain of the histology of the endometrium by gross examination of the curetting. If the symptoms warrant curettage, then the endometrium deserves a full histologic diagnosis under hysteroscopic visualization.

Curettage is also performed for bleeding from a cervical stump and is frequently performed as part of a cervical conization to rule out extension of cervical carcinoma into the endometrium. Helmkamp and associates found no evidence of endometrial abnormality in any of 114 curettage specimens removed at the time of 114 cervical conizations. These investigators recommend that curettage at the time of cervical conization should not be performed routinely but should be performed selectively in postmenopausal and perimenopausal patients when the cytology smear shows abnormal glandular cells or when an intrauterine abnormality is suspected.

The chief contraindication to curettage is infection. Acute endometritis and salpingitis are conditions under which curettage should be avoided. If curettage is necessary for removal of infected placental tissue, it should be preceded by a period of parenteral antibiotic therapy adequate to achieve therapeutic tissue levels. Endometritis associated with retained products of conception will remain unresolved until the infected necrotic material is removed. Curettage is also contraindicated when pyometra is present.

Technique of Curettage of the Uterus

After the patient is anesthetized and placed in the lithotomy position, the bladder is emptied with a catheter. The pelvic organs are examined thoroughly before the patient is prepped and draped. The procedure includes a bimanual rectovaginal–abdominal examination. The examination under anesthesia is one of the most informative features of this operation because it can provide anatomic details of the reproductive tract that are unrecognizable without anesthesia. The vagina and perineum are cleaned with the usual technique.

Fractional curettage is an attempt to remove tissue samples from the endocervical canal apart from tissue removed from the endometrial cavity. The cervical canal should be curetted before dilatation of the cervical canal and curettage of the endometrial cavity. The special shape of the small Gusberg curette makes it particularly useful for curetting the endocervix. Differential curettage of the endocervix, separate from the endometrium, is important for diagnosis of endometrial carcinoma that may have extended to the endocervix. All cases of perimenopausal bleeding should be fractionally curetted; this procedure is too often neglected. If the endocervical curettage is not performed, a second fractional curettage is required to determine the anatomic boundaries of endometrial carcinoma. The value of fractional curettage has been questioned, but Chen and Lee and others have emphasized the importance of cervical stromal invasion, rather than the finding of tumor tissue, as the crucial criterion in endocervical curetting affecting staging and prognosis.

The uterine cavity is then sounded to determine its size and to confirm the position determined from examination under anesthesia. The cervical canal is dilated with the Hegar or Hank-Bradley (Fig. 26.6) dilator. A dilatation to 8 or 9 mm by a Hegar dilator (Fig. 26.7) is sufficient for the usual diagnostic curettage. A gauze is placed in the posterior vaginal fornix along the posterior retractor so that the blood and the endometrium removed from the uterus can fall on it. Before the curettage is performed, the uterine cavity is explored for

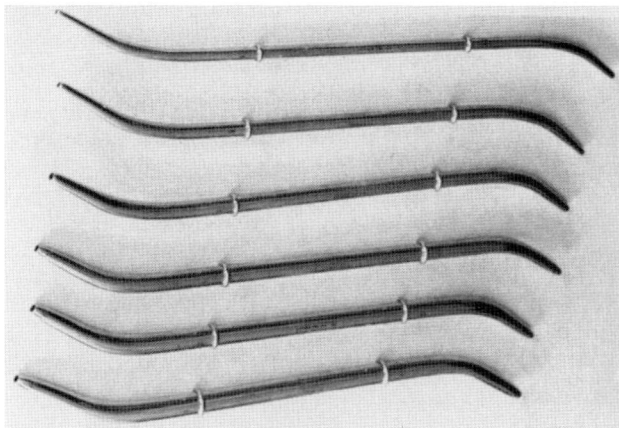

FIGURE 26.6 Hank-Bradley dilators in graduated sizes. Note central canal that extends through length of dilator.

endometrial polyps by use of a narrow stone forceps. This forceps can be opened and closed as the tip of the forceps is moved systematically across the dome of the uterus and the anterior and posterior walls. An endometrial polyp can be easily missed with an ordinary curette, and unnecessary hysterectomies have been performed because of supposed persistent

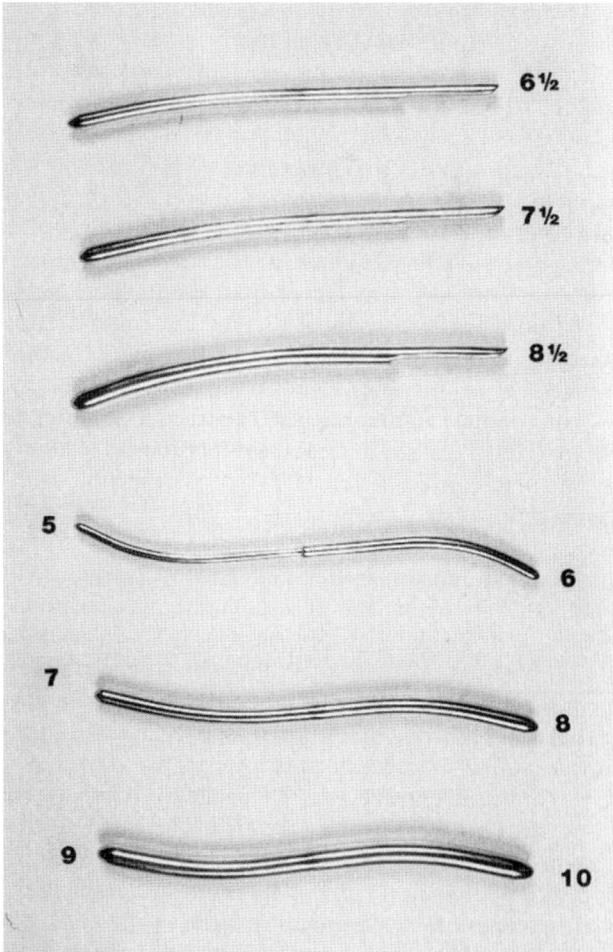

FIGURE 26.7 Graduated Hegar dilators and "half-size" Hegar dilators.

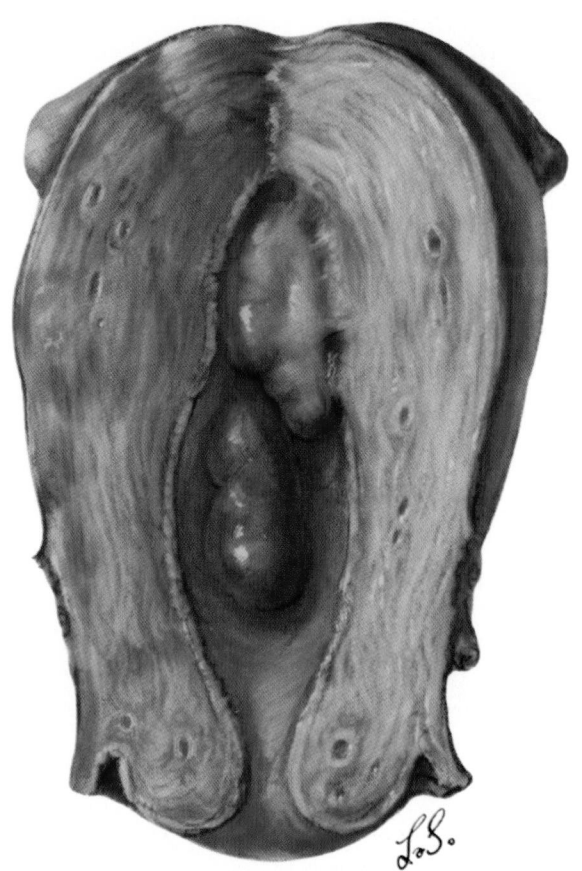

FIGURE 26.8 Opened uterus, showing two separate endometrial polyps.

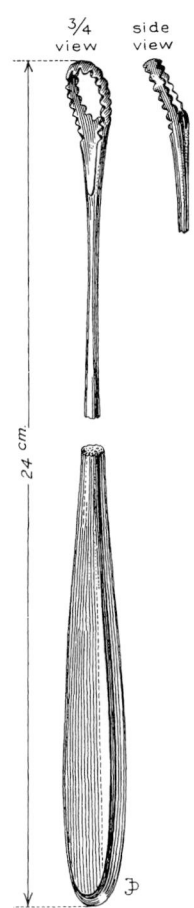

FIGURE 26.9 Small serrated curette for routine curettage.

or recurrent dysfunctional bleeding after curettage (**Fig. 26.8**). If polyp forceps are routinely used, such operations can be avoided. It is easier to identify and remove an endometrial polyp if the uterine cavity is explored with the stone forceps before the uterus is curetted. In a 28-month period during which forceps were used routinely at the Johns Hopkins Hospital, Josey found that endometrial polyp was diagnosed 130 times. In 83 of these cases, the polyp was removed by forceps. Although the sessile form of a submucous myoma is diagnosed easily by noting an irregularity of the uterine wall with the curette, the pedunculated variety, like the endometrial polyp, can escape detection because of its narrow stalk. Removal of pedunculated leiomyoma can sometimes be accomplished with the polyp forceps. A uterine septum can also sometimes be detected with the forceps, but imaging modalities such as saline sonohysterogram and hysterosalpingogram are more accurate diagnostic tests. The procedure is most likely to be diagnostic and therapeutic when it is combined with direct visualization of the uterine cavity through hysteroscopy. A small-sized or medium-sized, malleable, bluntly serrated curette (**Fig. 26.9**) is then introduced into the uterus, and the entire uterine cavity is systematically curetted. The anterior, lateral, and posterior walls should be sampled (**Fig. 26.10**). The handle of the curette should be held gently, as one would hold a pencil. The instrument is held loosely as it is inserted for the full distance. Pressure is then exerted against the uterine wall as the curette is drawn in an outward direction. Because the instrument is malleable, its curvature can be changed to conform to the contour of the uterine cavity. A uterine "cry," vibrations felt in the hand holding the curette, is often used as a sign that adequate tissue has been removed. It should be remembered, however, that overly aggressive curettage can lead to scarring of the endometrial cavity.

The unclotted blood is absorbed quickly by the gauze sponge, leaving the relatively clean endometrium to be placed in a prepared container with appropriate fixative. Again, the curettings should be removed carefully from the sponge with a pair of smooth-tipped forceps and placed immediately in the fixative. The curettings should be examined carefully at this time for fatty tissue or other unusual tissue.

When curettage is performed as a curative measure for removal of placental tissue, a large, blunt, smooth curette is used to lessen the possibilities of perforation and endometrial sclerosis. The larger and softer the uterus, the larger the curette should be and the more care one should exercise to avoid these complications. When large masses of placental tissue are present, ovum forceps are most useful when used in conjunction with the curette. High-vacuum suction is now used almost routinely for placental tissue removal.

Routine blind biopsy of the cervix is usually unrewarding if a negative cytologic smear has been obtained and there is no suspicious cervical lesion. A blind biopsy of the cervix at the time of curettage should not be performed unless an abnormal lesion is present. If a gross lesion is seen, directed biopsy of the lesion is indicated.

Complications of Cervical Dilatation and Uterine Curettage

If the position and the consistency of the uterus are carefully observed on bimanual examination under anesthesia before curettage is begun, perforation will rarely occur. Special care should be exercised with a uterus that is acutely anteflexed or

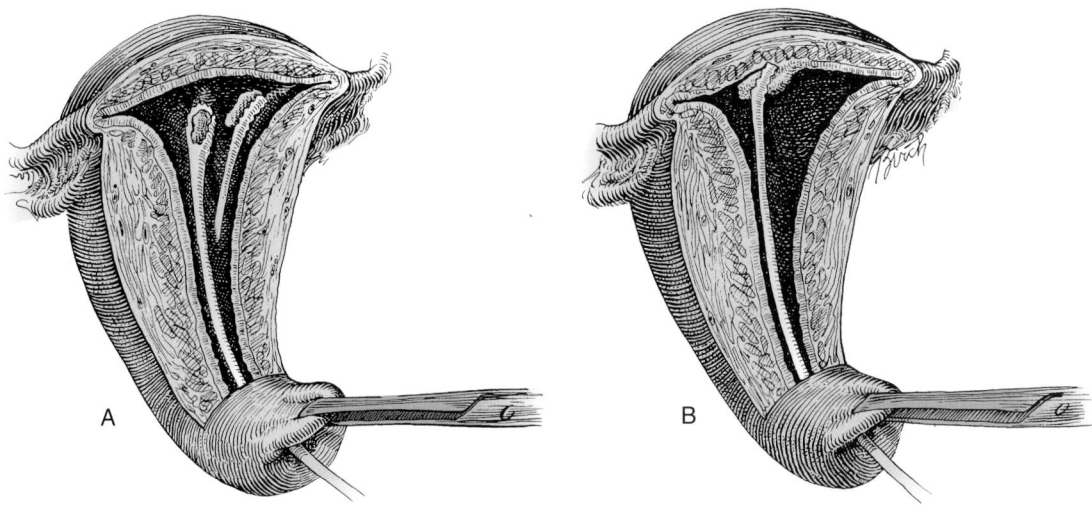

FIGURE 26.10 Method of curetting the uterine cavity systematically. **A:** The anterior, posterior, and lateral walls of the cavity are curetted systematically. **B:** The top of the cavity is then curetted thoroughly.

retroflexed (**Figs. 26.11** and **26.12**). With cervical stenosis, pregnancy, or intrauterine malignancy, perforation is more likely. The postmenopausal atrophic uterus can be perforated with only slight force applied to the uterine sound or the curette. Perforation is discovered when the sound or the curette fails to encounter resistance where it normally should, as judged by the palpated size of the uterus and initially measurement of the endometrial cavity by uterine sound. Abdominal ultrasound visualization of the uterus, cervix, and endocervical canal, which may require a distended bladder, can be useful in guiding the passage of either a dilator or a curette through the endocervical canal into the endometrial cavity in difficult cases. Ghosh and Chaudhuri found misoprostol in a dose of 400 µg twelve hours prior to the procedure can facilitate cervical dilation.

Perforation by the uterine sound or cervical dilator causes less damage than perforation by the sharp curette or suction cannula. Sharp curettage for legally induced abortion has a major complication rate that is two to three times higher than that for suction curettage, according to Grimes and Cates. The two principal dangers of uterine perforation are bleeding and trauma to the abdominal viscera. Lateral perforation through the uterine vessels is especially dangerous from the standpoint of intraperitoneal hemorrhage and broad ligament hematoma formation. Damage can occur to the bowel, omentum, mesentery, ureter, and fallopian tube. Perforation of the anterior or posterior wall of the uterus by a small curette in performing a diagnostic curettage is usually not a serious accident. However, it is usually necessary to discontinue curettage. One must

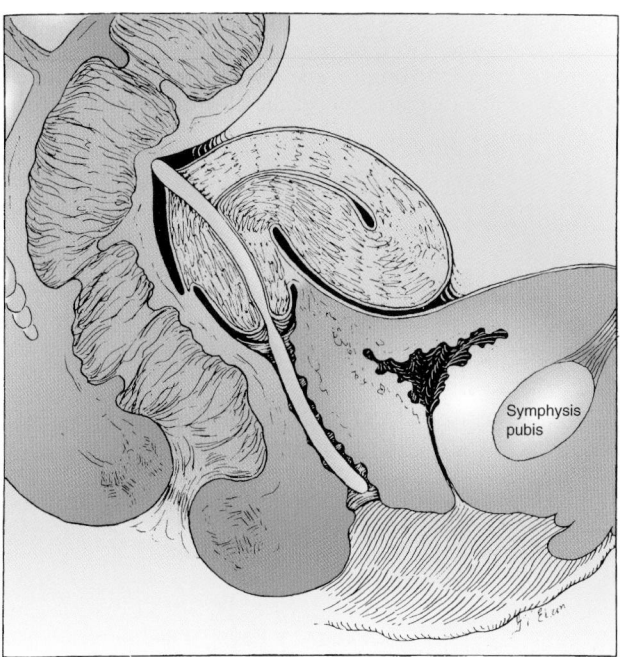

FIGURE 26.11 Perforation of the acutely anteflexed uterus. The uterus was thought to be in retroposition, and the Hegar dilator was erroneously directed posteriorly.

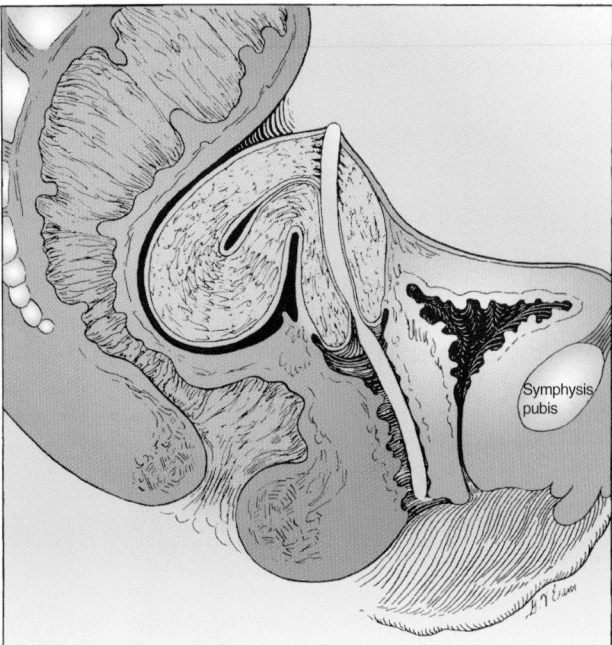

FIGURE 26.12 Perforation of the retroflexed uterus. The uterus was thought to be in anteposition, and the Hegar dilator was erroneously directed anteriorly.

watch carefully for signs of hemorrhage or infection. If signs of hemorrhage develop, the abdomen should be opened and the uterine wound sutured. If signs of infection occur, broad-spectrum antibiotics should be given. If a pelvic abscess develops, the abscess should be drained if possible. As described by Chappel and colleagues, this can sometimes be accomplished under radiographic guidance. Serious hemorrhage or infection occurs only rarely. When serious damage from perforation is suspected, laparoscopy can be performed to assess the extent of the damage and the needed repair. According to MacKenzie and Bibby, complications occurred in 1.7% of cases of D&C. McElin and colleagues reported that 0.5% of cases had postoperative febrile morbidity after D&C. Uterine perforation occurred in 0.63% of cases.

One should be absolutely certain that the endometrial cavity has been entered when D&C is performed for postmenopausal bleeding. A relatively stenotic internal cervical os and a fear of uterine perforation can prevent entry into the uterine cavity above the internal cervical os, resulting in failure to curette the uterine cavity and consequent failure to diagnose the cause of the bleeding. Again, ultrasound can be a valuable tool for confirming placement of the curette tip in the endometrial cavity. Many office hysteroscopes are small enough in diameter that they can be safely used in patients with cervical stenosis. It is also possible to use laminaria or misoprostol to facilitate cervical dilatation.

Perforation of a pregnant uterus is a more serious complication than is perforation of the nonpregnant uterus. First, there is the requirement that all remaining pregnancy tissue be completely removed to prevent sepsis. To accomplish this blindly when there is a defect in the uterine wall is unsafe. Second, the pregnant uterus is a much more vascular organ than is the nonpregnant uterus, and intraperitoneal bleeding can be profuse without significant external bleeding. Third, it often is difficult to be certain when the perforation occurred. If a high-vacuum suction Vacurect has passed through the myometrium and the vacuum has been activated, major bowel injury can be present. These considerations have led to the following protocol for D&C of the pregnant uterus:

1. Never activate the vacuum suction if there is any question about the safe location of the Vacurect within the uterine cavity.

2. Laparoscope any pregnant uterus that is possibly perforated. With the laparoscope in place, a second operator can evacuate remaining placental tissue while the laparoscopist monitors safety. Many perforations in which no other visceral damage has occurred are fundal. If laparoscopic observation confirms that bleeding is minimal, the perforation can be managed conservatively with antibiotics and serial hematocrit determination for 24 to 48 hours. If there is no evidence of continued bleeding or developing infection, the patient can be discharged.

3. During laparoscopy, if there is any evidence of intestinal injury or any suspicion of such injury, or if bleeding is significant, then laparotomy is mandatory. Unfortunately, bowel injury by high-vacuum suction may require bowel resection and anastomosis.

Figure 26.13 shows a uterus removed immediately after a perforation because of intraperitoneal bleeding. Word analyzed 70 accidental uterine perforations. Among these, an unplanned hysterectomy was performed on seven unprepared patients. In none of these cases did the intraperitoneal findings indicate the need for hysterectomy. In fact, hysterectomy compounded the surgical error. Fifty-five patients were treated conservatively, and only one developed a complication, in the form of a pelvic abscess that was drained by colpotomy. Forty-one of the 70 perforations occurred in postmenopausal women.

When a large, boggy, postabortion or puerperal uterus is perforated by a large curette or placental forceps in removing placental tissue, there is more danger of hemorrhage, infection, or injury to bowel. The treatment protocols and the procedures for these serious complications are discussed elsewhere in this textbook.

Asherman syndrome is a pathologic condition of intrauterine adhesions that can cause secondary amenorrhea, other menstrual irregularities, infertility, or recurrent abortion. Numerous investigators have shown a strong association between puerperal D&C and the formation of synechiae that can partially or completely obliterate the endometrial cavity. No incidence figures are available because no prospective studies have been performed, but factors other than pregnancy that increase the risk of endometrial sclerosis after D&C are infection, scant endometrium that exposes the basalis to trauma, and a hypoestrogenic state. Rarely, significant synechiae are seen in the absence of an antecedent

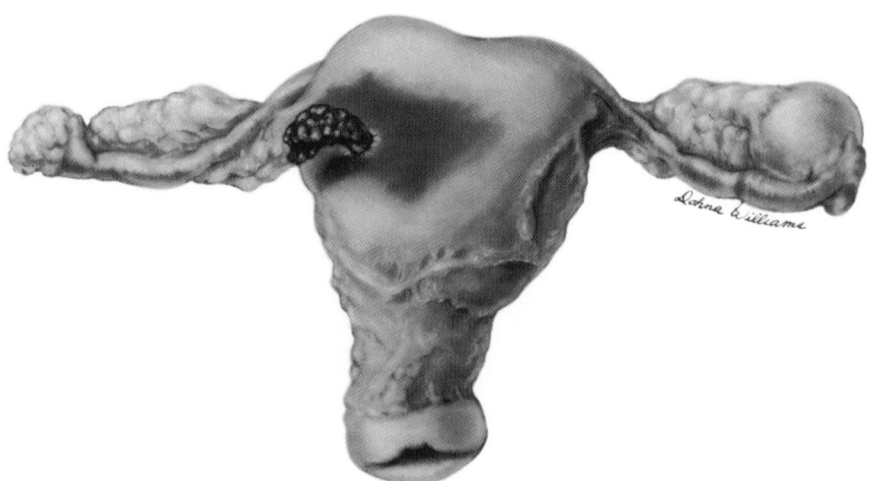

FIGURE 26.13 Result of uterine perforation. Specimen removed directly after perforation.

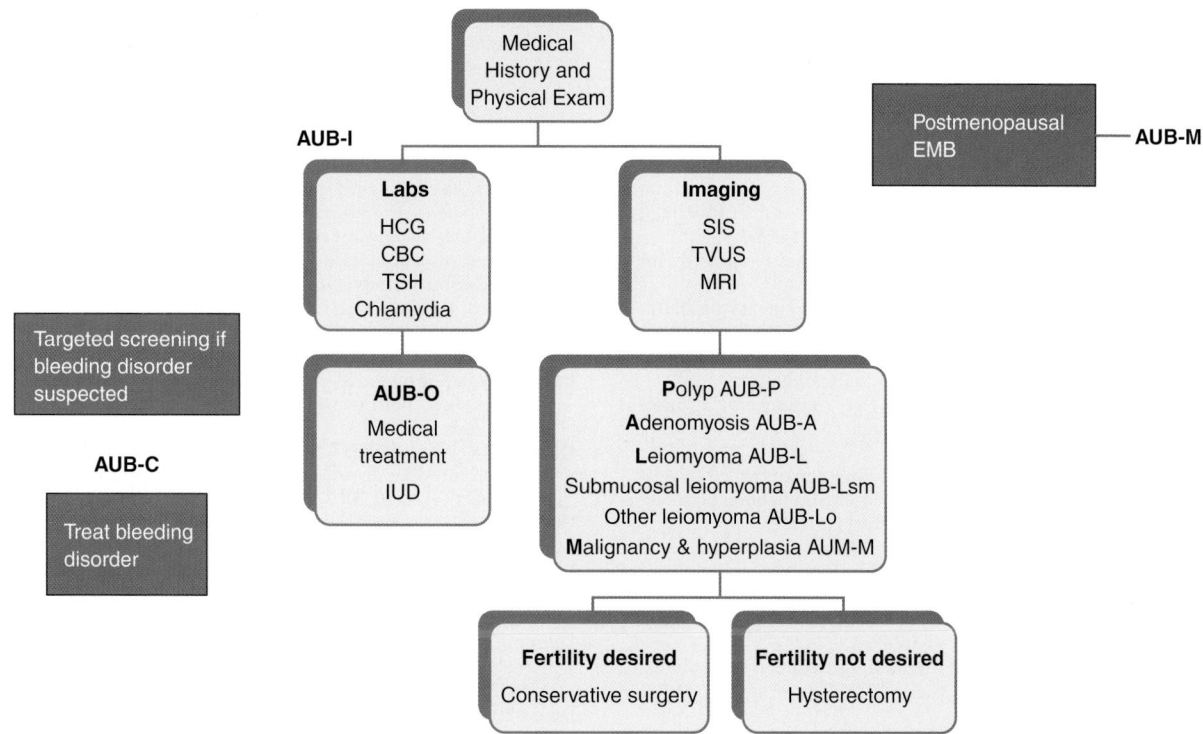

FIGURE 26.14 Diagnostic evaluation and treatment of AUB.

curettage. Cases have been reported after severe endometritis, tuberculosis, myomectomy, and cesarean section. Diagnosis is made by clinical history, hysterosalpingography, or hysteroscopy. Therapy requires lysis of adhesions by repeat curettage or, preferably, by hysteroscopic scissors.

Patency of the uterine cavity is maintained with an intrauterine device or balloon catheter, and endometrial regeneration is stimulated by oral estrogen therapy. Women with synechiae are significantly more likely to have placental abruption (2.1% vs. 0.6%), premature rupture of membranes (5.5% vs. 2.3%), and cesarean delivery for malpresentation (5.1% vs. 3.0%). In a recent review of 296 pregnancies with uterine synechiae and over 65,000 pregnancies without synechiae, Tuuli and colleagues did not find a significant increase in placenta previa, fetal growth restriction, stillbirth, and preterm delivery.

This chapter has reviewed normal menstruation, the pathophysiology underlying AUB, the evaluation of AUB, and current treatment modalities. It concludes with a detailed description of the technique of dilatation and curettage and management of complications of this procedure. Despite emerging medical and surgical therapies, AUB remains a common medical problem among women. An organized approach to the diagnosis and treatment of this problem is critical to the successful management of AUB. **Figure 26.14** provides an algorithm for the diagnosis and evaluation of AUB.

BEST SURGICAL PRACTICES

- Although hysteroscopy is the gold standard for evaluating endometrial cavity pathology, SIS has comparable sensitivity and is less invasive and less expensive.
- Historic data showed higher amenorrhea rates with endometrial ablation using endomyometrial resection. However, newer techniques of hydrothermablation, radiofrequency current, and microwaves have comparable amenorrhea rates. Hydrothermablation has the advantage of visualization of the endometrial cavity, radiofrequency

ablation does not require endometrial pretreatment, and microwave endometrial ablation has been reported to be successful in the presence of small submucous myomas.
- Endometrial sampling can be done by Pipelle, four-quadrant endometrial biopsy, or formal dilatation and curettage (D&C). All of these techniques can miss significant lesions, and the concurrent use of vaginal ultrasonography or SIS will improve sensitivity.
- Hysteroscopy is a valuable adjunct to D&C, particularly in the patient at higher risk for focal endometrial pathology that might be missed on endometrial sampling.
- Abdominal ultrasound guidance may reduce the risk of complications (e.g., perforation during difficult cervical D&C, such as in the stenotic postmenopausal patient or in the case of a large uterus).

BIBLIOGRAPHY

American Congress of Obstetricians and Gynecologists Practice Bulletin #128, July 2012 Diagnosis of Abnormal Uterine Bleeding in Reproductive-Aged Women.

American Congress of Obstetricians and Gynecologists Committee Opinion #557, April 2013 Management of Acute Abnormal Uterine Bleeding in Nonpregnant Reproductive-Aged Women.

Aksel S, Jones GS. Etiology and treatment of dysfunctional uterine bleeding. *Obstet Gynecol* 1974;44:1.

Ammerman SR, Nelson AL. A new progestogen-only medical therapy for outpatient management of acute, abnormal uterine bleeding: a pilot study. *Am J Obstet Gynecol* 2013;208:499.

Anderson ABM, Haynes PJ, Guillebaud J, et al. Reduction of menstrual blood loss by prostaglandin synthesis inhibition. *Lancet* 1976;1:774.

Andolf E, Dahlander K, Aspenberg P. Ultrasonic thickness of the endometrium correlated to body weight in asymptomatic postmenopausal women. *Obstet Gynecol* 1993;82:936.

Asherman J. Amenorrhea traumatica (atretica). *J Obstet Gynaecol Br Emp* 1948;55:23.

Atwood JT, Toth TL, Schiff I. Abnormal uterine bleeding in the perimenopause. *Int J Fertil* 1993;38:261.

Azziz R, Zacur HA. 21-Hydroxylase deficiency in female hyperandrogenemia. *J Clin Endocrinol Metab* 1989;69:577.

Barnett JM. Suction curettage on unanesthetized outpatients. *Obstet Gynecol* 1973;42:672.

Battacharya S, Cameron IM, Parkin DE, et al. A pragmatic randomized comparison of transcervical resection of the endometrium with endometrial laser ablation for the treatment of menorrhagia. *Br J Obstet Gynaecol* 1999;106:360.

Bayer SR, DeCherney AH. Clinical manifestations and treatment of dysfunctional uterine bleeding. *JAMA* 1993;269:1823.

Beller FK. Observations on the clotting of menstrual blood and clot formation. *Am J Obstet Gynecol* 1971;3:535.

Bettocchi S, Ceci O, Vicino M, et al. Diagnostic inadequacy of dilatation and curettage. *Fertil Steril* 2001;75:803.

Beyth Y, Yaffe H, Levii I, et al. Retrograde seeding of endometrium: a sequela of tubal flushing. *Fertil Steril* 1975;26:1094.

Bijen CB, deBock GH, ten Hoor KA, et al. Role of endocervical curettage in the preoperative staging of endometrial carcinoma. *Gynecol Oncol* 2009;112:521.

Bongers M, Bourdrez P, Mol B, et al. Randomised controlled trial of bipolar radio-frequency endometrial ablation and balloon endometrial ablation. *Br J Obstet Gynaecol* 2004;111:1095.

Brooks PG. Complications of operative hysteroscopy: how safe is it? *Clin Obstet Gynecol* 1993;35:256.

Brooks PG. Hysteroscopic surgery using the resectoscope: myomas, ablation, septae and synechiae: does pre-operative medication help?. *Clin Obstet Gynecol* 1993;35:249.

Brooks PG, Serden SP. Endometrial ablation in women with abnormal uterine bleeding aged fifty and over. *J Reprod Med* 1992;37:682.

Brooks-Carter GN, Killackey MA, Neuwirth RS. Adenocarcinoma of the endometrium after endometrial ablation. *Obstet Gynecol* 2000;96:836.

Busfield R, Farquhar C, Sowter M, et al. A randomized trial comparing the levonorgestrel intrauterine system and thermal balloon ablation for heavy menstrual bleeding. *Br J Obstet Gynaecol* 2006;113:257.

Bushnell DM, Martin LM, Moore KA, et al. Menorrhagia Impact Questionnaire: assessing the influence of heavy menstrual bleeding on quality of life. *Curr Med Res Opin* 2010;26:2745.

Cameron IT, Haining R, Lumsden M-A, et al. The effects of mefenamic acid and norethisterone on measured menstrual blood loss. *Obstet Gynecol* 1990;76:85.

Chappell CA, Wiesenfeld HC. Pathogenesis, diagnosis and management of severe pelvic inflammatory disease and tuboovarian abscess. *Clin Obstet Gynecol* 2012;55:893.

Chen SS, Lee L. Reappraisal of endocervical curettage in predicting cervical involvement by endometrial carcinoma. *Obstet Gynecol* 1986;31:50.

Chiazze L Jr, Brayer FT, Macisco JJ Jr, et al. The length and variability of the human menstrual cycle. *JAMA* 1968;203:377.

Claessens EA, Cowell CA. Acute adolescent menorrhagia. *Am J Obstet Gynecol* 1981;139:227.

Cohen CJ, Gusberg SB, Koffler D. Histologic screening for endometrial cancer. *Gynecol Oncol* 1974;2:279.

Cook J, Seman E. Pregnancy following endometrial ablation: case history and literature review. *Obstet Gynecol Surv* 2003;58:551.

Cooper J, Anderson T, Fortin C, et al. Microwave endometrial ablation vs. rollerball electroablation for menorrhagia: a multicenter randomized trial. *J Am Assoc Gynecol Laparosc* 2004;11:394.

Cooper J, Gimpelson R, Laberge P, et al. A randomized multicenter trial of safety and efficacy of the Novasure system in treatment of menorrhagia. *J Am Assoc Gynecol Laparosc* 2002;9:418.

Copperman AB, DeCherney AH, Olive DL. A case of endometrial cancer following endometrial ablation for dysfunctional uterine bleeding. *Obstet Gynecol* 1993;82:640.

Corson S. A multicenter evaluation of endometrial ablation by Hydro ThermAblator and rollerball for treatment of menorrhagia. *J Am Assoc Gynecol Laparosc* 2001;8:359.

Corson SL, Brill AI, Brooks PG, et al. Interim results of the American VESTA trial of endometrial ablation. *J Am Assoc Gynecol Laparosc* 1999;6:45.

Coulam CB, Annegers JF, Kranz JS. Chronic anovulation syndrome and associated neoplasia. *Obstet Gynecol* 1983;61:403.

Crosignani PG, Vercellini P, Mosconi P, et al. Levonorgestrel-releasing intrauterine device versus hysteroscopic endometrial resection in the treatment of dysfunctional uterine bleeding. *Obstet Gynecol* 1997;90:257.

Davies AJ, Anderson ABM, Turnbull AC. Reduction by naproxen of excessive menstrual bleeding in women using intrauterine devices. *Obstet Gynecol* 1981;57:74.

Denis R Jr, Barnett JM, Forbes SE. Diagnostic suction curettage. *Obstet Gynecol* 1973;42:301.

DeVore G, Owens O, Case NL. Use of intravenous Premarin in the treatment of dysfunctional uterine bleeding: a double-blind randomized control study. *Obstet Gynecol* 1982;59:285.

Dickson RB, Johnson MD, el-Ashry D, et al. Breast cancer: influence of endocrine hormones, growth factors and genetic alterations. *Adv Exp Med Biol* 1993;330:119.

Dickson RB, Lippman ME. Estrogenic regulation of growth and polypeptide growth factor secretion in human breast carcinoma. *Endocr Rev* 1987;8:39.

Dilley A, Drews C, Miller C, et al. Von Willebrand disease and other inherited bleeding disorders in women with diagnosed menorrhagia. *Obstet Gynecol* 2001;97:630.

Dodson MG. Use of transvaginal ultrasound in diagnosing the etiology of menometrorrhagia. *J Reprod Med* 1994;39:362.

Donnez J, Vilos G, Gannon MJ, et al. Goserelin acetate (Zoladex) plus endometrial ablation for dysfunctional uterine bleeding: a large randomized double-blind study. *Fertil Steril* 1997;68:29.

Donnez J, Tatarchuk TF, Bouchard P, et al. Ulipristal acetate versus placebo for fibroid treatment before surgery. *New Engl J Med* 2012;366:409.

Dueholm M, Lundorf E, Hansen ES, et al. Evaluation of the uterine cavity with magnetic resonance imaging, transvaginal sonography, hysterosonographic examination, and diagnostic hysteroscopy. *Fertil Steril* 2001;76:350.

Economos K, MacDonald PC, Casey ML. Endothelin-1 gene expression and protein biosynthesis in human endometrium: potential modulator of endometrial blood flow. *J Clin Endocrinol Metab* 1992;74:14.

Ejskjær K, Sørensen BS, Poulsen SS, et al. Expression of the epidermal growth factor system in human endometrium during the menstrual cycle. *Mol Hum Reprod* 2005;11:543.

Evans RM. The steroid and thyroid hormone receptor family. *Science* 1988;240:889.

Falcone T, Desjardins C, Bourgue J, et al. Dysfunctional uterine bleeding in adolescents. *J Reprod Med* 1994;39:761.

Fleming H, Oster AG, Pickel H, et al. Arteriovenous malformations of the uterus. *Obstet Gynecol* 1989;73:209.

Fraser IS, Baird DT. Blood production and ovarian secretion rates of estradiol-17, 3 and estrone in women and dysfunctional uterine bleeding. *J Clin Endocrinol Metab* 1974;38:727.

Fraser IS, Michie EA, Wide L, et al. Pituitary gonadotropins and ovarian function in adolescent dysfunctional uterine bleeding. *J Clin Endocrinol Metab* 1973;37:407.

Fraser IS, Pearse C, Shearman RP, et al. Efficacy of mefenamic acid in patients with a complaint of menorrhagia. *Obstet Gynecol* 1981;58:543.

Friedman AJ, Juneau-Norcross M, Rein MS. Adverse effects of leuprolide acetate depot treatment. *Fertil Steril* 1993;59:448.

Fritsch N. Ein Fall von volligen Schwund der gebarmutter Hohle nach Auskratzung. *Zentralbl Gumsrl* 1894;18:1337.

Galant C, Berlière M, Dubois D, et al. Focal expression and final activity of matrix metalloproteinases may explain irregular dysfunctional endometrial bleeding. *Am J Pathol* 2004;165:83.

Garry R, Shelly-Jones D, Mooney P, et al. Six hundred endometrial ablations. *Obstet Gynecol* 1995;85:24.

Ghosh A, Chaudhuri P. Misoprostol for cervical ripening prior to gynecological transcervical procedures. *Arch Gynecol Obstet* 2013;287:967.

Goldrath M. Evaluation of Hydro ThermAblator and rollerball endometrial ablation for menorrhagia 3 years after treatment. *J Am Assoc Gynecol Laparosc* 2003;10:505.

Gregg RH. The praxeology of the office dilatation and curettage. *Am J Obstet Gynecol* 1981;140:179.

Grimes D. Estimating vaginal blood loss. *J Reprod Med* 1979;22:190.

Grimes D, Cates W Jr. Complications from legally induced abortion: a review. *Obstet Gynecol Surv* 1979;34:177.

Guidice LC, Dsupin BA, Jin IH, et al. Differential expression of messenger ribonucleic acids encoding insulin-like growth factors and their receptors in human uterine endometrium and decidua. *J Clin Endocrinol Metab* 1993;76:1115.

Guido R, Kanbour-Shakir A, Rulin M, et al. Pipelle endometrial sampling: sensitivity in the detection of endometrial lesions. *J Reprod Med* 1995;40:553.

Guillebaud J, Barnett MD, Gordon YB. Plasma ferritin levels as an index of iron deficiency in women using intrauterine devices. *Br J Obstet Gynaecol* 1979;86:51.

Gull B, Carlsson SA, Karlsson B, et al. Transvaginal ultrasonography of the endometrium in women with postmenopausal bleeding: Is it always necessary to perform an endometrial biopsy? *Am J Obstet Gynecol* 2000;182:509.

Hallberg L, Hogdahl A, Nilsson L, et al. Menstrual blood and iron deficiency. *Acta Med Scand* 1966;180:639.

Hallberg L, Nilsson L. Constancy of individual menstrual blood loss. *Acta Obstet Gynecol Scand* 1964;43:352.

Hallberg L, Nilsson L. Determination of menstrual blood loss. *Scand J Clin Lab Invest* 1964;16:244.

Handwerger S, Richards RG, Markoff E. The physiology of decidual prolactin and other decidual protein hormones. *Trends Endocrinol Metab* 1992;3:91.

Haynes PJ, Hodgson H, Anderson ABM, et al. Measurement of menstrual blood loss in patients complaining of menorrhagia. *Br J Obstet Gynaecol* 1997;84:763.

Healy DL, Hogden GD. The endocrinology of human endometrium. *Obstet Gynecol Surv* 1983;38:509.

Helmkamp BF, Denslow BL, Boufiglio TA, et al. Cervical conization: when is dilatation and curettage indicated? *Am J Obstet Gynecol* 1983;146:893.

Hofmeister FJ. Endometrial biopsy: another look. *Am J Obstet Gynecol* 1974;118:773.

Hofmeister FJ. Endometrial curettage. In: Symmonds CM, Zuspan FT, eds. *Clinical and diagnostic procedures in obstetrics and gynecology.* New York: Marcel Dekker, 1984.

Hunt JS, Chen H-L, Hu X-L, et al. Tumor necrosis factor-a messenger ribonucleic acid and protein in human endometrium. *Biol Reprod* 1992;47:141.

Irvine G, Campbell-Brown M, Lumsden M, et al. Randomized comparative trial of the levonorgestrel intrauterine system and norethisterone for treatment of idiopathic menorrhagia. *Br J Obstet Gynaecol* 1998;105:592.

Jansen FW, Vredevoogd CB, Van Ulzen K, et al. Complications of hysteroscopy: a prospective multicenter study. *Obstet Gynecol* 2000;96:266.

Jensen J. Contraceptive and therapeutic effects of the levonorgestrel intrauterine system: an overview. *Obstet Gynecol Surv* 2005;60:604.

Jensen JA, Jensen JG. Abragio mucosae uteri e aspiratione. *Ugeskr Laeger* 1968;130:2121.

Jensen JG. Vacuum curettage. Outpatient curettage without anesthesia: a report of 350 cases. *Dan Med Bull* 1970;17:199.

Josey WE. Routine intrauterine forceps exploration at curettage. *Obstet Gynecol* 1958;11:108.

Joshi SG. Progestin-regulated proteins of the human endometrium. *Semin Reprod Endocrinol* 1983;1:221.

Kadir R, Lukes A, Kouides P, et al. Management of excessive menstrual bleeding in women with hemostatic disorders. *Fertil Steril* 2005;84:1352.

Karlsson B, Granberg S, Wikland M, et al. Transvaginal ultrasonography of the endometrium in women with postmenopausal bleeding: a Nordic multicenter study. *Am J Obstet Gynecol* 1995;172:1488.

Kaunitz AM, Portman DJ, Hait H, et al. Adding low-dose estrogen to the hormone-free interval: impact on bleeding patterns in users of a 91-day extended regimen oral contraceptive. *Contraception* 2009;79:350.

Kazandi M, Okmen F, Ergenoglu AM, et al. Comparison of histopathological diagnosis with dilatation- curettage and Pipelle endometrial sampling. *J Obstet Gynaecol* 2012;32:790.

Kelly HA. Curettage without anesthesia on the office table. *Am J Obstet Gynecol* 1925;9:78.

King RJB. Structure and function of steroid receptors. *J Endocrinol* 1987;114:341.

Klein SM, Garcia CR. Asherman's syndrome: a critique and current review. *Fertil Steril* 1973;24:722.

Kooy J, Taylor NH, Healy DL, et al. Endothelial cell proliferation in the endometrium of women with menorrhagia and in women following endometrial ablation. *Hum Reprod* 1996;11:1067.

Krettek JE, Arkin SI, Chaisilwattana P, et al. Chlamydia trachomatis in patients who used oral contraceptives and had intermenstrual spotting. *Obstet Gynecol* 1993;81:728.

Kubrinsky NL, Tulloch H. Treatment of refractory thrombocytopenic bleeding with desamino-8-D-arginine vasopressin (desmopressin). *J Pediatr* 1988;112:993.

Larsson PG, Bergman BB. Is there a causal connection between motile curved rods, *Mobiluncus* species and bleeding complications? *Am J Obstet Gynecol* 1986;154:107.

Laufer MR, Mitchell SR. Treatment of abnormal uterine bleeding with gonadotropin-releasing hormone analogues. *Clin Obstet Gynecol* 1993;36:668.

Leather A, Studd J, Watson N, et al. The prevention of bone loss in young women treated with GnRH analogues with "add-back" estrogen therapy. *Obstet Gynecol* 1993;81:104.

Lessey BA, Castelbaum AJ, Sawin SW, et al. Further characterization of endometrial integrins during the menstrual cycle and in pregnancy. *Fertil Steril* 1994;62:497.

Lessey BA, Damjanovich L, Cautifaris C, et al. Integrin adhesion molecules in the human endometrium: correlation with normal and abnormal menstrual cycle. *J Clin Invest* 1992;90:188.

Levens ED, Potlog-Nahari C, Armstrong AY, et al. CDB-2914 for uterine leiomyomata treatment: a randomized controlled trial. *Obstet Gynecol* 2008;111:1129.

Livingstone M, Fraser IS. Mechanisms of abnormal uterine bleeding. *Hum Reprod Update* 2002;8:60.

Lomano JM. Photocoagulation of the endometrium with the Nd:YAG laser for the treatment of menorrhagia: a report of 10 cases. *J Reprod Med* 1986;31:149.

Lukes A, Kadir R, Peyvandi F, et al. Disorders of hemostasis and excessive menstrual bleeding: prevalence and clinical impact. *Fertil Steril* 2005;84:1338.

Lukes AS, Moore KA, Muse KN, et al. Tranexamic acid treatment for heavy bleeding: a randomized controlled trial. *Obstet Gynecol* 2010;116:865.

Lutz MH, Underwood PB Jr, Kreutner A, et al. Vacuum aspiration: an efficient outpatient screening technique for endometrial disease. *South Med J* 1977;70:393.

MacKenzie IZ, Bibby JG. Critical assessment of dilatation and curettage in 1,029 women. *Lancet* 1978;2:566.

MacLennan AH, Taylor AW, Wilson DH. Hormone therapy use after the Women's Health Initiative. *Climacteric* 2004;7:138.

Mahoney S, Parker C, Nahari-Potlog C, et al. Abnormal uterine bleeding: a primary care perspective. *Consultant* 2006;46:225.

Manabe Y, Manabe A. Nelaton catheter for gradual and safe cervical dilatation: an ideal substitute for laminaria. *Am J Obstet Gynecol* 1981;140:465.

March CM. Hysteroscopy. *J Reprod Med* 1992;37:293.

Markee JE. Menstruation in intraocular endometrial transplants in the rhesus monkey. *Contr Embryol Carnegie Inst* 1940;28:219.

Martin PL, Rust JA. Surgical gynecology for the ambulatory patient. *Clin Obstet Gynecol* 1974;17:205.

McElin TW, Burd CC, Reeves BD, et al. Diagnostic dilatation and curettage. *Obstet Gynecol* 1969;33:807.

Mengert WF, Slate WG. Diagnostic dilatation and curettage as an outpatient procedure. *Am J Obstet Gynecol* 1960;79:727.

Meyer WR, Walsh BW, Grainger DA, et al. Thermal balloon and roller ball ablation to treat menorrhagia: a multicenter comparison. *Obstet Gynecol* 1998;92:98.

Milsom I, Andersson K, Andersch B, et al. A comparison of flurbiprofen, tranexamic acid and a levonorgestrel-releasing intrauterine contraceptive device in the treatment of idiopathic menorrhagia. *Am J Obstet Gynecol* 1991;164:879.

Mishell DR Jr, Connel E, Haney A, et al. Oral contraception for women in their 40s. *J Reprod Med* 1990;35:447.

Mularoni A, Mahfoudi A, Beck L, et al. Progesterone control of fibronectin secretion in guinea pig endometrium. *Endocrinology* 1992;131:2127.

Munro MG, Critchley HO, Broder MS, et al.; FIGO Working Group on Menstrual Disorders. FIGO classification system (PALM-COEIN) for causes of abnormal uterine bleeding in nongravid women of reproductive age. *Int J Gynaecol Obstet* 2011;113:3.

Munrow LA. Abnormal uterine bleeding and underlying hemostatic disorders: report of a consensus process. *Fertil Steril* 2005;84:1335.

Mylonas I, Jeschke U, Wiest I, et al. Inhibin/activin subunits alpha, beta-A and beta-B are differentially expressed in normal human endometrium throughout the menstrual cycle. *Histochem Cell Biol* 2004;122:461.

Narula RK. Endometrial histopathology in dysfunctional uterine bleeding. *J Obstet Gynaecol India* 1967;17:614.

Nasri MN, Shepherd JH, Setchell ME, et al. The role of vaginal scan in measurement of endometrial thickness in postmenopausal women. *Br J Obstet Gynaecol* 1991;98:470.

Nieman LK, Blocker W, Nansel T, et al. Efficacy and tolerability of CDB-2914 treatment for symptomatic uterine fibroids: a randomized, double-blind, placebo-controlled, phase IIb study. *Fertil Steril* 2011;95:767.

Nilsson L, Rybo G. Treatment of menorrhagia. *Am J Obstet Gynecol* 1971;110:713.

Novak E. Relation of hyperplasia of endometrium to so-called functional uterine hemorrhage. *JAMA* 1920;75:292.

Novak E. A suction curette apparatus and endometrial biopsy. *JAMA* 1935;104:1497.

O'Connor H, Magos A. Endometrial resection for the treatment of menorrhagia. *N Engl J Med* 1996;335:151.

Osmers R. Transvaginal sonography in endometrial cancer. *Ultrasound Obstet Gynecol* 1991;2:2.

Overton C, Hargreaves J, Maresh M. A national survey of the complications of endometrial destruction for menstrual disorders: the "the Mistletoe" study. *Br J Obstet Gynaecol* 1997;102:1351.

Pacheco JC, Kempers RD. Etiology of postmenopausal bleeding. *Obstet Gynecol* 1968;32:40.

Pines A. Guidelines and recommendations on hormone therapy in the menopause. *J Midlife Health* 2010;1:41.

Rauramo I, Elo I, Istre O. Long-term treatment of menorrhagia with levonorgestrel intrauterine system versus endometrial resection. *Obstet Gynecol* 2004;104:1314.

Reyniak JV. Dysfunctional uterine bleeding. *J Reprod Med* 1976;17:293.

Rodgers WH, Osteen KG, Matrisian LM, et al. Expression and localization of matrilysin, a matrix metalloproteinase, in human endometrium during the reproductive cycle. *Am J Obstet Gynecol* 1993;168:253.

Rubin MC, Davidson AR, Philliber SG, et al. Long-term effect of tubal sterilization on menstrual indices and pelvic pain. *Obstet Gynecol* 1993;82:118.

Rutherford TJ, Zreik TG, Troiano RN, et al. Endometrial cryoablation, a minimally invasive procedure for abnormal uterine bleeding. *J Am Assoc Gynecol Laparosc* 1998;5:23.

Sandmire HF, Austin SD. Curettage as an office procedure. *Am J Obstet Gynecol* 1974;119:82.

Schaedel Z, Dolan G, Powell M. The use of the levonorgestrel-releasing intrauterine system in the management of menorrhagia in women with hemostatic disorders. *Obstet Gynecol* 2005;193:1361.

Schranger S. Abnormal uterine bleeding associated with hormonal contraception. *Am Fam Physician* 2002;65:2073.

Schwab K, Chan R, Gargett C. Putative stem cell activity of human endometrial epithelial and stromal cells during the menstrual cycle. *Fertil Steril* 2005;84:1124.

Seeras RC, Gilliland GB. Resumption of menstruation after amenorrhea in women treated by endometrial ablation and myometrial resection. *J Am Assoc Gynecol Laparosc* 1997;4:305.

Sharp NC, Cronin N, Feldberg I, et al. Microwaves for menorrhagia: a new fast technique for endometrial ablation. *Lancet* 1995;346:1003.

Singer A, Almanza R, Rutierrez A, et al. Preliminary clinical experience with a thermal balloon ablation method to treat menorrhagia. *Obstet Gynecol* 1994;83:732.

Sivridis E, Giatromanolaki A. New insights into the normal menstrual cycle—regulatory molecules. *Histol Histopathol* 2004;19:511.

Smith SK, Abel MH, Kelly RW, et al. Prostaglandin synthesis in the endometrium of women with ovular dysfunctional uterine bleeding. *Br J Obstet Gynaecol* 1981;88:434.

Smith SK, Abel MH, Kelly RW, et al. A role for prostacyclin (PGI$_2$) in excessive menstrual bleeding. *Lancet* 1981;1:522.

Smith-Bindman R, Kerlikowske K, Feldstein V, et al. Endovaginal ultrasound to exclude endometrial cancer and other endometrial abnormalities. *JAMA* 1998;280:1510.

Southam AI, Richard RM. The prognosis for adolescents with menstrual abnormalities. *Am J Obstet Gynecol* 1966;94:637.

Spies JB, Coyne K, Guaou Guao N, et al. The UFS-QOL, a new disease-specific symptom and health-related quality of life questionnaire for leiomyomata. *Obstet Gynecol* 2002;99:290.

Speroff L, Glass RH, Kase NG. Dysfunctional uterine bleeding. In: *Clinical gynecologic endocrinology and infertility*, 6th ed. Baltimore, MD: Lippincott Williams & Wilkins, 1999:575.

Stefos T, Sotiriadis A, Tsanadis G, et al. Serum leptin and erythropoietin during menstruation. *Clin Exp Obstet Gynecol* 2005;32:41.

Stock RJ, Kanbour A. Pre-hysterectomy curettage: an evaluation. *Obstet Gynecol* 1975;45:537.

Summitt RJ Jr, Stovall TG, Steege JF, et al. A multicenter randomized comparison of laparoscopically assisted vaginal hysterectomy and abdominal hysterectomy candidates. *Obstet Gynecol* 1998;92:321.

Swartz DP, Jones GES. Progesterone in anovulatory uterine bleeding: clinical observations. *Fertil Steril* 1957;8:103.

Taylor PJ, Graham G. Is diagnostic curettage harmful in women with unexplained infertility? *Br J Obstet Gynaecol* 1982;89:296.

Teare AJ, Rippey JJ. Dilatation and curettage. *S Afr Med J* 1979;55:535.

Torry DS, Torry RJ. Angiogenesis and the expression of vascular endothelial growth factor in endometrium and placenta. *Am J Reprod Immunol* 1997;37:21.

Townsend DE, Fields G, McCausland A, et al. Diagnostic and operative hysteroscopy in the management of persistent postmenopausal bleeding. *Obstet Gynecol* 1993;82:419.

Tseng L, Gusberg SB, Gurpide E. Estradiol receptor and 17β-dehydrogenase in normal and abnormal human endometrium. *Ann N Y Acad Sci* 1977;286:190.

Tuuli MG, Shanks A, Bernhard L et al. Uterine synechiae and pregnancy complications. *Obstet Gynecol* 2012;119:810.

Van Eijkeren MA, Christiaens GC, Geuze JH, et al. Effects of mefenamic acid on menstrual hemostasis in essential menorrhagia. *Am J Obstet Gynecol* 1992;166:1419.

Van Eijkeren MA, Christiaens GC, Haspels AA, et al. Measured menstrual blood loss in women with a bleeding disorder or using oral anticoagulant therapy. *Am J Obstet Gynecol* 1990;162:1261.

Van Eijkeren MA, Christiaens GC, Sixma JJ, et al. Menorrhagia: a review. *Obstet Gynecol Surv* 1989;4:421.

Vercellini P, Oldani S, Yaylayan L, et al. Randomized comparison of vaporizing electrode and cutting loop for endometrial ablation. *Obstet Gynecol* 1999;94:521.

Vermeeren J, Chamberlain RR, Te Linde RW. Ten thousand minor gynecologic operations on an outpatient basis. *Obstet Gynecol* 1957;9:139.

Vilos GA, Pispidkis JT, Botz CK. Economic evaluation of hysteroscopic endometrial ablation versus vaginal hysterectomy for menorrhagia. *Obstet Gynecol* 1996;88:241.

Warner P, Critchley H, Lumsden M, et al. Menorrhagia II: is the 80-mL blood loss criterion useful in management of complaint of menorrhagia? *Am J Obstet Gynecol* 2004;190:1224.

Weisberg M, Goldrath MH, Berman J, et al. Hysteroscopic endometrial ablation using free heated saline for the treatment of menorrhagia. *J Am Assoc Gynecol Laparosc* 2000;7:311.

Whitehead MI, Frazier D. The effects of estrogens and progestogens on the endometrium. *Obstet Gynecol Clin North Am* 1987;14:299.

Whitehead MI, King RJ, McQueen J, et al. Endometrial histology and biochemistry in climacteric women during estrogen and estrogen/progestogen therapy. *J R Soc Med* 1979;72:322.

Wilansky DL, Greisman B. Early hypothyroidism in patients with menorrhagia *Am J Obstet Gynecol* 1989;160:673.

Wilborn WH, Flowers CE Jr. Cellular mechanisms for endometrial conservation during menstrual bleeding. *Semin Reprod Endocrinol* 1984;2:307.

Word B. Current concepts of uterine curettage. *Postgrad Med* 1960;28:450.

Word B, Gravlee LC, Wideman GL. The fallacy of simple uterine curettage. *Obstet Gynecol* 1958;12:642.

Xiao B, Wus C, Chong J, et al. Therapeutic effects of the levonorgestrel-releasing intrauterine system in the treatment of idiopathic menorrhagia. *Fertil Steril* 2003;79:963.

CHAPTER 27
Tubal Sterilization

Herbert B. Peterson, Jeffrey S. Warshaw,
Amy E. Pollack, and Barbara S. Levy

DEFINITIONS

Bipolar coagulation—Method of tubal occlusion usually performed via laparoscopy that causes electrocoagulation of the tube when current is applied by grasping forceps; one jaw of the forceps is an active electrode, and the other is a return electrode. There is less chance for unintended thermal injuries than with unipolar coagulation, and the chance of unintended thermal injury by capacitive coupling is virtually eliminated. However, less widespread thermal destruction of the tube increases the chance for sterilization failure relative to unipolar coagulation unless the surgeon uses techniques that maximize the likelihood of adequate tubal coagulation.

Capacitive coupling—Unintended consequence of laparoscopic use of unipolar coagulation, which under certain conditions can result in a charge being transferred to the operative laparoscope or conductive laparoscopic sheath. Subsequent occult transference of this charge to intestines can lead to thermal injury and subsequent perforation with infectious morbidity or mortality.

Cumulative failure rates—Contrary to previous beliefs, tubal sterilization failures are not isolated to a narrow window of time after the procedure but rather increase cumulatively with each passing year following sterilization. Younger women, who are more fecund at sterilization and for years after, have higher failure rates initially and over time.

Gas embolism—Potential complication of laparoscopic abdominal insufflation with the Veress needle, associated with "vapor lock" of the right ventricle, which occludes blood flow and results in cardiovascular collapse. A "cogwheel" murmur can sometimes be heard.

Hysteroscopic sterilization—Surgical approach in which an endoscope is introduced transcervically into the uterine cavity for the purpose of placing the Essure microinsert into the fallopian tubes across the uterotubal junction. It has the advantage of requiring no abdominal incision and only minimal analgesia. It can be performed in an outpatient or office surgery setting.

Irving method—Method of partial salpingectomy that buries the end of the proximal tubal stump in the myometrium of the uterus, in an attempt to reduce the rate of tuboperitoneal fistula.

Luteal phase pregnancy—Refers to pregnancies that occurred before sterilization but were detected after sterilization. Such pregnancies may be erroneously attributed to sterilization "failure."

Open laparoscopy—Laparoscopic procedure begun without prior insufflation by directly visualizing, elevating, and incising the layers of the abdominal wall near the umbilicus. Has the benefit of reducing vascular injuries and, potentially, bowel injuries associated with blind direct Veress needle and trocar insertion.

Parkland method—Method of partial salpingectomy that involves ligation of the tube in two places, followed by excision of the intervening segment of tube. Achieves immediate separation of severed tubal ends.

Pomeroy method—Method of partial salpingectomy that involves ligation, followed by excision, of a loop of tube. No attempt to bury the severed ends of the tube.

Poststerilization regret—Regret after the decision to undergo surgical sterilization can be related to several factors, including preexisting patient characteristics, subsequent changes in the patient's situation or attitudes, and dissatisfaction resulting from adverse side effects caused or perceived to be caused by the procedure. Studies have identified young age at tubal sterilization as a risk factor for later regret.

Posttubal ligation syndrome—Refers to the historic perception that menstrual disturbances could result from tubal sterilization. This term is outdated, as substantial evidence against such a syndrome now exists. Women who undergo sterilization are no more likely than are their nonsterilized counterparts to experience a syndrome of menstrual abnormalities.

Silicone rubber banding—Method of tubal occlusion usually performed via laparoscopy in which a silicone rubber band is applied to the isthmic portion of the tube. The technique is most effective when the tube has normal anatomy and the operator is experienced with the technique of application. The possibility of tubal transection, and resultant hemorrhage, appears to be highest with this technique.

Sterilization timing—Sterilization can be performed in relation to pregnancy (following vaginal delivery, cesarean section, or abortion) or remote from pregnancy (interval sterilization).

Tubal clips—Method of tubal occlusion usually performed via laparoscopy in which a Filshie or Hulka clip is applied to the isthmic portion of the tube. The technique is most effective when the tube has normal anatomy and the operator is experienced with the technique of application. These methods inflict the narrowest zone of tubal damage (3 to 5 mm), affording a greater chance of sterilization reversal when compared with other methods.

Tuboperitoneal fistula—Poststerilization communication of the proximal tubal stump with the peritoneal cavity, which can result in sterilization failure, including ectopic gestation. Theoretically, may be reduced by leaving a proximal tubal stump of 2 cm and by minimizing ligature-induced necrosis at the site of tubal interruption.

Uchida method—Method of partial salpingectomy that buries the end of the proximal tubal stump within the leaves of the mesosalpinx in an attempt to reduce the rate of tuboperitoneal fistula.

Unipolar coagulation—Method of tubal occlusion usually performed via laparoscopy that causes electrocoagulation of the tube when current is applied by grasping forceps; both jaws of the forceps serve as an active electrode. The high effectiveness rate observed with this method are a property of the wide zone of thermal destruction of the tube that results, but this same property increases the potential for morbidity from unintended thermal injuries. The surgeon must be vigilant regarding possibility of capacitive coupling.

In proposing the concept of tubal sterilization in 1842, James Blundell suggested the following:

> … the operator … ought to remove a portion, say one line, of the Fallopian tube, right and left, so as to intercept its caliber—the larger blood vessels being avoided. Mere divisions of the tube might be sufficient to produce sterility, but the further removal of a portion of the tube appears to be surer practice. I recommend this precaution, therefore, as an improvement of the operation.

Samuel Smith Lungren of Toledo, Ohio, is credited with having performed the first tubal sterilization in 1880, after having performed a cesarean section for a woman whose previous child was also born by cesarean section because of a contracted pelvis. During the second cesarean section, Lungren intended to remove the woman's ovaries to prevent future pregnancy, but instead decided that "the risk would be lessened and the same result would be accomplished by tying both Fallopian tubes with strong silk ligatures a one inch from the uterus." At the time of Lungren's successful tubal sterilization, laparotomy was a life-threatening procedure; thus, the performance of tubal sterilization at the time of cesarean section to prevent future pregnancy was potentially lifesaving. In 1919, Madlener reported on 85 tubal sterilizations performed at the time of laparotomy for other reasons, including cesarean section; 3 of the 85 women died postoperatively from infection. Because of the extreme risks, performing a laparotomy for the sole purpose of tubal sterilization remained an unpopular idea until the mid-20th century. Indeed, when three deaths occurred from 1936 to 1950 among 1,022 women who had postpartum Pomeroy sterilization, investigators Prystowsky and Eastman concluded that the risk for sterilization was comparable to that for multiparity and that "sterilization because of great multiparity alone cannot be justified on medical grounds."

In addition to concerns about safety, the early history of tubal sterilization included debate about the appropriateness of tubal sterilization for fertility control. At the 21st Annual Meeting of the American Gynecological Society in 1886, participants debated a woman's right to undergo surgical sterilization. During this debate, Edward P. Davis said, "I hold it [sterilization] to be the right of a woman who is in a condition to which natural delivery is impossible...." H. J. Garrigues objected by saying,

> We must leave that to Nature or to God. ... I do not think that the woman has a right of that kind. ... The mere fact that she does not want to have more children should not decide the question. (Speert)

The availability and acceptability of tubal sterilization as a method of fertility control remained limited until the mid-20th century, and, accordingly, tubal sterilization remained uncommon in the United States and around the world until the 1960s. In the 1970s, the worldwide popularity of tubal sterilization increased dramatically. Between 1970 and 1980, the estimated number of tubal sterilizations increased markedly in Europe, China, India, other parts of Asia, and Latin America. In the United States, the number of tubal sterilizations increased nearly fourfold—from approximately 200,000 in 1970 to approximately 700,000 in 1977. Among the factors affecting this increase were the availability and acceptability of two new surgical approaches—minilaparotomy and laparoscopy. In contrast to laparotomy for sterilization, these approaches were safer, allowed for surgery without hospitalization, reduced recovery time, and gave a better cosmetic result. Minilaparotomy has been used in many developing countries, and laparoscopy has been used in many developed countries, including in the United States.

Minilaparotomy for interval sterilization (i.e., sterilization at a time unrelated to pregnancy) requires a 2.5- to 3.0-cm suprapubic incision. The technique was first described by Uchida and colleagues in Japan in 1961. It was used in the early 1970s in Thailand by Vitoon and associates and then rapidly gained acceptance worldwide. Laparoscopy for tubal sterilization was first proposed by Anderson in 1937 and later described by Power and Barnes in 1941. The use of laparoscopy in Europe was encouraged by the work of Palmer (France), Steptoe (Britain), and Frangenheim (Germany), and use of the technique rapidly gained popularity in the 1970s, particularly in Europe and the United States.

In the United States, the increased use of tubal sterilization in the 1970s occurred concurrently with the widespread availability and acceptability of laparoscopy. In 1970, less than 1% of sterilizations were performed with a laparoscope, but by 1975, more than one third of the 550,000 women who had tubal sterilization had the procedure performed laparoscopically. This transition was associated with a marked reduction in length of hospital stay for tubal sterilization—from 6.5 nights in 1970 to 4 nights in the years 1975 to 1978. By 1987, one third of tubal sterilizations in the United States required no overnight hospital stay, and 79% of these were performed by way of laparoscopy. In 2002, the FDA approved a new even less invasive hysteroscopic approach for sterilization (Essure) that can be performed successfully in the office setting.

Sterilization is now the method of contraception most commonly used in the world. In 2009, about 251 million couples used sterilization (of themselves or their spouses) for contraception; 223 million were women using tubal sterilization and 28 million were men using vasectomy. Most of these sterilizations were performed in the developing world—229 million versus 22 million in the developed world.

In the United States, sterilization is also the most commonly used method of contraception. According to data from the National Center for Health Statistics, among women aged 15 to 44 in 2006–2010, about 14 million (22.7%) reported using either tubal sterilization (about 10 million) or vasectomy (about 4 million) for contraception. Among currently married women using contraception in 2006–2010, 47.3% were using either tubal sterilization (30.2%) or vasectomy (17.1%) for contraception. These percentages were very similar to those for 1995 (31.2% and 17.3%, respectively).

In 2006, of an estimated 643,000 tubal sterilizations, 351,000 (55%) were inpatient procedures and 292,000 (45%) were performed in an ambulatory setting. Nearly all of the former were postpartum procedures (either after vaginal delivery or concurrent with cesarean section). An increasing proportion of ambulatory procedures is being performed by hysteroscopy using the Essure device, but it is too early to determine the impact of such procedures on sterilization trends.

TIMING OF STERILIZATION

Tubal sterilization can be performed at the time of cesarean section, shortly after delivery or induced abortion, or at a time unrelated to pregnancy. About one half of tubal sterilizations in the United States are performed at a time unrelated to pregnancy. The timing of tubal sterilization can influence the choice of anesthetic, surgical approach, and method of tubal occlusion. For example, most sterilizations performed concurrently with cesarean section require no separate anesthesia and involve partial salpingectomy as the method of tubal occlusion. Most tubal sterilizations performed after vaginal delivery are done by minilaparotomy with subumbilical incisions and partial salpingectomy. Tubal sterilization not associated with birth usually is performed by laparoscopy (with use of coagulation, silicone rubber band application, or clip application), hysteroscopy (with use of Essure device), or minilaparotomy (with use of partial salpingectomy).

PREOPERATIVE EVALUATION

The candidate for sterilization should be extensively counseled. The intended permanence of the procedure, alternatives to sterilization, and risks of surgery should be discussed.

For couples desiring sterilization, no such discussion is complete without consideration of vasectomy as an alternative. Women also should be made aware that sterilization failure can occur and that the relative likelihood of ectopic pregnancy is increased when sterilization failure does occur.

The workup of women who are to undergo tubal sterilization includes a history and physical examination and a laboratory evaluation, as indicated. Consideration should be given to whether the woman might be pregnant at the time of sterilization, and pregnancy testing should be ordered as necessary.

A careful gynecologic history and examination also are necessary before sterilization. Women with gynecologic disease or symptoms may require additional diagnostic or therapeutic measures. Some ultimately may be better served by other surgical procedures, either instead of or in addition to sterilization. For example, some women with enlarged and symptomatic uterine leiomyomata, women with severe dysmenorrhea, and those with symptomatic pelvic relaxation may benefit more from hysterectomy than from tubal sterilization. Others, such as women with abnormal cervical cytology, need careful evaluation before a decision can be made about preventing or treating invasive cervical cancer.

ANESTHESIA

Complications of general anesthesia are the leading cause of death attributed to sterilization in the United States. The risks inherent in general anesthesia are exacerbated by its use postpartum and during laparoscopy. The special requirements of general anesthesia for laparoscopy have been well described.

Except for the use of conduction anesthesia postpartum, general anesthesia is the technique most often used for female sterilization by laparoscopy and minilaparotomy in the United States. A 1988 survey of members of the American Association of Gynecologic Laparoscopists revealed that the number of providers of tubal sterilization who used local anesthesia for laparoscopic sterilization had increased from 4% (in the 1982 survey) to 8%. Worldwide, more than 75% of tubal sterilization procedures are performed under local anesthesia. A discussion of the technology and regimen for administering general or conduction anesthesia is beyond the scope of this chapter. Instead, we focus on local anesthesia because of its increasing use in outpatient settings for many types of surgery.

Sterilization by laparoscopy, hysteroscopy, or minilaparotomy can be performed safely under local anesthesia, and hysteroscopic sterilization with the Essure device can be performed with minimal analgesia alone. The patient avoids the risks associated with general anesthesia, spends less time sedated or anesthetized, and has a more rapid recovery. Nausea and vomiting are less likely to occur, and the patient is awake to report symptoms that can indicate the occurrence of a complication. Furthermore, the overall expense often is reduced compared with procedures done under general anesthesia.

In the United States, the overall morbidity rate for female sterilization is so low that it is difficult to obtain a sample large enough to demonstrate a comparative safety advantage for local versus general anesthesia. One US study randomly assigned 100 women to either local or general anesthesia for laparoscopic sterilization. Serious or life-threatening events did not occur in either group. However, women who had general anesthesia were more likely to have intraoperative hypotension, hypertension, or tachycardia, which suggests that these women were hemodynamically less stable and may have been at increased risk for cardiovascular complications. In another study, 125 women were randomly allocated to the use of local or general anesthesia for laparoscopic sterilization. Women who had general anesthesia were more likely to

develop hypotension; hypertension was more common in the local anesthesia group. No women in either group had tachycardia.

Operating under local anesthesia incurs several possible disadvantages. The patient's anxiety may be increased; therefore, the surgeon must use a decisive and gentle surgical technique while talking with the patient. The patient may feel discomfort; thus, the physician must have a thorough understanding of the use of sedative and analgesic drugs. Although obesity can complicate the use of local anesthesia, several studies indicate that local anesthesia can be used successfully for obese women. Women with a history of multiple abdominal or pelvic surgical procedures or peritonitis may need additional anesthesia if the procedure is difficult or prolonged. Additional anesthesia also may be required during minilaparotomy if the abdominal incision needs to be extended. The hysteroscopic approach may be ideal for both obese women and those with multiple previous abdominal procedures as it avoids the necessity to access the tubes through the abdominal wall.

One US-based retrospective study reviewed 2,827 outpatient laparoscopic sterilizations performed under local anesthesia and mild sedation from 1980 to 1988. The mean operating time was 10.0 (±5.1) minutes, and the mean anesthesia time was 23.3 (±6.9) minutes. The hospital cost to the patient was reduced 65% to 85%. Another US study reported on 358 minilaparotomies for interval sterilization performed under local anesthesia. The average operating time was 21 minutes, and no complications were reported. In both series, the local anesthetic was 0.5% bupivacaine hydrochloride used alone or in combination with lidocaine. In one series, midazolam hydrochloride and fentanyl citrate were used for mild intravenous sedation; in the other series, meperidine hydrochloride and diazepam were used.

For local infiltration and paracervical block, agents of intermediate intrinsic potency (defined as the minimum concentration required to produce a block within 5 to 10 minutes), such as lidocaine or mepivacaine, have been found suitable. Both are amides with good stability and low toxicity. Onset of analgesic effects is rapid, even when a low concentration of medication is used, and the duration of the effect is sufficient for the procedure but not prolonged (about 1.5 hours when the medication is given in plain solution). Bupivacaine, a more potent and a longer-acting amide, is frequently used in the United States. However, the short duration of action provided by lidocaine or mepivacaine is preferred by some because it allows for awareness of any abnormal degree of persistent pain and early diagnosis of complications, such as hematoma formation.

SURGICAL APPROACH

Minilaparotomy

The minilaparotomy approach to tubal occlusion can be used in the interval or postpartum period. Although interval sterilization by minilaparotomy is the sterilization procedure most frequently performed in many countries, it is not a common procedure in the United States. Minilaparotomy in the United States often is used preferentially among women considered to be at increased risk for laparoscopy.

Interval minilaparotomy is performed with the use of a 2- to 3-cm midline vertical or transverse suprapubic incision. In patients with an enlarged uterus resulting from uterine leiomyomata or other benign conditions, the minilaparotomy incision should be made at the level of the uterine fundus to ensure access to the fallopian tubes. A uterine manipulator is placed through the cervix just before surgery and is used to bring the uterus toward the incision. Placement of a paracervical block before insertion of the uterine manipulator reduces discomfort for patients having surgery under local anesthesia. The abdomen is then entered with the approach that is used for laparotomy; small handheld retractors and the Trendelenburg position are used to enhance exposure. Once the uterus is identified, a tubal hook or a finger is placed posteriorly at the top of the fundus and moved along the uterus. The fallopian tube is identified first by the fimbriated end, and then the midportion of the fallopian tube is grasped with a small Babcock clamp and elevated through the abdominal incision. Tubal occlusion most often is performed by use of the modified Pomeroy or Parkland technique. However, clips or rings can be applied through the minilaparotomy incision with modified instruments originally developed for use through the operating laparoscope.

Postpartum minilaparotomy is performed in a manner similar to that of interval minilaparotomy. It is ideally performed before the onset of postpartum uterine involution while the uterine fundus is high in the abdomen (within 48 hours of delivery). A 2- to 3-cm subumbilical vertical or semicircular incision is made in the midline where the abdominal wall is thin. Because of the proximity of the enlarged uterus to the incision, access to the fallopian tubes is easier than it is with an interval approach. A uterine manipulator is unnecessary when minilaparotomy is performed in the postpartum period.

Laparoscopy

> The magic is in the magician, not in the wand. ... Entering the abdomen is the most dangerous part of the laparoscopic procedure. (Hulka and Reich)

The laparoscopic instrumentation, including laparoscope, light cables and light source, insufflator and tubing, and video camera and television, if used, should be set up and tested for proper functioning before any incisions are made. If a Veress needle is to be used, it is good practice to attach it to the insufflation tubing and test that gas flows freely through it. High line pressures (3 mm Hg or higher) during low-flow insufflation (1 L/min) through a Veress needle that has yet to be inserted into the abdominal cavity suggest that the needle has some occlusion. Checking for occlusion before inserting the needle can avoid the multiple attempts at needle placement that might occur in the belief that incorrect placement, rather than needle occlusion, is the cause of resistance to flow. It is convenient, while waiting for surgery, to have the end of the laparoscope bathing in warm sterile fluid to prevent it from fogging when it is inserted into the abdominal cavity.

A no. 11 scalpel blade is used to make a single vertical incision in the lower rim of the umbilicus. This must be done carefully because the aorta can lie just a few centimeters beneath the abdominal wall, particularly in a thin patient. The abdominal wall is lifted away from the aorta by pinching the skin beneath the umbilicus between thumb and index finger. The umbilicus is elevated with one hand or towel clips while the surgeon's other hand makes the controlled incision.

The Veress needle is disconnected from the insufflation tubing before insertion. The stopcock on the needle then is placed in the open position, and the spring action of the needle is tested for smooth operation. Elevating the abdominal wall and using the Veress needle with the stopcock open allows air to rush into the previously gas-free abdominal cavity when the end of the needle penetrates the peritoneal layer. The inrushing air, if heard, is one of the first indicators that successful abdominal entry has occurred. Outflow of blood likewise can serve as an immediate indicator of vessel injury. Allowing air to rush in also can cause the bowel to fall away from the abdominal wall.

The terminal aorta is palpated, even in a moderately obese patient, through the abdominal wall in the midline, just above or at the umbilicus. The pulsations of the aorta are lost in the midline just beneath the umbilicus, corresponding to the sacral hollow. The aorta bifurcates at the level of L4, which corresponds to the summits of the iliac crests. This is a more reliable landmark for bifurcation of the aorta than the umbilicus. The Veress needle is placed through the umbilical incision and is directed at an angle toward the sacral hollow or uterine fundus (to avoid the aorta) and in the midline (to avoid the iliac vessels). Elevating the abdominal wall during this placement increases the distance between the Veress needle and major vessels. While placing the Veress needle, the surgeon should hold the needle like a dart, being careful not to impede the action of the spring mechanism. Resistance at the tip of the needle causes the blunt cannula inside the needle to be pushed back, and the spring mechanism at the hub of the needle extends. When resistance at the tip of the advancing needle is lost, as occurs with successful penetration of the peritoneal cavity, the blunt cannula inside the needle advances back out to the tip, and the spring mechanism at the hub of the needle snaps back in. Observing the spring mechanism for this snap can serve as a sign to test for successful placement. Often, there are two snaps—the first when the fascia is penetrated and the second with peritoneal penetration. Continuing to advance the needle tip much beyond the point of penetration of the parietal peritoneum risks placing the needle tip between loops of bowel or under the omental apron, both of which can cause resistance to flow and can result in reinsertion of the needle. Continued advancement of the Veress needle also risks vascular injury. The needle tip should not be moved laterally once the tip is inserted in the abdomen; any simple vascular or intestinal puncture could be transformed into a major laceration if the needle tip is moved from side to side. Once abdominal penetration is made with the Veress needle, the needle should be stabilized carefully until the safety checks have been completed. The needle should not be moved, and a laparotomy should be performed immediately if major vascular injury is suspected.

The distance between skin and fascia can increase with increasing patient obesity. A given angle of entry of the Veress needle that successfully penetrates the peritoneal cavity in a thin patient might fall far short of the peritoneum in an obese patient. To bring the peritoneal cavity within the physical length of the Veress needle, it is often necessary to pursue entry with a trajectory closer to the vertical. However, this also directs the Veress needle toward the aorta and therefore should be attempted only by experienced surgeons, and with extreme care. Alternatively, open laparoscopy can be performed.

Several safety checks for correct intraabdominal placement can be performed while the Veress needle is held steady. The instillation of 5 to 10 mL of sterile saline through the needle, followed immediately by aspiration, can be helpful. The fluid should meet little resistance, and, more important, scant fluid should return on reaspiration. Reaspiration of fluid suggests that the needle tip is in a small enclosed space that does not allow immediate dispersion of the instilled fluid. Reaspiration of feculent fluid or bloody fluid suggests bowel or vascular penetration, respectively. Simple penetration of the bowel with a Veress needle does not mandate immediate exploratory laparotomy. Depending on the setting and the skill level of the surgeon, reinsertion of the needle or open laparoscopy, followed by laparoscopic visualization of the intestine, can be pursued.

A second safety check consists of attaching a filled 10-mL syringe to the hub of the Veress needle and then removing the plunger. Elevation of the abdominal wall at this point should cause an increased negative intraperitoneal pressure, which allows the fluid in the syringe to drain passively into the abdominal cavity through an open stopcock. Alternatively, a drop of saline (drip test) can be placed on the hub of the Veress needle, and, with the stopcock open, elevation of the abdominal wall should result in the drop flowing downward freely.

Once these safety checks are performed, insufflation is begun at 1 L/min or less. Initial insufflation pressures often are 5 mm Hg or less in thin patients and, even with correct needle placement, can be 10 mm Hg or more in obese patients. An intraabdominal pressure greater than 15 mm Hg during insufflation generally is avoided to prevent respiratory compromise and decreased venous return secondary to vena caval compression. Abdominal distention increases the distance between the abdominal wall and major pelvic vessels, and this increases the safety buffer when the trocar is inserted. However, the abdomen should not be distended so taut that it is difficult to manually elevate it for trocar insertion.

During insufflation, a shift from dullness to tympany with percussion over the liver is indicative of pneumoperitoneum formation. It also is prudent for the surgeon to pay attention to the electrocardiogram rhythm during insufflation, because the sudden appearance of premature ventricular contractions can be an indicator of intravascular insufflation. Sudden vascular collapse during insufflation can be caused by a gas embolism into the right side of the heart and, at times, this life-threatening event can be signaled by a new "cogwheel" or "mill wheel" murmur. Rapidly tilting the patient into Trendelenburg position and onto her left side and advancing a Swan-Ganz catheter into the right heart for aspiration can be lifesaving.

Once insufflation is complete, the Veress needle is removed, and the umbilical incision is widened to accommodate the trocar and sleeve. An incision that is too large can result in leakage of gas around the sleeve. An incision that is too small can restrict access. The trocar should be checked before insertion to ensure that it is sharp; a dull trocar potentially is dangerous because it requires increased force for abdominal entry.

The trocar is grasped as shown in Figure 27.1. If the surgeon's hand is large enough, the middle finger can serve as a stopper, preventing the forward momentum following fascial puncture from carrying the trocar deep into the pelvis. The precautions for insertion of the Veress needle pertain even more to insertion of the trocar; the abdominal wall is elevated, the trocar is directed toward the hollow of the sacrum or the uterine fundus, and a midline trajectory is followed. Slow, steady pressure with a sharp trocar will permit immediate recognition when the gas-filled cavity is penetrated.

Open laparoscopy is performed without previous creation of a pneumoperitoneum. The skin beneath the umbilicus is incised sufficiently with a scalpel in either a vertical or transverse direction to adequately visualize the underlying fascia. Small S retractors are most helpful in visualization—especially in obese patients. The skin is released, and the fascia is grasped and elevated. The fascia is then incised in the midline, and the opening is stretched with a hemostat or incised to a length just sufficient to visualize the underlying peritoneum, which in turn is elevated and incised. Keeping the incision in the central portion of the umbilicus where the peritoneum and fascia are fused is the easiest method for entry in obese patients. Each angle of the fascial incision is sutured with a no. 0 absorbable stitch but not tied. The Hasson blunt cannula and sleeve are then placed through the opening of the peritoneum. The blunt cannula then is removed, and the abdomen is insufflated through the port found on the sleeve.

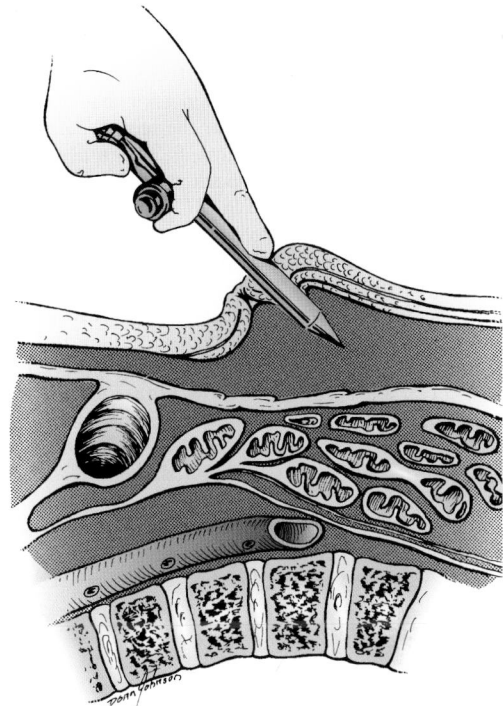

FIGURE 27.1 Trocar entry. When inserting the trocar through the abdominal wall, the trocar is "palmed" in the surgeon's dominant hand, with the extended middle finger serving as a stopper to prevent deep abdominal penetration. If the surgeon's hand is too small to accomplish this, open laparoscopy should be considered.

METHOD OF TUBAL OCCLUSION

All tubal sterilization methods rely on correct identification of the fallopian tube for success. With any of the transabdominal methods, the tube should be followed out to its fimbriated end to confirm that the correct structure has been identified.

Theoretically, the risk of tuboperitoneal fistula formation can be reduced by preserving a proximal tubal segment 1 to 2 cm in length. It is possible that the proximal tubal stump serves as a distensible reservoir for the small amount of uterine fluid that is normally forced through the interstitial portion of the tube by uterine contractions. This distensibility capacitance of the proximal stump might serve to dissipate the fluid pressure emanating from the uterus. Otherwise, this direct fluid pressure on the cut end of the tube might prevent complete closure of the tubal lumen during the healing process.

Irving Procedure

In 1924, and later in 1950, Irving reported on his method of achieving tubal sterilization. He attempted to reduce the risk of tuboperitoneal fistulae by extensively dissecting the ligated ends of the tubes and burying the proximal tubal segment. Although the extra dissection in this technique likely enhances effectiveness, it also carries the potential for greater blood loss, as well as increases the difficulty of performing the technique through a minilaparotomy incision. The procedure also takes slightly longer to perform than simpler methods.

The Irving technique is accomplished by first using a hemostat or scissors to create a window in the mesosalpinx just beneath the tube, about 4 cm from the uterotubal junction (**Fig. 27.2A**). Then, the tube is twice ligated (no. 1 chromic) and divided between the ties at this location. The free ends of the proximal stump ligature are held long. A 1-cm incision is made in the serosa of the posterior uterine wall near the uterotubal junction. A hemostat, or similar pointed instrument, is then used to bluntly deepen the incision, creating a pocket in the uterine musculature about 1 to 2 cm deep (**Fig. 27.2B**). The two free ends of the proximal stump ligature, previously held long, are then individually threaded onto a curved needle and brought deep into the myometrial tunnel and out through the uterine serosa (**Fig. 27.2C**). Traction on the sutures then draws the ligated proximal stump deep into the myometrial tunnel, and tying the free sutures fixes the tube in this buried location (**Fig. 27.2D**). Often, this can be accomplished without incising the mesosalpinx, but if extra mobilization of the proximal stump is needed, or if the proximal stump mesosalpinx appears in danger of being torn when traction is applied, then the mesosalpinx under the proximal tubal segment can be incised partly back toward the uterus. The serosal opening of the myometrial tunnel is then plicated closed around the tube with the use of a fine absorbable suture, but great care should be exercised to avoid compromising the tube as it enters the tunnel. Strangulation or damage to the tube with this stitch could cause necrosis and fistula formation in the extramyometrial portion of the proximal tube. No treatment of the distal tubal stump is necessary, but some surgeons choose to bury that segment in the mesosalpinx.

Modified Pomeroy Procedure

Bishop and Nelms, colleagues of Pomeroy, reported on the Pomeroy technique for tubal occlusion in 1930. They were careful to point out the importance of using absorbable suture as opposed to permanent suture.

In this method, the tube is grasped in its midportion, usually with a small atraumatic clamp such as the Babcock, and a loop of tube is elevated (**Fig. 27.3A**). The base of the loop is ligated with no. 1 plain catgut, leaving a 2-cm proximal stump of isthmus, and the sutures are held long. A 2- to 3-cm portion of tube in the ligated loop is transected and removed with scissors (**Fig. 27.3B**). Bishop and Nelms, in the original report on this method, pointed out that ligation was performed with a double strand of absorbable chromic catgut suture to allow the cut tubal ends to quickly separate after surgery. It was their belief that this would allow the ends to naturally fibrose and peritonealize without fistulization or communication. This also is the rationale for the common modification of the Pomeroy technique, in which the original chromic suture is replaced by plain catgut because of the more rapid degradation of the latter. Surgeons have a tendency to strenuously tighten the catgut ligature around the tube (as though the tighter the ligature, the better the occlusion), but this appears to go against the very principles of the procedure. This tightening can result in greater strangulation and necrosis of the adjoining tubal segments, potentially increasing the risk of fistula formation

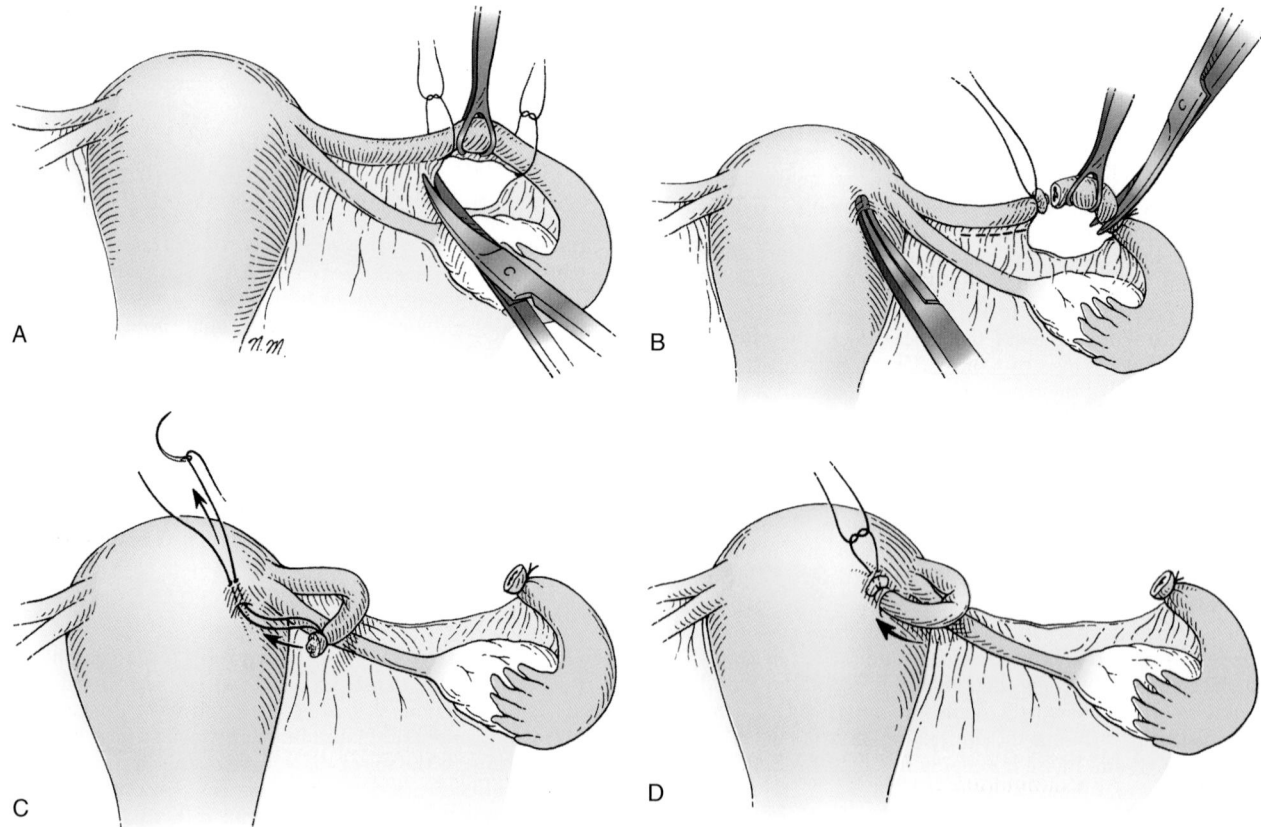

FIGURE 27.2 Irving method. **A:** A fenestration is made beneath the tube about 4 cm from the uterotubal junction using scissors or a hemostat. **B:** The tube is then twice ligated and a portion resected. A deep pocket is created in the myometrium on the posterior uterus. The *dashed line* shows the line of incision if added mobilization of the proximal tube is necessary to bury the end of the tube in the myometrium. **C:** The tagged ends of the tube are sutured deep into the myometrial tunnel and out through the uterine serosa. **D:** Tying these sutures secures the cut end of the proximal tube deep in the myometrial pocket.

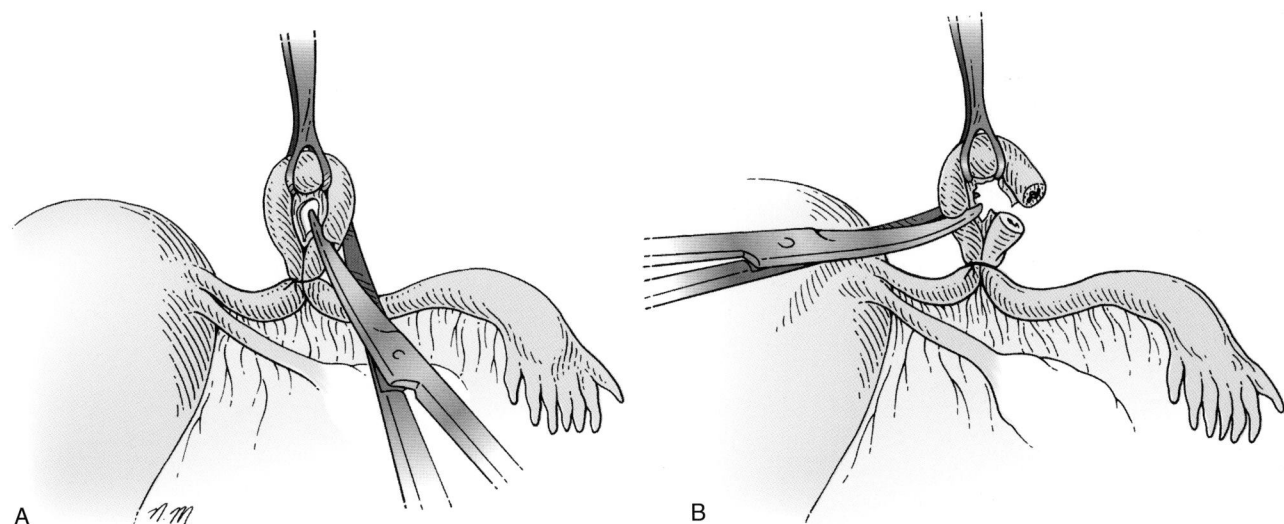

FIGURE 27.3 Pomeroy method. **A:** A loop of the isthmic portion of the tube is elevated and ligated at its base with one or two ties of no. 1 plain catgut suture. If performed through a minilaparotomy incision, these ties should be held long to prevent premature retraction of the tubal stumps into the abdomen when the loop of tube is transected. **B:** A fenestration is bluntly created through the mesentery within the tubal loop, and each limb of the tube on either side of this fenestration is individually cut. The cut ends of the tube are inspected for hemostasis and allowed to retract into the abdomen.

and failure. Taking time to identify the muscular tube, which is often seen pouting from each of the severed limbs of the ligated tube, is a good habit to develop, as is checking the tubal stumps for hemostasis. Resection of a limited amount of tube, restricted to the isthmic section, is ideal should unexpected future reanastomosis be requested. Making the knuckle of tube in the loop too small, however, can result in only a shave excision of the side of the tube, with incomplete transection of the lumen. To avoid incomplete resection, the mesosalpinx within the ligated loop should be perforated with scissors before the tubal limb on each side of this window is individually cut. It is important not to cut the loop so close to the suture that only short distal segments of tube remain beyond the tie. These short limbs can easily slip out of the ligature and cause delayed bleeding.

The Pomeroy method minimizes bleeding by compressing and sealing the vascular mesosalpinx before tubal transection. It is not unusual when performing tubal sterilization at the time of cesarean section to find the mesosalpinx greatly engorged with distended veins. Elevation of the uterus through the abdominal incision often facilitates tubal occlusion by allowing the vessels to drain and decompress. It is important when replacing the uterus into the peritoneal cavity to lead with one adnexa at a time while protecting the tubal ligation site on that side. Otherwise, when the uterus is replaced, a tight fit can cause the adnexa to be squeezed against the incision, with resultant avulsion of the ligature and postoperative bleeding. When a Pomeroy ligation is performed through a minilaparotomy incision, the ligation sutures are held while the tube is cut. This prevents retraction of the cut tubal stumps into the peritoneal cavity before they can be adequately examined and before hemostasis can be ensured. After examination is complete, the sutures are cut, and the tubal stumps are allowed to retract into the abdomen.

It is also possible to perform a modified Pomeroy tubal ligation as a laparoscopic interval procedure. In this technique, a laparoscope with an operating channel is placed through the umbilical port, and a 5-mm midline suprapubic cannula is introduced under direct vision. A plain gut Roeder loop (endoscopic slip knot) is introduced through the 5-mm port. A grasper is introduced through the operative channel of the laparoscope, advanced through the suture loop, and the appropriate portion of tube is grasped and retracted back through the loop. The slip knot of the loop is then tightened, ligating a knuckle of the tube. Scissors are then introduced through the operative scope, and the suture is cut. With the use of a grasper through the 5-mm port, the loop of tube is held on tension while the scissors are used through the operative channel to transect the tube above the ligature. When the procedure is complete and the tubal segment has been resected, the grasper is used through the operative channel to hold the specimen while the operative scope and grasper are removed together through the umbilical sleeve. In contrast to most other methods of laparoscopic sterilization, this technique has the advantage of producing a surgical specimen for evaluation.

Uchida Method

Originally reported on in 1961, and reported on in revised form in 1975, the Uchida method, like the Irving procedure before it, recognized the role of fistula formation in tubal sterilization failures and included steps to prevent this complication.

This method begins by having the surgeon grasp the tube in its midportion, about 6 to 7 cm from the uterotubal junction. A 1:1,000 epinephrine in saline solution is injected subserosally, creating a bleb over the tube that is then incised (**Fig. 27.4A**). The muscular tube, which often can be seen springing up through the serosal incision, then is divided between two hemostats. The serosa over the proximal tubal segment is dissected bluntly toward the uterus, exposing about 5 cm of the proximal tubal segment (**Fig. 27.4B**). The tube then is ligated with no. 0 chromic suture near the uterotubal junction, and this 5-cm segment of exposed tube is resected. The shortened proximal stump is allowed to retract into the mesosalpinx (**Fig. 27.4C**). The serosa around the opening in the mesosalpinx is sutured in a purse-string fashion with a fine absorbable

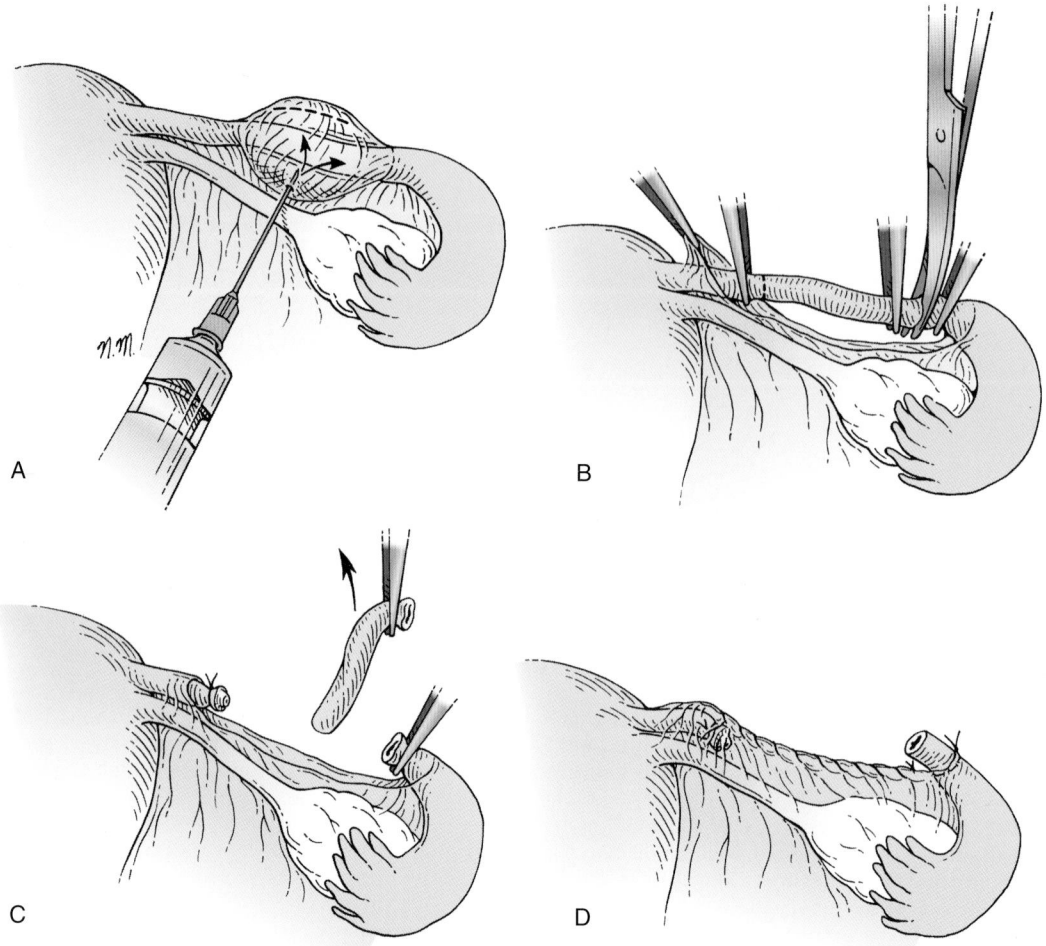

FIGURE 27.4 Uchida method. **A:** An injection of vasoconstricting solution is given beneath the serosa of the tube about 6 cm from the uterotubal junction. The serosa is then incised (*dashed line*). **B:** The antimesenteric edge of the mesosalpinx is pulled back toward the uterus, exposing about 5 cm of the tube. **C:** The tube is ligated proximally and cut, and the tied stump is allowed to retract into the mesosalpinx. The hemostat on the distal stump remains attached to facilitate exteriorization of this portion of the tube. **D:** The mesosalpinx is closed. A purse-string stitch of the mesosalpinx around the exteriorized tubal stump secures it in a position open to the abdomen, whereas the ligated proximal stump is buried within the mesosalpinx. Once the purse-string suture is tied, the hemostat can be removed.

stitch. Simultaneous ligation of the distal tube and gathering of the mesosalpinx around the distal stump are accomplished when the purse-string suture is tied (Fig. 27.4D). This step also fixes the distal stump in a position open to the peritoneal cavity while burying the proximal stump within the leaves of the mesosalpinx.

Uchida added fimbriectomy to the procedure in 1975 to enhance effectiveness. Some surgeons omit this step, and in addition excise only 1 to 2 cm of tube (rather than the recommended 5 cm) to permit future tubal anastomosis.

Parkland Method

In this method, made popular during the 1960s at Parkland Memorial Hospital, the tube is grasped in its midportion with a Babcock clamp, and a hemostat or scissors is used to create a window in an avascular area of the mesosalpinx just beneath the isthmic portion of the tube (Fig. 27.5A). The window is stretched to about 2.5 cm in length by opening the hemostat. Two ligatures of no. 0 chromic material are passed through the window, and the tube is ligated proximally and distally,

leaving a 2-cm proximal stump of isthmic tube (Fig. 27.5B). The intervening segment of tube between the ties then is resected (Fig. 27.5C). In contrast to the Pomeroy method, in which the resected portions of the tubes are ligated together and later separate when the suture weakens, immediate separation of the tubal ends is accomplished with the Parkland method. Care should be taken to avoid undue traction on the ligatures while resecting the tubal segments, because this could result in tearing of the mesosalpinx and excessive bleeding.

Unipolar Coagulation

Unipolar coagulation was the first method of laparoscopic tubal occlusion to achieve widespread use. However, reports of electrical complications, particularly thermal bowel injury, resulted in a significant decline in this method's popularity as soon as alternative methods of laparoscopic tubal occlusion became available in the mid-1970s. In unipolar coagulation, a specially designed insulated grasping forceps is introduced through the operating channel of the laparoscope or independently through a 5-mm second-puncture port. As a safety precaution, attachment of the

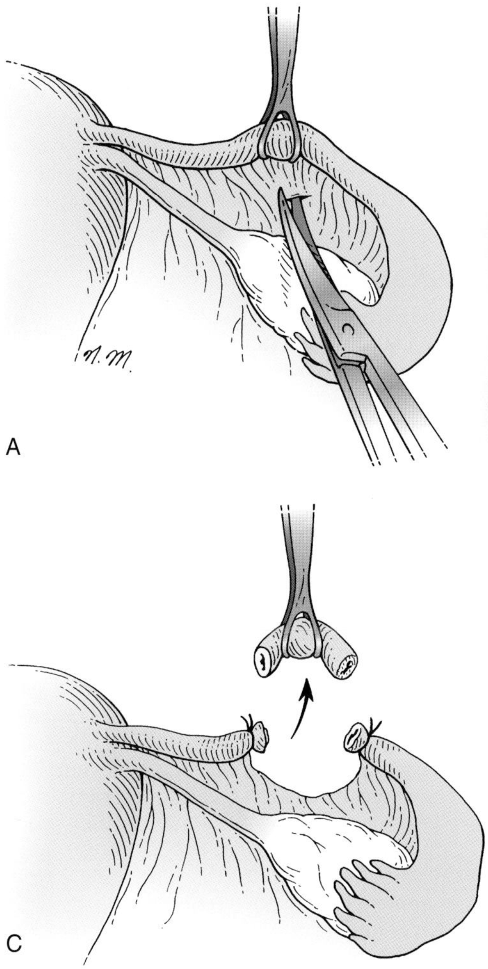

FIGURE 27.5 Parkland method. **A:** A 2- to 3-cm fenestration is made beneath the isthmic portion of tube either with scissors or bluntly with a hemostat. **B:** Ligation of the tube. Pulling up on the suture during ligation or during transection of the tube can shear the tube off the underlying mesentery, resulting in troublesome bleeding. **C:** Portion of tube removed.

electric cable to the grasping forceps should be delayed until the surgeon is ready to coagulate the fallopian tube.

With unipolar coagulation, as much as 3 to 5 cm of tube can be destroyed with a single burn, with occult damage occurring beyond the visual zone of desiccation. For this reason, the isthmic–ampullary portion of the tube should be carefully identified and grasped about 5 cm from the uterus to preserve some length of proximal tube. The jaws of the grasping forceps should completely encircle the fallopian tube and include a portion of the mesosalpinx as well. The tube should be elevated away from adjacent structures, such as bowel and bladder, before current is applied for about 5 seconds. If a second burn is required, it should be applied to the proximal rather than the distal portion of the tube. The current should be turned off before the tube is released and the grasping forceps are retracted into the laparoscope. Both jaws of the grasping forceps serve as active electrodes and will cause electrosurgical injury to any structure they touch while current is applied.

The thermal injuries to abdominal viscera that are seen with unipolar coagulation are, in some cases, likely attributable to the phenomenon of capacitive coupling. The current flowing down the unipolar probe creates an electromagnetic field that can transfer an electric charge to any conductor surrounding the probe. The greater the voltage being used with the probe, the greater this capacitive effect. In the case of laparoscopic unipolar coagulation for sterilization, the conductor surrounding the insulated unipolar probe is the operative laparoscope itself.

As long as the operative laparoscope is safely grounded (usually by contact with a metal trocar sleeve that, in turn, is in contact with the abdominal wall over a large surface area), then the capacitive charge on the laparoscope can be harmlessly dissipated. If, however, the laparoscope is prevented from safely grounding into the abdominal wall by a nonconducting trocar sleeve or by a nonconducting barrier around the trocar sleeve (e.g., a plastic collar with threads), then the capacitive charge that builds up on the scope discharges when and wherever any portion of that instrument touches the patient's tissues. Depending on the surface area of contact, the discharging current from the scope into the patient's tissues has either a high current density (small contact surface) or a low current density (large contact surface), resulting in either a large thermal effect or a minimal thermal effect, respectively. In the case of contact with bowel, this thermal effect easily can result in delayed necrosis and peritonitis. If the unipolar probe is brought into the abdomen by way of a second puncture trocar sheath, then it is the sheath itself that is capacitively charged (if it is made of a conducting material). If the charge on the conducting trocar sleeve is prevented from grounding through the abdominal wall (as could occur if a plastic collar with threads is being used around the trocar sleeve), then any bowel or other grounded tissue touching the trocar sleeve again has capacitive current flowing into it. The use of unmodulated cutting current minimizes the voltage required to create the desired tissue effect. Coagulation or modulated current relies on short bursts of much higher voltage and should be avoided in order to reduce the risk of capacitive coupling and unseen or unrecognized injury.

If thermal injury to the intestine is noticed during the laparoscopic procedure, then it is important to recognize that the injury can extend well beyond the visibly damaged area. Small burns of the bowel serosa may not require repair, but close observation for 5 to 7 days is recommended so the patient can be monitored for delayed peritonitis. A laparotomy is required if peritonitis occurs. A large area of superficial thermal bowel injury, or one that is thought to extend beyond the serosa, requires resection of that portion of intestine with a 5-cm margin on either side of the lesion. Oversewing the damaged area can result in stitches being placed in bowel that appears healthy visually but in reality is destined to necrose from occult thermal or electrical injury.

Bipolar Coagulation

The use of bipolar coagulation for tubal sterilization was reported by Rioux and Cloutier in 1974. With bipolar coagulation, current flows from one jaw of the grasper to the other, requiring only the intervening tissue of the patient within the jaws of the instrument to complete the circuit. This eliminates the need for a distant return electrode. Compared with unipolar coagulation, which uses the patient's body to complete the circuit, bipolar coagulation applies current in a more discrete manner (a 1.5- to 3-cm zone of thermal injury) and with a potentially increased element of safety. Capacitive coupling does not occur with bipolar forceps because the field effects from the equal but opposite currents that flow in both directions along the shaft of the instrument cancel out one another.

Once the fallopian tube is carefully identified, it is grasped in the distal isthmic section with the bipolar forceps in such a way that the tube is completely encircled, including a portion of the mesosalpinx (Fig. 27.6). The tube then is elevated away from any adjacent structures, and current is applied. Two additional contiguous areas similarly are coagulated to ensure at least a 3-cm area of desiccation. As with unipolar coagulation, an effort should be made to leave the proximal 2 cm of tube undisturbed to reduce the risk of tuboperitoneal fistula formation.

The visual end points of tubal blanching and swelling noted with bipolar coagulation cannot be used to ensure destruction of the endosalpinx. Desiccation of the outer one third of the fallopian tube can occur without desiccation of the inner one third. The use of an optical flowmeter has been recommended to evaluate cessation of current flow through the tube as an end point. Presumably, when complete desiccation occurs, there will be no further electrolytes in solution to carry current through the dehydrated tissue. Soderstrom and coworkers have demonstrated that complete desiccation of the fallopian tube with bipolar systems is more likely when a cutting waveform, as opposed to a coagulation or blended waveform, is used and when the power output is at least 25 W against a 100-V load.

Silicone Rubber Bands

Complications associated with the use of unipolar coagulation led to the pursuit of safer, nonthermal methods that could be applied laparoscopically. The first of these methods to gain popularity was the silicone rubber band, developed by Yoon and coworkers in the early 1970s.

The band is introduced with a specially designed endoscopic applicator that can be delivered through either the operating channel of a laparoscope or a separate second puncture port. The band is first stretched over the distal end of the applicator barrel (immediately before use to avoid extended deformation of the band). A transcervical uterine manipulator can be used to help achieve proper exposure. After the device is introduced into the abdominal cavity, grasping tongs are extended from within the applicator barrel. One of the tongs is used to gently hook and elevate the isthmic portion of the tube about 3 cm from the uterus. The tongs then are retracted into the applicator, which closes both arms of the tongs around the grasped tube while pulling the loop of tube up into the barrel (Fig. 27.7). The surgeon must take care in ensuring that the tube is completely encircled by the tongs as they are retracted into the applicator. Failure to do this can result in a band that is only tangentially applied to the tube (failing to occlude its lumen) or applied only to the mesosalpinx.

It is important to avoid excessive traction on the tube during retraction of the tongs. The surgeon should slowly advance the entire applicator toward the tube while gradually retracting

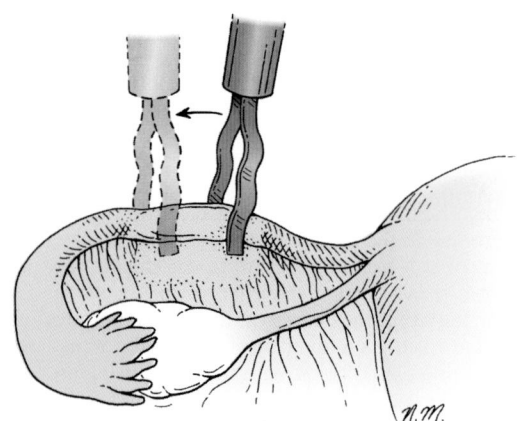

FIGURE 27.6 Bipolar method. A 3-cm minimum zone of isthmic tube is desiccated with bipolar forceps. The paddles of the forceps extend across the tube onto the mesosalpinx.

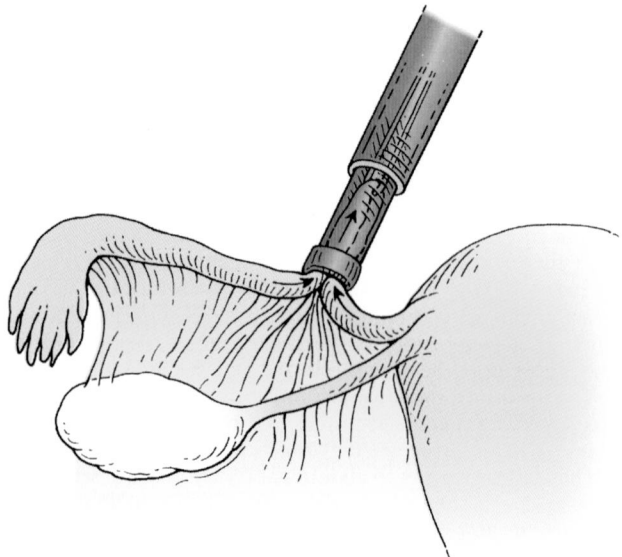

FIGURE 27.7 Silicone band method. The isthmic portion of the tube is retracted into the applicator barrel using grasping tongs, which should completely surround the tube. The applicator barrel is advanced toward the tube during this retraction process to avoid excessive traction on the tube and its mesentery.

the tongs and tube up into the applicator. Failure to do this can result in mesosalpingeal hemorrhage and tubal laceration. Once the loop is fully retracted into the device, the band is slid off the applicator barrel and onto the base of the loop.

Approximately 1.5 to 2 cm of tube is contained in the constricted loop. After devascularization, this portion of tube becomes anoxic and resorbs over time. Eventually, the band no longer encircles any tube; later it is often found in the mesosalpinx. Apart from the 2-cm loop of encircled tube, very little destruction is caused by the band, and 2 mm lateral to the area of constriction of the tube is relatively undisturbed.

It is difficult to apply a band to edematous or thickened fallopian tubes successfully. Tubal adhesions can reduce the mobility of the tube and preclude pulling an adequate loop of tube into the applicator. Additional rings can be applied to the cut edges if transection of the mesosalpinx or tube with accompanying hemorrhage occurs. Bipolar or unipolar coagulation can be used if this is unsuccessful.

Spring Clip

The use of a spring clip for tubal sterilization was reported by Hulka and colleagues in 1973. The introducer for the clip can be delivered into the abdomen through the operative channel of the laparoscope or a second puncture cannula (Fig. 27.8). Because the clip must be applied exactly perpendicular to the long axis of the fallopian tube, it is helpful at times to use the two-puncture method—placing the tube on stretch by use of a transcervical uterine manipulator and a grasping forceps inserted through the operating channel of the laparoscope and introducing the applicator through the second puncture port.

The clip is held in a cradle by the applicator and can be closed and opened on the tube multiple times until an acceptable application is achieved. At this point, further pressure on the thumb device of the applicator drives the spring mechanism over the jaws of the clip, locking it closed. If improper application is determined at this point, the clip cannot be removed, and another clip has to be placed. To be effective, the clip must be applied to the isthmic portion of the tube, approximately 2 cm from the uterus and exactly at right angles to the long axis of the tube. It must be applied fully advanced over the tube, with the hinge of the clip pressing against the tube

and with the tips of the jaws of the clip extending beyond the tube onto the mesosalpinx, creating a characteristic fold in the mesosalpinx when the clip is closed. The tube is not elevated when applying the clip, in contrast to the techniques used in coagulation and band application.

The clip, like the silicone rubber band, is most likely to be successful when applied to a normal tube. Tubal distortion, thickening, and adhesions make correct application difficult and often impossible.

A considerable advantage to the clip method of sterilization is that only 3 mm of tube is compressed by the clip, and minimal collateral damage occurs in the adjacent tissue. As a result, anastomosis procedures after clip sterilization often are highly successful.

Filshie Clip

The Filshie clip was first introduced in Europe in 1975, and the hinged Mark VI model was approved for use in the United States by the U.S. Food and Drug Administration (FDA) in 1996. The device has titanium jaws lined with silicone rubber and is used with specially designed applicators that are available in both single- and double-puncture versions for use with laparoscopy or minilaparotomy. The Filshie clip has a hinge on one end and a small curve on the other and is designed to be placed on the isthmic portion of the fallopian tube approximately 1 to 2 cm from the cornua (Fig. 27.9).

To be effective, the jaws of this clip, as with the spring clip, must include the entire circumference of the tube. Only one properly applied clip needs to be applied to each fallopian tube. Once the tube is occluded, both the tube and the silicone

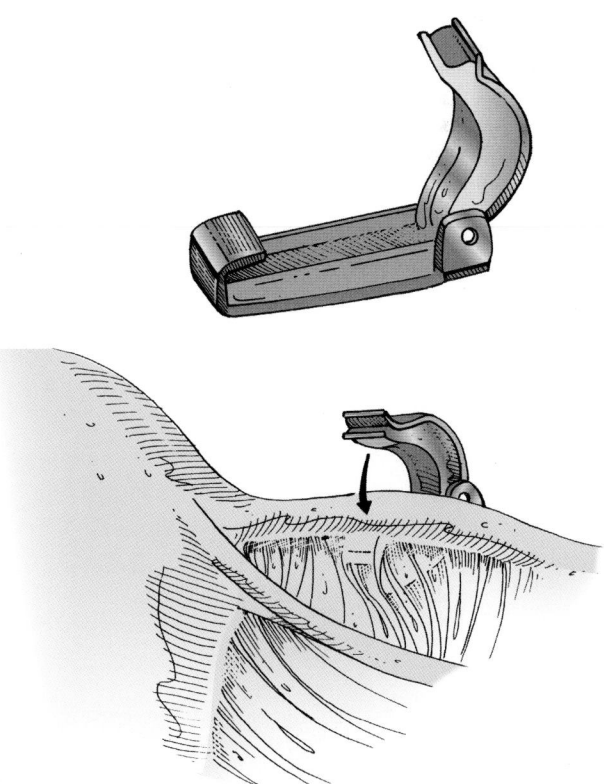

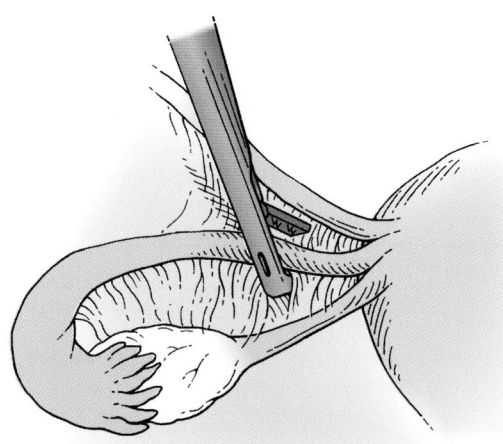

FIGURE 27.8 Spring clip method. The clip is applied to the midisthmus (approximately 2 cm from the cornua) at a 90-degree angle to the long axis of the tube. The hinge of the clip should be pressed against the tube, and the tips of the clip should extend onto the mesosalpinx.

FIGURE 27.9 Filshie clip method. The clip is applied to the midisthmus (approximately 1 to 2 cm from the cornua) with the lower jaw of the clip being visible in the mesosalpinx to assure that the entire circumference of the tube is included.

rubber lining of the clip are compressed. Over time, approximately 3 to 5 mm of the compressed tissue undergoes avascular necrosis, and the compressed silicone rubber expands. Eventually, plical attenuation and fibrosis of the adjacent tubal segments occurs, and the clips are peritonealized.

The clip is placed into the applicator, and the applicator and clip then are introduced through the cannula with the jaws of the clip in a partially closed position so that the instrument with the clip in place can be used to manipulate the fallopian tube into proper position. The clip may close prematurely if too much pressure is placed on the handle of the applicator. The lower jaw of the clip, with its small curve at the tip, should be seen through the mesosalpinx to assure that the clip includes the entire circumference of the isthmic portion of the tube before the clip is applied. Because of the clip's hinge and the silicone lining of the jaws, the tubes can be manipulated and released several times for better positioning of the clip. Gentle pressure is placed on the applicator handle once desired placement is obtained, which causes the upper jaw of the clip to flatten and lock under the curved tip of the lower jaw. The clip should be closed slowly to avoid transection of the fallopian tube, which is more likely with edematous tubes. A clip can be placed on each transected end if transection occurs. Many surgeons recommend the use of a double-puncture technique to assure proper placement.

Essure

The Essure microinsert was approved by the FDA for use as an interval tubal sterilization device in 2002. In 2007, the FDA approved the ESS 305 model, which was developed to improve bilateral placement rates. The device is inserted transcervically via hysteroscopy and thus avoids both entry into the abdominal cavity and the need for general or regional anesthesia. It is available as part of a disposable system that includes the microinsert, a delivery system, and a split introducer. The microinsert is comprised of a stainless steel inner coil, a nickel titanium alloy outer coil, and a layer of polyethylene terephthalate (PET) fibers around the inner coil. The microinsert is 4 cm in length and 0.8 mm in diameter before release from the insertion catheter; following release, it expands to 1.5 to 2.0 mm in diameter as the coils open up to anchor into the fallopian tube across the uterotubal junction (Fig. 27.10).

The Essure microinsert can be placed in an outpatient or office surgery setting with oral analgesia alone or using a paracervical block with or without intravenous sedation. Using a sterile standard 5-mm hysteroscope with a minimum 5-French operating channel and a 12- to 30-degree angled lens, the uterine cavity is distended adequately with 2 to 3 L of warmed physiologic saline to allow accurate identification of both tubal ostia. The procedure should be terminated if both tubal ostia are not visible, accessible, and considered likely to be patent. The manufacturer's package insert recommends that the risk of hypervolemia be reduced by immediately terminating the procedure if the fluid deficit of the physiologic saline distention medium exceeds 1,500 mL and by limiting the time of the hysteroscopic procedure to a maximum of 20 minutes.

The Essure microinsert is designed to be placed in the fallopian tube across the uterotubal junction where the tube exits the uterine wall but with 5 to 10 mm (the equivalent of three to eight coils) still trailing into the uterus. This is achieved by inserting the delivery catheter with the microinsert into the proximal tubal lumen to the level indicated by the black position marker on the catheter. When the device is correctly placed, the delivery catheter is withdrawn, and the delivery wire is separated from the microinsert. The trailing end of the coils aids in anchoring the device to decrease the risk of expulsion. The device is also anchored as it expands in the tube at placement, but occlusion is not considered adequate without tissue ingrowth from the tubal wall into the coils that occurs as a result of an inflammatory and fibrotic response to the PET fibers in the inner coil. A hysterosalpingogram (HSG) must be performed 3 months postinsertion to assure complete bilateral tubal occlusion. Transvaginal ultrasonography has also been used for microinsert localization but is not approved by the FDA as an alternative to HSG for this purpose. Alternate contraception should be used until occlusion is documented.

In early studies, 14% of microinsert attempts failed with the first attempt on one or both sides, using the original braided catheter. Although the rate of failed attempts was reduced as training improved, the insertion failure rate remained considerable at 10%. In a postapproval trial by Levie et al. of the ESS 305 model reported in 2011, the successful bilateral placement rate was 97.2%, but these encouraging findings require confirmation in the general population.

The Essure microinsert is indicated, as for other methods of sterilization, only for women who are certain about their desire to terminate future fertility. The effects of the microinserts on a desired subsequent pregnancy are unknown, but they are not removable once the fibrotic ingrowth is complete, and several coils may potentially project into the uterine cavity, making in vitro fertilization potentially less feasible than following sterilization by laparoscopy or minilaparotomy.

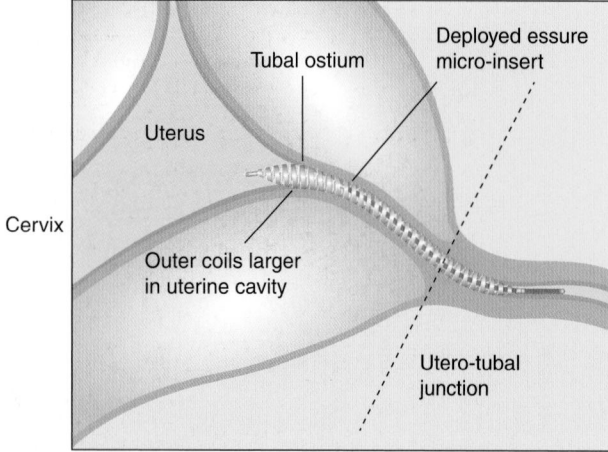

Uterus

Tubal ostium

Deployed essure micro-insert

Cervix

Outer coils larger in uterine cavity

Utero-tubal junction

FIGURE 27.10 Essure method. The Essure microinsert is designed to be placed in the fallopian tube across the uterotubal junction where the tube exits the uterine wall but with 5 to 10 mm (the equivalent of three to eight coils) still trailing into the uterus.

STEPS IN THE PROCEDURE

General Considerations

- Patient counseled on alternative options, permanence, risks, and failure rate of intended procedure
- Pregnancy test obtained preoperatively as indicated
- Procedure performed in follicular phase of cycle
- Sterilization procedures are performed on the area of tube, appropriate for the specific procedure approximately 2 cm from cornu

Minilaparotomy (Postpartum) Sterilization Pomeroy Technique

- Incision at umbilicus, with patient in Trendelenburg position
- Sweep tube up to incision using finger behind adnexa, Babcock clamp, and table tilt
- Elevate 2- to 3-cm knuckle of mid-isthmic portion of tube with Babcock clamp
- Ligate a 2- to 3-cm knuckle of tube with no. 1 plain catgut suture
- Bluntly create window in mesosalpinx of looped tube
- Excise the knuckle of the tube, cutting the tube to one side of window and then the other

Laparoscopic (Interval) Methods

Bipolar Coagulation

- Three contiguous burns (approximately 3 cm length) of fallopian tube using bipolar forceps, beginning 2 cm from cornu and progressing distally
- Bipolar at least 25 watts cutting current, and forceps grasp entire width of tube to include portion of underlying mesosalpinx
- Ammeter demonstrating cessation of current flow can help determine end point of desiccation

Clips

- Hulka or Filshie clips applied with device at right angle to the isthmic portion of tube, approximately 2 cm from cornu
- Clips should traverse entire width of tube and extend onto a portion of the mesosalpinx

Ring (Bands)

- One tong of the applicator gently hooks and elevates tube, approximately 3 cm from the cornu
- Ensure tongs completely encircle the tube as they are retracted into the applicator
- To avoid excessive traction that can sever tube, applicator should be advanced toward tube as tongs are retracted

Hysteroscopic Method

- Essure
- Gently introduce an operative hysteroscope through the cervix
- With adequate uterine distention using warmed normal saline, visualize both fallopian tube orifices
- Place the delivery catheter through the operating port of the scope and into the tubal orifice up to the level of the black marker
- Deploy the microinsert and separate it from the delivery catheter
- Remove the first catheter and repeat the procedure on the opposite side
- Visualize both tubal ostia and record the number of trailing coils visible on each side

Women with a known hypersensitivity to nickel should not have the Essure devices inserted because the outer coil is made of nickel–titanium alloy.

IMMEDIATE COMPLICATIONS

Mortality

In an international study of 41,834 sterilizations performed from 1971 to 1979 in 28 countries, the estimated case fatality rate was 13.4 per 100,000 interval tubal sterilization procedures, 53.3 per 100,000 postabortion sterilization procedures, and 43.4 per 100,000 sterilizations after vaginal delivery. At least some of the differences in case fatality rates between interval tubal sterilization and sterilization associated with pregnancy were likely attributable to complications of pregnancy termination or delivery rather than tubal sterilization per se.

The potential health impact of tubal sterilization in countries that have a high rate of maternal mortality can be assessed by analyzing sterilization-attributable deaths in Bangladesh. In the first of two epidemiologic investigations, 28 deaths were attributed to tubal sterilization in two geographic areas; the case fatality rate was 19 deaths per 100,000 tubal sterilizations. In the second investigation, 19 deaths were identified nationwide, for a case fatality rate of 12.4 deaths per 100,000 procedures. Anesthesia overdosage, tetanus, and hemorrhage were the leading causes of death in both investigations. On the basis of an estimated maternal mortality rate of 570 per 100,000 live births, more than 1,000 maternal deaths for each 100,000 tubal sterilizations performed would have been averted during the reproductive years of the cohort.

In the United States, deaths attributable to tubal sterilization are rare. Based on an assessment of tubal sterilizations performed in US hospitals in 1979 and 1980, the estimated case fatality rate for tubal sterilization is 1 to 2 per 100,000 procedures. Complications of general anesthesia are the leading cause of sterilization-attributable death. In a survey of deaths attributable to tubal sterilization in the United States from 1977 to 1981, 29 deaths were identified: Eleven followed complications of general anesthesia, seven were caused by sepsis, four were caused by hemorrhage, three were caused by myocardial infarction, and four were related to other causes.

At least some of these deaths are preventable. Safer use of general anesthesia or use of local anesthesia, particularly for interval laparoscopic and minilaparotomy procedures, should reduce the risk of death from anesthesia. Of the seven identified deaths caused by sepsis from 1977 to 1981, three were associated with the use of unipolar electrocoagulation. Safer use of unipolar coagulation or alternative methods of tubal occlusion reduces the risk of thermal bowel injury. Three of the four deaths attributable to hemorrhage occurred after major vessel laceration during abdominal entry for laparoscopy. Safer insertion of the Veress needle and trocar or use of alternative techniques, such as open laparoscopy or minilaparotomy, should reduce the risk of such major vessel injuries.

Morbidity

Morbidity attributable to tubal sterilization is uncommon but not rare. The risks for and types of morbidity vary somewhat by surgical approach and method of tubal occlusion. Direct comparisons of minilaparotomy and laparoscopy for tubal sterilization are limited, but studies suggest several differences. In a nonrandomized study in 23 countries, 7,053 women who had silicone rubber band application by way of laparoscopy were compared with 3,033 women who had silicone rubber band application by minilaparotomy and 5,081 women who had modified Pomeroy ligation by minilaparotomy. The surgical complication rates were 2.04%, 1.45%, and 0.79% for the three groups, respectively. In a smaller but randomized study in eight centers, 791 women who had modified Pomeroy occlusion by minilaparotomy were compared with 819 women who had occlusion from electrocoagulation (technique not specified) by way of laparoscopy. Major complications occurred in 1.5% of the women in the minilaparotomy group and 0.9% of the women in the laparoscopy group. Minor complications, which are more common, occurred in 11.6% of women in the former group and 6.0% in the latter group.

In a US multicenter, collaborative study, major complications were more common among women who had minilaparotomy (3.5%) than among those who had interval laparoscopic sterilization (1.6%). However, women in the study were not randomly assigned to groups, and the sterilization procedures were performed in institutions where most interval tubal sterilizations were done by way of laparoscopy. Thus, minilaparotomy sterilizations may have been performed selectively for women at increased risk for complications.

Although the overall complication rates are similar for minilaparotomy and laparoscopy, the types of complications appear to vary. Complications of minilaparotomy usually are not serious and typically include minor wound infection, longer operating time, slightly longer postoperative convalescence, and greater postoperative pain. Laparoscopic complications are more likely to include rare but life-threatening hemorrhage and viscus perforations during abdominal entry and thermal bowel injury during electrocoagulation. A study of 100,000 laparoscopies in France suggests that major vessel laceration occurs in three of 10,000 procedures. In a study conducted in the United Kingdom, major vessel laceration occurred in nine of 10,000 laparoscopies.

Some of the most serious complications of both interval minilaparotomy and laparoscopy occur during abdominal entry. Bladder laceration during suprapubic minilaparotomy can occur, but usually, it is recognized during surgery and is repaired easily. Major vessel and bowel laceration during needle or trocar insertion for laparoscopy are more difficult to recognize or repair, and delayed treatment of these injuries can be fatal. Meticulousness is required to reduce the risks of abdominal entry. Comparative studies of open versus conventional laparoscopy are limited and have insufficient power to assess the risk of life-threatening complications, but use of open laparoscopy should markedly reduce the risk of major vessel laceration and should reduce, to a lesser extent, the risk of bowel laceration. The use of open laparoscopy can be particularly advantageous for women known or strongly suspected to have multiple abdominal or pelvic adhesions. However, even open laparoscopy can result in bowel injury if the bowel is adherent to the anterior abdominal wall.

The method of tubal occlusion chosen influences the risk for and type of complications during laparoscopy. Thermal bowel injury is more common with unipolar than bipolar coagulation, but it can occur during the latter if the bowel is grasped and coagulated. Transection of the fallopian tube can occur with any technique, particularly when an attempt is made to mobilize the fallopian tube in the presence of thick peritubal adhesions. Tubal transection is most likely to occur when silicone rubber bands are used, but any resultant bleeding usually can be managed by the application of a second ring or by the use of coagulation.

Complications associated with insertion of the Essure device are generally related to the risks inherent in hysteroscopy, including hypervolemia, uterine perforation, and vasovagal syncope. Tubal spasm may occur precluding delivery of the microinserts beyond the tubal orifice. Patience while reducing intrauterine pressure and gentle pressure with the delivery catheter tip at the tubal orifice will usually result in relaxation of the spasm and successful microinsert placement. Intravascular delivery of local anesthetic solutions can occur. This may create the potential for seizures and cardiopulmonary arrest. Care should be taken when performing paracervical block anesthesia to infiltrate tissues superficially. Tubal perforation may also occur with placement of the microinserts across the uterotubal junction. This is typically unrecognized until the 3-month HSG confirmation test demonstrates poor positioning of the devices. Very rarely, patients may develop unrelenting crampy pain after insertion, which may necessitate removal of the devices if relief cannot be obtained with 7 to 10 days of medical management.

DELAYED COMPLICATIONS

Pregnancy

Tubal sterilization is highly effective in preventing pregnancy. A frequently cited failure rate is four pregnancies per 1,000 sterilization procedures. However, a range of failure rates is more likely to portray the risk of pregnancy after sterilization. The determinants of that range are likely to include the method of tubal occlusion, surgical technique, and the age of the woman at sterilization. In the US Collaborative Review of Sterilization, a multicenter, prospective, cohort study, 10,685 women undergoing tubal sterilization in medical centers in nine US cities from 1978 to 1987 were followed for up to 14 years. A total of 143 sterilization failures were identified with the 10-year cumulative probability of failure ranging from 7.5 per 1,000 procedures (for unipolar coagulation procedures and postpartum partial salpingectomy procedures) to 36.5 per 1,000 (for spring clip application procedures). The failure rates for most methods of tubal occlusion were higher for women aged 18 to 27 years at sterilization (as high as 54.3 and 52.1 per 1,000 bipolar coagulation and spring clip applications, respectively) than for women aged 34 to 44 years at sterilization (as low as 1.8 and 3.8 per 1,000 unipolar coagulation and postpartum partial salpingectomy procedures, respectively).

This large US multicenter study and two smaller studies in Thailand and Belgium have dispelled the widely held belief that nearly all pregnancies after sterilization occur in the first year or two after the procedure. In the Thai study, 418 women were followed for 6 to 10 years after sterilization, and only one of four pregnancies identified occurred within 2 years of the procedure. In the Belgian study, of 17 pregnancies after 1,437 sterilizations by bipolar coagulation, none occurred within 12 months of electrocoagulation, and eight occurred more than 24 months after the procedure. In the US study, the 10-year cumulative probability of pregnancy after bipolar coagulation (24.8 per 1,000 procedures) was approximately 10 times the probability (2.3 per 1,000) at 1 year. Further, pregnancies occurred in the 10th year after all four methods of laparoscopic sterilization studied (bipolar and unipolar coagulation, silicone rubber band application, and spring clip application).

The fact that the risk of pregnancy after sterilization only can be determined after long-term follow-up creates a dilemma in interpreting published failure rates. For example, the failure rates in the US Collaborative Review of Sterilization for six methods of tubal occlusion were based on procedures performed in the late 1970s and 1980s when laparoscopic sterilization was fairly new. Whether failure rates for procedures performed in the past reflect the risk for current procedures is unclear. In an analysis of bipolar coagulation procedures in the US Collaborative Review of Sterilization, the 5-year cumulative probability of pregnancy for women sterilized in 1978 to 1982 (19.5 per 1,000 procedures) was significantly greater than that for women sterilized in 1985 to 1987 (6.3 per 1,000 procedures). Further, most of the procedures evaluated in that study were performed in teaching institutions; it is unclear whether procedures performed in teaching institutions can be generalized outside such settings.

Luteal phase pregnancy, or pregnancy diagnosed after sterilization but conceived before sterilization, is estimated to occur in 2 to 3 per 1,000 sterilization procedures. The most effective strategy for reducing the risk for luteal phase pregnancy is to time the sterilization procedure to occur during the follicular phase of the menstrual cycle. Reliance on dilatation and curettage at the time of sterilization is substantially less effective. The likelihood of luteal phase pregnancy occurring also depends on the method of contraception used before tubal sterilization. Women who use steroid hormonal contraceptives or intrauterine devices are at substantially lower risk for luteal phase pregnancy than are women who use barrier methods or no method of contraception. Testing for pregnancy by using an enzyme-linked immunosorbent assay pregnancy test as indicated before sterilization also reduces the risk for luteal phase pregnancy.

The likelihood of ectopic pregnancy occurring is increased when pregnancy occurs after sterilization. In the US Collaborative Review of Sterilization, the highest proportion of ectopic pregnancies among all pregnancies after sterilization was among women who underwent bipolar coagulation (65%), followed by interval partial salpingectomy (43%), silicone rubber band application (29%), postpartum partial salpingectomy (20%), unipolar coagulation (17%), and spring clip application (15%). The proportion of pregnancies that were ectopic increased over time; for all methods combined, the proportion of ectopic pregnancies was three times greater in the 4th through 10th years after sterilization (61%) than in the first 3 years (20%). All pregnancies that occurred in the 10th year after unipolar and bipolar coagulation, silicone rubber band application, and spring clip application were ectopic. All but one (an ovarian pregnancy after bipolar coagulation) of the 47 ectopic pregnancies identified in the study were tubal pregnancies. The index of suspicion for ectopic pregnancy should be high when pregnancy is suspected after tubal sterilization. Pregnancy should be confirmed by use of a highly sensitive pregnancy test as soon as feasible.

A woman's individual risk for ectopic pregnancy can be considered in both absolute and relative terms. Her absolute risk is determined by the likelihood that the sterilization procedure can fail to prevent pregnancy and the likelihood that a resulting pregnancy will be ectopic. This risk is also relative to the risk for ectopic pregnancy that a woman had before tubal sterilization. Depending on the method of contraception used before sterilization, some women may be at greater risk for ectopic pregnancy after tubal sterilization. In a report from a case–control study in Seattle, both postpartum sterilization and interval sterilization were associated with a lower risk of ectopic pregnancy than was use of no contraception. However, women who had interval tubal sterilization had a higher risk of ectopic pregnancy than did women who were using oral contraceptives or barrier methods of contraception. In contrast, the risk for ectopic pregnancy was similar between women who had postpartum tubal sterilization and those who used oral contraceptives or barrier contraception.

Careful attention to surgical technique is required to maximize sterilization effectiveness. To reduce the risk of pregnancy

after bipolar coagulation, Soderstrom and colleagues identified determinants of complete electrocoagulation. In the US Collaborative Review of Sterilization, women undergoing bipolar coagulation later in the study who had three or more sites of coagulation had a 5-year cumulative probability of failure of 3.2 per 1,000 procedures. This is similar to the 5-year probability for unipolar coagulation (2.3 per 1,000) and substantially lower than that for women undergoing bipolar coagulation with fewer than three sites of coagulation (12.9 per 1,000). Stovall and coworkers reported on the use of silicone rubber bands and spring clips in a residency training program; all of 20 sterilization failures were associated with improper application of the occlusive device on gross and microscopic evaluation after subsequent bilateral salpingectomy. In the US Collaborative Review of Sterilization, the risks of pregnancy were significantly increased among women who had a silicone rubber band applied solely to the distal one third of at least one fallopian tube and among women who had a spring clip applied to a site other than the proximal one third of at least one tube.

The likelihood of sterilization failure depends not only on the sterilization technique but also on patient and physician factors. For example, proper application of silicone rubber bands and spring clips generally is difficult in the presence of thickened tubes or dense pelvic adhesions; under such circumstances, alternative techniques usually are preferred. As noted, failure rates generally are higher for women sterilized at younger ages, not only because they are more fecund at the time of sterilization than older women but also because they have a longer period after sterilization during which it would be feasible for pregnancy to occur. The latter consideration, which is an issue because it is now clear that pregnancy can occur for many years after sterilization, also applies to any temporary method of contraception that a woman chooses to use. For example, based on data from the US Collaborative Review of Sterilization, a woman sterilized at 28 to 33 years old has a 10-year chance of pregnancy of less than 1% to approximately 3%, depending on the method of tubal occlusion. The comparable risk for 10 years of use of the Copper T 380 intrauterine device is approximately 2%, but the typical failure rate for oral contraceptive use is approximately 6% to 8% in just the first 12 months of use. Data regarding the long-term failure rates of the Filshie clip and the Essure microinsert are less complete than those for the other commonly used techniques. However, based on data to date, both appear highly effective with proper placement.

In a 2012 systematic review that included 22 studies, 102 pregnancies were identified after Essure placement, but most of these pregnancies occurred when FDA's instructions for use were not followed. Especially noteworthy findings were not placing the microinserts during days 7 to 14 of the menstrual cycle, not having an imaging study at 3 months postinsertion to document successful placement, and not using effective contraception until tubal occlusion had been documented. Only 15 pregnancies occurred among women who had imaging confirmation of correct placement or tubal occlusion, highlighting not only the very low risk of pregnancy after successful bilateral tubal occlusion but also the importance of adequate follow-up imaging. Given the fundamentally different mechanism of tubal obstruction (fibrotic endosalpingeal ingrowth) with the hysteroscopic technique, the risk of ectopic pregnancy in sterilization failures may be quite different than with the laparoscopic or minilaparotomy approaches. Long-term careful follow-up studies will be needed to establish the long-term failure and ectopic risks with Essure.

Menstrual Changes

After nearly a half century of debate, questions regarding the existence of a posttubal ligation syndrome of menstrual abnormalities appear to be largely resolved. Questions arose initially when Williams and colleagues reported in 1951 that sterilized women had a higher-than-expected occurrence of menorrhagia and metrorrhagia. Studies in the 1970s appeared to support the existence of a poststerilization syndrome, but most of those studies had major methodologic shortcomings, including failure to account for factors other than sterilization per se that might have influenced poststerilization menstrual changes. One such factor was the use of oral contraceptives; in the United States, as many as 30% of women may use oral contraceptives immediately before tubal sterilization, and many of these women have menstrual changes after sterilization attributable solely to cessation of oral contraceptive use. Although one well-controlled study by Shain et al. in the 1980s identified poststerilization menstrual changes, nearly all other studies reported in the 1980s that controlled for factors such as cessation of oral contraceptive use found little or no evidence of a poststerilization syndrome at 1 to 2 years after sterilization.

Until the 1990s, questions remained about whether menstrual changes attributable to sterilization may occur several years after the procedure. Two US multicenter, prospective, cohort studies argue strongly against such an occurrence. In the first, reported in 1993, 500 women were evaluated at 6 to 10 months and 3 to 4.5 years after sterilization. When women who were taking oral contraceptives were excluded, no significant differences in seven menstrual parameters were found between sterilized women and two groups of nonsterilized women.

In the second, reported in 2000, 9,514 sterilized women enrolled in the US Collaborative Review of Sterilization were compared with 573 women whose husbands underwent vasectomy. All women were asked the same questions about six menstrual parameters before tubal sterilization or the husband's vasectomy and again at annual follow-up interviews for up to 5 years. The sterilized women were no more likely than the nonsterilized women to report changes in intermenstrual bleeding or cycle length. The sterilized women were more likely than the nonsterilized women to have decreases in the number of days of bleeding and the amount of bleeding and menstrual pain; they were also more likely to have an increase in cycle irregularity. When the risk of menstrual abnormalities was evaluated by method of tubal occlusion, there were no significant differences between the women sterilized by any of six methods and the women whose husbands underwent vasectomy in amount or duration of menstrual bleeding, intermenstrual bleeding, or menstrual pain. Women undergoing one of three methods of sterilization (silicone rubber band application, interval partial salpingectomy, and thermocoagulation) were more likely than nonsterilized women to have an increase in cycle irregularity, whereas women undergoing either of two other methods (unipolar and bipolar coagulation) were more likely to have decreases in cycle irregularity. This latter observation suggests strongly that the differences between sterilized and nonsterilized women in the likelihood of cycle irregularity and other menstrual features were attributable to chance or unmeasured differences between the study groups. Finally, sterilized women were compared with nonsterilized women for risk of a syndrome consisting of persistent increases in amount of bleeding, days of bleeding, or intermenstrual bleeding; no significant differences were identified.

Although sterilization procedures have been hypothesized to adversely affect ovarian function, laboratory studies have identified no consistent abnormalities that reflect ovarian dysfunction. Further, the biologic plausibility of such an occurrence is uncertain. The tubal branch of the uterine artery, which often is occluded during sterilization, connects with the ovarian branch of the uterine artery; thus, interrupting the tubal branch could affect the blood supply to the ovary. However, blood also is supplied to the ovary by the ovarian artery, which branches directly off the aorta and is remote from the site of tubal occlusion. The possibility has been raised that tubal occlusion could damage the ovary by acutely increasing pressure in the uteroovarian arterial loop. However, as noted, neither laboratory nor epidemiologic studies find changes consistent with acute injury to the ovary, and there is now strong evidence against the occurrence of sterilization-attributable menstrual abnormalities within 5 years of the procedure.

Some women who have no menstrual abnormalities before sterilization have them later, and for other women, menstrual abnormalities before sterilization resolve. To consider the former group as having a syndrome is inappropriate unless the latter group is considered to have an opposing syndrome. Although menstrual abnormalities are common among sterilized women, they also are common among nonsterilized women of similar ages. The balance of the evidence to date suggests strongly that sterilized women are no more likely than comparable nonsterilized women to have menstrual abnormalities.

Hysterectomy

Tubal sterilization and hysterectomy are common procedures in the United States, and any relation between the two has important consequences. Tubal sterilization could increase the risk for hysterectomy by increasing either the reality or the perception that a poststerilization syndrome occurs. As noted, the evidence against such a syndrome is now strong; thus, it should not be an indication for hysterectomy. Alternatively, the fact that a woman has had tubal sterilization could affect decision making about further surgery. At least three studies suggest that this effect can occur. Cohen studied 4,374 women 25 to 44 years old who had tubal sterilization in 1974 while enrolled in a universal health insurance plan in Canada. Women 25 to 29 years old at the time of sterilization were 1.6 times more likely than nonsterilized women to have a hysterectomy at a later time. However, women 30 years or older at the time of sterilization were no more likely than nonsterilized women to have a hysterectomy subsequently. Goldhaber and colleagues, who studied 39,502 women sterilized during 1971 to 1984, found that women sterilized at 20 to 24 years old were 2.4 times more likely than nonsterilized women to have a hysterectomy subsequently. For other sterilized women, the risk for hysterectomy steadily decreased with increasing age; women sterilized at 40 to 49 years old had no increased risk. Stergachis and associates studied 7,414 women sterilized during 1968 to 1983 and found that women sterilized at 20 to 29 years old were 3.4 times more likely than nonsterilized women to subsequently have a hysterectomy. Women sterilized at 30 years old or older had no increased risk for hysterectomy.

The fact that the increased risk for hysterectomy was concentrated among women sterilized at a young age in the noted studies suggests that any increased risk for hysterectomy after tubal sterilization is not biologic in etiology but attributable to other factors, such as removal of fertility preservation as a factor in decision making. In the US Collaborative Review of Sterilization, women sterilized at 34 years old and younger were four to five times more likely to undergo hysterectomy than women the same age whose husbands underwent vasectomy. However, women sterilized at 35 years old and older were also four to five times more likely to undergo hysterectomy than women whose husbands underwent vasectomy, suggesting that fertility preservation does not explain all differences in decision making between sterilized and nonsterilized women.

In the US Collaborative Review of Sterilization, the cumulative probability of undergoing hysterectomy within 14 years after sterilization was 17%. Although women with gynecologic disorders at the time of sterilization were at greater risk of hysterectomy, most women who reported gynecologic disorders at sterilization did not undergo hysterectomy within the follow-up period. For example, women who reported having a history of endometriosis at sterilization were more likely to undergo hysterectomy than women without a history of endometriosis; the probability of women reporting endometriosis undergoing hysterectomy within 14 years was 35% versus 15% for women without endometriosis. Similarly, women who reported having a history of uterine leiomyomata at sterilization were more likely to undergo hysterectomy than women without a history of leiomyomata; the 14-year cumulative probability of hysterectomy among women reporting leiomyomata was 27% versus 14% for women without leiomyomata.

Regret

The decision to undergo sterilization is serious to both men and women because the intent is to permanently terminate fertility. Although microsurgical methods of reversal are available, these methods require special skill, the procedures are complicated and lengthy, the costs are high, and none of the methods guarantees success.

Findings from studies of poststerilization regret provide useful information for presterilization counseling. Sterilization regret is a complex condition that is often causally linked to unpredictable life events. The risk factors for regret described here should not be used as reasons for restricting access to sterilization. Instead, they should be used to identify persons who may need extensive counseling. Presterilization counseling has been shown to correlate with poststerilization satisfaction.

Poststerilization regret can arise from several factors, including preexisting patient characteristics, subsequent changes in the patient's social situation or attitudes, and dissatisfaction resulting from adverse side effects caused or perceived to be caused by the procedure. Estimates of the prevalence of sterilization regret vary widely by measure of indication of regret and geographic region. During the last two decades, US-based studies have reported rates of poststerilization regret ranging from 0.9% to 26.0%. The wide range reflects, in part, differences in study design and questions asked of respondents. In general, the likelihood of a woman expressing regret after sterilization appears to increase over time. In the US Collaborative Review of Sterilization, the cumulative probability of regret increased from 4% at 3 years after sterilization to 8% at 7 years and 13% at 14 years. The 5-year cumulative probability of regret after tubal sterilization (7%) was similar to that for women whose husbands underwent vasectomy (6%).

In the 1982 National Survey of Family Growth, approximately 10% of women who had been sterilized reported that they would have the sterilization reversed if it were safe to do so. In the US Collaborative Review of Sterilization, 14% of sterilized women reported that they had sought information about tubal reanastomosis at least once within 14 years of sterilization; only 1% actually obtained a reversal.

At least five studies have identified young age at sterilization as the strongest predictor of later regret of sterilization. In the US Collaborative Review of Sterilization, young age at sterilization also was a strong predictor of regret, regardless of parity or marital status. After adjusting for other risk factors, women 30 years of age or younger at sterilization were

about twice as likely as older women to express regret within 14 years of sterilization. Similarly, the cumulative probability of expressing regret within 14 years was 20% for women 30 years old or younger versus 6% for women older than 30 years at sterilization. Likewise, the 14-year cumulative probability of requesting information about reversal was 40% among women sterilized at 18 to 24 years of age, and, after adjustment for other risk factors, women 18 to 24 years old were almost four times as likely as women 30 years old or older to request information about reversal. Although low parity has been identified as a risk factor for regret in some studies, it was not an independent risk factor in other studies after control for factors such as young age at the time of sterilization. The US Collaborative Review of Sterilization also found that women identifying substantial conflict with their husbands or partners before sterilization were more than three times as likely to regret their decision and more than five times as likely to request sterilization reversal.

Timing of the procedure in relation to pregnancy has been reported as a risk factor for regret. Several studies found that women who had tubal sterilization concurrent with cesarean section or following vaginal delivery or abortion were more likely to regret sterilization, but studies have been inconsistent in this regard. In the US Collaborative Review of Sterilization, the 14-year cumulative probability of regret was nearly identical for women whose sterilizations were concurrent with cesarean section (16%), after vaginal delivery (18%), and within 1 year of pregnancy (18%). The probability of regret decreased with time since the birth of the youngest child; women with 8 or more years since the birth of the youngest child had a probability of only 5%, a rate similar to that for women with no previous births (6%).

In summary, indicators of regret can vary significantly by cultural and individual circumstances. Most studies have found that age younger than 30 years is an independent risk factor for regret. The presterilization counseling for women in this age group should place special emphasis on the risk for regret. Other risk factors, such as time in relation to an obstetric event, ambivalence, or unstable life circumstances, should be assessed with each patient on an individual basis.

Sexual Function

In the US Collaborative Review of Sterilization, approximately 80% of women undergoing interval sterilization reported no consistent change in either sexual interest or pleasure in the first 2 years after the procedure. Of women reporting a consistent change, women were 10 and 15 times more likely to report positive changes in sexual interest or pleasure than negative ones.

Cancer

Although there is no evidence that tubal sterilization increases the risk for cancer at any site, studies are inconsistent regarding a possible reduction in risk of breast cancer after sterilization. One large prospective study by the American Cancer Society found that tubal sterilization reduced the risk of breast cancer mortality but only among women sterilized before 1975. It is unclear whether women who were sterilized had rates of screening mammography similar to those of nonsterilized women; thus, women who underwent tubal sterilization may have had greater access to screening services. A retrospective cohort study using data from the Ontario Cancer Registry found a reduced risk of breast cancer incidence among sterilized women, but that study was unable to control for potentially confounding variables. Two population-based case–control studies supported by NIH that did control for confounding found no effect of sterilization on breast cancer risk. Thus, at this point, it is unclear whether there is any biologic relationship between tubal sterilization and reduction in risk of subsequent breast cancer.

Several studies have identified a reduced risk of ovarian cancer after tubal sterilization. Hankinson and colleagues reported on the first large prospective cohort study of this relation; the risk of ovarian cancer for women who had tubal sterilization was one third that of nonsterilized women. In a pooled analysis of case–control studies, Whittemore and coworkers found a reduced risk of ovarian cancer after tubal sterilization. Whether the observed reduction in risk of ovarian cancer is a real protective effect or is attributable to some other factor remains unclear. However, there is reason for optimism that reduction in risk of ovarian cancer may be an important noncontraceptive health benefit of tubal sterilization.

VASECTOMY AS A SURGICAL ALTERNATIVE

Some couples who have chosen surgical sterilization for permanent contraception have difficulty in deciding whether vasectomy or tubal sterilization is most appropriate. Although numerous individual- or couple-related concerns can influence the decision, many couples include considerations about safety and effectiveness in their decision making. To assist such couples, we provide a brief overview of the health effects of vasectomy.

In regard to immediate surgical complications, vasectomy is a remarkably safe procedure. Serious morbidity and death are extremely rare. Fairly minor complications, such as scrotal swelling, ecchymosis, and pain, occur in up to 50% of men who have a vasectomy, but these symptoms usually resolve spontaneously within 1 to 2 weeks. Vasectomy generally has been performed through two incisions in the scrotum, one overlying each vas. Hematoma formation occurs in approximately 2% of such procedures; infections occur in less than 2%. In 1985, a new vasectomy technique was introduced, referred to as no-scalpel vasectomy. It reduced the already-low rate of minor complications. In most reports, pregnancy rates after vasectomy are less than 1%. Unlike tubal sterilization, vasectomy is not immediately effective. Three months are required to flush the vasa of viable sperm. This should be confirmed by a postvasectomy semen analysis at 3 months or more after the procedure.

In 1978, questions about the long-term health effects of vasectomy were raised when an increased risk for atherosclerosis was found among monkeys that had had a vasectomy. At least nine subsequent epidemiologic studies in men found no such increased risk, and later findings in monkeys did not support an increased risk. Thus, vasectomy does not affect the risk for subsequent cardiovascular disease. These studies also provided strong evidence that vasectomy does not increase overall mortality. More recently, questions were raised about the risk of prostate cancer after vasectomy. A 1998 metaanalysis of 14 observational studies concluded that the evidence for an association between vasectomy and prostate cancer was of low quality because of biases that overestimate the effect of vasectomy and that any association is likely not a causal one. Subsequently, a large population-based study in New Zealand found no relation between vasectomy and risk of prostate cancer. Thus, the evidence to date argues strongly against any causal relationship.

Questions remain regarding a potential syndrome of postvasectomy pain. The purported syndrome has been varyingly defined as chronic testicular, epididymal, or scrotal pain, and the proposed causes include epididymal congestion, nerve entrapment, and sperm granulomas. Although a few small, uncontrolled surveys found rates of such pain as high as 2% to 15%, the largest and best study found the incidence of epididymitis–orchitis more than 12 months after vasectomy to be 24.7 per 10,000 person-years versus 13.6 per 10,000 person-years among men who did not undergo vasectomy. Although uncertainties remain, it is likely that a small percentage of men will indeed experience chronic pain after vasectomy. It appears, based on limited information, that many such men will respond to conservative measures and that surgical management, including vasectomy reversal, may help others.

BEST SURGICAL PRACTICES

- Preprocedure assessment and counseling are essential elements in a successful sterilization procedure. Counseling regarding failure rates, risks, and risk factors for later regret should be performed. Preprocedure cytologic screening and day-of-surgery pregnancy testing are encouraged if indicated.
- General anesthesia is the leading cause of death from tubal sterilizations in the United States. Although tubal sterilizations can usually be performed safely under local anesthesia, general anesthesia is used more often in the United States. One of the reasons that vasectomy is safer than tubal sterilization is that general anesthesia is rarely required.
- A major portion of morbidity and mortality associated with laparoscopic methods of sterilization is related to entry into the abdominal cavity. Open laparoscopy can reduce the incidence of major vascular injury at entry. In closed laparoscopy technique, meticulous attention to details of entry can help reduce injury. Hysteroscopic sterilization eliminates both the need for general anesthesia and the risk of abdominal entry.
- With all the techniques of tubal sterilization, success is dependent on correct identification of the tube; hasty tubal identification, without taking the time to follow the tubes out to their fimbriated ends (if not distorted by adhesions), can result in procedural failure.
- Nearly all the techniques of tubal sterilization involve the isthmic portion of the fallopian tube, which is the narrowest and most uniform caliber portion of the extramural tube. However, it is suggested that 2 cm of the isthmic portion of the tube be left at the cornu, proximal to the site of tubal interruption, to theoretically reduce the incidence of tuboperitoneal fistula. Aggressive overtightening of ligatures, just as avoided in surgical technique elsewhere in the body, should likewise be avoided at the time of tubal interruption, as strangulation and necrosis of the tube can lead to fistulization and failure rather than success. Ligatures applied during partial salpingectomy methods of sterilization (e.g., Pomeroy, Parkland) at the time of cesarean delivery are at risk of dislodgement by shearing forces when the uterus is restituted into the abdominal cavity at the end of the procedure. Care should be exerted to protect the ligated areas as one and then the other adnexum is replaced into the abdomen.
- Laparoscopic unipolar coagulation of the fallopian tube is one of the most successful methods of sterilization, likely attributed to the approximately 5-cm zone of thermal destruction that results. However, the risk for thermal injuries is also highest with this method, unless the safe application of unipolar energy at laparoscopy and the concept of capacitive coupling are understood by the surgeon. Greater tubal destruction and sterilization success with this method go hand in hand with least likelihood that reversal could ever be achieved.

- Laparoscopic bipolar coagulation creates a smaller zone of thermal injury (approximately 3 cm) than unipolar and is also not likely to result in indirect thermal injury by capacitive coupling. Three contiguous burns over a 3-cm length of tube, beginning approximately 3 cm from the cornu and moving toward the fimbriated end, are recommended. Also recommended are the use of the cutting waveform, delivering at least 25 W of bipolar energy (continuous waveform by default), and the use of an optical flowmeter to estimate when coagulation (and flow of current) is complete.

- Silastic band application requires familiarity with the applicator and the tendency of its grasping tongs to transect the fallopian tube when trying to retract a knuckle of tube into the hollow applicator cannula. Tethered or thickened tubes are at greatest risk of transection, and an alternative method should be considered. A complete encirclement of the tube by the grasping tongs is necessary if a partial or tangential application of the ligating band is to be avoided.

- Hulka and Filshie clips are reliable methods of tubal interruption but require strict adherence to surgical technique to be successful. Application at right angles to the tube, 2 cm from the uterus, without excessive tubal elevation, and with the tips of the clips advanced onto the mesosalpinx are the key points of the application. Clips are associated with minimal tubal destruction (3 mm) and are therefore the most amenable to tubal reversal.

- Essure microinserts are placed transcervically via hysteroscopy. Care should be taken to create sufficient distention to identify both tubal ostia clearly and to insert the device into the proximal lumen to the level marked on the catheter. Hypervolemia should be avoided, and a confirmation HSG must be performed at 3 months postinsertion. Alternate contraception should be used until occlusion is documented.

BIBLIOGRAPHY

Allyn DP, Leton DA, Westcott NA, et al. Presterilization counseling and women's regret about having been sterilized. *J Reprod Med* 1986;31:1027.

Anderson ET. Peritoneoscopy. *Am J Surg* 1937;35:36.

Bernal-Delgado E, Latour-Perez J, Pradas-Arnal F, et al. The association between vasectomy and prostate cancer: a systematic review of the literature. *Fertil Steril* 1998;70:191.

Bhiwandiwala PP, Mumford SD, Feldblum PJ. A comparison of different laparoscopic sterilization occlusion techniques in 24,439 procedures. *Am J Obstet Gynecol* 1982;144:319.

Bhiwandiwala PP, Mumford SD, Kennedy KI. Comparison of the safety of open and conventional laparoscopic sterilization. *Obstet Gynecol* 1985;66:391.

Bishop E, Nelms WF. A simple method of tubal sterilization. *N Y State Med J* 1930;30:214.

Bordahl PE, Raeder JC, Nordentoft J, et al. Laparoscopic sterilization under local or general anesthesia? A randomized study. *Obstet Gynecol* 1993;81:137.

Boring CC, Rochat RW, Becerra J. Sterilization regret among Puerto Rican women. *Fertil Steril* 1988;49:973.

Brinton LA, Gammon MD, Coates RJ, et al. Tubal ligation and risk of breast cancer. *Br J Cancer* 2000;82:1600.

Calle EE, Rodriguez C, Walker KA, et al. Tubal sterilization and risk of breast cancer mortality in U.S. women. *Cancer Causes Control* 2001;12:127.

Chamberlain G, Brown JC, eds. *Gynaecological laparoscopy: the report of the confidential inquiry into gynaecological laparoscopy.* London, UK: The Royal College of Obstetricians and Gynaecologists, 1978.

Chan LM, Westhoff CL. Tubal sterilization trends in the United States. *Fertil Steril* 2010;94:1.

Cheng MCE, Cheong J, Ratnam SS, et al. Psychosocial sequelae of abortion and sterilization: a controlled study of 200 women randomly allocated to either a concurrent or interval abortion and sterilization. *Asia Oceania J Obstet Gynaecol* 1986;12:193.

Chi I-C, Feldblum PJ. Luteal phase pregnancies in female sterilization patients. *Contraception* 1981;23:579.

Choe JM, Kirkemo AK. Questionnaire-based outcomes study of non-oncological post-vasectomy complications. *J Urol* 1996;155:1284.

Cleary TP, Tepper NK, Cwiak C, et al. Pregnancies after hysteroscopic sterilization: a systematic review. *Contraception* 2013;87:539.

Cohen MM. Long-term risk of hysterectomy after tubal sterilization. *Am J Epidemiol* 1987;125:410.

Costello C, Hillis SD, Marchbanks PA, et al. The effect of interval tubal sterilization on sexual interest and pleasure. *Obstet Gynecol* 2002;100:511.

Cox B, Sneyd MJ, Paul C, et al. Vasectomy and risk of prostate cancer. *JAMA* 2002;287:3110.

DeStefano F, Greenspan JR, Ory HW, et al. Demographic trends in tubal sterilization: United States, 1970–1978. *Am J Public Health* 1982;72:480.

DeStefano F, Perlman JA, Peterson HB, et al. Long-term risks of menstrual disturbances after tubal sterilization. *Am J Obstet Gynecol* 1985;152:835.

Dueholm S, Zingenburg HJ, Sandgren G. Late sequelae after laparoscopic sterilization in the pregnant and nonpregnant woman. *Acta Obstet Gynecol Scand* 1987;66:227.

Emens JM, Olive JE. Timing of female sterilization. *Br Med J* 1978;2:1126.

Engender Health. *Contraceptive sterilization: global issues and trends.* New York: Engender Health, 2002:xii.

Escobedo LG, Peterson HB, Grubb GS, et al. Case-fatality rates for tubal sterilization in U.S. hospitals, 1979 to 1980. *Am J Obstet Gynecol* 1989;160:147.

Essure™ Permanent Birth Control System. *Instructions.* Conceptus, Inc., 2002.

Filshie GM, Casey D, Pogmore JR, et al. The titanium/silicone rubber clip for female sterilization. *Br J Obstet Gynaecol* 1981;88:655.

Fishburne JI. Anesthesia for laparoscopy: considerations, complications, and techniques. *J Reprod Med* 1978;21:37.

Gentile GP, Kaufman SC, Helbig DW. Is there any evidence for a post-tubal sterilization syndrome? *Fertil Steril* 1998;69:179.

Goldhaber MK, Armstrong MA, Golditch IM, et al. Long-term risk of hysterectomy among 80,007 sterilized and comparison women at Kaiser Permanente, 1971–1987. *Am J Epidemiol* 1993;138:508.

Grimes DA. Primary prevention of ovarian cancer. *JAMA* 1993;270:2855.

Grimes DA, Peterson HB, Rosenberg MJ, et al. Sterilization-attributable deaths in Bangladesh. *Int J Gynaecol Obstet* 1982;20:149.

Grimes DA, Satterthwaite AP, Rochat RW, et al. Deaths from contraceptive sterilization in Bangladesh: rates, causes, and prevention. *Obstet Gynecol* 1982;60:635.

Grubb GS, Peterson HB. Luteal phase pregnancy and tubal sterilization. *Obstet Gynecol* 1985;66:784.

Handa VL, Berlin M, Washington AE. A comparison of local and general anesthesia for laparoscopic tubal sterilization. *J Womens Health* 1994;3:135.

Hankinson SE, Hunter DJ, Colditz GA, et al. Tubal ligation, hysterectomy, and risk of ovarian cancer: a prospective study. *JAMA* 1993;270:2813.

Healy B. From the National Institutes of Health: does vasectomy cause prostate cancer? *JAMA* 1993;269:2620.

Henshaw SK, Singh S. Sterilization regret among U.S. couples. *Fam Plann Perspect* 1986;18:238.

Hillis SD, Marchbanks PA, Tylor LR, et al. Higher hysterectomy risk for sterilized than nonsterilized women: findings from the U.S. Collaborative Review of Sterilization. *Obstet Gynecol* 1998;91:241.

Hillis SD, Marchbanks PA, Tylor LR, et al. Poststerilization regret: findings from the United States Collaborative Review of Sterilization. *Obstet Gynecol* 1999;93:889.

Hillis SD, Marchbanks PA, Tylor LR, et al. Tubal sterilization and the long-term risk of hysterectomy: findings from the United States Collaborative Review of Sterilization. *Obstet Gynecol* 1997;89:609.

Holt VL, Chu J, Daling JR, et al. Tubal sterilization and subsequent ectopic pregnancy: a case–control study. *JAMA* 1991;226:242.

Hulka JF, Fishburne JI, Mercer JP, et al. Laparoscopic sterilization with a spring clip: a report of the first fifty cases. *Am J Obstet Gynecol* 1973;116:715.

Hulka JF, Peterson HB, Phillips JM. American Association of Gynecologic Laparoscopists' 1988 membership survey on laparoscopic sterilization. *J Reprod Med* 1990;35:584.

Hulka JF, Reich H. *Textbook of laparoscopy*, 2nd ed. Philadelphia, PA: WB Saunders, 1994:85.

Irving FC. Tubal sterilization. *Am J Obstet Gynecol* 1950;60:1101.

Irwin KL, Lee NC, Peterson HB, et al. Hysterectomy, tubal sterilization and the risk of breast cancer. *Am J Epidemiol* 1988;127:1192.

Jamieson DJ, Costello C, Trussell J, et al. The risk of pregnancy after vasectomy. *Obstet Gynecol* 2004;103:848.

Jamieson DJ, Hillis SD, Duerr A, et al. Complications of interval laparoscopic sterilization: findings from the United States Collaborative Review of Sterilization. *Obstet Gynecol* 2000;96:997.

Jamieson DJ, Kaufman SC, Costello C, et al. A comparison of women's regret after vasectomy versus tubal sterilization. *Obstet Gynecol* 2002;99:1073.

Jones J, Mosher W, Daniels K, et al. *Current contraceptive use in the United States, 2006–2010, and changes in patterns of use since 1995.* Hyattsville, MD: National Center for Health Statistics, 2012.

Kerin J, Munday D, Ritossa M, et al. Essure hysteroscopic sterilization: results based on utilizing a new coil catheter delivery system. *J Am Assoc Gynecol Laparosc* 2004;11:388.

Kjer JJ, Knudsen LB. Ectopic pregnancy subsequent to laparoscopic sterilization. *Am J Obstet Gynecol* 1989;160:1202.

Koetsawang S, Gates DS, Suwanichati S, et al. Long-term follow-up of laparoscopic sterilizations by electrocoagulation, the Hulka clip, and the tubal ring. *Contraception* 1990;41:9.

Kreiger N, Sloan M, Cotterchio M, et al. The risk of breast cancer following reproductive surgery. *Eur J Cancer* 1999;35:97.

Layde PM, Peterson HB, Dicker RC, et al. Risk factors for complications of interval tubal sterilization by laparotomy. *Obstet Gynecol* 1983;62:180.

Leader A, Galan N, George R, et al. A comparison of definable traits in women requesting reversal of sterilization and women satisfied with sterilization. *Am J Obstet Gynecol* 1983;145:198.

Levie M, Chudnoff SG. A comparison of novice and experience physicians performing hysteroscopic sterilization: an analysis of an FDA-mandated trial. *Contraception* 2011;96:643.

Levinson CJ, Daily HJ, Skinner SJ. Pathologic changes in the fallopian tube after Silastic ring occlusion. In: Phillips JM, ed. *Endoscopy in gynecology*. Downey, CA: American Association of Gynecologic Laparoscopists, 1978:180.

Lichter ED, Laff SP, Friedman EA. Value of routine dilation and curettage at the time of interval sterilization. *Obstet Gynecol* 1986;67:763.

Lipscomb GH, Spellman JR, Ling FW. The effect of same-day pregnancy testing on the incidence of luteal phase pregnancy. *Obstet Gynecol* 1993;82:411.

Liskin L, Pile JM, Quillin WF. Vasectomy—safe and simple. *Popul Rep D* 1983;4:D61.

Liskin L, Rinehart W. Minilaparotomy and laparoscopy: safe, effective, and widely used. *Popul Rep C* 1985;9:c-127.

Mackay AP, Kicke BA Jr, Koonin LM, et al. Tubal sterilization in the United States, 1994–1996. *Fam Plann Perspect* 2001;33:161.

Madlener M. γber sterilisierende operationen an den tuben. *Zentralbl Gynakol* 1919;20:380.

Makar AP, Vanderheyden JS, Schatteman EA, et al. Female sterilization failure after bipolar electrocoagulation: a six-year retrospective study. *Eur J Obstet Gynecol Reprod Biol* 1990;37:237.

Marcil-Gratton N. Sterilization regret among women in metropolitan Montreal. *Fam Plann Perspect* 1988;20:222.

Massey FJ Jr, Bernstein GS, O'Fallon WM, et al. Vasectomy and health: results from a large cohort study. *JAMA* 1984;252:1023.

McMahon AJ, Buckley J, Taylor A, et al. Chronic testicular pain following vasectomy. *Br J Urol* 1992;69:188.

Mintz M. Risks and prophylaxis in laparoscopy: a survey of 100,000 cases. *J Reprod Med* 1977;18:269.

Mumford SD, Bhiwandiwala PP, Chi I-C. Laparoscopic and minilaparotomy female sterilisation compared in 15,167 cases. *Lancet* 1980;2:1066.

Nirapathpongporn A, Huber DH, Krieger JN. No-scalpel vasectomy at the King's birthday vasectomy festival. *Lancet* 1990;335:894.

Nisanian A. Outpatient minilaparotomy sterilization with local anesthesia. *J Reprod Med* 1990;35:380.

Penfield AJ. The Filshie clip for female sterilization: a review of world experience. *Am J Obstet Gynecol* 2000;182:485.

Peterson HB, Curtis KM. Long-acting methods of contraception. *N Engl J Med* 2005;353:2169.

Peterson HB, DeStefano F, Rubin GL, et al. Deaths attributable to tubal sterilization in the United States, 1977 to 1981. *Am J Obstet Gynecol* 1983;146:131.

Peterson HB, Greenspan JR, DeStefano F, et al. The impact of laparoscopy on tubal sterilization in United States hospitals, 1970 and 1975 to 1978. *Am J Obstet Gynecol* 1981;140:811.

Peterson HB, Howards SS. Vasectomy and prostate cancer: the evidence to date. *Fertil Steril* 1998;70:201.

Peterson HB, Huber DH, Belker AM. Vasectomy: an appraisal for the obstetrician-gynecologist. *Obstet Gynecol* 1990;76:568.

Peterson HB, Hulka JF, Spielman FJ, et al. Local versus general anesthesia for laparoscopic sterilization: a randomized study. *Obstet Gynecol* 1987;70:903.

Peterson HB, Jeng G, Folger SG, et al. The risk of menstrual abnormalities after tubal sterilization. *N Engl J Med* 2000;343:1681.

Peterson HB, Xia Z, Hughes JM, et al. The risk of ectopic pregnancy after tubal sterilization. *N Engl J Med* 1997;336:762.

Peterson HB, Xia Z, Hughes JM, et al. The risk of pregnancy after tubal sterilization: findings from the U.S. Collaborative Review of Sterilization. *Am J Obstet Gynecol* 1996;174:1161.

Peterson HB, Xia Z, Wilcox LS, et al. Pregnancy after sterilization with bipolar electrocoagulation. *Obstet Gynecol* 1999;94:163.

Peterson HB, Xia Z, Wilcox LS, et al. Pregnancy after tubal sterilization with silicone rubber band and spring clip application. *Obstet Gynecol* 2001;97:205.

Pitaktepsombati P, Janowitz B. Sterilization acceptance and regret in Thailand. *Contraception* 1991;44:623.

Poindexter AN, Abdul-Malak M, Fast J. Laparoscopic tubal sterilization under local anesthesia. *Obstet Gynecol* 1990;75:5.

Power FH, Barnes AC. Sterilization by means of peritoneoscopic tubal fulguration. *Am J Obstet Gynecol* 1941;41:1038.

Prystowsky H, Eastman NJ. Puerperal tubal sterilization: report of 1,830 cases. *JAMA* 1955;158:463.

Rennie AL, Richard JA, Milne MK, et al. Post-partum sterilisation—an anaesthetic hazard? *Anaesthesia* 1979;34:267.

Rioux JE, Cloutier D. A new bipolar instrument for tubal sterilization. *Am J Obstet Gynecol* 1974;119:737.

Rochat RW, Bhiwandiwala PP, Feldblum PJ, et al. Mortality associated with sterilization: preliminary results of an international collaborative observational study. *Int J Gynaecol Obstet* 1986;24:275.

Ross JA, Frankenberg E. Sterilization. In: Ross JA, Frankenberg E, eds. *Findings from two decades of family planning research*. New York: Population Council, 1993:57.

Rulin MC, Davidson AR, Philliber SG, et al. Long-term effect of tubal sterilization on menstrual indices and pelvic pain. *Obstet Gynecol* 1993;82:118.

Rulin MC, Turner JH, Dunworth R, et al. Post-tubal sterilization syndrome—a misnomer. *Am J Obstet Gynecol* 1985;151:13.

Schmidt JE, Hillis SD, Marchbanks PA, et al. Requesting information about and obtaining reversal after tubal sterilization: findings from the U.S. Collaborative Review of Sterilization. *Fertil Steril* 2000;74:892.

Shain RN, Miller WB, Holden AEC. Married women's dissatisfaction with tubal sterilization and vasectomy at first-year follow-up: effects of perceived spousal dominance. *Fertil Steril* 1986;45:808.

Shain RN, Miller WB, Mitchell GW, et al. Menstrual pattern change one year after sterilization: results of a controlled, prospective study. *Fertil Steril* 1989;52:192.

Shy KK, Stergachis A, Grothaus LG, et al. Tubal sterilization and risk of subsequent hospital admission for menstrual disorders. *Am J Obstet Gynecol* 1992;166:1698.

Siegler AM, Grunebaum A. A short history of tubal sterilization. In: Phillips JM, ed. *Endoscopic female sterilization: a comparison of methods*. Downey, CA: American Association of Gynecologic Laparoscopists, 1983:3.

Soderstrom R. Electrical safety in laparoscopy. In: Phillips JM, ed. *Endoscopy in gynecology*. Downey, CA: American Association of Gynecologic Laparoscopists, 1978:306.

Soderstrom RM, Levy BS, Engel T. Reducing bipolar sterilization failures. *Obstet Gynecol* 1989;74:60.

Speert H. *Obstetrics and gynecology in America: a history*. Chicago, IL: American College of Obstetricians and Gynecologists, 1980:68.

Stergachis A, Shy KK, Grothaus LC, et al. Tubal sterilization and the long-term risk of hysterectomy. *JAMA* 1990;264:2893.

Stovall TG, Ling FW, O'Kelley KR, et al. Gross and histologic examination of tubal ligation failures in a residency training program. *Obstet Gynecol* 1990;76:461.

Trussell J, Hatcher RA, Cates W, et al. A guide to interpreting contraceptive efficacy studies. *Obstet Gynecol* 1990;76:558.

Trussell J, Kost K. Contraceptive failure in the United States: a critical review of the literature. *Stud Fam Plann* 1987;18:237.

Uchida H. Uchida tubal sterilization. *Am J Obstet Gynecol* 1975; 121:153.

Whittemore AS, Harris R, Itnyre J, et al. Characteristics relating to ovarian cancer risk: collaborative analysis of 12 U.S. case–control studies. II. Invasive epithelial ovarian cancers in white women. *Am J Epidemiol* 1992;136:1184.

Williams EL, Jones HE, Merrill RE. The subsequent course of patients sterilized by tubal ligation: a consideration of hysterectomy for sterilization. *Am J Obstet Gynecol* 1951;61:423.

World Health Organization Task Force on Female Sterilization, Special Programme of Research, Development and Research Training in Human Reproduction. Minilaparotomy or laparoscopy for sterilization: a multicenter, multinational, randomized study. *Am J Obstet Gynecol* 1982;143:645.

Wortman J. Female sterilization by minilaparotomy. *Popul Rep C* 1974;5:c-53.

Wortman J, Piotrow P. Laparoscopic sterilization—a new technique. *Popul Rep C* 1973;1:c-1.

Yoon IB, Wheeless CR, King TM. A preliminary report on a new laparoscopic sterilization approach: the silicone rubber band technique. *Am J Obstet Gynecol* 1974;120:132.

CHAPTER 28
Surgery for Benign Disease of the Ovary

Joseph S. Sanfilippo and John A. Rock

DEFINITIONS

Accessory ovary—An additional ovarian mass close to the normally placed ovary and connected to it by the utero-ovarian or infundibulopelvic ligament.

Fertility preservation prior to cancer therapy—Affording the patient prior to provision of chemoradiation therapy a host of options that provide for ovarian tissue, embryo, or oocyte cryopreservation as well as surgical procedures designed to protect the ovaries from radiation therapy.

Fimbria ovarica—The structure attaching the infundibulum of the fallopian tube to the distal pole of the ovary. It is vitally important to the fimbrial ovum capture mechanism.

Malpositioned ovary—An ovary located above the pelvic brim because of a lack of normal descent into the pelvis. It may be elongated, but it remains attached to the uterus by the utero-ovarian ligament and to the fallopian tube by the fimbria ovarica.

Ovarian cortex—The outer layer of the ovary consisting of an outer zone, which is mainly collagenous (tunica albuginea), and an inner zone, which is less fibrous and more cellular and contains the germ cells (primordial follicles).

Ovarian medulla—The inner region surrounding the hilum of the ovary. It contains no follicles, only blood vessels and the remnants of the tubular structures that are homologous to the male testis (rete testis).

Ovarian remnant—Persistent ovarian tissue unintentionally left behind following oophorectomy.

Prophylactic oophorectomy—In genetic mutation carriers, that is, BRCA1 or BRCA2, removal of both ovaries upon completion of childbearing in an effort to minimize chance of ovarian cancer.

Residual ovary—Symptomatic ovarian tissue following removal of the ovary.

Supernumerary ovary—An additional ovary that has no direct or ligamentous connection with a normally placed ovary. It is located at a distance from the normally placed ovaries.

Tumor markers—Substances identified in higher than normal amounts in blood, urine, or body tissues of patients with specific malignancies. They are produced directly by the tumor or as a response to the presence of cancer, that is, indirect marker.

Tunica albuginea—Condensed ovarian stroma that forms a fibrous capsule.

Evaluation and management of benign disease of the ovary continues to unfold with new and challenging clinical alternatives. Progress has occurred with regard to understanding the genetics of ovarian function, new surgical approaches to ovarian disease, and a host of knowledge that clinicians should be aware of. The population is living longer, and cancer survivors are increasing exponentially. All of this leads us to focus on enhancing our understanding of preservation of ovarian function; expanding the potential for conception, which includes determining treatment related to decreased postoperative adhesion formation; and addressing an array of other aspects related to ovarian activity.

It has been established that the ovaries and fallopian tubes are sensitive to ischemia from surgical trauma; adhesions may develop as a result; the normal anatomic relationship between fallopian tubes, ovaries, and uterus may be altered. Knowledge regarding anatomy and embryology of the ovaries and other reproductive organs complemented by mastery of the principles of microsurgery that can be applied to virtually any surgical procedure are the prerequisites for excellent results following ovarian reconstructive surgery. Embryology and anatomy are addressed in this chapter with emphasis on the importance of the anatomic relationship of the ovary to other pelvic organs in the section on the evaluation and management of an adnexal mass. State-of-the-art surgical procedures—both via minimally invasive, robotic-assisted and laparotomic approaches and techniques devised for the reconstruction of the ovary—for restoration of normal pelvic anatomy are presented in the context of specific pathology or other abnormal conditions that require surgical intervention. This chapter also focuses on pediatric and adolescent gynecologic surgical procedures that are performed when ovarian pathology is identified.

EMBRYOLOGY

The reproductive system is derived from mesoderm. The primordium of the urogenital ridge is divided into two segments. One is the nephrogenic ridge, that is, metanephros derivatives, the renal system; the other is the gonadal ridge for development of the reproductive tract. Gonads are a reflection of three origins: mesothelium, mesenchyme, and primordial germ cells. The paramesonephros gives rise to the fallopian tubes and the uterus. Two gonadal ridges arise early in gestation (4 to 5 weeks) in the developing embryo as thickening on the medial aspect of the coelomic cavity adjacent to the mesonephros. These gonadal outgrowths are composed of coelomic epithelium and underlying mesenchyme projecting into the future peritoneal cavity. The epithelial and mesenchymal cells of the gonadal primordia are of mesodermal origin (large, spherical ovoid germ cells that originate extragonadally in the wall of the yolk sac and migrate to the developing gonads). Until the 6th week of gestation, the gonads of the two sexes remain morphologically indistinguishable. The presumptive ovaries remain undifferentiated until the onset of meiosis at the end of the first trimester. The ovarian cortex is a single germinal epithelium. The tunica albuginea lies beneath the cortex and is composed of connective tissue. The stroma is composed of fibroblasts, smooth muscle, endothelium, and interstitial cells, including undifferentiated theca cells and corpora albicans.

Sexual differentiation requires initiation by various genes, along with a single gene determinant on the Y chromosome (testis-determining factor), which is necessary for testicular differentiation. In XX individuals (in the absence of a Y chromosome), the bipotential gonad develops into an ovary.

The mechanisms responsible for gonadal sex differentiation are largely unknown. Investigators have theorized the presence of a testis-determining factor (H–Y cell-surface antigen on the short arm of the Y chromosome) that is elaborated by a specific gene. Meiosis-inducing and meiosis-preventing substances, both of which are produced by cells derived from mesonephric structures adjacent to the gonad, are the agents of regulation of ovarian and testicular germ-cell differentiation. The balance between these two substances varies between the two sexes and at different stages of development. The meiosis-inducing substance predominates in the fetal ovary. Maternal ovarian hormone production is not required for differentiation of the germ cells or, apparently, for later development of the fetal reproductive tract. Various ultrastructural studies have shown no specific changes in fetal granulosa cells that can be definitely associated with steroid hormone secretion

such as is identified in the fetal Leydig cells. Thecal cells play an essential role in steroid synthesis in the adult ovary, but they do not appear until later in gestation and even then retain a relatively undifferentiated appearance. Fetal pituitary gonadotropin production begins as early as 10 weeks gestation and reaches peak levels at midgestation. Gonadotropins have a major influence on follicular development in the adult ovary, but evidence for a similar function in the fetus is lacking.

GENE EXPRESSION

Understanding of the genetics of the ovary continues to evolve. With the advent of polymerase chain reaction (PCR), real-time PCR, fluorescence in situ hybridization, single nucleotide polymorphism, and a host of other genetic advances, understanding of ovarian function has reached a new level (Fig. 28.1). Table 28.1 provides information regarding genes and associated phenotype.

Genes often are associated with specific clinical problems, for example, Kallmann syndrome, a genetic condition that results in the failure of pubertal development. Hypogonadism associated with a total lack of sense of smell (anosmia) or a heavily reduced sense of smell (hyposmia) characterizes the syndrome. Premature ovarian insufficiency (POI) is characterized by hypergonadotropic hypogonadism, which equates with the loss of ovarian function before age 40. The problem of POI overall is associated with a host of gene defects, all of which set the stage for genetic testing in patients in the reproductive age group with amenorrhea in association with hypergonadotropic state. Genes are also involved with cumulus expansion (GDF9 and BMP15) and endometriosis, and most recently serve as predictors of oocyte quality and successful embryo implantation and development. Specific follicular cell receptors bind growth factors, which are locally synthesized with the ultimate effect of intracellular signaling and protein kinase activation. This activity affects transcription of targeted genes. Gene expression is involved in follicle development, ovulation,

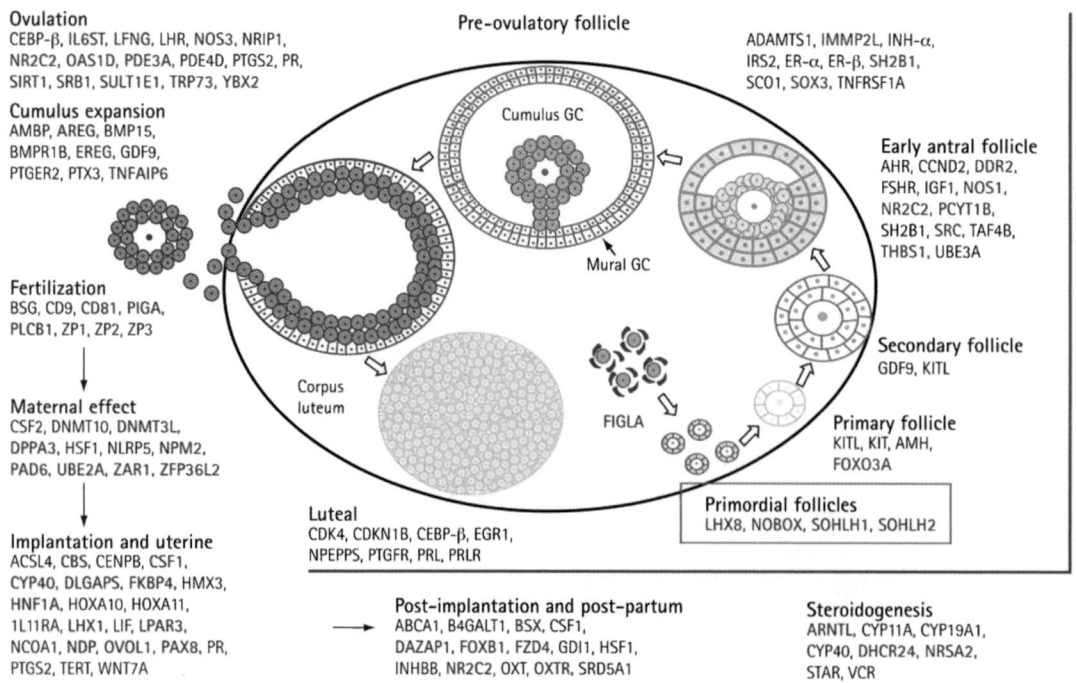

FIGURE 28.1 Model of ovarian genes recognized in 2008. (Reproduced from Fauser BC, Diedrich K, Bouchard P, et al. Contemporary genetic technologies and female reproduction. The Evian Annual Reproduction (EVAR) Workshop Group 2010. *Hum Reprod Update* 2011;17:829, with permission. Copyright © 2011 Oxford University Press.)

TABLE 28.1 Gene Mutations and Ovarian Activity	
Bone morphogenetic protein receptor 1 beta (BMPR 1Beta)	Ovarian dysfunction
Fibroblast growth factor beta (FGFBeta)	Kallmann syndrome (KAL2)
Fragile X mental retardation 1 (FMR1)	Premature ovarian insufficiency
Kallmann syndrome 1 (KAL1)	Hypogonadotropic hypogonadism and insomnia X-linked Kallmann syndrome
Premature ovarian failure 1 beta (POF1Beta)	Hypergonadotropic, primary amenorrhea (POF2Beta)
Prokineticin receptor 2 (PROKR2)	Kallmann syndrome (KAL3)

and corpus luteum and corpus albicans formation. Transcription factors include protooncogenes, c-Myc, and CCAAT/enhancer binding protein.

FEMALE FETAL DEVELOPMENT

The ovarian surface cortex, during the early prefollicular stage, is characterized by germ cells and granulosa cells organized in cords and sheets, but the cortex lacks specific conformation. The final distinctive change to occur in the fetal ovary is the onset of meiosis at the 11th or 12th week of gestation. Meiosis is preceded by differentiation of primitive germ cells into actively dividing mitotic cells called *oogonia*. The mitotic divisions of the oogonia are associated with complete separation at

telophase, leaving the daughter cells connected by intracellular bridges. After a series of mitotic divisions, there is progressive entry of cells into meiosis, beginning in the innermost cortex and gradually extending to the periphery. These cells passing through the various stages of the first meiotic prophase are then designated *oocytes*. By late gestation, all surviving oocytes have advanced to the diplotene stage. Further differentiation of the oocytes is arrested at this stage and does not resume until ovulation begins at menarche, approximately 12 years later.

Follicular formation begins at 18 to 20 weeks gestation and continues throughout the remaining weeks of fetal development. All the surviving oocytes are surrounded by adjacent granulosa cells; oocyte and follicular growth are well established by the late fetal and early neonatal period. The constant degeneration and loss of oocytes before their incorporation into the follicles reduces their numbers to only 1 to 2 million (follicles) in the newborn ovary.

ANATOMY

The dimensions of the adult ovary vary from individual to individual but average 3 to 5 cm in length, 2 to 3 cm in width, and 1 to 2 cm in diameter, with a weight of 3 to 8 g. The ovarian capsule is smooth in childhood, but its surface becomes pitted from follicular maturation and atresia.

The size, shape, and position of the ovary in the pelvis are somewhat variable, and both the consistency and the follicular changes taking place within the ovary vary with stage of the menstrual cycle. The ovary typically is anchored to the sidewall of the pelvis in the shallow peritoneal fossa of Waldeyer formed between the angles of proximity of the ovary to the ureter. This knowledge is important before dissecting the ovary off the pelvic sidewall.

The ovary is connected to the uterus by the utero-ovarian ligament, to the posterior aspect of the broad ligament by the mesovarium ligament, and to the lateral pelvic sidewall by the infundibulopelvic ligament (**Fig. 28.2**). The

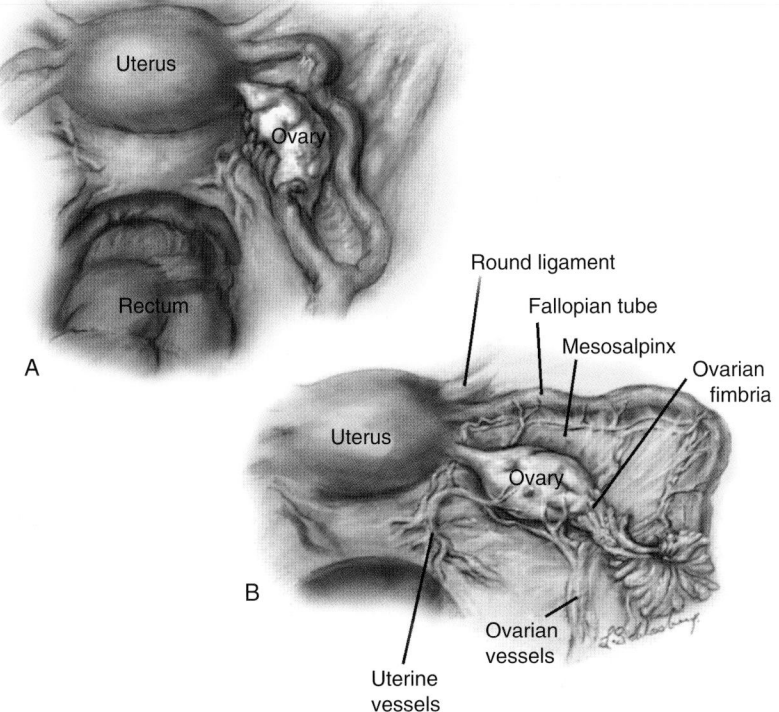

FIGURE 28.2 Normal anatomy of the ovary. **A:** Anatomic relations of the uterus, tube, and ovary. **B:** The infundibulum of the oviduct extends onto the ovary and is attached at its most distal pole (ovarian fimbria). The mesovarian suspends the ovary. Each ovary is attached at the hilum.

mesovarium ligament attaches to the mesentery of the ovary. The other two ligaments are attached at the hilum of the ovary.

The ovary migrates downward from high in the abdomen during embryonic life. The infundibulum of the fallopian tube extends onto the ovary and is attached to it at its most distal pole by the fimbria ovarica. The relation of the ovary to the fimbria ovarica and to the utero-ovarian ligament is crucial, and they should be carefully maintained during ovarian reconstruction.

During embryogenesis, the ovary may assume an unusual appearance (i.e., it may be septate) or assume an unusual position (Fig. 28.3). An accessory ovary (Fig. 28.3A) usually is close to or is connected to a normally placed ovary. An accessory ovary also may be attached to the broad, utero-ovarian, or infundibulopelvic ligaments. Unlike the accessory ovary, a supernumerary ovary (Fig. 28.3B) must have an independent embryologic origin. It may develop from a primordium such as arrested migrating gonadocytes. A supernumerary ovary consists of typical ovarian tissue but has no direct or ligamentous connection with a normally placed ovary. A supernumerary ovary is thus a true third ovary that has independent function and is located at a point that is distant to a normally placed ovary. Ovarian malposition (Fig. 28.3C) also may occur when the ovary fails to descend into the pelvis to assume its normal location. In ovarian malposition, the ovary is attached as it should be to the uterus by the utero-ovarian ligament and to the fallopian tube by the fimbria ovarica, but it may lie adjacent to the liver or spleen. The ovary is elongated and may measure up to 15 cm in length. The fallopian tube attaching to such a malpositioned ovary may be 20 to 26 cm in length, almost twice its normal length.

The normal ovary has a surface covering composed of a single layer of flattened, germinal epithelial cells. This layer is contiguous at the ovarian hilum, with the peritoneal epithelium of the posterior leaf of the broad ligament. Beneath the germinal epithelium is a second layer of condensed ovarian stroma that forms a fibrous capsule, the tunica albuginea. The area through which the vessels and nerves enter and exit is the hilum of the ovary. Immediately around the hilum and extending into the substance of the ovary is an area known as the medulla, which is covered by the cortex. The medulla is composed of fibrous tissue unlike the condensed stroma of the ovarian cortex. The medulla contains no follicles; it has only blood vessels and the remnants of the tubular structure that would have developed into a testis (i.e., the rete ovarii) had the fetus been male.

The ovarian artery arises from the renal arteries. The artery descends from the aorta and crosses the ureter obliquely to enter the infundibulopelvic ligament on its course to the ovary. When it reaches the broad ligament, the ovarian artery branches to supply the fallopian tube and ovary before it finally anastomoses directly with the uterine artery to form a continuous arcade in the broad ligament. The ovarian veins are situated mainly in the mesosalpinx, where they give rise to the pampiniform plexus. At the outer end of the broad ligament, this plexus coalesces to form a single, large ovarian vein. The ovarian vein runs adjacent to ovarian artery to terminate in the inferior vena cava on the right and the renal vein on the left.

The lymphatic vessels of the ovary drain in three directions. The main group accompanies the ovarian vessels in the infundibulopelvic ligament and eventually reaches the periaortic nodes in the vicinity of the kidney. Other lymphatic channels communicate with channels of the opposite ovary by crossing the fundus of the uterus through the ovarian ligament. Some channels drain through the ovarian and round ligaments into the superficial inguinal lymph nodes in the groin. The ovary is supplied by both motor and sensory parasympathetic and sympathetic nerves,

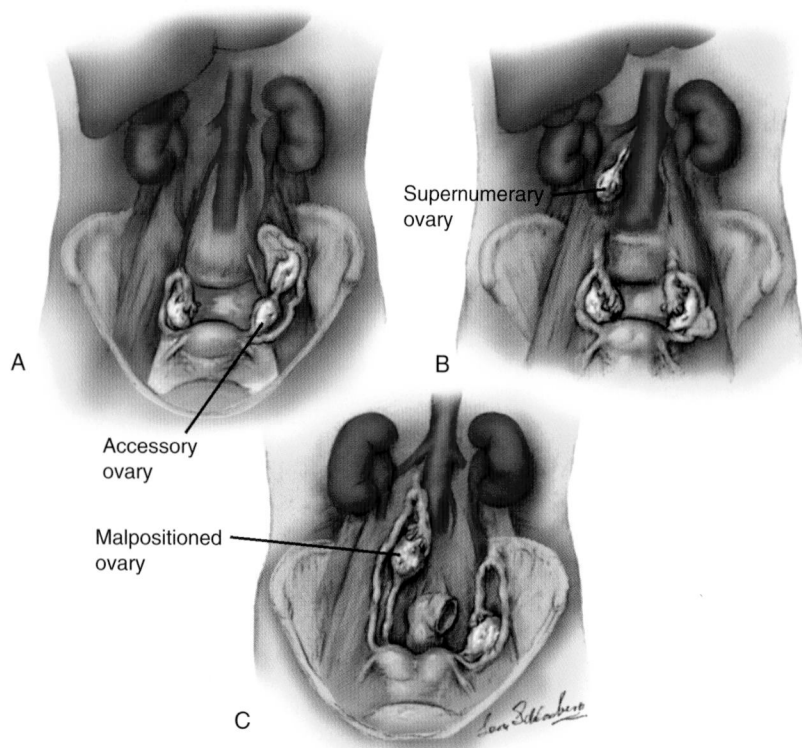

FIGURE 28.3 Ovarian anomalies. **A:** Accessory. **B:** Supernumerary. **C:** Malpositioned.

which accompany the ovarian vessels from the abdomen as they pass into the infundibulopelvic ligament to reach the hilum of the ovary. The segmented nerves supply the ovary from T10 and T11.

ADNEXAL MASS

The uterine adnexa (gynecologic origin) consist of the ovaries, the fallopian tubes, and the uterine ligaments. Although adnexal pathology often involves one of these structures, contiguous tissue of nongynecologic origin also may be involved. Adjunctive diagnostic techniques such as sonography, magnetic resonance imaging (MRI), and computed tomography (CT) may help delineate the nature of adnexal enlargement. Pelvic ultrasonography, especially three dimensional, is an accurate means of determining the location, size, extent, and consistency of pelvic masses and is also useful for detecting obstructive uropathy, ascites, and metastasis. Other more specialized diagnostic procedures also may be necessary for the evaluation of an adnexal mass (Table 28.1).

Computed tomography scanning has been particularly useful in gynecologic oncology because it helps define the extent of paracervical and parametrial involvement and allows a reasonable determination of the resectability of malignant neoplasms. Magnetic resonance imaging has surpassed CT in the precision of measurement of adnexal masses. Magnetic resonance imaging also allows a clear definition of the relationship of adjacent organs.

In a study conducted by Timmerman and coworkers, assessment was made of the use of both ultrasound and circulating levels of CA-125 antigen. Multivariate logistic regression analysis algorithms were used to distinguish benign adnexal masses from a malignant process. Transvaginal ultrasonography with color Doppler imaging was recorded in the 191 patients evaluated, aged 18 to 93 years. Of interest, 26.7% of the cohort of patients studied had malignant tumors. The authors believed that regression analysis could be used to accurately discriminate malignant from benign adnexal masses preoperatively.

An intriguing aspect of ultrasound assessment is the prediction of malignancy in adnexal masses using an artificial neural network. Taylor and colleagues reported generating a neural network algorithm that enabled computing of a probability of malignancy score for preoperative discrimination between malignant and benign adnexal masses. A retrospective analysis that included training in artificial neural network assessing transvaginal B-mode ultrasonography and color Doppler imaging was determined. The variables that were put into the artificial neural network included age, menopausal status, maximum diameter of the neoplasm, tumor volume, and papillary projections. The results identified four primary variables that were most effective in distinguishing benign versus malignant processes. These variables included age, time-averaged maximum velocity, papillary projection score, and maximum tumor diameter. The authors concluded that artificial neural networks are a useful clinical parameter to distinguish benign from malignant ovarian masses.

Surgical intervention ultimately may be necessary to determine the nature of the adnexal mass. Minimally invasive surgery is useful to exclude benign ovarian or nonovarian neoplasms. Indications for visualization and as indicated to obtain a tissue diagnosis of an adnexal mass with laparoscopy or exploratory laparotomy include the following:

- Ovarian mass greater than 6 cm in diameter
- Adnexal mass greater than 10 cm in diameter
- Any solid mass first developing after menopause
- Failure to discover the nature of the mass (e.g., leiomyoma) with radiologic or sonographic imaging techniques

One of the major goals of evaluation of the adnexal mass is to rule out malignancy. There is an age-dependent risk for a malignant adnexal mass. The incidence of malignant neoplasm increases significantly after age 50 years. Increased size of the adnexal mass is associated with an increased risk of malignancy.

Granberg and colleagues found that less than 1% of masses smaller than 5 cm were malignant, less than 11% of masses 5 to 10 cm were malignant, and 72% of masses larger than 10 cm were malignant. Sassone and associates, in an evaluation of women of all ages (mean age 41 years) by transvaginal sonography, found that 3% of masses smaller than 5 cm and 7% of masses 5 to 10 cm were malignant; the incidence of malignancy for masses larger than 10 cm was 13%.

Endometriosis is a common cause of an adnexal mass. An endometrial cyst of the ovary may develop into an endometrioma. Leakage of blood from the cyst may cause peritoneal irritation, pelvic adhesions, and pelvic organ fixation.

Tubo-ovarian inflammatory complex usually is the result of incompletely treated or unresolved subacute, chronic pelvic inflammatory disease (PID) in the walled-off area surrounding the pelvic structure.

Uterine leiomyomata cause nodularity and consequent irregular conformation of the uterus. The uterus may become enlarged and may present as an abdominal mass. The inability to distinguish a leiomyoma from an ovarian tumor on pelvic examination is an indication for further diagnostic evaluation.

Adnexal enlargement may be the result of carcinoma of the rectum, appendix, or bladder. Patients present with a variety of symptoms according to the organ involved. A complete and thorough evaluation is necessary to delineate the etiology of a neoplasm.

An adnexal mass may be noted in cases of acute abdomen. The differential diagnosis should include adnexal torsion, ruptured hemorrhagic cyst, degenerating leiomyomata, ectopic pregnancy, unruptured tubo-ovarian abscess, acute appendicitis with or without abscess formation, and diverticular disease of the sigmoid colon. A careful history, pelvic examination, and appropriate imaging studies often allow a prompt diagnosis.

Although every adnexal mass requires individual evaluation and management, it is possible to make a number of useful general recommendations. Expectant management is justified only when an asymptomatic physiologic cyst is suspected. Most cysts greater than 6 cm in diameter require a thorough evaluation. Imaging techniques are invaluable for characterizing the nature of the adnexal enlargement, but these procedures do not replace a careful medical history and thorough physical and pelvic examination.

ADNEXAL MASS DURING PREGNANCY

The incidence of adnexal mass in pregnancy requiring surgical intervention has been reported to occur at 1 in 81 to 2,500 pregnancies. When an adnexal mass is noted incidentally on ultrasound during pregnancy, the majority of small, simple cysts do not pose a risk to the pregnancy. Furthermore, most large or sonographically complex masses spontaneously resolve, as reported by Bernhard and colleagues; this study evaluated 18,391 ultrasound studies done in an obstetric population for which 432 women were identified with an adnexal mass. The incidence of adnexal masses was 2.3% in the pregnant population evaluated. In addition, the rate of torsion of the adnexal mass was 1%, and the rate of malignancy was also reported as 1%.

The majority of patients in one other study involving 320 pregnant patients with an adnexal mass were noted to have a simple cyst less than 5 cm, specifically 76%; the cysts were more commonly asymptomatic. The remaining patients were noted to have complex cycsts greater than 5 cm; of interest, of the complex cysts, 69% resolved spontaneously. The concern always remains regarding the potential for malignancy. Masses with increased blood flow or decreased resistance index and greater than 10 cm or a growth rate greater than 3.5 cm per week were noted to have a higher risk for malignancy.

Hoover and Jenkins addressed the incidence and differential diagnosis, benign cystic teratoma (7% to 37%), serous cystadenoma (5% to 28%), mucinous cystadenoma (3% to 24%), endometrioma (0.8% to 27%), paraovarian cyst (<5%), and leiomyoma (91% to 25%). Ovarian malignancy accounted for 1% to 8%, most of which were low malignant potential (LMP).

Other risks related to adnexal mass in pregnancy include rupture and obstruction regarding labor. Randomized prospective data focused are lacking with regard to pregnant patients with adnexal masses addressed surgically versus expectant management. Complications that include preterm labor and spontaneous abortion must be included in the overall assessment and management. Evaluation of oncofetal antigens includes alpha-fetoprotein, human chorionic gonadotropin (hCG), lactate dehydrogenase, estradiol, and testosterone.

Before operative intervention, a complete assessment of the fetus—including ultrasound to rule out a lethal anomaly and to document cardiac activity—is in order. The optimal time for elective surgery is during the second trimester. The patient should be informed of the increased risk of preterm labor and delivery. The patient should be placed in the left lateral tilt position to avoid inferior vena cava compression and associated uteroplacental insufficiency. Postoperatively, the fetus should be placed on continuous fetal heart rate monitoring.

The most effective approach in the management of adnexal masses during pregnancy remains a point of controversy (i.e., laparoscopy vs. laparotomy). In a series of 88 pregnant women who underwent 93 surgical procedures for suspected adnexal pathology, laparoscopy was performed during the first trimester in 39 patients. The remaining 54 patients underwent laparotomy, 25 during the first trimester and 29 during the second trimester. Neither intraoperative nor postoperative internal complications were reported in the series. Five of thirty-nine women undergoing the first-trimester surgery had a spontaneous abortion. During the first trimester, a Veress needle was used for insufflation, and the procedure was in essence conducted in a manner virtually identical to that in the nonpregnant state (i.e., closed laparoscopy). It was concluded that laparoscopic gynecologic surgery is safe during pregnancy when conducted in the first trimester.

ULTRASOUND

Ultrasound is useful in predicting malignancy (Table 28.2). Characteristic features of benign versus malignant neoplasms have been reported. Collated data from studies of ultrasound accuracy in the prediction of malignancy have an average positive predictive value of 74% and an average sensitivity of 88% (Tables 28.3 and 28.4).

Weiner and coworkers have used transvaginal color flow imaging before exploratory surgery to study the impedance to blood flow in women with an adnexal mass. Intramural blood vessels consistently demonstrated low impedance to flow with a pulsatility index less than 1:16 in women with malignant tumors. The sensitivity and specificity of the

TABLE 28.2 Special Diagnostic Procedures for the Evaluation of an Adnexal Mass
Nonoperative noninvasive
Abdominal and pelvic radiography
Barium enema
Excretory urography
Gastrointestinal series with small-bowel follow-through
Computed tomography scan
Magnetic resonance imaging
β-hCG
CA-125
Nonoperative invasive
Culdocentesis
Pelvic arteriography
Operative noninvasive
Abdominal and pelvic examination under anesthesia
Operative invasive
Culdoscopy
Laparoscopy
Exploratory posterior colpotomy
Exploratory laparotomy

preoperative pulsatility index in detecting malignant ovarian tumors were 94% and 97%, respectively. Kurjak and colleagues found that vessels with a low resistance index near the center of the mass or within papules or septa were highly correlated with malignancy. Therefore, transvaginal color flow imaging may be a useful clinical tool in the preoperative evaluation of ovarian masses.

Doppler resistance index has been used as a "vascular" scoring system. Color Doppler ultrasonography appears to be a reliable method in presurgically evaluating ovarian neoplasms.

Transvaginal color Doppler sonography has identified the following parameters as useful in determining malignant versus benign ovarian masses: number of vessels detected in each tumor, tumor vessel location (central vs. peripheral), peak systolic velocity, lowest resistance index, mean resistance index,

TABLE 28.3 Ultrasound Characteristics of the Ovary
Benign pattern
Simple cyst without internal echoes
Simple cyst with scattered echoes
Polycystic echoes
Polycystic echoes with thick septum
Sessile or polypoid smooth mural echoes
Central dense round echoes
Thin or thick multiple linear echoes
Thin or thick multiple linear echoes with dense part
Malignant pattern
Cystic echoes with papillary or indented mural part
Polycystic echoes with irregular thick septum and solid part
Solid pattern (50%) heterogeneous component with irregular cystic part
Completely solid with homogeneous component
Low impedance to flow (color Doppler)

TABLE 28.4 Ultrasound Accuracy in Prediction of Malignancy

AUTHOR	PATIENTS (n)	MALIGNANCY PREVALENCE	POSITIVE PREDICTIVE VALUE (%)	NEGATIVE PREDICTIVE VALUE (%)	SENSITIVITY	SPECIFICITY
Kobayashi (1976)	406	15	31	93	71	73
Meire et al. (1978)	51	35	83	91	83	91
Pussell (1980)	26	48	83	91	83	84
Herrmann et al. (1987)	241	21	75	95	82	93
Finkler et al. (1988)	102	36	88	81	62	95
Benacerraf et al. (1990)	100	30	72	91	80	87
Granberg et al. (1989)	180	21.5	74	95	82	92
Sassone et al. (1991)	143	10	87	100	100	83

lower pulsatility index, and mean pulsatility index. Color Doppler signals were detected in 100% of malignant masses and 75% of benign masses, with the difference being statistically significant as reported by Alcazar and associates. Tumor vessel location appears to be central in virtually all malignant masses. Overall, the receiver operating characteristic curves generated can be used to predict malignant processes. The lowest resistance index was associated with the majority of malignant tumors.

Three-dimensional ultrasonographic technology has been used to evaluate adnexal masses. Images are dissected in *XYZ* planes and can be focused especially on areas suggestive of malignancy. Three-dimensional ultrasonography facilitates real-time analysis of acquired image data and allows reassessment of the findings at the time of the original ultrasound. Three-dimensional transvaginal ultrasonographic technology appears to enhance and facilitate morphologic assessment of benign as well as malignant ovarian masses.

The appearance on ultrasound provides clinically useful information. Up to 95% of endometriomas exhibit diffuse homogenous low-level internal echoes. They can vary in appearance to include large cystic and solid components; thus, hemorrhagic cysts must be included in the differential. Teratomas on ultrasound demonstrate hyperechoic nodules with distal acoustic shadowing, often termed a "dermal plug." Hair and sebaceous contents are visualized as hyperechoic lines and dots, termed a "dermoid mesh." With regard to cystadenomas, serous are more common than mucinous and the former are noted to have thin septations; occasionally, papillary projections may be noted. Mucinous cysts are multilocular with varying amounts of fluid content; low-level internal echoes with multiple thin septa are commonly noted. Cystadenocarcinoma is characterized by thicker septations, papillary projections greater than 3 mm, and irregular walls. Tumors of LMP demonstrate an "ovarian crescent sign," equated with a rim of normal-appearing ovarian tissue adjacent to the tumor mass. Vascular mural nodules and papillary projection may be present. Paraovarian masses include paraovarian cysts and hydrosalpinx. Ovarian torsion is associated with a "ground-glass" appearance on ultrasound; a characteristic "whirlpool sign" is consistent with the appearance of vessels coiling in a twisted vascular pedicle on color Doppler studies. The latter may demonstrate arterial or venous flow, only arterial flow, or no flow at all to the torsed ovary.

In addition to the role of Doppler ultrasonography with regard to identifying a malignancy, it is also useful in following the progression or regression of the adnexal mass.

MAGNETIC RESONANCE IMAGING

Magnetic resonance imaging is a "second-line imaging modality." It is important that patients fast 4 hours before the planned MRI examination as this limits artifact from bowel peristalsis. Scanning in left lateral decubitus position may be necessary during pregnancy. A body array coil is frequently used over the pelvis in pregnant women undergoing MRI. Gadolinium-based contrast is a pregnancy category C drug.

TUMOR MARKERS

Tumor markers are substances that are identified in higher than normal amounts in blood, urine, or body tissues of patients with specific malignancies. Tumor markers are not unique to malignant processes and can be elevated with benign conditions. Tumor markers are not elevated in every patient with malignancy, especially in the early stages of the disease. Many tumor markers are not specific for a particular type of cancer; therefore, there are limitations to the use of tumor markers.

CA-125 is a tumor-associated antigen to an antibody expressed by approximately 80% of patients with epithelial ovarian cancer. It can be increased by nongynecologic malignancies with involvement of the pleura or peritoneum and by benign conditions that result in ascites. Because of the many medical diagnoses that give false-positive CA-125 results, CA-125 cannot be used for general population screening for ovarian cancer in either premenopausal or postmenopausal women. However, in menopausal women who present with a pelvic mass, CA-125 can help differentiate benign from malignant masses.

Because menopausal women have fewer gynecologic diseases that give false elevation of CA-125, the test is more sensitive and specific in this age group. Several authors have

TABLE 28.5 Tumor Markers: Adnexal Masses

MARKER	COMMENTS
CA-125	80% nonmucinous ovarian carcinomas have elevation of CA-125. Decreasing levels generally indicate response to therapy. Used to identify recurrences.
CEA	Primary use is to monitor recurrence of colon cancer. Oncofetal antigen–Ag complex glycoprotein, 20,000 d associated with plasma membrane of tumor cells. Increased with ovarian cancer and with melanoma, breast, pancreatic, stomach, cervical, bladder, kidney, thyroid, and liver cancer. Inflammatory bowel disease and smoking elevate CEA.
c-Myc	Amplified in 30%–50% of ovarian tumors. The protein is simultaneously overexpressed.
c-MycRA	Associated with aneuploidy in ovarian malignant cell progression.
BRCA1	Associated with mutations of breast tumor–related antigen. BRCA1 tumor suppressor gene has been identified; 63% risk of developing ovarian cancer with positive BRCA1 gene.

TABLE 28.6 Classification of the Adnexal Mass

GYNECOLOGIC ORIGIN	NONGYNECOLOGIC ORIGIN
Nonneoplastic	Nonneoplastic
Ovarian	Appendiceal abscess
Physiologic cysts	Diverticulosis
Follicular	Adhesions of bowel and omentum
Corpus luteum	
Theca lutein cyst	Peritoneal cyst
Luteoma of pregnancy	Feces in rectosigmoid
Polycystic ovaries	Urine in bladder
Inflammatory cysts	Pelvic kidney
Urachal cyst	Anterior sacral meningocele
Nonovarian	Neoplastic
Ectopic pregnancy	Carcinoma
Congenital anomalies	Sigmoid
Embryologic remnants	Cecum
Tubal	Appendix
Pyosalpinx	Retroperitoneal neoplasm
Hydrosalpinx	Presacral teratoma
Bladder	
Neoplastic	
Ovarian	
Nonovarian	
Leiomyomata	
Paraovarian cyst	
Endometrial carcinoma	
Tubal carcinoma	

Adapted from Hall DJ, Hurt WG. The adnexal mass. *J Fam Pract* 1982;14:135, with permission.

TABLE 28.7 Clinical Findings Suggesting Benign or Malignant Adnexal Mass

BENIGN	MALIGNANT
Unilateral	Bilateral
Cystic	Solid
Mobile	Fixed
Smooth	Irregular
No ascites	Ascites
Slow growth	Rapid growth
Younger patient	Older patient

demonstrated that a panel of assays can improve both sensitivity and specificity in the detection of ovarian malignancies. For example, Soper and associates demonstrated 100% specificity and predictive value for CA-125 with TAG 72 or CA-15-3. Table 28.5 provides specific markers and their clinical application.

The clinical findings listed in Tables 28.5 through 28.7 are often helpful in differentiating a malignant from a benign neoplasm. All ovarian neoplasms larger than 6 cm in diameter with a solid component should undergo investigation. The postmenopausal ovary is usually small and nonpalpable. Enlargement of the postmenopausal ovary requires appropriate investigation. Symptoms of ovarian neoplasms usually depend on their size, rate of growth, and position in the pelvis or abdomen. Symptoms may include vague lower abdominal fullness or pressure discomfort. Larger masses rise out of the true pelvis and may cause abdominal enlargement with varicosities and edema of the lower extremities. Most ovarian neoplasms are asymptomatic until they enlarge or affect adjacent organs and structures.

MINIMALLY INVASIVE APPROACH TO AN ADNEXAL MASS

STEPS IN THE PROCEDURE

Laparoscopic Excision of Adnexal Mass

- Preoperative assessment: Imaging studies and tumor markers as appropriate
- Intraoperative management:
  - Lithotomy position, Foley catheter in the bladder, drape perineum into sterile field
  - Laparoscopic placement of secondary trocar ports
  - Evaluation of the upper abdomen and pelvis
  - Identification of adnexal mass
  - Determine the most appropriate procedure
  - Obtain pelvic washings if appropriate
  - Restore normal anatomy
  - Identify ureter(s) in pelvis

- If cystectomy, plan resection to preserve normal ovarian tissue
- If adnexectomy, elevate adnexa; identify, isolate, and secure infundibulopelvic vasculature
- Divide uterine tube at isthmus
- Secure hemostasis along mesosalpinx/mesovarium
- Extirpate adnexa
- Reduce insufflation, and check for hemostasis
- Remove adnexa using Endo Catch bag or other techniques for removal

The pelvic (adnexal) mass may be of gynecologic or nongynecologic origin (Table 28.6). Specific clinical findings are helpful to differentiate a malignant from a benign neoplasm (Table 28.7). It is important to establish whether the mass is of ovarian origin and to understand that a solid mass causing an ovary to enlarge to greater than 6 cm in diameter should be considered potentially malignant until proven otherwise. The most common ovarian mass is the physiologic ovarian cyst, which is caused by failure of a follicle to rupture or to regress. Physiologic ovarian cysts normally are less than 6 cm in diameter, smooth, mobile, and may be slightly tender to palpation. They usually contain straw-colored fluid and may be associated with menstrual irregularity. Physiologic ovarian cysts smaller than 6 cm usually regress by absorption of the fluid or spontaneous rupture. The premenopausal patient may be managed conservatively over two menstrual cycles. If regression fails to occur over two periods of observation or if enlargement is noted, reassessment is indicated.

Oral contraceptives have been suggested as an alternative treatment for functional cysts. The combination-type oral contraceptives send negative feedback to the pituitary gland to decrease gonadotropin stimulation of the ovary, which causes regression of the cyst. Steinkampf and colleagues noted that the rate of disappearance of functional ovarian cysts was not affected by estrogen–progestin treatment; nevertheless, a patient taking oral contraceptives with an adnexal mass should be thoroughly investigated.

Failure of the corpus luteum to regress (in the nonpregnant patient) may cause development of a corpus luteum cyst. The size of the corpus luteum cyst varies according to the amount of blood contained within the cyst. A large corpus luteum may rupture and cause intraperitoneal hemorrhage. Amenorrhea or irregular uterine bleeding may accompany the development of a corpus luteum cyst. A sensitive pregnancy test, ultrasonography, and laparoscopy can be used to differentiate an ectopic pregnancy from a persistent corpus luteum.

A theca lutein cyst, which may be associated with gestational trophoblastic disease or pregnancy, is the result of luteinization of the ovary by hCG. Many of these cysts are bilateral and multicystic. A reduction in hCG levels usually leads to their spontaneous regression.

Polycystic ovarian (PCO) disease is associated with bilaterally enlarged ovaries with a smooth surface. The ovaries contain multiple follicular cysts; many patients are obese and hirsute and have accompanying anovulation (see below).

Congenital anomalies of the müllerian system and vestigial remnants of the wolffian system are of gynecologic, if not strictly ovarian, origin. Müllerian anomalies should be considered in the differential diagnosis of an adnexal mass. Uterine anomalies with outflow tract obstruction oftentimes are associated with cyclic pain from development of hematometra, whereas an enlarged paraovarian cyst may be asymptomatic.

OVARIAN REMNANT SYNDROME

The ovarian remnant occurs in patients who have had previous oophorectomy with or without hysterectomy. The patient may present with symptoms with or without a palpable mass or with a palpable pelvic mass but no symptoms. Pathologic investigation confirms the presence of ovarian tissue when there should be none.

The ovarian remnant syndrome differs from the residual ovarian syndrome in that with the latter, the ovary is purposely saved, and a pathologic process subsequently develops in the ovary. The ovarian remnant syndrome follows attempted oophorectomy.

Minke and associates demonstrated that devascularization of ovarian tissue can occur with reimplanting on intact or abraded peritoneal surfaces, where it may resume endocrine function. Thus, the authors suggest that great care should be exercised to remove all ovarian tissue, particularly when oophorectomy is performed through the laparoscope.

Ultrasonography remains a valuable tool in establishing the diagnosis of ovarian remnant syndrome. The use of both transabdominal sonography and transvaginal sonography with use of color Doppler identification of the mass acquires information with respect to both arterial and venous flow. This facilitates identification of ovarian tissue.

Symmonds and Petit identified three major factors that may complicate the initial surgery and make it difficult or impossible for the surgeon to ascertain whether all ovarian tissue has been removed: increased pelvic vascularity, which renders hemostasis difficult; adhesions, which distort the anatomy and make dissection difficult; and neoplasms, which also distort the anatomy. The most common preexisting disease is endometriosis, followed in frequency by PID. Patients with ovarian remnant syndrome often present with both pelvic pain and a mass. The quality of the pain varies, often cyclically, and ranges from a sensation of pressure or dull aching to a severe stabbing pain.

The clinical diagnosis of ovarian remnant syndrome can be difficult. A finding of premenopausal levels of follicle-stimulating hormone (FSH) may facilitate the diagnosis. Sonography (especially vaginal) may be of value, and a CT scan or MRI may be useful for defining the physical relation of the ovarian remnant to surrounding structures.

The treatment of choice is adequate excision of the ovarian remnant with removal of contiguous adherent tissue such as pelvic peritoneum, bowel serosa, the underlying involved ligament, and alveolar and vascular tissues (Fig. 28.4A, B). Excision of ovarian tissue may require a retroperitoneal dissection to define the relation of the ureter to the bowel and ovary.

Magtibay and colleagues addressed the surgical management of patients with ovarian remnant syndrome at the Mayo Clinic. All operations for residual ovary syndrome were performed by laparotomy. Of 186 patients who underwent a wide dissection and removal of the remnant, a moderate risk of bowel, bladder, or ureteral injury was noted; however, 90% of patients had complete resolution or marked improvement of symptoms after surgery.

Laparoscopic excision of ovarian remnant ovaries is feasible. A retroperitoneal approach that allows dissection of the course of the ureters with coagulation and dissection of the infundibulopelvic ligament and the uterine vessels can be accomplished. There is potential for ureteral injury as well as cystotomy and bowel injury.

RESIDUAL OVARY

Based on the clinical circumstance, the gynecologic surgeon should consider the value of ovarian conservation at the time of hysterectomy for benign disease. Some authors have noted the incidence of malignant neoplasm in retained ovaries as a reason for prophylactic oophorectomy, and others have noted

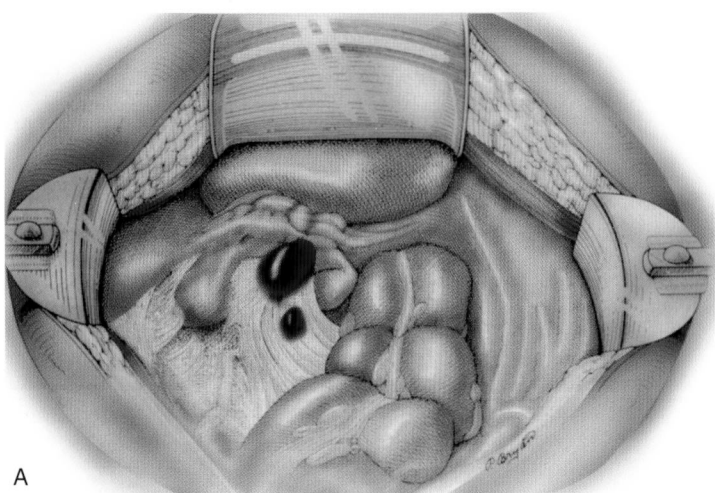

A

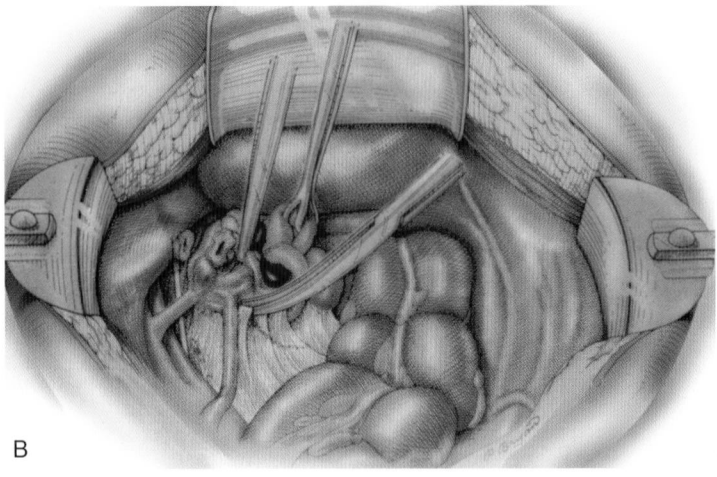

B

FIGURE 28.4 A: Not infrequently, the ovarian remnant may adhere to the bowel and the pelvic sidewall peritoneum. **B:** The ureter must be visualized and its relation to the bowel and ovarian remnant established. This may require development of the pararectal and rectovaginal spaces.

the presence of "residual ovary syndrome," characterized by either recurrent pelvic pain or a persistent pelvic mass (sonogram image) (Fig. 28.5). However, Funt followed 992 patients after conservation of one or both ovaries at the time of hysterectomy and reported that none developed ovarian malignancy, and only 1.4% required subsequent surgical intervention for adnexal pathology. The benefits of preserved ovarian function thus appear to substantially outweigh the risk of subsequent ovarian pathology requiring further surgery. Before surgery, the gynecologic surgeon should discuss the various risks and benefits of bilateral oophorectomy and should encourage the patient to participate in any decision concerning the fate of her ovaries.

Gonadotropin-releasing hormone (GnRH) agonists have been used to assess response of residual ovaries with chronic pelvic pain followed by surgical intervention to remove the residual ovarian tissue. Resolution of pelvic pain in six treated patients occurred with the analogize GnRH agonist and persisted with surgical extirpation of the ovarian tissue. Suppression of ovarian function by GnRH agonists allows differentiation of pelvic pain caused by residual ovary from other sources and thus should be a prerequisite to surgical intervention.

In a retrospective report of 20 years of experience with residual ovary syndrome in which 2,561 hysterectomies were performed, the incidence of residual ovary syndrome was 2.85%. Thus, 1 in 35 women who undergo hysterectomy with ovarian preservation become symptomatic—that is, they experience pelvic pain often with the presence of a benign cyst. Patients should be counseled preoperatively with respect to the potential for

residual ovary syndrome when the initial surgical intervention is anticipated. In addition to chronic pelvic pain, a pelvic mass and dyspareunia include the "cluster of symptoms" that can occur in patients who have undergone previous hysterectomy.

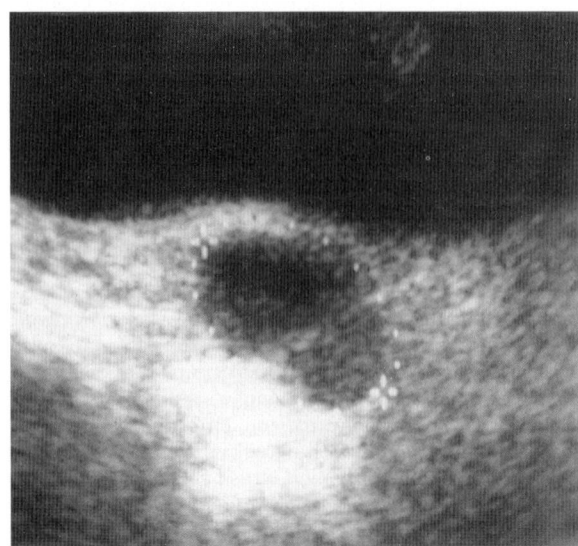

FIGURE 28.5 Abdominal sonogram showing a residual ovary with presumed follicular activity.

ADNEXAL TORSION

Torsion of the adnexa is an infrequent cause of pain in the lower abdomen. However, torsion is a common gynecologic surgical emergency, with a prevalence of 2.7%. Treatment of adnexal torsion is considered an emergency because peritonitis and death can result. Any portion of the adnexa (tube or ovary) may undergo torsion. It may occur in neoplastic ovaries or as a consequence of hyperstimulation.

The clinical findings of torsion are nonspecific. For this reason, delay in diagnosis and surgical intervention is common. The classic presentation is the acute onset of abdominal pain with clinical evidence of peritonitis and an adnexal mass. However, according to Bayer and Wiskind, the presenting findings in most patients are nonspecific and unimpressive. Torsion is more likely to occur during ovulation or as a premenstrual event associated with increased pelvic congestion; the authors found no correlation between the phase of the cycle and the onset of the symptoms.

Historically, the adnexa usually were removed because some authors suggested that untwisting the adnexa could increase the risk of thromboembolism. This has not been well substantiated. There is growing evidence that unwinding the involved adnexa to observe for tissue reperfusion and viability is safe. Nevertheless, a significant delay in surgical intervention may result in irreversible necrosis, requiring removal of the tube, ovary, or both.

The minimally invasive surgical management of adnexal torsion has been increasing in efficacy. Mage and colleagues found that untwisting the adnexa was possible in most patients in their series, and no further intervention was required. Likewise, Shalev and Peleg demonstrated that laparoscopic detorsion of the adnexa is safe and reliable as a primary treatment of this condition. Thus, the weight of evidence warrants conservation of the adnexa if there is evidence of reperfusion and if significant delay has not resulted in irreversible tissue necrosis. In most instances, detorsion may be accomplished through the laparoscope.

SURGERY OF THE OVARIAN SURFACE

Surgery to remove adhesions or endometriosis from the ovarian surface is not unusual and primarily accomplished via minimally invasive surgery. De novo adhesions or adhesions between the medial surface of the ovary and the broad ligament may be filmy and vascular (Fig. 28.6A) and may be excised by fine electrocautery or vaporized with the use of a laser (Fig. 28.6B). More extensive adhesions that completely cover the ovarian surface may be thick and avascular (Fig. 28.6C, D). The plane of dissection between the broad ligament or pelvic sidewall and the adherent ovarian surface must be developed with care so as not to remove or damage the peritoneum while excising the adhesion (Fig. 28.6D). Multiple, small adhesions distributed over the ovarian surface, once coagulated, can be gently removed from the ovary without trauma to the ovarian cortex.

If the lateral aspect of the ovary is densely adherent to the broad ligament, it may be necessary to dissect the ovary free. Some cases require that a large area of the sidewall or the broad ligament be denuded; reperitonealization can be accomplished with nonreactive absorbable suture material.

Small endometrial implants can be fulgurated or vaporized. The resulting small ovarian defect usually does not require closure. Care should be taken to ensure that the endometriosis is superficial and that the implant is not actually the tip of a large endometrioma within the substance of the ovary.

RECONSTRUCTION OF THE OVARY

Before ovarian reconstruction is begun, it is important that proper mobilization of the ovary be accomplished for reestablishment of normal anatomy. Once complete excision of the involved ovarian pathology has been accomplished, the main objectives of ovarian reconstruction are atraumatic closure of the stroma and cortex and prevention of adhesion formation. The principles for accomplishing this goal include gentle tissue handling, hemostasis, the use of fine (and ideally minimally reactive) suture material, and an effort to "bury knots" for the prevention of adhesions.

The restoration of normal-appearing anatomy is the most logical approach for creating maximal ovarian surface, which facilitates ovum pickup by the fallopian tube. Controversy continues as to whether it is more appropriate to completely excise or lyse paraovarian and peritubal adhesions.

The most important aspect of ovarian reconstruction whether done via laparotomy or with a minimally invasive, including robotic surgical, approach is excellent reapproximation of the cortex with the use of atraumatic techniques, including fine absorbable suture material and minimizing suture exposure on the cortex. On completion of the procedure, intraabdominal lavage should be used, ideally with a physiologic substance such as lactated Ringer solution. Every effort should be made to remove all blood from the peritoneal cavity, preferably with the patient taken out of the Trendelenburg position.

The approach to resection of an ovarian cyst should be planned so as to minimize adhesion formation. The incidence of de novo adhesion formation appears to be decreased when the initial approach is through laparoscopy. The Operative Laparoscopy Study Group assessed the issue of frequency and severity of adhesion reformation and of de novo adhesions after operative laparoscopy. In a multicenter collaborative approach that included early second-look intervention, 68 patients underwent operative laparoscopic procedures, including adhesiolysis as well as ovarian cystectomy. The scoring of adhesions noted during the second-look laparoscopy occurred at nine sites (each ovary, each fallopian tube, omentum, culde-sac, pelvic sidewall, and large and small bowel). The study concluded that adhesion reformation is a frequent occurrence and that de novo adhesion formation occurred less frequently after initial operative laparoscopy.

A number of agents have been advocated for preventing adhesions, including oxidized regenerated cellulose (Interceed [TC7], Johnson & Johnson Medical, Arlington, TX), which is an absorbable barrier that promotes reepithelialization of the affected area. Pagidas and Tulandi compared Interceed with lactated Ringer solution for adhesion prevention. Lactated Ringer solution was as effective as Interceed in decreasing adhesion formation. Haney and colleagues compared oxidized regenerated cellulose with expanded polytetrafluoroethylene (Gore-Tex surgical membrane). The results indicated that expanded polytetrafluoroethylene was associated with fewer postsurgical adhesions. Other agents include sodium hyaluronate carboxymethyl cellulose (Seprafilm). A number of adhesion barriers are currently being evaluated and include Hyalobarrier, SprayShield, Prevadh, and INTERCOAT. Further research may well provide clinicians with an extended armamentarium for adhesion prevention.

Functional Ovarian Cysts

Physiologic cyst enlargement of the ovary may occur as a sequela of failure of either follicular rupture or corpus luteum regression. The latter is termed Halban syndrome. The former has been associated with luteinized unruptured follicle syndrome, in which "intraovarian ovulation" is thought to occur; this is a diagnosis usually established with ultrasound. In general, functional ovarian cysts regress spontaneously; however, they may persist and become symptomatic, reaching dimensions as large as 10 cm in diameter. The obvious and most feasible approach is observation, because most such cysts are

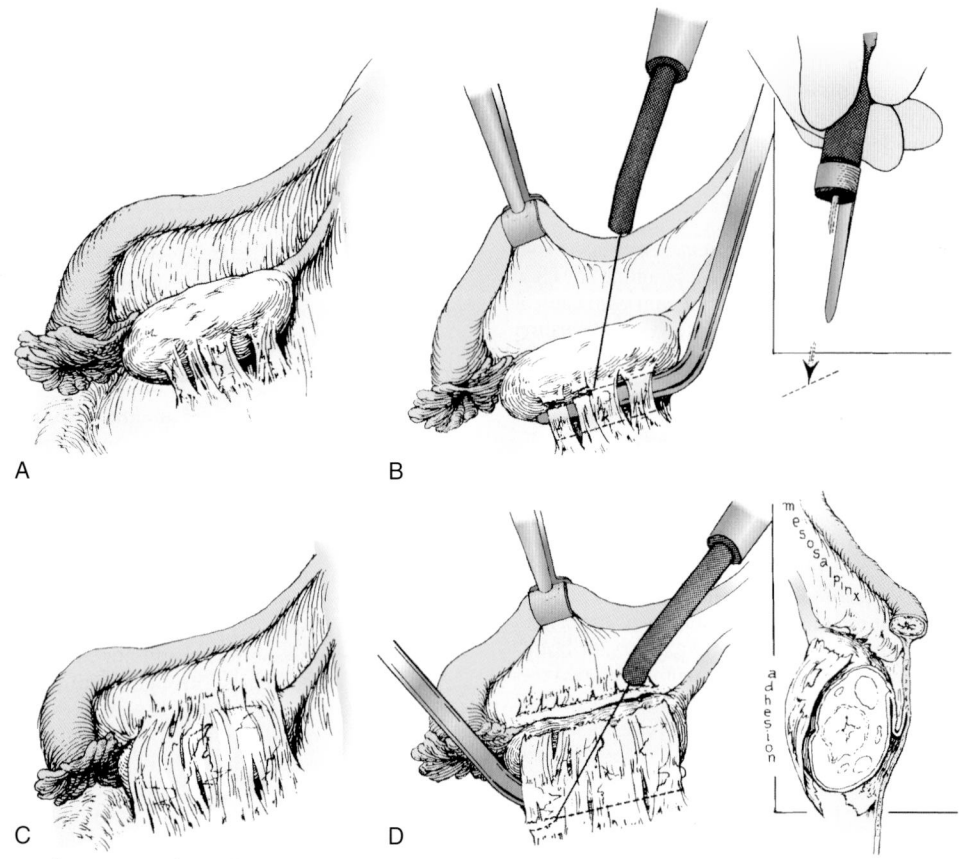

FIGURE 28.6 Ovarian adhesions. **A:** Filmy adhesions between the medial aspect of the ovary and the pelvic sidewall. **B:** These may be removed with laser or fine electrocautery with use of a quartz or glass rod, respectively, as a backstop. **C:** The ovary may be enveloped by adhesions. **D:** Care should be taken to tent up the adhesions so that the peritoneum is not damaged or incised.

self-limited. The cyst, however, may prove to be a source of continued pelvic pain or may adhere to the posterior broad ligament, producing persistent symptoms. The potential for adnexal torsion always exists with an ovarian cyst.

RESECTION OF BENIGN CYSTS

Surgical intervention often is initiated with a laparoscopic approach, which permits completion of fenestration of the nonneoplastic ovarian cyst. The cyst lining is stripped from the remaining "normal ovary," and ovarian reconstruction takes place. In several series of laparoscopic management of ovarian cysts, a simple follicular or luteal cyst was identified in most patients evaluated for pelvic pain. In a series by Kleppinger, 31 of 64 ovarian cysts were noted to fall into this category.

Surgical Techniques

Laparotomy

An elliptic incision is made through the thin ovarian cortex of a benign cyst (**Fig. 28.7**). The end of the knife handle is then inserted and a plane developed over the cyst wall. Alternatively, fine-needle electrocautery can be used to develop a plane, and microsurgical scissors can be used to separate the cyst wall from the ovarian cortex. Low-power magnification (i.e., surgical loupes) often assists the surgeon in identifying the correct plane between the cyst wall and the ovarian parenchyma. After the cyst wall has been completely separated from its adherent attachments to the thin ovarian cortex, it can be shelled out

without rupture. However, even with the gentlest technique, rupture can occur because of the friability of the cyst wall. Before the cyst is shelled out, it is important to pack the cul-de-sac with moist, lint-free pads so that, if rupture does occur, spillage does not contaminate the pelvic cavity. After the cyst has been removed, the dead space can be obliterated with a purse-string suture of fine-gauge nonreactive material. Alternatively, nonreactive vertical mattress sutures or figure-of-eight, or both, can be placed to approximate the lateral walls of the ovary. The ovarian surface is then neatly reapproximated with a subcortical running suture of fine-gauge nonreactive material (**Fig. 28.7A**). If the cortex is quite friable, it may be necessary to place interrupted fine-gauge sutures to achieve adequate approximation. Some authors advocate leaving the ovary open after cystectomy. To date, there have been no controlled trials evaluating postoperative adhesion formation when the incised ovarian surface is or is not reapproximated.

In some instances, there is excessive redundant thin cortex, which may present a special problem in ovarian reconstruction. The amount of cortex removed depends on the position of the cyst as well as its overall size. Careful assessment of the ovary is necessary before the initial incision is made. The incision in the ovarian cortex facilitates symmetric reconstruction. The redundant cortex can be removed and the dead space obliterated with an internal closure, with care taken to prevent suture material from penetrating the ovarian cortex. This prevents ischemia and adhesion formation. The infolding technique recommended by Kistner and Patton may result in anatomic distortion and puckering of the ovarian cortex. The

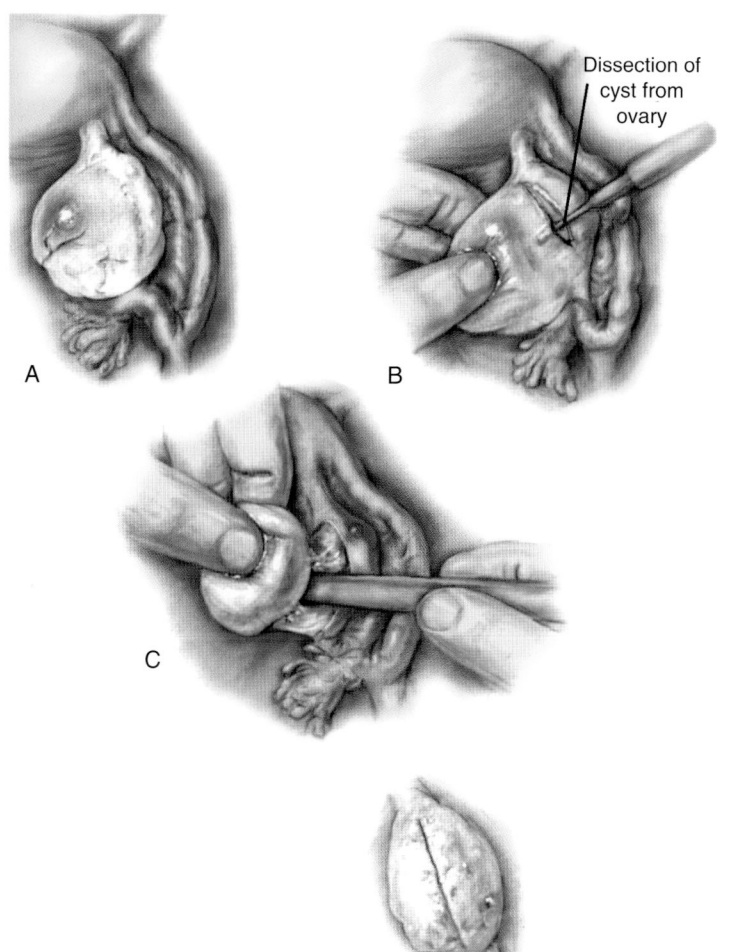

FIGURE 28.7 Resection of benign cyst. **A:** Thin-walled ovarian cyst. **B:** An incision is made through the cortex. **C:** A plane is developed by the use of blunt dissection. The inner ovarian stroma may be approximated with a purse-string suture of 5-0 nonreactive material. **D:** The ovarian cortex is approximated with 7-0 nonreactive suture material.

"baseball" closure allows careful approximation of cortical edges when redundancy is noted (Fig. 28.8).

Concern over ovarian surgery via laparotomy has been reported. In an older reference of 36 young women operated on for an ovarian cyst, 45% were noted subsequently to be infertile. The author, Van der Watt, conveyed the importance of not interfering with functional cysts in "normal ovaries," because resulting adhesion formation could compromise fertility. It was advocated that benign ovarian cysts should not be removed at the time of surgery for other indications unless they are sufficiently large to interfere with tubal function or cause discomfort to the patient.

Minimally Invasive and Robotic-Assisted Surgery

Overview

Specific skill levels reflecting both the degree of operator expertise and appropriate instrumentation provide clinicians with four levels of training. Level I stands for equipment needs and potential surgical procedures for basic operative laparoscopy, including such entities as diagnostic laparoscopy, tubal sterilization, lysis of filmy adhesions, and biopsy. Level II reflects the clinician's ability to perform linear salpingostomy for ectopic pregnancy, salpingectomy, lysis of vascular adhesions, and elimination of endometriotic implants. Level III includes the ability to perform salpingo-oophorectomy, lysis of extensive adhesions (including bowel adhesions), ovarian cystectomy, appendectomy, myomectomy, laparoscopic-assisted hysterectomy, and neosalpingostomy,

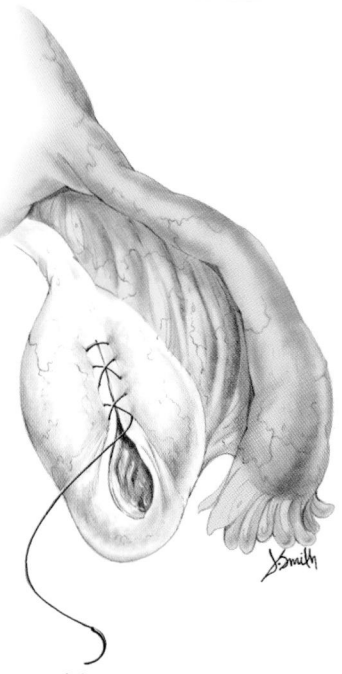

FIGURE 28.8 Closure of the ovary with a baseball stitch.

as well as the ability to treat tubo-ovarian abscess and uterine suspension. Level IV includes bowel resection, anastomosis, pelvic lymphadenectomy, presacral neurectomy, tubal reanastomosis, and excision of deep, infiltrating vaginal, paravaginal, and rectal endometriosis.

A number of principles should be followed as surgeons proceed with the correction of pelvic abnormalities that are amenable to a laparoscopic approach. The first is to restore normal anatomy. Once the ovary is stabilized, ideally with an atraumatic forceps, an appropriately planned ovarian incision can be made to correct the pathology encountered. Every effort should be made not to spill the contents.

Large amounts of irrigation solution should be used. In some instances, the cyst wall can be stripped, electrocoagulated, or vaporized. The ovarian incision can then be either left open to heal by primary intention or reapproximated with sutures with either extracorporeal or intracorporeal suture-tying techniques. When this procedure is completed, the pelvis is irrigated with large amounts of irrigation solution (Ringer lacate), and the patient is taken out of the Trendelenburg position to facilitate removal of any blood products that remain in the peritoneal cavity.

One alternative to suturing is to reapproximate incised segments of ovarian cortex with the use of bipolar coagulation to provide coaptation of the incised segment of the ovary. There is continued debate regarding the use of adhesion prevention materials.

A number of potential pitfalls continue to be of concern in the laparoscopic approach to ovarian lesions. These have been addressed by Seltzer and colleagues and include the following:

- The potential for disruption of an ovarian malignancy
- Whether observation-recommended surgical intervention would be the most feasible alternative
- Potential for increased duration of the surgical procedure if done endoscopically
- Total cost
- Potential for incomplete resection of an ovarian lesion laparoscopically

One can view laparoscopic approach to the adnexal mass based on age. Specifically, in the pediatric patient, problems such as torsion, hemorrhagic cysts, benign neoplasm (e.g., teratoma), as well as oophorectomy have been reportedly addressed via the laparoscope. One advantage over laparotomy is the ability to better visualize the entire lower abdomen and pelvis, including the opposite ovary. In the adult, depending on the clinical circumstance, cyst aspiration, cystectomy, or oophorectomy can be accomplished laparoscopically.

Predictors of clinical outcomes in the laparoscopic management of adnexal mass have been addressed by Havrilesky and coauthors. The authors noted that adnexal mass thought to be benign preoperatively were successfully managed laparoscopically in three fourths of the patients. Adverse events were attributable to concurrent hysterectomy rather than removal of the adnexal mass. Malignancy occurred in 2%, and laparoscopic management was not associated with adverse outcomes.

Concern is expressed for an ovarian neoplasm subsequently noted to be malignant. In a countrywide survey in Austria, Wenzl and colleagues reported on 54,198 laparoscopies; 16,601 were performed for adnexal masses, and 108 cases of ovarian tumors were subsequently found to be malignant. Of the 108 cases, 20 were managed laparoscopically, 22 by immediate laparotomy, and the rest by delayed laparotomy (3 to 1,415 days). The authors concluded that laparoscopic surgery with the finding of an ovarian malignancy is rare: 0.65% of all endoscopic surgical procedures.

The extent of damage to ovarian reserve associated with laparoscopic excision of endometriomas was studied by Ragni and coauthors. A reduced number of dominate follicles, oocytes, embryos, and high-quality embryos were observed in the operated gonad. Fertilization rate and rate of good-quality embryos were similar in operated and control groups. Laparoscopic excision of endometriomas is associated with a quantitative but not a qualitative damage to ovarian reserve.

Robotic-assisted intervention brings a 3D perspective to surgical procedures. Wrist movement of the surgeon at the console provides seven degrees of freedom (movement) and can provide an added dimension to pelvic surgical procedures. Nezhat and coworkers assessed robotic surgical intervention in 15 patients undergoing gynecologic surgery. These clinicians concluded that robotic-assisted laparoscopic surgical intervention had advantages in providing a 3-dimensional visualization of the operative field, decreasing operator fatigue and tension tremor, and added wrist motion for improved dexterity and greater surgical precision. The disadvantages include additional expense and added operating time for assembly (docking) and disassembly (undocking) and the bulkiness of the equipment.

MANAGEMENT OF POLYCYSTIC OVARIAN DISEASE

Signs and symptoms of PCO syndrome (PCOS) begin at puberty. Polycystic ovary is a sign, not a diagnosis. In a consensus meeting held in Rotterdam, the American Society for Reproductive Medicine (ASRM) and the European Society of Human Reproduction and Embryology (ESHRE) agreed that two of the following criteria must be met once other endocrinopathies have been ruled out (i.e., Cushing, adrenal hyperplasia):

- Oligomenorrhea
- Clinical and/or biochemical evidence for hyperandrogenemia
- Polycystic-appearing ovaries on ultrasound

The polycystic ovary may result from a virilizing ovarian or adrenal neoplasm or from congenital adrenal hyperplasia, or it may result from suboptimal hypothalamic–pituitary function at puberty. The exact mechanism for the development of ovulatory failure has been attributed to androgen overproduction and its effect on the hypothalamic–pituitary–ovarian axis.

Stein and Leventhal, during the period 1902 to 1935, noted that a group of women had evidence for what is currently called polycystic ovaries at the time of laparotomy. Specifically, in 1935, Stein and Leventhal reported seven patients with the hallmarks of PCO.

The histologic findings in a polycystic ovary cover a broad spectrum, ranging from the originally described typical "Stein-Leventhal" type of polycystic ovary with a large number of follicular cysts and few atretic cysts in which there is marked stromal hyperplasia and hyperthecosis to a smaller ovary with a few follicular cysts and atretic follicles. The polycystic ovary may exhibit microscopic islands of luteinized thecal cells, that is, hyperthecosis, scattered in the stroma, but usually, there is a thickened, fibrosed tunica with a large number of cystic follicles beneath this thickened capsule.

Methods of management of ovulation induction include use of clomiphene citrate, controlled ovarian hyperstimulation with gonadotropins–follicle-stimulating hormone, and the option of assisted reproductive technology (ART). With select indications use of metformin, in off-label indication, as management of associated insulin resistance-hyperinsulinemia. Ovarian drilling remains one additional option for management of PCOS in select patients. There are several hypotheses regarding the mechanism by which ovarian drilling (wedge resection) of the polycystic ovary resolves ovulatory failure. The theory stating that the fibrous capsule acts as a mechanical barrier to the ovulatory follicle has been refuted. Evidence against this theory consists of the observation that if one ovary is removed, ovulation occurs from the remaining ovary. In addition, the use of clomiphene citrate of letrozole results in ovulation through an intact capsule. Some have stated that neonatal androgens may cause an abnormal hypothalamic–pituitary axis, resulting in abnormal gonadal patterns. This theory is not widely accepted. Neonatal androgen treatment in rats is associated with masculinization of the hypothalamus and with ovulatory failure with polycystic ovaries.

The most popular theory explaining how ovarian drilling results in the resumption of ovulatory cycles notes that the removal of androgen-secreting stroma and theca reduces the amount of abnormal steroid production in the ovary. After wedge resection, there is usually a decrease in the mean level of 17α-hydroxyprogesterone, dehydroepiandrosterone, androstenedione, and testosterone, as well as a transitory decrease in estradiol. This reduction in the steroidogenesis of androgens, allowing normalization of the luteinizing hormone (LH) to follicle-stimulating hormone (LH:FSH) ratio, results in the resumption of ovulatory cycles. Ovarian renin–angiotensin activity is enhanced with PCO. This system—renin–angiotensin—remains unaltered following ovarian electrocautery (i.e., ovarian drilling), even though serum levels of LH, testosterone, and androstenedione decline.

Sex hormone–binding globulin (SHBG) concentrations following electrocautery with PCO have been evaluated. Whereas there were significant decreases in serum androgens and gonadotropins, the concentration of SHBG increased in the serum. Gjonnaess has reported that there is no change with respect to dehydroepiandrosterone sulfate with ovarian drilling. This is indicative of neural alteration in the pituitary–adrenal axis in comparison to the pituitary–ovarian axis.

A consensus (2007) regarding PCOS focused on treatment. The results noted better pregnancy rates with use of clomiphene citrate or clomiphene citrate plus the insulin sensitizer metformin in comparison to metformin alone. They also felt that there is a role for ovarian drilling.

There is some debate as to the amount of ovarian mass that should be removed at the time of wedge resection. Halbe and coworkers attempted to clarify this question by removing different amounts of ovarian cortex and medulla from a random selection of patients with PCO disease. Thirty-eight of sixty-two patients were interested in conception. The 38 patients were divided into three groups, the first of which underwent removal of not more than one fifth of the original ovarian size. The second group had one third of the ovarian mass removed, and the third group had one half to three fourths of the original ovarian size reduced. The resumption of ovulatory cycles was recorded at 53%, 71%, and 91%, respectively. The authors concluded that the best ovulatory rate and the best pregnancy rate resulted after removal of at least half of the ovarian medulla.

The introduction of clomiphene citrate and the oral antihyperglycemic drug and insulin sensitizer metformin has changed the management of PCO syndrome in patients who desire pregnancy. Depending on the clinical circumstance, the conception rate with clomiphene citrate has been reported at 50% to 60%. The incidence of post–clomiphene citrate birth defects (3.1%) is not increased over commonly quoted rates for populations at large. Some patients may not want to accept the risks of multiple births or hyperstimulation with administration of pure FSH or FSH and LH ovulation induction.

Antidiabetic agents have been advocated to reduce insulin resistance with PCO. Metformin has been shown to decrease insulin levels with resultant diminishing of circulating androgens. Hirsutism often improves. Metformin may enhance the efficacy of clomiphene and gonadotropin therapy with PCO. Metformin may also promote weight loss. Baseline and periodic liver function tests are recommended. Metformin is contraindicated with renal or hepatic disease. Patients have shown a response at dosages of 500 mg three times per day.

Surgical Technique of Laparoscopic Treatment of Polycystic Ovaries

STEPS IN THE PROCEDURE

Polycystic Ovaries-Minimally Invasive Surgical Approach-Ovarian Drilling

- Lithotomy position, Foley catheter in the bladder, prepped, and draped
- Laparoscope and secondary ports placed
- Inspection of upper and lower abdomen
- With monopolar 20 to 30 W cutting current (or analogous setting for bipolar), vaporize all visible subcapsular follicles
- Place 2 to 4 mm depth punctures over capsule, caution must be addressed at stroma
- Place 5 to 10 punctures in each ovary

The laparoscopic approach incorporates the use of monopolar cautery with a needlepoint applicator or bipolar cautery to drill holes several millimeters apart through the ovarian cortex (Fig. 28.9). Care should be exercised to avoid the hilum because bleeding could result if it is penetrated. It is important to achieve hemostasis over the drilled areas.

The ovarian drilling technique includes a 5-mm second puncture placed suprapubically, through which suction irrigation or grasping of tissues can be performed. All visible subcapsular follicles are vaporized, and a 2- to 4-mm–diameter crater is made randomly in the ovarian stroma. Hemostasis is accomplished with bipolar forceps.

Ovarian coagulation can be accomplished with unipolar electrode. The power setting is 20 to 30 W in a cutting mode. The cortex is usually penetrated at 10 to 15 sites for a depth of 3 to 5 mm. No study has correlated the number of drilling sites and incidence of ovulation or pregnancy. Different studies have recommended 5, 10, or 15 perforations per ovary. In general, 5 to 10 punctures are made in each ovary at a 40-W power setting for each puncture over a 2- to 3-second time frame. Caution is exercised to minimize thermal damage. Smaller ovaries may require fewer cauterization sites.

As noted above, the PCOS Consensus Workshop Group provided support for ovarian drilling in patient's refractory to medical methods of ovulation induction. The procedure has also been termed multiperforation as well as laparoscopic ovarian diathermy. Monopolar and laser techniques have been described.

Overall, ovarian drilling is a second-line treatment for PCOS patients who desire fertility. Benefits of ovarian drilling include low probability of multiple births and avoidance of ovarian hyperstimulation syndrome as is more common with gonadotropin ovulation induction. Preoperatively, patients should be apprised of the potential consequences of ovarian drilling, which include adhesion formation and damage to

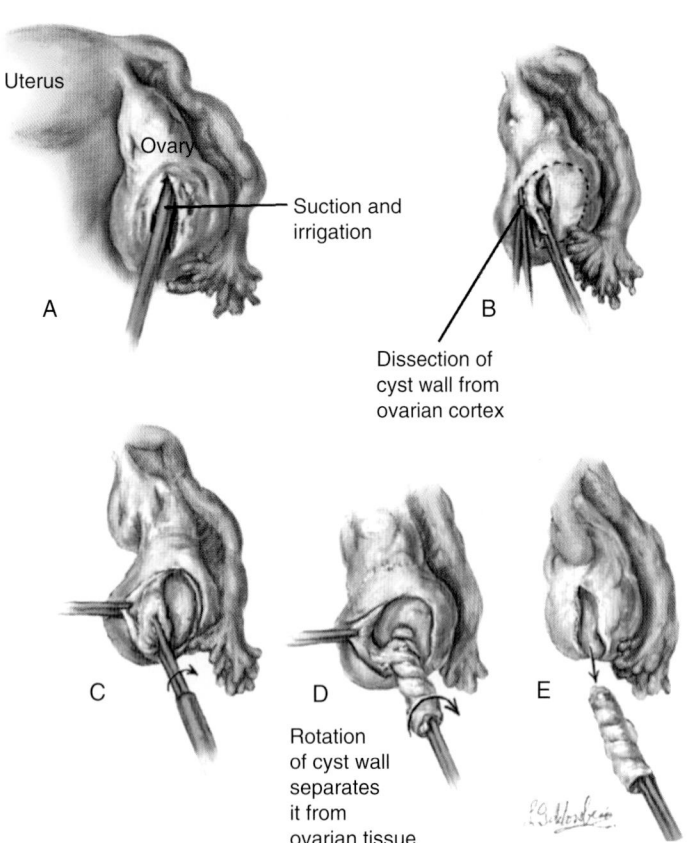

FIGURE 28.9 Removal of a small ovarian endometrial cyst through the laparoscope. **A:** After incision of the ovarian cortex, the contents of the endometrioma are removed with suction and irrigation. **B:** The plane between the ovary and the cyst wall is developed by using traction and twisting the forceps clockwise. **C:** The endometrial cyst wall is grasped with forceps. **D:** The cyst wall separates from the ovarian tissue by use of a twisting motion. The ovarian defect may be left open to heal by secondary intention or may be closed with vertical mattress sutures. **E:** The cyst wall is removed.

ovarian reserve. Incidence of ovulation with ovarian drilling is reported at 70% and pregnancy rates as high as 40% after three monitored cycles.

There are no randomized controlled studies addressing the efficacy of the laparoscopic approach to ovarian drilling. Twenty-seven studies were evaluated by Donesky and Adashi and involved a total of 729 patients. The ovulation rate was 84.2%, and the pregnancy rate was 55.7%. These authors emphasized that well-designed studies are needed in this area, which would encompass the PCO population proposed for laparoscopic drilling. This cohort of patients would require a well-documented clinical and biochemical finding of PCO, documented long-standing infertility (2 years or more), evidence for failure of clomiphene citrate, absence or correction of other infertility factors, randomization into a treatment group, and standardized documented follow-up, with particular attention to postovulatory patterns.

As noted above with regard to complications, the major concern is that of adhesion formation after either wedge resection or laparoscopic drilling. Toaff and associates noted extensive peritubular and periovarian adhesions in a small series (seven) of patients who did not conceive after bilateral wedge resection. One other concern is that of bilateral ovarian atrophy as a reflection of aggressive ovarian resection. This is a rare complication of the procedure. Thus, iatrogenic consequences of the surgical approaches must be discussed with the patient preoperatively (Fig. 28.10).

INCIDENTALOMA

Incidental adnexal masses (incidentaloma) are more common in postmenopausal women with a prevalence of 3% to 18% among asymptomatic women. More commonly, these present

as unilocular, benign-appearing ovarian cysts noted on ultrasonographic studies. Overall, 80% resolve spontaneously over several months. Persistent adnexal masses should be assessed which evaluation specific to the clinical circumstance, patient's age, sonographic findings, Doppler studies, etc. Masses greater than 10 cm should have a histopathologic diagnosis.

There does not appear to be consensus regarding methods of ovarian screening among major medical societies; ongoing studies continue to address this question from a cost-effective perspective. This includes use of CA-125 and pelvic sonography.

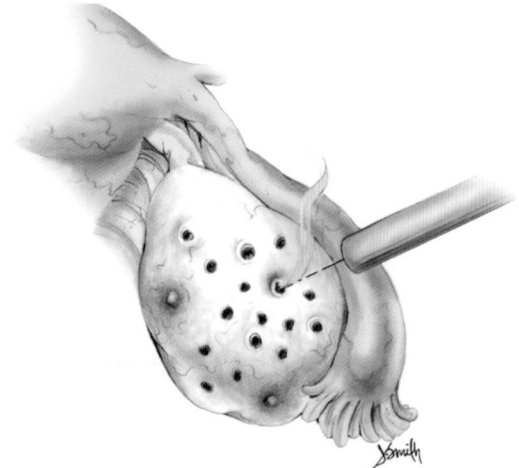

FIGURE 28.10 Laser drilling of ovary for surgical treatment of PCO disease.

PARADOXICAL OOPHORECTOMY

Paradoxical oophorectomy is the removal of severely pathologic adnexa to improve fertility in patients with strictly unilateral tubal disease. Consideration of removal of the contralateral ovary when there is single tubal patency (i.e., paradoxical oophorectomy) has perhaps taken on a new perspective with the advent of ART. From a historical point of view, it has been advocated that a patient with one functional tube would benefit from paradoxical oophorectomy, thus ensuring that ovulation would occur repeatedly on the appropriate side. Scott and coworkers reported a series of 24 patients with unilateral tubal patency diagnosed by retrograde injection at laparotomy. Contralateral oophorectomy or salpingo-oophorectomy was performed on all patients, and 16 women subsequently had 21 pregnancies, for a pregnancy rate of 67%. The authors suggested that the frequency with which transperitoneal migration occurs may be a factor. Hallet noted that one in five tubal ectopic pregnancies has a corpus luteum on the contralateral side; Jansen noted an intrauterine pregnancy rate of 18.7% ($n = 91$), contrasted with bilateral salpingostomy for hydrosalpinges in the presence of only one ovary wherein the pregnancy rate was 43.8% ($n = 16$). With unilateral salpingostomy or bilateral division of adhesions, pregnancy rates were comparable to those after bilateral salpingolysis. The mean surgery–pregnancy interval was longer after unilateral salpingostomy (104 weeks) than after bilateral salpingolysis (45 weeks). The author suggested that salpingo-oophorectomy may be preferable to salpingoneostomy for unilateral hydrosalpinx. With the provision of ART/in vitro fertilization (IVF), the management of tubal obstruction, especially in the absence of a hydrosalpinx, has led to a more conservative surgical approach.

Perhaps the major concern is for the patient who presents with tubal ectopic gestation in which the opposite (i.e., normal-appearing) adnexa appears to be unaffected. The paradoxical salpingo-oophorectomy approach has been advocated with this circumstance by Scott and coworkers. It has been advocated to wait at least 2 years after diagnostic laparoscopy reveals extensive unilateral disease before proceeding with paradoxical oophorectomy. From the other perspective, if the patient plans to proceed with IVF, the presence of two functional ovaries usually results in more oocytes recovered.

Randomized, carefully controlled clinical trials are necessary to further evaluate the efficacy of paradoxical oophorectomy. The risks and benefits must be carefully considered both preoperatively and intraoperatively, especially if the patient is a candidate for ART. There is clear evidence that increased numbers of ova can be recovered when both ovaries are in situ. Increased pregnancy success after superovulation is a reflection of the number of ovaries (one vs. two)—the total number of follicles available for stimulation.

Minimally Invasive Oophorectomy

The general principles of laparoscopic oophorectomy include placing the patient in the Trendelenburg position, with appropriate planning of ports for the proposed procedure and planning for removal of the affected adnexa. Pelvic washings and use of frozen section may be germane to the task at hand. After restoration of normal anatomy and adhesiolysis as indicated, the adnexa are gently placed on stretch. They are approached from either the infundibulopelvic ligament or the insertion of the round ligament. Regardless of the approach chosen, identification of the ureter is of paramount importance. The infundibulopelvic ligament is identified and coagulated. The broad ligament is incised, beginning at the round ligament, and

further dissection is performed into the retroperitoneal space. Every effort must be made to completely remove all ovarian tissue to prevent ovarian remnant syndrome.

With regard to tissue removal, once the adnexa have been completely freed, if benign disease is extremely likely, desiccation of the tissue and thus segmental removal are appropriate. However, if there is concern for the pathology, use of an endoscopic pouch is appropriate. In this circumstance, every effort is made to remove the ovary intact. Careful inspection of the operative site and a check for any bleeding are recommended. In addition, the end-point pressure of CO_2 insufflation should be reduced with suctioning of some of the CO_2 to check for any tamponade effect. As with all laparoscopic procedures, the patient should be monitored after surgery for any signs of intraperitoneal bleeding.

FERTILITY PRESERVATION WITH CANCER

As responses to both medical and surgical therapies continue to result in increasing numbers of cancer survivors, gynecologic surgeons must be kept abreast of current thinking in this field. Cryopreservation of ovarian tissue—nonfertilized, immature germ cells—is receiving increased attention including in prepubertal girls. Medical agents, including letrozole and tamoxifen, have been used prior to cryopreservation in women with breast cancer. Tamoxifen resulted in two to five times higher embryo yield than natural cycle IVF. The best prognosis for fertility appears to preserve gametes before initiation of chemotherapy for cancer. Ovarian transplantation with subsequent embryo generation has been reported after restoration of ovarian function by heterotopic transplantation. Ovarian transplantation remains an experimental technique at this point in time. Ovarian cortical tissue strip retrieval is amenable to a laparoscopic approach. Autologous, orthotopic transplantation after cryopreservation has been successfully used to restore fertility. Ovarian tissue banking and autografting of ovarian cortex are promising therapies for patients with ovarian failure. Kim and coauthors have verified the correlation between ischemic tissue damage and the duration of ischemia. The authors noted the ovarian cortex could tolerate ischemia for at least 3 hours. Thus, it appears that the future of ovarian transplantation depends on the postgrafting ischemia time by effective revascularization techniques.

Specific chemotherapeutic agents are proven to be toxic to the ovary. Resultant amenorrhea and infertility are the consequences. Patient age, drug dose, and dose and extent of disease are contributing factors (Table 28.8).

Fertility-sparing surgery includes oophoropexy–ovarian transposition (Table 28.9 and Fig. 28.11). This procedure temporarily relocates the ovaries as when pelvic radiation is planned. Cancers of the spine and colon and gynecologic cancers may require pelvic irradiation. The procedure of ovarian transposition (Fig. 28.11) can be done via a minimally invasive surgical approach. In general, such procedures reduce the ovarian exposure to radiation by 90% to 95%. On occasion, ovaries have been reported to migrate back to the pelvis.

Ovarian function remains intact in 60% to 89% of patients who undergo radiation therapy, while in the reproductive age, scattering of radiotherapy may account for the failures. Spontaneous pregnancies have been reported following oophoropexy. In addition, access for IVF has been successful in providing pregnancies following ovarian transposition. Complications include pelvic pain secondary to the ovarian relocation.

Tumors of LMP diagnosed in the reproductive age group can be managed, depending on the clinical circumstance, with unilateral salpingo-oophorectomy to preserve fertility (Table 28.9).

TABLE 28.8 Chemotherapy and Medical Diagnosis

AGENT	CANCERS IN THIS CATEGORY
High risk	
Cyclophosphamide	Leukemia lymphoma
Busulfan	
Intermediate risk	
Cisplatin	Breast cancer
Carboplatin	Ovarian endometrial
	Cervical
Low risk	
Doxorubicin	Hodgkin lymphoma
Bleomycin	Lymphoma
Vinblastine	Acute myelogenous leukemia
Dacarbazine	Breast cancer
Anthracycline	Multiple myeloma
Cytarabine	GI tract cancers
Methotrexate	
Dactinomycin	
Mercaptopurine	

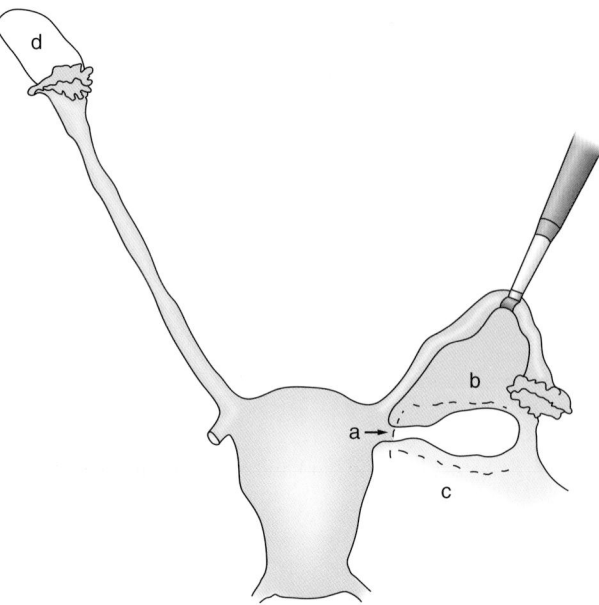

FIGURE 28.11 Laparoscopic ovarian transposition. Ovarian ligament (a) and mesovarium (b) are divided. If mobility is inadequate, relaxing incision on peritoneum inferior to ovary (c) may be needed. Final location of ovary is shown (d). (Reprinted from Bisharah M, Tulandi T. Laparoscopic preservation of ovarian function: an underused procedure. *Am J Obstet Gynecol* 2003;188:367. Copyright © 2003, with permission from Elsevier.)

Simultaneous administration of gonadotropin-releasing hormone agonists (GnRHa) with chemotherapy has been advocated in women in the reproductive age group but remains an area of controversy, the theory being to prevent or decrease the rate of ovarian damage. This may be more effective in the category of low-risk chemotherapeutic agents; however, there is a paucity of prospective studies assessing the efficacy of simultaneous GnRHa therapy with chemotherapy and ultimate effect on pregnancy rate. Detailed discussion of each option and specific indication is beyond the objective of this chapter. Suffice to say, it is important that patients be apprised of options prior to proceeding with chemo- and/or radiation therapy.

OVARIAN TRANSPOSITION BEFORE RADIOTHERAPY

Lemevel and coworkers reported laparoscopic transposition in a patient being treated for Hodgkin disease before receiving radiotherapy. The ovaries were laparoscopically suspended out of the field of radiation. Iatrogenic menopause did not occur in the four patients for which this was reported. Other authors have reported similar recommendations. Bisharah and Tulandi have recommended transection of the ovarian ligament and transposition of the ovaries without affecting the fallopian tubes. This is associated with positioning of the ovaries laterally and anteriorly at the level of the anterosuperior iliac spines.

Gonads are sensitive to irradiation. Whole-body, abdominal, or pelvic irradiation can cause ovarian damage and

adversely affect uterine function. It is estimated that the sensitivity of oocytes to radiation is an LD50 (the lethal dose required to eliminate 50% of the oocytes) of 2 Gy.

As noted in Table 28.8, cytotoxic drugs are classified as follows:

High risk: Cyclophosphamide, ifosfamide, chlormethine, busulfan, melphalan, procarbazine, and chlorambucil
Intermediate risk: Cisplatin and carboplatin
Low risk: Vincristine, methotrexate, dactinomycin, bleomycin, mercaptopurine, and vinblastine

Attempts have been made to assess ovarian function and "ovarian reserve." This has included evaluation of ovarian volume, serum inhibin B secreted by antral developing follicles, and antimüllerian hormone, a glycoprotein expressed in fetal tissue and preantral and small antral follicles, but in the adult, when levels are lowered (i.e., in cancer survivors), the ovarian reserve is decreased.

One alternative to oophoropexy is oocyte retrieval, fertilization, and cryopreservation—that is, ART/IVF. Preserving unfertilized oocytes remains an area of increasing success, as technology advances in cryopreservation continues to unfold.

Fertility outcome following ovarian transposition and pelvic irradiation for pelvic cancer has been addressed in a total of 37 consecutive cases by Morice and colleagues. Patients were treated for clear cell adenocarcinoma of the vagina or cervix, ovarian dysgerminoma, and sarcoma. The pregnancy rate was 15% (4/27) in patients attempting pregnancy with clear cell adenocarcinoma of the vagina or cervix. In the dysgerminoma and sarcoma group, 80% pregnancy occurred (8/10). Thus, the prognosis for future fertility following ovarian transposition and irradiation should be considered for discussion in selected patients before radiotherapy. The subject of fertility preservation in cancer survivors has been addressed by the Ethics Committee of the American Society for Reproductive Medicine, the main

TABLE 28.9 Options for Fertility Sparing

Fast-track ART/IVF
Embryo cryopreservation
Oocyte cryopreservation
In vitro maturation of oocytes
Donor oocyte
Donor embryo
Gestational carrier
Ovarian cortex cryopreservation and transplantation

focus of which is that physicians should inform cancer patients before treatment of their alternatives and include them in pretherapy discussion of alternatives before initiation of treatment.

PROPHYLACTIC OOPHOECTOMY IN ASSOCIATION WITH INCREASED CANCER RISK

Patients with a personal or family history that leads to assessment of genetic defects that include BRCA1 and BRCA2 mutation carrier status may benefit from prophylactic bilateral salpingo-oophorectomy (BSO), especially if childbearing is completed. No effective ovarian cancer screening exists. Tumor markers that include CA-125 and pelvic imaging done on a screening basis, as noted above, lack sensitivity and specificity. Overall, they are inefficient as a screening tool. Retrospective data support prophylactic BSO and lower occurrence of breast cancer in BRCA1 carriers (OR = 0.44, 95% CI: 0.28 to 1.15). Average interval between BSO and diagnosis of breast cancer was 7.2 years in those affected. The problem of primary peritoneal cancer remains a concern despite BSO. Thus, BSO does not completely eliminate the possibility of ovarian cancer. Primary peritoneal origin is associated with diffuse involvement of tumor on peritoneal surfaces and resembling papillary serous carcinoma of the ovary. This can occur with BRCA1 and BRCA2 mutations after BSO has occurred. Occult either ovarian or fallopian tube carcinoma has been noted at time of prophylactic BSO in 2% to 10% of patients with BRCA1 and BRCA2 mutations. Of note, use of hormone therapy following prophylactic BSO did not alter the reduction in breast cancer risk in BRCA1 and BRCA2 mutation carriers.

OVARIAN CYSTS IN NEONATE AND PREPUBERTAL CHILD

In a retrospective study of 65 fetal ovarian cysts noted by ultrasound, 57% were located on the left, 36% were on the right, and 7% were bilateral. In 17 patients, intervention was required after delivery because of persistence and/or enlargement. The histologic results included follicular cysts in 12 cases, a lymphangioma, and one teratoma; the remaining were amenable to aspiration. The authors, Mittermayer and colleagues, conclude that lack of regression requires intervention in the neonatal period. Ovarian cysts in the neonate greater than 5 cm in diameter have an increased chance of torsion.

Ovarian surgery in the premenarchal girl has been evaluated in a study from the University of Michigan in 52 patients, 50% of whom were less than 1 year old and 31% between 1 and 8 years of age. The most common presentation was abdominal/pelvic mass ($n = 24$), and the postoperative diagnoses included torsion in 18 and malignancy in 5 patients. Histopathologic evaluation included hemorrhagic infarction, dysgenetic gonads, simple cysts, teratoma, theca lutein cyst, fibroma, neuroblastoma, germ-cell tumor, gonadoblastoma, and metastatic Wilms tumor.

A general statement is that pathologic cysts in a newborn are equated with greater than 2 cm. There is no exact guideline for monitoring or management of neonatal ovarian cysts. Torsion of the intrauterine ovary can occur. Other problems to be considered included intracystic hemorrhage, rupture, and dystocia. A complex cyst is equated with increased chance of ovarian vascular dysgenesis or of a neoplasm. In general, neonatal ovarian cysts are predominately benign and self-limiting. There is a frequency of up to 5% of all abdominal masses in the 1st month of life. Overall, the earliest identification of

neonatal ovarian cyst formation is 19 weeks of gestation and more often noted at 32 to 26 weeks gestational age.

Aspiration of a neonatal ovarian cyst can be considered if the concern for interference with spontaneous delivery exists. Postnatal percutaneous aspiration of a large ovarian cyst may reduce the rate of torsion and other sequela. Separation of fetal–neonatal cysts into simple versus complex allows the clinician options for management, the former being of less concern. In general, cysts less than 5 cm may be observed especially if they have a simple cyst appearance. Laparoscopic approach and, when feasible, an ovarian cortex–preserving approach are advised, especially when it is thought to be a benign process. Expectant management over a 4- to 6-month period is acceptable especially if the cyst appears to be "simple." Malignancy of the neonatal ovary is rare. In childhood during the second decade, ovarian malignancy becomes of higher probability than in the neonate. In a series from Children's Hospital of Philadelphia reported by Brown and associates, one malignancy in 34 adnexal masses in children less than 8 years of age was noted (2.9%) in comparison to a 33% incidence in children greater than 8 years of age (18 of 58). Treatment options in large part depend on the clinical circumstance, whether the mass is simple, complex, symptomatic, etc. Surgical intervention should include the possibility of minimally invasive approach if feasible.

LAPAROSCOPIC OVARIAN SURGERY IN THE PEDIATRIC OR ADOLESCENT PATIENT

STEPS IN THE PROCEDURE

Laparoscopic Surgical Procedures in Pediatric and Adolescent Patient

- In pediatric patient, Crede bladder, prep, and drape abdomen
- Place Veress needle, and introduce 2- to 3-mm laparoscope and secondary ports
- CO_2 is introduced at 0.5 L/min with an end-point pressure of 6 to 8 mm Hg depending on age/size of patient
- In the adolescent, the pressure setting is 10 to 12 mm Hg; depending on age/size of patient, closed or open technique for abdominal insufflation and laparoscope placement is appropriate
- Port closure in the pediatric patient may require use of Steri-Strips
- In the adolescent, skin approximation at secondary ports can be accomplished with sutures

As noted above, a number of gynecologic problems from the neonatal period through adolescence can be addressed laparoscopically. Entities such as ovarian torsion, acute PID (diagnosis and treatment complementing antimicrobial therapy), torsion, and benign neoplasms must be considered in the latter age group. In addition, gonadectomy for problems such as male pseudohermaphroditism is amenable to a laparoscopic approach.

Follicular cysts appear to be of particular concern in both the pediatric and adolescent patient because they present with abdominal pain. An abdominal or pelvic mass can be identified on physical examination. The clinician must always keep in mind the importance of appropriate preoperative assessment (with the use of ultrasound and other clinical parameters) in deciding which patients are candidates for operative intervention. Depending on the clinical circumstance, a conservative approach in this age group is advocated; concern must be given (especially in the pediatric patient) to the potential for malignancy with ovarian masses, particularly if a solid component is identified.

The literature attests to operative intervention of ovarian cysts that appear to be nonfunctional. One of these was reported in a 1.5-month-old infant in whom ultrasound showed evidence of an ovarian mass. At laparotomy, the mass proved to be consistent with right ovarian torsion and necrosis, and it required adnexectomy. In one other reported case, a follicular-appearing cyst seen on ultrasound was associated with rapidly progressive virilization and a markedly elevated plasma testosterone level (289 ng/dL); histologic evaluation identified a granulosa cell tumor with mild luteinization.

The feasibility of aspirating an ovarian cyst continues to be controversial. In two case reports, laparoscopic puncture and aspiration of a malignant ovarian cyst were performed. Preoperative ultrasound indicated that the involved adnexal mass had a benign nature. Cytologically negative fluid was obtained from the aspirate. Eight weeks after operation, extensive disseminated ovarian carcinoma was noted at laparotomy.

Endoscopic surgery continues to broaden its horizon with expansion into laparoscopic surgical care beginning with the neonate. The use of 2-mm laparoscopes with the addition of 2- to 3-mm instrumentation has facilitated the diagnostic and therapeutic aspects of laparoscopy in this age group. Miniaturized video camera systems are necessary when one uses the 2-mm laparoscope telescope. When a decision is made to proceed with laparoscopy in a neonate or infant, general endotracheal anesthesia is used. Ideally, prophylactic antibiotics are administered preoperatively. The stomach is emptied with a suction catheter when the patient is asleep, and the bladder is emptied by use of the Crede maneuver. The abdominal wall is thinner and more elastic in the child than in the adolescent or adult. One must take this into consideration when introducing instrumentation, because it may be easier to insufflate in the subcutaneous space of the child than in the subcutaneous space of an adult. A Veress needle can be used with insufflation of carbon dioxide at 0.5 L/min. In infants, the end point of peritoneal-distending pressure should be set at 6 to 8 mm Hg; in the pediatric patient, 8 to 10 mm Hg; and in the older child or adolescent, 10 to 12 mm Hg.

After surgery, the trocar sites can be sutured in children, whereas in neonates and infants, the use of Steri-Strips (3 M, St. Paul, MN) or other wound closure bandages is usually adequate for reapproximation of the incised skin edges. Waldschmidt and Schier reported a series of 136 laparoscopic surgical procedures in neonates and infants. The most frequent indications were lysis of adhesions, abdominal cysts and neoplasms, gonadectomy, appendectomy, and cholecystectomy. A 1,400-g preterm infant was the only one in the series who suffered a complication (hernia at the incision site). Thus, adnexal pathology in this age group appears to be amenable to a laparoscopic approach.

Procedures such as transposition of an ovary before radiotherapy, bilateral gonadal excision in a male pseudohermaphrodite (i.e., Y-bearing chromosomal analysis), adnexal torsion, suspected salpingitis, and endometriosis all have been identified in this age group. The authors concluded that because the morbidity is low, a laparoscopic approach should be considered.

Although certain procedures in the child do not differ significantly from those in the adult, the early diagnosis of ovarian pathology (e.g., adnexal torsion) can result in a significant advantage in terms of managing the patient and preserving ovarian tissue.

BEST SURGICAL PRACTICES

- Minimally invasive surgery can be used to evaluate and manage ovarian masses ≥6 cm and adnexal masses ≥10 cm.
- Before operative intervention in a pregnant patient with a symptomatic adnexal mass, complete assessment of the fetus—including ultrasound to rule out any fetal anomalies—is recommended. The optimal time for elective intervention is during the second trimester. The patient should be informed regarding preterm labor and delivery. The surgical procedure ideally is performed in the left lateral decubitus position.
- Transvaginal color Doppler sonographic assessment of ovarian malignant masses includes vessels detected, location of tumor vessels (central vs. peripheral), determination of peak systolic velocity, low resistance index, mean resistance index, and lower pulsatility index.
- The major goal of the evaluation of a pelvic mass is to rule out malignancy. All ovarian neoplasms greater than 6 cm with a solid component should undergo a thorough evaluation to rule out cancer.
- In management of ovarian remnant syndrome, treatment of choice is adequate excision of the remnant ovarian tissue and contiguous adherent tissues: pelvic peritoneum, bowel serosa, and underlying involved alveolar and/or vascular tissues. Retroperitoneal dissection may be required.
- Prior to cancer therapy, whether it be chemo- or radiation therapy, patients should be counseled regarding option for fertility preservation.

BIBLIOGRAPHY

Abbott D, Dumesic D, Franks S. Developmental origin of polycystic ovary syndrome—a hypothesis. *J Endocrinol* 2002;174:1.

Adashi EY, Rock JA, Guzick D, et al. Fertility following bilateral ovarian wedge resection: a critical analysis of 90 consecutive cases of the polycystic ovary syndrome. *Fertil Steril* 1981;35:320.

Adhesion Barrier Study Group. Interceed (TC-7). Prevention of post surgical adhesions by Interceed (TC-7). *Fertil Steril* 1989;51:933.

Akin M, Akin L, Ozbek S, et al. Fetal-neonatal ovarian cysts-their monitoring and management: retrospective evaluation of 20 cases and review of the literature. *J Clin Res Pediatr Endocrinol* 2010;2:28.

Alborzi S, Momtahan M, Parsanezhad ME, et al. A prospective, randomized study comparing laparoscopic ovarian cystectomy versus fenestration and coagulation in patients with endometriomas. *Fertil Steril* 2004;82:1633.

Alcazar J, Ruiz-Perez M, Errasti T. Transvaginal color-Doppler sonography in adnexal masses: which parameter performs best?. *Ultrasound Obstet Gynecol* 1996;8:114.

American Society for Reproductive Medicine. Fertility preservation and reproduction in cancer patients. *Fertil Steril* 2005;83:1622.

Andolf E, Jorgensen C, Astedt B. Ultrasound examination for detection of ovarian carcinoma in high risk groups. *Obstet Gynecol* 1990;75:106.

Anttila L, Tenttila T, Matinlauri I, et al. Serum total renin levels after ovarian electrocautery in women with polycystic ovary syndrome. *Gynecol Endocrinol* 1998;12:327.

Babaknia A, Calfopoulos P, Jones HW Jr. The Stein-Leventhal syndrome and coincidental ovarian tumors. *Obstet Gynecol* 1976;47:223.

Bayer AI, Wiskind AK. Adnexal torsion: can the adnexa be saved? *Am J Obstet Gynecol* 1994;171:1506.

Benacerraf BR, Finkler NJ, Wojciechowski C, et al. Sonographic accuracy in the diagnosis of ovarian masses. *J Reprod Med* 1990;35:491.

Bernhard LM, Klebba PK, Gray DL, et al. Predictors of persistence of adnexal masses in pregnancy. *Obstet Gynecol* 1999;93:585.

Bisharah M, Tulandi T. Laparoscopic preservation of ovarian function: an underused procedure. *Am J Obstet Gynecol* 2003; 188:367.

Bromley B, Benacerraf B. Adnexal masses during pregnancy; accuracy of sonographic diagnosis and outcome. *J Ultrasound Med* 1997;16:337.

Brown M, Hebra A, McGeehin K, et al. Ovarian masses in children: a review of 91 cases of malignant and benign masses. *J Pediatr Surg* 1993;28:930.

Carmina E, Lobo R. Does metformin induce ovulation in normoandrogenic anovulatory women? *Am J Obstet Gynecol* 2004;191:1580.

Carey M, Slack M. GnRH analogue in assessing chronic pelvic pain in women with residual ovaries. *Br J Obstet Gynaecol* 1996;103:150.

Caruso A, Caforio L, Testa A, et al. Transvaginal color Doppler ultrasonography in the presurgical characterization of adnexal masses. *Gynecol Oncol* 1996;63:184.

Casper RF, Greenblatt EM. Laparoscopic ovarian cautery for induction of ovulation in women with polycystic ovary disease. *Semin Reprod Endocrinol* 1990;8:209.

Chan L, Lin W, Uerpairojkit B, et al. Evaluation of adnexal masses using three-dimensional ultrasonographic technology: preliminary report. *J Ultrasound Med* 1997;16:349.

Damewood M, Hesla H, Lowen M, et al. Induction of ovulation and pregnancy following lateral oophoropexy for Hodgkin's disease. *Int J Gynecol Obstet* 1990;33:369.

Davidoff AM, Hebra A, Kerr J, et al. Laparoscopic oophorectomy in children. *J Laparoendosc Surg* 1996;6:SIIS.

Dexel A, Efrat Z, Orvito R, et al. The residual ovary syndrome: a 20 year experience. *Eur J Obstet Gynecol Reprod Biol* 1996;68:159.

Diamond MP, Daniell JF, Feste J, et al. Adhesion reformation and de novo adhesion formation after reproductive pelvic surgery. *Fertil Steril* 1987;47:864.

Dolgin S. Ovarian masses in the newborn. *Semin Pediatr Surg* 2000; 9:121.

Domchek S, Rebbeck T. Prophylactic oophorectomy in women at increased cancer risk. *Curr Opin Obstet Gynecol* 2007;19:27.

Donesky BW, Adashi EY. Surgically induced ovulation in the polycystic ovary syndrome: wedge resection revisited in the age of laparoscopy. *Fertil Steril* 1995;63:439.

Ehrman DA. Medical progress: polycystic ovary syndrome. *N Engl J Med* 2005;352:1223.

Einhorn N, Bast RC Jr, Knapp RC, et al. Preoperative evaluation of serum CA 125 levels in patients with primary epithelial ovarian carcinoma. *Obstet Gynecol* 1986;67:414.

Eisen A, Lubinski J, Klijn J, et al. Breast cancer risk following bilateral oophorectomy I BRCA 1 and BRCA 2 mutation carriers: an international case-control study. *J Clin Oncol* 2005;23:7491.

Farquhar C, Vandekerckhove P, Lilford R. Laparoscopic drilling by diathermy or laser for ovulation induction in anovulatory polycystic ovary syndrome. *Cochrane Database Syst Rev* 2001;4:1.

Fauser BC, Diedrich K, Bouchard P, et al. Contemporary genetic technologies and female reproduction. The Evian Annual Reproduction (EVAR) Workshop Group 2010. *Hum Reprod Update* 2011;17:829.

Finkler NJ, Benacerraf B, Lavin PT, et al. Comparison of serum CA-125, clinical impression, and ultrasound in the postoperative evaluation of ovarian masses. *Obstet Gynecol* 1988;72:659.

Flyckt R, Goldberg J. Laparoscopic ovarian drilling for clomiphene-resistant polycystic ovary syndrome. *Semin Reprod Med* 2011;29:138.

Funt M. The residual adnexa: asset or liability? *Am J Obstet Gynecol* 1977;129:251.

Gailey A, Ginsburg E. Fertility preservation options for females. *Adv Exp Med Biol* 2012;732:9.

Gillman J. The development of the gonads in man with a consideration of the role of fetal endocrine and the histogenesis of ovarian tumors. *Carnegie Contrib Embryol* 1948;32:81.

Gjonnaess II. Late endocrine effects of electrocautery in women with polycystic ovary syndrome. *Fertil Steril* 1998;69:697.

Granberg S, Wickland M. A comparison between ultrasound and gynecologic examination for detection of enlarged ovaries in a group of women at risk for ovarian carcinoma. *J Ultrasound Med* 1988;7:59.

Granberg S, Wikland M, Jansson I. Macroscopic characterization of ovarian tumors and the relation to the histologic diagnosis: criteria to be used for ultrasound evaluation. *Gynecol Oncol* 1989;35:139.

Grogan RH. Reappraisal of the residual ovary. *Am J Obstet Gynecol* 1967;97:124.

Gurgan T, Yarali H, Urman B. Laparoscopic treatment of polycystic ovarian disease. *Hum Reprod* 1994;9:573.

Halbe HW, da Fonseca AM, Silva P deP, et al. Stein-Leventhal syndrome. *Am J Obstet Gynecol* 1972;114:280.

Hall DJ, Hurt WG. The adnexal mass. *J Fam Pract* 1982;14:135.

Hallet JC. Repeat ectopic pregnancy: a study of 123 consecutive cases. *Am J Obstet Gynecol* 1975;122:520.

Haney AF, Doty E. Murine peritoneal injury and de novo adhesion formation caused by oxidized-regenerated cellulose (Interceed [TC7]) but not expanded to polytetrafluoroethylene (Gore-Tex surgical membrane). *Fertil Steril* 1992;57:202.

Haney AF, Hesla J, Hurst BS, et al. Expanded polytetrafluoroethylene (Gore-Tex surgical membrane) is superior to oxidized regenerated cellulose (Interceed TC7) in preventing adhesions. *Fertil Steril* 1995;63:1021.

Havrilesky LJ, Peterson BL, Dryden DK, et al. Predictors of clinical outcomes in the laparoscopic management of adnexal masses. *Obstet Gynecol* 2003;102:243.

Heinrich U, Eberlein-Gonska M, Benz G, et al. Late-onset 30-hydroxysteroid dehydrogenase deficiency with virilization induced by a large ovarian cyst. *Horm Res* 1993;40:227.

Heloury Y, Guiberteau V, Sagot P, et al. Laparoscopy in adnexal pathology in the child: a study of 28 cases. *Eur J Pediatr Surg* 1993;3:75.

Hernandez E, Miyazawa K. The pelvic mass: patients' ages and pathologic findings. *J Reprod Med* 1988;33:361.

Herrmann UJ Jr, Locher GW, Goldhirsch A. Sonographic patterns of ovarian tumors: prediction of malignancy. *Obstet Gynecol* 1987;69:777.

Hoover K, Jenkins T. Evaluation and management of adnexal mass in pregnancy. *Am J Obstet Gynecol* 2011;205:97.

Horowitz N. Management of adnexal masses in pregnancy. *Clin Obstet Gynecol* 2011;54:519.

Huser M, Zakova J, Smardova L, et al. Combination of fertility preservation strategies in young women with recently diagnosed cancer. *Eur J Gynaecol Oncol* 2012;33:42.

Jansen RP. Surgery pregnancy time intervals after salpingolysis, unilateral salpingostomy and bilateral salpingostomy. *Fertil Steril* 1980;34:222.

Jawad A, Al-Meshari A. Laparoscopy for ovarian pathology in infancy and childhood. *Pediatr Surg Int* 1998;14:62.

Jeffcoate TA. *Principles of gynecology*. London, UK: Butterworths, 1975.

Jeremias E, Bedaiwy MA, Nelson D, et al. Assessment of tissue injury in cryopreserved ovarian tissue. *Fertil Steril* 2003;79:651.

Kamprath S, Possover M, Schneider A. Description of a laparoscopic technique for treating patients with ovarian remnant syndrome. *Fertil Steril* 1997;68:663.

Kim SS, Yang HW, Kang HG, et al. Quantitative assessment of ischemic tissue damage in ovarian cortical tissue with or without antioxidant (ascorbic acid) treatment. *Fertil Steril* 2004;82:679.

Kiran G, Kiran H, Coban YK, et al. Fresh autologous transplantation of ovarian cortical strips to the anterior abdominal wall at the Pfannenstiel incision site. *Fertil Steril* 2004;82:954.

Kistner RW, Patton GW. Surgery of the ovary. In: *Atlas of infertility surgery*. Boston, MA: Little, Brown, 1975:105.

Kleppinger RK. Ovarian cyst fenestration via laparoscopy. *J Reprod Med* 1978;21:16.

Kobayashi M. Use of diagnostic ultrasound in trophoblastic neoplasms and ovarian tumors. *Cancer* 1976;38:441.

Kojima E. Ovarian wedge resection with contract Nd:YAG laser irradiation used laparoscopically. *J Reprod Med* 1989;34:444.

Kurjak A, Predanic M, Kupesic-Urek S, et al. Transvaginal color and pulsed Doppler assessment of adnexal tumor vascularity. *Gynecol Oncol* 1993;50:3.

Larsen JF, Pedersen OD, Gregersen E. Ovarian cyst fenestration via the laparoscope. *Acta Obstet Gynecol Scand* 1986;65:539.

Laxman D, Burgman A, Sagi J, et al. The postmenopausal adnexal mass: correlation between ultrasonic and pathologic findings. *Obstet Gynecol* 1991;77:726.

Lemevel A, Bourdin S, Harousseau J, et al. Ovarian transposition by laparoscopy before radiotherapy in the treatment of Hodgkin's disease. *Cancer* 1998;83:1420.

Litos M, Furara S, Chin K. Supernumerary ovary: a case report and literature review. *J Obstet Gynaecol* 2003;23:325.

V

Mage G, Canis M, Mandes II, et al. Laparoscopic management of adnexal torsion: a review of 35 cases. *J Reprod Med* 1989;34:520.

Magtibay PM, Nyholm JL, Hemandez JL, et al. Ovarian remnant syndrome. *Am J Obstet Gynecol* 2005;193:2062.

Maiman M, Seltzer V, Boyce J. Laparoscopic excision of ovarian neoplasms subsequently found to be malignant. *Obstet Gynecol* 1991;77:563.

Malkasian G Jr, Knapp R, Lavin PT, et al. Preoperative evaluation of serum CA125 levels in premenopausal and postmenopausal patients with pelvic masses: discrimination of benign from malignant disease. *Am J Obstet Gynecol* 1988;159:341.

Meire HB, Farrant P, Guha T. Distinction of benign from malignant ovarian masses by ultrasound. *Br J Obstet Gynaecol* 1978;85:893.

Merritt DR. Torsion of the uterine adnexa: a review. *Adolesc Pediatr Gynecol* 1991;4:3.

Minke T, Depond W, Winkelmann T, et al. Ovarian remnant syndrome: study in laboratory rats. *Am J Obstet Gynecol* 1994;171:1440.

Mittermayer C, Blaicher W, Grassauer D, et al. Fetal ovarian cysts: developmental and neonatal outcome. *Ultraschall Med* 2003; 24:21.

Morice P, Thiam-Ba R, Castaige D, et al. Fertility results after ovarian transposition for pelvic malignancies treated by external irradiation or brachytherapy. *Hum Reprod* 1998;13:660.

Nezhat C, Saberi NS, Shahmohamady B, et al. Robotic-assisted laparoscopy in gynecological surgery. *JSLS* 2006;10:317.

Nooyes N, Knopman J, Long K, et al Fertility considerations in the management of gynecologic malignancies. *Gynecol Oncol* 2011;120:326.

Oehler M, Wain G, Brand A. Gynaecological malignancies in pregnancy: a review. *Aust N Z Obstet Gynaecol* 2003;43:414.

Oktay K. Fertility preservation: an emerging discipline in the care of young patients with cancer. *Lancet Oncol* 2005;6:192.

Oktay K, Alp Aydin B, Karlikaya G. A technique for laparoscopic transplantation of frozen-banked ovarian tissue. *Fertil Steril* 2001;75:1212.

Oktay K, Buyuk E, Rosenwaks Z, et al. A technique for transplantation of ovarian cortical strips to the forearm. *Fertil Steril* 2003;80:193.

Operative Laparoscopy Study Group. Postoperative adhesion development after operative laparoscopy: evaluation at early second-look procedures. *Fertil Steril* 1992;55:700.

Pabuccu R, Onalan G, Goktolga U, et al. Aspiration of ovarian endometriomas before intracytoplasmic sperm injection. *Fertil Steril* 2004;82:705.

Pagidas K, Tulandi T. Effects of Ringer's lactate, Interceed (TC7) and Gore-Tex surgical membrane on post-surgical adhesion formation. *Fertil Steril* 1992;57:199.

PCOS Consensus Workshop Group that included representation from the American Society for Reproductive Medicine and the European Society of Human Reproduction and Embryology. ESHRE/ASRM 2008 Consensus on infertility treatment related to polycystic ovary syndrome (PCOS). *Hum Reprod* 2008;23:462.

Pussell SJ, Cosgrove DO, Hinton J, et al. Carcinoma of the ovary—correlation of ultrasound with second look laparotomy. *Br J Obstet Gynaecol* 1980;87:1140.

Quint EH, Smith YR. Ovarian surgery in premenarchal girls. *J Pediatr Adolesc Gynecol* 1999;12:27.

Ragni G, Somigliana E, Benedetti F, et al. Damage to ovarian reserve associated with laparoscopic excision of endometriomas: a quantitative rather than a qualitative injury. *Am J Obstet Gynecol* 2005;193:1908.

Rane A, Ohizua O. "Acute" residual ovary syndrome. *Aust N Z J Obstet Gynaecol* 1998;38:447.

Rotterdam ESHRE/ASRM PCOS Consensus Workshop Group. Revised 2003 consensus on diagnostic criteria and long-term health risks related to polycystic ovary syndrome. *Fertil Steril* 2004;81:19.

Sassone AM, Timor-Tritsch IE, Artner A, et al. Transvaginal sonographic characterization of ovarian disease: evaluation of a new scoring system to predict ovarian malignancy. *Obstet Gynecol* 1991;78:70.

Schmeler K, Mayo-Smith W, Peipert J, et al. Adnexal masses in pregnancy: surgery compared with observation. *Obstet Gynecol* 2005;105:1098.

Schwobel MG, Stauffer UG. Surgery of the female gonads. *Z Kinderchir* 1988;43:289.

Scott JS, Lynch EM, Anderson JA. Surgical treatment of female infertility; value of paradoxical oophorectomy. *Br Med J* 1976;1:631.

Scott RT, Beatse SN, Illions EH, et al. Use of the GnRH agonist stimulation test in the diagnosis of ovarian remnant syndrome: a report of three cases. *J Reprod Med* 1995;40:143.

Seltzer V, Maiman M, Boyce J. Laparoscopic surgery in the management of ovarian cysts. *Female Patient* 1992;17:19.

Shalev E, Mann S, Romano S, et al. Laparoscopic detorsion of adnexa in childhood: a case report. *J Pediatr Surg* 1991;26:1145.

Shalev E, Peleg D. Laparoscopic treatment of adnexal torsion. *Surg Obstet Gynecol* 1993;176:448.

Sherard G, Hodson C, Williams HJ, et al. Adnexal masses and pregnancy: a 12 year experience *Am J Obstet Gynecol* 2003;189:358.

Solnik MJ, Alexander C. Ovarian incidentaloma. *Best Pract Res Clin Endocrinol Metab* 2012;26:105.

Soper JT, Hunter VJ, Daly L, et al. Preoperative serum tumor-associated antigen levels in women with pelvic masses. *Obstet Gynecol* 1990;75:249.

Soriano D, Wefet Y, Seidman D, et al. Laparoscopy versus laparotomy in the management of adnexal masses during pregnancy. *Fertil Steril* 1999;71:955.

Stein I, Leventhal ML. Amenorrhea associated with bilateral polycystic ovaries. *Am J Obstet Gynecol* 1935;29:181.

Steinkampf MP, Hammond KR, Blackwell RE. Hormonal treatment of functional ovarian cysts: a randomized prospective study. *Fertil Steril* 1990;54:775.

Symmonds RE, Petit P. Ovarian remnant syndrome. *Obstet Gynecol* 1979;54:175.

Tawa K. Ovarian tumors in pregnancy. *Am J Obstet Gynecol* 1964;90:5111.

Taylor A, Jurkovic D, Bourne T, et al. Sonographic prediction of malignancy in adnexal masses using an artificial neural network. *Br J Obstet Gynaecol* 1999;106:21.

Terz J, Barber H, Bronschwig A. Incidence of carcinoma in the retained ovary. *Am J Surg* 1967;113:511.

Timmerman D, Bourne T, Tailor A, et al. A comparison of methods for pre-operative discrimination between malignant and benign adnexal masses: the development of a new logistic regression model. *Am J Obstet Gynecol* 1999;181:57.

Toaff R, Toaff ME, Peyser MR. Infertility following wedge resection of the ovaries. *Am J Obstet Gynecol* 1976;124:92.

Trimbos-Kemper TC, Trimbos JB, van Hall EV. Management of infertile patients with unilateral tubal pathology by paradoxical oophorectomy. *Fertil Steril* 1982;37:623.

Tulandi T, Al-Took S. Laparoscopic ovarian suspension before radiation therapy. *Fertil Steril* 1998;70:381.

Van der Watt J. The mutilated ovary syndrome. *S Afr Med J* 1970;44:687.

Waldschmidt J, Schier F. Laparoscopic surgery in neonates and infants. *Eur J Pediatr Surg* 1991;1:145.

Wallace WH, Anderson R, Irvine DS. Fertility preservation for young patients with cancer: who is at risk and what can be offered? *Lancet Oncol* 2005;6:209.

Weiner Z, Thaler I, Beck D, et al. Differentiating malignant from benign ovarian tumors with transvaginal color flow imaging. *Obstet Gynecol* 1992;79:159.

Wenzl R, Lehner R, Husslein P, et al. Laparoscopic surgery in cases of ovarian malignancy: an Austria-wide survey. *Gynecol Oncol* 1996;63:57.

White M, Stella J. Ovarian torsion: 10 year perspective. *Emerg Med Australas* 2005;17:231.

Williams RS, Mendenhall N. Laparoscopic oophoropexy for preservation of ovarian function before pelvic node irradiation. *Obstet Gynecol* 1992;80:541.

Witschi E. Embryology of the ovary. In: *The ovary.* Baltimore, MD: Williams & Wilkins, 1963:1.

Witschi E. Migration of the germ cells of human embryos from the yolk sac to the primitive gonadal folds. *Contrib Embryol* 1948;32:69.

Yacobozzi M, Nguyen D, Rakita D. Adnexal masses in pregnancy. *Semin Ultrasound CT MRI* 2012;33:55.

CHAPTER 29
Persistent or Chronic Pelvic Pain

Matthew T. Siedhoff

DEFINITIONS

Allodynia—Pain resulting from a nonnoxious stimulus.
Hyperalgesia—Painful sensation of abnormal severity following noxious stimulation.
Neuropathic pain—Pain persisting after healing of disease or trauma-induced tissue damage.
Neuroplasticity—The malleability of central pain perception mechanisms in response to chronic pain states.
Nociceptor—A nerve receptor for pain.

There is not universal agreement on a single definition of chronic pelvic pain (CPP), but most practitioners accept the proposal of the American Congress of Obstetricians and Gynecologists: noncyclic pain of 6 or more months' duration that localizes to the anatomic pelvis, anterior abdominal wall at or below the umbilicus, or the lumbosacral back or the buttocks and is of sufficient severity to cause functional disability or lead to medical care. We are in need of deeper and updated investigation into the epidemiology of pelvic pain, but likely, at least 15% of women are affected by pelvic pain, most commonly during reproductive-age years. When last tabulated in 1996, it was estimated nearly $3 billion was spent annually in physician costs and out-of-pocket expenses. CPP accounts for at least 10% of outpatient visits to a gynecologist and is the indication for 40% of gynecologic laparoscopies.

Endometriosis and adhesions are some of the most common conditions assigned as an etiology of pelvic pain, but the connection between these problems and pain symptoms is actually more tenuous than has been traditionally taught. More and more data confirming the coexistence of multiple chronic pain disorders in patients—conditions such as interstitial cystitis (IC), painful bladder syndrome, irritable bowel syndrome (IBS), temporomandibular joint disorder, migraine headaches, vulvodynia, and fibromyalgia—suggest that perhaps we ought to be treating pelvic pain under an updated paradigm where the disease is pain itself rather than a manifestation of a specific etiology. In this chapter, we will apply the concept of central sensitization to CPP and point out common peripheral pain generators—nociceptive stimuli—than can be modulated by gynecologic interventions. We will review important elements in evaluation and describe the criteria for a chronic pain syndrome (CPS), offering a theoretical model to explain the evolution of chronic pain over.

HISTORY

Over the past 60 years, the study of CPP has gone through significant changes in approach. Investigations undertaken before the development of laparoscopy focused on correlations between pelvic pain and psychological distress. In the absence of palpable pathology, the gynecologist of the 1950s and 1960s was understandably reluctant to subject a patient to laparotomy to investigate pain. During this era, the prevailing cartesian theory of pain perception suggested that pain should be somewhat proportional to the degree of tissue damage found. Hence,

if the pathology was not big enough to palpate, it was seldom operated on. Although this model was sufficient to address most causes of acute pain, it fails to elucidate the majority of chronic pain disorders, in gynecology as well as other areas of medicine. The gate control theory, promulgated by Melzack and Wall in 1965, allowed integration of physical and psychological parameters and explained how chronic pain can be quite different from acute pain. The model also suggests that information flows in two directions regarding pain: (a) nociceptive signals from peripheral tissue ascend through the spinal cord to higher centers, and (b) central centers can modulate, via descending signals altering spinal cord neurotransmitter and interneuron activity, the transmission of these nociceptive signals from the periphery. Deterioration of these regulatory processes was thought to potentially account for development of chronic pain states by allowing too many peripheral signals to pass through the spinal cord "gates." Variation in patients' relative degree of gate opening could thus explain why similar amounts of physical tissue damage result in different degrees of pain perception. The concept is similar to the way we view differences in depth of sleep—for some, the brain can easily filter out stimuli; for others, it takes very little exposure (e.g., light, sound) to overcome unconsciousness and bring about wakefulness.

While these theory changes were stimulating the field of pain research, gynecologists were busy developing laparoscopy. Previously cherished myths soon fell by the wayside: for example, the incorrect assumption that endometriosis is seldom found in adolescents or women of African descent. With these observations came the hope that laparoscopic and medical treatment of encountered pathology would fix CPP. Reports of CPP from that era focused on "laparoscopy-negative" patients; indeed, some pelvic pain clinics required a negative laparoscopy as an entry criterion, implying that if some pathology were found, it must be a "real" cause for pain. Subsequent experience has shown that even though treatment

TABLE 29.1 Contributors to Pelvic Pain in Laparoscopy-Negative Patients

Gastrointestinal
Constipation
Irritable bowel syndrome
Inflammatory bowel disease
Diverticulitis
Urinary
Urethral syndrome
Interstitial cystitis/painful bladder syndrome
Musculoskeletal or neurologic
Pelvic floor tension myalgia
Piriformis syndrome
Nerve entrapment
Ventral hernia
Rectus tendon strain
Myofascial pain
Back or pelvic postural changes
Gynecologic
Pelvic vascular congestion
Cervical stenosis

Reprinted from Steege JF, Stout AL, Somkuti SG. Chronic pelvic pain: toward an integrative model. *Obstet Gynecol Surv* 1993;48:95, with permission. Copyright © 1993 Wolters Kluwer Health.

of laparoscopically diagnosed pathology is often helpful, the clinical reality is more complex:

1. In many instances, the organic pathology found at laparoscopy may be incidental and not related to the pain.
2. In those with pathology that does contribute to nociception, the pain experienced by the patient may differ from another patient with anatomically similar pathology.
3. Pain from a laparoscopic finding may be the sum of that contribution plus signals from some or all of the disorders listed in Table 29.1.

Consider the research of the 1980s that documented a distressingly high prevalence of physical and sexual abuse. Epidemiologic surveys of community samples revealed that as many as 25% to 30% of adult women reported having experienced sexual abuse during childhood. Studies of women attending pelvic pain clinics, especially those based in psychiatric settings, showed that up to 60% of these women had been abused. These observations led to the speculation that the experience of abuse may make a person more vulnerable to the development of CPP or perhaps be a specific cause for pain. Studies using positron emission tomography and functional magnetic resonance imaging suggest that the experience of abuse may indeed leave its neurophysiologic footprints: stressful stimuli produce different central response patterns in abused versus nonabused subjects. In relation to pain, abuse, particularly that which occurs in formative years, may serve to alter response to nociception and central pain processing. That said, not all abused patients go on to have chronic pain nor do all patients with pain have a history of abuse, so it might be the response to trauma that plays a key role in development of chronic pain. Health care providers need to take into account the presence of abuse in a patient's history when detected, but be careful to avoid necessarily concluding a causal relationship in that patient's pain.

Melzack neuromatrix theory is an expansion of his original work that includes the notion of neuroplasticity, among other elements. The concept of neuroplasticity suggests that experience can change the neurophysiologic behavior of the central nervous system in a manner that influences the subsequent processing of nociceptive stimuli. It may explain the apparent development of pain responses to stimuli usually thought of as nonpainful (allodynia), as well as exaggerated responses to painful stimuli (hyperalgesia). Every practicing gynecologist has seen patients whose pain responses seem out of proportion to the pathology found. This may reflect the emotional meaning of the problem for the patient, as well as past or present trauma, but it may also be the result of nociceptive mechanisms not yet fully understood (e.g., the exact mechanism of pain from endometriosis) or the result of sensitization of spinal cord interneurons that have become pain amplifiers as a result of being on the receiving end of peripheral nociceptive stimuli for prolonged periods. When nociception has been emanating from one organ system for a period of time, adjacent organs may join the chorus. This concept may help explain the common finding of coexistent somatosensory disorders in the same patient, an observation that has led some investigators to pursue potential genetic variations in central neurotransmitter networks that might predispose to the development of multiple such disorders. The above is the negative side of neuroplasticity. The positive side of the neuroplasticity concept is that, perhaps, given enough time and the right treatment, even seemingly intractable chronic pain problems may ameliorate to the point of allowing substantially improved function.

The concept of central sensitization adds another layer to theoretical understanding of chronic pain. This idea emphasizes the ramping up of pain signaling with repeated stimuli over time. The centralized pain hypersensitivity helps us understand how multiple organ systems can be recruited into the syndrome, incorporating genetic and social factors in pain amplification.

CONTRIBUTIONS OF PERIPHERAL PAIN GENERATORS

This section deserves an important caveat. Though we believe that types of tissue damage or other nociceptive input can generate pain, they cannot be viewed in isolation of the patient's individual central pain processing. Management strategies will be discussed in more detail, but, in general, the goal of the treating provider involves trying to dampen overall pain signaling sensitivity—"turning down the master volume"—and looking for areas in the periphery that can be "tuned up" toward better functioning. The following peripheral generators represent areas where we can intervene but should not be described to patients with CPP as *the* cause of their pain. These conditions can be completely asymptomatic in many patients, and thus the host where the disease manifests is much more important than the disease itself.

Endometriosis

A review summarized laparoscopic findings from 2,615 patients in 15 studies (nine retrospective, six prospective). Endometriosis was found in 2% to 51% of patients, suggesting that referral biases lead to very skewed samples. Clearly, not every woman with pain has endometriosis, nor does every woman with endometriosis have pain, although women with the disease had pain more often than those without it. A number of previous studies of CPP described only either patients without visible laparoscopic findings or stratified patients according to the presence or absence of such findings. The description of atypical (nonpigmented) endometriosis by Jansen and Russell in 1986 calls these classifications into question. Laparoscopy studies published before that time reported that 11% of women with CPP had endometriosis, whereas three similarly conducted studies published since 1986 reported a 41% prevalence of endometriosis in women undergoing laparoscopy for CPP. The pre-1986 literature on pelvic pain must be reevaluated with this information in mind. Many studies may have included women with endometriosis in the anatomically normal group, thus generating erroneous conclusions about the entirely psychogenic nature of their pain.

There are a variety of proposed mechanisms explaining pain associated with endometriosis, including inflammatory, nociceptive, and neuropathic. There is no pathognomonic symptom associated with endometriosis. Laparoscopic treatment of endometriosis improves pain symptoms more than diagnostic surgery alone, but many of the symptoms often assigned to the disease (e.g., dyspareunia, dysmenorrhea, abnormal bowel or bladder function) are commonly found in functional disorders such as IBS, making it difficult to understand the relevant contribution of endometriosis to CPP. The severity of the pain correlates poorly with the amount of superficial peritoneal disease, and such implants do not localize to the site of patients' symptoms. Deeply infiltrating endometriosis (DIE)—fibrotic, vascular, desmoplastic tissue destruction—is an exception to this rule. Nodular disease of the colon is associated with dyschezia and hematochezia; urologic tract disease with hematuria, dysuria, and obstruction; and cul-de-sac disease (uterosacral ligaments, rectovaginal septum, ovarian endometriomas) with deep dyspareunia. Fear of worsened pain, impaired fertility, or recurrent disease after treatment may increase pain levels. Of the women for whom we repeat laparoscopy for recurrent pain following complete hysterectomy and adnexectomy for endometriosis, only a small minority (3% to 5%) prove to have recurrent disease. Most cases of continued postoperative pain are interpreted in the context of the patient's overall sensitivity to pain and other peripheral stimuli functioning under that same sensitivity, such as pelvic floor tension myalgia, painful bladder, or functional gastrointestinal disease.

Those experienced in treating the disease can often detect DIE with clinical exam and imaging. When endometriosis is strongly suspected otherwise, and initial treatment with oral contraceptives (OCs) has failed, diagnostic laparoscopy should be the next step. One widely discussed study by Ling et al. concluded that a careful clinical history and physical examination can predict the presence of endometriosis in approximately 80% of cases. However, this was done in the setting of a strict research protocol; the diagnostic sensitivity of this approach in general clinical practice is likely much lower. Unfortunately, the study is often misinterpreted as implying that pain relief following gonadotropin-releasing hormone (GnRH) agonist treatment is not only a sensitive detector of endometriosis but is also *specific*—that is, it makes the diagnosis of endometriosis. Careful reading of the data reveals that this is not the case: the frequency of relief following GnRH treatment was the same in women with and without endometriosis. In addition, pain sensitivity is known to increase perimenstrually even in women without CPP. This may mean that nociception from pain disorders outside the reproductive tract may also improve when menstrual cyclicity is eliminated. For example, IBS symptoms also decline in women taking GnRH agonists. Hence, although *failure* to relieve pain with a GnRH agonist supports the notion that the reproductive organs are not involved, relief of pain with these medications does not prove that they are to blame.

Pelvic Adhesions

Early reviews supported the role of adhesions as a significant peripheral pain generator in CPP. In one, 6% to 55% of the 2,615 patients who underwent laparoscopy for pelvic pain had pelvic adhesions. In more recent investigation, Latthe et al. demonstrated a relatively weak correlation between adhesions and CPP, much less than factors such as psychosomatic symptoms and substance abuse. Correlation, of course, does not imply causality, and few, if any, well-designed studies demonstrate effective treatment of CPP with adhesiolysis. Unfortunately, in an effort to provide some explanation for complex pain disorders, providers often still posit adhesions as an etiology, even when a patient's surgical history includes only laparoscopy with findings of minimal or no endometriosis, pelvic inflammatory disease, or other conditions associated with meaningful adhesions. This explanation can happen even when the patient's pain escalation is remote from the last surgery. Adhesions may play some role in pain conditions in some women, but the relative contribution is probably small. Also, the putative treatment—repeat surgical intervention—can add new contributions to pain syndromes, such as the impact of surgical trauma, disappointment from lack of pain relief, feeding the psychological need of being "ill" with more surgery, and, in the worst case, generating a complication such as enterotomy.

Pelvic Support

Most women in pain clinics are in their third or fourth decade of life, while pelvic organ prolapse affects significantly older women, suggesting a very minimal role for support problems in CPP.

Pelvic relaxation usually leads to reports of heaviness, pressure, dropping sensations, or aching. In attempting to hold in prolapsing organs, the patient may tense the levator plate, leading to tenderness during daily activities and intercourse. Fear of (or actual) loss of urinary control during coitus can add to the discomfort by impairing physiologic sexual response.

Uterine retroversion is another potential etiology for CPP, particularly in the form of deep dyspareunia. Clearly for many women, retroversion is an innocent anatomic variant, but for those with pain, uncontrolled clinical series of uterine suspension procedures suggest changing the position of the uterus to an axial or anteverted position can improve dyspareunia by elevating a tender fundus out of the posterior cul-de-sac and allowing for better vaginal expansion as a natural part of the sexual response cycle.

Pelvic Congestion

Overfilling (congestion) of the pelvic venous system has been implicated as a cause of dull chronic aching pain that usually is unilateral and worse at the end of the day after prolonged standing, premenstrually, and postcoitally. Some studies suggest the condition is present in nearly one third of women with CPP, but there is no agreed-upon reference standard for diagnosis, despite individual technical regimens involving venography, MRI, and ultrasonography. Hormonal suppression, percutaneous embolotherapy, and surgery (vein ligation, hysterectomy, and salpingo-oophorectomy) represent available treatments, but study protocols involving these interventions are diverse, and few have been investigated in controlled trials.

Residual Ovary

When the uterus has been removed, with or without removal of one ovary, the remaining ovary or ovaries become symptomatic in 1% to 4% of women. Pain from the ovary can be increased by confinement within postoperative adhesions, rupture or leakage of a cyst prompting additional adhesion formation, or attachment of the ovary to the sigmoid colon or vaginal apex by postoperative adhesions. In the case of attachment to the vaginal apex, deep dyspareunia can result when the area is struck.

Ovarian Remnant

A more difficult situation can develop if a small fragment of ovarian tissue is left behind during attempted oophorectomy. In most instances, this happens when challenging dissection is required, such as cases of extensive pelvic adhesions and/or DIE. Within 1 to 3 years of the attempted oophorectomy, continued follicle-stimulating hormone (FSH) stimulation will result in growth of the ovarian fragment, often producing an intermittently symptomatic pelvic mass located along the course of the ovarian vascular supply. A postulated mechanism for pain generation includes the cystic enlargement of the mass confined within fibrotic adhesions. If the remnant developed because endometriosis is made for difficult oophorectomy, that disease is often found in the remnant and probably also serves as a pain generator. Ovarian remnants are uncommon, but not rare, as implied by early case series. Classic symptoms include absence of vasomotor symptoms when bilateral oophorectomy was intended and presence of cyclic unilateral pain. As in the case of the residual ovary, the remnant can produce dyspareunia if it is located close to the vaginal apex. When performing oophorectomy, it is best to open the pararectal space and completely skeletonize the infundibulopelvic (IP) ligament, not only to avoid complications such as ureteral injury but also to prevent ovarian remnant syndrome. In difficult cases, dividing the IP at or above the pelvic brim, as in risk reduction prophylactic oophorectomy, is prudent.

Vaginal Apex Pain

Following hysterectomy, pain may persist or recur because of intrinsic sensitivity of the vaginal apex. Although the cuff may appear to have healed perfectly well, gentle examination with a cotton-tipped applicator may reveal focal sensitivity of moderate-to-severe degree, many times located in one lateral fornix or the other and often replicating the reported pain of dyspareunia. When this is not done, the unaware examiner may then, noting pain upon traditional bimanual examination, mistakenly conclude that the source of nociception lies cephalad, for example, in a remaining ovary, pelvic scarring, or bowel adhesions.

The diagnosis may be confirmed by noting elimination of the pain following injection of local anesthetic. The condition is generally considered neuropathic, by virtue of the character of the pain (burning, stinging, sharp), and that neuropathic treatments (overnight application of lidocaine, oral medications such as nortriptyline, amitriptyline, gabapentin, etc.) seem to benefit some patients. Laparoscopic revision of the vaginal cuff may give good initial relief in approximately two thirds of patients, but pain tends to recur to a degree over the subsequent 2 to 3 years.

Musculoskeletal Problems

Musculoskeletal changes can become involved with CPP, either as the primary problem or as a secondary reaction to the pelvic pain. Dysmenorrhea can be referred to the midline of the low back, especially when the uterus is retroverted. Pain can also be referred to the midline of the low back in the presence of cul-de-sac endometriosis. An ovary fixed to the pelvic sidewall can refer pain to the ipsilateral low back, lower quadrant, and upper thigh.

The muscular problem that most often produces pelvic pain is pelvic floor tension myalgia. Intermittent or constant painful contraction of the levator plate can be present as a primary psychophysiologic problem, but contraction is more often a reaction to some other source of pain. Even when the primary source of pain is successfully treated, the reactive muscle contraction can persist as a learned response, in much the same way that vaginal introital muscle spasm (vaginismus) can persist after transient but repeated painful vaginal events. Pelvic floor tension myalgia is often found in the setting of generalized somatic hypersensitivity, a condition whose worst case includes fibromyalgia.

Lumbar musculature can become tender as a primary problem or in reaction to subtle changes in posture and motion. Trigger points can be present in the low back and gluteal areas in the muscles best inspected by pelvic examination (e.g., levator plate, piriformis, obturator internus).

The piriformis and obturator muscles warrant additional mention because they are seldom appreciated as possible sources of pain. These muscles are external rotators of the leg, and rotation against resistance can allow detection of tender spasm of the muscles during the pelvic examination. The sciatic nerve can traverse the belly of the piriformis as a normal anatomic variant, producing symptoms similar to sciatica when the muscle is in spasm.

Myofascial Pain

Focal lower quadrant abdominal wall pain can be produced by entrapment of the genitofemoral and ilioinguinal nerves, as described by Applegate. Such entrapment appears most often after Pfannenstiel abdominal incisions. Reiter and Gambone reported that 14% of 122 laparoscopy-negative women had myofascial pain probably related to a previous surgical incision. Myofascial trigger points—palpable taut bands of tender skeletal muscle—may be a primary problem or a later reaction to the long duration of pain from some other source.

Medical Comorbidity

Peripheral pain generation in CPP often involves nongynecologic systems (Table 29.1). A careful history and close physical examination of gastrointestinal, urologic, musculoskeletal, and neurologic systems are needed to evaluate these additional contributions to CPP. Most of the available literature examines these problems of other systems independently of each other and without reference to their relevance to CPP or to the overall prevalence of these disorders in CPP.

The gastrointestinal system is perhaps the most common nongynecologic contributor to CPP. Constipation and IBS occur most frequently, although inflammatory bowel disease and diverticulitis can at times present with pain alone. Women are proportionately more affected by IBS, and some have hypothesized increased relaxin levels produced by a dysfunctional corpus luteum as one of many possible contributing factors. As previously mentioned, treatment with a GnRH agonist may reduce symptoms of IBS.

Urologic problems, which are less easily confused with gynecologic disorders, are perhaps second in terms of prevalence. The urethral syndrome (frequency, urgency, and dysuria in the absence of bacteriuria), IC, and bladder spasms are all accompanied by significant anxiety and depression symptoms. The symptoms of these three disorders are very similar to those in a population of gynecologic CPP patients. Structured questionnaires (e.g., the Pelvic Pain and Urgency/Frequency [PUF] scale) help detect symptoms possibly emanating from the bladder. In some patients, however, a "positive" score can be achieved on the basis of other components of pelvic pain alone—without specific bladder symptoms—making the measure perhaps too *sensitive* and hence insufficiently *specific*. A history (whether pain occurs during micturition, daily activities, or coitus) does not always reveal the involved system, but careful pelvic examination with stepwise gentle palpation of the urethra, bladder base, and bladder may help the physician identify the site of the pain the patient is experiencing.

Many patients do not experience the problems described here in pure form, but rather in varying degrees of intensity, with varying contributions to an individual's total discomfort. Indeed, we suspect that shared innervation of pelvic organs may often lead to subsyndromal symptoms in an organ system that neighbors one with different pathology. Such patients have a multifaceted somatosensory disorder, as opposed to being the unfortunate victim of multiple unrelated organ-specific disease processes. Close attention to such nuances of detail is warranted both in clinical management and in published reports.

PSYCHOLOGICAL FACTORS

Personality

The links between chronic pain and individual psychology and personality style have been sought after and discussed in the psychiatric literature for many years. Some early reports implied that women who reported CPP had a high prevalence of feminine identity problems related to conflicts about adult sexuality, psychiatric disturbance characterized by mixed character disorder with predominant schizoid features, high neuroticism, and unsatisfactory relationships. Although these initial studies were an important beginning, the high prevalence of psychopathology in some reported samples did not seem applicable to significant numbers of CPP patients seen in practice. The findings are difficult to interpret, partly because there is a lack of clarity concerning the operational definition of CPP that was used. Biases in patient selection and interviewer information, inadequate control groups, and the absence of diagnostic laparoscopy also contribute to the confusion. Despite these shortcomings, it seems apparent that disorders of personality, especially borderline personality, are overrepresented both in the general population of severe chronic pain patients and in the population of those with CPP.

In primary care, such patients usually are seen less often. In any case, a label of personality disorder should not be applied indiscriminately to every angry patient by her frustrated physician. People who have difficulties maintaining satisfactory relationships and function in life, even when these difficulties are caused in part by subsyndromal personality problems, can be more vulnerable to nociceptive signals from tissue damaged by endometriosis, infection, or surgery. Unmet dependency needs may lead them to seek external solutions such as medications and further surgery, rather than to rely on their own impaired coping skills.

Depression

Focusing specifically on a CPP sample that had been evaluated by diagnostic laparoscopy, Walker and associates found that women with CPP (with and without positive laparoscopic findings) met criteria for lifetime major depression, current major depression, lifetime substance abuse, adult sexual dysfunction, and somatization more often than did control subjects. Stout and Steege found that 59% of 294 women seeking evaluation at a pelvic pain clinic scored in the depressed range (>16) on the Center for Epidemiologic Studies Depression Scale at the time of their initial visit. Slocumb and colleagues reported that patients with an abdominal pelvic pain syndrome scored higher on scales of anxiety, depression, anger–hostility, and somatization on the Hopkins Symptom Checklist.

Because no study of CPP has assessed its association with depression over time, no statement can be made as to whether depressive symptoms are a predisposing factor leading to, or a reaction to, the pain condition. There seem to be two distinct groups of CPP patients: one in which pain and depression are common final presentations reached by a number of pathways and another in which depression develops in reaction to pain, as is the case with many other acute and chronic medical diseases.

History of Sexual Abuse

Women seeking treatment for CPP have a high prevalence of sexual trauma in their personal histories. In Reiter's study of 106 women with CPP, 48% had a history of major psychosexual trauma (molestation, incest, or rape) compared with 6.5% of 92 pain-free control subjects presenting for annual routine gynecologic examination (P < 0.001). The high prevalence of reports of psychosexual trauma elicited from CPP patients supports the hypothesis that pelvic pain is specifically and psychodynamically related to sexual abuse. However, Rapkin and colleagues did not find a higher prevalence of childhood or adult sexual abuse in a group of women with CPP compared with women with chronic pain in other locations. These findings argue against a unique relation between sexual abuse and CPP and suggest that abusive experiences promote the chronicity of many different painful conditions.

When such a history is noted, the clinician and patient together must judge whether the feelings surrounding these events are intense enough to intrude upon the present. If so, psychotherapeutic help may be indicated. If not, although the memories may be painful, further emotional work on this area may not be beneficial. The literature on the sequelae of abuse and subsequent treatment is disappointing, especially when the abuse occurred in the distant past. In any case, it is difficult to judge whether these events are directly relevant to present pain and hence demand attention or whether they contribute to a psychologically vulnerable substrate influenced by subsequent physical and emotional events. In these circumstances, it may be worthwhile to suggest further mental health evaluation as an exploratory measure, being careful not to imply that the patient is being referred because the physician is certain that the abuse is related to the development of the pain.

Sexual Dysfunction

In clinical practice, women presenting with CPP often report a high incidence of marital distress and sexual dysfunction, particularly dyspareunia. Stout and Steege found that 56% of 220 married women scored in the maritally distressed range (<100) on the Locke-Wallace Marital Adjustment Scale at the time of initial visit. A high level of marital distress has also been reported in other chronic pain patients and their spouses. Although some women report satisfactory sexual functioning before the onset of pain symptoms, others appear to have long-standing impairments in sexual response. In our experience, sexual difficulties are often the problem that makes a person seek (or is encouraged by her partner to seek) help for her pain.

DIAGNOSTIC STRATEGIES

Recognizing a Chronic Pain Syndrome

Many women can experience pain for longer than 6 months without becoming debilitated; although their pain is chronic, such women are not described as having a CPS. The following are the common clinical hallmarks of true CPS:

1. Duration of 6 months or longer
2. Incomplete relief by most previous treatments
3. Significantly impaired physical function at home or at work
4. Signs of depression (sleep disturbance, weight loss, loss of appetite)
5. Hypersensitive response to nociceptive stimuli
6. Altered family roles

Of the signs of depression, sleep disturbance is usually the first to appear. Careful questioning is needed to distinguish awakening caused by pain from awakening that just happens. In the true vegetative sign, the person usually cannot get back to sleep even if pain is relieved (by medication or other means).

The alteration of family roles is perhaps the most important of those mentioned. This includes changed responsibilities for household, children, finances, and so forth. Initially intended as helpful, such changes may eventually diminish the patient's self-esteem and progressively reduce her family's interactions with her to little more than checking on her pain. Over time, this covertly reinforces the symptom of pain and imparts to it unintended value as a major means of maintaining communication within the family.

Simultaneous Medical and Psychosocial Evaluation

When the aforementioned markers of CPS are present, one should surrender the need to immediately discover how much of the pain problem is physical and how much is psychological. Rather than guess, it is useful to ask two separate questions: Is there physical disease that requires medical or surgical treatment? Is there emotional or psychological distress that requires treatment?

It is useful to directly state that the precise connection between these two cannot be measured; this can help diminish the patient's fear that she will be told "it's all in her head." In one sense, that statement is true: Pain is, by definition, a product of the brain, spinal cord, and peripheral nervous system, but few patients nefariously endorse nonexistent symptoms for secondary gain. A provider telling a patient he or she believes her pain symptoms are real—they might be modified by a host of psychological, experiential, or genetic factors that influence the interpretation of peripheral stimuli, but they are real—can establish an important therapeutic bond. The patient may then be more open to sharing her personal and emotional concerns. If this statement is made early in the evaluation, before all physical evaluations have been carried out, the patient is likely to be less defensive. In this framework, a mental health consultant has a better chance of developing rapport with the patient and will be a more helpful collaborator when needed.

History Taking

The site, duration, pattern during activities, relation to position changes, and association with bodily functions are all important elements of pain. For example, pain that is absent in the morning but worsens progressively during the day may be associated with pelvic floor muscle dysfunction, while a tender "spot" of dyspareunia might be related to nodular cul-de-sac endometriosis.

The chronology of a patient's pain is critical. As CPS develops, pain can be present over a progressively larger area despite stable visible pathology. Interpreting this as the breakdown or wearing out of physiologic systems that deal with pain signals has some biologic validity and may make sense to the patient. The clinician may need to counter the idea patients sometimes have that endometriosis "flares" like rheumatoid disease or spreads like a malignancy.

From a cognitive perspective, it is invaluable to discern the patient's and her family's ideas about the causes of and future for her pain. Fears of cancer can be discovered even if this diagnosis was never even remotely considered by the clinician. Less dramatic but equally powerful attributions of cause can emerge, such as pelvic infection that is due to sexual acts remote in time, arguments with a spouse, divine retribution, and so forth.

Physical Examination

It can be helpful to begin the exam with the back, evaluating for tenderness of the spine, paraspinous muscles, and sacroiliac joints. This may identify pain generators and sites for therapeutic intervention, but it also allows for touch to begin in a very nonthreatening way. Gynecologic assessment is uncomfortable to some degree for almost all women, but the patient with CPP is particularly vulnerable. Moving from back to abdomen to pelvis can establish trust and reduce fear. The abdominal wall is examined with and without flexed rectus muscles. A positive Carnett sign (increased tenderness when palpation is done in the presence of abdominal wall flexion) implies at least a contribution to the pain from abdominal wall myofascial sources. Decreased pain during this maneuver implies a higher contribution from visceral sources. On occasion, gentle fingertip palpation of the abdominal wall can detect such trigger points in the musculature. Rarely, a subcutaneous abdominal wall endometrioma is discovered, a diagnosis supported by a history of predictable, cyclic focal tenderness.

Pelvic exam then begins with external review of the vulva and vestibule. Gentle palpation with a cotton swab can detect areas of sensitivity consistent with vestibulitis in the introitus or trigger points higher in the vagina.

Guiding a patient through contraction–relaxation sequences of the abdominal, thigh, and vaginal introital muscles can reduce the discomfort of the examination and can indicate the patient's degree of control over muscle tension. Single-digit palpation of the levator plate, piriformis, and obturator muscles can elicit the tenderness of pelvic floor tension myalgia. This condition can present as a sequel to some other pelvic pain or a problem in itself. Discomfort is usually felt as pelvic pressure and radiation pain to the sacrum, near the insertions of the levator plate muscles.

Single-digit palpation should also be used to discover areas of tenderness in the cervix, uterus, and adnexa as well. Premature addition of the abdominal hand to the exam adds in nociceptive signals from abdominal wall myofascial components that may lead the examiner to overattribute pain to the viscera. Finally, the abdominal hand is added to assess size, shape, and mobility of pelvic structures. Adnexal thickening and mobility, pelvic relaxation, coccygeal tenderness, and foci of pain that reproduce dyspareunia should be noted. A rectovaginal exam is important when DIE is suspected.

During all components of the physical exam, it is important to not only ask the question "Does this hurt?" but also ask the questions "Do you feel pain where I am pressing or somewhere else?" and "Is this the pain you were describing earlier—is this *your* pain?" If a patient answers affirmatively to the final question, it can be helpful to point out what structure you are palpating (e.g., pelvic floor muscle vs. ovary).

Laboratory Tests

Imaging Studies

In the case of CPS, it has already been established that intensity of pain does not correlate well with extent of visible pathology. It follows that if the physical examination is relatively benign and is not severely limited by body habitus, extensive imaging usually adds little to the database needed before laparoscopy is performed. This is especially true in the case of organ-specific studies (intravenous pyelography, barium enema, colonoscopy) in the absence of symptoms or signs pointing to an explicit organ system (e.g., blood in the stools). Ultrasounds, CT scans, and MRIs can, at times, discover unrelated or nonspecific items misinterpreted by the patient and physician. Understandably limited by the setting, many patients have been told by emergency physicians her pain is due to ovarian cysts. This explanation is supported by an imaging study—either (a) a cyst (physiologic or not) is present or (b) a small amount of fluid is seen, interpreted as cystic rupture. Intervening for CPP on the basis of an imaging study finding alone is unlikely to be fruitful. On the other hand, with a specific question in mind—for example, pelvic sonography to confirm ovarian endometrioma, MRI when adenomyosis is suspected, or lower endoscopic ultrasound to rule out invasive rectal endometriosis—imaging can be quite helpful.

Blood Studies

Relatively few hematologic or chemical measures are of use in diagnosing CPP. An elevated leukocyte count and erythrocyte sedimentation rate may make the clinician suspect chronic pelvic inflammatory disease even when cervical probes are negative for the most common sexually transmitted infections. Serum cancer antigen 125 (CA 125) can confirm suspicions of DIE in those without prior surgical evaluation but is not sufficiently sensitive to detect early-stage disease. In those with advanced endometriosis, anti-müllerian hormone levels can help fertility counseling in a woman considering extirpative surgical treatment for her disease. In patients with post–bilateral oophorectomy with remnant ovarian tissue, FSH and estradiol levels remain in premenopausal ranges. Women using replacement estrogen therapy should stop 3 weeks before these levels are measured.

Anesthetic Blocks

Injection of small volumes of a local anesthetic, 1 to 5 mL of 1% lidocaine or 0.25% to 0.5% bupivacaine, blocks pain from either an entrapped segmental nerve (e.g., ilioinguinal) or an abdominal wall trigger point. Such blocks can be therapeutic as well as diagnostic. Many anesthesia pain clinics administer epidural or spinal anesthetics to distinguish pain arising from peripheral organs from pain that has become completely central in origin.

In some instances, it is useful to attempt diagnostic/therapeutic transvaginal blocks with the same local anesthetics for vaginal apex pain, as discussed above. A series of three or four blocks administered 1 to 2 weeks apart may provide durable relief in some instances.

In most cases, a history and careful routine physical examination distinguish central from lateral sources of pelvic pain. When this discrimination is difficult, it may be useful to administer a transvaginal uterosacral block (blocking most uterine innervation) and then repeat the pelvic examination. When this relieves the pain, the pain can be assumed to arise from the uterus. If the pain is not relieved, however, one cannot distinguish a failed block from pain of nonuterine origin.

Psychological Tests and Interviews

To distinguish physical from psychological contributions to pain, many studies of CPP have used traditional psychological instruments that were developed to measure general psychopathology or personality factors. In some studies, more psychological abnormalities are detected in women without visible pathology at laparoscopy. In other studies, women with positive laparoscopy who have had pain for a long time appear equally distressed in their questionnaire responses. These psychometric instruments generally have uncertain face value for chronic pain patients, and their use can support the patient's fears that the health care provider thinks she is "crazy" or that the pain is imagined. Once again, the question of whether the emotional distress identified by these instruments is an antecedent to or a consequence of persistent pain remains unanswered. Psychometric tests are most useful when they are interpreted by a psychologist who has interviewed the patient, and they serve best as a means to better understand the patient's strengths and weaknesses, rather than as a means to decide who has "organic" versus "psychological" pathology or who needs surgery.

Laparoscopy

Great strides have been made in operative laparoscopy in the past three decades. Laparoscopy can be useful diagnostically and therapeutically (even in the face of negative findings), but when a CPS is clinically evident, results of laparoscopic treatment alone, despite comparable pathology, are much less impressive. For a patient with the clinical markers of CPS listed earlier, the complete workup as described should be performed before laparoscopy.

In some puzzling cases, we have performed laparoscopy under local anesthesia to "pain map" the pelvis. A 2-mm laparoscope and a small suprapubic probe are placed with the use of short-acting, reversible intravenous analgesia (e.g., remifentanil) and local anesthetic. Having been oriented to the procedure beforehand, as each organ is touched, the patient is asked if the site is painful, to rate it on an ordinal scale from 1 to 10, and if the discomfort represents her pain. It is possible in some cases to block the superior hypogastric plexus during pain mapping to better predict benefit from presacral neurectomy. In this approach, mapping is done before and after injecting 10 mL of 1% lidocaine just underneath the peritoneum over the sacrum, using a 7-inch, 22-gauge spinal needle.

Limiting patient characteristics for using pain mapping include high states of anxiety and obesity, where the torque required to move an instrument against a thick abdominal wall can provide distracting nociceptive information. Once thought to be the "holy grail" of CPP diagnostics, better understanding of the central mechanisms of chronic pain and the relationship among various named pain disorders has led to diminished enthusiasm for laparoscopic pain mapping in routine practice.

MANAGEMENT

Relatively straightforward pain problems are not challenging to manage, such as treating isolated dysmenorrhea with hormonal suppression or a chronic tuboovarian abscess with adnexectomy. More often, however, CPP represents a complex and nuanced syndrome where treatment may vary considerably depending on the patient. When pain itself is the disease, the goal of treatment is not necessarily complete eradication of pain, but rather finding strategies that afford more functional living. Neuromodulatory medications (e.g., tricyclic antidepressants, neurotransmitter reuptake inhibitors, neuroleptics), psychological adjuncts (e.g., cognitive–behavioral therapy, pain psychotherapy, sexual counseling), and complementary strategies (e.g., mindfulness-based medication, yoga, acupuncture) can be useful to dampen central hypersensitivity. For the peripheral elements, physical therapy, diet modification, peripheral nerve blocks, and surgery can be helpful depending on the target pain generator. In all cases, good sleep hygiene, exercise, healthy eating, and social support are important foundational elements that improve the effectiveness of CPP treatment.

General Principles

A complete evaluation of CPS often reveals a number of contributing factors, such as bladder irritability, irregular bowel function, poor posture, and emotional and relationship stresses, in addition to laparoscopically visualized pathology. Treating each component sequentially is common practice but often ends in frustration because each treatment addresses only a part of the problem. Simultaneous treatments often begin with disquieting multimodal therapy but allow better relief. Close follow-up at regularly scheduled visits provides support and a coping mechanism for the patient. When the patient is essentially required to feel worse to be seen again, the pain may be tacitly reinforced.

Medication Use

Analgesics

Analgesics such as nonsteroidal anti-inflammatory drugs and opioid narcotics can be quite effective for acute conditions, but their use in chronic pain is marred by a host of adverse outcomes and limited efficacy associated with long-term use. Dose-related effects of medications such as acetaminophen (liver toxicity) and cyclooxygenase inhibitors (gastric and renal damage) are well known, but they are not major offenders in the realm of tolerance and withdrawal. Opioid narcotics, on the other hand, are notoriously dangerous in regard to these consequences, in addition to problems such as narcotic bowel syndrome and opioid-induced hyperalgesia. Some patients benefit from structured narcotic therapy, but, if they are to be used for CPP, clinicians should screen carefully for factors associated with high risk for misuse and set nonnegotiable ground rules, such as limiting prescriptions to one provider, not entertaining requests for early refills, mandating scheduled urine drug screens, and refraining from uncontrolled dose escalation. Newer opioid medications, such as oxymorphone and tapentadol, are considered less euphoria generating than the more commonly employed narcotics such as hydrocodone, oxycodone, and hydromorphone.

Antidepressants and Neuroleptics

This class of drugs is commonly employed in the treatment of chronic pain, including CPP, although few controlled trials have been carried out specifically in this population. While no longer first line for mood disorders, tricyclic antidepressants such as amitriptyline, nortriptyline, and desipramine have a long record of being effective in treating chronic pain. Newer-generation neurotransmitter reuptake inhibitors such as duloxetine and desvenlafaxine can also be useful. Neuroleptics such as gabapentin, pregabalin, and lamotrigine are generally employed when symptoms are more specifically neuropathic in nature. It is important to discuss with patients that, although they tend to diminish with continued use, all of these medications have central side effects, some of which are predictable and others quite idiosyncratic. When higher doses or multiple agents are used, it can be helpful to consult with a psychiatrist or psychopharmacologist to avoid complications such as severe mood dysregulation or serotonin syndrome.

Anxiolytics

Anxiolytic drugs are certainly widely prescribed by gynecologists, although it is uncertain how often they are given for pain. In one study, alprazolam, a triazolobenzodiazepine with mixed anxiolytic and antidepressant effects, had a surprising degree of analgesic effect in moderate-to-high doses in patients with chronic pain of malignant origin and concomitant mood changes or anxiety. These patients were already receiving narcotics, which may suggest that alprazolam potentiates the analgesic effect of narcotics. Their role in conjunction with nonnarcotic analgesics is uncertain, and the addiction potential is obvious.

Hormonal Medications

Oral contraceptives are effective in reducing dysmenorrhea and cyclic symptoms associated with endometriosis. It is not uncommon, however, to meet resistance to using these medications in women with CPP—either because they were previously used and did not cure the entirety of the pain syndrome and were thus deemed ineffective or because of sensitivity to side effects such as nausea, an understandable consequence in a viscerally hypersensitive group. Avoiding ultra–low-dose 20-mcg ethinyl estradiol formulations can help reduce unscheduled bleeding, important for women who may closely associate bleeding with pain. Outside of DIE, progestin-only formulations, by enteral or parenteral route, run the risk of exacerbating depressive symptoms in a vulnerable population. A notable exception includes the levonorgestrel intrauterine system (LNG-IUS), which has little systemic absorption and can control dysmenorrhea and pain from endometriosis in a low-risk, reversible, long-acting manner.

The use of GnRH agonists deserves special mention. They have been recommended to distinguish gynecologic from non-gynecologic sources of pain; however, these agents also relieve symptoms of other functional conditions. Furthermore, pain thresholds have been shown to be lower premenstrually, even in asymptomatic women. The impact of the menstrual cycle itself in chronic pain patients has not been well explored, but it seems likely that it may impart some cyclicity even to conditions unrelated to the reproductive tract. Cyclicity of symptoms must therefore be interpreted with caution, and the disappearance of symptoms or of their cyclicity by pharmacologically obliterating the menstrual cycle does not demonstrate a gynecologic cause. To address the most common clinical circumstance, relieving pain with a GnRH agonist does not prove that the pain is due to endometriosis, nor does it prove that pain comes from the reproductive tract, as discussed above. Gonadotropin-releasing hormone agonists can be useful when differential diagnosis includes ovarian remnant syndrome or residual ovary syndrome or in the treatment of DIE, but its utility in treating general CPP is limited by cost and morbidity. Contrary to popular belief, GnRH agonists are not more effective than other more benign hormonal manipulations directed at pelvic pain. For DIE, aromatase inhibitors may work similarly, without as significant hypoestrogenic effects.

Surgery

Two basic surgical approaches have been used to treat CPP: removing pelvic organs and treating visible disease while leaving the pelvic organs in place. The use of both approaches is guided by clinical experience, as scientific data regarding the role of surgery in pelvic pain are sparse. Expansion of literature on the topic, including stratification for characteristics that lead to strong or poor response, would be most welcome.

In the United States, approximately 12% of hysterectomies are performed with pelvic pain as the primary indication. An additional 6.1% are performed for endometriosis or adenomyosis, and 5.1% are performed for pelvic inflammatory disease; no doubt many in these two categories also involve symptoms of pain. In approximately one third of hysterectomies performed for pain, no pathology is found. Despite the frequency of pain as an indication for this procedure, data regarding efficacy are surprisingly sparse. One report notes relief in 78% of women after hysterectomy for pelvic pain of uterine etiology (women with adnexal or other pelvic disease were excluded). Interestingly, the presence or absence of uterine pathology (adenomyosis or leiomyomata) had no bearing on whether pain was relieved.

Others have suggested hysterectomy performed in primary care settings is very effective for the treatment of CPP. In a prospective observational study of private practices in Maine, Carlson and associates reported that at a 1-year follow-up, satisfaction with the outcome of surgical treatment was much higher than satisfaction with the outcome of medical therapy. However, approximately one third of women improved substantially on medical therapy; perhaps, women were more likely to undergo operation when visible pathology was apparent. In the Maryland Women's Health Study, 1,299 women were interviewed at length before hysterectomy for benign disease and at 3, 6, 12, and 24 months after surgery. In more than 90% of cases, the procedure was well tolerated and did not result in postoperative depression or a decline in sexual functioning. In the subset of women with pain as the primary indication for surgery, relief of pain occurred in more than 80%, indicating that the clinicians involved generally used good judgment and technique. In general, women with preoperative depression or sexual dysfunction did not fare as well as their less symptomatic counterparts, although even when hysterectomy is performed in women with both depression and CPP, slightly more than 80% are improved emotionally and in terms of pain at 2-year follow-up.

Rigorous study design is lacking regarding data on adhesiolysis, with reports essentially limited to little more than clinical case series. When treated by laparotomy, 28 of 42 (65%) patients reported cure or improvement of pain. In a sample of mostly primary care patients, 84% of 65 patients had relief of pain after laser laparoscopic adhesiolysis with follow-up intervals of 1 to 5 years. In Sutton's large series, 85% had pain relief at 1 year. Steege and Stout reported that 15 of 20 (75%) patients without a CPS who were undergoing laser laparoscopic adhesiolysis had good relief of pain at a follow-up 6 to 12 months after surgery. However, if a CPS was present, only 4 of 10 (40%) patients with equivalent adhesive disease obtained relief. The greater the emotional and behavioral disability, the greater the need for combined medical, surgical, and mental health management.

Endometriosis is a more common finding among women undergoing laparoscopy for pelvic pain than those for other indications. Peritoneal disease does not correlate with symptom site or stage of disease with symptom severity. Laparoscopic treatment, even of mild disease, is more effective than diagnostic surgery alone. Some studies suggest superiority of excision to ablation of endometriosis implants, and this approach probably makes good clinical sense, but there is insufficient evidence to conclude one is definitively superior to the other in pain reduction. Specific symptom improvement following DIE (gastrointestinal, urologic, cul-de-sac) resection is best documented in the literature. The benefits of surgical excision may be prolonged by subsequent medical therapy. Numerous studies have been done of postsurgical treatment with hormonal medications. Oral contraceptives, danazol, progestins, and GnRH agonists (with and without add-back estrogen/progestin) have all been shown to be effective. Although the GnRH agonists have become perhaps the most widely used of these, definitive evidence for their superiority is lacking. The more economical and less physiologically intrusive approach would seem to favor sex steroids over GnRH agonists. Most troublesome in reviewing all of these studies is the observation that dyspareunia is the symptom that is most refractory to treatment, testifying to its multifactorial nature.

Presacral neurectomy, as an adjunct to surgical excision of endometriosis, has been evaluated for its effect on pelvic pain. In a retrospective sample of 71 women undergoing conservative resection of endometriosis by way of laparotomy, 35 (50%) who also had presacral neurectomy enjoyed significantly greater improvement in both dysmenorrhea and dyspareunia. Two subsequent retrospective reports noted that similar percentages (approximately 75%) of women obtained pain relief after endometriosis surgery that included presacral neurectomy, compared with approximately 25% who obtained relief without neurectomy. Zullo et al. investigated the question with a double-masked randomized trial and demonstrated a 20% difference in pain improvement when presacral neurectomy was added to endometriosis excision in women with central pain.

An ovarian remnant should be removed if it is persistently symptomatic despite attempts at medical suppression and if menopause cannot be expected in the patient's near future. The dissection should be detailed and should include all the peritoneum surrounding the mass. The pararectal space, and paravesical space if needed, should be opened systematically, and the ureter and pelvic sidewall vessels exposed and carefully freed from the specimen. Usually, there is vascular supply along the tract of the IP, and it is prudent to divide the pedicle well above the pelvic brim. When a GnRH agonist has been used preoperatively for symptom control or to distinguish the relative contributions made by the remnant and other pelvic pathology, such as adhesions, the remnant tissue may become so small as to make it difficult to identify. Hence, if a palpable (or ultrasonically visible) mass disappears after GnRH agonist treatment, it may be wise to allow time for it to regrow before pursuing surgical excision. When the remnant is small, some surgeons have stimulated the remnant with clomiphene citrate to make it easier to find.

Psychological and Alternative Treatments

Psychological disorders should be treated in CPP, whether independently present or the result of a long-standing pain disorder. Some practitioners may find cognitive–behavioral or biofeedback therapy useful in reducing automatic responses to painful stimuli. Sexual counseling, couples counseling, and psychotherapy can be helpful adjuncts. Alternative strategies, such as mindfulness-based meditation, yoga, and acupuncture, all have their appropriate roles in individual cases, but none is so clearly applicable or effective that its automatic use is supported in cases of CPP.

Management Overview

The most effective clinical approach requires simultaneous treatment of as many factors as possible: anatomic, musculoskeletal, functional bowel and bladder, psychological, and so forth. The patient and physician must contract for the long term and work from a rehabilitation perspective, rather than hope that the latest single addition to the treatment will prove to be *the* answer. The physician, to prevent frustration and feelings of defeat, must often play the role of helping to manage and relieve the pain while helping to maximize function, even when pain persists. To the surgically trained gynecologist who prefers a clear-cut single answer to a clinical problem, this can be the most difficult part of dealing with the problem of CPP. It is important to free oneself from the responsibility of needing to "fix" a patient's CPP. While the compassionate provider can be an invaluable aide, much of the work in improving from pelvic pain is the burden of the patient herself.

THE EVOLUTION OF A CHRONIC PAIN SYNDROME

As is apparent from this discussion, CPP is a heterogeneous problem, not a single diagnosis, and no single etiologic hypothesis is clearly supported. Most of the hypotheses reviewed here have some credible evidence supporting them; none have been sufficiently validated.

Some patients appear to have a pure version of one or the other of the syndromes described, whereas many others present with several or many simultaneously. Psychological and neurologic mechanisms are proposed here to explain how the evolution of chronic pain may occur, regardless of the particular tissue damage or functional disorder that may first have provided nociceptive stimuli. We suggest the following elements (Fig. 29.1): biologic events sufficient to initiate nociception, alterations of lifestyles and relations over time, recruitment of neighboring organ systems, anxiety and affective disorders, and a circular interaction (vicious cycle) among these elements.

Biologic Events Sufficient to Initiate Nociception

Sexually transmitted diseases, endometriosis, recurrent bladder and vaginal infections, primary or secondary functional dyspareunia, alterations of bowel habit, muscular dysfunction, pelvic congestion, and gynecologic or other abdominal surgeries (Table 29.1) may contribute individually or in combination.

Alteration of Lifestyle and Relations

Physical activities at home and recreational pursuits can suffer. Believing that rest usually helps in the treatment of most causes of acute pain, the patient may assume that the same applies to chronic pain and may thus restrict herself more than actual discomfort dictates. Family members start to regard the patient as sick and leave her out of many activities, thus reducing her

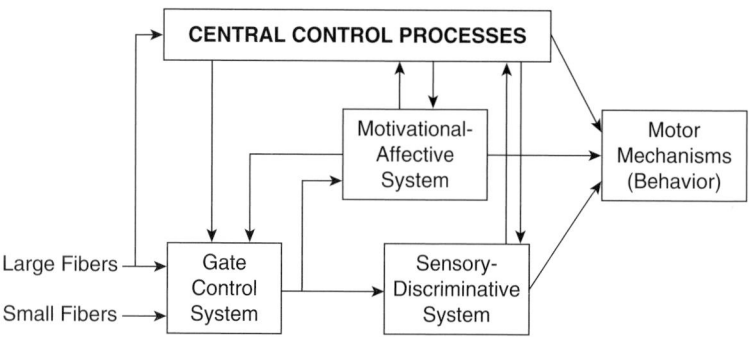

FIGURE 29.1 The gate control theory of pain perception.

roles within the family structure. With time, concern for and discussion of her pain can become the family's major pattern of communication with the pain victim. If sexual intimacy has been the major means of emotional sharing and smoothing over of differences, and if this intimacy is reduced, then the altered pattern of interactions may take hold more quickly.

Anxiety and Affective Disorders

Depression can occur as a cumulative result of the disability suffered, or the pain can bring on an episode of depression in a patient already biologically vulnerable. The observation most relevant here is that pain patients with a family history of depression can derive the most benefit from antidepressants.

The Vicious Cycle

Diminished activity, altered family roles and social supports, anxiety, and affective disturbances can influence nociception by a variety of central pathways, ultimately altering spinal cord "gating" of nociceptive signals. Cognitions about the pain can play an additional role.

Several important modifying influences can be present in addition to these major pathways (**Fig. 29.2**). Incest and other forms of sexual abuse have attracted the most attention as possible forerunners of CPP. However, CPP is clearly not a unique or specific sequel to sexual abuse, and a large proportion of CPP patients have not been abused in this manner. Victims of sexual abuse have many negative emotional sequelae; pain problems often occur after abuse, but they are not necessarily directly caused by the abuse.

A genetic predisposition to depression also allows the vicious cycle to become easily established and strengthened over time. Antidepressant medications play an important role

in the overall therapeutic plan in such cases. A relatively new area of research in pain is dealing with possible genetically determined variations in central neurotransmitter processes that may predispose to the development of pain syndromes.

Several authors have suggested that the concept of perceived control best explains the development of affective changes accompanying chronic pain, regardless of the location of the pain. The individual who sees herself as having little control over the physical and emotional events affecting her may be most vulnerable to development of a CPS. Another factor thought to influence pelvic pain is a patient's degree of catastrophization, a state of interpreting negative things are far worse than they are. It may be reasonable to consider these variables as a culmination of the effects of affective change, activity, family roles, sexual dysfunction, and previous victimization experiences.

The longer that pain has been a part of the person's life, and the more psychological vulnerabilities she carries forward to the present, the less likely it is that any treatment of the tissue damage itself will be effective in relieving pain and restoring physical and emotional function. However, as treatment studies show, the contribution of peripheral generators to chronic pain can seldom be dismissed entirely. The more difficult task is the selection of an efficient and cost-effective combination of treatment approaches aimed at the most important factors acting in the present.

BEST SURGICAL PRACTICES

- A complete medical and psychosocial history, as well as a pain-oriented physical and pelvic examination, should be completed before diagnostic laparoscopy is performed.
- Neuropathic and musculoskeletal components of CPP often require treatment both before and after appropriate pelvic surgery.
- A minimally invasive (laparoscopic) approach is especially appropriate for chronic pain patients.
- Laparoscopic treatment of endometriosis is more effective than diagnostic surgery alone.
- Presacral neurectomy can be an effective adjunct to endometriosis excision when a central component of pain is present.
- Resection of DIE is effective treatment of organ-specific symptoms.
- Complete skeletonization of the IP vessels, especially in difficult oophorectomy, reduces the risk of adjacent organ injury and ovarian remnant syndrome. Ovarian remnants should be removed with careful opening of avascular spaces and identification of retroperitoneal structures.
- Though not a cure for all components of a woman's CPP, hysterectomy can be an effective treatment, even in women with both depression and pain.

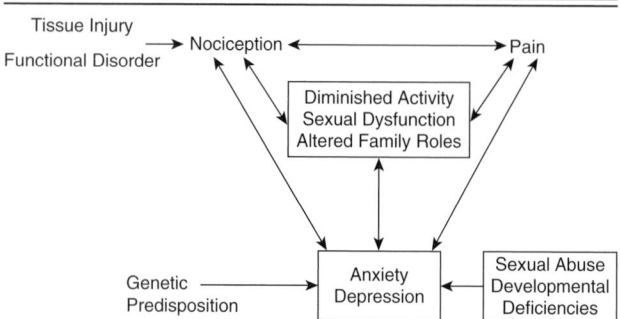

FIGURE 29.2 An integrative model for CPP, including elements of gate control theory, cognitive–behavioral theory, and the operant conditioning model.

BIBLIOGRAPHY

Abbott J, Hawe J, Hunter D, et al. Laparoscopic excision of endometriosis: a randomized, placebo-controlled trial. *Fertil Steril* 2004;82:878.

Abrao MS, Gonçalves MO, Dias JA Jr, et al. Comparison between clinical examination, transvaginal sonography and magnetic resonance imaging for the diagnosis of deep endometriosis. *Hum Reprod* 2007;22:3092.

Andrews J, Yunker A, Reynolds WS, et al. *Noncyclic chronic pelvic pain therapies for women: comparative effectiveness.* Rockville, MD: Agency for Healthcare Research and Quality (US), 2012, Report No.: 11(12)-EHC088-EF. AHRQ Comparative Effectiveness Reviews.

American Congress of Obstetricians and Gynecologists (ACOG) Committee on Practice Bulletins—Gynecology. ACOG Practice Bulletin No. 51. Chronic pelvic pain. *Obstet Gynecol* 2004;103:589.

Applegate WV. Abdominal cutaneous nerve entrapment syndrome. *Surgery* 1972;71:188.

Barbot J, Parent B, Dubuisson JB, et al. A clinical study of the CO_2 laser and electrosurgery for adhesiolysis in 172 cases followed by early second-look laparoscopy. *Fertil Steril* 1987;48:140.

Beard RW, Belsey EM, Lieberman BA, et al. Pelvic pain in women. *Am J Obstet Gynecol* 1977;128:566.

Beard RW, Highman JH, Pearce S, et al. Diagnosis of pelvic varicosities in women with chronic pelvic pain. *Lancet* 1984;2:946.

Carlson KJ, Miller BA, Fowler FJ. The Maine Women's Health Study: II. Outcomes of nonsurgical management of leiomyomas, abnormal bleeding, and chronic pelvic pain. *Obstet Gynecol* 1994;83:566.

Castelnuovo-Tedesco P, Krout BM. Psychosomatic aspects of chronic pelvic pain. *Int J Psychiatry Med* 1970;1:109.

Chan CLK, Wood C. Pelvic adhesiolysis: the assessment of symptom relief by 100 patients. *Aust N Z J Obstet Gynaecol* 1985;25:295.

Chapron C, Santulli P, de Ziegler D, et al. Ovarian endometrioma: severe pelvic pain is associated with deeply infiltrating endometriosis. *Hum Reprod* 2012;27:702.

Chatman DL, Zbella EA. Pelvic peritoneal defects and endometriosis: further observations. *Fertil Steril* 1986;46:711.

Crisson JE, Keefe FJ. The relationship of locus of control to pain coping strategies and psychological distress in chronic pain patients. *Pain* 1988;35:147.

Diamond MP, Daniell JF, Johns DA, et al. Postoperative adhesion development after operative laparoscopy: evaluation at early second-look procedures. *Fertil Steril* 1991;55:700.

Diamond MP, Daniell JF, Martin DC, et al. Tubal patency and pelvic adhesions at early second-look laparoscopy following intra-abdominal use of the carbon dioxide laser: initial report of the Intra-abdominal Laser Study Group. *Fertil Steril* 1984;42:717.

Dicker RC, Greenspan JR, Straus LT, et al. Complications of abdominal and vaginal hysterectomy among women of reproductive age in the United States: the collaborative review of sterilization. *Am J Obstet Gynecol* 1982;144:841.

Duncan CH, Taylor HC. A psychosomatic study of pelvic congestion. *Am J Obstet Gynecol* 1952;64:1.

Farquhar CM, Rogers V, Franks S, et al. A randomized controlled trial of medroxyprogesterone acetate and psychotherapy for the treatment of pelvic congestion. *Br J Obstet Gynaecol* 1989;96:1153.

Fauconnier A, Chapron C, Dubuisson JB, et al. Relation between pain symptoms and the anatomic location of deep infiltrating endometriosis. *Fertil Steril* 2002;78:719.

Fedele L, Parazzini F, Bianchi S, et al. Stage and localization of pelvic endometriosis and pain. *Fertil Steril* 1990;53:155.

Fenton BW, Durner C, Fanning J. Frequency and distribution of multiple diagnoses in chronic pelvic pain related to previous abuse or drug-seeking behavior. *Gynecol Obstet Invest* 2008;65:247.

Fernandez F, Adams F, Holmes VF. Analgesic effect of alprazolam in patients with chronic, organic pain of malignant origin. *J Clin Psychopharmacol* 1987;7:167.

Fordyce WE. *Behavioral methods of control of chronic pain and illness.* St. Louis, MO: CV Mosby, 1976.

Garcia C-R, David SS. Pelvic endometriosis: infertility and pelvic pain. *Am J Obstet Gynecol* 1977;129:740.

Gidro-Frank L, Gordon I, Taylor HC. Pelvic pain and female identity: a survey of emotional factors in 40 patients. *Am J Obstet Gynecol* 1960;79:1184.

Gross R, Doerr H, Caldirola D, et al. Borderline syndrome and incest in chronic pelvic pain patients. *Int J Psychiatry Med* 1980/81;10:79.

Grunkemeier DM, Cassara JE, Dalton CB, et al. The narcotic bowel syndrome: clinical features, pathophysiology, and management. *Clin Gastroenterol Hepatol* 2007;5:1126.

Gruppo Italiano per lo Studio dell'Endometriosi. Relationship between stage, site and morphological characteristics of pelvic endometriosis and pain. *Hum Reprod* 2001;16:2668.

Haber J, Roos C. Effects of spouse abuse and/or sexual abuse in the development and maintenance of chronic pain in women. *Adv Pain Res Ther* 1985;9:889.

Hartmann KE, Ma C, Lamvu GM, et al. Quality of life and sexual function after hysterectomy in women with preoperative pain and depression. *Obstet Gynecol* 2004;104:701.

Hornstein MD, Hemmings R, Yuzpe AA, et al. Use of nafarelin versus placebo after reductive laparoscopic surgery for endometriosis. *Fertil Steril* 1997;68:860.

Howard FM. Endometriosis and mechanisms of pelvic pain. *J Minim Invasive Gynecol* 2009;16:540.

Howard FM, El-Minawi AM, Sanchez RA. Conscious pain mapping by laparoscopy in women with chronic pelvic pain. *Obstet Gynecol* 2000;96:934.

Howard FM. The role of laparoscopy in chronic pelvic pain: promise and pitfalls. *Obstet Gynecol Surv* 1993;48:357.

Hsu AL, Sinaii N, Segars J, et al. Relating pelvic pain location to surgical findings of endometriosis. *Obstet Gynecol* 2011;118:223.

Jamieson DJ, Steege JF. The association of sexual abuse with pelvic pain complaints in a primary care population. *Am J Obstet Gynecol* 1997;177:1408.

Jansen RPS, Russell P. Nonpigmented endometriosis: clinical, laparoscopic, and pathologic definition. *Am J Obstet Gynecol* 1986;155:1154.

Keye WR, Hansen LW, Astin M, et al. Argon laser therapy of endometriosis: a review of 92 consecutive patients. *Fertil Steril* 1987;47:208.

Kjerulff KH, Langenberg PW, Rhodes JC, et al. Effectiveness of hysterectomy. *Obstet Gynecol* 2000;95:319.

Kresch AJ, Seifer DB, Sachs LB, et al. Laparoscopy in 100 women with chronic pelvic pain. *Obstet Gynecol* 1984;64:672.

Lamvu G, Robinson B, Zolnoun D, et al. Vaginal apex revision: a treatment option for vaginal apex pain. *Obstet Gynecol* 2004;104:1340.

Latthe P, Mignini L, Gray R, et al. Factors predisposing women to chronic pelvic pain: systematic review. *Br Med J* 2006;332:749.

Lee M, Silverman SM, Hansen H, et al. A comprehensive review of opioid-induced hyperalgesia. *Pain Physician* 2011;14:145.

Lee RB, Stone K, Magelssen D, et al. Presacral neurectomy for chronic pelvic pain. *Obstet Gynecol* 1986;68:517.

Ling FW; for the Pelvic Pain Study Group. Randomized controlled trial of depot leuprolide in patients with chronic pelvic pain and clinically suspected endometriosis. *Obstet Gynecol* 1999;93:51.

Longstreth GF, Drossman DA. Severe irritable bowel and functional abdominal pain syndromes: managing the patient and health care costs. *Clin Gastroenterol Hepatol* 2005;3:397.

Luciano AA, Maier DB, Koch EL, et al. A comparative study of postoperative adhesions following laser surgery by laparoscopy versus laparotomy in the rabbit model. *Obstet Gynecol* 1989;75:220.

Manchikanti L, Abdi S, Atluri S, et al. American Society of Interventional Pain Physicians (ASIPP) guidelines for responsible opioid prescribing in chronic non-cancer pain: Part I—evidence assessment. *Pain Physician* 2012;15:S1.

Manchikanti L, Abdi S, Atluri S, et al. American Society of Interventional Pain Physicians (ASIPP) guidelines for responsible opioid prescribing in chronic non-cancer pain: Part 2—guidance. *Pain Physician* 2012;15:S67.

Martin CE, Johnson E, Wechter ME, et al. Catastrophizing: a predictor of persistent pain among women with endometriosis at 1 year. *Hum Reprod* 2011;26:3078.

Mathias SD, Kuppermann M, Liberman RF, et al. Chronic pelvic pain: prevalence, health-related quality of life, and economic correlates. *Obstet Gynecol* 1996;87:321.

Mathias JR, Clench MH, Roberts PH, et al. Serum relaxin levels detected in women with functional bowel disease and reduced by leuprolide acetate (LA) therapy. *Gastroenterology* 1993;104: A549.

Mattingly RF, Thompson JD. Leiomyomata uteri and abdominal hysterectomy for benign disease. In: *Te Linde's operative gynecology*, 6th ed. Philadelphia, PA: JB Lippincott, 1985:227.

Melzack R. From the gate to the neuromatrix. *Pain* 1999;82:121.

Melzack R. Neurophysiologic foundations of pain. In: Sternbach RA, ed. *The psychology of pain*. New York, NY: Raven Press, 1986:1.

Melzack R, Wall PD. Pain mechanisms: a new theory. *Science* 1965;150:971.

Milingos S, Protopapas A, Kallipolitis G, et al. Endometriosis in patients with chronic pelvic pain: is staging predictive of the efficacy of laparoscopic surgery in pain relief? *Gynecol Obstet Invest* 2006;62:48.

Morrison J. Childhood sexual histories of women with somatization disorder. *Am J Psychiatry* 1989;146:239.

Nezhat CR, Nezhat FR, Metzger DA, et al. Adhesion reformation after reproductive surgery by videolaseroscopy. *Fertil Steril* 1990;53:1008.

Olive DL. Endometriosis. *N Engl J Med* 1993;328:1759.

O'Shaughnessy A, Check JH, Nowroozi K, et al. CA-125 levels measured in different phases of the menstrual cycle in screening for endometriosis. *Obstet Gynecol* 1993;81:99.

Porpora MG, Koninckx PR, Piazze J, et al. Correlation between endometriosis and pelvic pain. *J Am Assoc Gynecol Laparosc* 1999;6:429.

Portenoy RK, Foley KM. Chronic use of opioid analgesics in non-malignant pain: report of 38 cases. *Pain* 1986;25:171.

Prentice A, Deary AJ, Bland E. Progestins and anti-progestagens for pain associated with endometriosis (Cochrane Review). In: *The Cochrane Library, Issue 2*. Oxford, UK: Update Software, 2001.

Prentice A, Deary AJ, Goldbeck-Wood S, et al. Gonadotropin-releasing hormone analogues for pain associated with endometriosis (Cochrane Review). In: *The Cochrane Library, Issue 2*. Oxford, UK: Update Software, 2001.

Rapkin AJ, Kames LD, Darke LL, et al. History of physical and sexual abuse in women with chronic pain. *Obstet Gynecol* 1990;76:92.

Raskin DE. Diagnosis in patients with chronic pelvic pain [Letter]. *Am J Psychiatry* 1984;141:824.

Redwine DB. Conservative laparoscopic excision of endometriosis by sharp dissection: life table analysis of reoperation and persistent or recurrent disease. *Fertil Steril* 1991;56:628.

Reiter RC. Occult somatic pathology in women with chronic pelvic pain. *Clin Obstet Gynecol* 1990;33:154.

Reiter RC, Gambone JC. Demographic and historic variables in women with idiopathic chronic pelvic pain. *Obstet Gynecol* 1990;75:428.

Rudy TE, Kerns RD, Turk DC. Chronic pain and depression: toward a cognitive-behavioral mediation model. *Pain* 1988;35:129.

Seaman HE, Ballard KD, Wright JT, et al. Endometriosis and its coexistence with irritable bowel syndrome and pelvic inflammatory disease: findings from a national case-control study—Part 2. *Br J Obstet Gynaecol* 2008;115:1392.

Selak V, Farquhar C, Prentice A, et al. Danazol for pelvic pain associated with endometriosis (Cochrane Review). In: *The Cochrane Library, Issue 2*. Oxford, UK: Update Software, 2001.

Simons DG, Travell J. Myofascial trigger points: a possible explanation. *Pain* 1981;10:100.

Sinaki M, Merritt JL, Stillwell GK. Tension myalgia of the pelvic floor. *Mayo Clin Proc* 1977;52:717.

Sinaii N, Cleary SD, Ballweg ML, et al. High rates of autoimmune and endocrine disorders, fibromyalgia, chronic fatigue syndrome and atopic diseases among women with endometriosis: a survey analysis. *Hum Reprod* 2002;17:2715.

Slocumb J. Neurological factors in chronic pelvic pain: trigger points and the abdominal pelvic pain syndrome. *Am J Obstet Gynecol* 1984;149:536.

Slocumb JC, Kellner R, Rosenfeld RC, et al. Anxiety and depression in patients with the abdominal pelvic pain syndrome. *Gen Hosp Psychiatry* 1989;11:48.

Soysal ME, Soysal S, Vicdan K, et al. A randomized controlled trial of goserelin and medroxyprogesterone acetate in the treatment of pelvic congestion. *Hum Reprod* 2001;16:931.

Steege JF. Dyspareunia and vaginismus. *Clin Obstet Gynecol* 1984; 27:750.

Steege JF. Ovarian remnant syndrome. *Obstet Gynecol* 1987;70:64.

Steege JF, Metzger DA, Levy BS. *Chronic pelvic pain: an integrated approach*. Philadelphia, PA: WB Saunders, 1998.

Steege JF, Stout AL. Resolution of chronic pelvic pain following laparoscopic adhesiolysis. *Am J Obstet Gynecol* 1991;165:278.

Steege JF, Stout AL, Somkuti SG. Chronic pelvic pain: toward an integrative model. *Obstet Gynecol Surv* 1993;48:95.

Stout AL, Steege JF. *Psychosocial and behavioral self-reports of chronic pelvic pain patients*. Presented at the meeting of the American Society for Psychosomatic Obstetrics and Gynecology, Houston, TX, March 1991.

Stout AL, Steege JF, Dodson WC, et al. Relationship of laparoscopic findings to self-report of pelvic pain. *Am J Obstet Gynecol* 1991;164:73.

Stovall TG, Ling FW, Crawford DA. Hysterectomy for chronic pelvic pain of presumed uterine etiology. *Obstet Gynecol* 1990; 75:676.

Summitt RL, Ling FW. Urethral syndrome presenting as chronic pelvic pain. *J Psychosom Obstet Gynaecol* 1991;12:77.

Sutton CJ, Ewen SP, Whitelaw N, et al. Prospective, randomized, double blind controlled trial of laser laparoscopy in the treatment of pelvic pain associated with minimal, mild, and moderate endometriosis. *Fertil Steril* 1994;62:696.

Sutton C, MacDonald R. Laser laparoscopic adhesiolysis. *J Gynecol Surg* 1990;6:155.

Sutton CJ, Pooley AS, Ewen SP, et al. Follow-up report on a randomized, controlled trial of laser laparoscopy in the treatment of pelvic pain associated with minimal to moderate endometriosis. *Fertil Steril* 1997;68:1070.

Tu FF, Hahn D, Steege JF. Pelvic congestion syndrome-associated pelvic pain: a systematic review of diagnosis and management. *Obstet Gynecol Surv* 2010;65:332.

Tulandi T. Adhesion reformation after reproductive surgery with and without the carbon dioxide laser. *Fertil Steril* 1987;47:704.

Tulandi T. Salpingo-ovariolysis: a comparison between laser surgery and electrosurgery. *Fertil Steril* 1986;45:489.

Vercellini P, Fedele L, Aimi G, et al. Association between endometriosis stage, lesion type, patient characteristics and severity of pelvic pain symptoms: a multivariate analysis of over 1000 patients. *Hum Reprod* 2007;22:266.

Vercellini P, Trespidi L, Colombo A, et al. A gonadotropin-releasing hormone agonist versus a low-dose oral contraceptive for pelvic pain with endometriosis. *Fertil Steril* 1993;60:75.

Walker EW, Katon W, Harrop-Griffiths J, et al. Relationship of chronic pelvic pain to psychiatric diagnoses and childhood sexual abuse. *Am J Psychiatry* 1988;145:75.

Walters MD. Definitive surgery. In: Schenken RS, ed. *Endometriosis: contemporary concepts in clinical management*. Philadelphia, PA: JB Lippincott, 1989:267.

Warren JW, Morozov V, Howard FM. Could chronic pelvic pain be a functional somatic syndrome? *Am J Obstet Gynecol* 2011; 205:199.

Williams RE, Hartmann KE, Sandler RS, et al. Recognition and treatment of irritable bowel syndrome among women with chronic pelvic pain. *Am J Obstet Gynecol* 2005;192:761.

Winkel CA, Bray M. Treatment of women with endometriosis using excision alone, ablation alone, or ablation in combination with leuprolide acetate. *Proceedings of the 5th World Congress on Endometriosis*, Yokahama, Japan, 1996:55.

Zullo F, Palomba S, Zupi E, et al. Effectiveness of presacral neurectomy in women with severe dysmenorrhea caused by endometriosis who were treated with laparoscopic conservative surgery: a 1-year prospective randomized double-blind controlled trial. *Am J Obstet Gynecol* 2003;189:5.

CHAPTER 30
Pelvic Inflammatory Disease

Mark G. Martens

DEFINITIONS

Bacterial vaginosis (BV)—A vaginal condition demonstrated by a replacement of the normal lactobacillus-predominant vaginal flora with a mixture of facultative and obligate anaerobes, mycoplasma, and other species, resulting in a malodorous discharge. The presence of *Gardnerella vaginalis* without symptoms is not synonymous with BV.

Colpotomy—Incision into and through the vaginal epithelium into a cavity (often abscess or pelvic/abdominal cavity).

Febrile morbidity—Temperature equal to or greater than 100.4°F or 38°C on two separate occasions (>4 hours apart), starting 24 hours after the initiating event.

Fever—Temperature equal to or greater than 99.6°F or 37.5°C.

Lower genital tract infection (LGTI)—An alternative term used to describe infection limited to the cervix and/or vulva and vagina.

Mollicutes—Class of organisms that includes *Chlamydia, Mycoplasma, Ureaplasma,* and other species.

Outpatient therapy—Previously synonymous with oral therapy; however, the term now includes oral, ambulatory intravenous, or intermittent injectable therapies.

Parenteral therapy—Usually denotes intravenous (antibiotic) therapy, but not necessarily given while hospitalized.

Pelvic inflammatory disease (PID)—A general term used to refer to infection and inflammation of the upper genital tract in women.

Phlegmon—A massive infiltration of inflammatory cells into infected soft tissue resulting not in an abscess, but a "woody induration" sensation upon examination/palpation.

Prevotella—Newly named genus that now includes several species formerly called Bacteroides (e.g., *Bacteroides bivia*).

Salpingitis—Infection/inflammation of one or both of the fallopian tubes (often incorrectly used as an equivalent to all PID).

Tuboovarian abscess (TOA)—A term used to describe an abscess incorporating the fallopian tube and ovary.

Upper genital tract infection (UGTI)—A more descriptive term used alternatively to PID.

Pelvic inflammatory disease (PID) is one of the most serious infections faced by women today. Also, it is one of the most common gynecologic reasons for hospitalization and emergency department visits in the United States each year.

Untreated or unsuccessfully treated women may suffer life-threatening consequences, and even adequately treated women are at much higher risk for potentially serious sequelae. PID is a spectrum of diseases initially involving the cervix, uterus, and fallopian tubes. Acute PID, the acute clinical syndrome, is most often attributed to an ascending spread of microorganisms from the vagina and endocervix to the endometrium, fallopian tubes, and contiguous structures. The terms *acute PID* and *acute salpingitis* are often used interchangeably, but PID is not limited to tubal infection only. A more descriptive term to differentiate the severity and extent of various forms of PID was introduced by Hemsell and colleagues: *upper genital tract infection (UGTI)*. This is differentiated from *lower genital tract infection (LGTI)* because response to treatment appears to be different in these two entities. PID has also been categorized into inpatient or outpatient treatment groups. However, this may not accurately reflect the severity of illness, but rather the predictive accuracy of the caregiver for hospitalization.

EPIDEMIOLOGY

Sexually transmitted infections (STIs) have been reported at epidemic proportions in the United States, with the Centers for Disease Control and Prevention (CDC) estimating almost 20 million new infections each year at a cost of $6 billion each year. The incidence of *Chlamydia trachomatis* infections has increased 8% since 2010, to a rate of 458 per 100,000 people, with a total of 1,412,791 cases reported in 2011 (**Fig. 30.1**).

Neisseria gonorrhoeae incidence has also increased to 4% since 2010 with a rate of 104 per 100,000 people, with more than 320,000 cases reported in 2011 in the United States. For women, acute PID is the most common and important complication of STIs. Bell and Holmes in the 1980s estimated that 1 million women a year were treated for acute salpingitis in the United States, but recent estimates by Sutton and colleagues estimated a decrease in cases of PID to approximately 770,000 per year and a 68% decrease in hospitalized PID from 1995 to 2001.

The CDC estimates that of the 750,000 to 1 million women per year who experience an episode of PID, up to 15% will become infertile as a result of the infection. Hospitalization rates have been declining over the past decade. However, it is uncertain if this is due to decreasing incidence of the disease or a change in clinical management to treat more patients as outpatients. A consequence of the latter scenario is that despite

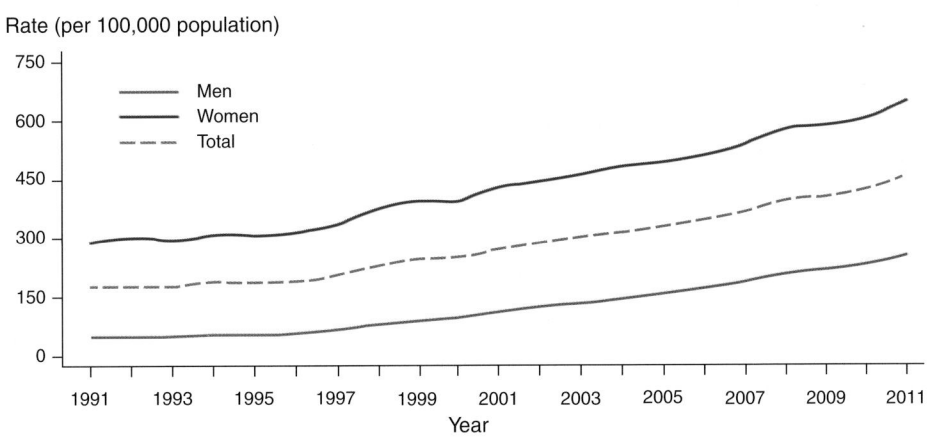

Rate (per 100,000 population)

FIGURE 30.1 Chlamydia rates by sex, United States, 1991–2011. (Data from the Centers for Disease Control.)

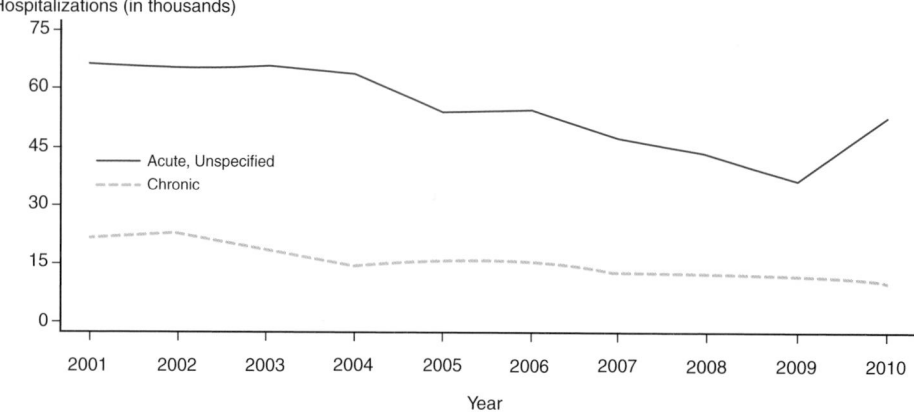

FIGURE 30.2 PID—Hospitalizations of women aged 15 to 44 years, United States, 2001–2010. (Data from the Centers for Disease Control.)

the long-term trend of decreased hospitalization, as confirmed by Sørbye and colleagues (35% reduction in hospitalized cases of PID), they also found that there was a 65% increase ($P = 0.013$) of tuboovarian abscesses in these patients.

However, after hitting an all-time low in hospitalizations for PID in 2009, there was a marked increase in 2009 to 2010, and we are anxious to see if this will become a long-term trend (Fig. 30.2).

In addition to the 200,000 women who are hospitalized each year with a diagnosis of salpingitis or PID, the disease also generates nearly 2.5 million visits to physicians and an estimated 150,000 surgical procedures for complications every year. In terms of overall incidence, acute PID occurs in 10% to 15% of women during their lifetime, with a diagnosis in 1% to 2% of young, sexually active women each year. Therefore, PID is the most common serious bacterial infection in women aged 16 to 25 years, and the resultant morbidity exceeds that produced by all other infections combined for this age group.

ETIOLOGY

Within certain geographic areas or populations, *N. gonorrhoeae* is a common cause of PID. However, most cases of acute PID are the result of a polymicrobial infection caused by organisms ascending from the vagina and cervix to infect the lining of the endometrium and fallopian tubes. Approximately 85% of cases are spontaneous, noniatrogenic infections that occur in sexually active women of reproductive age. The remaining 15% of infections occur after procedures that break the cervical mucous barrier, such as with the placement of an intrauterine device (IUD), endometrial biopsy, or uterine curettage, which allow vaginal flora to infect the upper genital tract.

In the United States, nontuberculous PID was traditionally separated into gonococcal and nongonococcal disease, depending on the isolation of *N. gonorrhoeae* from the endocervix. However, a variety of organisms can be isolated from the endocervix. Therefore, it is difficult to determine which of these organisms cause PID and which are coexistent cervicovaginal flora representing vaginal colonizers in the upper genital tract at time of diagnosis. While upper genital tract organisms are probably more indicative of the causative organisms, they are often difficult to obtain without suspecting endocervical contamination from the diagnostic procedure. However, studies by Martens and colleagues of transcervical cultures of the infected uterine cavities did not find significant contamination with this approach with either protected catheters or suction curettes. Bacterial organisms cultured directly from tubal fluid may commonly include *N. gonorrhoeae*, *C. trachomatis*,

endogenous aerobic and anaerobic bacteria, and genital *Mycoplasma* species. Laparoscopic studies have demonstrated a correlation of no more than 50% between endocervical and tubal cultures, but the presence of *N. gonorrhoeae* is almost always considered an important causative factor. Even in the presence of *N. gonorrhoeae*, direct fallopian tube cultures have demonstrated that tubal infections are often polymicrobial. The type and number of species vary depending on the stage of the disease. Gonorrhea, for example, is often cultured from the cervix during the first 24 to 48 hours of the disease but is often absent later. Similarly, fewer organisms are cultured late in the disease, and anaerobic bacteria such as *Prevotella*, *Bacteroides*, *Peptococcus*, and *Peptostreptococcus* species tend to predominate. Whether these anaerobes play a causative role or increase in number and frequency as a result of the inflammatory response is uncertain. Sweet has summarized the literature by stating that in approximately one third of women with PID, *N. gonorrhoeae* is the only organism recovered by direct tubal or cul-de-sac culture, one third have a culture positive for *N. gonorrhoeae* plus a mixture of endogenous aerobic and anaerobic flora, and the remaining third have only aerobic and anaerobic organisms. Chow and colleagues and Monif and colleagues have postulated that the intense inflammatory nature of gonococcus may initiate acute PID and produce tissue damage. This damage changes the local environment, which in turn allows anaerobic and aerobic organisms from the vaginal and cervical flora to invade the upper genital tract. Both Eschenbach and Sweet have suggested that not all PID follows gonococcal infection and that acute PID initially may also have a polymicrobial etiology.

According to Sweet and Gibbs, approximately 20% of all women with salpingitis have tubal cultures positive for *C. trachomatis*. Also, both *N. gonorrhoeae* and *C. trachomatis* are found in the same individual 25% to 40% of the time. Scandinavian studies by Eilard and coworkers have reported the recovery of *C. trachomatis* from the cervix in 22% to 47% of women with acute PID. *C. trachomatis* by itself produces a mild form of salpingitis with an insidious onset. In contrast to gonorrhea, *Chlamydia* can remain in the fallopian tubes for months or years after initial colonization of the upper genital tract. Svensson and colleagues found that women with *C. trachomatis* infection at laparoscopy had the most severe fallopian tube involvement, probably because of its clinically silent or minimally symptomatic nature, which results in difficult or delayed diagnosis and therefore delayed or absent treatment. The two major sequelae of acute PID are tubal infertility and ectopic pregnancy. These have been strongly associated with prior chlamydial infection as a consequence of intratubal and peritubal adhesions.

Although *C. trachomatis* is generally believed to be one of the most common causes of PID, its etiologic role is very different when compared to *N. gonorrhoeae*. *N. gonorrhoeae* is a Gram-negative diplococcus with rapid growth that is due to a short reproductive cycle of about 20 to 40 minutes to divide. This results in a logarithmic increase in the number of organisms once *N. gonorrhoeae* reaches a relatively sterile area such as the endometrium or fallopian tube, where growth is relatively unimpeded. This rapid increase in the number of Gram-negative bacteria usually results in a rapid and intense inflammatory response by the woman's host defenses. The response to this rapid bacterial growth is proliferation and aggregation of white blood cells (WBCs) and their inflammatory products. Migration of this bacterial and leukocytic mixture in two directions, both through the fallopian tube to the ovary and peritoneal cavity and back to the cervix and vagina, causes the symptoms that are pathognomonic of acute PID—abdominal/pelvic pain and cervicovaginal discharge.

For years, *N. gonorrhoeae* was thought to be the primary PID pathogen. Its often severe immunologic response, mostly due to its release of lipopolysaccharide, resulted in acute and severe pain, high fevers, and a marked WBC response. This triad resulted in an easily recognized clinical course, a prompt diagnosis and often early hospitalization, and initiation of antibiotic treatment.

Chlamydia trachomatis, however, is a slow-growing intracellular organism. Its lack of mitochondria results in its obligatory intracellular existence and also causes its growth cycle to be extremely slow compared with *N. gonorrhoeae* and other nonintracellular microorganisms. The growth cycle of *Chlamydia* is 48 to 72 hours; therefore, several weeks to months are required for the growth to reach numbers sufficient to cause clinical symptoms, if at all. Its slow growth does not induce a rapid or violent inflammatory response. This explains the slow and insidious nature of the symptoms of acute *C. trachomatis* infections. However, because of its intracellular growth cycle, the release of elementary bodies (its infectious vehicle) occurs by rupture of the cell that it has invaded. In addition, Linhares and Witkin have eloquently documented the serious immunopathologic consequences of the 60-kDa heat shock protein (hsp60) from *Chlamydia* on the fallopian tube.

Thus, the repeated occurrence of elementary body infection of susceptible cells—and their subsequent destruction by rupture—along with a chronic inflammatory response are the major mechanisms by which *C. trachomatis* causes disease in acute and chronic pelvic infections. Also, because the slow growth and the chronic inflammatory response often result in subtle clinical symptoms, treatment is often delayed or not started at all, adding to the extended tissue destruction and PID sequelae.

The lack of acute symptoms does not lessen the importance of *Chlamydia* as a PID pathogen. Not only does the tissue destruction result in severe complications such as ectopic pregnancy and infertility, but also the tissue damage provides fertile ground for the growth of secondarily infecting aerobic and anaerobic bacteria. This necrotic tissue is an excellent growth medium, and the epithelial damage enhances the breakdown of the surface defense mechanisms. The importance of *Chlamydia* was documented during the 1980s when treatment of acute PID during new antibiotic research trials was initially believed to be successfully accomplished with regimens not active against *C. trachomatis*. However, although success was evident at short-term follow-up, long-term follow-up demonstrated that treatment of *C. trachomatis* was necessary. PID regimens without *Chlamydia* coverage resulted in an increased incidence of recurrent episodes and long-term complications such as abscesses and chronic pelvic pain, with resultant increased

surgical intervention. Therefore, current treatment of PID includes *C. trachomatis* coverage, even though this organism may not be the cause of the acute symptoms. Therefore, despite the lack of immediate and acute symptoms, *Chlamydia* remains an important pathogen in PID, as subtle or absent symptoms are more difficult to diagnose and treat early, resulting in much of the serious long-term sequelae found with PID. This is supported by the high incidence of *Chlamydia* antibodies in patients with acute PID, ectopic pregnancy, and infertility in several studies.

Despite the focus on these two STIs, nongonococcal and nonchlamydial pathogens cause more than 60% of PID infections. Besides *N. gonorrhoeae* and *C. trachomatis*, aerobic and anaerobic bacteria and other microorganisms, particularly other mollicutes, have been implicated as etiologic agents in acute salpingitis.

Haggerty et al., Cohen et al., Short et al., and others have all demonstrated the clinical significance of *Mycoplasma genitalium* in PID. Other novel pathogens are certain to be identified as the Human Microbiome Project identifies new, difficult-to-culture organisms found to be associated with PID.

However, *M. genitalium* is the current pathogen generating much attention after recent studies by Clausen et al. and Svenstrup and colleagues have found an association with *M. genitalium* and tubal factor infertility. More importantly, current PID treatment regimens may not adequately treat *M. genitalium*. Since it is a mollicute similar to *Chlamydia*, it lacks a cell wall and thus is resistant to cell wall–inhibiting antibiotics such as the penicillins and cephalosporins.

Also, studies by Björnelius and Falk and their colleagues in men and women with *M. genitalium* have found persistence of the organism despite treatment with levofloxacin and tetracyclines. However, these same researchers have found azithromycin to have better activity against *M. genitalium*. Moxifloxacin, a newer quinolone, also appears to have good in vitro activity.

In the large National Institutes of Health (NIH) PID study called the PID Evaluation and Clinical Health trial, Haggerty reported that 41% of *M. genitalium*–positive women experience microbiologic failure to eradicate the organism with standard Centers for Disease Control (CDC) PID treatment regimens, and more importantly, 44% experienced clinical failure. These results will most certainly be addressed at the next CDC review of PID treatment guidelines scheduled for 2015.

Bacterial vaginosis (BV)-related organisms such as *Gardnerella*, *Mycoplasma hominis*, and *Ureaplasma urealyticum* have also been suggested as causal agents in acute salpingitis by Ness and colleagues. However, their role remains controversial, as other studies have not found an association with PID. Cervical cultures positive for both *M. hominis* and *U. urealyticum* have been recovered from women with PID. However, the rate of isolation can be as high as 75%, which is not statistically different from that of women who are sexually active but without PID (baseline rate of about 50%), as found by Lemeke and Lsonka. Also, Clarke et al. have published evidence that *Cytomegalovirus* (CMV) may be associated with PID, but additional confirmatory investigations are limited.

Group B streptococcus, *Escherichia coli*, and other facultative anaerobic agents are also associated with PID, but fortunately are generally adequately covered by current CDC guidelines. In light of all the new data, the main point to emphasize is that although *N. gonorrhoeae* and *C. trachomatis* are significant pathogens, they are still only associated with 30% to 40% of all PID episodes. Thus, while current standard of care requires testing for both these organisms, negative results do not mean the patient does not have PID, and treatment should be initiated or completed based on the patient clinical course or additional microbiologic testing if possible.

RISK FACTORS

Several factors that predispose to the development of acute PID have been identified. Risk factors are important considerations in both the clinical management and prevention of UGTIs. First and foremost, there is a strong correlation between exposure to STIs and PID. In the United States, recent studies have confirmed this association with the recovery of *N. gonorrhoeae* or *C. trachomatis* in 40% to 50% of patients hospitalized with acute PID. Age at first intercourse, frequency of intercourse, number of sexual partners, and marital status are all associated with the frequency of exposure to STIs and thus are associated with PID. Women with multiple partners have an increased risk (four to six times normal) for development of PID, compared with women who have monogamous sexual relations. Additional studies by Ness and colleagues have found significant factors including age at first sex, cervicitis, history of PID, family income, smoking, medroxyprogesterone use, and sex with menses.

The incidence of acute PID decreases with advancing age. Adolescent girls are at significant risk for development of acute salpingitis. Westrom reported that nearly 70% of women with PID were younger than 25 years of age, 33% experienced their first infection before the age of 19, and 75% were nulliparous. The risk for development of acute PID in a sexually active adolescent female patient was 1:8, whereas the risk was 1:80 for a sexually active woman 24 years of age or older. Several reasons have been suggested for this increased risk. The two microorganisms most commonly considered to be the inciting agents in cases of PID, *N. gonorrhoeae* and *C. trachomatis*, have a predilection for columnar epithelium. As suggested by Schaefer and by Sweet and colleagues, cervical columnar epithelium is exposed to a greater extent in younger individuals and recedes into the cervical canal with increasing age.

Clinical and laboratory studies have documented that the use of contraceptives change the relative risk for development of PID. Multiple case–control studies have shown an increased risk of acute PID in women who use an IUD. It has been estimated that IUD users have a threefold to fivefold increased risk for development of acute PID, with the greatest risk the first 20 days after insertion. The incidence of infection has recently been described by Sufrin and colleagues in over 57,000 IUD insertions in California from 2005 to 2009. They reported an overall rate of approximately 1 in 200 patients.

Barrier methods of contraception (condoms, diaphragms, and spermicidal preparations) are effective both as mechanical obstructive devices and as chemical barriers. A nearly 60% decrease in the risk of PID has been demonstrated among women using a barrier method of contraception. Ness and colleagues found a 30% to 60% decrease in recurrent PID in women using condoms consistently.

Oral contraceptives have also been shown to reduce the risk and severity of acute PID. The mechanism for such protection remains speculative. The thicker cervical mucus produced by the progestin component of oral contraceptives is believed to inhibit sperm and accompanying bacteria penetration into the upper genital tract. The decrease in duration of menstrual flow accompanying oral contraceptive use theoretically creates a shorter interval for bacterial colonization. Svensson and coworkers reported that in addition to protecting against PID, the use of oral contraceptive pills was associated with a better prognosis for future fertility than was seen in women with acute PID using other contraceptive methods or no contraceptive methods. The pill's ability to inhibit ovulation also helps prevent an open nidus for tuboovarian abscess formation.

Surgical procedures of the female genital tract also place the patient at risk for PID. About 15% of pelvic infections occur after procedures that break the cervical mucous barrier, allowing for colonization of the upper genital tract. Eschenbach and Holmes reported that these procedures include endometrial biopsy, curettage, IUD insertion, hysteroscopy, and hysterosalpingography. The incidence of UGTI associated with first-trimester abortions is approximately 1 in 200 cases. Recent practice has emphasized the use of prophylactic antibiotics in high-risk cases to attempt to decrease the incidence of iatrogenic acute PID. A randomized trial by Jackson and a randomized trial by the Luton and Dunstable Hospital Study Group have indicated that the treatment of BV with metronidazole substantially reduced postabortion PID.

Acute salpingitis occurring in a woman with a previous tubal ligation was once believed to be rare. However, Phillips and D'Abling reported that acute PID developed in the proximal stump of previously ligated fallopian tubes in 1 of 450 women hospitalized for acute salpingitis. In addition, it is suspected that many cases may be undiagnosed because of the absence of peritoneal signs from the prevention of retrograde spillage of bacteria and inflammatory exudate in the pelvic cavity.

Previous acute PID is also a risk factor for future episodes of the disease. Another acute tubal infection develops in approximately 25% of women who have had acute PID. The exact mechanism for this increased susceptibility has not been determined, but it may be loss of the natural protective mechanisms of the fallopian tube lining against microorganisms. This increased risk may also be related to the sexual habits of the woman involved, such as reinfection from an untreated male partner. Eschenbach has documented that more than 80% of male contacts are not treated.

Genetic factors for PID have been further delineated recently. Paavonen and Taylor et al. have demonstrated that variants in the genes that regulate toll-like receptors can interfere with the innate immune system and are associated with an increased progression of infection, especially with *C. trachomatis*.

DIAGNOSIS

Acute PID presents with a broad spectrum of clinical symptoms. The differential diagnosis of acute PID includes acute appendicitis, endometriosis, torsion or rupture of an adnexal mass, ectopic pregnancy, and cervicitis.

Common clinical manifestations include lower abdominal pain, cervical motion tenderness, and adnexal tenderness and may include fever, cervical discharge, and leukocytosis. Historically, the diagnosis of acute PID was not established unless the patient had the triad of lower abdominal and pelvic pain, fever, and leukocytosis.

Jacobson and Westrom have shown that all three criteria are present in only 15% to 30% of documented PID cases. In fact, 50% of patients initially present with a normal temperature and WBC count. Pain in the lower abdomen and pelvis is by far the most common symptom of acute PID. It occurs in more than 90% of patients at initial presentation. The pain is usually described as constant and dull and is accentuated by motion and sexual activity. Generally, the pain is of recent onset, usually less than 7 days. About 75% of patients with PID have an associated endocervical infection and coexistent purulent vaginal discharge. Nausea and vomiting are relatively late symptoms in the course of the disease. Abnormal vaginal bleeding, especially menorrhagia or spotting, is noted in about 40% of patients. The CDC has established the criteria for making the diagnosis of salpingitis based on clinical grounds. They specify that only signs of pelvic and abdominal pain are required for a potential diagnosis of PID and eliminate leukocytosis and fever as essential criteria (Table 30.1).

TABLE 30.1 Criteria for the Diagnosis of Acute PID

Empirical treatment of PID should be initiated in sexually active young women and other women at risk for STDs if they are experiencing pelvic or lower abdominal pain, if no cause for the illness other than PID can be identified, and if one or more of the following minimum criteria are present on pelvic examination:

- Cervical motion tenderness *or* uterine tenderness *or* adnexal tenderness

The requirement that all three minimum criteria be present before the initiation of empiric treatment could result in insufficient sensitivity for the diagnosis of PID. The presence of signs of lower genital tract inflammation (predominance of leukocytes in vaginal secretions, cervical exudates, or cervical friability), in addition to one of the three minimum criteria, increases the specificity of the diagnosis. Upon deciding whether to initiate empiric treatment, clinicians should also consider the risk profile of the patient for STDs.

More elaborate diagnostic evaluation frequently is needed because incorrect diagnosis and management might cause unnecessary morbidity. One or more of the following criteria can be used to enhance the specificity of the minimum criteria. The following additional criteria can be used to enhance the specificity of the minimum criteria and support a diagnosis of PID:

- Oral temperature >101°F (>38.3°C)
- Abnormal cervical or vaginal mucopurulent discharge
- Presence of abundant numbers of WBC on saline microscopy of vaginal secretions
- Elevated erythrocyte sedimentation rate (ESR)
- Elevated C-reactive protein
- Laboratory documentation of cervical infection with *N. gonorrhoeae* or *C. trachomatis*

Most women with PID have either mucopurulent cervical discharge or evidence of WBCs on a microscopic evaluation of a saline preparation of vaginal fluid (i.e., wet prep). If the cervical discharge appears normal and no WBCs are observed on the wet prep of vaginal fluid, the diagnosis of PID is unlikely, and alternative causes of pain should be considered. A wet prep of vaginal fluid offers the ability to detect the presence of concomitant infections (e.g., BV and trichomoniasis).

The most specific criteria for diagnosing PID include the following:

- Endometrial biopsy with histopathologic evidence of endometritis;
- Transvaginal sonography or magnetic resonance imaging techniques showing thickened, fluid-filled tubes with or without free pelvic fluid or tuboovarian complex, or Doppler studies suggesting pelvic infection (e.g., tubal hyperemia); or
- Laparoscopic abnormalities consistent with PID

A diagnostic evaluation that includes some of these more extensive procedures might be warranted in some cases. Endometrial biopsy is warranted in women undergoing laparoscopy who do not have visual evidence of salpingitis, because endometritis is the only sign of PID for some women.

Abdominal pain can also be associated with perihepatic inflammation and adhesions, more commonly known as the Fitz-Hugh-Curtis syndrome. It is believed to develop in 1% to 10% of patients with acute PID. Signs and symptoms include right upper quadrant pain, pleuritic pain, and tenderness in the right upper quadrant when the liver is palpated (Fig. 30.3). Usually, the symptoms and signs of this syndrome are preceded by the clinical onset of acute PID. Due to the upper abdominal pain, this condition is often mistakenly diagnosed as either acute cholecystitis or pneumonia. Fitz-Hugh-Curtis syndrome is believed to develop from vascular or transperitoneal dissemination of either *N. gonorrhoeae* or *C. trachomatis* to produce the perihepatic inflammation. Other organisms may be involved, but limited data exist on their causality.

Jacobson and Westrom attempted to correlate the clinical diagnosis of acute salpingitis with laparoscopic pelvic findings. Of 814 women in whom laparoscopy was performed for presumed acute PID, 512 (65%) had visual evidence of salpingitis, 184 (23%) had normal visual findings, and 98 (12%) had other pelvic pathology. Because of the positive clinical findings consistent with PID, many of the patients with normal findings were suspected to have early PID with endometritis and endosalpingitis, without the visual evidence of tubal or pelvic damage. Thus, *laparoscopy* is limited as a method of diagnosing the early stages of PID, but it is crucial to rule out the 12% "other" pathology, especially the non-PID surgical emergencies, such as appendicitis, and noninfectious entities requiring different treatment modalities, such as endometriosis or hemorrhagic cyst.

Despite these shortcomings of early diagnosis, laparoscopic visualization of the pelvis is still important as the most

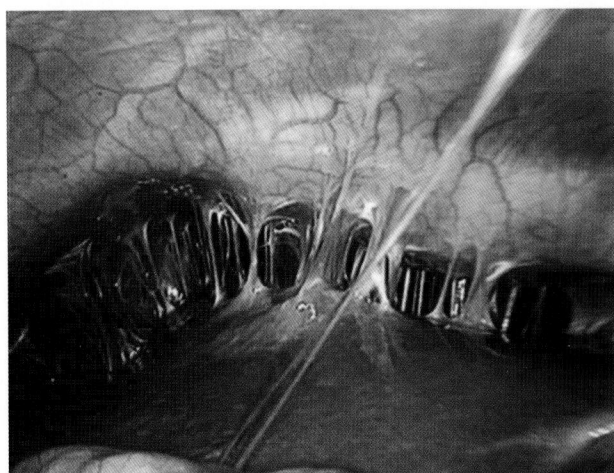

FIGURE 30.3 Violin-string adhesions of chronic Fitz-Hugh-Curtis syndrome. (Image reprinted from Medscape Reference, http://emedicine.medscape.com/, 2013, with permission, available at: http://emedicine.medscape.com/article/256448-overview)

accurate method of confirming the diagnosis and assessing the severity of acute PID. However, it is logistically and economically impractical for all patients suspected of having acute PID to undergo diagnostic laparoscopy in the United States. Therefore, the diagnosis of most episodes of acute PID is often made on the basis of clinical history and physical examination. Although it is suggested that laparoscopy be offered to all patients with an uncertain diagnosis, it is strongly indicated for patients who are not responding to therapy, to confirm the diagnosis, to obtain cultures from the cul-de-sac or fallopian tubes, or to drain pus if necessary. In summary, laparoscopic studies have shown the following:

1. The clinical diagnosis of acute PID may be inaccurate.
2. Acute PID is sometimes found in patients undergoing laparoscopy for other causes of pelvic pain.
3. Laparoscopy is a relatively safe method in most cases for making the visual diagnosis of the latter stages of PID and thus assessing future fertility prognosis and planning.
4. Laparoscopy is an excellent means of obtaining cultures directly from the tube and peritoneal cavity.

The appearance of the pelvic organs can vary from erythematous, indurated, edematous oviducts, to pockets of purulent material, to a large pyosalpinx or tuboovarian abscess. However, although no disease may be evident in early stages, it is imperative to render treatment to all stages to avoid long-term sequelae.

Other less invasive methods of diagnosis have been suggested for verifying a clinical diagnosis of acute PID.

Because most cases of UGTI are associated with and preceded by LGTI, examination of the endocervix for inflammation, Gram stain, and culture for both *N. gonorrhoeae* and *C. trachomatis* are important for proper evaluation. A negative Gram-stained smear of the endocervix does not absolutely rule out upper tract infection. However, most studies have found that acute PID is rare without a concomitant increase in inflammatory cells in the vagina and the cervix.

Endometrial biopsy is one alternative to laparoscopy. Paavonen and associates reported a 90% correlation between histologic endometritis and laparoscopically confirmed salpingitis. However, results may be delayed up to 2 to 3 days, making its clinical applicability limited.

Ultrasonography is of limited value for patients with mild or moderate pelvic PID. Thus, the routine use of sonography in patients with early PID is often not helpful. However, ultrasound is indicated in distinguishing an adnexal mass, especially in patients who demonstrate a lack of response to antimicrobial therapy in the initial 48 to 72 hours of therapy. Sonohysterography, an ultrasound examination using the instillation of saline to better define pelvic structures, is not indicated at this time for patients suspected of having PID, because no studies have been performed to demonstrate its safety in the event that pathogens are dispersed into the upper genital tract in the process of instilling the saline.

Culdocentesis, with evidence of purulent peritoneal fluid, is a helpful, but painful, method to help diagnose acute PID. With acute PID, the WBC count of peritoneal fluid is greater than 30,000 cells/mL, compared with a WBC count of 1,000 cells/mL in women without peritoneal inflammation. However, other infections, such as appendicitis and diverticulitis, among others, can also cause purulent pelvic fluid and a false diagnosis of PID.

Laboratory tests can be obtained, but their results lack sufficient sensitivity and specificity to make them an important factor in establishing the diagnosis. Leukocytosis is not a reliable indicator of acute PID, nor does it accurately correlate with the severity of tubal inflammation or need for hospitalization. Less than 50% of women with acute PID have a WBC count greater than 10,000 cells/mL. Similarly, the erythrocyte sedimentation rate (ESR), which for years was a routine laboratory test for women with acute PID, is nonspecific and is a crude indicator of severity of disease. The ESR is elevated higher than 15 mm/hour in about 75% of women with laparoscopically confirmed acute salpingitis. However, 53% of women with pelvic pain and normal-appearing pelvic organs also have an elevated ESR. Plasma proteins, such as C-reactive protein and antichymotrypsin, have been studied to determine whether they help in the diagnosis of acute PID. They have been found to be more sensitive than the ESR. Other investigators have found that *decreased or absent isoamylase in peritoneal fluid* in cases of acute PID is the best nonculture laboratory test for the disease. The major disadvantages of this test are that it requires several hours to complete and that peritoneal fluid must be obtained.

Other evaluations have revealed various inflammatory cytokines to be associated with pelvic infections; however, these tests are not yet commercially available to a useful extent.

SEQUELAE

Infertility

One fourth of all women who have had acute salpingitis experience one or more long-term sequelae. The most common is involuntary infertility, which occurs in about 20% of patients. Thus, PID ranks as one of the major causes of infertility. Before antibiotic therapy, 50% to 70% of women who had experienced UGTIs became sterile. The sequelae of infections vary from a patent oviduct, to peritubular and periovarian adhesions that may interfere with ovum pickup, and/or to complete tubal obstruction. The infertility rate increases directly with the number of episodes of acute pelvic infection. Also, women with mild disease are seven times less likely to suffer tubal obstruction than women with severe PID.

Ectopic Pregnancy

The chance of ectopic pregnancy is increased 6- to 10-fold in patients with a previous episode of acute salpingitis. Pathologic studies estimate that at least 50% of ectopic pregnancies occur in fallopian tubes damaged by previous salpingitis. The mechanism for the increased rate is believed to be interference of ovum transport through the tube or entrapment of the ovum secondary to intraluminal tubal damage.

Chronic Pelvic Pain

The chance that chronic pelvic pain will develop in a woman after acute salpingitis is four times that of control subjects without pelvic infection (20% vs. 5%). Chronic pelvic pain can be caused by a hydrosalpinx. A hydrosalpinx is presumably the end-stage development of a pyosalpinx. The pain can also be related to adhesions surrounding the tube and ovary. All patients with chronic pelvic pain believed to be caused by acute PID should undergo laparoscopy or laparotomy to establish the cause of the chronic pain and rule out other diseases such as endometriosis, which require different treatment, or the presence of pelvic adhesions, which can often be directly resolved.

A tuboovarian complex is a collection of pus within an anatomic space created by adherence to adjacent organs. The incidence of true adnexal abscess is about 10% in women with acute PID. Landers and Sweet noted a 20% rate of early treatment failure (after 48 to 72 hours) of antibiotic therapy as a result of persistent pain or enlargement of a tuboovarian abscess or complex. In addition, according to Landers and Sweet, 31% required an operation several weeks to months after their acute infections for persistent disease or pain.

MORTALITY

Before antibiotic therapy, the mortality rate associated with acute PID was 1%. Most of these deaths resulted from rupture of tuboovarian abscesses. Today, death associated with PID is rare, as effective antibiotic treatment is frequently initiated. However, the mortality rate can still be as high as 5% to 10% for ruptured tuboovarian abscesses, if treatment is delayed or inadequate. Death is mostly the result of subsequent development of adult respiratory distress syndrome (ARDS), a condition often associated with serious infection or delayed treatment after intra-abdominal spillage of pus and bacteria.

TREATMENT

The therapeutic goals in the management of acute PID include both elimination of the acute infection and symptoms and prevention of long-term sequelae such as infertility, ectopic pregnancy, and chronic pelvic pain. Antibiotic treatment should be started as soon as cultures have been obtained and diagnosis is confirmed or strongly suspected. Treatment is based on the consensus that PID is polymicrobial in cause. Empirical antibiotic protocols should cover a wide range of bacteria, including *N. gonorrhoeae, C. trachomatis,* anaerobic rods and cocci, Gram-negative aerobic rods, Gram-positive aerobes, and *Mycoplasma* species. Despite general agreement that broad-spectrum therapy is appropriate, questions persist regarding optimal therapeutic regimens.

Controversy has arisen over the issue of outpatient treatment with oral antibiotics versus inpatient treatment with parenteral antibiotics. There is limited data available to evaluate the efficacy of hospital versus ambulatory management of acute PID, due to the ethics of randomizing seriously ill PID patients to outpatient therapy. However, in the United States, three of four women with acute pelvic infection are treated as outpatients for their disease.

In Scandinavia, which has a different health care system, most women are treated as inpatients. In 2010, the CDC published recommended treatment guidelines for outpatient management of acute PID (Table 30.2). Some of the treatment regimens are based on the controversial premise that it may be adequate to cover just a few of the major etiologic agents (*N. gonorrhoeae* and *C. trachomatis*) involved in acute PID. As a result, studies have documented a 10% to 20% treatment failure rate for women receiving oral antibiotics as outpatients compared with a 5% to 10% failure rate for women without an abscess receiving intravenous antibiotics as inpatients, where broader coverage is used.

It is important to reevaluate patients within 48 to 72 hours of initiating outpatient therapy to determine the response of the disease. If a poor response has been obtained, the patient should be hospitalized with parenteral antibiotics and possible laparoscopic evaluation in the hope of preventing or limiting the sequelae of PID or discovering a different diagnosis, such as appendicitis or diverticulitis.

Ideally, every woman with acute PID should be hospitalized for the first few days for parenteral antibiotic treatment. Because this may not be practical because of limited economic or physical facility resources, the clinician who diagnoses acute PID in the office or emergency department is faced with the question of which patient to hospitalize. Indications for the hospitalization of patients with acute PID are also defined by the CDC in the 2010 guidelines (Table 30.3). In the past, the CDC has suggested that all adolescents with PID be hospitalized because of their high noncompliance rate and to optimize treatment to prevent damage to the reproductive tract, which could affect future fertility and/or result in chronic pelvic pain. Recently, Kelly and colleagues found a high incidence of recurrence in adolescents, perhaps related to poor compliance. However, the CDC's new policy is to use the same criteria for hospitalization as for older women. This recommendation is not agreed upon by all infectious disease groups because of the seriousness of inadequately treated PID in a younger, often noncompliant population.

Another indication for hospitalization is the presence of an adnexal or pelvic abscess. Outpatient therapy may not provide antibiotic levels high enough to penetrate an abscess, and rupture of the abscess may have serious consequences.

Also, women in whom the definitive diagnosis of acute PID is in question should also be hospitalized, and additional diagnostic measures should be instituted. As previously stated, at least 10% of all patients have other serious diagnoses, such as acute appendicitis, ectopic pregnancy, or adnexal torsion, and these should be ruled out. Patients with serious illness, patients with nausea and vomiting, patients who are unable to follow or tolerate outpatient therapy, and patients with a previously failed outpatient oral regimen also should be hospitalized and given parenteral antibiotics. A trial by Ness and colleagues investigating the outcomes in patients randomized to inpatient or outpatient did not find differences in short-term outcomes, but difficulties in patient selection and randomization may not permit these results to be applicable to all PID patients.

The 2010 CDC guidelines for inpatient treatment of acute PID describe two regimens (Table 30.4). Regimen A is a combination of oral or parenteral doxycycline plus intravenous cefoxitin or cefotetan. Other third-generation cephalosporins can be substituted, such as ceftizoxime (Cefizox) or cefotaxime (Claforan). All of these agents are effective against penicillinase-producing *N. gonorrhoeae, Peptostreptococcus,* and other anaerobic species, as well as *E. coli* and other aerobic (facultative) species. Ceftriaxone is recommended by the CDC; however, its poor anaerobic activity and lack of controlled trials in PID patients do not make it an acceptable alternative for several investigators. Doxycycline can be given intravenously if the patient is unable to tolerate oral therapy, but it must be infused very slowly to prevent pain and sclerosis of the vein. Oral doxycycline has been demonstrated to be equally effective as parenteral doxycycline because of the slow growth cycle of *Chlamydia* and the requirement of prolonged treatment.

A recent study by Viberga and colleagues investigating the microbiology of IUD-related infection found an increased recovery of *Fusobacterium* and *Peptostreptococcus* species, which generally are covered by both cephalosporin and clindamycin. A possible disadvantage of the cephalosporin–doxycycline combination is that these two antibiotics may be less than ideal for anaerobic infections such as in a pelvic abscess.

Regimen B is a combination of clindamycin and an aminoglycoside (gentamicin). This combination provides excellent activity against anaerobes, Gram-negative aerobes, and Gram-positive aerobes. Historically, it has been the preferred regimen for patients with an abscess, IUD-related infections, or pelvic infections after a diagnostic or operative procedure. However, there are few data to prove that it is significantly more effective than the cephalosporin regimens. A possible disadvantage of regimen B is that it may not provide optimal activity against *C. trachomatis* and *N. gonorrhoeae.* Clindamycin in high doses (900 mg in 8 hours) has good activity against *Chlamydia,* and in vitro studies by Martens and colleagues have demonstrated

TABLE 30.2 CDC-Recommended Treatment Regimen for Oral Therapy of Acute PID

Outpatient oral therapy can be considered for women with mild to moderately severe acute PID, because the clinical outcomes among women treated with oral therapy are similar to those treated with parenteral therapy. The following regimens provide coverage against the frequent etiologic agents of PID. Patients who do not respond to oral therapy within 72 h should be reevaluated to confirm the diagnosis and should be administered parenteral therapy on either an outpatient or inpatient basis.

Ceftriaxone 250 mg IM in a single dose

PLUS
Doxycycline 100 mg orally twice a day for 14 d

WITH OR WITHOUT
Metronidazole 500 mg orally twice a day for 14 d

OR
Cefoxitin 2 g IM in a single dose and probenecid, 1 g orally administered concurrently in a single dose

PLUS
Doxycycline 100 mg orally twice a day for 14 d

WITH OR WITHOUT
Metronidazole 500 mg orally twice a day for 14 d

OR
Other parenteral third-generation cephalosporin (e.g., ceftizoxime or cefotaxime)

PLUS
Doxycycline 100 mg orally twice a day for 14 d

WITH OR WITHOUT
Metronidazole 500 mg orally twice a day for 14 d
The optimal choice of a cephalosporin is unclear; although cefoxitin has better anaerobic coverage, ceftriaxone has better coverage against *N. gonorrhoeae*. A single dose of cefoxitin is effective in obtaining short-term clinical response in women who have PID. However, the theoretical limitations in its coverage of anaerobes may require the addition of metronidazole to the treatment regimen. Adding metronidazole also will effectively treat BV, which is frequently associated with PID. No data have been published regarding the use of oral cephalosporins for the treatment of PID.

Alternative Oral Regimens
Although information regarding other outpatient regimens is limited, other regimens have undergone at least one clinical trial and have demonstrated broad-spectrum coverage. In a single clinical trial, amoxicillin/clavulanic acid and doxycycline were effective together in obtaining short-term clinical response; however, gastrointestinal symptoms might limit compliance with this regimen. Azithromycin has demonstrated short-term effectiveness in one randomized trial, and in another study, it was effective when used in combination with ceftriaxone 250 mg IM single dose and azithromycin 1 g orally once a week for 2 wk. When considering alternative regimens, the addition of metronidazole should be considered, because anaerobic organisms are suspected in the etiology of PID and metronidazole will also treat BV.
As a result of the emergence of quinolone-resistant *Neisseria gonorrhoeae*, regimens that include a quinolone agent are no longer recommended for the treatment of PID. If parenteral cephalosporin therapy is not feasible, use of fluoroquinolones (levofloxacin 500 mg orally once daily or ofloxacin 400 mg twice daily for 14 d) with or without metronidazole (500 mg orally twice daily for 14 d) can be considered if the community prevalence and individual risk for gonorrhea are low. Diagnostic tests for gonorrhea must be performed before instituting therapy and the patient managed as follows if the test is positive.

• Laparoscopic abnormalities consistent with PID. If the culture for gonorrhea is positive, treatment should be based on results of antimicrobial susceptibility.
• If the isolate is determined to be quinolone-resistant *N. gonorrhoeae* or if antimicrobial susceptibility cannot be assessed (e.g., if only nucleic acid amplification testing is available), parenteral cephalosporin is recommended. However, if cephalosporin therapy is not feasible, the addition of azithromycin 2 g orally as a single dose to a quinolone-based PID regimen is recommended.

effectiveness against 90% of *C. trachomatis* strains. Doxycycline is the most effective chlamydial agent, according to in vitro testing, but needs to be used for at least 7 days to complete treatment when the patient is switched from parenteral to posthospitalization therapy. Also, the CDC recommendation of once-daily dosing for gentamicin is not based on any data on PID patients and should be used only if indicated for renal considerations until more studies are completed.

Each regimen stresses two concepts: the polymicrobial etiology of acute pelvic infection and the necessity of protecting against *C. trachomatis* and *N. gonorrhoeae*. With both regimens, the CDC recommends a minimum of at least 24 hours of intravenous treatment after clinical improvement. Both protocols also require completion of a 14-day course of oral antibiotics (doxycycline or clindamycin) to eradicate slow-growing organisms such as *C. trachomatis* and other mollicutes.

TABLE 30.3 Criteria for Hospitalization of Patients with Acute PID

In women with PID of mild or moderate clinical severity, outpatient therapy yields short- and long-term clinical outcomes similar to inpatient therapy. The decision of whether hospitalization is necessary should be based on the judgment of the provider and whether the patient meets any of the following suggested criteria:

- Surgical emergencies (such as appendicitis) cannot be excluded.
- The patient is pregnant.
- The patient does not respond clinically to oral antimicrobial therapy.
- The patient is unable to follow or tolerate an outpatient oral regimen.
- The patient has severe illness, nausea and vomiting, or high fever.
- The patient has a tuboovarian abscess.

No evidence is available to suggest that adolescents benefit from hospitalization for treatment of PID. The decision to hospitalize adolescents with acute PID should be based on the same criteria used for older women. Younger women with mild-to-moderate acute PID have similar outcomes with either outpatient or inpatient therapy, and clinical response to outpatient treatment is similar among younger and older women.

TABLE 30.4 CDC-Recommended Treatment Regimens for Parenteral Therapy of Acute PID

REGIMEN A
Cefotetan 2 g IV every 12 h

OR
Cefoxitin 2 g IV every 6 h

PLUS
Doxycycline 100 mg orally or IV every 12 h
Because of the pain associated with intravenous infusion, doxycycline should be administered orally when possible. Oral and IV administration of doxycycline provides similar bioavailability.
Parenteral therapy can be discontinued 24 h after clinical improvement, but oral therapy with doxycycline (100 mg twice a day) should continue to complete 14 d of therapy. When tuboovarian abscess is present, clindamycin or metronidazole with doxycycline can be used for continued therapy rather than doxycycline alone, because this regimen provides more effective anaerobic coverage.
Limited data are available to support the use of other second- or third-generation cephalosporins (e.g., ceftizoxime, cefotaxime, and ceftriaxone), which also might be effective therapy for PID and could potentially replace cefotetan or cefoxitin. However, these cephalosporins are less active than cefotetan or cefoxitin against anaerobic bacteria.

Regimen B
Clindamycin 900 mg IV every 8 h

PLUS
Gentamicin loading dose IV or IM (2 mg/kg of body weight) followed by a maintenance dose (1.5 mg/kg) every 8 h. Single daily dosing (3–5 mg/kg) can be substituted.
Although use of a single daily dose of gentamicin has not been evaluated for the treatment of PID, it is efficacious in analogous situations. Parenteral therapy can be discontinued 24 h after clinical improvement; ongoing oral therapy should consist of doxycycline 100 mg orally twice a day or clindamycin 450 mg orally four times a day to complete a total of 14 d of therapy. When tuboovarian abscess is present, clindamycin should be continued rather than doxycycline, because clindamycin provides more effective anaerobic coverage.

Alternative Parenteral Regimens
Limited data are available to support the use of other parenteral regimens. The following regimen has been investigated in at least one clinical trial and has broad-spectrum coverage.
Ampicillin/sulbactam 3 g IV every 6 h

PLUS
Doxycycline 100 mg orally or IV every 12 h
Ampicillin/sulbactam plus doxycycline is effective against *C. trachomatis*, *N. gonorrhoeae*, and anaerobes in women with tuboovarian abscess. One trial demonstrated high short-term clinical cure rates with azithromycin, either as monotherapy for 1 wk (500 mg IV for one or two doses followed by 250 mg orally for 5–6 d) or combined with a 12-day course of metronidazole.

V

Alternative inpatient parenteral regimens are included in the 2010 CDC PID guidelines (Table 30.4). The CDC lists only the β-lactamase inhibitor combination ampicillin–sulbactam (Unasyn), but piperacillin–tazobactam combination has been demonstrated by Hemsell and colleagues, Sweet and colleagues, and others to have excellent in vitro and in vivo activity against PID and its pathogens and does have an FDA-approved indication for the treatment of pelvic infections.

MANAGEMENT OF SEX PARTNERS

According to the CDC:

Male sex partners of women with PID should be examined and treated if they had sexual contact with the patient during the 60 days preceding the patient's onset of symptoms. If a patient's last sexual intercourse was less than 60 days before onset of symptoms or diagnosis, the patient's most recent sex partner should be treated. Patients should be instructed to abstain from sexual intercourse until therapy is completed and until they and their sex partners no longer have symptoms. Evaluation and treatment are imperative because of the risk for reinfection of the patient and the strong likelihood of urethral gonococcal or chlamydial infection in the sex partner. Male partners of women who have PID caused by *C. trachomatis* and/or *N. gonorrhoeae* frequently are asymptomatic.

Sex partners should be treated empirically with regimens effective against both of these infections, regardless of the etiology of PID or pathogens isolated from the infected woman. Even in clinical settings in which only women are treated, arrangements should be made to provide care or appropriate referral for male sex partners of women who have PID. Expedited partner treatment and enhanced patient referral are alternative approaches to treating male partners of women who have chlamydial or gonococcal infections.

HIV INFECTION

Differences in the clinical manifestations of PID between human immunodeficiency virus (HIV)-infected women and HIV-negative women have not been well delineated. In early observational studies, HIV-infected women with PID were more likely to require surgical intervention. In recent, more comprehensive observational and controlled studies, HIV-infected women with PID had similar symptoms when compared with uninfected controls. They were more likely to have a tuboovarian abscess, but responded equally to standard parenteral and oral antibiotic regimens when compared with HIV-negative women. The microbiologic findings for HIV-positive and HIV-negative women were similar, except for (a) higher rates of concomitant *M. hominis*, *Candida*, streptococcal, and HPV infections and (b) HPV-related cytologic abnormalities among those with HIV infection. Regardless of these data, whether the management of immunodeficient HIV-infected women with PID requires more aggressive interventions (e.g., hospitalization or parenteral antimicrobial regimens) had not been determined.

Intrauterine Contraceptive Devices

Also, per CDC guidelines:

IUDs are popular contraceptive choices for women. Both levonorgestrel and copper-containing devices are marketed in the United States. The risk for PID associated with IUD use is primarily confined to the first 3 weeks after insertion and is uncommon thereafter. Given the popularity of IUDs, practitioners might encounter PID in IUD users. Evidence is insufficient to recommend the removal of IUDs in women diagnosed with acute PID. However, caution should be exercised if the IUD remains in place, and close clinical follow-up is mandatory. The rate of treatment failure and recurrent PID in women continuing to use an IUD is unknown, and no data have been collected regarding treatment outcomes by type of IUD (e.g., copper or levonorgestrel).

SURGICAL MANAGEMENT

If the diagnosis is under question, or the patient is responding poorly, surgical evaluation and/or management are indicated.

Laparotomy should generally be reserved for patients with surgical emergencies such as ruptured abscesses or definitive treatment of failed medical management. Laparoscopy, however, is an underused but usually helpful procedure for diagnosis, prognosis, and possibly treatment of PID. Laparoscopic evaluation should be considered in all patients with a differential diagnosis of PID and without laparoscopic surgery contraindications.

Laparoscopy is important not only to diagnose PID but also to rule out surgical emergencies, such as appendicitis and ruptured abscesses. It also prevents inappropriate management of patients with noninfectious problems, such as endometriosis. These patients need additional surgical and medical management, not antibiotic therapy and delayed diagnosis. In addition, evaluation of the extent of the inflammatory process in confirmed PID is helpful in establishing a prognosis and further management plan if initial treatment fails. Patients with evidence of current or previous abscesses have a higher failure rate with antibiotic therapy. Also, treatment of unilateral abscesses may necessitate surgical management to avoid the spread of the infection to the other tube and ovary.

Cultures obtained from the peritubal region or from the peritoneal cavity can also be helpful for identifying organisms resistant to initial management. This has become increasingly important in light of the increasing rate of clindamycin-resistant anaerobes and the elimination of intravenous metronidazole from the CDC-recommended inpatient guidelines. Laparoscopic management of PID that appears helpful includes copious lavage of the pelvis with normal saline or preferably Ringer solution. Antibiotic inclusion in the lavage fluid has not been demonstrated to be helpful to date.

Laparoscopic manipulation or drainage of documented pelvic abscesses has been attempted by several investigators. Henry-Suchet and associates reported the successful use of laparoscopy to diagnose and drain tuboovarian abscesses in 50 women. Adhesions were lysed, and the abscesses were drained through the laparoscope. All patients received intravenous antibiotics. Forty-five of the fifty (90%) patients were cured. Reich and McGlynn had a similar experience in 25 women with pelvic abscesses treated laparoscopically. Four of seven women desiring pregnancy conceived, and two women had unplanned pregnancies. However, the diagnosis of abscesses was not uniform in these studies. Also, it is of concern that similar results will not necessarily be demonstrated in less experienced hands. Anatomically, drainage of abscesses within the pelvic cavity by laparoscope will not drain the entire abscess contents out of the pelvic cavity, and despite how extensive the lavage or laparoscopic removal is, pus and bacteria will be spilled and exposed to the pelvic cavity. This is contrary to the natural defense mechanism of the body of isolating and containing the inflammation-causing organisms within an abscess. Therefore, laparoscopic drainage of pelvic abscesses should be undertaken only by experienced laparoscopic surgeons and with the patient's full understanding of all other options.

Laparotomy with extensive pelvic surgery was often recommended in the past, before the development of broad-spectrum antibiotics.

If a patient has been hospitalized on several occasions for acute exacerbation of PID with bilateral tuboovarian abscesses to the point where the future surgical risk increases significantly, definitive surgical intervention may be indicated. The operation should be done when the infection is quiescent, if possible. The surgery may still be difficult, but there will be fewer complications than when patients are operated on in the acute phase of the infection. The timing of the operative intervention is important. There should be complete absorption of the inflammatory exudate surrounding the focus of the infection, as seen radiologically. Bimanual pelvic examination should be possible without producing a marked or persistent febrile response. It has been suggested that definitive surgery be delayed for 2 to 3 months after the recent exacerbation for more complete resolution of the infection. Ideally, the patient should have a normal ESR, WBC, and hematocrit, and relatively nontender pelvic organs, except possibly with motion.

Kaplan and associates recommended more aggressive management in patients who exhibit either no clinical response or only partial response after 24 to 72 hours. Their approach included a total abdominal hysterectomy and bilateral salpingo-oophorectomy and was thought to reduce the protracted period of intensive medical therapy in a group of patients who would eventually require surgery. They noted that conservative management of their cases usually resulted in protracted periods of intensive care and repeated hospital admissions, and rarely in subsequent pregnancies. However, the early surgical intervention described above was associated with several incidences of injury to the bowel and additional postoperative complications. Also, patients with acute pelvic abscess are frequently young, and future childbearing is often desired. Even with uterine and ovarian preservation, pregnancy is difficult without intervention such as in vitro fertilization for most patients. Conservation of ovarian function for these young women is an important benefit of medical management for the rest of their adult lives.

Older studies of the management of patients with pelvic abscess, which emphasized the early use of surgery, are no longer pertinent, because modern antibiotic drugs were not available then. Collins and Jansen in 1959 had an early failure rate of 10% for conservative medical therapy. However, 113 of their 174 patients required later surgery, which corresponds to a late failure rate of 65%. Two decades later, Ginsburg and associates reviewed cases of 160 patients treated for tuboovarian abscess during the years 1969 to 1979. The early failure rate with broad-spectrum antibiotics was high at 31%, but the late failure rate was only 21%. Thus, with an average follow-up period of 25.5 months, 48% did not require later surgery. Subsequent reports by Hager and colleagues and by Landers and Sweet support conservative management, as better antibiotics have been introduced.

POSTERIOR COLPOTOMY

When conservative management fails and a pelvic abscess is noted dissecting the rectovaginal septum, drainage by way of colpotomy may be possible.

In a classic article, Wharton described various techniques of vaginal drainage of pelvic abscess. Today, posterior colpotomy is done to evacuate pus and to establish drainage from a pelvic abscess that presents in the cul-de-sac.

There are three requirements for colpotomy drainage of a pelvic abscess:

1. The abscess must be predominantly midline.
2. The abscess should be adherent to the cul-de-sac peritoneum and should dissect the rectovaginal septum to assure the surgeon that the drainage will be extraperitoneal and that pus will not be disseminated transperitoneally.
3. The abscess should be cystic or fluctuant to ensure adequate drainage.

Occasionally, a cul-de-sac abscess can be successfully drained without dissecting the septum. However, the serosal surface of the abscess should be adherent to the cul-de-sac peritoneum. Ultrasonography may be helpful in locating the pockets of pus.

After adequate anesthesia, the patient is placed in the lithotomy position. It is essential that a thorough examination of the pelvis be performed under anesthesia so that the operator knows the size and position of the mass that is to be drained.

After preparation and draping in the dorsal lithotomy position, the posterior lip of the cervix is grasped with a tenaculum and drawn down and forward. The vaginal epithelium of the posterior vaginal fornix is incised just below the reflection of the vaginal mucosa onto the cervix, and the transverse incision is widened with a pair of long scissors (Fig. 30.4A). The incision must be large enough to allow adequate exploration and drainage of the abscess cavity with the index finger. The cul-de-sac peritoneum and abscess wall are punctured with a long Kelly clamp (Fig. 30.4B). As the abscess wall is perforated, there is a definite sensation of puncturing a cystic cavity. If blood or pus is present, this is soon seen coming into the upper vagina. The jaws of the clamp are spread, and the flow

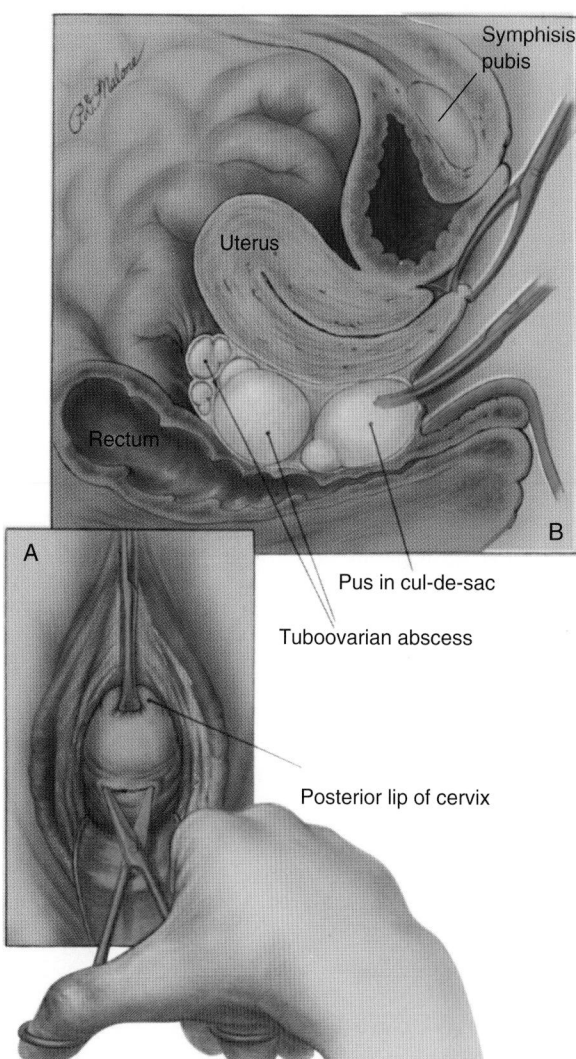

FIGURE 30.4 Posterior colpotomy. **A:** A transverse incision is made through the vaginal mucosa at the junction of the posterior vaginal fornix with the cervix. **B:** A Kelly clamp is thrust through the abscess wall.

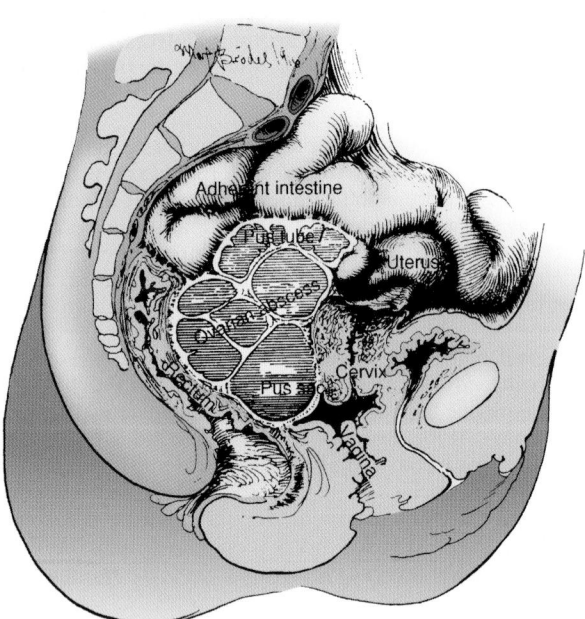

FIGURE 30.5 Pus may be contained within the tuboovarian abscess and within other pockets in the pelvic cavity.

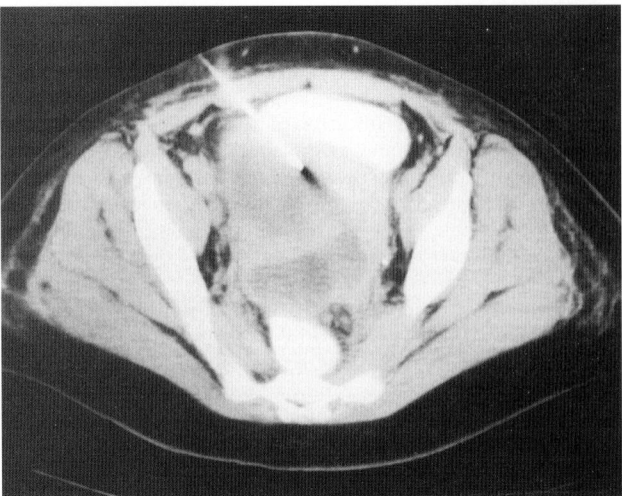

FIGURE 30.6 Transabdominal needle aspiration of a pelvic abscess under guidance of CT. Drainage tube is also placed.

of liquid from the cul-de-sac is increased. A sample of the purulent exudate is sent to the microbiology laboratory for appropriate culture and sensitivity. Collection of the specimen anaerobically with a capped syringe with rapid transport to the laboratory allows the more fastidious flora to be defined. A direct smear for Gram stain is also made from the pus examined for predominating organisms.

There may be more than one compartment in an abscess cavity (Fig. 30.5). It is desirable to insert an index finger in the cavity and explore. Fibrous adhesions within the cavity can be gently broken. If another abscess wall is felt, it can often be cautiously and safely punctured under the guidance of a finger. Exploration and manipulation should be done carefully to avoid intraperitoneal rupture of the abscess or perforation of the bowel. To allow adequate drainage, the vaginal incision should be at least 2 cm wide. If pus has been obtained, one or two drains are inserted into the abscess cavity and anchored by balloon or with fine absorbable suture to permit easy removal. Penrose or closed suction drainage systems can be used. These should be left for several days until drainage stops and to allow air to prevent the reaccumulation of anaerobic organisms. Wharton has emphasized the importance of prolonged drainage. A suture or two may be required to control bleeding from the vaginal mucosa. However, if a mushroom (Malecot) catheter is used for drainage, it should be removed in 48 to 72 hours to prevent significant fibrosis that could hinder removal.

Patients in whom the abscess does not meet the criteria for colpotomy drainage often require laparotomy and direct drainage. Transabdominal, transvaginal, and transrectal drainage has been attempted to avoid the expense and complications of laparotomy and for patients in whom laparotomy is contraindicated.

PERCUTANEOUS DRAINAGE

Experience with *percutaneous drainage* of intraabdominal and pelvic abscesses under ultrasonographic or computed tomographic (CT) guidance has been reported by Olak and

associates and by others. Worthen and Gunning used percutaneous catheter drainage of 11 abscesses in nine patients and achieved a cure rate of 77%. Two patients required surgical intervention subsequently. In 19 patients, simple percutaneous aspiration of 23 abscesses was successful, with a 94% cure rate. The attempt at aspiration failed in seven patients (Fig. 30.6). The Grady Memorial Hospital experience, as reported by Tyrrel and associates, is similar. CT-guided percutaneous drainage in eight patients with tuboovarian abscess resulted in recovery without surgery in seven. One patient had marked clinical improvement but still required a posterior colpotomy. No complications occurred. Loy and associates have reported that the simultaneous use of real-time pelvic ultrasonography can facilitate transvaginal drainage of a pelvic abscess. If patients do not respond to intravenous antibiotics and percutaneous drainage or aspiration, surgical intervention is required. MRI-assisted drainage has been utilized and is helpful when overlying gas patterns from the intestines or abscess cavity obscure ultrasonic imaging for needle placement.

The long-term effects of pus and organisms released into the pelvis from the puncture site are unknown. However, short-term success rates are good, and surgical drainage of acute abscess is the basic principle. Therefore, needle drainage can be considered with proper patient selection and appropriate informed consent, which includes other management options.

EXPLORATORY LAPAROTOMY

If *exploratory laparotomy* is necessary, the patient can be positioned in Allen universal stirrups. A lower abdominal transverse Maylard incision is ideal because it affords good exposure to the lateral adnexal pelvic organs and pelvic side walls. Pelvic adhesions should be released, and the bowel should be packed off before the pelvic dissection commences. During the dissection, free pus is often spilled, and the upper abdomen should be isolated from this, if possible. When a ruptured abscess is encountered, the exudate is collected and sent immediately to the laboratory for Gram stain, anaerobic and aerobic cultures, and antimicrobial sensitivity studies. The easiest way to obtain the material for anaerobic culture is simply to collect it in an airtight syringe and to submit a small piece of the abscess wall in an airtight container. The easiest place to begin the dissection is in the round ligament, which is the most consistently available and identifiable landmark. Following the round ligament medially always leads to the uterine corpus. Variations in the usual technique for the operation may be required because of extensive disease, dense adhesions, indurated and edematous tissue, and distorted anatomy. For example, it is sometimes convenient to perform the central dissection first (i.e., a subtotal hysterectomy). This allows more space and adequate exposure to perform the required adnexal surgery. Tuboovarian inflammatory masses may be found densely adherent in the cul-de-sac to the uterus, to the posterior surface of the broad ligament, and to the lateral pelvic sidewall. There is risk of injury to the ureters, sigmoid, rectum, and small intestines. The method of dissection used depends on the nature of the adhesions. Soft, fresh adhesions can be broken gently and easily with finger dissection. Dense fibrotic adhesions must be carefully dissected and cut with scissors. The dissection can be especially difficult and risky if pelvic tissues are intensely indurated, as in ligneous pelvic cellulitis. If the infundibulopelvic ligament can be clamped, cut, and securely ligated, one can gain access to the lateral retroperitoneal space and identify the ureter. This facilitates a safe dissection of the abscess wall away from the ureter. In cases with extensive disease involving one or both adnexa, the use of preoperative ureteral catheterization may be helpful in identifying the location of the pelvic ureters. With tuboovarian abscess, the anatomic limits of the ovary may be difficult to define. If the ovary is to be removed, it should be removed completely to prevent subsequent development of ovarian remnant syndrome.

When both adnexa must be removed, a hysterectomy should be entertained if extensive uterine involvement is suspected. In some cases, only a subtotal hysterectomy is feasible. However, if the lower uterine segment can be visualized, the cervix can usually be excised after removal of the adnexa and the uterine corpus. The operative field should be copiously irrigated. The vaginal vault should be left open for drainage. A Penrose drain can be inserted and then removed several days later. Suspension of the vaginal vault and reperitonization of the pelvis are accomplished in the usual manner, if possible. A routine closure of the abdominal incision is performed. Jackson-Pratt suction drains are often placed above the fascia and brought out through a separate incision.

Because the patient has been placed in the Allen universal stirrups for laparotomy, ureteral integrity can be confirmed as discussed elsewhere. Five milliliters of indigo carmine is given intravenously, and a cystoscope is placed in the bladder. Blue dye can then be seen flowing from each ureteral orifice.

In the past, it was standard practice to do a bilateral salpingo-oophorectomy in almost all patients who had a laparotomy for acute pelvic abscess. This practice was based on the belief that the disease is almost always severe in both adnexa. Recent studies have suggested that as many as 25% to 50% of patients will have a relatively normal tube and ovary on one side. This may be especially true of patients whose infection is associated with IUD use. Golde and associates reported that 37 of 85 patients (44%) with tuboovarian abscesses confirmed at operation had unilateral abscesses; 20 were using an IUD. The studies of Landers and Sweet, Hager and Majmudar, and Ginsburg and coworkers also found a higher percentage of unilateral adnexal disease than was previously reported. In light of these findings, conservative adnexal surgery may be possible in some patients. We have no hesitation in leaving a relatively normal tube and ovary at the time of hysterectomy with removal of the opposite adnexa for acute pelvic abscess. When the uterus is removed and the continuity between the conserved tube and the lower genital tract is interrupted, there is little risk of a new infection. If a strictly unilateral

pelvic abscess is found at laparotomy, removal of the affected tube and ovary only, leaving in the uterus and the opposite adnexa, is acceptable in a patient who wishes to preserve fertility. However, in vitro fertilization techniques may be required to accomplish pregnancy. Such a patient will then still have a risk of recurrent tuboovarian abscess. It is especially important that her sexual partner be examined and receive treatment when indicated.

In recent years, there have been advances in reproductive technology that allow infertile patients to conceive and carry pregnancies to term under the most extraordinary circumstances. It has been possible, for example, to accomplish a successful pregnancy in a woman who has a uterus but no ovaries by instillation of a donated fertilized ovum into a suitably prepared uterus. Such a sophisticated procedure is not available to a large number of patients. However, in light of the recent findings of the risk of estrogen plus progesterone treatment from the Women's Health Initiative Study, the option of leaving in the uterus when bilateral salpingo-oophorectomy is to be performed should be discussed with the patient, especially if she is young and nulliparous.

In summary, patients with an acute pelvic abscess should be hospitalized for treatment with parenteral broad-spectrum antibiotics. Surgery is indicated if the diagnosis is uncertain, if intraperitoneal rupture is diagnosed or suspected, or if the patient fails to respond to medical management.

RUPTURED PELVIC ABSCESS

A tuboovarian or pelvic abscess can rupture spontaneously into the rectum or sigmoid colon, into the bladder, or into the free peritoneal cavity. A pelvic abscess almost never ruptures spontaneously into the vagina unless the patient has previously damaged epithelium such as from a previous posterior colpotomy for drainage of an abscess. Under these circumstances, a recurrent pelvic abscess can dissect along the tract of the previous posterior colpotomy incision and drain spontaneously through the vagina.

Spontaneous drainage through the rectum or sigmoid colon usually occurs in a patient whose abscess is too high to drain with a posterior colpotomy. In other words, although the abscess is fluctuant and midline, it is not yet dissecting the rectovaginal septum. While waiting for the abscess to come down, a sudden unexpected improvement in the patient's condition is noted, and she will confirm that pus has begun to drain through the anus. Further improvement in her condition usually occurs. A posterior colpotomy is not needed and, indeed, is contraindicated because doing so could cause a rectovaginal fistula to form.

Spontaneous drainage through the bladder is rare. It occurs most commonly in elderly women with chronic abscesses developing from ruptured sigmoid diverticula. Only rarely does a chronic tuboovarian or pelvic abscess rupture and drain through the bladder, causing secondary infection of the bladder. When the abscess is removed with laparotomy, a defect in the bladder wall is noted. The indurated tissue around the defect should be removed and the defect closed with 3-0 delayed absorbable suture in two layers. A Foley catheter can be left in place for 10 to 14 days while healing of the bladder wall takes place.

Of all the complications that can result from PID, intraabdominal rupture of a tuboovarian abscess is the most life threatening. Mortality from this complication is due to septic shock and the complications of generalized peritonitis, and the mortality rate can approach up to 10% in patients with warm shock.

Abscesses can rupture spontaneously or iatrogenically after bimanual examination or accidental trauma. Bacteriologic study of the contents of the abscess has historically been unrewarding; a specific organism has been isolated in less than 50% of cases. The gonococcus is rarely identified in a pelvic abscess. Careful aerobic and anaerobic cultures often demonstrate the presence of a mixed infection that includes anaerobic organisms. McNamara and Mead reviewed the results of three separate studies that demonstrated 31 positive isolates of anaerobes in 30 patients with a pelvic abscess. Landers and Sweet have also confirmed similar findings in their series.

Diagnosis of Ruptured Tuboovarian Abscess

The major clinical symptom of ruptured tuboovarian abscess is acute, progressive pelvic pain that is usually so severe that the patient can accurately identify the time and place of its occurrence. In a classic series from the Johns Hopkins Hospital reported by Vermeeren and Te Linde, the average age of patients with a ruptured tuboovarian abscess was 33 years, which is at least 10 years older than the average age of patients with acute PID. Approximately 2% of these patients are postmenopausal. To our knowledge, only two cases of ruptured tuboovarian abscess in a pregnant patient have been reported. Often, there is a history of recurrent attacks of PID, with a sudden increase in the severity and extent of abdominal pain during a recent exacerbation of infection. On examination, the patient appears seriously ill and dehydrated, with rapid, shallow respirations. The abdomen is distended and quiet, with diminished or absent bowel sounds. Signs of generalized peritonitis, direct and rebound tenderness, muscle rigidity, and shifting dullness may be noted. A pelvic mass is palpable in only approximately 50% of cases. Tachycardia is common. Shock can be present or can develop while the patient is under observation. It is due to accumulation of fluids in peripheral tissues and later failure of compensatory vasoconstrictor mechanisms. The patient's temperature is usually greater than 101°F, but it can also be normal and even subnormal late in the course. The leukocyte count is likely to be more than 15,000, but it also can be normal, if the neutrophils are being depleted. Severe leukopenia is an ominous sign. A culdocentesis is a valuable diagnostic aid and was positive for purulent material in 70% of the cases in the Mickal and Sellmann series. An abdominal radiograph usually shows a paralytic ileus, sometimes evidence of free fluid in the peritoneal cavity, and atelectasis in the lung bases. A CT scan of the pelvis and abdomen is most helpful and will usually confirm the pelvic abscess with free purulent fluid in the upper abdomen. It may also suggest an alternative diagnosis such as a ruptured appendix or acute cholecystitis.

Treatment of Ruptured Tuboovarian Abscess

The longer the delay in the operative treatment of ruptured tuboovarian abscess, the greater the primary mortality rate. In the series by Vermeeren and Te Linde from the Johns Hopkins Hospital, death occurred less than 90 hours after the time of rupture in 88% of fatal cases, both operative and nonoperative.

As time passes after rupture of a tuboovarian abscess, septic peritonitis becomes more severe and generalized. The passage of time allows the development of septic shock from greater absorption of bacteria and bacterial endotoxins and secretion of great quantities of fluid into the peritoneal cavity across inflamed peritoneal surfaces. Fluid shifts from the intravascular compartment to interstitial spaces as a result of the increased vascular permeability of the inflamed peritoneal membrane. This leads to hypovolemia, decreased cardiac output, decreased central venous pressure, hypotension, vasoconstriction, increased peripheral resistance, decreased tissue perfusion, metabolic acidosis, ARDS, decreased renal glomerular perfusion and filtration with decreased urine flow, severe hypoxemia, multiple organ system failure, and ultimately death. The prompt diagnosis and treatment of intraperitoneal rupture of a tuboovarian abscess is essential to minimize the risk of mortality of generalized peritonitis.

The treatment of patients with ruptured tuboovarian abscess can be divided into three phases: preoperative, operative, and postoperative.

Preoperative Phase

Surgery should be undertaken after rapid but adequate preoperative preparation. The patient should be typed and crossmatched for 2 to 4 units of packed red blood cells. Monitoring of central venous pressure is essential for proper evaluation of the hemodynamics of this condition, because many patients are dehydrated, in shock, and anemic. Swan-Ganz catheter placement may be preferable because it allows pulmonary capillary wedge pressure and pulmonary artery pressure determinations that are helpful in assessing the adequacy of fluid replacement and in detecting fluid overload. Variable amounts of fluid, sometimes tremendous amounts, are lost into the peritoneal cavity and intestinal tract because of peritonitis. Blood chemistry determinations (e.g., serum electrolytes, creatinine, glucose, bilirubin, and alkaline phosphatase) should be obtained and intravenous fluids, preferably Ringer lactate, started immediately. Crystalloid solutions for fluid volume resuscitation are preferred for most patients with septic peritonitis. It may be advantageous to use partial colloid resuscitation in some patients with evidence of cardiopulmonary dysfunction, because a smaller total volume is required. An excess of intravenous crystalloid solution may result in fluid overload.

Vigorous broad-spectrum intravenous antibiotic therapy should be instituted. The most active antimicrobials with FDA approval for female pelvic infections include piperacillin–tazobactam 3.75 g every 6 hours and ertapenem 1 g every 24 hours. Dosage adjustments need to be made due to the patient's renal status. Changes can be made to single or combination therapies once culture results and sensitivities return.

An indwelling urethral catheter is used to monitor fluid intake with hourly urine output. Combating shock is a primary concern throughout treatment. Clinical assessment of respiratory function should be made. A distended tender abdomen may cause rapid, shallow respirations and use of accessory muscles for ventilation. Arterial blood gases may indicate mild hypoxemia, in which case oxygen should be administered. If anemia is severe, blood transfusion should be started before surgery.

When the patient has been properly prepared, immediate surgery should be undertaken. The results of treatment are better if major metabolic and hemodynamic problems are corrected before operation, but one cannot wait even a short amount of time in treating a critically ill patient with septic peritonitis.

Operative Phase

The anesthetic of choice depends on the preference and experience of the anesthesiologist and the medical condition of the patient.

The operation should be performed as rapidly as possible. Because speed as well as access to the upper abdomen may be required, a lower midline incision should be used. It can be quickly extended above the umbilicus if necessary. The patient should not be put in the Trendelenburg position until the abdomen is packed off, and no more of a dependent position should be used than is needed to prevent further dissemination of pus into the upper abdomen. When the abdomen is opened, any odor that is present should be noted. An unpleasant, putrid odor is indicative of infection with anaerobic organisms. Pus from the abdomen should be collected correctly for both aerobic and anaerobic culture and for Gram stain and should be promptly transported to the laboratory. Organisms grown should be tested for sensitivity to various antibiotics.

The operation of choice in a patient with a ruptured abscess is the removal of the free pus. In patients bordering or in shock, removal of the abscess, the uterus, the tubes, and usually the ovaries is often necessary. Occasionally, it is possible to leave an ovary in a patient with a ruptured pelvic abscess. However, reoperation in a seriously ill patient is often not an option, so all tissue suspected to be infected should be removed. If rupture has occurred from a strictly unilateral tuboovarian abscess, with a relatively normal tube and ovary on the opposite side, a unilateral salpingo-oophorectomy can be performed, especially if the patient is young. However, the risk of a recurrent abscess in the opposite tube and ovary is high if the uterus is also left in place. When the uterus is removed along with the tuboovarian abscess, the risk of recurrent abscess in the opposite adnexa is reduced. When hysterectomy is performed, usually a total hysterectomy can be done. However, even in the best surgical hands, a subtotal hysterectomy is faster than a total one and is sometimes justified. Although we believe firmly in total hysterectomy, we do not believe in performing it when the danger of total hysterectomy exceeds the danger from a retained cervix. Except in the young patient, it is often better to remove the corpus than to perform a unilateral adnexectomy alone. Furthermore, the opposite adnexa are significantly involved in most patients, and subsequent operation may be necessary if conservation of one side is practiced, as was required in 35% of Pedowitz and Bloomfield's cases. This is contrary to what has been described earlier in the surgical treatment of an unruptured abscess, because the risk of incomplete eradication of the immediate infection in an acutely ill patient with rupture, peritonitis, and possibly septic shock is much higher. Therefore, definitive surgical treatment is usually recommended in severely ill patients with ruptured abscess.

The technical performance of the procedure may be difficult, but it is similar to that described earlier for laparotomy followed by failed colpotomy drainage or suspected rupture. Anatomy is distorted, dependable landmarks are obscured, and tissues are thick, edematous, friable, and inflamed. Loops of densely adherent intestine must be separated carefully to avoid injury. Injury to the serosa of distended bowel occurs commonly and often requires repair. Any entry into the lumen of the bowel must be recognized and repaired. Retroperitoneal planes of dissection can be used to advantage in identifying the ureters and removing inflammatory adnexal masses. Otherwise, it is likely that a fragment of ovary will be left behind, which can subsequently cause signs and symptoms of the ovarian remnant syndrome. As much of the remaining abscess wall as possible should be removed without causing unnecessary additional bleeding. Pieces of the abscess wall can be left adherent to the pelvic sidewall and cul-de-sac.

The upper abdomen should be carefully explored for collections of pus in the subdiaphragmatic and subhepatic regions. If an upper abdominal abscess is found, it may be necessary to place a closed suction drain into the abscess cavity through the upper abdominal wall.

Before the incision is closed, the abdominal cavity should be irrigated with copious quantities of warm sterile saline to remove remaining bacteria and debris. There is always some fear of dissemination of the infection by copious irrigation. However, this disadvantage is far outweighed by the benefit of diluting and removing bacteria and necrotic debris. We do not add antiseptics or antibiotics to the irrigating solution. If hemostasis is poor or if considerable necrotic material is left behind, there may be some benefit from peritoneal drainage with closed suction catheters. Closed suction drains can be placed through a separate stab wound in the abdominal wall, through the cul-de-sac, or through the vaginal vault when a total hysterectomy has been done, but the drainage of free peritoneal exudate in the upper abdomen is of no therapeutic value.

The abdominal incision is closed with a Smead-Jones technique or with a continuous suture taking large bites of tissue. A monofilament suture of polypropylene or nylon should be used. Retention sutures can be placed but are not usually necessary. The incision should be irrigated with warm saline. When there has been gross contamination of the incision, the subcutaneous fat and skin should be left open and packed lightly with gauze soaked in an antibiotic or dilute acetic acid solution. The wound is repacked daily and inspected. In 4 to 5 days, if the tissues are healthy, the incision is closed secondarily with sutures. Alternatively, the edges can be drawn together with sterile adhesive strips.

Postoperative Phase

Postoperative care should consider shock, infection, ileus, and fluid imbalances. Complications of the late postoperative period include undrained or recurrent pelvic and abdominal abscesses, intestinal obstruction, intestinal fistulas, incisional breakdown with or without evisceration, pulmonary embolus, continued sepsis, and disseminated intravascular coagulation. Serious medical problems such as uncontrolled diabetes or renal or pulmonary failure (ARDS) further complicate recovery from this potentially lethal disease.

Septic shock should be combated with blood (when indicated for a hemoglobin less than 7.0 g), Ringer lactate, respiratory support, and, if necessary, vasoactive substances. Infection is controlled by the continued aggressive use of broad-spectrum intravenous antibiotics until the patient can take antibiotics orally. When the results of the antibiotic sensitivity studies on the operative specimen are available, a change to more effective or safer agents should be considered, but only if the patient shows evidence of continued sepsis. Antibiotics should not necessarily be changed on the basis of sensitivity studies if the patient is improving clinically. Sometimes, the patient's condition improves initially, only to show signs of recurring intraabdominal infection the 2nd week after operation. Under these circumstances, it is appropriate to change antibiotics. Antibiotics should be continued until the patient is afebrile with only a mild leukocytosis or mildly elevated C-reactive protein and is able to eat a regular diet. Too long a period of treatment with antibiotics may result in complications such as pseudomembranous enterocolitis or fungal superinfection.

The semi-Fowler position may help prevent subphrenic and subdiaphragmatic abscess formation. Patients with signs of continued intraabdominal sepsis should have CT scans to identify collections of pus. If found, CT-directed drainage may be possible.

Constant intestinal suction by means of a long intestinal tube is a very important feature of postoperative care. A dynamic ileus persists postoperatively for a variable period and is best treated with the long intestinal tube until there is evidence of peristalsis and the patient is passing flatus.

Close attention to fluid balance and blood chemistry determinations is mandatory. Frequently, patients with ruptured tuboovarian abscess may have poor kidney function. The fluid output and serum creatinine should be followed closely.

PRIMARY OVARIAN ABSCESS

A primary ovarian abscess is an entity distinctly different from tuboovarian abscess. A tuboovarian abscess is one in which the abscess wall is composed of fallopian tube and ovarian parenchyma. A primary ovarian abscess, on the other hand, is one in which the infection occurs in the parenchyma of the ovary. Unlike tuboovarian abscess, it is an unusual condition. Interest in primary ovarian abscess was stimulated by the 1964 report of Willson and Black. According to a review by Wetchler and Dunn, 120 cases had been reported by 1985. Its frequency may be increasing, although still rare, as Askenazi and colleagues in 1994 reported a 0.2% to 2.2% rate of ovarian abscesses following transvaginal oocyte retrieval and transcervical embryo transfer.

Although bacteria can gain access to the ovarian parenchyma by hematogenous or lymphatic spread, it is probable that most primary ovarian abscesses occur because bacteria present around the ovary gain access to the parenchyma through a break in the ovarian capsule. This can occur naturally by ovulation, or it can be broken by a surgical procedure. Bacteria come from the fallopian tube, from the vagina during or after hysterectomy or any colpotomy procedure, from intrauterine infection associated with an IUD or another transcervical procedure, or from appendicitis, diverticulitis, or any other condition that is associated with peritonitis. A primary ovarian abscess is usually unilateral. However, its occasional occurrence simultaneously in both ovaries and during pregnancy seems to support the rare hematogenous or lymphatic spread, or both. Primary ovarian abscess has been reported secondary to infections at distant sites (tonsillitis, typhoid, parotitis, and tuberculosis).

Diagnosis of an unruptured primary ovarian abscess can be difficult because of the variable clinical presentation. Lower abdominal pain and fever are usually present. Lower abdominal and pelvic tenderness and an adnexal mass may be present, but the pelvic examination is sometimes not helpful, due to pain and guarding. Although an event predisposing to primary ovarian abscess (e.g., surgery, IUD use, appendicitis, or systemic infection) may be uncovered in the history, the event is sometimes remote. Ultrasonography and CT can be helpful in identifying an abscess cavity. If an ovarian abscess ruptures, the clinical picture is much the same as in ruptured tuboovarian abscess, with abdominal distention, direct and rebound tenderness, ileus, and sometimes shock. The patient appears gravely ill, and the need for immediate surgery is usually obvious.

The management of patients with primary ovarian abscess is similar to the management of patients with acute tuboovarian abscess. If the abscess is not ruptured, medical management with antibiotics for both anaerobic and aerobic organisms plus supportive care is indicated. A failure to respond or deterioration in the patient's condition suggests alteration in antibiotic coverage or possible exploratory surgery, or both, to remove the abscess. Ruptured ovarian abscess requires immediate laparotomy after a brief but intense effort to stabilize the patient and start antibiotic therapy. At operation, only the affected ovary need be removed. The tubes and the uterus can be conserved.

If both ovaries are involved, they should be removed. For a patient who is not interested in conception in the future, the uterus and both tubes can also be removed to decrease the possibility of the need for reoperation. If the patient is interested in pregnancy, the uterus and fallopian tubes can be left in place for possible implantation of a donated egg in the future.

SURGERY FOR CHRONIC PELVIC INFLAMMATORY DISEASE

Although the gonococcus may be responsible for initiating acute salpingitis, which is short-lived, residual chronic salpingitis is usually due to secondary invaders, both aerobic and anaerobic, or perhaps to an initial infection with *C. trachomatis*. As a result of the initial infection or from subsequent secondary exacerbations, the fimbria can become occluded and the tubes bound to the ovaries with adhesions. In addition, the bowel can become adherent to the broad ligament and the adnexal structures, and the fascia and loose connective tissue of the broad ligament can be converted into an indurated, brawny structure typical of ligneous induration. This can extend to include tissues beneath the peritoneum on the lateral pelvic sidewall, where ligneous pelvic cellulitis can cause ureteral obstruction. If the chronic infection persists, serious effusion from the inflammatory process within the endosalpinx produces a hydrosalpinx that can ignite periodically with secondary subacute pelvic infection or can progress to produce a pyosalpinx and tuboovarian abscess. If the subacute infection is left untreated or is treated inadequately, spontaneous intraabdominal rupture or leakage of an old tuboovarian abscess can occur. In a review of this subject, Heaton and Ledger identified this problem principally in premenopausal women, with only 1.7% of patients with a tuboovarian abscess being postmenopausal. However, when tuboovarian abscess is diagnosed in postmenopausal women, Protopapas et al. found that 47% had a concomitant gynecologic malignity. They concluded, "Conservative treatment of TOAs has no place during the menopause."

The signs and symptoms of chronic PID that most often require surgical treatment include severe, persistent, progressive pelvic pain, usually bilateral, although occasionally localized in one of the lower abdominal quadrants; repeated exacerbations of PID requiring multiple hospitalizations and recurrent medical treatment; progressive enlargement of a tuboovarian inflammatory mass, especially if it cannot be distinguished from a neoplastic tumor of the ovary; severe dyspareunia related to the chronic pelvic infection; and bilateral ureteral obstruction from ligneous cellulitis. It was formerly accepted that a history of previous colpotomy for drainage of a pelvic abscess was sufficient reason in itself to justify definitive abdominal surgery later for removal of the uterus and adnexa. However, several patients have become pregnant after posterior colpotomy for drainage of a cul-de-sac abscess or have remained relatively free of symptoms for long periods. Today, previous posterior colpotomy for pelvic abscess drainage is not a sufficient indication by itself for definitive abdominal surgery later when the patient is stable.

Selection of Operative Technique

The final decision regarding the proper operation for the surgical management of chronic PID is usually made with the abdomen open. Consideration must be given not only to the pathologic lesions found at operation but also to the patient's age, parity, desire for children, previous history of pelvic disease, and other associated pelvic disease and symptoms. Because a knowledge of all these is essential to the best surgical judgment, the operator should be thoroughly familiar with the patient, her history, and her desires.

In the surgical management of chronic PID, the question of removal or retention of the ovary at the time of hysterectomy

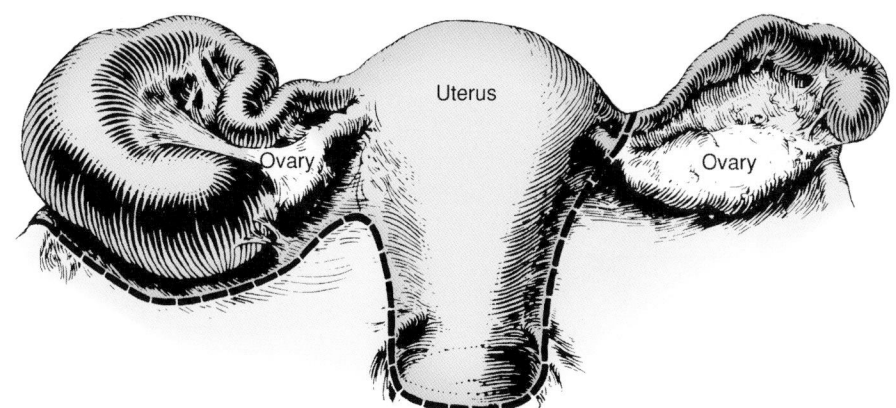

FIGURE 30.7 Total abdominal hysterectomy and unilateral salpingo-oophorectomy from extensive chronic salpingo-oophoritis. A small hydrosalpinx on the opposite side can be left in to preserve blood supply to the ovary.

and salpingectomy has been left open to conjecture and individual surgical opinion in most instances. This question was the subject of a study by Weiner and Wallach of the ovarian histology in ovaries removed from patients with PID. In 40 consecutive women who underwent oophorectomy during surgical treatment of PID, nearly 50% of the removed ovaries were free of inflammatory disease and demonstrated normal follicular activity. The study concluded that ovarian histology was usually normal among patients who gave no history of dysfunctional uterine bleeding. Therefore, the menstrual history of such patients should be helpful in the decision regarding ovarian conservation or ablation. Kirtley and Benigno have reviewed the Emory experience with ovarian conservation at the time of surgery for PID. In this series, 98 (82%) patients who required surgery had a total abdominal hysterectomy and bilateral salpingo-oophorectomy. In 22 patients (18%), either part or all of an ovary was retained. Of these 22 patients, 15 were available for follow-up hormonal assays. The mean follow-up time was 58 months. Cyclic ovarian function was confirmed in all but two patients. In the two patients with ovarian failure, other significant disease processes were also present. No patient suffered a complication as a result of adnexal conservation. We believe that normal ovarian tissue should be conserved at the time of definitive surgery for PID (Fig. 30.7). The release of peritubal adhesions in mild chronic PID is indicated occasionally in women in whom future childbearing is desired, as long as the tubes can be shown to be patent, usually by transfundal chromotubation after the lower uterine isthmus is occluded by a Ziegler clamp. This type of procedure provides the most rewarding pregnancy rate of all types of tubal reconstructive surgery. More often, one tube is hopelessly closed, and the opposite tube is patent after release of adhesions. In such a case, unilateral salpingectomy may be required if reconstructive surgery of the blocked tube is not possible (Fig. 30.8).

In most instances of surgery for chronic PID, total abdominal hysterectomy and bilateral salpingo-oophorectomy are necessary to remove the primary tubal pathology because of inflammatory damage of both tubes and ovaries. Total abdominal hysterectomy and bilateral salpingo-oophorectomy (Fig. 30.9) have been performed for severe actinomycosis infection.

If the uterus is removed and an ovary is preserved, it may be preferable to leave the entire adnexa in place in the absence of active tubal infection rather than compromise the venous drainage or the arterial blood supply to the ovary with subsequent cystic changes that may require an additional operative procedure later. Once the continuity of the tubal lumen from the uterine cavity is broken, the chronically inflamed tube does not usually produce subsequent symptoms, as shown by Falk in his series of cases with interstitial tubal resection. A small hydrosalpinx on the same side as the normal ovary can also be left in place so that ovarian blood supply is not disturbed during an attempt to remove the tube. When it is considered advisable to remove both adnexa because of the extent of the tuboovarian disease, a total hysterectomy may also be considered unless the uterus is hopelessly encased in pelvic scar tissue and densely adherent to the pelvic viscera.

In the optimum case, especially in a young woman who wishes to establish or maintain the possibility of future fertility, conservative surgery may be desirable, with the hope that pregnancy can be accomplished through in vitro fertilization techniques. In this situation, the uterus and one adnexa should be conserved, and the ovary should be positioned in the pelvis so an ovum can be harvested later through the laparoscope or through the vagina. As mentioned earlier, if the patient wishes, the uterus can be left in place even though both tubes and ovaries have been removed.

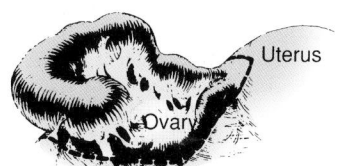

FIGURE 30.8 When significant chronic PID involves only one adnexum and preservation of uterine function is indicated, a unilateral salpingo-oophorectomy can be performed.

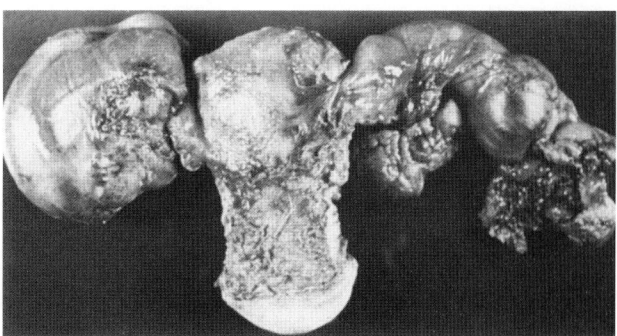

FIGURE 30.9 Total abdominal hysterectomy and bilateral salpingo-oophorectomy for severe pelvic actinomycosis.

Salpingectomy for Chronic Salpingitis

At the time of surgery for the treatment of chronic PID, every effort should be made to retain uninvolved organs. Unilateral salpingectomy should be considered when the oviduct is hopelessly destroyed by the disease process and presents as a large hydrosalpinx.

Once the abdomen has been opened and the extent of disease evaluated, the adhesions binding the tube are cut, and the tube is freed. It is held by a Kelly clamp placed on the mesosalpinx just beneath the fimbriated end. The mesosalpinx is then clamped and cut, with a succession of small bites taken as close to the tube as possible (Fig. 30.10A). Removal of a chronic hydrosalpinx can also be done laparoscopically.

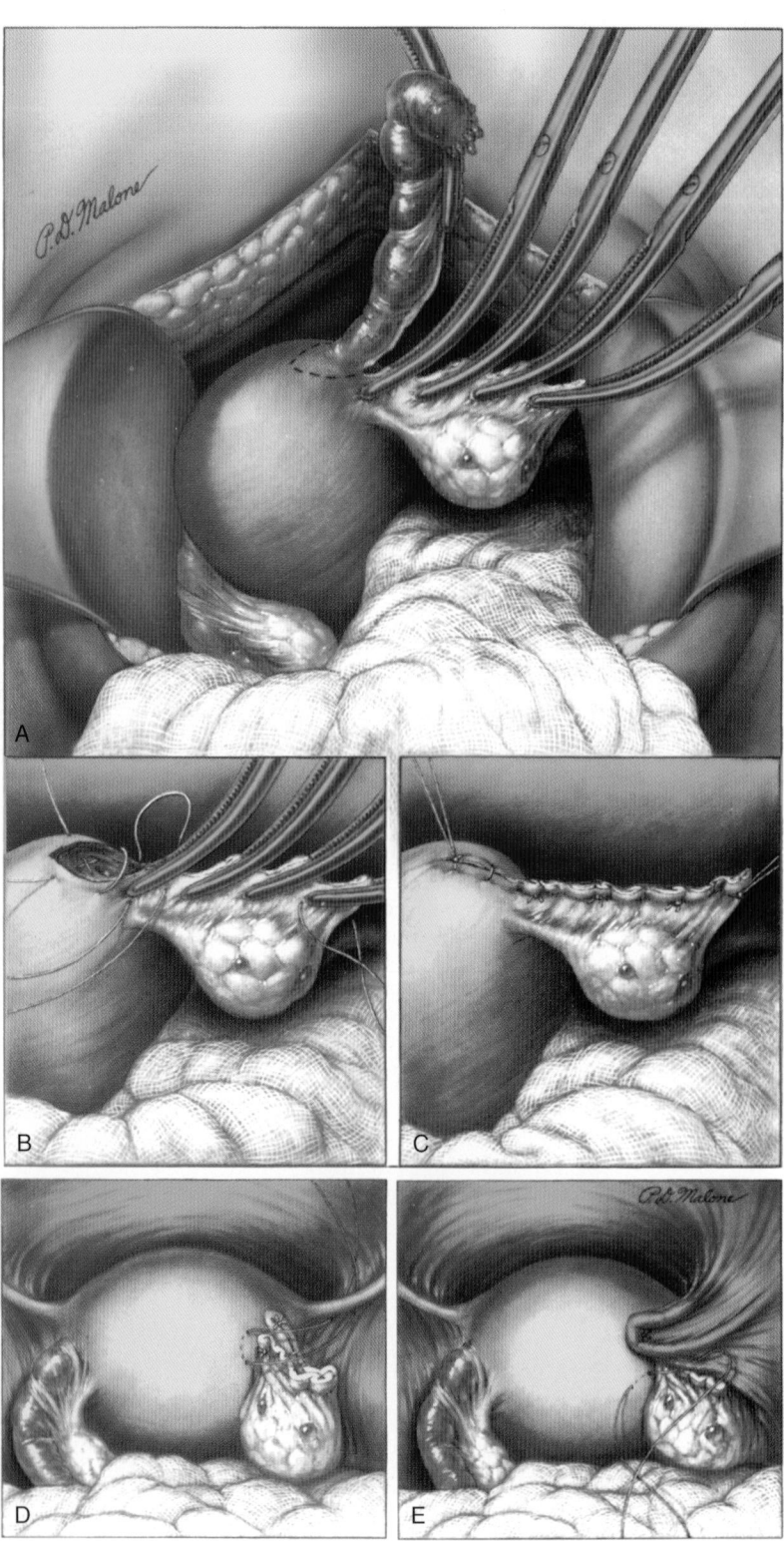

FIGURE 30.10 Salpingectomy. **A:** Mesosalpinx is clamped with multiple Kelly clamps and cut. *Dotted lines* indicate cornual excision, which is elective. **B:** Cornual wound is closed with 2-0 delayed absorbable suture. **C:** Mesosalpinx vessels are transfixed. **D:** Mattress suture is placed to cover operative area. **E:** Round ligament and broad ligament cover operative area.

Keeping the operative trauma as far as possible from the ovary that is to be retained lessens the danger of imperiling its blood supply. Experience has shown that the ovary whose tube has been removed is more apt to become cystic than the ovary whose tube has been left undisturbed.

The tube is excised at the uterine cornu in a wedge-shaped manner, as indicated in **Figure 30.10B**. A wide, figure-of-eight 2-0 delayed absorbable suture is placed in the cornu before the wedge is excised and is tightened as the interstitial portion of the tube is removed. If there is palpable extension of the inflammation at the uterine cornu (so-called salpingitis isthmica nodosa), the wedge may be large.

The wound in the uterus is closed with one or more 2-0 delayed absorbable figure-of-eight sutures (**Fig. 30.10B**). The vessels in the mesosalpinx are ligated with transfixion 3-0 delayed absorbable sutures. The advantage of the transfixion suture is that it does not slip off the tissue when tied as the clamp is withdrawn (**Fig. 30.10C**).

A mattress suture of 3-0 delayed absorbable material is used to bring the broad and round ligaments over the cornual wound (**Fig. 30.10D**). This suture passes just beneath the round ligament, so that the ligament is not strangulated when the suture is drawn tight. When this suture is tied, the cornual wound is covered with the broad ligament, and the uterus is suspended to some extent in a manner similar to that used in the Coffey suspension. Usually, a second mattress or interrupted suture is necessary to cover the mesosalpinx completely, as shown in **Figure 30.10E**.

Salpingo-Oophorectomy for Chronic Salpingitis

As in salpingectomy, the abdomen is entered through a transverse Maylard incision. The chronic tuboovarian inflammatory mass is first dissected free, and the infundibulopelvic ligament is identified. It is doubly clamped with Ochsner clamps, and a third clamp is applied to control back bleeding (**Fig. 30.11A**). The ureter must be identified before the infundibulopelvic ligament is clamped, cut, and ligated.

After the infundibulopelvic ligament is cut and ligated, the remainder of the broad ligament attachment of the tube and the ovary is clamped, cut, and ligated. The uterine end of the tube and the ovarian ligament are excised from the uterus in a wedge-shaped manner. The ascending uterine vessels are ligated just below the cornual wound, and the cornual incision is closed with a 2-0 delayed absorbable figure-of-eight suture (**Fig. 30.11B**).

The infundibulopelvic ligament is doubly ligated with 2-0 delayed absorbable sutures, and the vessels in the broad ligament are ligated with 3-0 delayed absorbable sutures. The cornual wound is peritonized, and the uterus is suspended to some degree by bringing the round and the broad ligaments over the uterine cornu with a mattress suture of 2-0 delayed absorbable material, as shown in **Figure 30.11C**. An attempt should be made to remove the tuboovarian inflammatory complex completely. If a fragment of ovary is left attached to the lateral pelvic peritoneum or the broad ligament, the ovarian remnant syndrome may develop later. To prevent this, a retroperitoneal approach may be required.

Identification of the Ureter

Identification of the course of the ureter in a pelvis in which the anatomy has become obliterated as a result of PID is one of the most important techniques for the gynecologic surgeon. In the surgical treatment of this disease, one may find a tuboovarian inflammatory mass that is located between

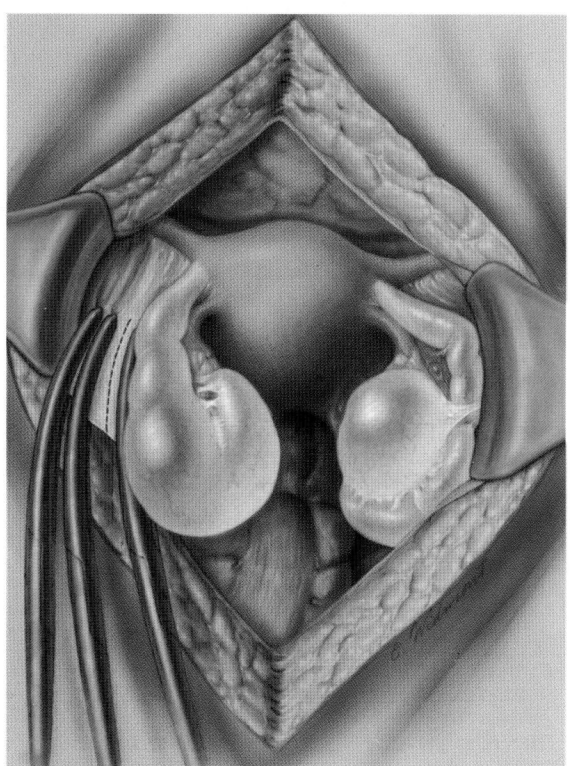
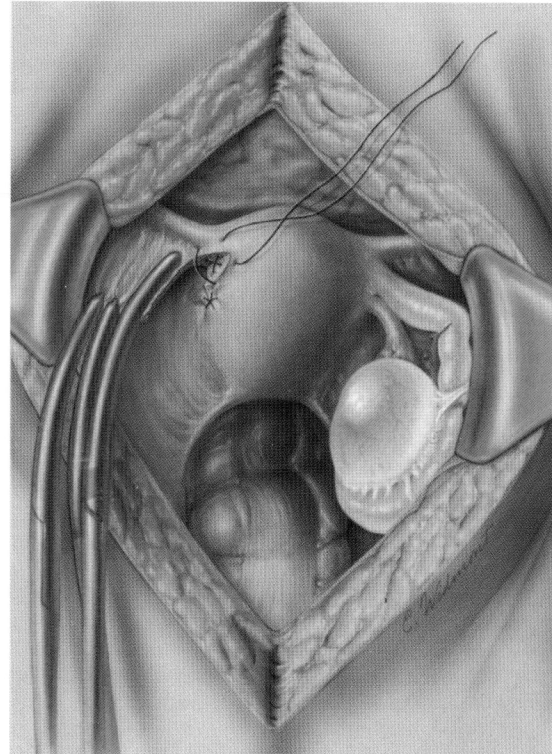

A   B

FIGURE 30.11 Salpingo-oophorectomy. **A:** The infundibulopelvic ligament is doubly clamped. Another clamp is placed to control back bleeding. *Dotted line* indicates incision. **B:** A suture has been placed to ligate the ascending uterine vessels just below the cornual incision. The cornual incision is closed with a figure-of-eight suture of 2-0 delayed absorbable material.

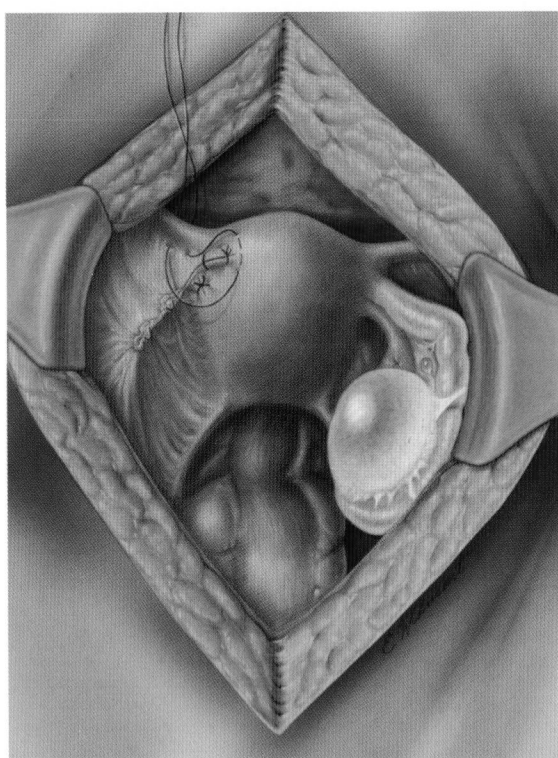

C

FIGURE 30.11 (*Continued*) **C:** The infundibulopelvic ligament and the rest of the broad ligament vessels have been ligated. The cornual wound is covered with the round and the broad ligament using a mattress suture of 2-0 delayed absorbable material.

the leaves of the broad ligament and extends to the lateral pelvic wall. It is not uncommon for the ligneous induration of the thickened parietal peritoneum to obscure completely the location and course of the pelvic ureter so that dissection of the diseased adnexa produces a surgical risk to the urinary tract, requiring great technical skill to avoid ureteral injury. Knowledge of the normal anatomic location of the pelvic ureters is essential so that these vital structures can be identified before an attempt is made to remove the adnexal masses. Division of the round ligament allows access to the lateral pelvic wall beneath the peritoneum. After the round ligament is divided, the peritoneum is incised inferiorly toward the internal cervical os and superiorly just lateral to the infundibulopelvic ligament. The peritoneum is easily reflected medially away from the pelvic sidewall with finger dissection, and the ureter is identified. It remains attached to the peritoneum. If there is difficulty with this procedure, the ureter can usually be identified as it crosses over the common iliac artery just above its bifurcation, and it can be traced downward.

Such patients may have a preoperative ureteral catheterization when there is clinical evidence of large, adherent adnexal masses. However, if such an anatomic problem is encountered at the time of laparotomy, an incision can be made in the dome of the bladder that allows the passage of ureteral catheters. If the patient has been positioned in the Allen universal stirrups for operation, intraoperative cystoscopy with passage of ureteral stents is easily accomplished. At the end of the operation, 5 mL of indigo carmine is given intravenously. With a cystoscope in the bladder, the dye can be seen effusing from both ureteral orifices, confirming that the ureters have not been injured or compromised.

PELVIC TUBERCULOSIS

Tuberculosis of the upper genital tract is a rare disease in the United States. However, it is a frequent cause of chronic PID and infertility in other parts of the world. For various reasons, the incidence of tuberculosis is again increasing in the United States. Therefore, cases of tuberculosis-associated PID may also become more evident. It should always be considered in the differential diagnosis of pelvic pain in immigrants, especially those from Asia, the Middle East, and Latin America, and in patients with HIV. Pelvic tuberculosis is produced primarily by either *Mycobacterium tuberculosis* or *Mycobacterium bovis*. The primary site of infection for tuberculosis is usually the lung, with lymphatic spread from the Ghon complex to regional lymph nodes at the hilum usually occurring within 1 to 2 years. More rapid dissemination is due to hematogenous spread, which results in miliary disease often within the 1st year. The fallopian tubes are the predominant site of pelvic tuberculosis, but the bacilli also spread to the endometrium and occasionally the ovaries.

No location in the body is immune to the development of metastatic foci of infection. Tuberculosis of the bone, meninges, kidney, epididymis, fallopian tubes, and other sites can develop. At some sites of miliary spread, the lesions can remain quiescent for long periods before reactivation and further spread of the disease. Direct extension from one organ or system to an adjacent organ or system can also occur. Organs of the female reproductive tract are usually infected by hematogenous miliary spread from a primary pulmonary lesion, by hematogenous spread from a secondary miliary site, by lymphatic spread from a primary pulmonary site to intestinal lymph nodes and then to the pelvis, or by direct extension from adjacent abdominal organs (small intestines, appendix, rectum, bladder) that are the site of tuberculous infection. Fistulas between the intestinal tract and the fallopian tubes have been reported with pelvic tuberculosis.

A venereal transmission of the disease has been reported, with primary genital infection in the woman occurring after coitus with a sexual partner who had tuberculosis of the genitourinary tract. According to Sutherland and MacFarlane, it is not possible to prove conclusively that genitourinary tuberculosis in the man can be transmitted to the woman through sexual intercourse. Because it has been shown that *M. tuberculosis* is present in the sperm of men with urogenital tuberculosis, the possibility of transmission to the pelvic organs of the woman through intercourse must be accepted. Sutherland presents five cases in which sexual transmission of genitourinary tuberculosis from man to woman presumably occurred. However, of 128 husbands of women with genital tuberculosis, only 5 (3.9%) were found to have active genitourinary tuberculosis. When tuberculosis of the vulva, vagina, and cervix is present without evidence of tuberculosis elsewhere in the body, venereal transmission should be suspected.

Pathology of Pelvic Tuberculosis

Both fallopian tubes are involved in almost all patients with pelvic tuberculosis. About one half of patients with tuberculous salpingitis have tuberculous endometritis. Tuberculosis of the cervix is present in 5% of cases. The vagina and vulva are rarely involved. At operation, one may find evidence of generalized tuberculous peritonitis with small, grayish white tubercles covering all peritoneal surfaces of the abdominal and pelvic organs. The epithelium of the fallopian tubes may not be involved in generalized serosal tuberculous infection. At a later stage of infection, tuberculous salpingitis may grossly resemble other forms of PID involving the adnexa. Unless tubercles are

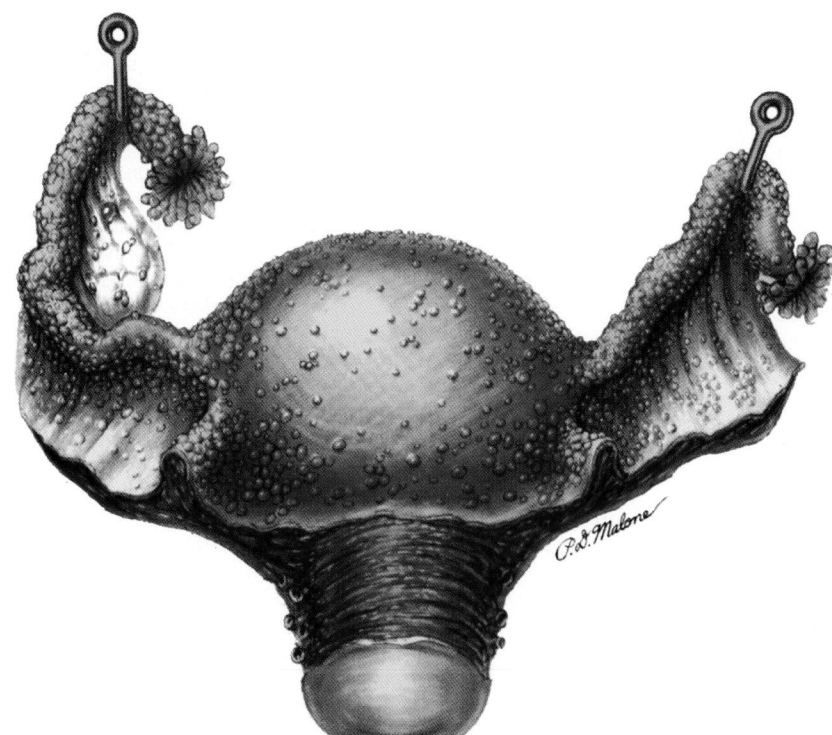

FIGURE 30.12 Typical specimen of tuberculosis of the reproductive organs as part of generalized tuberculous peritonitis.

seen, the diagnosis may not be apparent until microscopic sections are examined by the pathologist. A large pyosalpinx may contain the caseous material of a tuberculous infection but may also contain the purulent exudate of a secondary infection with other common organisms. Tubercles form in the lining of the tube. Some have caseation at the center, with giant cells and epithelioid cells. A proliferation of the mucosal lining of the fallopian tube may resemble a primary tubal carcinoma microscopically and may be confusing to the pathologist.

Tuberculous peritonitis is commonly associated with tuberculosis of the pelvis. Clinically, tuberculous peritonitis can be divided into two groups. In "wet" peritonitis, there is an outpouring of straw-colored fluid into the peritoneal cavity, producing ascites. The peritoneum of the parietal wall and viscera is covered with innumerable small tubercles (Fig. 30.12). The tubes, in addition to being covered with miliary tubercles on the serosal surface, are usually slightly enlarged and distended. In contrast to other forms of salpingitis, the fimbriae may be patent. Within the tubal wall and tubal mucosa, the histology is typical of tuberculosis, with tubercle formation, multinucleated giant cells, and epithelioid reaction (Fig. 30.13). In advanced cases, frank caseation is present. This pattern is usually associated with hematogenous spread of the tuberculous organism to the peritoneal surfaces and the pelvic organs.

Another type of tuberculous peritonitis encountered in women is the "dry" or adhesive type. Bowel adheres to bowel by innumerable dense adhesions that blend with the musculature. The muscle of the bowel is often invaded to some degree by the tuberculous process. Separation of these adhesions is extremely difficult surgically, and accidental injury to the bowel is common. The pelvic organs show evidence of tuberculous salpingitis with enlargement of the tubes and occasionally pyosalpinges and even tuboovarian abscess formation.

Tuberculous involvement of the myometrium is rare. Tuberculous endometritis, however, is common, occurring in 60% to 70% of women with pelvic tuberculosis. Microscopically,

tubercles are seen scattered throughout the endometrium, but they may be scanty. Tubercles are often seen in the endometrium removed by curettage in the premenstrual phase and are usually located in the endometrium adjacent to the

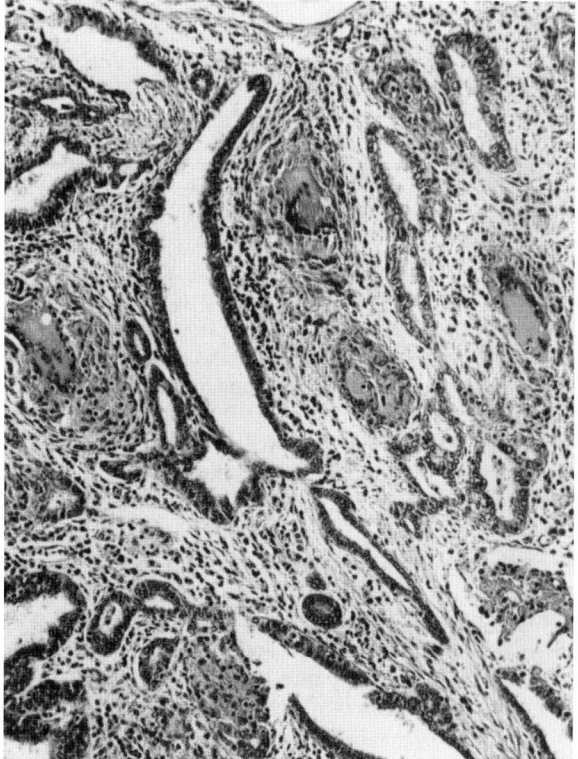

FIGURE 30.13 Tuberculosis of the fallopian tube. Note the multinucleated giant cells.

tubal ostia. Apparently, the uterine cavity is protected from advanced tuberculous infection by the cyclic shedding of endometrial tissue in the reproductive years. Even in advanced pelvic tuberculous infections, evidence of caseation, fibrosis, and calcification are rarely seen in the uterine cavity. Occasionally, the endometrial cavity is obliterated by extensive adhesions. Total destruction of the endometrium can result in amenorrhea. Tuberculous pyometra can also develop, especially in postmenopausal women with an occluded internal cervical os.

Tuberculous lesions of the cervix are rare. They can be either ulcerative or exophytic and can resemble a primary cervical malignancy or granuloma inguinale of the cervix. When there is a tuberculous lesion of the cervix, the cervical biopsy often reveals tubercles.

A tuberculous infection of the ovary usually involves only the surface of the ovary and represents simply an extension of infection from the peritoneal cavity and the adjacent fallopian tubes. The infection is usually limited to a perioophoritis. Tuberculous caseation can be found within the ovarian parenchyma, although this is uncommon. Presumably, it occurs as a result of hematogenous spread to the ovarian parenchyma rather than by direct extension through the ovarian capsule. However, a break in the ovary caused by ovulation may also allow the tubercular bacilli to gain access to the ovarian parenchyma. The ovaries are involved in about 25% of cases of pelvic tuberculosis.

It is uncommon for tuberculosis to involve the vulva and vagina. It is seen in only 2% of patients with pelvic tuberculosis. The gross appearance may be ulcerative with multiple sinuses, it may be hypertrophic with elephantiasis, or it may be similar to that of carcinoma.

Throughout the pelvic organs, the microscopic picture is similar, with tubercles of granulomatous inflammation, Langhans giant cells, epithelioid cells, and central caseation associated with chronic inflammation. With special stains, acid-fast bacilli (AFB) can be demonstrated on careful microscopic examination of the tubercles.

Clinical Features of Pelvic Tuberculosis

Pelvic tuberculosis occurs most often in patients between the ages of 20 and 40 years. The age of patients with gynecologic tuberculosis has changed in recent years; the proportion of patients older than 40 years of age is now much higher than it was in the past. Falk and associates found that the incidence of pelvic tuberculosis in postmenopausal Swedish women is increasing. This was also the opinion of Sutherland, who reported an investigation from Glasgow in which 26 of 701 patients (3.7%) with proven gynecologic tuberculosis were postmenopausal.

The most common clinical symptoms of pelvic tuberculosis include pelvic pain, general malaise, menstrual irregularity, and infertility. Brown and associates found that menstrual irregularity occurred in nearly 50% of patients, whereas amenorrhea or oligomenorrhea was present in 27%. A low-grade fever that on occasion can produce a fulminating septic course is noted in most cases of active or subacute disease. The failure of fever to subside with high doses of broad-spectrum antibiotics is a classic feature of pelvic tuberculosis. A clinical course that is refractory to antibiotic therapy for the usual PID should alert the clinician to the possibility of tuberculosis in a woman who previously resided in an endemic country.

Among patients with pulmonary tuberculosis, the incidence of pelvic tuberculosis generally varies between 10% and 20%. Falk and associates noted that 38% of women with genital tuberculosis had previously had tuberculosis in other organs, usually the lungs. Often, the patient's clinical course is that of a chronic indolent illness.

Diagnosis of Pelvic Tuberculosis

The clinical symptoms and signs of pelvic tuberculosis should direct the clinician to the diagnosis. However, the disease is so uncommon that it is seldom encountered in the gynecologist's usual practice; therefore, the clinical index of suspicion is generally low. In many cases, the clinical presentation is obscure, and the diagnosis is delayed. Howard Kelly once said that when competent gynecologists disagree about the diagnosis of an obscure pelvic condition, it usually is diagnosed as either an "old ectopic pregnancy or pelvic tuberculosis."

More than two thirds of the cases are diagnosed at the time of laparotomy performed for some other indication or at the time of investigation for infertility or abnormal uterine bleeding. The most common symptom is infertility, and the second most common symptom is lower abdominal and pelvic pain. Some patients are completely asymptomatic and are found to have pelvic tuberculosis during examination for other disorders such as infertility. A dilatation and curettage or endometrial biopsy is diagnostic in some cases, especially if performed in the late premenstrual phase of the menstrual cycle. In addition to standard microscopic sections, the specimen can be examined by fluorescent antibody technique. Acid-fast staining of tissue or culture of menstrual blood is effective in detecting the organism in only about 10% of cases, according to Overbeck. The menstrual blood can be collected in a cervical cap, but culture can be repeated many times before a positive result is obtained. Acid-fast stains of tissue suspected of tuberculous infection are important to confirm the diagnosis. Because some AFB are not tuberculous bacilli, it is important to obtain a positive culture whenever possible. A negative evaluation of the endometrium does not rule out pelvic tuberculosis, because the disease can be present in the fallopian tubes without tuberculous endometritis in 30% to 40% of cases.

On pelvic examination, bilateral adnexal tenderness is the rule. The tenderness is usually less marked than with acute gonococcal or streptococcal infections. Occasionally, a large tuberculous tuboovarian abscess is palpated on pelvic examination and even felt through the abdominal wall. The classic doughy feel of the broad ligament suggests a tuberculous inflammatory disease that is produced by a combination of thickening of the broad ligament, adherent bowel, and some ascitic fluid. On occasion, cul-de-sac nodules representing tubercles on the serosal surfaces of pelvic organs can be felt. The clinical detection of ascites is the strongest evidence obtainable in favor of pelvic tuberculosis. It was present in one fifth of the cases reported by Brown and associates. However, other causes of ascites must be considered, including ovarian carcinoma and cirrhosis of the liver. In differentiating tuberculous salpingitis from gonococcal infections, the finding of a virginal outlet in the presence of obvious tubal inflammation should lend strength to the diagnosis of pelvic tuberculosis.

The diagnosis of tuberculosis cannot be made with certainty from a hysterosalpingogram, but it may be helpful. The radiographic criteria for a suspicion of pelvic tuberculosis by hysterosalpingogram have been described by Klein and associates as follows: calcified lymph nodes or smaller, irregular calcifications in the adnexal areas; obstruction of the fallopian tube in the zone of transition between the isthmus and the ampulla; multiple constrictions along the course of the fallopian tube; endometrial adhesions or deformity or obliteration of the endometrial cavity in the absence of a history of curettage or abortion; and vascular or lymphatic extravasation of contrast material. Although a conclusive diagnosis of pelvic tuberculosis can be made only from a positive culture, these authors conclude that hysterosalpingography is a useful aid, especially in patients who are asymptomatic except for infertility.

When the diagnosis of pelvic tuberculosis cannot be made in other ways, laparoscopy has been used. Because numerous adhesions may be present, making the introduction of the trocar hazardous, we believe that laparoscopy should be used with particular care. If possible, biopsy specimens of tubal fimbriae or other suspicious areas should be examined histologically or cultured to confirm the diagnosis. In addition to disclosing numerous adhesions, laparoscopy may reveal widespread miliary tubercles involving the omentum and peritoneal surfaces. Matted adnexal masses may be seen. Microscopic examination of peritoneal fluid shows a predominance of lymphocytes.

Vaginal cytology is of limited value in diagnosing tuberculosis. The cytologist must be familiar with the morphology of epithelioid cells in the vaginal smear. Only in cases of tuberculosis of the cervix may cytology be helpful. Patients with pelvic tuberculosis should also have an examination and special diagnostic procedures to rule out tuberculous infections in the upper genital tract. Chest radiograph, tuberculin skin test, pelvic ultrasonography, intravenous pyelogram, and urine, gastric, and sputum cultures for *M. tuberculosis* should be done. In some patients, exploratory laparotomy is needed to make the diagnosis.

Treatment of Pelvic Tuberculosis

Before the advent of antituberculous drug therapy, surgery was often used in the treatment of pelvic tuberculosis. Primary surgical treatment was technically difficult, sometimes ineffective, and associated with a high risk of fistula formation and persistent draining sinuses. With the advent of effective drug therapy, the surgical treatment for genital tuberculosis has been restricted to specific indications. Beginning with streptomycin more than 30 years ago, and later isoniazid and para-aminosalicylic acid, it became evident that many cases of pelvic tuberculosis could be cured or controlled with antituberculous drug therapy. There have been major advances in the antibiotic treatment of this disease, including the use of isoniazid with rifampin, with or without ethambutol, given sometimes for a period of 2 years or longer. Sutherland analyzed the results obtained with various drug schedules. The drugs that have been used to treat tuberculosis are isoniazid, rifampin, streptomycin, ethambutol, and pyrazinamide. Isoniazid and rifampin are the most effective and have the lowest toxicity. They should be the foundation of most drug regimens. The addition of ethambutol may not be of benefit, at least not in pulmonary tuberculosis. Severe and sometimes fatal hepatitis, which can develop even after months of treatment, has been associated with isoniazid therapy. The risk of developing hepatitis increases with age and with the daily consumption of alcohol. Liver function studies should be done before treatment is started, and patients should be carefully monitored with liver function studies throughout the course of therapy and later. The regimen options and dosage recommendations of the American Thoracic Society, the Infectious Disease Society of America, and the CDC from 2003 for the treatment of tuberculosis can be found at http://www.cdc.gov with initial treatment outlines shown in Table 30.5.

The therapeutic success of modern antituberculous drug treatment regimens in pelvic tuberculosis is difficult to assess in view of the limited number of cases available in the literature. The cure rate varies in the literature from 65% to 95%. Kardos removed the fallopian tubes from 168 patients after medical treatment for 10 months and still found active tuberculosis in 35% of the surgical specimens. The experience of Sutherland suggests, however, that the results of treatment may be improved with newer drugs. The patients under treatment must be followed up closely for evidence of regression or remission of the pelvic tuberculosis. Only about 50% of patients with genital tuberculosis have the disease in the endometrial cavity; therefore, repeat endometrial biopsies and culture of menstrual egress provide only limited diagnostic information. The progress of the disease can be monitored closely by evaluating the size of adnexal masses with pelvic examinations and ultrasonography as well as tracking the ESR, WBC count, and temperature response. Prolonged follow-up is probably indicated in all cases, because recurrence of the tuberculous pelvic lesion 5 years and even later after the end of drug treatment has occasionally been found.

Surgery in the management of patients with pelvic tuberculosis should be reserved for specific indications, as outlined by Schaefer and by Sutherland. In general, surgery is reserved for

TABLE 30.5 Basic Tuberculosis Disease Treatment Regimens		
PREFERRED REGIMEN	**ALTERNATIVE REGIMEN**	**ALTERNATIVE REGIMEN**
Initial Phase		
Daily INH, RIF, PZA, and EMB[a] for 56 doses (8 wk)	Daily INH, RIF, PZA, and EMB[a] for 14 doses (2 wk), then twice weekly for 12 doses (6 wk)	Thrice-weekly INH, RIF, PZA, and EMB[a] for 24 doses (8 wk)
Continuation Phase		
Daily INH and RIF for 126 doses (18 wk) or Twice-weekly INH and RIF for 36 doses (18 wk)	Twice-weekly INH and RIF for 36 doses (18 wk)	Thrice-weekly INH and RIF for 54 doses (18 wk)

[a]EMB can be discontinued if drug susceptibility studies demonstrate susceptibility to first-line drugs.
Note: A continuation phase of once-weekly INH/rifapentine can be used for HIV-negative patients who do not have cavities on the chest film *and* who have negative AFB smears at the completion of the initial phase of treatment. INH, isoniazid; RIF, rifampin; EMB, ethambutol; PZA, pyrazinamide.

those patients who have failed to respond to an adequate trial of medical therapy. Our indications for the surgical treatment of pelvic tuberculosis include the following:

1. Persistence or enlargement of an adnexal mass after 4 to 6 months of antituberculous antibiotic therapy. The rare possibility of an ovarian tumor must always be considered, even though pelvic tuberculosis is also present. In a 1980 report by Sutherland, the persistence or development of substantial pelvic masses was the indication for surgery in 36 of 91 women with proven tuberculosis of the genital tract treated by surgery. Pelvic ultrasonography should be useful in following the response of adnexal masses to treatment.
2. Persistence of pelvic pain or recurrence of pelvic pain while on medical therapy. In Sutherland's report, 40 of 91 patients were operated on because of pain.
3. Primary unresponsiveness of the tuberculous infection to antibiotic therapy, as shown by persistent spiking temperature, leukocytosis, elevated ESR, and evidence on biopsy specimens of continued endometrial infection. Of the 91 women in Sutherland's report, 10 were operated on because of persistence of endometrial tuberculosis.
4. Difficulty in obtaining patient cooperation for continued long-term therapy. In these cases, we are accustomed to giving a brief course of streptomycin, 0.5 g every 12 hours intramuscularly for 1 week before surgery, to perform definitive surgery, and then to giving 0.5 g every 24 hours in the postoperative period for 2 weeks. A persistent effort should be made to obtain the patient's cooperation for continued antituberculous therapy postoperatively. It is advisable to continue treatment for a year or longer. Isoniazid and rifampin should be used if possible. A common reason for failure of treatment is a tendency for the physician to discontinue drugs after only a few months because the patient appears well.

The preferred surgical treatment includes total abdominal hysterectomy and bilateral salpingo-oophorectomy. The nature of this inflammatory disease may make this operative procedure technically difficult, with an increased risk of injury to bowel and bladder. Consequently, in the event of a frozen pelvis from pelvic tuberculosis, it is occasionally necessary to perform only a subtotal abdominal hysterectomy and adnexectomy.

Adhesions, which are invariably present and usually widespread, may make the dissection more difficult and injury more likely. However, it is usually possible to do this operation without a high incidence of bowel fistulas and other significant complications. Sutherland reported the results of surgery in 77 patients operated on while antituberculous therapy was administered. There were no deaths, no fistulas, and few late complications.

For young patients who are eager to attempt future childbearing, conservative adnexectomy should be carried out only if it is possible to do so after the extent of the adnexal disease is carefully evaluated and is found to be minimal. It is unwise for the surgeon to be committed to a specific operative procedure before the time of surgery, because conservative pelvic surgery for tuberculosis may constitute poor surgical judgment once the operative findings are known. The patient should be forewarned that conservative surgery will be performed only if the disease is minimal and such surgery is considered medically advisable and is consented to as such.

Conservation of an ovary at the time of operation for pelvic tuberculosis is occasionally possible if the ovary is involved only on its surface. However, if one finds gross evidence of ovarian enlargement or other gross evidence of infection deep in the ovarian parenchyma, the ovary should be removed.

Bisection of ovaries to assess the presence of disease deep in the ovarian parenchyma is not advisable.

Reactivation of silent pelvic tuberculosis after tubal reconstructive surgery has been reported by Ballon and associates and by others. We believe that reconstructive tubal surgery has no place in the management of patients whose infertility is the result of bilateral tubal obstruction from tuberculous salpingitis.

Pregnancy after Pelvic Tuberculosis

It is evident from the literature, including the studies of both Schaefer and Sutherland, that only about 5% of patients with genital tuberculosis are capable of becoming pregnant, and only 2% carry a pregnancy to term. It is also evident that in the presence of tuberculous tuboovarian abscesses, pregnancy is extremely rare, and conservative surgery for the purpose of preserving fertility is unwarranted. Only when there is minimal pelvic disease without adnexal masses should conservative surgery be considered.

BEST SURGICAL PRACTICES

- Laparoscopy should be discussed with all patients suspected of PID to confirm the diagnosis and to rule out other surgical emergencies such as appendicitis, ectopic pregnancy, or ruptured abscess. However, stable patients at high risk for complications or with contraindications to laparoscopy can be started on antimicrobial therapy and followed for 24 to 48 hours for a response. With the advent of very effective antimicrobial therapy, strong consideration should be given for surgical exploration if the patient fails initial therapy or symptomatology changes, suggesting an alternative diagnosis. If laparoscopy is not selected as initial management, an endometrial sampling for detection of inflammatory cells and bacterial culture is usually helpful.
- Sonohysterography is contraindicated in patients suspected of having PID. Culdocentesis with the finding of purulent peritoneal fluid may indicate PID but does not rule out appendicitis or diverticulitis.
- Posterior colpotomy requires a midline abscess, an abscess that is adherent to cul-de-sac peritoneum and dissects the rectovaginal septum, and a cystic or fluctuant abscess.
- Hysterectomy is no longer absolutely necessary if salpingo-oophorectomy is needed for treatment of tuboovarian abscesses. Copious irrigation with lactated Ringer is essential if an abscess has ruptured or if pus is present in the abdomen. Antibiotic irrigation has not demonstrated additional benefit or risk. If hysterectomy is necessary after bilateral salpingo-oophorectomy, the vaginal vault should be left open for drainage (with or without a Penrose drain).
- Swan-Ganz catheter placement is helpful in monitoring central venous pressure in patients undergoing surgery for ruptured tuboovarian abscess.

BIBLIOGRAPHY

Askenazi J, Farhi J, Dicker D, et al. Acute pelvic inflammatory disease after oocyte retrieval: adverse effects on the results of implantation. *Fertil Steril* 1994;61:526.

Ballon SC, Clewell WH, Lamb EJ. Reactivation of silent pelvic tuberculosis by reconstructive tubal surgery. *Am J Obstet Gynecol* 1975;122:991.

Bell TA, Holmes KK. Age-specific risks of syphilis, gonorrhea, and hospitalized pelvic inflammatory disease in sexually experienced U.S. women. *Sex Transm Dis* 1989;11:291.

Björnelius E, Anagrius C, Bojs G, et al. Antibiotic treatment of symptomatic Mycoplasma genitalium infection in Scandinavia: a controlled clinical trial. *Sex Transm Infect* 2008;84:72.

Brown AB, Gilbert RA, Te Linde RW. Pelvic tuberculosis. *Obstet Gynecol* 1953;2:476.

Centers for Disease Control and Prevention. Initial therapy for tuberculosis in the era of multidrug resistance. *JAMA* 1993;270:694.

Centers for Disease Control and Prevention. Sexually transmitted diseases: treatment guidelines. *MMWR Morb Mortal Wkly Rep* 2010;59:1.

Centers for Disease Control and Prevention. Division of tuberculosis elimination treatment for TB disease. Available at: http://www.cdc.gov/tb/topic/treatment/tbdisease.htm. September 2012.

Centers for Disease Control and Prevention. Sexually transmitted disease surveillance, 2011. Available at: http://www.cdc.gov/STD/stats11/default.htm

Centers for Disease Control and Prevention. Trends in reportable sexually transmitted diseases in the United States, 2004. Available at: http://www.cdc.gov/std/stats04/trends2004.htm. November 2005.

Chow AW, Pattern V, Marshall JR. The bacteriology of acute pelvic inflammatory disease. *Am J Obstet Gynecol* 1975;122:876.

Clarke LM, Duerr A, Yeung KA, et al. Recovery of Cytomegalovirus and Herpes Simplex Virus from upper and lower genital tract specimens obtained from women with pelvic inflammatory disease. *J Infect Dis* 1997;176:286.

Clausen HF, Fedder J, Drasbek M, et al. Serological investigation of Mycoplasma genitalium in infertile women. *Hum Reprod* 2001;16:1866.

Cohen CR, Mugo NR, Astete SG, et al. Detection of Mycoplasma genitalium in women with laparoscopically diagnosed acute salpingitis. *Sex Transm Infect* 2005;81:463.

Collins CG, Jansen FW. Management of tubo-ovarian abscess. *Clin Obstet Gynecol* 1959;2:512.

Eilard ET, Brorsson JE, Hanmark B, et al. Isolation of *Chlamydia* in acute salpingitis. *Scand J Infect Dis* 1976;9:82.

Eschenbach DA. Epidemiology and diagnosis of acute pelvic inflammatory disease. *Obstet Gynecol* 1980;55:142.

Eschenbach DA, Holmes KK. Acute PID: current concepts of pathogenesis, etiology and management. *Clin Obstet Gynecol* 1975;18:35.

Falk HC. Cornual resection for the treatment of recurrent salpingitis. *Am J Surg* 1951;81:595.

Falk V, Ludviksson K, Argen G. Genital tuberculosis in women. Analysis of 187 newly diagnosed cases from 47 Swedish hospitals during the ten-year period 1968 to 1977. *Am J Obstet Gynecol* 1980;138:974.

Falk L, Fredlund H, Jensen JS. Tetracycline treatment does not eradicate Mycoplasma genitalium. *Sex Transm Infect* 2003;79:318.

Fitz-Hugh T. Acute gonococcic peritonitis of the right upper quadrant in women. *JAMA* 1934;102:2084.

Franklin EW III, Hevron JE Jr, Thompson JD. Management of pelvic abscess. *Clin Obstet Gynecol* 1973;16:66.

Ginsburg DS, Stern JL, Hamod KA, et al. Tubo-ovarian abscess: a retrospective review. *Am J Obstet Gynecol* 1980;138:1055.

Golde SH, Israel R, Ledger WJ. Unilateral tubo-ovarian abscess: a distinct entity. *Am J Obstet Gynecol* 1977;17:807.

Hager WD, Majmudar B. Pelvic actinomycosis in women using intrauterine contraceptive devices. *Am J Obstet Gynecol* 1979;133:60.

Hager WD, McDaniel PS. Treatment of serious obstetric and gynecologic infections with cefoxitin. *J Reprod Med* 1983;28:337.

Hager WD, Eschenbach DA, Spence MR, et al. Criteria for diagnosis and grading of salpingitis. *Obstet Gynecol* 1983;61:113.

Haggerty CL, Totten PA, Astete SG, et al. Mycoplasma genitalium among women with nongonococcal, nonchlamydial pelvic inflammatory disease. *Infect Dis Obstet Gynecol* 2006;30184:1.

Haggerty CL, Totten PA, Astete SG, et al. Failure of cefoxitin and doxycycline to eradicate endometrial Mycoplasma genitalium and the consequence for clinical cure of pelvic inflammatory disease. *Sex Transm Infect* 2008;84:338.

Heaton FC, Ledger WJ. Postmenopausal tubal ovarian abscess. *Obstet Gynecol* 1976;47:90.

Hemsell DL, Wendel GD, Hemsell PG, et al. Inpatient treatment for uncomplicated and complicated acute pelvic inflammatory disease: ampicillin/sulbactam vs. cefoxitin. *Infect Dis Obstet Gynecol* 1993;1:123.

Hemsell DL, Ledger WJ, Martens M, et al. Concerns regarding the Centers for Disease Control's published guidelines for pelvic inflammatory disease. *Clin Infect Dis* 2001;32:103.

Henry-Suchet J, Soler A, Loffredo V. Laparoscopic treatment of tubo-ovarian abscesses. *J Reprod Med* 1984;29:579.

Jackson P, Ridley WJ, Pattison NS. Single dose metronidazole prophylaxis in gynaecological surgery. *N Z Med J* 1979;89:243.

Jacobson L, Westrom L. Objectivized diagnosis of acute pelvic inflammatory disease. *Am J Obstet Gynecol* 1969;105:1088.

Kaplan AL, Jacobs WM, Ehresman JR. Aggressive management of pelvic abscess. *Am J Obstet Gynecol* 1967;98:982.

Kaplan RL, Sahn SA, Petty TL. Incidence and outcome of the respiratory distress syndrome in gram-negative sepsis. *Arch Intern Med* 1979;1939:867.

Kardos F. Late results in women with genital tuberculosis. *Obstet Gynecol* 1967;29:247.

Kelly H. *Operative gynecology*. Vol. II. New York: Appleton, 1898.

Kelly AM, Ireland M, Aughey D. Pelvic inflammatory disease in adolescents: high incidence and recurrence rates in an urban teen clinic. *J Pediatr Adolesc Gynecol* 2004;17:383.

Kirtley L, Benigno BB. The residual adnexa following surgery for pelvic inflammatory disease. Resident Research Day. Atlanta, GA: Emory University School of Medicine, Gynecology and Obstetrics Department, 1979. Unpublished data.

Klein TA, Richmond JA, Mishell DR Jr. Pelvic tuberculosis. *Obstet Gynecol* 1976;48:99.

Landers DV, Sweet RL. Tubo-ovarian abscess: contemporary approach to management. *Rev Infect Dis* 1983;5:876.

Larsen B. Pelvic inflammatory disease in teenagers. *Clin Adv Treat Infect* 1991;5:1.

Lemeke R, Lsonka GW. Antibodies against pleuropneumonia-like organisms in patients with salpingitis. *Br J Vener Dis* 1962;38:212.

Linhares IM, Witkin SS. Immunopathogenic consequences of Chlamydia trachomatis 60 kDa heat shock protein expression in the female reproductive tract. *Cell Stress Chaperones* 2010;15:467.

Loy RA, Gallup DG, Hill JA, et al. Pelvic abscess: examination and transvaginal drainage guided by real-time ultrasonography. *South Med J* 1989;82:788.

Luton and Dunstable Hospital Study Group. Metronidazole in the prevention and treatment of bacteroides infections in gynaecological patients. *Lancet* 1974;304:1543.

Martens MG, Faro S, Phillips LE, et al. Comparison of two endometrial sampling devices: cotton-tipped swab and double-lumen catheter with a brush. *J Reprod Med* 1989;34:875.

Martens MG, Faro S, Hammill H, et al. Transcervical uterine cultures with a new endometrial suction curette: a comparison of three sampling methods in postpartum endometritis. *Obstet Gynecol* 1989;74:273.

Martens MG, Faro S, Maccato M, et al. In-vitro susceptibility testing of clinical isolates of *Chlamydia trachomatis*. *Infect Dis Obstet Gynecol* 1993;1:40.

McNamara MT, Mead PB. Diagnosis and management of the pelvic abscess. *J Reprod Med* 1976;17:299.

Mickal A, Sellmann AH. Management of tubo-ovarian abscess. *Clin Obstet Gynecol* 1969;12:252.

Mickal A, Sellmann AH, Beebe JL. Ruptured tubo-ovarian abscesses. *Am J Obstet Gynecol* 1968;100:432.

Monif GR. Significance of polymicrobial bacterial superinfection in the therapy of gonococcal endometritis-salpingitis-peritonitis. *Obstet Gynecol* 1980;55:1545.

Monif GR. Clinical staging of acute bacterial salpingitis and its therapeutic ramifications. *Am J Obstet Gynecol* 1982;143:489.

Monif GR, Welkos SL, Baer H, et al. Cul-de-sac isolates from patients with endometritis-salpingitis-peritonitis and gonococcal endocervicitis. *Am J Obstet Gynecol* 1976;126:158.

Ness RB, Hillier SL, Kip KE, et al. Bacterial vaginosis and risk of pelvic inflammatory disease. *Obstet Gynecol* 2004;104:761.

Ness RB, Randall H, Richter HE, et al. Condom use and the risk of recurrent pelvic inflammatory disease, chronic pelvic pain, or infertility following an episode of pelvic inflammatory disease. *Am J Public Health* 2004;94:1327.

Ness RB, Kip KE, Hillier SL, et al. A cluster analysis of bacterial vaginosis-associated microflora and pelvic inflammatory disease. *Am J Epidemiol* 2005;162:585.

Ness RB, Trautmann G, Soper DE. Effectiveness of treatment strategies of some women with pelvic inflammatory disease: a randomized trial. *Obstet Gynecol* 2005;106:573.

Ness RB, Smith KJ, Chang CC, et al. Prediction of pelvic inflammatory disease among young, single, sexually active women. *Sex Transm Dis* 2006;33:137.

Olak J, Christon NV, Stein LA, et al. Operative vs. percutaneous drainage of intra-abdominal abscesses. *Arch Surg* 1986;121:141.

Overbeck L. Is tuberculosis of the female urogenital tract an entity? *J Obstet Gynaecol Br Commonw* 1966;73:624.

Paavonen J. Chlamydia trachomatis infections of the female genital tract: state of the art. *Ann Med* 2012;44:18.

Paavonen J, Kiviat N, Brunham RC, et al. Prevalence and manifestations of endometritis among women with cervicitis. *Am J Obstet Gynecol* 1985;152:280.

Pedowitz P, Bloomfield R. Ruptured adnexal abscess (tubo-ovarian) with generalized peritonitis. *Am J Obstet Gynecol* 1964;88:721.

Peterson HB, Walker CK, Kahn JG, et al. Pelvic inflammatory disease: key treatment issues and options. *JAMA* 1991;266:2605.

Phillips AJ, D'Abling G. Acute salpingitis subsequent to tubal ligation. *Obstet Gynecol* 1986;67:55.

Protopapas AG, Diakomanolis ES, Milingos SD, et al. Tubo-ovarian abscesses in postmenopausal women: gynecological malignancy until proven otherwise? *Eur J Obstet Gynecol Reprod Biol* 2004;114:203.

Reich H, McGlynn F. Laparoscopic treatment of tuboovarian and pelvic abscess. *J Reprod Med* 1987;32:747.

Rivlin MR, Hunt JA. Ruptured tubo-ovarian abscess: is hysterectomy necessary?. *Obstet Gynecol* 1983;61:169.

Rossouw JE, Anderson GL, Prentice RL, et al.; Writing Group for the Women's Health Initiative Investigators. Risks and benefits of estrogen plus progestin in healthy postmenopausal women: principal results from the Women's Health Initiative randomized controlled trial. *JAMA* 2002;288:321.

Schaefer G. Female genital tuberculosis. *Clin Obstet Gynecol* 1976;19:223.

Short VL, Totten PA, Ness RB, et al. Clinical presentation of Mycoplasma genitalium infection versus Neisseria gonorrhoeae infection among women with pelvic inflammatory disease. *Clin Infect Dis* 2009;48:41.

Sørbye IK, Jerve F, Staff AC. Reduction in hospitalized women with pelvic inflammatory disease in Oslo over the past decade. *Acta Obstet Gynecol Scand* 2005;84:290.

Sufrin CB, Postlethwaite D, Armstrong MA, et al. Neisseria gonorrhea and Chlamydia trachomatis screening at intrauterine device insertion and pelvic inflammatory disease. *Obstet Gynecol* 2012;120:1314.

Sutherland AM. The management of genital tuberculosis in women. *Gazzet San* 1970;19:180.

Sutherland AM. Twenty-five years' experience of the drug treatment of tuberculosis of the female genital tract. *Br J Obstet Gynaecol* 1977;84:881.

Sutherland AM. Laparoscopy in diagnosis of pelvic tuberculosis. *Lancet* 1979;2:95.

Sutherland AM. Surgical treatment of tuberculosis of the female genital tract. *BJOG* 1980;87:610.

Sutherland AM. The treatment of tuberculosis of the female genital tract with rifampicin, ethambutol, and isoniazid. *Arch Gynecol* 1981;230:315.

Sutherland AM. Postmenopausal tuberculosis of the female genital tract. *Obstet Gynecol* 1982;59:545.

Sutherland AM. The changing pattern of tuberculosis of the female genital tract. A thirty year survey. *Arch Gynecol* 1983;234:95.

Sutherland AM, MacFarlane JR. Transmission of genitourinary tuberculosis. *Health Bull (Edinb)* 1982;40:87.

Sutton MY, Strenberg M, Zaida A, et al. Trends in pelvic inflammatory disease hospital discharges and ambulatory visits, United States, 1985–2001. *Sex Transm Dis* 2005;32:778.

Svensson L, Westrom L, Ripa KT, et al. Differences in some clinical laboratory parameters in acute salpingitis related to culture and serologic findings. *Am J Obstet Gynecol* 1980;138:1017.

Svensson L, Westrom L, Mardh PA. Contraceptives and acute salpingitis. *JAMA* 1987;251:2553.

Svenstrup HF, Fedder J, Kristoffersen SE, et al. Mycoplasma genitalium, Chlamydia trachomatis, and tubal factor infertility—a prospective study. *Fertil Steril* 2008;90:513.

Sweet RL. PID and infertility in women. *Infect Dis Clin North Am* 1987;1:199.

Sweet RL, Gibbs RS. *Infectious diseases of the female genital tract.* Baltimore, MD: Williams & Wilkins, 1990:241.

Sweet RL, Draper DL, Schacter J, et al. Microbiology and pathogenesis of acute salpingitis as determined by laparoscopy: what is the appropriate site to sample? *Am J Obstet Gynecol* 1980;138:985.

Sweet RL, Schacter J, Robbie M. Failure of beta-lactam antibiotics to eradicate *Chlamydia trachomatis* in the endometrium despite clinical care of acute salpingitis. *JAMA* 1983;250:2641.

Sweet RL, Roy S, Faro S, et al. Piperacillin-tazobactam versus clindamycin and gentamicin in the treatment of hospitalized women with pelvic infection. *Obstet Gynecol* 1994;83:280.

Tatum HJ, Schmidt FH, Phillips D, et al. The Dalkon shield controversy: structural and bacteriological studies of IUD trials. *JAMA* 1975;231:711.

Taylor BD, Darville T, Ferrell RE, et al. Variants in toll-like receptor 1 and 4 genes are associated with Chlamydia trachomatis among women with pelvic inflammatory disease. *J Infect Dis* 2012;205:603.

Tyrrel RT, Murphy FB, Bernardino ME. Tubo-ovarian abscesses: CT-guided percutaneous drainage. *Radiology* 1990;175:87.

Vermeeren J, Te Linde RW. Intraabdominal rupture of pelvic abscesses. *Am J Obstet Gynecol* 1954;68:402.

Viberga I, Odlind V, Lazdane G, et al. Microbiology profile in women with pelvic inflammatory disease in relation to IUD use. *Infect Dis Obstet Gynecol* 2005;13:183.

Washington AE, Cates W Jr, Zaidi AA. Hospitalization for PID: epidemiology and trends in the U.S., 1975 to 1981. *JAMA* 1984;251:2529.

Weiner S, Wallach EE. Ovarian histology in pelvic inflammatory disease. *Obstet Gynecol* 1974;43:431.

Westrom L. Incidence, prevalence and trends of acute pelvic inflammatory disease and its consequences in industrialized countries. *Am J Obstet Gynecol* 1980;138:880.

Westrom L. Introductory address: treatment of pelvic inflammatory disease in view of etiology and risk factors. *Sex Transm Dis* 1984;11:437.

Wetchler SJ, Dunn LJ. Ovarian abscess: report of a case and a review of the literature. *Obstet Gynecol Surv* 1985;40:476.

Wharton LR. Pelvic abscess: a study based on a series of 716. *Arch Surg* 1921;2:246.

Willson JR, Black JR. Ovarian abscess. *Am J Obstet Gynecol* 1964;90:34.

Worthen NJ, Gunning JE. Percutaneous drainage of pelvic abscesses: management of the tubo-ovarian abscess. *J Ultrasound Med* 1986;5:551.

CHAPTER 31
Leiomyomata Uteri and Myomectomy

Carla P. Roberts and Jennifer F. Kawwass

DEFINITIONS

Intravenous leiomyomatosis—Smooth muscle tumor that consists of polypoid intravascular projections into the veins of the parametrium and broad ligaments.

Leiomyomatosis peritonealis disseminata—A benign reparative process in which fibroblasts replace soft peritoneal decidua on subperitoneal surfaces of the uterus and other pelvic and abdominal viscera resulting in nodules with a pseudoleiomyomatous pattern.

Menorrhagia—Prolonged (>7 days) or heavy (>80 mL) menstrual bleeding occurring at regular intervals.

Metrorrhagia—Uterine bleeding occurring at irregular intervals, sometimes of prolonged duration.

Menometrorrhagia—Heavy, prolonged bleeding occurring at irregular intervals.

Submucosal—Present within the uterine myometrium just below the basal layer of the endometrial lining.

Subserosal—Present within the uterine myometrium just below the serosal or peritoneal covering of the uterus.

Leiomyomata are the most common tumors of the uterus and the female pelvis. This chapter discusses the pathologic and clinical features of uterine leiomyomata, the choice of treatment, and the indications and techniques for myomectomy.

Hysterectomy is sometimes required for the management of leiomyomata. It is also performed for many other indications, but leiomyomatous uteri are the most common indication for hysterectomy. Refer to Chapter 32 for a complete discussion of hysterectomy.

Advances in gynecologic surgery in the early 1900s finally brought this common, sometimes fatal, disease of women under reasonable control. Before the 20th century, no effective treatment was available. Uterine leiomyomata often grew to enormous size and caused great suffering from bleeding, pain, and emaciation (**Fig. 31.1**). Death from this benign disease was not uncommon. Progress in gynecologic surgery and anesthesia finally allowed the safe removal of these tumors by skilled gynecologic surgeons.

No one played a more important role in this endeavor than Drs. Kelly and Cullen. Working together at Johns Hopkins Hospital, they gradually developed surgical techniques that were successful in preventing and controlling intraoperative hemorrhage. Several illustrations from their magnificent treatise, *Myomata of the Uterus,* published in 1907, are included in this chapter. In the preface, Cullen wrote:

> It was my good fortune to come to Baltimore in 1891, shortly after the hospital opened. At that time many cases of myoma were considered inoperable, and even when hysterectomy was undertaken it was only in the cases in which a stout rubber ligature could be temporarily tied around the cervix and when, as happened in some cases, this ligature slipped, alarming hemorrhage followed. Then came the systematic controlling of each of the cardinal vessels; later the bisection, and finally the transverse severance of the cervix as a preliminary feature of the operation in exceptionally difficult cases, until at present a myomatous uterus that cannot be removed is almost unheard of. I have watched the gradual simplification of the surgical procedures with the greatest interest.

Many American surgeons have had much to do with the wonderful advance in this direction, but I know of no other man, either here or abroad, who has done as much toward this advancement as Howard A. Kelly.

The mortality rate for 1,373 operations performed for uterine leiomyomata at Johns Hopkins Hospital between 1889 and 1906 was 5.75%; it was less than 1% for 238 operations performed between 1906 and 1909. In 55 patients, no operation was attempted because of patients' refusal or weakened condition. Among these patients, 21 deaths occurred in the hospital. Death from uterine leiomyomata rarely occurs today. The near elimination of mortality secondary to uterine fibroids represents a major milestone in the health care of women.

During the past century, hysterectomy and myomectomy by the traditional and classic techniques have been the main treatment for women with uterine leiomyomata and significant symptoms; they continue to be so today. Each year in the United States, more than 200,000 hysterectomies are performed with uterine leiomyomata as the primary indication. However, this traditional management is currently evolving toward more conservative, less invasive techniques for several reasons:

1. Concern regarding the increasing costs of health care has focused on the need to use effective but less expensive methods of management of uterine leiomyomata.
2. Advances in surgical technology now allow certain patients to be treated with new, minimally invasive techniques, including robotic hysterectomy, laparoscopic hysterectomy, laparoscopic-assisted vaginal hysterectomy, robotic myomectomy, laparoscopic myomectomy, laparoscopic myoma coagulation (myolysis), and hysteroscopic resection of submucous myomata. Under proper circumstances, these procedures can be safe, effective, and less costly.
3. Interest in nonsurgical management also appears to be increasing with more data available regarding minimally invasive procedures, including uterine artery embolization (UAE). This procedure has emerged from an investigational realm to common clinical practice. As more long-term data become available, outcomes and prognosis are becoming more clearly delineated.
4. A medical approach to the management of patients with leiomyomata is now available. Gonadotropin-releasing hormone (GnRH) analogs, administered for 3 to 6 months, cause most uterine leiomyomata to shrink. However, the myomata regain their original size several months after the GnRH analog is discontinued. This medical regimen has

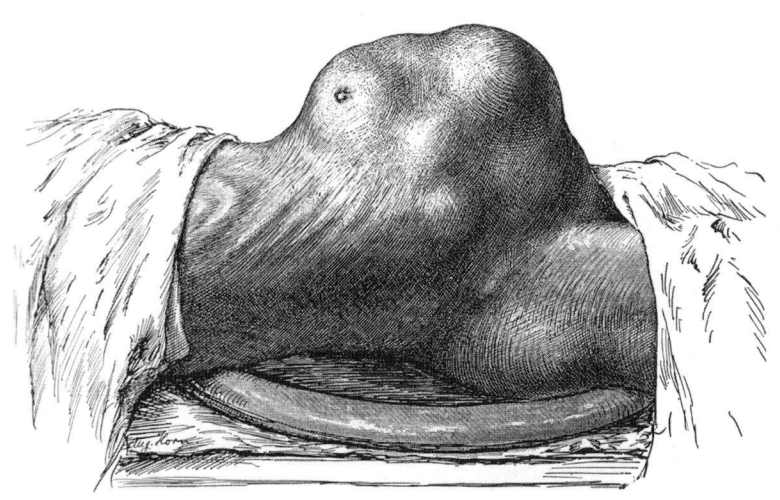

FIGURE 31.1 The patient is thin and emaciated, the outline of the ribs being prominent. Such advanced and neglected cases of multiple uterine leiomyomata are rarely seen today.

been useful as an adjunct to surgical management. Women who become symptomatic with leiomyomata just before menopause can be treated temporarily with GnRH analogs and can possibly avoid surgical therapy.

5. Uterine leiomyoma are a major public health and women's health care problem. Society has a legitimate reason for interest and concern and has questioned the advisability of hysterectomy for the management of most cases of uterine leiomyomata. Many women insist on the preservation of uterine function for future childbearing and sometimes even when future childbearing is not desired or not likely to occur. A greater emphasis has developed on expectant management, medical management, minimally invasive surgical procedures, and conservational management of uterine leiomyomata in the future.

In the future, the traditional and classic techniques of hysterectomy and myomectomy will be required less often for patients with symptomatic leiomyomata. At present, however, these operations are still appropriate in many situations.

ETIOLOGY, PATHOLOGY, AND GROWTH CHARACTERISTICS OF UTERINE LEIOMYOMATA

A leiomyoma is a benign tumor composed mainly of smooth muscle cells but containing varying amounts of fibrous connective tissue. The tumor is well circumscribed but not encapsulated. Various terms are used to refer to the tumor, such as *fibromyoma, myofibroma, leiomyofibroma, fibroleiomyoma, myoma, fibroma,* and *fibroid.* The latter designation is the one most commonly used, but it is the least accurate and acceptable. The term *leiomyoma* is a reasonably accurate one that emphasizes the origin of this tumor from smooth muscle cells and the predominance of the smooth muscle component. The tissue culture work of Miller and Ludovici suggested an origin from smooth muscle cells, and the studies of Townsend and associates affirm a unicellular origin for leiomyomata.

Leiomyomata are the most common tumors of the uterus and female pelvis. It is impossible to determine their true incidence accurately, although the frequently quoted incidence of 50% found at postmortem examinations seems reasonable. Leiomyomata are responsible for about one third of all hospital admissions to gynecology services. It is well recognized that the incidence is much higher in African American than in Caucasian women. In a careful study of leiomyomata among women in Augusta, Georgia, Torpin and associates found the incidence among African American women to be three and one third times that among Caucasian women. There is no known explanation for this racial difference. Leiomyomata also are larger and occur at a younger age in African Americans. In fact, many African American women develop leiomyomata before 30 years of age. However, development prior to age 20 is extremely rare, regardless of race. Patients with uterine leiomyomata often have a positive family history of uterine leiomyomata. This suggests the presence of a gene, which has yet to be discovered, encoding for their development.

About 40% to 50% of leiomyomas show karyotypically detectable chromosomal abnormalities that are both nonrandom and tumor specific. Identified chromosomal abnormalities include t(12;14) (q15;q23–24), del(7) (q22q32), rearrangements involving 6p21, 10q, trisomy 12, and deletions of 3q. Interestingly, a recent study of 217 myomas found a positive correlation between the presence of a cytogenetic abnormality and the anatomic location of the myoma. In this study by Brosens and colleagues, submucous myomas were consistently shown to have fewer cytogenetic abnormalities when compared with intramural and subserous lesions (12% vs. 35% and 29%, respectively). An increased prevalence in certain races, twin studies indicating higher correlation with hysterectomy in monozygotic twins, and increased incidence in first-degree relatives all seem to support an inherited predisposition. The true genetic contribution to the development of uterine leiomyoma remains to be defined.

Most of the data concerning the incidence of uterine leiomyomata are based on gross examination of the uterus, routine pathology reports, or the clinical diagnosis of uterine leiomyomata. Cramer and Patel subjected 100 uteri to gross serial sectioning at 2-mm intervals. They found 649 leiomyomata, roughly threefold the number identified by routine pathologic examination. Admittedly, some were only a few millimeters in diameter, but all were grossly visible. In 48 uteri with no mention of leiomyomata in the routine report, 27 were found to have small tumors. The incidence of leiomyomata was the same in premenopausal and postmenopausal uteri, although the average number of leiomyomata and the average size of the largest leiomyoma were greater in the premenopausal women. This work has important implications for future epidemiologic studies. It also suggests that it is almost never possible to surgically remove all leiomyomata when a myomectomy is performed.

The growth of leiomyomata is dependent on estrogen production. The tumors thrive during the years of greatest ovarian activity. Continuous estrogen secretion, especially when uninterrupted by pregnancy and lactation, is thought to be the most important underlying risk factor in the development of myomata. After menopause, with regression of ovarian estrogen secretion, growth of leiomyomata usually ceases. Actual regression in the tumor size may occur. There are rare instances, however, of postmenopausal growth of benign leiomyomata, suggesting the possibility of postmenopausal estrogen production either in the ovary or elsewhere. Postmenopausal ovarian cortical stromal hyperplasia may be associated with an increase in estrogen secretion by the ovary. The postmenopausal ovarian stroma in a variety of presumably inactive ovarian tumors, including mucinous cysts and Brenner tumors, can also produce estrogen. When a central pelvic tumor presumed to be uterine leiomyomata enlarges after menopause, one should think of the possibility of malignant change in the leiomyoma itself or in the adjacent myometrium, or of the growth of a new pelvic tumor of extrauterine origin.

Older nulliparous women have an increased risk of developing leiomyomata. However, in multiparous women, the relative risk decreases with each pregnancy. A woman who has had five term pregnancies has only one fifth the risk of a nulliparous woman of developing myomata. The risk is reduced in women who smoke and is increased in obese women; this is possibly related to the conversion of androgens to estrogen by fat aromatase.

The observation that leiomyomata may show significant enlargement during pregnancy provides further clinical evidence of the relation of estrogen and progesterone to the growth of these tumors. However, a better blood supply during pregnancy might also encourage their growth. In a prospective ultrasonographic study of 29 pregnant patients with uterine leiomyomata, Aharoni and associates found no evidence of enlargement of the myomata in 78%. Lev-Toaff and colleagues also confirmed that some but not all leiomyomata enlarge during pregnancy in response to estrogen and progesterone.

In the initial two decades following the introduction of oral contraceptives containing high-dose estrogen, there was a striking increase in the occurrence of large leiomyomata among young women of all racial backgrounds who took these pills. Although the growth of uterine leiomyomata is not invariably stimulated, oral contraceptives containing high-dose estrogen should not be prescribed for women with these tumors. Oral contraceptives with low-dose estrogen are less likely to stimulate growth. According to Parazzini and associates, there is no significant relation between the occurrence or growth of leiomyomata and the newer oral contraceptives that contain much smaller amounts of estrogens and progestins, and some believe that the risk of developing myomata is reduced with these low-dose pills.

Scientific investigators have been intrigued by the observation that leiomyomata develop during the reproductive years, sometimes grow during pregnancy, and regress after menopause. Nelson, Lipschutz, and others have produced multiple leiomyomata artificially on the serosal surface of the uterus and other peritoneal surfaces in guinea pigs given prolonged estrogen injections. Spellacy and coworkers found that levels of plasma estradiol were the same in patients with and without leiomyomata. However, Wilson and associates found a significantly higher concentration of estrogen receptors in leiomyomata than in myometrium. Farber and colleagues reported that these tumors bind about 20% more estradiol per milligram of cytoplasmic protein than does the normal myometrium of the same organ. This observation was not uniformly true for all leiomyomata, suggesting that different cellular components with a leiomyoma may be associated with different biologic activity. Otubu and coworkers found the concentration of estradiol to be significantly higher in leiomyomata than in normal myometrium, especially in the proliferative phase of the menstrual cycle. Soules and McCarty reported that leiomyomata had more estrogen receptors than did normal uterine tissues in the first phase (days 1 through 9) and in the second phase (days 10 through 18) of the menstrual cycle. Gabb and Stone found that the ability to convert estradiol to estrone was similar in leiomyomata and myometrium. However, Pollow and associates found the conversion of estradiol into estrone to be significantly lower in leiomyomata than in myometrium. This difference in conversion rate could result in a relative accumulation of estrogen in a leiomyoma, causing a hyperestrogenic state within the tumor and surrounding tissues. The enzyme 17β-hydroxy dehydrogenase accelerates the conversion of estradiol to estrone. Leiomyomata have a low concentration of 17β-hydroxy dehydrogenase, which results in a relative accumulation of estradiol in leiomyomatous tissue. These findings may explain the myometrial hypertrophy that is invariably present with leiomyomata.

Other abnormalities in endocrine function have also been suggested. Ylikorkala and colleagues found that pituitary function may be abnormal in women with leiomyomata. Patients with leiomyomata had a low follicle-stimulating hormone level and a diminished follicle-stimulating hormone response to pituitary GnRH. There was an excessive prolactin response to thyrotropin-releasing hormone. Spellacy and colleagues found that the peak levels of human growth hormone reached during a hypoglycemic test were twice as high in patients with leiomyomata as in the control group. Reddy and Rose suggested the possibility that 5α-reduced androgens may play a role in the pathophysiology of uterine leiomyomata, because a significant increase in 5α-reductase has been found in leiomyoma tissue as compared with the myometrium and endometrium. Influenced by the experimental investigations of Lipschutz and associates, Goodman in 1946 treated patients with uterine leiomyomata

with progesterone and noted a decrease in tumor size in all patients. However, Segaloff and colleagues reported no effect in their study. Goldzieher and coworkers produced histologic evidence of extensive degenerative changes in leiomyomata by administering high-dose progestin therapy (medrogestone in high doses for 21 days). Filiceri and associates have reported the regression of a uterine leiomyoma after long-term administration of a long-acting luteinizing hormone–releasing hormone agonist given to suppress ovarian estrogen secretion. Coutinho successfully used a potent 19-norsteroid antiestrogen–antiprogesterone to treat excessive uterine bleeding in 16 patients with uterine leiomyomata. A reduction in the size of the tumors was noted.

Although the exact etiology of uterine leiomyomata is not known, the puzzle may be solved bit by bit by the research of Kornyei and colleagues, Wilson and coworkers, Tamaya and associates, Buchi and Keller, Sadan and colleagues, and others who continue to investigate estrogen and progesterone as possible growth factors. Although some data are conflicting, evidence suggests that both estrogen and progesterone are involved in the growth of uterine leiomyomata. The possibility that progesterone may play a role in the growth of leiomyomata is suggested by the work of Kawaguchi and coworkers, who found a higher mitotic count in leiomyomata obtained in the proliferative phase of the menstrual cycle.

Anderson and associates have shown that medroxyprogesterone acetate, a progestin, causes a decrease in connexin-43 messenger ribonucleic acid levels in primary cultures of human myometrium and leiomyoma. Connexin-43 is a gap junction protein whose formation is stimulated by 17β-estradiol.

According to the research data of Brandon and colleagues, progesterone receptor messenger ribonucleic acid is overexpressed in uterine leiomyomata, compared with normal adjacent myometrium, suggesting that amplified progesterone-mediated signaling is instrumental in the abnormal growth of these tumors. It is possible that the increased amount of progesterone receptor is caused by an alteration of estrogen or estrogen receptors in leiomyomata. The work of Kastner and coworkers and Nardulli and associates has demonstrated that progesterone receptor expression is regulated by estrogen.

Research in recent years has also focused on polypeptide growth factors in the stimulation of growth of leiomyomata. Polypeptide growth factors that have been investigated include epidermal growth factor, transforming growth factor alpha and beta, insulin-like growth factor (IGF), platelet-derived growth factor, vascular endothelial growth factor, and basic fibroblast growth factor. Other growth factors may also be involved. Polypeptide growth factor research has been performed by Goustin and colleagues, by Hoffmann and coworkers, by Lumsden and associates, and by others. A brief review of this research has been written by Vollenhoven and associates, who have been involved in the study of IGFs in uterine leiomyomata.

Results from a study by Strawn and colleagues demonstrate that IGF-I stimulates leiomyoma growth in a dose-related manner over that of normal myometrial tissue in monolayer culture. This stimulatory effect, in the absence of sex steroid hormones or other growth factors, provides additional support that IGF-I may play an important direct role in the pathogenesis of these tumors, possibly by modulating the response of these tumors to various levels of sex steroids. Dawood and Kahn-Dawood were unable to find any significant elevation in peripheral levels of serum IGF-I in nonpregnant premenopausal women with uterine leiomyomata of 14 weeks gestational size. The authors state, "Nevertheless, the finding does not detract from the potential paracrine or autocrine role that

IGF-I produced by leiomyoma cells may have either on the growth of its own or adjacent myomas or on the vascular supply and blood flow of the uterus and myomas."

Rein and coworkers have proposed a hypothesis to explain the pathogenesis of myomata. This hypothesis suggests a critical role for progesterone in the growth of myomata. They state:

> The initiation and growth of myomas likely involves a multistep cascade of separate tumor initiators and promoters. The initial neoplastic transformation of the normal myocyte involves somatic mutations. Although the initiators of the somatic mutations remain unclear, the mitogenic effect of progesterone may enhance the propagation of somatic mutations. Myoma proliferation is the result of clonal expansion and likely involves the complex interactions of estrogen, progesterone, and local growth factors. Estrogen and progesterone appear equally important as promoters of myoma growth.

To treat patients with uterine leiomyomata properly, the gynecologic surgeon must be familiar with their pathology, growth characteristics, and clinical features. Leiomyomata may be single, but most are multiple. They develop most commonly in the uterine corpus and much less often in the cervix. They may develop in the round ligaments, but this is rare. Because they arise in the myometrium, they are all interstitial or intramural in the beginning. As they enlarge, they can remain intramural, but growth often extends in an internal or external direction. Thus, the tumor can eventually become subserous or submucous in location. A subserous tumor can become pedunculated and occasionally parasitic, receiving its blood supply from another source, usually the omentum. A submucous tumor can also become pedunculated and may gradually dilate the endocervical canal and protrude through the cervical os. Indeed, a submucous myoma may descend through the vagina. Rarely, chronic uterine inversion results if the prolapsing submucous leiomyoma is attached to the top of the endometrial cavity and pulls the uterine fundus downward through the cervix.

In general, subserous leiomyomata contain more fibrous tissue than submucous leiomyomata. However, submucous leiomyomata contain more smooth muscle tissue than subserous leiomyomata. Sarcomatous change is more common in submucous tumors.

The typical uterine leiomyoma is a firm multinodular structure of variable size. The largest tumor, reported by Hunt in 1888, weighed more than 65 kg. Tumors of 4 to 5 kg are not rare, but most are smaller. In the operating room, leiomyomata appear as nodular tumors of different sizes that distort the uterus in various ways, depending on their size, location, and direction of growth. Growth between the leaves of the broad ligament and origin from the cervix may make surgical removal difficult. Subserous and subserous pedunculated tumors, as well as intraligamentous tumors, may create problems in diagnosis because they are difficult to distinguish from tumors arising from the adnexal organs (Fig. 31.2). When tumors cause symmetric enlargement of the uterus, they may be mistaken for a pregnant uterus on bimanual examination.

The "normal" intramural leiomyoma on section protrudes from the surrounding compressed myometrium. Ordinarily, there is a clear distinction between the myoma and the myometrium so that dissection between the two is easy to accomplish. Myomata usually can be removed from surrounding myometrium with ease. Although these tumors are not encapsulated, a clear distinction can usually be made between a myoma and the myometrium that surrounds it. The cut surface appears as glistening pinkish white and gray. It is firm, and there is a whorllike arrangement of the muscle and the fibrous tissue. In contrast to this typical appearance, the myometrium may be thickened by a diffuse, ill-defined nodularity of smooth muscle. This so-called diffuse leiomyomatosis usually involves all parts of the myometrium and causes symmetric enlargement of the uterine corpus. The nodules of smooth muscle are not distinct, contain little collagen, and merge with one another and the surrounding hypertrophied myometrium.

The extracellular matrix of leiomyomata is composed mostly of collagen but also contains proteoglycans and fibronectin. According to Fujita, myomata contain 50% more collagen than does normal myometrium, and the ratio of collagen type I to collagen type III is increased in myomata. Proteoglycans provide hydrated spaces between myoma cells. Fibronectin is a glycoprotein that mediates adhesion between myoma cells and extracellular matrix.

The most common change in leiomyomata is hyaline degeneration. The cut surface of a hyalinized area is smooth and homogeneous and does not show the whorllike arrangement of the rest of the leiomyoma. Almost all leiomyomata, except the smallest, have scattered areas of hyaline degeneration. Eventually, these may become liquefied and form cystic cavities filled with clear liquid or gelatinous material

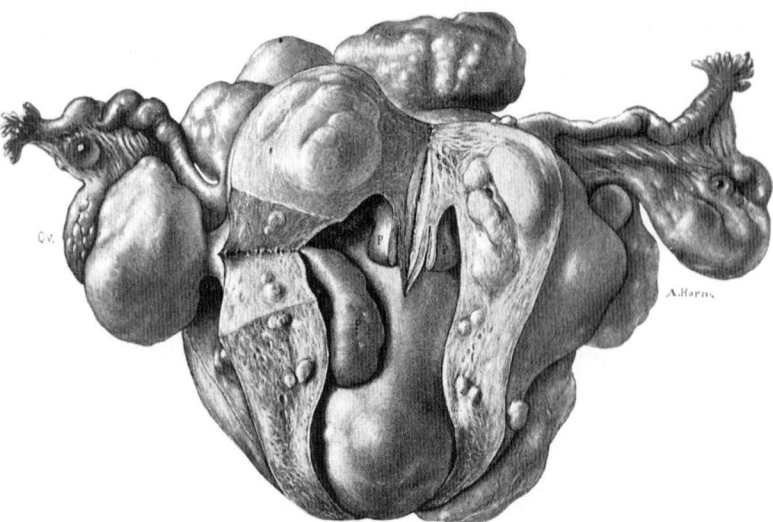

FIGURE 31.2 The uterine corpus is almost completely replaced by small and large myomas in intramural, subserous, and submucous positions. Some are pedunculated. A pedunculated submucous myoma is dilating the endocervical canal. A pedunculated subserous myoma is adjacent to the left ovary and will interfere with its palpation.

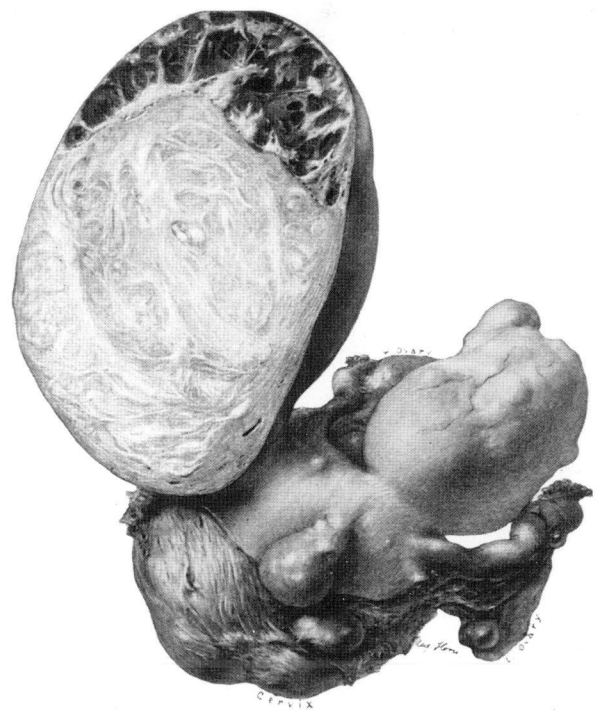

FIGURE 31.3 Multiple leiomyomata are present. A large subserous myoma has undergone partial cystic degeneration.

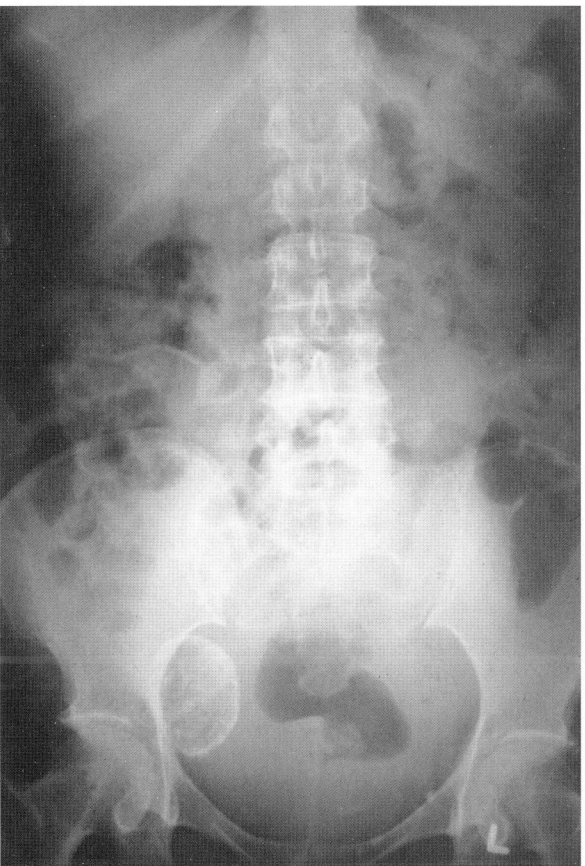

FIGURE 31.4 An abdominal radiograph shows typical calcification in a leiomyoma.

(**Fig. 31.3**). Sometimes, the cystic change is so great that the leiomyoma becomes a mere shell and is truly a cystic tumor. Softness of a tumor does not necessarily indicate cystic degeneration. Fleshy leiomyomata may be equally soft.

Over time, with continued diminished blood supply and ischemic necrosis of tissue, calcium phosphates and carbonates are deposited in myomata. Their presence is evidence of a continuum of degenerative changes. The calcium may be deposited in varying amounts. If it is deposited at the periphery of the tumor, the leiomyoma may resemble a calcified cyst. Other calcified leiomyomata may show an irregular or diffuse distribution throughout with a honeycomb or mulberry appearance. When the degenerative change is advanced, the leiomyoma may become solidly calcified. Such calcified tumors have been called "womb stones." Calcified leiomyomata are seen most often in elderly women, in African American women, and in women who have pedunculated subserous tumors. They are easily seen radiographically (**Fig. 31.4**).

Leiomyomata may undergo changes as a result of infection. Submucous leiomyomata are most commonly infected when they protrude into the uterine cavity, or especially into the vagina (**Fig. 31.5**). The pedunculated submucous leiomyoma thins out the endometrium as it grows inward, and eventually, the surface becomes ulcerated and infected (**Fig. 31.6**). An intramural leiomyoma in an involuting puerperal uterus can also become infected when endometritis is present. Microscopic abscesses can be found, and gross abscesses occasionally occur, particularly if the leiomyoma descends as low as the cervical canal. Such infections are usually streptococcal and may be virulent. *Bacteroides fragilis* infections also occur. Parametritis, peritonitis, and even septicemia may result.

Necrosis of a leiomyoma is caused by interference with its blood supply. Occasionally, a pedunculated subserous leiomyoma twists, and if an operation is not done immediately, infarction results. Necrosis sometimes occurs in the center of

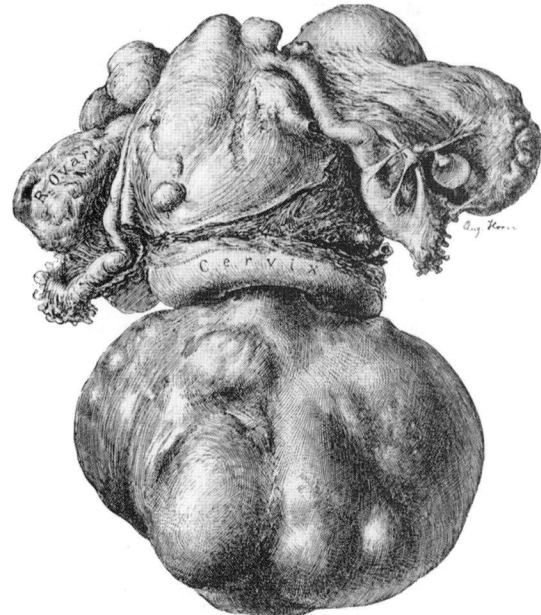

FIGURE 31.5 A large submucous pedunculated myoma has dilated the cervix and is now located in the vagina. Its pedicle is attached inside the uterine cavity. Morcellation of the myoma performed transvaginally allows clamping and ligation of the pedicle.

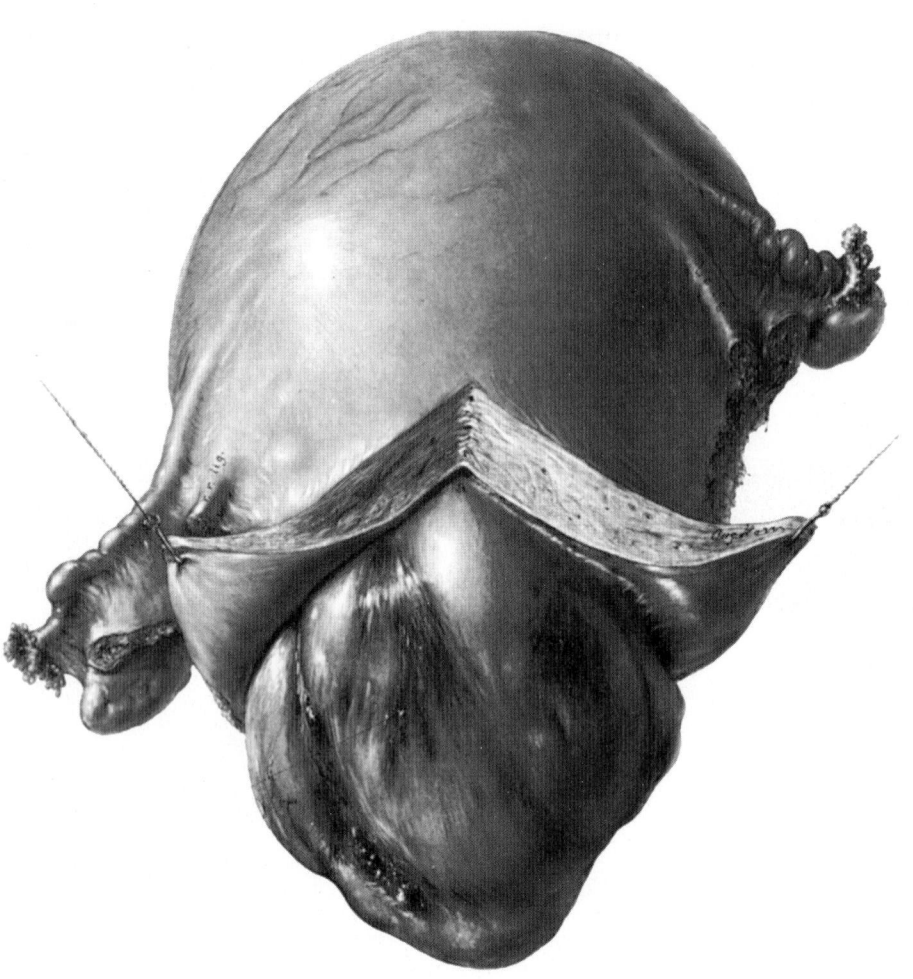

FIGURE 31.6 Pedunculated submucous myoma showing necrosis and ulceration.

a large tumor simply as a result of poor circulation. Necrotic leiomyomata are dark and hemorrhagic in the interior. Eventually, the tissue breaks down completely. So-called red or carneous degeneration is seen occasionally, especially in association with pregnancy. This condition is thought to result from poor circulation of blood through a rapidly growing tumor. Thrombosis and extravasation of blood into the myoma tissue are responsible for the reddish discoloration (**Fig. 31.7**).

A subserous and especially a subserous pedunculated myoma may gradually outgrow its blood supply (**Fig. 31.8**). To keep the myoma tissue from undergoing complete ischemic necrosis, the omentum becomes adherent to the peritoneal surface of a pedunculated subserous myoma and provides whatever blood supply is needed. Eventually, the pedicle may disappear or twist, and the myoma will become completely free from the uterus, wander in the upper abdomen, and receive its "parasitic" blood supply from the omentum and other sources.

On occasion, fat occurs in leiomyomata as true fatty degeneration. The cut surface may have a yellowish discoloration. Infrequently, a deposit of true fat may form a fibrolipoma; however, the presence of fat in a leiomyoma is rare. Indeed, if fat is seen grossly or microscopically in a curettage specimen, one should not assume that it represents fatty degeneration of a leiomyoma. One should assume that the uterus has been perforated and that fragments of fat have been curetted from the mesentery or omentum.

The most important, but rare, change in a leiomyoma is sarcomatous degeneration. There is much variation in the reported incidence of sarcoma in leiomyomata. The incidence given by

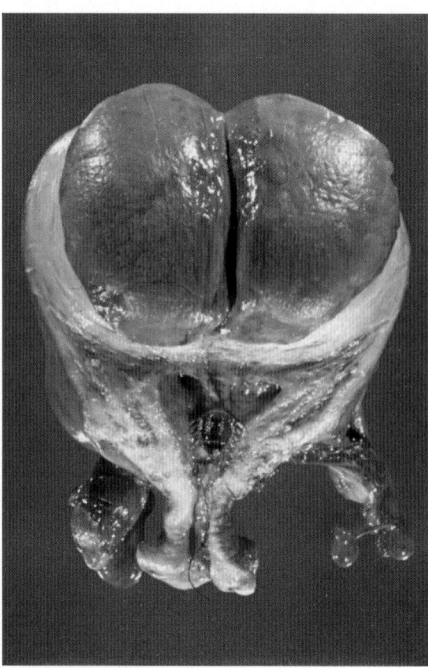

FIGURE 31.7 Degenerating leiomyoma showing carneous discoloration caused by thrombosis and extravasation of blood into the myoma tissue. A Dalkon shield can be seen in the endometrial cavity.

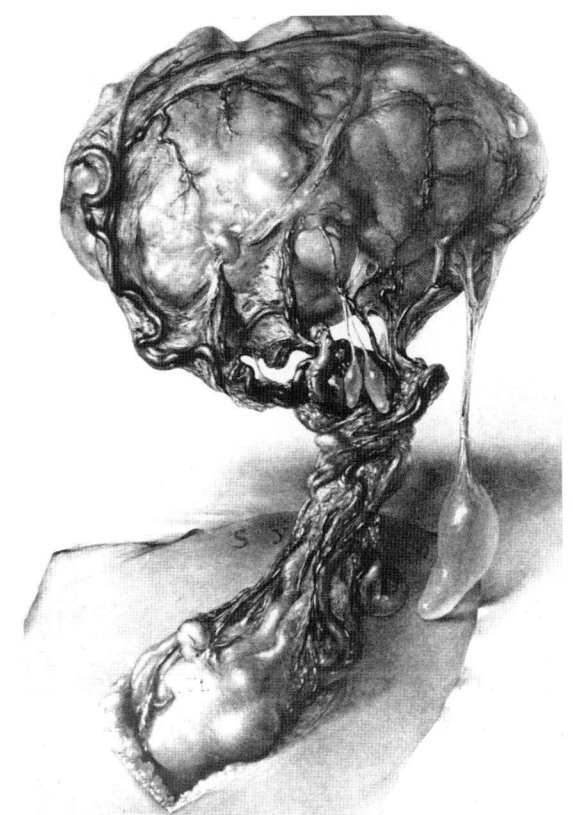

FIGURE 31.8 A subserous pedunculated myoma receives tenuous blood supply through its uterine pedicle. Such a myoma may wander in the upper abdomen and eventually receive its blood supply from other sources. It may also twist on its pedicle and undergo infarction.

Novak is 0.7%. However, a review of 13,000 myomata by Montague and associates at Johns Hopkins Hospital revealed 38 cases of malignant change, the incidence of sarcoma thus being 0.29%. Corscaden and Singh indicated by their study that the true incidence of sarcoma developing within uterine leiomyomata is no higher than 0.13% and is probably as low as 0.04%. It should be remembered that because most women with uterine leiomyomata do not undergo surgical removal, the true incidence of sarcoma in leiomyomata is probably much lower than 1 per 1,000 (0.1%).

After hysterectomy in 1,429 patients with presumed benign leiomyomata, the histologic diagnosis of leiomyosarcoma was made in seven (0.49%), according to a study by Leibsohn and coworkers. There was no evidence of malignancy in the endometrial sampling of any of these seven patients, and the diagnosis was suspected intraoperatively in only three. Uterine weights ranged from 120 to 1,100 g. In a woman between 41 and 50 years of age with presumed symptomatic leiomyomata, there is a 1 in 112 chance of a leiomyosarcoma being present, according to these authors. This information has important implications in the consideration of conservative or delayed treatment for these women. Parker and associates found that the total incidence of uterine sarcomas (leiomyosarcoma, endometrial stromal sarcoma, and mixed mesodermal tumor) among patients operated on for presumed benign uterine leiomyoma is lower (0.23%) than the 0.49% reported by Leibsohn and coworkers.

The difficulty in defining the true incidence of sarcomatous change is understandable if one is familiar with the histology of leiomyomata. Abundantly, cellular leiomyomata are relatively common, and at first glance, they suggest sarcoma; however, they lack a significant number of mitotic figures, and patients from whom such tumors are removed all remain well. Misinterpretation of the histologic picture of this type of cellular leiomyoma undoubtedly accounts for the increased incidence of leiomyosarcoma reported by some. When cutting into leiomyomata in the operating room, the surgeon finds that sarcomatous areas have a somewhat characteristic appearance, although the histologic diagnosis certainly cannot be made by gross examination. A sarcoma is likely to occur in a rather large leiomyoma and toward the center of the tumor, where the blood supply is poorest. Instead of being firm fibrous tissue that grates when scraped with a knife blade, the tissue is soft and homogeneous and is described as resembling raw pork. Later, as necrosis of the malignant tissue occurs, it becomes more friable and hemorrhagic.

It has been difficult to understand uterine leiomyosarcoma, because pathologists do not agree on the criteria necessary for diagnosis. Some pathologists rely on the mitotic count. All tumors with less than 5 mitotic figures per 10 high-power fields are considered benign. All tumors with more than 10 mitotic figures per 10 high-power fields are called malignant. Those in between can be called smooth muscle tumors of uncertain malignant potential.

Other pathologists believe the mitotic count may have some significance but choose to rely instead on the presence of nuclear hyperchromatism, nuclear pleomorphism, or giant cells and other bizarre cell forms to make the diagnosis. Corscaden and Singh believe that no combination of histologic features is reliable and that only smooth muscle tumors that metastasize or recur are definitely malignant. We believe that all of these features should be taken into consideration for diagnosis and prognosis. When the tumor is confined to the uterus, both mitotic grade and histologic grade are important in the diagnosis and prognosis. A poor prognosis is associated with high mitotic counts and extremely atypical and anaplastic cytologic features. Bell and colleagues at Stanford University Medical Center assessed a variety of histopathologic features of 213 problematic smooth muscle neoplasms for which there were at least 2 years of clinical follow-up data. From the wide variety of light microscopic features assessed, the important predictors that emerged were mitotic index, the degree of cytologic atypia, and the presence or absence of coagulative tumor cell necrosis. Previously, the mitotic index was relied on exclusively to determine whether a uterine smooth muscle tumor was benign or malignant, but currently, an approach is used that incorporates additional histopathologic features.

A normal chromosome complement (46,XX) was observed by Meloni and coworkers in about 50% of leiomyoma cases. About 50% showed clonal abnormalities, such as those of chromosomes 1, 7, and 13, and t(12;14). Interstitial deletions of chromosome 7 were the ones most often involved, suggesting that this abnormality may be of primary importance in the cellular proliferation of leiomyomata. A relation between more aggressive histology and chromosomal abnormalities was also suggested.

Tumors that show obvious evidence of blood vessel invasion or spread to contiguous organs are rarely cured. The extent of the disease at the time of initial diagnosis is of even greater significance. In other words, when the diagnosis is suspected for the first time by the pathologist when he or she examines routine sections from a uterine leiomyoma, the patient almost always survives. However, if the diagnosis is made preoperatively by the gynecologist or is suspected during the operative procedure because of invasion of surrounding organs, the prognosis is grave.

An unusual atypical smooth muscle tumor was first described in the stomach by Martin and associates in 1960. Variously called *bizarre leiomyoma, leiomyoblastoma, clear cell leiomyoma*, and *plexiform tumorlet*, these atypical smooth tumors probably all belong together. The term *epithelioid leiomyoma* was adopted by the World Health Organization. Kurman and Norris have proposed that this term be used for all atypical leiomyomata. Histologically, the characteristic feature is the mixture of rounded polygonal cells and multinucleated giant cells present in epithelioid clear cell and plexiform patterns. Clinically, in the uterus most of these tumors are benign. They may rarely exhibit malignant potential. Malignancy is difficult to predict from histologic criteria because some metastases occurred from tumors that demonstrated very few mitoses. Kurman and Norris have suggested, however, that epithelioid neoplasms having more than 5 mitotic figures per 10 high-power fields should be called *epithelioid leiomyosarcomas* and that the term *epithelioid leiomyoma* should be applied when there is a lower level of mitotic activity. Although combination therapy (surgery plus radiation therapy or chemotherapy) may not be indicated for a patient with an epithelioid leiomyoma, follow-up should be considered essential, as emphasized by Klunder and colleagues.

An unusual benign form of leiomyomata uteri, *intravenous leiomyomatosis*, was first recognized at the turn of the 20th century and has been reported sporadically since then. Before 1982, about 50 cases had been reported, according to Bahary and coworkers. Probably, at least that many have been reported since. Marshall and Morris presented the first detailed report of this entity in the American literature in 1959. The characteristic feature of this peculiar smooth muscle tumor is the extension of the polypoid intravascular projections into the veins of the parametrium and broad ligaments. Although there may be some difficulty in distinguishing such lesions from low-grade sarcoma, they are distinctly different histologically from stromatosis uteri because the intravenous plugs are mainly smooth muscle in origin. In 1966, Edwards and Peacock collected 32 cases of intravenous leiomyomatosis, including two cases of their own, and reviewed the clinical experience with this condition. In approximately 50% of the cases, the intravenous tumor was confined to the parametrium; in 75%, it extended no further than the veins of the broad ligament. The observations of Edwards and Peacock suggest that the severed intravenous extensions are probably incapable of independent parasitic existence and remain dormant after removal of the uterus. However, the cases presented by Bahary and associates tend to refute this idea. Total surgical excision of the tumor should be attempted for successful therapy. Some patients have survived for many years after incomplete resection of the tumor. A review of 14 cases of this rare uterine tumor from the file of the Armed Forces Institute of Pathology has been reported by Norris and Parmley. In this series, two of three patients with incomplete resection had a recurrence; the recurrent tumor was excised surgically, and the patients were alive and free of disease 5 and 11 years after operation. The authors concluded that this tumor behaves clinically like a benign neoplasm, although its wormlike extensions may involve uterine, vaginal, ovarian, and iliac veins. The uterine veins in the broad ligaments are the most common sites of extension. The mitotic index is quite low, with the most active lesions showing only one mitosis per 15 high-power fields. The material from the Armed Forces Institute of Pathology provides histologic evidence consistent with both theories of origin of intravenous leiomyomatosis, namely, that it may be the result of unusual vascular invasion from a leiomyoma or may arise de novo from the wall of veins within the myometrium.

Extension of benign leiomyomatosis up the vena cava and into the right atrium has been reported in several cases, with a fatal outcome in some. Before 1994, approximately 27 cases of intravenous leiomyomatosis extending to the heart were reported. Several recent cases requiring open heart surgery to remove the intracardiac tumor thrombosis have been successful and without recurrence. All reported cases occurred in women. Tierney and colleagues reported that substantial quantities of cytoplasmic estradiol and progesterone receptors were found in the right atrial tumor removed from a patient with intravenous leiomyomatosis. Their patient was treated with the antiestrogen tamoxifen because of residual tumor in the vena cava that could be estrogen dependent. Irey and Norris have presented evidence that female reproductive steroids can produce intimal proliferation of veins in predisposed persons. Interestingly, of the 30 patients with leiomyomata and leiomyosarcomas of the vena cava reviewed by Wray and Dawkins, 80% were female. Both intravenous leiomyomatosis and benign metastasizing leiomyoma have been reported to metastasize to the lung. As suggested by Banner and coworkers, by Horstmann and associates, and by Evans and colleagues, oophorectomy may be indicated in patients with these conditions, again because of the possibility that these tumors may be estrogen dependent or that estrogens may have the ability to stimulate their development, whether in a uterine or extrauterine location and whether they appear to be endothelial or mesenchymal in origin.

The possibility of metastases from a histologically benign uterine leiomyoma has been discussed by Idelson and Davids and by Clark and Weed. When such a case occurs, it is usually settled by finding a sarcomatous component in the leiomyoma or by finding evidence of intravenous leiomyomatosis. However, multiple cases have now been reported in which a benign uterine leiomyoma metastasized. Idelson and Davids' case showed metastases to the aortic lymph nodes. The patient reported by Cramer and associates had metastatic tumor to the omentum, ovary, periaortic lymph node, and lung. In each location, the histology and estrogen receptor content of the tumor resembled those of a benign leiomyoma. The recommended treatment consists of surgical removal with castration and little or no estrogen replacement.

Leiomyomatosis peritonealis disseminata is sometimes confused with intravenous leiomyomatosis. However, only subperitoneal surfaces of the uterus and other pelvic and abdominal viscera are involved with leiomyomatosis peritonealis disseminata, and invasion of the lumen of blood vessels does not occur. Only about 15 cases have been reported, according to Pearce. All occurred in patients in the reproductive years who often had large uterine leiomyomata and were usually pregnant or taking oral contraceptives. The condition is likely to be confused with a disseminated intraabdominal malignancy, but it is entirely benign histologically and clinically. Parmley and colleagues have demonstrated the histologic similarities between this peritoneal lesion and the decidual change of the mesothelium in the pelvis, and they propose that the condition represents a benign reparative process in which fibroblasts replace soft peritoneal decidua. They suggest that this fibrotic reaction occurs during pregnancy and especially in the postpartum period, resulting in nodules with a pseudoleiomyomatous pattern. Similar findings have been noted in patients with endometriosis treated with prolonged Enovid therapy. These findings indicate that prolonged and continuous stimulation of subperitoneal decidua by either endogenous or exogenous estrogen and progesterone is important in the pathogenesis of this condition. Parmley and coworkers suggest that the condition is more appropriately called *disseminated fibrosing deciduosis*. Goldberg and associates, on the other hand, on the basis of electron microscopy studies, believe that the tumors arise from smooth muscles of small blood vessels. This has been confirmed by Ceccacci and colleagues. It has been possible to show a continuum from fibroblastic cells through myofibroblasts to leiomyocytes. Although the cell of origin of this tumor is still controversial, the tumor is benign, and the acceptable treatment to date is total abdominal hysterectomy and bilateral salpingo-oophorectomy. If this tumor occurs in the omentum, an omentectomy should also be performed to define more clearly the histologic nature of the lesion.

In attempting to distinguish between benign and malignant disease in a patient with uterine leiomyomata who also has unusual clinical findings, it is appropriate to keep the entities mentioned earlier (intravenous leiomyomatosis, atypical bizarre leiomyoma, benign metastasizing leiomyoma, and disseminated intraperitoneal leiomyomatosis) in mind. Although they all have features similar to those of malignant disease, they are almost always benign and amenable to treatment. One should also remember that benign uterine leiomyomata have been associated with pseudo-Meigs syndrome in a few cases. Meigs reported five cases in 1954. In these cases, the ascites did not reappear after removal of the uterine leiomyomata.

There is a high frequency of endometrial hyperplasia when the uterus contains leiomyomata. Degligdish and Loewenthal reported that cystic glandular hyperplasia is often found in the endometrium at the margin of the leiomyoma. Yamamoto and coworkers have reported high concentrations of estrone and estrone sulfatase activity in the endometrium overlying a myoma. They suggest that the local hyperestrogenism in the endometrium overlying a leiomyoma may assist in the genesis or enlargement of these tumors.

Gynecologic surgeons are especially concerned about the vascularity of individual leiomyomata and about the blood flow to the uterus in the presence of multiple and sometimes very large leiomyomata. These considerations are pertinent when surgery, especially myomectomy, is contemplated.

According to Vollenhoven and associates, the vascularization of leiomyomata was studied by Vasserman and colleagues, and the findings were presented to the World Congress of Gynecology and Obstetrics in 1988. Using femoral arteriography, selective intraoperative angiography, radiography, and injection of surgical specimens, these investigators showed that leiomyomata have a rich vascular supply, including blood lakes within tumors. They found more than one nutrient vessel per myoma. Venous channels were predominantly peripheral, whereas the arterial supply was both internal and peripheral. Farrer-Brown and coworkers, using radiologic methods, demonstrated that myomata in various locations within the myometrium can cause congestion and dilatation of endometrial venous plexuses by obstructing venous return. These obstructions can result in ectasia of endometrial and myometrial venules (**Fig. 31.9**). The degree of vascularity of leiomyomata was also studied by Karlsson and Persson. Vascularity varied from many, to few, to no intrinsic vessels demonstrable. Generally, the sum of the width of the uterine arteries increases with the size of the uterus, but the diameter of the two sides sometimes differs markedly. A rich vascularity was found in 22 of 34 uteri with leiomyomata, but with increasing size, there is a tendency to less vascularity. In none of five cases with very large (20 cm or more) leiomyomata uteri was the vascularity rich. The intrinsic vessels were few in two cases and absent in three cases.

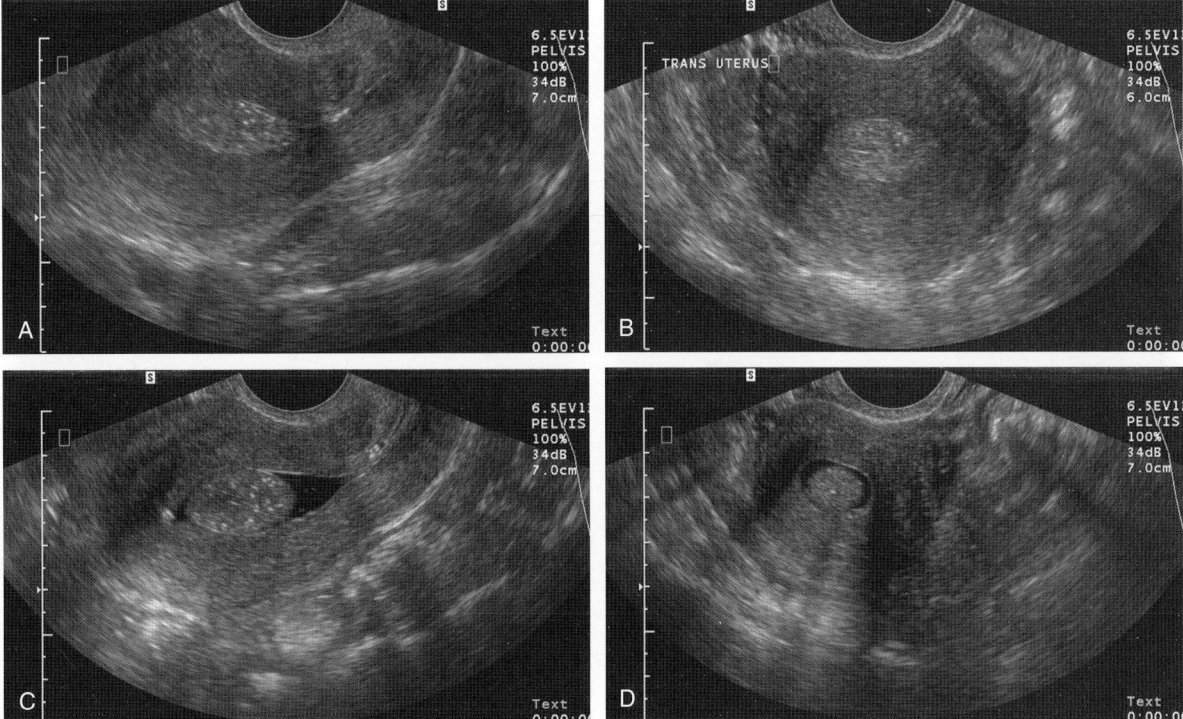

FIGURE 31.9 Sonographic images of a 48-year-old patient with a history of pelvic pain. Both transabdominal and transvaginal images were obtained on cycle day 8. Longitudinal (**A**) and transversely oriented (**B**) transvaginal images reveal a suspicious endometrial cavity, suggesting a thickened lining, endometrial polyp, or a submucosal myoma. **C and D:** Fluid-enhanced sonohysterographic studies clearly demonstrate a mass lesion and not generalized thickening of the endometrial lining. The patient underwent a hysteroscopy and uterine curettage, which revealed a histologically confirmed endometrial polyp. (Images courtesy of Jeff Dicke, MD.)

CLINICAL FEATURES OF UTERINE LEIOMYOMATA

Asymptomatic Leiomyomata

Most leiomyomata are asymptomatic. Untold numbers of such symptomless leiomyomata are removed surgically by either hysterectomy or myomectomy when they would have been better left undisturbed. The incidence of malignancy in leiomyomata is less than 0.1%, which is lower than the operative mortality rate of hysterectomy in the average hospital; therefore, unless there is some reason to suspect malignant change, the risk of the operation for asymptomatic leiomyomata may exceed the danger of malignancy. A history of rapid growth, however, particularly postmenopausal growth, does indicate removal, even when the tumor produces no symptoms. Signs of rapid enlargement are important in all patients but are even more ominous in older patients. In younger patients, the most common reason for rapid enlargement of a uterus with leiomyomata is pregnancy. If pregnancy can be ruled out, a leiomyosarcoma may be suspected but is rarely found.

Small leiomyomata that are asymptomatic need only to be observed from time to time, with pelvic examinations perhaps every 6 to 12 months and pelvic ultrasonography (US) when indicated. In the beginning, frequent examination may be indicated to determine the growth rate. Such tumors may remain remarkably constant in size for years. If small leiomyomata are discovered late in menstrual life, it is unusual for symptoms to appear or for surgical treatment to be required. Larger tumors can also be watched safely, but if a policy of watchful waiting is adopted, one should be very sure of the nature of the tumors. If there is uncertainty of the uterine or ovarian origin of a tumor, as may well be the case when the tumor fills the whole pelvis or when a pedunculated tumor is felt in the adnexal region (**Fig. 31.10**), special diagnostic procedures may be indicated. Pelvic examination by an experienced gynecologist can usually clear up the uncertainty. In difficult cases, an examination under anesthesia may be necessary. Laparoscopy may be of great value in determining the nature of an adnexal mass. Before invasive techniques are used, however, noninvasive diagnostic evaluation should be performed. These include radiographic studies of the abdomen and pelvis, US, and computed tomography (CT). The characteristic calcification in a leiomyoma may be seen on radiographs. The US and CT features of uterine leiomyomata have been well described. However, mistakes in the interpretation can still be made. Tada and associates reported that 5% of patients given the diagnosis of uterine leiomyomata by CT actually had an ovarian tumor at operation. Therefore, if uncertainty about the diagnosis persists, laparoscopy or laparotomy should still be performed.

When large asymptomatic leiomyomata occur in premenopausal women who have had their families or in whom future childbearing is not desired, a recommendation for removal may be made. It is impossible to predict which patients will become symptomatic in the remaining years before menopause. However, such tumors, with additional years to grow, are likely to require surgical removal eventually. Therefore, it is better to remove them when the patient is a good operative candidate of relatively low operative risk and when conservation of normal ovaries with a good blood supply can be easily accomplished. Such tumors should usually be 12 to 14 weeks in gestational size or larger. Depending on a variety of factors, either myomectomy or hysterectomy can be recommended to the patient. GnRH agonists may be useful in women approaching menopause to control symptoms or asymptomatic uterine myoma growth until menopause. The regrowth of tumors after the cessation of treatment limits the usefulness of these agents, however. Nakamura and Yoshimura reported their experience with GnRH agonists in the treatment of uterine leiomyomata in perimenopausal women. One third of patients reached menopause after 16 weeks of treatment, thus avoiding the need for surgery.

Reiter and colleagues studied 93 consecutive patients undergoing hysterectomy for leiomyomata. When the uterus was larger than 12 weeks gestational size, there was no increased incidence of surgical complications compared with women with smaller uteri. On the basis of this small series, the authors concluded that hysterectomy need not be recommended to women with large asymptomatic uterine leiomyomata to avoid a possible increased risk of surgical complications.

There is no uniform size of an asymptomatic leiomyomatous uterus that can be used as an indication for hysterectomy or myomectomy. When size is the only significant indication for surgery in an asymptomatic patient, the location of the tumors is more important than the total uterine mass. When the leiomyomata are located in the cornual area or in the lateral wall of the uterus and obscure the anatomy of the adnexa and broad ligament, the risk of error in the early recognition of an ovarian tumor is greater. In such cases, one must carefully weigh the advantages and disadvantages of the conservative approach to the management of uterine leiomyomata. When adnexal tumors are present, it is critical that the origin of these tumors be confirmed. The diagnostic studies mentioned earlier should be performed to establish clearly that the tumors are of uterine origin before a decision is made to follow up the patient rather than operate. It is unacceptable to wait to see whether an adnexal tumor enlarges before identifying the site of origin of the mass as either uterine or ovarian. Ovarian carcinoma remains the most lethal disease of the female reproductive tract and the most difficult to diagnose early. Every diagnostic and therapeutic effort must be made to avoid errors in the clinical evaluation of pelvic neoplasms (**Fig. 31.10**). In women who are approaching menopause, relatively large uterine leiomyomata can be kept under observation with the knowledge that after menopause, they will not increase in size and may actually regress somewhat. Still, one must be certain

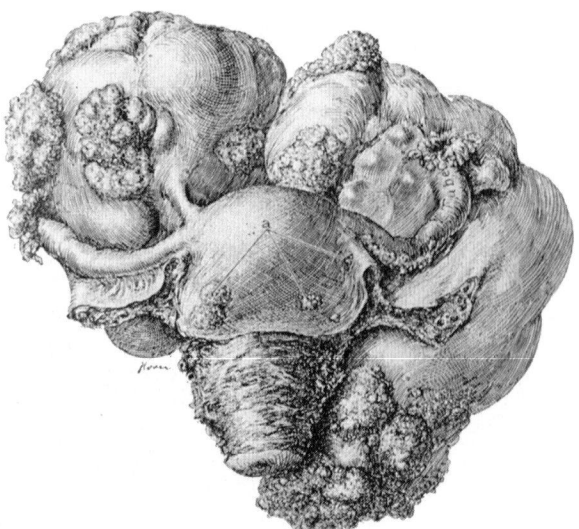

FIGURE 31.10 Although this central pelvic mass may feel like a multiple leiomyomatous uterus on bimanual pelvic examination, it is actually a bilateral ovarian malignancy. Differentiation between these two diagnoses may require special diagnostic procedures.

that the entire central pelvic mass is a leiomyomatous uterus. Patient management is largely dependent on knowledge of the exact location and size of leiomyomas. Imaging modalities play an important role in determining patient management, especially when differentiating a benign leiomyoma from other pathologic conditions that may require different therapies.

Uterine size as an indication for surgical intervention in women with leiomyomata has been thoughtfully discussed by Friedman and Haas. These authors point out that many gynecologists advocate surgical removal of leiomyomata when the uterus reaches 12 weeks gestational size or greater, regardless of the presence or absence of significant symptoms. Historical reasons given for surgical intervention include the following:

- The inability to accurately assess the ovaries by examination
- The possible malignancy of the pelvic mass
- The potential for compromise of adjacent organ function if the mass continues to enlarge
- The greater risk of surgical complications if the mass grows to a larger size
- The potential for better fertility if myomectomy is performed when the uterus is smaller
- The possibility of continued growth of uterine leiomyomata if hormone replacement therapy is given after menopause

Friedman and Haas find very little in the literature to support these indications for surgical intervention and believe the availability of modern high-resolution US and magnetic resonance imaging (MRI) allows for expectant management in many patients with large asymptomatic uterine leiomyomata. They prefer to give primary consideration to the presence and severity of myoma-related symptoms in deciding whether surgical intervention is indicated. We believe that such a course of expectant management is appropriate only when there is relative certainty regarding the benign nature of the central pelvic mass and all of its components and when it is possible to get the patient to return for periodic assessment of gynecologic symptoms and findings on pelvic examination. Repeat MRI may also be required occasionally.

If one elects to observe a patient with a relatively large asymptomatic uterine leiomyoma, it is a good rule to obtain an excretory urogram or renal ultrasound. Everett and Sturgis showed many years ago that ureteral compression at the pelvic brim may occur so that hydroureter and hydronephrosis develop (Fig. 31.11). It is usually the symmetrically enlarged uterus with intramural leiomyomata that extends near or above the umbilicus and rests on the pelvic brim that compresses the ureters, in the same way as a symmetrically enlarged gravid uterus. The process is usually slow and painless even when moderate to severe hydronephrosis has occurred. Pyelographic evidence of kidney damage may be the determining factor in a decision to operate on a patient with an entirely asymptomatic leiomyoma. The irregularly and asymmetrically enlarged uterus with subserous tumors usually does not produce pressure on the ureters.

After menopause, asymptomatic leiomyomata generally should be left undisturbed. Again, the gynecologist must be absolutely certain that an ovarian neoplasm can be ruled out. In the postmenopausal years, shrinkage of myomata and the myometrium occurs. However, the myometrial shrinkage may be disproportionately greater than the myoma shrinkage. Therefore, a myoma in an intramural location before menopause may become a submucous myoma after menopause and then become symptomatic for the first time, usually with postmenopausal bleeding.

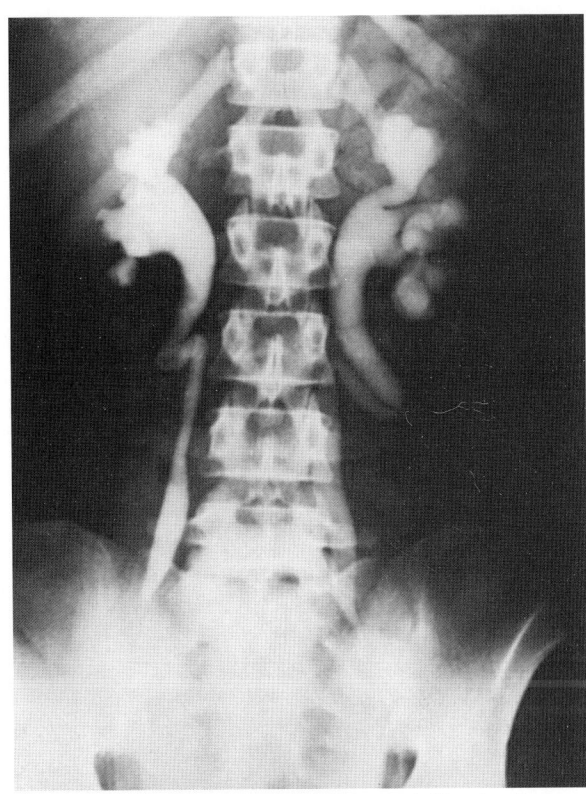

FIGURE 31.11 Bilateral ureteral obstruction and dilatation from pressure of large leiomyomata.

In menopausal women, the appearance of even the slightest trace of vaginal bleeding should make one suspect cervical or endometrial malignancy or the possibility of sarcomatous change in the leiomyoma (**Figs. 31.12** and **31.13**). Careful pelvic examination, Papanicolaou smear, and evaluation of the cervix by colposcopy or biopsy, pelvic US, fractional curettage, and perhaps hysteroscopy should be done. If the bleeding remains unexplained and the presence of atrophic vaginitis or the use of exogenous estrogens has been excluded, the leiomyomatous uterus should be removed because of the risk of sarcomatous change.

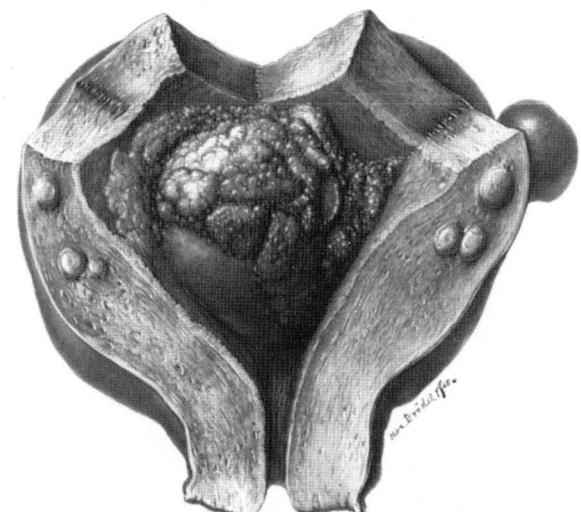

FIGURE 31.12 Adenocarcinoma of the endometrium is present in a symmetrically enlarged leiomyomatous uterus.

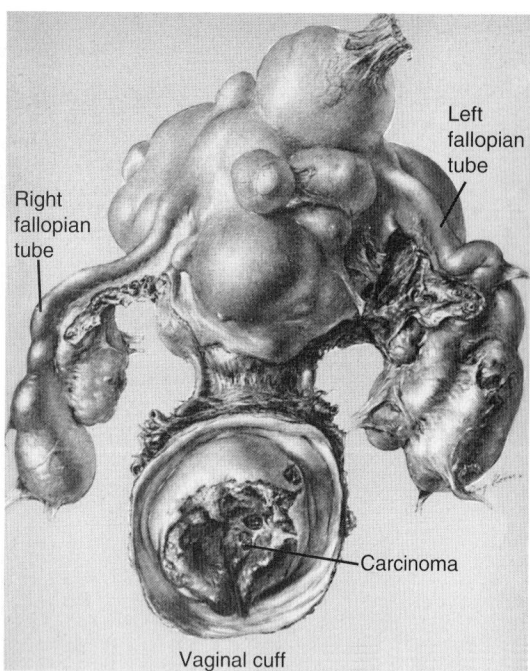

FIGURE 31.13 This specimen shows multiple uterine leiomyomata but also shows chronic pelvic inflammatory disease and cervical carcinoma. Patients with uterine leiomyomata may have abnormal bleeding, but a coexisting cervical carcinoma may also cause bleeding.

Transabdominal and endovaginal US are the standard imaging modalities for the detection of leiomyomas. Pelvic US by transvaginal and transabdominal techniques is most useful because of good patient tolerance, relatively low cost, availability, and accuracy when performed by well-trained and experienced ultrasonographers (**Fig. 31.14**). Ultrasonography is the most cost-effective screening mechanism for uterine masses suggestive of myomata. Sonographic criteria for diagnosis have been well described. Generally, abdominal US is unable to detect myomas less than 2 cm in diameter. Transvaginal probes have allowed for improved visualization of both the uterus and adnexa. With higher frequencies, sensitivity in the detection of small myomas has substantially increased. In a series evaluated by Fedele and colleagues using endovaginal ultrasound before hysterectomy, submucous leiomyomas were identified with a sensitivity of 100%. Difficulties may arise, however, if myomas are small or pedunculated, patients are obese, or the uterus is retroverted.

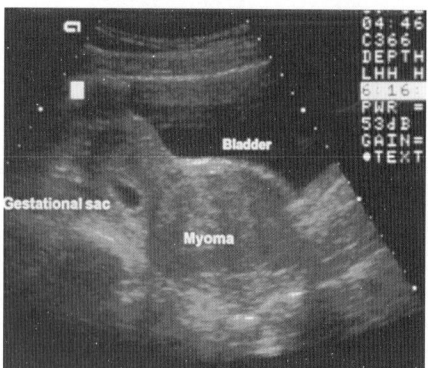

FIGURE 31.14 An US study shows a cervical myoma and a very early intrauterine pregnancy.

Transvaginal fluid-enhanced vaginal probe sonography (sonohysterography) is a useful technique to assess myomata that distort the endometrial cavity. This technique has little to no complications and is generally well tolerated with only mild cramping described by patients. The limitation of detection of leiomyomas with this modality is 0.5 cm diameter. In a study by Hoetzinger, the majority of intrauterine myomata (14 of 16, or 88%) were detected by sonohysterography. Ultrasound transducing catheters have been suggested as a potential tool to supplement abdominal and endovaginal sonography. Three-dimensional data display has recently undergone development and application in sonography; however, the role in evaluation and management of leiomyoma remains unclear (**Fig. 31.9**).

There is no technique that reliably identifies a leiomyosarcoma. Plain abdominal or pelvic radiographs and hysterosalpingography are older, standard techniques that are still useful in assessing uterine size, calcification in myomata, intrauterine filling defects caused by submucous myomata, and tubal patency. These techniques, combined with US, are the most useful for assessing patients with a central pelvic mass thought to be a leiomyomatous uterus. CA-125 levels may be elevated in women with uterine leiomyomata, but the levels are generally lower than those in patients with ovarian cancer.

Symptomatic Leiomyomata

Less than 50% of patients with uterine leiomyomata have symptoms. Symptoms may be single or multiple and depend on the location, size, and number of tumors present. A clinical and pathologic study of 298 patients with uterine leiomyomata by Persaud and Arjoon revealed no significant relation between the presenting symptoms and the presence of degenerative changes in the tumors. Some form of degeneration was demonstrated in 65% of the specimens, with hyaline degeneration accounting for 63% of all types of degeneration. Hyaline degeneration produces no characteristic symptoms. Symptoms, especially pain and fever, may be present in some patients with red degeneration of a leiomyoma during pregnancy, with torsion and infarction of a subserous pedunculated leiomyoma, or with an infected leiomyoma. A discussion of the signs and symptoms caused by uterine leiomyomata follows.

Abnormal Bleeding

It is surprising but not unusual that even patients with large uterine leiomyomata may have a history of normal menstruation. Such patients should be questioned carefully about recent slight increases in the amount, duration, and frequency of menstruation. Some patients with a history of normal menstruation are found to have iron deficiency anemia from a gradual increase in menstrual blood loss that even the patient has not recognized. If a case of uterine leiomyomata is to be followed, the patient should be asked to monitor her menstrual blood loss carefully and should be given instructions to keep a menstrual calendar and monthly record of the number of pads or tampons used each day. A more objective measurement of the amount of menstrual blood loss using the method of Hallberg and Nilsson may be helpful in doubtful cases. Iron depletion may not be evident by laboratory determination unless one checks serum ferritin levels. In the early months of increased menstrual blood loss, the hemoglobin and hematocrit values are normal. Heavy menstruation does not cause anemia until iron stores are first depleted.

Abnormal bleeding occurs in about one third of patients with symptomatic uterine leiomyomata and commonly indicates that treatment is necessary. The menstrual flow is usually heavy (menorrhagia) but can also occur for prolonged periods of time at irregular intervals (metrorrhagia). It may also be both heavy and prolonged (menometrorrhagia). Abnormal bleeding may be associated with submucous, intramural, and subserous tumors, but there is a distinct clinical impression that bleeding is more common and more severe in the presence of submucous tumors. The submucous leiomyoma bleeds freely at menstruation and may also bleed between periods as a result of passive congestion, necrosis, and ulceration of the endometrial surface over the tumor and ulceration of the contralateral uterine surface. If the submucous myoma is pedunculated, there is usually a constant, thin, blood-tinged discharge in addition to the menorrhagia. An intramural tumor that is just beginning to encroach on the uterine cavity can also be responsible for menorrhagia. Intramural leiomyomata near the serosal surface and pedunculated subserous tumors can also be associated with abnormal bleeding. When bleeding occurs with such tumors, however, one should search for some other lesions to account for it. The mere presence of leiomyomata in a woman who has abnormal uterine bleeding is not proof that the leiomyomata are causing the bleeding. This fact is important, particularly when there is intermenstrual bleeding. When a patient with leiomyomata has intermenstrual bleeding, it is a rule in our practice to examine and study the cervix carefully with special diagnostic procedures and to sample and evaluate the uterine cavity before we proceed with treatment of the leiomyomata. If an endometrial or cervical malignancy is detected, the treatment of the leiomyomata may need to be altered.

There are several mechanisms by which leiomyomata can cause abnormal bleeding, although a single specific mechanism may not be apparent in a particular patient. According to Sehgal and Haskins, the surface area of the endometrial cavity in a normal uterus is 15 cm². The surface area of the endometrial cavity in the presence of leiomyomata may exceed 200 cm². These authors demonstrated a correlation between the severity of the bleeding and the area of endometrial surface. In addition to an increased surface area from which to bleed, the endometrium may demonstrate local hyperestrogenism in areas immediately adjacent to submucous tumors, and endometrial hyperplasia and endometrial polyps are commonly found. Degligdish and Loewenthal noted a broad spectrum of histologic abnormalities in the endometrium associated with leiomyomata, ranging from atrophy to hyperplasia. Thinning and ulceration of the endometrial surface may be present over large submucous tumors; smaller ones may show slight thinning without ulceration. The presence of leiomyomata may interfere with myometrial contractility as well as contractility of the spiral arterioles in the basalis portion of the endometrium. Miller and Ludovici suggested that anovulation and dysfunctional uterine bleeding are more common in the presence of uterine leiomyomata.

Sampson in 1913 was the first to study the blood supply of uterine leiomyomata and its effect on uterine bleeding. More recent studies have been performed by Faulkner and by Farrer-Brown and associates. The most prominent and important change is the presence of endometrial venule ectasia. Tumors that are strategically located in the myometrium may cause obstruction and proximal congestion of veins in the myometrium and endometrium. Thrombosis and sloughing of these large dilated venous channels within the endometrium produce heavy bleeding (Fig. 31.15).

Makarainen and Ylikorkala have presented evidence that further supports the concept that prostanoids play a role in primary menorrhagia. They found that the production of 6-keto-prostaglandin F_1 alpha (6-keto-$PGF_{1\alpha}$), a metabolite of prostacyclin (PGI_2), and thromboxane B_2 (TXB_2), a metabolite of thromboxane A_2 (TXA_2), was normal in menorrhagic

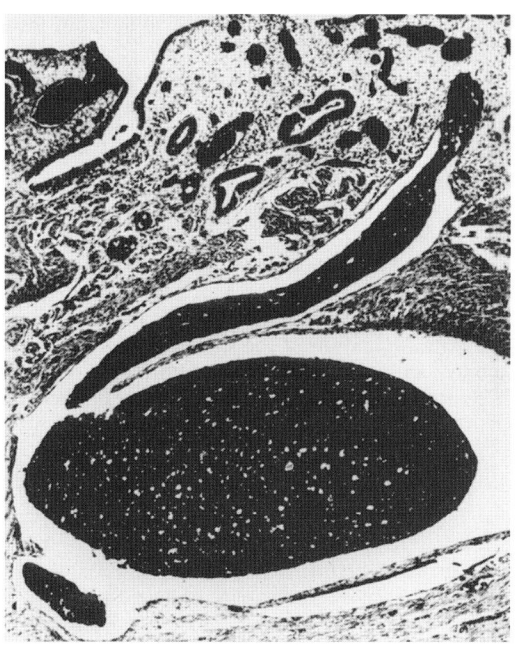

FIGURE 31.15 Dilated endometrial venous space communicating with a grossly enlarged vessel in the inner myometrium of a uterus with submucous leiomyomata. (Reprinted from Farrer-Brown G, Beilby JO, Tarbit MH. Venous changes in the endometrium of myomatous uteri. *Obstet Gynecol* 1971;83:743, with permission. Copyright 1971, The American College of Obstetricians and Gynecologists.)

endometrium. However, the balance between TXA_2 and PGI_2 shifted to a relative TXA_2 deficiency and was negatively related to blood loss in patients with menorrhagia. Although ibuprofen decreased the blood loss in patients with primary menorrhagia, it failed to reduce myoma-associated menorrhagia. The authors suggest that uterine factors other than prostanoids are more important in causing menorrhagia associated with uterine leiomyomata.

In most cases, when bleeding occurs postmenopausally and leiomyomata are discovered on bimanual examination, the bleeding is due to some other factors, such as cervical or endometrial abnormalities, atrophic vaginitis, or exogenous estrogen, and the leiomyomata are purely incidental. Occasionally, however, the postmenopausal leiomyoma can be responsible for the bleeding. As stated earlier, leiomyomata that do not bleed during the menstrual life of the patient have been found to migrate to a submucous position in later years. This occurs because after menopause, the myometrium atrophies and the uterine wall becomes thinner. Leiomyomata also shrink somewhat, but not as much as the surrounding myometrium. Thus, a leiomyoma that was intramural before menopause may work itself into a submucous position after menopause, become ulcerated, and bleed. Postmenopausal growth of uterine leiomyomata may indicate malignant change, especially if associated with postmenopausal bleeding. We have rarely observed postmenopausal growth in a leiomyoma without finding malignancy in the tumor; whenever there is enlargement of the leiomyoma after menopause, one should seriously consider the possibility of sarcomatous change and remove the leiomyoma.

Patients with heavy menstruation and uterine leiomyomata should be evaluated for the presence of submucous myomata. Even patients without palpable evidence of uterine leiomyomata or uterine enlargement who have heavy menstruation should be evaluated for the presence of submucous myomata. When endometrial curettage is performed, irregularity of the uterine cavity may suggest the presence of a submucous myoma. However, a submucous myoma may not be detected with the curette. An accurate diagnosis is more likely to be made by hysterosalpingography, conventional transvaginal or transabdominal US, sonohysterography, MRI, or hysteroscopy. Cincinelli and colleagues reported their experience with transabdominal sonohysterography, a technique that involves transabdominal ultrasonographic scanning while 30 mL of sterile isotonic saline is slowly injected into the uterine cavity. According to these investigators, this technique provided the most accurate evaluation of the size of submucous myomata, intracavitary and intramural growth, and location within the uterine cavity, with sensitivity, specificity, and predictive values of 100%.

Pressure

Evidence of pressure on nearby pelvic viscera may be an indication for treatment. The urinary bladder suffers most often from such pressure, giving rise to urgency and frequency of urination and sometimes even urinary incontinence (**Fig. 31.16**). Although this symptom is common with large leiomyomata, one frequently finds the pelvis filled with leiomyomata when there is no urinary frequency. Occasionally, acute retention of urine or overflow incontinence results from a leiomyoma and necessitates surgical intervention. These effects can occur as a result of rapid interior growth of the leiomyoma with compression of the urethra and bladder neck against the pubic bone. More often, a tumor the size of a 3-month pregnancy may become incarcerated in the cul-de-sac, wedging the cervix forward against the urethra and obstructing the flow of urine

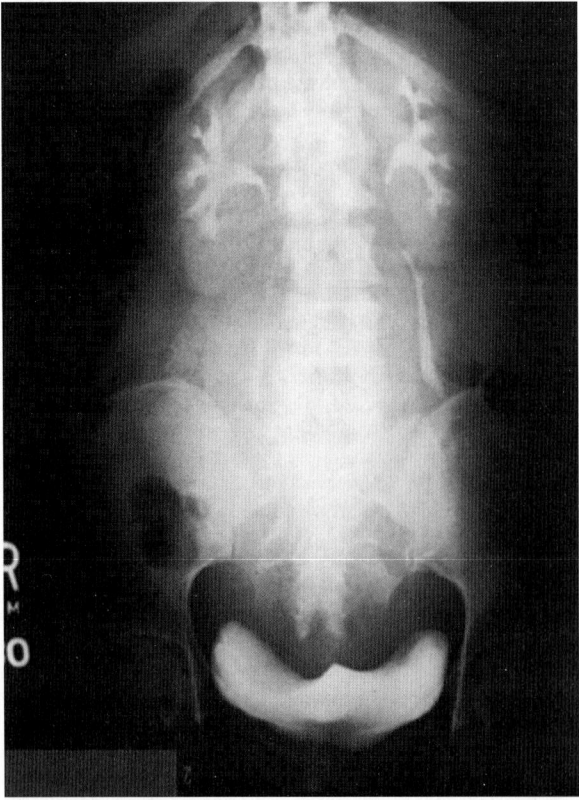

FIGURE 31.16 Cystogram and intravenous pyelogram showing distortion of the bladder by pressure from a leiomyoma.

through the urethra. A large pedunculated submucous tumor may fill and distend the vagina and press the urethra against the symphysis, causing urinary retention.

As pointed out by Mattingly, one can expect to encounter women who have uterine leiomyomata of significant size and in addition have protrusion of the bladder base and posterior urethra through a widened levator muscle hiatus and a weakened urogenital diaphragm. Both conditions are relatively common. In addition to the usual symptoms produced by the leiomyomata, socially disabling stress urinary incontinence may be present. When the anterior wall of the uterus is greatly distorted by the presence of these tumors, pressure against the bladder can cause urinary frequency. If anatomic pressure equalization incontinence is also present, it may be aggravated by the increased intravesical pressure caused by the leiomyomata. However, the presence of anatomic stress urinary incontinence has no etiologic relation to the uterine enlargement caused by the leiomyomata.

Silent ureteral obstruction from pressure against the pelvic brim is an uncommon complication of uterine enlargement caused by multiple large leiomyomata. Such an asymptomatic anatomic change occurs more often with a symmetrically enlarged leiomyomatous uterus that becomes large enough to fill the pelvis and compress the ureter against the pelvic sidewalls (**Fig. 31.11**). Although an infrequent complication, the obstruction can occur in either ureter, depending on the location of the uterine tumors. If there has been no infection or parenchymal damage to the kidney, this anatomic alteration is completely reversible with removal of the uterus and relief of the pressure against the ureter. However, if urinary tract obstruction from leiomyomata has been neglected, uremia may result. Removal of the tumor and relief of obstruction are necessary to restore kidney function. Chronic bladder neck obstruction from uterine leiomyomata can be so severe as to cause a remarkable increase in the thickness of the bladder wall and enlargement of the bladder resembling that seen in men with urethral obstruction from prostatic enlargement. Indeed, in these neglected cases, the bladder may fill the entire lower abdominal wall so that an incision above the umbilicus is required to enter the peritoneal cavity to remove the tumor without injury to the bladder.

The bowel is less apt to show symptoms from pressure than is the bladder, but constipation can be caused and aggravated by pressure of leiomyomata against the rectum. The small intestines can become entwined with subserous pedunculated tumors, causing intermittent intestinal obstruction.

Pain

Abdominal and pelvic pain or discomfort, a feeling of heaviness in the pelvis, and dyspareunia are present in about one third of patients with symptomatic uterine leiomyomata and may be an appropriate reason for intervention. There are several causes of pain with leiomyomata. However, the usual hyaline or cystic degeneration of these tumors does not produce symptoms. In rare instances, pedunculated subserous leiomyomata twist and give rise to a clinical picture of acute abdominal pain, much like that seen with a torsed ovarian tumor. These pedunculated tumors twist more often during pregnancy and after menopause. Acute carneous or red degeneration of a leiomyoma can occur at any period of reproductive life, although pain from this form of degeneration is more common during pregnancy. Dysmenorrhea, acquired in the fourth or fifth decade, may be the outstanding symptom of the growth of leiomyomata. A common symptom complex resulting from leiomyomata at this time of life is menstrual pain coupled with increased menstrual flow. Diffuse adenomyosis can also cause these symptoms, and the differentiation of this condition from a symmetrically enlarged intramural leiomyoma may be extremely difficult and may require MRI. The differentiation may be academic when surgery is planned; however, in cases when UAE is considered, this distinction is important because it may be less effective in cases of adenomyosis.

Patients who have uterine leiomyomata and pain may have concomitant pelvic disease such as ovarian pathology, pelvic inflammatory disease, tubal pregnancy, endometriosis, or urinary tract or intestinal pathology, including appendicitis. One must be careful to rule out other pathologies that may be obscured by uterine leiomyomata.

Abdominal Distortion

Distortion of the normal abdominal wall contour because of large tumors may justify their removal. Tumors of such size often give rise to other symptoms also, so there is ample reason for surgical interference. However, when no other symptoms are present, one may recommend removal of the tumors if the abdominal distortion is of such a magnitude as to be embarrassing to the patient.

Rapid Growth

Evidence of rapid growth of uterine leiomyomata, as observed by the same examiner over time or as confirmed by US, is an indication for surgical intervention. Such rapid growth in a premenopausal patient is only rarely due to sarcoma. Parker and others reviewed the medical records of 1,332 women admitted for surgical management of uterine leiomyoma. They found no correlation between rapid growth and the presence of uterine sarcoma. It may be due to pregnancy or to the use of oral contraceptives containing large amounts of estrogens. In the latter case, these drugs should be discontinued and an alternative method of contraception prescribed. In the postmenopausal patient, however, growth of a uterine leiomyoma is highly suggestive of a malignancy. The malignancy may be a sarcomatous change in the leiomyoma itself, a sarcoma or carcinoma in the endometrium causing uterine enlargement, or an ovarian neoplasm whose estrogen secretion is stimulating enlargement of the leiomyoma or whose growth may be mistaken for rapid enlargement of uterine leiomyomata. Although malignancy is not invariably found, the chances in its favor are so great that one must proceed on the assumption that it exists and should perform dilatation and curettage followed by removal of the enlarged uterus.

Rapid growth of a leiomyomatous uterus is difficult to define in exact terms. Buttram and Reiter have arbitrarily defined it as a gain of 6 weeks or more in gestational size within a year or less. Although this definition could apply in premenopausal women, it might be disastrous to wait for this amount of growth in a postmenopausal woman. It is important to have a definite method of documenting uterine size at periodic intervals. Repeated sounding of the uterine cavity may be of some benefit, although leiomyomatous growth is not always accompanied by concomitant enlargement of the uterine cavity. It is important to document the size of specific leiomyomata or the total uterine size in terms of centimeters or grams of uterine weight rather than in terms of gestational size of the uterus, although the latter method has become quite popular. Changes in a patient's weight can make evaluation of growth more difficult. Ultrasonography is a much more objective way of establishing the size of a uterine leiomyoma in the beginning and, when indicated, of evaluating its rate of growth. There is a need for more information about the natural growth patterns of myomata before and after menopause.

Although leiomyomata can increase dramatically in size during pregnancy, usually there is no appreciable growth. Winer-Muram and coworkers studied 89 pregnant women with uterine leiomyomata documented by US examination. In 83 of the patients, there was no demonstrable increase in the size of the leiomyomata. In 6 patients, there was an increase in size of up to 4 cm. Those myomata that increase in size during pregnancy will decrease in size a few weeks after the pregnancy is over.

Spontaneous Abortion and Other Pregnancy-Related Problems

Fibroid size and location affect the type and degree of patient symptoms and may also have reproductive consequences including pregnancy loss and infertility. The extent of uterine fibroids' effect on pregnancy rates and outcomes remains controversial.

Various mechanisms have been proposed to explain the occurrence of spontaneous abortion from uteri with leiomyomata. These include disturbances in uterine blood flow, alterations in blood supply to the endometrium, uterine irritability, rapid growth or degeneration of leiomyomata during pregnancy, difficulty in enlargement of the uterine cavity to accommodate for the growth of the fetus and placenta, and interference with proper implantation and placental growth by poorly developed endometrium or by subjacent leiomyomata. Implantation in a thin, poorly vascularized endometrium over a submucous leiomyoma is doomed to failure, because proper growth and development of the embryo and placenta are impossible (Fig. 31.17). Matsunaga and Shiota found a twofold increase in the number of malformed embryos recovered from patients with uterine leiomyomata having artificial termination of pregnancy.

Uterine leiomyomata may also be associated with other obstetrical concerns, including premature delivery, stillbirth, and interstitial pregnancy, as in the case reported by Starks. In a retrospective population-based study by Sheiner and colleagues, obstetrical outcomes appeared to be compromised by uterine leiomyoma. Compared with controls, women with myomata during pregnancy had an increase in intrauterine growth restriction (6.8% vs. 1.9%), placental abruption (2.8% vs. 0.7%), abnormal presentation (16.9% vs. 2.4%), cesarean section rate (57.7% vs. 10.8%), premature rupture of membranes (9.6% vs. 5.5%), and likelihood to receive a blood transfusion (4.2% vs. 1.4%). All of these outcomes were statistically significant ($P < 0.001$). Muram and associates have followed patients with leiomyomata through pregnancy with US. When a leiomyoma was in close proximity to the placental site, an increased incidence of pregnancy-related complications was seen. These were mainly bleeding complications, but pain, premature delivery, and postpartum hemorrhage also occurred. Exacoustos and Rosati reviewed the US scans of 12,708 pregnant patients. Four hundred ninety-two patients had myomata. A statistically significant increased incidence of threatened abortion, threatened preterm delivery, abruptio placentae, and pelvic pain was observed in patients with myomata. Abruptio placentae was particularly evident in women with myoma volumes greater than 200 cm³, submucosal location, or superimposition of the placenta. The authors suggest that US findings make it possible to identify women at risk for myoma-related complications of pregnancy. Factors responsible for spontaneous abortion in patients without uterine leiomyomata may also be responsible for spontaneous abortion in patients with leiomyomata.

Occasionally, pregnancy causes a remarkable growth of leiomyomata in the same way that the myometrium undergoes hypertrophy in pregnancy. Red or carneous degeneration of

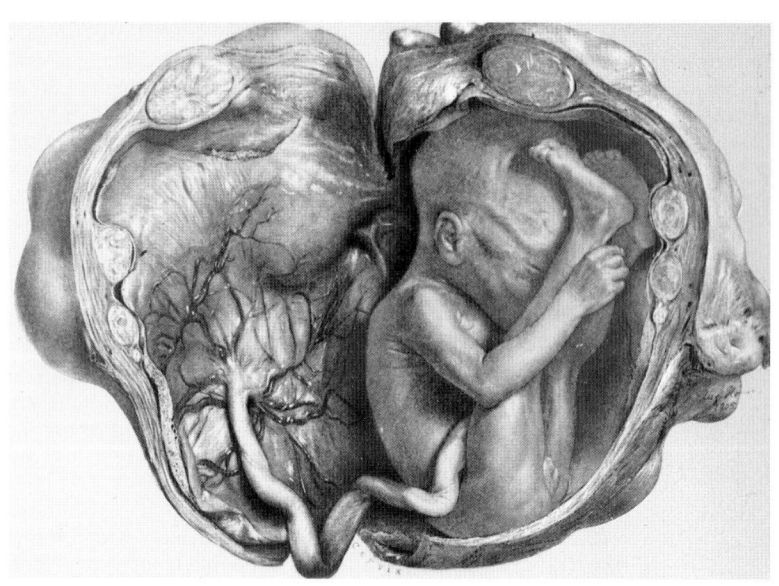

FIGURE 31.17 When the placenta is implanted over a myoma in the uterine wall, the blood supply to the fetus may be tenuous.

leiomyomata during pregnancy is associated with pain, tenderness over the tumor, low-grade fever, and leukocytosis. Management should be expectant with analgesic medications and bed rest. If premature uterine contractions occur, tocolytics may be given. Pain usually subsides within a few days. Operation is not indicated unless it is necessary to rule out other problems that require surgery for relief, because differentiation from appendicitis, placental abruption, torsed adnexa, and other problems may be difficult. After delivery, leiomyomata involute and generally return to their prepregnancy size by the third postpartum month.

Torsion with infarction of subserous pedunculated leiomyomata is more common in pregnancy. A leiomyoma may interfere with labor and delivery by causing an abnormal presentation, by causing dysfunctional labor, or by obstructing the pelvis. A submucous leiomyoma in the lower uterine segment may entrap the placenta, necessitating manual removal. Indeed, furious postpartum hemorrhage can result if a submucous leiomyoma is disturbed at delivery or during exploration of the uterine cavity. Immediate hysterectomy may be necessary to control the bleeding.

Most patients with uterine leiomyomata have no difficulty conceiving and carry their pregnancies to term without complications. The only problem encountered may be a difficulty in estimating gestational age from uterine size because of the presence of leiomyomata.

Infertility

When asymptomatic leiomyomata are discovered in young women, the question of how these tumors relate to sterility and pregnancy usually arises. A number of factors may be responsible for infertility in a patient with uterine leiomyomata. Anovulatory cycles may occur more commonly. There may be interference with sperm transport caused by distortion and an increased surface area within the uterine cavity, impingement of leiomyomata on the endocervical canal or interstitial portion of the fallopian tube, or interference with prostaglandin-induced uterine contractions, which are thought to enhance sperm migration. Endometrial changes (atrophy, ulceration, focal hyperplasia, and polyps), vascular alterations (venous congestion, venule ectasia, impaired blood flow), and enlargement of the uterine cavity may be present.

Because uterine leiomyomata occur in later reproductive years, relatively greater difficulty accomplishing conception can be expected in older couples.

The finding of small leiomyomata in sterile women is not an indication for immediate myomectomy. Quite often, an infertile patient with uterine leiomyomata is found to have some other causes of infertility. Tubal inflammatory disease with associated pelvic adhesions is especially common in patients with uterine leiomyomata. Both marital partners should have a complete infertility investigation, and the leiomyomata should initially be disregarded if it is asymptomatic. The ultimate decision regarding disposal of the tumors depends on their size and location. Usually, small subserous leiomyomata are not considered a factor in infertility. Even if the woman fails to become pregnant, removal of small subserous leiomyomata is not justified. When leiomyomata are intramural or submucous and of significant size, they may well be factors causing the infertility, and a myomectomy may be rewarded with a subsequent pregnancy.

When an unsuspected asymptomatic leiomyomatous uterus of significant size is found in a woman who is planning to become pregnant in the future, great tact is required in describing the problem to the patient. The best surgical and obstetric judgment is needed to make a proper recommendation. Should the patient be discouraged from attempting pregnancy because the risk of complications may be increased? Should a myomectomy be advised before pregnancy is attempted, with the knowledge that postmyomectomy adhesions may cause infertility? Such questions cannot be answered in a stereotypical manner. Each case presents its own problems, and the answers depend on the patient's age, her general physical health, her pelvic findings, and, most important, her own desires. All must be considered before a final recommendation can be made. In general terms, under these circumstances, an attempt to become pregnant will be rewarded with a satisfactory outcome in most cases. If pregnancy does not occur or is not successful, a myomectomy may be advised, but one must keep in mind that all causes of infertility, spontaneous abortion, and other pregnancy-related problems must also be investigated in patients with uterine leiomyomata; uterine leiomyomata represent an infrequent cause of infertility.

Eldar-Geva and colleagues performed a retrospective review of the treatment outcome of 106 assisted reproductive technology cycles in 88 patients with uterine myomata (subserosal, intramuscular without cavity distortion, and submucosal). Patients underwent controlled ovarian hyperstimulation and advanced reproductive technology. Not surprisingly, pregnancy (30.1%) and implantation (15.7%) rates were significantly lower in women with submucosal myomas; however, both pregnancy (16.4%) and implantation (6.4%) rates were also significantly lower in women with intramural myomas. In some advanced assisted reproductive technology patients, this information may influence the decision for surgical intervention regardless of menstrual pattern. A study by Olive et al. suggests that submucosal myomas that significantly distort or encroach on the uterine cavity may lower implantation and pregnancy rates in infertile women undergoing IVF. Several recent studies evaluated the effect of fibroids on in vitro fertilization cycles; the balance of data from independent studies by Farhi, Ramzy Jun, and Surrey suggests that pregnancy outcomes and implantation rates are adversely affected by submucosal myomas that enter the uterine cavity but not by subserosal or intramural fibroids that are less than 5 to 7 cm in size. Resection of submucosal fibroids clearly within the uterine cavity is likely warranted in patients with dysfunctional uterine bleeding, infertility, or pregnancy loss who desire to optimize future fertility.

A review of information about infertility and uterine leiomyomata was published by Wallach and Vu, by Vercellini and colleagues, and by Verkauf.

Miscellaneous Signs and Symptoms

A variety of other unusual problems may be associated with uterine leiomyomata and may require treatment. Ascites and uterine inversion have already been mentioned. Sudden intraperitoneal hemorrhage can result from rupture of a dilated vein beneath the serosal surface of a subserous leiomyoma. Although leiomyomata are more often associated with iron deficiency anemia from chronic uterine blood loss, occasionally, patients present with polycythemia. Islands of extramedullary erythropoiesis have been found in leiomyomata. Arteriovenous shunts within the tumors have been found and may be etiologically important in polycythemia. If the tumor obstructs the ureters and causes back pressure on the renal parenchyma, erythropoiesis can be stimulated. Weiss and coworkers and other investigators have found marked erythropoietin activity within uterine leiomyomata. The polycythemia in these cases is cured by hysterectomy.

CHOICE OF TREATMENT FOR UTERINE LEIOMYOMATA

According to statistics from the Centers for Disease Control, 600,000 hysterectomies are performed annually in the United States. Approximately 33% are performed with uterine leiomyomata as the primary indication. Nearly 35,000 myomectomies were reportedly performed annually in 2001, and it is believed that this number is increasing substantially. There are no statistics to indicate the number of hysteroscopic and laparoscopic myomectomies performed each year. Effective medical therapies are available to use as adjuncts to surgical treatment. Additional radiologic procedures may also be desirous in patients who may not be suitable surgical candidates. However, surgery is the preferred method of therapy in many circumstances.

Hysterectomy (abdominal, vaginal, and laparoscopic or robot assisted) is discussed in Chapter 32. In this chapter, surgical techniques that allow conservation of uterine function are discussed, as are medical therapies that can be used as adjuncts to surgical therapy.

Medical Management of Uterine Leiomyomata

Most (70% to 80%) uterine leiomyomata are asymptomatic and are discovered incidentally during a routine pelvic examination. Such patients require an explanation and reassurance and reexamination at periodic intervals. An initial baseline pelvic US examination or MRI study may be indicated for comparison with future examinations and to evaluate the adnexa if the ovaries cannot be felt on pelvic examination. An experienced pelvic examiner can be fairly certain that a central pelvic mass is a leiomyomatous uterus. However, pelvic US examinations and repeat pelvic examinations can add to the certainty of the diagnosis. If the diagnosis remains doubtful, however, visualization of the mass, usually by laparoscopy, may be indicated. Patients with an asymptomatic central pelvic mass should be followed up with periodic pelvic examination only when the mass is benign, usually a leiomyomatous uterus. Otherwise, expectant management is not appropriate.

Effective medical treatment that is likely to result in the permanent cure of uterine leiomyomata is not yet available. Surgical excision by a variety of techniques remains the most effective and widely used method of management for patients with significant symptoms. Medical therapies are available as an adjunct to surgical treatment or as a temporary substitute for definitive surgical treatment. The role of radiologic intervention continues to expand with UAE and recently U.S. Food and Drug Administration (FDA)–approved, MRI-guided, high-frequency focused ultrasonography.

Hormonal therapy for the management of uterine leiomyomata has been the subject of investigation for many years. There is no support for the use of danazol or progestins in view of the disappointing results reported. Antiprogestin therapy with mifepristone (RU-486) for 3 months has been shown by Murphy and colleagues to decrease leiomyoma volume by an average of 49%, with a variation of 0% to 87%. The immunoreactivity of progesterone, but not estrogen, receptors in the myoma and myometrial tissue was decreased significantly by RU-486 treatment, suggesting that regression of these tumors may be attained through a direct antiprogesterone effect. All patients became amenorrheic. Side effects were mild, and bone density was not diminished. An effective dose to cause a clinically significant (50%) decrease in leiomyoma volume appears to be 25 mg daily. Additional experience is needed to further evaluate these promising results. Reinsch and associates have demonstrated that RU-486 and leuprolide acetate are both effective in decreasing blood flow to the uterus. It is suggested that a decrease in uterine artery blood flow may provide a mechanism for a decrease in uterine size.

Gestrinone, a synthetic derivative of ethinyl-nortestosterone with antiestrogen and antiprogesterone properties, has been shown by Coutinho and associates to induce regression of leiomyomata. The treatment lasted 6 months to 1 year. The best results were obtained when the drug was administered intravaginally. Even the regression of large leiomyomata lasted up to a year after treatment. Side effects, though mildly androgenic, were well tolerated.

Many studies have been performed to investigate the treatment of patients with uterine leiomyomata with GnRH analogs. GnRH analogs bind to GnRH receptors, resulting in a biphasic response: a temporary increase in the levels of gonadotropins and gonadal steroids (agonist phase) is followed by chronic suppression of gonadotropin and gonadal steroid secretion (desensitization phase). In 1 to 3 weeks, a profound hypogonadotropic hypogonadal state begins and exists as long as the treatment lasts, but it is promptly reversed when treatment is discontinued. GnRH agonist treatment results in "medical oophorectomy" and "medical menopause" and is associated with the usual symptoms of a profound hypogonadal state (e.g., hot flashes, insomnia, mood lability, headaches, vaginal dryness, arthralgias, and myalgias). According to Friedman and associates, these adverse effects of treatment are self-limited and disappear within 3 to 6 months of cessation of GnRH agonist treatment. Dawood and colleagues describe a significant reduction in trabecular bone density after 24 weeks of GnRH agonist treatment that may not be completely reversible when treatment is discontinued. A mean reduction in trabecular bone density of 1% per month occurs in women treated for 6 months. Some of this bone loss may be permanent, but some is reversible.

Friedman and colleagues state that the average reduction in uterine and myoma volume is 40% to 50% after 3 to 6 months of GnRH agonist treatment; this is generally confirmed by others. Most of the response occurs in the first 12 weeks, and it is variable and unpredictable.

According to the analysis by these investigators, 4% of patients had an increase in uterine volume ranging from 0.1% to 25%, 24% had decreases in uterine volume ranging from 0.1% to 25%, 51% had decreases in uterine volume ranging from 25.1% to 50%, and 21% had decreases in uterine volume greater than 50%. No factors were found to predict the degree of uterine shrinkage. There were negative correlations with body weight, pretreatment uterine volume, age, height, and serum estradiol concentration.

It is commonly thought that GnRH analogs affect leiomyomata by reducing vascularity and the individual cell size within the tumor. The biochemical changes in leiomyomata obtained from women treated with the GnRH agonist leuprolide acetate depot for 3 months were studied by Rein and coworkers. The concentrations of amino acids contained in collagen were significantly greater in uterine myomata from treated patients than in myomata from placebo-treated controls. These investigators suggest that the reduction in uterine myoma volume associated with GnRH agonist therapy is due primarily to alterations in the extracellular matrix rather than to a reduction in the number or volume of cells in the myoma. Di Lieto and colleagues evaluated the clinical response; immunohistologic expression of the angiogenetic growth factors βFGF, VEGF, and PDGF; and vascular changes in uterine leiomyomas from women treated with GnRH agonist. They demonstrated that the GnRH agonist therapy caused a reduction in the synthesis of the three considered growth factors in leiomyomatous cells (βFGF, VEGF, and PDGF). The total number of vessels and angiogenetic vessels was also decreased after treatment with leuprolide acetate for 3 months.

Because uterine leiomyomata are hormone-sensitive neoplasms that can be stimulated to grow by estrogen, some clinicians have been reluctant to prescribe oral contraceptive pills in patients with leiomyomata. However, Friedman and Thomas and others have demonstrated conclusively that oral contraceptives containing 30 to 35 mg of ethinyl estradiol do not cause uterine leiomyomata to increase in size. Therefore, low-dose contraceptives can be used to manage menorrhagia in patients with uterine leiomyomata. Friedman and Thomas demonstrated a significant decrease in the mean duration of menstrual flow and a significant increase in hematocrit values in response to low-dose oral contraceptives in patients with uterine leiomyomata.

When myoma-associated menorrhagia is more severe, GnRH agonist and iron treatment may be more effective than oral contraceptives. In about two thirds of patients, GnRH agonist treatment induces amenorrhea. Most of the remaining patients experience very light, irregular vaginal bleeding or spotting, according to Friedman. A combination of menstrual suppression and iron therapy allows correction of iron deficiency and iron deficiency anemia during a 6-month treatment period. Ovulatory menses resume 3 to 24 weeks after the last depot GnRH agonist injection. Stovall and associates reported that a GnRH agonist plus iron was more effective than iron alone in treating anemia in patients with leiomyomata and in alleviating menorrhagia. With such effective treatment now available, there is rarely a need to use blood transfusions to correct anemia caused by myoma-associated menorrhagia. Only patients with significant symptoms from severe anemia may require transfusion.

Medical therapy may also be used transiently before surgery. By initiating the medication preoperatively, the maximum decrease in myoma volume may play a role in determining the route of surgery. If a hysterectomy is planned, the pharmacologic effect may facilitate a vaginal hysterectomy when the uterus is of borderline size. Vercellini and colleagues performed a multicenter, prospective, randomized, controlled study to assess if this shrinkage may increase the likelihood of a vaginal procedure. One hundred and twenty-seven premenopausal women with uterine volumes of 12 to 16 weeks were enrolled. After examination and disposition for an abdominal or vaginal hysterectomy, patients were randomized for GnRH therapy. Clinical assessment after the treatment course showed that abdominal hysterectomy was no longer indicated in 25 of 53 (47%) patients. No appreciable difference was found between the groups in postoperative complications. These findings are consistent with previously published studies, as well.

GnRH agonist treatment alone should not be given for periods longer than 6 months. A prolonged hypoestrogenic state is undesirable for a number of reasons, the most important being the loss of trabecular bone. If there are circumstances that require that GnRH treatment be extended beyond 6 months, consideration should be given to adding low-dose steroids after 3 months of GnRH therapy. The usual postmenopausal estrogen–progestin replacement regimen can be prescribed without interfering with the reduction in uterine volume anticipated. Loss of trabecular bone may not be as great. By adding estrogen–progestin replacement to GnRH agonist therapy, the adverse effects of a prolonged hypoestrogenic state may be prevented, and treatment with GnRH agonists may be prolonged. Friedman and colleagues treated 51 premenopausal women with large, symptomatic myomata with leuprolide acetate depot for 104 weeks. After the first 12 weeks, 0.75 mg of estropipate plus 0.7 mg of norethindrone was added on days 1 through 14 each month. Menorrhagia and other symptoms of uterine leiomyomata were controlled successfully. Hemoglobin and hematocrit levels increased. Symptoms of hypoestrogenism (hot flashes, vaginal dryness) were decreased significantly. Bone density decreased in the first 12 weeks, but only a small additional decrease occurred between weeks 12 and 52.

The use of GnRH analogs in the medical management of uterine leiomyomata is an emerging issue. How valuable it will be remains to be seen. Additional information and experience will define its use more exactly. For example, it may be possible for patients with symptomatic uterine leiomyomata who are approaching menopause to be managed medically through menopause without having a hysterectomy. It may be possible to improve fertility in some patients with uterine leiomyomata by treatment with GnRH analogs without myomectomy. With additional data, these and other questions can be answered.

Vaginal Myomectomy

In 1845, Atlee performed the first successful vaginal myomectomy on a patient with a submucous pedunculated myoma.

When a submucous myoma becomes pedunculated within the uterine cavity, there is a natural tendency for the uterus to try to expel it through the endocervical canal. Eventually, the cervix dilates. Even very large submucous pedunculated myomata can be delivered gradually through a markedly dilated cervix. Because adequate blood circulation through a long pedicle is difficult to maintain, the myoma becomes necrotic and infected (Figs. 31.5 and 31.6).

Patients report cramping lower abdominal pain; pressure and heaviness in the pelvis; a thin, bloody, foul discharge; difficulty with urination; and other symptoms. Episodes of profuse vaginal hemorrhage can occur. Such large submucous myomata may resemble a fetal head.

After satisfactory preoperative preparation, including broad-spectrum antibiotics and correction of anemia, vaginal myomectomy should be performed in the operating room. Morcellation may be required to remove very large tumors in many small pieces. Usually, there is very little bleeding. One should avoid too much downward traction on the tumor because the uterine fundus may invert. Eventually, the pedicle is identified. It should be clamped and ligated as high as possible within the uterine cavity. The use of a laparoscopic instrumentation, such as the Endoloop, can be advantageous to facilitate safe, secure ligation of the pedicle as high as possible. If ligation of the pedicle is not possible, the clamps can be left in place and safely removed 48 hours later.

Smaller submucous pedunculated myomata can be diagnosed by hysteroscopy, by hysterosalpingography, by sonohysterogram, or at the time of dilation and curettage. They can also be felt on digital exploration through a slightly dilated external cervical os. If the myoma can be grasped with an instrument (ring forceps or Allis clamp), it can be removed by twisting it free of its attachment. A tonsil snare can also be used. Bleeding is usually minimal. If brisk bleeding does occur, a 26-French, 30-mL Foley catheter can be inserted through the cervix and inflated for tamponade. If necessary, the cervix can be sutured around the catheter to hold it in place.

To gain access to submucous pedunculated myomata that are higher in the endocervical canal or uterine cavity, special procedures are required. An attempt at hysteroscopic removal may be successful. Alternatively, the cervix can be dilated with instruments or with *Laminaria japonica*, as described by Goldrath. Dührssen incisions can be made in the cervix. Also, the cervix can be incised by having the surgeon perform a vaginal hysterotomy (Fig. 31.18A, B). After the bladder is advanced, the cervix is dilated, and an anterior midline incision is made in the cervix high enough to identify the myoma. The pedicle of the myoma is ligated as high as possible (Figs. 31.18C, D). The incision in the cervix is repaired with 2-0 interrupted delayed absorbable sutures. The vaginal mucosa is reapproximated with 3-0 delayed absorbable sutures (Figs. 31.18E, F).

A submucous pedunculated myoma may be solitary, and there may not be other myomata in the uterus. In fact, many patients exhibit no evidence of uterine enlargement. After a successful vaginal myomectomy, most patients are asymptomatic and menstruate normally. A few even become pregnant and deliver vaginally without difficulty. Cervical incompetence has been reported. Hysterectomy or myomectomy is required only for those few patients who have multiple leiomyomata and continue to have significant symptoms.

Excellent results of vaginal removal of submucous pedunculated myomata in 151 patients were reported by Goldrath. Ben-Baruch and coworkers also achieved excellent results in 43 of 46 women in whom vaginal myomectomy was attempted. Vaginal myomectomy is recommended as the most appropriate initial treatment for pedunculated submucous myomata.

Vaginal myomectomy is traditionally used for submucosal myomata; however, it has been described for other myomata. Davies and colleagues reported a prospective study regarding the safety and efficacy of excision of intramural and subserosal leiomyoma by a vaginal route. Preoperative criteria included (a) uterine size less than or equal to 16 weeks gestation, (b) good uterine mobility, (c) adequate vaginal access, (d) the presence of intramural or subserosal myomata, and (e) the

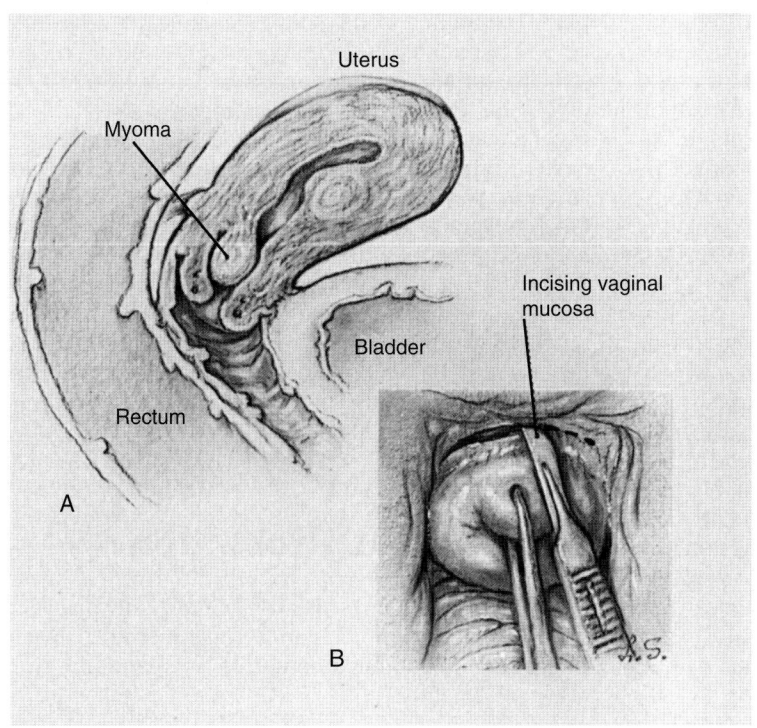

FIGURE 31.18 Transvaginal removal of a pedunculated submucous myoma that presents itself at the external cervical os. **A:** Sagittal view of uterus, demonstrating the location of the myoma originating on the posterior wall of the fundus just above the cervix. **B:** A transverse incision made anteriorly through the vaginal mucosa at the cervicovaginal junction.

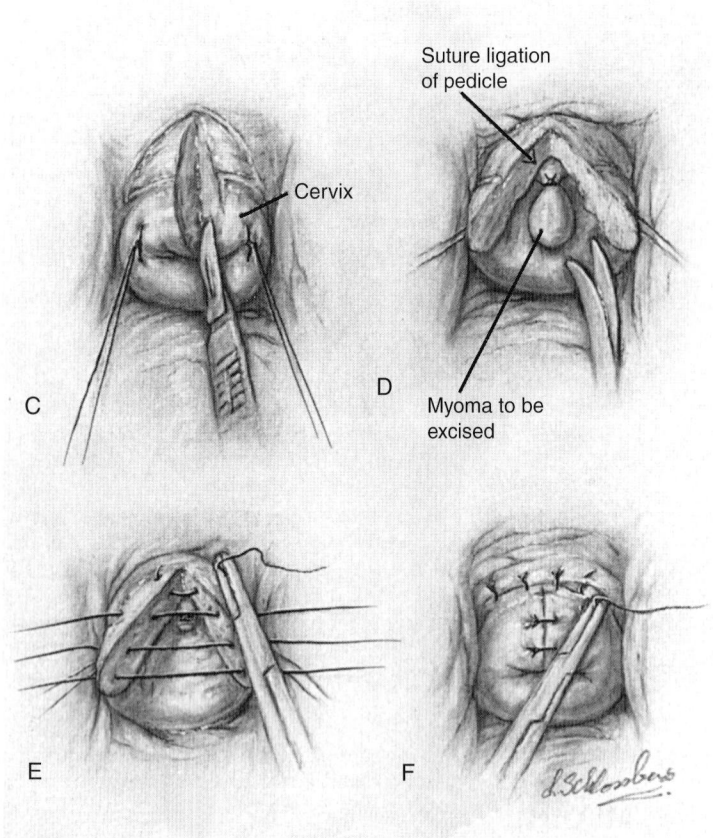

FIGURE 31.18 (*Continued*) **C:** After the bladder is advanced bluntly, the cervix is incised anteriorly in the midline. **D:** The myoma and its pedicle are exposed, and the pedicle is suture ligated for hemostasis. **E:** After the myoma is excised, the cervix is reapproximated with interrupted 2-0 absorbable, nonreactive sutures. **F:** The overlying vaginal mucosa is sutured with interrupted 3-0 absorbable sutures.

absence of adnexal pathology. Essentially, an open abdominal myomectomy technique was performed through an anterior or posterior colpotomy. The uterus was manipulated to bring the myoma into the colpotomy. The management of 35 women was described. The mean number of myomas removed was 2.5 per patient with mean mass of 113.8 g. Three patients (8.6%) required conversion to a laparotomy. Neither mean blood loss nor length of hospital stay was improved. Additionally, four (11.4%) patients developed pelvic hematomas postoperatively. At this time, this procedure does not seem to provide inherent benefits over an open abdominal myomectomy or a laparoscopic approach. With further review, better outcome data may demonstrate the advantages of this technique.

The tissue removed at vaginal myomectomy must be submitted for pathologic examination to rule out malignancy.

Hysteroscopic Resection of Submucous Myomata

Hysteroscopic resection of submucous myomata was first reported by Neuwirth and Amin in 1976 and was reported again by Neuwirth in 1978. A urologic resectoscope was used. In 1981, Goldrath and associates used "photocoagulation" of the endometrium with the neodymium-doped:yttrium–aluminum–garnet (Nd:YAG) laser to treat patients with menorrhagia. Many subsequent reports by Derman and associates, Donnez and colleagues, Goldenberg and coworkers, Corson, Indman, Hallez, Baggish and associates, Wamsteker and colleagues, and others have confirmed the advantages of hysteroscopic treatment of menorrhagia in women with and without submucous leiomyomata. The menorrhagia associated with submucous myomata can sometimes be managed with oral contraceptives as long as the bleeding is not too severe. A favorable response can also be expected with GnRH analogs, but the menorrhagia usually reappears when the treatment is discontinued. Friedman has reported three cases of severe menorrhagia with resultant anemia requiring transfusions in women with submucous leiomyomata treated with leuprolide acetate. Both oral contraceptives and GnRH analogs are counterproductive in women who are seeking relief from infertility. The uterine cavity can be curetted several times, but the benefit of this procedure is temporary at best.

When hysteroscopic resection of submucous myomata is performed, menorrhagia can be controlled in more than 90% of patients. According to Indman, the mean number of pads used during the heaviest day of menses decreased from 17.8 before treatment to 6.8 after treatment in women undergoing myoma resection only and from 21.4 to 1.7 pads per day in women whose treatment also included endometrial ablation. Dysmenorrhea was also reduced significantly. Forty-eight of fifty-one women (94%) with uterine leiomyomata who were seen with menorrhagia were able to avoid major gynecologic surgery for up to 5 years of follow-up. In the report of 156 patients by Derman and associates, 91.3% of patients did not require further surgery after 6 years of follow-up, and 83.9% did not require further surgery after 9 years of follow-up. Further review in recent papers supports Derman's results. Magos and colleagues performed a prospective observational study to identify factors that influence outcomes of hysteroscopic myomectomies by following up patients for almost 8 years. One hundred twenty-two patients enrolled in the study, and results suggest that hysteroscopic myomectomy is successful in treating menstrual symptoms in four of five cases. In addition, statistical analysis demonstrated that outcome is significantly better when the uterus is only slightly enlarged and if the myoma is mainly submucous in nature.

If endometrial ablation is performed with myoma resection, pregnancy is not likely to occur subsequently. Without simultaneous endometrial ablation, 21 patients became pregnant after myoma resection only, with 18 infants delivered in the series reported by Derman and colleagues. The pregnancy rates among women who wished to conceive varied between 47% and 66% in several reports. These rates are comparable to those reported for abdominal myomectomy.

Donnez and coworkers used a biodegradable GnRH agonist (Zoladex Implant ICI) preoperatively in a series of 60 women with large submucous myomata. Submucous myomectomy by hysteroscopy and Nd:YAG laser was easily performed. In 12 patients, the procedure was accomplished in two stages. Perino and associates used GnRH agonists in 58 women with submucous leiomyomata diagnosed during investigation for infertility or menstrual disorder. There was a significant reduction in operating time, intraoperative bleeding, infusion volume, and failure rate in the treated group compared with the control subjects. Myoma size is reduced and hemoglobin concentration is restored to normal preoperatively. Campo and colleagues collected data on 80 consecutive resectoscopic myomectomies performed on premenopausal women. Forty-two patients did not receive any preoperative medical therapy, whereas 38 patients received 2 months of intramuscular GnRH analog therapy. Perioperative results were recorded, followed by a 24-month follow-up period when recurrent symptoms, myoma recurrence, and the need for repeat surgery were collected. Surgical time for the pretreated group was significantly longer than that of the untreated patients. Although GnRH analog pretreatment may be beneficial in improving anemia in some patients, Campo and colleagues did not demonstrate any improvement in short- or long-term outcomes.

A hysteroscopic approach is reasonable if the majority of the fibroid is within the cavity or if subtotal hysteroscopic myomectomy is deemed preferable to total abdominal myomectomy. Hysteroscopic resection may be performed using a hysteroscopic morcellator or resectoscope. A resectoscope allows for the use of electrocautery at the time of resection but, as a result, requires electrolyte-poor distending media such as mannitol, sorbitol, or glycine. Morcellating devices resect using a rotating blade rather than electrocautery and allow for use of isotonic distending media such as normal saline or lactated Ringer, which have lower risk for fluid overload and subsequent electrolyte imbalance. The avoidance of electrocautery also has a theoretical benefit of avoiding thermal damage to the myometrium and decreasing the chance of future uterine rupture at time of pregnancy. Both methods incur a risk of procedure abortion secondary to bleeding. Prior to starting the hysteroscopy, injection of vasopressin into the cervical stroma can be used to help decrease myoma bleeding. If bleeding is encountered intraoperatively, conversion from morcellator to electrocautery or use of uterine balloon for tamponade and uterine compression can be used to help achieve hemostasis.

When submucous myomata extend deeply into the myometrium, it may not be possible to perform a complete resection for obvious technical reasons. However, it should be possible to remove most irregularities in the uterine cavity and to restore the contour of the cavity to almost normal in most cases. According to Wamsteker and colleagues, hysteroscopic resection of submucous myomata with more than 50% intramural extension should be performed only in selected cases. Repeat procedures may be needed in cases of initial incomplete resection.

To avoid the possibility of inadvertent uterine perforation or to allow its prompt diagnosis if it occurs, hysteroscopic resection is usually performed under laparoscopic guidance. However, as reported by Sullivan and coworkers, laparoscopy may be insufficient to evaluate fully the possible sequelae of uterine perforation. Laparotomy may be necessary to assess the pelvic viscera fully. Letterie and Kramer were able to safely substitute intraoperative transabdominal ultrasonographic guidance for laparoscopy. In their opinion, operative hysteroscopy with intraoperative ultrasonographic guidance provides an accurate and precise method to monitor intrauterine surgery, and it can be used to enhance the performance of hysteroscopic myomectomy and endometrial resection. Intraoperative US guidance provided sufficient details of the relation between the hysteroscope and the myoma and uterine walls to gauge the depth of resection and prevent uterine perforation. Lin et al. resected six submucous myomas under ultrasonographic guidance. All cases were completed in under 1 hour without any complications and resulted in improvement in menorrhagia and metrorrhagia. Postoperative hysteroscopy revealed no intrauterine adhesions, and the endometrium at the operative site appeared normal. Wortman and Dagget used ultrasonographic control to remove large submucous myomas and claimed that US may help prevent perforation and obviate laparoscopy.

The success and safety of the procedure depend on the experience and skill of the operator. During hysteroscopic resection, vascular spaces are opened in the endometrium and myometrium. Large volumes of fluid are instilled into the uterine cavity. Fluid balance must be monitored carefully by the surgeon and the anesthesiologist to avoid fluid overload.

All tissue must be submitted for pathologic examination. Among 92 patients undergoing hysteroscopic resection in the series reported by Corson and Brooks, two cases of leiomyosarcoma were diagnosed. Leiomyosarcoma is said to be more common in submucous leiomyomata than in intramural or subserous leiomyomata.

As time passes after hysteroscopic resection of submucous myomata, the possibility of recurrent problems increases because of regrowth of myomata. However, this is no more likely to occur than it is with standard abdominal myomectomy. The experience of many investigators has demonstrated that hysteroscopic management of menorrhagia in patients with submucous leiomyomata is a reasonable alternative to classic surgical hysterectomy or myomectomy. The occasional psychological problems and complications of hysterectomy are avoided. An abdominal incision is avoided, there is less discomfort, the procedure can often be performed in an outpatient setting, and the patient can usually resume normal activity after a very brief recovery period.

Hysteroscopic resection of a small submucous myoma is illustrated in **Figure 31.19**. Details of the indications, technique, complications, and results of hysteroscopic resection are also provided in Chapter 18.

Laparoscopic and Robotic-Assisted Myomectomy

When abdominal myomectomy is indicated, the laparoscopic or robotic-assisted approach can be offered as an alternative to the standard "open" abdominal myomectomy in selected patients. However, this procedure is appropriate in very few patients for several reasons. First, myomectomy is indicated in infertility patients only if there is significant distortion of the uterine wall or endometrial cavity or if there is obstruction or distortion of the fallopian tubes by myomata. Second, myomectomy is indicated in patients who wish to retain their uterus only if the myomata are significantly symptomatic. In both circumstances, the myomata are likely to be multiple and large, and laparoscopic/robotic-assisted myomectomy should only be considered if the uterine repair is comparable, or superior, to the uterine closure of an abdominal myomectomy.

Myoma

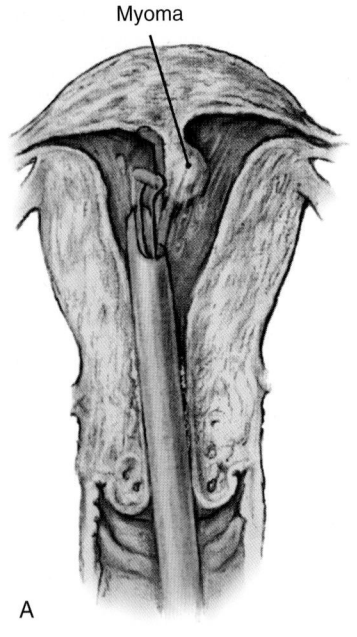

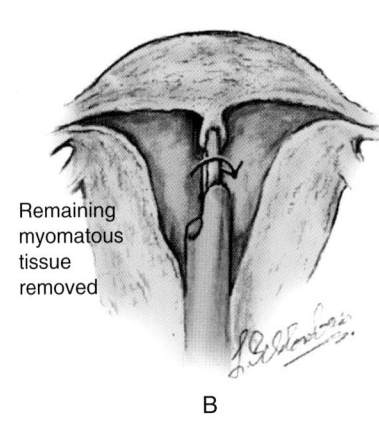

Remaining
myomatous
tissue
removed

A

B

FIGURE 31.19 Hysteroscopic removal of a submucous myoma. **A:** After insertion of the resectoscope, the submucous myoma is removed by progressive shaving. The loop of the resectoscope is placed at the most distant portion of the myoma, and the current is applied as the resectoscope is drawn toward the surgeon. Pressure is exerted by the loop against the myoma with each stroke. **B:** A grasping forceps is used to twist off the remaining tissue once the size has been appreciably reduced.

There are limitations to both laparoscopic and robotic-assisted myomectomies, and these are mostly technical. Myomata in certain locations are difficult to remove. When myomata are large or multiple, or both, operative time and blood loss may be unacceptable. When myomata are embedded deeply in the myometrium, proper repair of the uterine wall may be difficult or impossible, and uterine rupture may occur in a subsequent pregnancy. Retrieval of the resected myomata from the peritoneal cavity can also pose problems. Large myomata must be morcellated into smaller pieces for retrieval. Retrieval through the posterior vaginal fornix or through the abdominal wall requires separate additional incisions, which somewhat defeats the idea of a minimally invasive procedure. Only very skillful laparoscopists or trained robotic surgeons should attempt extensive myomectomy through the laparoscope. According to Mais and colleagues, operation time for myomectomy was significantly longer for laparoscopy than for laparotomy when more than four myomata had to be removed and the largest myoma was greater than 6 cm. Dubuisson and coworkers also reinforce the difficulty of the technique by reporting conversion to laparotomy at a rate of 7.5% (93.7% due to operative difficulties) and a complication rate of 3.8%. These authors echo similar intraoperative concerns: (a) the location of the hysterotomy, (b) the type of hysterotomy, (c) the uterine suture, and (d) removal of the myoma. In addition, they report that one third of patients developed adhesions at the uterine scar.

The robot, which provides additional degrees of freedom as compared to laparoscopy, was first approved by the U.S. FDA for use in gynecologic surgery in 2005. It improves potential surgical dexterity and allows for 3-dimensional visualization of the tissue. Several technical innovations have been developed to facilitate laparoscopic and robotic-assisted myomectomy. Electrosurgical and laser techniques are used in ingenious ways. Special traction devices, including corkscrews of various sizes, are required. The operator must be able to provide hemostasis using monopolar cutting current and bipolar forceps. The role of the Harmonic scalpel has also expanded for clean dissection and the potential for less blood loss. Aquadissection can be used to establish planes for dissection between myomata and the surrounding myometrium.

Special techniques of approximating myometrium with larger curved needles are used with either intracorporeal or extracorporeal suture tying, depending on the surgeon's expertise. Knowledge of available laparoscopic instrumentation is essential to maximize surgical outcome. Autologous blood donation with intraoperative transfusion when necessary reduces the risk of homologous transfusion. Larger myomata can be removed vaginally with morcellation through a posterior colpotomy incision. In cases of myomas of extreme size, Pelosi and colleagues proposed the use of hand-assisted laparoscopy to avoid a laparotomy. This technique allows the insertion of a hand into the abdomen to assist in dissection. This is accomplished through a glove-sized incision at laparoscopy while preserving the pneumoperitoneum. A cylindrical serrated morcellator can also be used to convert smaller myomata to small strips of tissue, which can then be removed abdominally through the trocar sleeve or through a minilaparotomy incision. Retrieval of all bits and pieces of myoma tissue from the peritoneal cavity can be a tedious challenge. Hirai and colleagues from Japan described a microwave coagulator and electromechanical tissue borer to minimize invasion of the myometrium and abdominal wall. The proposed advantage of this technique is that by morcellating the tissue before removal from the uterus, less myometrial trauma is sustained. Horizontal and perpendicular blades at the tip rotate and hollow out the myoma, allowing large myomas to be removed through a small uterine incision. The authors described the use in five patients with four of the five having myomas weighing less than 170 g. The blood loss and operating time were not substantially different than with conventional abdominal procedures. Long-term data regarding myometrial strength over time and pregnancy outcomes are not yet available. More experience with this procedure is necessary to determine its role in myomectomy. A recent review of robotic-assisted technique was published by Quaas and colleagues.

Another technical innovation called myolysis has been described by Goldfarb and is based on earlier experience in Europe. Either Nd:YAG laser or bipolar needles are used laparoscopically to penetrate the myomata at multiple sites at a 90-degree angle to the uterus. In response to treatment, the myomata ultimately atrophy. The technique is based on the theory that the coagulating effects of lasers or the bipolar needle can necrose myometrial stroma, denature protein, destroy vascularity, and result in substantial shrinkage of myomas when deprived of their blood supply. Goldfarb advises treatment with GnRH agonists before surgery. The ideal candidates for myolysis are perimenopausal women who have symptomatic leiomyomata measuring 3 to 10 cm or uterine size less than 14 weeks gestation. Goldfarb combines myolysis with endometrial ablation in patients with symptomatic myomas with persistent uterine bleeding. The addition of myolysis to endometrial ablation increased the rate of postsurgical amenorrhea from 36.5% to 57%, and second procedures, including hysterectomy, were reduced from 38% to 12.5%. Goldfarb described significant adhesions at follow-up laparoscopy in patients treated with the Nd:YAG laser technique because of excessive serosal injury from multiple punctures. A circumferential technique was later developed to destroy vasculature instead of the myomatous tissue. The devascularized myoma becomes cyanotic, loses viability, and fibroses. Phillips reported on women who underwent elective diagnostic laparoscopy to evaluate adhesions associated with previously performed myolysis. Mean adhesion score was only 1.15 ± 0.6 on a scale of 10.

Zreik and colleagues at Yale University modified the myolysis procedure to include cryotechnology to "freeze" uterine leiomyomas. The technique, *cryomyolysis,* was described in a prospective pilot study of 14 patients. All patients were pretreated with GnRH agonist therapy for 3 months. Thirteen of the fourteen endoscopic procedures were performed by laparoscopy and the remaining one by hysteroscopic visualization. Cryoprobe placement was verified, and freezing was performed at an internal probe temperature of $-180°C$ until the ice ball encompassed the entire fibroid or reached maximum size. A thaw cycle was then performed, followed by one more freeze–thaw cycle. A hollow track remained within the frozen myoma after removal of the cryoprobe. MRI studies were used to assess uterine and myoma size. The uterus enlarged by 22% after discontinuation of the GnRH therapy. Myoma volume decreased by 6% over 4 months postoperatively, with some patients having a decrease of more than 50%. Four of six women who underwent second-look office laparoscopy had adhesion formation at freezing sites. The authors attributed risk and severity of adhesion formation to the number of punctures with the cryoprobe. The role of this therapy in conservative treatment of uterine myomata remains to be defined.

Hysteroscopic myomectomy and endometrial resection can be performed simultaneously if submucous myomata are present. In more than 300 myolysis procedures, the author reported minimal morbidity with a 30% to 50% reduction in myoma size beyond the reduction achieved with GnRH agonist treatment. No regrowth occurred after several years of follow-up, even after estrogen replacement therapy. Bipolar coagulation myolysis may be less likely to cause damage to the uterine serosa and less likely to cause adhesion formation postoperatively. According to Goldfarb, "As a same-day procedure, myoma coagulation appears to be an extremely safe alternative to hysterectomy, allowing the patient to avoid major surgery and its subsequent recovery time, while providing an alternative solution for patients with symptomatic leiomyomas."

Nezhat and coworkers used a combination of laparoscopy and minilaparotomy to perform myomectomy in 57 women with uteri at 8 to 26 weeks in gestational size. In this laparoscopically assisted myomectomy procedure, the myomata were removed and the uterus repaired through the minilaparotomy incision. It was technically less difficult than laparoscopic myomectomy and allowed better closure of the uterine defects. This technique may be preferable in the case of large myomas in that it is easier to achieve conventional multilayer suturing and easier to extract myomas.

A recent retrospective review by Pitter et al. included 872 women who underwent robotic-assisted myomectomy and evaluated pregnancy outcomes among 127 of the women who conceived (92 of whom delivered) postoperatively. They found rates of miscarriage, preterm delivery, and uterine rupture to be comparable to those reported for laparoscopic myomectomy. A similar but smaller study by Göçmen including 38 patients noted comparable operative time, hospital stay, and estimated blood loss between patients undergoing laparoscopic and robot-assisted myomectomy. Moreover, several independent studies by Ranisavljevic, Mansour, and Nash suggest that robotic-assisted myomectomy appears to have similar advantages as laparoscopic myomectomy when compared to abdominal myomectomy. Behera, however, contends that, currently, robotic-assisted cases are less cost-efficient than laparoscopic or abdominal cases. This cost discrepancy may improve over time.

A significant disadvantage of myomectomy is the risk of postoperative pelvic adhesions. The adhesions may adversely affect fertility, give rise to pain, and increase the risk of ectopic pregnancy or even intestinal obstruction. Several studies have demonstrated that the risk of postoperative adhesions decreases when a laparoscopic approach is used in lieu of an open abdominal approach. Literature review demonstrates that the average rate of postoperative adhesions after laparoscopic myomectomy is 41% versus more than 90% after a myomectomy via laparotomy. Dubuisson and colleagues assessed adhesion formation after laparoscopic myomectomy in a prospective manner. Forty-five patients underwent a second look after laparoscopic myomectomy. Seventy-two sites were evaluated. The overall rate of postoperative adhesions was 35.6% per patient. The rate of adhesions per myomectomy site was 16.7%. The rate of adhesions on the adnexa was 24.4%. Associations with the occurrence of adnexal adhesions included an additional surgical procedure carried out at the same time, the existence of adhesions before the operation, and posterior location of the myoma. Several factors may increase the risk of postoperative adhesion formation after a laparoscopic myomectomy. Recognition of these factors may be helpful in limiting adhesion formation.

The use of uterine suture appears to increase the risk of uterine adhesions. In some studies, the frequency doubled after suturing. The suture induces local tissue ischemia with inflammatory changes, which slow the healing process and induce the formation of adhesions. Contradictory data have been published regarding adhesion formation and the use of bipolar coagulation during a laparoscopic procedure.

The location of the myoma also affects adhesion formation. Adhesions are more likely to form when the myomectomy site is located on the posterior uterine wall. During laparoscopy, a uterine incision must be made over each individual myoma. With laparotomy, a single anterior uterine incision may be used for polymyomectomy, even when posterior myomas are present.

The prior existence of pelvic adhesions significantly increases the risk of postoperative adnexal adhesions but has not been shown to affect adhesions at the myomectomy site.

Two prospective, randomized controlled studies have evaluated the efficacy of adhesion barriers during laparoscopic myomectomy, and both found intervention to be beneficial. Mais and colleagues evaluated the efficacy of oxidized regenerated cellulose, Interceed, on adhesion formation in a prospective randomized study of 50 women after laparoscopic myomectomy. Interceed was placed over all incisions and suture material with a 1 cm margin, and the barrier was then moistened with saline. During the second-look laparoscopy, 60% of the Interceed group was free of adhesions, compared with only 12% of patients in the control group. Interceed appeared to substantially reduce, but not prevent, adhesions after laparoscopic myomectomy. Pellicano and collaborators showed that hyaluronic acid gel reduced adhesions after laparoscopic myomectomy in a prospective randomized study of 36 infertile women. During second look, 72% of patients were adhesion free, with hyaluronic acid gel treatment versus an adhesion-free rate of only 22% in the control group.

Multiple published studies (Seracchioli et al., Bulletti et al., Stringer et al., and Campo et al.) suggest that laparoscopic myomectomy may be a viable option for women with leiomyomata and infertility. The best prognosis is for young women with otherwise unexplained infertility and myomas that distort the endometrial cavity. Pregnancy rates and spontaneous abortion rates are comparable to abdominal myomectomy. Data are currently insufficient to determine the appropriate recommendation regarding mode of delivery.

Laparoscopic myomectomy is further discussed in Chapter 17.

Abdominal Myomectomy

The first successful abdominal myomectomy was performed in the United States by the Atlee brothers, Washington and John, in 1844. The first abdominal multiple myomectomy was performed by W. Alexander of Liverpool in 1898. In the early part of the 20th century, the technique of abdominal myomectomy was refined by many notable gynecologic surgeons, including Kelly, Cullen, Mayo, Rubin, Bonney, and others. The procedure did not gain popularity until the middle of the 20th century. The incidence of complications, including hemorrhage, infection, and postoperative intestinal obstruction from adhesions, was considered to be too high. Advances in surgical techniques to control intraoperative bleeding during myomectomy, along with advances in anesthesia, blood transfusion therapy, and GnRH analogs, have made myomectomy a safe alternative to hysterectomy in women with symptomatic leiomyomata. The number of myomectomies performed in the United States is increasing.

Because myomectomy is rarely an emergency, time is available to prepare the patient for surgery. It is important that she be properly informed of the reasons myomectomy has been recommended. She should understand the nature of the procedure so she can know what to expect and what is expected of her. It is especially important that she be informed of the possibility that intraoperative findings may contraindicate myomectomy and require that hysterectomy be performed instead. For example, myomectomy may not be technically feasible if diffuse leiomyomatosis is found. The technical challenge of removing a large cervical myoma can also preclude myomectomy.

A preoperative hysterosalpingogram may indicate distortion of the fallopian tubes or uterine cavity, findings that are important in planning the technique of myomectomy. An assessment of fallopian tube patency is helpful in predicting fertility. If the tubes are occluded, however, myomectomy is not necessarily contraindicated. According to Seoud and associates, myomectomy does not interfere with in vitro fertilization performance in relation to overall and ongoing pregnancy rates. The patient whose tubes are occluded should understand that fertility may not be established by myomectomy, and assisted reproductive technologies may still be required after myomectomy. Tubal reconstruction procedures are uniformly unrewarding when performed at the same time multiple myomectomy is done. Indeed, tubal reconstruction may not always be necessary to

establish tubal patency. In a report by Lev-Toaff and associates, nonfilling of the fallopian tubes was present on the preoperative hysterosalpingogram unilaterally in two patients and bilaterally in another two. In all four patients, tubal patency was shown after myomectomy. In the experience of these authors, hysterosalpingography before myomectomy can assist the gynecologic surgeon in planning the surgical approach by showing the presence, size, and location of submucous leiomyomata and concomitant tubal disease.

Imaging modalities such as transabdominal, transvaginal US and MRI play an important role in the management of patients with leiomyomata, especially those patients who are being prepared for myomectomy. As explained by Mayer and Shipilov, US is the preferred method for screening and initial evaluation of the pelvis. In many cases, it is the only imaging study necessary. There are special cases for which US cannot provide all the diagnostic information required. In a study by Schwartz and colleagues, US results were inconclusive in 20% of cases and did not yield a definitive diagnosis in 59% of cases. MRI was more definitive in all cases (**Fig. 31.20**).

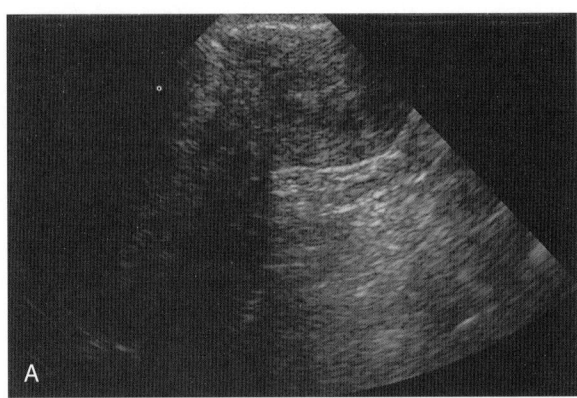

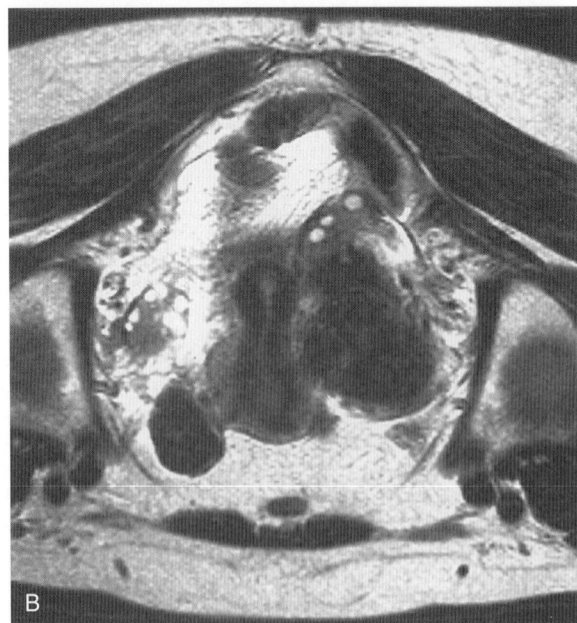

FIGURE 31.20 A: The ultrasound evaluation of this patient with a very large leiomyoma was not helpful in delineating the leiomyoma from the adnexa. **B:** The MRI study demonstrated multiple leiomyomas distinctly separate from the adnexa bilaterally. The ovaries are seen bilaterally with multiple cysts. (Image courtesy of Deborah Baumgarten, MD.)

The preoperative diagnosis of submucous leiomyomata by MRI may allow hysteroscopic resection and avoid abdominal myomectomy in some cases. Differentiation between uterine leiomyomata and adnexal pathology is more accurate with MRI and thus avoids the need for laparoscopy or laparotomy in some cases (**Fig. 31.21**). MRI studies can differentiate between uterine leiomyomata, diffuse and localized adenomyosis, and diffuse leiomyomatosis. MRI is the most accurate imaging technique for the detection and localization of leiomyomata (**Fig. 31.22**). Hricak and coworkers were able to identify accurately by MRI all subserosal (9 of 9), all intramural (37), and 10 of 11 submucosal leiomyomata. Leiomyomata as small as 0.3 cm can be detected. Various degrees of cellularity, degeneration, necrosis, and calcification can be identified by MRI, and sarcomatous change can be suspected. MRI provides imaging planes that are not available on transabdominal or transvaginal US, a feature that permits better visualization of the more lateral and posterior areas of the pelvis. MRI is the most accurate method for preoperative localization of leiomyomata and surgical planning for myomectomy. Given the greater costs of MRI, it should be used judiciously. However, as noted by Mayer and Shipilov, the effective cost differential between MRI and US is decreasing.

As discussed by Wiskind and Thompson, one of the most serious risks of surgical bleeding during myomectomy is the risk associated with homologous blood transfusion. The first rule in reducing or eliminating the need for transfusion is to bring the patient to the operating room with the highest possible hemoglobin and hematocrit level. About 30% of myomectomy patients have associated menorrhagia. These small, repeated menstrual hemorrhages deplete the body's iron stores over time and eventually result in iron deficiency anemia of various degrees of severity. Patients scheduled for myomectomy benefit from oral iron supplementation. In a study by Thompson, the liberal use of oral iron therapy preoperatively was shown to decrease the number of blood transfusions on the gynecologic surgical service at the Johns Hopkins Hospital. A blood transfusion is seldom necessary to correct iron deficiency anemia in a gynecologic patient. Blood transfusions should generally be reserved for patients with hypovolemic

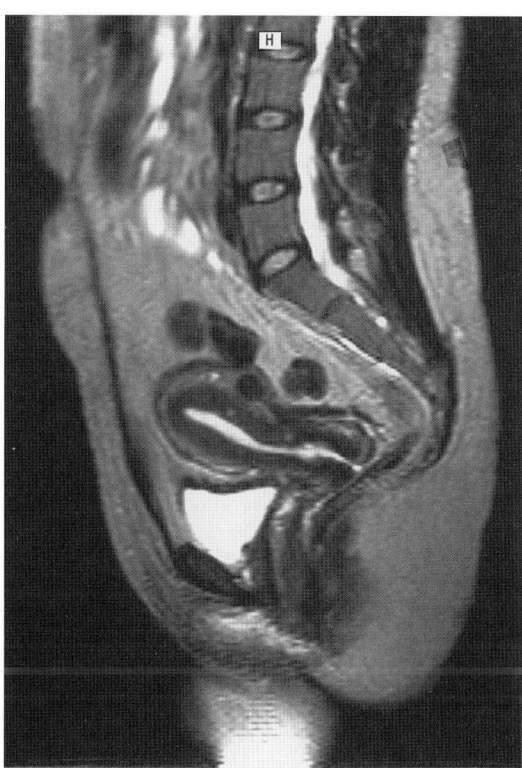

FIGURE 31.22 The location of this small posterior intramural leiomyoma is clearly delineated in this magnetic resonance image. The cervical canal is also easily visible. (Image courtesy of Deborah Baumgarten, MD.)

shock or aregenerative forms of anemia. In most other circumstances, elective surgery should be delayed until the anemia has been corrected by oral iron supplementation.

Occasionally, patients with a myomatous uterus have iron deficiency anemia because of menstrual bleeding that is too heavy or too continuous to allow a response to oral iron therapy. In this situation, it may be beneficial to induce amenorrhea with hormonal therapy to allow the anemia to be corrected more expeditiously. Amenorrhea can be induced with progestational agents such as norethindrone or medroxyprogesterone acetate, with danazol, or with GnRH agonists. Several studies have demonstrated a significant increase in hemoglobin and hematocrit values in patients with leiomyomata treated preoperatively for 8 to 24 weeks with GnRH analogs compared with matched control groups. Friedman and colleagues also found a significant increase in serum iron and total iron-binding capacity in a study group treated with the GnRH agonist leuprolide acetate. In some patients, oral iron was also given. In an evaluation of 265 patients, GnRH agonists plus iron were more effective than iron alone in treating the anemia of patients with uterine leiomyomata, according to Stovall and coworkers. In a double-blind, placebo-controlled, multicenter study, Friedman and associates reported resolution of menorrhagia in 97% of uterine leiomyomata patients treated with GnRH agonists.

Preoperative treatment with GnRH analogs can actually reduce the operative blood loss during myomectomy, according to studies by Friedman and colleagues, Andreyko and coworkers, Moghissi, and others. In a prospective randomized study of 50 patients undergoing hysterectomy for symptomatic leiomyomata, Stovall and colleagues found a significant decrease in operative blood loss between those patients who

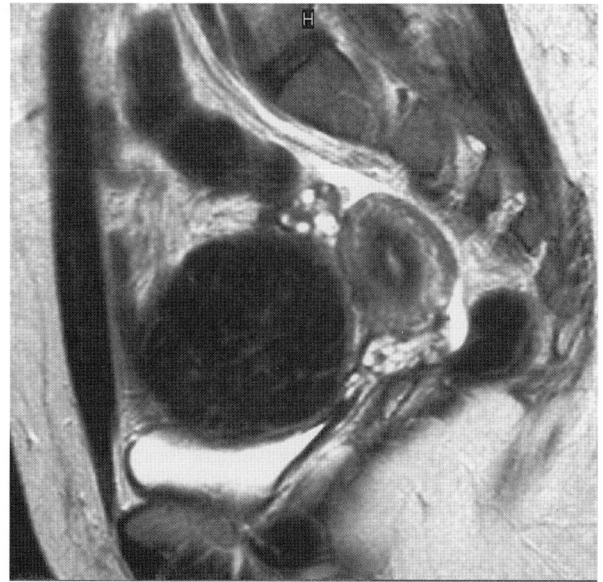

FIGURE 31.21 On MRI, a large anterior, pedunculated leiomyoma is shown as a separate entity from the ovary in this patient. The ovary is displaced superiorly. (Image courtesy of Deborah Baumgarten, MD.)

V

received 2 months of leuprolide acetate treatment preoperatively and matched control subjects. An elegant study by Friedman and associates demonstrated a significant decrease in operative blood loss during myomectomy between patients with pretreatment uterine volumes greater than 600 cm³ who were treated with depot leuprolide acetate for 12 weeks preoperatively and a matched control group. However, there was no significant difference in blood loss between the two groups when patients with smaller uterine volumes (150 to 600 cm³) were included in the analysis. It has been suggested that the hypoestrogenic environment caused by GnRH analog therapy reduces the vascular supply to uterine leiomyomata. However, even in patients not treated with GnRH agonists, blood flow has been observed to be lower in myomata and adjacent tissue.

Intraoperative autotransfusion and normovolemic hemodilution are also discussed. These techniques of reducing or avoiding the risk of homologous blood transfusion are discussed in detail by Wiskind and Thompson.

Perioperative antimicrobial prophylaxis is indicated with myomectomy. It is preferable to perform the operation in the follicular phase of the menstrual cycle. This avoids the chance of encountering an unknown or unsuspected pregnancy and reduces the problems encountered when a fresh corpus luteum is inadvertently traumatized.

Surgical Technique: Abdominal Myomectomy

After induction of anesthesia, the patient is placed in Allen universal stirrups, the bladder is emptied, and a careful pelvic examination, including a rectovaginal–abdominal bimanual examination, is performed under anesthesia. Preparation and draping are done to allow access to the vagina and cervix in case it is necessary to place an instrument through the cervix and into the endometrial cavity during the procedure. Cervical dilatation should be done to facilitate postoperative drainage from the endometrial cavity, especially for cases in which the endometrial cavity has been entered during the myomectomy.

Many of the general principles of pelvic surgery are applicable to myomectomy. Perhaps the most important of these is optimum exposure at the operative site. This is accomplished primarily by an adequate incision, but there must also be proper retraction, good lighting, and able assistants. Although a Pfannenstiel incision is considered adequate for myomectomy on a small uterus, we prefer the Maylard incision for larger uteri, even those that exceed a size equivalent to a 12-week pregnancy. A Maylard incision provides excellent exposure throughout the pelvis. Because it is a transverse incision, it is stronger and provides better cosmesis than a vertical midline incision. A Bookwalter retractor optimizes exposure of the operative site. A Pfannenstiel incision can be used for removal of a small, solitary myoma.

The importance of adequate exposure cannot be overemphasized. With proper exposure, operative time can be shortened and surgical bleeding can be more easily identified and controlled. Limited exposure may lengthen operative time, increase the risk of inadvertent injury to other pelvic structures, and force abandonment of a myomectomy in favor of a hysterectomy in especially difficult cases.

After the peritoneal cavity is entered, the abdomen is explored as usual. Adhesions in the pelvis must be carefully released or excised so that the intestines can be placed in the upper abdomen and held there with packs. The operation is performed according to microsurgical techniques and principles. For example, the laparotomy packs that are used to hold the intestines in the upper abdomen are placed in plastic bags to reduce the microscopic trauma to peritoneal surfaces caused by regular laparotomy packs. Lintless laparotomy packs are

preferred. Several laparotomy packs in plastic bags can be used to fill the cul-de-sac, thus elevating and stabilizing the uterus for easier access. Visualization of the operative site can be improved by the liberal use of suction to remove blood from the field. Suction should be used instead of sponges because it allows for a more accurate determination of blood loss and is less traumatic to tissues.

The operative field is kept moist and free of clots with a solution of lactated Ringer containing heparin. Very fine instruments and sutures are used when possible, and tissue is handled gently to avoid unnecessary trauma to serosal surfaces. Traumatic instrumentation (e.g., uterine elevators with teeth, Kocher clamps, or any instrument on the uterine serosa) must be avoided. Sutures on serosal surfaces should be of a fine absorbable nonreactive material. Running suture lines are preferable to avoid extra knot volume, which may contribute to adhesion formation. If pelvic adhesions develop after myomectomy, future fertility may be adversely affected. Performing the operation in a way that minimizes adhesion formation greatly improves the possibility of a successful result.

At this point in the operative procedure, one should pause and evaluate the size, location, and number of myomata present. Special note should be made of their proximity to the endocervical canal, uterine vessels, and fallopian tubes. One must decide if myomectomy is still feasible, how the leiomyomata will be removed (and in what sequence), and how the uterus will be reconstructed.

The conservation of uterine function with myomectomy requires control of bleeding from uterine incisions and myoma beds. Contrary to hysterectomy for leiomyomata, conservation of the uterus requires that the blood supply to the uterus through the uterine and ovarian vessels remains intact. Removing multiple myomata embedded deeply in a vascular myometrium can result in considerable blood loss. Proper application of special techniques to limit blood loss can allow multiple myomectomies even in uteri up to 20 weeks pregnancy size if satisfactory reconstruction is possible.

Controlled hypotensive anesthesia has become a useful adjunct to decrease surgical bleeding in selected patients. The main mechanism in the control of operative field bleeding with hypotensive anesthesia is the reduction of venous tone. This can be accomplished by specific vasodilating agents—such as nitroglycerin or sodium nitroprusside, epidural or spinal anesthesia, some inhalation anesthetic agents, and ganglionic blockade—to achieve and maintain a target mean blood pressure of 60 mm Hg. Our experience with this technique has been favorable. Venous bleeding can be further reduced if the patient is placed in a moderate Trendelenburg position. This facilitates venous drainage from the lower extremities and pelvis by gravity and may further reduce the blood pressure at the operative site.

Induced hypotension is contraindicated in patients with cerebrovascular disease, myocardial ischemia, peripheral vascular disease, severe renal or hepatic disease, and hypovolemia. None of these contraindications is seen very often in myomectomy patients. An anesthesiologist experienced with the technique is an essential requirement. The decision to use hypotension should be made jointly by the surgeon and the anesthesiologist. It is essential that the blood pressure be returned to normal before closure of the incision to ensure that adequate surgical hemostasis has been established.

Early proponents of myomectomy focused on methods to temporarily occlude uterine blood flow to control hemorrhage and provide a bloodless operative field. One of the earliest methods was simply to have an assistant grasp the broad ligaments firmly with each hand during myomectomy to impede blood flow through the uterine vessels. In the 1920s, Victor Bonney introduced a specially designed clamp that was placed around the uterine vessels and the round ligaments. The ovarian vessels were occluded with ring forceps. Using this technique, he was able on one occasion to remove more than 200 myomata from a single uterus. Rubin, in 1938, was the first to use an elastic rubber tourniquet through the broad ligament, encircling the cervix and occluding the uterine vessels during myomectomy. Rubber-shod clamps applied to the broad ligaments have also been used to occlude the uterine vessels and control bleeding.

Gynecologic surgeons do not often have the opportunity to use tourniquets to control bleeding; however, a myomectomy is particularly suited to their use. We prefer to use tourniquets fashioned in the manner of a Rumel-type tourniquet, which is used by vascular, thoracic, and trauma surgeons to occlude major vessels. Initially, a small hole is made in an avascular space in the broad ligament on either side of the uterine isthmus just lateral to the uterine vessels. A 5-French pediatric feeding tube is looped around the upper cervix through the holes in the broad ligament, and the two ends of the tube are

then threaded through a 4-inch length of 35-French Malecot catheter and held with a clamp. A loop tourniquet can then be placed around each infundibulopelvic ligament through the same holes in the broad ligaments (Fig. 31.23A).

As the tourniquets are being placed, controlled hypotension is induced by the anesthesiology staff. Before the tourniquets are tightened, the location of the uterine arterial blood flow is identified with a sterile Doptone. When everything is in readiness and the plan of operation has been selected by the surgical team, the tourniquets are snugged down and tightened progressively until the uterine arterial flow is no longer audible with the Doptone (Fig. 31.23B). It is very important that the arterial blood flow be occluded. If the venous flow is occluded while the arterial flow remains intact, blood loss could actually be increased with the tourniquets. The mean blood pressure should be reduced to the target hypotensive level (about 60 mm Hg) before the tourniquets are tightened. The higher the blood pressure, the tighter the tourniquets must be to occlude the uterine circulation.

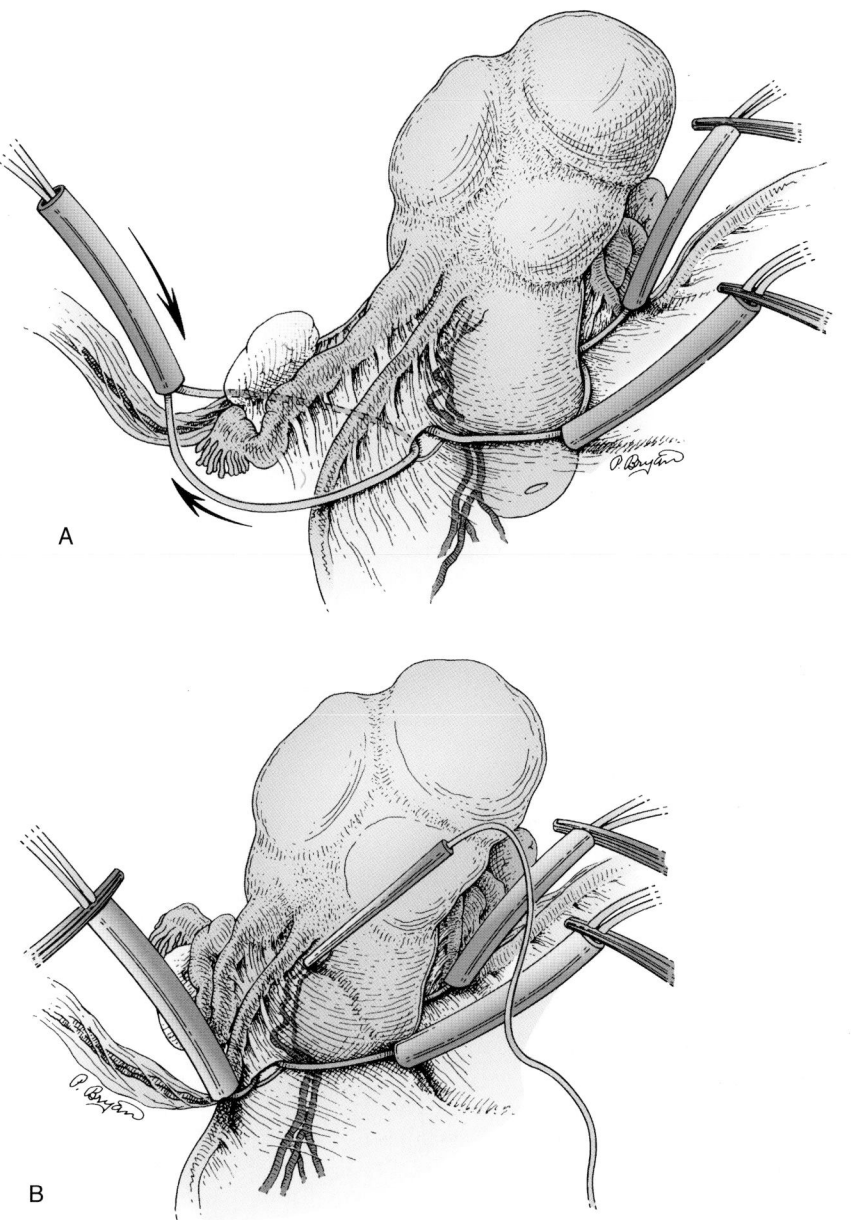

FIGURE 31.23 A: Through a small hole in the broad ligament on each side of the uterus, a Rumel tourniquet is placed around the lower uterus and around each infundibulopelvic ligament. **B:** When the tourniquets are tightened sufficiently, the blood flow to the uterus stops. The absence of arterial pulsations can be determined with the sterile Doptone.

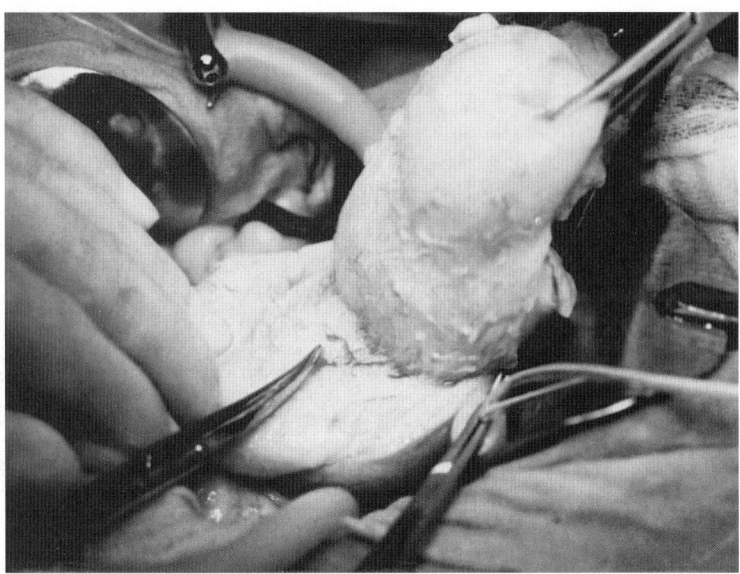

FIGURE 31.24 With tourniquets properly secured, myomectomy can be performed with minimal blood loss.

With the combination of properly applied tourniquets and controlled hypotensive anesthesia, the entire circulation to the uterus can be occluded. The myomectomy can then be performed in a bloodless field, greatly facilitating complete removal of all tumors and a neat reconstruction of the uterus (Figs. 31.24 and 31.25). Occasionally, a large cervical or broad ligament myoma prevents placement of the tourniquets. In this situation, the offending tumor should be removed first, the defects repaired when feasible, and the tourniquets applied for the remainder of the multiple myomectomy.

Once the tourniquets are tightened in place, the myomectomy should proceed expeditiously to prevent ischemic damage to the uterus, tubes, and ovaries. The length of time the pelvic structures can be without blood flow before irreversible damage occurs is unknown. We generally do not release the tourniquets until the myomectomy is complete (usually within an hour) and have not experienced any adverse events. Lock also agrees that intermittent release of the tourniquets is unnecessary. However, because the potential for injury does exist, tourniquet time should be monitored and kept to a minimum. The tourniquets should not be tightened

until the surgical team is ready to perform the myomectomy. Intermittent release of the tourniquets should be considered if the operating time becomes excessive. We usually release the tourniquets around the ovarian vessels as the uterine serosa is being closed to restore circulation to the tubes and ovaries and to restore some collateral flow to the uterus. After reconstruction of the uterus is complete, the determination of adequate hemostasis in the uterus cannot be made until all the tourniquets are released and the blood pressure has returned to normal. Sometimes, additional sutures are required for hemostasis. Before the abdomen is closed, the small holes in the broad ligament are repaired with figure-of-eight sutures.

Tourniquets are not necessary for every myomectomy, especially when the tumors are small or pedunculated. However, they are safe and inexpensive to use and can be of great benefit when large or multiple intramural myomata must be removed. A criticism of uterine tourniquets is that they are traumatic to pelvic structures. Our experience, to the contrary, is that soft plastic tubes used as tourniquets are quite atraumatic. No injuries attributable to these tourniquets have occurred in several hundred cases.

An alternative to the use of tourniquets to control bleeding during myomectomy is the local injection of vasoconstrictive agents. Perhaps, the most commonly used agent is vasopressin, a synthetic derivative of the antidiuretic hormone from the posterior lobe of the pituitary gland. In addition to this antidiuretic effect, vasopressin induces smooth muscle contraction of the gastrointestinal tract and the vascular bed. In particular, it has been found to have a potent vasoconstrictor effect on the nonpregnant uterus when injected locally. It has a plasma half-life of 10 to 20 minutes and has been used effectively as a hemostatic agent during myomectomy. Pharmacologic vasoconstriction can be accomplished with vasopressin (antidiuretic hormone), 20 U (Pitressin). Twenty units of vasopressin are diluted in 20 mL of normal saline and injected into the superficial myometrium and serosa overlying the myoma. The effect usually lasts for 30 minutes.

Dillon reported that with the use of vasopressin, 72% of patients requiring myomectomy did not need blood replacement compared with control subjects. Frederick and coworkers noted significantly less blood loss compared with an untreated group. Ginsberg and associates compared vasopressin with mechanical vascular occlusion and found that there were no demonstrable

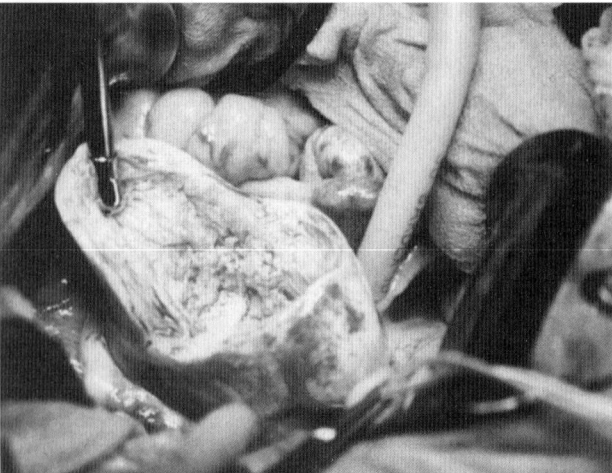

FIGURE 31.25 The use of tourniquets to control bleeding facilitates closure of the myoma bed and uterine incision.

differences in blood loss, morbidity, or transfusion requirements between the two techniques. A favorable experience with vasopressin has also been reported by Semm and Mettler.

The weight of evidence in current clinical investigation indicates that vasopressin is as effective as mechanical vascular occlusion in controlling blood loss with myomectomy. Nevertheless, careful dissection around myomata and prompt suturing with exertion of direct pressure to bleeding vessels by the operative assistant are necessary to minimize blood loss. Care should be taken to avoid injecting the solution directly into a vascular channel, and no more than 30 mL per patient is recommended because of potential side effects. Vasopressin should not be used in patients with vascular disease, especially disease of the coronary arteries. Inadvertent intravascular injection can cause anginal pain; larger doses can cause myocardial infarction. Water intoxication can also occur as a result of the antidiuretic effect of vasopressin. This effect is potentiated in patients taking tricyclic antidepressants.

Although late postoperative bleeding does occur with the use of vasopressin, it is not a common complication. Arterial bleeding masked by vasopressin still requires suture ligation. Because of the short half-life of vasopressin, the hemostatic effect is observed only for 20 to 30 minutes and should be over before the incisional closure is started. However, some do claim that vasopressin simply delays bleeding, gives a false sense of security, and is not particularly effective for larger myomata and very extensive myomectomies.

For a variety of reasons, epinephrine as a vasoconstrictive agent is not recommended for use in gynecologic surgery.

Since its introduction into clinical practice in 1972, the CO_2 laser has been touted as a tool that increases surgical precision and decreases bleeding, tissue injury, and adhesion formation. The laser can be used to make a single uterine incision through which multiple myomata are removed. An elliptical incision can also be made around the base of larger myomata to facilitate their removal. Myomata less than 1 cm in diameter can be vaporized directly with the laser, which destroys tissue by vaporizing cellular water. Despite the favorable results reported by Weather, Reyniak and Corenthal, McLaughlin,

and Starks, we believe that there is no clear advantage to using the CO_2 laser for abdominal myomectomy, especially considering the added cost to the patient.

Although the methods described earlier to control bleeding during myomectomy are helpful, they cannot substitute for good surgical techniques. Adherence to basic principles is essential for good results. Perhaps the most important of these is careful planning of the uterine incisions. Only a minimal number of incisions should be made. If possible, removal of all leiomyomata should be accomplished through a single incision in the anterior uterine corpus and in the midline, when feasible, to avoid the vascular areas of the uterus and broad ligaments laterally. Even intramural leiomyomata in the posterior uterine wall can be removed through anterior incisions. Incisions in the posterior uterine wall may be necessary, however, if posterior subserous tumors are being removed. If posterior uterine incisions are made, adhesions are more likely to develop and will likely involve the tubes and ovaries as well.

As many tumors as possible should be removed through a single incision. Methods of removing myomata through a single anterior incision have been described by Bonney. The linear or elliptic incision should usually be over the largest myoma. It should be carried through the superficial myometrium directly into the underlying myoma. The myoma is then grasped with a double-tooth tenaculum or a large Lahey thyroid clamp for traction. The plane of cleavage between the myoma and the surrounding myometrium is easily identified. Sometimes in patients who have been treated with GnRH analogs, the plane of cleavage may seem less distinct. Sharp dissection with the scalpel or Metzenbaum scissors, or blunt dissection with the finger or knife handle, is required to enucleate the myoma from its bed. Sometimes, the myoma is larger than expected. It may then be necessary to enlarge the incision or to remove the tumor by morcellation. Other adjacent tumors should be removed through the same incision. Any entry in the endometrial cavity should be noted, and a special attempt should be made to close it with sutures placed in the underlying supporting myometrium. Examples of the step-by-step planning and performance of a multiple myomectomy are illustrated in **Figures 31.26** and **31.27**.

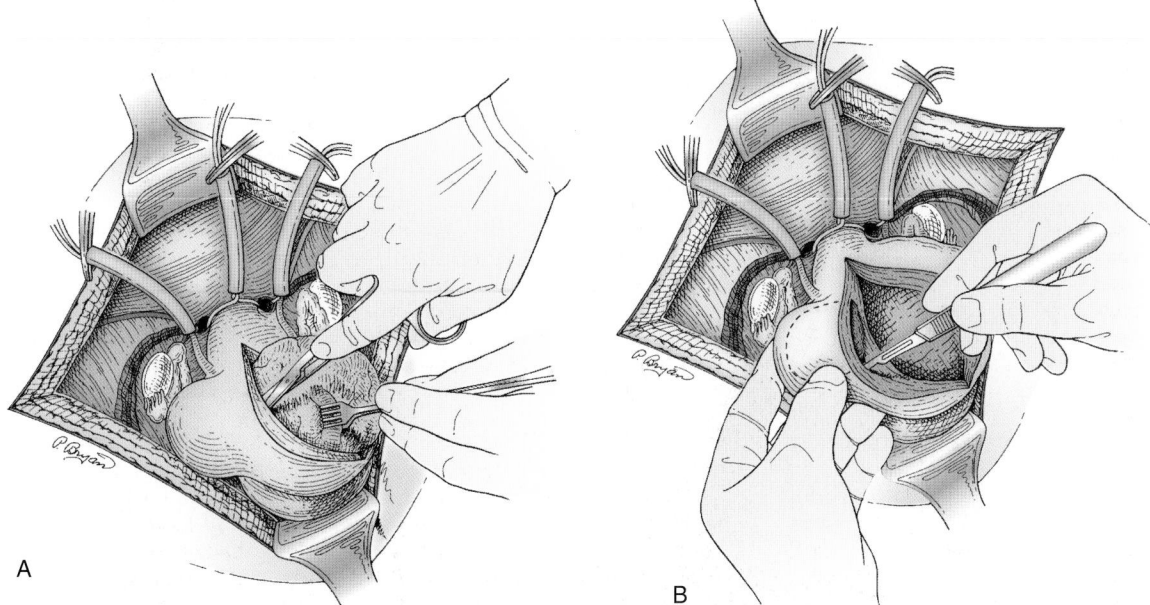

A   B

FIGURE 31.26 The sequence of steps in a multiple myomectomy is shown in these illustrations. **A:** Through a transverse Maylard incision, tourniquets are placed to occlude the uterine and ovarian artery flow. Through a single incision in the anterior myometrium, a large anterior myoma is removed first. All other myomas are removed through this incision. **B:** A smaller intramural myoma is removed through the same incision.

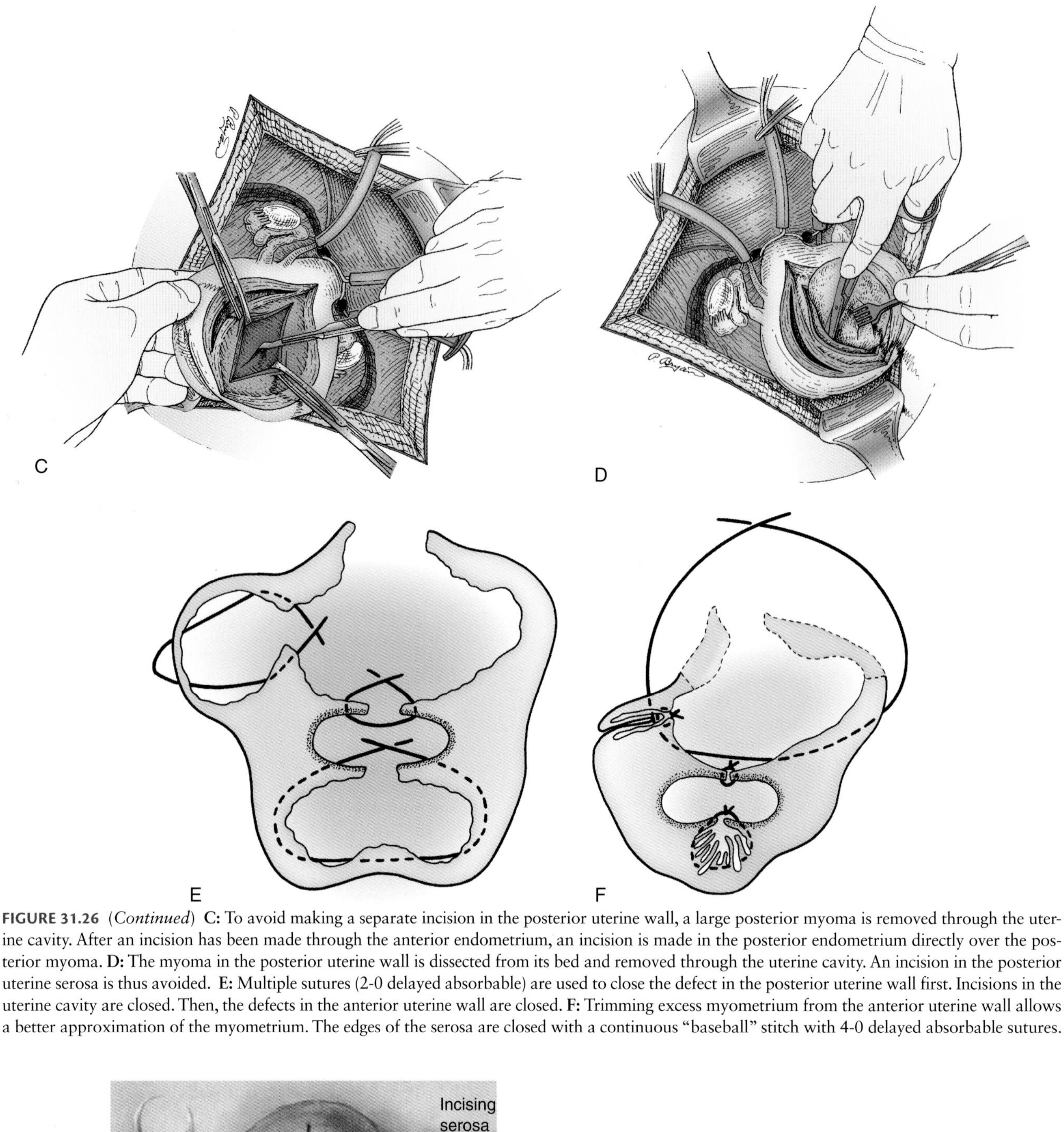

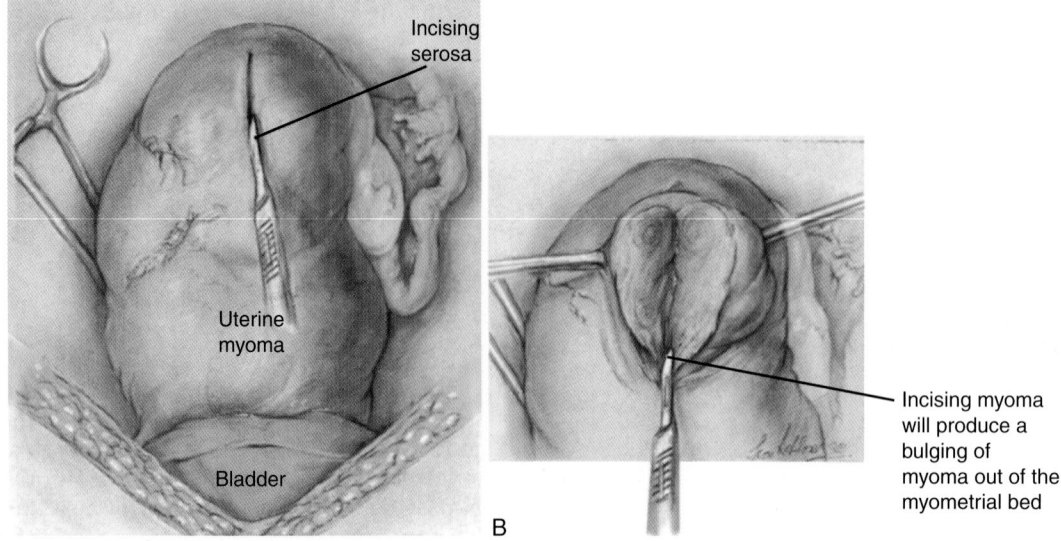

FIGURE 31.26 (*Continued*) **C:** To avoid making a separate incision in the posterior uterine wall, a large posterior myoma is removed through the uterine cavity. After an incision has been made through the anterior endometrium, an incision is made in the posterior endometrium directly over the posterior myoma. **D:** The myoma in the posterior uterine wall is dissected from its bed and removed through the uterine cavity. An incision in the posterior uterine serosa is thus avoided. **E:** Multiple sutures (2-0 delayed absorbable) are used to close the defect in the posterior uterine wall first. Incisions in the uterine cavity are closed. Then, the defects in the anterior uterine wall are closed. **F:** Trimming excess myometrium from the anterior uterine wall allows a better approximation of the myometrium. The edges of the serosa are closed with a continuous "baseball" stitch with 4-0 delayed absorbable sutures.

FIGURE 31.27 Techniques of multiple myomectomy. **A:** A vertical incision is made over a myoma on the anterior surface of the fundus as close to the midline as possible. Many myomas can be removed through this single incision. **B:** The incision is extended into the substance of the myoma.

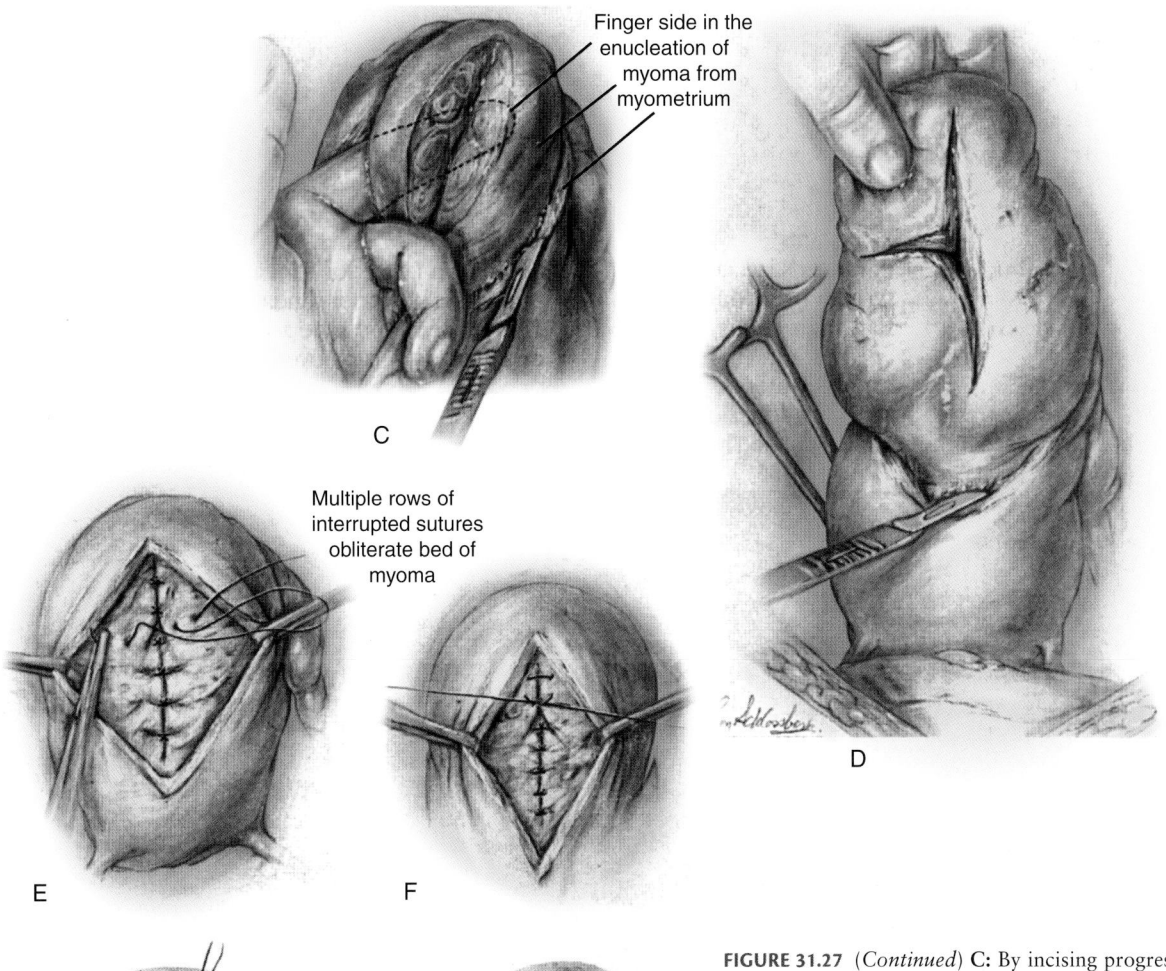

FIGURE 31.27 (*Continued*) **C:** By incising progressively deeper into the myoma, the surgeon can identify and bluntly dissect the plane between myoma capsule and myometrium. **D:** Sharp dissection may be necessary to separate the myoma from its capsule at its base. **E:** After the removal of as many myomas as possible, the remaining cavity is obliterated and hemostasis secured. **F:** Multiple rows of nonreactive interrupted absorbable suture material are used to close the cavity. **G:** When the "dead space" has been obliterated, the serosa is closed with a continuous "baseball" suture of 5-0 or 6-0 nonreactive absorbable material. **H:** This type of closure approximates the serosal edges.

The muscle fibers and blood vessels surrounding a myoma are compressed by its growth. This compression of surrounding tissue forms a pseudocapsule around the myoma. No large blood vessels enter the myoma, and there is no vascular pedicle. If the dissection can be carried out between the myoma and the pseudocapsule, blood loss can be minimized. If blood vessels are cut or left on the surface of the myoma, it usually means that the dissection has been carried out in an improper plane. Dissection in the proper plane may be more difficult if the patient received GnRH analog therapy preoperatively.

Several ingenious techniques for removing leiomyomata and for repairing defects have been described. For example,

Bonney hood can be used to remove a large leiomyoma in the uterine fundus. The myoma is first exposed through an elliptic incision made transversely across the anterior fundus, taking care to avoid the interstitial portion of the fallopian tube on each side (**Fig. 31.28A, B**). After the primary tumor is removed (**Fig. 31.28C**), other leiomyomata can also be removed through the same incision. Excess myometrium can be trimmed away (**Fig. 31.28D**). Interrupted sutures obliterate the dead space, approximate the myometrium, and accomplish satisfactory hemostasis. The sutures are placed in such a way that the posterior flap of myometrium is folded over the anterior uterine wall and sutured in place, thus fashioning Bonney hood (**Fig. 31.28D**).

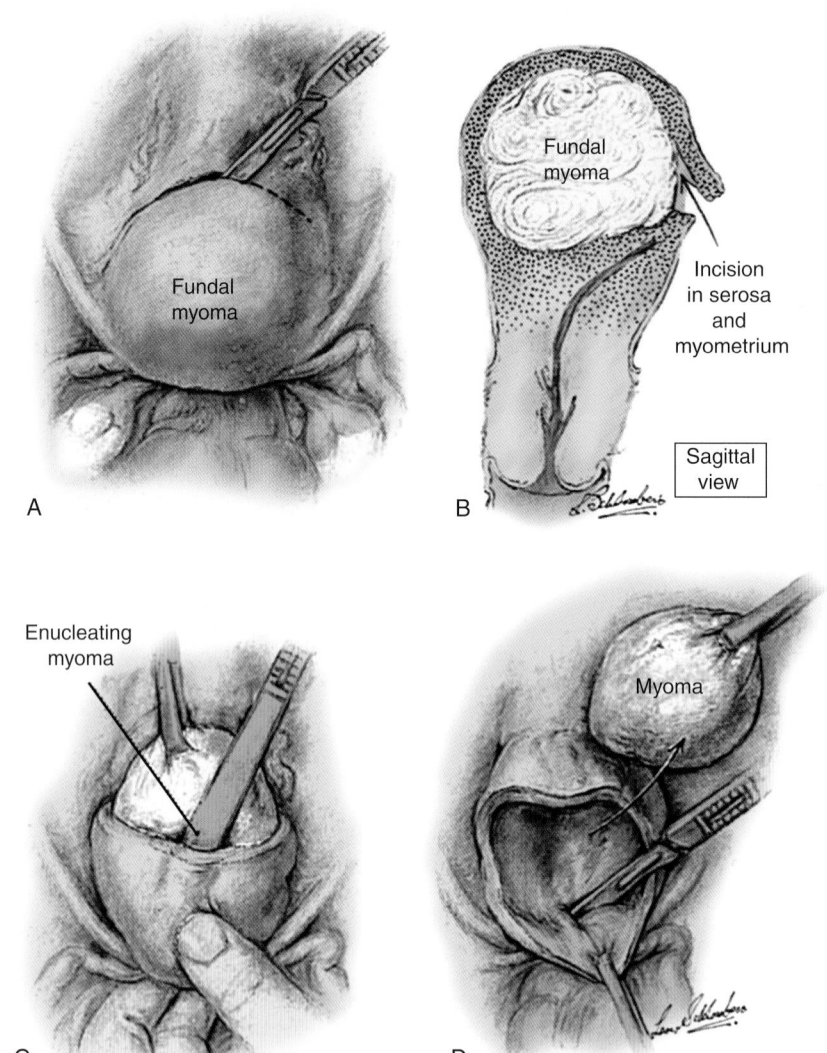

A

Fundal myoma

B

Fundal myoma

Incision in serosa and myometrium

Sagittal view

Enucleating myoma

C

Myoma

D

FIGURE 31.28 Technique of myomectomy using an anterior hood incision as described by Bonney. **A:** A transverse incision is made in the anterior fundal wall over the myoma. **B:** Sagittal view of the location of the incision. **C and D:** Using blunt and sharp dissection, the surgeon enucleates the myoma from its bed. Excess hypertrophied myometrium may be trimmed and removed before closure of myometrium and serosa.

Meticulous closure of defects from the enucleated myomata is essential to maintain hemostasis postoperatively, but this should be deferred until all the tumors are removed. Hypertrophy of the normal myometrium is always present with uterine leiomyomata. Some of this hypertrophied myometrium is considered excess and can be trimmed to facilitate a more normal reconstruction of the uterus. Involution of the myometrial hypertrophy is expected to occur in the first few months after myomectomy. Therefore, only a small amount of normal myometrial tissue should be removed. In reconstructing the uterus, the surgeon should refer to fixed points such as the attachments of the round ligaments and fallopian tubes on each side of the corpus. Symmetric reconstruction is preferred but is not always possible. The myoma beds are usually closed with interrupted figure-of-eight or mattress 2-0 delayed absorbable sutures. Large defects can be closed initially with a purse-string suture to obliterate the dead space. Several layers of sutures may be required. One must be careful to avoid occlusion of the uterine vessels, the endocervical canal, or the interstitial portion of the fallopian tubes. Transfundal or transcervical chromotubation to test fallopian tube patency after uterine reconstruction is complete is not usually possible because of leakage of the dye through the myometrial incisions.

In closing a myomectomy incision, the security of the closure comes from sutures placed in the myometrium. If possible, these sutures and knots must not be exposed. In **Figure 31.26E** and **F**, several techniques of closing myometrial defects are illustrated. The serosal edge of the uterine incision should be carefully approximated with a continuous 5-0 or 4-0 delayed absorbable "baseball" stitch.

The tourniquets are removed, the hypotensive anesthesia is reversed, and the uterus is carefully inspected for evidence of bleeding. Additional sutures are sometimes required. If a uterine suspension is needed, a modified Coffey or modified Gilliam technique along with uterosacral ligament plication is used.

Adhesion prevention can also be achieved by the use of absorbable or nonabsorbable barriers. The absorbable barrier Interceed (oxidized regenerated cellulose) can be placed over the uterine corpus to protect the tubes and ovaries from denuded peritoneal surfaces and uterine incision. Alternatively, a nonabsorbable barrier, Gore-Tex (polytetrafluoroethylene surgical membrane), can be sutured over the uterine incisions with 7-0 absorbable minimal reactive sutures. The use of Gore-Tex has been associated with a reduction in new adhesion formation. Diamond and the Seprafilm Adhesion Study Group assessed the efficacy of Seprafilm (HAL-F) bioresorbable membrane (sodium hyaluronate and carboxymethylcellulose) in reducing the incidence, severity, extent, and area of uterine adhesions after myomectomy. This prospective, randomized, blinded, multicenter study involved an independent gynecologic surgeon's review of each patient's second-look laparoscopy. One hundred twenty-seven women undergoing uterine myomectomy with at least one posterior uterine incision were randomized to treatment with Seprafilm or to no treatment at the completion of the myomectomy. All indices, including incidence, severity, and extent of adhesions, were decreased in the treatment group. This suggests that newer barriers may also have a role in adhesion prevention. Free grafts of peritoneum or omentum should not be used to cover uterine incisions.

In a randomized controlled trial, Imai found fewer adhesions with GnRH analogue pretreatment compared with no treatment after both laparoscopic and abdominal myomectomy. The utility of GnRH analogues in reducing adhesions has also been demonstrated in other clinical and animal studies.

Second-look laparoscopy may be indicated in patients with multiple incisions or in those with posteriorly located incisions adjacent to the adnexa. Early adhesions can be easily lysed, and an additional barrier membrane can be placed. The clinical role of second-look laparoscopy, outside of research, is not well defined, and conflicting studies can be found in the literature regarding the efficacy of this procedure.

A comprehensive review of methods to prevent adhesion formation in gynecologic surgery has been published by Damario and Rock and by diZerega.

Results of Myomectomy

An extensive multiple myomectomy is a major operation with the potential for a higher morbidity than that found with hysterectomy. The major immediate postoperative complications after myomectomy are febrile morbidity and intraperitoneal bleeding.

Postoperative febrile morbidity may be related to extensive tissue trauma or to infection for a variety of reasons. Perioperative antibiotics are routinely given, but antibiotics are not usually continued beyond the day of operation. Any evidence of infection in the recovery period should be treated vigorously and promptly because infection in the operative site may be adhesiogenic and may have devastating effects on future fertility. Unfortunately, subclinical infection in the operative site may not be recognized and therefore may not be treated, but it can also have adverse effects on fertility because of de novo adhesion formation. For these reasons, meticulous and sterile surgical technique during myomectomy must be impeccable.

Intraperitoneal bleeding after myomectomy is usually due to failure to achieve hemostasis of the myometrial vessels during closure of the myoma beds and uterine incisions. Although we do use a heparin solution (5,000 U of heparin per 1,000 mL of lactated Ringer solution) for irrigation during myomectomy, there is no evidence to suggest that this contributes to occult intraperitoneal bleeding.

The diagnosis of intraperitoneal bleeding in the postoperative patient may be difficult. The vital signs can remain stable for several hours before rapidly deteriorating. Peritoneal signs are often subtle and may be masked by incisional pain and analgesic medications. In addition, the peritoneal cavity has an enormous capacity for accommodating occult blood loss. Indeed, as much as 3,000 mL of blood can be shed into the peritoneal cavity with only a 1-cm increase in the abdominal radius.

Therefore, patients must be carefully monitored for the first 24 hours after myomectomy. Vital signs are routinely checked every 15 minutes for the first 2 hours after surgery, then every 30 minutes until stable. Subsequently, they are monitored every 2 to 4 hours for the first 24 hours postoperatively. A hematocrit is usually performed 6 hours after the operation is completed and again on the first postoperative morning. It can also be performed whenever there is a suspicion of intraperitoneal bleeding, anemia, or hypovolemia. Any sign of restlessness, tachycardia, or tachypnea may be an indication of blood loss, especially when associated with hypotension.

When occult postoperative intraperitoneal bleeding is suspected, peritoneal lavage can be a valuable diagnostic tool. If the lavage solution yields a red blood cell count of $100,000/mm^3$, intraperitoneal bleeding is likely, and reexploration is indicated without delay. Lavage is unnecessary when the diagnosis of intraperitoneal bleeding is unequivocal and associated with definite hypovolemia. In this situation, immediate return to the operating room for reexploration is indicated.

Postoperative bleeding after myomectomy can be devastating. Intraoperative control of bleeding during an extensive multiple myomectomy often requires that the uterine blood flow be impeded with tourniquets, clamps, or the local injection of vasoconstrictive agents. However, the demonstration of adequate surgical hemostasis in the uterus cannot be made until the uterine circulation has been fully restored. Assiduous attention to this principle intraoperatively prevents postmyomectomy bleeding in almost all cases.

Reports by Smith and Uhlir, Rosenfield, and LaMorte and associates indicate that the morbidity of myomectomy is no greater than the morbidity of hysterectomy. Verkauf reviewed current published reports and found that the operative risk of myomectomy does not exceed that of hysterectomy. One case of disseminated intravascular coagulation, hemolytic anemia, and acute renal failure associated with extensive multiple myomectomy was reported by Sacks and Hoyne.

Myomectomy has an excellent record in reducing heavy menstruation in patients reporting menorrhagia. In more than 80% of patients, menorrhagia is cured or significantly improved. Pelvic pain and discomfort and dysmenorrhea can also be relieved, but the results are not as dramatic because leiomyomata are often associated with other gynecologic diseases (e.g., endometriosis and pelvic inflammatory disease) that can also cause pelvic pain.

The impact of abdominal myomectomy on infertility is difficult to assess. Other factors besides leiomyomata may be present to a varying degree. The extent to which the uterine cavity or the fallopian tubes are distorted also varies. The percentage of patients in each series who wish to conceive after myomectomy is not the same. There is also considerable variation in the surgical technique and skill of the gynecologic surgeon. Prospective, randomized, controlled studies are lacking. These and other factors make it difficult to assess the impact of abdominal myomectomy on infertility.

There are a number of published reports regarding women who experience recurrent pregnancy wastage or prior infertility with another cause and who undergo myomectomy. According to Verkauf's review, conception occurs in more than half of such women who were not previously pregnant. A comprehensive review of 23 studies by Vercellini and colleagues regarding leiomyomas and reproduction reported an overall conception rate of 57% after myomectomy among prospective studies. Among women with otherwise unexplained infertility, the conception rate was 61% after myomectomy. The conception rate is approximately 53% to 70% after myomectomy for submucous myomas and 58% to 65% after myomectomy with intramural or subserosal leiomyomas. The conception rate among women older than age 35 may not be as good. Also, the postmyomectomy conception rate may be lower when the uterus is greater than 12 weeks gestational size and when more than four myomata are removed. When abdominal myomectomy includes removal of submucous myomata, Garcia and Tureck report that 53% of patients attempting to establish a pregnancy conceive. Both Li and colleagues and Vercellini and coworkers published retrospective reviews supporting excellent conception and pregnancy rates following abdominal myomectomies. Vercellini's work suggests that certainly age at the time of the procedure is important, as it was one of three independent variables (age, duration of infertility before surgery, and the presence of other infertility factors) associated with postoperative cumulative conception rate.

An ultrasonographic study of uterine remodeling after conservative myomectomy was reported by Beyth and associates. There was a gradual decrease in uterine volume in all patients during the 6 months after myomectomy, with the most remarkable decrease occurring in the first 2 to 3 months. Presumably, this represents an involution of myometrial hypertrophy and postoperative healing of uterine incisions. We recommend that all patients use local methods of contraception (diaphragm, condoms, and spermicidal jelly or foam) for at least 3 months to avoid conception until the myomectomy incisions are healed.

Finally, there is the matter of recurrence of myomata after myomectomy. In Verkauf's review, leiomyomata recurred in 7.5% of patients, and 6.8% required reoperation. Most recurrences appeared more than 3 years after myomectomy, thus allowing sufficient time for conception to occur before recurrence. Friedman and associates investigated a concern that GnRH agonist–induced myoma shrinkage would make some small intramural and submucosal tumors "invisible" at myomectomy, causing early "recurrence" of leiomyomata once gonadal suppression ceased and estrogen production returned. In their study, there was no difference in myoma recurrence between women pretreated with GnRH agonists (67%) and those treated with placebo (56%) 27 to 38 months after myomectomy. Their myoma recurrence rate of 61% is much higher than that previously reported in combined myomectomy series. The authors believe that this discrepancy is most likely due to the use of high-resolution US to diagnose small myomata that would otherwise be missed on bimanual examination. Rosetti and colleagues reported long-term follow-up of 81 patients randomized to abdominal or laparoscopic myomectomy plus 84 nonrandomized patients and found similar recurrence rates, 23% and 27% respectively, between the laparoscopic and abdominal myomectomy, with most recurrences seen within 24 months of surgery.

Matta and colleagues reported that after GnRH analog treatment, the US outline of some myomata was lost or obscured. Such myomata are probably more difficult to identify and remove with myomectomy and may be more likely to reappear when GnRH analog treatment is discontinued after myomectomy.

Embolotherapy

With current technology progressing toward less invasive therapies, the minimally invasive procedure of UAE is gaining popularity. This procedure can potentially obviate the need for surgical procedures in patients who suffer from symptomatic leiomyomas.

In the female genital tract, embolotherapy for control of hemorrhage from malignancy was first reported in the late 1970s. In 1980, Pais and colleagues described successful embolization for postpartum hemorrhage. Many more reports followed in the mid-1980s. In the early 1990s, Ravina and coworkers began using embolotherapy as a preoperative maneuver to decrease intraoperative blood loss during surgery for myomas. The protocol generally included embolization about 24 hours before the surgery; however, some occurred a few days or weeks before surgery. Such an improvement in symptoms occurred that many surgeries were canceled altogether. This serendipitous discovery led to the performance of UAE as a primary procedure. UAE for leiomyomas was first performed in the United States by Goodwin and colleagues in 1995. Since then, several large series have been reported, and experience continues to grow.

UAE is appropriate for patients with symptomatic leiomyomata and a preference for treatment other than surgical. Clinical findings, therapeutic goals, and overall medical conditions factor into the decision making. Several concerns have developed in treating patients who may desire future conception. Hypotheses include reduced fertility as a consequence of injury to the uterus or ovaries, placental insufficiency resulting from inadequate blood flow through the uterus, or uterine rupture during pregnancy from UAE-induced myoma necrosis. A limited number of deliveries have been reported after UAE for uterine myomata. Reports of obstetric outcomes following embolization are mixed. Although previous studies have suggested that embolization therapy may increase the risk of miscarriage, postpartum hemorrhage, preterm delivery, and malpresentation compared with laparoscopic myomectomy, a recent retrospective review by McLucas including 28 pregnancies following UAE found no significant difference in preterm delivery or miscarriage as compared to the general population. Nonetheless, desire for future pregnancy remains a contraindication for UAE until more comprehensive long-term outcome data are available.

Interestingly, amenorrhea has been reported in 1% to 2% of patients after UAE; however, some authors have attributed this to the coincidental onset of menopause. Contraindications to this procedure include pregnancy, active pelvic infection, severe contrast medium allergy, arteriovenous malformations, desire for future pregnancy, a strong suspicion of adenomyosis or pedunculated leiomyoma, and undiagnosed pelvic mass. The technique is generally preceded by preprocedural testing, and patients are pretreated with intravenous antibiotics. Many perform preliminary arteriographic mapping of the pelvis. A review by Hutchins and Worthington-Kirsch provides an excellent description of the procedure.

The technical success rate is consistently reported in the 96% to 98% range with experienced teams. Eighty percent to ninety percent of embolized patients have reported improvements in menorrhagia, bulk-related symptoms, or both. Reduction in overall uterine volume peaks at more than 60% by 6 to 9 months after the procedure because of the gradual nature of the process. Individual myomas show average volume reductions of 60% to 65%.

The Fibroid Registry for Outcomes Data was established by the Society of Interventional Radiology and includes 25 core sites and 50 to 60 other participating sites. This clinical registry has enrolled more than 3,300 patients in an effort to obtain rapid and reliable data regarding patient outcomes. Based on 30-day and 1-year data, near 90% of patients responded favorably to UAE. Recurrence of symptoms and repeat procedures occur in about 10% of patients by 3 years. Worthington-Kirsch, a leading member of the steering committee, estimates that by 5 years postprocedure, as many as 20% of patients will have another procedure. Approximately 1,300 to 1,500 patients continue to provide annual data through self-reported questionnaires, permitting continued long-term follow-up of the UAE procedure.

Forty percent of patients develop a syndrome of fever and malaise in the first 10 to 14 days after UAE. This is also associated with leukocytosis. This entity is well described as postembolization syndrome. It is typically self-limited and resolves in 3 to 5 days and rarely requires treatment except antipyretics. Other complications include those that may be attributed to the angiographic component and target or nontarget organ embolization. Groin infections, groin bleeding or hematoma, contrast-induced renal damage, and vascular damage may be attributed to the angiographic component. Uterine infection or perforation, sexual dysfunction, and myoma sloughing may be attributed to the target organ effects. Reported nontarget organ embolization complications include ovarian sequelae, sciatic nerve effects, and gluteal muscle pain. Current experience confirms a major complication rate of less than 1%.

BEST SURGICAL PRACTICES

- Women with symptomatic or problematic uterine leiomyomata should be considered candidates for surgical or radiologic intervention.
- Management options, including medical, radiologic, and surgical, should be discussed with patients, emphasizing risks and benefits of each option.
- Careful preoperative evaluation for women who undergo surgical treatment of leiomyomata should include radiographic evaluation to determine the extent, location, and size of leiomyomata.
- In patients with infertility, myomectomy—performed by either an abdominal or a laparoscopic approach—should only be performed after complete evaluation of other potential causes of infertility.
- Adhesion barriers are advantageous in reducing adhesions during both abdominal and laparoscopic myomectomies.
- Pregnancy rates and outcomes after laparoscopic myomectomy compare favorably with those after abdominal myomectomy.
- Meticulous repair of the uterine myometrium is essential for patients desiring pregnancy after a myomectomy.
- Hysteroscopic myomectomy is an effective surgical alternative to relieve symptoms associated with submucosal myomas.
- Current information regarding UAE is promising, but patients should be made aware that limited long-term data are available regarding outcomes, especially relating to fertility and pregnancy.

ABDOMINAL MYOMECTOMY CHECKLIST

- Position the patient in Allen stirrups.
- Perform exam under anesthesia, paying careful attention to uterine size and mobility.
- Prep and drape the patient.
- Place Foley.
- Perform cervical dilation, and consider staining the endometrial cavity.
- Make an abdominal incision (consider Maylard for uteri >12-week size), and enter the abdominal cavity.
- Optimize exposure (incision type and size, lighting, packing of intestines, retractors).
- Evaluate number, size, and location of fibroids.

- Minimize blood loss.
  - Make use of delicate surgical technique (avoid traumatic instruments).
  - Consider hypotensive anesthesia.
  - Consider use of a tourniquet.
  - Consider use of dilute Pitressin.
- Make a linear uterine incision over the largest myoma.
  - Dissect along the natural tissue plane, and excise the myoma.
- Meticulously close all uterine defects.
- Confirm hemostasis.
- Close abdominal cavity, fascial, and skin incisions.

BIBLIOGRAPHY

Adamson G. Myomectomy: GnRH analogs and adhesions. *Prog Clin Biol Res* 1993;381:155.

Aharoni A, Reiter A, Golan D, et al. Patterns of growth of uterine leiomyomata during pregnancy: a prospective longitudinal study. *BJOG* 1988;95:510.

American College of Obstetricians and Gynecologists, ACOG Committee Opinion. Uterine artery embolization. *Obstet Gynecol* 2004;103:403.

Amussat JZ, quoted by Rubin IC. Progress in myomectomy. *Am J Obstet Gynecol* 1942;44:197.

Anderson J, Grine E, Eng CLY, et al. Expression of connexin-43 in human myometrium and leiomyoma. *Am J Obstet Gynecol* 1993;169:1266.

Andreyko J, Blumenfeld Z, Marshall L. Use of an agonistic analog of gonadotropin-releasing hormone (nafarelin) to treat leiomyomas: assessment by magnetic resonance imaging. *Am J Obstet Gynecol* 1988;158:903.

Ariel IM, Trinidad S. Pulmonary metastases from a uterine "leiomyoma." *Am J Obstet Gynecol* 1966;94:110.

Babaknia A, Rock JA, Jones HW Jr. Pregnancy success following abdominal myomectomy for infertility. *Fertil Steril* 1978;30:644.

Baggish MS, Sze EH, Morgan G. Hysteroscopic treatment of symptomatic submucous myomata uteri with the Nd:YAG laser. *J Gynecol Surg* 1989;5:27.

Bahary CM, Gorodeski IG, Nilly M, et al. Intravascular leiomyomatosis. *Obstet Gynecol* 1982;59:735.

Baines RE. Problems associated with myomectomy in Cape Town. *S Afr Med J* 1971;45:668.

Baird DT, Bramley TA, Hawkins TA, et al. Effect of treatment with LHRH analog Zoladex on binding of oestradiol, progesterone and epidermal growth factor to uterine fibromyomata. *Horm Res* 1989;32:154.

Banner AS, Carrington CB, Emory WB, et al. Efficacy of oophorectomy in lymphangio-leiomyomatosis and benign metastasizing leiomyoma. *N Engl J Med* 1981;305:204.

Beacham WD, Webster HD, Lawson EH, et al. Uterine and/or ovarian tumors weighing 25 pounds or more. *Am J Obstet Gynecol* 1971;109:1153.

Behera MA, Likes CE III, Judd JP, et al. Cost analysis of abdominal, laparoscopic, and robotic-assisted myomectomies. *J Minim Invasive Gynecol* 2012;19:52.

Bell SW, Kempson RL, Hendrickson MR. Problematic uterine smooth muscle neoplasm. *Am J Surg Pathol* 1994;18:535.

Ben-Baruch G, Schiff E, Menashe Y, et al. Immediate and late outcome of vaginal myomectomy for prolapsed pedunculated submucous myoma. *Obstet Gynecol* 1988;72:858.

Berkeley AS, DeCherney AH, Polan ML. Abdominal myomectomy and subsequent fertility. *Surg Gynecol Obstet* 1983;156:319.

Beyth Y, Jaffe R, Goldberger S. Uterine remodelling following conservative myomectomy: ultrasonographic evaluation. *Acta Obstet Gynecol Scand* 1992;71:632.

Bonney V. The technique and results of myomectomy. *Lancet* 1931;220:171.

Bonney V. Abdominal myomectomy. In: Berkeley AS, Bonney V, eds. *A textbook of gynaecological surgery*, 5th ed. New York: Paul B. Hoeber, 1948.

Brandon DD, Bethea CL, Strawn EY, et al. Progesterone receptor messenger ribonucleic acid and protein are overexpressed in human leiomyomas. *Am J Obstet Gynecol* 1993;169:78.

Brosens I, Deprest J, Dal Cin P, et al. Clinical significance of cytogenetic abnormalities in uterine myomas. *Fertil Steril* 1998;69:232.

Brown AB, Chamberlain R, Te Linde RW. Myomectomy. *Am J Obstet Gynecol* 1956;71:759.

Brown JM, Malkasian GD, Symmonds RE. Abdominal myomectomy. *Am J Obstet Gynecol* 1967;99:126.

Buchi KA, Keller PJ. Estrogen receptors in normal and myomatous human uteri. *Gynecol Obstet Invest* 1980;11:59.

Buchi KA, Keller PJ. Cytoplasmic progestin receptors in myomal and myometrial tissues. *Acta Obstet Gynecol Scand* 1983;62:487.

Bulletti C, DeZiegler D, Polli V, et al. The role of leiomyomas in infertility. *J Am Assoc Gynecol Laparosc* 1999;6:441.

Buttram VC, Reiter RC. Uterine leiomyomata: etiology, symptomatology, and management. *Fertil Steril* 1981;36:433.

Campo S, Garcea N. Laparoscopic myomectomy in premenopausal women with and without preoperative treatment with gonadotropin-releasing hormone analogues. *Hum Reprod* 1999;14:44.

Campo S, Campo V, Gambadauro P. Short-term and long-term results of resectoscopic myomectomy with and without pretreatment with GnRH analogs in premenopausal women. *Acta Obstet Gynecol Scand* 2005;84:756.

Ceccacci L, Jacobs J, Powell A. Leiomyomatosis peritonealis disseminata: report of a case in a nonpregnant woman. *Am J Obstet Gynecol* 1982;144:105.

Cincinelli E, Romano F, Anastasio PS, et al. Transabdominal sonohysterography, transvaginal sonography, and hysteroscopy in evaluation of submucous myomas. *Obstet Gynecol* 1995;85:42.

Clark DH, Weed JC. Metastasizing leiomyoma: a case report. *Am J Obstet Gynecol* 1977;127:672.

Cohen LS, Valle RF. Role of vaginal sonography and hysterosonography in the endoscopic treatment of uterine myomas. *Fertil Steril* 2000;73:197.

Cole P, Berlin J. Elective hysterectomy. *Obstet Gynecol* 1977;129:117.

Colgan T, Pendergast S, LeBlanc M. The histopathology of uterine leiomyomas following treatment with gonadotropin-releasing hormone analogs. *Hum Pathol* 1993;24:1073.

Corscaden JA, Singh BP. Leiomyosarcoma of the uterus. *Am J Obstet Gynecol* 1958;75:149.

Corson SL. Hysteroscopic diagnosis and operative therapy of submucous myoma. *Obstet Gynecol Clin North Am* 1995;22:739.

Corson SL, Brooks PG. Resectoscopic myomectomy. *Fertil Steril* 1991;55:1041.

Coutinho E. Treatment of large fibroid with high doses of gestrinone. *Gynecol Obstet Invest* 1990;30:44.

Coutinho E, Boulanger G, Goncalves M. Regression of uterine leiomyomas after treatment with gestrinone, an antiestrogen, antiprogesterone. *Am J Obstet Gynecol* 1986;155:761.

Cramer SF, Patel A. The frequency of uterine leiomyomas. *Am J Clin Pathol* 1990;94:435.

Cramer SF, Meyer JS, Kraner JF, et al. Metastasizing leiomyoma of the uterus: S-phase fraction, estrogen receptor, and ultrastructure. *Cancer* 1980;45:932.

Damario M, Rock J. Methods to prevent postoperative adhesion formation in gynecologic surgery. *J Gynecol Technol* 1995;1:1.

Daniell J, Gurley L. Laparoscopic treatment of clinically significant symptomatic uterine fibroids. *J Gynecol Surg* 1991;7:37.

Darai E, Dechaud H, Benifla JL, et al. Fertility after laparoscopic myomectomy: preliminary results. *Hum Reprod* 1997;12:1931.

Davids A. Myomectomy: surgical techniques and results in a series of 1,150 cases. *Am J Obstet Gynecol* 1952;63:592.

Davies A, Hart R, Magos AL. The excision of uterine fibroids by vaginal myomectomy: a prospective study. *Fertil Steril* 1999;71:961.

Dawood MY, Khan-Dawood FS. Plasma insulin-like growth factor-I, CA-125 estrogen and progesterone in women with leiomyomas. *Fertil Steril* 1994;61:217.

Dawood M, Lewis V, Ramos J. Cortical and trabecular bone mineral content in women with endometriosis: effect of gonadotropin-releasing hormone agonist and danazol. *Fertil Steril* 1989;52:21.

DeCherney A, Maheux R, Polan M. A medical treatment for myomata uteri. *Fertil Steril* 1983;39:429.

Degligdish L, Loewenthal M. Endometrial changes associated with myomata of the uterus. *J Clin Pathol* 1970;23:677.

Derman SG, Rehustrom J, Neuwirth RS. The long-term effectiveness of hysteroscopic treatment of menorrhagia and leiomyomas. *Obstet Gynecol* 1991;77:591.

Di Lieto A, De Falco M, Pollio F, et al. Clinical response, vascular change, and angiogenesis in gonadotropin-releasing hormone analogue-treated women with uterine myomas. *J Soc Gynecol Investig* 2005;12:123.

Diamond MP. Reduction of adhesions after uterine myomectomy by Seprafilm membrane (HAL-F): a blinded, prospective, randomized, multicenter clinical study. *Fertil Steril* 1996;66:904.

Dillon T. Control of blood loss during gynecologic surgery. *Obstet Gynecol* 1962;19:428.

diZerega G. Contemporary adhesion prevention. *Fertil Steril* 1994;61:219.

Donnez J, Gillerot S, Bourgoujon D, et al. Neodymium:YAG laser hysteroscopy in large submucous fibroids. *Fertil Steril* 1990;54:999.

Dubuisson JB, Lecuru F, Foulot H, et al. Myomectomy by laparoscopy: preliminary report of 43 cases. *Fertil Steril* 1991;56:828.

Dubuisson JB, Chapron C, Fauconnier A. Laparoscopic myomectomy: operative technique and results. *Ann N Y Acad Sci* 1997;828:326.

Dubuisson JB, Chapron C, Fauconnier A, et al. Laparoscopic myomectomy and myolysis. *Curr Opin Obstet Gynecol* 1997;9:233.

Dubuisson JB, Fauconnier A, Chapron C, et al. Second look after laparoscopic myomectomy. *Hum Reprod* 1998;13:2102.

Edwards DR, Peacock JF. Intravenous leiomyomatosis of the uterus: report of 2 cases. *Obstet Gynecol* 1966;27:176.

Eldar-Geva T, Meagher S, Healy DL, et al. Effect of intramural, subserosal, and submucosal uterine fibroids on the outcome of assisted reproductive technology treatment. *Fertil Steril* 1998;70:687.

Evans AT, Symmonds RE, Gaffey TA. Recurrent pelvic intravenous leiomyomatosis. *Obstet Gynecol* 1981;57:260.

Everett HS, Sturgis WJ. The effect of some common gynecological disorders upon the urinary tract. *Urol Cutaneous Rev* 1940;44:638.

Exacoustos C, Rosati P. Ultrasound diagnosis of uterine myomas and complications in pregnancy. *Obstet Gynecol* 1993;82:97.

Farber M, Conrad S, Heinrichs WL, et al. Estradiol binding by fibroid tumors and normal myometrium. *Obstet Gynecol* 1972;40:479.

Farhi J, Bar-Hava I, Homburg R, et al. Induced regeneration of endometrium following curettage for abortion: a comparative study. *Hum Reprod* 1993;8:1143.

Farquhar C, Vandekerckhove P, Watson A, et al. Barrier agents for preventing adhesions after surgery for subfertility. *Cochrane Database Syst Rev* 2000;(2):CD000475.

Farrer-Brown G, Beilby JO, Tarbit MH. The vascular patterns in myomatous uteri. *J Obstet Gynaecol Br Commonw* 1970;77:967.

Farrer-Brown G, Beilby JO, Tarbit MH. Venous changes in the endometrium of myomatous uteri. *Obstet Gynecol* 1971;38:743.

Faulkner RL. The blood vessels of the myomatous uterus. *Am J Obstet Gynecol* 1944;47:185.

Fedele L, Bianchi S, Dorta M, et al. Transvaginal sonography versus hysteroscopy in the diagnosis of uterine submucous myomas. *Obstet Gynecol* 1991;77:745.

Feeney JG, Basu SB. *Bacteroides* infection in fibroids during the puerperium. *BMJ* 1979;2:1038.

Filiceri M, Hall D, Loughlin J, et al. A conservative approach to the management of uterine leiomyoma: pituitary desensitization by a luteinizing hormone releasing hormone analog. *Am J Obstet Gynecol* 1983;147:726.

Floridon C, Lund N, Thomsen SG. Alternative treatment for symptomatic fibroids. *Curr Opin Obstet Gynecol* 2001;13:491.

Frederick J, Fletcher A, Simeon D, et al. Intramyometrial vasopressin as a hemostatic agent. *BJOG* 1994;101:435.

Friedman AJ. Vaginal hemorrhage associated with degenerating submucous leiomyomata during leuprolide acetate treatment. *Fertil Steril* 1989;52:152.

Friedman A. The biochemistry, physiology and pharmacology of gonadotropin releasing hormone (GnRH) and GnRH analogs. In: Barbieri RL, Friedman F, eds. *Gonadotropin releasing hormone analogs: applications in gynecology.* New York: Elsevier, 1991:10.

Friedman A. Acute urinary retention after gonadotropin-releasing hormone agonist treatment for leiomyomata uteri. *Fertil Steril* 1993;59:677.

Friedman A. Use of gonadotropin-releasing hormone agonists before myomectomy. *Clin Obstet Gynecol* 1993;36:650.

Friedman AJ, Haas ST. Should uterine size be an indication for surgical intervention in women with myomas? *Am J Obstet Gynecol* 1993;168:751.

Friedman A, Thomas P. Does low-dose combination oral contraceptive use affect uterine size or menstrual flow in premenopausal women with leiomyomas? *Obstet Gynecol* 1995;85:631.

Friedman A, Barbieri R, Benacerraf B, et al. Treatment of leiomyomata with intranasal or subcutaneous leuprolide, a gonadotropin-releasing leuprolide, a gonadotropin-releasing hormone agonist. *Fertil Steril* 1987;48:56.

Friedman A, Barbieri R, Doubilet P, et al. A randomized double-blind trial of a gonadotropin-releasing hormone agonist (leuprolide) with or without medroxy progesterone acetate in the treatment of leiomyomata uteri. *Fertil Steril* 1988;49:404.

Friedman A, Harrison-Atlas D, Barbieri R, et al. A randomized, placebo-controlled, double-blind study evaluating the efficacy of leuprolide acetate depot in the treatment of uterine leiomyomata. *Fertil Steril* 1989;51:251.

Friedman A, Rein M, Harrison-Atlas D, et al. A randomized, placebo-controlled, double-blind study evaluating leuprolide acetate depot treatment before myomectomy. *Fertil Steril* 1989;52:728.

Friedman A, Lobel S, Rein M, et al. Efficacy and safety considerations in women with uterine leiomyomas treated with gonadotropin-releasing hormone agonist: the estrogen threshold hypothesis. *Am J Obstet Gynecol* 1990;163:111.

Friedman A, Hoffman D, Canite F, et al.; for the Leuprolide Study Group. Treatment of leiomyomata uteri with leuprolide acetate depot: a double-blind, placebo-controlled, multicenter study. *Obstet Gynecol* 1991;77:720.

Friedman A, Daly M, Juneau-Norcross M, et al. Predictors of uterine volume reduction in women with myomas treated with a gonadotropin-releasing hormone agonist. *Fertil Steril* 1992;58:413.

Friedman A, Daly M, Juneau-Norcross M, et al. Recurrence of myomas after myomectomy in women pretreated with leuprolide acetate depot or placebo. *Fertil Steril* 1992;58:205.

Friedman A, Daly M, Juneau-Norcross M, et al. A prospective randomized trial of gonadotropin-releasing hormone agonist plus estrogen-progestin or progestin "add-back" regimens for women with leiomyomata uteri. *J Clin Endocrinol Metab* 1993;76:1439.

Friedman A, Juneau-Norcross M, Rein M. Adverse effects of leuprolide acetate depot treatment. *Fertil Steril* 1993;59:448.

Fujita M. Histological and biochemical studies of collagen in human leiomyomas. *Hokkaido Igaku Zasshi* 1985;60:602.

Gabb RG, Stone GM. Uptake and metabolism of tritiated oestradiol and oestrone by human endometrial and myometrial tissue *in vitro*. *J Endocrinol* 1974;62:109.

Gal D, Buchsbaum HJ, Voet R, et al. Massive ascites with uterine leiomyomas and ovarian vein thrombosis. *Am J Obstet Gynecol* 1982;144:729.

Garcia CR, Tureck RW. Submucosal leiomyomas and infertility. *Fertil Steril* 1984;42:16.

Gehlback D, Sousa R, Carpenter S, et al. Abdominal myomectomy in the treatment of infertility. *Int J Gynaecol Obstet* 1993;40:45.

Gilbert HA, Kagan AR, Lagasse L. The value of radiation therapy in uterine sarcoma. *Obstet Gynecol* 1975;45:84.

Ginsberg E, Benson C, Garfield J, et al. The effect of operative technique and uterine size on blood loss during myomectomy: a prospective randomized study. *Fertil Steril* 1993;60:956.

Göçmen A, Şanlıkan F, Uçar MG. Comparison of robotic-assisted laparoscopic myomectomy outcomes with laparoscopic myomectomy. *Arch Gynecol Obstet* 2013;287:91.

Golan A, Bukovsky I, Pansky M, et al. Pre-operative gonadotropin-releasing hormone agonist treatment in surgery for uterine leiomyomata. *Hum Reprod* 1993;8:450.

Goldberg MF, Hurt G, Frable WJ. Leiomyomatosis peritonealis disseminata. *Obstet Gynecol* 1977;49:46s.

Goldberg J, Pereira L, Berghella V, et al. Pregnancy outcomes after treatment for fibromyomata: uterine artery embolization versus laparoscopic myomectomy. *Am J Obstet Gynecol* 2004;191:18.

Goldenberg M, Sivan E, Sharabi Z, et al. Outcome of hysteroscopic resection of submucous myomas for infertility. *Fertil Steril* 1995;64:714.

Goldfarb HA. Nd:YAG laser laparoscopic coagulation of symptomatic myomas. *J Reprod Med* 1992;37:636.

Goldfarb HA. Removing uterine fibroids laparoscopically. *Contemp Obstet Gynecol* 1994;39:50.

Goldfarb H. Laparoscopic coagulation of myoma (myolysis). *Obstet Gynecol Clin North Am* 1995;22:807.

Goldfarb HA. Myoma coagulation (myolysis). *Obstet Gynecol Clin North Am* 2000;27:421.

Goldrath MH. Vaginal removal of the pedunculated submucous myoma: historical observations and development of a new procedure. *J Reprod Med* 1990;35:921.

Goldrath MH, Fuller TA, Segal S. Laser photovaporization of endometrium for the treatment of menorrhagia. *Am J Obstet Gynecol* 1981;140:14.

Goldzieher JW, Maqueo M, Ricaud L, et al. Induction of degenerative changes in uterine myomas by high-dosage progestin therapy. *Am J Obstet Gynecol* 1966;96:1078.

Gomel V. From microsurgery to laparoscopic surgery: a progress. *Fertil Steril* 1995;63:464.

Goodman AL. Progesterone therapy in uterine fibromyoma. *J Clin Endocrinol Metab* 1946;6:402.

Goodwin SC, Vedantham S, McLucas B, et al. Uterine artery embolization for uterine fibroids: results of a pilot study. *J Vasc Interv Radiol* 1997;8:517.

Goustin AS, Leof EB, Shipley GD, et al. Growth factors and cancer. *Cancer Res* 1986;46:1015.

Grow DR, Coddington CC, Hsiu JG, et al. Role of hypoestrogenism or sex steroid antagonism in adhesion formation after myometrial surgery in primates. *Fertil Steril* 1996;66:140.

Gutmann J, Thornton K, Diamond M, et al. Evaluation of leuprolide acetate treatment on histopathology of uterine myomata. *Fertil Steril* 1994;61:622.

Hallberg L, Nilsson L. Determination of menstrual blood loss. *Scand J Clin Lab Invest* 1964;43:352.

Hallez JP. Single-stage hysteroscopic myomectomies: indications, techniques, and results. *Fertil Steril* 1995;63:703.

Hanson H, Rotman C, Rana N, et al. Laparoscopic myomectomy. *Obstet Gynecol* 1992;80:885.

Harris W. Uterine dehiscence following laparoscopic myomectomy. *Obstet Gynecol* 1992;80:545.

Hart R, Molnar BG, Magos A. Long term follow-up of hysteroscopic myomectomy assessed by survival analysis. *BJOG* 1999;106:700.

Healy D, Frazer H, Lawson S. Shrinkage of a uterine fibroid after subcutaneous infusion of a LHRH agonist. *BMJ* 1984;289:1267.

Healy D, Lawson S, Abbott M, et al. Toward removing uterine fibroids without surgery: subcutaneous infusion of a luteinizing hormone-releasing hormone agonist commencing in the luteal phase. *J Clin Endocrinol Metab* 1986;63:619.

Hehenkamp WJ, Volkers NA, Donderwinkel PF, et al. Uterine artery embolization versus hysterectomy for fibroids. *Am J Obstet Gynecol* 2005;193:1618.

Hirai K, Kanaoka Y, Isshiko O, et al. A novel technique for myomectomy: intranodal surgery with an elctromechanical tissue borer. *J Reprod Med* 2000;45:813.

Hoetzinger H. Hysterosonography and hysterography in benign and malignant diseases of the uterus: a comparative *in vitro* study. *J Ultrasound Med* 1991;10:259.

Hoffmann GE, Rao V, Barrows GH, et al. Binding sites for epidermal growth factors in human uterine tissues and leiomyomas. *J Clin Endocrinol Metab* 1984;17:44.

Horstmann JP, Pietra GG, Harman JA, et al. Spontaneous regression of pulmonary leiomyomas during pregnancy. *Cancer* 1977;39:314.

Hricak H, Tscholakoff D, Heinrichs L. Uterine leiomyomas: correlation of MR, histopathological findings, and symptoms. *Radiology* 1986;158:385.

Hunt SH. Fibroid weighing one hundred and forty pounds. *Am J Obstet Gynecol* 1888;21:62.

Hurst BS, Matthews ML, Marshburn PB. Laparoscopic myomectomy for symptomatic uterine myomas. *Fertil Steril* 2005;83:1.

Hutchins F. Myomectomy after selective preoperative treatment with a gonadotropin-releasing hormone analog. *J Reprod Med* 1992;37:699.

Hutchins FL. Uterine fibroids: diagnosis and indications for treatment. *Obstet Gynecol* 1992;80:545.

Hutchins FL, Worthington-Kirsch R. Embolotherapy for myoma-induced menorrhagia. *Obstet Gynecol Clin North Am* 2000;27:397.

Idelson MG, Davids AM. Metastasis of uterine fibroleiomyomata. *Obstet Gynecol* 1963;21:78.

Imai A, Sugiyama M, Furui T, et al. Gonadotropin-releasing hormone agonist therapy increases peritoneal fibrinolytic activity and prevents adhesion formation after myomectomy. *J Obstet Gynaecol* 2003;23:660.

Indman PD. Hysteroscopic treatment of menorrhagia associated with uterine leiomyomas. *Obstet Gynecol* 1993;81:716.

Ingersoll FM, Malone LJ. Myomectomy: an alternative to hysterectomy. *Arch Surg* 1970;100:557.

Interceed (TC7) Adhesion Barrier Study Group. Prevention of postsurgical adhesions by Interceed (TC7), an absorbable adhesion barrier: a prospective, randomized multicenter clinical study. *Fertil Steril* 1989;51:933.

Irey NS, Norris HJ. Intimal vascular lesions associated with female reproductive steroids. *Arch Pathol* 1973;96:227.

Jones HW Jr, Andrew MC. Congenital anomalies and infertility. In: Ridley JH, ed. *Gynecologic surgery*, 2nd ed. Baltimore, MD: Williams & Wilkins, 1981.

Jun SH, Ginsburg ES, Racowsky C, et al. Uterine leiomyomas and their effect on in vitro fertilization outcome: a retrospective study. *J Assist Reprod Genet* 2001;18:139.

Karlsson S, Persson P. Angiography in uterine and adnexal tumors. *Acta Radiol Diagn* 1980;21:11.

Kastner P, Krust A, Turcotte B, et al. Two distinct estrogen-regulated promoters generate transcripts encoding the two functionally different human progesterone receptor forms A and B. *EMBO J* 1990;9:1603.

Kawaguchi J, Fujii S, Konishi I, et al. Mitotic activity in uterine leiomyomas during the menstrual cycle. *Am J Obstet Gynecol* 1989;160:637.

Kelly HA, Cullen TS. *Myomata of the uterus*. Philadelphia, PA: WB Saunders, 1907.

Kettel L, Murphy A, Morales A, et al. Rapid regression of uterine leiomyomas in response to daily administration of gonadotropin-releasing hormone antagonist. *Fertil Steril* 1993;60:642.

Kiltz R, Rutgers J, Phillips J, et al. Absence of a dose–response effect of leuprolide acetate on leiomyomata uteri size. *Fertil Steril* 1994;61:1021.

Klunder KB, Svanholm H, Frimodt-Moller PC. Uterine bizarre leiomyoma. *Acta Obstet Gynecol Scand* 1982;61:121.

Környei J, Csermely T, Székely JA, et al. Two types of nuclear oestradiol binding sites in human myometrium and leiomyoma during the menstrual cycle. *Exp Clin Endocrinol* 1986;87:256.

Kumakiri J, Takeuchi H, Kitade M, et al. Pregnancy and delivery after laparoscopic myomectomy. *J Minim Invasive Gynecol* 2005;241.

Kurman RJ, Norris HJ. Mesenchymal tumors of the uterus VI. Epithelioid smooth muscle tumors including leiomyoblastoma and clear cell leiomyoma. *Cancer* 1976;37:1853.

LaMorte A, Lalwani S, Diamond M. Morbidity associated with myomectomy. *Obstet Gynecol* 1993;82:897.

Lapan B, Solomon L. Diffuse leiomyomatosis of the uterus precluding myomectomy. *Obstet Gynecol* 1979;53:825.

Leibsohn S, D'Ablaing G, Mishell DR, et al. Leiomyosarcoma in a series of hysterectomies performed for presumed uterine leiomyomas. *Am J Obstet Gynecol* 1990;162:968.

Letterie GS, Kramer DJ. Intraoperative ultrasound guidance for intrauterine endoscopic surgery. *Fertil Steril* 1994;62:654.

Lev-Toaff AS, Coleman BG, Arger PH, et al. Leiomyomas in pregnancy: sonographic study. *Radiology* 1987;164:375.

Lev-Toaff AS, Karasick S, Toaff ME. Hysterosalpingography before and after myomectomy: clinical value and imaging findings. *AJR Am J Roentgenol* 1993;160:803.

Li TC, Mortimer R, Cooke ID. Myomectomy: a retrospective study to examine reproductive performance before and after surgery. *Hum Reprod* 1999;14:1735.

Ligon AH, Morton CC. Genetics of uterine leiomyomata. *Genes Chromosomes Cancer* 2000;28:235.

Lin CC, Ou MC, Hsiao SM, et al. Myomectomy through the uterine cervix using forceps under sonographic guidance. *Ultrasound Obstet Gynecol* 2009;33:228.

Lipschutz A. Experimental fibroids and the antifibromatogenic action of steroid hormones. *JAMA* 1942;120:171.

Lipschutz A, Murillo R, Vargas L. Antitumorigenic action of progesterone. *Lancet* 1939;2:420.

Lock FR. Multiple myomectomy. *Am J Obstet Gynecol* 1969;104:642.

Loeffler FE, Noble AD. Myomectomy at the Chelsea Hospital for Women. *J Obstet Gynaecol Br Commonw* 1970;77:167.

Lumsden MA, West CP, Bromley J, et al. The binding of epidermal growth factor to the human uterus and leiomyomata in women rendered hypo-oestrogenic by continuous administration of an LHRH-agonist. *BJOG* 1988;95:1299.

Magos AL, Bournas N, Sinha R, et al. Vaginal myomectomy. *BJOG* 1994;101:1092.

Maheux R, Guilloteau C, Lemay A, et al. Regression of leiomyomata uteri following hypo-oestrogenism induced by repetitive luteinizing hormone-releasing hormone agonist treatment: preliminary report. *Fertil Steril* 1984;42:644.

Maheux R, Guilloteau C, Lemay A, et al. Luteinizing hormone-releasing hormone agonist and uterine leiomyomata: a pilot study. *Am J Obstet Gynecol* 1985;152:1034.

Mais V, Ajossa S, Piras B, et al. Prevention of *de novo* adhesion formation after laparoscopic myomectomy: a randomized trial to evaluate the effectiveness of an oxidized regenerated cellulose absorbable barrier. *Hum Reprod* 1995;10:3133.

Mais V, Ajossa S, Guerriero S, et al. Laparoscopic versus abdominal myomectomy: a prospective, randomized trial to evaluate benefits in early outcome. *Am J Obstet Gynecol* 1996;174:654.

Makarainen L, Ylikorkala O. Primary and myoma-associated menorrhagia: role of prostaglandins and effects of ibuprofen. *BJOG* 1986;93:974.

Malone LJ, Ingersoll FM. Myomectomy in infertility. In: Bermen SG, Kistner RW, eds. *Progress in infertility*. Boston, MA: Little Brown, 1975.

Mansour FW, Kives S, Urbach DR, et al. Robotically assisted laparoscopic myomectomy: a Canadian experience. *J Obstet Gynaecol Can* 2012;34:353.

Marschburn PB, Meek JM, Gruber HE, et al. Preoperative leuprolide acetate combined with Interceed optimally reduces uterine adhesions and fibrosis in a rabbit model. *Fertil Steril* 2004;81:194.

Marshall JF, Morris DS. Intravenous leiomyomatosis of the uterus and pelvis: case report. *Ann Surg* 1959;149:126.

Martin JF, Bazin P, Feroldi J, et al. Tumeurs myoides intramurales de l'estomac: considerations microscopiques apropos de 6 cas. *Ann Anat Pathol* 1960;5:484.

Matsunaga E, Shiota K. Ectopic pregnancy and myoma uteri: teratogenic effects and maternal characteristics. *Teratology* 1980;21:61.

Matta W, Shaw R, Hesp R, et al. Reversible trabecular bone density loss following induced hypo-estrogenism with GnRH analog buserelin in premenopausal women. *Clin Endocrinol (Oxf)* 1988;29:45.

Matta W, Stabile I, Shaw RW, et al. Doppler assessment of uterine blood flow changes in patients with fibroids receiving the gonadotropin-releasing hormone agonist buserelin. *Fertil Steril* 1988;49:1083.

Mattingly RF. Large myomata uteri and stress urinary incontinence. In: Nichols DH, ed. *Clinical problems, injuries, and complications of gynecologic surgery*. Baltimore, MD: Williams & Wilkins, 1983.

Mayer D, Shipilov V. Ultrasonography and magnetic resonance imaging of uterine fibroids. *Obstet Gynecol Clin North Am* 1995;22:667.

Mayo WJ. Some observations on the operation of abdominal myomectomy for myomata of the uterus. *Surg Gynecol Obstet* 1911;12:97.

McLaughlin D. Metroplasty and myomectomy with CO_2 laser for maximizing the preservation of normal tissue and minimizing blood loss. *J Reprod Med* 1985;30:1.

McLucas B. Pregnancy following uterine artery embolization: An update. *Minim Invasive Ther Allied Technol* 2013;22:39.

McLucas B, Goodwin S, Adler L, et al. Pregnancy following uterine fibroid embolization. *Int J Gynaecol Obstet* 2001;74:1.

Meigs JV. Pelvic tumors other than fibromas of the ovary with ascites and hydrothorax. *Obstet Gynecol* 1954;3:471.

Meloni AM, Surti U, Contento AM, et al. Uterine leiomyomas: cytogenetic and histologic profile. *Obstet Gynecol* 1992;80:209.

Meyer W, Mayer A, Diamond M, et al. Unsuspected leiomyosarcoma: treatment with a gonadotropin-releasing hormone analog. *Obstet Gynecol* 1990;75:529.

Miller NF, Ludovici PP. On the origin and development of uterine fibroids. *Am J Obstet Gynecol* 1955;70:720.

Mixson W, Hammond D. Response of fibromyomas to a progestin. *Am J Obstet Gynecol* 1961;82:754.

Moghissi K. Hormonal therapy before surgical treatment for uterine leiomyomas. *Surg Gynecol Obstet* 1991;172:497.

Montague A, Swartz DP, Woodruff JD. Sarcoma arising in leiomyoma of uterus: factors influencing prognosis. *Am J Obstet Gynecol* 1965; 92:421.

Muram D, Gillieson MS, Walters JH. Myomas of the uterus in pregnancy: ultrasonographic follow-up. *Am J Obstet Gynecol* 1980;138:16.

Murphy A, Kettel L, Morales A, et al. Regression of uterine leiomyomata in response to the anti-progesterone RU 486. *J Clin Endocrinol Metab* 1993;76:513.

Murphy A, Morales A, Kettel L, et al. Regression of uterine leiomyomata to the antiprogesterone RU486: dose–response effect. *Fertil Steril* 1995;64:187.

Nakamura Y, Yoshimura Y. Treatment of uterine leiomyomas in perimenopausal women with gonadotropin-releasing hormone agonists. *Clin Obstet Gynecol* 1993;36:660.

Nardulli AM, Greene GL, O'Malley BW, et al. Regulation of progesterone receptor messenger ribonucleic acid and protein levels in MCF-cells by estradiol: analysis of estrogen's effect on progesterone receptor synthesis and degradation. *Endocrinology* 1988; 122:935.

Nash K, Feinglass J, Zei C, et al. Robotic-assisted laparoscopic myomectomy versus abdominal myomectomy: a comparative analysis of surgical outcomes and costs. *Arch Gynecol Obstet* 2012;285:435.

Nelson WO. Endometrial and myometrial changes including fibromyomatous nodules, induced in the uterus of the guinea pig by the prolonged administration of oestrogenic hormone. *Anat Rec* 1937;68:99.

Neuwirth RS. A new technique for and additional experience with hysteroscopic resection of submucous fibroids. *Am J Obstet Gynecol* 1978;131:91.

Neuwirth RS. Hysteroscopic management of symptomatic submucous fibroids. *Obstet Gynecol* 1983;62:509.

Neuwirth RS, Amin HK. Excision of submucous fibroids with hysteroscopic control. *Am J Obstet Gynecol* 1976;126:95.

Nezhat C, Nezhat F, Bess O, et al. Laparoscopically assisted myomectomy: a report of a new technique in 57 cases. *Int J Fertil* 1994; 39:39.

Nisolle M, Smets M, Malvaux V, et al. Laparoscopic myolysis with the Nd:YAG laser. *J Gynecol Surg* 1993;9:95.

Nordic Adhesion Prevention Study Group. The efficacy of Interceed (TC7) for prevention of reformation of postoperative adhesions on ovaries, fallopian tubes, and fimbriae in microsurgical operations for fertility: a multicenter study. *Fertil Steril* 1995;63:709.

Norris HJ, Parmley T. Mesenchymal tumors of the uterus versus intravenous leiomyomatosis: a clinical and pathologic study of 14 cases. *Cancer* 1975;36:2164.

Novak ER. Benign and malignant changes in uterine myomas. *Clin Obstet Gynecol* 1958;1:421.

Olive DL. The surgical treatment of fibroids for infertility. *Semin Reprod Med* 2011;29:113.

Otubu JA, Buttram VC, Besch NF, et al. Unconjugated steroids in leiomyomas and tumor-bearing myometrium. *Am J Obstet Gynecol* 1982;143:130.

Pais SO, Glickman M, Schwartz PE, et al. Embolization of pelvic arteries for control of postpartum hemorrhage. *Obstet Gynecol* 1980;55:741.

Parazzini F, Negri E, La Vecchia C, et al. Oral contraceptive use and risk of uterine fibroids. *Obstet Gynecol* 1992;79:430.

Parker W. Myomectomy: laparoscopy or laparotomy? *Clin Obstet Gynecol* 1995;38:392.

Parker WH, Fu YS, Berek JS. Uterine sarcomas in patients operated on for presumed leiomyoma and rapidly growing leiomyoma. *Obstet Gynecol* 1994;83:414.

Parmley TH, Woodruff JD, Winn K. Histogenesis of leiomyomatosis peritonealis disseminata (disseminated fibrosing deciduosis). *Obstet Gynecol* 1975;46:511.

Pearce PH. Leiomyomatosis peritonealis disseminata. *Am J Obstet Gynecol* 1982;144:133.

Pelage JP, Jacob D, Fazel A, et al. Midterm results of uterine artery embolization for symptomatic adenomyosis: initial experience. *Radiology* 2005;234:948.

Pellicano M, Bramante S, Cirillo D, et al. Effectiveness of autocrosslinked hyaluronic acid gel after laparoscopic myomectomy in infertile patients: a prospective, randomized, controlled study. *Fertil Steril* 2003;80:441.

Pelosi MA, Pelosi MA 3rd, Eim J. Hand-assisted laparoscopy for megamyomectomy. *J Reprod Med* 2000;45:519.

Perino A, Chianchiano N, Petronio M, et al. Role of leuprolide acetate depot in hysteroscopic surgery: a controlled study. *Fertil Steril* 1993;59:507.

Persaud V, Arjoon PD. Uterine leiomyoma: incidence of degenerative change and a correlation of associated symptoms. *Obstet Gynecol* 1970;135:432.

Phillips D. Laparoscopic leiomyoma coagulation (myolysis). *Gynecol Endosc* 1995;4:5.

Pitter MC, Gargiulo AR, Bonaventura LM, et al. Pregnancy outcomes following robot-assisted myomectomy. *Hum Reprod* 2013;28:99.

Pollow K, Geilfub J, Boquoi E, et al. Estrogen and progesterone binding proteins in normal human myometrium. *J Clin Chem Clin Biochem* 1978;16:503.

Prayson RA, Hart W. Pathologic considerations of uterine smooth muscle tumors. *Obstet Gynecol Clin North Am* 1995;22:637.

Quaas AM, Einarsson JI, Srouji S, et al. Robotic myomectomy: a review of indications and techniques. *Rev Obstet Gynecol* 2010; 3:185.

Ramzy AM, Sattar M, Amin Y, et al. Uterine myomata and outcome of assisted reproduction. *Hum Reprod* 1998;13:198.

Ranisavljevic N, Mercier G, Masia F, et al. Robot-assisted laparoscopic myomectomy: comparison with abdominal myomectomy. *J Gynecol Obstet Biol Reprod (Paris)* 2012;41:439.

Ranney B, Frederick I. The occasional need for myomectomy. *Obstet Gynecol* 1979;53:437.

Ravina JH, Aymard A, Ciraru-Vigneron N, et al. Value of preoperative embolization of uterine fibroma: report of a multicenter series of 31 cases. *Contracept Fertil Sex* 1995;23:45.

Ravina JH, Vigneron NC, Aymard A, et al. Pregnancy after embolization of uterine myoma: report of 12 cases. *Fertil Steril* 2000;73: 1241.

Razavi MK, Hwang G, Jahed A, et al. Abdominal myomectomy versus uterine fibroid embolization in the treatment of symptomatic uterine leiomyomas. *AJR Am J Roentgenol* 2003;180: 1571.

Reddy VV, Rose LI. Δ^4-3-Ketosteroid 5 α-oxidoreductase in human uterine leiomyoma. *Am J Obstet Gynecol* 1979;135:415.

Reich H. Laparoscopic myomectomy. *Obstet Gynecol Clin North Am* 1995;22:757.

Rein MS, Barbieri RL, Welch W, et al. The concentrations of collagen-associated amino acids are higher in GnRH agonist-treated uterine myomas. *Obstet Gynecol* 1993;82:901.

Rein MS, Barbieri RL, Friedman AJ. Progesterone: a critical role in the pathogenesis of uterine myomas. *Am J Obstet Gynecol* 1995;172:14.

Rein MS, Powell WL, Walters FC, et al. Cytogenetic abnormalities in uterine myomas are associated with myoma size. *Mol Hum Reprod* 1998;4:83.

Reinsch R, Murphy A, Morales A, et al. The effects of RU 486 and leuprolide acetate on uterine artery blood flow in the fibroid uterus: a prospective, randomized study. *Am J Obstet Gynecol* 1994;170:1623.

Reiter RC, Wagner PL, Gambone JC. Routine hysterectomy for large asymptomatic uterine leiomyomata: a reappraisal. *Obstet Gynecol* 1992;79:481.

Reyniak J, Corenthal L. Microsurgical laser techniques for abdominal myomectomy. *Microsurgery* 1987;8:92.

Riley P. Treatment of prolapsed submucous fibroids. *S Afr Med J* 1982;62:22.

Rosenfield DC. Abdominal myomectomy for otherwise unexplained infertility. *Fertil Steril* 1986;46:328.

Ross R, Pike M, Vessey M, et al. Risk factor for uterine fibroids: reduced risk associated with oral contraceptives. *BMJ* 1986;293:359.

Rossetti A, Sizzi O, Soranna L, et al. Long-term results of laparoscopic myomectomy: recurrence rate in comparison with abdominal myomectomy. *Hum Reprod* 2001;16:770.

Rubin I. Progress in myomectomy. Surgical measures and diagnostic aids favoring lower morbidity and mortality. *Am J Obstet Gynecol* 1942;44:196.

Rubin I. Uterine fibromyomas and sterility. *Clin Obstet Gynecol* 1958;1:501.

Sacks P, Hoyne P. Disseminated intravascular coagulation, hemolytic anemia, and acute renal failure associated with multiple myomectomy. *Obstet Gynecol* 1992;79:835.

Sadan O, Vauiddekinge B, Van Gelderen CJ, et al. Oestrogen and progesterone receptor concentrations in leiomyoma and normal myometrium. *Ann Clin Biochem* 1987;24:263.

Sampson JA. The influence of myomata on the blood supply of the uterus with special reference to abnormal uterine bleeding. *Surg Gynecol Obstet* 1913;16:144.

Schlaff WD, Zerhoun E, Huth J, et al. A placebo-controlled trial of a depot gonadotropin-releasing hormone analog (leuprolide) in the treatment of uterine leiomyomata. *Obstet Gynecol* 1989;74:856.

Schwartz L, Panageas E, Lange R, et al. Female pelvis: impact of MR imaging on treatment decisions and net cost analysis. *Radiology* 1994;192:55.

Segaloff A, Weed JC, Sternberg WH, et al. The progesterone therapy of human uterine leiomyomas. *J Clin Endocrinol Metab* 1919;9:1273.

Sehgal N, Haskins AL. The mechanism of uterine bleeding in the presence of fibromyomas. *Am J Surg* 1960;26:21.

Semm K, Mettler L. Local infiltration of ornithine 8-vasopressin (POR8) as a vasoconstrictive agent in surgical pelviscopy. *Endoscopy* 1988;20:298.

Seoud M, Patterson R, Muasher S, et al. Effects of myomas or prior myomectomy on *in vitro* fertilization (IVF) performance. *J Assist Reprod Genet* 1992;9:217.

Seracchioli R, Rossi S, Govoni F, et al. Fertility and obstetric outcome after laparoscopic myomectomy of large myomata: a randomized comparison with abdominal myomectomy. *Hum Reprod* 2000;15:2663.

Sheiner E, Bashiri A, Levy A, et al. Obstetric and perinatal outcome of pregnancies with uterine leiomyomas. *J Reprod Med* 2004; 49:182.

Singhabhandhu B, Akin JJ Jr, Ridley JH, et al. Giant leiomyoma of the uterus: report of a case and review of the literature. *Am Surg* 1973;39:391.

Smith DC, Uhlir J. Myomectomy as a reproductive procedure. *Am J Obstet Gynecol* 1990;162:1476.

Soto E, Flyckt R, Falcone T. Endoscopic management of uterine fibroids: an update. *Minerva Ginecol* 2012;64:507.

Soules MR, McCarty KS Jr. Leiomyomas: steroid receptor content. Variation within normal menstrual cycles. *Am J Obstet Gynecol* 1982;143:6.

Spellacy WN, LeMaire WJ, Buhi WC, et al. Plasma growth hormone and estradiol levels in women with uterine myomas. *Obstet Gynecol* 1972;40:829.

Spies JB, Cooper JM, Worthington-Kirsch R, et al. Outcome of uterine artery embolization and hysterectomy for leiomyomas: results of a multicenter study. *Am J Obstet Gynecol* 2004;191:22.

Spies JB, Myers ER, Worthington-Kirsch R, et al.; FIBROID investigators. The FIBROID Registry: symptom and quality-of-life status 1 year after therapy. *Obstet Gynecol* 2005;106:1309.

Starks GC. Unilateral twin interstitial ectopic pregnancy: a case report. *J Reprod Med* 1980;25:79.

Starks GC. CO_2 laser myomectomy in an infertile population. *J Reprod Med* 1988;33:184.

Stovall T. Gonadotropin-releasing hormone agonists: utilization before hysterectomy. *Clin Obstet Gynecol* 1993;36:642.

Stovall T, Ling F, Henry L, et al. A randomized trial evaluating leuprolide acetate before hysterectomy as treatment for leiomyomas. *Am J Obstet Gynecol* 1991;164:1420.

Stovall T, Muneyyirei-Delale O, Summitt R, et al.; for the Leuprolide Acetate Study Group. GnRH agonist and iron versus placebo and iron in the anemic patient before surgery for leiomyomas: a randomized controlled trial. *Obstet Gynecol* 1995;86:65.

Stovall TG, Summit RL, Washburn SA, et al. Gonadotropin-releasing hormone agonist before hysterectomy for leiomyomas: results of a multicentre, randomised controlled trial. *BJOG* 1998;105:1148.

Strawn EY, Novy MF, Burry KA, et al. Insulin-like growth factor I promotes leiomyoma cell growth *in vitro*. *Am J Obstet Gynecol* 1995;172:1837.

Stringer NH, Walker JC, Meyer PM. Comparison of 49 laparoscopic myomectomies with 49 open myomectomies. *J Am Assoc Gynecol Laparosc* 1997;4:457.

Sullivan B, Kenney P, Seibel M. Hysteroscopic resection of fibroid with thermal injury to sigmoid. *Obstet Gynecol* 1992;80:546.

Surrey ES, Lietz AK, Schoolcraft WB. Impact of intramural leiomyomata in patients with a normal endometrial cavity on in vitro fertilization-embryo transfer cycle outcome. *Fertil Steril* 2001;75:405.

Tada S, Tsukioka M, Ishii C, et al. Computed tomographic features of uterine myoma. *J Comput Assist Tomogr* 1981;5:866.

Tamaya T, Fujimoto J, Okada H. Comparison of cellular levels of steroid receptors in uterine leiomyoma and myometrium. *Acta Obstet Gynecol Scand* 1985;64:307.

Thompson J. Anemia due to gynecologic disease. *South Med J* 1957;50:679.

Tierney WN, Ehrlich CE, Bailey JC, et al. Intravenous leiomyomatosis of the uterus with extension into the heart. *Am J Med* 1980; 69:471.

Torpin R, Pond E, Peoples WJ. The etiologic and pathologic factors in a series of 1,741 fibromyomas of the uterus. *Am J Obstet Gynecol* 1942;44:569.

Townsend DE, Sparkes RS, Baluda MC, et al. Unicellular histogenesis of uterine leiomyomas as determined by electrophoresis of glucose-6-phosphate dehydrogenase. *Am J Obstet Gynecol* 1970;107:1168.

Tulandi T, Murray C, Guralneck M. Adhesion formation and reproductive outcome after myomectomy and second-look laparoscopy. *Obstet Gynecol* 1993;82:213.

Upadhyaya N, Doddy M, Googe P. Histopathologic changes in leiomyomata treated with leuprolide acetate. *Fertil Steril* 1990;54:811.

Vasserman J, Baracat E, Bondu KC, et al. Vascularization of uterine myomata. *Abstracts of the 12th World Congress of Obstetrics and Gynecology* 1988;108.

Vercellini P, Bocciolone L, Rognoni M, et al. Fibroids and infertility. *Adv Reprod Endocrinol* 1992;4:47.

Vercellini P, Crosignani PG, Mangioni C, et al. Treatment with a gonadotrophin releasing hormone agonist before hysterectomy for leiomyomas: results of a multicentre randomised controlled trial. *BJOG* 1998;105:1148.

Vercellini P, Maddalena S, De Giorgi O, et al. Determinants of reproductive outcome after abdominal myomectomy for infertility. *Fertil Steril* 1999;72:109.

Vercellini P, Zaina B, Yaylayan L, et al. Hysteroscopic myomectomy: long-term effects on menstrual pattern and fertility. *Obstet Gynecol* 1999;94:341.

Verkauf B. Myomectomy for fertility enhancement and preservation. *Fertil Steril* 1992;58:1.

Verkauf B. Changing trends in treatment of leiomyomata uteri. *Curr Opin Obstet Gynecol* 1993;5:301.

Vollenhoven BJ, Lawrence AS, Healy DL. Uterine fibroids: a clinical review. *BJOG* 1990;97:285.

Wallach EE, Vlahos NF. Uterine myomas: an overview of development, clinical features, and management. *Obstet Gynecol* 2004;104:393.

Wallach E, Vu K. Myomata uteri and infertility. *Obstet Gynecol Clin North Am* 1995;22:791.

Wamsteker K, Emanuel MH, deKruif JH. Transcervical hysteroscopic resection of submucous fibroids for abnormal uterine bleeding: results regarding the degree of intramural extension. *Obstet Gynecol* 1993;82:736.

Watanabe Y, Nakamura G. Effects of two different doses of leuprolide acetate depot on uterine cavity area in patients with uterine leiomyomata. *Fertil Steril* 1995;63:487.

Weather L. Carbon dioxide laser myomectomy. *J Natl Med Assoc* 1986;78:933.

Weiss DB, Aldor A, Aboulafia Y. Erythrocytosis due to erythropoietin-producing uterine fibromyoma. *Am J Obstet Gynecol* 1975;122:358.

West C, Lumsden M, Lawson S, et al. Shrinkage of uterine fibroids during therapy with goserelin (Zoladex): a luteinizing hormone-releasing hormone agonist administered as a monthly subcutaneous depot. *Fertil Steril* 1987;48:45.

Wilson EA, Yang F, Rees ED. Estradiol and progesterone binding in uterine leiomyomata and in normal uterine tissues. *Obstet Gynecol* 1980;55:20.

Winer-Muram HT, Muram D, Gillieson MS, et al. Uterine myomas in pregnancy. *Can Med Assoc J* 1983;128:949.

Wiskind A, Thompson J. Abdominal myomectomy: reducing the risk of hemorrhage. *Semin Reprod Endocrinol* 1992;10:358.

Wong GC, Muir SJ, Lai AP, et al. Uterine artery embolization: a minimally invasive technique for the treatment of uterine fibroids. *J Womens Health Gend-Based Med* 2000;9:357.

Worthington-Kirsch R, Spies JB, Myers ER, et al.; FIBROID investigators. The Fibroid Registry for outcomes data (FIBROID) for uterine embolization: short term outcomes. *Obstet Gynecol* 2005;106:52. Erratum in: *Obstet Gynecol* 2005;106:869.

Wortman M, Dagget A. Hysteroscopic myomectomy. *J Am Assoc Gynecol Laparosc* 1995;3:39.

Wray RC Jr, Dawkins H. Primary smooth muscle tumors of the inferior vena cava. *Ann Surg* 1971;174:1009.

Yamamoto T, Urabe M, Naitoh K, et al. Estrone sulfatase activity in human leiomyoma. *Gynecol Oncol* 1990;37:315.

Ylikorkala O, Kauppila A, Rajala T. Pituitary gonadotrophins and prolactin in patients with endometrial cancer, fibroids or ovarian tumours. *BJOG* 1979;86:901.

Zawin M, McCarthy S, Scoutt LM, et al. High-field MRI and US evaluation of the pelvis in women with leiomyomas. *Magn Reson Imaging* 1990;8:371.

Zreik TG, Rutherford TJ, Palter SF, et al. Cryomyolysis: a new procedure for the conservative treatment of uterine fibroids. *J Am Assoc Gynecol Laparosc* 1998;5:33.

CHAPTER 32A
Abdominal Hysterectomy

Howard W. Jones III

DEFINITIONS

Incidental oophorectomy—When clinically normal ovaries are removed at the time of a hysterectomy. This is an older term. *Prophylactic oophorectomy* is now preferred.

Prophylactic oophorectomy—The preferred term for removing clinically normal ovaries at the time of hysterectomy. This terminology emphasizes the risk reduction of ovarian and possibly breast cancer as a result of oophorectomy.

Supracervical hysterectomy—Also referred to as a *subtotal hysterectomy*. This operation removes the uterine fundus, transecting the upper portion of the cervix below the level of the uterine vessels. The cervix is left in situ.

Trendelenburg position—With the patient on the operating table in the supine position, the head is lowered below the level of the pelvis.

Hysterectomy is the most common operation performed by the gynecologist, and it is the second most common major surgical procedure done in the United States. Only cesarean section is more common. There are many indications for hysterectomy, and the uterus can be removed using any of a variety of techniques and approaches, including abdominal, vaginal, laparoscopic, and, more recently, robotic hysterectomy. In most cases, a total hysterectomy with removal of the uterine corpus and cervix is done; but in recent years, there has been a resurgence in the popularity of supracervical hysterectomy. The ovaries and tubes may or may not be removed along with the uterus, depending on the patient's age and a variety of other factors. The gynecologic surgeon not only should be technically adept at these various procedures but also should use history, physical examination, and discussion with the patient to match the surgical procedure to the patient to obtain the most satisfactory outcome.

The three sections of this chapter discuss abdominal, vaginal, and laparoscopic hysterectomy. Robotically assisted hysterectomy or robotic hysterectomy is discussed in Chapter 17 on Robotic Surgery.

HISTORY

The history of hysterectomy is long and varied. Although significant advances in the technique of hysterectomy did not occur until the 19th century, earlier attempts are known. Some references to hysterectomy even date to the fifth century BC, in the time of Hippocrates. The earliest attempts at removal of the uterus were made vaginally for indications of uterine prolapse or uterine inversion. By the 16th century, a number of hysterectomies already had been done in Europe, including Italy, Germany, and Spain. In 1600, Schenck of Grabenberg cataloged 26 cases of vaginal hysterectomy.

Vaginal hysterectomies were done sporadically through the 17th and 18th centuries. In 1810, Wrisberg presented a paper to the Vienna Royal Academy of Medicine recommending vaginal hysterectomy for uterine cancer. Three years later, the German surgeon Langenbeck successfully performed a vaginal hysterectomy for uterine cancer. The first vaginal hysterectomy performed in the United States was in 1829 by John Collins Warren at Harvard University; however, the patient expired on the fourth postoperative day. Three years following Warren's attempt, Herman and Werneberg in Pittsburgh successfully performed a vaginal hysterectomy for uterine cancer. By the late 19th century, techniques for vaginal hysterectomy were systematically studied and developed by Czerny, Billroth, Mikulicz, Schroeder, Kocher, Teuffel, and Spencer Wells.

The earliest abdominal hysterectomy attempts usually involved uterine leiomyomata that had been misdiagnosed as ovarian cysts. In the early 19th century, laparotomy for ovarian cysts still was considered dangerous, despite initial successes by McDowell in the United States and Emiliami in Europe in 1815. Abdominal hysterectomy for any reason was considered impossible to accomplish successfully. Many of the earliest myomectomies involved pedunculated tumors. Washington L. Atlee of Lancaster, Pennsylvania, performed the first successful abdominal myomectomy in 1844; although in a series of 125 surgeries, he did not attempt to remove the uterus.

The first reported abdominal hysterectomy was attempted by Langenbeck in 1825. The 7-minute operation for advanced cervical cancer resulted in the patient's demise several hours later. Abdominal surgery was commonly complicated by postoperative hemorrhage that was often lethal. In the mid-19th century, an English surgeon, A.M. Heath from Manchester, was the first to ligate the uterine arteries, but it would be nearly 50 years before his technique became common practice.

Successful surgery depends on control of bleeding, infection, and pain. Ligatures were known to be used to tie off bleeding vessels as early as 1090, and artery forceps were invented in the mid-16th century by Ambroise Pare. However, information regarding the pathophysiology of hemorrhage, shock, and blood transfusions was not available until the 20th century. The importance of infection control was first recognized by Austrian Ignaz Semmelweiss in his work with childbed fever. His 1840s work was furthered by Joseph Lister in the 1860s and aided by notable discoveries by Louis Pasteur and Robert Koch.

It was not until 1864 that the Frenchman Koeberle introduced his method of securing the large vascular pedicle of the lower uterus with his tool, the serrenoeud. This ligature en masse around the lower uterus with the corpus amputated above was the usual technique of controlling bleeding with hysterectomy in the earliest years. The stump thus formed was such a large mass of tissue that it could not always be safely returned to the peritoneal cavity owing to risk of intraperitoneal bleeding; often, the stump was fixed extraperitoneally in the incision so that it could be clamped later if necessary.

American Crawford W. Long first used ether as anesthesia in 1842, and Scotsman Sir James Y. Simpson initiated the use of chloroform in his obstetric practice. W.A. Freund of Germany further refined hysterectomy techniques in 1878 using anesthesia, antiseptic technique, Trendelenburg position, and ligature around ligaments and major vessels. The bladder was dissected from the uterus, and the cardinal and uterosacral ligaments were detached; the pelvic peritoneum then was closed. Late in the 19th century, further refinements were made to abdominal hysterectomy techniques by the surgeons of the Johns Hopkins Hospital, where they reduced their mortality to 5.9%.

In the early decades of the 20th century, hysterectomy became more commonly used as treatment for gynecologic disease and symptoms. Gynecology as a specialty was developing, and little else but surgery was available to gynecologists to help their patients. Major discoveries and concepts of reproductive organ physiology and pathology were just beginning. Estrogen and progesterone were not discovered until the late 1920s and early 1930s.

As gynecology matured as a specialty, knowledge of reproductive organ function and disease became more complete. Special and more accurate diagnostic techniques were developed, and effective nonsurgical methods of therapy were discovered. In the modern practice of gynecology, appropriate use of this knowledge and advanced modern diagnostic technologies allow more accurate diagnosis, and conditions such as uterine fibroids or abnormal uterine bleeding, which used to be treated primarily by surgery, can now often be managed with hormones or other medications. In addition, surgical techniques have evolved and minimally invasive or even noninvasive approaches to uterine pathology have been developed. Focused ultrasound destruction of uterine fibroids and vascular embolization of fibroids are two examples of modern techniques (done primarily by radiologists) that have replaced traditional gynecologic surgical procedures.

Advances in anesthetic techniques, blood transfusions and fluid management, and the use of prophylactic antibiotics have made surgery safer and appropriate for more women with medical comorbidities. But the gynecologic surgical procedures themselves have changed significantly in the modern era. Laparoscopy, hysteroscopy, and robotically assisted techniques have added new technology to manage gynecology pathology and new platforms to accomplish a hysterectomy.

INCIDENCE

Hysterectomy is a very common surgical procedure. In the United States, more than half a million women undergo hysterectomy each year, and it is estimated that by age 65, one third of women in this country will have had their uterus surgically removed. Annual medical costs related to hysterectomy exceed $5 billion in the United States. However, there are significant variations in hysterectomy rates within the United States and throughout the world. In a study from the Kaiser health care plan in California, Jacobson and colleagues reported an overall hysterectomy rate of 3.41 per 1,000 women older than age 20 in 2003. This is similar to but somewhat lower than the rate of 4.7 per 1,000 women reported from Olmsted County, Minnesota, from 1995 to 2002. In a nationwide sample, Farquhar and Steiner reported an overall hysterectomy rate of 5.6 per 1,000 women in the United States in 1997. In Western Australia, Spilsbury and colleagues recently reported an age-standardized rate of 4.8 per 1,000 women. In Italy, Mataria has reported a rate of 3.7, and a very low rate of 1.2 per 1,000 eligible women was reported from Norway.

This variation in rates from one location to another is due to several factors, including patient expectations and availability of medical care. But it is primarily related to the training and practice patterns of the local gynecologic surgeons. In some areas, abnormal uterine bleeding may be managed primarily by hormonal therapy, whereas in other locations, hysterectomy may be quickly recommended. Alternatives to hysterectomy have decreased the rate of hysterectomy in recent years. Systemic hormonal therapies have been effective for managing menorrhagia; recently, a progestational intrauterine system has been shown to be similarly effective. Intrauterine thermal balloons, microwave, and electrical instruments are all effective outpatient techniques for endometrial ablation as an alternative to hysterectomy for symptomatic uterine bleeding. Leiomyomata can now be treated with transcervical hysteroscopic resection and also by transcatheter uterine artery embolization. These new management techniques, together with an overall desire to decrease the use of major surgery, have decreased the use of hysterectomy in recent years.

In addition, today's gynecologic surgeon has several techniques for hysterectomy from which to choose. Although abdominal hysterectomy is still the most commonly used approach, there has been a definite increase in the use of both vaginal and laparoscopic hysterectomy in recent years. Table 32A.1 shows

TABLE 32A.1 Worldwide Comparison of Hysterectomy Technique

	ABDOMINAL (%)	VAGINAL (%)	LAPAROSCOPIC (%)
USA, nationwide	63	29	11
USA, California	71	25	4
USA, Minnesota	44	56	<1
England	75	23	1.4
Australia	40	45	15
Denmark	80	14	6
Finland	58	18	24

the frequency of the various techniques in recent reports from around the world. For the first time, this edition of the hysterectomy chapter is subdivided into sections on abdominal, vaginal, and laparoscopic hysterectomy. In this section, we concentrate on the abdominal approach to hysterectomy.

INDICATIONS FOR HYSTERECTOMY

Table 32A.2 lists commonly accepted indications for hysterectomy. As discussed above, a variety of new surgical and nonsurgical techniques or treatments are now available to manage many of the symptoms or conditions for which hysterectomy has been required in the past. These approaches are often a compromise. Alternative management approaches may be less invasive, less morbid, and possibly less expensive, but symptoms, although improved, may persist. Eventually, hysterectomy may be elected as a secondary management option for some patients, such as those who continue to have more bleeding than they are willing to tolerate after transcervical endometrial ablation.

In some cases, hysterectomy may be done in conjunction with other abdominal procedures, such as removal of a benign or malignant ovarian tumor or treatment of chronic pelvic inflammatory disease or endometriosis. There may be no pathologic changes in such a uterus, and some have contended that these are examples of an "unnecessary hysterectomy." This is certainly not true, but it is important that the surgeon clearly explain why the uterus is being removed as a part of the surgical procedure. Because abdominal hysterectomy is the most common major gynecologic operation done in the United States, it is under careful scrutiny by a variety of regulatory agencies and public health care policy groups. The surgeon should carefully evaluate each patient and consider the diagnosis and management options before recommending hysterectomy and, specifically, abdominal hysterectomy. Numerous studies have shown that women who have undergone hysterectomy show a significant improvement in their quality-of-life indices. But care must be taken to make the correct diagnosis, be sure that the patient's condition will benefit from hysterectomy, and recommend the most appropriate type of hysterectomy for that specific patient.

TABLE 32A.2 Indications for Hysterectomy

BENIGN DISEASE	MALIGNANT DISEASE
Abnormal bleeding	Cervical intraepithelial neoplasm
Leiomyoma	
Adenomyosis	Invasive cervical cancer
Endometriosis	Atypical endometrial hyperplasia
Pelvic organ prolapse	Endometrial cancer
Pelvic inflammatory disease	Ovarian cancer
	Fallopian tube cancer
Chronic pelvic pain	Gestational trophoblastic tumors
Pregnancy-related conditions	

The late Richard W. Te Linde, professor of gynecology at the Johns Hopkins University and the original author of this text, wrote:

> The ease with which the average hysterectomy may be done has proven both a blessing and a curse to womankind. There is no doubt that a hysterectomy done with proper indications may restore a woman to health and even save her life. However, in the practice of gynecology, one has ample opportunity to observe countless women who have been advised to have hysterectomies without proper indications … I am inclined to believe that the greatest single factor in promoting unnecessary hysterectomies is a lack of understanding of gynecologic pathology. The greatest need today among those who are performing pelvic surgery is a better knowledge of gynecologic pathology.

CHOICE OF APPROACH: ABDOMINAL, VAGINAL, OR LAPAROSCOPIC

Today, there are many different approaches to hysterectomy. The uterus can be removed via the abdominal route, transvaginally, or laparoscopically. Combinations of several techniques can be selected, such as a laparoscopically assisted vaginal hysterectomy. Although abdominal hysterectomy continues to be the most common approach used worldwide, there is good evidence from multiple randomized, prospective trials that vaginal and laparoscopic hysterectomies are associated with fewer complications, a shorter hospital stay, a more rapid recovery, and lower overall costs (Table 32A.3). In addition, Kovac and others have shown that most patients who require hysterectomy can have it performed vaginally. Who, then, is a proper candidate for an abdominal hysterectomy? Most patients with gynecologic malignancy are still operated on with an abdominal incision. Although this will undoubtedly continue to be true for women with ovarian cancer who frequently have extensive pelvic and upper abdominal metastases, laparoscopic techniques and more recently robotic surgical techniques are being used more and more frequently in women with endometrial and cervical cancer.

Another indication for abdominal hysterectomy is a large uterus that prevents safe and reasonable vaginal hysterectomy. This is obviously very dependent on the skills and experience of the surgeon, because there are various techniques that allow a very large benign uterus to be removed from below. Nevertheless, most gynecologists would agree that a uterus larger than 12 weeks' gestational size is a reasonable size to qualify for an abdominal approach. The shape and size of the pelvic outlet are also key factors. Although the degree of prolapse is not an absolute factor, patients with limited uterine prolapse are more difficult to do transvaginally. Cervical fibroids or cervical enlargement for any reason may compromise vaginal exposure and make it difficult to place clamps laterally.

An unknown adnexal mass, extensive pelvic endometriosis, or adhesions from prior surgery or pelvic infection may also be an indication for an open abdominal approach including a hysterectomy. In some cases, a diagnostic laparoscopy will clarify the situation and may allow the procedure to be converted to a laparoscopically assisted vaginal hysterectomy. A careful preoperative evaluation—starting with a thoughtful history and physical examination and supplemented, where indicated, by imaging studies such as a pelvic ultrasound or computerized tomography scan of the pelvis and abdomen—will usually enable the gynecologist to decide on the most appropriate type of hysterectomy. The diagnosis and reason for the approach selected should be thoroughly explained and discussed with the patient and any appropriate family or friends. In rare cases, the final decision concerning the type of hysterectomy will depend on the findings of the exam under

TABLE 32A.3 Characteristics of Hysterectomy by Different Approaches

	ABDOMINAL	VAGINAL	LAPAROSCOPICALLY ASSISTED VAGINAL
Number of patients	1,184	530	839
Uterine weight (average)	216 g	113 g	129 g
Operative time (average)	82 min	63 min	102 min
Blood loss[a] (average)	5.35%	5.19%	6.0%
Complications			
Fever 101 °F	9.1%	3.2%	2.0%
Transfused	2.5%	0.9%	0.6%
Bowel, bladder, or ureteral injury	1.0%	0.9%	0.7%
Death	0	1	0
Hospital stay	60 h	40 h	40 h
Hospital charges	$6,552	$5,879	$6,431

[a]Blood loss is percent change in preoperative versus postoperative hematocrit.
From Johns DA, Carrera B, Jones J, et al. The medical and economic impact of laparoscopically assisted vaginal hysterectomy in a large, metropolitan, not-for-profit hospital. *Am J Obstet Gynecol* 1995;172:1709, with permission.

anesthesia or the findings at laparoscopy. In those cases, all the "what ifs …" should be carefully reviewed with the patient before the surgery and the family kept informed as decisions are made during the operation.

Subtotal versus Total Hysterectomy for Benign Conditions

In the United States, and throughout most of the world, hysterectomy—whether done transvaginally or through an abdominal incision—usually includes removal of the cervix. Over the past 50 years, subtotal or supracervical hysterectomy has come to be viewed as a suboptimal procedure reserved for those rare instances when concern over blood loss or anatomic distortion dictates limiting the extent of dissection.

More recently, however, the routine practice of removing the cervix at the time of hysterectomy for benign disease is now being challenged as many traditional surgical procedures are being modified to accommodate minimally invasive techniques. Total laparoscopic hysterectomy has been associated with an increased risk of ureteral and bladder injury so that laparoscopic supracervical hysterectomy has been introduced to avoid these complications. The introduction of a powered laparoscopic tissue morcellator has allowed gynecologic surgeons to perform a supracervical hysterectomy rapidly and efficiently, even on an enlarged uterus. The rapidity of the procedure, the quick postoperative recovery, and the popularity of cervical preservation among the lay public have now resulted in an increased use of abdominal supracervical hysterectomy.

In a study from California involving almost 650,000 women who underwent hysterectomy between 1991 and 2004, Smith et al. reported that the incidence of subtotal, supracervical hysterectomy increased from negligible to 21% of all hysterectomies in 2004. It is doubtful that this technique is as common in other regions of the United States and throughout the world, but the advantages of speed and a low complication rate plus the reduced risk of cervical cancer in the retained cervix due to improved screening and conservative management of cervical intraepithelial neoplasia make supracervical hysterectomy attractive to many patients and surgeons.

There is clearly a market for this procedure, but all of the recent prospective, randomized trials have not found any long-term advantage of supracervical abdominal hysterectomy

compared with total abdominal hysterectomy. However, several recent prospective, randomized studies in the United States and abroad have shown no difference in sexual satisfaction, bowel or bladder function, or vaginal prolapse after simple total hysterectomy compared with supracervical hysterectomy for benign disease. My own clinical experience over 30 years also confirms this impression.

Management of Normal Ovaries

Should normal ovaries be removed at the time of hysterectomy for benign disease? The term *prophylactic oophorectomy* is preferred when referring to the removal of clinical normal ovaries at the time of hysterectomy. The use of *incidental oophorectomy* is not recommended because it suggests that an oophorectomy is done without planning or consideration and has no consequences. There is no doubt that bilateral oophorectomy reduces the risk of ovarian cancer and the need for future surgery for benign conditions of the ovaries. However, the ovaries continue to produce low levels of androgens even after the menopause, and although the benefits, if any, of this hormone production are unknown, the psychological effect of oophorectomy on some women is significant.

Prophylactic oophorectomy is done in 50% to 66% of women aged 40 to 65 who undergo hysterectomy in the United States. Averette and Nguyen have estimated that 1,000 of the approximately 24,000 new cases of ovarian cancer in the United States would be prevented if prophylactic bilateral salpingo-oophorectomy was done at the time of hysterectomy on all women older than age 40. In a more recent prospective cohort study of 30,117 women in the Nurses' Health Study, Parker et al. confirmed a very significant risk reduction in death from ovarian cancer and death from breast cancer for those women who underwent bilateral oophorectomy before age 47.5 years. However, they also observed that there was a significant (1.15 hazard ratio) increased risk of death from all causes in those women who underwent bilateral oophorectomy before age 50. This increased risk of death from all causes (especially cardiovascular disease and lung cancer) was not observed in those women who used estrogen replacement therapy. The significance and implications of these findings have been discussed and questioned, but it is clear that while removing the ovaries and fallopian tubes will decrease the subsequent risk of cancer of these organs, the hormonal effects of premenopausal oophorectomy have implications more life threatening than hot flashes or night sweats. It behooves the gynecologic surgeon to keep up with this ongoing controversy so that we can counsel our patients based on the most recent facts and concepts.

Clearly, there are some significant potential benefits to oophorectomy at the time of any pelvic surgery in women with a known BRCA1 or BRCA2 gene mutation, a strong family history of ovarian or breast cancer, or women of Eastern European Jewish heritage. Recent studies also have clearly shown a decrease in the risk of breast cancer in women who have undergone bilateral oophorectomy. This is of particular importance in women from families with a history of ovarian or breast cancer and those with known BRCA gene mutations. In a series of 177 women with BRCA1 or BRCA2 mutations who were enrolled prospectively and followed for up to 6 years, Kauf and associates reported a 4% incidence of breast cancer among the 69 women who underwent prophylactic oophorectomy compared with a 13% incidence among those who elected follow-up surveillance only. In a similar retrospective review of 259 women compared with matched controls, the risk of breast cancer was reduced by 50% in the women who had bilateral oophorectomy. In both series, the risk of peritoneal or ovarian cancer was decreased by 95%. In a follow-up study of 4,931 women who underwent hysterectomy without oophorectomy at 10, 20, and 30 years with a control group of women who had not had hysterectomy, the risk of additional surgery to remove the ovaries was 3.5% (1.9% rate of oophorectomy in the women who had not has a hysterectomy). By 20 years, 6.2% of the women who had previously undergone hysterectomy had required oophorectomy, and by 30 years, 9.2% had undergone oophorectomy. Removing one ovary at the time of hysterectomy did reduce the risk of subsequent surgery for oophorectomy, but even without any pelvic surgery, 7.3% of the age-matched control group required oophorectomy during 30 years of follow-up.

Four case–control studies that found a lower risk of ovarian cancer among women who had a history of previous hysterectomy with ovarian conservation have been analyzed by Weiss and Harlow. The authors felt the reduction in ovarian cancer risk was explained by incidental screening for visible ovarian malignancy at the time of hysterectomy in those women in whom the ovaries are not removed. Those women with grossly normal ovaries have a reduced risk of developing symptomatic ovarian cancer over the next few years. In a large, prospective cohort study of 238,130 married, female nurses in the United States, Rice et al. found that hysterectomy was associated with a 20% reduction in the rate of subsequent ovarian cancer. Tubal ligation resulted in a 24% decreased risk of ovarian cancer. Unilateral oophorectomy was found to reduce the risk of ovarian cancer by 30%. The mechanism by which hysterectomy and tubal ligation reduce ovarian cancer is not known, but it is possible that the interruption of the pathway of unknown pathogens from the vagina to the ovary may be involved.

Traditionally, many gynecologists have recommended against prophylactic oophorectomy in women younger than the age of 40 and offered oophorectomy to postmenopausal women. There is no consensus for the management of women between 40 and 50. There are no data to support these approaches. It seems reasonable to discuss the possibility of oophorectomy before planned hysterectomy for benign disease in women older than age 45. However, it should be made clear to those women that there are some definite disadvantages to oophorectomy, especially if they will not or cannot use estrogen replacement therapy postoperatively. Each patient brings her own ideas and experiences to this discussion, and the surgeon should try to counsel the patient and her family so she will be happy with her decision about oophorectomy.

PREOPERATIVE COUNSELING

The gynecologist needs to talk with the patient while trying to decide whether a hysterectomy is indicated. Fortunately for the patient and the gynecologist, time for talking is available in almost every instance. A hysterectomy is rarely an emergency. Unfortunately, the time may not be used properly. In a survey of women who underwent hysterectomy, Neefus and Taylor found that there is an urgent need for patient education on the physical, psychological, and sexual aspects of hysterectomy.

Often, the need for hysterectomy is obvious. There is a complete prolapse, or a large and symptomatic leiomyomatous uterus, or a pelvic cancer. However, under all circumstances, the indications for hysterectomy should be carefully explained. It is important that whenever possible, not only the patient but, in addition, her family and/or those who will support her during the perioperative period be involved in these discussions. The "informed consent" should be explained clearly and in language that the patient and her family can understand. Treatment alternatives should be discussed and the reasons for recommending one approach over another should be explained. The risks, benefits, and side effects, specifically including the possibility of transfusion, must be reviewed, but in such a way that the patient is not unduly alarmed. Then, the patient and the physician should spend the time necessary to discuss any questions that the patient or family may have. Additionally, the patient should be encouraged to ask questions about the operation: how long it will take, the recuperation period in the hospital and at home, whether ovarian function should be conserved, and possible hormone replacement therapy. Patient information pamphlets and videos also are useful for preoperative education. The expectations of the patient and her family are very important in her postoperative view of the success (or failure) of the operation.

Because the uterus is the main organ associated with reproduction, it is an important part of a woman's self-image; in some cultures, a woman's sexuality and reproductive potential are viewed as important parts of her value or status in her family or society as a whole. For these reasons, it is absolutely necessary for the gynecologic surgeon to understand and help patients cope with the emotional turmoil that may accompany hysterectomy. For some women who have had their children and need a hysterectomy for prolonged heavy bleeding and cramping associated with uterine fibroids or those with a diagnosis of endometrial cancer, the indications are clear, the benefits are obvious, and the loss of reproductive capacity often is not of great concern. The emotional stress of hysterectomy on these women is usually minimal, and psychological adjustment often is rapid and complete. However, the young woman needing a hysterectomy for cervical cancer or a complication of pregnancy may have considerable difficulty adjusting to the loss of her uterus. Even the 32-year-old woman with three children and severe uterovaginal prolapse may not be comfortable with the idea of hysterectomy. The gynecologist must be sensitive to these possible concerns and anxiety. Even when the patient does not express any emotional distress, the gynecologist can provide an opening for the patient to discuss her feelings by statements such as "Most studies have shown no change in sexuality and sexual function after hysterectomy, but I know many patients have concerns about this. Do you have any questions?" The support of the patient's husband or partner and her family and friends are very useful elements to prevent and manage depression and the emotional stress of hysterectomy. The wise surgeon includes members of this support group in preoperative discussions and encourages them to ask questions or express opinions that actually may be questions or opinions of the patient that she may be hesitant to express.

Despite improvements in preoperative counseling in recent years, some women are depressed after hysterectomy. In most instances, this depression is short-lived and self-limiting, but the gynecologist should be alert for severe or prolonged symptoms of continued lack of energy, inability to return to normal activities of daily living, sleep difficulties, or other indicators of depression following surgery. Occasionally, antidepressants and/or psychiatric consultation may be necessary. The psychological aspects of pelvic surgery are extensively reviewed in Chapter 3.

PREPARATION FOR HYSTERECTOMY

A complete history and physical examination is indicated before any operative procedure. This evaluation is detailed in Chapter 8, but a few points deserve emphasis. Although it is appropriate to ensure that all gynecologic symptoms have been evaluated carefully and a pelvic examination performed, a complete physical evaluation is necessary to be sure the patient can safely tolerate anesthesia and major surgery. Appropriate consultation should be sought where indicated to assure safe anesthesia administration and anticipation of any perioperative medical problems. In addition to a preoperative hematocrit or hemoglobin and other laboratory tests as indicated by the patient's medical condition, it is important to have a recent Pap or HPV test to rule out cervical neoplasia. A pregnancy test in reproductive-age women is recommended before surgery.

Preoperative chest x-rays are no longer routinely recommended but may be indicated in women with a history of cardiorespiratory disease or malignancy. An intravenous pyelogram, ultrasound, or computed tomography scan of the abdomen and pelvis may be useful in women with uterine or extrauterine pelvic masses, but these are not indicated routinely.

Mechanical bowel preparation before simple hysterectomy has been largely abandoned in recent years. However, when the uterus is large or extensive adhesiolysis is anticipated, we prefer to have the colon evacuated before pelvic surgery to facilitate exposure and reduce trauma to the bowel caused by retraction and packing. In these patients, we recommend a clear liquid diet on the day before surgery, and 250 mL of oral magnesium citrate is an effective laxative on the afternoon before surgery. A bisacodyl suppository immediately on arising on the morning of surgery will evacuate any residual feces or fluid in the sigmoid and prevent contamination of the field during surgery. A complete mechanical or antibiotic bowel preparation is indicated only when intestinal surgery is a possibility (see Chapter 47).

Surgical site infection risk is decreased by routine use of prophylactic intravenous antibiotics given approximately 30 minutes before the skin incision. First- or second-generation cephalosporins, such as cefazolin or cefoxitin, are commonly used. Recommended antibiotic regimens are shown in Table 32A.4. Prospective, randomized trials have shown a significant reduction in the risk of febrile morbidity and infection in both abdominal and vaginal hysterectomy. Studies have shown no benefit of continuing antibiotics postoperatively, although a second dose of antibiotics generally should be given during hysterectomy procedures that last longer than 3 hours. Some have suggested that bacterial vaginosis increases the risk of postoperative infections after vaginal hysterectomy, but preoperative evaluation and treatment remain controversial. Although povidone–iodine douches and antibiotic scrubs

TABLE 32A.4 Recommended Prophylactic Antibiotic Regimens for Hysterectomy

ANTIBIOTIC	DOSAGE	HALF-LIFE
Cefoxitin	2 g IV	0.5–1.1 h
Cefazolin	1–2 g IV	1.2–2.5 h
Cefotetan	1–2 g IV	2.8–4.6 h
For patients with an immediate sensitivity to penicillin		
Metronidazole[a]	1 g IV	6–14 h
OR		
Metronidazole[b] + gentamicin or a quinolone	1 g IV 1.5 mg/kg or 500 mg	
OR		
Clindamycin[b]	900 mg IV	2–5 h

IV, intravenously.
[a]American College of Obstetricians and Gynecologists. ACOG Practice Bulletin No. 74. *Antibiotic prophylaxis for gynecologic procedures.* Washington, DC: ACOG, 2006.
[b]Surgical Care Improvement Project recommendation, October 2006. Surgical Care Improvement Project. *Prophylactic antibiotic regimen selection for surgery.* Available at: http://www.mediqic.org/scip. Accessed April 16, 2007.

before surgery have been widely used in the past, studies have shown no added benefit when perioperative intravenous antibiotics are employed.

If necessary, the pubic and/or vulvar hair should be clipped with an electric clipper or even scissors rather than shaved. The patient should be instructed not to shave the operative site before surgery because it has been shown to increase the risk of wound infection and cellulitis.

TOTAL ABDOMINAL HYSTERECTOMY: SURGICAL TECHNIQUE

Previous editions of Te Linde's text have described gradually evolving modifications of Edward H. Richardson's technique for abdominal hysterectomy with which thousands of gynecologic surgeons have been trained over the years. The operative technique was first published in 1929, and because Te Linde felt it was a classic, he quoted it word for word in the fourth edition of this textbook with two added "modifications." This was the edition on my bedside table when I was a resident. I have had the good fortune to operate with many fine surgeons, including E. Stewart Taylor and Felix Rutledge, and have been challenged by many young residents over the years. These experiences have been further enhanced by discussions of surgical technique with gynecologists from around the world, who have suggested changes or ideas that I have tried and sometimes incorporated into my basic technique for abdominal hysterectomy. Although it is important to learn a basic technique for standard abdominal hysterectomy, every surgeon should be interested in observing new and different techniques or modifications to be tried from time to time when appropriate. As a resident, you should try all of the different techniques used by the different attending physicians, always asking why this clamp is used or that suture or needle is selected or why the cuff is left open or closed. Having tried many different ideas, each gynecologic surgeon gradually evolves her or his own basic techniques that feel comfortable, work for him or her, and make sense. Because each patient is unique, it also is useful to have experience with different techniques and various modifications of the basic operation so that when the occasion calls for it, an alternative technique that is more suitable for the particular situation can be employed. Our basic technique for abdominal hysterectomy and several modifications are described in the following.

On the day of surgery, the surgeon always attempts to see the patient and her family and supporters before she is brought into the operating room. Although surgery may be routine to the gynecologist, major surgery is often a once-in-a-lifetime, frightening experience for the patient. The calm reassurance of the surgeon and the professional and caring nature of the entire operative team are very helpful to the patient and her family at this point. The focus of attention should be on the patient and her surgery. A certain amount of relaxed chatter about someone's birthday or hospital gossip is reasonable, but the patient should feel that the concentration of the surgical team is focused on the surgery at hand. Remarks about other patients or how the surgeon had to stay up all night with a difficult patient in labor are not appropriate. An equipment problem or technical difficulties that affect the operation certainly should be discussed with the surgeon before starting the procedure; however, it is inappropriate to talk about these in front of the patient. Remarks such as "The table is broken and won't go down" or "We weren't able to get your favorite retractor today" may not affect the performance of the operation, but such statements just before a patient is ready to be anesthetized may raise serious doubts as to whether the operative team is optimally prepared for this operation and may raise uncomfortable questions later if complications or unexpected results occur.

Positioning

The patient is brought into the operating room and placed in the supine position on the operating table. It is nice to place a warm blanket on the bed immediately before the patient's arrival and to cover the patient with a blanket from the warmer or use a warm air circulating blanket when she is positioned on the operating table because most operating rooms are somewhat cool and the patient is only lightly clothed.

When the patient has been anesthetized, a careful examination under anesthesia is done. At this point, the surgeon should concentrate on potential problems affecting resectability. Is there nodularity from endometriosis in the cul-de-sac that may make dissection of the rectum off of the posterior cervix difficult? Is the myoma in the broad ligament really wedged into the pelvic sidewall or does it move freely with the uterus? The mobility and descent of the uterus under anesthesia are particularly important when a vaginal hysterectomy is being considered. These potential problems and possible solutions should be considered and possibly discussed with the operative team while the surgeon scrubs. By consideration and discussion of potential problems and possible solutions, difficulties

that arise during surgery may have already been contemplated and plans and solutions already developed.

The vagina and perineum are prepped with antiseptic solutions, and a Foley catheter is inserted. I prefer to position the patient supine on the operative table with a soft pillow under her knees to provide gentle flexion. The patient's legs provide a table on which instruments can be placed. These days, it is common for the patient to be positioned in the low Allen stirrups with her legs slightly apart. This allows an assistant to stand between the legs and provides ready access to the vagina for examination or manipulation and the urethra for cystoscopy, which is routine in most pelvic surgery.

The abdomen then is prepped from the anterior thighs to the xiphoid, and sterile drapes are applied. In most instances, abdominal hysterectomy for benign disease can be done through a low transverse incision; most gynecologists prefer a Pfannenstiel incision, which is cosmetically appealing and strong. If more exposure is required, a Cherney or Maylard incision can be used. A midline incision is usually done if malignant disease is present or exposure to the upper abdomen may be required. The choice of abdominal incision is discussed in Chapter 14.

Once the abdomen is opened, the pelvic pathology is carefully evaluated and the abdomen explored. The operating surgeon should examine the appendix and palpate the upper abdominal organs, including the kidneys, liver, gallbladder, stomach, spleen, diaphragm, bowel, and omentum. The retroperitoneal nodes in the pelvic and paraaortic area should be palpated and the area of the pancreas gently examined to identify any abnormalities. The status of these organs should be recorded in the operative note, and an intraoperative consultation may be indicated if abnormalities are identified.

After the abdomen has been explored, a slight Trendelenburg position should be requested, a self-retaining retractor placed, and the bowel packed superiorly to afford good exposure of the pelvis. Any adhesions of the small bowel or rectosigmoid may need to be divided at this time so that the bowel can be mobilized out of the operative field. In relatively thin patients with benign disease, I prefer to use a Kirschner retractor, which is light and simple and provides a choice of several fairly wide, shallow blades that fit on a square frame, allowing adjustable retraction laterally, inferiorly, and superiorly. The cecum and sigmoid are packed first with separate packs, and a third rolled or folded pack is placed in the center behind the superior retractor blade to hold back the small bowel. In larger patients, or patients with a longer midline incision, a Bookwalter or Omni-Tract retractor, with many options of blades and variable positioning, is invaluable. These large retractor systems are screwed onto the operating table and provide excellent retraction in almost any situation. They are particularly useful in obese patients.

Hysterectomy

When the bowel has been packed away and exposure to the pelvis is satisfactory, the round ligaments and uteroovarian ligaments are grasped on each side with a Kocher clamp, elevating the uterus out of the pelvis. In some cases of extensive inflammatory disease, endometriosis, malignancy, or very large fibroids, uterine mobility is limited; but in most benign conditions, uterine mobility is satisfactory. The operator is generally on the patient's left side so that the right-handed surgeon can use her or his dominant hand to extend down into the pelvis. The first assistant is on the opposite side. The uterus is retracted to the patient's left side, and the right round ligament is stretched taut. A 0 delayed absorbable suture is placed under the round ligament approximately halfway between the uterus and the pelvic sidewall. The small artery of Sampson runs just under the round ligament and, in many cases, transilluminating this area allows the surgeon to easily visualize the artery and be sure that the suture is passed under it so that the artery will be ligated. A second suture is placed approximately 1 cm medial to the first suture; these two sutures are now tied simultaneously by the surgeon and first assistant. Clamping the round ligament is an extra step that is rarely necessary.

With traction on these sutures, the round ligament is held taunt and divided with Metzenbaum scissors between the two suture ligatures (**Fig. 32A.1**). This opens the retroperitoneal space, which is almost always a free space for blunt dissection, even in the patient with extensive tumor, inflammatory disease, or endometriosis. *If the ovaries are to be removed at the time of hysterectomy*, the peritoneal incision then is extended superiorly, lateral to the ovary and parallel with the infundibulopelvic ligament. The peritoneal incision also can be extended anteriorly down to the bladder reflection, but the peritoneum over the anterior cervix does not need to be divided at this time because exposure of this area is not yet required and bleeding may be encountered. With the index finger and the tip of the suction or the back of a tissue forceps, the surgeon gently divides the loose areolar tissue of the retroperitoneum, identifying the external iliac artery on the medial surface of the psoas muscle. In most cases, the artery can be identified very easily, and blunt dissection is used to extend the exposure superiorly to the level of the bifurcation of the common iliac artery. The ureter always crosses the pelvic brim at this location and should be identified easily on the inside of the medial leaf of the peritoneum at this point. The internal iliac or

hypogastric artery dives into the pelvis at this location parallel to the ureter, and it should be identified also. This retroperitoneal exploration may seem awkward at first, but with practice, the external and internal iliac arteries and ureter can be visualized easily in 10 to 20 seconds.

If the ovary is to be removed, a hole in the peritoneum between the ureter and the ovarian vessels superior to the ovary can be made under direct vision. We use a fairly fine sharp-pointed 9-inch clamp that can be passed gently through the peritoneum from lateral to medial against and between two fingers, supporting the medial side of the peritoneum. Alternatively, the peritoneum may be divided sharply or with the electrosurgical blade. We prefer to use a fairly delicate tonsil clamp on the infundibulopelvic ligament because it reminds us to isolate the vessels and take a fairly small pedicle. If there is significant inflammation or edema, a larger clamp, such as a Heaney clamp, may be used on the infundibulopelvic ligament pedicle (**Fig. 32A.2**). A second back clamp then is placed distally and the ovarian vessels divided between the two clamps. This pedicle then is ligated with a free tie, and then, a second transfixion suture ligature is placed for safety between the free tie and the clamp. Zero-gauge delayed absorbable sutures and ties are used throughout. The suture ligature is placed distal to the free tie so that if the needle happens to puncture one of the ovarian vessels, the vessel has already been ligated by the more proximal free tie. The back clamp is ligated with a single free tie, and the posterior peritoneum then is torn or cut above the ureter toward the back of the uterus, mobilizing the ovary, which is then tied to the clamp on the right side of the uterus to keep it from flopping around and obscuring the operative field. The sutures on the round ligaments and infundibulopelvic

Round ligament

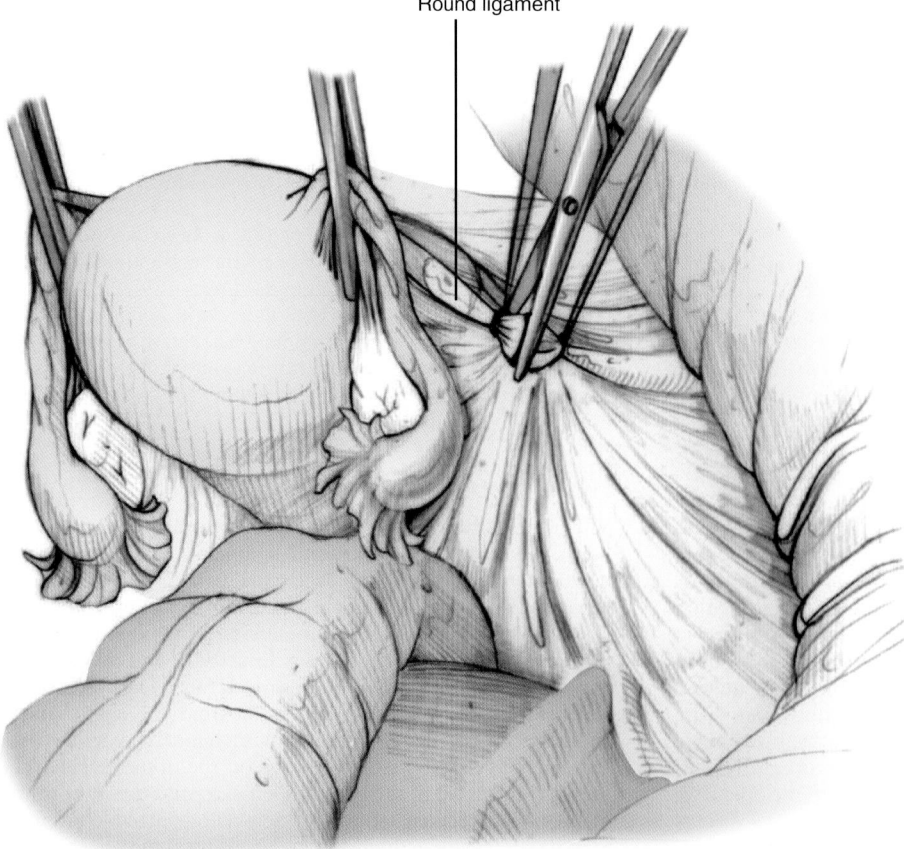

FIGURE 32A.1 The technique of abdominal hysterectomy begins with the round ligament. The ligament is ligated with transfixion sutures and cut. The broad ligament is opened.

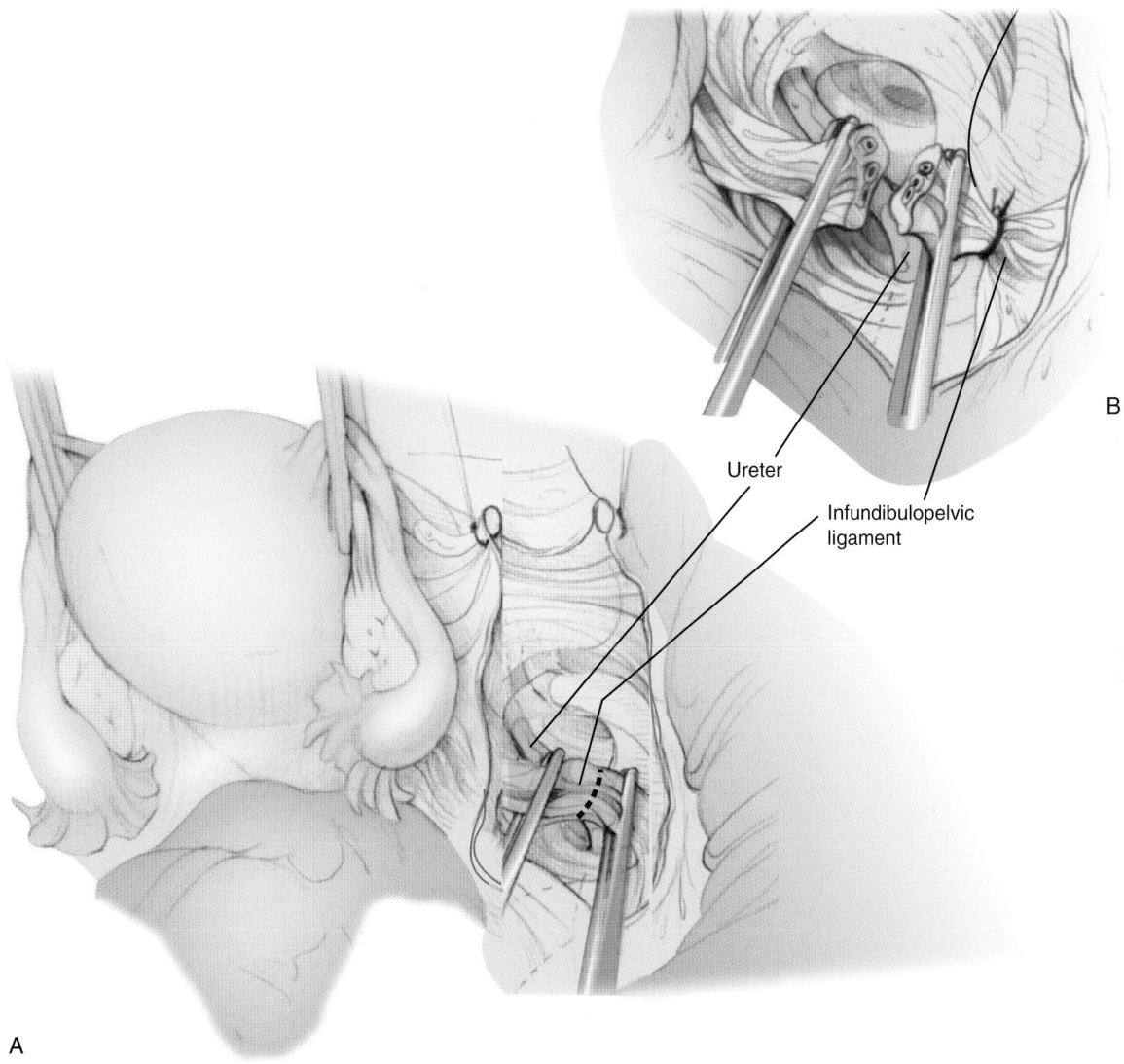

Ureter

Infundibulopelvic
ligament

A

B

V

FIGURE 32A.2 A: The infundibulopelvic ligament is doubly clamped, and the ovarian vessels are cut between the clamps. Care is taken to be sure the ureter is clear as the clamps are applied. **B:** The proximal pedicle is ligated with a free tie followed by a transfixion suture ligature.

ligament then are cut. The procedure is repeated on the patient's left side.

If the ovary and tube are to be left in situ at the time of hysterectomy, a window in the peritoneum beneath the fallopian tube between the uterus and ovary is made sharply or bluntly, and a heavy clamp—such as a Heaney, Kocher, or similar clamp—is used to clamp the uteroovarian pedicle (**Fig. 32A.3**). The round ligament should not be included in this clamp. The clamp that was initially placed on the round ligament and fallopian tube just lateral to the uterine fundus at the beginning of the procedure serves as the back clamp for this pedicle. The tube and uteroovarian ligament are divided and the pedicle ligated as previously noted with a free tie followed by a suture ligature. The ovary and tube may be left in the posterior pelvis if exposure is adequate or gently packed in the paracolic gutter, with care being taken to ensure that the blood supply is not compromised.

The next step is the dissection of the bladder from the anterior cervix. With the uterus elevated out of the pelvis by traction on the clamps on the tube and round ligament, the

bladder peritoneum is divided just inferior to its attachment to the lower uterine segment. If the peritoneum is divided 5 to 10 mm below its uterine attachment, it is usually mobile, and an avascular plane of loose areolar tissue can be identified between the posterior bladder wall and the anterior cervix. We begin this dissection sharply using the Metzenbaum scissors. With upward traction on the bladder peritoneum and the uterine fundus stretched tightly out of the pelvis, the tips of the Metzenbaum scissors should rest lightly on the fascia overlying the cervix and small bites used to develop this tissue plane, dissecting the bladder from the anterior cervix (**Fig. 32A.4**). This dissection should take place over the cervix, because if it is carried too far laterally, bleeding may be encountered, and the uterine vessels or ureters could be injured. Except in patients with a previous cesarean section or an adherent bladder for other reasons, this bladder dissection often can be done bluntly, but it is good practice to do it sharply from time to time so that in those patients in whom the bladder is adherent and sharp dissection is required, the technique will be familiar. Blunt dissection of the bladder can be accomplished easily by

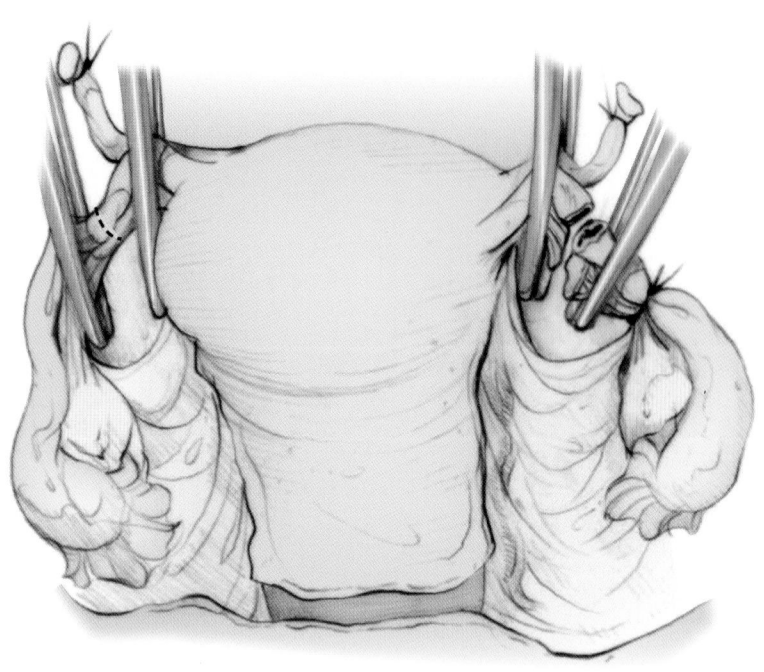

FIGURE 32A.3 When the ovary is to be conserved, a peritoneal window is made above the ureter and the tube and utero-ovarian ligament are clamped. This pedicle is divided and doubly ligated.

grasping the uterus and lower uterine segment between both hands and gently using the first one or two fingers to advance the bladder, as illustrated in Richardson's classic paper (Fig. 32A.5). It also is possible to grasp the uterus with your dominant hand, placing the thumb in front on the anterior cervix and the fingers behind the uterus. The thumb is gently pushed downward toward the cervix and inferiorly toward the vagina, gently dissecting the bladder off of the cervix and lower uterine segment. With this technique, the pressure is against the cervix rather than against the bladder, which should minimize

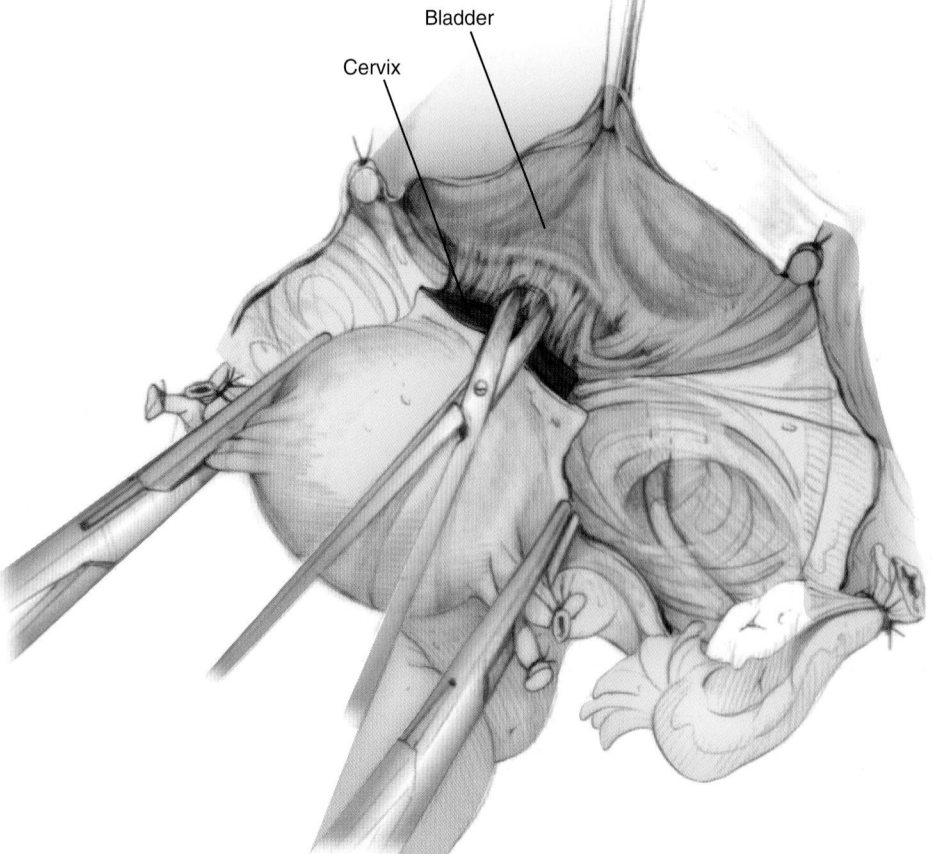

Bladder

Cervix

FIGURE 32A.4 The bladder is mobilized inferiorly by sharp dissection away from the cervix. To avoid unnecessary bleeding, this step may be done in stages as necessary.

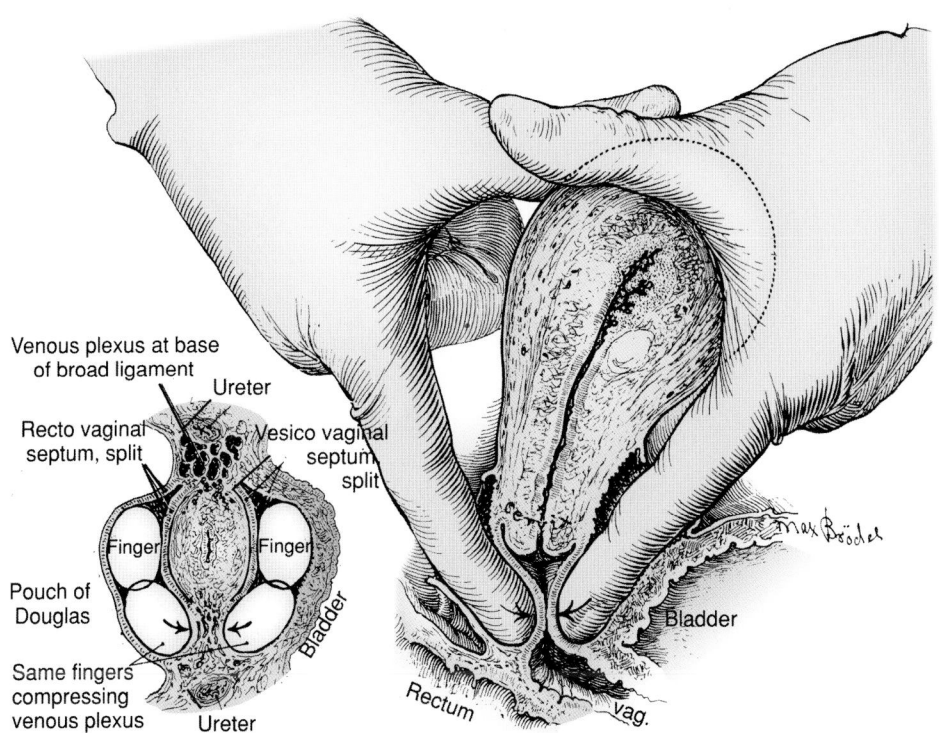

Venous plexus at base of broad ligament

Ureter

Recto vaginal septum, split

Vesico vaginal septum split

Finger   Finger

Pouch of Douglas

Bladder

Same fingers compressing venous plexus

Ureter

Bladder

Rectum   Vag.

FIGURE 32A.5 The bladder and, if necessary, the rectum can be gently advanced with blunt dissection. The depth of this dissection can be checked by squeezing the anterior and posterior fingers together below the cervix. (From Richardson EH. A simplified technique for abdominal panhysterectomy. *Surg Gynecol Obstet* 1929;48:248, with permission.)

the risk of bladder injury. Excessive force should not be used. As the bladder is dissected below the cervix, the thumb in front and the fingers behind come into closer opposition because they now have only the vaginal wall between them. The dissection is extended laterally to encompass the full cervix. Usually, it is not necessary to dissect the rectum off of the posterior cul-de-sac; but if adherent rectum prevents good posterior exposure, it should be dissected free after the uterine vessels have been divided.

Once the bladder has been freed from the anterior cervix, the uterine artery and vein are skeletonized (**Fig. 32A.6A**). The uterus is pulled sharply to the patient's left side, and the surgeon gently dissects the loose fatty tissue adjacent to the lateral lower uterine segment on the right. The uterine artery is usually found immediately adjacent to the uterus at the level of the internal cervical os. In most patients, the uterine artery is easily exposed by holding the tissue laterally and gently "raking" with the Metzenbaum scissors slightly opened from medial to lateral. "Skeletonizing" the uterine artery and vein allows them to be clamped more accurately, with less adjacent tissue, and a smaller vascular pedicle, which allows more precise and more secure ligation. However, good surgical judgment should be used so that excessive attempts to isolate the vessels do not produce unnecessary bleeding. When the vessels are exposed, a fairly heavy, slightly curved clamp then is used to clamp the vessels just adjacent to the uterus (**Fig. 32A.6B**). We prefer to use a Heaney, Zeppelin, or Masterson clamp for these pedicles. The tip of the clamp should be around the vessels, and the clamp should come across the pedicle as close to a right angle as possible, rather than at the diagonal, so that the least amount of tissue will be incorporated in the pedicle. The tip of the clamp should not include too much cervical or uterine tissue because this makes application of subsequent clamps more difficult. A second clamp can be placed above the first for added safety, if desired, and a third or back clamp used to prevent annoying back bleeding from the uterus after the

vessels have been cut if the uterus is enlarged or the other vascular pedicles to the uterus have not been secured.

If exposure is satisfactory after a single clamp has been placed on the right uterine artery and vein, we skeletonize the uterine vessels on the patient's left side and place a clamp on these vessels as well. If the uterus is small, no back clamp is required because the four major vessels supplying the uterus have now been clamped or ligated. Next, the uterine vessels are cut with scissors or a knife and the pedicle doubly ligated with 0 delayed absorbed sutures. We prefer to use a small tapered point needle (CT-2, Ethicon) for these pedicles because we feel that large needles are more difficult to place in the small confines of the deep pelvis. If a back clamp has been used, it is now ligated and removed so that the field is not obscured by an excessive number of clamps. The technique illustrated here starts with the right side, but the patient's anatomy and surgical preference should guide which side is skeletonized and clamped first.

Hemostasis should be good at this point. If not, any bleeding should be controlled. The bladder is again checked to ensure it is well below the cervix. If the rectum needs to be dissected from the posterior cervix, this should be done now. This is usually not necessary for a simple abdominal hysterectomy for benign disease. The peritoneum of the posterior cul-de-sac between the uterosacral ligaments can be divided easily, and blunt dissection of the posterior vaginal wall from the anterior rectum usually is easy, although the rectosigmoid occasionally may be densely adherent to the posterior uterine segment or cervix by endometriosis or pelvic inflammatory disease. If the bladder and/or rectum is too densely adherent and there is concern that further attempts at dissection may damage them or cause troublesome bleeding, a supracervical hysterectomy should be considered.

Once the bladder has been freed from the cervix anteriorly and the rectum posteriorly, the uterus is placed on tension, exposing the deeper portions of the broad ligament and

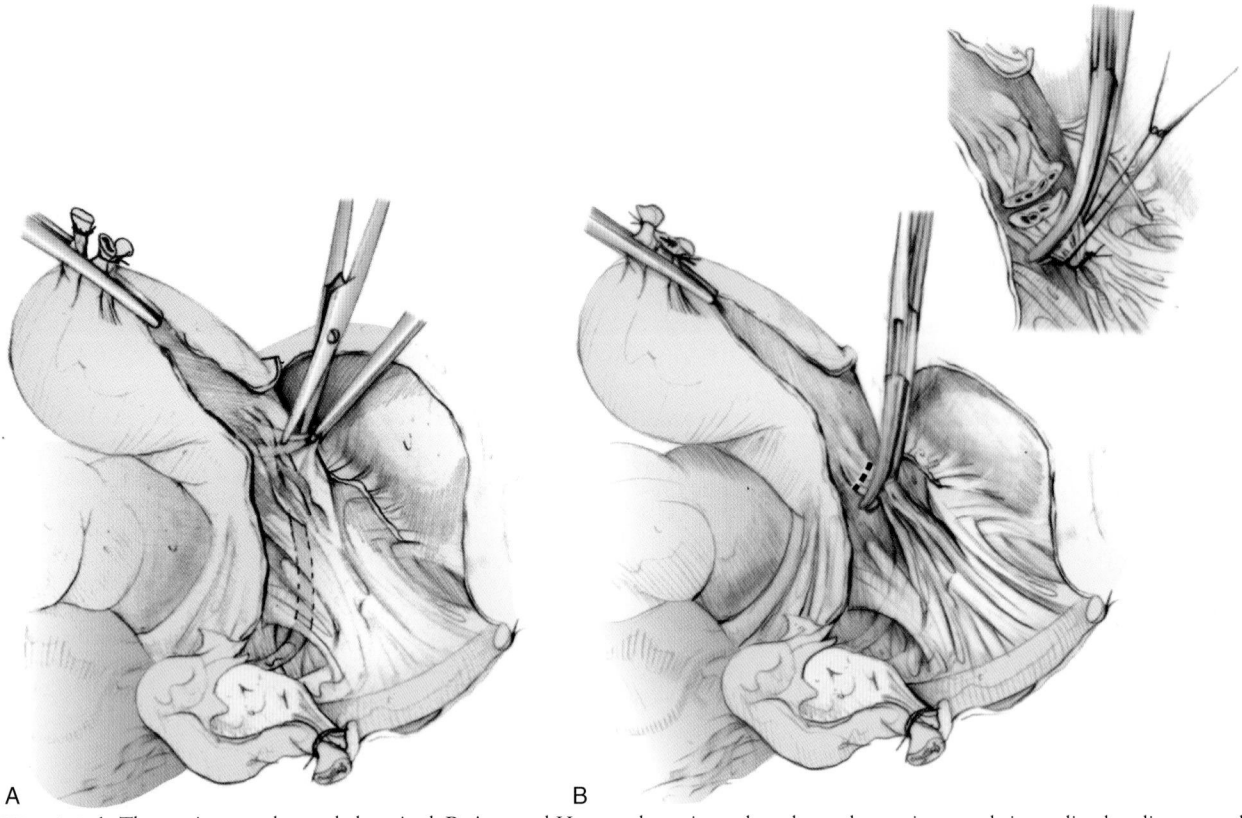

FIGURE 32A.6 **A:** The uterine vessels are skeletonized. **B:** A curved Heaney clamp is used to clamp the uterine vessels immediately adjacent to the uterus. They are ligated by two suture ligatures.

pulling the lower uterine segment away from the ureter. A medium-width malleable retractor may be useful to retract the bladder anteriorly; if necessary, a wide malleable retractor in the posterior cul-de-sac will provide deep exposure posteriorly. In most cases, a series of straight Heaney or Zeppelin clamps can now be used to successfully clamp the remaining portion of the broad ligament (**Fig. 32A.7**). The tips of these clamps should be placed on the lateral portion of the cervix, and the upper portion of the jaw should lie immediately adjacent to the previous pedicle. As the clamp is gently squeezed closed, the tip slides off of the firm cervix, finally closing snugly against the lateral wall of the muscular cervix. By staying close to the cervix in this way, the risk of damaging the ureter, which is not too far away laterally, is minimized. The pedicle then is cut with heavy scissors or a knife. A millimeter or two of tissue may be left medial to the clamp as insurance, but this is not necessary. The tip of the transfixion suture needle is placed at the lateral tip of the clamp jaw; if the pedicle is longer than 1 cm, we recommend using a Heaney suture ligature so that the upper end of the pedicle is secondarily transfixed to prevent it from slipping out of the ligature. While good exposure is maintained, one or two pedicles are tied on each side, and then the procedure is repeated on the opposite side until the level of the cervical–vaginal junction has been reached. Once again, the bladder and rectum are checked and advanced if necessary to be sure that they are well clear and the anterior and posterior vaginal walls exposed.

Sharply angled large Zeppelin clamps are used to clamp across the vagina below the cervix. These clamps include the base of the cardinal ligaments laterally, the uterosacral ligament posteriorly, and the vaginal wall anteriorly and posteriorly. A clamp is applied from each side; in most cases, the

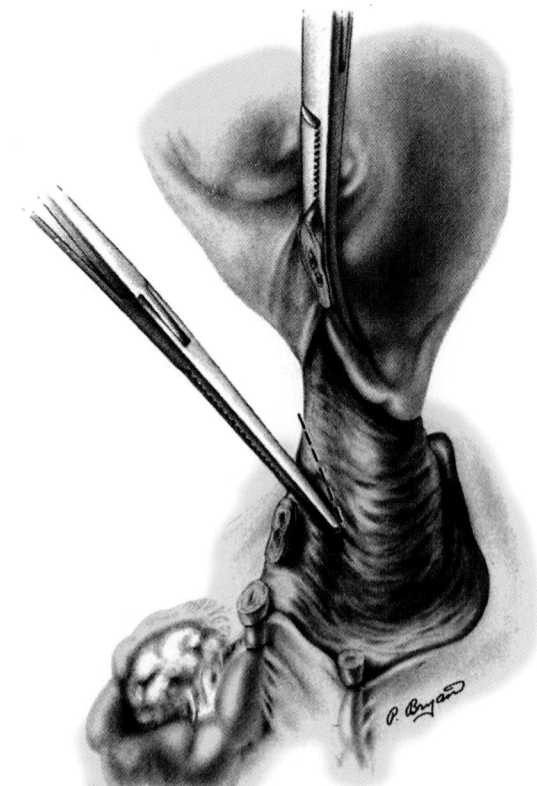

FIGURE 32A.7 After the uterine artery and vein have been ligated, the remaining lower portion of the broad ligament is clamped with a series of straight clamps. The tips are placed on the edge of the cervix and the back of the jaw immediately adjacent to the previous pedicle.

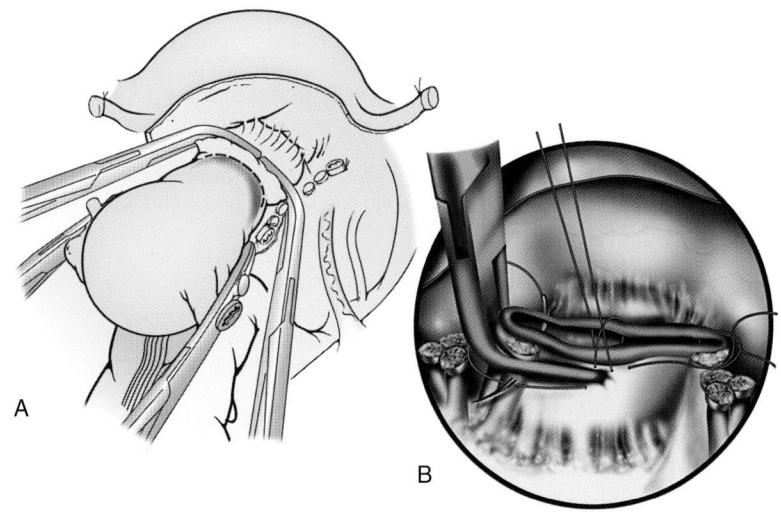

A

B

FIGURE 32A.8 A: After checking to be sure the bladder and rectum are clear, the vagina is cross clamped with long, sharply curved Zeppelin clamps just below the cervix (*dotted line*). The vagina is divided just above the clamps with a knife or angled scissors. **B:** The vaginal cuff then is closed with a figure-of-eight suture in the middle and Heaney suture ligatures on the angles, including the uterosacral and cardinal ligaments for support.

tips of these clamps meet in the middle just below the cervix (**Fig. 32A.8**). A knife or heavy, sharply angled Jorgenson scissors is used to divide the vagina above these clamps and below the cervix. The uterus is removed and placed in a pan on the back table for later examination. Care is taken not to contaminate the surgical field by touching the vagina or vaginal portion of the cervix or dripping vaginal fluid in the pelvis. A single figure-of-eight suture is placed between the tips of the two clamps to close the midportion of the vagina. The ends of this suture are held initially and not tied. A Heaney suture ligature is placed on each of the lateral clamps with the second bite going through the uterosacral ligament posteriorly. Inclusion of the uterosacral and cardinal ligament in this pedicle provides excellent support of the vaginal apex. When these lateral sutures have been tied, the figure-of-eight suture in the middle then is tied also. The lateral sutures are cut and the figure-of-eight in the middle of the cuff is held to provide traction on the vaginal apex. With this closed cuff technique, the vagina is never exposed, which reduces contamination of the pelvis. However, there may be instances, such as a large cervical myoma, when there is a very deep vaginal fornix, and a closed technique would remove too much vagina. Entry into the vagina with the electrosurgical blade and then carefully opening the vagina circumferentially under direct vision is an option in such cases. As the vagina is opened, the full-thickness vaginal edges are grasped with Kocher clamps as the dissection proceeds. In this instance, we generally close the vaginal cuff with a series of figure-of-eight stitches of 0 delayed absorbable suture, taking care to incorporate the uterosacral and cardinal ligaments into the cuff for support. Since the advent of prophylactic antibiotics for hysterectomy many years ago, we have not run the vaginal wall with a locking stitch for hemostasis and left the cuff open for drainage (closing the pelvic peritoneum over the open cuff).

In the classic Richardson technique, the peritoneum over the posterior cervix is divided, the peritoneum is dissected off the cul-de-sac, and the rectovaginal septum is entered to reflect the rectum posteriorly. In our experience, this has not been necessary in the vast majority of patients with benign disease. In contrast to the anterior bladder dissection, this posterior peritoneum is much more adherent. There is usually some bleeding associated with this dissection, making it both bloody and time-consuming. With the

Richardson technique, the uterosacral ligaments also are clamped separately and subsequently attached to the vaginal cuff for support. In the technique described above, this is accomplished in a single step.

STEPS IN THE PROCEDURE

Abdominal Hysterectomy

1. Open the abdomen and visualize and/or palpate the pelvis, abdomen, and retroperitoneal area to evaluate the presence of normal or abnormal findings and anatomy.

2. Place a retractor if needed to provide adequate exposure for safe pelvic surgery.

3. Grasp the round ligament, utero-ovarian ligament, and fallopian tube with a large bite of a straight clamp (Kocher) where they arise from each side of the uterus. One clamp on each side will provide an easy way to manipulate the uterus.

4. Elevating the uterus out of the pelvis, the anatomy is reevaluated and any adhesions to adjacent bowel or omentum are freed.

5. The round ligament on one side is ligated and divided, opening the retroperitoneal space.

6. If the ovaries are to be preserved, the utero-ovarian pedicle is clamped, divided, and ligated.

7. If the ovary is to be removed, the retroperitoneal space is opened, the ureter is identified, and the infundibulopelvic ligament (containing the ovarian artery and vein) is isolated, clamped, divided, and ligated.

8. Steps 5, 6, and 7 are then repeated on the opposite side.

9. The bladder is then dissected free from the anterior wall of the lower uterine segment and cervix so that the anterior vaginal wall is exposed.

V

10. The uterine vessels are skeletonized on both sides at the level of the lower uterine segment.

11. The uterine vessels are clamped bilaterally. The uterine vessels are then divided and suture ligated (usually with two sutures on each side).

12. The exposure of the anterior and posterior vaginal wall just below the cervix is again checked, and the bladder and rectum are dissected still more if additional exposure is needed to safely clamp across the vagina below the cervix.

13. The remaining portion of the broad ligament on each side of the cervix is then clamped, divided, and ligated using a series of clamps until the cervix is reached, and the broad ligament on each side has been detached from the lateral cervix and upper vagina is well exposed.

14. With the uterus strongly elevated out of the pelvis, large right angle clamps are placed across the vagina just below the cervix—one from each side with the tips meeting the middle.

15. The vagina is divided with a knife or long heavy curved scissors above the clamps, and the uterus and cervix are passed off the operative field.

16. The vaginal apex is closed. Heaney suture ligatures can be used on each side incorporating the uterosacral and cardinal ligaments into the cuff for support.

17. The pelvis is irrigated with warm, sterile saline and hemostasis is checked. The packs and retractors are removed, and the sigmoid colon is carefully replaced in the pelvis.

18. The abdominal wall is closed.

Closure

After the pelvis has been copiously irrigated with warm saline, the pedicles are inspected carefully to be sure that hemostasis is present. Electrocautery or suture ligatures with 3-0 absorbable sutures on fine needles are used to control small bleeders. The location of the ureters, bladder, and major vessels should be known when placing these sutures. Common sites of ureteral injury during abdominal hysterectomy include the infundibulopelvic ligament where the ovarian vessels are ligated, the area of the uterine artery ligation, and the bladder base. Distorted anatomy associated with fibroids, endometriosis, and malignancy is a signal for special care to avoid ureteral injury. The pelvis is not reperitonealized, but the rectosigmoid colon is gently laid over the vaginal cuff to cover this raw surface and minimize the risk of small bowel adhesions. The packs and retractor are removed, the abdomen checked again for hemostasis, and the omentum placed anteriorly to minimize the risk of intestinal adhesions to the abdominal incision. The anterior peritoneum is closed with delayed absorbable suture, although some surgeons today feel that it is unnecessary to close the abdominal peritoneum. The fascial closure should be commensurate with the patient's risk of infection and hernia. Generally, a running monofilament delayed absorbable suture such as PDS (Ethicon) on a larger, curved, tapered needle (CT-1, Ethicon) can be used. If there is a significant risk of dehiscence secondary to infection, obesity, or other medical problems, interrupted sutures or a mass closure technique may be used. Closure techniques are illustrated in Chapter 14. Because patients are often discharged by the third or fourth postoperative day, we generally prefer to close the skin with a subcuticular absorbable suture, which eliminates the necessity for a return to the office for suture or staple removal.

After the patient has been taken to the recovery room, the surgeon should speak with the family, preferably face to face, to assure them that the patient is doing well and to review the operative findings with them. We also strongly recommend that the surgeon ask the circulating nurse to contact the family about once an hour to update them on the progress of the operation during the surgical procedure. This especially is helpful if there were any unknown questions going into the operation (Did the ovaries look normal? Was the endometriosis involving the ureter?). A brief operative note must be immediately recorded in the patient's chart describing the procedure, blood loss, fluid replacement, and if any packs or drains were left in the patient. Postoperative orders are written. A full and complete operative note should be prepared with emphasis on any unusual findings or variations from standard techniques.

SUBTOTAL ABDOMINAL HYSTERECTOMY

The technique of subtotal or supracervical abdominal hysterectomy is similar to the technique for abdominal hysterectomy as described, until the uterine vessels have been clamped and ligated. At this point, care should be taken to be sure that the bladder and rectum have been advanced at least far enough so that the cervix can be clearly visualized both anteriorly and posteriorly. The uterine fundus is strongly retracted out of the pelvis, and electrocautery is used to cut the cervix anteriorly just above the level of the ligated uterine vessels (Fig. 32A.9). A shallow V-shaped incision is used both anteriorly and posteriorly until the uterine fundus is excised. The "coagulate" mode of the electrosurgical unit is used, and hemostasis usually is excellent. An attempt to cut across the upper cervix should not be made until the uterine vessels have been ligated bilaterally. Bleeding will be prohibitive. Once the fundus has been amputated, several generous figure-of-eight sutures on a large needle then are used to close the upper endocervix in a hemostatic fashion. The top of the cervix is checked for bleeding, and the bladder peritoneum may be used to cover this cervical stump to minimize the risk of adhesions.

POSTOPERATIVE CARE

Although routine postoperative care is thoroughly reviewed in Chapter 9, there are several facets that should be emphasized following hysterectomy.

Studies over the past few years have indicated that early feeding after hysterectomy is safe and actually results in earlier discharge. In many cases, patients are able to tolerate solid food on the first postoperative day following abdominal hysterectomy. The surgeon should nevertheless take into account the amount of dissection and bowel trauma that occurred during the operative procedure and be conservative with the diet orders if a postoperative ileus is anticipated. Patients and their caregivers always should be cautioned not to eat or drink if they feel nauseous or are vomiting. Having a bowel movement or even the passage of flatus are no longer requirements for hospital discharge as long as the patient has normal, active bowel sounds, is tolerating solid food, and is not distended.

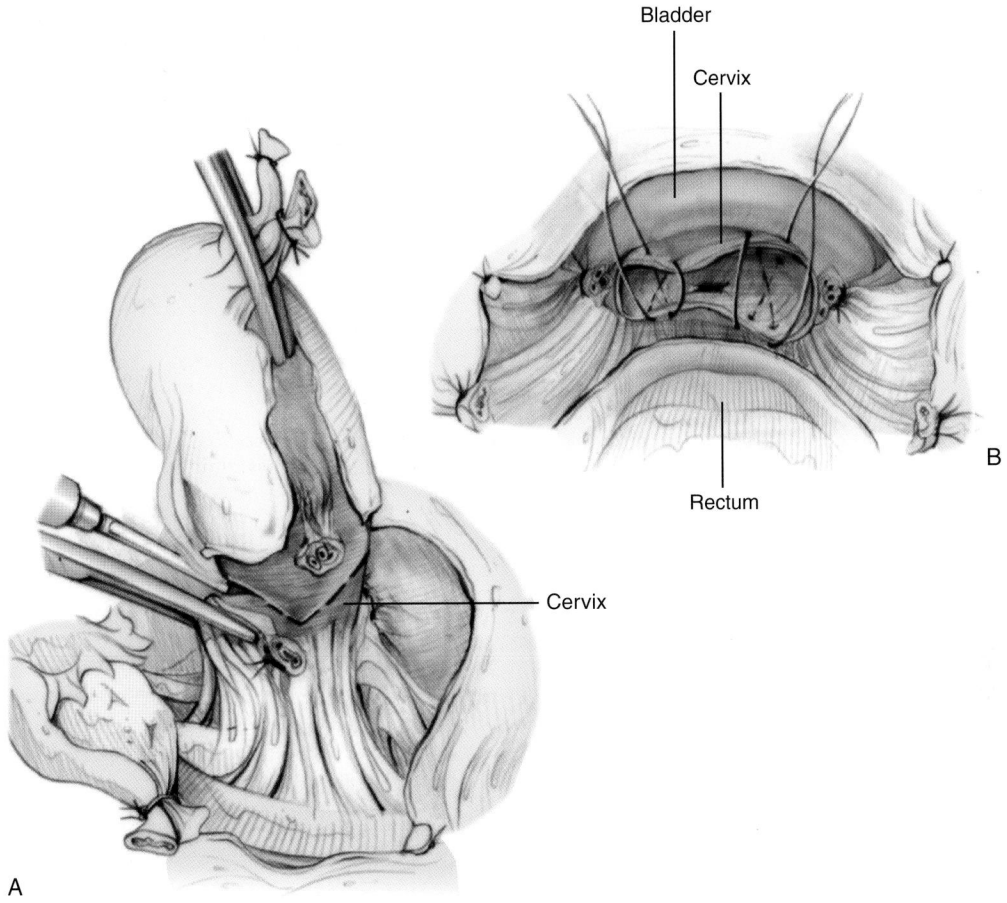

Bladder

Cervix

B

Rectum

Cervix

A

FIGURE 32A.9 Subtotal or supracervical hysterectomy. **A:** After the uterine vessels have been ligated, the fundus is amputated using the electrocautery in a shallow cone-shaped technique. **B:** The cervix or lower uterine segment then is closed with several large figure-of-eight sutures.

Most patients have a Foley catheter for bladder drainage overnight following abdominal hysterectomy, although Richardson and many gynecologic surgeons have shown it is possible to avoid this in many patients with the help of a good, enthusiastic nursing staff. In most situations, however, a catheter is inserted before hysterectomy and removed on the first postoperative day. In patients with bladder injury or continuous epidural for postoperative pain relief, more prolonged catheter drainage may be indicated.

The length of postoperative hospitalization has decreased dramatically in the last 20 years. Although it was common in the past for women to remain in the hospital for 7 to 10 days after abdominal hysterectomy, most patients are now discharged home in 3 or 4 days. This trend toward a shorter hospital stay requires better patient education and a reasonable home environment to which the patient can be safely and comfortably discharged. The surgeon must also carefully evaluate the patient before discharge and resist pressure from insurance companies and hospital administrators when the patient's condition indicates that she is not suitable for an early discharge. The patient and her family must be instructed on proper care. Can she take a bath? Can she go up and down the stairs? Can she pick up her grandchild? How soon can she drive a car? A printed set of instructions for home care as well as answers to frequently asked questions are good ideas. Liberal use of home visiting nurses is also recommended, especially in older

or more debilitated patients or in those whose home situation may be less than ideal.

COMPLICATIONS

Complications from hysterectomy can be diagnosed intraoperatively or postoperatively. In a thorough review, Harris found an overall complication rate of up to 50% associated with abdominal hysterectomy, but serious complications requiring reoperation or long-term disability are relatively uncommon. Reoperation rates of 4% to 4.3% have been reported by Gambone and associates and Browne and Frazer. The most common complications include infection, hemorrhage, and injuries to adjacent organs (Table 32A.5). Prevention and management of hemorrhage, infection, and operative injury complications are extensively discussed in several chapters of this text. Good surgical training, proper patient selection, knowledge of the anatomy, and good surgical judgment—which includes knowing your personal skills and limits—are all keys to minimizing complications.

Several factors have been consistently shown to be associated with an increased risk of complications related to hysterectomy. These are increasing age, medical illness, obesity, and malignancy. These conditions are beyond the control of the gynecologic surgeon, but they should be considered in the risk:benefit ratio when considering surgery, and every effort

TABLE 32A.5 Complications of Hysterectomy

COMPLICATION	ABDOMINAL	VAGINAL	LAPAROSCOPICALLY ASSISTED VAGINAL
Bleeding			
Hemorrhage	1%–2%	1%–5%	1%
Transfusion	2%–12%	2%–8.3%	1.58%
Infection			
Unexplained fever	10%–20%	5%–8%	2.14%
Operative site	6.6%–24.7%	3.9%–10%	0.54%
Wound	4%–8%	NA	NA
Pelvic	3.2%–10%	3.9%–10%	1.27%
Urinary tract	1.1%–5%	1.7%–5%	0.81%
Pneumonia	0.4%–2.6%	0.29%–2%	0.11%
Injuries			
Bladder	1%–2%	0.5%–1.5%	1%
Bowel	0.1%–1%	0.1%–0.8%	0.1%–1%
Ureter	0.1%–0.5%	0.05%–0.1%	0.19%
Vesicovaginal fistula	0.1%–0.2%	0.1%–0.2%	0.22%
Trocar injuries	—	—	0.5%

From Harris WJ. Early complications of abdominal and vaginal hysterectomy. *Obstet Gynecol Surv* 1995;50:795, with permission.

should be made to have the patient in the best possible condition at the time of surgery.

BEST SURGICAL PRACTICES

- Hysterectomy is one of the most common major operations performed in the United States. The most common indications are uterine leiomyoma, endometriosis, abnormal uterine bleeding, and malignancy. There are many techniques to perform a hysterectomy, including abdominal, vaginal, laparoscopic and laparoscopically assisted, total, and subtotal. Before surgery, the surgeon should discuss the indications, other management options, choice of surgical approach, risks and potential complications of surgery, and expected outcomes with the patient and her supporters and obtain a fully informed operative consent.
- Numerous prospective randomized studies have shown that total abdominal hysterectomy results in the same or better postoperative sexual function, urinary tract and bowel function, and pelvic support as does supracervical hysterectomy.
- Prophylactic antibiotics administered within 1 hour before the initial incision significantly reduce the risk of a surgical site infection. There is no advantage to continuing antibiotics after surgery in an uninfected patient.
- The surgeon and the surgical team should be completely focused on the operation. Thoughtful preoperative preparation, careful surgical technique, well-reasoned judgment intraoperatively, and attentive postoperative care by a well-trained and interactive team will result in the best outcomes. Good communication between all members of the team is of great importance.
- We have found that the surgical techniques described in this chapter have been highly effective, but each surgeon should be familiar with a number of variations of standard hysterectomy technique and use appropriate variations that might suit the anatomy or pathology of a specific patient.

BIBLIOGRAPHY

Abdel-Fattah M, Barrington J, Yousef M, et al. Effect of total abdominal hysterectomy on pelvic floor function. *Obstet Gynecol Surv* 2004;59:299.

Adelman MR, Bardsley TR, Sharp HT. Urinary tract injuries in laparoscopic hysterectomy: a systematic review. *J Minim Invasive Gynecol* 2014;21:558. pii: S1553-4650(14)00036-3.

Alessandri F, Mistrangelo E, Lijoi D, et al. A prospective, randomized trial comparing immediate versus delayed catheter removal following hysterectomy. *Acta Obstet Gynecol Scand* 2006;85:716.

Allen WM, Masters WH. Traumatic laceration of uterine support: the clinical syndrome and the operative treatment. *Am J Obstet Gynecol* 1955;70:500.

American College of Obstetricians and Gynecologists. *ACOG Practice Bulletin No. 96: Alternatives to hysterectomy in the management of leiomyomas*. Washington, DC: ACOG, 2008.

American College of Obstetricians and Gynecologists. *ACOG Practice Bulletin No. 104: Antibiotic prophylaxis for gynecologic procedures*. Washington, DC: ACOG, 2009.

American College of Obstetricians and Gynecologists. *ACOG Practice Bulletin No. 578: Elective surgery and patient choice*. Washington, DC: ACOG, 2013.

American College of Obstetricians and Gynecologists. *ACOG Practice Bulletin No. 464: Patient safety in the surgical environment*. Washington, DC: ACOG, 2012.

American College of Obstetricians and Gynecologists. *ACOG Practice Bulletin No. 21: Prevention of deep vein thrombosis and pulmonary embolism*. Washington, DC: ACOG, 2000.

American College of Obstetricians and Gynecologists. *ACOG Practice Bulletin No. 7: Prophylactic oophorectomy*. Washington, DC: ACOG, 1999.

American College of Obstetricians and Gynecologists. *ACOG Practice Bulletin No. 571: Solutions for surgical preparation of the vagina*. Washington, DC: ACOG, 2013.

Asante A, Whiteman MK, Kulkarni A, et al. Elective oophorectomy in the United States: trends and in-hospital complications, 1998–2006. *Obstet Gynecol* 2010;16:1088.

Azari L, Santoso JT, Osborne SE. Optimal pain management in total abdominal hysterectomy. *Obstet Gynecol Surv* 2013;68:215.

Averette HE, Nguyen HN. The role of prophylactic oophorectomy in cancer prevention. *Gynecol Oncol* 1994;55:S38.

Babalola EO, Bharucha AE, Schleck CD, et al. Decreasing utilization of hysterectomy: a population-based study in Olmsted County, Minnesota, 1965–2002. *Am J Obstet Gynecol* 2007;196:214.

Bhattacharya S, Middleton LJ, Tsourapas A, et al. Hysterectomy, endometrial ablation and Mirena® for heavy menstrual bleeding: a systematic review of clinical effectiveness and cost-effectiveness analysis. *Health Technol Assess* 2011;15:iii, 1.

Bottle A, Aylin P. Variations in vaginal and abdominal hysterectomy by region and trust in England. *BJOG* 2005;112:326.

Bridgman S, Dobbins J, Casbard A. The VALUE national hysterectomy study: description of the patients and their surgery. *BJOG* 2002; 109:302.

Broder MS, Kanouse DE, Mittman BS, et al. The appropriateness of recommendations for hysterectomy. *Obstet Gynecol* 2000;95:199.

Brooks P, Clouse J, Morris L. Hysterectomy vs. resectoscopic endometrial ablation for the control of abnormal uterine bleeding: a cost-comparative study. *J Reprod Med* 1994;39:755.

Brummer TH, Heikkinen AM, Jalkanen J, et al. Antibiotic prophylaxis in hysterectomy, a prospective cohort study: cefuroxime, metronidazole, or both? *BJOG* 2013;120:1269.

Brummer TH, Jalkanen J, Fraser J, et al. FINHYST, a prospective study of 5279 hysterectomies: complications and their risk factors. *Hum Reprod* 2011;26:1741.

Bukovsky I, Liftshitz Y, Langer R, et al. Ovarian residual syndrome. *Surg Gynecol Obstet* 1988;167:132.

Carlson K, Miller B, Flowler F. The Maine Women's Health Study: I. Outcomes of hysterectomy. *Obstet Gynecol* 1994;83:556.

Carlson K, Miller B, Flowler F. The Maine Women's Health Study: II. Outcomes of non-surgical management of leiomyomas, abnormal bleeding, and chronic pelvic pain. *Obstet Gynecol* 1994;83:566.

Carlson K, Nichols D, Schiff I. Indications for hysterectomy. *N Engl J Med* 1993;328:856.

Casiano ER, Trabuco EC, Bharucha AE, et al. Risk of oophorectomy after hysterectomy. *Obstet Gynecol* 2013;121:1069.

Castelo-Branco C, Figueras F, Sanjuan A, et al. Long-term compliance with estrogen replacement therapy in surgical postmenopausal women: benefits to bone and analysis of factors associated with discontinuation. *Menopause* 1999;6:307.

Ceccaroni M, Berretta R, Malzoni M, et al. Vaginal cuff dehiscence after hysterectomy: a multicenter retrospective study. *Eur J Obstet Gynecol Reprod Biol* 2011;158:308.

Chamsy DJ, Louie MY, Lum DA, et al. Clinical utility of postoperative hemoglobin level testing following total laparoscopic hysterectomy. *Am J Obstet Gynecol* 2014;211:224.e1. pii: S0002-9378(14)00341-X. doi:10.1016/j.ajog.2014.04.003

Clarke A, Black N, Rowe P, et al. Indications for and outcome of total abdominal hysterectomy for benign disease: a prospective cohort study. *BJOG* 1995;102:611.

Clarke-Pearson DL, Geller EJ. Complications of hysterectomy. *Obstet Gynecol* 2013;121:654.

Clifford V, Daley A. Antibiotic prophylaxis in obstetric and gynaecological procedures: a review. *Aust N Z J Obstet Gynaecol* 2012;52:412.

Darai E, Soriano D, Kimata P, et al. Vaginal hysterectomy for enlarged uteri, with or without laparoscopic assistance: randomized study. *Obstet Gynecol* 2001;97:712.

Dickson E, Argenta PA, Reichert JA. Results of introducing a rapid recovery program for total abdominal hysterectomy. *Gynecol Obstet Invest* 2012;73:21.

Dorsey J, Steinberg E, Holtz P. Clinical indications for hysterectomy route: patient characteristics or physician preference? *Am J Obstet Gynecol* 1995;173:1452.

Dorsey JH, Holtz PM, Griffiths RI, et al. Costs and charges associated with three alternative techniques of hysterectomy. *N Engl J Med* 1996;335:476.

Duhan N. Current and emerging treatments for uterine myoma—an update. *Int J Womens Health* 2011;3:231.

Einarsson JI, Suzuki Y, Vellinga TT, et al. Prospective evaluation of quality of life in total versus supracervical laparoscopic hysterectomy. *J Minim Invasive Gynecol* 2011;18:617.

Ewen S, Sutton C. Initial experience with supracervical laparoscopic hysterectomy and removal of the cervical transformation zone. *BJOG* 1994;101:225.

Fatania K, Vithayathil M, Newbold P, et al. Vaginal versus abdominal hysterectomy for the enlarged non-prolapsed uterus: a retrospective cohort study. *Eur J Obstet Gynecol Reprod Biol* 2014; 174:111.

Fong YF, Lim FK, Arulkumaran S. Prophylactic oophorectomy: a continuing controversy. *Obstet Gynecol Surv* 1998;53:493.

Franchi M, Ghezzi F, Zanaboni F, et al. Nonclosure of peritoneum at radical abdominal hysterectomy and pelvic node dissection: a randomized study. *Obstet Gynecol* 1997;90:622.

Garry R. The future of hysterectomy. *BJOG* 2005;112:133.

Gill SE, Mills BB. Physician opinions regarding elective bilateral salpingectomy with hysterectomy and for sterilization. *J Minim Invasive Gynecol* 2013;20:517.

Gimbel H. Total or subtotal hysterectomy for benign uterine diseases? A meta-analysis. *Acta Obstet Gynecol Scand* 2007;86:133.

Gimbel H, Zobbe V, Andersen BM, et al. Randomised controlled trial of total compared with subtotal hysterectomy with one-year follow up results. *BJOG* 2003;110:1088.

Goldman JA, Feldberg D, Dicker D, et al. Femoral neuropathy subsequent to abdominal hysterectomy: a comparative study. *Eur J Obstet Gynecol Reprod Biol* 1985;20:385.

Grosse-Drieling D, Schlutius JC, Altgassen C, et al. Laparoscopic supracervical hysterectomy (LASH), a retrospective study of 1,584 cases regarding intra- and perioperative complications. *Arch Gynecol Obstet* 2012;285:1391.

Harris M, Olive D. Changing hysterectomy patterns after introduction of laparoscopically assisted vaginal hysterectomy. *Am J Obstet Gynecol* 1994;171:340.

Hasson HM. Cervical removal at hysterectomy for benign disease: risks and benefits. *J Reprod Med* 1993;38:781.

Hillis S, Marchbanks P, Peterson H. The effectiveness of hysterectomy for chronic pelvic pain. *Obstet Gynecol* 1995;86:941.

Hillis S, Marchbanks P, Peterson H. Uterine size and risks of complications among women undergoing abdominal hysterectomy for leiomyomas. *Obstet Gynecol* 1996;87:539.

Horbach NS, Lee TTM, Levy BS, et al. Unraveling the myths of laparoscopic supracervical hysterectomy. *Cont OB/GYN* 2006.

Howard F. The role of laparoscopy in chronic pelvic pain: promise and pitfalls. *Obstet Gynecol Surv* 1993;48:357.

Irwin KL, Weiss SN, Lee NC, et al. Tubal sterilization, hysterectomy, and the subsequent occurrence of epithelial ovarian cancer. *Am J Epidemiol* 1991;134:363.

Islam MS, Protic O, Giannubilo SR, et al. Uterine leiomyoma: available medical treatments and new possible therapeutic options. *J Clin Endocrinol Metab* 2013;98:921.

Jacobs I, Oram D. Prevention of ovarian cancer: a survey of the practice of prophylactic oophorectomy by fellows and members of the Royal College of Obstetricians and Gynaecologists. *BJOG* 1989;96:510.

Jacobson GF, Shaber RE, Armstrong MA, et al. Hysterectomy rates for benign indications. *Obstet Gynecol* 2006;107:1278.

Janssen PF, Brölmann HA, van Kesteren PJ, et al. Perioperative outcomes using LigaSure compared with conventional bipolar instruments in laparoscopic hysterectomy: a randomised controlled trial. *BJOG* 2011;118:1568.

Johnson N, Barlow D, Lethaby A, et al. Surgical approach to hysterectomy for benign gynaecological disease. *Cochrane Database Syst Rev* 2006;(19):CD003677.

Kauf ND, Satagopan JM, Robson ME, et al. Risk-reducing salpingo-oophorectomy in women with a BRCA1 or BRCA2 mutation. *N Engl J Med* 2002;356:1609.

Kelly HA. *Operative gynecology*. New York, NY: Appleton, 1896.

Kelly HA, Cullen TS. *Myomata of the uterus*. Philadelphia, PA: WB Saunders, 1909.

Kelly HA, Noble CP. *Gynecology and abdominal surgery*, vol. 1. Philadelphia, PA: WB Saunders, 1907.

Kerber IJ, Turner RJ. Ovaries, estrogen, and longevity and long-term mortality associated with oophorectomy compared with ovarian conservation in the Nurses' Health Study and variation in ovarian conservation in women undergoing hysterectomy for benign indications. *Obstet Gynecol* 2013;122:397.

Kohli N, Mallipeddi PK, Neff JM, et al. Routine hematocrit after elective gynecologic surgery. *Obstet Gynecol* 2000;95:847.

V

Korkontzelos I, Gkioulekas N, Stamatopoulos C, et al. Complicated abdominal hysterectomy subsequent to uterine embolization for large fibroids. *Clin Exp Obstet Gynecol* 2012;39:122.

Kovac SR. Clinical opinion: guidelines for hysterectomy. *Am J Obstet Gynecol* 2004;191:635.

Kovac SR. Hysterectomy outcomes in patients with similar indications. *Obstet Gynecol* 2000;95:787.

Krizova A, Clarke BA, Bernardini MQ, et al. Histologic artifacts in abdominal, vaginal, laparoscopic, and robotic hysterectomy specimens: a blinded, retrospective review. *Am J Surg Pathol* 2011; 35:115.

Kuppermann M, Varner RE, Summitt RL, et al. Effect of hysterectomy versus medical treatment on health-related quality of life and sexual function. *Obstet Gynecol Surv* 2004;59:706.

Landeen LB, Bell MC, Hubert HB, et al. Clinical and cost comparisons for hysterectomy via abdominal, standard laparoscopic, vaginal and robot-assisted approaches. *S D Med* 2011;64:197, 201, 203 passim.

Learman LA. Hysterectomy 2014: indications and techniques. *Clin Obstet Gynecol* 2014;57:1.

Learman LA, Summitt RL Jr, Varner RE, et al. Total or Supracervical Hysterectomy (TOSH) Research Group. A randomized comparison of total or supracervical hysterectomy: surgical complications and clinical outcomes. *Obstet Gynecol* 2003;102:453.

Lofgren M, Poromaa IS, Stjerndahl JH, et al. Postoperative infections and antibiotic prophylaxis for hysterectomy in Sweden: a study by the Swedish National Register for Gynecologic Surgery. *Acta Obstet Gynecol Scand* 2004;83:1202.

Lonnee-Hoffmann RA, Schei B, Eriksson NH. Sexual experience of partners after hysterectomy, comparing subtotal with total abdominal hysterectomy. *Acta Obstet Gynecol Scand* 2006;85:1389.

Lykke R, Blaakær J, Ottesen B, et al. Hysterectomy in Denmark 1977–2011: changes in rate, indications, and hospitalization. *Eur J Obstet Gynecol Reprod Biol* 2013;171:333.

Lynch HT, Lynch PM. Tumor variation in the cancer family syndrome: ovarian cancer. *Am J Surg* 1979;138:439.

Lyons TL. Laparoscopic supracervical hysterectomy. *Obstet Gynecol Clin North Am* 2000;27:441.

Mahdi H, Goodrich S, Lockhart D, et al. Predictors of surgical site infection in women undergoing hysterectomy for benign gynecologic disease: a multicenter analysis using the National Surgical Quality Improvement Program data. *J Minim Invasive Gynecol* 2014;21:901. pii: S1553-4650(14)00249-0. doi:10.1016/j.jmig.2014.04.003

Mamik MM, Antosh D, White DE, et al. Risk factors for lower urinary tract injury at the time of hysterectomy for benign reasons. *Int Urogynecol J* 2014;25:1031.

Matteson KA, Peipert JF, Hirway P, et al. Factors associated with increased charges for hysterectomy. *Obstet Gynecol* 2006;107:1057.

Mikhail E, Miladinovic B, Finan M. The relationship between obesity and trends of the routes of hysterectomy for benign indications. *Obstet Gynecol* 2014;123:126S. doi:10.1097/01.AOG.0000447087.18352.06

Morgan K, Thomas E. Nerve injury at abdominal hysterectomy. *BJOG* 1995;102:665.

Muffly TM, Ridgeway B, Abbott S, et al. Small bowel obstruction after hysterectomy to treat benign disease. *J Minim Invasive Gynecol* 2012;19:615.

Munro MG. Management of heavy menstrual bleeding: is hysterectomy the radical mastectomy of gynecology? *Clin Obstet Gynecol* 2007;50:324.

Myers ER, Steege JF. Risk adjustment for complications of hysterectomy: limitations of routinely collected administrative data. *Am J Obstet Gynecol* 1999;181:567.

Nichols DH, Willey PS, Randall CL. Significance of restoration of normal vaginal depth and axis. *Obstet Gynecol* 1970;36:251.

Nieboer TE, Hendriks JC, Bongers MY, et al. Quality of life after laparoscopic and abdominal hysterectomy: a randomized controlled trial. *Obstet Gynecol* 2012;119:85.

Ostrzenski A. A new, simplified posterior culdoplasty and vaginal vault suspension during abdominal hysterectomy. *Int J Obstet Gynecol* 1995;49:25.

Ouldamer L, Rossard L, Arbion F, et al. Risk of incidental finding of endometrial cancer at the time of hysterectomy for benign condition. *J Minim Invasive Gynecol* 2014;21:131.

Parazzini F, Negri E, Vecchia C, et al. Hysterectomy, oophorectomy, and subsequent ovarian cancer risk. *Obstet Gynecol* 1993;81:363.

Park MJ, Kim YS, Rhim H, Lim HK. Safety and therapeutic efficacy of complete or near-complete ablation of symptomatic uterine fibroid tumors by MR imaging-guided high-intensity focused US therapy. *J Vasc Interv Radiol* 2014;25:231.

Peipert JF, Weitzen S, Cruickshank C, et al. Risk factors for febrile morbidity after hysterectomy. *Obstet Gynecol* 2004;103:86.

Perera HK, Ananth CV, Richards CA, et al. Variation in ovarian conservation in women undergoing hysterectomy for benign indications. *Obstet Gynecol* 2013;121:717.

Pinion S, Parkin D, Abramovich D, et al. Randomized trial of hysterectomy, endometrial ablation, and transcervical endometrial resection for dysfunctional uterine bleeding. *BMJ* 1994;309:979.

Pynnä K, Vuorela P, Lodenius L, et al. Cost-effectiveness of hysterectomy for benign gynecological conditions: a systematic review. *Acta Obstet Gynecol Scand* 2013;93:225. doi:10.1111/aogs.12299

Ramirez PT, Klemer DP. Vaginal evisceration after hysterectomy: a literature review. *Obstet Gynecol Surv* 2002;57:462.

Rebbeck TR, Lynch HT, Neuhausen SL, et al. Prophylactic oophorectomy in carriers of BRCA1 or BRCA2 mutations. *N Engl J Med* 2002;346:1616.

Ribeiro SC, Ribeiro RM, Santos NC, et al. A randomized study of total abdominal, vaginal and laparoscopic hysterectomy. *Int J Gynecol Obstet* 2003;83:37.

Rice MS, Hankinson SE, Tworoger SS. Tubal ligation, hysterectomy, unilateral oophorectomy, and risk of ovarian cancer in the Nurses' Health Studies. *Fert Steril* 2014;102:192.

Richardson EH. A simplified technique for abdominal panhysterectomy. *Surg Obstet Gynecol* 1929;48:248.

Robertson D, Lefebvre G, Leyland N, et al. Adhesion prevention in gynaecological surgery. *J Obstet Gynaecol Can* 2010;32:598.

Schollmeyer T, Elessawy M, Chastamouratidhs B, et al. Hysterectomy trends over a 9-year period in an endoscopic teaching center. *Int J Gynaecol Obstet* 2014;126:45. pii: S0020-7292(14)00192-1.

Semm K. Endoscopic subtotal hysterectomy without colpotomy: classic intrafascial SEMM hysterectomy. A new method of hysterectomy by pelviscopy, laparotomy, per vaginam or functionally by total uterine mucosal ablation. *Int Surg* 1996;81:362.

Sharon A, Auslander R, Brandes-Klein O. Cystoscopy after total or subtotal laparoscopic hysterectomy: the value of a routine procedure. *Obstet Gynecol Surv* 2006;61:511.

Smorgick N, Patzkowsky KE, Hoffman MR, et al. The increasing use of robot-assisted approach for hysterectomy results in decreasing rates of abdominal hysterectomy and traditional laparoscopic hysterectomy. *Arch Gynecol Obstet* 2014;289:101.

Solnik MJ, Munro MG. Indications and alternatives to hysterectomy. *Clin Obstet Gynecol* 2014;57:14.

Solomon ER, Muffly TM, Barber MD. Common postoperative pulmonary complications after hysterectomy for benign indications. *Am J Obstet Gynecol* 2013;208:54.e1.

Song H, Lu D, Navaratnam K, Shi G. Aromatase inhibitors for uterine fibroids. *Cochrane Database Syst Rev* 2013;(10):CD009505. doi:10.1002/14651858.CD009505.pub2

Spilsbury K, Semmens JB, Hammond I, et al. Persistent high rates of hysterectomy in Western Australia: a population-based study of 83,000 procedures over 23 years. *BJOG* 2006;113:804.

Stovall T, Muneyyirci-Delale O, Summitt R, et al.; for the Leuprolide Acetate Study Group. GnRH agonist and iron versus placebo and iron in the anemic patient before surgery for leiomyomas: a randomized controlled trial. *Obstet Gynecol* 1995;86:65.

Surgical Care Improvement Project. *Prophylactic antibiotic regimen selection for surgery.* Available at: http://www.mediqic.org/scip

Symmonds RE, Pettit PDM. Ovarian remnant syndrome. *Obstet Gynecol* 1979;54:174.

Vierhout ME. Influence of nonradical hysterectomy on the function of the lower urinary tract. *Obstet Gynecol Surv* 2001;56:381.

Watson T. Vaginal cuff closure with abdominal hysterectomy: a new approach. *J Reprod Med* 1994;39:903.

Wijk L, Franzen K, Ljungqvist O, Nilsson K. Implementing a structured Enhanced Recovery After Surgery (ERAS) protocol reduces length of stay after abdominal hysterectomy. *Acta Obstet Gynecol Scand* 2014;93:749. doi:10.1111/aogs.12423

V

Wright JD, Ananth CV, Tergas AI, et al. An economic analysis of robotically assisted hysterectomy. *Obstet Gynecol* 2014;123:1038. doi:10.1097/AOG.0000000000000244

Wright JD, Herzog TJ, Tsui J, et al. Nationwide trends in the performance of inpatient hysterectomy in the United States. *Obstet Gynecol* 2013;122:233.

Zimmermann A, Bernuit D, Gerlinger C, et al. Prevalence, symptoms and management of uterine fibroids: an international internet-based survey of 21,746 women. *BMC Womens Health* 2012;12:6.

CHAPTER 32B
Vaginal Hysterectomy

Carl W. Zimmerman

DEFINITIONS

Endopelvic fascia—The layer of fibroelastic connective endopelvic tissue surrounding the bladder, vagina, and rectum. By investing the central pelvic organs in a continuous fashion from the vaginal introitus to the axial skeleton (sacrum), this tissue furnishes suspension to the entire uterovaginal complex and surrounding organs. Division of the paracolpium portion of this continuum is necessary for the completion of a vaginal hysterectomy.

Enterocele—Formed from a separation of the rectovaginal fascia or the pubocervical fascia from the posterior cervix or anterior cervix, respectively. An enterocele is a pelvic hernia that descends through the posterior vaginal fornix or anterior vaginal fornix. The most common location for an enterocele is the posterior superior vaginal segment.

Intramyometrial coring—A surgical technique useful for removal of a large uterus during vaginal hysterectomy. After the uterine vessels have been divided, the myometrium can be circumferentially incised with a scalpel placed parallel to the long axis of the uterus and beneath the serosal covering of the uterus. In effect, coring converts the normal spherical shape of the uterus into an elongated cylindrical or rod shape, enhancing the surgeon's ability to facilitate uterine removal.

Morcellation—A surgical technique that is useful in reducing the size of an enlarged uterus after the paracolpium and uterine vasculature are ligated. The cervix is divided in a vertical fashion until the enlarged fundus is encountered. At that point, leiomyomata or myometrial segments can be removed using various types of sharp and blunt dissection until the fundus is sufficiently reduced in size to allow completion of extirpation of the organ.

McCall culdoplasty—The most commonly employed technique to reattach the uterosacral ligaments to the posterior vaginal cuff. This technique is useful in posterior enterocele prophylaxis.

The technique of operating through the vagina is a prerogative of the gynecologic surgeon. Vaginal surgery is an essential prerequisite in the cultural and surgical training of a qualified gynecologist. However, in the United States, the most common operation gynecologists perform, the hysterectomy, is predominantly done abdominally or with one of the various endoscopic techniques.

Vaginal hysterectomy is the signature operation of the gynecologic profession. Ample evidence shows that the vaginal approach results in lower morbidity, less pain, more rapid recovery, more rapid return to normal activities, consumption of fewer health care dollars and resources, and a host of other benefits. A gynecologic surgeon should have the ability to perform abdominal, endoscopic, and vaginal hysterectomies. However, vaginal hysterectomy is, and should remain, the hallmark of gynecologic extirpative hysterectomy surgery, and the ability to perform hysterectomy via the vaginal route is a measure of surgical excellence. Vaginal hysterectomy is the "gold standard" for the surgical removal of the uterus because it is minimally invasive when compared to all other routes and techniques. The vaginal route should be considered primary unless a specific contraindication to that approach is recognized. Surgeons' preference of route is not an indication for avoiding the vaginal approach.

INDICATIONS

With the advent of evidence-based research and outcome studies, several randomized controlled trials have documented the advantages of the vaginal approach to hysterectomy. A 2010 Cochrane review concluded that vaginal hysterectomy, rather than abdominal, should be performed whenever technically feasible to reduce complications, shorten hospital stays, and accelerate the patient's return to normal activities. Endoscopic approaches were recommended only in those cases where the vaginal approach was not practical. Unfortunately, these clear evidence-based recommendations have not stimulated a change in physician practice patterns. Several authors have addressed the reasons for the continued dominance of the abdominal route for hysterectomy. Johns and colleagues suggested that the route of hysterectomy is usually determined by the skill, experience, and preference of the operating gynecologist. Unfortunately, few other parameters really matter in day-to-day practice. Dorsey and associates stated that the hysterectomy patient is best served by a surgeon who selects the route with which he or she is most confident and comfortable; however, ideal surgical care remains the responsibility of the surgeon. With that in mind, training programs should do whatever is necessary to provide graduates with skill sets that give patients access to evidence-based care. Julian has addressed this concept in detail.

Suggesting that the competency and comfort of the surgeon to perform a vaginal hysterectomy is a requisite to selection of that route may restrict its implementation as a primary technique. Surgeons who prefer to use abdominal or laparoscopic techniques may therefore not choose the route that is most minimally invasive to the patient. Hysterectomy guidelines have been developed in order to identify when abdominal hysterectomy is truly mandated (Fig. 32B.1). Using these guidelines, expert gynecologic surgeons have achieved vaginal hysterectomy rates in excess of 90% without sacrificing quality of care. In contrast, the overall US average for the vaginal approach is approximately 30%, with that figure including laparoscopically assisted vaginal hysterectomy. More recent data indicate that the advent of robotic techniques will further complicate the selection of hysterectomy route in a way that does not rely on outcome data. In an era of pressure to consume fewer health care dollars, the more expensive abdominal, laparoscopic, and robotic approaches continue to flourish despite incontrovertible evidence that vaginal hysterectomy provides as good or better outcomes at less cost.

Vaginal hysterectomy traditionally has been indicated for women with uterine or pelvic organ prolapse, and traditional indications for abdominal hysterectomy have included an

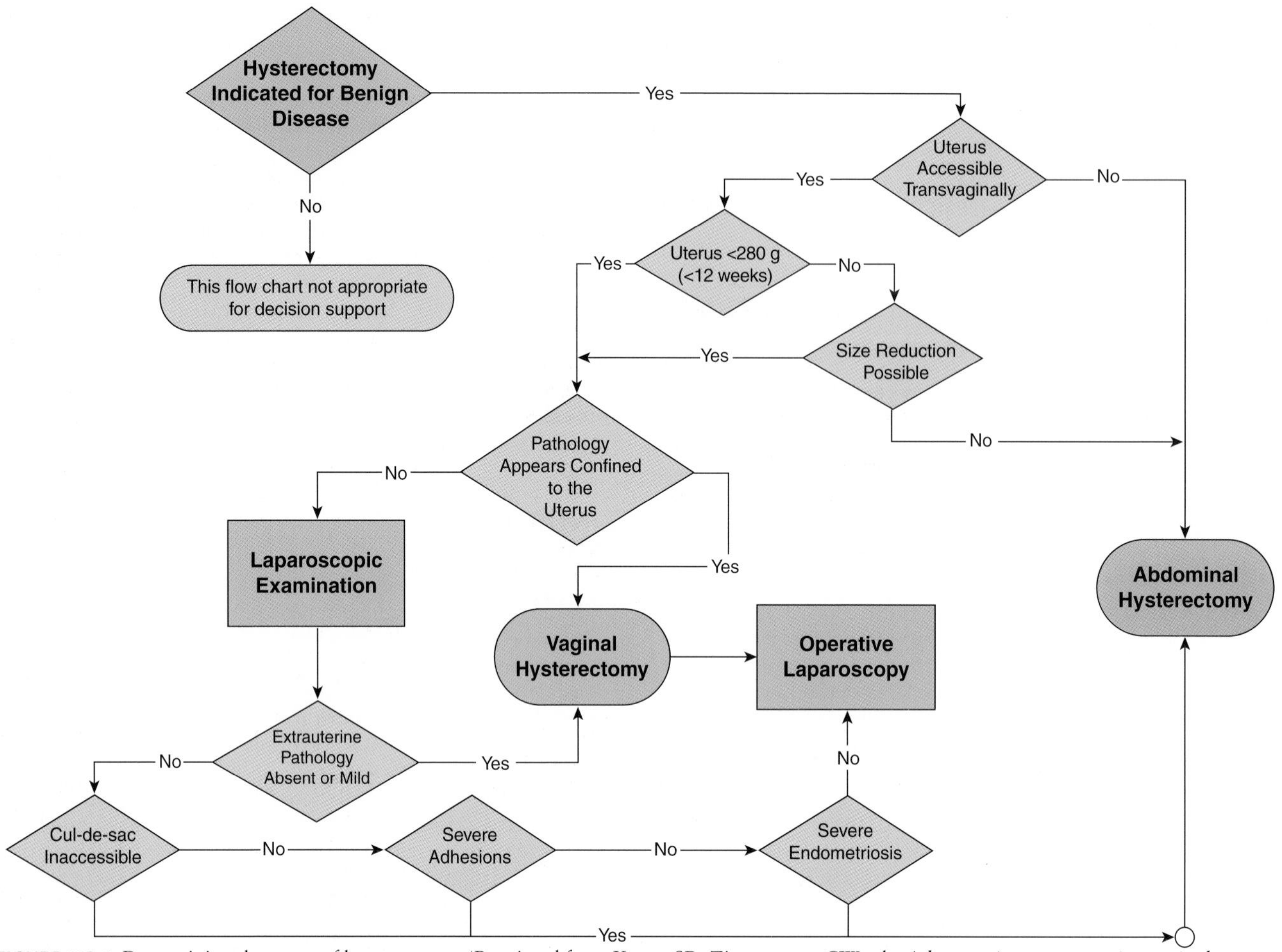

FIGURE 32B.1 Determining the route of hysterectomy. (Reprinted from Kovac SR, Zimmerman CW, eds. *Advances in reconstructive vaginal surgery*. Philadelphia, PA: Lippincott Williams & Wilkins, 2007;95, with permission. Copyright © 2007 Lippincott Williams & Wilkins.)

enlarged uterus, prior pelvic surgery, malignancy, and extrauterine disease, such as endometriosis or pelvic inflammatory disease. We now know that successful vaginal hysterectomy can be done in most of these patients; however, special techniques, such as uterine coring or morcellation, are often helpful, and such ancillary techniques as laparoscopic lymphadenectomy may be required in women with cervical or endometrial cancer. Laparoscopy may also be useful to help evaluate an adnexal mass prior to removal or the extent of endometriosis before completing the surgery with a vaginal hysterectomy and oophorectomy. Laparoscopy may also be used as an aid to reassure and give confidence to the less experienced vaginal surgeon to objectify the pelvic anatomy so that vaginal hysterectomy, in many cases, can be accomplished. With increasing confidence and skill that comes from experience, there are very few patients with indications for hysterectomy in whom the procedure cannot be performed vaginally.

PREOPERATIVE PREPARATION

If the surgeon is concerned about unintentionally injuring the rectum, it may be important for the patient to cleanse the rectum with an electrolyte purgative or a Phospho soda enema given the evening before surgery. Bowel cleansing evacuates solid stool from the rectum, reduces the bacterial load of the intestinal tract, and reduces the incidence of postoperative ileus and constipation.

A single-dose antibiotic as a prophylactic measure, usually a first-generation cephalosporin, should be given within 1 hour before the operation is started. Prophylactic antibiotics have been documented to reduce the risk of postoperative infections. The vaginal pH may be checked at a preoperative visit and prior to prepping the patient. If the pH is elevated above normal (3.8 to 4.2), the normal vaginal ecosystem has been altered. A vaginal pH in the range of 5.0 or greater suggests the potential for bacterial vaginosis and the likelihood that the facultative bacteria normally present in the vagina at concentrations of 10^3 have reached concentrations of 10^8. This finding strongly suggests that the vagina is infected before the start of the operation. These patients may not be protected by routine prophylactic antibiotics but may benefit from postoperative therapeutic antibiotics and ideally correction prior to arrival in the operating room. In such patients, consider administration of 500 mg of metronidazole orally twice daily from the second to the seventh postoperative day. This practice reduces the postoperative infection rate following vaginal hysterectomy.

Gynecologists have long believed that a Betadine solution used as a preoperative vaginal scrub will remove most potential pathogens in the vagina, but this has recently been questioned. Some surgeons prep patients with 70% ethanol, even in the vagina, and use a self-adherent surgical drape that covers the rectum and conveniently keeps pubic hair and the labia from interfering with the operative field. Shaving of the pubic hair is unnecessary, and shaven patients are more uncomfortable postoperatively. Clipping of pubic hair is preferred if hair removal is desired.

Copious lavage of the vaginal vault before, during, and after vaginal hysterectomy may also help to prevent postoperative infections by removing nonadherent bacteria from the vaginal epithelium. Lavage is not used as frequently in the vaginal approach as in other surgical approaches despite the fact that the vagina is a clean contaminated operative field.

The type of stirrups used for the lithotomy position is solely at the discretion of the surgeon. No matter what type is used, careful attention is required to protect vulnerable vascular, bony, and neurologic points in the lower extremities. Some surgeons prefer candy cane–type stirrups. The patient should be positioned with the buttocks at the end of the surgical table or just beyond. The table is placed at a zero horizontal position without Trendelenburg. In this manner, the surgeon can look directly into the vagina without having to look over the weighted speculum. Boot-type stirrups have achieved popularity and may also be used with the patient in the standard lithotomy position. Here, the femur is vertical, and the tibia/fibula horizontal and oriented toward the contralateral shoulder. Hyperflexion of the femur is discouraged with either type of stirrup. If a procedure lasts more than 4 hours, the risk of neurovascular injury increases. For that reason, every 90 minutes to 2 hours, lowering the legs from the standard lithotomy position into a low lithotomy position for a period of approximately 10 minutes should be considered. Also, final positioning of the patient should protect the patient, allowing the surgeon to operate comfortably, and provide adequate room for surgical assistants to be effective. Assistants need to stand inside the stirrups to see the operative field to both observe and learn the operation. Pneumatic compression stockings are also recommended.

OPERATIVE TECHNIQUE

An examination under anesthesia before initiating the operation to confirm the preoperative findings is recommended in all cases. Undetected pathology may be appreciated during an anesthetized exam along with a more complete assessment of the subtleties of the patient's anatomy. Placement of a tenaculum for applying traction on the cervix can document the degree of descensus. If more descensus is desired, strong traction on the cervix with vigorous massage of the uterosacral ligaments, especially the left uterosacral ligament, for approximately 30 seconds results in a further descensus of the cervix of approximately 2 to 3 cm.

Although some surgeons prefer to stand during vaginal hysterectomy, others prefer to sit. Assistants to the surgeon should be as comfortable as possible during the operation. The height of the operating table and the surgeon's chair should be adjusted accordingly. If sitting, an instrument tray may be placed on the surgeon's lap, making it easier to have access to the desired instruments during the operation. The number of instruments used during vaginal surgery should be kept at a minimum to prevent instruments from obscuring the surgeon's vision.

Catheterization of the bladder before the initiation of vaginal hysterectomy is performed at the preference of the surgeon. Sometimes, it is easier to identify unintentional cystotomy when the bladder is moderately distended (approximately 200 mL) with urine, dyed fluid, or sterile infant milk. If the bladder becomes too distended, catheter drainage of the bladder may improve the visibility within the restricted operative space. If a cystotomy occurs, it is usually best to complete

the vaginal hysterectomy before proceeding with repair of the bladder. In many cases, the cystotomy may make the bladder dissection easier because now, the location of the bladder is clear and the correct plane of dissection is more easily visualized. Sometimes, a finger in the bladder may also facilitate a difficult vesicocervical or vesicouterine dissection. The bladder must be mobilized adequately around the area of operative injury so that the surgeon can completely evaluate the extent of the cystotomy and be certain that the repair is completed without excess tension on the injured site.

The initial anterior vaginal incision should be made through the full thickness of the vaginal epithelium at the border of the vaginal rugae and the smooth epithelium covering the cervix (**Fig. 32B.2**). An initial circumscribing cervical incision made on the cervix at the junction of rugae and smooth epithelium preserves vaginal length and helps avoid unintentional entry into the bladder anteriorly and rectum posteriorly. In addition, an incision at the point where the vaginal rugae begin to reflect away from the smooth epithelium of the cervix appropriately places the epithelial incision closer to the point of entry into the posterior and anterior peritoneum (**Fig. 32B.3**). An incision in this location allows the surgeon to avoid excessive dissection of the connective tissues between the vagina and the peritoneum, reduces blood loss from cervical artery branches, shortens operative time, and facilitates identification of the peritoneal entry points.

Julian has reported on the benefit of infiltrating the vaginal wall with a mixture of 1:200,000 epinephrine diluted in normal saline to control small blood vessel bleeding from the vagina. However, in our experience, oozing from the incised

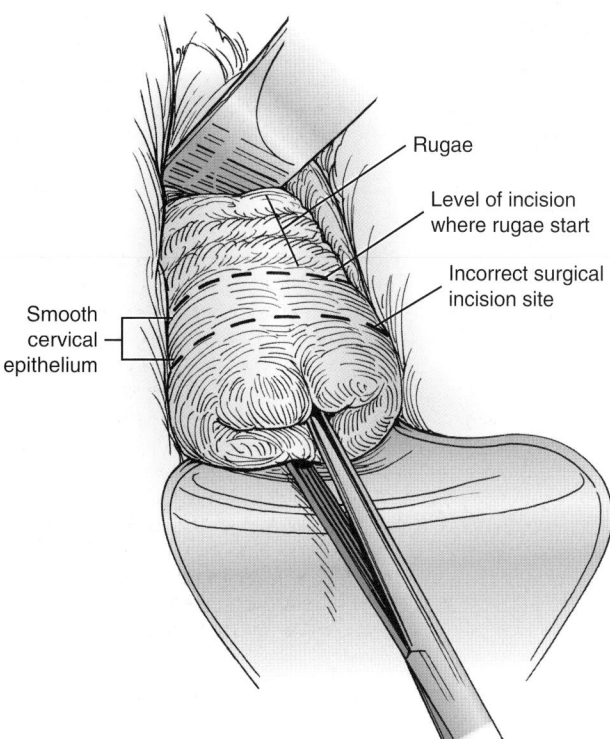

FIGURE 32B.2 Initial incision should be a full-thickness incision at the border where the vaginal rugae begin and the smooth cervical epithelium on the cervix ends. (Reprinted from Kovac SR, Zimmerman CW, eds. *Advances in reconstructive vaginal surgery.* Philadelphia, PA: Lippincott Williams & Wilkins, 2007, with permission. Copyright © 2007 Lippincott Williams & Wilkins.)

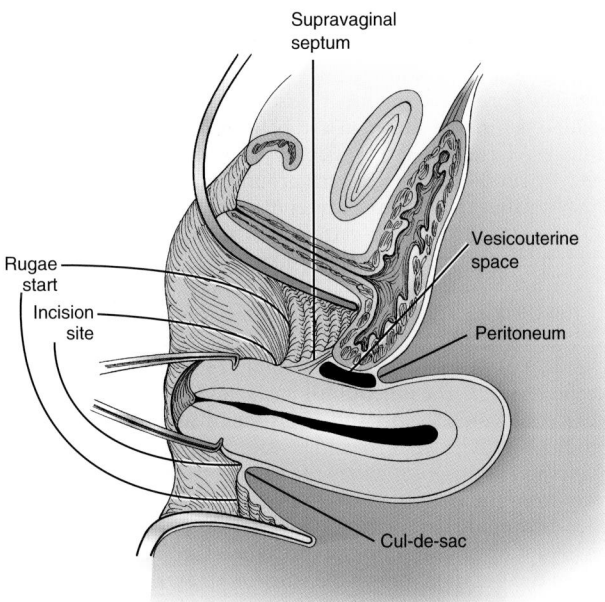

FIGURE 32B.3 Relationship between the vaginal rugae and the anterior and posterior peritoneum. (Reprinted from Kovac SR, Zimmerman CW, eds. *Advances in reconstructive vaginal surgery*. Philadelphia, PA: Lippincott Williams & Wilkins, 2007, with permission. Copyright © 2007 Lippincott Williams & Wilkins.)

vaginal epithelium rarely results in significant blood loss when the incision is made where the vaginal rugae start. If oozing from the incised edges of the vagina becomes a problem, it is easy to control with electrocautery.

At the beginning of the operation, when the cervix is still within the vagina, a circumscribing incision around the cervix is difficult to perform with a scalpel or electrocautery instrument because it is difficult to maintain either device perpendicular to the circumscribing vaginal incision. This issue is not a concern when the cervix protrudes from the vagina. However, when the cervix cannot be brought out of the vagina with traction, the initial incision should be made on the anterior vaginal wall from approximately the 10- to 2-o'clock position and on the posterior vaginal wall between the 8- and 4-o'clock positions. These incisions provide adequate space for transection of the paracolpium allowing the cervix to descend for subsequent entry into the posterior and anterior peritoneum and ligation of the uterine vasculature at the appropriate time (Fig. 32B.4A, B).

After completing the vaginal incisions, the cervical tenaculum is replaced on the posterior lip of the cervix with taut traction of the cervix achieved by elevating the tenaculum anteriorly. If the posterior incision in the vagina is placed at the appropriate level where rugae are not present and at the point where the uterosacral ligaments join the cervix, the posterior cul-de-sac and peritoneum can readily be identified with an Allis clamp or tissue forceps. This step is facilitated by putting the vaginal epithelium and accompanying peritoneum on stretch as the peritoneum bulges outward

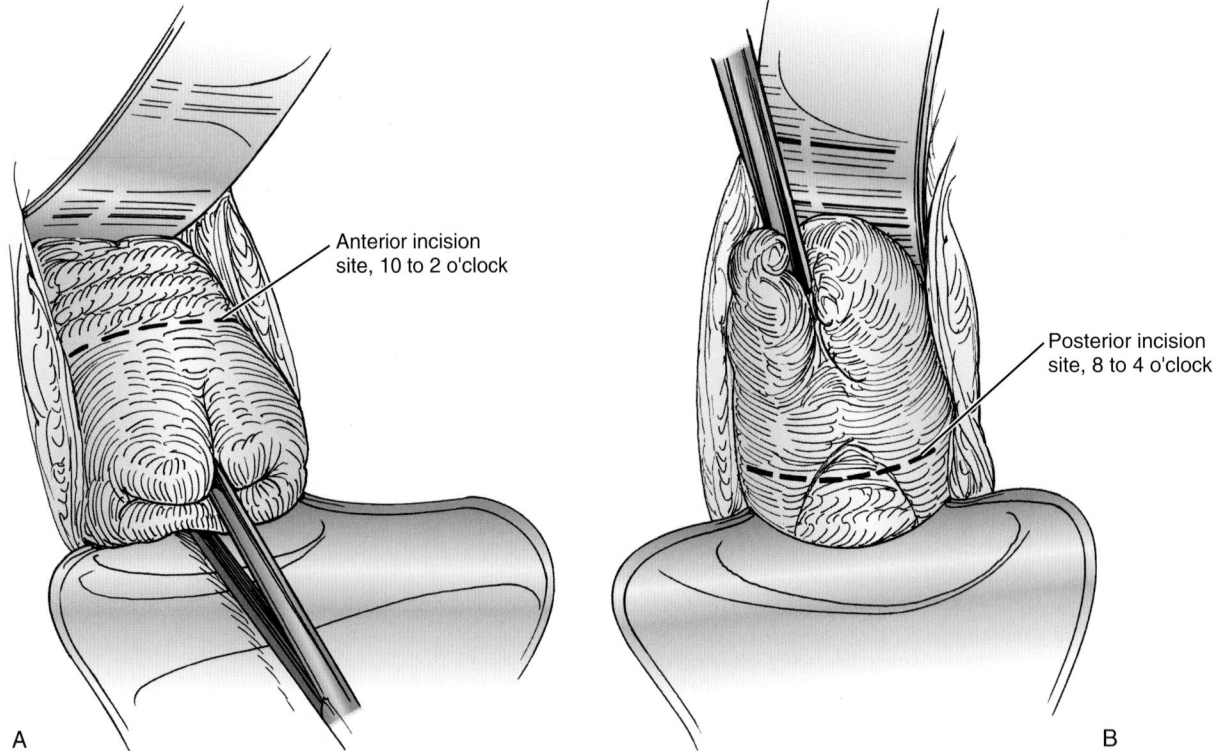

FIGURE 32B.4 A: When the cervix remains within the vagina when traction is applied with a tenaculum, the anterior full-thickness vaginal incision needs only to be performed between 10 and 2 o'clock. **B:** Initial full-thickness vaginal incision needs only to be performed between the 8- and 4-o'clock position. Note this incision is placed posteriorly where the vaginal rugae begin and where the uterosacral ligaments attach to the cervix. (Reprinted from Kovac SR, Zimmerman CW, eds. *Advances in reconstructive vaginal surgery*. Philadelphia, PA: Lippincott Williams & Wilkins, 2007:106, with permission. Copyright © 2007 Lippincott Williams & Wilkins.)

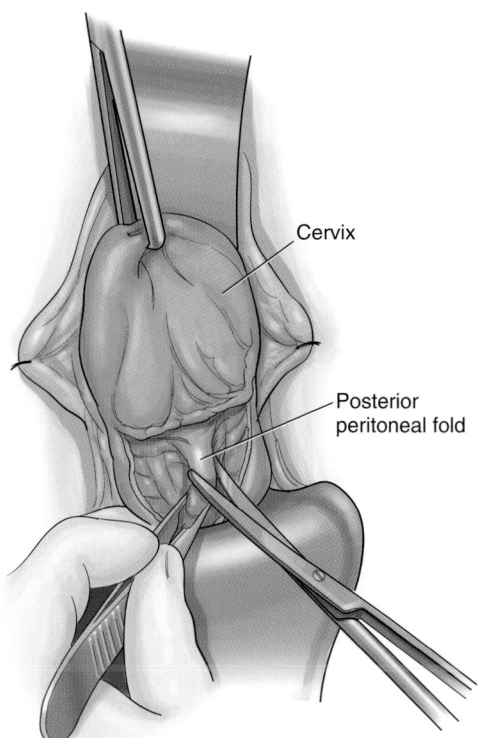

FIGURE 32B.5 With traction on the cervix anteriorly, the posterior peritoneal fold is grasped with tissue forceps, and the peritoneum is entered by incising with scissors the peritoneal fold directly above the tissue forceps. (Reprinted from Kovac SR, Zimmerman CW, eds. *Advances in reconstructive vaginal surgery.* Philadelphia, PA: Lippincott Williams & Wilkins, 2007:107, with permission. Copyright © 2007 Lippincott Williams & Wilkins.)

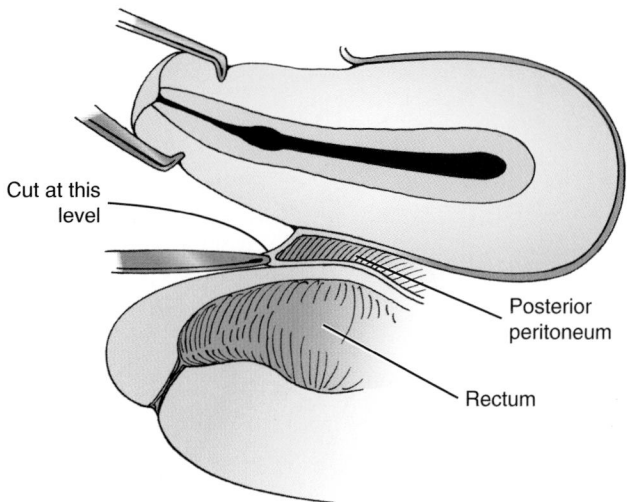

FIGURE 32B.6 Transverse view of entering the peritoneal cavity. (Reprinted from Kovac SR, Zimmerman CW, eds. *Advances in reconstructive vaginal surgery.* Philadelphia, PA: Lippincott Williams & Wilkins, 2007:107, with permission. Copyright © 2007 Lippincott Williams & Wilkins.)

toward the surgeon (**Fig. 32B.5**). The importance of properly performing this step cannot be overstated. Entry into the posterior peritoneum is best accomplished by an incision directly above the tissue forceps that grasps the outward U-shaped bulge of the peritoneal fold (**Fig. 32B.6**). If the incision is placed closer to the cervix in an attempt to prevent injury to the rectum, the dissection often proceeds into the posterior cervical stroma. Unfortunately, an incision placed nearer to the cervix frequently results in a retroperitoneal dissection, which continues in this plane and ultimately pushes the peritoneum superiorly and posteriorly, obscuring identification of the peritoneum and frustrating the surgeon. Should this occur, the posterior lip of the cervix and vagina can be cut in a vertical direction that exposes the peritoneum at a higher level so it can be recognized and entered directly. This procedure is a cervicocolpotomy (**Fig. 32B.7**).

The posterior peritoneum is then opened with curved scissors, and a long-bladed Steiner Auvard weighted speculum is introduced into the posterior peritoneal cavity. Examination of the cul-de-sac can reveal further pathology, for example, endometriosis, leiomyomata, or adnexal pathology—that may need to be addressed later in the operation. Identification of the uterosacral ligaments by palpation can be accomplished during examination of the cul-de-sac by placing a digit medial to the ligament and identifying the rectouterine fold through the posterior colpotomy incision.

Oozing of blood from the posterior incision between the vagina and peritoneum may occur. Placement of a weighted speculum into the posterior peritoneal cavity will compress

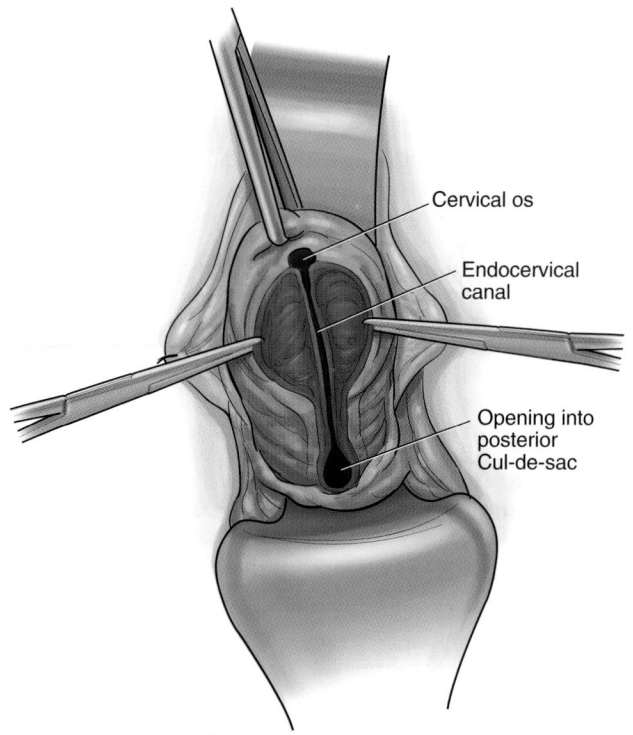

FIGURE 32B.7 Cervical colpotomy for entry into the posterior peritoneum. The posterior cervix is grasped with Allis clamps approximately at 4- and 8-o'clock positions. The cervix is incised starting at the 6-o'clock position and incising the cervix and posterior wall of the uterus until the posterior peritoneum is entered. Once the peritoneum is entered, a weighted speculum is placed into the posterior peritoneal cavity. (Reprinted from Kovac SR, Zimmerman CW, eds. *Advances in reconstructive vaginal surgery.* Philadelphia, PA: Lippincott Williams & Wilkins, 2007:108, with permission. Copyright © 2007 Lippincott Williams & Wilkins.)

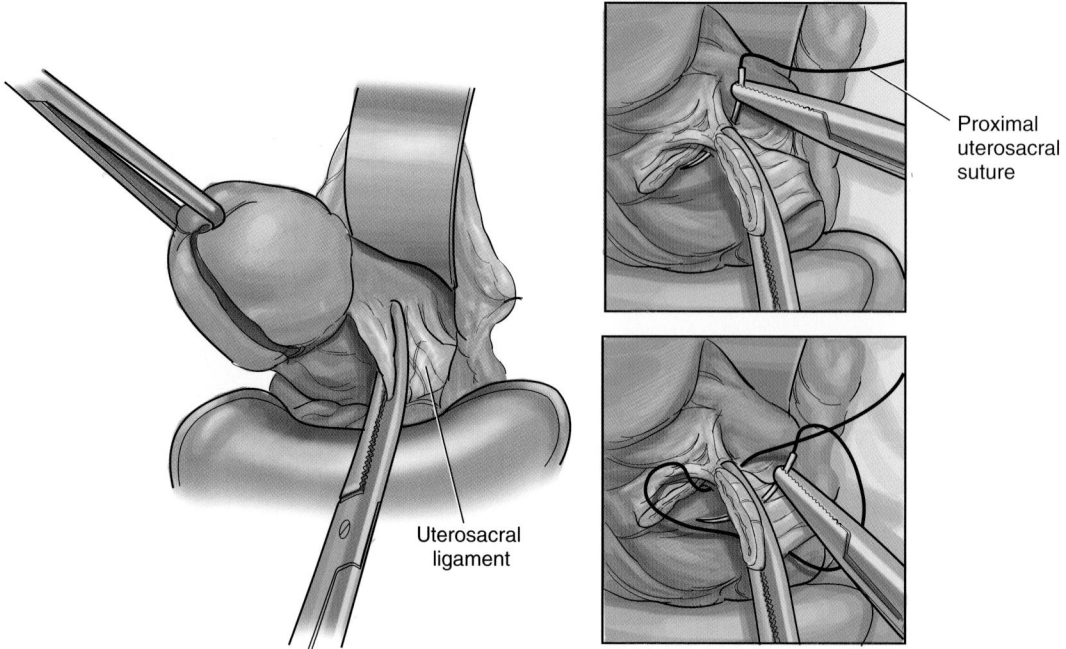

Proximal
uterosacral
suture

Uterosacral
ligament

FIGURE 32B.8 The uterosacral ligament is clamped, cut and ligated. Note that the tip of the clamp closely approximates the cervix. The suture ligature is initially placed with the clamp in an almost vertical orientation for maximum exposure to the anterior blade of the clamp but as the needle comes through the pedicle, the clamp is rotated more horizontally to provide better exposure to the underside of the pedicle for easy retrieval of the needle. (Reprinted from Kovac SR, Zimmerman CW, eds. *Advances in reconstructive vaginal surgery*. Philadelphia, PA: Lippincott Williams & Wilkins, 2007:109, with permission. Copyright © 2007 Lippincott Williams & Wilkins.)

most bleeding points in this area until completion of the surgery and cuff closure. If the vaginal epithelium has not been completely circumscribed, once posterior dissection has been developed, the vaginal epithelial incision should be completed by connecting the previous anterior and posterior incisions before the supportive ligaments of the uterus can be clamped.

Transection of the uterosacral ligaments is the single most important step in successfully completing a vaginal hysterectomy. The uterosacral ligament pedicle should be completed by placing the medial jaw of the clamp within the rectouterine fold while holding the clamp vertical and not try to swing around the cervix in a more horizontal plane. The medial tip of each clamp should be placed within the peritoneal cavity in the rectouterine fold and the lateral tip around the outside of the ligament. Special hysterectomy clamps have been developed to improve on the traditional Heaney clamp (**Fig. 32B.8A–C**). After transection of the pedicle, rotating the handles of the clamp laterally and superiorly facilitates suturing at the tip of the clamp. This rotation brings the tip of the clamp into full view and exposes a triangular area beneath the clamp for easier retrieval of the needle. Placement of a double clamp for uterine supportive or vascular structures is not necessary. Each uterosacral ligament should be secured by a transfixation suture to the posterolateral surface of the vagina and tied behind the clamp at about the 4- and 8-o'clock positions. Lateral traction on this suture provides the best exposure to the remaining structures that need to be transected to complete hysterectomy (**Fig. 32B.9**). This traction and the use of large hysterectomy clamps largely replace the need for lateral retractors in the vagina. Clamping and tagging the uterosacral ligaments separately allows for their identification, later use in cuff repair, and, if desired, a McCall culdoplasty at the end of the procedure. The uterosacral ligament pedicle is the only one that needs to be tagged during

a vaginal hysterectomy and the only one that may safely be placed under traction.

After making sure the tips of the clamps are within the posterior peritoneal cavity, the cardinal and pubocervical (bladder pillar) ligaments are clamped by placing a clamp horizontally

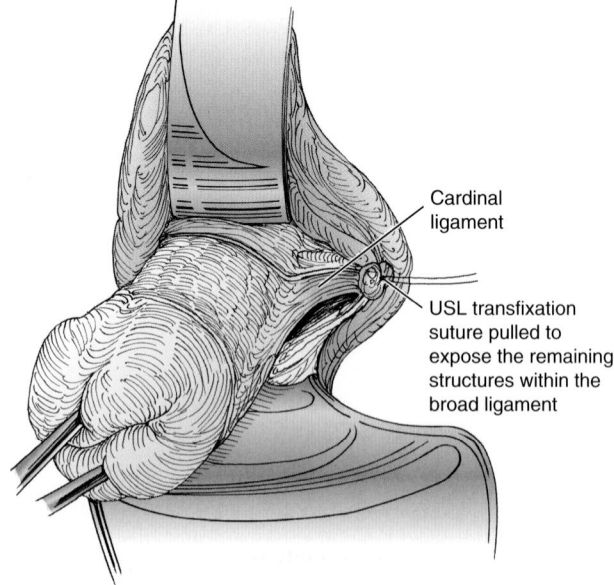

Cardinal
ligament

USL transfixation
suture pulled to
expose the remaining
structures within the
broad ligament

FIGURE 32B.9 Traction on the uterosacral ligament suture laterally exposes the cardinal ligament. (Reprinted from Kovac SR, Zimmerman CW, eds. *Advances in reconstructive vaginal surgery*. Philadelphia, PA: Lippincott Williams & Wilkins, 2007:116, with permission. Copyright © 2007 Lippincott Williams & Wilkins.)

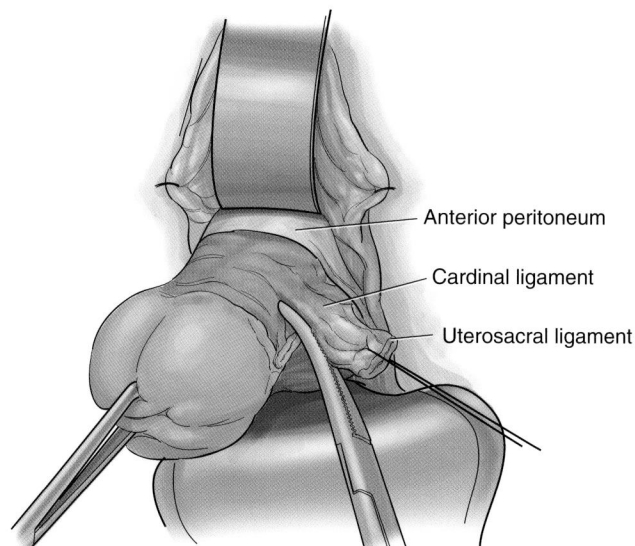

FIGURE 32B.10 With traction on the uterosacral pedicle, the cardinal ligament is exposed and can be clamped with the posterior jaw of the clamp in the posterior peritoneal cavity and the tip of the anterior jaw at the edge of the cervix. (Reprinted from Kovac SR, Zimmerman CW, eds. *Advances in reconstructive vaginal surgery.* Philadelphia, PA: Lippincott Williams & Wilkins, 2007:110, with permission. Copyright © 2007 Lippincott Williams & Wilkins.)

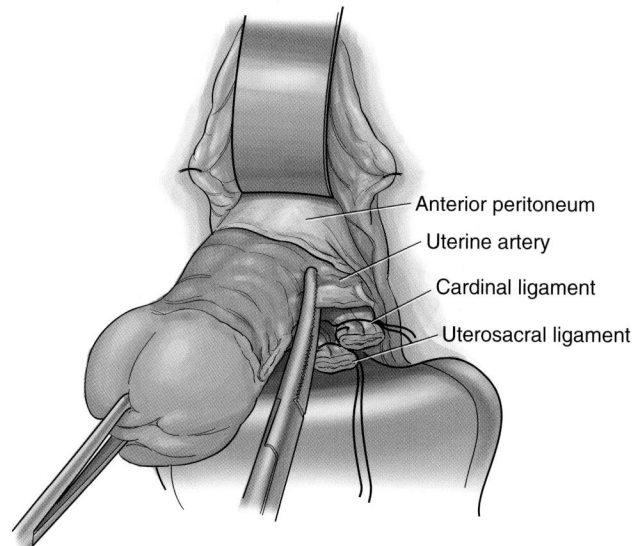

FIGURE 32B.11 If exposure is good after the cardinal ligaments have been divided, the uterine vessels may be clamped before the anterior peritoneum is entered. (Reprinted from Kovac SR, Zimmerman CW, eds. *Advances in reconstructive vaginal surgery.* Philadelphia, PA: Lippincott Williams & Wilkins, 2007:136, with permission. Copyright © 2007 Lippincott Williams & Wilkins.)

and clamping from the apex of the uterosacral pedicle to a point on the anterior cervix medial to the bladder pillar encompassing all the remaining connective tissue of the paracolpium (Fig. 32B.10). If already entered, the anterior peritoneum should not be pulled into this clamp at this point of the operation. A complete anterior dissection is needed to safely complete this pedicle. Bringing the anterior and posterior peritoneal edges together should only be accomplished with the uterine artery pedicle as this maneuver serves to seal off the broad ligament and effectively prevents bleeding from the vascular plexus located within the leaves of the broad ligament. Because the anterior peritoneum usually begins at the level of the uterine vessels, there is not enough peritoneal mobility to bring both the anterior and posterior peritoneal surfaces together at the level of the cardinal ligaments. Therefore, to be certain that the surgeon can seal both leaves of the broad ligament together with the uterine artery, it is best to avoid any attempt to bring the peritoneal edges together when the uterosacral or cardinal ligament is clamped. A simple suture ligature first at the tip and then around the end of the clamp is usually sufficient for hemostasis of the cardinal ligament without the need for transfixation. This suture ligature is not tagged or held.

If exposure is good, the uterine arteries may be clamped, divided, and ligated at the point before entering the peritoneum anteriorly under the bladder. They are best clamped in their entirety and under direct visualization. In contrast to the uterosacral and cardinal/pubocervical clamps that are placed perpendicular to the body of the cervix, the uterine artery clamp is placed parallel to the long axis of the uterus as the tip of the clamp secures the uterine artery as it bifurcates into ascending and descending branches (Fig. 32B.11). As traction is placed on the uterus when the artery is cut, there is a definite sensation that the uterus descends signifying that the entire uterine vascular bundle has been transected, including the ascending and descending branches. If descent of the

uterus is not noted, often an additional portion of the uterine artery remains and must be secured with another clamp. A single well-tied suture is all that is required for the uterine artery pedicle. Limiting the tissue within the clamp to the vascular bundle helps to make the pedicle manageable and the suture ligature more secure. Many surgeons try to include middle portions of the broad ligament with the uterine artery because they feel a need to place clamps on the remaining portions of the broad ligament as they proceed up on each side of the uterus.

Complete development by dissection of the vesicocervical and vesicouterine spaces is a prerequisite to identifying and opening the anterior peritoneum. This step is perceived to be the most difficult portion of the vaginal hysterectomy procedure. Adequate exposure, by division of the paracolpium and full dissection of the anterior avascular spaces, makes this key step of hysterectomy much easier to complete.

The cervix should then be retracted downward and inferiorly, and the anterior subvaginal tissue, including the supravaginal septum and the bladder, elevated in the midline and placed on a small amount of tension with an Allis clamp or tissue forceps and elevated. The supravaginal septum is part of the pericervical ring and is identified and incised using curved scissors with the tips pointing downward toward the body of the cervix. The handles of the scissors are not elevated above the horizontal axis because that maneuver would increase the likelihood of dissection into the body of the cervix (Fig. 32B.12). Dissection in the proper plane using gentle traction and countertraction exposes the vesicouterine space, the proper avascular cleavage plane to bloodlessly elevate the bladder away from the anterior uterus and thereby gain access to the anterior peritoneum. Gentle push and spread of the blades of the scissors will allow identification of the proper plane of dissection. Bleeding is a warning sign of deviation anteriorly toward the bladder, posteriorly toward the cervix, or laterally toward the bladder pillars. After the vesicouterine

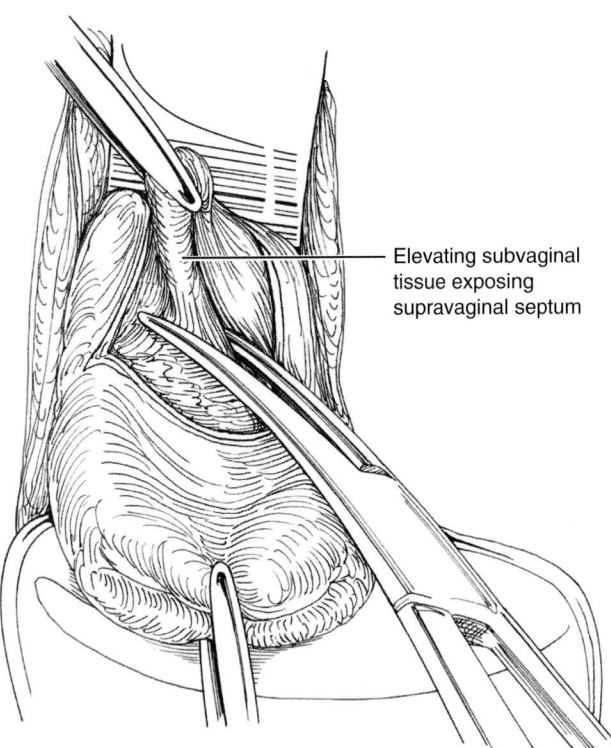

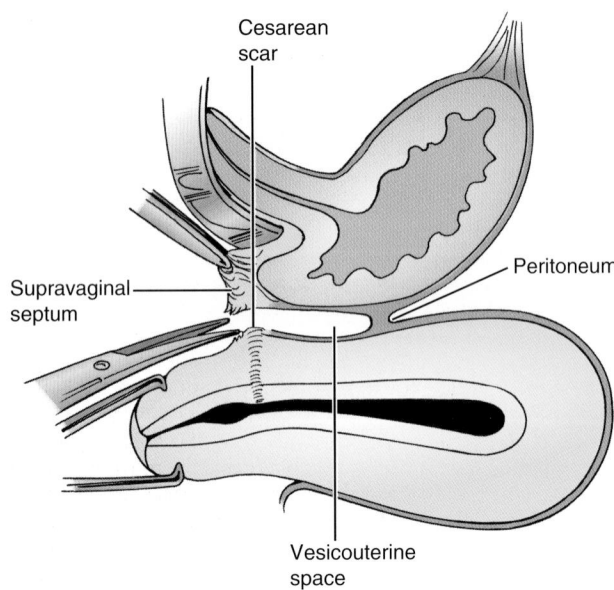

FIGURE 32B.13 Relationship between the supravaginal septum, vesicouterine space, cesarean section scar, and anterior peritoneal fold. (From Kovac SR, Zimmerman CW, eds. *Advances in reconstructive vaginal surgery*. Philadelphia, PA: Lippincott Williams & Wilkins, 2007:109. Copyright © 2007 Lippincott Williams & Wilkins.)

FIGURE 32B.12 Entry into the anterior peritoneum involves incising the supravaginal septum to gain entry into the vesicouterine space. Once the vesicouterine space has been entered, the space is developed by spreading the dissecting scissors for placement of a retractor to elevate the bladder. (From Kovac SR, Zimmerman CW, eds. *Advances in reconstructive vaginal surgery*. Philadelphia: Lippincott Williams & Wilkins; 2006:109.)

plane is fully developed, a lightweight right-angled retractor can be placed into this space to elevate the bladder and expose the anterior peritoneal fold.

If the patient had a previous cesarean section, the scar of this procedure can be readily visualized and identified separately from the bladder (Fig. 32B.13). Controlled dissection of a cesarean section scar is easier and more directly visible from the vaginal than from the abdominal or endoscopic approach. A low transverse cervical cesarean section incision is made in the portion of the cervix near the isthmus of the uterus. For that reason, in the nonpregnant state, the scar is close to the anterior vaginal incision used to develop the vesicocervical and vesicouterine avascular spaces in vaginal hysterectomy and can be readily identified and dissected. A cesarean section scar distorts the anatomy by occluding the vesicouterine space between the scar and the urinary bladder. Further dissection above the scar can be performed by identifying the scar, the bladder, and the peritoneum as independent structures. On occasion, it is also possible to dissect under the scar, which keeps the dissection even further from the urinary bladder (Fig. 32B.14). Sheth has described the utility of the broad ligament space in the presence of cesarean scar. Gentle lateral pressure along the side of the cervix and uterine body will allow the anterior leaf of the broad ligament to separate lateral to the cesarean scar. At that point, digital or instrument dissection can proceed medially above the scar and often allow complete isolation of the scar. Classical and low vertical cesarean and myomectomy scars present further

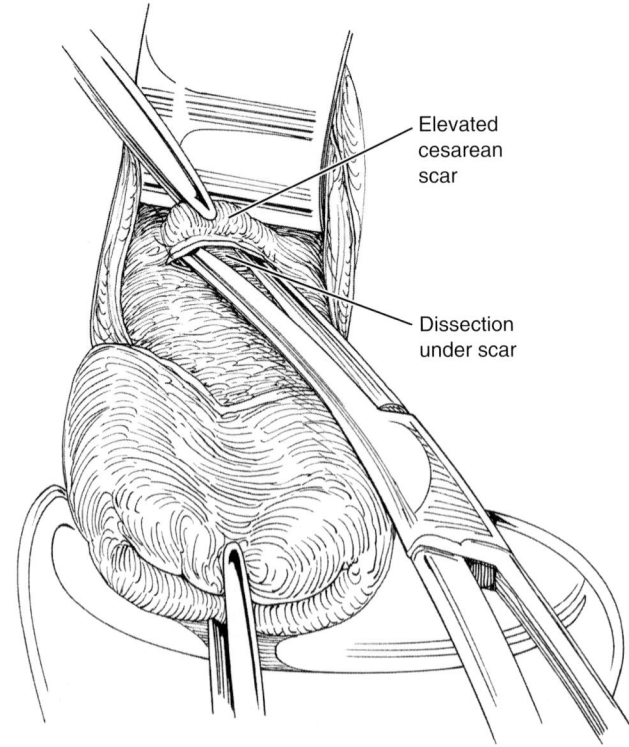

FIGURE 32B.14 Sometimes it is possible to dissect beneath the cesarean section scar to gain entry into the superior part of the vesicouterine space to identify the anterior peritoneal fold. (From Kovac SR, Zimmerman CW, eds. *Advances in reconstructive vaginal surgery*. Philadelphia: Lippincott Williams & Wilkins; 2006:110.)

challenges that must be individualized based on case-by-case findings.

After dissection of the vesicouterine space, the anterior peritoneum is grasped under direct vision and entered via a 1-cm opening with the scissors. The shining surface of the peritoneum is recognizable after all adventitial tissue is dissected away and may be identified visually or with the so-called silk sac sign prior to incision. Upon confirmation of entry into the peritoneal cavity by seeing intraperitoneal fat, the opening is further stretched by spreading of the scissors into this space to allow insertion of the right-angle retractor into the anterior cul-de-sac. This retractor should remain in this position for the remainder of the hysterectomy in order to safely elevate the bladder out of the operative field. Proper dissection and peritoneal entry reduce the risk of operative injury to the bladder and ureters (Fig. 32B.15A, B). Because of the surgeon's desire to avoid injury to the bladder, there is the tendency to dissect as far as possible from the bladder. This move may cause the surgeon to enter into the connective tissue capsule of the cervix and myometrium of the lower uterine segment. Further retroperitoneal dissection in this area will cause bleeding and further delay anterior peritoneal entry. Similar to the posterior dissection, this problem is more likely when the initial incision into the vagina is made too close to the cervix. Further dissection beneath the peritoneum covering of the anterior uterine segment results in failure to enter the anatomic vesicouterine space between the bladder and uterus. Excessive

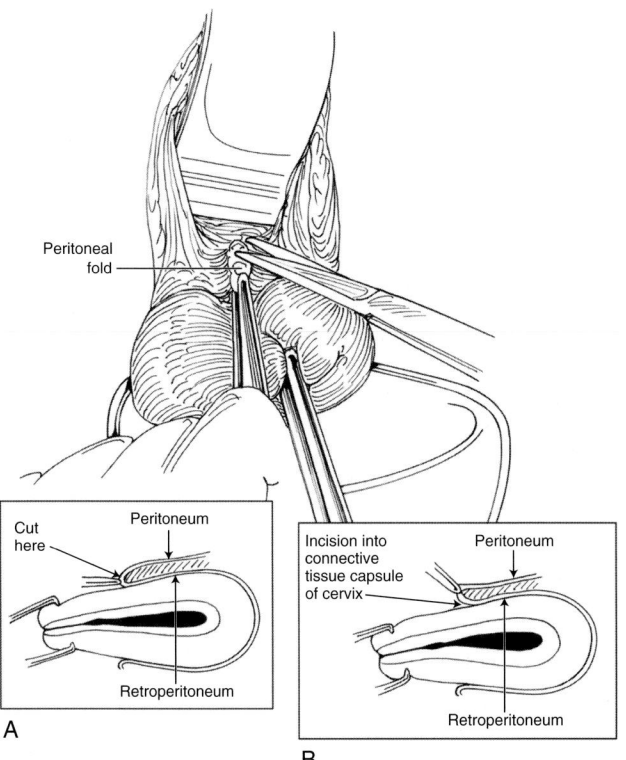

FIGURE 32B.15 Entry into the anterior peritoneum. Peritoneal fold is grasped with tissue forceps and pulled downward. Scissors incise peritoneal fold just above tissue forceps. **A:** Lateral view demonstrating the method for entering the anterior peritoneum. **B:** Retroperitoneal dissection with elevation of the peritoneal fold. (From Kovac SR, Zimmerman CW, eds. *Advances in reconstructive vaginal surgery.* Philadelphia: Lippincott Williams & Wilkins; 2006:110.)

bleeding, frustration, and a lack of progress will occur. Failure to identify the correct tissue plane or a lack of caution results in either further retroperitoneal dissection or unintentional bladder penetration. Cystoscopy may be performed at any point in the process of anterior dissection to confirm integrity or injury to the bladder and ureters.

If an injury to the bladder results, it will likely occur well above the trigone of the bladder and not near the ureteral orifices. Cystoscopy will reveal the exact location. This injury is simple to repair after the uterus has been removed. Unintentional operative cystotomy is a risk of any type of hysterectomy with any technique or approach. The overall incidence of operative cystotomy while performing and teaching this technique has resulted in a cystotomy rate of 1.2% with vaginal hysterectomies. Gilmour and others have documented the value of cystoscopy at the time of hysterectomy in recognizing urinary tract injury during the operation rather than later after the patient has left the operating room. Additionally, the overall rate of urinary tract injury was lower for the vaginal approach than in any other route of hysterectomy.

The use of a sponge on the surgeon's finger to push through the supravaginal septum and bluntly dissect the vesicouterine space superiorly to expose the anterior peritoneum is frequently taught. This technique could be considered as more of a technique of *accomplir forcee* (i.e., to accomplish with force) than a surgical dissection, as the cleavage plane becomes indistinguishable from the supravaginal septum up to the anterior peritoneal fold. No effort is made to visually or surgically identify any of the involved planes or tissues. The risk of tearing the bladder with this technique is potentially increased, especially if the patient had a previous cesarean section. Furthermore, the risk of not recognizing the injury is likely increased. The anterior peritoneum should always be opened under direct vision, never blindly, as unintentional entry into the bladder frequently results from an attempt to enter the peritoneum blindly.

Persistent attempts to open the anterior peritoneum if there is doubt that the peritoneal fold is clearly identified are unnecessary. Transecting the uterosacral and cardinal ligaments and perhaps the uterine vascular bundle prior to entering the anterior peritoneum will bring the uterus and peritoneal fold closer to the surgeon providing better exposure, thus simplifying this step of the procedure. Eventually, during this sequence of steps, the peritoneum will be identified and entry will be possible at some later point in the operation than is customary. Anterior peritoneal entry can also be safely facilitated, especially when the uterus is enlarged by adenomyosis or leiomyomata, with a vertical incision in the vaginal epithelium similar to the one used in an anterior colporrhaphy (Fig. 32B.16). This additional room for dissection of the bladder away from the cervix allows accurate identification of the bladder from the peritoneal fold. The surgeon may use a finger or a malleable uterine sound or retractor inserted through the posterior cul-de-sac and bent over the fundus of the uterus into the anterior cul-de-sac to help identify the exact location of the peritoneal fold. This step is especially useful in difficult cases or those in which the proper plane of dissection has not developed.

After both the posterior and anterior peritonea have been successfully entered, detachment of the uterus from its supportive ligaments can be accomplished if they have not already been surgically transected. As stated earlier, we prefer to secure and divide the uterosacral and cardinal ligaments before attempts to enter the anterior peritoneum. This extraperitoneal approach provides significant additional exposure for anterior peritoneal entry. Separating the cervix

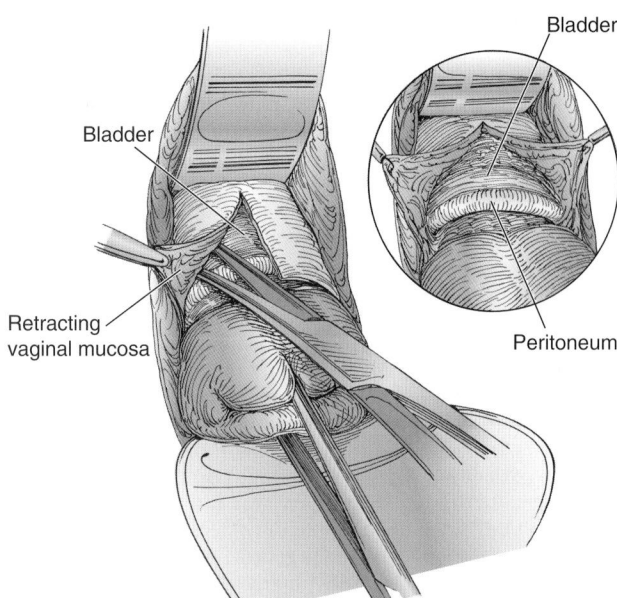

FIGURE 32B.16 Opening the anterior vaginal wall to expose the bladder and anterior peritoneal fold. (Reprinted from Kovac SR, Zimmerman CW, eds. *Advances in reconstructive vaginal surgery.* Philadelphia, PA: Lippincott Williams & Wilkins, 2007, with permission. Copyright © 2007 Lippincott Williams & Wilkins.)

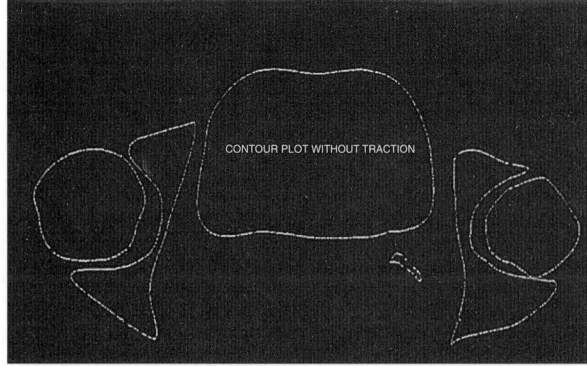

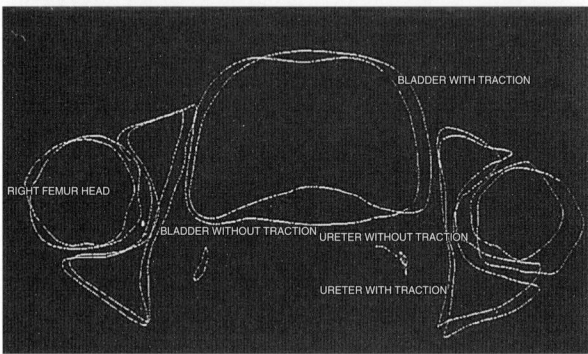

FIGURE 32B.17 A: Magnetic resonance imaging (MRI) studies of ureteral movement when downward traction is placed on the uterus. Ureter position is seen on the right. **B:** Overlay of MRI films. Traction on the uterus with a brass tenaculum is applied to the cervix. Note indentation to the bladder from the uterus and lateral and upward displacement of the ureter compared with the position of the ureter without traction to the uterus. (Reprinted from Kovac SR, Zimmerman CW, eds. *Advances in reconstructive vaginal surgery.* Philadelphia, PA: Lippincott Williams & Wilkins, 2007:112, with permission. Copyright © 2007 Lippincott Williams & Wilkins.)

from the paracolpium, along with the resulting descent of the uterus, increases visibility. This exposure is significant and makes the peritoneal identification/entry process less troublesome. The uterine artery can also be divided before anterior peritoneal entry, allowing even greater exposure. The key to successful vaginal hysterectomy is not to proceed in lock step through a draconian set of tasks but to identify structures and manipulate them surgically in the order that they present.

The exact location of the ureter during abdominal, laparoscopic, and vaginal hysterectomy is always a concern. Nichols and Randall suggested that the risk of ureteral injury during a vaginal hysterectomy is greater because the ureters may be pulled downward and medially by the tethering effect of the uterine artery. By studying the surgical anatomy of the ureter during vaginal hysterectomy, it has been determined with the use of imaging that the uterine artery is not the primary factor drawing the ureter closer to the uterus. Instead, traction on the cardinal ligament is the chief factor affecting movement of the ureter, suggesting there is a margin of safety during each step of a vaginal hysterectomy. This concept was confirmed by magnetic resonance imaging studies with a brass tenaculum placed on the cervix in a resting state and under traction. When traction was applied to the cervix, the ureter's position was displaced upward and lateral to the position of the ureter at rest (**Fig. 32B.17A, B**). This movement confirmed radiographically that the ureters were displaced further laterally and superiorly from the cervix to a position of surgical safety. When bladder retraction was used, this effect was more pronounced. During surgical identification of the ureter at the time of radical vaginal hysterectomy, it can be observed that once the uterosacral and cardinal ligament complex has been cut, the ureter actually moves further out of harm's way. If the ureters have not been dissected and identified before the cutting of uterosacral and cardinal ligaments, it is difficult to dissect and visualize them vaginally once the ligaments have

been cut during a vaginal hysterectomy because of this movement. Thus, it is evident that the uterosacral and cardinal ligaments, not the uterine artery, play a major role in determining the ureter's position during vaginal hysterectomy. Once these ligaments have been divided, the ureter will retract out of the operative field and make division of the uterine artery safer (**Fig. 32B.18A, B**).

Entry into the posterior peritoneum before clamping the uterosacral and cardinal ligaments is desirable. Anterior cervical and uterine plane dissection and placement of a retractor under the bladder also elevate the ureter out of the operative field (**Fig. 32B.19A, B**). Once the retractor is placed under the bladder, it should not be removed during any stage of the vaginal hysterectomy. During vaginal hysterectomy, if forceful traction is applied to the uterus with no retraction of the bladder, the ureter can be pulled medially and potentially placed in harm's way.

After posterior and anterior entry into the peritoneum and completely ligating the vascular pedicle, the remainder of the broad ligament may be dissected in the same manner familiar to the abdominal or endoscopic surgeon. Continued clamping up each side of the remaining broad ligament is not usually required for successful uterine removal. When the vaginal surgeon continues to place clamps above the uterine artery, the space to place each clamp becomes more restrictive, and placing sutures around these clamps becomes more difficult. This is

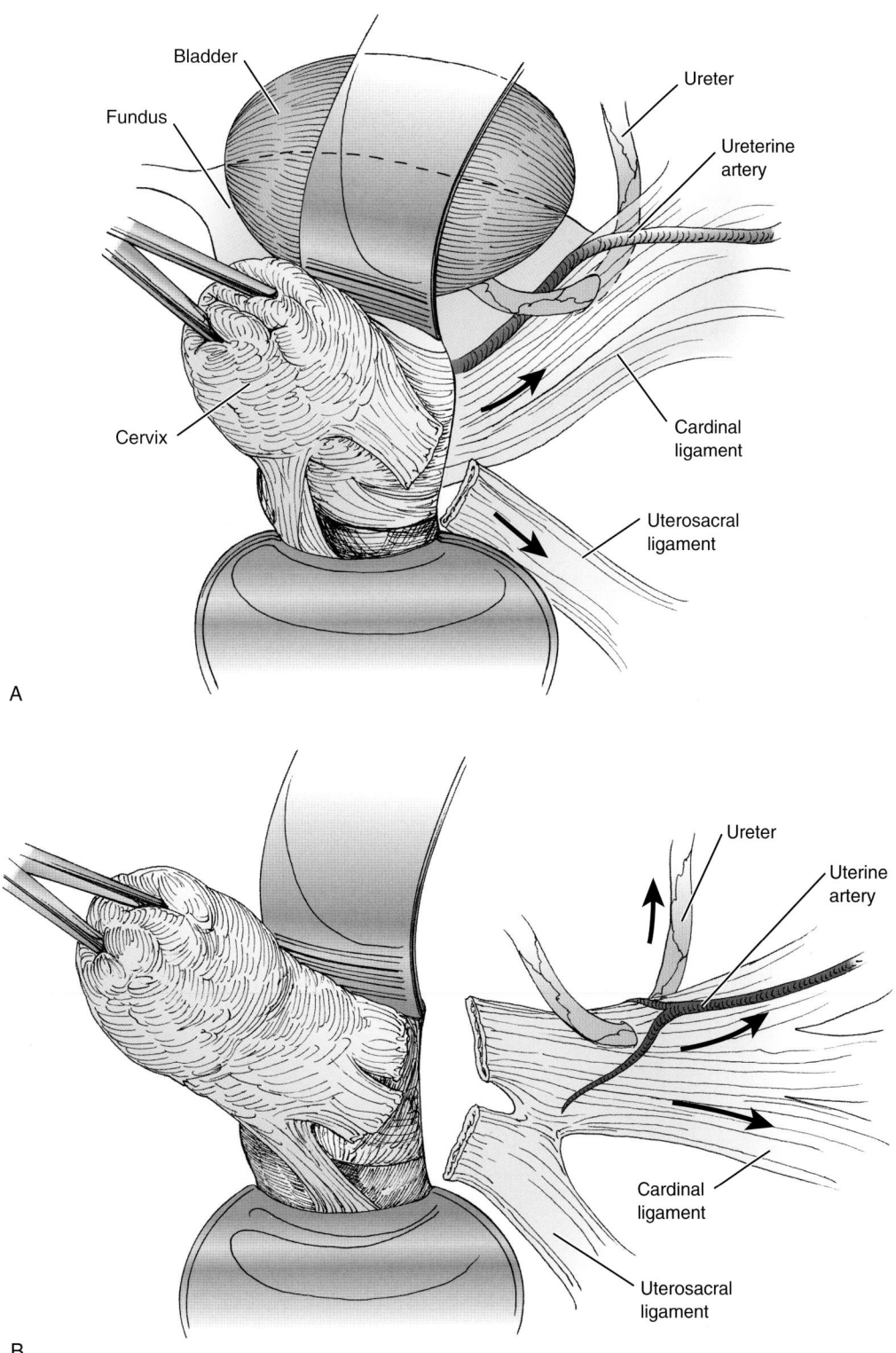

Bladder

Fundus

Cervix

Ureter

Ureterine artery

Cardinal ligament

Uterosacral ligament

A

Ureter

Uterine artery

Cardinal ligament

Uterosacral ligament

B

V

FIGURE 32B.18 A: Transection of the uterosacral ligament returns this structure to its original position. **B:** After both uterosacral and cardinal ligaments have been transected, ureters are displaced upward and lateral out of harm's way. (Reprinted from Kovac SR, Zimmerman CW, eds. *Advances in reconstructive vaginal surgery*. Philadelphia, PA: Lippincott Williams & Wilkins, 2007:113, with permission. Copyright © 2007 Lippincott Williams & Wilkins.)

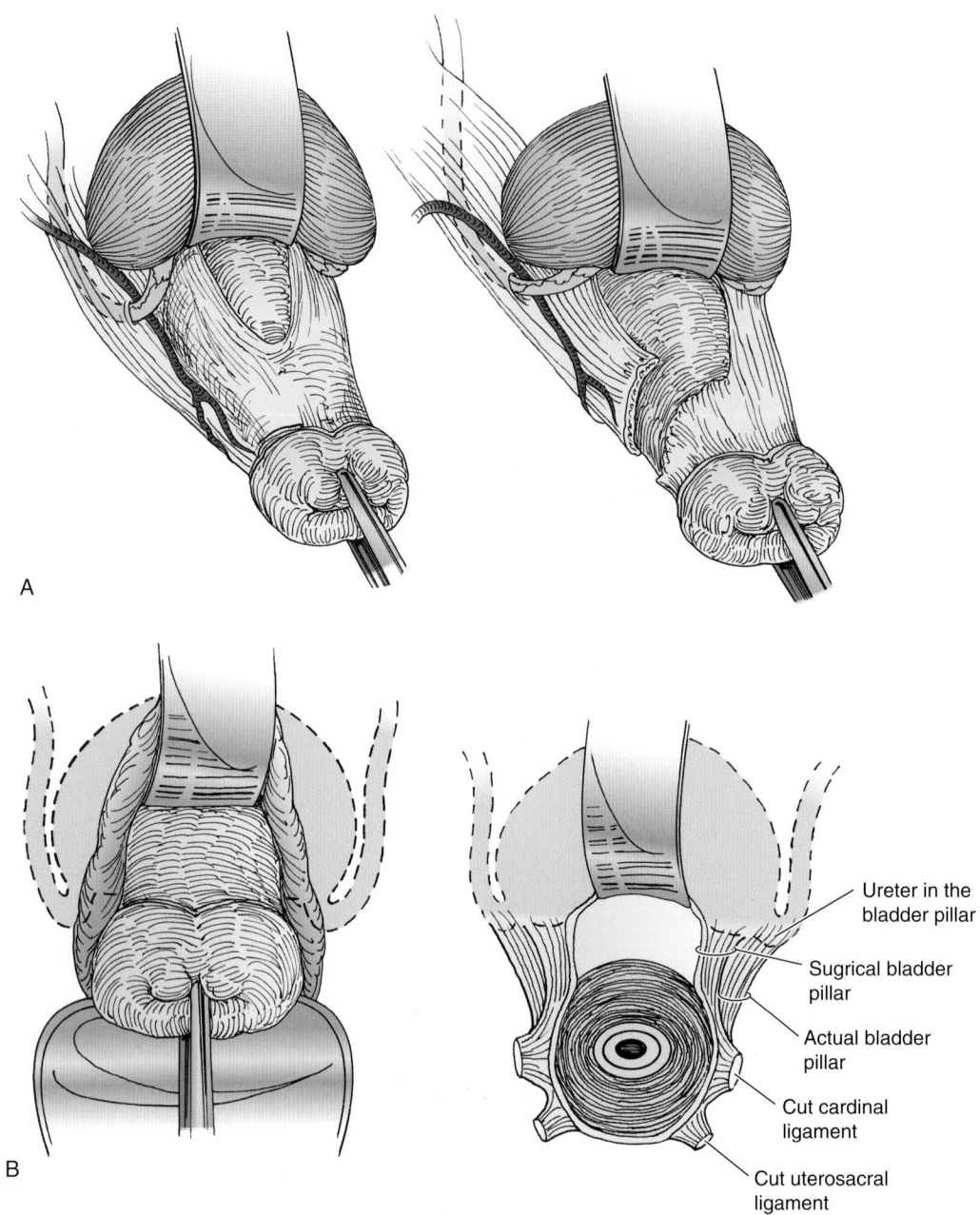

Ureter in the
bladder pillar

Sugrical bladder
pillar

Actual bladder
pillar

Cut cardinal
ligament

Cut uterosacral
ligament

A

B

FIGURE 32B.19 A, B: Note elevation of the ureters out of harm's way with upward traction on the bladder during vaginal hysterectomy. (Reprinted from Kovac SR, Zimmerman CW, eds. *Advances in reconstructive vaginal surgery*. Philadelphia, PA: Lippincott Williams & Wilkins, 2007:114, with permission. Copyright © 2007 Lippincott Williams & Wilkins.)

the type of problem that can create the conception that vaginal hysterectomy is a more difficult operation because of restrictive access and visibility. Clamping and suturing of the broad ligament above the uterine artery are unnecessary because there are only occasional significant blood vessels within the leaves of the broad ligament. There is no need to place clamps above the uterine artery until the round ligaments, fallopian tubes, and utero-ovarian pedicles are encountered, visualized, and prepared for ligation. Once the entire vascular bundle has been transected, a sufficient amount of tissue has been transected to allow rotation of the uterus posteriorly.

If the uterus is small and the uterine artery has been secured, the next step in uterine removal is to deliver the fundus

through the posterior or occasionally the anterior colpotomy (Döderlein technique). With a small, mobile uterus, simple traction may result in delivery of the uterus without the need for rotating the fundus one way or the other. If delivery of the uterus (regardless of the size) is challenging, the organ may be brought closer to the surgeon and out of the vagina by using the alternate technique of *intramyometrial coring*. This technique was introduced by Lash in 1941 and reintroduced in 1986 by Kovac for removal of large uteri; however, it may be used on uteri of any size. In this simple technique, the myometrium can be circumferentially incised with a scalpel placed parallel to the long axis of the uterus and beneath the serosal covering of the uterus with continuous traction on the cervix and direct

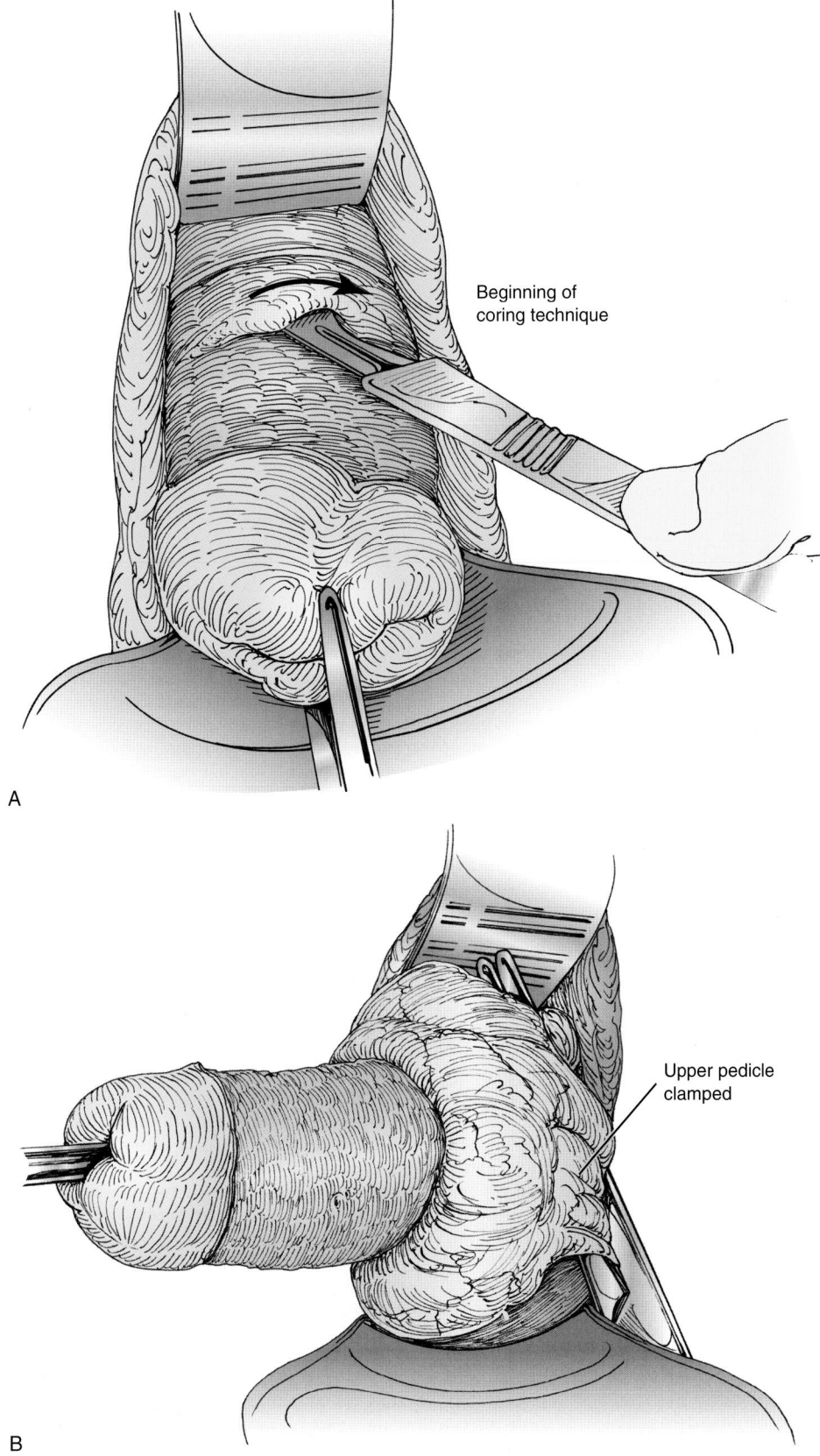

Beginning of
coring technique

A

Upper pedicle
clamped

B

FIGURE 32B.20 A: Coring incision is
started just below the serosal covering of the uterus anteriorly. **B:** Coring
of a small uterus to facilitate exposure and clamping of the upper pedicle. No sutures were placed above
the uterine artery to bring the uterus
closer to the surgeon for removal of
the uterus. (Reprinted from Kovac
SR, Zimmerman CW, eds. *Advances
in reconstructive vaginal surgery.*
Philadelphia, PA: Lippincott Williams
& Wilkins, 2007:118, with permission. Copyright © 2007 Lippincott
Williams & Wilkins.)

V

vision at all times (**Fig. 32B.20A, B**). This maneuver removes a core inside the uterus without violating the integrity of the endometrial cavity or uterine serosa. Ligation of the uterine artery is absolutely necessary prior to coring. The Lash or coring incision reduces the size of the uterus by decreasing its width, thereby increasing its length, similar to the way a baby's head becomes more cylindrical and less spherical as it becomes molded during childbirth. In effect, coring converts a spherical structure into an elongated cylindrical or rod shape, enhancing the surgeon's ability to facilitate transvaginal removal of a wide uterine fundus (**Fig. 32B.21A–C**). This process is a surprisingly bloodless maneuver once the uterine arteries have been secured. Strong traction is placed on the uterus during the coring, which restricts blood flow from the ovarian pedicles.

During the coring procedure, the uterus will begin to descend through the vagina, allowing the surgeon to visualize the cornual portion of the uterus and exposing the utero-ovarian ligament, round ligament, and fallopian tube. Once these structures become visible, the surgeon is assured that the uterus can be removed vaginally.

Some surgeons prefer bivalving the uterus with *morcellation*. Morcellation is especially useful if multiple leiomyomata are present. A thyroid vulsellum clamp may be placed on either side of the cervix, and with strong downward traction, the cervix may be incised with a knife vertically until the fundus of the uterus is reached. Once the fundus is reached, wedges of myometrium or specific leiomyomata may be removed in a nearly bloodless field until the uterine size is sufficiently reduced to allow removal. Individual selection of technique for each case is needed. Coring is most useful in the presence of adenomyosis while morcellation is most useful in the presence of leiomyomata although neither technique is restricted to those respective clinical situations. No effort should be made to use either morcellation or coring until the uterine artery pedicles are secure.

Once the cornual pedicles are visualized, they can either be clamped individually. Depending on the surgeon's preference and experience, the clamp may be left on the pedicle or a suture may be placed around the tip of the clamp and tied or transfixed behind is appropriate. This suture may be tagged. The clamp or suture may be used to provide gentle traction on the pedicle and expose the ovary for evaluation or removal.

Once the uterus has been removed, it is appropriate to evaluate each pedicle to confirm hemostasis. If the ovaries are removed before confirmation that all pedicles are hemostatic, the surgeon may spend considerable operative time finding the source of such bleeding, as it frequently appears to be from a higher point but may actually be from one of the uterine pedicles. Each pedicle can be evaluated by starting at the 12-o'clock position within the peritoneal cavity and proceeding in a clockwise manner. The use of a surgical sponge folded longitudinally on sponge forceps may be very helpful as is an auxiliary light source. If brisk bleeding is noted, most often it can be found by placing traction on the uterosacral tag and looking between the uteroovarian and uterine artery pedicles. Bleeding from this area of the broad ligament is usually a result of the anastomosis of vessels between the ovarian and uterine artery. Because this is the most frequent site of this type of bleeding, the surgeon should direct his or her search to this area first. Placement of a long Kelly or Allis clamp at the site of bleeding without undue traction may be followed by a helical suture or a figure-of-eight suture passed through the vagina into the peritoneum from outward to inward will rapidly control this bleeding (**Fig. 32B.22**). Care should be taken to specifically identify sites of bleeding, to not suture blindly, and to control the depth of suturing in this area due to the proximity of the ureters.

If no bleeding points are discovered from any of the hysterectomy pedicles, the posterior vaginal epithelium will most likely be determined to be the source of bleeding. Posterior cuff bleeding may sometimes be rather brisk from the separation of the vagina and the peritoneal edge. It is likely to be more brisk in premenopausal patients especially those younger than 40 years of age. Before proceeding with any concurrent procedure, blood loss from this area should be controlled with electrosurgery or absorbable suture. Once hysterectomy pedicle and posterior cuff hemostasis is complete, further examination of the peritoneal cavity should reveal complete hemostasis from all potential bleeding sites. The anterior cuff is rarely a source of troublesome bleeding.

If only the uterus is to be removed, support of the vaginal apex becomes the next most important decision. If a salpingo-oophorectomy is planned in conjunction with the hysterectomy, it should be performed at this point.

VAGINAL OOPHORECTOMY

There appears to be some reluctance to combine vaginal hysterectomy with oophorectomy because vaginal oophorectomy is thought to be a risky and difficult procedure. Factors that seem to foster this perception are fear of restricted access to the ovaries and the belief that there is inadequate visibility of the adnexa along with safe access to the infundibulopelvic ligament during conventional vaginal surgery.

To obtain objective evidence regarding these perceptions, a prospective study was designed by Baden and Walker to determine whether there is adequate visibility and accessibility for transvaginal oophorectomy in most patients undergoing vaginal hysterectomy. After the uterus was removed, accessibility of the ovaries for transvaginal removal was assessed by stretching the infundibulopelvic ligament, placing traction on the suture tag used to ligate the uteroovarian ligament, round ligament, and fallopian tube and grading the position of the ovaries in relation to the long axis of the vagina. The degree of ovarian descent and visibility was graded with a system used to grade pelvic organ prolapse (**Fig. 32B.23; Table 32B.1**). The grade corresponded to the minimal degree of descent of either ovary.

To determine what grade would be considered accessible and visible for transvaginal oophorectomy by most gynecologic surgeons, the experience of other surgical specialties was considered. For example, the distance from the hymenal ring to the ischial spine is approximately 8 cm. In dentistry, the distance from the front teeth to the last molar is 6 cm; in otolaryngology, the distance from the front teeth to the tonsil for tonsillectomy is 10 cm. Therefore, it was postulated that any ovary that was positioned at grade I or lower in the vagina should be visible and accessible for transvaginal removal by most gynecologic surgeons. Of the 875 patients between 29 and 69 years of age who were evaluated for ovarian descent after hysterectomy, 92.9% had ovarian mobility to at least the midportion of the vagina (grade II). In another 4.6%, the ovary could be pulled down outside the hymenal ring (grade II). Only 2.5% of these patients had very little ovarian mobility, which would have made vaginal oophorectomy very difficult (2.4% grade I and 0.1% grade 0). Although this study provided objective evidence that the ovaries may be more visible and accessible for transvaginal removal than previously perceived, there may be times that the ovary may be inaccessible for transvaginal removal as a result of adhesive disease, endometriosis, suspected significant pathology, or other conditions. However, the ovary should not be presumed to be inaccessible at the start of any vaginal hysterectomy. Smale and colleagues, Davies and associates, and Sheth have reported

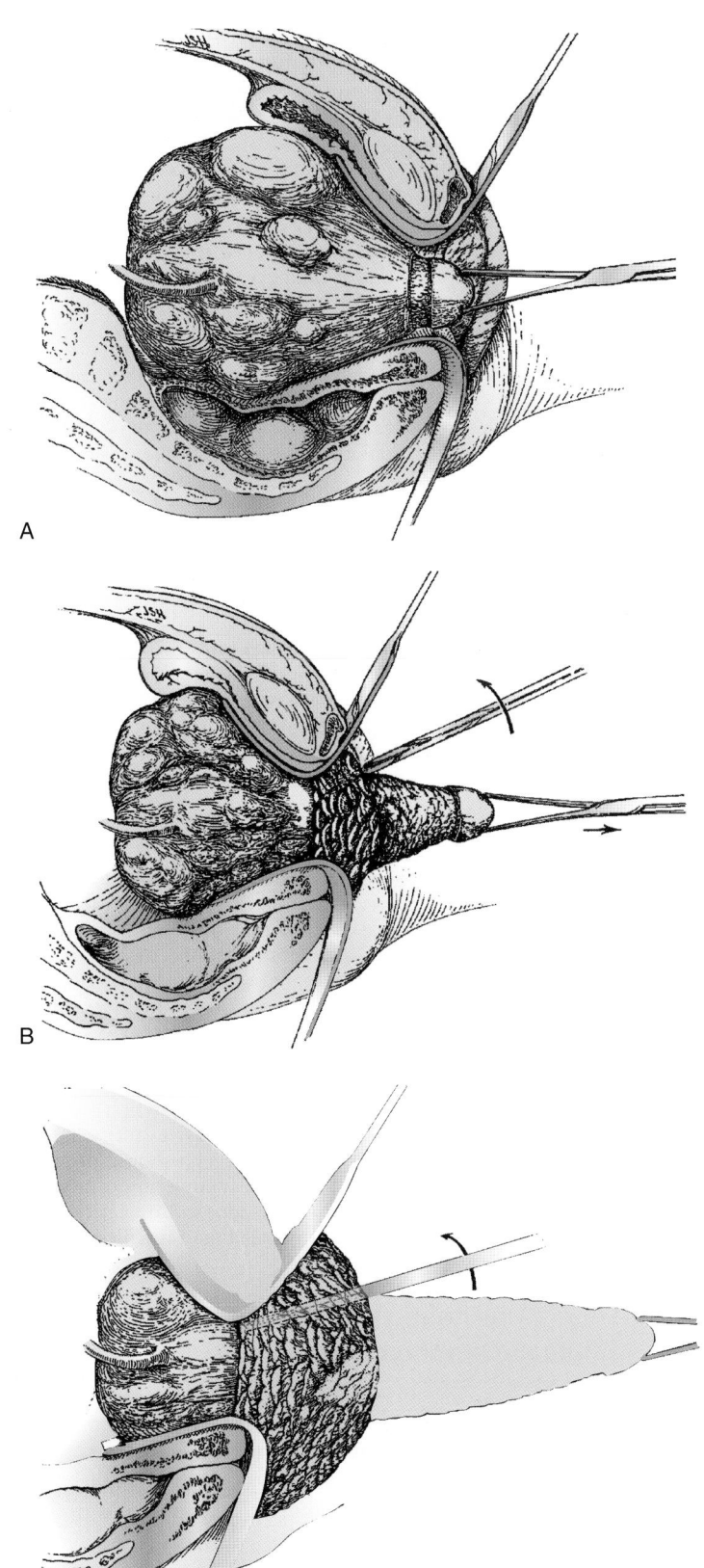

FIGURE 32B.21 A: The cervix has been circumscribed through the full thickness of the vagina around the cervix, the posterior and anterior peritoneum entered, and the uterosacral and cardinal ligaments secured. **B:** After ligation of the uterine arteries, an incision is made in a circumferential fashion parallel to the endometrial cavity and into the outer superficial myometrium in the same plane. Constant traction on the tenaculum while coring assists in developing the proper plane. **C:** Continued coring and traction reduce the size of the uterus by exteriorizing the inside of the uterus with an intact endometrial cavity through the introitus. Intramural myomas are sometimes transected during the coring process. (Reprinted from Kovac SR. Intramyometrial coring as an adjunct to vaginal hysterectomy. *Obstet Gynecol* 1986:76;131, with permission. Copyright © 2007 Lippincott Williams & Wilkins.)

V

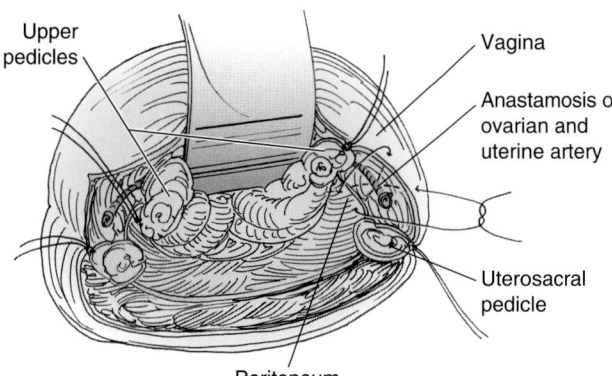

FIGURE 32B.22 The most common source of bleeding after removal of the uterus is the anastomosis between uterine and ovarian arteries. Suture placed through the lateral vagina into the lateral peritoneum in a figure-of-eight fashion and tied resolves most, if not all, bleeding from this area. (Reprinted from Kovac SR, Zimmerman CW, eds. *Advances in reconstructive vaginal surgery.* Philadelphia, PA: Lippincott Williams & Wilkins, 2007:120, with permission. Copyright © 2007 Lippincott Williams & Wilkins.)

that planned vaginal salpingo-oophorectomy is successful in 94% to 97% of women undergoing vaginal hysterectomy. The routine use of the laparoscope to perform an oophorectomy before a vaginal hysterectomy has been heralded as safe and comfortable and therefore has become commonplace. "To be sure we can get the ovaries" is a phrase too often heard worldwide to justify the use of abdominal, laparoscopic, or even robotic approaches to hysterectomy. For too many years, the belief that the ovaries were inaccessible because they are "too high" for transvaginal removal has been prevalent. This

TABLE 32B.1 The Baden-Walker Halfway System for Grading the Degrees of Ovarian Descent After Hysterectomy	
GRADE	**FINDINGS**
0	No descent was defined. The infundibulopelvic ligament has little or no stretchability, and the ovaries are positioned at the lateral pelvic wall at or above the ischial spines and cannot, with traction, be brought into the long-axis plane of the vagina.
I	Infundibulopelvic ligament stretchability brings the descent of the ovaries into the long axis of the vagina with traction halfway between the ischial spines and the mid-vagina.
II	Infundibulopelvic ligament stretchability brings the descent of the ovaries into the long axis of the vagina with traction between the midportion of the vagina and the hymenal ring.
II	Infundibulopelvic ligament stretchability brings the descent of the ovaries into the longitudinal plane of the vagina with traction past the hymenal ring.

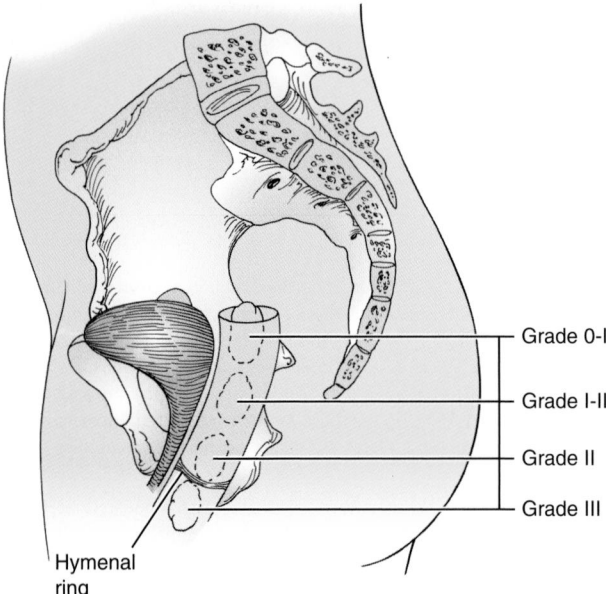

FIGURE 32B.23 Grading ovarian descent after vaginal hysterectomy with Baden-Walker Halfway System. Grade corresponds to the position of the ovary at the ischial spine superiorly and the hymenal ring inferiorly. (Reprinted from Kovac SR, Zimmerman CW, eds. *Advances in reconstructive vaginal surgery.* Philadelphia, PA: Lippincott Williams & Wilkins, 2007:120, with permission. Copyright © 2007 Lippincott Williams & Wilkins.)

misconception has erroneously guided the selection of abdominal or endoscopic hysterectomy.

Good surgical practice dictates that objective determination of the visibility and accessibility of the ovaries is the primary criteria for selecting a particular route of oophorectomy. Thus, if the ovaries are found to be inaccessible at the time of vaginal hysterectomy, ovarian removal can be performed with the laparoscope or by a simple laparotomy once the initial vaginal operation is complete. The correct paradigm substantiated by clinical evidence is to first attempt ovarian removal by the minimally invasive transvaginal approach. If that is not possible, the surgeon should proceed with laparoscopy or laparotomy after completion of a vaginal hysterectomy for removal of the adnexa. Indications for salpingo-oophorectomy should not change regardless of the route of surgery.

Surgical Technique of Vaginal Salpingo-Oophorectomy

STEPS IN THE PROCEDURE

Vaginal Hysterectomy Bilateral Salpingo-Oophorectomy

1. History and physical exam for assessment of indications for surgery and appropriateness of patient for surgery, including medical and anesthesia clearance as needed.

2. Preoperative and examination under anesthesia to document adequate access to the cervix and apical vaginal structures, especially the uterosacral ligaments.

3. Careful positioning of the patient in the standard lithotomy position with the femur vertical and tibia/fibula close to the horizontal plane and oriented toward the opposite shoulder.

4. Debate and variation exist among experts regarding preparation of the bladder for surgery. Some surgeons, including the author, prefer catheter placement prior to surgery. Others prefer leaving fluid in the bladder in order to alert the surgeon of the presence of bladder injury.[1]

5. Grasp the cervix firmly, and in cases that do not include an adequate degree of prolapse, firmly massage the uterosacral ligaments to establish maximum descent prior to proceeding.

6. Grasp the posterior cul-de-sac. With downward traction on the vaginal epithelium and upward traction on the cervix, incise the posterior cul-de-sac and document peritoneal entry.

7. Complete circumscription of the vaginal epithelium around the cervix.

8. Dissect the vesicocervical space, transect the pericervical ring/supravaginal septum, and dissect the vesicouterine space. Place a retractor in the anterior dissection to elevate the bladder. Note that there is no compelling reason to complete entry into the anterior cul-de-sac at this point unless specifically desired.

9. Identify, clamp, transect, and ligate the uterosacral ligament pedicle separately. This pedicle will be used in cuff closure.

10. Identify, clamp, transect, and ligate the cardinal/pubocervical ligament pedicle.

11. Identify, clamp, transect, and ligate the uterine vasculature.

12. Identify and enter the anterior cul-de-sac of not already accomplished.

13. Clamp and ligate the lower portion of the broad ligament (often including the ascending portion of the uterine vasculature) including the anterior and posterior peritoneum.

14. Deliver the fundus of the uterus posteriorly. An alternative is to deliver the fundus of the uterus anteriorly; however, posterior delivery is usually the more efficient method.

15. If uterine size does not permit fundal delivery, uteroreductive techniques (e.g., morcellation, coring, cervicectomy, or bivalving) may be helpful at this stage of the procedure.

16. Identify, clamp, and transect the adnexal pedicle (fallopian tube, round ligament, and utero-ovarian ligament) to remove the uterus.

17. If adnexectomy is desired, identify and divide the round ligament to begin the process. Then identify, clamp, divide, and ligate the mesovarium.

18. Identify, clamp, divide, and ligate the infundibulopelvic ligament to complete the removal of the adnexa.

19. Carefully inspect all pedicles for hemostasis.

20. Irrigate the surgical field.

21. If appropriate, perform one of the variations of culdoplasty (e.g., McCall) incorporating the uterosacral ligaments into the cuff to help prevent future prolapse.

22. Perform cystourethroscopy to document bladder and ureteral integrity.

23. Perform cuff closure. Several variations exist. Most surgeons prefer interrupted sutures rather than a running closure because of potential hematoma or abscess formation.

24. Vaginal packing is optional. It is not necessary in the absence of concomitant pelvic reconstructive surgery.

Vaginal salpingo-oophorectomy may be accomplished if sufficient descent is found in the following manner. Downward traction is applied to the surgical clamp or suture ligating the uteroovarian ligament, round ligament, and fallopian tube or the clamp securing that pedicle. The initial step in vaginal adnexal removal is a digital and visual exam of the structures in order to assess size and eliminate any adhesions that may be present. After those tasks have been accomplished, the end of the fallopian tube is directed toward the ovary with tissue forceps and a long, sharply angled clamp is placed between the round ligament, the uteroovarian ligament, and tube across the infundibulopelvic ligament. Under direct vision, the tube and ovary may be excised. A suture is placed approximately 2 cm from the tip of the clamp, and a single throw tie is tightened around the tip, which usually secures the ovarian artery (Fig. 32B.24). The suture is then placed behind the clamp for suture transfixation and firmly tied with several throws. As the suture is tied, the surgeon can appreciate the security of this suture around the infundibulopelvic ligament. Alternatively, some surgeons have used an Endoloop (Ethicon Endo-Surgery, Cincinnati, OH) to secure the infundibulopelvic pedicle. If the Endoloop is used, at least the round ligament should be divided to debulk the pedicle prior to application of the suture.

An alternative method of salpingo-oophorectomy is the three-step technique described by Zimmerman and others. This technique is especially useful when descent of the adnexa is not pronounced; however, routine use of these steps makes difficult cases more manageable when they are encountered. The surgical steps mimic the same maneuvers that are used to remove the adnexa abdominally. After removal of the uterus, the utero-ovarian pedicle is held with a clamp, and the handle is rotated laterally and the tip pointed medially. This maneuver exposes the round ligament that can be clamped, transected, and ligated or divided with electrocautery. Division of the round ligament gives the surgeon access to the retroperitoneal

---

[1]Author's note: The specific steps of vaginal hysterectomy do not necessarily proceed in a predetermined order, they all must be accomplished; however, the exact order is somewhat variable from case to case and from surgeon to surgeon. For example, some surgeons prefer anterior dissection first and others prefer posterior dissection initially. No evidence clearly favors one approach over the others; therefore, surgeon discretion is paramount. The steps outlined below are the ones favored by the author.

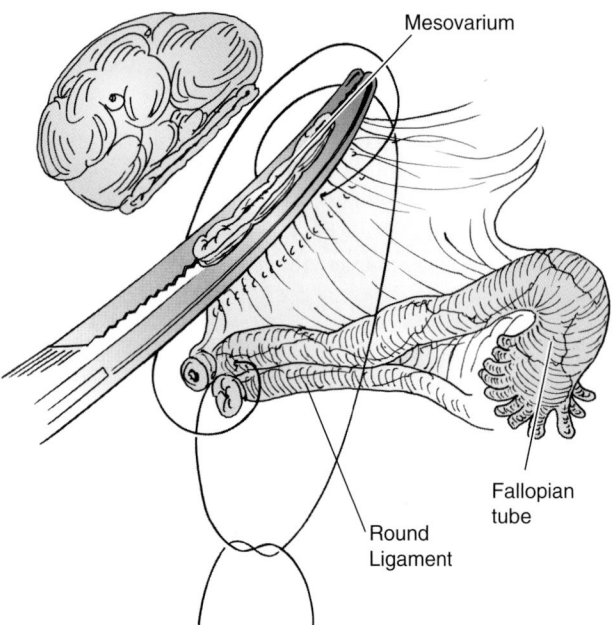

FIGURE 32B.24 The infundibulopelvic ligament has been clamped and the ovary and the tube removed. There is a single penetration of the infundibulopelvic ligament and its midpoint and tied around the end of the clamp. This transfixation suture usually occludes the ovarian artery. The suture is then passed around the end of the clamp and transfixed into the tissues behind the heel of the clamp and tied again. (Reprinted from Kovac SR, Zimmerman CW, eds. *Advances in reconstructive vaginal surgery*. Philadelphia, PA: Lippincott Williams & Wilkins, 2007:122, with permission. Copyright © 2007 Lippincott Williams & Wilkins.)

space between the leaves of the broad ligament. Gentle dissection of this space makes it possible to isolate, clamp, and ligate the mesovarium as a separate pedicle. Elimination from the adnexal complex of these two structures results in an additional and significant amount of descent of the tube and ovary. After division of the mesovarium, the only remaining tissue connected to the adnexa is the infundibulopelvic ligament. This ligament can be clamped and suture ligated or secured with an Endoloop. Division of the adnexectomy into three manageable steps increases surgical control, decreases the bulk of attachment, and decreases the likelihood of a complication during suture application. Transection of the round ligament and mesovarium as separate pedicles significantly increases descent of the adnexa, resulting in increased visibility of the infundibulopelvic ligament.

Consideration of salpingectomy only has recently become more prevalent. This idea is based on the emerging idea that many malignancies that have been labeled as ovarian in the past are now suspected to have a salpingeal origin. Obviously, if the ovary was left in place, the surgery would be easier to accomplish. At this time, there is no definitive evidence to either support or refute this idea.

CLOSURE AND SUPPORT OF THE VAGINAL CUFF

Closure of the peritoneum with vaginal hysterectomy is not routinely necessary for healing and rarely is indicated as a part of the procedure. Leaving the peritoneum open may help to expose any immediate intraperitoneal postoperative bleeding.

The remaining part of the vaginal hysterectomy is to support the vaginal cuff so that the chance that an enterocele or vaginal vault prolapse will develop later in life is reduced. Compensation for the connective tissue defect and disruption of the vaginal suspensory axis created by the removal of the cervix is best accomplished at the time of hysterectomy. Failure to adequately compensate for the cervical defect may expose the patient to an increased risk for posthysterectomy vaginal vault prolapse in the form of a posterior enterocele or apical anterior vaginal wall prolapse (anterior enterocele). Enterocele repair and suspension of the prolapsed posthysterectomy vagina are among the most technically demanding of all pelvic surgery procedures. Closure of the cervical defect along with reestablishment of the suspensory axis of the vagina by incorporating the uterosacral ligaments into the cuff is effective prophylaxis reducing the risk of future prolapse. As a general rule, closure of the cuff and correction of the cervical defect should consume approximately as much time as extirpation of the uterus.

The incidence of enterocele after hysterectomy can range between 0.1% and 16%. Nichols and Randall described a technique of excising excess peritoneum in the cul-de-sac to prevent future development of an anterior enterocele (Fig. 32B.25). Because this technique only removes excess peritoneum and does not address the cause of an enterocele after hysterectomy, subsequent enterocele formation has not been prevented because no musculofascial defect has been corrected or reinforced.

Several other methods to repair the posterior vaginal cuff for prolapse prophylaxis have been described. These procedures emphasize the use of the uterosacral ligaments in any repair. Inclusion of the uterosacral ligaments in cuff repair is very important because of their role as the primary suspensory elements in

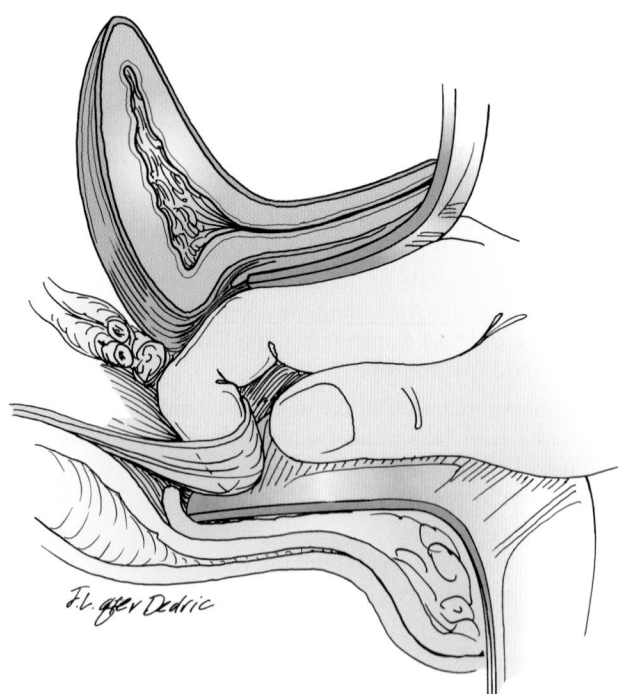

FIGURE 32B.25 Identification of excess peritoneum in cul-de-sac. Excision of excess peritoneum will not prevent future enterocele formation, as the cause of the enterocele is not determined. (Reprinted from Kovac SR, Zimmerman CW, eds. *Advances in reconstructive vaginal surgery*. Philadelphia, PA: Lippincott Williams & Wilkins, 2007:122, with permission. Copyright © 2007 Lippincott Williams & Wilkins.)

the uterovaginal continuum of structures. Connecting the uterosacral ligaments to the cuff reestablishes the posterior arm of the suspensory axis of the vagina and should be considered during all hysterectomies regardless of route. The most commonly employed technique to close the posterior vaginal cuff is the McCall culdoplasty. This technique is designed to obliterate the cul-de-sac while it suspends the posterior superior vagina and its fascial attachments to the uterosacral ligaments. Bringing these supporting ligaments together in the midline is common; however, it is no longer believed to be necessary. Care should be taken to document ureteral patency after this procedure. The risk of ureteral occlusion is directly proportional to the number of uterosacral plication sutures placed. This type of prolapse prophylaxis technique is a marked improvement over previous beliefs that the only thing necessary after the uterus was removed was to close the vagina. Simple closure of the vagina resulted in a high incidence of vaginal vault prolapse and associated enterocele formation. More recently, simple closures such as those used by abdominal, laparoscopic, and robotic surgeons have resulted in an unacceptably high incidence of vaginal cuff dehiscence. Some form of McCall culdoplasty after all vaginal hysterectomies should be considered routine. Some modification of this step should also be considered if another approach to hysterectomy is used.

Recent advancements in pelvic reconstructive techniques, as well as an understanding of the cause of enteroceles, have brought us to a new method of preventing enteroceles and vault prolapse at the time of hysterectomy, especially with those patients who have a rectocele. Rectoceles and enteroceles result from an apical separation of the rectovaginal septum from the uterosacral ligaments. This distal displacement of the rectovaginal septum allows both of these vaginal defects to develop contiguously through the same fascial defect. Because enteroceles are routinely associated with rectoceles, they may not both be suspected during the vaginal hysterectomy. This idea suggests that failure to identify and manage the presence of an enterocele at the time of vaginal hysterectomy might be the cause of the increased incidence of rectocele and enterocele formation in later years.

Enteroceles may also form as a result of the separation of the rectovaginal fascia from the pubocervical fascia (Fig. 32B.26). As a result of hysterectomy and removal of the cervix, there is an iatrogenic separation of the rectovaginal septum and the fibers that normally connect this structure to the anterior vaginal fascia through the connective tissue that forms the pericervical ring. This separation widens the cul-de-sac and separates the normal fascial attachments thus allowing the peritoneum and accompanying intra-abdominal structures, to potentially protrude through this weakness with any increase in intra-abdominal pressure. This concept likely explains the fact that most posthysterectomy vaginal vault prolapse is located apically or on the apical anterior segment of the vagina (cervical defect). Proper cuff closure reduces this possibility by reconnection of all connective tissue elements by incorporation within the suture lines.

An effort to restore normal anatomy from the disruption of these support and suspensory structures created by hysterectomy is the obligation of the hysterectomy surgeon regardless of route. McCall culdoplasty is intended to prevent incipient recto-enteroceles. If a true rectoenterocele is identified at hysterectomy, a repair should be considered.

Surgical Techniques

Cuff repair is as much a part of hysterectomy as removal of the uterus and adnexa. If a rectocele has not been identified, management of the vaginal cuff is performed by reducing the defect left by the absence of the cervix. Options include incorporation of the cardinal ligament pedicles in the repair particularly in the presence of a sizeable cervical defect. The cardinal ligament pedicles may actually be tied together across the midline with safety. Traditional McCall culdoplasty incorporates suture(s) in each uterosacral ligament accessed intraperitoneally and sutured into the posterior cuff. In the traditional technique, one or more sutures are placed and tied across the midline in order to occlude the posterior cul-de-sac. With recognition of the importance of the integrated suspensory axes, it is sufficient to incorporate the intraperitoneal portion of the uterosacral ligaments into the vaginal cuff ipsilaterally without plication into the midline. Simply securing this attachment is enough to allow the apex of the vaginal vault to remain suspended over the sacrococcygeal raphe. An effort should also be made to incorporate both the anterior and posterior fasciae into the repair of the cuff by suturing through the full thickness of the vaginal epithelium. Apical attachment of the anterior pubocervical fascia and the rectovaginal fascia posteriorly to the cuff is critical to successful cuff closure. Those two attachments close the space vacated by the absence of the cervix. The difference between the shorter anterior pubocervical fascia and the longer posterior rectovaginal fascia is resolved with soft tissue occlusion. Permanent suture may be used on the uterosacral sutures so long as they are not exposed intravaginally.

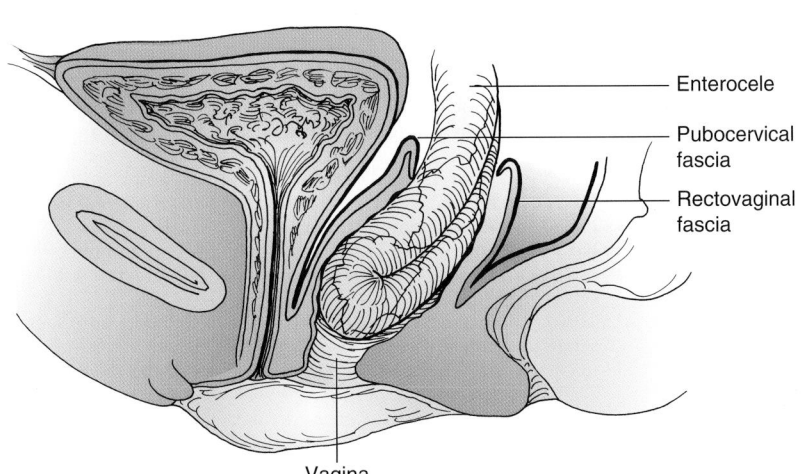

Enterocele

Pubocervical fascia

Rectovaginal fascia

Vagina

FIGURE 32B.26 Separation of the pubocervical and rectovaginal fascia with enterocele formation. (Reprinted from Kovac SR, Zimmerman CW, eds. *Advances in reconstructive vaginal surgery.* Philadelphia, PA: Lippincott Williams & Wilkins, 2007:124, with permission. Copyright © 2007 Lippincott Williams & Wilkins.)

Debate exists regarding specific techniques of cuff closure. Some surgeons prefer running suture, others interrupted. Some prefer vertical closure, others horizontal. No definitive data exist to resolve these issues. Much more important are the concepts of reintegration of the suspensory axes of the vagina.

The presence of a rectocele requires the posterior vaginal wall be opened in the midline up to the level of the newly formed cul-de-sac. The defect from separation of the rectovaginal fascia from the uterosacral ligaments is identified. If an enterocele sac is identified, opening of the sac with high ligation of the sac is unnecessary, as the mesothelial lining of the peritoneal sac has little supportive value. The sac is simply pushed upward by reattachment of the uterosacral ligaments to the posterior cuff and the rectovaginal septum. The vagina can be closed vertically or horizontally, as neither is superior in preserving vaginal length. Cruikshank and Pixley demonstrated that vaginal length depended on the support of the vaginal cuff, not any specific method of epithelial closure. They concluded that as long as there is good restoration of vault suspension, vaginal length is not affected by the vertical versus horizontal orientation of the vaginal epithelial closure. If the cuff has been adequately suspended, the cuff closure is positioned toward the anterior vagina wall, leaving more depth to the posterior vaginal wall for accommodation of coitus.

Some investigators have recommended that the vaginal cuff be left open or a drain placed within the vaginal (closure) incision to reduce the morbidity of vaginal cuff cellulitis or abscess formation. With the widespread use of prophylactic antibiotics and the recognition that irrigation during a vaginal procedure is required, there is no longer any need for those techniques. In addition, leaving the cuff open may lead to an increased incidence of enterocele formation and vaginal vault prolapse.

The decision to place packing into the vagina postoperatively is an optional one. A vaginal pack need not be used after vaginal hysterectomy unless concomitant pelvic reconstructive surgery is performed. Complete hemostasis should be achieved after vaginal hysterectomy and prior to cuff closure. Significant postoperative bleeding will rarely occur from the single vascular pedicle on each side of a hysterectomy bed. If that type of bleeding does occur, it is important to become aware of this problem as soon as possible and vaginal packing will only delay the diagnosis and not prevent the problem. Vaginal packing compresses the vaginal walls much more effectively than the apex of the vagina where there is no structure against which packing may compress the vaginal tissues. It is important to be aware of postoperative bleeding sooner rather than later while the patient is still hemodynamically stable, so a pelvic arteriogram or surgical intervention can be performed early in the course of any such bleeding. The arteriogram may demonstrate the bleeding site and allow arterial occlusion, thus preventing the need for a return to the operating room or laparotomy.

For some surgeons, it is not routine practice to insert an indwelling transurethral catheter following the removal of a normal-size uterus. Removal of an enlarged uterus may cause occasional transient insult to the bladder and transient postoperative voiding problems; therefore, in such patients, bladder drainage is usually suggested, at least overnight.

Routine cystoscopy following vaginal hysterectomy significantly increases the incidence of recognition of both bladder and ureteral injury. Before cystoscopy, 5 mL of indigo carmine is administered intravenously by the anesthesiologist. Alternatively, a single tablet of Pyridium 200 mg can be administered prior to the start of the procedure. The strong efflux of blue or ochre dye through each ureteral orifice following hysterectomy with or without pelvic reconstruction implies the integrity of the ureters. Although this routine may not be absolutely necessary with each vaginal hysterectomy, it certainly makes the surgeon more comfortable and helps protect the patient from unacceptable consequences.

BEST SURGICAL PRACTICES

- Randomized controlled trials have demonstrated that women treated by vaginal hysterectomy experience lower morbidity, less pain, more rapid recovery, and a more rapid return to normal activities compared with abdominal, endoscopic, or laparoscopically assisted vaginal hysterectomy. They also consume fewer health care dollars and resources. Little evidence is available to compare robotic and vaginal surgeries.
- Using guidelines to determine the route of hysterectomy adopted by the National Guideline Clearinghouse, and with maximum development of surgical technique, it is feasible to perform 90% of hysterectomies for benign disease indications via the vaginal route.
- Following the National Guideline Clearinghouse guidelines for selecting the route of hysterectomy, even for a resident training environment, has been shown to decrease the number of abdominal and consequently endoscopic hysterectomies.
- To minimize bladder and rectal injuries, the anterior and posterior peritoneum should always be entered under direct vision.
- The risk of ureteral injury can be minimized by retracting the bladder anteriorly at all times after completion of the dissection of the vesicocervical and vesicouterine spaces and dividing the cardinal ligament before cutting, clamping, or suturing in the anterolateral area above the cervix.
- The only vascular pedicle above the uterine vessels contains the round ligament, utero-ovarian ligament, and fallopian tube. These structures can generally be clamped in a single pedicle.
- Transvaginal removal of the ovaries at the time of vaginal hysterectomy should be technically feasible in more than 90% of patients.
- Following vaginal hysterectomy, the presence of preexisting pelvic support defects should be carefully evaluated and repaired if present. The vaginal vault should always be resuspended to the uterosacral ligaments.

ACKNOWLEDGMENT

This chapter is based on material from Kovac SR, Zimmerman CW. *Advances in vaginal reconstructive surgery*. Philadelphia, PA: Lippincott, 2007.

BIBLIOGRAPHY

Amstey MS, Jones AP. Preparation of the vagina for surgery: a comparison of povidone-iodine and saline solution. *JAMA* 1981;245:839.

Baden WF, Walker T. Fundamentals, symptoms, and classification. In: Baden WF, Walker T, eds. *Surgical repair of vaginal defects*. Philadelphia, PA: Lippincott, 1992:51.

Ballard LA, Walters MD. Transvaginal mobilization and removal of ovaries and Fallopian tubes after vaginal hysterectomy. *Obstet Gynecol* 1996;87:35.

Colaco J, Campos AP, Nunes F, et al. Route of hysterectomy: vaginal versus abdominal. *J Pelvic Med Surg* 2003;9:69.

Cruikshank SH, Kovac SR. Anatomic changes of the ureter during vaginal hysterectomy. *Contemp Obstet Gynecol* 1993;38:38.

Cruikshank SH, Kovac SR. Role of the uterosacral-cardinal ligament complex in protecting the ureter during vaginal hysterectomy. *Int J Gynaecol Obstet* 1993;40:141.

Cruikshank SH, Pixley RL. Methods of vaginal cuff closure and preservation of vaginal depth during transvaginal hysterectomy. *Obstet Gynecol* 1987;70:61.

Culligan PJ, Kubik K, Murphy M, et al. A randomized trial that compared povidone iodine and chlorhexidine as antiseptics for vaginal hysterectomy. *Am J Obstet Gynecol* 2005;192:422.

Davies A, O'Connor H, Magos AL. A prospective study to evaluate oophorectomy at the time of vaginal hysterectomy. *BJOG* 1996;103: 915.

Dorsey JH, Steinberg EP, Holtz PM. Clinical indications for hysterectomy route: patient characteristics or physician preference. *Am J Obstet Gynecol* 1995;173:1452.

Emergency Care Research Institute (ECRI). Laparoscopy in hysterectomy for benign conditions. *Technology Assessment Custom Report Level 2.* Plymouth Meeting, PA: ECRI, 1995:1.

Garry R, Fountain J, Mason S, et al. The eVALuate study: two parallel randomised trials, one comparing laparoscopic with abdominal hysterectomy, the other comparing laparoscopic with vaginal hysterectomy. *BMJ* 2004;328:129.

Gilmour DT, Das S, Flowerdew G. Rates of urinary tract injury from gynecologic surgery and the role of intraoperative cystoscopy. *Obstet Gynecol* 2006;107:1366.

Jelen I, Bachmann G. An anatomical approach to oophorectomy during vaginal hysterectomy. *Obstet Gynecol* 1996;87:137.

Johns DA, Carrera B, Jones J, et al. The medical and economic impact of laparoscopically assisted vaginal hysterectomy in a large, metropolitan, not-for-profit hospital. *Am J Obstet Gynecol* 1995;172:1709.

Julian TM. Vaginal hysterectomy: an apparent exception to evidence-based decision making. *Obstet Gynecol* 2008;111:812.

Julian TM. Vasopressin use during vaginal surgery. *Contemp Obstet Gynecol* 1993;38:82.

Kovac SR. A technique for reducing the risk of intentional cystotomy during vaginal hysterectomy. *J Pelvic Surg* 1999;5:32.

Kovac SR. Intramyometrial coring as an adjunct to vaginal hysterectomy. *Obstet Gynecol* 1986;67:131.

Kovac SR, Barhan S, Lister M, et al. Guidelines for the selection of the route of hysterectomy: application in a resident clinic population. *Am J Obstet Gynecol* 2002;187:1521.

Kovac SR, Cruikshank SH. Guidelines to determine the route of oophorectomy with hysterectomy. *Am J Obstet Gynecol* 1996;175:1483.

Kovac SR, Zimmerman CW, eds. *Advances in reconstructive vaginal surgery.* Baltimore, MD: Lippincott Williams & Wilkins, 2006.

Lash AF. A method for reducing the size of the uterus in vaginal hysterectomy. *Am J Obstet Gynecol* 1941;42:452.

McCall MH. Posterior culdoplasty, surgical correction of enterocele during vaginal hysterectomy: a preliminary report. *Obstet Gynecol* 1957;10:595.

Nichols DH, Randall CL. *Vaginal surgery,* 2nd ed. Baltimore, MD: Williams & Wilkins, 1983:548.

Nieboer T, Johnson N, Lethaby A, et al. Surgical approach to hysterectomy for benign gynaecological disease. *Cochrane Database Syst Rev* 2010;12.

Pelosi II MA, Pelosi III. Simplified technique of vaginal hysterectomy. In: Seth S, Studd J, eds. *Vaginal hysterectomy.* The Livery House UK: Martin Dunitz, 2002:59.

Sheth SS. The place of oophorectomy at vaginal hysterectomy. *Br J Obstet Gynaecol* 1991;98:662.

Sheth SS. Vaginal hysterectomy following previous cesarean section. *Int J Gynecol Obstet* 1995;50:165.

Sizzi O, Paparella P, Bonito C, et al. Laparoscopic assistance after vaginal hysterectomy and unsuccessful access to the ovaries or failed uterine mobilization: changing trends. *JSLS* 2004;8:339.

Smale LE, Smale ML, Wilkening RL, et al. Salpingo-oophorectomy at the time of vaginal hysterectomy. *Am J Obstet Gynecol* 1978;131:122.

Turner LC, Shepherd JP, Wang L, et al. Hysterectomy surgical trends: a more accurate depiction of the last decade? *Am J Obstet Gynecol* 2013;208:277.e1.

Zimmerman CW. Oophorectomy at vaginal hysterectomy. *OBG Management* 1990;11:50.

Zimmerman CW. Vaginal hysterectomy: is skill the limiting factor? *OBG Management* 2006;18:21.

CHAPTER 32C
Laparoscopic Hysterectomy

Ted L. Anderson

DEFINITIONS

Colpotomy ring—A device placed into the vagina prior to total laparoscopic hysterectomy to lateralize the ureters, delineate the vaginal fornices, and aid in the colpotomy incision. It may be a hollow or solid cup, or a rotating molded form, made of plastic or metal.

Laparoscopic supracervical hysterectomy (LSH)—Hysterectomy that is performed completely by laparoscopy. The uterine corpus is amputated from the cervix at the level of the isthmus. The cervical stump will remain in situ.

Laparoscopically assisted vaginal hysterectomy (LAVH)—Variant of vaginal hysterectomy in which laparoscopy is employed for adnexectomy (if indicated) and the superior portions of the hysterectomy, but not ligation of the uterine vessels.

Morcellation—The process of dividing a large uterus into small strips or pieces in order to remove it through the vagina, through a minilaparotomy or extended umbilical incision, or using an electromechanical (power) morcellator placed through a laparoscopic incision.

Pneumoperitoneum (vaginal) occluder—A device inserted into the vagina prior to total laparoscopic hysterectomy designed to maintain the pneumoperitoneum after the colpotomy incision is made until the vaginal cuff is closed.

Total laparoscopic hysterectomy (TLH)—Total hysterectomy that is performed completely by laparoscopy with no vaginal component. The vaginal cuff is closed via the laparoscopic approach.

INTRODUCTION

Hysterectomy is the most common gynecologic procedure performed in the United States with approximately 500,000 being performed annually, although the numbers seem to be trending downward slightly for the past few years. The vast majority of benign hysterectomies (over 65%) are still performed through a laparotomy incision despite the urging of professional societies like the American College (Congress) of Obstetricians and Gynecologists (ACOG) and the American Association of Gynecologic Laparoscopists (AAGL) to employ minimally invasive approaches to hysterectomy, including vaginal and laparoscopic techniques. Laparoscopic hysterectomy was first described by Harry Reich in 1989 and has slowly gained popularity from less than 0.5% of hysterectomies in 1990 to a current rate of approximately 15%. Failure of laparoscopic hysterectomy to ascend to the primary approach for hysterectomy may be due, in part, to the technical challenges associated with the large uterus or concomitant intra-abdominal pathology. Additionally, the yielding of advanced surgical training time in residencies to other necessary components of the general obstetrics and gynecology curriculum (e.g., high-risk pregnancies and primary care) creates what Reich has called "a formidable obstacle to promotion of this technique." Indeed, most gynecologic surgeons who gain proficiency in laparoscopic hysterectomy have done so, and will likely continue to do so, during fellowship programs or other postresidency training.

The term laparoscopic hysterectomy includes a family of procedures that vary in degree to which the procedure is performed laparoscopically. This ranges from simple treatment of endometriosis or adhesiolysis and division of ovarian vasculature to completion of the entire procedure laparoscopically, including cuff closure. In 2000, the AAGL published a detailed classification system for total (Table 32C.1) and supracervical (Table 32C.2) laparoscopic hysterectomy in order to standardize terminology and reporting of outcomes. In this chapter, the techniques of total laparoscopic hysterectomy (TLH) and laparoscopic supracervical hysterectomy (LSH) are addressed. A logical and systematic surgical approach is described, based on "honoring the anatomy" and highlighting similarities to comparable steps of the abdominal hysterectomy approach, further supporting the mantra that laparoscopy is an access, not a procedure. Laparoscopically assisted vaginal hysterectomy (LAVH) is not described here, as it is basically a variant of vaginal hysterectomy that employs the laparoscopic approach simply to mobilize adnexal structures and treat relevant abdominal pathology such as adhesions. Nor is robotic-assisted laparoscopic hysterectomy discussed. Robotic technology applied to laparoscopic surgery has stimulated the adoption of TLH by many gynecologists previously hesitant to perform that procedure. By adding three-dimensional vision and instruments with articulating tips, clearer identification of tissue planes and easier laparoscopic suturing are facilitated. However, robotic-assisted laparoscopy is neither a technique nor an access, but rather a tool for performing laparoscopic hysterectomy.

TABLE 32C.1 The American Association of Gynecologic Laparoscopists Classification System for Laparoscopic Hysterectomy

TYPE	DESCRIPTION
0	Laparoscopic preparation for vaginal hysterectomy, including diagnostic only, treatment of intraperitoneal disease, and/or adhesiolysis
I	Laparoscopic occlusion and division of ovarian pedicle, unilateral or bilateral, and dissection up to but not including the uterine artery
II	Type I + occlusion and division of the uterine artery, unilateral or bilateral
III	Type II + dissection of a portion but not all of the cardinal–uterosacral ligament complex, unilateral or bilateral
IV	Type III + complete transection of the cardinal–uterosacral ligament complex, unilateral or bilateral, with or without entry into the vagina

Types I through IV are further divided into subgroups (A) dissection or division of pedicles or vessels as described; (B) dissection of bladder including anterior colpotomy; (C) posterior colpotomy; and (D) both anterior dissection and posterior colpotomy. Type IV also includes subgroup (C) with anterior dissection and colpotomy, posterior colpotomy, amputation of the uterus from the vagina, and laparoscopic-directed extirpation of the uterus (total laparoscopic hysterectomy).
Adapted from Olive DL, Parker WH, Cooper JM, et al. The AAG classification system for laparoscopic hysterectomy. *J Am Assoc Gynecol Laparosc* 2000;7:9–15, with permission. Copyright © 2000, Elsevier.

TABLE 32C.2 The American Association of Gynecologic Laparoscopists Classification System for Laparoscopic Supracervical Hysterectomy

TYPE	DESCRIPTION
LSH I	Laparoscopic occlusion and division of ovarian pedicle, unilateral or bilateral; occlusion and division of the superior branches of the uterine vessels above the level of the internal os; with or without dissection but not occlusion of the main uterine artery, unilateral or bilateral
LSH II	Type LSH I + occlusion but not division of the main uterine artery, unilateral or bilateral
LSH III	Type LSH II + division of the main uterine artery, unilateral or bilateral

Types LSH I through LSH III are further divided into subgroups, based on treatment of the cervical stump, including (A) without excision or ablation of the cervical canal; (B) with ablation of the cervical canal; and (C) with excision of the cervical canal.
Adapted from Olive DL, Parker WH, Cooper JM, et al. The AAG classification system for laparoscopic hysterectomy. *J Am Assoc Gynecol Laparosc* 2000;7:9–15, with permission. Copyright © 2000, Elsevier.

Historical Perspective

Laparoscopy was incorporated into gynecologic practice in the 1950s by Raoul Palmer in France, followed by Kurt Semm in Germany. After gaining popularity in Europe, it was spread to the United States by Melvin Cohen in the 1960s. Although there was increased utilization over the ensuing decades, early descriptions of laparoscopic appendectomy, ovarian cystectomy, and treatment of ectopic pregnancy were often refused publication in American journals as they were considered "unethical" surgical adventures. It was not until the development of microchip video cameras enabled projection of images onto television monitors in the mid-1980s, ushering in the so-called era of videolaparoscopy, that the techniques of laparoscopy became more integrated into gynecologic surgery.

Harry Reich and John DeCaprio published their landmark description of the first TLH in 1989. They used bipolar current to coagulate blood vessels, monopolar current to amputate the uterus from the vagina, and running Vicryl to close the vaginal cuff after delivering the specimen through the vagina. Viewing it as a substitute for abdominal hysterectomy and not for vaginal hysterectomy, they noted that this approach "may avoid the increased morbidity associated with abdominal surgery while retaining the surgical advantages of the abdominal approach, that is, thorough visualization and easy access to the vascular pedicles." Shortly thereafter, Kurt Semm described the classic intrafascial supracervical hysterectomy (CISH) procedure that involved coring out the endocervical canal including the squamocolumnar junction. About this same time, Thomas Lyons described a technique for LSH that was more similar to its laparotomy counterpart. This, in part, stimulated a renewed interest in supracervical hysterectomy. Although LSH was touted initially as preserving pelvic support and improving posthysterectomy sexual satisfaction, subsequent studies have shown no difference in either sexual function or pelvic support between supracervical and total hysterectomy. However, the technique of LSH did gain increased popularity among many gynecologic surgeons as it was easier and quicker to perform, was associated with less blood loss, allowed the surgeon to stay farther away from the ureter while securing vascular pedicles, decreased infectious complications by avoiding vaginal entry, and did not require suturing the vaginal cuff.

Today's high definition and even 3D video cameras, advanced electrosurgical instruments with interactive generators, innovative devices for safe colpotomy while protecting the ureters, and enabling tools for laparoscopic suturing should continue to enhance the acceptance of laparoscopic hysterectomy as part of our surgical armamentarium.

Advantages and Disadvantages of Laparoscopic Hysterectomy

The decision for appropriateness of hysterectomy as a therapeutic intervention is the same regardless of the approach being considered, although the access for hysterectomy is generally a function of patient pathology and surgeon skill and preference. A 2006 Cochrane database systematic review including over 3,600 patients in 27 randomized studies pointed to significant advantages of laparoscopic hysterectomy (LH) over abdominal hysterectomy (AH), including less blood loss, fewer wound infections or fevers, smaller incisions with less pain, shorter hospital stay, and speedier recovery. However, LH was associated with longer operating time and greater likelihood of urinary tract injuries. The eVALuate trial is one of the largest randomized trials comparing different approaches to hysterectomy. Conclusions pointed to LH as being associated with less pain, quicker recovery, and better quality of life compared with AH but as taking longer to perform. The report also concluded that total vaginal hysterectomy (TVH) was the preferred approach, when possible, as it offered similar benefits as LH with less cost and shorter operating times.

While TVH may be the preferred hysterectomy route for a variety of reasons, there are definitely patients in whom this approach is less than ideal. Specifically, a laparoscopic approach may be favored in patients who are morbidly obese, who have a constricted pelvic anatomy, who have no uterine descensus, or who have known or suspected concomitant pelvic disease (e.g., adhesions, endometriosis, etc). Indeed, there are few contraindications to laparoscopic hysterectomy, and most are relative contraindications related to the patient's comorbidities, including deficiencies in main physiologic functions and elevated body mass index. These would include the following:

- Medical conditions that would limit pneumoperitoneum, adequate ventilation, or Trendelenburg positioning (e.g., morbid obesity, increased intracranial pressure, ventriculoperitoneal shunt, portal or pulmonary hypertension, hemorrhagic shock)
- Severe abdominal or pelvic adhesive disease or other conditions that preclude safe entry or adequate operating space (e.g., advanced pregnancy, bulky uterine or fibroid size that precludes access to uterine vessels)
- Malignancy or other tumors in which a large specimen needs to be removed intact (e.g., ovarian cancer, dermoid, leiomyoma with necrotic degeneration or other findings suspicious for leiomyosarcoma)

On the other hand, there are recognizable challenges to performing laparoscopic hysterectomy, including the following:

- Reduced range of motion through laparoscopic ports and with conventional (straight) laparoscopic instruments resulting in reduced dexterity

- Reduced field of view in which only the tissues actively being manipulated are generally seen by the surgeon
- Reduced depth perception in converting a 3D surgical field to a 2D video image
- Reduced haptics and difficulty in assessing degree of force needed or being applied to tissues
- Reduced intuitive movements due to the fulcrum effect in which the tool tips move in the opposite direction as the surgeon's hands

In all cases, a decision regarding route of hysterectomies is largely dependent on the surgeon's capabilities. Insufficient knowledge, skill, and experience of the surgeon remain the most common reasons for assigning or converting any hysterectomy to the abdominal route.

Supracervical Versus Total Hysterectomy

Supracervical hysterectomy was first performed by Wilhelm Alexander Freund in 1878 and remained the leading technique of hysterectomy for over 80 years. At that time, there was a recognized association between cervicectomy and complications such as peritonitis, fistula, hemorrhage, ureteral injury, cystotomy, and enterotomy. In fact, the mortality rate associated with total hysterectomy through the 1930s was up to 50% higher compared with the supracervical approach. By the late 1940s, supracervical hysterectomy was largely abandoned in favor of total hysterectomy. This trend reflected the considerable refinement of surgical instruments and techniques, introduction of safer and more effective antibiotics, progression of blood banking technology with transfusions becoming more routine, and subsequent occurrence of cervical cancer in almost 2% of patients following supracervical hysterectomy.

In the early 1990s, after descriptions of successful laparoscopic techniques for supracervical hysterectomy by Kurt Semm and Thomas Lyons, there was a resurgence of interest in supracervical hysterectomy. Some have suggested this was driven equally by surgeon interest in a laparoscopic hysterectomy that was easier, quicker, and safer to perform than TLH as well as industry supply of instruments and devices to facilitate advanced laparoscopic procedures and tissue extraction. Conventional wisdom would assume that preservation of the cervix during LSH reduces the potential for intraoperative injury to the ureter, bladder, and rectum that would more likely occur during the transection of the cardinal ligament complex required to isolate and remove the cervix. Furthermore, hemorrhage most often occurs below the level of the uterine isthmus. Despite a plethora of studies comparing laparoscopic, vaginal, and abdominal approaches to hysterectomy, comparatively, few studies have focused on the role of the cervix. A meta-analysis of 47 studies published in 2006 reported the rate of urinary tract injury in all gynecologic surgery to be approximately 0.33%. In this report, the incidence in TLH was noted to be approximately 1.3% but fell to under 0.1% with LSH. More recent studies have demonstrated that, when performing concomitant laparoscopic sacrocolpopexy, LSH has been shown to offer an almost fivefold decrease in mesh erosion compared with TVH. Accordingly, there is objective evidence that leaving the cervix does indeed offer protection from complications in selected patients.

Another driver of LSH has been patient perception that pelvic support and sexual satisfaction would be preserved or enhanced over TLH. However, a systematic review of randomized trials comparing LSH with TLH documented no differences in rates of incontinence, prolapse, dyspareunia, sexual satisfaction, transfusion rate, recovery times, and readmission rates. Interestingly, a 2-year prospective study demonstrated significant overall improvement in sexual functioning, including increased libido, coital activity, and orgasm with decreased dyspareunia after TLH. Although several other studies have suggested increased orgasmic frequency after LSH, subsequent studies have failed to confirm these findings. Nonetheless, perception is a powerful motivating force. Many women contemplating elective hysterectomy consider preservation of the cervix a pivotal factor in the decision whether to undergo this procedure.

During the past decade, many gynecologists have reassessed the value of supracervical hysterectomy. The rationale for routine cervicectomy to prevent cervical cancer has been largely eliminated by the effectiveness of present-day cytologic and molecular screening for cervical disease, the natural history of human papillomavirus (HPV) infections in immunocompetent patients, and changes in treatment algorithms for preinvasive disease. Further, development of cervical dysplasia is rare in appropriately selected low-risk patients, and there is no evidence that supracervical hysterectomy increases the risk of cervical cancer. The incidence of cancer of the cervical stump appears to be equal to that of an intact uterus, as is the prognosis.

Finally, removal of the uterine corpus alone is often adequate treatment for women suffering from abnormal uterine bleeding or benign uterine fibroids. Nonetheless, many surgeons remain reluctant to offer this approach to women requiring hysterectomy for benign disease, citing the risk for persistent pain and cyclic vaginal bleeding necessitating subsequent trachelectomy. The incidence of persistent cyclic bleeding or spotting remains low (between 2% and 12%) and may be associated more with younger patients and those having preexisting endometriosis. In fact, some have considered the presence of extensive endometriosis to be a relative contraindication as these women may have persistence of dyspareunia if the cervix is retained.

The only absolute contraindication to supracervical hysterectomy is the presence of a malignant or premalignant condition of the uterine corpus or cervix. Supracervical hysterectomy is indicated for select patients who choose this procedure after appropriate counseling, and occasionally in surgical emergencies. Supracervical hysterectomy should not be performed simply because of the surgeon's lack of comfort with removing the cervix. Instead, assistance from more skilled surgeons should be sought.

PREPARING FOR HYSTERECTOMY

Preoperative Preparation

Prior to any elective surgical intervention, patients should be optimized with respect to comorbidities such as diabetes, hypertension, pulmonary compromise, and underlying disease processes that may affect performance of the procedure and postoperative healing; this is no different with laparoscopic hysterectomy. Special attention should be made to coordinate care with the anesthesia team in light of physiologic stresses that abdominal insufflation and prolonged Trendelenburg positioning can have on critical cardiopulmonary physiology, including peak inspiratory pressures and cardiac preload. Few objective criteria guide this assessment; it is the product of the surgeon's experience in consultation with the anesthesiologist.

In consideration of the Surgical Care Improvement Project (SCIP) protocol of the Joint Commission, plans for prophylactic antibiotics and deep vein thrombosis prophylaxis should be addressed, the latter of which may extend into the postoperative interval. Although there is no compelling objective evidence that a cathartic bowel preparation is indicated for benign gynecologic surgery, many surgeons find that decompression of the bowel through clear liquid diet or a mild laxative on the day prior to surgery is beneficial in keeping the bowel out of the surgical field.

Any discussion of patient preparation would be incomplete without mentioning the importance of informed consent. Notably, this is a process of patient counseling that is usually documented by a consent form. The process of informed consent should include a discussion of those risks that will be incurred by the patient related to any surgical procedure in general (e.g., complications of anesthesia, infection, bleeding, pain, scarring), related to the specific surgical procedure being performed (e.g., damage to the bowel, bladder, or ureters), and related to the instrumentation that will be used (e.g., thermal injury from electrosurgical devices or intraperitoneal dissemination of benign or previously undetected malignant tissue from the use of a morcellator). Further, the downstream consequences of those risks should be discussed (e.g., possible need for transfusion in cases of excessive blood loss or need for additional surgical procedures to address a ureteral injury). Finally, the potential need for conversion to a laparotomy should always be a part of the consent process for any laparoscopic procedure. In summary, the informed consent process is an educational process that should inform the patient, in terms she can understand, of all the relevant information a reasonable patient would want to know in order to make decisions related to the planned procedure.

Positioning and Port Placement

There are no specific variants from the basic principles of patient positioning for laparoscopic surgery that must be adapted for laparoscopic hysterectomy. However, a few key elements merit special attention. First, the patient should be situated sufficiently far down on the table. I find this critical concept to be underestimated often, only to encounter challenges with maneuvering the uterus when the table interferes with range of motion of the uterine manipulator after the procedure is well underway. One useful trick that can help address this is to rock the patient's hips forward to reduce lordosis, which can stabilize the patient's pelvis. Secondly, it is imperative that arm and leg position and padding relieve pressure points that could lead to nerve injury. A draw sheet placed across the operating table wrapped under well-padded arms and tucked back under the patient's back can provide excellent arm stability, maintain good function of iv's and blood pressure cuff, and allow for maximum mobility of the surgeon throughout the procedure. Third, extra measures should be taken to prevent patients from sliding cranially on the operating table with steep Trendelenburg positioning. A gel or egg crate foam pad, or a surgical beanbag, can stabilize even larger patients. Although shoulder braces are discouraged due to the increased potential for brachial plexus injury, placing them laterally over the acromioclavicular joint rather than medially on the shoulder may minimize that risk. Finally, prior to the surgical scrub, the patient should be placed in maximum Trendelenburg position to confirm adequate positioning and stability prior to starting the surgical procedure (tilt test).

Objective guidelines for optimal laparoscopic port placement are limited; the decision is usually influenced more by habit than logic. Importantly, although a surgeon may be comfortable with a particular port distribution, there needs to be flexibility in number and location of ports to accommodate procedure, pathology, and preference. Adding 1 to 2 more strategically positioned ports does not contribute significant morbidity, but may dramatically improve the ergonomics of the procedure while reducing surgical time.

The camera port is typically placed through the umbilicus in uncomplicated patients with a smaller uterus. This can be placed using a traditional closed technique before or after abdominal insufflation, with or without an optical trocar to visualize passing through abdominal wall layers. Alternatively, an open (Hasson) technique or a left upper quadrant (Palmer point) entry might be chosen. While these alternative modes of initial entry are often recommended in patients with prior surgery where periumbilical adhesions are suspected, there is no evidence that any specific entry technique always prevents injury to underlying viscera. However, the Hasson method has been associated with decreased incidence of vascular injury. A 1999 study of 814 patients undergoing left upper quadrant entry for laparoscopy described the incidence of infraumbilical adhesions depending on prior surgical history, including no prior incision (0.68%), prior laparoscopic procedure (1.6%), prior Pfannenstiel incision (19.8%), and prior vertical midline incision (51.7%). They also described the rates of "severe adhesions with potential risk for bowel injury" during trocar insertion in these same four groups as 0.42%, 0.80%, 6.87%, and 31.46%, respectively. However, they did not report the incidence of upper abdominal adhesions, nor did they include patients with prior splenectomy or bariatric surgery in whom the incidence of left upper quadrants adhesions may be increased. There is strong evidence to support using the surgeon's most common initial entry method regardless of the underlying pathology.

All subsequent accessory ports should be placed under laparoscopic guidance. Typical port placement is illustrated in Figure 32C.1. It is usually helpful for at least one port to be a 10-to 12-mm size (often the midline port) to facilitate use of a 10-mm laparoscope, passing suture, introducing adhesion barriers, or passing specimen bags for tissue removal as needed. In most cases, all other ports can be 5 mm to minimize postoperative pain and reduce the chance of trocar site hernia. With a small uterus less than 10 weeks in size, a three-port technique is often adequate with umbilical placement of a camera port and a primary accessory port in the left and right lower abdominal quadrant. If the uterus is slightly larger, up to about 14 weeks in size, umbilical placement of a port for the camera still usually permits adequate visualization. However, additional

(secondary) accessory ports placed higher and slightly more medial than the lower (primary) accessory ports may aid significantly with uterine manipulation and access to intended operative sites (Fig. 32C.1A). In addition to using 10-mm angled telescopes, using a 5-mm straight, angled, or flexible telescope through well-positioned accessory ports at different times during the procedure can be very useful for optimal visualization of the operative field. The primary lower lateral ports should be positioned to provide a good angle for access to ipsilateral pelvic structures and to provide retraction for access to the contralateral pelvic structures. Caution should be taken not to place these ports too low on the abdominal wall close to the pelvic bones. Such a choice of port placement, which is often driven by concern for cosmesis rather than functionality, usually results in an insufficient angle to access to the ipsilateral deep pelvic structures and increases the chance of injury to the ilioinguinal, iliohypogastric, and superficial circumflex vessels. A point at least 2-cm cephalad to the anterior superior iliac spine and at least 2 cm lateral to the rectus sheath is generally a safe starting point for placement choice. Secondary accessory ports become more important contributors to the surgical procedure as uterine size increases. When used, they should be placed cephalad and medial enough to assist with both ipsilateral and contralateral surgical maneuvers and/or retraction and to provide adequate triangulation for suturing. With a larger uterus approximating 20 weeks' size or more, port placement, including the midline camera port, will typically need to be displaced more cephalad but not necessarily more lateral as illustrated in Figure 32C.1B.

Uterine Manipulation

Selection of the ideal device for uterine manipulation depends on the nature of the hysterectomy being performed (LSH or TLH), the uterine size, and occasionally the patient size. The larger the uterus, the less effective any uterine manipulator will be in true manipulation of the uterine corpus and greater reliance will be placed on instruments placed through primary and especially secondary accessory ports. For LSH, delineation of the vaginal fornices and maintaining pneumoperitoneum after a colpotomy

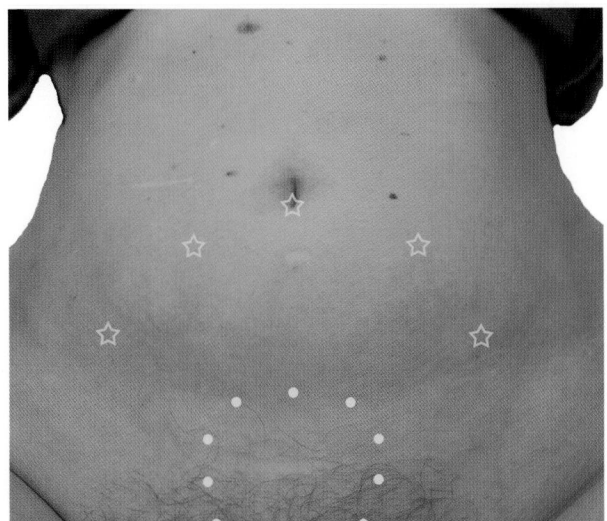
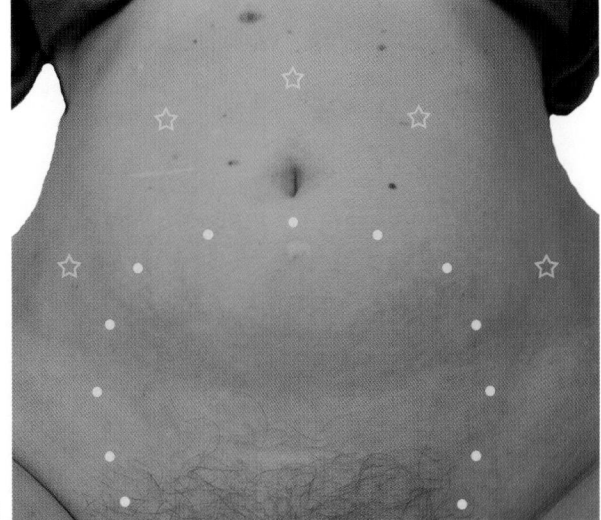

FIGURE 32C.1 Trocar placement. With a uterus less than 14 weeks' size, umbilical placement of a port for the camera usually permits adequate visualization (**A**). Positions of the primary lower lateral ports and secondary accessory ports (when needed) should be chosen to optimize access for surgical maneuvers, retraction, and triangulation for suturing. With a larger uterus approximating 20 weeks' size or more, port placement typically needs to be displaced superiorly but not necessarily laterally (**B**).

incision are not primary concerns; a Hulka tenaculum or Valchev manipulator is usually adequate. However, both of these features are critical in performing TLH, where the colpotomy ring lateralizes and protects the ureters and identifies the vaginal fornices as a guide for colpotomy. A pneumo-occluder, which may be incorporated into the design of the manipulator or may be added as a separate component, maintains the pneumoperitoneum after colpotomy and amputation of the specimen from the vagina until the cuff is closed. Choice of manipulator can contribute significantly to ease of operation and shorten operating time. A wide variety of choices are available; some commonly used manipulators are depicted in Figure 32C.2. Although selection of specific combinations of devices may vary with surgeon preference and experience, choosing the appropriate straight or curved manipulator and the right size and shape colpotomy ring for manipulation of the cervix and fornix when securing the blood supply and amputating the uterus from the vagina is critical to success and safety. It has been my experience that the combination of ZUMI manipulator with a Koh colpotomy ring and a balloon pneumo-occluder (Fig. 32C.2A) works well in most situations. However, when operating on patients with a greater body mass index, or with a very large uterus, I find the more rigid Advincula Arch (RUMI) manipulator with a molded colpotomy ring and occluder unit (Fig. 32C.2B) to be more useful to achieve necessary uterine elevation and manipulation.

OPERATIVE TECHNIQUE

It is often useful to think of TLH as having five components: (1) separation of the adnexal structures from the uterine corpus for subsequent preservation or removal; (2) dissecting, occluding, and dividing the blood supply prior to extirpation of the uterine corpus; (3) transection of the cardinal ligament complex with colpotomy and amputation of the cervix from the vaginal apex; (4) removing the specimen; and (5) closing the vaginal cuff. For LSH, the first two components are essentially identical. However, step 3 involves amputation of the uterine corpus from the cervix above the cardinal ligament, step 4 incorporates fewer options, and step 5 is not needed. In the case of TLH for a very large fibroid uterus, or in the case of significantly distorted anatomy, I frequently find it quite helpful to perform an LSH first (in the absence of endometrial neoplasm) and then address the colpotomy and cervical amputation with the uterine corpus out of the operative field. All of

the steps of TLH mimic or correlate with a comparable step in abdominal hysterectomy. There are some options for modification owing to the increased magnification and proximity of visual field to the surgical target appreciated with laparoscopy.

The Adnexa

Regardless of whether the ultimate goal is to remove or preserve the adnexal structures, I uniformly find it expedient to begin the laparoscopic hysterectomy by separating ovaries and fallopian tubes from the uterine fundus. This serves two distinct purposes. First, and most obvious, the adnexa are not dangling from the corpus for the remainder of the procedure potentially obscuring visual and operative access while securing the uterine vessels, amputating the uterine corpus (LSH), or performing a colpotomy (TLH). Second, and less appreciated, any subsequent procedure involving the adnexa can be deferred until the uterus can first be removed from the operative field. This provides unencumbered views of, and access to, the pelvic sidewall from both ipsilateral and contralateral approaches, thus facilitating even the most challenging of adnexal procedures involving distorted anatomy, adhesions, or endometriosis.

As with abdominal hysterectomy, separation of the adnexa can be accomplished by coagulating and dividing the round ligament first, dissecting the retroperitoneal space beneath the broad ligament to identify and isolate the ureter, then sealing and dividing the proximal fallopian tube and utero-ovarian ligament. It is important to recognize that, with laparoscopic approach, the ureter can usually be identified through the intact peritoneum crossing the pelvic brim at the bifurcation of the external and internal iliac vessels and coursing across the pelvic sidewall inferior to the infundibulopelvic ligament but superior to the uterosacral ligament (Fig. 32C.3). If this is the case, a retroperitoneal dissection at this point in the procedure does not add any benefit to the laparoscopic hysterectomy and might even result in unnecessary bleeding. Accordingly, while keeping the location of the ureter in view, the proximal fallopian tube and the utero-ovarian ligament can be coagulated and transected, preferably from the contralateral approach (Fig. 32C.4A). Tissue transection is continued parallel to the round ligament until the adnexa are completely isolated from the uterine corpus (Fig. 32C.4B).

Next, the round ligament is coagulated and transected, thus entering the broad ligament for subsequent dissection of

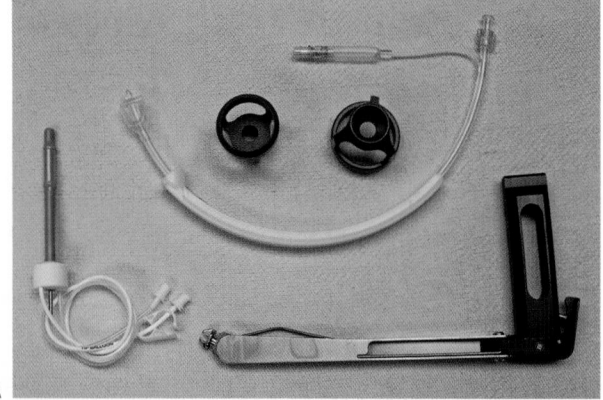

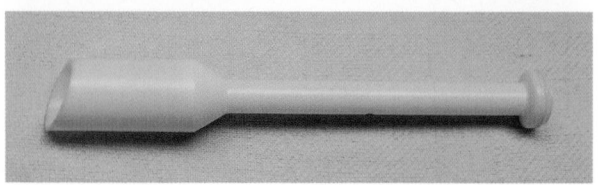

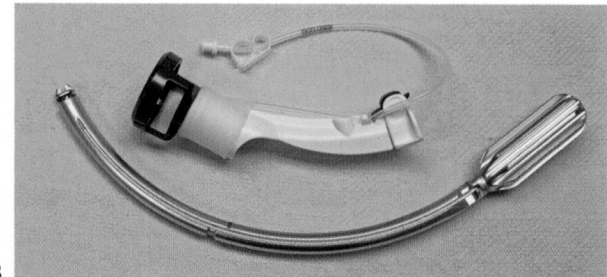

FIGURE 32C.2 Uterine manipulator examples. **A:** ZUMI curved uterine manipulator (*top*) with different sizes of Koh colpotomy rings and RUMI straight uterine manipulator (*bottom*) with attachable uterine probe. **B:** Advincula arch uterine manipulator with KohEfficient colpotomy ring including attached pneumo-occluder. **C:** ColpoProbe. All available from CooperSurgical (Trumbull, CT).

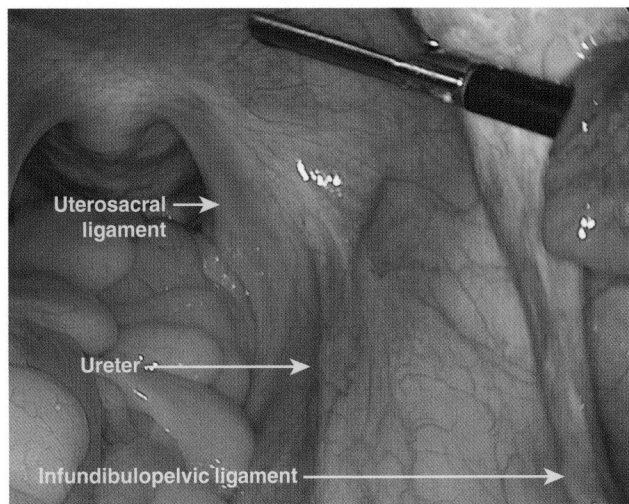

FIGURE 32C.3 Identification of the ureter. The ureter can usually be identified crossing the pelvic brim and coursing across the pelvic sidewall inferior to the infundibulopelvic ligament and superior to the uterosacral ligament. Understanding and identifying this anatomic relationship can prevent the need for retroperitoneal dissection for ureter identification prior to adnexectomy.

the uterine vessels. If the uterus is small enough, or if secondary accessory ports have been placed high enough, the round ligament should be grasped from the contralateral side to retract the uterus medially and stabilize the round ligament. Coagulation of the round ligament to open the leaves of the broad ligament and enter the retroperitoneal space, and subsequent dissection within the broad ligament, can then be accomplished from an ipsilateral approach (Fig. 32C.4C). Conversely, in cases where the uterus is larger, distorted by fibroids, or otherwise conformed in a manner where retraction using instruments through the contralateral ports is suboptimal, then "retraction" can be attained by pushing the uterus medially using an instrument through one ipsilateral port and coagulating, cutting, and dissecting through the other ipsilateral port, as illustrated in Figure 32C.4D. Note that the blades of the grasper are opened to add stability to the "retraction," which can be aided by using existing features of the uterus (in this case a fibroid). Although it cannot be fully appreciated in this image, the "retracting" instrument has been placed through the left primary (lower) accessory port for optimal manipulation of the uterus both cephalad and medial. Then the instrument used for manipulation, coagulation, and cutting has been placed through left secondary (upper) accessory port in order to achieve the best angle for dissection of the broad ligament toward the uterine isthmus.

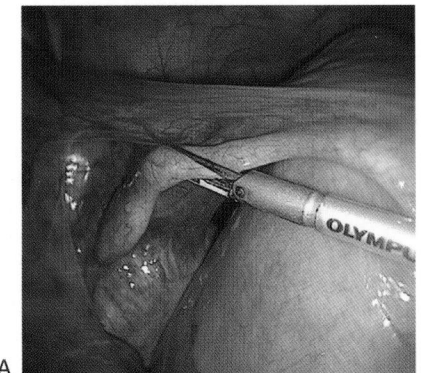
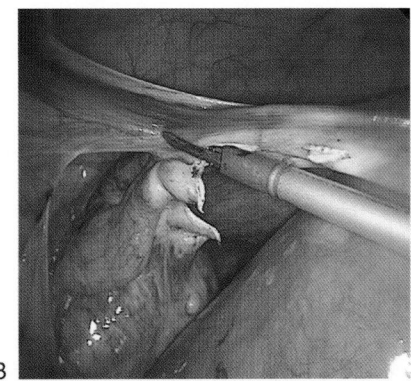
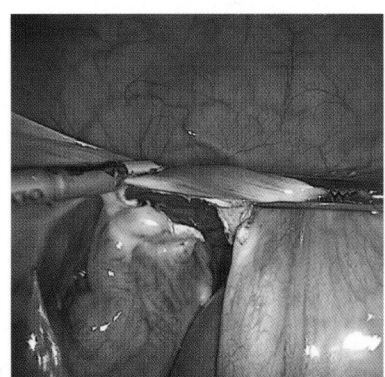

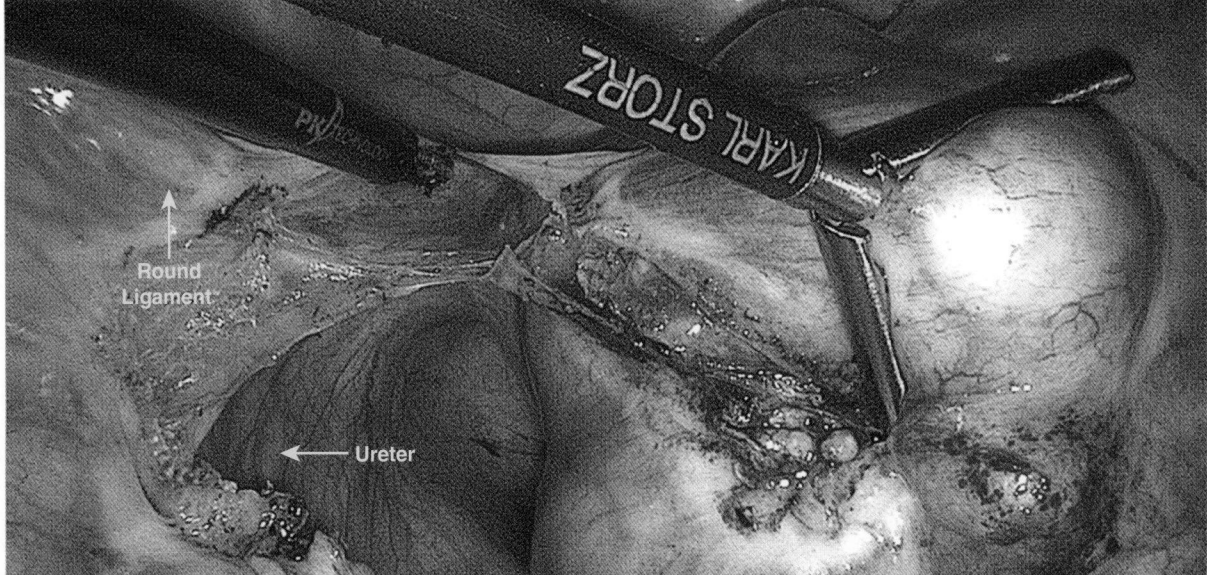

FIGURE 32C.4 Isolate adnexal structures. The proximal fallopian tube (**A**) and utero-ovarian ligament (**B**) are usually best transected from the contralateral approach. The round ligament is best transected from the ipsilateral approach (**C**). Retraction for transection of the round ligament and subsequent dissection of the broad ligament space can be accomplished from either a contralateral approach (**C**) or an ipsilateral approach (**D**), depending on the size of the uterus and port placement.

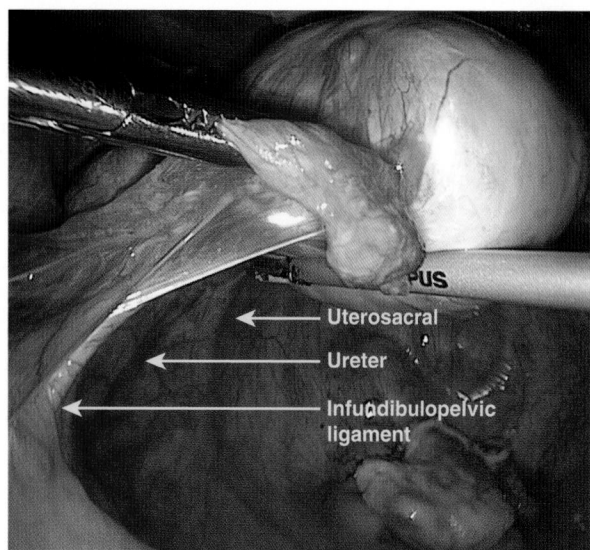

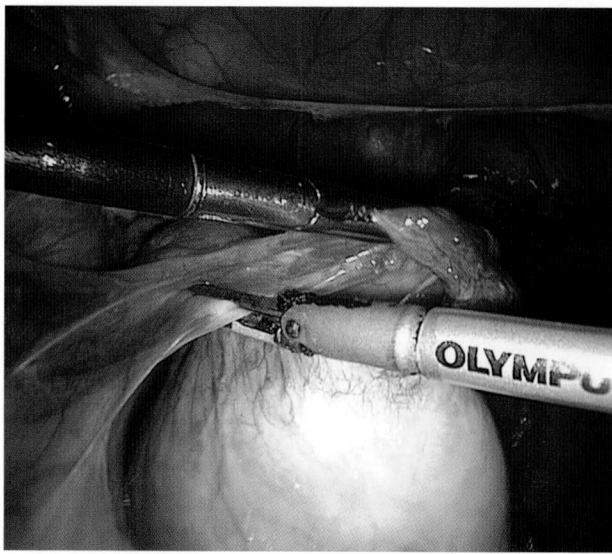

FIGURE 32C.5 Salpingo-oophorectomy. After removal of the uterine corpus, there is unobstructed access to the adnexal structures. The infundibulopelvic ligament is easily distinguished from the ureter (**A**) for safe coagulation and transection (**B**).

In cases of distorted anatomy, the more traditional approach of entering the retroperitoneal space through the round ligament, identifying the ureter, and dissecting its course toward the uterine artery prior to isolating the adnexal structures is often preferred.

If the ultimate goal is ovarian preservation, then adnexa can be ignored at this point. Alternatively, when the intent is to remove the fallopian tubes and/or ovaries, to treat ovarian pathology (e.g., remove a dermoid cyst or endometrioma), and/or to address pelvic sidewall issues (e.g., adhesions or endometriosis), this action can usually be deferred until after the uterine corpus is out of the way. At that time, the mesosalpinx or the infundibulopelvic ligament can be isolated, coagulated, and transected. Ergonomically, it is preferable to retract the adnexal structures medially from the ipsilateral side while securing and transecting the pedicles from the contralateral side (Fig. 32C.5). This approach permits an application of

your energy source that is perpendicular to the pedicle, which maximizes efficient performance of the instrument and minimizes collateral thermal tissue damage.

The Uterine Corpus and Cervix

Once the round ligament has been transected and the leaves of the broad ligament have been separated, dissection can continue to the level of the uterine vessels at the junction of the lower uterine segment with the cervix. Subsequently, a bladder flap can be created (Fig. 32C.6A) and the uterine vessels skeletonized (Fig. 32C.6B). These steps are identical to their abdominal hysterectomy counterparts and require minimal application of energy. In fact, cold sharp dissection (or only very brief pulses of bipolar current to maintain hemostasis of superficial peritoneal vessels) is preferred during this step until the anatomic limits of the bladder are defined.

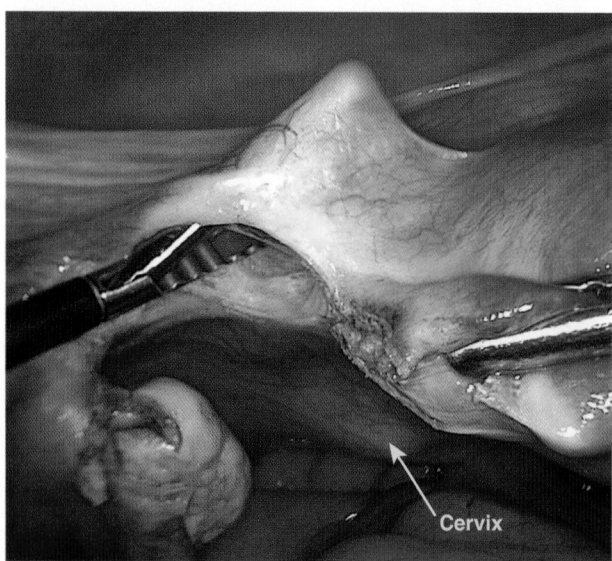

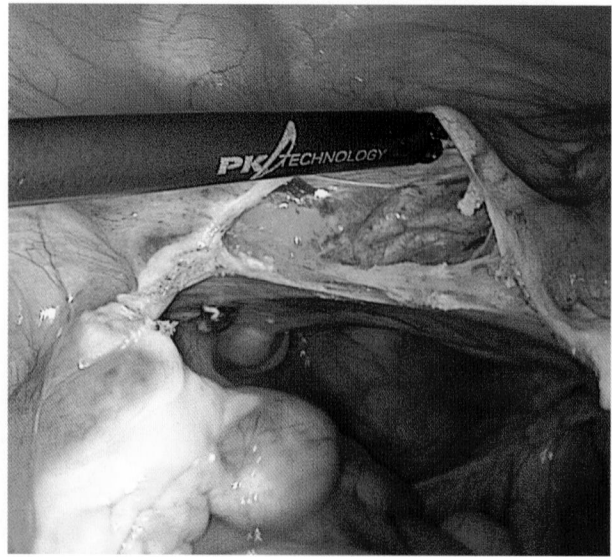

FIGURE 32C.6 Creation of bladder flap and amputation of the uterus. The anterior and posterior leaves of the broad ligament are separated to create a bladder flap (**A**), which allows the surgeon to expose and skeletonize the ascending uterine vessels (**B**).

When skeletonizing, coagulating, and transecting the uterine vessels, retraction of the uterus from the contralateral side is preferred as this allows the more efficient use of two operative instruments by the surgeon. However, in situations where contralateral retraction is not possible, the ipsilateral retraction technique described above can be employed. Either way, care should be taken not to twist the uterus, which can cause distortion of the anatomy and disorientation of the surgeon. It is still possible to accomplish these maneuvers effectively even if only one operative instrument can be employed. Most advanced electrosurgical instruments used in laparoscopic procedures today are designed to permit tissue dissection, sealing, and transection. A skilled experienced surgeon can use a single instrument to develop the bladder flap and skeletonize, coagulate, and transect the uterine vessels. Understanding the specific properties of your electrosurgical instrument of choice is critical.

LAPAROSCOPIC SUPRACERVICAL HYSTERECTOMY

When performing LSH, the ascending branches of the uterine vessels should be coagulated and transected at the junction of the lower uterine segment with the cervix (Fig. 32C.7A). This is also the level at which the uterus is amputated from the cervical stump. This is perhaps the most critical step in performing LSH. The optimal level of vessel transection and fundal amputation can be identified in most uteri where the curvature of the fundus "flattens out" into the cervix. This is the isthmus. You should be certain that you have coagulated the uterine vessels just inferior (toward the cervix) to where you plan to amputate the fundus. Additionally, if you continue to coagulate the uterine vessels in an ascending manner up the lateral edge of the uterus, this will not only decrease back bleeding from the uterus, but it will also accentuate the angle of the junction between the uterine fundus and cervix as a guide for amputation plane.

It has been my experience that many surgeons attempt to amputate the uterine fundus too low on the cervix. Whether it is related to difficulty in ascertaining the optimal plane for amputation, or whether it stems from a belief that excising more cervix will decrease the likelihood of subsequent cyclic bleeding, this seems to be especially characteristic of surgeons

that are learning and perfecting the technique of LSH. The incidence of post-LSH cyclic bleeding does not appear to be related to length of cervix left. However, what definitely will happen if the surgeon is too aggressive in estimating the amount of tissue to amputate is that increased bleeding will be encountered associated with the rich plexus of vascular supply to the cervix and upper vagina, necessitating further efforts to achieve hemostasis. If electrosurgical energy application is employed to this end, there is an increased risk of thermal injury to the ureter or compromise of the vascular supply to the remaining cervical stump, both of which are likely not to be recognized until several days after the procedure with fistula formation or necrosis of the cervical stump, respectively. To mitigate this risk, the cervical stump should be elevated out of the pelvis using a sponge stick or other transvaginal manipulator and energy applied sparingly. Alternatively, other mechanisms for hemostasis could be considered, including vascular clips or suturing.

Subsequent to fundal amputation, the endocervical canal can be fulgurated, preferably using bipolar current, or it can be left untreated. Although it seems intuitive that fulguration of the endocervical canal would decrease the incidence of post-LSH cyclic bleeding, there is no evidence to support that belief. Rather, the probability of bleeding may be more related to patient age and/or the presence of preexisting endometriosis.

TOTAL LAPAROSCOPIC HYSTERECTOMY

When performing TLH, once the bladder flap is created, the skeletonized ascending branches of the uterine vessels can be identified crossing the colpotomy ring (Fig. 32C.7B). The vessels should be coagulated and transected at this level. As with LSH described above, this step and subsequent colpotomy and amputation of the uterus from the vagina are the most critical steps when performing TLH. Also, similar to the technique described for LSH, continued coagulation of the uterine vessels in an ascending manner up the lateral edge of the uterus will decrease back bleeding from the uterus at the time of vessel transection. However, in contrast with the LSH, the presence of a previously placed colpotomy ring usually delineates the vaginal fornix, providing an excellent guide for exactly where to transect the vessels and exactly where to amputate the uterus from the vagina.

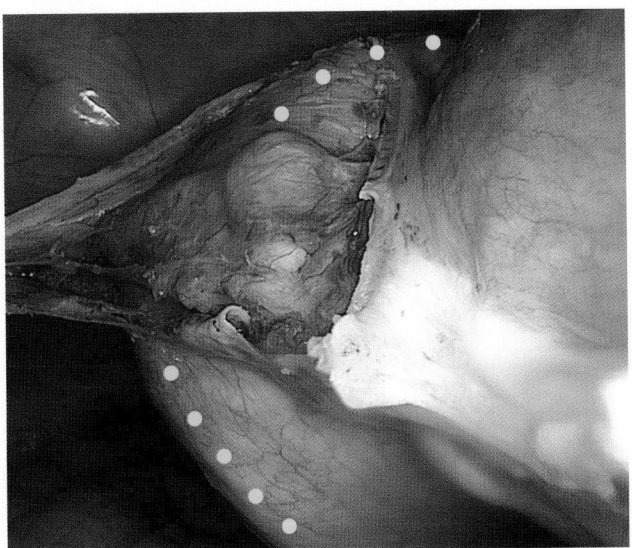
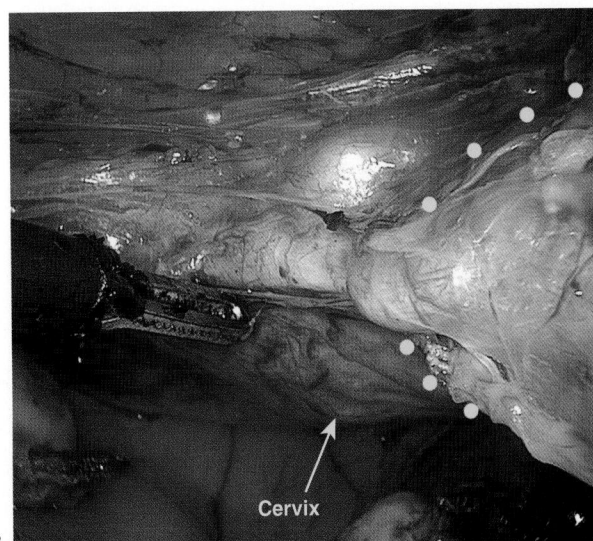

FIGURE 32C.7 Colpotomy and cervical amputation. When performing LSH, the vessels are coagulated and transected at the junction of the lower uterine segment with the cervix (**A**) and the uterine corpus is amputated by transecting the cervix at this location (*dotted line*). When performing TLH, the ascending branch of the uterine vessels can be coagulated and transected as they are crossing the colpotomy ring (**B**), which also serves as a guide for subsequent amputation (*dotted line*).

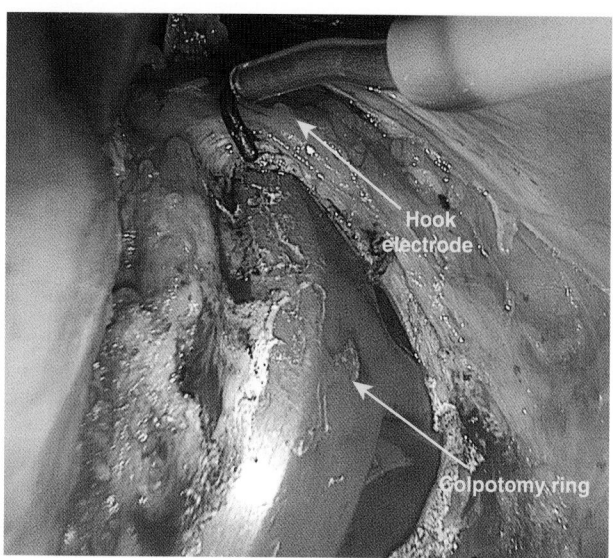

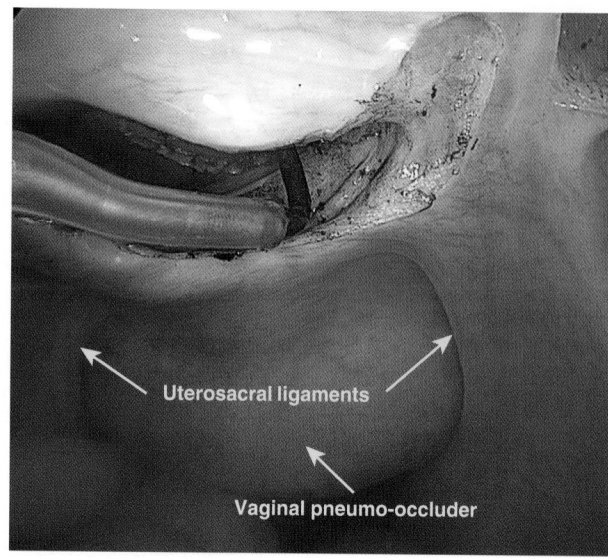

FIGURE 32C.8 Amputation of the uterus. A thin monopolar electrode (e.g., hook) is recommended for amputation of the uterus using the colpotomy ring as a guide (**A**). This applies the lowest voltage energy and minimizes the risk of thermal injury to the ureter or bladder. Amputation of the uterus and cervix at the level of the colpotomy ring transects the cardinal ligament complex, leaving the uterosacral ligaments attached to the fascia of the vaginal apex (**B**).

The colpotomy incision and amputation of the uterus are the most important steps in performing TLH with respect to potential urinary tract injury. There is no single electrosurgical instrument that has been shown to be superior in mitigating this risk. However, each instrument does have distinctive electrical and mechanical properties related to spread of thermal energy, tissue sealing, and cutting. Regardless of which instrument is chosen, a comprehensive understanding of its unique properties is critical. While bipolar current is typically used to coagulate the uterine vessels, a variety of instruments can be used to perform the colpotomy incision. Attention should be paid to minimize electrosurgical energy at this step. A monopolar hook electrode attached to a "Bovie pencil" using continuous (cutting) current is particularly useful. Using the colpotomy ring as a backstop, it has the ability to deliver very focused electrosurgical energy with low voltage (Fig. 32C.8A). Any oozing that is encountered can usually be handled with short bursts of monopolar discontinuous (coagulation) current. This minimizes thermal spread that results in devitalization of tissue at the cuff over time and minimizes the risk of inadvertent electrosurgical injury to the bladder or ureter.

It does not matter whether the anterior or posterior colpotomy incision is made first. It is more important to choose whichever is most identifiable and accessible so that the edge of the colpotomy ring can be identified when the tissue is divided. Once this is achieved, the amputation is simply a matter of "following the ring" circumferentially using the tip of the hook electrode for precise focal energy delivery (Fig. 32C.8A). Importantly, when the colpotomy ring is placed and identified appropriately, the level of cervical amputation is at the cardinal ligament. Accordingly, when the posterior colpotomy incision is made, the uterosacral ligaments remain attached to the fascia of the vaginal apex (Fig. 32C.8B). This facilitates incorporation of the uterosacral ligaments into the subsequent cuff closure for pelvic support.

In cases where the uterus is particularly bulky, or there is distortion of the pelvic anatomy due to adhesions, endometriosis, or other concomitant pathology, amputation of the fundus from the cervix can be accomplished prior to attempting colpotomy and amputation of the cervix. In fact, it is often preferable to do so. In this case, the same steps described above with LSH are followed, usually amputating even higher on the cervix or even lower uterine segment. Subsequently, the plane delineated by the colpotomy ring is easier to identify and to access for cervical amputation.

STEPS IN THE PROCEDURE

Laparoscopic Hysterectomy

- Place the patient in lithotomy position, and perform tilt test to ensure stability on table.
- Drape into sterile field, uterine manipulator, colpotomy ring, pneumoperitoneum occluder (depending on procedure), and Foley catheter.
- Peritoneal insufflation and port placement depending on size of uterus.
- Identification of anatomic landmarks including ureters, uterosacral ligaments, bladder edge, and colpotomy ring.
- Coagulate and transect proximal fallopian tube(s) and utero-ovarian ligament(s) to separate adnexal structures from uterine corpus.
- Coagulate and transect round ligament and dissect broad ligament to the level of the uterine isthmus.
- Create bladder flap and skeletonize uterine vessels.
- For supracervical hysterectomy:
- Coagulate uterine vessels at the level of the uterine isthmus.
- Amputate the uterus from the cervix at the level of the isthmus.
- For total laparoscopic hysterectomy:
- Coagulate uterine vessels at the level of the colpotomy ring.

- Transect cardinal ligament and amputate the uterus and cervix from the vaginal apex, using colpotomy ring as a guide, with monopolar continuous (cutting) current
- Isolate, coagulate, and transect infundibulopelvic ligaments (if salpingo-oophorectomy is desired).
- Coagulate and transect mesosalpinx (if only salpingectomy is desired).
- Remove adnexal tissue intact and uterus (with morcellation, if indicated).
- Close the vaginal cuff incorporating the uterosacral ligaments.
- Secure hemostasis and close trocar sites in usual fashion.

Tissue removal

When performing TLH, the uterus, cervix, and adnexal structures can usually be removed through the vagina prior to closing the cuff. This becomes more challenging with increasing uterine size, but vaginal morcellation offers an excellent technique for removal of larger specimens. Each surgeon will have to determine his or her own skill level with respect to vaginal morcellation and the size at which alternative tissue removal techniques will need to be employed. When performing LSH, tissue removal options are more limited.

Aside from extraction of tissue through the vagina, removal options include making a small laparotomy incision to remove the tissue intact or with manual morcellation, extending the umbilical incision enough to accomplish the same, or using electromechanical morcellation. Recent controversy has arisen regarding the safety of tissue morcellation. Use of electromechanical morcellation has been shown in some cases to disseminate benign tissue, or neoplastic tissue in the rare case of an undiagnosed malignancy, with potential adverse downstream consequences. Importantly, manual morcellation has not been proven to avoid this possibility; it simply has not been studied.

Clearly, morcellation should not be employed when a malignant or premalignant diagnosis is known or if preoperative assessment of the patient is suspicious for the same. In these cases, tissue needs to be removed intact, even if it means converting to a laparotomy. Critical reviews of relevant literature by different professional organizations, including AAGL and ACOG, support that tissue morcellation can be performed safely and effectively by properly trained and experienced surgeons in appropriately screened and selected patients.

After the uterus has been removed through the vagina or an alternative mechanism, a pneumo-occluder in the vagina can maintain pneumoperitoneum until the vaginal cuff is closed (Fig. 32C.9A). When necessary, a ring forcep can be introduced transvaginally around the pneumo-occluder to grasp and retrieve the ovaries and/or tubes prior to closing the vaginal cuff.

Cuff Closure

With laparoscopic hysterectomy, the vaginal cuff can be closed laparoscopically or vaginally, depending on the skill of the surgeon, but the former defines a true TLH. The basic tenets of cuff closure that are considered with abdominal and vaginal hysterectomy apply to TLH, only the visual perspective and magnification changes. Both intracorporeal and extracorporeal knot-tying techniques have been described using absorbable suture. Notably, the advent of barbed suture has facilitated laparoscopic suturing because it does not require knot typing, which is the most technically challenging and skill limiting component.

There is a statistically increased incidence of cuff dehiscence with TLH. A 2007 study of over 7,200 hysterectomies reported the rates of cuff dehiscence to be 0.12% with abdominal hysterectomy, 0.29% with vaginal hysterectomy, and 4.93% with laparoscopic hysterectomy. Barbed suture was not included in this study. There is no evidence that use of barbed suture increases the incidence of cuff dehiscence. In fact, there is evidence that cuff closure in two layers using barbed sutures decreases the incidence of cuff dehiscence in TLH. Two factors that are thought to contribute to the increased cuff dehiscence rate after TLH include (1) increased magnification of the surgical field with the laparoscope, leading the surgeon to think the tissue included in the suture is more than it really is, and (2) progressive devitalization of tissue with time due to thermal effect during colpotomy, possibly extending to or beyond the suture line. Accordingly, the

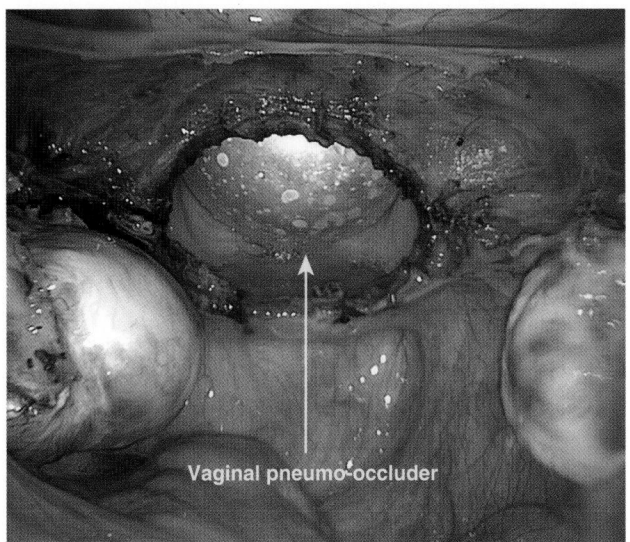

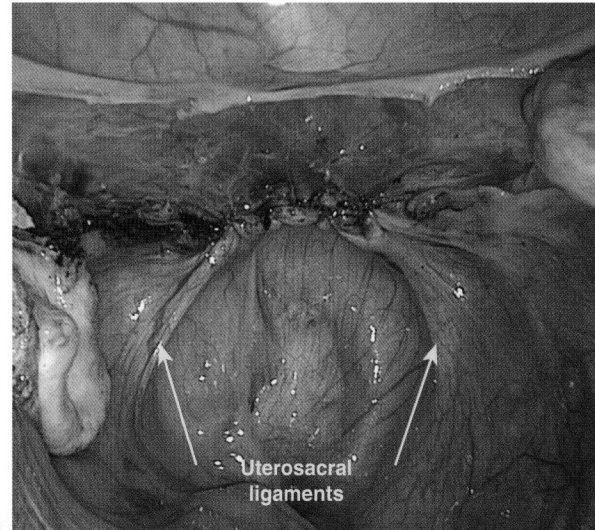

FIGURE 32C.9 Closure of the vaginal cuff. After amputation of the uterus, a pneumo-occluder balloon in the vagina can maintain peritoneal insufflation (**A**) until the vaginal cuff is closed. Cuff closure should incorporate the uterosacral ligaments (**B**).

greatest steps that can be taken during cuff closure to mitigate dehiscence, in addition to basic surgical principles of hemostasis and "approximation, not strangulation" of tissue, are minimizing application of thermal energy during colpotomy and incorporating adequate healthy tissue in the suture line.

Incorporation of the uterosacral ligaments into cuff closure has become relatively standard with abdominal or vaginal hysterectomy and has been demonstrated to decrease the incidence of posthysterectomy vaginal vault prolapse from 25% to 5%, with or without culdoplasty. Although there have been no long-term trials to show comparable results after TLH, there is every expectation for similar outcomes and incorporation of the uterosacral ligaments into the cuff closure is recommended (Fig. 32C.9B); laparoscopy is a different access, not a different procedure.

COMPLICATIONS

The nature of complications occurring with TLH is similar to that of those reported for abdominal and vaginal hysterectomy. Complications related to medical comorbidities, anesthesia, or the hysterectomy procedure may occur, as well as those related specifically to laparoscopy. Regardless of access, hysterectomy remains a relatively safe procedure with a mortality rate estimated between 0.12 and 0.34 per 1,000 procedures.

Postoperative wound complications such as infection after laparoscopic hysterectomy appear to be less frequent than with abdominal hysterectomy, largely owing to the smaller size. However, complications do occur specifically related to the use of trocars. These are related to trocar insertion (specifically, abdominal wall vasculature or nerve injury and intra-abdominal vascular or intestinal injury) or to trocar site hernia (which is <1%). Trocars should be removed under visualization at the conclusion of the hysterectomy to watch for bleeding. The fascia should be closed separately from the skin at trocar sites 10 mm or greater. This can be accomplished using traditional suturing technique or by using a variety of commercially available products available for this purpose (Carter-Thomason device, Endoclose device, etc.).

Two large studies have compared complications rates with different routes of hysterectomy. Both were published in 2004. The Vaginal Abdominal Laparoscopic Uterine Excision (VALUE) study was a prospective cohort examination of severe complications related to hysterectomy in over 37,000 women. "Severe complications" (e.g., visceral injury, hemorrhage, thromboembolic disease, myocardial infarction, stroke, end-organ failure) were noted to be low (4.4%) overall, but the risk was doubled in younger patients undergoing a laparoscopic procedure for fibroids and those with significant comorbidities, compared with similar patients undergoing abdominal or vaginal hysterectomies. Unfortunately, hysterectomies involving laparoscopy comprised only 3% of the study population and were limited to LAVH (no TLH or LSH).

The eVALuate study was actually two parallel prospective randomized trials including over 1,300 patients that compared complications of laparoscopic hysterectomy with either abdominal hysterectomy or vaginal hysterectomy. Significant findings are listed in Table 32C.3. In this study, laparoscopic

TABLE 32C.3 Reported Complications in Both Arms of the eVALuate Trial

	ABDOMINAL TRIAL		VAGINAL TRIAL	
	ABDOMINAL HYSTERECTOMY	**LAPAROSCOPIC HYSTERECTOMY**	**VAGINAL HYSTERECTOMY**	**LAPAROSCOPIC HYSTERECTOMY**
At least one complication[a]	6.2%	7.2%	5.4%	6.7%
Conversion to laparotomy	—	3.9%	4.2%	2.7%
Bowel injury	1%	0.2%	0%	0%
Ureter injury	0%	0.9%	0%	0.3%
Bladder injury	1%	2.1%	1.2%	0.9%
Deep vein thrombosis	0%	0.3%	0%	0%
Pulmonary embolus	0.7%	0.2%	0%	0.6%
Wound dehiscence	0.3%	0.2%	0%	0.3%
Hematoma	0.7%	0.7%	1.2%	2.1%
Major hemorrhage	2.4%	4.6%	2.9%	5.1%
Anesthesia problem	0%	0.9%	0%	0.6%
Return to operating room	0.3%	0.5%	0%	0.3%

[a]Excludes "conversion to laparotomy" as a complication.
A patient may have had more than one complication.
Adapted from Garry R, Fountain J, Mason S, et al. The eVALuate study: two parallel randomised trials, one comparing laparoscopic with abdominal hysterectomy, the other comparing laparoscopic with vaginal hysterectomy. *BMJ* 2004;328(7432):129, with permission.
Copyright © 2004, British Medical Journal Publishing Group.

hysterectomy encompassed LAVH, LSH, and TLH. In the abdominal hysterectomy arm, advantages of a laparoscopic approach were noted to include fewer infections, smaller drop in hemoglobin, less pain, shorter hospital stay, quicker recovery, and improved short-term quality of life when compared with an abdominal approach. There was an increased incidence of bladder and ureter injuries with the laparoscopic approach. The study reported an overall complication rate in laparoscopic hysterectomy increased over abdominal hysterectomy (11.1% vs. 6.2%, respectively). However, they included "conversion to laparotomy" (which is not possible in abdominal hysterectomy) as a complication of laparoscopy. When this is more appropriately considered an exercise of good surgical judgment rather than a complication, the overall rate complication rate between the laparoscopic and abdominal groups becomes nonsignificant (7.2% vs. 6.2%, respectively). Similarly, there was no significant difference in overall complication rates between laparoscopic and vaginal hysterectomy, although vaginal hysterectomies were performed in half the time. Of note, this arm of the study contained cases of "low technical challenge" and was underpowered.

Gynecologic surgery, specifically hysterectomy, is the most common cause of iatrogenic urinary tract injury. Several studies have reported an increased rate of urinary tract injuries in laparoscopic hysterectomy compared with abdominal or vaginal hysterectomy. Most of those studies included only LAVH (not TLH or LSH) and even then represented a small percentage of the study population.

A common risk factor for bladder injury is the presence of prior cesarean section, pelvic adhesive disease, or endometriosis involving the bladder. On the other hand, greater than 90% of ureteral injuries during laparoscopic hysterectomy can be attributed to thermal injury related to division of the cardinal ligament. A case controlled study of over 5,000 hysterectomies demonstrated that the risk of urinary tract injury is increased in vaginal (1.3%) or laparoscopic (1.8%) hysterectomy when compared with abdominal hysterectomy (0.76%). Further, a 2009 study involving over 800 patients described bladder injury during hysterectomy in 2.9% of patients and ureteral injury in 1.8% of patients, 75% of which were unsuspected. Interestingly, evidence from a 2006 meta-analysis demonstrated that when cystoscopy is performed immediately after hysterectomy, 89% of ureteral and 95% of bladder injuries are detected intraoperatively. Conversely, in the absence of cystoscopy, intraoperative detection drops to 43% of bladder and only 7% of ureteral injuries.

Although overall urinary tract injury rates are low, overall postoperative morbidity is not increased when bladder injuries are recognized and repaired at the time of surgery. Indeed, intraoperative identification may help to avoid additional surgery and loss of renal function. The role of routine cystoscopy after hysterectomy continues to be debated, but fiscal analysis suggests intraoperative cystoscopy becomes cost-effective when the injury rate exceeds 2%.

Finally, the role of surgeon experience in reducing complications of laparoscopic hysterectomy cannot be overemphasized. Multiple studies have demonstrated decreased complications rates that plateau after about 100 cases and with high volume laparoscopic surgeons.

CONCLUSIONS

After performing the first total laparoscopic hysterectomy, Harry Reich envisioned its role as decreasing the need for abdominal hysterectomy by "avoiding the increased morbidity associated with abdominal surgery while retaining the surgical advantages of the abdominal approach." Not only did his words ring true, his efforts launched an era of advanced laparoscopic gynecologic surgery enjoyed today. Indeed, laparoscopy simultaneously provides superior exposure to the adnexa and upper abdomen, which is not available to the vaginal surgeon, but simultaneously avoids a large abdominal wall incision, thus reducing the associated risk of infection, postoperative pain, and hernia. Thus, with appropriate training, skill, and experience, the surgeon performing laparoscopic hysterectomy enjoys vision and access advantages that are superior to abdominal hysterectomy while retaining the decreased morbidity of the vaginal approach.

BEST SURGICAL PRACTICES

- The choice of access for and type of hysterectomy should be based on the patient's anatomy and pathology. Supracervical hysterectomy should not be performed simply because of the surgeon's lack of comfort with removing the cervix. Instead, assistance from more skilled surgeons should be sought.
- The patient should be counseled thoroughly regarding anticipated outcomes, potential complications, preoperative preparation, and postoperative care. Risks and benefits of using energy-based instruments and morcellators should be included in the informed consent process. Discuss alternatives for tissue removal, including vaginal morcellation or laparotomy.
- Preprocedure optimization of comorbidities, especially cardiovascular, should be coordinated with the anesthesia team to minimize medical complications.
- An appropriate uterine manipulator and vaginal fornix delineator should be used for total laparoscopic hysterectomy to improve procedural ergonomics and decrease complications.
- Anatomy should be respected. Clearly identify ureters, bladder, and other anatomic landmarks. Isolate or skeletonize vessels to be coagulated.
- Understand the electrosurgical and mechanical characteristics of energy-based instruments you are using, and apply those principles to minimize undesired thermal tissue effects.
- Prevent or minimize bleeding as much as possible during laparoscopic hysterectomy. Blood absorbs light and hinders full visualization by decreasing light intensity in the surgical field.

BIBLIOGRAPHY

American Association of Gynecologic Laparoscopists. AAGL Practice Report: Morcellation during uterine tissue extraction. *J Minim Invasiv Gynecol* 2014;21:517.

American Association of Gynecologic Laparoscopist. AAGL position statement: route of hysterectomy to treat benign uterine disease. *J Minim Invasive Gynecol* 2011;18:1.

American College of Obstetricians and Gynecologists. ACOG committee opinion No. 388: supracervical hysterectomy. *Obstet Gynecol* 2007;110:1215.

American College of Obstetricians and Gynecologists. ACOG committee opinion No. 444: choosing the route of hysterectomy for benign disease. *Obstet Gynecol* 2009;114:1156.

American College of Obstetricians and Gynecologists. Power morcellation and occult malignancy in gynecologic surgery. *Obstet Gynecol* 2014.

Audebert AJ, Gomel V. Role of microlaparoscopy in the diagnosis of peritoneal and visceral adhesions and in the prevention of bowel injury associated with blind trocar insertion. *Fertil Steril* 2000;73:631.

Duoung TH, Gellasch TL. Incidental cystotomy at the time of a hysterectomy. *Female Pelvic Med Reconstr Surg* 2010;16:129.

V

Berner E, Qvigstad E, Myrvold AK, et al. Pelvic pain and patient satisfaction after laparoscopic supracervical hysterectomy: prospective trial. *J Minim Invasive Gynecol* 2014;21:406.

Falcone T, Paraiso MF, Mascha E. Prospective randomized clinical trial of laparoscopically assisted vaginal hysterectomy versus total abdominal hysterectomy. *Am J Obstet Gynecol* 1999;180:955.

Falcone T, Walters MD. Hysterectomy for benign disease. *Obstet Gynecol* 2008;111:753.

Garry R. A consensus document concerning laparoscopic entry techniques. *Gynecol Endosc* 1999;8:403.

Garry R, Fountain J, Mason S, et al. The eVALuate study: two parallel randomised trials, one comparing laparoscopic with abdominal hysterectomy, the other comparing laparoscopic with vaginal hysterectomy. *BMJ* 2004;328:129.

Ghomi A, Hantes J, Lotze EC. Incidence of cyclical bleeding after laparoscopic supra-cervical hysterectomy. *J Minim Invasive Gynecol* 2005;12:201.

Gilmour DT, Das S, Flowerdew G. Rates of urinary tract injury from gynecologic surgery and the role of intraoperative cystoscopy. *Obstet Gynecol* 2006;107:1366.

Gimbel H, Zobbe V, Andersen BM, et al. Randomised controlled trial of total compared with subtotal hysterectomy with one-year follow-up results. *BJOG* 2003;110:1088.

Hannoun-Lévi JM, Peiffert D, Hoffstetter S, et al. Carcinoma of the cervical stump: retrospective analysis of 77 cases. *Radiother Oncol* 1997;43:147.

Hasson HM. Cervical removal at hysterectomy for benign disease. Risks and benefits. *J Reprod Med* 1993;38:781.

Hur HC, Guido RS, Mansuria SM, et al. Incidence and patient characteristics of vaginal cuff dehiscence after different modes of hysterectomies. *J Minim Invasive Gynecol* 2007;14:311.

Ibeanu OA, Chesson RR, Echols KT, et al. Urinary tract injury during hysterectomy based on universal cystoscopy. *Obstet Gynecol* 2009;113:6.

Jasmine Tan-Kim J, Menefee SA, Luber KA, et al. Prevalence and risk factors for mesh erosion after laparoscopic-assisted sacrocolpopexy. *Int Urogynecol J* 2011;22:205.

Johnson N, Barlow D, Lethaby A, et al. Surgical approach to hysterectomy for benign gynaecological disease. *Cochrane Database Syst Rev* 2006;CD003677.

Kilkku P, Grönroos M, Hirvonen T, et al. Supravaginal uterine amputation vs. hysterectomy. Effects on libido and orgasm. *Acta Obstet Gynecol Scand* 1983;62:147.

Kovalic JJ, Grigsby PW, Perez CA, et al. Cervical stump carcinoma. *Int J Radiat Oncol Biol Phys* 1991;20:933.

Learman LA, Summitt RL Jr, Varner RE, et al. A randomized comparison of total or supracervical hysterectomy: surgical complications and clinical outcomes. *Obstet Gynecol* 2003;102:453.

Lethaby A, Ivanova V, Johnson NP. Total versus subtotal hysterectomy for benign gynaecological conditions. *Cochrane Database Syst Rev* 2006;CD004993.

Lyons TL. Laparoscopic supracervical hysterectomy. *Obstet Gynecol Clin North Am* 2000;27:441.

Lyons TL. Laparoscopic supracervical hysterectomy: a comparison of morbidity and mortality results with laparoscopically assisted vaginal hysterectomy. *J Reprod Med* 1993;38:763.

McPherson K, Metcalfe MA, Herbert A, et al. Severe complications of hysterectomy: the VALUE study. *BJOG* 2004;111:688.

Munro MG. Supracervical hysterectomy: … a time for reappraisal. *Obstet Gynecol* 1997;89:133.

Okaro EO, Jones KD, Sutton C. Long term outcome following laparoscopic supracervical hysterectomy. *BJOG* 2001;108:1017.

Olsson JH, Ellstrom M, Hahlin M. A randomised prospective trial comparing laparoscopic and abdominal hysterectomy. *BJOG* 1996;103:345.

Perino A, Cucinella G, Venezia R, et al. Total laparoscopic hysterectomy versus total abdominal hysterectomy: an assessment of the learning curve in a prospective randomized study. *Hum Reprod* 1999;14:2996.

Pillet M-CL, Leonard F, Chopin N, et al. Incidence and risk factors of bladder injuries during laparoscopic hysterectomy indicated for benign uterine pathologies: a 14.5 years experience in a continuous series of 1501 procedures. *Hum Reprod* 2009;24:842.

Reich H, DeCaprio J, McGlynn F. Laparoscopic hysterectomy. *J Gynecol Surg* 1989;5:216.

Rhodes JC, Kjerulff KH, Langenberg PW, et al. Hysterectomy and sexual functioning. *JAMA* 1999;282:1934.

Richardson RE, Bournas N, Magos AL. Is laparoscopic hysterectomy a waste of time? *Lancet* 1995;345:36.

Rogo-Gupta LJ, Lewin SN, Kim JH, et al. The effect of surgeon volume on outcomes and resource use for vaginal hysterectomy. *Obstet Gynecol* 2010;116:1341.

Rooney CM, Crawford AT, Vassallo BJ, et al. Is previous cesarean section a risk for incidental cystotomy at the time of hysterectomy? A case-controlled study. *Am J Obstet Gynecol* 2005;193:2041.

Seracchioli R, Venturoli S, Vianello F, et al. Total laparoscopic hysterectomy compared with abdominal hysterectomy in the presence of a large uterus. *J Am Assoc Gynecol Laparosc* 2002;9:333.

Scheib SA, Tanner E, Green IC, et al. Laparoscopy in the morbidly obese: physiologic considerations and surgical techniques to optimize success. *J Minim Invasive Gynecol* 2014;21:182.

Scott JR, Sharp HT, Dodson MK, et al. Subtotal hysterectomy in modern gynecology: a decision analysis. *Am J Obstet Gynecol* 1997;176:1186.

Siedhoff MT, Yunker AC, Steege JF. Decreased incidence of vaginal cuff dehiscence after laparoscopic closure with bidirectional barbed suture. *J Minim Invasive Gynecol* 2011;189:218.

Tamussino KF, Lang PF, Breinl E. Ureteral complications with operative gynecologic laparoscopy. *Am J Obstet Gynecol* 1998;178:967.

Thakar R, Ayers S, Clarkson P, et al. Outcomes after total versus subtotal abdominal hysterectomy. *N Engl J Med* 2002;347:1318.

The Joint Commission. *The Surgical Care Improvement Project (SCIP).* http://www.jointcommission.org/surgical_care_improvement_project

Visco AG, Taber KH, Weidner AC, et al. Cost-effectiveness of universal cystoscopy to identify ureteral injury at hysterectomy. *Obstet Gynecol* 2001;97:685.

Wiskind AK, Thompson JD. Should cystoscopy be performed at every gynecologic operation to diagnose unsuspected ureteral injury? *J Pelvic Surg* 1995;11:134.

Wright JD, Herzog TJ, Tsui J, et al. Nationwide trends in the performance of inpatient hysterectomy in the United States. *Obstet Gynecol* 2013;122:233.

Wright JD, Ananth CV, Lewin SN, et al. Robotic assisted vs laparoscopic hysterectomy among women with benign gynecologic disease. *JAMA* 2013;309:689.

Yunker AC, Curlin H, Banet N, et al. Cervix innervation after subtotal hysterectomy and its association with future trachelectomy for pain and non-pain indications. *J Minim Invasive Gynecol* 2011;18:S25.

CHAPTER 33
Management of Abortion

Eva Lathrop and Carrie Cwiak

DEFINITIONS

Anembryonic pregnancy—A pregnancy in which trophoblast develops without development of embryonic tissue.

Dilation and evacuation—A surgical technique for pregnancies beyond 12 to 14 weeks gestation, utilizing advanced cervical dilation and evacuation of fetus and placenta via suction and forceps.

Early pregnancy loss—Loss of a pregnancy before 24 weeks gestation.

Electric vacuum aspiration—A surgical technique for pregnancies less than 12 to 14 weeks gestation, utilizing cervical dilation and aspiration of the fetus and placenta via suction.

Embryonic death—The finding of no cardiac activity in an embryo at least 5 mm and up to 15 mm (8 weeks) in length.

Fetal death—The finding of no cardiac activity in a fetus over 8 weeks (15 mm) gestation.

Incomplete abortion—Clinical and ultrasonic evidence of retained tissue in the uterus after an early pregnancy loss or induced abortion.

Induced abortion—Medical or surgical termination of an ongoing pregnancy.

Inevitable abortion—Dilation of the cervix without passage of pregnancy-related tissue.

Manual vacuum aspiration—Aspiration of the fetus and placenta via suction generated by a handheld syringe.

Missed abortion—Clinical or ultrasonic evidence of a nonviable pregnancy without cervical dilation or passage of pregnancy-related tissue.

The management of abortion remains a principal focus of gynecology. In the United States, each year, more than 1 million pregnancy losses occur and more than 1 million induced abortions are performed. With minimal modification, the surgical management of early pregnancy loss (EPL) is the same as for induced abortion, making uterine aspiration one of the most frequently performed operations in gynecology and one of the most thoroughly studied. In addition, the medical techniques effective for induced abortion are typically as effective for EPL. This chapter focuses on the surgical management of abortion but also summarizes other treatment options. It reviews the incidence, risk factors, preoperative assessment, and evidence-based treatment for spontaneous, illegal, and legal abortion. Readers should keep in mind that abortion technology is rapidly evolving, and new protocols may supplant those described here.

EARLY PREGNANCY LOSS

Incidence

Pregnancy loss is a common reproductive outcome. National Vital Statistics estimated that 1,118,000 total pregnancy losses occurred in 2008 in the United States (17% of all pregnancies). The incidence of EPL is dependent on the definitions utilized for EPL and for recognized pregnancy but is typically quoted as between 10% and 15% of all pregnancies. The contemporary definition for EPL is the loss of a pregnancy before 24 weeks estimated gestational age (EGA), recognizing the typical limits of fetal viability when resources are available. The greatest percentage—over 85%—of EPL occurs before 13 weeks gestation.

Fetal death is defined as no cardiac activity in a fetus over 8 weeks gestation and is uncommon after the first trimester. The U.S. National Vital Statistics System utilizes the World Health Organization (WHO) categories for fetal death: early (<20 weeks EGA), intermediate (20 to 28 weeks), and late (28 weeks or more), the latter corresponding to the international definition for stillbirth. The 2006 data from the U.S. National Center for Health Statistics report a fetal death rate of 6.05 per 1,000 live births. The incidence of fetal death decreases with increasing gestational age. Of the fetal deaths over 20 weeks in 2006, greater than 50% occurred between 20 and 27 weeks, with over one third occurring between 20 and 23 weeks. These categories overlap with the definition commonly used for EPL. In addition, individual states vary in the gestational ages at which they begin collecting data on pregnancy loss or fetal death. However, determining the upper limit by which to define EPL may be more an argument of necessity for statistical records than for clinical practice.

The true incidence of EPL is also uncertain because of the difficulty in recognizing early conceptions and losses. When Wilcox and associates monitored daily urinary β-human chorionic gonadotropin (β-hCG) in the 1980s, they found that 31% of pregnancies resulted in spontaneous abortion after implantation, but approximately 70% of these—22% of all losses—were not yet clinically identified. Wang and colleagues published data in 2003 in which 8% of all conceptions in their study were recognized pregnancies followed by spontaneous loss. Twenty-six percent of all conceptions in that study were losses before knowledge of the pregnancy. The ability to confirm pregnancy at an earlier EGA has significantly improved with the clinical use of highly sensitive urine pregnancy tests that can detect levels as low as 15 mIU/mL or 10 days after the last menstrual period. However, home pregnancy tests remain highly variable and can require levels as high as 100 mIU/mL before testing positive. Therefore, a significant amount of EPL may still be unreported.

Terminology

EPL has been previously referred to as *early pregnancy failure* and *spontaneous abortion*. In addition to sensitive urine pregnancy tests, the availability of transvaginal ultrasound has enabled the diagnosis of EPL at very early EGAs. Terminology has thus evolved to reflect the pathophysiology of the loss. Anembryonic pregnancy occurs when the trophoblast develops in the uterus without subsequent development of embryonic tissue. The diagnosis is confirmed by the ultrasonic finding of no yolk sac or embryonic pole and intrauterine gestational sac with mean sac diameter (MSD) of 16 mm or more, though utilizing an MSD cutoff of 20 mm in clinical practice can increase the specificity of diagnosis. Embryonic death is diagnosed by the ultrasound finding of no cardiac activity in an embryo at least 5 mm and up to 15 mm (8 weeks) in length. Fetal death is diagnosed by the ultrasound finding of no cardiac activity in a fetus over 8 weeks (15 mm) gestation. The first trimester of pregnancy is generally defined as either the first 12 or 14 weeks of pregnancy.

Once the diagnosis of a nonviable pregnancy has been made by abnormal trend in β-hCG or ultrasound, then terminology is also used to describe the clinical presentation of EPL. Missed abortion refers to a nonviable pregnancy in which dilation of the cervix and passage of pregnancy-related tissue have not yet occurred. Although missed abortion was associated in the past with complications from delayed diagnosis and retained products of conception, currently, it is often made when a patient is asymptomatic. Inevitable abortion can be considered the next stage in a continual process, in which a woman has a dilated cervix but passage of tissue has not yet occurred. Incomplete abortion refers to EPL in which some, but not all, of the tissue has passed. As a clinical definition, incomplete abortion refers to a woman who is symptomatic with abnormal bleeding, pain, or signs of infection due to retained tissue in the uterus. However, after passage of the gestational sac, it can be difficult to determine if the remaining tissue in the uterus is clinically significant in the woman with mild to no symptoms.

Risk Factors

EPL has several important risk factors. Over two thirds of EPL prior to 12 weeks EGA are associated with chromosomal anomalies, the most frequent of which are autosomal trisomies, followed by polyploidies, and then monosomy X. The earlier the gestational age at loss, the higher the frequency of chromosomal anomaly. Almost all anomalies, including some that would not appear to handicap survival (such as cleft lip), increase the likelihood of EPL. These anomalies are typically the result of random mutations, though a predisposition due to a balanced translocation or family history of a genetic defect can increase maternal or paternal risk.

Demographic details point to some other nonmodifiable risk factors. In a large study published by Nybo Anderson and colleagues, the rates of EPL increased with maternal age. Women aged 20 to 30 years, 35 years, 40 years, and 45 years saw a 9% to 17%, 20%, 40%, and 80% EPL rate, respectively. Previous studies reported an increase from 12% at ages less than 20 to 26% at age 40. Likewise, the risk increases with advancing paternal age. Race also plays a role. At each stage of pregnancy, black and Hispanic women in the United States have higher rates of pregnancy loss overall and of fetal death than do white women.

Independent of the effect of age, the risk of EPL changes with previous pregnancy history. Increasing rates are seen with increasing gravidity or parity. Personal history of one or more spontaneous losses increases the risk of recurrence. This effect is seen at all gestational ages. The risk of EPL was reported to increase with each documented loss in one study, increasing from 20% after one loss to 43% after three or more. Alternatively, the risk of EPL is lower for a woman who has not had a previous pregnancy or whose last pregnancy was successful. The length of the interval between pregnancies appears to have little impact.

Modifiable risk factors for EPL have also been identified. Overall, poor diet and obesity have each been associated with increased risk of EPL. Smoking may increase the risk of EPL. Because smoking is not teratogenic, its effect on spontaneous abortion rates may be via abortion of normal conceptuses. In one study, the risk of loss doubled; in other studies, the increase in risk was slight. Recent studies have not confirmed this increased risk. Alcohol consumption is associated with EPL as well as teratogenicity. The effects of alcohol on EPL risk appear to be greatest for those whose alcohol consumption is greater. Additionally, the risk appears to be greater with increased intake in the earlier gestational ages. Alcohol consumption as a teratogen has a dose-dependent effect and can result in mental retardation, microcephaly, midface hypoplasia, and renal and cardiac defects. Caffeine intake has been evaluated in many studies regarding EPL. Several studies had suggested an increased risk for spontaneous abortion in women who drank greater than 500 mg—or the equivalence of 5 cups—of coffee per day. However, a systematic review by Signorello and McLaughlin indicates that there is insufficient evidence supporting a causal relationship.

Certain maternal comorbidities are associated with an increased risk of EPL. Women with poorly controlled diabetes have higher levels of pregnancy loss as well as congenital anomalies. Increased rates of EPL are seen in women with other endocrine imbalances such as thyroid disease and polycystic ovarian syndrome, autoimmune disease, hypercoagulable states such as antiphospholipid antibody syndrome and thrombophilias, and chronic infections.

Cervical incompetence can lead to EPL. Cervical incompetence is more accurately defined as premature cervical dilation in midtrimester of pregnancy without uterine contractions, but the diagnosis is often made retrospectively in the women with unexplained repetitive midtrimester EPL without labor. Incidence rates range from 0.05 to 1 per 100 pregnancies. Though cervical loop electrocautery excision procedure is associated with EPL, data are otherwise lacking to confirm or refute other potential causes, such as previous cervical laceration or excessive mechanical dilation; the occurrence of this condition in primigravidas suggests alternative causes. These may include associated uterine anomalies, prenatal exposure to diethylstilbestrol, or abnormal histology of the cervix. In addition, premature cervical dilation without labor may be inheritable.

The presence of uterine anomalies can lead to EPL as well. Uterine synechiae, or Asherman syndrome, may permit insufficient surface area to support a pregnancy and lead to spontaneous loss. Uterine septa and abnormalities of müllerian fusion can also result in pregnancy loss if the pregnancy implants on the septum and outgrows its blood supply. Although no effect is seen in the first trimester, the incidence of EPL due to uterine anomalies after 13 weeks gestation may be 20% to 25%. Leiomyomata, specifically submucosal or large myomata, can interfere with implantation and make sustained pregnancy difficult.

Prevention

It is largely unknown how to prevent EPL. A meta-analysis of four studies suggests that oral or vaginal progesterone can prevent fetal loss when given to women with threatened abortion (bleeding, but with a viable fetus). Because the studies were small and of poor quality, further study is warranted before this can be accepted as proven therapy. One study by Mills and colleagues indicated that women with diabetes with excellent glycemic control early in pregnancy had the same rate of spontaneous abortion as did controls. Optimization of maternal health and avoidance of substances may be advisable for all women to prevent EPL as well as encourage maternal well-being. However, Cochrane reviews of randomized trials have found insufficient evidence for EPL prevention from vitamin supplementation, Chinese herbal medicine, bed rest, HCG, or beta-agonists.

Surgery may benefit some women with cervical incompetence or uterine abnormalities. For cervical incompetence, vaginal or abdominal cerclage can be performed, and those techniques are described elsewhere in this text. A Cochrane review of randomized trials concluded that cerclage reduces preterm delivery, though not perinatal mortality, in women at high risk for recurrent preterm delivery. Benefits for low-risk women are unproven. If uterine synechiae are diagnosed, hysteroscopic lysis of adhesions is recommended. Women with müllerian anomalies who experience EPL at 13 weeks gestation or later may be candidates for reconstructive operations, described elsewhere in this text. Removal of uterine fibroids, if performed only because of infertility, may help little; the effect of myomectomy on pregnancy loss rates is unknown.

Evaluation

A majority of the time, viability concerns in early pregnancy are preceded by vaginal bleeding. Bleeding in early pregnancy is common, reported in up to 25% of early pregnancies, and ensuring appropriate evaluation and management is essential for women's health. In addition to the history and physical exam, ultrasonography and serial measurement of β-hCG are important diagnostic tools to differentiate threatened, incomplete, and complete abortion. These are also important in the diagnosis of ectopic pregnancy, as an intrauterine pregnancy identified on ultrasound virtually excludes the diagnosis of ectopic pregnancy.

The average rise of β-hCG is 100% over 48 hours, but the lower limit of β-hCG rise in normal pregnancies has been shown to be as low as 53% in 48 hours. Conversely, once trophoblastic development has stopped, β-hCG clears the serum at about the same rate of 100% in 2 days. β-hCG serum levels clear faster after EPL than after induced abortion, though levels can similarly be seen to plateau toward the end of clearance. Therefore, depending on the level of β-hCG at the time of EPL, β-hCG may remain positive for up to 8 weeks thereafter.

Although persistent β-hCG levels might alert the provider to abnormal trophoblastic tissue and an increasing trend to a continuing or new pregnancy, a single β-hCG level cannot assist in diagnosis of retained products of conception because if trophoblastic development has been interrupted, whether by EPL or induced abortion, then a positive β-hCG may be present, trending down, without retention of a clinically significant amount of tissue. Conversely, clinically significant but nonviable, retained tissue can be present with a negative β-hCG value since trophoblastic development is no longer occurring.

Increasing use of vaginal ultrasound has improved diagnostic validity, especially at early gestational ages. When an embryo is visible, management is straightforward. However, most abnormal pregnancies stop developing before an embryo is visible by sonography. The discriminatory zone is the β-hCG serum level at which an intrauterine gestational sac can be seen via ultrasound for a viable pregnancy. The discriminatory zone for vaginal ultrasound can range from 1,500 to 2,000 mIU/mL depending on laboratory and sonographic resources and has a specificity of 95% to 100%. Two additional sonographic findings have high specificity: a gestation sac at least 25 mm in mean diameter without an embryo and distorted sac shape. On the other hand, the sensitivity of these criteria appears to be low. Presence of fetal heart activity is more accurate in predicting EPL than are morphologic criteria. Several reports concur that once fetal cardiac activity is documented

by ultrasonography in the first 12 weeks of pregnancy, the likelihood of subsequent fetal loss is low: about 2% to 4.5%. This does not hold true, however, for women older than age 35 or those with a history of recurrent pregnancy loss. Furthermore, studies have noted that fetal heart rates less than 100 beats per minute in the embryonic stage are associated with a significantly lower survival rate than those with normal fetal heart rates.

Given the lack of medical need for intervention in the majority of cases of EPL, clinicians need not act on a single abnormal clinical finding in a desired pregnancy, such as a falling β-hCG level or failure to observe fetal cardiac activity. Following the β-hCG trend can establish the diagnosis of normal versus abnormal (EPL or ectopic) pregnancy. Alternatively, repeating the ultrasound at an appropriate interval improves the diagnostic accuracy of this procedure.

The traditional approach to threatened abortion, characterized by uterine bleeding without cervical dilation or expulsion of tissue and demonstration of a potentially viable fetus, has been watchful waiting. The chance of EPL after threatened abortion can be as high as 50%. Reliably predicting fetal outcomes in such situations is not yet possible, and serial β-hCG levels or ultrasound examinations may be necessary to determine viability of a pregnancy that is not actively being passed.

In the case of missed abortion and in the absence of gestational trophoblastic disease, little to no trophoblastic tissue proliferation occurs after the pregnancy loss, and so, the current uterine size or ultrasound findings typically indicate the EGA at the time of loss. The discrepancy between current EGA and expected EGA based on last menstrual period or previous normal ultrasound suggests how long ago the loss actually occurred and, in extreme cases, may suggest whether infection, hemorrhage, and/or disseminated intravascular coagulation (DIC) is likely. Missed abortion in which the pregnancy is retained for 8 weeks or more has been associated with hemorrhage and DIC.

Diagnosis of incomplete abortion has come full circle from a basis of clinical symptoms, to detection of retained tissue in the uterus on ultrasound, back to clinical diagnosis. Harwood et al. noted that the endometrial thickness after EPL was as high as 29 mm in asymptomatic women. Similar studies have concluded that no cutoff value could predict which patients would require surgical management after medical or expectant management of EPL. Follow-up studies after early medical and surgical abortion have found similar results, leading to the conclusion that the thickness of the endometrium after completion of a pregnancy has a wide range of normal variability. Therefore, the diagnosis of incomplete abortion is typically made on clinical grounds and then confirmed by ultrasound findings. In other words, a thickened endometrium in an asymptomatic woman need not be acted upon.

Management

After confirmation of EPL, the first, and perhaps most important, step is to counsel the women and her partner. Helping the couple to grieve appropriately can minimize psychological sequelae from what can be a devastating loss. Subsequent clinical management is largely discretionary. Historically, surgical management was recommended for EPL due to a higher incidence of infectious and bleeding complications associated with delayed diagnosis, or the misclassification of illegal abortion as incomplete abortion. However, for women with missed, inevitable, or incomplete abortion, several options are available. Patient preference should generally determine the management as long as there is hemodynamic stability and absence of infection.

VI

Many women faced with the disappointing diagnosis of EPL prefer prompt surgical evacuation. Surgical management of EPL is dependent upon EGA determined by current uterine examination and ultrasound and upon clinical diagnosis. EPL up to 12 to 14 weeks EGA should be performed by uterine aspiration, via either manual vacuum aspiration (MVA) or electric vacuum aspiration. As with induced abortion, sharp curettage is no longer standard of care for EPL as it is associated with more blood loss, postoperative hemorrhage, anemia, pain, and operative time compared to manual or electric aspiration. The safe limits of EGA for uterine aspiration are dependent on clinician experience and available equipment, but it can be safely performed up to 14 weeks EGA if the appropriate-sized cannula is available for use with either manual syringe or electric vacuum. As with induced abortion, cannula size in mm should typically correspond to uterine size in weeks gestation, plus or minus 1 mm in cannula size. Utilizing a cannula that is too small can result in increased operative time, bleeding, and risk of retained products, especially in the case of EPL that has occurred several weeks before. Although nonviable fetal tissue frequently softens over time, placental and trophoblastic tissue can become indurated and less likely to pass through a too-small cannula. For missed abortion, the guidelines for preoperative cervical preparation for induced abortion can be followed (see "Preoperative Cervical Preparation"). For inevitable and incomplete abortion, minimal to no cervical dilation may be necessary if the cervix is already dilated enough to admit the correct-sized cannula. The technique of uterine aspiration, via manual or electric vacuum, is identical to that for induced abortion (see "Manual Vacuum Aspiration" and "Electric Vacuum Aspiration").

Site of uterine aspiration may depend on time of day, staff and equipment resources available, local protocols for sedation, and clinical presentation. The syringe used for MVA is portable, inexpensive, and convenient for outpatient use. The technique is described in detail later in this chapter. Blumenthal and Remsburg found that for surgical management of EPL, MVA in the clinic or emergency room was more cost-effective than was uterine aspiration in an operating room. Development of a protocol for MVA in an office or emergency room can decrease patient cost and increase patient satisfaction. Many women prefer in-office MVA for surgical management of EPL. As with other in-office procedures, patients must be clinically stable, without multiple comorbidities, and otherwise appropriate candidates for in-office sedation and surgical management. Clinicians who are contemplating provision of in-office MVA may be more comfortable initially offering it to patients with incomplete abortion or at an early EGA and then increasing the range as their comfort level allows.

Dependent on the skill of the physician, EPL past 12 to 14 weeks EGA can also be managed surgically, via dilation and evacuation (D&E). For women with a closed cervix, preoperative cervical preparation is essential. The guidelines for cervical preparation for induced abortion can be followed for fetal loss in the second trimester as well. For D&E, larger cannulas are available for use with electric vacuum aspiration. But for an EGA larger than the size of the suction cannula available, Bierer forceps should be utilized for safe evacuation of fetus and placenta. Even with retained placenta after second- or third-trimester loss or delivery, use of Bierer forceps for evacuation is safer and more efficient than the traditional horseshoe curette. The technique of D&E for fetal loss or retained placenta is identical to that for induced abortion (see "Dilation and Evacuation").

Antibiotics should be administered as soon as possible for women with infectious complications of EPL, and timely uterine evacuation is recommended. However, perioperative antibiotic prophylaxis has not been found to decrease infection when used for incomplete abortion. It is unknown whether antibiotic prophylaxis is effective in other presentations of EPL like inevitable or missed abortion.

There are no studies that specifically address venous thromboembolism (VTE) associated with surgical management of EPL or induced abortion. The guidelines for VTE prophylaxis for gynecologic surgery may be followed in either situation (see "Venous Thromboembolism Prophylaxis").

Analgesia should be used and can be provided via paracervical anesthesia, sedation, or combination of the two. Sedation is more likely to be associated with postoperative nausea and vomiting than paracervical block (PCB) alone. For sedation regimens, anxiolytic and narcotic medications are effective, whether via oral or intravenous administration. For the surgical management of EPL, randomized trials have concluded that adding an NSAID to a narcotic sedation regimen provides no additional benefit. And in comparison to sedation, general anesthesia provided no additional relief from postoperative pain but was associated with higher patient satisfaction. Whether this is due to the patient's emotional state or her perception of increased pain relief with general anesthesia, preoperative patient counseling may increase satisfaction with sedation. Any benefit must be balanced against the potential complications of induction of anesthesia in addition to the fact that anesthesia is associated with more need for blood transfusion. The WHO Safe Abortion Guidelines recommend that general anesthesia not be routinely used first line for management of abortion, suggesting that the risks of general anesthesia outweigh the benefits in most cases.

Another option to expedite the expulsion of the pregnancy after EPL is medical management via the prostaglandin analogue, misoprostol. For missed abortion in the first or second trimester, randomized trials have shown that medical management is a safe and effective option for women desiring to avoid surgery. When compared to immediate surgical management, Graziosi et al. noted a cost savings to offering initial misoprostol management followed by surgery if the abortion was not complete by 24 hours. Though patient satisfaction was 58% in each arm of the trial, satisfaction was significantly decreased for women who started misoprostol treatment but eventually required surgical aspiration. When randomized versus placebo, misoprostol resulted in higher rates of complete abortion for fetal loss, at shorter time intervals, without an increase in side effects. Compared to smaller doses, 800 µg of misoprostol is most effective without additional side effects. At this dose, vaginal is similar to oral administration in overall success rates (70% to 90%) but superior in time to successful completion of abortion with less vomiting. Sublingual administration is also similar in efficacy to vaginal but with higher incidence of diarrhea. A randomized, controlled multicenter study by Zhang and colleagues comparing medical management with surgical evacuation found an 84% completion rate by day 8 when vaginal dosing of 800 µg of misoprostol was repeated at 48 hours if passage had not yet occurred, without increase in side effects. In that study, 83% of the woman stated they would recommend the medical treatment to others.

For EPL, only one of two trials has found the addition of mifepristone to the misoprostol regimen increases rates of complete abortion. Laminaria, methotrexate, and the practice of moistening misoprostol prior to vaginal insertion did not increase success. In comparison to other prostaglandins, misoprostol is superior to prostaglandin E but similar to gemeprost. Pain management should be provided and may include NSAIDs or narcotics, with more pain control required at higher EGAs.

For incomplete abortion in the first trimester, medical management with vaginal misoprostol had success rates of 80% to 91% in randomized trials compared to 89% to 100% success with surgical management. As expected, vaginal misoprostol was associated with less use of surgical aspiration overall but higher incidence of unplanned surgery for completion of abortion. Vaginal misoprostol was also associated with more days of bleeding, more need for pain relief, and slightly less patient satisfaction, but no difference in gastrointestinal symptoms, need for blood transfusion, anemia, infection, death, or serious complication. As for missed abortion, vaginal misoprostol provides the same efficacy as oral but with less gastrointestinal side effects. For incomplete abortion, repeated oral doses did not significantly increase the success of abortion completion but did increase side effects. There are no studies comparing medical management to surgical or expectant management for incomplete abortion in the second trimester.

A third option is to await spontaneous expulsion of the pregnancy. Expectant management has been found to have a wide range of success for missed abortion (56% to 98%) and incomplete abortion (52% to 85%) in the first trimester, as defined by no need for surgical intervention. When randomized to surgical management, expectant management was associated with a greater incidence of unplanned surgery for completion of abortion, bleeding, and blood transfusion. However, cost was decreased, and rates of infection, return to normal activity level, and psychological outcome were similar. Rates of success at 6 to 8 weeks were not significantly improved compared to 2 weeks, suggesting that 2 weeks is a reasonable time period to allow complete abortion to occur before intervening. When randomized to misoprostol management, expectant management has similar outcomes for incomplete abortion but inferior efficacy for missed abortion. When categorized by sonographic criteria, Luise et al. noted that 91% of incomplete abortions resolved spontaneously compared with 66% of anembryonic pregnancies. If choosing expectant management, a woman deserves counseling that several days or weeks may pass before resolution and that medical or surgical intervention may ultimately be necessary. Women with a diagnosis of anembryonic pregnancy may be counseled that their success rates may be lower with expectant management. Conversely, women at later gestational ages may not be good candidates for expectant management due to the longer time interval required for expulsion as well as the higher risk of bleeding and need for intervention.

According to a recent meta-analysis, there is insufficient evidence to prescribe one of the above management plans in any given clinical situation. Surgical management is more likely to result in completion than medical management, and medical management is more likely to result in completion than expectant management, but the inverse is true of costs incurred. Patient safety and satisfaction are equivalent with any of these management plans, with the exception that expectant management for EPL in the second trimester has not been studied in randomized trials. Certainly in the face of severe anemia, hemodynamic instability, pain, or infection, surgical evacuation should be performed. Without these, patient preference should be strongly considered. There is no evidence to support the use of antibiotic prophylaxis with medical or expectant management of EPL.

Aftercare for EPL includes surveillance for signs of abnormal grieving reactions or depression, preconception or contraceptive care depending on future fertility desires, and return to regular preventive reproductive care. In the absence of complications, contraception can be initiated immediately, following the same guidelines as for induced abortion (see "Postoperative Care"). Routine follow-up visits are not necessary after uncomplicated management of EPL.

Complications

Early diagnosis of EPL has reduced the risk of complications. In the 1970s, the maternal case fatality rate was estimated to be 4.5 deaths per 100,000 fetal deaths. The most frequent causes of maternal death from fetal death were uterine perforation and coagulopathy. As with induced abortion, advances in care have made mortality from EPL a rare event. The Centers for Disease Control and Prevention (CDC) identified 62 maternal deaths from pregnancy loss in the United States between 1981 and 1991. This represented a case fatality rate of 0.7 deaths per 100,000 pregnancy loss. In 2002, there were two maternal deaths that were due to pregnancy loss. Infection, hemorrhage, and embolism were the leading causes of death. The mortality risk increased with gestational age; women who were older and of minority races also were at increased risk of death.

EPL is a potentially sensitizing event for Rh-negative women. Rates of use of Rh immunoglobulin (RhIG) after EPL are significantly lower than after induced abortion. RhIG candidates at 12 weeks gestation or earlier should receive a 50-μg dose; later abortions mandate a 300-μg dose.

The profound grief that frequently accompanies EPL often receives insufficient attention. Women and men experience the stages of grief. Guilt may be a difficult stage to resolve without help, and counseling plays an important role.

ILLEGAL ABORTION

Incidence

Despite the availability of legal abortions, small numbers of illegal procedures continue to occur in the United States. Estimates of the incidence of illegal abortion in the United States before 1970 or legalization ranged from 200,000 to 1.2 million per year; estimates for the late 1970s ranged from 5,000 to 23,000 per year. More recent estimates are not available; however, a national survey of US abortion patients demonstrated 1.2% of patients reported using misoprostol for self-induction of abortion and 1.4% reported self-inducing with other substances. Illegal abortions occur in large numbers in developing countries, where, according to WHO estimates, close to 50,000 women continue to die of illegal abortion complications each year, and deaths from unsafe abortion account for approximately 13% of all maternal deaths.

Risk Factors

Lack of access to safe, legal abortion is the most important risk factor for having an illegal procedure in the world today. Little is known about characteristics of women in the United States who may still obtain illegal abortions, although in a national survey assessing abortion patients' reports of previous self-induction, women who have self-induced live in geographically diverse areas in the United States, the majority are not foreign born, but the level of use overall appears to be higher among foreign-born women.

Techniques

Although a wide variety of illegal abortion methods are used around the world, two methods dominate in the United States: oral abortifacients and intrauterine instrumentation. Orally administered substances include self-obtained misoprostol, turpentine, laundry bleach, large doses of quinine, and various herbs. Intrauterine techniques were less common, more effective, and more dangerous; these ranged from intrauterine injection of soap or phenol disinfectants to insertion of foreign objects. Self-induction of abortion, by any technique in the United States, while difficult to estimate, appears to be very rare.

Complications

Transcervical administration of toxic substances carries a high risk of serious complications. The most frequently reported complication of illegal abortion is retained products of conception, although the incidence of such complications is unknown. In many countries in Latin America, Africa, and Asia where elective abortion is illegal or highly restricted, the black-market or private pharmacy availability of misoprostol has increased dramatically and led to important improvements in abortion safety, because misoprostol has reduced reliance on instrumentation of the cervix.

The number of illegal abortion deaths in the United States declined dramatically during the 1970s. During the 1975 to 1979 interval, women in both extremes of the reproductive age span had higher death rates from illegal abortion than did other women. The racial discrepancy in death rate was more striking: The mortality rate for black and Hispanic women was more than 10 times greater than for white women.

As with morbidity, the likelihood of mortality is strongly related to the abortion technique. Of the 17 illegal abortion deaths from 1975 to 1979, only one followed ingestion of an abortifacient (pennyroyal oil). The other deaths were related to intrauterine techniques, ranging from injection of cleaning solutions to insertion of foreign bodies (e.g., catheters, cotton swabs, thermometers, and coat hangers). Sepsis (10 cases) and air embolism (three cases) accounted for most of these deaths. The last reported death from illegal abortion in the United States was in 2004.

Management of Septic Abortion

Most women with septic abortion respond rapidly to uterine evacuation plus broad-spectrum antibiotics. Before beginning treatment, intrauterine and blood cultures should be obtained. An upright radiograph of the abdomen may identify a residual foreign body, gas bubbles in the uterus, or free air under the diaphragm; these findings direct management.

Antibiotic administration should begin immediately upon identification of septic abortion. Coverage should include gram-positive, gram-negative, and anaerobic bacteria. Ideally, in a case of septic abortion, the patient should go directly from the emergency department to the operating room. Peak serum levels of antibiotics will be present within an hour of their administration. Further delay of uterine evacuation is unwarranted and can compromise recovery. Prompt elimination of the necrotic infected tissue is critical. Tissue obtained during curettage should quickly go for microbiologic cultures. The yield of organisms, especially anaerobes, is often higher from a tissue specimen than from a swab inserted into the uterus.

Subsequent management is governed by the response of the woman and by microbiologic findings. All women with septic abortions should be closely observed after surgery, with special attention to vital signs and urine output, to detect incipient shock. Prompt aggressive therapy is essential if septic shock develops.

Postabortal sepsis from *Clostridium perfringens* has become rare. When this infection occurs, however, it can be catastrophic. In the absence of hemolysis, *C. perfringens* bacteremia can be managed by uterine aspiration and antibiotics. In the presence of hemolysis, hysterectomy and more aggressive medical therapy may be indicated.

LEGAL ABORTION

Incidence

Legal abortion is one of the most frequently performed operations in the United States. In 2009, 784,507 induced abortions were reported. The national abortion ratio was 227 abortions per 1,000 live births in that year. The abortion rate was 15.1 abortions per 1,000 women aged 15 to 44. The total number of induced abortions and the rate of induced abortion both declined by 5% from 2008 to 2009, the most recent year for which data are available.

Demographic Characteristics

The majority of women having induced abortions in the United States tend to be young, white, single, and of low parity. Non-Hispanic white women had the lowest rate of induced abortion at 8.5/1,000 women aged 15 to 44, and non-Hispanic black women had the highest rate of induced abortion at 32.5/1,000 women aged 15 to 44. In 2009, most (64%) abortions took place at 8 weeks gestation or earlier; 92% occurred at 13 weeks gestation or earlier. Only 7% of procedures were done between 14 and 20 weeks gestation and 1.3% at more than 21 weeks. Before 1990, provision of very early (<6 weeks of gestational age) abortions was rare. Between 2000 and 2009, the percentage of abortions performed at 6 weeks or less increased by 47%. Most abortions take place safely in free-standing clinics (93%) and physician's offices (2%). In-hospital procedures (5%) are necessary when women have a higher risk of medical or surgical complications.

Preoperative Counseling

In a recent large study, the reasons most often cited by US women for choosing abortion were that having a baby would interfere with her education, work, or ability to care for her other dependents. A majority (73%) could not afford a baby, and almost half were having relationship problems and did not want to be single mothers. Preoperative counseling should include a nonjudgmental discussion of all alternatives available, including continuing the pregnancy and adoption. Abortion procedures are reviewed and compared, including the risks, benefits, and expected experience with each method. Women choose surgical abortion to avoid the perceived involvement, awareness, pain, or emotional impact of medical abortion. Women choose early medical abortion in order to avoid surgery or anesthesia, to experience a simpler or more natural process, or in situations in which medical abortion was available sooner. Conversely, in comparison to surgical abortion, early medical abortion is associated with a longer duration of bleeding, and patients should be counseled accordingly. Contraceptive options, eligibility, and desires should also be reviewed during preoperative counseling.

Legal Considerations

It is important for clinicians to know the legal restrictions to abortion in their state. State regulations include, but are not limited to, waiting periods, counseling requirements, parental involvement for minors, ultrasound requirements, specific scripted consents, and insurance regulations.

Preoperative Medical Evaluation

The preoperative evaluation should include counseling, informed consent, a brief history, and a limited physical examination. The history taking should focus on relevant data, such as gynecologic problems (e.g., leiomyomata, uterine anomalies,

VI

cervical stenosis) or medical problems (e.g., cardiac disease, asthma, morbid obesity) that might influence the course of the operation. Physical examination should include the heart and lungs (if anesthesia is to be used), abdomen, and pelvis. Although ultrasonography is not necessary on a routine basis, it is useful in several scenarios. Ultrasound is recommended if the size, shape, or position of the uterus is unclear as in the case of very early pregnancy, when uterine size is inconsistent with EGA per last menstrual period, and in preparation for most second-trimester cases. If ectopic pregnancy or a uterine anomaly is suspected, ultrasound should also be utilized. Ultrasound is a routine component of early medical abortions, which requires exclusion of ectopic pregnancy before use of most regimens. It is imperative to be aware of the legal requirements regarding ultrasound and abortion in a given state in order to be in compliance with these requirements when possible. Routine laboratory tests include the hematocrit (or hemoglobin) and Rh type. Additional laboratory tests may be indicated in patients with medical disorders that could influence surgical approach, anesthesia options, or the decision to perform a hospital-based procedure. Many clinicians perform a urine pregnancy test on all patients requesting abortion. Screening for chlamydia and gonorrhea need not be routine but should be targeted based on risk factors, symptoms, or examination. If bacterial vaginosis is detected preoperatively, it should be treated.

Preoperative Cervical Preparation

Osmotic dilators help to prepare the cervix for D&E abortions and can occasionally be used for earlier aspiration abortions in certain circumstances (Fig. 33.1). Osmotic dilators currently available in the United States include laminaria, Lamicel, and Dilapan. Laminaria are hygroscopic sticks of seaweed that dilate the cervix over several hours. The mode of action is not well understood, but the principal mechanism appears to be desiccation of the cervix. This drying can alter the ratio of collagen to ground substance, thus changing collagen cross-linkages. Alternatively, laminaria can alter the elaboration, release, or degradation of uterine prostaglandins. Laminaria cause the cervix to dilate the areas not in physical contact with the laminaria; whatever the mechanism, it is more complex than mere passive stretching, as previously thought. Maximum dilation is achieved at 12 and 24 hours after placement. Laminaria is made of natural resources, and there have been historical concerns of potential increased infection risk. There are no

studies that show an increased risk of infection with laminaria and several studies that demonstrate the safety of and lack of increased infection with laminaria use.

Lamicel is a cylinder of polyvinyl alcohol sponge impregnated with magnesium sulfate. It works within several hours, achieving maximum dilation by 6 hours postplacement, and has the advantage of uniform size (either 5 or 3 mm diameter), assured sterility, and easy insertion and removal. Lamicel is effective as a cervical preparation agent a few hours before procedures up to 16 weeks and can be used overnight in preparation for procedures up to 17 to 18 weeks, but Lamicel is rarely used as a sole agent for cervical preparation for later procedures given the limits of its dilation capabilities. Dilapan-S is another available synthetic osmotic dilator, made of a polyacrylate-based proprietary hydrogel, and is available in 3 and 4 mm diameters and lengths of 55 and 65 mm. Dilapan-S swells rapidly demonstrating significant dilation by 2 hours. Most of the dilation is completed by 4 to 6 hours after placement, but it continues to expand up to 24 hours. Dilapan-S does have some potential problems; it shortens as it expands, prompting the recommendation to choose the longer length to ensure continuous dilation of the internal os, and it can be difficult to remove.

Osmotic dilators are convenient in an outpatient setting. Placement of any of the available brands for 3 to 4 hours before abortion frequently dilates the cervix sufficiently for abortion. Women can be sent home with laminaria in place overnight, allowing for maximal dilation. In-facility admission for observation is not necessary. Compared with use of metal dilators, use of laminaria dramatically reduces the risk of cervical injury and uterine perforation. This protection against trauma can be especially important for young teenagers with immature cervices who are at increased risk for cervical injury. Disadvantages include the cost, inconvenience, and occasional cramping involved. Instances of extramural delivery after placement of osmotic dilators are rare.

Alternatively, preoperative preparation of the cervix with misoprostol can facilitate abortion. Misoprostol, a prostaglandin E derivative, is safe, inexpensive, stable at room temperature, and effective in improving the Bishop score of the cervix. It is superior in cost efficacy and side effect profile in comparison to gemeprost. The drug can be given orally, vaginally, buccally, or sublingually. In general, misoprostol is better tolerated when given by the vaginal route versus the oral route; this probably relates to different pharmacokinetics when absorbed through the vagina versus through the gut. Both the sublingual and buccal routes demonstrate effectiveness similar to that of the vaginal route, while the side effect profile remains slightly higher than that of the vaginal route. Buccal use generally has fewer side effects than the sublingual route. Women often prefer an oral route to vaginal self-administration, but when placed in the vagina by the clinician at the end of the pelvic examination, most patients find this manner of administration acceptable. A randomized controlled trial (RCT) by Singh and colleagues suggests that misoprostol 400 μg per vagina 3 to 4 hours before the operation may be the optimal dose. Administration 1 hour before a procedure has been found not to be effective, and short intervals without proven efficacy should be discouraged. This has been reiterated by the Society of Family Planning (SFP) in the clinical guidelines for cervical preparation for procedures 14 weeks or below. In this guideline, cervical preparation with misoprostol can be considered for women who may be at increased risk of complications from cervical dilation: women in the late first trimester, adolescents, and women in whom cervical dilation is expected to be difficult due to either patient factors or provider experience. Recent data show an inferior

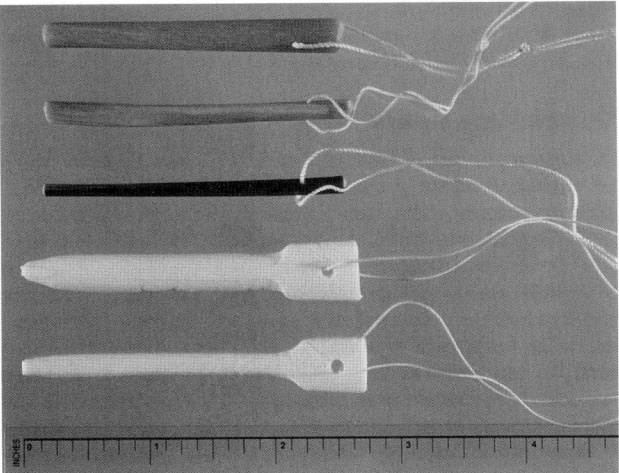

FIGURE 33.1 Osmotic dilators. **Top:** Laminaria of various sizes. **Bottom:** Lamicel in 5- and 3-mm sizes.

VI

effect of same-day misoprostol for preoperative cervical priming in second-trimester procedures as compared with laminaria administered the day before the procedure. In the SFP guideline addressing cervical preparation for second-trimester abortions, misoprostol can be considered as an alternative to laminaria for early second-trimester cases (13 to 16 weeks) in women considered at low risk for cervical injury but should not routinely replace laminaria. After 16 weeks, misoprostol can be used in conjunction with laminaria in select cases but provides inadequate dilation alone at later gestations. Disadvantages of cervical preparation with misoprostol include the delay required, spotting and cramping, and occasional expulsion of the pregnancy in the waiting room.

Prophylactic Antibiotics

Induced abortion patients should receive prophylactic antibiotics. A meta-analysis of the RCTs on this topic by Sawaya and colleagues showed decreased risk for postabortal endometritis for women deemed low and high risk for infection when prophylactic antibiotics were given as part of routine abortion care. The choice of antibiotic and duration of therapy are unclear. Both tetracyclines and nitroimidazoles have been shown to be effective. Doxycycline is the most commonly recommended prophylactic antibiotic in the setting of surgical abortion and has been shown to substantially reduce the risk of postabortal infection. The regimen of 100 mg of doxycycline preoperatively followed by 200 mg immediately postoperatively has been shown to decrease infection risk by 87%. Alternatives to this include azithromycin or metronidazole in prophylactic doses. However, if one administers antibiotics for more than 24 hours, prophylaxis ends and presumptive treatment of *C. trachomatis* begins. In high-risk populations, presumptive treatment of all patients for chlamydial infection (or bacterial vaginosis with metronidazole) may be a reasonable course of action.

Venous Thromboembolism Prophylaxis

As for EPL, there are no studies that specifically address VTE associated with surgical management of induced abortion. The Society of Gynecologic Surgeons' systematic review concluded that, other than early ambulation, no prophylaxis is required for minor surgeries in patients without significant risk factors for VTE, as they are considered low risk for VTE. Patients having minor surgery who have two or more risk factors for thromboembolism (previous VTE, thrombophilia, malignancy, etc.) are at moderate risk, and prophylaxis can be provided via intermittent compression devices, with the addition of heparin if the risk is particularly high. Although based on limited numbers of trials of gynecologic surgery, these recommendations are feasible for the management of high-risk abortion patients who would typically be managed in an operating room.

Preoperative Preparation

If local anesthesia is to be used alone, no preoperative fasting is necessary, but if conscious sedation is a possibility, the patient should fast for at least 6 hours before the procedure. Similarly, if conscious sedation is used, the patient should be instructed to bring someone with her to escort her home. She should empty her bladder before being placed in the dorsal lithotomy position; catheterization is unnecessary. An antiseptic is applied to the cervix and vagina (e.g., povidone–iodine or chlorhexidine). Routine sterile precautions (e.g., drapes, caps, masks, and gowns) are unnecessary. The clinician should use a "no-touch" technique: He or she wears sterile gloves and does not touch those ends and portions of the sterile instruments

inserted into the uterus. Use of local anesthesia predominates in the United States. Although local anesthesia does not completely relieve discomfort, it is less expensive and safer than general anesthesia. As with EPL, the benefits as well as the risks must be considered before using general anesthesia. It is a good general rule, when performing abortions under local anesthesia, to use slow, controlled movements. A support person who can talk to the patient also helps alleviate anxiety and discomfort.

Paracervical Anesthesia

To perform a PCB, the clinician should use the smallest volume of the lowest concentration of local anesthetic. Local anesthetics vary in their toxicity; for example, chloroprocaine is substantially less toxic than lidocaine. With lidocaine, a 0.5% concentration is safer than a 1% solution and is equally effective. The total dose of lidocaine should not exceed 5 mg/kg or 300 mg, whichever is less. Maximum is approximately 20 mL of 1% lidocaine or 0.25% bupivacaine for a 50-kg woman, with 10 mL being typically sufficient. Alternatively, use of local anesthesia with vasoconstrictor (e.g., epinephrine 1:200,000) slows systemic absorption of anesthetic and allows a larger total dose, although the epinephrine has additional risks and side effects. Some clinicians buffer the lidocaine solution with sodium bicarbonate to decrease burning. Vasovagal episodes occur rarely and can be treated with atropine.

Paracervical anesthesia is widely used prior to abortion procedures and has been shown to decrease pain from cervical dilation and uterine aspiration. Approaches include infiltration of the cervix at the 12-o'clock position (for application of the tenaculum) and then injection at four sites (at the 2-, 4-, 8-, and 10-o'clock positions) or two sites (at the 4- and 8-o'clock positions) at the junction of the cervix and vagina. Submucosal injection precludes inadvertent intravascular injection. Despite its widespread use, a systematic review of pain control for first-trimester abortions found insufficient evidence of a clear benefit to PCB and was not able to support its use without further well-designed RCTs. This systematic review did find evidence of decreased pain with first-trimester procedures in women who were given conscious sedation and general anesthesia or who listened to music during the procedure. In 2012, Renner et al. performed an RCT, single blinded with a sham arm to minimize confounders with adequate power to detect differences in perceived pain, and were able to demonstrate a clear decrease in pain in the PCB group and higher satisfaction overall with the abortion experience. Deep injection (3 cm) and a delay of a few minutes between injection and dilation may maximize the benefits of the PCB.

Hemorrhage Prophylaxis

Intraoperative blood loss is typically minimal with surgical management for induced abortion (as well as for EPL). Although many clinicians routinely provide misoprostol, methylergonovine maleate (methergine), or oxytocin with first- or second-trimester uterine evacuation, evidence for use of uterotonics to prevent significant blood loss is limited. For first-trimester procedures, one study has shown that intramuscular methergine significantly decreases uterine atony and need for reaspiration. However, oral methergine is unstable at room temperature and utilizing it for prophylaxis is not recommended. Prophylactic oxytocin does not significantly decrease blood loss in the first trimester. And there are no studies of misoprostol use in this setting.

In the second trimester, an RCT found that vasopressin administered with paracervical anesthesia significantly decreases blood loss with D&E, most notably at later EGAs. As little as 4 U (0.2 mL) mixed in with the anesthetic lowers the blood loss significantly; overall, vasopressin lowers four-fold the risk of a hemorrhage of 500 mL or more. It is important to remember to administer vasopressin when opting to administer regional or general anesthesia, in which case the vasopressin can be mixed with saline and injected paracervically. The SFP guideline for postabortion hemorrhage recommends its routine use with D&E to decrease blood loss. 400 μg of misoprostol, when studied alone or with osmotic dilators for preoperative cervical preparation, was found to have little to no effect on blood loss. Larger misoprostol doses, as are typical for controlling postpartum hemorrhage, have not been studied for postabortion hemorrhage. Administration of oxytocin during D&E procedures after 20 weeks, when oxytocin receptors are present to some degree, may be helpful in preventing excess blood loss, and its use is determined by provider preference. Lack of evidence for prophylactic use does not preclude the use of uterotonics for treatment of hemorrhage (see "Immediate Complications").

Manual Vacuum Aspiration

As with EPL, sharp curettage is an obsolete method for induced abortion, supplanted by uterine aspiration, which usually involves dilation of the cervix, followed by manual or electric vacuum (suction) aspiration at 12 to 14 weeks gestation or earlier. *Menstrual regulation, menstrual extraction,* and *minisuction* are euphemisms for early uterine aspiration and are used widely in many parts of the world. The most common technique used for this early "regulation," as well as later procedures done by manual vacuum with syringe, is MVA. This technique uses a plastic cannula as small as 3 mm in diameter and as large as 12 mm, with a self-locking syringe (50 to 60 mL) as a source of suction (**Fig. 33.2**). A large series using MVA in early pregnancy reported a 99% success rate on nearly 2,400 abortions done at less than 6 weeks gestation. MVA has been shown to be as safe and effective as electric

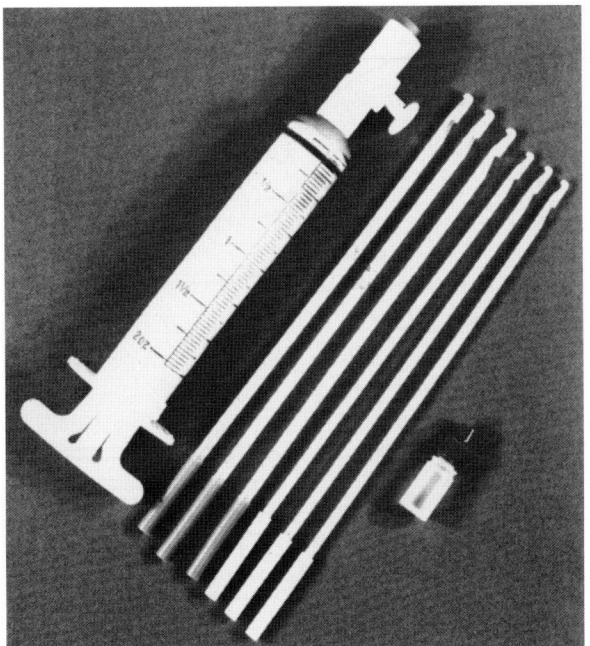

FIGURE 33.2 Karman cannulas, self-locking syringe with pinch valve. (Copyright IPAS, Chapel Hill, NC, with permission.)

vacuum through 10 weeks of gestation and can be used in conjunction with forceps in later procedures. For early MVA procedures, dilation is often unnecessary. Consequently, anesthesia may not be necessary, although analgesia can ease the cramping that occurs toward the end of the aspiration. After insertion of the appropriate cannula, the clinician attaches the syringe and releases the pinch valve to create a vacuum and begin suctioning. Alternatively, some clinicians connect the cannula to the syringe before insertion. The abortion involves rotary and in-and-out cannula movement, allowing blood and tissue flow into the syringe. This should be repeated until the gritty feel of the endometrium occurs and bubbles appear in the syringe, indicating completion of the procedure. The clinician should not remove the cannula from the uterus while a vacuum exists in the syringe, because the endocervical canal should not be aspirated; likewise, the clinician should not advance the plunger of the syringe while the cannula is connected and is within the uterus. Air embolism can result. The syringe and cannula are technically disposable, although standard instructions are available for providers to disinfect the syringe and use it multiple times.

Electric Vacuum Aspiration

Electric vacuum aspiration requires few instruments. It is useful to have an ultrasound machine available in case one is not able to enter the uterus or suction adequate tissue; however, ultrasound is not necessary to perform abortions. Most clinicians prefer to use a bivalve speculum. A speculum with standard-length blades, however, prevents the cervix from being drawn toward the introitus during the procedure and makes the operation more difficult. The commercially available Moore modification of the Graves speculum, which has 1-inch shorter blades of standard width, prevents this. Some clinicians prefer an atraumatic tenaculum; however, these tend to slip off more readily than does the single-toothed variety. Alternatively, having an extra single-toothed tenaculum can sometimes be helpful. If difficulty during dilation occurs, the clinician can place the second tenaculum on the posterior cervix to stabilize it. Sounding before the procedure is unnecessary and should not be done, as it increases the risk of perforation. If the direction of the cervical canal is in question, then the clinician can gently probe with a small dilator. Pratt dilators are preferable to Hegar dilators for abortion because they require less force to dilate the cervix. A useful modification of the Pratt dilators is the Denniston dilator; this is similar to the Pratt dilator but is plastic. Hence, it is light, slightly flexible, and inexpensive, yet it is capable of being autoclaved.

Traction on the cervix is important during suction aspiration; it both stabilizes the uterus and straightens the angle between the cervix and corpus, which should reduce the risk of perforation. The tenaculum should have a firm purchase on the cervix. High vertical placement at the 12-o'clock position, with one tooth in the canal and one on the anterior cervix, almost eliminates the risk of the tenaculum tearing through during dilation. In contrast, a superficial horizontal application of the tenaculum is more likely to allow the tenaculum to pull off but will not obscure the vision and movement of instruments for the provider. If the uterus is retroverted, some clinicians prefer to place the tenaculum on the cervix at the 6-o'clock position (**Fig. 33.3**). If the puncture site on the cervix bleeds after tenaculum removal, direct pressure nearly always stops the bleeding. Silver nitrate or Monsel solution can be used if pressure does not achieve hemostasis. While use of the tenaculum straightens the angle of the uterus, the operator must remain cognizant of the anatomy. For an anteverted uterus, instruments used for the procedure often need to be at an angle, with the intrauterine

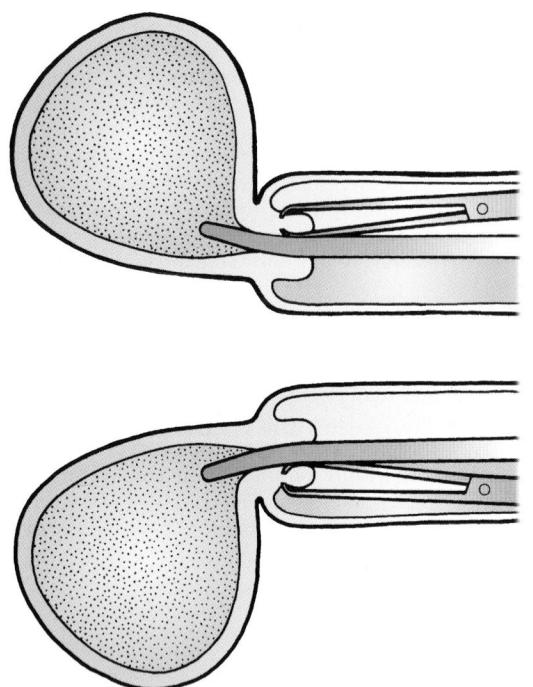

FIGURE 33.3 Traction on the cervix during dilation. **Top:** Tenaculum placed vertically on the anterior lip. **Bottom:** Tenaculum placed vertically on the posterior lip for a retroverted uterus. Note posterior direction of dilator.

tip of the instrument pointing upward. If the instrument was inserted straight back in a patient like this, there would be an increased risk for posterior perforation.

Gentleness is the key to safe cervical dilation. Dilation should allow insertion and rotation of the desired cannula. Pratt dilators are measured in French units or mm of circumference. Hence, to determine the diameter, the clinician needs to divide by pi or approximately 3. For example, to insert an 8-mm cannula, dilation with Pratt dilators to 25 F allows free rotation. The clinician should hold the dilator between the thumb and index finger to limit the force applied. In addition, the other fingers can remain extended to prevent plunging forward in case of sudden loss of resistance. No-touch technique or protecting ends of dilators and cannulas that enter into the uterine cavity should be practiced meticulously throughout the procedure. Dilation need not start with the smallest dilator on the set; starting with a larger size (e.g., 15 F instead of 13 F) may reduce the risk of perforating the uterus or creating a false channel.

If more than two fingers of force is necessary during dilation, the clinician should stop and reassess the situation, rather than risk injuring the cervix. One option is to use a smaller cannula than originally planned. Alternatively, the clinician can pack the cervix with one or more osmotic dilators, interrupt the procedure, and then complete the operation several hours later, by which time adequate dilation will have been achieved. Another treatment option is to administer oral or vaginal misoprostol and complete the procedure in several hours. Performance of the procedure in two stages is far preferable to forceful dilation.

After adequate dilation, the clinician inserts the cannula. In general, the diameter of the cannula in millimeters should be equal to the weeks of gestation from last menses, plus or minus 1 week. For example, an 8-mm cannula may be adequate for evacuating a pregnancy of 9 weeks 0 days' gestation,

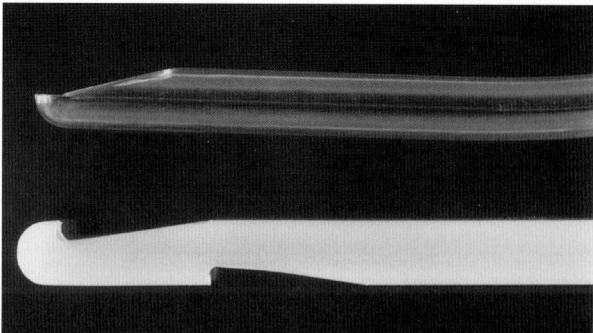

FIGURE 33.4 Distal ends of rigid curved 8-mm cannula and flexible 8-mm cannula with twin whistle-tip ports.

but a 10-mm cannula may be used to evacuate a pregnancy of 9 week 6 days if cervical dilation allows. The exception is for patients with uterine fibroids, in which added uterine size is not related to intrauterine tissue. Skilled clinicians often prefer to use even smaller cannulas than this guideline suggests; the clinician must weigh the advantage of needing less dilation against the potential disadvantages of longer operating time and an increased risk of incomplete abortion.

The most frequently used cannulas in the United States are clear plastic, with a slight angulation (Fig. 33.4). The clinician should insert the cannula into the lower uterine segment. For electric vacuum aspiration, a hose with a swivel handle attaches to the cannula and then to the vacuum machine. The clinician then turns on the suction machine and aspirates the uterus with the cannula (Fig. 33.5). One of the principles of abortion technique is to start working in the lower uterine segment. The fundal contents of the uterus are brought down by suction and the involution of the uterus as it empties. The flexible plastic cannula (Fig. 33.5) suctions opposite sides of the cavity simultaneously and provides a distinct gritty sensation when the evacuation is complete. Bubbles will also appear in the suction tubing when the procedure is complete. Some clinicians use a sharp curette to check for completeness at the

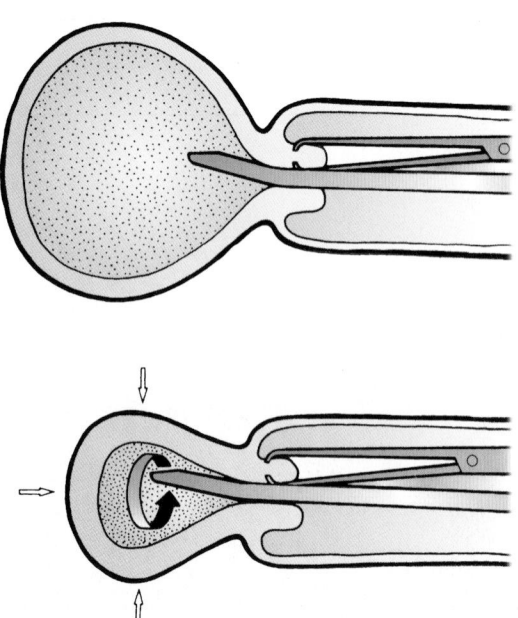

FIGURE 33.5 Uterine aspiration. **Top:** Cannula inserted just beyond internal os. **Bottom:** Aspiration with rotating motion.

end of the operation; however, completion of the procedure can be determined by the grittiness of the endometrium and the pink bubbles in the tubing, and routine use of the sharp curette should be avoided to maximally decrease the risk of perforation. If the gritty sensation is not appreciated with a rigid plastic cannula, a small (e.g., 8-mm-diameter) Karman-type double-port cannula provides the same gritty sensation as a metal curette and is far safer.

The operation is not finished until the clinician or another trained observer has examined the aspirated tissue. This is to confirm the presence of fetal tissue, which usually excludes the possibility of an ectopic pregnancy. Since 1972, more than 20 women in the United States have died from ectopic pregnancies undetected at the time of attempted suction aspiration. This tissue inspection will not detect the rare twin ectopic pregnancy, commonly termed "heterotopic."

Pregnancies of 9 weeks gestation and later will have recognizable fetal parts; earlier pregnancies may not. Identification of chorionic villi and membranes in these earlier pregnancies is essential. The clinician rinses the aspirated tissue in a fine mesh strainer under tap water to remove blood and clots. A glass dish is useful for examining the tissue suspended in water (Fig 33.6). For early pregnancies, white vinegar (instead of water) may facilitate the recognition of villi. Back lighting from a horizontal x-ray viewing box is especially useful (Fig. 33.6). Villi appear soft, fluffy, and feathery, with discernible fingerlike projections; in contrast, decidua appears coarse and shaggy (Fig. 33.7). Amnion and chorion are filmy and transparent; decidua is translucent. With early pregnancies, a magnifying glass, dissecting microscope, colposcope, or standard microscope (3,100) can help identify villi (Fig. 33.8). It is essential to learn the difference between the appearance of villi and decidua; this is useful in the management of EPL, as well as in distinguishing between bleeding from EPL and ectopic pregnancy.

When the clinician cannot confirm fetal tissue, he or she should reevaluate the patient, with special attention to the adnexa. Repeat aspiration (perhaps with ultrasound guidance) is often appropriate. A sensitive urine pregnancy test or a quantitative β-hCG can be helpful. Ultrasound can sometimes identify a gestational sac. Failure to identify villi in the presence of a positive pregnancy test suggests several possibilities: recent spontaneous abortion, failed attempted abortion,

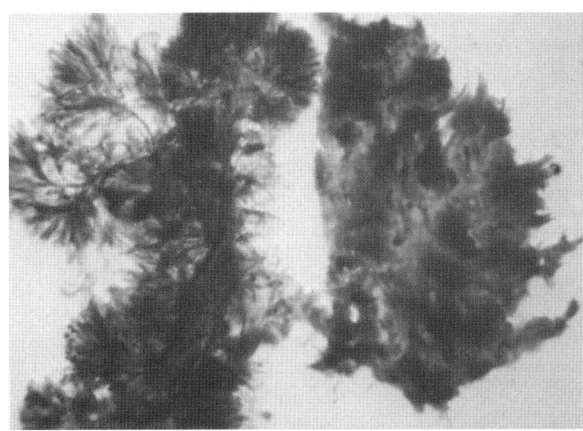

FIGURE 33.7 Left: Typical fluffy villi of placenta. Right: Shaggy decidua. (Reprinted from Munsick RA. Clinical test for placenta in 300 consecutive menstrual aspirations. *Obstet Gynecol* 1982;60:738, with permission. Copyright © 1982 The American College of Obstetricians and Gynecologists.)

perforation with aspiration outside the uterus, or ectopic pregnancy. The clinician must carefully evaluate these possibilities.

Women with uterine anomalies, such as a bicornuate uterus, have a high risk of failed attempted abortion. Sometimes, the unique anatomy makes it difficult to enter the horn with the pregnancy. One useful approach is to perform the aspiration under ultrasound guidance. If the clinician can insert a bent sound into the cavity with the pregnancy, he or she can then place the bent sound inside a flexible 8-mm plastic cannula as a stent or guide. With ultrasound guidance, the clinician then inserts the cannula into the cavity and removes the sound, connects the cannula adapter, and then aspirates the cavity. Another alternative is to use medical abortion. Rarely, hysterotomy may be needed if aspiration and medical abortion fail in the setting of müllerian anomalies.

Dilation and Evacuation

D&E is the surgical technique recommended for pregnancies beyond 12 to 14 weeks gestation, utilizing advanced cervical

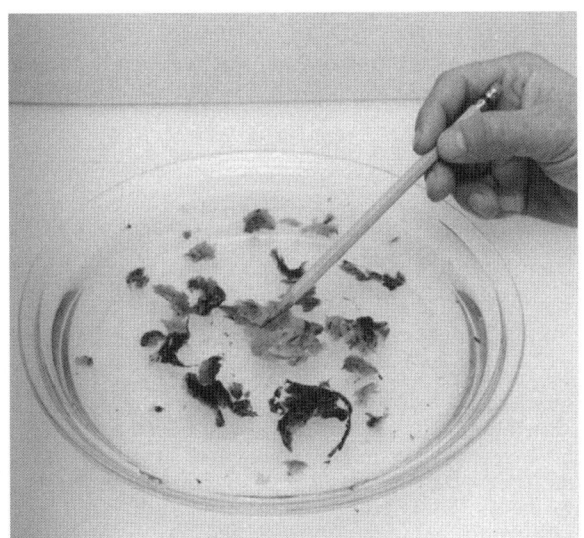

FIGURE 33.6 Examination of aspirated tissue over x-ray viewing box for back lighting.

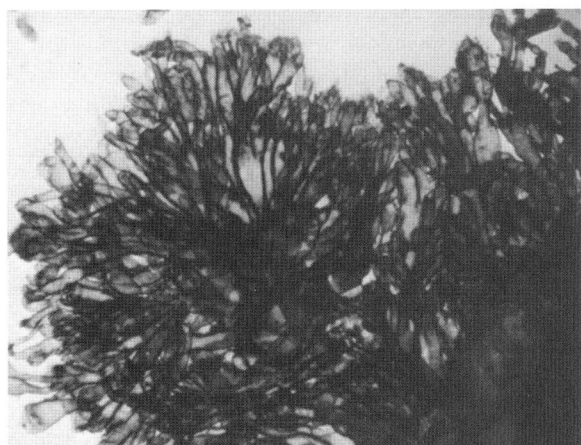

FIGURE 33.8 Wet-mount microscopic appearance of placental villi. (Reprinted from Munsick RA. Clinical test for placenta in 300 consecutive menstrual aspirations. *Obstet Gynecol* 1982;60:738, with permission. Copyright © 1982 The American College of Obstetricians and Gynecologists.)

TABLE 33.1 Percentages of Reported Legal Abortions, by Method and Gestational Age, Selected States, United States, 2009

TYPE OF PROCEDURE	%		
Suction aspiration (≤13 wk)	74.4		
D + E (>13 wk)	8.0		
Medical (≤8 wk)	15.3		
Medical (>8 wk)	0.9		
Other (includes hysterotomy, hysterectomy, and others)	1.6	100.0	100.0

From Pazol K, Creanga AA, Zane SB, et al.; Centers for Disease Control and Prevention. Abortion Surveillance–2009. *MMWR Surveill Summ* 2012;61:1.

dilation, followed by evacuation of fetus and placenta via suction and forceps. During the 1970s, D&E emerged as the most frequently used method for second-trimester abortions. The proportion of abortions performed by surgical (aspiration or evacuation) techniques is inversely related to gestational age (Table 33.1). Even at gestations greater than 20 weeks, D&E remains the dominant method of abortion in the United States. In April 2007, the U.S. Supreme Court upheld a decision to ban an abortion procedure called D&X, in which there is a partial breech delivery of a fetus and decompression of the calvarium to complete the delivery. The law does not contain an exception to permit the procedure to protect the health and life of the mother. Broader repercussions of this ruling are unknown.

STEPS IN THE PROCEDURE

Surgical Abortion Care

- Understand state-specific legal requirements for abortion provision.
- Preoperative medical evaluation:
  - Options counseling
  - Informed consent
  - Brief history and limited physical exam
  - Establishment of gestational age
  - Decide upon most appropriate surgical procedure
  - Hb and Rh status
- Preoperative cervical preparation if indicated.
- Administration of prophylactic antibiotics.
- Administration of anesthesia if other than local anesthesia indicated.
- Dorsal lithotomy position.
- Empty the bladder if the patient has not already done so.
- If suction aspiration (MVA or EVA):
  - Bimanual exam if not done in preoperative evaluation or different provider.

- Follow no-touch technique for remaining steps.
- Insert speculum.
- Apply antiseptic to cervix.
- Apply tenaculum to cervix.
- Administer paracervical block if indicated.
- Gently perform cervical dilation appropriate for gestational age and chosen cannula size.
- Gently insert cannula, attach syringe or suction tubing, and gently begin repetitive rotary and in-and-out motions to evacuate tissue.
- Limit number of passes through the cervix.
- The procedure is complete when the endometrium has a gritty feel in all quadrants, no further tissue is evacuated, and pink foamy bubbles appear in the cannula.
- Examine the aspirate and ensure it correlates with expected findings for gestational age.
- Remove tenaculum.
- Assess for hemostasis.
- Remove speculum.
- Return to dorsal supine position.
- If dilation and extraction:
  - Remove vaginal gauze and laminaria if placed, and ensure the number removed correlates with the number placed.
  - Insert speculum.
  - Place ring forceps on anterior lip of the cervix.
  - Administer vasopressin.
  - Assess cervix for adequate dilation.
  - Insert 14- or 16-mm cannula, attach to suction tubing, and drain amniotic fluid.
  - Insert forceps (under ultrasound guidance if preferred), and remove tissue. Evacuation should occur from the lower uterine segment whenever possible and in as few passes as possible through the cervix and uterus to minimize risk of perforation and cervical trauma.
  - Confirm complete evacuation with 1 pass with the cannula.
  - Examine tissue to confirm removal of all fetal parts.
  - Ensure hemostasis, and remove ring forceps and speculum.
  - Return to dorsal supine position.

Based on data from the 1970s, D&E is clearly safer than alternative methods through 16 weeks gestation. At later gestational ages, the distinction blurs between D&E and labor induction methods in terms of morbidity and mortality. Patients often prefer D&E because they avoid experiencing labor. However, many physicians have not been surgically trained to provide later D&E procedures. Often, the choice of abortion method at this later stage depends on access to abortion services, the presence of skilled personnel, and whether the fetus needs to be intact for autopsy after fetal loss. When fetal cardiac activity is present, some physicians prefer to administer feticidal agents, such as digoxin or potassium chloride, under ultrasound guidance preoperatively. A randomized, controlled trial by Jackson and colleagues found that doing so had no operative benefit. The use of feticidal agents, either intra-amniotic or intrafetal digoxin or fetal intracardiac potassium chloride, has not been shown to improve the safety of second-trimester medical or surgical abortions, and its routine use is not recommended. In select instances, such as a medical induction after 20 weeks gestation, women and/or providers may prefer feticide to avoid any transient fetal survival after expulsion. For D&E procedures, accurate preoperative determination of gestational age by ultrasound is essential. Underestimation of gestational age can lead to inadequate dilation, which complicates the procedure. D&E differs from uterine aspiration in two principal ways: D&E requires wider cervical dilation, and physicians need forceps to evacuate more advanced pregnancies.

Dilating the cervix to a large diameter over several minutes manually can damage the cervix. Indeed, the first large study of this question revealed a higher incidence of low-birth-weight infants in subsequent desired pregnancies. Hence, D&E procedures beyond about 14 weeks gestation should use osmotic dilators or misoprostol or both for cervical preparation. Patients must understand that once osmotic dilators have been inserted, the abortion needs completion. Occasionally, the patient may abort just from the dilator, but out-of-facility expulsion is rare. Rarely, a patient changes her mind about abortion after placement of an osmotic dilator. Although some women have continued their pregnancies uneventfully after removal of the devices, others have developed infections and/or aborted.

To achieve adequate dilation, many clinicians insert osmotic dilators several hours to several days before D&E (Fig. 33.9). For example, five laminaria placed overnight result in 1.5- to 2-cm dilation with minimal discomfort for most women. Use of a single Lamicel for about 4 hours produces as much dilation as do several laminaria at 14 to 16 weeks gestation, and the same is true for the use of a single Dilapan-S.

In the 13- to 16-week interval, vacuum aspiration alone is often adequate; thereafter, forceps evacuation predominates. A cannula 14 mm in diameter can evacuate pregnancies through

about 16 menstrual weeks gestation. For later pregnancies, the cannula primarily drains amniotic fluid at the beginning of the evacuation and draws tissue into the lower uterus for forceps evacuation. Specially designed Bierer forceps for D&E are far superior to standard sponge forceps, as they are designed to cause minimal trauma to the surrounding endometrium. As with suction aspiration, evacuation should occur from the lower uterus to minimize the risks of perforation. Some physicians use the cannula with suction at the end of the procedure to confirm complete evacuation. Some physicians routinely perform D&E procedures under ultrasound guidance, although this is not a requirement.

The physician must confirm completion by identifying all major fetal parts (four extremities, spine, and calvarium). The calvarium is the component most frequently missed during the initial evacuation. Gentle exploration of the fundal and cornual areas with the forceps usually enables location and removal of the calvarium. Intraoperative ultrasonography can be helpful. If ultrasonography is not available, the physician may be able to remove the speculum and insert one digit into the uterine cavity to locate the missing part.

If the abortion cannot be completed with ease, the physician should interrupt the procedure. If the patient is hemodynamically stable, a safe and simple remedy is to discontinue the operation and administer misoprostol or oxytocin for 2 to 3 hours in the recovery room. After the patient returns to the operating room, the physician usually finds the retained tissue at the internal os, from which it can be easily removed. No D&E abortion needs to finish in a single session; time often helps. Once membranes rupture, the uterus contracts to expel its contents.

In D&E abortions, the skill of the physician is critical. D&E abortion requires specific training that is often not routinely acquired in a US OB/GYN residency. The likelihood that a physician will offer abortion services is highly correlated with whether he or she was trained in residency. The physician should study operative technique. He or she should then observe and assist skilled physicians and then perform D&E procedures only under direct supervision. Use of ultrasound guidance for residents learning D&E was associated with a dramatic lowering of the perforation rate and a reduction in operating time. The gestational age range can advance as skill grows. In summary, D&E is a specialized surgical technique that can be learned with appropriate training.

Hysterotomy and Hysterectomy

Neither hysterotomy nor hysterectomy should be a primary method of abortion. The morbidity, mortality, expense, and pain associated with these operations are greater than with alternative methods. Hysterotomy for abortion should be used only when usual surgical and medical approaches fail. **Figure 33.10** depicts a hysterotomy to evacuate a 14-week pregnancy in the left horn of a bicornuate uterus; both labor induction and attempts to enter to pregnant horn through the cervix with ultrasonography and laparoscopy guidance had failed in this primigravida. Hysterectomy is appropriate in rare cases in which preexisting pathology, such as large leiomyomata (**Fig. 33.11**) or carcinoma in situ of the cervix, justifies hysterectomy. Counseling regarding loss of future fertility and increased risk of complications compared to other approaches to abortion, that is, D&E or labor induction, should accompany any decision to perform a gravid hysterectomy for abortion.

Postoperative Care

Women should expect some spotting and bleeding after the procedure that improves with time and usually stops by 1 to

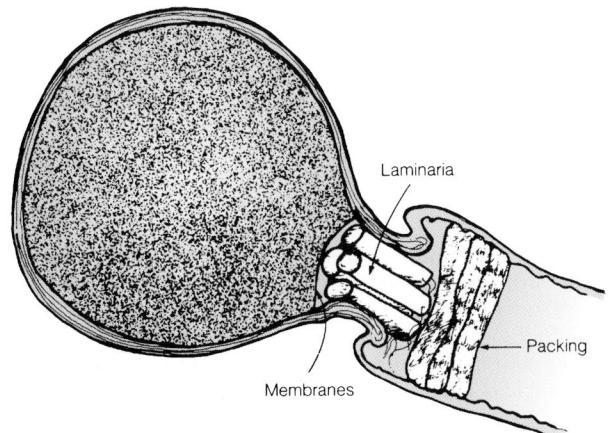

FIGURE 33.9 Laminaria in place after overnight preparation of the cervix. (Reprinted from Grimes DA, Hulka JF. Midtrimester dilatation and evacuation abortion. *South Med J* 1980;73:448, with permission. Copyright © 1980 Southern Medical Association.)

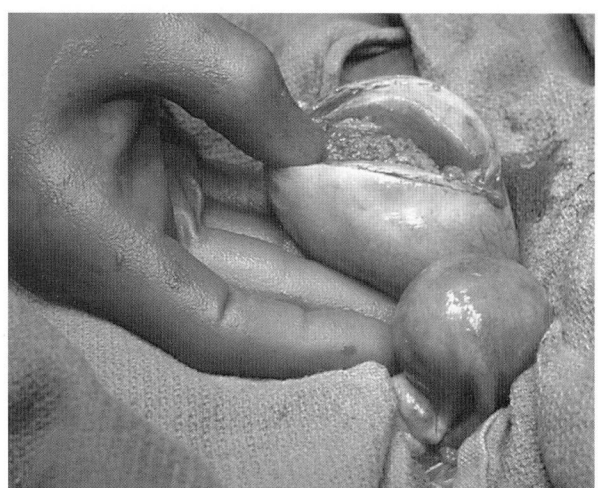

FIGURE 33.10 Hysterotomy incision in left uterine cavity, 14 weeks gestation, after failed labor induction abortion and failed attempted dilation and evacuation. The patient had a single cervix and two cavities. Nonpregnant cavity seen at right.

2 weeks. They should be instructed to notify the clinician with any signs of a complication: fever, pain, prolonged bleeding or bleeding more than a period, dizziness or weakness, passage of tissue, and ongoing symptoms of pregnancy. Pregnancy symptoms that do not dissipate within 1 week or normal menses not returning within 6 weeks are reasons to return. They should be given 24-hour emergency phone numbers. Any woman whose procedure did not definitely identify tissue should be actively managed to rule out ectopic pregnancy. Women may resume work the day following an abortion or when they feel up to it.

Almost all forms of contraception may be started on the day of an abortion procedure, including the placement of intrauterine devices. Commonly, a postoperative visit is scheduled 2 to 3 weeks after the procedure to ensure complete abortion and rule out any complications. However, there is no medical need for a routine follow-up after a surgical abortion. If women are thoroughly educated regarding the signs and symptoms of an ongoing pregnancy or other complications, and encouraged to

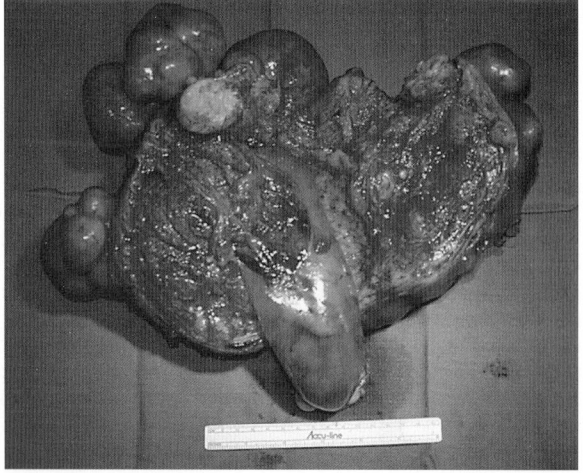

FIGURE 33.11 Total abdominal hysterectomy for abortion at 15 weeks gestation in a patient with multiple symptomatic leiomyomata with resultant anemia. Gestational sac and fetus visible in situ. **Bottom:** 15-cm ruler.

follow up with any of these issues, questions, or concerns, routine postoperative visits can be avoided. Alternatively, many providers find this visit useful to assess contraceptive use and satisfaction, as well as to provide regular gynecologic care that may not be a routine part of the preoperative abortion care—for example, cervical cytology. Routine β-hCG testing should not be done at this visit. After an uncomplicated procedure, β-hCG can be detected for a mean of 30 days and up to 60 days. Therefore, it is not useful for ruling out retained tissue and causes confusion when found to be positive.

Early Medical Abortion

Early medical abortion has also begun to play a significant role in provision of abortion, accounting for 16.5% of procedures in 2009. As an alternative to surgical abortion, early medical abortion has allowed for increased access to abortion at earlier gestations and via more nontraditional providers such as family medicine physicians. The most effective regimen for early medical abortion is the antiprogesterone mifepristone plus the prostaglandin misoprostol. Mifepristone is a derivative of norethindrone; it binds to the progesterone receptor but does not activate it. When bound, it blocks progesterone activity and acts to alter the decidua, allowing trophoblast separation. This alone can lead to bleeding and in vivo prostaglandin release that can cause an abortion in early pregnancy. Mifepristone alone, however, results in completed abortion 64% to 85% of the time. For induced abortion, success rates are significantly increased when mifepristone is combined with a prostaglandin analogue that dilates the cervix and contracts the uterine muscle to expel the pregnancy. The regimen approved by the U.S. Food and Drug Administration (FDA) calls for a single oral dose of mifepristone 600 mg, followed in 48 hours by misoprostol 400 mg orally, both doses given in the clinician's office. This has been approved for use up to 49 days' gestation. Success rates with this regimen range from 92% to 97%.

Several RCTs have investigated this regimen. Data currently support alternative dosage, route, timing, and gestational age criteria than those established by the FDA guidelines. These changes result in improved efficacy and patient convenience, decreased cost, and sustained safety.

Several studies have shown that 200 mg of mifepristone effect abortion at rates equivalent to 600 mg. El-Refaey and colleagues first reported this finding in 1995. This was confirmed by a study by WHO, reporting in 2000 that there was found no difference in the completed abortion rate between women given 200 mg of mifepristone compared with those given 600 mg. Additionally, this study included women up to 63 days' gestation. This equivalence in dosing is secondary to nonlinear pharmacokinetics. The binding site for the mifepristone is rapidly saturated. Women given 100 mg, 200 mg, and 800 mg have a peak serum concentration of 2.0 to 2.5 μg/mL approximately 2 hours after ingestion, regardless of dosage given. Therefore, pharmacology and economics support use of 200 mg mifepristone.

Several studies have also investigated misoprostol dosing and route of administration. As with cervical preparation, vaginal dosing of misoprostol has superior efficacy with less side effects overall when compared with oral dosing. Schaff and colleagues compared oral (400 μg and 800 μg) versus vaginal (800 μg) misoprostol following 200 mg mifepristone. Compared to either dose of oral misoprostol, they found a statistically significant higher level of completed abortions in those who received vaginal misoprostol (84%, 92%, and 96%, respectively). Randomized trials have found that buccal or sublingual dosing was equivalent to vaginal dosing in efficacy, but with more side effects.

Investigators have also questioned the timing of the misoprostol dosing and where it should be administered. Acceptability of women to self-administer the misoprostol at home has been shown repeatedly. Schaff and colleagues also explored efficacy of different schedules of prostaglandin administration. Following 200 mg of mifepristone, more than 2,000 subjects were randomized to self-administration of 800 μg misoprostol vaginally 24, 48, and 72 hours later. Completed abortions were found in 98%, 98%, and 96%, respectively. Patient satisfaction decreased with increasing time interval. However, decreasing the time interval further to 6 hours post mifepristone has been associated with decreased success in two randomized trials. With patient acceptability and convenience of avoiding additional clinic visits, self-administration of misoprostol at home 24 to 48 hours after mifepristone allows for an effective but flexible regimen for patients.

Lastly, the upper limit of gestational age can be extended to 63 days. When mifepristone 200 mg is followed in 24 to 48 hours by misoprostol 800 mg vaginally, complete abortion rates 95% or greater can be achieved through 63 days' gestation; this has been supported by several trials. Some small studies have found success using the combination of mifepristone and misoprostol for gestations up to 91 days; however, most agree that the likelihood of success declines with advancing gestational age.

If the alternative, evidence-based regimen is chosen, appropriate patient consent and education about variance from the FDA regimen are required in order to dispense mifepristone. NSAIDs, antiemetics, and antidiarrheals can decrease associated side effects. Narcotic prescriptions can be provided for additional pain control as needed. Women undergoing medical abortion who do not bleed within 24 hours of receiving misoprostol should contact their provider, as they may be at higher risk of ectopic pregnancy. Follow-up can be accomplished as early as one week post mifepristone, using repeat ultrasound or serum β-hCG to rule out a continuing pregnancy. Alternative follow-up protocols utilize clinical symptoms and low sensitivity urine pregnancy tests to determine which women need further evaluation for unsuccessful abortion. An inability to follow up in the time frame specified or in the event of an emergency should preclude provision of a medical abortion. In the few percent of women who fail to abort or who have incomplete abortions, observation or repeated dosing of misoprostol can be offered. For women who continue to have vaginal bleeding, in-office completion of the process with a handheld syringe and cannula (Fig. 33.4) is an option. If aspiration is needed, no additional dilation is usually required. Patients should be counseled before starting that in the rare event of ongoing pregnancy after medical abortion, suction aspiration is recommended because of the teratogenic effects of misoprostol.

Medical abortion is safe, effective, and well tolerated. With current regimens, cramping and bleeding are common, but infection and bleeding heavy enough to require transfusion are rare. Data collected from postmarketing experience since the FDA approval of mifepristone in the United States in September 2000 have demonstrated the safety. More than 460,000 women have undergone medical abortion in the United States between 2000 and mid-2005. Serious complications have included seventeen ectopic pregnancies, hemorrhage requiring blood transfusion (in < 0.03%), and seven serious bacterial infections, including five deaths from *Clostridium sordellii* sepsis. In light of potential complications and the abortion experience occurring outside of the provider's office, thorough counseling and patient understanding are imperative.

Before the marketing of mifepristone in the United States, physicians relied on other medical abortifacient regimens. One regimen included a single intramuscular injection of methotrexate, 50 mg/m^2 body surface area, followed 3 to 7 days later by vaginal administration of misoprostol, 800 μg. The efficacy of the combined regimen was 90%. In a randomized, controlled trial, this regimen proved superior to the same dose of misoprostol given alone. At 49 days' gestation or less, methotrexate and misoprostol can achieve success rates similar to those with mifepristone and misoprostol, but the process is slower with methotrexate: Providing the misoprostol at 7 days postmethotrexate rather than 3 days has been shown to increase efficacy to as high as 98%. From 20% to 30% of women require 1 to 5 weeks to complete the abortion. On the other hand, methotrexate remains an option when mifepristone is not available or when ectopic pregnancy cannot be ruled out. Methotrexate works as an antimetabolite; it continues to be used in the medical management of ectopic pregnancy.

Another alternative is use of misoprostol alone. The success rates with misoprostol alone have consistently been shown to be lower than when misoprostol is used as an adjunct with mifepristone or methotrexate. Although gastrointestinal side effects increase with multiple doses, success rates with multiple doses approach 93%, and therefore, a multidose regimen is a viable option when mifepristone is not available. Similar to when misoprostol is used with mifepristone, buccal or sublingual dosing is as effective as vaginal dosing but tends to lead to more side effects.

Medical approaches may be especially useful for challenging abortions. These include patients with müllerian anomalies, large cervical leiomyomata, prior failed attempted abortion, or obesity. Should the medical regimen not effect abortion, surgical completion is made substantially easier by this preparation of the cervix.

Labor Induction

Although D&E has supplanted many labor induction abortions, the need for such abortions continues, particularly at later gestational ages. In contrast to D&E, the proportion of abortions performed by labor induction increases with gestational age (Table 33.1). However, available resources or provider training typically dictates whether both D&E and induction can be offered, as D&E is more cost-effective than is induction but requires specialized surgical training. For settings and clinical presentations in which woman can self-select the method used, grief processes are unaffected by method chosen. Medical abortifacients in the United States used for induction of labor in the second trimester include uterotonic drugs, such as prostaglandins and oxytocin, with or without mifepristone. Uterotonics act directly on the myometrium to stimulate contractions. Prostaglandins available in the United States include misoprostol, vaginal prostaglandin E$_2$ (PGE$_2$) preparations, and 15-methyl PGF$_{2\alpha}$ for extra-amniotic use. Extra-amniotic administration of ethacridine lactate is an induction method that is infrequently used. The practice of intrauterine instillation of hypertonic solutions (saline, urea) has significantly decreased since the 1990s. Because of the increased induction time, the potential serious side effects, and the availability of safe and effective alternatives, the use of this method is not recommended.

Misoprostol as a second-trimester induction agent has emerged as a safe and effective agent. Its ease of use, affordability, and stability at room temperature make it a first-line prostaglandin option. The first study by Jain and Mishell used 200 μg vaginally every 12 hours, which was found to be as effective as vaginal PGE$_2$ suppositories and was associated with fewer side effects. As with early medical abortion, efficacy is significantly increased when 200 mg of mifepristone is combined with misoprostol. Starting misoprostol dosing 48 hours versus 24 hours after mifepristone results in shorter induction time, though the overall success rate is not affected. In RCTs, dosing intervals for misoprostol seem to affect induction times more so than the dose itself: Three-hour intervals result in shorter induction times. Misoprostol doses lower than 400 mcg are effective when preceded by mifepristone or a loading dose of 600 to 800 μg misoprostol. Oral, vaginal, and sublingual dosing appear to be equally effective when preceding by a loading dose, with the exception of nulliparous women who may benefit more from continued vaginal dosing. Studies have not been consistent as to whether women prefer nonvaginal over vaginal administration. Neither moistening the misoprostol nor adding laminaria dilators improves efficacy. The regimen recommended by the Royal College of Obstetricians & Gynaecologists and the WHO is based on a trial by Ashok et al. Thirty-six to forty-eight hours following 200 mg of mifepristone, 800 μg misoprostol was given vaginally followed by 400 μg orally every 3 hours, with a maximum of four oral doses. If abortion did not occur, patients rested for 12 hours before the misoprostol dosing was repeated. This regimen resulted in 97% successful abortion with a mean induction to abortion time of 6.25 hours (in those that were successful). Of the 1,002 patients in the study, complications were seen in 11 (0.01%): Ten had significant bleeding, and seven of these women required transfusion. One woman had significant hemorrhage and was found to have a myometrial tear upon laparotomy. She had received one dose of prostaglandin. Both mifepristone and misoprostol are not currently labeled for second-trimester termination.

Clinical trials of induction regimens have varied in terms of gestational age range, definition of success (delivery of the fetus vs. fetus and placenta), and medication combination or dose utilized, often preventing direct comparison between regimens. The high success rates observed in several of these trials suggest that regimens may be safely adjusted to fit the clinical presentation. When mifepristone is not available or infection requires immediate induction, misoprostol alone still results in high success rates. Although feticide with digoxin or potassium chloride does not improve success rates, it may be used to prevent the possibility of a live birth. Other prostaglandin regimens can be safely and feasibly administered. If prostaglandins are not available or are contraindicated, oxytocin alone can result in completed abortion up to 90% of the time, though induction time is longer. The frequency of fever, vomiting, and diarrhea was significantly lower with oxytocin compared with PGE$_2$ and misoprostol, but more attention is required in order to avoid complications. One regimen includes oxytocin, 50 U in 500 mL of dextrose and normal saline administered intravenously over 3 hours; maintenance fluid (dextrose in normal saline) then follows for 1 hour. In stepwise fashion, the concentration of oxytocin increases by 50 U every 4 hours to a maximum of 300 U/500 mL. The investigators administered oxytocin in isotonic fluid and interrupted the oxytocin infusion every 4 hours for diuresis. With prolonged high-dose oxytocin infusion in hypotonic solutions, water intoxication and death can result.

The decision about labor induction in women with a previous uterine scar remains a difficult one for clinicians. There are reports of uterine rupture both with and without previous cesarean delivery and with almost all induction methods. A systematic review of uterine rupture associated with misoprostol induction in the second trimester found that the rupture rate was 0.28% in women with a previous hysterotomy compared with 0.04% in women with an unscarred uterus. Conversely, a case series of 100 women at 14 to 28 weeks with previous cesarean delivery undergoing induction with

misoprostol reported no uterine ruptures. Further study is necessary. Women with a uterine scar require detailed counseling about the risk of rupture. If induction is chosen, it should be completed in a hospital setting where complications can be managed appropriately.

One of only two RCTs that compared D&E to induction included intrauterine instillation and misoprostol induction, as well as later gestational ages in the induction arm only; there were higher rates of complications and surgery related to retained placenta with induction. When limited to just misoprostol induction, complication rates were still higher than with D&E, again predominantly related to retained placenta. However, Green et al. demonstrated a low (6%) curettage rate with misoprostol induction when they allowed women *who were not bleeding* up to 4 hours to deliver the placenta, suggesting there are ways to further increase the safety of induction. Women undergoing labor induction need the same meticulous, attentive obstetric care as do women in labor with childbirth, even if the need for cervical exams may not be as frequent. NSAIDs, antiemetics, and antidiarrheals can decrease associated side effects. Pain control can be successfully achieved with patient-controlled analgesia (PCA) pumps. If the membranes rupture, then labor must conclude within a reasonable period. In many cases, the preferred means of concluding a slow induction abortion is D&E. Twenty-four hours is a reasonable limit for labor induction abortions. Frequently, the cervix is open several centimeters, and D&E proceeds quickly. If significant bleeding is present, then active management of a retained fetus or placenta prevents morbidity. If spontaneous delivery of the placenta has not occurred within a few hours after delivery, the placenta should be removed by suction aspiration. Notably, misoprostol is associated with a significantly lower rate of retained placenta when compared with PGE$_2$ or oxytocin (2% vs. 15%).

Complications

Morbidity

Legal abortion in the United States is safe. Less than 1 woman in 100 develops a serious complication, and less than 1 in 100,000 dies as a result of the operation. This mortality rate is far below the rate for women who elect to continue their pregnancy, which ranges from 10 to 14 times higher for women who progress to deliver a live infant.

Gestational age is one of two important determinants of the likelihood of morbidity. In Table 33.2, which lists serious complication rates for abortion by gestational age, the term *serious complication rates* is defined as fever of 38°C or higher for 3 or more days, hemorrhage requiring transfusion, or unintended surgery. These data, derived from a 1970s multicenter study including 84,000 abortions, relate to those women without concurrent sterilization or preexisting medical conditions and for whom follow-up information was available. Abortions performed at the 7 to 10 weeks gestation interval had the lowest incidence of serious complications. Thereafter, complications increased progressively with advancing gestational age. The method of abortion is the second principal determinant of the likelihood of complications. Table 33.3, derived from the same study as Table 33.2, demonstrates that suction aspiration is the safest available abortion method. The risk of serious complications with D&E at 13 weeks gestation or later is higher than that with suction aspiration and lower than that with labor induction abortion.

Abortion complications have three temporal categories: immediate, delayed, and late complications. Immediate complications are those that develop during or within 3 hours of the operation. Delayed complications occur more than 3 hours

TABLE 33.2 Serious Complication Rates for Legal Abortions by Gestational Age: United States, 1975–1978[a]

GESTATIONAL AGE (WK)	RATE[b]
6	0.4
7–8	0.2
9–10	0.1
11–12	0.3
13–14	0.6
15–16	1.3
17–20	1.9

[a]For women with follow-up and without concurrent sterilization or preexisting conditions. Serious complications include temperature of 38°C or higher for 3 days or more, hemorrhage requiring blood transfusion, and any complication requiring unintended surgery (excluding aspiration).
[b]Per 100 abortions.

and up to 28 days after the procedure. Late complications develop thereafter.

Immediate Complications

Hemorrhage Reported rates of hemorrhage vary widely, reflecting both diverse definitions (100 to 1,000 mL blood loss) and imprecision in estimating volumes of blood loss. Rates of hemorrhage range from 0.05 to 4.9 per 100 abortions in large case series reports. The best index of clinically important hemorrhage is probably the rate of blood transfusion. The rate of transfusion associated with suction aspiration in a large multicenter study was 0.06 per 100 abortions. For abortions performed later in pregnancy, investigators have reported hemorrhage and transfusion rates of up to 1 and 0.26 per 100, respectively, for D&E.

TABLE 33.3 Serious Complication Rates for Legal Abortions by Method: United States, 1975–1978[a]

METHOD	RATE[b]
Suction aspiration	0.2
Dilation and evacuation	0.7
Saline instillation	2.1
Prostaglandin instillation	2.5
Urea–prostaglandin instillation	1.3

[a]For women with follow-up and without concurrent sterilization or preexisting conditions. Serious complications include temperature of 38°C or higher for 3 days or more, hemorrhage requiring blood transfusion, and any complication requiring unintended surgery (excluding aspiration).
[b]Per 100 abortions.

When hemorrhage occurs after suction aspiration, physical exam is necessary to determine if cervical laceration, uterine perforation, or atony is the most likely etiology. For uterine atony, administration of uterotonic agents and manual compression usually resolve the problem. Vasopressin can be injected intra- or paracervically. As with labor-related atony, methylergonovine maleate may be given (0.2 mg intramuscularly) as well as prostaglandins: carboprost 250 µg intramuscularly or misoprostol 1,000 µg per rectum. Administration of oxytocin during D&E, when oxytocin receptors are present to some degree, may be helpful in controlling hemorrhage. Should bleeding persist, reassessment of the endometrial cavity by suction aspiration, with ultrasound if available, should be done to rule out retained tissue. Occasionally, internal compression of the cavity by a large Foley catheter or a Bakri balloon can be helpful. If these measures fail, uterine artery embolization can be done in a stable patient, with the last resort being hysterectomy.

With the increasing cohort of women who have had cesarean deliveries, the risk of encountering placenta accreta during abortion is increasing as well. In a series of more than 16,000 D&E abortions, the incidence of placenta accreta leading to hysterectomy was 4 per 10,000 cases.

Cervical Injury Cervical injury encompasses a broad spectrum of trauma. The most common type is a superficial laceration caused by the tenaculum tearing off during dilation. At the other extreme are the cervicovaginal fistula and the longitudinal laceration ascending to the level of the uterine vessels. Rates of cervical injury range from 0.01 to 1.6 per 100 suction aspiration abortions and increase up to 3% for D&E.

Several risk factors for cervical injury during suction aspiration have emerged. Among factors within the control of the physician, use of laminaria and performance of the abortion by an attending physician (rather than a resident) lower the risk significantly, whereas use of general anesthesia raises the risk significantly. Use of laminaria and performance of the abortion under local anesthesia by an attending physician together yield a 27-fold protective effect. Cervical preparation with misoprostol may confer similar benefits as laminaria at early gestations, although more extensive experience will be needed to confirm this. Among factors beyond the control of the physician, later gestational age, previous cesarean delivery, and age of 17 years or younger increase the risk.

Acute Hematometra Also termed the *postabortal syndrome*, acute hematometra is an important complication of suction aspiration; its cause is unknown. The incidence of this syndrome ranges from 0.1 to 1.0 per 100 suction aspiration abortions, according to the available literature.

Women with this condition develop severe cramping, usually within 2 hours of the abortion. Vaginal bleeding is less than expected. The woman may be weak and sweaty and her uterus large and markedly tender. Treatment consists of prompt repeat aspiration, usually without anesthesia or dilation. Evacuation of both liquid and clotted blood leads to rapid resolution of the symptoms. The clinician can aspirate the blood with a suction cannula, a Karman cannula and syringe, or even a catheter attached to wall suction. Administration of a uterotonic after the repeat evacuation is standard. Whether routine prophylactic use of a uterotonic would reduce the incidence of acute hematometra is unknown.

Anesthesia Complications Pain experienced during abortion relates not only to the choice of anesthesia but also to the characteristics of the patient. Young women (13 to 17 years

VI

old) and those with depression before the abortion report more pain than do other women.

Local anesthesia is safer than general anesthesia for both first- and second-trimester abortions. In an Italian study, use of general anesthesia had a relative risk for all complications combined of 1.8 (95% confidence interval, 1.4 to 2.5). The largest effect occurred with hemorrhage. Similarly, use of general anesthesia for D&E abortion in the United States increases the risk of serious complications. Overall, the attributable risk related to general anesthesia is low, and many women are willing to assume incremental risks in order to have no discomfort during the operation.

Perforation Perforation is a potentially serious but infrequent complication of abortion. The incidence of perforation is about 0.2 per 100 suction aspiration abortions.

Several risk factors for perforation exist. Performance of an aspiration abortion by a resident rather than by an attending physician increases the risk more than fivefold; on the other hand, cervical dilation by laminaria decreases the risk about fivefold. The risk of perforation increases significantly with advancing gestational age. Multiparous women have three times the risk of nulliparous women. The use of routine ultrasound guidance for D&E was noted to reduce the risk of perforation in one study.

The two principal dangers of perforation are hemorrhage and damage to the abdominal contents. Lateral perforations in the cervicoisthmic region are particularly hazardous because of the proximity of the uterine vessels. Perforations of the fundus are more likely to be innocuous. Indeed, most perforations are not suspected or detected. In a series of patients undergoing combined abortion and sterilization by laparoscopy, the investigators found a sixfold higher rate of uterine perforation than they had suspected clinically (20 vs. 3 per 1,000 abortions).

Not all perforations require treatment. Many suspected or documented perforations require only observation. Perforation with a dilator or sound is unlikely to damage abdominal contents. If the perforation occurs before suction, the procedure can be completed under either ultrasound or laparoscopic guidance with extra observation after the procedure. On the other hand, a recognized perforation with a suction cannula or forceps warrants further surgery to rule out organ injury. It is recommended to administer broad-spectrum prophylactic antibiotics when perforation occurs.

If the clinician suspects a perforation, the procedure should stop immediately. If unmanageable hemorrhage, expanding hematoma, or injury to abdominal contents occurs, prompt laparotomy is necessary. In a stable patient, laparoscopy can be useful in documenting perforation and assessing damage; if necessary, the physician can complete the abortion under laparoscopic visualization. Any woman with severe pain within hours after the abortion should be evaluated for possible perforation with bowel injury.

Delayed Complications

Retained Tissue Although retained tissue after abortion can pass without incident, it can also lead to hemorrhage, infection, or both. This complication occurs infrequently, however. Its incidence after suction aspiration abortion is less than 1 per 100 abortions.

This complication usually manifests itself within several days of the abortion. Women present with cramping and bleeding, with or without fever. As with management of EPL, β-hCG levels are typically not helpful for diagnosis once an ongoing pregnancy has been ruled out. Similarly, the need for reaspiration is determined based on clinical symptoms and

then confirmed by ultrasound findings, since the thickness of the endometrium after successful abortion is variable. Prompt administration of antibiotics along with outpatient suction aspiration is needed. Close follow-up is necessary.

Infection Postabortal infection can result simply from the procedure or from retained tissue. The organisms responsible for postabortal infection are similar to those responsible for other gynecologic infections. Administration of broad-spectrum antibiotics and uterine reaspiration (if retained tissue is present) are the cornerstones of therapy. The likelihood of febrile morbidity after abortion depends on the method used. The incidence of fever of 38°C or higher for 1 or more days is usually less than 1 per 100 abortions by suction aspiration. Corresponding figures for D&E are 1.5 per 100 abortions and for urea–prostaglandin, 6.3.

A number of risk factors for infection exist. Women are at increased risk if they have untreated endocervical gonorrhea or chlamydial infection. Later gestational age abortions also increase the risk. Likewise, use of local rather than general anesthesia for suction aspiration increases the risk. Preoperative prophylactic antibiotics decrease the incidence of infection.

Late Complications

Rh Sensitization Legal abortion is a potentially important cause of Rh sensitization for women at risk. The likelihood of sensitization increases with advancing gestational age (and, hence, larger volumes of fetal erythrocytes). One study has quantified the risk of Rh sensitization from first-trimester suction aspiration without RhIG prophylaxis. A total of 3.1% of women whose first pregnancy terminated by suction aspiration without RhIG prophylaxis had antibodies in their second pregnancy. Subtracting 0.5% (the percentage of women estimated to have become sensitized primarily during the second pregnancy), the investigators estimated the risk of sensitization from suction aspiration to be 2.6%. Thus, on a nationwide basis, the clinical impact of failure to administer RhIG to candidates after abortion may be substantial. Candidates should receive 50 μg of RhIG after abortions performed at 12 weeks gestation or earlier or 300 μg after abortions performed later in pregnancy.

Adverse Pregnancy Outcomes Investigators have linked induced abortion with a broad array of adverse reproductive outcomes, ranging from infertility to ectopic pregnancy. Most published reports, however, suffer from serious methodologic shortcomings that limit their usefulness. To examine the potential association between first-trimester induced abortion and subsequent reproductive performance, epidemiologists have performed an exhaustive review and analysis of the world literature. This includes more than 150 epidemiologic studies published in 11 languages. The findings of this analysis are largely reassuring. No increase in the risk of secondary infertility and ectopic pregnancy appears, even in studies with substantial power to detect differences in rates. Midtrimester pregnancy loss is no more common among women who have had one previous abortion than among women pregnant for the first time. Similarly, the risk of premature delivery does not increase for women having undergone induced abortion. On the other hand, low birth weight is more frequent in first births after abortion by sharp curettage performed under general anesthesia compared with first-pregnancy births. This does not occur after other methods of abortion, such as suction aspiration. The question of the effect of repeat induced abortion and second-trimester abortion remains unresolved, but the increased risk associated with sharp curettage provides an additional reason why this method should be avoided. Firstborn infants of women who had one induced abortion

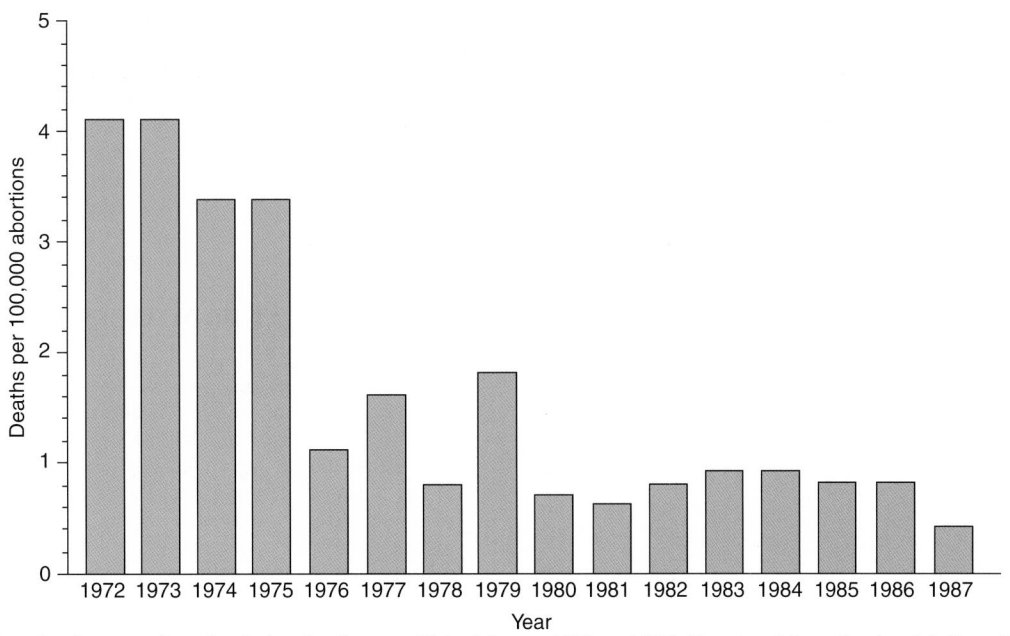

FIGURE 33.12 Case fatality rates from legal abortion by year, United States, 1972 to 1987. (Reprinted from Bartlett LA, Berg CJ, Shulman HB, et al. Risk factors for legal induced abortion-related mortality in the United States. *Obstet Gynecol* 2004;103:729, with permission. Copyright © 1982 The American College of Obstetricians and Gynecologists.)

have risks of morbidity and mortality similar to those of other firstborn children.

Additional studies have corroborated the absence of adverse effects of induced abortion on subsequent reproduction. Outcomes studied included infertility, ectopic pregnancy, spontaneous abortion, and adverse obstetric outcomes. One unresolved issue is placenta previa. Sophisticated studies have found either no or a marginally significant increase in the risk (relative risk, 1.3; 95% confidence interval, 1.0 to 1.6), which was comparable to that with EPL.

Induced abortion does not threaten a woman's emotional health. In contrast, the most common emotional reactions to induced abortion are a sense of relief accompanied by sadness and loss. In several studies, abortion appeared to improve the emotional well-being of women by resolving an intense personal crisis. Specifically, claims of a postabortion trauma syndrome lack scientific merit. Studies to date have failed to adequately assess or control for any preexisting mental illness in women who have had an abortion.

The putative association between induced abortion and breast cancer remains controversial. Although a number of case–control studies have found an association, this appears because of recall bias among controls. Women who are well (controls) are less likely to report prior induced abortions than are women with breast cancer (cases). This type of information bias has been documented in studies from Sweden. Two large cohort studies, which are less likely to be biased than are case–control studies, have shown either no effect or a protective effect of induced abortion on later breast cancer. No firm evidence links abortion to other cancers.

Mortality

Since 1972, when the CDC first began nationwide surveillance of abortion deaths, the safety of abortion has improved dramatically. As shown in **Figure 33.12**, the overall death rate fell from 4.1 deaths per 100,000 abortions in 1972 to 0.7 in the data published for the decade between 1988 and 1997. In an extensive review by Raymond and Grimes

in 2012, estimating the mortality rate associated with live births and legal abortions in the United States from 1998 to 2005 found the pregnancy-associated mortality rate for women who delivered a live neonate to be 8.8/100,000 live births and the mortality rate related to induced abortion to be 0.6/100,000 legal induced abortions. This demonstrates the risk of death to be 14 times higher for women continuing with pregnancy to a live birth than for women undergoing legal induced abortion. The most recent abortion surveillance report from the CDC, based on US data, reports a case fatality rate of 0.64 deaths per 100,000 reported legal abortions.

The causes of death from legal abortion have changed as well. After abortion became legal in 1973, abortion-related deaths declined because of an increase in the skill and experience of providers. When the abortion surveillance system identified procedures that increased risks, practitioners changed their procedures to increase safety. For example, this led to the decline of instillation procedures identified as riskier in the 1970s and the use of general anesthesia in the 1980s. For the 1998 to 2005 time period, the main causes of death were hemorrhage, infection, and complications from anesthesia, which accounted for nearly three fourths of deaths. Embolism, noncardiovascular conditions, cardiovascular conditions, and other causes accounted for the rest.

The risk of death from legal abortion, as reported by Bartlett and colleagues, increases exponentially with increasing gestational age: The earlier the abortion, the safer the abortion (Table 33.4). The risks from 1988 to 1997 (and therefore not including mifepristone abortions) are as follows: The risk with gestational age ≤8 weeks is 1 per million, at 12 weeks is 0.4 per 100,000, at 16 to 20 is 3.4, and at ≥21 weeks is 8.9 per 100,000 procedures (76 times higher than with the earliest procedures). Given the fact that earlier abortions are safer, issues such as access to abortion are medically relevant. These include number of trained providers, cost, and gestational age limit of particular institutions.

The risk of death for women of black and other races was about twice that of white women. For women having

TABLE 33.4 Legal Abortion Case Fatality Rates and Relative Risks by Selected Categories: United States, 1988–1997

RISK CATEGORY	N[a]	RATE[b]	RELATIVE RISK AND 95% CONFIDENCE INTERVAL
Age group (y)			
≤19	0.7	20	1.2 (0.6–2.2)
20–24	0.7	29	1.1 (0.6–2.0)
25–29	0.6	18	Referent
30–34	0.9	16	1.5 (0.7–2.9)
≥35	0.8	10	1.3 (0.6–2.9)
Race			
White	38	0.5	Referent
Black and other	56	1.1	2.4 (1.6–3.6)
Parity[c]			
0	16	0.3	Referent
1–2	27	0.5	1.9 (1.0–3.5)
≥3	7	0.5	2.1 (0.9–5.2)
Gestational age (wk)[d]			
≤8	8	0.1	Referent
9–10	5	0.2	1.4 (0.5–4.2)
11–12	6	0.4	3.4 (1.2–9.7)
13–15	15	1.7	14.7 (6.2–34.7)
16–20	19	3.4	29.5 (12.9–67.4)
≥21	15	8.9	76.6 (32.5–180.8)
Time period			
1972–1979	163	2.2	3.1 (2.4–4.0)
1980–1987	80	0.8	1.1 (0.8–1.4)
1988–1997	94	0.7	Referent

[a]Number of legal abortion-related deaths.
[b]Rate of legal abortion deaths as number per 100,000 abortions.
[c]Denominators for calculating rates by parity use previous live birth data from abortion surveillance. Deaths with unknown parity are excluded.
[d]Deaths with unknown gestational age are excluded.
Reprinted from Bartlett LA, Berg CJ, Shulman HB, et al. Risk factors for legal induced abortion-related mortality in the United States. *Obstet Gynecol* 2004;103:729–737, with permission. Copyright © 2004 The American College of Obstetricians and Gynecologists.

second-trimester procedures, mortality rates for D&E were 2.5 times lower than those for instillation and other procedures, although this was not statistically significant. No statistically significant difference in risk related to maternal age or parity was found in this last time period of record.

CONCLUSION

Abortion is a frequent outcome of human conception; thus, management of abortion and its complications is an important responsibility for clinicians. Chromosomal anomalies are the single most important cause of EPL. For women with threatened abortion, use of ultrasonography and β-hCG monitoring can help predict the outcome of the pregnancy. For women who either require or desire prompt evacuation after EPL, either aspiration or labor induction may be appropriate.

Small numbers of illegal abortions continue to occur in the United States. Legally induced abortion, however, is one of the most frequently performed—and one of the safest—operations in contemporary practice. Less than 1 per 100 of those having an abortion suffers a major complication, and less than 1 per 100,000 dies from causes associated with the procedure. The marketing of mifepristone in the United States for early abortion has broadened the options available to women, and use of misoprostol for cervical preparation before aspiration represents an important advance in gynecology.

BEST SURGICAL PRACTICES

- Management of EPL includes surgical management, medical management with misoprostol, or expectant management. Suction aspiration at early EGAs can be accomplished with a manual syringe or an electric vacuum source. D&E is a safe technique for later EGAs. Intervention is not required in the absence of symptoms. Patient preference can direct management plan in most cases.
- Septic abortion requires aggressive management. This includes obtaining intrauterine and blood cultures, administration of broad-spectrum antibiotics, and prompt surgical evacuation of the uterus.
- Suction aspiration is the most frequent method of legal abortion in the United States. MVA is increasing in use as an alternative to using electric vacuum. Both may safely be done in outpatient facilities.
- Preoperative medical evaluation for induced abortion should include patient's medical, surgical, and anesthetic history, confirmation of gestational age, and thorough counseling about all available options, including continuing pregnancy, adoption, and medical and surgical abortion. Abortion regulations vary by state and should be followed by providers.
- Cervical dilation necessary for first-trimester suction aspiration can be achieved with osmotic dilators, medical preparation with misoprostol, or manual dilation. If manual dilation is necessary, a variety of dilators are available. Gentle dilation is imperative in prevention of uterine perforation.
- Prophylactic measures can be adopted into routine practice in order to decrease complication rates. Prophylactic antibiotic use is indicated for all surgical management of induced abortion, including MVA, electric vacuum aspiration, and D&E. The use of vasopressin decreases the risk of hemorrhage during D&E. The incidence of retained products of conception after surgical abortion can be decreased if aspirated tissue is inspected for presence of fetal tissue or chorionic villi.
- Pain control is essential in abortion care. This is most easily achieved with paracervical anesthesia. Additional measures include relaxation techniques, sedation, and general anesthesia. Risks and benefits of all options must be considered with respect to the patient's emotional or physical status.
- Second-trimester abortion can be achieved surgically via D&E. D&E is generally safer and faster, but only in the hands of a properly trained physician. Adequate preoperative cervical preparation is essential and can be achieved with osmotic dilators or misoprostol. Intraoperative ultrasound may decrease operative time as well as complications. Special forceps are used to facilitate evacuation of later gestations.
- Medical abortion with mifepristone and misoprostol is a safe way to terminate early gestations. The most effective regimens administer misoprostol at least 24 hours after mifepristone and in high doses. Thorough patient counseling will increase patient satisfaction and decrease complications. In order to be a candidate for medical abortion, a

patient must be able to understand the regimen, have access to emergency care if needed, and be able to follow up to ensure completion of the procedure.

- Labor induction can be performed using prostaglandins (misoprostol, $PGF_{2\alpha}$, PGE_2) or oxytocin. Multiple regimens for prostaglandins exist; the most effective regimens utilize mifepristone and short dosing intervals of misoprostol. Clinicians must weigh efficacy and speed of abortion against side effects like fever, nausea, vomiting, and diarrhea. Use of prostaglandins in women with scarred uteri remains an area that requires further study.
- Complications of abortion include hemorrhage, cervical injury, uterine perforation, retained products, infection, anesthetic complications, and Rh sensitization. Morbidity and mortality from legal abortion are very rare.

BIBLIOGRAPHY

Achilles SL, Reeves MF; Society of Family Planning. Prevention of infection after induced abortion: release date October 2010: SFP guideline 20102. *Contraception* 2011;83:295.

Adler NE, David HP, Major BN, et al. Psychological responses after abortion. *Science* 1990;248:41.

Aleman A, Althabe F, Belizan JM, et al. Bedrest during pregnancy for preventing miscarriage. *Cochrane Database Syst Rev* 2005;2:CD003576.

Alfirevic Z, Stampalija T, Roberts D, et al. Cervical stitch (cerclage) for preventing preterm birth in singleton pregnancy. *Cochrane Database Syst Rev* 2012;4:CD008991.

American College of Obstetricians and Gynecologists. *ACOG Practice Bulletin No. 48: Cervical insufficiency.* Washington, DC: American College of Obstetricians and Gynecologists, 2003.

American College of Obstetricians and Gynecologists. *ACOG Committee Opinion No. 245: Mifepristone for medical pregnancy termination.* Washington, DC: American College of Obstetricians and Gynecologists, 2000.

ACOG practice bulletin: second trimester abortion, 2013. Unpublished at the time of writing.

Ashok PW, Templeton A, Wagaarachchi PT, et al. Midtrimester medical termination of pregnancy: a review of 1002 consecutive cases. *Contraception* 2004;69:51.

Atrash HK, MacKay HT, Hogue CJR. Ectopic pregnancy concurrent with induced abortion: incidence and mortality. *Am J Obstet Gynecol* 1990;162:726.

Bartlett LA, Berg CJ, Shulman HB, et al. Risk factors for legal induced abortion-related mortality in the United States. *Obstet Gynecol* 2004;103:729.

Berg CJ, Callaghan WM, Syverson C, et al. Pregnancy related mortality in the United States: 1998–2005. *Obstet Gynecol* 2010;116:1302.

Blanchard K, Winikoff B, Ellertson C. Misoprostol used alone for the termination of early pregnancy: review of the evidence. *Contraception* 1999;59:209.

Blumenthal PD, Remsburg RE. A time and cost analysis of the management of incomplete abortion with manual vacuum aspiration. *Int J Gynaecol Obstet* 1994;45:261.

Borgatta L, Kapp N. Labor induction abortion in the second trimester. SFP guideline 20111. *Contraception* 2011;84:4.

Bugalho A, Bique C, Almeida L, et al. Pregnancy interruption by vaginal misoprostol. *Gynecol Obstet Invest* 1993;36:226.

Calvache JA, Delgado-Noguera MF, Lesaffre E, et al. Anaesthesia for evacuation of incomplete miscarriage. *Cochrane Database Syst Rev* 2012;4:CD008681.

Chen BA, Creinin MD. Contemporary management of early pregnancy failure. *Clin Obstet Gynecol* 2007;50:67.

Cnattinguis S, Signorello LB, Anneren G, et al. Caffeine intake and the risk of first-trimester spontaneous abortion. *N Engl J Med* 2000;343:1839.

Creinin MD, Edwards J. Early abortion: surgical and medical options. *Curr Probl Obstet Gynecol Fertil* 1997;20:6.

Creinin MD, Vittinghoff E. Methotrexate and misoprostol vs. misoprostol alone for early abortion: a randomized controlled trial. *JAMA* 1994;272:1190.

Creinin MD, Vittinghoff E, Keder L, et al. Methotrexate and misoprostol for early abortion: a multicenter trial. I: Safety and efficacy. *Contraception* 1996;53:321.

Cunningham FG, Leveno KL, Bloom SL, et al. *Williams obstetrics.* New York, NY: McGraw-Hill, 2005.

Dalton VK, Harris LH, Clark SJ, et al. Treatment patterns for early pregnancy failure in Michigan. *J Womens Health* 2009;18:787.

Daskalakis GJ, Mesogitis SA, Papantoniou NE, et al. Misoprostol for second trimester pregnancy termination in women with prior cesarean section. *Br J Obstet Gynaecol* 2005;115:97.

Devaseelan P, Fogarty PP, Regan L. Human chorionic gonadotrophin for threatened miscarriage. *Cochrane Database Syst Rev* 2010;5:CD007422.

Diedrich J, Drey E; Society of Family Planning. Induction of fetal demise before abortion. *Contraception* 2010;81:462.

Doubilet PM, Benson CB, Chow JS. Long-term prognosis of pregnancies complicated by slow embryonic heart rates in early first trimester. *J Ultrasound Med* 1999;18:537.

Edwards J, Carson SA. New technologies permit safe abortion at less than six weeks' gestation and provide timely detection of ectopic gestation. *Am J Obstet Gynecol* 1997;176:1101.

El-Refaey H, Rajasekar D, Abdalla M, et al. Induction of abortion with mifepristone (RU 486) and oral or vaginal misoprostol. *N Engl J Med* 1995;332:983.

Finer LB, Frohwith LF, Dauphinee LA, et al. Reasons U.S. women have abortions: quantitative and qualitative perspectives. *Perspect Sex Reprod Health* 2005;37:110.

Finer LB, Henshaw SK. Abortion incidence and services in the United States in 2000. *Perspect Sex Reprod Health* 2003;35:6.

Fox MC, Hayes JL; Society for Family Planning. Cervical preparation for second trimester surgical abortions prior to 20 weeks of gestation. *Contraception* 2007;76:486.

Goldberg AB, Dean G, Kang MS, et al. Manual versus electric vacuum aspiration for early first-trimester abortion: a controlled study of complication rates. *Obstet Gynecol* 2004;103:101.

Goldberg AB, Drey EA, Whitaker AK, et al. Misoprostol compared with laminaria before early second-trimester surgical abortion: a randomized trial. *Obstet Gynecol* 2005;106:234.

Graziosi GC, van der Steeg JW, Reuwer PH, et al. Economic evaluation of misoprostol in the treatment of early pregnancy failure compared to curettage after an expectant management. *Hum Reprod* 2005;20:1067.

Green J, Borgatta L, Sia M, et al. Intervention rates for placental removal following induction abortion with misoprostol. *Contraception* 2007;76:310.

Grimes DA, Hulka JF. Midtrimester dilatation and evacuation abortion. *South Med J* 1980;73:448.

Grossman D, Ellertson C, Grimes DA, et al. Routine follow-up visits after first-trimester induced abortion. *Obstet Gynecol* 2004;103:738.

Hamoda H, Ashok PW, Flett GM, et al. Medical abortion at 64 to 91 days of gestation: a review of 483 consecutive cases. *Am J Obstet Gynecol* 2003;188:1315.

Harper CC, Henderson JT, Darney PD. Abortion in the United States. *Annu Rev Public Health* 2005;26:501.

Harwood B, Meckstroth KR, Mishell DR, et al. Serum beta-human chorionic gonadotropin levels and endometrial thickness after medical abortion. *Contraception* 2001;63:255.

Jackson RA, Teplin VL, Drey EA, et al. Digoxin to facilitate late second-trimester abortion: a randomized, masked, placebo-controlled trial. *Obstet Gynecol* 2001;97:471.

Jain JK, Mishell DR Jr. A comparison of intravaginal misoprostol with prostaglandin E_2 for termination of second-trimester pregnancy. *N Engl J Med* 1994;331:290.

Jones RK. How commonly do US abortion patients report attempts to self-induce? *Am J Obstet Gynecol* 2011;204:23.e1.

Kapp N, Whyte P, Tang J, et al. A review of evidence for safe abortion care. *Contraception* 2012;88:350.

Kerns J, Steinauer J. Management of postabortion hemorrhage. SFP guideline 20131. *Contraception* 2013;87:331.

Kochanek KD, Murphy SL, Anderson RN, et al. *Deaths: final data for 2002, National Vital Statistics Report,* vol. 53, No. 5. Hyattsville, MD: National Center for Health Statistics, 2004.

Koonin LM, Strauss LT, Chrisman CE, et al.; Centers for Disease Control and Prevention (CDC). Abortion surveillance—United States, 1997. *MMWR CDC Surveill Summ* 2000;49:1.

Kulier R, Kapp N, Gulmezoglu AM, et al. Medical methods for first trimester abortion. *Cochrane Database Syst Rev* 2011;11:CD002855.

Lawson HW, Frye A, Atrash HK, et al. Abortion mortality, United States, 1972 through 1987. *Am J Obstet Gynecol* 1994;171:1365.

Lede R, Duley L. Uterine muscle relaxant drugs for threatened miscarriage. *Cochrane Database Syst Rev* 2005;3:CD002857.

Levi CS, Lyons EA, Zheng XH, et al. Endovaginal US: demonstration of cardiac activity in embryos of less than 5.0 mm in crown-rump length. *Radiology* 1990;176:71.

Lichtenberg ES, Paul M, Jones H. First trimester surgical abortion practices: a survey of National Abortion Federation members. *Contraception* 2001;64:345.

Li L, Dou L, Leung PC, et al. Chinese herbal medicines for threatened miscarriage. *Cochrane Database Syst Rev* 2012;5:CD008510.

Luise C, Jermy K, May C, et al. Outcome of expectant management of spontaneous first trimester miscarriage: observational study. *BMJ* 2002;324:873.

MacDorman MF, Kimeyer SE, Wilson EC. *Fetal and perinatal mortality, United States, 2006. National vital statistics reports*, vol. 60, no. 8. Hyattsville, MD: National Center for Health Statistics, 2012.

May W, Gulmezoglu AM, Ba-Thike K. Antibiotics for incomplete abortion. *Cochrane Database Syst Rev* 2007;4:CD001779.

Mills JL, Simpson JL, Driscoll SG, et al. Incidence of spontaneous abortion among normal women and insulin-dependent diabetic women whose pregnancies were identified within 21 days of conception. *N Engl J Med* 1988;319:1618.

Munsick RA. Clinical test for placenta in 300 consecutive menstrual aspirations. *Obstet Gynecol* 1982;60:738.

Nanda K, Lopez LM, Grimes DA, et al. Expectant care versus surgical management for miscarriage. *Cochrane Database Syst Rev* 2012;3:CD003518.

National Abortion Federation. *Early medical abortion with mifepristone or methotrexate: overview and protocol recommendations*. Washington, DC: National Abortion Federation, 2001.

Neilson JP, Hickey M, Vazquez JC. Medical treatment for early fetal death (less than 24 weeks). *Cochrane Database Syst Rev* 2006;3:CD002253.

Neilson JP, Gyte GML, Hickey M, et al. Medical treatments for incomplete miscarriage (less than 24 weeks). *Cochrane Database Syst Rev* 2010;1:CD007223.

Ness RB, Grisso JA, Hirshinger, et al. Cocaine and tobacco use and the risk of spontaneous abortion. *N Engl J Med* 1999;340:333.

Newhall EP, Winikoff B. Abortion with mifepristone and misoprostol: regimens, efficacy, acceptability and future directions. *Am J Obstet Gynecol* 2000;183:S44.

Nybo Anderson MA, Wohlfahrt J, Christens P, et al. Maternal age and fetal loss: population based register linkage study. *BMJ* 2000;320:1708.

Osborn JF, Arisi E, Spinelli A, et al. General anaesthesia: a risk factor for complication following induced abortion? *Eur J Epidemiol* 1990;6:416.

Owen J, Hauth JC, Winkler CL, et al. Midtrimester pregnancy termination: a randomized trial of prostaglandin E_2 versus concentrated oxytocin. *Am J Obstet Gynecol* 1992;167:1112.

Paul M, Lichtenberg ES, Borgatta L, et al. *Management of unintended and abnormal pregnancy: comprehensive abortion care*. Hoboken: Wiley-Blackwell, 2009.

Pazol K, Creanga AA, Zane SB, et al.; Centers for Disease Control and Prevention. Abortion Surveillance—2009. *MMWR Surveill Summ* 2012;61:1.

Peyron R, Aubeny E, Targosz V, et al. Early termination of pregnancy with mifepristone (RU-486) and the orally active prostaglandin misoprostol. *N Engl J Med* 1993;328:1509.

Rahn DD, Mamik MM, Sanses TVD, et al. Venous thromboembolism prophylaxis in gynecologic surgery: a systematic review. *Obstet Gynecol* 2011;118:1111.

Rasch V. Cigarette, alcohol, and caffeine consumption: risk factors for spontaneous abortion. *Acta Obstet Gynecol Scand* 2003;82:182.

Rashbaum WK, Gates EJ, Jones J, et al. Placenta accreta encountered during dilation and evacuation in the second trimester. *Obstet Gynecol* 1995;85:701.

Raymond EG, Grimes DA. The comparative safety of legal induced abortion and childbirth in the United States. *Obstet Gynecol* 2012;119:215.

Regan L, Braude PR, Trembath PL. Influence of past reproductive performance on risk of spontaneous abortion. *BMJ* 1989;299:541.

Regan L, Rai R. Epidemiology and the medical causes of miscarriage. *Baillieres Best Pract Res Clin Obstet Gynaecol* 2000;14:839.

Remennick LI. Induced abortion as cancer risk factor: a review of epidemiological evidence. *J Epidemiol Community Health* 1990;44:259.

Renner MR, Jensen JT, Nichols MD, et al. Pain control in first trimester abortions: a systematic review of randomized controlled trials. *Contraception* 2010;81:372.

Renner MR, Nichols MD, Jensen JT, et al. Paracervical block for pain control in first trimester surgical abortion: a randomized controlled trial. *Obstet Gynecol* 2012;119:1030.

Rumbold A, Middleton P, Pan N, et al. Vitamin supplementation for preventing miscarriage. *Cochrane Database Syst Rev* 2011;1:CD004073.

Saraiya M, Green CA, Berg CJ, et al. Spontaneous abortion–related deaths among women in the United States: 1981–1991. *Obstet Gynecol* 1999;94:172.

Sawaya GF, Grady D, Kerlikowske K, et al. Antibiotics at the time of induced abortion: the case for universal prophylaxis based on a meta-analysis. *Obstet Gynecol* 1996;87:884.

Say L, Brahmi D, Kulier R, et al. Medical versus surgical methods for first trimester termination of pregnancy. *Cochrane Database Syst Rev* 2002;4:CD003037.

Schaff EA, Fielding SL, Westhoff C. Randomized trial of oral versus vaginal misoprostol 2 days after mifepristone 200 mg for abortion up to 63 days of pregnancy. *Contraception* 2002;66:247.

Schaff EA, Fielding SL, Westhoff C, et al. Vaginal misoprostol administered 1, 2, or 3 days after mifepristone for early medical abortion: a randomized trial. *JAMA* 2000;284:1948.

Schaff EA, Wortman M, Eisinger SH, et al. Methotrexate and misoprostol when surgical abortion fails. *Obstet Gynecol* 1996;87:450.

Schreiber C, Creinin MD. Mifepristone in abortion care. *Semin Reprod Med* 2005;23:82.

Sharma S, Refaey H, Stafford M, et al. Oral versus vaginal misoprostol administered one hour before surgical termination of pregnancy: a randomized, controlled study. *BJOG* 2005;112:456.

Signorello LB, McLaughlin JK. Maternal caffeine consumption and spontaneous abortion: a review of the epidemiologic evidence. *Epidemiology* 2004;15:229.

Signorello LB, Nordmark A, Granath F, et al. Caffeine metabolism and the risk of spontaneous abortion of normal karyotype fetuses. *Obstet Gynecol* 2001;98:1059.

Singh K, Fong YF, Prasad RN, et al. Randomized trial to determine optimal dose of vaginal misoprostol for preabortion cervical priming. *Obstet Gynecol* 1998;92:795.

Sotiriadis A, Makrydimas G, Papatheodorou S, et al. Expectant, medical, or surgical management of first-trimester miscarriage: a meta-analysis. *Obstet Gynecol* 2005;105:1104.

Stephenson P, Wagner M, Badea M, et al. The public health consequences of restricted induced abortion: lessons from Romania. *Am J Public Health* 1992;82:1328.

Stotland NL. The myth of the abortion trauma syndrome. *JAMA* 1992;268:2078.

Strauss LT, Herndon J, Chang J, et al. Abortion surveillance—United States, 2001. *MMWR Surveill Summ* 2004;53:1.

Strauss LT, Herndon J, Chang J, et al. Abortion surveillance—United States, 2002. In: CDC surveillance summaries, November 25, 2005. *MMWR Surveill Summ* 2005;54.

Stubblefield PG, Carr-Ellis S, Borgotta L. Methods for induced abortion. *Obstet Gynecol* 2004;104:174.

Tang OS, Ho PC. Medical abortion in the second trimester. *Best Pract Res Clin Obstet Gynaecol* 2002;16:237.

Taylor VM, Kramer MD, Vaughan TL, et al. Placenta previa in relation to induced and spontaneous abortion: a population-based study. *Obstet Gynecol* 1993;82:88.

Townsend DE, Barbis SD, Mathews RD. Vasopressin and operative hysteroscopy in the management of delayed postabortion and postpartum bleeding. *Am J Obstet Gynecol* 1991;165:616.

Tuncalp O, Gulmezoglu AM, Souza JP. Surgical procedures for evacuating incomplete miscarriage. *Cochrane Database Syst Rev* 2010;9:CD001993.

Ulmann A, Silvestre L, Chemama L, et al. Medical termination of early pregnancy with mifepristone (RU-486) followed by a prostaglandin analogue: study in 16,369 women. *Acta Obstet Gynecol Scand* 1992;71:278.

Unsafe Abortion Mortality. *World Health Organization.* http://www.who.int/reproductivehealth/topics/unsafe_abortion/magnitude/en/index.html

Ventura SJ, Curtin SC, Abma JC, et al. *Estimated pregnancy rates and rates of pregnancy outcomes for the United States, 1990–2008. National vital statistics reports*, vol. 60, no. 7. Hyattsville, MD: National Center for Health Statistics, 2012.

Von Hertzen H, Honkanen H, Piaggio G, et al. WHO multinational study of three misoprostol regimens after mifepristone for early medical abortion. I: Efficacy. *BJOG* 2003;110:808.

Wahabi HA, Fayed AA, Esmaeil SA, et al. Progestogen for treating threatened miscarriage. *Cochrane Database Syst Rev* 2011;12:CD005943.

Wilcox AJ, Weinberg CR, O'Connor JF, et al. Incidence of early loss of pregnancy. *N Engl J Med* 1988;319:189.

Wang X, Chen C, Wang L, et al. Conception, early pregnancy loss, and time to clinical pregnancy: a population-based prospective study. *Fertil Steril* 2003;79:577.

Winkler CL, Gray SE, Hauth JC, et al. Mid-second-trimester labor induction: concentrated oxytocin compared with prostaglandin E$_2$ vaginal suppositories. *Obstet Gynecol* 1991;77:297.

Wisborg K, Kesmodel U, Henriksen TB, et al. A prospective study of maternal smoking and spontaneous abortion. *Acta Obstet Gynecol Scand* 2003;82:936.

World Health Organization. *Medical methods for termination of pregnancy.* WHO technical report series 871. Geneva: World Health Organization, 1997.

World Health Organization. *Safe abortion: technical and policy guidance for health systems*, 2nd ed. Geneva: World Health Organization, 2012.

World Health Organization. *Spontaneous and induced abortion.* WHO technical report series 461. Geneva: World Health Organization, 1970.

Yapar EG, Senoz S, Urkutur M, et al. Second trimester pregnancy termination including fetal death: comparison of five different methods. *Eur J Obstet Gynecol Reprod Biol* 1996;69:97.

Zhang J, Giles JM, Barnhart K, et al. A comparison of medical management with misoprostol and surgical management for early pregnancy failure. *N Engl J Med* 2005;353:761.

Zieman M, Fong SK, Benowitz NL, et al. Absorption kinetics of misoprostol with oral or vaginal administration. *Obstet Gynecol* 1997;90:88.

CHAPTER 34
Ectopic Pregnancy

Mark A. Damario

DEFINITIONS

Abdominal pregnancy—A pregnancy that develops in the peritoneal cavity. Most abdominal pregnancies are secondary, the result of early tubal abortion or rupture with secondary implantation of the pregnancy into the peritoneal cavity. A primary abdominal pregnancy is one that implants directly into the peritoneal cavity.

Arias-Stella reaction—A reaction in endometrial cells associated (but not exclusively) with ectopic pregnancy, showing nuclear enlargement, irregularity, and hyperchromasia with cytoplasmic vacuolization.

β-hCG assay—A quantitative determination of the serum concentration of the human chorionic gonadotropin hormone obtained using a highly sensitive immunoassay that is specific for the β-subunit of human chorionic gonadotropin. Useful in the early diagnosis of ectopic pregnancy.

Cervical pregnancy—A pregnancy developing in the cervical canal below the level of the internal os.

Culdocentesis—Aspiration of fluid from the cul-de-sac (pouch of Douglas) via a needle puncturing the vaginal wall between the uterosacral ligaments.

Dilatation and curettage—A surgical procedure in which the endometrial cavity contents are removed and submitted for histologic study. Useful in the early diagnosis of ectopic pregnancy when β-hCG assays and transvaginal ultrasonography are nondiagnostic and a nonviable pregnancy is suspected.

Ectopic pregnancy—A pregnancy that develops following implantation anywhere other than the endometrial cavity of the uterus.

Heterotopic pregnancy—Combined intrauterine and extrauterine pregnancy.

Interstitial pregnancy—A pregnancy developing in the interstitial portion of the oviduct.

Laparoscopy—A surgical technique that allows for both diagnosis and treatment of an ectopic pregnancy. Remains the "gold standard" method of diagnosis.

Ovarian pregnancy—A pregnancy developing in the ovary. Criteria for diagnosis include the following: (a) The ipsilateral tube is intact and clearly separate from the ovary, (b) the gestational sac definitely occupies the normal position of the ovary, (c) the sac is connected to the uterus by the utero-ovarian ligament, and (d) ovarian tissue is unquestionably demonstrated in the wall of the sac.

Persistent ectopic pregnancy—Continued presence of viable trophoblastic tissue after conservative surgical treatment of an unruptured ectopic pregnancy. The typical presentation includes persistence of β-hCG concentrations that do not fall appropriately following conservative surgery.

Salpingectomy—Operative removal of an oviduct.

Salpingotomy—Operative opening made in the oviduct that is used to remove an unruptured tubal pregnancy for the purpose of retaining the oviduct.

Serum progesterone assay—A quantitative determination of the serum concentration of progesterone hormone. Useful in the early diagnosis of ectopic pregnancy.

Transvaginal ultrasonography—Ultrasound imaging of the female pelvis using an endoscopic probe placed in the vagina. Useful in the early diagnosis of an ectopic pregnancy.

Tubal pregnancy—The most common type of ectopic pregnancy. May involve the ampullary, fimbrial, or isthmic portion of the oviduct.

Ectopic pregnancy was first recognized in 1693 by Busiere when he was examining the body of a prisoner executed in Paris. Gifford of England made a more complete report in 1731 that described the condition of a fertilized ovum implanted outside the uterine cavity. Ectopic pregnancy has since become recognized as one of the more serious complications of pregnancy. One of the leading causes of maternal morbidity and mortality in the United States, it still accounted for 6% of all maternal deaths from 1991 to 1999, according to the Centers for Disease Control and Prevention (CDC). Despite significant advances in diagnosis and treatment, ectopic pregnancy remains the leading cause of maternal death in the first trimester.

Today, early diagnosis of ectopic pregnancy is possible with highly sensitive and rapid β-human chorionic gonadotropin (β-hCG) assays and the aid of advanced vaginal ultrasonographic equipment. The benefit of early diagnosis is that expectant medical therapy or conservative surgery becomes possible.

VI

Conservative management in the case of a small ectopic pregnancy that is present without rupture is usually successful when preservation of the oviduct to maintain or enhance fertility is important. Physicians should maintain a high index of suspicion for ectopic pregnancy and should be cognizant of the importance of early diagnosis and early intervention. This chapter summarizes the contemporary methods for diagnosis and treatment of ectopic pregnancy.

EPIDEMIOLOGY OF ECTOPIC PREGNANCY

Although the total number of pregnancies has declined over the past four decades, the rate of ectopic pregnancy increased in most Western nations. In the United States, the incidence of ectopic pregnancy increased from 4.5 per 1,000 pregnancies in 1970 to 19.7 per 1,000 pregnancies in 1992. In Norway, an increase from 12.5 to 18.0 per 1,000 pregnancies was reported from 1976 to 1993. One contributing factor for the rising ratio of extrauterine to intrauterine pregnancies is felt to be the rising incidence of sexually transmitted diseases as well as the efficacy of modern antibiotic treatments for pelvic inflammatory disease (PID). A second factor may be the increased ability to detect the disease. Although the risk of death from ectopic pregnancy declined among all races and ages in the United States, women of black and other minority races remained at significantly increased risk of death from ectopic pregnancy compared with white women. Although the overall incidence of ectopic pregnancy in the United States during 1970 to 1989 increased approximately fivefold, the risk of death from ectopic pregnancy declined by 90%. This decline in mortality from ectopic pregnancies may have been related both to the increased awareness of the condition and improved diagnostic and therapeutic methods.

Tracking trends in the incidence and outcomes of ectopic pregnancy has been more difficult in the past two decades due to changes in diagnosis and treatment, including a larger proportion of patients treated as surgical outpatients or medically with methotrexate (MTX) (as opposed to hospital discharge surveys). Utilizing computerized data systems in a large managed care organization, Van Den Eeden et al. identified an annual rate of 20.7 per 1,000 pregnancies between 1997 and 2000. Utilizing administrative claims data, Hoover et al. identified an annual rate equivalent to 6.4 per 1,000 pregnancies between 2002 and 2007.

PATHOLOGY

A tubal gestation traditionally has been defined as one that implants and grows within the tubal lumen. Budowick and associates have suggested that tubal implantation actually occurs in the lumen but is soon followed by penetration into the lamina propria and muscularis to become extraluminal. Pauerstein and colleagues demonstrated that trophoblastic infiltration can be predominantly intraluminal or predominantly extraluminal, or, occasionally, mixed. It is impossible to ascertain in the operating room the predominant pattern of growth of a given tubal pregnancy. In any event, fimbrial expression usually is an unacceptable method for removal of ectopic pregnancy. Not only is the method traumatic, but it frequently does not remove all of the trophoblastic tissue. The resultant persistent ectopic pregnancy may therefore require additional therapy.

ETIOLOGY OF ECTOPIC PREGNANCY

Tubal Damage Secondary to Inflammation

Both the increased incidence of sexually transmitted disease resulting in salpingitis and the efficacy of antibiotic therapy in preventing total tubal occlusion after an episode of salpingitis are related to the increasing incidence of ectopic pregnancy. Levin and associates have demonstrated that the risk of ectopic pregnancy is increased in women with a primary history of PID. Westrom compared women with PID confirmed by laparoscopy with healthy women, matched by age and parity, and found a sixfold greater incidence of ectopic pregnancy in women with PID, an alarming rate of 1 ectopic pregnancy out of every 24 gestations. Similar statistics have been reported by other authors. Many of the patients in these studies had received antibiotic treatment for salpingitis.

Before antibiotics became available for the treatment of PID, salpingitis was usually so acute that the inflamed tube became totally occluded, and permanent sterility was the result. Women who attempted to conceive after a pelvic infection were successful less than 40% of the time. Today, the rate of pregnancy exceeds 60% for patients adequately treated with antibiotics. After initial appropriate treatment of an infection with antibiotics, agglutination of the cilia can still occur, and synechial bands can form within the tubal lumen to cause partial tubal obstruction. Westrom has demonstrated by laparoscopy that bilateral tubal occlusion occurs in approximately 12.8% of patients after treatment for the first tubal infection, in 35% after two infections, and in 75% after three or more infections. In addition, Westrom found that approximately 4% of all pregnancies subsequent to salpingitis were ectopic.

Fallopian tubes containing a gestation are frequently normal on macroscopic visualization and gross histologic examination. Vasquez and colleagues, using scanning electron microscopy and light microscopy studies of tubal biopsies from five groups of women, discovered marked differences in their ciliated surfaces. The proportion of ciliated cells was significantly lower in biopsy specimens taken from 25 women with tubal pregnancies as compared with biopsy specimens from seven women with intrauterine pregnancies at the same stage of gestation. Marked deciliation was likewise seen in eight women who had undergone biopsies during tubal reconstructive surgery. In another study, Gerard and colleagues found that seven of ten fallopian tube samples from patients with ectopic pregnancy were PCR positive for *C. trachomatis* DNA. Therefore, the increased occurrence of sexually transmitted diseases contributing to subclinical tubal epithelial damage may be an important contributor to ectopic pregnancy. Comprehensive programs to prevent sexually transmitted diseases undertaken in Sweden and Wisconsin have been found to decrease not only the incidence of *C. trachomatis* infections and other sexually transmitted diseases but also the rate of ectopic pregnancies.

Contraceptive Devices

The use of intrauterine devices (IUDs) has been associated with an increased incidence of ectopic pregnancy. In a summary of published reports on ectopic pregnancy, Tatum and Schmidt observed that 4% of the pregnancies that occurred with an IUD in place were ectopic. In a recent meta-analysis, Mol and associates reported a range of odds ratios from 4.2 to 45 from heterogeneous studies of IUD use and ectopic pregnancy. Subtle tubal epithelial damage or actual PID episodes are likely responsible for the observed association between IUDs and ectopic pregnancy.

Oral Contraceptives

The overall risk of an ectopic pregnancy is lowered in women using oral contraceptives. When oral contraceptives fail, however, the risk of an ectopic pregnancy is slightly increased. This increase is presumed secondary to the inhibitory progestin effect on tubal motility. This hypothesis is supported by several studies implicating progestin-only oral contraceptives in the etiology of ectopic pregnancies.

Prior Tubal Surgery

An operative procedure on the oviduct, whether a sterilization procedure or tubal reconstructive surgery, can cause an ectopic pregnancy. The incidence of ectopic pregnancies occurring after neosalpingostomy for distal tubal obstruction ranges from 2% to 18% (Table 34.1). The rate of ectopic pregnancy after a microsurgical reversal of a sterilization procedure is only about 4%, presumably because the tubes have not been damaged by prior infection.

The U.S. Collaborative Review of Sterilization Working Group followed a total of 10,685 women undergoing tubal sterilization in a multicenter, prospective cohort study. The overall cumulative probability of pregnancy in the study cohort 10 years after sterilization was 18.5 per 1,000 procedures (failure rate of 1.85%). The 10-year cumulative probability of ectopic pregnancy for all methods of tubal sterilization was 7.3 per 1,000 procedures. From these data, one can therefore estimate that in the setting of a positive pregnancy following tubal sterilization, there is an approximately 40% risk that the pregnancy will be ectopic. The type of sterilization procedure and age of the patient at the time of sterilization appear to be relevant factors. Women sterilized by bipolar tubal coagulation before the age of 30 years had a probability of ectopic pregnancy that was 27 times as high as that of women of similar age who underwent postpartum partial salpingectomy (31.9 vs. 1.2 ectopic pregnancies per 1,000 procedures). In addition, ectopic pregnancy was often seen many years after the sterilization procedure. The annual rates of ectopic pregnancy in the 4th through 10th years after sterilization were no lower than that seen in the first 3 years.

The pathophysiology of ectopic pregnancy after elective tubal sterilization is not clear. It is possible that a tuboperitoneal fistula in a previously coagulated segment of fallopian tube may allow spermatozoa to escape and reach the oocyte. Such fistulae have been demonstrated radiographically by Shah and colleagues in 11% of 150 women after laparoscopic electrocoagulation. Improper surgical technique (such as incomplete coagulation or misplacement of a mechanical device) may also influence the sterilization failure rate and incidence of ectopic pregnancy, although their likelihood is presumably low.

Assisted Reproductive Technologies

Ectopic pregnancies are known to occur after in vitro fertilization (IVF) and related techniques, although the incidence may be decreasing. The Society for Assisted Reproductive Technology (SART) reported that 2.1% of pregnancies established after IVF in the United States during 2000 were ectopic, although the CDC reported that only 0.7% of pregnancies established after IVF utilizing fresh, nondonor oocytes were ectopic in 2010. Several theories have been proposed regarding the occurrence of ectopic implantation after transcervical intrauterine embryo transfer. Potential factors include the possibility of direct injection of embryos into the fallopian tube, uterine contractions provoked by the transfer catheter that propel the embryos retrograde, position or depth of the transfer catheter in the uterine cavity, and the volume of transfer medium. Verhulst and colleagues reported that tubal damage was a major risk factor. These researchers found that the ectopic pregnancy rate after IVF was significantly greater in patients with tubal disease (3.65% of pregnancies) than in those without tubal disease (1.19% of pregnancies). Strandell and associates found that a history of a previous ectopic pregnancy and a history of a previous myomectomy also appear to be risk factors for ectopic pregnancies following IVF.

A couple of recent reports suggest that the rate of ectopic pregnancy may be significantly lower following frozen transfers rather than fresh transfers utilizing blastocyst-stage embryos. Ishihara and colleagues reported an ectopic pregnancy rate of 0.81% following frozen-thawed single blastocyst transfers as opposed to 1.8% following fresh IVF single blastocyst transfers and 1.4% following fresh intracytoplasmic sperm injection single blastocyst transfers. Shapiro and associates reported no ectopic pregnancies following frozen-thawed blastocyst transfers as compared to 1.5% in fresh cycles. Possible speculative etiologies for these findings include a potential difference in endometrial receptivity as well as uterine contractility between fresh and frozen transfer cycles.

Assisted reproductive technologies may also be associated with higher incidences of less common forms of ectopic pregnancy, including heterotopic pregnancies and tubal stump

VI

TABLE 34.1 Summary: Ectopic Pregnancy after Tubal Surgery

PROCEDURE	TECHNIQUE	TOTAL PREGNANCY (%)	PREGNANCY RANGE (%)	ECTOPIC (%)	ECTOPIC RANGE (%)
Salpingoscopy	Macrosurgery	42	35–65	3.4	1–20
	Microsurgery	52	31–69	1.8	0–16
Fimbrioplasty	Macrosurgery	42	36–50	14	10–18
	Microsurgery	59	26–68	6	4–11
Neosalpingostomy	Macrosurgery	27	20–38	4.2	2–10
	Microsurgery	26	17–44	7.7	0–18
Tubal anastomosis	Macrosurgery	44	25–83	9.2	0–15
	Microsurgery	62	35–78	2.3	1–6.2
Removal of ectopic pregnancy	Salpingectomy	42	38–49	12	8–17
	Salpingostomy	57	39–73	11	0–20

TABLE 34.2 Risk Factors for Ectopic Pregnancy
Chronic PID
Prior tubal surgery
Surgical sterilization
Use of an IUD
Previous ectopic pregnancy
DES exposure
Progestin-only contraceptives
Assisted reproductive technologies
Infertility
Developmental tubal anomalies
Multiple sex partners
Early age at first intercourse
Cigarette smoking
Vaginal douching

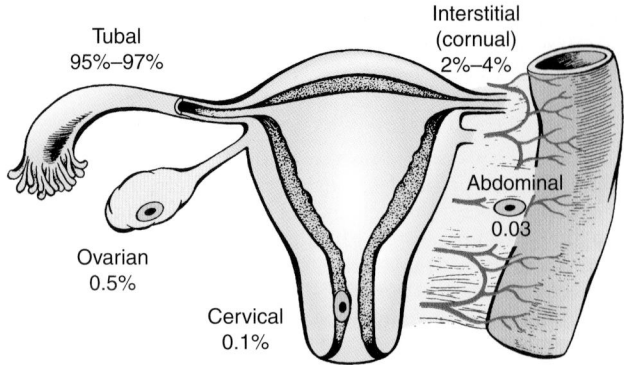

FIGURE 34.1 Sites and incidence of ectopic pregnancy.

portion accounts for 20% to 25%, implantation in the infundibulum and fimbria accounts for 17%, and implantation in the interstitial segment (cornua) accounts for 2% to 4%. Ectopic implantations occur less often in the ovary, the cervix, and the peritoneal cavity (Fig. 34.1).

Walters and colleagues reported that 16% of tubal pregnancies result from a contralateral ovulation. Transmigration of the ovum in the peritoneal cavity can occur because the oviducts and ovaries may be situated close together in the cul-de-sac. Alternatively, this phenomenon could also result from transmigration of the embryo through the endometrial cavity into the opposite oviduct.

pregnancies. Tummon and coworkers reported a 2% risk of heterotopic pregnancy in women undergoing IVF who had distorted tubal anatomy. This is about 100 to 200 times the reported incidence of combined intrauterine and extrauterine pregnancies occurring spontaneously. These authors found that the risk of heterotopic pregnancy appeared to increase proportionately with the number of embryos transferred. Ko and coauthors reported six tubal stump (postsalpingectomy) pregnancies among 1,466 ectopic pregnancies occurring in patients undergoing assisted reproductive technology ART (including ovulation induction and IVF-ET).

Developmental Anomalies

Intramural polyps and tubal diverticula can block or alter tubal transport of fertilized ova. Congenital absence of segments of the fallopian tube with peritoneal fistulae can also predispose to tubal pregnancy. Women exposed to diethylstilbestrol (DES) in utero are at higher risk of ectopic pregnancy. These women may have absent or minimal fimbriae and fallopian tubes that are shorter and thinner than normal.

Other Causal Factors

Several studies have demonstrated that cigarette smoking seems to be an independent, dose-related risk factor for ectopic pregnancy. Other lifestyle factors, such as multiple sex partners and early age at first intercourse, are associated with an increased risk. Vaginal douching has also been associated with a slightly increased risk of ectopic pregnancy, probably by increasing the overall risk of pelvic infections and resultant tubal damage. A summary of risk factors related to ectopic pregnancy is summarized in Table 34.2.

SITES OF ECTOPIC PREGNANCY

About 95% of extrauterine implantations occur in the oviduct. About 55% of these tubal implantations occur in the ampulla, the most common site: Implantation in the isthmic

EFFECTS OF ECTOPIC PREGNANCY ON FUTURE REPRODUCTION

Tubal pregnancy is associated with a poor prognosis for subsequent reproduction. In most cases, an extrauterine pregnancy represents an impairment of the fertilized ovum's ability to migrate through the deep rugae of the oviduct as a result of altered tubal function. The morphologic abnormality is usually bilateral and irreversible and can produce repeated ectopic pregnancies or permanent sterility. In a 1975 study, Shoen and Nowak concluded that about 70% of patients who have an ectopic first pregnancy are unable to produce a living child. As many as 30% of the patients who have an ectopic first pregnancy will have a repeat ectopic pregnancy, which compares with the total repeat ectopic rate of 10% to 15% for the overall population of reproductive-age women. More than half of the subsequent extrauterine pregnancies will occur within a 2-year period, and 80% will occur within 4 years of the initial ectopic pregnancy. In reviewing the experience of the Kaiser Foundation hospitals, Hallatt reported a 9.2% overall incidence of repeat ectopic pregnancies among 1,330 women who had extrauterine pregnancies. The potential reproductive capacity for a patient who has had an ectopic pregnancy therefore depends on her reproductive history. If an ectopic pregnancy was the result of her first reproductive effort, then the prognosis for future pregnancies is much worse than if the complication occurred after one or more successful pregnancies.

In a recent publication utilizing the Danish national health registries, Karhus et al. reported on the long-term reproductive outcomes in women whose first pregnancy was ectopic. They reported that women who had a first ectopic pregnancy between 1977 and 2009 had a long-term rate of deliveries of 69% and overall 17.6% risk of further ectopic pregnancies. They mentioned that the emergence of IVF may have improved the delivery chance for latter cohorts of women in their study as compared to previous studies.

Mueller and associates have estimated that 92% of infertility in women who have had a tubal pregnancy results from tubal damage that is due to the tubal pregnancy itself or other factors that had predisposed to its occurrence. A history of infertility itself is a risk factor for ectopic pregnancy. A twofold increase in the risk of tubal pregnancy exists among infertile women with no evident abnormality during infertility evaluation.

TUBAL ECTOPIC PREGNANCY

The morbidity and mortality associated with extrauterine pregnancy are directly related to the length of time required for diagnosis. In a CDC survey, two thirds of all patients who were later proven to have an ectopic pregnancy were previously seen by a physician, and either the diagnosis was deferred or the condition was incorrectly assessed. For a successful outcome, an ectopic pregnancy must be diagnosed early. In some clinics where the condition is treated frequently, a high proportion of cases are diagnosed and treated before tubal rupture occurs. In some cases, however, the symptoms that bring a patient to seek medical care are caused by an already-leaking or ruptured ectopic pregnancy. As many as 15% of all tubal pregnancies rupture before the first missed menstrual period, particularly if a patient's usual menstrual pattern is very irregular.

Diagnostic accuracy is often improved in repeat ectopic pregnancies. The vast majority of patients with repeat ectopic pregnancies will be diagnosed and treated before tubal rupture. A difference with a repeat ectopic pregnancy is that the patient herself often raises the question of an extrauterine pregnancy. Being suspicious, the patient may seek medical care earlier and provide a more specific medical history than does a patient experiencing her first ectopic pregnancy. The result is often an earlier diagnosis and an improved chance for a successful outcome.

Some form of vaginal bleeding occurs around the expected time of menses in more than 50% of women with an ectopic pregnancy, so that many patients and their physicians are unaware that a pregnancy has occurred. The vaginal bleeding may be followed by a period of amenorrhea. Clinical symptoms of an ectopic pregnancy usually appear 6 to 10 weeks after the last normal menstrual period.

DIAGNOSIS

Classic Symptoms: Pain, Bleeding, and Adnexal Mass

The classic presentation of pain and uterine bleeding with the finding of an adnexal mass has been the clinical hallmark of an extrauterine pregnancy, but even classic presentations can be misleading. Schwartz and DiPietro observed that of the patients who presented with the classic signs and symptoms, only 14% had an ectopic pregnancy. The severity of the symptoms and signs depends on the stage of the condition, but in the early stages of an ectopic gestation, symptoms are less predictive than in the more advanced stages of the disease. A discrete, unilateral mass separate from the adjacent ovary has been detected in less than one third of all proven ectopic pregnancies. Locating a mass depends on many factors, including the diagnostic skill of the examiner, the degree of pelvic peritonitis present, the presence or absence of tubal rupture, and the degree of stoicism and cooperation of the patient. Even when all factors are optimal, an adnexal mass can be felt in only half of the cases.

Diagnostic Studies

Three major advances have made early diagnosis of extrauterine pregnancy possible: (a) the development of highly sensitive and rapid β-hCG assays, (b) the ability to use ultrasound to evaluate the uterus and the adnexa (vaginal sonography further increases the accuracy of diagnosis), and (c) the application of laparoscopy as a diagnostic tool. Suction curettage can be useful under certain circumstances (e.g., to help establish the presence of a nonviable intrauterine pregnancy). Other diagnostic methods, such as serum progesterone assays or color Doppler flow analyses, can also provide useful information.

β-hCG Assays

The principal endocrine marker of pregnancy is hCG, which is synthesized by the trophoblast. hCG is a glycoprotein consisting of two subunits: α and β. The α-subunit has significant homology with other glycoprotein hormones, such as follicle-stimulating hormone, luteinizing hormone, and thyroid-stimulating hormone. The β-subunit, on the other hand, is specific to hCG, and antibodies against the β-subunit form the basis for current immunoassays. Current commercial automated β-hCG immunoassays use enzyme fluorometry, enzyme spectrometry, or chemiluminescence methods, as opposed to the traditional radioimmunoassay methods commonly used in the past. An immunoassay for β-hCG can detect levels of hCG as low as 5 IU/L of serum with less than a 0.2% incidence of false-negative results. β-hCG can be detected in maternal serum as early as 7 to 8 days after ovulation or approximately the day after blastocyst implantation.

The quantification of serum β-hCG levels is useful in determining the viability of pregnancy. To optimally use β-hCG data in treating a patient with a problematic pregnancy, one should first have a thorough understanding of the particular assay used. The World Health Organization has established reference standards for β-hCG assays. The Third or Fourth International Standards (Third or Fourth IS) are the most commonly used reference standards used by the available commercial kits of today. These standards are roughly equivalent to the First International Reference Preparation (First IRP) but are quite a bit different from the Second International Standard (Second IS). The Second IS contains about 20% intact hCG and was initially developed for use in hCG bioassays. One international unit of β-hCG based on the First IRP is equal to approximately 0.58 IU of β-hCG using the Second IS. Fortunately, the Second IS has been exhausted and is no longer used. The First IRP, Third IS, and Fourth IS are highly purified preparations that were developed to overcome the deficiencies seen in the use of a heterogeneous standard. This notwithstanding, due to the continuing variation of assay methodologies and β-hCG standards, there remains considerable between-method variation in β-hCG assay results.

Serum hCG concentrations increase in an exponential fashion in early pregnancy. During the period of gestation in which the hCG concentration is less than 10,000 IU/L (First IRP), or about 25 to 30 days postovulation, the time required for doubling of hCG levels remains relatively constant, with a mean of 1.9 days. Kadar and colleagues reported that 87% of women with ectopic pregnancies and 15% of women with normal intrauterine pregnancies could expect to have hCG doubling times of more than 2.7 days when the hCG concentration measured less than 6,000 IU/L. The lower limits of the increase in serum hCG for viable intrauterine pregnancies have been established by Barnhart and colleagues in a large cohort study. In this study, the serial β-hCG titers of 287 women who presented with pain and/or bleeding in the first trimester and were ultimately diagnosed with a viable intrauterine pregnancy were evaluated. For viable intrauterine gestations less than 10 weeks from last menstrual period or those with an initial β-hCG titer less than 5,000 mIU/mL, the investigators noted that the curve generated for serial hCG concentrations best fit a log-linear model. Overall, β-hCG concentrations tended to double every 2 days. The median rise of hCG after 1 day was 50% and after 2 days was 124%. The slowest or minimal rise for a normal viable intrauterine pregnancy, however, was 24% at 1 day and 53% at 2 days. Interval β-hCG determinations interpreted within the context of several values can therefore be of prognostic significance in the differentiation between normal intrauterine and extrauterine pregnancies. A normal rise in hCG production, however, does not always differentiate an ectopic from a viable intrauterine pregnancy. Shepherd and associates reported that, in their experience, a normal rise in hCG production did not reliably differentiate an ectopic from a viable intrauterine pregnancy in the symptomatic patient. Early ectopic pregnancies can initially secrete appropriate amounts of hCG because of a well-vascularized placental bed.

Serum Progesterone Assay

Serum progesterone levels reflect the production of progesterone by the corpus luteum in early pregnancy. During the first 8 to 10 weeks of gestation, serum progesterone concentrations change little; as pregnancy fails, the levels decrease. Matthews and colleagues reported progesterone levels in 29 patients with ectopic pregnancy using a direct radioimmunoassay that offers results within 4 hours. Patients with normal intrauterine pregnancies had serum progesterone levels greater than 20 ng/mL, and all patients with ectopic pregnancies had progesterone levels less than 15 ng/mL. Yeko and associates proposed that all ectopic pregnancies could be potentially diagnosed at the first emergency visit with a single serum progesterone determination using a discriminatory value of 15 ng/mL. Other authors, however, have demonstrated significant overlap in the serum progesterone concentrations in ectopic and normal intrauterine pregnancies. One large study by Gelder and colleagues reported that 98% of patients with a normal intrauterine pregnancy had progesterone levels greater than 10 ng/mL and that 98% of patients with ectopic pregnancies not associated with ovulation induction had progesterone levels less than 20 ng/mL. Unfortunately, 31% of viable intrauterine pregnancies, 23% of abnormal intrauterine pregnancies, and 51% of ectopic pregnancies in this series had progesterone levels that fell between 10 and 20 ng/mL, which greatly limited the clinical usefulness of the test. Hahlin and colleagues reported that a serum progesterone value of less than 9.4 ng/mL combined with an abnormal hCG increase had a positive predictive value of 1.0 for pathologic pregnancy. In 1992, Stovall and colleagues reported that in a group of more than 1,000 first-trimester pregnant patients, the lowest serum progesterone level associated with a viable pregnancy was 5.1 ng/mL. Therefore, these investigators established the lower cutoff limit of serum progesterone levels of 5 ng/mL; patients below this threshold had a nonviable pregnancy with 100% certainty and therefore underwent curettage. Patients with serum progesterone levels greater than 25 ng/mL had a 97% likelihood of having a viable intrauterine pregnancy in this study.

Transvaginal Ultrasonography

Pelvic ultrasound has revolutionized the diagnostic process of ectopic pregnancy. Transvaginal ultrasonography, in particular, may identify masses in the adnexa as small as 10 mm in diameter and can provide more detail about the character of the mass than clinical exam (Fig. 34.2). At the same time, transvaginal ultrasonography can evaluate the contents of the endometrial cavity and can document the presence of a viable intrauterine pregnancy with great accuracy. In addition, transvaginal ultrasonography allows for the simultaneous assessment for the presence of free peritoneal fluid.

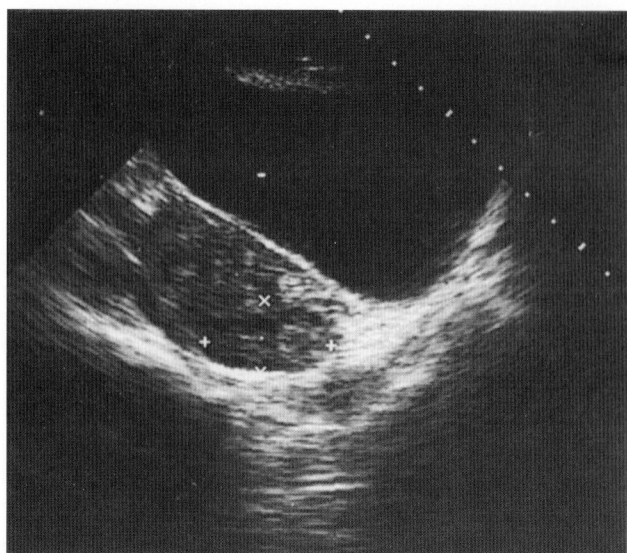

FIGURE 34.2 Tubal ectopic pregnancy documented by endovaginal sonography.

Transvaginal ultrasonography is usually considered superior to transabdominal ultrasonography in the diagnosis of ectopic pregnancy. Although the latter provides a broader perspective of the abdominal cavity and pelvis, transvaginal ultrasonography generally provides better resolution of the internal female genitalia. A 5-MHz transvaginal transducer allows for a deeper penetration of the pelvis than transducers of higher frequency, whereas a 7.5-MHz transvaginal transducer provides for better near-resolution at the cost of shallower penetration. On rare occasions, an ectopic pregnancy may be located beyond the reach of the transvaginal transducer's scanning field. On these particular occasions, incorporation of transabdominal ultrasonography may be an important adjunctive step.

Jain and colleagues compared endovaginal and transabdominal ultrasound results in 90 patients with a positive serum pregnancy test (Table 34.3). The specific diagnosis of ectopic pregnancy was impossible using only transabdominal ultrasound before 7 gestational weeks. Normal intrauterine pregnancies could be detected earlier with endovaginal ultrasound because the yolk sac, fetal pole, and fetal heart motion could be seen sooner. Fetal heart motion was detected as early as 34 days after the last menstrual period in patients with identifiable fetal poles at the time the crown-to-rump length was 0.3 cm.

Although diagnosis by transvaginal ultrasound can be quite useful, it may at times be confusing. One problem is that a pseudogestational sac that is due to a decidual cast can be mistaken for an amniotic sac. A useful differentiating feature is the "double-line" image, caused by the faint hypoechoic decidual lining of the uterus and the hyperechogenic rim of the trophoblast surrounding the gestational sac. The double-line image can be seen as early as 5 weeks after the last menstrual period. Even in the presence of the double-line image, however, it is important to further follow the course of pregnancy and subsequently confirm a viable intrauterine pregnancy with the ascertainment of ultrasonographically imaged intrauterine cardiac motion.

Although not always seen, Frates and Laing reported that the presence of a noncystic extraovarian adnexal mass, extrauterine cardiac motion, or a "tubal ring" by transvaginal ultrasonography is highly specific for ectopic pregnancy (98.9%), with a high positive predictive value (96.3%). These

TABLE 34.3 Pregnancy Earliest Seen with Ultrasonography

EARLY INTRAUTERINE PREGNANCY	ENDOVAGINAL	TRANSABDOMINAL
Gestational sac seen		
Gestational sac size	0.5 cm	0.5 cm
Gestational sac age	4.3 wk	4.3 wk
Double decidual outline		
Gestational sac size	0.6–0.7 cm	1.0 cm
Gestational sac age	4.4 wk	5.0 wk
Yolk sac seen		
Gestational sac size	0.7 cm	1.0 cm
Gestational sac age	4.6 wk (34 d)	5.0 wk (35 d)
Fetal pole seen		
Gestational sac size	0.7 cm	1.7 cm
Gestational sac age	4.6 wk	6.0 wk
Fetal heart motion seen		
Crown–rump length	0.3 cm	0.6 cm
Gestational sac age	4.6 wk (34 d)	.5 wk (47 d)

Reprinted with permission from the *American Journal of Roentgenology*; Jain K, Hamper VM, Sanders RC. Comparison of transvaginal and transabdominal sonography in the detection of early pregnancy and its complications. *Am J Radiol* 1988;151:1139.

authors described that the direct imaging of the ectopic pregnancy using any of these differentiating features is possible in 84% of cases.

Many authors have reported on correlations between threshold levels of hCG above which an intrauterine gestational sac is expected by ultrasonography in a normal pregnancy (discriminatory zone). Early on, Kadar and colleagues described a threshold level of hCG above which an intrauterine gestational sac was expected by abdominal sonography in a normal pregnancy (discriminatory zone). This threshold hCG level was initially characterized as a titer of 6,500 IU/L or higher using the First IRP. Presently, transvaginal ultrasonography reliably detects intrauterine gestations as early as 1 week after missed menses (β-hCG > 1,500 IU/L; 5 to 6 weeks gestation). Barnhart and associates reported that with a β-hCG concentration of 1,500 IU/L or higher, an empty uterus on transvaginal ultrasonography identified an ectopic pregnancy with 100% accuracy. Even using a discriminatory serum β-hCG concentration of 1,000 IU/L, Cacciatore and associates identified an intrauterine gestation in all intrauterine pregnancies and in none of the ectopic pregnancies. Furthermore, these investigators reported that the detection of an adnexal mass in combination with an empty uterus had a sensitivity of 97%, specificity of 99%, positive predictive value of 98%, and negative predictive value of 98%, provided that serum β-hCG concentrations exceeded 1,000 IU/L. The coupling of hCG titers with transvaginal ultrasonographic findings has therefore greatly facilitated the early diagnosis of ectopic gestation. It must be stressed, however, that considering the variations in β-hCG assays, ultrasound equipment, and sonographer experience, each institution must determine their own discriminatory thresholds for the sonographic detection of an intrauterine pregnancy.

The advent of color-flow Doppler technology may potentially further improve the accuracy of noninvasive diagnostic methods. Kurjak and colleagues reported that ectopic pregnancies are characterized by the identification of peritrophoblastic flow associated with an adnexal mass by color Doppler techniques. Kirchler and coworkers showed that color Doppler qualitative blood flow analyses of the tubal arteries can help localize the side of a tubal ectopic pregnancy. These investigators reported a between-side difference in tubal blood flow of 20% to 45%, with increased blood flow seen on the side of the ectopic pregnancy. Emerson and colleagues demonstrated that color-flow Doppler capability can help differentiate between viable intrauterine pregnancy, completed abortion, incomplete abortion, and ectopic pregnancy by analyzing uterine color Doppler appearance, intrauterine venous flow, the presence or absence of intrauterine peritrophoblastic flow, corpus luteal flow, and the presence or absence of peritrophoblastic flow in the adnexa. Pellerito and associates reported that color-flow imaging increased the sensitivity of detecting an ectopic pregnancy. Of 65 patients with surgically confirmed ectopic pregnancies, 36 (sensitivity 54%) cases were detected by endovaginal sonography alone, whereas 62 (sensitivity 95%) cases were detected by a combination of endovaginal sonography and color-flow imaging.

Dilation and Curettage

At one time, the histologic changes in the endometrium that accompany an ectopic gestation were routinely confirmed by dilatation and curettage (D&C). Today, more accurate diagnostic methods—such as the immunoassay for β-hCG, transvaginal ultrasonography, and laparoscopy—exist. In this setting, a D&C may therefore not always be necessary. If, however, the plateau level of β-hCG is low, a D&C can be helpful to establish the presence of degenerating villi, and if a patient is bleeding excessively, a D&C may also be required. In either case, assessment of the removed material and findings of decidua without chorionic villi suggests the diagnosis of ectopic pregnancy. Such findings do not provide absolute proof, however, because they also occur with spontaneous abortion. To distinguish between an ectopic pregnancy and spontaneous abortion, Stovall and colleagues reported that if β-hCG concentrations did not decline ≥15% within 8 to 12 hours following curettage, an ectopic pregnancy was likely.

If available, a frozen section may be obtained immediately after curettage, providing an opportunity to confirm the diagnosis within minutes while the patient is still in the operating room under anesthesia. If no chorionic villi are present, further assessment and treatment by laparoscopy may be considered. In a recent report of 87 consecutive frozen section samples taken from uterine curettings, Spandorfer and colleagues found that 93.1% of these specimens were identified correctly after further analyses of the tissue by permanent section.

The atypical epithelial changes of the gestational endometrium in a case of tubal pregnancy were first described by Polak and Wolfe in 1924, and these changes were further expanded on by Arias-Stella in 1954 (Fig. 34.3). These comprise a highly controversial set of histologic criteria that depend, for accuracy, on the precise definition of the particular cell type involved in the morphologic change, together with ill-defined physiologic events that reportedly produce the changes. Arias-Stella and others were convinced that these histologic changes are a progressive phenomenon resulting from the exaggerated proliferative and secretory endometrial responses to the elevated hormonal levels of pregnancy. Lloyd and Fienberg disagreed, maintaining that these endometrial changes are regressive and involutional and are the result of declining hormonal levels. Whichever hypothesis is ultimately proven, similar endometrial changes may be seen with a normal pregnancy, spontaneous abortion, or ectopic pregnancy. Histologic endometrial criteria, therefore, seem to have limited value in the specific diagnosis of extrauterine pregnancies.

Culdocentesis

Culdocentesis is a diagnostic tool for identifying the presence of intraperitoneal bleeding. This simple procedure of inserting an 18-gauge spinal needle attached to a 50-mL aspirating

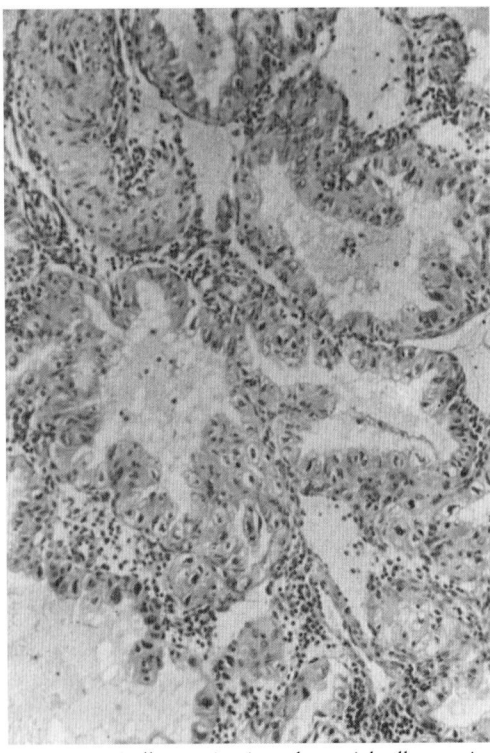

FIGURE 34.3 Arias-Stella reaction in endometrial cells associated with ectopic pregnancy, showing nuclear enlargement, irregularity, and hyperchromasia with cytoplasmic vacuolization.

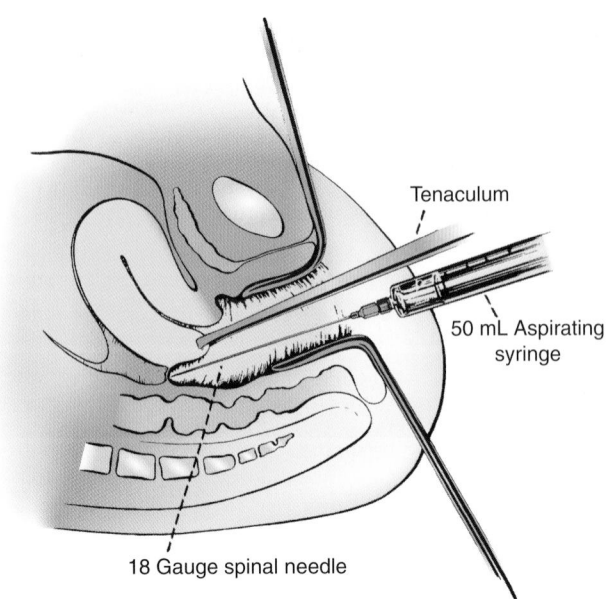

FIGURE 34.4 Culdocentesis. An 18-gauge spinal needle is inserted through the posterior fornix and enters the cul-de-sac between the uterosacral ligaments.

syringe into the cul-de-sac between the uterosacral ligaments (Fig. 34.4) provides immediate clinical information when unclotted blood is aspirated from the cul-de-sac. The procedure cannot be used for a definitive diagnosis, of course, because a tubal pregnancy may not have ruptured or leaked into the peritoneal cavity. In addition, a culdocentesis does not provide information concerning whether the blood is from an ectopic pregnancy or from some other cause of intra-abdominal bleeding. The rupture of a corpus luteal hemorrhagic cyst, for instance, may cause a similar bleeding pattern.

The availability of sensitive transvaginal ultrasonographic technology presently limits the usefulness of the culdocentesis procedure, such that it is rarely presently performed. Free intraperitoneal blood has a characteristic ultrasonographic appearance and can be seen in nearly all cases in which a significant intraperitoneal hemorrhage has occurred. In the absence of the immediate availability of transvaginal ultrasonography or in an emergency setting, however, a culdocentesis may still be of potential value.

Laparoscopy

Laparoscopy remains the gold standard in the detection of ectopic pregnancy, although noninvasive diagnostic methods continue to improve. In addition to permitting the diagnosis of an ectopic pregnancy, it enables surgical treatment. Laparoscopy also provides an opportunity to visualize the entire pelvis and other peritoneal organs. In particular, the condition of the unaffected fallopian tube can be assessed, as well as the presence of pelvic adhesions and endometriosis. This information may be particularly valuable for those patients interested in future fertility. The disadvantage of laparoscopy is that it is an invasive procedure that carries some risk of complications. Using standard methods, it requires general anesthesia and an operating room setting, thereby contributing to increased medical costs. Recent investigators, however, have been exploring the potential of "microlaparoscopy," in which improved optics and smaller-diameter laparoscopes and trocars allow for a definitive diagnosis and possible treatment in the nonoperating room setting. Several authors have reported the encouraging use of microlaparoscopy in the office setting, using local rather than general anesthesia. The specific utility of microlaparoscopy, however, for the primary evaluation and treatment of ectopic pregnancy remains to be established.

Laparoscopy may be useful when an ectopic pregnancy is suspected, but no signs of an ultrasonographically visualized extrauterine gestational sac are evident. This includes situations in which there is an inability to visualize an intrauterine gestational sac and serial β-hCG determinations are rising inappropriately. This also includes situations in which a D&C fails to identify products of conception. One must be careful, however, in settings in which the β-hCG determinations are very low or the gestational age is limited. In these settings, the ectopically implanted gestational mass may be so small that it is still not able to be seen at laparoscopy. The clinician and patient might therefore be falsely reassured by negative laparoscopic findings. All patients without a definitive diagnosis established at laparoscopy should continue to be followed closely.

Other Potential Diagnostic Aids

Gleicher et al. described the use of hysterosalpingography and selective salpingography in differentiating early (biochemical) intrauterine from failing intratubal gestations. A characteristic tubal opacification pattern was seen in the cases of early tubal pregnancy. Confino and coworkers reported that selective salpingography was useful in diagnosing early tubal pregnancies in some patients with equivocal clinical, laboratory, and sonographic findings. In addition, these investigators injected a single dose of MTX through the selective salpingography catheter after cannulation of the tubal ostia and identification of a characteristic ampullary radiolucency in seven patients. Each had subsequent complete resolution of the pregnancy without complication. Risquez and colleagues reported the successful visualization of two ectopic pregnancies by transcervical tubal cannulation and falloposcopy. The falloposcope is a microendoscopic instrument 0.5 mm in external diameter that is introduced by a 1-mm coaxial catheter. Although limited by the presence of blood in the tubal lumen, direct visualization of the ectopic pregnancies was accomplished in both cases and confirmed by concurrent laparoscopy. Other investigative teams have explored the potential of other imaging methods, such as magnetic resonance imaging (MRI), in the diagnostic workup for ectopic pregnancy. MRI might be useful if the sonographic image is inconclusive, although it is likely to be rarely needed, particularly if laparoscopy is generally considered in uncertain cases.

Summary of Diagnostic Methods for Detecting Tubal Ectopic Pregnancy

When a patient is seen with a clinical history suggestive of ectopic pregnancy, a careful examination is performed (Fig. 34.5). Quantitative serum β-hCG and rapid serum progesterone

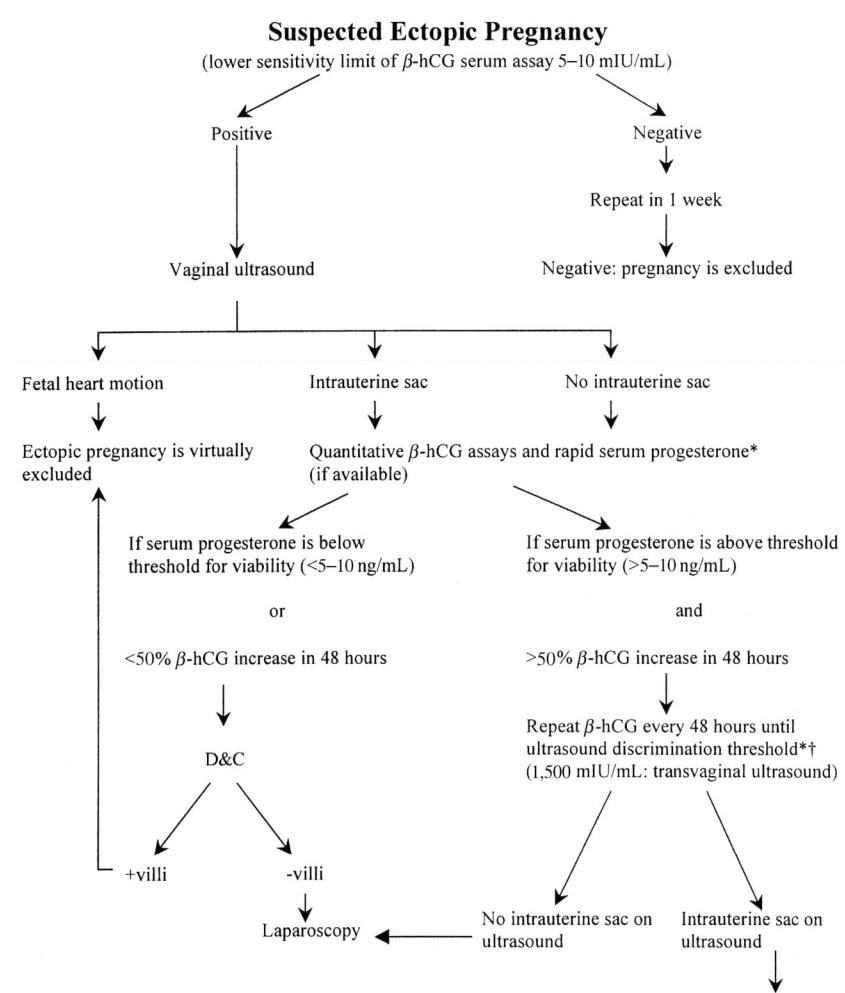

FIGURE 34.5 Evaluation of the stable patient with suspected ectopic pregnancy. *Hormonal parameters can vary depending on the assay technique and reference standard used. †The discriminatory threshold for sonographic detection of an intrauterine gestational sac must be established by each institution.

levels (if available) are obtained. If the β-hCG titer is positive, a transvaginal ultrasound is performed. If an intrauterine sac is visualized with fetal heart activity, then the diagnosis of intrauterine pregnancy is established. If, however, there are no intrauterine sacs or there is a questionable intrauterine sac without fetal heart activity, then the asymptomatic patient may be expectantly treated awaiting further testing. If the serum progesterone level is, with certainty, below the threshold level for viability, then a uterine curettage can be performed. The subsequent failure to find chorionic villi on curettage is very suggestive, but not diagnostic, of an ectopic pregnancy. If the serum progesterone level is more than 25 ng/mL in the absence of ovulation induction, then there is a strong likelihood that a viable pregnancy is present. If the quantitative serum β-hCG level is above the discriminatory zone for a particular institution and no intrauterine gestational sac is apparent using transvaginal ultrasonography, then an ectopic pregnancy is likely. The level of hCG at which an intrauterine gestational sac should be visible varies, however, depending on the β-hCG assay and the method of pelvic ultrasonography. Many contemporary investigators report that with transvaginal ultrasonography, an intrauterine gestational sac should be identified at a β-hCG level of 1,500 IU/L (Third or Fourth IS) with high sensitivity and specificity.

Commonly, results from initial testing are equivocal. The ectopic pregnancy can produce a low level of β-hCG from the aborting or degenerating trophoblast. The differential diagnosis should include spontaneous abortion or blighted ovum. When the diagnosis is uncertain and the patient is in an unstable condition or significant intraperitoneal fluid is seen, then evaluation should proceed immediately by laparoscopy and, if necessary, by laparotomy. If the patient is in stable condition, tests for serial β-hCG levels should be taken at 48-hour intervals, and the assays should be correlated with the patient's previous values. If the hCG level increases more than 50% within a 48-hour period, then the patient may have a normal intrauterine pregnancy and nonsurgical care (expectant management) is indicated. If the increase in the serial hCG level is less than 50% of the original value, then a nonviable pregnancy should be suspected. Ultrasound can often then corroborate the diagnosis of an ectopic pregnancy with the demonstration of a gestational sac in the adnexa or fluid in the cul-de-sac.

Initially, a normal increase in the β-hCG level may be observed. Over time, however, the level may slowly plateau, never reaching the discriminatory zone. If a potential intrauterine pregnancy is thought to be nonviable, then a D&C can be performed. If there is any question of viability, however, laparoscopy is preferred to rule out ectopic pregnancy first. Once fetal heart motion is observed within the uterine cavity, the possibility of a tubal ectopic pregnancy is virtually excluded. Certain patients should continue to be observed closely, however, particularly after a superovulation regimen, which is associated with an increased risk of a simultaneous intrauterine and ectopic pregnancy. Nevertheless, the overall risk of the two existing simultaneously, even after a superovulation regimen, is quite small.

The use of vaginal ultrasonography with improved resolution and the potential addition of color Doppler flow analysis will invariably further define a lower discriminatory zone in the future. Both modalities appear to complement each other in attaining improved sensitivity and specificity in the diagnosis of ectopic pregnancy. Other investigative diagnostic techniques, such as selective salpingography and falloposcopy, should be considered strictly experimental.

TREATMENT FOR ECTOPIC PREGNANCY

Expectant Therapy

Before the advent of effective therapy for ectopic pregnancy, it was noted that the condition was not uniformly fatal and that some patients had spontaneous resolution of the ectopic gestation, through either spontaneous regression or tubal abortion. The natural history of ectopic pregnancy therefore suggests that a number of tubal pregnancies can resolve without treatment. In 1988, Fernandez and associates reported a spontaneous resolution of ectopic pregnancy in 64% of carefully selected patients. The mean time for resolution was 20 ± 13 days. Spontaneous resolution occurred more frequently when the initial hCG concentration was less than 1,000 mIU/mL. The authors observed that a β-hCG threshold of 1,000 mIU/mL and a hemoperitoneum of less than 50 mL with a hematosalpinx of less than 2 cm appeared to be most compatible with successful expectant management.

Subsequent larger studies have demonstrated similar results with expectant therapy. Korhonen and colleagues have published the largest series to date. Criteria for patient selection included decreasing β-hCG levels, an absent intrauterine pregnancy by transvaginal ultrasonography, and an adnexal mass of less than 4 cm without an embryonic heartbeat. Seventy-seven (65%) of one hundred and eighteen patients had spontaneous resolution of the ectopic pregnancy. The remaining patients had laparoscopy for increasing abdominal pain, increasing culde-sac fluid volume, or plateauing or increasing β-hCG levels. One patient required a salpingectomy for a ruptured ectopic pregnancy. Similar to other reports, these authors also noted an increased success rate with lower initial β-hCG concentrations.

Medical Treatment

Systemic Medical Therapy

MTX is a folic acid antagonist that can be administered to eradicate trophoblastic tissue in an ectopic pregnancy. MTX is the chemotherapeutic agent of choice in the treatment of gestational trophoblastic disease. Long-term follow-up of women who have taken MTX for gestational trophoblastic disease has failed to demonstrate an increase in congenital malformations, spontaneous abortions, or second tumors after chemotherapy.

Tanaka and colleagues reported the first use of systemic MTX for an ectopic pregnancy in 1982. This group successfully treated an interstitial pregnancy with a course of systemic MTX. Shortly thereafter, Farabow and coworkers described the use of systemic MTX in the treatment of a cervical pregnancy. Ory and associates reported the use of high-dose, short-course MTX therapy (plus citrovorum factor [CF]) to resolve small unruptured ectopic pregnancies without the need for conservative surgery. Six patients with ampullary pregnancies were treated, and resolution of the ectopic pregnancy was achieved in five patients. Surgical intervention was required in the sixth patient. Two of the five patients who experienced resolution, however, had protracted courses and required blood transfusions. Sauer and associates also reported the use of systemic MTX and CF in 21 patients with ectopic pregnancy. Inclusion criteria included β-hCG levels that were reaching a plateau or slightly rising, laparoscopic confirmation of the ectopic pregnancy, and a tubal diameter of less than 3 cm with the tubal serosa intact and no evidence of bleeding. Treatment consisted of 1.0 mg/kg MTX administered intramuscularly on postoperative days 1, 3, 5, and 7, along with 0.1 mg/kg CF administered intramuscularly on postoperative days 2, 4, 6, and 8. Twenty of twenty-one pregnancies resolved without the need for laparotomy. Two patients required blood transfusions, including one patient who required laparotomy and salpingectomy for a hemoperitoneum. In both of these cases, fetal heart activity in the adnexa was identified initially on ultrasound examination. This led the authors to suggest that MTX + CF can be safely used in selected cases of unruptured ectopic pregnancies that have not formed fetal elements that can be visualized by ultrasound.

In 1991, Stovall and colleagues reviewed the results of several series of tubal ectopic pregnancies treated with MTX + CF. Of 100 cases, 50 were diagnosed by laparoscopy, and 50 were diagnosed by a nonlaparoscopic algorithm. Complete resolution was achieved in 96 patients over a range of 14 to 92 days. In four patients, laparotomy was necessary because of tubal rupture; in one case, rupture occurred as late as 23 days after MTX administration. In five patients, cardiac activity was observed on ultrasound, and treatment was successful in four of them. Three patients experienced minor side effects. In 49 of 58 (84%) women who underwent subsequent hysterosalpingograms, tubal patency was demonstrated on the ipsilateral side. Of 56 patients desiring to conceive, 37 subsequently became pregnant; 33 of these were intrauterine pregnancies and 4 were repeat ectopic pregnancies.

Stovall and Ling later studied the efficacy and safety of a simplified regimen of single-dose systemic MTX. All patients were diagnosed with a nonlaparoscopic algorithm by the use of serial hCG titers, serum progesterone, transvaginal ultrasonography, and curettage. Patients were treated with a single dose of 50 mg/m^2 MTX intramuscularly if they were hemodynamically stable and the unruptured ectopic pregnancy did not exceed 3.5 cm in diameter. In the initial report, 120 patients were treated, including 14 (11.7%) with visualized cardiac activity. One hundred thirteen (94.2%) patients had complete resolution with treatment, with a mean time to resolution of 35.5 days. Four (3.3%) of the successfully treated patients required a second course of MTX on day 7. Seven (5.8%) patients required surgical management of the ectopic pregnancy, including two of the patients with cardiac activity. No major chemotherapy-related side effects were seen. Posttreatment hysterosalpingograms demonstrated tubal patency on the ipsilateral side in 51 of 62 (82.3%) patients. Of those attempting pregnancy, 79.6% subsequently became pregnant; 87.2% of these were intrauterine and 12.8% were ectopic.

Lipscomb and colleagues further reported on the expanded Memphis cohort of patients treated with single-dose MTX. They used similar inclusion criteria, with the exception of further allowing pregnancies up to 4.0 cm in diameter provided that ectopic cardiac activity was not present. In this series, 287 of 315 (90.1%) patients were successfully treated with MTX. Forty-four patients with positive ectopic cardiac activity were treated with an 87.5% success rate. Of note, however, is that approximately 20% of these patients required more than one cycle of treatment. The authors' protocol reported that following the MTX dosing on day 1, serum chorionic gonadotropin was measured on days 1, 4, and 7. In many patients, they noted that β-hCG levels frequently continued to rise until day 4. If the chorionic gonadotropin levels then declined less than 15% between days 4 and 7, the MTX protocol was repeated. If the levels declined 15% or more between days 4 and 7, serum β-hCG was measured weekly until the level was less than 15 IU/L. If the chorionic gonadotropin level declined less than 15% during any subsequent week of follow-up, the MTX protocol was also then repeated. Other potentially difficult issues with single-dose MTX therapy include the management of "resolution pain" (which may occur in 20% of patients) and the prolonged time to resolution sometimes seen.

A further review by Lipscomb and colleagues regarding the variables related to the success of single-dose MTX in the treatment of singleton ectopic pregnancy has been compiled. In this review, logistic regression analysis demonstrated that the serum chorionic gonadotropin level before treatment was the only factor that contributed significantly to the failure rate. Success rates were reported to be as high as 98% when serum chorionic gonadotropin concentrations were less than 1,000 IU/L, although were only 68% when serum chorionic gonadotropin concentrations were greater than 15,000 IU/L. Interestingly, the size and volume of the mass, the volume of hematoma, and the presence or absence of free peritoneal blood in the pelvis were not associated with a significant risk of treatment failure.

Comparisons of the multidose MTX and single-dose MTX regimens suggest that the multidose regimen may be slightly more effective although associated with greater side effects. Barnhart and coworkers reported a meta-analysis of 26 studies and reported an odds ratio for successful treatment of 1.71 (1.04 to 2.82 95% confidence intervals) favoring multidose MTX over single-dose MTX. The crude overall success rates for multidose MTX and single-dose MTX regimens were 92.7% and 88.1%, respectively. Clinical superiority of multidose MTX, however, was not demonstrated in two small prospective, randomized trials to date (Alleyassin and associates, Guven and coworkers). Barnhart and colleagues additionally described a hybrid protocol in which two equal doses of MTX (50 mg/m^2) are administered intramuscularly on days 1 and 4 without leucovorin, which may offer an intermediate approach as compared to the multidose and single-dose MTX regimens.

Use of mifepristone as an adjunct to MTX treatment for ectopic pregnancy has also been assessed in two randomized controlled trials. In the first trial, Gazvani and colleagues reported both treatment approaches were successful, although the time to resolution was significantly faster in the group receiving MTX and mifepristone in comparison to the MTX alone group. In the subsequent multicenter randomized trial, Rozenberg and colleagues failed to demonstrate an overall benefit from the addition of mifepristone to MTX. These investigators, by contrast, demonstrated a higher efficacy of MTX and mifepristone in the subgroup of patients with higher initial serum progesterone levels ($\geq$10 ng/L). Further studies are needed to define the role of mifepristone in combination with MTX in the treatment of ectopic pregnancy.

MTX has also been used to treat persistent ectopic pregnancy after conservative surgery. In these patients, persistent ectopic pregnancy results from proliferation of residual trophoblastic tissue remaining after a conservative surgical procedure. The trophoblast can be located within the muscular layer of the oviduct or between the muscularis and the serosa such that at the time of salpingotomy, only the portion of the trophoblast within the tubal lumen is removed. In those patients with persistent ectopic pregnancy described in the literature, the majority have been managed by a second operation and salpingectomy. Some patients, however, have been treated with either expectant management or MTX. Hoppe and colleagues have reported the largest MTX experience to date for persistent ectopic pregnancy. These authors noted successful treatment in all 19 patients treated following linear salpingotomy. All patients should therefore have a follow-up β-hCG titer 1 to 2 weeks after conservative surgery. If the titer is elevated, then serial β-hCG titers are indicated. If the titer then continues to fall, the patient can be treated expectantly. If the β-hCG level remains the same or increases, however, consideration should be given to a single dose of MTX or perhaps further surgery to remove the remaining portion of the ectopic pregnancy.

Systemic MTX is an alternative that can be used for the treatment of patients with small unruptured ectopic pregnancies or patients with persistent ectopic pregnancies following conservative surgery. Safeguards are necessary to enhance the success and minimize the toxicity of therapy. Patients should be carefully monitored with hematologic indices and liver chemistries. A history of active hepatic, renal, or peptic ulcer disease, elevated baseline liver enzyme concentrations, and thrombocytopenia or neutropenia are contraindications to therapy. Patients should avoid exposure to the sun, because photosensitivity can be a complication. Patients should refrain from sexual intercourse during therapy. Patients should also avoid folate-containing vitamins. Appropriate candidates for systemic medical therapy should also be willing to accept a small risk of tubal rupture and participate in closely monitored follow-up.

Care and diligent effort should be made to definitively diagnose an ectopic pregnancy prior to MTX treatment. Medical treatment of an abnormal pregnancy of unknown location as a presumed ectopic pregnancy may expose a patient to MTX and its side effects unnecessarily, may result in future pregnancies being viewed as high risk for ectopic pregnancy, and may expose an intrauterine pregnancy to a known teratogen and abortifacient. Utilizing data derived from three North American Teratology Information Services between 2002 and 2010, Nurmohamed and associates reported the outcome of eight women exposed to high-dose MTX for the treatment of a presumed ectopic pregnancy and later identified to have a viable intrauterine pregnancy. Three patients miscarried shortly after exposure, three patients elected to terminate their pregnancies, and two patients had newborns with severe malformations.

Medical Therapy by Local Injection

In 1987, Feichtinger and Kemeter reported the direct injection of MTX under transvaginal ultrasound guidance into an ectopic gestational sac. They instilled 10 mg of MTX and observed resolution of the pregnancy within 2 weeks. Other investigators, including Kojima and colleagues, have reported the successful application of local MTX administered by direct injection at the time of laparoscopy. In 1993, Fernandez and colleagues reported a large series of patients who underwent intratubal MTX at a dose of 1 mg/kg under transvaginal sonographic control. Eighty-three of one-hundred patients were successfully cured; however, twenty-eight of the eighty-three successfully cured patients required additional MTX, which was subsequently given intramuscularly.

Direct injection of MTX has theoretic advantages over systemic treatment. The concentration of MTX at the site of implantation is many times higher after local injection than after systemic administration. With less systemic distribution of the drug, a smaller therapeutic dose might be necessary and toxicity would be less. Schiff and associates, however, evaluated the pharmacokinetics of MTX after local tubal injection and found that the peak serum level of MTX after local injection was not significantly lower than that of patients who were treated systemically with a similar dose of the drug. In addition, the success rates in practice appear to be unacceptably low. A review by Carson and Buster revealed that only 83% of the direct tubal injection procedures reported were successful.

Several trials have been conducted evaluating other intratubal agents administered for the treatment of ectopic pregnancy. Studies using prostaglandins (prostaglandin $F_{2\alpha}$, 15-methyl-prostaglandin $F_{2\alpha}$) were discouraging because of poor efficacy and serious adverse effects, including cardiac arrhythmia, malignant hypertension, and gastrointestinal symptoms. Other investigators have studied the use of hyperosmolar glucose, a less toxic agent, injected locally into the gestational sac of the ectopic gestation by either laparoscopy or transvaginal ultrasound-guided needle puncture. Lang and colleagues reported a 92% success rate using hyperosmolar glucose by laparoscopic puncture. Gjelland and associates reported successful treatment in 32 (82%) of 39 patients using local hyperosmolar glucose administered by transvaginal ultrasound guidance. They noted an inverse relationship between initial serum hCG concentrations and successful outcomes. Further larger trials are needed, however, to determine the precise clinical role, if any, of local injection therapies for ectopic pregnancy.

Surgical Treatment

Conservative Surgical Treatment

Conservative management of an unruptured ectopic pregnancy usually consists of one of two possible procedures: linear salpingotomy or segmental resection. A conservative surgical approach is possible when the diagnosis of ectopic pregnancy is made sufficiently early so that rupture of the oviduct has not yet occurred.

Linear Salpingotomy
In women who wish to preserve their fertility, conservative surgery by linear salpingotomy is considered the gold standard for the management of a distal tubal pregnancy. Recent studies have reported that the uninvolved tube may be abnormal, either grossly or subclinically, in at least 50% of cases of ectopic pregnancy. Although there have been no randomized studies comparing the fertility outcome after conservative and radical surgery for ectopic pregnancy, most of the available information suggests that the subsequent intrauterine pregnancy rate is higher after conservative surgery (linear salpingotomy).

In 1898, Kelly was among the first to advocate conservative surgery for tubal gestation. He recommended drainage of the pregnancy per vaginum, particularly for chronic hemorrhage and formation of a pelvic hematoma. More than half a century elapsed before Stromme reported the first successful use of salpingotomy to treat a patient with tubal pregnancy. In 1973, Stromme reported his surgical experience with 36 cases of unruptured tubal pregnancy, 21 of which were treated by conservative salpingotomy. Five were performed when there was only one tube remaining. Only one term pregnancy ensued from the five single-tube procedures, but Stromme's work led to the development of more effective conservative surgical procedures. Stromme reported a rate of 13.5% repeat ectopic pregnancies, which was no higher than the repeat ectopic rate at the time for more radical procedures.

Since the time of Stromme's report, physicians have achieved good success with conservative linear salpingotomy. According to the review by Yao and Tulandi, of the 1,514 patients attempting to conceive following linear salpingotomy, 61.2% had a subsequent intrauterine pregnancy, whereas 15.5% had an ectopic recurrence. On the other hand, only 38.1% of the 3,584 patients attempting to conceive following salpingectomy had a subsequent intrauterine pregnancy, although the ectopic recurrence risk was likewise lower (9.8%). In 1993, Silva and colleagues reported a prospective cohort study in which the intrauterine pregnancy rates were 60.0% and 53.8% and recurrent ectopic rates were 18.3% and 7.7% in the conservative and radical surgery groups, respectively. Many of the available reports on linear salpingotomy unfortunately do not describe the condition of the uninvolved oviduct. Langer and associates did include a description of the uninvolved oviduct in their report of 30 patients undergoing salpingotomy. Of the patients in whom the contralateral tube was normal, 80% subsequently had normal pregnancies. When the contralateral tube was damaged or contained peritubal adhesions, only 11 (55%) patients later achieved a viable pregnancy.

Among recent reports of salpingotomy performed on a single remaining oviduct, an intrauterine pregnancy rate of about 50% has been achieved by several investigators, although the results are quite variable, and some reports have only a limited number of patients treated. The repeat ectopic pregnancy rate in the single-tube salpingotomy patients appears to be about 20%, a slightly higher rate than that in series of patients with both oviducts.

In general, conservative salpingotomy is the preferred treatment for patients who desire further pregnancies. For results to be optimal, the oviduct should be unruptured and without serosal invasion, and the patient should be in a surgically stable condition.

STEPS IN THE PROCEDURE

Laparoscopic Salpingotomy

- Patient in dorsal lithotomy position following induction of general endotracheal anesthesia
- Placement of Foley catheter into bladder to gravity drainage
- Placement of intrauterine manipulator
- Establishment of pneumoperitoneum
- Placement of laparoscopic trocars (three-puncture technique) with patient additionally placed in moderate Trendelenburg position
- Evacuation of hemoperitoneum with large-bore suction irrigator, if present
- Infiltration of intended salpingotomy incision site with dilute solution of vasopressin (prepared by mixing 20 U of vasopressin with 100 mL of physiologic saline), utilizing a 22-gauge needle inserted either through the abdominal wall or through a 5-mm portal

- Performance of the salpingotomy incision in the area of maximal bulge on antimesenteric side of fallopian tube utilizing laser, unipolar needle electrocautery, or scissors
- Spontaneous extrusion of products of conception from the fallopian tube, or following hydrodissection or gentle tubal compression
- Removal of trophoblastic tissue in an endoscopic bag
- Careful irrigation of the fallopian tube and inspection for hemostasis
- Fallopian tube left to heal by secondary intention or sutured with fine suture

Transabdominal Conservative Procedure The procedure for linear salpingotomy starts by exposing, elevating, and stabilizing the tube. A linear incision is then made over the distended segment of the tube (Figs. 34.6 and 34.7). The incision is extended through the antimesenteric wall until entry is made into the lumen of the distended oviduct. When gentle pressure is exerted from the opposite side of the tube, the products of gestation are gently expressed from the lumen. Because a

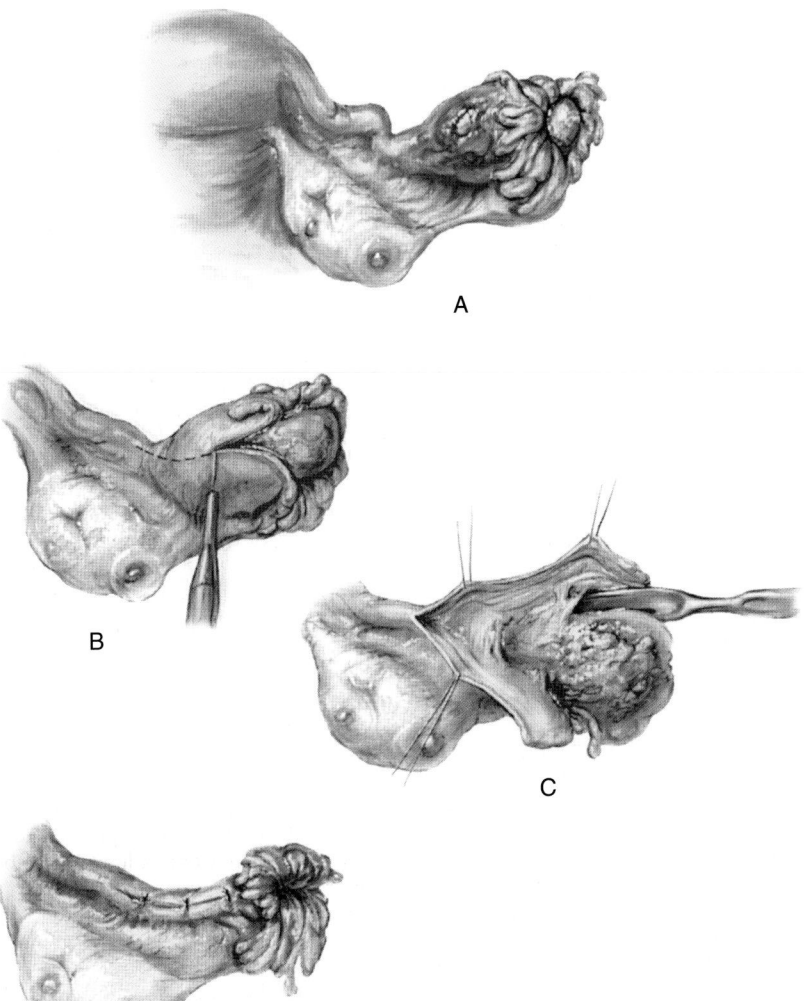

FIGURE 34.6 Removal of ectopic pregnancy of the distal ampulla. **A:** Distal ampulla involved with ectopic pregnancy. **B:** Initial incision on the antimesenteric border. **C:** The gestational contents are carefully removed by use of blunt dissection. **D:** Tubal serosa and muscularis are closed as a single layer with 5-0 nonreactive suture material.

VI

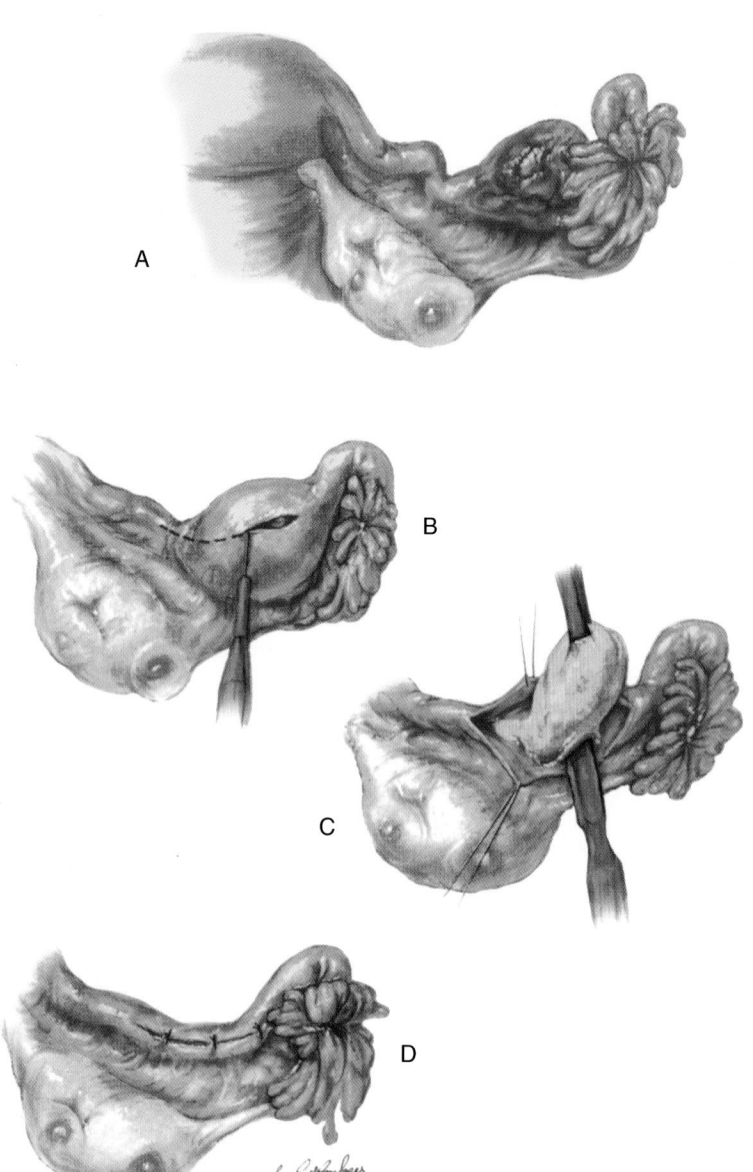

FIGURE 34.7 Removal of a midampullary ectopic pregnancy. **A:** Midampullary ectopic pregnancy. **B:** Antimesenteric incision with fine microdiathermy needle. **C:** The pregnancy is carefully removed by grasping the tissue and lifting while bluntly teasing the trophoblastic tissue away from the endosalpinx. **D:** The serosa and muscularis are closed with interrupted 5-0 nonreactive suture material.

certain amount of separation of the trophoblast has usually occurred, the conceptus generally can be easily removed from the lumen. Gentle traction by suction or by forceps teeth can be used if necessary, but care should be taken to avoid trauma to the mucosa. Any remaining fragments of the anchoring trophoblast should be removed by profuse irrigation of the lumen with warm lactated Ringer solution to prevent further damage to the mucosa.

Care must be taken to provide complete hemostasis in the tubal mucosa; failure to do so results in troublesome postoperative bleeding, which can lead to the formation of intraluminal adhesions. The small tubal vessels are easily identified while the tube is being irrigated, and loupe magnifying glasses can be used if necessary for better resolution. An operating microscope is usually not needed.

The mucosal margins are then closed with interrupted sutures, taking care that only the serosa and muscularis are approximated and that there is no undue tension. Care should be taken also to ensure that no suture material is retained on the mucosal surface, because even a small amount can produce a secondary inflammatory reaction with subsequent adhesion formation.

Laparoscopic Conservative Procedure Currently, most ectopic pregnancies are treated by laparoscopic surgery. In fact, most studies have suggested that laparoscopic surgery is superior to laparotomy in hemodynamically stable patients. Advantages of laparoscopy include lower cost, shorter hospital stay, less surgical blood loss, less analgesia requirement, and a shorter postoperative convalescence. Not all patients, however, may be suitable for laparoscopic treatment. These include patients with an unstable hemodynamic status, those with severe pelvic adhesions, and those with a specific contraindication to laparoscopy.

The presence of a hemoperitoneum should not preclude laparoscopic treatment. Using a large-bore suction irrigator, the blood can be evacuated, and the pelvic organs irrigated with a crystalloid solution. Once the ectopic has been documented, two auxiliary puncture sites are made suprapubically to allow manipulation of the fallopian tube (Fig. 34.8). Using a 22-gauge injection needle inserted either directly through the abdominal wall or through a 5-mm portal, a dilute solution of vasopressin (prepared by mixing 20 U of vasopressin with 100 mL of physiologic saline) is injected into the tubal wall

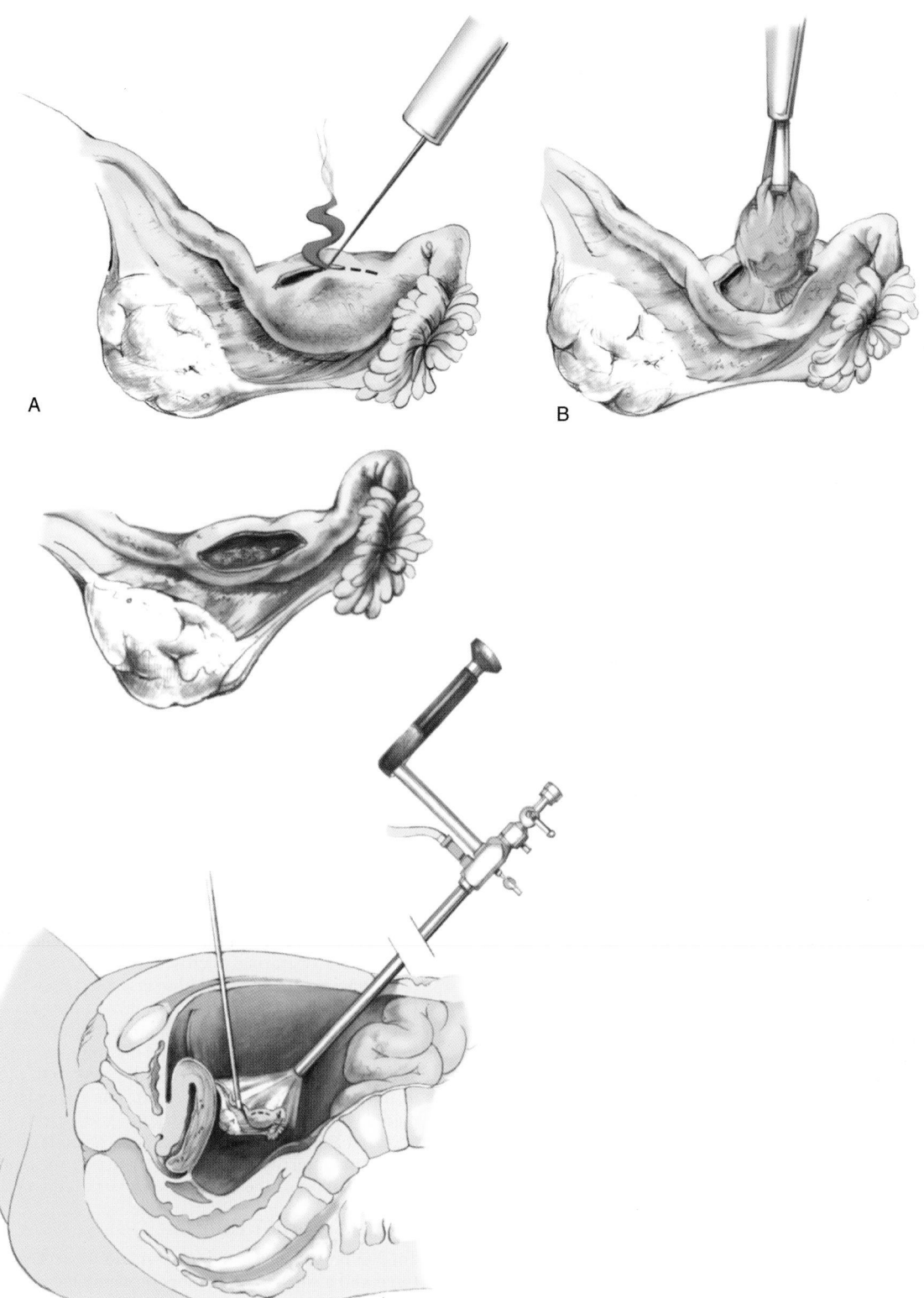

FIGURE 34.8 Laparoscopic salpingostomy for ectopic pregnancy. **A:** An incision is made with the fine monopolar diathermy needle along the antimesenteric border of the oviduct. **B:** The trophoblastic mass is removed with forceps. **C:** The lumen is allowed to heal by secondary intention.

at the area of maximal bulge. This step is crucial and allows for minimal bleeding and the precise removal of the ectopic pregnancy without damaging the surrounding mucosa. Laser, unipolar needle electrocautery, or scissors can then be used to make the salpingotomy incision. It is important to make the

incision along the antimesenteric wall of the tube in the area of maximal distension and large enough to allow for complete extrusion of the products of conception without difficulty. It is also important to keep the fallopian tube taut. If the products of conception do not spontaneously extrude following completion of the incision, either hydrodissection or gentle tubal compression with a blunt probe or suction irrigator will usually work. The tissue is then placed in an endoscopic bag and removed from the abdominal cavity. Special care is taken to remove all of the placental tissue, as it is known that persistent peritoneal implants of trophoblastic tissue following laparoscopic salpingotomy may occur. After the tissue is removed, the tube is irrigated carefully and checked for hemostasis. The tube is then either left to heal by secondary intention or sutured, with secondary intention being appropriate for most cases. A laparoscopic salpingotomy study by Fujishita and colleagues failed to demonstrate any benefit from suturing over the nonsuturing technique.

The results of salpingotomy are very similar, whether performed by either laparotomy or laparoscopy. Yao and Tulandi reported that among the 811 patients attempting to conceive after the laparotomy approach, the intrauterine pregnancy rate was 61.4%, and the recurrent ectopic pregnancy rate was 15.4%. Similarly, of the 703 patients attempting to conceive following laparoscopy, 61.0% had an intrauterine pregnancy, and 15.5% had a repeat ectopic pregnancy.

Persistent Tubal Ectopic Gestation Persistent trophoblastic tissue can remain after linear salpingotomy. Although there can be an initial decrease in the β-hCG level after surgery, the level can then slowly rise, ultimately resulting in symptoms. For this reason, it is recommended to obtain weekly β-hCG measurements after linear salpingotomy. Yao and Tulandi reported that persistent ectopic pregnancy was encountered in 8.3% of patients treated by laparoscopic salpingotomy and in 3.9% of patients treated by a similar procedure at laparotomy. The incidence of persistent ectopic pregnancy following laparoscopy, however, was quite variable, ranging from 3.5% to 20.0%. Pouly and colleagues achieved a relatively low 3.5% incidence of recurrent ectopic pregnancy in their series. Indeed, in many current practices, the incidence of persistent ectopic pregnancy appears to be low. There is a tendency for persistent trophoblastic tissue to be found in the proximal portion of the tube; therefore, special attention to this area is important. The use of hydrodissection to flush out the gestational products rather than removal of trophoblastic tissue piecemeal with forceps is recommended. One must, however, never assume that the chance for persistent trophoblast is entirely mitigated by the characteristics and ease of the procedure.

Risk factors for persistent ectopic pregnancy include small ectopic pregnancies (<2 cm diameter), early therapy (<42 days from last menstrual period), and high concentrations of β-hCG preoperatively. Rabischong and associates reported the outcome of 1,306 laparoscopic salpingotomy procedures and noted that a pretherapeutic hCG level of at least 1,960 IU/L was the only factor related to treatment failure. In high-risk cases, a single dose of MTX (1 mg/kg) can be administered postoperatively for prophylaxis. Graczykowski and Mishell demonstrated that the rate of persistent ectopic pregnancy was reduced to a rate of 1.9% using MTX prophylaxis in comparison with a rate of 14.5% among controls. Spandorfer and associates suggested that the postoperative day 1 serum β-hCG concentration can be used as a predictor of persistent ectopic pregnancy. They reported that a day 1 serum β-hCG decrease of less than 50% from preoperative levels may be predictive of persistent ectopic pregnancy. If day 1 serum β-hCG concentrations decreased greater than 50% of the preoperative value, there was more than an 85% probability that a persistent ectopic pregnancy would not occur.

Options for treatment of persistent ectopic pregnancy include reoperation and medical therapy. The choice of treatment can also include expectant therapy if the patient is asymptomatic

and β-hCG levels are not rapidly increasing. MTX appears to be particularly effective in the setting of persistent ectopic pregnancy following linear salpingotomy. In the largest series reported to date, all 19 patients with persistent ectopic pregnancies were successfully treated with a single intramuscular dose of systemic MTX (50 mg/m^2). The patient's reproductive prognosis does not appear to be particularly lessened following a persistent ectopic pregnancy. In a review of 50 cases, Seifer and colleagues reported that after 36 months of follow-up, there were 19 (59%) intrauterine pregnancies and no recurrent ectopic pregnancies in 32 such women attempting to conceive.

Because of the chance for persistent ectopic pregnancies to present relatively late following initial appropriate decreases in β-hCG concentrations, it is recommended to obtain weekly β-hCG measurements until they return to the normal range.

Segmental Resection The optimal surgical approach to the isthmic ectopic pregnancy remains controversial. Three conservative operations have been described: segmental resection of the involved portion of oviduct with primary microsurgical anastomosis, segmental resection with reanastomosis at a later operation, and linear salpingotomy. In Sweden, Swolin initially advocated for segmental resection in 1967. Subsequently, other surgeons, including Stangel and Gomel as well as DeCherney and Boyers, have found segmental resection to be preferable to salpingotomy in most cases of isthmic pregnancy. In the isthmus, the tubal lumen is narrower and the muscularis is thicker than in the ampulla. Thus, the isthmus is more predisposed to severe postoperative damage, and the rate of proximal tubal obstruction seems to be higher following linear salpingotomy.

With segmental resection and end-to-end reanastomosis, the implantation site is removed so that it cannot be involved in a subsequent tubal pregnancy. A more normal architecture for the oviduct is consequently achieved. The anatomic restoration is a time-consuming process requiring special expertise and extensive microsurgical experience; *it should not be undertaken by an inexperienced surgeon.* The success of future pregnancies depends on the skill and precision of technique used in the procedure, and, once begun, the only alternative is total salpingectomy.

Segmental resection is best performed with loupe magnification or the operating microscope; the required microsurgical techniques are identical to those discussed elsewhere in this text. Care must be taken to avoid trauma to the very vascular oviduct; only patients with minimal bleeding should be considered for the operation. The adjacent mesosalpinx must be incised and removed with care to avoid the formation of a hematoma in the broad ligament (Fig. 34.9). The muscularis sutures are placed with the use of magnification and no. 6-0 or 7-0 delayed absorbable material, and the serosa is secondarily supported by additional interrupted sutures. Patency of the oviduct is tested by insufflation of the uterine cavity with indigo carmine dye.

Radical Surgical Treatment

Total salpingectomy is required when a tubal pregnancy has ruptured and a substantial hemoperitoneum has occurred. In these cases, the intra-abdominal hemorrhage must be quickly controlled, and a conservative operation should not be attempted. Extensive hemoperitoneum places a patient in serious jeopardy of cardiopulmonary crises.

A salpingectomy may also be indicated for other reasons. These include a recurrent ectopic pregnancy in the same fallopian tube, an ectopic pregnancy in a severely damaged tube, and an ectopic pregnancy in a woman who has completed her family.

Some earlier reports advocated for the combined use of a prophylactic oophorectomy with salpingectomy. Theoretically,

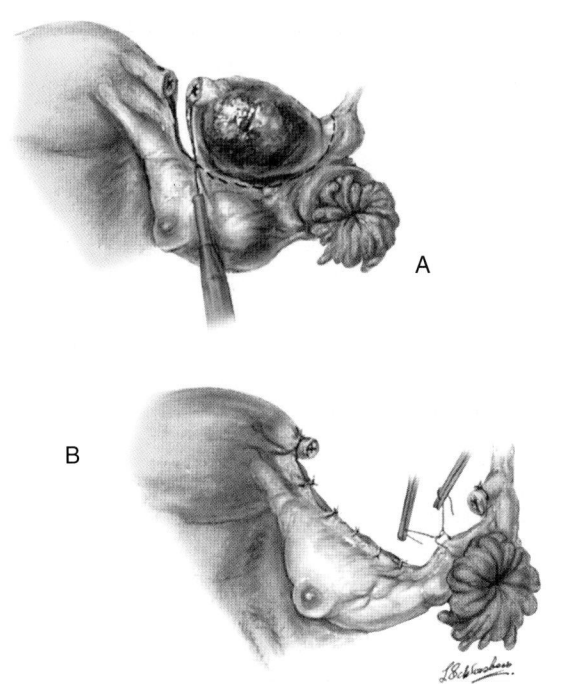

FIGURE 34.9 Segmental resection of midtubal ectopic pregnancy. **A:** A needle cautery is useful to resect the pregnancy. **B:** Care should be taken to approximate the mesosalpinx. Reanastomosis can be performed either immediately or in 3 to 5 months.

removal of the ipsilateral ovary would cause the other ovary to ovulate more frequently, perhaps favoring future pregnancy. In reality, the benefits of removal of the contralateral ovary are outweighed by the consideration that any future oophorectomy would then mean castration. The high success rate of IVF is a further incentive to maintain functioning of both ovaries.

As stated earlier, most patients with an ectopic pregnancy currently are candidates for laparoscopic surgery. Radical surgical procedures, such as salpingectomy, are also easily adapted to laparoscopic surgery. Of course, certain patients remain noncandidates for laparoscopic surgery, including those with unstable hemodynamic status or severe pelvic adhesions. The latter patients are still best treated by laparotomy.

At laparotomy, total salpingectomy with partial cornual resection has been criticized for providing a residual sinus tract that allows development of a subsequent interstitial pregnancy. This problem may not lie in the procedure per se but rather the surgeon's performance of the procedure. Complete peritonealization of the cornual incision and advancement of the round and broad ligaments over the uterine cornua (the modified Coffey technique of uterine suspension) should provide complete protection from recurrent interstitial pregnancy (Fig. 34.10). A too-vigorous resection of the uterine cornua can also cause problems. A residual myometrial defect can cause uterine rupture, interstitial recanalization, or placental encroachment during a subsequent intrauterine pregnancy and should be avoided by making certain that the interstitial resection includes less

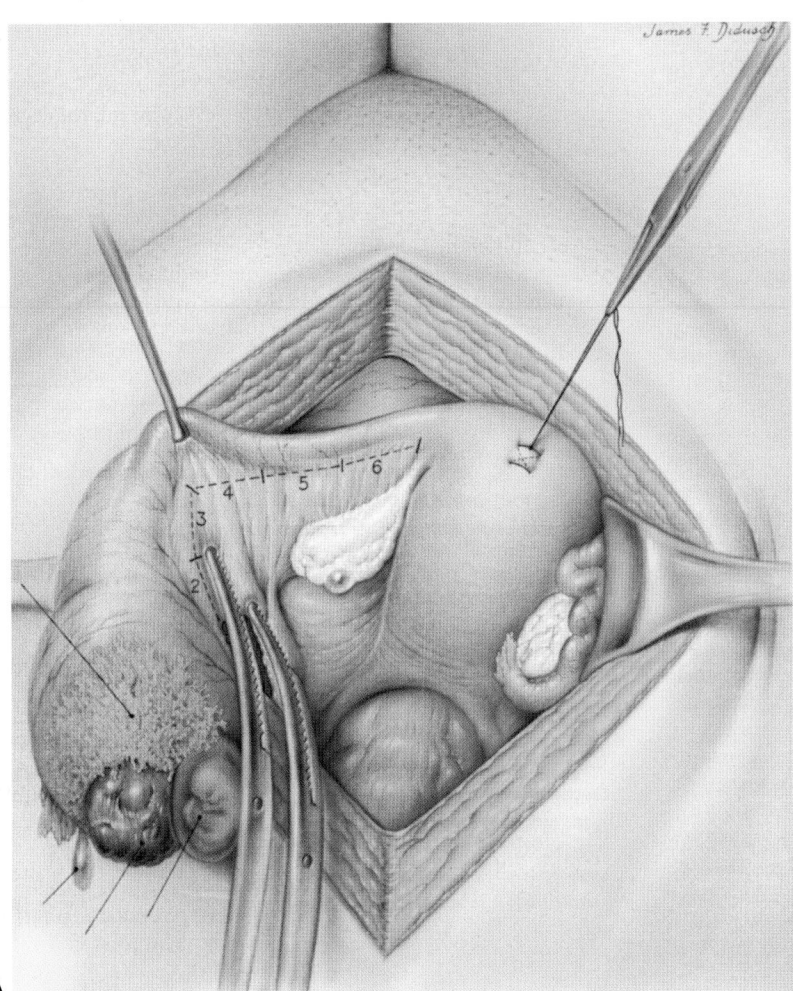

FIGURE 34.10 Salpingectomy for tubal pregnancy. **A:** The tube has been delivered, and the mesosalpinx is being clamped and cut with a succession of Kelly clamps.

VI

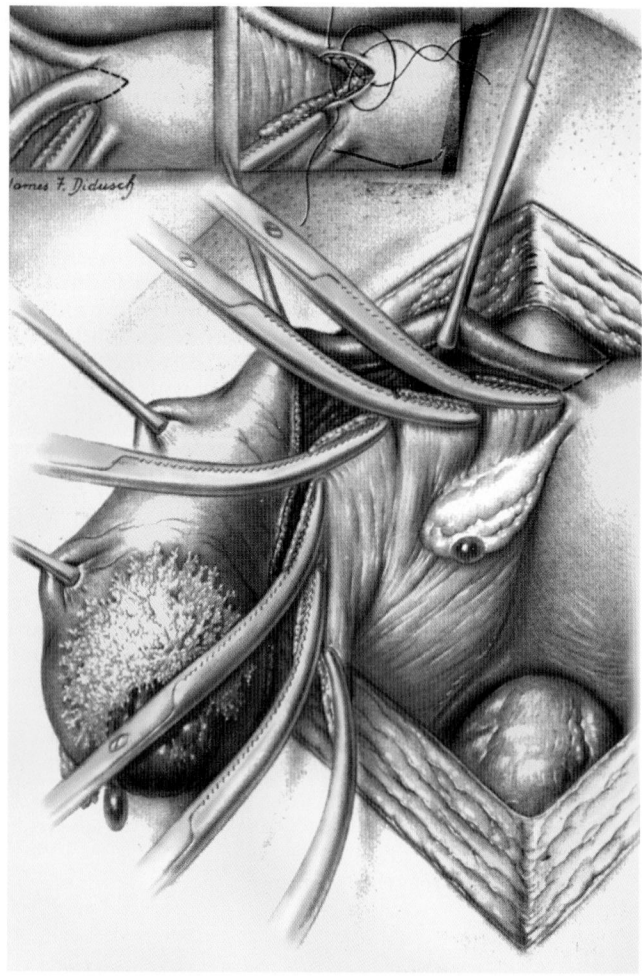

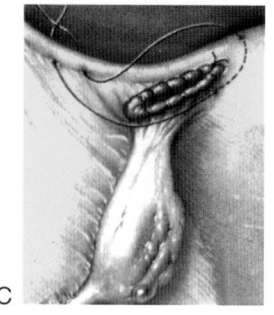
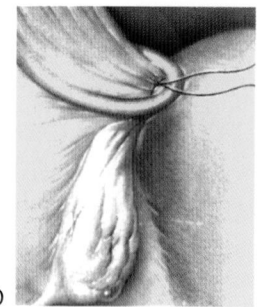

B

FIGURE 34.10 (*Continued*) **B:** The mesosalpinx has been completely clamped and cut. The *dashed line* indicates the line of excision of the tube at the cornu. **Inset** shows the superficial wedge resection of the interstitial portion of the tube and the suture of the cornu. **C:** The method of placing a mattress suture for peritonealization is shown with anchoring of the medial portion of the broad ligament to the uterus, a little posterior and superior to the uterine incision. **D:** Peritonealization is completed by tying the mattress suture, which brings the broad and the round ligaments over the uterine cornu.

than one third the thickness of the cornual portion of the myometrium.

Dubuisson and colleagues reported the first large series of patients treated by total salpingectomy at laparoscopy for ampullary ectopic pregnancies. They used a three-puncture laparoscopic technique. They thermocoagulated the tubal isthmus, mesosalpinx, and tubo-ovarian ligament, followed by excision with hook scissors. The tube was subsequently removed with polyp forceps through one of the suprapubic punctures. They reported no immediate complications in 98 patients successfully treated at laparoscopy, although one patient experienced a postoperative deep venous thrombosis. Two patients initially intended for laparoscopy, however, required laparotomy because of either severe pelvic adhesions or significant intraperitoneal blood. In a later report, Dubuisson and associates advised opening the tube first to aspirate the trophoblast in cases in which the tube is large to more easily remove the tissue through a 12-mm trocar.

Technique of Salpingectomy at Laparotomy A suprapubic Pfannenstiel or low midline vertical abdominal incision is used, and the distended tube is elevated. The mesosalpinx is clamped with a succession of Kelly clamps as close to the tube as possible (Fig. 34.10A). The tube is then excised by cutting a small myometrial wedge at the uterine cornu (Fig. 34.10B). Care should be taken to avoid a deep incision into the myometrium. A figure-of-eight mattress suture of no. 0 delayed

absorbable material is used to close the myometrium at the site of the wedge resection. The mesosalpinx is closed with interrupted ligatures of no. 2-0 delayed absorbable suture. Complete hemostasis is essential to avoid a hematoma of the broad ligament.

The fundus is held forward, and the round and broad ligaments are sutured over the uterine cornu (Fig. 34.10C). This procedure, the modified Coffey suspension, accomplishes complete peritonealization. Mattress sutures anchor the broad ligament to the uterus. The no. 0 delayed absorbable suture first penetrates the broad ligament from its anterior surface, just below the round ligament, at a distance of 2 to 3 cm from the cornu. The next "bite" is taken into the fundus of the uterus, a little posterior and superior to the uterine incision. The suture is then placed through the posterior aspect of the broad ligament, about 1 cm lateral to the previous suture. When this suture is tied, the cornual incision and the mesosalpinx are covered with mesothelium (Fig. 34.10D). If there is excessive tension on this suture, or if peritonealization is incomplete, then supporting sutures can be placed in the myometrium and the round ligament to ensure that the peritonealization suture will remain in place.

Technique of Salpingectomy at Laparoscopy Several methods have been successfully used for laparoscopic salpingectomy, including endoscopic stapling devices, endocoagulation, bipolar cautery, and pretied endoscopic ligatures. Following

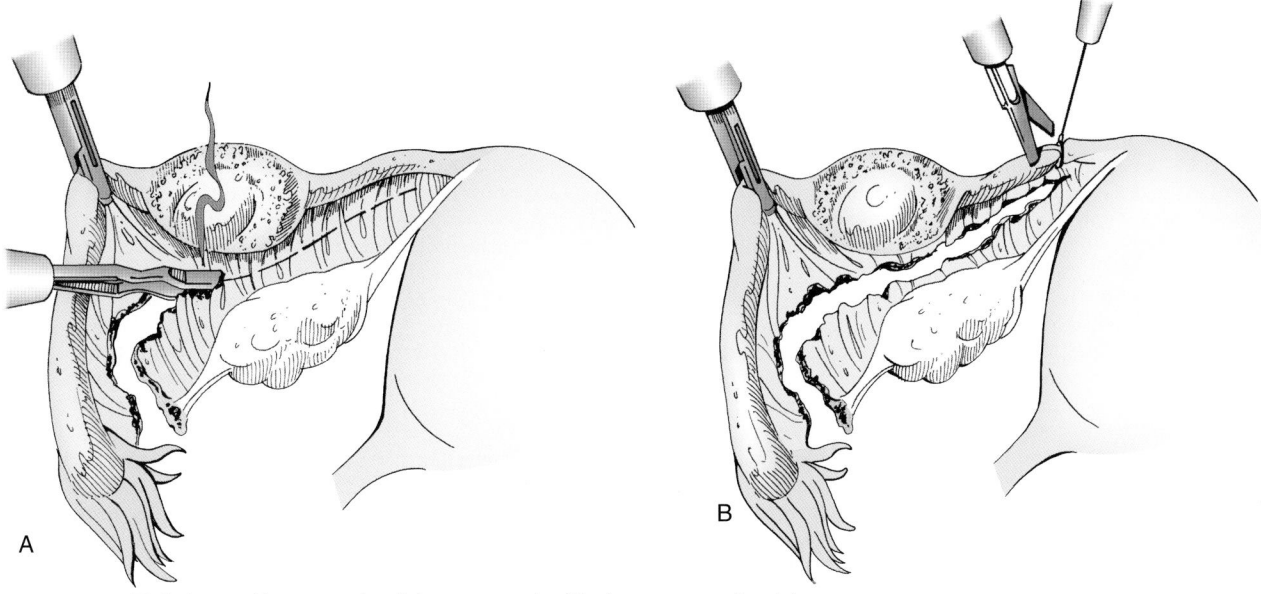

FIGURE 34.11 Techniques of laparoscopic salpingectomy using bipolar cautery and excision.

placement of laparoscopic trocar ports (usually three-puncture technique), irrigation of the pelvis, and the evacuation of all blood clots, the involved tube is then grasped with a toothed grasper. One method then includes cauterizing the tubo-ovarian ligament first with bipolar forceps, followed by transection with scissors (Fig. 34.11) or the blade of a coagulation-cutting device. The mesosalpinx is similarly cauterized and transected, taking care to stay as close as possible to the fallopian tube. The proximal tubal isthmus is then cauterized and transected. Care should be taken such that excess cauterization of the uterine cornu does not occur because of concerns about the potential of interstitial sinus tracts or diminished myometrial integrity. The specimen is then placed in an endoscopic specimen retrieval bag and removed through a 12-mm port. Alternatively, the tube can be excised distal to a no. 0 polyglactin 910 (Vicryl) Endoloop ligature secured proximal to the ectopic implantation site, although this technique works optimally if the entire mesosalpinx is transected such that the Endoloop ligatures can be placed precisely at the tubal insertion at the cornua. Consideration may also be given to covering the proximal tubal pedicle with an absorbable adhesion prevention barrier.

Comparisons of Surgical and Medical Therapy

Several studies have compared conservative laparoscopic treatment with systemic MTX in the management of ectopic pregnancy. Saraj and associates reported a randomized trial comparing single-dose intramuscular MTX (1 mg/kg) with laparoscopic salpingotomy. They reported similar immediate treatment success rates: 94.7% for MTX and 91.4% for laparoscopic salpingotomy. Additional MTX injections were required in 15.8% of women who were randomized to the single-dose MTX group. Initial serum hCG titers were higher for the patients who required additional MTX doses than for those who required only one dose. The mean times for serum progesterone and hCG concentrations to decrease to less than 1.5 ng/mL and 15 IU/L, respectively, were significantly less for laparoscopic salpingotomy. Fernandez and colleagues also reported a randomized trial of conservative laparoscopic treatment and MTX administration (by either transvaginal or intramuscular injection) and found similar immediate treatment success. Additional studies have also suggested that despite the increased number of posttreatment visits that are necessary, MTX therapy results in appreciable cost savings in comparison with laparoscopic treatment.

Hemodynamically stable patients who meet strict criteria, without excessively large or advanced ectopic pregnancies, may therefore be offered either medical or conservative surgical therapy. The immediate clinical and long-term outcomes in these selected patients appear to be similar.

INTERSTITIAL PREGNANCY

Interstitial (cornual) pregnancy is a rare condition that accounts for no more than 2% to 4% of all tubal pregnancies. The condition occurs once every 2,500 to 5,000 live births. An interstitial pregnancy should first be differentiated from an angular pregnancy. The latter entity was first described by Kelly in 1898. It occurs when an embryo implants in the lateral angle of the uterine cavity medial to the internal ostium of the fallopian tube. The clinical course of an angular pregnancy varies, although in many instances leads to asymmetric and symptomatic enlargement of the uterus.

Because the gestational sac is better protected in the interstitial than in other portions of the tube, it was felt that symptoms of interstitial ectopic pregnancies may manifest later (>12 gestational weeks). This general belief has recently been disputed, however, by Tulandi and Al-Jaroudi, who reported the results of an Interstitial Pregnancy Registry sponsored by the Society of Reproductive Surgeons (SRS). In this registry, 14 cases (43.7%) of rupture of interstitial pregnancy were reported, all at the time of initial diagnosis. Pelvic pain and vaginal spotting are common early symptoms. The developing chorionic villi may eventually erode into the blood vessels of the uterine cornu, causing a severe hemorrhage. Because the pregnancy occurs at the most richly vascularized area of the female pelvis—the junction of the uterine and ovarian vessels—rupture usually causes profound and sudden shock.

Before 1893, the only available reports on interstitial pregnancies were from autopsies. Since then, numerous cases have been reported. Most of the same risk factors for interstitial pregnancy are similar to those for ectopic pregnancy in general, including PID, previous pelvic surgery, and the use of assisted reproductive technologies. Ipsilateral salpingectomy may be a unique risk factor for interstitial pregnancy, occurring in 37.5% of patients, according to the SRS Interstitial Pregnancy Registry. Earlier diagnosis and more experience in treating this disorder have reduced the present maternal mortality rate to approximately 2% to 2.5% of all interstitial pregnancies.

The diagnosis of interstitial pregnancy is made by critical evaluation of all the criteria used for other types of tubal pregnancy. The presentation often includes acute abdominal pain, intraperitoneal bleeding, a low hematocrit, and a positive serum or urine pregnancy test. Diagnostic tests include the sensitive β-hCG immunoassay and vaginal ultrasonography.

Asymmetry of the uterus, often indicative of an interstitial pregnancy, can be misinterpreted as a pregnancy in a bicornuate uterus or a myoma in a pregnant uterus instead of an interstitial pregnancy. Knowledge of the previous shape of the uterus can help to confirm or exclude the existence of a bicornuate or myomatous uterus. A firm protrusion on the uterus suggests a myoma; a soft, tender asymmetric enlargement suggests an interstitial pregnancy.

Timor-Tritsch and colleagues established transvaginal ultrasonic criteria for interstitial pregnancy. These criteria include (a) an empty uterine cavity, (b) a chorionic sac seen separately and greater than 1 cm from the most lateral edge of the uterine cavity, and (c) a thick myometrial layer surrounding the chorionic sac. All of these parameters were relatively specific (88% to 93%) but lacked high sensitivity (only about 40%) for the diagnosis of interstitial pregnancy. Other investigators have described an "interstitial line sign." This sign refers to the visualization of an echogenic line extending from the endometrial cavity into the cornual region and abutting the interstitial mass or gestational sac. Ackerman and associates reported that the "interstitial line sign" was 80% sensitive and 98% specific for the diagnosis of interstitial pregnancy.

Often, the difference between an interstitial pregnancy and an angular pregnancy is subtle. In addition, it may be easy to confuse an angular pregnancy with a pregnancy in a septated or bicornuate uterus. Because ultrasound cannot always confirm the position of the pregnancy, laparoscopy may be required to confirm the diagnosis. In cases of massive intra-abdominal bleeding, an immediate laparotomy should be performed.

Treatment for Interstitial Pregnancy

The choice of treatment for an interstitial (cornual) pregnancy depends on the extent of trauma that has occurred in the uterine wall and on the interest of the patient in preserving her childbearing function. Systemic MTX has been used in a limited number of patients with unruptured interstitial pregnancies. Tanaka and coworkers reported the first successful treatment of an interstitial pregnancy with systemic MTX. Since this report, according to Lau and Tulandi, there have been 40 additional published cases of interstitial pregnancies treated with the use of systemic or local MTX, or a combination of both. An overall success rate of 83% was reported.

If an interstitial pregnancy is observed when it is still small, it might be excised using conservative laparoscopic techniques. In their review, Lau and Tulandi noted 22 successful cases of laparoscopic treatment of interstitial pregnancy. Techniques used varied from cornuostomy with careful extraction of the products of conception to a more formal cornual resection. Hemostatic methods have included ligation of the ascending branches of the uterine vessels, intracorporeal and extracorporeal suturing, and surgical stapling. A further review by

Moawad et al. reported 164 successful cases of laparoscopic management of interstitial pregnancies out of 192 attempted procedures. Although the immediate efficacy of laparoscopic conservative procedures for interstitial pregnancy is high, the risk of uterine rupture in a subsequent pregnancy is unknown. Uterine rupture can occur at the site of a previous interstitial pregnancy. Patients treated by conservative laparoscopic techniques should therefore be carefully counseled about this risk. The risk of uterine rupture also emphasizes the importance of proper suturing of the uterine cornu during conservative surgical treatment of an interstitial pregnancy.

For many surgeons, cornual resection and repair of the defect by laparotomy remains the standard conservative surgical procedure for interstitial pregnancy. Provided that uterine rupture has not occurred, this is technically feasible in most cases. Unfortunately, in many cases in which uterine rupture has occurred or a very large interstitial pregnancy is present, a hysterectomy may be required. Hysterectomy remains the treatment of choice for pregnancies advanced to such a stage that repair of the cornu would be technically difficult and medically hazardous.

Excision of Interstitial Pregnancy by Cornual Resection and Salpingectomy

Whenever possible, the ovary should be saved. A cornual resection and salpingectomy are performed by first ligating the ascending uterine vessels where they approach the cornu (Fig. 34.12A). Each is ligated separately with a figure-of-eight suture. One may also consider the use of a dilute solution of vasopressin (prepared by mixing 20 U of vasopressin with 30 mL of physiologic saline) injected in the intended myometrial incisional line to further optimize intraoperative hemostasis. The interstitial pregnancy is excised in a V-shaped manner, and the myometrium is approximated with a figure-of-eight closure using no. 0 delayed absorbable suture (Fig. 34.12B). The remainder of the fallopian tube is excised. If it becomes necessary, the round ligament can be cut and resutured to the cornu and the uterine serosa by use of interrupted sutures (Fig. 34.12C). The round and broad ligaments are brought over the incision with mattress sutures (the modified Coffey suspension) (Fig. 34.12D), and additional interrupted sutures of no. 2-0 or no. 3-0 delayed absorbable material can be used to secure the serosa of the round ligament to the serosa of the uterus to maintain the operative site in a permanent retroperitoneal position.

OVARIAN ECTOPIC PREGNANCY

Because IUDs protect the endometrium and, to a lesser extent, the proximal oviducts from implantation, it was expected that when IUDs were introduced, future reports of extrauterine pregnancies might show an increased rate of ovarian involvement. Data from the Cooperative Statistical Program of the Population Council show that 1 of every 9 ectopic pregnancies among IUD users is an ovarian pregnancy. Of total pregnancies among IUD users, 4.3% are extrauterine.

There are several reviews in the English literature on the subject of primary ovarian pregnancy. Boronow and associates summarized 62 cases in a review of the literature between 1950 and 1963. Campbell and associates brought the list up to date through 1973 with 91 cases, including three new cases of their own. Pratt-Thomas and colleagues reported an additional 10 new cases in 1974. Grimes and associates summarized the major reviews through 1980 and added 18 previously unreported cases of primary ovarian pregnancy from the records of six hospitals. Their combined data from this review,

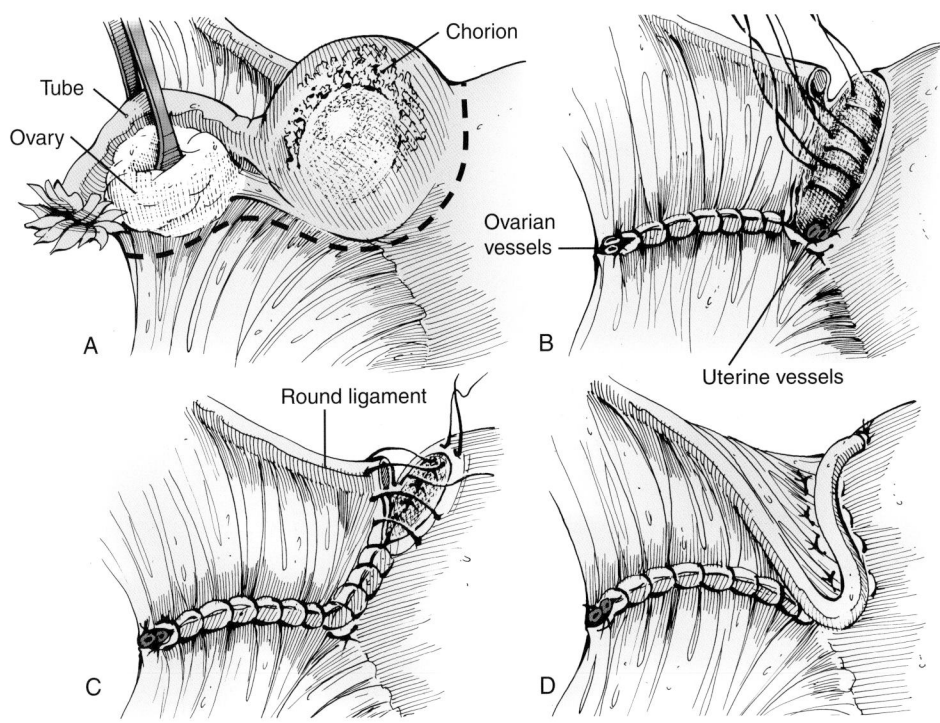

FIGURE 34.12 Salpingo-oophorectomy with resection of interstitial pregnancy. **A:** The dotted line denotes the line of excision. **B:** Tube, ovary, and the cornual pregnancy have been excised. The myometrium is being approximated with figure-of-eight sutures of no. 0 delayed absorbable suture. Note that the uterine vessels have been ligated separately. **C:** The round ligament, which was cut, is being resutured to the cornu. The ovarian vessels have been ligated, and the broad ligament has been closed with a continuous lock stitch. Serosa of the uterine wound is closed with a simple continuous stitch. **D:** The cornual wound is covered with the round and broad ligaments.

the hospital cases, and four other recent reports totaled 34 cases of primary ovarian pregnancy among 236,983 deliveries, a rate of 1 ovarian pregnancy in 7,000 deliveries.

In an intrafollicular ovarian pregnancy, the second stage of meiosis, ovum capacitation, and fertilization each occur within the follicle. Only 15% of cases of ovarian pregnancy are intrafollicular in origin. In an intrafollicular pregnancy, a well-preserved corpus luteum can be identified in the wall of the gestational sac. Four other criteria presented by Spiegelberg for identifying an intrafollicular pregnancy are that the tube, including the fimbria ovarica, is intact and is clearly separate from the ovary; that the gestational sac definitely occupies the normal position of the ovary; that the sac is connected to the uterus by the utero-ovarian ligament; and that ovarian tissue is unquestionably demonstrated in the wall of the sac.

Diagnosis of Ovarian Pregnancy

Early diagnosis of an ovarian pregnancy, of all the diagnoses relating to extrauterine gestations, is perhaps the most difficult. As stated previously, the classic symptoms of a tubal gestation are abdominal pain, amenorrhea, and bleeding; however, persistent pelvic pain alone, a symptom not always easily related to its cause, is the most frequent clinical manifestation of an ovarian gestation. Although an adnexal mass is palpable in as many as 60% of ovarian pregnancies, the mass is frequently confused with a leaking corpus luteum hematoma.

All of the test criteria used for diagnosing a tubal pregnancy are helpful in diagnosing a primary ovarian pregnancy. In particular, the highly sensitive β-hCG immunoassay is effective for identifying the presence of low hCG levels. The test can confirm the presence of a gestational process, but knowing the β-hCG level does not help to precisely locate the gestation. Incomplete spontaneous abortion with a leaking corpus luteum hematoma, one of the most common complications of pregnancy, mimics an ovarian pregnancy. In such cases, a D&C

will often show the remnants of trophoblastic villi responsible for the low levels of β-hCG.

A tubal pregnancy can easily be ruled out with laparoscopy, but an ovarian pregnancy is sometimes difficult to differentiate from a leaking corpus luteum hematoma by gross appearance. Ultrasonography can be helpful, but only in advanced ovarian pregnancy will the ultrasound image show a discrete gestational sac, therefore confirming an ovarian pregnancy.

Critical evaluation of all of the diagnostic studies, particularly the sensitive β-hCG immunoassay and vaginal ultrasonography, is necessary in making the diagnosis. When the β-hCG is positive, ultrasonography shows no intrauterine gestational sac, and free blood exists in the peritoneal cavity, a laparoscopy should be performed to confirm or refute a diagnosis of suspected ovarian pregnancy.

Treatment for Ovarian Pregnancy

Raziel and Golan, as well as Chelmow and colleagues, reported cases in which an intact ovarian pregnancy was diagnosed by laparoscopy and systemic MTX treatment was successful. In many cases, an ovarian pregnancy is diagnosed after a significant hemoperitoneum has occurred and medical therapy is contraindicated. An ovarian pregnancy is easily confused with a leaking corpus luteum hematoma. For this reason, a safe approach is to proceed with localized surgical resection of the bleeding mass with conservation of the ovary, if possible. Unless the diagnosis is made late, the ovary can usually be preserved. In 1997, Seinera and colleagues reported successful laparoscopic treatment of ovarian pregnancy in eight patients over a 12-year time span. Einenkel and associates even reported the successful conservative resection of an ovarian pregnancy in a patient with ovarian hyperstimulation. The concomitant increased ovarian size, fragility, and vascularity presented an additional surgical challenge for these authors, although the use of intraoperative ultrasound greatly facilitated the precise localization of the ectopic pregnancy within the ovary.

Only rarely is the hemorrhage so profuse that oophorectomy is required to control bleeding. Even if the last trophoblastic villus cannot be removed in the ovarian resection, the ovary should be preserved. Any remaining trophoblastic tissue will usually degenerate rapidly or respond to postoperative MTX therapy and therefore should produce no long-standing clinical problem.

ABDOMINAL ECTOPIC PREGNANCY

An abdominal pregnancy is perhaps both the rarest and the most serious type of extrauterine gestation. Reports of the frequency of abdominal pregnancy vary, ranging from 1 in 3,371 deliveries to greater than 1 in 10,200 deliveries. Stafford and Ragan reported an incidence of 1 abdominal pregnancy in 7,269 deliveries, a figure that is representative of the reports in the literature.

Abdominal pregnancies are classified as primary or secondary. Most are secondary, the result of early tubal abortion or rupture with secondary implantation of the pregnancy into the peritoneal cavity. To be considered a primary abdominal pregnancy, the pregnancy must meet the three criteria defined by Studdiford in 1942:

1. Both tubes and ovaries must be in normal condition with no evidence of recent or remote injury.
2. No evidence of uteroperitoneal fistula should be found.
3. The pregnancy must be related exclusively to the peritoneal surface and be early enough to eliminate the possibility that it is a secondary implantation following a primary implantation in the tube.

Secondary abdominal pregnancy occurs when a tubal gestation attaches itself to other viscera as the enlarging placenta spreads through the wall of the tube or is aborted through the fimbriated end. The placenta probably retains some tubal attachment, which supplies blood for the gestation to continue developing in the new peritoneal site. Rare types of secondary abdominal pregnancies have occurred after spontaneous separation of an old cesarean section scar, after uterine perforation during a therapeutic or elective abortion, and after subtotal or total hysterectomy.

Diagnosis of Abdominal Pregnancy

Early diagnosis of an abdominal pregnancy is difficult but critical, because a catastrophic hemorrhage can result from separation of the placenta later in pregnancy. A history of recurrent abdominal discomfort, fetal movement beneath the abdominal wall, and the presence of fetal movements high in the upper abdomen should alert the clinician to the possibility of an abdominal implantation. Other clinical clues include cessation of fetal movement, vomiting late in pregnancy, fetal malposition, a closed and uneffaced cervix, or the failure of oxytocin to stimulate the gestational mass.

Confirmation of the diagnosis requires demonstration of the fetus outside the uterine cavity. In their review of 199 cases, Costa and colleagues reported that only in 68 cases (40.2%) was a mass adjacent to or distinct from the uterus found. The radiologic finding of fetal small parts in the lateral position overlying the maternal spine was first noted by Weinberg and Sherwin in 1956; this finding is a fairly reliable sign of an abdominal pregnancy. A radiologic examination of the abdomen, including anterior, posterior, and lateral views, is also helpful in defining malposition of the fetus, which is most often discovered to

be in the transverse position. Ultrasound, however, is the most effective method for diagnosing an abdominal pregnancy. Ultrasound can usually identify an abdominal gestation as separate from the nonpregnant uterus. Ultrasonography can be expected to have high diagnostic accuracy in most cases. In those cases in which ultrasonography is equivocal, MRI may be useful.

The maternal mortality risk from abdominal pregnancy in the United States is 7.7 times greater than the maternal mortality risk from tubal ectopic pregnancy and 90 times greater than that with intrauterine pregnancy. Reported maternal mortality rates in the literature have varied in the past from 4% to 29%. Maternal morbidity can also be substantial, with high incidences of pelvic abscess, peritonitis, and sepsis caused by retained placental remnants. Rare instances of massive rectal bleeding or rectal passage of fetal bones secondary to the formation of celo-intestinal fistulae have also been reported. Fetal mortality is notoriously high, ranging from 75% to 95% of all cases.

Management of Advanced Abdominal Pregnancy

Recent techniques of fetal monitoring serve as diagnostic adjuncts to the management of the advanced abdominal pregnancy. Fetal assessment—including repeated ultrasonography to measure biparietal diameter, nonstress testing, monitoring of fetal movements, and biophysical profiles—can provide clinical evidence of fetal maturity and fetal welfare. Despite the use of these diagnostic tools, fetal death occurred in all of the 15 cases of abdominal pregnancy reported by Martin and associates. Clark and Jones reported a fetal salvage rate of only 11.4% in a study of 35 advanced abdominal pregnancies.

One of the major factors in fetal survival is the condition of the fetal membranes. If the membranes rupture, the fetus usually dies from respiratory distress in the peritoneal cavity within a short time of the rupture. When the volume of amniotic fluid is significantly decreased or absent, the incidence of fetal malformations increases significantly, pressure deformities occur, and pulmonary hypoplasia precludes the possibility of delivering a viable fetus. In situations in which the pregnancy is advanced and there is sufficient volume of amniotic fluid, there exists a reasonable possibility of a good fetal outcome. In rare instances, there may be justification for postponed surgery to allow for further fetal maturity and a better perinatal prognosis.

Preoperative preparation of a patient with an advanced abdominal pregnancy should include an adequate supply of compatible blood and blood products and appropriate intravenous infusion lines that can deliver large amounts of fluid quickly. The use of a cell-saver or MAST (military antishock trouser) suit has been reported in the management of patients experiencing massive hemorrhage and shock. A surgical team should be standing by that is capable of handling the possible bowel, vascular, or genitourinary complications that may arise.

Following incision into the amniotic sac and delivery of the fetus, the management of the placenta still remains a controversial issue. Most clinicians believe the best treatment is to clamp the cord, to leave the placenta in situ, and to close the abdomen, but to allow retroperitoneal drainage if possible. The placenta can be removed after complete cessation of function is demonstrated by quantitative β-hCG titers. The placenta should be removed during laparotomy only if it is accessible and if its removal can be accomplished without excessive blood loss. In case of doubt, the placenta should be left in place. Thompson has reported leaving the placenta in the peritoneal cavity for a period of 13 years without physical harm to the patient. MTX has been used occasionally to hasten trophoblastic degeneration, but it leads to the accelerated accumulation of necrotic placental tissue, which may become infected. For this reason, it is currently felt best not to administer MTX in this clinical setting.

CERVICAL ECTOPIC PREGNANCY

The cervix is a rare but hazardous site for placental implantation because the trophoblast can penetrate through the cervical wall and into the uterine blood supply. Cervical gestations have, until recently, received little attention in the literature, but increased awareness of the condition has resulted in a number of recent reports.

The following three criteria for the diagnosis of cervical pregnancy were established by Rubin in 1911:

1. Cervical glands must be opposite the placental attachment.
2. Placental attachment to the cervix must be situated below the entrance of the uterine vessels or below the peritoneal reflection of the anterior and posterior surfaces of the uterus.
3. Fetal elements must be absent from the corpus uteri.

Because strict anatomical and histologic criteria necessitate a hysterectomy for a complete study of the entire uterus, Paalman and McElin proposed five more clinically practical criteria for the diagnosis of this condition:

1. Uterine bleeding without cramping pain following a period of amenorrhea
2. A soft, enlarged cervix equal to or larger than the fundus (the "hourglass" uterus)
3. Products of conception entirely confined within and firmly attached to the endocervix
4. A closed internal cervical os
5. A partially opened external cervical os

The incidence of this rare entity varies. The Mayo Clinic reported 1 in 16,000 pregnancies. The highest incidence, 1 in 1,000 pregnancies, was reported from Japan. The high incidence of elective abortion in Japan is probably a factor in the higher rates. D&C seems to be a predisposing factor for cervical pregnancy. Shinagawa and Nagayama noted that in 18 of 19 cases of cervical pregnancy, there was a history of legal abortion. In the review by Ushakov and associates, 68.6% of patients with a cervical pregnancy had a previous uterine curettage. It has also been suggested that a previous cesarean section may play a role in the etiology of cervical pregnancy.

Cervical gestation is frequently confused with a neoplastic process because of the marked vascularity and friable appearance of the cervix. Profuse bleeding can occur if the placenta is mistaken for a tumor and a biopsy is taken. A cervical gestation also can be mistaken for a spontaneous abortion in which the products of conception were retained within the cervical canal (Fig. 34.13).

Treatment for Cervical Pregnancy

The treatment for a cervical pregnancy is surgical, and the condition often requires an abdominal hysterectomy. In selected patients, conservative evacuation of an early cervical pregnancy may be accomplished by skillful D&C, although the procedure has the potential to be complicated by profuse hemorrhage. Further preoperative preparations directed to reduce the vascularity of the uterine cervix—such as transvaginal ligation of cervical branches of the uterine arteries, a Shirodkar-type cerclage, angiographic uterine artery embolization (UAE), or intracervical vasopressin injection—may reduce operative morbidity. In a review by Ushakov and colleagues, of the 16 cases in which one of these methods was employed, 15 had minimal (50 to 200 mL) blood loss, one patient had a hemorrhage of 1,200 mL requiring transfusion, and no patient required laparotomy or hysterectomy. Among 41 cases in which D&C was performed without cervical preparation, minimal bleeding occurred in just five cases (12.2%),

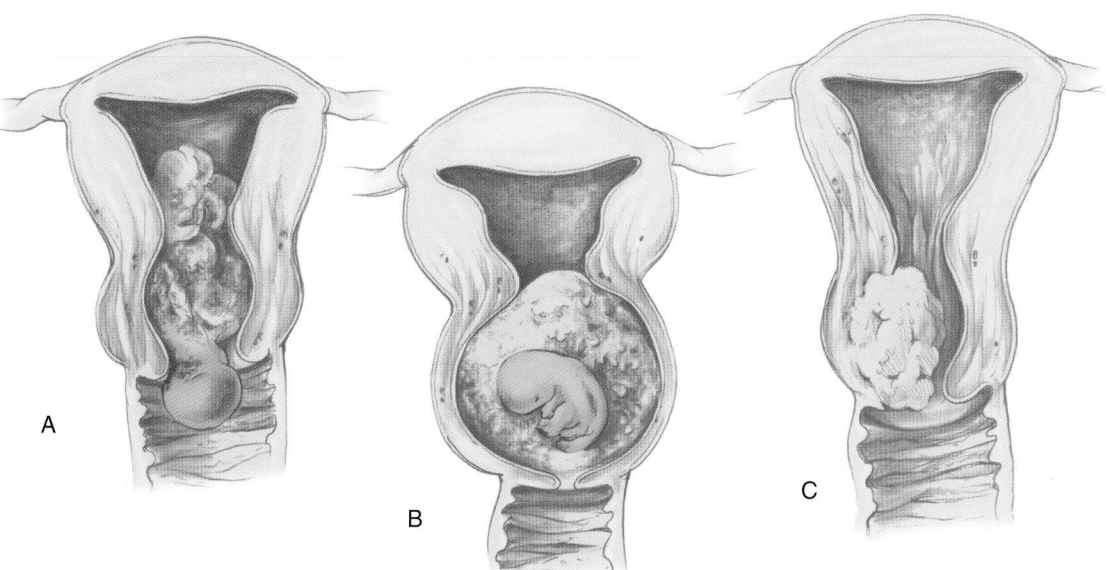

FIGURE 34.13 Differential diagnosis of cervical pregnancy. **A:** In the cervical phase of uterine abortion, the placenta is mainly within the expanded cervix, and the external and internal ora are dilated. **B:** In a cervical abortion (abortion into the cervix), because of stenosis of the external os, spontaneous rupture of the cervical wall can cause severe hemorrhage. **C:** Ragged, friable cervix seen in cervical pregnancy mimics carcinoma of the cervix. (Redrawn from Rothe DJ, Birnbaum SJ. Cervical pregnancy: diagnosis and management. *Obstet Gynecol* 1973;42:675, with permission. Copyright © 1973 The American College of Obstetricians and Gynecologists.)

massive bleeding (1,200 to 5,000 mL) occurred in 70.7%, and hysterectomy was performed in seven cases (17.1%). Laparotomy with bilateral internal iliac artery ligation or bilateral uterine artery ligation was also required in an additional five (12.2%) of these patients. To control postevacuation bleeding, several authors, including Kuppuswami and colleagues and Werber and associates, have described the successful use of a Foley catheter balloon to tamponade the cervical implantation site in patients who continued to have blood loss after cervical pregnancy evacuation. A 26-French Foley catheter with a 30-mL balloon is preferably used and left inflated for 0.5 to 6 days, as clinically indicated.

Medical therapy can also be considered for the primary treatment of cervical pregnancy or as an adjunct to surgical therapy through decreased vascularization of the mass. Kung and Chang reviewed the use of MTX administration for cervical ectopic pregnancy from 1983 to 1997. Among 35 cases of viable cervical ectopic pregnancies less than 12 weeks gestation, 63% of patients received either systemic MTX alone or a combination of systemic MTX with a local (intra-amniotic or intracervical) injection of either MTX or potassium chloride. Among the 23 cases of nonviable cervical pregnancy less than 12 weeks gestation, 96% of women required systemic MTX alone. The ultimate success rate of uterine preservation was similar (94% for the viable pregnancy group; 91% for the nonviable pregnancy group), although the patients in the viable pregnancy group required a significantly higher number of concomitant additional surgical procedures (43% vs. 13%).

Zakaria and associates reported successful nonsurgical conservative management of 15 cases of cervical ectopic pregnancy. Five patients were treated with multidose MTX and leucovorin rescue, six patients were treated with multidose MTX and bilateral UAE, and four patients were treated with multidose MTX and bilateral UAE with intra-amniotic potassium chloride additionally administered prior to UAE.

CESAREAN SCAR PREGNANCY

With the increasing utilization of cesarean section for delivery, there has been recent identification of an increasing number of abnormal (ectopic) pregnancies in which there is implantation of the gestational sac in the hysterotomy scar. It is felt that endometrial and myometrial disruption due to poor healing can predispose to abnormal pregnancy implantation in this area, although it has also been speculated that implantation may occur through a microscopic tract into the myometrium. Fylstra reported a review of the English literature from 1966 until 2002 and identified 19 cases. Since this time, numerous additional reports have appeared in the literature, including a series of 96 cases reported by Zhang and associates.

The diagnosis may be difficult, and a false-negative diagnosis has the potential for a major complication, including profound hemorrhage and the need for hysterectomy. Timor-Tritsch and colleagues proposed the following transvaginal ultrasonographic criteria for cesarean scar pregnancy:

1. Visualization of an empty uterine cavity as well as an empty endocervical canal.
2. Detection of the placenta and/or a gestational sac embedded in the hysterotomy scar.
3. In early gestations (≤8 weeks), a triangular gestational sac that fills the niche of the scar; at ≥ 8 postmenstrual weeks, this shape may become rounded or even oval.
4. A thin (1 to 3 mm) or absent myometrial layer between the gestational sac and the bladder.

5. A closed and empty cervical canal.
6. The presence of embryonic/fetal pole and/or yolk sac with or without heart activity.
7. The presence of prominent and at times rich vascular pattern at or in the area of cesarean delivery scar in the presence of a positive pregnancy test.

Treatment for Cesarean Scar Pregnancy

A wide variety of conservative, fertility-sparing treatment approaches for cesarean scar pregnancy have been reported, including resection and uterine scar dehiscence repair by both laparotomy and laparoscopy approaches. Successful resection by either hysteroscopy or curettage has also occurred following bilateral UAE and systemic MTX. Curettage alone has been attempted, but secondary salvage treatments were necessary to resolve these pregnancies. Curettage alone appears contraindicated due to the trophoblast location being outside of the realm of the uterine cavity (beyond the reach of the curette) as well as due to the potential risk of uterine rupture and hemorrhage. Systemic MTX as primary treatment, bilateral UAE alone, and bilateral UAE combined with systemic MTX have all also been reported in the treatment of cesarean scar pregnancy.

Timor-Tritsch and colleagues reported on a series of 19 patients between 6 and 14 postmenstrual weeks who were successfully treated for cesarean scar pregnancy. Each patient had 50 mg of MTX injected into the gestational sac, with 25 mg into the area of the embryo and 25 mg into the placental area. An additional 25 mg of MTX was administered intramuscularly. It was speculated that intragestational sac injection may be more effective, as a cesarean scar pregnancy may potentially have inefficient drug delivery following systemic MTX alone due to its being surrounded by fibrous scar rather than a normally vascularized myometrium.

HETEROTOPIC PREGNANCY

Heterotopic pregnancy (coexistence of intra- and extrauterine pregnancies) is rare. The incidence has been estimated to be about 1 in 30,000 spontaneous pregnancies. With the use of assisted reproductive technologies, the incidence is higher, as high as 0.75% to 1.5% of pregnancies.

Although the precise cause of a combined pregnancy is frequently obscure, most of the risk factors are the same as those associated with other forms of ectopic pregnancy. The use of ovulation-inducing agents has increased the incidence of multiple gestations and heterotopic pregnancies. Berger and Taymor reported an incidence of combined pregnancy in as many as 1 in 100 stimulated patients. The most common predisposing anatomic finding associated with heterotopic pregnancies is preexisting tubal disease.

Abdominal pain, an adnexal mass, peritoneal irritation, and an enlarged uterus together constitute the major clinical features associated with a heterotopic pregnancy. Additional diagnostic findings include the presence of two corpora lutea found at the time of laparotomy or laparoscopy, hemoperitoneum, acute abdominal pain after the termination of an intrauterine pregnancy, and the persistence of an enlarged uterus with amenorrhea after excision of an ectopic pregnancy.

As opposed to solely extrauterine pregnancies, which are presently diagnosed and treated electively at an early preclinical stage, heterotopic pregnancies are still mostly diagnosed after clinical signs develop. In their review, Rojansky and Schenker report that nearly half of the cases present with rupture, hemorrhage, and emergency intervention. This is due to the fact that serial β-hCG determinations and transvaginal ultrasonography are often not helpful in establishing an early diagnosis of heterotopic pregnancy.

The majority of heterotopic pregnancies consist of a single tubal gestation combined with an intrauterine pregnancy. Rarer varieties include combined cervical–intrauterine, ovarian–intrauterine, abdominal–intrauterine, and interstitial–intrauterine pregnancies.

Treatment for Heterotopic Pregnancy

Laparoscopy has been employed with reasonable success for the treatment of combined tubal and intrauterine pregnancies. Louis-Sylvestre and associates reported treating 13 patients laparoscopically, 10 by salpingectomy and 3 by salpingostomy. Subsequently, 60% of the patients with a viable intrauterine pregnancy at the time of surgery had a favorable outcome. On the other hand, in cases in which hemodynamic instability or an interstitial–intrauterine pregnancy is present, a laparotomy is indicated. Expectant management does not seem to have a role in the care of a patient with a heterotopic pregnancy. This is due to the fact that the specific course of the extrauterine component cannot be monitored by serial β-hCG determinations. Likewise, either local or systemic MTX therapy would be contraindicated in the presence of a viable intrauterine gestation. The use of a local injection of potassium chloride into the extrauterine gestational sac, however, has been used successfully in a few cases. There are very rare cases in which extrauterine abdominal pregnancies progress simultaneously with intrauterine pregnancies to viability. In their review of the world's literature, Reece and associates found only 13 cases in which both pregnancies reached term and both infants were delivered and survived the neonatal period. In the absence of such rare circumstances, the outcome for the intrauterine pregnancy is optimized by immediate therapy of the extrauterine pregnancy.

Rh IMMUNOGLOBULIN USE AFTER ECTOPIC PREGNANCY

Grimes has reported that Rh-negative mothers were recognized and administered Rh immunoglobulin in only 36% of cases. Fetomaternal hemorrhage associated with ectopic pregnancy can sensitize Rh-negative women at risk. A dose of 50 μg Rh immunoglobulin is usually sufficient to prevent Rh sensitization.

BEST SURGICAL PRACTICES

- The benefits derived from the early diagnosis of an ectopic pregnancy include the potential use of medical and conservative surgical procedures that optimize future fertility. Early diagnosis may also preclude ectopic pregnancy rupture and therefore result in lower patient morbidity and mortality.
- The astute clinician is aware of the risk factors for ectopic pregnancy, thereby increasing the level of suspicion in the appropriate clinical context. Risk factors for ectopic pregnancy include chronic PID, prior tubal surgery, surgical sterilization, use of an IUD, previous ectopic pregnancy, DES exposure, progestin-only contraceptives, assisted reproductive technologies, infertility, tubal developmental anomalies, multiple sex partners, early age at first intercourse, cigarette smoking, and vaginal douching.

- The classic presentation of pain and uterine bleeding with the finding of an adnexal mass is present in only 14% of patients with ectopic pregnancy. Even when present, these classic signs and symptoms are not entirely specific for ectopic pregnancy.
- Highly sensitive β-hCG assays have greatly aided in the early diagnosis of ectopic pregnancies. Serum hCG concentrations increase in an exponential fashion in early pregnancy. During the period of gestation in which the hCG concentration is less than 10,000 IU/L, the time required for doubling of hCG levels remains consistent, with a mean of 1.9 days. The slowest minimal hCG rise for a normal viable intrauterine pregnancy is 53% in 2 days. Transvaginal ultrasonographic evidence of an intrauterine pregnancy can be expected to be seen with very high sensitivity when β-hCG concentrations exceed 1,500 IU/L.
- Serum progesterone assays are useful in the early diagnosis of an ectopic pregnancy. In one large study, 98% of patients with a normal intrauterine pregnancy had progesterone levels greater than 10 ng/mL, and 98% of patients with an ectopic pregnancy had progesterone levels less than 20 ng/mL. Diagnostic limitations of the serum progesterone assay included the fact that 31% of viable intrauterine pregnancies, 23% of abnormal intrauterine pregnancies, and 51% of ectopic pregnancies had progesterone levels between 10 and 20 ng/mL in this study. In another large trial, the lowest serum progesterone concentration associated with a viable pregnancy was 5.1 ng/mL.
- A D&C procedure is helpful when β-hCG assays and transvaginal ultrasonography are nondiagnostic and a nonviable pregnancy is suspected. Appropriate indications include (a) a failure of β-hCG concentration rise of greater than 50% in 2 days, (b) a serum progesterone level less than 5 ng/mL, and (c) a failure to visualize an intrauterine gestational sac by transvaginal ultrasonography when the β-hCG concentrations exceed 1,500 IU/L. An ectopic pregnancy is suspected after uterine curettage if chorionic villi are not present on frozen section or if β-hCG concentrations do not fall by at least 15% 8 to 12 hours after the procedure.
- Laparoscopy remains the gold standard for the diagnosis of ectopic pregnancy, although it still has a low rate of false-negative and false-positive outcomes.
- Systemic MTX is an alternative that can be used for the treatment of patients with small, unruptured ectopic pregnancies or patients with persistent ectopic pregnancies following conservative surgery. A history of active hepatic, renal, or peptic ulcer disease; elevated liver enzyme concentrations; and thrombocytopenia or neutropenia are contraindications to MTX therapy. Appropriate candidates for systemic MTX therapy should be willing to accept a small risk of tubal rupture and participate in closely monitored follow-up.
- In women who wish to preserve their fertility, conservative surgery by linear salpingotomy is the preferred treatment of a distal unruptured tubal pregnancy. Contraindications to conservative tubal surgery include an extensive hemoperitoneum and potentially compromised cardiovascular status, a recurrent ectopic pregnancy in the same fallopian tube, an ectopic pregnancy in a severely damaged tube, and an ectopic pregnancy in a woman who has completed her family.
- During laparoscopic salpingotomy, it is important to make the incision along the antimesenteric wall of the tube in the area of maximal distension and large enough to allow for complete extrusion of the products of conception without difficulty. Following laparoscopic salpingotomy, healing by secondary intention is felt appropriate in most cases.

- During laparoscopic salpingectomy, take care to stay as close as possible to the fallopian tube during transection of the tubo-ovarian ligament and mesosalpinx. If cautery and transection of the proximal tubal isthmus are used, care should be taken such that excess cauterization of the uterine cornu does not occur because of concerns about the potential of interstitial sinus tracts or diminished myometrial integrity.
- All Rh-negative patients with an ectopic pregnancy should be offered at least 50 µg of Rh immunoglobulin to prevent Rh sensitization caused by fetomaternal hemorrhage.

BIBLIOGRAPHY

Ackerman TE, Levi CS, Dashefsky SM, et al. Interstitial line: sonographic finding in interstitial (cornual) ectopic pregnancy. *Radiology* 1993;189:83.

Alleyassin A, Khademi A, Aghahosseini M, et al. Comparison of success rates in the medical management of ectopic pregnancy with single-dose and multiple-dose administration of methotrexate: a prospective, randomized clinical trial. *Fertil Steril* 2006;85:1661.

Ankum WM, Mol BWJ, Van der Veen R, et al. Risk factors for ectopic pregnancy: a meta-analysis. *Fertil Steril* 1996;65:1093.

Arias-Stella J. Atypical endometrial changes associated with the presence of chorionic tissue. *Arch Pathol* 1954;58:112.

Atrash HK, Friede A, Hogue CJR. Abdominal pregnancy in the United States: frequency and maternal mortality. *Obstet Gynecol* 1987;69:333.

Atrash HK, Friede A, Hogue CJ. Ectopic pregnancy mortality in the United States: 1970–1983. *Obstet Gynecol* 1987;70:817.

Auslender R, Arodi J, Pascal B, et al. Interstitial pregnancy: early diagnosis by ultrasonography. *Am J Obstet Gynecol* 1983;146:717.

Barnhart K, Mennuti M, Benjamin J, et al. Prompt diagnosis of ectopic pregnancy in an emergency department setting. *Obstet Gynecol* 1994;84:1010.

Barnhart KT, Gosman G, Ashby R, et al. The medical management of ectopic pregnancy: a meta-analysis comparing "single-dose" and "multidose" regiments. *Obstet Gynecol* 2003;101:778.

Barnhart K, Sammel MD, Rinaudo PF, et al. Symptomatic patients with an early viable intrauterine pregnancy: hCG curves redefined. *Obstet Gynecol* 2004;104:50.

Barnhart KT, Sammel HS, Hummel A, et al. A novel "two dose" regimen of methotrexate to treat ectopic pregnancy. *Fertil Steril* 2005;84: S130.

Berger MJ, Taymor ML. Simultaneous intrauterine and tubal pregnancies following ovulation induction. *Am J Obstet Gynecol* 1972;113:812.

Boronow RC, McElin TW, West RH, et al. Ovarian pregnancy: a report of 4 cases and a 13-year survey of the English literature. *Am J Obstet Gynecol* 1965;91:1095.

Budowick M, Johnson TRB Jr, Genadry R, et al. The histopathology of the developing tubal ectopic pregnancy. *Fertil Steril* 1980;34:169.

Cacciatore B, Stenman U, Ylostalo P. Diagnosis of ectopic pregnancy by vaginal ultrasonography in combination with a discriminatory serum hCG level of 1000 IU/L (IRP). *BJOG* 1990;97:904.

Campbell JS, Hacquebard S, Mitton DM, et al. Acute hemoperitoneum, IUD, and occult ovarian pregnancy. *Obstet Gynecol* 1974;43:438.

Carson SA, Buster JE. Ectopic pregnancy. *N Engl J Med* 1993;329:1174.

Centers for Disease Control and Prevention. Current trends ectopic pregnancy—United States, 1990–1992. *MMWR Morb Mortal Wkly Rep* 1995;44:46.

Centers for Disease Control and Prevention. Pregnancy-related mortality surveillance—United States, 1991–1999. *MMWR Morb Mortal Wkly Rep* 2003;52:1.

Centers for Disease Control and Prevention. *2010 Assisted reproductive technology report.* http://www.cdc.gov/ART/ART2010

Chelmow D, Gates E, Penzias AS. Laparoscopic diagnosis and methotrexate treatment of an ovarian pregnancy: a case report. *Fertil Steril* 1994;62:879.

Clark JF, Jones SA. Advanced ectopic pregnancy. *J Reprod Med* 1975; 14:30.

Confino E, Binor Z, Molo MW, et al. Selective salpingography for the diagnosis and treatment of early tubal pregnancy. *Fertil Steril* 1994;62:286.

Costa SD, Presley J, Bastert G. Advanced abdominal pregnancy. *Obstet Gynecol Surv* 1991;46:515.

De Voe RW, Pratt JH. Simultaneous intrauterine and extrauterine pregnancy. *Am J Obstet Gynecol* 1948;56:1119.

DeCherney AH, Boyers SP. Isthmic ectopic pregnancy: segmental resection as treatment of choice. *Fertil Steril* 1985;44:307.

Dor J, Seidman DS, Levran D, et al. The incidence of combined intrauterine and extrauterine pregnancy after in vitro fertilization and embryo transfer. *Fertil Steril* 1991;55:833.

Dubuisson JB, Aubriot FX, Cardone V. Laparoscopic salpingectomy for tubal pregnancy. *Fertil Steril* 1987;47:225.

Dubuisson JB, Morice P, Chapron C, et al. Salpingectomy: the laparoscopic surgical choice for ectopic pregnancy. *Hum Reprod* 1996;11:1199.

Egger M, Low N, Smith GD, et al. Screening for chlamydia infections and the risk of ectopic pregnancy in a county in Sweden: ecological analysis. *BMJ* 1998;316:1776.

Einenkel J, Baier D, Horn LC, et al. Laparoscopic therapy of an intact primary ovarian pregnancy with ovarian hyperstimulation syndrome: case report. *Hum Reprod* 2000;15:2037.

Emerson DS, Cartier MS, Altieri LA, et al. Diagnostic efficacy of endovaginal color Doppler flow imaging in an ectopic pregnancy screening program. *Radiology* 1992;183:413.

Faber BM, Coddington CC. Microlaparoscopy: a comparative study of diagnostic accuracy. *Fertil Steril* 1997;67:952.

Farabow W, Fulton J, Fletcher V, et al. Cervical pregnancy treated with methotrexate. *N C Med J* 1983;44:91.

Feichtinger W, Kemeter P. Conservative treatment of ectopic pregnancy by transvaginal aspiration under sonographic control and methotrexate injection. *Lancet* 1987;1:381.

Fernandez H, Benifla JL, Lelaidier C, et al. Methotrexate treatment of ectopic pregnancy: 100 cases treated by primary transvaginal injection under sonographic control. *Fertil Steril* 1993;59:773.

Fernandez H, Capella S, Vincent AY, et al. Randomized trial of conservative laparoscopic treatment and methotrexate administration in ectopic pregnancy and subsequent fertility. *Hum Reprod* 1998;13:3239.

Fernandez H, Rainhorn JD, Papiernik E, et al. Spontaneous resolution of ectopic pregnancy. *Obstet Gynecol* 1988;71:171.

Frates MC, Laing FC. Sonographic evaluation of ectopic pregnancy: an update. *AJR Am J Roentgenol* 1995;165:251.

Fujishita A, Masuzaki H, Khan KN, et al. Laparoscopic salpingotomy for tubal pregnancy: comparison of linear salpingotomy with and without suturing. *Hum Reprod* 2004;19:1195.

Fylstra DL. Ectopic pregnancy within a cesarean scar: a review. *Obstet Gynecol Surv* 2002;57:537.

Gazvani MR, Baruah DN, Afirevic Z, et al. Mifepristone in combination with methotrexate for the medical treatment of tubal pregnancy: a randomized, controlled trial. *Hum Reprod* 1998;13:1987.

Gelder MS, Boots LR, Younger JB. Use of a single random serum progesterone value as a diagnostic aid for ectopic pregnancy. *Fertil Steril* 1991;55:497.

Gerard HC, Branigan PJ, Balsara GR, et al. Viability of *Chlamydia trachomatis* in fallopian tubes of patients with ectopic pregnancy. *Fertil Steril* 1998;70:945.

Giuliani A, Panzitt T, Schoell W, et al. Severe bleeding from peritoneal implants of trophoblastic tissue after laparoscopic salpingostomy for ectopic pregnancy. *Fertil Steril* 1998;70:369.

Gjelland K, Hordnes K, Tjugum J, et al. Treatment of ectopic pregnancy by local injection of hyperosmolar glucose: a randomized trial comparing administration guided by transvaginal ultrasound or laparoscopy. *Acta Obstet Gynecol Scand* 1995;74:629.

Gleicher N, Parrilli M, Pratt DE. Hysterosalpingography and selective salpingography in the differential diagnosis of chemical intrauterine versus tubal pregnancy. *Fertil Steril* 1992;57:553.

Goldner TE, Lawson HW, Xia Z, et al. Surveillance for ectopic pregnancy–United States, 1970–1989. *MMWR CDC Surveill Summ* 1993;42:73.

Graczykowski JW, Mishell DR. Methotrexate prophylaxis for persistent ectopic pregnancy after conservative treatment by salpingostomy. *Obstet Gynecol* 1997;89:118.

Grimes DA. The morbidity and mortality of pregnancy: still risky business. *Am J Obstet Gynecol* 1995;170:1489.

Grimes DA, Geary FH Jr, Hatcher RA. Rh immunoglobulin utilization after ectopic pregnancy. *Am J Obstet Gynecol* 1981;140:246.

Grimes HG, Nosal RA, Gallagher JC. Ovarian pregnancy: a series of 34 cases. *Obstet Gynecol* 1983;61:174.

Guven ESG, Dilbaz S, Dilbaz B, et al. Comparison of single and multiple dose methotrexate therapy for unruptured tubal ectopic pregnancy: a prospective randomized study. *Acta Obstet Gynecol* 2010;89:889.

Hahlin M, Sjoblom P, Lindblom B. Combined use of progesterone and human chorionic gonadotropin determinations for differential diagnosis of very early pregnancy. *Fertil Steril* 1991;55:492.

Hallatt JG. Tubal conservation in ectopic pregnancy: a study of 200 cases. *Am J Obstet Gynecol* 1986;54:1216.

Hillis SD, Nakashima A, Amsterdam L, et al. The impact of a comprehensive chlamydia prevention program in Wisconsin. *Fam Plann Perspect* 1995;27:108.

Hoover KW, Tao G, Kent CK. Trends in the diagnosis and treatment of ectopic pregnancy in the United States. *Obstet Gynecol* 2010;115:495.

Hoppe DE, Bekkar BE, Nager CW. Single-dose systemic methotrexate for the treatment of persistent ectopic pregnancy after conservative surgery. *Obstet Gynecol* 1994;83:51.

Ishihara O, Kuwahara A, Saitoh H. Frozen-thawed blastocyst transfer reduces ectopic pregnancy risk: an analysis of single embryo transfer cycles in Japan. *Fertil Steril* 2011;95:1966.

Jain K, Hamper VM, Sanders RC. Comparison of transvaginal sonography in the detection of early pregnancy and its complications. *Am J Radiol* 1988;151:1139.

Jauchler GW, Baker RL. Cervical pregnancy: review of the literature and a case report. *Obstet Gynecol* 1970;35:870.

Kadar N, Caldwell BV, Romero R. A method of screening for ectopic pregnancy and its indications. *Obstet Gynecol* 1981;58:162.

Kadar N, DeVore G, Romero R. Discriminatory hCG zone: its use in the sonographic evaluation for ectopic pregnancy. *Obstet Gynecol* 1981;58:156.

Karhus LL, Egerup P, Skovlund CW, et al. Long-term reproductive outcomes in women whose first pregnancy is ectopic: a national controlled follow-up study. *Hum Reprod* 2013;28:241.

Kataoka ML, Togashi K, Kobayashi H, et al. Evaluation of ectopic pregnancy by magnetic resonance imaging. *Hum Reprod* 1999;14:2644.

Kelly H. *Operative gynecology*, vol. 2. New York: Appleton, 1898:453.

Kirchler HC, Seebacher S, Alge AA, et al. Early diagnosis of tubal pregnancy: changes in tubal blood flow evaluated by endovaginal color Doppler sonography. *Obstet Gynecol* 1993;82:561.

Ko PC, Liang CC, Lo TS, et al. Six cases of tubal stump pregnancy: complication of assisted reproductive technology? *Fertil Steril* 2011;95:2432.e1.

Kojima E, Abe Y, Morita M, et al. The treatment of unruptured tubal pregnancy with intratubal methotrexate injection under laparoscopic control. *Obstet Gynecol* 1990;75:723.

Korhonen J, Stenman UH, Ylostalo P. Serum human chorionic gonadotropin dynamics during spontaneous resolution of ectopic pregnancy. *Fertil Steril* 1994;61:632.

Kung FT, Chang SY. Efficacy of methotrexate treatment in viable and nonviable cervical pregnancies. *Am J Obstet Gynecol* 1999;181:1438.

Kuppuswami N, Vindekilde J, Sethi CM, et al. Diagnosis and treatment of cervical pregnancy. *Obstet Gynecol* 1983;61:651.

Kurjak A, Zalud I, Schulman H. Ectopic pregnancy: transvaginal color Doppler of trophoblastic flow in questionable adnexa. *J Ultrasound Med* 1991;10:685.

Lang PF, Tamussino K, Honigi W, et al. Treatment of unruptured tubal pregnancy by laparoscopic instillation of hyperosmolar glucose solution. *Am J Obstet Gynecol* 1992;166:1378.

Langer R, Bukovsky I, Herman A, et al. Conservative surgery for tubal pregnancy. *Fertil Steril* 1982;38:427.

Lau S, Tulandi T. Conservative medical and surgical management of interstitial ectopic pregnancy. *Fertil Steril* 1999;72:207.

Lavy G, Diamond MP, DeCherney AH. Ectopic pregnancy: relationship to tubal reconstructive surgery. *Fertil Steril* 1987;47:543.

Lecuru F, Robin F, Chasset S, et al. Direct cost of single dose methotrexate for unruptured ectopic pregnancy: prospective comparison with laparoscopy. *Eur J Obstet Gynecol Reprod Biol* 2000;88:1.

Levin AA, Schoenbaum SC, Stubblefield PG, et al. Ectopic pregnancy and prior induced abortion. *Am J Public Health* 1982;72:253.

Lipscomb GH, Bran D, McCord ML, et al. Analysis of three hundred fifteen ectopic pregnancies treated with single-dose methotrexate. *Am J Obstet Gynecol* 1998;178:1354.

Lipscomb GH, McCord ML, Stovall TG, et al. Predictors of success of methotrexate treatment in women with tubal ectopic pregnancies. *N Engl J Med* 1999;341:1974.

Louis-Sylvestre C, Morice P, Chapron C, et al. The role of laparoscopy in the diagnosis and management of heterotopic pregnancies. *Hum Reprod* 1997;12:1100.

Lloyd HE, Feinberg R. The Arias-Stella reaction: a non-specific involutional phenomenon in intra- as well as extrauterine pregnancy. *Am J Clin Pathol* 1965;43:428.

Marcus SF, Macnamee M, Brinsden P. Heterotopic pregnancies after in-vitro fertilization and embryo transfer. *Hum Reprod* 1995;10:1232.

Martin JN Jr, Sessums JK, Martin RW, et al. Abdominal pregnancy: current concepts of management. *Obstet Gynecol* 1988;71:549.

Matthews CP, Coulson PB, Weld RA. Serum progesterone levels as an aid in the diagnosis of ectopic pregnancy. *Obstet Gynecol* 1986;68:390.

Moawad NS, Mahajan ST, Moniz MH, et al. Current diagnosis and treatment of interstitial pregnancy. *Am J Obstet Gynecol* 2010;202:15.

Mol BW, Ankum WM, Bossuyt PM, et al. Contraception and the risk of ectopic pregnancy: a meta-analysis. *Contraception* 1995;52:337.

Morlock RJ, Lafata JE, Eisenstein D. Cost-effectiveness of single-dose methotrexate compared with laparoscopic treatment of ectopic pregnancy. *Obstet Gynecol* 2000;95:407.

Mueller BA, Daling JR, Weiss NS, et al. Tubal pregnancy and the risks of subsequent infertility. *Obstet Gynecol* 1987;69:722.

Nurmohamed L, Moretti ME, Schecter T, et al. Outcome following high-dose methotrexate in pregnancies misdiagnosed as ectopic. *Am J Obstet Gynecol* 2011;205:533.e1.

Ory SJ, Villanueva AL, Sand PK, et al. Conservative treatment of ectopic pregnancy with methotrexate. *Am J Obstet Gynecol* 1986;154:1299.

Paalman R, McElin T. Cervical pregnancy. *Am J Obstet Gynecol* 1959;77:1261.

Pauerstein CJ, Hodgson BJ, Kramen MA. The anatomy and physiology of the oviduct. *Obstet Gynecol Annu* 1974;3:137.

Pellerito JS, Taylor KJW, Quedens-Case C, et al. Ectopic pregnancy: evaluation with endovaginal color flow imaging. *Radiology* 1992;183:407.

Peterson HB, Xia Z, Hughes JM, et al. The risk of ectopic pregnancy after tubal sterilization. *N Engl J Med* 1997;336:762.

Peterson HB, Xia Z, Hughes JM, et al. The risk of pregnancy after tubal sterilization: findings from the U.S. Collaborative Review of Sterilization. *Am J Obstet Gynecol* 1996;174:1161.

Polak JO, Wolfe SA. A further study of the origin of uterine bleeding in tubal pregnancy. *Am J Obstet Gynecol* 1924;8:730.

Pouly JL, Mahnes H, Mage G, et al. Conservative laparoscopic treatment of 321 ectopic pregnancies. *Fertil Steril* 1986;46:1093.

Pratt-Thomas HR, White L, Messer HH. Primary ovarian pregnancy: presentation of ten cases including one full-term pregnancy. *South Med J* 1974;67:920.

Rabischong B, Larrain D, Pouly JL, et al. Predicting success of laparoscopic salpingostomy for ectopic pregnancy. *Obstet Gynecol* 2010;116:701.

Raziel A, Golan A. Primary ovarian pregnancy successfully treated with methotrexate [letter; comment]. *Am J Obstet Gynecol* 1993;169:1362.

Reece EA, Petrie RH, Sirmans MF, et al. Combined intrauterine and extrauterine gestations: a review. *Am J Obstet Gynecol* 1983;146:323.

Risquez F, Pennehouat G, Foulot H, et al. Transcervical tubal cannulation and falloposcopy for the management of tubal pregnancy. *Fertil Steril* 1992;7:274.

Risquez F, Pennehoaut G, McCorvey, et al. Diagnostic and operative microlaparoscopy: a preliminary multicentre report. *Hum Reprod* 1997;12:1645.

Rojansky N, Schenker JG. Heterotopic pregnancy and assisted reproduction: an update. *J Assist Reprod Genet* 1996;13:594.

Rothe DJ, Birnbaum SJ. Cervical pregnancy: diagnosis and management. *Obstet Gynecol* 1973;42:675.

Rozenberg P, Chevret S, Camus S, et al. Medical treatment of ectopic pregnancies: a randomized clinical trial comparing methotrexate-mifepristone and methotrexate-placebo. *Hum Reprod* 2003;18:1802.

Rubin IC. Cervical pregnancy. *Surg Gynecol Obstet* 1911;13:625.

Sandberg EC, Pelligra R. The medical antigravity suit for management of surgically uncontrollable bleeding associated with abdominal pregnancy. *Am J Obstet Gynecol* 1983;146:519.

Saraiya M, Berg CJ, Kendrick JS, et al. Cigarette smoking as a risk factor for ectopic pregnancy. *Am J Obstet Gynecol* 1998;178:493.

Saraj AJ, Wilcox JG, Najmabadi S, et al. Resolution of hormonal markers of ectopic gestation: a randomized trial comparing single-dose intramuscular methotrexate with salpingostomy. *Obstet Gynecol* 1998;92:989.

Sauer MV, Gorrill MJ, Rodi LA, et al. Nonsurgical management of unruptured ectopic pregnancy: an extended clinical trial. *Fertil Steril* 1987;48:752.

Schiff E, Shalev E, Bostan M, et al. Pharmacokinetics of methotrexate after local tubal injection for conservative treatment of ectopic pregnancy. *Fertil Steril* 1992;57:688.

Schwartz RO, DiPietro DL. Beta-hCG as a diagnostic aid for suspected ectopic pregnancy. *Obstet Gynecol* 1980;56:197.

Seifer DB, Silva PD, Grainger DA, et al. Reproductive potential after treatment for persistent ectopic pregnancy. *Fertil Steril* 1994;62:194.

Seinera P, DiGregorio A, Arisio R, et al. Ovarian pregnancy and operative laparoscopy: report of eight cases. *Hum Reprod* 1997;12:608.

Shah A, Courey NG, Cunanan RG. Pregnancy following laparoscopic tubal electrocoagulation and excision. *Am J Obstet Gynecol* 1977;129:459.

Shapiro BS, Daneshmand ST, De Leon ST, et al. Frozen-thawed embryo transfer is associated with a significantly reduced incidence of ectopic pregnancy. *Fertil Steril* 2012;98:1490.

Shepherd RW, Patton PE, Novy MJ, et al. Serial beta-hCG measurements in the early detection of ectopic pregnancy. *Obstet Gynecol* 1990;75:417.

Shinagawa S, Nagayama M. Cervical pregnancy as a possible sequela of induced abortion: report of 19 cases. *Am J Obstet Gynecol* 1969;105:282.

Shoen JA, Nowak RJ. Repeat ectopic pregnancy: a 16-year clinical survey. *Obstet Gynecol* 1975;45:542.

Silva PD, Schaper AM, Rooney B. Reproductive outcome after 143 laparoscopic procedures for ectopic pregnancy. *Obstet Gynecol* 1993;81:710.

Smith M, Vessey MP, Bounds W, et al. Progestogen-only oral contraception and ectopic gestation. *BMJ* 1974;4:104.

Society for Assisted Reproductive Technology and American Society for Reproductive Medicine. Assisted reproductive technology in the United States: 2000 results generated from the American Society for Reproductive Medicine/Society for Assisted Reproductive Technology Registry. *Fertil Steril* 2004;81:1207.

Spandorfer SD, Menzin A, Barnhart KT, et al. Efficacy of frozen-section evaluation of uterine curettings in the diagnosis of ectopic pregnancy. *Am J Obstet Gynecol* 1996;175:603.

Spandorfer SD, Sawin SW, Benjamin I, et al. Postoperative day 1 serum human chorionic gonadotropin level as a predictor of persistent ectopic pregnancy after conservative surgical management. *Fertil Steril* 1997;68:430.

Spiegelberg O. Zur Casuistik den Ovarial-Schwangerschaft. *Arch Gynaek* 1878;13:73.

Stafford JC, Ragan WD. Abdominal pregnancy: review of current management. *Obstet Gynecol* 1977;50:548.

Stangel JJ, Gomel V. Techniques in conservative surgery for tubal gestation. *Clin Obstet Gynecol* 1980;23:1221.

Storeide O, Veholmen M, Eide M, et al. The incidence of ectopic pregnancy in Hordaland county, Norway 1976–1993. *Acta Obstet Gynecol Scand* 1997;76:345.

Stovall TG, Ling FW. Single-dose methotrexate: an expanded clinical trial. *Am J Obstet Gynecol* 1993;168:1759.

Stovall TG, Ling FW, Carson SA, et al. Nonsurgical diagnosis and treatment of tubal pregnancy. *Fertil Steril* 1990;54:537.

Stovall TG, Ling FW, Carson SA, et al. Serum progesterone and uterine curettage in differential diagnosis of ectopic pregnancy. *Fertil Steril* 1992;57:456.

Stovall TG, Ling FW, Gray LA, et al. Methotrexate treatment of unruptured ectopic pregnancy: a report of 100 cases. *Obstet Gynecol* 1991;77:749.

Strandell A, Thorburn J, Hamberger L. Risk factors for ectopic pregnancy in assisted reproduction. *Fertil Steril* 1999;71:282.

Stromme WB. Conservative surgery for ectopic pregnancy: a twenty-year review. *Obstet Gynecol* 1973;41:215.

Stromme WB. Salpingotomy for tubal pregnancy: report of a successful case. *Obstet Gynecol* 1953;1:472.

Studdiford WE. Primary peritoneal pregnancy. *Am J Obstet Gynecol* 1942;44:487.

Swolin K, Fall M. Ectopic pregnancy; recurrence, postoperative fertility and aspects of treatment based on 182 patients. *Acta Eur Fertil* 1972;3:147.

Tanaka T, Hayashi J, Kutsuzawa T, et al. Treatment of interstitial ectopic pregnancy with methotrexate: report of a successful case. *Fertil Steril* 1982;37:851.

Tatum HJ, Schmidt FH. Contraceptive and sterilization practices and extrauterine pregnancy: a realistic perspective. *Fertil Steril* 1977;28:407.

Thompson LR. Abdominal pregnancy at term with later removal of placenta. *Am J Surg* 1966;111:272.

Timor-Tritsch IE, Monteagudo A, Matera C, et al. Sonographic evolution of cornual pregnancies treated without surgery. *Obstet Gynecol* 1992;79:1044.

Timor-Tritsch IE, Monteagudo A, Santos R, et al. The diagnosis, treatment and follow-up of cesarean scar pregnancy. *Am J Obstet Gynecol* 2012;207:44e1.

Tulandi T, Al-Jaroudi D. Interstitial pregnancy: results from the Society of Reproductive Surgeons Registry. *Obstet Gynecol* 2004;103:47.

Tummon IS, Whitmore NA, Daniel SAJ, et al. Transferring more embryos increases risk of heterotopic pregnancy. *Fertil Steril* 1994;61:1065.

Ushakov FB, Elchalal U, Aceman PJ, et al. Cervical pregnancy: past and future. *Obstet Gynecol Surv* 1996;52:45.

Vasquez G, Winston RML, Brosens IA. Tubal mucosa and ectopic pregnancy. *BJOG* 1983;90:468.

Van Den Eeden SK, Shan J, Bruce C, et al. Ectopic pregnancy rate and treatment utilization in a large managed care organization. *Obstet Gynecol* 2005;105:1052.

Verhulst G, Camus M, Bollen N, et al. Analysis of the risk factors with regard to the occurrence of ectopic pregnancy after medically assisted procreation. *Hum Reprod* 1993;8:1284.

Walters MD, Eddy C, Pauerstein CJ. The contralateral corpus luteum and tubal pregnancy. *Obstet Gynecol* 1987;70:823.

Weinberg A, Sherwin AS. A new sign in roentgen diagnosis of advanced ectopic pregnancy. *Obstet Gynecol* 1956;7:99.

Weissman A, Fishman A. Uterine rupture following conservative surgery for interstitial pregnancy. *Eur J Obstet Gynecol Reprod Biol* 1992;44:237.

Werber J, Prasadarao PR, Harris VJ. Cervical pregnancy diagnosed by ultrasound. *Radiology* 1983;149:279.

Westrom L. Effect of acute pelvic inflammatory disease on fertility. *Am J Obstet Gynecol* 1975;121:707.

WHO Task Force. A multinational case-control study of ectopic pregnancy. *Clin Reprod Fertil* 1985;3:131.

Yao M, Tulandi T. Current status of surgical and nonsurgical management of ectopic pregnancy. *Fertil Steril* 1997;67:421.

Yeko TR, Gorrill MJ, Hughes LH, et al. Timely diagnosis of early ectopic pregnancy using a single blood progesterone measurement. *Fertil Steril* 1987;48:1048.

Zakaria MA, Abdallah ME, Shavell, VI, et al. Conservative management of cervical ectopic pregnancy: utility of uterine artery embolization. *Fertil Steril* 2011;95:872.

Zhang Y, Chen YS, Wang JJ, et al. Analysis of 96 cases with cesarean scar pregnancy. *Zhonghua Fe Chan Ke Za Zhi* 2010;45:664.

CHAPTER 35A
Surgical Management of Obstetric Complications

Kelly A. Bennett

DEFINITIONS

B-Lynch stitch—A uterine body compression suture used to control postpartum hemorrhage resulting from uterine atony. A deep suture is placed vertically on the side of the uterus from 3 cm below the end of the uterine incision to 3 cm above the incision. The suture is then taken over the fundus, and a horizontal bite is taken on the posterior wall of the uterus below the level of the uterine vessels entering the myometrium on the same side as the anterior stitch. The suture is again passed over the fundus on the opposite side, and a deep suture is placed starting 3 cm above the other end of the anterior uterine incision and exiting 3 cm below the incision. This large four-corner mattress suture is then tightly tied down, compressing the fundus.

Cervical insufficiency—Premature, painless dilation of the cervix leading to midtrimester delivery if not treated. The etiology of the condition is poorly understood and may be due to prior cervical trauma and/or an inherent cervical defect.

Cerclage—A purse-string suture placed around the cervix to treat or prevent premature cervical dilation without labor.

Late postpartum hemorrhage—Hemorrhage occurring more than 24 hours following delivery.

McDonald suture—Surgical treatment for cervical insufficiency. A purse-string suture of heavy caliber is placed around the cervix at the level of the internal os.

Placenta accreta—Abnormal invasion of the placenta into the decidual layer lining of the endometrial cavity with no plane of separation.

Placenta increta—The placenta penetrates into the myometrium.

Placenta percreta—The placenta penetrates through the whole thickness of the myometrium up to the serosal surfaces or beyond to surrounding organs.

Postpartum hemorrhage—Blood loss is difficult to estimate accurately; the American Congress of Obstetricians and Gynecologists has arbitrarily defined postpartum hemorrhage as blood loss of greater than 500 mL with a vaginal delivery or greater than 1,000 mL with a cesarean section. Other definitions describe a 10% drop in the hematocrit or the need for blood transfusion (as defined by CA Combs in 1991).

Shirodkar suture—A thick suture or mesh band is placed submucosally around the cervix to treat cervical insufficiency.

Surgery in the pregnant patient presents several unique challenges. There is, of course, the added complexity of caring for two patients simultaneously. Illness and surgery both affect the fetus and the mother, and every decision to recommend surgery and when that surgery should be done requires weighing the risks and benefits to both patients. In many cases, there may be some urgency required to prevent or reduce maternal or fetal morbidity or mortality. In addition, the physiologic and anatomic changes of pregnancy may complicate diagnosis and alter the surgeon's normal operative field. The size of the uterus and increased vascularity of the pelvis may make it significantly more difficult to perform routine gynecologic procedures during pregnancy.

PHYSIOLOGIC CHANGES OF PREGNANCY

Profound physiologic changes of the cardiovascular, respiratory, renal, and coagulation systems occur during pregnancy. It is important for the surgeon to understand these changes in order to understand normal from abnormal findings because they can affect laboratory interpretation, blood product replacement, and surgical approach.

Cardiovascular System

During pregnancy, maternal blood volume increases by 45% to 50% above nonpregnant volumes. Placental hormone production stimulates maternal erythropoiesis, increasing red cell mass by approximately 20%. Because plasma volume increases disproportionately to the increase in red blood cell mass, physiologic hemodilution occurs, manifested as a physiologic anemia. Pregnancy should be considered a hypervolemic state. A mild increase in maternal heart rate begins early in pregnancy and continues until term. In late pregnancy, maternal heart rate is increased by approximately 20% over antepartum values, often resulting in mild tachycardia.

Systemic vascular resistance decreases by 20%, but gradually increases near term. This results in a decrease in systolic and diastolic blood pressure during pregnancy, with a gradual recovery to nonpregnant values by term. As there is increased pressure in the venous system, there is decreased return from the lower extremities, resulting in dependent edema.

Respiratory System

In pregnancy, minute volume is increased, while functional residual volume is decreased. This is primarily the result of upward displacement of the diaphragm. It seems intuitive that lung volume would be decreased during pregnancy, but an increase in minute volume in association with an expansion of the anterior and posterior diameter of the chest results in increased tidal volume, thereby also increasing minute ventilation. These changes result in a compensated respiratory alkalosis. Normal PCO_2 in pregnancy ranges from 28 to 35 mm Hg. PO_2 is usually greater than or equal to 100 mm Hg. Oxygen consumption and basal metabolic rate are also increased during pregnancy by approximately 20%.

These physiologic changes result in less pulmonary reserve for the acutely ill pregnant patient; therefore, this reduces the time interval from respiratory distress to respiratory failure. Because of this, early recognition and intervention in patients with respiratory challenge is mandatory.

Gastrointestinal Tract

During pregnancy, there is a decrease in gastrointestinal motility. This is caused by mechanical changes in the abdomen with the enlarging uterus and smooth muscle relaxation induced by high production of progesterone in pregnancy. Gastric emptying may be delayed for up to 8 hours; therefore, pregnant women should be considered to have a functionally full stomach at all times. In addition, a decrease in large intestine motility may result in constipation severe enough to cause significant abdominal pain.

Coagulation Changes

Pregnancy is a hypercoagulable state. Fibrinogen is increased approximately 30% over baseline values. The hypercoagulable

VI

state of pregnancy is associated with increased risk of deep venous thrombosis and pulmonary embolus. This is particularly compounded when bed rest or immobilization occurs during the gestational period.

Renal Changes

Pregnancy increases blood flow to the renal pelvis approximately 60% to 80%. This results in an increased glomerular filtration rate accompanied by frequent urination. Serum creatinine is approximately 40% less than in a nonpregnant state. Therefore, a creatinine of 1 mg/dL during gestation should be considered to be at the upper limits of normal.

Ureteral diameter increases in pregnancy secondary to compression and smooth muscle relaxation. Peristalsis is delayed, and reflux occurs freely from the bladder into the lower ureteral segment. This results in an increased incidence of pyelonephritis during pregnancy, making treatment of significant asymptomatic bacteriuria mandatory.

IMAGING TECHNIQUES

The most common imaging technique used during pregnancy is *ultrasonography*. Ultrasound is considered safe and primarily is used for fetal assessment. In patients with abdominal pain, an ultrasound should be considered the first-line diagnostic imaging test. During ultrasound, the presence of an intrauterine pregnancy should be documented and the size and other pertinent parameters of fetal well-being should be recorded. Evaluation of the cul-de-sac for fluid, the ureter for dilatation or stones, the gallbladder for the presence of gallstones, and the placenta for abnormalities should also be noted in the report.

Magnetic resonance imaging can be safely used during pregnancy. There are no data to suggest any increased fetal risk from this modality. Magnetic resonance imaging is now used to diagnose fetal abnormalities, especially abnormalities of the central nervous system. It may be particularly important for the diagnosis of appendicitis in pregnancy.

Although there are theoretical risks associated with ionizing radiation, fortunately, most *diagnostic x-ray procedures* are associated with minimal or no risk to the fetus. While unnecessary, multiple, or recurrent x-ray exposure should be avoided, existing evidence suggests that there is no increased risk of fetal congenital malformations, growth restriction, or abortion from x-ray procedures that expose the fetus to doses of 5 rads or less. The American Congress of Obstetricians and Gynecologists has published guidelines regarding diagnostic imaging during pregnancy. Women should be reassured that concern about radiation exposure should not prevent medically indicated diagnostic procedures. It cannot be stressed enough that maternal well-being is of the utmost importance, and appropriate diagnostic procedures should be obtained to facilitate a rapid diagnosis.

POSTPARTUM HEMORRHAGE

Postpartum hemorrhage is poorly defined by estimation of blood loss; therefore, it is difficult to accurately determine actual or percentage of blood loss at the time of delivery. Additionally, blood volume expansion is variable during pregnancy and can be affected by several factors including hypertension, renal disease, maternal body mass index, and the presence of multifetal gestations. The potential effects of blood loss largely depend on the degree of blood volume expansion. For example, blood loss of 1,000 mL during cesarean section is generally well tolerated by healthy pregnant women. A blood loss of 500 to 750 mL, however, may not be tolerated in a woman with minimal volume

expansion or one who is hemoconcentrated secondary to severe preeclampsia or eclampsia. The American Congress of Obstetricians and Gynecologists has noted that a number of definitions have been used to define hemorrhage, including a blood loss greater than 500 mL with a vaginal delivery or greater than 1,000 mL during a cesarean section or a drop in hematocrit of 10% regardless of the amount of documented blood loss.

Gilstrap and Ramin have defined clinically significant hemorrhage as that amount of bleeding "that produces signs and symptoms of hemodynamic instability or that is likely to produce such if left unabated."

Incidence and Etiology

Although the exact incidence of hemorrhage associated with pregnancy is unknown, it remains one of the leading causes of maternal mortality in this country. Kaunitz and associates reported that 13% of more than 2,000 maternal deaths were secondary to hemorrhage, and one third of these occurred postpartum. Rochat and colleagues reported a similar incidence of 11% of maternal deaths resulting from hemorrhage.

In a randomized trial conducted in the United States, birth weight, labor induction and augmentation, chorioamnionitis, use of magnesium sulfate, and a maternal history of previous obstetrical hemorrhage were associated with increased risk of postpartum hemorrhage. A large population-based study supported these findings, with significant risk factors identified using multivariate analysis. Risk factors associated with an increased risk of postpartum hemorrhage were retained placenta (odds ratio [OR] 3.5; 95% confidence interval [CI]: 2.1 to 5.8), failure to progress during the second stage of labor (OR 3.4; 95% CI: 2.4 to 4.7), placenta accreta (OR 3.3; 95% CI: 1.7 to 6.4), vaginal or perineal lacerations (OR 2.4; 95% CI: 2.0 to 2.8), instrumental delivery (OR 2.3; 95% CI: 1.6 to 3.4), large-for-gestational-age newborn (OR 1.9; 95% CI: 1.6 to 2.4), hypertensive disorders (OR 1.7; 95% CI: 1.2 to 2.1), induction of labor (OR 1.4; 95% CI: 1.1 to 1.7), and augmentation of labor with oxytocin (OR 1.4; 95% CI: 1.2 to 1.7).

Diagnosis and Medical Management

The most important aspects in the management of postpartum hemorrhage are prompt recognition and treatment of the condition. Recognition of external bleeding is straightforward and almost always can be controlled with medical or minor surgical means. Tachycardia, decreased urine output, and, finally, hypotension without obvious external blood loss are important signs of potential internal bleeding, and many such instances will require surgical intervention to arrest the hemorrhage. If the etiology of the hemorrhage is not determined quickly, coagulopathy may complicate the clinical presentation, thereby making diagnosis and treatment more difficult.

Uterine atony is readily recognizable by palpation of the uterus. If atony it not present, the cervix and vagina should be carefully inspected for lacerations. The placenta also should be inspected for missing fragments, and careful manual palpation of the uterine cavity should be performed. If the source of bleeding still is not obvious or if bleeding is seen around venipuncture or catheter sites, then the patient should be evaluated for coagulopathy. A thrombin clot (clot retraction test) tube will reveal gross disruption in coagulation within minutes. Useful laboratory tests include prothrombin time, partial thromboplastin time, platelet count, fibrinogen, and fibrin degradation product levels. The clinician should note that d-dimer levels may be abnormal during pregnancy even in patients without coagulopathy. Before surgical intervention, an ultrasound examination of the uterine cavity may prove useful for the identification of an accessory placental lobe or fragment.

Medical management of postpartum hemorrhage consists of volume replacement and uterotonics, including intravenous oxytocin and parenteral methylergonovine and prostaglandins. Volume can be maintained with crystalloid and blood or blood products. Invasive monitoring, such as with a pulmonary artery catheter, generally is not necessary and may be dangerous in the presence of a coagulopathy. Its use should be reserved for those patients who do not respond to usual and expected therapy. As a general rule, monitoring of urine output, vital signs, and oxygen saturation will be sufficient. Volume replacement generally is adequate when the blood pressure is maintained at 90 to 100 mm Hg systolic, pulse rate is less than 100 beats per minute, and urine output is at least 25 to 30 mL per hour. When a patient has required transfusion of packed red blood cells, it is important to transfuse coagulation factors to replace those lost in the hemorrhage. Calcium also should be replaced in these patients because of risk of complications such as hypotension related to hypocalcemia in patients receiving massive transfusions. Fluid overload generally can be detected with a stethoscope and an oxygen monitor in conjunction with clinical signs and symptoms. Diuretics should only be used to remove excess fluid if the patient becomes hypoxic related to volume overload. A medical management protocol for postpartum hemorrhage is summarized in Table 35A.1.

Surgical Management

Lower genital tract lacerations usually are best managed by suturing. The rare case of uterine rupture also is managed surgically. Other techniques to control hemorrhage include uterine and utero-ovarian artery ligation, hysterectomy, or uterine or hypogastric artery embolization.

Uterine packing, which until recently had been abandoned by most clinicians, may allow adequate time for blood and fluid replacement before surgical intervention. Maier described the use of a packing device called a Torpin packer. The device uses a plunger to place several yards of 4-inch-wide gauze into the uterine cavity and has been used successfully to control postpartum hemorrhage. Uterine packing allows time for volume

---

TABLE 35A.1 Medical Management Protocol for Postpartum Hemorrhage

General
  Large-bore intravenous line
  Foley catheter

Drugs
  Oxytocin, dilute solution of 20 U in 1,000 mL of normal saline or Ringer solution, given as IV infusion
  Methylergonovine, 0.2 mg IM
  15-Methyl PGF$_{2\alpha}$, 0.25 mg IM or intramyometrially every 15–60 min as indicated

Volume Replacement
  Crystalloid, 3 mL/mL of estimated blood loss (maintain urine output ≥30 mL/h)
  Packed red blood cells
  Fresh frozen plasma, platelets, or cryoprecipitate, as indicated

IM, intramuscularly; IV, intravenously.
Reprinted from American College of Obstetricians and Gynecologists. *ACOG Technical Bulletin No. 143: Diagnosis and management of postpartum hemorrhage.* Washington, DC: ACOG, 1990, with permission. Copyright © 1991, Elsevier.

---

replacement and slows bleeding enough to allow for surgical techniques short of hysterectomy. In many cases, it may stop the bleeding so that no further treatment is necessary. Other methods of uterine tamponade reported in the literature have included the use of a Foley catheter with a 30- to 50-mL balloon or a Sengstaken-Blakemore tube with the esophageal balloon inflated with 50 mL of normal saline and, more recently, the use of the Bakery balloon. The choice of a specific surgical technique to control bleeding depends on several factors, including the degree of hemorrhage, the hemodynamic status of the patient, parity, and the desire for future childbearing. An undoubtedly important factor in achieving a favorable outcome in control of postpartum hemorrhage is the experience of the surgeon.

Arterial Embolization

Angiographic arterial embolization has been described for the successful control of obstetric and gynecologic bleeding. Small metal coils, Gelfoam, polyvinyl alcohol dehydrated particles, and other substances have been used for such embolizations. Pelage and associates, in two separate reports, describe use of arterial embolization in patients with primary or secondary postpartum hemorrhage, defining primary postpartum hemorrhage as that which occurs within 24 hours after delivery. Twenty-seven women were identified, including two who had already undergone hysterectomy in an unsuccessful attempt to control the hemorrhage. Following transcatheter embolization, immediate decrease or cessation of bleeding occurred in all patients. Two patients required repeat embolization the next day with no further complications. Fourteen women were diagnosed with secondary postpartum hemorrhage after the first 24 hours following delivery. All of these patients had complete resolution of bleeding with embolization with no further complications. Arterial embolization can be performed quickly and safely; therefore, it should be strongly considered in patients with postpartum hemorrhage who are stable enough to be managed in the radiology suite. There have been reports of successful pregnancies following embolization, which makes it an especially attractive alternative to hysterectomy in the patient who desires preservation of fertility.

Uterine Artery Ligation

STEPS IN THE PROCEDURE

Uterine Artery and Utero-Ovarian Artery Ligation (O'Leary Stitch)

- First-line treatment to control postpartum hemorrhage at the time of cesarean delivery.

- Advance bladder before placement of sutures is important to avoid bladder injury.

- Absorbable suture no. 0 chromic or polyglycolic acid suture is placed through the lateral aspect of the lower uterine segment, 2 to 3 cm medial to the uterine vessels through the myometrium, and then back through the broad ligament just lateral to the uterine vessels.

- The suture is tied *to compress the vessels.*

- Placement of second ligature at junction of the utero-ovarian ligament and uterus.

Uterine artery ligation is a relatively safe procedure that can be performed by most obstetricians. It also allows for future childbearing. The technique consists of ligating the uterine artery and vein at the lower uterine segment 2 to 3 cm below the level of the transverse uterine incision. An

VI

absorbable ligature is placed 2 to 3 cm medial to the uterine vessels through the myometrium (to obliterate any intramyometrial ascending branches) and then lateral to the vessels through the broad ligament. It is imperative that the bladder be advanced before placement of the suture to prevent bladder injury. Because of collateral flow from the ovarian artery, some recommend that a second ligature be placed at the junction of the utero-ovarian ligament and uterus. The technique of uterine artery ligation is shown in Figures 35A.1 and 35A.2.

In a review of 90 women who underwent uterine artery ligation (30 were for uterine atony), O'Leary reported that only six (7%) procedures resulted in failure. There were no major complications from the procedure itself. In a follow-up review of 265 women who underwent uterine artery ligation, O'Leary reported a greater-than-95% success rate.

This technique is most useful (and successful) when hemorrhage is of a moderate degree and originates from the lower uterine segment. Such an example is bleeding from a low placental implantation site. Uterine artery ligation also can prove beneficial for lower segment extensions or lacerations, in addition to slowing bleeding for a uterine artery laceration. Philippe and associates reported a vaginal approach to ligation of the uterine arteries in two patients after vaginal delivery, but a larger case series would have to be performed to determine the feasibility of this approach.

B-Lynch Suture

STEPS IN THE PROCEDURE

B-Lynch Suture Placement

- The B-Lynch suture is an effective method for reducing uterine blood loss related to uterine atony.
- A large Mayo needle with absorbable suture is used to enter and exit the uterine cavity laterally in the lower uterine segment.
- The initial placement is anteriorly at one angle of the uterine incision.
- The suture is passed over the uterine fundus.
- A deep transverse bite is taken in the posterior lower uterine segment.

- The suture is then passed back over the fundus to enter the anterior lower uterine segment opposite and parallel to the initial bite.
- The free ends are pulled tightly and tied down securely to compress the uterus.

B-Lynch and colleagues also described five cases in which hemorrhage was controlled by placing an absorbable suture vertically from 3 cm below the uterine incision to 3 cm above the uterine incision on the right side of the uterus (Fig. 35A.3). The stitch is then taken vertically over the fundus and placed horizontally in the posterior uterus at the same level as the anterior suture. The suture is threaded over the left side of the uterus to place another stitch on the left from 3 cm above the uterine incision to 3 cm below the uterine incision. The long suture is tied, compressing the fundus. A large suture, such as no. 1 Prolene on a large needle, is used. The uterine incision is closed in the usual fashion. There are several case series in the literature supporting the efficacy of the B-Lynch stitch for the treatment of uterine atony. In all series, the suture has been reported to be effective. It has been suggested that the B-Lynch be considered in all cases of severe postpartum hemorrhage before resorting to hysterectomy.

Hypogastric Artery Ligation

STEPS IN THE PROCEDURE

Hypogastric Artery Ligation: Ligation Performed Bilaterally

- Open the peritoneum overlying the common iliac artery.
- Identify the ureter and retract medially.
- Longitudinally open the sheath covering the internal iliac (hypogastric) artery.
- A right angle clamp is passed lateral to the medial direction with blunt dissection.
- Two nonabsorbable 2-0 silk sutures are placed 2 cm distal to the bifurcation.
- Hypogastric artery ligation should be performed bilaterally to adequately decrease pressure to the uterus.

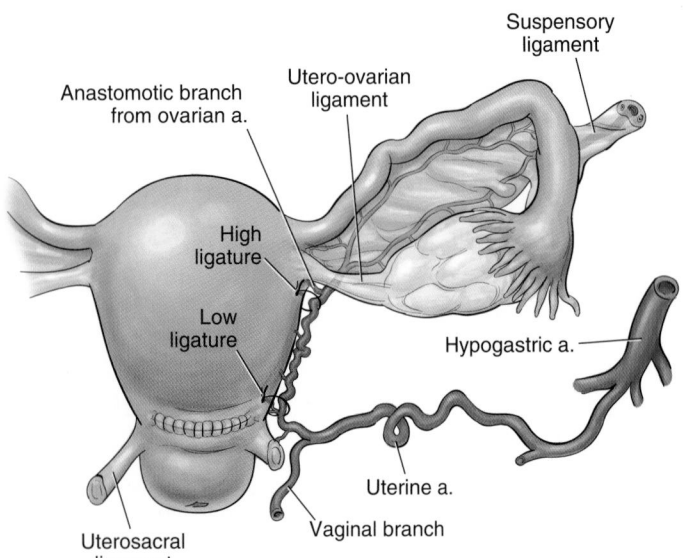

FIGURE 35A.1 Uterine artery ligation.

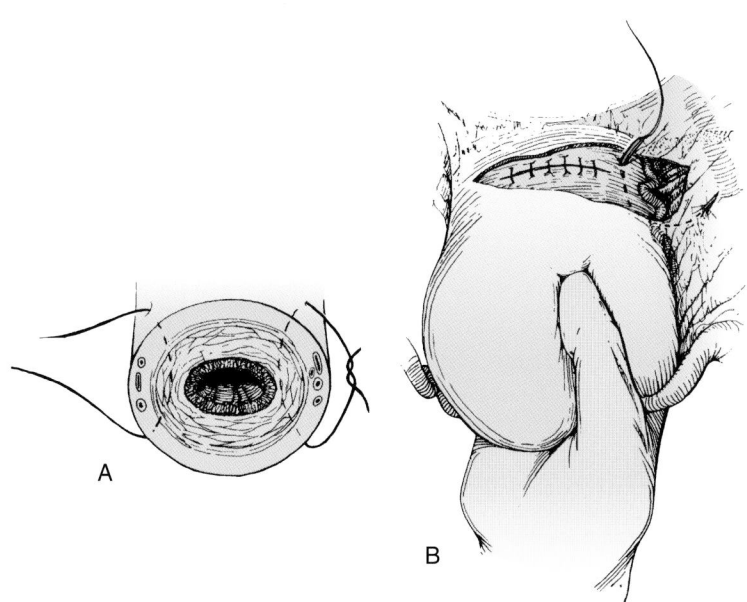

FIGURE 35A.2 Uterine artery ligation. A: Lateral view demonstrating ligature placement. B: Anatomic relation of ligature to uterine wall and vessels. (Reprinted from Floyd RC, Morrison JC. Postpartum hemorrhage. In: Plauche WC, Morrison JC, O'Sullivan MJ, eds. *Surgical obstetrics.* Philadelphia, PA: WB Saunders, 1992:272, with permission. Copyright © 1992, Elsevier.)

The major blood supply to the uterus and pelvis comes from the internal iliac artery, often called the hypogastric artery. Bilateral ligation of this artery can effectively control significant bleeding and thus prevent the need for hysterectomy and permanent sterilization. Burchell has aptly described the physiology of internal iliac artery ligation. It appears that ligation of this artery controls bleeding by converting an arterial system into a venous system, which decreases the pulse pressure by as much as 85%. This allows pressure and packing to produce clotting. Hypogastric artery ligation probably interferes little, if at all, with subsequent pregnancies. Mengert and colleagues reported successful pregnancies in five women who had undergone internal iliac artery ligation. This technique also may prove useful for controlling bleeding in patients with large hematomas of the broad ligament or for a lacerated artery that has retracted into the broad ligament.

Such vessels or active bleeding sites often are difficult to identify. If the bleeding is from the hypogastric vein, ligation of the hypogastric artery will decrease venous pressure which makes the bleeding easier to control.

The technique of hypogastric artery ligation is illustrated in Figure 35A.4. The peritoneum overlying the external iliac artery is divided directly above the artery between the infundibulopelvic ligament and the round ligament of the uterus. The internal iliac (hypogastric) artery is identified as it arises and runs from the common iliac artery posteriorly into the pelvis just beneath the infundibulopelvic ligament. The ligation should be performed about 2 cm distal to the bifurcation to avoid disrupting the posterior division of the hypogastric, which can lead to ischemia and necrosis of the skin and subcutaneous tissue of the gluteus. A right angle clamp is gently passed under the artery in the lateral to medial direction with blunt dissection. Great care must

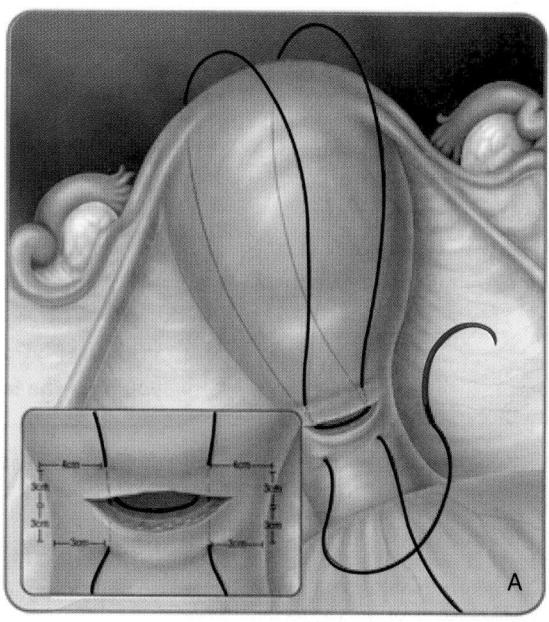

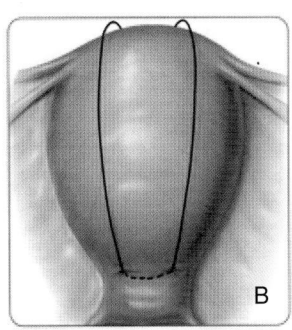

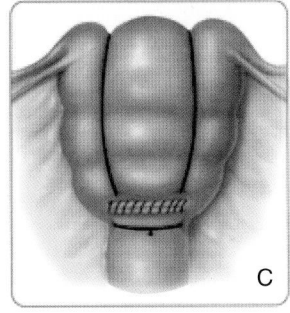

FIGURE 35A.3 Technique of B-Lynch suture placement. A: The initial bite is placed anteriorly at one angle of the uterine incision (see **inset**). B: After the anterior B-Lynch suture is placed, the suture is passed over the fundus, a deep transverse bite is taken in the posterior lower uterine segment, and the suture is passed back over the fundus.

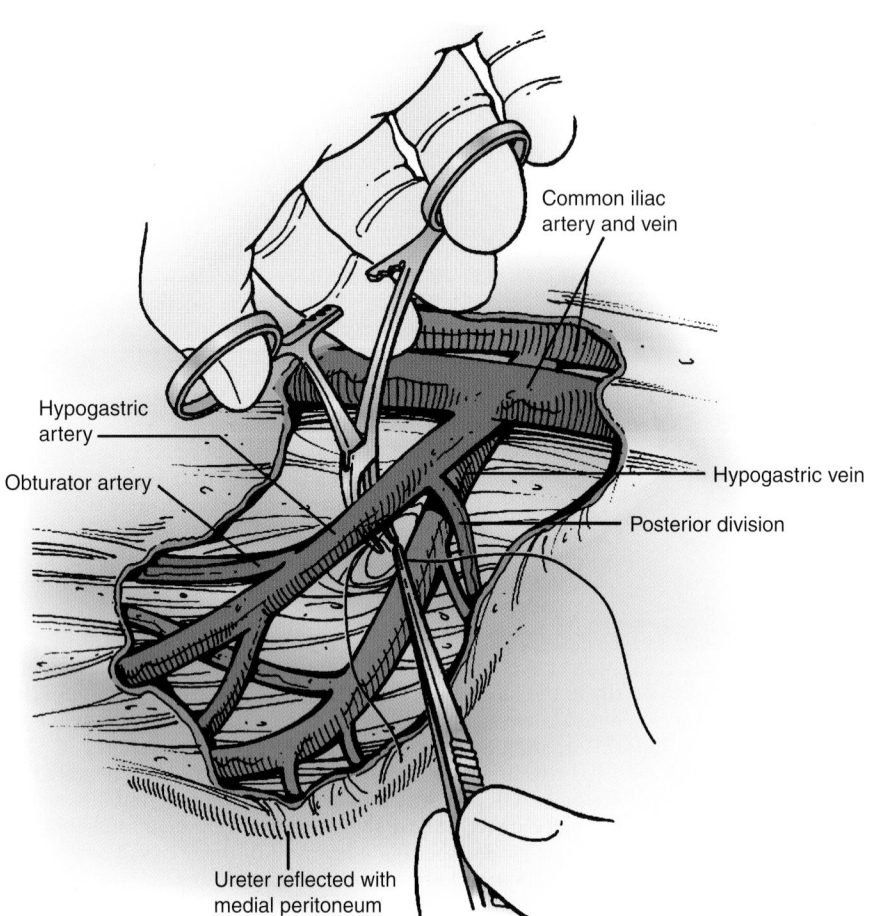

FIGURE 35A.4 Ligation of the right hypogastric artery. The clamp is passed laterally to medial, and the ligature is placed around the anterior division of the hypogastric artery. Note the ureter is attached to the peritoneum, which is reflected medially.

be taken not to perforate the internal iliac vein, and the clamp is passed lateral to medial to avoid injury to the vein by the tip of the clamp. Two nonabsorbable sutures of 2-0 silk should be used for ligation. It is important that hypogastric artery ligation be performed bilaterally to adequately decrease systolic pressure to the uterus. Clark and associates reported on the successful control of bleeding in 8 (42%) of 19 women who underwent hypogastric artery ligation. In a review of hypogastric artery ligation from three series, Clark reported that this procedure prevented hysterectomy in about half of the patients associated with uterine atony and placenta accreta. Interestingly, in this series, the success of hypogastric artery ligation did not appear to be related directly to the conditions for which it was performed. It must be noted, however, that the number of patients in each category is small.

Although this procedure is successful in about 50% of patients and does not interfere with subsequent fertility, it is not technically easy to perform and requires special skill and experience. Many obstetricians have little, if any, experience with this procedure, especially in the presence of a surgical emergency. Moreover, potential complications of hypogastric artery ligation include laceration of the iliac vein, ligation of the external iliac artery, ureteral injury, and death.

Hysterectomy

Because of the lack of experience and skill with the technique of hypogastric artery ligation, many clinicians prefer to do a hysterectomy to control postpartum hemorrhage. Peripartum hysterectomy is extensively discussed later in this chapter.

Hysterectomy usually is the safest procedure and also the quickest that can be performed for refractory bleeding. For example, Clark and associates reported that patients undergoing hypogastric artery ligation who subsequently required hysterectomy had an increased incidence of cardiac arrest secondary to blood loss. The increased morbidity associated with hypogastric artery ligation followed by hysterectomy may be secondary to a delay resulting from attempted conservative management short of hysterectomy. Hypogastric artery ligation was attempted before hysterectomy 64% of the time in nulliparous women, compared with 10% of the time for multiparous patients. Lack of experience with hypogastric artery ligation adds to the overall time required to attempt the procedure and overall blood loss.

In a review of 70 women who underwent emergency hysterectomy for postpartum hemorrhage, Clark and colleagues reported that almost all required blood transfusion, and 50% had postoperative febrile morbidity. The most common indication for hysterectomy in this series was uterine atony, followed by placenta accreta. Of the 70 procedures, 60 were performed after cesarean delivery. Mean operating time was 3.1 hours, and mean blood loss was 3,575 mL.

ABNORMAL PLACENTATION

Placenta accreta occurs when the placenta attaches abnormally to the underlying uterine wall. It is believed to occur due to an abnormal attachment of the chorionic villi to the myometrium due to an absence of decidua basalis and incomplete development of the fibrinoid layer. Placenta increta occurs when the placenta extends in to the myometrium, and placenta percreta occurs when the placenta invades through the myometrium and serosa with possible involvement of adjacent organs. Because of the abnormal attachment to the myometrium, there is a risk of life-threatening hemorrhage often requiring massive transfusion of blood products and hysterectomy. The maternal mortality rate was reported in 1996 by O'Brien and his group to be as high as 6% to 7%.

Flood and his group reported in 2009 that the incidence of placenta accreta has increased from approximately 0.8 per 1,000 deliveries in the 1980s to 3 per 1,000 in the past decade. The rising incidence of placenta accreta parallels the rising cesarean section rate. Important risk factors include prior history of placenta previa, previous cesarean delivery, increasing parity and maternal age, and prior uterine surgery. Antepartum diagnosis of placenta accreta is best accomplished by ultrasound, with a reported sensitivity of 77%, specificity of 71%, and a positive predictive value of 65%. Sonographic findings that may be associated with accreta include loss of normal hypoechoic retroplacental myometrial zone, thinning of the uterine serosa–bladder interface, and increased vascularity at the interface of the uterus and bladder. Magnetic resonance imaging may be helpful if there is suspicion that the placenta has invaded the parametrium or surrounding organs.

LATE POSTPARTUM HEMORRHAGE

Late postpartum hemorrhage is defined as occurring more than 24 hours after delivery. The etiology of such bleeding includes placental site subinvolution, infection, coagulopathy, and retained products of conception. Initial therapy for this complication is the same as for early hemorrhage. If infection is present, antibiotics should be used. Endometrial curettage may be necessary for retained placental fragments. Angiographic embolization may prove especially useful in the case of late postpartum hemorrhage. Uterine artery ligation, hypogastric artery ligation, and hysterectomy are rarely required for control of late postpartum hemorrhage.

PERIPARTUM HYSTERECTOMY

Horatio Storer performed the first cesarean hysterectomy in 1869. Initially, the procedure was performed only for emergency situations, but in the early 20th century, it became an accepted means of sterilization. In the modern obstetrical age, elective cesarean hysterectomy is rarely performed, except in cases of cervical neoplasia.

Peripartum hysterectomy can be performed in conjunction with a cesarean delivery (e.g., cesarean hysterectomy) or after a vaginal delivery for complications such as postpartum hemorrhage. In a recent review of a nationwide sample of deliveries from 1998 to 2003, Whiteman and colleagues estimated that the rate of peripartum hysterectomy in the United States is 0.77 per 1,000 deliveries.

Although there is little controversy regarding peripartum hysterectomy for emergency conditions, there is significant debate in modern obstetrics regarding an elective hysterectomy performed at the time of cesarean delivery. There has been legitimate concern about increased morbidity related to peripartum hysterectomy—including damage to the ureters, bladder, and rectum—and an increased rate of reoperation. However, Plauche has pointed out that morbidity often is associated with the conditions leading to the hysterectomy and not necessarily the procedure itself. Lower morbidities have been reported for elective cesarean hysterectomies when compared

with emergency hysterectomies. However, there is inherent bias in these retrospective reviews. Emergent surgery for life-saving maternal indications would be expected to have higher morbidities, such as blood loss and injury to surrounding structures. In a retrospective study, Castaneda and colleagues observed that over the years the indications for peripartum hysterectomy have changed from predominantly elective to almost exclusively emergent indications. In their series, the average blood loss was 3,009 mL in emergent cases and 1,262 mL in nonemergent cases. They concluded that, at the present time, peripartum hysterectomy is almost always emergent in nature and associated with a significant blood loss. As might be expected, there are no randomized prospective studies of elective cesarean hysterectomy, and it is unlikely that such a study could ever be done given the ethical dilemma involved.

Emergency Peripartum Hysterectomy

Obstetric hemorrhage secondary to a variety of etiologies is a common indication reported for peripartum emergency hysterectomy. The three most common reasons are uterine rupture, abnormal placentation, and uterine atony. Although the exact incidence of emergency peripartum hysterectomy is not known, several authors have reported widely varying rates of 0.004 to 1.5 per 1,000 deliveries.

Clark and associates reviewed 70 cases of emergency hysterectomy for obstetric hemorrhage and found that 60 (86%) of these procedures were performed after cesarean delivery and 10 (14%) were performed after vaginal delivery. Uterine atony and placenta accreta accounted for almost three fourths of the cases. Other indications were uterine rupture, extension of the uterine incision, and fibroids precluding closure of the uterine incision.

It is clear from the literature that *abnormal adherent placentation or placenta accreta (with or without hemorrhage) is emerging as the most common condition leading to an emergency hysterectomy.* In three studies from 1993 to the present, 156 (56%) of the 279 emergent peripartum hysterectomies were performed for placenta accreta. These studies are outlined in Table 35A.2. *The increase in placenta accreta is related to the high rate of cesarean deliveries,* which has risen in the United States from 5% in the early 1960s to 30% at the present time. A recent study of more than 60,000 deliveries at the University of Chicago by Wu et al. found that the rate of placenta accreta had increased to 3 per 1,000 deliveries in 2003. They observed that this was directly associated with the increase in cesarean section rate. Clarke and colleagues found that in the presence of a placenta previa, the risk of having placenta accreta increased from 24% in women with one prior cesarean delivery to 67% in women with 3 or more prior cesareans.

Cesarean Hysterectomy

STEPS IN THE PROCEDURE

Cesarean Hysterectomy

- Midline skin incision.
- Cesarean delivery with dissection of bladder flap.
- Placenta removal unless placental invasion exists.
- If accreta is suspected, clamp cord and leave placenta in situ.
- Close the uterine incision with a no. 1 suture placed in a running locking fashion.

VI

TABLE 35A.2 Indications for Emergency Hysterectomy for Obstetric Hemorrhage

INDICATION	CLARK ET AL. (1984) (*n* = 70)	BAKSHI ET AL. (2000) (*n* = 39)	STANCO ET AL. (1993) (*n* = 123)	ZELOP ET AL. (1993) (*n* = 117)
Uterine atony/hemorrhage	30 (43%)	11 (28%)	44 (35.9%)	25 (21.3%)
Placenta accreta/percreta	21 (30%)	20 (51%)	61 (49%)	75 (64.1%)
Uterine rupture	9 (13%)	5 (15%)	14 (11.5%)	—
Extension of uterine incision	7 (10%)	—	—	—
Leiomyomata	3 (4%)	2 (5%)	3 (2.4%)	—
Uterine infection	—	—	—	17 (14.5%)
Other	—	1 (1%)	1 (1.2%)	—

- Ligate the round ligament close to the uterus using 0 Vicryl.
- Open the peritoneum superiorly.
- Identify the ureters crossing the iliac artery at the level of the bifurcation in the medial leaf of the broad ligament.
- Identify the utero-ovarian ligaments, then clamp, cut, and ligate bilaterally.
- With upward traction on the uterus, identify and clamp the uterine vessels bilaterally (using a Heaney or Zeppelin clamp); vascular pedicles are double ligated.
- Using a straight or slightly curved clamp, clamp, cut, and tie the cardinal and uterosacral ligaments at the level of the cervix.
- Remove the uterus by clamping across the vagina on each side and incising the vaginal mucosa.
- Secure the lateral vaginal fornix to the cardinal and uterosacral ligaments.
- Close the vaginal cuff with interrupted figure-of-eight sutures.
- Inspect all pedicles for bleeding.
- Close the abdominal incision.

Although a number of conditions have been reported as indications for elective cesarean hysterectomy, currently accepted indications are usually limited to microinvasive or invasive cervical cancer. In retrospective reviews that go back to the 1950s and 1960s, sterilization, menstrual abnormalities, and uterine fibroids are listed as indications; however, most practitioners would not consider these appropriate indications for such an invasive surgical procedure in the 21st century.

Morbidity and Mortality of Hysterectomy

The conditions leading to emergency hysterectomy also are responsible for much of the morbidity reported with the procedure. Two other important factors associated with morbidity, both of which are difficult to quantify, are training and experience (or surgical skill) of the surgeon. Chestnut and associates reported statistically significant reductions in operative time, estimated blood loss, intraoperative and total blood replacement, and length of hospital stay if the patient was in the care of an experienced surgeon. It seems reasonable, however, to conclude that morbidity and complications are also higher in women undergoing emergency versus elective procedures despite the skill of the surgeon.

Zelop and associates reported 102 (87%) of the patients in their series required transfusion of blood products. Complications of three series, totaling 279 cases of emergency peripartum hysterectomy, are summarized in Table 35A.3. Maternal mortality rates in these studies varied between 0% and 4.5%. As with morbidity, mortality is better correlated with the specific complication than with the hysterectomy per se.

In a review of 80 women undergoing elective cesarean hysterectomy, McNulty reported that only 5 (6%) experienced febrile morbidity and 15 (19%) received blood transfusion. Four (5%) women sustained bladder injuries, and 4 (5%) women developed broad ligament hematomas. Yancey and colleagues compared the outcomes in 43 women undergoing scheduled cesarean hysterectomy with those of 86 women who underwent cesarean delivery and subsequent scheduled delayed postpartum hysterectomy. Although women in the cesarean hysterectomy group were more likely to need a blood transfusion than were women in the subsequent hysterectomy group (OR 3.4; 95% CI: 1.4 to 8.4), they were less likely to have other complications, such as infection (OR 0.34; 95% CI: 0.25 to 0.45). The overall postoperative complication rate was the same in both groups (51%). Thus, it appears from the older literature that *elective* cesarean hysterectomy is not associated with an increased risk of complications or morbidity compared with a cesarean delivery followed by an elective hysterectomy at a later time. However, in a healthy population, one must weigh the risk of blood transfusion versus the benefit of the combined procedure. As pointed out by Baker and D'Alton, there is little doubt that elective cesarean hysterectomy is associated with increased morbidity when compared with a cesarean delivery and a tubal ligation.

Emergency versus Elective Hysterectomy

In two studies comparing emergency with elective peripartum hysterectomy, morbidity was greater with the emergency procedure. Estimated blood loss, number of women transfused, and operating time were all higher in the emergency group.

TABLE 35A.3 Complications of 279 Cases of Emergency Peripartum Hysterectomy

	COMPLICATION INCIDENCE (%)			
	CLARK ET AL. (*n* = 70)	BAKSHI ET AL. (*n* = 39)	STANCO ET AL. (*n* = 123)	ZELOP ET AL. (*n* = 117)
Infection	50	20.5	9	50
Wound infection	12	—	9	3.4
Blood transfusion	96	80	82	87
Coagulopathy	6	2.5	5.7	27
Urologic injury	4	7.7	13	10.2
Death	1	0	0	0

It is important to remember that many of the patients who undergo emergent delivery have already had significant blood loss and hemorrhage before the decision is made to proceed with hysterectomy.

Cesarean Hysterectomy Technique

Elective cesarean hysterectomy can be accomplished through either a midline or low transverse (Pfannenstiel) skin incision. Often, it is more prudent to use a midline skin incision, which affords better surgical exposure.

After the cesarean delivery, the placenta is quickly removed unless there is a contraindication to do so. *No attempt is made to remove the placenta in cases of placenta accreta because significant life-threatening hemorrhage can ensue.* In cases of placenta percreta involving the posterior wall of the bladder, a partial cystectomy may be required. In these cases, the bladder trigone and ureteral orifices must be carefully identified, and urologic consultation may be needed. In cases of anterior placenta previa and suspected placenta accreta, it is prudent to arrange for urologic support preoperatively. In cases of suspected accreta, some interventional radiologists may place bilateral hypogastric artery balloons preoperatively. When inflated, these balloons have significantly decreased operative blood loss in our experience.

The uterine incision can be closed with a running no. 1 suture in a locking fashion. The bladder flap should be dissected well down before the start of the hysterectomy. This is best accomplished at the time of the cesarean delivery. The bladder should be dissected off the anterior, lower uterine segment with sharp dissection if firm adhesions are encountered. Firm adhesions often are present in patients who have undergone multiple cesarean deliveries. If bleeding is a problem, further dissection of the bladder from the lower uterine segment can be accomplished after ligation of the uterine artery. If significant difficulty or bleeding is encountered in dissection of the bladder flap, a supracervical hysterectomy should be considered. Bleeding many also be diminished after the uterine arteries have been ligated bilaterally, so another attempt to dissect the bladder off of the anterior cervix may be considered at this time.

The actual hysterectomy is begun by ligating the round ligament close to the uterus and ligating the distal stump with a 0 Vicryl suture ligature. The vesicouterine serosa, where the bladder was attached before its dissection, then is extended laterally to the severed round ligaments.

The peritoneal incision should be extended superiorly. Because the ureters are dilated in pregnancy, they should

be identified quickly to avoid injury. The ureter can be seen crossing the iliac artery at the level of the bifurcation in the medial leaf of the broad ligament and is most easily identified at this location. The utero-ovarian ligaments can be secured by first making a "window" through the posterior leaf of the broad ligament and then doubly clamping, cutting, and ligating the utero-ovarian ligament bilaterally (Fig. 35A.5). This step is easy and uncomplicated in the nonpregnant patient, but the dilated vasculature of pregnancy requires the surgeon to carefully select a clear window and handle the tissues gently to avoid troublesome bleeding from easily torn veins. The uterine vessels are skeletonized as in the nonpuerperal

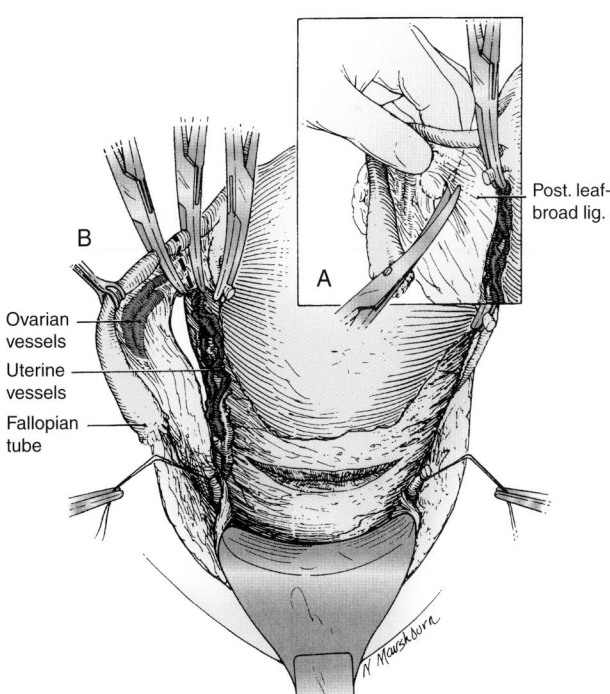

FIGURE 35A.5 A: The posterior leaf of the broad ligament adjacent to the uterus is perforated just beneath the fallopian tube, utero-ovarian ligaments, and ovarian vessels. **B:** These are then doubly clamped close to the uterus and severed. (From Cunningham FG, MacDonald PC, Gant NF, et al. Caesarean section and caesarean hysterectomy. In: *Williams obstetrics*, 19th ed. Norwalk, CT: Appleton & Lange, 1993:591, with permission from The McGraw-Hill Companies, Inc.)

hysterectomy. These vessels are large and easy to identify. Dissection is made easier with continuous upward traction of the uterus. If possible, the uterine vessels are clamped bilaterally (usually with a Heaney or Zeppelin clamp) before the vessels are cut. If there is room, we prefer to place three large clamps on each side and divide the pedicle between the first and second clamp (Fig. 35A.6). This provides two clamps on the active vessels for security and one back clamp to prevent back bleeding from the enlarged, blood-engorged uterus. The vascular pedicles are doubly ligated with 0 synthetic absorbable sutures, and we generally prefer to suture ligate the back bleeders also, so that the back camps can be removed from the field. This provides better exposure and reduces the risk of tearing the uterine tissues by excessive traction on these clamps. Once the uterine vessels are secured bilaterally, bleeding should be decreased and the situation should be reevaluated. Taking into account the indication for the hysterectomy in the first place, the stability of the patient, the blood loss to this point and an estimation of additional blood loss, and the pelvic anatomy, the surgeon may elect to complete the total hysterectomy or decide that, if the bleeding is now well controlled but the patient is unstable or further pelvic dissection risks urinary tract injury or hemorrhage, a supracervical hysterectomy may be advisable. As with all hysterectomies, care must be exercised in identifying and avoiding the ureter.

The next pedicles encountered should be the broad ligament, the base of which is the cardinal ligament. A slightly curved or a straight clamp, whichever fits the anatomy best, can be used for these ligaments. It is better to take several small pedicles instead of one large bite, because an excessively large pedicle can slide out of a clamp or suture. This is especially true with the edematous tissues associated with pregnancy. Once the cardinal and uterosacral ligaments have been clamped, cut, and tied at the level of the cervix, the specimen can be removed by clamping across the vagina on each side and incising the vaginal mucosa (Fig. 35A.7). It may be difficult to identify the lower extent of the cervix, especially if the cervix is effaced. The cervix can be grasped with a thumb anteriorly and the hand wrapping around the cervix with the fingers posteriorly. The cervix is then pinched between the thumb and middle finger as the hand slowly slides down the cervix toward the vagina. Usually, it is possible to feel the lower end of the cervix in this way. If there is any doubt, it may also be helpful to make an incision into what is believed to be the anterior vagina just below the cervix using the electrosurgical blade. A finger can be inserted into the vagina, and the cervix palpated directly to confirm its location. Once the specimen has been removed, the cervix should be inspected to ensure that it has been removed completely.

After removal of the uterus and cervix, each of the angles of the lateral vaginal fornix is secured to the cardinal and uterosacral ligaments with a figure-of-eight 0 delayed absorbable suture. There is no unanimity of opinion regarding whether the vaginal cuff should be run and left open or closed. The vaginal cuff can be closed with interrupted figure-of-eight sutures. If there is continued oozing, as with a coagulopathy or in the presence of purulent amniotic fluid, then the vaginal cuff is left open to allow for adequate drainage. Hemostatic agents such as Gelfoam, with or without topical thrombin, or Surgicel can be considered. Reperitonization of the pelvis is not necessary in most cases. All pedicles should be closely inspected for bleeding before the abdominal incision is closed.

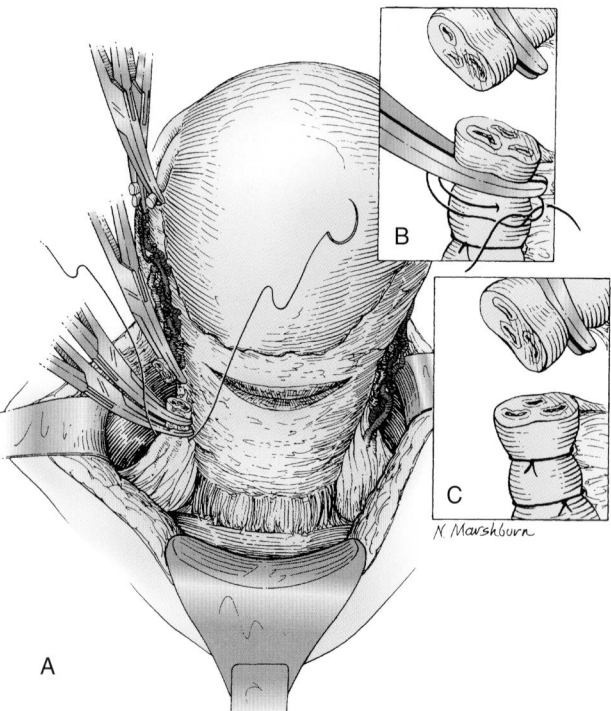

FIGURE 35A.6 **A:** The uterine artery and veins on either side are doubly clamped immediately adjacent to the uterus and divided. **B, C:** The vascular pedicle is doubly suture ligated. (From Cunningham FG, MacDonald PC, Gant NF, et al. Caesarean section and caesarean hysterectomy. In: *Williams obstetrics*, 19th ed. Norwalk, CT: Appleton & Lange, 1993:591, with permission from The McGraw-Hill Companies, Inc.)

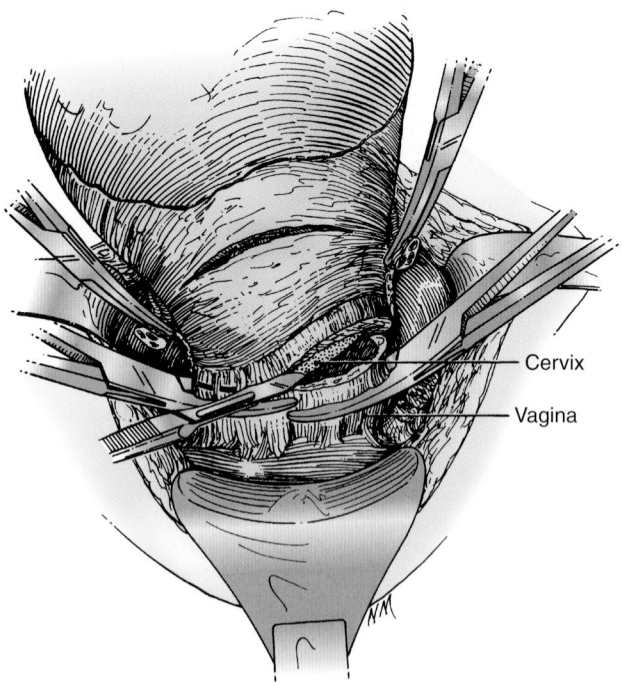

Cervix

Vagina

FIGURE 35A.7 A curved clamp is swung in across the lateral vaginal fornix below the level of the cervix, and the tissue is incised medially to the point of the clamp. (Reprinted from Cunningham FG, MacDonald PC, Gant NF, et al. Caesarean section and caesarean hysterectomy. In: *Williams obstetrics*, 19th ed. Norwalk, CT: Appleton & Lange, 1993:591, with permission from The McGraw-Hill Companies, Inc.)

Subtotal versus Total Hysterectomy

Some clinicians have a tendency to perform a subtotal or supracervical hysterectomy in most cases of emergency peripartum hysterectomy. There is a general belief that both operating time and blood loss are significantly lower with the subtotal technique. In addition, the risk of bladder or ureteral injury may be decreased. There is no question that in the select patient who has been or is hemodynamically unstable, it may be prudent to perform a supracervical hysterectomy, especially if all bleeding has been controlled to that point. However, it is necessary to remove the cervix in cases of placenta previa or placenta accreta involving the lower uterine segment.

Despite the reputed advantages of a supracervical hysterectomy, there is evidence that performance of a complete hysterectomy with removal of the cervix adds little to either operating time or blood loss. Clark and associates reported no significant differences in mean values for blood loss and operating time in obstetric patients undergoing emergency total hysterectomy versus supracervical hysterectomy. Mean hospital stay also was not significantly different. However, the women in this study were not randomized to supracervical versus total hysterectomy. In 1998, Zorlu and associates also reported no significant difference between total and supracervical hysterectomy in operative time, blood transfusion, and mean hospital stay. It is important to separate emergency cesarean hysterectomy for hemorrhage, and so on, from elective peripartum hysterectomy for indications such as microinvasive cervical cancer because the blood loss and other morbidity are generally significantly greater for the emergency procedure. It is important for the surgeon to appreciate his or her experience; the stability of the patient; the operative team, including the anesthesiologists and the availability of operative consultation such as other gynecologic surgeons or urologists; and the postoperative support of a good intensive care unit and possible interventional radiology. A combination of good surgical judgment as well as surgical skill is required to achieve the best result.

EPISIOTOMY

An episiotomy is a surgical incision into the perineal body for the purpose of either aiding the actual delivery process or preventing tears and lacerations.

Indications

The routine use of episiotomy with vaginal delivery has been strongly challenged. A recent Practice Bulletin from the American Congress of Obstetricians and Gynecologists stated that the previously held ideas that episiotomy facilitated vaginal delivery, especially difficult or operative vaginal delivery, or improved neonatal outcome when expeditious delivery was indicated are *not* supported by current evidence. Studies by Myles and Santolaya and Bodner-Adler and colleagues failed to show any reduction in anal sphincter damage, rectal mucosal tears, or improved neonatal outcomes in women who underwent episiotomy.

In the past, it was thought that episiotomy prevented vaginal and perineal damage that led to subsequent pelvic relaxation. However, there is little evidence to support the premise that "prophylactic" episiotomy prevents cystocele, rectocele, enterocele, uterine prolapse, vaginal prolapse, or stress urinary incontinence. Röckner and associates evaluated pelvic floor muscle strength using vaginal cones and found that women with episiotomies had less strength than those with spontaneous vaginal deliveries. Neural testing of the perineal musculature in other studies showed that the amount of denervation was associated with weight of the baby and the length of the second stage of labor and was unrelated to episiotomy. Sleep and Grant looked at deliveries in those who restricted use of episiotomy and those who reported liberal use of episiotomy. Over 3 years of follow-up, there was little difference between the two groups in severity of incontinence or the reported incidence of incontinence. These studies indicate that episiotomy does not appear to prevent the physical/anatomic or symptomatic changes of pelvic relaxation.

In addition, there are no good data to support prophylactic episiotomy for the prevention of "trauma" to the fetus, especially the preterm fetus. Although there is no evidence that the risk of shoulder dystocia can be decreased by the use of an episiotomy, many experts feel that a generous episiotomy may help in the management of a shoulder dystocia when it presents.

In summary, current opinion does not support the routine use of episiotomy for vaginal delivery. Previous ideas that suggested episiotomy decreased the risk of perineal injury, reduced trauma of operative delivery, or improved neonatal outcome have not been supported by recent studies. An episiotomy undoubtedly provides more room for a difficult vaginal delivery. Such deliveries are inherently associated with an increased risk of fetal distress and maternal trauma. The obstetrician must individualize each patient and weigh the potential advantages of an episiotomy against the known risks of episiotomy or vaginal delivery without an episiotomy or even cesarean delivery.

Midline versus Mediolateral Episiotomy

There is little question that the midline perineal incision is easier to perform and repair and is associated with less postoperative pain than is the mediolateral episiotomy. In general, it is also associated with less blood loss and better anatomic results. Midline perineal incisions are used more frequently in the United States, whereas mediolateral episiotomy is used more commonly in Europe. The major disadvantage of midline episiotomy is an increased risk of third- and fourth-degree lacerations. Owen and Hauth report that 20% of primiparous women with a midline episiotomy had a third- or fourth-degree laceration, compared with 9% of women with a mediolateral incision and only 1% when no episiotomy was performed. Of interest, multiparous women with a midline episiotomy had fewer third- and fourth-degree lacerations than those with a mediolateral episiotomy. Although these data appear to favor performing either a mediolateral episiotomy or no episiotomy at all, caution must be exercised when interpreting the data because this was not a randomized, prospective study, and it does not control for possible confounding factors. For example, patients who underwent episiotomy may well have had larger babies, a higher incidence of forceps assistance, or other characteristics resulting in an increased risk of laceration.

Although the mediolateral episiotomy may be associated with fewer third- and fourth-degree lacerations (at least in the primiparous patient) (Table 35A.4), there are several disadvantages to this technique. Blood loss is greater, and mediolateral episiotomies are more difficult to repair. Postoperative pain also is more common and can be very troublesome.

In the absence of good, prospective, randomized trials, the decision to perform a mediolateral or midline episiotomy must be based on clinical judgment and experience. A mediolateral episiotomy may provide more room for a difficult delivery

VI

TABLE 35A.4 Relation of Lacerations to Type of Episiotomy in 7,675 Primiparous Women

	TYPE OF EPISIOTOMY		
LACERATION TYPE	**MIDLINE (*n* = 4,822)**	**MEDIOLATERAL (*n* = 79)**	**NONE (*n* = 2,774)**
Second degree	1,425 (30%)	26 (33%)	375 (14%)
Third or fourth degree	968 (20%)	7 (9%)	52 (1%)
Other	295 (6%)	7 (9%)	274 (10%)
Totals	2,688 (56%)	40 (51%)	701 (25%)

Reprinted from Owen J, Hauth JC. Episiotomy infection and dehiscence. In: Gilstrap LC III, Faro S, eds. *Infections in pregnancy*. New York, NY: Alan R. Liss, 1990:61, with permission. Copyright © 1997, John Wiley and Sons.

with a lower risk of third- and fourth-degree laceration, but it also results in more blood loss and a greater risk of long-term dyspareunia.

Episiotomy Repair

STEPS IN THE PROCEDURE

Episiotomy Repair

- Closure of the vaginal mucosa and submucosa with a continuous running locking 2-0 absorbable suture.
- Closure of the fascia and muscle of the perineal body with interrupted sutures using absorbable suture material.
- Closure of the skin of the perineum can be closed with a continuous subcuticular stitch using 3-0 or 4-0 suture. An alternate method to close skin is to use interrupted sutures of 3-0 or 4-0 absorbable suture.
- For sphincter repair, carefully approximate with several interrupted 2-0 sutures through the muscle and fibrous capsule.
- For repair of the rectum, approximate the edges of the rectal mucosa with a running submucosal 3-0 or 4-0 delayed absorbable suture, followed by a second reinforcement layer of the rectovaginal septal tissue.

An episiotomy can be repaired in numerous ways. One popular method is to close the vaginal mucosa and submucosa with a continuous locking suture of 2-0 synthetic delayed absorbable suture, followed by closure of the fascia and muscle of the perineal body with three or four interrupted sutures of similar suture material. The skin of the perineum can then be closed with a continuous subcuticular stitch or by interrupted sutures of 3-0 or 4-0 synthetic absorbable or chromic suture through the subcutaneous tissue and skin. In cases of fourth-degree lacerations, it is important to approximate the edges of the rectal mucosa with a running submucosal 3-0 or 4-0 delayed absorbable or chromic suture, followed by a second reinforcing layer of the rectovaginal septal tissue. If the external anal sphincter is severed, it should be carefully reapproximated with several interrupted 2-0 sutures through the

muscle and fibrous capsule. The technique for primary episiotomy closure is illustrated later in this chapter and is also discussed in Chapter 40.

Complications of Episiotomy

Extensions and Fistula Formation

The major complications of episiotomy include infection, hematoma, breakdown, and fistula formation. Probably the single most common complication is extension (i.e., third- or fourth-degree laceration). Extensions in turn can lead to incontinence of flatus and stool, rectovaginal fistula, and infection. The association of extensions with the type of episiotomy has been discussed already. In the report by Harris, 11.6% of the more than 7,000 women with midline episiotomies had a third- or fourth-degree laceration. In the women with these lacerations, 2% subsequently had poor sphincter tone, and 0.1% developed a rectovaginal fistula. Signorello and colleagues performed a retrospective cohort study to evaluate the relationship between midline episiotomy and anal incontinence postpartum. Women with episiotomies had a higher risk of fecal incontinence 3 months and 6 months postpartum. Episiotomy tripled the risk of fecal incontinence at 3 months and 6 months postpartum and doubled the risk of flatus incontinence compared with women with spontaneous lacerations. In a prospective evaluation of 16,583 deliveries, Walsh and colleagues found that 0.56% of deliveries were complicated by third-degree lacerations. Lacerations were not prevented by episiotomy but were associated with forceps delivery. Of the 81 patients followed, 30 had abnormal anorectal examination, 7% were incontinent of stool, and 12% were incontinent of flatus.

Fistula is fortunately an uncommon complication of episiotomy. Causes include unrecognized lacerations in the rectovaginal septum at the time of episiotomy repair or infected hematoma. Risk factors for fistula formation include obesity, poor hygiene, malnutrition, anemia, history of inflammatory bowel disease, connective tissue disease, or prior exposure to radiation therapy. Half of these fistulae spontaneously heal, but repair should be considered if the patient is bothered by symptoms.

Dehiscence

The exact incidence of episiotomy dehiscence is unknown, but it appears to occur infrequently. In a review of 390 women with fourth-degree perineal lacerations, 18 (4.6%) experienced a dehiscence, and 11 of these were associated with infection.

Several predisposing factors have been reported to be associated with episiotomy dehiscence, including infection, human papillomavirus, cigarette smoking, hematoma, or trauma. Infection is probably the most common factor. In the study by Ramin and associates, 86% of patients with midline episiotomy dehiscence and 69% of patients with mediolateral episiotomy dehiscence had evidence of infection that was based on the presence of fever or purulent discharge. Infection with human papillomavirus also has been reported by some to be associated with dehiscence. Although inadequate or "faulty" repair has been reported to be associated with dehiscence, this is a rare cause.

Early Repair of Dehiscence In the past, it had been taught that repair of episiotomy dehiscence should be delayed for several months to allow for revascularization and healing. However, current surgical opinion supported by recent data strongly favors early repair. Delayed repair is an inconvenience for the woman and may be associated with fecal incontinence and loss of sexual function. Delay also can increase the hospital stay and cost, and increase risk of litigation.

There are many advantages to early repair of episiotomy dehiscence. Hauth and colleagues reported on the efficacy and safety of early repair in eight women who had a dehiscence of a fourth-degree midline episiotomy. Early repair was successful in seven of the eight women. One woman developed a pinpoint rectovaginal fistula 4 days after early repair. This was fixed with a 1-cm rectal flap 4 months later.

Monberg and Hammen reported on the successful resuturing of episiotomy breakdown in 20 women with infection, dehiscence, or both. Although four of the women had superficial reseparation, all subsequently healed spontaneously.

Hankins and associates updated the initial report by Hauth and colleagues to include 22 women with dehiscence of an initial fourth-degree repair, 4 with dehiscence of a third-degree repair, and 5 with breakdown of a mediolateral repair. Initial success of early repair was achieved in 29 (94%) of 31 women. Two women with a pinpoint rectovaginal fistula were subsequently repaired with a rectal flap procedure. Of the 27 women with a follow-up of 1 year or greater, all were continent and had resumption of normal coital activity. The follow-up of the 22 women with early repair of episiotomy dehiscence revealed no complications in 18 patients. Occasional incontinence of flatus and stool, dyspareunia, dyschezia, and numbness occurred in the remaining patients. All of the symptoms resolved by 9 months, except for 2 patients who had persistent dyspareunia.

Ramin and coworkers reported on the early repair of 34 women with episiotomy dehiscence, most of whom were infected (Table 35A.5). These women received care from a large urban hospital serving primarily an indigent population. The timing of repair for dehiscence ranged from 3 to 13 days. Two women with initial third-degree episiotomy dehiscence had unsuccessful repairs. Thus, successful repairs were accomplished in 32 (94%) of the women. The average time from delivery to subsequent discharge after repair of the dehiscence was 15.5 days. This is similar to the time reported by Hankins and colleagues. This time probably can be shortened significantly with outpatient management of the wound and repair in ambulatory care units.

Secondary Repair Technique Before attempting a closure, it is important to prepare the wound for repair. The first step is cleaning and debridement of the episiotomy site. This can be accomplished either on the ward with intravenous sedation or local anesthesia or in the operating room under regional anesthesia. All necrotic tissue and suture fragments should be removed

TABLE 35A.5 Characteristics of 34 Patients with Episiotomy Dehiscence and Subsequent Early Repair		
CHARACTERISTIC	**MIDLINE**	**MEDIOLATERAL**
Total number of patients	21	13
Type of delivery		
Spontaneous	11	0
Outlet forceps	3	3
Low forceps	7	10
Extension		
None	1	5
Third degree	9	6
Fourth degree	11	2
Evidence of infection	18 (86%)	9 (69%)
Early repair failures	1	1

Reprinted from Ramin SM, Ramus RM, Little BB, et al. Early repair of episiotomy dehiscence associated with infection. *Am J Obstet Gynecol* 1992;167:1104, with permission. Copyright © 1992, Elsevier.

and the wound irrigated with a diluted povidone–iodine solution or half-strength Dakin solution. Broad-spectrum antibiotics are indicated for overt infection or significant cellulitis. After initial debridement, the wound should be scrubbed and cleaned at least twice daily. Scrub brushes impregnated with povidone–iodine or gauze dressing pads can be used. A 1% lidocaine jelly is applied to the wound several minutes before cleansing, and analgesics should be used as necessary. The liberal use of sitz baths helps keep the wound clean.

Secondary repair of the episiotomy is not attempted until the wound is free of exudate and covered by granulation tissue. A mechanical bowel preparation with an oral electrolyte solution should be administered the evening before surgery for fourth-degree breakdowns. Prophylactic antibiotics are recommended for all repairs. One to three doses of a first-generation cephalosporin generally proves satisfactory.

The first step in the surgical repair of dehiscence is debridement of granulation tissue and dissection to ensure good tissue mobility. If the anal sphincter muscle has been severed, extensive retraction usually has occurred. It is important to identify the fibrous capsule and mobilize the muscle and capsule for successful reapproximation. If the rectal mucosa has been lacerated, it should be reapproximated as described in this chapter. In a prospective, randomized trial, Fitzpatrick and colleagues compared 55 women who underwent a sphincter overlap procedure with 57 women who underwent staple approximation repair of third-degree lacerations. In this study, there were no significant differences in anal manometry or endoanal ultrasound in the two groups. Therefore, either approach is acceptable. The rest of the closure is the same as for a secondary episiotomy repair. The secondary repair of a fourth-degree episiotomy breakdown is shown in Figures 35A.8 to 35A.11.

Postoperatively, women can be placed on a regular diet if the rectal mucosa is not involved. If the rectal mucosa is involved, a low-residue diet should be used for several days and advanced to a regular diet. Stool softeners are recommended, but diarrhea should be avoided because of the increased likelihood of infection. Postoperative care should also include sitz baths and a heat lamp.

The care and repair of a mediolateral episiotomy dehiscence are the same as for a midline repair. More extensive tissue mobilization may be required with the repair of a mediolateral episiotomy dehiscence.

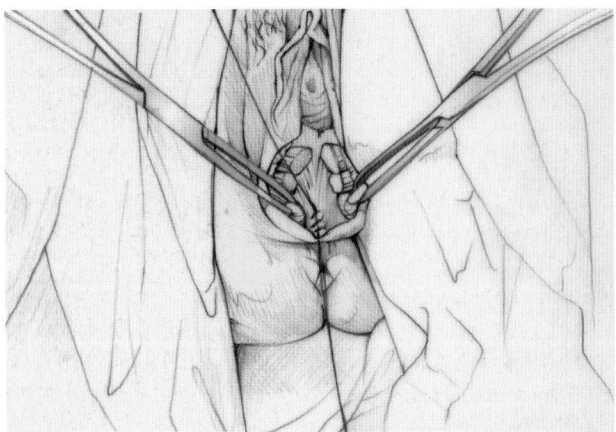

FIGURE 35A.8 Secondary closure of fourth-degree episiotomy breakdown. The rectal mucosa has been closed with 4-0 running chromic submucosal suture and reinforced with a second layer of 3-0 chromic suture through the rectovaginal septum.

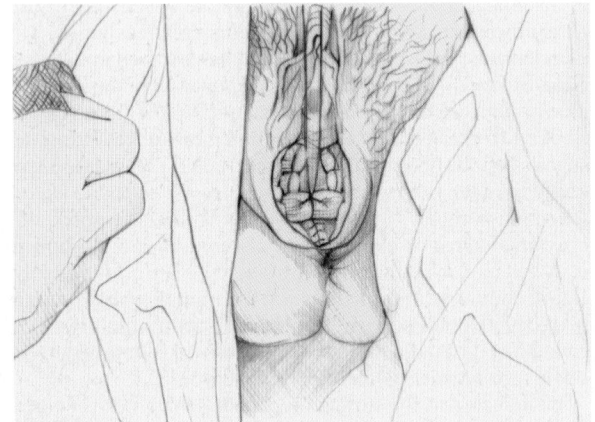

FIGURE 35A.9 The anal sphincter muscle has been reapproximated end to end with several interrupted 2-0 chromic sutures through the muscle and capsule.

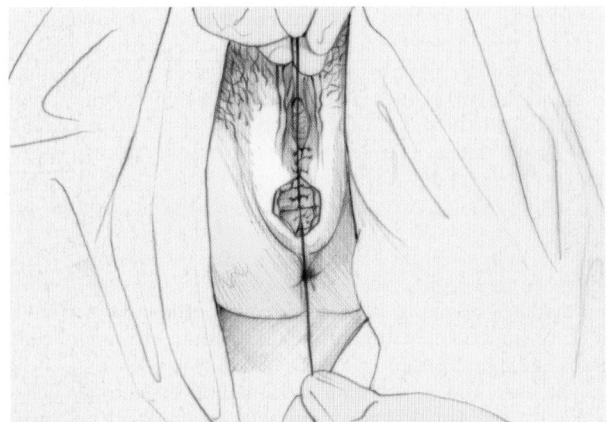

FIGURE 35A.10 The vaginal mucosa and bulbocavernosus muscle have been closed with 2-0 chromic suture.

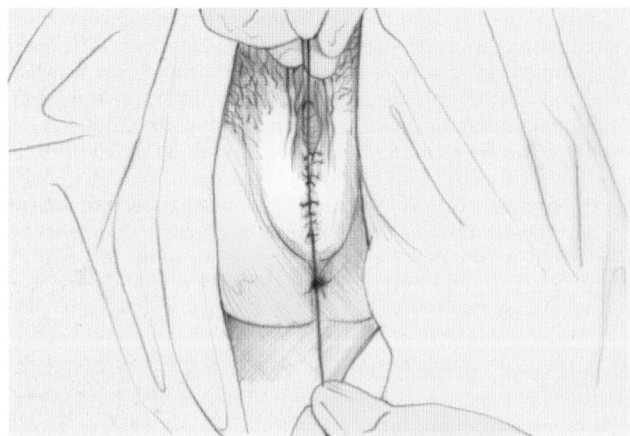

FIGURE 35A.11 Secondary repair of fourth-degree episiotomy dehiscence is completed. (Courtesy of Susan Ramin, University of Texas, Dallas.)

CERVICAL CERCLAGE

Premature dilation of the uterine cervix is a major cause of loss or delivery in midpregnancy. Although the pathophysiology of *cervical insufficiency* is poorly understood and the diagnosis challenging, concepts continue to evolve regarding this complex situation. The concept of cervical insufficiency, its diagnosis, and its management have been well reviewed in a Practice Bulletin issued by the American Congress of Obstetricians and Gynecologists. Although a variety of diagnostic criteria—including prior midtrimester losses and history of cervical surgery (including loop electrode excision procedure or cone biopsy) and painless dilatation of the cervix—have been used in the past and serve as useful clinical risk factors, today *ultrasound monitoring of cervical length and funneling are usually used to make a diagnosis of cervical insufficiency.*

Shirodkar first described cerclage placement in 1955 as a new method to prevent habitual abortion in the second trimester. McDonald, in 1957, reported a simplified technique. The technique for the abdominal approach for cerclage was described by Benson and Durfee in 1965. Data regarding the efficacy of cerclage placement has been conflicting. The Cervical Incompetence Prevention Randomized Cerclage Trial (CIPRACT) concluded that serial ultrasounds for evaluation of cervical insufficiency with secondary intervention are a safe alternative to traditional prophylactic cerclage. Studies have supported the uses of cerclage for pregnancy prolongation in singleton gestations; however, there are conflicting data about its utility in multiple gestations. Cerclage is rarely performed after 24.5 weeks gestation because the risks of surgery are outweighed by the benefits of bed rest for a few weeks to achieve improved fetal survival.

Zaveri and colleagues noted that transabdominal cerclage may be associated with a lower risk of perinatal death, but has a higher risk of intraoperative complications. Data suggest that an abdominal cerclage may be preferable in patients in whom a transvaginal cerclage has failed. The abdominal approach is also indicated in patients whose cervix has been shortened significantly by cone biopsy or other surgery. Laparoscopic transabdominal suture insertion during and before pregnancy has recently been described. Recent case reports suggest that placement of the abdominal cerclage by a laparoscopic approach is safe and may reduce maternal recovery time; however, its efficacy over the additional abdominal approach has not been examined.

Technique

STEPS IN THE PROCEDURE

Cervical Cerclage: Transvaginal

- Modified Shirodkar
  - Make a transverse incision in the vaginal mucosa of the anterior cervix to allow for displacement of the bladder upward.
  - A posterior incision is made in a similar fashion to avoid entry into the rectum.
  - The lateral angles of the anterior and posterior incisions are then expanded with blunt dissection of the lateral cervix.
  - A 5-mm woven Mersilene tape on a large needle is then passed through the submucosal tunnel from anterior to posterior on both sides of the cervix, then tied posteriorly.
- McDonald approach
  - Placement of a suture of 5-mm Mersilene or other type of heavy monofilament suture (Prolene) around the cervix in a purse-string fashion and securely tied anteriorly

STEPS IN THE PROCEDURE

Cervical Cerclage: Abdominal

- Low, transverse abdominal incision (Pfannenstiel technique)
- Transverse incision of the vesicouterine peritoneum to allow for bladder retraction
- Placement of 5-mm Mersilene suture through the broad ligament close to the cervical stroma and tied securely
- Delivery by cesarean section

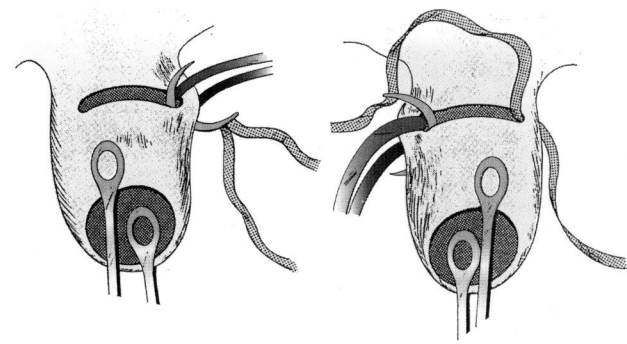

FIGURE 35A.12 Modified Shirodkar cerclage. An incision in the mucosa is made anteriorly and posteriorly to advance the bladder and rectum. A 5-mm Mersilene suture on a large needle is placed in a submucosal tunnel around the cervix and tied posteriorly.

The modified Shirodkar and the McDonald procedure are performed using the transvaginal approach. In the *modified Shirodkar approach*, a transverse incision is made in the vaginal mucosa of the anterior cervix to allow for upward displacement of the bladder to avoid injury. A posterior incision is made in similar fashion to avoid entry into the rectum. The lateral angles of the anterior and posterior incisions are then expanded with blunt fingertip dissection of the lateral cervix (Fig. 35A.12). A 5-mm woven Mersilene tape on a large needle (Ethicon, USA) is then passed through the submucosal tunnel from anterior to posterior on both sides of the cervix. It is preferable to avoid entering the cervical canal because the tape may irritate the fetal membranes; this can be done by placing an index finger in the cervical canal as the needle is passed through the lateral cervix. The lateral cervical mucosa at 3 and 9 o'clock can also be grasped with an Allis clamp or ring forceps as shown in Figure 35A.12 to facilitate placement of the sutures. After the suture is placed on both sides of the cervix, the knot is tied in the posterior defect. The defects are then closed with 3-0 Vicryl in figure-of-eight fashion. We usually leave a whisker of the Mersilene band extending through the closure so that it can be grasped and the suture exposed and cut when the patient goes into labor.

The *McDonald* approach requires no dissection into the cervical tissues. A suture of braided Mersilene or a heavy monofilament suture (Prolene) may be placed around the cervix in purse-string fashion and tied securely (Fig. 35A.13).

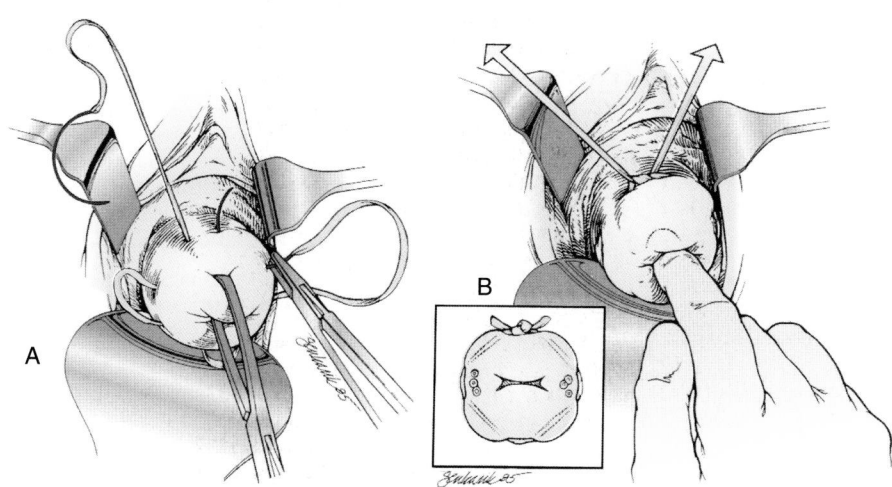

FIGURE 35A.13 Placement of suture for McDonald cervical cerclage. **A:** We use a double-headed Mersilene band with four "bites" in the cervix, avoiding the vessels. **B:** The suture is placed high upon the cervix close to the cervical–vaginal junction, approximately the level of the internal os.

VI

Proponents of the modified Shirodkar feel that cervical dissection assists in placing a higher cerclage, but Rozenburg and associates noted that the anterior colpotomy associated with the modified Shirodkar cerclage only increased the distance from the external os by 2.7 mm. Rust and colleagues noted that the length of the cervix below the level of the cerclage does not affect the rate of preterm delivery.

Placement of the *abdominal cerclage* traditionally has required a low transverse abdominal incision, usually performed by Pfannenstiel technique. The vesicouterine peritoneum is incised in transverse fashion to allow for retraction of the bladder inferiorly. A suture of 5-mm Mersilene is placed through the broad ligament close to the cervical stroma with care taken to avoid the uterine vessels. The suture is then tied securely. Unlike the transvaginal cerclage, the suture cannot be removed vaginally; thus, the patient requires a cesarean delivery. This suture may be left in place until childbearing is complete.

BEST SURGICAL PRACTICES

- The anatomic and physiologic changes of pregnancy may make diagnosis and surgical management more complex. Ultrasound and magnetic resonance imaging are safe and useful diagnostic imaging techniques that can be used in the pregnant patient.
- Postpartum hemorrhage may be a life-threatening emergency. It may be due to an obstetric laceration, retained products of conception, uterine atony, or coagulation defects. Aggressive fluid replacement and oxytocic agents are indicated while a diagnostic evaluation is undertaken. Uterine packing has recently been rediscovered as an effective way to treat hemorrhage from uterine atony.
- Transcatheter arterial embolization may be very effective to control postpartum hemorrhage. Bilateral uterine artery or hypogastric artery embolization is recommended. This technique is highly effective, preserves the uterus, and does not preclude future pregnancies.
- Surgical techniques for the management of peripartum hemorrhage include uterine artery ligation, hypogastric artery ligation, B-Lynch compression sutures, and hysterectomy. Emergency hysterectomy for hemorrhage is associated with a significantly increased risk of complications, including urinary tract injury and infection. It is not clear whether elective hysterectomy performed at the time of a scheduled cesarean delivery is associated with increased morbidity, but blood loss and risk of transfusion are increased, and delivery followed by hysterectomy 3 to 6 months later may be considered as an alternative.
- The use of episiotomy has declined significantly in recent years. Recently, studies have not shown any benefit of episiotomy in reducing the risk of third- and fourth-degree lacerations, reducing the risk of long-term pelvic support defects, or improving neonatal outcome. Episiotomy should not be used routinely. Median episiotomy is associated with a higher risk of anal sphincter and rectal injury. Mediolateral episiotomy is associated with increased blood loss and perhaps an increase in postpartum pain and long-term dyspareunia. Repair of episiotomy, especially if there is rectal or sphincter injury, should be done meticulously, using good surgical technique with adequate anesthesia and sterile technique.
- Surgical treatment of cervical insufficiency is complicated by a poor understanding of the pathophysiology of the condition. Painless dilatation and effacement of the cervix in the second trimester, usually documented by ultrasound,

is an indication for treatment. Both the McDonald and Shirodkar techniques have been used successfully. An abdominal cerclage may be considered if the cervix has been shortened or damaged by surgery or trauma.

ACKNOWLEDGMENTS

The author would like to acknowledge Cornelia Graves for her work in the previous editions of this text.

BIBLIOGRAPHY

Alamia V Jr, Meyer BA. Peripartum hemorrhage. *Obstet Gynecol Clin North Am* 1999;26:385.

Allahdin S, Aird C, Danielian P. B-Lynch sutures for major primary postpartum haemorrhage at caesarean section. *J Obstet Gynaecol* 2006;26:639.

Allen RE, Hoster GL, Smith ARB, et al. Pelvic floor damage and childbirth: a neurophysiologic study. *BJOG* 1990;97:770.

Althuisius SM, Dekker GA, Hummel P, et al. Cervical in competence prevention randomized cerclage trial. *Am J Obstet Gynecol* 2003;189:907.

Amant F, Spitz B, Timmerman D, et al. Misoprostol compared with methylergometrine for the prevention of postpartum haemorrhage: a double-blind randomised trial. *BJOG* 1999;106:1066.

American College of Obstetricians and Gynecologists. *ACOG Practice Bulletin No. 48: Cervical insufficiency.* Washington, DC: ACOG, 2003.

American College of Obstetricians and Gynecologists. *ACOG Technical Bulletin No. 76: Diagnosis and management of postpartum hemorrhage.* Washington, DC: ACOG, 2006.

American College of Obstetricians and Gynecologists. *ACOG Practice Bulletin No. 71: Episiotomy.* Washington, DC: ACOG, 2006.

American College of Obstetricians and Gynecologists. *ACOG Technical Bulletin No. 299: Guidelines for diagnostic imaging during pregnancy.* Washington, DC: ACOG, 2004.

Angioli R, Gomez-Marin O, Cantuaria G, et al. Severe perineal lacerations during vaginal delivery: the University of Miami experience. *Am J Obstet Gynecol* 2000;182:1083.

Arona AJ, Al-Marayati L, Grimes DA, et al. Early secondary repair of third- and fourth-degree perineal lacerations after outpatient wound preparation. *Obstet Gynecol* 1995;86:294.

Argentine Episiotomy Trial Collaborative Group. Routine vs selective episiotomy: a randomised controlled trial. *Lancet* 1993;342:1517.

Baker ER, D'Alton ME. Caesarean section and caesarean hysterectomy. *Clin Obstet Gynecol* 1994;37:806.

Bakshi S, Meyer BA. Indications for and outcomes of emergency peripartum hysterectomy. A five-year review. *J Reprod Med* 2000;45:733.

Bamigboye AA, Hofmeyr GJ, Merrell DA. Rectal misoprostol in the prevention of postpartum hemorrhage: a placebo-controlled trial. *Am J Obstet Gynecol* 1998;179:1043.

Bauman P, Hammond AO, McNeeley SG, et al. Factors associated with anal sphincter laceration in 40,923 primiparous women. *Int Urogynecol J Pelvic Floor Dysfunct* 2007;18:985.

Benson RC, Durfee RB. Transabdominal cervico uterine cerclage during pregnancy for the treatment of cervical incompetency. *Obstet Gynecol* 1965;25:145.

B-Lynch C, Coker A, Lawai A, et al. The B-Lynch surgical technique for the control of massive postpartum haemorrhage: an alternative to hysterectomy? Five cases reported. *BJOG* 1997;104:372.

Bodner-Adler B, Bodner K, Kimberger O, et al. Management of the perineum during forceps delivery: association of episiotomy with the frequency and severity of perineal trauma in women undergoing forceps delivery. *J Reprod Med* 2003;48:239.

Burchell RC. Physiology of internal iliac artery ligation. *J Obstet Gynaecol Br Commonw* 1968;75:642.

Casele HL, Laifer SA. Successful pregnancy after bilateral hypogastric artery ligation: a case report. *J Reprod Med* 1997;42:306.

Castaneda S, Karrison T, Cibilis LA. Peripartum hysterectomy. *J Perinat Med* 2000;28:472.

Chan C, Razvi K, Tham KF, et al. The use of a Sengstaken-Blakemore tube to control post-partum hemorrhage. *Int J Gynecol Obstet* 1997;58:251.

Chang CY, Wu MT, Shih JC, et al. Preservation of uterine integrity via transarterial embolization under postoperative massive vaginal bleeding due to caesarean section pregnancy. *Taiwan J Obstet Gynecol* 2006;45:183.

Christianson LM, Bovbjerg VE, McDavitt EC, et al. Risk factors for perineal injury during delivery. *Am J Obstet Gynecol* 2003;189:255.

Clark SL. Uterine and hypogastric artery ligation. In: Phelan JP, Clark SL, eds. *Caesarean delivery.* New York, NY: Elsevier, 1988:238.

Clark SL, Phelan JP, Yeh SY, et al. Hypogastric artery ligation for obstetric hemorrhage. *Obstet Gynecol* 1985;66:353.

Clark SL, Yeh SY, Phelan JP, et al. Emergency hysterectomy for obstetric hemorrhage. *Obstet Gynecol* 1984;64:376.

Connolly AM, Thorp JM Jr. Childbirth-related perineal trauma: clinical significance and prevention. *Clin Obstet Gynecol* 1999;42:820.

Craig S, Chau H, Cho H. Treatment of severe postpartum hemorrhage by rectally administered gemeprost pessaries. *J Perinat Med* 1999;27:231.

Cunningham FG, MacDonald PC, Gant NF, et al., eds. Abnormalities of the third stage of labor. In: *Williams obstetrics,* 19th ed. Norwalk, CT: Appleton & Lange, 1993:615.

Cunningham FG, MacDonald PC, Gant NF, et al., eds. Caesarean section and caesarean hysterectomy. In: *Williams obstetrics,* 19th ed. Norwalk, CT: Appleton & Lange, 1993:591.

Cunningham FG, MacDonald PC, Gant NF, et al., eds. Conduct of normal labor. In: *Williams obstetrics,* 19th ed. Norwalk, CT: Appleton & Lange, 1993:371.

Cunningham FG, MacDonald PC, Gant NF, et al., eds. Injuries to the birth canal. In: *Williams obstetrics,* 19th ed. Norwalk, CT: Appleton & Lange, 1993:543.

De Loor JA, van Dam PA. Foley catheters for uncontrollable obstetric or gynecologic hemorrhage. *Obstet Gynecol* 1996;88:737.

Dildy GA, Scott JR, et al. Pelvic pressure pack for catastrophic postpartum hemorrhage. *Obstet Gynecol* 2000;95:7S.

Ding CD, Hsu S, Chu TW, et al. Emergency peripartum hysterectomy in a teaching hospital in Eastern Taiwan. *J Obstet Gynaecol* 2006;26:635.

Eason E, Feldman P. Much ado about a little cut: is episiotomy worthwhile? *Obstet Gynecol* 2000;95:616.

Eason E, Labrecque M, Wells G, et al. Preventing perineal trauma during childbirth: a systematic review. *Obstet Gynecol* 2000;95:464.

Eniola OA, Bewley S, Waterstone M, et al. Obstetric hysterectomy in a population of South East England. *J Obstet Gynaecol* 2006;26:104.

Ferguson II JE, Bourgeois FJ, Underwood PB Jr. B-Lynch suture for postpartum hemorrhage. *Obstet Gynecol* 2000;95:1020.

Fitzpatrick M, Behan M, O'Connell PR, et al. A randomized clinical trial comparing primary overlap with approximation repair of third-degree obstetric tears. *Am J Obstet Gynecol* 2000;183:1220.

Flood KM, Said S, Geary M, et al. Changing trends in peripartum hysterectomy over the last 4 decades. *Am J Obstet Gynecol* 2009;200:632.e1.

Floyd RC, Morrison JC. Postpartum hemorrhage. In: Plauche WC, Morrison JC, O'Sullivan MJ, eds. *Surgical obstetrics.* Philadelphia, PA: WB Saunders, 1992:272.

Ghomi A, Rodgers B. Laparoscopic abdominal cerclage during pregnancy: a case report and a review of the described operative techniques. *J Minim Invasive Gynecol* 2006;4:337.

Gilstrap LC, Hauth JC, Hankins GDV, et al. Effect of type of anesthesia on blood loss at caesarean section. *Obstet Gynecol* 1987;69:328.

Gilstrap LC, Ramin SM. Postpartum hemorrhage. *Clin Obstet Gynecol* 1994;37:824.

Goldaber KG, Wendel PJ, McIntire D, et al. Postpartum perineal morbidity after fourth-degree perineal repair. *Am J Obstet Gynecol* 1993;168:489.

Gonsoulin W, Kennedy RT, Guidry KH. Elective versus emergency caesarean hysterectomy cases in a residency program setting: a review of 129 cases from 1984 to 1988. *Am J Obstet Gynecol* 1991;165:91.

Handa VL, Harris TA, Ostergard DR. Protecting the pelvic floor: obstetric management to prevent incontinence and pelvic organ prolapse. *Obstet Gynecol* 1996;88:470.

Hankins GDV, Hauth JC, Gilstrap LC III, et al. Early repair of episiotomy dehiscence. *Obstet Gynecol* 1990;75:48.

Hansch E, Chitkara U, McAlpine J, et al. Pelvic arterial embolization for control of obstetric hemorrhage: a five year experience. *Am J Obstet Gynecol* 1999;180:1454.

Harris RE. An evaluation of the median episiotomy. *Am J Obstet Gynecol* 1970;106:660.

Hauth JC, Gilstrap LC III, Ward SC, et al. Early repair of an external sphincter ani muscle and rectal mucosal dehiscence. *Obstet Gynecol* 1986;67:806.

Henriksen T, Bek KM, Hedegaard M, et al. Episiotomy and perineal lesions in spontaneous vaginal deliveries. *BJOG* 1992;99:950.

Homsi R, Daikoku NH, Littlejohn J, et al. Episiotomy: risks of dehiscence and rectovaginal fistula. *Obstet Gynecol Surv* 1994; 49:803.

Hsu YR, Wan YL. Successful management of intractable puerperal hematoma and severe postpartum hemorrhage with DIC through transcatheter arterial embolization—two cases. *Acta Obstet Gynecol Scand* 1998;77:129.

Hueston WJ. Factors associated with the use of episiotomy during vaginal delivery. *Obstet Gynecol* 1996;87:1001.

Jackson KW Jr, Allbert JR, Schemmer GK, et al. A randomized controlled trial comparing oxytocin administration before and after placental delivery in the prevention of postpartum hemorrhage. *Am J Obstet Gynecol* 2001;185:873.

Kaunitz AM, Hughes JM, Grimes DA, et al. Causes of maternal mortality in the United States. *Obstet Gynecol* 1985;65:605.

Klein MC, Gauthier RJ, Jorgensen SH, et al. Does episiotomy prevent perineal trauma and pelvic floor relaxation? Online. *J Curr Clin Trials* 1992;2 [document no. 10].

Klein MC, Gauthier RJ, Robbins JM, et al. Relationship of episiotomy to perineal trauma and morbidity, sexual dysfunction, and pelvic floor relaxation. *Am J Obstet Gynecol* 1994;171:591.

Klein MC, Janssen PA, MacWilliam L, et al. Determinants of vaginal-perineal integrity and pelvic floor functioning in childbirth. *Am J Obstet Gynecol* 1997;176:403.

Kovavisarach E. Obstetric hysterectomy: a 14-year experience of Rajavithi Hospital, 1989–2002. *J Med Assoc Thai* 2006;89:1817.

Larsson PG, Platz-Christensen JJ, Bergman B, et al. Advantage or disadvantage of episiotomy compared with spontaneous perineal laceration. *Gynecol Obstet Invest* 1991;31:213.

Lede RL, Belizan JM, Carroli G. Is routine use of episiotomy justified? *Am J Obstet Gynecol* 1996;174:1399.

Liu CM, Hsu JJ, Hsieh TT, et al. Postpartum hemorrhage of the uterine artery rupture. *Acta Obstet Gynecol Scand* 1998;77:695.

Lotgering FK, Gaugler-Senden IP, Lotgering SF. Outcome after transabdominal cervicoisthmic cerclage. *Obstet Gynecol* 2006;107:779.

Maier RC. Control of postpartum hemorrhage with uterine packing. *Am J Obstet Gynecol* 1993;169:317.

Marcovici I, Scoccia B. Postpartum hemorrhage and intrauterine balloon tamponade: a report of three cases. *J Reprod Med* 1999;44:122.

McNulty JV. Elective caesarean hysterectomy revisited. *Am J Obstet Gynecol* 1984;149:29.

Mengert WF, Burchell RC, Blumstein RW, et al. Pregnancy of the bilateral ligation after internal iliac and ovarian arteries. *Obstet Gynecol* 1969;34:664.

Monberg J, Hammen S. Ruptured episiotomies resutured primarily. *Acta Obstet Gynecol Scand* 1987;66:163.

Mousa H, Alfirevic Z. Treatment for primary postpartum haemorrhage. *Cochrane Database Syst Rev* 2007;(1):CD003249.

Myers-Helfgott MG, Helfgott AW. Routine use of episiotomy in modern obstetrics. Should it be performed? *Obstet Gynecol Clin North Am* 1999;26:305.

Myles TD, Santolaya J. Maternal and neonatal outcomes in patients with prolonged second stage of labor. *Obstet Gynecol* 2003; 102:52.

O'Brien JM, Barton JR, Donaldson ES. The management of placenta percreta: conservative and operative strategies. *Am J Obstet Gynecol* 1996;175:1632.

Oei PL, Chua S, Tan L, et al. Arterial embolization for bleeding following hysterectomy for intractable postpartum hemorrhage. *Int J Gynaecol Obstet* 1998;62:83.

VI

O'Leary JA. Stop OB hemorrhage with uterine artery ligation. *Contemp Obstet Gynecol* 1986;28:13.

O'Leary JA. Uterine artery ligation in the control of postcaesarean hemorrhage. *J Reprod Med* 1995;40:189.

Owen J, Andrews WW. Wound complications after caesarean sections. *Clin Obstet Gynecol* 1994;37:842.

Owen J, Hauth JC. Episiotomy infection and dehiscence. In: Gilstrap LC III, Faro S, eds. *Infections in pregnancy*. New York, NY: Alan R. Liss, 1990:61.

Patino JF, Castro D. Necrotizing lesions of the soft tissue: a review. *World J Surg* 1991;15:235.

Payne TN, Carey JC, Rayburn WF. Prior third- or fourth-degree perineal tears and recurrence risks. *Int J Gynaecol Obstet* 1999;64:55.

Pelage JP, Le Dref O, Mateo J, et al. Life-threatening primary postpartum hemorrhage: treatment with emergency selective arterial embolization. *Radiology* 1999;208:359.

Pelage JP, Soyer P, Repiquet D, et al. Secondary postpartum hemorrhage: treatment with selective arterial embolization. *Radiology* 1999;212:385.

Philippe HJ, d'Oreye D, Lewin D. Vaginal ligature of uterine arteries during postpartum hemorrhage. *Int J Gynaecol Obstet* 1997;56:267.

Plauche WC. Caesarean hysterectomy: indications, technique, and complications. *Clin Obstet Gynecol* 1986;29:318.

Plauche WC. Peripartal hysterectomy. In: Plauche WC, Morrison JC, O'Sullivan MJ, eds. *Surgical obstetrics*. Philadelphia, PA: WB Saunders, 1992:447.

Price N, B-Lynch C. Technical description of the B-Lynch brace suture for treatment of massive postpartum hemorrhage and review of published cases. *Int J Fertil Womens Med* 2005;50:148.

Ramin SM, Gilstrap LC III. Episiotomy and early repair of dehiscence. *Clin Obstet Gynecol* 1994;37:816.

Ramin SM, Ramus RM, Little BB, et al. Early repair of episiotomy dehiscence associated with infection. *Am J Obstet Gynecol* 1992;167:1104.

Reynders FC, Senten L, Tjalma W, et al. Postpartum hemorrhage: practical approach to a life-threatening complication. *Clin Exp Obstet Gynecol* 2006;33:81.

Roberts WE. Emergent obstetric management of postpartum hemorrhage. *Obstet Gynecol Clin North Am* 1995;22:283.

Robinson JN, Norwitz ER, Cohen AP, et al. Episiotomy, operative vaginal delivery, and significant perineal trauma in nulliparous women. *Am J Obstet Gynecol* 1999;181:1180.

Rochat RW, Koonin LM, Atrash HK, et al. Maternal mortality in the United States: report from the Maternal Mortality Collaborative. *Obstet Gynecol* 1988;72:91.

Röckner G, Jonasson A, Blund A. The effect of mediolateral episiotomy at delivery on pelvic floor muscle strength evaluated with vaginal cones. *Acta Obstet Gynecol Scand* 1991;70:51.

Rozenberg P, Sénat MV, Gillet A, et al. Comparison of two methods of cervical cerclage by ultrasound cervical measurement. *J Matern Fetal Neonatal Med* 2003;13:314.

Reist OA, Atlas RO, Meyer J, et al. Does cerclage location influence perinatal outcome? *Am J Obstet Gynecol* 2003;189:1688.

Selo-Ojeme DO, Okonofua FE. Risk factors for primary postpartum haemorrhage. *Arch Gynecol Obstet* 1997;259:179.

Sheiner E, Sarid L, Levy A, et al. Obstetric risk factors and outcome of pregnancies complicated with early postpartum hemorrhage: a population-based study. *J Matern Fetal Neonatal Med* 2005;18:149.

Signorello LB, Harlow BL, Chekos AK, et al. Midline episiotomy and anal incontinence: retrospective cohort study. *BMJ* 2000;320:86 [comment].

Sleep J, Grant A. West Berkshire perineal management trial: three year follow-up. *BMJ* 1987;295:749.

Smith J, Mousa HA. Peripartum hysterectomy for primary postpartum haemorrhage. *J Obstet Gynaecol* 2007;27:44.

Snyder RR, Hammond TL, Hankins GDV. Human papillomavirus associated with poor healing of episiotomy repairs. *Obstet Gynecol* 1990;76:664.

Stanco LM, Schrimmer DB, Paul RH, et al. Emergency peripartum hysterectomy and associated risk factors. *Am J Obstet Gynecol* 1993;168:879.

Strickland JL, Griffen WT, Llorens AS, et al. Caesarean hysterectomy: a procedure for modern obstetrics? *South Med J* 1989;82:1245.

Sturdee DW, Rushton DI. Caesarean and post-partum hysterectomy 1968–1983. *BJOG* 1986;93:270.

Thorp JM Jr, Bowes WA Jr. Episiotomy: can its routine use be defended? *Am J Obstet Gynecol* 1989;160:1027.

Thorp JM Jr, Bowes WA Jr, Brame RG, et al. Selected use of midline episiotomy: effect on perineal trauma. *Obstet Gynecol* 1987;70:260.

Van Selm M, Kanhai HH, Keirse MJ. Preventing the recurrence of atonic postpartum hemorrhage: a double-blind trial. *Acta Obstet Gynecol Scand* 1995;74:270.

Varma A, Gunn J, Gardiner A, et al. Obstetric anal sphincter injury: prospective evaluation of incidence. *Dis Colon Rectum* 1999;42:1537.

Varma A, Gunn J, Lindow SW, et al. Do routinely measured delivery variables predict anal sphincter outcome? *Dis Colon Rectum* 1999;42:1261.

Vedantham S, Goodwin SC, McLucas B, et al. Uterine artery embolization: an underused method of controlling pelvic hemorrhage. *Am J Obstet Gynecol* 1997;176:938.

Viktrup L, Lose G, Rolff M, et al. The symptom of stress incontinence caused by pregnancy or delivery in primiparas. *Obstet Gynecol* 1992;79: 945.

Wagaarachchi PT, Fernando L. Fertility following ligation of internal iliac arteries for life-threatening obstetric haemorrhage. *Hum Reprod* 2000;15:1311.

Walsh CJ, Mooney EF, Upton GJ, et al. Incidence of third-degree perineal tears in labour and outcome after primary repair. *Br J Surg* 1996;83:218.

Whiteman MK, Kuklina E, Hill SD, et al. Incidence and determinants of peripartum hysterectomy. *Obstet Gynecol* 2006;108:1486.

Woolley RJ. Benefits and risks of episiotomy: a review of the English-language literature since 1980. Part I. *Obstet Gynecol Surv* 1995;50:806.

Woolley RJ. Benefits and risks of episiotomy: a review of the English language literature since 1980. Part II. *Obstet Gynecol Surv* 1995;50:821.

Wu S, Kocherginsky M, Hibbard JU. Abnormal placentation: twenty-year analysis. *Am J Obstet Gynecol* 2005;192:1458.

Yancey MK, Harlass FE, Benson W, et al. The perioperative morbidity of scheduled caesarean hysterectomy. *Obstet Gynecol* 1993;81:206.

Zaveri V, Aghajafari F, Amankwah K, et al. Abdominal versus vaginal cerclage after failed transvaginal cerclage: systemic review. *Am J Obstet Gynecol* 2002;187:868.

Zelop CM, Harlow BL, Frigoletto FD, et al. Emergency peripartum hysterectomy. *Am J Obstet Gynecol* 1993;168:1443.

CHAPTER 35B
Ovarian Tumors Complicating Pregnancy

Jack Basil, Kristin Coppage, and James Pavelka

DEFINITIONS

Hyperreactio luteinalis—A benign, frequently large (15 to 20 cm), usually bilateral ovarian enlargement caused by an increased sensitivity to human chorionic gonadotropin (hCG). These masses are composed of numerous luteinized follicular cysts and are more common in conditions in which the hCG is increased (e.g., hydatidiform mole, multiple gestation). This condition is benign and resolves spontaneously after pregnancy.

Luteoma of pregnancy—A benign neoplasm of the ovary caused by the hormonal effects of pregnancy. It is usually solid and unilateral. It is most often asymptomatic and found incidentally. It may cause virilization and complications if torsion occurs. It resolves spontaneously after pregnancy.

Pulsatility index (PI)—An arterial waveform index that has been shown to be useful in discriminating benign from malignant adnexal masses. A PI > 1.0 is almost always associated with a benign mass. A PI < 1.0 is suggestive of malignancy but can be seen in a corpus luteum cyst or an inflammatory mass.

The coexistence of an adnexal mass with pregnancy presents problems to both the clinician and the patient, the most serious being that of malignancy. The care of the patient must balance the competing risks and benefits of the mother and fetus. Through a multidisciplinary approach of specialists in gynecologic oncology, maternal fetal medicine, pathology, and neonatology, the best plan of action, observation versus intervention, can be determined. Therapeutic implications including loss of the current pregnancy and loss of future fertility result in an emotionally charged environment, which must be skillfully navigated by all members of the health care team.

EPIDEMIOLOGY

Cancer complicates 1:1,000 pregnancies in the United States. The most common malignancies seen in pregnancy include malignant melanoma (2.6:1,000), Hodgkin lymphoma (1:1,000–6,000), breast cancer (1:3,000–10,000), cervical cancer (1.2:10,000), ovarian cancer (1:10,000–100,000), colorectal cancer (1:13,000), and leukemias (1:75,000–100,000).

The lifetime risk of developing ovarian cancer is 1.4% (14 per 1,000), the highest risk occurring after menopause. Women of reproductive age have a low risk approximating 0.2% to 0.4%. Benign ovarian tumors are the most common complicating pregnancy. The exact incidence, however, depends on whether one considers simple cysts noted on ultrasound examination (1 in 50 live births), during pelvic examination (1 in 80 live births), or those that ultimately require laparotomy (1 in 1,000 to 1 in 1,500 live births). Hill and colleagues reported findings for ovarian cysts found at the time of second- and third-trimester ultrasound. Ovarian cysts were diagnosed in 4.1% of second- or third-trimester ultrasounds. Most of these cysts were less than 3 cm and resolved spontaneously. Eighteen of the 7,996 patients had an exploratory laparotomy, which was equivalent to one surgery in 444 deliveries. All of these lesions were benign on pathologic examination. Ueda and Ueki reported 106 patients who required ovarian surgery during pregnancy. Of these patients, 31 (29.2%) had physiologic ovarian cysts, 70 (66%) were benign tumors, and 5 (4.7%) were malignant. More recent observations by Schlemer et al. have noted that adnexal masses greater than 5 cm were observed in 63 patients (0.05%), with 4 patients (6.8% of masses and 0.0032% of deliveries) diagnosed as malignant. Finally, these tumors may also be an incidental finding at the time of cesarean. Koonings and colleagues noted the incidence of ovarian tumors complicating cesarean section to be about 1 in 200 cesarean births. Dede et al. also observed a 0.8% incidence of masses greater than 5 cm at the time of cesarean section.

DIAGNOSIS

The definitive diagnosis of an ovarian tumor can only be made by pathologic examination. This places the clinician in a difficult dilemma during pregnancy. Until the widespread use of ultrasound, ovarian masses often remained unrecognized, as their symptoms frequently mimic common symptoms of pregnancy. Over time, clinicians have realized that there are windows of opportunity to evaluate the adnexa. These include the initial pelvic examination in the first trimester (palpable masses), any ultrasound performed, and careful evaluation at the time of operative intervention (cesarean section or postpartum tubal ligation). A thorough pelvic examination at the time of termination of pregnancy is another opportunity to evaluate the ovaries.

The increasing (nearly routine) use of ultrasound examination in pregnancy affords an excellent opportunity for the diagnosis of coexistent ovarian pathology; it is for this reason that such an examination should always include the adnexa (**Fig. 35B.1**). The results of ultrasound, although potentially very useful in the relatively rare patient with an ovarian malignancy, may create a difficult dilemma for the clinician who must decide how to proceed when an ovarian cyst is diagnosed in pregnancy. Perkins and coworkers evaluated 1,001 patients with first-trimester ultrasound and determined that a simple ovarian cyst was seen in 29% of these patients. The incidence of ovarian cysts decreased after 8 weeks, and absence of a cyst was more often associated with blighted ovum.

Bromley and Benacerraf evaluated the accuracy of sonographic diagnosis of adnexal masses during pregnancy. They evaluated all patients with an adnexal mass measuring 4 cm or greater noted beyond 12 weeks gestation. One hundred and thirty-one lesions were noted; of these, 89.3% were accurately diagnosed as benign. Fourteen of the 131 lesions (10.7%) had sonographic characteristics of malignancy. One of 14 (7%) of these patients had ovarian cancer, for a 0.8% malignancy rate in this study. Lavery and colleagues, in a review of 3,918 ultrasound examinations at 20 weeks gestation, noted cyst formation greater than 2 cm in 2.4% of examinations. Only nine patients (0.23%) required surgical intervention. Hogston and Lifford, in a review of 26,000 patients who received routine ultrasound, noted an incidence of cyst formation of 0.52%. All complex cysts and those greater than 6 cm were operated on primarily (10%). Eighty-five percent of the remaining patients who were followed conservatively showed spontaneous resolution, with the exception of 5 patients who ultimately required laparotomy.

Doppler sonography has been evaluated for use in complex adnexal masses in pregnancy. Wheeler and Fleischer evaluated 34 pregnant patients with complex adnexal masses. Diagnosis made by color Doppler sonography was compared with actual

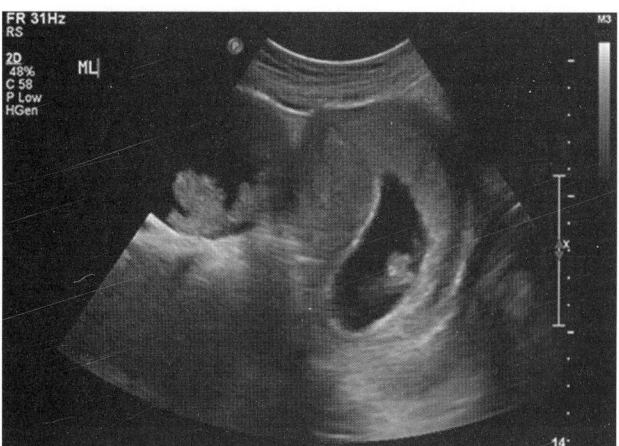

FIGURE 35B.1 This is a midline picture from a first-trimester ultrasound. Both the intrauterine pregnancy on the right and maternal adnexal mass on the left are visualized.

histopathologic diagnosis. Three malignant and five low malignant potential tumors were correctly identified with a sensitivity of 0.89 and a mean pulsatility index (PI) of 0.71. The mean PI for benign lesions was greater than 1, and the negative predictive value for PI > 1 was 0.93. The positive predictive value for PI < 1 was 0.42, indicating that some benign lesions were incorrectly classified as malignant when a PI < 1 is used as a cutoff for possibly malignant tumors. However, color Doppler appears to be highly predictive of a benign lesion when the PI is greater than 1.

Epithelial tumor markers such as CA-125, CEA, CA-19-9, and CA-15-3 demonstrate some fluctuation during pregnancy and should be interpreted with caution. However, median levels are still typically within established norms for premenopausal women. Alpha-fetoprotein levels rise during pregnancy. High MSAFP (maternal serum alpha fetoprotein) levels can be seen with germ cell tumors. These levels are significantly higher (MoM of 24) than are those seen in neural tube defects or abdominal wall defects as shown in a study by Elit and colleagues. Alpha-fetoprotein is heterogeneous, and the yolk sac variant can be separated by affinity chromatography to determine if the elevation is due to the yolk sac or liver variant. Another chemical marker is LDH (lactate dehydrogenase). Ovarian dysgerminomas may have significantly elevated levels of LDH in pregnancy as shown by Buller and colleagues. Pregnancy LDH is usually in normal range unless preeclampsia/HELLP syndrome has been diagnosed. Inhibin is a chemical made by the placenta and can be used to assess risk for chromosomal anomalies. Therefore, inhibin cannot be used during pregnancy to help to diagnose cell tumors, as it does in a nonpregnant patient. Finally, human chorionic gonadotropin (hCG) is used to follow some germ cell tumors such as choriocarcinoma; however, it again is not useful in pregnancy. Composite tests, such as the newer OVA-1 test, have no established data in pregnant women; include components such as transferrin, which are altered in pregnancy; and are therefore not recommended.

From a treatment standpoint, the first trimester is clearly the best time to diagnose an adnexal mass complicating pregnancy. Because tumors are rarely symptomatic during this period, most such tumors are discovered by ultrasound examination. With the increasing incidence of ultrasound evaluation and use of cesarean section, recent articles suggest that only about 50% of ovarian tumors complicating pregnancy are symptomatic. When symptomatic, the patient typically presents with abdominal pain, abdominal distention, and vague gastrointestinal symptoms. All these symptoms can be directly attributable to pregnancy itself; therefore, it is not surprising that most pregnant women with these symptoms are not evaluated for an ovarian tumor.

A successful outcome for both mother and fetus depends on a high index of suspicion with early diagnosis. One should consider an ovarian mass in any woman who experiences abdominal pain in pregnancy. Furthermore, torsion, rupture, infection, or hemorrhage of an ovarian tumor should be included in the differential diagnosis of any catastrophic abdominal obstetric event. This is particularly true during times of rapid change in uterine size or position (e.g., 8 to 16 weeks), during termination of pregnancy, during labor and delivery, or in the immediate postpartum period.

The incidence of torsion complicating an ovarian tumor in the nonpregnant state is about 2%. Torsion complicating an ovarian tumor during pregnancy is much higher. One report by Ueda and Ueki showed a 21.8% rate of torsion in ovarian tumors in pregnancy. Further, it is clear that the previously

unrecognized symptomatic ovarian tumor complicating pregnancy can become catastrophic. Wang and colleagues retrospectively evaluated 174 patients who underwent surgery for ovarian masses during pregnancy. These patients were divided into two groups: those with emergency surgery (32 patients) and those with elective surgery (142 patients). They found in the emergency surgery group that half of the surgeries occurred in the first trimester, they contributed to 75% of total fetal wastage and 87% of spontaneous fetal loss, and tumor sizes were significantly larger. In their experience, tumors less than 5 cm in size never caused symptoms requiring surgery. Therefore, size of tumor, ultrasound characteristics, color Doppler flow, serum analytes, and symptoms are important in determining the management of pregnant patients with adnexal masses.

PATHOLOGY

Benign neoplasms complicating pregnancy include two tumor-like conditions with which every gynecologist should be familiar. *Hyperreactio luteinalis* (first described by Burger in 1938 as a grossly multicystic, usually bilateral ovarian enlargement, often 15 to 20 cm in size) is a term used to describe numerous luteinized follicular cysts of the ovary complicating pregnancy. Microscopically, one notes extensive luteinization of the theca and granulosa cell layers. Bradshaw and associates suggest that the hyperandrogenicity seen in this condition is related to increased ovarian sensitivity to hCG. Therefore, it is seen in conditions in which the hCG is elevated, such as hydatidiform mole, multiple gestations, choriocarcinoma, and erythroblastosis fetalis. Hyperreactio luteinalis also has been associated with normal pregnancy, and, in these patients, it has not been associated with fetal virilization. These tumors spontaneously regress after delivery but may take up to 6 months to resolve. Hyperreactio luteinalis also may occur in subsequent pregnancies.

Luteoma of pregnancy is a specific benign, usually unilateral, solid lutein cell tumor of the ovary found in late pregnancy, often noted at cesarean section (Fig. 35B.2A, B). First described by Sternberg in 1966, this tumor is grossly bosselated, soft, fleshy, yellow, or hemorrhagic. Microscopically, it exhibits an acidophilic granular cytoplasm with sparse lipid formation and a distinctive reticular pattern. It is likely the most common cause of maternal virilization during pregnancy. The etiology is unknown, but theories have included luteinized stromal cells present before pregnancy that respond to hCG or "hyperluteinized" theca cells, granulosa cells, or a combination of the two. Fifty percent of female infants born to virilized mothers with pregnancy luteoma exhibit signs of virilization.

The important clinical implication with both of these lesions is that if they are recognized or suspected, simple biopsy without further surgery is adequate therapy, because both invariably resolve spontaneously.

The most common benign neoplasm of the ovary in pregnancy is the *benign cystic teratoma*, which accounts for about one third of all benign ovarian tumors seen in pregnancy (Fig. 35B.3A, B). The second most common group of ovarian tumors complicating pregnancy is that of cystadenomas (Fig. 35B.4). These represent about 15% of tumors. Endometriomas, simple cysts, corpus luteal cysts, tubal cysts, myomas, and other miscellaneous lesions constitute the remaining types of tumors seen in pregnancy (Table 35B.1).

Malignant ovarian tumors constitute only about 1% to 2% of all adnexal masses that complicate pregnancy and require

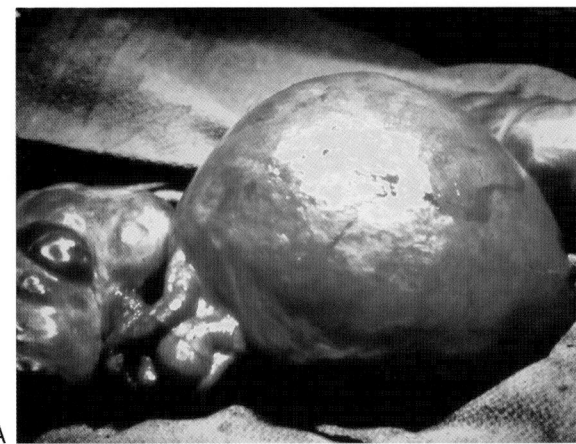

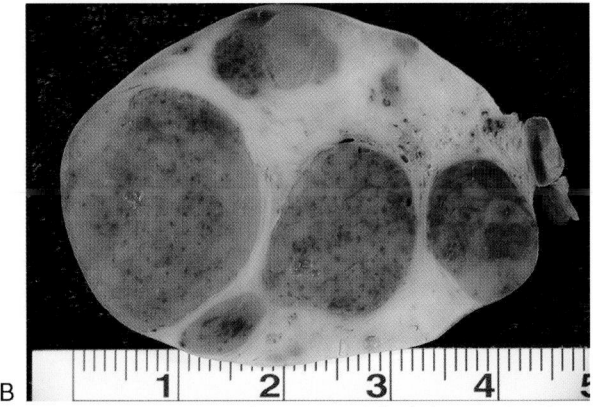

FIGURE 35B.2 A: Luteoma of pregnancy. The left ovary is enlarged with a lobulated smooth surface. These are usually unilateral. **B:** In this gross photograph, the ovary is bivalved and 5 reddish-brown leuteomas are clearly visible within the yellowish ovarian stroma. Leuteomas usually resolve spontaneously within several weeks of delivery. (With permission of Ed Uthman, MD.)

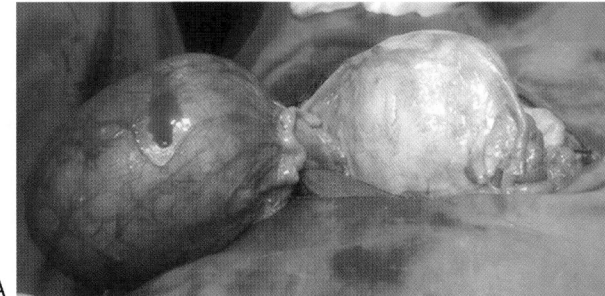

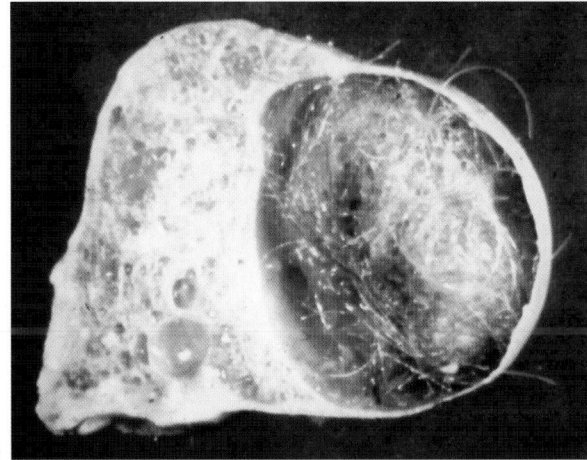

FIGURE 35B.3 A: Benign cystic teratoma (dermoid cyst) of the right ovary in a 15-week pregnant woman. (Reprinted from Shah K, Anjurani S, Bhat P, et al. Ovarian mass in pregnancy: a review of six cases treated with surgery. *Internet J Gynecol Obstet* 2000;14, with permission. Available at http://www.ispub.com.) **B:** Gross appearance of a bisected benign cystic teratoma with a large amount of oily hair. The small cyst contained oil and thick sebaceous material.

surgical exploration. The single most common malignant ovarian tumor complicating pregnancy probably is *dysgerminoma*. Malignant tumors of epithelial origin as a group, however, are more common (Fig. 35B.5); tumors of low malignant potential occur most frequently (Fig. 35B.6). Sex-cord stromal tumors are the third most common primary malignant ovarian neoplasms, representing about 17% to 20% of such tumors. Krukenberg and other metastatic tumors represent about 12% to 13% of malignant ovarian neoplasms complicating pregnancy (Fig. 35B.7).

Whether malignant or benign, most ovarian tumors complicating pregnancy are unilateral. Karlen and associates reported 90% of dysgerminomas in pregnancy to be unilateral, and Young and colleagues reported 35 of 36 sex-cord stromal tumors to be unilateral when complicating pregnancy. Even malignant tumors of epithelial origin noted during pregnancy are unilateral in 90% of cases. The rarer germ cell tumors, such as endodermal sinus tumors, virtually always are unilateral as well. It is also interesting that most bilateral tumors occurring in pregnancy are not malignant; these include benign cystic teratoma, endometriosis, and hyperreactio luteinalis. The most common bilateral malignant ovarian tumors are the metastatic Krukenberg types. Somewhat less common are primary malignant tumors of epithelial origin.

Virilization secondary to an ovarian tumor sometimes complicates pregnancy. The classic painting titled *Magdalena*

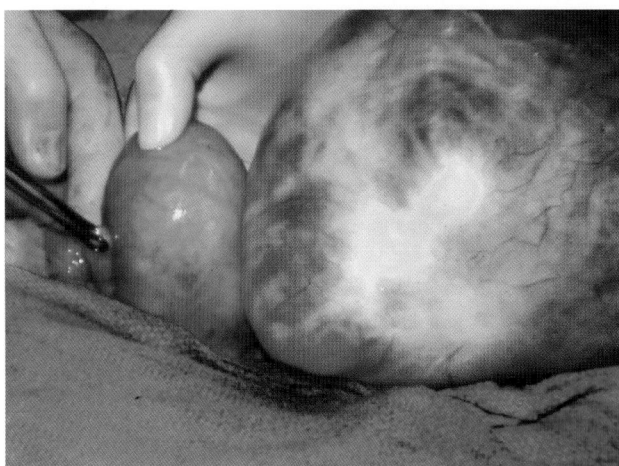

FIGURE 35B.4 Serous cyst adenoma of the left ovary. This patient presented to the emergency department with severe lower abdominal pain. She reported several missed periods and on exam had a tender mass up to the umbilicus. Ultrasound demonstrated a 10-week pregnancy plus a separate 22-cm smooth-walled, simple cystic mass with no ascites. *Note:* The pregnant uterus should be manipulated as little as possible during surgery.

TABLE 35B.1 Pathology of Pelvic Masses Complicating Pregnancy

	BROMLEY AND BENACERRAF $n = 131$	HILL ET AL. $n = 19$	WHEELER AND FLEISCHER $n = 34$	UEDA AND UEKI $n = 106$	TOTAL 290
Dermoid	40	8	8	48	104 (36%)
Endometrioma	15	1	2	10	28 (9.7%)
Functional cysts	14	1	0	6	21 (7.2%)
Cystadenomas	13	4	10	18	45 (15.5%)
Tubal cyst	9	2	0	0	11 (3.8%)
Fibroids	4	0	2	0	6 (2.1%)
Adenocarcinoma of the ovary	1	0	1	2	4 (1.4%)
Corpus luteum	0	2	2	15	19 (6.6%)
Serous cystadenoma/ endometrioma	1	0	0	0	1 (0.3%)
Cystadenofibroma	2	0	0	0	2 (0.6%)
Fibrothecoma	1	0	0	0	1 (0.3%)
Serous	1	0	0	0	1 (0.3%)
Cystadenofibroma	1	0	0	0	1 (0.3%)
Dermoid/fibrothecoma	1	0	0	0	1 (0.3%)
Fibroma	0	1	0	4	5 (1.7%)
Tarlov cyst	1	0	0	0	1 (0.3%)
Struma ovarii	2	0	0	0	2 (0.6%)
Luteoma of pregnancy	1	0	1	0	2 (0.6%)
Echinococcal cyst	1	0	0	0	1 (0.3%)
Dysgerminoma	0	0	1	1	2 (0.6%)
Lymphoma	0	0	1	0	1 (0.3%)
Low malignant potential tumors	0	0	6	1	7 (2.4%)
Embryonal carcinoma	0	0	0	1	1 (0.3%)
Normal ovaries	24	0	0	0	

Ventura with Husband and Son, painted in 1631 by Ribera, documents such a problem (Fig. 35B.8). Magdalena, after having several children, became virilized at age 37, with apparent infertility thereafter. However, when she was 52, a son was born. One would speculate that she probably had an ovarian Sertoli-Leydig cell tumor. Young and colleagues have noted that although about 50% of Sertoli-Leydig cell tumors in the nonpregnant state are functional, only about 15% of those complicating pregnancy result in maternal virilization. They proposed two possible explanations for this apparent decrease in virilization. The first is that the most active of such tumors result in anovulation; therefore, women with virilizing tumors rarely become pregnant. The second is that the placenta may aromatize the tumor-produced androgens into estrogens. In any event, Sertoli-Leydig cell tumors are not the most common tumors in pregnancy associated with

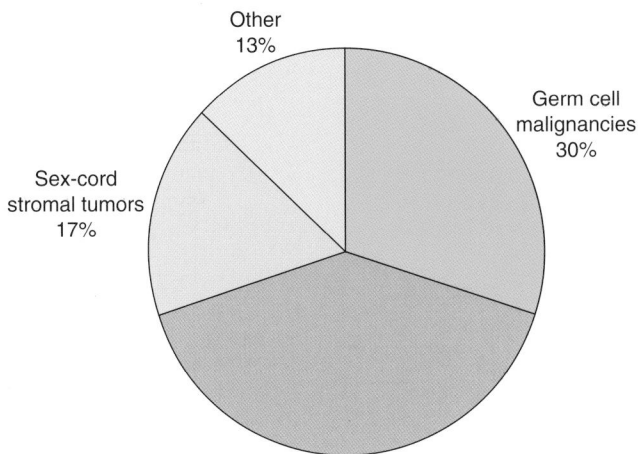

FIGURE 35B.5 The approximate relative frequency of the most common malignant ovarian tumors.

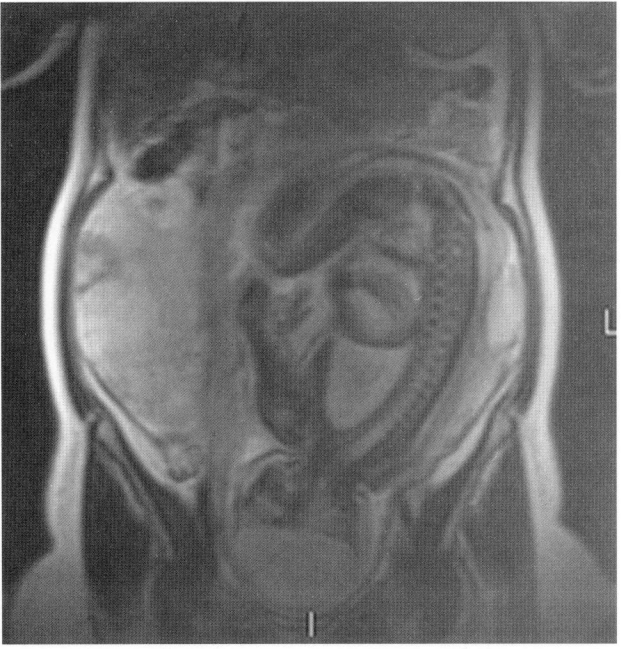

FIGURE 35B.7 This MRI depicts a fetus and intrauterine pregnancy at 32 weeks. Anterior to the uterus is a large adnexal mass that was removed at the time of cesarean section. Final pathology revealed a Krukenberg tumor.

virilization. This distinction falls to those tumors associated with a functioning ovarian stroma. The most common virilizing ovarian tumor that complicates pregnancy is the luteoma, followed by Krukenberg tumors and mucinous epithelial tumors (Table 35B.2).

The clinical implications of virilizing tumors complicating pregnancy are somewhat different from those of such tumors in the nonpregnant state. Virilization usually occurs late in pregnancy, is of short duration, and usually is reversible. The majority of such cases, as mentioned, are secondary to luteoma; therefore, they resolve spontaneously. If sex-cord stromal or epithelial tumors are present, the ultimate outcome remains quite good. However, patients with Krukenberg lesions have a poor outcome.

Malignancies also can be metastatic to the placenta or products of conception. Although this is an uncommon occurrence, tumors that may metastasize to the placenta include malignant melanoma, leukemias and lymphomas, breast carcinoma, lung carcinoma, and some sarcomas.

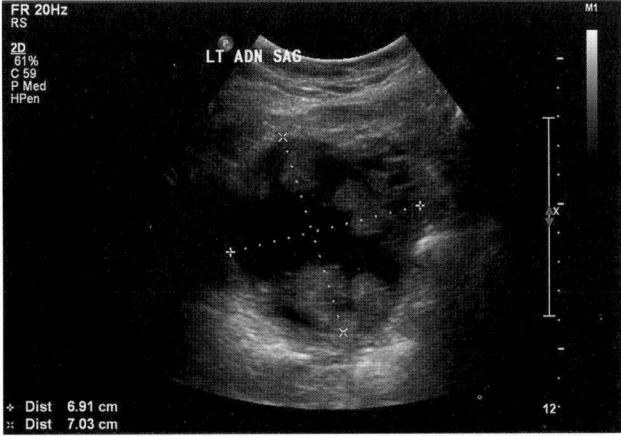

FIGURE 35B.6 Ultrasound of a complex 7-cm left adnexal mass that was noted during pregnancy. The size of the mass and the ultrasound characteristics of papillary projections were concern for malignancy. Final pathology revealed a mucinous tumor of low malignant potential.

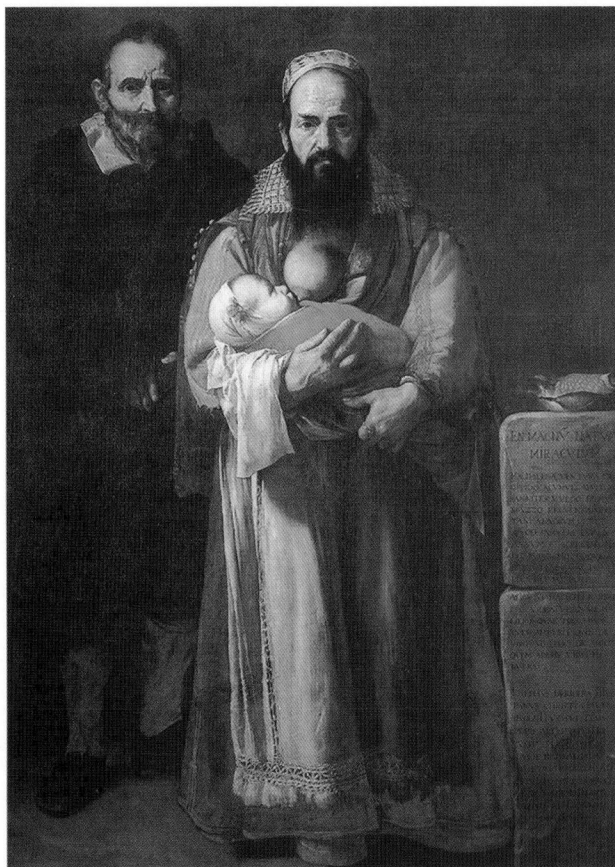

FIGURE 35B.8 The painting by Ribera titled *Magdalena Ventura with Husband and Son* (1631). The most common virilizing tumors of the ovary complicating pregnancy are those with functioning stroma.

VI

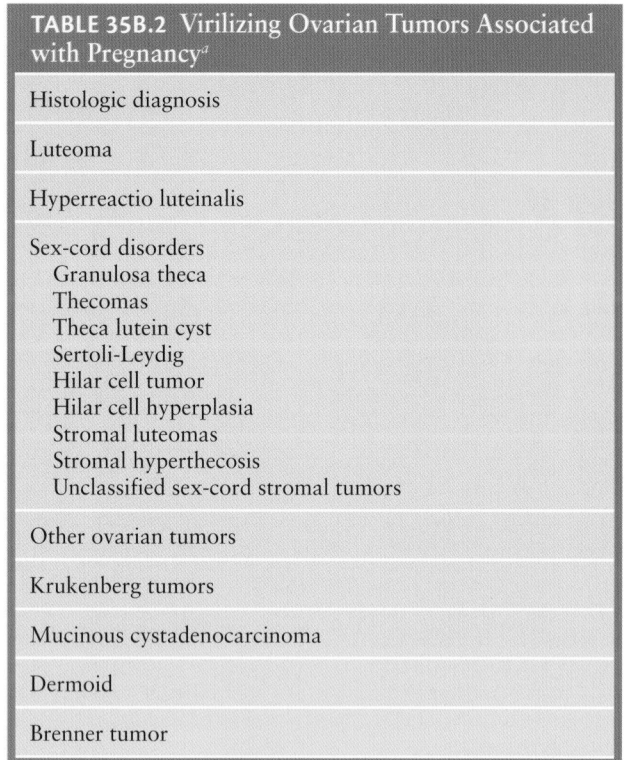

TABLE 35B.2 Virilizing Ovarian Tumors Associated with Pregnancy[a]

Histologic diagnosis
Luteoma
Hyperreactio luteinalis

Sex-cord disorders
  Granulosa theca
  Thecomas
  Theca lutein cyst
  Sertoli-Leydig
  Hilar cell tumor
  Hilar cell hyperplasia
  Stromal luteomas
  Stromal hyperthecosis
  Unclassified sex-cord stromal tumors

Other ovarian tumors
Krukenberg tumors
Mucinous cystadenocarcinoma
Dermoid
Brenner tumor

THERAPY

The first successful oophorectomy for an ovarian tumor complicating pregnancy was performed in 1846 by Bund. Although the woman survived, the fetus aborted at 12 weeks gestation. At about the same time, J. Marion Sims was the first to successfully remove an ovarian tumor in a pregnant woman and to have both the woman and fetus survive. As late as 1906, McKerran reported a 21% maternal mortality rate and a 50% fetal mortality rate with surgical management of ovarian tumors in pregnancy. While contemporary surgical management of adnexal masses in pregnancy carries significantly lower risk to both the patient and her fetus, a thorough understanding of potential pitfalls will improve outcomes.

In general, one should avoid elective surgery in the first trimester, because many ovarian lesions represent the cystic corpus luteum of pregnancy and resolve spontaneously. Therefore, ultrasound should be repeated in 6 weeks to determine if the mass is persistent before considering surgical intervention. Buttery and colleagues noted an abortion rate of about 30% in those patients operated on in the first trimester, so first-trimester procedures are high risk. Nevertheless, highly symptomatic masses with suspicion of torsion or masses with solid and cystic conformation or other findings such as ascites, which would correlate with a high suspicion of malignancy, should be operated on immediately (**Fig. 35B.9**). Preoperative evaluation should include careful clinical evaluation and pelvic ultrasound examination. Studies relying on ionizing radiation such as barium enema, computed tomography, and other such studies are best avoided. Magnetic resonance imaging has a well-established track record of safety in pregnancy and, with newer imaging techniques, can help in the evaluation of adnexal masses and other abdominal pathologies.

The optimum time for surgical intervention is 16 to 18 weeks. In general, the first trimester should be avoided

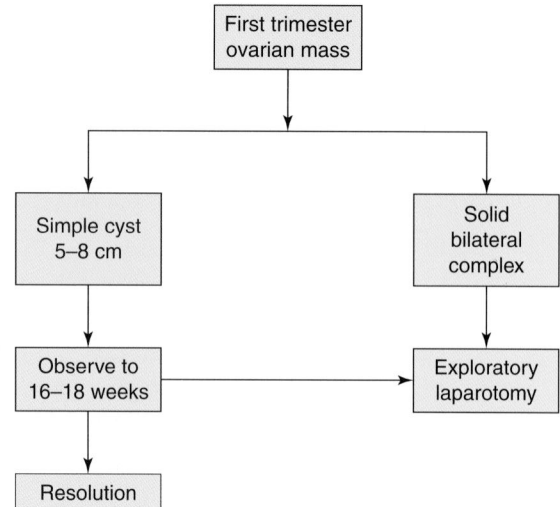

FIGURE 35B.9 Algorithm for the surgical management of ovarian tumors complicating pregnancy in the first trimester. Symptomatic, solid, bilateral, and complex lesions should be operated on when discovered.

if possible because of the naturally occurring high rate of spontaneous abortion. Additionally, disruption of the corpus luteum in the first trimester could lead to fetal wastage unless progesterone supplementation is provided. In any case, it is difficult to avoid the conclusion that any pregnancy loss occurring within a short time of surgery is related to the surgery, so that if it is possible to wait until the second trimester, the risk of an unrelated spontaneous abortion is decreased. Patients in whom the asymptomatic mass is noted at or near term may be considered for delivery by cesarean section with careful intraoperative evaluation of the adnexa. Vaginal delivery in this situation has been associated with torsion, rupture, and hemorrhage that can occur during labor or immediately postpartum. The size and ultrasound characteristics of the mass will help to guide the clinician's decision concerning the best route of delivery. Caspi and colleagues described *conservative management* of 63 patients who had dermoid cysts ≤6 cm. None of these patients had an increase in size of the dermoid during pregnancy. In this study, 55 patients had normal vaginal deliveries, and none had complications related to the cyst.

General anesthesia is the anesthesia of choice, although a combination of epidural and general anesthesia can be considered. One should remember that delayed gastric emptying and esophageal reflux can occur in pregnancy; therefore, appropriate precautions are necessary. One also should be aware of and prevent compression of the vena cava and aorta by proper patient positioning.

The next consideration is *laparoscopy versus laparotomy* as primary surgical management. Several case series have evaluated the safety and efficacy of laparoscopic management of adnexal masses in pregnancy. These studies have shown that a laparoscopic approach can be employed without increased risk to mother or fetus. Laparoscopy should be considered early in the second trimester if the mass is mobile and accessible and does not have characteristics of malignancy such as ascites or carcinomatosis. Left upper quadrant or open laparoscopic entry should be considered to minimize risk of unintentional uterine or adnexal trauma. If laparotomy is the chosen surgical approach, a vertical incision is preferred due to the flexibility it offers to complete staging, if necessary, and because after 16 weeks gestation the ovary becomes an abdominal rather than pelvic structure. The incision should be placed higher than usual.

Regardless of surgical approach, thorough evaluation of peritoneal cavity and all contents should be performed, along with pelvic washings. The involved ovary should be sent for frozen section to establish a preliminary diagnosis. The contralateral ovary should be carefully inspected. Biopsy or wedge resection of the contralateral ovary should be avoided if no gross evidence of involvement is present. One possible exception is if the primary tumor is a dysgerminoma, because these tumors can involve the contralateral ovary in a clinically undetectable, microscopic manner. If the frozen section demonstrates a malignant germ cell tumor, an epithelial ovarian cancer, or low malignant potential tumor, staging should be performed to include omentectomy, peritoneal biopsies, and pelvic and aortic lymph node dissection. Malignant ovarian stromal tumors rarely spread to retroperitoneal nodes, and the value of routine lymphadenectomy in these patients is questioned. While it has been argued historically that routine appendectomy should be performed in the case of a mucinous ovarian tumor, recent data suggest that a visibly normal appendix is extremely unlikely to harbor pathology.

The uterus should be handled gently in any case, and frequent irrigation should be used to prevent the tissue from drying. When ovarian cystectomy is required, simple hemostasis is sufficient, and ovarian closure is unnecessary and may lead to iatrogenic bleeding. If closure is required, an internal closure with use of a 4-0 absorbable is recommended.

Before the decision is made to perform oophorectomy, one must always consciously exclude hyperreactio luteinalis and luteoma of pregnancy. Furthermore, because most malignant ovarian tumors are unilateral, total abdominal hysterectomy and bilateral salpingo-oophorectomy are rarely indicated (Fig. 35B.10). Total hysterectomy and removal of ovaries should never be performed on the basis of a frozen section diagnosis of borderline or low-grade malignancy unless the patient has clearly expressed a desire to abort this pregnancy and does not wish to preserve fertility and ovarian function.

When faced with a clearly malignant bilateral or metastatic tumor, one usually treats the patient as if she were nonpregnant, with bilateral salpingo-oophorectomy, pelvic and abdominal washings, omentectomy, and pelvic and aortic node biopsies. Hysterectomy should be performed in a desired pregnancy only when gross involvement of the uterus is appreciated and after appropriate preoperative consultation. Although other tumors are known to metastasize rarely to either the placenta or fetus, primary ovarian tumors almost never do so.

Preoperative discussion with the patient and her family is of paramount importance. All the possible findings at surgery and possible surgical management options should be carefully discussed, and a good understanding of the planned therapy should be agreed on by all. A complete preoperative note about the discussion should be made in the patient's chart. The family should be informed of the findings and plans during

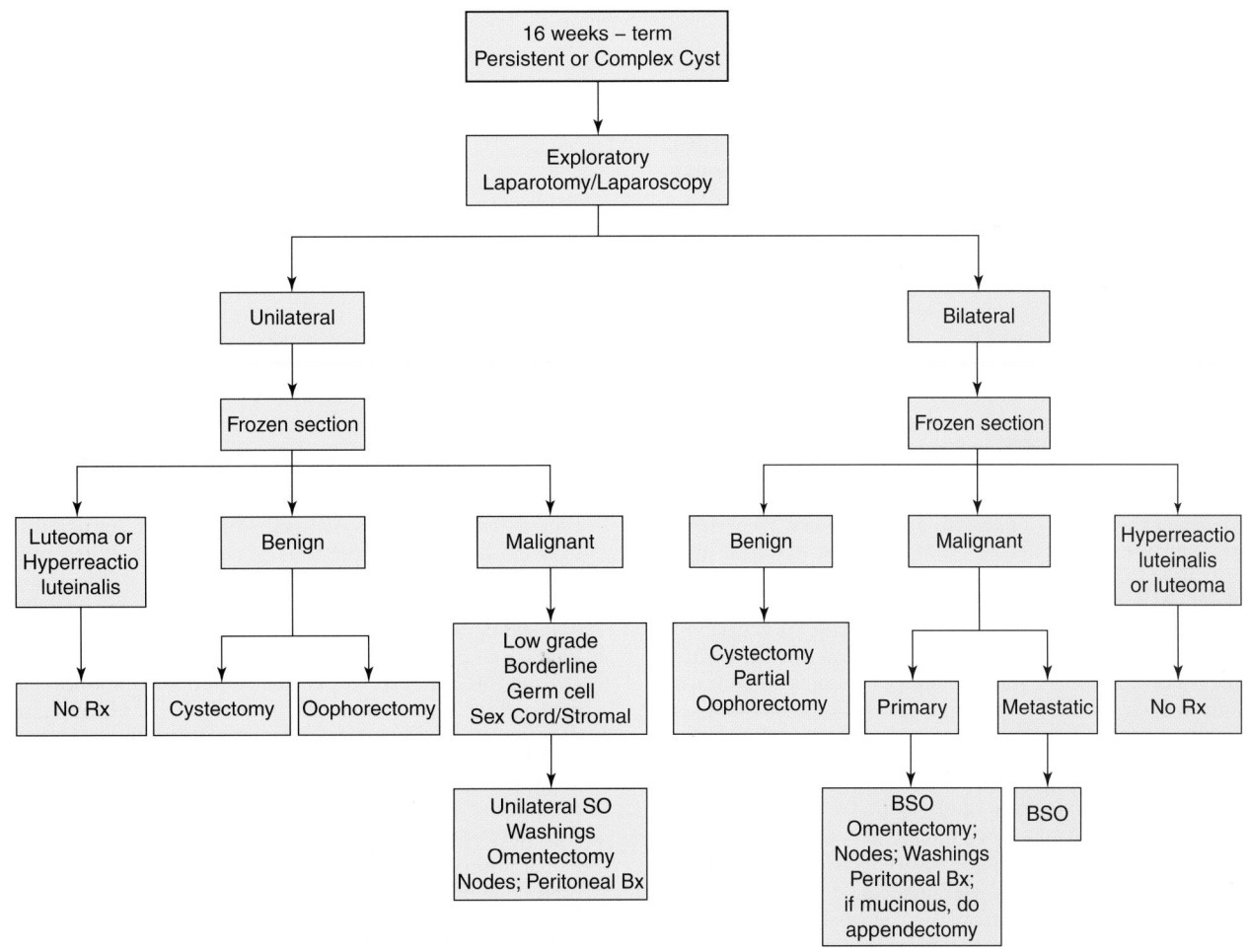

FIGURE 35B.10 Algorithm for the surgical management of ovarian tumors occurring after 16 weeks gestation. (BSO, bilateral salpingo-oophorectomy; SO, salpingo-oophorectomy; TAH, total abdominal hysterectomy; Bx, biopsy; Rx, treatment.)

the course of surgery, and consultation should be obtained if necessary.

The role of progesterone to prevent labor in the postoperative period is unclear but should be considered if the surgery occurs in the first trimester and the corpus luteum is disrupted. The patient should have fetal heart tones checked preoperatively, immediately postoperatively, and periodically through the postoperative period. If contractions occur, these can be treated with hydration, indomethacin (if before 32 weeks), or standard tocolytic therapy for symptom relief.

TREATMENT OUTCOME

For benign disease, the patient's surgical outcomes should be excellent. With malignant disease, the overall 5-year survival rate depends on histology, stage, and treatment choices. In a classic paper on ovarian cancer in pregnancy, Novak and associates reported a 5-year survival rate of 75% from the Johns Hopkins Hospital. In a review of 27 dysgerminomas, Karlen and associates reported a tendency toward local recurrence with conservative treatment but an overall 5-year survival rate of 90%. Young and coworkers, in a review of 36 sex-cord stromal tumors, noted a 5-year survival rate of 100%, although they cautioned that granulosa cell tumors are prone to late recurrence. However, patients with Krukenberg tumors or metastatic disease have a poor prognosis.

Fetal mortality also should be minimal with early diagnosis and appropriate surgical intervention. Although Karlen and associates reported a fetal mortality rate of 25%, two of the five deaths were secondary to hysterotomy. Young and colleagues reported three fetal deaths in 36 cases, two of which resulted from hysterectomy. Ueda and Ueki reported on 106 surgeries with a spontaneous abortion rate of 10%. Two patients desired termination of pregnancy in the second trimester owing to ovarian diagnosis, and one fetus died despite intensive efforts.

CYTOTOXIC CHEMOTHERAPY DURING PREGNANCY

At no time is the treatment of cancer during pregnancy more complicated than when adjunctive therapy is indicated. Can such therapy be given safely during pregnancy? The relative safety of cytotoxic chemotherapy to a developing fetus depends on many variables, including choice of drug, relative dose intensity and dose density, maternal metabolism, and especially gestational age. Although single-agent or combination chemotherapy may be teratogenic in the first trimester, it is now apparent that cytotoxic chemotherapy can for the most part be used safely in the second and third trimesters.

Antimetabolite therapy, including both aminopterin and methotrexate, seems to pose the greatest risk to a developing fetus and has been reported to be associated with a fairly high rate of congenital abnormalities. The aminopterin syndrome—which consists of cranial dysostosis, hypertelorism, anomalies of the external ear, micrognathia, and cleft palate—has occurred in the fetuses of about 20% of patients treated in the first trimester. In the reported literature, when methotrexate is given in the early first trimester for an erroneous diagnosis of ectopic pregnancy, spontaneous abortion or severe malformations will occur in a majority of cases. The alkylating agent chlorambucil has been associated with congenital abnormalities—namely, renal aplasia, cleft palate, and skeletal anomalies—but only with first-trimester exposure.

If drugs outside the antimetabolite class are administered in the second or third trimester, the safety profile is fairly sound.

Cisplatin and carboplatin have a well-established record of use in this setting, with no apparent teratogenicity significantly above the baseline observed. Some hearing loss and transient renal effects have been reported with in utero exposure to cisplatin. Antitumor antibiotics such as bleomycin, doxorubicin, and daunorubicin have shown no adverse fetal outcomes. Vincristine and vinblastine cause malformations in animals, but the effects have not been reported in humans. Paclitaxel is very effective in treatment of epithelial ovarian malignancies, and there are several reports in the literature of its successful use during pregnancy without significant negative fetal effects.

Besides such congenital abnormalities and spontaneous abortions, other concerns with the use of chemotherapy in pregnancy include sterility, low birth weight, pancytopenia, delayed cognitive development, and carcinogenesis. The risk and benefits to the fetus and mother must be considered before beginning therapy. Of course, cytotoxic chemotherapy has other effects, including hematopoietic depression and infection. For this reason, the timing of chemotherapy in relation to anticipated delivery must be assessed carefully so that delivery does not occur when the patient is pancytopenic.

OTHER ISSUES SURROUNDING MALIGNANCY

Symptom control is very important in pregnant patients with malignancy. Symptoms commonly seen in malignancy include pain, nausea, vomiting, anorexia, dyspnea, fatigue, and depression. Oxycodone and hydrocodone with acetaminophen can be used safely for pain. Codeine should be avoided in the first trimester because of possible fetal malformation. Opiates can be used, but with long-term usage or usage in close proximity to delivery, the neonate should be monitored for withdrawal. For nausea, options include ondansetron, chlorpromazine, prochlorperazine, prednisone, and metoclopramide. Morphine and albuterol have been successfully used to control dyspnea in patients with malignancy. Many patients with advanced cancer have depression. Tricyclic antidepressants, bupropion, and selective serotonin reuptake inhibitors with the exception of paroxetine have been used safely in pregnancy; the risks and the benefits should be discussed with these patients before starting them on medications. The use of monoamine oxidase inhibitors is discouraged in pregnant patients.

BEST SURGICAL PRACTICES

- Symptomatic adnexal masses may require surgery at any time during pregnancy. Women with asymptomatic masses may be diagnosed at the time of routine second-trimester ultrasound examination. Color Doppler blood flow characteristic, size, and morphology on ultrasound may be helpful in deciding which masses need surgical management.
- Elective surgery is best avoided in the first trimester. Benign corpus luteum cysts are common and so is spontaneous miscarriage unrelated to the adnexal mass. Many masses detected in the first trimester will resolve spontaneously; therefore, ultrasound should be repeated in 6 weeks to determine if the mass is persistent before considering surgical intervention.
- The best time for surgery is 16 to 18 weeks gestation. General anesthesia is recommended. Laparoscopy may be preferable if laparoscopy would be used for similar findings in a nonpregnant patient. If laparotomy is the chosen surgical approach, a vertical incision is preferred due to the flexibility it offers to complete staging, if necessary, and because after 16 weeks gestation the ovary becomes an abdominal

rather than pelvic structure. A conservative approach is advised. Most ovarian masses in pregnancy are benign. In the absence of obvious metastatic cancer, if a malignancy is found, unilateral oophorectomy with conservative staging should be performed, and final treatment plans are deferred pending a definitive pathology diagnosis.

- Even if unilateral dysgerminoma or a sex-cord stromal tumor is diagnosed, conservative therapy offers a good prognosis. Delivery may be delayed, and further surgery may be unnecessary.

- If metastatic cancer is diagnosed, a debulking surgery can be performed and pregnancy continued while the patient is started on chemotherapy. Careful consideration of all options should be discussed with a multidisciplinary approach including the gynecologic oncologist, the maternal fetal specialist, the pathologist, the neonatologist, and the patient and her family.

BIBLIOGRAPHY

Agarwal N, Parul K, Bhalta N, et al. Management and outcome of pregnancies complicated with adnexal masses in pregnancy. *Arch Gynecol Obstet* 2003;267:148.

Aiman J. Virilizing ovarian tumors. *Clin J Obstet Gynecol* 1991; 34:835.

Antonelli NM, Dotters DJ, Katz VL, et al. Cancer in pregnancy: a review of the literature. Part I–II. *Obstet Gynecol Surv* 1996; 51:125.

Borgfeldt C, Iosif C, Masback A. Fertility-sparing surgery and outcome in fertile women with ovarian borderline tumors and epithelial invasive ovarian cancer. *Eur J Obstet Gynecol Reprod Biol* 2006;134:110.

Boulay R, Podczaski E. Ovarian cancer complicating pregnancy. *Obstet Gynecol Clin North Am* 1998;25:385.

Bradshaw KD, Santos-Ramos R, Rawlins SC, et al. Endocrine studies in a pregnancy complicated by ovarian theca lutein cysts and hyperreactio luteinalis. *Obstet Gynecol* 1986;67:66S.

Bromley B, Benacerraf B. Adnexal masses during pregnancy: accuracy of sonographic diagnosis and outcome. *J Ultrasound Med* 1997;16:447.

Buller RE, Darrow V, Manetta A, et al. Conservative surgical management of dysgerminoma concomitant with pregnancy. *Obstet Gynecol* 1992;79:887.

Carter JR, Lau M, Fowler JM, et al. Blood flow characteristics of ovarian tumors: implications for ovarian cancer screening. *Am J Obstet Gynecol* 1995;172:901.

Caspi B, Ben-Arie A, Appelman Z, et al. Aspiration of simple pelvic cysts during pregnancy. *Gynecol Obstet Invest* 2000; 49:102.

Caspi B, Levi R, Appelman Z, et al. Conservative management of ovarian cystic teratoma during pregnancy and labor. *Am J Obstet Gynecol* 2000;182:503.

Check JH, Choe JK, Nazari A. Hyperreactio luteinalis despite absence of a corpus luteum and suppressed serum follicle stimulating concentrations in a triplet pregnancy. *Hum Reprod* 2000; 15:1043.

De Palma P, Wronski M, Bifernino V, et al. Krukenberg tumor in pregnancy with virilization. *Eur J Gynaecol Oncol* 1995;16:59.

Dede M, Yenen MC, Yilmaz A, et al. Treatment of incidental adnexal masses at cesarean section: a retrospective study. *Int J Gynecol Cancer* 2007;17:339.

Dgani R, Soham Z, Atar OE, et al. Ovarian carcinoma during pregnancy. *Gynecol Oncol* 1989;33:326.

Dildy GA, Moise KJ, Carpenter RJ, et al. Maternal malignancy metastatic to the products of conception: a review. *Obstet Gynecol Surv* 1989;44:535.

Donegan WL. Cancer and pregnancy. *CA Cancer J Clin* 1983;33:194.

Ebert U, Loffler H, Kirch W. Cytotoxic therapy and pregnancy. *Pharmacol Ther* 1997;74:207.

Elerding SC. Laparoscopic surgery in pregnancy. *Am J Surg* 1993; 165:625.

Elit L, Bocking A, Kenyon C, et al. An endodermal sinus tumor diagnosed in pregnancy: case report and review of the literature. *Gynecol Oncol* 1999;72:123.

Ercan Ş, Kaymaz Ö, Yücel N, et al. Serum concentrations of CA 125, CA 15-3, CA 19-9 and CEA in normal pregnancy: a longitudinal study. *Arch Gynecol Obstet* 2012;285:579.

Farahmand SM, Marchetti DL, Asirwatham JE, et al. Ovarian endodermal sinus tumor associated with pregnancy: a review of the literature. *Gynecol Oncol* 1991;41:156.

Ferrandina G, Distefano M, Testa A, et al. Management of an advanced ovarian cancer at 15 weeks of gestation: case report and literature review. *Gynecol Oncol* 2005;97:693.

Fleischer AC, Shah DM, Entman SS. Sonographic evaluation of maternal disorders during pregnancy. *Radiol Clin North Am* 1990; 28:51.

Frederiksen MC, Casanova L, Schink JC. An elevated maternal serum alpha-fetoprotein leading to the diagnosis of an immature teratoma. *Int J Gynaecol Obstet* 1991;35:343.

Garcia-Bunuel RG, Berek JS, Woodruff JD. Luteomas of pregnancy. *Obstet Gynecol* 1975;45:407.

Ghaemmaghami F, Hasanzadeh M. Good fetal outcome of pregnancies with gynecologic cancer conditions: cases and literature review. *Int J Gynecol Cancer* 2006;16:225.

Giuntoli RL II, Vang RS, Bristow RE. Evaluation and management of adnexal masses during pregnancy. *Clin Obstet Gynecol* 2006;49:492.

Greskovich JF Jr, Macklis RM. Radiation therapy in pregnancy: risk calculation and risk minimization. *Semin Oncol* 2000;27:633.

Henderson CE, Giovanni E, Garfinkel D, et al. Platinum chemotherapy during pregnancy for serous cystadenocarcinoma of the ovary. *Gynecol Oncol* 1993;49:92.

Hermans RH, Fischer DC, van der Putten HW, et al. Adnexal masses in pregnancy. *Onkologie* 2003;26:167.

Hill LM, Connors-Beatty DJ, Nowak A, et al. The role of ultrasonography in the detection and management of adnexal masses during the second and third trimesters of pregnancy. *Am J Obstet Gynecol* 1998;179:703.

Hogston P, Lifford RJ. Ultrasound study of ovarian cysts in pregnancy: prevalence and significance. *BJOG* 1986;93:625.

Hopkins MP, Duchon MA. Adnexal surgery in pregnancy. *J Reprod Med* 1986;31:1035.

Illingworth PJ, Johnstone FD, Steel J, et al. Luteoma of pregnancy: masculinisation of a female fetus prevented by placental aromatisation. *BJOG* 1992;99:1019.

Karlen JR, Akbari A, Cook WA. Dysgerminoma associated with pregnancy. *Obstet Gynecol* 1979;53:330.

Kier R, McCarthy SM, Scoutt LM, et al. Pelvic masses in pregnancy: MR imaging. *Radiology* 1990;176:709.

King LA, Nevin PC, Williams PP, et al. Treatment of advanced epithelial ovarian carcinoma in pregnancy with cisplatin-based chemotherapy. *Gynecol Oncol* 1991;41:78.

Kobayashi H, Yoshida A, Kobayashi M, et al. Changes in size of the functional cyst on ultrasonography during early pregnancy. *Am J Perinatol* 1997;14:1.

Koonings PP, Platt LD, Wallace R. Incidental adnexal neoplasms at caesarean section. *Obstet Gynecol* 1988;72:767.

Koren G, Lishner M, Farine D, eds. *Cancer in pregnancy. Maternal and fetal risks.* Cambridge, UK: Cambridge University Press, 1996.

Lavery JP, Koontz WL, Layman L, et al. Sonographic evaluation of the adnexa during early pregnancy. *Surg Gynecol Obstet* 1986;163:319.

Leiserowitz GS, Xing G, Cress R, et al. Adnexal masses in pregnancy: how often are they malignant? *Gynecol Oncol* 2006;101:315.

Lin JE, Seo S, Kushner DM, et al. The role of appendectomy for mucinous ovarian neoplasms. *Am J Obstet Gynecol* 2013; 208:46.

Luisi S, Florio P, Reis FM, et al. Inhibins in female and male reproductive physiology: role in gametogenesis, conception, implantation and early pregnancy. *Hum Reprod Update* 2005;11:123.

MacDougall M, LeGrand SB, Walsh D. Symptom control in the pregnant cancer patient. *Semin Oncol* 2000;27:704.

Machado F, Vegas C, Leon J, et al. Ovarian cancer during pregnancy: analysis of 15 cases. *Gynecol Oncol* 2007;105:446.

Malfetano JH, Goldkrand JW. Cis platinum combination chemotherapy during pregnancy for advanced epithelial ovarian carcinoma. *Obstet Gynecol* 1990;75:545.

Manganiello PD, Adams LV, Harris RD, et al. *Obstet Gynecol Surv* 1995;50:404.

Mantovani G, Mais V, Parodo G, et al. Use of chemotherapy for ovarian cancer during human pregnancy: case report and literature review. *Eur J Obstet Gynecol Reprod Biol* 2007;131:238.

Marhhom E, Cohen I. Fertility preservation options for women with malignancies. *Obstet Gynecol Surv* 2007;62:58.

Matsuyma T, Tsukamoto N, Matsukuma K, et al. Malignant ovarian tumors associated with pregnancy. *Int J Gynecol Oncol* 1989;28:61.

Mendez LE, Mueller A, Salom E, et al. Paclitaxel and carboplatin chemotherapy administered during pregnancy for advanced epithelial ovarian cancer. *Obstet Gynecol* 2003;102:1200.

Metz SA, Day TG, Pursell SH. Adjuvant chemotherapy in a pregnancy patient with endodermal sinus tumor of the ovary. *Gynecol Oncol* 1989;32:371.

Mir O, Berveiller P, Ropert S, et al. Use of platinum derivatives during pregnancy. *Cancer* 2008;113:3069.

Mooney J, Silva E, Tornos C, et al. Unusual features of serous neoplasms of low malignant potential during pregnancy. *Gynecol Oncol* 1997;65:30.

Nawa A, Obata N, Kikkawa F, et al. Prognostic factors of patients with yolk sac tumors of the ovary. *Am J Obstet Gynecol* 2001;184:1182.

Nezhat F, Nezhat C, Silfen SL, et al. Laparoscopic ovarian cystectomy during pregnancy. *J Laparoendosc Surg* 1991;1:161.

Nicklas AH, Baker ME. Imaging strategies in the pregnant cancer patient. *Semin Oncol* 2000;27:623.

Nieminen V, Remes N. Malignancy during pregnancy. *Acta Obstet Gynecol Scand* 1970;49:315.

Novak ER, Lambrose CD, Woodruff JD. Ovarian tumors in pregnancy. *Obstet Gynecol* 1975;46:401.

Nurmohamed L, Moretti ME, Schechter T, et al. Outcome following high-dose **methotrexate** in pregnancies misdiagnosed as ectopic. *Am J Obstet Gynecol* 2011;205:533.e1.

Pavlidis NA. Cancer and pregnancy. *Ann Oncol* 2000;11(suppl 3):247.

Pavlidis NA. Coexistence of pregnancy and malignancy. *Oncologist* 2002;7:279.

Perkins KY, Johnson JL, Kay HH. Simple ovarian cysts: clinical features on a first-trimester ultrasound scan. *J Reprod Med* 1997; 42:440.

Piana S, Nogales FF, Corrado S, et al. Pregnancy luteoma with granulosa cell proliferation: an unusual hyperplastic lesion arising in pregnancy and mimicking an ovarian neoplasia. *Pathol Res Pract* 1999;195:859.

Picone O, Lhomme C, Tournaire M, et al. Preservation of pregnancy in a patient with a stage IIIB ovarian epithelial carcinoma diagnosed at 22 weeks of gestation and treated with initial chemotherapy: case report and literature review. *Gynecol Oncol* 2004;94:600.

Rodriguez M, Harrison TA, Nowazki MR, et al. Luteoma of pregnancy presenting with massive ascites and markedly elevated CA-125. *Obstet Gynecol* 1999;94:854.

Sandmeier D, Lobrinus JA, Vial Y, et al. Bilateral Krukenberg tumor of the ovary during pregnancy. *Eur J Gynaecol Oncol* 2000;21:58.

Sarandakou A, Protonotariou E, Rizos D. Tumor markers in biological fluids associated with pregnancy. *Crit Rev Clin Lab Sci* 2007;44:151.

Sasa H, Komatsu Y, Kobayashi M. Ovarian carcinoma in the first trimester. *Int J Gynaecol Obstet* 1998;60:283.

Schapira DV, Chudley AE. Successful pregnancy following continuous treatment with combination chemotherapy before conception and throughout pregnancy. *Cancer* 1984;54:800.

Schmeler KM, Mayo-Smith WW, Peipert JF, et al. Adnexal masses in pregnancy: surgery compared with observation. *Obstet Gynecol* 2005;105:1098.

Schover L. Psychosocial issues associated with cancer in pregnancy. *Semin Oncol* 2000;27:699.

Schumer ST, Cannistra SA. Granulosa cell tumor of the ovary. *J Clin Oncol* 2003;21:1180.

Schwartzberg BS, Conyers JA, Moore JA. First trimester of pregnancy laparoscopic procedures. *Surg Endosc* 1997;11:1216.

SEER Cancer Statistics. 1975–2005. www.cancer.gov/cancertopics/factsheet/risk/BRCA

Shibahara H, Wakimoto E, Mitsuo M, et al. A case of a patient diagnosed with malignant mixed mullerian tumor of the ovary who conceived after conservative surgery and adjuvant chemotherapy. *Gynecol Oncol* 1997;65:363.

Silva PD, Proto M, Moyer DL, et al. Clinical and ultrastructural findings of an androgenizing Krukenberg tumor in pregnancy. *Obstet Gynecol* 1988;71:432.

Smith LH, Dalrymple JL, Leiserowitz GS, et al. Obstetrical deliveries associated with maternal malignancy in California, 1992 through 1997. *Am J Obstet Gynecol* 2001;184:1504 [discussion 1512].

Stedman CM, Kline RC. Intraoperative complications and unexpected pathology at the time of c-section. *Obstet Gynecol Clin North Am* 1988;15:745.

Sternberg WH, Barclay DL. Luteoma of pregnancy. *Am J Obstet Gynecol* 1966;95:195.

Tawan K, Baker TH. Ovarian tumors in pregnancy. *J Int Coll Surg* 1964;41:60.

Telischak NA, Yeh BM, Joe BN, et al. MRI of adnexal masses in pregnancy. *AJR Am J Roentgenol* 2008;191:364.

Tewari K, Brewer C, Cappuccini F, et al. Advanced-stage small cell carcinoma of the ovary in pregnancy: long-term survival after surgical debulking and multiagent chemotherapy. *Gynecol Oncol* 1997;66:531.

Tewari K, Cappuccini F, Disaia PJ, et al. Malignant germ cell tumors of the ovary. *Obstet Gynecol* 2000;95:128.

Thornton JF, Wells M. Ovarian cysts in pregnancy: does ultrasound make traditional management inappropriate? *Obstet Gynecol* 1987;69:717.

Thrall MM, Paley P, Pizer E, et al. Patterns of spread and recurrence of sex cord-stromal tumors of the ovary. *Gynecol Oncol* 2011;122:242.

Ueda M, Ueki M. Ovarian tumors associated with pregnancy. *Int J Gynaecol Obstet* 1996;55:59.

Van der Zee AG, deBruijn HW, Bouma J, et al. Endodermal sinus tumor of the ovary during pregnancy. *Am J Obstet Gynecol* 1991;164:504.

Wang PH, Chao HT, Yuan CC, et al. Ovarian tumors complicating pregnancy: emergency and elective surgery. *J Reprod Med* 1999;44:279.

Weinreb JC, Brown CE, Lowe TW, et al. Pelvic masses in pregnant patients: MR and US imaging. *Radiology* 1986;159:717.

Wheeler TC, Fleischer AC. Complex adnexal mass in pregnancy: predictive value of color Doppler sonography. *J Ultrasound Med* 1997;16:425.

Williams SF, Schilsky RL. Antineoplastic drugs administered during pregnancy. *Semin Oncol* 2000;27:618.

Wingo PA, Tong T, Bolden S. Cancer statistics, 1995. *Cancer J Clin* 1995;45:8 [erratum 127].

Young RH, Dudley AG, Scully RE. Granulosa cell, Sertoli-Leydig cell, and unclassified sex cord stromal tumors associated with pregnancy: a clinicopathological analysis of thirty-six cases. *Gynecol Oncol* 1984;18:181.

Yuen PM, Chang AMZ. Laparoscopic management of adnexal mass during pregnancy. *Acta Obstet Gynecol Scand* 1997; 76:173.

Zanotti KM, Belinson JL, Kennedy AW. Treatment of gynecologic cancers in pregnancy. *Semin Oncol* 2000;27:686.

Zhao XY, Huang HF, Lian LJ, et al. Ovarian cancer in pregnancy: a clinicopathologic analysis of 22 cases and review of the literature. *Int J Gynecol Cancer* 2006;1.

VI

CHAPTER 36
Pelvic Organ Prolapse: Basic Principles

Carl W. Zimmerman

The judgment as to surgical correction should depend upon a correlation of the history and physical findings. Even marked prolapse in the absence of complaint should rarely be corrected. The patient should ask the gynecologist for relief; the gynecologist should not urge the patient to have corrective surgery if she does not feel sufficiently uncomfortable to request it.

—Richard Te Linde, 1966

DEFINITIONS

Endopelvic fascia—The deep endopelvic connective tissue located between the dependent portion of the pelvic peritoneum and the superior fascia of the pelvic diaphragm. This continuum of tissue serves to support, suspend, and separate the central pelvic organs.

Kegel exercise—Voluntary contraction of the pelvic diaphragm, primarily the puborectalis muscle, and the external anal sphincter.

Interspinous diameter—The distance between the ischial spines. The narrowest diameter in the human pelvis. The components of the deep endopelvic connective tissue suspend the cervix and pericervical ring within this plane in normal anatomy.

Pelvic diaphragm—The skeletal muscles of the pelvic floor and their parietal fasciae. These muscles cover the majority of the pelvic outlet. These muscles originate on the pelvic sidewall and insert on the sacrum, coccyx, or sacrococcygeal raphe.

Rugae—Transverse creases in the vaginal wall that signify the presence of deep endopelvic connective tissue. Conversely, the absence of rugae implies the absence or a disruption of deep endopelvic connective tissue.

Urogenital hiatus—The large central opening in the pelvic diaphragm. The vagina, urethra, and anus exit the pelvis through this area.

Uterosacral ligaments—A named component of the endopelvic fascia. The primary apical suspensory elements of the uterovaginal complex. They extend from the pericervical ring to the presacral periosteum and probably the anterior parietal fascia of the piriformis muscles. These ligaments hold the cervix behind the posterior margin of the urogenital hiatus and over the sacrococcygeal raphe.

Valsalva maneuver—Pressure exerted downward on the pelvic floor by fixing the respiratory diaphragm and the anterior abdominal wall.

BASIC CONCEPTS

Pelvic organ prolapse is the downward displacement of central pelvic organs that are normally located at the level of or adjacent to the vaginal vault. Because these displacements are each associated with defects in integrated connective tissue structures, they may each be considered a pelvic hernia. These conditions are common and affect a progressively larger percentage of women as age advances especially in the postmenopausal years. Whereas mortality from this condition is negligible, significant morbidity or deterioration of lifestyle may be associated with prolapse. Women in developed countries who have access to modern health care can benefit from the advances that have been made in nonsurgical and surgical treatments for pelvic organ prolapse. If the problem is viewed from a worldwide perspective, however, the scope of suffering is much greater. In areas of high parity and little or no access to health care, countless women suffer from problems associated with pelvic organ prolapse with no real possibility of resolution. The direct effect that these conditions have on urinary, gastrointestinal, and sexual functions can only be appreciated by those women burdened with these problems on a daily basis.

Treatment of pelvic organ prolapse and the associated symptoms constitutes a major subject in gynecology. Especially in the advanced state, management of these conditions is one of the most challenging problems a pelvic surgeon can face. Indeed, success in treating prolapse is frequently used to judge the overall skill of those surgeons. Providing permanent relief from this classic malady by restoring normal anatomy and maximum physiologic function always tests the ingenuity of gynecologists. As medical sophistication has progressed, so has the ability to understand more completely and better treat pelvic organ prolapse.

A brief review of the history of treatment of prolapse is helpful in understanding modern treatments and current concepts of these conditions. Because it was mentioned in the writings of Hippocrates and Galen, prolapse was clearly known to the ancients. Early treatments may seem quaint by today's standards. Yet some of these interventions continue to be used today. Fortunately, others have not survived. Vaginal packing, tampons, massages, and exercises were used with some success. Other patients were suspended from their feet for a period of 24 hours to treat prolapse. Rodericus A. Castro advised that prolapse should be attacked with a red hot iron as if to burn it, "when fright would cause it to recede into the vagina." Various caustics were used, including silver nitrate, nitric acid, acid nitrate of mercury, hot metal, and sulfuric acid.

Perhaps, the first real advance in treatment was the development of pessaries. These devices functioned as trusses. Their fitting and placement became a desirable skill. They continue to bring relief to a large number of women and seldom do any serious harm. They were especially popular in the middle of the 19th century. Some were held in place by waistbands. In some cases, pessaries were deliberately left in place until erosions of the vaginal epithelium occurred. The subsequent healing was expected to reduce the caliber of the vagina with scarification adding to support, but serious complications could occur. Reports exist of neglected pessaries being retrieved from the peritoneal cavity and bladder. Fistulae may also occur in various locations, especially the bladder and anorectum.

The earliest surgical attempts to relieve prolapse were relatively simple. These procedures included labial suturing and removing portions of the vaginal epithelium to reduce the caliber of the vagina. Although Heming operated on the anterior vaginal wall in 1831, surgery for uterovaginal prolapse was not common until the advent of anesthesia and antisepsis later in the 19th century. The first vaginal hysterectomy for prolapse was performed by Samuel Choppin of New Orleans in 1861. Many years passed before this surgical technique became common. By the beginning of the 20th century, European and American reports of hysterectomy, colporrhaphy, cervical amputation, transposition/interposition operations (Manchester-Fothergill), cervical ligament plications, colpocleisis (Le Fort), ventral fixation of the uterus to the abdominal wall, and trachelorrhaphy for procidentia were being published. The timing of this ingenious variety of operations is certainly consistent with the development of anesthesia and various surgical techniques in all fields of medicine.

During the 20th century, advances in understanding and treatment of prolapse have progressed at an ever-increasing rate. In 1909, George R. White of Georgia published an account of cystocele repair using a transvaginal paravaginal approach. His correct perspective on the importance of lateral vaginal support took nearly 50 years to be rediscovered by mainstream gynecologic surgeons. The paravaginal repair was not widely known and accepted at the time because it was overshadowed by the work of Howard A. Kelly of Johns Hopkins. This great and influential surgeon popularized the concept of fascial attenuation. Midline anterior and posterior plications were touted as the correct surgical approach to the problem of prolapse. The Kelly-Kennedy anterior plication and levator ani plication of the posterior vaginal wall remain as commonly performed procedures today, despite the fact that more contemporary surgical techniques described in this chapter more effectively correct the anatomic defects of pelvic prolapse and achieve better clinical results with fewer long-term side effects.

In the 1950s, Milton L. McCall of Louisiana developed a culdoplasty technique that emphasized the important suspensory function of the uterosacral ligaments. He believed this operation prevented enteroceles and posthysterectomy vaginal vault prolapse when it was performed at the time of hysterectomy. Currently, the restitution of vaginal vault support at the time of any type of hysterectomy is considered a very important step in prevention of future prolapse.

In the 1960s, Baden and Walker of Texas began to systemize a new defect-specific approach to pelvic organ prolapse repair. Page 1 of their 1992 book, *Surgical Repair of Vaginal Defects*, stated: "In a sense, the defect approach reverses the prior evolution toward 'compensatory' reparative techniques—our goal is to return all vaginal supports to their original anatomic status." Many other surgeons have contributed to this powerful concept of pelvic reconstructive surgery. A. Cullen Richardson and associates of Georgia developed the concept of classifying fascial defects as proximal, distal, central, and lateral. This observation and the teaching of such master surgeons as David H. Nichols of New England encouraged gynecologists to not only identify and repair each vaginal defect but to return support attachments to their original anatomic location. Emphasis was focused on the hernial nature of prolapse and led to the abandonment of absorbable suture in favor of permanent suture in critical locations in these repairs. In the 1990s, pelvic anatomist, John O.L. DeLancey

of Michigan, published a biomechanical analysis of normal vaginal anatomy. His observations have the precision of an engineer's work and identify specific structural goals for each of three vaginal levels of support. Proximal (apical) vaginal suspension, midvaginal lateral attachment, and distal vaginal fusion to the perineum and urogenital diaphragm are the basic concepts that modern pelvic surgeons must satisfy to successfully complete a prolapse surgery.

In the 1980s, hernia repair literature began to demonstrate better long-term results with the use of bolsters. For that reason, autografts, allografts, xenografts, and various synthetic meshes achieved frequent use in surgical techniques for prolapse in the first decade of the 2000s. Because of an increasing number of reported problems and lack of strong data to support their use, the Food and Drug Administration has issued two statements urging caution in the use of these bolsters, especially polypropylene meshes. Considerable debate exists regarding the indications for their use (if at all) and the type, amount, and best location for pelvic support grafts.

A fusion of anatomic, physiologic, and biomechanical principles has allowed surgeons to offer their patients better treatments for prolapse than have historically been available. This brief and incomplete historical discussion outlines the evolution of our current understanding of a complex topic. Historically ineffective treatments of the presurgical era gave way to surgical approaches for advanced cases. As surgical sophistication has increased, anatomically distorting operations have gradually been replaced by anatomically restoring procedures. Many interesting aspects of the historical development of this subject are described in previous editions of this book and in the bibliographic selections at the end of this section.

A better understanding of a problem always leads to more questions that deserve answers. For example, the process of childbirth is regarded as an important cause of vaginal prolapse. Little or no effort has been made to analyze the forces of childbirth as they relate to specific patterns of damage to the deep endopelvic connective tissue. Delineation of these patterns would assist the surgeon in recognizing defects and undoubtedly improving operative outcome. Precise knowledge of the effects of labor and delivery on the pelvic floor would likely lead to new surgical techniques and create the potential for better obstetrical decisions designed to reduce the potentially damaging effects of childbirth. The concept of prolapse prevention is underused in the practice of gynecology. Teaching patients about physical therapy of the pelvic floor, better lifestyle, and proper evacuation habits should be part of the gynecologist's job. The long-term benefits of an organized program of prolapse prevention have never been evaluated.

Controversy exists as to the best surgical management for specific cases of female pelvic organ prolapse. In fact, now that reparative options are no longer limited to midline plications, more procedures are available than ever before. Vaginal, abdominal, laparoscopic, robotic, minimally invasive devices, and combined approaches each have their advocates. The necessary randomized trials with matched controls will likely never be done to generate true evidence-based outcomes, especially because two of the most powerful variables are surgical skill and experience. The necessary long-term follow-up is rarely available in the pelvic surgery literature. New concepts and techniques appear before the older ones can properly be compared in studies. Surgical techniques for prolapse must be carefully evaluated so that anatomic and functional results will continue to improve.

The authors of the following chapters of this section describe interventions and operations that gynecologic surgeons should consider when managing pelvic organ prolapse. Each of these surgeons possesses a combination of operative skill, experience, and special interest in their topics that have led to their selection. The operative techniques presented should be combined with appropriate clinical evaluation and skillful technical performance to obtain maximum benefit for the patients.

ANATOMIC CONSIDERATIONS

The normal position, support, and suspension of the uterus, vagina, bladder, and rectum rely on an interdependent system of bony, muscular, and connective tissue elements. This entire system is three dimensional, and even subtle alterations in one part may lead to stresses in other parts that eventually lead to alteration or failure of normal anatomy. An understanding of normal applied pelvic anatomy is imperative in the repair of pelvic organ prolapse.

The bony pelvis has a central opening that is necessary for reproductive function. During evolutionary transition to upright bipedal posture, the potential for prolapse became more likely because of gravitational stress. In the human female, a lordosis of the lumbosacral portion of the spine places the pelvic inlet in an oblique orientation reminiscent of the pelvic posture of a quadruped. The physical result of this shift is that the posterior aspect of the pelvic inlet is approximately 60 degrees above the anterior aspect with the promontory of the sacrum placed in a vertical plane above the pubic symphysis (Fig. 36.1). This partially vertical orientation of the pelvic inlet deflects force onto the superior symphysis pubis rather than directly on the pelvic outlet and urogenital hiatus. Consequently, the pelvic outlet is partially shielded from downward stresses in the anatomically normal woman.

The muscles of the pelvic diaphragm primarily provide pelvic support. These muscles form a basin or covering of the pelvic outlet and are often grouped together as the levator ani or levator sling (Fig. 36.2). Within this diaphragm is the urogenital hiatus, an opening large enough to allow childbirth. This large central opening in the muscular pelvic floor explains why prolapse is such a significant problem in humans. The most medial portion of the pelvic diaphragm is formed by the puborectalis muscle, the muscular boundary of the urogenital hiatus. The obstetric axis of the pelvis passes through the urogenital hiatus medial to the puborectalis muscle. In the standing patient, the puborectalis muscle is horizontal and is palpable as a 2- to 2.5-cm band of voluntary muscle on each lateral side of the distal one third of the vagina. When well innervated and

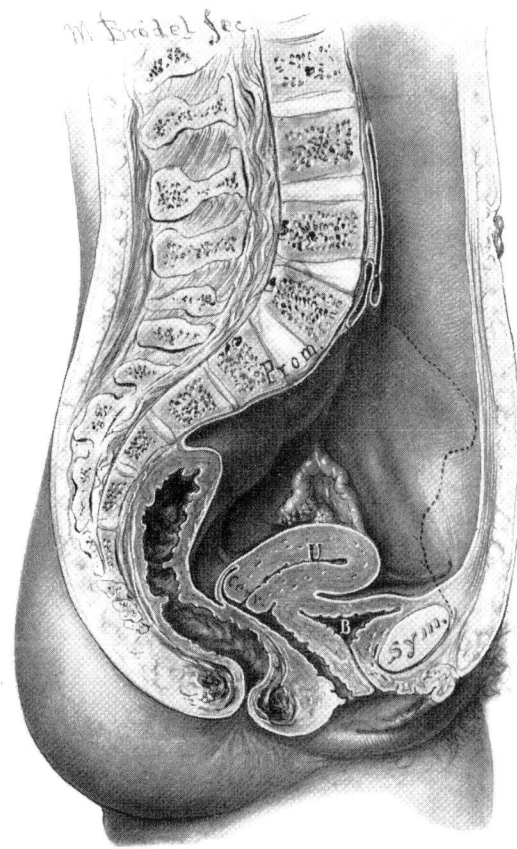

FIGURE 36.1 The relationship between the pelvic floor and the abdominal cavity. Notice the lordosis of the lumbosacral spine and the almost vertical orientation of the pelvic inlet. (The original illustration is in the Max Brödel Archives in the Department of Art as Applied to Medicine, The Johns Hopkins University School of Medicine, Baltimore, MD. Used with permission.)

contracted, the puborectalis muscle closes the distal vagina and displaces the posterior wall of the rectum anteriorly creating the anorectal angle. Forming the bulk of the pelvic diaphragm, the

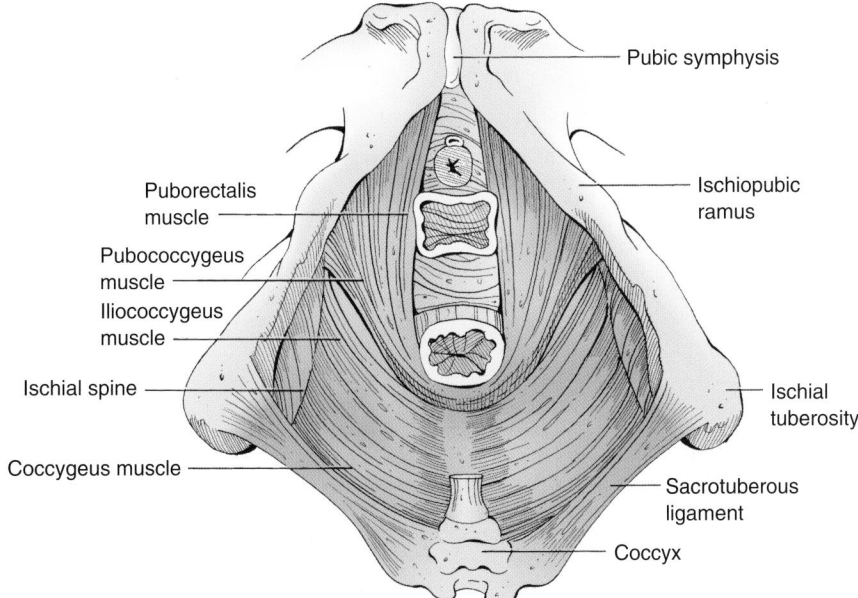

FIGURE 36.2 The pelvic diaphragm viewed from below.

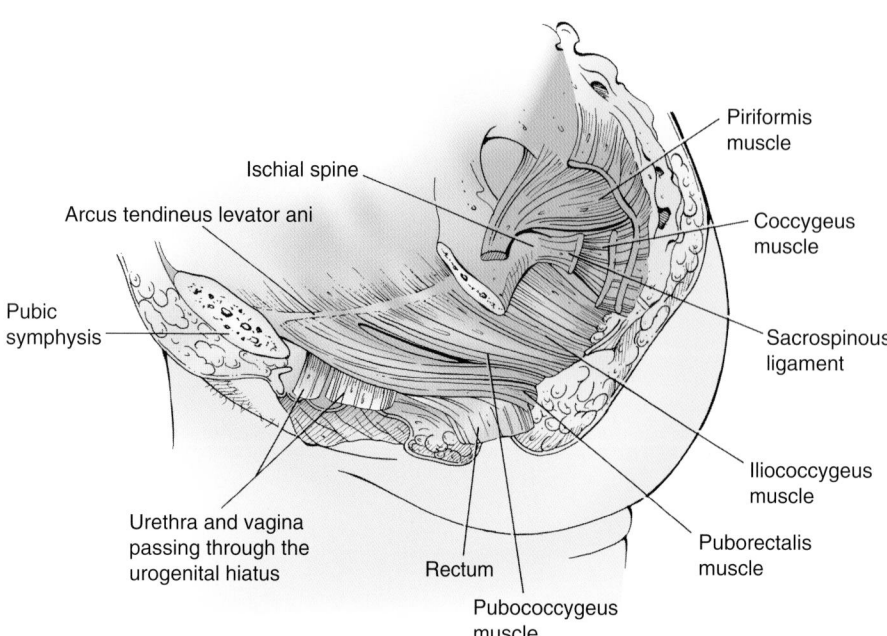

FIGURE 36.3 Muscles of the pelvic floor, lateral view.

pubococcygeus and iliococcygeus muscles cover the posterior and lateral portions of the pelvic outlet (Fig. 36.3). The superior insertion of the iliococcygeus muscles is an important landmark in pelvic support anatomy. These insertions are thickenings of the pelvic sidewall parietal fascia of the obturator internus muscle that extend from the ischial spines posteriorly to points on the pubic bone known as the pubic tubercles. These lines of insertion are known as the arcus tendineus levator ani or muscular arches (Figs. 36.4 and 36.5). Immediately inferior to the muscular arches are thickenings of the parietal fascia of the bellies of the iliococcygeus muscles known as the arcus tendineus fasciae pelvis (fascial arches) or white lines. These structures are

the lateral attachment points for the pubocervical septum and apical rectovaginal septum. The white line serves the function of midvaginal lateral support. Paravaginal and apical pararectal defects are located immediately medial to the white line. In the standing patient, the white line is nearly horizontal; in the standard lithotomy position, it is nearly vertical.

During paravaginal repair, the white lines are palpable as stringlike structures that extend between the ischial spines and the pubic arch. Another fascial thickening has been described that runs posteriorly from the white line to the structures of the lateral perineal body and serves as lateral support for the distal rectovaginal septum of the posterior vagina. This structure

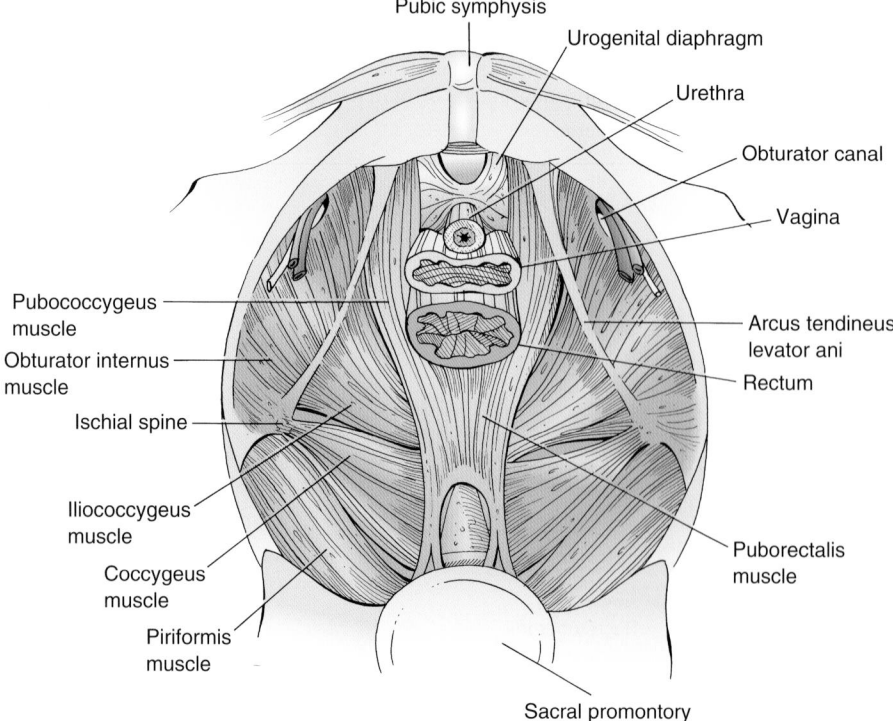

FIGURE 36.4 The pelvic diaphragm viewed from above.

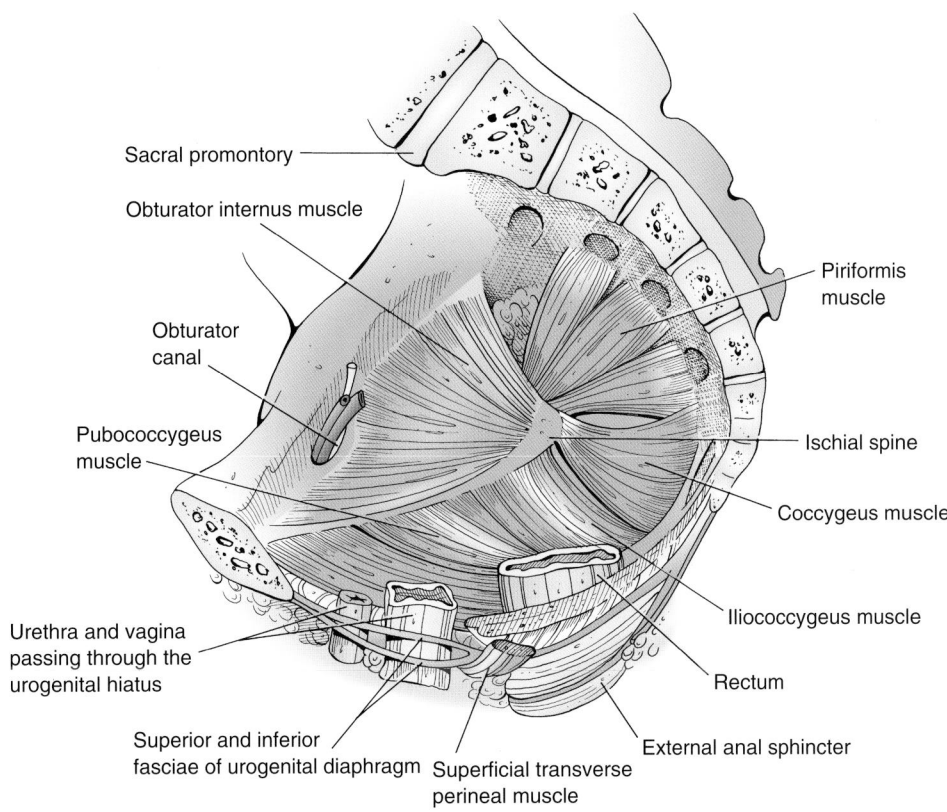

Sacral promontory

Obturator internus muscle

Obturator canal

Pubococcygeus muscle

Urethra and vagina passing through the urogenital hiatus

Superior and inferior fasciae of urogenital diaphragm

Superficial transverse perineal muscle

Piriformis muscle

Ischial spine

Coccygeus muscle

Iliococcygeus muscle

Rectum

External anal sphincter

FIGURE 36.5 Sagittal view of the pelvis.

has been named the arcus tendineus fasciae rectovaginalis (Fig. 36.6). The lateral supports of the anterior and posterior vaginal septa merge and are not separate in the apical half of the vagina. Superior to the muscular arch is the uppermost portion of the obturator internus muscle and the parietal obturator fascia. The obturator internus muscles qualify as pelvic muscles because they form the lateral borders of the upper portion of the pelvic basin. Posterior to the iliococcygeus, the pelvic floor is

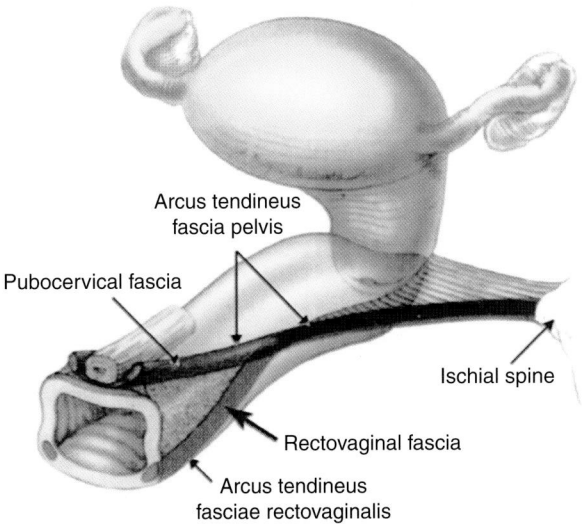

Arcus tendineus fascia pelvis

Pubocervical fascia

Ischial spine

Rectovaginal fascia

Arcus tendineus fasciae rectovaginalis

FIGURE 36.6 The lateral attachments of the pubocervical fascia (PCF) and the rectovaginal fascia (RVF) to the pelvic sidewall. Also shown are the arcus tendineus fascia pelvis (ATFP), arcus tendineus fasciae rectovaginalis (ATFRV), and ischial spine (IS).

covered by the coccygeus muscle and the closely associated sacrospinous ligament (Fig. 36.5). These structures pass between the ischial spine and the terminal sacrum and coccyx. The most posterior portion of the pelvis is bounded by the piriformis muscle. The midline confluence of the levator muscles forms a particularly strong band of connective tissue between the coccyx and the posterior anus known as the levator plate or sacrococcygeal raphe. This plate is oriented horizontally in the standing patient. The vagina and the rectum are suspended by the endopelvic fascia (primarily the uterosacral ligaments) directly over the levator plate. Myopathies or neuropathies cause weakness of the pubococcygeus and iliococcygeus muscles and may allow the levator plate to sag and descend permanently. This descent causes the genital hiatus to remain open as it does during defecation. This increased opening changes the normal horizontal axis of the apical vagina to a more vertical orientation and predisposes the central pelvic organs to prolapse.

The pudendal nerve is an important motor and sensory nerve of the pelvic floor and perineum. It descends through the pelvic diaphragm between the coccygeus and piriformis muscles in the area posterior to the ischial spine into Alcock canal. Alcock canal is located in the ischiorectal fossa immediately adjacent to the fascia of the obturator internus muscle on the lateral wall of this space. Because of its location, the pudendal nerve is subjected to significant stretch and pressure particularly in the area adjacent to the ischial spines during the descent of a fetus through the pelvis. The muscles of the pelvic diaphragm are also subjected to great pressure and stretch during labor. Magnetic resonance imaging studies have demonstrated atrophy and breaks in the levator muscles of parous women. Neuropathy of the pudendal nerve and myopathy of the levator muscles are believed to be significant contributing factors in the development of pelvic organ prolapse.

VII

Unfortunately, at this time, no treatments are available for myopathies and neuropathies of this type. For that reason, surgical treatment of pelvic organ prolapse is limited largely to manipulation of the deep endopelvic connective tissues.

The connective tissues of the pelvis are collectively known as the endopelvic fascia. This fibroelastic connective tissue matrix contains varying amounts of smooth muscle. It supports and invests all the midline organs and structures of the pelvis. Only the ovaries and fallopian tubes lie outside this investment. At various locations, the endopelvic fascia manifests different characteristics. These forms include loose areolar tissue capable of distention; neurovascular sheaths; septa and ligaments that support, suspend, and separate the pelvic organs; and dense skeletal muscle investments. In the central pelvis, the visceral peritoneum drapes over the midline structures, dipping into recesses but not descending into direct contact with the muscular pelvic floor. The irregular space between the pelvic diaphragm, the muscular pelvic sidewall, and the visceral peritoneum is the location of the endopelvic fascia. The endopelvic fascia may be divided into three parts: parietal fasciae, visceral fasciae, and deep endopelvic connective tissue.

The parietal fasciae of the endopelvic fascia are relatively dense membranes investing the pelvic surface of the skeletal muscles of the pelvic sidewall (Table 36.1). They are similar in structure, form, and function to other parietal fasciae of the body, for example, the rectus abdominis fasciae. At muscular margins, they blend with the various periostea of the bony pelvis.

The visceral pelvic fasciae are loose, highly elastic, and relatively ill-defined encasements of the central pelvic organs, taking the form of sheaths and sleeves (Table 36.2). These structures allow for the high degree of physiologic distention necessitated by the intestinal, urinary, and reproductive functions of the pelvic organs. The visceral fasciae blend intimately with the organs that they encase, are not easily separable from those organs, and are not useful for support and suspension purposes in surgery.

The deep endopelvic connective tissue is of central importance in the clinically applied anatomy of the pelvis and is especially significant to the pelvic reconstructive surgeon. This structure is part of a continuum of retroperitoneal connective tissue that extends from the respiratory diaphragm in the upper abdomen to the pelvic diaphragm. Included in this continuum of structures

are the mesenteries and ligaments of the upper abdomen. Anatomists debate whether the condensations of this connective tissue should be considered as true ligaments and fasciae or septa. Part of this debate stems from the fact that some of these structures contain a significant muscular component and others serve as neurovascular conduits. Certainly, from a functional standpoint in the pelvis, they meet criteria for being so named. The endopelvic connective tissue is continuous from one part to the other. Separate portions serve different functions, take various forms, and therefore are given different names. The named structures of the deep endopelvic connective tissue include six ligaments, two septa, and one ring. Important anatomic details of these elements are summarized in the following tables.

The six pericervical ligaments form the paracolpium (Tables 36.3, 36.4, and 36.5). The net effect of these structures is the suspension of the cervix in the posterior pelvis and the consequent placement of the vagina directly over the levator plate and away from direct exposure to the urogenital hiatus. In the normal anatomic position, pressure from above tends to close

---

TABLE 36.1 Parietal Pelvic Fasciae

Obturator fascia
Particularly well defined in the area superior to the arcus tendineus levator ani and below the linea terminalis. This fascia may represent a vestigial portion of the levator ani whose origin has been lowered through evolution to the level of the muscular arch.

Levator ani fascia (Superior fascia of the pelvic diaphragm)
This fascia is continuous across the pelvic floor, blending laterally with the obturator fascia at the arcus tendineus levator ani and centrally with the levator plate and the visceral fasciae at the urogenital hiatus.

Coccygeus fascia (Sacrospinous ligament)
This important pelvic support structure extends from the ischial spine laterally to the sacrum medially and is an important alternative source of proximal support when the uterosacral ligament is unavailable or insufficient.

Piriformis fascia
This fascia is the thinnest and most posterior of the parietal fasciae of the pelvis.

TABLE 36.2 Visceral Pelvic Fasciae

Pelvic organs and structures invested by visceral fasciae
Vagina
Uterus
Bladder
Rectum

Pelvic organs and structures not invested by visceral fasciae
Fallopian tubes
Ovaries

TABLE 36.3 Components of the Deep Endopelvic Connective Tissue: Uterosacral Ligaments

Origin
Periosteum of sacral vertebrae 2, 3, and 4

Insertion
The points of insertion are on the posterior and lateral supravaginal cervix at the 5-o'clock and 7-o'clock positions. The ligaments are continuous with and form part of the pericervical ring.

Neurologic content
Uterosacral plexus of autonomic nerves

Vascular content
Minimal

Muscular content
Rectouterine muscle

Function
These structures are the primary proximal suspensory elements of the uterovaginal complex. They hold the cervix behind the urogenital hiatus in the posterior pelvis at the level of the ischial spines with the uterus in anteflexion and the vagina suspended over the levator plate.

Synonym
Rectal pillar
At their insertion into the pericervical ring, the uterosacral ligaments blend as continuous structures superiorly and laterally with the cardinal ligaments and distally with the proximal rectovaginal septum.

TABLE 36.4 Components of the Deep Endopelvic Connective Tissue: Cardinal Ligaments

Origin
The hypogastric root with fibrous connections to the lateral abdominal and pelvic walls

Insertion
The points of insertion are on the lateral supravaginal cervix at the 3-o'clock and 9-o'clock positions. This insertion is continuous with and forms part of the pericervical ring.

Neurologic content
Portions of the uterosacral plexus

Vascular content
Uterine artery and veins

Muscular content
Minimal smooth muscle content with no named component

Urinary
The distal ureter passes under the uterine artery within the superior portion of the cardinal ligament.

Function
These ligaments are the primary vascular conduits of the uterus and vagina, providing lateral stabilization to the cervix at the level of the ischial spines. They are similar in structure, content, and function to the mesenteries of the abdomen.

Synonyms
Mackenrodt ligament, lateral cervical ligament, and proper cervical ligament

---

TABLE 36.5 Components of the Deep Endopelvic Connective Tissue: Pubocervical Ligaments

Origin
Inferior surface of the superior pubic ramus medially and the arcus tendineus fascia pelvis laterally

Insertion
The points of insertion are on the anterior and lateral supravaginal cervix at the 11-o'clock and 1-o'clock positions. This insertion is continuous with and forms part of the pericervical ring.

Vascular component
Artery and veins of the bladder pillar

Function
These ligaments are the least well developed of the pericervical ligaments, serving as a vascular conduit and for a minimal degree of cervical stabilization.

Synonym
Bladder pillar

TABLE 36.6 Components of the Deep Endopelvic Connective Tissue: Pubocervical Septum or Fascia

Shape
Trapezoidal with the narrow end located distally

Contents
Fibroelastic connective tissue and smooth muscle

Function
Anterior vaginal support, including support of the bladder

Synonyms
Vesicovaginal septum or fascia, pubovesicocervical septum or fascia

Boundaries
Distal: Pubic tubercles laterally and the pubic arch centrally fusing with the urogenital diaphragm
Lateral: Arcus tendineus fascia pelvis or white line
Proximal: Pericervical ring centrally and both pubocervical and cardinal ligaments laterally
Superior: Visceral fascia of the bladder
Inferior: Epithelium of the vagina

---

with the vaginal epithelium and visceral fasciae of the adjacent organs. Clinically, they are separate from their adjacent structures. When the septa and their supports are intact, the vaginal and rectal axes have a posterior angle of approximately 130 degrees at the anterior point of their suspension over the levator plate due to the action of the puborectalis muscle. Distal to the puborectalis muscle, the vagina is nearly vertical as it

---

TABLE 36.7 Components of the Deep Endopelvic Connective Tissue: Rectovaginal Septum or Fascia

Shape
Trapezoidal with the narrow end located distally

Contents
Fibroelastic connective tissue and smooth muscle

Function
Posterior vaginal support and suspension, stabilization of the rectum, and perineal suspension. The vaginal suspensory axis consists of the perineum, rectovaginal septum, pericervical ring, uterosacral ligaments, and presacral periosteum. The rectovaginal septum also guides the leading edge of a descending bowel movement into the anus.

Synonym
Denonvilliers fascia

Boundaries
Distal: Fusion with the proximal perineal body at the central tendon of the perineum
Lateral: In the distal half of the vagina, the lateral boundary is the arcus tendineus fasciae rectovaginalis; in the proximal half of the vagina, the lateral boundary is the arcus tendineus fascia pelvis.
Proximal: Uterosacral ligaments laterally and the pericervical ring centrally
Superior: Epithelium of the vagina
Inferior: Visceral fascia of the rectum

---

the apical vaginal vault by compressing it against the sacrococcygeal raphe with no tendency toward prolapse. This compression of the vagina is a flap valve type of mechanism and is aided by the anchoring of the cervix by the uterosacral ligaments.

Two septa or fasciae (Tables 36.6 and 36.7) are located within the deep endopelvic connective tissue. These condensations of fibroelastic connective tissue are in close contact

TABLE 36.8 Components of the Deep Endopelvic Connective Tissue: Pericervical Ring

Shape
Collar of connective tissue encircling the supravaginal cervix

Contents
Fibroelastic connective tissue

Function
Cervical stabilization within the interspinous diameter by connecting with all other named components of the deep endopelvic connective tissue

Synonym
Supravaginal septum

Connections
Anterior: The pericervical ring is located between the base of the bladder and the anterior cervix, where it connects with the pubocervical ligaments at the 11-o'clock and 1-o'clock positions and the proximal pubocervical septum centrally.
Lateral: Cardinal ligaments at the 3-o'clock and 9-o'clock positions
Posterior: The pericervical ring is located between the rectum and the posterior cervix, where it connects with the uterosacral ligaments at the 5-o'clock and 7-o'clock positions and the proximal rectovaginal septum centrally.

TABLE 36.9 Avascular Spaces of the Pelvis

Prevesical
Paravesical
Vesicovaginal
Vesicocervical
Rectovaginal
Pararectal
Retrorectal

passes through the urogenital hiatus. The apical or proximal two thirds of the vagina is nearly horizontal and is suspended over the levator plate. The normal vaginal axis is oriented posteriorly toward a point just above the center of the fourth sacral vertebra. This area of the anterior sacrum corresponds to the exact area of the origin of the uterosacral ligaments.

The pericervical ring (Table 36.8) is the single location where all deep endopelvic connective tissue support structures converge. *Simply stated, the goal of the defect-specific pelvic reconstructive surgeon is the restitution of the anatomical connections of the pericervical ring within the interspinous diameter.* If the dissection and reconstructive efforts during such a surgery do not extend apically to the interspinous diameter, the surgery is likely to fail because that diameter is the normal location of the pericervical ring. Because the cervix is located on the apical anterior vaginal wall, the pubocervical septum is shorter than the rectovaginal septum by a length equal to the diameter of the pericervical ring. If one carries this line of reasoning further, an inherent structural problem is present in the posthysterectomy prolapse patient. If the cervix and its surrounding support tissues are absent, no completely anatomic method to reconstruct the proximal anterior vaginal support exists. Some form of anatomic distortion (e.g., shortening of the vagina or plication) or bolstering is necessary to compensate for this defect. Likely, this dilemma is the reason that the most frequently encountered support defect in the posthysterectomy patient is most frequently in the apical anterior location.

The three-dimensional structure of the endopelvic fascia has another distinguishing anatomic characteristic that is of interest to the pelvic surgeon. Outside the confines of the named condensations of this tissue are avascular potential spaces (Table 36.9). When properly used, these spaces give the surgeon access to important support structures deep within the pelvis. Gynecologic oncologists base their surgical training around mastering the surgical manipulation of these spaces, usually from the abdominal approach. These spaces are not only available to the vaginal reconstructive surgeon, but they are also critical in identification of pelvic support landmarks.

DeLancey's biomechanical analysis of normal uterovaginal support by the deep endopelvic connective tissue helps to unify the anatomic principles pertinent to pelvic organ prolapse (Fig. 36.7). These concepts of support and suspension also help to define a set of goals for the reconstructive

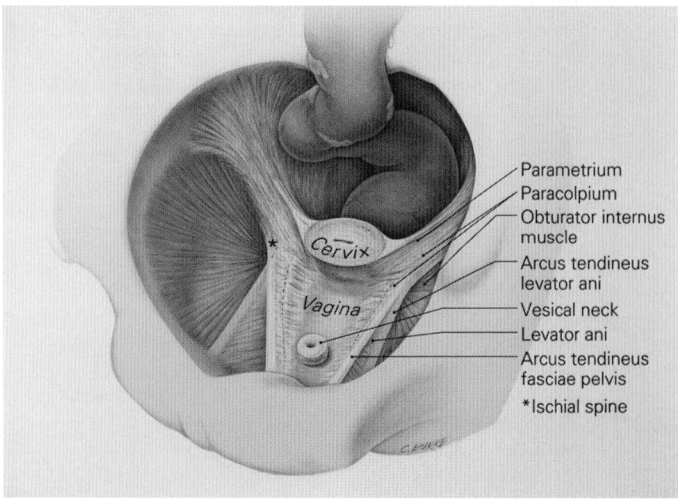

FIGURE 36.7 Three-dimensional view of the endopelvic fascia. Notice the location of the cervix in the proximal anterior vaginal segment. (Adapted from DeLancey JO. Anatomic aspects of vaginal eversion after hysterectomy. *Am J Obstet Gynecol* 1992;166:1717, with permission. Copyright © 1992, Elsevier.)

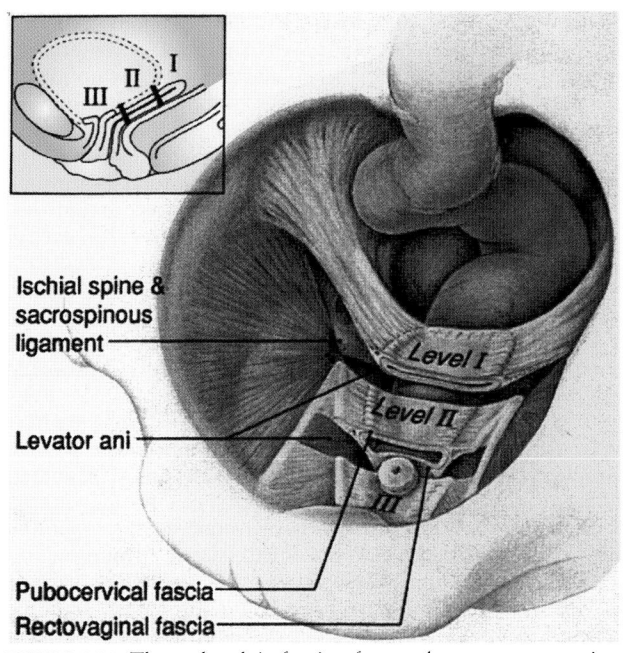

FIGURE 36.8 The endopelvic fascia of a posthysterectomy patient divided into DeLancey's biomechanical levels: level I, proximal suspension; level II, lateral attachment; level III, distal fusion. (Adapted from DeLancey JO. Anatomic aspects of vaginal eversion after hysterectomy. *Am J Obstet Gynecol* 1992;166:1717, with permission. Copyright © 1992, Elsevier.)

surgeon. Each goal must be satisfied for the long-term success of a prolapse surgery. DeLancey divided vaginal support into three levels (Fig. 36.8). *Proximal or apical vaginal level I support is attributed to suspension by the ligaments of the paracolpium primarily the uterosacral ligaments.* Damage to level I support results in uterovaginal prolapse, posthysterectomy

vaginal prolapse, and enterocele. The cause for level I support problems is necessarily at or above the level of the ischial spines. The primary load-bearing elements are the uterosacral ligaments and, to a lesser extent, the cardinal ligaments. This fact is consistent with cadaver observations made many years ago by Mengert showing that prolapse occurred only after 85% of the integrity of the paracolpium was severed. *Midvaginal level II support is due to lateral attachment of the fascial septa to the pelvic sidewalls.* The septa attach to the arcus tendineus fascia pelvis and the arcus tendineus fasciae rectovaginalis. Damage at this level results in paravaginal and pararectal defects. *Distal Level III support is attributed to fusion of the deep endopelvic connective tissue septa to the urogenital diaphragm anteriorly and to the proximal perineum posteriorly.* Damage at these sites can result in urinary incontinence anteriorly and in perineal body deficits and defecatory dysfunction posteriorly. Historically, cystocele and rectocele were believed to be central defects within the fabric of the pubocervical and rectovaginal septa. These defects are now believed to be due to displacements of the respective endopelvic septa originating at the margins of those structures, not centrally.

Another useful concept is the suspensory axis of the uterovaginal complex. This concept is consistent with DeLancey's various levels, but views the connective tissue structures as a continuum. The posterior suspensory axis includes the structures between the perineum and presacral periosteum. From inferior to superior, these elements are the perineal body, rectovaginal septum, posterior pericervical ring, uterosacral ligaments, and presacral periosteum. The posterior axis is the primary load-bearing structure of the uterovaginal complex. The anterior axis extends from the urogenital diaphragm, through the pubocervical septum, cervix, and pericervical ring merging with the posterior suspensory axis at the level of the ischial spines. Disruption of this continuum occurs due to childbirth at the level of the interspinous diameter during the process of childbirth (Fig. 36.9).

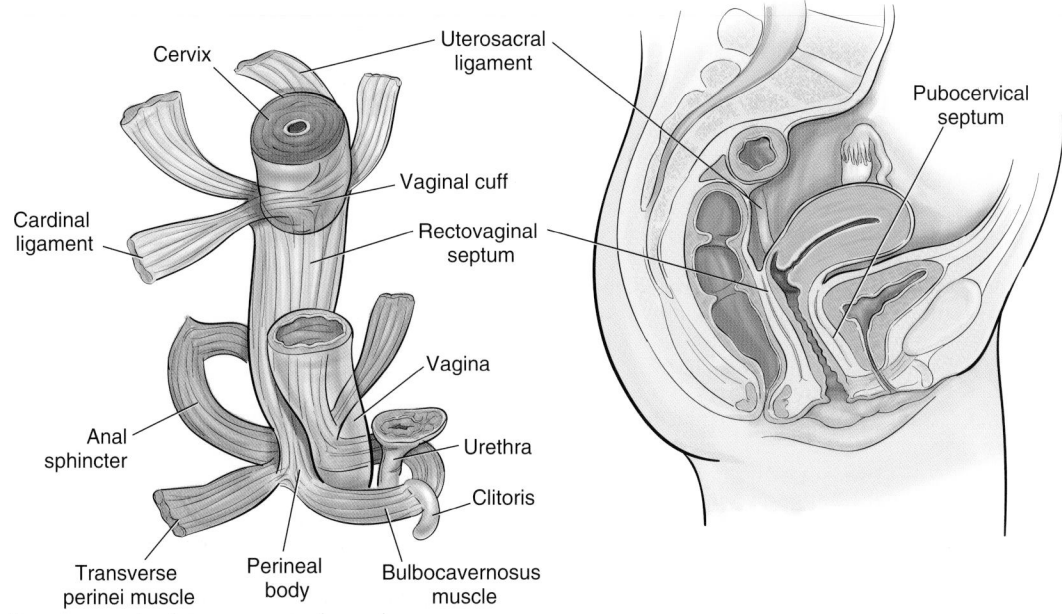

FIGURE 36.9 Suspensory axis of the uterovaginal complex.

VII

ETIOLOGY AND PREVENTION

In the vast majority of women who will develop pelvic organ prolapse, the process begins with their first *vaginal delivery*. Each subsequent vaginal delivery contributes to the likelihood that a clinically symptomatic prolapse will occur at some point in her lifetime. The normal process of labor and vaginal delivery are certainly desired, necessary, and important physiologic events. Nonetheless, childbirth does have a traumatic aspect by contributing to the development of pelvic organ prolapse. Commonly, many years pass, and other factors contribute to the progression of prolapse before such patients present for evaluation.

During labor, the fetal presenting part (about 95% are vertex) must overcome a significant amount of soft tissue resistance presented by the lower uterine segment and cervix, the endopelvic fascia, and the muscular pelvic floor. Because of the lordosis of the lumbosacral spine, the obstetric axis of the pelvis is noticeably angled, differing by 90 degrees between the inlet and outlet. This right angle occurs at the level of the ischial spines and causes the baby's head to extend sharply beginning at the level of the interspinous diameter in order to rotate under the pubic arch while following the anterior concavity of the sacrum. Thus, the fetus is driven by strong uterine contractions through a low-velocity, high-pressure, arcing transit through the pelvis. Labor aided by maternal pushing and, at times, by physician traction has a damaging effect on the intricately constructed support structures of the pelvis. Fortunately, the majority of women who deliver are capable of overcoming the stresses on their internal pelvic structures and never experience prolapse.

In the initial phase of a nulliparous labor, the fetal head engages, flexes, and descends to a point immediately apical to the interspinous diameter. Clinical examination at this stage commonly finds the cervix held in a far posterior position as a result of the strength and suspensory function of the uterosacral ligaments. In this situation, great pressure is placed on the anterior vaginal segment. The most common fetal presentation, the left occipitoanterior position, places the rotating arc of the fetal head in the maternal right hemipelvis. As the fetal head overcomes the resistance of the pubocervical septum, significant downward pressure is placed on the maternal right pelvic sidewall. This event likely explains the preponderance of full-length right paravaginal paravesical defects and apical transverse separation of the pubocervical septum as the most common fascial defects in anterior vaginal relaxation. As further fetal descent occurs, the cervix rotates anteriorly, representing uterosacral ligament damage apical to the interspinous diameter. The fetus then usually rotates into the occipitoanterior position as it encounters the interspinous diameter. This diameter is the narrowest in the female human pelvis and therefore is the plane of greatest pressure during labor and delivery. The fetal head then flexes to allow passage under the pubic symphysis. The anterior sacrococcygeal curvature is concave. As the fetus passes under the pubic arch, this concavity makes it necessary for the fetal head to extend to complete labor. This change in orientation places intense pressure on the posterior pericervical ring. The result is further uterosacral stress and a transverse apical detachment of the rectovaginal septum at its junction with the pericervical ring and uterosacral ligaments. As extension of the head progresses, displacement of the rectovaginal septum toward the perineum results in the creation of a nidus for apical vaginal enterocele and midvaginal rectocele formation. If the rectovaginal septum is displaced far enough distally, pararectal defects form as the septum is sheared away from its lateral attachments. The process of rectovaginal detachment and displacement also

weakens the apical support for the perineal body and predisposes to perineal descent. Note that rectocele, enterocele, and perineal descent are all explained by the disruption of the posterior suspensory axis at the level of the interspinous diameter. Subsequent deliveries progressively contribute damage to the endopelvic fascia. During complete dilation of the uterine cervix, descent and extension, the fetus passes through the urogenital hiatus. During this process, pressure is transmitted to the levator muscles and the pudendal nerve. If a patient dilates completely, pushes in an attempt to deliver, and then receives a cesarean section, she may have much of the same fascial damage as a woman with a successful vaginal delivery. A nulliparous patient with prolapse would likely suffer from isolated failure of the paracolpium, with the pericervical ring and fascial septa remaining intact.

A major shortcoming of the profession is that the effect of labor and delivery on the female pelvis has not been more completely objectified. Only recently has the study of pudendal neuropathy and levator myopathy been brought under scientific scrutiny. Even less has been done to determine the most common overall patterns of fascial and ligament damage during parturition. The pattern described in the previous paragraph is simply the most common one encountered. Other fetal presentations would result in different patterns of damage. Any experienced prolapse surgeon recognizes the variations in pattern of herniation, leading to the adage that no two patients are exactly alike. However, knowledge of the common pattern does help the surgeon who is new to the defect-specific approach know where to look to identify fascial edges and visually discriminate between the various tissues in the dissection field.

Fortunately, most women who bear children will not suffer a significant symptomatic degree of prolapse. Parturition then is a necessary cause but not a sufficient cause for the vast majority of prolapse cases. Other factors work over time and in combination with the damage caused by childbirth to convert incipient prolapse into a clinically apparent problem.

Prolapse becomes more common with *advancing age*. The likely cause is general weakening of tissues, including the pelvic floor muscles. Passage of time increases the cumulative effect of contributing causes on the pelvic floor. Most cases of prolapse become evident after the age of menopause. Virtually all the tissues of the pelvis possess estrogen receptors, and the *atrophic changes* that occur in the absence of estrogen are a contributing cause for prolapse. With age and a prolonged hypoestrogenic state, osteoporosis may develop. The kyphotic changes in the spine that result from osteoporosis displace the pelvic inlet into a more horizontal plane. This change in the pelvic inlet allows the weight of the abdominal contents to act more directly on the pelvic floor and on the urogenital hiatus.

Lifestyle may contribute to prolapse. Lifting objects heavy enough to require a Valsalva maneuver or fixation of the respiratory diaphragm displaces stress directly down on the pelvic floor. This process may be aided by shoulder, back, and extremity weakness. Defecation and micturition are commonly assisted with straining. This straining occurs when the pelvic diaphragm is intentionally relaxed. This action places substantial force on a passive pelvic floor and open urogenital hiatus several times a day. Straining has essentially the same effect as heavy lifting. Obesity, which is epidemic in the United States, directly increases the load on the pelvic floor and decreases mobility as well as the ability to do muscle strengthening exercises.

Medical conditions and their complications may contribute to the development of prolapse. A few examples suffice to illustrate how a *chronic medical condition* or the treatments for medical problems may affect the pelvic floor. The natural history of diabetes mellitus includes neuropathy and obesity, both of which contribute to the tendency to prolapse. Chronic cough accompanying asthma, bronchitis, or smoking places repeated stresses on the pelvic floor. The effects of repeated or paroxysmal coughing help to convert incipient prolapse into a clinical problem. Smoking also has antiestrogenic properties, contributes to vascular disease, and creates a chronic hypoxic state. Corticosteroid therapy is used in many chronic medical conditions. The weakening effect of these medications on connective tissue is well known. People with constitutional connective tissue disorders have been shown to be at increased risk for prolapse. Ehlers-Danlos syndrome, for example, is characterized by generalized fascial and connective tissue weaknesses. The pelvic floor is also affected by these deficits. More subtle connective tissue weakness, such as joint hypermobility, has been suspected to increase the long-term risk for prolapse. Development of ascites may cause a rapid increase in the degree of prolapse. This list is by no means complete. Any condition that affects the physical load on the pelvic floor or the integrity of the muscular and connective tissues of the pelvis will increase the likelihood that symptomatic prolapse will develop.

Some medical conditions may reduce the tendency to develop prolapse. This is the case for any condition that causes an inflammatory reaction in the paracervical or parametrial tissues with subsequent tissue fibrosis. Pelvic inflammatory disease, puerperal or postabortal sepsis, endometriosis, and pelvic radiation therapy are conditions that could lead to such a circumstance. Pelvic adhesions, regardless of the cause, might be dense and numerous enough to secondarily suspend a prolapse. Large uterine leiomyomata or other pelvic masses can mechanically prevent the development and descent of prolapse.

The list of contributing causes to pelvic organ prolapse is varied. *Prevention* should begin early in a woman's life and be continued into the later years. Many of the measures discussed as preventions also have a positive effect on a woman's general health. Any discussion of pelvic organ prolapse prevention must include the obstetric management of childbirth. Vaginal delivery undoubtedly has a primary and profound effect on pelvic support anatomy. Debates have occurred for decades about the wisdom of operative vaginal deliveries, optimal length for the second stage of labor, management of macrosomia, usefulness of episiotomy, and multiple other obstetric practices. In truth, little evidence-based information exists regarding these concepts as they relate to the subsequent development of prolapse. The most likely major contributing factor is simply vaginal delivery. The pelvis is contoured so that even in a normal labor and delivery, substantial forces are applied to the endopelvic fascia, muscular floor of the pelvis, and pudendal nerve. The greatest forces generated are at the level of the interspinous diameter. This plane is the location of the singularly important pericervical ring and its junction with every other septa and ligament associated with normal vaginal support and suspension. For example, an episiotomy may shorten the second stage of labor but is unlikely to have any effect on the stresses generated in the interspinous diameter. Does prophylactic cesarean section represent the ultimate in prolapse prevention? This tactic certainly has attained popularity in some parts of the world. One might argue that if vaginal delivery is a necessary cause for prolapse, then this strategy would be preventative. This topic has generated an active and emerging debate in obstetrics and gynecology. Evidence-based resolutions to these questions are unlikely to ever be available. In my opinion, prophylactic cesarean section will never be widely applied. Replacing a desired physiologic process with a major surgery is illogical when the consequence to

be prevented is relatively uncommon and not life threatening. However, occasional patients may present convincing arguments in favor of prophylactic cesarean section. The individual practitioner and patient must resolve the course of action in the privacy of the consultation room.

In the adult parous woman, strategies to prevent the development of prolapse center on efforts that decrease physical stress on the urogenital hiatus and strengthen the pelvic floor. Physical therapists have known for years that protection of the lower back is improved by strengthening the shoulder girdle, quadriceps muscles, and abdominal muscles, as well as the muscles of the low back. These same concepts are valid for protection of the pelvic floor. A program of exercise that develops strength in all these muscle groups allows women to accomplish the activities they desire without straining or using the assistance of a Valsalva maneuver. Care must be taken to respect the urogenital hiatus so that during such training, undue stress is not repeatedly placed on the pelvic floor. Likewise, in daily activity, the proper techniques to lift, push, and pull objects should be learned and practiced. The control of obesity must be considered part of the effort to reduce the load placed on the pelvic floor. Osteoporotic spinal changes cause a gradual kyphosis, replacing the normal lumbosacral lordosis. The net effect is to rotate the pelvic brim into a more horizontal position. This shift places more stress on the pelvic floor. Estrogen therapy not only helps to prevent osteoporosis but also has positive effects on the various estrogen-sensitive tissues of the pelvis. Hormone replacement therapy is complicated, controversial, and beyond the scope of this discussion. Other effective treatments for osteoporosis exist.

Pelvic floor strengthening by voluntary contraction of the muscles innervated by the pudendal nerve was popularized by Arnold Kegel. The associated exercises have been known by his name ever since. Many women know this term because it is used frequently in postpartum instructions. Several different strategies help to remind patients to do their Kegel exercises. One of the most effective techniques is briefly outlined below. The Kegel contraction should be confirmed during a pelvic examination to ensure that the patient understands the correct muscles to contract. Frequently, patients will either perform a Valsalva maneuver or tighten the gluteus maximus muscle instead of the external anal sphincter and levator ani muscles. The proper time to Kegel is after micturition. After the bladder is emptied, the patient is instructed to lean as far forward as her stability allows. While leaning forward, she performs three or more isometric Kegel exercises by tightening the muscles until they voluntarily relax on their own. The dependent portion of a cystocele is below the level of the internal urethral orifice. The forward tilt physically elevates the bladder floor and allows for more complete emptying. The muscular action of the Kegel contractions also aids the process of emptying. Coupling this activity with voiding habituates the patient to perform the exercises several times a day. The result is the combination of more complete emptying and a strengthened pelvic floor, both of which are advantageous for the patient. The patient may then be able to use the Kegel contraction during physical stress to prevent incontinence or to protect against the pelvic floor impact of sudden increases in abdominal pressure. If the patient knows how to use Kegel muscles that are strong and easily controlled, they become an asset in her daily life.

Splinting is particularly effective in alleviating the dysfunctional defecation related to symptomatic rectoceles. If a significant rectocele/enterocele herniation is present, patients frequently experience entrapment of the leading edge of the descending bowel movement in the resulting anterior rectal pocket. Entrapment leads to straining, which further enhances the entrapment. Often, patients in this circumstance will strain until the bowel movement fragments and allows partial defecation and descent of another segment of stool into the rectal pocket. Several trips to the toilet and a large segment of the day may be required to complete this process. This unfortunate problem may be avoided if the patient simply places upward pressure with her fingertips against the perineum or the area lateral to the perineum during the initial urge to defecate. Occasionally, the patient needs to place one or two fingers against the posterior vaginal wall. These maneuvers effectively reduce the rectocele pocket, allowing the stool to evacuate while bypassing the rectocele. This "digital defecation" or splinting technique may avoid surgery and certainly empowers the patient to be in better control of her daily activities. I encourage the use of this technique postoperatively to protect the suspended posterior vaginal segment against undue strain. This protective maneuver is particularly important while acute healing is under way.

Control of chronic diseases and habits are helpful preventative strategies. Effective treatment of persistent cough may decrease incontinence and prevent progression of prolapse. Cessation of smoking certainly may be considered part of the preventative effort. Diabetic complications such as obesity, myopathy, and neuropathy may be prevented by modern management strategies.

The prevention of pelvic organ prolapse involves care of the entire body. A healthy, fit, and well-nourished patient who is aware of ways to actively protect her pelvic floor is less likely to experience this potentially disabling problem. Many of the strategies outlined in this section should be part of the care of patients from their obstetric years onward. Prevention is always preferable to intervention in the operating room.

CLINICAL EVALUATION

The correct management of pelvic organ prolapse depends on a careful evaluation of each patient. Only after a thorough history and physical examination is the practitioner able to develop an effective treatment plan for the individual patient.

The *history* should begin with the patient's perception of the problem. This information helps to determine what specific goals the patient may have. The patient might be afraid that the prolapse could rupture or that it may be caused by a malignant growth. Reassurance may suffice if any of these are her major concern. Patients may or may not be interested in coital function, further childbearing, or simply knowing that the vagina is present if social circumstances change. Some women have grown accustomed to advanced prolapse and may describe very little inconvenience related to the herniation. These people may simply want to know if the prolapse represents any threat to their longevity. Other women are very conscious of an anatomically minor prolapse or may have pain unrelated to the prolapse. The patient may have unrealistic expectations or may be ready for intervention before the physician's operative criteria are met. In this situation, the pelvic reconstructive surgeon needs to be honest and forthright in discussing what will or will not improve after a surgery. A careful micturition, defecation, and sexual history may be invaluable in developing a treatment plan. Validated evaluation forms are available for each of these aspects of function. Patients must be placed at ease and reassured during the evaluation before a full history concerning the details of pelvic functions can be obtained. Stress, urge, and neurogenic urinary incontinence may be differentiated by history. Obviously, the evaluations and treatments differ for each of these conditions. The complex topic of urinary incontinence is covered in detail elsewhere in this book. The mechanics

involved in defecation are important. Determine the number of trips to the toilet and the compensatory measures necessary to complete evacuation. Fecal incontinence is a condition that patients are notoriously reluctant to discuss. This condition may or may not be due to physical damage to the anal continence control mechanism. The patient may be continent or incontinent of gas, liquid, or solids. Each patient may safely be presumed to desire urinary and bowel continence. Marked variation exists in patients' sexual goals. The practitioner should learn about these goals in a respectful and nonjudgmental way. Collecting sexual function information is an art, critical to the development of a management plan.

The past surgical history helps the surgeon assess the status of the patient in general and of the pelvis in particular. Specific interest should be placed on previous attempts to correct pelvic organ prolapse. Before her visit, the patient may be asked to prepare a list of previous surgeries so that none are overlooked. The route of hysterectomy and the indications for the procedure may be helpful. If previous prolapse surgery has been performed, the physician should try to obtain the operative notes. The anatomic details, type of suture used, and other details of the operative technique may help predict problems such as the likely location of anatomic distortion (previous plications) or the location of previously placed foreign bodies (e.g., meshes). Multiple previous attempts at repair necessitate a combination of caution and experience to achieve a successful outcome.

The medical history should be used to determine whether medical conditions exist that would likely interact with surgery or recovery. A complete pelvic reconstructive surgery may last several hours, involve significant blood loss, and even require combined vaginal and abdominal or endoscopic approaches. Obviously, the patient needs the physical reserve to withstand this degree of stress. Patients with morbid obesity, limited pulmonary and cardiac function, thromboembolic risks, entrenched tobacco addiction, or limited mobility are not ideal candidates for this type of surgery. A complete list of current medications, including herbals and over-the-counter preparations, and treating physicians is also helpful.

The proper *physical examination* of the prolapse patient requires that the examining physician have a working knowledge of normal pelvic anatomy. Older systems for recording physical findings related to prolapse relied on subjective terms such as *mild*, *moderate*, and *severe*. These terms have a limited ability to accurately describe prolapse and restrict effective communication between examiners. Two systems are currently in use that encourage a complete prolapse examination and that more objectively record anatomic detail. Each of these systems has strengths and weaknesses. The Baden-Walker Halfway System is user friendly, is easy to record, and maximizes the amount of detail that can be recorded in a very brief space. Proponents of this system maintain that the essence of the prolapse examination is recorded after writing six numbers and some editorial notes. Critics note that the abbreviation of detail means that some compromises are made along the way. The second system is the Pelvic Organ Prolapse-Quantification or POP-Q system. This is a more complex system incorporating more specific detail of the physical findings. Even for those clinicians accustomed to its use, the number of measurements needed requires additional time to acquire. The beauty of this system is that, theoretically, physician-to-physician variation is minimized. The POP-Q is currently used in many academic papers on the subject of prolapse. Interested physicians should become familiar with both of these systems. More important than any system is an accurate and anatomically based assessment of the patient at the time of examination.

TABLE 36.10 Primary and Secondary Symptoms at Each Site Used in the Baden-Walker Halfway System

ANATOMIC SITE	PRIMARY SYMPTOMS	SECONDARY SYMPTOMS
Urethral	Urinary incontinence	Falling out
Vesical	Voiding difficulties	Falling out
Uterine	Falling out	Heaviness and so forth
Cul-de-sac	Pelvic pressure (standing)	Falling out
Rectal	True bowel pocket	Falling out
Perineal	Anal incontinence	Too loose (gas/feces)

Reprinted from Baden WF, Walker T. *Surgical repair of vaginal defects*. Philadelphia, PA: JB Lippincott, 1992:12, with permission. Copyright © 1992 Wolters Kluwer Health.

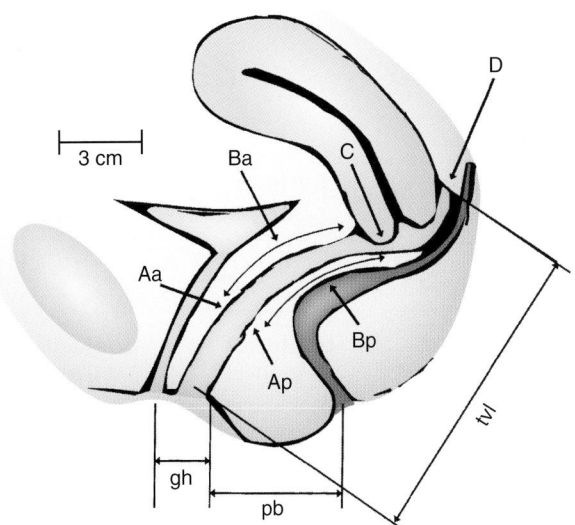

FIGURE 36.10 The nine specific sites of measurement used in the Pelvic Organ Prolapse-Quantification (POP-Q) system. (gh, genital hiatus; pb, perineal body; tvl, total vaginal length.) (Adapted from Bump RC, Mattiasson A, Bø K, et al. The standardization of terminology of female pelvic organ prolapse and pelvic floor dysfunction. *Am J Obstet Gynecol* 1996;175:10, with permission. Copyright © 1996, Elsevier.)

Baden-Walker Halfway System

The extent of prolapse is recorded using a number (0 to 4) at each of six defined sites in the vagina. There are two sites on the anterior, superior, and posterior walls of the vagina. Table 36.10 lists the anatomic sites and the associated symptoms. The six numbers are recorded as a measure of descent. For all sites except the perineum, the hymen is used as a fixed anatomic reference point. Zero indicates normal anatomic position for a site, whereas 4 represents maximum prolapse. Between these extremes, the intervening numbers grade descent using a halfway system. The examination is performed with the patient straining so that maximum descent is attained. The patient may wish to stand or use other maneuvers in order to demonstrate maximum descent.

The perineum is graded with the familiar perineal laceration system used in obstetrics. The patient is asked to hold or Kegel to evaluate the amount of muscular and fascial compensatory support. Editorial comments may include the site of dominant prolapse, location of scars, palpable plications from previous surgery, and the type of efforts necessary to demonstrate maximum prolapse. Strength of the levator contraction may be recorded as 0 to 4.

Example: 12/44/32. A dominant complete apical prolapse is noted with enterocele, significant cystocele and rectocele, and perineal attenuation to the level of the external anal sphincter. 2/4 levator strength is present.

Although this type of notation encodes much information in a small space, no specific location of fascial defects is indicated.

Pelvic Organ Prolapse-Quantification (POP-Q) System

This system was developed as an effort to introduce more objectivity into the quantification of pelvic organ prolapse. For example, measurements in centimeters are used instead of subjective grades. Nine specific measurements are recorded as indicated in Figure 36.10. Point Aa is defined as being 3 cm proximal or apical to the external urethral meatus on the anterior vaginal wall. Point Ap is defined as being 3 cm proximal to the hymen on the posterior vaginal wall. Points Ba and Bp are defined as points of maximum prolapse excursion on the

anterior and posterior vaginal walls, respectively. Measurements are recorded as negative numbers when proximal or apical to the hymen and positive numbers when distal to the hymen. POP-Q sites C (cervix or hysterectomy scar) and D (cul-de-sac of Douglas) are identical in location to Baden-Walker sites 3 and 4 in the apical vagina. In addition, measurements of the total vaginal length, genital hiatus, and perineal body are taken. All measurements are recorded on a tic-tac-toe style grid (Fig. 36.11). When combined with sagittal line drawings, a fairly complete picture of prolapse is attained (Fig. 36.12). Ordinal stages of pelvic organ prolapse are then assigned from stage 0 (no prolapse) to stage IV (complete prolapse) so that the outcome of cases of like magnitude may be compared.

This system is a physical examination tool and does not assign the specific location of fascial defects.

Pelvic Examination

After a general physical examination is performed, the prolapse may be evaluated. Any surgical scars on the abdomen should be correlated with the surgical history. Patients frequently forget procedures that may have an impact on the treatment plan. The physician should pay particular attention to the suprapubic region where previous incontinence procedure incisions may be located.

The pelvic examination is initiated with the patient in the lithotomy position. Hip mobility should be evaluated because adequate abduction and flexion of the thighs is required for a vaginal procedure. Thigh and buttock obesity may also be limiting factors related to surgical access. If exposure is limited, an extended procedure performed vaginally is not in the patient's or surgeon's best interest.

The labia are opened for introital inspection. Prolapse may be internal or incomplete (proximal to the hymen) or external, that is, complete (distal to the hymen), at rest. The extent of the prolapse may change considerably if the patient is asked to

anterior wall	anterior wall	cervix or cuff
Aa	**Ba**	**C**
genital hiatus	perineal body	total vaginal length
gh	**pb**	**tvl**
posterior wall	posterior wall	posterior fornix
Ap	**Bp**	**D**

FIGURE 36.11 The tic-tac-toe grid used to record measurements in the Pelvic Organ Prolapse-Quantified (POP-Q) system. (Adapted from Bump RC, Mattiasson A, Bø K, et al. The standardization of terminology of female pelvic organ prolapse and pelvic floor dysfunction. *Am J Obstet Gynecol* 1996;175:10, with permission. Copyright © 1996, Elsevier.)

strain or stand. This difference may be especially pronounced in patients with healthy pelvic floor muscles and an undescended levator plate. These two structures may help hold a prolapse in place. The patient may give a history of a prolapse that is not apparent on examination or not as large as she describes. In such a case, the patient is examined while she is in the standing position; or she may be asked to perform the maneuvers necessary to demonstrate the full extent of the prolapse.

The dominant prolapse is considered to be the first hernia to descend or the most dependent part of a prolapse that has previously descended. Proper identification of the dominant prolapse provides key clues about where the most significant fascial damage is located. The dominant prolapse is located and replaced to examine the remainder of the vaginal vault. A large dominant prolapse often fills the urogenital hiatus and

introitus, preventing incipient hernias from fully developing. Usually, an anterior prolapse is easily replaced by placing a tongue blade or Ayre spatula in each anterior lateral sulcus. If an apical transverse or lateral paravaginal defect is present, this maneuver replaces the anterior vaginal wall. If this maneuver does not reduce the hernia, a central anterior defect is likely present. A dominant posterior segment prolapse may be replaced with the posterior blade of a disjoined Sims speculum. A dominant superior segment prolapse may be replaced with a large cotton swab or a sponge stick or, in advanced cases, by attaching a tenaculum to the cervix. After replacement of the dominant prolapse, the secondary sites of prolapse become more apparent. An isolated single-site prolapse is not the norm. The location of the cervix or hysterectomy scar helps determine the location of the dominant prolapse. Frequently displaced, either anteriorly or posteriorly, these sites are often not at the most dependent part of the prolapse. The posthysterectomy scar is commonly a transverse fibrous band that may be slightly retracted. To either side of the band are dimples in the epithelium corresponding to the location of the insertion of cardinal and uterosacral ligament remnants. Incomplete prolapse evaluation may lead to incomplete repair and result in recurrent prolapse in a different location and multiple trips to the operating room. The support structures of all vaginal segments and levels are interdependent. Complete restoration of all defects is necessary for a successful outcome.

Careful inspection of the vaginal epithelium reveals the location of rugae. The presence of these transverse folds implies that endopelvic fascia is adherent to the epithelium in that location. The lateral vaginal sulci are the location of the junction of the pubocervical and rectovaginal septa to their respective lateral arcuate attachments. The pattern of rugae and the condition of the sulci should correlate with the pattern of fascial breaks found at surgery. The vaginal epithelium should also be inspected for atrophy created by the absence of the effects of estrogen. Local or systemic administration of estrogen before surgery assists in dissection and subsequent healing. Occasionally, an external prolapse may develop pressure ulcers as a result of entrapment when the patient is sitting. These lesions must be properly evaluated to rule out malignancy.

Rectovaginal examination assists in the evaluation of the posterior and superior vaginal segments. The uterosacral

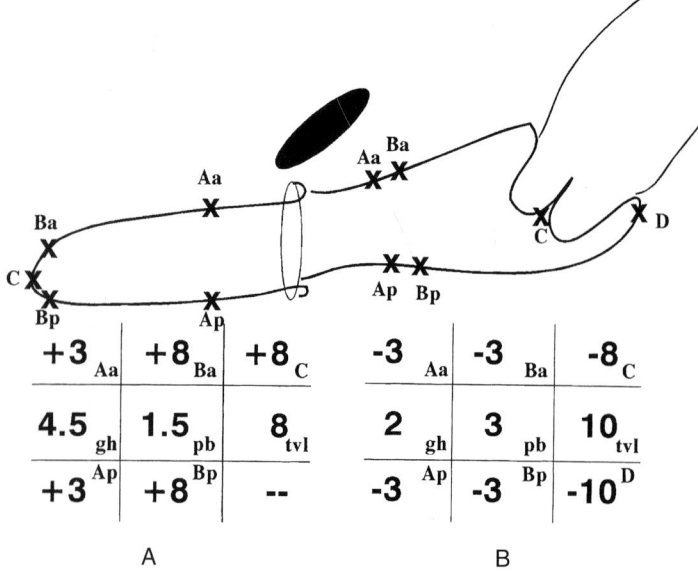

+3 Aa	+8 Ba	+8 C		-3 Aa	-3 Ba	-8 C
4.5 gh	1.5 pb	8 tvl		2 gh	3 pb	10 tvl
+3 Ap	+8 Bp	--		-3 Ap	-3 Bp	-10 D

| A | B |

FIGURE 36.12 Two examples of the Pelvic Organ Prolapse-Quantified (POP-Q) system. (Adapted from Bump RC, Mattiasson A, Bø K, et al. The standardization of terminology of female pelvic organ prolapse and pelvic floor dysfunction. *Am J Obstet Gynecol* 1996;175:10, with permission. Copyright © 1996, Elsevier.)

VII

ligaments may be palpable immediately medial to each ischial spine, especially if the uterus is present. The uterosacral ligaments are usually more easily palpated with traction placed on the cervix. Anterior displacement of the rectal examining finger toward the vagina helps to distinguish between rectocele and enterocele. During the rectal examination, the patient is asked to strain. If an enterocele is present, it bulges down in the nonrugated vaginal epithelium proximal to the tip of the examining finger. Palpating the transversely detached proximal edge of the rectovaginal septum is possible during this maneuver. This sharp border may retract distally all the way to the perineum. Perineal descent is also evaluated at the time of rectal examination. The levator plate is immediately posterior to the rectum and should be horizontal and immovable. The perineum is evaluated last. The perineum is triangular in the sagittal plane. The base is on the rectal side and the apex at the hymen. Perineal attenuation is very common in parous women. Apposition of the thumb of the examining hand while the index finger is in the rectum proximal to the anterior aspect of the external anal sphincter allows for evaluation of the integrity of this muscle. Voluntary contraction of the sphincter may be helpful. The S3 neurologic segment is necessary to contract this muscle and controls the ability to spread and dorsiflex the toes. If the patient cannot perform these tasks, the integrity of that neural segment is in question. The mechanical strength of the pelvic diaphragm is directly correlated with the ability to voluntarily contract these muscles. This ability is best tested clinically with light pressure placed on the posterior vaginal wall by the examining digits. The patient may need coaching to elicit a response. This time is an excellent opportunity to instruct the patient in the importance of postvoiding Kegel exercises and perineal support (splinting) during defecation.

If muscle activity is elicited, it may be subjectively graded from 0 to 4. If no muscle activity is detected, a more formal neurologic and medical workup should be considered. Pudendal nerve motor latency studies may reveal significant neuropathies. Magnetic resonance imaging of these patients has revealed the presence of advanced muscle atrophy and muscular detachments as well. Neuropathy and myopathy erode the surgeon's ability to correct prolapse. If the patient cannot properly move her toes and cannot contract the levator muscles, a spinal cord or central nervous system lesion must be considered.

The presence of urinary incontinence should be noted during any part of the evaluation of prolapse. In an advanced prolapse, assessment of incontinence should be conducted with the prolapse in a reduced state. A pessary or loose vaginal packing may be helpful in accomplishing this goal. Incontinence may be masked by a hypotonic bladder or reverse kinking of the urethra if a cystocele is large. Repair of a large prolapse may be followed by the appearance of urinary incontinence if the preoperative evaluation is not performed with the prolapse reduced.

When a large prolapse is present, the trigone of the bladder is often located outside the vaginal introitus. In this degree of displacement, one may deduce the location of the trigone as being directly adjacent to the location of a Foley catheter bulb. The course of the ureter in a large prolapse arcs from the superior and lateral aspect of the anterior prolapse to the area of the trigone. The ureter may often be palpated in this location. If the prolapse is chronic and advanced, hydroureter and even hydronephrosis may be present. In this circumstance, the ureters lose their cordlike consistency and are more difficult to palpate or recognize at the time of surgery. A large external prolapse makes the ureter more susceptible to surgical injury. Intraoperative placement of ureteral catheters may be helpful in such a patient. Postoperative documentation of ureteral patency is required.

A patient may present with the cervix near the level of the hymen. If no other signs of prolapse are present, the alert examiner is aware of the possibility of an elongated cervix. Sometimes, surgery is not necessary in these patients. If surgery is performed, the technique of hysterectomy needs to take into consideration the elongation of the cervix. Often, the paracolpium is properly placed in the interspinous diameter in these patients.

The examiner should not underestimate the value of an examination under anesthesia prior to the initiation of a planned surgical procedure to supplement information that has been gathered preoperatively. With the patient and her pelvic diaphragm relaxed, the full extent of prolapse may become more apparent. Deep structures of importance, such as the ischial spines and uterosacral ligaments, may be more easily palpated. An examination under anesthesia should be performed before initiating a prolapse surgery.

A number of ways may be used to summarize the array of clinical findings discussed in this section. My preference is to use a pelvic organ prolapse map (**Figs. 36.13** and **36.14**). Key anatomic landmarks are schematically outlined. The three-dimensional structure of the vagina is reduced to two dimensions as if the vagina were divided at the 3-o'clock and 9-o'clock positions. A Baden-Walker profile can be recorded vertically on the map with numbers placed beside the appropriate anatomic location. As seen in **Figure 36.15**, fascial defects can be sketched on the map at their suspected or known location. Editorial notes regarding the prolapse can be recorded in the space provided. A POP-Q evaluation may be used as well. The pattern that is noted in **Figure 36.15** is the one most commonly seen in pelvic organ prolapse surgery; however, many

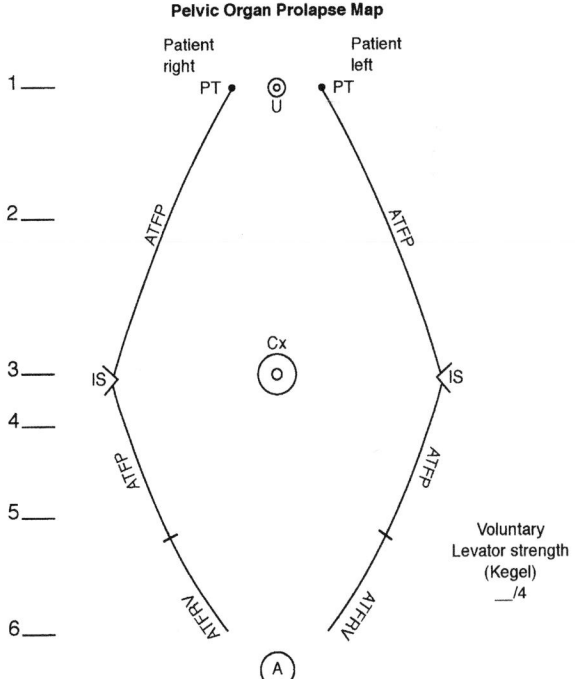

Pelvic Organ Prolapse Map

FIGURE 36.13 Key elements of pelvic support anatomy. Three dimensions are reduced to two by dividing the vagina at the 3-o'clock and 9-o'clock positions. Baden-Walker vaginal support profile sites: 1, urethral; 2, vesical; 3, uterine; 4, cul-de-sac; 5, rectal; 6, perineal. (PT, pubic tubercle; ATFP, arcus tendineus fascia pelvis; ATFRV, arcus tendineus fasciae rectovaginalis; IS, ischial spines; U, urethra; Cx, cervix; A, anus.)

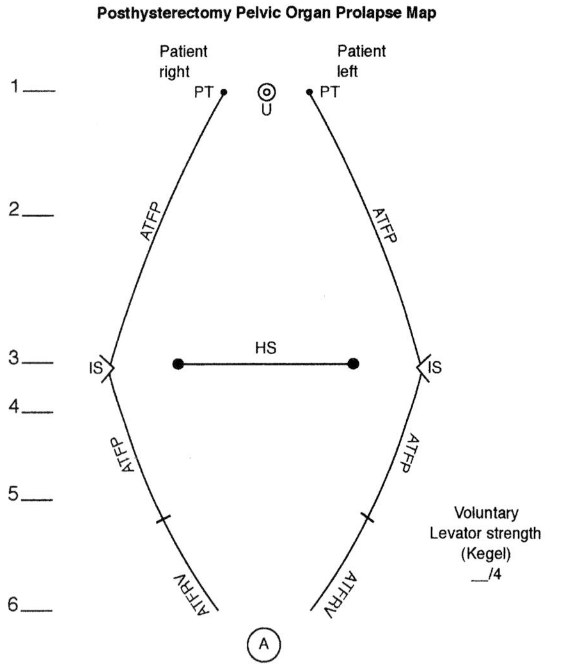

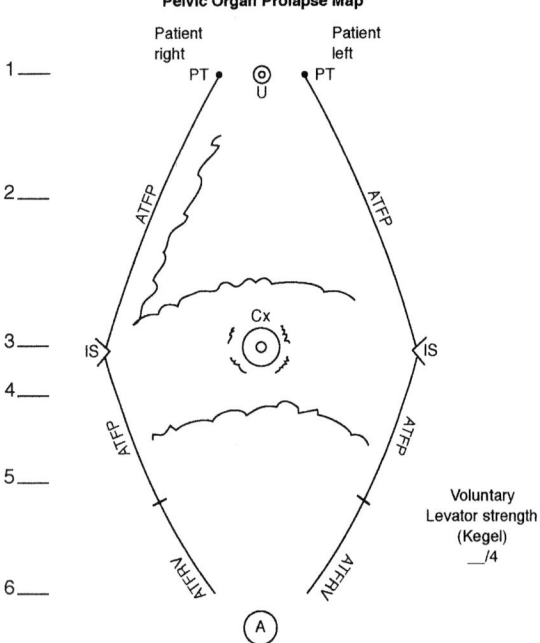

FIGURE 36.14 Key elements of posthysterectomy pelvic support anatomy. Three dimensions are reduced to two by dividing the vagina at the 3-o'clock and 9-o'clock positions. Baden-Walker vaginal support profile sites: 1, urethral; 2, vesical; 3, uterine; 4, cul-de-sac; 5, rectal; 6, perineal. (PT, pubic tubercle; ATFP, arcus tendineus fascia pelvis; ATFRV, arcus tendineus fasciae rectovaginalis; IS, ischial spines; U, urethra; HS, hysterectomy scar; A, anus.)

FIGURE 36.15 The most frequently encountered pattern of fascial damage in pelvic organ prolapse: (a) full-length right paravaginal defect; (b) transverse proximal detachment of the pubocervical septum; (c) transverse proximal detachment of the rectovaginal septum. This pattern of damage is consistent with the mechanics of a left occipitoanterior delivery. Baden-Walker vaginal support profile sites: 1, urethral; 2, vesical; 3, uterine; 4, cul-de-sac; 5, rectal; 6, perineal. (PT, pubic tubercle; ATFP, arcus tendineus fascia pelvis; ATFRV, arcus tendineus fasciae rectovaginalis; IS, ischial spines; U, urethra; Cx, cervix; A, anus.)

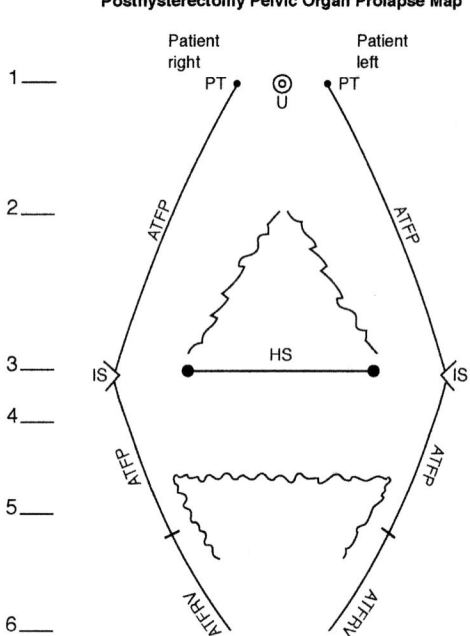

FIGURE 36.16 An infrequently encountered inverted "V" anterior central fascial defect. Posteriorly, the proximal detachment of the rectovaginal septum has retracted toward the perineum, creating an enterocele and rectocele. Notice the bilateral pararectal defects. Baden-Walker vaginal support profile sites: 1, urethral; 2, vesical; 3, uterine; 4, cul-de-sac; 5, rectal; 6, perineal. (PT, pubic tubercle; ATFP, arcus tendineus fascia pelvis; ATFRV, arcus tendineus fasciae rectovaginalis; IS, ischial spines; U, urethra; HS, hysterectomy scar; A, anus.)

variations on this theme are encountered (Fig. 36.16). Another diagram may be drawn to indicate the exact locations of fascial defects at the time of surgery.

A thorough history and physical examination improves the treatment of the prolapse patient. The physical findings must be recorded in an anatomically accurate and understandable way.

CHOICE OF TREATMENT

Vaginal reconstructive surgery is concerned with the return of abnormal organ relationships to a usual or normal state. There is no one site or degree of damage that must be repaired or restored; there are many and they occur in various combinations at various times of life, from different etiologic factors, in varying degrees, and with varying degrees of symptoms and disability.
—Nichols and Randall, 1989

Patients with pelvic organ prolapse have highly individualized perceptions of their situation. The single most important concept in the treatment of these conditions is to understand the patient's symptoms, concerns, and limitations related to the prolapse. Her quality of life should be of paramount concern in the decision-making process. The patient's expectations and her ability to tolerate surgery should be expertly evaluated. The physician's job is to educate the patient regarding options of treatment. After informed consent is given, the appropriate course of action is usually obvious to both the doctor and the patient. If the chosen course of action fails or becomes inappropriate over the course of time, the clinical evaluation and decision process can be revisited.

Nonsurgical Management

Regardless of the degree of prolapse, no surgery should be done unless the patient experiences a sufficient degree of morbidity. Most symptoms relate to quality-of-life issues. Generally, preventative measures should be the most widely applied techniques. Pelvic floor exercises, weight loss, treatment of chronic diseases, physical therapy, cessation of smoking, and estrogen therapy are all considerations in the conservative treatment of pelvic organ prolapse. These interventions have been discussed in the previous section of this chapter and should be used regardless of whether expectant management or surgical intervention is the plan. During expectant management, periodic examinations should be done to determine the status of pelvic organ support and the degree of progression. Symptoms and the ability to participate in daily activities may be reviewed to reinforce the patient's motivation to continue preventative measures.

Pessaries are ingenious devices that have been used in one form or another for much of recorded history. They were originally the product of an age when surgery was not an option for the prolapse patient. They are available in a variety of shapes and sizes, depending on the needs of the patient. In general, the greater the degree of prolapse and the more strenuous the daily activities of the patient, the less likely it is for a pessary to be a permanent solution. As the prolapse expands, occupies the urogenital hiatus, and dilates the introitus, the pressure of the prolapse tends to expel the pessary. A pessary may be valuable for a patient to wear to feel more comfortable during a specific activity, such as exercise. If a patient of limited activity and acute-onset advanced prolapse can be successfully fitted with a pessary, it may prevent progression and result in long-term improvement in intestinal and urinary function. Pessaries are discussed in detail in Chapter 40.

Surgical Principles and Management

The management of advanced and symptomatic prolapse is primarily surgical. In 1997, 226,000 women underwent pelvic organ prolapse surgery in the United States. This condition is one of the most common indications for major surgery. Eleven percent of all women will experience some type of prolapse surgery during their lifetimes, and 30% of these women will undergo another operation for recurrence of prolapse or a complication related to surgery. Prolapse is a high-incidence problem that commands a substantial expenditure of health care dollars. Only those patients who request relief should be considered surgical candidates. Once the decision is made to operate, quality-of-life goals need to be established. If the patient can tolerate a lengthy operation and especially if she desires coital function, a reconstructive operation should be considered. The restoration of normal anatomy (form) maximizes the potential that symptoms and limitations (function) will be corrected or significantly improved. Restoration of normal anatomy automatically addresses the questions of vaginal axis, caliber, and depth. If the patient does not desire coital function, an occlusive procedure, such as colpocleisis, might be the best choice. Colpocleisis, with or without vaginectomy, has a very low failure rate; however, the end does not justify the means in all patients because these operations render the patient permanently acoital.

Choosing the correct operation for prolapse is critical for success. The general plan for the procedures that will best correct the problems of the individual patient may be developed from details gathered during the preoperative history and pelvic examination and even the examination under anesthesia. Specific details become evident only during the intraoperative dissection. The goals of the operation are the restoration of normal form and function. Isolated areas of prolapse are uncommon. Childbirth places damaging pressure on all segments of suspension and support during the various phases of labor and delivery. Restricting an operative procedure to the repair of a single dominant or symptomatic site of prolapse may simply transfer the physical stress to a different vaginal segment. An incomplete reconstruction may result in a secondary prolapse descending as a new dominant prolapse. Sometimes, prolapse can return quickly postoperatively. Perhaps, the best known example of this phenomenon was the observation by Burch that many patients developed an enterocele after his anterior urethropexy procedure. An active search for potential and undeveloped defects must be done at the time of prolapse surgery. Site-specific repair of all segments and levels is the best insurance against failure.

The route of operation is a matter of debate. Vaginal surgery is the historical hallmark of the gynecologic surgeon. Although surgical training in vaginal techniques has eroded in recent years, a resurgence of interest in these operations is occurring. The vaginal approach requires either limited or no access to the peritoneal cavity and is surgically less stressful on the patient.

During the last three decades, a significant change has occurred in the way prolapse surgery is conceptualized and performed. Anatomically distorting distal plications have been replaced by defect-specific anatomic restorations. Several aspects of the defect-specific method favor the vaginal approach. Fascial defects can be best identified when the full extent of the vaginal segment to be repaired is dissected and exposed. Such dissections are only possible vaginally. The detached fascial edge of a paravaginal defect may retract across the midline to the contralateral side of the body. This retraction leaves the fascial edge in a position that is impossible to reach from the abdominal or endoscopic approach. No one questions that a paravaginal defect can be seen from the abdominal or endoscopic operative approach. A question does remain about whether the retracted fascial edge can be accessed and reattached to the white line using the abdominal or endoscopic approach. Likewise, a proximal rectovaginal septal defect that has retracted distally to the perineum would be very difficult to find and resuspend from above. All the major support anatomic landmarks and tissues are accessible vaginally. These points include the arcus tendineus fascia pelvis, arcus tendineus fasciae rectovaginalis, ischial spines, uterosacral ligaments, sacrospinous ligaments, and virtually all components of the deep endopelvic connective tissue. During childbirth, the named components of the endopelvic fascia are displaced away from the interspinous diameter. Reconstructive efforts must be centered in this diameter for a permanently successful outcome. Access to torn fascial edges is best attained by complete dissections of the vesicovaginal and rectovaginal spaces. Midvaginal lateral defects can easily be repaired by this route. Additionally, apical suspension can also be performed to complete the restoration of central pelvic organ suspension. For most primary reconstructions, the vaginal operative route is superior to any other approach. The vaginal route is also preferred for patients with failures from previous operations. This approach is especially useful when a previous operation did not use the defect-specific approach and did not include the use of permanent suture for critical support sites.

The discussion and opinions in the previous paragraphs do not preclude the use of abdominal and endoscopic techniques for certain problems in pelvic reconstructive surgery. Procedures to correct stress urinary incontinence are discussed extensively in Chapter 41. Anterior urethropexy approached through the prevesical space with a suprapubic incision or endoscopic technique has some advantages when compared with a suburethral sling urethropexy. No iatrogenic paravaginal defect is necessary during anterior urethropexy, for example. Such defects are made with pubovaginal sling

VII

procedures of all types. Some intentionally created defects are larger than others. To spend time and effort to reconstruct the pubocervical fascia anatomically from white line to white line and then to destroy part of the paravaginal support intentionally to allow passage of the sling material into the prevesical space does not make good sense. The primary prevesical space approach avoids this destructive necessity. Kelly-Kennedy plications and paravaginal repairs have been shown to be ineffective as incontinence procedures. New minimally invasive sling operations represent an effective totally vaginal operation to cure stress incontinence. Vaginal incontinence operations that avoid iatrogenic paravaginal damage and an abdominal or laparoscopic incision are ideal.

The abdominal approach is useful in some cases of prolapse in which one or more previous pelvic support operations have failed. Abdominal sacral colpopexy is an option in this situation. This operation also has its proponents as a primary procedure. Outcome data have generally been good with low recurrence rates. Colpopexy may be useful in a circumstance in which considerable scar is present from previous surgery. For example, consider a patient with a previous aggressive distal plication and a proximal support failure. Significant adhesiolysis would be necessary to gain access to the proximal structures necessary to repair the prolapse. A rescue abdominal sacral colpopexy may more easily and effectively correct the prolapse. Occasional patients whose support has failed following a site-specific operation with permanent suture may also benefit from this operation. Abdominal sacral colpopexy is not a site-specific operation; however, it provides substantial proximal apical support and protects vaginal length. Sacral colpopexy may be accomplished laparoscopically with or without robotic assistance in a less invasive manner, but should be considered equivalent only if the technique is not substantially altered.

During a prolapse surgery, the surgeon may determine that adequate support or repair is not attainable through the primary approach. No harm is done in using a combined approach. If support is not satisfactory after a vaginal procedure, an abdominal sacral colpopexy can be done at that time. Conversely, a vaginal examination should be performed after an abdominal sacral colpopexy to determine if the vaginal axis, caliber, and depth have been restored to an acceptable state. The patient with proper informed consent would likely prefer a combined procedure to subsequent surgery.

Suture selection for pelvic reconstruction has changed with the realization that prolapse surgery is really a series of herniorrhaphies. No surgeon would consider performing a repair of an inguinal or ventral hernia with absorbable suture. In the days of distal plications, the use of absorbable suture was common. Today, fascial defects are repaired with permanent suture. In an attempt to compromise, some surgeons use delayed absorbable sutures. They reason that the suture material is not needed after healing has been completed. No evidence exists in the hernia literature to support the use of anything other than permanent suture for these repairs. Monofilament and polyfilament sutures are acceptable. Monofilament sutures occasionally erode and cause an unpleasant whisker effect in the vagina. If erosion occurs, the suture can be removed. My choice of suture is interwoven braided polyester for fascial repairs. This suture is affordable and easily tied, has no sharp end, and infrequently causes a reaction or exposure. If exposure occurs, suture material should be removed in its entirety.

All prolapse patients should be carefully evaluated for concomitant vaginal, uterine, adnexal, pelvic, or abdominal disease. Coexisting pathology may change the operative approach selected for correction of prolapse. Orthopedic problems and obesity must be factored into the decision-making process because adequate surgical access is important.

Young patients with uterovaginal prolapse may request preservation of their fertility. Unless the problem is severe, these patients should be advised to complete their childbearing so that a definitive operation can be performed. Ring-type pessaries may provide temporary relief. They permit intercourse and may be worn at the discretion of the patient during exercise or strenuous activity and on other occasions. A unilateral sacrospinous ligament fixation with the uterus in place may be beneficial and does not prohibit subsequent vaginal childbirth. Various abdominal or endoscopic uterine suspensions may also be considered. In general, retention of the uterus when a significant degree of prolapse is present compromises the long-term operative result. The cervix limits access to the structures of the paracolpium that are necessary to achieve proper proximal suspension of the vaginal vault. At the same time, removal of the cervix creates an inherent defect in the proximal anterior vaginal wall. The posthysterectomy vault prolapse is in many instances a result of this cervical defect. Care must be taken to compensate for this weakness at the time of hysterectomy. This area is the location of the pericervical ring whose proper attachments are so important to normal vaginal suspension. No totally anatomic method to close this space exists. To achieve a satisfactory result is easier at hysterectomy than at subsequent posthysterectomy repair. Plication of the cardinal ligaments and McCall culdoplasty are necessary components of hysterectomy cuff repair. Permanent suture material may be used for McCall culdoplasty.

Various grafts, bolsters, and synthetic meshes can be valuable tools in prolapse surgery. For example, in a posthysterectomy prolapse, a small piece of foreign material used to bolster the weak area left by the absence of the cervix may decrease the amount of anatomic distortion needed to support the apical anterior vaginal wall. These materials are useful and often necessary in abdominal sacral colpopexy. However, the overzealous use of grafts and meshes is unnecessary and may predispose to the troublesome problems of exposure and erosion. Procedures that require the use of foreign materials to compensate for absent fasciae should be viewed with suspicion. Even in an advanced prolapse, the fascia is present in most cases. Fasciae, unlike muscles, do not atrophy. They may be retracted and scarred but are available for dissection and reattachment if the surgeon is trained in the proper techniques. Bolstering of site-specific repairs is acceptable. At no time should bolsters, grafts, and meshes be used as a substitute for meticulous surgical technique. Foreign materials should be used to strengthen anatomically restorative repairs. The Food and Drug Administration has issued two notifications indicating that complications related to bolsters used to correct prolapse are not rare and that care should be exercised in the use of these materials. Informed consent is essential.

Complications occurred in 15.5% of prolapse surgeries performed in the United States in 1997 (Table 36.11). The majority of these complications can be addressed in the operating room. Gynecologic surgeons have been well trained to irrigate inside the abdomen. The same principles are applicable when operating vaginally. In the operating room after the surgical prep and draping are completed, a vaginal lavage rinses the vagina of nonadherent bacteria. Intraoperative irrigation at frequent intervals also helps to prevent infection. Irrigation as described and prophylactic antibiotics greatly help reduce the incidence of postoperative infection. A vaginal pack may help initial adherence of the vaginal epithelium to the endopelvic fascia and may reduce hematoma formation. Packs should be removed the day after surgery.

The pelvis is a busy place anatomically. The deep dissections necessary for the correction of prolapse predispose the patient to injury to adjacent structures. Development of proper surgical planes helps to minimize the potential for such injuries.

TABLE 36.11 Frequency and Percentage of Morbidity Associated with Pelvic Organ Prolapse Surgery, 1997

MORBIDITY	FREQUENCY	PERCENT OF ALL SURGERIES[a]
Infections	14,824	5.4
Bleeding complications	13,945	5.4
Surgical injury	9,546	4.2
Pulmonary complications	3,024	1.3
Cardiovascular complications	2,407	1.1
Wound complications	1,368	0.6
Cerebrovascular complications	249	<0.1
Other complications	165	<0.1
Total morbidity	45,528	15.5

[a]$N = 225,964$ women undergoing prolapse surgery.
Reprinted from Brown JS, Waetjen LE, Subak LL, et al. Pelvic organ prolapse in the United States, 1997. *Am J Obstet Gynecol* 2001;186:712, with permission. Copyright © 2002, Elsevier.

Vascular injuries are usually immediately apparent and can be corrected during the operation. Intestinal and urinary injuries are often more subtle. The surgeon should not conclude the operative procedure without some reassurance of the integrity of these structures. Cystoscopy is a valuable skill that should be used by the pelvic support surgeon. A high rectal examination may suffice for intestinal reassurance unless damage is suspected higher than the examination extends.

Preoperative and postoperative care is discussed elsewhere in this text. Early ambulation and thrombosis prophylaxis are particularly important in the usual prolapse patient. The patient should be at sexual pelvic rest for approximately 6 weeks. The patient may be quite anxious about sexual activity. Sexual rehabilitation may require time, reassurance, and the helpful advice of the physician. Straining to void and defecate should be minimized. The act of perineal splinting postoperatively helps to protect the perineum from downward displacement during defecation. Lifting should be restricted to those things that can be accomplished with available strength in the shoulders, back, and legs.

The care of patients with pelvic organ prolapse can be equally challenging and rewarding. Attention to the details of anatomy, physical diagnosis, reconstructive surgical techniques, and good medical care will yield the best results.

BEST SURGICAL PRACTICES

- Pelvic organ prolapse affects a patient's quality of life. Any decision regarding treatment of prolapse should ultimately be made with significant input from the patient.
- A careful physical examination documenting the defects in pelvic supportive structures is useful in selecting the appropriate treatment to correct the anatomic defect responsible for the patient's symptoms and physical exam findings.

- Pelvic reconstructive surgeries should be designed to restore maximally the normal biomechanical support and suspension of the central pelvic organs. This concept is called site-specific repair of pelvic support defects. Restoration of normal anatomy maximizes the potential for normal urinary, intestinal, and sexual functions.
- Principles of hernia repair should be followed in prolapse surgery. Use of permanent suture is standard. Judicious use of meshes, bolsters, and grafts may be indicated; however, these products should be used to enhance rather than replace sound surgical technique.
- Complex pelvic surgery and dissection into the deep pelvic spaces require that ureteral patency be documented before leaving the operating room.
- Precise anatomical knowledge of deep pelvic anatomy is necessary for performance of pelvic organ prolapse surgery.

BIBLIOGRAPHY

Abitbol MM. *Birth and human evolution*. Westport, CT: Bergin & Garvey, 1996.
Baden WF, Walker T. *Surgical repair of vaginal defects*. Philadelphia, PA: JB Lippincott, 1992.
Barber MD, Visco AG, Weidner AC, et al. Bilateral uterosacral ligament vaginal vault suspension with site-specific endopelvic fascia defect repair for treatment of pelvic organ prolapse. *Am J Obstet Gynecol* 2000;183:1402.
Barber MD, Brubaker L, Nygaard I, et al. Defining success after surgery for pelvic organ prolapse. *Obstet Gynecol* 2009;114:600.
Bamberg C, Radermacher G, Güttler F, et al. Human birth observed in real-time open magnetic resonance imaging. *Am J Obstet Gynecol* 2012;206:505.e1.
Bonney V. An address on genital displacements. *BMJ* 1928;1:432.
Bonney V. The principles that should underlie all operations for prolapse. *J Obstet Gynaecol Br Emp* 1934;41:669.
Bradley CS, Nygaard IE. Vaginal wall descensus and pelvic floor symptoms in older women. *Obstet Gynecol* 2005;106:759.
Brown JS, Waetjen LE, Subak LL, et al. Pelvic organ prolapse in the United States, 1997. *Am J Obstet Gynecol* 2002;186:712.
Brubaker L. Vaginal delivery and the pelvic floor. *Int Urogynecol J* 1998;9:363.
Buller JL, Thompson JR, Cundiff GW. Uterosacral ligament: description of anatomic relationships to optimize surgical safety. *Obstet Gynecol* 2001;97:873.
Bump RC, Mattiasson A, Ba K, et al. The standardization of terminology of female pelvic organ prolapse and pelvic floor dysfunction. *Am J Obstet Gynecol* 1996;175:10.
Bump RC, Norton PA. Epidemiology and natural history of pelvic floor dysfunction. *Obstet Gynecol Clin North Am* 1998;25:723.
Burch JC. Cooper's ligament urethrovesical suspension for stress incontinence. Nine years' experience—results, complications, techniques. *Am J Obstet Gynecol* 2002;187:512, discussion 513.
Clark AL, Gregory T, Smith VJ, et al. Epidemiologic evaluation of reoperation for surgically treated pelvic organ prolapse and urinary incontinence. *Am J Obstet Gynecol* 2003;189:1261.
Clayden CS. The evaluation of pelvic organ prolapse. *J Pelvic Med Surg* 2004;10:173.
Cunningham F, Gant N, Gilstrap L, et al. *Williams obstetrics*, 21st ed. New York: McGraw-Hill, 2001.
Danforth KN, Townsend MK, Lifford K, et al. Risk factors for urinary incontinence among middle-aged women. *Am J Obstet Gynecol* 2006;194:339.
Davis K, Kumar D, Stanton SL. Pelvic floor dysfunction: the need for a multidisciplinary team approach. *J Pelvic Med Surg* 2003;9:23.
DeLancey JO. Anatomy and biomechanics of genital prolapse. *Clin Obstet Gynecol* 1993;36:897.
DeLancey JO. Structural anatomy of the posterior pelvic compartment as it relates to rectocele. *Am J Obstet Gynecol* 1999;180:815.
Dietz HP, Lanzarone V. Levator trauma after vaginal delivery. *Obstet Gynecol* 2005;106:707.
Emge LA, Durfee RB. Pelvic organ prolapse: four thousand years of treatment. *Clin Obstet Gynecol* 1966;9:997.

VII

Francis CC. *The human pelvis.* St. Louis, MO: CV Mosby, 1952.

Gershenson DM, ed. Reconstructive pelvic surgery. *Operat Tech Gynecol Surg* 1996;1:2.

Ghetti C, Gregory WT, Edwards SR, et al. Pelvic organ descent and symptoms of pelvic floor disorders. *Am J Obstet Gynecol* 2005;193:53.

Grody MH. *Benign postreproductive gynecologic surgery.* New York: McGraw-Hill, 1995.

Grody MH, Nyirjesy P, Kelley LM, et al. Paraurethral fascial sling urethropexy and vaginal paravaginal defects cystopexy in the correction of urethrovesical prolapse. *Int Urogynecol J* 1995;6:80.

Handa VL, Garrett E, Hendrix S, et al. Progression and remission of pelvic organ prolapse: a longitudinal study of menopausal women. *Am J Obstet Gynecol* 2004;190:27.

Harris RL, Cundiff GW, Theofrastous JP, et al. The value of intraoperative cystoscopy in urogynecologic and reconstructive pelvic surgery. *Am J Obstet Gynecol* 1997;177:1367.

Hollinshead WH, Rosse C. *Textbook of anatomy,* 4th ed. Philadelphia, PA: Harper & Row, 1985.

Hoyte L, Schierlitz L, Zou K. Two- and 3-dimensional MRI comparison of levator ani structure, volume, and integrity in women with stress incontinence and prolapse. *Am J Obstet Gynecol* 2001;185:11.

Jenkins VR II. Uterosacral ligament fixation for vaginal vault suspension in uterine and vaginal vault prolapse. *Am J Obstet Gynecol* 1997;177: 1337.

Kegel AH. Physiologic therapy for urinary stress incontinence. *JAMA* 1952;10:915.

Kovac SR. Guidelines to determine the route of hysterectomy. *Obstet Gynecol* 1995;85:18.

Leffler KS, Thompson JR, Cundiff GW. Attachment of the rectovaginal septum to the pelvic sidewall. *Am J Obstet Gynecol* 2001;185:41.

Lien K-C, Mooney B, DeLancey JO, et al. Levator ani stretch induced by simulated vaginal birth. *Obstet Gynecol* 2004;103:31.

McCall ML. Posterior culdoplasty. *Obstet Gynecol* 1957;10:595.

Mengert WF. Mechanics of uterine support and position. *Am J Obstet Gynecol* 1936;31:775.

Mutone MF, Colin T, Hale DS, et al. Factors which influence the short-term success of pessary management of pelvic organ prolapse. *Am J Obstet Gynecol* 2005;193:89.

Nguyen JK, Lind LR, Choe JY, et al. Lumbosacral spine and pelvic inlet changes associated with pelvic organ prolapse. *Obstet Gynecol* 2000;95:332.

Nichols DH, Clarke-Pearson DL. *Gynecologic, obstetric, and related surgery,* 2nd ed. St. Louis, MO: CV Mosby, 2000.

Nichols DH, Milley PS. Surgical significance of the rectovaginal septum. *Am J Obstet Gynecol* 1970;108:215.

Nichols DH, Milley PS, Randall CL. Significance of restoration of normal vaginal depth and axis. *Obstet Gynecol* 1970;36:251.

Nichols DH, Randal CL. *Vaginal surgery,* 3rd ed. Baltimore, MD: Lippincott Williams & Wilkins, 1989.

Nichols DH, Randall CL. *Vaginal surgery,* 4th ed. Baltimore, MD: Williams & Wilkins, 1996.

Peham H, Amreich J. *Operative gynecology.* Philadelphia, PA: JB Lippincott, 1934.

Reiffenstuhl G, Platzer W, Knapstein P-G. *Vaginal operations: surgical anatomy and technique,* 2nd ed. Baltimore, MD: Williams & Wilkins, 1994.

Retzy SS, Rogers RM, Richardson AC. Anatomy of female pelvic support. In: Brubaker LT, Saclarides TJ, eds. *The female pelvic floor: Disorders of function and support.* Philadelphia, PA: FA Davis, 1996:3.

Richardson AC, Lyon JB, Williams NL. A new look at pelvic relaxation. *Am J Obstet Gynecol* 1976;126:568.

Shull B. Clinical evaluation and physical examination of the incontinent woman. *J Pelvic Med Surg* 2000;6:334.

Shull BL, Bachofen C, Coates KW, et al. A transvaginal approach to repair of apical and other associated sites of pelvic organ prolapse with uterosacral ligaments. *Am J Obstet Gynecol* 2000;183:1365.

Singh K, Reid WM, Berger LA. Magnetic resonance imaging of normal levator ani anatomy and function. *Obstet Gynecol* 2002;99:433.

Subak LL, Quesenberry CP, Posner SF, et al. The effect of behavioral therapy on urinary incontinence: a randomized controlled trial. *Obstet Gynecol* 2002;100:72.

Strohbehn K, Ellis JH, Strohbehn JA, et al. Magnetic resonance imaging of the levator ani with anatomic correlation. *Obstet Gynecol* 1996;87:277.

Swift S, Woodman P, O'Boyle A, et al. Pelvic organ support study (POSST): the distribution, clinical definition, and epidemiologic condition of pelvic organ support defects. *Am J Obstet Gynecol* 2005;192:795.

Sze EH, Karram MM. Transvaginal repair of vault prolapse: a review. *Obstet Gynecol* 1997;89:466.

Sze EH, Sherard GB, Dolezal JM. Pregnancy, labor, delivery, and pelvic organ prolapse. *Obstet Gynecol* 2002;100:981.

Te Linde RW. Prolapse of the uterus and allied conditions. *Am J Obstet Gynecol* 1966;94:444.

Toglia MR, DeLancey JO. Anal incontinence and the obstetrician-gynecologist. *Obstet Gynecol* 1994;84:731.

Tunn R, DeLancey JO, Quint EE. Visibility of pelvic organ support system structures in magnetic resonance images without an endovaginal coil. *Am J Obstet Gynecol* 2001;184:1156.

Uhlenhuth E. *Problems in the anatomy of the pelvis.* Philadelphia, PA: JB Lippincott, 1953.

Uhlenhuth E, Nolley GW. Vaginal fascia, a myth? *Obstet Gynecol* 1957;10:349.

Ulfelder H. The mechanism of pelvic support in women: deductions from a study of the comparative anatomy and physiology of the structures involved. *Am J Obstet Gynecol* 1956;72:856.

Umek WH, Morgan DM, Ashton-Miller JA. Quantitative analysis of uterosacral ligament origin and insertion points by magnetic resonance imaging. *Obstet Gynecol* 2004;103:447.

U.S. Food and Drug Administration. *Surgical placement of mesh to repair pelvic organ prolapse poses risks.* Available at: http://www.fda.gov/NewsEvents/Newsroom/PressAnnouncements [July 13, 2011].

Wall LL. Birth trauma and the pelvic floor: lessons from the developing world. *J Womens Health* 1999;8:149.

Weber AM, Richter HE. Pelvic organ prolapse. *Obstet Gynecol* 2005;106:615.

Whiteside JL, Weber AM, Meyn LA, et al. Risk factors for prolapse recurrence after vaginal repair. *Am J Obstet Gynecol* 2004; 191:1533.

Wu JM, Ward RM, Allen-Brady KL, et al. Phenotyping clinical disorders: lessons learned from pelvic organ prolapse. *Am J Obstet Gynecol* 2013;208:360.

CHAPTER 37
Reconstruction of the Anterior Vagina for Prolapse

Mark D. Walters and Matthew D. Barber

DEFINITIONS

Anterior vaginal wall prolapse—Descent of the anterior vaginal wall. Most commonly, this would be due to bladder prolapse (cystocele: either central, paravaginal, or a combination). Higher-stage anterior vaginal wall prolapse will generally involve uterine or vaginal vault (if uterus is absent) descent. Occasionally, there might be anterior enterocele (hernia of peritoneum and possibly abdominal contents) after prior reconstructive surgery.

Arcus tendineus fasciae pelvis—The white line of the pelvic sidewall. This thickening of the pelvic sidewall fascia extends from the ischial spine posteriorly to the pubic tubercle anteriorly. It is the site of lateral attachment of the pubocervical fascia.

Paravaginal defect—When the pubocervical fascia becomes detached from, or torn just medial to, its lateral attachment to the arcus tendineus fasciae pelvis (white line).

Pelvic organ prolapse—The descent of one or more of the anterior vaginal wall, posterior vaginal wall, the uterus (cervix), or the apex of the vagina (vaginal vault or cuff scar after hysterectomy). The presence of any such sign should be correlated with relevant prolapse symptoms. More commonly, this correlation would occur at the level of the hymen or beyond.

Pubocervical fascia—A trapezoid-shaped fascia that provides support for the anterior vagina under the bladder. It is attached superiorly to the pericervical ring, distally to the pubic ramus, and laterally to the arcus tendineus fasciae pelvis (white line).

Anterior vaginal wall prolapse occurs commonly and may coexist with disorders of micturition. Mild anterior vaginal prolapse often occurs in parous women but usually presents few problems. As the prolapse progresses, symptoms may develop and worsen, and treatment becomes indicated. The anterior vaginal wall is the most common segment of the vagina to prolapse and the segment that is most likely to fail long term after surgical correction. This chapter reviews the anatomy and pathology of anterior vaginal wall prolapse, with and without stress incontinence, and describes methods of surgical repair.

TERMINOLOGY

Anterior vaginal wall prolapse (cystocele) is defined as pathologic descent of the anterior vaginal wall and overlying bladder base. According to the International Continence Society (ICS) standardized terminology for prolapse grading, the term "anterior vaginal prolapse" is preferred to "cystocele." This is because information obtained at the physical examination does not allow the exact identification of structures behind the anterior vaginal wall, although it usually is, in fact, the bladder. A more recent joint report on terminology by the International Urogynecological Association (IUGA) and International Continence Society (ICS) states that anterior vaginal wall prolapse is most commonly due to bladder prolapse (cystocele: either central, paravaginal, or a combination). Higher stage of anterior vaginal prolapse generally involves some amount of uterine or vaginal apex descent. Rare anterior enteroceles can also be found. Most gynecologists are generally comfortable with the terms cystocele, rectocele, vaginal vault prolapse, and enterocele. Coupled with the brevity of these terms and their clinical usage for up to 200 years, the inclusion of these terms is appropriate.

Some regard it as important to surgical strategy to differentiate between a central cystocele (central defect with loss of rugae due to stretching of the pubocervical and subvesical connective tissue and the vaginal wall) and a paravaginal defect (rugae preserved due to detachment of the lateral vagina from the arcus tendineus fasciae pelvis). Surgical procedures for each of these types of anterior vaginal wall prolapse are presented, although data specifically addressing the comparative efficacy of these various repairs are scarce.

ANATOMY AND PATHOLOGY

The etiology of anterior vaginal wall prolapse is not completely understood, but it is probably multifactorial, with different factors implicated in prolapse in individual patients. Normal support for the vagina and adjacent pelvic organs is provided by the interaction of the pelvic muscles and connective tissue. The upper vagina rests on the levator plate and is stabilized by superior and lateral connective tissue attachments. The midvagina is attached to the arcus tendineus fasciae pelvis (ATFP; white lines) on each side, and the apical portion of the anterior vagina is attached to the web of the endopelvic fascia, including pubocervical fascia, and the cardinal and uterosacral ligaments. Pathologic loss of lateral and/or apical support may occur with damage to or impairment of the pelvic muscles, connective tissue attachments, or both.

Nichols and Randall described two types of anterior vaginal prolapse: distension and displacement. Distension was thought to result from overstretching and attenuation of the anterior vaginal wall, caused by overdistention of the vagina associated with vaginal delivery or atrophic changes associated with aging and menopause. The distinguishing physical feature of this type was described as diminished or absent rugal folds of the anterior vaginal epithelium caused by thinning or loss of midline vaginal fascia. The other type of anterior vaginal prolapse—displacement—was attributed to pathologic detachment or elongation of the anterolateral vaginal supports to the ATFP. It may occur unilaterally or bilaterally and often coexists with some degree of distension cystocele, with urethral hypermobility, or with apical prolapse. Rugal folds may or may not be preserved.

Another theory ascribes most cases of anterior vaginal prolapse to disruption or detachment of the lateral connective tissue attachments at the ATFP, resulting in a paravaginal fascial defect and corresponding to the displacement type discussed earlier. This was first described by White in 1909 and 1912, but disregarded until reported by Richardson in 1976. Richardson also described transverse defects, midline defects, and defects involving isolated loss of integrity of pubourethral ligaments. Transverse defects were said to occur when the pubocervical fascia separated from its insertion around the cervix, whereas midline defects represented an anteroposterior separation of the fascia between the bladder and the vagina. A contemporary conceptual representation of vaginal and paravaginal defects is shown in **Figure 37.1**.

There have been few systematic or comprehensive descriptions of anterior vaginal prolapse based on physical findings and correlated with findings at surgery to provide objective evidence for any of these theories of pathologic anatomy. In a study of 71 women with anterior vaginal wall prolapse and stress incontinence who underwent retropubic operations, DeLancey described paravaginal defects in 87% on the left and 89% on the right. The ATFP were usually attached to the pubic bone but detached from the ischial spine for a variable distance. The pubococcygeal muscle was visibly abnormal with localized or generalized atrophy in over half of the women.

Improvements in pelvic imaging are leading to a greater understanding of normal pelvic anatomy and the structural and functional abnormalities associated with prolapse. Magnetic resonance imaging (MRI) holds great promise, with its excellent ability to differentiate soft tissues and its capacity for multiplanar imaging. The pelvic organs, pelvic muscles, and connective tissues can be identified easily with MRI. Various measurements can be made that may be associated with anterior vaginal prolapse or urinary incontinence, such as the urethrovesical angle, descent of the bladder base, quality of the levator muscles, and the relationship between the vagina and its lateral and apical connective tissue attachments. Aronson et al. used an endoluminal surface coil placed in the vagina to image pelvic anatomy with MRI and compared four continent nulliparous women with four incontinent women with anterior vaginal prolapse. Lateral vaginal attachments were identified in all continent women. In **Figure 37.2**, the "posterior pubourethral ligaments" (bilateral attachment of ATFP to posterior aspect of the pubic symphysis) are clearly seen. In the two subjects with clinically apparent paravaginal defects, lateral detachments were evident (**Fig. 37.3**). More recent studies

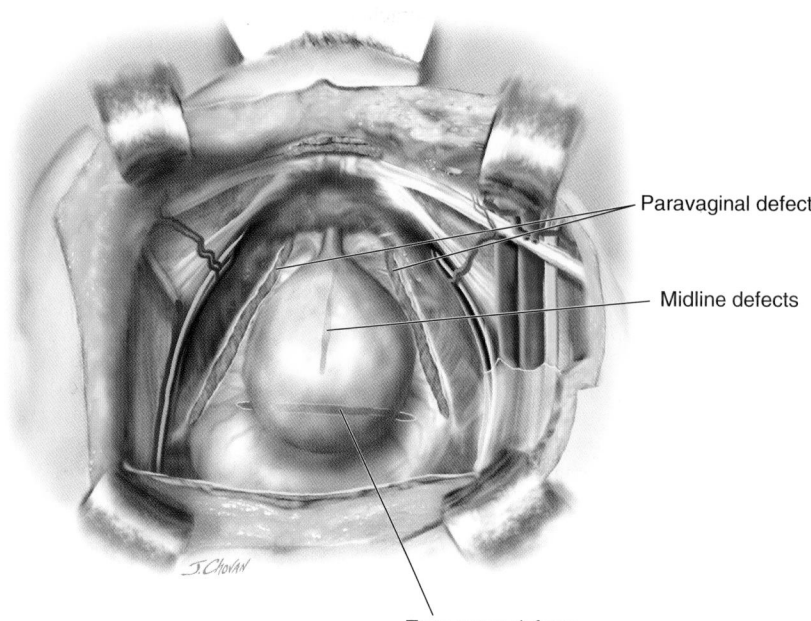

Paravaginal defects

Midline defects

Transverse defects

FIGURE 37.1 Three different defects can result in anterior vaginal wall prolapse. Lateral or paravaginal defects occur when there is a separation of the pubocervical fascia from the ATFP, midline defects occur secondary to attenuation of fascia supporting the bladder base, and transverse defects occur when the pubocervical fascia separates from the vaginal cuff or uterosacral ligaments and represents paravaginal, midline, and transverse defects. (Reprinted from Karram MM. *Surgical management of pelvic organ prolapse*. Philadelphia, PA: Elsevier/Saunders, 2013, with permission. Copyright 2013 Saunders, an Inprint of Elsevier, Inc.)

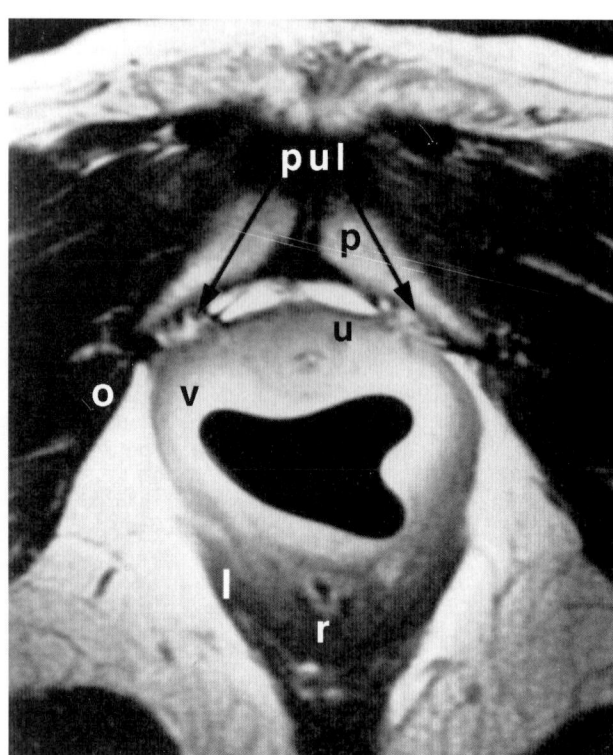

FIGURE 37.2 Axial T$_1$-weighted image from a continent 38-year-old nulliparous woman, showing the connection of the anterior vaginal wall (v) to the posterior pubic symphysis (p) by the pubourethral ligaments (pul). The anterior vaginal wall and endopelvic fascia function as a sling or hammock for support of the urethra (u). (o, obturator internus muscle; r, rectum; l, levator ani musculature.) (Reprinted from Aronson MP, Bates SM, Jacoby AF, et al. Periurethral and paravaginal anatomy: an endovaginal magnetic resonance imagining study. *Am J Obstet Gynecol* 1995;173:1702, with permission. Copyright © 1995, Elsevier.)

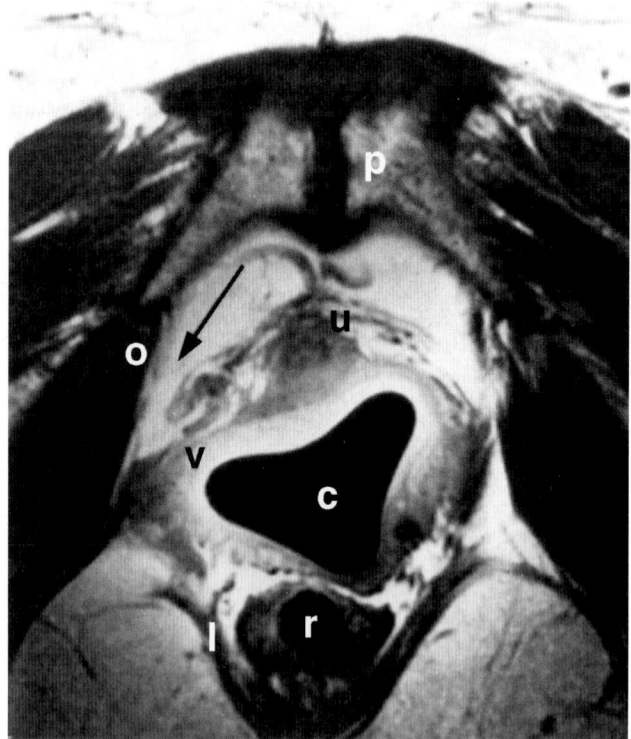

FIGURE 37.3 Axial T$_1$-weighted image from a 57-year-old woman, para 5, with stress urinary incontinence. The paravaginal detachment (*arrow*) is seen at the level of the urethrovesical junction. (v, anterior vaginal wall; p, posterior pubic symphysis; u, urethra; o, obturator internus muscle; c, endovaginal coil; r, rectum; l, levator ani musculature.) (Reprinted from Aronson MP, Bates SM, Jacoby AF, et al. Periurethral and paravaginal anatomy: an endovaginal magnetic resonance imagining study. *Am J Obstet Gynecol* 1995;173:1702, with permission. Copyright © 1995, Elsevier.)

based on MRI analysis and computer modeling suggest that apical support abnormalities are at least as important as, if not more important than, paravaginal defects; the degree of apical decent can explain about half of anterior wall descent. Other factors, such as levator muscle impairment, levator avulsion, greater anterior wall length, and widened levator hiatus, also contribute to anterior vaginal prolapse.

Anterior vaginal prolapse commonly coexists with stress urinary incontinence (SUI). Some features of pathophysiology may overlap, such as loss of anterior vaginal support with bladder-base descent and urethral hypermobility; other features, such as sphincteric dysfunction, may occur independent of vaginal and urethral support. The pathophysiology and surgical treatments of stress incontinence are covered more fully in Chapter 41.

EVALUATION

History

When evaluating women with pelvic organ prolapse or urinary or fecal incontinence, attention should be paid to all aspects of pelvic organ support. The reconstructive surgeon must determine the specific sites of damage for each patient, with the ultimate goal of restoring both anatomy and function.

Patients with anterior vaginal prolapse complain of symptoms directly related to vaginal protrusion or of associated symptoms such as urinary incontinence or voiding difficulty. Symptoms related to prolapse may include the sensation of a vaginal mass or bulge, pelvic pressure, low back pain, and sexual difficulty. SUI commonly occurs in association with anterior vaginal prolapse, particularly when it is mild. In contrast, women with anterior vaginal prolapse that extends beyond the hymen are less likely to complain of stress incontinence and more likely to have obstructed voiding symptoms such as urinary hesitancy, intermittent flow, weak or prolonged stream, feeling of incomplete emptying, the need to manually reduce (splint) the prolapse to initiate or complete urination, and, in rare cases, urinary retention. The mechanism for this appears to be mechanical obstruction resulting from urethral kinking that occurs with progressively worsening anterior vaginal prolapse.

Physical Examination

The physical examination should be conducted with the patient in the lithotomy position, as for a routine pelvic examination. The examination is first performed with the patient supine. If physical findings do not correspond to symptoms or if the maximum extent of the prolapse cannot be confirmed, the woman is reexamined in the standing position.

The genitalia are inspected, and if no displacement is apparent, the labia are gently spread to expose the vestibule and hymen. The integrity of the perineal body is evaluated, and the approximate size of all prolapsed parts is assessed. A retractor or Sims speculum can be used to depress the posterior vagina to aid in visualizing the anterior vagina. After the resting examination, the patient is instructed to strain down forcefully or to cough vigorously. During this maneuver, the order of descent of the pelvic organs is noted, as is the relationship of the pelvic organs at the peak of straining.

It may be possible to differentiate lateral defects, identified as detachment or effacement of the lateral vaginal sulci, from central defects, seen as midline protrusion but with preservation of the lateral sulci, by using a pair of curved forceps placed in the anterolateral vaginal sulci directed toward

the ischial spine. Bulging of the anterior vaginal wall in the midline between the forceps blades implies a midline defect; blunting or descent of the vaginal fornices on either side with straining suggests lateral paravaginal defects. Studies have shown that the physical examination technique to detect paravaginal defects is not particularly reliable or accurate. In a study by Barber et al. of 117 women with prolapse, the sensitivity of clinical examination to detect paravaginal defects was good (92%), yet the specificity was poor (52%); despite an unexpectedly high prevalence of paravaginal defects, the positive predictive value was poor (61%). Less than two thirds of women believed to have a paravaginal defect on physical examination were confirmed to possess the same at surgery. Another study by Whiteside et al. demonstrated poor reproducibility of clinical examination in detecting specific anterior vaginal wall defects. Thus, the clinical value of determining the location of midline, apical, and lateral paravaginal defects remains unknown.

Anterior vaginal wall descent usually represents bladder descent with or without concomitant urethral hypermobility. In 1.6% of women with anterior vaginal prolapse, an anterior enterocele mimics a cystocele on physical examination (Tulikangas et al., 2004). Other uncommon conditions, such as anterior vaginal cysts or myomas, can also mimic anterior vaginal prolapse.

Diagnostic Tests

After a careful history and physical examination, a few diagnostic tests are needed to evaluate patients with anterior vaginal prolapse. A urinalysis should be performed to evaluate for urinary tract infection if the patient complains of any lower urinary tract dysfunction. Hydronephrosis occurs in a small proportion of women with severe prolapse; however, even if identified, it usually does not change management in women for whom surgical repair is planned. Therefore, routine imaging of the kidneys and ureters is not necessary.

If urinary incontinence is present, further diagnostic testing is indicated to determine the cause of the incontinence. Urodynamic (simple or complex), endoscopic, or radiologic assessments of filling and voiding function are generally indicated only when symptoms of incontinence or voiding dysfunction are present. Even if no urologic symptoms are noted, voiding function should be assessed to evaluate for completeness of bladder emptying. This procedure usually involves a timed, measured void, followed by urethral catheterization or bladder ultrasound to measure postvoid residual urine volume.

In women with severe prolapse, it is important to check urethral function after the prolapse is repositioned. Women with severe prolapse may be paradoxically continent because of urethral kinking; when the prolapse is reduced, urethral dysfunction may be unmasked with occurrence of incontinence (occult stress incontinence). A pessary, vaginal retractor, or vaginal packing can be used to reduce the prolapse before office bladder filling or electronic urodynamic testing. If urinary leaking occurs with coughing or Valsalva maneuvers after reduction of the prolapse, the urethral sphincter may be incompetent, even if the patient is normally continent. This is reported to occur in 17% to 69% of women with stage III or IV prolapse. In this situation, the surgeon should choose an antiincontinence procedure in conjunction with anterior vaginal prolapse repair. If stress incontinence is not present even after reduction of the prolapse, an antiincontinence procedure probably is not indicated, although this is a subject of ongoing research.

VII

SURGICAL REPAIR TECHNIQUES

General Considerations

The transvaginal operative procedures begin with the patient supine, with the legs elevated and abducted in stirrups and the buttocks placed just past the edge of the operating table. Antibiotics should be given within 60 minutes of incision to achieve minimal inhibitory concentrations in the skin and tissues by the time the incision is made. This typically means a first-generation cephalosporin (cefazolin) or combination regimens (500-mg metronidazole and 400-mg ciprofloxacin) if the patient has an allergy to penicillin. In general, all patients undergoing apical prolapse surgery are at moderate risk for thromboembolic events and require a prevention strategy. Low-dose unfractionated heparin (5,000 units every 12 hours) or low molecular weight heparins (e.g., 40-mg enoxaparin or 2,500 units of dalteparin), an intermittent pneumatic compression device, or a combination of these are recommended. Either form of heparin should be started 2 hours before surgery and the compression stockings placed on the patient in the operating room before incision. These treatment approaches should be continued until the patient is ambulatory.

Paravaginal Defect Repair: Transvaginal Approach

The aim of paravaginal defect repair for anterior vaginal prolapse is to reattach the detached lateral vagina to its normal place of attachment at the level of the ATFP. This can be accomplished using a vaginal or open or laparoscopic retropubic approach.

The preparation for vaginal paravaginal repair and for anterior colporrhaphy is similar. The abdomen, vagina, and perineum are sterilely prepped and draped, and a 16-French Foley catheter with a 10-mL balloon is inserted for easy identification of the bladder neck. A weighted speculum is placed into the vagina. Hemostatic solution (such as 0.5% lidocaine with 1:200,000 epinephrine) or saline may be injected below the epithelium along the midline of the anterior vaginal wall to decrease bleeding and to aid in dissection. If a vaginal hysterectomy has been performed, the incised apex of the anterior vaginal wall is grasped transversely with two Allis clamps and elevated. Otherwise, a transverse or diamond-shaped incision may be made in the vaginal epithelium near the apex. A third Allis clamp is placed about 2 cm below the posterior margin of the urethral meatus and pulled up. If a midurethral sling is to be done, then the incision is only made to the bladder neck. Additional Allis clamps may be placed in the midline between the urethra and the apex.

Marking sutures are placed on the anterior vaginal wall on each side of the urethrovesical junction, identified by the location of the Foley balloon after gentle traction is placed on the catheter. In patients who have had a hysterectomy, marking sutures are also placed at the vaginal apex. If a culdoplasty or apical suspension procedure is being performed, the stitches are placed but not tied until completion of the paravaginal repair and closure of the anterior vaginal wall. As for anterior colporrhaphy, vaginal flaps are developed by incising the vagina in the midline and dissecting the vaginal muscularis laterally. The dissection is performed bilaterally until a space—the paravaginal space—is developed between the vaginal wall and obturator internus muscle. Blunt dissection using the surgeon's index finger is used to extend the space anteriorly along the ischiopubic rami, medially to the pubic symphysis, and laterally toward the ischial spine. If the defect is present and dissection is occurring in the appropriate

plane, one should easily enter the retropubic space, visualizing retropubic and paravaginal adipose tissue. The ischial spine then can be palpated on each side. The ATFP coming off the spine can be followed to the back of the symphysis pubis (Fig. 37.4B). After dissection is complete, midline plication of the bladder adventitia is usually performed, either at this point or after placement and tying of the paravaginal sutures.

On the lateral pelvic sidewall, the obturator internus muscle and the ATFP are identified by palpation and then visualization. Retraction of the bladder and urethra medially is best accomplished with a Breisky-Navratil retractor, and posterior retraction could be provided with a lighted right-angle retractor. Using No. 0 nonabsorbable or delayed absorbable suture on a CT-2 needle, the first stitch is placed around the tissue of the white line just anterior to the ischial spine. Alternatively, a Capio device (Boston Scientific, Natick, MA) works well to facilitate suture placement. If the white line is detached from the pelvic sidewall or clinically not felt to be durable, then the attachment should be to the fascia overlying the obturator internus muscle. The placement of subsequent sutures is aided by placing tension on the first suture. A series of three to six stitches are placed and held, working anteriorly along the white line from the ischial spine to the level of the urethrovesical junction (Fig. 37.4A). Starting with the most anterior stitch, the surgeon picks up the edge of the periurethral tissue (vaginal muscularis or pubocervical fascia) at the level of the urethrovesical junction and then the tissue from the undersurface of the vaginal flap at the previously marked sites. Subsequent stitches move posteriorly until the last stitch closest to the ischial spine is attached to the vagina nearest the apex, again using the previously placed marking sutures for guidance. Stitches in the vaginal wall must be placed carefully to allow adequate tissue for subsequent midline vaginal closure. After all the stitches are placed on one side, the same procedure is carried out on the other side. The stitches are then tied in order from the urethra to the apex, alternating from one side to the other. This repair is a three-point closure involving the vaginal epithelium, vaginal muscularis and endopelvic fascia (pubocervical fascia), and lateral pelvic sidewall at the ATFP (Fig. 37.4B, C). There must be tissue-to-tissue approximation between these structures. Suture bridges must be avoided by careful planning of suture placement. Vaginal tissue should not be trimmed until all the stitches are tied. The vaginal flaps are trimmed and closed with a running subcuticular or interlocking delayed absorbable suture.

Paravaginal Defect Repair: Retropubic Approach

The object of the retropubic paravaginal defect repair is to reattach, bilaterally, the anterolateral vaginal sulcus with its overlying endopelvic fascia to the pubococcygeus and obturator internus muscles and fascia at the level of the ATFP. The retropubic space is entered laparoscopically or through a small, low transverse incision, and the bladder and vagina are depressed and pulled medially to allow visualization of the lateral retropubic space, including the obturator internus and levator muscles, and the fossa containing the obturator neurovascular bundle. Blunt dissection can be carried dorsally from this point until the ischial spine is palpated. The ATFP is often visualized as a white band of tissue running over the pubococcygeus and obturator internus muscles from the back of the lower edge of the symphysis pubis toward the ischial spine. A lateral paravaginal defect representing avulsion of the vagina

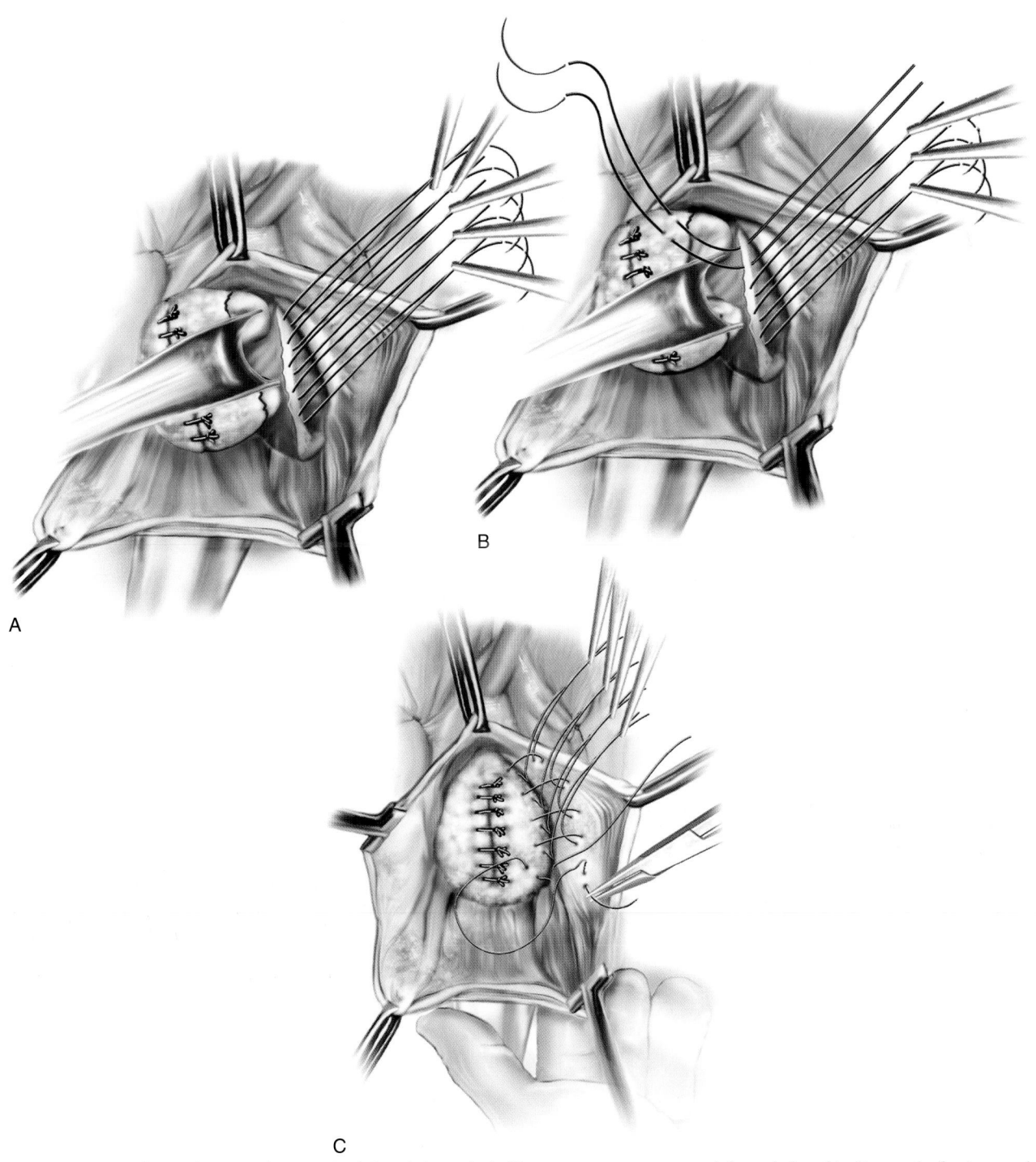

FIGURE 37.4 Surgical steps for vaginal paravaginal (3-point) repair. **A:** Numerous sutures are passed through the white line on the fascia over the obturator internus muscle (point 1). **B:** Each suture is passed through the lateral edge of the detached fascia (point 2). **C:** Each suture is passed through the full thickness of the vaginal wall excluding the epithelium (point 3). (Reprinted from Karram MM. *Surgical management of pelvic organ prolapse*. Philadelphia, PA: Elsevier/Saunders, 2013, with permission. Copyright 2013 Saunders, an Inprint of Elsevier, Inc.)

off the ATFP or of the ATFP off the obturator internus muscle may be visualized (Fig. 37.5).

The surgeon's nondominant hand is inserted into the vagina. While gently retracting the vagina and bladder medially, the surgeon elevates the anterolateral vaginal sulcus. Starting near the vaginal apex, a suture is placed, first through the full thickness of the vagina (excluding the vaginal epithelium) and then

deep into the obturator internus fascia or ATFP, 1 to 2 cm anterior to its origin at the ischial spine. After this first stitch is tied, additional (three to five) sutures are placed through the vaginal wall and overlying fascia and then into the obturator internus at about 1-cm intervals toward the pubic ramus (Fig. 37.5). The most distal sutures should be placed as close as possible to the pubic ramus, into the pubourethral ligament; alternatively,

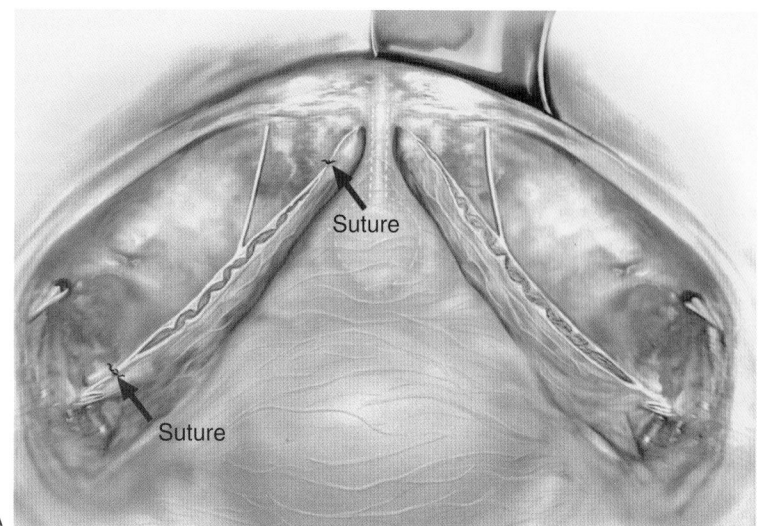

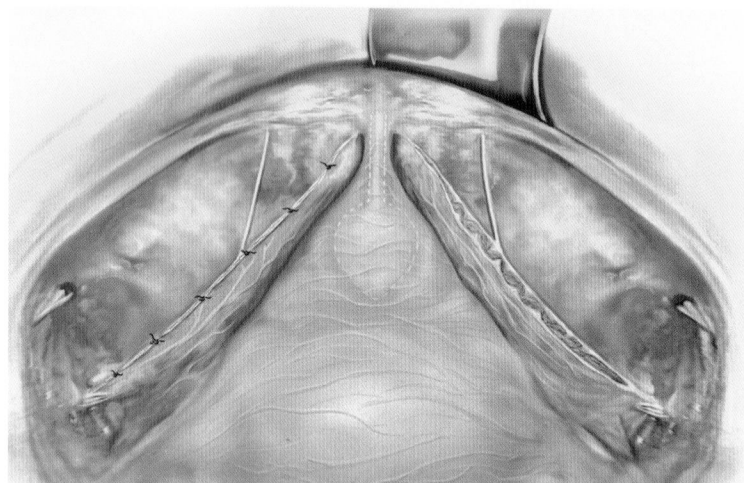

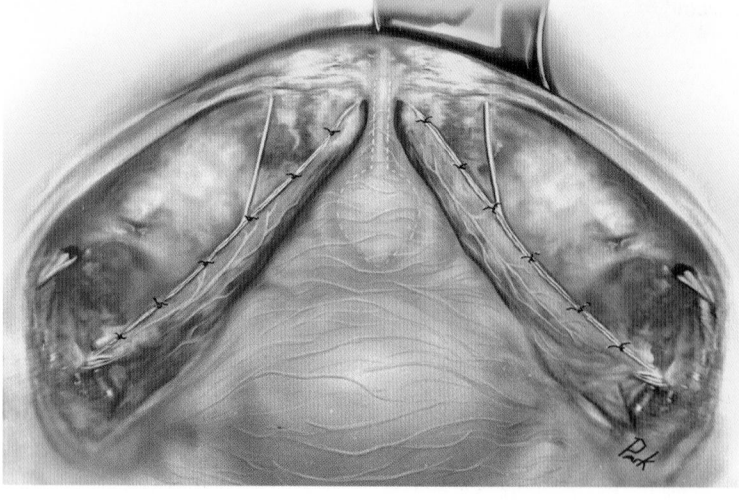

FIGURE 37.5 Abdominal paravaginal defect repair reattaches the pubocervical fascia to the white lines bilaterally. **A:** A patient with bilateral paravaginal defects. The repair has been started on the left with sutures at the two extremes of the defect. **B:** The repair is complete on the left side. **C:** Both sides are repaired. (Reprinted from Shull BL. How I do abdominal paravaginal repair. *J Pelvic Surg* 1995;1:43, with permission. Copyright © 1995 Wolters Kluwer Health.)

Burch colposuspension sutures can be placed bilaterally at the level of the bladder neck and urethra if the patient has stress incontinence. No. 2-0 or 0 nonabsorbable suture on a medium-sized, tapered needle usually is used for the paravaginal repair.

This procedure leaves free space between the symphysis pubis and the proximal urethra but secure support so that rotational descent of the proximal urethra and bladder base is prevented with sudden increases in intra-abdominal pressure. According to Turner-Warwick, it avoids overcorrection and fixation of the periurethral fascia, which might compromise the functional movements of the urethra and bladder base and lead to obstruction and voiding difficulty. This principle may explain why the paravaginal defect repair usually results in spontaneous voiding on the first or second postoperative day.

Anterior Colporrhaphy

The objective of anterior colporrhaphy is to plicate the layers of vaginal muscularis and adventitia overlying the bladder ("pubocervical fascia") or to plicate and reattach the paravaginal tissue in such a way as to reduce the central protrusion of the bladder and vagina. Modifications of the technique depend on how lateral the dissection is carried, where the plicating sutures are placed, and whether additional layers (natural or synthetic grafts) are placed in the anterior vagina for extra support.

Operative setup and preparation are as for a vaginal paravaginal defect repair. A scalpel is used to open the anterior wall in the midline (Fig. 37.6A). Alternatively, the points of a pair of curved Mayo scissors are inserted between the vaginal epithelium and the vaginal muscularis, or between the layers of the vaginal muscularis, and gently forced upward while being kept half-opened/half-closed (Fig. 37.6B). Countertraction during this maneuver is important to minimize the likelihood of perforation of the bladder. The vagina is incised in the midline, and the incision is continued to the level of the midurethra (or bladder neck if a sling is being done). As the vagina is incised, the edges are grasped with Allis or T-clamps and drawn laterally for further mobilization. Dissection of the vaginal flaps is then accomplished by turning the clamps back across the forefinger and incising the vaginal muscularis with a scalpel or Metzenbaum scissors, as shown in Figure 37.6C. An assistant maintains constant traction medially on the remaining vaginal muscularis and underlying

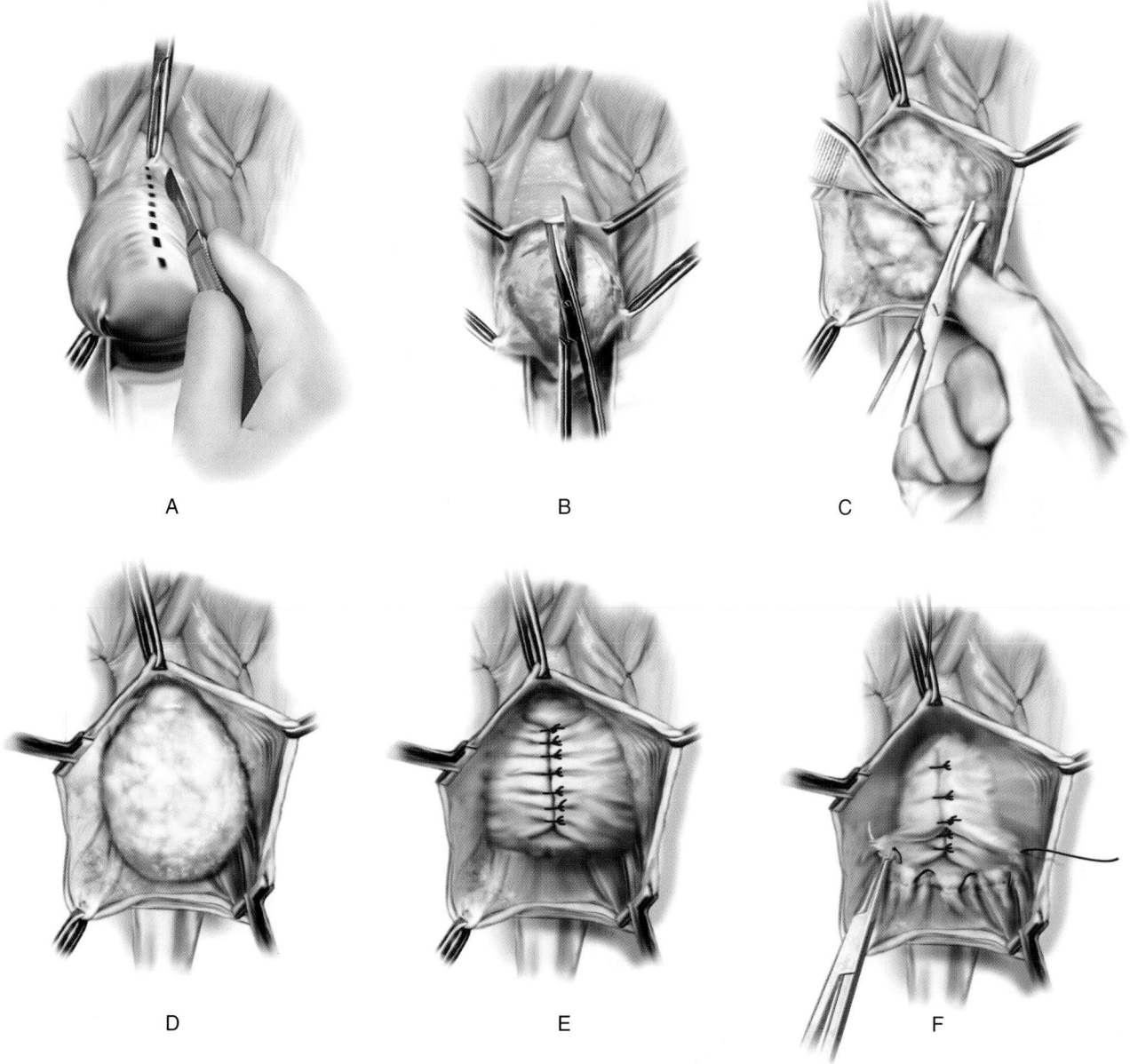

FIGURE 37.6 Classic anterior colporrhaphy. **A:** Initial midline anterior vaginal wall incision is demonstrated. **B:** The midline incision is extended using scissors. **C:** Sharp dissection of the bladder off the vaginal wall should be lateral to the superior pubic ramus, and the base of the bladder should be dissected off the vaginal cuff or cervix to the level of the preperitoneal space of the anterior cul-de-sac. **D:** The bladder has been completely mobilized off the vagina. **E:** Initial plication layer is placed. **F:** Second plication layer is placed, which commonly requires further mobilization of vaginal muscularis off of the vaginal epithelium. The most proximal stitch involves plication of the inside of the vaginal wall at the level of the vaginal apex or upper portion of the cervix.

VII

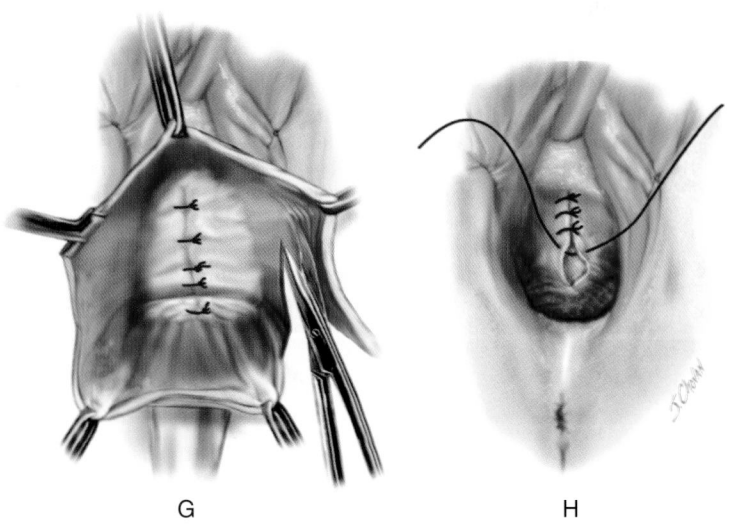

G   H

FIGURE 37.6 (*Continued*) **G:** The completed second plication layer and the trimming of excess vaginal mucosa are demonstrated. **H:** Closure of vaginal mucosa is demonstrated. (Reprinted from Karram MM. *Surgical management of pelvic organ prolapse.* Philadelphia, PA: Elsevier/Saunders, 2013, with permission. Copyright 2013 Saunders, an Inprint of Elsevier, Inc.)

vesicovaginal adventitia. This procedure is performed bilaterally until the entire extent of the anterior vaginal prolapse has been dissected; in general, the dissection should be carried further laterally with more advanced prolapse (**Fig. 37.6D**). The spaces lateral to the urethrovesical junction are sharply dissected toward the ischiopubic rami. It is also important to use sharp dissection to mobilize the bladder base from the vaginal apex, if necessary.

Some surgeons routinely perform a bladder neck plication (Kelly-Kennedy plication; **Fig. 37.7**) at the time of anterior colporrhaphy, particularly when a concurrent midurethral sling is not planned. Vesical neck plication was used to treat mild SUI in the past, but is no longer done for that indication. It may, however, help to prevent the later development of de novo stress incontinence in the patient. Once the vaginal flaps have been completely developed, the urethrovesical junction can be identified visually or by pulling the Foley catheter downward until the bulb obstructs the vesical neck. Repair should begin at the urethrovesical junction, using No. 2-0 or 0 delayed absorbable suture. The first plicating stitch is placed into the periurethral endopelvic fascia and tied. One or two additional stitches are placed to support the length of the urethra and urethrovesical junction.

In a standard anterior colporrhaphy, stitches using No. 2-0 or 0 delayed absorbable sutures are placed in the vaginal tissue (muscularis and adventitia) medial to the vaginal flaps and plicated in the midline without excessive tension. Depending on the severity of the prolapse, one or two rows of plication sutures or a purse-string suture followed by plication sutures are placed (**Fig. 37.6E–G**). Excess vaginal epithelium is then trimmed from the flaps bilaterally, and the remaining anterior vaginal wall is closed with a running No. 2-0 subcuticular or locking suture (**Fig. 37.6H**).

Anti-incontinence operations are often performed at the same time as anterior vaginal prolapse repair to treat coexistent or occult stress incontinence. More advanced anterior vaginal prolapse often also has anterior–apical prolapse and requires a concurrent colpopexy procedure. Surgical judgment is required to perform the bladder plication tightly enough to reduce the anterior vaginal prolapse sufficiently, yet preserve some mobility of the anterior vagina. If anterior colporrhaphy is combined with a sling procedure (midurethral or bladder neck), the cystocele should be repaired before the final tension is set for the sling. A midurethral sling, such as a tension-free vaginal tape or transobturator sling, is best done through a separate midurethral incision after the cystocele repair is complete.

Anterior Prolapse Repair with Grafts

A prosthetic material can be used to provide support in the anterior vagina, but this remains controversial. This can be done in a number of ways, and the surgical techniques continue to evolve. Graft materials may include synthetic absorbable grafts (e.g., polyglactin 910 mesh), synthetic permanent meshes (e.g., polypropylene), and biologic materials. Biologic materials that have been used include autografts of harvested rectus fascia and fascia lata, human allografts including fascia lata and dura mater, and xenografts such as porcine dermis, porcine small intestinal submucosa, and bovine pericardium. In 2010, approximately 25% of surgeries for pelvic organ prolapse in the United States included transvaginal placement of biologic or synthetic mesh, but this rate of use has decreased in recent years. Many surgeons use transvaginal graft placement in an attempt to increase the efficacy and durability of their surgical repair. For anterior prolapse, studies have demonstrated improved anatomic outcomes after transvaginal placement of permanent synthetic mesh when compared to anterior colporrhaphy without mesh ("native tissue repair"). However, this comes at the expense of an increased rate of complications unique to synthetic mesh placement including vaginal mesh exposure or extrusion, mesh erosion or perforation into an adjacent organ (bladder, urethra, or rectum), and vaginal mesh tension or contraction with associated pain and dyspareunia. Concerns over increased adverse events from transvaginal mesh placement led to two separate FDA notifications. In October 2008, the FDA issued a Public Health Notification (PHN) to inform clinicians and patients of adverse events related to urogynecologic use of surgical mesh and to provide recommendations on how to mitigate risks and counsel patients. In July 2011, the FDA provided an updated PHN on urogynecologic surgical mesh and reported that the complications of mesh used transvaginally are not rare.

When considering the use of transvaginal mesh for anterior prolapse, surgeons and patients must balance improved anatomic support of the anterior vaginal wall against the cost of the devices and increased complications such as mesh erosion, exposure, or extrusion; pelvic pain; groin pain; and dyspareunia. In a joint Committee Opinion published in December 2011, the American Urogynecologic Society and the American Congress of Obstetricians and Gynecologists recommended that pelvic organ prolapse vaginal mesh repair should

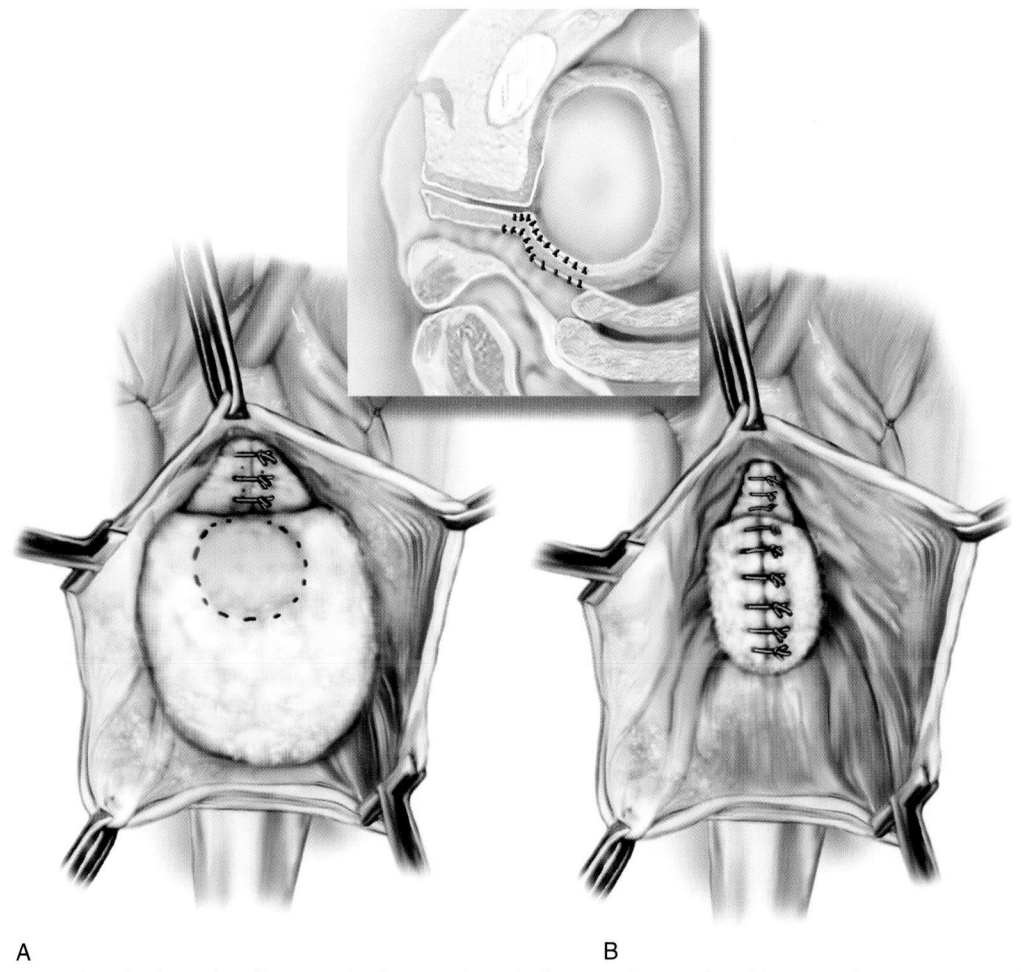

A   B

FIGURE 37.7 Anterior colporrhaphy with Kelly-Kennedy plication: **A:** Vaginal mucosa is opened, and interrupted sutures are started under the urethra; **B:** Completed colporrhaphy uses midline plication with interrupted sutures. Preferential support is provided to the proximal urethra over that provided to the bladder. (Reprinted from Karram MM. *Surgical management of pelvic organ prolapse.* Philadelphia, PA: Elsevier/Saunders, 2013, with permission. Copyright 2013 Saunders, an Inprint of Elsevier, Inc.)

be reserved for high-risk individuals in whom the benefit of mesh placement may justify the risk, such as individuals with recurrent anterior prolapse or with medical comorbidities that preclude more invasive and lengthier open and endoscopic procedures. They also noted that surgeons placing vaginal mesh should undergo training specific to each device and have experience with reconstructive surgical procedures and a thorough understanding of pelvic anatomy.

Prior to considering treating anterior vaginal prolapse with graft or mesh, patients should undergo a thorough informed consent process including discussion of risks, benefits, and both surgical and nonsurgical alternative treatments. There are several situations where mesh use is contraindicated. Many surgeons would not consider the use of mesh in a patient who has had a previous mesh complication. Mesh augmentations should not be used in pregnant women or women who are contemplating future pregnancy, as the mesh does not stretch significantly as the patient grows. In patients who have had pelvic radiation, mesh placement is not recommended because of the risk of poor wound healing. Similarly, preexisting local or systemic infection is a contraindication for vaginal mesh placement, particularly nonabsorbable synthetic mesh. Many surgeons would not recommend the use of nonabsorbable synthetic mesh if colorectal surgery is being performed concurrently. Chronic steroid use, smoking, uncontrolled diabetes

mellitus, or other causes of a compromised immune system can impair wound healing, and many would consider these conditions to be relative contraindications to vaginal mesh placement. Pelvic pain syndromes such as endometriosis, vulvodynia, interstitial cystitis, fibromyalgia, and dyspareunia should be evaluated preoperatively to allow for comprehensive counseling as to the best surgical and nonsurgical form of treatment.

Currently, there are three general categories of transvaginal mesh or graft placement options for the management of anterior vaginal prolapse: (a) self-tailored mesh, (b) commercially available trocar-guided mesh kits that use a transobturator approach, and (c) commercially available mesh kits that use a transvaginal fixation method rather than a trocar (nontrocar kits). No matter what placement option is used, the general surgical approach to treat anterior vaginal wall prolapse is fixation of mesh to the ATFP or the coccygeus muscle. The initial incision for anterior vaginal mesh placement usually involves significant hydrodissection and a deeper colpotomy incision than usually performed for a traditional native tissue anterior colporrhaphy so that the perivesical space is entered. The mesh is spread laterally toward the ATFP proximally and distally and, in many of the newer nontrocar kits, attached apically to the sacrospinous ligament. Despite the lack of evidence that any one placement technique is best in managing a

VII

patient's symptoms, most experts would agree on some basic perioperative tenets:

- The bladder should be drained with a transurethral catheter.
- A well-estrogenized vaginal wall is preferred prior to surgery. (We use intravaginal estrogen cream daily [0.5 to 1.0 g/day] for 2 to 3 weeks preoperatively if the patient is eligible and willing to use estrogen.) A vaginal pessary should be removed 1 to 2 weeks prior to surgery to limit vaginal epithelium irritation.
- All patients require perioperative prophylactic antibiotics and efforts to prevent venous thromboembolic events, as noted earlier.
- Avoid making inverted "T-shaped" incisions from a concurrent hysterectomy and colporrhaphy, if possible.
- Exposure of the correct vesicovaginal space is performed with hydrodissection of 20 to 80 mL of 0.5% lidocaine with 1:200,000 epinephrine, dilute Pitressin (20 units in 60 to 100 mL of saline), or normal saline. The correct space for dissection is found using a "loss of resistance" technique similar to that used by an anesthesiologist placing an epidural. A wheal or blanching illustrates incorrect intraepithelial placement of the fluid. Hydrodissection in the correct plane will create a fluid bubble in the avascular vesicovaginal and rectovaginal spaces.
- As opposed to an anterior colporrhaphy where the vaginal epithelium and muscularis are split for plication, mesh should be placed underneath the vaginal muscularis. It is vital that the surgeon perform a full-thickness dissection deep into the vesicovaginal and rectovaginal spaces to avoid erosion of the mesh postoperatively. Proper hydrodissection, as described above, facilitates the identification of the proper dissection plane.
- It is unknown whether or not the bladder wall should be plicated in the midline below the graft.
- Place the graft loosely because mesh can contract by up to 20% following placement, compromising vaginal length and caliber. Allow enough room for Mayo scissors to be easily placed between the mesh and the vagina. Also, ensuring that the mesh is placed flat and with minimal tension will improve fibroblast growth and minimize complications of pain or erosion.
- The vaginal epithelium should not be trimmed. Trimming the vaginal epithelium can lead to discomfort, and it may also contract. The colpotomy incision is closed utilizing a nonlocking continuous absorbable suture.
- Cystourethroscopy with assessment of urine flow from both ureters should be performed routinely after anterior mesh placement to identify potential urethral, bladder, or ureteral injury.

Self-Tailored Mesh Placement

Self-tailored mesh can be customized by the surgeon to match the size and shape of each patient's individual pelvic anatomy. Mesh is cut into a trapezoid multiarmed shape for compartment augmentation and fixed to sacrospinous ligaments, obturator fascia, ATFP, and/or the distal bladder neck (**Fig. 37.8**). This type of surgery requires a strong set of vaginal surgical skills as it involves dissections similar to sacrospinous ligament fixation, iliococcygeus suspension, uterosacral suspension, and vaginal paravaginal defect repair. No studies have compared standard repair techniques using self-tailored mesh with other mesh placement techniques.

Trocar-Based Mesh Kits

Trocar-guided devices can be used to suspend mesh by passing needles through the transobturator and/or ischiorectal fossa. Trocar-based mesh kits were the first commercially available transvaginal mesh products, but some are no longer marketed by their respective companies. In general, the technique for placement of these products is similar, and the vesicovaginal spaces are dissected as described previously. First, a weighted speculum, self-retaining retractor, or Deaver retractors are placed in the vagina. As the vesicovaginal dissection plane is advanced superiorly, loose areolar tissue is encountered until the ischial spine, the ATFP, and, depending upon the kit, the sacrospinous ligaments are exposed. A number of different trocar types are available including helical shaped trocars similar to those for transobturator slings and flexible straight trocars. Cutaneous incisions that are 4 to 7 mm in length are made over the appropriate locations for the obturator foramen and/or gluteus trocars. When placing multiple mesh arms through the transobturator space, the superior and inferior puncture sites should be at least 3 cm apart so the mesh can lay flat. Two fingers placed into the vagina can retract the colon, elevate the bladder, and minimize deviation of the trocar tip with direct palpation. For anterior compartment mesh, the surgeon immediately identifies the incoming trocar passing through the ATFP. The prosthesis is loosely placed in a "tension-free" manner because mesh can contract by up to 20% following placement, creating tension and compromising vaginal length and caliber. A finger should be kept inside the vagina whenever tensioning the graft. This provides countertraction and splints the tissue at the points of fixation. Stay sutures can be used to help the mesh lay flat against the vagina. If the surgeon conserves the uterus, then permanent sutures can be placed into the cervical stroma to stabilize the mesh and prevent enterocele. Cystoscopic and rectal examinations before, during, and after each portion of the surgery can be helpful. Once adequate hemostasis is obtained, the vaginal epithelium is closed with a continuous nonlocking stitch of delayed absorbable suture. Placing a lubricated vaginal pack may minimize bleeding and keep the mesh flat during healing. After desired tensioning, all ends of the mesh arms should be trimmed below the surface of the skin, and the incisions closed. Concurrent procedures, such as a midurethral sling, should be done through a separate vaginal incision at this time.

Nontrocar Mesh Kits

The nontrocar or "single-incision" mesh kits have become increasingly popular and have largely replaced trocar-based kits. The products avoid the potential complications associated with blind trocar passage through the transobturator space and ischiorectal fossa and allow mesh fixation via direct visualization. Additionally, most currently available nontrocar kits provide apical fixation to the sacrospinous ligaments bilaterally as well as anterior vaginal support. The technique for the nontrocar kits begins similarly to the technique for trocar-guided kit placement. After the vesicovaginal space is dissected, pertinent fixation points are identified including the ischial spines, ATFP, and sacrospinous ligaments. For apical fixation, the surgeon palpates the location of interest then identifies the sacrospinous ligament at least one fingerbreadth medial to the ischial spine. The ligament is penetrated using the surgeon's device of choice. The ATFP mesh arms provide lateral fixation. An index finger placed into the vagina palpates the ATFP from the ischial spine to the posterior pubis. The mesh can be passed through the upper third of the ATFP using the same fixation methods. The mesh arms are slowly and individually adjusted to a loose tension; then, the mesh is sutured flat. Cystoscopy is performed to ensure integrity of the bladder and ureters. The colpotomy is closed and the vagina packed as described above.

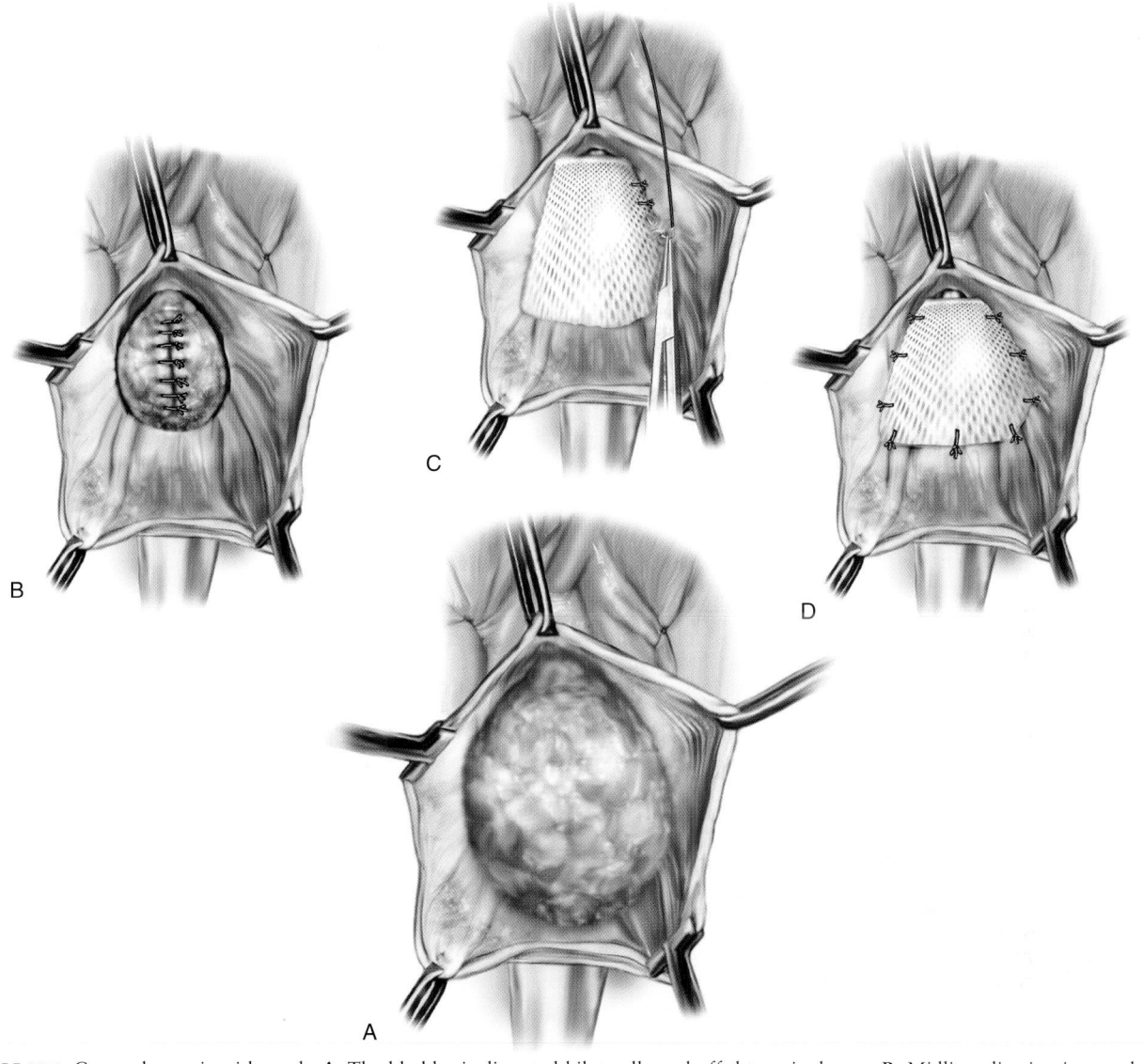

FIGURE 37.8 Cystocele repair with mesh: **A:** The bladder is dissected bilaterally and off the vaginal apex. **B:** Midline plication is completed. **C:** After entering the left paravaginal space and exposing the ATFP (*white line*) if desired, the self-styled prosthetic mesh is sewn in place. **D:** The mesh is attached bilaterally, and all sutures are tied, supporting the bladder. (Reprinted from Karram MM. *Surgical management of pelvic organ prolapse*. Philadelphia, PA: Elsevier/Saunders, 2013, with permission. Copyright 2013 Saunders, an Imprint of Elsevier, Inc.)

VII

Cystoscopy

Cystoscopy with direct observation of urine flow from both ureters is usually performed after cystocele repair, especially if slings, mesh, or apical suspension procedures are also being performed. The purpose is to ensure that no sutures or mesh have been placed in the bladder and to verify patency of both ureters. The rate of ureteral obstruction after simple anterior colporrhaphy is only about 0.4%, but the rate increases with the addition of some types of apical suspension. Intraoperative release of the offending sutures almost always releases the ureteral obstruction without further sequelae.

RESULTS

The main indication for surgical repair of anterior vaginal prolapse is to relieve symptoms when they exist or as part of a comprehensive pelvic reconstructive procedure for multiple sites of pelvic organ prolapse, with or without SUI. Few studies have addressed the long-term success of surgical treatments for anterior vaginal wall prolapse. While the majority of studies evaluating anterior vaginal prolapse repairs are uncontrolled series, an increasing number of randomized surgical trials have been done in recent years. Success rates vary considerably depending upon the outcome measure used to define success. Historically, most studies evaluating the treatment of pelvic organ prolapse have focused exclusively on anatomic success without considering other important areas such as symptoms, vaginal compliance, quality of life, sexual function, or socioeconomic outcomes. For an individual patient, the most important outcome of a surgical procedure is the relief of her symptoms and improvement in her quality of life, yet until recently these areas have largely been ignored. Reported success rates for native tissue anterior colporrhaphy range from 37% to 100% with most cohorts reporting success rates greater than 80%.

No randomized trials have been performed evaluating the efficacy of paravaginal defect repair for the treatment of anterior vaginal wall prolapse. Single-center uncontrolled case series suggest good anatomic results for both open retropubic (success rate 75% to 97%) and vaginal (success rate 67% to 100%) approaches. However, the vaginal approach appears to be associated with high risk of hemorrhage, with one series reporting a 21% blood transfusion rate. Few data are available on the efficacy or safety of the laparoscopic or robotic paravaginal defect repair.

In 2001, Weber et al. studied three variations of anterior colporrhaphy using a prospective randomized study design and a strict definition of success (Aa and Ba points at –3 or –2 cm; stage 0 or I). Standard anterior colporrhaphy resulted in 30% of patients with an optimal or satisfactory anatomic result, anterior colporrhaphy with polyglactin 910 mesh overlay had a 42% optimal or satisfactory result, and ultralateral plication under tension had a 46% optimal or satisfactory result. No difference was seen in anatomic or functional outcomes, and most patients reported satisfaction with their symptom improvement. The low success rates found in the trial are used as evidence that anterior colporrhaphy should either be augmented by synthetic mesh or another approach used (e.g., sacrocolpopexy) for treatment of anterior vaginal prolapse. More recently, Chmielewski et al. reanalyzed the data from this trial using more clinically relevant definitions of success and reported considerably better outcomes with only 10% of subjects developing anatomic recurrence beyond the hymen, 5% of subjects developing symptomatic recurrence, and less than 1% having another surgery for prolapse at 23 months' follow-up. In general, it appears that native tissue anterior colporrhaphy commonly results in asymptomatic anterior vaginal descent to within 1 cm of the hymen (POPQ stage 2); however, prolapse beyond the hymen, development of symptomatic prolapse (e.g., vaginal bulging symptoms), and reoperation for recurrent prolapse are uncommon events in the first 2 to 3 years after surgery. Long-term results of anterior colporrhaphy are largely unknown, although Gotthart et al. reported only 13 reoperations for prolapse (2.9%) after 10 years in 456 patients who

had vaginal hysterectomy and colporrhaphy. The median interval from the fist surgery to the second was 5.5 years.

Two studies evaluated the use of absorbable polyglactin 910 mesh to augment anterior colporrhaphy and reported mixed results. The Weber et al. trial described above found no benefit, while a randomized trial by Sand et al. found a 75% success rate 1 year after surgery in those receiving absorbable mesh compared with a 57% success in those receiving native tissue anterior colporrhaphy. To date, six trials have compared biologic graft overlay to anterior colporrhaphy, and two trials have compared biologic graft to permanent synthetic graft. Based on a meta-analysis of these trials, a Cochrane review concluded that overall use of a biologic graft overlay is associated with a lower risk of anatomic failure than anterior colporrhaphy alone (failure rate, anterior colporrhaphy 25% vs. biologic graft 14%; RR 1.44 [95% CI: 1.20 to 2.63]), but no difference was found in subjective cure or improvement in quality of life. Given the different characteristics of many of the biologic grafts, it seems likely that results will vary depending upon the specific biologic graft used; however, no head-to-head comparisons have been performed. Two clinical trials have found inferior anatomic outcomes for porcine dermis when compared to polypropylene graft.

Six randomized trials have compared the efficacy of mesh augmentation with polypropylene to native tissue anterior colporrhaphy for the treatment of anterior vaginal prolapse (see Table 37.1). The 2012 Cochrane review concluded that use of permanent synthetic mesh for anterior prolapse repair was associated with a decreased anatomic failure rate when compared to anterior colporrhaphy alone (14% vs. 49%; RR 3.50, 95% CI: 2.71 to 4.52), but no differences were found in the reoperation rate for prolapse or for improvement in quality of life measures. Of note, use of mesh in the anterior vaginal wall appeared to predispose to prolapse in the apical and posterior segments in these trials compared to native tissue repair. The Cochrane reviewers also found that anterior vaginal mesh placement was

TABLE 37.1 Randomized Trials of Transvaginal Synthetic Permanent Mesh-Augmented Anterior Vaginal Repair to Anterior Colporrhaphy

AUTHOR	YEAR	GRAFT	NO.	REVIEW MONTHS	SUCCESS	COMPLICATIONS
Nguyen et al.	2008	AC Perigee	38 38	24	18/38 (47%) 32/38 (87%)	Blood loss greater for mesh, 6% exposure
Sivaslioglu et al.	2008	AC Self-styled obturator	42 43	12	30/42 (71%) 39/43 (91%)	9% mesh exposure
Carey et al.	2009	AC + PC Self-styled Gynemesh overlay	60 62	12	40/60 (67%) 51/62 (82%)	6.5% mesh exposure
Nieminen et al.	2010	AC Self-styled obturator	96 104	36	57/97 (59%) 90/104 (86%)	19% mesh exposure, no difference in symptomatic recurrence
Altman et al.	2011	AC Polypropylene Prolift	182 186	12	64/182 (35%) 113/186 (61%)	Mesh: ↑operating time, blood loss, cystotomy, de novo SUI, dyspareunia, reoperation rate
Vollebregt et al.	2011	AC Polypropylene Avaulta	58 56	12	24/58 (41%) 51/56 (91%)	AC: 5% reoperation rate for prolapse Mesh: No reoperation for prolapse, 4% exposure

SUI, stress urinary incontinence; PC, posterior colporrhaphy; AC, anterior colporrhaphy.
Adapted from Maher C, Baessler K, Barber M, et al. Surgery for pelvic organ prolapse. In: Abrams P, Brubaker L, Cardozo C, Wein A, eds. *5th International Consultation on Incontinence*. Paris: Health Publications, Ltd., 2013.

associated with greater operating time, greater blood loss, and a tendency for more cystotomies and de novo SUI.

Vaginal mesh erosions can be a particularly difficult problem, and a small but significant number require reoperation for mesh removal due to chronic discharge, bleeding, pain, and other serious complications. The average rate of mesh exposure reported in the literature in the 1st year after transvaginal mesh placement for pelvic organ prolapse is 10.9%. More than half of the women who experienced erosion or exposure from nonabsorbable synthetic mesh after transvaginal placement require surgical excision in the operating room with some women requiring multiple operations. Creation of thicker vaginal flaps with an attached fibromuscularis, limiting vaginal trimming and avoiding inverted "T" colpotomy incisions or concurrent vaginal hysterectomy, probably decreases the mesh erosion rate. Treatment of vaginal atrophy and cessation of smoking may also help to decrease the mesh erosion rate.

It is worth emphasizing that the great majority of clinical trial evidence available for anterior transvaginal mesh placement studied trocar-based mesh products that are no longer commercially available. In recent years, there has been a significant shift toward the non–trocar-based mesh kits for which there are currently few data. As of the writing of this chapter, no clinical trials comparing nontrocar-based mesh kits for anterior vaginal prolapse have been published.

Risk factors for failure of anterior vaginal prolapse repair have not been specifically studied separate from studies of total prolapse. Vaginal prolapse in general recurs with increasing age and length of follow-up, but the actual frequency is unknown and tends to vary with different definitions of prolapse. Recurrence of anterior prolapse is more likely to occur with more severe initial prolapse and probably with transvaginal, compared to abdominal, repairs. Recurrence may represent a failure to identify and repair all support defects, or weakening, stretching, or breaking of patients' tissues, as occurs with advancing age and after menopause. Sacrospinous ligament suspension of the vaginal apex, with exaggerated retrosuspension of the vagina, may predispose patients to recurrence of anterior vaginal prolapse. Other characteristics that may increase chances of recurrence are genetic predisposition, subsequent pregnancy, heavy lifting, chronic pulmonary disease, chronic straining at stool, smoking, and obesity.

COMPLICATIONS

Intraoperative complications are uncommon with native tissue anterior vaginal prolapse repair. Excessive blood loss may occur, requiring blood transfusion, or a hematoma may develop in the anterior vagina; this is probably more common after vaginal paravaginal repair than anterior colporrhaphy. The lumen of the bladder or urethra may be entered in the course of dissection. Accidental cystotomy should be repaired in layers at the time of the injury. After repair of cystotomy, the bladder is generally drained for 7 to 14 days to allow adequate healing. Ureteral damage or obstruction occurs rarely (0% to 2%), usually with very large cystoceles or with apical prolapse. Other rare complications include intravesical or urethral suture placement (and associated urologic problems) and fistulae, either urethrovaginal or vesicovaginal.

Complications unique to synthetic mesh use in the vagina include vaginal mesh exposure or extrusion; mesh erosion or perforation into an adjacent organ including the bladder, urethra, and rectum; and vaginal mesh contraction with associated pain and dyspareunia. Complications that can occur with any reconstructive pelvic surgery but that can be made more severe or complicated by the presence of synthetic mesh include bleeding, infection, fistulas, pelvic pain, sexual dysfunction, and dysfunction of the lower urinary and lower gastrointestinal tract.

While many of these complications can be managed nonsurgically, a significant proportion will require surgical excision of some or all of the mesh. The incidence of these complications varies from 3% to 39%. A systematic review of 110 studies by Abed et al. found the average rate of graft erosion or exposure to be 10.3% with permanent synthetic grafts and 10.1% after biologic grafts. Wound granulation was seen in 7.8%. Approximately two thirds of women with a mesh exposure after permanent synthetic mesh placement require some surgery to correct the exposure; in some cases, multiple procedures are required.

De novo stress incontinence occurs in 15% to 59% of women after anterior vaginal prolapse repair. This risk is higher in women who demonstrate a positive cough stress test with prolapse reduction prior to surgery than those who do not. However, performance of an antiincontinence procedure such as a midurethral sling or Burch colposuspension decreases this risk whether the preoperative stress test is positive or not.

Voiding difficulty can occur after anterior vaginal prolapse repair. This problem may occur more often in women with subclinical preoperative voiding dysfunction, especially if a suburethal plication is done. Treatment is bladder drainage or intermittent self-catheterization until spontaneous voiding resumes, usually within 6 weeks. Urinary tract infections are common (especially with concurrent catheter usage), but other infections such as pelvic or vaginal abscesses are uncommon.

Sexual function may be positively or negatively affected by vaginal operations for anterior vaginal prolapse. Most prospective studies demonstrate that sexual function either does not change or improves in the majority of women after vaginal reconstructive surgery for pelvic organ prolapse; however, worsening sexual function can be seen in some patients. As many as 50% of patients with advanced prolapse report dyspareunia prior to surgery. In general, dyspareunia rates go down after prolapse surgery; however, de novo dyspareunia can be seen in as many as 18%, especially if a posterior colporrhaphy is also performed. Vaginal length and caliber appear to have little relationship with postoperative sexual satisfaction. In a comprehensive study by Kuhn et al. of male and female sexual function after primary repair of vaginal prolapse without the use of mesh, female patients reported improvement in sexual desire, arousal, lubrication, pain, and overall satisfaction, but not orgasm. De novo dyspareunia only occurred in 2 of 70 women. Male partner function improved as well in domains of interest, sexual desire, and overall satisfaction. One prospective comparison of patients undergoing vaginal versus nonvaginal (open or robotic) prolapse repair found that sexual function improved overall after surgery with no difference between groups. Comparisons of sexual outcomes between native tissue and mesh-augmented repairs have had mixed results with some showing worse sexual function after mesh repairs, and others show no difference between the groups. The Cochrane reviewers found no difference in postoperative de novo dyspareunia between native tissue prolapse repair and those augmented with synthetic or biologic grafts.

BEST SURGICAL PRACTICES

- Anterior vaginal wall prolapse can involve prolapse of the bladder, prolapse of the uterus or vaginal apex, and even anterior enterocele.
- Anterior vaginal wall prolapse can adversely affect quality of life, sexuality, voiding function, and urinary continence.
- The goal of the operative repair of a paravaginal defect is to reattach the pubocervical fascia to the ATFP and to the fascia overlying the obturator internus muscle.
- Using an open retropubic technique, the bony landmarks of the pelvis are identified by palpation; then, tissue forceps are used to develop the space between the pelvic sidewall

VII

fascia and the bladder and urethra. Care is taken to avoid venous bleeding in this area. After the white line and the lateral edge of the pubocervical fascia have been identified, a series of interrupted 2-0 permanent sutures are placed about 1 to 2 cm apart to reapproximate the fascial edge to the white line of the pelvic sidewall fascia.

- When a transvaginal approach is used, the retropubic space is opened and cleared back to the ischial spine and the important landmarks visualized as with an anterior retropubic approach. Starting near the ischial spine, a series of sutures are placed in the white line and held with the needles in place. Then, in reverse order, starting with the most distal suture, a bite is taken in the edge of the pubocervical fascia and the undersurface of the vaginal mucosa. The process is repeated, advancing deeper into the pelvis until the highest suture is placed. The sutures are then tied, starting with the one closest to the vaginal introitus and proceeding to the vaginal apex. The vaginal mucosa is then closed in the midline.
- Women with anterior vaginal prolapse should be evaluated for symptomatic or occult SUI, and, if SUI is found, consideration of placing a concurrent antiincontinence procedure should be made.
- Cystoscopy with assessment of both ureters is usually performed after cystocele repair, especially if slings, mesh, or apical suspension procedures are also being performed. The purpose is to ensure that no sutures or mesh have been placed in the bladder and to verify patency of both ureters.
- The 2012 Cochrane review concluded that use of permanent synthetic mesh for anterior prolapse repair was associated with a decreased anatomic failure rate when compared to anterior colporrhaphy alone (14% vs. 49%; RR 3.50, 95% CI: 2.71 to 4.52), but no differences were found in the reoperation rate for prolapse or for improvement in quality-of-life measures. Also, the overall rate of reoperations including reoperation for recurrent prolapse, de novo stress incontinence, or mesh exposure is almost two times higher after anterior vaginal mesh than native tissue repair (10.2% vs. 5.8%).

BIBLIOGRAPHY

Abed H, Rahn DD, Lowenstein L, et al. Incidence and management of graft erosion, wound granulation, and dyspareunia following vaginal prolapse repair with graft materials: a systematic review. *Int Urogynecol J Pelvic Floor Dysfunct* 2011;22:789.

ACOG Practice Bulletin No. 104. Antibiotic prophylaxis for gynecologic procedures. *Obstet Gynecol* 2009;113:1180.

ACOG Committee on Gynecologic Practice. Committee Opinion No. 513: vaginal placement of synthetic mesh for pelvic organ prolapse. *Obstet Gynecol* 2011;118:1459.

Altman D, Vayrynen T, Engh ME, et al. Anterior colporrhaphy versus transvaginal mesh for pelvic-organ prolapse. *N Engl J Med* 2011;364:1826.

Aronson MP, Bates SM, Jacoby AF, et al. Periurethral and paravaginal anatomy: an endovaginal magnetic resonance imaging study. *Am J Obstet Gynecol* 1995;173:1702.

Barber MD, Brubaker L, Nygaard I, et al. Defining success after surgery for pelvic organ prolapse. *Obstet Gynecol* 2009;114:600.

Barber MD, Cundiff GW, Weidner AC, et al. Accuracy of clinical assessment of paravaginal defects in women with anterior vaginal wall prolapse. *Am J Obstet Gynecol* 1999;181:87.

Barber MD. Symptoms and outcome measures of pelvic organ prolapse. *Clin Obstet Gynecol* 2005;48:648.

Bump RC, Fantl JA, Hurt WG. The mechanism of urinary continence in women with severe uterovaginal prolapse: results of barrier studies. *Obstet Gynecol* 1988;72:291.

Bump RC, Mattiasson A, Bø K, et al. The standardization of terminology of female pelvic organ prolapse and pelvic floor dysfunction. *Am J Obstet Gynecol* 1996;175:10.

Carey M, Higgs P, Goh J, et al. Vaginal repair with mesh versus colporrhaphy for prolapse: a randomized controlled trial. *BJOG* 2009;116:1380.

Chen CH, Wu WY, Sheu BC, et al. Comparison of recurrence rates after anterior colporrhaphy for cystocele using three different surgical techniques. *Gynecol Obstet Invest* 2007;63:214.

Chen L, Ashton-Miller JA, DeLancey JOL. A 3D finite element model of anterior vaginal wall support to evaluate mechanisms underlying cystocele formation. *J Biomech* 2009;42:1371.

Chmielewski L, Walters MD, Weber AM, et al. Reanalysis of a randomized trial of 3 techniques of anterior colporrhaphy using clinically relevant definitions of success. *Am J Obstet Gynecol* 2011;205:69.

Clarke-Pearson DL, Abaid LN. Prevention of venous thromboembolic events after gynecologic surgery. *Obstet Gynecol* 2012;119:155.

Colombo M, Vitobello D, Proietti F, et al. Randomised comparison of Burch colposuspension versus anterior colporrhaphy in women with stress urinary incontinence and anterior vaginal wall prolapse. *BJOG* 2000;107:544.

DeLancey JO. Fascial and muscular abnormalities in women with urethral hypermobility and anterior vaginal wall prolapse. *Am J Obstet Gynecol* 2002;187:93.

DeLancey JOL. Anatomic aspects of vaginal eversion after hysterectomy. *Am J Obstet Gynecol* 1992;166:1717.

Feldner PC Jr, Castro RA, Cipolotti LA, et al. Anterior vaginal wall prolapse: a randomized controlled trial of SIS graft versus traditional colporrhaphy. *Int Urogynecol J Pelvic Floor Dysfunct* 2010;21:1057.

Gandhi S, Goldberg RP, Kwon C, et al. A prospective randomized trial using solvent dehydrated fascia lata for the prevention of recurrent anterior vaginal wall prolapse. *Am J Obstet Gynecol* 2005;192:1649.

Ganj FA, Okechukwu AI, Bedestani A, et al. Complications of transvaginal monofilament polypropylene mesh in pelvic organ prolapse repair. *Int Urogynecol J Pelvic Floor Dysfunct* 2009;20:919.

Glazener CMA, Cooper K. Anterior vaginal repair for urinary incontinence in women (Cochrane Review). In: *The Cochrane Library*, Issue 3. Oxford, UK: Update Software, 2002.

Goldberg RP, Koduri S, Lobel RW, et al. Protective effect of suburethral slings on postoperative cystocele recurrence after reconstructive pelvic operation. *Am J Obstet Gynecol* 2001;185:1307.

Gotthart PT, Aigmueller T, Lang PF, et al. Reoperation for pelvic organ prolapse within 10 years of primary surgery for prolapse. *Int Urogynecol J Pelvic Floor Dysfunct* 2012;23:1221.

Guerette NL, Peterson TV, Aguirre OA, et al. Anterior repair with or without collagen matrix reinforcement: a randomized controlled trial. *Obstet Gynecol* 2009;114:59.

Gustilo-Ashby AM, Jelovsek JE, Barber MD, et al. The incidence of ureteral obstruction and the value of intraoperative cystoscopy during vaginal surgery for pelvic organ prolapse. *Am J Obstet Gynecol* 2006;194:1478.

Haase P, Skibsted L. Influence of operations for stress incontinence and/or genital descensus on sexual life. *Acta Obstet Gynecol Scand* 1988;67:659.

Haylen BT, de Ridder D, Freeman RM, et al.; International Urogynecological Association; International Continence Society. An International Urogynecological Association (IUGA)/International Continence Society (ICS) joint report on the terminology for female pelvic floor dysfunction. *Neurourol Urodyn* 2010;29:4.

Hsu Y, Chen L, Summers A, et al. Anterior vaginal wall length and degree of anterior compartment prolapse seen on dynamic MRI. *Int Urogynecol J Pelvic Floor Dysfunct* 2008;19:137.

Hviid U, Hviid TV, Rudnicki M. Porcine skin collagen implants for anterior vaginal wall prolapse: a randomised prospective controlled study. *Int Urogynecol J Pelvic Floor Dysfunct* 2010;21:529.

Jia X, Glazener C, Mowatt G, et al. Efficacy and safety of using mesh or grafts in surgery for anterior and/or posterior vaginal wall prolapse: systematic review and meta-analysis. *BJOG* 2008;115:1350.

Kapoor DS, Nemcova M, Pantazis K, et al. Reoperation rate for traditional anterior vaginal repair: analysis of 207 cases with a median 4-year follow-up. *Int Urogynecol J Pelvic Floor Dysfunct* 2010;21:27.

Karp DR, Peterson TV, Mahdy A, et al. Biologic grafts for cystocele repair: does concomitant midline fascial plication improve surgical outcomes? *Int Urogynecol J Pelvic Floor Dysfunct* 2011;22:985.

Kobak WH, Walters MD, Piedmonte MR. Determinants of voiding after three types of incontinence surgery. *Obstet Gynecol* 2001;97:86.

Kuhn A, Brunnmayr G, Stadimayr W, et al. Male and female sexual function after surgical repair of female organ prolapse. *J Sex Med* 2009;6:1324.

Kwon CH, Goldberg RP, Koduri S, et al. The use of intraoperative cystoscopy in major vaginal and urogynecologic surgeries. *Am J Obstet Gynecol* 2002;187:1466.

Maher C, Baessler K, Barber M, et al. Surgery for pelvic organ prolapse. In: Abrams P, Brubaker L, Cardozo C, et al., eds. *5th International Consultation on Incontinence*. Paris, France: Health Publications, Ltd., 2013.

Maher CF, Qatawneh AM, Dwyer PL, et al. Abdominal sacral colpopexy or vaginal sacrospinous colpopexy vaginal vault prolapse: a prospective randomized study. *Am J Obstet Gynecol* 2004;190:20.

Maher CM, Feiner B, Baessler K, et al. Surgical management of pelvic organ prolapse in women: the updated summary version Cochrane review. *Int Urogynecol J Pelvic Floor Dysfunct* 2011;22:1445.

Mallipeddi PK, Steele AC, Hohli N, et al. Anatomic and functional outcome of vaginal paravaginal repair in the correction of anterior vaginal prolapse. *Int Urogynecol J Pelvic Floor Dysfunct* 2001;12:83.

Medina CA, Candiotti K, Takacs P. Wide genital hiatus is a risk factor for recurrence following anterior vaginal repair. *Int J Gynaecol Obstet* 2008;101:184.

Menefee SA, Dyer KY, Lukacz ES, et al. Colporrhaphy compared with mesh or graft-reinforced vaginal paravaginal repair for anterior vaginal wall prolapse: a randomized controlled trial. *Obstet Gynecol* 2011;118:1337.

Meschia M, Pifarotti P, Bernasconi F, et al. Porcine skin collagen implants to prevent anterior vaginal wall prolapse recurrence: a multicenter, randomized study. *J Urol* 2007;177:192.

Meschia M, Pifarotti P, Spennacchio M, et al. A randomized comparison of tension-free vaginal tape and endopelvic fascia plication in women with genital prolapse and occult stress urinary incontinence. *Am J Obstet Gynecol* 2004;190:609.

Moore RD, Mitchell GK, Miklos JR. Single-incision vaginal approach to treat cystocele and vault prolapse with an anterior wall mesh anchored apically to the sacrospinous ligament. *Int Urogynecol J Pelvic Floor Dysfunct* 2012;23:85.

Morse AN, O'dell KK, Howard AE, et al. Midline anterior repair alone vs anterior repair plus vaginal paravaginal repair: a comparison of anatomic and quality of life outcomes. *Int Urogynecol J Pelvic Floor Dysfunct* 2007;18:245.

Muffly TM, Barber MD. Insertion and removal of vaginal mesh for pelvic organ prolapse. *Clin Obstet Gynecol* 2010;53:99.

Natale F, La Penna C, Padoa A, et al. A prospective, randomized, controlled study comparing Gynemesh, a synthetic mesh, and Pelvicol, a biologic graft, in the surgical treatment of recurrent cystocele. *Int Urogynecol J Pelvic Floor Dysfunct* 2009;20:75.

Nguyen JN, Burchette RJ. Outcome after anterior vaginal prolapse repair: a randomized controlled trial. *Obstet Gynecol* 2008;111:891.

Nichols DH, Randall CL. *Vaginal surgery*, 4th ed. Baltimore, MD: Williams & Wilkins, 1996.

Nieminen K, Hiltunen R, Takala T, et al. Outcomes after anterior vaginal wall repair with mesh: a randomized, controlled trial with a 3 year follow-up. *Am J Obstet Gynecol* 2010;203:235.

Nüssler EK, Greisen S, Kesmodel US, et al. Operation for recurrent cystocele with anterior colporrhaphy or non-absorbable mesh: patient reported outcomes. *Int Urogynecol J Pelvic Floor Dysfunct* 2013;24:1925.

Richardson AC, Lyon JB, Williams NL. A new look at pelvic relaxation. *Am J Obstet Gynecol* 1976;126:568.

Ridgeway B, Walters MD, Paraiso MF, et al. Early experience with mesh excision for adverse outcomes after transvaginal mesh placement using prolapse kits. *Am J Obstet Gynecol* 2008;199:703.

Sand PK, Koduri S, Lobel RW, et al. Prospective randomized trial of polyglactin 910 mesh to prevent recurrence of cystoceles and rectoceles. *Am J Obstet Gynecol* 2001;184:1357.

Shull BL, Baden WF. A six-year experience with paravaginal defect repair for stress urinary incontinence. *Am J Obstet Gynecol* 1989;160:1432; discussion 1439–1440.

Shull BL, Benn SJ, Kuehl TJ. Surgical management of prolapse of the anterior vaginal segment: an analysis of support defects, operative morbidity, and anatomic outcome. *Am J Obstet Gynecol* 1994;171:1429; discussion 1436.

Siddiqui NY, Fulton RG, Kuchibhatla M, et al. Sexual function after vaginal versus nonvaginal prolapse surgery. *Female Pelvic Med Reconstr Surg* 2012;18:238.

Sivaslioglu AA, Unlubilgin E, Dolen I. A randomized comparison of polypropylene mesh surgery with site-specific surgery in the treatment of cystocoele. *Int Urogynecol J Pelvic Floor Dysfunct* 2008;19:467.

Summers A, Winkel LA, Hussain HK, et al. The relationship between anterior and apical compartment support. *Am J Obstet Gynecol* 2006;194:1438.

Sung VW, Rogers RG, Schaffer JI, et al. Graft use in transvaginal pelvic organ prolapse repair: a systematic review. *Obstet Gynecol* 2008;112:1131.

Tulikangas PK, Lukban JC, Walters MD. Anterior enterocele: a report of three cases. *Int Urogynecol J Pelvic Floor Dysfunct* 2004;15:350.

Vollebregt A, Fischer K, Gietelink D, et al. Primary surgical repair of anterior vaginal prolapse: a randomised trial comparing anatomical and functional outcome between anterior colporrhaphy and trocar-guided transobturator anterior mesh. *BJOG* 2011;118:1518.

Vu MK, Letko J, Jirschele K, et al. Minimal mesh repair for apical and anterior prolapse: initial anatomical and subjective outcomes. *Int Urogynecol J Pelvic Floor Dysfunct* 2012;23:1753.

Weber AM, Walters MD, Piedmonte MA, et al. Anterior colporrhaphy: a randomized trial of three surgical techniques. *Am J Obstet Gynecol* 2001;185:1299.

Weber AM, Walters MD. Anterior vaginal prolapse: review of anatomy and techniques of surgical repair. *Obstet Gynecol* 1997;89:311.

White GR. A radical cure by suturing lateral sulci of vagina to white line of pelvic fascia. *JAMA* 1909;21:1707.

White GR. An anatomical operation for the cure of cystocele. *Am J Obstet Dis Women Child* 1912;65:286.

Whiteside JL, Barber MD, Paraiso MF, et al. Clinical evaluation of anterior vaginal wall support defect: interexaminer and intraexaminer reliability. *Am J Obstet Gynecol* 2004;191:100.

Whiteside JL, Weber AM, Meyn LA, et al. Risk factors for prolapse recurrence after vaginal repair. *Am J Obstet Gynecol* 2004;191:1533.

Young SB, Daman JJ, Bony LG. Vaginal paravaginal repair: one-year outcomes. *Am J Obstet Gynecol* 2001;185:1360.

CHAPTER 38
Posterior Compartment Defects

Oz Harmanli and Keisha Jones

DEFINITIONS

Constipation—The following criteria must be present for the last 3 months with symptom onset at least 6 months before diagnosis and must include two or more of the following being present during at least 25% of defecations: straining during defecation, lumpy or hard stools, sensation of incomplete evacuation, sensation of anorectal obstruction/blockage, manual maneuvers to facilitate at least 25% of defecations (e.g., digital evacuation, support of the pelvic floor), or fewer than three defecations per week. Loose stools are rarely present without the use of laxatives. There are insufficient criteria for irritable bowel syndrome.

Defecatory dysfunction (DD)—A heterogeneous term used to describe any difficulty with defecation, excluding anal incontinence. DD is often used synonymously with constipation.

Defecatory dyssynergia—A phenomenon whereby the puborectalis and external anal sphincter muscles contract paradoxically during defecation or fail to relax.

Defecography—A dynamic evaluation that provides a two-dimensional view to assess defecation in real time, using fluoroscopy. It may identify a rectocele, sigmoidocele, rectal intussusception, and rectal prolapse and can help to exclude pelvic floor dysynergy.

Endopelvic fascia—A network of connective tissue composed of collagen, elastin, and nonvascular smooth muscle strands that connect pelvic support structures.

Incomplete emptying—Complaint that the rectum does not feel empty after defecation.

Midline plication/traditional posterior colporrhaphy—The operation that plicates the posterior vaginal wall fibromuscular layer, usually from the vaginal apex to the perineal body.

Pelvic diaphragm—The muscular support structure, which forms the pelvic floor posteriorly and laterally and includes the levator ani and coccygeus muscles that originate from the pubic and ischial rami at the level of the arcus tendineus levator ani.

Pericervical ring—The location where the endopelvic connective tissue connects to support the structures surrounding the cervix and vaginal apex.

Perineal body—A midline, fibromuscular confluence between the urogenital and anal triangles where perineal membrane and several muscles including the bulbocavernosus and deep and superficial transverse perineal and external anal sphincter muscles are attached.

Perineal descent—A bulge in the perineum where the perineum descends greater than or equal to 2 cm below the ischial tuberosities at rest or with straining.

Perineal membrane—The inferior fascia of the urogenital diaphragm, which is dense and instrumental in the stability of perineal body and support of the rectum. Some recent anatomic descriptions have begun using the terms, perineal membrane and urogenital diaphragm, interchangeably.

Perineorrhaphy—Reapproximation of torn dense perineal connective tissue including the bulbocavernosus and perineal muscles in an effort to restore the perineal body.

Rectocele and enterocele—The terms used historically to describe protrusion of rectum (rectocele) and other intestines (enterocele) through posterior vaginal wall defects. This is no longer the preferred terminology as the examiner cannot identify the origin of the prolapse accurately with physical examination alone.

Rectovaginal septum (RVS) or fascia—A misnomer for the dense fibromuscular layer of the vaginal wall between the vaginal epithelium and the rectal wall. This structure, which is not a true histologic fascia or septum, is dense distally and becomes adipose with bundles of fibrous tissue and elastic fibers toward the vaginal apex.

Site-specific repair of the posterior vaginal compartment—Identification of the specific defects of the posterior vaginal wall and subsequent repair of these localized defects.

Splinting/digitation—Complaint of need to digitally replace the prolapse or to otherwise apply pressure, for example, to the vagina or perineum (splinting) or to the vagina or rectum (manual evacuation/digitation) to assist voiding or defecation.

Urogenital diaphragm—The fibromuscular structure that spans from one ischiopubic ramus to the other. It is divided in the middle by the genital hiatus, which contains the urethra and the vagina. Urogenital diaphragm includes deep transverse perineal and sphincter urethra muscles and is covered by fascia on both sides like other muscles in the body.

EPIDEMIOLOGY

Pelvic floor disorders are a prevalent problem that increases cumulatively with age. It is the indication for over 400,000 surgeries annually, representing only a small fraction of those affected by prolapse. The reported prevalence of rectocele varies from 13% to 20% depending on the population studied. Posterior vaginal wall descent is found in approximately 80% of women who have documented prolapse, with isolated rectoceles occurring in 7% of women. Posterior compartment repair is performed in about 40% to 70% of all pelvic floor repairs.

Posterior compartment prolapse can present with symptoms of impaired structure and/or function. Structural abnormalities may manifest as bulge symptoms or sensation of pressure, while functional disorders will usually include defecatory dysfunction (DD). DD is generally used synonymously with constipation, the prevalence of which is estimated as 10% to 15% in most studies and between 9% and 60% in women seen in urogynecology practices. Anal incontinence may also be present but is not typically related to posterior compartment prolapse. The term anorectal dysfunction includes anal incontinence and DD. For the purposes of this chapter; we will focus on DD because anal incontinence is not a typical symptom of posterior compartment prolapse.

Posterior vaginal wall prolapse, the recommended term for bulging that presents in the posterior wall of the vagina, could potentially lead to a protrusion of the anterior wall of the rectum into the vagina (rectocele), small bowel (enterocele), perineal body (perineocele), or the rare entity of the sigmoid colon (sigmoidocele). Bump et al. recommended the term posterior vaginal wall prolapse as the examiner cannot identify with certainty the organs that are protruding through the posterior vaginal wall. This distinction can generally be made once the patient is brought to the operating room.

HISTOLOGY

The vaginal wall is comprised of four layers: a nonkeratinized stratified squamous epithelium; subepithelium, which contains collagen and elastin; lamina propria, a smooth muscle layer; and a loose connective tissue layer, the adventitia. Multiple researchers have investigated the potential alterations that occur in collagen that may result in prolapse; studies have variably concluded that there was overall a lower amount of collagen or a change in the predominant type of collagen in patients with prolapse. In addition, the smooth muscle content of the posterior vaginal wall is disorganized and significantly reduced in women with pelvic organ prolapse.

Histologic studies of the posterior vaginal wall reveal that the rectum with its outer and inner muscular layers, lamina propria and rectal mucosa, lies immediately adjacent to the vaginal adventitia. There is no evidence of a continuous sheet of dense collagen that would qualify histologically as fascia (Figs. 38.1 and 38.2). The layer that supports the vaginal walls is the fibromuscular layer of the vagina, which is rich in elastin. Though technically inaccurate, it has been commonly named "rectovaginal fascia," "rectovaginal septum," or "Denonvilliers fascia." In the proximal vagina, this so-called rectovaginal septum contains mostly adipose tissue, while the most distal 3 to 3.5 cm is dense connective tissue without a true cleavage plane.

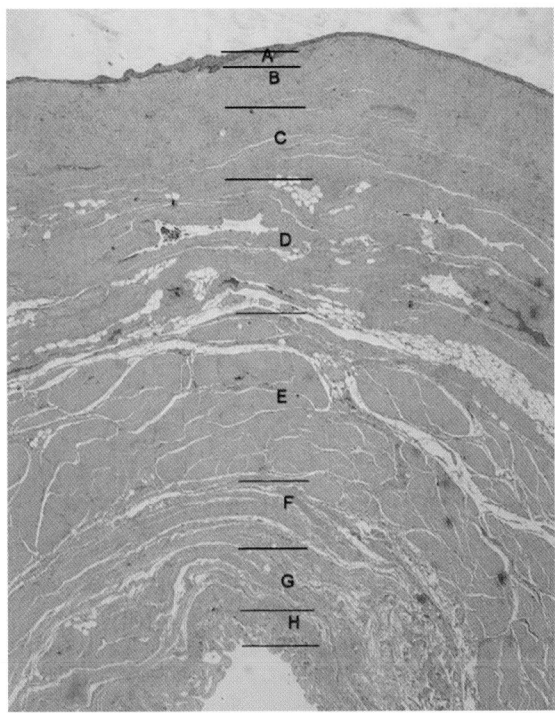

FIGURE 38.1 Histologic layers of the posterior vaginal wall. Hematoxylin and eosin (H&E) horizontal section. (*A*) Vaginal epithelium, (*B*) lamina propria of the vagina, (*C*) fibromuscular wall of the vagina, (*D*) adventitia, (*E*) outer muscular wall of the rectum, (*F*) inner muscular wall of the rectum, (*G*) lamina propria of the rectum, (*H*) rectal mucosa. (Reprinted from Kleeman SD, Westermann C, Karram MM, et al. Rectocele and the anatomy of the posterior vagina wall: revisited. *Am J Obstet Gynecol* 2005;193:2050–2055, with permission. Copyright © 2005, Elsevier.)

ANATOMY

Due to the interdependent nature of the tissues of the pelvic floor, a thorough understanding of the anatomy of posterior vagina is prudent for the gynecologic surgeon planning repair of the posterior compartment. Identification of all anatomic defects is essential when planning surgery for durable outcomes. Pelvic organ support is provided by the vagina, which is supported by the physiologically complex interactions between the levator ani muscles, surrounding fascia, the arcus tendineus fascia pelvis, the uterosacral ligaments, the connective tissue attachments of the vagina to the bony pelvis, the perineal body, and the perineal membrane (Fig. 38.3). The network of connective tissue that envelops the pelvic structures including the vagina is known as the endopelvic fascia. Its integrity is critical for pelvic floor support. It is made of collagen, elastin, and smooth muscle fibers. The smooth muscle strands in the endopelvic fascia are long and wavy unlike those that form part of the intestinal and bladder wall. The pelvic diaphragm provides the muscular support and includes the levator ani muscles and coccygeus muscles, which originate at the pubic rami at the level of the arcus tendineus levator ani and create the pelvic floor posteriorly and laterally.

In the presence of normal support, the vagina is pulled posteriorly toward the sacrum by uterosacral ligaments and to a lesser degree cephalad by cardinal ligaments, resulting in an almost horizontal orientation in its proximal two thirds

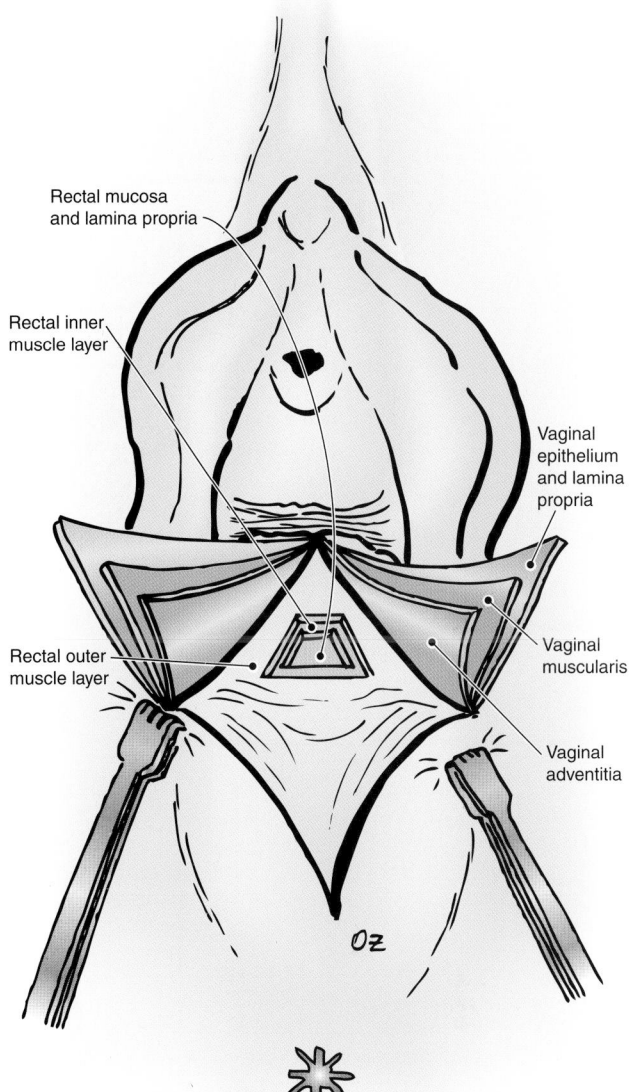

FIGURE 38.2 Layers of posterior vaginal wall.

(Fig. 38.4). Damage to any of the apical vaginal support will lead to a more vertical position of the vagina over the levator ani muscles, predisposing to abnormal distribution of pressures to the these muscles, and the subsequent development of prolapse.

The urogenital diaphragm closes the anterior portion of the pelvic outlet. It spans from one ischiopubic ramus to the other and is divided in the middle by genital hiatus, which contains the urethra and the vagina. The urogenital diaphragm, which includes deep transverse perineal and sphincter urethra muscles, is covered by fascia on both sides similar to other muscles in the body. The fascia on the superior surface is thin and unremarkable, whereas the inferior fascia is dense and deserves a specific name, the perineal membrane (Fig. 38.5).

As described by DeLancey, support of the posterior vaginal wall can also be divided into three levels. The perineal body and its lateral attachments make the most distal level, level III. The perineal body is the key anchoring point where

VII

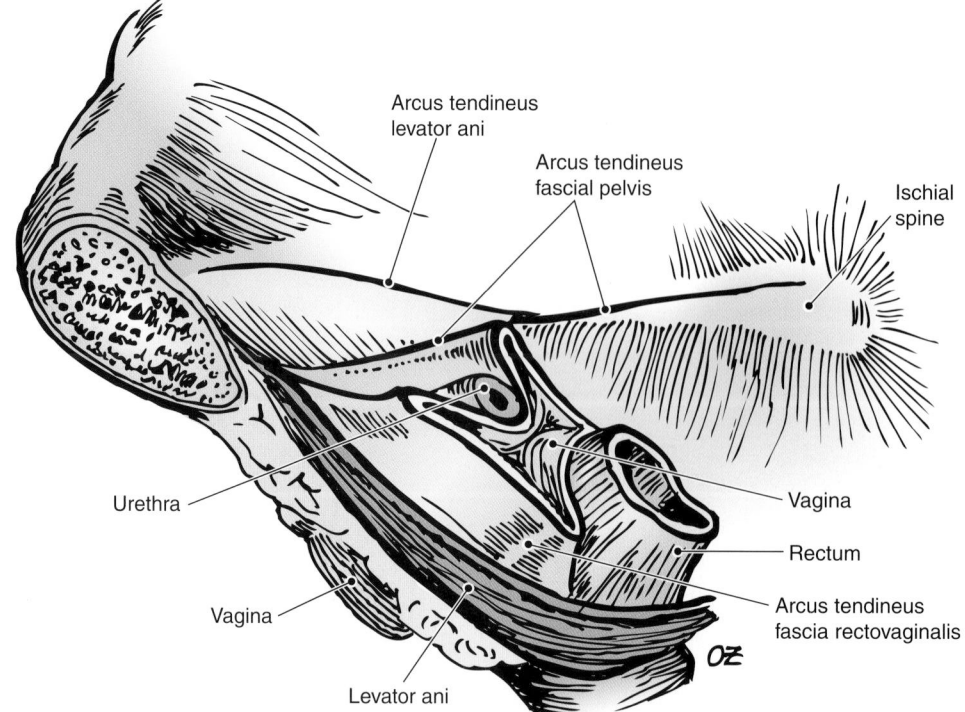

FIGURE 38.3 Pelvic floor support demonstrating the levator ani muscles and the lateral attachments of the vagina.

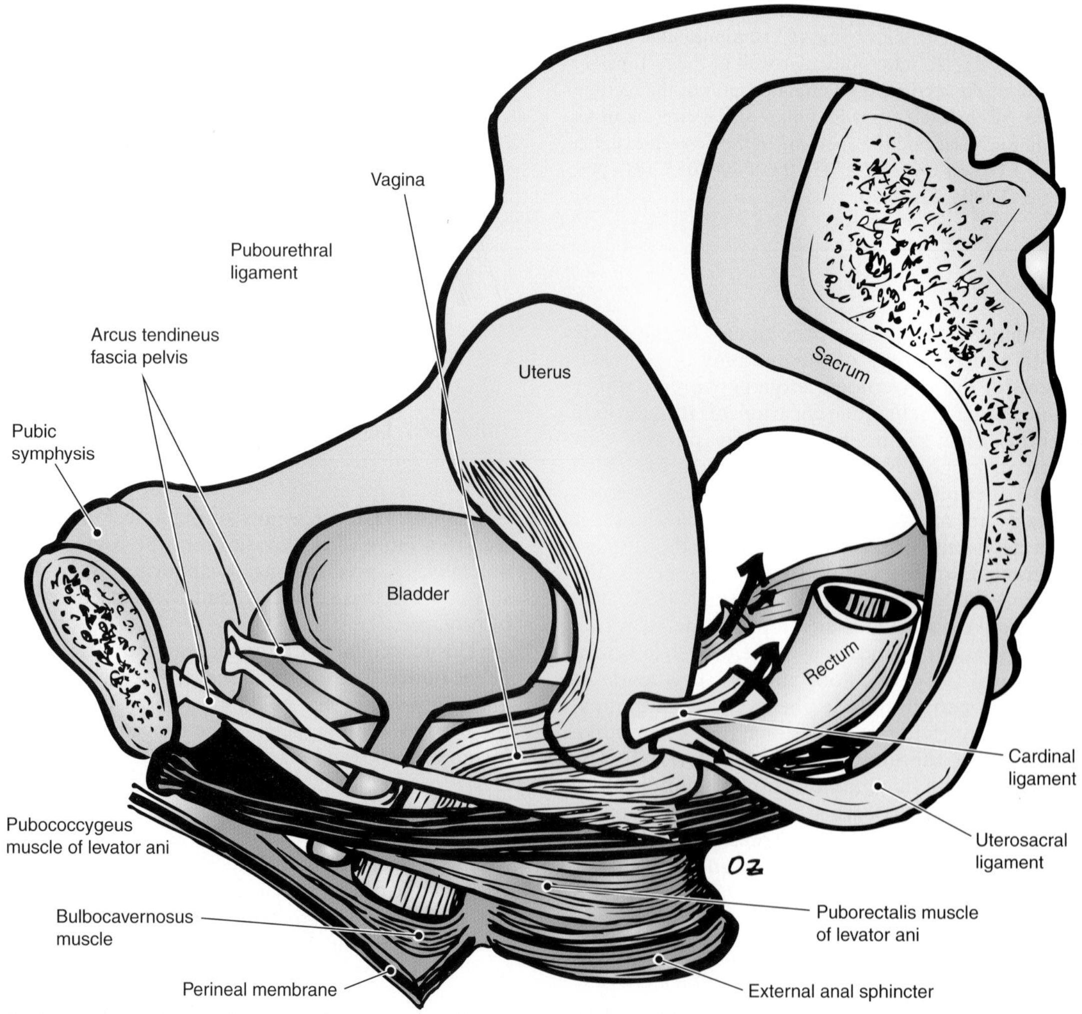

FIGURE 38.4 In the presence of normal support, the vagina is pulled posteriorly toward the sacrum by uterosacral ligaments and to a lesser degree cephalad by cardinal ligaments, resulting in an almost horizontal orientation in the proximal two thirds.

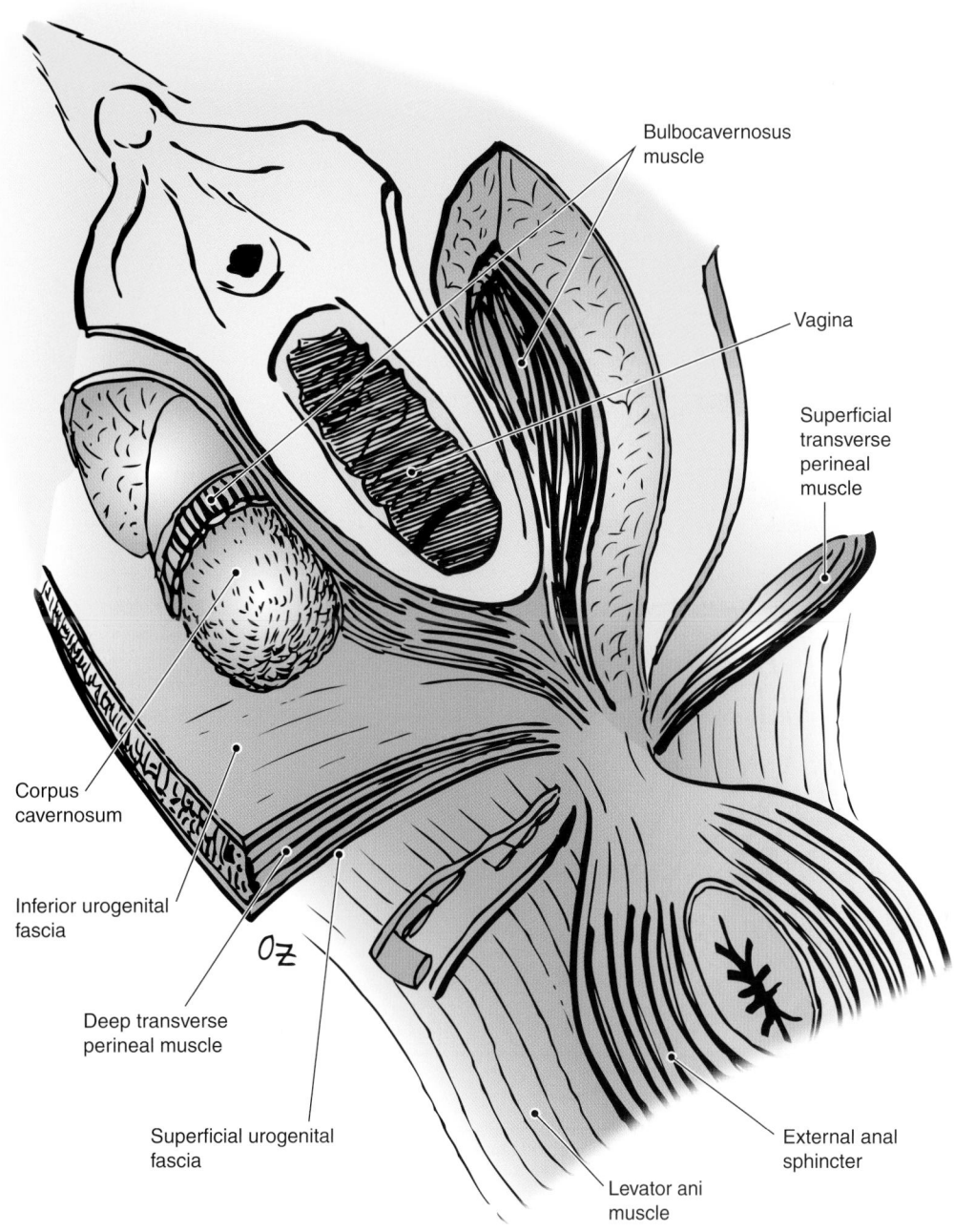

FIGURE 38.5 Urogenital diaphragm and perineal membrane.

the perineal membrane and deep transverse perineal muscles attach from each side. There is a debate among anatomists whether deep transverse perineal muscles truly exist because it is difficult to dissect a distinct striated muscle in the dense connective tissue of the urogenital diaphragm, which contains significant amount of smooth muscle fibers as well. The distal rectum lies against the dense connective tissue of the perineal body. The fibers of the perineal membrane contract and resist further displacement when the distal rectum is subjected to increased downward force. The structural integrity of the perineal body is crucial in maintaining resistance to downward displacement as it connects the right and left sides of the perineal membrane. When the perineal body is attenuated, as is often seen following obstetrical trauma, the distal

rectum becomes vulnerable to pressure and may prolapse (Fig. 38.6). The bulbocavernosus muscle, which in some anatomic descriptions is referred to as the urethrovaginal sphincter, is a thin, flat muscle with an about 5-mm width that extends dorsally along the lateral vaginal introitus immediately deep to the cephalic edge of the vestibular bulb. Its fibers interdigitate with its counterpart dorsal to the vagina within the perineal body, and as a result, level III support maintains a U configuration. Individual muscles of the perineum are not always easy to identify even in a nulliparous woman. The perineal body is thickest at the distal end of the vagina, but continues as a substantive structure for a distance of approximately 2 to 3 cm cephalad to the hymenal ring (Fig. 38.7).

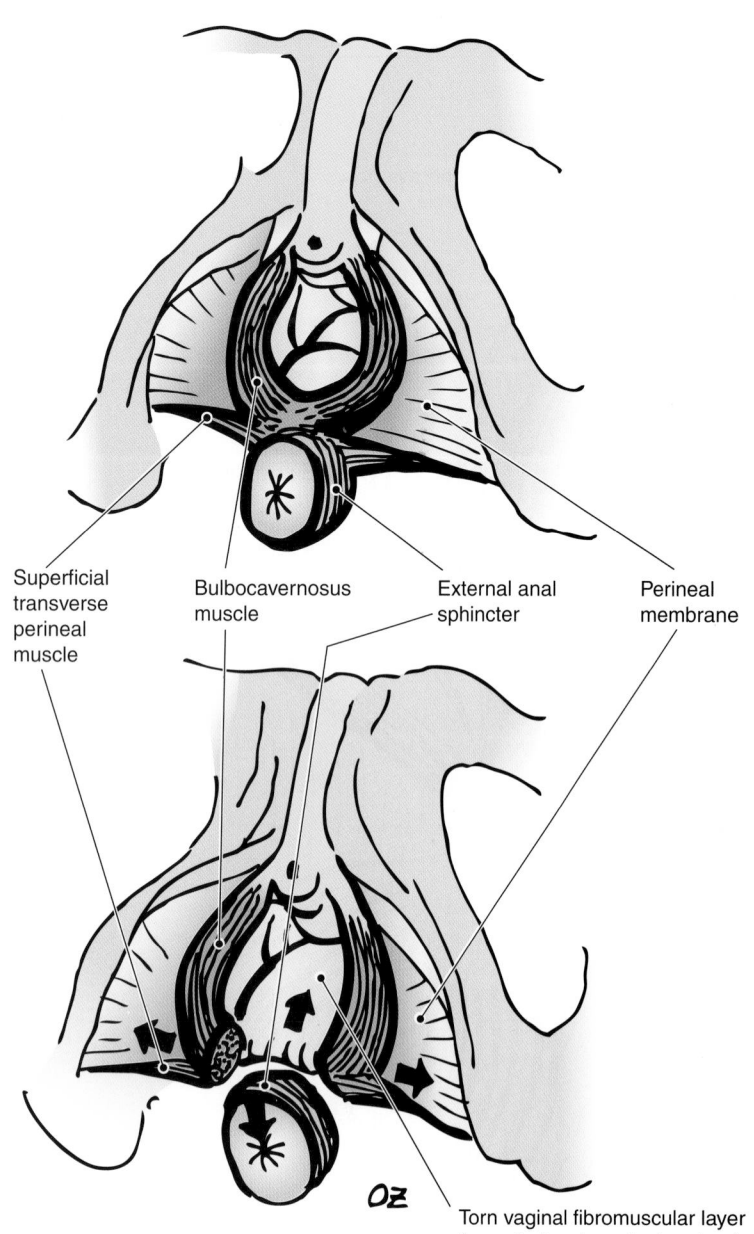

Superficial transverse perineal muscle

Bulbocavernosus muscle

External anal sphincter

Perineal membrane

Torn vaginal fibromuscular layer (so-called rectovaginal septum)

FIGURE 38.6 The perineal body is the anchoring point where the perineal membrane and deep transverse perineal muscles attach from each side. When perineal body is attenuated, as is often seen with obstetrical trauma, the distal rectum becomes vulnerable to pressure and may protrude.

The support of the posterior midvagina (level II) is continuous with the level III support. Level II support is provided by the endopelvic fascia fibers that extend from the superior surface of the pelvic diaphragm on either side of the rectum. Tension generated by these fibers in a dorsal direction creates bilateral posterior vaginal sulci and a W configuration in level II posterior compartment. Together with the levator plate formed by the pubococcygeus component of levator ani muscles, these endopelvic fascia fibers keep the posterior midvagina in a horizontal plane. A rectocele may form if these fibers are detached, as may occur with birth trauma. Any damage to the levator muscles may also result in rectocele by weakening these lateral attachments. Finally, the upper portion of the posterior vagina is attached to the lateral condensations of the endopelvic fascia, namely, the uterosacral and cardinal ligaments or level I support. The final shape of the vagina is determined by the interaction of these three levels of support.

Contrary to the general perception, the vagina is not a cylinder. Level I support makes the vagina wider at its proximal end. The vagina becomes narrower as it extends distally. Its upper two thirds is flattened horizontally due to the intricate balance of the forces controlled by level II support. In addition, the bulbocavernosus muscles practically behave almost as a sphincter at the introitus, making the distal vagina the narrowest portion. Pendergrass and her colleagues demonstrated this well by casting the vaginas of women without pelvic floor defects. Most women were shown to have conical-shaped vaginas with a width of 5 to 6 cm at the apex and 3 cm at the introitus (Fig. 38.8). The average vaginal length is 10 cm with a range from 9 to 12 cm, and it is distensible to approximately 11.5 cm.

Through cadaver studies and clinical analysis, Richardson identified various locations in the posterior vaginal wall where breaks were commonly observed. He concluded that breaks of the fibromuscular network would cause pelvic

VII

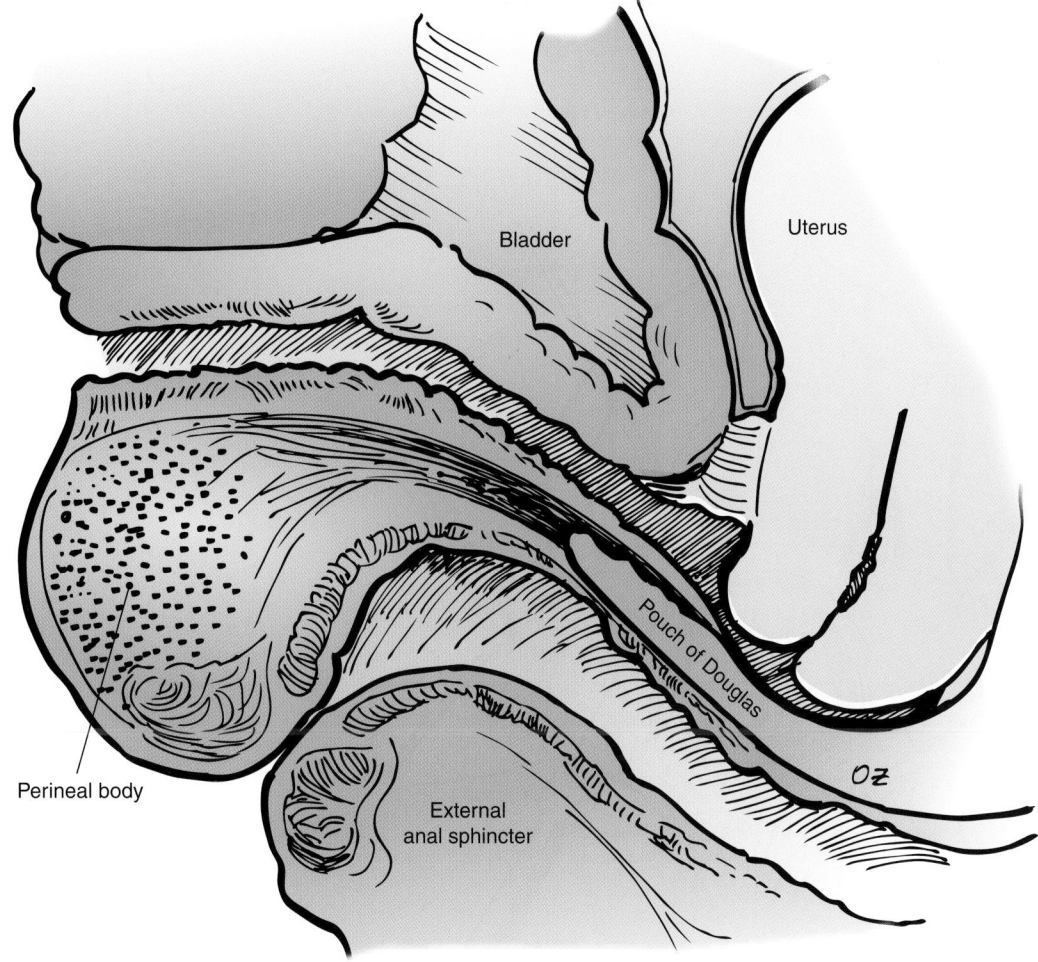

Bladder

Uterus

Pouch of Douglas

OZ

Perineal body

External
anal sphincter

FIGURE 38.7 Sagittal view of the perineal body.

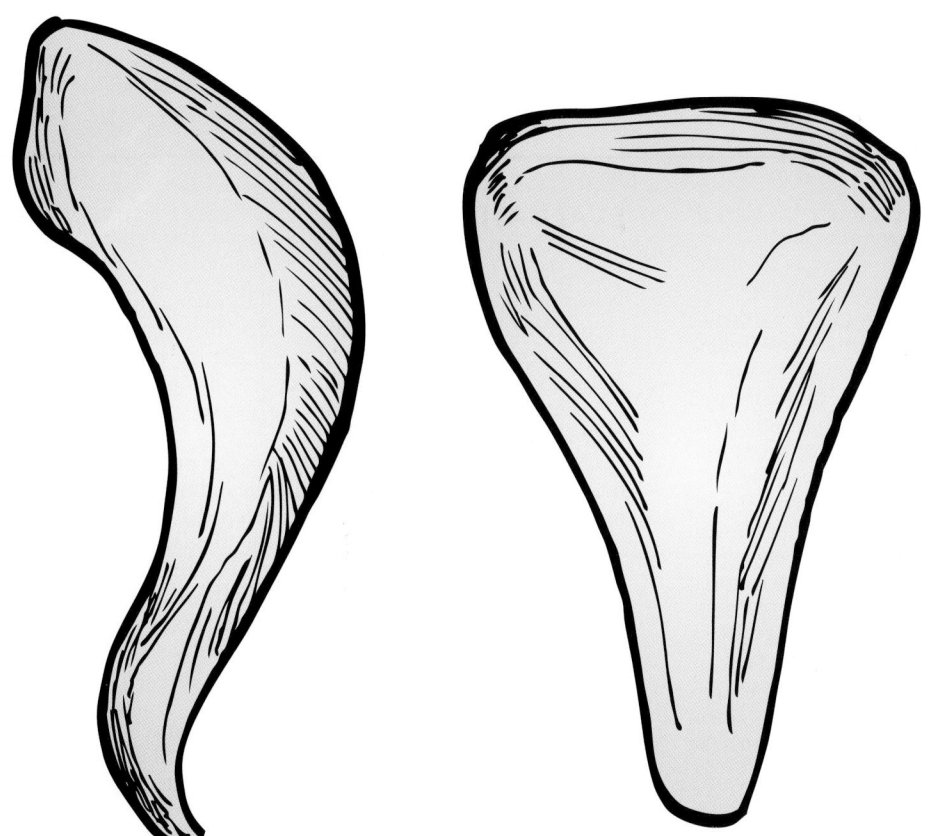

FIGURE 38.8 Most women were shown to have conical-shaped vaginas with a width about 5 to 6 cm long at the apex and 3 cm at the introitus. (After Pendergrass PB, et al. Comparison of vaginal shapes in Afro-American, Caucasian, and Hispanic women as seen with vinyl polysiloxane casting. *Gynecol Obstet Invest* 2000;50(1):54–59.)

VII

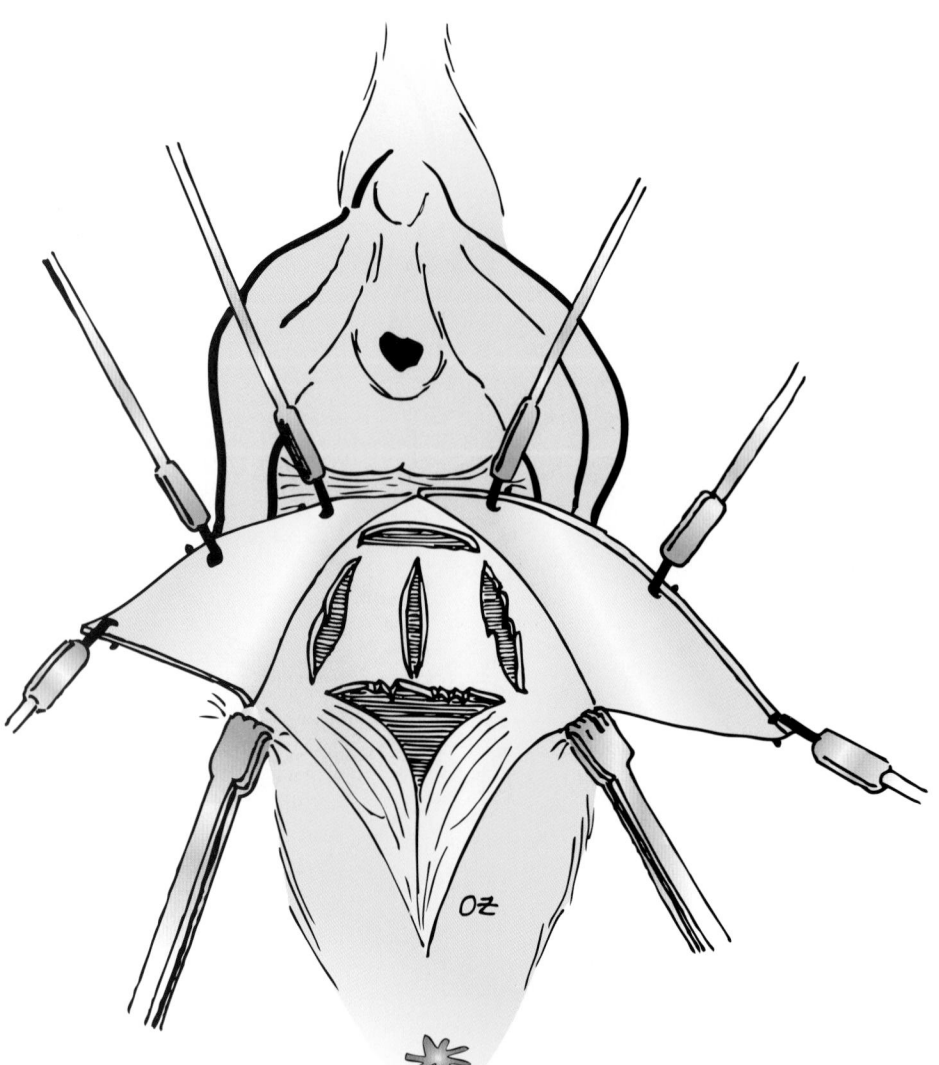

FIGURE 38.9 The formation of rectocele most likely results from discrete tears occurring in the rectovaginal fascia at various points along the posterior vagina.

organ prolapse (Fig. 38.9). Rectoceles were formed as a result of discrete "rectovaginal fascia" tears at various points along the posterior vagina. His work demonstrated that the most common defect was a transverse separation of the rectovaginal fascia from the perineal body, resulting in a low (distal) rectocele. With similar frequency, he and other researchers identified midline vertical defects that were caused by poorly repaired or healed lacerations or episiotomies. In addition, a high (proximal) rectocele or an enterocele may result from detachment of the vaginal fibromuscular layer from the pericervical ring.

The anatomic findings of Richardson's work correlate well with the different types of rectoceles encountered in clinical practice. Identification of these defects intraoperatively is paramount for a lasting, successful repair. Defects in midvaginal support can give rise to a rectocele, which may occur in the middle of the vagina despite normal levator function and an intact perineal body. This condition must be addressed not by plicating the rectovaginal fascia but by retrieving and reuniting the separated fibers of the perineal body. If the perineal body has separated from the level II support, they must be reunited.

EVALUATION

History

Pelvic organ prolapse is usually mildly symptomatic or even asymptomatic. It is often discovered by the gynecologists during a routine visit or an encounter for another reason. Prolapse generally becomes symptomatic once it has passed the hymenal ring. Severely symptomatic prolapse usually represents only a small group of patients.

Prior to the first visit, all patients in our practice are sent an intake form for general information including medical history, medications, previous surgeries, obstetrical and gynecologic history, and social history along with standardized condition specific questionnaires. This is reviewed by the physician prior to the patient encounter. Obtaining initial patient data through these forms facilitate the discussion at the first visit as patients with pelvic organ prolapse often have a difficult time discussing some of their symptoms and concerns due to their sensitive nature.

Patients with posterior vaginal wall prolapse usually complain of a sense of pelvic pressure or bulge and difficulty with initiating and completing evacuation. They often report a need for digitation for bowel movements and pressure on the posterior vagina or perineum in an effort to complete rectal evacuation. Pain during intercourse may also be a consequence of a posterior vaginal wall prolapse.

Symptoms of DD should be carefully delineated in all women with pelvic organ prolapse, especially in the posterior compartment. When the patient reports constipation, a thorough understanding of stool frequency and consistency is important as the definition of constipation can vary. When evaluating a patient with DD, one must first exclude systemic causes including metabolic, neurologic, endocrine, or psychiatric abnormalities. In addition, if a functional disorder, that is, dysmotility, irritable bowel syndrome, colonic inertia, or functional constipation, is suspected, the appropriate studies should be performed with referral to a gastroenterologist. In cases of obstructed defecation, it is prudent to exclude gastrointestinal abnormalities that could result in these symptoms including rectal prolapse, colorectal tumors, hemorrhoids, or fecal impaction. Defecatory dyssynergia should also be ruled out in patients with a functional abnormality. On defecography or anal manometry, the findings would include contraction or failure to relax the puborectalis and/or the external anal sphincter muscles with attempted defecation. The gynecologic surgeon is then left with a patient with obstructed defecation that is likely due to the anatomical abnormalities associated with posterior compartment prolapse. In many cases, symptoms generally do no correlate with the severity of prolapse. It is not unusual to see a severely symptomatic woman with only mild anatomic defects. A recent cross-sectional study failed to identify an association between symptoms of incomplete evacuation and straining. In addition, the patient should understand that surgery may not improve chronic constipation, and, in fact, constipation may contribute to the return of a rectocele if not managed aggressively after surgery.

Information regarding fecal incontinence, which may present with pelvic organ prolapse, is not always volunteered due to embarrassment. When it is present, the physician must consider appropriate investigation to rule out dysfunction of the anorectal sphincteric mechanism, neurologic abnormality, a bowel lesion, or a rectal mass. Patients may also describe coital discomfort or a sensation of obstruction in the vagina by their partner. This can be due to prolapse in any compartment, but may often be seen when the couple attempts intercourse in the presence of a rectocele and hard stool in the vault. It is important to remember that pelvic organ prolapse is frequently complex; in addition to a careful history of DD, a complete history of any urinary voiding dysfunction should be obtained.

Physical Examination

Physical examination should begin with a brief mental status exam, assessment of cranial nerve integrity, and cerebellar control. Deep tendon reflexes and muscle strength should be assessed in the lower extremities. Once this is complete, the remainder of the exam takes place in a dorsal lithotomy position. Sensory function may be quickly evaluated from dermatomes L2 through S3 by testing for sensation to pinprick or light touch. The integrity of S3 is elicited by swabbing the perineum and observing for a contraction of the external anal sphincter. The Pelvic Organ Prolapse-Quantification exam is performed using a measuring spatula, which can be marked with centimeter markings to improve precision. First, the genital hiatus and perineal body are measured. Then, a lubricated speculum is inserted in the vagina for inspection of the entire vagina and the cervix. At this time, the measuring spatula is placed in the posterior fornix to measure total vagina length when the patient is at rest. The patient is then asked to perform a Valsalva maneuver with the spatula in the vaginal apex to quantify vaginal apical descent. This is followed by inspection and measurement of the descent of each vaginal wall under maximum Valsalva effort when the posterior blade of the split speculum is used to support the opposite compartment.

The examiner should avoid excessive support, especially apically, as this can lead to underestimation of the extent of the prolapse. A bimanual examination is then performed to assess the size and position of the uterus and the adnexa; this can also be used to reassess apical descent as it is of paramount importance in any surgical planning for pelvic organ prolapse. Before the fingers are removed, they are rotated 180 degrees to evaluate the integrity and strength of the levator muscles. The patient is asked to perform a "Kegel" contraction for assessment of the patient's ability to control these muscles. It is important that the patient believes that the extent of prolapse demonstrated in the office is consistent with what she feels on a regular basis. If the examiner is unable to elicit the maximum extent of her prolapse, the exam should be repeated in a standing position with Valsalva. It may sometimes be helpful to leave the patient alone in the room for her to reproduce a physical activity or position that aggravates the prolapse. If these efforts fail, the exam can be repeated on a different day.

Once the maximum descent of each compartment is ascertained, the focus is turned to delineate exact location of the defects of each compartment. Typically, smoothening and loss of rugae in any part of the posterior wall may indicate an area that lacks fibromuscular support. As reviewed in the anatomy section of this chapter, a common defect seen in the posterior compartment occurs because of separation and retraction of perineal muscles and disruption of so-called rectovaginal septum from the perineal body. This is reflected on physical examination as a finding of skin-fold-like perineal body that has lost its fibromuscular elements including bulbocavernosus muscles in the midline; formation of a dimple between this fold and the most protruding part of the distal posterior vaginal wall; and, commonly, an increased genital hiatus measurement, which often occurs at the expense of perineal body (Fig. 38.10). A longitudinal defect along the rectovaginal fascia, with lateral disruption of the fascia on either side, may present itself as a false and asymmetric longitudinal sulcus. Proximal posterior vaginal wall prolapse, which is a result of an apical detachment of the rectovaginal fascia from the pericervical fascia, also causes loss of rugae and flattening of vaginal surface in the defective area. The perineum is then carefully examined at rest and with straining. If a 2-cm or more descent of the perineum below the ischial tuberosities is identified, there is perineal body descent. A shortened distance between hymenal ring and rectum indicates perineal body deficiency.

Posterior vaginal wall examination is incomplete until a thorough bimanual rectovaginal examination is performed. Rectal examination begins with inspection of the anus. Then, the examiner inserts one index finger into the rectum first to assess the internal and external anal sphincter tone. Identification of any incidental rectal masses or lesions is crucial. The rectal examination should also include palpation of the rectal wall with simultaneous palpation and observation of the posterior vagina with the other index finger (Fig. 38.11). If the rectal-examining finger contains the entire posterior vaginal bulge, a rectocele is likely present. However, a significant defect above the examining finger likely represents an enterocele or possibly a sigmoidocele.

VII

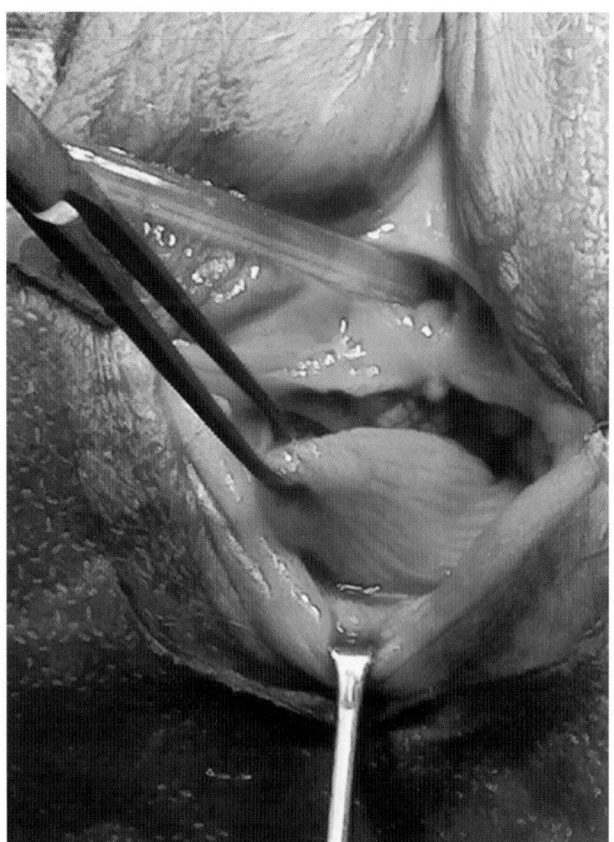
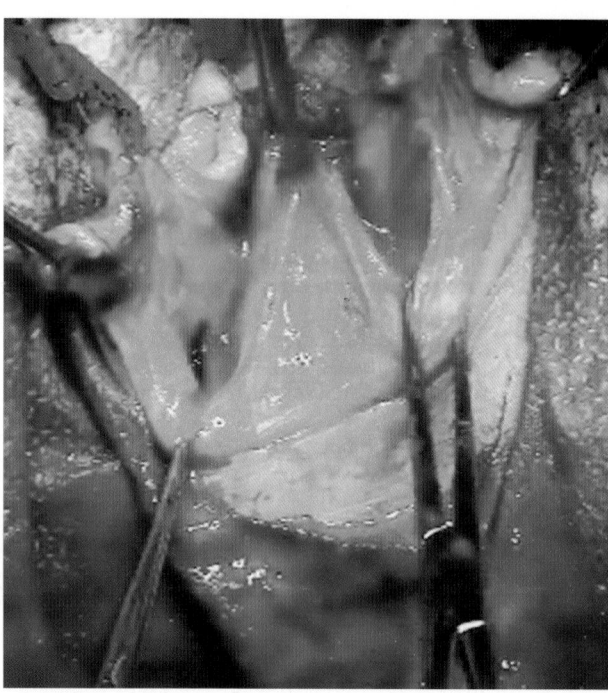

A   B

FIGURE 38.10 The most common defect is a transverse separation of the rectovaginal fascia from the perineal body, resulting in a low (distal) rectocele. **A:** This is reflected on physical examination as a finding of skin-fold-like perineal body and formation of a dimple between this fold and most protruding part of the distal posterior vaginal wall. **B:** Shows the same defect dissected. Allis clamp is pulling the torn edge of vaginal muscularis.

Ancillary Testing

Identification of a rectocele is generally made clinically. Ancillary testing is not a standard part of the rectocele evaluation. We perform simple cystometry on all patients with advanced prolapse, including those without urinary loss as occult incontinence may often be present. With the bladder filled to capacity, after the rectocele is reduced with two scopettes or a half speculum, stress testing with Valsalva maneuver and a cough is performed in the supine and standing position. When apical or anterior descent is also identified, urodynamic studies are performed on patients prior to surgery because urinary incontinence is often coincident in these cases.

Multiple ancillary tests may be appropriate in patients with surgical failure or atypical presentations. For any patient with DD, collaboration with a gastroenterologist is prudent in order to assess problems associated with endocrine or metabolic conditions, malabsorption, colonic motility, and dietary issues. Consultation with a colorectal surgeon and colonoscopy may be indicated for rectal abnormalities such as hemorrhoids, prolapse, and anal fissures.

Imaging studies that can be useful in posterior vaginal wall prolapse include defecography and dynamic magnetic resonance imaging; however, radiologic diagnosis of rectocele has not been standardized. Defecography is a fluoroscopic study performed after insertion of radiopaque contrast material into the colon. Defecography provides dynamic visualization of defecation under fluoroscopy. It may assist identification of the location and size of a rectocele, rectal prolapse, intussusception, and sigmoidocele. In addition, there should be a coordinated relaxation of the puborectalis and external anal sphincter muscles with defecation, the absence of which may indicate dysynergy of the pelvic floor. There are, however, no studies indicating that the information obtained with defecography will alter management or clinical outcomes.

Dynamic magnetic resonance imaging (MRI) will provide the highest-quality images of the posterior vagina and surrounding structures, without exposure to radiation. However, this test may not demonstrate the true extent of prolapse as it is performed in a supine position. The clinical utility of MRI, which is costly and not performed at all centers, is also debatable.

Anal manometry is used to assess rectal function by measuring the resting and squeeze sphincter pressure as well as the functional length of the anal canal. Functional anal canal length is the length of the anal canal over which resting pressure exceeds that of the rectum by greater than 5 mm Hg. Rectal compliance reflects the capacity and distensibility of the rectum. Higher compliance indicates lower resistance to distention.

Electrophysiologic studies of bowel function such as electromyography and nerve conduction velocity, especially those measuring individual muscle responses, have generally been abandoned by physical therapists and gastroenterologists because of the tests' inability to measure clinically significant parameters.

Endoanal ultrasound can be used for the diagnosis of anal sphincter defects in patients presenting with fecal incontinence but has limited utility for managing rectoceles.

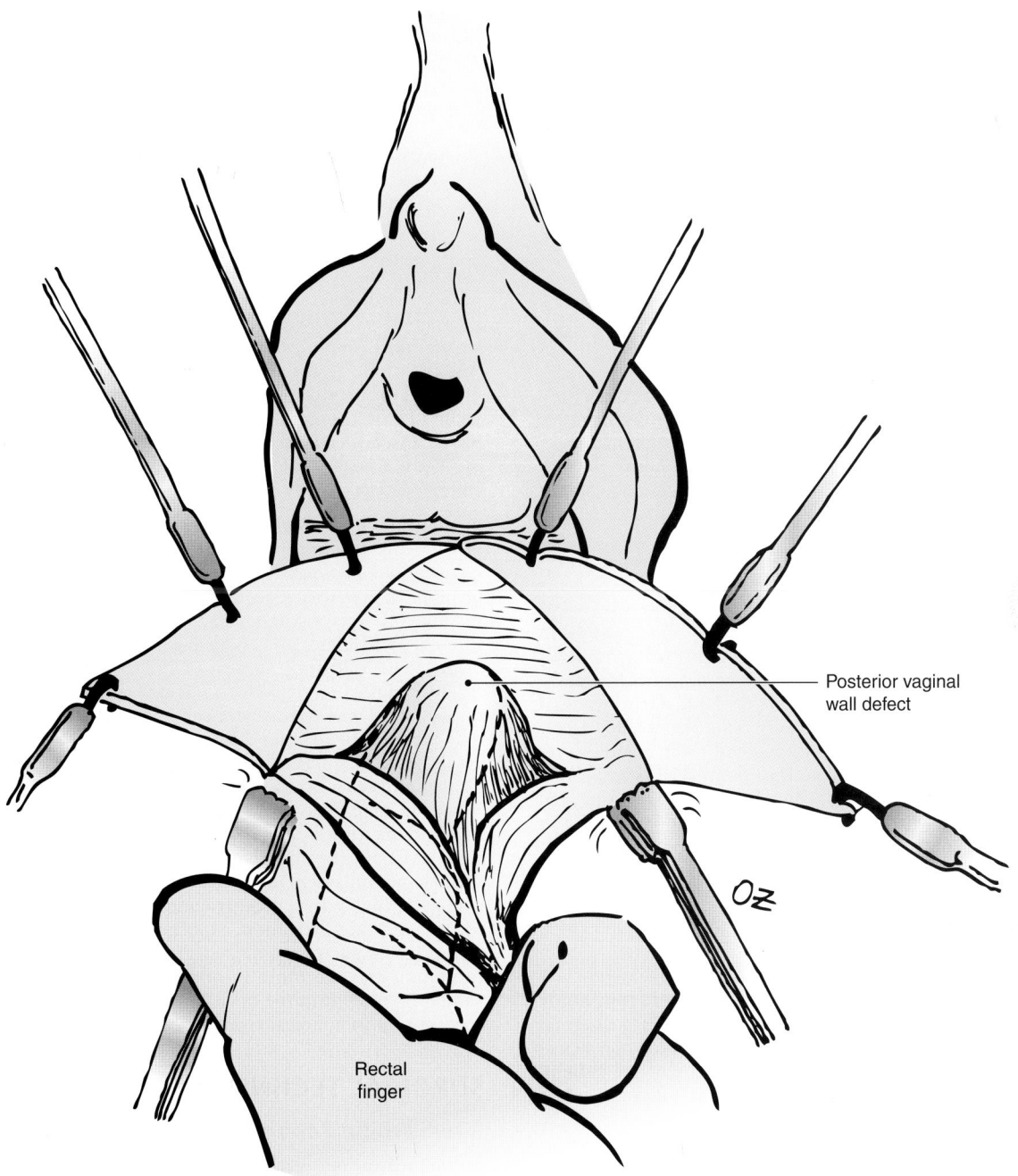

Posterior vaginal
wall defect

Rectal
finger

FIGURE 38.11 The rectal examination should also include palpation of the rectal wall with simultaneous palpation and observation of the posterior vagina with the other index finger. If the rectal examining finger contains the entire posterior vaginal bulge, a rectocele is likely present. However, a significant defect above the examining finger likely represents an enterocele or possibly a sigmoidocele.

MANAGEMENT

Conservative Management

Asymptomatic patients may be managed expectantly. For most patients, reassurance and review of precautions and lifestyle changes, which may prevent progression of prolapse, is sufficient. We recommend a follow-up visit to monitor the changes in the symptoms and pelvic floor in 6 to 12 months.

For patients who have symptoms related to pelvic organ prolapse, the most common nonsurgical approach is use of a pessary. Unfortunately, data on pessaries are limited. There is

no specific pessary that works best for patients with rectoceles. The examiner should decide which pessary is appropriate based on the patient's vaginal length, genital hiatus, sexual activity, and severity of prolapse. Clemons et al. found that a vaginal length of 6 cm or less and an introitus greater than 4 fingerbreadths were risk factors for an unsuccessful pessary trial. In addition, prior pelvic surgery and previous hysterectomy were also associated with increased failure of pessary trial. We generally begin with a supportive pessary such as a ring pessary with a platform and attempt multiple sizes. If the patient cannot retain the pessary, it is uncomfortable, or the pessary does not provide enough support, we generally will move to the Gellhorn pessary, a space-occupying pessary. Donut and cube pessaries are rarely used, if ever, in our practice as we find they often result in ulcerations and copious vaginal discharge and are very difficult to insert and remove.

Pelvic floor physical therapy and biofeedback have both been shown to improve symptoms from pelvic organ prolapse, especially in early stages. Its greatest role may be in the treatment of dysergy of the pelvic floor. It should also be utilized for patients with fecal incontinence with the addition of biofeedback.

SURGICAL MANAGEMENT

Informed Consent

The preoperative office visit is crucial for a detailed discussion of natural history, treatment options including conservative and surgical methods, and risks and benefits of each treatment alternative. It is advisable to ask the patient to come to the visit with family members in an effort to provide a clear understanding of the procedure not only by the patient but also those who may potentially be affected by the surgery or participate in her care during her recovery. Explaining prolapse and the procedure with simplified visuals can make it easier for the patients to differentiate between facts and fallacies in this sensitive era since the warning of the Food and Drug Administration. In our practice, we continue judicial use of grafts for pelvic floor reconstruction in women who present with an isolated stage III proximal posterior compartment prolapse with proximal rectocele and/or enterocele, especially if they have failed a previous native tissue repair. We recommend using a procedure-specific consent form, which lists the potential risks associated with surgery in addition to the one required by the hospital in all surgical cases whether graft material will be introduced or not. Detailed guidelines for the consent can be found on the American Urogynecologic Society Web site using the consent toolkit (www.augs.org).

Bowel Preparation

Although some pelvic surgeons advise a light lunch and clear liquids for dinner followed by a fleet enema, there is no study to guide us regarding bowel preparation before transvaginal pelvic floor repair. Therefore, surgical preparation for a posterior wall repair can be minimal on the part of the patient. Patients can simply be instructed to discontinue oral intake at midnight the night before surgery. Simple evacuation of the rectum at the time of surgery may be sufficient for posterior vaginal repair.

Anesthesia and Preoperative Preparation

Regional anesthesia with spinal or epidural approach is very suitable and may even be more appropriate for vaginal procedures. Local anesthesia with conscious sedation may also be utilized when general or regional anesthesia is considered too risky. Although there is no strong evidence for guidance, preoperative single-dose intravenous antibiotic has been the standard for all vaginal procedures. Prevention for venous thromboembolism with sequential compression boots or subcutaneous heparin is routine.

Patient Positioning

Posterior compartment repairs are performed with the patient in a dorsal lithotomy position. We prefer stirrups that support the entire lower extremity for these cases, but the surgeon should use the stirrup of his or her choice. During positioning, the minimum angles should be 60 degrees between the thighs and the torso and 90 degrees at the knee in an effort to prevent any tension or pressure on any aspect of the lower extremities. The patient's buttocks should extend slightly over the edge of the table for best access. Although helpful in the anterior compartment procedures, Trendelenburg position may hinder ergonomic dissection during posterior repairs in the distal vagina. The bladder is generally emptied and drained throughout the case as not to obstruct visibility. A self-retaining retractor can be used to improve visualization. We prefer the Lone Star Retractor System (CooperSurgical, Trumbull, CT) for this purpose and generally use at least six retraction hooks during the procedure. We find the rectangular-shaped retractor to be the most helpful, but other shapes may also be adopted. Additional retractors are needed only occasionally when self-retaining retraction systems are in use. Initial retraction can be facilitated by placing the first two hooks at the hymenal ring, which also holds the self-retaining retractor in place.

Instruments

In addition to the self-retaining retractors, several surgical instruments facilitate the identification of tissue layers, dissection, and hemostasis. In addition to at least six to eight medium and at least two long Allis clamps to grasp the epithelium or other tissue layers, we recommend including six to eight Pratt clamps (T-shaped grasping clamps) in the surgical set to hold the edges of epithelial incisions. The blunt rounded tips of curved Mayo scissors are ideal for dissection of vaginal planes. When necessary, Metzenbaum scissors also may be used for delicate dissection. Versatility of ribbon malleable retractors makes them very suitable for vaginal surgery. Deaver and wide Breisky-Navratil retractors also can be used. When an apical suspension procedure such as sacrospinous ligament fixation is also planned, a suture placement device such as Capio (Boston Scientific, Marlborough, MA) and its special monofilament delayed absorbable sutures should be available. Lighted suction–irrigation devices are very helpful for visualization, irrigation, exposure, and hemostasis. Hemostatic agents such as oxidized regenerated cellulose, topical thrombin, and the other thrombin products in gelatin foam should be present in the operating room particularly for procedures requiring apical repairs.

SURGICAL TECHNIQUES

Site-Specific Repair

In our institution, we have adopted a site-specific approach. This technique requires identification and repair of discrete tears in the rectovaginal wall. Intraoperative examination under anesthesia is essential for confirmation of the findings in the outpatient setting and ascertainment of the specific defects in the posterior compartment. It also will determine the appropriate plane of dissection during the surgery once the surgeon decides between native tissue and graft-augmented repair in a woman with advanced posterior compartment prolapse who has permitted the use of grafts, if deemed necessary. Full-thickness dissection is imperative if graft use is decided.

After a careful inspection of the rugae and palpation of the rectovaginal wall with rectovaginal examination as described above, the defects may be identified with improved accuracy under anesthesia before any incision is made. If the surgeon decides that apical disruption has resulted in a severe displacement of the most proximal end of the rectovaginal tear from the apical support structures and significant shortening of the fibromuscular layer, graft use is considered. Because the possibility of graft utilization is discussed at length during the informed consent process, the surgeon should feel comfortable proceeding with graft application. The other important determinants of graft use include a previous failed attempt, chronic constipation, patient's current sexual activity, and functional expectations from the surgery.

Injection of local anesthetics with epinephrine into the surgical field is commonly recommended in an effort to hydro-dissect vaginal tissue planes and provide hemostasis. In our opinion, this is not necessary and may potentially complicate identification of correct tissue planes. If the dissection is performed accurately, there will not be any significant bleeding as the vascular elements reside in the fibromuscular layer. Minor bleeding due to perforators between the layers can easily be controlled with judicious use of cautery.

If intraoperative assessment of the posterior vaginal wall concludes that native tissue repair is to be performed, the surgeon should start the dissection between the epithelial and fibromuscular layers (so-called "rectovaginal septum") of the vagina. The procedure starts with placement of Allis clamps on each side of the hymenal ring at approximately 4 o'clock and 8 o'clock. Approximation of the Allis clamps in the midline will give the surgeon a good estimate of vaginal caliber after the

procedure. The reconstructed vagina should be able accommodate three fingers comfortably. These two Allis clamps remain in place for the entire duration of the repair. If these clamps are held by an assistant during dissection and suture placement, the direction and force of the traction applied on these clamps should be equal to maintain symmetry.

Restoration of perineal body anatomy is integral to all posterior vaginal repairs in our practice. As described above, its role in rectal support and normal pelvic function as the level III support is critical. Perineal body repair may also add 2 to 3 cm to the vaginal length. Therefore, our initial incision is made to accommodate a perineorrhaphy as well. With this goal in mind, another Allis clamp is placed at the perineal end of the posterior fourchette. These three clamps represent the corners of a triangular skin incision, which will be made in this location (Fig. 38.12). These incisions can be made with cautery. This triangular skin portion is then removed with particular attention to preserve the perineal connective tissue and maintain hemostasis. Then, another Allis clamp is placed on the posterior vagina at the midline, approximately 3 to 4 cm proximal from the hymenal ring. After one Allis is placed on each side of the midpoint of the vaginal side of the transverse incision for outward traction, Mayo scissors with their tips up are used to start the dissection of the vaginal epithelium

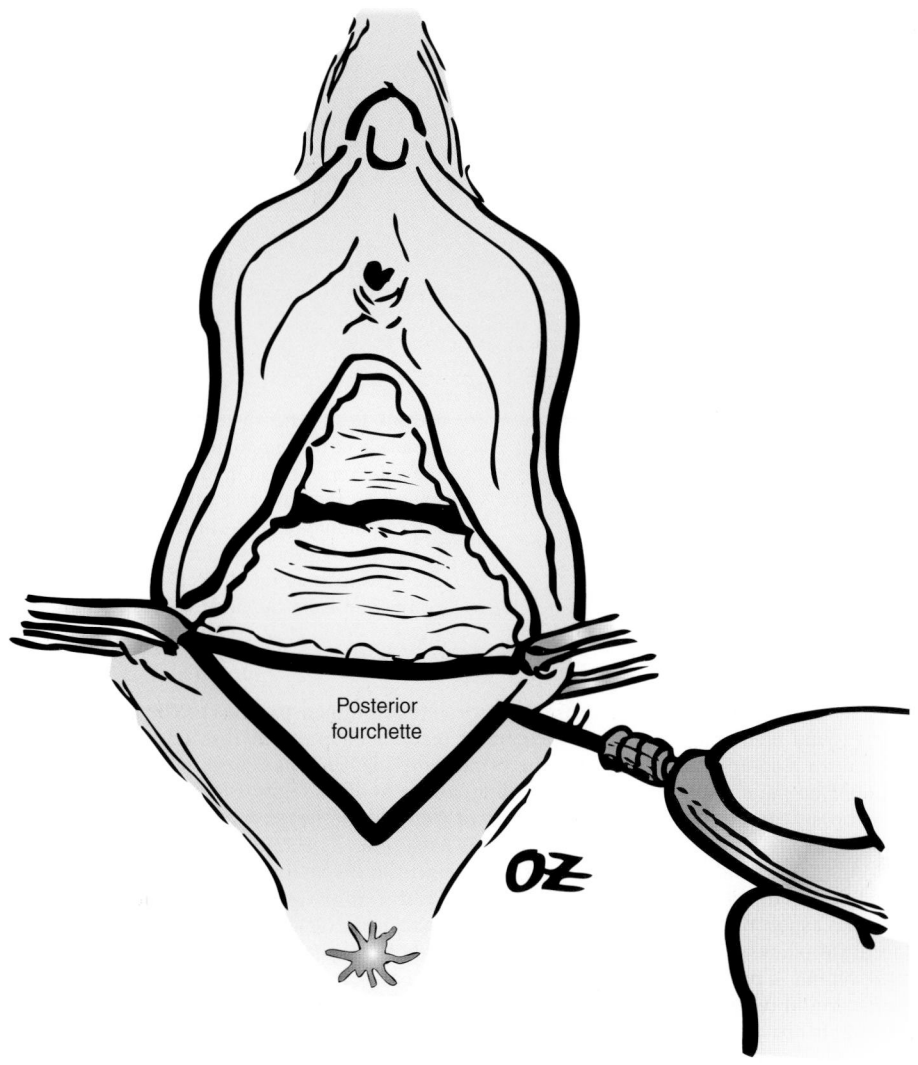

Posterior fourchette

FIGURE 38.12 After assessment of targeted introital dimensions by placing Allis clamps on each side of the posterior hymenal ring, a triangular skin incision is made on the posterior fourchette and the skin within this triangle is removed.

VII

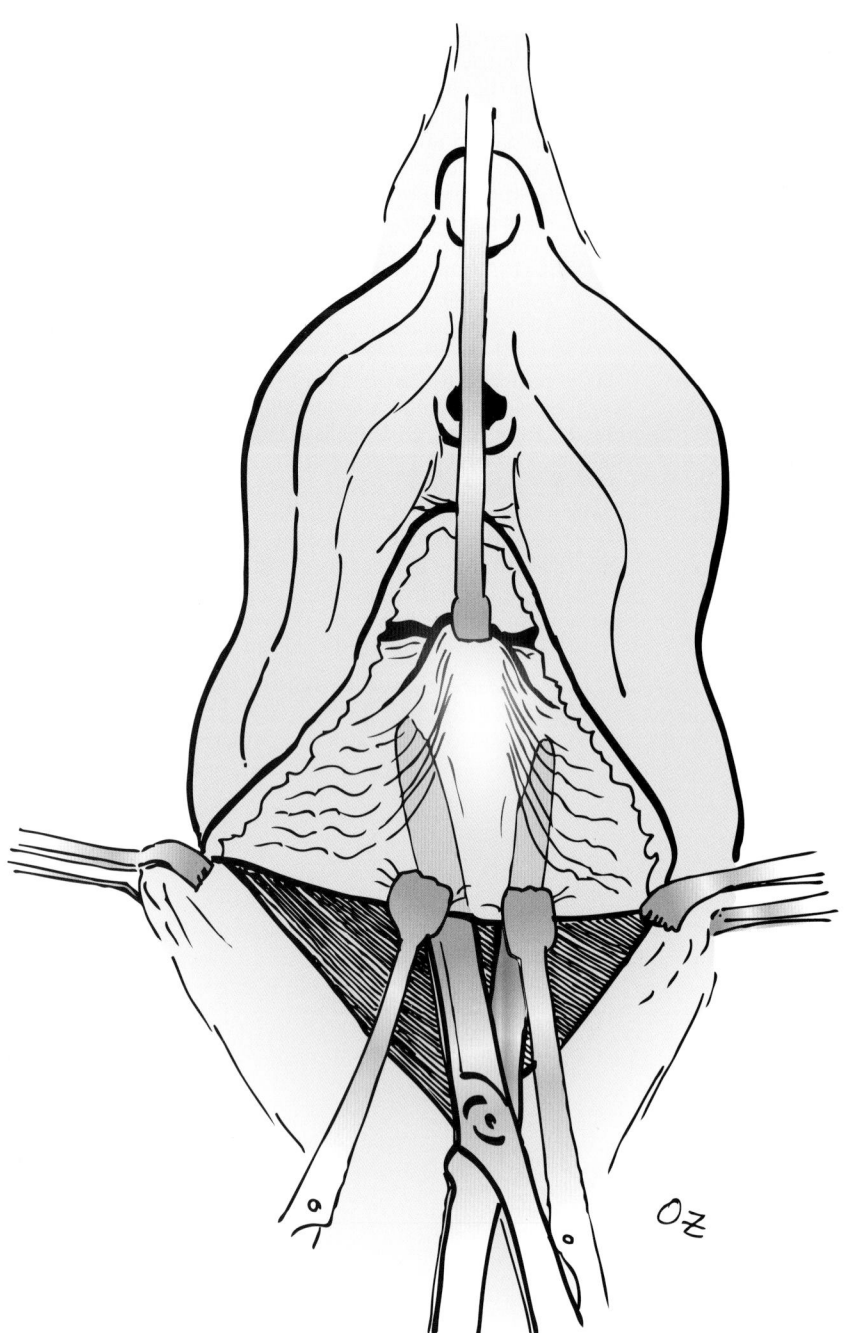

FIGURE 38.13 After one Allis clamp is placed on each side of the midpoint of the vaginal side of the transverse incision, another Allis clamp is placed on the posterior vagina at the midline, approximately 3 to 4 cm proximal from the hymenal ring. Mayo scissors with their tips up are used to start the dissection of the vaginal epithelium from the underlying fibromuscular tissue.

from the underlying fibromuscular tissue (Fig. 38.13). Identification of the correct plane between the vaginal epithelial and fibromuscular layers at the onset is crucial for a complete and hemostatic dissection. The surgeon should be patient as this plane may not be easily entered due to fibrosis caused by previous obstetrical trauma or repair or pelvic floor repairs in the distal posterior vagina. Placing the nondominant index finger on the vaginal epithelium may add tactile feedback at this point (Fig. 38.14). Blanching on the vaginal aspect of this dissection plane ensures entry into the accurate plane. Once the commonly fibrotic portion in the distal vagina is passed, the dissection becomes easier. Mayo scissors should never be pushed bluntly when previous repairs or mesh are present in this area. Inadvertent rectal entry can be avoided if the

dissecting scissors is maintained parallel to the vaginal wall. Once the correct plane is entered, the dissection is continued toward the proximally placed Allis clamp, which elevates the vaginal midline, and a midline sagittal incision can be made. The cut edges of the midline incision are then grasped with Pratt clamps on each side. The midline Allis clamp is then moved cephalad, and the dissection is continued for another 3 cm. A pair of Pratt clamps is placed on each side. This approximately 6-cm incision is typically sufficient to complete any posterior repair because the rest of the dissection toward the vaginal apex can easily be accomplished without any further midline incision.

Once the midline incision is complete, the rest of the dissection in the apical and lateral direction is performed with Mayo

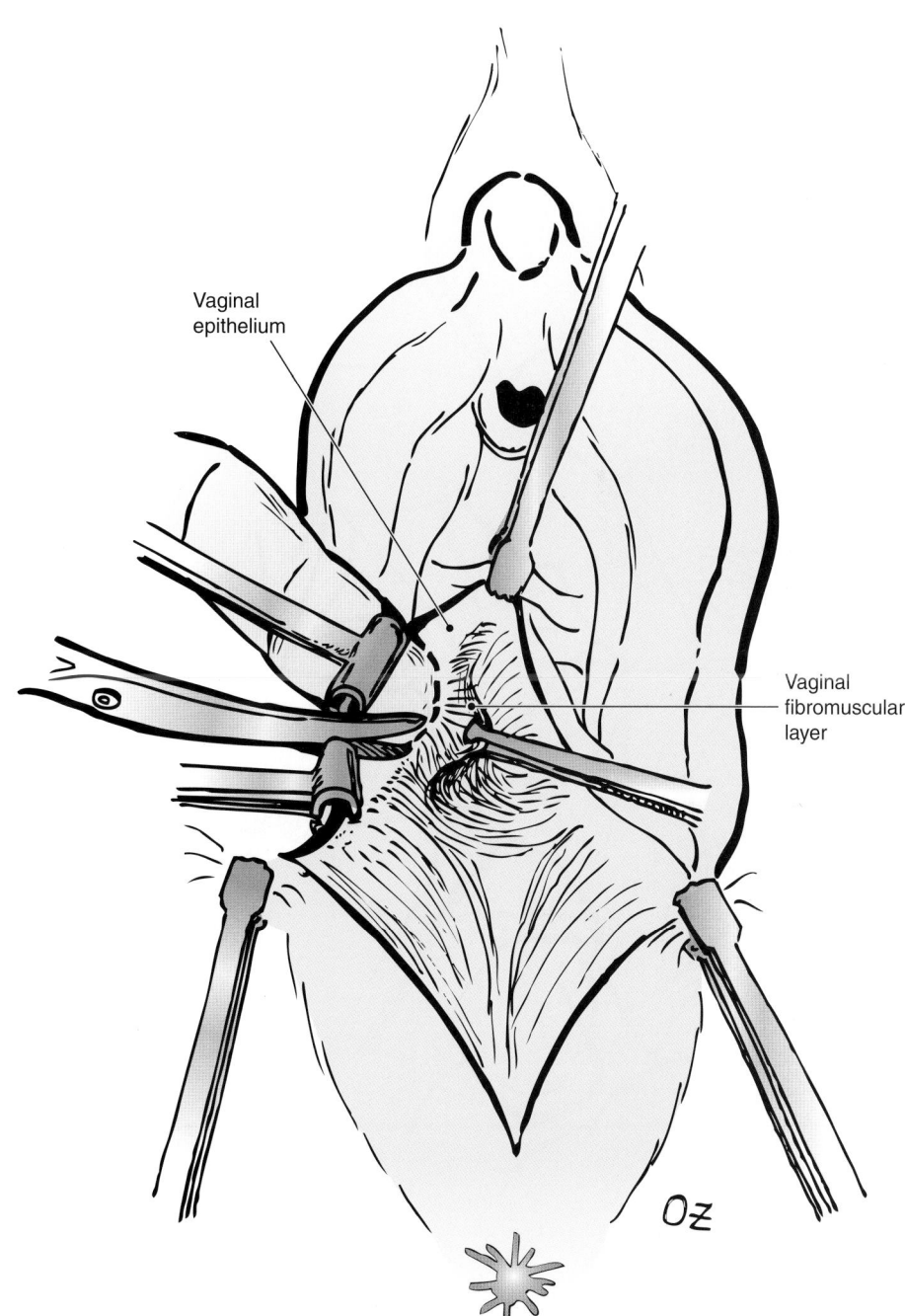

Vaginal
epithelium

Vaginal
fibromuscular
layer

FIGURE 38.14 Once the midline incision is complete, the rest of the dissection in the apical and lateral direction is performed with Mayo scissors using spread and snip technique with the help of Pratt clamps applying traction on the incision to facilitate dissection.

VII

scissors using spread and snip technique with the help of Pratt clamps applying traction on the incision (Fig. 38.14). In addition, countertraction provided by an assistant on the fibromuscular layer is helpful. For best results, the concave side of the scissors is pressed against the convex curve of the nondominant index finger lying on the vaginal epithelial surface during this dissection. Starting the dissection at the apex of the midline incision is helpful as tissue planes are easier to identify in this area where scarring is rarely encountered unless the repair is for recurrent prolapse. A white undersurface on the vaginal wall against the pink- and red-colored vascular fibromuscular layer represents the correct dissection plane. Bleeding is often a sign that the fibromuscular layer has been invaded. The dissection is continued laterally to the attachment of the fibromuscular layer to the inner levator fascia and until all the defects

are exposed. This dissection leaves an inverted T-shaped incision. Premenopausal women will have abundant venous lakes especially at the perineal body on either side. Energy should be used judiciously to allow for a hemostatic dissection. At this point, the Pratt clamps are replaced with retraction hooks. It is important to maintain symmetry during the placement of these hooks. Typically, there will be no need for a manual retractor once the retraction hooks of the self-retaining system are placed.

After careful evaluation of the entire rectovaginal wall between two opposing index fingers, one in the rectum and the other in the vagina, all the defects are identified and labeled with Allis clamps or sutures (Fig. 38.15). Torn and retracted perineal fibromuscular structure on both sides distal at the level of the introitus should also be visualized.

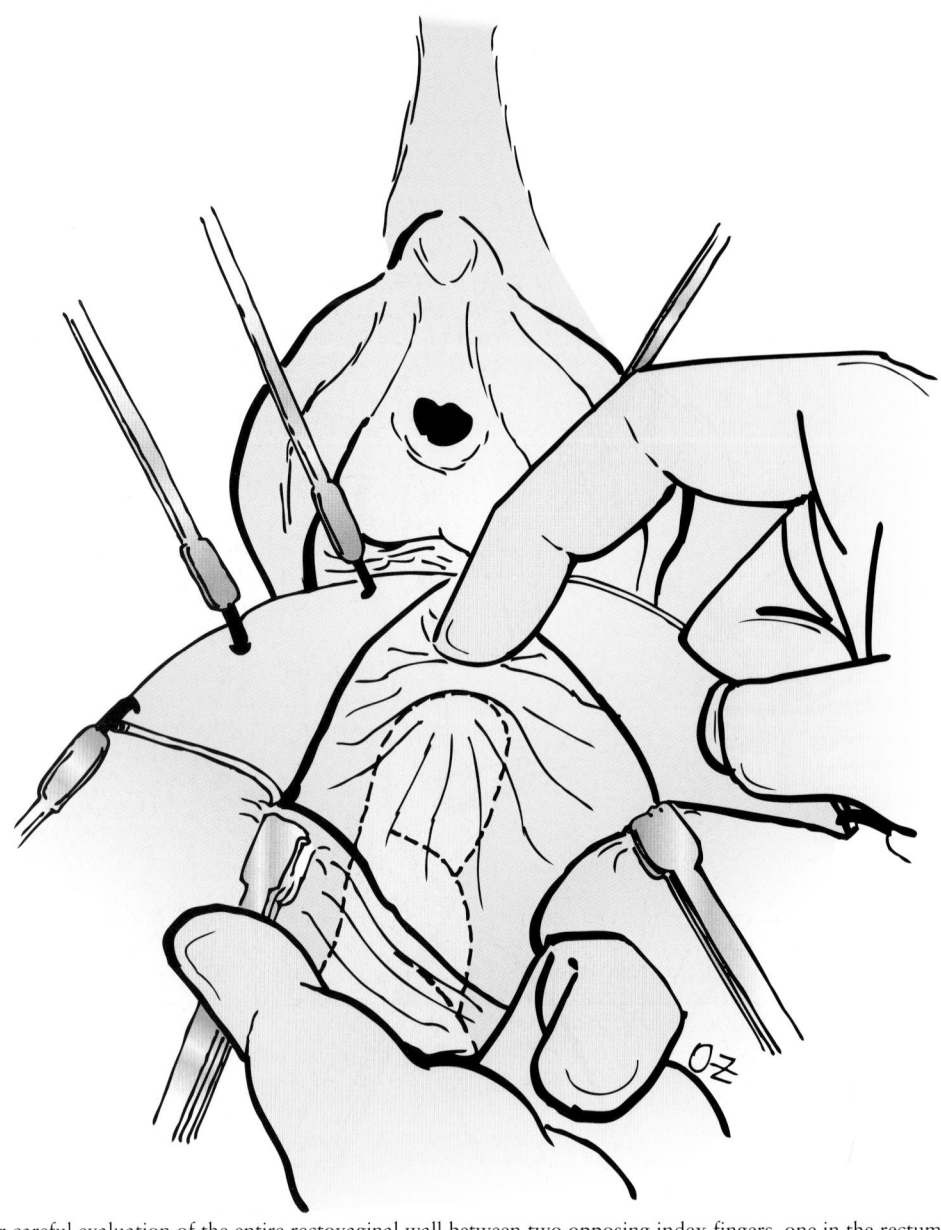

FIGURE 38.15 After careful evaluation of the entire rectovaginal wall between two opposing index fingers, one in the rectum and the other in the vagina, all the defects are identified and labeled with Allis clamps or sutures.

For almost all posterior vaginal repairs, we use zero polyglactin 910 sutures, as we noted that monofilament polydioxanone sutures delayed return to comfortable coital activity. This is more because the large knot, created with the six to seven throws required for a secure knot with polydioxanone suture material, takes at least 6 months to absorb.

No vaginal repair will be durable without addressing the apical prolapse. It has been shown that posterior compartment prolapse may be relieved with an effective apical repair per se in 30% of women. If an entirely vaginal repair is planned, bilateral sacrospinous or extraperitoneal uterosacral ligament suspension sutures are placed and turned into pulley stitches at this time; however, these sutures are not tied until all but the most distal transverse defects are corrected. If concomitant vaginal hysterectomy is to be performed, uterosacral ligaments can be accessed with an intraperitoneal approach. Identification of the intermediate segment of ligaments is

crucial for prevention of ureteral injury with this intraperitoneal technique. Applying outward traction on the cut end of the uterosacral ligament and the posterior cuff edge with Allis clamps, an index finger placed in the rectum may help locate the safe zone.

We start with the correction of the most apical defect, which occurs as a result of a transverse tear of the fibromuscular layer from the cervical ring and uterosacral ligaments. If the uterus is in situ, this edge is attached to the posterior cervix and the uterosacral ligaments with interrupted sutures. In a patient with a history of hysterectomy, the most apical end of the fibromuscular layer of the anterior vaginal wall, so-called pubovesicocervical fascia, is carefully identified and integrity of pericervical ring is restored by suturing the fibromuscular layers of anterior and posterior vaginal walls. Combination of this technique with a vaginal apical repair procedure such as sacrospinous ligament or extraperitoneal uterosacral ligament suspension restores the level I defect. In order to correct the level II posterior compartment support, the edges of each defect in the midvagina are reapproximated with the same technique until the distal posterior vagina is reached. Rectal examination is necessary after each defect repair to confirm effective restitution of the posterior vaginal wall support.

Before repairing the most common defect, which is a transverse separation of the fibromuscular layer from the perineal fibromuscular tissue, the perineal body should be restored. It is helpful to label the distal edge of the detached fibromuscular layer first (Fig. 38.16). Bulbocavernosus muscles are identified with careful dissection on each side of the vestibule and held with Allis clamps similar to the technique used to locate the torn edges of the external anal sphincter muscle. Of note, deep transverse perineal muscles are not easily identified, but they lie within the dense connective tissue of the perineal body torn and retracted laterally. When placing these sutures, the needle should enter perpendicularly into these structures. No suture is tied until three of these are placed sequentially starting from inside to the outside of the introitus (Fig. 38.17A). Attention is paid not to begin too cephalad from the hymenal ring in an effort to prevent inclusion of the pubococcygeus muscles, which are adjacent to these perineal structures. The surgeon should also ensure that sutures, although placed

deep into the muscle, are not ending high in the vagina as this will compromise the vaginal caliber. Vaginal caliber should be assessed after these sutures are tied. This is followed by suturing the torn fibromuscular layer to the restored perineal body with approximately four to five sutures (Fig. 38.17B, C). Another rectal examination is performed at this time to ensure that the defects have been appropriately addressed and the rectocele has been reduced. Occasionally, a few distal plication sutures are placed on the fibromuscular layer if site-specific repair does not produce the desired vaginal caliber.

Once the repair is complete, the vaginal epithelium can be reapproximated in a running fashion with a 2-0 absorbable suture. Before this closure, the edges of the vaginal epithelium may be slightly trimmed as needed (Fig. 38.18). It is not unusual to find excess vaginal epithelium at the most proximal end of the midline incision line; this can be managed by trimming 0.5 to 1 cm further apically. At the distal end of this incision, only rounding up the corners will be sufficient. We place one to two interrupted 3-0 absorbable sutures on each side of the midline at the introitus in a transverse fashion in an effort to prevent introital constriction before completion of the sagittal midline closure.

If the rectum is entered inadvertently during dissection, it is prudent to complete the dissection with the rectum open, providing a good reference. This area should be copiously irrigated

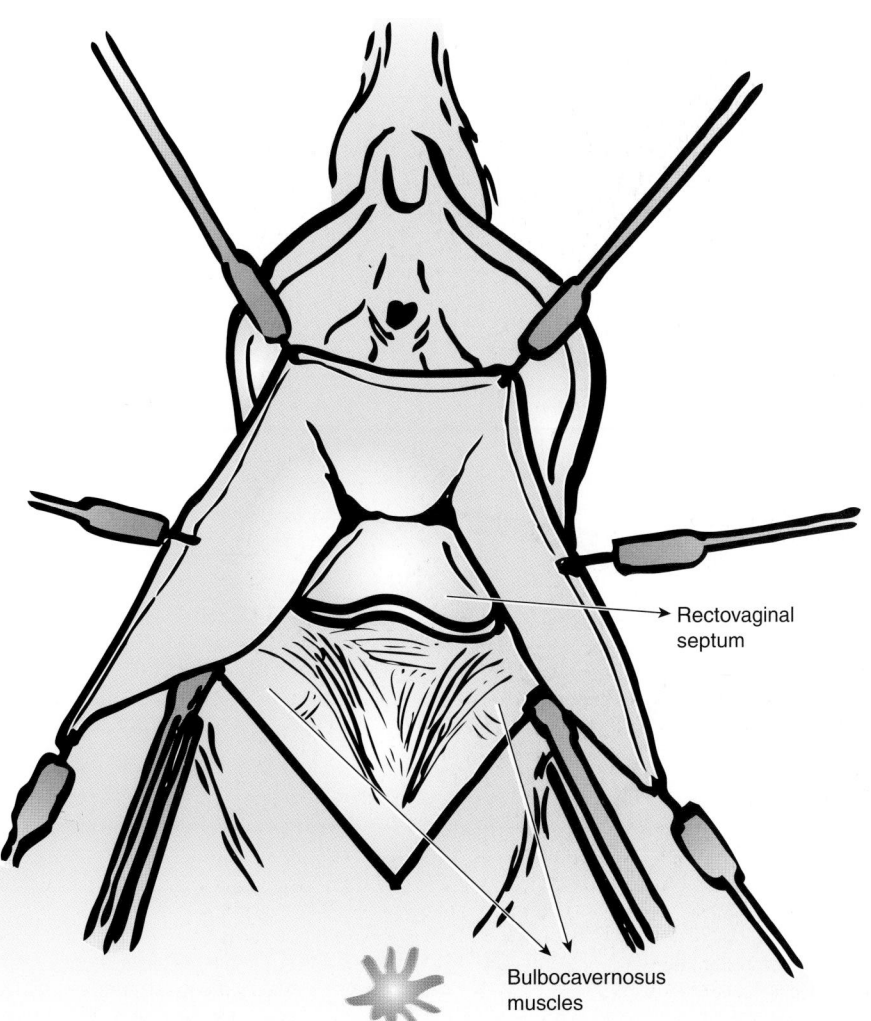

Rectovaginal septum

Bulbocavernosus muscles

FIGURE 38.16 Before repairing transverse separation of the fibromuscular layer from the perineal body, torn perineal fibromuscular tissue should be identified.

VII

during this time and after closure. Most teaching texts finish description of a posterior vaginal repair by advising performance of a rectal examination to ensure the rectal lumen is not invaded by any suture. We choose to do this after completion of all reparative sutures before the closure of the vaginal epithelium and perineal skin, as it is the best time to replace any suture that penetrates into the rectal lumen. When the rectum is accidentally entered, graft material should not be used and an alternate native tissue repair should be implemented. Cystoscopy is not necessary for any type of posterior compartment repair as the bladder or ureters are not at risk during this procedure unless any additional procedure such as intraperitoneal uterosacral ligament suspension, anterior compartment repair, or an anti-incontinence procedure is performed.

Site-Specific Repair with Graft

With little data to guide the surgeon regarding use of graft material in the posterior compartment, the decision to augment the repair should be made with careful thought and appropriate patient counseling. Indeed, there are patients that present with large apical defects and severely attenuated posterior vaginal walls where graft use may be appropriate. When pre- and intraoperative assessment suggests displacement of the torn apical edge of fibromuscular layer distally by about 5 to 6 cm, we offer a repair with synthetic graft to well-informed women who have previous failures and chronic constipation and are not sexually active. Patients should be counseled on the lack of data regarding graft use.

We begin the procedure with a triangular-shaped incision over the perineal body. Once again, the hymenal ring is grasped with two Allis clamps. The posterior vagina is grasped approximately 3 cm proximal to the hymen with an Allis clamp in the midline. The critical difference in these cases is the plane of dissection. The surgeon must separate the entire vaginal wall including its fibromuscular layer from the rectal wall as opposed to splitting the epithelial and fibromuscular layers as in native tissue techniques. Once the full-thickness vaginal wall is dissected from the rectum, a 5-cm midline sagittal incision is made. It is important to keep the incision short and away from the vaginal apex, since most graft exposures occur due to infection or dehiscence of incisional wounds.

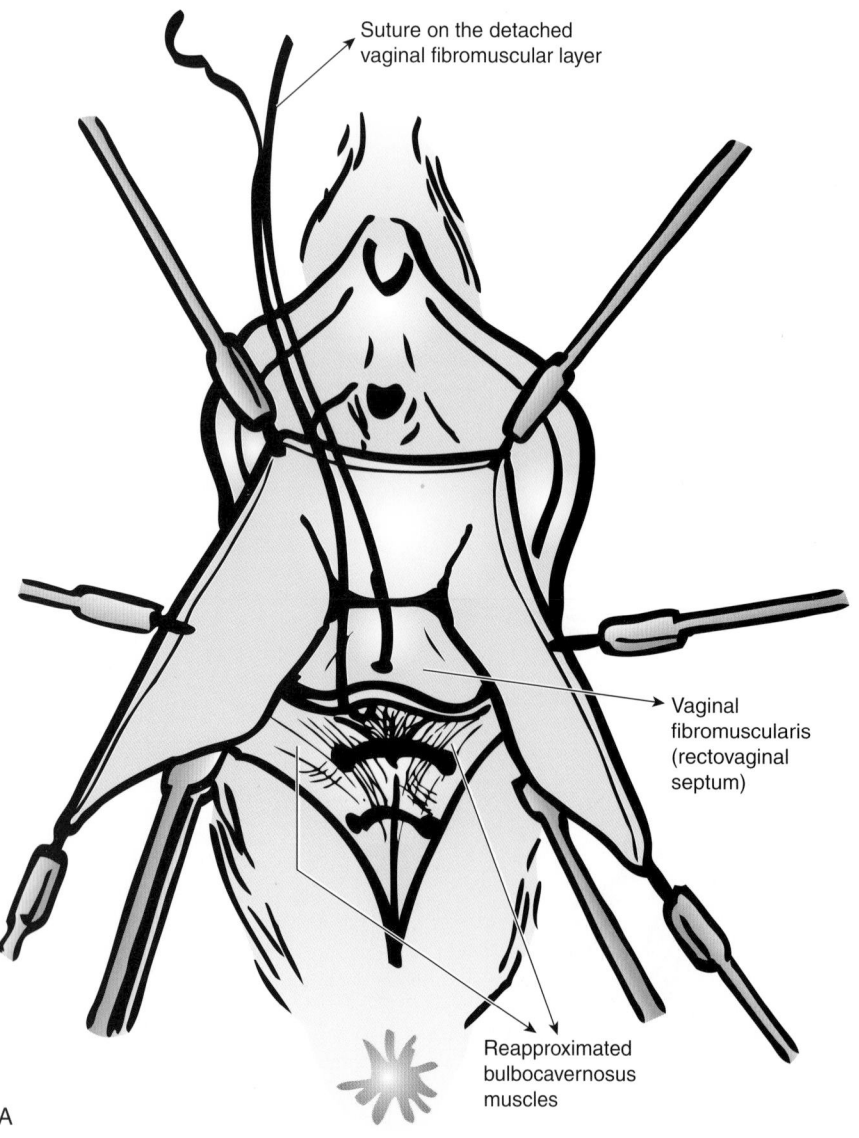

Suture on the detached vaginal fibromuscular layer

Vaginal fibromuscularis (rectovaginal septum)

Reapproximated bulbocavernosus muscles

A

FIGURE 38.17 A: After perineal fibromuscular tissue including the bulbocavernosus muscles is reunited.

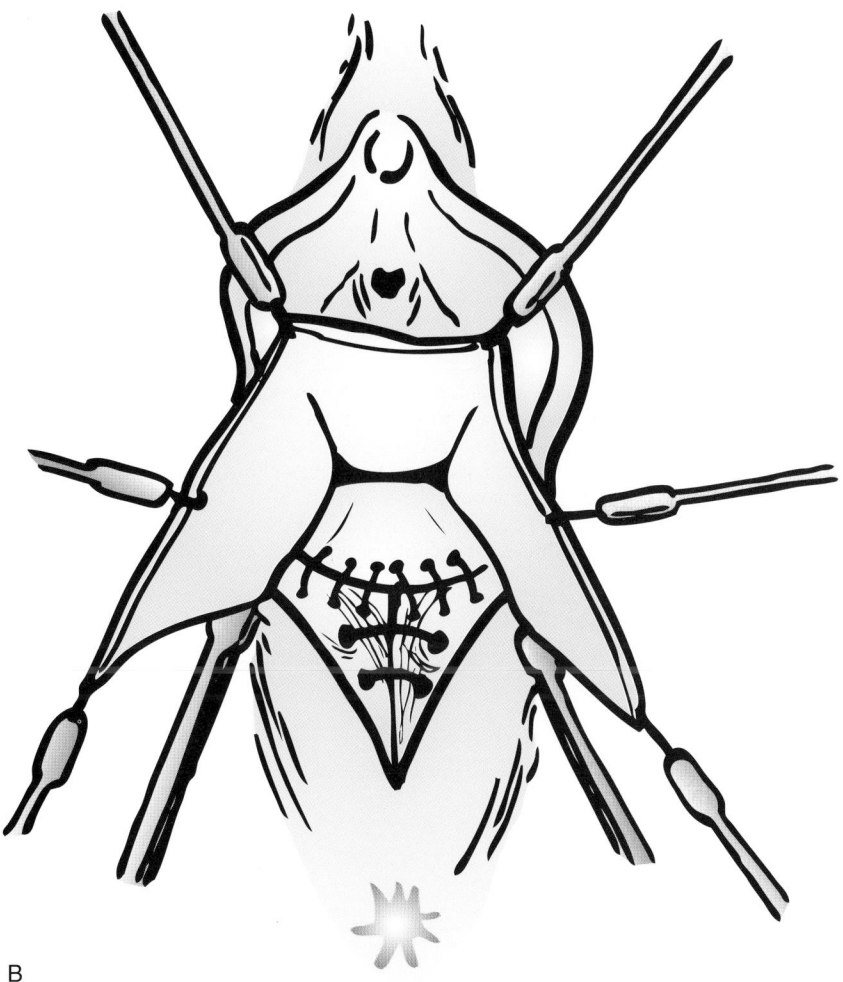

B

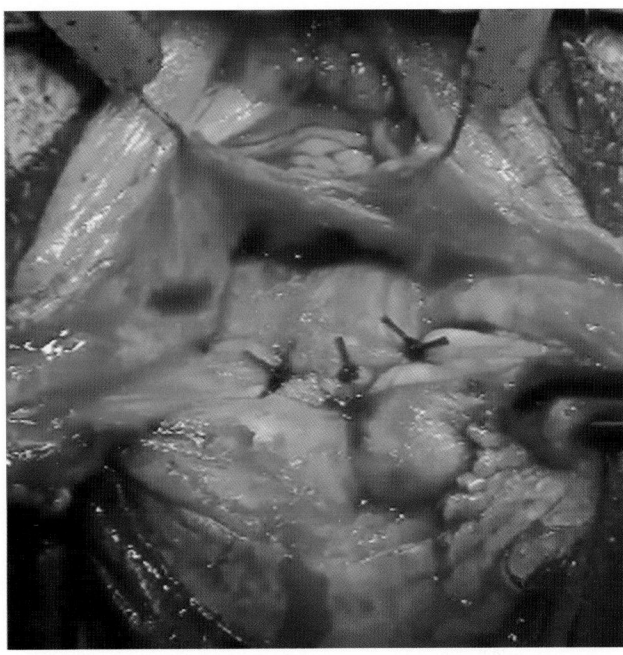

C

FIGURE 38.17 (*Continued*) **B:** The detached edge of the vaginal fibromuscular layer is sutured to the restored perineal body with approximately four to five sutures. **C:** Shows this technique applied during a surgery.

VII

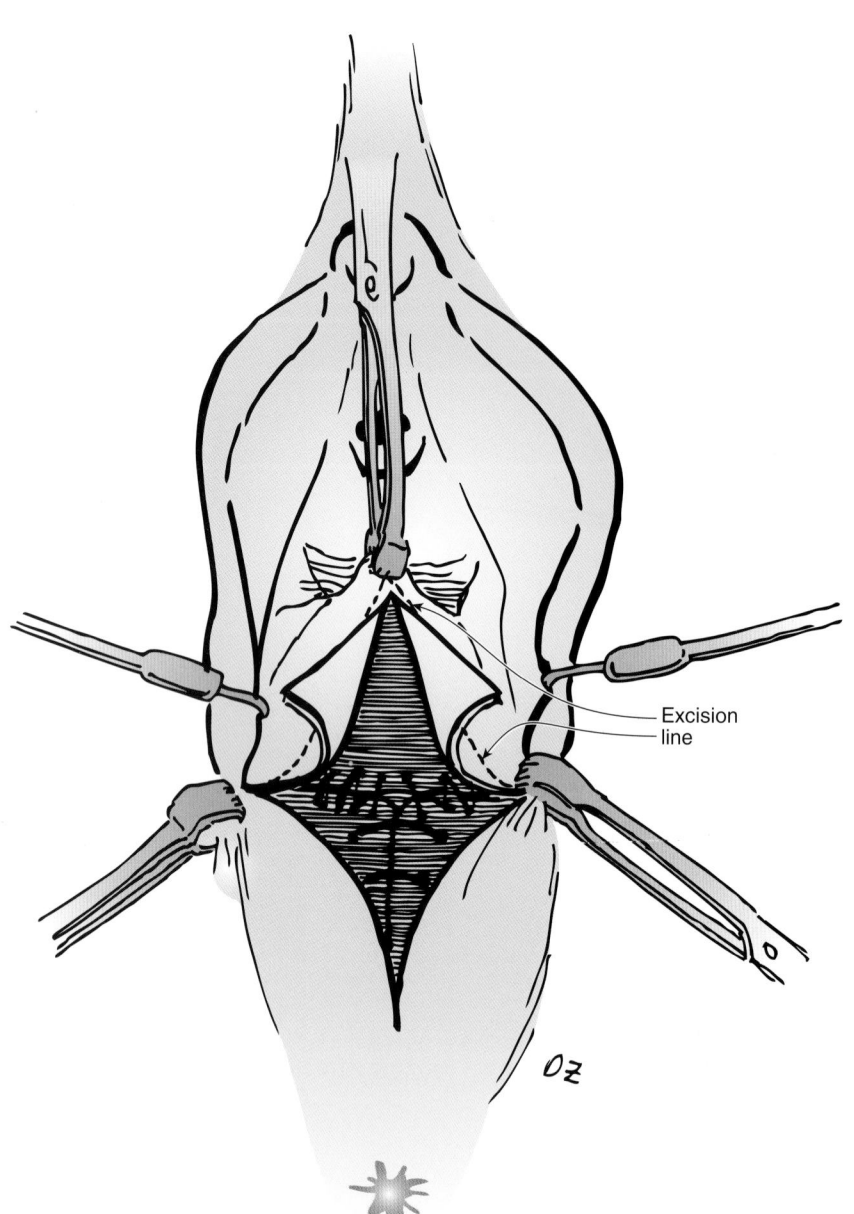

Excision
line

FIGURE 38.18 Before the closure of the vaginal epithelium, its edges may be trimmed slightly as needed. It is not unusual to find excess vaginal epithelium at the most proximal end of the midline incision line; this can be managed by trimming 0.5 to 1 cm further apically. Sometimes, rounding up the corners of the perineal end of the midline incision may be sufficient.

Some surgeons trained to use pelvic floor systems marketed by medical device companies are accustomed to utilizing local anesthetic with epinephrine for hemostasis and hydrodissection. We do not think this approach is necessary. In fact, the tissue planes may be more precisely identified without local infiltration with this local anesthetic solution. If the correct plane is entered, there should be no bleeding. Alternatively, the dissection can be further facilitated with the nondominant finger in the rectum. The initial 3 cm of this dissection is the most difficult in women with previous repair due to dense fibrosis in this area. However, once the correct plane is entered, the rest of the dissection becomes easier. The entire posterior vaginal wall is separated from the rectum. At the apical part of dissection, there is a risk of entering the peritoneal cavity as many patients have an enterocele component. If this occurs, the enterocele is ignored and peritoneum is simply closed with 2-0 absorbable suture. The surgeon must then palpate the ischial spine and sacrospinous ligament/coccygeus complex

bilaterally. The ligament is exposed with clearing soft tissue and separation of coccygeal muscle fibers bluntly. A suture is placed through the ligament approximately 1 to 1.5 cm medial to the ischial spine using a suture placement device such as Capio™ and a delayed absorbable suture with the rectum deviated contralaterally. Once the suture is placed, the surgeon should tug on the suture to evaluate the strength of the purchase into the ligament. When performing a posterior repair with graft, we use a 10 × 15 cm sheet of type I macroporous monofilament polypropylene mesh cut into a Y shape and customized for each patient (**Fig. 38.19**). The top part of the Y-shaped graft represents its apical part. The graft should be secured apically with one absorbable suture on each side of the midline so that the entire defect is covered and the mesh does not migrate. In a woman who has a uterus, it is attached to the posterior cervix and the uterosacral ligaments. If the patient is posthysterectomy, it is sutured to the most apical end of the fibromuscular layer of the anterior vaginal wall. At this time,

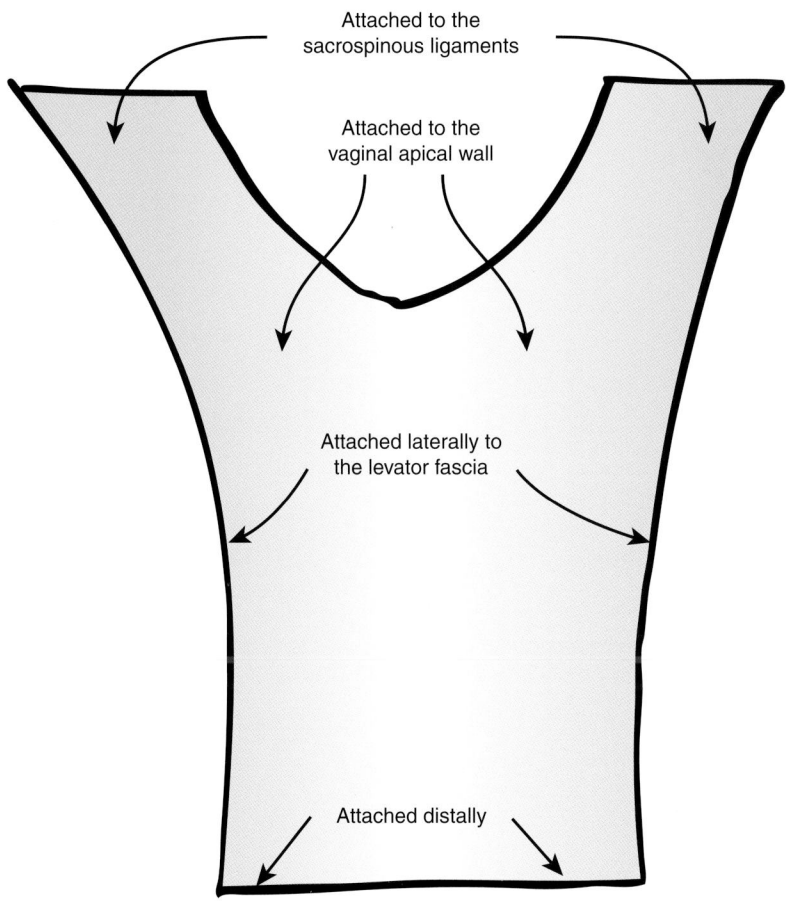

Attached to the
sacrospinous ligaments

Attached to the
vaginal apical wall

Attached laterally to
the levator fascia

Attached distally

FIGURE 38.19 When performing a posterior repair with graft, we use a 10 × 15 cm sheet of type I macroporous monofilament polypropylene mesh cut into a Y shape and customized for each patient.

sacrospinous ligament sutures are passed through the tips of the Y-shaped graft and tied in a pulley fashion. Then, they are tied down without any suture bridging, with an assistant bringing the vaginal apex closer to that side using an instrument. The graft is then sutured laterally to the levator fascia at several locations. Its distal end is trimmed so that it ends about 3 cm cephalad to the introitus, where the perineal body is supposed to start. This procedure not only corrects an apical posterior defect but also repairs an apical prolapse by elevating the vaginal apex toward the sacrospinous ligaments. The surgeon should ensure that the graft lays flat without tension. The procedure ends with a perineorrhaphy as described in the site-specific repair section. These perineal sutures may provide an additional layer of coverage over the distal end of the graft, which has the highest risk of exposure as it is the only part that corresponds to the midline incision line. A Foley catheter is inserted, and the vagina is packed for one night.

Midline Plication/Traditional Colporrhaphy

An alternate approach to the site-specific repair is the posterior midline plication technique (Fig. 38.20). This traditional posterior repair method was developed to address obstetric lacerations. It included plication of pubococcygeus and the posterior vaginal fibromuscular layer with perineal body reconstruction.

There is no doubt that traditional posterior colporrhaphy with plication of the fibromuscular layer improves objective and subjective outcomes as shown in case series and comparative studies. However, like many surgical procedures that were developed empirically, it was shown to achieve anatomic and

functional goals in most patients. It can be likened to sacrocolpopexy, which is not an anatomically correct procedure but serves as one of the best apical prolapse approaches available.

The incisions and dissection for this technique are similar to that described above for site-specific repair. The fibromuscular layer is then plicated in the midline in one or two layers with 0 absorbable sutures. Care must be taken not to restrict the vaginal caliber. The surgeon should avoid plication of the pubococcygeus muscles and plication in the proximal 5 cm of the posterior vaginal wall because these may cause significant dyspareunia by compromising the vaginal caliber in sexually active women. Perineorrhaphy is also performed by continuation of the plication onto the torn bulbocavernosus and deep transverse perineal muscles and connective tissue in the manner described above. The process of trimming and closure of the vaginal epithelium is also the same. The surgeon should ensure that the vagina can easily accommodate three fingers at completion of the surgery.

Our reservation for midline plication technique includes the possibility of conversion of the vagina into a tube and tendency to plicate the pubococcygeus muscles overzealously with this approach. As reviewed above, the vagina is not a tube. Turning it into a tube may have functional consequences. Similarly, plication of the levator muscles in the midline between the vagina and the rectum may also cause dyspareunia.

Transanal Repair

According to a recent Cochrane review, transvaginal posterior wall repairs performed better than the transanal repair of rectocele. There was significantly lower recurrence rate of

VII

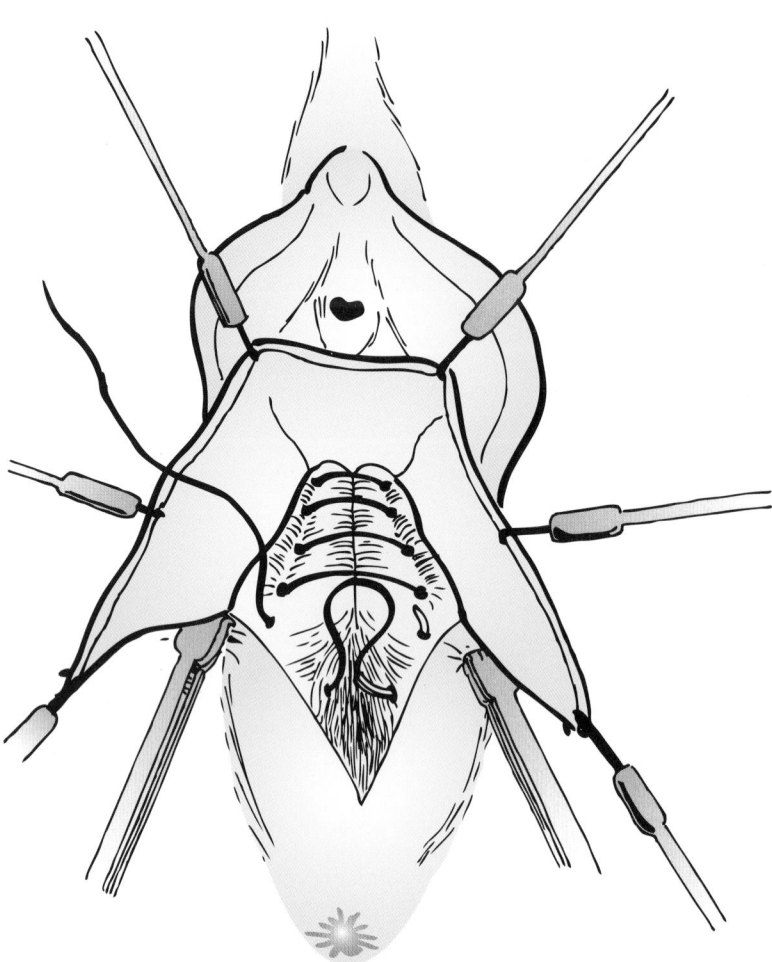

FIGURE 38.20 Midline plication/traditional posterior colporrhaphy.

rectocele in two trials comparing transvaginal to transanal approach, despite a higher blood loss and greater use of pain medication with the transvaginal approach.

Sacrocolpoperineopexy

Abdominal or laparoscopic sacroperineopexy is very suitable in women who present with both apical and posterior pelvic organ prolapse. By extending the posterior part of the sacro-colpopexy graft down to the distal vagina, both level I and II defects of the posterior vaginal wall can be corrected. However, it is not uncommon that the genital hiatus may remain enlarged with this approach as the distal 3 cm of the posterior wall support is provided by the perineal structures described above in detail. Posterior wall support cannot be restored completely without a level III repair, that is, perineorrhaphy.

OUTCOMES

Success Rate

Anatomic success rates have been reported to be 82% to 100% for site-specific repair. Similarly, anatomic cure was achieved in 80% to 96% of the patients with traditional posterior colporrhaphy. In a well-designed randomized study, Paraiso et al. compared these two native tissue methods with graft-augmented repair. At 1 year, they did not find any significant difference between 37 women who underwent traditional posterior colporrhaphy with midline plication (86%) and

37 women who were assigned to site-specific rectocele repair (78%). Abramov et al. retrospectively compared 124 women who underwent site-specific rectocele repair with 183 women who had midline plication with at least 1-year follow-up. They reported a significantly higher recurrence and symptomatic bulge rate in women who underwent site-specific repair (11% vs. 4% for both outcome measures).

Biologic and synthetic graft materials have been used in pelvic floor repairs in conjunction with both traditional and site-specific repairs to enforce the attenuated posterior vaginal wall. Although there have been large randomized trials of graft use in the anterior compartment repairs, there is insufficient evidence for guidance in the posterior compartment. There have been only two randomized trials that addressed graft use to the posterior compartment; however, both utilized porcine graft and did not show any benefit over native tissue repair. In fact, in the trial by Paraiso et al., anatomic outcomes were significantly worse for the graft arm (46%). In a subsequent larger randomized double-blinded trial of 137 women that compared native tissue repair, either midline plication or site-specific techniques at the discretion of the surgeon, with those undergoing site-specific or traditional repair, augmented with porcine dermis. At 1 year, statistically similar anatomic success (about 90%) was accomplished in both groups. In both of these trials, surgical technique for graft placement such as the size, anchoring sites, and the plane of insertion of the graft was different from the method described in this chapter. Moreover, the outcomes may be different for polypropylene graft, which is a permanent implant, compared to the results from biologic grafts, which are usually degraded by the immune system. Undoubtedly, more evidence is needed for guidance regarding graft use in the posterior vaginal compartment.

In the aforementioned randomized study by Paraiso et al., DD, splinting to defecate, straining, and fecal incontinence were significantly improved in all patients regardless of the approach at 1 year after the repair, but new-onset symptoms developed in 11% of the study participants. Of note, anatomic cure was associated with a reduced risk of straining or feeling of incomplete emptying. Sung et al. found that the prevalence of bowel symptoms including splinting, straining, incomplete evacuation, and obstructed defecation were all significantly improved. However, incomplete evacuation (19%), splinting (23%), and straining (37%) symptoms persisted in a considerable group of subjects. Those women who had the longest duration of splinting were found to have over a twofold increased risk for persistent splinting.

Sexual function has been an important concern for the surgeon performing posterior vaginal compartment repair. However, the studies reporting on sexual function have shown conflicting results. Even though traditional midline plication has been associated with postoperative dyspareunia (8% to 26%), especially in the setting of levator plication, a study on 38 women who underwent midline plication for a stage II or greater rectocele and obstructed defecation found dyspareunia significantly improved from 37% at baseline to 5% postoperatively.

In some studies, postoperative dyspareunia has been associated with native tissue repairs of the posterior compartment regardless of the technique utilized. In the retrospective cohort study by Abramov et al., both site-specific (17%) and midline plication arms (16%) had similar postoperative dyspareunia rates. Of note, levator plication was not used in any arm of this study. In a cohort of 73 women undergoing surgery for urinary incontinence and/or pelvic organ prolapse, 30 women who had posterior repair with either type of native tissue techniques reported higher dyspareunia rates than those who did not. However, sexual function scores based on a validated sexual questionnaire indicated similar improvement in both groups. Graft use has always been associated with dyspareunia; however, in the randomized trial by Paraiso et al. mentioned above, sexual function significantly improved in all groups similarly regardless of the repair technique.

Although the place of perineorrhaphy has always been a subject of heated debate, little evidence exists for guidance in this area. The trial conducted by Paraiso et al. generated some evidence. They performed perineorrhaphy in 82 (78%) women across the study arms. Although it was not independently associated with anatomic success, postoperative dyspareunia, postoperative DD, or "any" postoperative splinting, women who had a perineorrhaphy reported about 12 times (odds ratio, 0.08) less bothersome splinting at 1-year postoperative assessment after controlling for treatment group and baseline symptoms.

Complications

Though uncommon, complications such as bleeding, rectal injury, hematoma, temporary urinary retention, and infection may occur after rectocele repair in the short term. In most studies on the posterior compartment including the randomized trials, the patients had other pelvic floor procedures; therefore, the rates of these complications attributable to posterior wall repairs are not clear. Across the studies, bleeding complications were approximately 1% to 3% and wound-related complications were about 5% to 10%.

In the immediate postoperative period, intractable pain in the posterior aspect of the thighs may be a sign of nerve entrapment of a branch of sacral roots in women who underwent concomitant sacrospinous or uterosacral ligament suspension. De novo dyspareunia is a delayed complication of posterior wall repairs. A detailed review of this is presented in the outcomes section above. Though very rare, complications such as rectovaginal fistula and fecal incontinence may also occur.

There are also complications specific to graft use such as graft exposure. Because biologic grafts were used in the aforementioned randomized trials, graft exposure was not a problem and, therefore, not reported. In one of these trials, wound-related problems were reported with no significant difference between the groups although the study was possibly not powered to analyze this outcome. The studies conducted to evaluate the outcomes of synthetic graft–based kits from medical device companies have not been very helpful to guide us for posterior vaginal wall repairs, as most of the available data come from studies performed on the anterior vaginal compartment.

POSTOPERATIVE CARE

Postoperative management will vary based on training and experience. After our procedures, the vagina is packed with either plain packing or packing lubricated with bacitracin ointment for easy removal the following morning. A Foley catheter is placed for overnight gravity drainage. It may be appropriate to use 1 to 2 g of estrogen cream with packing; however, we feel that using a large amount of estrogen, that is, an entire tube of 42 g of equine estrogen, immediately after pelvic surgery, may potentially increase the risk of thromboembolism in an elderly woman undergoing pelvic reconstructive surgery. The vaginal packing is removed just prior to the removal of the Foley catheter and voiding trial. Patients are discharged with narcotic pain medication, ibuprofen, docusate, and recommendations to take fiber supplements twice daily in efforts to avoid constipation and straining. All postmenopausal women are advised to use vaginal estrogen starting a few months prior to the procedure and continue this medication postoperatively unless there is a contraindication to estrogen use.

All patients are contacted by phone 2 days after the procedure. Posterior vaginal repair, especially with perineorrhaphy, can be accompanied by significant perineal discomfort. The patient should be counseled extensively to set appropriate expectations about this problem. Often surprised by the degree of discomfort that is "normal" for these procedures, some patients need more reassurance. We advise, if tolerated, the use of ibuprofen every 6 to 8 hours for the first few days after surgery. Sitz baths may be helpful in alleviating some of this perineal discomfort. Since constipation is often an issue, we are very aggressive with the bowel regimen after surgery and in the postoperative period; docusate, fiber, polyethylene glycol, and magnesium-based laxatives can all be utilized in this time period. Patients should be advised to refrain from prolonged narcotic use because it may delay the first bowel movement and complicate postoperative recovery. It is important to prepare the patients for possible buttock pain in the pericoccygeal area when sacrospinous ligament suspension is utilized. Early ambulation is encouraged, but intercourse and any weight-bearing activity or exercise should be avoided for 6 weeks.

In women who continue to have severe pain at 2 weeks after the procedure, a gentle rectovaginal exam should be performed to rule out hematoma formation. If this is the case, conservative care with pain medication and close observation will be sufficient. If the hematoma is too large to allow regular bowel movements, vaginal evacuation by separating the vaginal incision slightly, followed by placement of a packing to stay overnight, is appropriate. Nerve entrapment should be closely monitored. If further neurologic evaluation confirms this condition, it should be relieved surgically by removing the suture causing the entrapment. For refractory pain, neuroleptics, physical therapy, trigger point injections, and finally suture or graft removal should be considered.

The most common site for graft exposure, though rare, is the distal vagina and likely due to wound separation or infection. It may also occur if the graft is placed too superficially between the epithelial and fibromuscular layers of the posterior vaginal wall. This may cause pain for the patient or her partner, spotting, and discharge. Vaginal estrogen occasionally may help for very small exposures. If the patient is asymptomatic, as may be the case in women who are not sexually active, and there is no recurrent prolapse, no further intervention may be necessary. When the patient requires a procedure for graft removal due to bothersome symptoms and there is no ongoing infection, the exposed graft with 1- to 2-cm margins should be removed after mobilization of the surrounding vaginal tissue. A layered closure over this site may be appropriate.

BEST SURGICAL PRACTICES

- A thorough history and physical examination assessing the patient's symptoms, anatomic abnormalities, goals, and expectations from the treatment is essential for successful surgical planning in women with posterior compartment defects.
- DD is multifactorial. Not all defecatory problems arise from posterior compartment defects.
- Patients should be well prepared for postoperative perineal discomfort prior to posterior compartment repairs with perineorrhaphy.
- Posterior compartment repairs improve defecatory outcomes in most women; however, at least a third of women may continue to have DD.
- Rectoceles are caused by discrete tears of the fibromuscular layer at various points along the posterior vagina. Best efforts have to be made to identify all anatomic defects of the posterior compartment for a successful and durable repair.
- Rectal examination prior to, during, and before vaginal closure is critical for identification of the defects and confirmation of restoration of normal anatomy.
- No vaginal reconstruction will be effective without addressing apical support.
- The perineal body constitutes level III support to the vagina. It is the site where most posterior compartment defects occur. Perineal restoration is an integral part of the posterior compartment repair.
- Although traditional plication of the vaginal fibromuscular layer has been shown to provide anatomic success rates similar to site-specific repair, the risk of dyspareunia is increased especially if levator plication is used. There may be functional consequences of turning a naturally conical vagina into a tube.
- Data on graft use in the posterior compartment derive from two randomized trials and are limited to porcine dermis. Though insufficient to make meaningful conclusions, these studies did not show any benefit of porcine graft in the posterior compartment repairs.
- Insufficient evidence exists for guidance regarding polypropylene graft use for posterior compartment defects. In addition, complications due to mesh insertion include, but are not limited to, mesh exposure and dyspareunia. Surgeons must counsel patients extensively with visual tools before surgery if they plan the use of polypropylene mesh in the posterior compartment.
- Selective use of polypropylene grafts may be appropriate in well-informed patients who have a history of previous surgical failure or have infrequent coital activity. Grafts must be inserted beneath full-thickness vagina through a short incision.

BIBLIOGRAPHY

Abramov Y, Gandhi S, Goldberg RP, et al. Site-specific rectocele repair compared with standard posterior colporrhaphy. *Obstet Gynecol* 2005;105:314.

ACOG Committee on Practice Bulletins-Gynecology. ACOG practice bulletin No. 104: antibiotic prophylaxis for gynecologic procedures. *Obstet Gynecol* 2009;113:1180.

Alperin M, Moalli PA. Remodeling of vaginal connective tissue in patients with prolapse. *Curr Opin Obstet Gynecol* 2006; 18:544.

Arnold MW, Stewart WR, Aguilar PS. Rectocele repair: four years' experience. *Dis Colon Rectum* 1990;33:684.

Berglas B, Rubin IC. Study of the supportive structure of the uterus by levator myorrhaphy. *Surg Gynecol Obstet* 1953;97:677.

Boreham MK, Wai CY, Miller RT, et al. Morphometric properties of the posterior vaginal wall in women with pelvic organ prolapse. *Am J Obstet Gynecol* 2002;187:1501.

Brandt LJ, Prather CM, Quigley EM, et al. Systematic review on the management of chronic constipation in North America. *Am J Gastroenterol* 2008;100:s5.

Bump RC, Mattiasson A, Bo K, et al. The standardization of terminology of female pelvic organ prolapse and pelvic floor dysfunction. *Am J Obstet Gynecol* 1996;175:10.

Clemons JL, Aguilar VC, Tillinghast TA, et al. Risk factors associated with an unsuccessful pessary fitting trial in women with pelvic organ prolapse. *Am J Obstet Gynecol* 2004;190:345.

Cundiff GW, Fenner D. Evaluation and treatment of women with rectocele: focus on associated defecatory and sexual dysfunction. *Obstet Gynecol* 2004;104:1403.

Cundiff GW, Weidner AC, Visco AG, et al. An anatomic and functional assessment of the discrete defect rectocele repair. *Am J Obstet Gynecol* 1998;179:1451.

DeLancey JO. Structural anatomy of the posterior pelvic compartment as it relates to rectocele. *Am J Obstet Gynecol* 1999; 180:815.

Donnelly MJ, Powell-Morgan S, Olsen AL, et al. Vaginal pessaries for the management of stress and mixed urinary incontinence. *Int Urogynecol J Pelvic Floor Dysfunct* 2004;15:302.

Erekson EA, Jassis NC, Washington BB, et al. The association between stage II or greater prolapse and bothersome obstructive bowel symptoms. *Female Pelvic Med Reconstr Surg* 2010;16:59.

Flynn MK, Weidner AC, Amundsen CL. Sensory nerve injury after uterosacral ligament suspension. *Am J Obstet Gynecol* 2006;195:1869.

Glavind K, Madsen H. A prospective study of the discrete fascial defect rectocele repair. *Acta Obstet Gynecol Scand* 2000;79:145.

Grimes CL, Lukacz ES. Posterior vaginal compartment prolapse and defecatory dysfunction: are they related? *Int Urogynecol J* 2012;23:537.

Gustilo-Ashby AM, Paraiso MFR, Jelovsek JE, et al. Bowel symptoms 1 year after surgery for prolapse: further analysis of a randomized trial of rectocele repair. *Am J Obstet Gynecol* 2007;197:76.e1.

Handa VL, Garrett E, Hendrix S, et al. Progression and remission of pelvic organ prolapse: a longitudinal study of menopausal women. *Am J Obstet Gynecol* 2004;190:27.

Hendrix SL, Clark A, Nygaard I, et al. Pelvic organ prolapse in the Women's Health Initiative: gravity and gravidity. *Am J Obstet Gynecol* 2002;186:1160.

Jones KA, Moalli PA. Pathophysiology of pelvic organ prolapse. *Female Pelvic Med Reconstruct Surg* 2010;16:79

Kahn MA, Stanton SL. Posterior colporrhaphy: its effects on bowel and sexual function. *Br J Obstet Gynaecol* 1997;104:82.

Kahn MA, Stanton SL, Kumar D, et al. Posterior colporrhaphy is superior to the transanal repair for treatment of posterior vaginal wall prolapse. *Neurourol Urodyn* 1999;18:70.

Kenton K, Shott S, Brubaker L. Outcome after rectovaginal fascia reattachment for rectocele repair. *Am J Obstet Gynecol* 1999;181:1360.

Kleeman SD, Westermann MD, Karram MK. Rectocele and the anatomy of the posterior vagina wall: revisited. *Am J Obstet Gynecol* 2005;193:2050.

Komesu YM, Rogers RG, Kammerer-Doak DN, et al. Posterior repair and sexual function. *Am J Obstet Gynecol* 2007;197:101.e1.

Kudish BI, Iglesia CB. Posterior vaginal wall and repair. *Clin Obstet Gynecol* 2010;53:59.

Longstreth GF, Thompson WG, Chey WD, et al. Functional bowel disorders. *Gastroenterology* 2006;130:1480.

Maher C, Feiner B, Baessler K, et al. Surgical management of prolapse in women. *Cochrane Syst Rev* 2010, Accessed February 2013.

Mellgren A, Anzen B, Nilsson BY, et al. Results of rectocele repair: a prospective study. *Dis Colon Rectum* 1995;38:7.

Nieminen K, Hiltunen KM, Laitinen J, et al. Transanal or vaginal approach to rectocele repair: a prospective, randomized pilot study. *Dis Colon Rectum* 2004;47:1636.

Oelrich TM. The striated urogenital sphincter muscle in the female. *Anat Rec* 1983;205:223.

Olsen AL, Smith VJ, Bergstrom JO, et al. Epidemiology of surgically managed pelvic organ prolapse and urinary incontinence. *Obstet Gynecol* 1997;89:501.

Paraiso MDR, Barber MD, Muir TW, et al. Rectocele repair; randomized trial of three surgical techniques including graft augmentation. *Am J Obstet Gynecol* 2006;195:1762.

Pendergrass PB, Reeves CA, Belovicz MW, et al. Comparison of vaginal shapes in Afro-American, Caucasian and Hispanic women as seen with vinyl polysiloxane casting. *Gynecol Obstet Invest* 2000;50:54.

Porter WE, Steele A, Walsh P, et al. The anatomic and functional outcomes of defect-specific rectocele repairs. *Am J Obstet Gynecol* 1999;181:1353.

Rao SS, Welcher KD, Leistikow JS. Obstructive defecation: a failure of rectoanal coordination. *Am J Gastroenterol* 1998;93:1042.

Richardson AC. The rectovaginal septum revisited: its relationship to rectocele and its importance in rectocele repair. *Clin Obstet Gynecol* 1993;36:976.

Roshanravan SM, Wieslander CK, Schaffer JI, et al. Neurovascular anatomy of the sacrospinous ligament region in female cadavers: implications in sacrospinous ligament fixation. *Am J Obstet Gynecol* 2007;197:660.e1.

Sand PK, Koduri A, Lobel RW, et al. Prospective randomized trial of polyglactin 910 mesh to prevent recurrence of cystoceles and rectoceles. *Am J Obstet Gynecol* 2001;184:1357.

Singh K, Cortes E, Reid WMN. Evaluation of the fascial technique for surgical repair of isolated posterior vaginal wall prolapse. *Obstet Gynecol* 2003;101:320.

Sung VW, Rardin CR, Raker CA, et al. Porcine subintestinal submucosal graft augmentation for rectocele repair: a randomized controlled trial. *Obstet Gynecol* 2012;119:125.

Sung VW, Rardin CR, Raker CA, et al. Porcine submucosal graft augmentation and rectocele repair: a randomized controlled trial. *Obstet Gynecol* 2012;119:125.

Swift SE, Tate SB, Nicholas J. Correlation of symptoms with the degree of pelvic organ support in a general population: what is pelvic organ prolapse? *Am J Obstet Gynecol* 2003;189:372.

Varma MG, Hart SL, Brown JS, et al. Obstructive defecation in middle aged women. *Dig Dis Sci* 2008;53:2702.

Weber AM, Walters MD, Piedmonte MR. Sexual function and vaginal anatomy in women before and after surgery for pelvic organ prolapse and urinary incontinence. *Am J Obstet Gynecol* 2000;182:1610.

Whitcomb EL, Lukacz ES, Lawrence JM, et al. Prevalence of defecatory dysfunction in women with and without pelvic floor disorders. *Female Pelvic Med Reconstr Surg* 2009;15:179.

CHAPTER 39
Vaginal Vault Prolapse

Victoria L. Handa

DEFINITIONS

End-to-end anastomosis (EEA) sizer—One of a series of metal instruments that are used primarily to evaluate the size of the end-to-end bowel anastomosis. It is also an excellent instrument for distending and manipulating the vaginal apex from below, allowing the abdominal surgeon to easily feel the vagina and dissect against a firm surface (**Fig. 39.1**).

Levels of support defects (according to DeLancey classification)—Level I, apical defects caused by loss of support of the uterosacral ligaments, paracolpium, and parametrium; level II, disruption of the normal lateral attachments of the midvagina; and level III, lower vaginal defects in the perineal body or fusion of the distal urethra to the pubic bone.

Occult urinary stress incontinence—Stress incontinence that becomes apparent after treatment of apical vaginal prolapse. The presumed mechanism is resolution of urinary obstruction with correction of prolapse.

Uterine/cervical prolapse—Descent of the uterus or uterine cervix.

Vaginal vault prolapse—Descent of the vaginal vault (cuff scar after hysterectomy).

As women live longer and healthier lives, pelvic floor disorders continue to become even more prevalent and are an important health and social issue. The prevalence of symptomatic prolapse increases with increasing age. The lifetime risk of surgery for pelvic prolapse has been estimated at 7%. Clark et al. found that 12% of women undergo a second surgery within 6 years of the first procedure due to recurrence, and Denman et al. found the recurrence rate was 17% at 10 years. Thus, prolapse surgery is common, and reoperation is an important concern.

The management of pelvic organ prolapse can be challenging because different support defects often coexist and because of the variable effects on bowel, bladder, and sexual function. The pelvic surgeon must be adept in the thorough evaluation and management of these issues. An understanding of the anatomy and the relationship of the vagina to surrounding structures is imperative.

Our understanding of pelvic prolapse and the treatment thereof has changed in recent years. A number of theories have been proposed to explain the development of pelvic prolapse. It was formerly taught that prolapse resulted from attenuation or stretching of endopelvic fascia. Richardson, Lyon, and Williams challenged this theory by introducing the concept of discrete breaks in endopelvic fascia. However, microscopic studies have failed to identify a distinct histologic "fascia" along the anterior and posterior vaginal wall. Currently, it is now generally accepted that the dense tissue under the vaginal epithelium is muscularis rather than fascia. Also, Richardson's description of an enterocele as a separation of pubocervical fascia from rectovaginal fascia is at odds with microscopic studies of patients with enteroceles, which

VII

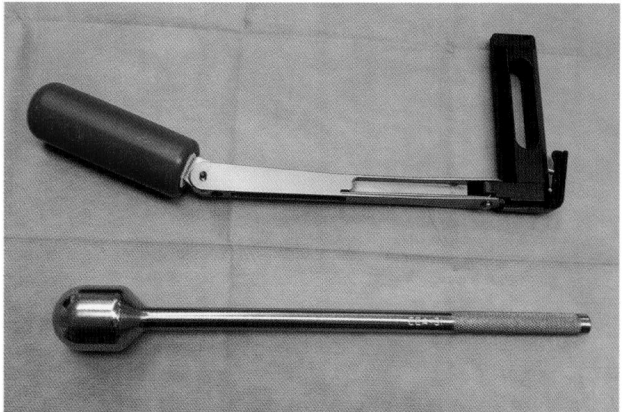

FIGURE 39.1 Instruments useful for the manipulation of the vagina during sacral colpopexy. Shown are a commercially available disposable plastic stent (RUMI handle and Sacrocolpopexy Tip, CooperSurgical, Trumbull CT) and an end-to-end anastomosis (EEA) sizer. (Photo courtesy of Victoria L. Handa.)

have failed to identify peritoneum in contact with vaginal epithelium (**Fig. 39.2**). Work by DeLancey and colleagues has suggested that pelvic muscle weakness may play a critical role in the genesis of prolapse. Specifically, poor function of the levator ani muscle complex or detachment of the levator ani from the pubis may contribute to the development of prolapse for some women. Each of these theories contributes to our overall understanding of vaginal support.

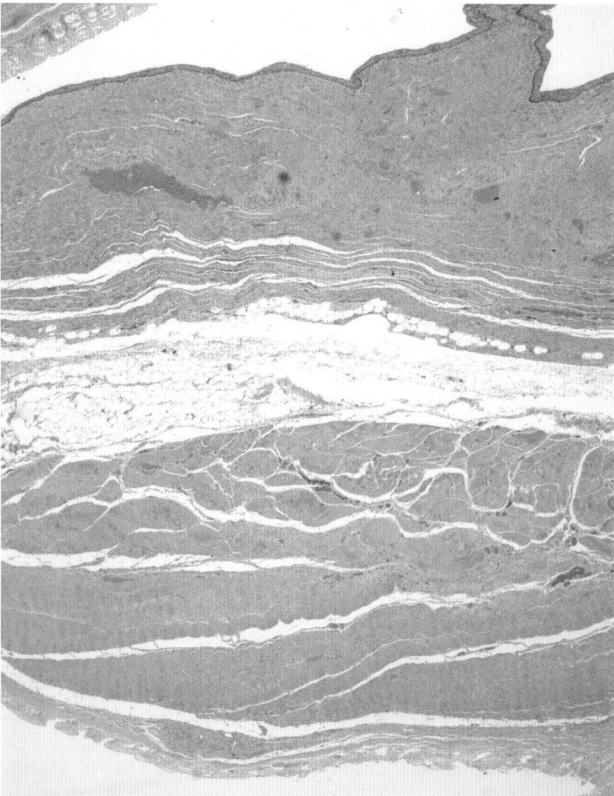

FIGURE 39.2 Microscopic hematoxylin and eosin stain of the upper third of the vagina. The vaginal epithelium is at the top, and the rectal mucosa at the bottom.

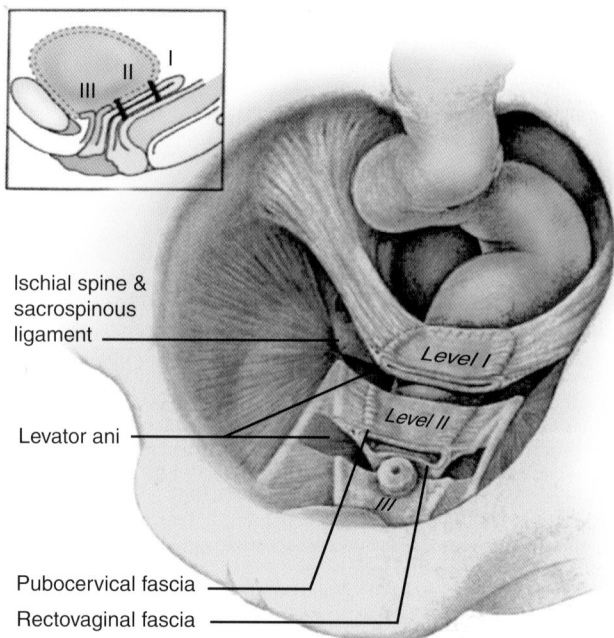

FIGURE 39.3 Levels of support. DeLancey's biomechanical levels: level I, proximal suspension; level II, lateral attachment; and level III, distal fusion. (Reprinted from DeLancey JOL. Anatomic aspects of vaginal eversion after hysterectomy. *Am J Obstet Gynecol* 1992;166:1717, with permission. Copyright © 1992, Elsevier.)

DeLancey divided the support of the vagina into three levels (**Fig. 39.3**). This concept is helpful in understanding normal anatomic relationships and appreciating why certain repairs may work in some patients and not in others. Level I support defects are apical defects, which correspond to loss of support of the uterosacral ligaments, paracolpium, and parametrium. Level II support defects may represent loss of normal lateral attachment of the midvagina. Level III support defects correspond to loss in the support of the perineal body or distal urethra.

The goals of surgery for pelvic organ prolapse should be to restore anatomy and minimize symptoms. With respect to restoring anatomy, the main goal should be to suspend the vaginal vault as near as possible to its normal anatomic position. Magnetic resonance imaging (**Figs. 39.4** and **39.5**) demonstrates that the normal position of the vaginal apex is approximately 5 cm inferior to the second sacral vertebral body and approximately 5 cm medial to the ipsilateral ischial spine. Surgeries that recreate this anatomy will also accomplish the goal of suspending the vaginal apex over the levator plate. Distortion of the position of the vaginal apex, whether in an anterior or posterior direction, can contribute to dyspareunia and could contribute to recurrent prolapse opposite the vaginal vault.

It is extremely important to determine preoperatively whether lower urinary tract dysfunction, sexual dysfunction, and defecatory dysfunction exist. Surgery for pelvic organ prolapse may offer an opportunity to address other pelvic floor problems, including stress urinary incontinence and rectal prolapse. Stress urinary incontinence may be masked in patients with advanced pelvic organ prolapse by obstructing or kinking the urethra. Thus, assessment for "occult" stress incontinence (with reduction maneuvers) has been proposed to identify those patients who would benefit from an anti-incontinence procedure in conjunction with their pelvic reconstructive

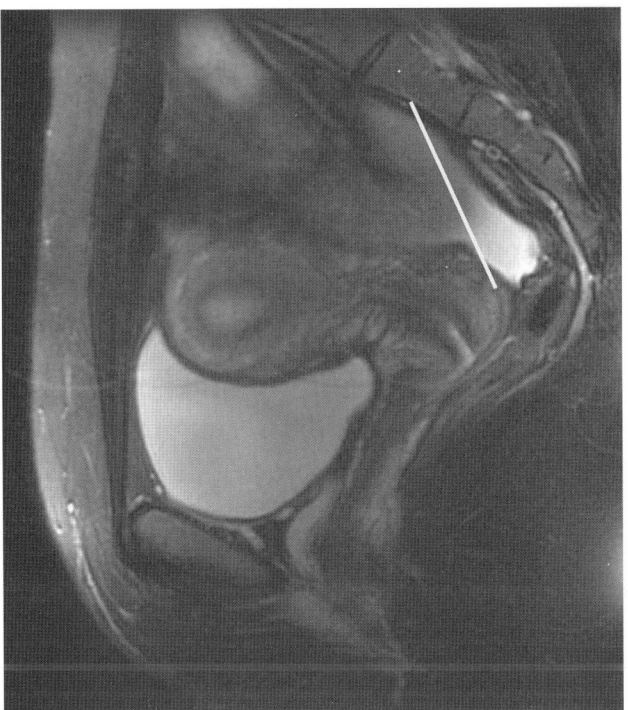

FIGURE 39.4 Sagittal MRI illustrating the relationship between the posterior vaginal fornix and the anterior surface of the middle of the second sacral vertebra.

surgery. However, the value of testing for "occult" incontinence remains controversial.

Another controversy is the value of initiating local estrogen therapy preoperatively in patients who have urogenital atrophy. Cytologic and histologic changes in the vaginal epithelium are seen after as little as 3 weeks of therapy,

and therefore, 3 to 6 weeks of preoperative vaginal estrogen may be recommended by some surgeons. However, the benefits of preoperative estrogen therapy have not been demonstrated.

Many operations have been described for suspending the prolapsed vaginal vault. There is no general consensus on what is the best procedure. The choice of procedure is influenced by many factors, including the comfort and skill of the surgeon; whether the prolapse is primary or recurrent; the patient's age, state of health, and sexual activity; anticipated outcome; and overall state of the tissues.

PROCEDURES TO SUSPEND THE VAGINAL APEX

McCall Culdoplasty

Several operations have been described and used by surgeons for vaginal vault suspension with correction of concurrent enterocele. McCall (in 1957) described his technique of surgical correction of enterocele at the time of vaginal hysterectomy. He used several nonabsorbable sutures to obliterate the enterocele (internal McCall sutures) by approximating both uterosacral ligaments and a running suture through the posterior peritoneum (**Fig. 39.6**). Delayed absorbable sutures are then inserted through the full thickness of the posterior vagina just lateral to the midline and passed through each uterosacral ligament and back out the posterior vaginal wall. Additional external sutures are placed as required by the amount of prolapse. The internal sutures are then tied, and the external sutures are tied after the vaginal cuff is closed. This simple procedure obliterates the cul-de-sac, supports the vaginal apex, and lengthens the posterior vaginal wall. McCall originally reported on 45 cases and stated there was no incidence of enterocele recurrence.

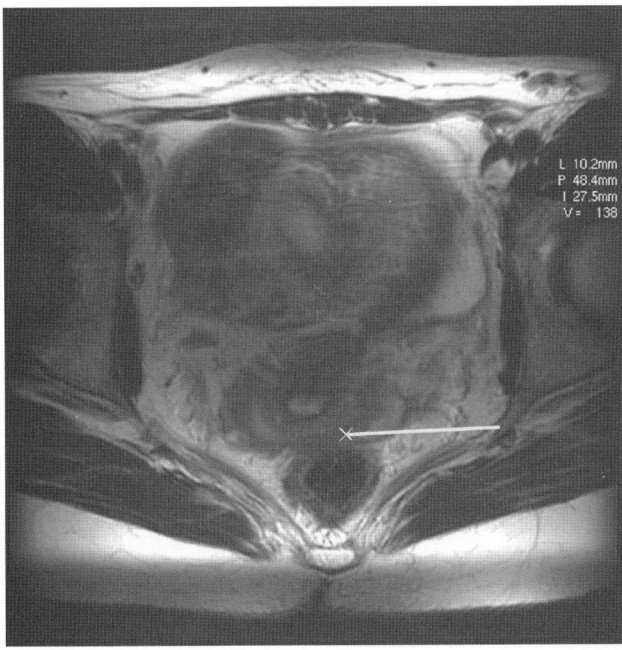

FIGURE 39.5 Axial MRI illustrating the relationship between the left cervical vaginal junction (×) and the left ischial spine.

STEPS IN THE PROCEDURE

McCall Culdoplasty

- The patient is positioned in high lithotomy position.

- The bladder is drained.

- If the procedure is done in the setting of vaginal hysterectomy, the hysterectomy is completed. If a hysterectomy was previously performed, the apex is grasped with Allis clamps and a colpotomy created.

- The enterocele is obliterated with nonabsorbable sutures, plicating the uterosacral ligaments and intervening peritoneum.

- A delayed absorbable suture is inserted through the full thickness of the posterior vagina (just lateral to the midline). The suture is then passed through each uterosacral ligament and back out the posterior vaginal wall.

- The permanent sutures are tied, obliterating the cul-de-sac.

- The delayed absorbable suture is tied, suspending the apex to the uterosacral ligaments.

- Cystoscopy is performed to evaluate ureteral patency and to exclude lower urinary tract injury.

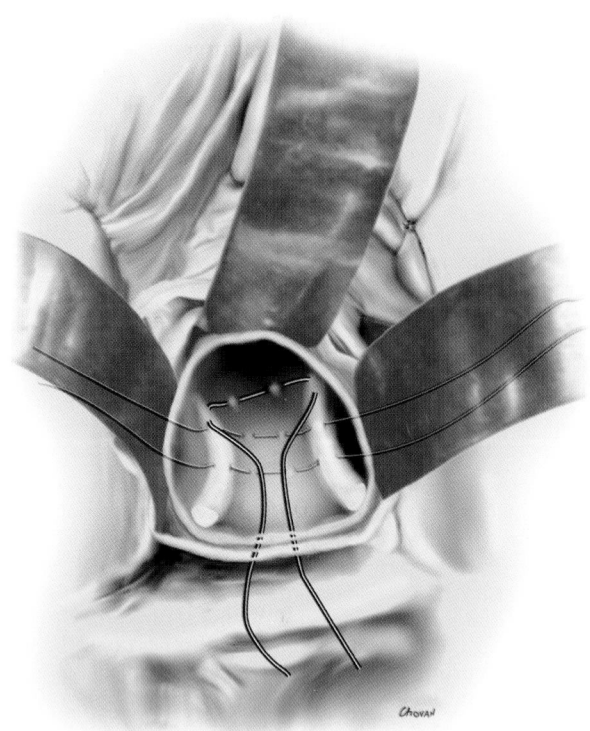

FIGURE 39.6 McCall culdoplasty. Two internal sutures (permanent) and one external suture (delayed absorbable) have been placed. (Reprinted from Baggish MS, Karram MM. *Atlas of pelvic anatomy and gynecologic surgery*. New York, NY: Saunders, 2001, with permission. Copyright © 2001, Elsevier).

Several modifications of McCall technique have been described, most notably the modified endopelvic fascia repair, also known as a "Mayo culdoplasty." The enterocele is delineated, and the sac is then dissected free and excised at the neck (Fig. 39.7). A wedge of vaginal mucosa is removed from the anterior and posterior vaginal wall. This narrows the vault when closed. The ureters are identified by palpation bilaterally. One to three internal McCall sutures are placed as described above, using nonabsorbable suture. After these sutures are placed and tagged, modified external McCall sutures are placed by passing delayed absorbable sutures through the posterior vaginal wall and peritoneum, through remnants of uterosacral and cardinal ligaments on the patient's left. Several bites of peritoneum overlying the rectosigmoid are taken, and then the right perirectal fascia and uterosacral ligament are incorporated into the suture (Fig. 39.8). Last, the suture is passed back out through the posterior vaginal wall. The number of internal and external sutures placed depends on the size of enterocele and redundancy of the upper vagina. After these sutures are tied, the vaginal cuff is closed. There is a risk of ureteral injury or kinking, and therefore, ureteral patency should be confirmed at the conclusion of surgery.

In 1998, Webb reported on 693 women who underwent primary repair of posthysterectomy vaginal vault prolapse at the Mayo Clinic, including 660 who were treated with a Mayo culdoplasty. Among women followed for a mean of 7.4 years, 36/529 (7%) underwent further surgery for prolapse. Of 504 who completed a follow-up questionnaire, 80 (16%) reported symptoms of bulging or protrusion. While these results are encouraging, they are difficult to interpret without information regarding the severity of prolapse before surgery. It is also of note that 42 of 189 sexually active women (22%) reported dyspareunia at the time of follow-up.

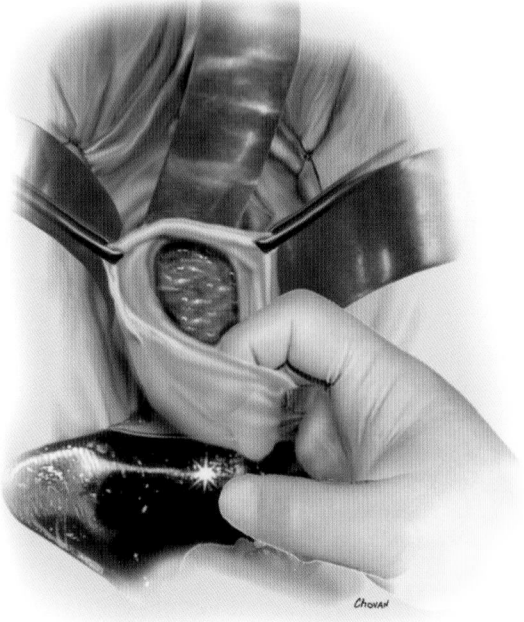
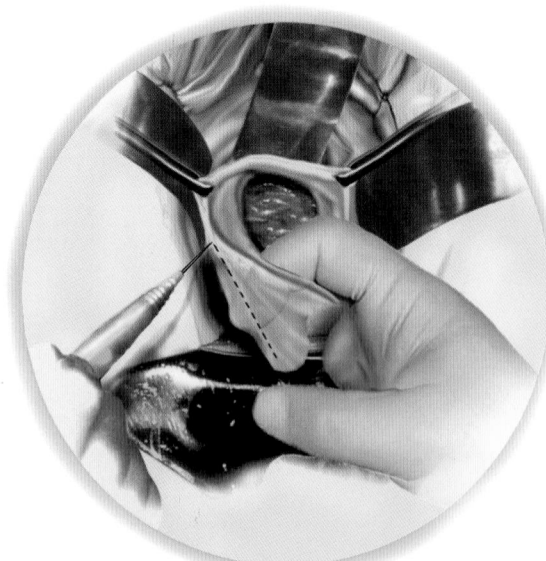

FIGURE 39.7 With the vaginal cuff open, the surgeon palpates the posterior cul-de-sac and enterocele. **Inset:** The redundant wedge of posterior vaginal wall and peritoneum is removed. (Reprinted from Baggish MS, Karram MM. *Atlas of pelvic anatomy and gynecologic surgery*. New York, NY: Saunders, 2001, with permission. Copyright © 2001, Elsevier.)

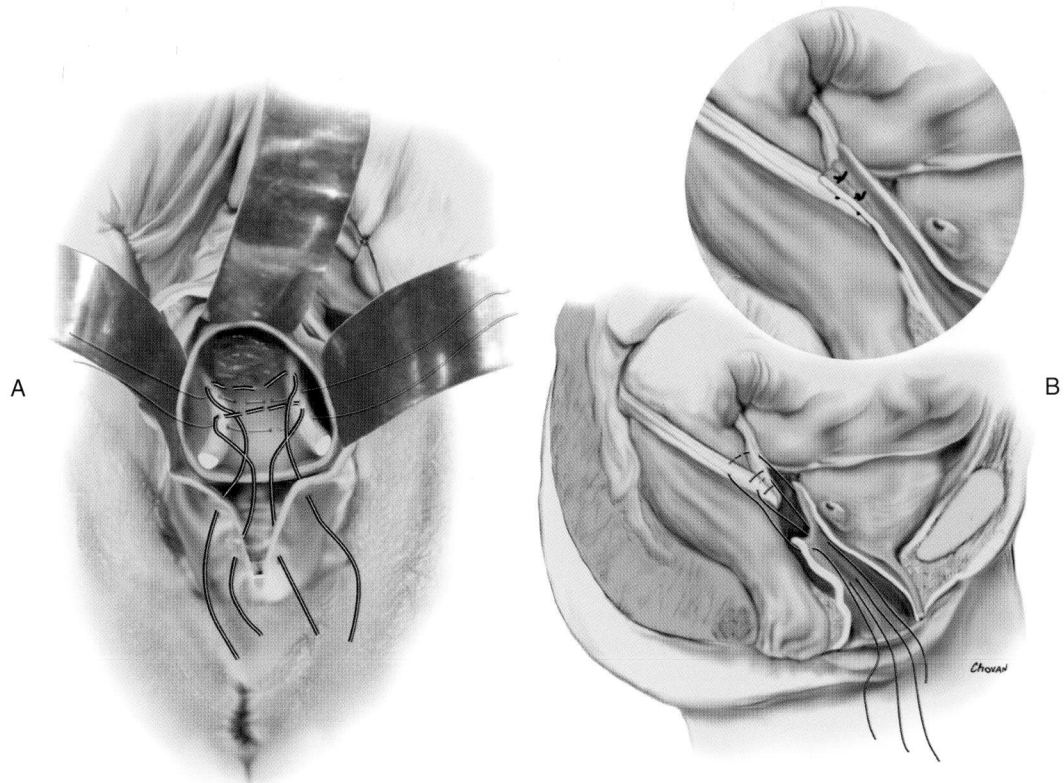

A

B

FIGURE 39.8 A: Placement of internal (nonabsorbable) and external (delayed absorbable) McCall sutures. A wedge of posterior vaginal wall was previously removed. **B:** Cross section of the upper vagina and vaginal vault before tying these sutures. The **inset** illustrates the final result, after the sutures are tied. (Reprinted from Baggish MS, Karram MM. *Atlas of pelvic anatomy and gynecologic surgery.* New York, NY: Saunders, 2001, with permission. Copyright © 2001, Elsevier.)

Sacrospinous Ligament Fixation

The sacrospinous ligament is a cordlike structure that exists within the body of the coccygeus muscle. The sacrospinous ligament attaches medially to the sacrum and coccyx and attaches laterally to the ischial spine (Fig. 39.9). The complex is collectively called the coccygeus–sacrospinous ligament (CSSL) complex. The CSSL is best identified by palpating the ischial spine and tracing the fingerlike ligamentous structure

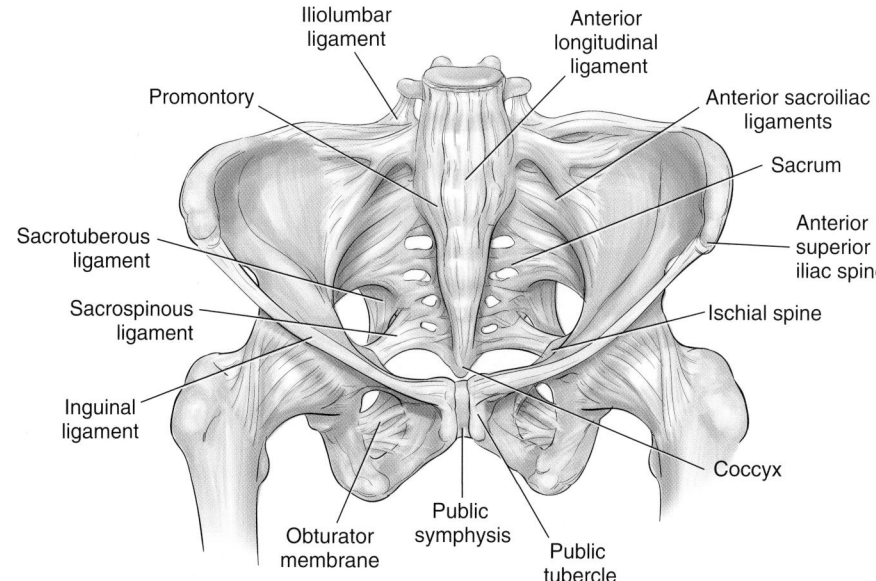

Iliolumbar ligament

Anterior longitudinal ligament

Promontory

Anterior sacroiliac ligaments

Sacrum

Sacrotuberous ligament

Anterior superior iliac spine

Sacrospinous ligament

Ischial spine

Inguinal ligament

Coccyx

Obturator membrane

Public symphysis

Public tubercle

FIGURE 39.9 Ligaments of the bony pelvis. The sacrospinous ligament extends from the ischial spine to the sacrum. The ligament is wider medially and narrows as it inserts on the ischial spine. The ligament lies within the coccygeus muscle (not shown).

VII

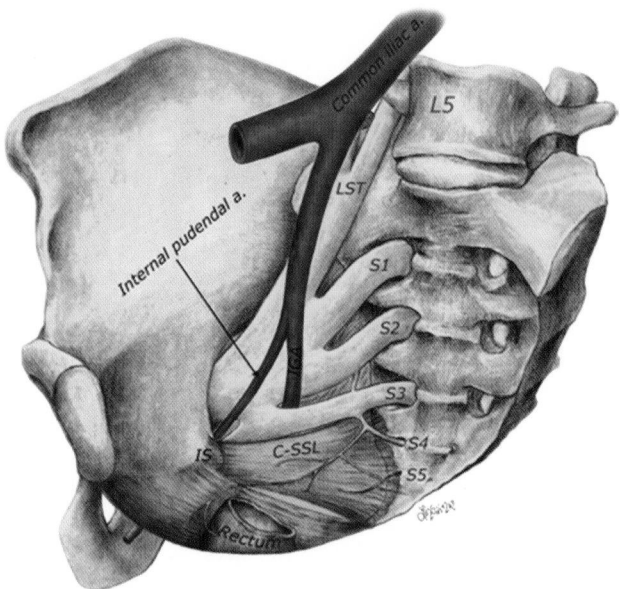

FIGURE 39.10 The right CSSL complex and ischial spine (IS) are shown with respect to the course and relationships of the internal pudendal artery, inferior gluteal artery (IGA), lumbosacral trunk (LST), and sacral nerves (S1 to S5). (Reprinted from Roshanravan SM, Wieslander CK, Schaffer JI, et al. Neurovascular anatomy of the sacrospinous ligament region in female cadavers. *Am J Obstet Gynecol* 2007, with permission. Copyright © 2007, Elsevier.)

medially and posteriorly toward the sacrum. To perform sacrospinous ligament fixation, it is imperative that the surgeon be familiar with the anatomy of the sacrospinous ligament complex and of the pararectal space (Fig. 39.10). Obtaining adequate exposure is critical, and vascular complications, when encountered, may be life threatening. Superior to the ligament lie the inferior gluteal vessels and the hypogastric venous plexus. The pudendal nerve and vessels pass directly posterior to the ischial spine. The sciatic nerve, derived from the lumbosacral nerve roots, passes superior and lateral to the sacrospinous ligament. To avoid trauma to these structures, it is important to place the fixation sutures two fingers medial to the ischial spine.

STEPS IN THE PROCEDURE

Sacrospinous Ligament Suspension

- The patient is positioned in high lithotomy position.
- The bladder is drained.
- If the procedure is done in the setting of vaginal hysterectomy, the hysterectomy is completed and the vaginal cuff is closed.
- The surgeon identifies the intended vaginal apex.
- The posterior vagina is incised longitudinally. The vaginal epithelium is dissected away to expose the rectovaginal space. If present, an enterocele is identified and repaired.
- A window is created in the rectal pillar, and the pararectal space is entered.

- A pair of Breisky-Navratil retractors is used to expose the CSSL complex.
- Using a Miya hook or similar instrument, a permanent suture is passed through the CSSL, two fingers medial to the ischial spine. The loop of the suture is retrieved with a nerve hook, pulled through, and tagged. A second suture is placed, 1 cm medial to the first.
- One end of each suspension suture is sewn into the undersurface of the vagina apex and tied by a half hitch.
- The upper aspect of the posterior vaginal incision is closed.
- Traction on the free end of each suspension suture pulls the vagina directly onto the ligament. The surgeon then ties a square knot to anchor the apex to the ligament.
- Cystoscopy is performed to evaluate ureteral patency and to exclude lower urinary tract injury.
- The vagina may be packed for up to 24 hours after the procedure.

Most surgeons prefer to use the sacrospinous ligament opposite their dominant hand; that is, the right-handed surgeon uses the right sacrospinous ligament, although some surgeons prefer to perform a bilateral fixation. The first step of the surgery is to identify the intended vaginal apex by elevating the vagina to the ligament using an Allis clamp. It may be necessary to choose a different fixation point than the original vaginal cuff scar. This is best illustrated in a patient with a foreshortened anterior segment and a large enterocele. In this case, the new fixation point would be moved to an area over the enterocele. After identifying the intended vaginal apex, marking sutures are helpful to identify this site throughout the operation.

A posterior vaginal incision is made and extended to the vaginal apex. The rectovaginal space is developed. Almost always an enterocele sac is present. The enterocele sac should be mobilized off the posterior vaginal wall up to its neck; the sac is then opened and the peritoneum excised. The defect is then closed with purse-string sutures.

The next step is entry into the perirectal space (Fig. 39.11). The rectal pillar separates the rectovaginal space from the perirectal space. A window must be created through the rectal pillar, which is best accomplished by blunt dissection just lateral to the enterocele sac over the ischial spine. The window can also be created with the tips of scissors, a tonsil clamp, or a hemostat. The window should be gently enlarged to accommodate the vagina. The sacrospinous ligament can then be palpated by palpating the spine and moving the fingers dorsal and medial. It may be necessary to use blunt dissection to remove excess tissue from the CSSL.

Once the window has been created and the ligament is identified, a Breisky-Navratil retractor is used to displace the rectum medially and to expose the CSSL complex (Fig. 39.12). Great care must be taken to avoid raking the retractor over the anterior surface of the sacrum and causing damage to presacral nerves and vessels. Traditionally, the Deschamps ligature carrier was used to pass the suture through the sacrospinous ligament, but this may be more cumbersome than are other methods. We recommend a Miyazaki hook (Miya hook; Fig. 39.13) for placement of the suspension sutures. The Miya ligature carrier is easy to operate and facilitates penetration of the sacrospinous ligament under direct visualization.

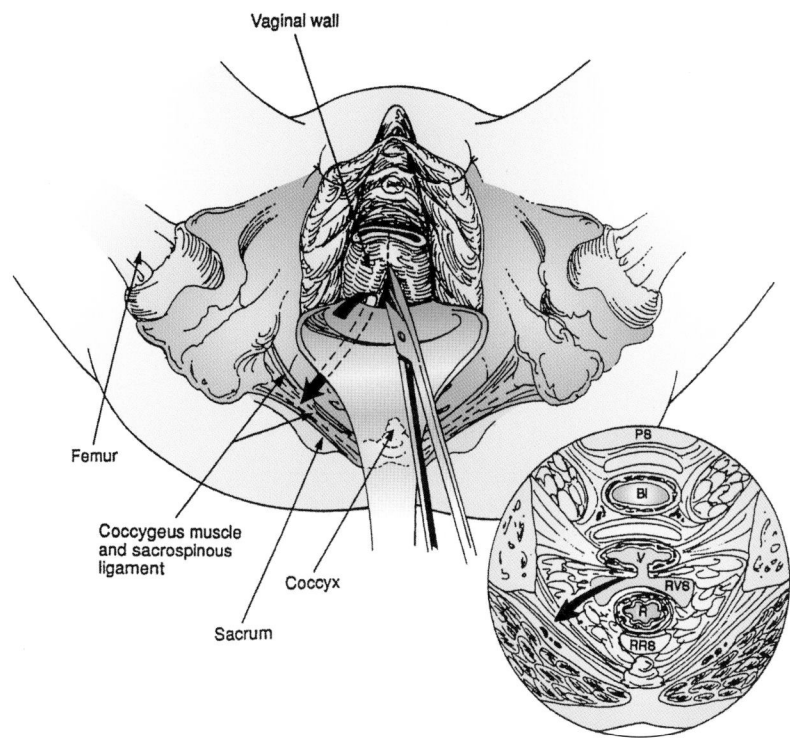

Vaginal wall

Femur

Coccygeus muscle
and sacrospinous
ligament

Coccyx

Sacrum

FIGURE 39.11 After dissecting the rectovaginal space, the surgeon perforates the rectal pillar to enter the pararectal space. (Reprinted from Cruikshank SH, Cox DW. Sacrospinous ligament fixation at the time of transvaginal hysterectomy. *Am J Obstet Gynecol* 1990;162:1611–1619, with permission. Copyright © 1990, Elsevier.)

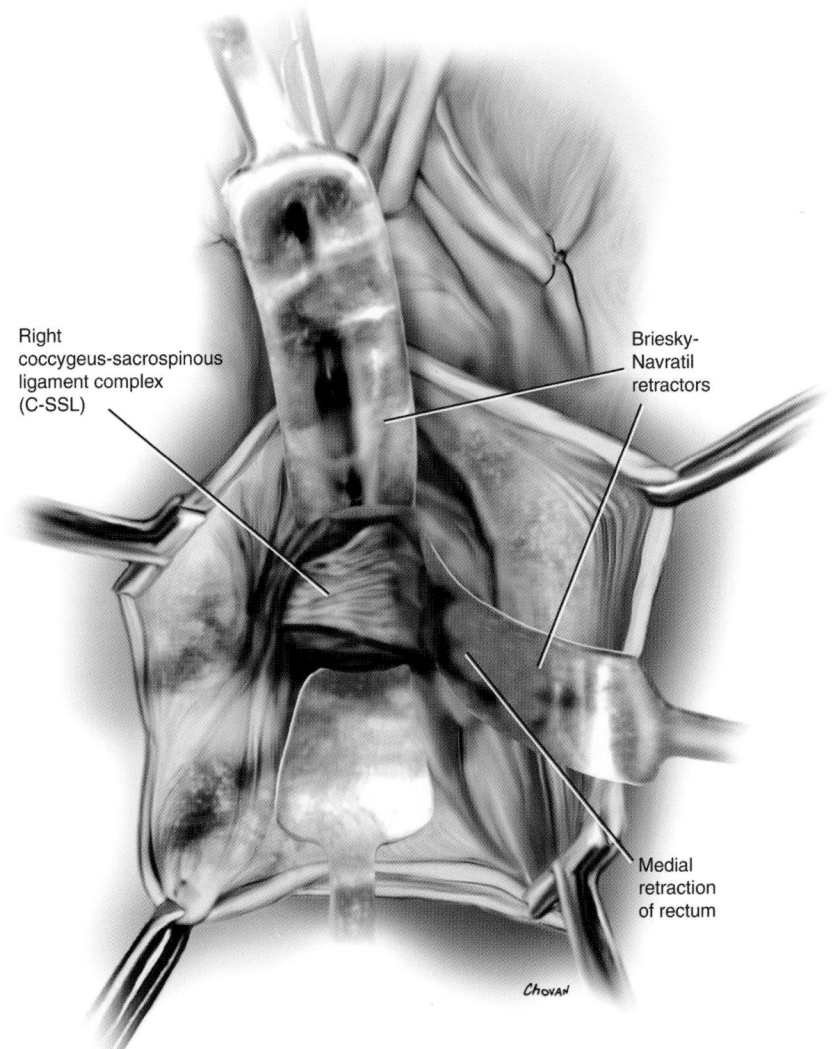

Right
coccygeus-sacrospinous
ligament complex
(C-SSL)

Briesky-
Navratil
retractors

Medial
retraction
of rectum

Chovan

FIGURE 39.12 Two Breisky-Navratil retractors are used to expose the CSSL complex. One retractor is placed anteriorly. A second is used to retract the rectum medially. In this figure, a third retractor is placed inferiorly. Alternatively, a notched speculum (Fig. 39.13) can be used inferiorly. (Reprinted from Baggish MS, Karram MM. *Atlas of pelvic anatomy and gynecologic surgery.* New York, NY: Saunders, 2001, with permission. Copyright © 2001, Elsevier.)

VII

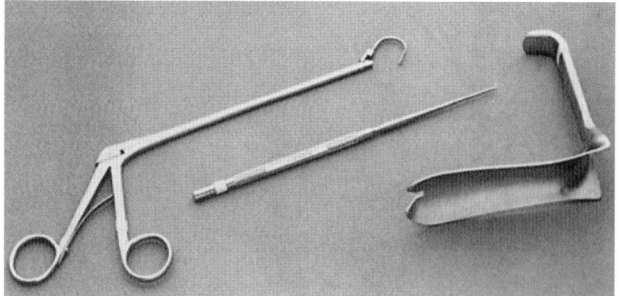

FIGURE 39.13 Instruments for sacrospinous ligament suspension. Miya hook, notched speculum, and suture hook. (Reprinted from Walters MD, Karram MM. *Urogynecology and reconstructive pelvic surgery*, 2nd ed. St. Louis, MO: CV Mosby, 1999, with permission. Copyright © 1999, Elsevier.)

Palpation of the ischial spine identifies the correct location for the placement of the sutures, along the inferior half of the sacrospinous ligament, two fingers medial to the ischial spine. The ligament is exposed using a pair of Breisky-Navratil retractors, and a notched speculum is inserted. The notch can be used to guide placement of the suture. Nonabsorbable suture is used. There should be considerable resistance as the carrier is pushed through the body of the ligament. If no resistance is felt, the surgeon should suspect that the carrier either passed in front of or around the ligament. After the suture has been passed, the loop of the suture is retrieved with a nerve hook, pulled through, and tagged. A second suture is placed in a similar fashion approximately 1 cm medial to the first (**Fig. 39.14**). If a good purchase of tissue has been taken, the surgeon should be able to gently move the patient with traction of the suture.

Once the surgeon has the two sutures through the sacrospinous ligament, the vaginal vault can be suspended. There are two ways for the surgeon to attach the sutures to the vagina. The first is to use a pulley stitch. Here, one end of the suture is sewn into the full thickness of the fibromuscular layer on the undersurface of the vagina (excluding the epithelium) and then tied by a half hitch. Traction on the free end of the suture will pull the vagina directly onto the ligament. Suture bridging should be avoided, since this could predispose to recurrent prolapse. Once pulled into position, a square knot is used to fix the suture in place. A second technique involves passing each end of the sutures through the full thickness of the vagina. This technique requires the use of absorbable suture, however.

The upper portion of the posterior vaginal wall should be closed with interrupted or running 3-0 absorbable sutures before tying the colpopexy sutures. If the colpopexy sutures are tied before the proximal posterior wall is closed, the visibility of the vault is reduced, and this segment of the posterior vaginal incision is difficult to close.

After the colpopexy sutures are tied, a posterior colporrhaphy and perineorrhaphy are usually performed. If an anterior colporrhaphy is planned, this step is most easily accomplished prior to the sacrospinous suspension. At the conclusion of surgery, the vagina is then packed with moist gauze for 12 to 24 hours.

Injury to the ureter or obstruction due to ureteral kinking has been reported after sacrospinous suspension. Therefore, cystoscopy with assessment of ureteral patency should be performed at the conclusion of surgery.

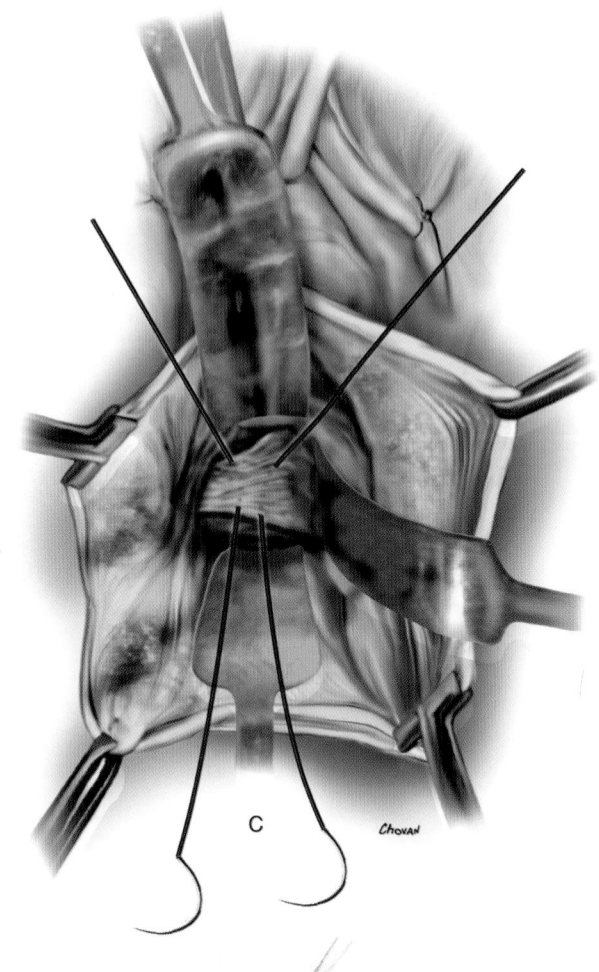

FIGURE 39.14 Two sutures are passed through the sacrospinous ligament. (Reprinted from Baggish MS, Karram MM. *Atlas of pelvic anatomy and gynecologic surgery*. New York, NY: Saunders, 2001, with permission. Copyright © 2001, Elsevier.)

The overall results from sacrospinous fixation have been good. A 2007 systematic review suggested a low rate of apical prolapse beyond Baden-Walker grade 1 (7.2%, 95% confidence interval: 4.0% to 10.4%). Symptom relief was noted in approximately 90% of women across seven studies. However, recurrent prolapse of the anterior wall remains a long-term challenge after sacrospinous suspension. Specifically, one third of patients may experience recurrent prolapse to or beyond the hymen if all vaginal segments are considered.

Complications can occur, and the more common complications are discussed here. It is important to do a rectal examination during this procedure to make sure that no inadvertent proctotomy has occurred. If there is evidence of suture penetration, the offending suture should be removed and replaced. Lacerations should be closed in a standard two-layer fashion.

Hemorrhage can result from injury to the hypogastric venous plexus, inferior gluteal vessels, and internal pudendal vessels. Barksdale described the rich collateral circulate of these vessels, which also anastomose with the superior gluteal, vertebral, and sacral arteries. Vascular injury can occur from overzealous dissection, from inappropriate needle passage, or from an improperly placed retractor. If bleeding occurs, pressure should be applied to the bleeding area. Continued bleeding should be addressed with suture ligation, hemoclips, and possibly embolization. It has been noted that hypogastric artery ligation would likely be ineffective because the anterior division of the internal iliac artery is preferentially ligated during this procedure, and thus, the blood flow could actually increase to the branches of the posterior division (including the inferior gluteal artery). Thus, every effort should be made to control bleeding transvaginally.

Sutures that are placed too close to the ischial spine risk injury to the pudendal nerves and the sciatic nerve (Fig. 39.10). A patient who reports postoperative gluteal pain may have a pudendal nerve injury. Injury to the branches of the sciatic nerve will result in pain that also radiates down the posterior leg. In some cases, symptoms may be self-limiting or may resolve with conservative measures. However, prompt removal of permanent sutures should be considered if pain is severe or is associated with weakness, or if symptoms do not resolve. Improvement in buttock pain after removal of permanent sutures has been reported up to two years after surgery.

According to a 2010 Cochrane review, dyspareunia may be more likely after sacrospinous suspension than other apical suspensions. This may be due to narrowing of the vagina. Vaginal stenosis can occur if too much vaginal tissue is removed before closing the vaginal incision. An aggressive posterior repair can also cause a constriction ring. If a constriction ring is present while the patient is still under anesthesia, it should be addressed at that time. Also, there is some evidence that sacrospinous suspension is associated with a shorter vagina and a change in the vaginal axis. These factors could potentially contribute to dyspareunia.

Uterosacral Ligament Suspension

In 1997, Jenkins published a technique for transvaginal, intraperitoneal suspension of the prolapsed vagina from the uterosacral ligaments. A distinction between this technique and the earlier technique of McCall is that each uterosacral ligament is used to suspend the ipsilateral vaginal cuff and there is no attempt to plicate the ligaments across the midline. A second distinction is that the fixation of the vagina to the uterosacral ligament is at or above the level of the ischial spine. This technique presumes that the ligaments are detached from the vaginal apex but are preserved in their more proximal segments, allowing for a secure attachment of the vaginal apex. This technique is based on Richardson's theory of site-specific defect repair. After Jenkins published results in 1997, a similar technique was described in case series by Shull et al., Barber et al., and Karram et al.

STEPS IN THE PROCEDURE

Uterosacral Ligament Suspension

- The patient is positioned in high lithotomy position.
- The bladder is drained.
- If the procedure is done in the setting of vaginal hysterectomy, the hysterectomy is completed. If a hysterectomy was previously performed, the apex is grasped with Allis clamps and a colpotomy created.

- A Deaver retractor is placed anteriorly, and the abdominal contents are packed up and out of the pelvis with a moist, 4-inch Kerlix sponge.
- The uterosacral ligament is identified and grasped with a long Allis clamp. To identify the ligament, the surgeon may place traction on the vaginal cuff at 5 o'clock or 7 o'clock. Alternatively, the ligament may be palpated, medial and posterior to the ischial spine.
- By palpation, the surgeon confirms that the location grasped with the Allis is at the level of the ischial spine. A nonabsorbable suture is placed through the ligament, and a second suture is placed approximately 1 cm proximally.
- The same steps are repeated on the contralateral side.
- An anterior colporrhaphy is performed if indicated.
- One arm of each suspensory suture is placed through the anterior cuff and the other arm placed through the posterior cuff, with the superior sutures placed more medially.
- The sutures are tied down. The vaginal cuff is closed over the permanent suspension sutures.
- Cystoscopy is performed to evaluate ureteral patency and to exclude lower urinary tract injury.
- The vagina may be packed for up to 24 hours after the procedure.

Uterosacral vaginal vault suspension is performed with the patient in high lithotomy position. It can be performed immediately following a vaginal hysterectomy or in the setting of posthysterectomy prolapse. In the latter setting, two Allis clamps are used to grasp the vaginal apex. With traction on the Allis clamps, the vaginal epithelium overlying the vaginal apex is incised. The cul-de-sac is palpated for adhesions and any unsuspected pathology. If adhesions are present, they should be carefully taken down. The excess peritoneum is excised.

A Heaney retractor or Deaver is then placed anteriorly. The abdominal contents are carefully packed out of the pelvis with a moist, 4-inch Kerlix sponge. The retractor is withdrawn and then replaced so as to elevate the sponge and abdominal contents out of the pelvis, exposing the cul-de-sac (Fig. 39.15). Two Allis clamps are then placed where the remnants of uterosacral ligaments are believed to insert into the vaginal cuff, usually the 5-o'clock and 7-o'clock positions. With tension on the Allis clamp directed outward, the pelvic sidewalls are palpated. The ischial spine is palpated transperitoneally, and an attempt is made to palpate the ureter. If the uterosacral ligament is difficult to find, the Allis clamp can be repositioned. The ureter is usually found 2 to 5 cm ventral and lateral to the ischial spine. The ureter is best found by applying pressure to the pelvic sidewall with the tip of the index or middle finger and sweeping from an anterosuperior to a posteroinferior position.

The uterosacral ligament is identified at the level of the ischial spine. The ligament is grasped with a long Allis clamp and elevated (Fig. 39.15). By palpation, the surgeon confirms that the location grasped with the Allis is medial and posterior to the ischial spine. Then, under direct visualization, sutures are placed through the ligament with a long, straight needle

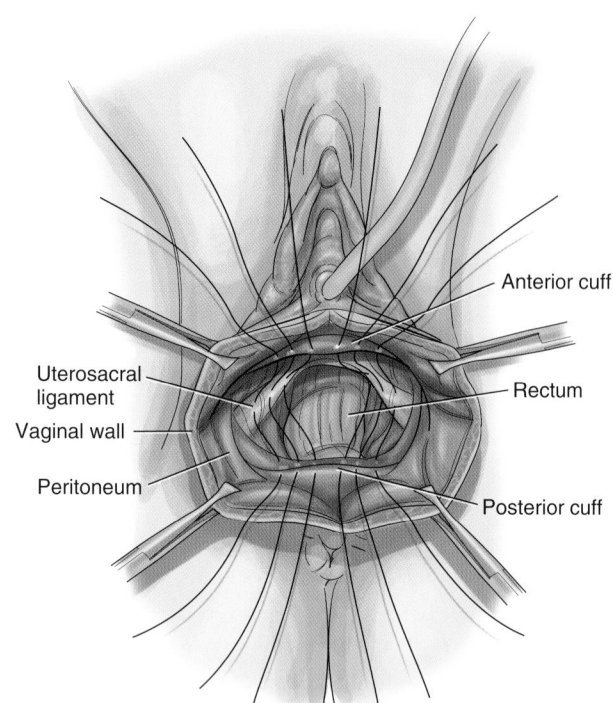

FIGURE 39.15 The uterosacral ligament sutures are placed through the vaginal cuff. One end of each suture is placed through the anterior cuff and one through the posterior cuff, including the peritoneum and the entire thickness of the vaginal wall with the exception of the epithelium. The suture that was placed more superiorly on the ligament is passed through the vaginal cuff more medially.

driver. The most distal suture is placed at the level of the ischial spine, and a second suture is placed approximately 1 cm proximally. This location is optimal for safety and also approximates the normal position of the vaginal apex. Once placed, these sutures are tagged and set aside. The packing is removed from the pelvis.

At this point, the surgeon should perform an anterior colporrhaphy if indicated. The tagged uterosacral sutures are then passed through the vaginal wall at the cuff, including the peritoneum and the entire vaginal wall with the exception of the epithelium. The superior sutures are placed through the vaginal cuff more medially, with the inferior suspensory sutures placed more laterally (Fig. 39.15). After one arm of each suspensory suture has been placed through the anterior cuff and the other arm placed through the posterior cuff, the two medial sutures are tied down, bringing the cuff into high apposition with the uterosacral ligament on either side. After the suspension, cystoscopy is performed. Administration of a coloring agent, such as preoperative oral phenazopyridine or interoperative intravenous methylene blue, is recommended to demonstrate ureteral patency. The final step is closure of the vaginal cuff over the suspensory sutures. A meticulous closure is necessary to minimize the risk of suture exposure.

Some surgeons elect to perform the uterosacral suspension with delayed absorbable suture. A rationale for using delayed absorbable suture is the incidence of exposure or erosion of permanent sutures after uterosacral suspension. Suture exposure may be asymptomatic or may present with bleeding, discharge, dyspareunia, or pain. The incidence

of this complication is unknown. Yazdany et al. reported suture erosion in 37 out of 83 patients (44%). In contrast, Kasturi et al. observed suture erosion in 22%, while Chung et al. reported an incidence of 9%. Typically, suture exposure is relatively easy to address in an office setting, with excision of the exposed suture. This complication can be prevented through the use of delayed absorbable suture for the suspension. However, there is controversy regarding whether the effectiveness of the surgery is reduced by the use of delayed absorbable suture. Chung and colleagues reported a higher incidence of prolapse recurrence in the first year if delayed absorbable sutures were used. If delayed absorbable suture is used, the suspension sutures can be passed through the full thickness of the posterior vaginal wall.

A recent systematic review by Margulies suggested a high success rate for uterosacral suspension of the vaginal vault. Specifically, "optimal" (POP-Q stage 0) or "satisfactory" (POP-Q stage 1) at the apex was observed in 98.3% (95% confidence interval: 95.7% to 100%). Support of the anterior vagina was achieved less often: stages 0 to 1 in 81.2% (95% confidence interval: 67.5% to 94.5%). Also, in the anterior compartment, preoperative prolapse severity was noted to influence postoperative success. Specifically, success for women presenting with preoperative stage II prolapse was 92% versus a success rate of only 66.8% for women presenting with stage III prolapse. Based on these observations, it is our preference to reserve this procedure for women with stage II prolapse.

A potential complication of high uterosacral suspension is ureteral injury or kinking. Karram and colleagues reported a 2.4% risk, Barber and colleagues reported an 11% risk, and Shull and colleagues reported a 1% risk. It is imperative that intraoperative cystoscopy be done to ensure ureteral patency. If ureteral spill is not observed, then the suspension sutures on that side should be cut and removed and the ureter reevaluated. Often, the suture can be replaced using a more medial placement into the uterosacral ligament complex.

Another potential complication of uterosacral suspension is injury to the sacral nerve roots (Fig. 39.16). This should be suspected in patients presenting with new-onset buttock and/or thigh pain, numbness, or weakness. Chung and colleagues observed this complication in 8 out of 515 patients (1.6%) after uterosacral suspension. A significantly higher incidence was reported by Montoya (19 out of 278 women [6.8%]). Anatomic studies have demonstrated that the sacral nerve roots pass under the uterosacral ligament and are potentially vulnerable to suture entrapment. The risk of nerve injury may be minimized by elevating the ligament with an Allis clamp prior to placing the suspension sutures and by placing sutures within 1 to 2 cm of the ischial spine, rather than more proximally. When recognized, symptoms suggestive of nerve injury may be managed conservatively. However, removal of suspension sutures should be considered if pain is severe or persistent.

Abdominal Sacral Colpopexy

Suspension of the vagina to the sacral promontory or into the hollow of the sacrum with an intervening mesh has been shown to be an effective treatment for vault prolapse. This procedure restores the vaginal apex close to the normal anatomic position, approximately 1 cm anterior and 5 cm inferior to the second sacral vertebra.

STEPS IN THE PROCEDURE

Sacrocolpopexy

- The patient is positioned in Allen stirrups.

- The bladder is drained.

- A low transverse abdominal incision is created, and the peritoneal cavity is entered. The abdominal contents are packed out of the pelvis. If a uterus is present, a total or supracervical hysterectomy is performed.

- An EEA sizer or similar manipulator is placed in the vagina. The surgeon dissects the bladder and rectum off the vagina.

- A 2- to 3-cm-wide graft of polypropylene is attached to the vagina, with one anterior and one posterior arm. The graft is sewn in place with interrupted sutures of nonabsorbable monofilament.

- The presacral space is entered and the peritoneal incision extended from the cul-de-sac to sacral promontory, keeping the right ureter in view.

- The ventral surfaces of the S1 and S2 vertebral bodies are exposed. Two to three nonabsorbable sutures are placed through the anterior ligament, with care to avoid injury to the middle sacral vessels. The sutures are tagged.

- Both ends of each suture are passed through the polypropylene graft and tied down. The graft should be in contact with the ligament (without intervening suture bridges). When the sutures are tied down, the vagina should be elevated without tension on the graft.

- Cystoscopy is performed to evaluate ureteral patency and to exclude lower urinary tract injury.

- Before the abdomen is closed, the peritoneum is closed over the graft.

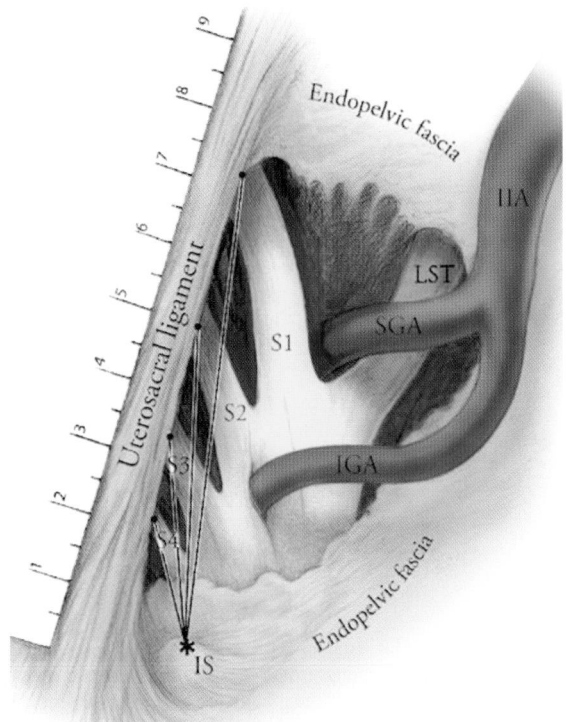

FIGURE 39.16 The sacral nerve roots course under the uterosacral ligament as they pass laterally to exit the greater sciatic foramen. The S4 nerve root passes under the ligament less than 1 cm from the ischial spine, while the S3 root and S2 root pass under the ligament 1.5 cm and 2.6 cm cephalad to the spine, respectively. (Reprinted from Siddique SA, Gutman RE, Schön Ybarra MA, et al. Relationship of the uterosacral ligament to the sacral plexus and to the pudendal nerve. *Int Urogynecol J Pelvic Floor Dysfunct* 2006;17:642, with permission. Copyright © 2006, Springer.)

The patient is placed in Allen stirrups and is prepped and draped. A Foley catheter is placed; a three-way Foley may be useful if the surgeon anticipates distending the bladder to aide in the dissection of the bladder away from the adjacent vagina.

A laparotomy incision is made via a low transverse or vertical midline approach. Moist laparotomy sponges are then used to pack the bowel into the upper abdomen. Any adhesions should be carefully taken down. The course of the ureters and the cul-de-sac should be inspected and palpated. If the patient has a uterus, a hysterectomy should be done first and the cuff closed. It is our practice to perform total hysterectomy, although some surgeons recommend supracervical hysterectomy as a strategy to minimize mesh exposure at the vaginal cuff. Variations of the sacrocolpopexy in which the uterus is retained have been described, but the outcomes of "sacral hysteropexy" are not established.

The vagina is then elevated using an EEA sizer or similar instrument (Fig. 39.1). The peritoneum is then dissected off the anterior vaginal wall. The peritoneum on the posterior aspect of the vagina is incised in the midline and carried down into the cul-de-sac. The peritoneum is then dissected free laterally. A synthetic polypropylene mesh is then prepared. The mesh is prepared as two separate straps, each 2 to 3 cm wide. Additional width increases the total surface of synthetic material without any proven benefit. Although we prefer two separate straps of mesh, other potential configurations have also been described. For example, some surgeons prefer using a "Y" mesh.

The sizer is then used to direct the vagina toward the S1 or S2 vertebra. This will allow the surgeon to identify the site along the vaginal wall that will be the new apex. A critical point is that the apex should be selected to provide adequate elevation to both the anterior and posterior vaginal walls without putting excessive tension on either vaginal wall.

A strap of mesh is then sutured to the anterior vagina using interrupted nonabsorbable sutures, placed 1 to 2 cm apart. We prefer monofilament sutures, as these may reduce the risk of graft/suture erosion when compared to braided sutures. We suture the distal aspect of the mesh first. In some cases, it may be easier to place the first (most distal) suture through the vaginal wall, tag the free ends, and then feed both ends of the suture through the mesh. The suture can then be tied. A second mesh strap is fixed to the posterior vagina using a similar technique. The suture should incorporate the full thickness of the vaginal wall without entering the vaginal lumen. The benefit of the EEA sizer is that penetration into the vagina is easily detected by the tactile sensation of the needle on the metal sizer. If two independent straps of mesh are used, the anterior mesh is sewn to the posterior mesh just proximal to the vaginal apex.

VII

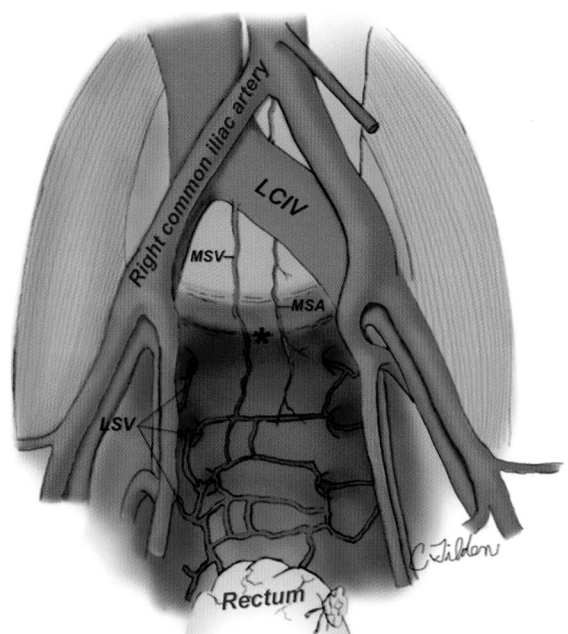

FIGURE 39.17 Vascular anatomy of the presacral space. The vessel closest to the sacral promontory (*) is the left common iliac vein (LCIV), which is 2.7 cm from the midline. Also adjacent to the promontory is the middle sacral artery (MSA), middle sacral vein (MSV), and lateral sacral veins (LSV). (Reprinted from Wieslander CK, Rahn DD, McIntire DD, et al. Vascular anatomy of the presacral space in unembalmed female cadavers. *Am J Obstet Gynecol* 2006;195:1736, with permission. Copyright © 2006, Elsevier.)

The point of attachment for the suspension graft is the anterior longitudinal ligament (Fig. 39.9). Ideally, the graft is attached at the level of S1 or S2. To expose the ligament, the peritoneum over the sacral promontory is opened and this incision carried down over the anterior surface of the sacrum. The surgeon should be mindful of the position of the bifurcation of the vena cava; the left iliac vein is typically within 2 cm of the sacral promontory and is the structure most vulnerable as the peritoneum is opened at the promontory (Fig. 39.17). The hypogastric plexus may be present at the sacral promontory, although it is not typically grossly evident. With the peritoneum reflected, the middle sacral artery and vein are identified. The sacral promontory and the anterior longitudinal ligament are then exposed by blunt and delicate dissection.

The peritoneum is opened into the cul-de-sac. Alternatively, a subperitoneal tunnel can be created into the cul-de-sac by blunt and sharp dissection. The goal is to place the graft retroperitoneally.

Two to four sutures of 0 nonabsorbable sutures are placed through the longitudinal ligament over the sacral promontory (Fig. 39.18). The polypropylene graft is elevated, and the surgeon adjusts tension on the graft to provide adequate elevation of the vagina without excessive tension. The sutures are placed through the graft and tied to bring the graft to the surface of the sacrum without an intervening suture "bridge" (Fig. 39.19). Excessive graft material is trimmed.

The peritoneum is then closed with a 2-0 or 3-0 absorbable suture, continuing over the anterior vaginal wall (thereby covering the mesh). Cystoscopy is performed to confirm ureteral patency as well as an absence of suture material in the bladder. The abdomen is then closed.

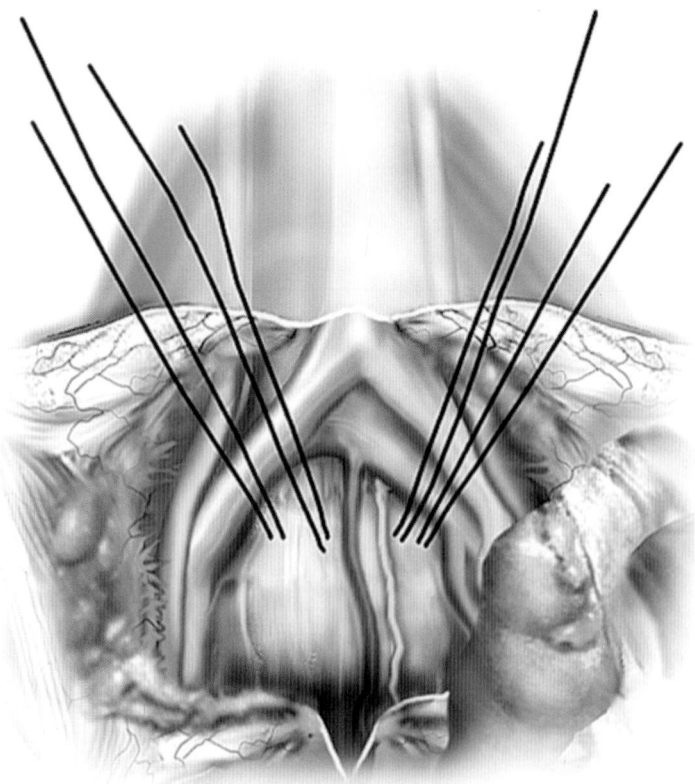

FIGURE 39.18 The sacral promontory, with permanent sutures placed through the longitudinal ligament of sacrum. (Reprinted from Baggish MS, Karram MM. *Atlas of pelvic anatomy and gynecologic surgery.* New York, NY: Saunders, 2001, with permission. Copyright © 2001, Elsevier.)

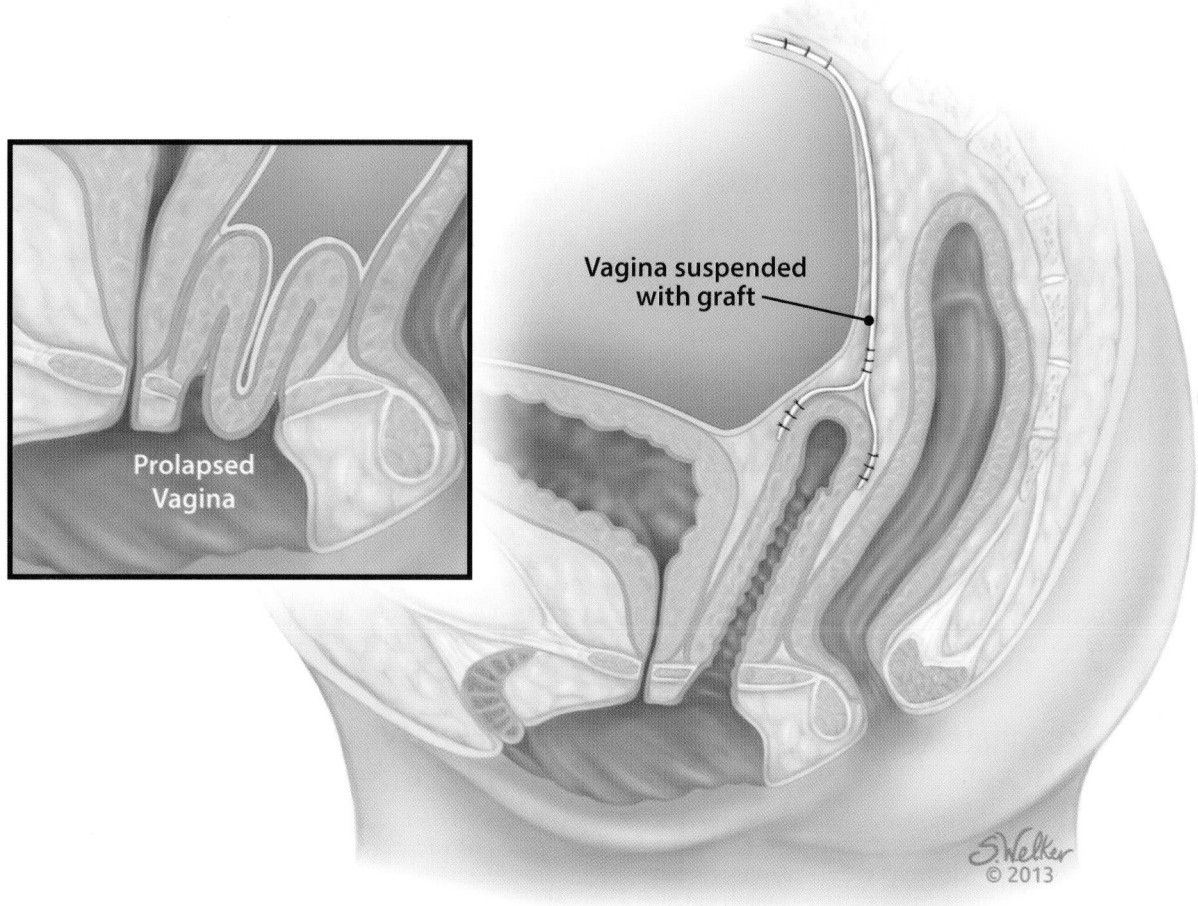

FIGURE 39.19 Attachment of the mesh to the sacrum. The peritoneum has been closed over the entire length of the graft. (Preoperative vault prolapse is shown in the inset.) (Illustrated by Samantha Welker.)

The vagina is inspected and evaluated for any remaining support defects. Occasionally, a posterior colporrhaphy and a perineoplasty are also required.

Although the exact indications for abdominal sacral colpopexy are controversial, many surgeons use it as their primary surgery for all cases of posthysterectomy vault prolapse. We typically recommend abdominal sacral colpopexy for patients with stage III support, young patients with advanced prolapse, patients who have previously failed a vaginal approach, patients who have a foreshortened vagina, or patients who have other coexisting conditions that predispose to subsequent failure.

It has been shown by multiple investigators that abdominal sacral colpopexy is a durable and strong surgical correction for vaginal vault prolapse. Excellent results have been reported by many centers. A 2004 review suggested that durable support at the vaginal apex is obtained in more than 90%, although most studies have less than 2 years of follow-up and few have used validated instruments to assess symptoms. Recent long-term data were provided by the Pelvic Floor Disorders Network. Investigators followed 215 women for up to 7 years after sacropexy. Of the 215 women, 149 underwent physical examinations for prolapse assessment. By 7 years, 31 of 149 women (21%) had anatomic prolapse recurrence; 11 women (7%) had apical

recurrence. Of 31 with anatomic prolapse recurrence, 16 (52%) were symptomatic. This suggests that the process of deteriorating pelvic support is not completely prevented by sacrocolpopexy and that long-term studies are required to identify the best approaches.

Perioperative complications of sacrocolpopexy include ileus, small bowel obstruction, and wound complications, as would be expected from any procedure addressed via laparotomy. Bladder and ureteral injury are rare (<3%). Hemorrhage, especially from presacral vessels, can be life-threatening. Hemostasis can be difficult because damaged presacral vessels tend to retract beneath the bony surface. Sutures, hemoclips, and bone wax should be used initially. If these measures fail, then sterile thumbtacks can be employed. These stainless steel thumbtacks should be placed on the retracted bleeding vessel.

The most common long-term complication has been exposure of synthetic mesh in the vagina, which occurs in 3% to 4%. Exposure can present years after sacropexy. Removal of the eroded mesh can be done via an abdominal or vaginal route. We prefer a vaginal approach, because approximately 50% of mesh exposures resolve with excision of the exposed mesh via the vaginal route. With the patient prepped and draped, as much of the mesh as possible is exposed. The mesh is cut as high as possible and removed. The vaginal edges are then trimmed and closed in layers. Vaginoscopy (with a zero-degree scope, such as a 5-mm laparoscope) can improve visibility, especially when the vaginal apex is high.

LAPAROSCOPIC AND ROBOTIC APPROACH TO VAGINAL SUSPENSION

The techniques and concepts described for sacral colpopexy can also be approached via laparoscopy, with or without robotic assistance. The laparoscopic approach to the patient for positioning, port placement, and equipment is described elsewhere. The laparoscopic approach to these procedures requires patience, attention to detail, and the realization that there is a steep learning curve. Studies comparing robotic, laparoscopic, and open sacrocolpopexy suggest similar short-term outcomes with respect to pelvic organ support, although costs and short-term complications may differ between these approaches. A critical point is that the route of surgery is not as important to patient outcomes as are the underlying surgical principles. It is our belief that the operation and subsequent outcomes should not be compromised for the purpose of having achieved the operation by this approach. Therefore, the surgical measures taken to achieve the underlying concepts should not be significantly altered or changed.

THE OPTIMAL APPROACH TO PELVIC PROLAPSE

Expert opinion differs as to the most appropriate approach to pelvic organ prolapse. Benson and colleagues randomized patients with prolapse to abdominal sacral colpopexy versus bilateral sacrospinous ligament fixation. They found superior results with abdominal sacral colpopexy. The reoperation rate was 16% in the abdominal group and 33% in the vaginal group. Optimal results were obtained in only 29% of the vaginal group and 58% of the abdominal group. The time of operation was longer for the abdominal group. Lo and Wang also reported higher success rates with abdominal sacral colpopexy than sacrospinous fixation, and Maher and associates reported similar success rates. In summary, these three prospective trials found that sacrocolpopexy has a higher success rate than sacrospinous suspension.

Based on a review of these trials, a recent Cochrane review concluded that recurrent vault prolapse was significantly less common after sacrocolpopexy than sacrospinous suspension (relative risk, 0.23; 95% confidence interval, 0.07 to 0.77). However, this conclusion is based on only three randomized trials, with relatively short-term outcomes and limited information about quality-of-life and subjective patient outcomes. Also, when compared to sacrocolpopexy, the sacrospinous suspension was found to be quicker, cheaper, and associated with an earlier return to activities of daily living. In selected cases, a potential advantage of the sacrospinous suspension is that the procedure does not require entry into the peritoneal cavity. We are not aware of randomized trials comparing sacrocolpopexy versus McCall culdoplasty or uterosacral suspension procedures. However, Denman and colleagues found that an abdominal approach to prolapse repair significantly reduced the odds of reoperation compared with the vaginal approach (hazard ratio, 0.37; 95% confidence interval, 0.17 to 0.83; $P = 0.02$).

It is our opinion that no one surgical approach is appropriate for all patients. Surgeons must be adept at multiple approaches and procedures to effectively care for all patients. In general, given the available evidence, we prefer to approach most cases of stage II prolapse transvaginally, reserving abdominal sacral colpopexy for patients with stage III support and for those who have failed a previous vaginal approach. Obliterative procedures including partial Le Fort or complete colpocleisis are highly effective options for women who are no longer sexually active.

ROLE OF HYSTERECTOMY IN PROLAPSE REPAIRS

Hysterectomy with repair of pelvic support defects is standard practice for most parts of the world. However, more attention has been placed on uterine preservation when undergoing surgery for prolapse repairs. It is not known whether the surgical modifications required to perform these surgeries with uterine preservation would impact surgical results or complications. Three studies by Maher and associates, Hefni and colleagues, and van Brummen and associates failed to show a decrease in prolapse recurrence if hysterectomy was performed. There are no prospective studies comparing sacrocolpopexy with and without hysterectomy. More research is needed to understand the impact of hysterectomy on anatomic and functional outcomes when performing prolapse surgery.

OBLITERATIVE PROCEDURES

Le Fort Partial Colpocleisis

At times, patients may be sufficiently bothered by uterovaginal or vault prolapse, but they are poor candidates for major reconstructive surgery because of their overall medical condition. An obliterative procedure may then be a good approach for these women. A Le Fort procedure is an option if the patient has her uterus and is no longer sexually active. Because the uterus is retained, it will be difficult to evaluate any future uterine bleeding or cervical pathology. Therefore, evaluation for upper genital tract pathology (potentially including transvaginal ultrasound and/or endometrial biopsy) and Papanicolaou smear must be done before surgery. It is our practice to pursue a different approach for women who require surveillance of upper tract pathology, such as women with a history of preinvasive conditions of the cervix or endometrium.

STEPS IN THE PROCEDURE

Le Fort Colpocleisis

- The patient is positioned in high lithotomy position.

- The bladder is drained.

- The cervix is grasped, and rectangles are marked on the anterior and posterior vagina. The proximal edge of each rectangle should typically be 2 cm distal to the cervix (to allow room for the cervix once the walls are approximated). The distal edge of the anterior rectangle is at the bladder neck, with a corresponding location selected posteriorly. Lateral channels should be left.

- These rectangular areas are injected with a dilute solution of vasopressin, and the marked segments of vaginal epithelium are removed by sharp dissection.

- The edges of the rectangle and denuded vaginal wall are closed in successive rows, using delayed interrupted sutures. As successive rows of sutures are placed and tied, proceeding from proximal to distal vagina, the uterus and vaginal apex are gradually turned inward.
- An aggressive perineorrhaphy should be done to narrow the introitus.
- Cystoscopy is performed to evaluate ureteral patency and to exclude lower urinary tract injury.

The procedure is started by placing the cervix on traction to evert the vagina. A marking pen or scalpel is used to mark out the areas that are to be denuded both anteriorly and posteriorly (Fig. 39.20). Anteriorly, a rectangle of vaginal epithelium should be marked from approximately 2 cm distal to the cervix to the level of the bladder neck. A mirror image on the posterior vaginal wall should also be marked out. It is critical that these rectangles be selected such that there is sufficient room proximally for the cervix (e.g., after suturing the proximal edges to each other). In addition, a channel should be left on either side of the vagina, with a diameter that is sufficient to allow drainage of blood and cervical secretions but small enough that the cervix cannot prolapse through the channel.

The previously marked areas are injected with a dilute solution of vasopressin (such as 20 units in 30 mL sterile saline). The marked segments of vaginal epithelium are removed by sharp dissection (Fig. 39.21). The surgeon should leave the maximum amount of fibromuscular vaginal wall behind on the bladder and rectum. Hemostasis is an absolute must.

The cut edges of the anterior and posterior vaginal wall are sewn together with rows of interrupted delayed absorbable

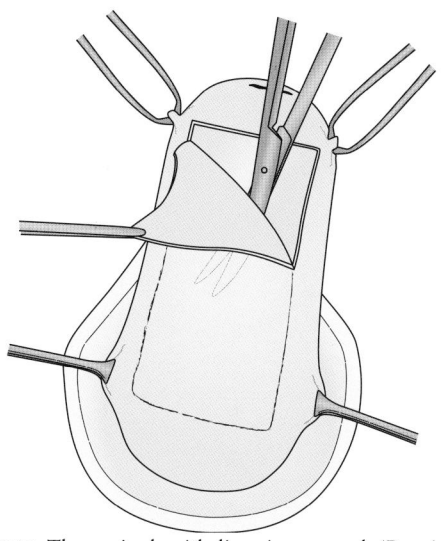

FIGURE 39.21 The vaginal epithelium is removed. (Reprinted from Bent AE, Cundiff GW, Swift SE. *Ostergard's urogynecology and pelvic floor dysfunction*, 6th ed. Philadelphia, PA: Lippincott Williams & Wilkins, 2007, with permission. Copyright © 2007, Lippincott Williams & Wilkins.)

sutures (Fig. 39.22). The knot should be turned into the epithelium-lined tunnels that were created bilaterally. As successive rows of sutures are placed and tied, the uterus and vaginal apex are gradually turned inward (Fig. 39.23). After the vagina has been inverted, the distal margins of the rectangle can be sutured. In some cases, an anti-incontinence procedure may be indicated to treat stress incontinence or to prevent postoperative stress incontinence. Also, an aggressive perineorrhaphy should be done to narrow the introitus.

Due to the potential for ureteral or bladder injury, intraoperative cystoscopy is recommended. Other perioperative

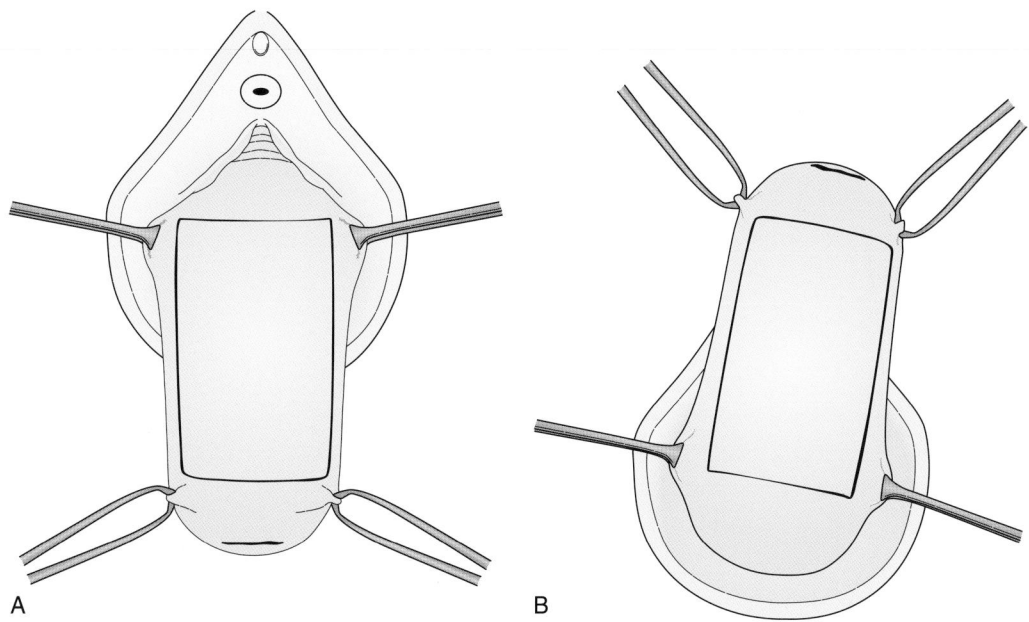

FIGURE 39.20 Rectangles of vaginal mucosa are marked on the (A) anterior vagina and (B) posterior vagina. A 2-cm gap is left between the rectangles to allow for the creation of drainage channels. (Reprinted from Bent AE, Cundiff GW, Swift SE. *Ostergard's urogynecology and pelvic floor dysfunction*, 6th ed. Philadelphia, PA: Lippincott Williams & Wilkins, 2007, with permission. Copyright © 2007, Lippincott Williams & Wilkins.)

VII

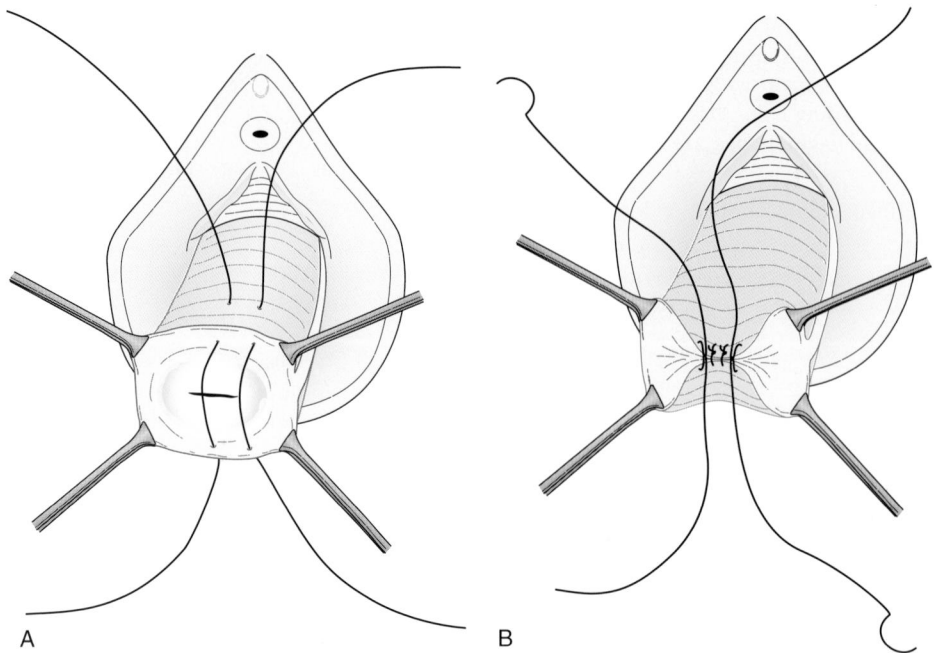

FIGURE 39.22 The colpocleisis is closed in rows. **A:** The first row of interrupted delayed absorbable sutures is placed along the proximal edge of the dissection. **B:** As sutures are tied down, the excised rectangles are brought together. (Reprinted from Bent AE, Cundiff GW, Swift SE. *Ostergard's urogynecology and pelvic floor dysfunction*, 6th ed. Philadelphia, PA: Lippincott Williams & Wilkins, 2007, with permission. Copyright © 2007, Lippincott Williams & Wilkins.)

complications are rare. Because Le Fort colpocleisis is typically reserved for elderly or medically compromised women, the most common perioperative complications are related to their underlying medical and surgical risks. Surgical site infection is rare, although cases of pyometra have been reported months or years after colpocleisis.

Long-term results of colpocleisis are excellent. Case series have suggested a cure rate of 90% to 100%. In a recent multicenter study, colpocleisis was associated with high patient satisfaction among 152 women. One year after surgery, 73% had stage 0 to 1 support and an additional 20% had stage 2 support. Ninety-five percent were "satisfied" or "very satisfied."

Colpectomy and Colpocleisis

For patients with posthysterectomy vault prolapse who do not desire coital function and for whom operative time is to be kept at a minimum, a colpectomy and colpocleisis can be done to treat the prolapse.

The distinction between this approach and a Le Fort colpocleisis is that the former technique does not require the creation of lateral drainage channels. Thus, the entire vaginal epithelium is removed (Fig. 39.24). It is our practice to limit the dissection to the vaginal segment superior to the bladder neck. This allows future suburethral access if needed. After the vaginal mucosa is completely excised from the underlying

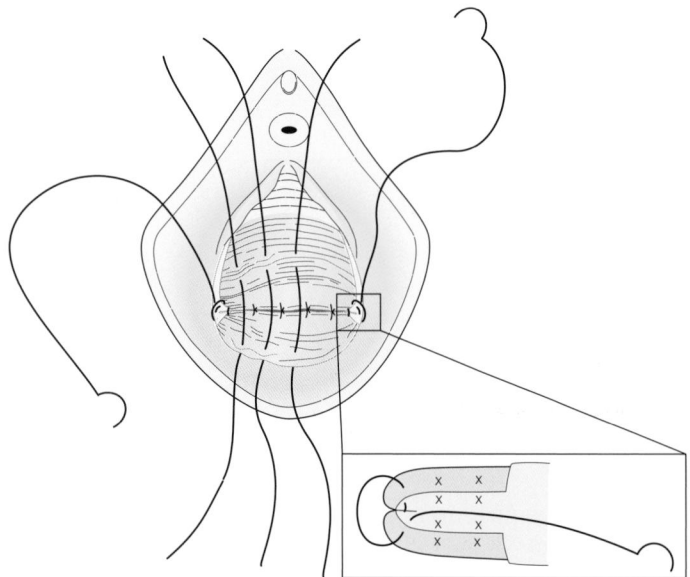

FIGURE 39.23 Interrupted absorbable sutures are placed in rows to reapproximate the vaginal muscularis. As each row is placed, the vagina gradually inverts. Laterally, the vaginal drainage channels are preserved. (Reprinted from Bent AE, Cundiff GW, Swift SE. *Ostergard's urogynecology and pelvic floor dysfunction*, 6th ed. Philadelphia, PA: Lippincott Williams & Wilkins, 2007, with permission. Copyright © 2007, Lippincott Williams & Wilkins.)

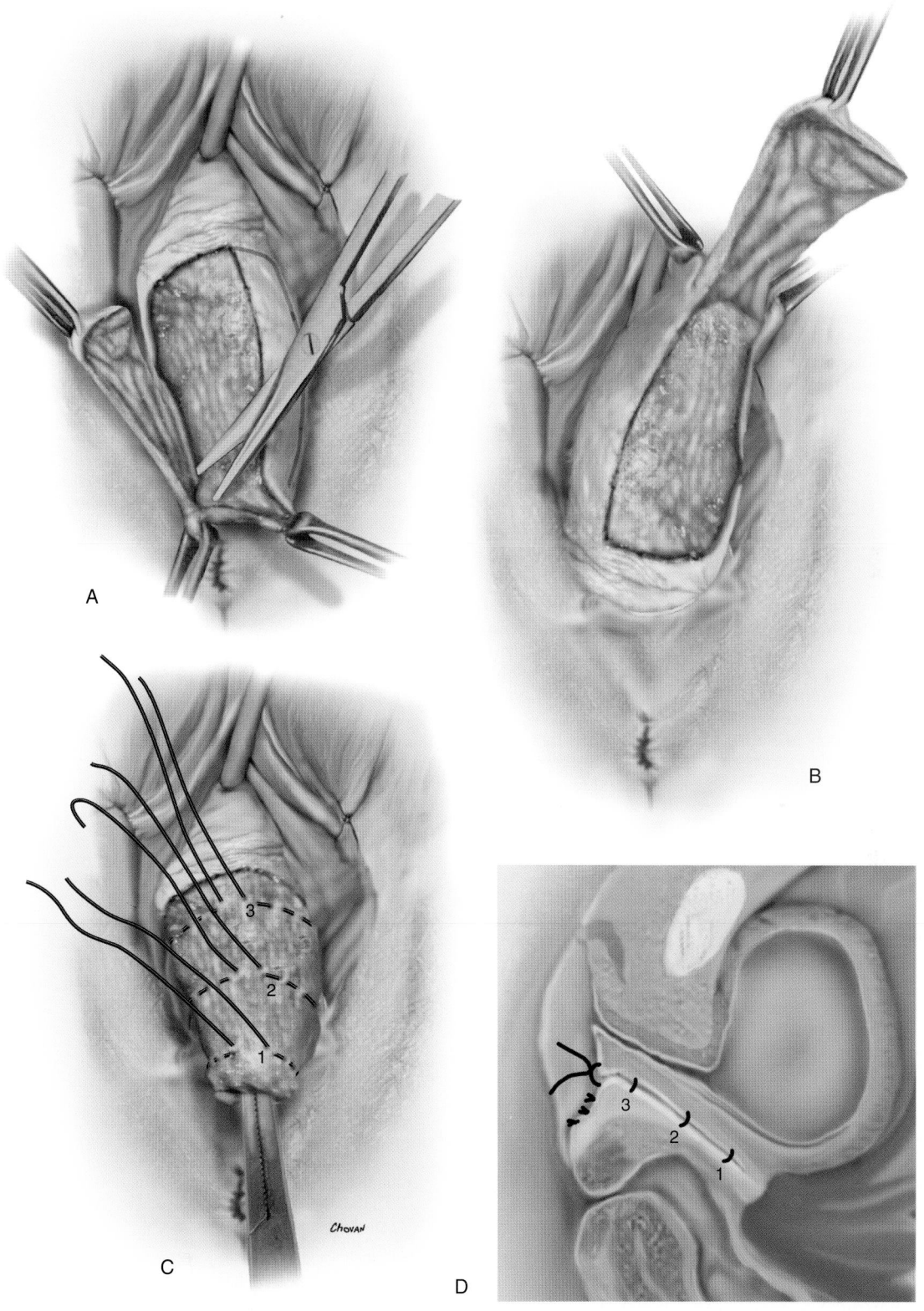

FIGURE 39.24 Colpectomy and complete colpocleisis. **A and B:** After subcutaneous infiltration with lidocaine or bupivacaine hydrochloride in 1/200,000 epinephrine solution, the vagina is circumscribed by an incision at the site of the hymen and marked into quadrants. Each quadrant is removed by sharp dissection. **C:** Purse-string delayed absorbable sutures are placed. The leading edge of the soft tissue is inverted by the tip of a forceps. Purse-string sutures are tied *1* before *2* and *2* before *3*, with progressive inversion of the soft tissue before the tying of each suture. **D:** The final relationship is shown in cross section. A perineorrhaphy is also usually performed. (Reprinted from Baggish MS, Karram MM. *Atlas of pelvic anatomy and gynecologic surgery*. New York, NY: Saunders, 2001, with permission. Copyright © 2001, Elsevier.)

endopelvic fibromuscular vaginal wall, series of purse-string sutures are used to invert the prolapse (Fig. 39.24). Once the prolapse is reduced, an aggressive perineorrhaphy is done to narrow the introitus. Cystoscopy should be performed at the conclusion, with verification of ureteral patency.

CONCLUSION

Our understanding of the anatomy and concepts of pelvic organ prolapse and its treatments are constantly evolving. This evolution will and must continue to facilitate our understanding of the complex and varied etiologies of pelvic organ prolapse. Surgical treatments must restore both anatomy and address functional derangements. This evolution will also provide insight into preventive measures for women at risk for pelvic organ prolapse and pelvic floor dysfunction. We, as pelvic surgeons, must continue to evaluate and apply new principles and techniques to established surgical dictums. There must be continued research, education, and a thoughtful, honest comparison of long-term surgical outcomes if we are going to continue to improve our care to a growing number of afflicted but active patients.

BEST SURGICAL PRACTICES

- The ultimate goal of pelvic reconstructive surgery is to restore anatomy, maintain or restore visceral function, and maintain or restore sexual function.
- The McCall culdoplasty and its various modifications are well-established transvaginal techniques to suspend the vaginal apex. Approximately two to three permanent sutures are used to plicate the uterosacral ligaments. The Mayo Clinic technique excises a wedge of vaginal wall, with repair of any enterocele that is present.
- For stage II vaginal prolapse, the sacrospinous ligament fixation is a useful extraperitoneal technique. Surgeons should be very familiar with the anatomy and experienced with the procedure. Injury to the pudendal nerve or vessels can cause serious injury or life-threatening hemorrhage. One third of patients may experience recurrent prolapse, especially pertaining to the anterior vaginal wall.
- An alternative is transvaginal uterosacral suspension of the vagina. The surgeon fixes the vaginal cuff to the uterosacral ligaments at the level of the ischial spine. Long-term outcomes are excellent, although preoperative prolapse severity affects postoperative success.
- Abdominal sacral colpopexy may be preferred by some surgeons for the treatment of severe (stage 3 to 4) prolapse and recurrent prolapse after a prior surgical failure and for women felt to be at high risk for recurrence. The anterior and posterior vaginal walls are supported to the longitudinal ligament of the sacrum using synthetic mesh.

BIBLIOGRAPHY

Alevizon SJ, Finan MA. Sacrospinous colpopexy: management of postoperative pudendal nerve entrapment. *Obstet Gynecol* 1996;88:713.

Baden WB, Walker TA, Lindsey JH. The vaginal profile. *Tex Med* 1968;64:56.

Baggish MS, Karram MM. *Atlas of pelvic anatomy and gynecologic surgery*. New York, NY: Saunders, 2001.

Barber MD, Visco AG, Weidner AC, et al. Bilateral uterosacral ligament vaginal vault suspension with site-specific endopelvic fascia defect repair for treatment of pelvic organ prolapse. *Am J Obstet Gynecol* 2000;183:1402.

Barksdale PA, Elkins TE, Sanders CK, et al. An anatomic approach to pelvic hemorrhage during sacrospinous ligament fixation of the vaginal vault. *Obstet Gynecol* 1998;91:715.

Benson JT, Lucente V, McClellan E. Vaginal versus abdominal reconstructive surgery for the treatment of pelvic support defects: a prospective randomized study with long-term outcome evaluation.

Bent AE, Cundiff GW, Swift SE. *Ostergard's urogynecology and pelvic floor dysfunction*, 6th ed. Philadelphia, PA: Lippincott Williams & Wilkins, 2007.

Brizzolara S, Pillai-Allen A. Risk of mesh erosion with sacral colpopexy and concurrent hysterectomy. *Obstet Gynecol* 2003;102:306.

Brubaker L, Nygaard I, Richter HE, et al. Two-year outcomes after sacrocolpopexy with and without burch to prevent stress urinary incontinence. *Obstet Gynecol* 2008;112:49.

Buller JL, Thompson JR, Cundiff GW, et al. Uterosacral ligament: description of anatomic relationships to optimize surgical safety. *Obstet Gynecol* 2001;97:873.

Chen L, Ashton-Miller JA, Hsu Y, et al. Interaction among apical support, levator ani impairment, and anterior vaginal wall prolapse. *Obstet Gynecol* 2006;108:324.

Chung CP, Kuehl TJ, Larsen WI, et al. Recognition and management of nerve entrapment pain after uterosacral ligament suspension. *Obstet Gynecol* 2012;120:292.

Chung CP, Miskimins R, Kuehl TJ, et al. Permanent suture used in uterosacral ligament suspension offers better anatomical support than delayed absorbable suture. *Int Urogynecol J* 2012;23:223.

Clark AL, Gregory T, Smith VJ, et al. Epidemiologic evaluation of reoperation for surgically treated pelvic organ prolapse and urinary incontinence. *Am J Obstet Gynecol* 2003;189:1261.

Cruikshank SH, Cox DW. Sacrospinous ligament fixation at the time of transvaginal hysterectomy. *Am J Obstet Gynecol* 1990;162:1611.

DeLancey JOL, Morley GW. Total colpocleisis for vaginal eversion. *Am J Obstet Gynecol* 1997;176:1228.

DeLancey JOL, Starr RA. Histology of the connection between the vagina and levator ani muscles; implications for urinary tract function. *J Reprod Med* 1990;35:765.

DeLancey JOL. Anatomic aspects of vaginal eversion after hysterectomy. *Am J Obstet Gynecol* 1992;166:1717.

Denman MA, Gregory WT, Boyles SH, et al. Reoperation 10 years after surgically managed pelvic organ prolapse and urinary incontinence. *Am J Obstet Gynecol* 2008;198:555.e1.

Farrell SA, Dempsey T, Geldenhuys L. Histologic examination of "fascia" used in colporrhaphy. *Obstet Gynecol* 2001;98:794.

Fialkow MF, Newton KM, Lentz GM, et al. Lifetime risk of surgical management for pelvic organ prolapse or urinary incontinence. *Int Urogynecol J Pelvic Floor Dysfunct* 2008;19:437.

Fitzgerald MP, Richter HE, Bradley CS, et al. Pelvic support, pelvic symptoms, and patient satisfaction after colpocleisis. *Int Urogynecol J Pelvic Floor Dysfunct* 2008;19:1603.

Given FT Jr, Muhlendorf IK, Browning GM. Vaginal length and sexual function after colpopexy for complete uterovaginal eversion. *Am J Obstet Gynecol* 1993;169:284.

Goldman J, Ovadia J, Feldberg D. The Neugebauer-LeFort operation: a review of 118 partial colpocleises. *Eur J Obstet Gynaecol Reprod Biol* 1985;12:31.

Goldman HB. SUI surgery at the time of vaginal POP repair: is a surgical algorithm possible or desirable? *Neurourol Urodyn* 2011;30:758.

Gutman RE, Pannu HK, Cundiff GW, et al. Anatomic relationship between the vaginal apex and the bony architecture of the pelvis: a magnetic resonance imaging evaluation. *Am J Obstet Gynecol* 2005;192:1544.

Hefni M, El-Toukhy T, Bhaumik J, et al. Sacrospinous cervicocolpopexy with uterine conservation for uterovaginal prolapse in elderly women: an evolving concept. *Am J Obstet Gynecol* 2003;188:645.

Jenkins VR. Uterosacral ligament fixation for vaginal vault suspension in uterine and vaginal vault prolapse. *Am J Obstet Gynecol* 1997;177:1337.

Karram MM, Goldwasser S, Kleeman S, et al. High uterosacral vaginal vault suspension with fascial reconstruction for vaginal repair of enterocele and vaginal vault prolapse. *Am J Obstet Gynecol* 2001;185:1339.

Kasturi S, Bentley-Taylor M, Woodman PJ, et al. High uterosacral ligament vaginal vault suspension: comparison of absorbable versus permanent suture for apical fixation. *Int Urogynecol J* 2012;23:941.

VII

Leone Roberti Maggiore U, Alessandri F, Remorgida V, et al. Vaginal sacrospinous colpopexy using the Capio suture-capturing device versus traditional technique: feasibility and outcome. *Arch Gynecol Obstet* 2013;287:267.

Lo TS, Wang AC. Abdominal colposacropexy and sacrospinous ligament suspension for severe uterovaginal prolapse: a comparison. *J Gynecol Surg* 1998;14:59.

Maher C, Feiner B, Baessler K, et al. Surgical management of pelvic organ prolapse in women. *Cochrane Database Syst Rev* 2010;(4) [Art. No.: CD004014].

Maher CF, Cary MP, Slack MC, et al. Uterine preservation or hysterectomy at sacrospinous colpopexy for Uterovaginal prolapse? *Int Urogynecol J Pelvic Floor Dysfunct* 2001;12:381.

Maher CF, Qatawney AM, Dwyer PL, et al. Abdominal sacral colpopexy or vaginal sacrospinous colpopexy for vaginal vault prolapse: a prospective randomized study. *Am J Obstet Gynecol* 2004;190:20.

Margulies RU, Rogers MA, Morgan DM, et al. Outcomes of transvaginal uterosacral ligament suspension: systematic review and metaanalysis. *Am J Obstet Gynecol* 2010;202:124.

McCall ML. Posterior culdoplasty. *Obstet Gynecol* 1957;10:595.

Miyazaki FS. Miya Hook ligature carrier for sacrospinous ligament suspension. *Obstet Gynecol* 1987;70:286.

Montoya TI, Luebbehusen HI, Schaffer JI, et al. Sensory neuropathy following suspension of the vaginal apex to the proximal uterosacral ligaments. *Int Urogynecol J* 2012;23:1735.

Morgan DM, Rogers MA, Huebner M, et al. Heterogeneity in anatomic outcome of sacrospinous ligament fixation for prolapse: a systematic review. *Obstet Gynecol* 2007;109:1424.

Morley GW, DeLancey JO. Sacrospinous ligament fixation for eversion of the vagina. *Am J Obstet Gynecol* 1988;158:872.

Nichols DH, Randall CL. *Vaginal surgery*, 3rd ed. Baltimore, MD: Williams & Wilkins, 1989.

Nichols DH. Sacrospinous fixation for massive eversion of the vagina. *Am J Obstet Gynecol* 1982;142:901.

Nygaard I, Brubaker L, Zyczynski HM, et al. Long-term outcomes following abdominal sacrocolpopexy for pelvic organ prolapse. *JAMA* 2013;309:2016.

Nygaard IE, McCreery R, Brubaker L, et al. Abdominal sacrocolpopexy: a comprehensive review. *Obstet Gynecol* 2004;104:805.

Olsen AL, Smith VJ, Bergstrom JO, et al. Epidemiology of surgically managed pelvic organ prolapse and urinary incontinence. *Obstet Gynecol* 1997;89:501.

Patsner B. Mesh erosion into the bladder after abdominal sacral colpopexy. *Obstet Gynecol* 2000;95:1029.

Quiroz LH, Gutman RE, Fagan MJ, et al. Partial colpocleisis for the treatment of sacrocolpopexy mesh erosions. *Int Urogynecol J Pelvic Floor Dysfunct* 2008;19:261.

Randall C, Nichols D. Surgical treatment of vaginal inversion. *Obstet Gynecol* 1971;38:327.

Rane A, Lim YN, Withey G, et al. Magnetic resonance imaging findings following three different vaginal vault repair procedures: a randomised study. *Aust N Z J Obstet Gynaecol* 2004;44:135.

Richardson AC, Lyon JB, Williams NL. A new look at pelvic relaxation. *Am J Obstet Gynecol* 1976;126:568.

Richter K, Albright W. Long-term results following fixation of the vagina on the sacrospinal ligament by the vaginal route. *Am J Obstet Gynecol* 1981;151:811.

Roshanravan SM, Wieslander CK, Schaffer JI, et al. Neurovascular anatomy of the sacrospinous ligament region in female cadavers: implications in sacrospinous ligament fixation. *Am J Obstet Gynecol* 2007;197:660.e1.

Shepherd JP, Higdon HL III, Stanford EJ, et al. Effect of suture selection on the rate of suture or mesh erosion and surgery failure in abdominal sacrocolpopexy. *Female Pelvic Med Reconstr Surg* 2010;16:229.

Shull BL, Bachofen C, Coates KW, et al. A transvaginal approach to repair of apical and other associated sites of pelvic organ prolapse with uterosacral ligaments. *Am J Obstet Gynecol* 2000;183:1365; discussion 1373.

Siddique SA, Gutman RE, Schön Ybarra MA, et al. Relationship of the uterosacral ligament to the sacral plexus and to the pudendal nerve. *Int Urogynecol J Pelvic Floor Dysfunct* 2006;17:642.

Silva WA, Pauls RN, Segal JL, et al. Uterosacral ligament vault suspension: five-year outcomes. *Obstet Gynecol* 2006;108:255.

Sylvester T, Bond V, Johnson HW Jr, et al. Radiologic images of retrograde ureterography before and after release of bilateral sacrospinous ligament fixation sutures. *Female Pelvic Med Reconstr Surg* 2012;18:168.

Sze EH, Meranus J, Kohli N, et al. Vaginal configuration on MRI after abdominal sacrocolpopexy and sacrospinous ligament suspension. *Int Urogynecol J Pelvic Floor Dysfunct* 2001;12:375.

Thompson JR, Gibb JS, Genadry R, et al. Anatomy of pelvic arteries adjacent to the sacrospinous ligament: importance of the coccygeal branch of the inferior gluteal artery. *Obstet Gynecol* 1999;94:973.

Toglia MR, Fagan MJ. Pyometra complicating a LeFort colpocleisis. *Int Urogynecol J Pelvic Floor Dysfunct* 2009;20:361.

Tulikangas PK, Walters MD, Brainard JA, et al. Enterocele: is there a histologic defect? *Obstet Gynecol* 2001;98:634.

Van Brummen HJ, Van de Pol G, Aalders CI, et al. Sacrospinous hysteropexy compared to vaginal hysterectomy as primary surgical treatment for a descensus uteri: effects on urinary symptoms. *Int Urogynecol J Pelvic Floor Dysfunct* 2003;14:350.

Verdeja AM, Elkins TE, Odoi A, et al. Transvaginal sacrospinous colpopexy: anatomic landmarks to be aware of to minimize complications. *Am J Obstet Gynecol* 1995;173:1468.

Von Pechmann WS, Mutone M, Fyffe J, et al. Total colpocleisis with high levator plication for the treatment of advanced pelvic organ prolapse. *Am J Obstet Gynecol* 2003;189:121.

Walters MD, Karram MM. *Urogynecology and reconstructive pelvic surgery*, 2nd ed. St. Louis, MO: CV Mosby, 1999.

Webb MJ, Aronson MP, Ferguson LK, et al. Posthysterectomy vaginal vault prolapse: primary repair in 693 patients. *Obstet Gynecol* 1998;92:281.

Wieslander CK, Rahn DD, McIntire DD, et al. Vascular anatomy of the presacral space in unembalmed female cadavers. *Am J Obstet Gynecol* 2006;195:1736.

Wieslander CK, Roshanravan SM, Wai CY, et al. Uterosacral ligament suspension sutures: anatomic relationships in unembalmed female cadavers. *Am J Obstet Gynecol* 2007;197:672.e1.

Wu JM, Wells EC, Hundley AF, et al. Mesh erosion in abdominal sacral colpopexy with and without concomitant hysterectomy. *Am J Obstet Gynecol* 2006;194:1418.

Yazdany T, Yip S, Bhatia NN, et al. Suture complications in a teaching institution among patients undergoing uterosacral ligament suspension with permanent braided suture. *Int Urogynecol J* 2010;21:813.

CHAPTER 40

Nonsurgical Management of Pelvic Organ Prolapse: The Use of Vaginal Pessaries and Pelvic Floor Muscle Training

Chi Chiung Grace Chen and Jaime B. Long

DEFINITIONS

Occult and de novo stress urinary incontinence—Although occult incontinence refers to preexisting incontinence that only becomes symptomatic after prolapse reduction and de novo incontinence refers to new incontinence symptoms that develops after an intervention, these terms are often used interchangeably in the literature.

Pelvic organ prolapse—Descent/herniation of the anterior vaginal compartment (cystocele, urethrocele), apical compartment (uterine or vaginal vault prolapse), and/or posterior compartment (rectocele, sigmoidocele, perineocele, enterocele).

Pelvic floor muscle training—Exercises aimed to improve the strength and function of the pelvic floor muscles.

Pelvic Organ Prolapse-Quantification (POP-Q) system—Validated and widely accepted standardized scoring system used to measure the degree and type of pelvic organ prolapse; includes an assessment of vaginal length, genital hiatus, and perineal body; see Chapter 36.

Pessary—Device inserted into the vagina for reduction of pelvic organ prolapse.

Stress urinary incontinence—Involuntary urinary leakage with effort or exertion or with sneezing or coughing as defined by the International Consultation on Incontinence.

Urge urinary incontinence—Involuntary urinary leakage accompanied by or immediately preceded by urgency as defined by the International Consultation on Incontinence.

Vaginal splinting—Digital reduction of prolapse tissue to facilitate urination and/or defecation.

Pelvic floor disorders such as pelvic organ prolapse (POP) are common and costly conditions that will be encountered by any practitioner who cares for women, especially older women. From the 2005 to 2006 National Health and Nutrition Examination Survey of 1961 nonpregnant women, Nygaard et al. reported that the prevalence of symptomatic POP was noted to be 2.87% (3.3 million). Wu et al. in 2009 reported that Due to the aging population, the prevalence of symptomatic prolapse is estimated to increase 46% (4.9 million) by 2050.

According to Olsen et al., in the United States it is currently estimated that by the age of 80, women have an 11% chance of undergoing surgery for POP or urinary incontinence with a reoperation rate of 30%. Subak et al. estimated that over 1 billion dollars are spent and over 300,000 procedures are performed annually to surgically treat prolapse; however, surgery is just one approach, and providers caring for women with this condition should be familiar with conservative options. In comparing the prevalence estimates and the number of surgeries that are performed, it is clear that many women with prolapse either choose conservative strategies or go without treatment. This observation, coupled with the high rates of surgical failure and reoperation, underscores the importance of understanding conservative management options for prolapse and discussing these options with patients. This chapter reviews the available data and recommendations on pessary use and pelvic floor muscle training (PFMT) for POP.

Pessaries have been in use for thousands of years, and although vigorous scientific trials regarding their use are only beginning to emerge, years of expert opinion and experience continue to support and guide clinical decisions. Pessaries are also utilized for urinary incontinence, uterine retroversion, and obstetric indications such as cervical insufficiency; however, this chapter focuses specifically on their use for POP.

PFMT involves exercises aimed to improve the strength and function of the pelvic floor muscles. These exercises are often performed with a physical therapist and may also involve education on lifestyle modifications such as weight loss and avoidance of heavy lifting. Although these interventions are well researched and considered first-line treatment in other pelvic floor disorders such as stress, urge, and mixed urinary incontinence, this chapter focuses specifically on the use of PFMT for POP.

HISTORY OF PESSARY

The term "pessary" is derived from the Greek word "pessós," which is an oval stone used in certain games. This term was originally used to describe oval stones that were inserted into the uteri of camels for contraception and later was used to describe other intrauterine devices.

Throughout history and into modern times, there has been a clear consensus that the ideal conservative treatment for prolapse involves reducing the prolapse with a lubricating substance followed by placement of an object inside the vagina to prevent reprolapse. What has changed are the methods and materials involved in this process. According to Shah and colleagues and Oliver and colleagues, the first reference of uterine/vaginal prolapse and "remedies to allow the womb of a woman to slip into its place" was from the Ebers papyrus, which dates back to as early as 1550 BC. Some of these remedies include the use of honey and petroleum to reduce the prolapse as well as the use of fumes and astringents to penetrate the uterine cavity so that it would revert back into the body.

At the time of Hippocrates (400 BC), many physicians prescribed succussion therapy, which involved hanging the patient upside down from her feet and moving her up and down as to return the prolapsed organ back into the body. Various agents were used to facilitate this process, including hot oil. Earliest pessaries were fashioned from a variety of materials such as an astringent-soaked plug of wool and half a pomegranate soaked in wine. Several methods were described to hold the prolapse and/or pessary in place, including leg binding and bed rest with the foot raised above the level of the head.

In addition to the above methods, Soranus of Ephesus (98 AD) in his treatise *Gynaecology* believed that placing herbs that emit pleasant odors around the patient's head would entice the prolapse to ascend. This was coupled with placing astringents that emit foul odors around the vagina to force the prolapse back into the body. He recommended that surgery not be performed unless the uterus was gangrenous. In the Middle Ages, other methods reported included frightening the prolapse with hot iron so that it would retreat back into the body. Cupping has also been advocated for prolapse reduction.

Until the 16th century, most of the materials used for pessaries were naturally occurring materials or objects that had been repurposed. It was not until the end of the 16th century that devices were purposely made to address prolapse. Notably, Ambrose Pare, a royal surgeon in the French court, made oval-shaped pessaries from materials such as brass or cork covered in wax. These pessaries were often held in place with a belt-like device worn across the waist. Hendrik van Roonhuyse (1625–1672), the Dutch gynecologist who is credited with writing one of the earliest textbooks of operative gynecology, devised a pessary made of cork with a hole in it to allow for passage of discharge. The late 17th century saw a considerable number of medical therapies and pharmaceutical concoctions promoted for the treatment of genital prolapse, which persisted even into the 18th century. Specifically, soft rubber pessaries that resembled contraceptive diaphragms with a perforated gold tip to allow for the escape of discharge were devised to address prolapse and the issue of vaginal wall injuries, which were a common result of metal pessaries. In the mid-19th century, the American Medical Association documented 123 different pessaries. Hugh Lennox Hodge (1796–1873) recommended metal, glass, and porcelain pessaries instead of wood, cork, or sponge due to his belief that the harm attributable to pessaries stems from the material, the form, and the size. Modern pessaries are primarily made of silicone and are rarely made of latex, rubber, or acrylic. These materials have completely replaced the hard plastic and polystyrene used previously. Silicone is advantageous because it is flexible yet sturdy, durable, hypoallergenic, and noncarcinogenic. It is also inert, does not absorb secretions or odors, and can be repeatedly cleaned and autoclaved, if needed for resterilization.

INDICATIONS AND THERAPEUTIC BENEFITS OF PESSARY

Pessaries are used to alleviate the symptoms of prolapse and delay or eliminate the need for surgery. As discussed below, there may also be some evidence that pessaries may retard prolapse progression. In recent surveys of gynecologists and female pelvic medicine and reconstructive surgeons/urogynecologists in the United States and United Kingdom, 86% to 98% of respondents prescribe pessaries in their practice. Cundiff et al. reported that specifically, among members of the American Urogynecologic Society (AUGS), 77% of respondents used pessaries as first-line therapy for prolapse, whereas 12% offered them only to women who are not considered good surgical candidates. Ninety-two percent believed that pessaries alleviated prolapse symptoms while 48% believed that pessaries also improved pelvic support.

The 2004 Cochrane Review concluded that there are no published randomized controlled trials addressing pessary use for POP. Although there is still no consensus on the indication for use, the use of different types of pessaries, or the ideal follow-up regimen, as discussed below, there is at least one randomized controlled trial (by Cundiff et al.) comparing the use of two different pessaries for prolapse. It is also important not to discount findings from numerous published series and experience from thousands of years of pessary use.

As most women with prolapse do not tend to experience symptoms until the prolapse extends beyond the vaginal introitus, the primary goal of pessary placement is to prevent the vaginal prolapse from extending beyond the vaginal opening. Although pessary can be offered as a treatment option to most patients with prolapse, managing the patient's expectations regarding the likelihood of successful placement, continued use, alleviation of symptoms, and improvement of quality of life is important and may save both the provider and patient time and frustration. Pessary placement is associated with improvements in vaginal and bladder symptoms. Clemons et al. reported that compared with symptoms at baseline, pessary users were significantly less likely to experience sensation of vaginal bulge (90% to 3%), pressure (49% to 3%), presence of vaginal discharge (12% to 0%), and vaginal splinting (14% to 0%). Pessary placement has also been associated with improvement of bowel symptoms, although this was not a consistent finding in all studies. In addition to overall improvements in quality of life, body image and sexual function are also improved after pessary placement.

Because women with severe prolapse may have voiding dysfunction from the prolapse kinking the urethra leading to bladder neck obstruction, by correcting the vaginal axis, pessaries may improve obstructive and urinary urgency symptoms. In one study by Fernando et al., after pessary placement, fewer women reported difficulty voiding (77% to 48%), urinary urgency (93% to 58%), and urge incontinence (84% to 65%). Similarly, in a small retrospective review of 24 women with prolapse and elevated postvoid residuals (>100 mL) who planned to undergo surgery, Lazarou et al. reported that 75% of women had normal postvoid residuals after pessary placement. Of these women, only 1 had persistence of elevated postvoid residuals after surgery. However, due to the "unkinking" of the urethrovesical angle, pessary placement has also been associated with de novo/occult stress urinary incontinence. One prospective study by Clemons et al. found occult/de novo stress incontinence to occur in 21% of women with symptomatic prolapse fitted with a pessary.

In addition to pessary use for ongoing management of prolapse, pessary placement may also have a diagnostic role in women who desire surgery for prolapse but whose symptoms, such as pelvic or back pain, may not directly result from prolapse. In this group of women, symptom improvement during a trial of pessary may aid the clinician in counseling the patient regarding symptom improvement after surgery.

Although it is beyond the scope of this chapter to discuss pessary placement for obstetric indications such as cervical insufficiency, it is pertinent to mention that pessaries can be used for vaginal prolapse during pregnancy. In this setting, pessary use can result in similar benefits seen in nonpregnant women, such as decreased vaginal bulge symptoms and improved voiding. Although there are no data on the prevalence of prolapse during pregnancy, some experts postulate that pregnant women, may be less likely to experience prolapse later in pregnancy due to the displacement of the gravid uterus outside of the pelvis, while others hypothesize that prolapse may become more severe with pregnancy progression due to the weight of the uterus.

In addition to the symptomatic benefits of pessary use, there are some data by Handa and Jones, Matsubara and Ohki, and Jones et al. to suggest that pessary use may lead to improvement of prolapse stage and decrease in the size of genital hiatus. However, it is unclear if the observed benefit is durable or merely a more transient effect of pessary placement. It is also not evident if the change in anatomy is correlated with a significant change in symptom. These case series were limited by small sample size with short follow-up periods, and most of the observed changes were modest. What is equally or more significant is that pessary use does not appear to be associated with an increase in the severity of prolapse.

Pessary use has also been compared to surgery with mixed results. In one prospective study by Abdool et al. that compared a cohort of women who chose surgery to women who chose pessary, there were similar improvements in urinary, bowel, and sexual function, and quality of life. In a study by Barber et al. addressing the responsiveness of two condition-specific quality-of-life questionnaires (Pelvic Floor Distress Inventory [PFDI] and Pelvic Floor Impact Questionnaire [PFIQ]), women who underwent vaginal reconstructive surgery experienced significantly greater improvement in the above scales than did women enrolled in a pessary trial. Although women in the pessary trial experienced significant improvement in the prolapse and urinary subscales of the PFDI after pessary placement, there were no significant changes in the colorectal subscale of the PFDI or any of the PFIQ subscales (prolapse, urinary, colorectal). As of this publication, there are no randomized controlled trials comparing pessary and surgery in patients with POP. There is one cost-effective analysis, by Hullfish et al., that demonstrated pessary use may be more cost-effective than vaginal reconstructive surgery or expectant management in women with posthysterectomy POP.

PATIENT CONSIDERATIONS AND SELECTION FOR PESSARY USE

A pessary trial is a low-risk option for women experiencing symptomatic POP and should be considered and offered routinely. According to Pott-Grinstein and Newcomer, a 1998 survey of randomly selected members of the American College of Obstetricians and Gynecologists showed that although 86% of respondents prescribed pessaries, most felt that they underwent minimal to no training during residency. Learning the skills necessary to successfully fit and manage pessaries is fortunately not difficult and improves rapidly with experience.

Research by Heit et al., Kapoor et al., and Chan et al. shows that 30% to 60% of women diagnosed with POP will initially choose conservative management. Patients who were more likely to choose pessary tended to be older; patients with greater degree of prolapse, impairment in sexual activity, stress urinary incontinence, difficulty with bowel emptying, or previous prolapse surgery were more likely to select surgery. Additionally, those who previously encountered complications related to pessary use were more likely to choose surgery.

Research by Clemons et al., Hanson et al., Maito et al., Cundiff et al., and Komesu et al. shows that most patients (73% to 92%) can be successfully fitted with a pessary with rates of continued pessary use ranging from 16% to 89% at 6 months to 1 year. Patient characteristics that have consistently been associated with unsuccessful fitting include short vaginal length (<6 cm) and wide introitus (>4 fingerbreadths) and previous hysterectomy or reconstructive surgery (Table 40.1). Systemic and local hormone replacement therapy prior to fitting may improve the ability to successfully fit a pessary. Degree or predominant compartment of prolapse was not found to negatively impact the ability to successfully fit a pessary in most studies, but one small study did demonstrate that posterior vaginal wall prolapse was associated with increased fitting failure. Being sexually active also does not impact pessary fitting.

Long-term pessary use is related to the degree that the pessary corrects bothersome symptoms without creating new symptoms. According to Clemons et al., Komesu et al., and Friedman et al., after one year, most women (56% to 77%) will continue pessary use. Older age (>65 years) is the greatest predictor of continued use. Discontinuation of pessary use was associated with preexisting and de novo stress urinary incontinence, previous prolapse surgery, desire for surgery at first visit, and severe posterior vaginal prolapse. Being sexually active does not preclude long-term pessary use.

Pessary use is associated with few complications, and as such, there are few contraindications for usage. The most important contraindication is noncompliance with follow-up, as this can result in severe complications as described below. It is important to consider any medical condition or social situation that may predispose a patient to noncompliance,

such as dementia or difficulty accessing health care routinely. Additionally, pessary use should be delayed in women with active pelvic/vaginal infection until these issues are treated and resolved. Patients with latex allergy should not use Inflatoball pessary (CooperSurgical, Inc., Trumbull, CT), but this is the only commonly available pessary made with latex. In the 1997 survey of AUGS members, although 64%, 42%, and 45% of respondents believed hypoestrogenism, prior hysterectomy, or sexual activity, respectively, to be contraindications for pessary placement/use, we do not believe that any of these factors prohibit a trial of pessary based on the existing literature and our experience.

PESSARY SELECTION AND FITTING

Although more than 100 pessaries have been described, 13 styles are most commonly used, each with many different sizes (Fig. 40.1). Pessaries used for prolapse can be broadly classified as support pessaries, such as the ring with or without support or space-filling pessaries such as Gellhorn or Donut (Table 40.2). Support pessaries theoretically use a spring mechanism and are thought to rest between the pubic symphysis and posterior vaginal fornix; however, in actuality, with the patient upright, these pessaries rest just inside the introitus (Fig. 40.2). Space-filling pessaries either occupy the space within the vagina or create suction and adhere to the vaginal tissue. In the standing patient, these pessaries also sit just inside the vaginal introitus (Fig. 40.3).

In the 1997 survey of AUGS members, the most commonly used pessaries were the ring and Gellhorn; 22% of respondents reported using the same pessary, usually a ring pessary, for all vaginal prolapse; 78% tailored the pessary to the prolapse and were more likely to use support pessaries for anterior and apical vaginal prolapse, and space-filling pessaries for posterior vaginal prolapse and total prolapse/complete procidentia. In studies addressing pessaries used to treat prolapse, most analyses examined ring and/or Gellhorn pessaries. In a multicenter, randomized crossover trial comparing Gellhorn with ring to support pessaries, Cundiff et al. reported that both pessaries were found to be similar in decreasing prolapse symptoms as well as associated urinary and bowel symptoms. Pessary fitting is a trial and error process and involves selecting

TABLE 40.1 Patient Factors Impacting Pessary Fitting and Long-Term Use

ASSOCIATED WITH SUCCESS	ASSOCIATED WITH FAILURE	NOT SIGNIFICANT
• Hormone replacement (systemic or local)	• Short vaginal length (<6 cm) • Wide introitus (>4 fingerbreadths) • Previous hysterectomy • Previous reconstructive surgery • Predominant compartment of prolapse	• Degree of prolapse • Parity • Age • Sexual activity
ASSOCIATED WITH LONG-TERM USE	**ASSOCIATED WITH DISCONTINUATION**	**NOT SIGNIFICANT**
• Age > 65 y	• Stress urinary incontinence • Previous prolapse surgery • Desire for surgery at initial visit • Severe posterior prolapse	• Sexually active • Hormone replacement • Smoking • Body Mass Index • Medical comorbidities • Parity

Clemons (2004), Brincat (2004), Mutone (2005), Maito (2006), Hanson (2006), Komesu (2007), Markle (2011), and Friedman (2010).

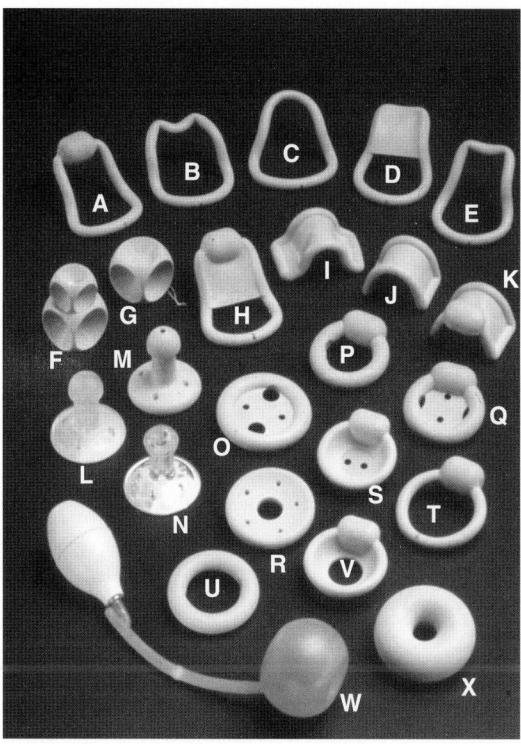

FIGURE 40.1 Types of pessaries. *A:* Hodge with knob (silicone); *B:* Risser (silicone); *C:* Smith (silicone); *D:* Hodge with support; *E:* Hodge (silicone); *F:* Tandem-cube (silicone); *G:* Cube (silicone); *H:* Hodge with support plus knob (silicone); *I:* Regula (silicone); *J:* Gehrung (silicone); *K:* Gehrung with knob (silicone); *L:* Gellhorn 95% rigid (silicone); *M:* Gellhorn flexible (silicone); *N:* Gellhorn rigid (silicone); *O:* Ring with support (silicone); *P:* Ring with knob (silicone); *Q:* Ring with support plus knob (silicone); *R:* Shaatz (silicone); *S:* Incontinence dish with support (silicone); *T:* Ring incontinence (silicone); *U:* Ring (silicone); *V:* Incontinence dish (silicone); *W:* Inflatoball (latex); *X:* Donut (silicone).

the ideal type of pessary as well as the correct size. In our experience, it is reasonable to start with a ring (with or without support) pessary, as this is generally the easiest for the patient to manage herself. If the patient cannot retain a ring pessary, we recommend a Gellhorn pessary followed by the Donut or cube pessary.

Both the ring and the Gellhorn, as well as most other pessaries, are available in different sizes. Generally, the smallest size pessary that is retained by the patient and results in alleviation of prolapse symptoms is best. There are pessary fitting kits available, such as the ring pessary sizer; however, it is not clear if these kits are needed to improve pessary fitting success. Most women can be successfully fitted with a pessary after one attempt, with most studies reporting an average of 2 to 3 pessaries tried over 1 to 3 attempts. Not surprisingly, pessary fitting success was highest with the first attempt; however, many women may still benefit from repeat trial of pessary fitting; one study by Clemons et al. reported that 45% of women who initially failed pessary placement were able to be successfully fitted at subsequent visits. After successful fitting, the pessary should be comfortable and relieve prolapse symptoms; it should be retained with Valsalva, ambulation, and urination and defecation.

Women with POP who are contemplating pessary placement should undergo a careful evaluation by history and physical examination as outlined in Chapter 36. As the goal of pessary placement is the alleviation of prolapse symptoms, particular attention should be placed on the assessment of symptoms attributable to prolapse, including sensation of vaginal bulge as well as bowel and urinary symptoms such as voiding/defecatory symptoms and incontinence. The degree of bother resulting from these symptoms as well as the impact on quality of life can also be determined from using validated questionnaires such as the PFDI short form 20 and the PFIQ short form 7. Additionally, it may be important to have the patient self-identify goals of pessary treatment, as attainment of those goals has been shown to be associated with continued pessary use. Although this is not essential, the Pelvic Organ Prolapse-Quantication (POP-Q) system, which is discussed in Chapter 36, can be used to identify and quantify the specific pelvic support defects present in terms of anterior, posterior, and apical vaginal compartments. As patients with severe prolapse may also have incomplete bladder emptying with urinary retention, assessment of postvoid residual before and after pessary placement can be performed. Evaluation of the vaginal epithelium to assess for urogenital atrophy and presence of abnormal lesions or discharge is necessary.

Other evaluations that should be considered include testing the patient for occult/de novo stress urinary incontinence, as one series by Clemons et al. showed 21% of women without previous incontinence symptoms developing de novo incontinence after pessary placement. This can be demonstrated by having the patient perform provocative maneuvers such as Valsalva and/or coughing while reducing the prolapse at the time of pessary placement or with instruments such as a half speculum or sponge stick. It is important to counsel and manage patients with baseline and de novo stress incontinence, as patients with continued stress incontinence after pessary placement may be more likely to discontinue pessary use. In addition to other conservative measures for stress incontinence as discussed in Chapter 41, prolapse patients with preexisting stress incontinence as well as occult/de novo incontinence may benefit from an incontinence pessary.

If the patient is deemed an appropriate pessary candidate following the above evaluation, the patient is next fitted for a pessary. To accomplish this task, the examiner places two fingers within the vagina as would be done at the time of a bimanual examination to estimate the vaginal depth. The index and middle fingers are spread as wide as comfortably possible to estimate the vagina width, which should approximate the diameter of the pessary (Fig. 40.4). The vaginal length and width will impact the type and size of pessary the patient may be able to tolerate and retain.

To insert the pessary, apply a small amount of water-based lubricant to the leading edge of the pessary. Insert the pessary into the vagina by applying pressure gently toward the posterior vagina and placing the pessary at an oblique angle so as to minimize pressure on the base of the urethra. Tips on pessary insertion and removal of a few commonly used pessaries are described in Table 40.2. It is beyond the scope of this chapter to discuss techniques involved in the placement of every pessary. For detailed instructions, consult the pessary company website or the detailed instructions provided with every commercially available pessary.

After the pessary is placed, one finger should easily fit between the pessary and the vagina. The patient should feel no discomfort and may often not feel the pessary at all. Mild vaginal irritation may occur as a result of the fitting process or urogenital atrophy. To increase the success of pessary fitting, patients with urogenital atrophy and other vulvar pathology such as lichen sclerosus may benefit from appropriate treatment before pessary placement. Lidocaine

VII

TABLE 40.2 Commonly Used Pessaries

PESSARY	TYPE	PROS	CONS	TIPS
Ring	Support	• Easy to insert/remove • Compatible with intercourse	• May not support severe prolapse	• Fold like a taco for insertion/removal or simply insert, unfolded, at an oblique angle
Gellhorn	Space filling	• Works well for severe prolapse	• Self-care difficult • Must remove for intercourse	• Fold knob against base for insertion • To remove, first break suction separating pessary base from vaginal wall, then use ring forceps or single tooth tenaculum to remove, if needed • Short knob versions available
Donut	Space filling	• Works well for severe prolapse	• Self-care difficult • Must remove for intercourse	• Use large-bore needle, and withdraw air to maximally compress pessary for removal and insertion
Cube	Space filling	• Works well for severe prolapse, often used as a last resort	• Foul discharge, erosions common • Must remove for intercourse	• Must be frequently removed and cleaned (every 1 to 2 night)

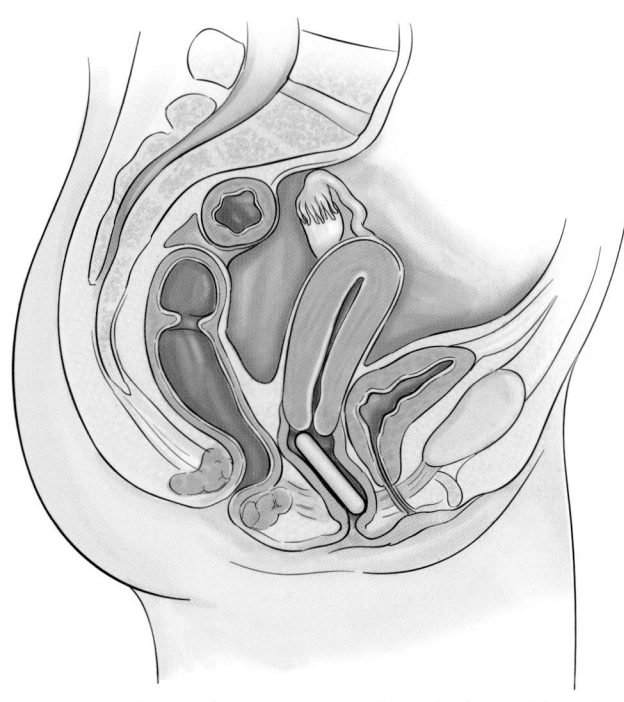

FIGURE 40.2 Ring with support pessary shown in the upright patient.

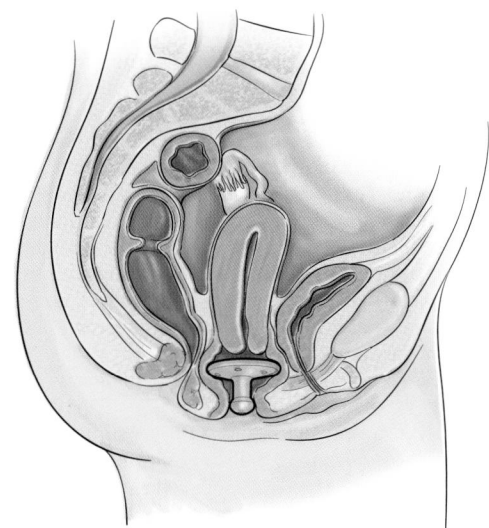

FIGURE 40.3 Gellhorn pessary shown in the upright patient.

gel may also be placed at the introitus several minutes prior to pessary placement to decrease discomfort. Voiding and/ or defecating before pessary placement to optimize room in the vagina may also ease pessary fitting for patients in whom placement is difficult.

With the patient still in dorsal lithotomy position, the patient should be asked to perform maneuvers that increase the intra-abdominal pressure such as Valsalva or coughing to ensure that the pessary is retained and that there is not significant prolapse beyond the pessary. This process should be repeated with the patient standing and squatting. The patient should also try to void with the pessary in place. While on the toilet, the patient may perform Valsalva maneuvers to mimic defecation to confirm that the pessary will be retained. A plastic urimeter/"nun's hat" can be placed on the toilet to catch the pessary in case it is not retained. If the patient is not able to successfully retain even large space-filling pessaries, some experts recommend placing two pessaries (e.g., two rings or Donut and Gellhorn).

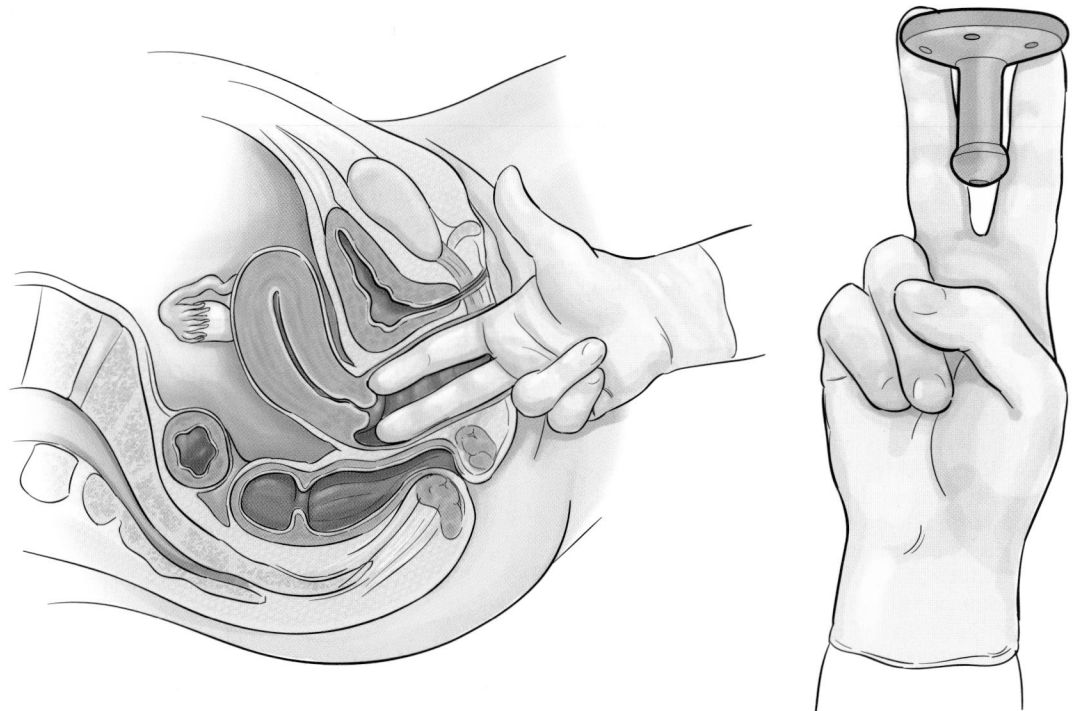

FIGURE 40.4 Digital measurement of vaginal width and length to approximate pessary size. (Adapted from *Urol Nurs* 2012;32:114. Reprinted with permission of the publisher, the Society of Urologic Nurses and Associates, Inc. (SUNA), East Holly Avenue, Box 56, Pitman, NJ 08071-0056; 856-256-2300; FAX 856-589-7463; Email: uronsg@ajj.com; Web site: www.suna.org)

VII

MANAGEMENT/FOLLOW-UP OF PESSARY

Although most experts would agree that routine follow-up is essential after successful pessary placement, there is no clear evidence or consensus on the optimal interval. According to Cundiff et al., in the 1997 survey of AUGS members, common follow-up schedules included evaluating the patient at 1 week or 1 month after initial pessary placement followed by visits every 1 to 3 months. The follow-up interval is dependent upon whether the patient is able to remove and replace the pessary herself. In general, we recommend a visit 1 week to 1 month after initial fitting to confirm that the patient is comfortable and satisfied with the pessary and, if applicable, able to successfully remove and replace the pessary.

Ideally, pessary removal and replacement should be taught to all patients or their caretakers to maximize patient autonomy. Typically, the ring (with and without support) pessaries are the easiest to self-manage; however, other types of pessaries such as Gellhorn have also been successfully self-managed by patients. For these women who are able to perform self-care, annual visits are typically sufficient.

For women unable to perform self-care, routine follow-up is typically every 3 to 4 months. During these visits, questions regarding comfort of use, vaginal bleeding, malodorous discharge, urinary tract infection, and defecation or voiding problems should be elicited and further evaluation performed as needed. The pessary should be removed and cleaned and the vagina thoroughly inspected.

There is no consensus or clear evidence on the optimal frequency of pessary removal. With the exception of the cube and Inflatoball (CooperSurgical, Inc., Trumbull, CT) pessaries, which most experts recommend removal every 1 to 2 nights with pessary replacement the next morning, other types of pessaries can be removed daily, weekly, or monthly and can be tailored to the individual needs of the patient. It is pertinent to consider that the amount of vaginal discharge may be dependent on the duration of continuous pessary use, with less discharge associated with more frequent pessary removal. The more frequent a woman removes her pessary, the less she may also be at risk for development of vaginal erosions. Although a woman can technically engage in vaginal intercourse with certain types of pessaries such as the ring with and without support, typically pessaries should be removed before intercourse.

In terms of concurrent therapies, there is limited evidence recommending the routine use of local or systemic hormone replacement therapy or other vaginal preparations in pessary users. It is important to individualize concurrent therapies based on patient needs and abilities. Vaginal preparations such as estrogen may often be expensive, messy, and difficult to place for some patients. Therefore, mandating their use may unnecessarily deter a patient from using a pessary. The rationale behind estrogen use in postmenopausal women is the improvement of urogenital atrophy by promoting epithelial cell growth and maturation leading to increased vaginal wall thickness and elasticity and decreasing vaginal pH to premenopausal levels (3.5 to 4.5) to promote continued or recolonization with normal flora—lactobacilli. Estrogens used vaginally are more effective than are estrogens taken systemically at correcting urogenital atrophy. In the 1997 survey of AUGS members, Cundiff et al. reported that 94% of respondents recommended estrogen replacement for pessary users. As mentioned above, there is some evidence to suggest that vaginal estrogen use may have a role in the success of initial pessary placement and may decrease vaginal irritation/abrasion. As discussed further in the complications section, vaginal estrogen may also have a role in the treatment of vaginal abrasion.

Some experts also recommend over-the-counter agents such as Trimo-San vaginal jelly (hydroxyquinoline topical) (CooperSurgical, Inc., Trumbull, CT) or vaginal moisturizers that contain polycarbophil (RepHresh, Lil' Drug Store Products, Inc., Cedar Rapids, IA) 2 to 3 times per week for lubrication and to maintain a vaginal pH of 4 to decrease malodorous discharge and patient discomfort. Although there are presently no published efficacy data, there is an ongoing randomized controlled trial addressing the effects of using this gel on the development of bacterial vaginosis and patient satisfaction in pessary users.

Complications

Serious complications of pessary use are rare and can typically be avoided with regular follow-up examinations. A literature review by Arias, Ridgeway, and Barber of major complications from 1950 to 2007 reported 39 published complications that required surgical interventions. These included 8 vesicovaginal fistulae, 5 other urologic complications, 4 rectovaginal fistulae, 3 bowel complications, and 19 impacted pessaries. Only 2 of the 39 patients who developed complications were followed regularly by a health care professional. Therefore, prevention of most major complications can be avoided by educating the patient on the importance of regular follow-up and self-care, if applicable.

More commonly, pessary patients may experience minor, transient complications. These may include, but are not limited to, pessary expulsion, urinary incontinence, rectal pressure, vaginal discharge or bleeding, and mechanical pressure ulcers. A long-term study of ring pessary users (median duration of use was 7 years) by Sarma, Ying, and Moore found that 56% of women experienced bleeding, extrusion, vaginal discharge, pain, or constipation at some point during their pessary use. Although these symptoms are generally not serious, they may limit a woman's ability to tolerate a pessary and desire for continued pessary use, and should be avoided if possible and managed effectively when they occur (Table 40.3).

TABLE 40.3 Management of Common Issues Associated with Pessary Use

ISSUE	MANAGEMENT
Expulsion or rectal pressure	• Change pessary size or type
Urinary incontinence	• Use an incontinence pessary with support at urethrovesical junction
Vaginal discharge	• Inspect the vagina to exclude ulceration • More frequent pessary removal • Acidification gel or douches • Antimicrobial treatment • Vaginal estrogen
Vaginal bleeding	• Inspect vagina to exclude ulceration • Consider vaginal or endometrial biopsy or ultrasound if uterus present
Vaginal abrasion/ ulceration	• Remove the pessary for 2 to 4 weeks. • Vaginal estrogen • Consider biopsy if persistent

A commonly encountered minor complication with pessary use is vaginal abrasion/ulceration. The patient may be asymptomatic or may experience heavier vaginal discharge or bleeding. Atrophic vaginal epithelium may contribute to a higher rate of vaginal abrasion, and therefore, many practitioners prescribe vaginal estrogen both as a preventative and a treatment measure. Vaginal abrasions may lead to higher pessary discontinuation rates and therefore are important to prevent. Vaginal estrogen therapy is utilized to promote epithelial cell growth and maturation, and increase vaginal wall thickness and elasticity. When abrasions occur, it is generally recommended to remove the pessary and apply topical estrogen for 2 to 4 weeks before reinsertion. If abrasions do not promptly resolve after relief of mechanical pressure, they should be biopsied, as cases of cervical and vaginal cancer have occurred in patients with pessaries.

Another common pessary-related issue is increased vaginal discharge and/or odor. Inspection of the vagina to exclude vaginal ulceration is mandatory. If bleeding is reported, it is important to consider an endometrial biopsy even if vaginal abrasion is found. In one study by Alnaif and Drutz, pessary users were significantly more likely to develop bothersome bacterial vaginosis compared with controls (32% vs. 10%, odds ratio [OR] 4.37, 95% confidence interval [CI]: 2.15 to 9.32). Therefore, appropriate antimicrobial or antifungal treatment should be prescribed based on findings of the wet mount/wet prep. If there are no pathologic organisms on wet mount, vaginal estrogen and/or acidifying products (Trimo-San vaginal jelly [CooperSurgical, Inc., Trumbull, CT] or vinegar douches) can be used as well as recommending more frequent pessary removal.

Pelvic Floor Muscle Training

Women with POP are more likely to have pelvic floor muscle weakness and atrophy, major defects of the levator ani muscles, and/or significantly decreased vaginal closure force when compared to women without prolapse. Greater pelvic floor muscle weakness is associated with larger genital hiatus measurements and more advanced stages of prolapse. Significantly fewer women with prolapse were able to achieve an effective involuntary muscle contraction during cough compared to women without prolapse. These findings are also consistent with the pelvic floor muscle function of women with urinary incontinence.

Pelvic Floor Muscle Training essentially consists of exercises to improve the strength and function of the pelvic floor muscles. Proper identification and contraction of the pelvic floor muscles is essential for women with prolapse. However, with verbal instruction alone, 68% of women with prolapse actually depressed (rather than contracted) their pelvic floor muscles, according to Thompson and O'Sullivan. To ensure proper technique of the pelvic floor muscle contraction, PFMT is ideally performed with guidance from a pelvic floor physical therapist. Besides verifying correct contraction of the pelvic floor muscles, the therapist ensures that a moderate to maximum level of intensity is produced, without contracting accessory muscles including the gluteal, rectus abdominis, or adductor muscles.

Although there are different PFMT regimens and interventions without consensus on the optimal regimen or duration of therapy, the integral components of most programs include assessment of and exercises to improve voluntary muscle strength and endurance, as well as timing of involuntary muscle contraction with increases in intra-abdominal pressure. Patients are prescribed individualized pelvic floor exercise programs to improve any and all of the deficits identified. Functional strategies are also taught, including contraction of the pelvic floor

against anticipated increases in intra-abdominal pressure events (also known as "the Knack"). The goal of pelvic floor muscle exercise and functional training is to ultimately improve support of the pelvic organs, especially during certain activities that may increase intra-abdominal pressure. Although there are limited data regarding increase in efficacy, electrical stimulation and biofeedback are commonly used adjuncts for these programs.

As is the case with other pelvic floor disorders such as urinary incontinence, emerging evidence suggests PFMT may be an effective conservative management for both anatomic and symptomatic improvements of POP. In a large trial by Braekken et al., 109 women with POP-Q stages 1, 2, and 3 prolapse were randomized to PFMT for 6 months (including both individual sessions with physical therapy and home exercise regimen) versus control (who were only given instruction to avoid straining and to utilize "the Knack"). Compared to women in the control group, those in the PFMT group were significantly more likely to have reduced frequency (74% vs. 31%, relative risk [RR] 0.37, 95% CI: 0.21 to 0.65) and bother (67% vs. 42%, RR 0.56, 95% CI: 0.33 to 0.97) from prolapse symptoms. Additionally, more women from the PFMT groups improved one POP-Q stage on physical examination compared with controls (19% vs. 8%, $P = 0.035$). No adverse events were reported in either group.

Other studies involving women with POP-Q stages 1 and 2 found significant anatomic and symptomatic improvement in women randomized to 14 to 16 weeks of PFMT and lifestyle advice compared with the control group who only received lifestyle advice. A Cochrane Review published in 2011 concluded that there is some evidence to support a beneficial effect of PFMT on prolapse symptom and severity. The improvement in prolapse stage anatomically may be more likely seen in women with less severe prolapse. Given the conclusions of level I evidence supporting the use of PFMT for treatment of POP as well as the lack of harm from this intervention, it should be offered to patients desiring conservative management.

PFMT can also be used in conjunction with pessary placement. Although there are limited data on the effects of pelvic floor muscle exercises in pessary users, in the 1997 survey of AUGS members, Cundiff et al. reported that 61% of respondents recommended pelvic floor muscle exercises for pessary users.

SUMMARY

POP is a common, bothersome, and costly condition and is suspected to become more prevalent as the aging population increases. Most women that present with bothersome prolapse symptoms should be offered conservative management with pessary placement and/or PFMT, especially as these interventions are usually not associated with significant adverse events. Although there are limited level I evidence, the findings from numerous published series and the experiences from years of pessary use suggest pessaries are an effective treatment of prolapse symptoms, and pessary use with routinely scheduled follow-up typically does not result in significant complications. Selection of the ideal type and size of pessary is a trial and error process, which improves with provider experience. Moreover, factors such as patient selection, specific follow-up regimen, and use of concomitant therapies including vaginal agents and pelvic floor muscle exercises should be individualized. Although there is limited data on the optimal duration of physical therapy and the durability of results, there is emerging level I evidence demonstrating the beneficial effects of PFMT on prolapse symptom and possibly anatomic prolapse stage in women with mild to moderate prolapse.

VII

BEST CLINICAL PRACTICES

- Nonsurgical management of POP including pessary placement and PFMT should be considered in all patients with symptomatic POP.
- Pessary use may improve vaginal, bladder, and possibly bowel symptoms.
- Although pessary use may improve voiding and defecation, it may also exacerbate stress urinary incontinence or result in de novo/occult stress incontinence.
- Patient characteristics that have consistently been associated with unsuccessful fitting include short vaginal length (<6 cm) and wide introitus (>4 fingerbreadths) and previous hysterectomy or reconstructive surgery; sexual activity and the degree or compartment of prolapse do not negatively impact pessary placement.
- Older patients (>65 years) were more likely to continue with pessary use, while preexisting and de novo/occult stress incontinence, previous prolapse surgery, desire for surgery, and severe posterior vaginal prolapse were associated with discontinuation of pessary. Being sexually active does not preclude long-term use of pessary.
- Using vaginal estrogen in patients with urogenital atrophy may improve the success of pessary fitting as well as long-term use.
- Pessary fitting is a trial and error process and should be individualized to the patient.
- Patients should be followed routinely after pessary placement and should be examined with pessary removal at regular intervals.
- Minor complications of long-term pessary use are common and include discharge and mucosal erosion/abrasion, while serious complications including fistulae, cancer, and pessary incarceration are rare, especially with routine follow-up.
- PFMT performed under the supervision of a pelvic floor physical therapist should be offered to prolapse patients, as there has been level I evidence demonstrating this treatment to be effective with no adverse outcomes.
- Although there is limited evidence on efficacy, pessary placement and PFMT can be offered concurrently to women with symptomatic prolapse.

BIBLIOGRAPHY

Abdool Z, Thakar R, Sultan AH, et al. Prospective evaluation of outcome of vaginal pessaries versus surgery in women with symptomatic pelvic organ prolapsed. *Int Urogynecol J* 2011;22:273.

ACOG Committee on Practice Bulletins—Gynecology. ACOG Practice Bulletin No. 85: pelvic organ prolapse. *Obstet Gynecol* 2007;110:717.

Adams E, Thomson A, Maher C, et al. Mechanical devices for pelvic organ prolapse in women. *Cochrane Database Syst Rev* 2004:CD004010.

Albertsen PC. Patient satisfaction and changes in prolapse and urinary symptoms in women who were fitted successfully with a pessary for pelvic organ prolapsed. *J Urol* 2005;173:942.

Alnaif B, Drutz HP. Bacterial vaginosis increases in pessary users. *Int Urogynecol J* 2000;11:219.

Arias BE, Ridgeway B, Barber MD. Complications of neglected vaginal pessaries: case presentation and literature review. *Int Urogynecol J Pelvic Floor Dysfunct* 2008;19:1173.

Atnip SD. Pessary use and management for pelvic organ prolapse. *Obstet Gynecol Clin North Am* 2009;36:541.

Bai SW, Yoon BS, Kwon JY, et al. Survey of the characteristics and satisfaction degree of the patients using a pessary. *Int Urogynecol J Pelvic Floor Dysfunct* 2005;16:182.

Barber MD, Walters MD, Cundiff GW, et al. Responsiveness of the Pelvic Floor Distress Inventory (PFDI) and Pelvic Floor Impact Questionnaire (PFIQ) in women undergoing vaginal surgery and pessary treatment for pelvic organ prolapse. *Am J Obstet Gynecol* 2006;194:1492.

Berger J, Van den Bosch T, Deprest J. Impaction after partial expulsion of a neglected pessary. *Obstet Gynecol* 2009;114:468.

Borello-France DF, Handa VL, Brown MB, et al. Pelvic-floor muscle function in women with pelvic organ prolapse. *Phys Ther* 2007;87:399.

Braekken IH, Majida M, Engh ME, et al. Can pelvic floor muscle training reverse pelvic organ prolapse and reduce prolapse symptoms? An assessor-blinded, randomized, controlled trial. *Am J Obstet Gynecol* 2010;203:170.

Brincat C, Kenton K, Pat Fitzgerald M, et al. Sexual activity predicts continued pessary use. *Am J Obstet Gynecol* 2004;191:198.

Bugge C, Hagen S, Thakar R. Vaginal pessaries for pelvic organ prolapse and urinary incontinence: a multiprofessional survey of practice. *Int Urogynecol J* 2012;21.

Chan SS, Cheung RY, Yiu KW, et al. Symptoms, quality of life, and factors affecting women's treatment decisions regarding pelvic organ prolapse. *Int Urogynecol J* 2012;23:1027.

Cheung WK, Ho MP, Wei MC, et al. Association between uterine prolapse and cervical squamous cell carcinoma in an elderly adult. *J Am Geriatr Soc* 2012;60:1775.

Clemons JL, Aguilar VC, Sokol ER, et al. Patient characteristics that are associated with continued pessary use versus surgery after 1 year. *Am J Obstet Gynecol* 2004;191:159.

Clemons JL, Aguilar VC, Tillinghast TA, et al. Patient satisfaction and changes in prolapse and urinary symptoms in women who were fitted successfully with a pessary for pelvic organ prolapse. *Am J Obstet Gynecol* 2004;190:1025.

Clemons JL, Aguilar VC, Tillinghast TA, et al. Risk factors associated with an unsuccessful pessary fitting trial in women with pelvic organ prolapse. *Am J Obstet Gynecol* 2004;190:345.

Cooke TJ, Gousse AE. A historical perspective on cystocele repair—from honey to pessaries to anterior colporrhaphy: lessons from the past. *J Urol* 2008;179:2126.

Culligan PJ. Nonsurgical management of pelvic organ prolapse. *Obstet Gynecol* 2012;119:852.

Cundiff GW, Amundsen CL, Bent AE, et al. The PESSRI study: symptom relief outcomes of a randomized crossover trial of the ring and Gellhorn pessaries. *Am J Obstet Gynecol* 2007;196:405.e1–405.e8.

Cundiff GW, Weidner AC, Visco AG, et al. A survey of pessary use by members of the American Urogynecologic Society. *Obstet Gynecol* 2000;95:931.

DeLancey JOL, Morgan DM, Fenner DE, et al. Comparison of levator ani muscle defects and function in women with and without pelvic organ prolapse. *Obstet Gynecol* 2007;109:295.

Di Benedetto P, Coidessa A, Floris S. Rationale of pelvic floor muscles training in women with urinary incontinence. *Minerva Ginecol* 2008;60:529.

Fernando RJ, Thakar R, Sultan AH, et al. Effect of vaginal pessaries on symptoms associated with pelvic organ prolapse. *Obstet Gynecol* 2006;108:93.

Friedman S, Sandhu KS, Wang C, et al. Factors influencing long-term pessary use. *Int Urogynecol J* 2010;21:673.

Gorti M, Hudelist G, Simons A. Evaluation of vaginal pessary management: a UK-based survey. *J Obstet Gynaecol* 2009;29:129.

Hagen S, Stark D. Conservative prevention and management of pelvic organ prolapse in women. *Cochrane Database Syst Rev* 2011;7: CD003882.

Hagen S, Stark D, Glazener C, et al. A randomized controlled trial of pelvic floor muscle training for stages I and II pelvic organ prolapse. *Int Urogynecol J Pelvic Floor Dysfunct* 2009;20:45.

Hanavadi S, Durham-Hall A, Oke T, et al. Forgotten vaginal pessary eroding into rectum. *Ann R Coll Surg Engl* 2004;86:W18.

Handa VL, Jones M. Do pessaries prevent the progression of pelvic organ prolapse? *Int Urogynecol J Pelvic Floor Dysfunct* 2002;13:349.

Hanson LA, Schulz JA, Flood CG, et al. Vaginal pessaries in managing women with pelvic organ prolapse and urinary incontinence: patient characteristics and factors contributing to success. *Int Urogynecol J* 2006;17:155.

Heit M, Rosenquist C, Culligan P, et al. Predicting treatment choice for patients with pelvic organ prolapse. *Obstet Gynecol* 2003;101:1279.

Hullfish KL, Trowbridge ER, Stukenborg GJ. Treatment strategies for pelvic organ prolapse: a cost-effectiveness analysis. *Int Urogynecol J* 2011;22:507.

Jain A, Majoko F, Freites O. How innocent is the vaginal pessary? Two cases of vaginal cancer associated with pessary use. *J Obstet Gynaecol* 2006;26:829.

Jones K, Yang L, Lowder JL, et al. Effect of pessary use on genital hiatus measurements in women with pelvic organ prolapse. *Obstet Gynecol* 2008;112:630.

Kapoor DS, Thakar R, Sultan AH, et al. Conservative versus surgical management of prolapse: what dictates patient choice? *Int Urogynecol J Pelvic Floor Dysfunct* 2009;20:1157.

Ko PC, Lo TS, Tseng LH, et al. Use of a pessary in treatment of pelvic organ prolapse: quality of life, compliance, and failure at 1-year follow-up. *J Minim Invasive Gynecol* 2011;18:68.

Komesu YM, Rogers RG, Rode MA, et al. Pelvic floor symptom changes in pessary users. *Am J Obstet Gynecol* 2007;197:620.e1.

Komesu YM, Rogers RG, Rode MA, et al. Patient-selected goal attainment for pessary wearers: what is the clinical relevance? *Am J Obstet Gynecol* 2008;198:577.e1.

Kuhn A, Bapst D, Stadlmayr W, et al. Sexual and organ function in patients with symptomatic prolapse: are pessaries helpful? *Fertil Steril* 2009;91:1914.

Lazarou G, Scotti RJ, Mikhail MS, et al. Pessary reduction and post-operative cure of retention in women with anterior vaginal wall prolapse. *Int Urogynecol J Pelvic Floor Dysfunct* 2004;15:175.

Lone F, Thakar R, Sultan AH, et al. A 5-year prospective study of vaginal pessary use for pelvic organ prolapse. *Int J Gynaecol Obstet* 2011;114:56.

Maito JM, Quam ZA, Craig E, et al. Predictors of successful pessary fitting and continued use in a nurse-midwifery pessary clinic. *J Midwifery Womens Health* 2006;51:78.

Markle D, Skoczylas L, Goldsmith C, et al. Patient characteristics associated with a successful pessary fitting. *Female Pelvic Med Reconstr Surg* 2011;17:249.

Matsubara S, Ohki Y. Can a ring pessary have a lasting effect to reverse uterine prolapse even after its removal? *J Obstet Gynaecol Res* 2010;36:459.

Mokrzycki ML, Hatangadi SB, Zaccardi JE, et al. Preexisting stress urinary incontinence: a predictor of discontinuation with pessary management. *J Low Genit Tract Dis* 2001;5:204.

Mutone MF, Terry C, Hale DS, et al. Factors which influence the short-term success of pessary management of pelvic organ prolapse. *Am J Obstet Gynecol* 2005;193:89.

Nygaard I, Barber MD, Burgio KL, et al. Prevalence of symptomatic pelvic floor disorders in US women. *JAMA* 2008;300:1311.

Oliver R, Thakar R, Sultan AH. The history and usage of the vaginal pessary: a review. *Eur J Obstet Gynecol Reprod Biol* 2011;156:125.

Olsen AL, Smith VJ, Bergstron JO, et al. Epidemiology of surgically managed pelvic organ prolapse and urinary incontinence. *Obstet Gynecol* 1997;89:501.

Patel MS, Mellen C, O'Sullivan DM, et al. Pessary use and impact on quality of life and body image. *Female Pelvic Med Reconstr Surg* 2011;17:298.

Pott-Grinstein E, Newcomer JR. Gynecologists' patterns of prescribing pessaries. *J Reprod Med* 2001;46:205.

Sampselle CM, Burns PA, Dougherty MC, et al. Continence for women. *J Obstet Gynecol Neonatal Nurs* 1997;26:375.

Sarma S, Ying T, Moore KH. Long-term vaginal ring pessary use: discontinuation rates and adverse events. *Br J of Obstet Gynaecol* 2009;116:1715.

Shah SM, Sultan AH, Thakar R. The history and evolution of pessaries for pelvic organ prolapse. *Int Urogynecol J Pelvic Floor Dysfunct* 2006;17:170.

Slieker-ten Hove M, Pool-Goudzwaard A, Eijkemans M, et al. Pelvic floor muscle function in a general population of women with and without pelvic organ prolapse. *Int Urogynecol J* 2010;21:311.

Stephan WB, Zaaijman Jdu T. Retention of a vaginal ring pessary in a postmenopausal patient. *S Afr Med J* 2007;97:552.

Stüpp L, Resende AP, Oliveira E, et al. Pelvic floor muscle training for treatment of pelvic organ prolapse: an assessor-blinded randomized controlled trial. *Int Urogynecol J* 2011;22:1233.

Subak LL, Waetjen LE, van den Eeden S, et al. Cost of pelvic organ prolapse surgery in the United States. *Obstet Gynecol* 2001;98:646.

Thompson JA, O'Sullivan PB. Levator plate movement during voluntary pelvic floor muscle contraction in subjects with incontinence

and prolapse: a cross-sectional study and review. *Int Urogynecol J* 2003;14:84.

Wu V, Farrell SA, Baskett TF, et al. A simplified protocol for pessary management. *Obstet Gynecol* 1997;90:990.

Wu JM, Hundley AF, Fulton RG, et al. Forecasting the prevalence of pelvic floor disorders in US women. *Obstet Gynecol* 2009;114:1278.

Yamada T, Matsubara S. Rectocoele, but not cystocoele, may predict unsuccessful pessary fitting. *J Obstet Gynaecol* 2011;31:441.

CHAPTER 41
Stress Urinary Incontinence

Victoria L. Handa

DEFINITIONS

Cotton swab test—Measure of urethral mobility; with the patient in supine lithotomy position, a lubricated cotton swab (or other similar device) is placed into the urethra, allowing a measurement of the rotational descent of the bladder neck with Valsalva; an angle of ≥30 degrees (with respect to the horizontal) is classically defined as a hypermobile urethra.

Cystometry—Tests of the pressure/volume relationship during bladder filling; "simple" cystometry is a manometric evaluation, while "complex" cystometry involves an electronic measurement and recording of bladder pressure during filling, often with simultaneous measurement of intra-abdominal pressure (and sometimes urethral pressure).

Intrinsic sphincter deficiency (ISD)—Urinary incontinence that is due to dysfunction of the urethral sphincter mechanism, presumably related to loss of smooth muscle tone and/or coaptation of the urethral lumen.

Occult stress incontinence—Stress incontinence only observed after the reduction of coexistent prolapse (e.g., after surgical correction of prolapse).

Stress urinary incontinence—The symptom of involuntary leakage of urine from the urethra at the time of increased intra-abdominal pressure (e.g., coughing, straining).

Urethral hypermobility—Descent of the bladder neck with increased intra-abdominal pressure, typically defined as a cotton swab angle greater than 30 degrees from the horizontal.

Urodynamic stress incontinence—The involuntary leakage of urine during filling cystometry, associated with increased intra-abdominal pressure, in the absence of a detrusor contraction.

Urinary incontinence is a condition that affects 30% to 40% of older American women, with the majority afflicted with stress urinary incontinence (SUI). The management of SUI has changed dramatically over the past two decades, due in part to the introduction of synthetic midurethral slings and due also to the accumulation of evidence from clinical trials to guide therapy. Surgeries that were once the standard of care, such as Pereyra needle suspensions and anterior colporrhaphy with Kelly placation, are now known to be less effective than are other options and are therefore no longer recommended for treatment of SUI.

VII

The phrase "stress urinary incontinence" is used to refer to a symptom, a physical finding, and a urodynamic diagnosis. The symptom of SUI is the complaint of involuntary loss of urine on effort or physical exertion (e.g., exercise), or on sneezing or coughing. The sign of SUI is the observation, on physical examination, of incontinence from the urethra synchronous with effort similar provocation, such as coughing. Urodynamic stress incontinence is defined as the involuntary leakage of urine during increased abdominal pressure in the absence of a detrusor contraction.

INITIAL EVALUATION

The history and physical examination are critical in the assessment of SUI. Typically, a thorough history will distinguish SUI from other types of urinary incontinence. The initial assessment should also include an evaluation of the impact of SUI on quality of life, as treatment is indicated only if the woman considers her symptoms to be bothersome or to interfere with her activities. Other goals for the initial assessment include the identification of other factors that could exacerbate or precipitate symptoms, such as neurologic disease, polyuria, and many medications (especially those with effects on the autonomic nervous system). A voiding diary may be appropriate to assess normal voiding habits. The physical examination should include a measure of postvoid residual. Laboratory studies can be limited to screening for urinalysis to exclude hematuria and pyuria.

Among women planning surgical treatment of SUI, urethral hypermobility should be assessed on physical examination. A variety of methods can be used to assess urethral mobility, although this is traditionally evaluated with a cotton swab test. For this test, a lubricated cotton swab is inserted into the urethra with the patient in the supine lithotomy position (**Fig. 41.1**). As the patient strains or coughs, the angle formed by the cotton swab with respect to the horizontal is measured. Women with a straining cotton swab angle of at least 30 degrees above the horizontal are said to have a hypermobile urethra. Most women with SUI will have evidence of a hypermobile urethra, but it is important

TABLE 41.1 Criteria for Surgical Management of Stress Urinary Incontinence without Urodynamic Evaluation

- Clear symptoms of SUI in the absence of frequency, urgency, and other significant urge-related symptoms
- Postvoid residual volume less than 150 mL
- Hypermobile urethra
- Positive "stress test" (visual evidence of urine loss with cough or Valsalva)
- No history of anti-incontinence surgery
- No history of radical pelvic surgery or radiation
- No neurologic disease

to note that a hypermobile urethra is neither necessary nor sufficient for the diagnosis of SUI. However, this finding has been associated with surgical outcomes, and it is therefore important to assess patients for urethral hypermobility if surgery is planned.

Urodynamic investigation, including cystometry, has historically played an important role in the preoperative assessment of women with SUI. The goals of urodynamic investigation are to confirm the diagnosis of SUI and to exclude conditions that could either impact the success of therapy or signify an increased risk of adverse outcomes. However, many women with uncomplicated SUI may not benefit from testing. Those unlikely to benefit from testing (Table 41.1) include women with clear symptoms of SUI in the absence of significant urge-related symptoms, a postvoid residual volume less than 150 mL, a hypermobile urethra, and a positive "stress test" (visual evidence of urine loss with cough or Valsalva). In general practice, most women with SUI probably meet these criteria and can therefore be managed without urodynamic testing. However, in a tertiary setting, Nager and colleagues found that only 1,375 of 4,083 women with SUI (33%) fell into this "low-risk" category. Indications for urodynamic testing or referral to a specialist include those who do not meet the criteria above; those with a history of prior anti-incontinence surgery, prior radical pelvic surgery, or radiation; and those with neurologic disease. Cystoscopy may also be indicated in the evaluation of women with these risk factors.

There is controversy surrounding the value of preoperative assessment for "intrinsic sphincter deficiency (ISD)" in women with SUI. This concept refers to a poorly functioning urethra. The contemporary view is that urethral function is a spectrum and that all women with SUI have at least some component of poor urethral function. In theory, the "intrinsic" sphincter function of the urethra is provided by smooth muscle tone and coaptation of the urethral lumen. Thus, presumably, ISD is related to a deficiency in one or both of these continence mechanisms. Some experts argue that women with SUI who do not have urethral hypermobility must have ISD. Others consider ISD to be a measure of more severe SUI (measured either by symptom severity or with a leak point pressure, an indication of the ease with which SUI is demonstrated on physical examination). Yet a third classification scheme assigns a diagnosis of ISD in cases of low urethral closure pressure or an "open" bladder neck at rest (e.g., during urethroscopy or contrast imaging; **Fig. 41.2**). With contemporary treatment of SUI, the distinction between ISD and other types of SUI has become less important. It is not clear that the diagnosis of ISD has an impact on the management of SUI.

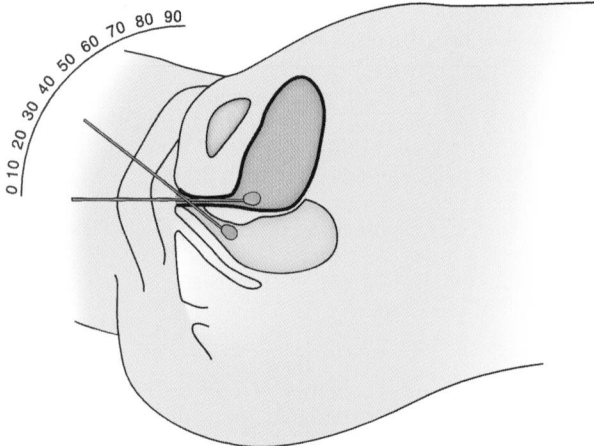

FIGURE 41.1 The cotton swab test demonstrates a resting angle close to 0 degrees and a straining angle of approximately 40 degrees. A straining angle greater than 30 degrees above the horizontal is considered "hypermobile." (Reprinted from Bent AE, Cundiff GW, Swift SE. *Ostergard, Ostergard's urogynecology and pelvic floor dysfunction*, 6th ed. Philadelphia, PA: Lippincott, Williams & Wilkins, 2007, with permission. Copyright © 2007 Wolters Kluwer Health.)

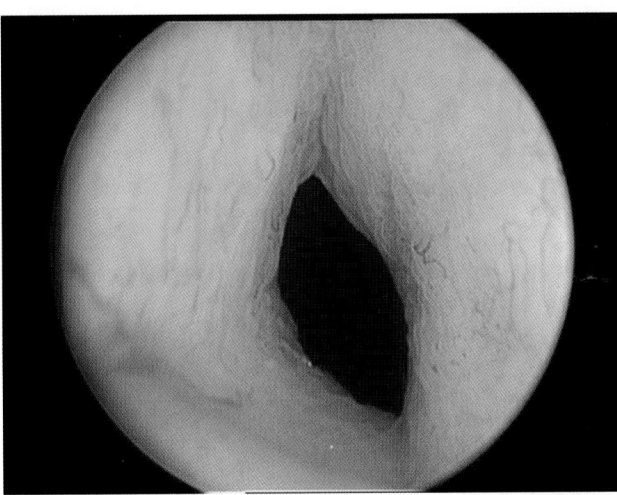

FIGURE 41.2 Photograph from urethroscopy, illustrating a function-less urethra. The bladder neck is passively open at rest. In a woman with stress incontinence, this appearance may signify intrinsic sphincter deficiency. (Reprinted from Bent AE, Cundiff GW, Swift SE. *Ostergard, Ostergard's urogynecology and pelvic floor dysfunction,* 6th ed. Philadelphia, PA: Lippincott, Williams & Wilkins, 2007, with permission. Copyright © 2007 Wolters Kluwer Health.)

INITIAL MANAGEMENT

Randomized clinical trials have demonstrated the effectiveness of anti-incontinence pessaries and pelvic muscle physical therapy. Conservative therapy helps a large number of these patients. However, a recent multicenter trial by Richter and colleagues suggested that only 50% of women with SUI will be satisfied with the outcome of these nonsurgical approaches. Nevertheless, all women with bothersome SUI should be offered nonsurgical options. Surgery should be reserved for women who decline or fail nonsurgical therapies.

SURGICAL TECHNIQUES FOR THE TREATMENT OF STRESS INCONTINENCE

More than 200 procedures have been described in the literature for the treatment of stress incontinence. This reflects a combination of the evolution of established and effective procedures as well as the introduction of newer technologies and materials. Most of these surgeries, including the anterior colporrhaphy with Kelly placation and Pereyra needle suspensions, are now of historical interest only. This chapter focuses on retropubic and transobturator midurethral sling procedures, which have become the mainstays of surgical therapy for SUI. Other options, appropriate for selected populations, include the retropubic urethropexy, rectus fascia suburethral sling procedures, and the injection of bulking agents. These also are addressed.

Retropubic Midurethral Sling Procedures

The retropubic midurethral sling was first described by Ulmsten and colleagues. The appeal of a tension-free midurethral sling is that it is an effective, minimally invasive technique that can be applied to a day-surgery setting. Thus, this approach was an important innovation when it was introduced in the 1990s.

The patient is typically positioned in low lithotomy, with Allen stirrups (**Fig. 41.3**). The bladder is emptied with an 18-F

catheter. Suprapubic sites are marked approximately 2 to 3 cm lateral to the midline. These sites are selected to be medial to the pubic tubercle; they represent the lateral boundary for safe perforation of the abdominal wall. More lateral sling placement will increase the risk of neurovascular injury.

A 1- to 2-cm incision is made under the midurethra (Fig. 41.4A). Typically, the distal aspect of the incision is 1 to 1.5 cm from the urethral meatus. The midurethral location can be confirmed via palpation of the Foley bulb while gentle traction is placed on the Foley. After the creation of the incision, a 2-cm tunnel is made with Metzenbaum scissors at a 45-degree angle toward the descending pubic ramus on each side (Fig. 41.4B). Minimal vaginal dissection is recommended to limit bleeding from the paraurethral vascular plexus, to maintain the sling in its position under the midurethra (e.g., minimizing the probability that it will be displaced to the proximal or distal urethra), and to minimize the risk of mesh exposure.

Some surgeons inject the vaginal wall and retropubic space with a dilute solution of local anesthetic (such as a 3:1 dilution of 1% xylocaine or ¼% bupivacaine). A spinal needle is advanced through the abdominal wall, immediately along the pubis, and into the retropubic space. Traditionally, 5 to 10 mL of solution is injected suprapubically on each side. Then, 10 mL

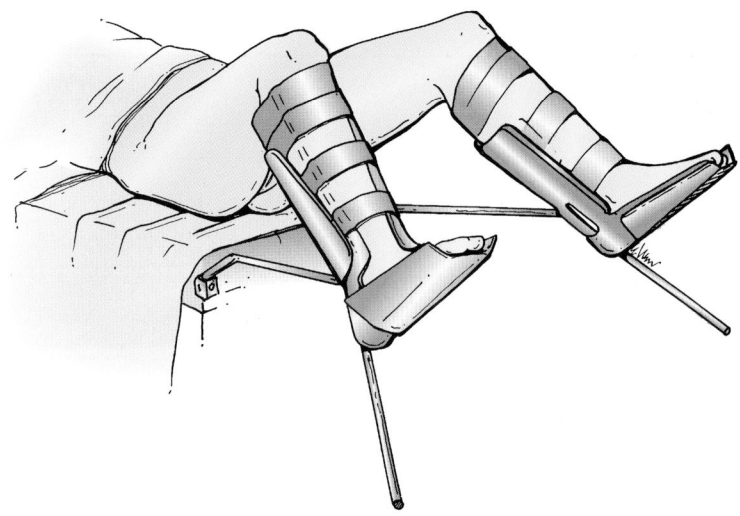

FIGURE 41.3 Positioning the patient in Allen universal stirrups to allow vaginal and abdominal access.

Mucosal incision

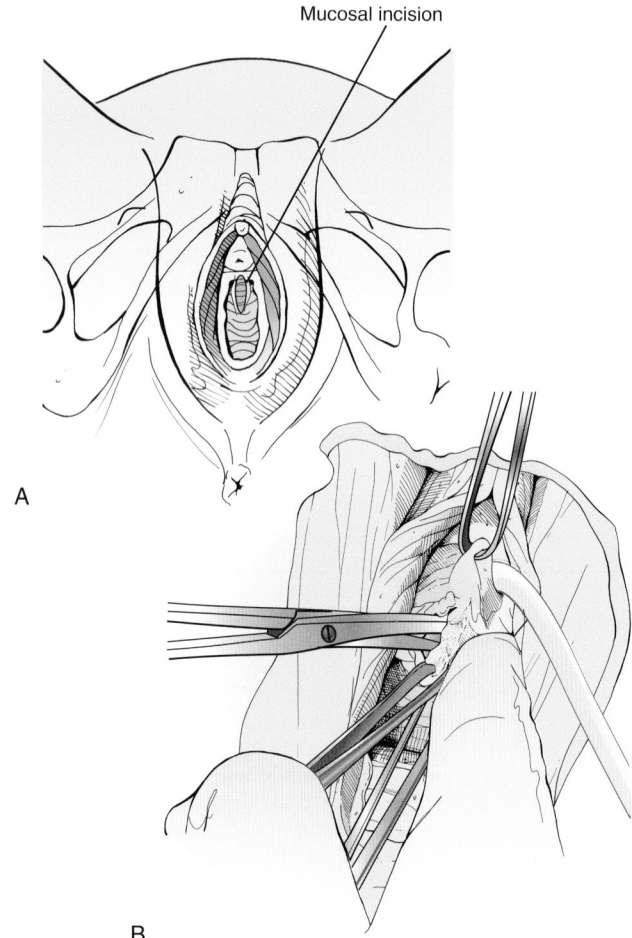

FIGURE 41.4 A: The vaginal incision for a midurethral sling procedure is approximately 1.5 cm in length and is located at the midurethra, typically 1 to 1.5 cm from the urethral meatus. **B:** For a retropubic midurethral sling, fine scissors are used to dissect a subepithelial tunnel, typically 2 cm in length. The angle of the tunnel is typically at 45 degrees, aimed toward the junction of the descending pubic ramus and the pubis.

of the solution is placed in the retropubic space bilaterally by a vaginal approach. The needle is advanced through the vaginal incision and under the vaginal epithelium, injecting small amounts along the intended path of the sling trocar, entering the retropubic space at the junction of the descending pubic ramus and the pubis. Five to ten milliliters is placed on each side. Injection of saline or local anesthetic into the retropubic space ("hydrodissection") is thought to distend the space, facilitating safe placement of the trocars. Some experts prefer injections of saline (for hydrodissection of the retropubic space) rather than a local anesthetic. This is because the benefits of local anesthetic injection are limited to the first few hours after surgery.

Commercially available midurethral slings consist of a polypropylene strap and rigid trocars for insertion (**Fig. 41.5**). Prior to placement of the trocar, a rigid catheter guide is placed through the 18-F catheter. Using the rigid guide, the bladder can be directed away from the side on which the surgeon is working, so as to minimize the risk of bladder injury. The retropubic sling is passed into the retropubic space using the curved trocar (**Fig. 41.6**). A knowledge of retropubic anatomy is critical to the safe placement of the sling. The trocar should be advanced into the retropubic space at the junction of the descending pubic ramus and the pubis, immediately along the inferior surface of the bone. This is a relatively avascular zone of the retropubic space (**Fig. 41.7**). If the trocar perforates in this location, the trocar will be lateral to the retropubic branches of the internal pudendal vessels and medial to the inferior epigastric, obturator, and accessory obturator vessels. If the trocar is directed away from the surface of the bone, a bladder perforation is more likely, as is an injury to branches of the perivesical venous plexus and vesical vessels. The pubic veins, branches of the obturator vessels that course medially along the ventral surface of the pubis, are the only vessels likely to be along the path of the needle placed in this fashion. After initial insertion through vaginal wall, the trocar may also pass close to (or through) the paraurethral vascular plexus, which arise from the internal pudendal and superior vesical arteries. Shobeiri found that injury to these paraurethral vessels is likely, but the related bleeding is of limited clinical significance and can typically be controlled by pressure or vaginal packing. He recommended minimal vaginal dissection to reduce risk of significant bleeding from the paraurethral vessels.

As the trocar is passed into the retropubic space, it hugs the pubic ramus as the endopelvic fascia is penetrated and then is advanced until the tip appears suprapubically, immediately

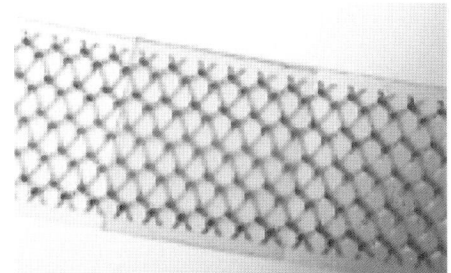
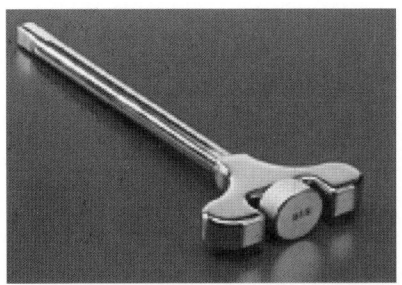
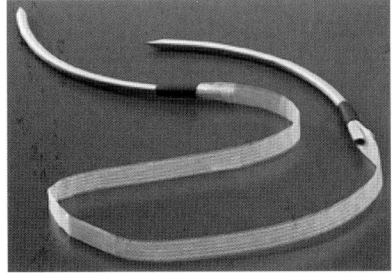
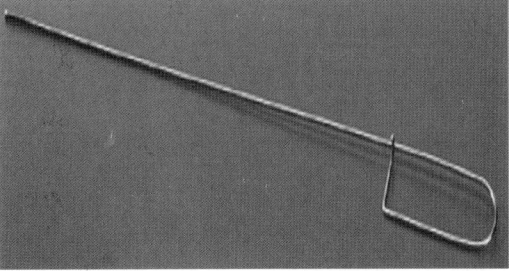

FIGURE 41.5 Vaginal approach for tension-free vaginal tape procedure. Gynecare TVT Obturator System Tension-Free Support for Incontinence. Materials include a catheter guide to retract the bladder away from the working area, the tape material attached to two insertion needles, and the handle to attach to the needles for insertion. (Copyright © Ethicon, Inc. 2010–2013. Reproduced with permission).

medial to the site previously marked (**Fig. 41.8**). The needle tip is passed just through the skin. The tape is passed on the opposite side using a similar technique. Cystoscopy is performed after each pass or, alternatively, after both passes have been made (**Fig. 41.9**). If there is no bladder perforation, the needles are advanced and pulled completely through the abdominal

wall. The needles are detached from the sling device. The sling with protective sheath is tightened over a number 9/10 Hegar dilator or other instrument, which is held in place until the sling is secured. The plastic sheaths are pulled free from the mesh, and excess sling material is cut flush to the skin surface. At this point, the Hegar dilator can be removed. The vaginal and skin incisions are closed. The sling is not sutured to any underlying tissue, and the composition of the mesh allows tissue ingrowth to fix the sling in place.

Anatomic studies have identified several techniques that minimize the risk to obturator and iliac vessels. For example, during passage of the retropubic trocars, the surgeon should not laterally divert the tip of the trocar; rotation of the trocar is a safer technique. Shobeiri demonstrated that if the surgeon rotates the needle without lateral diversion, injury to the external iliac vessels cannot except in cases of extreme rotation (>75 degrees). Injury may be increased if the trocar is both laterally diverted and rotated. The surgeon should also be familiar with the corona mortis, an anastomosis between the obturator and inferior epigastric vessels. This anastomosis is typically greater than 6 cm lateral to the midline and is reliably 3 cm lateral to the midline. Experienced retropubic surgeons are aware that this anastomosis is almost invariably present in a fat pad at the lateral aspect of Cooper ligament. Injury to the corona mortis can easily be avoided if the trocar does not pass more than 3 cm lateral to the midline. Finally, Rahn and colleagues have shown that perforation of the pubococcygeus muscle can occur if the retropubic trocar is deviated laterally (**Fig. 41.10**), although perforation of the muscle is of uncertain consequence.

A vaginal pack is not usually placed unless there has been considerable bleeding. A Foley catheter is placed, or, alternatively, the patient may go to recovery without a catheter. A voiding trial is initiated in the recovery room; if the patient cannot void adequately, she performs self-catheterization, or a Foley catheter is placed. In the first week after surgery, voiding dysfunction is common. Patients discharged with an indwelling Foley catheter are scheduled to return to clinic for assessment of voiding function. About half of patients will void adequately by the time of discharge from day surgery. Of those who require catheterization, many are voiding well by the following day, and almost all have recovered normal voiding function within the first week.

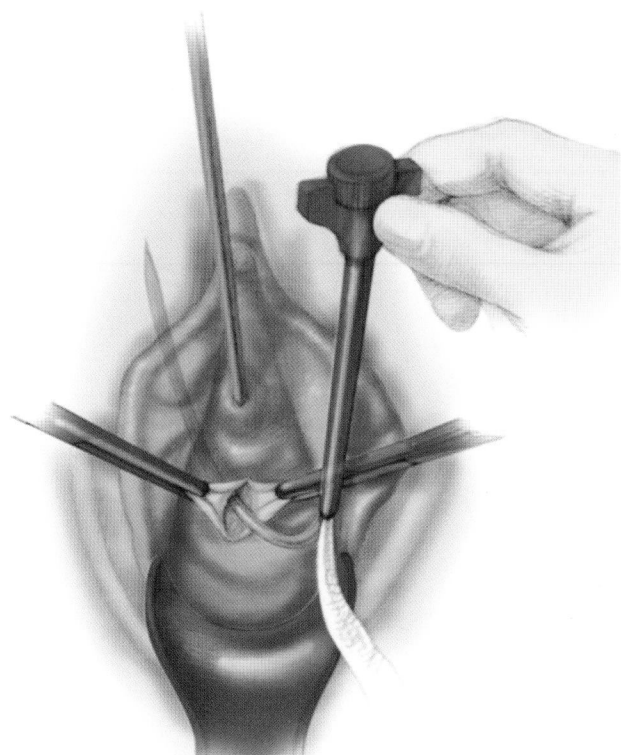

FIGURE 41.6 With the rigid catheter guide deviating the bladder to the left, the curved trocar is inserted in the retropubic position. The trocar perforates the retropubic space at the junction of the descending pubic ramus and the pubis, immediately along the surface of the bone.

VII

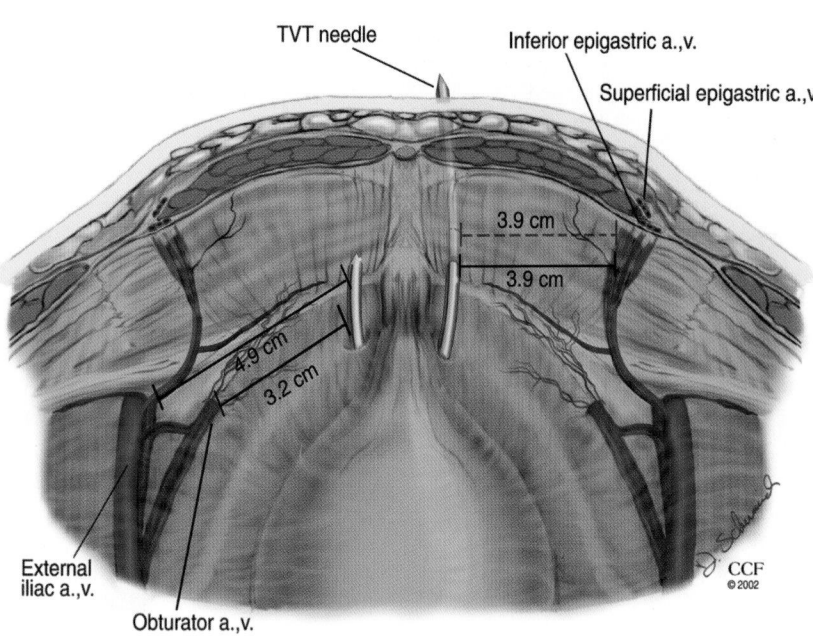

FIGURE 41.7 Retropubic trocars in the space of Retzius. The trocars enter the retropubic space approximately 2 to 3 cm from the midline. In this position, they are medial to the inferior epigastric, obturator, and accessory obturator vessels. The pubic branches of the obturator vessels are seen to course medially along the surface of the pubis.

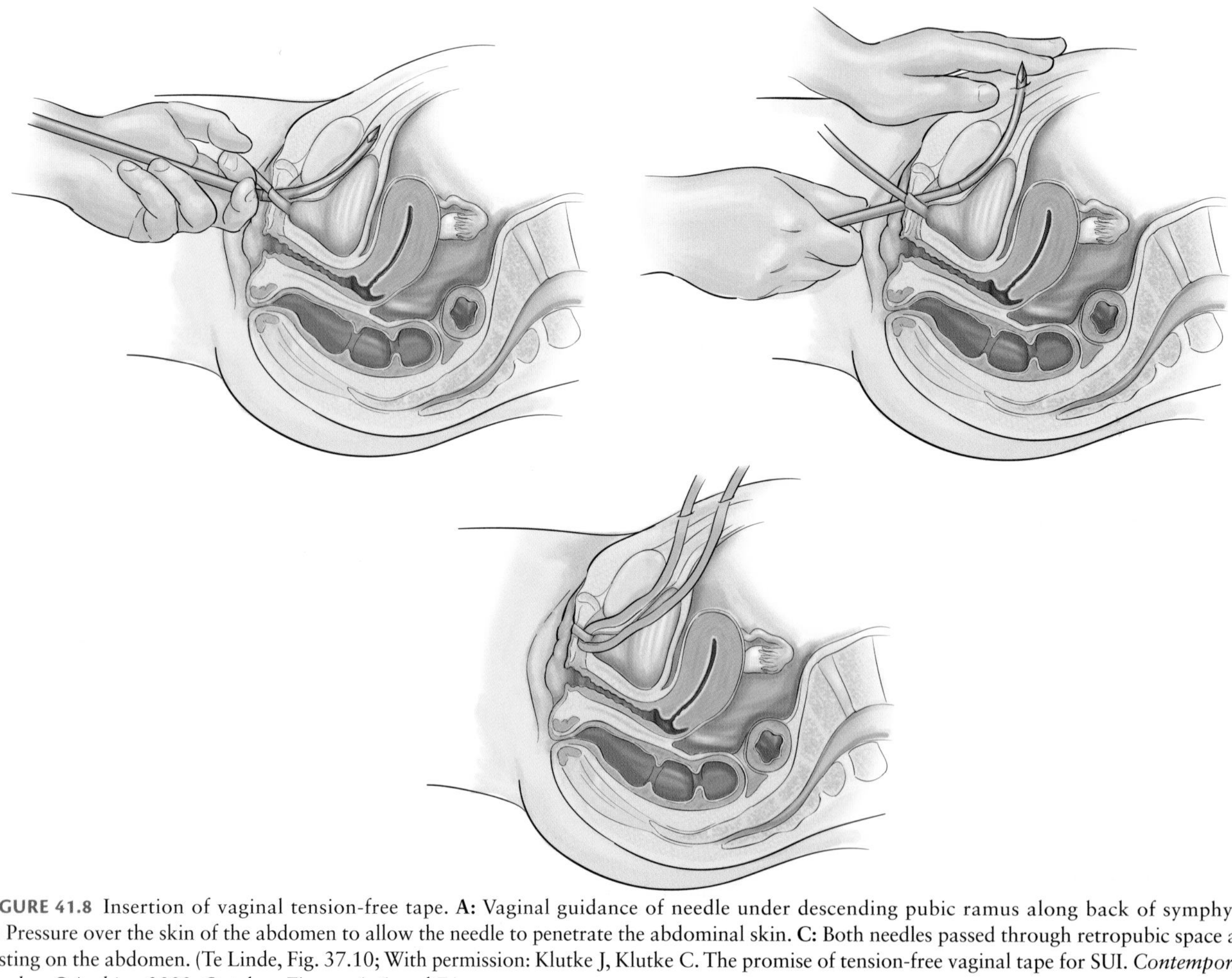

FIGURE 41.8 Insertion of vaginal tension-free tape. **A:** Vaginal guidance of needle under descending pubic ramus along back of symphysis. **B:** Pressure over the skin of the abdomen to allow the needle to penetrate the abdominal skin. **C:** Both needles passed through retropubic space and resting on the abdomen. (Te Linde, Fig. 37.10; With permission: Klutke J, Klutke C. The promise of tension-free vaginal tape for SUI. *Contemporary Urology®Archive*. 2000; October: Figures 4, 6, and 7.)

The most serious complications from the retropubic midurethral sling procedure pertain to the percutaneous passage of the trocar (Table 41.2). There have been rare deaths from undiagnosed bowel perforation. Major vascular injury is rare and will be minimized by ensuring that the insertion needle does not stray laterally. Smaller venous channels are frequently penetrated and are managed by pressure for 5 minutes or placement of a vaginal pack. Occasionally, a retropubic space hematoma will develop, but it is self-limited, and the usual treatment is observation.

Bladder perforation occurs in 2% to 4%; the incidence decreases with surgeon experience. Once identified, this event is usually managed by withdrawal and reinsertion of the needle (Table 41.3). When this occurs, a Foley catheter is recommended for bladder drainage. The optimal duration for bladder drainage in this setting is not known. Assuming that the sling is replaced after a perforation, it is our practice to continue drainage for 1 week, given that the perforation is almost always adjacent to the permanent implant. Bladder perforation may be minimized by hydrodissection of the retropubic space, keeping the bladder empty and directing the bladder away from the operative site with the rigid catheter guide.

There is a 2% to 3% risk of persistent urinary retention requiring sling revision. This is best performed in the first 4 to 6 weeks after surgery (e.g., before advanced scarring around the mesh). Sling revision includes exposure of the sling by sharp dissection, with midline transsection to allow retraction of the mesh away from the underside of the urethra. In some cases of retention, the tape will be found to have migrated somewhat proximally along the urethra. After sling transsection, continence is maintained in most patients, and the release of the sling allows normal voiding in most cases.

De novo urinary urgency occurs in 10% to 12%, although this symptom is typically self-limited. However, a number of patients require medical intervention. Release or loosening of the sling may help resolve severe urgency symptoms.

Exposure of the permanent sling material is a delayed complication, occurring in approximately 4% of patients within 24 months. Possible symptoms include bleeding, discharge, and dyspareunia. This complication is usually managed by excision of the exposed mesh and resuturing of the vagina.

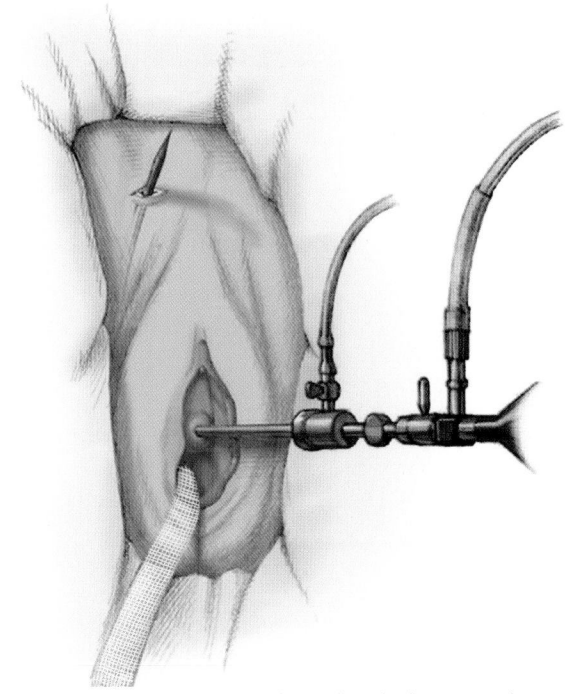

FIGURE 41.9 Cystoscopy is performed with the retropubic trocar in place. (Reprinted from Zubke W, Gruber IV, Gardanis K, et al. Tension-free vaginal tape (TVT): our modified technique—effective solutions for postoperative TVT correction. *Gynecol Surg* 2004;1:111, with permission. Copyright © 2004, Springer-Verlag Berlin/Heidelberg.)

The success rate of the retropubic midurethral sling is approximately 85%. Risk factors for failure include prior incontinence surgery, coexistent urge incontinence, and the absence of preoperative urethral hypermobility. Age also appears to be a risk factor for persistent SUI symptoms. Urodynamic parameters, such as low maximum urethral closure pressure and leak point pressure, may reduce objective success of midurethral slings; however, the predictive value of these parameters is relatively poor.

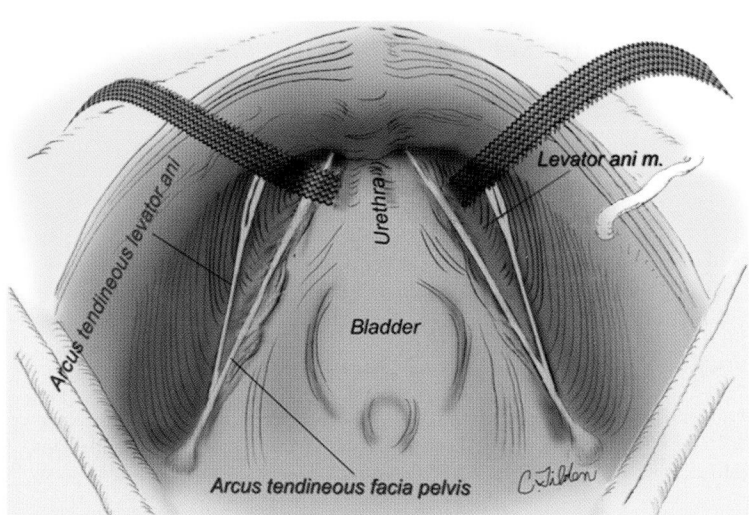

FIGURE 41.10 Retropubic space illustration showing location a retropubic sling. The sling on the right passes lateral to the arcus tendineus fascia pelvis (ATFP), perforating the levator ani muscle complex. The sling on the left is in the more typical location, medial to the ATFP. (Reprinted from Rahn DD, Marinis SI, Schaffer JI, et al. Anatomical path of the TVT: reassessing current teachings. *Am J Obstet Gynecol* 2006;195;1809, with permission. Copyright © 2006, Elsevier.)

VII

TABLE 41.2 Reported Major Tension-Free Vaginal Tape Complications[a] Based on 500,000 Cases

COMPLICATION	UNITED STATES	OUTSIDE UNITED STATES	TOTAL	PERCENT
Vascular injury	7	37	44	0.009
Vaginal mesh exposure	43	17	60	0.012
Urethral erosion	20	0	20	0.004
Bowel perforation[b]	16	12	28	0.006
Nerve injury	3	1	4	0.0008
Urinary retention	48	45	93	0.019
Hematoma formation	4	16	20	0.004

[a]Gynecare report to Food and Drug Administration as of September 26, 2003.
[b]Seven deaths have been reported, six associated with bowel perforation.

Transobturator Midurethral Sling Procedures

Compared to the retropubic sling, the transobturator sling has the advantage of minimizing the risk to the urinary tract (such as bladder perforation) because the procedure is theoretically below the level of the levator muscles. Thus, risk of injury to the bladder or bowel is theoretically avoided. A second argument in favor of transobturator approach is that the procedure is somewhat quicker: Operative times are approximately 10 minutes shorter with this approach. However, this difference is primarily due to exclusion of cystoscopy in many series.

STEPS IN THE PROCEDURE

Transobturator Midurethral Sling (Inside Out)

- The patient is positioned in Allen stirrups.
- The bladder is drained.
- An anterior vaginal wall incision (1 to 2 cm) is made over the midurethra.
- Using Metzenbaum scissors, a tunnel is created under the vaginal wall, oriented at 45 degrees, until the obturator membrane is penetrated with the scissor tips.
- The winged guide is inserted into the incision.
- The helical trocar is placed through the vaginal incision, following the winged guide. The handle is rotated and moved inferiorly to a vertical position such that the trocar exits 1 cm lateral to the groin fold and at the level of the clitoris.
- The sling is tensioned with a spacer (such as a 9 Hegar dilator) between the sling and the urethra.
- Cystoscopy is performed.
- The same procedure is repeated on the contralateral side.
- The bladder is drained and a voiding trial performed before discharge.

There have been several randomized controlled trials comparing outcomes after transobturator and retropubic slings. A recent Cochrane review of published studies concluded that cure rates were higher with the retropubic (vs. transobturator) approach, but with higher rates of complications. Specifically, cure rates were 88% after retropubic midurethral sling versus 84% after transobturator midurethral sling (relative risk 0.96, 95% confidence interval: 0.93 to 0.99). With respect to complications, the transobturator sling was associated with lower rates of bladder perforation (5.5% vs. 0.3%) and voiding dysfunction (7.0% vs. 4.4%). Although some have argued that symptoms of overactive bladder are more likely after the retropubic approach, the Cochrane review concluded that there is no significant difference in de novo urgency or urge incontinence. Thus, the slightly higher probability of cure after the retropubic sling is balanced by a slightly higher risk of bladder perforation and voiding dysfunction. Similar conclusions were drawn

TABLE 41.3 Minor Complications in 1,455 Tension-Free Vaginal Tape Cases[a]

INCIDENCE	N/1,000	PERCENT
Minor voiding difficulty	76	7.6
Urinary tract infection	41	4.1
Bladder perforation	38	3.8
Postoperative urinary retention	23	2.3
Retropubic hematoma	19	1.9
Wound infection	8	0.8

[a]A nationwide analysis of complications associated with the TVT. Reprinted from Kuuva N, Nilsson CG. A nationwide analysis of complications associated with the TVT procedure. *Acta Obstet Gynecol Scand* 2002;81:72, with permission. Copyright © 2002, John Wiley and Sons.

by Dyrkorn, Kulseng-Hanssen, and Sandvik, who analyzed data from a registry of 5,942 Swedish women. Thus, weighing the pros and cons, both procedures are reasonable options for the surgical treatment of SUI.

The transobturator sling may be placed with either the "inside-out" or the "outside-in" technique. In either case, the manufacturer supplies the sling with a mechanism to attach the sling to a helical insertion trocar. For the inside-out transobturator sling, the vaginal incision is created under the midurethra. Scissor dissection proceeds on one side until the obturator membrane is penetrated with the scissor tips. A metal winged guide is placed into the vaginal incision and advanced to the defect in the obturator membrane. The helical trocar is placed along the direction of the winged guide and then rotated while the handle is moved inferiorly to a vertical position. The trocar exits 1 cm lateral to the groin fold about 2 cm superior to the urethral meatus and parallel to the clitoris (Fig. 41.11). The tape is retrieved, and tightening follows the same pattern as with the retropubic technique.

For the "outside-in" approach, the vaginal incision needs to be larger, such that the surgeon can insert a finger under the vaginal mucosa to reach to the ischiopubic ramus. The thumb of the same hand grasps the outline of the ramus in the genitofemoral fold between labium majus and the thigh. A point in the groin fold level with the clitoris is selected and a 5-mm incision made on each side. The helical trocar is inserted

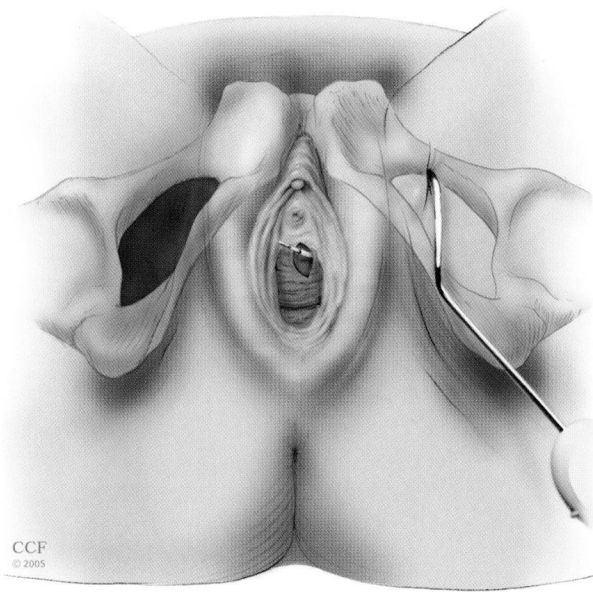

FIGURE 41.12 Outside-in transobturator sling. The passage of the helical needle is shown, beginning at a 5-mm skin incision created approximately 1 cm lateral to the groin fold and at the level of the clitoris. The surgeon's finger, inserted via the vaginal incision to the ischiopubic ramus, guides the trocar into the vaginal incision.

perpendicularly, and the handle of the helical trocar is at a 45-degree angle (from the horizontal) to accomplish the correct passage (Fig. 41.12). The trocar is then rotated under the pubic ramus, and the vaginal index finger guides it into the vaginal incision (Fig. 41.13). The sling is drawn back through

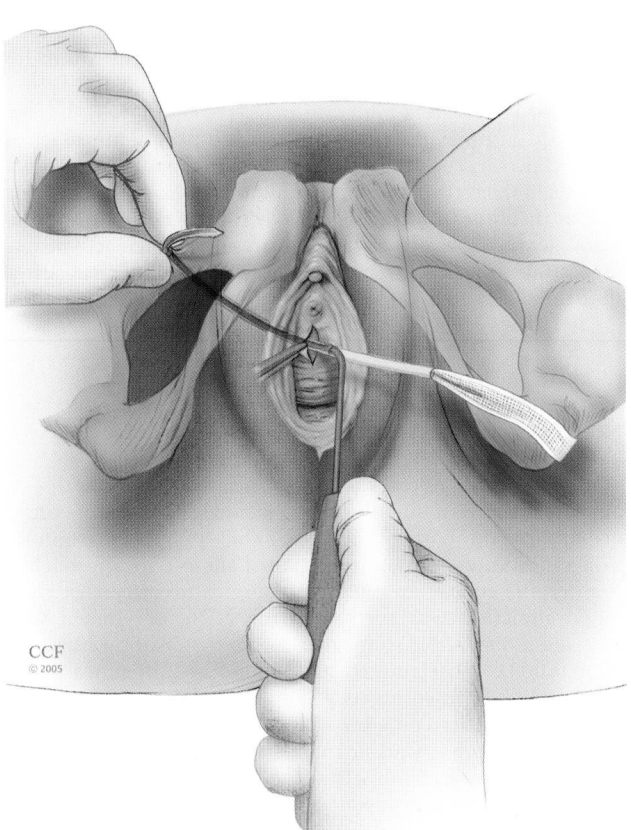

FIGURE 41.11 Inside-out transobturator sling. The passage of the helical needle is shown, exiting the skin approximately 1 cm lateral to the groin fold about 2 cm superior to the urethral meatus and parallel to the clitoris. (Reproduced with permission from Cleveland Clinic Foundation.)

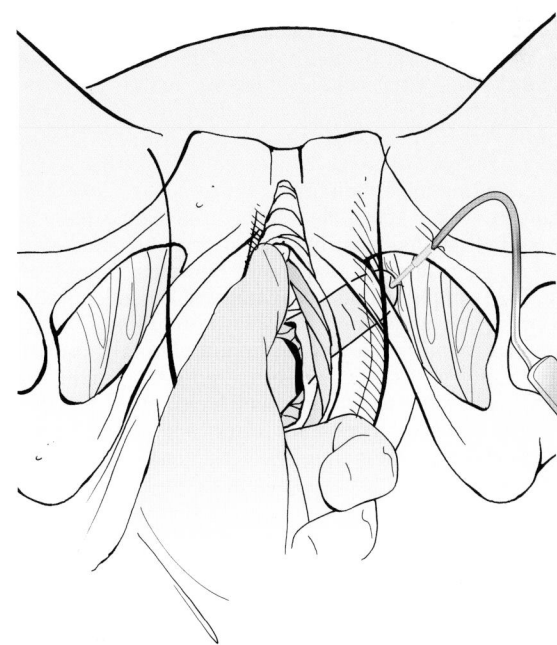

FIGURE 41.13 The trocar for the outside-in transobturator sling is guided into the vaginal incision. The end of the sling will be attached to the trocar and then withdrawn to the skin incision. (Reproduced with permission from Cleveland Clinic Foundation.)

VII

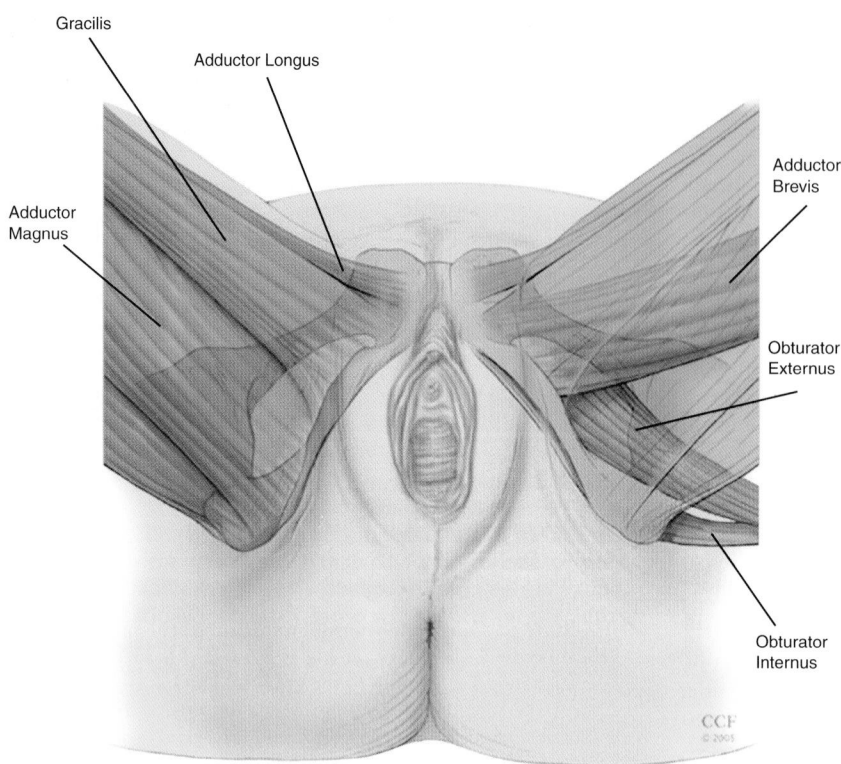

Gracilis

Adductor Longus

Adductor Magnus

Adductor Brevis

Obturator Externus

Obturator Internus

CCF © 2008

FIGURE 41.14 Along the path of the transobturator sling, potentially vulnerable structures include the muscles of the medial thigh, including the gracilis, adductor brevis, adductor longus, and adductor magnus. (Reproduced with permission from Cleveland Clinic Foundation.)

the path of the trocar. The identical procedure is performed on the opposite side. The tightening of the sling is the same as the retropubic approach.

There have been isolated reports of bladder perforation and urethral injury after transobturator sling placement. Therefore, it is appropriate to perform cystoscopy (with urethral inspection) at the end of the procedure, especially in women with significant prolapse. Vaginal perforation can also occur. The surgeon should diligently assess the vaginal fornices at the conclusion of surgery to ensure the mesh is not exposed. Risk factors for failure of the transobturator sling are similar to those for the retropubic sling: prior incontinence surgery, coexistent urge incontinence, age, and the absence of preoperative urethral hypermobility.

Similar to the retropubic sling, urodynamic parameters, such as low maximum urethral closure pressure and leak point pressure, may signify a lower cure rate after transobturator sling. For example, in one recent multicenter randomized comparison of retropubic and transobturator slings, Nager and colleagues found that a low maximum urethral closure pressure or Valsalva leak point pressure almost doubled the odds of surgical failure in each group. Some have argued that women with poor urethral function are better candidates for retropubic than transobturator slings. Schierlitz and colleagues randomized women with low maximum urethral closure pressure or Valsalva leak point pressure to retropubic or transobturator slings and found a superior cure rate in the retropubic sling group. However, Nager and colleagues could not demonstrate a difference between these two approaches for women with poor urethral function.

The transobturator approach minimizes the risk of retroperitoneal vascular injury, bowel injury, and bladder perforation. However, the trade-off is the possibility of damage to the obturator vessels and nerves. Potentially vulnerable structures (some of which are not familiar to the gynecologist)

include the anterior and posterior branches of the obturator nerve and several thigh muscles (gracilis, adductor brevis, adductor longus, and adductor magnus; Fig. 41.14). In fact, the main argument against the transobturator approach is that pelvic surgeons are more comfortable managing complications in the retropubic space than the transobturator space. The transobturator trocars pass within 1 cm of the obturator nerve, especially if the legs are not sufficiently flexed. One study in cadavers by Hubka and colleagues suggested that the distance to the obturator nerve can be increased to greater than 2 cm if the legs are flexed to 90 degrees with 30 degrees of abduction. The transobturator approach can result in the same postoperative complications of bleeding, hematoma, urgency, and bladder infections as with the retropubic approach. Abscess formation in the ischiorectal fossa has been reported, but it is very uncommon.

As previously noted, the transobturator midurethral sling appears to have a slightly lower incidence of postoperative urinary retention than the retropubic sling. For example, in a multicenter randomized trial of these two approaches, Richter and colleagues found that surgical treatment of voiding dysfunction was performed for 2.7% of women who received a retropubic sling and 0% after transobturator sling ($P = 0.004$). Most authors have found no difference in the incidence of de novo urgency symptoms. Leg and groin pain seems to be more common after transobturator sling placement. For example, Cadish and colleagues reported postoperative groin pain in 34 of 219 (15.5%) at a median follow-up of 1.6 months. The incidence of long-term or persistent groin pain is unknown.

Retropubic Urethropexy

Until midurethral slings became the mainstay of therapy for SUI, the gold standard for the surgical treatment of

SUI was the retropubic urethropexy (either a Burch or Marshall-Marchetti-Krantz [MMK] procedure). In the past decade, these approaches have largely been abandoned, due to evidence suggesting that midurethral sling procedures are equally effective, with less postoperative voiding dysfunction, shorter operative time, and reduced costs. Nevertheless, these procedures remain effective alternatives for selected patients.

The traditional approach to the retropubic space has been through a low transverse incision. A Foley catheter keeps the bladder empty and helps identify the bladder neck. Entry into the peritoneal cavity is avoided unless there is a surgical indication. After opening the rectus fascia, the rectus muscles are separated, and then, gentle downward pressure just behind and lateral to the symphysis allows approach to the pelvic sidewall and endopelvic fascia (Fig. 41.15). If there has been prior surgery in this area, sharp dissection is required to separate the rectus muscle from the underlying preperitoneal tissue and bladder. Depending on the incision size, a self-retaining retractor may be used. The bladder is retracted superiorly with the aid of a moist pack, and the inferior part of the incision is retracted to expose the bladder. Following exposure of the retropubic space, the bladder neck is identified by palpation of a Foley catheter bulb, and it may be marked with hemoclips if desired. The anatomic landmarks and points of attachment of endopelvic fascia can then be identified.

When performing a Burch retropubic urethropexy, the paraurethral tissue is exposed either with a "daisy sponge" (three 4 × 4 sponges fanned out on a sponge stick) or by using a moist sponge and narrow retractor. Some surgeons prefer to use a Miyazaki all-purpose lighted retractor. The paraurethral areas may be cleared of fat that overlies the pubocervical fascia (fibromuscular layer of the vagina). The pubocervical tissue is elevated with a vaginal finger, and the overlying tissue and bladder are mobilized medially and superiorly away from the site of suture placement using a small dissecting sponge or "peanut" (Fig. 41.16). The large veins in this area are avoided, if possible, but may require control with suture, hemoclips, or cautery. The most important aspects of the development of the retropubic space dissection are exposure and retraction and identification of the white endopelvic fascia (also called pubocervical fascia or fibromuscular layer of the vagina). Permanent sutures are placed on either side of the bladder neck. The

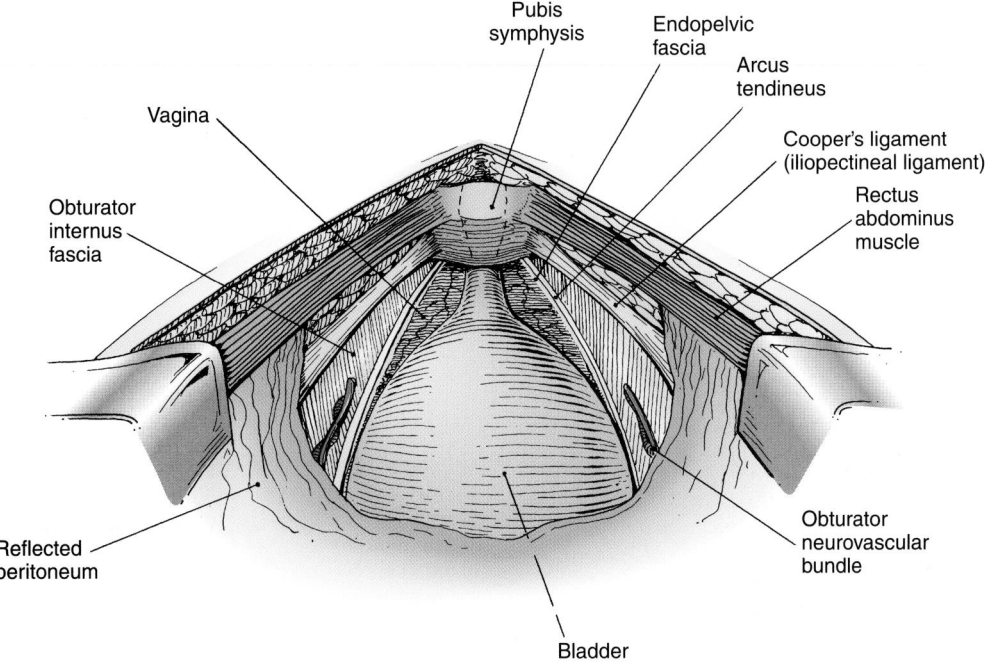

FIGURE 41.15 Anatomic landmarks in the space of Retzius.

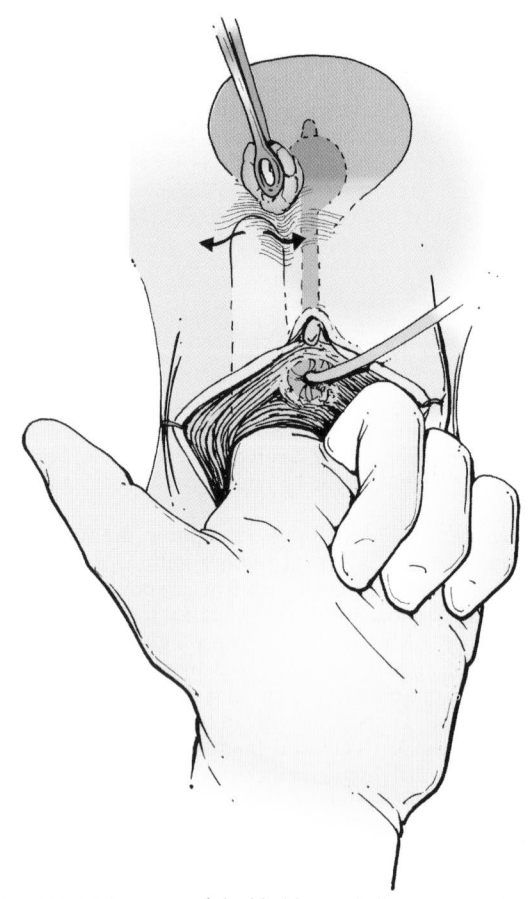

FIGURE 41.16 Dissection of the bladder medially to expose the endopelvic fascia. The finger of the vaginal hand elevates the vagina while the instrument pushes medially against the finger.

more proximal pair of sutures are placed 2 cm lateral to the urethra, into the endopelvic fascia (avoiding full thickness). The more distal pair of sutures are placed at the level of the midurethra (**Fig. 41.17**). For each of these sutures,

a figure-of-eight suture is preferred and will provide additional hemostasis.

One arm of each suture is placed through the ipsilateral Cooper ligament. The proximal sutures are placed through the more lateral aspect of the Cooper ligament with the distal sutures placed more medially. Recommendation for tensioning of the sutures varies. We prefer to tie the sutures such that the endopelvic fascia is seen to lift slightly. Some surgeons tie the sutures with an assistant's fingers in the vagina, tightening the sutures until the assistant feels the vaginal wall lift off the vaginal fingers. Cystoscopy is performed to exclude injury to the bladder and to verify ureteral patency.

An MMK procedure is performed by identifying the urethra with the aid of the Foley catheter (**Fig. 41.18**). Sutures are placed on either side of the urethra in a paraurethral location quite close to the urethra (**Fig. 41.19**). Bilateral permanent sutures are placed at the bladder neck, and usually, at least one set is placed more distally. These sutures are attached to the fibrocartilage of the symphysis pubis. Some surgeons open the bladder dome to locate the bladder neck by direct vision for exact suture placement at the bladder neck. Cystoscopy is performed at the conclusion of the procedure.

The aim of both procedures is to reestablish the intra-abdominal location of the proximal urethra and urethrovesical junction and to minimize descent of the bladder neck, thus allowing normal pressure transmission to this crucial area during times of increased intra-abdominal pressure. Cure rates for these procedures range from 85% to 90% at 1 to 5 years and greater than 70% at 10 years. Cure rates are lower among women without preoperative urethral hypermobility, those with recurrent incontinence after prior incontinence surgery, and among those with coexistent urge incontinence.

The Burch urethropexy can also be accomplished laparoscopically. The approach could be either intra-abdominal or extraperitoneal. To facilitate the laparoscopic approach, numerous modifications to the original Burch procedure were described (including using only two sutures; substituting mesh; or using tacks, anchors, and other tools to elevate the bladder neck), but these variations significantly lowered

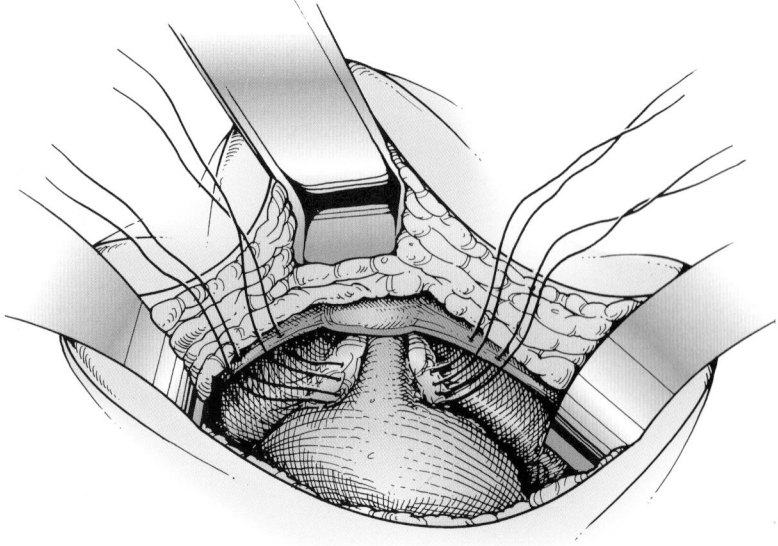

FIGURE 41.17 Permanent sutures on either side of the bladder neck for the Burch urethropexy. The more proximal pair of sutures are lateral to the bladder neck, and the more distal pair of sutures are at the level of the midurethra. The proximal sutures are placed through the more lateral aspect of Cooper ligament with the distal sutures placed more medially. (Adapted from Tanagho EA. Colpocystourethropexy: the way we do it. *J Urol* 1976;116:751. Copyright © 1976, Elsevier.)

Suburethral Slings

The concept of placing a material under the urethra and suspending it to the abdominal wall was introduced as early as 1907 when Giordano used gracilis muscle transposed beneath the bladder neck. Goebell in 1910 used pyramidalis muscles transposed through the space of Retzius, and first Frangenheim in 1914 and then Stoeckel in 1917 described using a strip of anterior abdominal fascia with the pyramidalis muscles. Price in 1933 harvested fascia lata, which he passed beneath the urethra and then retropubically, and attached it to the anterior rectus fascia on either side of the midline. This technique and its modifications became known as the Goebell-Stoeckel-Frangenheim procedure, or fascia lata sling, but the named surgeons never used fascia lata. Aldridge in 1942 used strips of rectus fascia from a transverse abdominal incision, passed them retropubically, and secured them beneath the urethra. McGuire and Lytton in 1978 described a sling procedure using rectus fascia supported by sutures extending through the space of Retzius and attached to the rectus fascia.

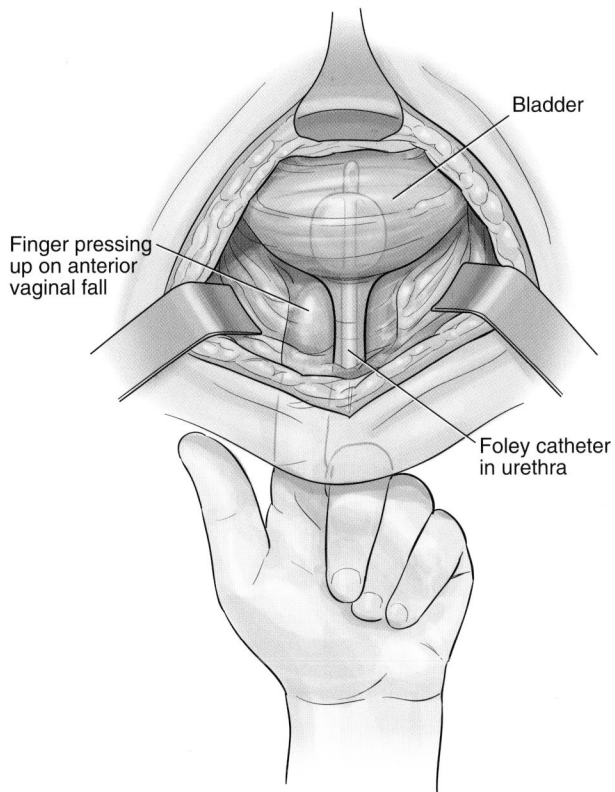

FIGURE 41.18 For the Marshall-Marchetti-Krantz procedure, the surgeon's finger, in the vagina, allows palpation of the Foley catheter and bulb, assisting with the identification of the urethra and bladder neck.

cure rates as compared with traditional open urethropexy. A laparoscopic approach with placement of four permanent sutures, identical to an open procedure, has yielded similar 1- and 2-year cure rates as an open Burch (93% and 89%, respectively). However, the more recent introduction of tension-free tape procedures made the laparoscopic Burch less popular.

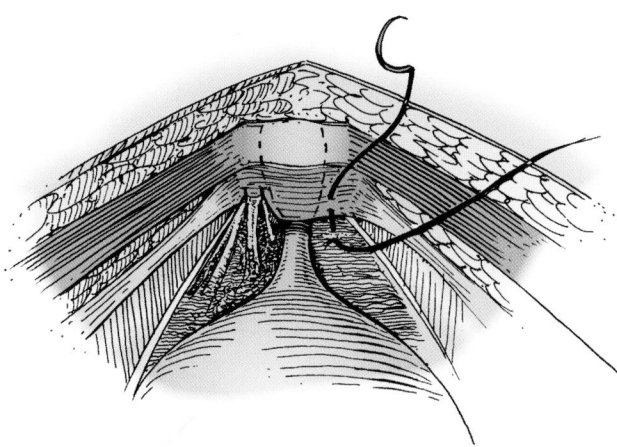

FIGURE 41.19 Suture placement for Marshall-Marchetti-Krantz operation. Sutures are placed into the endopelvic fascia along the urethra and fixed into the periosteum or fibrocartilage along the back of the symphysis pubis.

STEPS IN THE PROCEDURE

Suburethral Sling

- The patient is positioned high lithotomy. The bladder is drained with a Foley catheter. If rectus fascia is harvested, Allen stirrups may be preferred.

- A suprapubic transverse abdominal incision is made and continued to the fascia. The surgeon may elect to harvest rectus fascia at this point.

- Subcutaneous fat is cleared from the surface of the fascia at the location where the sling arms (or sutures) will be passed through the fascia (above the symphysis and 2 cm lateral to the midline).

- A midline vaginal incision is created, and the vaginal epithelium is dissected off the fibromuscular layer to the descending pubic ramus.

- The surgeon enters the retropubic space and uses a finger to mobilize the bladder and retropubic fat medially and superiorly.

- A long pair of packing forceps is inserted via the abdominal incision, perforating the rectus and entering the retropubic space. The surgeon's finger, placed into the retropubic space via the vagina, meets the advancing clamp (minimizing the potential risks of blind passage).

- Each sling arm is thus passed from the vaginal to the abdominal field. The central portion of the sling is tacked to the bladder neck to prevent movement from the placement site.

- Tension on the sling arms is adjusted. If the sling is of sufficient length, the sling arms are sutured to the rectus fascia. If the sling is not sufficiently long, permanent sutures, placed through the end of each sling arm, are sutured to the rectus fascia.

- Cystoscopy is performed.

VII

There are several critical differences between the traditional *suburethral* sling and newer *midurethral* sling procedures. The most obvious difference is that a midurethral sling is positioned at the midurethra, while a suburethral sling is placed at the proximal urethra or bladder neck. Also, suburethral slings are not "tension free," while the suburethral sling is intended to both elevate the urethrovesical junction into an intra-abdominal location and to provide partial compression of the urethra. Another distinction between the suburethral and midurethral sling is that the ends of the suburethral sling are fixed to the rectus fascia. During periods of increased abdominal pressure, the abdominal wall moves outward and the sling is thus drawn upward. This compresses the urethra and increases intraurethral resistance.

Since the original introduction of the suburethral sling procedure, a variety of materials have been employed, including rectus fascia, fascia lata, grafts of vaginal wall, gracilis muscle, round ligaments, pyramidalis muscle, and rectus muscle. Our preference is to use rectus fascia. However, because of additional operative time and morbidity to harvest autologous materials, a variety of synthetic materials have also been used. Synthetic materials are now almost completely confined to polypropylene mesh. Other biomaterials, including human allografts and xenografts (such as porcine and bovine tissues), have also been used, but their use has largely been abandoned due to variability in inflammatory response and evidence to suggest poorer treatment outcomes.

Sling length has varied in the many procedures described. Our preference is to harvest an autologous fascial sling of sufficient length to attach directly to the rectus fascia. A full-length sling is greater than 10 cm long; a sling of this length is usually sufficiently long to pass underneath the urethra, through the endopelvic fascia and retropubic space, all the way to the point of fixation at the rectus fascia, where it is secured with sutures. An alternative is a sling that is sufficiently long to extend into the retropubic space (at least 6 cm length) but not to the rectus fascia. This "half-sling" is anchored to the rectus fascia via suspending sutures and secured to the sling arms. Shorter slings ("patch slings") are similar to the Pereyra procedure and other needle suspension procedures that have been abandoned due to lack of efficacy. Thus, patch slings are not recommended.

The traditional suburethral sling procedure includes both abdominal and vaginal incisions. The retropubic space can be entered from either route, but our preference is to enter this space from the vaginal field. The abdominal incision should be created first if rectus fascia is harvested. The suprapubic incision is typically transverse, approximately 1 to 2 cm above the pubic bone. The goal is to harvest a fascial strip 2 cm wide (Fig. 41.20). After excision, the graft is wrapped in saline-soaked gauze or placed in an antibiotic solution. The fascia is mobilized sharply off the underlying muscle to avoid tension in the closure. The fascial incision is then closed. After the rectus fascia strip is harvested, subcutaneous fat is cleared from the surface of the fascia at sites 2 cm above the symphysis and 2 cm lateral to the midline. This is the location where the sling arms (or sutures) will be passed through the fascia.

The vaginal dissection commences with an inverted T midline incision along the anterior vaginal wall. The epithelium is dissected off the fibromuscular layer laterally until access through the endopelvic fascia is readily available beneath the descending pubic ramus. Sharp dissection to the level of the pubic ramus allows easy access to perforate the endopelvic

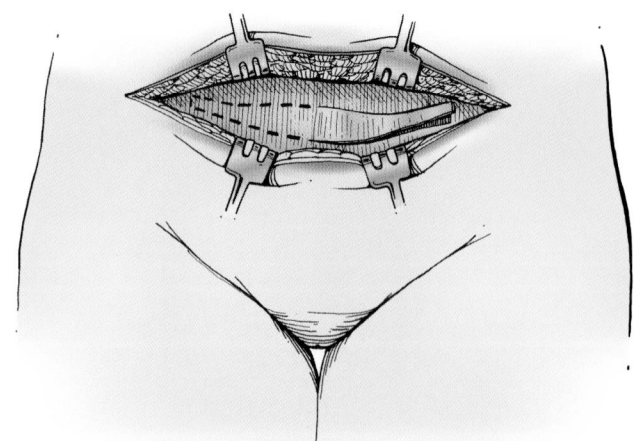

FIGURE 41.20 Incision for harvest of rectus fascia.

fascia. The surgeon may perforate into the retropubic space sharply or bluntly, directing the instrument or finger toward the ipsilateral shoulder (Fig. 41.21). Once the endopelvic fascia has been perforated, the surgeon uses a finger to mobilize the bladder and retropubic fat medially and superiorly, clearing the tissue away from the bone.

At this point, the fibromuscular layer of the vaginal wall can be plicated if extra thickness is desired under a synthetic sling or there is a central anterior vaginal wall support defect.

From the abdominal incision, a long pair of packing forceps or similar instrument or a Stamey needle is used to pass the sling from the vaginal to the abdominal incision.

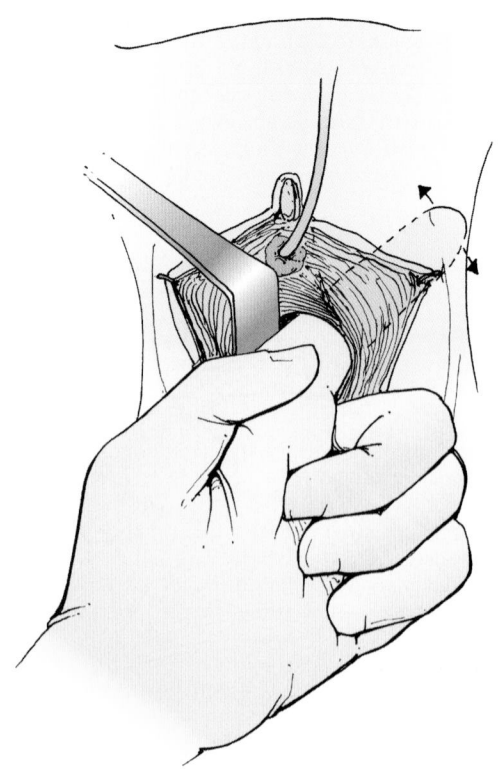

FIGURE 41.21 Perforation of the endopelvic fascia to open the space of Retzius and mobilize the periurethral tissues.

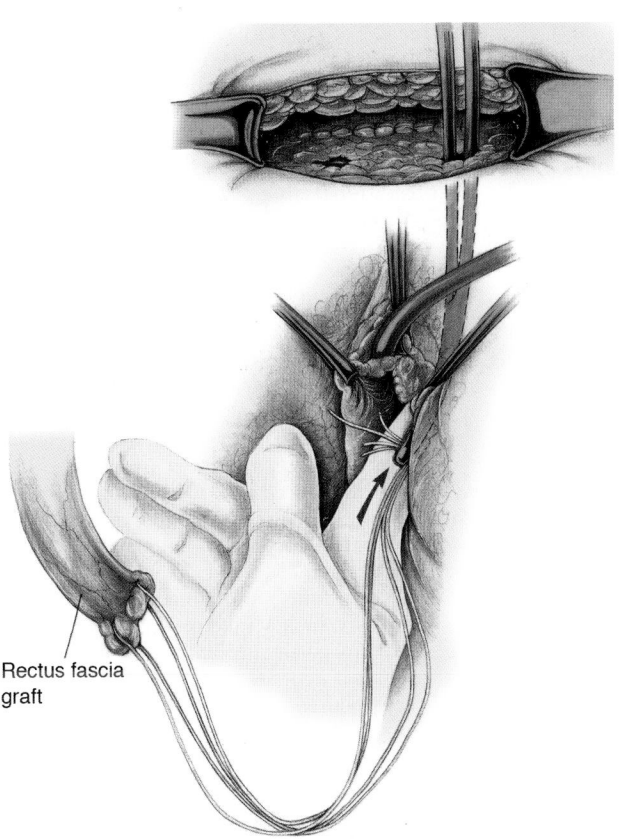

Rectus fascia
graft

FIGURE 41.22 Passage of sling material through the space of Retzius from vaginal to abdominal site. Rectus fascia partial sling with attached sutures. (Reprinted from Brubaker L. Suburethral sling procedures. *Oper Tech Gynecol Surg* 1997;2:48, with permission. Copyright © 1997, Elsevier.)

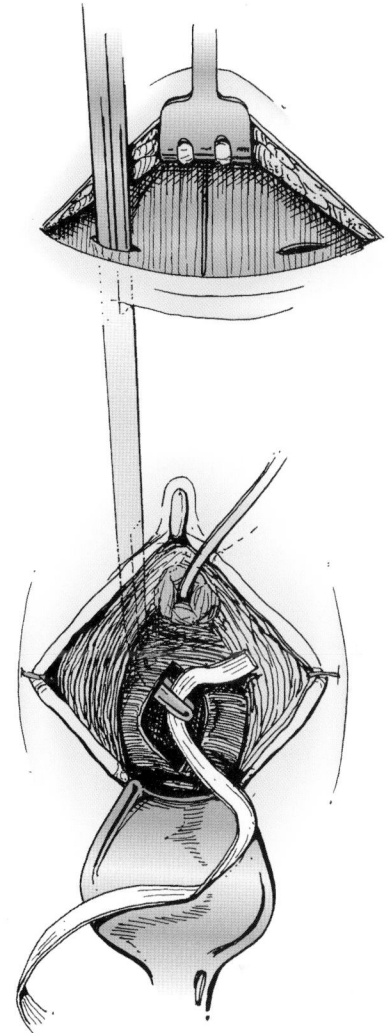

FIGURE 41.23 Passage of fascia lata strip through space of Retzius. Under guidance from the surgeon's hand in the vaginal incision through the endopelvic fascia into the space of Retzius, a clamp is passed from the abdominal incision to the vaginal incision. The end of the fascia is grasped and retrieved to the abdominal site.

The instrument perforates the rectus fascia just superior to the pubis, approximately 2 cm lateral to the midline. A finger placed in the vaginal dissection reaches to the retropubic space to meet the advancing clamp or needle, minimizing the potential risks of blind passage (Figs. 41.22 and 41.23). On each side, one arm of the sling is grasped and passed to the abdominal field and held. If the sling is short and the surgeon believes the sling arms cannot reach the abdominal wall fascia, permanent sutures are passed through each sling arm, and these sutures are then passed to the abdominal field.

After the sling arms are passed, the midportion of the sling is sutured under the bladder neck and proximal urethra to prevent movement from the placement site. A Foley catheter bulb is used to identify the bladder neck. Traditionally, the sling was placed at the bladder neck. However, as surgeons have gained experience with slings placed at the midurethra, many have also moved traditional suburethral sling placement more distally, to the proximal urethra or midurethra.

At the abdominal field, the sling arms are sutured to the rectus fascia (Fig. 41.24). The arms of the sling or suspending sutures may also be secured to each other, across the midline. Sling tension has been variably described. Some surgeons intentionally leave the sling loose (tension-free). Our practice has been to place a lubricated cotton swab in the urethra and to elevate the sling arms until there is a very

slight deflection of the swab (indicating very slight tension on the sling arms). The vaginal and abdominal incisions are closed. A vaginal pack is placed at the discretion of the surgeon.

The duration of voiding dysfunction is longer after a suburethral sling procedure than after the retropubic urethra or midurethral sling procedures. Thus, a suprapubic catheter may be preferred in this setting. However, a suprapubic catheter, Foley catheter, and intermittent self-catheterization are acceptable options. In our experience, the duration of hospitalization is one night.

Complications (Table 41.3) include retropubic bleeding. Large veins under the descending pubic ramus may be avulsed during the vaginal portion of the procedure, and there are often vessels on the medial side of the vaginal dissection into the retropubic space. The latter can be isolated and cauterized or sutured, but bleeding from under the pubis is best controlled by pressure, completion of the procedure, and placement of a vaginal pack. Significant bleeding is rare.

VII

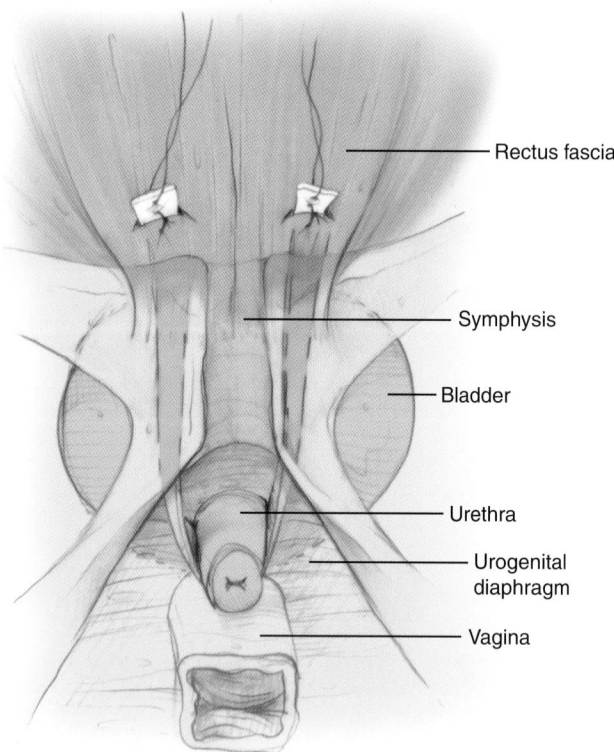

Rectus fascia

Symphysis

Bladder

Urethra

Urogenital
diaphragm

Vagina

FIGURE 41.24 Sling positioned at proximal urethra, extending through the space of Retzius, and fixed to the rectus fascia.

Bladder perforation can occur during retropubic dissection. Cystoscopy at the completion of the procedure is critical to identify injury to the urinary tract and ureteral compromise; urethroscopy is sometimes used to assess for obstruction due to excessive tension on the sling arms.

Short-term complications include continued voiding difficulty, bladder infection, and overactive bladder symptoms. A wound seroma or infection may occur at either the abdominal incision site or at the fascial harvest site. If a significant hematoma has occurred, abscess formation may follow. Vaginal healing may be compromised by delayed healing of the anterior vaginal wall, oozing or bleeding from the suture sites, and failure of the incision to close properly over the sling.

Long-term complications include voiding dysfunction, overactive bladder symptoms, and procedure failure. If the patient is unable to void at all, the sling may need to be incised. The occurrence of a vaginal exposure of a synthetic sling is usually a delayed event.

The cure rate for sling procedures is more than 80%. Traditionally, suburethral slings were reserved for cases of recurrent incontinence (after prior anti-incontinence surgery) or in cases complicated by ISD. However, suburethral sling procedures may also be considered for the surgical treatment of primary SUI. In a multicenter clinical trial, Albo and colleagues found that the suburethral sling resulted in a higher cure rate compared to retropubic urethropexy (66% vs. 49%, where cure was defined as a negative cough and Valsalva stress test, no self-reported symptoms, and no retreatment for the condition; $P < 0.001$). However, the same investigators found that the suburethral sling was associated with a greater risk of voiding dysfunction at 6 weeks (14% vs. 3%)

and a greater incidence of surgical revision due to voiding difficulty (6% vs. 0%). A Cochrane review identified 12 studies comparing traditional suburethral slings with minimally invasive midurethral slings. Effectiveness was similar, but the traditional slings had longer operative time and more complications. Also, postoperative voiding dysfunction was more likely higher after traditional sling procedures. Thus, suburethral sling procedures are typically reserved for recurrent or complicated SUI.

Periurethral Bulking Procedures

In 1993, the U.S. Food and Drug Administration approved the use of cross-linked bovine collagen (Contigen) for the treatment of SUI complicated by ISD (defined by Medicare as a low Valsalva leak point pressure). Although this product is no longer commercially available, a number of other bulking agents have since been introduced. At this writing, the commercially available urethral bulking products in the United States include carbon-coated zirconium oxide beads (Durasphere [Coloplast; Minneapolis, MN]), calcium hydroxylapatite (Coaptite; Boston Scientific), and polydimethylsiloxane, (Macroplastique [Uroplasty, Inc.; Minnetonka, MN]). Because there is no advantage of any particular bulking agent, selection is usually based on operator experience, ease of injection, cost, and availability of the product.

STEPS IN THE PROCEDURE

Transurethral Injection of Bulking Agent

- This procedure may be done in the office or clinic.
- The patient empties her bladder and is placed in the lithotomy position.
- Topical anesthetic gel can be applied to the urethra.
- Using a cystoscope with a 12-degree or 25-degree lens, the urethra is inspected. The bladder neck is identified, and the scope is withdrawn to visualize the proximal urethra.
- The desired bulking agent is injected via an appropriate needle (usually gauge), approximately 2 cm distal to the bladder neck.
- The usual injection sites are 3 and 9 o'clock.
- Bulking material is injected until visible closure of the urethral lumen.
- A voiding trial should be performed before the patient leaves the clinic. This can be facilitated by leaving the bladder comfortably full at the conclusion of the procedure.

Urethral bulking agents are traditionally a choice for women with limited urethral mobility. Indeed, the initial labeling for Contigen specified that the product was intended for use in the absence of urethral hypermobility. The ideal patient for treatment with a bulking agent is one who has documented SUI with a fixed bladder neck (cotton swab straining angle 30 degrees or less). A bulking agent may also be preferred in women with SUI who are poor surgical candidates and for those who prefer to use a less invasive technique.

VII

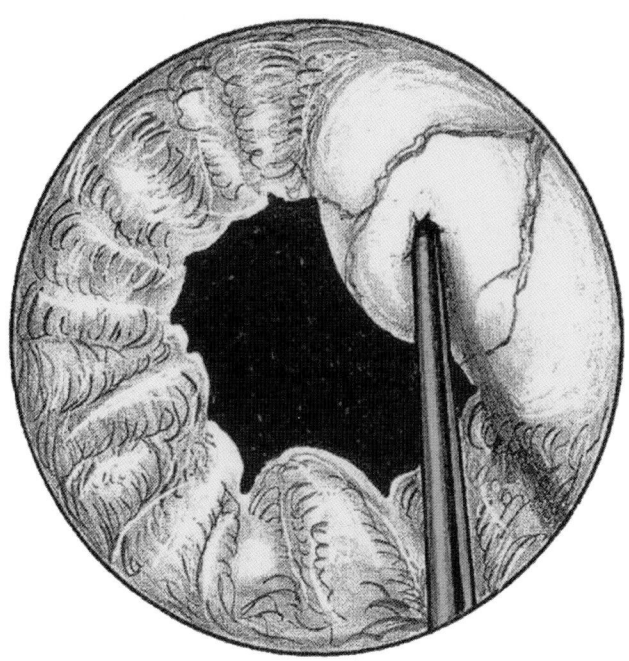

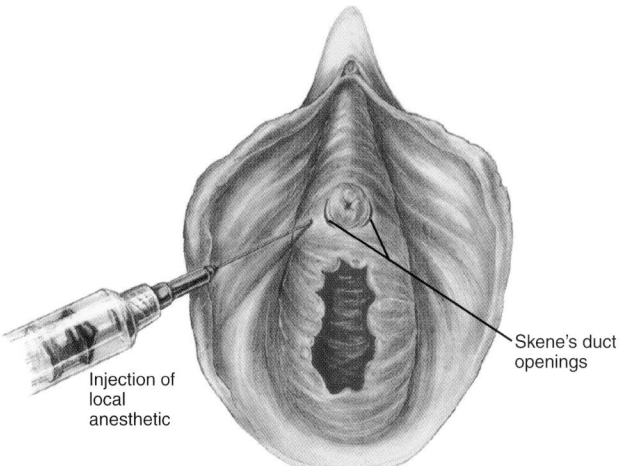

FIGURE 41.26 Periurethral bulking technique. Injection of local anesthetic lateral to Skene duct openings. (Te Linde figure 37.22; Reprinted from Bent AE. Periurethral collagen injections. *Oper Tech Gynecol Surg* 1997;2:52, with permission. Copyright © 1997 Elsevier.)

FIGURE 41.25 Transurethral needle placement in urethral submucosa. (Reprinted from Bent AE. Periurethral collagen injections. *Oper Tech Gynecol Surg* 1997;2:54, with permission. Copyright © 1997 Elsevier.)

Bulking agents can be injected via either a periurethral or transurethral technique. The ideal setting for injection is the office or clinic. No sedation is required. The injection is performed in a sterilized field by using no-touch technique. We typically prefer the transurethral technique when the procedure is performed in the office setting because of patient comfort. Before the procedure, some surgeons administer a single dose of fluoroquinolone or trimethoprim/sulfamethoxazole, although the benefit of prophylactic antibiotics has not been demonstrated.

Prior to the procedure, the patient empties her bladder and is placed in lithotomy position. Topical anesthetic gel can be applied to the urethra. The transurethral method is best accomplished using a cystoscope with a 12-degree or 25-degree lens. The sheath should have an operating channel that allows the passage of an injection needle, and the tip should not be fenestrated. If a local anesthetic is desired, the needle may be prefilled with lidocaine 1% solution. If no local anesthetic injection is planned, the syringe with bulking material is attached, and the cystoscope with injection needle retracted is placed into the bladder. The bladder neck is identified, and the scope is withdrawn to visualize the proximal urethra. The usual injection sites are 3 and 9 o'clock, but this can be varied, depending on user preference and number of injection sites selected (up to four). The injection needle is advanced into the urethra submucosa approximately 2 cm distal to the bladder neck (Fig. 41.25), and the bulking material is injected. The goal is to achieve coaptation, with visible closure of the urethral lumen.

For the periurethral technique, local anesthesia using 0.5 to 1.0 mL of lidocaine hydrochloride is injected 0.5 cm on either side of the urethral meatus (Fig. 41.26). Under endoscopic guidance, lidocaine 1% solution is injected lateral to the urethra, using a spinal needle. The needle is advanced, parallel to the urethra, while endoscopic guidance is used to direct the injection. Lidocaine is injected in small amounts as the needle

is advanced until reaching 1 cm distal to the bladder neck (Fig. 41.27). At this point, the syringe with lidocaine is replaced with a syringe of bulking agent (e.g., without withdrawing the needle), and the material is injected until the entire syringe has been injected or there has been adequate effect noted with urethral bulking. To achieve the desired coaptation, the process may be repeated on the opposite site. The second side may be more difficult to inject because of the distortion caused by the initial injection.

Injection needles vary in diameter according to the ease of injection of the selected material, and the implant manufacturers typically recommend their own proprietary needles for this purpose. Durasphere and Macroplastique are injected through an 18-gauge needle, while Coaptite can be injected through a 21-gauge needle. Macroplastique injection is accomplished using a proprietary high-pressure administration device that allows the surgeon to deliver the implant by pulling on a trigger-like lever.

A voiding trial should be performed before the patient leaves the clinic. This can be facilitated by leaving the bladder comfortably full at the conclusion of the procedure. If the patient is unable to void adequately, she should be instructed in self-catheterization. After injection, the patient may experience dysuria or urethral burning. This symptom typically lasts for only part of a day and can be controlled with phenazopyridine (Pyridium).

One or two additional injections may be required to obtain a satisfactory result; we typically assess the need for a second injection 4 to 6 weeks after the first. After 1 to 3 initial injections, the success rate is generally quoted to be about 70%. However, there is substantial controversy about the durability of the effect achieved with bulking agents. Chrouser et al. found that the initial success declined by about one half over the first year of observation. In a longitudinal study of women treated with Macroplastique, Ghoniem found that two thirds of those successfully treated remained "dry" at 24 months. Thus, the effectiveness of bulking agents declines over time. Women treated successfully with an injection of bulking agent often experience recurrence; repeat injections can be employed. There is no limit to the number of injections, provided that improvement occurs after each injection and lasts a reasonable period of time.

VII

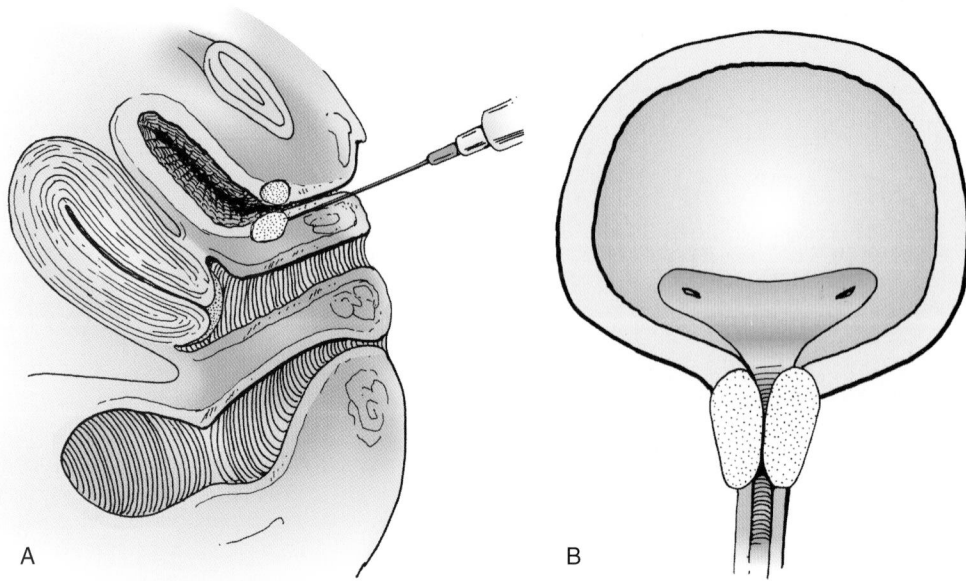

FIGURE 41.27 A: Periurethral injection at the bladder neck. **B:** Bulking of bladder neck and proximal urethra.

The success of bulking agents does not appear to depend on the presence of urethral hypermobility. Thus, this option is the most attractive for women with a well-supported urethra (because the success of more invasive methods, such as sling procedures, is relatively low in this setting). However, there have been relatively few clinical trials comparing bulking agents with other surgical treatments for SUI. Corcos and colleagues performed a randomized comparison of Contigen injection versus surgery (a variety of surgical procedures were included). In this study, the majority of participants had urethral hypermobility. The investigators found no significant difference in the proportion of women with a "dry" pad test at 1 year. However, 25% of women did not receive the randomized treatment assignment, thus decreasing the probability that a difference would be detected. In another study, Maher et al. randomized women with SUI and low urethral closure pressure to injection of Macroplastique versus rectus fascia sling. Approximately 10% of the participants had urethral hypermobility. At 6 months, objective but not subjective cure rate was significantly higher in the sling group.

Complications of bulking agents are limited to transient urinary retention (best managed with intermittent self-catheterization) and rare cases of granuloma or erosion of the material into the urethra.

SUMMARY

The surgical management of SUI has developed over almost 100 years. In the past two decades, high-quality randomized controlled trials have been conducted, providing evidence-based options for the surgical treatment of SUI. As a result, less effective surgeries (such as Kelly placation and needle suspensions) have largely been abandoned. The contemporary approach to treatment of SUI begins with a very careful clinical evaluation and the selective use of urodynamic testing. A positive stress test should be demonstrated before surgery. Referral to a subspecialist is appropriate for women with more complicated incontinence, such as those with

mixed incontinence (e.g., significant urge-related symptoms), absent urethral hypermobility, urinary retention (postvoid residual volume >150 mL), prior anti-incontinence surgery, prior radical pelvic surgery or irradiation, and those with neurologic disease. Nonsurgical options, such as anti-incontinence pessaries and supervised physiotherapy programs, result in satisfactory outcomes for 50% of women and should be encouraged. For those who elect surgical treatment, midurethral sling procedures (either retropubic or transobturator) provide high success rates. More invasive options, which might be appropriate in certain clinical situations, include the retropubic urethropexy and suburethral sling procedures.

BEST SURGICAL PRACTICES

- Evaluation before surgery for SUI includes history, physical examination, pelvic examination, voiding diary, symptom questionnaire, residual urine determination, cotton swab test for urethral mobility, and urinalysis. If there is any concern regarding symptoms or prior procedure failure, then cystometry (and often cystoscopy) should be performed. Referral to a subspecialist is appropriate for women with more complicated incontinence, such as those with mixed incontinence (e.g., significant urge-related symptoms), absent urethral hypermobility, urinary retention (postvoid residual volume >150 mL), prior anti-incontinence surgery, prior radical pelvic surgery or irradiation, and those with neurologic disease.
- Women who elect surgical treatment of primary SUI may be offered a tension-free midurethral sling (either retropubic or transobturator). Other effective options include Burch retropubic urethropexy or suburethral sling.
- After an anti-incontinence procedure, cystoscopy is recommended to assure there is no bladder injury.
- Urethral bulking agents may be a good choice in the treatment of women with SUI who are poor surgical candidates and those with minimal mobility of the bladder neck, that is, cotton swab test less than 30 degrees straining.

TEST QUESTIONS

1. Which of the following women are least likely to benefit from a urodynamic evaluation prior to surgical treatment of stress incontinence?
   A. A 45-year-old with a history of a prior sling procedure
   B. A 55-year-old with a well-supported bladder neck
   C. A 68-year-old who did not experience improvement in symptoms after a course of supervised behavioral therapy
   D. A 44-year-old who has mixed symptoms of stress and urgency incontinence
   (The answer is C.)

2. Which of the following vascular structures are most vulnerable in a retropubic midurethral sling procedure?
   A. The inferior epigastric artery
   B. The internal pudendal artery
   C. The perineal branch of the external pudendal artery
   D. The internal iliac artery
   (The answer is A.)

3. Which of the following is not true?
   A. The incidence of persistent voiding dysfunction requiring surgical revision is approximately 3% after retropubic midurethral sling.
   B. Women with voiding dysfunction can be reassured that continence is usually maintained after sling transsection.
   C. Among women with voiding dysfunction after midurethral sling procedure, urinary retention resolves in a majority of cases treated with sling transsection.
   D. The incidence of postoperative voiding dysfunction is the same after retropubic versus transobturator midurethral sling.
   (The answer is D.)

BIBLIOGRAPHY

Abrams P, Andersson KE, Brubaker L, et al. Recommendations of the International Scientific Committee. In: Abrams P, Cardozo L, Khoury S, et al., eds. *Incontinence.* Paris, France: Health Publications, Ltd., 2005:1606.

Albo ME, Richter HE, Brubaker L, et al. Burch colposuspension versus fascial sling to reduce urinary stress incontinence. *N Engl J Med* 2007;356:2143.

Aldridge AH. Transplantation of fascia for relief of urinary stress incontinence. *Am J Obstet Gynecol* 1942;44:398.

American College of Obstetricians and Gynecologists. *ACOG Practice Bulletin Number 63. Urinary incontinence in women: clinical management guidelines for obstetricians–gynecologists.* Washington, DC: ACOG, 2005.

Bent AE. Periurethral collagen injections. *Oper Tech Gynecol Surg* 1997;2:54.

Bracken JN, Huffaker RK, Yandell PM, et al. A randomized comparison of bupivacaine versus saline during placement of tension-free vaginal tape. *Female Pelvic Med Reconstr Surg* 2012;18:93.

Brubaker L. Suburethral sling procedures. *Oper Tech Gynecol Surg* 1997;2:48.

Brubaker L, Norton PA, Albo ME, et al. Adverse events over two years after retropubic or transobturator midurethral sling surgery: findings from the Trial of Midurethral Slings (TOMUS) study. *Am J Obstet Gynecol* 2011;205:498.e1.

Burch JC. Cooper's ligament urethrovesical suspension for stress incontinence: nine years' experience—results, complications, technique. *Am J Obstet Gynecol* 1968;100:764.

Burch JC. Urethrovaginal fixation to Cooper's ligament for correction of stress incontinence, cystocele, and prolapse. *Am J Obstet Gynecol* 1961;81:281.

Cadish LA, Hacker MR, Dodge LE, et al. Association of body mass index with hip and thigh pain following transobturator midurethral sling placement. *Am J Obstet Gynecol* 2010;203:508.e1.

Chrouser KL, Fick F, Goel A, et al. Carbon coated zirconium beads in beta-glucan gel and bovine glutaraldehyde cross-linked collagen injections for intrinsic sphincter deficiency: continence and satisfaction after extended followup. *J Urol* 2004;171:1152.

Corcos J, Collet JP, Shapiro S, et al. Multicenter randomized clinical trial comparing surgery and collagen injections for treatment of female stress urinary incontinence. *Urology* 2005;65:898.

Crystle CD, Charme LS, Copeland WE. Q-tip test in stress urinary incontinence. *Obstet Gynecol* 1971;38:313.

DeLancey JOL. Structural support of the urethra as it relates to stress incontinence: the hammock hypothesis. *Am J Obstet Gynecol* 1994;170:1713.

DeLorme E. Transobturator urethral suspension: mini-invasive procedure in the treatment of stress urinary incontinence in women. *Prog Urol* 2001;11:1306.

Dunivan GC, Parnell BA, Connolly A, et al. Bupivacaine injection during midurethral sling and postoperative pain: a randomized controlled trial. *Int Urogynecol J* 2011;22:433.

Dyrkorn OA, Kulseng-Hanssen S, Sandvik L. TVT compared with TVT-O and TOT: results from the Norwegian National Incontinence Registry. *Int Urogynecol J* 2010;21:1321.

Frangenheim P. Zu operative behandlung der inkontinenz der mannlichen harnohre. *Ver Dtsch Ges Chir* 1914;43:149.

Fritel X, Fauconnier A, Bader G, et al. Diagnosis and management of adult female stress urinary incontinence: guidelines for clinical practice from the French College of Gynaecologists and Obstetricians. *Eur J Obstet Gynecol Reprod Biol* 2010;151:14.

Ghoniem G, Corcos J, Comiter C, et al. Durability of urethral bulking agent injection for female stress urinary incontinence: 2-year multicenter study results. *J Urol* 2010;183:1444.

Goebell R. Zur operativen beseitigung der angeborenen. *Incontinentia Vesicae Z Gynakol Urol* 1910;2:187.

Haylen BT, de Ridder D, Freeman RM, et al. An International Urogynecological Association (IUGA)/International Continence Society (ICS) joint report on the terminology for female pelvic floor dysfunction. *Neurourol Urodyn* 2010;29:4.

Houwert RM, Venema PL, Aquarius AE, et al. Risk factors for failure of retropubic and transobturator midurethral slings. *Am J Obstet Gynecol* 2009;201:202.e1.

Hubka P, Nanka O, Martan A, et al. Anatomical study of position of the TVT-O to the obturator nerve influenced by the position of the legs during the procedure: based upon findings at formalin-embalmed and fresh-frozen bodies. *Arch Gynecol Obstet* 2011;284:901.

Jaburek L, Jaburkova J, Lubusky M, et al. Risk of haemorrhagic complications of retropubic surgery in females: anatomic remarks. *Biomed Pap Med Fac Univ Palacky Olomouc Czech Repub* 2011;155:75.

Karram MM, Segal JL, Vassallo BJ, et al. Complications and untoward effects of the tension-free vaginal tape procedure. *Obstet Gynecol* 2003;101:929.

Kelly HA. Incontinence of urine in women. *Urol Cutan Rev* 1913;17:291.

Krambeck AE, Dora CD, Sebo TJ, et al. Time-dependent variations in inflammation and scar formation of six different pubovaginal sling materials in the rabbit model. *Urology* 2006;67:1105.

Krofta L, Feyereisl J, Otcenásek M, et al. TVT and TVT-O for surgical treatment of primary stress urinary incontinence: prospective randomized trial. *Int Urogynecol J* 2010;21:141.

Kuuva N, Nilsson CO. A nationwide analysis of complications associated with the tension free vaginal tape (TVT) procedure. *Acta Obstet Gynecol Scand* 2002;81:72.

Lapitan MCM, Cody JD. Open retropubic colposuspension for urinary incontinence in women. *Cochrane Database Syst Rev* 2012; [Art. No.: CD002912].

Maher CF, O'Reilly BA, Dwyer PL, et al. Pubovaginal sling versus transurethral Macroplastique for stress urinary incontinence and intrinsic sphincter deficiency: a prospective randomised controlled trial. *BJOG* 2005;112:797.

Marshall VF, Marchetti AA, Krantz KE. The correction of stress incontinence by simple vesicourethral suspension. *Surg Gynecol Obstet* 1949;88:509.

VII

McGuire EJ, Appell RA. Transurethral collagen injection for urinary incontinence. *Urology* 1994;43:413.

McGuire EJ, Lytton B. Pubovaginal sling procedure for stress incontinence. *J Urol* 1978;119:82.

Muir TW, Tulikangas PK, Fidela Paraiso M, et al. The relationship of tension-free vaginal tape insertion and the vascular anatomy. *Obstet Gynecol* 2003;101:933.

Nager CW, Brubaker L, Litman HJ, et al. A randomized trial of urodynamic testing before stress-incontinence surgery. *N Engl J Med* 2012;366:1987.

Nager CW, FitzGerald M, Kraus SR, et al. Urodynamic measures do not predict stress continence outcomes after surgery for stress urinary incontinence in selected women. *J Urol* 2008; 179:1470.

Nager CW, Sirls L, Litman HJ, et al. Baseline urodynamic predictors of treatment failure 1 year after mid urethral sling surgery. *J Urol* 2011;186:597.

Nilsson CG, Rezapour M, Falconer C. Seven-year follow-up of the tension free vaginal tape procedure. *Int Urogynecol J* 2003;14:35.

Ogah J, Cody JD, Rogerson L. Minimally invasive synthetic suburethral sling operations for stress urinary incontinence in women. *Cochrane Database Syst Rev* 2009;(4):CD006375.

Price PB. Plastic operations for incontinence of urine and feces. *Arch Surg* 1933;26:1043.

Rahn DD, Marinis SI, Schaffer JI, et al. Anatomical path of the tension-free vaginal tape: reassessing current teachings. *Am J Obstet Gynecol* 2006;195:1809.

Rehman H, Bezerra CCB, Bruschini H, et al. Traditional suburethral sling operations for urinary incontinence in women. *Cochrane Database Syst Rev* 2011;(1) [Art. No.: CD001754].

Richter HE, Albo ME, Zyczynski HM, et al. Retropubic versus transobturator midurethral slings for stress incontinence. *N Engl J Med* 2010;362:2066.

Richter HE, Burgio KL, Brubaker L, et al. Continence pessary compared with behavioral therapy or combined therapy for stress incontinence: a randomized controlled trial. *Obstet Gynecol* 2010;115:609.

Richter HE, Goode PS, Brubaker L, et al. Two-year outcomes after surgery for stress urinary incontinence in older compared with younger women. *Obstet Gynecol* 2008;112:621.

Richter HE, Litman HJ, Lukacz ES, et al. Demographic and clinical predictors of treatment failure one year after midurethral sling surgery. *Obstet Gynecol* 2011;117:913.

Rovner ES, Goudelocke CM. Which injectable to use in the treatment of intrinsic sphincter deficiency? *Curr Opin Urol* 2010; 20:296.

Schierlitz L, Dwyer PL, Rosamilia A, et al. Effectiveness of tension-free vaginal tape compared with transobturator tape in women with stress urinary incontinence and intrinsic sphincter deficiency: a randomized controlled trial. *Obstet Gynecol* 2008; 112:1253.

Shobeiri SA, Gasser RF, Chesson RR, et al. The anatomy of midurethral slings and dynamics of neurovascular injury. *Int Urogynecol J Pelvic Floor Dysfunct* 2003;14:185.

Stoeckel W. Uber die verwendung der musculi pyridimale beider operative behandlung der incontinentia urinae. *Gynakol* 1917; 41:11.

Tamussino K, Hanzal E, Kölle D, et al. Transobturator tapes for stress urinary incontinence: results of the Austrian Registry. *Am J Obstet Gynecol* 2007;197:634.e1.

Tanagho EA. Colpocystourethropexy: the way we do it. *J Urol* 1976; 116:751.

Ulmsten U, Henriksson L, Johnson P, et al. An ambulatory surgical procedure under local anesthesia for treatment of female urinary incontinence. *Int Urogynecol J* 1996;7:81.

Wu JM, Gandhi MP, Shah AD, et al. Trends in inpatient urinary incontinence surgery in the USA, 1998–2007. *Int Urogynecol J* 2011;22:1437.

Yurteri-Kaplan LA, Gutman RE. The use of biological materials in urogynecologic reconstruction: a systematic review. *Plast Reconstr Surg* 2012;130:242S.

Zubke W, Gruber IV, Gardanis K, et al. Tension-free vaginal tape (TVT): our modified technique–effective solutions for postoperative TVT correction. *Gynecol Surg* 2004.

CHAPTER 42
Operative Injuries to the Ureter

E. James Wright and Victoria L. Handa

DEFINITIONS

Cystotomy—Incision into the urinary bladder.

Psoas hitch—A technique to facilitate repair of mid- and distal ureteral injuries. The bladder is mobilized and anchored to the ipsilateral psoas muscle to facilitate tension-free ureteroneocystostomy.

Spatulate—To incise the cut end of a tubular structure longitudinally and splay it open to allow creation of an elliptical anastomosis of greater circumference than would be possible with conventional transverse or oblique end-to-end anastomoses.

Tampon test—A test used to differentiate vesicovaginal from uterovaginal fistula in the setting of postoperative vaginal fluid leak. Saline colored with methylene blue dye is instilled into the bladder and a tampon inserted into the vagina. If the tampon is unstained, a ureteral injury is suspected.

Ureteroileoneocystomy—Restoration of continuity of the urinary tract by anastomosis of the upper segment of the ureter to a segment of ileum, the lower end of which is then implanted into the bladder.

Ureteroneocystostomy—Reimplantation of the ureter into the bladder.

Ureteroureterostomy—Anastomosis between two segments of the ipsilateral ureter. When done between contralateral ureteral segments, this is termed transureteroureterostomy.

Urinoma—A fluid collection containing urine.

Ureteral injuries have been recognized as a potential complication of gynecologic surgery since the inception of our discipline. Over the years, numerous unique surgical modifications of procedures have been offered with the specific intent of decreasing the probability of ureteral injury. Despite these efforts, ureteral injury remains a very real complication of abdominal–pelvic surgery in the female patient.

The incidence of ureteral injury during gynecologic surgery is commonly cited as 1% to 2%, although the incidence varies with the nature of the surgery, the skill of the surgeon, and the complexity of the patient's anatomy. Ibeanu and colleagues reported injury to the ureter in 15 of 839 hysterectomies performed at a teaching hospital in which universal cystoscopy was employed (incidence 1.8%, 95% confidence interval: 1.0%, 2.9%). Therefore, it is important for the gynecologic surgeon to be cognizant of ways to minimize the occurrence of this potentially disastrous complication, and to be facile in the diagnosis and management of such an injury should it occur.

The goals of this chapter are to (a) outline the functional anatomy of the ureter and illustrate how this leads to the ureter being in harm's way during gynecologic surgery, (b) review the unique issues surrounding ureteral injury during the performance of specific groups of gynecologic surgical procedures, and (c) summarize the basic principles of injury avoidance and, should injury occur, recognition and management.

FUNCTIONAL ANATOMY OF THE URETER

When viewed in cross section, the ureter can be divided into distinct layers: the lumen with transitional epithelium; the mucosa—the muscular layer—which is made up of longitudinal, circular, and spiral smooth muscle fibers; and the adventitia, which contains an intercommunicating network of blood vessels (Fig. 42.1). The peritoneum lies over the ureter, making it a completely retroperitoneal structure.

In normal adults, the ureter is between 25 and 30 cm in length from the renal pelvis to the trigone of the bladder. By convention, the pelvic brim divides the ureter into the abdominal and pelvic segments; each of these components is approximately 12 to 15 cm in length.

The abdominal ureter runs along the ventral surface of the psoas muscle and posterior to the ovarian vessels to the level of the pelvic brim. The right ureter lies slightly lateral to the inferior vena cava and descends into the pelvis over the common iliac artery at approximately the site of the latter's bifurcation. In rare instances, the right ureter can be over the vena cava; therefore, if one is performing a paraaortic node sampling, the ureter must be identified before removing any nodes. The left ureter runs lateral to the aorta and posterior to the inferior mesenteric artery, ovarian vessels, and colon. The left ureter mirrors

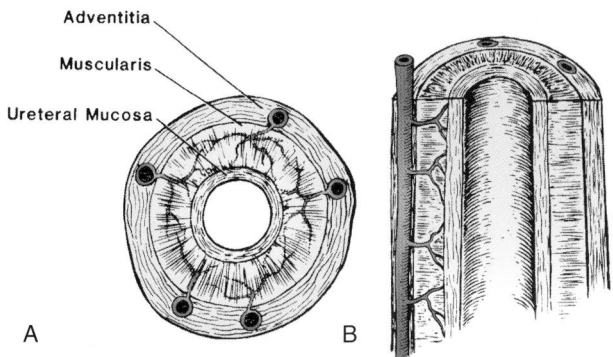

FIGURE 42.1 Cross-sectional (**A**) and sagittal (**B**) views of the longitudinal arteries and veins in the adventitia. These arteries and veins provide the important collateral circulation along the course of the ureter.

the right at the pelvic brim, entering the pelvis over the bifurcation of the left common iliac artery (Fig. 42.2). The left ureter is commonly obscured by the sigmoid colon at the pelvic brim.

There is little variance between the positions taken by the pelvic ureters. They descend into the posterior lateral pelvis

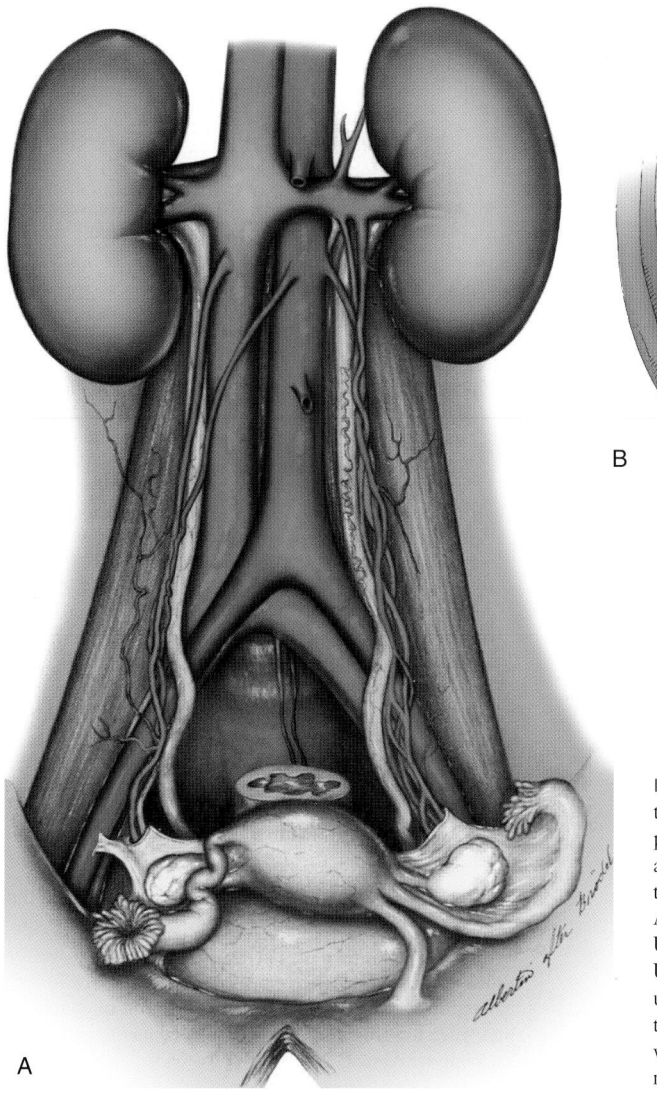

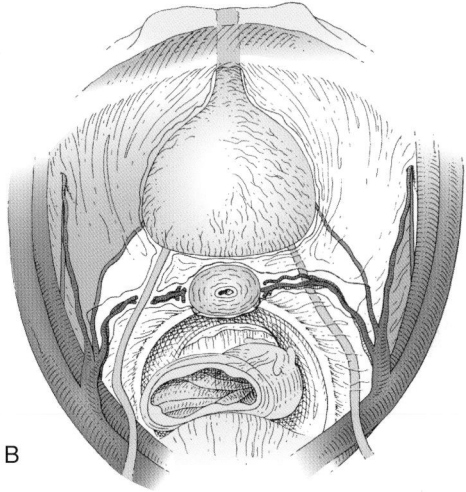

FIGURE 42.2 A: Abdominal and pelvic portions of the ureter showing relation to aorta, psoas muscle, vena cava, and common iliac artery and vein. (The original illustration is in the Max Brödel Archives in the Department of Art as Applied to Medicine, the Johns Hopkins University School of Medicine, Baltimore, MD. Used with permission.) **B:** Pelvic portion of the ureter showing its course along the sidewall of the pelvis and its relation to the common iliac vessels, hypogastric vessels, uterosacral ligaments, uterine vessels, and cervix.

VII

lateral to the sacrum and immediately ventral to internal iliac (hypogastric) artery. The ureters then course medial to the internal iliac artery and its anterior branches. The ureters subsequently pass beneath the uterine artery (often referred to as *water under the bridge*). The ureter is approximately 1.5 cm lateral to the cervix where it enters the paracervical tissues. The ureter passes through this paracervical tissue, often referred to as "the tunnel" of the cardinal ligament/anterior bladder pillar (also referred to as the web or the tunnel of Wertheim). Once through this tunnel, the ureter travels medially and anteriorly over the vaginal fornix to enter the trigone of the bladder.

When inflammatory or adhesive changes are not present, the ureters can usually be visualized through the peritoneum from the pelvic brim to this parametrial tissue. Once the ureters have entered this tunnel, they cannot be easily seen or palpated; if identification is required, they must be mobilized out of this tissue. Although the peristaltic activity that occurs in the normal ureter may be helpful in its identification, it is not uncommon that the ureter, following any degree of trauma, will have transient paralysis. Therefore, the skill of accurately identifying the ureter is based on understanding its anatomy, not its motion. The ureter is unique in that it has a "snap" feeling when passed between the fingers during laparotomy. This may be helpful in massively obese women with poor exposure. This "snap" will also permit one to follow the ureter to the tunnel without actually exposing it. This technique is not applicable to laparoscopic or robot-assisted procedures. In these cases, identification of the ureter is enhanced by camera magnification but may require surgical exposure for confirmation of its course. Having defined the general anatomy of the

ureter, one must appreciate that there is a significant degree of interpatient variability, even in a pelvis free of inflammatory, infectious, neoplastic, congenital, or postsurgical changes. Direct visualization of the ureter is the only sure way to know its location in any given patient.

Along its course, the vascular supply of the ureter is derived from a variety of sources. Above the pelvic brim, the blood supply of the ureter is derived from medial vessels; more distally, the blood supply originates laterally (Fig. 42.3). Thus, cephalad to the pelvic brim, dissection and mobilization of the ureter should be approached from its lateral aspect, and the converse is true distal to the pelvic brim. The ureter is perfused by a rich network, with anastomoses within the adventitial sheath. The ureter is therefore relatively resistant to devascularization. However, such injuries may occur and can be difficult to diagnose, as the sequelae may not be apparent until the postoperative period.

INJURY TO THE URETER IN GYNECOLOGIC SURGERY

Hysterectomy

The ureter is vulnerable to injury during hysterectomy when the uterine artery is divided (Fig. 42.4). This is because the ureter passes under the uterine artery, lateral to the uterosacral ligaments, as it travels medially and ventrally to terminate in the bladder. The risk of injury to the ureter can be minimized by careful dissection of the bladder off the cervix, by upward traction on the uterus during the placement of clamps, and by clamping the uterine artery immediately along the cervix (rather than more laterally). At the conclusion of hysterectomy, the surgeon should be particularly vigilant when addressing bleeding from pedicles, especially at the vaginal angles. Bleeding from the pedicles or vaginal angle should be controlled by a "superficial" 3-0 suture so as not to incorporate the ureter.

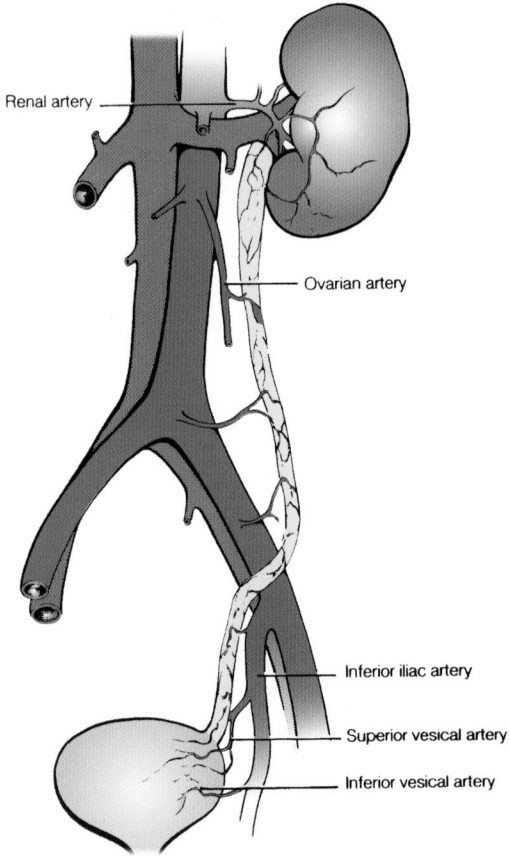

Renal artery

Ovarian artery

Inferior iliac artery

Superior vesical artery

Inferior vesical artery

FIGURE 42.3 Blood supply of the ureter.

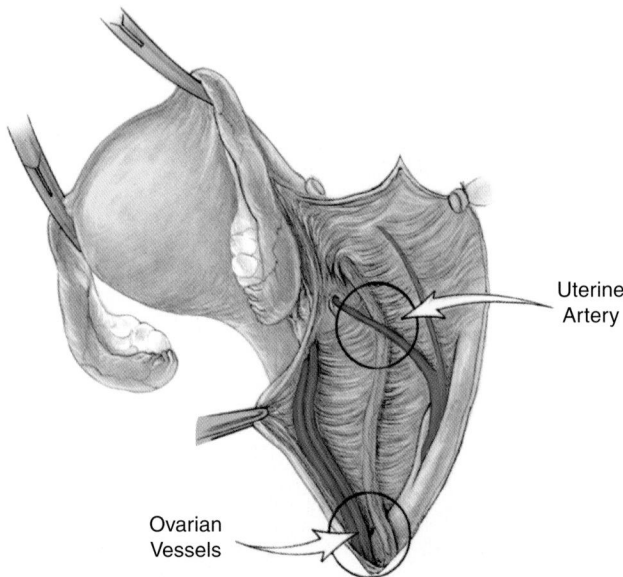

Uterine Artery

Ovarian Vessels

FIGURE 42.4 The ureter may be injured during hysterectomy. The uterine artery is divided adjacent to the cervix, where the ureter is in close proximity to uterine artery. The ureter may also be injured during ligation of the infundibulopelvic ligament, as it passes adjacent to the ovarian vessels.

Hysterectomy in the setting of cervical or broad ligament fibroids can be particularly challenging. The ureter can be anterior, lateral, or posterior to the fibroid. Clamping pedicles around the fibroid imposes significant risk for ureteral injury. In such cases, it may be prudent to perform a myomectomy by incision adjacent to the uterus or cervix. This can be done without risk of ureteral injury by staying within the myometrial capsule of the fibroid. Bleeding may occur, but once the fibroid is out, such bleeding is easily controlled by clamping adjacent to the uterus. In the rare case when this is impossible, the entire course of the ureter must be identified before clamping or cutting.

Ureteral injury during vaginal hysterectomy is remarkably uncommon. To some extent, this may be because vaginal hysterectomy is not typically performed for conditions most likely to distort ureteral anatomy, such as endometriosis or malignancy. In addition, the risk of ureteral injury is reduced during vaginal hysterectomy (compared to abdominal hysterectomy) because traction on the cervix pulls the uterus farther from the ureter. Tension on the cervix is therefore critical during the clamping of pedicles.

Ureteral injuries that occur during laparoscopic hysterectomy may be the result of thermal injury. When performing laparoscopic hysterectomy, it is imperative to know the location of the ureter. It can usually be visualized through the peritoneum; when not visible, it should be identified retroperitoneally and followed to the site of operative interest. Extreme caution should be used with cautery near or over the ureter, as thermal spread can cause occult injury that does not become apparent until 2 to 5 days after surgery.

Adnexal Surgery

Ureteral injury at the time of adnexectomy is worthy of specific comment. Especially in cases of an adnexal mass and distortion of the anatomy, the ureter is particularly vulnerable and it is in this setting that the ureter is commonly injured. These injuries can be avoided by using a retroperitoneal approach.

Every pelvic surgeon must be able to quickly and safely enter the retroperitoneum (which continues deep into the pelvis as the pararectal space). This surgical skill is necessary to (a) access the pelvic vessels for the purpose of establishing hemostasis and (b) use the retroperitoneum as an adhesion- and pathology-free "space" in which to operate. Access is obtained most commonly for the latter purpose. Once this retroperitoneal space has been developed, the ureter should be visible on the medial leaf of the broad ligament.

If an adnexal mass is adherent to the peritoneum overlying the ureter, the ureter can safely be dissected from the peritoneum. Distal to the pelvic brim, the dissection should be approached from the medial aspect of the ureter to minimize the risk of devascularizing the ureter. Once the ureter has been mobilized and is out of harm's way, resection of the mass and the inflamed, scarred, or fibrotic peritoneum can be performed safely (Fig. 42.5). There are rare instances when it is impossible to mobilize the ureter from the pathology. In this setting, the surgeon must decide whether to leave residual tissue on the ureter (risking subsequent ureteral obstruction) or to resect a segment of ureter and repair accordingly.

Retropubic Surgery

Injury to the distal ureter may occur with high elevation of Burch colposuspension sutures. The ureter may also be injured by excessive lateral mobilization of the bladder. Mobilization exposes the dorsal surface of the bladder in the vicinity of the trigone and may bring the ureter into the operative field.

There are specific steps that can be taken to avoid such injuries. Dissection into and through the space of Retzius should be done under direct visualization, remaining as close to the symphysis pubis as possible. The amount of dissection that occurs over the lateral paravaginal tissues should be kept to the minimal amount needed to guarantee accurate and appropriate placement of the sutures. Finally, the urethrovesical junction must not be elevated excessively as this can cause kinking not only of the urethra but also the ureters in certain patients.

Surgery for Pelvic Organ Prolapse

The ureter may be ligated or kinked with surgery to correct prolapse. The risk appears to be highest with uterosacral ligament suspensions of the vagina. Barber and colleagues

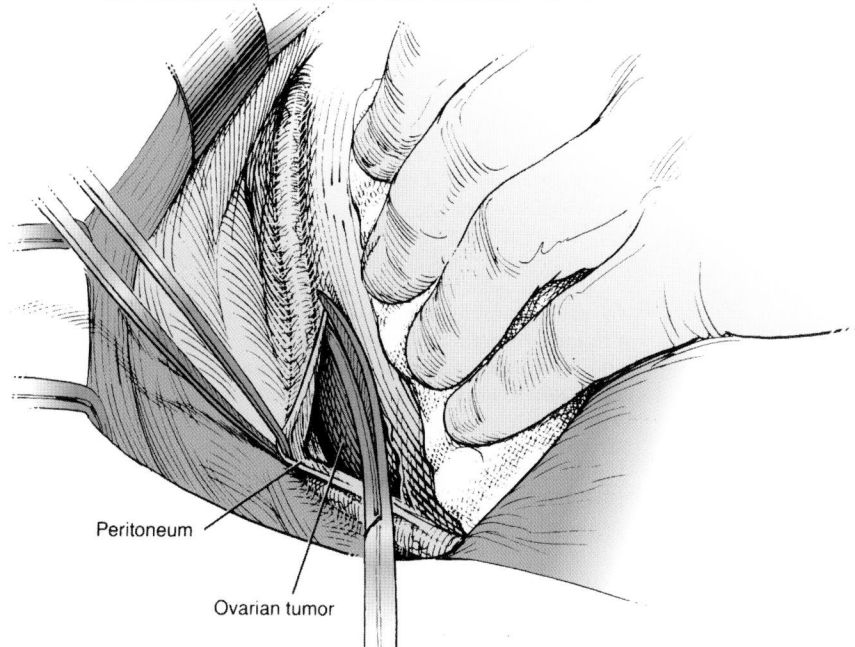

Peritoneum

Ovarian tumor

FIGURE 42.5 The ureter is dissected away from the peritoneum to permit resecting of ovarian mass/remnant.

VII

reported ureteral obstruction in 11% (5/46) of cases (treated with release of the suspension sutures or ureteral reimplantation). Karram and colleagues reported ureteral injury in 5/202 (2.4%), and Shull and colleagues reported ureteral injury in 3/302 (1%).

Anatomic studies by Buller and colleagues demonstrated that the distance from ureter to uterosacral ligament is 4.1 ± 0.6 cm at the sacral origin of the uterosacral ligament, decreasing to 0.9 ± 0.4 as the uterosacral ligament approaches the cervix. Placement of the suspension sutures at or slightly above the level of the ischial spine (in the intermediate portion of the uterosacral ligament) is therefore recommended to minimize the risk of injury. Ureteral injury has also been reported with sacrospinous suspension, midurethral sling, and anterior colporrhaphy. Thus, confirmation of ureteral patency via cystoscopy should be routinely performed at the conclusion of these procedures to verify ureteral integrity.

Radical Pelvic Surgery

Of all the groups of surgical procedures performed, those performed for the treatment of cancers affecting the female reproductive tract are the most likely to involve either intentional ureteral surgery or have the highest risk of an associated ureteral injury. It is important to differentiate between intentional ureteral disruption and unintended or inadvertent injury. The MD Anderson type IV radical hysterectomy, a total or anterior pelvic exenteration, and resection of a fixed pelvic sidewall mass involving the ureter may include ureteral resection and reconstruction by design. As a result of the nature of gynecologic malignancies and the procedures performed to treat those diseases, intentional and sometimes unintentional ureteral injuries occur. Additionally, the need to explore a radiated field, or one in which multiple operations have been performed, compounds cofactors that put the ureter at risk. It is evident that the surgeon must not only be expert in pelvic anatomy but also have the judgment to establish how and when to address a problem while minimizing the probability of injury.

How common are ureteral injuries in association with radical pelvic surgery? Recent data from the National Hospital Discharge Survey suggest that ureteral injury during radical hysterectomy occurs in 7.7 per 1,000 cases. Historically, the average rate of ureteral injury at the time of radical hysterectomy has approximated 1%, with a concomitant similar rate of bladder injury. Interestingly, these rates have been consistent over time and among different surgical groups. In contradistinction to these relatively low rates of ureteral injury, when radical resection is performed following radiation therapy there is an associated risk of ureteral dysfunction of approximately 30%. Ureteral injury associated with lymph node dissection or when performing "radical" oophorectomy is remarkably uncommon when those injuries occurring near the entrance to and through the tunnel of Wertheim are excluded from the data.

DIAGNOSING URETERAL INJURY

Diagnosis of Ureteral Injury during Surgery

As noted, pelvic surgery risks injury to the ureter at a number of sites along its course (Table 42.1). A clear understanding of ureteral anatomy and its potential variability is critical to avoiding injury. The surgeon should make a habit of confirming ureteral integrity during and at the conclusion of any pelvic procedure, regardless of whether the surgery is done by the vaginal, open, laparoscopic, or robot-assisted approach. This will require direct visualization of the ureter (or palpation, in the setting of laparotomy). For both open and laparoscopic procedures,

TABLE 42.1 Common Sites of Ureteral Injuries

Cardinal ligament where the ureter crosses under the uterine artery
Tunnel of Wertheim
Intramural portion of the ureter
Dorsal to the infundibulopelvic ligament near or at the pelvic brim
Lateral pelvic sidewall above the uterosacral ligament

opening of the parietal peritoneum may at times be necessary to allow for accurate inspection or to allow for mobilization and separation from the site of operative interest. This is especially important in the setting of inflammatory conditions such as endometriosis, malignancy, or adhesions from prior surgery.

If ureteral injury is suspected, visualizing peristalsis is inadequate to exclude occlusion or extravasation. Ureteral integrity can be confirmed during intra-abdominal surgery by intravenous administration of a coloring agent and observation for intrapelvic extravasation. In vaginal surgery, direct visualization of the at-risk ureteral segments is seldom possible. For this reason, we advocate intraoperative cystoscopy for confirmation of urine efflux from the ureteral orifices at the conclusion of transvaginal procedures accessing the anterior or apical vagina. This may be facilitated by an intravenous coloring agent. Following abdominal procedures, cystoscopy may also be performed to confirm ureteral patency. The use of a flexible cystoscope allows this procedure to be done with the patient in supine position if necessary.

To the extent possible, acute ureteral injuries are best recognized and managed intraoperatively. Many of these occurrences may rely on collaborative assistance from colleagues in urology or urogynecology. This would include decisions regarding the nature of the repair and the decision to proceed with intracorporeal repair versus conversion to laparotomy in the setting of laparoscopic and robot-assisted procedures. Successful intraoperative repair of ureteral injuries minimizes the risk of sequelae, including stricture, fistulae, loss of renal function, and need for subsequent reoperation.

With the common and generous use of cautery devices in pelvic surgery, ureteral injury may not be apparent until the postoperative period. Cautery devices must be used with care, as diffusion of thermal energy can cause occult ureteral injury resulting in delayed stricture or urine leak presenting days to weeks postoperatively. A high index of suspicion must be carried through the postoperative period to insure early diagnosis and management if necessary.

It is unclear whether preoperative ureteral stenting helps to prevent ureteral injury. The data generally suggest that presence of a ureteral stent facilitates identification of injury should it occur, rather than prevention of such injuries. Complications related to stent placement (including ureteral perforation, stent malposition, extravasation, hematuria, and stricture) are rare. However, preoperative stent placement is typically considered in complex cases. In this setting, stent placement can be uniquely challenging, with an increase in the probability of complications.

Postoperative Diagnosis of Ureteral Injury

The sequelae of unrecognized ureteral injuries commonly present in the immediate postoperative period, but the related complications may develop several weeks following surgery. This is especially true for thermal injuries resulting in intraperitoneal or retroperitoneal urine leak (e.g., urinoma) or ureteral stricture. Common manifestations of urinoma include fever, unexplained leukocytosis, peritonitis, or vaginal fluid leakage. Hematuria may also be seen. Rarely, urinoma may present as a palpable pelvic or abdominal mass. It should be noted that changes in serum creatinine are not a reliable indicator of ureteral injury. Postoperative elevations in serum creatinine should prompt further investigation, but normal values do not adequately exclude ureteral injury.

Accurate diagnosis of a delayed ureteral injury relies primarily on appropriate imaging studies, such as computed tomography with administration of intravenous contrast and delayed image acquisition. This study can delineate ureteral obstruction as well as urine extravasation. In cases presenting with unilateral flank pain postoperatively, a renal ultrasound study may be obtained initially to assess for obstruction (hydroureteronephrosis) as well as urinoma. This study may identify obstruction and urinoma but may fail to detect a urine leak.

Retrograde ureteropyelography is also useful in the diagnosis and initial therapy of a ureteral injury. Contrast injection and opacification of the ureter can define the site and severity of leakage or obstruction and facilitates possible ureteral stenting. This can allow for control and resorption of a urinoma and in many cases may result in spontaneous healing of the ureter. If stenting is not possible, a nephrostomy tube can be placed to facilitate urine drainage and prevent renal injury. If a large urinoma is present, a percutaneous drain can be placed. If surgical intervention is necessary to repair a ureteral injury, this is best done within the first 3 to 5 days postoperatively. Beyond this window, reconstruction is optimal after 6 to 8 weeks to allow resolution of postsurgical inflammation.

In cases presenting with vaginal drainage, it is important to differentiate ureteral injury from bladder injury. Recognition that it is possible for these injuries to occur simultaneously is also important. The bladder can be filled through a catheter with a dilute solution of methylene blue and saline, with a tampon placed in the vagina. Staining of the tampon indicates a vesicovaginal fistula. If this initial test is negative, oral phenazopyridine or an intravenous colorant (methylene blue) can be administered and the test repeated. Staining of the tampon indicates a ureteral vaginal fistula. It is also possible to collect the fluid and analyze its creatinine content. If the value is any greater than the serum level, the fluid contains urine. Urine typically has a creatinine content greater than 10 mg/dL. Imaging studies would follow in order to localize the site of injury.

TECHNIQUES FOR URETERAL REPAIR

Several common elements associated with ureteral injury are listed in Table 42.2. Successful management of surgical ureteral injury requires an understanding of ureteral anatomy as well as the mechanism of injury. The ureter can be divided anatomically into thirds, with the upper segment defined by the ureteropelvic junction and proximal 5 cm. High in the retroperitoneum, this segment is seldom injured during pelvic surgery. The midureter defines the segment from below the ureteropelvic junction to the pelvic brim. The lower ureter includes the segment from the pelvic brim to the ureteral orifice. Selection of repair strategy is based on the location of ureteral injury.

General principles of ureteral repair include spatulation ≥1 cm to create a wide-caliber lumen, judicious ureteral mobilization to allow for tension-free anastomosis, and use of fine absorbable suture (4-0, 5-0) to minimize inflammatory

TABLE 42.2 Ureteral Injury Associated with Gynecologic Surgery

Most common site: Pelvic brim near the infundibulopelvic ligament
Most common procedure: Simple abdominal hysterectomy
Most common type of injury: Obstruction
Most common "activity" leading to injury: Attempts to obtain hemostasis
Most common time of diagnosis: None: 50–50 split between intraoperative and postoperative

response and subsequent stricture. The ureter is typically stented at the time of reconstruction and a suction drain placed near to but not in contact with the repair. A stent is left in place for at least 14 days. There is little evidence to suggest a longer period of stenting is either necessary or helpful. Strategies for ureteral repair are based on the location of injury and its mechanism (Table 42.3).

Acute Ureteral Injury

The ureter may be injured by transection, ligation, or thermal conduction. In cases in which the ureter is partially transected, it can be closed loosely with fine (5-0) absorbable suture and stented. This applies along the entire length. In such cases, placement of the stent can be accomplished over a flexible guidewire using intraoperative cystoscopy (flexible cystoscopy is useful if the patient is supine) or directly through a small anterior cystotomy. The bladder is typically drained for 7 to 10 days following repair.

Ureteroureterostomy

In cases of complete ureteral transection, the level of injury should guide the method of repair. In the midureter, ureteroureterostomy is often the procedure of choice. The proximal and distal ends of the ureter are carefully mobilized with preservation of the adventitia and feeding blood vessels. The exposed ureteral ends should be viable, with a bleeding edge. If thermal injury is suspected, the involved edges should be debrided or resected

TABLE 42.3 General Guidelines for Management of Ureteral Injuries Identified at Time of Surgery

Ureteral ligation: Suture release, assessment of viability, stent placement
Partial transection: Primary repair over ureteral stent
Total transection • Uncomplicated upper and middle thirds: Ureteroureterostomy over ureteral stent • Complicated upper and middle thirds: Ureteroileal interposition • Lower third: Ureteroneocystostomy with psoas hitch over ureteral stent
Thermal injury: Resection with management as per a transection

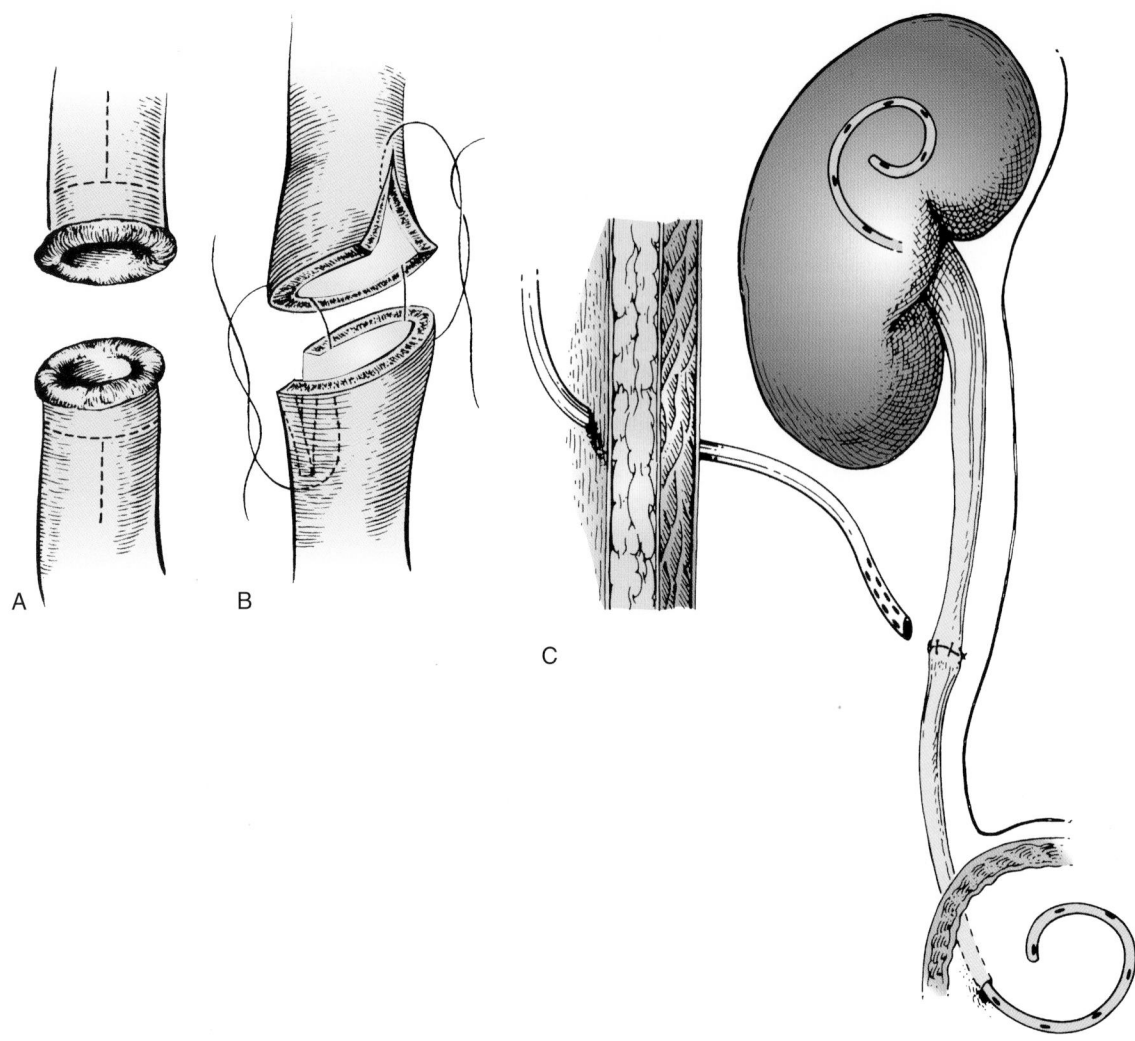

FIGURE 42.6 Ureteral reanastomosis. **A:** The ends of the ureters are trimmed obliquely and spatulated. **B:** Fine delayed absorbable sutures are used to approximate the ends of the ureter. **C:** The anastomosis is done over a double-J or pigtail stent. A suction catheter is placed retroperitoneally at the site of anastomosis.

to healthy tissue. The ends of the ureter are spatulated for at least 1 cm to allow for a wide-caliber tension-free anastomosis (Fig. 42.6). Fine absorbable suture should be used to minimize risk of stricture. The ureter is stented. A stent of 24 to 26 cm in length is usually sufficient. Stent placement is facilitated by advancing a guidewire into the proximal ureter and renal collecting system and advancing the stent over the wire. The distal end of the stent can be uncoiled, threaded into the ureter with forceps, and advanced into the bladder. Alternatively, the bladder can be opened and a guidewire passed into the ureteral orifice on the side of the injury. The anastomosis may be supported by an omental wrap if available. If transection has occurred in the lower ureter, simple ureteroneocystostomy may be elected.

If the ureter has been ligated, release of the constricting suture or clip is first undertaken and a judgment made as to the integrity of the injury site. If the ureter is not deformed, it can be treated conservatively. It may be helpful to wrap the injured area with omentum to facilitate healing. This type of injury can be associated with a delayed ureteral stricture, and one should have a low threshold to place a stent for 10 to 14 days. In the mid ureter, if the site remains blanched or has

evidence of crush injury, it should be resected and repaired with ureteroureterostomy over a stent. If injury occurs in the distal ureter, direct ureteroneocystostomy or psoas hitch repair is indicated.

An obvious acute thermal injury poses the greatest challenge, in that the extent of damage can be difficult to assess. We recommend wide resection of the damaged ureter and consideration of ureteroureterostomy only if tension-free anastomosis is possible. Otherwise, thermal injury in the mid ureter should be repaired immediately with neocystostomy and psoas hitch.

Acute injury to the mid or upper ureter may occasionally require complex repair due to a significant gap between the proximal ureter and the bladder. These techniques are reviewed in the sections that follow and may include Boari flap reconstruction, ileal interposition, or possibly renal autotransplantation. Another alternative is transureteroureterostomy, with mobilization of the injured ureter to the contralateral side for end-to-side ureteral anastomosis (Fig. 42.7). While this technique can be effective, critics highlight the risk of subsequent stricture at the site of repair, putting both kidneys at risk for obstruction and functional compromise. Transureteroureterostomy is contraindicated in patients with a history of kidney

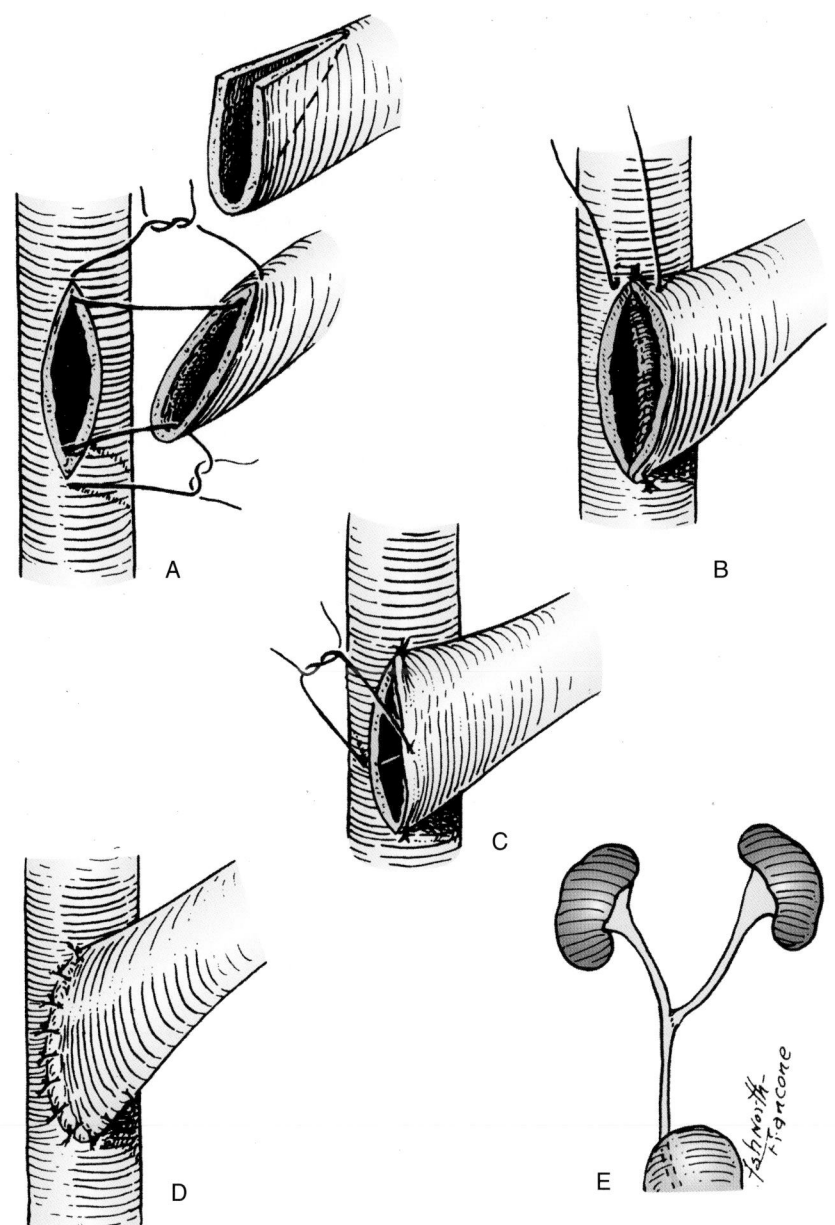

A

B

C

D

E

FIGURE 42.7 Transureteroureterostomy. The injured ureter is mobilized to the contralateral side for end-to-side ureteral anastomosis (**A–E**). The anastomosis is accomplished with interrupted sutures of fine absorbable suture.

VII

stone formation. In cases involving long ureteral defects, it is advisable to ligate the ureter above the site of injury and arrange for postoperative nephrostomy tube placement. This allows for staged repair after adequate patient counseling and additional evaluation.

STEPS IN THE PROCEDURE

Ureteroureterostomy

- The site of ureteral injury is identified. If this is an acute injury in the midportion (below the ureteropelvic junction and above the pelvic brim), ureteroureterostomy is a suitable option.

- The proximal and distal aspects of the ureter are dissected from the surrounding attachments sharply with care taken to preserve the periureteral sheath and periureteral blood supply.

- The exposed ureteral lumen is debrided until a healthy edge is obtained. This is essential in the setting of either a crush injury (from clip, clamp, or suture) or thermal insult, and may require tissue resection.

- The proximal and distal ends of the ureter are spatulated using fine scissors for 1 cm or more to allow for an overlapping, tension-free anastomosis.

- Ureteroureterostomy is complete using fine (4-0, 5-0) absorbable suture using either a running or interrupted technique.

- Prior to completing the anastomosis, a double-J ureteral stent is placed. A stent of 24 to 26 cm in length is usually sufficient. This is facilitated by advancing a guide wire into the proximal ureter and renal collecting system and advancing the stent over the wire. The distal end of the stent can be uncoiled, threaded into the ureter with forceps, and advanced into the bladder. Alternatively, the bladder can be opened and a guidewire passed into the ureteral orifice on the side of the injury. After the stent is advanced over the wire, the wire is removed and the bladder is subsequently closed with absorbable suture (2-0, 3-0) in one or two layers.

- After the ureteroureterostomy is complete, a portion of the omentum, if available, can be dissected free and wrapped around the ureter to minimize leak and adhesion.

- A suction drain is left in the pelvis for 2 to 3 days following repair. The bladder is drained postoperatively for 7 to 10 days and the stent left in place for at least 14 days.

Ureteroneocystostomy

Injuries to the distal ureter can be corrected with direct anastomosis to the bladder. The simplest technique is an extravesical, refluxing reimplant (Fig. 42.8). The distal ureter is freshened and spatulated for 1 cm. The bladder is distended with saline through a Foley catheter and the catheter clamped. This allows for selection of a suitable reimplant site on the posterolateral aspect of the bladder and confirmation of adequate ureteral length for tension-free anastomosis. While it may seem suitable, one should avoid reimplantation to the dome of the bladder as this mobile section may allow the ureter to become kinked with filling leading to obstruction. At the reimplant site, the peritoneum and detrusor muscle are incised with cautery for 1 to 2 cm. The detrusor muscle can be dissected free from the bladder epithelium using fine scissors. This is aided by the bladder distension, and the epithelium becomes readily visible. Fine absorbable suture can be used to complete half of the anastomosis, incorporating the epithelium, ureter, and detrusor muscle. The epithelium is then incised, allowing the bladder to decompress. A ureteral stent is placed and the anastomosis completed using the stent as a guide. The bladder can be refilled to insure a watertight connection, and the serosa and peritoneum closed loosely over the ureter with fine absorbable suture to provide additional security (Fig. 42.8).

It is also possible to perform ureteroneocystostomy using an intravesical technique (Fig. 42.9). A midline cystotomy is made and a suitable site for reimplant identified. A hiatus is made in the bladder wall and the ureter transferred to the interior. The ureter can be matured to the full thickness of the bladder using fine absorbable suture (Fig. 42.9).

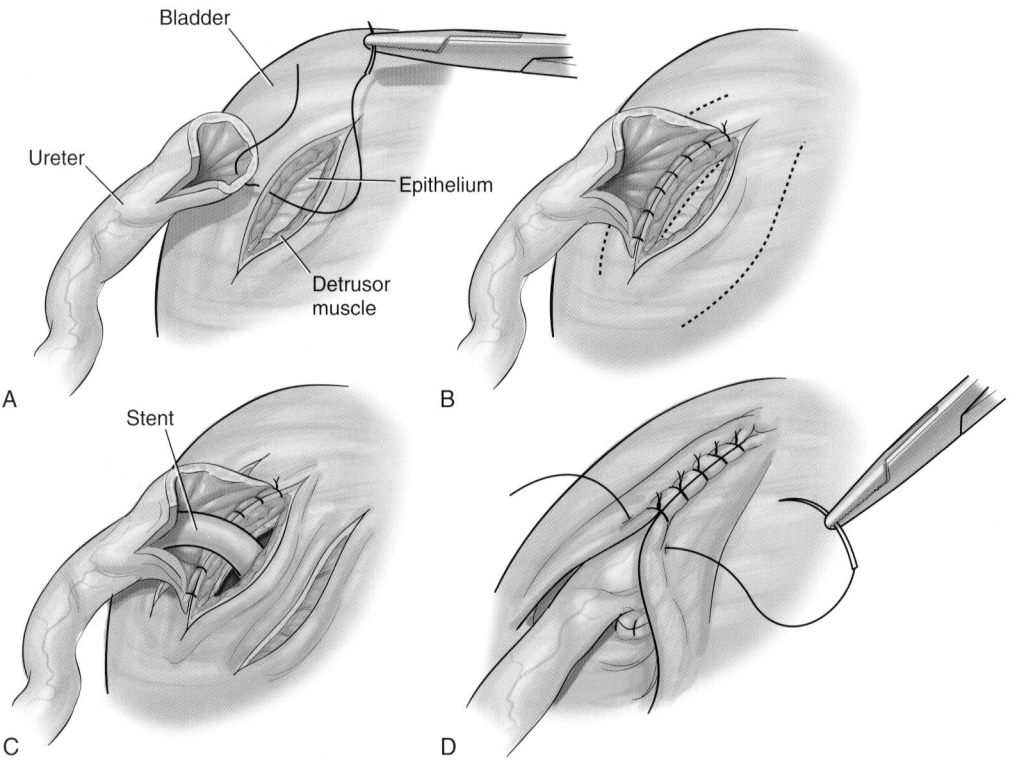

FIGURE 42.8 Extravesical technique for ureteroneocystostomy. **A:** The distal ureter is freshened and spatulated for 1 cm. The detrusor muscle is incised for 1 to 2 cm on the posterolateral aspect of the bladder to expose the epithelium. **B:** The lateral aspect of the anastomosis is completed before incising the urothelium. **C:** The epithelium is incised and a stent introduced across the anastomosis. **D:** The ureteral anastomosis is completed, and the serosa is closed over the ureter.

Ureteroneocystostomy with Psoas Hitch

- The peritoneum over the ipsilateral psoas muscle is opened sharply at the level of the pelvic brim.

- Three 2-0 nonabsorbable sutures are placed in the psoas muscle, parallel to the muscle fibers (to avoid injury to the underlying genitofemoral nerve), and set aside.

- The bladder is distended with saline through the Foley catheter to near full capacity.

- An incision is made in the bladder diagonally across the anterior dome. Full-thickness stay sutures are placed at the midpoint of this incision to provide traction.

- The nonabsorbable sutures are placed through the detrusor muscle. Care should be taken not to perforate the bladder epithelium with the anchoring sutures to avoid bladder stone formation. These are tied in sequence to anchor the bladder.

- Bladder closure is undertaken perpendicular to the original incision. If desired, the bladder closure can incorporate the site of ureteral reimplantation without the need for separate neocystostomy.

- Prior to implantation, the proximal ureter is mobilized sharply and spatulated for at least 1 cm. Ureteral vesical anastomosis is completed using fine absorbable suture in a tension-free fashion. The remainder of the bladder wall is closed using 2-0 or 3-0 absorbable suture in one or two layers.

- The perivesical fat and peritoneum can be closed over the ureterovesical suture line to provide additional coverage.

- Prior to completion of the bladder closure, a double-J ureteral stent 24 to 26 cm in length is passed into the ureter over a guide wire.

- Postoperatively, the pelvic is drained for 2 to 3 days, the bladder is drained for 7 to 10 days, and the stent kept in place for at least 14 days.

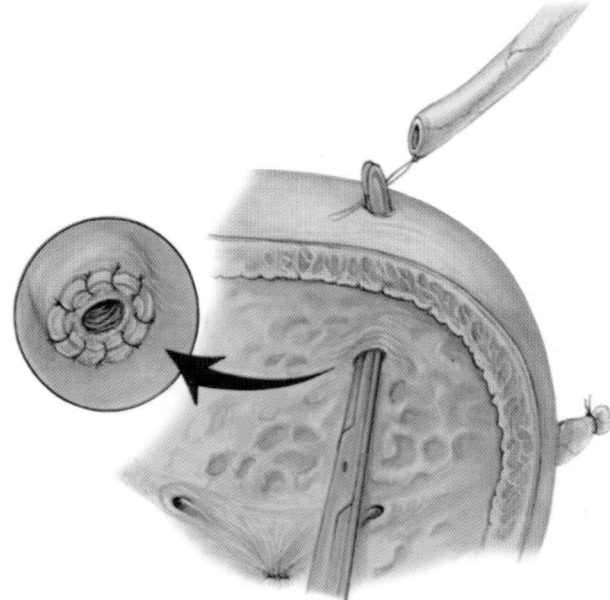

FIGURE 42.9 Intravesical technique for ureteroneocystostomy. After cystotomy, an incision is made in the urothelium and a tunnel created in the bladder wall. The distal ureter is then pulled through this hiatus and fixed to the bladder wall using fine absorbable suture.

nonabsorbable sutures are fixed to the posterior aspect of the detrusor for anchorage to the psoas muscle, thereby shortening the gap to the distal ureter. The ureteroneocystostomy can be incorporated into the bladder closure, which is undertaken perpendicular to the original incision. Care should be taken not to perforate the bladder epithelium with the anchoring sutures so as to avoid bladder stone formation.

Boari Flap

This technique can be used to repair injury to the proximal aspect of the mid ureter. It is best used in a delayed fashion after additional workup and patient counseling. This should include a cystogram and possible cystometrogram to insure adequate bladder capacity and compliance. Functional and anatomic bladder capacity can be reduced following Boari flap reconstruction, and patients should be counseled regarding these outcomes.

The bladder is distended and the gap between ureter and bladder measured. A suitable wide-based flap (4 to 5 cm) originating from the cephalad margin of the bladder is outlined along a diagonal toward the contralateral side. The distal aspect of the flap should not be less than 2 to 3 cm in width. The flap is raised and extended to the spatulated ureter and sewn into a tube over a 16- to 18-French catheter using absorbable suture (3-0, 4-0). The spatulated ureter can then be fixed end to end to the bladder tube with fine absorbable suture. The repair is stented prior to completion and a pelvic drain placed. The bladder should be drained with a Foley catheter for 7 to 10 days. The stent can be removed after 2 weeks.

Ureteroileal Interposition

Injuries to the upper mid or proximal ureter often require bridging a gap longer than the bladder can extend with psoas hitch or Boari flap construction. In these cases, a segment of ileum can be interposed between the ureter and bladder

Psoas Hitch

Reimplantation of the ureter high in the pelvis can often be accomplished by incorporation of a psoas hitch to the bladder (**Fig. 42.10**). This procedure secures the bladder to the ipsilateral psoas muscle allowing for tension-free ureteroneocystostomy. The psoas muscle is exposed by opening the posterior peritoneum and three 2-0 nonabsorbable sutures are placed in the psoas muscle belly. We prefer to place these parallel to the muscle fibers to avoid injury to the underlying genitofemoral nerve. The white band of the psoas minor tendon can often serve as a good anchorage. These sutures are set aside and the bladder distended to confirm adequate capacity and mobility. Peritoneal attachments to the bladder can be extensively divided to improve necessary mobility. The contralateral vascular pedicle can also be divided, but this is not routine. The bladder is then incised diagonally along the anterior dome to allow the posterolateral aspect to reach to the psoas muscle (**Fig. 42.10**). Full-thickness stay sutures are placed at the midpoint of this incision to provide traction. The previously placed

VII

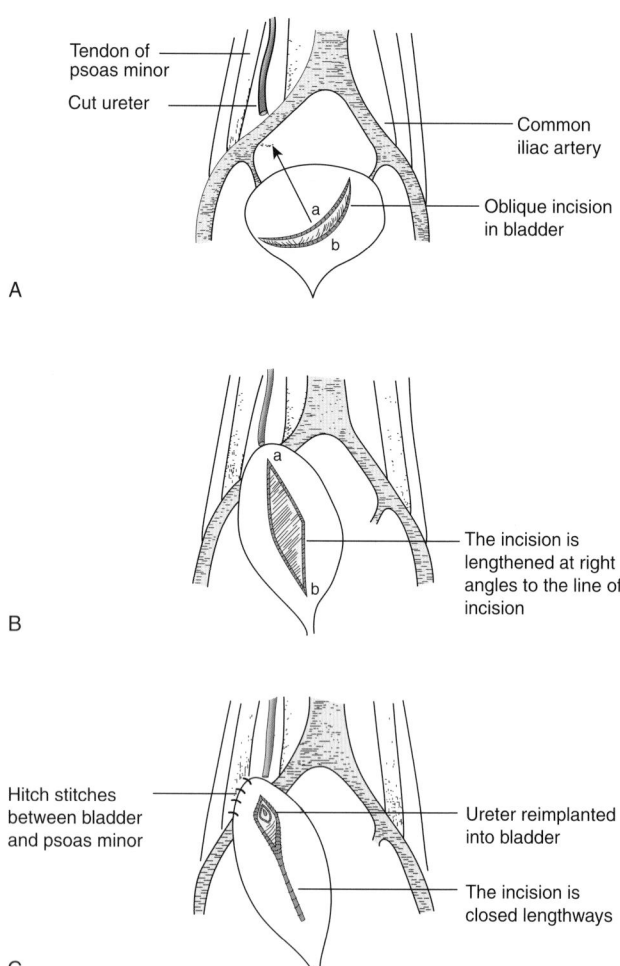

FIGURE 42.10 A: An incision is made in the bladder obliquely. **B:** This allows the superior aspect of the bladder (*a*) to elongate towards the ureter perpendicular to the original cystotomy. **C:** The bladder is anchored to the psoas muscle with permanent suture. Neocystostomy is completed and the bladder closed with absorbable suture. (Reproduced with permission from Hashim H, Reynard J, Cowan NC. Urological Emergencies in Clinical Practice. London: Springer-Verlag London LTD, 2005: 78.)

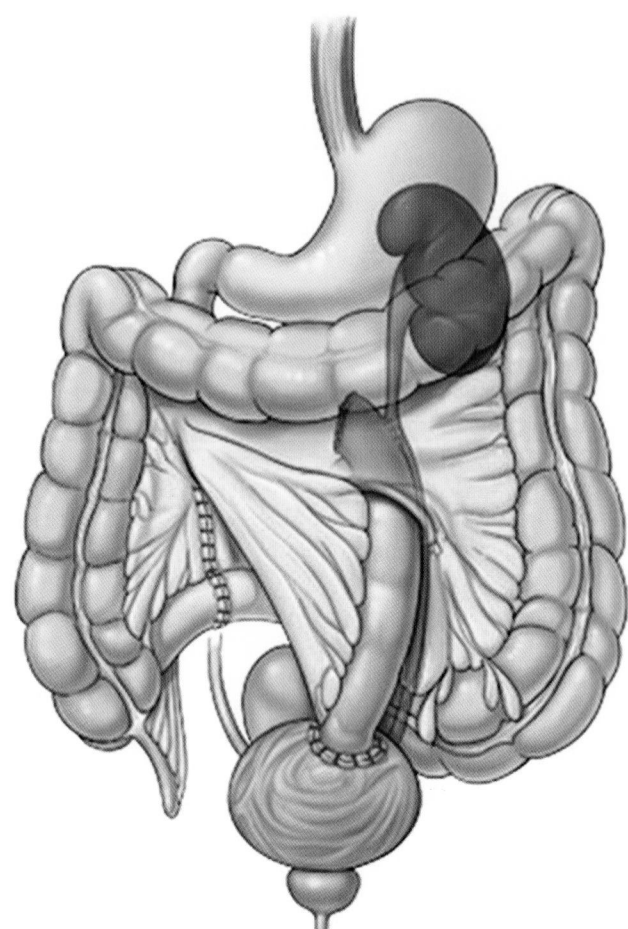

FIGURE 42.11 Ileal interposition. (Reprinted from Stein RJ, Turna B, Patel NS, et al. Laparoscopic assisted ileal ureter: technique, outcomes and comparison to the open procedure. *J Urol* 2009;182:1032, with permission. Copyright © 2009, Elsevier.)

to reestablish continuity (**Fig. 42.11**). This procedure is best suited for delayed repair following patient counseling regarding the need for bowel anastomosis, extended postoperative recovery, effects on ipsilateral renal function, and the persistence of mucous in the urine.

Following mobilization and spatulation of the distal ureter, the gap from ureter to bladder is measured. A psoas hitch can be incorporated in this procedure to shorten the segment of bowel needed for repair. Use of the shortest ileal segment possible minimizes metabolic derangement from urine resorption as well as mucous discharge with voiding. A segment of ileum adequate to bridge the ureteral defect is identified. This segment should be 12 to 15 cm proximal to the ileocecal valve in order to avoid malabsorption. The mesentery to the ileal segment is preserved and bowel continuity reestablished. It is recommended to place the ileal–ileal anastomosis cephalad to the segment for ureteral replacement. The ureter is brought through the posterior peritoneum and anastomosis

to the ileum completed with fine absorbable suture over a stent extending to the bladder. The ileum is typically placed in a properistaltic orientation to facilitate urine drainage and minimize reflux. An end-to-side ileal–vesical anastomosis is completed over the ureteral stent. The pelvis is drained postoperatively. A Foley catheter is kept in place for 7 to 10 days and a cystogram obtained prior to removal to insure absence of extravasation. The ureteral stent can be removed after 2 weeks.

SUMMARY

Sound knowledge of ureteral anatomy is critical to the avoidance of injury. In the event that the ureter is damaged during gynecologic surgery, intraoperative diagnosis allows for immediate repair in most cases. For this reason, intraoperative confirmation of ureteral integrity should be routine, whether the surgical approach is transvaginal or transabdominal through the open, laparoscopic, or robot-assisted approach. The ureter may be assessed visually, by palpation, or cystoscopically. Identification of the mechanism of injury and its location guides immediate or delayed repair. With proper recognition and therapy, ureteral function can be restored and renal function maintained.

BEST SURGICAL PRACTICES

- Knowledge of ureteral anatomy is critical for avoidance of injury.
- Injury most commonly occurs at the following sites: within the cardinal ligament as it crosses below the uterine arteries, the tunnel of Wertheim, near the infundibulopelvic ligament at or above the pelvic brim, and lateral to the uterosacral ligament in the pelvic sidewall.
- Hysterectomy is the procedure most commonly associated with ureteral injury.
- Intraoperative assessment of ureteral integrity should be a routine part of gynecologic surgery. This may be done by palpation, visually, or cystoscopically.
- Successful ureteral repair relies on careful mobilization, wide spatulation, use of fine absorbable suture (4-0, 5-0), and temporary stenting.
- Transection of the ureter at or below the pelvic brim can often be repaired with simple ureteroneocystostomy.
- Psoas hitch ureteroneocystostomy and Boari flap construction may facilitate ureteral reimplantation.
- Postoperative signs and symptoms of ureteral injury may include unilateral flank pain, fever, prolonged ileus, and abdominal or pelvic fluid collection (urinoma).

BIBLIOGRAPHY

Barber MD, Visco AG, Weidner AC, et al. Bilateral uterosacral ligament vaginal vault suspension with site-specific endopelvic fascia defect repair for treatment of pelvic organ prolapse. *Am J Obstet Gynecol* 2000;183:1402.

Brandes S, Coburn M, Armenakas NA, et al. Diagnosis and management of ureteric injury: an evidence-based analysis. *BJU Int* 2004;94:277.

Boxer RJ, Fritzsche P, Skinner DG, et al. Replacement of the ureter by small intestine: clinical application and results of the ileal ureter in 89 patients. *J Urol* 1979;121:728.

Buller JL, Thompson JR, Cundiff GW, et al. Uterosacral ligament: description of anatomic relationships to optimize surgical safety. *Obstet Gynecol* 2001;97:873.

Cosson M, Lambaudie E, Boukerrou M, et al. Vaginal, laparoscopic, or abdominal hysterectomies for benign disorders: immediate and early postoperative complications. *Eur J Obstet Gynecol Reprod Biol* 2001;98:231.

Daly JW, Higgens KA. Injury to the ureter during gynecologic surgical procedures. *Surg Gynecol Obstet* 1988;167:19.

Drake MJ, Noble JG. Ureteric trauma in gynecologic surgery. *Int Urogynecol J Pelvic Floor Dysfunct* 1998;9:108.

Eisenberg ML, Lee KL, Zumrutbas AE, et al. Long-term outcomes and late complications of laparoscopic nephrectomy with renal autotransplantation. *J Urol* 2008;179:240.

Ehrlich RM, Skinner DG. Complications of transureteroureterostomy. *J Urol* 1975;113:467.

Elkins TE. Ureteral injury at time of abdominal hysterectomy for benign disease. *Oper Tech Gynecol Surg* 1998;3:108.

Flynn JT, Tiptaft RC, Woodhouse CR, et al. The early and aggressive repair of iatrogenic ureteric injuries. *Br J Urol* 1979;51:454.

Frankman EA, Wang L, Bunker CH, et al. Lower urinary tract injury in women in the United States, 1979–2006. *Am J Obstet Gynecol* 2010;202:495.e1.

Gomel V, James C. Intraoperative management of ureteral injury during operative laparoscopy. *Fertil Steril* 1997;55:416.

Goodno JA Jr, Powers TW, Harris VD. Ureteral injury in gynecologic surgery: a ten-year review in a community hospital. *Am J Obstet Gynecol* 1995;172:1817.

Gustilo-Ashby AM, Jelovsek JE, Barber MD, et al. The incidence of ureteral obstruction and the value of intraoperative cystoscopy during vaginal surgery for pelvic organ prolapse. *Am J Obstet Gynecol* 2006;194:1478.

Harris RL, Cundiff GW, Theofratous JP, et al. The value of intraoperative cystoscopy in urogynecologic and reconstructive surgery. *Am J Obstet Gynecol* 1997;177:1367.

Ibeanu OA, Chesson RR, Echols KT, et al. Urinary tract injury during hysterectomy based on universal cystoscopy. *Obstet Gynecol* 2009;113:6.

Karram M, Goldwasser S, Kleeman S, et al. High uterosacral vaginal vault suspension with fascial reconstruction for vaginal repair of enterocele and vaginal vault prolapse. *Am J Obstet Gynecol* 2001;185:1339.

Leonard F, Fotso A, Borghese B, et al. Ureteral complications from laparoscopic hysterectomy indicated for benign uterine pathologies: a 13-year experience in a continuous series of 1,300 patients. *Hum Reprod* 2007;22:2006.

Matlaga BR, Shah OD, Hart LJ, et al. Ileal ureter substitution: a contemporary series. *Urology* 2003;62:998.

Mauck RJ, Hudak SJ, Terlecki RP, et al. Central role of Boari bladder flap and downward nephropexy in upper ureteral reconstruction. *J Urol* 2011;186:1345.

Middleton RG. Routine use of the psoas hitch in ureteral reimplantation. *J Urol* 1980;123:352.

Monk BJ, Solkh S, Johnson MT, et al. Radical hysterectomy after pelvic irradiation in patients with high risk cervical cancer or uterine sarcoma: morbidity and outcome. *Eur J Gynaecol Oncol* 1993;14:506.

Musch M, Hohenhorst L, Pailliart A, et al. Robot-assisted reconstructive surgery of the distal ureter: single institution experience in 16 patients. *BJU Int* 2013;111:773.

Nezhat C, Nezhat F. Laparoscopic repair of ureter resected during operative laparoscopy. *Obstet Gynecol* 1992;80:543.

Nezhat C, Nezhat FR, Nezhat F. Laparoscopic ureteroneocystostomy vesicopsoas hitch for infiltrative ureteral endometriosis. *Fertil Steril* 1999;71:376.

Ogan K, Abbott JT, Wilmot C, et al. Laparoscopic ureteral reimplant for distal ureteral strictures. *JSLS* 2008;12:13.

Oh BR, Kwon DD, Park KS, et al. Late presentation of ureteral injury after laparoscopic surgery. *Obstet Gynecol* 2000;95:337.

Ozdemir E, Ozturk U, Celen S, et al. Urinary complications of gynecologic surgery: iatrogenic urinary tract system injuries in obstetrics and gynecology operations. *Clin Exp Obstet Gynecol* 2011;38:217.

Papanikolaou A, Tsolakidis D, Theodoulidis V, et al. Surgery for ureteral repair after gynaecological procedures: a single tertiary centre experience. *Arch Gynecol Obstet* 2013;287:947.

Rafique M, Arif MH. Management of iatrogenic ureteric injuries associated with gynecological surgery. *Int Urol Nephrol* 2002;34:31.

Rao D, Yu H, Zhu H, et al. The diagnosis and treatment of iatrogenic ureteral and bladder injury caused by traditional gynaecology and obstetrics operation. *Arch Gynecol Obstet* 2012;285:763.

Rassweiler JJ, Gözen AS, Erdogru T, et al. Ureteral reimplantation for management of ureteral strictures: a retrospective comparison of laparoscopic and open techniques. *Eur Urol* 2007;51:512.

Riedmiller H, Becht E, Hertle L, et al. Psoas-hitch ureteroneocystostomy: experience with 181 cases. *Eur Urol* 1984;10:145.

Sandberg EM, Cohen SL, Hurwitz S, et al. Utility of cystoscopy during hysterectomy. *Obstet Gynecol* 2012;120:1363.

Seideman CA, Huckabay C, Smith KD, et al. Laparoscopic ureteral reimplantation: technique and outcomes. *J Urol* 2009;181:1742.

Shull BL, Bachofen C, Coates KW, et al. A transvaginal approach to repair of apical and other associated sites of pelvic organ prolapse with uterosacral ligaments. *Am J Obstet Gynecol* 2000;183:1365.

Steele AC, Goldwasser S, Karram M. Failure of intraoperative cystoscopy to identify partial ureteral obstruction. *Obstet Gynecol* 2000;96:847.

Vabili B, Chesson RR, Kyle BL, et al. The incidence of urinary tract injury during hysterectomy and a prospective analysis based on universal cystoscopy. *Am J Obstet Gynecol* 2005;192:1599.

Vakili B, Chesson RR, Kyle BL, et al. The incidence of urinary tract injury during hysterectomy: a prospective analysis based on universal cystoscopy. *Am J Obstet Gynecol* 2005;192:1599.

Verduyckt FJ, Heesakkers JP, Debruyne FM. Long-term results of ileum interposition for ureteral obstruction. *Eur Urol* 2002;42:181.

Visco AG, Taber KH, Weidner AC, et al. Cost-effectiveness of universal cystoscopy to identify ureteral injury at hysterectomy. *Obstet Gynecol* 2001;97:685.

Wolff B, Chartier-Kastler E, Mozer P, et al. Long-term functional outcomes after ileal ureter substitution: a single-center experience. *Urology* 2011;78:692.

VII

CHAPTER 43
Vesicovaginal and Urethrovaginal Fistulas

Rony A. Adam

TABLE 43.1 Anatomic Classification of Genitourinary Fistulas

- Vesicovaginal
- Urethrovaginal
- Vesicouterine
- Vesicocervical
- Ureterovaginal
- Ureterouterine
- Combination fistulas
  Vesicoureterovaginal
  Vesicoureterouterine
  Vesicovaginorectal

DEFINITIONS

Fistula—An abnormal passage or communication that leads from one hollow organ to another.

Interposition graft—Placement of tissue attached to its own blood supply into the space between two viscera to enhance the likelihood of successful repair. Examples include a Martius graft or omental flap.

Retropubic vesicovaginal fistula repair—Access to the fistula and its closure involves dissection in the retropubic space (space of Retzius). This may be accomplished by an open laparotomy, by laparoscopy, or robotically.

Transperitoneal vesicovaginal fistula repair—Access to the fistula and its closure involves entry into the peritoneal cavity. This may be accomplished by an open laparotomy, by laparoscopy, or robotically.

Transvesical vesicovaginal fistula repair—Access to the fistula and its closure involves separate entry into the bladder (excluding entry through the fistula itself). This may be accomplished via a retropubic or a transperitoneal approach.

Urethrovaginal fistula—An abnormal communication between the urethra and the vagina.

Vaginal vesicovaginal fistula repair—Access to the fistula and its closure is accomplished through the vagina.

Vesicovaginal fistula—An abnormal communication between the bladder and the vagina.

INTRODUCTION

It is likely that women have suffered from urogenital fistulas throughout human existence as a consequence of childbirth. From an anthropologic perspective, humans experience difficult birthing requiring assistance primarily due to pelvic adaptations resulting from a trade-off between the evolutionary pressures of large brain size and bipedal biomechanics. Findings of a vesicovaginal fistula (VVF) have been identified in mummified remains from ancient Egypt. Since the mid-19th century, the evolution of surgical management of urogenital fistulas as described by Marion Sims, Thomas Emmet, Howard Kelly, and others has had a lasting influence on the development of our specialty.

It has long been recognized that women with VVF are severely afflicted physically, socially, and emotionally owing to the constant uncontrollable dribbling of urine. In the developing world, VVFs are most commonly noted as a consequence of prolonged labor. Perhaps a hundred years ago the situation was very similar in the (currently) developed world; however, due to dramatically improved access to expert obstetrical care, VVFs are now primarily acquired iatrogenically, mostly following hysterectomy. Providers and patients experience a vastly different set of circumstances in these two settings. In the latter, which is the primary focus of this chapter, patients are often litigious, yet they remain among the most grateful once their condition is explained and cured. Although the published literature regarding urogenital fistulas is extensive, it remains dominated by retrospective case series and expert opinion. The various types of urogenital fistulas are listed in Table 43.1 based upon anatomic involvement. This chapter primarily discusses vesicovaginal and urethrovaginal fistulas encountered in gynecologic and urogynecologic practice with a brief overview of obstetrical fistulas.

ETIOLOGY AND EPIDEMIOLOGY

Genitourinary fistulas can be congenital or acquired. Congenital fistulas are exceedingly rare, with only a few case reports in the literature. Most reported cases are associated with other urogenital anomalies. Acquired fistulas may be the result of childbirth, pelvic surgery, malignancy, irradiation, infection, and an assortment of unusual presentations (Table 43.2). This section discusses obstetrical and nonobstetrical urogenital fistulas. The nonobstetrical fistula portion will further discuss the following issues associated with urogenital fistula etiology and epidemiology: hysterectomy-associated cystotomies, urogynecologic and other gynecologic procedures, urethrovaginal fistulas, and an assortment of miscellaneous circumstances that have been reported in the literature.

Obstetrical Urogenital Fistulas

In the developing world, the most common predisposing factor is prolonged, obstructed childbirth, accounting for over 80% of genitourinary fistulas in these regions. These fistulas develop from the resulting necrosis of the vaginal and bladder wall and, therefore, are large and often associated with other related damages. These circumstances have become exceedingly rare in developed countries owing to improvements in access to and delivery of skilled obstetric care. Ibrahim et al. report that the mean age at diagnosis was 15 years, patients were in labor for 4 days on average, and the fetus died in 87% of cases. These findings are similar to another single-institution series from Nigeria, where 79% of fistula patients had labors that lasted over 2 days, and 21% had been in labor for 4 or more days during the index pregnancy associated with the injury. The fetal fatality rate in these cases was 92%. In a rural, population-based study of parturients in Senegal, the incidence rate was 124 per 100,000 deliveries, whereas no fistulas were noted in six major cities in West Africa. It is estimated that over 33,400 new cases of obstetric fistulas occur annually in sub-Saharan Africa, with an incidence of over 120 per 100,000 births. Constitutional risk factors include short stature, lower

TABLE 43.2 Conditions Associated with Development of Urogenital Fistulas

Obstetric conditions or procedures
Prolonged, obstructed labor
Placenta percreta
Cesarean section (especially repeat cesarean section)
Cesarean hysterectomy
Operative vaginal delivery
Cervical cerclage

Gynecologic and urogynecologic procedures
Hysterectomy
Myomectomy
Loop excision of the cervix
Voluntary interruption of pregnancy
Suburethral slings
Anterior colporrhaphy
Periurethral bulking
Burch colposuspension
Urethral diverticulum repair
Ureteral wall stent

Pelvic/medical conditions
Endometriosis
Gynecologic cancer
Pelvic irradiation
Behçet syndrome
Bladder stone
Infection
   Schistosomiasis
   Tuberculosis
   Lymphogranuloma venereum
Intrauterine device
Neglected pessary
Retention of other vaginal foreign objects
Accidental trauma
Sexual trauma
Mitomycin C instillation

family and social support structures, worsening economic hardship, isolation, and malnutrition being commonplace.

Surgical correction is curative in the first operation for obstetric VVF in about 80% of cases. Multiple attempts may be necessary to achieve a success rate over 95% for large fistulas. As the reality and complexity of this global tragedy is realized, solutions are suggested for its prevention that include improving the stature of women and access to competent routine and emergency obstetrical care as well as family planning services. Both global and regional economic and political actions will be necessary to effect meaningful and lasting change.

Other obstetric events and procedures have been noted to be associated with urogenital fistula formation worldwide. Cesarean section, especially in patients who have had prolonged, obstructed labor, may result in formation of a vesicouterine fistula (Youssef syndrome). The classic presentation is that of cyclical hematuria (menouria), amenorrhea, and urinary continence, but it may also present with total urinary incontinence with normal menstruation and represents 1% to 4% of all genitourinary fistulas. Vesicovaginal fistulas have also been reported following cesarean section, with or without associated hysterectomy. Even more rarely reported are vesicocervical, urethrovaginal, ureterovaginal, and ureterouterine fistulas following cesarean section. Operative vaginal delivery may rarely result in vesicouterine fistula in a patient undergoing vaginal birth delivery after cesarean section. Similarly, cervical cerclage placed for the treatment of cervical insufficiency has been associated with vesicovaginal and vesicocervical fistulas. A recent case series and pooled analysis suggests that previous cervical procedures (prior cerclage or cervical conization), prior cesarean delivery, and use of the McDonald technique (which does not involve a bladder dissection as with the Shirodkar technique) may play a role in the formation of urogenital fistula in these cases.

Although not an obstetrical practice, the traditional tribal practice of "gishiri cutting" is associated with formation of urogenital fistulas and is common in many parts of northern Nigeria. It involves cutting the anterior vagina with a razor or knife blade and has been noted to be the primary cause of fistula formation in 13% to 15% of cases. In more recently reported series in areas where gishiri cutting was reported, urogenital fistula was noted in 2.3% to 6.2% of cases.

Nonobstetrical Urogenital Fistulas

Nonobstetric urogenital fistulas have been reported as a consequence of gynecologic, urologic, and general surgical procedures and are the most commonly seen in developed countries. Various manifestations of urogenital trauma, certain medical conditions, and even medication instilled into the bladder have also been associated with subsequent development of urogenital fistulas.

Hysterectomy is the most common surgical procedure associated with a VVF. In a retrospective review of the Mayo Clinic experience regarding the treatment of 303 women with genitourinary fistulas, 190 were vesicovaginal. Of these, 156 (82%) were associated with hysterectomy (mostly abdominal), 19 (10%) with cesarean section or forceps delivery, and 6 (3%) each with radiation and with trauma.

Harkki-Siren et al. reviewed the incidence of urinary tract injuries from a Finnish national database of 62,379 hysterectomies with a VVF prevalence of 0.8 per 1,000. In a nationwide registry-based cohort study from Sweden that included all hysterectomies performed for benign indications over 30 years (n = 182,641), the prevalence of surgically managed genitourinary fistulas was 1.1 per 1,000. This is the same rate reported in a retrospective study of two institutions in the

education and socioeconomic levels, and young maternal age. Circumstantial contributing factors include a very high rate of home births attended to by unskilled birth attendants, wherein only 35% of deliveries in Nigeria are attended by trained personnel. Late presentation in northern Nigeria is primarily related to lack of husband's permission followed by transportation difficulties (distance, nonavailability of vehicle, and bad roads). The general lack of hospital resources including surgical supplies and reliable electrical power have been cited as contributing to delayed cesarean section for those who need it.

Hilton reviewed VVFs in developing countries and outlined management strategies to include immediate catheter drainage as long as the tract has not yet epithelialized, perhaps even prophylactically following obstructed labor with evident vaginal sloughing. Attention to adequate vulvar skin care, nutrition, lower extremity rehabilitation, and counseling are important adjuncts in the care of obstetrical fistula patients. Arrowsmith et al. similarly remind us of the spectrum of additional trauma sustained by the fistula patient and the need to address more than just the "hole in the bladder." Additional concurrent injuries may include and result in amenorrhea, total urethral loss, stress incontinence, hydronephrosis, renal failure, anorectal injury, cervical destruction, vaginal stenosis, nerve damage affecting mobility, and other physical maladies. The psychosocial toll is equally devastating with divorce, separation from

United States but has been reported as high as 3.0 per 1,000 in one of those institutions.

In a retrospective cohort study of 343,771 hysterectomies in the English National Health Service from 2000 until 2008, the overall urogenital fistula (vesicovaginal and urethrovaginal) rate was reported to be 1.3 per 1,000 within the year following surgery. Rates were noted to vary by the procedure type and the indication, with the highest rate in patients undergoing radical hysterectomy due to cervical cancer (11.5 per 1,000) and the lowest for vaginal hysterectomy due to prolapse (0.26 per 1,000). Most interesting was a subanalysis of abdominal hysterectomy for benign conditions excluding prolapse, where a 46% increase in the risk of fistula rates was noted over the course of the study itself from 1.5 per 1,000 in the first 2 years to 2.2 per 1,000 in the last 2 years of the study. See Table 43.3 for a summary of the various epidemiologic studies discussed.

As previously noted, hysterectomy for cancer is associated with an increased risk of fistula formation. In a retrospective study of 536 patients who underwent a radical hysterectomy due to cervical cancer, a VVF rate of 2.6% and a ureterovaginal fistula rate of 2.4% were reported. Risk factors included cancer stage, intraoperative bladder injury, diabetes, and postoperative surgical site infection. Vaginal cancer shows a high likelihood of fistula development (both vesicovaginal and rectovaginal) with no association to radiation therapy.

Hysterectomy-Associated Cystotomy and Vesicovaginal Fistula Formation

The association of a cystotomy sustained at the time of hysterectomy (recognized or not) and subsequent development of a VVF has long been noted but is nonetheless complex (see further discussion under Pathogenesis). A review of published articles reporting on cystotomies during gynecologic surgery showed that the rate of cystotomy is significantly increased in series that employed routine cystoscopy rather than the traditional intra- or postoperative diagnosis on which the other studies relied. These disparate rates of bladder injury continue with two distinct single-institution studies that employed routine cystoscopy at the time of hysterectomy, reporting a cystotomy rate of 2.6% to 2.9%, while estimates from a US national hospital discharge database–derived study

reported bladder injury rates of only 0.7% to 1.4% depending on the type of hysterectomy. Although one cannot conclude that the two- to threefold difference in cystotomy rates is due to detection bias, it is not unreasonable to consider that some bladder injuries may go undetected during hysterectomy, which may contribute to the overall posthysterectomy VVF rate.

Even when a cystotomy is immediately recognized and repaired, a subsequent VVF may still occur. In their data on over 43,000 total abdominal hysterectomies, Harkki-Siren et al. report failure of primary bladder repair 18% of the time. In a case–control single-institution study of 1,317 benign hysterectomies, which included routine cystoscopic evaluation, 34 cystotomies were recognized and repaired, but among those, four patients (11.8%) developed a VVF. The degree of bladder injury retrospectively assessed by using the American Association for the Surgery of Trauma (AAST) system was found to be strongly associated with subsequent fistula formation despite cystotomy repair. The AAST grading system is used to describe the degree of injury to the bladder using the location and size of the defect with higher grades denoting worse trauma. Of highest risk are larger extraperitoneal (>2 cm) injuries, any intraperitoneal bladder injuries, and injuries involving the bladder neck or the trigone. Additional associated risk factors for occurrence of a VVF following cystotomy and repair include larger uterus, longer operative time, and longer hospital stay. A trend was noted when the hysterectomy was associated with greater than 1 L blood loss and for tobacco use. The strong association of bladder injury severity with subsequent VVF formation persisted in a subsequent expansion of this original study. There were 5,698 hysterectomies in the combined cohort where 102 cystotomies were diagnosed and repaired. Of these, there were six VVFs (5.9%) identified.

Urogynecologic Procedures

Due to the immediate proximity of the lower urinary tract to the operative field in surgeries for the treatment of urinary incontinence, pelvic organ prolapse, and other pelvic floor disorders, there have been reports of both vesicovaginal and urethrovaginal fistulas with these types of surgery. Surgeries for the treatment of stress urinary incontinence have been implicated, including Burch colposuspension, bone-anchored cystourethropexy, Stamey bladder neck suspension, transobturator tape, and retropubic tension-free vaginal tape procedures.

TABLE 43.3 Prevalence of Vesicovaginal Fistula by Type of Hysterectomy

	OVERALL	LAPAROSCOPIC	TAH	SAH	TVH
Harkki-Siren et al. (1998)	0.8/1,000 (n = 62,379)	2.2/1,000 (n = 2,741)	1/1,000 (n = 43,149)	0 (n = 10,854)	0.2/1,000 (n = 5,636)
Forsgren et al. (2009)	1.1/1,000 (n = 182,641)	3.3/1,000 (n = 1,783)	1.5/1,000 (n = 117,242)	0.2/1,000 (n = 44,754)	0.5/1,000 (n = 18,828)
Duong et al. (2009)	3.0/1,000 (n = 1,317)	12.6/1,000 (n = 79)	3.3/1,000 (n = 606)	N/A	1.6/1,000 (n = 632)
Duong et al. (2011)	1.1/1,000 (n = 5,698)	2.2/1,000 (n = 456)	0.6/1,000 (n = 3,305)	N/A	1.5/1,000 (n = 1,937)
Hilton and Cromwell (2012)*	1.2/1,000 (n = 286,053)	N/A	1.8/1,000 (n = 149,227)	0.4/1,000 (n = 20,511)	0.5/1,000 (n = 116,315)

TAH, total abdominal hysterectomy; SAH, supracervical abdominal hysterectomy; TVH, total vaginal hysterectomy.

*Vesicovaginal and urethrovaginal fistulas are combined, data are a subset of hysterectomies for benign indications, excluding prolapse.

Surgery for anterior prolapse occurs adjacent to the bladder and may result in immediate or delayed injury to the lower urinary tract. Anterior colporrhaphy has been associated with VVF only in case reports regarding fistula repairs. In a single surgeon case series of 519 anterior colporrhaphy patients (with Kelly-Kennedy urethropexy for the treatment of stress incontinence), the authors reported two urethrovaginal fistulas but no VVFs. Mesh kit procedures for the treatment of anterior prolapse have been associated with VVFs by several investigators. The incidence of VVF from trocar-based mesh kit surgery for the treatment of anterior prolapse has been noted to be 0.3% in a large series. A recent case report noted a ureterovaginal fistula 28 days following a transobturator mesh kit surgery for anterior prolapse. A case report of a VVF following total abdominal hysterectomy with sacrocolpopexy for uterine prolapse noted that the fistula was adjacent to the distal edge of the colpopexy mesh.

Urethrovaginal fistulas have been associated with each of the various forms of midurethral (mesh) slings, vaginal urethropexies, and even periurethral bulking injections. With the increasing popularity of midurethral slings for the treatment of stress incontinence, reports of associated urethral injury and urethrovaginal fistulas have been accumulating. A literature review identified 3 VVFs and 11 urethrovaginal fistulas with retropubic and transobturator approaches implicated in both fistula types. The reviewed literature was insufficient to estimate the rates of urethrovaginal fistulas.

Urethrovaginal fistulas may occur as a consequence of urethral diverticulum repair. Review of available series, ranging from 18 to 85 patients each, reveals that urethrovaginal fistula develops in 1.2% to 7.8% of patients undergoing vaginal repair of a urethral diverticulum.

Other Gynecologic Procedures

Additional gynecologic procedures associated with urogenital fistulas, although with greater rarity (see Table 43.2), include myomectomy, loop excision of the cervical transformation zone for cervical intraepithelial neoplasia, and voluntary interruption of pregnancy. Fistulas are noted following radiation therapy for gynecologic cancers and uterine artery embolization for leiomyomatous uteri.

Urethrovaginal Fistula

Urethrovaginal fistulas are less common than are VVFs, with an incidence ratio of 1 per 8.5. In the developed world, the most common predisposing event is surgery for urethral diverticulum, anterior vaginal prolapse and incontinence, radiation therapy, or trauma. Operative vaginal delivery and cesarean section also have been reported to precede urethrovaginal fistula formation. There has been an increase in urethrovaginal fistula formation related to the increased use of suburethral slings in the treatment of stress incontinence (please see subsection on Urogynecologic Procedures).

Miscellaneous Circumstances

An assortment of presentations and conditions can be found in the literature associated with urogenital fistulas mostly in the form of case presentations. These include Behçet syndrome; infections such as schistosomiasis, tuberculosis, lymphogranuloma venereum; endometriosis; accidental trauma; sexual trauma; masturbation; and a variety of retained foreign objects. Bladder calculi are found to be rarely associated with long-standing fistulas but not considered etiologic. Additional gynecologic associations include neglected diaphragm, neglected pessary, intrauterine device, and a ureteral wall stent used to treat a ureteral stricture. Intravesical instillation of mitomycin C has been reported to be associated with urogenital fistula formation.

PATHOGENESIS

The pathophysiologic mechanism of fistula formation is not completely understood. Etiologies have been proposed based on interpretation of the epidemiologic data and risk factors previously discussed. Vascular compromise and subsequent epithelial necrosis of the intervening vaginal walls are indisputable in cases of prolonged obstructed labor where the presenting fetal vertex compresses the vaginal walls against the pubic symphysis. If this pressure is present for a sufficient period of time, even once relieved, the affected vaginal, bladder, and/or urethral walls undergo necrosis and sloughing, thus creating the abnormal (often large) communication between adjoining viscera.

The precise pathophysiology of nonobstetrical urogenital fistulas is somewhat less obvious, but can likely also be understood in terms of abnormal healing associated with microvascular compromise coincident with posterior bladder/anterior vaginal wall injury. From empirical evidence, we know that small-sized bladder perforation in the non–gravity-dependent areas of the bladder rarely if ever results in any fistula formation. Consider suprapubic catheters that are removed with initial formation of a vesicocutaneous tract that almost inevitably heals without further intervention, as well as retropubic tension-free tapes that are found perforating the anterior and anterolateral bladder only to be repositioned with little to no consequence, even without prophylactic catheter drainage. On the other hand, the dependent area of the bladder is more prone to fistula formation due to its closer proximity to the vagina and possibly the effect of gravity and the near-constant presence of urine in this part of the bladder.

Experimental evidence further shows that not all injuries result in VVF formation, even in the dependent portion of the bladder. Meeks et al. demonstrated in a rabbit model that fistula formation did *not* occur when figure-of-eight absorbable sutures were placed incorporating full-thickness bladder wall and vaginal cuff during a hysterectomy. In a laparoscopic dog model, none developed a fistula after bipolar cautery injury to the bladder base nor when absorbable sutures were placed through the bladder and vaginal cuff during a laparoscopic hysterectomy. Fistula formation, however, was noted in the dogs that had a monopolar cautery-induced bladder base laceration and had repair either with single-layer absorbable suture in the normal fashion or with suture that incorporated the anterior vaginal wall. No differences were found histologically in the specimens that primarily showed inflammation, fibrosis, foreign body giant cell reaction, and recanalization of thrombus. It should be noted that these animal models of hysterectomy, because of anatomic differences, do not require any dissection of the bladder off the uterus and in that respect may be different from humans undergoing total hysterectomy.

From the aforementioned data, vascular or microvascular compromise may be the common pathway to fistula formation, which then leads to localized impairment of healing that allows the formation of an epithelialized tract between the two adjacent organs. Such microvascular compromise may aid in the understanding of urogenital fistulas caused by local infection or even subacute infection when foreign materials (suture, mesh, etc.) or electrocautery are used, as well as aid in the understanding of radiation-associated fistulas. Thus, in posthysterectomy urogenital fistulas, the mechanisms involved may be more complex than the previously assumed "undiagnosed bladder injury" or "inadvertently placed suture" that many have previously suggested. Further research into the pathophysiology is needed to elucidate the mechanisms at work in such circumstances.

VII

CLINICAL PRESENTATION

The classic presentation of urogenital fistula is continuous urinary leakage from the vagina several days or weeks following pelvic surgery. This may occur in the absence of urinary urgency, Valsalva maneuvers, or changes in body position. The degree to which leakage presents depends primarily on the precise location and size of the fistula, perhaps the pliability and healing of the surrounding tissue, and the condition of the rest of the vagina. Patients have a spectrum of leakage from truly continuous to intermittent primarily at bladder capacity with attendant urinary odor. Although it is generally accepted that the larger the fistula, the worse the leakage, even small fistulas leak significantly. In developed countries, an antecedent gynecologic, urologic, or general surgical procedure involving the pelvis will often be noted. Delivery by the operative vaginal or, more commonly, cesarean section route may precede the onset of symptoms.

The majority of cases will present in 1 to 10 days following surgery and nearly all by 30 days, although the author has seen patients manifest symptoms as much as 3 months postoperatively. The increasing prevalence of multiple procedures undertaken at the same time for complex pelvic floor disorders (often by multiple surgeons) may complicate the diagnosis of subsequent fistula formation, related to multiple potential sites of injury, preexisting symptoms, and added potential postoperative urinary complications. Indeed, subsequent anti-incontinence procedures have been mistakenly done believing the cause of leakage is stress incontinence. Other potential causes of postoperative urinary leakage should be considered and ruled out, as listed in Table 43.4.

Many patients develop coexisting urinary tract infections and symptoms of frequency, urgency, and dysuria. The predominant organism is *Escherichia coli* in most cases. Urinary leakage from any genitourinary fistula may be accompanied by hematuria and rarely may have associated stones.

Vesicouterine fistulas tend to present with cyclic hematuria, and if the fistula is located above the cervix, amenorrhea may occur if all the menstrual blood is redirected into the bladder because of a closed cervical canal. Patients with coexistenting mesh erosion into the bladder experience urgency, frequency, voiding dysfunction, and pain. If there is concurrent erosion into the vagina, coital discomfort and a vaginal discharge may occur as well.

Urethrovaginal fistula may present either as continuous vaginal leakage or vaginal voiding either during or just following micturition. This depends primarily on the location of the fistula whether it affects the continence mechanism or not. Vaginal bleeding and dyspareunia may also present concurrently regardless of the fistula's location and may be exacerbated by foreign material associated with the preceding surgery (mesh, graft, suture, etc.).

Any significant urine leakage for even a short period of time may result in significant irritation of the vagina, the skin of the vulva, or perineum. This often occurs, despite the patient's attempt at frequent cleansing. Among obstetrical fistula patients, dermatitis symptoms were noted in 20% of patients. If urine leakage persists, severe perineal dermatitis may result owing to exposure of the skin to ammonia. Phosphate crystallization may precipitate on the vagina and vulva, further irritating the area.

PREVENTION

Since the occurrence of a cystotomy is considered a risk factor for subsequent fistula formation, prevention is discussed primarily in terms of preventing a cystotomy (primary prevention) or adequately detecting and repairing one if it occurs (secondary prevention). Careful consideration of the bladder, trigone, and ureteral anatomy in relation to the anterior vagina, uterus, and cervix is important to maintain during each step of any hysterectomy, but especially with a total hysterectomy (Fig. 43.1).

Anatomically, the bladder base overlies the uterine isthmus and the cervix, the bladder trigone is positioned anterior to the upper third of the vagina, and the external cervical os is proximal to the base of the trigone (the interureteric ridge). During a simple hysterectomy, mobilization of the bladder does not involve the upper third of the vagina and therefore rarely puts the trigone at risk. A subtotal (supracervical) hysterectomy requires no bladder mobilization and indeed results in dramatically fewer fistulas even in large series (see Table 43.3). This is not the case, however, with anterior colporrhaphy or vaginal paravaginal repair, where the anterior vaginal dissection is carried more distally and laterally upon the vagina, indeed involving its middle and upper thirds.

The likelihood of cystotomy is reduced by avoiding blunt dissection at the time of bladder mobilization during hysterectomy (or anterior repair), especially when the vesicovaginal space is scarred from prior cesarean section or other surgery. The precise direction of forces cannot be controlled as accurately when blunt dissection is used, when compared with sharp dissection. Gentle traction and countertraction are helpful in dissecting the correct plane and thereby preventing direct bladder injury, as is utilizing an intrafascial hysterectomy technique. Another cause of bladder injury may be direct trauma by retractors, particularly during vaginal hysterectomy; retractors should always be used with appropriate caution. As previously reviewed (see Pathogenesis section), experimental data suggest a detrimental effect of using monopolar electrocautery. As such, one should consider electrocautery with monopolar current in the vesicovaginal space only after carefully considering the risks and benefits.

If during the course of a hysterectomy or any pelvic surgery, a bladder injury (cystotomy) occurs, it is critical to diagnose and properly manage it prior to the conclusion of the surgery so as to minimize the likelihood of subsequent fistula formation (secondary prevention). See Steps in the Procedure for the surgical steps of cystotomy repair. In addition to careful inspection of the operative field, cystoscopy is often recommended to assess for bladder and ureteral injury following hysterectomy and routinely recommended after surgery for pelvic prolapse or urinary incontinence. The routine use of cystoscopy at the time of hysterectomy remains controversial by some, yet recommended by others. The alternative to routine cystoscopy is performing it as needed when a suspicion for injury arises as may occur with new-onset gross hematuria, while the bladder is catheterized or visualization of fluid in the operative field. Studies in which routine cystoscopy has been performed report a bladder injury detection rate of only 35% to 50% when relying on visualization alone.

TABLE 43.4 Differential Diagnosis of Postoperative Urinary Incontinence
• Urogenital fistula
• Stress incontinence
• Urge incontinence
• Overflow incontinence
• Vaginal discharge/erosion of mesh

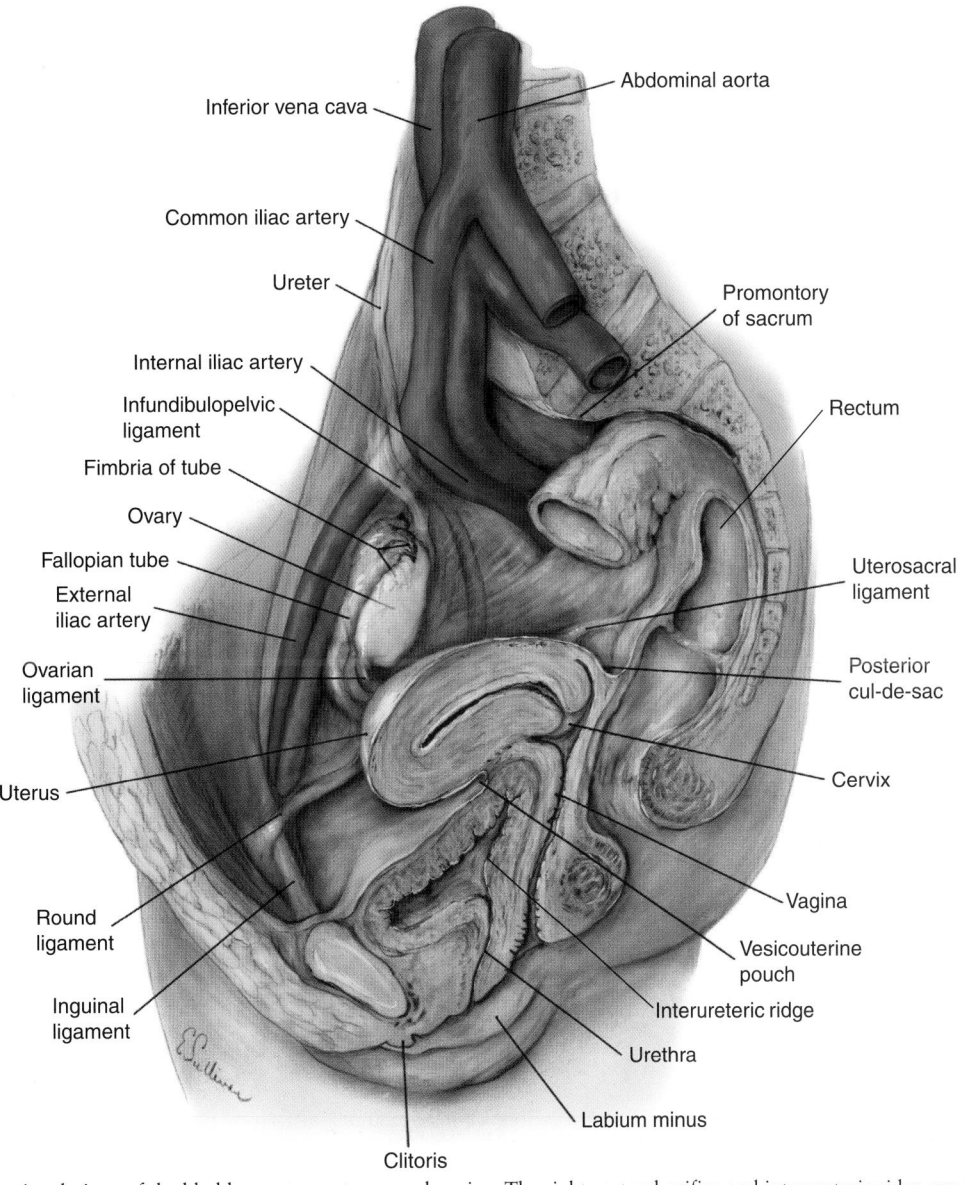

FIGURE 43.1 Anatomic relations of the bladder, rectum, uterus, and vagina. The right ureteral orifice and interureteric ridge are denoted. Note that the cervix and the anterior cervicovaginal sulcus are at a position higher than the interureteric ridge, which explains why the simple posthysterectomy vesicovaginal fistulas are supratrigonal at the level of the vaginal cuff.

STEPS IN THE PROCEDURE

Cystotomy Closure

- Recognize that a cystotomy has occurred.

- Evaluate cystoscopically and vaginally to assess size, location relative to known landmarks (trigone and ureters), and the quality of the injured tissue.

- If injury deemed needing repair and safe from present or potential ureter injury, simple cystotomy closure is indicated: (1) ureteral catheterization as needed if close to ureter(s); (2) bladder should be catheterized with a transurethral Foley.

- Carefully and accurately identify the margins of the bladder injury (beware, there often is a hidden invagination). Use fine surgical technique and delicate tissue handling while optimizing visualization, using suction and irrigation as needed. Avoid prolonged clamping of the injured tissue during the repair, and avoid electrocautery near the injury.

- Sharply dissect the vesicovaginal space sufficiently to allow tension-free closure.

- Close the urothelial (lamina propria) layer with interrupted or running fine 3-0 delayed absorbable suture.

- Reapproximate the muscular layer with running or interrupted 2-0 or 3-0 delayed absorbable suture. Ensure hemostasis in the vesicovaginal space.

- Bring a third layer of peritoneum to further reinforce the repair if available using interrupted 3-0 delayed absorbable suture.

VII

- Perform cystoscopy to ensure intravesical hemostasis the and ensure integrity of the repair by looking vaginally for spillage; assess for injury or obstruction to the ureter using intravenous indigo carmine. Remove any blood clots that may obstruct catheter drainage.

- If there is an adjacent vaginal injury or opening (e.g., vaginal cuff), ensure it is closed separately by the end of the surgery, making certain that the vaginal closure does not incorporate the bladder in any way.

- Determine how long bladder catheterization is needed, and ensure orders are written to avoid inadvertent routine catheter removal on the following day.

In the event of a cystotomy, the location, extent, and size as categorized in the AAST grading system previously discussed may be an important factor in assessing prognosis of the repair of a posterior bladder injury. Also, as previously discussed in the Pathogenesis section, a small anterior bladder injury does not result in urogenital fistula formation as observed following removal of suprapubic catheters or trocar injuries from retropubic midurethral slings. Since these injuries are approximately 0.5 cm in diameter, any bladder injury greater than that may be considered for primary repair versus longer catheter drainage to allow for spontaneous healing. Owing to the dependent position of the bladder base however, any significant injury in the posterior bladder requires consideration of suture closure and bladder drainage.

Once a cystotomy is recognized, it may be repaired immediately or delayed until the hysterectomy or other surgical procedure is completed. The benefit of immediate repair is that blood and urine do not continually flow into the surgical field; however, with continued surgery and retraction, there may be potential compromise to the fresh suture line, and this should be meticulously avoided. Cystoscopy, when an injury is first suspected, is helpful in delineating the exact location and extent of the injury as well as distance to the ureters and trigone. Adequate dissection of the bladder off the vagina is usually necessary to ensure tension-free closure and allow sufficient mobilization for a second layer. Careful inspection of the cystotomy is critical to identify the true borders of the defect. Due to the inherent pliability and redundancy of the bladder, repair without careful delineation of the edges may miss a particularly well-hidden portion of the defect, which could lead to nonhealing and subsequent VVF formation. The first layer can be accomplished with 2-0 or 3-0 absorbable suture placed in an interrupted or running fashion (**Fig. 43.2A**). There is controversy regarding whether this first layer can be placed through the mucosa or should remain extramucosal. It is thought that the extramucosal technique may decrease the likelihood of subsequent fistula formation and perhaps prevent bladder stone formation, although this has not been demonstrated, whereas excluding the urothelial edge may result in bleeding from it. Results from an experimental laparoscopic hysterectomy model of electrocautery-induced bladder injury with laparoscopic repair in dogs suggest that double-layer closure is superior to single-layer closure in preventing VVF. The second layer placed to imbricate the first is thought to diminish tension on the suture line. A third layer of closure usually can be achieved with the peritoneum either vaginally or abdominally (**Fig. 43.2B, C**). Cystoscopy is important to evaluate ureteral and bladder integrity following completion

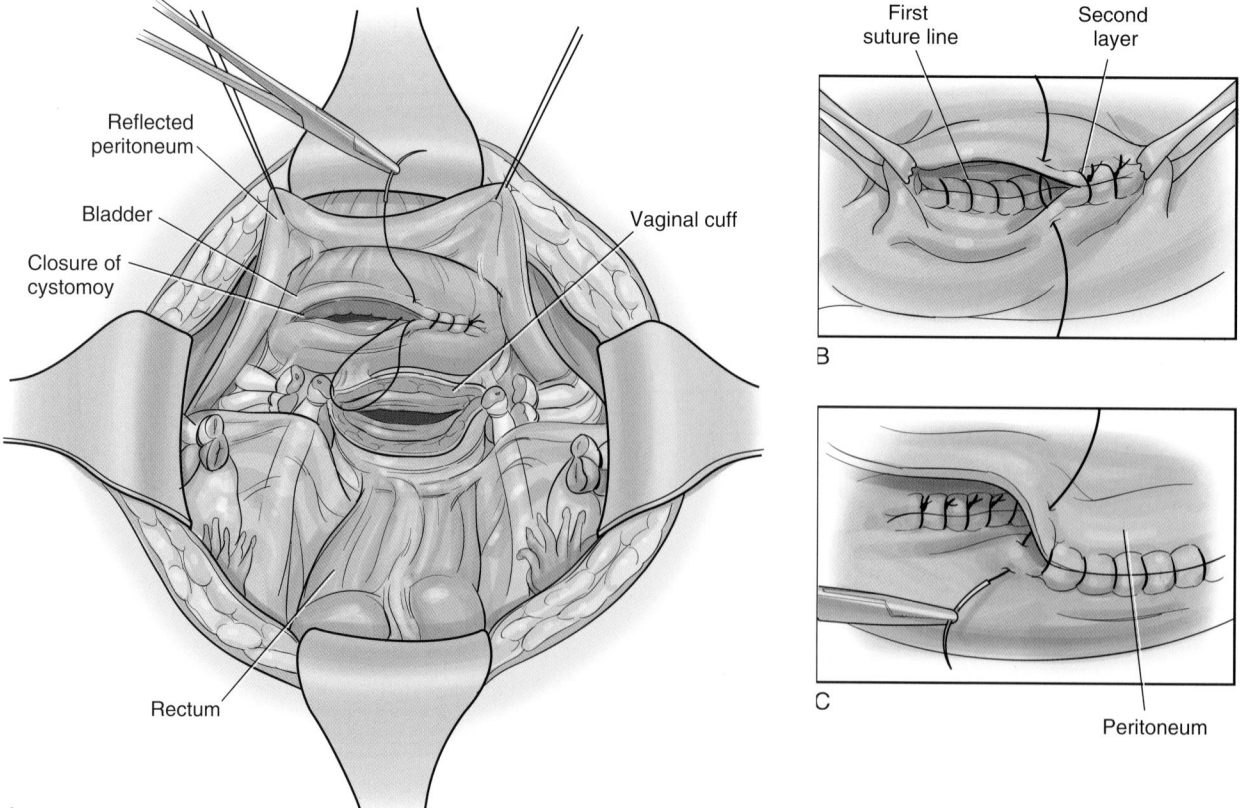

FIGURE 43.2 Closure of cystotomy associated with total abdominal hysterectomy (abdominal view). **A:** Initial layer is closed with a running suture. **B:** An imbricating second layer is being placed using interrupted stitches. **C:** A third layer covering the repair with peritoneum.

of the repair and to ensure there is no significant hematuria, which can obstruct catheter drainage with the formation of clots. Cystoscopy should be done with minimal bladder filling to avoid tension on the suture line.

Transurethral or suprapubic catheter drainage must prevent bladder filling to avoid exerting tension on the suture line that would otherwise occur when the bladder fills. The lack of reliable postoperative catheter drainage as a significant cause of failure of fistula repair was discussed at length in 1852 by Sims in his landmark paper regarding urogenital fistulas. Judgment should be exercised regarding duration of drainage, based on the extent of injury, its location, the security of the closure, and any factors that may impact the normal healing process, but generally should be for 7 to 10 days. Some advocate use of a cystogram prior to catheter removal; however, subsequent VVF in the face of a normal cystogram has been noted anecdotally, calling this extra step into question. A retrospective study of bladder injury in the trauma setting concluded that in patients undergoing simple intraperitoneal bladder injury management, routine follow-up cystograms did not affect clinical management, while all extraperitoneal and complex intraperitoneal injuries required follow-up cystograms.

DIAGNOSIS AND EVALUATION

Often, the diagnosis of nonobstetrical urogenital fistula is straightforward based on history and demonstrable pooling of urine in the vaginal vault; occasionally, however, the diagnosis is elusive. In all cases, it is necessary to evaluate the fistula with regard to its size, precise location, degree of epithelialization, whether it is simple or complex, accessibility, and the overall health status and mobility of the surrounding tissues. In the instance of a recurrent fistula, precise knowledge of prior conservative management and review of the surgical description of prior repair attempts are extremely helpful for choosing the most appropriate route, type, and timing of the repair.

In the case of clinical suspicion of a urogenital fistula that cannot be verified on initial speculum examination, the physician can try concurrent Valsalva maneuvers and partial closure of the speculum to reduce the tension on the vaginal walls. If this is not helpful in visualizing vaginal leakage, then a dye test should be tried. Sterile water dyed with indigo carmine or methylene blue is instilled via a transurethral Foley catheter (16 French) with great care taken to avoid spilling the dye externally. Once the vagina and vulva are cleaned, a tampon is placed and the patient is asked to ambulate and wait for one-half hour. The tampon is removed and inspected for the presence of blue dye; if the tampon is wet with urine but not dyed, then a ureterovaginal fistula is suspected and is best diagnosed by appropriate radiologic studies. On rare occasions, these office diagnostic procedures are nondiagnostic despite a compelling history. In this case, the patient is asked to take phenazopyridine (Pyridium) and wear a series of tampons at home over a longer period of time with varying degrees of physical activity. The tampons are placed individually in plastic bags and brought in to be inspected. The patient must be counseled regarding careful use of the tampons to eliminate the possibility of dye contamination during insertion or removal.

Regarding urogenital fistula, radiologic studies are not routinely helpful in the actual diagnosis. However, it is often necessary to evaluate the upper urinary tracts once a fistula is identified. This may be accomplished by an intravenous pyelogram or contrast computed tomography scan. Cystourethrography may be utilized to show a vesicovaginal or urethrovaginal fistula, but it is rarely needed to make an initial diagnosis. It has been occasionally helpful in delineating

a complex fistula with multiple channels and openings. The use of Doppler ultrasound has been described to diagnose VVFs, with a sensitivity of 92%. Although this modality may be useful in the follow-up of patients undergoing conservative bladder drainage (one of four such patients demonstrated resolution of the fistula after 6 weeks), it too is rarely necessary to make an initial diagnosis.

All patients suspected of having a nonobstetrical urogenital fistula should undergo cystourethroscopy. This may be done as a separate procedure, allowing for improved surgical planning, discussion, and informed consent prior to the definitive operation, especially in complex or recurrent cases. Alternatively, the evaluation may be done just prior to operative management of the fistula and associated complications, but then surgical consenting must be done assuming all reasonable options.

Information to be sought during cystourethroscopy includes delineating the fistula's precise location and size; noting any surrounding induration, edema, and/or scarring; determining whether it is simple, complex, or multiple; and evaluating ureteral patency, location, and proximity to the fistula. It is preferable to examine the patient under anesthesia when possible, thus allowing improved determination of fistula accessibility to the vaginal route of repair. If the fistula is large enough to prevent adequate distention of the bladder during fluid-filled cystourethroscopy, placing a vaginal pack is helpful in allowing better visualization. When there is clinical suspicion of a vesicouterine fistula, hysterography or hysteroscopy may be helpful in making the diagnosis. If the patient is taken for examination under anesthesia and cystourethroscopy, then diagnostic hysteroscopy may help further delineate the course of such a fistula.

Some have advocated urodynamics testing prior to repair of a urogenital fistula on clinical and medicolegal grounds. Abnormalities on preoperative urodynamics have been reported in most patients. Urodynamic stress incontinence was noted in 75% of patients with urethral or bladder neck fistulas ($n = 12$) and 36% with VVFs ($n = 14$), with detrusor instability, impaired bladder compliance, and voiding dysfunction noted frequently as well. Of the 24 patients who were anatomically cured in this series, 1 (4%) had stress incontinence and 9 (38%) had urgency or urge incontinence. Preoperative urodynamics should be performed only if surgical management will be influenced by the results. Others do not routinely perform urodynamics preoperatively, preferring instead to provide counseling that if bladder symptoms occur and are bothersome to the patient, further diagnostic workup would then be indicated following an appropriate period of healing.

There have been several urogenital fistula classification systems devised in hopes of providing a prognostic indicator prior to intervention. Unfortunately, the prognostic ability of these classification systems has thus far been noted fair to poor. At this time, careful assessment of the type, nature, condition, location, and size of the fistula; condition of the bladder itself (including the trigone); the ureteral orifices and their patency; and the condition of the vagina should be noted and documented.

The classification of fistula is determined by which anatomic structures are found abnormally communicating (see Table 43.1). The nature of the fistula includes whether it represents a single or multiple channel fistula, while the condition denotes the appearance of the mucosa in the region of the fistula, whether indurated, edematous, necrotic, scarred, etc. The same components of condition should be assessed regarding the bladder in general. Any foreign material or objects in the bladder cavity or exposed through the mucosa should be noted as well, describing its location in the bladder and relative to the fistula.

VII

Fistula location should be described in terms of distance from known landmarks, such as the (left or right) ureter orifice, interureteric ridge, trigone, bladder neck (or proximal urethra), and/or the urethral meatus as appropriate. Finally, from the cystourethroscopic view, an estimate of the fistula's size (diameter) should be recorded. Similarly, a determination of the size and location of the fistula from the vaginal perspective is useful in the detailed description of a fistula. Specify laterality, distance to the cuff or urethral meatus, condition of the vaginal epithelium (scarring, induration, etc.), and mobility/vaginal accessibility of the fistula.

MANAGEMENT OF UROGENITAL FISTULAS

Nonsurgical Management

Once a urogenital fistula has been diagnosed, a trial of conservative management should be offered, although there is no consensus regarding when this should be offered and for what duration. This is particularly true for small fistulas that present early and have no evidence of epithelialization of the tract. Transurethral bladder drainage may help small (<0.5 cm and certainly <1 cm) and early (<3 weeks) VVFs resolve without further intervention and may be tried for 4 to 6 weeks as long as catheterization resolves the vaginal leakage. Medical management should include optimizing nutrition, correcting anemia, and improving vaginal estrogenization. In a retrospective case series of 558 urogenital fistulas (72% associated with obstructed labor), a trial of conservative treatment was done in 42 patients with successful closure of the fistula in 8 (19%) patients. All patients with successful conservative management had a supratrigonal fistula that was less than 4 mm with healthy surrounding mucosa as assessed by cystoscopy.

The use of collection devices has been tried with varying success but may be offered for temporary relief of constant urinary leakage until a more permanent solution is performed. Most are based on a Foley catheter or preferably a Malecot drain inserted into the center of a well-fitted contraceptive diaphragm and placed in the upper vagina to temporarily collect urine and avoid the distress of constant leakage.

Conservative Surgical Management

Some success has been reported in small series with cystoscopic laser treatment of VVF, primarily limited to small (2 to 4 mm) supratrigonal fistulas as well as electrocoagulation. Successful occlusion of a large complex postoperative VVF with fibrin was first reported in 1979. Since then, fibrin glue has been used successfully in the treatment of VVFs. Most recently, autologous platelet-rich plasma has been injected transvaginally with interposition of platelet-rich fibrin to successfully treat 11 of 12 iatrogenic VVFs. A small randomized trial comparing interposition of fibrin glue to the use of a Martius flap during complicated obstetrical VVF repair concluded that the outcomes were similar and operative time was decreased with self-made fibrin glue. A recent case report of ureteral obstruction and urinary fistula associated with fibrin glue used at the time of partial nephrectomy is an appropriate general reminder of the potential for risk as well. Experience with all these modalities continues to be sparse but potentially useful pending further long-term data.

Surgical Correction of Urogenital Fistula

When conservative therapy fails or the patient is not a candidate for conservative therapy, surgical repair is the only alternative to relieve the patient of her symptoms. The pelvic surgeon must determine the optimal timing, technique, and route of repair, as well as determine what suturing technique to use, how many layers of closure are sufficient for repair, and whether or not to use an interposition graft. No definitive trials adequately address any of these dilemmas at this time. Several general principles may apply and are discussed, emphasizing the care for iatrogenic rather than obstetrical fistulas. A synopsis of the literature regarding principles related to repair and surgical outcomes is presented, followed by an outline of the technical details of the operations discussed.

Principles of Surgical Repair

Traditionally, delayed repair of VVFs for several months was standard to allow the surrounding tissue to heal from the inciting injury. These recommendations were formulated primarily from what was and still is experienced in cases of obstetrical fistulas where there is often a large amount of tissue necrosis. Since that time, several case series have shown the safety and efficacy of earlier repair as long as there is no evidence of concurrent infection, inflammation, or necrosis in the tissue bed and when the fistula is not associated with radiation. The definition of what constitutes an early repair varies and has not been determined, but the previously referenced series report the interval to be from 1 to 6 weeks after the original insult, with another series specifically reporting excellent results when repair is undertaken 2 weeks or less from the inciting procedure. Obstetric (particularly if the fistula is not supratrigonal) and radiation injuries, however, require more time to heal prior to an attempt at fistula repair. In a large series from England, the first surgical attempt at repair of urogenital fistulas was noted to give the best chance of anatomic cure (98.2% vs. 88.2%) or reduce the chance of repeat surgery.

In Sims' classic article regarding the surgical treatment of VVFs, he emphasized the need to excise all scar tissue within the fistula and create fresh tissue edges for reapproximation. Additional surgical principles include tension-free closure of the wound by widely mobilizing the bladder and atraumatic handling of tissues to preserve the vascular supply needed for subsequent wound healing, including the absolute minimal use of electrocautery. Additional critical elements of success include ensuring excellent hemostasis of the surgical site, fine suture material (silver wire "drawn down to about the size of a horsehair"), avoidance of too much force on the suture closure, and maintaining good postoperative bladder drainage until healing is established. Of note, since the silver wire had to be subsequently cut and removed, the original operation left the vagina open without any surgical reapproximation.

Despite these original tenets, there is currently no consensus about whether to excise the margins of the fistula. Several series have reported success with preservation of the fistula tract (primarily during vaginal route of repair), with some being concerned about making the fistulous opening larger, as occurs when the fistulous tract is excised. Others have continued to report their experiences with excision of the tract with little concern about the enlargement of the defect in the process. The purported benefit of tract excision is allowing fresh tissue edges to be approximated, thus promoting healing of these surfaces to each other and reducing the likelihood of nonunion of the fistula's epithelialized lining. A randomized trial of 64 obstetrical fistula patients revealed no difference in surgical success with or without trimming of the fibrous fistula edge on the bladder side once the vesicovaginal space was developed. With an average fistula size of 1 to 1.3 cm, the authors voiced concern regarding enlarging the fistula further when the fistula edges were trimmed. It remains unknown how these findings may be interpreted in the management of posthysterectomy VVFs, which tend to be significantly smaller.

Another technical dilemma is whether to permit through-and-through suture placement or insist on excluding the mucosal layer from the suture bite. Concern over incorporating the mucosal layer stems from the possibility that it would increase the likelihood of failure and may lead to stone formation given that this region is the most dependent portion of the bladder and is therefore continuously in contact with urine, and how urine solutes would interact with the exposed suture material. The potential benefits of a through-and-through stitch are its ease and better hemostasis at the incision site. It remains for the operating surgeon to decide individually how to balance the pros and cons and how best to close the bladder aspect of the incision.

Similarly, the choice of suture type or caliber in urogenital fistula repair has not been compared in the literature and, therefore, no specific comment regarding the use of braided or nonbraided and absorbable or delayed absorbable suture type can be recommended. However, given the risk of bladder stone formation reported around permanent sutures, these should be avoided in the repair of urogenital fistulas. Many prefer the use of small-caliber fine sutures for repair, particularly on the bladder aspect of the repair, but no data are available regarding this issue. Although rarely noted in the literature since Sims's original description, there are those that only repair the bladder while leaving the vaginal side open.

In Sims's original article, the closure was described as a single-layer closure, which was necessitated by the need to remove the silver sutures postoperatively. In modern surgical practice, many advocate multilayer closure, primarily to reduce the forces that tend to pull the first layer of closure apart but also to add additional tissue bulk between the bladder and vagina. Although data in an animal model have suggested that multilayer closure of a cystotomy is superior to single-layer closure in preventing a subsequent VVF, there are no data comparing the two options in the repair of a VVF once it is established.

Reported techniques also vary concerning whether suturing is interrupted or continuous, with no clear consensus as to which is the better approach in urogenital repair. The reported benefits of a continuous closure are primarily related to convenience, speed, and perhaps use of less suture. The theorized benefit of interrupted suture placement is that it provides a perpendicular orientation of the vector forces, keeping the wound together with the least tension for a given closing force. Increased tension leads to more pressure on the surrounding tissue and may lead to reduced blood flow at the incision where it is most needed for successful healing.

Perhaps the most intense debate has been regarding the route of vesicovaginal repair—transabdominal or transvaginal. There is general agreement that the vaginal repair is more convenient for the patient in terms of recovery, length of hospital stay, and cosmetic issues, but little agreement regarding which is the better operation. Absolute indications for an abdominal approach include conditions that require bladder augmentation (a small capacity or poorly compliant bladder, as may occur following irradiation), a fistula involving or very close to a ureter that requires ureteral reimplantation, a combination fistula involving other intra-abdominal organs, inability to adequately expose the fistula transvaginally due to positioning, or other access problems (Table 43.5).

The debate over the route of repair is now further complicated by increasing numbers of laparoscopic series both with and without robotic assistance. The scarcity of VVFs and the absence of specified centers in developed countries will likely result in the continued absence of large well-designed randomized prospective trials in this setting. Ultimately, this is a

TABLE 43.5 Indications for Abdominal Vesicovaginal Fistula Repair

- Small capacity or poorly compliant bladder requiring bladder augmentation
- Fistula involving or very close to a ureter requiring ureteral reimplantation
- Combination fistula involving other intra-abdominal organs
- Inability to adequately expose the fistula transvaginally

decision best made between a patient who is well informed regarding the various options, their advantages, and disadvantages and an experienced pelvic surgeon capable of tailoring the approach to the specific circumstances at hand.

Repair of urethrovaginal fistulas is different from VVF repair given the added issues related to whether the sphincter complex is affected as well as the possibility that urethral stenosis may develop with consequent urinary retention. Reconstruction of the urethra often involves less readily available tissue when compared to VVF repair; thus, some advocate the frequent use of the Martius graft. An added level of complexity is noted in recent increases of fistulas associated with synthetic suburethral slings. The periurethral scarring frequently requires more extensive and difficult urethral repair, which is further complicated by the need to remove the surrounding graft material. Despite these apparent complicating factors, it seems that the overall success rates for both vesicovaginal and urethrovaginal fistula repairs are similar.

When preparing patients for surgical correction of a urogenital fistula, detailed informed consent and discussion are very important. Patients with urogenital fistulas as complications of benign pelvic surgery have already experienced an adverse outcome that they may or may not have been prepared for. They invariably have some degree of frustration, anxiety, and suspicion. All aspects of operative risk should be discussed with the patient prior to fistula repair, including the likelihood of fistula recurrence. Even in the event of successful anatomic repair, the occurrence or persistence of lower urinary tract symptoms such as incontinence, overactive bladder, voiding dysfunction, and bladder pain should be discussed. Discussing the expected recovery course of the various available approaches and potential adverse consequences of associated procedures such as episiotomy or Schuchardt incisions, disfigurement from flaps, and discomfort from suprapubic and transurethral catheters seems to prepare patients for some of the difficulties that may lie ahead. This information should be incorporated into the discussion to decide on the route of repair—a discussion in which the patient should ideally be an active participant. When ureteral reimplantation may be required, the need for stenting and subsequent cystoscopic stent removal should be discussed, as well as the need for drains, the risk of ureteral stenosis, and the need for subsequent radiologic follow-up. Patients undergoing a vaginal repair should be made aware of the possibility of conversion to an abdominal procedure, although this is a rare occurrence.

Outcomes of Surgical Repair

In a contemporary retrospective cohort study spanning 10 years and derived from the English National Health Service inpatient database, 905 urogenital fistula repairs were noted and 11.9% required a repeat operation. This report did not differentiate the route of the surgical approach.

VII

Through the abdomin, the physician can utilize the transperitoneal–transvesical approach made popular by O'Conor and Sokol, which involves bivalving of the bladder or avoid entering the peritoneal cavity by a retropubic transvesical repair introduced by Landes, which involves entering the bladder through an anterior cystotomy that does not communicate contiguously with the fistula. Success rates for the transperitoneal–transvesical approach have been between 86% and 100% for benign, nonirradiated fistulas. Furthermore, a technique termed a mini-O'Conor that involves a less extensive bladder incision than originally described reported 100% success in 26 supratrigonal VVFs. In data pooled from three studies reporting variations of the retroperitoneal transvesical technique, with a total of 91 fistula patients (primary and recurrent), the success rate is 100%. In a series comparing a center's experience between vaginal and abdominal approaches for the repair of supratrigonal VVFs, the rates of successful repair were comparable (94.8% vs. 100%, respectively, $n = 48$).

A number of laparoscopic series have been published since Nezhat et al. first published their case report of laparoscopic repair of a VVF in 1994, with reported success rates that are comparable to the open approaches with benefits demonstrated that are inherent to a minimally invasive approach. The vast majority of these reports are transperitoneal–transvesical in the manner of a traditional O'Conor technique, although primarily through smaller cystotomy incisions, thus avoiding bivalving the bladder while maintaining the ability to place an interposition flap when needed. Laparoscopic case series are numerous, mostly consisting of 10 patients or less (some much less) with success rates of 93% to 100%.

In the largest published series thus far, Shah reported on 25 patients with planned laparoscopic transperitoneal–transvesical management of VVFs. Of these fistulas, 64% were posthysterectomy with the rest related to various obstetrical circumstances. Of the 22 patients that had undergone laparoscopic management (three required laparotomy due to dense adhesions), the success rate was 86%.

A transperitoneal extravesical laparoscopic technique is also described in which entry into the bladder is made through the fistula itself once the vesicovaginal space has been developed to the area of the fistula. Fistula cure rates of 91% to 100% were reported using this particular approach, including an omental flap.

Even fewer reports are found in the literature regarding laparoendoscopic single-site surgery (LESS) for the repair of VVFs. One such report involved 5 patients with a transperitoneal extravesical approach with success. A single case report of LESS using a suprapubic transvesical access similar to the open version reported by Landes has been described as well.

The experience in the literature regarding robotically assisted laparoscopic repair of VVFs is again dominated by very small case series (all are seven patients or less, and most had no more than three patients) since the first case report by Melamud et al. in 2005. These case reports and series demonstrate the technique and feasibility of the transperitoneal robotic approach using either a transvesical or extravesical technique, but represent very early experiences utilizing this new technology. A retrospective study compared open versus robotically assisted laparoscopic O'Conor-type repair of recurrent VVF. Gupta et al. report 100% success in their 12 robotic cases, which were a result of obstetrical as well as gynecologic etiologies, compared to 90% among their 20 open cases. This difference was not statistically significant.

Vaginal repairs of VVFs have reported success rates of 92% to 97% in the larger series in the literature. These vaginal procedures encompass various techniques with the variations as discussed previously. No comparative studies are available to determine which specific vaginal procedure, if any, is superior. As such, it is clearly advantageous that surgeons who repair these lesions be comfortable with several different approaches and individualize their techniques to the particular case at hand.

Various techniques have been described to augment fistula repairs, both for the transabdominal and transvaginal approaches. This is thought to bring additional tissue to interpose between the bladder and the vagina but more importantly, a healthy blood supply. Occasionally, such grafts also serve to fill in lost tissue space, as with large fistulas where a large amount of tissue is lost. The routine use of interposition grafts has been advanced by some; however, most surgeons use these adjuncts based on individualized clinical judgment. It is generally agreed that tissue interposition is needed in irradiation-induced fistulas or in other instances where there is local vascular compromise, such as recurrent, severely scarred, or previously infected fistulas. Transabdominally, the omentum is most often used with excellent results. In one series, a 100% (10/10) success rate with such interposition grafts compared with 63% (12/19) when grafts were not used in benign VVFs repaired transabdominally.

Rangnekar et al. report on Martius bulbocavernosus fat pad grafting to reinforce 21 obstetric urethrovaginal and VVF repairs performed transvaginally. Seven patients of 8 (87%) were cured of their urethrovaginal fistula, whereas all 13 patients (100%) with VVFs were cured with use of the Martius graft. For extremely large defects, a myocutaneous modification of the Martius bulbocavernosus graft has been described. The island of skin after sublabial transfer was sutured to the defect in the vaginal wall. Such modified repair has been suggested for large obstetric or irradiation-induced fistulas. Eilber et al. report long-term results of transvaginal repair of complex or recurrent VVFs with either peritoneal interposition graft for fistulas high in the vault or Martius flap or labial flap for distal defects. Cure rates were 96% of 83 patients with peritoneal graft and 97% of 34 patients with Martius fat pad graft.

Fistulas that form within a previously irradiated field are more prone to recurrence, and most surgeons would agree that additional pedicled flaps are needed in their surgical repair because of the inherent microvascular compromise. In a large series of 210 cases, the primary approach was vaginal (97%). Martius fat pad transposition was used in 41% of the cases. The overall primary repair success rate was 48%, and with multiple interventions the cumulative success rate was 80%.

Alternative vascular flaps have been described in difficult cases. In six patients who failed urethrovaginal fistula closure with Martius transposition, Bruce et al. report 100% successful resolution of the fistula when treated with a pedicled, tubularized rectus abdominis muscle flap interposed suburethrally. In a more recent small series by Svaerdborg et al., such a vascular muscle flap was used to successfully manage postradiation VVF without closure of the bladder or vaginal aspects of the fistula. Myocutaneous flaps have also been described, including gracilis and rectus abdominis.

Urethrovaginal fistula repair outcomes are often reported in terms of anatomical and continence cure rates. Anatomic cure rates in surgical series have been reported to be 82% to 92%, while continence cure rate is 80%. Urethral obstruction related to stenosis has been reported in about 10% of cases.

UROGENITAL FISTULA REPAIR—TECHNICAL DETAILS

Vesicovaginal Fistula Repair

See the Steps in the Procedure box for general surgical steps required in the repair of a VVF. This is followed by a detailed discussion of the surgeries described in the literature.

STEPS IN THE PROCEDURE

Vesicovaginal Fistula Repair

- Evaluate fistula cystoscopically and vaginally to assess size, location relative to known landmarks (urethra, trigone, and ureters), and the quality of the injured tissue.

- If timing deemed appropriate, proceed with VVF repair as outlined below. Ureteral catheterization is needed if the fistula is close to the ureter(s). Place transurethral Foley catheter.

- Access the fistula vaginally, intraperitoneally, and/or transvesically (see text for details). Use fine instruments and surgical technique as well as delicate tissue handling while optimizing visualization using gentle suction and copious irrigation. Avoid prolonged clamping of the vagina or bladder during the repair, and avoid electrocautery near the injury.

- Circumscribe the fistula, and sharply dissect the vesicovaginal space sufficiently to allow tension-free closure, keeping ureteral anatomy and safety constantly in mind.

- Excise the fistula tract, and send it for histopathologic evaluation. The tract is not excised if a Latzko procedure is performed.

- Reassess tissue for significant fibrosis and, if appropriate, further excise until healthy, well-vascularized tissue is encountered.

- Reassess the vesicovaginal dissection to ensure adequate separation of bladder from vagina and a tension-free repair. Approximately 1 cm circumferentially beyond the edges to be reapproximated is needed.

- The order of closure depends upon the route of VVF repair. Depicted in Figure 43.3 is a transvaginal repair; if transperitoneal or transvesical, the vaginal closure is completed first.

- Close the urothelial (lamina propria) layer with interrupted or running fine 3-0 delayed absorbable suture.

- Reapproximate the muscular layer with interrupted 2-0 or 3-0 delayed absorbable suture. Place the sutures in a staggered fashion, thus avoiding overlapping sutures one atop the other. Ensure hemostasis in the vesicovaginal space.

- A third imbricating layer of bladder muscularis to further reinforce the repair may be possible using interrupted 3-0 delayed absorbable suture.

- Perform cystoscopy to ensure the following:
  - Intravesical hemostasis. Irrigate with small volumes of fluid, and remove any blood clots that may obstruct catheter drainage.
  - Integrity of the repair by looking vaginally for spillage of cystoscopy fluid.
  - Absence of injury or obstruction to the ureter using intravenous indigo carmine.

- Determine whether an interposition graft is needed (see text for details), and if perrformed, ensure adequate vascularity and stable interposition into the vesicovaginal space.

- Close the vaginal side of the fistula separately with interrupted 2-0 or 0 delayed absorbable suture. It is preferable to perform the bladder and vaginal closures in different orientations, one vertical and the other horizontal. If the same orientation is chosen, place the sutures in a staggered fashion, thus avoiding overlapping sutures.

- Determine whether a three-way Foley is needed for postoperative bladder irrigation in the face of hematuria.

Vaginal Approach

The patient is placed in the dorsal lithotomy position using candy-cane stirrups. Examination under anesthesia is performed with water cystoscopy. The 30 degrees or 70 degrees lens is used to best visualize the fistula intravesically and identify any associated abnormalities. Identify the intravesical and vaginal openings, and assess the tract's angle and rule out multiple tracts. The fistula's proximity to the ureters is assessed, and transvaginal repair is continued if it is not too close. Ureteral stenting may be done to continuously identify the ureters if needed. Dilation of the fistulous tract allows an 8-French Foley catheter to be inserted and the balloon inflated. Appropriate traction allows the fistula to be brought distally for better access and exposure. When the tissue surrounding the fistula is extensively scarred, subepithelial injection of saline may be used to facilitate dissection of the vaginal flap. Some authors advocate the injection of epinephrine or vasopressin to diminish surgical bleeding; some concern may be delayed bleeding into the vesicovaginal space once the vasoconstrictive activity is past, which can undermine the repair.

The vaginal mucosa is incised circumferentially around the fistulous opening; the vaginal mucosa is then carefully dissected off the bladder to a distance that will allow tension-free multiple-layer closure, approximately 1 to 2 cm radially around the incision. All tissue must be handled delicately with fine instruments that are of sufficient length to reach all levels of the fistula and the dissected tissues. Excellent hemostasis is best achieved with liberal use of pressure and subsequent suture closure, avoiding the use of electrocautery if at all possible. The fistula collar is excised and sent for pathologic evaluation. Repeat cystoscopy verifies the location of the ureters in relation to the somewhat larger fistulous opening. A suprapubic catheter is then placed. The bladder mucosa is closed in the direction of least tension (side to side or proximal to distal) with interrupted 3-0 or 4-0 delayed absorbable sutures, placed approximately 0.5 cm apart. Proximal-to-distal orientation is chosen if the ureters are in close proximity to the defect once the fistula is excised. If extramucosal suturing is possible, it is preferred; however, if desired or if mucosal edge bleeding is encountered, through-and-through suturing may be considered. A second layer consisting of bladder muscularis is brought

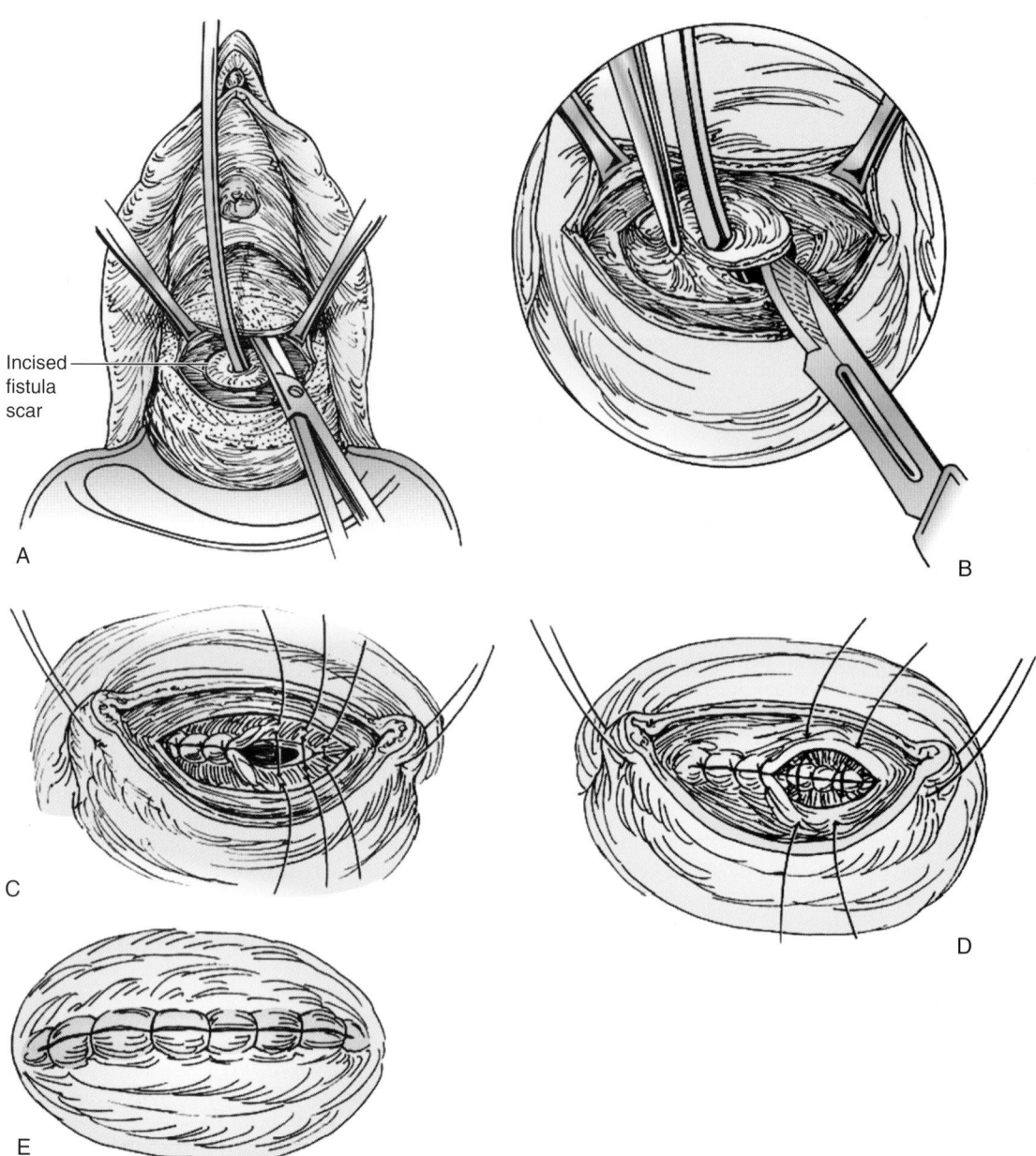

FIGURE 43.3 Traditional vesicovaginal fistula repair. **A:** Initial incision of a circumferential collar around the fistulous opening. The vaginal epithelium is sharply dissected radially from the collar. **B:** The fistula is excised sharply, making sure that healthy tissue is left to be reapproximated. Excessive trimming, increasing the loss of tissue, should be avoided. **C:** Interrupted fine, delayed absorbable suture on a small tapered needle is used, extramucosally if possible, to close the first layer. Stitches are placed approximately 0.5 cm apart with sufficient purchase of tissue to securely close the defect. **D:** The second layer imbricates over the first with suture being placed in a staggered fashion into the bladder muscularis so as not to overlap the sutures of these layers. **E:** The vaginal epithelium is closed with interrupted delayed absorbable suture after ensuring proper hemostasis in the vesicovaginal space. (Adapted with permission from Kovac SR, Zimmerman CW. *Advances in reconstructive vaginal surgery.* Philadelphia, PA: Lippincott, Williams & Wilkins, 2006.)

together over the first suture line, so it imbricates over it. This is achieved with interrupted suture that is placed staggered in between the underlying stitches on the first layer (Fig. 43.3). If the bladder peritoneum can be mobilized over the repair, it is accomplished at this point. If a Martius fat pad transposition is desired, this may be done instead of the peritoneal layer at this time. The vaginal mucosa is then closed with interrupted suture preferably in a different orientation than that of the bladder closure. At all stages of the

closure, the absence of tension on each level is paramount to successful repair, as is hemostasis and verification of healthy, well-vascularized tissue for apposition. Cystoscopy may be used to verify watertight closure of the fistula, suture line hemostasis, and integrity of the ureters, but care must be taken to limit retrograde filling to avoid placing the fresh suture line under tension.

The Latzko procedure begins in a similar fashion with a circumscribing incision and dissection of the vagina off the

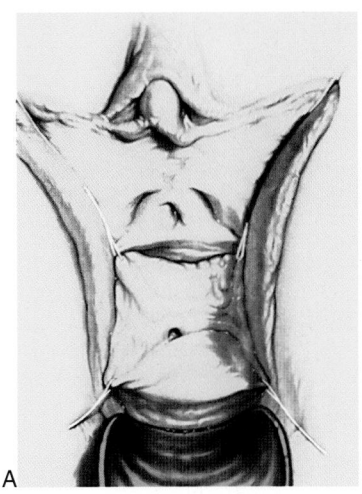
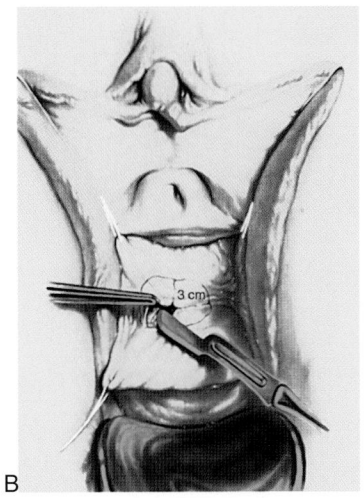
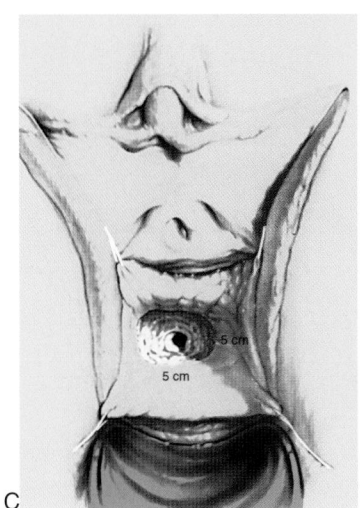

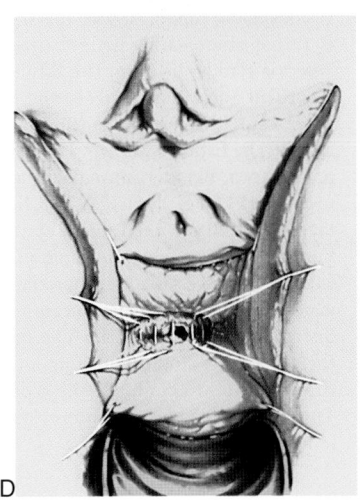
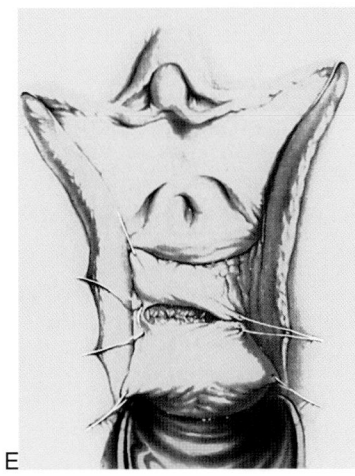

FIGURE 43.4 Latzko procedure. **A:** Stay sutures are placed to help stabilize and bring the fistula distally towards the operating surgeon. **B:** Vaginal epithelium is sharply dissected and excised circumferentially about the fistula. **C:** Completed epithelial excision around the fistula. **D:** First extramucosal layer of closure. **E:** Closure of the vaginal epithelial layer. (Adapted with permission from Ostergard DR, Bent AE, Cundiff GW, et al. *Ostergard's urogynecology and pelvic floor dysfunction*, 6th ed. Philadelphia, PA: Lippincott, Williams & Wilkins, 2007.)

cervicovaginal fascia (Fig. 43.4). Instead of excising the fistulous tract, it is imbricated into the bladder cavity with sequential layers of interrupted 3-0 or 4-0 delayed absorbable suture on a small tapered needle. Care should be taken to stagger the sutures so none lay atop the next layer. Cystoscopy should be used to verify watertight closure of the fistula and integrity of the ureters, but care must be taken to limit retrograde filling to avoid placing the fresh suture line under tension.

Abdominal Approach
Retropubic Transvesical Vesicovaginal Fistula Repair
This procedure is indicated for simple posthysterectomy VVF when adequate vaginal exposure cannot be obtained or can be obtained only with a Schuchardt or episiotomy incision and the patient prefers an abdominal approach. A Cherney or midline abdominal wall incision is made, the retropubic space is entered, and a midline vertical incision is made in the anterior bladder. The ureteral orifices are inspected and catheterized if needed. The fistula is identified and dilated to admit an 8-French pediatric Foley catheter after the position of the ureters is verified and the balloon inflated. A pediatric Foley catheter is placed through the fistula and the balloon inflated. Traction on the Foley allows improved access, and a circumscribing incision is made 2 to 3 mm from the fistula

and the vesicovaginal space dissected circumferentially 1 to 2 cm outward. The fistula may be excised or kept in situ (as originally described by Landes) and the defect closed in layers with the vaginal layer first using interrupted delayed absorbable 3-0 suture and the knots placed within the vaginal lumen. The bladder muscularis is closed next with knots placed in the vesicovaginal space. A third row incorporating bladder muscularis and mucosa is closed with 4-0 suture (Fig. 43.5). Ureteral integrity is verified. If a suprapubic catheter is used, it is placed through a separate incision. The bladder incision is closed with running delayed absorbable suture in two layers. Cystoscopy is used to verify watertight closure and ureteral integrity prior to wound closure, but care must be taken to limit retrograde filling to avoid placing the fresh suture line under tension.

Transvesical–Transperitoneal Vesicovaginal Repair
Intraperitoneal access is obtained by laparotomy, laparoscopy, or robotically, and the bladder is vertically bisected in the midline. Ureteral catheterization is particularly helpful with laparoscopic and robotic access. The original description depicted starting this incision at the retropubic anterior portion of the bladder, but a less extensive bisection is possible and may be used according to the specific circumstance

VII

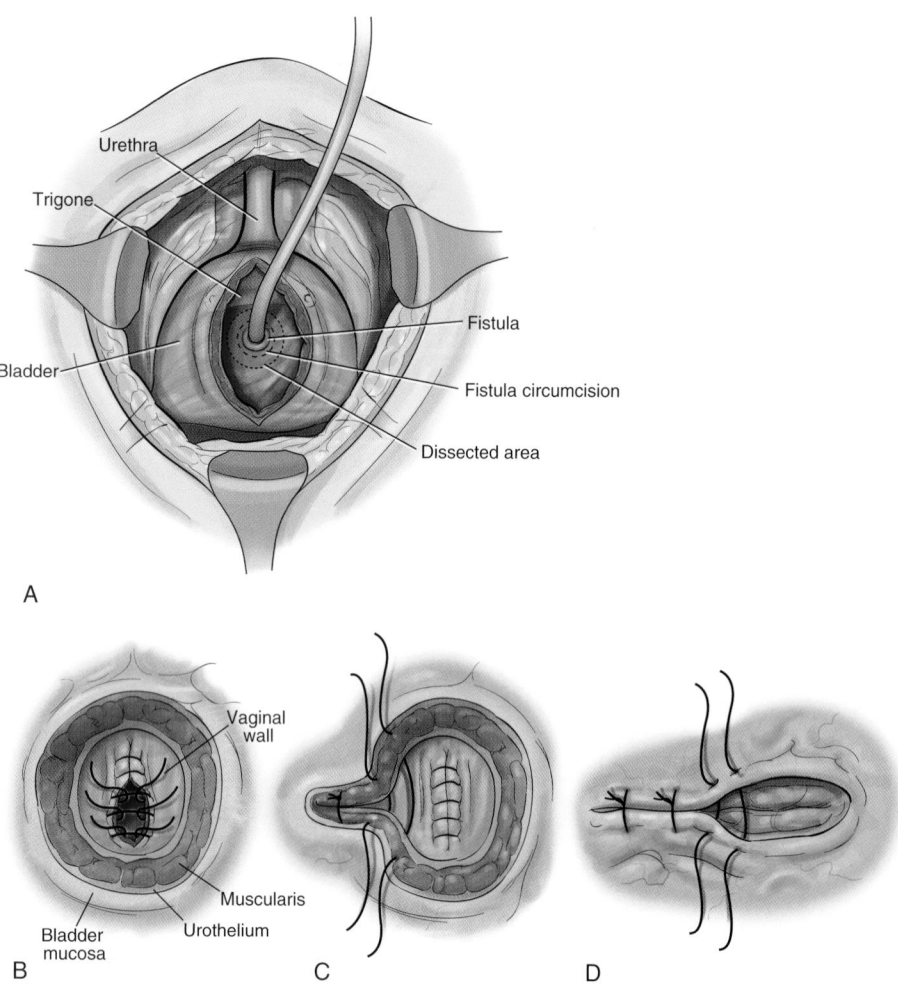

A

B

C

D

FIGURE 43.5 Retropubic intravesical vesicovaginal repair. **A:** The approach is retropubic, with retroperitoneal anterior bladder incision. The fistula is identified and circumscribed, and the vesicovaginal space is dissected radially. **B:** The fistula is shown with vaginal mucosa, bladder muscularis, and urothelial layers depicted. The first layer incorporates the vaginal epithelium in a vertical closure using interrupted suture. **C:** Bladder muscularis is closed with interrupted suture in a horizontal orientation. **D:** The urothelial layer is closed with fine interrupted suture to complete the repair. The anterior bladder incision is closed in layers.

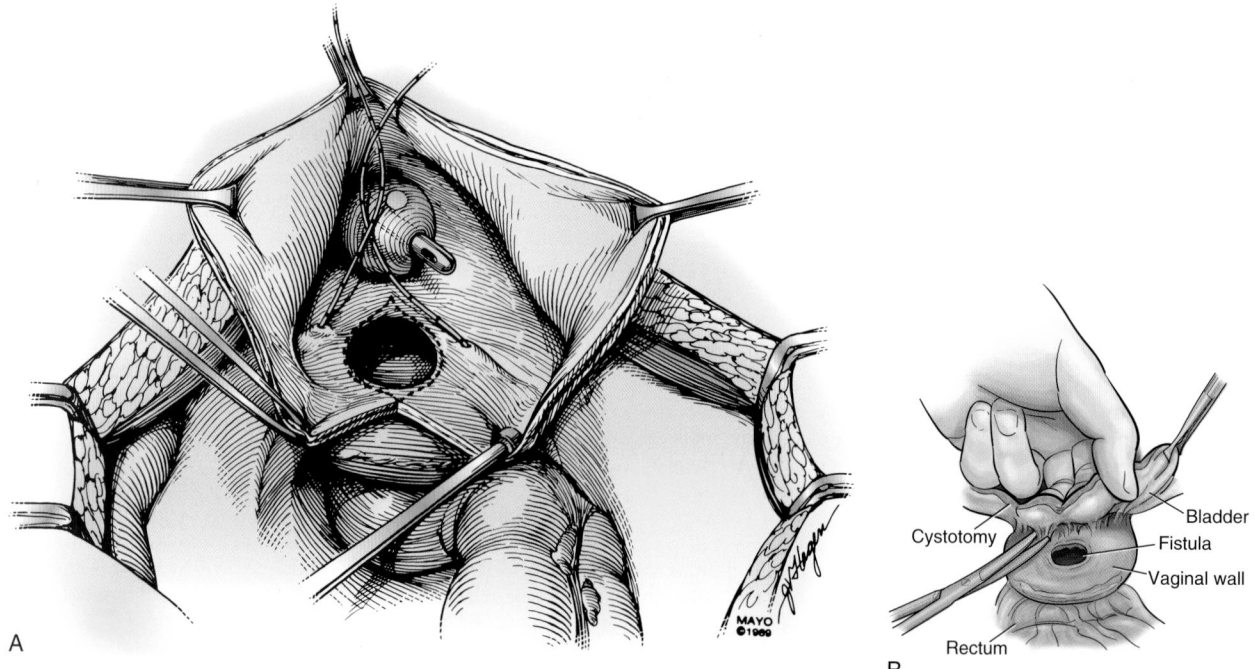

A

B

FIGURE 43.6 Transperitoneal–transvesical vesicovaginal fistula repair. **A:** The bladder is incised midline from its anterior portion back posteriorly until the fistula is reached; the fistula is excised, and the ureters are protected. **B:** Dissection is continued in the vesicovaginal space distal to the fistula to allow tension-free closure in layers.

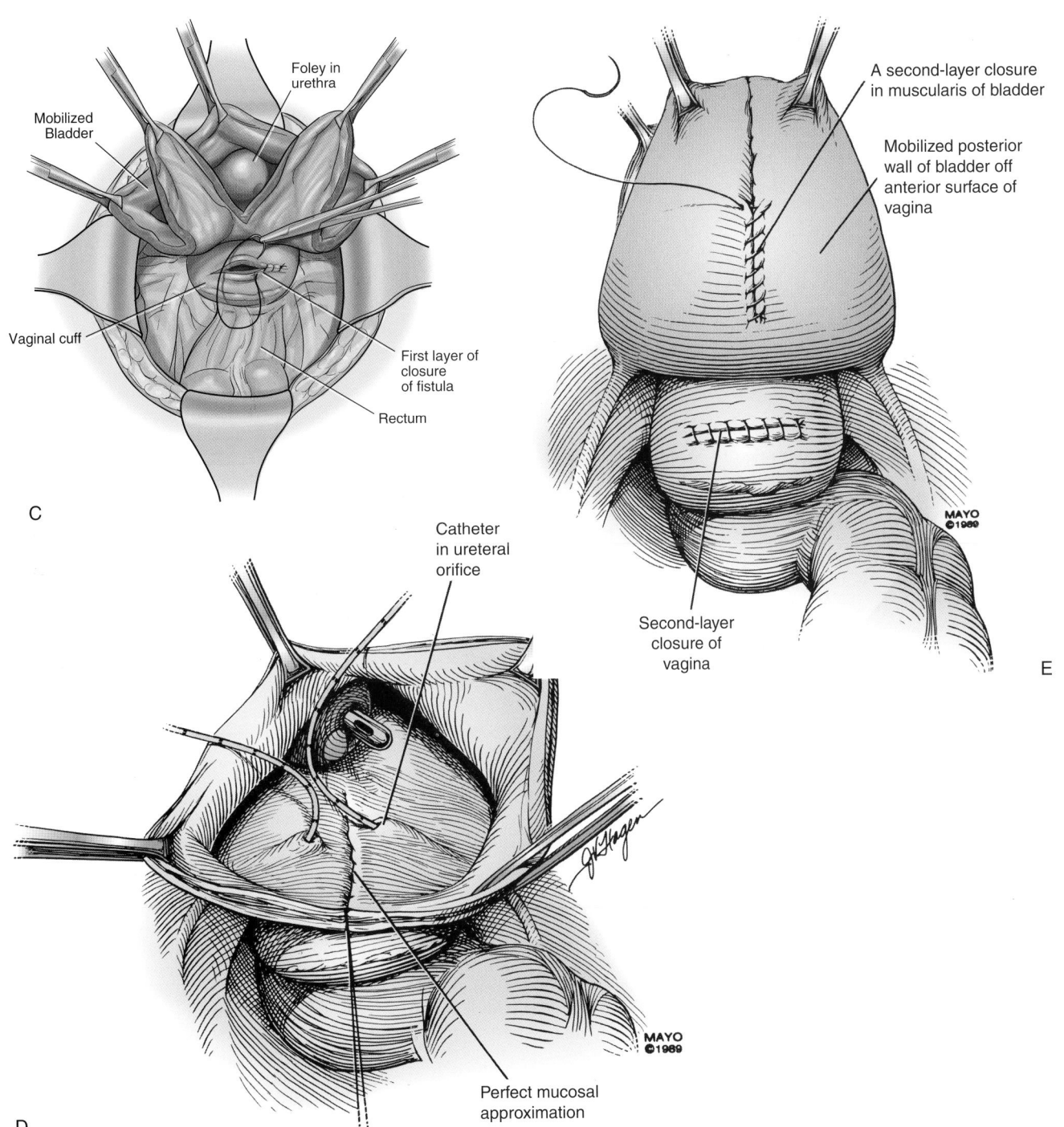

FIGURE 43.6 (*Continued*) **C:** The vagina is closed with interrupted delayed absorbable suture with the knots located inside the vagina. A second layer of closure is depicted in the insert. **D:** The dependent portion of the bladder is usually closed with interrupted double-layer closure of the bladder. Depicted in the figure is a single-layer submucosal running suture that was elected due to the very large size of the fistula and its proximity to the ureters. **E:** The rest of the bladder incision is closed with running suture in two layers. (From Lee RA. *Atlas of gynecologic surgery.* Philadelphia, PA: WB Saunders, 1992. By permission of Mayo Foundation for Medical Education and Research. All rights reserved.)

at hand (**Fig. 43.6**). Regardless, the incision is continued to the posterior bladder until it reaches the vesicovaginal space, which is then sharply dissected laterally and distally until the fistula is encountered, using gentle anterior bladder traction with posterior vaginal stabilization. The fistula is identified, and the tract is excised, while ureteral integrity is verified and continually visualized during the surgery. The vagina is closed transversely with interrupted delayed

absorbable suture with the knots within the vaginal lumen. A second layer of vagina is used to imbricate the first if sufficient tissue is found. The bladder is closed in two layers side to side with fine absorbable suture to reapproximate the urothelial and muscular layers without tension. Prior to complete closure of the bladder, a suprapubic catheter may be placed through a separate stab incision. If an omental flap is deemed necessary, it is suggested to place the anchoring

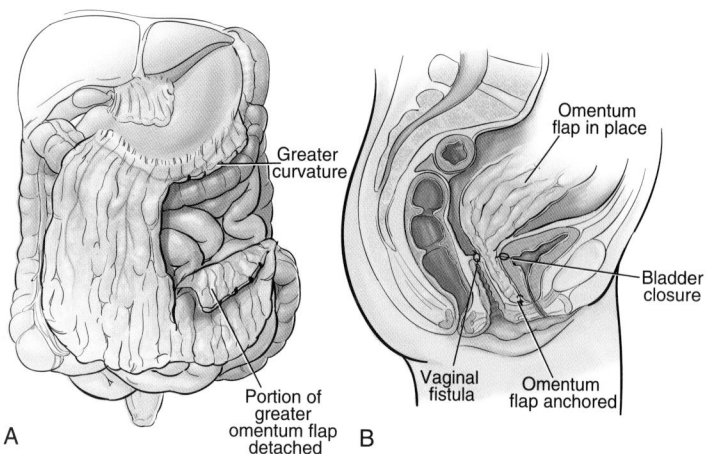

FIGURE 43.7 Omental flap. **A:** The omentum is partially detached by severing its vasculature on the left along the greater curvature of the stomach. **B:** This results in extra length so the flap will reach the vesicovaginal space, and is anchored by absorbable suture as depicted.

sutures after vaginal closure but prior to bladder closure to improve accessibility. Once the bladder closure is complete, these sutures are attached to the omental flap and tied into the vesicovaginal space (Fig. 43.7). Cystoscopy with small-volume distension is used to verify watertight closure, and care is taken to avoid having any significant blood clots in the bladder that may impede catheter drainage.

When the fistula is adjacent to the ureteral orifice, ureteroneocystostomy must be performed at the time of fistula repair (see Chapter 39). Once the dependent portion of the repair is complete, attention is turned to performing the ureteroneocystostomy. The implantation site should be placed in the posterior aspect of the bladder but sufficiently distant from the repair site. A double-J stent is placed and left for 4 to 6 weeks. The anastomosis site is drained with a Jackson-Pratt drain brought out through a separate stab incision.

Urethrovaginal Fistula Repair

STEPS IN THE PROCEDURE

Repair of a Urethrovaginal Fistula

- Evaluate the fistula cystoscopically and vaginally to assess size, location relative to known landmarks (urethra, trigone, and ureters), and the quality of the injured tissue.
- Place transurethral Foley.
- Circumscribe the urethrovaginal fistula with proximal and distal midline extensions. Then, carefully dissect the urethrovaginal space laterally on both sides avoiding any electrocautery and sufficient to allow for tension-free closure and expose the paraurethral tissue.
- If severe fibrosis noted, carefully excise the fistulous tract until significant scar is removed.
- Close the urethra by placing interrupted fine, 3-0 or 4-0 delayed absorbable suture on a small tapered needle through the muscularis while avoiding intramucosal placement if possible.
- The second layer is closed with interrupted 3-0 delayed absorbable suture utilizing the paraurethral tissue (pubocervical fascia) previously exposed. Place

the sutures in a staggered fashion, thus avoiding overlapping sutures.
- Martius fat pad transposition is recommended to further support these repairs, particularly if recurrent, there is significant scarring (such as occurs associated with mesh), or the paraurethral second layer closure is absent or deficient in any way.
- Close the vaginal incision with 3-0 or 2-0 delayed absorbable suture in an interrupted and staggered fashion to avoid overlapping sutures.

The same principles of careful handling of tissues, good hemostasis, and tension-free apposition of tissues must be maintained with surgical correction of urethrovaginal fistulas. A distal fistula may rarely be closed in a proximal-to-distal orientation to limit the possibility of urethral stenosis; otherwise, these defects are closed side to side in layers. Eversion of the fistula edges into the limited space of the urethral lumen is not recommended, and transmucosally placed sutures are to be avoided. If there is adequate substance, the fistula is minimally excised, but often, there is enough loss of urethral wall that this may be impossible without resultant stricture formation (Fig. 43.8). A second layer is often created by imbricating paraurethral tissue over the first layer. Liberal use of the Martius flap to support these repairs is advocated by many, particularly if a second layer is not feasible (Fig. 43.9).

Postoperative Care Ensuring proper bladder drainage is of utmost importance. If a suprapubic catheter is chosen, then combined transurethral and suprapubic drainage is performed early on. The transurethral catheter is removed once significant gross hematuria has cleared, usually 1 to 2 days. This often takes longer with the transvesical–transperitoneal (especially if done open) than with the vaginal approach. The suprapubic catheter is left for 2 to 3 weeks depending on the complexity of the repair. Some advocate routine evaluation with a cystogram prior to its removal; others do not. The option of having catheter drainage that is exclusively transurethral is also feasible and may be associated with less potential for complications.

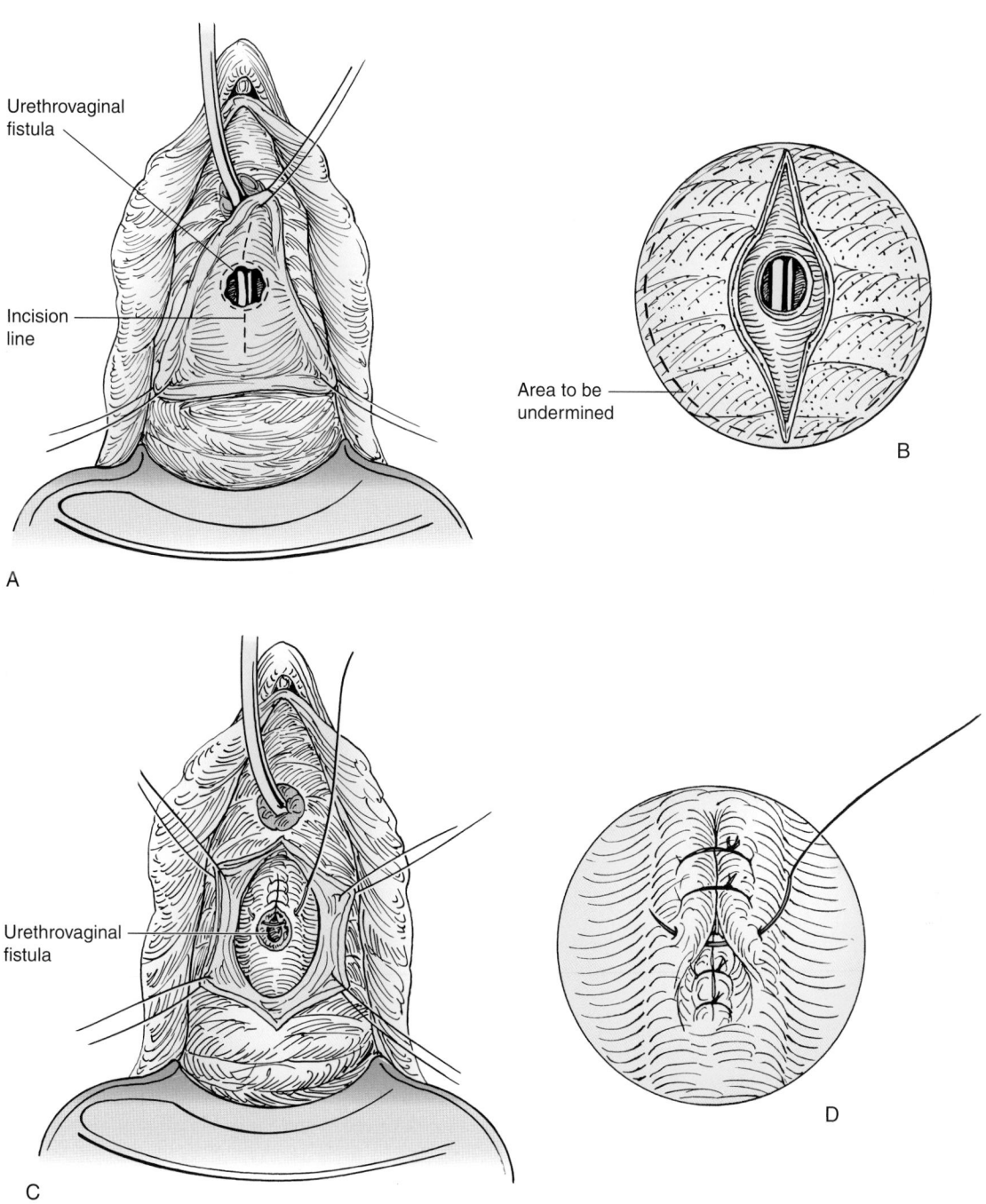

FIGURE 43.8 Urethrovaginal fistula repair. **A:** Note the initial circumferential incision with midline extension proximally and distally. **B:** Further lateral dissection exposes paraurethral tissue and allows for tension-free closure. **C:** The first layer is closed by interrupted fine, delayed absorbable suture on a small tapered needle, avoiding intramucosal placement. **D:** The second is an interrupted imbricating layer of paraurethral tissue. Martius fat pad transposition is occasionally needed to further support these repairs. If not, the vaginal epithelium is closed to complete the repair. (Adapted with permission from Kovac SR, Zimmerman CW. *Advances in reconstructive vaginal surgery*. Philadelphia, PA: Lippincott, Williams & Wilkins, 2006.)

Avoiding bladder spasms is considered important in preventing recurrence, although this has not been well studied. Some patients have severe pain associated with bladder spasms, and these may require belladonna and opioid suppositories. For most patients, standard anticholinergic medication is sufficient to prevent these spasms and detrusor overactivity if needed.

Vaginal packing rarely seems necessary following fistula surgery. Vaginal intercourse is prohibited for 2 to 3 months, to allow complete healing of the suture line. The use of vaginal estrogen cream is encouraged preoperatively to allow for reepithelialization of the incision in patients with vaginal atrophy.

VII

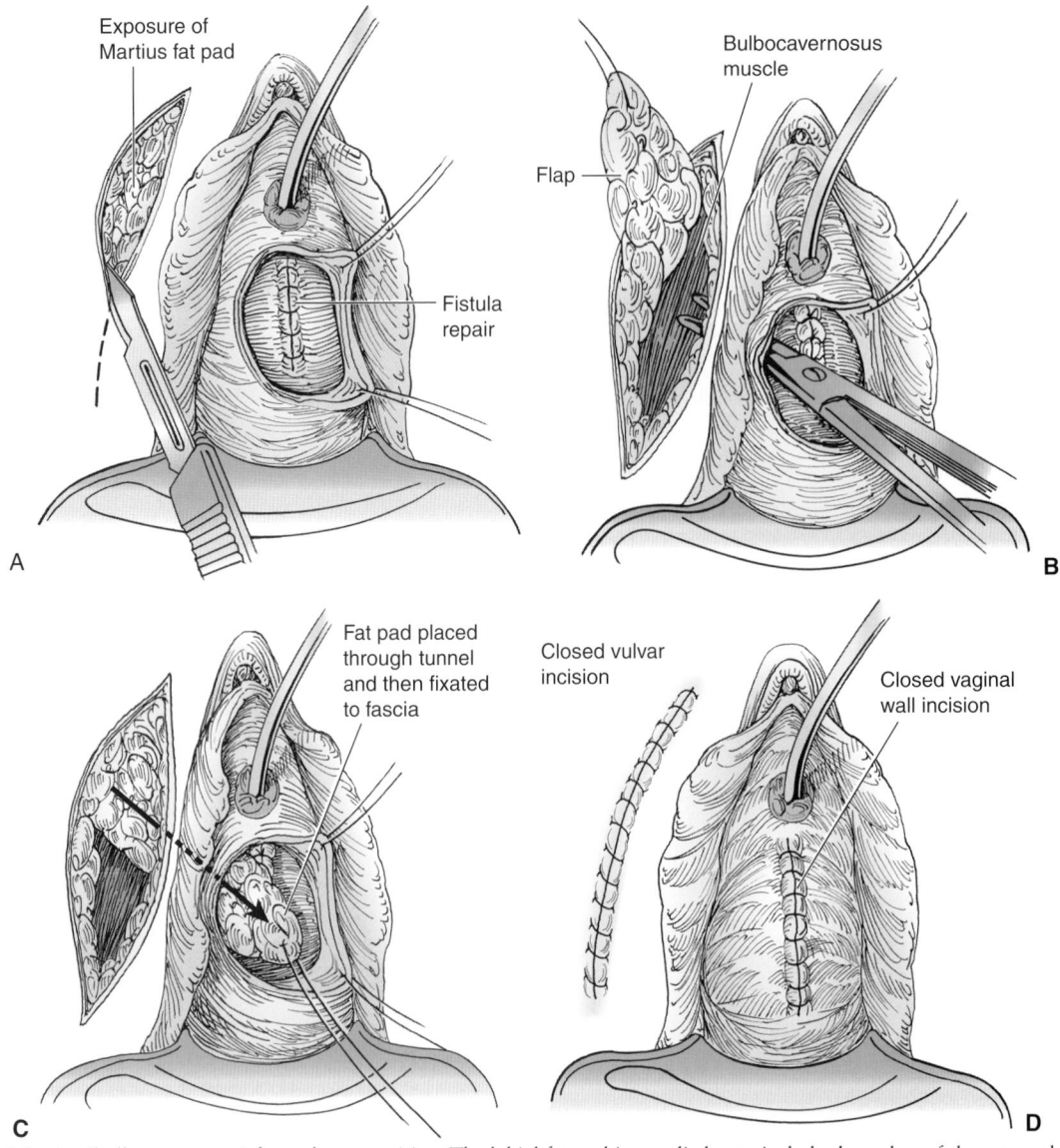

FIGURE 43.9 Martius (bulbocavernosus) fat pad transposition. The labial fat pad is supplied anteriorly by branches of the external pudendal and obturator arteries, and posteriorly by branches of the internal pudendal artery. Although traditionally the posterior blood supply was thought to be of superior quality, the graft may be swung anteriorly or posteriorly depending on the need of the surgeon. **A:** An incision is made over the labial fat pad, and it is dissected bluntly and with electrocautery ensuring adequate hemostasis and a continued adequate blood supply from the chosen pedicle. **B:** Once the labial fat pad is partially detached, a submucosal tunnel is created and enlarged to ensure adequate blood flow to the tip of the graft. **C:** The graft is carefully pulled through the tunnel to the area needed. Once the graft is pulled through the tunnel, it is sutured in place. **D:** Hemostasis of the donor site is verified, the skin and vaginal mucosal incisions are closed. (Adapted with permission from Kovac SR, Zimmerman CW. *Advances in reconstructive vaginal surgery*. Philadelphia, PA: Lippincott, Williams & Wilkins, 2006.)

BIBLIOGRAPHY

Abdel-Karim AM, Mousa A, Hasouna M, et al. Laparoscopic transperitoneal extravesical repair of vesicovaginal fistula. *Int Urogynecol J* 2011;22:693.

Abdel-Karim AM, Moussa A, Elsalmy S. Laparoendoscopic single-site surgery extravesical repair of vesicovaginal fistula: early experience. *Urology* 2011;78:567.

Abrams P, Andersson KE, Birder L, et al. Fourth International Consultation on Incontinence Recommendations of the International Scientific Committee: evaluation and treatment of urinary incontinence, pelvic organ prolapse, and fecal incontinence. *Neurourol Urodyn* 2010;29:213.

Arias BE, Ridgeway B, Barber MD. Complications of neglected vaginal pessaries: case presentation and literature review. *Int Urogynecol J Pelvic Floor Dysfunct* 2008;19:1173.

Arrowsmith S, Hamlin EC, Wall LL. Obstructed labor injury complex: obstetric fistula formation and the multifaceted morbidity of maternal birth trauma in the developing world. *Obstet Gynecol Surv* 1996;51:568.

Asanuma H, Nakai H, Shishido S, et al. Congenital vesicovaginal fistula. *Int J Urol* 2000;7:195.

Bai SW, Kim SH, Kwon HS, et al. Surgical outcome of female genital fistula in Korea. *Yonsei Med J* 2002;43:315.

Bajory Z, Fekete Z, Kiraly I, et al. Consecutive vesicovaginal fistula for transobturator sling perforations and successful repairs with skin flap. *Neurourol Urodyn* 2011;30:1530.

Bazi T. Spontaneous closure of vesicovaginal fistulas after bladder drainage alone: review of the evidence. *Int Urogynecol J Pelvic Floor Dysfunct* 2007;18:329.

Beck RP, McCormick S, Nordstrom L. A 25-year experience with 519 anterior colporrhaphy procedures. *Obstet Gynecol* 1991;78:1011.

Bekker MD, Bevers RF, Elzevier HW. Transurethral and suprapubic mesh resection after prolift bladder perforation: a case report. *Int Urogynecol J* 2010;21:1301.

Bettez M, Tu le M, Carlson K, et al. 2012 update: guidelines for Adult Urinary Incontinence Collaborative Consensus document for the Canadian Urological Association. *Can Urol Assoc J* 2012; 6:354.

Billmeyer BR, Nygaard IE, Kreder KJ. Ureterouterine and vesicoureterovaginal fistulas as a complication of cesarean section. *J Urol* 2001;165:1212.

Blaivas JG, Heritz DM, Romanzi LJ. Early versus late repair of vesicovaginal fistulas: vaginal and abdominal approaches. *J Urol* 1995;153:1110.

Bland KG, Gelfand M. The influence of urinary bilharziasis on vesicovaginal fistula in relation to causation and healing. *Trans R Soc Trop Med Hyg* 1970;64:588.

Blandy JP, Badenoch DF, Fowler CG, et al. Early repair of iatrogenic injury to the ureter or bladder after gynecological surgery. *J Urol* 1991;146:761.

Bouya PA, Odzebe AW, Ondongo Atipo MA, et al. Stones associated with vesicovaginal fistulas. *Prog Urol* 2012;22:549.

Bouya PA, Odzebe AW, Otiobanda FG, et al. Urological complications of gynecologic surgery. *Prog Urol* 2011;21:875.

Bruce RG, El-Galley RE, Galloway NT. Use of rectus abdominis muscle flap for the treatment of complex and refractory urethrovaginal fistulas. *J Urol* 2000;163:1212.

Caquant F, Collinet P, Debodinance P, et al. Safety of trans vaginal mesh procedure: retrospective study of 684 patients. *J Obstet Gynaecol Res* 2008;34:449.

Carlin BI, Klutke CG. Development of urethrovaginal fistula following periurethral collagen injection. *J Urol* 2000;164:124.

Cass AS, Luxenberg M. Management of extraperitoneal ruptures of bladder caused by external trauma. *Urology* 1989;33:179.

Cogan S, Bedaiwy MA, Paraiso MF, et al. Healing patterns of bladder injuries incurred at laparoscopic hysterectomy: a histologic assessment. *Int Urogynecol J Pelvic Floor Dysfunct* 2007; 18:49.

Cogan SL, Paraiso MF, Bedaiwy MA. Formation of vesicovaginal fistulas in laparoscopic hysterectomy with electrosurgically induced cystotomy in female Mongrel dogs. *Am J Obstet Gynecol* 2002;187:1510.

Conrad S, Pieper A, De la Maza SF, et al. Long-term results of the Stamey bladder neck suspension procedure: a patient questionnaire based outcome analysis. *J Urol* 1997;157:1672.

Cromwell D, Hilton P. Retrospective cohort study on patterns of care and outcomes of surgical treatment for lower urinary-genital tract fistula among English National Health Service Hospitals between 2000 and 2009. *BJU Int* 2013;111:E257.

D'Arcy FT, Jaffry S. The treatment of vesicovaginal fistula by endoscopic injection of fibrin glue. *Surgeon* 2010;8:174.

Dalela D, Goel A, Shakhwar SN, et al. Vesical calculi with unrepaired vesicovaginal fistula: a clinical appraisal of an uncommon association. *J Urol* 2003;170:2206.

Dalela D, Ranjan P, Sankhwar PL, et al. Supratrigonal VVF repair by modified O'Connor's technique: an experience of 26 cases. *Eur Urol* 2006;49:551.

Dangle PP, Wang WP, Pohar KS. Vesicoenteric, vesicovaginal, vesicocutaneous fistula—an unusual complication with intravesical mitomycin. *Can J Urol* 2008;15:4269.

Das Mahapatra P, Bhattacharyya P. Laparoscopic intraperitoneal repair of high-up urinary bladder fistula: a review of 12 cases. *Int Urogynecol J Pelvic Floor Dysfunct* 2007;18:635.

Dass AK, Lo TS, Khanuengkitkong S, et al. A delayed type of ureteric injury developed after transobturator mesh procedure for massive prolapse. *Female Pelvic Med Reconstr Surg* 2013;19:179.

Dennis N, Wilkinson J, Robboy S, et al. Schistosomiasis and vesicovaginal fistula. *Afr J Reprod Health* 2009;13:137.

Dodero D, Corticelli A, Caporale E, et al. Endometriosis arises from implant of endometriotic cells outside the uterus: a report of active vesicouterine centrifugal fistula. *Clin Exp Obstet Gynecol* 2001;28:97.

Dogra PN, Saini AK. Laser welding of vesicovaginal fistula—outcome analysis and long-term outcome: single-centre experience. *Int Urogynecol J* 2011;22:981.

Dorairajan LN, Khattar N, Kumar S, et al. Latzko repair for vesicovaginal fistula revisited in the era of minimal-access surgery. *Int Urol Nephrol* 2008;40:317.

Drutz HP, Mainprize TC. Unrecognized small vesicovaginal fistula as a cause of persistent urinary incontinence. *Am J Obstet Gynecol* 1988;158:237.

Duong TH, Gellasch TL, Adam RA. Risk factors for the development of vesicovaginal fistula after incidental cystotomy at the time of a benign hysterectomy. *Am J Obstet Gynecol* 2009;201:512.e1.

Duong TH, Taylor DP, Meeks GR. A multicenter study of vesicovaginal fistula following incidental cystotomy during benign hysterectomies. *Int Urogynecol J* 2011;22:975.

Eilber KS, Kavaler E, Rodriguez LV, et al. Ten-year experience with transvaginal vesicovaginal fistula repair using tissue interposition. *J Urol* 2003;169:1033.

El-Hefnawy AS, El-Nahas AR, Osman Y, et al. Urinary complications of migrated intrauterine contraceptive device. *Int Urogynecol J Pelvic Floor Dysfunct* 2008;19:241.

El-Shalakany AH, Nasr El-Din MH, Wafa GA, et al. Massive vault necrosis with bladder fistula after uterine artery embolisation. *Br J Obstet Gynaecol* 2003;110:215.

Elkins TE. Fistula surgery: past, present and future directions. *Int Urogynecol J Pelvic Floor Dysfunct* 1997;8:30.

Evans DH, Madjar S, Politano VA, et al. Interposition flaps in transabdominal vesicovaginal fistula repairs: are they really necessary? *Urology* 2001;57:670.

Firoozi F, Ingber MS, Moore CK, et al. Purely transvaginal/perineal management of complications from commercial prolapse kits using a new prostheses/grafts complication classification system. *J Urol* 2012;187:1674.

Flisser AJ, Blaivas JG. Outcome of urethral reconstructive surgery in a series of 74 women. *J Urol* 2003;169:2246.

Flores-Carreras O, Cabrera JR, Galeano PA, et al. Fistulas of the urinary tract in gynecologic and obstetric surgery. *Int Urogynecol J Pelvic Floor Dysfunct* 2001;12:203.

Forsgren C, Lundholm C, Johansson AL, et al. Hysterectomy for benign indications and risk of pelvic organ fistula disease. *Obstet Gynecol* 2009;114:594.

Fourie T, Ramphal S. Aerosol caps and vesicovaginal fistulas. *Int J Gynaecol Obstet* 2001;73:275.

Frajzyngier V, Li G, Larson E, et al. Development and comparison of prognostic scoring systems for surgical closure of genitourinary fistula. *Am J Obstet Gynecol* 2013;208:112.e1.

Franciscus RG. When did the modern human pattern of childbirth arise? New insights from an old Neandertal pelvis. *Proc Natl Acad Sci U S A* 2009;106:9125.

Frankman EA, Wang L, Bunker CH, et al. Lower urinary tract injury in women in the United States, 1979–2006. *Am J Obstet Gynecol* 2010;202:495.e1.

Galczynski K, Futyma K, Bar K, et al. Bladder injury during sling operation in the treatment of Sui—review of literature and case report. *Ginekol Pol* 2012;83:784.

Ganabathi K, Leach GE, Zimmern PE, et al. Experience with the management of urethral diverticulum in 63 women. *J Urol* 1994;152: 1445.

Gaurish S, Prakash PS, Padmanabha Bhat A, et al. Tuberculosis as a cause of vesicovaginal fistula. *J Assoc Physicians India* 2009;57: 343.

Gharoro EP, Agholor KN. Aspects of psychosocial problems of patients with vesico-vaginal fistula. *J Obstet Gynaecol* 2009;29:644.

Ghatak DP. A study of urinary fistulae in Sokoto, Nigeria. *J Indian Med Assoc* 1992;90:285.

Gil-Vernet JM, Gil-Vernet A, Campos JA. New surgical approach for treatment of complex vesicovaginal fistula. *J Urol* 1989;141:513.

Gil A, Sultana CJ. Vesicouterine fistula after vacuum delivery and two previous cesarean sections. A case report. *J Reprod Med* 2001; 46:853.

Gilmour DT, Das S, Flowerdew G. Rates of urinary tract injury from gynecologic surgery and the role of intraoperative cystoscopy. *Obstet Gynecol* 2006;107:1366.

Goel A, Dalela D, Gupta S, et al. Pediatric tuberculous vesicovaginal fistula. *J Urol* 2004;171:389.

Goh JT, Howat P, de Costa C. Oestrogen therapy in the management of vesicovaginal fistula. *Aust N Z J Obstet Gynaecol* 2001;41:333.

Golomb J, Ben-Chaim J, Goldwasser B, et al. Conservative treatment of a vesicocervical fistula resulting from Shirodkar cervical cerclage. *J Urol* 1993;149:833.

Grody MH, Nyirjesy P, Chatwani A. Intravesical foreign body and vesicovaginal fistula: a rare complication of a neglected pessary. *Int Urogynecol J Pelvic Floor Dysfunct* 1999;10:407.

Gunderson CC, Nugent EK, Yunker AC, et al. Vaginal cancer: the experience from 2 large academic centers during a 15-year period. *J Low Genit Tract Dis* 2013;17:409.

Gupta NP, Mishra S, Hemal AK, et al. Comparative analysis of outcome between open and robotic surgical repair of recurrent supra-trigonal vesico-vaginal fistula. *J Endourol* 2010;24:1779.

Harkki-Siren P, Sjoberg J, Tiitinen A. Urinary tract injuries after hysterectomy. *Obstet Gynecol* 1998;92:113.

Hasan M, Firoozabadi D, Abedinzadeh M, et al. Genitourinary system trauma after 2003 Bam earthquake in Kerman, Iran. *Ther Clin Risk Manag* 2011;7:49.

Hemal AK, Kumar R, Nabi G. Post-cesarean cervicovesical fistula: technique of laparoscopic repair. *J Urol* 2001;165:1167.

Hilton P. Urodynamic findings in patients with urogenital fistulae. *Br J Urol* 1998;81:539.

Hilton P. Urethrovaginal fistula associated with 'sterile abscess' formation following periurethral injection of dextranomer/hyaluronic acid co-polymer (Zuidex) for the treatment of stress urinary incontinence—a case report. *Br J Obstet Gynaecol* 2009;116:1527.

Hilton P. Vesico-vaginal fistulas in developing countries. *Int J Gynaecol Obstet* 2003;82:285.

Hilton P. Urogenital fistula in the UK: a personal case series managed over 25 years. *BJU Int* 2012;110:102.

Hilton P, Cromwell DA. The risk of vesicovaginal and urethrovaginal fistula after hysterectomy performed in the English National Health Service—a retrospective cohort study examining patterns of care between 2000 and 2008. *Br J Obstet Gynaecol* 2012;119:1447.

Hilton P, Ward A. Epidemiological and surgical aspects of urogenital fistulae: a review of 25 years' experience in Southeast Nigeria. *Int Urogynecol J* 1998;9:189.

Holden D, Vere M, Manyonda I. Vesico-uterine fistula occurring in a woman with a previous caesarean section and two subsequent normal vaginal deliveries. *Br J Obstet Gynaecol* 1994;101:354.

Horch RE, Gitsch G, Schultze-Seemann W. Bilateral pedicled myocutaneous vertical rectus abdominis muscle flaps to close vesicovaginal and pouch-vaginal fistulas with simultaneous vaginal and perineal reconstruction in irradiated pelvic wounds. *Urology* 2002;60:502.

Huang CR, Sun N, Wei P, et al. The management of old urethral injury in young girls: analysis of 44 cases. *J Pediatr Surg* 2003;38:1329.

Ibeanu OA, Chesson RR, Echols KT, et al. Urinary tract injury during hysterectomy based on universal cystoscopy. *Obstet Gynecol* 2009;113:6.

Ibrahim T, Sadiq AU, Daniel SO. Characteristics of VVF patients as seen at the Specialist Hospital Sokoto, Nigeria. *West Afr J Med* 2000;19:59.

Ijaiya MA, Rahman AG, Aboyeji AP, et al. Vesicovaginal fistula: a review of Nigerian experience. *West Afr J Med* 2010;29:293.

Ikechebelu JI, Ugboaja JO, Okeke CF. Post-cesarean vesicouterine fistula (Youssef syndrome): report of two cases. *J Obstet Gynaecol Res* 2011;37:912.

Inaba K, McKenney M, Munera F, et al. Cystogram follow-up in the management of traumatic bladder disruption. *J Trauma* 2006;60:23.

Jelovsek JE, Chiung C, Chen G, et al. Incidence of lower urinary tract injury at the time of total laparoscopic hysterectomy. *JSLS* 2007;11:422.

Kleeman SD, Vasallo B, Segal J, et al. Vesicocervical fistula following insertion of a modified McDonald suture. *Br J Obstet Gynaecol* 2002;109:1408.

Kumar A, Goyal NK, Das SK, et al. Our experience with genitourinary fistulae. *Urol Int* 2009;82:404.

Landes RR. Simple transvesical repair of vesicovaginal fistula. *J Urol* 1979;122:604.

Langkilde NC, Pless TK, Lundbeck F. Surgical repair of vesicovaginal fistulae—a ten-year retrospective study. *Scand J Urol Nephrol* 1999;33:100.

Lee RA. Diverticulum of the female urethra: postoperative complications and results. *Obstet Gynecol* 1983;61:52.

Lee RA, Symmonds RE, Williams TJ. Current status of genitourinary fistula. *Obstet Gynecol* 1988;72:313.

Leng WW, Amundsen CL, McGuire EJ. Management of female genitourinary fistulas: transvesical or transvaginal approach? *J Urol* 1998;160:1995.

Likic IS, Kadija S, Ladjevic NG, et al. Analysis of urologic complications after radical hysterectomy. *Am J Obstet Gynecol* 2008;199:644.e1.

Lodh U, Kumar S, Arya MC, et al. Ureterouterine fistula as a complication of an elective abortion. *Aust N Z J Obstet Gynaecol* 1996;36:94.

Lovatsis D, Drutz HP. Persistent vesicovaginal fistula associated with endometriosis. *Int Urogynecol J Pelvic Floor Dysfunct* 2003;14:358.

Lovatsis D, Easton W, Wilkie D. Guidelines for the evaluation and treatment of recurrent urinary incontinence following pelvic floor surgery. *J Obstet Gynaecol Can* 2010;32:893.

Mahapatra TP, Rao MS, Rao K, et al. Vesical calculi associated with vesicovaginal fistulas: management considerations. *J Urol* 1986;136:94.

Margulies RU, Lewicky-Gaupp C, Fenner DE, et al. Complications requiring reoperation following vaginal mesh kit procedures for prolapse. *Am J Obstet Gynecol* 2008;199:678.e1.

Massengill JC, Baker TM, Von Pechmann WS, et al. Commonalities of cerclage-related genitourinary fistulas. *Female Pelvic Med Reconstr Surg* 2012;18:362.

Meeks GR, Sams JO 4th, Field KW, et al. Formation of vesicovaginal fistula: the role of suture placement into the bladder during closure of the vaginal cuff after transabdominal hysterectomy. *Am J Obstet Gynecol* 1997;177:1298.

Melamud O, Eichel L, Turbow B, et al. Laparoscopic vesicovaginal fistula repair with robotic reconstruction. *Urology* 2005;65:163.

Meyer S, Fahlbusch M, Thon WF. Fistula between the bladder and vagina and perforation after implantation of a wall stent for ureteral stricture. *Urologe A* 2010;49:543.

Mokrzycki ML, Hampton BS. Vesicouterine fistula presenting with urinary incontinence after primary cesarean section: a case report. *J Reprod Med* 2007;52:1107.

Mondet F, Chartier-Kastler EJ, Conort P, et al. Anatomic and functional results of transperitoneal-transvesical vesicovaginal fistula repair. *Urology* 2001;58:882.

Monteiro H, Nogueira R, de Carvalho H. Behcet's syndrome and vesicovaginal fistula: an unusual complication. *J Urol* 1995;153:407.

Morita T, Tokue A. Successful endoscopic closure of radiation induced vesicovaginal fistula with fibrin glue and bovine collagen. *J Urol* 1999;162:1689.

Morton HC, Hilton P. Urethral injury associated with minimally invasive mid-urethral sling procedures for the treatment of stress urinary incontinence: a case series and systematic literature search. *Br J Obstet Gynaecol* 2009;116:1120.

Nagraj HK, Kishore TA, Nagalaksmi S. Early laparoscopic repair for supratrigonal vesicovaginal fistula. *Int Urogynecol J Pelvic Floor Dysfunct* 2007;18:759.

Nesrallah LJ, Srougi M, Gittes RF. The O'Conor technique: the gold standard for supratrigonal vesicovaginal fistula repair. *J Urol* 1999;161:566.

Nezhat CH, Nezhat F, Nezhat C, et al. Laparoscopic repair of a vesicovaginal fistula: a case report. *Obstet Gynecol* 1994;83:899.

O'Conor VJ, Sokol JK. Vesicovaginal fistula from the standpoint of the urologist. *J Urol* 1951;66:579.

Ojanuga Onolemhemhen D, Ekwempu CC. An investigation of socio-medical risk factors associated with vaginal fistula in Northern Nigeria. *Women Health* 1999;28:103.

Park KE, Ku SY, Kim HS, et al. Vesicovaginal fistula following large-loop excision of the transformation zone in a chronic systemic glucocorticoid user. *J Obstet Gynaecol Res* 2011; 37:1459.

Pettersson S, Hedelin H, Jansson I, et al. Fibrin occlusion of a vesicovaginal fistula. *Lancet* 1979;1:933.

Porcaro AB, Zicari M, Zecchini Antoniolli S, et al. Vesicouterine fistulas following cesarean section: report on a case, review and update of the literature. *Int Urol Nephrol* 2002;34:335.

Porpiglia F, Destefanis P, Fiori C, et al. Preoperative risk factors for surgery female urethral diverticula. Our experience. *Urol Int* 2002;69:7.

Punekar SV, Buch DN, Soni AB, et al. Martius' labial fat pad interposition and its modification in complex lower urinary fistulae. *J Postgrad Med* 1999;45:69.

Puppo A, Naselli A, Centurioni MG. Vesicovaginal fistula caused by a vaginal foreign body in a 72-year-old woman: case report and literature review. *Int Urogynecol J Pelvic Floor Dysfunct* 2009; 20:1387.

Puri M, Goyal U, Jain S, et al. A rare case of vesicovaginal fistula following illegal abortion. *Indian J Med Sci* 2005;59:30.

Pushkar DY, Dyakov VV, Kasyan GR. Management of radiation-induced vesicovaginal fistula. *Eur Urol* 2009;55:131.

Rajamaheswari N, Chhikara AB, Seethalakshmi K, et al. Transvaginal repair of gynecological supratrigonal vesicovaginal fistulae: a worthy option! *Urol Ann* 2012;4:154.

Rajamaheshwari N, Seethalakshmi K, Varghese L. Menouria due to congenital vesicovaginal fistula associated with complex genitourinary malformation. *Indian J Urol* 2009;25:534.

Ramaiah KS, Kumar S. Vesicovaginal fistula following masturbation managed conservatively. *Aust N Z J Obstet Gynaecol* 1998; 38:475.

Rangnekar NP, Imdad Ali N, Kaul SA, et al. Role of the martius procedure in the management of urinary-vaginal fistulas. *J Am Coll Surg* 2000;191:259.

Ravi B, Schiavello H, Abayev D, et al. Conservative management of vesicouterine fistula. A report of 2 cases. *J Reprod Med* 2003;48:989.

Ridgeway B, Walters MD, Paraiso MF, et al. Early experience with mesh excision for adverse outcomes after transvaginal mesh placement using prolapse kits. *Am J Obstet Gynecol* 2008;199: 703.e1.

Rizvi SJ, Gupta R, Patel S, et al. Modified laparoscopic abdominal vesico-vaginal fistula repair—mini-O'Conor vesicotomy. *J Laparoendosc Adv Surg Tech A* 2010;20:13.

Roca Edreira A, Gutierrez Banos JL, Martin Garcia B, et al. Stress urinary incontinence. Comparative study of suprapubic and vaginal surgical techniques. *Arch Esp Urol* 1994;47:711.

Rosenblatt P, Adams S, Adelowo A. An Improved Urinary Drainage Device for Management of Vesicovaginal Fistula. Presented at the American Urogynecology Society (AUGS) 33rd Annual Scientific Meeting, October 2012.

Roslan M, Markuszewski MM, Baginska J, et al. Suprapubic transvesical laparoendoscopic single-site surgery for vesicovaginal fistula repair: a case report. *Wideochir Inne Tech Malo Inwazyjne* 2012;7:307.

Roy KK, Vaijyanath AM, Sinha A, et al. Sexual trauma—an unusual cause of a vesicovaginal fistula. *Eur J Obstet Gynecol Reprod Biol* 2002;101:89.

Rubinstein C, Russell WJ. Wound closure and suturing patterns: a vector analysis of suture tension. *Aust N Z J Surg* 1992; 62:733.

Ryan JA Jr., Gibbons RP, Correa RJ Jr. Urologic use of gracilis muscle flap for nonhealing perineal wounds and fistulas. *Urology* 1985;26:456.

Sandberg EM, Cohen SL, Hurwitz S, et al. Utility of cystoscopy during hysterectomy. *Obstet Gynecol* 2012;120:1363.

Schwarz JK, Wahab S, Grigsby PW. Prospective phase I-II trial of helical tomotherapy with or without chemotherapy for postoperative cervical cancer patients. *Int J Radiat Oncol Biol Phys* 2011;81:1258.

Shah SJ. Laparoscopic transabdominal transvesical vesicovaginal fistula repair. *J Endourol* 2009;23:1135.

Shah SJ. Role of day care vesicovaginal fistula fulguration in small vesicovaginal fistula. *J Endourol* 2010;24:1659.

Shaker H, Saafan A, Yassin M, et al. Obstetric vesico-vaginal fistula repair: should we trim the fistula edges? A randomized prospective study. *Neurourol Urodyn* 2011;30:302.

Sharma SK, Madhusudnan P, Kumar A, et al. Vesicovaginal fistulas of uncommon etiology. *J Urol* 1987;137:280.

Sharma SK, Perry KT, Turk TM. Endoscopic injection of fibrin glue for the treatment of urinary-tract pathology. *J Endourol* 2005;19:419.

Shelbaia AM, Hashish NM. Limited experience in early management of genitourinary tract fistulas. *Urology* 2007;69:572.

Shirvan MK, Alamdari DH, Ghoreifi A. A novel method for iatrogenic vesicovaginal fistula treatment: autologous platelet rich plasma injection and platelet rich fibrin glue interposition. *J Urol* 2013;189:2125.

Siddiqui NY, Paraiso MF. Vesicovaginal fistula due to an unreported foreign body in an adolescent. *J Pediatr Adolesc Gynecol* 2007;20:253.

Sims JM. On the treatment of vesico-vaginal fistula. 1852. *Int Urogynecol J Pelvic Floor Dysfunct* 1998;9:236.

Sokol AI, Paraiso MF, Cogan SL, et al. Prevention of vesicovaginal fistulas after laparoscopic hysterectomy with electrosurgical cystotomy in female Mongrel dogs. *Am J Obstet Gynecol* 2004;190:628.

Sotelo R, Mariano MB, Garcia-Segui A, et al. Laparoscopic repair of vesicovaginal fistula. *J Urol* 2005;173:1615.

Starkman JS, Meints L, Scarpero HM, et al. Vesicovaginal fistula following a transobturator midurethral sling procedure. *Int Urogynecol J Pelvic Floor Dysfunct* 2007;18:113.

Staskin D, Malloy T, Carpiniello V, et al. Urological complications secondary to a contraceptive diaphragm. *J Urol* 1985;134:142.

Stav K, Dwyer PL. Urinary bladder stones in women. *Obstet Gynecol Surv* 2012;67:715.

Stelmachow J, Borkowski A, Zawada E, et al. Late vesico-vaginal fistula after colporrhaphy for urinary incontinence. *Ginekol Pol* 1992;63:204.

Sultana CJ, Goldberg J, Aizenman L, et al. Vesicouterine fistula after uterine artery embolization: a case report. *Am J Obstet Gynecol* 2002;187:1726.

Sundaram BM, Kalidasan G, Hemal AK. Robotic repair of vesicovaginal fistula: case series of five patients. *Urology* 2006;67:970.

Svaerdborg M, Birke-Sorensen H, Bek KM, et al. A modified surgical technique for treatment of radiation-induced vesicovaginal fistulas. *Urology* 2012;79:950.

Tahzib F. Epidemiological determinants of vesicovaginal fistulas. *Br J Obstet Gynaecol* 1983;90:387.

Tahzib F. Vesicovaginal fistula in Nigerian children. *Lancet* 1985;2:1291.

Tancer ML. Observations on prevention and management of vesicovaginal fistula after total hysterectomy. *Surg Gynecol Obstet* 1992;175:501.

Tancer ML. A report of thirty-four instances of urethrovaginal and bladder neck fistulas. *Surg Gynecol Obstet* 1993;177:77.

Tenggardjaja CF, Goldman HB. Advances in minimally invasive repair of vesicovaginal fistulas. *Curr Urol Rep* 2013;14:253.

Thomas K, Williams G. Medicolegal aspects of vesicovaginal fistulae. *BJU Int* 2000;86:354.

Tsivian A, Shtricker A, Levin S, et al. Bone anchor 4-corner cystourethropexy: long-term results. *J Urol* 2003;169:2244.

Vakili B, Chesson RR, Kyle BL, et al. The incidence of urinary tract injury during hysterectomy: a prospective analysis based on universal cystoscopy. *Am J Obstet Gynecol* 2005;192:1599.

Vangeenderhuysen C, Prual A, Ould el Joud D. Obstetric fistulae: incidence estimates for sub-Saharan Africa. *Int J Gynaecol Obstet* 2001;73:65.

Viennas LK, Alonso AM, Salama V. Repair of radiation-induced vesicovaginal fistula with a rectus abdominis myocutaneous flap. *Plast Reconstr Surg* 1995;96:1435.

Villasanta U. Complications of radiotherapy for carcinoma of the uterine cervix. *Am J Obstet Gynecol* 1972;114:717.

Volkmer BG, Kuefer R, Nesslauer T, et al. Colour Doppler ultrasound in vesicovaginal fistulas. *Ultrasound Med Biol* 2000;26:771.

Wall LL. Thomas Addis Emmet, the vesicovaginal fistula, and the origins of reconstructive gynecologic surgery. *Int Urogynecol J Pelvic Floor Dysfunct* 2002;13:145.

VII

Wall LL. Preventing obstetric fistulas in low-resource countries: insights from a Haddon matrix. *Obstet Gynecol Surv* 2012;67:111.

Wall LL, Karshima JA, Kirschner C, et al. The obstetric vesicovaginal fistula: characteristics of 899 patients from Jos, Nigeria. *Am J Obstet Gynecol* 2004;190:1011.

Wall LL, Khan F, Adams S. Vesicovaginal fistula formation after cervical cerclage mimicking premature rupture of membranes. *Obstet Gynecol* 2007;109:493.

Wang AC, Wang CR. Radiologic diagnosis and surgical treatment of urethral diverticulum in women. A reappraisal of voiding cystourethrography and positive pressure urethrography. *J Reprod Med* 2000;45:377.

Wang CJ, Kong DB, Shen BH, et al. Ureteral obstruction and urinary fistula due to fibrin glue after partial nephrectomy: a case report and review of the literature. *Oncol Lett* 2013;5:825.

Wang PT, Su SC, Hung FY, et al. Huge pelvic mass, cutaneous and vaginal fistulas, and bilateral hydronephrosis: a rare presentation of actinomycosis with a good response to conservative treatment and with long-term sequelae of renal atrophy and hydronephrosis. *Taiwan J Obstet Gynecol* 2008;47:206.

Wild TT, Bradley CS, Erickson BA. Successful conservative management of a large iatrogenic vesicovaginal fistula after loop electrosurgical excision procedure. *Am J Obstet Gynecol* 2012; 207:e4.

Yamamoto Y, Nishimura K, Ueda N, et al. Vesicovaginal fistula caused by abdominal hysterectomy and sacrocolpopexy with polypropylene mesh (gynemesh): a case report. *Hinyokika Kiyo* 2010;56:517.

Yip SK, Fung HY, Wong WS, et al. Vesico-uterine fistula—a rare complication of vacuum extraction in a patient with previous caesarean section. *Br J Urol* 1997;80:502.

Zhang Q, Ye Z, Liu F, et al. Laparoscopic transabdominal transvesical repair of supratrigonal vesicovaginal fistula. *Int Urogynecol J* 2013;24:337.

CHAPTER 44
Anal Incontinence and Rectovaginal Fistula

James Unger

DEFINITIONS

Anal incontinence—Involuntary loss through the anus of flatus, liquid stool, or solid stool that is perceived as a social or hygienic problem.

Anal manometry—A diagnostic test that provides information regarding function, sensation, compliance, and the presence of intact reflexes within the anal canal and distal rectum.

Anal ultrasonography—An imaging modality used to define the anatomy of the sphincter complex. It is the simplest, most reliable, least invasive test for definition of anatomic defects in external and internal anal sphincter.

Closing reflex—Exaggerated increase in muscle contraction allowing for anal closure at the end of defecation.

Defecography—A diagnostic test that involves imaging of the rectum with contrast material and observation of the process, rate, and completeness of rectal evacuation using fluoroscopic techniques.

External anal sphincter—Striated muscle sphincter, under voluntary control, that is responsible for much of the squeeze pressure in the anal canal.

Extra-anal incontinence—Involuntary loss through a fistula of flatus, liquid stool, or solid stool.

Fecal incontinence—Involuntary loss through the anus of liquid or solid stool only; excludes flatal incontinence.

Fourth-degree laceration—Complete rupture of the external anal sphincter and laceration of the anorectal mucosa.

Internal anal sphincter—Thickened continuation of the circular smooth muscle layer of the bowel, under autonomic control, that is responsible for much of the resting pressure in the anal canal.

Noble procedure—Transperineal approach to anal sphincteroplasty and perineoplasty in patients with chronic perineal laceration. Since it involves mobilization of the anterior rectal wall outside the anal orifice, it can also be used for anal–vaginal fistula repair. Major advantage is the lack of sutures in the anorectal canal.

Pelvic floor electromyography—A diagnostic test that evaluates the pelvic floor muscles for evidence of nerve injury. It is performed for three purposes: to identify areas of sphincter injury by mapping the sphincter, to determine whether the muscle contracts or relaxes, and to identify denervation–reinnervation potential indicative of nerve injury.

Puborectalis muscle—Striated muscle medial portion of the levator ani that is responsible for maintaining and increasing the anorectal angle and contributes to the squeeze pressure in the anal canal.

Pudendal nerve terminal motor latency (PNTML)—Operator-dependent technique to measure the response of the external anal sphincter to stimulation of the pudendal nerve. Prolongation of response has been associated with anal sphincter weakness due to pudendal nerve damage, although this is very controversial.

Rectovaginal fistula—Epithelial-lined connection between the rectosigmoid or anal canal and the vagina or perineum.

Rectoanal inhibitory reflex (RAIR)—Complex process in which sampling of rectal contents by the anal canal occurs every 8 to 10 minutes in response to rectal filling. This reflex primarily occurs through relaxation of the upper internal anal sphincter with continued pressure maintained by the lower internal anal sphincter. Concurrent contraction of the external anal sphincter and puborectalis muscle force the sampled contents back into the rectum.

Resting pressure—Reflects the tonic activity of both internal anal sphincter and external anal sphincter; approximately 75% to 85% of this pressure is derived from the internal anal sphincter.

Sacral neuromodulation—Stimulation of S2–S4 nerve roots via an implanted electrode introduced through selected sacral foramina, which in turn is connected to an implanted electrostimulator in order to cause contraction of levator muscles and external anal sphincter.

Secca procedure—Transanal delivery of temperature-controlled radiofrequency energy to the sphincter complex, which results in tissue remodeling and improved anal sphincter function.

Third-degree laceration—A partial or complete laceration of the external anal sphincter without involvement of the anorectal mucosa.

INTRODUCTION

Obstetricians and gynecologists have an important role to play in the diagnosis, management, and prevention of anal incontinence in women. Women with anal incontinence may bring this problem to the attention of their obstetrician–gynecologist as a primary complaint or in many cases discuss it only after close questioning about symptoms. This is because many women are understandably reluctant to mention such problems on their own due to feelings of embarrassment. This discussion may occur with the acute onset of symptoms shortly after a pregnancy or much later in life unrelated to recent childbirth. While in the first case such incontinence may be the direct result of acute childbirth injury, in the latter case, it may be related to chronic injury due to childbirth injury years ago or unrelated to any childbirth event. In either case, the gynecologist is often the first consulted to provide evaluation and management.

In addition, the prevention of obstetric trauma and its adverse effects on pelvic floor function including anal continence has become a major public health question. It seems clear that sphincter injury at the time of vaginal delivery significantly increases the odds of anal incontinence even years later beyond the postpartum period. Pollack and coworkers reported a 53% anal incontinence rate at 5 years in women who had undergone an anal sphincter tear compared to 32% in women without a tear. They calculated an odds ratio of 2.3 (95% CI 1.1 to 5.0) for anal sphincter tear and later incontinence. More recently, Evers and coworkers also calculated an odds ratio of 2.3 (95% CI 1.27 to 4.26) for anal incontinence women 5 to 10 years following an anal sphincter laceration. They also concluded that vaginal delivery in the absence of an anal sphincter laceration was not a risk factor for anal incontinence.

Surgical repair of chronic anal sphincter injury, the major subject of this chapter, is by no means uniformly successful, and results seem to deteriorate with time. Gutierrez and colleagues reported on 191 patients at 10 years after anal sphincter repair and found that only 6% of the 130 patients who returned questionnaires had full continence. In addition, 58% were incontinent of solid stool. Zutshi and coworkers reported on 31 patients with a median age of 44 years at the time of overlapping sphincter repair with a median follow-up of 129 months. No patients were fully continent at 129 months. Patients who were older at the time of surgery and those who had undergone multiple vaginal births had the worse outcomes. Dudding and coworkers in a systematic review of the literature in 2008 determined that only 20% of patients were continent to liquid and/or solid stool at 10 years after overlapping sphincter repair.

Likewise, obstetric lacerations involving the rectum may result in rectal/anal–vaginal fistulae even when expertly repaired. Although childbirth-related fistulae can usually be successfully repaired with surgery, they are physically and emotionally distressing. Sometimes, more than one surgical attempt is required. It is also evident that certain obstetric practices such as midline episiotomy and operative vaginal delivery may contribute to later adverse effects on fecal continence, most likely by increasing the risks of anal sphincter and rectal injury. This has generated considerable discussion and debate regarding the appropriate use of episiotomy, operative vaginal delivery, and even cesarean section on demand for the sole purpose of preventing pelvic floor injury as noted in a recent commentary by Nygaard.

Approximately 1.4% of normal community-dwelling adults are incontinent to liquid or solid stools. Perry and coworkers reported on a total sample of 10,116 adults over age 40 years a major fecal incontinence rate of 1.4%. There was no significant difference between men and women, although incontinence was more prevalent and more severe in older people. Walter and colleagues in a random sample of 2,000 community-dwelling individuals between the ages of 31 and 76 reported a rate of leakage of solid stools of 1.4% in women and 0.4% for men. The prevalence increases with normal aging to 6% to 7% of elderly adults over age 60 years

living independently according to a study performed in the Netherlands by Teunissen and colleagues. On the other hand, Tobin and Brocklehurst reported that 10.3% of residents in 30 different residential homes for the elderly had fecal incontinence at least once weekly. Therefore, anal incontinence is a symptom that affects millions of women and has many causes in addition to childbirth trauma (Table 44.1). In fact,

TABLE 44.1 Causes of Anal Incontinence

ABNORMAL PELVIC FLOOR
Congenital anorectal malformations
Obstetric injury
  Third- of fourth-degree perineal lacerations
  Episiotomy breakdown
  Forceps delivery
Operative procedures
  Colpoperineorrhaphy
  Vulvectomy
  Difficult hysterectomy
  Colpotomy drainage of pelvic abscess
  Excision of Bartholin gland
  Hemorrhoidectomy
Trauma
  Impalement
  Pelvic fracture
  Foreign body
  Anal intercourse
Inflammatory bowel disease
  Crohn disease
  Tuberculosis
  Granulomatous venereal disease
  Ulcerative colitis
  Diverticulitis
  Perirectal abscess
Malignancy
  Carcinoma of the cervix
  Carcinoma of the vagina
  Carcinoma of the vulva
  Carcinoma of the rectum
Pelvic floor denervation (idiopathic neurogenic incontinence)
  Vaginal delivery
  Chronic straining at stool
  Rectal
Aging

NORMAL PELVIC FLOOR
Diarrheal states
  Infectious diarrhea
  Inflammatory bowel disease
  Short-gut syndrome
  Laxative abuse
  Radiation enteritis
Overflow
  Impaction
  Encopresis
  Rectal neoplasms
Neurologic conditions
  Congenital anomalies (i.e., myelomeningocele)
  Multiple sclerosis
  Dementia, stroke, and tabes dorsalis
  Neuropathy (i.e., diabetes)
  Neoplasms of brain, spinal cord, and cauda equina
  Injuries to brain, spinal cord, and cauda equina

VII

Whitehead and coworkers demonstrated that after adjusting for age, neither vaginal delivery nor gender was predictive of anal incontinence. Like Perry, they reported that increasing age is the major determinant of fecal incontinence. However, many cases in women do seem to be strongly associated with pelvic floor injury, especially injury to the anal sphincter sustained either overtly or covertly during childbirth as previously noted. These injuries may result from direct traumatic disruption to some component of the anal sphincter mechanism or functional deterioration over time as a result of occult nerve injury and aging. Identifying the role of childbirth and risk factors associated with delivery that are linked to later incontinence is important since some of these factors may be modifiable by altering certain childbirth practices and thus lowering the risk of subsequent incontinence. Women with either acute or chronic anatomic injury as a cause of their incontinence are the ones most likely to benefit from care of the well-trained surgical gynecologist. The obstetrician–gynecologist not only will be the first one to be involved in the prevention of such injuries but also will be responsible for the surgical repair required in the delivery room. In addition, the obstetrician and gynecologist may be the first one consulted to evaluate women with chronic fecal incontinence and must be able to carefully assess such women with a thorough history, physical examination, and appropriate imaging or testing, in order to arrive at a precise etiology of this condition. At this point, patients may be referred to other specialists such as those in female pelvic medicine and reconstructive surgery, gastroenterologists, colorectal surgeons, physical therapists, and others if treatment of the underlying condition is outside the expertise of the patient's obstetrician–gynecologist.

FUNCTIONAL ANATOMY OF ANAL CONTINENCE

The mechanisms and structures involved in defecation and preservation of anal continence are reviewed in detail in the following section. A summary of the structures and processes involved is illustrated in Figures 44.1 and 44.2.

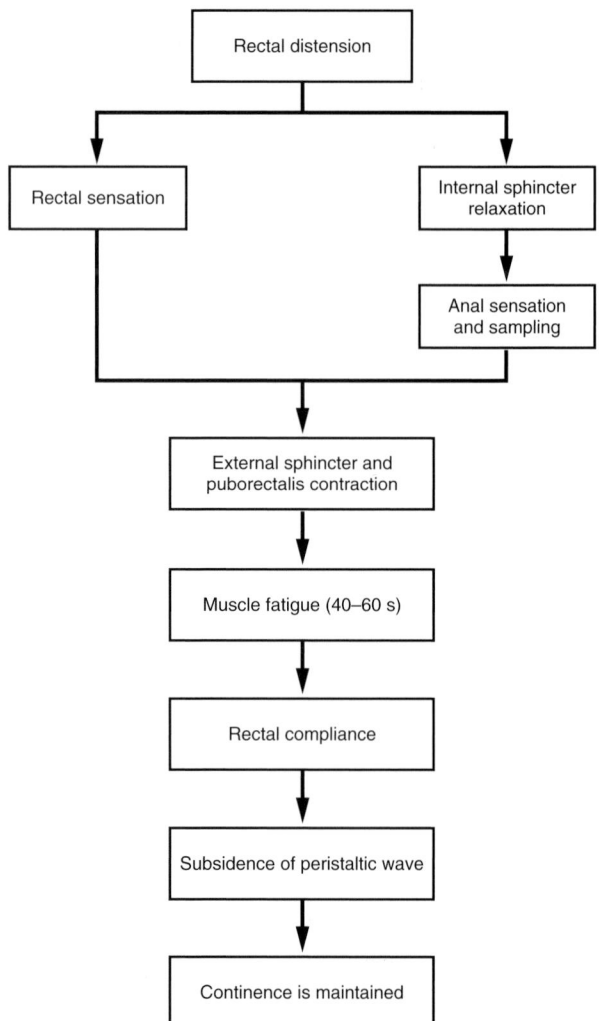

FIGURE 44.2 Algorithm for anal continence mechanism. Diagrammatic illustration of the anal canal and sphincters.

Rectum

Adequate knowledge of the anatomy of the rectum and the anorectal canal and its normal function in defecation is critical to understanding the mechanisms of anal continence (Table 44.2). The rectum lies posterior to the vagina as it descends below the cul-de-sac peritoneum. Here, it accomplishes one of its major functions contributing to continence, that of a temporary appropriate storage unit when defecation needs to be delayed. The puborectalis muscle, which encircles the rectum and pulls

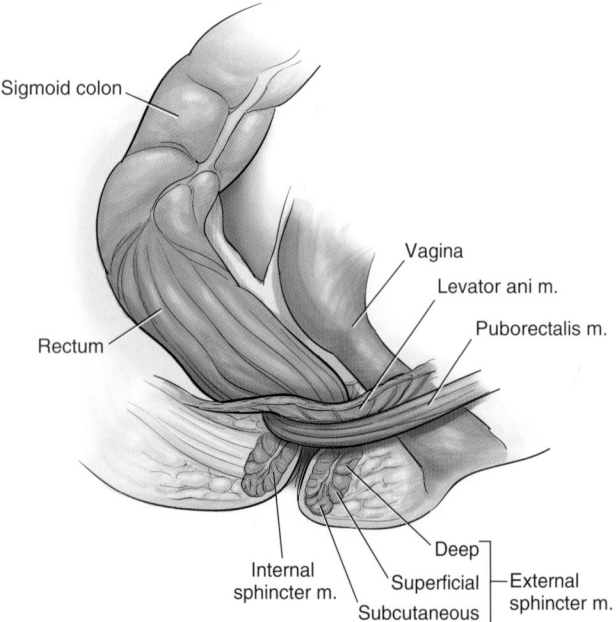

FIGURE 44.1 Location of the anal sphincter in relation to other structures of the female pelvic floor.

TABLE 44.2 Mechanisms of Anal Continence
Anatomic
Anal sphincter mechanisms
Puborectalis sling/anorectal angle
Neurologic
Intact pudendal enervation
Anorectal reflex and sensory mechanisms
Functional
Stool volume and consistency
Colonic transit time
Rectal capacity, distensibility, and tone

it forward toward its own attachment at the symphysis pubis, marks the distal margin of the rectum and the beginning of the anal canal. In addition to the external and internal anal sphincters, it is an important muscular component of the continence mechanism. In addition to its storage role, the rectum functions as a very important sensory unit responsible for the initiation of the continence mechanism. Finally, when the appropriate time arrives, the rectum also has dynamic propulsive activity allowing complete emptying of its contents until it is empty.

The process of storage and appropriate evacuation of stool begins when the rectum senses the presence of material within its lumen. Not unlike the bladder, the cerebral cortex is responsible for interpreting this information as regards its precise nature and the problem of what to do about it. Fortunately, also like the bladder, the rectum is a high-volume, low-pressure system when healthy. It can accommodate increasing volumes of material, that is, feces, until a critical volume, and thus ultimately critical pressure is reached. This compliance of the rectum can be compromised due to inflammation of the rectum as in inflammatory bowel disease or with fibrosis as occurs with radiation. Compliance can be measured clinically with anorectal manometry with balloon distention as is discussed later in the section on testing. Patients with urgency, incontinence, and even constipation may have issues with abnormal compliance and/or abnormal sensation. When normal sensation and compliance exists, the sensation of rectal filling allows one to consciously initiate the anal continence mechanism, which is discussed further below. However, without normal rectal compliance, even an otherwise intact continence mechanism will be severely compromised.

Rectal expulsion of its contents when appropriate is the final event in defecation. It seems to be under both voluntary and reflex control. The voluntary nature involves the willful relaxation of the muscular components of the continence mechanism followed by the reflex propulsive contractions of the rectum usually assisted by a voluntary increase in intra-abdominal pressure. This continues until the rectum is completely empty as determined by sensory input from the anal canal.

Anal Canal

The actual structures involved in the anal continence mechanism include the anal canal and its surrounding muscular structures. However, not to be forgotten is the important role of the rectum as it interacts with the continence process as described above. For the obstetrician and gynecologist, it is the anal canal and its related structures such as the anal sphincters that will be most directly linked to the problem of fecal incontinence.

The anal canal in the female is approximately 2.5 to 4 cm in length and normally remains completely collapsed because of the tonic contraction of the sphincters. The lining of the anal canal is nonuniform. The proximal 1 cm is lined by rectal-type columnar mucosa, followed by modified or stratified columnar epithelium for about 1.5 cm. The distal half of the anal canal is lined by squamous epithelium, which is richly supplied by branches of the inferior hemorrhoidal nerves and is exquisitely sensitive. The anal mucosa, like the rectum, is also surrounded by the inner circular layer of smooth muscle, which is in turn surrounded by the outer longitudinal layer. The main blood

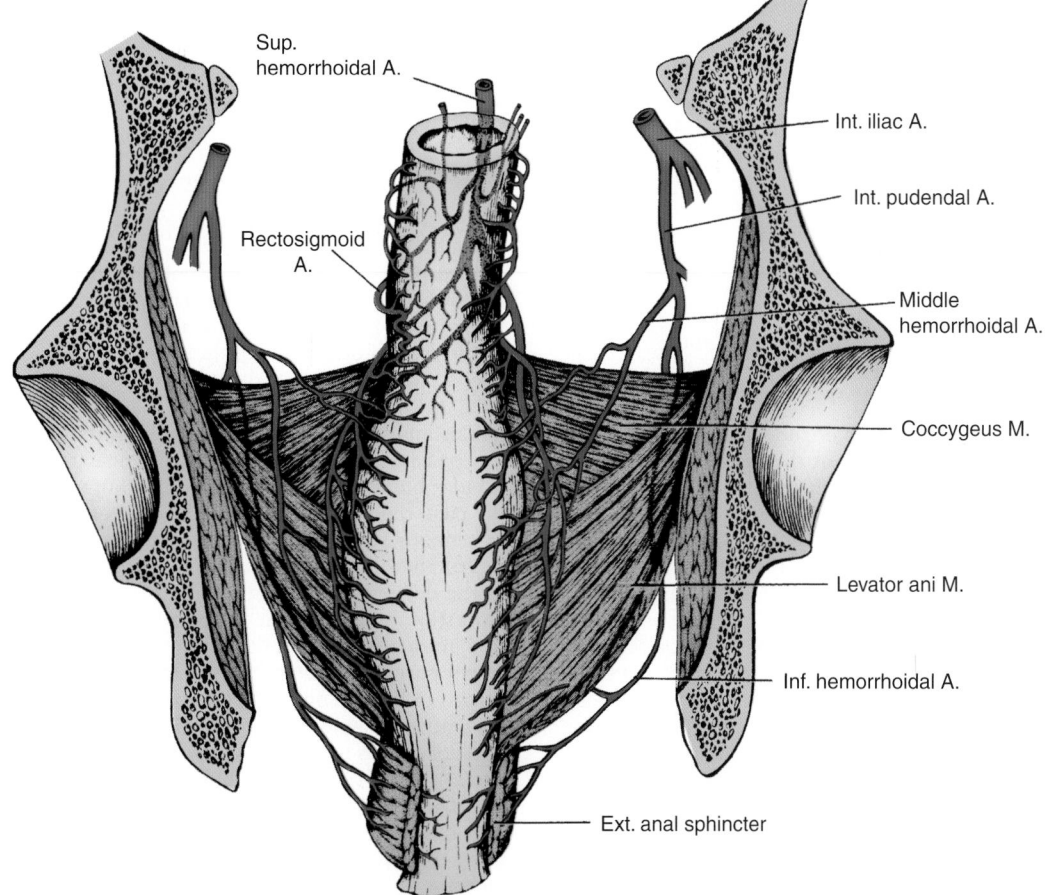

FIGURE 44.3 Rectosigmoid colon and anal canal showing collateral arterial circulation from superior hemorrhoidal (inferior mesenteric), middle hemorrhoidal (hypogastric or internal iliac), and inferior hemorrhoidal (internal pudendal) arteries.

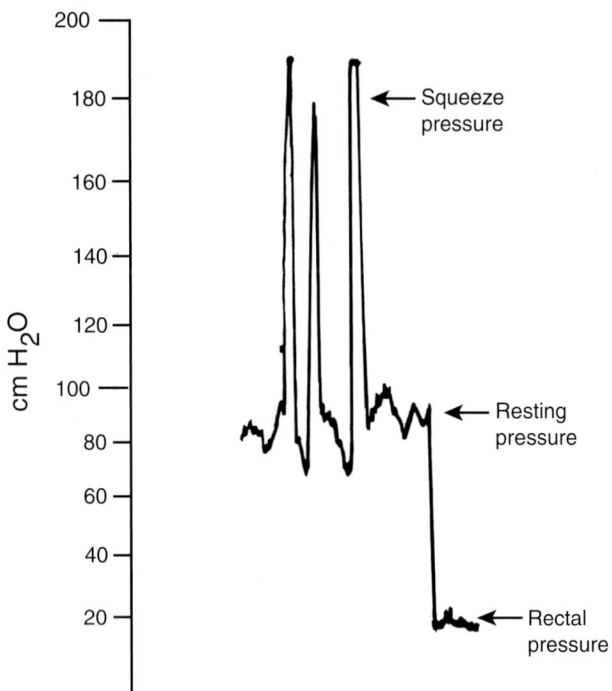

FIGURE 44.4 Anal manometry demonstrating pressures in the anal canal. Rectal pressure reflects intra-abdominal baseline pressure recorded in the rectal reservoir. Resting pressure essentially reflects the effect of the involuntary, smooth muscle internal anal sphincter. Squeeze pressure largely reflects the transient contractile effort of the voluntary, striated external anal sphincter.

supply to the rectum and the anal canal is from branches of the superior and inferior hemorrhoidal arteries (Fig. 44.3).

The muscular portions of the anal continence mechanism or anal sphincter consist of three separate muscular structures surrounding the anal canal: the internal anal sphincter, the external anal sphincter, and the puborectalis muscle. The internal anal sphincter provides most of the involuntary resting tone to the anal canal, while the external anal sphincter and the puborectalis muscle are under voluntary control and contribute the most when we call upon the need to delay defecation.

The Internal Anal Sphincter

The circular smooth muscle layer of the rectal wall, which is under autonomic control, thickens at the proximal anal canal to form the internal anal sphincter. It triples in thickness and is approximately 3 cm in length and 3 mm wide. It is longer in men and thickens with age. It provides about 85% of the resting anal tone with the remainder supplied by the hemorrhoidal vessels and external sphincter. These pressures can be shown by anal manometry demonstrated in Figure 44.4. The internal sphincter terminates just short of the most caudal portion of the external anal sphincter and is separated from it by the longitudinal smooth muscle layer of the bowel. The internal anal sphincter seems to have two major functions: prevention of passive leakage of anal contents and initiation of the rectoanal inhibitory reflex (RAIR) or anorectal sampling as demonstrated in the anal manometry study illustrated in Figure 44.5.

Injury to the internal anal sphincter may result in passive leakage of anal contents, which may be continuous or intermittent. It should also be suspected when patients complain of loss of stool completely without warning or awareness. Injury to the internal anal sphincter can be diagnosed by endoanal sonography as is discussed in the section on childbirth injury.

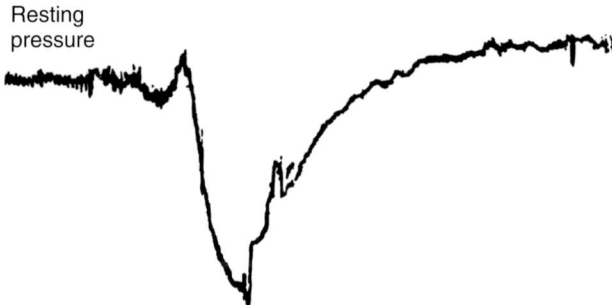

FIGURE 44.5 Rectoanal inhibitory reflex. Arrival of stool in the rectum triggers reflex relaxation of the internal anal sphincter, allowing the bolus to enter the proximal anal canal, where discrimination of the solid, liquid, or gaseous nature of the bolus by the sensory-rich upper anal canal occurs.

Anorectal sampling or the RAIR occurs every 8 to 10 minutes in response to rectal filling. The upper internal anal sphincter relaxes in response to rectal filling to allow the sensory epithelium of the anal canal to determine the nature of the rectal contents. The amount of relaxation of the internal sphincter is directly related to the degree of rectal distention. Incontinence does not occur because the lower internal sphincter maintains higher pressure all the while this is occurring. Concurrent contraction of the external anal sphincter and the puborectalis muscle forces the sampled contents back into the rectum. Clearly, damage to the internal anal sphincter, which allows for a larger volume of sampling contents to enter an anal canal that is further compromised by a lack of opposing pressure, may result in leakage. This compromise will be further worsened if there is a lack of voluntary action on the part of the external anal sphincter and puborectalis to force the contents back into the rectum.

The External Anal Sphincter

The external anal sphincter extends approximately 1 cm beyond the internal sphincter. It is generally but somewhat arbitrarily divided into three components: deep, superficial, and subcutaneous (Fig. 44.1). The deep part blends with the fibers of the puborectalis as its fibers encircle the undersurface of the rectum on its way to the symphysis pubis. The subcutaneous portion is attached to the perianal skin, and the superficial portion forms the bulk of the muscle. Classically, the female anal sphincter complex has been thought of as forming a broad band of tissue posteriorly but narrowing to a small tubular bundle of tissue anteriorly within the perineal body. In the past, the internal sphincter has been most often portrayed as a minor structure. These concepts came from many centuries of anatomic study of cadavers augmented by observations in the delivery room, at the time of third- and fourth-degree laceration repairs, of the transected ends of the anterior portion retracted into round holes in the perineal body. In the recent past, it has become possible to view this anatomy undisturbed in living, continent, nulliparous subjects with magnetic resonance imaging (MRI). In an early MRI study, Aronson and colleagues found the shape of the combined internal and external anal sphincter complex to be nearly cylindrical as it encircles the anal canal. Measured in the midline, the anterior portion of the anal sphincter complex appeared as a broad band of tissue, not a narrow tube. In this study, 54% of the anterior thickness was smooth muscle of the internal anal sphincter. Subsequent studies, including the cadaver studies of DeLancey et al., found a similar shape with a substantial contribution from the internal anal sphincter. This substantial

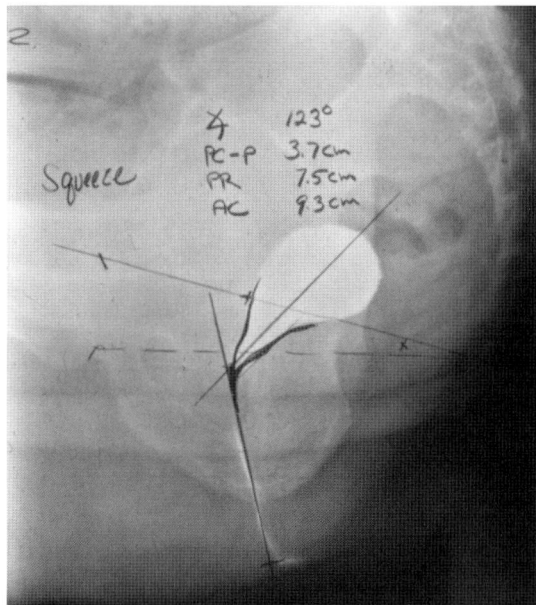 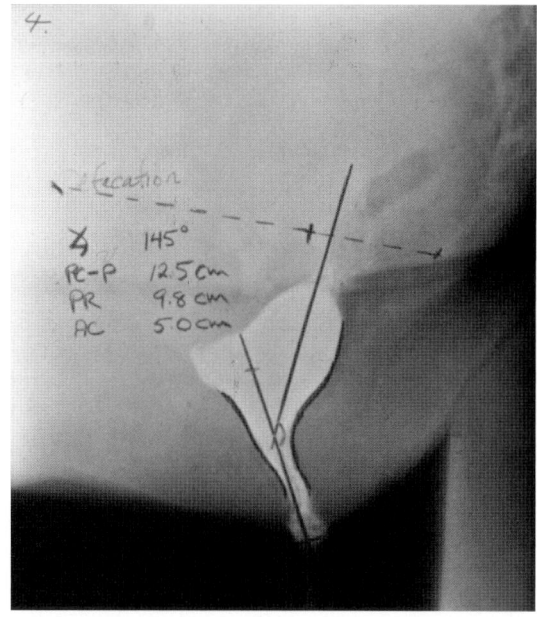

FIGURE 44.6 A: Lateral defecography of normal continent patient deferring defecation by contracting puborectalis sling, increasing anorectal angle, and exerting squeeze pressure in the anal canal. Note how barium bolus is supported over the levator plate and away from the fatigable anal sphincter complex. **B:** Lateral defecography of normal continent patient willfully defecating by relaxing puborectalis sling, decreasing anorectal angle, and decreasing pressure in the anal canal. Note how barium bolus becomes lined up over the anal canal.

anterior anal sphincter length and thickness, as well as the contribution from the internal sphincter, is important to keep in mind during primary repair of obstetric lacerations as well as in surgical correction of anal incontinence secondary to chronic perineal laceration. The external anal sphincter is a striated muscle that is under voluntary control via the pudendal nerve. It provides a certain degree of constant tone to the anal canal due to its slow-twitch muscle fibers. However, it can undergo muscle fatigue due to its "fast-twitch" fibers as well. Its primary function is to generate adequate pressure in the anal canal when needed to allow for postponement of defecation. It accomplishes this by allowing the rise in anal pressure to exceed that in the rectum, until rectal accommodation occurs through normal rectal compliance, and rectal pressure falls (Fig. 44.6).

As previously mentioned, the external anal sphincter also plays a vital role in the RAIR by helping to generate opposing pressure when the internal anal sphincter relaxes and along with the puborectalis returns the sampled contents into the rectum. This response of the external anal sphincter is critical in preventing passive fecal loss.

Finally, the external anal sphincter is important in protecting against postdefecation incontinence. This is demonstrated by the so-called closing reflex. When traction is released on the external anal sphincter as fecal material is evacuated, there is an exaggerated increase in muscle contraction. This allows for anal closure at the end of defecation.

The Puborectalis Muscle

The puborectalis muscle is the most medial portion of the levator ani. The puborectalis muscle encircles the anorectal junction pulling it toward its insertion on the inner surface of the pubis. It thus forms a sling that creates the anorectal angle. The anorectal angle is an approximately 90-degree angle that closes the rectal inlet and maintains the rectum over the levator plate rather than directly over the anal canal (Fig. 44.7A). It does this by tonic contraction utilizing its slow-twitch muscle fibers.

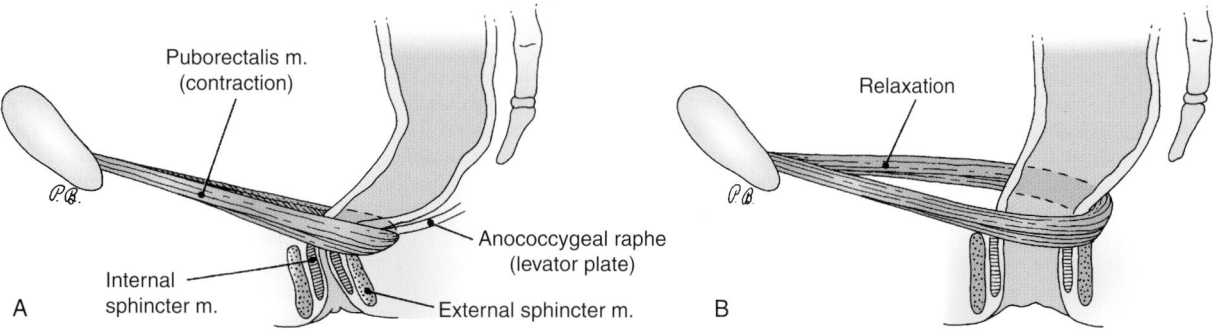

FIGURE 44.7 Function of the anal sphincter and puborectalis muscle. **A:** At rest, the constant tone of the puborectalis muscle pulls the anorectal junction anteriorly to create an approximately 90-degree angle between the rectum and anal canal, closing the rectal inlet and maintaining continence of solid stool. At moments of need, this muscle can be contracted further, increasing the angle and supporting the stool bolus over the levator plate. **B:** During defecation, the puborectalis muscle relaxes, opening the rectal inlet, while intestinal peristalsis and the voluntary increase in intraabdominal pressure move stool into the anal canal. The anorectal angle is decreased, and the stool bolus is lined up over the anal canal.

VII

When there is a need to delay defecation, it can contract further under voluntary control and further increase the anorectal angle. When defecation is permitted, the puborectalis relaxes, decreasing the anorectal angle, allowing the rectum to line up directly over the anal canal (Fig. 44.7B). The role of puborectalis injury in anal incontinence is unclear.

THE EFFECT OF PREGNANCY AND CHILDBIRTH ON THE PELVIC FLOOR

In this section, we review some of the effects of pregnancy and childbirth on the function of the pelvic floor and also the direct effects of childbirth trauma on the anal sphincter mechanism. This is an area of much conflicting data that are difficult to interpret in terms of developing a clear understanding of the natural history of pregnancy and childbirth and how they relate to anal incontinence. It is hard to tease out the effects of pregnancy itself, vaginal delivery with or without sphincter injury, occult sphincter injury, neurologic injury, efficacy of sphincter repair, and other issues contributing to incontinence. However, it is an area of intense current investigation, and hopefully, many of these questions will be answered in the future. For obstetricians–gynecologists and the women they care for, childbirth-related injuries will be the most common cause of anal incontinence they will have to deal with.

General Effects on the Pelvic Floor and Continence

Signs of pelvic floor dysfunction often develop during pregnancy itself. This adds to the difficulty of trying to differentiate pregnancy-related pelvic floor dysfunction as to its timing—antepartum versus intrapartum. These problems include both urinary incontinence and fecal incontinence. King and coworkers reported that 65% of their nulliparous patients reported anal (flatus and/or fecal) incontinence during the third trimester. Fourteen percent complained of fecal incontinence. By 2 weeks postpartum, the anal incontinence rate had dropped to 47%, while the fecal incontinence rate had risen to 17%, including 10 women who had new-onset fecal incontinence by the 2-week visit. Of these 10 subjects, 3 had spontaneous vaginal delivery, 3 delivered by forceps, and 4 had delivered by cesarean delivery after labor. At 6 months postpartum, 49% still complained of incontinence of flatus and 11% of fecal incontinence. Solans-Domenech reporting for the Catalan Agency for Health Technology Assessment and Research found that 39.1% of previously continent pregnant women developed urinary incontinence at some time during their pregnancy. Ten percent of women in this study developed anal incontinence at some point during the pregnancy. This was incontinence of flatus only in 90%, although during the postpartum period nearly one third of these women noted some loss of liquid or solid stool. For both urinary incontinence and fecal incontinence during pregnancy, risk factors were related to increased weight and age over 35 years. The major risk factor for the persistence of incontinence at the 7-week postpartum visit was vaginal delivery. However, in the case of anal incontinence, this was true only if anal incontinence was also present during pregnancy. Instrumental delivery and episiotomy were not significant risk factors for postpartum incontinence. Overall, 7.3% of women continued to complain of fecal incontinence at their postpartum visit. This is very similar to the 11.2% prevalence of anal incontinence noted in the vaginal delivery group and the 10.3% prevalence in the cesarean delivery group reported by Borello-France for the Pelvic Floor

Disorders Network. At 6 months after delivery, the anal incontinence rate had dropped to 8.2% and 7.6% in the vaginal and cesarean groups, respectively. However, women who had sustained a known sphincter injury reported much higher prevalence of fecal incontinence at both the 6-week postpartum visit and at 6 months, 26.6% and 17%, respectively.

Stretch and compression injury to the pudendal nerve, which innervates the external anal sphincter, and to the S2, S3, and S4 nerve fibers, which directly innervate the levator muscles, may be responsible for incontinence not associated with direct muscle trauma. This may be due to the normal descent of the fetal head or by trauma from forceps. Snooks and coworkers have identified such other risk factors as length of the second stage of labor, multiparity, and high birth weight. Allen and colleagues studied 96 nulliparous women and found electromyography (EMG) evidence of reinnervation in the pelvic floor muscles after vaginal delivery in 80% of those studied. Women with a prolonged second stage and larger babies had the most evidence of nerve damage. Surprisingly, forceps deliveries and perineal tears did not affect nerve damage. None of these studies included neurophysiologic testing during pregnancy itself, and therefore, it is not possible to tease out the role pregnancy itself apart from delivery may have played. However, even though it appears these denervation injuries are common, occurring in up to 80% of women, they seem to be minor and to resolve in most. However, Snooks in a follow-up study in 1990 found evidence of persistent neuropathy in some women even at 5 years.

Another area that may contribute to pelvic floor dysfunction due to childbirth is a direct effect on pelvic muscle strength. This may or may not be due to direct injury to the levator. A recent study by Friedman and coworkers in parous women revealed decreased muscle strength in women with anal incontinence and pelvic organ prolapse 6 to 11 years following vaginal delivery. Vaginal delivery overall was associated with a significant reduction in pelvic muscle strength compared to cesarean delivery. The greatest reduction in strength was in women who had forceps delivery. However, in the study noted above by King, which demonstrated a very high prevalence of anal incontinence in pregnant nulliparous women, they were not able to demonstrate a difference in pelvic muscle strength between those with and without symptoms during the antepartum or postpartum period. Finally, DeLancey and coworkers have reported an association between defects in the levator ani muscle demonstrated by MRI and pelvic organ prolapse. However, the exact role these injuries may play in the etiology of anal incontinence is unknown.

Anal Sphincter Injury and Incontinence

Clinically recognizable anal sphincter injury occurs in from 3.3% to 19% of vaginal deliveries. Handa and coworkers in a large population-based study of over 2 million vaginal deliveries in California reported a frequency of anal sphincter lacerations of 5.85%. Faltin and colleagues reported occult injuries detectable by ultrasound in up to 28% of women without a clinically suspected injury. Direct disruption injury to the external anal sphincter during childbirth has been commonly associated with anal incontinence in women. Farrell and coworkers in a prospective observational study found that incontinence of flatus at 6 months postpartum was higher in women who had sustained a third- or fourth-degree laceration compared to those women without anal sphincter injury. Likewise, earlier, Sultan and coworkers reported higher rates of anal incontinence in women with demonstrable external anal sphincter defects postpartum. Pollack and colleagues reported a 5-year prospective study where 53% of women with a sphincter injury reported anal incontinence compared to 32% without a sphincter injury. Likewise, as reported above by Borello-France for the Pelvic Floor Disorders Network, there was an 11.2% prevalence of anal incontinence noted in the vaginal delivery group and the 10.3% prevalence in the cesarean delivery group. At 6 months after delivery, the anal incontinence rate had dropped to 8.2% and 7.6% in the vaginal and cesarean groups, respectively, in this study. However, women who had sustained a known sphincter injury reported much higher prevalence of fecal incontinence at both the 6-week postpartum visit and at 6 months, 26.6% and 17%, respectively.

More recently, Evers and coworkers, using anal incontinence and quality-of-life scores to define incontinence, reported on 937 women 5 to 10 years after first delivery, 90 of whom had sustained a clinically diagnosed sphincter injury at the time of delivery. Nineteen percent of women with a sphincter injury had anal incontinence as defined by the score, compared to 10% in the vaginal delivery without injury group and 9% in the cesarean group. Sultan also raised the issue of the effectiveness of primary end-to-end repair of the external anal sphincter performed at the time of delivery by reporting that 82% of women still had a sphincter defect present by ultrasound 7 weeks later. Of note, 33% of women who did not have a recognized anal sphincter injury at delivery were noted to have a defect present at 7 weeks. Subsequently, Sultan and his team reported retrospective case series of 32 women who underwent overlapping sphincter repair in the operating room under anesthesia, of whom only 7% had incontinence of flatus and none had fecal incontinence at 5 months postpartum. However, three subsequent randomized studies (Fitzpatrick et al., 2000; Williams et al., 2006; Fernando et al., 2006) as well as a Cochrane review in 2006 all failed to demonstrate a difference in fecal incontinence between repair types.

In 2010, Farrel and coworkers reported a prospective randomized study on nulliparous women assigned to either end-to-end or overlapping repair after sustaining third- or fourth-degree lacerations. By confining their study to nulliparous women, they hoped to eliminate bias generated by those cases of multiparous women who may have a preexisting injury. They reported a significantly increased rate of incontinence of flatus at 6 months in women undergoing overlapping repair compared to those undergoing end-to-end repair (61% vs. 39%). However, there was not a significant difference in fecal incontinence between the two groups (15% vs. 8%). Ultrasound findings of sphincter defects did not correlate with flatal or fecal incontinence except for those women who demonstrated both internal and external anal sphincter defects. Combined disruption noted on ultrasound was significantly associated with fecal incontinence with an odds ratio of 6.5. There was also no significant difference in rates of isolated internal, external, or combined sphincter defects in either group. Internal anal sphincter defects were present in 46% of the end-to-end repair group versus 38% in the overlapping repair; external anal sphincter defects in 53% versus 62%, respectively; and both sphincters in 32% for each. Rates for incontinence following repair were not statistically different whether there was an intact sphincter on ultrasound or not except as noted above for fecal incontinence in the women with persistent combined defects versus no defect (incontinence of flatus 52% vs. 54%, respectively; fecal incontinence 30% vs. 6%, respectively). Women with a persistent internal anal sphincter defect had a 60% rate of incontinence of flatus versus 50% of those with an intact internal anal sphincter, while fecal incontinence was present in 23% versus 7%, respectively. Finally, women with a persistent external anal sphincter defect had a 51% rate of incontinence of flatus versus 57% with an intact sphincter, while fecal incontinence occurred in 20% versus 7%, respectively. The authors concluded that the primary cause of incontinence following a third- or fourth-degree laceration was denervation injury rather than persistent structural defects following repair. Likewise, it is interesting to note that Frudinger and coworkers failed to demonstrate a link between anal sphincter disruption diagnosed in asymptomatic postpartum women by ultrasound only and anal incontinence 10 years later. The issue of the true relationship between endoscopically defined anal sphincter defects, denervation injury, and symptoms of incontinence later remains unclear.

There are known risk factors for anal sphincter trauma at vaginal delivery. A recent review by Dudding and colleagues in which 451 articles and abstracts were studied concluded that major risk factors for injury included instrumental delivery, prolonged second stage of labor, birth weight greater than 4 kg, fetal occipitoposterior presentation, and episiotomy. The population-based study of over 2 million vaginal deliveries by Handa and coworkers noted earlier identified primiparity, macrosomia, and operative vaginal delivery as major risk factors. In addition, episiotomy, especially midline episiotomy, is an important risk factor for sphincter lacerations as demonstrated by Angioli and colleagues as well as by FitzGerald and coworkers.

Finally, obstetric lacerations can extend into the rectum resulting in a so-called fourth-degree laceration. Although these usually also involve a complete tear through the anal sphincter, this is not always the case. At times, there may be an isolated laceration through the rectum or anal canal with an intact external anal sphincter. Therefore, these isolated injuries must be looked for and are usually diagnosed by digital rectal exam at the time of delivery. On occasion, the rectal mucosal portion of a repair will break down with or without concomitant disruption of the sphincter and perineum, which can result in rectovaginal fistula. In Hibbard's series of 24 rectovaginal fistulae and 27 chronic perineal lacerations, 47 (92%) were caused by obstetric trauma. Even meticulously repaired lacerations will occasionally completely break down. This leaves the patient with an open cloacal deformity or an isolated rectal/anal–vaginal fistula with an intact perineum and sphincter. Anal incontinence usually is a problem for these patients until the tissues are healed sufficiently to allow secondary repair. Surgical repair will be discussed in detail in the section on fistula repair.

Obviously, the issue of anal incontinence during and following pregnancy and delivery is complex as to its etiology and treatment. Especially confusing is the role of neurologic injury versus structural damage to the anatomic sphincter mechanism. The best surgical method to repair sphincter injury and the effect of the adequacy of the repair on overall continence later is equally unclear. Finally, the overall contribution of childbirth injury to the ultimate development of long-term anal incontinence is uncertain as well, although the significance of intrapartum injury appears to decrease with age. This subject is particularly important when it comes to counseling older patients with anal incontinence and who are also found to have clinical or imaging evidence of sphincter disruption remote from delivery.

Other Causes

A promoter of anal incontinence over time is the fact that the normal process of aging results in decreased efficiency of the anal sphincter complex. Haadem and associates showed a natural decline with aging in resting and squeeze pressures in the anal canal of continent subjects. With increasing age, the

VII

internal sphincter generates a lower resting pressure, and the proportion of fibrous tissue increases. The squeeze pressure able to be exerted by the external sphincter suffers a natural decline as well. Vaccaro and coworkers found pudendal neuropathy to be an age-related phenomenon as well in patients with anal incontinence and constipation. Because of this, many patients with damaged continence mechanisms may be able to compensate for a period of time, but they go on to decompensate secondary to these age-related changes and become incontinent.

Functional problems of the bowel, such as constipation or diarrhea, can result in incontinence. Chronic constipation with its repeated straining at stool can cause stretch-induced injury to pudendal enervation. Overall, the most common cause of anal incontinence in the elderly, particularly those who are institutionalized, is fecal impaction with overflow incontinence. A diarrheal state can result in anal incontinence even in a patient with normal anorectal function, owing to the presence of large quantities of liquid stool that may overwhelm a normally functional mechanism. Neurologic disorders affecting sphincter control also may result in anal incontinence. Usually, the neurologic defect is widespread, and anal incontinence is but one manifestation.

Traumatic injury, more often a side-straddle injury in young girls, may result in simple or extensive laceration of the perineum. The extent of the injury may be difficult to determine because of pain, fear, edema, hemorrhage, and hematoma formation. Examination under anesthesia is advisable so that appropriate repair can be made, looking carefully for lacerations of the anal sphincter and rectum as well as other structures. Hematoma dissection above the levator muscles must be ruled out with pelvic ultrasound and with careful rectovaginal examination under anesthesia. Above the levator muscles, there is nothing to impede the progression of a hematoma until the diaphragm is reached.

Rectal trauma from operative procedures can affect rectal capacity and compromise anal continence or perhaps lead to extra-anal incontinence through a rectovaginal fistula. Entry into the rectum may occur during posterior colpoperineorrhaphy, especially when the anterior rectal wall and posterior vaginal skin are closely adherent with little, if any, intervening connective tissue. Such an enterotomy should be repaired transversely if longitudinal closure would compromise rectal capacity. A difficult hysterectomy, either abdominal or vaginal, may result in injury to the rectum, especially when dissection behind the cervix is difficult because of dense adhesions, indurated tissue from infection, or involvement of the cul-de-sac and anterior rectal wall with endometriosis. If the rectal defect does not heal properly or is not closed properly, a high rectovaginal fistula may develop through the newly closed vaginal apex. Partial excision of anal sphincter and other muscles involved in maintaining anal continence may be required in extensive vulvectomy for cancer resulting in anal incontinence, as reported by Berek and others. Injury to the anterior rectal wall may occur during hemorrhoidectomy, excision of a Bartholin gland, or colpotomy for pelvic abscess drainage.

Forty to sixty percent of patients with rectal or rectal mucosal prolapse also have some degree of anal incontinence. Although this was originally thought to be secondary to a dilatation effect on the internal anal sphincter, there is often evidence of associated neurogenic damage to the external sphincter muscles as well. These individuals may present with a patulous anal sphincter, passive stretching of the puborectalis muscles, and a long history of straining with constipation. The tissue prolapse may be related to prolapsing internal hemorrhoidal tissue or rectal mucosa or complete (full-thickness) rectal prolapse. Questions such as the frequency of occurrence of the prolapse, association with activity or defecation, estimated distance of the prolapsed tissue from the anus, spontaneous or manual reducibility, and history of incarceration may be helpful in better defining the type of problem. Patients may have relatively occult prolapse of tissue, which can manifest as mucous or brownish staining in the undergarments with occasional blood.

On physical examination, it is important to note the following: a patulous anus, which may indicate that chronic tissue prolapse has been occurring. The presence of enlarged external hemorrhoidal tissue may suggest the presence of enlarged internal hemorrhoidal complexes; however, they may be found in relative isolation and may be mistaken as prolapsed tissue. Patients should be asked to bear down as if defecating to manifest any prolapsed tissue. Concentric circular folds and a large protruding mass suggest the presence of complete prolapse, which often extends well beyond the anus. Noncircumferential folds may be either mucosal prolapse or hemorrhoidal tissue. If the patient's history suggests the presence of prolapse and it is not visualized with the patient in the left lateral or lithotomy position, it is often helpful to have the patient sit on a commode with subsequent examination in this position. Correction of prolapsing tissue such as hemorrhoids may lead to improvement in anal continence, if this is the primary cause of the problem. In patients with complete rectal prolapse undergoing surgical repair, the rate of some degree of residual incontinence ranges from 40% to 90%, depending on the type of repair used.

Crohn disease is the most important of the variety of inflammatory bowel diseases that may cause extra-anal incontinence through a rectovaginal fistula. Among 138 patients with rectovaginal fistulae seen at Duke University Medical Center, Bandy and associates reported that 15 (11%) were caused by Crohn disease. The diagnosis, perioperative management, and surgical technique chosen for these patients constitute a special challenge for the gynecologic surgeon. Crohn disease must be considered as a possible cause of rectovaginal fistula in any patient in whom other causes are not clear, particularly if the fistula orifice is tender to palpation. Crohn disease also should be considered in the patient who has failed multiple attempts at fistula repair because the fistula tends to recur at the operative site in these individuals.

The role of diverticulitis as a cause of sigmoidovaginal fistulae has been highlighted by Tancer and Veridiano, who report on 130 such cases. These fistulae usually present with a malodorous vaginal discharge in women older than 50 years of age, some years after a hysterectomy. Such fistulae commonly develop between the inflamed bowel segment and the apical vaginal scar from the previous hysterectomy, although they may infrequently occur through a retained cervix. Often, the diverticular disease is silent and is only discovered with further investigations of the fistula tract. A diverticular abscess may have formed and found drainage though the path of least resistance, which in this case is the thinned out scar of the vaginal cuff.

Malignant tumors may erode through the tissues between the vagina and the rectum. When a patient with tumor involvement of the rectovaginal wall receives radiation, sloughing of the tumor may result in a rectovaginal fistula. Radiation also may cause a rectovaginal fistula without tumor erosion.

Rarely, anal incontinence may be congenital, as seen in one of 5,000 newborn girls who have an imperforate anus with associated fecal incontinence through a congenital rectovaginal or rectoperineal fistula. Total rectal agenesis is rare. Paul and Lloyd reported hindgut duplication with a congenital rectovaginal fistula; however, most anal incontinence is acquired.

Finally, although anal incontinence may be termed idiopathic in about 10% of women, the mechanism of incontinence in these women is usually secondary to pelvic floor denervation.

In summary, although an intact and functional anal sphincter complex and puborectalis sling are important in the maintenance of anal continence, it must be remembered that a variety of other factors are involved, including intact anorectal sensation and reflexes, rectal capacity and distensibility, reasonable colonic transit time, appropriate stool volume and consistency, and adequate patient mental function and mobility.

EVALUATION OF ANAL INCONTINENCE

The most common cause of anal incontinence that the obstetrician–gynecologist will encounter is that related to obstetric injury. As noted previously, these patients may present shortly after childbirth or many years later. In the latter case, this may be because of failure of compensatory mechanism with time and aging. It is these later cases that require the most extensive diagnostic workup and which are the most resistant to surgical repair of the structural defect.

History and Physical Examination

Most often, history alone provides strong clues as to the etiology of the incontinence. The temporal relationship between a recent traumatic vaginal delivery and the postpartum onset of incontinence, especially urgency, will quickly lead one to suspect an undiagnosed sphincter injury or a failed sphincter repair. This will be quickly confirmed by pelvic examination without the need for additional testing. Likewise, flatal or fecal incontinence without urgency in this context should lead one to carefully search for a rectovaginal or anovaginal fistula. These are usually located in the lower one third of the vagina and are often identified as a red area of what appears to be granulation tissue. This usually represents an isolated small disruption of the previously repaired anal or rectal suture line. Fecal material is usually present near the fistula opening within the vagina. These fresh injuries are usually easy to identify as opposed to some small older fistulae for which patients seek care years later.

Patients who present remote from childbirth with anal incontinence require a more extensive workup both due to the possibility of a cause unrelated to childbirth and to develop a rational plan for repair, if indicated, with reasonable patient expectations for success. It may be helpful in these cases especially to attempt to quantify the degree of incontinence using one of a number of scoring systems. Scoring systems should include the effect of incontinence on the patient's quality of life and allow for monitoring the response to treatment. There are a variety of these validated questionnaires available. Avery and coworkers have published a very helpful review of these with graded recommendations. Although no questionnaires received an "A" grade for anal incontinence, three were recommended with grades of "B." These were the Fecal Incontinence Quality of Life Scale (Rockwood et al., 2000), Manchester Health Questionnaire (Bug et al., 2001), and Birmingham Bowel and Urinary Symptoms Questionnaire (Hiller et al., 2002).

Pelvic examination should include a careful inspection of the posterior vaginal wall, perineum, anal sphincter, anal canal, and rectum, including assessment of the patient's function as well as anatomy. A patulous anus indicates a major loss of sphincter function and can be associated with rectal prolapse. Most obstetric injuries are associated with an anterior segmental defect in the external anal sphincter and may appear as the loss of the perineal body, loss of the corrugated appearance

surrounding the anus, or attenuation of the rectovaginal septum in some instances. In more subtle cases in which the perineal body appears intact but the external sphincter is actually separated, only the dimples of the laterally retracted ends of the anal sphincter muscles may be apparent. This produces a "dovetail" appearance, as described by Toglia and DeLancey, in which the normal radial distribution of the anal creases is absent anteriorly but is present laterally and inferiorly. If there is a question as to the presence of a segmental defect, endoanal or transperineal ultrasound can be useful in delineating the anatomy. Next, a screening evaluation of the perineal reflexes to assess the integrity of the S2–S4 dermatomes should be performed. Perception of pinpoint and light touch over the perineal skin and buttocks can be tested easily with the broken end of a wooden cotton swab or a safety pin. Light stroking of the inferolateral margin of the labia majora should cause a reflex contraction of the bulbocavernosus muscle within the labia. The anal wink reflex can be elicited by lightly stroking the perianal skin or touching it with a pin to cause a reflex contraction of the external anal sphincter. Asking the patient to cough also should elicit the reflex contraction of the external anal sphincter. With both of these maneuvers, the anal canal should constrict concentrically owing to contraction of the external sphincter, and the anus should be pulled inward secondary to the contraction of the puborectalis muscle. In women with separation of the external anal sphincter, voluntary contraction of the pelvic floor muscles can cause an accentuation in the lateral perineal dimpling of the retracted ends. In patients with a denervated sphincter, there is no retraction of the anal skin during voluntary contraction. Patients who demonstrate abnormalities of these pelvic floor reflexes may require more in-depth neurologic evaluation.

Extra-anal incontinence may result from a fistulous tract. A rectovaginal fistula is usually easily diagnosed by careful inspection of the posterior vaginal wall. By spreading the labia, a low fistula can be revealed, usually involving the area of a previous episiotomy or obstetric laceration. A high fistula can be seen using a bivalve speculum and often appears at the vaginal cuff scar. A straight-handled speculum can be useful as it can be rotated to allow full visualization of both the anterior and posterior vaginal walls. The vaginal opening of a fistula may be localized by the presence of feces in the vagina or by the dark red rectal mucosa seen protruding at the fistulous opening contrasting with the lighter pink vaginal mucosa. Colposcopic examination of the vagina sometimes assists in the identification of a small fistula orifice. When the fistula is small, it may be difficult to locate both the vaginal and rectal ends of the fistula, but both orifices must be located for complete care to be given. A small probe can be pushed gently from the vaginal side of the fistula and the tip felt on a rectally placed finger. Instillation of methylene blue through the vaginal orifice of the fistula may aid in the proctoscopic visualization of the rectal orifice. Carey describes the following examination technique to identify a suspected rectovaginal fistula. A Foley catheter with a 10-mL balloon is inserted into the anus, while the posterior vaginal wall is painted with a concentrated solution of soap and water, or, alternatively, the vagina can be filled with water. As the rectum is distended with air by a syringe attached to the Foley catheter, the vaginal orifice of the fistula may be localized by the presence of bubbles forming at the fistula site. A small probe may then be passed along the fistula tract.

Alternatively, when a rectovaginal fistula is suspected but cannot be identified, radiologic studies such as a vaginogram or fistulogram may identify a fistulous tract. These studies are superior to barium enema for identifying a fistula because they use a thin, water-soluble radiopaque medium rather than a thick barium solution. As such, although fistulae occasionally may be identified by barium enema, the intraluminal pressure of the bowel often is inadequate to force the barium solution through a small fistula opening. In addition, the presence of barium in the lower bowel may obscure a fistula tract. Likewise, a tampon test may be performed in which a tampon is placed in the vagina and the patient is given a small enema with methylene blue–colored water, which she is asked to retain for 20 minutes. Blue discoloration of the tampon is noted in the presence of a fistula.

When a rectovaginal fistula is diagnosed, it is important to complete a thorough assessment of the anal sphincter and pelvic floor as well because these patients may have multiple defects. If not properly evaluated preoperatively, the patient may undergo successful repair of her fistula only to become anally incontinent postoperatively. Her compromised sphincter function may have been adequate preoperatively when excess pressure was bypassing the sphincter through the fistula. After her fistula is repaired and the full force of rectal contents is delivered to the sphincter complex, there may not be adequate function to maintain continence. A full treatment of rectovaginal fistula management appears later in this chapter.

A thorough digital rectal examination should be performed. Any rectal mass must be noted and the stool consistency assessed. A gross assessment of the patient's resting and squeeze pressures within the anal canal and her ability to contract her levator ani muscles should be included. Anal sphincter tone should be evaluated with the patient at rest and during sphincter contraction. An anterior sphincter defect may be easily detectable as the loss of the palpable muscular ring within the perineal body. Even in the absence of external anal sphincter muscle anteriorly, a scarified band of tissue can remain that completes the contractile ring and helps the patient maintain continence. Next, the anorectal axis can be assessed. On rectal examination, the puborectalis muscle is palpable posteriorly at the junction between the rectum and the anal canal. By directing the examining finger posteriorly, the angle between the anus and rectum can be estimated and should approximate 90 degrees in a normal woman. More important, when the patient is asked to squeeze the sphincter, the puborectalis muscle should pull the examiner's finger anteriorly toward the pubic bone.

Finally, some patients may complain of passive incontinence, or the loss of stool without their awareness. This may indicate damage to the internal anal sphincter. It cannot be assessed adequately by physical examination alone, but can be determined by radiologic and physiologic tests only. A defect of the internal sphincter can be assumed, however, if there is significant thinning of the rectovaginal septum. In many of these cases, both the internal and external anal sphincters are injured. Certainly, the patient with a chronic perineal laceration or cloacal deformity by definition has a segmental defect in both sphincters. From a practical and technical viewpoint, the internal anal sphincter cannot be repaired unless the external sphincter also is repaired. Surgery is rarely effective for an isolated defect of the internal sphincter. When surgical repair of the external anal sphincter is indicated, however, one should consider repairing defects in the internal sphincter as well.

Testing

Clearly, many patients will have a diagnosis and be ready to proceed to treatment after their history and physical examination. For others, the picture will be less clear. There may be questions about a particular patient that thoughtful use of testing can answer. Is a segmental defect present in the internal or external anal sphincter? What is the functional status within the anal canal? Is rectal sensation normal? Is the innervation to the striated musculature of the continent mechanism intact? How does the patient actually defecate? Judicious use of testing based on the information needed to arrive at an accurate diagnosis and to plan successful treatment can be important. The American Gastroenterological Association guidelines (March, 1999) for anorectal testing techniques are available through their Web site at www.gastro.org/practice/medical-position-statements. Procedures of value in addition to symptom diary and rectal examination include (a) anal ultrasonography, (b) anorectal manometry, (c) rectal and anal sensory testing, and (d) rectal compliance testing. These are now covered in detail.

Endoanal, transvaginal, and transperineal ultrasound techniques have made it simple and relatively inexpensive to identify defects in both the internal and external anal sphincters (**Fig. 44.8**). These defects can go clinically unrecognized, but may be amenable to surgical repair if the patient is symptomatic. Anal endosonography is one radiologic technique for assessing posttraumatic defects of the internal and external anal sphincters. High-resolution images of the separate sphincter muscles are obtained using a rotating Endoprobe, and anatomic defects can be identified as a loss of continuity of the muscle rings. Several studies have found that anal endosonography correlates well with needle EMG mapping of sphincter defects, manometric mapping of sphincter defects, and intraoperative findings. Ultrasound is less time-consuming than EMG or manometry and much more comfortable for the patient. Other studies have established that transvaginal ultrasound is equally efficacious to endoanal ultrasound in identifying sphincter defects. Peschers and colleagues described normal sphincter and puborectalis anatomy as well as defects in both the internal and external sphincters using exoanal ultrasonography: a conventional 5-MHz convex transducer placed on the perineum. Ultrasound currently is the study of choice for establishing the presence or absence of a segmental anal sphincter defect. The approach chosen—endoanal, transvaginal, or transperineal—may depend on the equipment available and operator expertise.

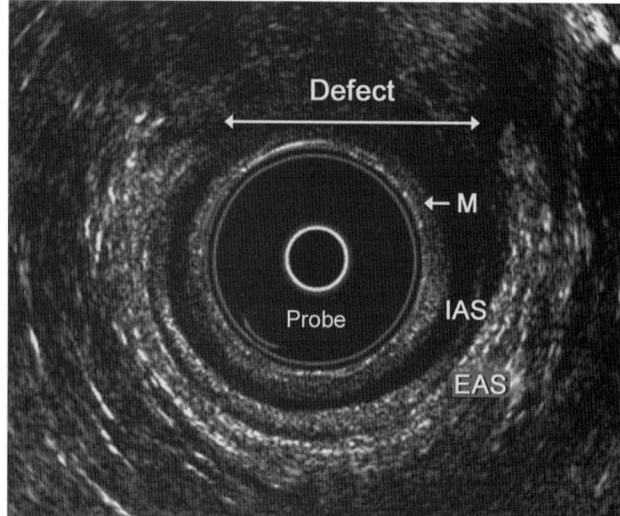

FIGURE 44.8 Endoanal ultrasound image of an anally incontinent patient with a segmental external anal sphincter defect. *Probe*, endoanal ultrasound probe; *M*, anal mucosa; *IAS*, internal anal sphincter; *EAS*, external anal sphincter; *defect*, segmental defect of external anal sphincter. (Photograph courtesy of Justin A. Maykel, MD.)

Endoanal ultrasound identifies anatomic defects or thinning of the internal anal sphincter, but Heyer and associates showed that interpretation of external sphincter images is much more subjective and confounded by normal anatomic variations in the external anal sphincter. Indeed, the external anal sphincter and perirectal fat are both echogenic and frequently indistinguishable; the external sphincter may be asymmetrical in the upper anal canal, particularly in women. A new imaging modality with better soft tissue definition may be desirable. MRI may prove to be superior to endoanal ultrasound because of high tissue contrast between the external anal sphincter and the perirectal fat. DeSouza and associates reported 100% concordance between MRI performed with an endoanal coil and surgical findings for presence, size, and location of anal sphincter tears in seven patients with obstetric trauma. Additionally, Lienemann and colleagues and Healy and associates have demonstrated that MRI also can define dynamic pelvic floor motion during defecation and squeeze. Rapid image acquisition is crucial for optimal visualization of dynamic motion, particularly because patients cannot maintain rectal expulsion or puborectalis contraction for more than 15 to 30 seconds.

Anal manometry provides information regarding function, sensation, compliance, and the presence of intact reflexes within the anal canal and distal rectum. It is most useful in defining functional sphincter weakness. Here, it is complementary to endoanal ultrasonography in determining whether this weakness is secondary to an anatomic defect. The first part of this test is essentially a pressure profile of the anal canal, providing information on the functional status of the internal and external anal sphincters. Some computer-based, multichannel manometry equipment can provide graphic cross-sectional analysis of the anal canal to help detect the presence of segmental sphincter defects.

The test usually is performed with the patient in the left lateral decubitus position without any special bowel preparation. There are many different protocols for performing anal manometry. Most commonly, a fluid-filled pressure catheter with radial side ports located 90 degrees apart circumferentially is connected to pressure transducers, and a recording device is used to measure the anal canal pressures during rest and during voluntary contraction of the anal sphincter (**Fig. 44.9**). These pressures may be recorded either as the pressure catheter is slowly pulled through the anal canal—a station pull-through technique—or at static points along the anal canal as the pressure catheter is pulled out in certain increments, usually every 0.5 cm. The average pressure measured at rest in the anal canal is the resting pressure, and the highest pressure recorded along the anal canal with the patient at rest is the maximum resting pressure. The increase in pressure over the basal canal pressure initiated by voluntary contraction of the anal sphincter is the squeeze pressure, and the highest such increment is the maximum squeeze pressure. The resting anal canal length is measured from the point at which the anal sphincter pressure continuously exceeds the average intrarectal pressure by 4 mm Hg. The resting pressure is largely a reflection of the internal anal sphincter function, whereas the squeeze pressure reflects the strength of the external anal sphincter voluntary contraction (**Fig. 44.4**).

"Normal" range for maximum resting pressure is 40 to 80 cm H_2O and for maximum squeeze pressure is 100 to 200 cm H_2O; however, there is tremendous overlap in values between patients who are continent and those who are incontinent. As a group, incontinent patients have lower values on anal manometry testing than continent patients, although there is no discriminatory level that can be used to predict incontinence. It has been suggested that patients with a maximum resting pressure of less than 20 cm H_2O and a maximum squeeze pressure of less than 40 cm H_2O are unlikely to be continent. Sentovich and colleagues found decreased resting and squeeze pressures in 90% of patients with a history of anal sphincter injury. Poen and associates also reported significantly decreased maximum squeeze pressures and in addition observed that the first sensation of filling was significantly increased in 40 subjects who had third-degree lacerations primarily repaired compared with controls. They also found that 35 (88%) of these subjects still had sphincter defects present

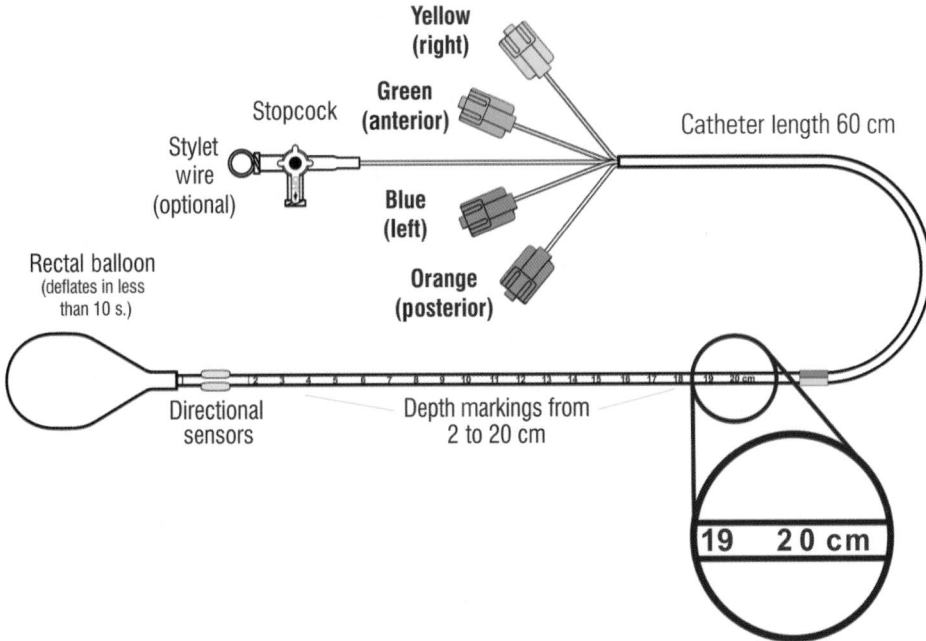

GIM-6000D Directional anorectal catheter

FIGURE 44.9 Drawing of an anorectal manometry catheter. (Courtesy of Sandhill Scientific.)

on endoanal ultrasound despite apparently successful healing of their repair. Gearhart and colleagues were unable to demonstrate any single preoperative manometric parameter that was predictive of outcome following sphincteroplasty.

A second part of anal manometry testing is the evaluation of rectal sensation. A balloon is placed in the rectum and incrementally distended. The minimum perceived volume, the volume causing the urge to defecate, and the maximum tolerable volume are recorded. Balloon distention is commonly used to detect threshold volumes for three different sensations: (a) the first detectable sensation (rectal sensory threshold), (b) sensation of the urgency to defecate, and (c) sensation of pain (maximum tolerable volume). Most healthy patients have a minimal perceived volume of about 30 mL and a maximum tolerable volume of about 300 to 350 mL, although this can be highly variable. A rectal maximum tolerable volume of less than 100 mL may indicate the presence of hypersensitivity, poor rectal compliance, or rectal irritability.

Measurements of pressures within the balloon allow the calculation of rectal compliance. The presence of a reflex rectal contraction after a bolus of air is introduced into the balloon, followed by the return to normal baseline pressures as the rectum accommodates, also is noted.

According to the American Gastroenterological Association, EMG of the external anal sphincter and pelvic floor muscles is performed for three purposes: (a) to identify areas of sphincter injury by mapping the sphincter, (b) to determine whether the muscle contracts or relaxes by the number of motor neuron units firing, and (c) to identify denervation–reinnervation potentials indicative of nerve injury. However, anal endosonography has largely replaced EMG in the first instance, defining sphincter trauma. Although neurologic injury may be identified by careful physical examination, information obtained from EMG may be helpful. This is important since patients with neurologic injury are less likely to have a good functional response to operations designed to restore anal incontinence, even when the anatomic result appears completely successful. Knowledge of a patient's pelvic floor neurologic status can be particularly useful for counseling her on prognosis.

The smallest functional neuromuscular unit is the motor unit, and injury to nerves or muscles produces characteristic changes recorded in the motor unit action potential. EMG can be performed using a needle electrode, a surface electrode on the perianal skin, or an anal plug. Concentric needle EMG involves placing a small needle with a recording electrode into the muscle being studied. The firing pattern of the motor units is assessed as the needle is being inserted, during spontaneous muscle activity, and during maximum voluntary contraction of the muscle. The characteristics of the recordings can then be evaluated. Single-fiber EMG allows the recording of action potentials from individual muscle fibers of a motor unit. When nerve injury occurs, there is often reinnervation but with a change in fiber density. The reinnervation is more diffuse and results in less effective muscle contraction than the original active enervation. When these studies indicate nerve reinnervation, therefore, it reflects prior nerve damage that has healed. Osterberg and associates found a correlation between fiber density and clinical and manometric variables in 72 incontinent patients.

Finally, nerve conduction velocities, which are the actual speed of conduction of the action potential along the nerve, are another measure of nerve function. The nerve conduction velocity can be calculated by measuring the nerve latency, which is the delay between the stimulation of the nerve at a specific point and the response in the target muscle supplied by the nerve. Standardized latencies for most peripheral nerves

have been established. Evaluation of the pudendal nerve terminal motor latency (PNTML), as developed by Snooks and colleagues, is of interest in patients with anal incontinence. The pudendal nerve is stimulated as it courses behind the ischial spine into Alcock canal, and the time is measured until a response is detected in the external anal sphincter. Prolonged PNTMLs indicate nerve damage; however, this test only reflects the conduction time of the healthiest axon remaining in a nerve. Therefore, normal PNTMLs do not confirm a lack of damage to the whole nerve, only that at least one axon remains intact that can conduct a response normally. Cheong and colleagues found pudendal neuropathy in 36% (21% bilateral and 15% unilateral) of 225 patients (174 women) presenting with anal incontinence. Chen and colleagues found in a small group of patients undergoing sphincteroplasty that, based on continence scores, the one patient with no neuropathy had an excellent result; of seven patients with unilateral pudendal neuropathy, 70% had a good to excellent result and 30% had a fair to poor result; whereas in four patients with bilateral neuropathy, half had a good to excellent result and the other half scored fair to poor. Gilliland and colleagues looked at a large group of patients who had undergone an overlapping sphincteroplasty with a median follow-up of 2.4 years. They found that 62% of 59 patients with normal pudendal function had a successful outcome, compared with only 17% of the 12 patients with unilateral or bilateral prolonged PNTMLs. Although the presence of pudendal neuropathy implies a poorer prognosis for the potential sphincteroplasty patient as noted earlier, it does not mean that some patients may not derive significant improvement in their continence. The American Gastroenterological Association's (AGA) medical position statement on anorectal testing techniques states that "although interesting from a research point of view, the clinical usefulness of this test is controversial. … The PNTML cannot be recommended for evaluation of patients with fecal incontinence."

Defecography is a radiologic evaluation of the lower gastrointestinal tract. It was used initially in the evaluation of patients with defecation disorders; but more recently, it has been used as part of the evaluation of anal incontinence. The rectum of the patient is filled with a barium–oatmeal or barium–potato starch paste mixed to a consistency to approximate semisolid stool. The patient then is seated on a special commode chair and asked to defecate during fluoroscopy. Lateral radiographs usually are taken before, during, and after evacuation of the rectum. Alternatively, cinedefecography can be performed, which is a videotaped dynamic fluoroscopic study.

The anorectal angle can be observed, as can the effect of willful contraction of the puborectalis muscle on this angle. It also provides information about rectal emptying and the mobility of the rectal wall. Indeed, its major value may be in identifying those patients with incomplete evacuation leading the patient's physician to consider overflow incontinence as the cause of the patient's incontinence. Anatomic abnormalities of the gastrointestinal tract not previously identified, such as intussusception, rectal prolapse, and rectal ulcers, can be detected by defecography. Now, it is possible to perform a triple contrast study wherein the rectosigmoid, small bowel, and bladder are all opacified with contrast. These studies often reveal disturbances of dynamic pelvic floor motion and interaction of support defects in more than one compartment, for example, rectoceles, sigmoidoceles, enteroceles, and cystoceles.

In relation to anal incontinence, however, the clinical relevance of many of these findings is questionable because there are no findings that are specific for anal incontinence. Many anatomic abnormalities are also found in asymptomatic controls. Although the anorectal angle may be more obtuse in incontinent patients both at rest and during squeezing than in continent patients, recent studies have questioned the significance of the anorectal angle because of the wide overlap in measurements between the two groups. In addition, there is a significant intraobserver variation in the measurement of the anorectal angle from the same set of radiographic films among different radiologists. Last, surgical restoration of the angle with a postanal repair, or retrorectal levatorplasty, is poorly correlated with a return of continence. Therefore, the role of defecography in the evaluation of patients with anal incontinence is unclear.

In summary, because anal continence depends on multiple mechanisms, no one test is ideal for clinical evaluation of the incontinent patient. There is not a standard testing protocol for the anally incontinent patient. Testing should be individualized. Studies should be obtained only to gather specific information needed in the evaluation of an individual patient. As noted above, procedures thought by the American Gastroenterological Association to be of value in selected patients are (a) symptom diary for diagnosis and monitoring of progress, (b) digital examination for basic qualitative assessment of resting and squeeze pressures, (c) anal ultrasound to assess anatomic integrity of the sphincters, (d) anorectal manometry to define sphincter weakness and predict response to biofeedback training, (e) rectal and anal sensory testing, and (f) testing of rectal compliance. Procedures of possible value for an individual patient might include (a) surface EMG for evaluation of sphincter function and evacuation proctography or (b) cinedefecography, when rectal prolapse is suspected. Testing procedures that are controversial for the clinical evaluation of anally incontinent individuals at present include (a) PNTML testing for assessment of pudendal nerve function and (b) MRI, because of its expense.

TREATMENT

Nonsurgical Treatment

Nonsurgical treatment of anal incontinence includes a variety of methods directed at a number of conditions. In some cases, medical treatment may be directed at the primary underlying cause of the incontinence, such as chronic diarrhea or as an attempt to compensate for functional or structural defects of the continence mechanism by altering the rectal contents into a more suitable solid form for bowel control. Other nonsurgical treatment may be directed at improving actual function of the compromised but intact sphincter mechanism through biofeedback or by augmentation of structural weakness without surgery with injectable bulk-adding agents or radiofrequency tissue remodeling procedures. Perianal electrical stimulation has been used to generate anal contractions in spinal injury patients and as an adjunct to biofeedback in postpartum women. Finally, staged sacral neuromodulation with implantable electrodes has been utilized to provide direct stimulation of the sacral nerves in patients with anal sphincter dysfunction with either intact or structurally damaged anal sphincters.

Patients with chronic diarrhea may suffer from fecal incontinence even with intact and functional sphincter mechanisms. Obviously, if there is an underlying cause of the diarrhea as in irritable bowel syndrome or ulcerative colitis, it should be treated. Otherwise, attempts to improve the consistency of the stool into a more solid form should be undertaken with the use of bulk-adding agents such as fiber or constipating medications such as loperamide. This type of therapy aimed at producing a more solid stool may also be helpful in those patients with mild fecal incontinence due to neurologic injury or those with

structural damage who either do not wish attempted surgical repair or who are poor candidates for successful repair. Finally, individuals with overflow fecal incontinence due to chronic fecal impaction may find some degree of relief with the regular use of enemas or scheduled disimpaction.

Both an NIH consensus statement and the American Gastroenterological Association (AGA) have recommended biofeedback therapy in patients with fecal incontinence when it occurs within the first year following childbirth (NIH) or when it is associated with an intact sphincter or decreased rectal sensation due to nerve injury (AGA). Biofeedback is used to train patients to achieve improved striated muscle contraction with their pelvic floor or improve their ability to perceive rectal distention. A variety of techniques have been used. However, the effectiveness of biofeedback especially compared to standard therapy of patient education along with dietary measures and use of medications as needed to improve stool consistency is not settled. A Cochrane review in 2006 of randomized trials of a variety of biofeedback procedures failed to demonstrate an advantage to biofeedback.

A variety of injectable bulking agents and anal submucosal injection techniques have been used since 2001 in an attempt to treat passive fecal incontinence secondary to a damaged or weak internal anal sphincter with variable results. These materials have included silicone-based biomaterials (Malouf et al., 2001; Maeda et al., 2007; Soerensen et al., 2009), hyaluronic acid and dextranomer (Dehli, 2007; Graf et al., 2011; Schwandner et al., 2011), carbon-coated microbeads (Altomare et al., 2008; Aigner et al., 2009), calcium hydroxylapatite (Ganio et al., 2008), and collagen (Ullah et al., 2011). In 2011, the FDA approved Solesta (Salix Pharmaceuticals, Inc., Raleigh, NC), a sterile, injectable dextranomer hyaluronic gel to treat fecal incontinence. This is an office procedure consisting of four submucosal injections just proximal to the dentate line in the anal canal resulting in narrowing of the anal canal (Fig. 44.10).

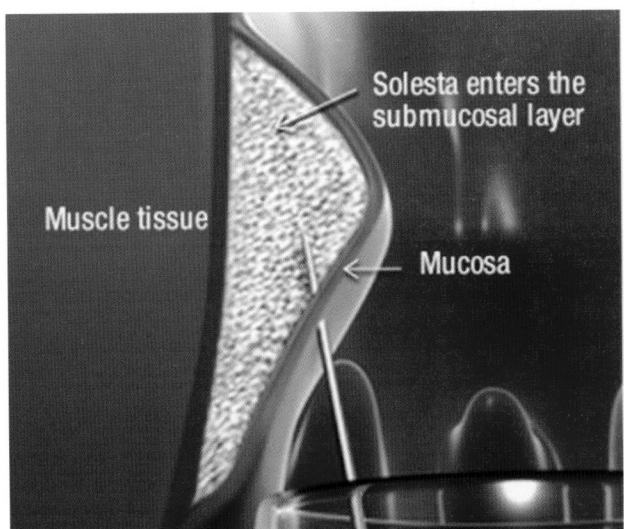

FIGURE 44.10 FDA approved Solesta, a sterile, injectable dextranomer hyaluronic gel, to treat fecal incontinence. This is an office procedure consisting of four submucosal injections just proximal to the dentate line in the anal canal resulting in narrowing of the anal canal. (Solesta is under license from and manufactured by Q-Med AB for Salix Pharmaceuticals, Inc. Used with permission of the copyright owner, Salix Pharmaceuticals.)

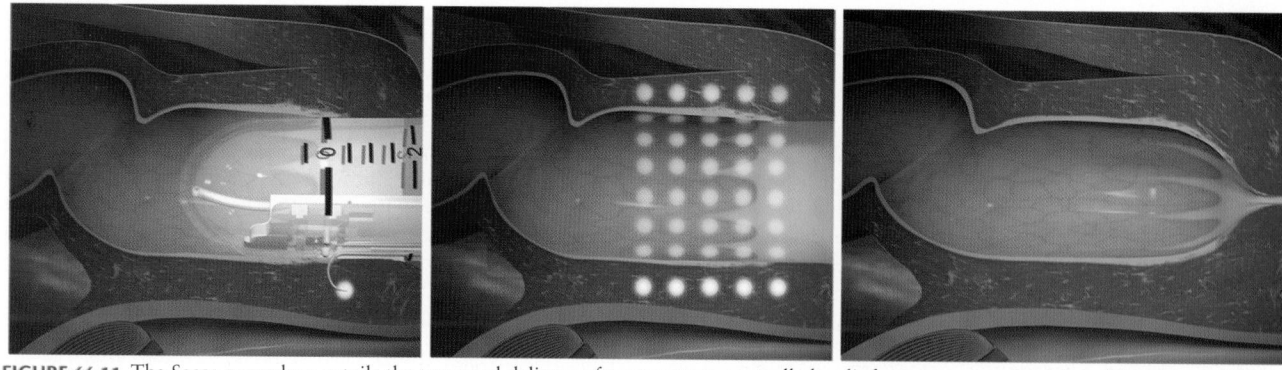

FIGURE 44.11 The Secca procedure entails the transanal delivery of temperature-controlled radiofrequency energy to the sphincter complex. It is an outpatient procedure usually performed under conscious sedation. An endoscopic device (**left panel**) uses four electrodes to deliver controlled radiofrequency energy to the sphincter muscles (**middle panel**). This results in precise, submucosal burn lesions ultimately resulting in tissue remodeling and improvement in anal sphincter function (**right panel**). (Copyright © Mederi Therapeutics, Inc. 2013. Used with permission.)

The randomized, double-blind, sham-controlled study by Graf demonstrated a decrease in incontinence episodes by 50% in the Solesta group compared to 31% in the sham treatment group in the short term. However, many questions yet remain about the long-term efficacy and patient selection criteria of this therapy. A Cochrane review done in 2010 examining the effectiveness of perianal injection of a variety of bulking agents up to that point reported that most trials demonstrated a short-term benefit regardless of the material used. No long-term evidence on outcomes is available. It is considered an investigational therapy by most insurance companies.

The Secca procedure (Mederi Therapeutics, Inc., Greenwich, CT), which received FDA clearance through Investigational Device Exemption in 2002, entails the transanal delivery of temperature-controlled radiofrequency energy to the sphincter complex (**Fig. 44.11**). It is an outpatient procedure usually performed under conscious sedation. An endoscopic device uses four electrodes to deliver controlled radiofrequency energy to the sphincter muscles. This results in precise, submucosal burn lesions ultimately resulting in tissue remodeling and improvement in anal sphincter function. Studies mostly consisting of short-term small case series by Takahashi and coworkers and by Efron and colleagues have demonstrated inconsistent effects on symptoms and quality of life. There have been no demonstrable objective effects such as increased anal canal manometry pressures or sphincter muscle thickness. A follow-up study by Takahashi-Monroy demonstrated sustained improvements in incontinence symptoms and quality-of-life scores at 5 years. However, Kim and associates recently failed to demonstrate either subjective or objective incontinence improvement at 6 months while at the same time reporting significant complications associated with the procedure. Most insurance companies consider the transanal application of radiofrequency energy for the treatment of incontinence to be investigational.

Perianal electrical stimulation has been shown to cause anal contraction in spinal cord injury patients as reported by Riedy and coworkers. A Cochrane review in 2000 of trials attempting to treat fecal incontinence was unable to make any reliable conclusions as to its efficacy. In addition, a randomized controlled trial using electrical stimulation of the anal sphincter as part of a biofeedback program for women with postpartum incontinence failed to demonstrate any benefit in outcome compared to standard biofeedback. There does not seem to be a role for perianal electrical stimulation for fecal incontinence treatment or prevention.

Sacral neuromodulation or sacral nerve stimulation (Inter-Stim, Medtronic, Minneapolis, MN) involves the placement

of electrodes under fluoroscopic guidance for stimulation of the S2, S3, and S4 nerve roots via their foramina (**Fig. 44.12**). This stimulation results in the contraction of the levator muscles and external anal sphincter. Kenefick and Christeansen reported that sacral neuromodulation seems to act by recruiting additional inactive motor units in the sphincter and pelvic floor muscles resulting in improved muscle strength and an increase in resting anal pressure. Originally, it was used only in the presence of intact although weakened sphincters. However, there are now multiple studies documenting improvement in

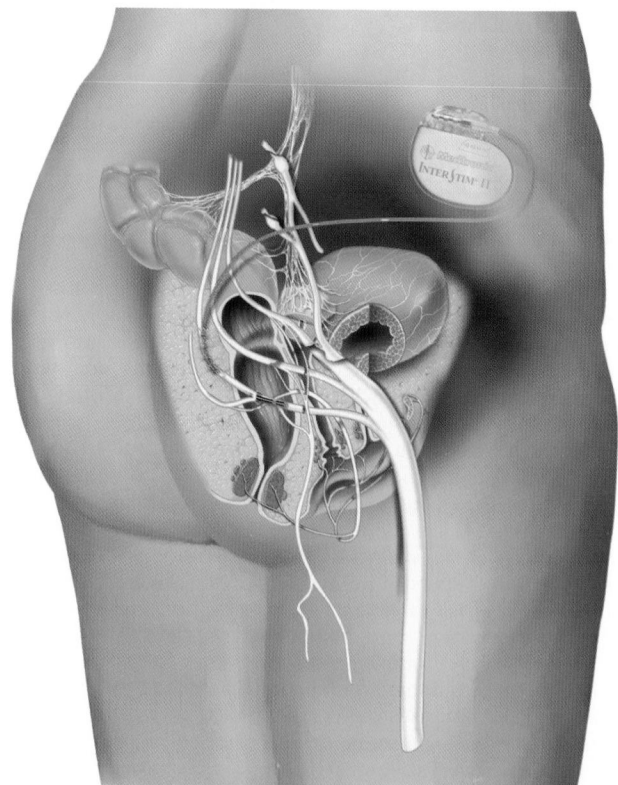

FIGURE 44.12 Sacral neuromodulation or sacral nerve stimulation involves the placement of electrodes under fluoroscopic guidance for stimulation of the S2, S3, and S4 nerve roots via their foramina. This stimulation results in the contraction of the levator muscles and external anal sphincter. (Copyright of 2011, image provided by Medtronic, Inc.)

fecal incontinence in those with anatomic sphincter defects (Chan et al., 2008; Boyle et al., 2009; Ratto et al., 2010; Brouwer & Duthie, 2010). It is a two-staged procedure involving the placement of a temporary percutaneous electrode attached to an external stimulator. If significant benefits are demonstrated over a 2- to 3-week period, then a permanent stimulator is placed. Wexner and colleagues, in a recent multicenter prospective randomized trial of 120 patients over 36 months, demonstrated a 50% decrease in weekly incontinence episodes in over 75% of individuals. Likewise, a meta-analysis in 2011 by Tan and coworkers of 34 studies involving 944 patients demonstrated significant improvements in objective and subjective outcome measures. Weekly incontinence episodes (weighted mean difference) decreased by 6.83 in the sacral neuromodulation groups compared to conservative management. Likewise, quality-of-life scores were also significantly improved. Both resting anal pressure and squeeze pressure were also significantly improved. Although there was greater improvement seen in sphincter intact patients, there was still significant improvement in the sphincter impaired group. Finally, Hull and colleagues recently reported on 5- to 8-year follow-up on 76 patients who underwent sacral neuromodulation device implantation for severe fecal incontinence. Fecal incontinence episodes per week decreased from a mean of 9.1 at baseline to 1.7 at 5 years, with 89% having a greater than 50% improvement and 36% having complete continence. Improvement in quality-of-life scores was also maintained over this 5-year period. Sacral neuromodulation must be considered in the treatment algorithm in patients with and without an intact sphincter. Its drawbacks are its expense and the need for a two-staged procedure. Matzel has recently published a treatment algorithm for fecal incontinence, which includes sacral nerve stimulation as a therapeutic alternative to surgical repair especially in those patients with a sphincteric defect of ≤180 degrees. The InterStim device received FDA approval in April 2011 for the treatment of chronic fecal incontinence.

Surgical Repair

STEPS IN THE PROCEDURE

Layered Approach to Anal Sphincteroplasty and Perineal Repair for Chronic Perineal Laceration

- Preoperative bowel preparation and antibiotics.
- Use of Lone Star Retractor for adequate perineal exposure.
- Transverse perineal incision at the junction of the posterior vaginal wall and anal mucosa.
- Sharp dissection to create a midline incision of the posterior vagina followed by further sharp dissection to free the distal vagina from the rectum.
- Dissection lateral to anal canal to identify ends of retracted external anal sphincter. Grasp ends of sphincter with Allis clamps.
- After excising scar from margins of anorectal mucosa, repair the defect in the anal mucosa with a continuous 3-0 delayed absorbable monofilament suture. If tissue is friable and won't hold the suture, place sutures full thickness through the mucosa;
  otherwise, try to stay submucosal.

- Repair the internal anal sphincter in a similar manner. This usually appears as a white layer of tissue well lateral to the anal mucosa you just repaired. Carry this repair distally for at least 3 to 4 cm all the way to the end of the anal mucosal suture line.
- Repair the external anal sphincter either through simple end-to-end reapproximation or overlapping repair. In the end-to-end repair, use 2-0 delayed absorbable monofilament suture, making sure that all four quadrants of the muscle are repaired. In the overlapping repair, dissect enough sphincter out so that the ends can overlap. Repair with 2-0 delayed absorbable monofilament suture in two rows of two horizontal mattress sutures.
- Narrow the genital hiatus by plicating the most distal ends of the puborectalis muscle together as part of the perineal body reconstruction. Do not allow this placation to extend above the perineal body and into the vaginal canal. Use 2-0 monofilament absorbable suture.
- Further repair the perineal body by suturing together the disrupted ends of the superficial transverse perineal muscles and the bulbocavernosus muscles using 2-0 delayed absorbable monofilament suture.
- Excise excess vaginal mucosa and repair with 3-0 delayed absorbable monofilament suture including a subcuticular closure of the perineal skin.
- Postoperatively every effort should be made to avoid stool passage through the repair for at least 3 to 4 days. However, avoid constipation. Keep stools soft for the next 6 to 8 weeks.

Patients with a demonstrable external sphincter defect may be considered for a surgical repair with either end-to-end repair or overlapping sphincteroplasty. Overlapping repair of the muscle seems to be preferred although differences in success rate between procedures seem small whether performed at the time of acute injury or delayed repair. The anal sphincter complex is a surgical challenge to repair because both the internal and external sphincters have a constant tone that begins pulling against the healing area almost immediately. Functional results from this surgery are far from perfect. The overlapping repair was proposed for the external anal sphincter in the hopes that the scarified ends of the torn sphincter would bolster support for the reparative sutures and not allow them to pull through, resulting in a better anatomic result and, it is hoped, better functional results. The advantage in terms of outcome seems to favor the overlapping approach over the end-to-end approximation method; however, more data from modern, well-designed, prospective studies clearly are needed in this area.

Many of these patients for delayed repair with a prior obstetrical injury will present with complete disruption of the perineal body along with an injury to the external anal sphincter and require separate repair of the anal canal mucosa and perineal body as well. This is usually performed through the standard layered approach to perineal repair and anterior sphincteroplasty. However, older operations such as the Warren flap or Noble procedure can also be performed.

The advantage of these two older procedures is the lack of a suture line in the anal mucosa. Regardless of the approach, it is the anterior sphincteroplasty that is most important in determining successful restoration of continence. Oliveira and colleagues demonstrated that in 55 women undergoing anterior sphincteroplasty of whom 39 had a successful outcome, the most important factor correlating with regained continence was the increase in mean and maximal resting and squeeze pressures obtained after surgery.

Blaisdell, in an older report, and Arnaud and associates, more recently, reported success rates of approximately 60% using the end-to-end approach. Using the overlapping technique, Sitzler and Thomson reported a 74% success rate in 27 women, most of whom had obstetric sphincter injuries. The continence rates after anal sphincteroplasty appear to diminish with time from the surgical correction. Rothbarth and colleagues reported on 39 patients who had obstetric injuries and underwent overlapping sphincteroplasty. Their success rates were 77%, 67%, and 62% at 3, 9, and 12 months, respectively. Multiple long-term follow-up studies of the degree and quality of continence after overlapping sphincteroplasties reflect the difficulty of the task at hand and that success rates diminish with time. Malouf and associates studied patients with a minimum of 5-year follow-up (median 77 months) and reported that 23 of 46 patients (50%) had a successful outcome defined as no further surgery and episodes of urge fecal incontinence occurring once a month or less. Of these, 23 patients were judged to have a successful outcome, 15 had passive soiling, 17 had fecal urgency, 19 were incontinent of solid and liquid stool, and none were fully continent of stool and flatus. In a study of 71 consecutive patients with long-term follow-up treated by overlapping sphincteroplasty, Halverson and Hull found that 54% were incontinent of solid or liquid stool, and only 14% remained totally continent. Median follow-up was 69 months with a range of 48 to 141 months. Gutierrez and colleagues reported on 130 patients with a median follow-up of 10 years. Sixty-one percent continued to have incontinence or required further surgery. Eight patients (6%) were totally continent. Zutshi and coworkers reported on 31 patients with a median age of 44 years at the time of overlapping sphincter repair with a median follow-up of 129 months. No patients were fully continent at 129 months. Patients who were older at the time of surgery and those who had undergone multiple vaginal births had the worst outcomes. Finally, Dudding and coworkers in a systematic review of the literature in 2008 determined that only 20% of patients were continent to liquid and solid stool at 10 years after overlapping sphincter repair. They reviewed 10 studies of secondary overlapping sphincter repair each with greater than 30 subjects with more than 12-month follow-up. The percentage of patients with incontinence to liquid and/or solid stool was significantly greater the longer the duration of the study ($r^2 = 0.71$; $P = 0.0024$).

As previously mentioned, success rates for anal sphincter repair in patients with concurrent pudendal neuropathy are generally worse than for those with intact innervation. Gilliland and colleagues looked at a large group of patients who had undergone an overlapping sphincteroplasty with a median follow-up of 2.4 years. They found that 62% of 59 patients with normal pudendal function had a successful outcome, compared with only 17% of the 12 patients with unilateral or bilateral prolonged PNTMLs.

Karoui and associates also observed that success rates deteriorated with time and that poor results were associated with the presence of an internal sphincter defect. The importance of the internal anal sphincter to continence is a subject of recent interest. It has long been known that this structure contributes most of the resting tone in the anal canal and helps to maintain day-to-day continence. Purposeful lateral disruption of the internal sphincter to aid with anal fissure healing has been shown to be associated with the development of at least transient incontinence. Vaizey and associates have identified primary degeneration of the internal sphincter as an independent cause of passive anal incontinence in some women with normal neurologic function and no obstetric trauma. It follows that repair of a disrupted internal sphincter should contribute to continence.

Little attention has been paid in the past to repair of the internal sphincter either at the time of initial obstetric injury or at the time of reconstruction of a long-standing injury. Repair of the internal anal sphincter should be attempted at the time of anterior sphincteroplasty although this seems to be much more difficult to achieve. A recent report by Farrell and associates on primary repair of obstetrical third- and fourth-degree lacerations demonstrated a persistent defect of the internal anal sphincter in 90% of the 27 women studied. This high incidence of persistent postrepair defect was despite what the author characterized as a heightened emphasis on the identification and repair of the sphincter.

Layered Method of Repair and Anterior Sphincteroplasty

Preoperatively, a mechanical bowel preparation is important. An oral bowel preparation should be given the evening before surgery is scheduled. If such a preparation is given the day of surgery, the patient may still be releasing stool during the operation. Preoperative parenteral prophylactic antibiotics should be given. The optimal postoperative diet for these patients is a matter of much controversy but little scientific study. Decades ago, these patients were given diverting colostomies to keep the fecal stream away from the repair until healing was complete. Patients would then have another procedure to close their colostomy. Most postoperative feeding regimens are based on the concept of keeping fecal material from the repair site for at least 4 to 5 days until the mucosal suture line has healed adequately and the reparative process is well established. A regimen of clear liquids for 3 to 5 days, with progression to a soft, low-residue diet for the next several weeks, can be given. Constipating agents are sometimes used immediately postoperatively, but should not be used for a prolonged period of time because one wants the first bowel movement to be soft so as not to distend the repair. The use of an elemental liquid diet for 1 week postoperatively can be useful, but is poorly tolerated by many patients and can lead to diarrhea in some. Alternatively, fiber supplementation and adequate hydration can be used to give patients more bulky but deformable stool so as not to traumatize the repair. Stool softeners and a high-fiber diet are advisable for 6 weeks postoperatively.

A transverse or crescent perineal incision is used at the junction of the posterior vaginal wall and anal mucosa. The lateral margins of the incision are extended to the region of the perineal dimple created by the retracted external sphincter, and a midline incision is made along the lower half of the posterior vaginal wall (**Fig. 44.13A**).

The edges of the vaginal and rectal mucosa are grasped separately with Allis clamps, and the anterior rectal wall is separated in the midline from the posterior vaginal wall with careful scissors dissection. The dissection is carried laterally by sharp dissection to the region of the external anal sphincter. The internal anal sphincter, which is the thickened distal condensation of the circular smooth muscle layer of the rectum, can be seen between the external anal sphincter and the anorectal

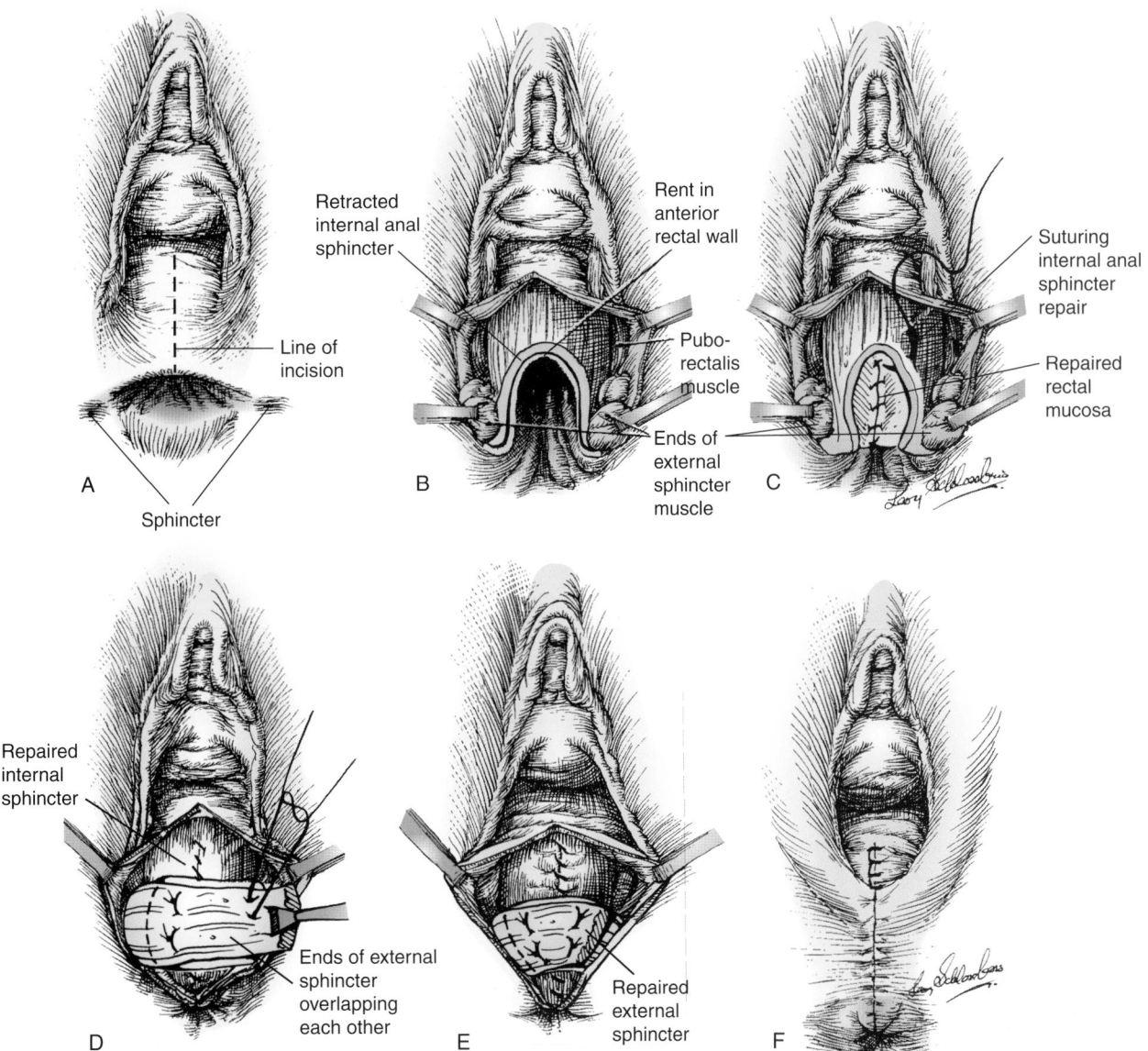

FIGURE 44.13 Layered closure of a chronic complete perineal laceration with overlapping sphincteroplasty. **A:** A transverse incision is made at the junction of the vaginal and rectal mucosa and extended up the midline of the posterior vaginal wall. **B:** The rectal wall has been separated from the posterior vaginal wall with careful sharp dissection. The ends of the external sphincter have been identified and grasped with Allis clamps. The internal anal sphincter can be seen between the external anal sphincter and the anorectal mucosa as an area of white fibrous tissue. **C:** The defect in the anal mucosa has been closed with a continuous 3-0 delayed absorbable suture. The internal anal sphincter then is reapproximated over a length of 3 to 5 cm. This layer also serves to imbricate and isolate the mucosal layer and take tension off of it to help it heal and seal against infection. **D:** The ends of the external anal sphincter are widely mobilized with the scar tissue left on. Care should be taken not to dissect beyond the 3-o'clock and 9-o'clock position as that is where the pudendal enervation to the sphincter enters laterally. The external sphincter then is brought together over the repaired internal sphincter with two rows of two horizontal mattress sutures of delayed absorbable or permanent suture material. **E:** After the external sphincter has been repaired, the genital hiatus is narrowed by bringing the puborectalis muscles closer together with interrupted delayed absorbable sutures placed in the fascia overlying them. **F:** The bulbocavernosus and superficial transverse perineal muscles have been reattached to the perineal body, and the vaginal mucosa was closed with a continuous locking stitch of 3-0 delayed absorbable suture that was continued subcuticularly to approximate the perineal skin.

mucosa as an area of white fibrous tissue (Fig. 44.13B). Meticulous hemostasis and wide mobilization to allow closure without tension are crucial to success with this operation.

A fibrous scar that is retracted lateral to the wall of the anal canal often identifies the external sphincter. The exact anatomic margins of the external sphincter frequently are difficult to ascertain. A nerve stimulator can be used to identify contractile skeletal muscle. Alternatively, the Allis clamps

containing the ends of the external sphincter can be brought together in the midline and a circumferential sphincter tested for by inserting a double-gloved index finger into the rectum. If necessary, the clamps should be readjusted to incorporate more of the retracted muscle bundles until the constricted effect of the reapproximated sphincter can be demonstrated.

All scar tissue is excised from the margins of the anorectal mucosa, and the defect in the anal mucosa is closed using a

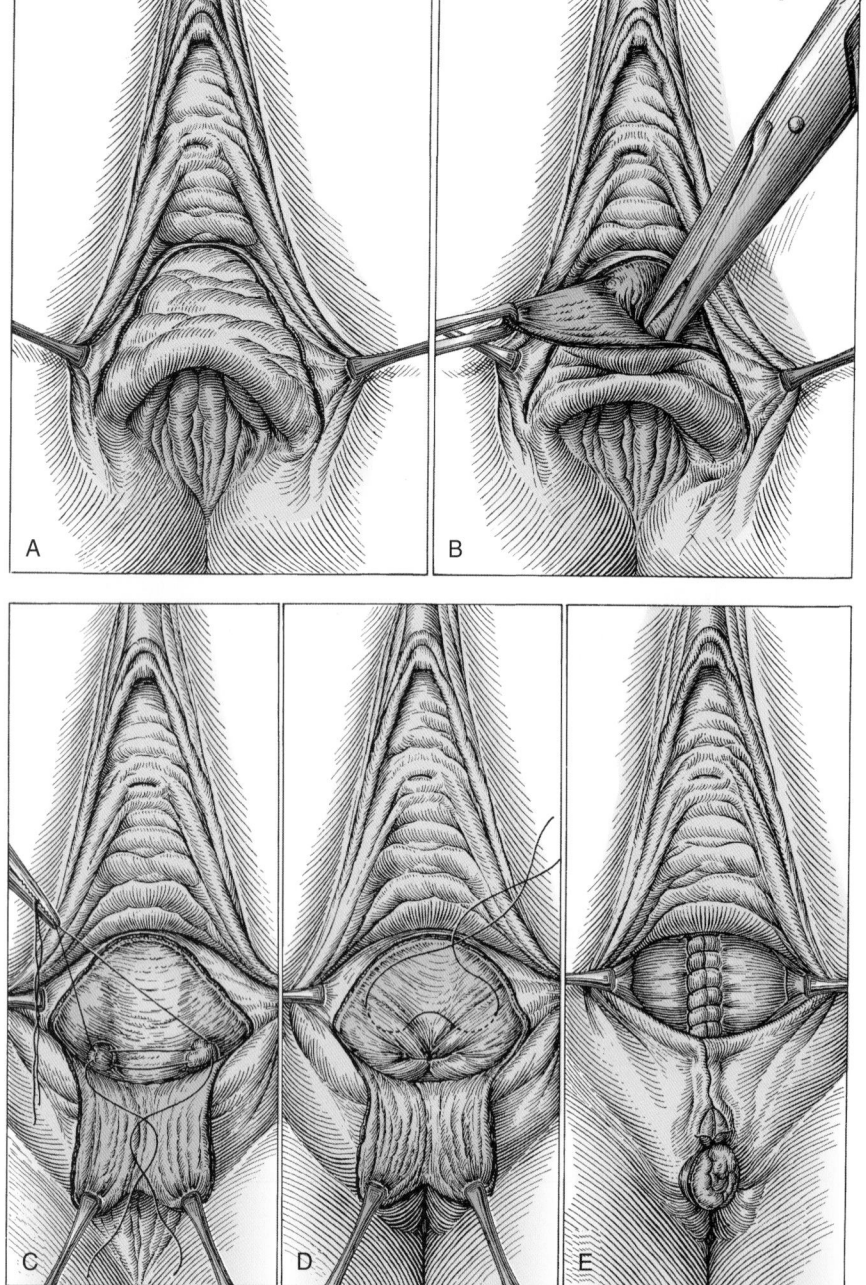

FIGURE 44.14 Warren flap operation for complete perineal laceration. **A:** The line of incision outlines the flap of vaginal mucosa. **B:** The flap is dissected free and turned back. **C:** The flap is retracted downward. The ends of the sphincter are delivered and are either sutured end to end as pictured or with an overlapping technique as described. **D:** The external sphincter has been repaired, and the puborectalis muscles are then brought closer together taking care to not create a posterior band of tissue. **E:** The vaginal incision is closed with a continuous locking stitch that is continued subcuticularly over the perineum. The margins of the flap are included in the continuous suture, which may temporarily create a peaked appearance in the perineal skin. If the margins of the vaginal mucosal flap are redundant, it may be trimmed.

continuous or interrupted suture of 3-0 delayed absorbable material. A running suture may have the advantage of distributing tension along the entire suture line and helping prevent a gap in the closure that could occur from ischemia if an interrupted suture is tied too tight. A submucosally placed suture is ideal. Sometimes, this tissue is quite friable, and a full-thickness suturing of the mucosa is the safest method.

After the mucosal margins are approximated, a second supporting layer inverts the initial mucosal suture line (Fig. 44.13C). This layer often has been thought of in the past as "perirectal fascia," but in fact, it is the thickened downward continuation of the circular smooth muscle layer of the rectum that is the internal anal sphincter. This appears as a white smooth layer of tissue between the anorectal mucosal closure

and the external anal sphincter. Care should be taken in reapproximating this layer over a length of 3 to 5 cm as this muscle is responsible for most of the resting pressure in what is normally a 4-cm high-pressure zone in the anal canal. This layer also serves to imbricate and isolate the mucosal layer and take tension off of it to help it heal and seal against infection.

In an approximation-type external anal sphincteroplasty, the external anal sphincter ends are completely trimmed of scar tissue and united in the midline with interrupted 0 or 2-0 delayed absorbable sutures. Although some surgeons prefer a permanent suture, such as a braided silicone-treated polyester, a delayed absorbable monofilament suture such as polydioxanone has the advantage of maintaining excellent tensile strength for an extended period while avoiding the presence of a permanent foreign body. This becomes particularly important in the event of wound infection. Four or five sutures are used to approximate the sphincter muscle. These can be placed 1 cm apart, full thickness, with the nondominant index finger in the anal canal to aid in acquiring excellent purchase on both ends while assuring no penetration of the anal canal itself.

In an overlapping approach to the external anal sphincter, the scarified ends of the sphincter are important to the repair itself and are left in place. The concept of the overlapping sphincteroplasty is to use the scarred ends of the torn sphincter to help hold the sutures that reconstitute the circumferential sphincter. The ends are widely mobilized with the scar tissue left on. Care should be taken to not dissect beyond the 3-o'clock and 9-o'clock position because the pudendal innervation to the sphincter enters laterally. The external sphincter then is brought together over the repaired internal sphincter with two rows of two horizontal mattress sutures of delayed absorbable or permanent suture material (**Fig. 44.13D**).

An important part of the perineal reconstruction is the restoration of a narrower genital hiatus by bringing the puborectalis muscles closer together. One must remember that the arms of the puborectalis muscle do not normally come in contact with each other between the rectum and the vagina. Overzealous plication of the puborectalis muscle can constrict the vaginal introitus and create posterior tissue banding that can lead to dyspareunia. Dissection should be carried out laterally to the fascia overlying the medial border of the puborectalis muscle. This fascia should then be brought together by a series of interrupted, delayed absorbable sutures. Each suture should be held tightly and the vagina tested before tying to assure that posterior banding is not created. If it is, that suture should be removed and another placed (**Fig. 44.13E**).

Further support and elevation of the perineal body are provided by bringing together the disrupted ends of the superficial transverse perineal muscles and the bulbocavernosus muscles. These muscles normally insert on the perineal body and play a part in pelvic floor support. They should be included in perineal reconstruction, including obstetric repair, to reestablish and support the perineal body. After this step, the redundant vaginal mucosa is excised, and the remaining mucosa is approximated in the midline with a continuous 2-0 or 3-0 delayed absorbable suture. This is followed by a subcuticular closure of the perineal skin (**Fig. 44.13F**).

Warren Flap Operation for Complete Third-Degree Tear

An inverted V-shaped incision is made in the posterior vaginal mucosa, outlining the flap that is to be turned down. The lower ends of the incision should be just lateral to the dimples caused by retracted sphincter ends (**Fig. 44.14A**). The length of the flap should measure a minimum of 3 cm to provide sufficient vaginal mucosa to be incorporated into the anal canal and cover the reconstructed perineal body.

Taking care to avoid injuring the bowel wall, the surgeon dissects the flap of mucosa free from the top downward (**Fig. 44.14B**), stopping short of the margin between the vaginal and anal mucosa. If this margin is perforated, then the blood supply to the mucosal flap is compromised, thereby nullifying the advantage of the flap technique. The properly demarcated flap allows the areas overlying the sphincter ends to be denuded. The flap is grasped with two mucosal Allis clamps and is turned down to hang over the anus. The external anal sphincter ends are then dissected free, using Allis clamps for traction. An approximation- or overlapping-type external anal sphincteroplasty then is performed (**Fig. 44.14C**). Although an

approximation-type sphincteroplasty is pictured, an overlapping procedure as described above could be incorporated into this procedure.

The fascia overlying the medial aspect of the puborectalis muscles is identified, and this tissue is brought together with a series of interrupted sutures for reinforcement in the manner described for the layered technique, using 0 or 2-0 delayed absorbable sutures (**Fig. 44.14D**). Each suture should be tested before tying to assure that the caliber of the vagina is not compromised.

Closure of the vaginal mucosa is carried out as in an ordinary perineal repair. Interrupted plication stitches of 2-0 delayed absorbable suture are used to advance the fascia and shorten the muscle fibers of the perineal body, which strengthens the external sphincter as well. The margins of the vaginal mucosa and graft are approximated in the midline by a continuous locking stitch of 3-0 delayed absorbable suture. The tip end of the vaginal mucosal flap should not be trimmed too closely, even though it protrudes somewhat from the repaired perineal body. It retracts as healing occurs (**Fig. 44.14E**).

Noble Procedure for Complete Perineal Laceration

The torn perineal, anal, and rectal tissues in patients with a complete perineal laceration form a "butterfly" appearance across the perineum (**Fig. 44.15A**). The "wings" of the butterfly are the lateral perineal dimples of the retracted ends of the external anal sphincter. The initial incision is outlined around the margins of this area following the margin of the anal mucosa along the anatomic defect in the rectovaginal septum. The perineal skin is left attached and held with Allis clamps to facilitate later dissection of the retracted ends of the external sphincter. A small margin of vaginal mucosa is also left attached to the anal wall for traction because the anal mucosa is so friable.

Atraumatic clamps are placed along the margin of the anal canal, and sharp dissection is used to carefully separate the anal wall from the overlying vaginal mucosa. The external anal sphincter remnants should be sharply mobilized and separated from the underlying anal wall (**Fig. 44.15B**). The vaginal mucosa is widely mobilized from the anal canal and lower rectal wall laterally to the underlying levator muscles and proximally into the middle or upper one third. Adequate mobilization of the anterior anorectal wall allows it to be pulled outside the margin of the anal orifice without difficulty, thus avoiding sutures in the anorectal canal.

Once the ends of the external anal sphincter are mobilized to meet in the midline with traction on the Allis clamps, the overlying skin previously left attached is excised, and the sphincter ends are approximated end to end in the midline (**Fig. 44.15C**). Alternatively, one could perform an overlapping sphincteroplasty as previously described. Several of these sphincteroplasty sutures also should include the muscular layers of the anterior rectal wall to prevent it from retracting inward and to avoid tension on the suture line between the advanced anterior anorectal wall and the perineal skin. The genital hiatus should be narrowed by bringing the puborectalis muscles closer together as previously described (**Fig. 44.15D**). The transverse perineal muscles and the inferior margins of the bulbocavernosus muscles then are reapproximated, further reconstituting and supporting the perineal body.

The vaginal mucosa is trimmed, if necessary, and the margins of the posterior vaginal wall are approximated with a continuous locking stitch of 3-0 delayed absorbable suture.

VII

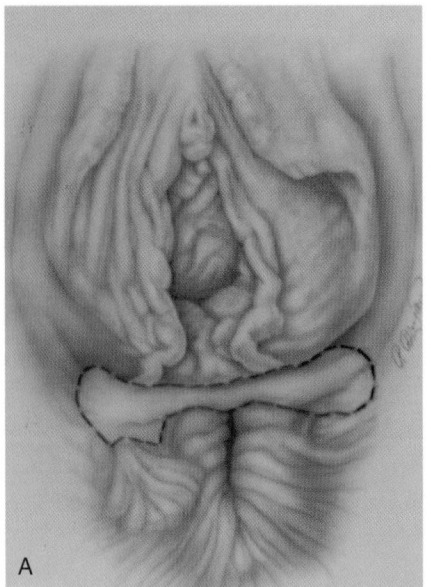
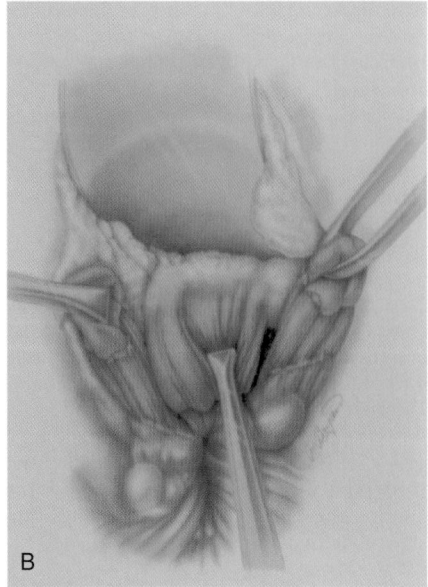
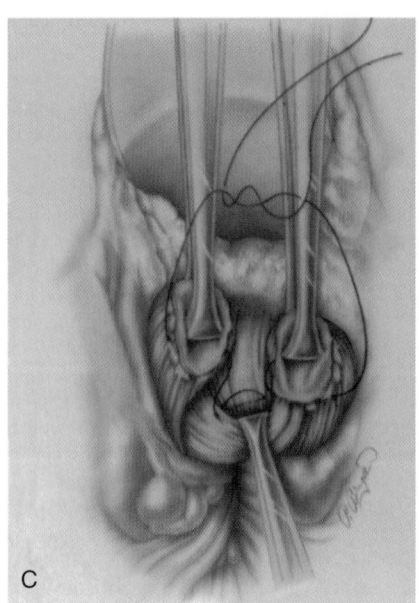

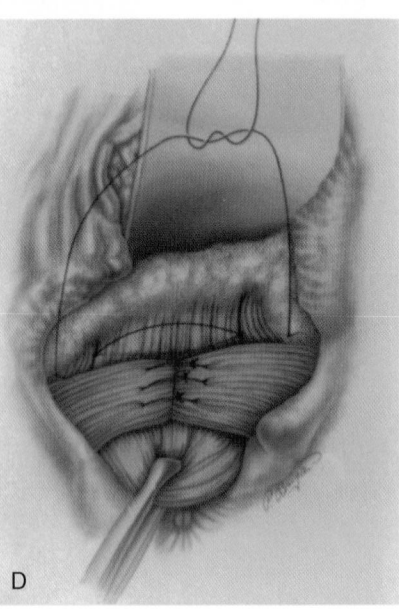
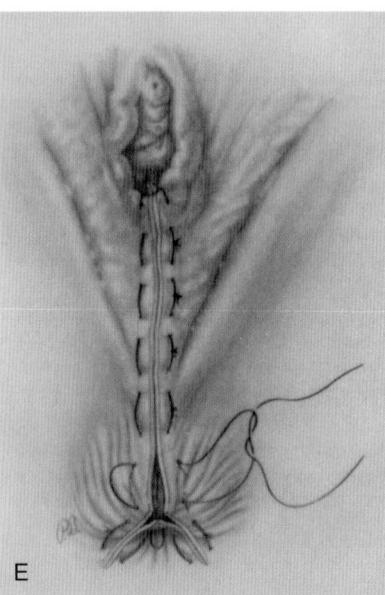

FIGURE 44.15 The Noble operation for complete perineal laceration. **A:** A "butterfly-shaped" scar is noted across the perineum, where there are torn perineal, anal, and rectal tissues. The ends of the external anal sphincter can be recognized by lateral perineal dimpling. **B:** The anterior rectal wall is mobilized extensively from the posterior vaginal wall to allow it to be pulled down without tension. The wings of the butterfly are left attached to facilitate dissection of the retracted ends of the sphincter. **C:** Ends of the anal sphincter are trimmed and sutured together and to the pararectal fascia of the advanced anterior rectal wall. Several delayed absorbable sutures are used. **D:** The levator muscles and pararectal fascia are brought closer together in the midline. **E:** The transverse perineal muscles and the inferior margins of the bulbocavernosus muscles are brought together to reconstitute the perineal body, and the vaginal mucosa and perineal skin are closed. The mobilized anterior wall of the anal canal is sutured without tension to the perineal skin.

The continuous suture closing the posterior vaginal mucosa is carried over the perineal body as a subcuticular stitch, and the perianal skin then is approximated at the midline. The mobilized anterior wall of the anal canal is drawn outside the reconstructed anal orifice and sutured without tension to the perianal skin (Fig. 44.15E). The excess anal mucosa is trimmed. Care should be taken to remove as little of the distal anal canal as possible because this tissue contains the internal anal sphincter. Vertical mattress sutures of 3-0 delayed absorbable suture are used to approximate the broad surface of the

anal submucosa to the perianal skin. Any residual separation of the margins of the anal mucosa and perianal skin can be approximated with interrupted sutures.

Muscle Transposition, Artificial Sphincters, and Diversion

The following advanced procedures are largely reserved for patients with difficult anal incontinence problems or multiple operative failures. Muscle transposition procedures exist in which the gracilis muscle, sartorius muscle, or gluteus muscle is swung a flap to encircle the anal canal. Dynamic muscleplasty procedures involve stimulation of this muscle with an intramuscular neurostimulator to induce it to convert to the characteristics of normal external anal sphincter muscle. The muscle is continuously stimulated at a low frequency for 8 to 10 weeks until the transformation from a fast-twitch to a slow-twitch muscle has been achieved. At this point, the frequency of stimulation is increased so that the muscle contracts around the anal canal and occludes it continuously. When the patient wishes to defecate, the pulse generator can be turned off by a magnet. Once defecation is complete, the stimulator can be turned on again by the magnet. In a series of 20 patients reported by Hallan and associates, 12 have a functioning neoanal sphincter. Madoff and colleagues found a 70% reduction in solid stool incontinence in two thirds of patients undergoing a dynamic graciloplasty. However, one third of these patients experienced a major wound complication with their surgery. Penninckx studied 60 consecutive patients undergoing dynamic graciloplasty. The operation failed in 27, 7 of whom went on to have stoma construction. There were 75 complications that required 61 reoperations in 44 patients.

Some investigators have used an artificial bowel sphincter, ABS (Acticon Neosphincter, American Medical Systems, Minneapolis, MN), around the anal canal in patients with severe anal incontinence (**Fig. 44.16A, B**). It restores physiologic anal canal pressures through the transfer of fluid pressures between components. Although the initial results were good in a small series of patients, cuff erosion into the anal canal and infection have been significant problems that have caused a number of the sphincters to be removed. In a small randomized controlled trial of artificial sphincter versus supportive care, O'Brien and associates found a significant improvement in continence scores in the operative group. Unfortunately, in

a review in 2004, Mundy and associates reported revision and removal rates to be between 12.5% to 50% and 16.7% to 41.2%. Revisions seem to be most often due to leaks from the anal cuff from microperforations attributable to repeated cycles of inflation and deflation, while removal is usually due to localized infections around the device components.

More recently, Lehur and coworkers have reported on a magnetic anal sphincter (MAS) device like that used in gastroesophageal reflux disease (Bonavina et al., 2008; Ganz et al., 2008) implanted in a small number of patients with fecal incontinence. This implantable device (FENIX, Torax Medical, Inc., Shoreview, MN) consists of a series of titanium beads with magnetic cores hermetically sealed inside (**Fig. 44.17**). The beads are interlinked together with independent titanium wires to form a flexible ring around the external anal sphincter in a circular fashion. The purpose of the device is to reinforce the sphincter and prevent episodes of incontinence. Defecation is accomplished by having the patient push as in normal defecation such that a number of beads separate allowing stool to move through the device. Results from an early feasibility study by Lehur and associates involving 14 patients were encouraging with 5 completing at least 6 months of follow-up. There was a mean reduction of weekly incontinence episodes of over 90%, improvement in continence scores, and quality-of-life scores. Wong and coworkers have recently reported comparable results with this device to the ABS noted earlier. This retrospective study involving 10 patients in each group demonstrated improved quality-of-life scores and continence scores in each group. The advantage of the MAS device so far seems to be simpler implantation procedure compared to the artificial sphincter. Obviously, the exact role this device will play in the future will depend on long-term outcomes.

For the patient with uncontrollable anal incontinence that cannot be addressed by any other procedure, a permanent

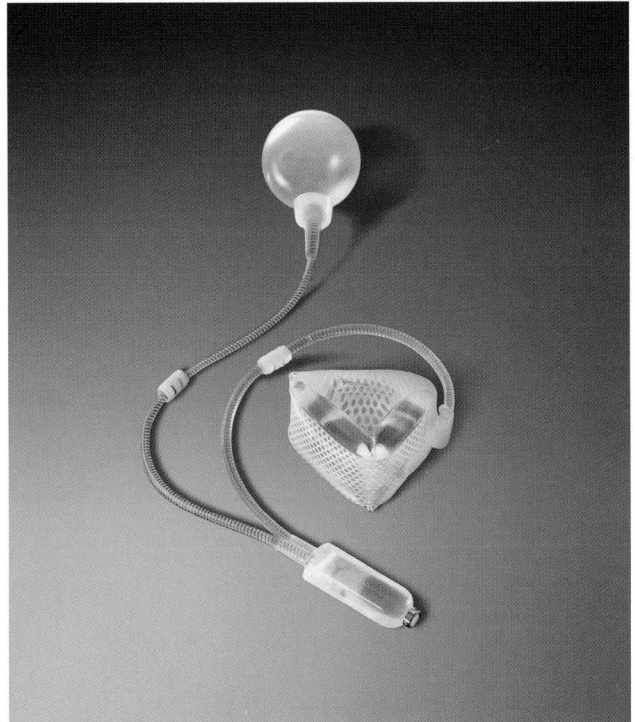

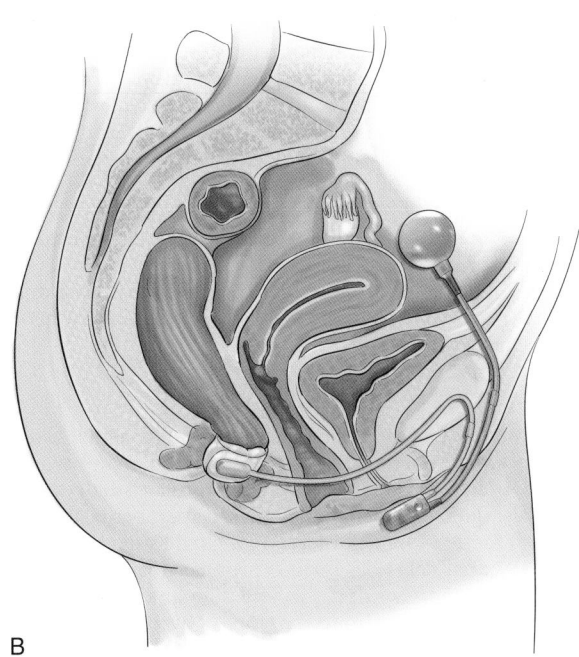

A   B

FIGURE 44.16 A: Artificial bowel sphincter, ABS (Acticon Neosphincter, American Medical Systems, Minneapolis, MN) illustrating its three major components: pressure-regulating balloon, anal cuff, and pump. It restores physiologic anal canal pressures through the transfer of fluid pressures between components. **B:** Implanted ABS device. (Reprinted with permission of American Medical Systems, Inc.)

VII

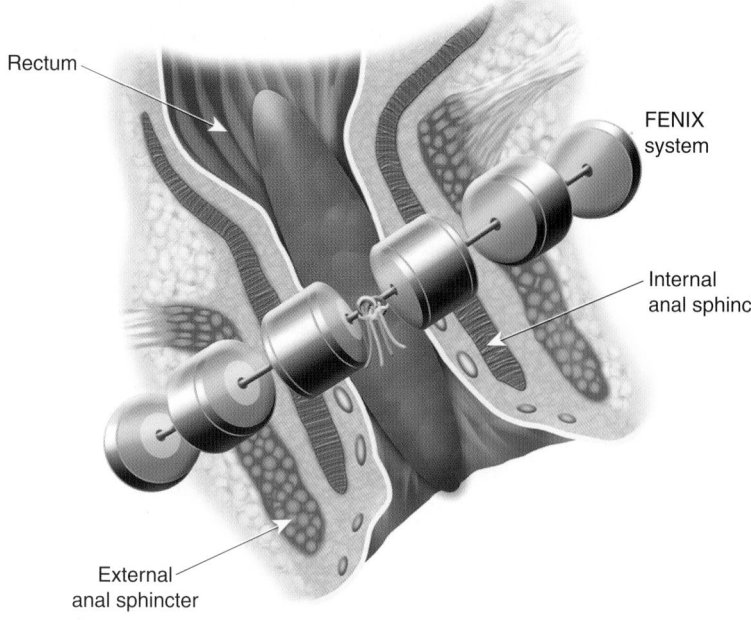

Rectum

FENIX system

Internal anal sphincter

External anal sphincter

FIGURE 44.17 Implanted (FENIX, Torax Medical, Inc., Shoreview, MN) device consists of a series of titanium beads with magnetic cores hermetically sealed inside. The beads are interlinked together with independent titanium wires to form a flexible ring around the external anal sphincter in a circular fashion. Defecation is accomplished by having the patient push as in normal defecation such that a number of beads separate allowing stool to move through the device. (Reprinted with permission from Torax Medical, Inc.)

diverting colostomy may be a more manageable and preferable alternative to constant perineal soiling with the hygienic and social problems it brings. Stoma problems, however, occur in as many as one quarter of patients.

RECTOVAGINAL FISTULAE

A rectovaginal fistula resulting in extra-anal fecal incontinence is a distressing condition for the patient and a challenge to her physician. Most fistulae actually arise in the anal canal beginning distal to the pectinate line and should more accurately be considered anovaginal fistulae. The result of this condition often is the uncontrolled passage of flatus or stool from the anorectal canal through the fistulous tract into the vagina. It can be a socially disabling condition. Further, the difficulties of treatment leading to failure (contaminated operative site, high-pressure anal canal, usually without diversion) challenge both the patience of the affected individuals and the surgeon's skill.

Rectovaginal fistulae are usually classified as to their size, location, and cause. A simple system is as follows:

Simple—low or mid vaginal, less than 2.5 cm in diameter, due to trauma or infection
Complex—high vaginal, greater than 2.5 cm in diameter, due to previous inflammatory bowel disease, radiation, or neoplasm, and previous failed repairs

Etiology

Although there are many different causes of rectovaginal fistulae (Table 44.3), numerous series report that the majority are caused by obstetric trauma. Rectovaginal fistulae usually arise as a complication of a repaired fourth-degree perineal tear. Risk factors for development of a rectovaginal fistula in association with vaginal deliveries include prolonged labor, difficult forceps delivery, shoulder dystocia, and a midline episiotomy.

A rectovaginal fistula may develop as a result of direct surgical injury to the rectum or vagina, ischemia, or postoperative infection. Other less common causes include blunt instrumentation or penetrating trauma caused by an accident. Occasionally, rectovaginal fistulae follow an infectious

process such as a perianal abscess or an infected Bartholin duct cyst abscess. The most common cause of high rectovaginal fistulae is repeated bouts of diverticulitis with abscess formation followed by development of a sigmoidovaginal fistula or a combined sigmoidovesicovaginal fistula. Inflammatory bowel disease such as ulcerative colitis or Crohn disease may result in complex rectovaginal fistulae. Crohn disease is a transmural condition of the bowel that often results in a rectovaginal fistula.

Radiation is a relatively infrequent cause of fistula formation today. These fistulae usually begin as a proctitis with ulceration and fistula formation followed by a stricture. Fistulae may occur several years after completion of radiation therapy. Primary or metastatic disease in surrounding organs (rectum, cervix, uterus, or vagina) may result in rectovaginal fistulae. Because congenital rectovaginal fistula is usually managed at a young age and is associated with other anomalies, it is usually not managed by the gynecologic surgeon.

Clinical Evaluation

The most common symptoms are the passage of flatus and stool into the vagina. The severity of those symptoms may be affected by the size of the fistula. There is usually a foul-smelling vaginal discharge with periodic, uncontrolled escape of gas. Occasionally, the fistula may develop immediately following

TABLE 44.3 Causes of Rectovaginal Fistula

Congenital
Acquired
 Trauma
  Obstetric
  Operative
  Violent
 Infectious
 Inflammatory bowel disease
 Radiation
 Carcinoma

obstetrical trauma. More commonly, it appears 7 to 10 days after delivery. The breakdown of a primary repair, inadequate repair, or infection at the primary site may explain this delayed presentation. Because of antepartum fecal incontinence associated with pregnancy, perineal pain associated with delivery or episiotomy, and/or stool softeners prescribed in pregnancy or postpartum, the patient may not seek medical attention for some time. Diarrhea, rectal bleeding, mucus discharge, and abdominal pain may be caused by the underlying status of the bowel and usually do not result from the fistula per se.

The history frequently suggests the underlying cause of the fistula and may greatly influence the timing and route of repair. On physical examination, the location, size, and number of openings can be identified. On vaginal exam, the granulation-like tissue of the fistula may be noted. The route of the fistula may be outlined by the passage of a thin probe from the vagina through the fistulous tract into the anal or rectal canal. Placing an examining finger in the rectum aids this process. Contraction of the puborectalis and external anal sphincter should be evaluated for competency. Multiple studies have demonstrated that associated sphincter injury is present in nearly 100% of patients where obstetrical trauma is the cause of the fistula. The perineal body is examined, and the tissues about the fistula are delineated to gain more insight into the cause of the underlying fistula. Multiple perianal fistulae should raise the suspicion of Crohn disease. A proctosigmoidoscopic examination usually is done to ensure that the mucosa of the intestinal tract is normal.

In patients with a history compatible with a fistula but in whom no fistula opening can be identified, a simple office examination can be helpful. With the patient in a slight Trendelenburg position with a size 20 Foley urinary catheter, a 5-mL balloon is placed in the anal canal. Air is instilled through the catheter while the water-filled or soap-covered vagina is observed for any escape of air bubbles originating from the anal canal. Likewise, a tampon test may be performed in which a tampon is placed in the vagina and the patient is given a small enema with methylene blue–colored water, which she is asked to retain for 20 minutes. Blue discoloration of the tampon is noted in the presence of a fistula. However, this test may be negative if there is a very low fistula. Contrast studies may be necessary to define the sigmoidovaginal fistula or fistulae associated with primary bowel disease.

Surgical Management

Numerous operative procedures have been described for repair of rectovaginal fistula, including transvaginal, transanal, and abdominal approaches. Gynecologists usually use a transvaginal approach, whereas colon and rectal surgeons prefer the transanal technique. The transvaginal technique allows for a layered closure of the fistula and sphincteroplasty with or without a perineoproctotomy. Also, the vaginal advancement or Noble procedure is an option with the transvaginal approach. Transanal techniques include the layered closure, endorectal flap advancement, and anocutaneous flap advancement. The determining factors to be considered include the cause of the fistula, its location and accessibility, and the status of the anal sphincter. Overall, the success rate for repair seems to be more related to the type of fistula than to the type of repair. Pinto and colleagues in a recent case series of 184 procedures of various types including transanal, transvaginal, gracilis interposition, and transperineal approaches carried out in 125 patients with fistulae of various etiologies from the Cleveland Clinic Florida found that the overall success rate per procedure was 60% with no difference in recurrence rates

based on type of repair. Patients with obstetrical injuries had a success rate per procedure of 66.7%. Overall, there was a success rate of 89% with an average of 1.3 procedures per patient for obstetric patients. On the other hand, patients with Crohn disease had more recurrent fistulae with an only 44.2% success per procedure, although eventually 78% of these patients eventually healed with an average of 1.8 procedures.

Early Repair

Hankins and colleagues described early repair of carefully selected rectovaginal fistulae and episiotomy breakdowns using a technique of early return to the operating room for debridement followed by daily cleansing of the wound area. After a 6- to 7-day interval, their patients were returned to the operating room for surgical repair of the fistula. With this approach, successful healing occurred in 90% of their patients. We prefer to wait 8 to 12 weeks to allow the surrounding inflammation to resolve before surgical intervention. Preoperative mechanical bowel preparation should be given. On the morning of operation, tap water enemas can be given until clear.

Appropriate treatment of a rectovaginal fistula requires consideration of the cause and location of the fistula and the condition of the involved tissues. For fistulae located in the lower portion of the anal canal, we prefer to use the lithotomy position to carry out the operative repair. For fistulae at the very apex of the vagina, an abdominal approach generally is required. This may include needed resection of the involved bowel side of the fistula as in the case of a malignant or radiation-induced fistula.

Low Rectovaginal Fistula: Layered Repair

A transvaginal technique for small rectovaginal fistula repair involves a circular incision about the fistulous opening (Fig. 44.18). With traction on the vaginal wall and

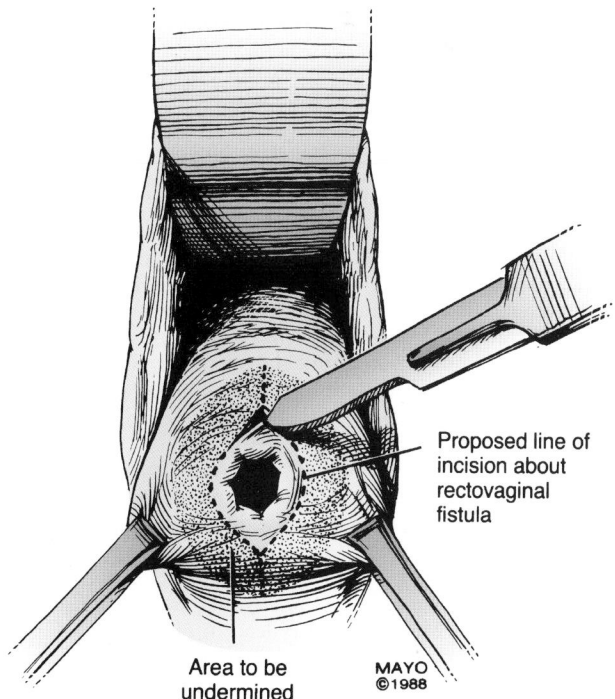

Proposed line of incision about rectovaginal fistula

Area to be undermined

MAYO ©1988

FIGURE 44.18 Small rectovaginal fistula with proposed line of initial incision. (Adapted from Lee RA. *Atlas of gynecologic surgery.* Philadelphia, PA: WB Saunders, 1992. By permission of Mayo Foundation for Medical Education and Research. All rights reserved.)

VII

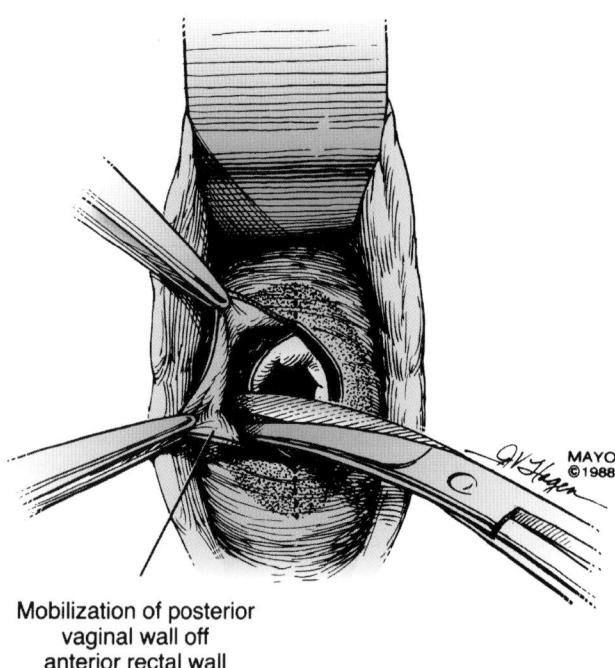

Mobilization of posterior
vaginal wall off
anterior rectal wall

FIGURE 44.19 Incision of vaginal wall, mobilizing posterior vagina from underlying anterior anal canal. (Adapted from Lee RA. *Atlas of gynecologic surgery*. Philadelphia, PA: WB Saunders, 1992. By permission of Mayo Foundation for Medical Education and Research. All rights reserved.)

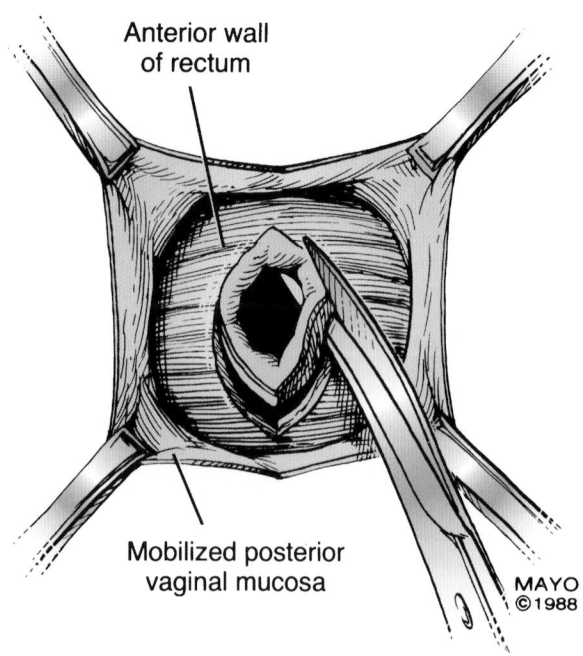

Anterior wall
of rectum

Mobilized posterior
vaginal mucosa

FIGURE 44.20 Excision of fistulous tract. (Adapted from Lee RA. *Atlas of gynecologic surgery*. Philadelphia, PA: WB Saunders, 1992. By permission of Mayo Foundation for Medical Education and Research. All rights reserved.)

countertraction applied to the edge of the fistulous tract, the vagina is separated from the underlying rectal wall with sharp dissection, and this proceeds circumferentially (Fig. 44.19). This wide mobilization permits later approximation of the fresh injury free of tension. Once the vaginal walls are mobilized from the underlying rectum, the entire fistulous tract is excised to include a small rim of the rectal mucosa (Fig. 44.20), converting the fistula to a fresh injury. With the surgeon's nondominant index finger lifting and supporting the anterior rectal wall, the initial sutures are placed extramucosally, including a portion of the muscularis and submucosa, with 3-0 delayed absorbable sutures (Fig. 44.21). We frequently place all sutures throughout the length of the fistula, after which they are individually tied in the order in which they were placed. The initial suture line begins and is extended a full 5 to 8 mm above and below the site of the fistulous tract to assure complete closure. A second layer (Fig. 44.22) begins 5 mm above the previously closed suture line and extends 5 mm distal to the fistulous closure, inverting the initial suture line into the rectum, and no sutures are located within the rectal lumen.

Once the wall of the rectum is reconstructed, the lower portions of the puborectalis muscle and the external anal sphincter are approximated to add a third layer in the closure (Fig. 44.23A), which helps to reconstitute the anterior rectal wall. Care should be taken that approximation is not carried so far superiorly that it results in a transverse bar across the posterior vaginal wall, which may lead to dyspareunia. Once the muscular walls are approximated, the vaginal wall is approximated with 3-0 delayed absorbable sutures, accurately placed so as to promote primary apposition of the fresh edge of the vaginal wall (Fig. 44.23B).

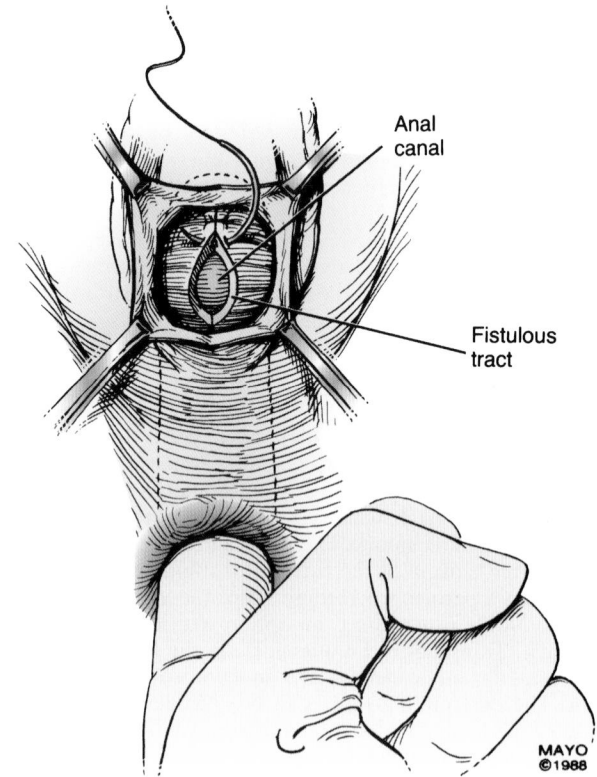

Anal
canal

Fistulous
tract

FIGURE 44.21 Extramucosal placement of sutures in the wall of the anterior anal canal. (Adapted from Lee RA. *Atlas of gynecologic surgery*. Philadelphia, PA: WB Saunders, 1992. By permission of Mayo Foundation for Medical Education and Research. All rights reserved.)

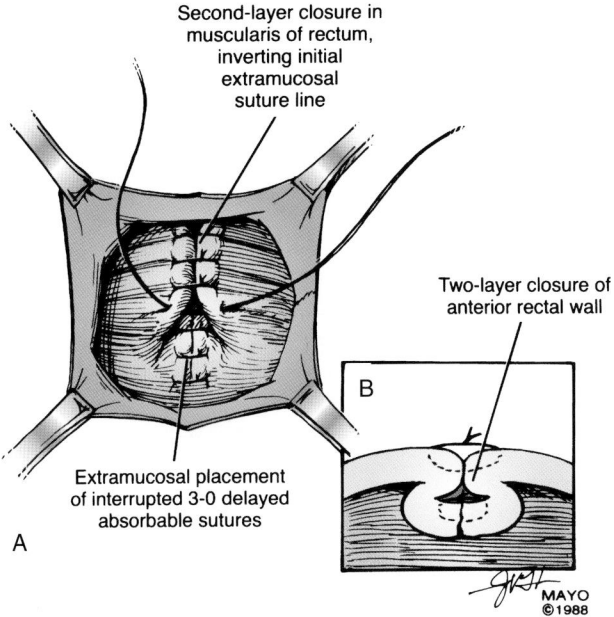

FIGURE 44.22 **A:** Inversion of initial suture line with approximation of the muscularis of the anal canal. This thickened smooth muscle layer is the internal anal sphincter. **B:** Side view representing closure of the first and second layers in the anal canal. (Adapted from Lee RA. *Atlas of gynecologic surgery.* Philadelphia, PA: WB Saunders, 1992. By permission of Mayo Foundation for Medical Education and Research. All rights reserved.)

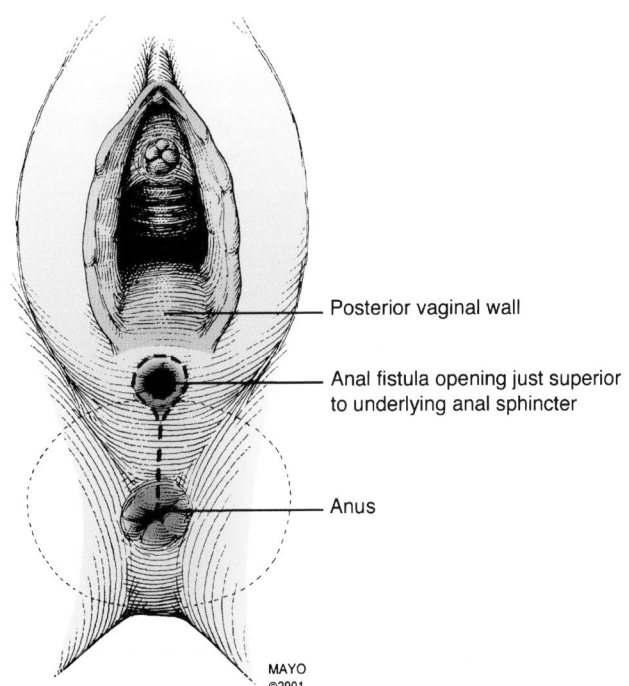

FIGURE 44.24 Proposed incision of the perineal body and posterior vaginal wall with excision of fistulous tract. (Adapted from Lee RA. *Atlas of gynecologic surgery.* Philadelphia, PA: WB Saunders, 1992. By permission of Mayo Foundation for Medical Education and Research. All rights reserved.)

Occasionally, the fistulous tract is so close to the external anal sphincter that closure is difficult. In this situation, a perineoproctotomy in which the bridge of skin, sphincter, and perineal body are divided, and the fistula is thus essentially converted to a fourth-degree tear (**Fig. 44.24**). The fistulous tract is excised, and the posterior vaginal wall is mobilized from the anterior anal wall (**Fig. 44.25**). The anal canal is

then reconstructed with interrupted or running fine delayed absorbable sutures approximating the mucosa of the anal canal. This initial suture line then is inverted with a second layer of interrupted fine delayed absorbable sutures approximating the retracted tissues of the internal anal sphincter, resulting in reconstruction of the anal canal (**Fig. 44.26**). The retracted ends of the external anal sphincter are approximated

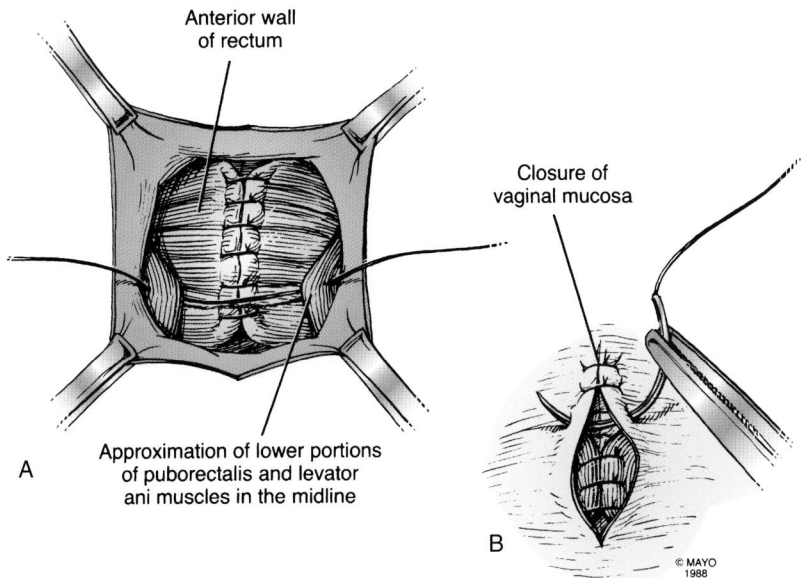

FIGURE 44.23 **A:** Reconstruction of the anal canal with approximation of portions of the puborectalis and external anal sphincter. **B:** Interrupted sutures approximating the posterior vaginal wall. (Adapted from Lee RA. *Atlas of gynecologic surgery.* Philadelphia, PA: WB Saunders, 1992. By permission of Mayo Foundation for Medical Education and Research. All rights reserved.)

VII

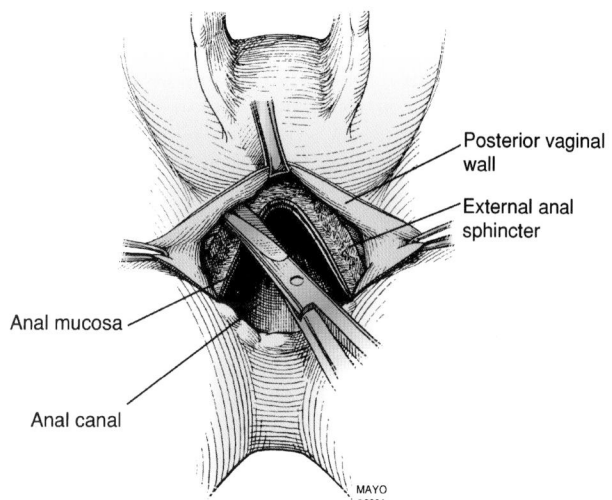

FIGURE 44.25 Mobilization of the posterior vagina off the anterior anal canal with conversion of rectovaginal fistula to fourth-degree injury. (By permission of Mayo Foundation.)

in the midline in an end-to-end fashion with fine delayed absorbable sutures (Fig. 44.27). This results in a snug closure that is resistant to the passage of the surgeon's little finger. Alternatively, at this point, one could perform an overlapping sphincteroplasty as described earlier. The perineal body is reconstructed in such a fashion that there is significant support to the reconstructed anal sphincter, and yet entrance to the vagina is not compromised (Fig. 44.28).

Considerable experience exists with the transanal flap approach to rectovaginal fistulae involving the lower portion of the rectovaginal septum. Rothenberger and colleagues reported on a technique that uses an endorectal flap consisting of mucosa, submucosa, and circular muscle fibers. The flap is twice as wide at the base as it is at the apex. They achieved successful repair in 32 of 35 patients with rectovaginal fistulae. Hoexter and associates reported a similar high rate of fistula healing and improvement in anal continence, emphasizing several points for successful repair via

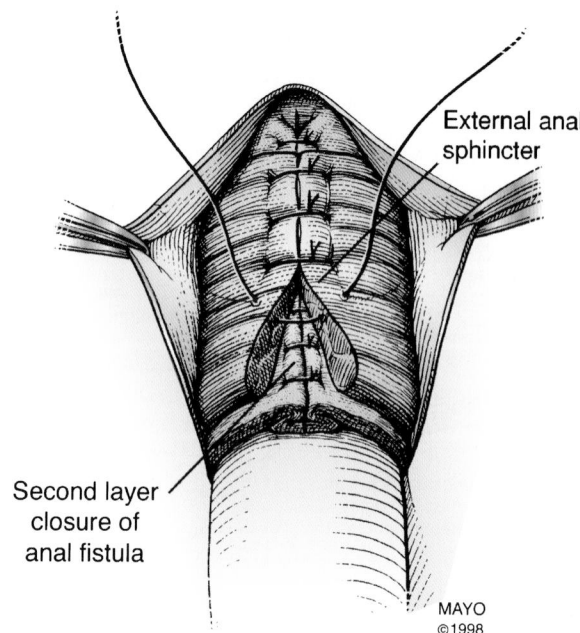

FIGURE 44.27 Reanastomosis of retracted external anal sphincter with the surgeon's left index finger in the anal canal. (Adapted from Lee RA. *Atlas of gynecologic surgery*. Philadelphia, PA: WB Saunders, 1992. By permission of Mayo Foundation for Medical Education and Research. All rights reserved.)

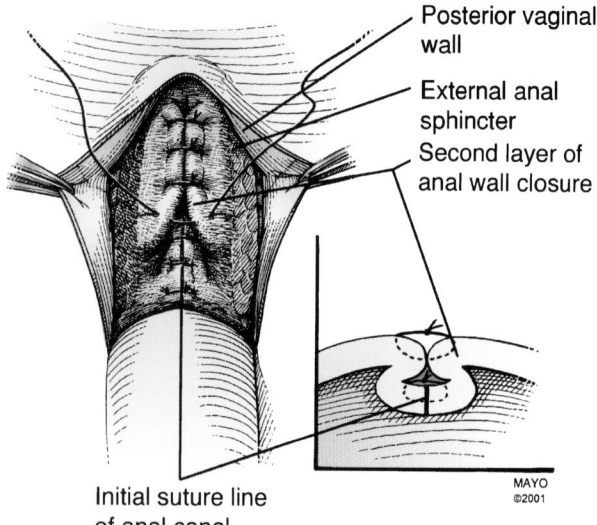

FIGURE 44.26 Two-layer reconstruction of anal canal. (By permission of Mayo Foundation.)

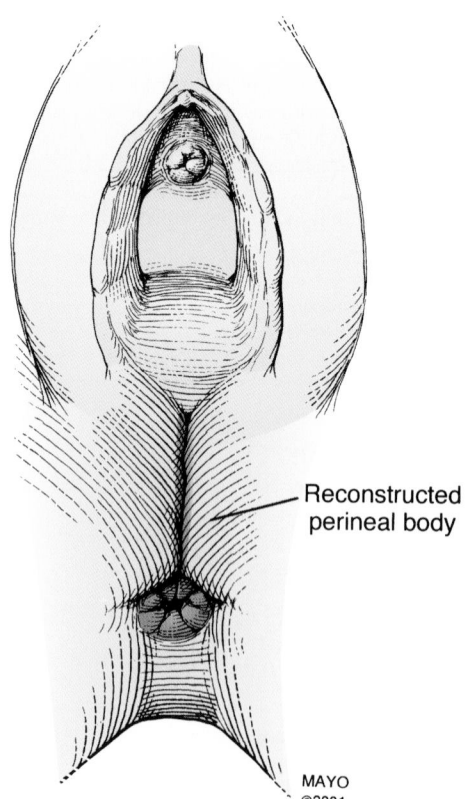

FIGURE 44.28 Reconstructed perineal body with subcuticular approximation of skin of perineum. (Adapted from Lee RA. *Atlas of gynecologic surgery*. Philadelphia, PA: WB Saunders, 1992. By permission of Mayo Foundation for Medical Education and Research. All rights reserved.)

endorectal flap: (a) elevating the rectal flap for at least 4 cm to the fistula, (b) excising the fistulous tract, (c) leaving the vaginal wound open for drainage, and (d) using an elliptic flap to avoid devascularization of the flap apex. Others have reported a high degree of efficacy of the endorectal flap for achieving both fistula healing and repair of any associated anal sphincter disruptions.

Tissue Interposition

A variety of techniques have been described to transpose healthy muscle tissue between the vagina and the rectum in order to successfully repair a rectovaginal fistula. Tissue interposition is intended to interpose normal healthy tissue between suture lines and bring well-vascularized tissue into the area. This may be needed in cases of previous failed repairs or radiation injury with resulting fibrosis and poor vascularity of the tissues. Tissue interposition with either the labial fat pad (Martius procedure) or gracilis muscle has been described. However, since successful closure of a radiation fistula requires aggressive excision of the surrounding tissues, the fistula is often best managed with a primary resection and anastomosis of the rectosigmoid through a lower abdominal incision.

Lefevre and coworkers recently reported on eight patients who underwent a gracilis muscle transposition for recurrent fistulae after an average of three prior failed repairs. The etiology was Crohn disease in 5, iatrogenic injury in 2, and obstetrical injury in 1. Six of the eight patients (75%) healed after the gracilis muscle transplant alone.

Boronow has used bulbocavernosus–labial tissue graft (Martius procedure) to successfully treat radiation-induced rectovaginal fistulae. He reported on 25 radiation-induced vaginal fistulae in 22 patients. There were 16 rectovaginal fistulae, 3 vesicovaginal fistulae, and 3 combined vesicovaginal and rectovaginal fistulae. Successful closure was accomplished in 84% of the patients with rectovaginal fistulae.

A description of the Martius procedure follows. Figure 44.29 depicts the usual location of a radiation fistula, high in the posterior vaginal wall. The potential sites from which the pedicled bulbocavernosus Martius-type flap are obtained are illustrated in Figure 44.30. Initially, an incision is made in the vagina to separate the scarred vagina from the underlying anterior wall of the rectum circumferentially. The edge of the scarred vaginal epithelium adjacent to the edge of the rectal mucosa is excised in anticipation of this being the site of the initial suture line approximating the squamous epithelium from the vulvar flap to the rectum in order to fill the defect in the rectum. With a Mayo scissors, a subcutaneous tunnel is made from the labium majus to the fistula under the labium and vaginal mucosa (Fig. 44.31). The free end of the muscle is guided through the subcutaneous tunnel with a single absorbable suture placed along its edge to assist in passage through the tunnel. The rectal defect is such that it cannot be closed primarily. Thus, the edge of the squamous epithelium from the vulvar graft is sutured to the edge of the rectal mucosa with 4-0 delayed absorbable sutures. Occasionally, a Schuchardt incision is required in the vagina to obtain adequate exposure for the dissection.

The pedicled graft is used to close the fistulous defect, beginning at the 3-o'clock position, in a synchronous fashion such that the entire edge of the fistulous tract is in immediate proximity to the edge of the skin from the vulva (Fig. 44.32). Once in place, the muscle and subcutaneous tissue of the graft are sutured to the surrounding connective tissue.

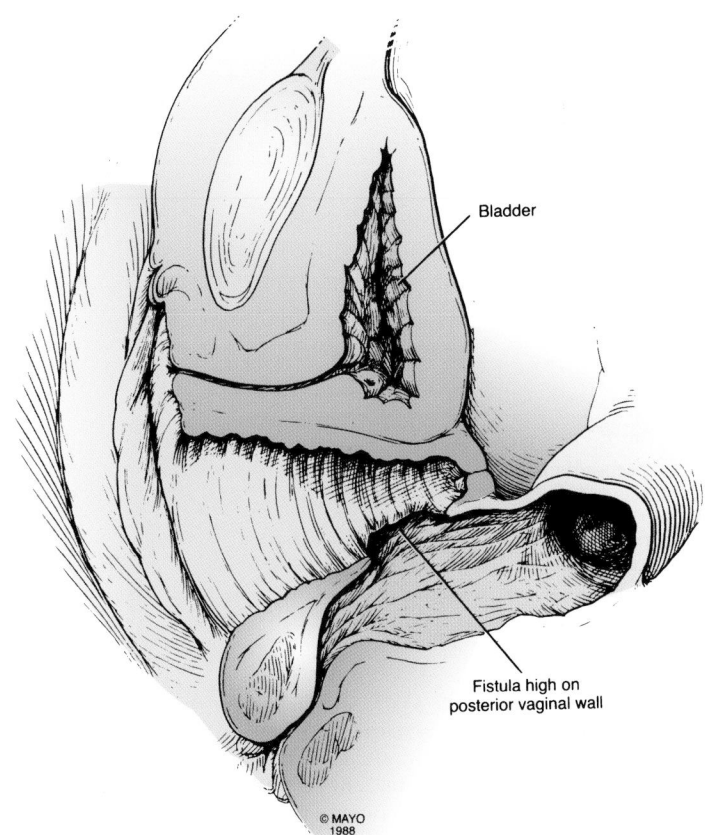

Bladder

Fistula high on
posterior vaginal wall

© MAYO
1988

FIGURE 44.29 Radiation-induced fistula. (By permission of Mayo Foundation.)

VII

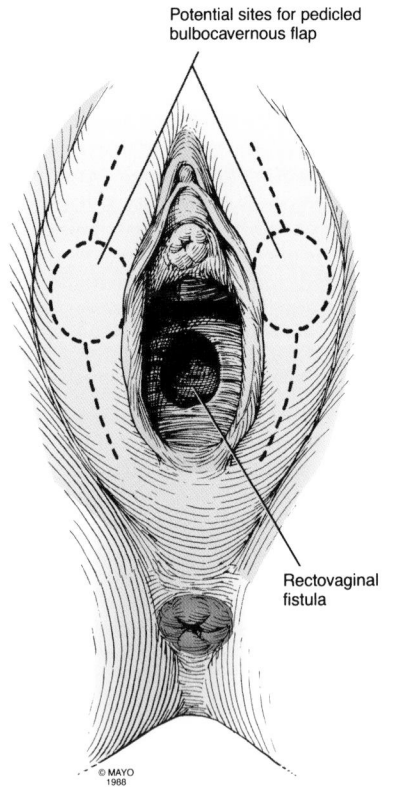

FIGURE 44.30 Proposed sites to harvest the skin and subcutaneous tissue in preparation to fill hole of rectovaginal fistula. (Adapted from Lee RA. *Atlas of gynecologic surgery*. Philadelphia, PA: WB Saunders, 1992. By permission of Mayo Foundation for Medical Education and Research. All rights reserved.)

To provide coverage for the exposed Martius flap, which has been inserted as a plug into the rectum, a similar pedicled graft is developed from the patient's right side; this is placed so that the skin of the vulva is approximated to the skin of the vagina (Fig. 44.33). The edges are placed such that there is no exposed source for granulation tissue (Fig. 44.34).

A small suction catheter is placed between the two pedicled grafts and brought out through a stab wound lateral to the perineal incision. The vulvar incision is closed in layers and the skin approximated with fine interrupted delayed absorbable suture. In patients requiring a pedicled graft, the repair may result in a narrowing of the vagina and a degree of stenosis. This results not only from the encroachment on the vaginal lumen by the pedicled grafts but also from the associated contracture caused by the underlying cause of the fistula: pelvic radiation. There is a tendency for further contracture and stenosis of the vagina, which may result in significant dyspareunia or apareunia. These potential outcomes should be carefully discussed with the patient and her family prior to attempted surgical correction of a radiation-induced rectovaginal fistula.

Sigmoidovaginal Fistula: Sigmoid Resection with Sigmoidorectostomy

Fistulae between the sigmoid colon and vagina occur infrequently, but the overwhelming majority result from diverticulitis of the sigmoid colon (Fig. 44.35) in a patient who has previously had a hysterectomy. Generally, the sequence of events consists of the patient experiencing repeated bouts of acute diverticulitis that finally result in perforation of a diverticulum and abscess formation with a fistulous tract communicating to the vagina. Passage of fecal material or gas through the vagina in the absence of a rectal communication should

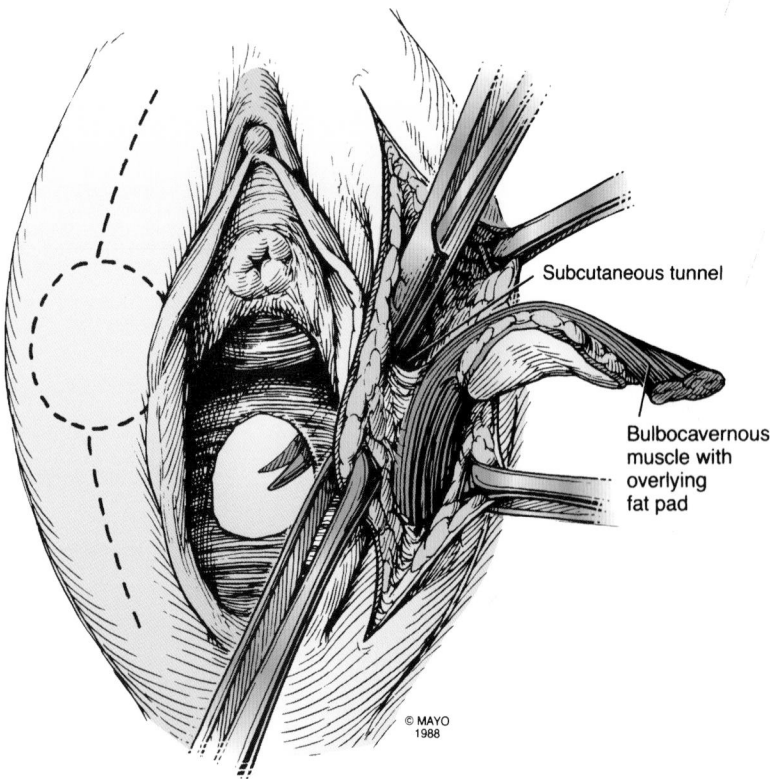

FIGURE 44.31 Mobilization of the bulbocavernosus muscle with overlying fat pad. (Adapted from Lee RA. *Atlas of gynecologic surgery*. Philadelphia, PA: WB Saunders, 1992. By permission of Mayo Foundation for Medical Education and Research. All rights reserved.)

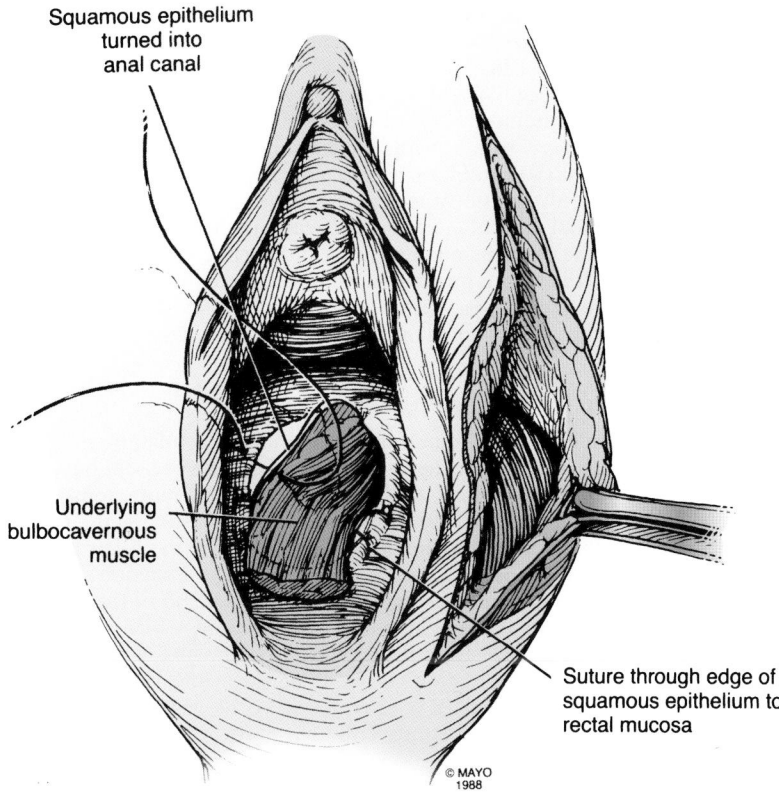

Squamous epithelium turned into anal canal

Underlying bulbocavernous muscle

Suture through edge of squamous epithelium to rectal mucosa

© MAYO 1988

FIGURE 44.32 Suture fixation of the pedicled skin to rectal mucosa. (Adapted from Lee RA. *Atlas of gynecologic surgery*. Philadelphia, PA: WB Saunders, 1992. By permission of Mayo Foundation for Medical Education and Research. All rights reserved.)

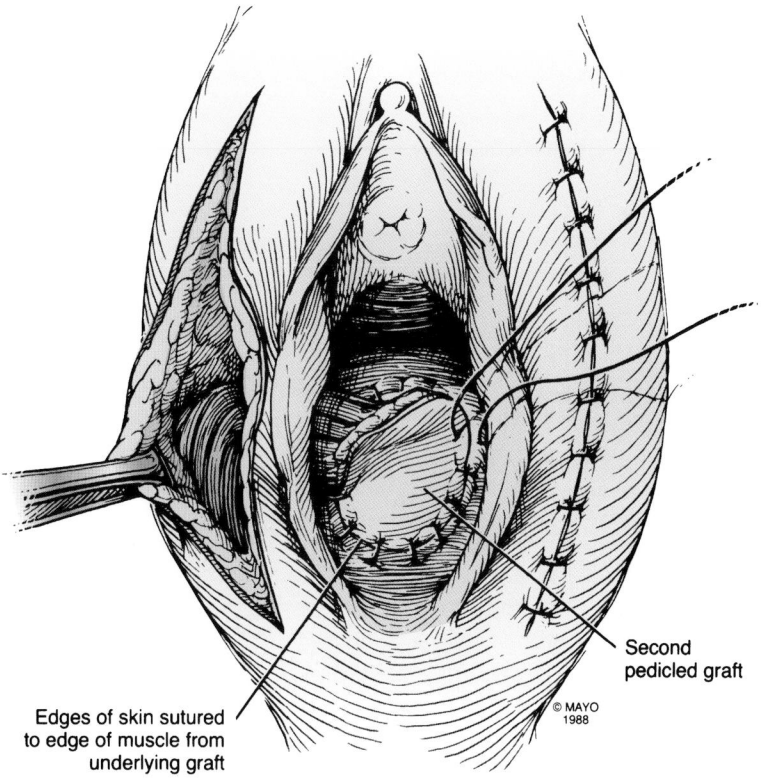

Second pedicled graft

Edges of skin sutured to edge of muscle from underlying graft

© MAYO 1988

FIGURE 44.33 Approximation of the skin of the vulvar flap to the skin of the vaginal wall. (Adapted from Lee RA. *Atlas of gynecologic surgery*. Philadelphia, PA: WB Saunders, 1992. By permission of Mayo Foundation for Medical Education and Research. All rights reserved.)

VII

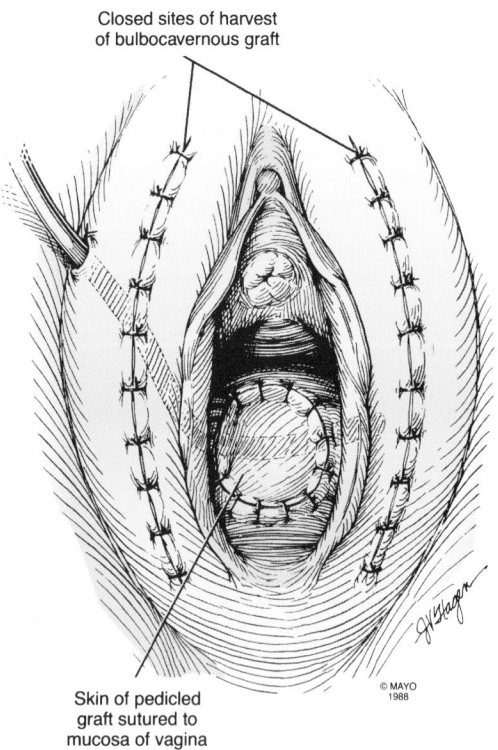

FIGURE 44.34 Reconstructed perineum in completed repair of fistula. (Adapted from Lee RA. *Atlas of gynecologic surgery*. Philadelphia, PA: WB Saunders, 1992. By permission of Mayo Foundation for Medical Education and Research. All rights reserved.)

lead one to suspect a fistula arising from the sigmoid colon or small intestine. A proctoscopic examination should be done, although often it is impossible to visualize the fistulous orifice because of narrowing or fixation resulting from the inflammatory condition. Surgical intervention is indicated for a sigmoidovaginal fistula that is large enough to permit the passage of fecal material. In a few selected patients, a colostomy may be the only treatment, or the fistula may be divided and the sigmoidal defect closed with or without a temporary colostomy. In the overwhelming majority of patients, we prefer a sigmoid resection with primary anastomosis and closure of the opening into the vagina. The need for a temporary protective colostomy is determined on an individual basis.

Hartmann Procedure

Under some circumstances, the infected, inflammatory process is such that the sigmoid mass may be excised, but a primary anastomosis is ill advised. It may be more appropriate to excise the diseased colon and close the fistula in the vagina, leaving the defunctionalized rectal stump in the pelvis for later reanastomosis (Fig. 44.36). Omentum and a suction drain are usually placed over the stump. The distal end of the descending colon is brought out as a colostomy, which is matured at the initial surgical procedure. Later, usually after 2 to 3 months, reoperation can be done through the previous incision. Placement of a gauze pack in the vagina and an EEA sizer in the anal stump will help to identify these structures. Once identified, the descending colon is freed from the splenic flexure in a sufficient fashion to permit the primary descending colorectostomy in a noninfected field as a closing step in this two-stage procedure.

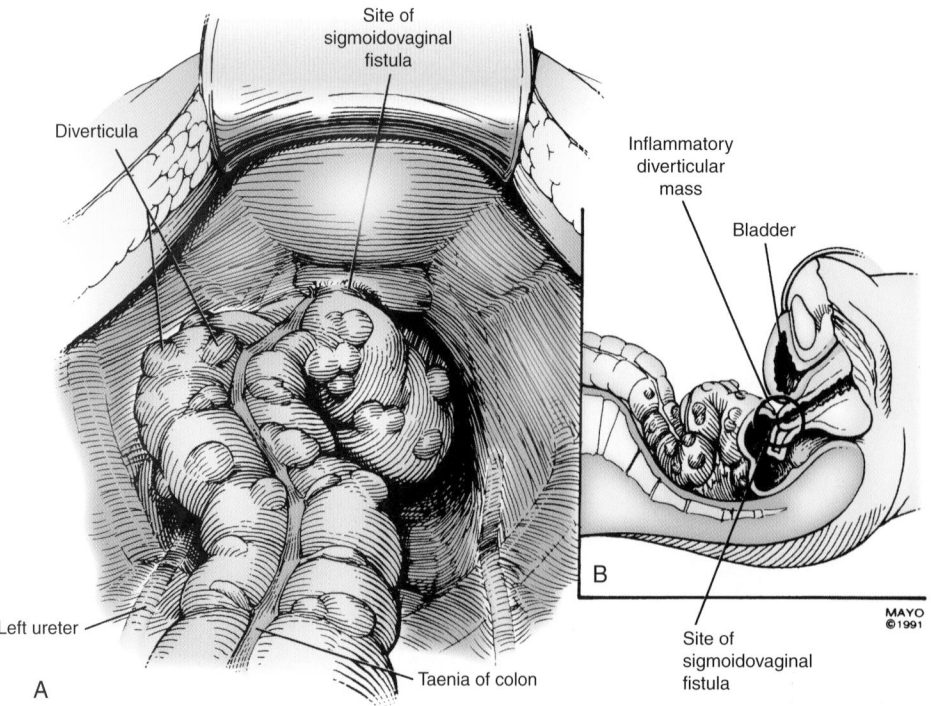

FIGURE 44.35 **A:** Sigmoid with multiple diverticula and site of sigmoidovaginal fistula. **B:** Site of sigmoidovaginal fistula at the apex of the vagina. (Adapted from Lee RA. *Atlas of gynecologic surgery*. Philadelphia, PA: WB Saunders, 1992. By permission of Mayo Foundation for Medical Education and Research. All rights reserved.)

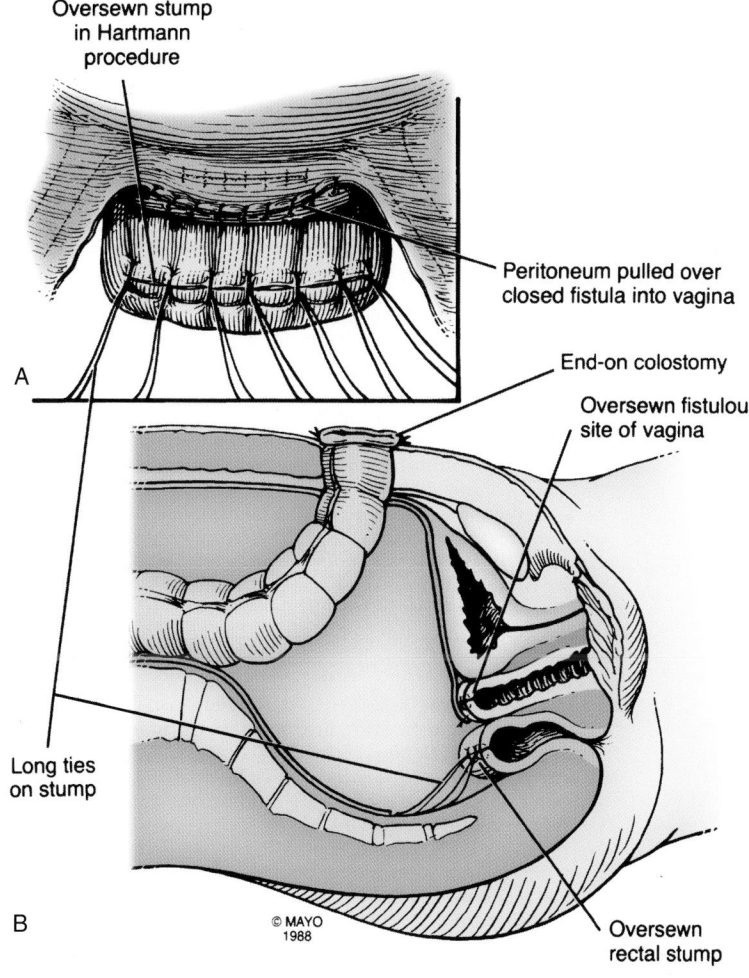

FIGURE 44.36 A: Separate closures of top of vagina and remnant of rectum. **B:** Matured colostomy and oversewn site of sigmoidovaginal fistula. (Adapted from Lee RA. *Atlas of gynecologic surgery.* Philadelphia, PA: WB Saunders, 1992. By permission of Mayo Foundation for Medical Education and Research. All rights reserved.)

SUMMARY

The management of the anally incontinent patient is a complex undertaking whether that incontinence is transanal or extraanal through a rectovaginal fistula. Care must be taken in the assessment and diagnosis of these patients with testing judiciously used where it will provide clinically useful information. Because surgical results in anally incontinent patients are less than perfect, consideration should be given to initially trying nonsurgical management. In those who fail conservative therapy, and in those who go directly to surgical therapy, a thoughtful preoperative workup with extensive preoperative counseling regarding expectations and possible outcomes is crucial for the ultimate satisfaction of the patient. Surgery for anal incontinence and rectovaginal fistula repair requires thorough surgical planning, careful attention to detail, and a meticulous operative technique to provide the patient with optimal results.

BEST SURGICAL PRACTICES

- Preoperative evaluation of the anally incontinent patient should include a careful assessment of her symptoms and their impact on her quality of life.
- Success rates of surgical procedures for anal incontinence, especially as they relate to specific diagnoses, should be explained preoperatively to patients. Patients need to understand that results are rarely perfect and even good results may deteriorate with time.

- Consideration should be given to the use of nonsurgical therapy including diet and lifestyle modification before a decision for surgery is made. Physicians must keep up to date regarding newer, nonsurgical options that may be available.
- Judicious use of preoperative testing can aid in the diagnosis of the etiology of incontinence and thus provide assistance when advising patients about prognosis especially as it relates to surgery.
- Mechanical bowel preparation, perioperative antibiotic prophylaxis, and attention to postoperative diet and stool consistency management seem to be important but not well studied or defined.
- The anal sphincteroplasty is the most important part of any perineal reconstruction for the patient with anal incontinence.
- Current data remain unclear as to whether overlapping sphincter repair may yield greater functional improvement than an end-to-end sphincter reapproximation.
- Rectovaginal fistula repair requires careful attention to sharp dissection, gentle tissue handling, wide mobilization, meticulous hemostasis, and a tension-free closure.

ACKNOWLEDGMENTS

The author would like to acknowledge the continued valuable contributions of the previous authors of this chapter, Drs. Raymond Lee and Michael Aronson, and also thank Soumia Brakta, MD, and Teuta Shemshedini, MD, for their assistance with this new edition.

VII

BIBLIOGRAPHY

Aartsen EJ, Sindram IS. Repair of the radiation induced rectovaginal fistula without or with interposition of the bulbocavernosus muscle (Martius procedure). *Eur J Surg Oncol* 1988;14:171.

Abramov Y, Sand PK, Botros SM, et al. Risk factors for female anal incontinence: new insight through Evanston-Northwestern twin sisters study. *Obstet Gynecol* 2005;106:726.

Abrams P, Cardozo L, Khoury S, et al., eds. *Incontinence.* 3rd International Consultation on Incontinence, Monaco 2004. Pub Health Publications Ltd., 2005:286.

Aigner F, Conrad F, Margreiter R, et al. Coloproctology Working Group. Anal submucosal carbon bead injection for treatment of idiopathic fecal incontinence: a preliminary report. *Dis Colon Rectum* 2009;52:293.

Allen RE, Hosker GL, Smith ARB, et al. Pelvic floor damage and childbirth: a neurophysiological study. *BJOG* 1990;97:770.

Altomare D, La Torre F, Rinaldi M, et al. Carbon-coated microbeads anal injection in outpatient treatment of minor fecal incontinence. *Dis Colon Rectum* 2008;51:432.

American Gastroenterological Association. American Gastroenterological Association medical position statement on anorectal testing techniques. *Gastroenterology* 1999;116:732.

Angioli R, Gomez-Marin O, Cantuaria G, et al. Severe perineal lacerations during vaginal delivery: the University of Miami experience. *Am J Obstet Gynecol* 2000;182:1083.

Arnaud A, Sarles JC, Sielezneff I, et al. Sphincter repair without overlapping for fecal incontinence. *Dis Colon Rectum* 1991;34:744.

Aronson MP, Lee RA, Berquist TH. Anatomy of anal sphincters and related structures in continent women studied with magnetic resonance imaging. *Obstet Gynecol* 1990;76:846.

Avery K, Bosch J, Gotoh M, et al. Questionnaires to assess urinary and anal incontinence: review and recommendations. *J Urol* 2007;177:39.

Bajwa A, Emmanuel A. The physiology of continence and evacuation. *Best Pract Res Clin Gastroenterol* 2009;23:477.

Bartolo DCC, Roe AM, Locke-Edmunds JC, et al. Flap-valve theory of anorectal incontinence. *Br J Surg* 1986;73:1012.

Barton JR. A rectovaginal fistula cured. *Am J Med Sci* 1840;26:305.

Berek JS, Lagasse LD, Hacker NF, et al. Levator ani transposition for anal incompetence secondary to sphincter damage. *Obstet Gynecol* 1982;59:108.

Bielefeldt K, Enck P, Erckenbrecht JF. Sensory and motor function in the maintenance of anal continence. *Dis Colon Rectum* 1990;33:674.

Bielefeldt K, Enck P, Zamboglou N, et al. Anorectal manometry and defecography in the diagnosis of fecal incontinence. *J Clin Gastroenterol* 1991;13:661.

Birnhaum W. A method of repair for a common type of traumatic incontinence of the anal sphincter. *Surg Gynecol Obstet* 1948;87:716.

Blaisdell PC. Repair of the incontinent sphincter ani. *Surg Gynecol Obstet* 1940;70:692.

Bonavina L, Saino G, Bona D, et al. Magnetic augmentation of the lower esophageal sphincter: results of a feasibility clinical trial. *J Gastrointest Surg* 2008;12:2133.

Boreham MK, Richter HE, Kenton KE, et al. Anal incontinence in women presenting for gynecologic care: prevalence, risk factors, and impact on quality of life. *Am J Obstet Gynecol* 2004;192:1637.

Borello-France D, Burgio K, Richter H, et al. Fecal and urinary incontinence in primiparous women. *Obstet Gynecol* 2006;108:863.

Boronow RC. Repair of the radiation-induced vaginal fistula using the Martius technique. *World J Surg* 1986;10:237.

Boyle D, Knowles C, Lunniss P, et al. Efficacy of sacral nerve stimulation for fecal incontinence in patients with anal sphincter defects. *Dis Colon Rectum* 2009;52:1234.

Brouwer R, Duthie G. Sacral nerve neuromodulation is effective treatment for fecal incontinence in the presence of a sphincter defect, pudendal neuropathy, or previous sphincter repair. *Dis Colon Rectum* 2010;53:272.

Bug G, Kiff E, Hosker G. A new condition-specific health-related quality of life questionnaire for the assessment of women with anal incontinence. *BJOG* 2001;108:1057.

Chan M, Tjandra J. Sacral nerve stimulation for fecal incontinence: external anal sphincter defect vs. intact anal sphincter. *Dis Colon Rectum* 2008;51:1015.

Chassagne P, Landrin I, Neveu C, et al. Fecal incontinence in the institutionalized elderly: incidence, risk factors, and prognosis. *J Urol* 1999;161:1813.

Chen AS, Luchtefeld MA, Senagore AJ, et al. Pudendal nerve latency. Does it predict outcome of anal sphincter repair? *J Clin Gastroenterol* 1998;27:108.

Cheong DM, Vaccaro CA, Salanga VD, et al. Electrodiagnostic evaluation of fecal incontinence. *JAMA* 1995;274:559. [Published erratum appears in *Muscle Nerve* 1995;18:1368].

Cundiff GW, Nygaard I, Bland DR, et al. Proceedings of the American Urogynecologic Society Multidisciplinary Symposium on Defecatory Disorders. *Eur J Obstet Gynecol Reprod Biol* 2000;89:159.

Dalley AF II. The riddle of the sphincters: the morphophysiology of the anorectal mechanism reviewed. *Am J Surg* 1987;53:298. [Published erratum appears in *Am J Surg* 1987;53:398].

Deen KI, Oya M, Ortiz J, et al. Randomized trial comparing three forms of pelvic floor repair for neuropathic faecal incontinence. *Br J Surg* 1993;80:794.

Dehli T, Lindsetmo R, Mevik K, et al. Anal incontinence—assessment of a new treatment. *Tidsskr Nor Laegeforen* 2007;127:2934.

DeLancey JOL, Hurd WW. Size of the urogenital hiatus in the levator ani muscles in normal women and women with pelvic organ prolapse. *Obstet Gynecol* 1998;91:364.

DeLancey JO, Kearney R, Chou Q, et al. The appearance of levator ani muscle abnormalities in magnetic resonance images after vaginal delivery. *Obstet Gynecol* 2003;101:46.

DeLancey JO, Morgan D, Fenner D, et al. Comparison of levator ani muscle defects and function in women with and without pelvic organ prolapsed. *Obstet Gynecol* 2007;109:295.

DeLancey JOL, Toglia MR, Perucchini D. Internal and external anal sphincter anatomy as it relates to midline obstetric lacerations. *Obstet Gynecol* 1997;90:924.

DeSouza NM, Puni R, Zbar A, et al. MR imaging of the anal sphincter in multiparous women using an endoanal coil: correlation with in vitro anatomy and appearances in fecal incontinence. *AJR Am J Roentgenol* 1996;167:1465.

Diamant N, Kamm M, Wald A, et al. AGA technical review on anorectal testing techniques. *Gastroenterology* 1999;116:735.

Dietz HP, Lanzarone V. Levator trauma after vaginal delivery. *Obstet Gynecol* 2005;106:707.

Dudding T, Vaizey C, Kamm M. Obstetric anal sphincter injury: incidence, risk factors, and management. *Ann Surg* 2008;247:224.

Eason E, Labrecque M, Marcoux S, et al. Anal incontinence after childbirth. *CMAJ* 2002;166:326.

Efron J, Corman M, Fleshman J, et al. Safety and effectiveness of temperature-controlled radio-frequency energy delivery to the anal canal (Secca procedure) for the treatment of fecal incontinence. *Dis Colon Rectum* 2003;46:1606.

Elkins TE, DeLancey JOL, McGuire EJ. The use of modified Martius graft as an adjunctive technique in vesicovaginal and rectovaginal fistula repair. *Obstet Gynecol* 1990;75:727.

Enck P, Daublin G, Lubke HJ, et al. Long-term efficacy of biofeedback training for fecal incontinence. *Dis Colon Rectum* 1995;38:370.

Engel A, Kamm M, Bartram C, et al. Relationship of symptoms in faecal incontinence to specific sphincter abnormalities. *Int J Colorectal Dis* 1995;10:152.

Evers E, Blomquist J, McDermott K, et al. Obstetrical anal sphincter laceration and anal incontinence 5–10 years after childbirth. *Am J Obstet Gynecol* 2012;207:425e1.

Faltin D, Boulvain M, Irion M, et al. Diagnosis of anal sphincter tears by postpartum endosonography to predict fecal incontinence. *Obstet Gynecol* 2000;95:643.

Faltin DL, Sangalli MR, Curtin F, et al. Prevalence of anal incontinence and other anorectal symptoms in women. *Int Urogynecol J* 2001;12:117.

Farrell S, Allen V, Baskett T. Anal incontinence in primiparas. *J Obstet Gynaecol Can* 2001;23:321.

Farrell S, Gilmour D, Turnbull G, et al. Overlapping compared with end-to-end repair of third- and fourth-degree obstetric anal sphincter tears: a randomized controlled trial. *Obstet Gynecol* 2010;116:16.

Fenner D, Genberg B, Brahma P, et al. Fecal and urinary incontinence after vaginal delivery with anal sphincter disruption in an obstetrics unit in the United States. *Am J Obstet Gynecol* 2003;189:1543.

Fernando R, Sultan AH, Kettle C, et al. Methods of repair for obstetric anal sphincter injury. *Cochrane Database Syst Rev* 2006;(3). [Art. No.: CD002866. DOI; 10.1002/14651858.CD002866.pub2].

Fernando RJ, Sultan AH, Kettle C, et al. Repair techniques for obstetric anal sphincter injuries: a randomized controlled trial. *Obstet Gynecol* 2006;107:1261.

FitzGerald M, Weber A, Howden N, et al. Risk factors for anal sphincter tear during vaginal delivery. *Obstet Gynecol* 2007;109:29.

Fitzpatrick M, Behan M, O'Connell PR, et al. A randomized clinical trial comparing primary overlap with approximation repair of third degree obstetric tears. *Am J Obstet Gynecol* 2000;183:1220.

Fornell EU, Matthiesen L, Sjödahl R, et al. Obstetric anal sphincter injury ten years after: subjective and objective long term effects. *BJOG* 2005;112:312.

Friedman S, Blomquist J, Nugent J, et al. Pelvic muscle strength after childbirth. *Obstet Gynecol* 2012;120:1021.

Frudinger A, Ballon M, Taylor S, et al. The natural history of clinically unrecognized anal sphincter tears over 10 years after first vaginal delivery. *Obstet Gynecol* 2008;111:1058.

Ganio E, Marino F, Giani I, et al. Injectable synthetic calcium hydroxylapatite ceramic microspheres (Coaptite) for passive fecal incontinence. *Tech Coloproctol* 2008;12:99.

Ganz R, Gostout C, Grudem J, et al. Use of a magnetic sphincter for the treatment of GERD: a feasibility study. *Gastrointest Endosc* 2008;67:287.

Gearhart S, Hull T, Floruta C, et al. Anal manometric parameters: predictors of outcome following anal sphincter repair? *J Gastrointest Surg* 2005;9:115.

Gilliland R, Altomare DF, Moreira H, et al. Pudendal neuropathy is predictive of failure following anterior overlapping sphincteroplasty. *Dis Colon Rectum* 1998;41:1516.

Gold D, Bartram C, Halligan S, et al. Three-dimensional endoanal sonography in assessing anal canal injury. *Br J Surg* 1999;86:365.

Goligher JC, Leacock AG, Brossy JJ. Surgical anatomy of anal canal. *Br J Surg* 1955;43:51.

Gordon D, Groutz A, Goldman G, et al. Anal incontinence: prevalence among female patients attending a urogynecologic clinic. *AJR Am J Roentgenol* 1999;173:179.

Graf W, Mellgren A, Matzel K, et al., NASHA Dx Study Group. Efficacy of dextranomer in stabilized hyaluronic acid for treatment of faecal incontinence: a randomized, sham-controlled trial. *Lancet* 2011;377:997.

Gutierrez AB, Madoff RD, Lowry AC, et al. Long term results of anal sphincteroplasty. *Dis Colon Rectum* 2004;47:727.

Haadem K, Dahlström JA, Ling L. Anal sphincter competence in healthy women: clinical implications of age and other factors. *Obstet Gynecol* 1991;78:823.

Hallan RI, George B, Williams NS. Anal sphincter function: fecal incontinence and its treatment. *Surg Annu* 1993;25:85.

Halversen AL, Hull TL. Long-term outcomes of overlapping anal sphincter repair. *Dis Colon Rectum* 2002;45:345.

Handa V, Blomquist J, Knoepp L, et al. Pelvic floor disorders 5–10 years after vaginal or cesarean childbirth. *Obstet Gynecol* 2011;118:777.

Handa VL, Danielsen BH, Gilbert WM. Obstetric anal sphincter lacerations. *Obstet Gynecol* 2001;98:225.

Hankins GDV, Hauth JC, Gilstrap LC, et al. Early repair of episiotomy dehiscence. *Obstet Gynecol* 1990;75:48.

Healy JC, Halligan S, Reznek RH, et al. Dynamic MR imaging compared with evacuation proctography when evaluating anorectal configuration and pelvic floor movement. *AJR Am J Roentgenol* 1997;169:775.

Heyer T, Enck P, Grantke B, et al. Anal endosonography: are morphometric measurements of the anal sphincter reproducible? *Gastroenterology* 1995;108:A613.

Hiller L, Radley S, Mann C, et al. Development and validation of a questionnaire for the assessment of bowel and lower urinary tract symptoms in women. *BJOG* 2002;109:413.

Hosker G, Norton C, Brazzelli M. Electrical stimulation for faecal incontinence in adults. *Cochrane Database Syst Rev* 2000;2: CD001310.

Hull T, Giese C, Wexner S, et al. Long-term durability of sacral nerve stimulation therapy for chronic fecal incontinence. *Dis Colon Rectum* 2013;56:234.

Jackson SL, Weber AM, Hull TL, et al. Fecal incontinence in women with urinary incontinence and pelvic organ prolapse. *Obstet Gynecol* 1997;89:423.

Jacobs PPM, Scheuer M, Kuijpers JHC. Obstetric fecal incontinence: role of pelvic floor denervation and results of delayed sphincter repair. *Dis Colon Rectum* 1990;33:494.

Johanson JF, Laferty J. Epidemiology of fecal incontinence: the silent affliction. *Am J Gastroenterol* 1996;91:33.

Kammerer-Doak DN, Wesol AB, Rogers RG, et al. A prospective cohort study of women after primary repair of obstetric anal sphincter laceration. *Am J Obstet Gynecol* 1999;181:1317.

Karoui S, Leroi AM, Koning E, et al. Results of sphincteroplasty in 86 patients with anal incontinence. *Dis Colon Rectum* 2000;43:813.

Kearney R, Miller JM, Ashton-Miller JA, et al. Obstetric factors associated with levator ani muscle injury after vaginal birth. *Obstet Gynecol* 2006;107:144.

Kenefick N, Christiansen J. A review of sacral nerve stimulation for the treatment of faecal incontinence. *Colorectal Dis* 2004;6:75.

Khanduja K, Yamashita H, Wise W, et al. Delayed repair of obstetric injuries of the anorectum and vagina. A stratified surgical approach. *Dis Colon Rectum* 1994;37:344.

Kim D, Yoon H, Park J, et al. Radiofrequency energy delivery to the anal canal: is it a promising new approach to the treatment of fecal incontinence? *Am J Surg* 2009;197:14.

King V, Boyles S, Worstell T, et al. Using the brink score to predict postpartum anal incontinence. *Am J Obstet Gynecol* 2010;203: 486.e1.

Kodner IJ, Mazor A, Shemesh EI, et al. Endorectal advancement flap repair of rectovaginal and other complicated anorectal fistulas. *Surgery* 1993;114:682.

Kwon S, Visco AG, Fitzgerald MP et al. Validity and reliability of the Modified Manchester Health Questionnaire in assessing patients with fecal incontinence. *Dis Colon Rectum* 2005;48:323.

Laurberg S, Swash M, Henry MM. Delayed external sphincter repair for obstetric tear. *Br J Surg* 1988;75:786.

Law PJ, Kamm MA, Bartram CI. A comparison between electromyography and anal endosonography in mapping external anal sphincter defects. *Dis Colon Rectum* 1990;33:370.

Law PJ, Kamm MA, Bartram CI. Anal endosonography in the investigation of faecal incontinence. *Br J Surg* 1991;78:312.

Lefevre J, Bretagnol F, Maggiori L, et al. Operative results and quality of life after gracilis muscle transposition for recurrent rectovaginal fistula. *Dis Colon Rectum* 2009;52:1290.

Lehur P, McNevin S, Buntzen S, et al. Magnetic anal sphincter augmentation for the treatment of fecal incontinence: a preliminary report from a feasibility study. *Dis Colon Rectum* 2010;53:1604.

Leroi AM, Weber J, Menard JF, et al. Prevalence of anal incontinence in 409 patients investigated for stress urinary incontinence. *Obstet Gynecol* 1999;94:689.

Lienemann A, Anthuber C, Baron A, et al. Dynamic MR colpocystorectography assessing pelvic-floor descent. *Eur J Radiol* 1997;7:1309.

Lotze M, Wietek B, Birbaumer N, et al. Cerebral activation during anal and rectal stimulation. *Neuroimage* 2001;14:1027.

Lowry AC, Thorson AG, Rothenberger DA, et al. Repair of simple rectovaginal fistulas: influence of previous repairs. *Dis Colon Rectum* 1988;31:676.

Macmillan AK, Arend MB, Merrie AE, et al. The prevalence of fecal incontinence in community-dwelling adults: a systematic review of the literature. *Dis Colon Rectum* 2004;47:1341.

Madoff RD, Rosen HR, Baeten CG, et al. Safety and efficacy of dynamic muscle plasty for anal incontinence: lessons from a prospective, multicenter trial. *Eur J Radiol* 1999;9:436.

Madoff RD, Williams JG, Caushaj PF. Fecal incontinence. *N Engl J Med* 1992;326:1002.

Maeda Y, Laurberg S, Norton C. Perianal injectable bulking agents as treatment for faecal incontinence in adults. *Cochrane Database Syst Rev* 2010;5:CD007959.

Maeda Y, Vaizey C, Kamm M. Long-term results of perianal silicone injection for faecal incontinence. *Colorectal Dis* 2007;9:357.

VII

Malouf AJ, Norton CS, Engel AF, et al. Long-term results of overlapping anterior anal-sphincter repair for obstetric trauma. *Lancet* 2000;355:260.

Malouf AJ, Vaizey CJ, Nicholls RJ, et al. Permanent sacral nerve stimulation for fecal incontinence. *Ann Surg* 2000;232:143.

Malouf A, Vaizey C, Norton C, et al. Internal anal sphincter augmentation for fecal incontinence using injectable silicone biomaterial. *Dis Colon Rectum* 2001;44:595.

Martius H. Die operative Wiederherstel-lung der vollkommen fehlenden. Harnrohare und des Schliessmuskels derselben. *Zentralb Gynakol* 1928;52:480.

Matsuoka H, Mavrantonis C, Wexner SD, et al. Postanal repair for fecal incontinence—is it worthwhile? *Dis Colon Rectum* 2000;43:1561.

Matzel KE. Sacral nerve stimulation for faecal incontinence: its role in the treatment algorithm. *Colorectal Dis* 2011;13:10.

Matzel KE, Kamm MA, Stosser M, et al. Sacral spinal nerve stimulation for faecal incontinence: multicentre study. *Lancet* 2004;363:1270.

Mazier WP, Senagore AJ, Schiesel EC. Operative repair of anovaginal and rectovaginal fistulas. *Dis Colon Rectum* 1995;38:4.

McCrea G, Miaskowski C, Stotts N, et al. Pathophysiology of constipation in the older adult. *World J Gastroenterol* 2008;14:2631.

McIntosh LJ, Frahm JD, Mallett VT. Pelvic floor rehabilitation in the treatment of incontinence. *J Reprod Med* 1993;38:662.

Miller NF, Brown W. The surgical treatment of complete perineal tears in the female. *Am J Obstet Gynecol* 1937;34:196.

Miner PB, Donnelly TC, Read NW. Investigation of mode of action of biofeedback in treatment of fecal incontinence. *Dig Dis Sci* 1990;35:1291.

Mundy L, Merlin T, Maddern G, et al. Systematic review of safety and effectiveness of an artificial bowel sphincter for faecal incontinence. *Br J Surg* 2004;91:665.

Nichols CM, Gill EJ, Nguyen T, et al. Anal sphincter injury in women with pelvic floor disorders. *Obstet Gynecol* 2004;104:690.

Norton C, Hosker G, Brazzelli M. Biofeedback and/or sphincter exercises for the treatment of fecal incontinence in adults. *Cochrane Database Syst Rev* 2000;(3):CD002111.

Nyam DC, Pemberton JH. Long-term results of lateral internal sphincterotomy for chronic anal fissure with particular reference to incidence of fecal incontinence. *Dis Colon Rectum* 1999;42:1306.

Nygaard IE, Roa SS, Dawson JD. Anal incontinence after anal sphincter disruption: a 30-year retrospective cohort study. *Obstet Gynecol* 1997;89:896.

Nygaard I. Vaginal birth: a relic of the past in bulldogs and women? *Obstet Gynecol* 2011;118:774.

O'Brien PE, Dixon JB, Skinner S, et al. A prospective, randomized, controlled clinical trial of placement of the artificial bowel sphincter for the control of fecal incontinence. *Dis Colon Rectum* 2004;47:1852.

Oliveira L, Pfeifer J, Wexner S. Physiological and clinical outcome of anterior sphincteroplasty. *Br J Surg* 1996;83:502.

Osterberg A, Graf W, Edebol Eeg-Olofsson K, et al. Results of neurophysiologic evaluation in fecal incontinence. *Dis Colon Rectum* 2000;43:1256.

Penninckx F. Belgian experience with dynamic graciloplasty for faecal incontinence. *Br J Surg* 2004;91:872.

Perry S, Shaw C, McGrother C, et al. Prevalence of faecal incontinence in adults aged 40 years or more living in the community. *Gut* 2002;50:480.

Peschers UM, DeLancey JO, Schaer GN, et al. Exoanal ultrasound of the anal sphincter: normal anatomy and sphincter defects. *Dis Colon Rectum* 1997;40:1430.

Pinto R, Peterson T, Shawki S, et al. Are there predictors of outcome following rectovaginal fistula repair? *Dis Colon Rectum* 2010;53:1240.

Poen AC, Felt-Bersma RJ, Strijers RL, et al. Third-degree obstetric perineal tear: long-term clinical and functional results after primary repair. *Br J Surg* 1998;85:1433.

Pollack J, Nordenstam J, Brismar S, et al. Anal incontinence after vaginal delivery: a five-year prospective cohort study. *Obstet Gynecol* 2004;104:1397.

Ratto C, Litta F, Parello A, et al. Sacral nerve stimulation is a valid approach in fecal incontinence due to sphincter lesions when compared to sphincter repair. *Dis Colon Rectum* 2010;53:264.

Richter H, Fielding J, Bradley C, et al. Endoanal ultrasound findings and fecal incontinence symptoms in women with and without recognized anal sphincter tears. *Obstet Gynecol* 2006;108:1394.

Riedy L, Chintam R, Walter J. Use of a neuromuscular stimulator to increase anal sphincter pressure. *Spinal Cord* 2000;38:724.

Roberts RO, Jacobsen SJ, Reilly WT, et al. Prevalence of combined fecal and urinary incontinence: a community-based study. *Dis Colon Rectum* 1999;42:857.

Rock JA, Woodruff JD. Surgical correction of a rectovaginal fistula. *Int J Gynecol Obstet* 1982;20:413.

Rockwood TH, Church JM, Fleshman JW, et al. Fecal Incontinence Quality of Life Scale: quality of life instrument for patients with fecal incontinence. *Dis Colon Rectum* 2000;43:813.

Rosenshein NB, Genadry RR, Woodruff JD. An anatomic classification of rectovaginal septal defects. *Am J Obstet Gynecol* 1980;137:439.

Rothbart J, Bemelman WA, Mierjerink WJ, et al. Long-term results of anterior anal sphincteroplasty repair for fecal incontinence due to obstetric injury/with invited commentaries. *Dig Surg* 2000;17:390.

Russo A, Sun, W, Sattawatthamrong Y, et al. Acute hyperglycemia affects motor and sensory function in normal subjects. *Gut* 1997;41:494.

Sangwan YP, Coller JA, Barrett RC, et al. Unilateral pudendal neuropathy: impact on outcome of anal sphincter repair. *Dis Colon Rectum* 1996;39:686.

Santoro GA, Eitan BZ, Pryde A, et al. Open study of low-dose amitriptyline in the treatment of patients with idiopathic fecal incontinence. *Dis Colon Rectum* 2000;43:1676.

Sartore A, DeSeta F, Maso G, et al. The effects of mediolateral episiotomy on pelvic floor function after vaginal delivery. *Obstet Gynecol* 2004;103:669.

Schwandner O, Brunner M, Dietl O. Quality of life and functional results of submucosal injection therapy using dextranomer hyaluronic acid for fecal incontinence. *Surg Innov* 2011;18:130.

Setti Carraro P, Kamm MA, Nicholls RJ. Long-term results of postanal repair for neurogenic faecal incontinence. *Br J Surg* 1994;81:140.

Shafik A, Doss S. Surgical anatomy of the somatic terminal enervation to the anal and urethral sphincters: role in anal and urethral surgery. *J Urol* 1999;161:85.

Shiono P, Klehanoff MA, Carey JC. Midline episiotomies: more harm than good? *Obstet Gynecol* 1990;75:765.

Sitzler PJ, Thomson JP. Overlap repair of damaged anal sphincter: a single surgeon's series. *Dis Colon Rectum* 1996;39:1356.

Snooks SJ, Swash M, Mathers S, et al. Effect of vaginal delivery on the pelvic floor: a 5-year follow-up. *Br J Surg* 1990;77:1358.

Soffer EE, Hull T. Fecal incontinence: a practical approach to evaluation and treatment. *Am J Gastroenterol* 2000;95:1873.

Solans-Domenech M, Sanchez E, Espuna-Pons M. Urinary and anal incontinence during pregnancy and postpartum: incidence, severity, and risk factors. *Obstet Gynecol* 2010;115:618.

Soerensen M, Lundby L, Buntzen S, et al. Intersphincteric injected silicone biomaterial implants: a treatment for faecal incontinence. *Colorectal Dis* 2009;11:73.

Stewart LK, Wilson SR. Transvaginal sonography of the anal sphincter: reliable, or not? *J Am Geriatr Soc* 1999;47:837.

Strohbehn K, Ellis JH, Strohbehn JA, et al. MRI of the levator ani with anatomic correlation. *Obstet Gynecol* 1996;87:277.

Sultan AH. Anal incontinence after childbirth. *Curr Opin Obstet Gynecol* 1997;9:320.

Sultan AH, Kamm MA, Hudson CN, et al. Anal-sphincter disruption during vaginal delivery. *N Engl J Med* 1993;329:1905.

Sultan A, Kamm M, Hudson C, et al. Third-degree obstetric anal sphincter tears: risk factors and outcomes of primary repair. *BMJ* 1994;308:887.

Sultan AH, Monga AK, Kumar D, et al. Primary repair of obstetric anal sphincter rupture using the overlap technique. *BJOG* 1999;106:318.

Swash M, Snooks SJ, Henry MM. A unifying concept of pelvic floor disorders and incontinence. *J R Soc Med* 1985;78:906.

Takahashi T, Garcia-Osogobio S, Valdovinos M, et al. Extended two-year results of radio-frequency energy delivery for the treatment of fecal incontinence (the Secca procedure). *Dis Colon Rectum* 2003;46:711.

Takahashi-Monroy T, Morales M, et al. SECCA procedure for the treatment of fecal incontinence: results of five-year follow-up. *Dis Colon Rectum* 2008;51:355.

Tan E, Ngo N, Darzi A, et al. Meta-analysis: sacral nerve stimulation versus conservative therapy in the treatment of faecal incontinence. *Int J Colorectal Dis* 2011;26:275.

Tancer ML, Veridiano NP. Genital fistulas secondary to diverticular disease of the sigmoid colon. *Obstet Gynecol Surv* 1996;51:67.

Teunissen T, van der Bosch W, van der Hoogen H, et al. Prevalence of urinary and faecal incontinence among community-dwelling elderly patients in Nijmegen, The Netherlands, January 1999–July 2001. *Ned Tijdschr Geneeskd* 2006;150:2430.

Thacker SB, Banta HD. Benefits and risks of episiotomy: an interpretive review of the English language literature, 1860–1980. *Obstet Gynecol Surv* 1983;38:322.

Thakar R, Sultan A. Anal endosonography and its role in assessing the incontinent patient. *Best Pract Res Clin Obstet Gynaecol* 2004;18:157.

Thorp JM, Bowes WA, Brame RG, et al. Selected use of midline episiotomy: effect on perineal trauma. *Obstet Gynecol* 1987;70:260.

Tjandra JJ, Lim JF, Hiscock R, et al. Injectable silicone biomaterial for fecal incontinence caused by internal anal sphincter dysfunction is effective. *Dis Colon Rectum* 2004;47:2138.

Tjandra JJ, Milsom JW, Schroeder T, et al. Endoluminal ultrasound is preferable to electromyography in mapping anal sphincter defects. *Dis Colon Rectum* 1993;36:689.

Toglia MR, DeLancey JOL. Anal incontinence and the obstetrician-gynecologist. *Obstet Gynecol* 1994;84:731.

Tsang C, Madoff R, Wong, W et al. Anal sphincter integrity and function influences outcome in rectovaginal fistula repair. *Dis Colon Rectum* 1998;41:1141.

Ullah S, Tayyab M, Arsalani-Zadeh R, et al. Injectable anal bulking agent for the management of faecal incontinence. *J Coll Physicians Surg Pak* 2011;21:227.

Vaizey CJ, Kamm MA, Bartram CI. Primary degeneration of the internal anal sphincter as a cause of passive faecal incontinence. *Lancet* 1997;349:612.

Varma A, Gunn J, Gardiner A, et al. Obstetric anal sphincter injury: prospective evaluation of incidence. *Am J Obstet Gynecol* 2000;182:S1.

Vernava AM III, Longo WE, Daniel GL. Pudendal neuropathy and the importance of EMG evaluation of fecal incontinence. *Dis Colon Rectum* 1993;36:23.

Veronikas DK, Nichols DH, Spino C. The Noble-Mengert-Fish operation revisited: a composite approach for persistent rectovaginal fistulas and complex perineal defects. *Am J Obstet Gynecol* 1998;179:1411.

Walter S, Hallbook O, Gotthard R, et al. A population-based study on bowel habits in a Swedish community: prevalence of faecal incontinence and constipation. *Scand J Gastroenterol* 2002;37:911.

Warren JC. A new method of operation for the relief of rupture of the perineum through the sphincter and rectum. *Trans Am Gynecol Soc* 1882;7:322.

Wexner S, Coller J, Devroede G, et al. Sacral nerve stimulation for fecal incontinence: results of a 120-patient prospective multicenter study. *Ann Surg* 2010;251:441.

Whitehead W, Borrud L, Goode P, et al. Fecal incontinence in US adults: epidemiology and risk factors. *Gastroenterology* 2009;137:512.

Wilcox LS, Strobino DM, Baruffi G, et al. Episiotomy and its role in the incidence of perineal lacerations in a maternity center and a tertiary hospital obstetric service. *Am J Obstet Gynecol* 1989;160:1047.

Williams A, Adams E, Tincello D, et al. How to repair an anal sphincter injury after vaginal delivery: results of a randomized controlled trial. *BJOG* 2006;113:201.

Williams JG, Wong WD, Jensen L, et al. Incontinence and rectal prolapse: a prospective manometric study. *Dis Colon Rectum* 1991;34:209.

Wise WE, Aguilar PS, Padmanabhan A, et al. Surgical treatment of low rectovaginal fistulas. *Dis Colon Rectum* 1991;34:271.

Wiskind AK, Thompson MD. Transverse transperineal repair of rectovaginal fistulas in the lower vagina. *Am J Obstet Gynecol* 1992;167:694.

Wong M, Meurette G, Stangherlin P, et al. The magnetic anal sphincter versus the artificial bowel sphincter: a comparison of 2 treatments for fecal incontinence. *Dis Colon Rectum* 2011;54:773.

Yee L, Birnbaum E, Read T, et al. Use of endoanal ultrasound in patients with rectovaginal fistulas. *Dis Colon Rectum* 1999;42:1057.

Zetterstrom J, Lopez A, Anzen B, et al. Anal sphincter tears at vaginal delivery: risk factors and clinical outcome of primary repair. *Obstet Gynecol* 1999;94:21.

Zutshi M, Hull T, Bast J, et al. Ten-year outcome after anal sphincter repair for fecal incontinence. *Dis Colon Rectum* 2009;52:1089.

VII

CHAPTER 45
Diseases of the Breast

Joseph L. Kelley III and Paniti Sukumvanich

DEFINITIONS

Axillary lymph node dissection—Surgical removal of lymph nodes from the pyramidal space in the axilla. The extent of dissection is defined in relationship to the pectoralis minor muscles: level I nodes lateral, level II posterior, and level III medial to this structure. Modern dissection involves the level I and level II nodal groups.

BRCA—One of two tumor suppressor genes (BRCA1 and BRCA2) that, when mutated, are associated with an increased risk of breast and ovarian cancer.

Breast-specific gamma imaging (BSGI)—Imaging modality in which technetium-99m (^{99m}Tc) sestamibi is used to highlight areas of increased metabolic activity in the breast to delineate possible areas of carcinoma from normal tissue.

Computer-aided detection (CAD)—Computer-based algorithms used in the second reading of mammographic films to increase sensitivity and reduce false-negative rates.

Diagnostic mammogram—Imaging utilized when a woman presents with symptoms, which may include multiple views and immediate interpretation by a radiologist. Additional testing, including sonography, tomosynthesis, magnetic resonance imaging (MRI), and percutaneous tissue sampling, may be advised at the radiologist's discretion.

Digital mammogram—An imaging technique that stores an x-ray image as a data file. This technique allows for digital magnification, manipulation of the image contrast, facilitation of storage, and use of telemedicine.

Ductal carcinoma in situ (DCIS)—Carcinoma of the lactiferous ducts that has not spread beyond the basement membrane; several subtypes and histologic grades exist.

Ductogram (galactography)—Contrast-enhanced mammographic imaging of the breast used in the evaluation of nipple discharge. The technique involves cannulation of duct openings in the nipple and injection of contrast dye.

Fibrocystic lesions—Spectrum of benign histopathologic changes in the breast associated with stromal fibrosis and with variable degrees of intraductal epithelial hyperplasia and sclerosing adenosis.

Fine needle aspiration (FNA) biopsy—Percutaneous sampling in which a cytologic specimen is obtained for analysis. This is accomplished through suction applied to a syringe and a fine needle. This can be therapeutic in drainage of a benign cyst and diagnostic in the evaluation of solid masses.

Intraductal papilloma—A benign hyperplastic breast mass within the duct that may present with spontaneous unilateral bloody nipple discharge; can be solitary when in the central ducts and multiple when located in the periphery of the breast.

Lobular carcinoma in situ (LCIS)—Also known as lobular intraepithelial neoplasia (LIN). A benign lesion characterized by distortion of the terminal ductal lobular unit with small cells. This entity is not a malignancy; rather, it is a risk factor for the development of breast cancer in either breast.

Magnetic resonance imaging (MRI)—Noninvasive imaging technique that generates computerized images of internal body tissues and is based on nuclear magnetic resonance of atoms within the body induced by the application of radio waves. A large magnet polarizes hydrogen atoms in the tissues and then monitors the summation of the spinning energies within cells.

Nipple-sparing mastectomy—Surgical removal of the breast, generally through an inframammary incision with preservation of the nipple–areolar complex. Generally reserved for patients undergoing prophylactic surgery but can be used in select circumstances for patients with known malignancy.

Microcalcifications—Calcium deposits visible on the mammogram that may appear alone or in clusters. To judge the likelihood of malignant change, a radiologist uses the shape and appearance of the clusters. Pleomorphism and clustering are concerning findings that warrant additional investigation.

Modified radical mastectomy—Surgical removal of the breast, pectoralis fascia, and axillary lymph nodes (generally levels I and II) with preservation of the pectoralis major muscle.

Paget disease—Changes in the nipple–areolar complex often mistaken for eczema, dermatitis, or mastitis. The condition is associated with an underlying malignancy of the breast, either an invasive or noninvasive cancer.

Partial mastectomy—Also known as "lumpectomy" or "segmental mastectomy." Surgical procedure in which only the portion of the breast in which the cancer is located is removed, along with a margin of normal breast tissue.

Percutaneous core biopsy—Percutaneous sampling using a hollow needle with or without vacuum assistance in which a cylindrical portion(s) of tissue is obtained for histologic analysis.

Positron emission mammography (PEM)—Imaging technique involving a pair of gamma radiation detectors placed above and below the breast to detect high metabolic activity via gamma ray emission after administering 18-flurodeoxyglucose (^{18}FDG) and identify probable sites of carcinoma.

Quadrantectomy—A procedure in which a full quadrant of the breast containing the tumor is excised with or without the overlying skin.

Radical mastectomy—En bloc removal of the breast tissue, associated skin, nipple, areola, axillary lymph nodes, and the underlying pectoralis major and minor muscles.

Screening mammogram—Traditional two-view images of each breast in asymptomatic women performed annually beginning between the ages of 40 and 50 years and continued as long as the woman is in good health.

VIII

Sentinel lymph node biopsy/mapping—Currently considered conventional treatment of the axilla in breast cancer patients without clinical or radiographic evidence of nodal involvement. The surgeon uses a visible blue dye and/or a radioisotope tracer to identify the key lymph node(s). These lymph nodes are used to predict the status of the nodal basin and help direct additional therapy.

Skin-sparing mastectomy—Surgical removal of the breast through a small periareolar incision maintaining the majority of the skin envelope.

Stereotactic needle biopsy—Use of mammogram images taken at two angles to map in three dimensions the location of lesions or microcalcifications. The patient lies prone on a dedicated table, and an automated core needle or vacuum-assisted device is used to biopsy the tissue.

Thermography—Imaging technique in which cutaneous temperatures of the breast and infrared radiation from the breast are measured through electronic detectors to aid in the diagnosis of breast disorders.

TNM staging—A system of clinicopathologic evaluation of tumors based on the extent of tumor involvement in the primary site (T), lymph nodes (N), and metastasis (M).

Tomosynthesis—Three-dimensional mammography in which multiple images of the breast are obtained by arcing the x-ray source around the breast. In this manner, multiplanar images are obtained that can enhance detection of masses within dense breast tissue that can be missed by conventional mammography. Other benefits include more accurate sizing, shape, and location of lesions. The digital nature of the technique may result in less radiation exposure.

Total (simple) mastectomy—Surgical removal of the breast tissue and associated skin, nipple, and areola without removing the underlying muscle.

Transverse rectus abdominis myocutaneous (TRAM) flap—Muscle flap procedure using the transverse rectus abdominus muscle as a method of breast reconstruction. The flap may remain attached to its blood supply (rotational flap) or reanastomosed to regional blood vessels (free flap).

Triple test—Correlation of the results of the breast physical examination, imaging, and tissue sampling technique to determine the malignant potential of a lesion. In instances in which a lesion is believed to be benign, all three results must be concordant or surgical excision must be performed.

Ultrasound (sonography)—Imaging technique for the breast that uses high-frequency soundwave transmission to aid in identification of breast lesions.

INTRODUCTION

Breast cancer is the most common cancer in women and, after lung cancer, is the second leading cause of cancer-related death. Data from the Centers for Disease Control and Prevention estimate 232,670 breast cancer diagnoses and 40,000 related deaths in 2014. The commonly reported statistic is that 1 in 8 women will develop breast cancer in their lifetime.

As providers of primary health care to women in all phases of their life, the obstetrician–gynecologist can be instrumental in the management of breast health concerns. The American Congress of Obstetricians and Gynecologists (ACOG) advocates for the obstetrician–gynecologist to have a working knowledge of the diagnosis of breast disease and cancer, to advise patients to perform self–breast examination, and to refer patients for screening mammography. These recommendations have resulted in increased ability to detect breast diseases and cancer. In the event of a malignant diagnosis, the obstetrician–gynecologist should be able to counsel the patient concerning the general treatment of the disease and facilitate a smooth transition to a breast cancer specialist. The Society of Gynecologic Oncology recently has recognized the expanding role of their specialty in the management of breast cancer. Several fellowship programs now include one additional year of training in the management of breast cancer and allied diseases. The American Board of Obstetrics and Gynecology Guide to Learning in Gynecologic Oncology indicates fellows are expected to have a working knowledge of breast diseases and be able to advise patients with regard to incidence of breast cancer, high-risk lesions, staging of the disease, and the role of multimodal therapy in the management of the disease process.

This chapter discusses basic strategies for the evaluation, diagnosis, and treatment of both benign and malignant breast diseases. The multidisciplinary approach for the evaluation of breast cancer is addressed, including surgical, radiotherapeutic, and adjuvant medical management.

EMBRYOLOGY

The mammary glands are specialized skin derivatives of ectodermal origin. During the 4th week of gestation, a pair of ectodermal thickenings—also known as the mammary ridges or milk line—form on the ventral surface of the embryo and extend in a curvilinear fashion from the axilla to the medial thigh. During the 5th week of gestation, an ingrowth of the ridge in the pectoral region at the fourth intercostal space occurs and forms a primary tissue bud. The remaining milk line regresses. Failure of regression of the milk line can lead to accessory nipples (polythelia) or breasts (polymastia) (Fig. 45.1). Subsequently, over the course of weeks, 15 to 20 secondary buds develop and become the breast lobules.

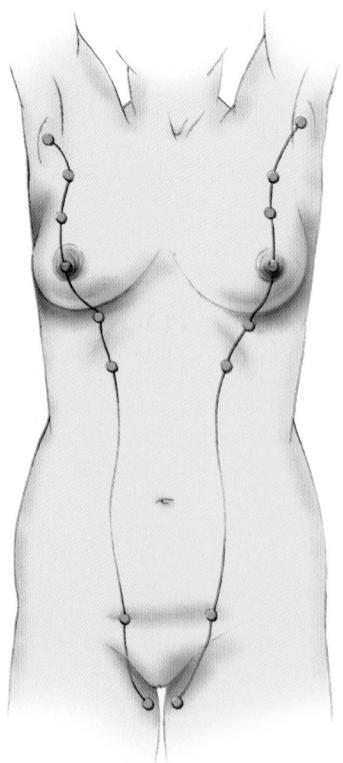

FIGURE 45.1 Mammary milk line.

TABLE 45.1 Tanner Stages of the Breast

STAGE	AGE	CLINICAL FINDINGS
I	Prepubescent	Elevation of the nipple without palpable glandular tissue or areolar pigmentation
II	11 ± 1.1 y	Presence of glandular tissue in the subareolar area. Nipple and breast project as single mound. Areola darkens.
III	12.2 ± 1 y	Increased amount of breast tissue. Widening of the areola and single plane between nipple/areola and the breast
IV	13.1 ± 1.2 y	Enlarging of areola, increasing pigmentation. Nipple–areolar complex forms a secondary mound above the breast.
V	15.3 ± 1.7 y	Mature adult breast. Breast covers most of the chest wall. Secondary mound disappears and nipple projects.

From Tanner J. *Wachstun und Reifung des Menschen.* Stuttgart, Germany: Georg Thieme Verlag; 1962; Tanner J. Physical growth and development. In: Forfar JO, Arnell GC, eds. *Textbook of paediatrics.* Edinburgh, Scotland: Churchill Livingston; 1984:292.

Lactiferous ducts form at approximately the 20th week as a result of luminae that develop within the buds. At term, there are 15 to 20 breast lobes and associated lactiferous ducts. The ducts drain into ampullae located beneath the developing nipple–areolar complex. The nipple forms as a result of mesenchymal proliferation and the formation of circular and longitudinally oriented smooth muscle fibers.

In both the male and female neonates, the breast contains radially arranged breast lobes that drain into the nipple via the lactiferous ducts. The female breast undergoes rapid changes, known as thelarche, during puberty. Exposure to rising levels of estrogen and progesterone induces changes in the ductal epithelium and breast acini. Other circulating agents, including growth hormone, cortisol, insulin, thyroxine, and prolactin, help the breast achieve complete functional status. To gauge pubertal development of the breast, Tanner staging can be assessed. Table 45.1 lists staging criteria. Failure to progress in accordance with established criteria can help identify hormone deficiencies and lead to early evaluation and treatment.

ANATOMY

The mammary gland is a modified sweat gland and is an accessory to reproduction in the female. The breast is located between the second rib and the sixth intercostal space in the vertical axis and extends horizontally from the sternum to beyond the anterior axillary fold. A portion of the breast—the axillary tail of Spence—extends into the axillary basin. It has a dome shape with a conical contour in a nulliparous female and may become pendulous in the mature or parous individual. The gland is composed of skin, subcutaneous tissue, epithelial glandular structures, and supporting stroma (Fig. 45.2).

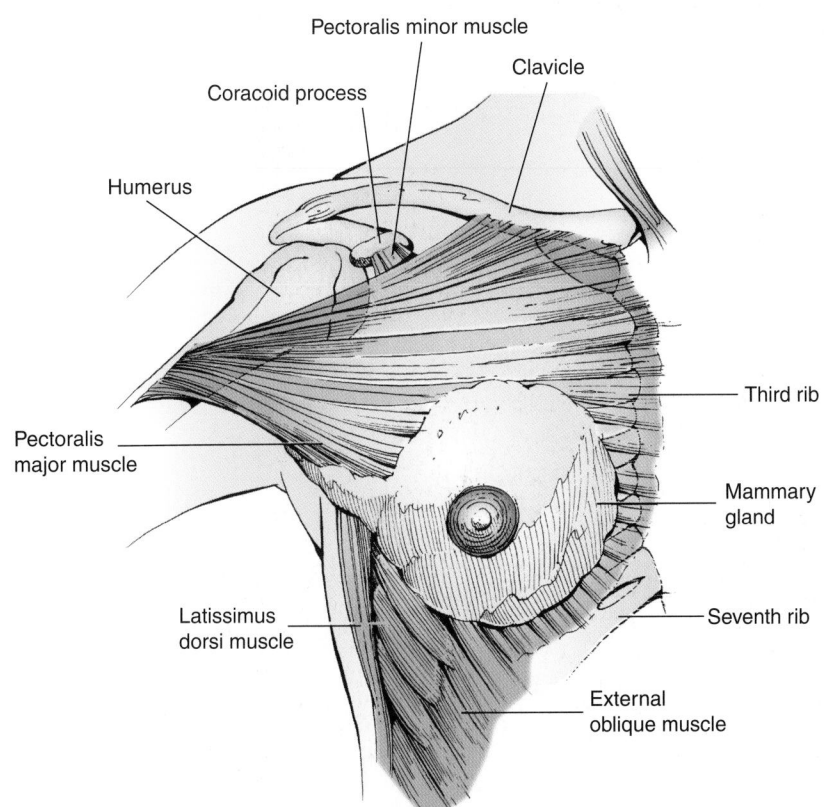

FIGURE 45.2 General anatomy of the breast.

VIII

The breast is composed of 15 to 20 lobes with each lobe being an irregular, flattened pyramid of glandular tissue with the apex directed toward the nipple–areolar complex. From each lobe, a single lactiferous duct extends to the nipple. Within the lobes, these ducts have multiple divisions beginning with branches to 20 to 40 lobules and subsequent branching to 10 to 100 alveoli units. The ducts, referred to as the lactiferous sinuses, are 1 to 2 mm in diameter but dilate to 4 to 5 mm beneath the nipple–areolar complex. The lactiferous sinuses drain to collecting ducts that have openings within the nipple (**Fig. 45.3**). Nomenclature for the epithelial system is highlighted in **Table 45.2**.

The stroma consists of connective tissue, adipose tissue, blood vessels, nerves, and lymphatics. The superficial pectoral fascia envelops the entire gland. The superficial pectoral fascia is in continuity with superficial fascia of the abdominal wall (Camper fascia). The posterior surface of the breast abuts the deep pectoralis fascia.

The nipple and areola are pigmented, covered with keratinized squamous epithelium, and contain smooth muscle fibers, which causes wrinkling of the skin and associated with nipple erection. Within the nipple are two receptor-type nerve endings, Ruffini-like bodies and bulb of Krause, that detect tactile stretch and pressure. The areola has sebaceous and apocrine sweat glands and accessory areolar glands also known as Montgomery glands. In the latter, these glands open onto the areola as small elevations known as Morgagni tubercles.

The major muscles proximate to the breast and axilla include the pectoralis major and minor, serratus anterior, and the latissimus dorsi. The pectoralis major has two parts: the clavicular portion and the sternocostal portion. This muscle forms the fullness of the upper chest and helps flex and adduct

the arm. Innervation is from the medial (C8, T1) and lateral pectoral nerves (C5, C6, and C7) that course from the brachial plexus and are named based on their cord of origin rather than anatomic location. The pectoralis minor arises from the third, fourth, and fifth rib and inserts into the coracoid process of the scapula. Motor function is from the medial pectoral nerve (C8, T1). The serratus anterior muscle arises from the first eight ribs and inserts into the vertebral border of the scapula on its costal surface. It is innervated by the long thoracic nerve of Bell

TABLE 45.2 Nomenclature of the Breast Epithelial System	
MAJOR DUCTS	**TERMINAL DUCTS**
Collecting ducts	Extralobular
Lactiferous sinuses	Intralobular
Segmental ducts	Lobules
Subsegmental ducts	Alveoli
Terminal duct–lobular unit	

From Osborne MP. Breast anatomy and development. In: Harris LM Jr, Morrow M, Osborne CK, eds. *Diseases of the breast.* Philadelphia, PA: Wolters Kluwer/Lippincott Williams & Wilkins; 2010:1–11; and Woodburne R. *Essentials of human anatomy.* New York, NY: Oxford University Press; 1979.

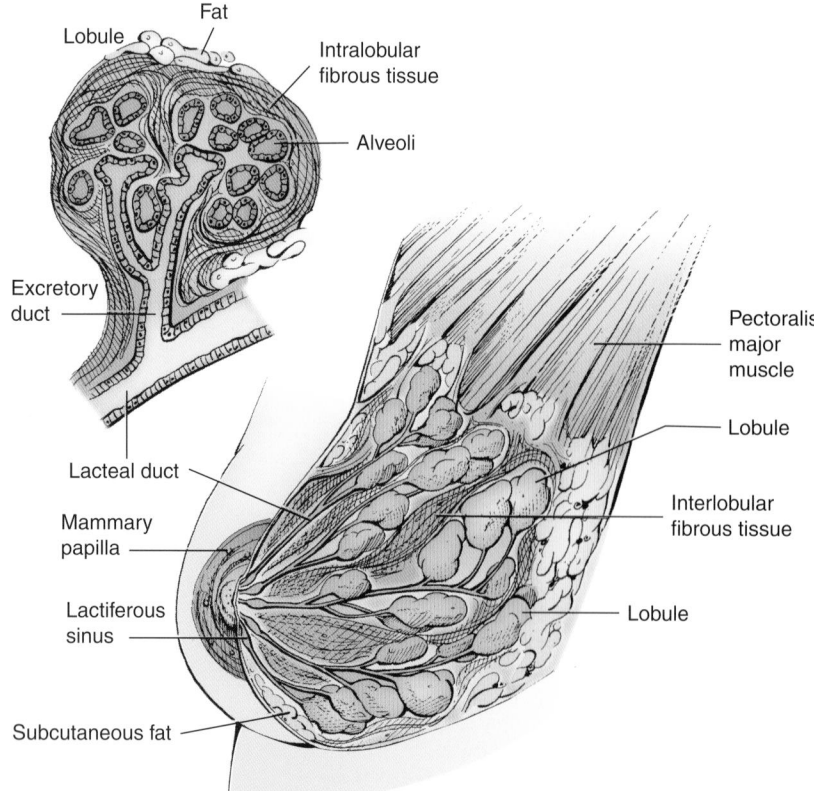

Fat
Lobule
Intralobular fibrous tissue
Alveoli
Excretory duct
Lacteal duct
Mammary papilla
Lactiferous sinus
Subcutaneous fat
Pectoralis major muscle
Lobule
Interlobular fibrous tissue
Lobule

FIGURE 45.3 Internal structure of the breast. The breast is a large apocrine gland. The secreting parenchyma is composed of lobules containing acini, fat, and fibrous tissue. The ducts drain centrally toward large lacunae located directly beneath the nipple.

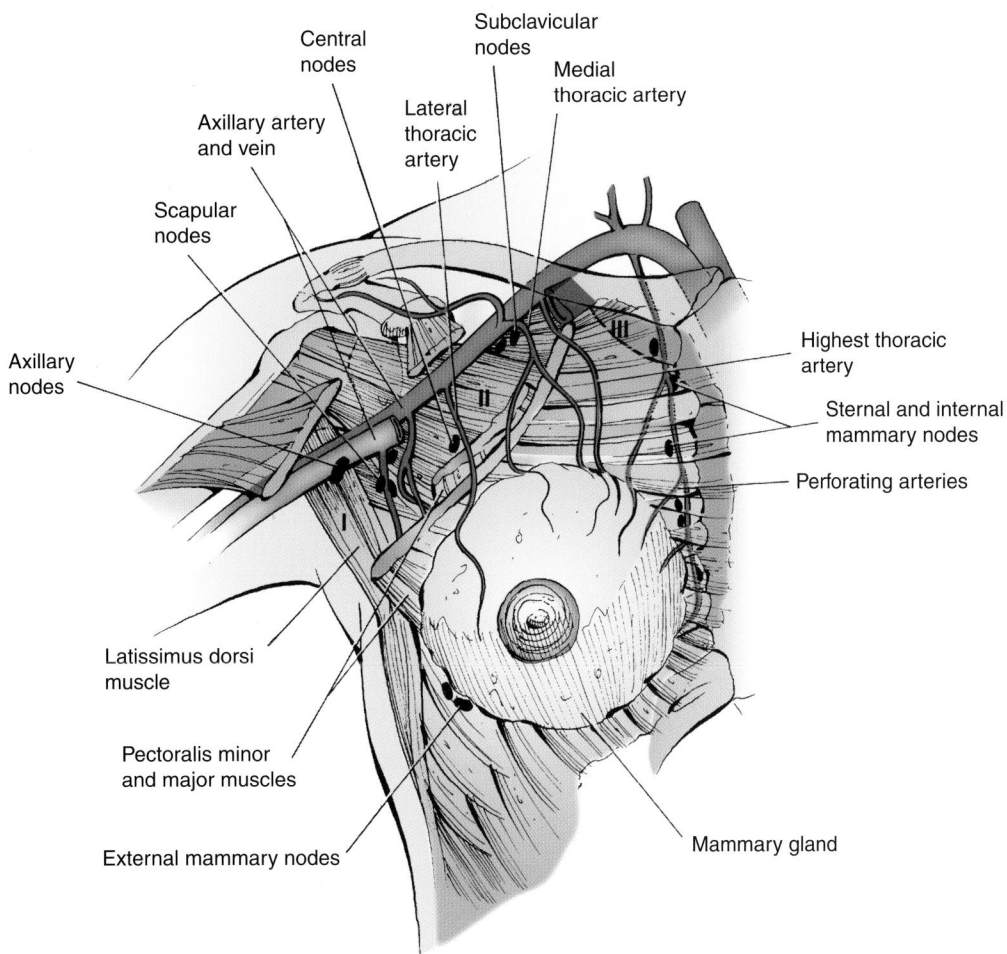

FIGURE 45.4 Lymphatics and blood supply of the breast. Over 97% of lymphatic drainage from the breast is to the axillary nodal basin.

that originates from the posterior roots of C5, C6, C7, and C8 of the brachial plexus. This nerve traverses the posterior aspect of the axilla and courses along the superficial aspect of the fascia of the serratus anterior. Injury to the nerve leads to the clinical presentation of a "winged" scapula and impairment of the shoulder.

The blood supply to the mammary gland is primarily derived from the internal mammary artery and the lateral thoracic artery. The anterior perforating branches of the internal mammary artery supply the medial and central breast, whereas the lateral thoracic artery supplies the upper outer portion of the gland. Additional vascular supply is derived from branches of the thoracoacromial, intercostal, subscapular, and thoracodorsal arteries (Fig. 45.4).

Venous drainage follows the course of the superficial and deep arterial supply. The medial quadrants primarily drain to the internal thoracic vein, whereas the lateral quadrants drain via branches of the axillary vein and posterior branches of the intercostal vein.

Over the past decade, the routine use of sentinel lymphatic mapping in the treatment of breast cancer has significantly enhanced the understanding of lymphatic drainage of the mammary gland. The subepithelial lymphatic plexus is confluent with the subepithelial plexus over the surface of the body. These vessels merge with the subdermal lymphatic vessels and

drain to Sappey plexus beneath the nipple–areolar complex. Lymph then flows through these valveless ducts in only one direction into lymphatics along the lactiferous ducts to the perilobular and deep subcutaneous plexus. Lymph flow then moves in a centrifugal manner toward the axillary and internal mammary nodes. Approximately 97% of the drainage is to the ipsilateral axilla with the remaining 3% of the effluent to the internal mammary nodes.

Approximately 20 to 30 lymph nodes are located within the axillary basin. They consist of five subgroups denoted by their relationship to the axillary structures. The subgroups include the *apical nodes* located medial to the pectoralis minor muscle, the *axillary vein group* located along the axillary vein extending from the pectoralis minor muscle to the lateral extent of the vein, *interpectoral (Rotter)* nodes located between the pectoralis major and minor muscles, the *scapular group* located along the subscapular vessels, and the *central nodes* located beneath the lateral border of the pectoralis major muscle. An alternative approach to the nodal basin nomenclature is to divide the nodal groups into three levels in relation to the pectoralis minor muscle. Level I nodes are lateral to the lateral border of the pectoralis minor muscle, level II nodes are located beneath this muscle, and level III nodes are located medial to the medial border of the pectoralis minor muscle (Fig. 45.5).

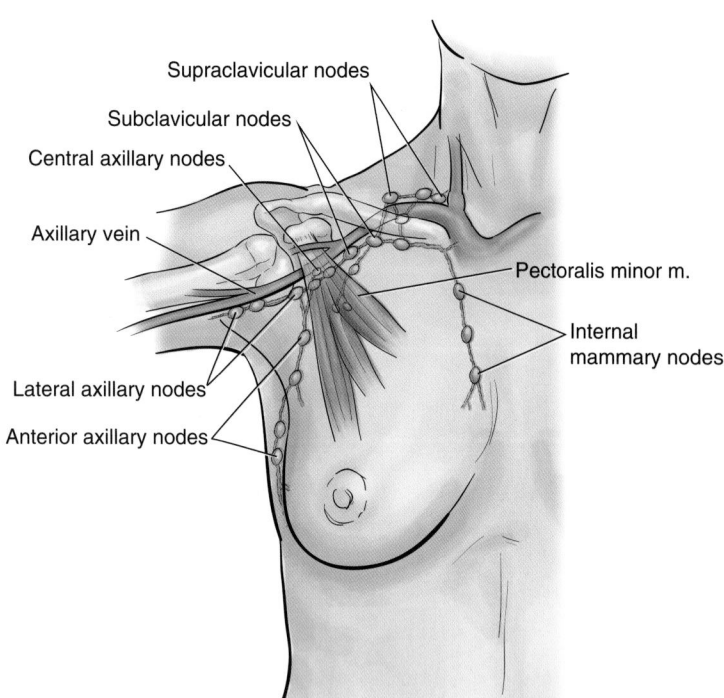

Supraclavicular nodes
Subclavicular nodes
Central axillary nodes
Axillary vein
Pectoralis minor m.
Internal mammary nodes
Lateral axillary nodes
Anterior axillary nodes

FIGURE 45.5 Axillary lymph nodes and level designations. Axillary lymph node levels according to the AJCC. 1: low axillary, level I; 2: midaxillary, level II; 3: high axillary, apical, level III; 4: supraclavicular; 5: internal mammary nodes. (Reprinted from Husarik DB, Steinert HC. Single-photon emission computed tomography/computed tomography for sentinel node mapping in breast cancer. *Sem Nucl Med* 2007;37(1):29–33, with permission. Copyright © 2007 Elsevier, Inc. All rights reserved.)

BREAST HEALTH ASSESSMENT

An intake history should be obtained in which the patient describes her concerns. Care should be taken to elicit information that can help identify a woman at risk for breast cancer.

Breast cancer cannot be excluded by any single fact within the patient's history; rather, the history can help focus attention on risk factors for the development of breast cancer. The practitioner should obtain detailed information about the patient's symptoms and other pertinent related positive and negative signs or concerns. Age, menstrual status, use of oral contraceptives, and postmenopausal hormone replacement therapy (HRT) (including the regimen and duration) are important parts of risk assessment. A detailed family history spanning three generations on both the maternal side and paternal side may identify an individual with a possible genetic predisposition. It is important to elicit and document the timing and specific nature of the concerns, whether any cyclic changes have occurred, change in site, and the presence of pain.

All previous breast diagnostic and surgical procedures should be documented. Past medical and surgical history, current medications, and social history (including tobacco use, alcohol intake, and educational level) should also be reviewed.

In the past, the traditional approach for early detection of breast cancer used a combination of breast self-examination (BSE), clinical breast examination (CBE), and mammography. For women with average risk of breast cancer, current guidelines from the American Cancer Society (ACS), the American Congress of Obstetricians and Gynecologists (ACOG), and the U.S. Preventive Services Task Force (USPSTF) are shown in Table 45.3. Both ACS and ACOG advise annual mammography beginning at the age of 40, CBE beginning in the 20s, and BSE beginning at age 20. Both groups encourage women to know what their breasts look and feel like and promptly report any changes to their health care providers.

BREAST EXAMINATION

Traditionally, BSE and CBE have been considered important facets of a breast screening program. Controversy surrounds the use of both of these physical examinations.

Breast Self-Examination

Recently, the role of BSE has been called into question, as it has been associated in two major studies with increased rates of radiographic imaging and invasive procedures. Controversy exists regarding the utility of routine BSE for increasing the rate of breast cancer detection. A study from Shanghai involving more than 250,000 women, who were randomly assigned to no instruction or intensive BSE instruction, failed to demonstrate any difference in the number of cancers detected or in the stage or size at which they were found (RR 0.97, 95% CI: 0.88 to 1.06). No reduction in mortality was seen, but more than twice as many benign lesions were found in the BSE group. In breast disease, wherein early detection is so clearly related to improved survival, the value of this relatively simple, economical, and minimally invasive technique cannot be overemphasized. ACOG and the ACS support BSE performed monthly beginning at age 20 as optional approach for early detection.

If BSE is advised, a discussion of the benefits, risks, and limitations for the individual patient should take place. Effective instruction of patients in the technique of BSE incorporates description of the procedure while the patient views the health care provider's performance of the examination. The patient should be encouraged to reiterate her understanding of what has been taught and then demonstrate her mastery of the technique using manufactured breast models to further solidify compliance. The patient should be informed of the significance of breast inspection in various positions and the utility of breast palpation in the standing and supine positions. The circular

TABLE 45.3 Screening Recommendations for Women at Average Risk

ORGANIZATION	BREAST SELF-EXAMINATION (BSE)	CLINICAL BREAST EXAM (CBE)	MAMMOGRAPHY
American Cancer Society	Women should know how their breasts normally look and feel and report any breast change promptly to their health care provider. BSE is an option for women starting in their 20s.	Annually for women 40 and older Every 2–3 y for women 20–39	Annual mammogram beginning at age 40 and continued as long as in good health
American Congress of Obstetricians and Gynecologists	Breast self-awareness should be encouraged and can include BSE. Women should report any changes in their breasts to their health care providers.	Annually for women 40 and older Every 2–3 y for women aged 20–39	Annual mammogram beginning at age 40[a,b]
U.S. Preventive Services Task Force	Advises against teaching BSE	Insufficient evidence to demonstrate benefits or risks of CBE	Biennial screening mammography between ages 50 and 74 y Insufficient evidence to assess the additional benefits and harms of screening mammography in women 75 y or older Prior to age 50, biennial screening mammography should be an individual one and take patient context into account, including the patient's values regarding specific benefits and harms.

[a]Women should be educated on the predictive value of screening mammography and the potential for false-positive results and false-negative results. Women should be informed of the potential for additional imaging or biopsies that may be recommended based on screening results.
[b]Women who are estimated to have a lifetime risk of breast cancer of 20% or greater, based on risk models that rely largely on family history (such as BRCAPRO, BODACEA, or Claus), but who are either untested or test negative for *BRCA* gene mutations, can be offered enhanced screening. For women with known BRCA1/BRCA2 deleterious mutations, enhanced screening should be recommended and risk reduction methods discussed.

method of breast palpation using the pads of her fingers is the easiest to master, although for patients with pendulous breasts, positional changes to ensure positioning of the breast tissue on the chest wall must be emphasized. The best time to perform the examination is usually after the week after the end of the menstrual cycle, although menopausal women should pick a convenient time of the month, such as their birth date or the first day of each month. After hysterectomy, patients with continued estrogenic support of the ovaries should observe for breast fullness or tenderness. Breast examination should then be performed 7 to 10 days after cessation of menstrual breast symptoms.

Clinical Breast Examination

The CBE is an important part of early detection of breast cancer. The ACS, ACOG, and others recommend CBE beginning in the mid-20s for women at average risk for breast cancer. The USPSTF states that insufficient evidence exists concerning the risk or benefit of this practice. CBE has a sensitivity of 57% to 70% in detecting breast cancer.

Strategies to improve a practitioner's ability to detect a mass include developing a systematic, consistent search mode, increasing the time devoted to the examination, and using a technique with variable degrees of pressure. The more facile and practiced the examiner, the greater the rates of detection of breast lesions.

CBE should be a routine part of the examination of gynecologic and obstetrical patients. Obstetrician–gynecologists should not abdicate their responsibilities by relying on previous examinations performed by other specialists. The practitioner must be mindful of the legal ramifications of errors of omission.

CBE is ideally performed 1 week after the end of the menstrual cycle to diminish the impact of luteal phase breast congestion, which can obscure mass detection. Each portion of the breast examination should be performed with the patient in both the sitting and supine positions because positional changes often expose a lesion that can be masked by the patient's normal anatomy.

The initial part of the examination should focus on breast inspection, viewing for symmetry, skin retraction, rashes, and nipple retraction or deviation (Fig. 45.6). Inspection should continue with the patient's arms raised overhead. This allows visualization of the inferior and lateral aspects of the breast. Inspection with the patient placing her hands on her hips while contracting the pectoralis muscles will highlight any changes in the upper quadrants of the breast. In patients with rheumatoid arthritis or other conditions preventing pressure on the hip joint, other more comfortable options may be used. One may have the patient either grasp her fingertips at a level near the waistline while pulling laterally or press her palms together while extended above the head. Because the breast lies on the pectoralis muscle and Cooper ligaments are attached to the muscle and the skin, tension on the muscle accentuates carcinoma invading these structures. An inspection of the breast for nipple retraction or inversion, which can result from either stromal contraction or direct attachment to the tissues beneath

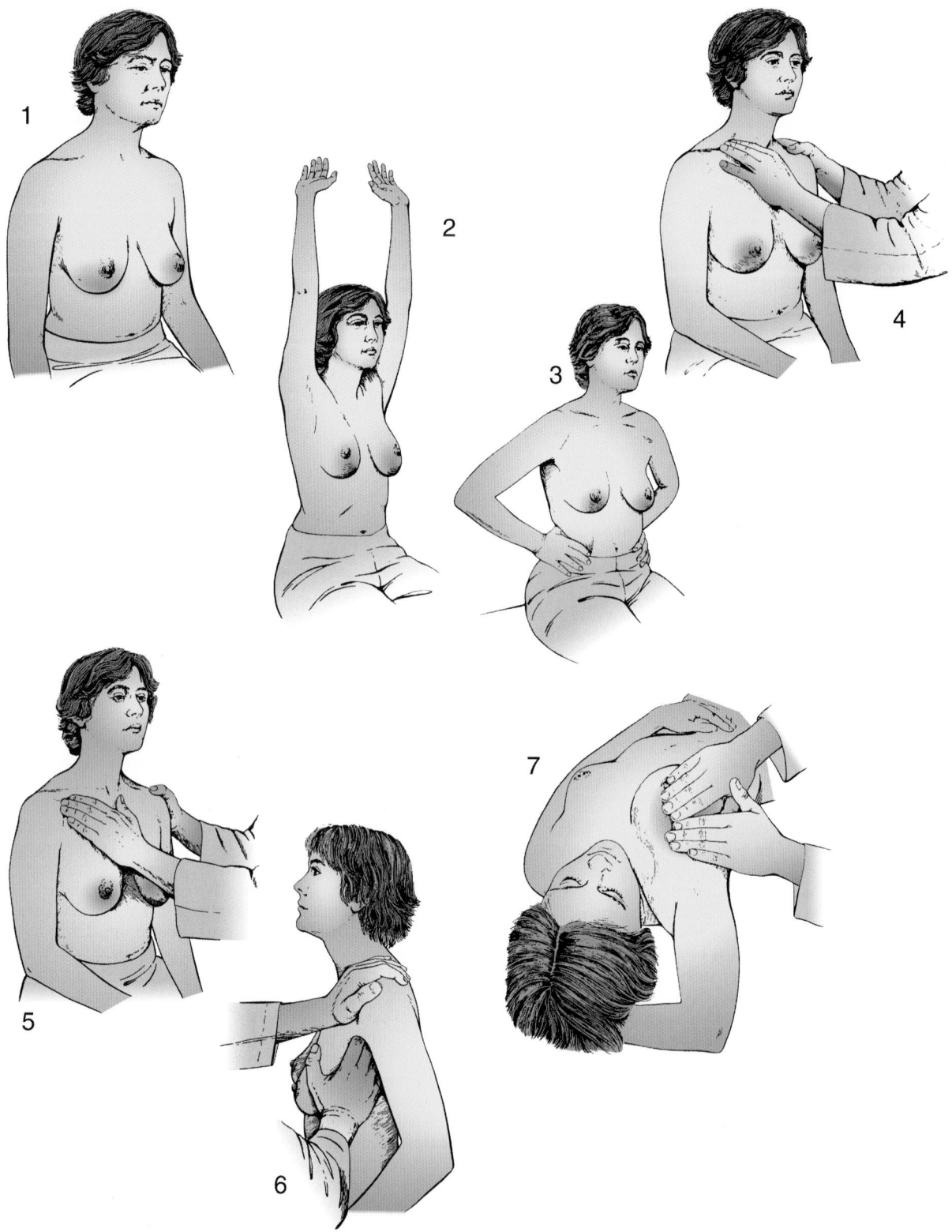

FIGURE 45.6 (*1*) Examination of the breasts begins with inspection. The patient is disrobed to the waist and comfortably seated facing the examiner. Asymmetry, prominent veins, and skin changes may be signs of disease. (*2*) The patient raises her arms above her head, thereby altering the position of the breasts. Immobility or abnormal cutaneous attachments may become evident. (*3*) Inward pressure on the hips tenses the pectoralis major muscle. Abnormal attachments to its overlying fascia and skin can produce retraction or dimpling of the skin. (*4*) Supraclavicular lymph nodes are examined by palpation. (*5*) The deltopectoral triangle is palpated for evidence of infraclavicular nodal enlargement. (*6*) Each axilla is examined for nodal enlargement. Proper placement of the examiner's hands and of the patient's arm is important. (*7*) Thorough examination of the entire breast for abnormalities is performed with the patient in the supine position. A fine rotational movement of the hands is useful to appreciate the consistency of the underlying tissues. The examiner should check for nipple discharge by compressing the ducts in a clockwise manner toward the nipple. (Reprinted from Scott JR, DiSaia PJ, Hammond CB, et al. *Danforth's obstetrics and gynecology*, 7th ed. Philadelphia, PA: JB Lippincott, 1994:700, with permission. Copyright © 1994, Lippincott Williams & Wilkins.)

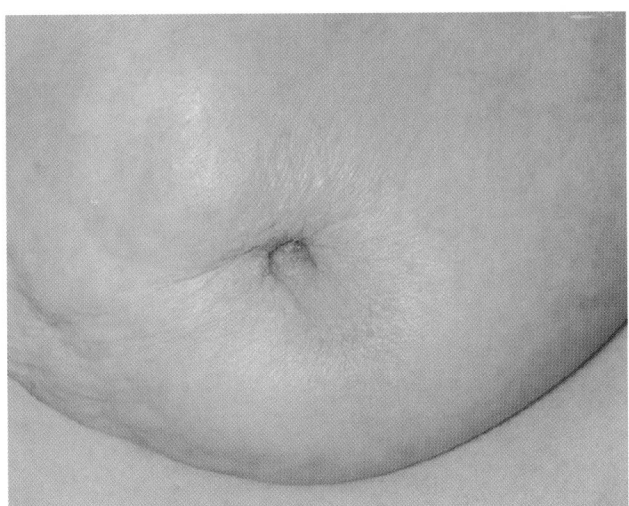

FIGURE 45.7 Nipple inversion due to cancer. (Reprinted from Harris JR, Lippman ME, Morrow M, et al. *Diseases of the breast*, 4th ed. Philadelphia, PA: Lippincott Williams & Wilkins, 2009, with permission. Copyright © 2009, Lippincott Williams & Wilkins.)

the nipple, should be performed (Fig. 45.7). Nipple inversion can be normal, and if with gentle manipulation eversion occurs, it is considered a normal variant. New onset of nipple inversion is concerning and warrants additional evaluation.

Inspection of the breast is followed by palpation. The patient should be properly gowned, with only the area being examined exposed. The patient must be positioned (by tilting her hips and torso) to allow the portion of the breast tissue being examined to lie directly upon the chest wall. For patients with pendulous breasts, this may require positional changes for each breast. The pads of the fingers and not the fingertips are the most sensitive and should be used in examination. Three circular motions are made with three levels of pressure (superficial, medium, and firm) on each 1-cm square area of the breast. Not only does this improve mass detection but it also prevents masking a mass through excessive pressure.

The circular pattern is the most frequently used; however, the "vertical-strip" and radial or "wheel and spoke" patterns are acceptable techniques. With the circular method of palpation, the examination proceeds clockwise around the full circumference of the breast at its perimeter and gradually moves inward toward the nipple.

During the vertical-strip search pattern, the provider will begin overlapping circular motions in the axilla extending inferiorly (1 cm at a time) to one to two ribs below the breast tissue. The fingers are then moved inward 1 cm, and the pattern of search is extended superiorly, in a straight line, to the clavicle. This pattern is continued until the sternum is reached. The patient's position may have to be changed several times during this portion of the exam to assure the tissue being examined lies directly upon the chest wall.

The wheel and spoke method requires radially palpating to the clavicle, sternum, and other bony margins and palpating from the nipple or vice versa. Each method should be mastered, as they may be helpful in certain clinical and diagnostic situations, such as patients with large breasts. Regardless of the pattern of breast examination used, the importance of using a consistent and methodical pattern of evaluation and allowing sufficient time for a thorough examination cannot be overemphasized.

Concurrently, the axilla is evaluated for masses. To allow proper assessment of the axilla in the sitting position, the arm should be extended at a 90-degree angle from the chest wall.

This maneuver relaxes the area to be examined for a more thorough evaluation. Next, the patient should be placed in a comfortable supine position with her arm—on the same side as the breast being examined—raised above her head to evenly distribute the breast over the chest wall, thereby making its deeper regions of the axillary basin more accessible.

Palpation should extend beyond the actual breast tissue to encompass the supraclavicular and infraclavicular lymph nodes, the area adjacent to the sternum, approximately 1 to 2 cm below the inframammary ridge, and the axillary tail of Spence. In this manner, all the borders of the breast and associated nodal basins are examined. Gentle pressure on the nipple and areolar area can be used to elicit discharge. Excessive breast manipulation can lead to a nipple discharge. Using a milking technique improves the examiner's ability to elicit a nipple discharge. Each quadrant of the breast is "milked" by sliding the fingers from the outer quadrant in a clockwise fashion toward the nipple and documenting the location of any fluid accumulation.

Careful and comprehensive documentation of the history, examination, and disposition of the case should be filed in the patient's record. A clear and legible note should record all findings. The use of a diagram is also helpful (Fig. 45.8). Although positive or abnormal findings are important, it also is valuable to list negative findings in the medical record.

Radiologic Breast Assessment

Imaging tests of the breast can be considered screening or diagnostic in nature. Screening tests are done in asymptomatic patients, while diagnostic tests are performed in patients with clinical findings such as breast masses, pain, or nipple discharge. Screening tests include mammograms, breast MRI, and tomosynthesis. Screening with breast ultrasounds is not commonly performed and is rarely indicated; however, increasing information suggests benefit from the use of ultrasound when mammography demonstrates dense breast tissue. Diagnostic tests include mammogram, breast ultrasound, breast MRI, tomosynthesis, and breast-specific gamma imaging.

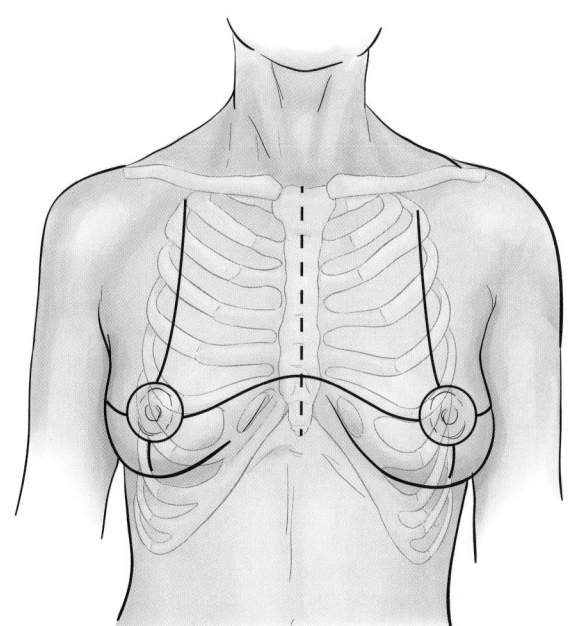

FIGURE 45.8 Breast diagram for documentation.

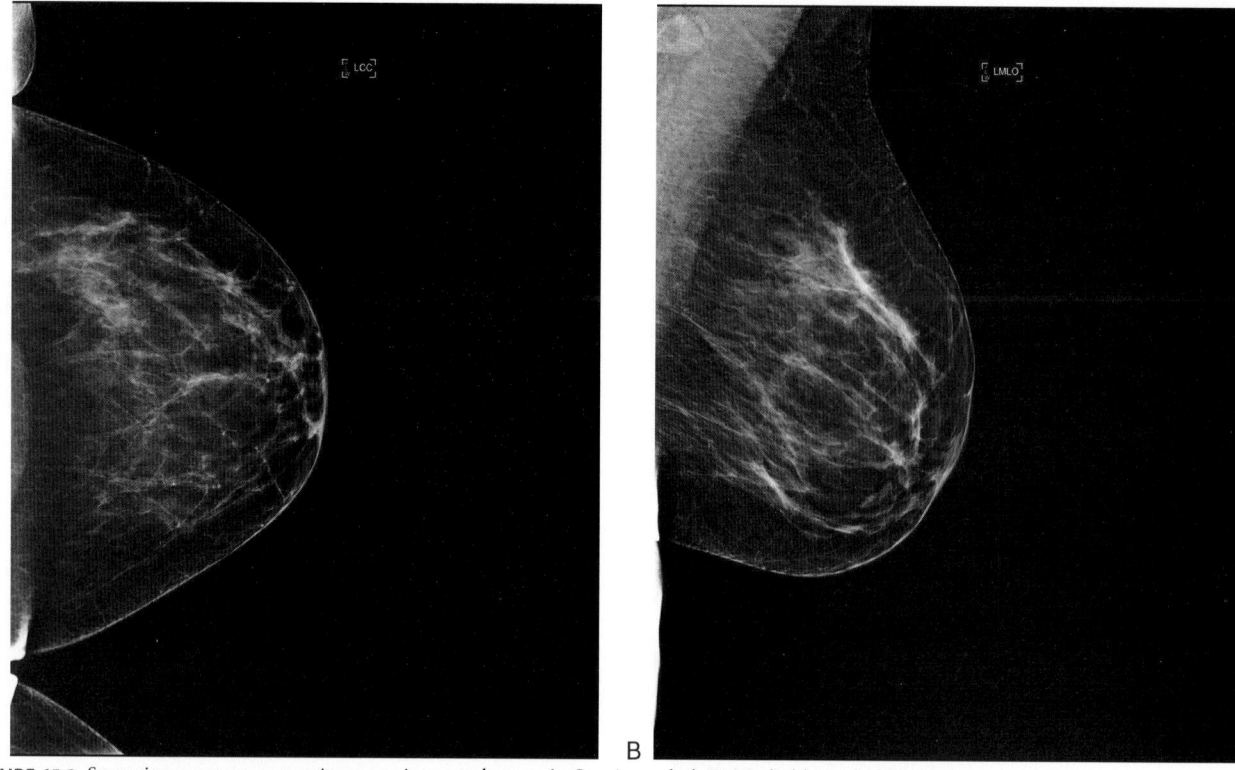

FIGURE 45.9 Screening mammogram using two views per breast. **A:** Craniocaudad. **B:** Medial lateral oblique views.

Mammography

The most common imaging test used for screening is mammography (Fig. 45.9A, B). Albert Salomon published the first study documenting that x-rays can be used to image breast cancer in 1913; however, many decades passed before mammograms were accepted as standard means of imaging the breast. The first randomized controlled trial of breast cancer screening with mammography, the health insurance plan (HIP) study was initiated in the 1960s. The first data were published in 1971; since then, a total of nine major randomized control trials have been completed and reported. A summary is presented in Table 45.4.

It is important to note that these trials have been performed in many countries with varying schedules of screening, study population age, and mammographic technique. The HIP study was one of the few studies in which the control group had no screening mammograms. This study enrolled 62,000 patients aged 40 to 64 years and found that 30% fewer deaths in the study group compared to the control group. A major issue with this study is that the prestudy breast cancer prevalence was unclear in the control group. The screening group underwent examinations at study entry and excluded patients with breast cancer, while the control group did not have equivalent assessment. Whether or not the patient had breast cancer prior to entry into the study was determined retrospectively in the control group; thus, it is possible that the control group had more undiagnosed breast cancer at entry. This bias may favor the screening group with regard to breast cancer mortality rate. Another issue is that the trial used outdated mammographic equipment compared to today's equipment. In Malmo, Sweden, another large randomized controlled trial was initiated in 1976. This trial had two cohorts that were randomized by birth year. This trial enrolled approximately 42,000 patients aged 45 to 69 years who subsequently underwent two-view mammograms

every 18 to 24 months for a total of five screening examinations. This study did not find any reduction in deaths between the study and control groups, although a nonsignificant 20% lower breast cancer death rate occurred in the study group for women greater than age 55 years. Lack of a positive finding may have been due to the high number of women in the control group undergoing at least one mammogram (24% for the entire cohort, 35% in women aged 45 to 49 years). Only 70% to 74% of the patients in the study group underwent screening examinations. The Swedish two-county study was a large trial that enrolled patients in two counties in Sweden, Östergötland and Kopparberg. More than 133,000 women between ages 40 and 74 years were enrolled in this study. This trial was different from previous trials in that the four screening intervals were varied by age, every 24 months for women aged 40 to 49 and every 33 months for ages 50 years and older. Data reported after 8, 11, 14, and 20 years of follow-up revealed 30% to 32% fewer breast cancer deaths in the study group compared to the controls. Unlike the HIP and Malmo trials, the Swedish two-county study used a single-view mammogram—a screening test that is not comparable to the current standards of screening mammography in the United States. Another issue with this study is approximately 13% of the control group had mammograms as part of routine care. In Stockholm, Sweden, in 1981, a large trial randomly assigned approximately 40,000 patients aged 40 to 64 years to two rounds of screening every 28 months with a single-view mammogram. The screening group was found to have 29% to 26% fewer breast cancer deaths compared to the controls at 7.4 and 11.4 years of follow-up, respectively. However, these differences were not statistically significant. There were concerns about the randomization methods in this study, and the number of patients in each arm varied significantly. In 1979, a randomized controlled trial was initiated in Edinburgh, United Kingdom, and enrolled approximately 25,000 patients aged 45 to 64 years. The screening strategy consisted

TABLE 45.4 Randomized Controlled Studies of Screening Mammography

TRIAL	STUDY POPULATION AGE	SIZE OF STUDY GROUP	SIZE OF CONTROL GROUP	INTERVENTION IN STUDY GROUP	CONTROL GROUP	DURATION OF FOLLOW-UP	RELATIVE RISK OF DEATH, SCREENING VERSUS CONTROL (95% CI)
HIP study	40–64	31,092	30,765	Annual two-view MMG and CBE for 3 y	No MMG	18 y	0.71 (0.55–0.93) at 10 y 0.77 (0.61–0.97) at 15 y
Malmo	45–69	21,088	21,195	Two-view MMG every 18–24 mo × 5	Usual care, MMG at the end of the study	12 y	0.81 (0.62–1.07)
Östergötland	40–74	38,405–39,034	37,145–37,936	Single-view MMG every 2 y for women <50 yo × 3 And every 33 mo for women >50 yo	Usual care, MMG at the end of the study	12 y	0.82 (0.64–1.05)
Kopparberg	40–74	38,562–39,051	18,478–18,846	Single-view MMG every 2 y for women <50 yo × 3 And every 33 mo for women >50 yo	Usual care, MMG at the end of the study	12 y	0.68 (0.52–0.89)
Edinburgh	45–64	23,226	21,904	Two-view MMG and CBE, then single-view MMG in years 3, 5, and 7	Usual care	10 y	0.84 (0.63–1.12)
NBSS-1	40–49	25,214	25,216	Annual two-view MMG and CBE for 4–5 y	Usual care	13 y	0.97 (0.74–1.27)
NBSS-2	50–59	19,711	19,694	Annual two-view MMG	Annual CBE	11–16 y (median 13 y)	1.02 (0.78–1.33)
Stockholm	40–64	38,525–40,318	19,943–20,978	Single-view MMG every 28 mo × 2	MMG at year 5	8 y	0.80 (0.53–1.22)
Gothenburg	39–59	21,650	29,961	Initially 2-view MMG then single-view MMG every 18 mo × 4	MMG × 1 3–8 mo after final screen in the study group	12–14 y	0.77 (0.60–1.00)
AGE trial	39–51	53,884	106,956	2-view MMG initially then single MLO view annually	Usual care	10.7 y	0.83 (0.66–1.04)

MMG, mammogram; CBE, clinical breast exam; MLO, medial lateral oblique view.

VIII

of a two-view mammogram and clinical breast exam and then annual CBE followed by a single-view mammogram in years 3, 5, and 7. Socioeconomic differences found between the general medical practices were not recognized until the study ended; adjustments were then made for these differences. A nonsignificant 21% reduction in deaths from breast cancer was found between the study and control group. A significant 29% reduction in deaths from breast cancer was noted when breast cancer deaths that occurred 3 years after the end of the study were censored. Only 61% of the screening group underwent screening. A randomized controlled trial performed in Gothenburg, Sweden, in over 51,000 women aged 39 to 59 years randomly assigned participants to five rounds of screening. The screening group underwent a two-view mammogram every 18 months unless a prior screening test indicated that a single-view mammogram was sufficient (this accounted for 30% of the women screened). At 11 years of follow-up, the study group had a 44% statistically significant reduction in breast cancer mortality among women aged 39 to 49 years. Issues with this study included a delay of 3 to 8 months in the end-of-study mammogram in the control group compared to the study group and a complex randomization scheme that resulted in unequal numbers of patients in the study and control groups. Two large Canadian randomized controlled trials, National Breast Screening Study (NBSS) I and II trials, were initiated in 1980. These trials were designed to evaluate the role of screening mammograms in women aged 40 to 49 years and 50 to 59 years, respectively. The NBSS I trial is unique in that it was the first trial designed specifically to test the efficacy of mammographic screening in women younger than 50 years. In this trial, approximately 50,000 patients were randomly assigned to an annual two-view mammogram or CBE for 4 to 5 years. Compliance in the study group was good, with 85.5% of patients undergoing screening mammograms by year 5. In the control group, noncompliance was high: Only 26.4% of patients had at least one mammogram. Surprisingly, this trial revealed more breast cancer–related deaths in the screening group at 7 and 10.5 years of follow-up, 36% breast cancer–related deaths in the study group compared to 14% in the control group. At 11 to 16 years of follow-up, the increase in breast cancer–related mortality persisted, with 7% more breast cancer–related deaths in the study group. The NBSS II study had similar results in the 50- to 59-year-old cohort, with 3% and 2% more breast cancer–related deaths in the study group at 7 and 13 years of follow-up, respectively. There has been much speculation as to why these results have differed from all the other randomized controlled trials. One possible explanation was the statistically significant higher number of advanced cancers in the study group. While this may account for the high death rates, it is not clear why this occurred. Concerns have been expressed with regard to the equipment, technical adequacy of the mammograms, and training of the radiologists. An external independent review found some inadequacy with regard to the mammographic views from 1980 to 1985. The last randomized controlled trial published to date is the UK Age Trial designed to evaluate the role of mammographic screening starting at the age of 40 years. This trial was unique in that it avoided contamination that can occur by screening episodes after the age of 50 years by starting annual screening at the age of 39 to 41 years and comparing this group to women who were screened beginning at age 50 years. At 10.7 years of follow-up, a statistically nonsignificant reduction occurred in breast cancer mortality in both relative and absolute terms, with a relative risk of 0.83 (95% CI: 0.66 to 1.04) and absolute risk reduction of 0.40 per 1,000 women invited for screening (95% CI: 0.07 to 0.87). The major issue with this trial was that patients underwent a two-view mammogram at entry; subsequent screenings utilized single-view mammograms.

The study was stopped early due to funding issues with lower post hoc power analysis than expected (72% vs. 80%).

Controversies with Regard to Mammographic Screening

There has been much debate over when mammographic screening should be initiated. The main issues with all randomized trials have been the heterogeneity of the type of screening (single- vs. two-view mammograms), length of time between screening exams (range of 12 to 28 months), and variation in the age of the study population. Due to these issues, there have been multiple meta-analyses of the randomized controlled trial data to date, all confirmed that mammographic screening decreased breast cancer mortality rate in patients who were invited for screening. The analysis by Wald and colleagues found a 26% reduction in breast cancer mortality in patients older than 50 years. Hendrick and colleagues found an 18% reduction in mortality rate in patients aged 40 to 49 years. The same authors found a 24% reduction in mortality rate in patients aged 50 to 74 years. The most recent update of the meta-analysis of the Swedish trials found a 21% reduction in breast cancer mortality between the study and control group; however, when various age groups were taken into account, the reduction in breast cancer mortality was not significant in patients younger than 50 years. In a 2004 meta-analysis of all the randomized controlled trials, Smith and colleagues found a 20% reduction in breast cancer mortality in women aged 40 to 74 years, a 15% reduction ($P < 0.05$) in women aged 40 to 49 years, and a 22% reduction ($P < 0.05$) in women aged 50 to 74 years. Given that many women who were invited to have mammographic screening did not have any screening done, the authors went on to analyze the actual effect of having a mammographic screen. When the results were analyzed only for women undergoing screening, the overall effect of mammographic screening was even higher, with a 40% reduction in mortality. Recently, the National Cancer Institute applied mathematical modeling with regard to outcomes of mammographic screening using six models with varying assumptions. All the models found that screening starting at the age of 40 years will lead to reductions in breast cancer mortality from 2% to 10% (median 3%) with annual mammographic screening. This would result in one breast cancer–related death averted per 1,000 women screened and 33 life years gained per 1,000 women. The life years gained per 1,000 women was lower at 25 years if biennial screening was done, but there was a reduction of approximately 50% in false-positive rates and unnecessary biopsies.

Overall, these data suggest that screening starting at the age of 40 years leads to reductions in breast cancer mortality rates but at increased cost. The National Cancer Institute (NCI) mathematical models suggest there would be approximately 1,250 false-positive results per 1,000 women screened. This has the potential to lead to approximately 88 unnecessary biopsies per 1,000 women. There is also a risk of radiation-induced mortality. It is estimated that that risk of radiation-induced breast cancer death is about 0.22 to 0.50 per 1,000 women screened. With regard to absolute benet-to-risk ratio, screening starting at age 40 years would still be expected to be of benefit; 1,894 women would need to be screened to prevent one breast cancer–related death, and one radiation-induced breast cancer–related death would likely occur per 6,456 women screened. The recent recommendation from the USPSTF states that screening should start at age 50 years and be conducted biennially. Although starting breast cancer screening at age 40 may result in increase in life years gained, the most efficient means of reducing the breast cancer mortality rate on the analysis of the ratio of benefits to screening exams was to start to screening at

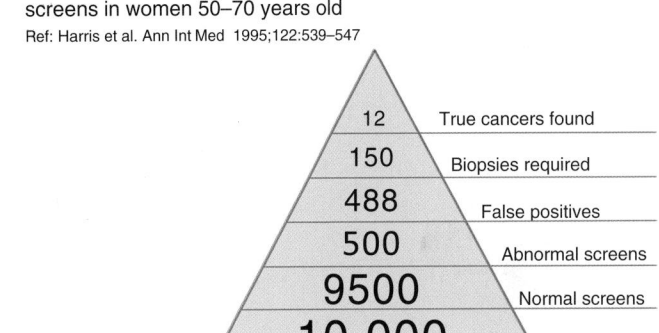

Hypothetical outcome of 10,000
screens in women 40–49 years old
Ref: Harris et al. Ann Int Med 1995;122:539–547

Hypothetical outcome of 10,000
screens in women 50–70 years old
Ref: Harris et al. Ann Int Med 1995;122:539–547

30	True cancers found
150	Biopsies required
475	False positives
500	Abnormal screens
9500	Normal screens
10,000	Initial screens

12	True cancers found
150	Biopsies required
488	False positives
500	Abnormal screens
9500	Normal screens
10,000	Initial screens

FIGURE 45.10 Outcome of screening evaluation in women aged 40 to 49 (**A**) and 50 to 70 (**B**).

age 50 years; hence, this was the basis for the recommendation. Additionally, biennial screening examinations maintained 81% of the benefit compared to annual exams while reducing the number of false-positive exams by nearly 50%. These recommendations are controversial as breast cancers in women younger than age 50 years are thought to be more aggressive and faster growing; thus, a biennial screening schedule may be too long. A recent analysis of the Surveillance, Epidemiology and End Results (SEER) database found that the biennial screening interval was associated with an increased risk of late stage disease (odds ratio 1.35, 95% CI: 1.01 to 1.81). Another study attempted to use the SEER database to evaluate the effect of screening mammogram on breast cancer incidence between 1976 and 2008. The authors found a significant increase in the number of early-stage breast cancer cases (112 to 234 cases per 100,000 women, i.e., absolute increase of 122 cases), while there has been a decrease of 8% in the number of late-stage disease (decrease of 102 to 94 cases per 100,000 women, i.e., absolute decrease of 8 cases). The authors concluded that only 8 of the 122 additional cases were expected to progress to advanced cancer; therefore, screening mammograms may be leading to an overdiagnosis of breast cancer. The main issue

with this paper is that the SEER database does not record how the cancers were diagnosed or who within this dataset had screening mammograms. In a different analysis, the authors looked at the utility of mammographic screening in absolute numbers (Fig. 45.10). In this analysis, one life may be extended per 1,700 to 5,000 women screened and followed for 15 years for women aged 50 to 70 years. The same analysis would predict that one or two lives may be extended per 5,000 to 10,000 mammograms in women aged 40 to 49 years. Recommendations from various national organizations are highlighted in Table 45.5. All of these various screening recommendations are reasonable with varying risks and benefits.

Breast Magnetic Resonance Imaging for Screening

Breast magnetic resonance imaging (MRI) is typically used for diagnostic evaluation, that is, workup of breast masses or physical findings (Fig. 45.11). The best data for using breast MRI as a screening test come from studies in high-risk populations. In 2004, Kriege and colleagues reported on 1,909 women at high risk for breast cancer (358 of whom were

TABLE 45.5 Screening Guidelines by Various Organizations					
ORGANIZATION	**INITIAL AGE FOR MAMMOGRAMS**	**UPPER AGE LIMIT FOR MAMMOGRAMS**	**SCHEDULE FOR MAMMOGRAMS**	**CLINICAL BREAST EXAMS**	**SELF-BREAST EXAMS**
American Congress of Obstetricians and Gynecologists (ACOG)	40 years old	75 years old (older than 75 should be based on patient's life expectancy)	Annually	Aged 20–39 every 1–3 y Aged 40 and older annually	Recommended
American Cancer Society	40 years old	No upper limit (continue as "long as a woman is in good health")	Annually	Optional for women older than 20 years old	Recommended
National Comprehensive Cancer Network	40 years old	No upper limit (patient's "overall health and estimated longevity" should be taken into consideration)	Annually	Recommended	Recommended
National Cancer Institute	40 years old	No statement on upper age limit	1–2 y	Not recommended	No statement
U.S. Preventive Services Task Force	50 years old	74 years old	Biennially	Insufficient evidence	No statement

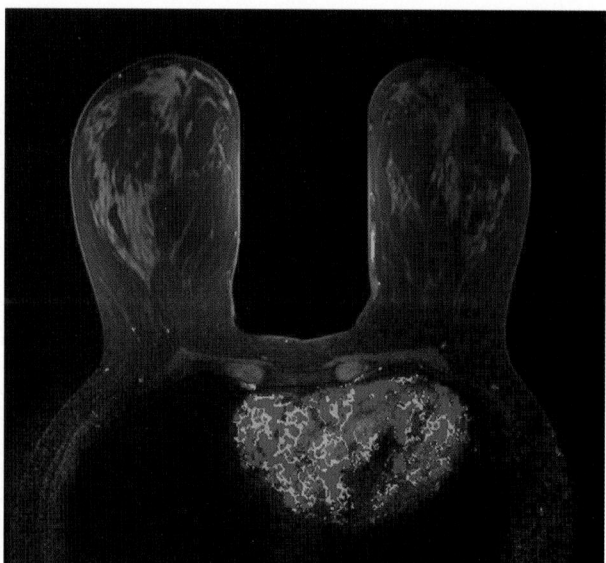

FIGURE 45.11 Normal MRI of patient at high risk.

carriers of germline mutations) who were screened with both breast MRI and mammograms. The authors found that the sensitivities of mammography and MRI in detecting breast tumors were 33.3% and 79.5%, respectively. It is important to note that while breast MRI sensitivity is higher than that of mammography, the tests were considered complementary as some breast cancers that were missed by breast MRI were detected by mammography. The overall sensitivity of testing was higher when the results of both tests were used, resulting in a combined sensitivity of 88%. This study demonstrated breast MRI had lower sensitivity for picking up DCIS compared to mammography (17% vs. 83%, respectively). A large study in Canada found that breast MRI was more sensitive than was mammography in the high-risk population. In this study, 236 women underwent screening with breast ultrasound, mammography, and MRI all on the same day. The authors found that breast MRI was the most sensitive test at 77% followed by mammography at 36% and ultrasound at 33%. Again, these tests appeared to be complementary as the sensitivity was improved to 95% when results from all three modalities were combined. Other studies have confirmed these results, and at present, the addition of breast MRI as part of a screening regimen is recommended for patients at high risk for developing breast cancer. The American Cancer Society's most recent guidelines state that women should undergo screening with breast MRI if they have a BRCA1 or BRCA2 mutation or have a first-degree relative (parent, sibling, child) with a BRCA1 or BRCA2 mutation (even if they have yet to be tested themselves), if their lifetime risk of breast cancer has been scored at 20% to 25% or greater based on one of several accepted risk assessment tools for evaluating family history and other factors, if they have received radiation to the chest between the ages of 10 and 30, if they have a male relative with history of breast cancer at any age, or if they have Li-Fraumeni syndrome, Cowden syndrome, or Bannayan-Riley-Ruvalcaba syndrome or may have one of these syndromes based on history in a first-degree relative. The presence of dense breast tissue is not a reason for using breast MRI for screening despite the lower sensitivity of mammography in these patients. It may be reasonable to use breast MRI as a screening test for women with a personal history of lobular carcinoma of the breast as these cancers are difficult to detect

via mammography. Another scenario in which screening with breast MRI may be appropriate is in women whose original cancer was not visible on mammography.

Breast Ultrasound

The most common use of breast ultrasound is as an adjunct to mammography. In one analysis of the six studies of screening ultrasounds with a total of 42,838 exams, only 150 (0.35%) additional cancers were only visible via ultrasonography. The largest study to date was performed by the American College of Radiology Imaging Network (ACRIN Protocol 6666). This study enrolled 2,809 women with dense breasts who had elevated risk of breast cancer (i.e., a personal history of breast cancer, lifetime risk >25% by Gail or Claus model, atypical ductal hyperplasia [ADH], atypical lobular hyperplasia [ALH], lobular carcinoma in situ [LCIS], atypical papilloma, presence of BRCA mutation, elevated 5-year Gail model risk, or history of chest radiation). This study found that the addition of screening ultrasound will increase the detection of breast cancer by 4.2 per 1,000 women screened, but will substantially increase the number of false-positive exams. At present, the most common use of breast ultrasound is to further evaluate abnormal findings on mammography and not necessarily as a primary screening tool. It may be of benefit in women with dense breasts; however, the American College of Radiology states that "the addition of ultrasound to screening mammography may be useful for incremental cancer detection." Due to the increase in false-positive rates and decrease in positive predictive value, it is not considered the standard of care for primary screening in women with dense breasts.

Digital Mammography

Digital mammography is a newer technology in which a digital detector is used in place of standard film. The images are then processed by a computer and displayed on a monitor. This results in images with greater resolution that can be easily magnified on a workstation. The contrast can also be adjusted to greater degree than in standard film. The ease in which the images can be manipulated is thought to lead to potential improvements in sensitivity. One of the largest studies to date is the Digital Mammographic Imaging Screening Trial (DMIST). The study compared film with digital mammography in over 49,000 women. Overall, the sensitivities of digital versus film mammography were similar (70% vs. 66%, respectively). Digital mammography was found to be 15% to 30% more sensitive for the detection of breast cancer in premenopausal women and in women with dense breasts (improvement in sensitivity from 51% to 55% to 70% to 78%, respectively). In another study that randomly assigned over 25,000 women aged 45 to 69 years old to either digital mammography or film mammography, a higher prevalence of breast cancer was found with digital mammography (0.59% vs. 0.38%, respectively). Recall rates were higher with digital mammography in comparison to film mammography (4.2% vs. 2.5%, respectively), but no difference in positive predictive value was observed between the two types of mammography. Unlike the DMIST trial, overall sensitivity was higher in the digital mammography arm at 77.4% versus 61.5% seen in the film mammography group. At the present time, digital mammography appears to be useful for breast cancer screening especially in younger patients and patients with dense breasts.

Breast Tomosynthesis

Breast tomosynthesis is a modification of digital mammography that utilizes a moving x-ray source and digital detector. This allows for three-dimensional images to be generated using computer algorithms (similar to CT images of the body) that can overcome the limitation of overlapping tissue that can decrease the sensitivity of traditional film mammography. This technique can avoid additional compression views and recall mammograms. A number of studies have compared breast tomosynthesis to routine two-view mammography with the majority of studies consisting of small case series. At the present time, there is no consensus of whether or not the sensitivity of breast tomosynthesis is higher than that of the traditional two-view mammography as some studies have shown decreased sensitivity while others have shown increased sensitivity. Notably, all of these studies demonstrated the specificity of breast tomosynthesis to be higher than that of two-view mammography. In one study, the use of breast tomosynthesis reduced false-positive recalls by 40%. The best role for breast tomosynthesis may be to use it in conjunction with two-view mammography. When breast tomosynthesis is performed in combination with two-view mammography, superior accuracy can be achieved.

Breast-Specific Gamma Imaging

Breast-specific gamma imaging (BSGI) is a nuclear medicine technique that measures the mitochondrial density of breast tissue through the use of technetium-99m sestamibi as a tracer. It is expected when there is increased mitochondrial density in breast cancer tissue, and by tagging the mitochondria at a cellular level, breast cancers can be detected. This technology is still relatively new in comparison to the other breast imaging techniques, and as such, there are still limited data on its utility. In general, the majority of the studies have found BSGI to have similar sensitivity to that of breast MRI. In one retrospective review, 159 women with a concerning physical exam and/or mammograms underwent additional testing with BSGI to assess for occult disease; BSGI was able to detect additional suspicious lesions in 29% of the women of whom 3% had occult cancer in the contralateral breast. In a study of 146 women at high risk for breast cancer, BSGI was found to have an overall sensitivity of 96.4% and specificity of 59.5%. A more recent study of 149 women also demonstrated a similar sensitivity rate of 98.0%. In one study that directly compared BSGI to breast MRI, the sensitivities were similar (88.8% vs. 92.3%, respectively), but BSGI appears to have improved the specificity to 90% compared to 39.4% in breast MRI. The main advantage of BSGI is that the study does not require the patient to lie in a prone position and it may be easier to perform in a patient with severe claustrophobia. However, the data are limited given the small cohorts in these studies. More studies are needed to determine the true sensitivity and specificity of BSGI to establish its role in breast imaging.

Positron Emission Mammography

Positron emission mammography (PEM) was designed as a way to use typical whole-body PET technology in breast imaging. Whole-body PET scanning is not particularly useful in imaging the breast due to its low resolution. Resolution with PEM is increased through the use of two detectors that are arranged in similar fashion to conventional mammogram. The dye used is the same as that used in PET scans, a positron-emitting isotope of fluorine, ^{18}F-2-deoxy-2-fluoro-D-glucose (FDG). Early small studies of PEM demonstrated sensitivities of 80% to 86%. One of the larger studies conducted in 94 women found that PEM had a sensitivity of 91% and specificity of 93% when interpreted with mammographic and clinical findings. However, the role of PEM in breast imaging requires further investigation; a recent study found PEM to be inferior to breast MRI in detecting contralateral breast cancers.

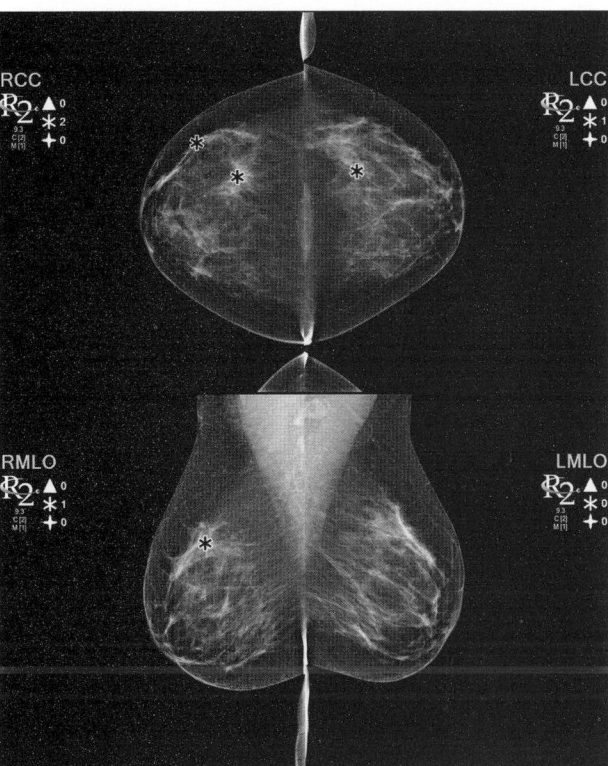

FIGURE 45.12 Computer-aided detection. Note the highlighted areas of concern. Additional evaluation was normal.

Thermography

This test is designed to measure the skin temperature over the breast, as it is thought that the presence of breast cancer may cause elevated localized skin temperature. No data exist to support the use of breast thermography, and such testing is not supported by guidelines from any major organizations. The U.S. Food and Drug Administration issued a communication in June of 2011 stating that breast thermography is not a replacement for mammography as a means of breast cancer screening and is not considered to be an effective screening tool.

Computer-Aided Detection

Computer-aided detection (CAD) uses software-based artificial intelligence to function as a "second reader" of mammographic films (Fig. 45.12). Second or double reading of films can improve sensitivity but with some loss of specificity. Improved detection rates upward of 15% have been reported but with an associated increase in false-positive or recall rates up to 45%. It functions as a second reader by identifying areas of concern that the radiologist must then characterize. It is estimated that CAD can correctly identify approximately 80% of cancers. Like double reading, CAD was shown to increase sensitivity but with a decline in specificity.

BENIGN PATHOLOGY

Fibrocystic Change

Fibrocystic change (FCC) of the breast is the most frequently encountered benign breast disorder. It occurs most often in women of reproductive age between 30 and 50 years. FCC does not increase the risk of developing breast cancer, but it can make the physical examination of the patient more difficult.

VIII

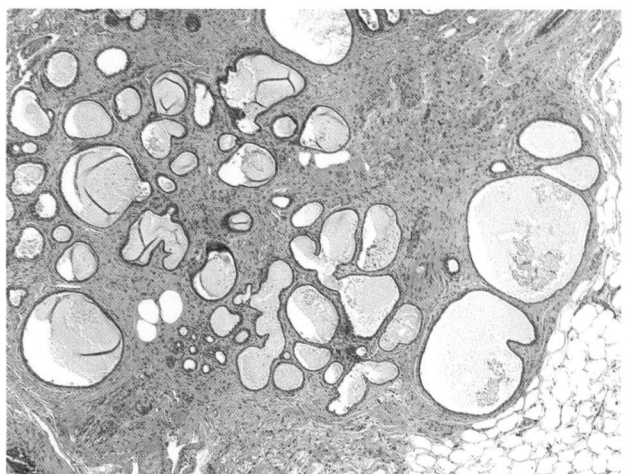

FIGURE 45.13 Histology of fibrocystic changes with extensive cyst formation, stromal hyperplasia, and apocrine metaplasia (H&E 4×). (Courtesy of Jing Yu, MD, University of Pittsburgh School of Medicine, Pittsburgh, PA.)

In 85% to 90% of cases of significant FCC, breast discomfort is the leading symptom. Women often present with a history of bilateral, menstrual-related, painful, tender, and nodular breasts, most often localized to the upper outer quadrants. Typically, the pain is most severe just before menses as a result of the normal physiologic stromal edema and ductal dilation.

FCC encompasses several histopathologic categories, including microcyst and macrocyst formation, hyperplasia of ductal epithelium, apocrine metaplasia, papillomatosis, duct ectasia, sclerosing adenosis (dense fibrotic tissue surrounds the acini), and stromal fibrosis. In essence, it has no single defining histologic entity (**Fig. 45.13**). Providing no atypia is identified, there is no increased risk of developing breast cancer when FCC is present. Table 45.6 lists benign pathologic findings and subsequent risk of breast cancer development. An explanation of relative risk is provided in Table 45.7.

Fibroadenoma

Fibroadenomas are benign tumors that consist of both fibrous and stromal elements. These are common lesions particularly

TABLE 45.6 Breast Lesions and Risk of Developing Invasive Breast Cancer

PATHOLOGY	RR
Nonproliferative changes (cysts, fibrocystic changes, fibroadenoma, adenosis)	No increased risk
Proliferative changes (hyperplasia, sclerosing adenosis, complex fibroadenoma, papilloma)	1.2–2.0
Hyperplasia with atypia (atypical ductal hyperplasia, atypical lobular hyperplasia)	4.0–5.0
Lobular carcinoma in situ	8.0–10.0

Data from Dupont WD, Page DL. Risk factors for breast cancer in women with proliferative breast disease. *N Engl J Med* 1985;312(3):146–151.

TABLE 45.7 Relative Risk

	DISEASE PRESENT	DISEASE ABSENT
Exposed	A	B
Nonexposed	C	D

Relative risk (RR) is a statistical assessment of developing disease as a result of exposure. It is a ratio comparing those exposed who develop the condition compared to those who were not exposed and developed the condition.

$$RR = a/(a+b)/c/(c+d)$$

in adolescents but can be seen in woman of all ages particularly prior to menopause. These lesions are thought to represent an exaggerated response to estrogen. Clinically, the patient presents with a palpable mass that is well circumscribed, rubbery in consistency, and often multilobulated. Lesions are generally 2 to 3 cm. They are commonly found in the upper outer quadrant, and in approximately 25% of cases, there are additional lesions that are present in either breast. Imaging modalities can include ultrasound and, if age appropriate, mammography. On sonography, the lesions are avascular and well circumscribed. Mammogram will often detect a solitary nodule with smooth borders with a halo around the mass. In the adolescent population, mammography should be avoided unless the index of suspicion for malignancy exists. Fine needle aspirate or core needle biopsy can confirm the diagnosis. Observation and reassurance are reasonable options for management. Excision should be considered for enlarging masses or discordant imaging or pathology finding or if the patient desires removal. Histologic evaluation demonstrates a well-circumscribed lesion with both epithelial and stromal elements. One or the other element often dominates. The epithelial component has well-defined, glandlike, and ductlike spaces, whereas the stromal component consists of bands of collagen (**Fig. 45.14**).

Phyllodes

These fibroepithelial lesions have diverse biologic behavior. Originally, this entity was termed cystosarcoma phyllodes,

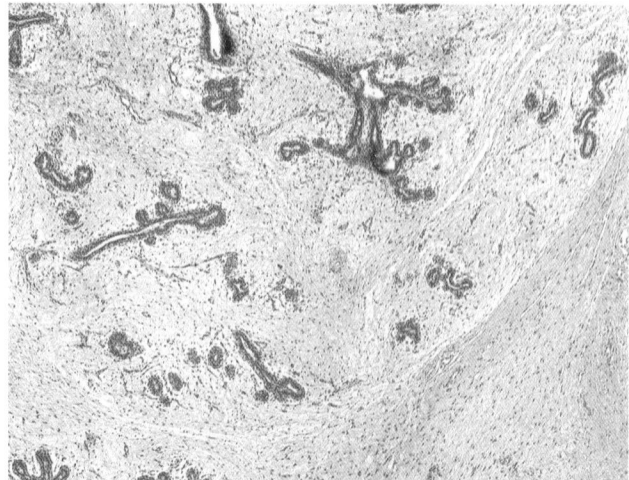

FIGURE 45.14 Histologic section of fibroadenoma with gland formation and well circumscribed by surrounding stroma (H&E 4×). (Courtesy of Jing Yu, MD, University of Pittsburgh School of Medicine, Pittsburgh, PA.)

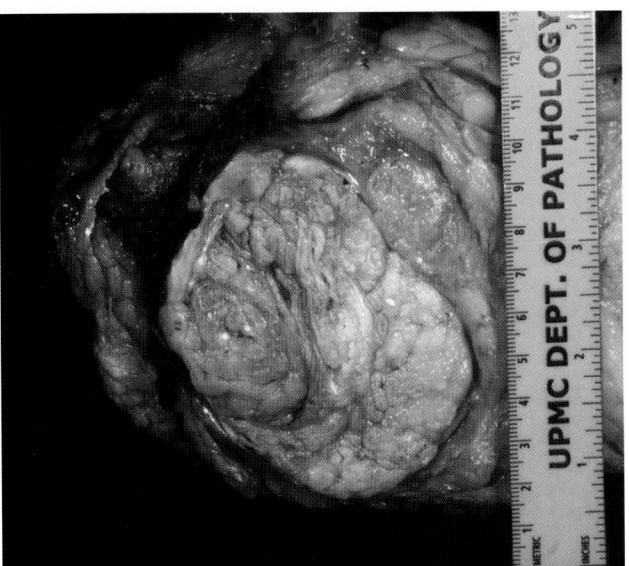

FIGURE 45.15 Gross picture of phyllodes tumor. Note leaflike pattern, lack of a capsule, and the fleshy nature of the lesion. (Courtesy of Jing Yu, MD, University of Pittsburgh School of Medicine, Pittsburgh, PA.)

but this terminology was deemed confusing as less than 5% of these lesions actually behave in a malignant fashion. Clinically, they are more common in women in their 30s and 40s, but presentation can mimic fibroadenomas with the findings of a solitary, well-circumscribed, mobile, multilobulated mass with a rubbery to firm texture. Phyllodes tumors tend to be larger and exhibit more rapid growth. Radiographic imaging with ultrasound and mammography can be similar to fibroadenomas. Determination of the diagnosis on percutaneous sampling can be difficult given similarity to fibroadenomas. On gross examination, the lesions can be gray or tan and tend to be plump and fleshy in texture, and a branching pattern can be seen (Fig. 45.15). On histologic inspection of the lesions, they lack a true capsule. A leaflike pattern involving both the epithelial and stromal components is diagnostic (Fig. 45.16). The stromal component determines the grading of the tumor

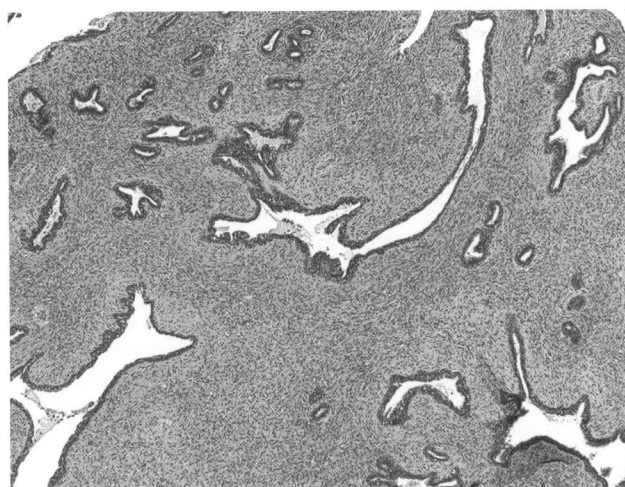

FIGURE 45.16 Histology of phyllodes tumor. There is increased stromal cellularity, cleft, and leaflike structures and no true capsule (H&E 4×). (Courtesy of Jing Yu, MD, University of Pittsburgh School of Medicine, Pittsburgh, PA.)

to include benign, borderline, and malignant entities. Stromal cellularity, atypia, pushing or infiltrative borders, and the presence of stromal overgrowth can be useful in evaluating prognosis and predicting behavior. Surgical excision with a margin of normal breast tissue is recommended. Local recurrence rates of 20% have been reported in instances of inadequate margins with less risk of recurrence for those with benign features.

Adenomas

Adenomas are well-circumscribed benign lesions primarily composed of epithelium with rare stroma. This distinguishes them from the diagnosis of fibroadenoma. Radiographic imaging findings with ultrasound and mammography can be similar to fibroadenomas. There are two basic types: tubular adenomas and lactating adenomas. Generally seen in young women, tubular adenomas tend to ovoid with a pseudocapsule and minimal stroma. An inner epithelial layer and an outer myoepithelial layer line the tubules. Clinical presentation is similar to fibroadenomas with a localized well-defined lesion. Lactating adenomas are seen in pregnancy or postpartum state. In these circumstances, there may be more than one lesion. On gross examination, they are tan in color and softer in texture than a tubular adenoma. Microscopically, cuboidal cells with secretory activity line the tubules. Diagnosis of these entities can be made on percutaneous biopsy. Radiographic imaging in a pregnant woman should be restricted to sonography unless a high suspicion of malignancy exists. Additionally, mammographic imaging of the breast of gravid or lactating women will be compromised due to increased density. Percutaneous or excisional biopsy during pregnancy or lactation is difficult due to increased vascularity. The presence of milk enhances risk of infection and milk fistula formation.

Papilloma

Papillomas are hyperplastic lesions categorized as central (solitary) or peripheral (multiple). Solitary papillomas are found in the major lactiferous ducts and are most often associated with the bloody nipple discharge. These are commonly seen in women between 30 and 50 years of age. They vary in size from a few millimeters to 1 cm, are attached to the duct walls by a thin stalk, and are prone to infarction. Histologically, they are composed of multiple, branching, and interanastomosing papillae arranged around a fibrovascular core. There can be areas of atypia that will classify them as atypical papilloma; on rare occasions, they are associated with DCIS or invasive cancer. From an epidemiologic point of view, solitary papillomas do not appear to markedly elevate the risk of subsequent breast cancer development.

Peripheral intraductal papillomas tend to be multiple and bilateral. The condition affects younger women and is not usually associated with nipple discharge. The condition itself raises the individual's risk of developing breast cancer, suggesting they are subject to malignant transformation.

Atypical Hyperplasia

Atypical hyperplasia encompasses both ADH and ALH. ADH is often found on percutaneous biopsy where the targeted lesion contains microcalcifications. ALH is often an incidental finding without discrete radiographic changes.

On histologic inspection, ADH has a proliferation of uniform epithelial cells with round nuclei filling part of the duct (Fig. 45.17). ALH has proliferation of monomorphic, evenly spaced cells filling part but not all of the lobules and sometimes the surrounding ducts. Both ALH and ADH share similar architectural and cytologic features with their in situ counterparts.

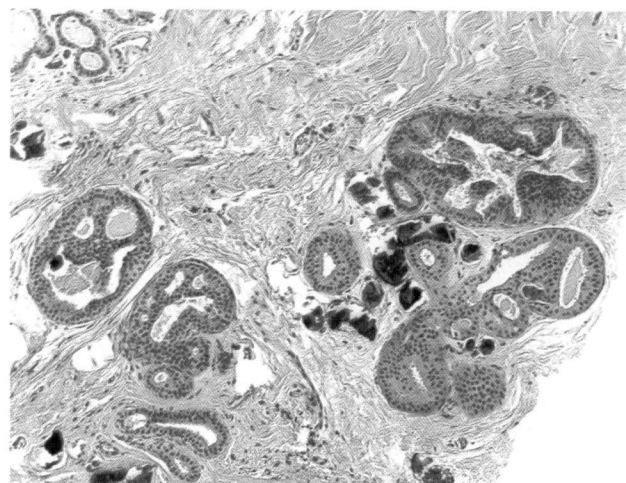

FIGURE 45.17 Atypical ductal hyperplasia (ADH) note proliferation of uniform epithelial cells with round nuclei filling part of the duct (H&E 10×). (Courtesy of Jing Yu, MD, University of Pittsburgh School of Medicine, Pittsburgh, PA.)

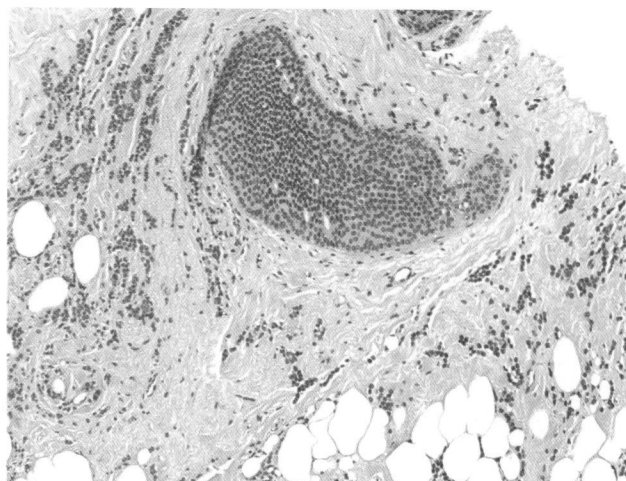

FIGURE 45.18 LCIS and infiltrating lobular cancer. The lobule is filled with small, uniform cells with a high nuclear-to-cytoplasmic ratio. Within the surrounding stroma is infiltrating lobular cancer with its typical pattern of linear infiltration (H&E 10×). (Courtesy of Jing Yu, MD, University of Pittsburgh School of Medicine, Pittsburgh, PA.)

When ADH is found on percutaneous core biopsy, the recommendation is for excisional biopsy. Ideally, the site has been previously marked at the time of biopsy with a titanium clip. Utilizing dye, wire, or radioactive seed localization can help the surgeon identify the site of concern. The basis of excisional biopsy is the concern of upgrading to either DCIS or invasive cancer, which occurs in 10% to 20% of cases. Larger core needles and a larger number of cores are associated with a lower incidence of DCIS and invasive cancer at excisional biopsy.

The presence of ADH increases the individual's personal risk of breast cancer (RR 3.7 to 5.5). This is conferred to either the ipsilateral or contralateral breast. Risk reduction strategies including the use of chemopreventative agents and lifestyle modification can be employed.

For ALH found on percutaneous biopsy, a similar approach to the management for ADH is utilized. Recently, the role of additional excision for areas of ALH has been called into question. For some women with concordant mammogram and pathologic findings, additional excision may be unnecessary.

Lobular Carcinoma In Situ

Originally described in 1941 as a rare form of mammary cancer, LCIS is now considered a benign condition. It is histologically characterized by the involvement of terminal duct lobular unit with small cells with round nuclei that distorts these spaces (Fig. 45.18). The condition tends to be multifocal in the affected breast and often an incidental finding. At the time of this initial report, recommendation for this condition was at least a total mastectomy. Contralateral breast involvement has been reported to be approximately 30%. The condition is often an incidental finding on percutaneous core needle biopsy and has no mammographic or clinical correlate. At times, mammographic microcalcifications can be an indicator of its presence. Average age of diagnosis is between 40 and 50 years. The lesion is associated with increasing an individual's breast cancer risk estimated to be 1% to 2% per year with a lifetime risk of 30% to 40%. The cancer may be ductal or lobular in nature and involve either breast. The term LCIS is often associated with the diagnosis of carcinoma; hence, there have been efforts to group both ALH and LCIS into the term lobular intraepithelial neoplasia (LIN), which accounts for a spectrum of conditions and is graded LIN1, LIN2, and LIN3

depending on morphology and clinical outcome. This classification system has not been universally accepted. Current clinical management of LCIS is individualized and includes the use of observation, chemopreventative agents, and surgical management of bilateral total mastectomy.

COMMON CLINICAL SCENARIOS

Several clinical scenarios occur in the evaluation of a patient for breast-related issues. Patients may present with complaints of a mass or thickening, abnormal mammogram, nipple discharge, or breast pain. Management and workup of each of these clinical scenarios is described below.

Evaluation of a Breast Mass

Many potential causes of breast mass exist, most of which are not related to a breast malignancy. One should always consider the patient's menopausal status during the evaluation of a breast mass. The likelihood that a mass is malignant is based on the patient's history. A thorough history and physical examination should be performed as part of the initial workup of a breast mass. The main point in the history-taking process is to get a sense of how long the mass has been present and whether it fluctuates with her menstrual cycle (if she is premenopausal) or mass has increased in size or whether any trauma to her breast has occurred. Masses that fluctuate with the patient's menstrual cycle are more likely to be benign. Breast trauma leading to fat necrosis can also lead to a breast mass; a commonly overlooked cause of breast trauma is a shoulder strap/seatbelt injury. Surgeries to the breast can cause scarring and fat necrosis that mimics a carcinoma. Patients with a personal history of breast cancer are at risk for recurrence of breast cancer. It is estimated that the risk of recurrence is approximately 0.7% per year and this risk is considered to be cumulative. Careful attention should be paid to the patient's family history and ethnicity. Ashkenazi Jewish patients have higher risks for harboring a BRCA mutation as it is estimated that the baseline risk in this population can be as high as 1 in 40. This risk can increase markedly depending on what age breast cancer is diagnosed. Strong family history with multiple members with breast and/or ovarian cancer also increases the patient's

TABLE 45.8 Key Questions in the Evaluation of a Breast Mass

Features of the Mass
1. When did the patient first notice the mass (i.e., length of time the lesion has been present)?
2. Does the mass seem to fluctuate in size with her menstrual cycle?
3. If the mass does not fluctuate with her menstrual cycle, has the mass grown over this period of time?
4. Any other masses that she has noticed, any masses in her axilla?
5. Any trauma to her breast?

Surgical History
1. Any surgical procedures on either breast?

Medical History
1. Any personal history of breast cancer?

Family History
1. Any family history of breast, ovarian, or colon cancer?
2. What is the patient's ethnicity?

risk for harboring BRCA mutations. Table 45.8 is a summary of the salient points to consider in the history taking process. Enlarging masses are concerning as are masses in patients with strong family histories of breast cancer.

A thorough physical examination should be conducted, identifying the location of the area of concern and documenting the size of the mass, the presence of any skin retraction/changes, nipple discharge, presence or absence of axillary and/or supraclavicular adenopathy, whether the lesion is mobile, whether the mass is firm or rubbery, and whether there is breast symmetry. Physical findings concerning for malignancy include a hard, irregularly shaped mass, presence of axillary and/or supraclavicular adenopathy, retraction or redness of the overlying skin, or an associated bloody nipple discharge. While breast cancer can present as a fixed mass, this is an uncommon finding as most breast tumors, unless very posterior, are not fixed to the pectoralis major until late in their course. At times, especially in a patient with very firm breasts, the tumor can be deceptively difficult to palpate and the only obvious finding is breast asymmetry with the involved breast being either larger or smaller (if there is retraction of the surrounding tissue). See Table 45.9 for the summary of the salient parts of the physical exam. Typically, masses that are concerning for malignancy are firm masses with associated skin retraction, masses in axilla, or masses causing breast asymmetry.

Once the history and physical examination is complete, the next part of the evaluation is to determine the role of imaging

TABLE 45.9 Key Physical Examination Points in Evaluating a Breast Mass

PHYSICAL ASSESSMENT

1. Location, consistency, and size of the mass
2. Presence of associated skin retraction or changes
3. Presence of nipple discharge
4. Presence of any associated masses in either breast, axilla, or supraclavicular region

tests. This assessment is based on the patient's menopausal status. Imaging tests are appropriate in patients who are postmenopausal even if the mass does not seem to be suspicious. Mammographic evaluation is the initial step, even if the patient has had a mammogram within the past year. Additional testing with breast ultrasound may be helpful especially in patients with dense breasts or if breast cysts are suspected. In a premenopausal patient, a nonsuspicious mass (smooth, mobile, ballotable) can be observed over one menstrual cycle. If the mass persists, imaging tests are recommended. In young patients (<25 years), mammograms are of little use due to the high breast density. In these patients, ultrasound should be the initial test. Regardless of menopausal status, if the mass on ultrasound is a cyst, a fine needle aspiration (FNA) of the cyst is indicated only if it is complex in nature or if the patient is symptomatic. Repeat imaging with ultrasound should be performed in 6 months to assess for cyst recurrence. If aspiration does not resolve the cyst completely, if it returns in 6 months, or if the aspirated fluid is bloody in nature, then an excisional biopsy should be performed. Simple cysts are not associated with malignancy, and no further workup is required. If the mass in not found to be a cyst, then either a percutaneous core or excisional biopsy (when a core is not possible) of the mass should be performed. In patients younger than 40 years, FNA can be utilized if examination and imaging test indicate a benign process. If the FNA is negative, the risk of the patient for having a breast malignancy is extremely low as the physical examination and imaging tests are concordant with the biopsy results. If the patient is 40 years old or older, then an image-guided core biopsy with either mammographic guidance (stereotactic core biopsy) or ultrasound guidance is recommended. Subsequent treatment is dependent on the results of the core biopsy. In general, most benign lesions do not require additional treatment unless atypical or papillary cells are found. These lesions are hyperplastic and can be associated with underlying malignancy; therefore, an excisional biopsy is required. The other "benign" lesion that requires an excisional biopsy is LCIS. While these lesions are not malignant, concurrent cancer may be found at the time of the excisional biopsy. Additionally, excisional biopsy should be performed if the results of the physical exam, pathology, and imaging results are not concordant; this is called the "triple test." The radiologist should review all imaging tests after the pathology report is issued to assess for concordance. If the radiologist does not feel that the biopsy explains the radiographic findings, an excisional biopsy is mandated. See Figure 45.19 for algorithm of workup of a breast mass.

Abnormal Screening Evaluation

A common clinical scenario is a patient presenting with an abnormal screening mammogram. Further evaluation and treatment of such abnormal mammographic findings should be based on Breast Imaging Reporting and Data System (BI-RADS) score. This American College of Radiology classification lexicon should be included in all mammogram reports. Table 45.10 details the BI-RADS classification system. Further workup is dependent on the BI-RADS category associated with the mammogram. BI-RADS 0 signifies that further work with spot compression views, breast ultrasound, or other imaging modalities are required to complete the evaluation. BI-RADS 1 indicates that the mammogram looks completely normal without any mammographic findings. BI-RADS 2 indicates a mammographic finding associated with benign disease (e.g., fibroadenoma, simple cyst). An inherent false-negative rate exists, and a negative mammogram (i.e., BI-RADS 1 or BI-RADS 2) does not rule out malignancy if a palpable mass

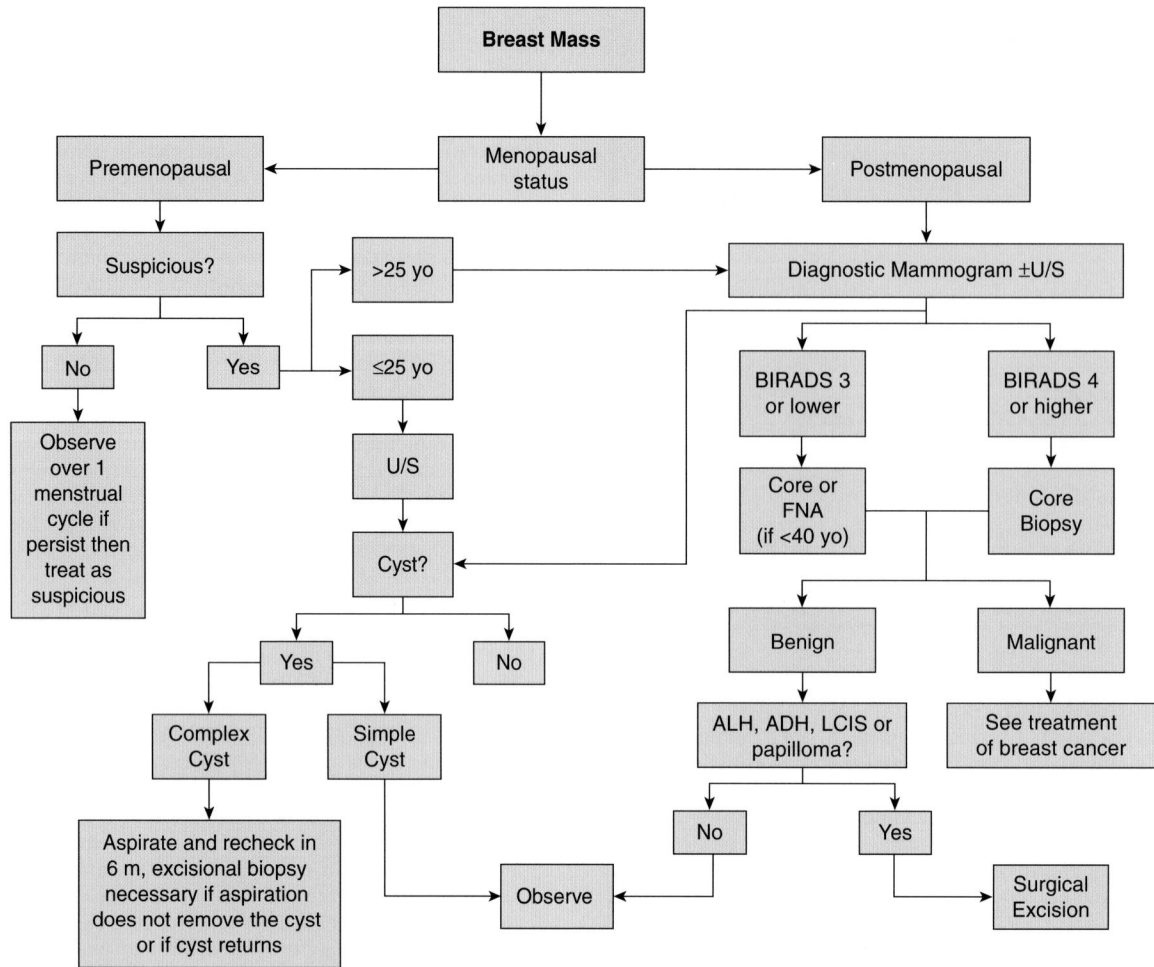

FIGURE 45.19 Algorithm for evaluation of a breast mass.

TABLE 45.10 BIRADS Reporting System

BIRADS CATEGORY	ASSESSMENT	RISK OF MALIGNANCY	RECOMMENDED FOLLOW-UP (MANAGEMENT)
0	Incomplete—need additional imaging evaluation and/or prior mammograms for comparison	N/A	Recall for additional imaging and/or comparison with prior examination(s).
1	Negative	0%	Routine mammography screening
2	Benign	0%	Routine mammography screening
3	Probably benign	≤2%	Short-interval (6-mo) follow-up or continued surveillance mammography
4	Suspicious	>2% to <95% (a) Low suspicion for malignancy (b) Moderate suspicion for malignancy (c) High suspicion for malignancy	Tissue diagnosis
5	Highly suggestive of malignancy	≥95%	Tissue diagnosis
6	Known biopsy-proven breast Malignancy	N/A	Surgical excision when clinically appropriate

Reprinted from Sickles EA, D'Orsi CJ, Bassett LW, et al. ACR BI-RADS® mammography. In: *ACR BI-RADS® Atlas, breast imaging reporting and data system*, 5th ed. Reston, VA: American College of Radiology; 2013, with permission. (http://www.acr.org/~/media/ACR/Documents/PDF/QualitySafety/Resources/BIRADS/01%20Mammography/02%20%20BIRADS%20Mammography%20Reporting.pdf) is present. (Refer to **Fig. 45.19** for evaluation of a palpable mass.) A mammogram interpreted as having findings that do not appear suspicious is classified as BI-RADS 3; by definition, these findings should have a 2% or less risk of malignancy; a repeat mammogram in 6 months is reasonable given the very low risk of malignancy. A BI-RADS 4 report indicates findings that are suspicious for malignancy. This category is further divided into 4A, 4B, and 4C. The risk of malignancy can be as high as 95% based on the subcategory. In these cases, a core biopsy should be considered in order to rule out an underlying malignancy. The same workup should be performed for BI-RADS 5, which indicates the findings are highly suspicious for malignancy (**Fig. 45.20**).

In general, when a biopsy is warranted as part of the additional workup, a percutaneous core biopsy should be performed as it provides histopathology. Ideally, the biopsy should be done with the imaging modality in which the mass was discovered. Studies have shown a concordance rate close to 100% between an open excisional biopsy and a core biopsy. Core biopsies have the advantage of being less invasive and resulting in a smaller scar. Even in cases of BI-RAD 5 in which underlying cancer is almost a certainty, a core biopsy allows the surgeon to strategize the operative approach; a diagnosis of DCIS in a patient undergoing breast-conserving surgery does not require sentinel mapping where an invasive cancer would require both partial mastectomy and a sentinel lymph node biopsy (SLNB).

Stereotactic core biopsies may not be possible in some cases (e.g., the breast size is small and compresses to less than 17 mm or if the lesion is superficial or close to the chest wall). Given that the core needle mechanism extends at least 1.5 cm beyond the needle tip, the issue of a through and through injury exists in this circumstance. In these cases, if the lesion is visible on ultrasound, an assessment of feasibility of core biopsy without compression is an option versus a localization and excisional biopsy procedure.

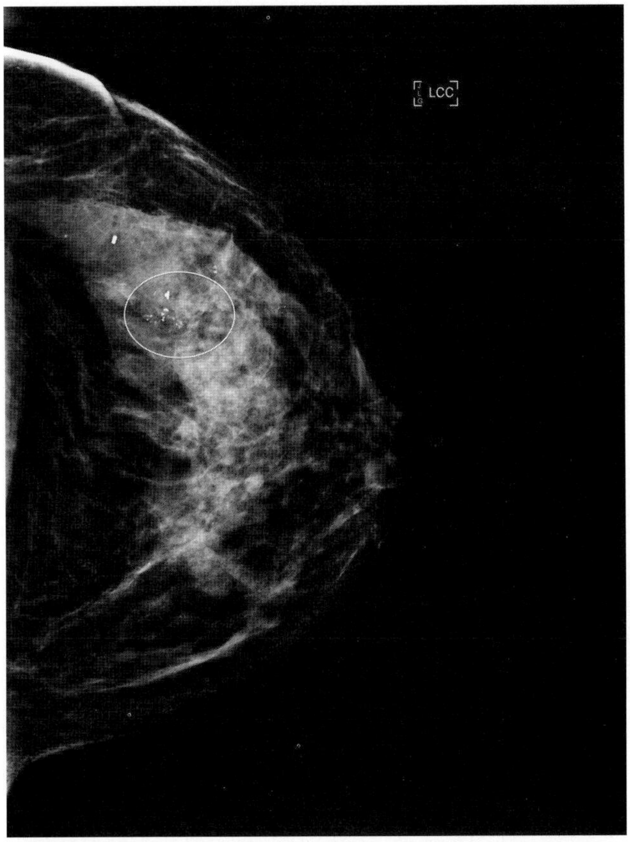

Further treatment depends on the histologic diagnosis. High-risk proliferative lesions such as atypical lobular/ductal hyperplasia, papillary lesions, and LCIS should be treated with an excisional biopsy. Treatment of breast cancer is discussed elsewhere in this chapter.

Evaluation of Nipple Discharge

One of the most common breast complaints is nipple discharge with up to 80% of women reporting this symptom. Of note, manipulation of the breast and nipple can yield a small amount of clear discharge in most premenopausal women. This section will discuss the management of galactorrhea and pathologic nipple discharge.

An estimated 10% to 15% of patients who present with nipple discharge have an underlying malignancy. Discharge can be classified as related to lactation, physiologic or pathologic (**Table 45.11**). Nipple discharge that is concerning can present as unilateral, bloody, and/or spontaneous discharge arising from a single duct. Discharges that come from multiple ducts or those that are bilateral tend to be less often associated with malignancy. Discharge from breast can be milky, clear, green, yellow, brown, or bloody. Intraductal papillomas are the most common cause of nipple discharge followed by ductal ectasia and cancer. These anatomic lesions present with unilateral nipple discharge, while physiologic causes such as galactorrhea will present with bilateral nipple discharge. Physiologic causes of galactorrhea include prolactinomas, pharmacologic agents, and any condition that can lead to increased prolactin production. Breast infections can also lead to nipple discharge. The initial workup of nipple discharge entails a thorough history and physical examination. One should get a sense of how long the discharge has been present and whether it was spontaneous, bloody, or unilateral. One also should ask if the discharge was seen coming from one or more ducts. Questions concerning headaches and vision changes should be considered as a

FIGURE 45.20 Mammogram interpreted as BIRADS 5 (highly suspicious for malignancy) based on malignant calcifications that are clustered and pleomorphic.

TABLE 45.11 Classification of Nipple Discharge

CLASSIFICATION	DESCRIPTION	ETIOLOGY
Lactation related	Milky Bilateral Multiple ducts Nonspontaneous	Pregnancy
Physiologic	Milky, straw colored, gray, brown, green Bilateral Multiple ducts Nonspontaneous/ spontaneous	Prolactinoma Medication related Chronic irritation
Pathologic	Bloody, clear, straw colored, brown, green Unilateral Single duct Spontaneous	Papilloma Duct ectasia Fibrocystic disease Ductal carcinoma in situ Invasive cancer

TABLE 45.12 Medications Associated with Galactorrhea

CATEGORY	EXAMPLES
Antihypertensives	Verapamil, reserpine, methyldopa
Antipsychotics	Phenothiazines, haloperidol, risperdal
Antidepressants	Desipramine, clomipramine
GI medications	Cimetidine, metoclopramide
Analgesics	Opioids–codeine, morphine

means to check for the presence of a symptomatic prolactinoma. A thorough evaluation of the patient's medications is important as common medications such as cimetidine, metoclopramide, and some antipsychotics can also lead to galactorrhea (Table 45.12). In examining the breast, one should pay attention to how many ducts the discharge is coming from, whether or not the discharge is reproducible, and if it is unilateral or bloody. An evaluation should also be made to see if a mass is present and whether or not there are skins changes consistent with Paget disease by the nipple (i.e., scaly rash originating from the center of the nipple spreading outward) or if any signs of infection are present. Guaiac assessment for occult blood (Hemoccult test) may be helpful in the evaluation, but the absence of does not preclude an underlying malignancy. A mammogram and ultrasound should be ordered as part of the workup. A ductogram may help localize the lesion more accurately. Breast MRI may be helpful, but normal imaging

cannot rule out an underlying malignancy. If any lesion is found on these imaging tests, an image-guided biopsy should be performed. If no lesions are found, duct excision is still considered standard treatment. If the duct with the discharge can easily be identified, a limited resection of the duct can be done by placing a lacrimal duct probe or fine suture in the affected duct and performing a directed excision. Approximately 2 to 5 cm of tissue distal from the nipple should be removed at the time of surgery. Figure 45.21 demonstrates an algorithm for evaluation of nipple discharge.

Evaluation of Mastalgia

Breast pain or mastalgia is one of the most common breast complaints. In one survey of premenopausal women, 75% of respondents stated that they had this symptom; 30% stated it was moderate to severe in nature. Typically, mastalgia is not considered to be a sign of breast cancer as the frequency of underlying breast cancer in women with breast pain is between 1.2% and 6.7%. Of note, the literature indicates that breast pain is a presenting symptom in 5% to 17% of patients with breast cancer. In one series, mastalgia was the only symptom in 7% of patients. The evaluation of the patient with breast pain should begin with the determination of whether or not the pain is cyclical in nature. Cyclical mastalgia is thought to be due to hormonal stimulation of the breasts. It is not uncommon to have some minor breast discomfort toward the latter half of the menstrual cycle, and this presents as diffuse bilateral breast pain. Cyclic mastalgia is not associated with cancer, and unless there are physical findings of concern, further workup is not necessary. By definition, noncyclical breast pain is not associated with the menstrual cycle. Despite a thorough workup, etiology of the pain often is not found. Noncyclical breast pain may be due to the stretching of the Cooper ligament, mastitis,

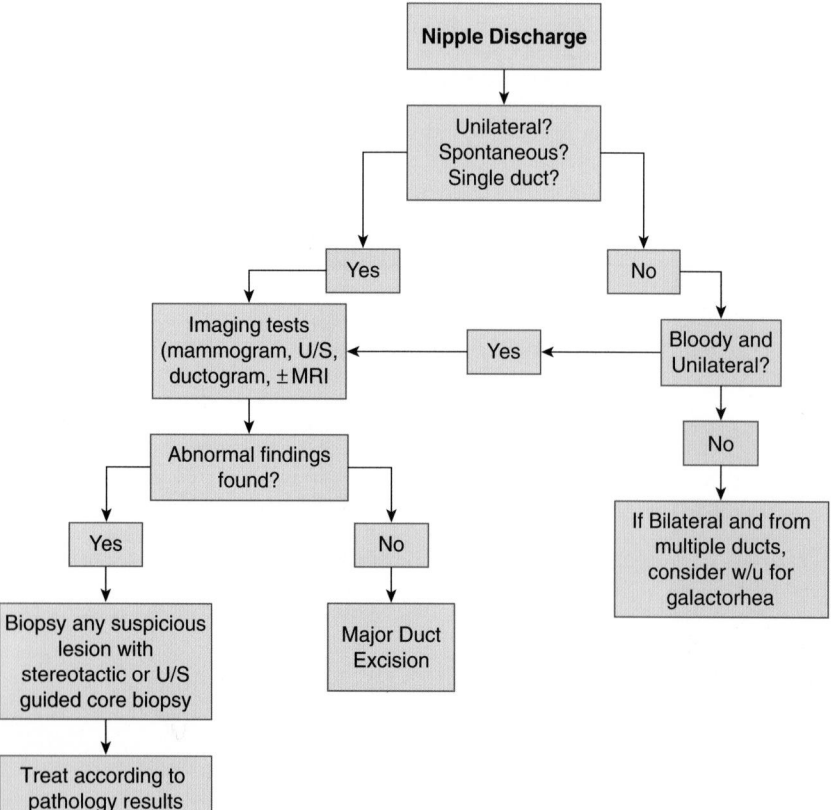

FIGURE 45.21 Algorithm for evaluation of nipple discharge.

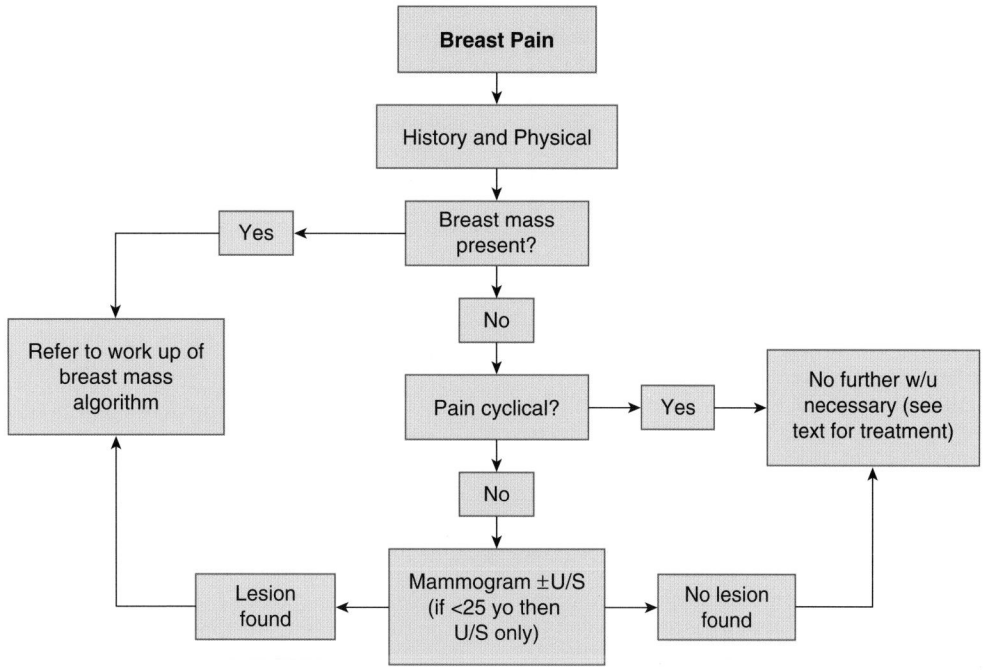

FIGURE 45.22 Algorithm for evaluation of breast pain.

ductal ectasia, hidradenitis suppurativa, medications (e.g., hormone replacement), increased intake of caffeine, chest musculoskeletal issues, previous surgery to the breast, or in rare circumstances inflammatory breast cancer (IBC).

The workup for breast pain begins with a thorough history and physical examination. Assessment should include the location, severity, and duration of the pain, whether it is bilateral, associated skin changes, previous breast surgery and/or other trauma, and if the pain limits her ability to perform daily activities. The patient's medications should be reviewed with particular attention given to oral contraceptive pills or hormone replacement medications, which can cause breast pain. Physical examination should assess the patient for any signs of trauma, skin changes, masses, or nipple discharge. The axillary and supraclavicular area should be examined for signs of adenopathy. Figure 45.22 depicts an algorithm for evaluation of mastalgia.

Patients with IBC can present with a firm, tender, and erythematous breast. Often, the onset is rapid, and the skin may have the typical peau d'orange appearance (dimpling and thickening of the skin) with or without an underlying mass. Mastitis or breast abscess can be associated with mastalgia. This often occurs in lactating women although subareolar abscesses also can occur in nonlactating women. Typically, the abscess will present as a painful mass close to the nipple or with skin changes over the nipple consistent with cellulitis. On occasion, painful masses can be due to hidradenitis suppurativa. This is thought to be due to occlusion of the terminal parts of the follicular acroinfundibulum and can present either on the breast or in the axilla. The lesions can present as solitary painful nodules without an area of central necrosis and can have secondary cellulitis.

Attention to the chest wall during physical examination is essential, as costochondritis can mimic breast pain. Costochondritis pain is parasternal and reproduced by pressing on the costochondral junctions. Most often, the physical exam will be normal with no masses or skin changes found to suggest breast cancer, cellulitis, breast abscess, or hidradenitis suppurativa. It is reasonable to order a breast mammogram and a targeted ultrasound of the tender area, though the yield of such testing is low; one study in 987 women found only four

cancers (a prevalence of 0.4%). Breast MRI is not indicated, as no studies suggest any clinical utility at this time.

Treatment of mastalgia will be dependent on the underlying cause. Antibiotics treatment for a breast abscess and cellulitis is generally successful, but refractory cases may require incision and drainage. If possible, a culture of the infected area can be taken and antibiotics regimens adjusted accordingly. In cases in which no underlying cause is found, treatment should be aimed at improving support of the breast through the use of better fitting bras. In patients with large pendulous breasts, a bra with steel underwire may provide relief. Reducing caffeine intake may benefit some patients; however a large case–control study did not find an association between caffeine and breast pain. Several medications have been prescribed for mastalgia. Medical management with nonsteroidal anti-inflammatory drugs (NSAIDs) or acetaminophen should be the first line of treatment. In cases in which medications have not been effective, a topical NSAID such as Aspercreme (Sanofi, Chattanooga, TN) or the Flector Patch (diclofenac epolamine topical patch (13%) Pfizer, Mission, KS) can be tried. Evening primrose oil at 3,000 mg/day or vitamin E at 1,200 IU/day also can be prescribed; however, efficacy may be due to a placebo effect as multiple randomized trials have not proven them to be effective treatment. Randomized trials have demonstrated that tamoxifen 10 mg/day decreases mastalgia, but this drug can be associated with side effects such as hot flashes, vaginal dryness, leg cramps, increased risk of venous thrombolic events, and development of endometrial cancer. Danazol, a synthetic testosterone (100 to 400 mg/day in two divided doses), also has proved effective for the treatment of mastalgia but can have significant androgenic side effects.

TREATMENT OF BENIGN BREAST DISEASE

Most benign lesions can be treated with observation alone, providing there is concordance between the clinical findings, radiographic imaging, and the cytologic or histologic results. Using these three criteria is referred to as the "triple test." Cytopathology and histology can be obtained through

VIII

TABLE 45.13 Advantages of Fine Needle Aspiration
Outpatient procedure
Minimal discomfort
Local anesthetic may or may not be utilized
Negligible complication rate
Rapid diagnosis

percutaneous fine needle aspirate and core biopsy, respectively. If all components of the test are concordant with a benign entity, the chance of breast cancer is low (0.7%). Indeterminate or suspicious findings in any one of the components is an indication for further evaluation until confirmation of either a benign or malignant entity is found. Excisional biopsy without percutaneous sampling is a reasonable alternative when the patient desires removal of a mass with benign features.

Fine Needle Aspiration

Fine needle aspiration (FNA) is an established diagnostic method in the evaluation of palpable breast lesions. In response to the increasing frequency with which women are consulting their obstetrician–gynecologists about concerns related to their breasts, the American Board of Obstetrics and Gynecology (ABOG) has specific educational requirements for resident training in the various aspects of diagnosing and treating breast disease. Technical proficiency in this procedure is recommended. In most areas where dedicated breast imaging centers exist, it is often the radiologist that performs this procedure.

FNA has a sensitivity of 96% and specificity of 98% (similar to core biopsies) as well as a 99% positive predictive value and 94% negative predictive value. It has a false-negative rate as high as 20% most notably in the detection of lobular cancers and carcinoma in situ. Performance of the procedure, preparation of the material for analysis, and the facility of the pathologist can affect these rates.

FNA has multiple advantages (Table 45.13) over excisional biopsy and is helpful in confirming the clinical impression of both benign and malignant breast disease. Nevertheless, a negative cytologic report, as with a negative mammographic report, must not be relied on to rule out malignancy in a clinically suspicious lesion. Any clinically suspicious mass in a patient with negative FNA findings requires additional evaluation, including core or excisional biopsy.

FNA is an easily mastered technique, but the adequacy of specimens is improved with experience and training. Table 45.14 lists suggested equipment for this approach. Procedure risks include infection, bleeding, and bruising at the site. Because the chest wall is immediately beneath the site, pneumothorax is a potential complication. The small size of the needle and assuring the mass is stabilized over a rib during the procedure significantly decreases this complication.

TABLE 45.14 Equipment for Fine Needle Aspiration
Fine needle aspiration gun or 10- to 20-mL syringe
21- to 23-gauge needle
Syringe holder (if desired)
Clear frosted-end glass slides
Alcohol/betadine pads
Fixative
Gauze pads
Adhesive bandage
0.5%–1% lidocaine in separate syringe with 25-gauge needle

After the procedure is explained to the patient and consent has been obtained, the skin is cleansed. The lesion is identified and stabilized, preferably over a rib, between the fingers of the nondominant hand. The area can be anesthetized by injecting and raising a wheal of 0.5% to 1.0% lidocaine in the skin over the mass. A 21- to 23-gauge needle with a clear hub attached to a 5- to 20-mL syringe is then inserted into the central portion of the mass; the smaller the syringe, the greater the pressure that can be generated during aspiration. Increasing the needle gauge does not necessarily increase the sample size as it can raise the risk of bleeding and hematoma formation. Two fingers are placed under the piston of the syringe, and the thumb is used against the body of the syringe to pull the piston toward the examiner, applying negative pressure (Fig. 45.23). A syringe pistol grip holder may be used to facilitate this procedure. With use of the holder, the grips of the holder are pulled together to apply negative pressure.

When a breast cyst is encountered, complete drainage of the mass should be attempted. During the aspiration, the fluid will appear in the hub and then fill the syringe. Most often, the fluid is clear but at times can be cloudy, gray, or green. This fluid can be appropriately discarded. By employing this approach, an immediate diagnosis of cyst can be made and the patient relieved of her concern of over the mass. If the cyst aspirate is bloody, the mass does not disappear, or reoccurs, the patient should be considered a candidate for excisional biopsy. It is important to reinforce to the patient the benefits of following recommended screening guidelines.

After complete sampling along each axis of the mass, suction is released and the needle is removed from the lesion. Releasing the suction *before* removing the needle is a critical aspect of this procedure. Continued negative pressure upon removing the needle (without release of suction) results in aspiration of the specimen into the body of the syringe that can be difficult to retrieve. Once the needle is removed, pressure is applied to the puncture site. A sterile dressing is then applied to the site.

The material should be expelled onto a glass slide with the needle bevel facing down to prevent scatter of the specimen. To release additional sample, the needle is detached, air is drawn into the syringe, the needle is reattached, and further expulsive efforts are accomplished. The "detach, draw air, and reattach" process is repeated until all the cellular material has been expelled. A second slide is placed on top, and the material is smeared between the two slides. Immediate fixation with 95% ethanol or a spray fixative should occur to prevent drying of the cells. The examiner must provide the cytopathologist with an accurate clinical history.

In the instance of a solid mass, the lesion is sampled by moving the needle up and down within the mass several times. Several passes should be made into every portion of the mass to prevent false-negative samples. Valuable cytologic material is harbored within the needle and hub and is then used for evaluation (Fig. 45.24).

Although FNA is cost-effective, several factors have led to diminished use of this technique, including the inability to diagnosis invasive versus in situ disease, the variability in sampling based on the provider's abilities, the limited training of pathologists in cytopathology interpretation, and the rising rates of percutaneous core biopsy. Current preference is for histologic assessment, and this can be obtained through large core needle biopsy.

Core Needle Breast Biopsy

It is estimated that approximately one million breast biopsies are performed yearly to diagnose approximately 200,000 breast cancers. Percutaneous core needle biopsy may spare many of these women the need for more deforming, invasive, and expensive surgical procedures. With this procedure, a

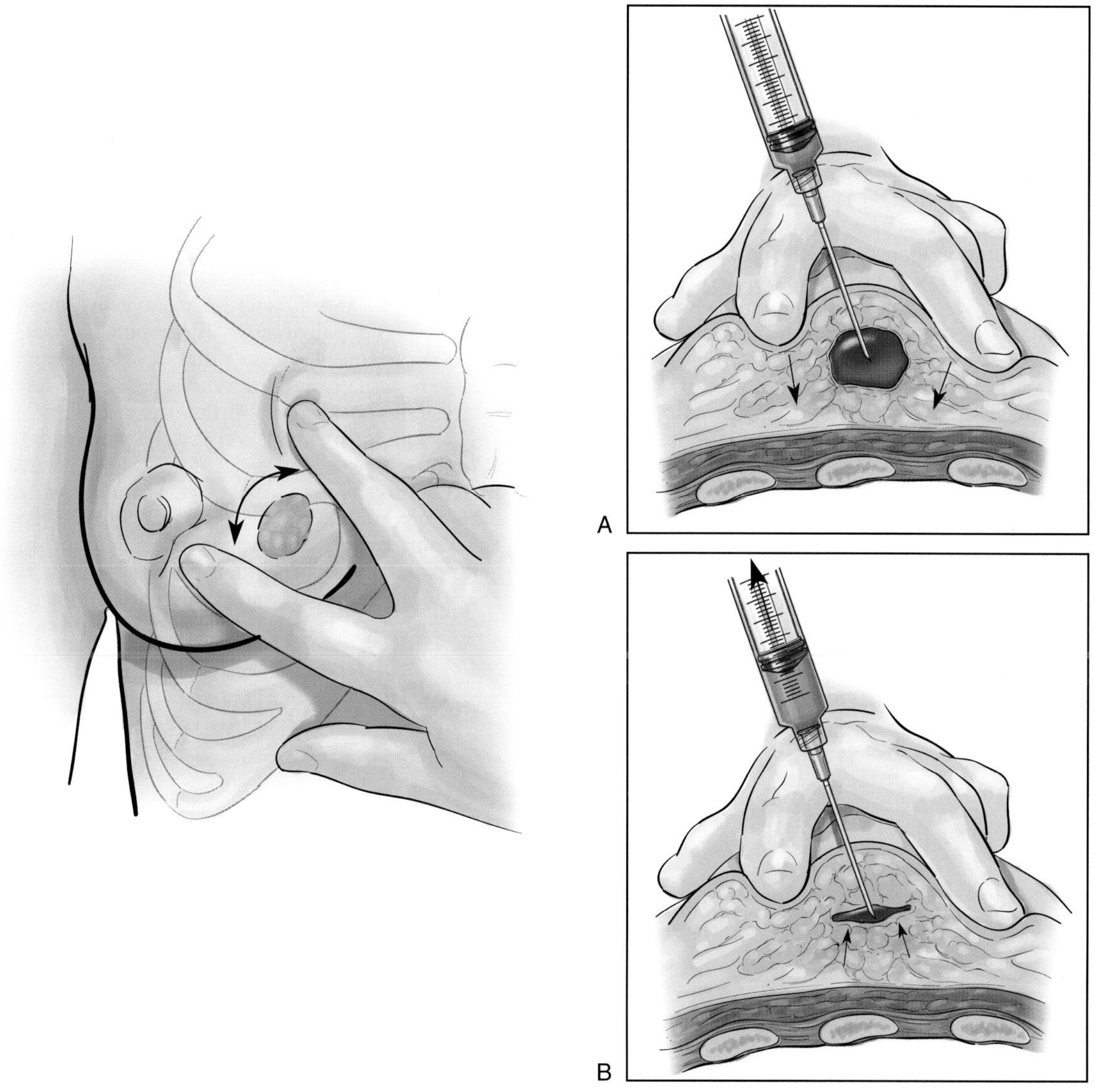

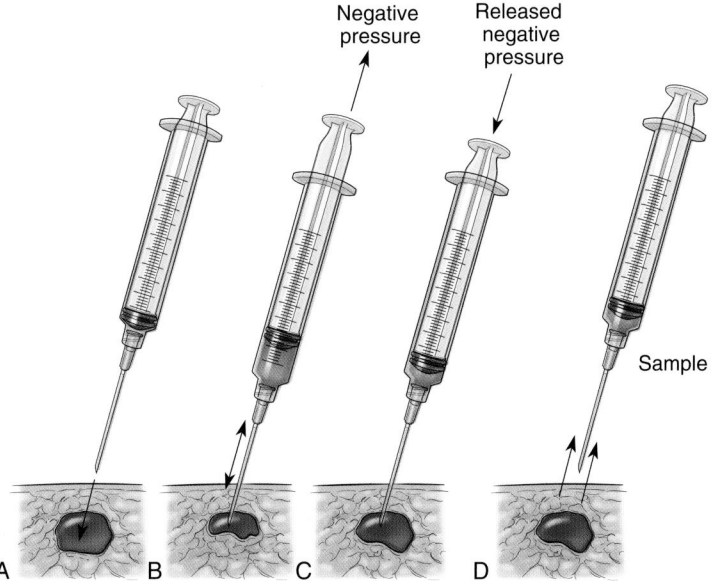

FIGURE 45.23 Technique of fine-needle aspiration. **A:** The mass is stabilized with the nondominant hand (preferably over a rib). After the needle is inserted into the mass, negative pressure is applied. **B:** As a cyst is aspirated, it collapses and the walls adhere and it resolves completely.

FIGURE 45.24 Fine-needle aspiration of a solid mass. **A:** The mass is located and the needle is inserted into the mass without negative pressure. **B:** Negative pressure is applied while the needle is moved in an up-and-down fashion within the mass. **C:** Negative pressure is released. **D:** The needle is removed from the mass.

VIII

histopathologic diagnosis is rendered compared with cytologic evaluation with FNA. Studies indicate a high degree of accuracy, with a sensitivity of 89%, specificity of 100%, positive predictive value of 98%, and an 80% negative predictive value in confirming invasive disease. False-negative results may occur, but false-positive results are rare except with radial scars. Increasing the number and the size of core specimens has increased the accuracy of the procedure.

Core needle biopsy may be performed under tactile, stereotactic, or ultrasound guidance. Less tissue is removed during core needle biopsy compared with excisional biopsy, resulting in no deformity in the breast and minimal to no scarring on subsequent mammograms. Another advantage is the ability to distinguish between invasive and in situ carcinoma. Because special training is not required to interpret the histologic material obtained from core needle biopsy, this obviates the need for skills of a cytopathologist. Given the larger needle size, local anesthesia is required, higher rates of postprocedure bleeding and hematoma formation occur, and there have been instances in which the track of the biopsy has been "seeded" with tumor leading to recurrences at the skin puncture sites. The use of an introducer needle has minimized the latter risk.

At times, core needle biopsy may not be possible due to lesions that are close to the nipple, lesions that are very posterior or superficial, or when the breast compresses to less than 1.7 cm.

This biopsy procedure is often used in the assessment of BI-RADS category 4 and 5 lesions. If core biopsy of a category 4 lesion yields a benign diagnosis concordant with the imaging characteristics, the woman is spared a diagnostic surgical biopsy. Although most often performed for nonpalpable lesions, percutaneous image-guided core biopsy also can be helpful in the evaluation of palpable breast masses, particularly those that are deep, mobile, or vaguely palpable. An advantage of image guidance is the ability to obtain radiographic documentation of the procedure. For select health care providers, this procedure can be performed in their office with or without ultrasound guidance.

Stereotactic core needle biopsy requires dedicated equipment but is helpful in evaluating suspicious mammographic findings that have no palpable or ultrasound correlates. Ultrasound-guided core needle biopsy has several advantages, including real-time visualization of the needle, lack of ionizing radiation, accessibility to all parts of the breast and axilla, multipurpose use of equipment, and lower cost. However, it is limited in detection of lesions less than 1 cm and has decreased sensitivity in detection of microcalcifications. Vacuum-assisted devices (e.g., Mammotome, Cincinnati, OH) may improve tissue sampling by obtaining larger intact samples. The choice of approach depends on several factors, including lesion visibility and accessibility, equipment availability, and preferences of the radiologist.

The area is cleansed and administration of local anesthesia is performed. An introducer needle is placed into the site of interest, and then the coring device is inserted through this conduit (Fig. 45.25). This can minimize the risk of seeding

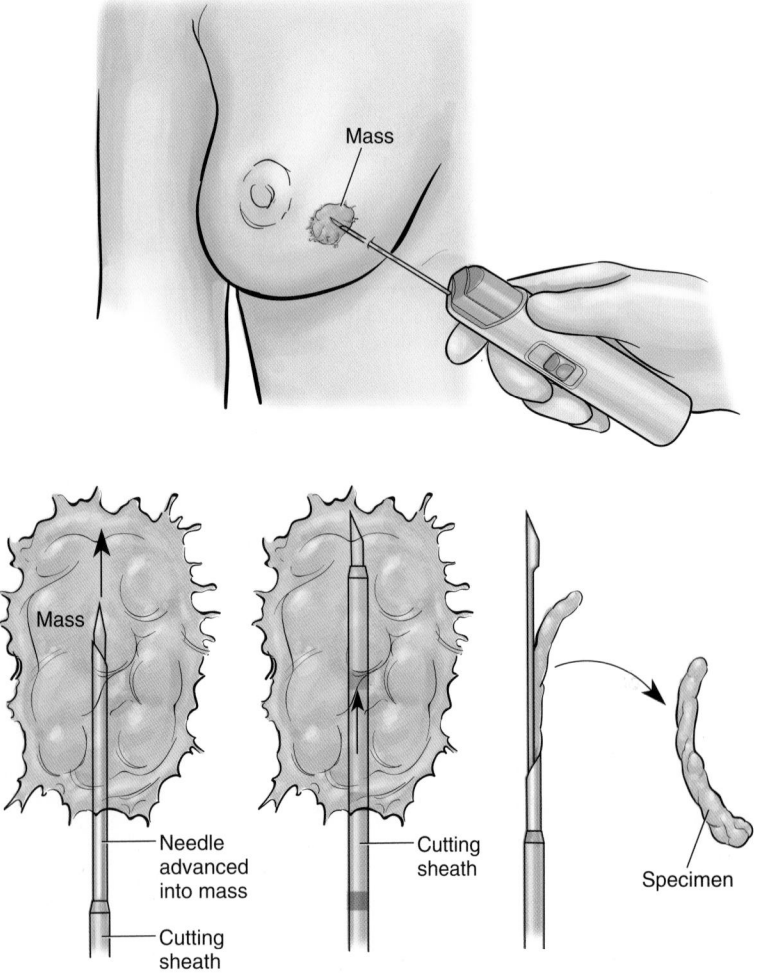

FIGURE 45.25 Core needle biopsy technique.

the biopsy track with malignant cells and allows for the core needle to be reintroduced multiple times without increasing the risk of further tissue disruption. As the core needle is introduced into the mass, the tissue inside the core of the needle is cut from the surrounding tissue as the outer sheath is advanced. The core needle device is spring loaded allowing for a mechanized capture of the tissue. After removal of the sheath and core needle, a pressure dressing is applied. In some circumstances, the entire lesion can be removed. After the core biopsies are obtained, a titanium clip is deployed into the biopsy site to identify the area for future localization if excisional biopsy is required. A variety of shapes of clips are available, allowing the radiologist to perform multiple biopsies to aid in further identification of these sites. The histopathologic findings then dictate whether observation or further assessment should occur. Disconcordant histology, that is, the imaging is concerning for malignancy but the biopsy is benign, is an indication for excisional biopsy. The radiologist should provide an addendum to the report when the pathology from the biopsy is available stating what the findings are and whether they confirm a benign entity and observation is acceptable or if further assessment is required. In instances where a cancer has been diagnosed, the core specimen can be assessed to determine the hormone and HER2 receptor status.

Excisional Biopsy

This procedure is primarily employed when a benign lesion such as a fibroadenoma or papilloma is present. The technique may be used with or without a localization procedure. The lesion in question is removed in its entirety often without additional breast tissue or margin. The surgeon should choose an incision that offers ready access to the site with minimal cosmetic disturbance (Fig. 45.26). Curvilinear, circumareolar, and radial incisions are chosen depending on location and the size of the lesion. If the incision is made along Langer lines, an improved cosmetic outcome is achieved (Fig. 45.27A, B).

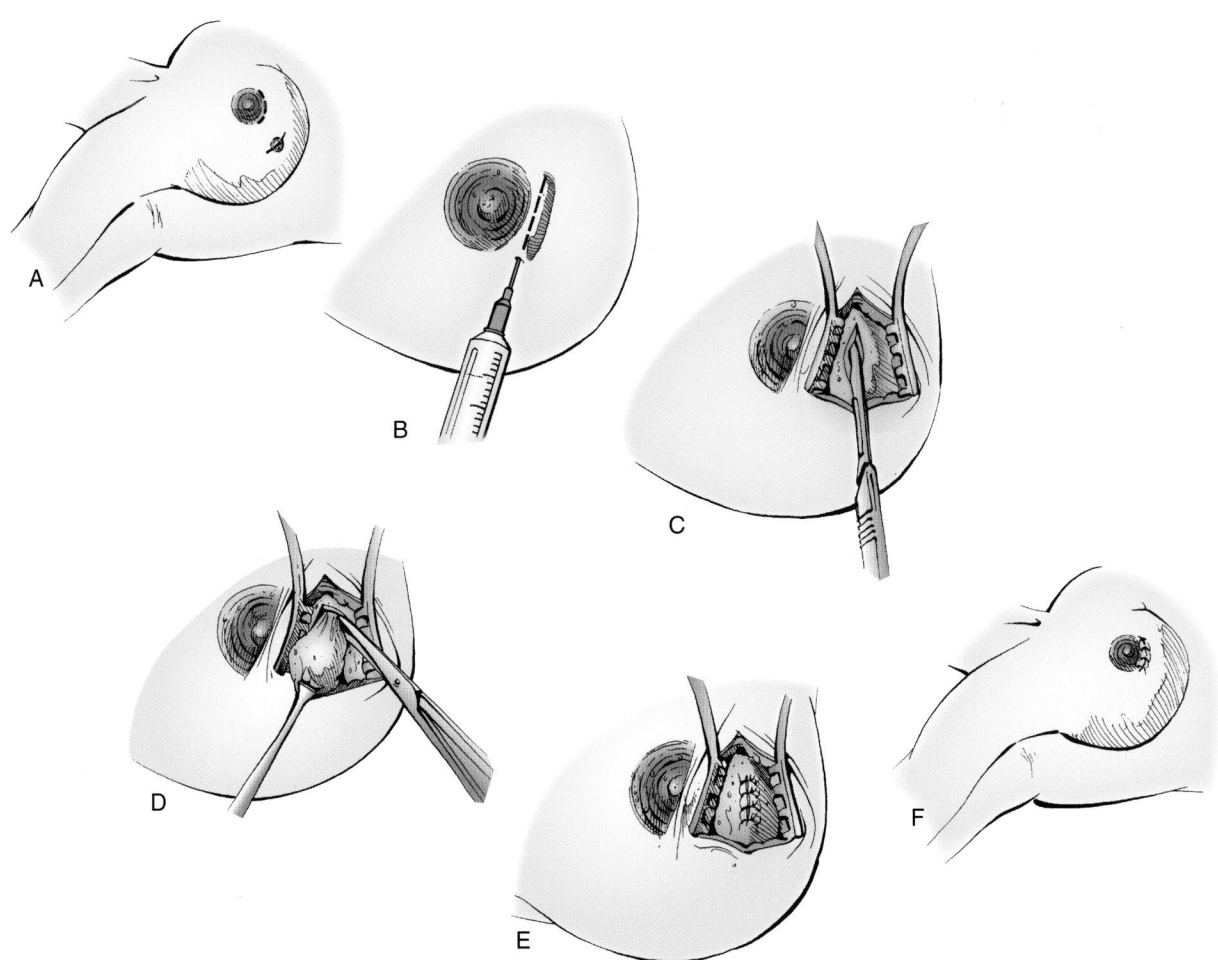

FIGURE 45.26 Technique of excisional biopsy. **A:** For cosmetic reasons, circumareolar incisions are preferable when the lesion is thought to be within 2 or 3 cm of the areola. Not more than one half of the areolar margin should be incised. A curvilinear incision parallel to the areola along Langer lines is made over lesions further out from the center. **B:** A local anesthetic is given in the proposed incision using 1% lidocaine and a hypodermic (no. 25) needle. From the wheal, deeper injections of anesthetic are made around the circumference of the lesion and beneath it. **C:** The incision is carried down through the dense subcutaneous tissue and into the lobule containing the lesion. Self-retaining retractors are helpful when an assistant is not available. **D:** If the lesion is small or easily mobilized, it should be sharply dissected and excised. **E:** The lobular defect can be sutured with fine absorbable suture material if the closure places no tension on the overlying skin or the cavity can be left open. Bleeding is controlled with absorbable ligatures or electrocoagulation. **F:** The skin is closed within two layers, approximately the deep and superficial subcuticular edges. A pressure dressing for 24 to 48 hours is desirable if a significant amount of dead space has been left behind.

VIII

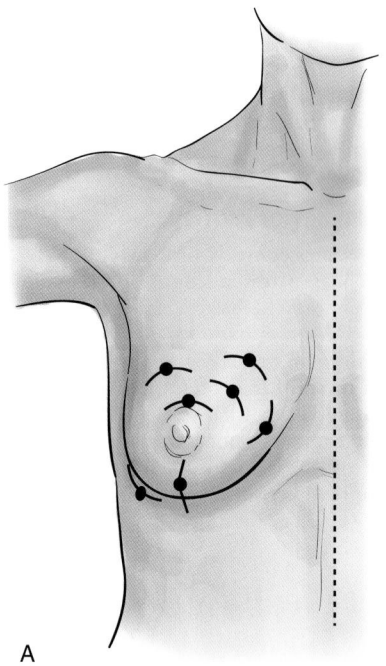
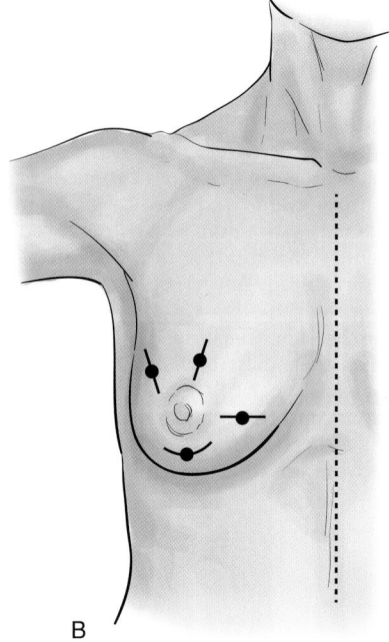

FIGURE 45.27 A: Preferred incision choices. **B:** Incisions to be avoided.

The procedure can be accomplished with sharp dissection, with the aid of an electrosurgical diathermy or high-frequency ultrasound (Harmonic Scalpel, Ethicon Endo-Surgery, New Brunswick, NJ). Meticulous attention to the resultant biopsy cavity is undertaken to assure adequate hemostasis. Most surgeons do not approximate the underlying breast tissue but rather allow a seroma cavity to form to maintain the normal contour of the breast. Subcuticular closure of the skin is then performed using monofilament fine sutures. (See Steps in the Procedure.)

STEPS IN THE PROCEDURE

Excisional Biopsy

- This procedure can be performed under local anesthesia, sedation and local anesthesia, or general anesthesia.
- Identify Langer line proximate to the lesion.
- Infiltrate the incision and surrounding tissue with 1% lidocaine.
- Use a scalpel to make the incision.
- Develop with either sharp dissection or with an electrocoagulation device skin flaps around the incision site.
- Excise the lesion completely.
- Size of excisional biopsy will be dependent on size of the lesion.
- Orient the specimen for pathologist to allow for margin assessment.
- If a radiographic localization was performed, obtain a specimen radiograph to confirm removal of the lesion(s).

- Make the operative bed hemostatic with either sutures or electrocoagulation.
- Leave the operative bed open to allow for seroma formation as this will maintain the normal contour of the breast.
- Skin closure in two layers using both an interrupted and running fine (3-0, 4-0) subcutaneous absorbable suture.

Ablative Techniques

Nonsurgical options currently exist for benign lesions and are being studied for use in known malignancies. Fibroadenomas are responsive to ablative techniques given their indolent nature. Cryoablation has been used successfully for lesions less than 4 cm. A probe is inserted under ultrasound guidance and then activated to achieve –40°C. Two freeze–thaw cycles are required to satisfactorily induce intracellular ice formation and membrane rupture. Over the course of several months, the lesions will resorb. The procedure can be performed in the office, and only local anesthesia to skin site is required.

Other ablative techniques exist including radiofrequency ablation and microwave thermography. Advantages of ablative approaches include minimal scarring, improved cosmesis, and the ability to accomplish the procedure under local anesthesia in the outpatient setting. Lack of complete histologic evaluation, delayed reabsorption of the mass, and incomplete response are some of the concerns surrounding these approaches.

Major Duct Excision

For evaluation of nipple discharge, duct excision can be performed. A technique described by Urban uses a radial or circumareolar skin incision to assess and remove the major ducts of

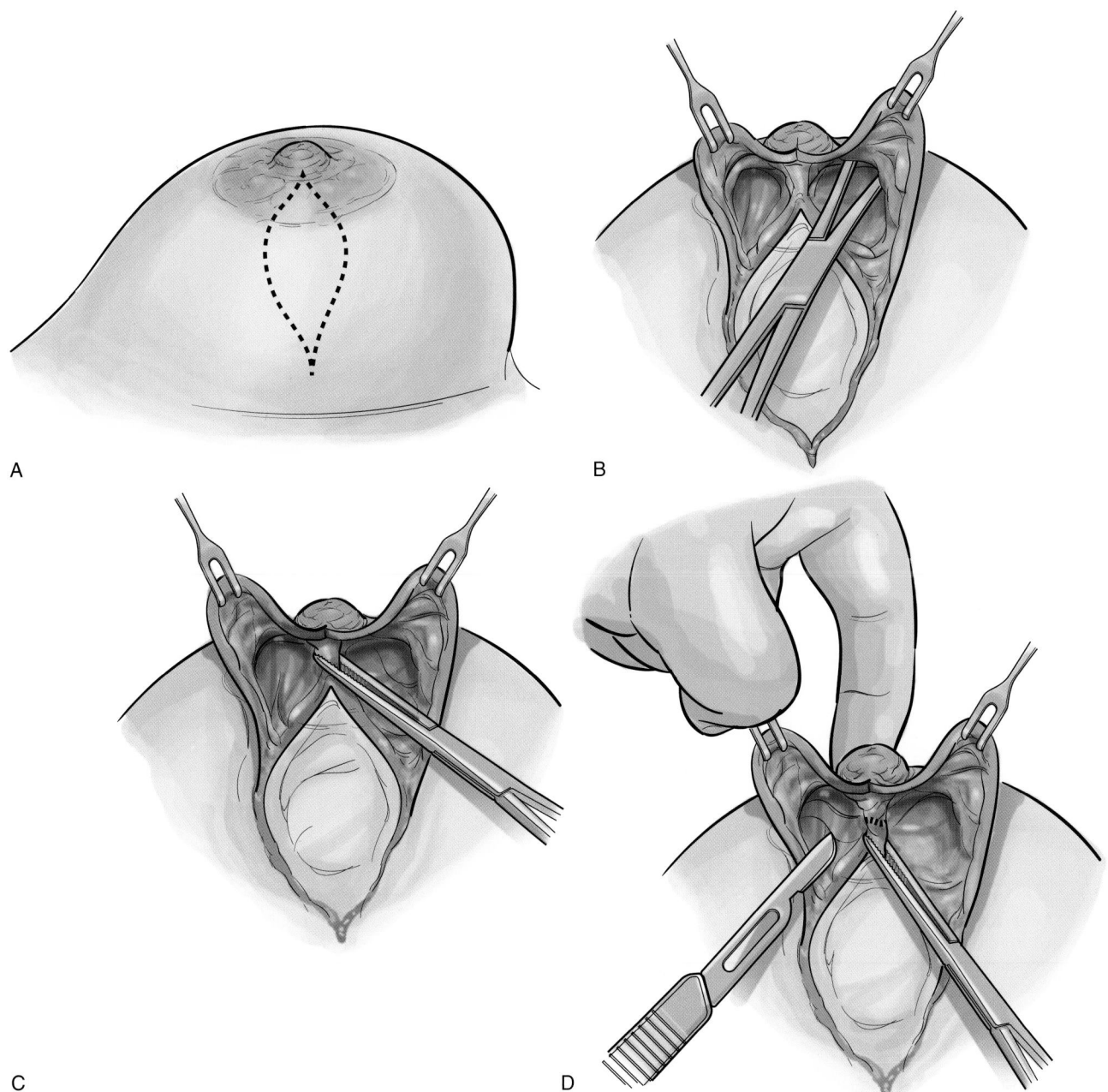

A

B

C

D

FIGURE 45.28 Technique of major duct excision (**A–D**). (Reprinted from Urban J. Excision of the major duct system of the breast. *Cancer* 1963;16: 515, with permission. Published by John Wiley and Sons. Copyright © 1963 American Cancer Society.)

the breast (Fig. 45.28). The overlying areolar skin is separated from the underlying breast parenchyma. As the base of the nipple is approached, the ductal system is visualized. The individual duct can then be isolated either by direct visualization or if previously localized by placing a fine suture or injecting dye into the affected nipple opening. The involved duct is traced for a minimal distance of 2 to 5 cm prior to being truncated. Five centimeters is chosen as the major ducts are present within this distance, and almost 95% of the lesions are located within this region. The ductal attachments to the base of the nipple are severed. In instances of ductal ectasia or where a solitary duct cannot be identified, the surgeon dissects

a minimal of 5 cm in a 360-degree manner and in this fashion develops a pyramidal portion of breast tissue, which is then released from the underlying stroma. The operative bed is made hemostatic and skin approximated in two layers. Some surgeons will place a fine (4-0 or 5-0) suture at the base of the nipple to prevent nipple invagination. (See Steps in the Procedure.) A similar approach is used when the patient has nonpuerperal breast abscess formation with or without sinus formation (Fig. 45.29). When a draining sinus is present, it is excised with a portion of the nipple. Risks of this surgical approach include denervation of the nipple, nipple necrosis as a result of ischemia, and cosmetic change.

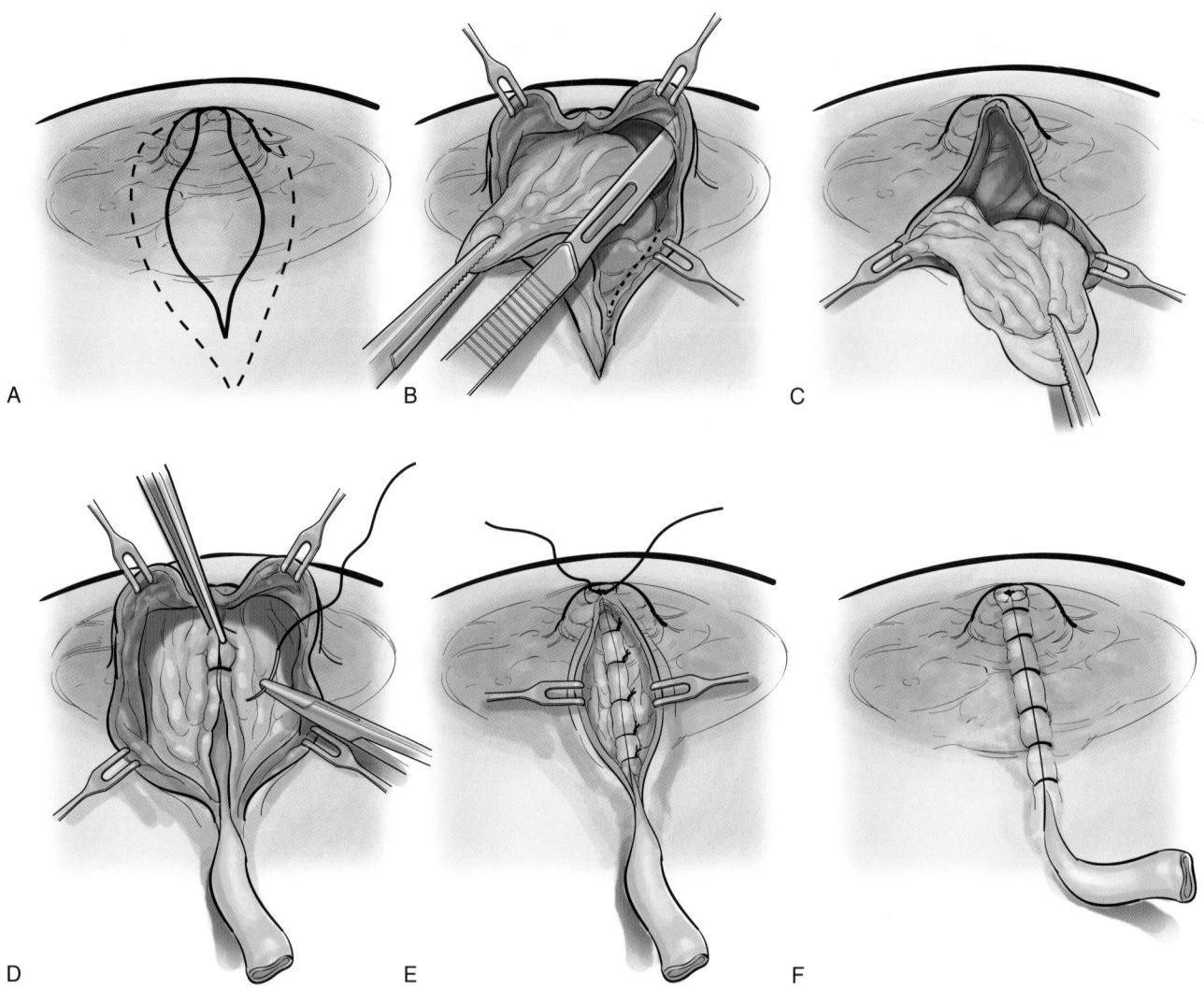

FIGURE 45.29 Major duct excision for periductal abscess (**A–F**). The procedure includes excising the sinus site and a portion of the nipple. (Reprinted from Urban J. Excision of the major duct system of the breast. *Cancer* 1963;16:515, with permission. Published by John Wiley and Sons. Copyright © 1963 American Cancer Society.)

STEPS IN THE PROCEDURE

Duct Excision

- This can be performed under local anesthesia, sedation and local anesthesia, or general anesthesia.
- Identify the duct with the discharge (if there is only one duct with discharge).
- Infiltrate the nipple areolar complex with 1% lidocaine.
- Using a duct probe, cannulate the duct with the discharge.
- Make a circumareolar incision along the edge of the areola that is closest to the duct with the discharge.
- Dissect the breast tissue off the nipple using electrocoagulation device or Metzenbaum scissors.
- If possible, resect the tissue under the nipple around the duct probe, and be sure to take at least 2 to 3 cm of tissue below the nipple.

- Orient the specimen for margin assessment.
- Make the area hemostatic with either sutures or electrocoagulation.
- If all of the tissue below the nipple is removed as part of major duct excision, then a purse-string stitch with a permanent suture such as 3-0 silk can be placed under the nipple in order to prevent the nipple from inverting.
- Skin closure using a running fine (4-0) subcutaneous absorbable suture.

Localization Techniques

In circumstances where the lesion is nonpalpable, localization of the lesion with ultrasound, mammogram, or MRI is warranted. Different techniques can be used to identify and guide the surgeon to the site of interest. Dye injection, wire localization, and seed localization are the current modes utilized. In the instances of dye and wire localization, using imaging guidance, a visual

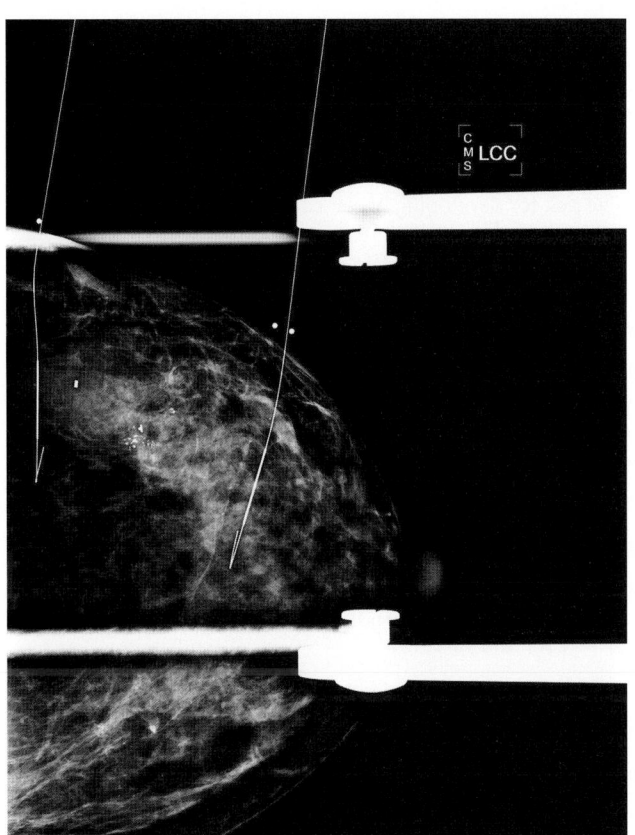

FIGURE 45.30 Example of wire localization. The patient has known DCIS, and two wires were used to bracket the areas of concern. Refer to Figure 41.26 for original mammogram.

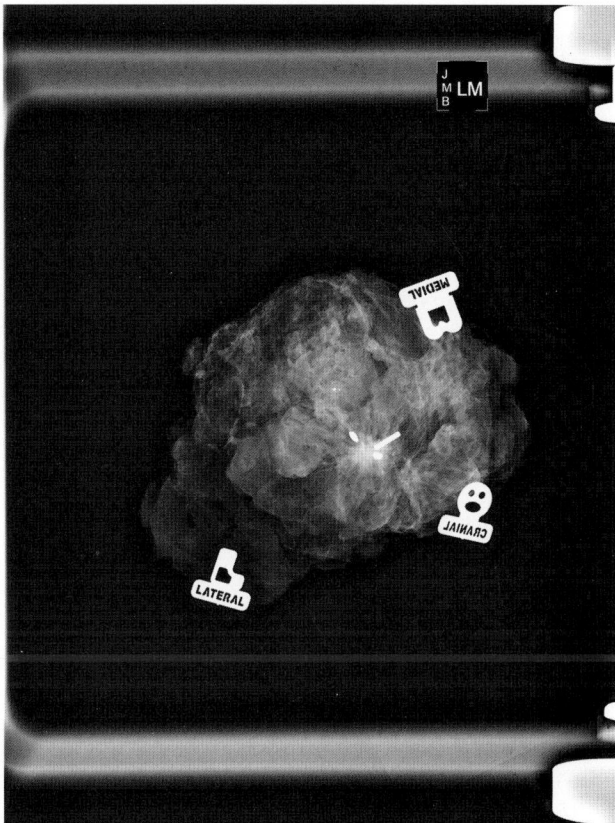

FIGURE 45.31 Specimen radiograph with speculated lesion and use of the Margin Map. (Beekley Corporation, Boston, MA.)

dye (methylene blue) can be injected or a Kopans (hook) wire placed in the area of concern. The dye can be placed up to a day in advance, whereas the wire procedure is performed on the day of the surgical excision. The use of the wire and placement mammograms can guide the surgeon to the site by visualizing in three dimensions the location of the wire tip (Fig. 45.30). As a matter of convention, the wire tip is placed beyond the lesion to help the surgeon achieve a margin around the mass. The use of the hook wire is the most commonly employed approach. A radiograph of the surgical specimen is then obtained to confirm removal via identification of the lesion or a previously placed clip. The use of radiopaque markers (Margin Map, Beekley Corporation, Boston, MA) can identify the margins of the specimen, and then when two orthogonal radiographs are performed, margin assessment can be obtained.

An alternative approach, which we employ at our institution, for high-risk lesions and known cancer is radioactive seed localization. This approach has been shown to be highly effective in localizing nonpalpable breast lesion. An iodine-125 seed is inserted into the lesion of interest via one of three imaging modalities. The surgeon then uses a gamma probe to identify the seed and allows for rapid identification in three dimensions of the site during the surgical event. The seed can be placed up to 5 days in advance of the procedure. Given the inverse square law, radioactivity detection rapidly declines as distance from the seed is increased. This allows the surgeon to assess the margins in all dimensions during the procedure. A specimen radiograph is obtained after the tissue is removed, and the remaining cavity is assessed for residual activity in event the seed has been cut and a portion left within the breast

(Fig. 45.31). We have noted diminished tissue removal and improvement in obtaining clean margins. Special training including radiation safety training and proctoring for the first several procedures is required. Given concerns of radioactive contamination, training of the operating room, radiology, and pathology staff is mandated.

BREAST CANCER

Worldwide, breast cancer is the most commonly diagnosed malignancy in women and a leading cause of cancer-related mortality. In the United States in 2014, it accounts for 29% of all cancer site diagnoses, and it is estimated that there will be in excess of 232,000 women diagnosed with this malignancy. In addition, breast cancer will be the second most common cause of cancer-related deaths accounting for approximately 40,000 deaths, with lung cancer being the leading cause.

Epidemiology

A large body of literature exists examining risk factors associated with the development of breast cancer. The etiology of breast cancer is likely multifactorial. Numerous risk factors have been identified; however, nearly three fourths of women with breast cancer have no known risk factors other than sex and age.

Risk factors for breast cancer include female sex, increasing age, nulliparity, delayed childbearing, personal or family history of breast cancer, atypical proliferative breast disease, obesity in postmenopausal women, a long menstrual history (menarche before age 12 and menopause after age 51), LCIS, prior radiation exposure, and higher education and socioeconomic status.

VIII

TABLE 45.15 Risk Factors for Breast Cancer Development

RISK FACTOR	RR
Female gender	150
Increasing age > 60	17
Inherited genetic mutation	3–7
Personal history of breast cancer	3–7
≥ 2 first-degree relatives with early onset of breast cancer	2.6
Atypical hyperplasia	3.7
Ionizing radiation to the chest	7
Early menarche ≤ 12	1.5
Late menopause ≥ 55	2.0
Nulliparity	1.4
Delayed childbearing ≥ 30	1.9–3.5
No history of lactation	1.4
Postmenopausal obesity	1.4–1.6
Alcohol consumption (2–5 drinks/d)	1.4
Combination hormone replacement therapy	1.2
Tall stature	1.2
Personal history of ovary, endometrial, or colon cancer	
Jewish heritage	

Data from Costanza ME, Chen W. Factors that modify breast cancer risk in women. In: Dizon DS, ed. *UpToDate*. Waltham, MA: UpToDate; 2013; Clemons GP. Estrogen and the risk of breast cancer. *N Engl J Med* 2001;344:276–285; Guibout C, Adjadj E, Rubino C, et al. Malignant breast tumors after radiotherapy for a first cancer during childhood. *J Clin Oncol* 2005;23(1):197–204; Kelsey JL. Breast cancer epidemiology: summary and future directions. *Epidemiol Rev* 1993;15(1):256–263.

Factors such as fat intake, smoking, and alcohol intake have all been suggested to contribute to breast cancer risks. Table 45.15 lists risk factors for breast cancer development.

Late onset of menarche, early menopause, multiparity, and breast-feeding are associated with risk reduction. Healthy lifestyle with maintenance of ideal body weight, avoidance of alcohol and tobacco, and a well-balanced diet with minimal processed foods and low fat are linked to lower rates of breast cancer.

Gender

Breast cancer is one hundred times more common in women. Male breast cancer is rare with an estimated 2,360 cases in the United States in 2014, accounting for 430 cancer-related deaths. The finding of breast cancer in a male should raise awareness of a possible genetic predisposition. Mutations of BRCA2 are associated with a 100-fold increased risk for the development of male breast cancer.

Age

The risk for developing breast cancer increases with advancing age and reaches its peak in the sixth decade. Between the ages of 20 and 34 years, breast cancer incidence is 2% and rises to 24% between the ages of 55 to 64 years. Subsequently, the risk falls in the elderly population to 6% for women 85 and older.

Ethnicity

Caucasian race has the highest rates of breast cancer, but breast cancer is the most common cancer in women in all ethnic groups. Black women present with more advanced disease and have higher breast cancer–specific mortality. Some factors may be related to lifestyle and access to the health care system, but other risks do exist. Black women have a higher incidence of early-onset breast cancer and rates of "triple-negative" disease. Women with Ashkenazi Jewish ancestry have a higher likelihood of harboring one of the founder mutations of BRCA1 and BRCA2.

Obesity

In and of itself, obesity is associated with increased morbidity and mortality. The Nurses' Health Study reported that a 10-kg weight gain in the postmenopausal period was associated with a relative risk of 1.18 of developing breast cancer. In other studies, elevated body mass index (BMI) has been shown to increase breast cancer risk. The association may be due to peripheral conversion of estrogen precursors within adipose tissue leading to higher levels of circulating estrogens. Women with BMI in excess of 33 kg/m^2 have an elevated breast cancer risk compared to women of ideal body weight.

Tall Stature

Higher risk of breast cancer is seen with increased height. One study reported a 20% increased risk in women whose heights exceeded 69 inches compared to those with heights less than 63 inches. Underlying association is not yet delineated. A possible explanation may be related to increased bone mineral density in taller women, suggesting exposure to higher levels of endogenous estrogen exposure.

Oral Contraceptives

The use of oral contraceptive pills (OCP) was initially reported to elevate an individual's risk of breast cancer. Subsequent reports fail to demonstrate a relationship between use and breast cancer risk. Three large series, including the Nurses' Health Study, fail to demonstrate an adverse relationship. Use of OCPs in women with a family history of breast cancer is not associated with increased risk. Interaction of OCPs in women who carry a deleterious mutation of BRCA1/BRCA2 is currently unknown.

Reproductive Factors

The longer exposure to endogenous hormonal milieu is associated with greater risk of breast cancer development. Early-onset menarche and later menopause are both associated with increased risk of breast cancer. For each year of delayed menopause, risk increases by approximately 1%. For each 2-year delay in the onset in menarche, the risk is reduced by 10%. Nulliparity, late ages at first pregnancy, and infertility also have been shown to have a relationship to increased risk.

Childbirth before age 18 years portends one third the risk of breast cancer than in a woman delivering at age 35 years. Multiparity is associated with reduced breast cancer risk. Breast-feeding has been demonstrated to have a beneficial effect on cancer risk reduction. An analysis in *Lancet* in 2002 of 47 epidemiologic studies demonstrated 4.3% risk reduction for every 12 months of breast-feeding. The common theme for risk elevation or risk reduction is exposure to ovulatory cycles. Benefits are seen with fewer or delayed onset of ovulatory events, whereas risks are increased with more frequent ovulatory cycles.

Family History

A family history of breast cancer increases the individual's risk. Level of risk depends on the number of relatives, degree of separation, and age at onset of disease in the affected individuals. The presence of breast cancer in a premenopausal relative should raise awareness for genetic predisposition. A collaborative reanalysis published in 2001 in *Lancet* of 52 epidemiologic studies on family history and breast cancer revealed risk of breast cancer is raised twofold when one first-degree relative is affected and threefold if there are two first-degree relatives who are affected by the disease. Identification of patients at increased risk for breast cancer can be obtained through a comprehensive three-generation family history and lead to referral for genetic assessment and modification of screening recommendations.

Personal History of Breast Cancer

A previous history of DCIS or invasive carcinoma increases the risk of developing a contralateral breast cancer. Reported rates are 0.5% to 1% per year after diagnosis. A woman diagnosed at the age of 40 years would have a 30% chance of contralateral breast cancer by the time she reaches age 70.

Atypical Hyperplasia

The proliferation of the ductal or lobular epithelium with cellular atypia imparts an increased relative risk of developing breast cancer. Dupont and colleagues reported on a retrospective cohort study the risk of estrogen replacement therapy in women with atypical proliferative breast disease and noted an increased risk of breast cancer development in patients who did and did not receive estrogen therapy with relative risks of 2.53 and 2.87, respectively.

If the diagnosis of ADH/ALH is made on percutaneous biopsy, it is advised that formal excisional biopsy is performed given that upstaging to in situ or invasive cancer occurs 10% to 20% of the time. Recently, the role of additional excision for areas of ALH has been called into question by McGhan and others.

Lobular Carcinoma In Situ

Often diagnosed as an incidental finding, LCIS places an individual at a higher than average risk of developing breast cancer. It is considered a marker for the future development of breast cancer. Estimated lifetime risk is between 30% and 40% (up to 1% per year) and depends on the age at diagnosis. This compares to unaffected individuals who have a 12.5% risk (1 in 8 individuals).

Lifestyle

Lack of physical activity, alcohol consumption, smoking, high fat intake, processed foods, and red meat ingestion have been linked to the development of breast cancer. In some circumstances, there is a dose–response relationship.

Night shift work has been correlated with breast cancer risk. A recent study in nurses reported an elevated odds ratio of 1.8 (95% CI: 1.2 to 2.8) working rotating shifts after midnight. In a subset analysis, odds ratio increased to 2.6 (95% CI: 1.8 to 3.8) when nurses worked rotating long-term day and night shifts. A possible hypothesis is the relationship to nocturnal light exposure and its effects on melatonin production as low melatonin levels have been associated with increased breast cancer risk.

Radiation Exposure

Ionizing radiation is directly linked to the development of breast cancer. Data from individuals treated for Hodgkin lymphoma and those who have received exposure as a result of nuclear plant accidents support this finding. An area of current investigation is the risk of exposure to diagnostic levels of radiation during chest radiography, mammography, CT, and others. Patients with BRCA1/BRCA2 deleterious mutations may be more prone to radiation-related risks.

Hereditary Breast Cancer Syndromes

Less than 10% of breast cancers and less than 15% of ovarian cancers are associated with known inherited (germline) genetic mutations. Currently, the majority of hereditary breast cancer syndromes are linked to mutations of breast cancer type 1 and 2 susceptibility genes also known as BRCA1 and BRCA2. Phosphatase and tensin homolog (PTEN) and tumor protein 53 (TP53) mutations identified in Cowden and Li-Fraumeni syndromes also are associated with breast cancer susceptibility.

BRCA1/BRCA2 Mutations

BRCA1 and BRCA2 are tumor suppressor genes. Mutations are linked to hereditary breast and ovarian syndromes. Approximately 5% of breast cancer cases are due to these germline mutations. BRCA1 gene is located on the long arm of chromosome 17, consists of 22 coding exons, and is located in region 2 band 1 (17q21). BRCA2 is located on the long arm of chromosome 13 at position 12.3 (13q12.3).

These tumor suppressor genes encode a protein that combines with other tumor suppressors, DNA damage sensors, and signal transducers to form a large protein complex that assists in the repair of DNA strand breaks. BRCA1 interacts with a number of genes including BARD1, CHK1, and RAD51, whereas BRCA2 interacts with RAD51, which is the strand invasion recombinase. Mutations of BRCA1/BRCA2 can prevent DNA damage repair and increase an individual's risk of cancer.

Mutations of the BRCA1/BRCA2 genes involve either insertion or deletions of DNA base pairs. These genes are inherited in an autosomal dominant manner. Founder mutations are alterations of a gene or genes of one or more individuals who are founders of a distinct population, such as the Ashkenazi Jewish population, which has high penetrance of two specific mutations, 185delAG and 5382insC, seen in 1 in 8 and 1 in 12 individuals, respectively.

Carriers of mutations of BRCA1/BRCA2 gene have a high penetrance of breast cancer up to 85% by the age of 70 years. Risk of ovarian cancer in this group is as high as 40% by the same age. BRCA2 mutation carriers may have a lower ovarian cancer risk. Basal-like or triple-negative tumors are more frequently observed in patients who have mutations of the BRCA1 gene. Luminal A/B lesions are more common in the population with BRCA2 mutations.

VIII

Prevalence of these genetic alterations varies between ethnic groups and geographic location. As noted, there is higher incidence in the Ashkenazi Jews. Other founder mutations have been seen in populations from French Canada, the Netherlands, Sweden, Hungary, and Iceland.

The diagnosis of early age of onset breast cancer, having multiple family members with either breast or ovarian cancer, and having a personal diagnosis of ovarian cancer and basal-like or triple-negative breast cancer are among the reasons to consider genetic assessment. Ideally, the individual should be referred to a genetic counselor who will obtain a comprehensive family and personal history and estimate the individual's chance of carrying a mutation. Several models to estimate risk exist, including Bayesian probability model BRCAPRO and the Penn II risk model that utilizes logistic regression. An estimated risk of 10% is the threshold for consideration of testing. The National Comprehensive Cancer Network (NCCN) criteria for consideration of testing are listed in Table 45.16. Individuals of Ashkenazi Jewish descent should be assessed for the founder mutations first and if need be full sequencing

considered if the original assessment is unrevealing. In addition, an important component of testing is both the pre- and, if appropriate, posttest counseling. The absence of a known mutation in an individual from a family with a known mutation is a true negative and can be used to counsel and reassure the individual that their risk is not greater than that of the general population. However, a negative test in an individual of whom no family member has an identified mutation is considered uninformative. Several possibilities exist, including a deleterious mutation that has not been detected, a gene mutation that is present but not identifiable at present, or the presence of mutation with unknown significance (termed "variant of uncertain significance"). Additionally, a sporadic (as opposed to hereditary) cancer may have developed.

Phosphatase and Tensin Homolog Mutations

PTEN mutations have been described in multiple rare syndromes collectively referred to as PTEN hamartoma tumor syndromes (PHTS). Cowden syndrome (multiple hamartoma syndrome) is linked to germline mutations of PTEN and is the most well known of the PHTS. It is inherited in an autosomal dominant manner and associated with oral fibromas, palmoplantar keratosis, multiple hamartomas of various tissues, and increased risk of breast, endometrial, thyroid, renal, and colorectal cancers.

Tumor Protein 53 Mutation

Li-Fraumeni syndrome is linked to aberrations in the TP53 gene located on the short arm of chromosome 17 (17p13.1). TP53 is a tumor suppressor gene involved in the management of cells containing damaged DNA. The syndrome is an inherited disorder that manifests itself with a wide range of early-onset malignancies including breast cancer. This syndrome is also known as the sarcoma, breast, leukemia, and adrenal gland (SBLA) syndrome.

Pathology of Breast Cancer

Breast cancer is most common in the upper outer quadrant of the breast followed by the central, upper inner, lower outer, and lower inner quadrants (Table 45.17). The pattern of distribution correlates with breast tissue distribution in these areas. Regional spread of disease is most common to the ipsilateral axillary basin, and often, the first site of metastases is the nodes most lateral to the pectoralis minor.

Ductal carcinoma in situ (DCIS) and lobular carcinoma in situ (LCIS) make up this class of histologic changes. While DCIS is considered a cancer with potential to transform into

---

TABLE 45.16 National Comprehensive Cancer Network Criteria for Consideration of BRCA1/BRCA2 Genetic Testing

INDIVIDUAL FROM A FAMILY WITH KNOWN DELETERIOUS MUTATION OF BRCA1/BRCA2 MUTATION

Personal history of breast cancer (invasive or in situ) plus one or more of the following:
Diagnosed age ≤45
Diagnosed age ≤50 with ≥1st-, 2nd-, or 3rd-degree blood relative with breast cancer ≤50 y and/or 1st-, 2nd-, or 3rd-degree blood relative with epithelial ovarian/fallopian tube/primary peritoneal cancer at any age
Two breast primaries (ipsilateral or contralateral) when first breast cancer diagnosis occurred ≤50 y
Diagnosed ≤60 y with triple-negative breast cancer
Diagnosed ≤50 y with a limited family history
Diagnosed at any age with ≥2 first-, second-, or third-degree blood relatives with breast and/or epithelial ovarian/fallopian tube/primary peritoneal cancer at any age
Diagnosed at any age with ≥2 first-, second-, or third-degree blood relatives with pancreatic cancer at any age
First-, second-, or third-degree male blood relative with breast cancer
For an individual of ethnicity associated with higher mutation frequency (e.g., Ashkenazi Jewish), no additional family history may be required.

Personal history of epithelial ovarian/fallopian tube/primary peritoneal cancer

Personal history of male breast cancer

Personal history of pancreatic cancer at any age with ≥2 first-, second-, or third-degree blood relatives with breast and/or ovarian cancer and/or pancreatic cancer at any age

Family history
First- or second-degree relative meeting any of the above criteria
Third-degree blood relative with ≥ first-, second-, or third-degree blood relatives with breast cancer (at least one breast cancer ≤50 y) and/or ovarian cancer/fallopian tube/primary peritoneal cancer

---

TABLE 45.17 Breast Cancer Site Distribution

QUADRANT	FREQUENCY OF BREAST CANCER
Upper outer	45%
Central	24%
Upper–inner	14%
Lower–outer	9%
Lower–inner	5%
Multifocal	3%

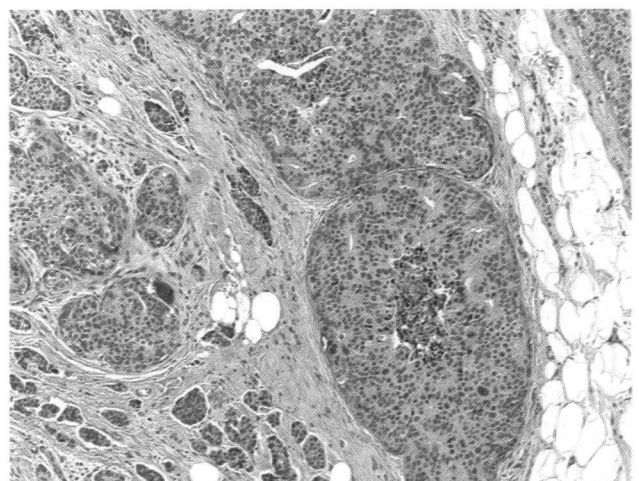

FIGURE 45.32 Ductal carcinoma in situ. The ducts are filled with pleomorphic and atypical cells with central areas of comedo necrosis. In the surrounding stroma, there are nests of infiltrating ductal carcinoma (H&E 10×). (Courtesy of Jing Yu, MD, University of Pittsburgh School of Medicine, Pittsburgh, PA.)

an invasive entity, the same is not true for LCIS, which is considered benign but predictive for the future development of breast cancer.

Ductal Carcinoma In Situ

DCIS is a noninvasive histologic variant of breast cancer. The histopathology of DCIS includes the proliferation of malignant cells within the ductal system of the breast but without invasion of the stromal tissue (Fig. 45.32). DCIS has a broad histologic presentation that includes traditional grading of well, moderate, and poor differentiation and includes subclassifications such as comedo, noncomedo, and micropapillary. These factors and the degrees of differentiation correlate with aggressiveness and likelihood of recurrence.

Widespread use of screening mammography coincides with a shift in the stage at presentation of breast cancer toward earlier-stage disease, particularly for DCIS. Data from the SEER program of the National Cancer Institute show nearly 300% change in incidence of DCIS in women aged 50 years and older and greater than 100% increase in the incidence of stage I disease in the same group. DCIS is considered a nonobligatory precursor to invasive ductal carcinoma (IDC) with variable rates of progression, depending on histology, size, and margin status. Radiographically, the most common finding is pleomorphic, clustered calcifications. Almost diagnostic is the finding of linear calcifications within the duct. DCIS detected based on palpation has up to a 25% incidence of associated invasive carcinoma.

Lobular Carcinoma In Situ

LCIS refers to proliferation of cells within the breast lobules. Typically, they comprise acini filled with small round cells with a thin rim of clear cytoplasm and a high nuclear-to-cytoplasmic ratio (Fig. 45.18). LCIS is considered a predictive marker of future cancer rather than a cancer precursor. The cancer risk applies to both breasts. It is often found *incidentally* at the time of breast biopsy performed for another indication and does not present characteristic clinical or mammographic findings. LCIS may be associated with clustered microcalcifications on imaging. It is typically multicentric. Studies of women with LCIS managed with biopsy alone demonstrate a risk of cancer development of approximately 1% per year.

TABLE 45.18 Histologic Types of Invasive Breast cancer	
HISTOLOGY TYPE	**%**
Ductal	50–70%
Lobular	5–16%
Medullary	3–6%
Mucinous	1–2%
Tubular	1–2%
Mixed	2–30%

Adapted from Dillon DA, Guidi AJ, Schnitt SJ. In: Harris JA, Lippman ME, Morrow M, et al., eds., *Pathology of invasive breast cancer in diseases of the breast*, 4th ed. Philadelphia, PA: Wolters Kluwer/Lippincott Williams & Wilkins; 2010.

Management of LCIS is discussed early in this chapter in the section on benign diseases.

Invasive Breast Cancer

Invasive breast cancers are a highly diverse group of tumors. More than 90% of breast cancers arise with the ducts. Infiltrating or invasive ductal carcinoma (IDC) is the most common histologic pattern of breast cancer accounting for greater than 70% of diagnoses. Infiltrating lobular carcinoma (ILC) is the second most frequent cancer with small contributions from the remaining subtypes. See Table 45.18 for breast histology classifications.

IDC accounts for the majority of breast cancers. No clinical or radiographic characteristics distinguish these lesions from the other histologic subtypes. Lesions are hard masses and tend to have stellate borders often with associated reaction of fibrous tissue surrounding the lesion. The histopathology is heterogenous to include cytologic atypia, mitotic activity and stromal desmoplasia. The tumor cells are arranged as glandular structures and exhibit varying degrees of cellular atypia, mitosis and stromal desmoplasia (Fig. 45.33).

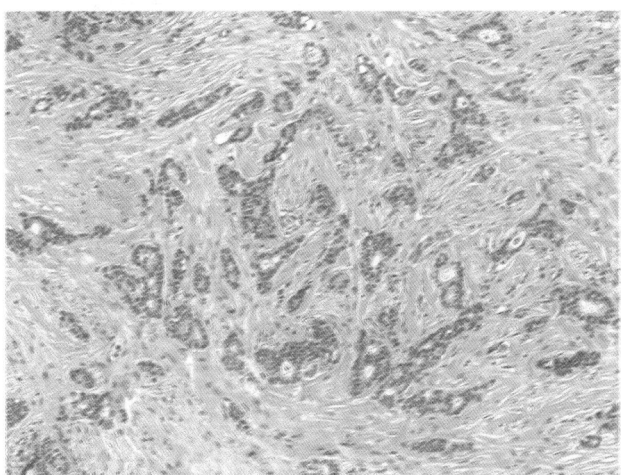

FIGURE 45.33 Infiltrating ductal cancer forming glands with varying degrees of cellular atypia and stromal desmoplasia (H&E 10×). (Courtesy of Jing Yu, MD, University of Pittsburgh School of Medicine, Pittsburgh, PA.)

VIII

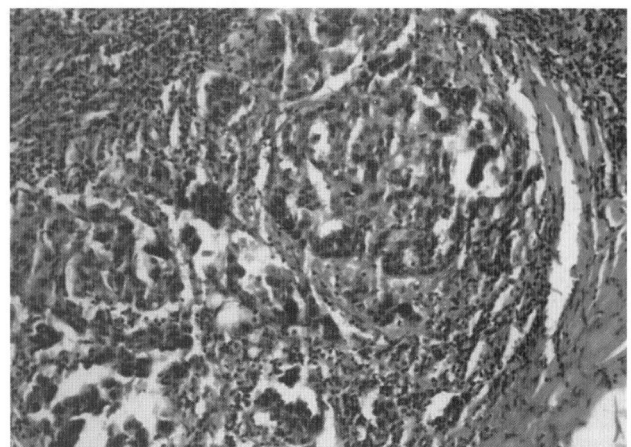

FIGURE 45.34 Histologic section of medullary carcinoma showing smooth margins, primitive malignant cells in syncytial growth surrounded by lymphoplasmacytic infiltrate (H&E 240×). (Courtesy of Taalat Tadros, MD, Emory University, School of Medicine, Atlanta, GA.)

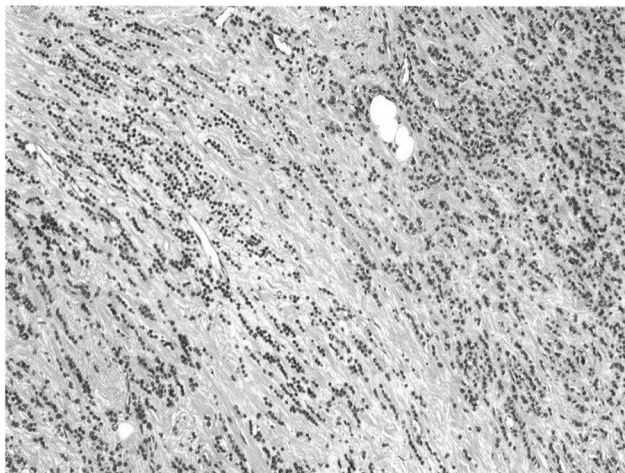

FIGURE 45.35 Infiltrating lobular carcinoma. The tumor cells are small and uniform and infiltrate the surrounding stroma in a linear fashion (H&E 10×). (Courtesy of Jing Yu, MD, University of Pittsburgh School of Medicine, Pittsburgh, PA.)

Tubular carcinoma is a variant of ductal carcinoma and has limited metastastic potential and excellent prognosis. It was commonly diagnosed in the early 1960s and was originally described in the literature as a palpable mass. It now accounts for 10% to 20% of cancers detected in a screened population. These tan or white lesions are typically 1.0 cm or smaller and infiltrate the surrounding tissue. Microscopic appearance demonstrates proliferation of well-formed glands or tubules lined by a single layer of epithelial cells. Nuclei are low grade and are pushed toward the lumen of the gland.

Medullary carcinoma has a propensity to be located in the upper outer quadrant of the breast. The tumors tend to be well circumscribed. Imaging echoes the clinical exam findings. The histopathologic appearance exhibits a predominance of syncytial cells, lymphocytic infiltrate, grade 2 and 3 nuclei, and an absence of glandular structure (**Fig. 45.34**). These tumors have a better prognosis than do the other IDC variants.

Mucinous or colloid carcinoma appears as a large, slow-growing, gelatinous mass usually found in older women. These lesions are associated with improved prognosis and are often diagnosed in the seventh or eighth decade of life. On exam, they are poorly defined or lobulated. On mammographic assessment, a mass lesion with irregular borders is identified; associated microcalcifications are rare. The histologic findings include tumor cells in small clusters, sheets, or papillary configurations with an abundance of extracellular mucin.

ILC often has a more subtle clinical presentation on both clinical and radiographic examinations and often is underestimated based on physical and mammographic examination. The use of MRI may be more valuable in patients with this disease process. The cancer tends to be multifocal and have a higher incidence of bilateral disease. Most often, the finding in the contralateral breast is LCIS. Histologically, the cells are small and uniform and infiltrate the surrounding stroma in a linear fashion. Multiple variants of the disease exist (**Fig. 45.35**).

Metastatic Disease to the Breast (Extramammary Malignancies)

Metastatic deposits to the breast from distant sites have been reported. Often, these lesions are multiple, bilateral, and well circumscribed. The sites of origin include the contralateral breast, melanoma, lung, choriocarcinoma, cervix, ovary, and many others. An unusual clinical, radiographic, or pathologic finding should raise the possibility of metastatic disease to the breast, and the clinician should provide adequate historical information to the pathologist to assist in diagnosis.

Nottingham Score

Histologic grading has been used to correlate with prognosis. The Elston-Ellis modification of the Scarff-Bloom-Richardson system, also known as "Nottingham Score," is the system most often employed. The current tumor grading system employs nuclear grade, tubule formation, and mitotic rate. Each element is on a scale of 1 to 3. The components are added together and can range from 3 to 9, whereby low is 3 to 5, moderate 6 to 7, and high-grade scores 8 to 9. Nottingham Scoring System is demonstrated in Table 45.19.

Molecular Tumor Classification

Gene expression profiling has aided in the identification of subtypes of breast cancer. The four basic subtypes include luminal

TABLE 45.19 Nottingham Scoring System

Nuclear Pleomorphism	Score
Small regular uniform cells	1
Moderate nuclear size and variation	2
Marked nuclear variation	3

Mitotic Count	Score
0–9 mitoses/10 HPF	1
10–19 mitoses/10 HPF	2
20 or > mitoses/10 HPF	3

Tubule Formation	Score
Majority of tumor (>75%)	1
Moderate degree (10%–75%)	2
Little or none (<10%)	3

Grading	Score
Low grade	3–5
Intermediate grade	6–7
High grade	8–9

A, luminal B, HER2, and basal-like. The subtypes have different patterns of gene expression, behavior, and response to therapy. Identification of subtypes can be beneficial in guiding therapy decisions and lead to individualized or personalized treatment.

Luminal A and B cancers have high rates of hormone receptor expression and improved prognosis. Together, they account for approximately 70% of all breast cancers. Both show high response rates to endocrine therapy, with luminal A demonstrating a slightly higher response. Luminal B has higher rates of response to cytotoxic chemotherapy.

HER2 cancers have higher rates of HER2 expression and are less likely to have estrogen (ER) and progesterone receptors (PR). They account for 15% of all breast cancers. Higher response rates are seen with combination of anthracycline-based chemotherapy with trastuzumab (Herceptin, Genentech, San Francisco, CA). Basal-like cancers are also known as "triple-negative" cancers and do not express ER, PR, or HER2 genes. They account for 15% of breast cancers and have a poorer prognosis than do the other three subtypes. This phenotype is most often seen in BRCA1 mutation–associated cancers and also is more common in the African American population.

Staging

Staging allows for assessment of extent of disease and correlates with the individual's prognosis. Clinical and pathologic assessment of the tumor (T), regional lymph nodes (N), and the presence of metastatic (M) disease allow for stage assignment. The American Joint Commission on Cancer determines the current TNM staging system. The latest addition was issued in 2009 and takes into account sentinel node evaluation and extent of involvement; it also downstaged the supraclavicular node metastasis from M1 to N3 disease. Stage is assigned after surgery and comprehensive pathologic review. For patients receiving preoperative chemotherapy, clinical staging is assigned until surgery can be accomplished. When surgery is completed, a "y" prefix is used with the TNM assignment. See Tables 45.20 and 45.21 for the most recent staging guidelines.

TABLE 45.20 American Joint Committee on Cancer: Breast Cancer Staging

Definition of TNM

Primary Tumor (T)

Definitions for classifying the primary tumor (T) are the same for clinical and for pathologic classification. If the measurement is made by physical examination, the examiner will use the major headings (T1, T2, or T3). If other measurements, such as mammographic or pathologic measurements, are used, the subsets of T1 can be used. Tumors should be measured to the nearest 0.1-cm increment.

TX	Primary tumor cannot be assessed.
T0	No evidence of primary tumor
Tis	Carcinoma in situ
Tis (DCIS)	Ductal carcinoma in situ
Tis (LCIS)	Lobular carcinoma in situ
Tis (Paget's)	Paget disease of the nipple NOT associated with invasive carcinoma and/or carcinoma in situ (DCIS and/or LCIS) in the underlying breast parenchyma. Carcinomas in the breast parenchyma associated with Paget disease are categorized based on the size and characteristics of the parenchymal disease, although the presence of Paget disease should still be noted.
T1	Tumor ≤20 mm or less in greatest dimension
T1mi	Tumor ≤1 mm in greatest dimension
T1a	Tumor >1 mm but ≤5 mm in greatest dimension
T1b	Tumor >5 mm but ≤10 mm in greatest dimension
T1c	Tumor >10 mm but ≤20 mm in greatest dimension
T2	Tumor >20 mm but ≤50 mm in greatest dimension
T3	Tumor >50 mm in greatest dimension
T4	Tumor of any size with direct extension to the chest wall and/or to skin (ulceration or skin nodules)
T4a	Extension to chest wall, not including only pectoralis muscle adherence/invasion
T4b	Ulceration and/or ipsilateral satellite nodules and/or edema (including peau d'orange) of the skin, which do not meet the criteria for inflammatory carcinoma
T4c	Both T4a and T4b
T4d	Inflammatory carcinoma

Regional Lymph Nodes/Clinical

NX	Regional lymph nodes cannot be assessed (e.g., previously removed).
N0	No regional lymph node metastasis
N1	Metastasis to movable ipsilateral level I, II axillary lymph nodes(s)
N2	Metastases in ipsilateral level I and II axillary lymph nodes that are clinically fixed or matted, or in clinically detected[a] ipsilateral internal mammary nodes in the absence of clinically evident lymph node metastases
N2a	Metastasis in ipsilateral level I and II axillary lymph nodes fixed to one another (matted) or to other structures
N2b	Metastasis only in clinically detected[a] ipsilateral internal mammary nodes and in the absence of clinically evident level I and II axillary lymph node metastasis
N3	Metastases in ipsilateral infraclavicular (level III axillary) lymph node(s) with or without level I and II axillary lymph node involvement, or in clinically detected[a] ipsilateral internal mammary lymph node(s) with clinically evident level I and II axillary lymph node metastases, or metastases in ipsilateral supraclavicular lymph node(s) with or without axillary or internal mammary lymph node involvement
N3a	Metastasis in ipsilateral infraclavicular lymph node(s)
N3b	Metastasis in ipsilateral internal mammary lymph node(s) and axillary lymph node(s)
N3c	Metastasis in ipsilateral supraclavicular lymph node(s)

VIII

(Continued)

TABLE 45.20 American Joint Committee on Cancer: Breast Cancer Staging *(Continued)*

Pathologic (PN)[b]

pNX	Regional lymph nodes cannot be assessed (e.g., previously removed or not removed for pathologic study).
pN0	No regional lymph node metastasis identified histologically

Note: Isolated tumor cells clusters (ITCs) are defined as small clusters of cells not greater than 0.2 mm, or single tumor cells, or a cluster of fewer than 200 cells in a single histologic cross section. ITCs may be detected by routine histology or by immunohistochemical (IHC) methods. Nodes containing only ITCs are excluded from the total positive node count for purposes of N classification but should be included in the total number of nodes evaluated.

pN0(i-)	No regional lymph node metastasis histologically, negative IHC
pN0(i+)	Malignant cells in regional lymph node(s) not greater than 0.2 mm (detected by H&E or IHC including ITC)
pN0(mol-)	No regional lymph node metastasis histologically, negative molecular findings (RT-PCR)
pN0(mol+)	Positive molecular findings (RT-PCR), but no regional lymph node metastases detected by histology or IHC
pN1	Micrometastases, or metastases in 1–3 axillary lymph nodes, and/or in internal mammary nodes with metastases detected by SLNB but not clinically detected[c]
pN1mi	Micrometastases (>0.2 mm and/or more than 200 cells, but none >2.0 mm)
pN1a	Metastases in 1–3 axillary lymph nodes, at least one metastasis >2.0 mm
pN1b	Metastases in internal mammary nodes with micrometastases or macrometastases detected by SLNB but not clinically detected[c]
pN1c	Metastases in 1–3 axillary lymph nodes and in internal mammary lymph nodes with micrometastases or macrometastases detected by SLNB but not clinically detected
pN2	Metastases in 4–9 axillary lymph nodes, or in clinically detected[§] internal mammary lymph nodes in the absence of axillary lymph node metastases
pN2a	Metastases in 4–9 axillary lymph nodes (at least one tumor deposit >2.0 mm)
pN2b	Metastases in clinically detected[§] internal mammary lymph nodes in the absence of axillary lymph node metastases
pN3	Metastases in 10 or more axillary lymph nodes, or in infraclavicular (level III axillary) lymph nodes, or in clinically detected[§] ipsilateral internal mammary lymph nodes in the presence of one or more positive level I and II axillary lymph node(s), or in more than three axillary lymph nodes and in internal mammary lymph nodes with micrometastases or macrometastases detected by SLNB but not clinically detected,[c] or in ipsilateral supraclavicular lymph nodes
pN3a	Metastases in 10 or more axillary lymph nodes (at least one tumor deposit larger than 2.0 mm), or metastases to the infraclavicular (level III axillary) lymph nodes
pN3b	Metastases in clinically detected[§] ipsilateral internal mammary lymph nodes in the presence of one or more positive axillary lymph nodes, or in more than three axillary lymph nodes and in internal mammary lymph nodes with micrometastases or macrometastases detected by sentinel lymph node biopsy but not clinically detected[d]
pN3c	Metastasis in ipsilateral supraclavicular lymph nodes

Distant Metastasis (M)

M0	No clinical or radiographic evidence of distant metastases
cM0(i+)	No clinical or radiographic evidence of distant metastases, but deposits of molecularly or microscopically detected tumor cells in circulating blood, bone marrow, or other nonregional nodal tissue that are no larger than 0.2 mm in a patient without symptoms or signs of metastases
M1	Distant detectable metastases as determined by classic clinical and radiographic means and/or histologically proven larger than 0.2 mm

RT-PCR, reverse transcriptase polymerase chain reaction.

[a]Clinically detected is defined as detected by imaging studies (excluding lymphoscintigraphy) or by clinical examination and having characteristics highly suspicious for malignancy or a presumed pathologic macrometastasis based on fine needle aspiration biopsy with cytologic examination. Confirmation of clinically detected metastatic disease by fine needle aspiration without excision biopsy is designated with an (f) suffix, for example, cN3a(f). Excisional biopsy of a lymph node or biopsy of a sentinel node, in the absence of assignment of a pT, is classified as a clinical N, for example, cN1. Information regarding the confirmation of the nodal status will be designated in site-specific factors as clinical, fine needle aspiration, core biopsy, or sentinel lymph node biopsy. Pathologic classification (pN) is used for excision or sentinel lymph node biopsy only in connection with a pathologic T assignment.

[b]Classification is based on axillary lymph node dissection with or without sentinel lymph node biopsy. Classification based solely on sentinel lymph node biopsy without subsequent axillary lymph node dissection is designated (sn) for "sentinel node," for example, pN0(sn).

[c]"Not clinically detected" is defined as not detected by imaging studies (excluding lymphoscintigraphy) or by clinical examination.

[d]"Clinically detected" is defined as detected by imaging studies (excluding lymphoscintigraphy) or by clinical examination and having characteristics highly suspicious for malignancy or a presumed pathologic macrometastasis based on fine needle aspiration biopsy with cytologic examination.

Reprinted from Edge SB, Byrd D, Compton CC, et al. *AJCC cancer staging manual.* New York, NY: Springer; 2009, with permission. Copyright 2009 Springer-Verlag New York, Inc.

TABLE 45.21 Stage by Tumor, Node, Metastasis (TNM)

STAGE	TNM
0	Tis, N0, M0
I	T1,[a] N0, M0
IIA	T0, N1, M0 T1,[a] N1, M0 T2, N0, M0
IIB	T2, N1, M0 T3, N0, M0
IIIA	T0, N2, M0 T1,[a] N2, M0 T2, N2, M0 T3, N1, M0 T3, N2, M0
IIIB	T4, N0, M0 T4, N1, M0 T4, N2, M0
IIIC[b]	Any T, N3, M0
IV	Any T, any N, M1

[a]T1 includes T1mic.
[b]Stage IIIC breast cancer includes patients with any T stage who have pN3 disease. Patients with pN3a and pN3b disease are considered operable and are managed as described in the section on stage I, II, IIIA, and operable IIIC breast cancer. Patients with pN3c disease are considered inoperable and are managed as described in the section on inoperable stage IIIB or IIIC or inflammatory breast cancer.
Reprinted from Edge SB, Byrd D, Compton CC, et al. *AJCC cancer staging manual.* New York, NY: Springer; 2009, with permission. Copyright 2009 Springer-Verlag New York, Inc.

The majority of patients are diagnosed with stage I disease, followed in frequency by stages II and 0. Table 45.22 lists stage distribution at the time of diagnosis.

TABLE 45.22 Breast Cancer Stage at Diagnosis, 2010

STAGE	CASES	PERCENTAGE
0	41,708	20.6%
I	82,245	40.6%
II	48,021	23.7%
III	17,285	8.5%
IV	7,819	3.9%
	202,675[a]	18% of cancer diagnoses

[a]Includes 5,579 cases not assigned stage.
Data from American College of Surgeons, The National Cancer Data Base (NCDB), http://www.facs.org/cancer/ncdb/

TABLE 45.23 5-Year Survival Rate by Stage

STAGE	5-YEAR SURVIVAL
0	96%
I	92.1%
IIA	85.3%
IIB	74%
IIIA	67%
IIIB	41%
IIIC	49%
IV	20.9%

Data from American College of Surgeons, The National Cancer Data Base (NCDB) for patients diagnosed with breast cancer between 2003 and 2005 http://www.facs.org/cancer/ncdb; Surgeons CoCotACo. National Cancer Data Base Benchmark Reports. 2003–2005; cromwell.facs.org/BMarks/BMCmp/ver10/Docs/. Accessed March 18, 2013.

Prognosis

Survival rates after the diagnosis of breast cancer are dependent on a number of factors, including age at diagnosis, stage, molecular subtype of the tumor, medical comorbidities, and performance status. A patient diagnosed with stage 0 (DCIS) has virtually a 100% likelihood of survival from the disease. As the stage of the disease advances, the likelihood of recurrence increases and overall and disease-free survival decreases. Lymph node status (reflected in stage) is the most significant prognostic factor. Table 45.23 lists stage and survival rates. Figure 45.36 demonstrates Kaplan-Meir survival curves by stage.

BREAST CANCER MANAGEMENT

Clinical Presentation

Patients with DCIS are generally without symptoms. The majority of patients are diagnosed with percutaneous biopsy after an abnormal mammogram. If the disease is palpable, there is a high likelihood of associated invasive cancer. Paget disease with its associated nipple areolar erythema and crusting may be an indicator of the presence of this disease process.

Fortunately, the majority of invasive breast cancer is now found on screening mammography without palpable evidence of disease; however, due to mammographic screening failures, rapidly growing disease, or lack of access to the health care system, patients sometimes present with clinical evidence of disease. A patient may present with an irregularly shaped mass with a firm consistency, fixed in position to surrounding tissue, and associated dimpling or retraction of the overlying skin and/or nipple. In advanced disease, peau d'orange skin changes occur due to obstruction of the dermal lymphatics (Fig. 45.37).

In general, breast cancer is slightly more common in the left breast than in the right. In most women, the left breast is slightly larger than the right. The upper outer quadrant is more frequently involved in malignant changes (this is the site of the highest distribution of breast tissue), with the central and subareolar regions being second (Table 45.17).

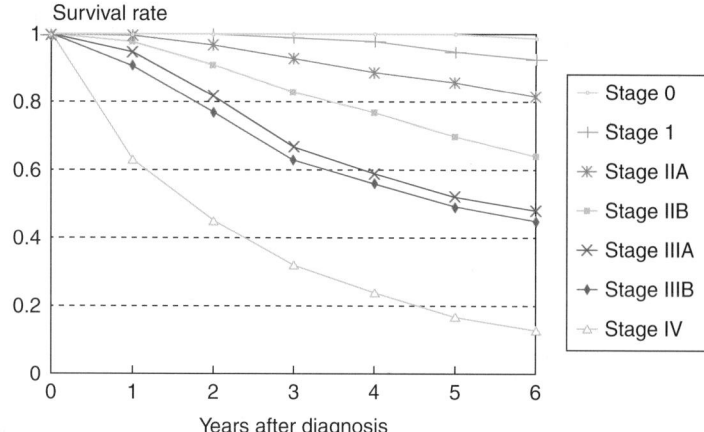

FIGURE 45.36 Kaplan-Meir survival curve by stage of breast cancer.

Management of Ductal Carcinoma In Situ

This category represents 20% of all newly diagnosed breast cancers and has a 20-year survival rate of 97%. In at least 90% of patients, the diagnosis is made with mammography. Approximately 10% of patients have a palpable mass. Comprehensive management includes a detailed history and physical examination, bilateral diagnostic mammography, pathology review, and ascertainment of hormone receptor status. A detailed family history can help identify patients who are at high risk for genetic mutations or family cancer syndromes. MRI is recommended for high-grade DCIS and in patients with dense breasts that preclude accurate assessment of disease extent. For patients in whom accelerated partial breast irradiation (APBI) is being considered, MRI is used at our institution to identify individuals with large volume disease and those with multifocal disease who would be ineligible for this treatment.

DCIS is usually identified on mammogram and presents as an area of pleomorphic, clustered calcifications. Linear calcifications tracking toward the nipple are virtually diagnostic for the entity. Percutaneous core biopsy is the most common method to confirm the diagnosis. At the time of surgical excision, associated invasive cancer is found in 25% of specimens and is more common when the DCIS is palpable.

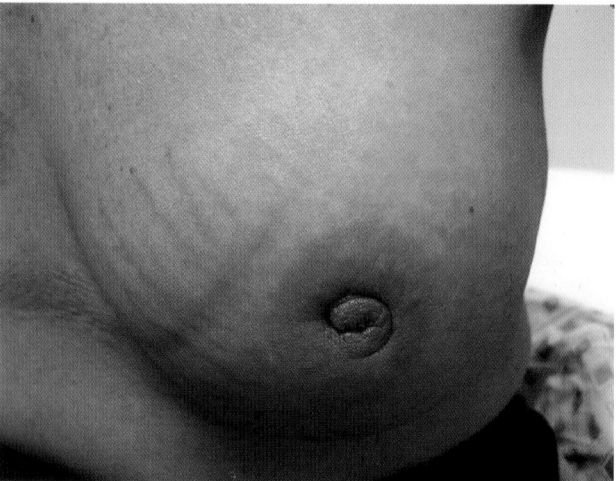

FIGURE 45.37 Inflammatory breast cancer. A 56-year-old who presented with a 2-week history of breast erythema and edema. There is visible nipple inversion from the underlying mass. Marked edema and peau d'orange are visible. (Courtesy of Emilia Diego, MD, University of Pittsburgh School of Medicine, Pittsburgh, PA.)

Surgical management for unifocal disease is surgical excision with a wide margin. Providing free margins are obtained, the patient is eligible for breast-conserving treatment. Whole breast radiation has been demonstrated to decrease local recurrence rate. In women 50 years of age or younger, a boost to the surgical bed is the traditional approach. No difference in overall survival occurs in patients treated with breast conservation and radiation compared to those treated with mastectomy. In the National Surgical Adjuvant Breast and Bowel Project (NSABP) B-17 study, patients with DCIS were randomly assigned to lumpectomy alone or lumpectomy with radiation therapy. For the radiation-treated cohort, the study demonstrated a 52% reduction in ipsilateral breast tumor recurrence rates. Additionally, the majority of the recurrences were DCIS. In patients treated with lumpectomy alone, recurrences were more common and evenly divided between invasive and in situ disease. The addition of radiation decreases both recurrence rate and invasive disease compared to patients treated with surgery alone.

Retrospective data suggest that radiation therapy is not warranted in all patients treated with breast-conserving surgery. Predictors for recurrence include grade and margin width. Attempts have been made to identify a subset of patients who can avoid postoperative radiotherapy. One such group appears to be those with low- or intermediate-grade lesions smaller than 2 cm with more than 1-cm margins. Margin width appears to be the single most prognostic factor for local recurrence; however, no clear definitions of margin adequacy exist. In reviewing the literature, the range of adequate margins is reported from larger than 1 mm up to 10 mm. Wider margins are associated with poorer cosmetic outcome.

The NSABP B-24 study assessed the role of tamoxifen therapy in patients with DCIS. The use of tamoxifen was associated with a 3.2% absolute reduction in ipsilateral breast tumor recurrence and a decreased incidence of contralateral cancer. The benefit in reducing ipsilateral tumor recurrence was restricted to patients with ER-positive DCIS, but the reduction in contralateral breast cancer was seen regardless of receptor status.

For patients with DCIS that is not amenable to breast conservation, total mastectomy with or without reconstruction is advised. Breast conservation surgery may not be feasible when lesions are multicentric (two or more foci of disease in different quadrants) and multifocal (two or more foci within the same quadrant) and cover a wide expanse such that the margins cannot be achieved or if a poor cosmetic outcome is likely. It is our practice to perform concurrent sentinel lymph node mapping at the time of mastectomy in event invasive cancer is found on final pathology analysis. Given the pathways of lymph drainage are altered by mastectomy, if sentinel lymph node evaluation was not performed, the finding of invasive cancer will obligate the patient to undergo an axillary dissection.

Invasive Breast Cancer Management

As recently as three decades ago, the management of breast cancer relied on local–regional treatments to achieve the best chance for cure. Surgical therapy consisted of radical mastectomy and the use of radiation therapy in a select subset of patients. The notion that radical local regional therapy was the key to preventing systemic failure has been challenged through the use of clinical trials proposing less radical surgery and focusing on the role of adjuvant therapy at diagnosis to treat occult metastatic disease and was a focus of an NIH consensus conference.

Today, all patients diagnosed with breast cancer are approached with multimodal therapy. When possible, breast-conserving surgery combined with radiation therapy has achieved equivalent outcomes to mastectomy in terms of local–regional control and overall survival. The use of adjuvant endocrine and chemotherapy has improved both disease-free and overall survival.

In patients with more advanced disease, multimodal therapy has proven beneficial. Again, the traditional approach of using radical local–regional therapy has been altered through clinical trials. The combination of surgery, radiation therapy, and adjuvant therapy has improved outcomes. Altering the traditional order of therapy to allow for upfront endocrine and/or cytotoxic chemotherapy can often allow a patient destined for mastectomy to undergo a breast-conserving surgery instead.

As knowledge has advanced and molecular profiling of tumors has become available, treatment based on subtypes and specific targets has altered recurrence rates. Genomic testing has come of age and allowed for risk stratification and individualization of treatment based on analysis of the tumor genome.

Comprehensive management includes a detailed history, family history, and physical examination. Evaluation should include bilateral diagnostic mammography, pathology review, and ascertainment of hormone receptor and HER2 status. A detailed family history can help identify patients who are at high risk for genetic mutations or family cancer syndromes. Chest radiograph and liver chemistries should be performed to assess for metastatic spread of disease. Patients with abnormal liver function assessment should have directed imaging with either hepatic ultrasound or abdominal CT scan. For patients in whom surgical management is contemplated, preoperative blood tests can be obtained including complete blood count, electrolytes, renal function, and coagulation profile. Patients who present with symptoms suggesting bone involvement should undergo a radionuclide bone scan (bone scintigraphy) or directed plain film radiographs. No role exists for routine use of bone scan, CT scan, PET–CT scan, or tumor markers.

MRI is optional and if performed should be on a machine with a dedicated breast coil. Patients who appear to benefit for MRI assessment are those with dense breasts in whom suspicion for disease extent is not adequately assessed on diagnostic mammography and/or ultrasound, in whom involved axillary nodes and a suspicion of an occult breast primary tumor exists, and in patients with known BRCA1/BRCA2 deleterious mutations for whom breast conservation is being considered. For patients deemed candidates for APBI, MRI can be helpful in assessing multicentric or multifocal disease that would preclude the technique. MRI detects contralateral breast disease in approximately 3% of patients with normal clinical and mammographic examinations. The finding of multicentric/multifocal disease is more common and found in some studies to be 15%. MRI is highly sensitive but not specific; therefore, patients should not be deemed ineligible for breast-conserving surgery without tissue confirmation of multiquadrant involvement.

For patients with locally advanced tumors, preoperative chemotherapy is a reasonable approach. Prior to initiating treatment, the site should be marked with a localization clip in event a complete clinical response is achieved. Radiographic imaging before and after induction therapy should be obtained to document objective response. For patients with ER-, PR-, and HER2-negative (basal-like or "triple-negative") tumors, preoperative therapy regardless of tumor size is a reasonable approach given its aggressive nature.

Axillary assessment with ultrasound is reasonable in patients with clinically negative nodes to identify patients who would not meet the criteria for sentinel lymph node mapping.

SURGICAL MANAGEMENT OF BREAST CANCER

Breast Conservation Surgery

Breast conservation is the favored mode of management of early breast cancer. The march toward breast conservation took almost 100 years. Several sentinel randomized studies demonstrated similar survival outcomes in patients treated with radical mastectomy, total mastectomy, and breast-conserving surgery. A leader in the field of breast cancer care has been Dr. Bernard Fisher and the National Surgical Adjuvant Breast and Bowel Project cooperative group. The NSABP B-4 study randomly assigned over 1,500 patients based on nodal status to radical mastectomy, total mastectomy with postoperative chest wall and axillary radiation, or total mastectomy for patients with clinically negative nodes at diagnosis. For patients with clinically involved lymph nodes, randomization was between radical mastectomy and total mastectomy with postoperative chest wall and axillary radiation. With 72 months of follow-up, no difference in overall survival or distant recurrence was noted. For patients not treated with axillary dissection, 16% demonstrated subsequent disease in this region and were managed with delayed axillary dissection. This landmark study was first published in 1977 and has had interim reports, the latest in 2002 with 25 years of follow-up demonstrating no difference in overall and disease-free survival. Advancing on this study, NSABP B-6 compared total mastectomy to lumpectomy with or without radiation. Entry criteria were restricted to early-stage disease with tumor size less than 4 cm, free margins in the case of lumpectomy, and patients with involved lymph nodes. All patients underwent an axillary dissection. Patients with node involvement received postoperative chemotherapy (melphalan and 5-fluorouracil). Overall survival and disease-free survival were equivalent in all arms of the study, demonstrating equivalency to breast removal. Concurrently, Veronesi and colleagues at the Milan Cancer Institute published their results on quadrantectomy and postoperative radiation therapy, demonstrating similar overall survival to patients treated with radical mastectomy. The procedure involved excision of the overlying skin and the involved quadrant of the breast.

Breast conservation surgery employs the use of wide local excision of the tumor with a margin of normal-appearing breast tissue. Various terms, including "lumpectomy," "tumorectomy," or "segmental mastectomy," have been used to describe the procedure. Multiple studies have demonstrated equivalency to total or radical mastectomy. Table 45.24 lists

TABLE 45.24 Prospective Randomized Trials Comparing BCS/RT with Mastectomy

TRIAL	TX PERIOD	N	STAGE	SURGERY	OS % BCS/R (P VALUE)	OS % MASTECTOMY	DFS % BCS/R (P-VALUE)	DFS % MASTECTOMY	ADJUVANT TX
Milan Cancer Inst. Trial I[3]	1973–1980	701	I	Quadrantectomy, rad. mastectomy	65 (NS)	65	NA	NA	CMF
Institut Gustave-Roussy	1972–1980	179	I	Wide excision, mod. rad. mast.	73 (0.19)	65	NA	NA	None
NSABP B-6	1976–1984	1,219	I–II	Wide excision, mod. rad. mast.	63 (0.12)	59	50 (0.21)	49	Melphalan, 5 FU
NCI	1979–1987	237	I–II	Local excision, mod. rad. mast.	77 (0.89)	75	72 (0.93)	69	AC
EORTC	1980–1986	874	I–II	Local excision, mod. rad. mast.	54 (NS)	61	NA	NA	CMF
Danish Breast Cancer Group	1983–1989	904	I–III	Quadrantectomy, wide excision, mod. rad. mast.	79 (NS)	82	70 (NS)	66	CMF, T

CMF, cyclophosphamide, methotrexate, and 5-fluorouracil; AC, doxorubicin and cyclophosphamide; T, tamoxifen; EORTC, European Organization for Research and Treatment of Cancer; NSABP, National Surgical Adjuvant Breast and Bowel Project.
Adapted from Winchester DP, Cox JD. Standards for diagnosis and management of invasive breast cancer. CA *Cancer J Clin* 1998:48:83–107, with permission. Published by and John Wiley and Sons. Copyright © 1998 American Cancer Society.

trials that compared breast-conserving surgery and radiation to mastectomy. Interestingly, each trial had a different definition of margins. Many studies specified a 1- to 2-cm minimal margin, whereas the NSABP trials required only "enough normal tissue removed to ensure that the specimen margins were tumor-free."

Breast-conserving surgery relies on the use of radiation therapy to reduce in-breast recurrences. In patients treated with lumpectomy alone, ipsilateral breast tumor recurrence rates were 40% compared to 14% in patients treated with breast conservation and postoperative radiation. Radiotherapeutic approaches are described in the next section of this chapter.

Contraindications to BCS can be classified as absolute and relative. When the concept of breast conservation was first introduced, absolute contraindications were numerous. As an understanding of the pathophysiology of the disease became apparent, and techniques of radiation therapy and neoadjuvant therapy improved, the use of breast-conserving surgery has become feasible in the majority of patients. Table 45.25 lists proposed absolute and relative contraindications.

Partial Mastectomy/Lumpectomy

Partial mastectomy/lumpectomy is the surgical technique employed most often for a known diagnosis of breast cancer. It involves the removal of a portion of the breast containing the known cancer along with additional 1 to 2 cm of normal-appearing breast tissue surrounding the lesion. The terms tumorectomy or segmental mastectomy are often used interchangeably for this procedure. Although varying definitions exist for segmental mastectomy, the description should be reserved for when one or more of the 12 to 16 segments of the breast are excised. Quadrantectomy involves removal of a full quarter of the breast in which the cancer is located (the initial description also included the overlying skin).

Surgical approach in partial mastectomy/lumpectomy is similar to excisional biopsy and is performed with or without a localization procedure. The incision site and size is chosen based on the location of the lesion. Care should be taken to choose existing skin lines (Langer) to achieve the best cosmetic outcome. The surgeon envisions the location by reviewing the radiographs and removes a margin of normal tissue around the cancer. The specimen is then carefully oriented in case additional margins are required. The pectoral fascia should be left intact whenever possible because exposure of the pectoral muscle causes the remaining breast tissue to adhere and cause dimpling of the overlying skin. It is important to assess margins while the surgical site is still open. If a radiographic localization took place, a specimen radiograph in two

TABLE 45.26 Protocol for Pathology Margin Assessment

PROCEDURE	MARGIN	COLOR
Excisional biopsy Segmental mastectomy	Anterior	Orange
	Posterior	Black
	Medial	Blue
	Lateral	Yellow
	Superior	Red
	Inferior	Green
Mastectomy	Anterior	Orange
	Inner upper quadrant	Black
	Inner lower quadrant	Blue
	Outer lower quadrant	Red
	Outer upper quadrant	Green

planes can provide margin information. Additionally, pathologic inspection of the margins should occur. The surgeon should communicate pertinent information to the pathologist, including the clinical size of the tumor, number of tumors, location, whether preoperative therapy was employed, and orientation of the specimen. Orientation is achieved by the use of a Margin Map® (Beekley Corp, Bristol, CT) or placement of sutures following protocol: long suture lateral, short suture superior, medium suture medial, and double sutures for the deep margin. The specimen is then inked with different colors for each margin to aid in microscopic assessment (Table 45.26). The specimen is divided in 1-cm intervals and the tumor and margins assessed. If any margin appears to be compromised, it is advantageous to excise additional margin at this point, as it will obviate the need for a second surgery. Aesthetic outcome is best if only one procedure is performed. Percutaneous drains should be avoided to prevent cosmetic deformity (Fig. 45.38).

Total Mastectomy

This procedure is performed in patients with multifocal DCIS, margin involvement after breast-conserving therapy for either DCIS or invasive cancer, or as risk-reducing surgery for genetic predisposition or LCIS. The initial approach can be either an

TABLE 45.25 Contraindications to Breast Conservation

Absolute
Multicentric disease
Diffuse, malignant-appearing calcifications
Inability to achieve clean margins around the tumor
Prior breast conservation surgery and radiation

Relative
Tumor to breast ratio unfavorable
Collagen vascular disease
Prior breast radiation (i.e., Hodgkin lymphoma mantle radiation)
Pregnancy

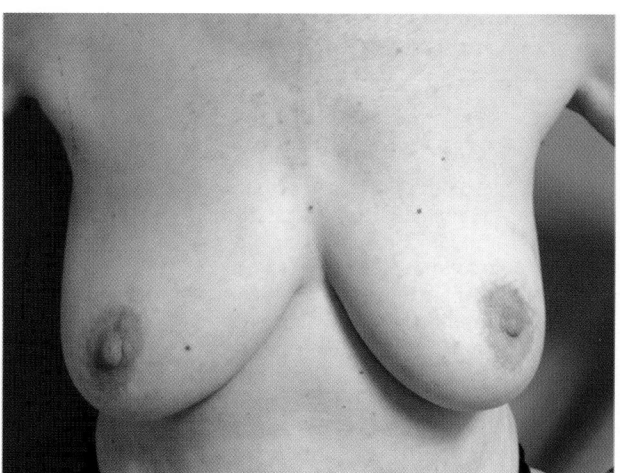

FIGURE 45.38 A 52-year-old stage I (T1, N0, M0) invasive ductal cancer status post left breast–conserving surgery and sentinel mapping.

VIII

elliptical skin paddle or circumareolar incision. The dissection separates the superficial fascia of the breast from the skin. The surgeon dissects superiorly to the clavicle, laterally to the latissimus dorsi muscle, inferiorly to the inframammary fold, and medially to the sternal border. The pectoralis fascia can be removed at the same time, but no attempt is made to remove the axillary lymph nodes. A single closed suction drain is placed, and the wound is closed using subcuticular sutures. The operation can be combined with immediate reconstruction and sentinel lymph node mapping. If an axillary dissection is performed, the operation is properly termed a modified radical mastectomy. (See Steps in the Procedure.)

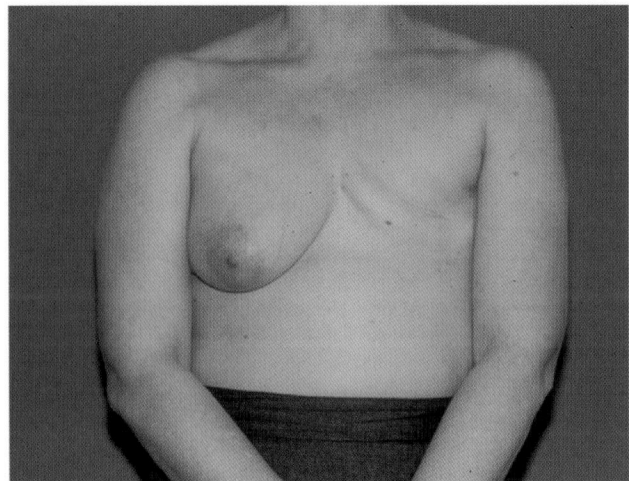

FIGURE 45.39 A 61-year-old with stage II (T2, N1, M0) invasive lobular cancer. The disease was multifocal, and she underwent a modified radical mastectomy. Note there is no chest wall deformity and the pectoralis major muscle adds definition to the shoulder.

STEPS IN THE PROCEDURE

Mastectomy

- This procedure is done under general anesthesia.

- This can be combined with sentinel lymphatic mapping, axillary dissection, and/or immediate breast reconstruction.

- For a skin-sparing procedure, the preferred incision is made around the nipple–areolar complex (NAC); otherwise, an elliptical incision is made to encompass the (NAC) and the surrounding skin to allow for closure of the skin without having skin tags (incision length should be twice the length of the width).

- Dissection takes place using sharp dissection or an electrocoagulation device. The superficial fascia of the breast is separated from the skin.

- Borders of the dissection include the clavicle, the inframammary fold, the sternal border, and the latissimus dorsi.

- The breast is released by separating the pectoralis fascia from the muscle.

- The specimen is oriented to allow for margin assessment.

- The wound is made hemostatic with either sutures or electrocoagulation.

- A closed suction drain is placed in the operative bed.

- The wound is then closed in two layers with subcuticular sutures.

Modified Radical Mastectomy

Originally described by Patey and Dyson, modified radical mastectomy involved a total mastectomy with preservation of the pectoralis major muscle but removal of the pectoralis minor muscle to allow for access to all three levels of axillary nodes. This modification maintained the contour of the thorax. The current modification of Patey's procedure is dividing the origin of the muscle at the insertion of the coracoid process. The modern modified radical mastectomy was further refined by Madden and colleagues, who reported on the preservation of both the pectoralis major and minor muscles.

The operation involves an elliptical skin incision incorporating the nipple–areolar complex (**Fig. 45.39**). To avoid the appearance of excess tissue also known as a "dog ear," the length of the incision should be double the width at the level

of the nipple–areolar complex. A flap is developed between the superficial fascia of the breast and the overlying skin. Flaps that are too thin will develop skin necrosis leading to infection and wound separation. Flaps that are too thick will predispose the patient to local recurrence as a result of residual breast tissue. The flaps are developed superiorly to the clavicle, medially to the sternal border, inferiorly to the insertion of the rectus muscle, laterally to the latissimus dorsi muscle, and posteriorly to the pectoralis fascia. The fascia is removed en bloc with the breast. Laterally, the dissection extends to axillary basin. The fat pad located between the pectoralis major and minor muscle and the latissimus dorsi contains the node-bearing tissue. The dissection continues along the latissimus dorsi until the axillary vein is encountered. The axillary vein is the superior border of the node dissection. Located above this vein are the nerves of the brachial plexus; injury to these structures can occur if the operator is too zealous in his or her approach. Care is taken to preserve as many intercostal brachial nerves as possible as they traverse the axillary fat pad. The surgeon must identify and preserve the thoracodorsal neurovascular complex to the latissimus dorsi. The vascular components are best preserved, as they can be utilized during free flap reconstruction. Additionally, the long thoracic nerve to the serratus anterior muscle is identified on the chest wall and preserved. Injury to the nerve leads to the appearance of a winged scapula. Finally, care is taken to identify the medial pectoral nerve as it courses along the lateral border of the pectoralis minor muscle. Injury to the nerve will cause denervation of the lateral portion of the pectoralis major muscle and lead atrophy and the appearance of loss of the muscle along the thorax. During the course of the dissection, the pectoralis muscles are elevated and the level II nodes are excised. Hemostasis is obtained by the use of electrocoagulation, clips, or individual suture ties. This completes the dissection.

The specimen is removed and oriented with a long suture for the lateral extent and a short suture for the superior margin. The pathologists then ink the specimen according to a protocol to help assess margin status on histopathologic assessment (Table 45.26). After obtaining hemostasis, one or two closed suction drains are placed to prevent seroma formation in the mastectomy bed and axillary basin and to allow for the skin to adhere to the underlying tissues. The wound is then closed using

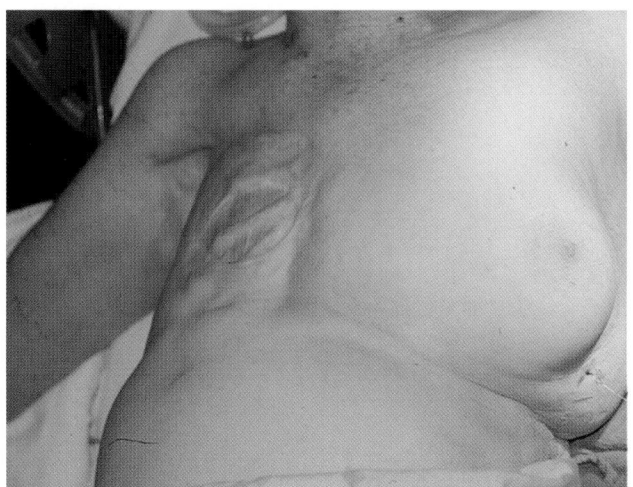

FIGURE 45.40 Patient treated with radical mastectomy and the use of a skin graft. Note the loss of chest wall and shoulder definition. The patient's ribs are also visualized.

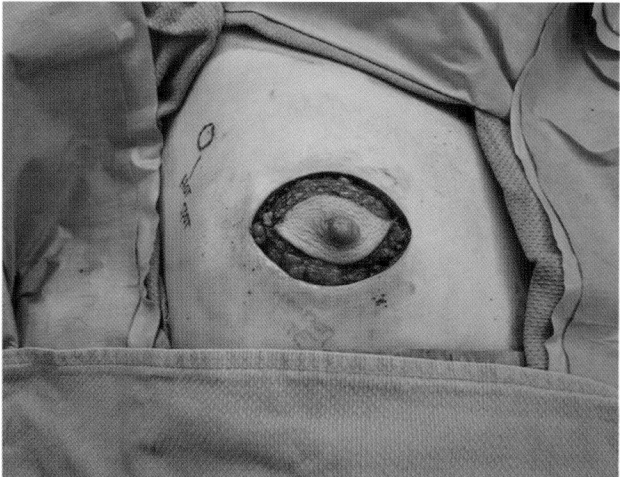

FIGURE 45.41 Circumareolar incision for skin-sparing mastectomy.

a two-layer subcuticular closure, skin staples, or a single-layer barbed suture such as the V-loc (Covidien, Mansfield, MA).

Radical Mastectomy

The radical mastectomy was the standard treatment for breast cancer for almost 100 years. Dr. William Halsted theorized that breast cancer spread in an orderly, stepwise manner from the breast via intervening lymphatics to the axillary lymph nodes and then finally to distant sites. His surgical approach was directed toward local–regional control by removing en bloc the breast, the pectoralis muscles, and the regional lymph nodes (Fig. 45.40). In 1894, he reported his results on 50 patients treated in this manner. Overall, a 6% local recurrence rate occurred, compared to known rates of 50% and no operative mortality. Considered the father of modern surgery, Halsted developed several tenets of surgery that improved surgical outcome. Halsted's tenets of surgery are listed in Table 45.27. In the same year, Meyer reported his experience with the radical mastectomy at his institution, echoing the findings of Halsted. The operation fell out of favor as a better understanding of the pathophysiology of breast cancer became evident.

In 1895, Röntgen reported on the discovery of x-rays. In addition to aiding in diagnoses, it was discovered that x-rays served a role in the management and treatment of cancer. Over the ensuing decades, less radical or no surgery for breast cancer combined with radiation therapy was investigated and reported. By the mid-1980s, the use of radical mastectomy as primary surgical management for breast cancer was abandoned.

Skin-Sparing Mastectomy

Skin-sparing mastectomy is a modification of the total mastectomy. This technique involves removal of the nipple–areolar

complex with preservation of the majority of the skin that serves as an envelope for the underlying reconstruction. This technique can be employed with either prosthetic implant-based or autogenous tissue transfer reconstruction. Long-term follow-up has not demonstrated an increased rate of local–regional recurrence compared to the traditional non–skin-sparing mastectomy, hence allowing for an excellent cosmetic outcome without compromising oncologic principles or outcome (Figs. 45.41, 45.42, and 45.43).

Nipple-Sparing Mastectomy

An extension of the skin-sparing mastectomy is the nipple-sparing mastectomy. This procedure allows for preservation of the nipple, the areola, and the skin of the breast with concomitant removal of the underlying parenchyma. The procedure is gaining acceptance as an alternative to skin-sparing or non–skin-sparing mastectomy in the settings of prophylactic/risk-reducing surgery and in selective circumstances for treatment of breast cancer.

Original attempts at a nipple-sparing operation were popularized with the subcutaneous mastectomy; however,

TABLE 45.27 Halsted's Principles of Surgery
Gentle tissue handling
Meticulous hemostasis
Aseptic techniques—preop, op, and post-op
Preoperative, intra-operative, postoperative
Obliteration of dead space and tension-free closure
Deliberate surgical pace

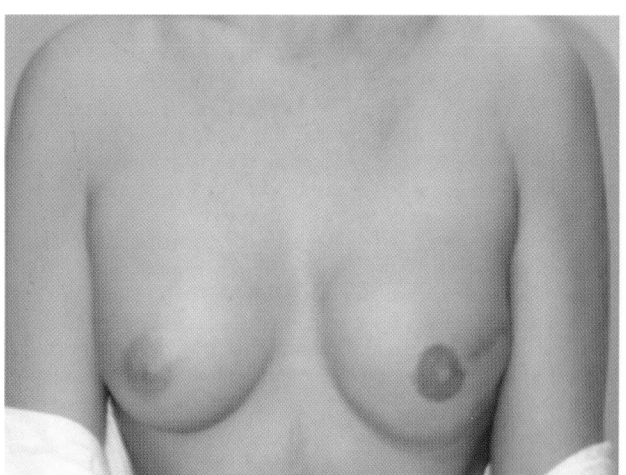

FIGURE 45.42 Left skin-sparing mastectomy with implant-based reconstruction. (Photo courtesy of Dr. Kenneth Shestak, University of Pittsburgh School of Medicine, Pittsburgh, PA.)

VIII

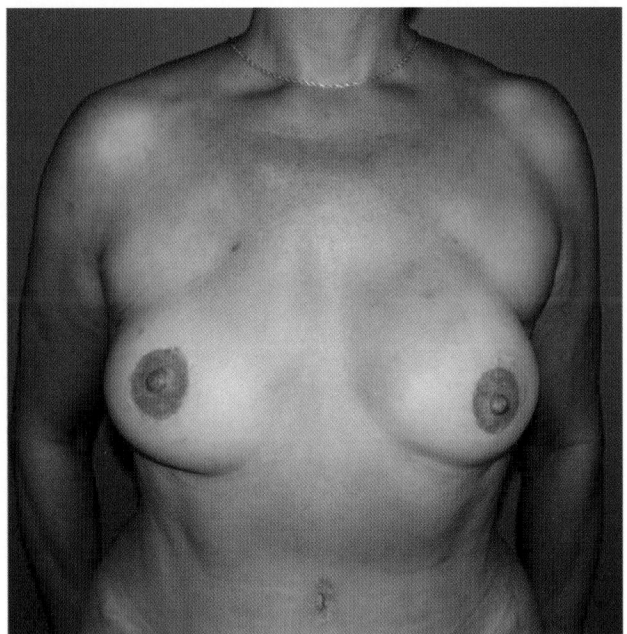

FIGURE 45.43 Bilateral skin-sparing mastectomy with autogenous tissue transfer (TRAM flap) and nipple–areolar reconstruction. (Photo courtesy of Dr. Kenneth Shestak, University of Pittsburgh School of Medicine, Pittsburgh, PA.)

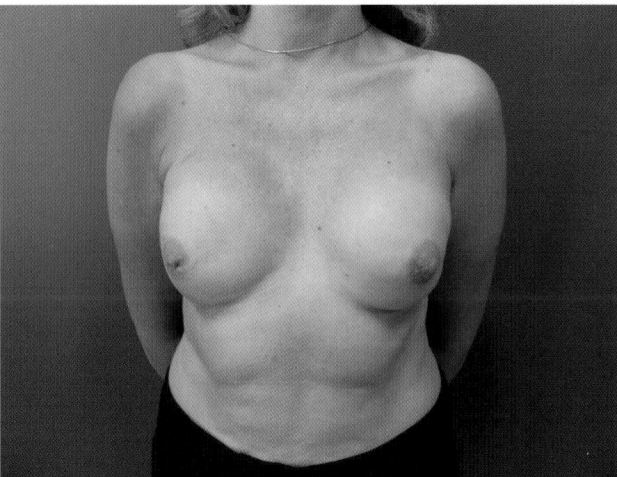

FIGURE 45.44 Bilateral nipple-sparing mastectomies with inframammary incisions. Acellular dermal matrix–assisted placement of tissue expanders and subsequent silicone gel breast implants with 2-year P.O. appearance. (Photo courtesy of Kenneth Shestak, MD, University of Pittsburgh School of Medicine, Pittsburgh, PA.)

the procedure was not optimal given high complication rates, limited reconstructive options, and retention of significant amounts of breast tissue. In 1999, a published report on the efficacy of prophylactic mastectomy in women with a family history of breast cancer reintroduced the concept of this approach. Subsequently, an additional report from the same institution demonstrated benefit in women with known BRCA mutations. Multiple reports have since demonstrated similar results. Varied surgical approaches exist, including the use of a periareolar incision with lateral extension, transareolar incision with medial or lateral extensions, inframammary incision (favored at our institution), and a lateral inframammary incision (Fig. 45.44).

Nipple-sparing mastectomy has been employed in patients as part of therapeutic management of a known breast cancer. General consensus is that the following criteria should be met in order to employ this technique: (a) the lesion should be 3 cm or less in size and at least 2 cm from the nipple–areolar complex, (b) clinically negative axillary nodes, (c) no evidence of skin involvement, and (d) preferably preoperative MRI imaging to rule out occult lesions. During the procedure, consideration should be given to obtaining a biopsy of the subareolar region to rule out occult spread.

If a patient meets oncologic criteria for risk-reducing or therapeutic mastectomy, an assessment should be made by the plastic surgeon with regard to role of nipple-sparing mastectomy. Patients with large and/or ptotic breasts are poor candidates for this operation. Common complications include flap necrosis, nipple–areolar necrosis, and loss of tactile sensation of the nipple.

Oncoplastic Breast Surgery

The use of a variety of techniques to maintain the volume, contour, and symmetry of the breast can be employed as part of breast-conserving surgery. As the name implies, it is used as part of the surgical treatment for breast cancer but also involves plastic surgery techniques to gain the optimum cosmetic outcome.

Patients with less than optimal tumor-to-breast ratios or large or ptotic breasts can have improved outcomes through wise choice of incisions, tissue rearrangement, and contouring of the contralateral breast. Partial mastectomy can result in marked volume reduction, dimpling, and nipple–areolar displacement. By employing these techniques, improved cosmetic results can be achieved. In some cases, muscle or myocutaneous flaps for partial reconstruction of the breast can be employed.

SENTINEL LYMPHATIC MAPPING

Sentinel node identification and lymphatic mapping had its genesis in other disease sites. In 1960, Gould and colleagues originally proposed the concept of a sentinel node for head and neck cancer in their description of the key node being identified at the junction of anterior and posterior veins of the neck. In gynecologic cancer, DiSaia and colleagues utilized the superficial inguinal lymph nodes as the "sentinel nodes" in the treatment of cancer of the vulva, to help identify patients who would not benefit from the more morbid complete lymphadenectomy. In the 1990s, Morton and colleagues described what is now modern lymphatic mapping in the treatment of melanoma in which a colloidal gold was used to identify the primary nodal basin drainage.

The premise of SLNB is that tumor cells from the primary lesion will migrate to one or a few lymph nodes prior to disseminating to others within the region. These key lymph nodes can be identified via the use of a vital blue dye (isosulfan blue/methylene blue) and/or a radiolabeled colloid. Key to the utilization of this technique is validation that identification of the sentinel lymph node accurately predicts the status of the remaining lymph nodes.

The status of the axillary lymph nodes is the strongest prognostic factor for breast cancer recurrence. As tumor size increases, so does the risk of metastatic disease to the lymph nodes. See Table 45.28. For patients with early-stage breast cancer and clinically negative nodes, sentinel lymphatic mapping has replaced axillary dissection as the standard of care. If suspicious nodes are detected on clinical or mammographic exam, ultrasound evaluation with percutaneous core biopsy or FNA can be performed. If an ultrasound reveals that lymph nodes are morphologically normal and/or core needle biopsy

TABLE 45.28 Tumor Size and Rates of Nodal Metastases

TUMOR SIZE	INCIDENCE OF NODAL SPREAD
Tis	0.8%
T1a	5%
T1b	16%
T1c	28%
T2	47%
T3	68%
T4	86%

Adapted from Weaver DL, Rosenberg RD, Barlow WE, et al. Pathologic findings from the Breast Cancer Surveillance Consortium: population-based outcomes in women undergoing biopsy after screening mammography. *Cancer* 2006;106(4): 732–742, with permission. Published by and John Wiley and Sons. Copyright © 1998 American Cancer Society.

or FNA is benign or indeterminate, sentinel lymphatic mapping should be employed.

A great benefit of this technique is that patients with uninvolved sentinel lymph nodes can avoid a completion axillary dissection and, hence, have a lower risk of upper extremity lymphedema. Two recent studies demonstrated the rate of lymphedema as a result of SLNB to be approximately 2% to 8% compared to 14% after SLNB and axillary dissection. Historically, rates as high as 40% have been reported.

For the treatment of breast cancer, this technique has been rapidly accepted and is now considered the standard approach for women with invasive or microinvasive breast cancer. It may also have applications in the treatment of DCIS when there is clinical concern for invasion or if the primary treatment will be mastectomy that then precludes a delayed SLNB procedure.

Sentinel lymph node identification is successful in more than 95% of surgical cases. The false-negative rate ranges from 5% to 10% as demonstrated in studies in which a completion axillary dissection was performed following SLNB. NSABP B-32 enrolled 5,611 patients with clinically negative nodes. Patients were randomly assigned to SLNB followed by axillary dissection to SLNB alone with axillary dissection performed in instances of SLNB involvement. SLNB detection rates were 97% with a 9.8% false-negative rate. No significant differences were noted in regard to overall and disease-free survival and importantly no difference in regional control. The later finding suggests that regional control is not achieved by surgical intervention alone, but rather adjuvant therapy is the key component of management. In NSABP B-4, in which one of the randomization arms was total mastectomy with or without postoperative chest wall and axillary radiation, approximately 16% of cancers recurred in the axilla and were managed by a delayed axillary dissection. No difference occurred in survival compared to individuals treated by modified radical mastectomy, suggesting axillary dissection does not improve outcomes in patients with clinically negative nodes.

A learning curve exists with this procedure. Improved detection rates are seen with increased experience of the surgeon. In the initial trials, recommendations were to perform 20 to 30 SLNBs with concurrent axillary dissection. Now that

SLNB is considered a standard approach and has been widely adopted, use of backup axillary dissection is not indicated. For surgeons just learning the technique, proctoring with an experienced colleague is advised.

Most institutions use both a visual blue dye and the radiocolloid technetium-99m to identify the sentinel node. More often, radiocolloid is more sensitive in identifying the sentinel node. The site of injection of the tracers has been extensively studied. Peritumoral, intraparenchymal, subdermal, subareolar, and intradermal all seem to have similar success.

Isosulfan blue (Lymphazurin, Covidien, Mansfield, MA) is approved for use in lymphatic mapping. It is a monosodium salt of 2,5-disulfonated triphenyl methane dye. It has a reported 1% incidence of allergic reactions including anaphylaxis. Alternative dyes include Patent Blue V dye (sodium salt of disulfonated triphenyl methane) and methylene blue (methylthioninium chloride). Patent Blue V dye is widely used outside of the United States and has reported allergic reaction rates of 0.2%.

Given a worldwide shortage of isosulfan blue dye in the early 2000s, methylene blue dye was studied and found to be an acceptable alternative. Dilution of methylene blue from full strength of 10 mg/mL to 1.25 mg/mL and giving the injection in the subareolar region was associated with the highest sentinel node detection rate (92%). Hypersensitivity reactions were rare, and the most frequent complication was skin necrosis, which occurred in 1.25% of patients and resolved in 4 of 5 patients without intervention. Allergic reactions to this drug are rare. Methylene blue injection is the drug of choice at our institution unless we are unable to discern radioactivity in the axilla prior to the surgery, in which circumstance, we use isosulfan blue dye.

At our institution, our preference is to perform the injections for sentinel lymphatic mapping in the operating room. This requires additional training of the surgeon to assure adequate technique and radiation training for patient and operating room personnel safety. After induction of anesthesia, the breast is prepped and 0.3 mL of Tc-99m sulfur colloid (0.45 microns with 0.5 millicuries activity) is injected intradermally at the 12-o'clock position of the breast. Three milliliters of the blue dye is injected into the subareolar region. Care is taken with methylene blue to avoid intradermal injection as this can cause skin necrosis. At the dilution of 1.25 mg/mL (1 mL dye to 7 mL of sterile saline), we have not observed instances of this adverse event.

For patients who have undergone previous breast surgery, particularly when incisions are present in the upper outer quadrant, deep parenchymal injections are preferred in addition to periareolar intradermal/subareolar injections. The normal pathways of drainage can be altered as a result of damage to the main trunks that traverse the upper outer quadrant.

Lymphoscintigraphy was used on a regular basis during the early phases of this technique (Fig. 45.45). As sentinel node detection rates exceed 95%, the role of this added procedure is diminished. Lymphoscintigraphy may have a role in the initial learning phase to assist the surgeon in identifying the number of sentinel nodes to be removed. At our institution, we no longer employ this nuclear medicine evaluation.

Sentinel lymph nodes receive a more intense evaluation using step sectioning to assess for metastatic disease. The lymph node is sectioned at 2-mm intervals along its long axis. If a previous frozen section was obtained (routine approach is to divide the node in half along its long axis), the two pieces of the lymph node are sectioned in a similar manner. A 4-micron section is cut from each block, and hematoxylin and eosin (H&E) staining is performed. Cytokeratin staining is not routinely performed unless the cancer is of the lobular cell type

VIII

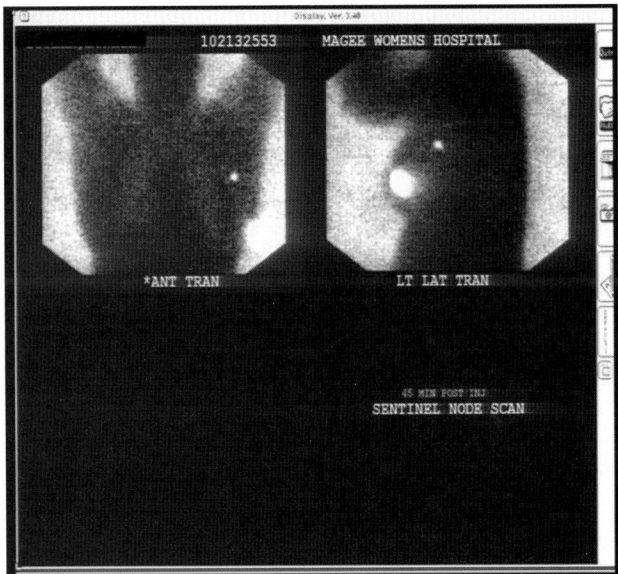

FIGURE 45.45 Lymphoscintigram for sentinel node mapping demonstrating one lymph node with marked radioisotope uptake.

that can be difficult to identify on routine H&E staining. We have utilized this approach at our institution for many years, and it is a well-accepted approach.

More intense evaluation of the sentinel node has led to more frequent findings of occult metastatic disease within the lymph nodes, but the prognostic significance is uncertain. Isolated tumor cells are small clusters not greater than 0.2 mm or nonconfluent or nearly confluent clusters of cells not exceeding 200 cells in single histologic node cross section. Although the current staging system takes this into account, in this situation, prognosis is considered similar to that of patients with node-negative cancers and no additional axillary surgery is advised. Micrometastases are defined as a cluster of tumor cells greater than 0.2 mm but not greater than 2.0 mm. Separate designation in staging is pN1mi. The finding of micrometastatic disease impacts prognosis, but whether there is a benefit from further axillary surgery is debatable. At present, NCCN guidelines recommend completion axillary dissection in this setting.

Occult micrometastases are not seen on traditional H&E staining but rather detected by the additional use of immunohistochemistry (IHC) or by reverse transcriptase polymerase chain reaction (RT-PCR). Initially employed in the evaluation of the sentinel node, a prospective study by the American College of Surgeons Oncology Group (ACOSOG) demonstrated no impact of IHC-detected metastases on overall survival. In a substudy of NSABPB-32, in patients treated with SLNB alone, initial pathologically negative sentinel lymph nodes were reevaluated. Paraffin-embedded tissue blocks were assessed using routine staining and immunohistochemical staining for cytokeratin. Occult metastases were detected in 15.9% of patients. A slight calculated overall 5-year survival difference of 1.2% (94.6% vs. 95.8%) was noted between those with and those without occult metastases. They concluded no clinical benefit derived from IHC staining of initially negative sentinel nodes. Current guidelines from the American Society of Clinical Oncology and NCCN do not support the routine use of IHC or RT-PCR in the evaluation of sentinel lymph nodes. The exception to this rule is in the setting of lobular cancer in order to discern metastatic cells by cytokeratin staining.

As a rule of thumb, if a sentinel lymph node harbors metastases, the risk of additional lymph node involvement is approximately 40%. Various nomograms exist to help predict possible involvement of the remaining axillary lymph nodes. At our institution, the commonly used site is the Memorial Sloan Kettering Cancer Center nomogram (www.mskcc.org/cancer-care/adult/breast/prediction-tools). The nomogram takes into account the size of the primary tumor, presence of lymph vascular space invasion, grade, nodal involvement, extranodal spread, number of sentinel nodes (SN) removed, and the number of involved SNs. The Z0011 study by ACOSOG examined the role of completion axillary dissection in patients with early-stage breast cancer in whom SN metastases were detected. Entrance criteria included T1 or T2 lesions, clinically negative nodes, and 3 or fewer involved sentinel nodes. Randomization was to observation or completion of axillary dissection. Overall 5-year survival was the same between the groups, and no difference was noted with regard to local–regional recurrence. Criticism of the study includes premature closure due to low accrual rates. These findings add to the growing body of literature demonstrating an advantage to adjuvant therapy. Clinical judgment and an informed discussion with the patient should guide the clinician in determining the role of axillary dissection.

For patients receiving preoperative endocrine/chemotherapy who have clinically negative nodes, controversy exists as to whether to perform sentinel mapping prior to initiating therapy to determine the role of axillary dissection at the time of local therapy. Alternatively, sentinel mapping can be performed at the time of postoperative local therapy. At our institution, if the nodes are clinically and radiographically normal, we delay the sentinel lymphatic mapping procedure until the time of definitive breast surgery.

Technique of SNLB

The site is marked in advance of surgery. After induction of anesthesia, the affected breast is cleansed with an alcohol wipe. At the 12-o'clock position, a dermal injection of the radioisotope is performed. Subsequently, 3 mL of the blue dye is injected into the subareolar area at the lateral extent of the nipple–areolar complex. The patient is then prepped and draped for surgical intervention. Using the gamma probe, an area of increased radioactivity is identified; the majority of the time, this is in the ipsilateral axilla. Using an indelible marker, the area is demarcated. An incision line is drawn between the anterior and posterior axillary lines 1 to 2 cm beneath the axillary hairline. We routinely infiltrate the incision line with 0.5% bupivacaine hydrochloride as preemptive analgesia. Incision length can vary depending on the comfort of the surgeon. Dissection takes place through the subcutaneous tissue until the clavipectoral fascia is encountered and incised. This exposes the axillary fat pad. At this point, the surgeon attempts to identify afferent lymphatics bearing blue dye and begins to trace them to the lymph node. Concurrently, the surgeon should employ the gamma probe to direct the surgical dissection and identify the area of highest activity. Once this lymph node is identified, care is taken to remove the lymph node without removing any additional tissue. Approximately 95% of the time, the sentinel lymph node is both blue and radioactive. An ex vivo count is performed and recorded, and the hunt begins anew to identify additional SNs. Any lymph node that has an afferent lymphatic with blue dye or has a radioactivity count of 10% or more of the highest count is considered sentinel. Any node that is clinically suspicious regardless of the presence of radioactivity or blue dye should be removed. Intraoperative assessment of the lymph node(s) is left to the discretion of the surgeon. We advise assessment only if this alters operative events. If the node is clinically suspicious, it is our practice to obtain intraoperative assessment and if the node is involved to perform an immediate axillary dissection to avoid a second operative event. The operative bed is made hemostatic and closed in subcuticular manner without the use of a closed suction drain. (See Steps in the Procedure.)

STEPS IN THE PROCEDURE

Sentinel Lymphatic Mapping

- This procedure is performed under general anesthesia.
- Inject the radioactive tracer (technetium-99m-human colloid albumin) in the subdermis at the 12-o'clock position of the areola.
- Inject the isosulfan blue/methylene blue dye in a subdermal manner by the areola.
- Wait several minutes, and then use a gamma probe to identify in the axilla the highest radiation activity. Also assess the internal mammary nodes for activity.
- Make a mark over the area.
- Infiltrate the skin with 1% lidocaine.
- Incise the skin over the area; the incision site should allow for conversion of the sentinel node biopsy into an axillary dissection if gross disease is found. This incision site is typically by the axillary fold just beneath the hair line.
- Using the gamma probe, identify the hot nodes and remove them. These nodes are often found below the clavipectoral fascia. Visual inspection and removal of any blue nodes should be done at this point as well.
- Take note of the radioactivity of the hottest sentinel node as the background count after removal of all of the sentinel nodes should not be greater than 10% of the hottest node.
- Once all the hot and blue nodes have been removed, the axilla should be palpated in order to inspect for any firm nodes. These nodes should be removed as well.
- The fat tissue can be closed under the skin using a fine (3-0) absorbable suture.
- Skin closure using a running subcutaneous absorbable suture. A drain is not necessary.

The role of SLNB in patients undergoing neoadjuvant therapy is evolving. NCCN guidelines advise SLNB prior to induction chemotherapy as this can provide prognostic information to aid in determination of local–regional therapy. This is an area of active investigation with some institutions performing SNLB at the time of definitive surgical intervention if the patient has a clinically and radiographically negative axillary node at the onset of therapy. A recent trial by ACOSOG Z1071 was designed to define the accuracy of SNLB after neoadjuvant therapy. Women with prechemotherapy clinical T0-4, N1-2, M0 breast cancer were enrolled. At time of surgery, all patients underwent sentinel lymph node surgery followed by axillary dissection. Primary endpoint was false-negative rate. Majority of women underwent

dual tracer identification of the sentinel node. Over a 2-year period, 756 women were enrolled. Sentinel node was identified in 84% of patients; false-negative rate was 12.8%, with 40% of the patients having a complete pathologic response in the lymph nodes. These findings demonstrate that SLNB is feasible after neoadjuvant therapy and may help identify a subset of patients who do not require completion axillary dissection.

Axillary reverse sentinel mapping (ARM) may have some feasibility in preventing the development of upper extremity lymphedema. In this technique, the tracers are injected intradermally into the upper extremity and identification of the nodes responsible for the drainage of the extremity can be identified and preserved. The inherent risk is in leaving metastatic disease behind in the basin.

In patients previously treated with breast-conserving surgery and SLNB who have a subsequent in-breast recurrence, the current recommendation is to perform an axillary dissection. Emerging studies are demonstrating the feasibility of a second mapping procedure. In our own experience, aberrant drainage to the contralateral axillary basin has been identified.

Axillary Dissection

In circumstances of known axillary lymph node involvement based on preoperative assessment, disease detected in the course of sentinel lymph node mapping, or on postoperative analysis of IBC, an axillary dissection is employed. For patients with early-stage breast cancer and clinically negative nodes, axillary dissection is contraindicated and the correct management is the use of sentinel lymphatic mapping. If on clinical or radiographic exam, suspicious nodes are detected, cytologic or histopathologic confirmation should be obtained. If the ultrasound, pathology, or cytology is normal, sentinel lymphatic mapping should be employed.

The patient should be positioned to allow adequate visualization of the axillae. The upper extremity should be at no more than a 90-degree angle from the chest wall. Abduction beyond 90 degrees will introduce the potential for stretching the nerves of the brachial plexus and resultant injury.

In cases in which the axillary dissection is performed in concert with a partial mastectomy, a separate 2- to 3-cm incision is made in the axilla between the anterior and posterior axillary fold along Langer lines, 1 to 2 cm below the axillary hairline. When a skin-sparing or nipple-sparing mastectomy operation is performed and inadequate visualization of the axilla is anticipated, a separate incision can be made. Often, a lateral extension of the existing incisions can improve visualization. Dissection takes place through the subcutaneous tissue until the clavipectoral fascia is encountered. It is then divided to expose the underlying axillary fat pad. The borders of the axilla are defined by identifying the pectoralis major and minor muscle medially, the latissimus dorsi laterally, and the axillary vein at the superior aspect of the dissection. In the course of the operation, both sharp and blunt dissections are utilized to aid in identification and preservation of the sensory (intercostobrachial) and motor nerves. The three major motor nerves are the medial pectoral, the thoracodorsal, and the long thoracic nerves. The medial pectoral nerve is bundled with both a venous and arterial blood supply that supplies the pectoralis minor and lateral aspect of the pectoralis major muscles. Approximately 60% of the time, this complex passes through the pectoralis muscle; 40% of the time, it courses along the lateral border of the pectoralis minor muscle. Injuring this complex will lead to atrophy of these muscles and subsequent loss of chest wall definition. The long thoracic nerve can be found beneath the medial aspect of the axillary vein and passes along the chest wall. This nerve provides motor function to the

VIII

serratus anterior muscle, and injury leads to the clinical finding of a winged scapula. Finally, the thoracodorsal neurovascular complex is identified in the midaxilla. Anterior to this complex is a superficial vein, the thoracoepigastric vein, which can be divided once confirmation of the integrity of the neurovascular complex is confirmed. Once the major nerve bundles are identified and secured, the fat pad can be removed en bloc.

The extent of the nodal dissection is defined by levels I to III in relationship to the anatomic location of the pectoralis minor muscle. The more comprehensive the dissection, the higher the rates are of postoperative morbidity.

A closed suction drain is then placed in the axillary basin and remains in place until the amount is less than 30 mL in 24 hours to prevent seroma formation. This allows for adherence of the surrounding structures. Some surgeons opt against placing a drain and will aspirate any seroma that forms. (See Steps in the Procedure.)

STEPS IN THE PROCEDURE

Axillary Dissection

- This procedure is performed under general anesthesia. Paralysis should be avoided to alert the surgeon of proximity to the major motor nerves.

- The procedure can be combined with either a segmental resection or mastectomy.

- Local anesthesia can be injected into the proposed incision site to reduce postoperative pain.

- When performed with a segmental resection, a separate incision is made between the anterior and posterior axillary fold just distal to the axillary hairline. If the operation is performed with a mastectomy, the operation is accomplished through the existing incision.

- Dissection takes place to identify the clavipectoral fascia.

- The borders of the axilla are identified—the medial border is the pectoralis major muscle, the lateral border is the latissimus dorsi, and the superior border is the axillary vein.

- Care is taken to preserve the intercostal brachial sensory nerves. The major motor nerves include the long thoracic nerve, which is located medially along the chest wall; the thoracodorsal neurovascular complex, which is identified medially to the latissimus dorsi; and the medial pectoral nerve, which either courses along the lateral border of the pectoralis major muscle or is located beneath the pectoralis minor muscle and traverses through both the minor and major muscles.

- The nodal tissue is gently dissected free to accomplish a level I and II dissection (removing nodal tissue lateral to and beneath the pectoralis minor muscle).

- Hemostasis is obtained with clips, ties, or electrocoagulation.

- Palpation of the basin should be performed to assess for any concerning lymph nodes.

- A closed suction drain is placed and secured to the skin.

- The wound is then closed in two layers with subcuticular sutures.

Postoperative complications include wound infection, hematoma and seroma formation, lymphedema, sensory loss, and motor injury. Rates of these complications vary from 1% to 10%. The most disturbing long-term complication is the development of lymphedema that can be seen in varying degrees depending on the extent of dissection.

Lymphedema

The most morbid outcome from breast cancer–related surgery is lymphedema. This is most often encountered as a result of breast-conserving surgery with axillary dissection, SLNB followed by completion axillary dissection, or modified radical mastectomy. Lymphedema is the result of disruption of the drainage pathways and manifests by swelling of the affected extremity. The degree of swelling is directly related to the extent of the axillary surgery, but similar to sentinel surgery, "key" lymph nodes or lymphatics, when disrupted, trigger this condition. Reported incidences range from 10% to 20% but can be as high as 40% if postoperative axillary radiation is employed.

Whenever possible, SLNB should be the procedure of choice, as multiple studies have demonstrated a low incidence (2%) of lymphedema when employed. If an axillary dissection has been performed, secondary prevention of lymphedema is the best defense. Meticulous skin and nail hygiene is recommended with prompt intervention if any signs of infection are noted. The patient should be taught to monitor for lymphedema and promptly report any changes in diameter, color, or temperature changes of their extremity. Avoiding tight-fitting garments that can impede lymph flow and not allowing the affected extremity to be maintained in a gravity-dependent position can help prevent the development of this condition. The patient should be instructed to avoid needle punctures and intravenous catheter placement in their upper extremity. Finally, maintaining an ideal body weight can prevent the development of lymphedema.

If lymphedema develops, early intervention has higher rates of success. The most commonly employed approach is complex decongestive therapy that has multiple components and involves physiotherapeutic techniques. The initial phase of treatment includes meticulous skin and nail care coupled with treatment of any signs of infection. Subsequently, manual lymphatic drainage coupled with compression garments is utilized on a frequent basis until the desired effect is reached. The patient is then placed on a maintenance program with use of compression garments to prevent recurrence.

BREAST RECONSTRUCTION

For patients not amenable to breast conservation surgery, breast reconstruction offers an option. Mastectomy not only carries physical changes but also has been associated in survivors with poor body image, depression, feelings of diminished self-worth, and alterations in occupational and social functioning. Breast reconstruction has been demonstrated to minimize these effects. Legislation introduced in 1998, in the Women's Health and Cancer Rights Act, mandated health care payer coverage for breast and nipple reconstruction, contralateral breast surgery to achieve symmetry, and surgical treatments for the sequelae of mastectomy.

Breast reconstructive techniques can use autogenous tissue, prosthetic placement, or a combination of both. The reconstruction can take place at the time of mastectomy or delayed to a later time.

It is preferred to offer the reconstruction at the same time as mastectomy. An advantage to this approach is the combination of both procedures into one setting, thereby minimizing the number of operative interventions, anesthetic risk, and cost. Additionally, a skin-sparing approach and the retention of the inframammary fold provide enhanced cosmetic outcome. Data exist to suggest psychosocial benefits. Potential disadvantages include prolonged operative time that may affect rates of infection and skin necrosis. Immediate reconstruction also carries the risk of identifying postoperatively the patient who should undergo postmastectomy chest wall radiation (tumor size 5 cm or larger, skin or chest wall involvement, or involvement of four or more lymph nodes). Fortunately, with the use of preoperative MRI, the incidence of this entity is low. Patients with locally advanced disease and multiple medical comorbidities (i.e., insulin-dependent diabetes, chronic obstructive pulmonary disease, smoking, obesity) are not ideal candidates for immediate reconstruction. Higher rates of skin necrosis, infection, donor site complications, and flap necrosis are seen when these medical issues exist.

In the past, delayed reconstruction was the usual approach. The basis of this was the belief that this allowed time for psychological adjustment to the loss of the breast. Advantages of delayed reconstruction include assessment of margins and nodal involvement, management of comorbidities to optimize the patient for surgery, and, in instances of advanced disease, allowance for neoadjuvant chemotherapy and postmastectomy radiation. Disadvantages include a second surgical procedure and less than optimal cosmetic result.

Options for reconstruction include prosthetic devices and autogenous tissue transfer utilizing skin, muscle, and fat. Determination of reconstruction is dependent on the patient's body habitus, type of therapy received or to be administered, and ability to achieve an optimal aesthetic outcome. Extensive counseling and discussion between the plastic surgeon and the patient is required.

Implant Reconstruction

Implant-based reconstruction utilizes a two-phase technique. In the first phase, a tissue expander, which is a silicone shell, is inserted at the initial operative event and incrementally expanded over several months with saline via an integrated port. In the second phase, after the desired breast size has been achieved from skin distention, the tissue expander is removed and a silicone or saline-based implant is placed. In women with an A cup sized breast, it may be feasible to avoid tissue expansion and immediately place the implant. To achieve symmetry, contralateral breast contouring may be required.

Autogenous Tissue Transfer

For patients who have large and/or ptotic breasts, have a large tissue deficit, or have undergone previous radiation therapy, myocutaneous flaps are often the best option. Aesthetically, the use of the patient's own tissue to develop the breast mound provides a more nature feel and appearance to the reconstructed site.

Flap placement can either utilize a pedicle-based transfer (moving the flap while keeping the vascular supply intact) or be completely mobilized and freed from the blood supply (free flap) and a microsurgical anastomosis performed to the internal mammary or thoracodorsal vessels.

The most common approach is the transverse rectus abdominis myocutaneous (TRAM) flap. It may be either pedicle based or developed as a free flap. Other techniques include the latissimus dorsi reconstruction, deep inferior epigastric pedicle flap (DIEP), and superficial inferior epigastric flap (SIEP). The DIEP and SIEP flaps use the same skin and fat island as a TRAM flap without the underlying rectus muscle. For patients who do not have sufficient abdominal fat, options include use of the superior gluteal artery (SGAP), inferior gluteal artery flap (IGAP), and a transverse upper gracilis (TUG) flap. These three types of flaps also place the scars in the less visible locations of the buttock or thigh.

RADIATION THERAPY

Breast conservation therapy relies on the use of postoperative radiation to achieve local control within the breast. For invasive cancer, NSABP B-6 demonstrated recurrence rates approaching 20% in patients treated with lumpectomy alone compared to 14% when treated with lumpectomy and radiation. For DCIS, postlumpectomy radiation therapy decreased ipsilateral breast tumor recurrence rates from 19.4% to 8.9%. Traditional radiation is delivered via two tangential planes to the breast in 1.8 to 2 gray (Gy) fractions daily, 5 days per week for 5 to 6 weeks for a total of 50 Gy. This amount has been shown to treat microscopic disease.

Newer techniques of delivering radiation therapy include intensity modulated radiation therapy (IMRT) and accelerated partial breast irradiation (APBI). Studies are ongoing to improve outcomes in an efficient manner and to decrease damage to surrounding tissues.

IMRT uses high-precision radiotherapy utilizing computer-controlled linear accelerators to treat the breast and minimize treatment of the surrounding tissues. IMRT allows for the radiation beams to conform to the breast and minimize treatment of the underlying lung and heart. Treatment involves 3D CT or MRI coupled with computerized dose calculations to modulate the dosing to the tumor bed and breast.

APBI can be given by external beam irradiation to a portion of the breast or by a directed, localized form of brachytherapy that involves the afterloading of radioactive sources (iridium-192) into catheters placed into the surgical bed. Interest in this technique was generated based on the findings that most in-breast cancer recurrences are near the prior lumpectomy site, thus calling into question the value of whole breast radiation. This technique delivers effective dosing and reduces treatment time. Treatment is usually twice a day for a period of 5 to 10 days. Prior to the advent of single-insertion site devices, multiple catheters were threaded through the lumpectomy bed at the time of surgical intervention. Newer devices are utilized via a single site and conform to the bed by either encasing catheters into a balloon or deploying the catheters to encompass the lumpectomy site. They can be placed either at the time of surgery or 1 to 4 weeks postsurgery. The advantages of postsurgical placement include the adequate assessment of the margins and sufficient time for regression of the surgical site to allow for a more adequate fit.

Several devices exist, including MammoSite or MammoSite ML (Hologic, Inc., Marlborough, MA) balloon apparatus with either a central single lumen or 4 lumens for afterloading radioactive sources, the Strut Assisted Volume Implant (SAVI) (Cianna Medical, Aliso Viejo, CA) device with 7 to 11 struts or catheters that conform to the cavity, and the Contura (Bard, Tempe, AZ) balloon device that contains 5 catheters.

Criteria for use include patient age older than 50 years, tumor size less than 3 cm, clear margins, and no evidence of lymph node metastases. Patients not meeting these criteria have a higher incidence of recurrence. The device must conform to the cavity, and adequate skin thickness is necessary to limit dosing to the skin to prevent necrosis.

VIII

Overlying skin thickness should be approximately 0.7 cm to avoid skin necrosis.

This treatment is not universally accepted, and ongoing randomized trials are comparing its effectiveness to standard whole breast irradiation. A recent retrospective population cohort review of 92,735 women aged 67 years or older demonstrated higher rates of subsequent mastectomy in patients treated with APBI compared to traditional whole breast irradiation. Additionally, patients treated with breast brachytherapy had high rates of complications, including breast infection, breast pain, fat necrosis, and rib fracture. Notably, overall survival was the same in both cohorts.

Alternative techniques to both whole and APBI are being investigated including intraoperative radiation therapy (IORT), permanent seed implantation, and electronic brachytherapy.

Intraoperative radiation therapy is attractive in that it is a one-time treatment, delivers the radiation directly to the tumor bed, and minimizes toxicity to the skin, chest wall, muscles, and ribs as it utilizes electron beam or low-energy x-ray. Criteria for treatment include unifocal disease, negative nodes, intraoperative assessment, and confirmation of clean margins. This approach requires retooling of the operating room suite and close coordination with the radiation oncologist. In addition, these changes require significant increases in treatment costs. Several studies evaluating this approach show promising results but, at present, should not be accepted as standard of care.

SYSTEMIC THERAPY

The use of both chemotherapy and hormone management has improved outcomes in individuals afflicted by breast cancer. These therapies can be engaged in different settings to include adjuvant therapy for early-stage disease, neoadjuvant therapy as opposed to immediate surgical intervention, and in the management of late-stage and metastatic breast cancer.

Adjuvant therapy is given after primary surgical therapy for breast cancer with the goal of preventing recurrence of disease and improving overall survival. Adjuvant therapy includes chemotherapy, endocrine therapy, targeted therapy, and radiation therapy.

The use of oophorectomy as adjuvant therapy for breast cancer was reported in the late 1880s. An initial observation of the effect of ovarian function on breast cancer was noted by Thomas Nunn who reported on perimenopausal women whose breast cancer began to regress within months of menopause. Others suggested oophorectomy would be of benefit for patients with advanced disease and to protect against local recurrence. In 1895, Beatson performed a bilateral oophorectomy on a woman with extensive soft tissue recurrence. This patient experienced a complete remission and survived 4 years after surgery.

As success in the treatment of patients with advanced breast cancer with endocrine and/or chemotherapy became apparent, these agents were introduced in early-stage disease. Adjuvant chemotherapy for breast cancer came of age in the late 1970s with the use of tamoxifen as single- and multiagent chemotherapy. The NIH had multiple consensus conferences to develop guidelines for care of pre- and postmenopausal women with or without nodal spread of disease. In May 1988, the National Cancer Institute issued a clinical alert advising adjuvant therapy for both pre- and postmenopausal women with stage I or stage II node-negative disease.

Initially, the decision-making process was based on the patient's age, menopausal status, presence of either estrogen receptor (ER) or progesterone receptor (PR) on the tumor, and the status of the axillary nodes. As understanding of the pathophysiology of the disease has increased, further stratification became possible based on subset analyses. Genomic testing has come of age and as a result is now being employed to identify patients who may receive the most benefit from additional therapy.

Adjuvant Therapy

Multiple randomized trials have demonstrated that use of adjuvant chemotherapy and/or endocrine therapy improves outcomes in patients with breast cancer. Several resources exist to help the clinician determine the therapeutic approach that will provide the most benefit to the individual patient. NCCN guidelines (www.nccn.org) and Adjuvant!online (a benefit/risk calculator) (www.adjuvantonline.com) are excellent guides for making therapy decisions. Regardless of recommendations from these guidelines, clinical judgment with regard to the benefits and risks should direct therapy.

Factors to consider when determining adjuvant therapy include tumor histology, tumor size, nodal status, presence or absence of estrogen and/or progesterone receptors, and human epidermal growth factor receptor 2 (HER2). The use of a risk to benefit calculator and genomic profiling may be of benefit in selecting appropriate candidates for the type of adjuvant therapy. Patients with favorable histology (tubular, colloid) and small tumors ($\leq$2 cm) that are ER and/or PR positive and HER2 negative without nodal involvement may not receive great benefit from additional cytotoxic or endocrine therapy.

Patients with early-stage, hormone receptor–positive/HER2-negative, node-negative (or microscopic nodal disease pN1mi $\leq$2 mm) are excellent candidates for endocrine therapy. The use of chemotherapy should be individualized based on patient and tumor characteristics. The NCCN guidelines suggest for tumors greater than 5 mm to utilize 21-gene RT-PCR assay (Oncotype DX, Redwood City, CA) to stratify risk of recurrence and consider adjuvant chemotherapy for scores greater than 18. For individuals with hormone receptor–positive, node-positive (>2 mm disease) HER2-negative disease, adjuvant chemotherapy and endocrine therapy should be offered. A subset of these patients may benefit from genomic analysis to determine the role of adjuvant cytotoxic therapy; however, this group is yet to be defined.

Patients with early-stage, ER-, PR-, HER2-negative node-negative disease should be stratified for treatment based on tumor size. For patients with lesions $\leq$5 mm, no adjuvant therapy is recommended; patients with lesions greater than 5 mm or with pN1mi disease should be offered adjuvant cytotoxic therapy.

The Early Breast Cancer Trialists' Collaborative Group (EBCTCG) meets every 5 years to review data from global breast cancer trials. The most recent publication occurred in 2012. Chemotherapy commonly employed included doxorubicin (or related anthracycline) and cyclophosphamide with or without 5-flurouracil (AC/FAC) or cyclophosphamide, methotrexate, and 5-fluorouracil (CMF). These regimens have demonstrated improvements in the risk of recurrence and reductions in breast cancer mortality and overall mortality. Patients who received the greatest benefit from cytotoxic therapy were those with estrogen receptor–negative disease. Furthermore, at standard dosing of doxorubicin-based regimens, AC and CMF were equivalent, but dose-dense AC (higher dose with shorter treatment interval) had an advantage over CMF. The most recent edition also reported that adjuvant taxanes (paclitaxel, docetaxel) were considered the most effective single agents in the treatment of early breast cancer.

General recommendation is for adjuvant cytotoxic therapy utilizing an anthracycline-based regimen for patients with node-negative disease with tumors that are greater than 0.5 cm and are ER, PR, and HER2 negative. Regardless of tumor size, if there is nodal involvement, the same regimen is recommended. For patients with ER-positive and/or PR-positive tumors, the use of genomic assessment should be applied for node-negative or microscopic nodal spread. In patients with hormone receptor–positive, HER2-negative tumors, large tumor size, high-grade, presence of lymph vascular space invasion, and macroscopic nodal involvement, chemotherapy in addition to endocrine therapy should be employed. For the same patient profile without nodal involvement and a high recurrence score (>31) on the 21-gene recurrence assay, adjuvant cytotoxic chemotherapy should be considered in addition to endocrine therapy.

Patients with HER2-positive breast cancers will benefit from the use of trastuzumab (Herceptin, Genentech, San Francisco, CA). In approximately 30% of patients, HER2 is overexpressed. Only patients who overexpress HER2 will benefit from this drug. HER2 expression is detected by immunohistochemical assays and is considered to be present if 3+, equivocal if 2+, and negative if 1+ or 0. In instances of equivocal findings, the gold standard is fluorescent in situ hybridization (FISH) to identify HER2 amplification. Trastuzumab is a monoclonal antibody that interferes with the HER2 receptor, blocks intracellular signaling, and interferes with cell proliferation. Several prospective adjuvant trials have demonstrated consistent benefit from the use of trastuzumab. For individuals with tumors greater than 5 mm that express hormone receptors, the use of endocrine therapy and trastuzumab should be considered. For individuals with tumors that do not express hormone receptors, adjuvant chemotherapy and trastuzumab should be considered for all tumors greater than 5 mm. In addition, adjuvant chemotherapy should be considered for if there is nodal involvement, if the tumor size is greater than 1.0 cm, or both. Ventricular dysfunction occurs in up to 7% of patients and may be exacerbated by left chest or breast irradiation. Lapatinib (Tykerb, GlaxoSmithKline, Brentford, United Kingdom) is a dual tyrosine kinase inhibitor that interrupts the HER2 and epidermal growth factor receptor (EGFR) pathways. This agent is used in patients whose tumors overexpress HER2 that are either chemotherapy naïve or previously failed other agents including anthracyclines, taxanes, or trastuzumab.

Molecular Profiling Tests

The knowledge of the genomic makeup of tumors has advanced and is now being employed in decision making for adjuvant therapy. Previously, factors such as age, ER/PR receptor status, tumor size, tumor grade, and nodal involvement were key components to determine therapy choices. The three distinct breast cancer subtypes of basal-like (also known as triple-negative), luminal A/luminal B, and ERBB2 type have different molecular footprints and have distinctly different prognostic and therapy response profiles. To help the health care provider make clinical decisions, a variety of molecular assays exist. The most commonly employed tests include Oncotype DX, MammaPrint, and Mammostrat. The test results, when combined with an assessment of traditional risk factors for recurrence,

can help the clinician and the patient make a more informed decision regarding adjuvant therapy.

Oncotype DX (Genomic Health, Redwood City, CA) is used to calculate the risk of recurrence and the benefits of cytotoxic chemotherapy for early-stage, ER-positive breast cancer. It utilizes a 21-gene set assay and an algorithm to assign a recurrence score. The testing is done on paraffin-embedded tissue. Scoring is as follows: less than 18 low risk, 18 to 30 intermediate risk, and greater than 30 high risk. The test is considered prognostic in the ability to estimate recurrence and predictive as it assesses likely benefit from chemotherapy. It is included in three clinical guidelines: the NCCN, ASCO, and St. Gallen Consensus Guidelines.

Recently, a new assay has been developed for patients with DCIS that utilizes a subset of the gene assay and a different algorithm to assess risk of recurrence of either DCIS or invasive cancer and the benefit of tamoxifen in hormone receptor–positive disease.

MammaPrint (Agendia, Irvine, CA) analyzes 70 genes involved in the molecular pathways of the metastatic cascade and provides a prediction of 10-year recurrence of either low or high. It is utilized in early-stage (I, II) ER-positive or ER-negative tumors that are less than 5 cm and do not have involved nodes. Fresh/frozen or paraffin-embedded tissue is required, and the 70 genes are analyzed to give a risk recurrence prediction in the absence of either hormone or cytotoxic chemotherapy. The results are dichotomous, whereby low risk signifies a 10% or less chance of recurrence within 10 years and high risk signifies at least a 29% chance of recurrence without adjuvant therapy during the same time period. There is no intermediate result. Another product, Symphony (Agendia, Irvine, CA), includes MammaPrint assay along with Blueprint (molecular subtyping assay), TargetPrint (ER/PR and HER2 status), and TheraPrint (56 gene assay) to provide a comprehensive molecular profile of the individual's tumor.

Mammostrat (Clarient Diagnostic Services, Aliso Viejo, CA) assesses the level of five biomarkers for early-stage (I, II), hormone receptor–positive breast cancer. This test can help identify patients at high risk who may benefit from cytotoxic chemotherapy in addition to hormonal therapy. The test was validated against NSABP B-20, which identified a subset of patients with ER-positive disease who benefited from cytotoxic chemotherapy. The test is additive to ER, PR, HER2, and Ki-67 testing. Paraffin-embedded tissue is used in the assay assessment. Biomarkers evaluated include p53 and HTF9C, CEACAM5, NDRG1, and SLC7A5, which assess cell cycle regulation, differentiation, hypoxia, and nutrient supply. The biomarker levels are assessed in a mathematical algorithm and a risk level assigned. Patient stratification is as follows: low risk 7.6%, moderate risk 16.3%, and high risk 20.9%. Utilizing the risk assignment along with the age of the patient, grade of the tumor, hormone receptor levels, and nodal involvement can help the patient and provider make an informed decision.

Neoadjuvant Therapy

For patients with locally advanced disease, multimodal systemic and local–regional therapy is utilized. Neoadjuvant therapy can be employed for locally advanced disease to induce tumor regression and may allow a patient to convert to breast conservation surgery. Regardless of tumor size or nodal involvement, neoadjuvant chemotherapy can be used in patients with triple-negative breast cancer. Most often, chemotherapy is utilized, even in patients with hormone receptor–positive disease. In patients in whom HER2 is overexpressed, there is a role for trastuzumab. Once a maximal or complete clinical response has been achieved, surgical intervention should occur. Indications for breast conservation surgery have been discussed elsewhere in this chapter. NSABP B-18 randomly assigned patients to either upfront AC chemotherapy or postoperative AC chemotherapy and demonstrated feasibility of this approach and noted 80% of patients experiencing regression of their primary tumors and decreased incidence of nodal metastases. Thirty-six percent of patients had a complete clinical response, and of those patients, approximately one fourth had a complete pathologic response. Upfront therapy increased the rate of lumpectomies by 175% in patients with tumors larger than 5 cm. As such, preoperative therapy should be considered for patients with tumors too large to be considered for primary breast-conserving surgery. Subsequently, NSABP B-27 evaluated the addition of docetaxel. Randomization was between upfront AC, upfront AC followed by four cycles of docetaxel, and upfront AC followed by surgery then postoperative docetaxel. By utilizing all three drugs prior to surgery, the complete pathologic response rate was doubled compared to those treated with AC alone. Despite improvements in breast conservation, no statistical improvement occurred in overall survival or disease-free survival. Patients receiving the additional taxane therapy had a trend toward increased disease-free and overall survival.

Treatment of Recurrent Disease

Treatment of recurrent disease varies depending on the location and extent of the disease. A local or regional recurrence can be managed by either surgical intervention or, when appropriate, radiation therapy. Careful history taking and comprehensive physical examination combined with radiographic assessment with a bone scan and CT of the chest/abdomen/pelvis should ensue in this circumstance. The use of fluorodeoxyglucose (^{18}F) (FDG) PET–CT is approved when looking for metastatic foci in patients with recurrent breast cancer. This test has decreased sensitivity for bone metastases; hence, plain radiographs, a bone scan, or a sodium fluoride PET–CT should be considered.

For individuals who have an in-breast recurrence after undergoing breast-conserving surgery, the recommendation is total mastectomy with or without reconstruction. Management of the axilla for individuals who have sentinel mapping is to perform a level I or II axillary dissection. Isolated nodal recurrences can be treated with resection of the involved node or, in cases of previous SLNB, a completion axillary dissection. The role of postoperative chemotherapy in the absence of known metastases is not clear at this time.

Treatment of Metastatic Disease

Patients with metastatic disease are unlikely to be cured of their disease. Hence, the goals of therapy are palliation of symptoms with minimal toxicity from treatment. In patients with hormone receptor–positive disease, endocrine therapy should be the first line of therapy. In patients who are premenopausal, ovarian oblation or suppression should be considered. Metastatic disease to the bone places patients at increased risk for debilitating fractures. Drugs that help maintain bone integrity, denosumab, zoledronic acid, or pamidronate (given with calcium and vitamin D supplementation), should be added to the regimen. In the absence of hormone receptor–positive disease, chemotherapy is employed. If visceral metastases within the liver, lung, or other organs are encountered, cytotoxic chemotherapy is considered front-line treatment. When chemotherapy is employed, a risk-to-benefit

assessment should take place and single-agent therapy given in a sequential fashion should be considered over combination therapy.

Endocrine Therapy

Endocrine therapy can be achieved through either ovarian oblation or the use of pharmacologic agents. Either selective estrogen receptor modifiers (SERMs) or aromatase inhibitors (AIs) are the current class of agent used to achieve endocrine suppression.

Ovarian Ablation

The role of ovarian ablation was first reported in 1896 by Beatson who demonstrated regression of recurrent breast cancer in premenopausal women whom he treated with bilateral oophorectomy. Until the advent of estrogen receptor modifiers, either surgical removal or radiation therapy was used to suppress ovarian function. For patients who are perimenopausal, the use of luteinizing hormone–releasing hormone (LHRH) analogs such as leuprolide and goserelin can bridge the patient to menopause and avoid the morbidity of surgery. LHRH analogs down-regulate receptors for LHRH and lead to decreased FSH and LH production and a resultant decrease in ovarian production of estrogen and progesterone. Data suggest that these agonists also may exert a direct effect on tumor cells.

In 1996, the EBCTCG reported a meta-analysis of 12 studies in which ovarian ablation was utilized. In women younger than 50 years, an improvement was seen in patients treated with ovarian ablation, with the most profound effect noted in patients with positive nodes. The same group published an analysis of 55 studies employing tamoxifen as adjuvant therapy. The analysis found tamoxifen to be efficacious for the reduction of recurrence in patients with ER-positive tumors. Survival benefit was greater in node-positive versus node-negative disease, with almost doubling of the reduction of recurrence risk in node-positive disease. Tamoxifen benefit was greater in the postmenopausal patients but was present in the pre- and perimenopausal group as well. An almost 50% reduction in contralateral breast cancer was observed in the tamoxifen-treated patients. Compared to historical controls, tamoxifen and ovarian ablation were equally efficacious. Patients with familial or genetic predisposition to ovarian cancer also benefit from surgical bilateral salpingo-oophorectomy.

Selective Estrogen Receptor Modulators

SERMs have a unique role in the management of breast cancer. The two most well-known drugs are tamoxifen and raloxifene.

Tamoxifen is a nonsteroidal triphenylethylene derivative that binds the ER. It has both estrogenic and antiestrogenic actions depending on the target tissue. In the breast, it has strong antiestrogenic effects but exerts estrogenic effects on the endometrium, as evidenced by the development of hyperplasia and on rare occasions carcinoma, and on the bone where it improves both osteoporosis and osteopenia. The mechanism of action is not completely delineated, but one pathway is the blockage of the ER in mammary epithelium and estrogen-driven proliferation of breast epithelium. This drug has a role in both advanced and early breast cancer. In the initial trials, a decreased risk of contralateral breast cancer was noted leading to a chemoprevention trial in which the drug was found to have significant activity in preventing both invasive and in situ diseases. Side effects include hot flashes, vaginal dryness, non–vision-threatening cataracts, venous thromboembolic events, and, as noted, endometrial hyperplasia and carcinoma. The Adjuvant Tamoxifen: Longer Against Shorter (ATLAS) trial demonstrated that 10 years of tamoxifen use for women with ER-positive disease was associated with decreased reduction in recurrence in mortality compared to 5 years of use.

Unlike tamoxifen, raloxifene is a benzothiophene. One mechanism of action is the binding of the estrogen receptor of breast epithelium that prevents estrogen stimulation and proliferation. Other pathways are still being elucidated. Unlike tamoxifen, it does not exert an estrogenic effect on uterine epithelium and, as such, does not increase risk of endometrial hyperplasia or cancer. Like tamoxifen, the drug helps to maintain bone density. When the drug was initially introduced, its primary focus was for treatment of osteoporosis in postmenopausal women. During the Multiple Outcomes of Raloxifene Effects (MORE) trial, usage was noted to decrease the incidence of breast cancer. Subsequently, a randomized trial demonstrated raloxifene to be of benefit in breast cancer risk reduction. Side effects are similar to those of tamoxifen with the exception of uterine cancer risk. It is not currently used as adjuvant therapy for breast cancer.

Aromatase Inhibitors

AIs inhibit the action of the enzyme aromatase that converts androgens to estrogens and thereby lowers levels of circulating estrogen. There are two basic types of AIs, steroidal (anastrozole, letrozole) and nonsteroidal (exemestane). Both types are equally efficacious with no clear advantage with regard to adverse events. The drugs are indicated for use in the treatment of hormone receptor–positive postmenopausal breast cancer. Most frequent side effects are musculoskeletal (myalgias and arthralgias), increased risk of hypercholesteremia, cardiovascular disease, and osteoporosis. This class of drugs is not used in premenopausal women as it can stimulate ovulation and increase endogenous estrogen levels due to ovarian stimulation. At present, no role exists for these drugs in the chemoprevention setting.

Anastrozole has proven superior to tamoxifen in the Arimidex, tamoxifen, alone, or in combination (ATAC) trial of treatment of 9,366 postmenopausal women with localized breast cancer with respect to disease-free survival, time to recurrence, incidence of contralateral breast primary tumors as first events, and a number of important tolerability parameters. Fewer patient withdrawals from the study occurred with anastrozole than with tamoxifen. Anastrozole was associated with fewer vascular and gynecologic side effects, including thromboembolism, hot flashes, vaginal bleeding, endometrial cancer, and vaginal discharge.

Letrozole also has shown effectiveness in ovulation induction and is one of the only safe options for breast cancer patients wishing to undergo in vitro fertilization and ovarian stimulation to assist in cryopreservation of embryos before their cancer therapy. Although the product's label states there is a contraindication in premenopausal women because of "the potential for maternal and fetal toxicity," many intrauterine insemination programs have replaced the standard clomiphene citrate with letrozole because of its superior pregnancy success rates and ability to decrease gonadotropin requirements.

Exemestane is an irreversible, steroidal aromatase inactivator. It is structurally related to androstenedione. It acts as false substrate for the enzyme and binds irreversibly to the active site of the enzyme. It has not been demonstrated to be superior to anastrozole. A recent study was completed comparing the steroidal AI exemestane to the nonsteroidal AI anastrozole. A total of 7,576 women were enrolled and randomly assigned to one of the two drugs. At 4 years of follow-up, event-free, distant disease-free, and disease-specific survival were the same with both drugs. Exemestane was associated with lower rates of osteoporosis, osteopenia, vaginal bleeding, hypertriglyceridemia, and hypercholesterolemia compared to anastrozole.

The Early Breast Cancer Trialists' Collaborative Group reported a meta-analysis comparing AIs to tamoxifen and noted an absolute 3% decrease in recurrence in the AI-treated patients. The report concluded that either monotherapy or introduction of AIs after 2 to 3 years of tamoxifen is beneficial. In 2003, the National Cancer Institute (NCI) issued a clinical alert recommending patients with ER-positive disease receive letrozole 2.5 mg daily for 5 years after concluding 5 years of tamoxifen therapy. The recommendation was based on the outcome of the NCI of Canada Clinical Trial MA27 that demonstrated an increase in both disease-free and overall survival when treated in this manner.

Cytotoxic Chemotherapy

Common cytotoxic multiagent chemotherapy regimens are listed in Table 45.29. Table 45.30 lists chemotherapy agents, mechanisms of action, dosages, and common adverse effects.

TABLE 45.29 Adjuvant Chemotherapy Regimens

REGIMEN		DOSING
AC-T	Doxorubicin, cyclophosphamide followed by taxol	60/600 mg/m² × 4 followed by 175 mg/m² × 4
TAC	Doxorubicin, docetaxel, and cyclophosphamide	50/75/500 mg/m² × 6
CMF	Cyclophosphamide, methotrexate, and 5-flurouracil	600/40/600 mg/m² × 6
FEC	5-Flurouracil, epirubicin, cyclophosphamide	500/100/500 mg/m² × 6
FEC-T	5-Flurouracil, epirubicin, cyclophosphamide followed by paclitaxel	500/100/500 mg/m² × 3 followed by 100 mg/m² × 3
TC	Docetaxel, cyclophosphamide or carboplatin	75 mg/m²/600 mg/m² or AUC 5-6

TABLE 45.30 Chemotherapy Agents

DRUG	CLASS	MECHANISM OF ACTION	DOSE	TOXICITY
Doxorubicin	Antitumor antibiotic	Topoisomerase II inhibition, DNA intercalation, free radical formation	50–60 mg/m² Lifetime max 450–550 mg/m²	Myelosuppression, nausea, vomiting, alopecia, cardiomyopathy Hepatic dysfunction Vesicant
Epirubicin	Antitumor antibiotic	Topoisomerase II inhibition, DNA intercalation, free radical formation	60–100 mg/m² q3wk	Myelosuppression, nausea, vomiting, alopecia, cardiomyopathy Hepatic dysfunction Vesicant
Carboplatin	Alkylating agent	DNA adduct formation DNA intercalation DAN single- and double-stranded breaks	AUC 5–6 q3wk	Myelosuppression Neuropathy Nephrotoxicity
Cyclophosphamide	Alkylating agent	DNA adduct formation DNA intercalation	500–600 mg/m² IV q3wk Oral dose: 50–100 mg/m² days 1–14	Myelosuppression Hemorrhagic cystitis Alopecia Secondary leukemia Nausea, vomiting
Methotrexate	Antimetabolite	Inhibition of dihydrofolate reductase leading to decreased DNA synthesis	50 mg/m² q3wk	Mucositis Myelosuppression Nail changes Alopecia Nausea, vomiting
5-Fluorouracil	Antimetabolite	Inhibition of thymidylate synthase leading to decreased DNA synthesis	500 mg/m² q3wk	Mucositis Myelosuppression Nail changes Alopecia Nausea, vomiting
Taxol	Agent derived from plants (bark of western yew)	Stabilizing intracellular microtubules	135–225 mg/m² q3wk	Neuropathy Myelosuppression Alopecia Nausea, vomiting Hypersensitivity reaction from cremophor carrier
Taxotere	Agent derived from plant (now synthetic, originally needle of European yew)	Promotes assembly and inhibits depolymerization of microtubules	60–100 mg/m² q3wk	Myelosuppression Neuropathy Alopecia Nausea, vomiting Hypersensitivity from Tween 80 carrier

UNUSUAL CLINICAL SCENARIOS

In addition to the presentation of a palpable mass, clinicians should be familiar with the patient who presents with either Paget disease of the breast or IBC. Prompt diagnosis of both conditions leads to improved outcomes.

Paget Disease

Paget disease presents as an eczematoid lesion or ulceration of the nipple–areolar complex and is associated with an underlying malignancy. The lesions tend to be erythematous and have associated scaling of the skin, crusting, erosion, or ulceration of the skin that tends to occur late in the disease process. "Cake-icing" appearance of an erythematous nipple–areolar complex covered with translucent, scaling skin should alert the clinician to this disease process (Fig. 45.46). A high index of suspicion is necessary to aid in the diagnosis. There should be a low threshold to perform a skin punch biopsy. The prognosis depends on extent of underlying malignancy. Both IDC and DCIS can be associated with Paget disease. On clinical examination, the majority of patients will not have a palpable underlying mass; in these cases, the most common underlying process is DCIS. The presence of a palpable mass should raise suspicion of an underlying invasive malignancy.

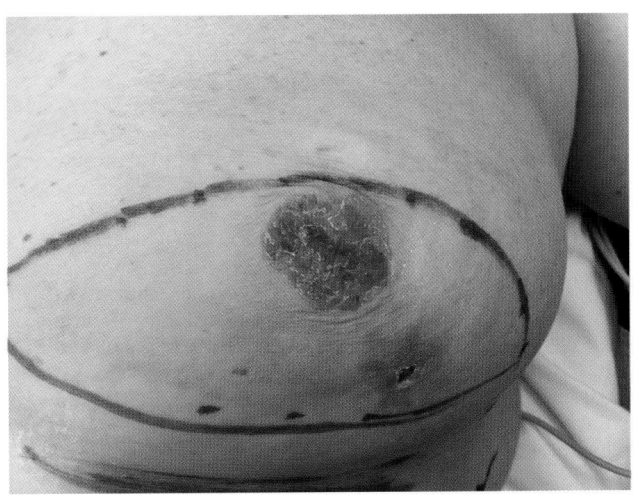

FIGURE 45.46 Paget disease of the nipple. Note the erythema and shiny covering over the epidermis. (Courtesy of Emilia Diego, MD, University of Pittsburgh School of Medicine, Pittsburgh, PA.)

Histologically, Paget cells appear in the epidermis as large anaplastic cells surrounded by a clear halo (Fig. 45.47). Immunohistochemical staining for periodic acid Schiff (PAS) and carcinoembryonic antigen (CEA) are useful in establishing the diagnosis. In order to distinguish the entity from melanoma, negative results from S100 protein and human melanoma black are useful.

Treatment depends on findings from radiographic and pathologic evaluation. Originally treated with total mastectomy with or without axillary lymphadenectomy, the option of breast conservation exists for subsets of patients. The use of central lumpectomy with removal of the nipple–areolar complex is feasible in the majority of patients.

Inflammatory Breast Cancer

IBC is an aggressive form of locally advanced breast cancer that requires prompt recognition and management. It accounts for up to 5% of breast cancers in the United States. The symptoms of the disease process appear rapidly over the course of

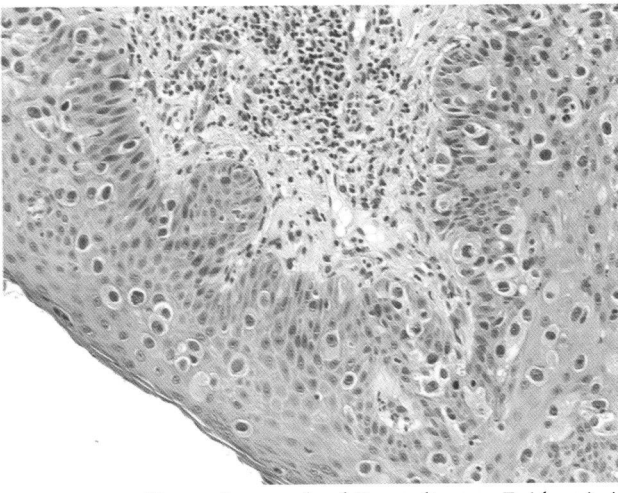

FIGURE 45.47 Photomicrograph of Paget disease. Epidermis is involved with large malignant cells with abundant clear cytoplasm and nuclei with prominent nucleoli (H&E 20×). (Courtesy of Jing Yu, MD, University of Pittsburgh School of Medicine, Pittsburgh, PA.)

weeks and are often confused with mastitis. The condition is clinically characterized by erythema or discoloration of the skin of at least one third of the breast, edema with fine dimpling (peau d'orange), warmth, and the presence of a palpable ridge at the edge of edema. Many of the changes are due to dermal lymphatic invasion (Fig. 45.37). Skin punch biopsy may aid in the diagnosis, but histopathologic finding of tumor cells within the lymphatics is not necessary to make the diagnosis.

Systemic signs of infection are absent. Lack of an elevated white count, fever, and a low incidence of mastitis in women who are not lactating should raise the clinician's index of suspicion to this entity. In addition to a comprehensive history and physical examination, use of mammography, ultrasonography, and MRI aids in assessing the extent of local–regional involvement. At presentation, the majority of patients will have nodal metastases and up to 25% will have evidence of systemic spread of disease. Laboratory and radiographic testing to include liver function tests, CT of the chest/abdomen/pelvis, or PET–CT imaging should be considered to determine disease extent.

Treatment involves a multimodal approach with close coordination between the surgeon, the medical oncologist, and the radiation oncologist. Given the known rapid growth and propensity for distant metastases, neoadjuvant therapy should be promptly initiated. The choice of cytotoxic agents will depend on the particular profile of the tumor. Many studies utilizing anthracycline-based therapy have shown great success. Up to 90% complete clinical response rates have been reported with four cycles of doxorubicin-based chemotherapy. Pathologic response does not mimic clinical response, with pathologic response rates only as high as 13% to 30%.

The advent of molecular targeted therapy also has altered the approach to these patients. Great success has been observed in patients with a known HER2-positive disease when they are given the combination of epirubicin, paclitaxel, and the targeted agent trastuzumab.

Subsequent to induction chemotherapy, a modified radical mastectomy is advised, followed by chest wall and axillary radiation. The addition of radiation therapy reduced the local failure rate to 4% compared to 27% in the control group in a the Eastern Cooperative Group Trial of 332 women with locally advanced breast cancer treated with neoadjuvant therapy who were randomly assigned to postoperative radiation therapy.

Breast Cancer Risk Reduction

Women with BRCA, PTEN, and TP-53 mutations as well as other family cancer syndromes are at increased risk for the development of breast cancer. Risk reduction options for breast cancer include chemoprevention, lifestyle modifications, and prophylactic (or risk-reducing) surgeries.

Chemoprevention

Both ASCO and the USPSTF developed guidelines for the initiation of endocrine therapy for breast cancer prevention. The guidelines recommend endocrine therapy in women over age 60 years, age over 35 years with LCIS or atypical ductal or lobular hyperplasia, between the ages of 35 and 59 years with a Gail model (statistical model that estimates risk of breast cancer development) risk of breast cancer of ≥1.66% (equivalent to the risk of a 60-year-old female), or in patients with known BRCA1 or BRCA2 deleterious mutation who have not undergone prophylactic mastectomy.

The Gail model is a multivariate logistic regression formula taking into account race, age, age at menarche, age at first live birth, number of breast biopsies, finding of atypia or LCIS, and number of first-degree relatives with breast cancer. Risk is low if less than 1.66 and high if greater than 1.66. The risk calculator is available online at several sites (e.g., http://www.cancer.gov/bcrisktool).

Chemoprevention became an option for risk reduction based on information from the Breast Cancer Prevention Trial (BCPT), which launched on 1992. This clinical trial (NSABP P-1) randomly assigned 13,207 healthy women at increased risk for breast cancer (based on Gail model score ≥1.66, age older than 60 years, or history of LCIS) in a double-blind manner to receive either placebo or tamoxifen 20 mg/day. The short-term risk of invasive breast cancer was reduced by 43% and that of noninvasive cancer reduced by 37%, particularly in women with a history of atypical hyperplasia ($P < 0.00001$). Tamoxifen significantly reduced the rate of ER-positive tumors but had no effect on ER-negative tumors. Tamoxifen use was associated with decreased hip fractures but with an increased risk of thromboembolic disease, endometrial cancer, and cataracts. Endometrial cancer risk was significantly increased in women over 50 years of age with a relative risk of 3.28. It accounted for 2.24 cases per 1,000 women compared to 0.69 per 1,000 women in the placebo group.

It is unclear how effective tamoxifen is in reducing breast cancer risk in women with hereditary breast cancer. Because the majority of cancers in BRCA1 mutation carriers are ER negative, one would not expect tamoxifen to be effective. However, BRCA2 carriers often have ER-positive tumors and thus are more likely to be responsive to tamoxifen chemoprophylaxis. Conversely, bilateral oophorectomy has been shown to reduce the risk of both ovarian and breast cancers in these individuals.

At the same time as the P-1 trial, two additional clinical trials were evaluating the role of tamoxifen for breast cancer prevention. The Royal Marsden Hospital Tamoxifen Randomised Chemoprevention Trial and the Italian Tamoxifen Prevention Trial both failed to demonstrate a benefit from the use of tamoxifen in women at risk for breast cancer. In the evaluation of these trials, the study populations were distinctly different. Both trials were smaller in scope; the Italian Trial enrolled 5,408 women and the Royal Marsden study enrolled 2,471 women. In the Italian trial, individuals had undergone premenopausal hysterectomy with or without bilateral salpingo-oophorectomy that, in and of itself, could lead to breast cancer risk reduction. Additionally, patients were allowed to take postmenopausal HRT that could negate the benefits of the selective estrogen receptor modulator. In the Royal Marsden trial, HRT also was allowed for this small population.

The multicenter, randomized, double-blind MORE trial revealed a 76% decreased risk of breast cancer among postmenopausal women with osteoporosis during 3 years of treatment with raloxifene. The effect was only on ER-positive breast cancer. The trial was not designed to assess breast cancer risk reduction but served as a basis for additional studies.

The subsequent chemoprevention trial, Study of Tamoxifen and Raloxifene (STAR) Trial, randomly assigned 19,747 postmenopausal women to one of the drugs for 5 years. Both tamoxifen and raloxifene were effective in reducing the incidence of invasive breast cancer by almost 50%. Raloxifene was associated with higher risks of invasive (310 vs. 247) and noninvasive breast cancer (137 vs. 111) but had a more favorable side effect profile with decreased incidence of endometrial hyperplasia and cancer (hyperplasia 0.84 events vs. 4.4 events per thousand, cancer 1.2 vs. 2.3 events/1,000 women).

The literature includes a report on the use of an aromatase inhibitor for breast cancer reduction. National Cancer Institute of Canada MAP.3 trial randomly assigned postmenopausal

patients at risk for developing breast cancer to exemestane (25 mg) or placebo for 5 years. A reduction in ER-positive invasive breast cancer was seen in the exemestane arm compared to placebo; however, there was no effect on DCIS. Patients on exemestane had increased menopausal symptoms, including hot flashes, musculoskeletal pain, and arthralgias.

Other risk reduction strategies include the use of suppressants of prostaglandin synthesis. Based on epidemiologic observations, use of aspirin and other NSAIDs resulted in up to a 30% breast cancer risk reduction. In preclinical models, COX-2 inhibitors reduced the incidence and growth of ER-positive tumors. NSAIDs function through inhibition of the cyclooxygenase enzyme (COX). The COX-2 enzyme is induced in both in situ and invasive breast cancers resulting in overexpression. COX-2 catalyzes the conversion of arachidonic acid to prostaglandin E_2. This prostaglandin in turn up-regulates a number of intracellular growth pathways, resulting in increased angiogenesis, induction of aromatase activity, cell growth, and division. It is postulated that inhibition of COX-2 may have a general anticancer effect via decreased blood vessel formation, decreased cell growth, and enhanced apoptosis.

Lifestyle

Lack of physical activity, alcohol consumption, smoking, high fat intake, processed foods, and red meat ingestion have been linked to the development of breast cancer. In some circumstances, there are dose–response relationships. Maintaining an ideal body weight after menopause has been associated with breast cancer risk reduction. Data continue to evolve, but, overall, regular physical exercise, smoking cessation, limiting alcohol intake, low fat diets, and avoidance of processed foods and red meat are promoters of a healthy lifestyle and provide benefits above and beyond limiting cancer risk. Individuals also should be encouraged to avail themselves of regular physical examinations and participate in screening evaluations as recommended by the American Cancer Society.

Prophylactic/Risk-Reducing Surgeries

Risk-reducing surgeries include the use of bilateral salpingo-oophorectomy and mastectomy. The primary goal is to prevent the future development of either ovarian or breast cancer. Patients with known deleterious BRCA1/BRCA2 mutations most often undergo these procedures given higher risks of developing these cancers. Timing of the procedures is generally after childbearing has been completed, by the age of 40, or prior to menopause given the escalating risk with age. The sequence of the surgical interventions may be important; patients with BRCA2 mutations may have a predilection for the development of ER-positive breast cancers, and they appear to have risk reduction for both breast and ovarian cancers with premenopausal prophylactic bilateral salpingo-oophorectomy. Analysis of case control data from women with BRCA mutations demonstrated not only a 90% reduction in ovarian cancer risk but also a 60% reduction in breast cancer risk with risk-reducing salpingo-oophorectomy. The role of HRT for women undergoing risk-reducing salpingo-oophorectomy is not yet defined. Patients with BRCA1 mutations tend to have ER-negative tumors so hypothetically should not be at increased risk with HRT.

A retrospective study by the Mayo Clinic reviewed data from women who underwent bilateral prophylactic subcutaneous mastectomy because of a strong family history of breast cancer. The authors demonstrated a 90% reduction in the risk of breast cancer and decreased mortality during 14 years of follow-up. The same group demonstrated 90% risk reduction in known BRCA1/BRCA2 mutation carriers. The costs (both emotional and financial) and benefits of these options must be carefully explained to the individual.

Surgical approaches include total mastectomy, skin-sparing mastectomy with reconstruction, and nipple–areolar or areolar-sparing mastectomies. Initially, subcutaneous mastectomy was performed wherein breast tissue is removed with preservation of the nipple–areolar complex; however, subsequent cases of breast cancer development were noted. This procedure has been largely abandoned because only 90% to 95% of the breast parenchyma is removed, residual ductal tissue remains adherent to the undersurface of the nipple–areolar complex, and nipple sensation was not preserved. Recently, the approach has been revised to include removing a portion of the base of the nipple. At our institution, the procedure has been reserved for women choosing to undergo risk reduction surgery and who have been counseled with regard to the risk of residual breast tissue. The procedure is limited to patients with minimal ptotic changes and breast cup size A or B, as this increases the surgeon's ability to visualize and remove the breast tissue. Nipple denervation is common, but the cosmetic outcome is superior to most reconstructive techniques.

Pregnancy-Associated Breast Cancer

Pregnancy-associated breast cancer (PABC) is defined as breast cancer diagnosed during pregnancy or within 1 year of delivery. Most experts believe that the majority of breast cancers have been present for 2 years before clinical detection. Hence, breast cancers diagnosed up to 1 year postpartum likely were present while the patients were pregnant. Approximately 10% of all women diagnosed with breast cancer who are younger than 40 years old will be pregnant. This makes PABC the second most common cancer in pregnancy with a frequency ranging from 1 in 3,000 to 1 in 10,000 deliveries. Women who have their first term pregnancy after the age of 30 years will have a two- to three-time higher risk of developing breast carcinoma than do women who have their first pregnancy before the age of 20 years. It is expected that breast cancer during pregnancy will become increasingly more common as women delay childbearing until later in life. Refer to treatment of breast cancer section in this chapter for patients who are diagnosed postpartum, as their treatment generally can follow protocols for any other breast cancer. The majority of the discussion in this section focuses on patients whose cancers were diagnosed during pregnancy.

Presentation and Evaluation

PABC is challenging to diagnose. Yearly mammographic screenings are generally performed only in women 40 years of age or older, and since PABC only occurs in young premenopausal women, these tumors generally are detected only on a clinical exam. The increase in breast density that occurs during pregnancy makes examination of the breast more difficult, leading to delays in detection from 1.5 to 6 months. Distinguishing benign from malignant masses can be difficult. Approximately 70% to 80% of masses detected during pregnancy are benign. Breast cancers may not present as a mass and may be subtle breast thickening. If discovered as a mass, these malignant masses are more likely to be mobile. It is important also to exam the axilla, as PABC is more likely to be discovered in later stages. Any masses palpated during pregnancy should undergo further evaluation with imaging modalities. Options for evaluation include the use of ultrasound and mammography. The first step in the evaluation should be breast ultrasonography. In the three published series on the use of this modality in this population, ultrasonography was able to detect the breast cancer in

all patients. However, it should be noted that all three series had less than 25 patients for evaluation. With regard to mammography, the sensitivity of using the latest digital mammography technology can be as high 72% to 78% in nonpregnant premenopausal patients and patients with dense breasts. Data from the small series utilizing mammograms on patients with PABC found similar sensitivities of 78% to 90%. If breast cancer is suspected, ultrasonography and mammography should both be used for evaluation, as these tests are complementary to each other. Ultrasound alone is insufficient as 30% to 90% of patients will have calcifications that can only be seen with mammography, and, therefore, mammography may be helpful in assessing the true size of these tumors. Other testing, such as bone scans, chest x-rays, and abdominal CT, may be indicated in patients with clinical stage IIIA or higher.

Radiologic Tests in Pregnancy

Two potential risks to the fetus exist with radiation exposure: teratogenesis and carcinogenesis. The exact dose at which teratogenesis occurs in pregnancy is unclear but is thought to be from 0.05 to 0.15 Gy. The greatest risk of teratogenesis occurs between the 2nd and 20th week of gestation. Within the first week of pregnancy, radiation exhibits an "all or none" effect in which levels that are too high can lead to a spontaneous abortion. With regard to carcinogenesis, even doses of 0.02 to 0.05 Gy can increase the risk of childhood cancer by twofold. However, it should be kept in mind that because the baseline risk of cancer is low, a twofold increase in the risk of dying of cancer only changes the actual incidence from 1 in 2,000 to 2 in 2,000. The doses of radiation exposure to the fetus with the commonly used tests in pregnancy are shown in Table 45.31. The amount of radiation exposure with routine imaging studies is low. In general, the use of mammography, bone scan, and chest x-ray poses minimal risk to the fetus and should be considered in the workup of a patient with PABC when warranted. Mammograms can help detect areas of calcifications and can be a useful adjunct to breast ultrasounds; hence, mammograms should be used in the workup of a patient with known PABC. Lead shielding to the patient's abdomen should be utilized when possible. The NCCN Guidelines recommend using a chest x-ray, CT of the abdomen with or without pelvis,

TABLE 45.31 Radiation Exposure from Radiographic Imaging to the Fetus

TEST	RADIATION EXPOSURE TO FETUS (cGy)
CXR	0.0005
Bone scan	0.076/0.13
Mammogram	<0.10
CT of chest	0.03
CT of abdomen	0.250

*Dose with/without urinary catheter in place.
Berlin L. Radiation exposure and the pregnant patient. *AJR Am J Roentgenol* 1996;167:1377; Ginsberg JS, Hirsh J, Rainbow AJ, et al. Risks to the fetus of radiologic procedures used in the diagnosis of maternal venous thromboembolic disease. *Thromb Haemost* 1989;61:189.

VIII

and a bone scan in the evaluation of patients with clinical stage IIIA (i.e., patients with tumors >5 cm and positive axillary nodes) or higher. Any patients with symptoms that suggest metastatic disease (e.g., bone pain, abdominal mass, enlarged liver, pulmonary symptoms) also should undergo targeted evaluation of these organs. Doses of radiation from CTs and bone scans are low enough that the benefits outweigh the risks.

Breast MRI is generally not recommended for PABC at this time. The Food and Drug Administration–required labeling for MRI states the safety of MRI during pregnancy to the fetus "has not been established." Several studies in patients who have undergone MRI during pregnancy suggest that MRI is safe; these studies have follow-up as long as 9 years. The use of gadolinium in pregnancy is generally contraindicated. Gadolinium is considered to be a class C drug and is known to be teratogenic at high levels in animal studies. The American College of Radiology states that gadolinium should be avoided in pregnancy.

Risk of Genetic Mutations and Role of Genetic Testing

Little information exists with regard to the prevalence of BRCA mutation carriers in PABC. One study evaluated breast cancer tissue from nine patients with PABC for BRCA1 and BRCA2 mutations. This study found allelic deletion at the *BRCA2* locus in 8 of 9 samples. A significant limitation of this study is that only tumor tissues were evaluated; tissue expression of BRCA does not correlate with an individual having a deleterious mutation of BRCA1/BRCA2. In another study, the prevalence of PABC in 39 families with BRCA1/BRCA2 mutations was evaluated. The patients were compared to an age-matched control group. An elevated risk of PABC was found in both BRCA1 and BRCA2 families. Statistically, more women were found to have PABC in the BRCA1 families (odds ratio 3.9 [95% CI 1.4 to 10.8]). The number of patients with BRCA2 mutations was too small to have any meaningful data. Despite these small numbers and significant limitation in both studies, a thorough family history should be taken in these patients as they may be at elevated risk for carrying either a BRCA1 or BRCA2 mutation. Genetic testing for deleterious mutations of BRCA1/BRCA2 on the basis of having PABC alone may be reasonable despite the limited data.

Pathology

Pathologic features of PABC tend to be high-grade invasive ductal carcinomas. Lymphovascular space invasion also is common. This population has a higher percentage of the hormone-independent tumors, with 50% to 72% of these tumors considered to be estrogen-receptor negative. Increased expression of HER2 was also common with a prevalence of 28% to 58%; the majority of these reports consist of case series.

Treatment Algorithm

PABC diagnosed after delivery is treated the same way as in the nonpregnant patient. If a postpartum patient is being treated with chemotherapy, breast-feeding would be contraindicated. A pregnant patient diagnosed with breast cancer must first decide whether or not to continue with the pregnancy. No data exist suggesting that termination improves survival outcomes in the patient, especially since the majority of these tumors are estrogen-receptor negative. In a series of 24 patients in the 1960s, Holleb and Farrow did not find any improvement in survival with patients who underwent abortions prior to

radical mastectomies. This has been confirmed in other small series. Termination of the pregnancy in the first trimester allows for the use of breast conservation surgery and removes the teratogenic risk of chemotherapy.

If the decision is made to continue with the pregnancy, the plan for treatment is dependent on the timing of diagnosis. Patients diagnosed with small operable tumors in the first trimester (≤12 weeks) are candidates for lumpectomies or mastectomies. It is preferable to wait until the second trimester before operating, since the risk of anesthesia is higher in the first trimester. If the patient opts for lumpectomy, radiation should be delayed until after the delivery. Delays of radiation therapy longer than 6 months after surgery may have significant impact on local recurrence, therefore is not recommended. Mastectomy obviates the need for postoperative radiation therapy especially in patients with small tumors (<5 cm) who have less than four positive lymph nodes. Adjuvant chemotherapy is not contraindicated during pregnancy and can be considered in patients with tumors greater than 1 cm or with lymph node involvement. In patients found to have estrogen receptor–positive tumors with negative nodes, the use of genomic assessment assays (Oncotype DX, MammaPrint) has not been examined in PABC.

In patients who have large tumors, removal of the mass without performing a mastectomy is difficult; if the patient desires breast conservation, neoadjuvant chemotherapy is a treatment option. Treatment typically will last 4 to 6 months. Surgery can then be performed at the end of treatment or can be delayed until after delivery. Delivery can be considered after the 35th week of gestation in order to facilitate any further treatment. Delivery should be delayed at least 3 to 4 weeks after the last dose of chemotherapy to decrease the risk of complications from possible neutropenia and thrombocytopenia. If the patient opts for a breast conservation therapy, then radiation therapy is given after delivery. A summary of the treatment plan is shown in **Figure 45.48.**

Role of Surgery

Surgical excision of breast cancer can be accomplished by either a partial or total mastectomy. For many years, a modified radical mastectomy was considered to be the standard treatment for PABC. Modified radical mastectomy would obviate the need for radiation therapy that is contraindicated during pregnancy and, therefore, can be used as initial treatment for clinical stage I–III breast cancer at any gestation. The initial treatment for stage IV breast cancers should be chemotherapy and not surgical excision.

Breast-conserving surgery consists of a lumpectomy and a 6-week course of radiation therapy to the breast. This 6-week course of radiation can expose the fetus to radiation doses ranging from 0.1 Gy early in pregnancy to 2 Gy later in the pregnancy. This amount of radiation is well above the acceptable threshold of radiation exposure of 0.15 Gy that would lead to increased risk of teratogenesis. There are no studies with regard to the APBI in pregnancy. Radiation therapy can be delayed up 4 months without increased risk of recurrence. If chemotherapy is indicated after lumpectomy, then a radiation treatment delay of 6 months may be possible. Recent recommendations from an international panel of experts state that even if patients are treated in the first trimester or early second trimester, breast irradiation can be delayed until after delivery. However, the local recurrence rate after breast-conserving surgery in pregnant women is unknown. The rates of local recurrence in women younger than 43 years have been reported to be as high as 30% in 8 years of follow-up.

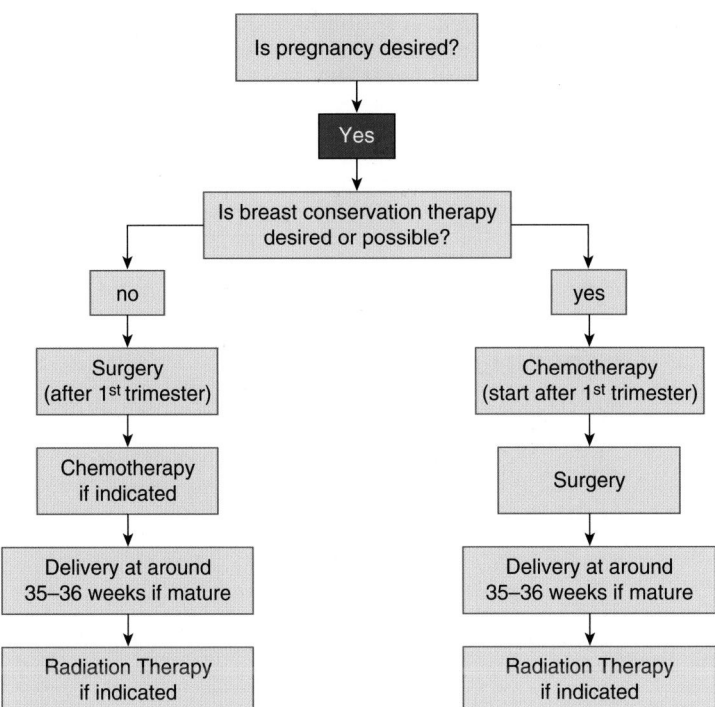

FIGURE 45.48 Treatment algorithm for pregnancy-associated breast cancer.

This information should be discussed with the patient to inform her decision to have breast-conserving surgery versus modified radical mastectomy.

The current standard of care for evaluation of the axilla in a nonpregnant patient with early-stage breast cancer is to perform an SLNB. Sentinel node biopsies involve the use of ^{99}Tc-labeled sulfur colloid and isosulfan blue dye. Keleher calculated the amount of radiation exposure to the fetus with either 0.5- or 2.5-mCi injections of ^{99}Tc and found the dose to be lower than the 0.15-Gy teratogenic threshold. Mondi and colleagues were able to show in a small series that sentinel node biopsies were feasible and safe. At this time, isosulfan blue dye is not approved by the Food and Drug Administration for use in pregnant women. A possible alternative to isosulfan blue dye if an SLNB is being considered is to use indigo carmine. Indigo carmine can safely be used in pregnancy. Indigo carmine is routinely employed in sentinel lymphatic mapping procedures in Japan. A recent review of the Japanese experience has shown that the use of ^{99}Tc along with indigo carmine can result in detection rates of 98% to 100%, which is similar to the results that can be obtained with isosulfan blue. The use of SLNB in PABC requires a thorough discussion with the patient with regard to the risks and benefits of such surgery given the paucity of data on the use of sentinel lymph node dissection in PABC.

Chemotherapy

Limited data exist on the use of chemotherapy for PABC. All chemotherapeutic agents are teratogenic in animals. The timing of chemotherapy administration impacts greatly on risk of fetal malformation and spontaneous abortion. Organogenesis occurs during the first semester. Chemotherapy in the first trimester can result in neural tube defects, cleft lip, amelia, cardiac defects, fetal loss, and other defects. The risk of fetal malformation is diminished when used in the second and third trimesters. Data from the Breast Cancer During Pregnancy Registry found that patients treated with chemotherapy did not have increased risk of intrauterine growth restriction, preterm delivery before 37 weeks, or obstetrical complications.

The majority of studies of chemotherapy in PABC consist of small case series. The University of Texas M.D. Anderson Cancer Center has reported the largest prospective series of PABC treated with chemotherapy. A total of 57 patients were treated in either the adjuvant ($n = 32$) or neoadjuvant ($n = 25$) setting. All patients were treated with FAC (5-fluorouracil, doxorubicin, and cyclophosphamide) for a total of 4 to 6 cycles. In the neoadjuvant group, 32% of the patients had a complete pathologic response. Breast-conserving surgery was more likely in the neoadjuvant group compared to the adjuvant group (37% vs. 19%). With a median follow-up of 38.5 months, 40 patients (70%) are alive without evidence of disease, 13 patients (23%) have died of disease, 3 patients (5%) are alive with disease, and 1 patient is of unknown status. The use of the FAC regimen appears to be safe with minimal neonatal complications. Of the patients who delivered after chemotherapy ($n = 40$), there was one case each of subarachnoid hemorrhage, clubfoot, and Down syndrome. The numbers in this series are too small to conclude if these outcomes were the result of chemotherapy administration, though the risk of subarachnoid hemorrhage in the general population is only 0.8/1,000 births.

Another large series reported on 28 patients treated with three different regimens: doxorubicin/cyclophosphamide (AC), epirubicin/cyclophosphamide (EC), and cyclophosphamide/methotrexate/5-fluorouracil (CMF). These regimens were initiated at 15 to 33 weeks' gestation. One patient was given CMF in the first trimester and had a spontaneous abortion after the first cycle. Overall, all three regimens were well tolerated with no fetal anomalies attributed to the chemotherapy. The combined survival for this cohort of patients was 67% at a median of 40.5 months of follow-up. The disease-free survival rate was 63%.

There are only case reports of other regimens used for PABC. The largest report of the use of taxanes in PABC comes

VIII

from the Breast Cancer During Pregnancy Registry in a total of 14 patients; however, data are limited, and taxanes should be used with caution.

In recent years, newer chemotherapeutic agents targeting growth receptors such as HEr2/*neu* have been part of standard treatment for patients with breast cancer who overexpress these receptors. Seven published case reports of PABC patients undergoing treatment with trastuzumab, a monoclonal antibody that blocks the human epidermal growth factor receptor 2 protein, indicate these patients were able to tolerate trastuzumab, except for the oligohydramnios or anhydramnios that was seen in five out of the seven patients. This decrease in amniotic fluid appears to be reversible with the discontinuation of trastuzumab. All patients were able to deliver a viable infant with the exception of one patient who had a twin pregnancy with loss of one twin secondary to chronic renal failure and lung disease after delivery at 31 weeks.

Hormonal therapy such as tamoxifen has been shown to be highly effective in premenopausal estrogen receptor–positive breast cancer and is routinely used once initial treatment with surgery, radiation therapy, and chemotherapy has been completed. Several case reports of patients treated with tamoxifen during pregnancy suggest that treatment is safe with no side effects; others have reported cases of Goldenhar syndrome (oculoauriculovertebral dysplasia) or ambiguous genitalia. It appears prudent to hold off treatment with tamoxifen until the patient has delivered, given the paucity of data.

Prognosis

It is unclear whether pregnancy is an independent adverse risk factor for outcomes in PABC. Early studies reported poor overall survival in patients diagnosed with PABC. These results may have been attributable to the fact that patients with PABC tend to present with higher stages and more advance disease. When PABC patients were compared to non-PABC cancer patients and controlled for stage, some studies have not shown any differences in outcome. In one series reported by Petrek and colleagues, patients with early-stage PABC with node-negative disease had similar survival to non-PABC patients (10-year survivals of 77% and 75%, respectively). Small numbers have hampered many studies of analysis of survival in patients with PABC. More recently, a large series using the California Cancer Registry was reported. A total of 797 PABC patients were compared to a cohort of 4,177 non-PABC patients. These authors found that even when controlled for stage, race, tumor size, type of surgery, and hormonal status, pregnancy status appears to have modest effect for poorer survival. The hazard ratio was 1.14 (95% CI: 1.0 to 1.29, $P = 0.46$) when PABC patients were compared to non-PABC patients. If one combines all the data from published studies that have reported 5-year survival, a total of 742 patients have been reported. Combining all the reported cases series, the overall 5-year survival for node-negative and node-positive PABC is 69% and 34%, respectively.

Follow-Up

Follow-up of the patient with PABC is no different than any other patient who has been diagnosed with breast cancer. The American Society of Clinical Oncology published their most recent guidelines in 2013. The guidelines recommend routine history and physical examination every 3 to 6 months in the first 3 years, every 6 to 12 months in the ensuing 2 years, and

annually 5 years after treatment. In patients who have undergone breast-conserving surgery, a posttreatment mammogram should be obtained 1 year after the initial mammogram and at least 6 months after completion of radiation therapy. Thereafter, unless otherwise indicated, a yearly mammographic evaluation should be performed. Other testing such as complete blood count, chemistry panels, bone scans, chest radiographs, liver ultrasounds, computed tomography scans, [^{18}F]fluorodeoxyglucose-positron emission tomography scanning, MRI, or tumor markers (CEA, CA 15-3, and CA 27.29) are not recommended by ASCO unless the patient is symptomatic.

SURVEILLANCE

Surveillance for patients treated for either in situ or invasive disease is directed at determining local and/or regional recurrence and identifying the development of a contralateral breast cancer. The risk of contralateral breast cancer varies depending on the age at initial diagnosis of breast cancer.

For patients with DCIS, a comprehensive physical examination every 6 to 12 months is recommended. In patients treated with breast-conserving surgery, an initial postsurgical mammogram should be conducted within 12 months. Assessment with MRI is recommended only for patients with dense breasts or for those in whom the initial diagnosis was made with this modality. Most recurrences occur in the ipsilateral breast near the previous segmental site. If the patient has undergone excisional surgery as the only therapy, this approach with or without radiation therapy is an option. If the patient previously received whole breast radiation, mastectomy is the preferred approach. In patients previously treated with APBI, decision on the surgical approach is individualized. In patients who have undergone irradiation, the majority of recurrences are in situ disease. Patients treated with mastectomy who experience a local recurrence should be treated with local excision and chest wall irradiation. If the patient is receiving tamoxifen therapy and has an intact uterus, an annual gynecologic assessment is recommended. Prompt evaluation of abnormal or postmenopausal bleeding is advised.

For patients with invasive cancer, a more intensive program of surveillance is recommended. In addition to assessing for local–regional recurrence and contralateral breast cancer, the issue of systemic recurrence exists in this population. In 2013, ASCO made recommendations for surveillance in asymptomatic women. These recommendations include a comprehensive history and physical examination every 3 to 6 months for the first 3 years, followed by every 6 to 12 months for years 4 and 5, and annually thereafter. Annual diagnostic mammographic surveillance is advised. MRI is not recommended unless the initial diagnosis was made with MRI, the patient is considered at high risk for in-breast or contralateral breast cancer as in patients with deleterious BRCA1/BRCA2 mutations, and in patients in whom breast density precludes adequate assessment. Routine radiographic testing such as CT scans, PET scans, chest radiographs, pelvic ultrasounds, and liver ultrasounds is not recommended. Comprehensive blood testing, including complete blood count, chemistries, tumor markers, and liver function testing, is not recommended if the patient is asymptomatic. Directed tests should be performed based on patient symptomatology.

For patients on adjuvant endocrine therapy, compliance with the medication should be assessed and adjustments made to increase adherence. For a patient on tamoxifen therapy and with an intact uterus, annual gynecologic evaluation is recommended. If the patient is experiencing abnormal or post-menopausal bleeding, an immediate evaluation with either endometrial biopsy or dilatation and curettage should occur. An ultrasound of the pelvis does not provide a histopathologic assessment and should not be used in place of obtaining a tissue diagnosis.

There is evidence that a healthy lifestyle provides benefits; hence, patients should be counseled to maintain or achieve an ideal body weight associated with improved health and survival. As previously described, smoking cessation, low fat intake, high fruit and vegetable intake, alcohol reduction, and avoidance of processed foods and red meat also have health benefits.

Individuals receiving aromatase inhibitors are at risk for osteopenia and osteoporosis. Appropriate surveillance with bone density assessment and use of bisphosphonate or other appropriate therapy should be used.

Hormone Replacement Therapy

As more breast cancers are detected at an earlier stage, resulting in increased survival, attention has been directed toward the use of HRT in breast cancer survivors. Caution is still advised, but a subset of patients may exist for whom, with appropriate counseling, placing on HRT may be an option. Premenopausal patients with ER-negative breast cancer who have lost ovarian function as a result of adjuvant therapy and menopausal breast cancer survivors may benefit from HRT to prevent long-term sequelae of estrogen depravation. Postmenopausal women who have symptomatic estrogen deficiency and are disease-free for at least 2 years (highest risk for recurrence) may be considered candidates for HRT. A patient with localized node-negative breast cancer who is at low risk for recurrent disease may be a candidate for long-term HRT. Women with unexplained vaginal bleeding, acute vascular thrombosis, or significant liver function impairment would remain ineligible for HRT. All women should be counseled concerning the potential risk of disease recurrence.

Vasomotor symptoms can be managed through nonhormonal approaches. Gabapentin (Neurotin, Pfizer, New York, NY) has been shown in a randomized double-blind placebo-controlled trial of 420 women to control hot flashes in breast cancer patients at 900 mg/day, demonstrating greater reduction in the posttreatment hot flash severity score compared with placebo and lower doses of gabapentin. Gabapentin is approved for the treatment of epileptic seizures but often is used for treatment of migraine headaches, restless legs syndrome, and bipolar disorder. Venlafaxine, a commonly used antidepressant, and SSRI appear to be effective treatment for hot flashes. An extended release preparation at an initial dose of 37.5 mg daily can reduce hot flashes in 50% to 60% of patients. If no response occurs within 2 weeks of starting the medication, the dose can be doubled.

Acupuncture has been reported to be of benefit for relief of vasomotor symptoms, but this has been questioned in the medical literature. Avoidance of triggers to hot flashes is a reasonable approach, such as cool and breathable clothing and minimizing hot and spicy food ingestion, hot tub and sauna use, and caffeine intake, and avoidance of smoking.

Atrophy of the urogenital epithelium can occur as a result of treatment for breast cancer. Particularly prone are premenopausal patients who enter menopause as a result of systemic use of SERMs and AIs and cytotoxic chemotherapy. Vaginal dryness can be managed using topical estrogens or with a time-released estradiol vaginal ring device (Estring, Pfizer, New York, NY). Systemic absorption of estrogen with this approach is reported to be minimal. Most of the effect is exerted locally and increases vaginal epithelium thickness and moisture. Limited data exist to guide the patient and health care provider. Additional studies should shed light on the safety of this approach.

Pregnancy after Treatment for Breast Cancer

Although oncologists generally caution patients to avoid pregnancy until 2 years after completing treatment for breast cancer, several investigators have shown no adverse effects or decreased survival for women who become pregnant after cancer therapy. Moreover, although lactation is decreased in the treated breast, radiation therapy appears to have no effect on the contralateral breast.

For patients who are premenopausal at diagnosis, a discussion should occur concerning the impact of adjuvant therapy on future fertility. Patients who desire childbearing should be afforded the opportunity to meet with a reproductive endocrinologist to review options for fertility preservation, including ovarian suppression and egg harvesting. The most efficacious approach appears to be cryopreservation of embryos.

Contraceptive options for premenopausal patients include barrier methods, surgical sterilization with tubal ligation (or vasectomy for the male partner), or use of an intrauterine device. The safety of oral contraceptives in patients, regardless of ER status of the tumor, is not known.

BEST SURGICAL PRACTICES

- Obstetrician–gynecologists, as primary providers of women's health care, are in a unique position to identify individuals at risk for breast cancer and to aid in the early diagnosis of the disease.
- One in eight women in the United States will develop breast cancer in their lifetime.
- Percutaneous sampling via FNA can aid in the diagnosis of benign and malignant masses, but the cytology cannot delineate between invasive and noninvasive breast cancer.
- Iatrogenic pneumothorax is a rare complication that may be reduced by stabilizing the lesion over a rib before needle introduction.
- Percutaneous core needle biopsy provides tissue samples for histologic analysis and can aid in the diagnosis of both invasive and noninvasive lesions. Core needle biopsy is the preferred management for palpable and nonpalpable lesions to help stratify operative interventions.
- Masses within 2 cm of the areolar margin can be removed through a circumareolar incision at the areolar margin with an excellent cosmetic outcome.
- The presence of a palpable mass and a normal or negative mammogram mandates additional evaluation.
- The most cosmetically acceptable scars result from incisions that follow the contour of Langer lines.
- Randomized controlled trials have demonstrated breast-conserving surgery and radiation therapy to be equivalent to radical mastectomy with regard to overall, disease-free, and distant disease-free survival.
- For a patient with breast cancer and a clinically negative axilla, sentinel lymphatic mapping is the operation of choice to assess nodal status.
- Multimodality therapy with surgery, chemotherapy, or endocrine therapy and postlumpectomy radiation therapy are effective means of treating breast cancer.

VIII

- IBC is a rare and highly aggressive form of breast cancer. Often, the patient will present with what appears to be mastitis but lacks systemic signs of fever and leukocytosis. Prompt diagnosis and treatment with cytotoxic chemotherapy followed by modified radical mastectomy and chest wall irradiation has improved survival from this disease.
- Most patients who undergo mastectomy are candidates for either immediate or delayed breast reconstruction.
- In a patient diagnosed with breast cancer associated with a pregnancy, careful coordination of care should occur between the surgeon, medical oncologist, and the obstetrician–gynecologist. The trimester of diagnosis determines the sequence of care.
- In a patient with PABC, referral for genetic assessment to identify either a BRCA deleterious mutation or family cancer syndrome is appropriate.
- Risk-reducing breast procedures include total mastectomy, skin-sparing mastectomy, and nipple-sparing mastectomy.

BIBLIOGRAPHY

Ader DN, Shriver CD. Cyclical mastalgia: prevalence and impact in an outpatient breast clinic sample. *J Am Coll Surg* 1997;185:466.

Alexander FE, Anderson TJ, Brown HK, et al. 14 years of follow-up from the Edinburgh randomised trial of breast-cancer screening. *Lancet* 1999;353:1903.

Alexander FE, Anderson TJ, Brown HK, et al. The Edinburgh randomised trial of breast cancer screening: results after 10 years of follow-up. *Br J Cancer* 1994;70:542.

Allred DC, Anderson AS, Paik S, et al. Adjuvant tamoxifen reduces subsequent breast cancer in women with estrogen-receptor positive ductal carcinoma in situ: a study based on NSABP protocol B-24. *J Clin Oncol* 2012;30:1268.

Anderson BO, Calhoun KE, Rosen EL. Evolving concepts in the management of lobular neoplasia. *J Natl Compr Cancer Netw* 2006;4:511.

Baines CJ, Miller AB, Kopans DB, et al. Canadian National Breast Screening Study: assessment of technical quality by external review. *AJR Am J Roentgenol* 1990;155:743.

Bear HD, Anderson S, Brown A, et al. The effect on tumor response of adding sequential preoperative docetaxel to preoperative doxorubicin and cyclophosphamide: preliminary results from National Surgical Adjuvant Breast and Bowel Project Protocol B-27. *J Clin Oncol* 2003;21:4165.

Beatson C. On treatment of inoperable cases of carcinoma of the mamma: suggestions for a new method of treatment with illustrative cases. *Lancet* 1896;2:104.

Berg JW. The significance of axillary node levels in the study of breast carcinoma. *Cancer* 1955;8:776.

Berg WA, Blume JD, Cormack JB, et al. Combined screening with ultrasound and mammography vs mammography alone in women at elevated risk of breast cancer. *JAMA* 2008;299:2151.

Berg WA, Weinberg IN, Narayanan D, et al. High-resolution fluorodeoxyglucose positron emission tomography with compression ("positron emission mammography") is highly accurate in depicting primary breast cancer. *Breast J* 2006;12:309.

Berg WA. Supplemental screening sonography in dense breasts. *Radiol Clin North Am* 2004;42:845.

Berlin L. Radiation exposure and the pregnant patient. *AJR Am J Roentgenol* 1996;167:1377.

Bijker N, Meijnen P, Peterse JL, et al. Breast-conserving treatment with or without radiotherapy in ductal carcinoma-in-situ: ten-year results of European Organisation for Research and Treatment of Cancer randomized phase III trial 10853—a study by the EORTC Breast Cancer Cooperative Group and EORTC Radiotherapy Group. *J Clin Oncol* 2006;24:3381.

Blechman KM, Karp NS, Levovitz C, et al. The lateral inframammary fold incision for nipple-sparing mastectomy: outcomes from over 50 immediate implant-based breast reconstructions. *Breast J* 2013;19:31.

Bleyer A, Welch HG. Effect of three decades of screening mammography on breast-cancer incidence. *N Engl J Med* 2012;367:1998.

Bordeleau L, Pritchard KL, Loprinzi CL, et al. Multicenter, randomized, cross-over clinical trial of venlafaxine versus gabapentin for the management of hot flashes in breast cancer survivors. *J Clin Oncol* 2010;28:5147.

Boughey J, Sunman VJ, Mittendord EA, et al. The role of sentinel lymph node surgery in patients presenting with node positive breast cancer. (T0-4, N1-2) who receive neoadjuvant chemotherapy results from the ACOSOG Z1071 Trial. *Paper presented at: 2012 CTRC-AACR San Antonio Brest Cancer Symposium 2012*, San Antonio, TX.

Boyle CA, Berkowitz GS, LiVolsi VA, et al. Caffeine consumption and fibrocystic breast disease: a case–control epidemiologic study. *J Natl Cancer Inst* 1984;72:1015.

Collaborative Group on Hormonal Factors in Breast Cancer. Breast cancer and breastfeeding: collaborative reanalysis of individual data from 47 epidemiological studies in 30 countries, including 50302 women with breast cancer and 96973 women without the disease. *Lancet* 2002;360:187.

Brem RF, Floerke AC, Rapeleya JA, et al. Breast-specific gamma imaging as an adjunct imaging modality for the diagnosis of breast cancer. *Radiology* 2008;247:651.

Brem RF, Shahan C, Rapleyea JA, et al. Detection of occult foci of breast cancer using breast-specific gamma imaging in women with one mammographic or clinically suspicious breast lesion. *Acad Radiol* 2010;17:735.

Burstein HJ, Kuter I, Campos SM, et al. Clinical activity of trastuzumab and vinorelbine in women with HER2-overexpressing metastatic breast cancer. *J Clin Oncol* 2001;19:2722.

Burstein H. Adjuvant chemotherapy for hormone receptor-positive or negative, HER2-negative breast cancer. In: Basow D, ed. *UpToDate*. Waltham, MA: UpToDate; 2013.

Calhoun KE, Kim JN, Lehman CD, et al. Phyllodes tumor. In: Harris LM Jr, Morrow M, Osborne CK, eds. *Diseases of the breast*, 4th ed. Philadelphia, PA: Wolter Kluwers/Lippincott Williams & Wilkins; 2010:781.

Carlson GW, Styblo TM, Lyles RH, et al. The use of skin sparing mastectomy in the treatment of breast cancer: the Emory experience. *Surg Oncol* 2003;12:265.

Casabona F, Bogliolo S, Valenzano Menada M, et al. Feasibility of axillary reverse mapping during sentinel lymph node biopsy in breast cancer patients. *Ann Surg Oncol* 2009;16:2459.

Chang S, Parker SL, Pham T, et al. Inflammatory breast carcinoma incidence and survival: the surveillance, epidemiology, and end results program of the National Cancer Institute, 1975–1992. *Cancer* 1998;82:2366.

Chen W. Selective estrogen receptor modulators and aromatase inhibitors for breast cancer prevention. In: Basow D, ed. *UpToDate*. Waltham, MA: UpToDate; 2013.

Clements H, Duncan KR, Fielding K, et al. Infants exposed to MRI in utero have a normal paediatric assessment at 9 months of age *Br J Radiol* 2000;73:190.

Costanza ME. Factors that modify breast cancer risk in women. In: Basow D, ed. *UpToDate*. Waltham, MA: UpToDate; 2013.

Cummings SR, Krueger KA, Grady D, et al. The effect of raloxifene on risk of breast cancer in postmenopausal women: results from the MORE randomized Trial. Multiple Outcomes of Raloxifene Evaluation. *JAMA* 1999;282:2124.

De Silva NK, Brandt ML. Disorders of the breast in children and adolescents. Part 2: breast masses. *J Pediatr Adolesc Gynecol* 2006;19:415.

Deneve JL, Hoefer RA Jr, Harris EE, et al. Accelerated partial breast irradiation: a review and description of an early North American surgical experience with the intrabeam delivery system. *Cancer Control* 2012;19:295.

Dickler MN. The MORE trial: multiple outcomes for raloxifene evaluation—breast cancer as a secondary end point: implications for prevention. *Ann N Y Acad Sci* 2001;949:134.

Dillon DA, Guigi AJ, Schnitt SJ. Pathology of invasive breast cancer. In: Harris LM Jr, Morrow M, Osborne CK, eds. *Diseases of the breast*, 4th ed. Philadelphia, PA: Wolter Kluwer/Lippincott Williams & Wilkins; 2010:374.

DiSaia PJ, Creasman WT, Rich WM. An alternate approach to early cancer of the vulva. *Am J Obstet Gynecol* 1979;133:825.

Djulbegovic B, Lyman GH. Screening mammography at 40–49 years: regret or no regret? *Lancet* 2006;368:2035.

Dowsett M, Cuzick J, Ingle J, et al. Meta-analysis of breast cancer outcomes in adjuvant trials of aromatase inhibitors versus tamoxifen. *J Clin Oncol* 2010;28:509.

Duijm LE, Guit GL, Hendriks JH, et al. Value of breast imaging in women with painful breasts: observational follow up study. *Br Med J* 1998;317:1492.

Dupont WD, Page DL, Parl FF, et al. Estrogen replacement therapy in women with a history of proliferative breast disease. *Cancer* 1999;85:1277.

Dupont WD, Page DL. Risk factors for breast cancer in women with proliferative breast disease. *N Engl J Med* 1985;312:146.

Early Stage Breast Cancer—NIH Consensus Conference. *JAMA* 1991;265:391.

Edge SB, Compton CC, Fritz A, et al. *AJCC cancer staging manual*, 7th ed. New York, NY: Springer; 2009.

Eliassen AH, Colditz GA, Rosner B, et al. Adult weight change and risk of postmenopausal breast cancer. *JAMA* 2006;296:193.

Elkhuizen PH, van Slooten HJ, Clahsen PC, et al. High local recurrence risk after breast-conserving therapy in node-negative premenopausal breast cancer patients is greatly reduced by one course of perioperative chemotherapy: a European Organization for Research and Treatment of Cancer Breast Cancer Cooperative Group Study. *J Clin Oncol* 2000;18:1075.

Elledge RM, Ciocca DR, Langone G, et al. Estrogen receptor, progesterone receptor, and HER-2/neu protein in breast cancers from pregnant patients. *Cancer* 1993;71:2499.

Elston CW, Ellis IO. Pathological prognostic factors in breast cancer. I. The value of histological grade in breast cancer: experience from a large study with long-term follow-up. *Histopathology* 1991;19:403.

Evans ML, Pritts E, Vittinghoff E, et al. Management of postmenopausal hot flushes with venlafaxine hydrochloride: a randomized, controlled trial. *Obstet Gynecol* 2005;105:161.

Familial breast cancer: collaborative reanalysis of individual data from 52 epidemiological studies including 58,209 women with breast cancer and 101,986 women without the disease. *Lancet* 2001;358:1389.

Fisher B, Dignam J, Wolmark N, et al. Lumpectomy and radiation therapy for the treatment of intraductal breast cancer: findings from National Surgical Adjuvant Breast and Bowel Project B-17. *J Clin Oncol* 1998;16:441.

Fisher B , Jeong JH, Bryant J, et al. Twenty-five year follow-up of a randomized trial comparing radical mastectomy, total mastectomy, and total mastectomy followed by irradiation. *N Engl J Med* 2002;347:567.

Fisher B, Anderson S, Bryant J, et al. Twenty-year follow-up of a randomized trial comparing total mastectomy, lumpectomy, and lumpectomy plus irradiation for the treatment of invasive breast cancer. *N Engl J Med* 2002;347:1233.

Fisher B, Bauer M, Margolese R, et al. Five-year results of a randomized clinical trial comparing total mastectomy and segmental mastectomy with or without radiation in the treatment of breast cancer. *N Engl J Med* 1985;312:665.

Fisher B, Brown A, Mamounas E, et al. Effect of preoperative chemotherapy on local-regional disease in women with operable breast cancer: findings from National Surgical Adjuvant Breast and Bowel Project B-18. *J Clin Oncol* 1997;15:2483.

Fisher B, Costantino JP, Wickerham DL, et al. Tamoxifen for prevention of breast cancer: report of the National Surgical Adjuvant Breast and Bowel Project P-1 Study. *J Natl Can Inst* 1998;90:1371.

Fisher B, Montague E, Redmond C, et al. Comparison of radical mastectomy with alternative treatments for primary breast cancer. A first report of results from a prospective randomized clinical trial. *Cancer* 1977;39:2827.

Fisher B, Redmond C, Poisson R, et al. Eight-year results of a randomized clinical trial comparing total mastectomy and lumpectomy with or without irradiation in the treatment of breast cancer. *N Engl J Med* 1989;320:822.

Foote FW, Stewart FW. Lobular carcinoma in situ: a rare form of mammary cancer. *Am J Pathol* 1941;17:491.

Gennaro G, Toledano A, di Maggio C, et al. Digital breast tomosynthesis versus digital mammography: a clinical performance study. *Eur Radiol* 2010;20:1545.

Gilleard O, Goodmen A, Cooper M, et al. The significance of the Van Nuys prognostic index in the management of ductal carcinoma in situ. *World J Surg Oncol* 2008;6:61.

Ginsberg JS, Hirsh J, Rainbow AJ, et al. Risks to the fetus of radiologic procedures used in the diagnosis of maternal venous thromboembolic disease. *Thromb Haemost* 1989;61:189.

Giuliano AE, Hawes D, Ballman KV, et al. Association of occult metastases in sentinel lymph nodes and bone marrow with survival among women with early-stage invasive breast cancer. *JAMA* 2011;306:385.

Good WF, Abrams GS, Catullo VJ, et al. Digital breast tomosynthesis: a pilot observer study. *AJR Am J Roentgenol* 2008;190:865.

Goss PE, Ingle JN, Ales-Martinez JE, et al. Exemestane for breast-cancer prevention in postmenopausal women. *N Engl J Med* 2011;364:2381.

Gould EA, Winship T, Philbin PH, et al. Observations on a "sentinel node" in cancer of the parotid. *Cancer* 1960;13:77.

Gray RJ, Pockaj BA, Karstaedt PJ, et al. Radioactive seed localization of nonpalpable breast lesions is better than wire localization. *Am J Surg* 2004;188:377.

Gray RJ, Salud C, Nguyen K, et al. Randomized prospective evaluation of a novel technique for biopsy or lumpectomy of nonpalpable breast lesions: radioactive seed versus wire localization. *Ann Surg Oncol* 2001;8:711.

Green V. Breast disease: benign and malignant. In: Rock JA, Thompson JE, eds. *Telinde's operative gynecology*, 10th ed. Philadelphia, PA: Lippincott Williams & Wilkins; 2011.

Greydanus DE, Matytsina L, Gains M. Breast disorders in children and adolescents. *Prim Care* 2006;33:455.

Guide to learning in gynecologic oncology. The Division of Gynecologic Oncology ABOG, Inc.; 2013. http://www.abog.org/publications/2013%20Guide%20to%20Learning-GO.pdf.

Guiliano AE, Hunt KK, Ballman KV, et al. Axillary dissection vs no axillary dissection in women with invasive breast cancer and sentinel node metastasis: a randomized clinical trial. *JAMA* 2011;305:569.

Guiliano AE, McCall L, Beitsch P, et al. Locoregional recurrence after sentinel lymph node dissection with or without axillary dissection in patients with sentinel lymph node metastases: The American College of Surgeons Oncology Group Z0011 randomized trial. *Ann Surg Oncol* 2010;252:426.

Hahn KM, Johnson PH, Gordon N, et al. Treatment of pregnant breast cancer patients and outcomes of children exposed to chemotherapy in utero. *Cancer* 2006;107:1219.

Hajdu SI, Espinosa MH, Robbins GF. Recurrent cystosarcoma phyllodes: a clinicopathologic study of 32 cases. *Cancer* 1976;38:1402.

Halsted T. The results of operations for the cure of cancer of the breast performed Johns Hopkins Hospital from June 1989 to January 1984. *Ann Surg* 1894;20:497.

Hankinson SE, Colditz GA, Manson JE, et al. A prospective study of oral contraceptive use and risk of breast cancer (Nurses' Health Study, United States). *Cancer Causes Control* 1997;8:65.

Hannaford PC, Selvaraj S, Elliott AM, et al. Cancer risk among users of oral contraceptives: cohort data from the Royal College of General Practitioner's oral contraception study. *Br Med J* 2007;335:651.

Hansen J, Stevens RG. Case–control study of shift-work and breast cancer risk in Danish nurses: impact of shift systems. *Eur J Cancer* 2012;48:1722.

Harlow SP WD. Sentinel lymph node biopsy for breast cancer: indications and outcomes. In: Basow D, ed. *UpToDate*. Waltham, MA: UpToDate; 2013.

Harris R, Leininger L. Clinical strategies for breast cancer screening: weighing and using the evidence. *Ann Intern Med* 1995;122:539.

Hartmann LC, Schaid DJ, Woods JE, et al. Efficacy of bilateral prophylactic mastectomy in women with a family history of breast cancer. *N Engl J Med* 1999;340:77.

Hartmann LC, Sellers TA, Schaid DJ, et al. Efficacy of bilateral prophylactic mastectomy in BRCA1 and BRCA2 gene mutation carriers. *J Natl Cancer Inst* 2001;93:1633.

Hayes D. Systemic-treatment for metastatic breast cancer: selection of chemotherapy regimen. In: Basow D, ed. *UpToDate*. Waltham, MA: UpToDate; 2013.

Helvie M. Imaging analysis: mammography. In: Harris LM Jr, Morrow M, Osborne CK, eds. *Diseases of the breast*, 4th ed. Philadelphia, PA: Wolters Kluwer/Lippincott Williams & Wilkins; 2009:116.

Helvie M. Improving mammographic interpretation: double reading and computer-aided diagnosis. *Radiol Clin North Am* 2007;45:801.

Henderson TO, Amsterdam A, Bhatia S, et al. Systematic review: surveillance for breast cancer in women treated with chest radiation for childhood, adolescent, or young adult cancer. *Ann Intern Med* 2010;152:444.

Hendrick RE, Smith RA, Rutledge JH, III, et al. Benefit of screening mammography in women aged 40–49: a new meta-analysis of randomized controlled trials. *J Natl Cancer Inst Monogr* 1997;87.

Hendrick RE, Helvie MA. Mammography screening: a new estimate of number needed to screen to prevent one breast cancer death. *AJR Am J Roentgenol* 2012;198:723.

Holleb AI, Farrow JH. Breast cancer and pregnancy. A report of 283 patients. *Acta Unio Inter Contra Cancrum* 1964;20:1480.

Holleb AI, Farrow JH. The relation of carcinoma of the breast and pregnancy in 283 patients. *Surg Gynecol Obstet* 1962;115:65.

Isaacs JH. Other nipple discharge. *Clin Obstet Gynecol* 1994; 37:898.

Issacs C FS, Penskin BN. Genetic testing for hereditary breast and ovarian cancer syndrome. In: Basow D, ed. *UpToDate*. Waltham, MA: UpToDate; 2013.

Jin H, Tu D, Zhao N, et al. Longer-term outcomes of letrozole versus placebo after 5 years of tamoxifen in the NCIC CTG MA.17 trial: analyses adjusting for treatment crossover. *J Clin Oncol* 2012;30:718.

Johannsson O, Loman N, Borg A, et al. Pregnancy-associated breast cancer in BRCA1 and BRCA2 germline mutation carriers. *Lancet* 1998;352:1359.

Kaufman CS, Littrey PJ, Freeman-Gibb LA, et al. Office-based cryoablation of breast fibroadenomas with long-term follow-up. *Breast J* 2005;11:344.

Keleher A, Wendt R, III, Delpassand E, et al. The safety of lymphatic mapping in pregnant breast cancer patients using Tc-99m sulfur colloid. *Breast J* 2004;10:492.

Kelley J. Evaluation of a breast lump. *Atlas Office Proced* 2001;4:397.

Kerlikowske K, Grady D, Rubin SM, et al. Efficacy of screening mammography. A meta-analysis. *JAMA* 1995;273:149.

Khatcheressian JL, Hurley P, Bantug E, et al. Breast cancer follow-up and management after primary treatment: American Society of Clinical Oncology clinical practice guideline update. *J Clin Oncol* 2013;31:961.

Kim T, Giuliano AE, Lyman GH. Lymphatic mapping and sentinel lymph node biopsy in early-stage breast carcinoma: a metaanalysis. *Cancer* 2006;106:4.

King RM, Welch JS, Martin JK, Jr, et al. Carcinoma of the breast associated with pregnancy. *Surg Gynecol Obstet* 1985;160:228.

Kok RD, de Vries MM, Heerschap A, et al. Absence of harmful effects of magnetic resonance exposure at 1.5 T in utero during the third trimester of pregnancy: a follow-up study. *Magn Reson Imaging* 2004;22:851.

Krag DN, Anderson SJ, Julian TB, et al. Sentinel-lymph-node resection compared with conventional axillary-lymph-node dissection in clinically node-negative patients with breast cancer: overall survival findings from the NSABP B-32 randomised phase 3 trial. *Lancet Oncol* 2010;11:927.

Krag DN, Anderson SJ, Julian TB, et al. Technical outcomes of sentinel-lymph-node resection and conventional axillary-lymph-node dissection in patients with clinically node-negative breast cancer: results from the NSABP B-32 randomised phase III trial. *Lancet Oncol* 2007;8:881.

Kriege M, Brekelmans CT, Boetes C, et al. Efficacy of MRI and mammography for breast-cancer screening in women with a familial or genetic predisposition. *N Engl J Med* 2004;351:427.

Land SR, Kopec JA, Julian TB, et al. Patient-reported outcomes in sentinel node-negative adjuvant breast cancer patients receiving sentinel-node biopsy or axillary dissection: National Surgical Adjuvant Breast and Bowel Project phase III protocol B-32. *J Clin Oncol* 2010;28:3929.

Lee CH, Dershaw DD, Kopans D, et al. Breast cancer screening with imaging: recommendations from the Society of Breast Imaging and

the ACR on the use of mammography, breast MRI, breast ultrasound, and other technologies for the detection of clinically occult breast cancer. *J Am Coll Radiol* 2010;7:18.

Lehman CD, Gatsonis C, Kuhl CK, et al. MRI evaluation of the contralateral breast in women with recently diagnosed breast cancer. *N Engl J Med* 2007;356:1295.

Levine EA, Freimanis RI, Perrier ND, et al. Positron emission mammography: initial clinical results. *Ann Surg Oncol* 2003;10:86.

Li C, Daling JR, Porter PL, et al. Relationship between potentially modifiable lifestyle factors and risk of second primary contralateral breast cancer among women diagnosed with estrogen receptor-positive invasive breast cancer. *J Clin Oncol* 2009;27:5312.

Liede A, Karlan BY, Narod SA. Cancer risks for male carriers of germline mutations in BRCA1 or BRCA2: a review of the literature. *J Clin Oncol* 2004;22:735.

Llombart-Cussac A, Ruiz A, Anton A, et al. Exemestane versus anastrozole as front-line endocrine therapy in postmenopausal patients with hormone receptor-positive, advanced breast cancer: final results from the Spanish Breast Cancer Group 2001–03 phase 2 randomized trial. *Cancer* 2012;118:241.

Loibl S, Han SN, von Minckwitz G, et al. Treatment of breast cancer during pregnancy: an observational study. *Lancet Oncol* 2012;13:887.

Loibl S, von Minckwitz G, Gwyn K, et al. Breast carcinoma during pregnancy. International recommendations from an expert meeting. *Cancer* 2006;106:237.

Loprinzi CL, Kugler JW, Sloan JA, et al. Venlafaxine in management of hot flashes in survivors of breast cancer: a randomised controlled trial. *Lancet* 2000;356:2059.

Love RR, Philips J. Oophorectomy for breast cancer: history revisited. *J Natl Cancer Inst* 2002;94:1433.

Lucci A, McCall LM, Beitsch PD, et al. Surgical complications associated with sentinel lymph node dissection (SLND) plus axillary lymph node dissection compared with SLND alone in the American College of Surgeons Oncology Group Trial Z0011. *J Clin Oncol* 2007;25:3657.

Lyman G, Giuliano AE, Somerfield MR, et al. American Society of Clinical Oncology guideline recommendations for sentinel lymph node biopsy in early-stage breast cancer. *J Clin Oncol* 2005;23:7703.

Madden JL, Kandalaft S, Bourque RA. Modified radical mastectomy. *Ann Surg* 1972;175:624.

Mandelblatt JS, Cronin KA, Bailey S, et al. Effects of mammography screening under different screening schedules: model estimates of potential benefits and harms. *Ann Intern Med* 2009;151:738.

Marchant D. Role of the obstetrician/gynecologist in the management of breast disease in contemporary management of breast disease 1: benign disease. *Obstet Gynecol* 1994;21:421.

Marchbanks PA, McDonald JA, Wilson HG, et al. Oral contraceptives and the risk of breast cancer. *N Engl J Med* 2002;346:2025.

Margenthaler J. Technique of axillary dissection. In: Basow D, ed. *UpToDate*. Waltham, MA: UpToDate; 2013.

Mathelin C, Croce S, Brasse D, et al. Methylene blue dye, an accurate dye for sentinel lymph node identification in early breast cancer. *Anticancer Res* 2009;29:4119.

McGhan LJ, McKeever SC, Pockaj BA, et al. Radioactive seed localization for nonpalpable breast lesions: review of 1,000 consecutive procedures at a single institution. *Ann Surg Oncol* 2011; 18:3096.

McGhan LJ, Pockaj BA, Wasif N, et al. Atypical ductal hyperplasia on core biopsy: an automatic trigger for excisional biopsy? *Ann Surg Oncol* 2012;19:3264.

Merajver SD, Sabel MS. Inflammatory breast cancer. In: Harris LM Jr, Morrow M, Osborne CK, eds. *Diseases of the breast*, 4th ed. Philadelphia, PA: Wolter Klower/Lippincott Williams & Wilkins; 2010:762.

Mevissen M, Buntenkotter S, Loscher W. Effects of static and time-varying (50-Hz) magnetic fields on reproduction and fetal development in rats. *Teratology* 1994;50:229.

Meyer W. An improved method of the radical operation for carcinoma of the breast. *Med Rec N Y* 1984;46:746.

Michell MJ, Iqbal A, Wasan RK, et al. A comparison of the accuracy of film-screen mammography, full-field digital mammography, and digital breast tomosynthesis. *Clin Radiol* 2012;67:976.

Middleton LP, Amin M, Gwyn K, et al. Breast carcinoma in pregnant women: assessment of clinicopathologic and immunohistochemical features. *Cancer* 2003;98:1055.

Miller AB, Baines CJ, To T, et al. Canadian National Breast Screening Study: 1. Breast cancer detection and death rates among women aged 40 to 49 years. *CMAJ* 1992;147:1459.

Miller AB, Baines CJ, To T, et al. Canadian National Breast Screening Study: 2. Breast cancer detection and death rates among women aged 50 to 59 years. *CMAJ* 1992;147:1477.

Miller AB, To T, Baines CJ, et al. Canadian National Breast Screening Study-2: 13-year results of a randomized trial in women aged 50–59 years. *J Natl Cancer Inst* 2000;92:1490.

Miller AB, To T, Baines CJ, et al. The Canadian National Breast Screening Study: update on breast cancer mortality. *J Natl Cancer Inst Monogr* 1997:37.

Mohler ER MT. *Prevention and treatment of lymphedema.* Waltham, MA: *UpToDate;* 2013.

Moja L, Tagliabue L, Balduzzi S, et al. Trastuzumab containing regimens for early breast cancer. *Cochrane Database Syst Rev* 2012; 4:CD006243.

Mondi MM, Cuenca RE, Ollila DW, et al. Sentinel lymph node biopsy during pregnancy: initial clinical experience. *Ann Surg Oncol* 2007;14:218.

Morton DL, Wen DR, Wong JH, et al. Technical details of intraoperative lymphatic mapping for early stage melanoma. *Arch Surg* 1992;127:392.

Moss SM, Cuckle H, Evans A, et al. Effect of mammographic screening from age 40 years on breast cancer mortality at 10 years' follow-up: a randomised controlled trial. *Lancet* 2006;368:2053.

Murray MP, Luedtke C, Liberman L, et al. Classic lobular carcinoma in situ and atypical lobular hyperplasia at percutaneous breast core biopsy: outcomes of prospective excision. *Cancer* 2012;119:1073.

Murthy K, Aznar M, Thompson CJ, et al. Results of preliminary clinical trials of the positron emission mammography system PEM-I: a dedicated breast imaging system producing glucose metabolic images using FDG. *J Nucl Med* 2000;41:1851.

Nahabedian M. Breast reconstruction in women with breast cancer. In: Basow D, ed. *UpToDate.* Waltham, MA: UpToDate; 2013.

Network NCC. *Breast cancer v1.2013*; 2013: http://www.nccn.org/professionals/physician_gls/pdf/breast.pdf, Accessed on 24 February, 2013.

Network NCC. *Breast cancer 1.2013*; 2013: http://www.nccn.org/professionals/physician_gls/pdf/breast.pdf. Accessed on 12 March, 2013.

Nonmalignant conditions of the breast: ACOG Technical Bulletin. Washington, DC: The American College of Obstetricians and Gynecologists Compendium of Selected Publications; 2001.

Nugent P, O'Connell TX. Breast cancer and pregnancy. *Arch Surg* 1985;120:1221.

Oktay K, Buyuk E, Libertella N, et al. Fertility preservation in breast cancer patients: a prospective controlled comparison of ovarian stimulation with tamoxifen and letrozole for embryo cryopreservation. *J Clin Oncol* 2005;23:4347.

Oktay K. Fertility preservation: an emerging discipline in the care of young patients with cancer. *Lancet Oncol* 2005;6:192.

Olson JE, Neuberg D, Pandya KJ, et al. The role of radiotherapy in the management of operable locally advanced breast carcinoma: results of a randomized trial by the Eastern Cooperative Oncology Group. *Cancer* 1997;79:1138.

Osborne MP. Breast anatomy and development. In: Harris LM Jr, Morrow M, Osborne CK, eds. *Diseases of the breast.* Philadelphia, PA: Wolters Kluwer/Lippincott Williams & Wilkins; 2010:1.

Ovarian ablation in early breast cancer: overview of the randomised trials. Early Breast Cancer Trialists' Collaborative Group. *Lancet* 1996;348:1189.

Page DL, Dupont WD, Rogers LW, et al. Atypical hyperplastic lesions of the female breast. A long-term follow-up study. *Cancer* 1985;55:2698.

Page DL, Kidd TE, Jr, Dupont WD, et al. Lobular neoplasia of the breast: higher risk for subsequent invasive cancer predicted by more extensive disease. *Hum Pathol* 1991;22:1232.

Patey DH, Dyson WH. The prognosis of carcinoma of the breast in relation to the type of operation performed. *Br J Cancer* 1948;2:7.

Peto R, Davies C, Godwin J, et al. Comparisons between different polychemotherapy regimens for early breast cancer: meta-analyses

of long-term outcome among 100,000 women in 123 randomised trials. *Lancet* 2012;379:432.

Petrek JA, Dukoff R, Rogatko A. Prognosis of pregnancy-associated breast cancer. *Cancer* 1991;67:869.

Pierce JP, Stephanick ML, Flatt SW, et al. Greater survival after breast cancer in physically active women with high vegetable-fruit intake regardless of obesity. *J Clin Oncol* 2007;25:2345.

Pijpe A, Andrieu N, Easton DF, et al. Exposure to diagnostic radiation and risk of breast cancer among carriers of BRCA1/2 mutations: retrospective cohort study (GENE-RAD-RISK). *Br Med J* 2012;345:e5660.

Polat AK, Kanbour-Shakir A, Andacoglu O, et al. Atypical hyperplasia on core biopsy: is further surgery needed? *Am J Med Sci* 2012;344:28.

Polgar C, Major T, Fodor J, et al. Accelerated partial-breast irradiation using high-dose-rate interstitial brachytherapy: 12-year update of a prospective clinical study. *Radiother Oncol* 2010;94:274.

Polgar C, Strnad V, Kovacs G. Partial-breast irradiation or whole-breast radiotherapy for early breast cancer: a meta-analysis of randomized trials. *Strahlenther Onkol* 2010;186:113.

Polgar C, Van Limbergen E, Potter R, et al. Patient selection for accelerated partial-breast irradiation (APBI) after breast-conserving surgery: recommendations of the Groupe Europeen de Curietherapie-European Society for Therapeutic Radiology and Oncology (GEC-ESTRO) breast cancer working group based on clinical evidence (2009). *Radiother Oncol* 2010;94:264.

Poplack SP, Tosteson TD, Kogel CA, et al. Digital breast tomosynthesis: initial experience in 98 women with abnormal digital screening mammography. *AJR Am J Roentgenol* 2007;189:616.

Powles T, Eeles, R, Ashley S, et al. Interim analysis of the incidence of breast cancer in the Royal Marsden Hospital tamoxifen randomised chemoprevention trial. *Lancet* 1998;352:98.

Preece PE, Baum M, Mansel RE, et al. Importance of mastalgia in operable breast cancer. *Br Med J* 1982;284:1299.

Pruthi S, Wahner-Roedler DL, Torkelson CJ, et al. Vitamin E and evening primrose oil for management of cyclical mastalgia: a randomized pilot study. *Altern Med Rev* 2010;15:59.

Rakha EA, El-Sayed ME, Lee AH, et al. Prognostic significance of Nottingham histologic grade in invasive breast carcinoma. *J Clin Oncol* 2008;26:3153.

Reed W, Sandstad B, Holm R, et al. The prognostic impact of hormone receptors and c-erbB-2 in pregnancy-associated breast cancer and their correlation with BRCA1 and cell cycle modulators. *Int J Surg Pathol* 2003;11:65.

Ring AE, Smith IE, Jones A, et al. Chemotherapy for breast cancer during pregnancy: an 18-year experience from five London teaching hospitals. *J Clin Oncol* 2005;23:4192.

Riveros M, Garcia R, Cabanas R. Lymphadenography of the dorsal lymphatics of the penis. Technique and results. *Cancer* 1967;20:2026.

Roberts JE, Oktay K. Fertility preservation: a comprehensive approach to the young woman with cancer. *J Natl Cancer Inst Monogr* 2005:57.

Roberts MM, Alexander FE, Anderson TJ, et al. The Edinburgh randomised trial of screening for breast cancer: description of method. *Br J Cancer* 1984;50:1.

Rodriguez AO, Chew H, Cress R, et al. Evidence of poorer survival in pregnancy-associated breast cancer. *Obstet Gynecol* 2008; 112:71.

Röntgen WC. On a new kind of rays. Sitzungsberichte de Würsburgher Physik-medik. Gesellschaft,1895. Role of the Obstetrician-Gynecologist in the Screening and Diagnosis of Breast Masses. ACOG Committee Opinion 334. *Obstet Gynecol* 2006;107: 1213.

Rosen EL, Turkington TG, Soo MS, et al. Detection of primary breast carcinoma with a dedicated, large-field-of-view FDG PET mammography device: initial experience. *Radiology* 2005;234:527.

Salama M, Winkler K, Murach KF, et al. Female fertility loss and preservation: threats and opportunities. *Ann Oncol* 2013;24:598.

Sardanelli F, Giuseppetti GM, Panizza P, et al. Sensitivity of MRI versus mammography for detecting foci of multifocal, multicentric breast cancer in fatty and dense breasts using the whole-breast pathologic examination as a gold standard. *AJR Am J Roentgenol* 2004;183:1149.

VIII

Schernhammer ES, Laden F, Speizer FE, et al. Rotating night shifts and risk of breast cancer in women participating in the nurses' health study. *J Natl Cancer Inst* 2001;93:1563.

Schnitt SA. Pathology of benign breast disorders. In: Schnitt SA, ed. *Diseases of the breast*, 4th ed. Philadelphia, PA: Wolters Kluwer/Lippincott Williams & Wilkins; 2010:116.

Schoenwolf GC, Brauer DR, Francis-West PH. *Larsen's human embryology*. Philadelphia, PA: Churchill Livingstone Elsevier; 2009.

Schott A. Systemic treatment for HER-2 positive metastatic disease. In: Hayes DF, ed. UpToDate. Waltham, MA: UpToDate; 2014.

Shah C, Wobb J, Grills I, et al. Use of intensity modulated radiation therapy to reduce acute and chronic toxicities of breast cancer patients treated with traditional and accelerated whole breast irradiation. *Pract Radiat Oncol* 2012;2:e45.

Shapiro S, Venet W, Strax P, et al. Ten- to fourteen-year effect of screening on breast cancer mortality. *J Natl Cancer Inst* 1982;69:349.

Shapiro S, Venet W, Strax P. *Periodic screening for breast cancer: the Health Insurance Plan project and its sequelae*. Baltimore, MD: Johns Hopkins Press; 1988.

Shen T, Vortmeyer AO, Zhuang Z, et al. High frequency of allelic loss of BRCA2 gene in pregnancy-associated breast carcinoma. *J Natl Cancer Inst* 1999;91:1686.

Shestak KC, Johnson RR, Greco RJ, et al. Partial mastectomy and breast reduction as a valuable treatment option for patients with macromastia and carcinoma of the breast. *Surg Gynecol Obstet* 1993;177:54.

Shousha S. Breast carcinoma presenting during or shortly after pregnancy and lactation. *Arch Pathol Lab Med* 2000;124:1053.

Siegel R, Ma J, Zou Z, et al. Cancer statistics, 2014. *CA: Cancer J Clinicians* 2014;64;9.

Sikov WM, Wolf AC.Neoadjuvant therapy for breast cancer: Rationale, pretreatment evaluation, and therapeutic options. In: Gralow JR, Hayes DF ed. UpToDate. Waltham, MA: UpToDate; 2014.

Silverstein MJ, Lagios MD, Craig PH, et al. A prognostic index for ductal carcinoma in situ of the breast. *Cancer* 1996;77:2267.

Skaane P, Gullien R, Bjorndal H, et al. Digital breast tomosynthesis (DBT): initial experience in a clinical setting. *Acta Radiol* 2012;53:524.

Skaane P, Hofvind S, Skjennald A. Randomized trial of screen-film versus full-field digital mammography with soft-copy reading in population-based screening program: follow-up and final results of Oslo II study. *Radiology* 2007;244:708.

Smith BD, Smith GL, Buchholz TA. Brachytherapy vs whole-breast irradiation: trial by data. *Int J Radiat Oncol Biol Phys* 2012;83:1078.

Smith RA, Duffy SW, Gabe R, et al. The randomized trials of breast cancer screening: what have we learned? *Radiol Clin North Am* 2004;42:793.

Smith RL, Pruthi S, Fitzpatrick LA. Evaluation and management of breast pain. *Mayo Clin Proc* 2004;79:353.

Spangler ML, Zuley ML, Sumkin JH, et al. Detection and classification of calcifications on digital breast tomosynthesis and 2D digital mammography: a comparison. *AJR Am J Roentgenol* 2011;196:320.

Spear SL, Hannan CM, Willey SC, et al. Nipple-sparing mastectomy. *Plast Reconst Surg* 2009;123:1665.

Srivastava A, Mansel RE, Arvind N, et al. Evidence-based management of Mastalgia: a meta-analysis of randomised trials. *Breast* 2007;16:503.

Svahn TM, Chakraborty DP, Ikeda D, et al. Breast tomosynthesis and digital mammography: a comparison of diagnostic accuracy. *Br J Radiol* 2012;85:e1074.

Svane G, Azavedo E, Lindman K, et al. Clinical experience of photon counting breast tomosynthesis: comparison with traditional mammography. *Acta Radiol* 2011;52:134.

Tabar L, Chen HH, Fagerberg G, et al. Recent results from the Swedish Two-County Trial: the effects of age, histologic type, and mode of detection on the efficacy of breast cancer screening. *J Natl Cancer Inst Monogr* 1997:43.

Tabar L, Fagerberg CJ, Gad A, et al. Reduction in mortality from breast cancer after mass screening with mammography. Randomised trial from the Breast Cancer Screening Working Group of the Swedish National Board of Health and Welfare. *Lancet* 1985;1:829.

Tabar L, Fagerberg G, Duffy SW, et al. The Swedish two county trial of mammographic screening for breast cancer: recent results and calculation of benefit. *J Epidemiol Community Health* 1989;43:107.

Tabar L, Vitak B, Chen HH, et al. The Swedish Two-County Trial twenty years later. Updated mortality results and new insights from long-term follow-up. *Radiol Clin North Am* 2000;38:625.

Tadwalkar RV, Rapelyea JA, Torrente J, et al. Breast-specific gamma imaging as an adjunct modality for the diagnosis of invasive breast cancer with correlation to tumour size and grade. *Br J Radiol* 2012;85:e212.

Taghian A, El-Ghamry M, Merajver SD. Overview of the treatment of newly diagnosed, non-metastatic breast cancer. In: Basow D, ed. UpToDate. Waltham, MA: UpToDate; 2013.

Early Breast Cancer Trialists' Collaborative Group. Tamoxifen for early breast cancer: an overview of the randomised trials. *Lancet* 1998;351:1451.

Tanner J. Physical growth and development. In: Forfar JO, Arnell GC, eds. *Textbook of paediatrics*. Edinburgh, Scotland: Churchill Livingston; 1984:292.

Tanner J. *Wachstun und Reifung des Menschen*. Stuttgart, Germany: Georg Thieme Verlag; 1962.

Thomas DB, Gao DL, Ray RM, et al. Randomized trial of breast self-examination in Shanghai: final results. *J Natl Cancer Inst* 2002;94:1445.

Toth BA, Forley BG, Calabria R. Retrospective study of the skin-sparing mastectomy in breast reconstruction. *Plast Reconstr Surg* 1999;104:77.

Toth BA, Lappert P. Modified skin incisions for mastectomy: the need for plastic surgical input in preoperative planning. *Plast Reconstr Surg* 1991;87:1048.

Uhara H, Takata M, Saida T. Sentinel lymph node biopsy in Japan. *Int J Clin Oncol* 2009;14:490.

Urban J. Excision of the major duct system of the breast. *Cancer* 1963;16:515.

Vaidya JS, Baum M, Tobias JS, et al. Long-term results of targeted intraoperative radiotherapy (Targit) boost during breast-conserving surgery. *Int J Radiat Oncol Biol Phys* 2011;81:1091.

Vaidya JS, Joseph DJ, Tobias JS, et al. Targeted intraoperative radiotherapy versus whole breast radiotherapy for breast cancer (TARGIT-A trial): an international, prospective, randomised, non-inferiority phase 3 trial. *Lancet* 2010;376:91.

Vaidya JS, Wenz F, Bulsara M, et al. Risk-adapted targeted intraoperative radiotherapy versus whole-breast radiotherapy for breast cancer: 5-year results for local control and overall survival from the TARGIT-A randomised trial. *Lancet* 2014;383:603.

Vaidya JS, Wenz F, Bulsara M, et al. Radiotherapy for breast cancer, the TARGIT—a trial. Authors' reply. *Lancet* 2014;383:1719.

van den Brandt PA, Spiegelman D, Yaun SS, et al. Pooled analysis of prospective cohort studies on height, weight, and breast cancer risk. *Am J Epidemiol* 2000;152:514.

Vargas C, Keslin L, Go N, et al. Factors associated with local recurrence and cause-specific survival in patients with ductal carcinoma in situ of the breast treated with breast-conserving therapy or mastectomy. *Int J Radiat Oncol Biol Phys* 2005;63:1514.

Vargas HI. Blue dye of choice for lymphatic mapping. *J Clin Oncol* 2005;23:3648.

Veronesi U, Saccozzi R, Del Vecchio M, et al. Comparing radical mastectomy with quadrantectomy, axillary dissection, and radiotherapy in patients with small cancers of the breast. *N Engl J Med* 1981;305:6.

Vincent A, Barton DL, Mandrekar JN, et al. Acupuncture for hot flashes: a randomized, sham-controlled clinical study. *Menopause* 2007;14:45.

Vogel VG Constantino J, Wickerham DL, et al. Update of the National Surgical Adjuvant Breast and Bowel Project Study of Tamoxifen and Raloxifene (STAR) P-2 trial: preventing breast cancer. *Cancer Prev Res* 2010;3:696.

Vogel VG, Costantino JP, Wickerham DL, et al. Effects of tamoxifen vs raloxifene on the risk of developing invasive breast cancer and other disease outcomes: the NSABP Study of Tamoxifen and Raloxifene (STAR) P-2 trial. *JAMA* 2006;295:2727.

Wald N, Chamberlain J, Hackshaw A. Report of the European Society of Mastology Breast Cancer Screening Evaluation Committee. *Tumori* 1993;79:371.

Wallis MG, Moa E, Zanca F, et al. Two-view and single-view tomosynthesis versus full-field digital mammography: high-resolution X-ray imaging observer study. *Radiology* 2012;262:788.

Wapnir IL, Dignan J, Fisher B, et al. Long-term outcomes of invasive ipsilateral breast tumor recurrences after lumpectomy in NSABP B-17 and B-24 randomized clinical trials for DCIS. *J Natl Cancer Inst* 2011;103:478.

Warner E, Plewes DB, Hill KA, et al. Surveillance of BRCA1 and BRCA2 mutation carriers with magnetic resonance imaging, ultrasound, mammography, and clinical breast examination. *JAMA* 2004;292:1317.

Weaver DL, Ashikaga T, Krag DN, et al. Effect of occult metastases on survival in node-negative breast cancer. *N Engl J Med* 2011;364:412.

White E, Miglioretti DL, Yankaskas BC, et al. Biennial versus annual mammography and the risk of late-stage breast cancer. *J Natl Cancer Inst* 2004;96:1832.

Wingo PA, Jamison PM, Young JL, et al. Population-based statistics for women diagnosed with inflammatory breast cancer (United States). *Cancer Causes Control* 2004;15:321.

Woodburne R. *Essentials of human anatomy.* New York, NY: Oxford University Press; 1979.

Zakaria S, Hoskin TL, Degnim AC. Safety and technical success of methylene blue dye for lymphatic mapping in breast cancer. *Am J Surg* 2008;196:228.

CHAPTER 46
The Vermiform Appendix in Relation to Gynecology

Amanda C. Yunker

DEFINITIONS

Appendicitis—Inflammation of the appendix, usually caused by obstruction of the appendiceal lumen, with subsequent distention of the appendix with secretions, venous congestion, bacterial proliferation, ischemia, and necrosis.

McBurney point—A point on the anterior abdominal wall, located 1/3 the distance between the right anterior superior iliac spine and the umbilicus.

Obturator sign—Increased pain in the abdomen, specifically the right lower quadrant, with passive internal rotation and flexion of the right lower extremity at the hip joint.

Psoas sign—Increased pain in the abdomen as the right lower extremity is moved into extension, with the patient in the left lateral decubitus position, and asking the patient to actively flex the leg at the hip joint against resistance.

Rovsing sign—Pain reported by the patient in the right lower quadrant of the abdomen while applying pressure to the left lower quadrant.

Fecalith—An intestinal stone formed around a central core of fecal matter.

The vermiform appendix, named for its wormlike appearance, is part of the gastrointestinal tract and usually falls in the purview of general surgeons. However, there are several gynecologic and obstetric associations with the appendix, some of which could be fatal, requiring the obstetrician–gynecologist to be mindful of this organ, its potential diseases, and its effects on other gynecologic structures.

The appendix is most commonly evaluated for acute abdominal pain, which could be the result of acute appendicitis. This occurs in 7% of the population over a lifetime, resulting in the most commonly performed emergent surgical procedure: appendectomy. It is estimated that approximately 300,000 emergent appendectomies are performed annually in the United States. The majority of cases occur in young patients, usually under age 20. However, appendicitis can occur even in elderly patients, and these patients have much higher morbidity and mortality rates associated with appendicitis and appendectomy, compared with their younger counterparts.

As an obstetrician–gynecologist, the appendix is of interest for many reasons. First, women presenting with acute-onset abdominal pain will likely be referred to a gynecologist for evaluation. Appendicitis should be included in the differential, along with pelvic inflammatory disease, ectopic pregnancy, ovarian cyst, ovarian torsion, and urinary tract infection. Second, acute appendicitis, especially if the appendix is ruptured, can have a negative impact on fertility given the anatomic proximity of the appendix to the fallopian tubes (**Fig. 46.1**). Third, though infrequent, appendicitis can occur during pregnancy and is associated with a higher morbidity in pregnant females

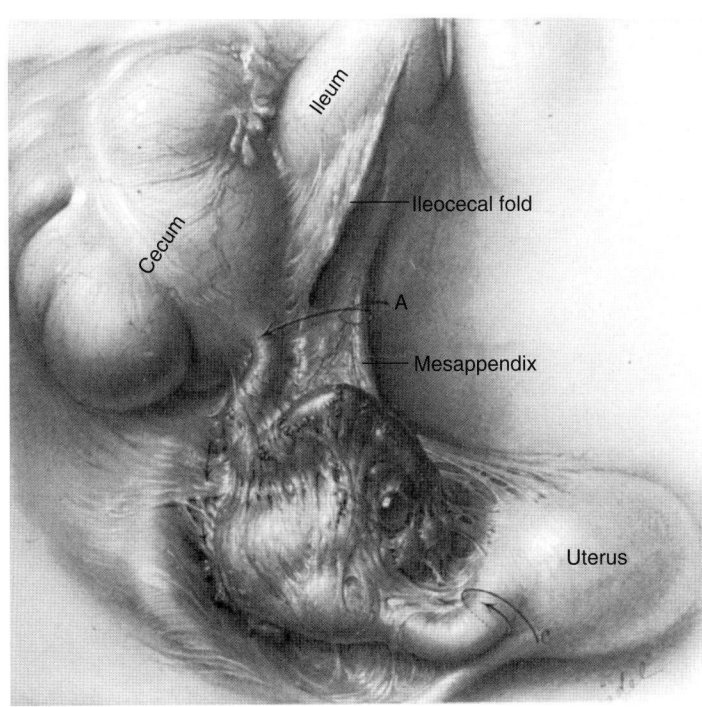

FIGURE 46.1 As illustrated in this original Max Brödel drawing, inflammatory disease of the appendix can involve the fallopian tube or vice versa. Extensive adhesions can form. The tube and the appendix can be removed as a single mass. (The original illustration is in the Max Brödel Archives in the Department of Art as Applied to Medicine, The Johns Hopkins University School of Medicine, Baltimore, MD, USA. Used with permission.)

VIII

compared to nonpregnant females. Pregnancy can complicate the differential diagnosis of abdominal pain simply because the pregnancy itself adds multiple etiologies for abdominal pain, and the anatomic location of the appendix can shift cephalad due to the gravid uterus. This can delay diagnosis. Finally, several gynecologic conditions—endometriosis, mucinous tumors, and ectopic pregnancy—can involve the appendix, thus compelling the obstetrician–gynecologist to include the appendix in the evaluation for chronic and acute gynecologic conditions.

ANATOMY AND FUNCTION OF THE APPENDIX

The appendix begins in infancy as a cone-shaped diverticulum at the base of the cecum. As the cecum grows in length and repeatedly distends with bowel function, the appendix eventually elongates and emerges 2 to 3 cm below the ileocecal valve. At full maturation, it is approximately 10 cm in length and 3 to 5 mm in width. The teniae coli travel along the cecum and then converge at the appendix, creating the outer longitudinal muscle of the appendix. This is helpful, in that the teniae may be followed to locate an appendix that may be hidden from view. One instance in which that occurs is a retrocecal appendix, which is found in 16% of adults. In the rest, the appendix is freely mobile and usually easily seen upon mobilization of the cecum (**Fig. 46.2**). The location of the appendix thus can vary and may influence the location of perceived pain during acute appendicitis.

Early in life, the appendix is composed of large collections of lymphoid follicles that then atrophy and decrease over time. This occurs with simultaneous fibrosis of the wall of the appendix and possible obliteration of the lumen. The lumen itself is lined with colonic mucosa, and the wall of the appendix is composed of smooth muscle, similar to the large and small bowel.

The appendix is supplied by two arterial branches. The main artery for the appendix is the appendicular artery, a branch of the ileocolic artery. It runs parallel to the appendix, in the mesoappendix. The base of the appendix is also supplied by a branch of the posterior cecal artery.

Thought to be primarily a vestigial organ, current general consensus is the appendix serves no function in humans. Due to the large presence of lymphoid tissue in childhood, the hypothesis exists that the appendix once played a role in immune protection of the intestinal tract. Additionally, the appendix does secrete immunoglobulin A, a mucosal surface antibody, thus bolstering the idea that it serves some immune function. However, the amount of secretion is minimal, and

the majority is not likely to breach the lumen into the cecum. Thus, removal of the appendix results in no obvious negative physiologic consequence.

ACUTE APPENDICITIS

Pathology arises within the appendix usually as a result of lumen obstruction. The most common cause of obstruction is fecaliths (50%), but other possibilities include lymphoid hyperplasia, malignancy, parasitic infections, endometriosis, and ingested foreign bodies (such as gum, teeth, nails, fruit pits, etc.). Once the lumen is blocked, the appendiceal secretions have no exit, resulting in venous congestion, ischemia, and necrosis. The bacteria, which are already present within the appendix lumen, become trapped and replicate, resulting in local tissue inflammation and pus formation. If untreated, rupture and abscess formation can occur. Leakage of the bacteria through the perforation and into the abdominal cavity leads to peritonitis (Fig. 46.3).

The lifetime risk for developing appendicitis is around 7%, with the majority of patients presenting in the second and third decade of life. The risk of mortality is this group is low, less than 1%, due to appropriate detection and early treatment. However, in individuals over age 50, although the incidence of appendicitis is extremely low, the risk of mortality from acute appendicitis is higher—5% to 15%. This group is also at risk for increased morbidity (50% to 60%) from the disease, such as longer hospitalization, wound infection, higher rates of perforation, sepsis, and other organ failure.

The diagnosis of appendicitis is usually delayed in the elderly, thus resulting in a far-advanced disease process when treatment is eventually started. This delay is likely a result of many factors: The elderly tend to delay seeking care, their symptoms are less specific than are those of their younger counterparts, and they have decreased febrile response and less prominent leukocytosis.

Clinical Presentation

The most common presenting symptom of acute appendicitis is abdominal pain, which is present in more than 95% of patients with appendicitis. The pain usually begins as diffuse and mild and is located in the periumbilical region. Once the disease process has progressed, the pain typically moves to the right lower quadrant, specifically to an area called McBurney point. The pain can be associated with fever, nausea, vomiting, and anorexia. Many times, there will be aggravation of the pain with movement. This has led to the development of many named physical exam tests, which are aimed at eliciting peritoneal stretch and irritation. These tests will be discussed below.

It should be stressed that the typical physical symptoms—pain, fever, nausea, and anorexia—are only present in 50% of patients, leaving an atypical presentation in the remaining 50%. The location of abdominal pain is variable, depending on the location of the appendix and the stage of the disease process. Although the location of the cecum is fairly constant, the appendiceal tip can be in the right upper quadrant (retrocecal), cul-de-sac, or anywhere between these two locations. As mentioned above, age also can affect the severity of pain felt by the patient. Elderly patients tend to report less severe and more diffuse abdominal pain. In a similar manner, abdominal pain is difficult to diagnose in children and infants because of the lack of ability to effectively communicate their symptoms. The incidence of appendiceal perforation is higher in these two groups for these reasons; thus, the vigilant practitioner must rely on other signs and symptoms and have a higher degree of suspicion when evaluating these patient populations. The presence of associated signs and symptoms is even more variable.

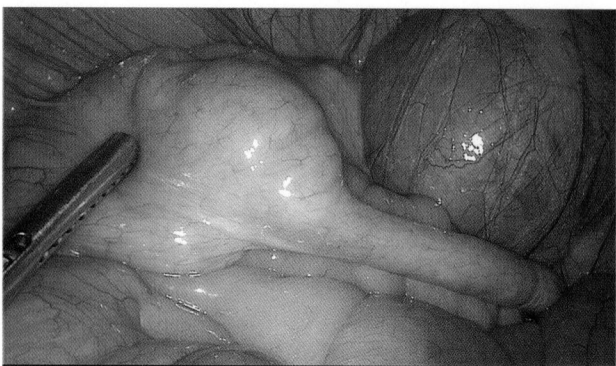

FIGURE 46.2 Mobile appendix easily seen upon mobilization of the cecum.

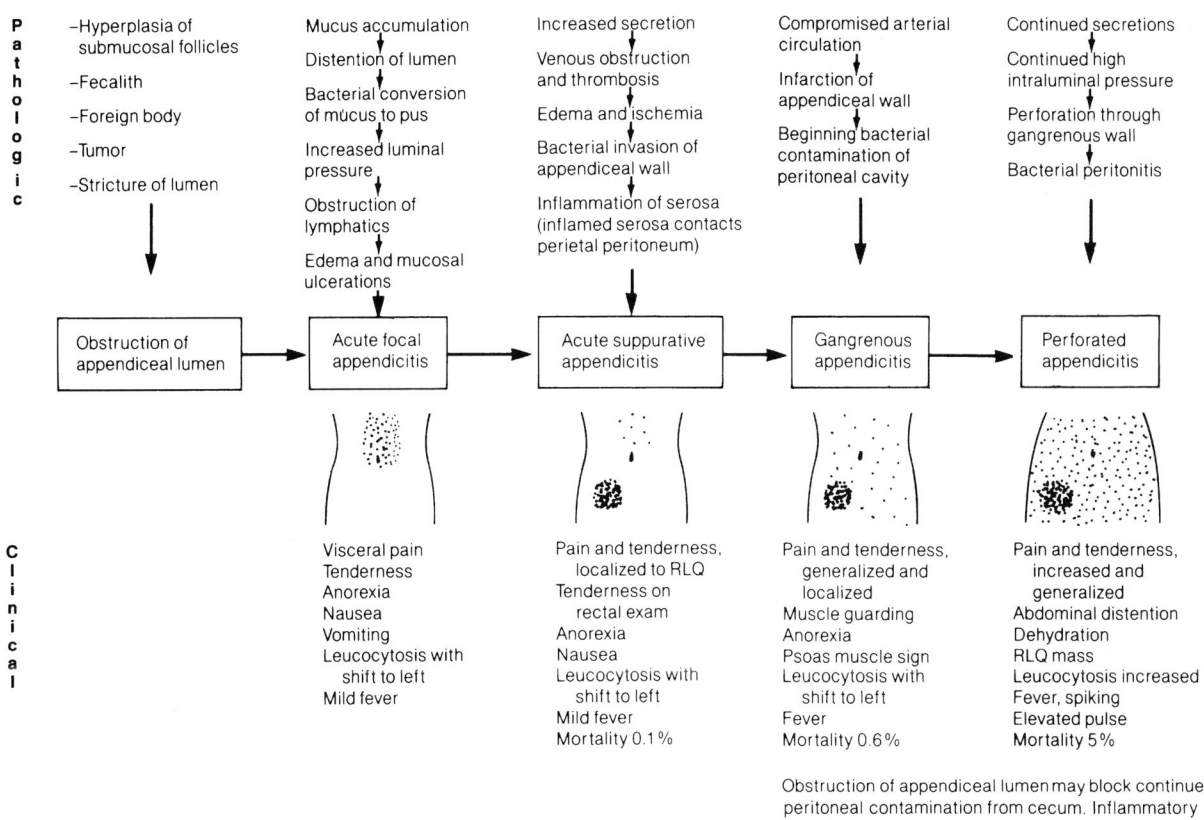

FIGURE 46.3 The clinical–pathologic correlations of appendicitis. RLQ, right lower quadrant. (From: Sabiston DC Jr, ed. *Textbook of surgery*, 14th ed. Philadelphia, PA: WB Saunders, 1991, with permission of Elsevier.)

Evaluation

Evaluation for appendicitis begins with the history and physical exam, then usually also includes several laboratory and imaging tests. The physical exam typically focuses on the abdomen and includes several "signs" that indicate peritoneal inflammation. Patients with appendicitis usually have tenderness to direct palpation (especially over McBurney point—located 1/3 the distance from the right anterior superior iliac spine to the umbilicus), rebound tenderness, and guarding of the abdomen. The Rovsing sign is often present and is described as pain in the right lower quadrant when pressure is applied to the left lower quadrant. Additionally, the patient may be positive for the psoas sign (increased pain in the abdomen as the right lower extremity is moved into extension, with the patient in the left lateral decubitus position, and asking the patient to actively flex the leg at the hip joint against resistance) or the obturator sign (increased pain in the abdomen, specifically the right lower quadrant, with passive internal rotation and flexion of the right lower extremity at the hip joint). A complete exam should include rectal and pelvic exams, which, in addition to identifying peritoneal tenderness, also can help rule in the presence of a mass or pelvic abscess.

The most common abnormal laboratory finding in a patient with appendicitis is leukocytosis. The average increase is to 15,000 WBC/mL; however, elevations in WBC are not specific for only appendicitis. Thus, leukocytosis is significant for appendicitis in the setting of the above classical presenting symptoms. Alone, leukocytosis, even with fever, is not a reliable test for appendicitis. Other causes of infection should be ruled out. Other laboratory tests that have been used included C-reactive protein and erythrocyte sedimentation rate. Because these two tests are nonspecific indicators for inflammation, they also are not helpful as individual tests for appendicitis.

Radiologic evaluation for appendicitis has increased over time and has come to include multiple different modalities. Imaging studies can be helpful in that they can image not only the appendix but also the adjacent abdominal structures, thus ruling in or out other diagnoses that can cause abdominal pain. Currently, computed tomography (CT) is usually the initial imaging technique used in emergency departments across the United States. Its diagnostic ability has been reported to be as high as 87% to 100% sensitivity and 95% to 99% specificity. Findings on CT that indicate acute appendicitis include enlarged appendix (≥6 mm), appendiceal wall thickening, periappendiceal fat stranding, and appendiceal wall enhancement (**Fig. 46.4**). CT may also diagnose an appendicolith, abscess, or the presence of free air. The Surgical Infection Society and Infectious Disease Society of America recommend helical CT with IV contrast only as the test of choice in patients with suspected appendicitis, if imaging is indicated and necessary. One benefit of preoperative imaging in patients with suspected appendicitis is the reduction in negative appendectomies (those with no pathology).

Ultrasound, unlike CT, is operator dependent, and its accuracy for diagnosis of appendicitis varies from institution to institution. However, in a comparison between the two imaging types, both CT and US were highly specific (93% to 95%) in both adults and children, whereas CT was more sensitive.

VIII

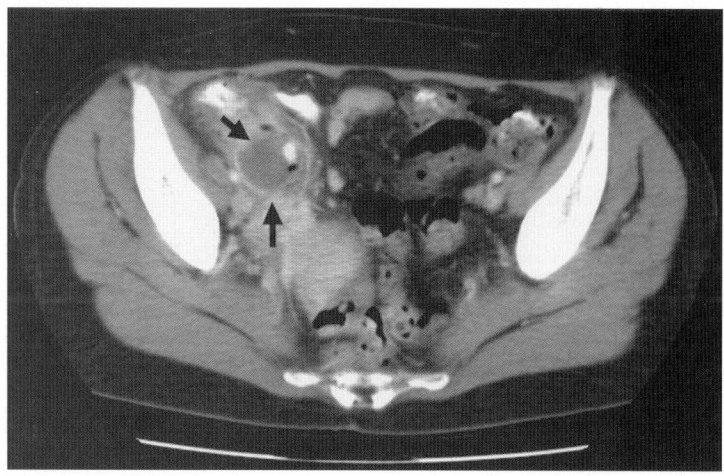

FIGURE 46.4 Computed tomography of appendiceal abscess. Note complex fluid mass with an enhancing rim in the right lower quadrant (*arrows*). (Courtesy of Ronald Arildsen, MD, Vanderbilt University.)

Ultrasound is beneficial in that it does not expose patients to ionizing radiation and thus can be used safely in pregnant patients. Most young women presenting for acute abdominal/pelvic pain, even those who are not pregnant, usually undergo US evaluation of the reproductive organs. Thus, performing US evaluation of the appendix is efficient, convenient, and cost-effective. The technique involves directing gradual pressure over the right lower quadrant in an attempt to collapse the overlying bowel and visualize the appendix. A typical "target appearance" identifies the appendix by characteristic changes within its wall (Fig. 46.5). Findings on US that are associated with acute appendicitis include increased appendiceal diameter (≥6 to 7 mm), loculated pericecal fluid, luminal distention, lack of compressibility, prominent pericecal fat, and loss of the submucosal layer.

Magnetic resonance imaging (MRI) is currently being investigated as a potential diagnostic tool for acute appendicitis. Its disadvantages include its much higher cost, when compared to CT or US, and its decreased availability to smaller/more rural institutions. However, there may be some advantages in special patient populations, such as pregnancy, which is discussed later.

Laparoscopy can be both diagnostic and therapeutic for acute appendicitis. If clinical suspicion is high enough, then surgical evaluation is justified. However, appendectomy for a nonpathologic appendix is not without risk. The goal of the presurgical evaluation—history, physical exam, and laboratory and imaging tests—is to determine who will most benefit from surgery and to decrease the negative appendectomy rate, which still hovers between 10% and 20%. Close inpatient observation may be indicated when there is an atypical presentation to allow progression of the clinical picture and completion of the diagnostic workup. If the gynecologist is the admitting attending physician, the consultation of the general surgery service should occur during this time interval.

Patients with persistently confusing findings may benefit from laparoscopy. In almost all circumstances, a laparoscopy with negative findings is preferable to delaying while an appendix ruptures or pelvic inflammatory disease progresses or an ovarian torsion results in a necrotic ovary. An unnecessary delay increases the likelihood of perforation, peritonitis, abscess formation, and sepsis. In a young woman, this also increases her risk of future adhesions, pelvic pain, and infertility. When surgery is performed within 24 hours of the onset of symptoms, less than 20% of infected appendices are perforated, compared with 70% when appendectomy occurs greater than 48 hours after symptom onset.

Treatment

As a rule, the best treatment of appendicitis is appendectomy. However, there are circumstances in which appendectomy can be or should be delayed. In those instances, other options include antibiotic therapy and interventional radiologic drainage of abdominal abscess.

Antibiotic therapy should be initiated promptly and include broad-spectrum coverage. A common combination of antibiotic treatment is cefazolin and metronidazole. Patients should remain nil per os during antibiotic treatment, in the event that the clinical picture worsens and immediate surgery is required. Antibiotics given prior to surgery have been shown to reduce the incidence of postoperative wound infections. The duration of antibiotic treatment after appendectomy varies. If the appendix was not ruptured at the time of surgery, then antibiotics can be discontinued immediately after. If perforation occurred, most surgeons advocate continued use of wide-spectrum antibiotics for several days after appendectomy, until the patient shows significant clinical improvement and resolution of the infection.

Several studies have been reported over the last few years comparing nonoperative versus operative management of

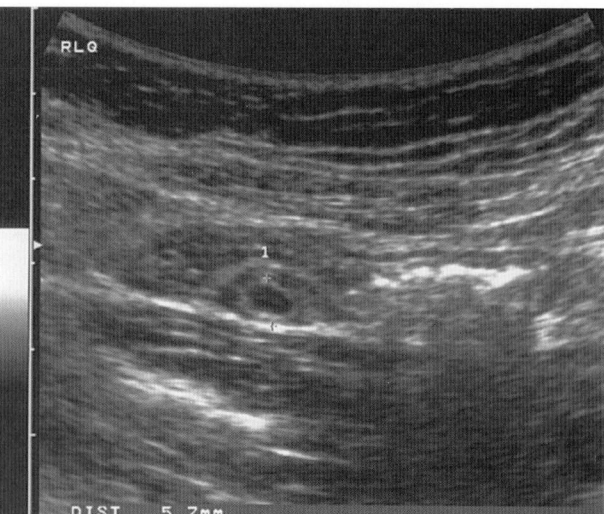

FIGURE 46.5 Transabdominal ultrasound of acute appendicitis. Note the "target-like" appearance produced by the thickened, inflamed wall of the appendix. (Courtesy of Arthur Fleischer, MD, Vanderbilt University.)

acute, uncomplicated appendicitis. In many of these studies, patients were offered antibiotics as their sole therapy if they desired and their surgeons agreed. If their symptoms improved on intravenous antibiotics, they were discharged on oral antibiotics with close follow-up. Failure of antibiotic therapy, either by physical exam or laboratory, resulted in immediate appendectomy. The majority of patients who were treated with antibiotics alone was adequately treated and did not require subsequent surgery. While overall the data look somewhat promising, there is still great hesitancy to adopt this antibiotic-only strategy as the primary treatment for appendicitis.

Another nonsurgical option for treatment of acute appendicitis is catheter drainage of periappendiceal abscess under CT or US guidance. This treatment option may be helpful in controlling the spread of infection prior to appendectomy. Limitations of percutaneous drainage include the inability to drain multiloculated abscesses, inaccessible location, and the possible need for anesthesia. If possible, once the abscess is drained and antibiotics have allowed the infectious process to "cool," an interval appendectomy can be performed. Most surgeons wait 6 to 12 weeks after nonoperative therapy to perform an interval appendectomy.

Open Appendectomy

STEPS IN THE PROCEDURE

Open Appendectomy
- Dorsal supine position.
- Foley catheter.
- Prep for RLQ incision over McBurney point.
- Divide muscles and adjacent fascia.
- Enter the peritoneum.
- Obtain any abnormal-appearing fluid for culture.
- Identify the cecum and bring to the incision (may need to incise attachment to lateral peritoneum for mobilization).
- Use moist lap sponges for tissue handling and to protect wound (if ruptured).
- Deliver the appendix through the incision.
- Separate the mesoappendix from the appendix to the base of the appendix (may use suture/cautery).
- Place clamp at the base of the appendix to "crush" the stump and repeat 1 cm distally.
- Ligate the base of the appendix with suture at proximal crushed edge.
- Place a purse-string stitch in serosa of cecum at base of appendix.
- Transect the appendix above the ligature and send for pathology.
- Bury the stump through purse-string suture and tie down.
- Check for hemostasis, and replace the cecum into the abdomen with omentum overriding.
- Irrigate and place a drain if needed.
- Close the incision in layers.

As mentioned above, the best treatment for appendicitis is surgical removal (appendectomy). Prior to the technical advances of modern laparoscopic surgery, open appendectomy was the norm. Open appendectomy is advantageous for several reasons. In the patient with an uncertain diagnosis, it provides wide exposure for evaluation and surgical management of pathologic conditions of the bowel, fallopian tube, and ovary; it is quick and simple and does not require sophisticated equipment or set up by experienced personnel.

After adequate general anesthesia, field preparation, and draping, the open technique is begun by making a small right lower quadrant incision. A modification may be made in the location of the incision if a palpable abdominal mass is noted. If this is the case, then it is presumed the mass is a loculated abscess, and the incision should override the mass to allow easier drainage. The right lower quadrant incision should be centered over McBurney point, can be made transversely or obliquely, and then extended medially a few centimeters over the underlying rectus muscles, if necessary (Fig. 46.6). The incision is then carried through the subcutaneous tissue. The external oblique fascia is incised in the same direction that the muscle fibers course, and the muscle fibers then separately bluntly. There should be no incision involving the rectus muscles. The peritoneum is then easily identified and incised transversely. Upon entry into the abdominal cavity, cultures are obtained of the peritoneal fluid.

After an initial cautious sweep of the abdominal cavity, retractors are placed around the incision and the cecum is brought to the wound. Adhesions can be bluntly or sharply dissected in order to free the appendix and allow it to be delivered through the incision and grasped with an atraumatic clamp. If this maneuver still does not result in easy access to the appendix, the incision can be extended medially into the

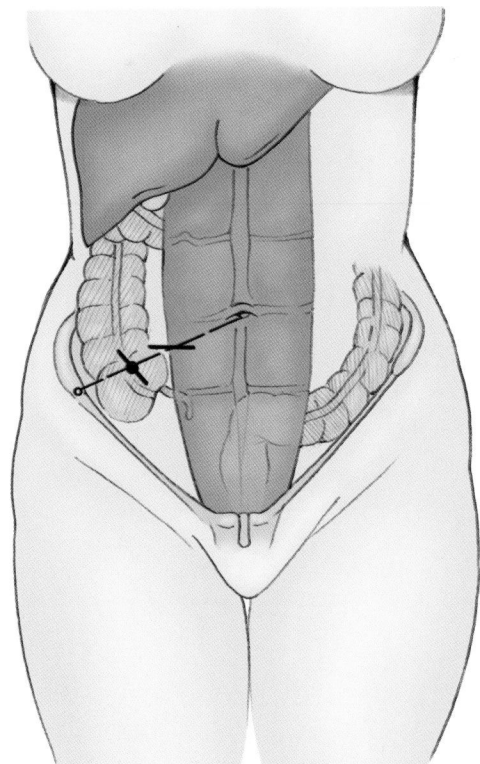

FIGURE 46.6 Common incisions for appendectomy. The classic McBurney incision over the cecum is not as easily extended to perform gynecologic procedures if needed.

rectus abdominis sheath to allow medial retractor of the muscles. Also, the lateral attachment of the cecum to the abdominal side wall can be lysed to further mobilize the cecum.

The appendix can be located by following the tenia coli as they converge at the base of the cecum. The appendix is elevated through the incision and the mesoappendix grasped at the base with a Kelly clamp. The mesoappendix is then serially clamped with a series of Kelly or hemostat clamps and ligated with delayed absorbable suture (**Fig. 46.7A**). The ligation of the mesoappendix is necessary in that the blood supply to the appendix, the appendicular artery, runs parallel to the appendix within the mesoappendix. Additionally, in some instances, there may be an additional vessel, an accessory branch of the posterior cecal artery, which requires ligation. This branch is

typically located at the base of the appendix, very near its exit from cecum. If bleeding is encountered in this area, a suture can be placed through the muscularis of the cecal wall near the base of the appendix.

The surgeon has several options when approaching ligation and excision of the appendiceal stump. Traditionally, this has been accomplished by placing two clamps across the base of the appendix, with sufficient spacing between the clamps to allow passage of a scalpel or scissors (**Fig. 46.7B**). The appendix is then passed off the field, with the attached clamp, to prevent contamination. The stump is doubly ligated with delayed absorbable suture (**Fig. 46.7C**). Some advocate using a small amount of electrocautery on the residual mucosa at the stump, thereby preventing a future mucocele.

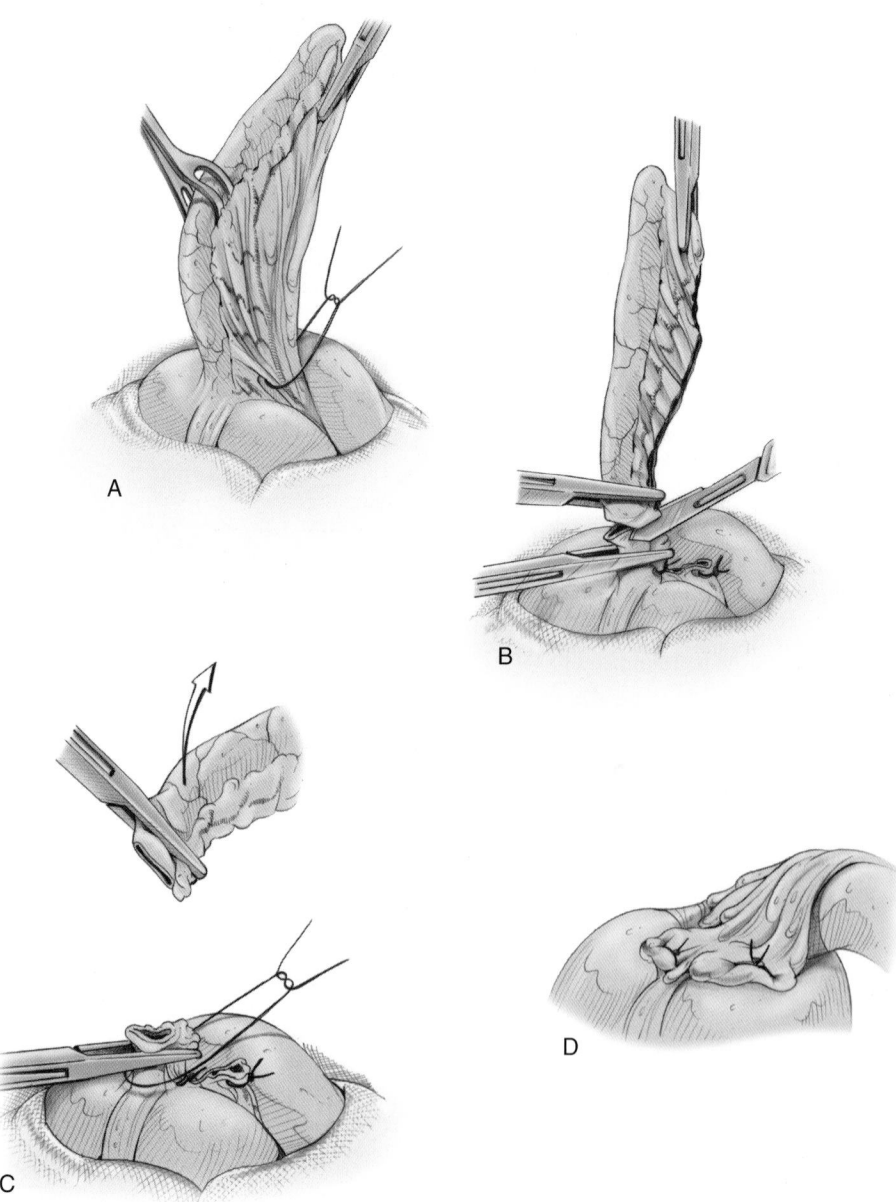

FIGURE 46.7 Technique of open appendectomy. **A:** The appendix is elevated by a Babcock clamp, and the mesoappendix is ligated. Alternatively, small clamps may be used to clamp, cut, and tie the mesoappendix. **B:** The operative field is isolated with gauze packs, and the appendix is cross-clamped and divided between the two closely placed clamps. **C:** The stump of the appendix is ligated with a 2.0 absorbable ligature. **D:** The stump is usually cauterized and covered with the adjacent mesoappendix.

At this point, the surgeon may choose to invert the stump with a purse-string or Z-stitch in the cecum, placed 1 cm from the stump, or leave the stump as is (Fig. 46.7D). One randomized trial of ligation and invagination versus ligation alone found no differences in wound infection, fever, or hospital stay. There is a small increased risk of early small-bowel obstruction after invagination.

Another option for ligation/excision of the appendix at the stump is a stapling device. Several handheld stapling devices are available on the market. The stapler crushes, seals, and transects the tissue in a single pass, making it very efficient and easy to use. It requires that the operator include a small portion of the distal cecum in the transection to ensure removal of the entire appendix. Care must be taken to avoid including too much of the cecum—and potentially the ileocecal valve—in the device.

Once the appendix is removed, the surgical field is copiously irrigated, and the abdominal incision is closed in layers. If an abscess is encountered at the beginning of the surgery, then a drain should be left in place at the time of closure.

Laparoscopic Appendectomy

STEPS IN THE PROCEDURE

Laparoscopic Appendectomy

- Lithotomy or dorsal supine position.
- Foley catheter and NG/OG tube.
- Trendelenburg with left lateral tilt.
- Three trocars: supraumbilical, LLQ or suprapubic, and RUQ.
- Obtain fluid for culture.
- Retract the cecum in the direction of the left upper quadrant.
- Identify and elevate appendix.
- Create a window through the mesoappendix at the base of the appendix.
- If using stapler: one pass at base of appendix and one pass across mesoappendix.
- If using suture: divide and ligate mesoappendix with cautery/clips, place double ligation at base of appendix, and transect with laparoscopic scissors.
- Remove the appendix through trocar or place in laparoscopic bag/pouch for removal.
- Irrigate and check for hemostasis.
- Place a drain in pelvis through small port site or new incision if abscess/rupture is encountered.
- Remove instruments and close port sites.

Removal of the appendix via the laparoscopic route was first described by Kurt Semm in 1983; however, widespread use of this technique did not occur until the 2000s. In 1999, 20% of appendectomies were performed laparoscopically. This increased to 43% in 2003. A recent pediatric surgery study revealed an even more striking trend, with an increase from 22% laparoscopic appendectomies in 1999 to 91% in 2010. The laparoscopic approach is favored in the pediatric population for similar reasons as the adult population: ease of recovery, decreased risk of wound infection, shorter hospitalizations, and cosmesis.

Initially, laparoscopic appendectomy was performed as an incidental procedure during another planned surgery. Since then, multiple studies, including randomized controlled trials and meta-analyses, have compared laparoscopic versus open appendectomy, both in the acute and nonacute settings. Laparoscopic appendectomy is associated with decreased incidence of wound infection, less postoperative pain, shorter hospital stay, and quicker return to normal activities. The disadvantages of the laparoscopic approach include longer operative times (adding approximately 10 minutes) and higher rates of intra-abdominal abscess. Laparoscopic equipment and experienced surgical nurses to set up and operate the equipment are widely available these days. Laparoscopy also allows the experience surgeon to evaluate and, in most cases, surgically manage nonappendiceal causes of right lower quadrant pain. Overall, the clinical differences between the two approaches are very small.

Laparoscopic appendectomy can usually be accomplished with a 3-trocar technique, using a combination of 5- and 10-mm trocars. After general anesthesia is induced, the patient is prepped and draped in sterile fashion, and a urinary catheter and orogastric tube are placed. Entrance is gained to the peritoneal cavity through trocar or Veress needle placement, and the abdomen is insufflated with carbon dioxide gas. The initial trocar can either be 5 or 10 mm (depending on the laparoscope diameter) and is usually placed in the umbilicus. A second trocar is placed under direct visualization in the right upper quadrant and a third in suprapubic regions. If a stapling device is planned, the suprapubic trocar should be 10 to 12 mm in size in order to accommodate it. Placing trocars in these locations allows the surgeon to "triangulate" around the appendix.

Initially, the abdominal cavity is surveyed to look for other abnormalities or causes of pain. The patient may be placed in Trendelenburg position with a left lateral tilt in order to facilitate visualization of the cecum and appendix. With an atraumatic grasper, the cecum is elevated and retracted superiorly and medially. If this retraction does not produce the appendix, it is possible that the appendix is in a retrocecal location. Lysing the peritoneal attachment of the cecum to the lateral abdominal wall may help reveal the appendix. Once seen, the appendix is grasped and extended anteriorly. With a Maryland grasper (or similar), a window is created between the appendix and the mesoappendix near the base (Fig. 46.8). Through this window, the mesoappendix is sealed/ligated and divided with a stapler, bipolar cautery,

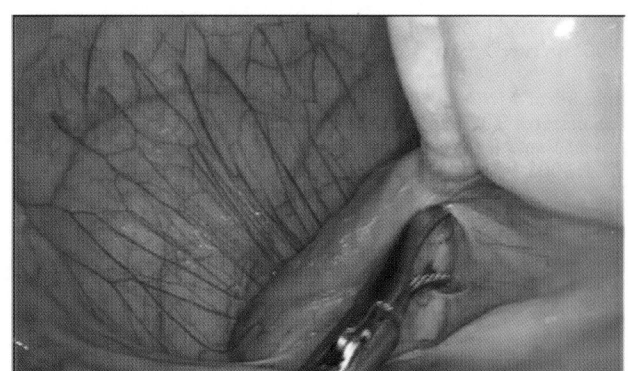

FIGURE 46.8 Creation of a window between the appendix and the mesoappendix near the base.

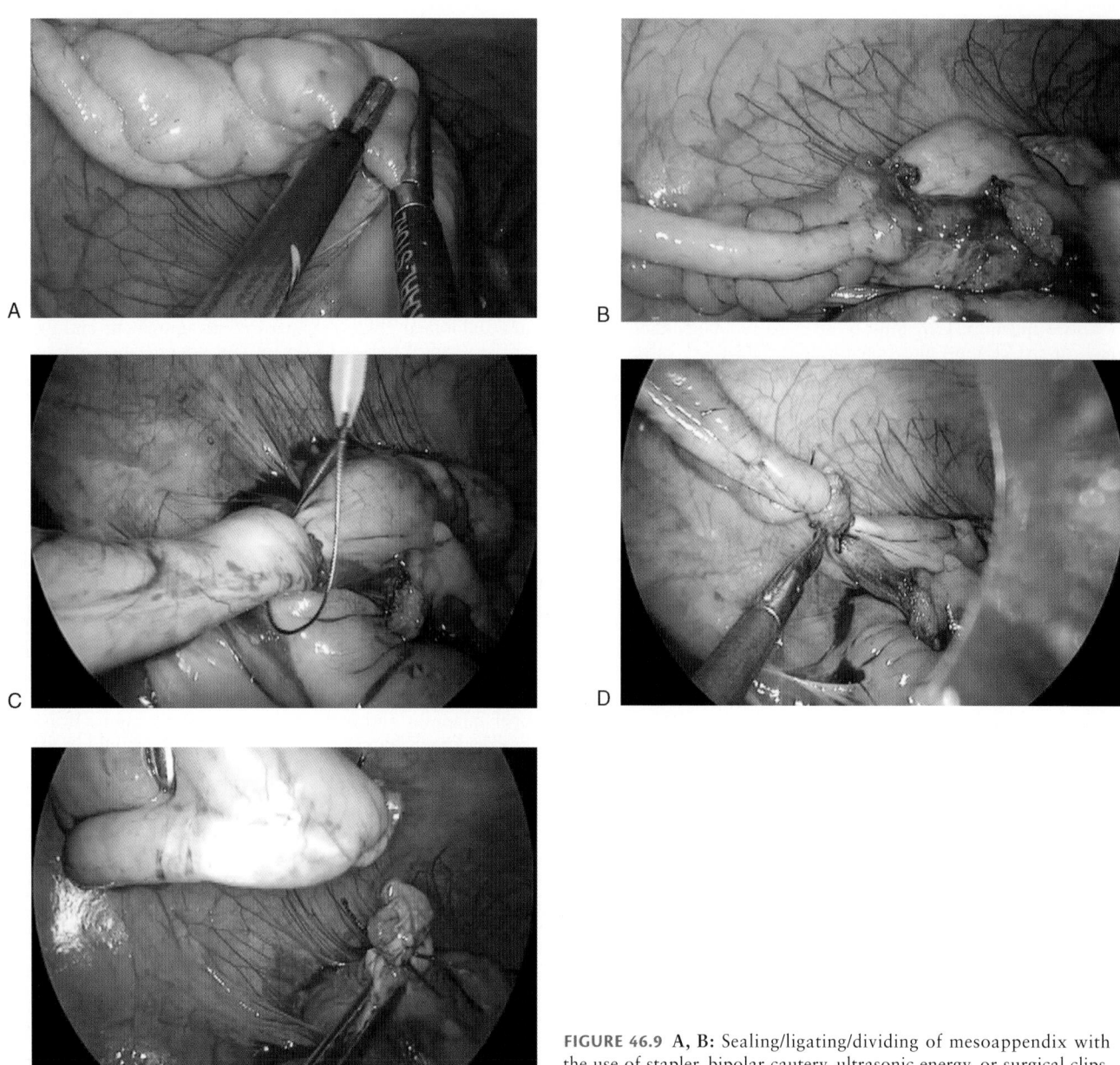

FIGURE 46.9 A, B: Sealing/ligating/dividing of mesoappendix with the use of stapler, bipolar cautery, ultrasonic energy, or surgical clips. **C–E:** Transecting of appendix using ligating suture loops and scissors.

ultrasonic energy, or surgical clips (Fig. 46.9A, B). The appendix is then transected, using either a stapling device or ligating suture loops and scissors (Fig. 46.9C–E). If a stapler is used, the transection should include a short cuff of cecum as well. If loops are used, then three loops are placed at the base of the appendix, and the incision is made between the middle and distal loop. There is no invagination performed with the laparoscopic approach.

For removal, an endoscopic bag is passed through one of the larger trocars, the appendix placed in the bag, and then both removed from the abdomen (Fig. 46.10A). The procedure is completed with irrigation of the surgical site, removal of the trocars, and closure of the incisions (Fig. 46.10B).

Single Incision

A novel method for appendectomy recently described in the literature is the single-incision laparoscopic approach. The first single-incision laparoscopic appendectomy was reported in 1992. This first report was in the adult population; however, soon after initial report, the pediatric surgeons were quick to adopt the technique. Single-incision appendectomy is comparable to the traditional 3-port technique in lower infection rates, decreased pain, faster recovery times, and improved cosmesis. A large, U-shaped incision is typically made at the umbilicus, allowing a multichannel port to be secured to the abdominal wall. The camera and laparoscopic instruments are passed through this port simultaneously. Often, a flexible scope is used to allow more operative space between the scope and instruments. Initially, there were longer operative times reported (during the period when this technique was novel), compared to traditional laparoscopy, but the surgery times for single-incision approach have decreased as the technique has gained momentum and surgeons have become more proficient with this technology.

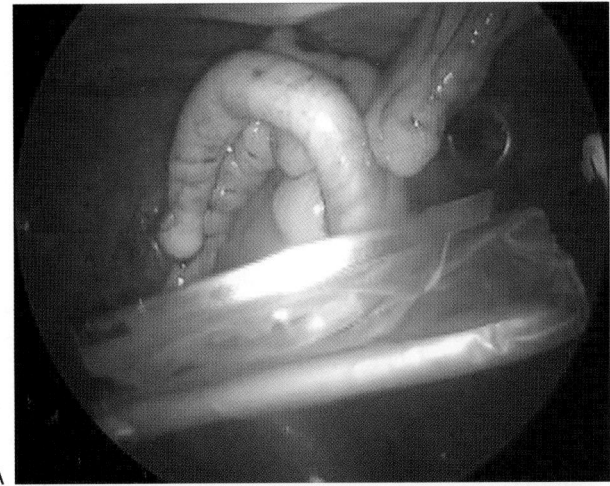

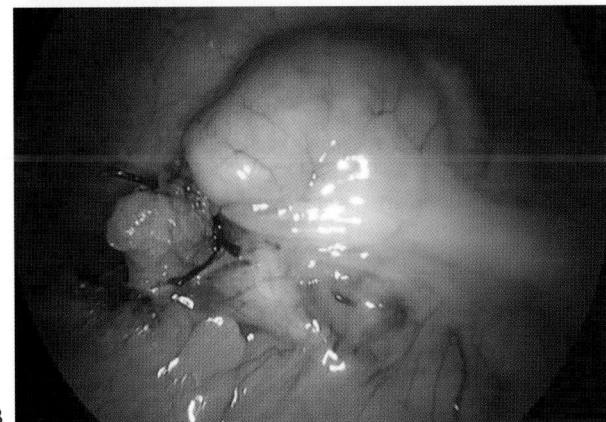

FIGURE 46.10 A, B: The appendix is removed with the use of an endoscopic bag and irrigation of the surgical site.

APPENDICITIS IN PREGNANCY

Appendectomy is the most common nonobstetrical operation in the pregnant patient. Acute appendicitis occurs in 1/1,400 to 1/6,600 pregnancies. In addition to the baseline risks of appendectomy and acute appendicitis in a nonpregnant patient, pregnancy itself exposes the patient to delayed diagnosis, risk of fetal effects, and preterm birth, difficulties with surgery, and increased risk of postoperative complications.

Delayed diagnosis of appendicitis in pregnant women occurs as a result of multiple factors. First, there are many pregnancy-related causes of abdominal and pelvic pain that typically distract the clinician from nonpregnancy-related causes. Ectopic pregnancies, threatened abortion, preterm/term labor, urinary tract infection/pyelonephritis, and uterine rupture are just a few of the pregnancy-related causes of abdominal pain that are typically ruled out first. Thus, the appendix, though on the list of differential diagnoses, is usually not the primary focus in the workup.

To confuse matters more, the typical clinical presentation of appendicitis may be altered in a pregnant patient. Acute appendicitis occurs more often in the second trimester (42%) compared with the first (32%) or third (26%) trimester. Thus, the majority of appendicitis occurs after the gravid uterus has moved out of the pelvis. The location of the appendix may move cephalad as the gravid uterus grows and displaces most pelvic structures with it; however, this theory is somewhat

controversial. In a study by Baer et al. in the 1930s, the appendix was shown to be above the level of the iliac crest in 88% of women after the 7th month of pregnancy. More recent studies have disproved this idea and demonstrated that pain in the right lower quadrant (the typical presentation of appendicitis), regardless of gestational age, is the most common presenting symptom of appendicitis in pregnant women. It is possible, though, that the location of appendicitis-related pain in a pregnant female can be anywhere in the right abdomen, thus confusing the diagnosis. Additionally, pregnancy-driven physiologic changes may result in leukocytosis and tachycardia, thus confusing the clinical and laboratory evaluation for acute appendicitis.

Typically, ultrasound and CT imaging studies are the methods of choice for radiologic diagnosis of acute appendicitis. In pregnancy, diagnostic abilities with ultrasound are limited due to changes in body habitus (i.e., increase in maternal BMI, soft tissue edema, and overriding gravid uterus), and CT is relatively contraindicated due to potential radiation exposure to the developing fetus. Several studies have evaluated MRI as the preferred imaging modality for acute abdominal conditions in pregnant women. The sensitivity of MRI for acute appendicitis is 80% to 100%, with a specificity of 94% to 99%. MRI has been show to decrease the number of unnecessary laparotomies in pregnant patients.

When appendicitis is diagnosed, or strongly suspected, then appendectomy must be performed, regardless of gestational age. Delay of treatment puts both the mother and fetus at risk. While laparoscopic surgery is often the route of choice in a nonpregnant patient, it is not always feasible or recommended in the pregnant patient. Two major considerations of laparoscopic surgery in pregnancy are (a) the effects of increased abdominal pressure, uterine and maternal circulation, and fetal acidosis with CO_2 pneumoperitoneum and (b) risk of trocar or instrument perforation into the gravid uterus. The potential fetal effects of pneumoperitoneum have been studied, and the results suggest there is no substantial negative effect on the fetus at intra-abdominal pressures below 12 mm Hg and operative times under 30 minutes. The risk of trocar or instrument injury to the uterus is decreased if laparoscopic surgeries are limited to pregnancies under 18 weeks' gestational age (although safe laparoscopic appendectomies have been reported at every stage of pregnancy). A recent systematic review and meta-analysis of laparoscopic versus open appendectomy in pregnant patients found that the risk of fetal loss was significantly worse in the laparoscopic group with no differences in risk of preterm labor, hospital stay, wound infection, birth weight, operative times, or Apgar scores. Based on the above concerns and often later gestational ages at diagnosis, most appendectomies in pregnant women are performed via the open route.

Overall, the diagnosis of appendicitis during pregnancy is associated with low birth weight, preterm delivery, small for gestational age infants, congenital anomalies (when appendicitis occurs in the first trimester), and cesarean delivery. Premature labor and delivery are the most serious fetal risks with up to 30% fetal mortality reported if perforation occurs. Because there is often a delay of diagnosis of appendicitis in pregnant women, these patients are more likely to have preoperative systemic infections before they undergo a treating procedure. Compared to their nonpregnant counterparts, some studies have shown they are also more likely to undergo an emergent procedure and have postoperative pneumonia. Although maternal mortality is rare, obstetric complications still occur in 10% to 20% of patients.

If a pregnant woman presents with suspected appendicitis, she should be immediately admitted with the plan for appendectomy. Appropriate antibiotic treatment should be initiated. The decision for route of appendectomy should be made based on gestational age, stage of appendicitis, body habitus, preexisting abdominal scars, and surgeon preference. A McBurney incision allows for easy access to the appendix in the first and early second trimesters. In the late second and third trimesters, this incision should be made higher in the abdominal wall to allow for manipulation of the cecum around the gravid uterus. A high midline incision may be used as well.

If the laparoscopic route is chosen, trocars are placed similarly as in the nongravid patient. The level of the trocars on the abdominal wall may be moved superiorly to adjust for gestational age. In the later stages of pregnancy, the three trocars can be grouped together toward the right of the gravid uterus. The abdominal pressure from CO_2 insufflation should remain below 12 mm Hg. Prior to any trocar or Veress needle placement, the surgeon should confirm the location of the uterine fundus either by palpation or ultrasound. Retraction or mobilization of the uterus (if absolutely necessary) should be performed by grasping the round ligament or utero-ovarian ligament, rather than the uterus itself.

Antithrombus prophylaxis may be indicated based on patient characteristics, length of procedure, gestational age, and type of surgery. Some authors advocate the use of tocolytic therapy during the procedure in all patients greater than 12 weeks' gestation. Others only recommend its use in patients showing signs of uterine irritability or preterm labor. Tocolytic therapy should be used with caution as it can increase the risk for pulmonary edema, which can compromise pulmonary status if systemic infection and pneumonia are already present.

If appendicitis occurs in the third trimester, concomitant cesarean delivery should only be performed for emergent obstetric indications. In the absence of fetal distress, the pregnancy should remain intact; otherwise, a hysterotomy exposes the fetus to infection and the mother to postoperative endometritis/parametritis.

The most important tenet of treating appendicitis in this special patient population is expediency. Delay in operating can result from concern about harming the pregnancy; however, removal of a normal appendix is rarely associated with negative maternal or fetal effects. Thus, the benefits of appendectomy, even if not completely assured of the diagnosis, outweigh the risks of delaying treatment. Heightened suspicion, early detection, lower treatment threshold, and performance of appendectomy within the first 24 hours of symptom onset are associated with markedly improved overall outcome, for both patient and fetus.

APPENDIX AND CHRONIC PELVIC PAIN

The appendix has long been considered a key component in the evaluation of chronic pelvic pain in women. Appendix-driven etiologies of chronic pain include endometriosis, chronic appendicitis, carcinoid tumors, and mucinous cystadenomas, with endometriosis being the most common in women.

The prevalence of appendiceal endometriosis on pathology specimens ranges between 0.05% and 0.6% in all patients to 1% to 5% in patients with pelvic pain. In patients with known pelvic endometriosis, the prevalence of appendiceal endometriosis has been reported in up to 22%. Similar to pelvic/gonadal endometriosis, preoperative diagnosis of appendiceal endometriosis is difficult, and imaging often yields negative results. Thus, evaluation during diagnostic laparoscopy is the gold standard. The appearance of serosal lesions, such as endometriotic lesions or periappendiceal inflammation/adhesions, is an indication for appendectomy. However, most cases of appendiceal endometriosis cannot be seen grossly and require microscopic evaluation and diagnosis. This creates a conundrum for the surgeon who desires to treat the patient's pain without exposing the patient to unnecessary surgical risk.

At the minimum, expert consensus recommends visual evaluation of the appendix during diagnostic laparoscopy for pelvic pain. In addition, there is evidence to suggest appendectomy is warranted in those patients with no other obvious source of pelvic pain and symptoms suspicious for appendix involvement (i.e., right lower quadrant pain), those with severe pelvic or bowel endometriosis, and those with obvious appendix pathology on gross inspection. Some studies have shown that up to 40% to 50% of women undergoing surgery for pelvic pain will have an appendiceal pathology.

INCIDENTAL APPENDECTOMY IN GYNECOLOGIC AND OBSTETRIC SURGERY

Now called an elective coincidental appendectomy by the American Congress of Obstetricians and Gynecologists, removal of an otherwise normal-appearing appendix during an unrelated surgical procedure is still somewhat controversial. The main advantage of removing an appendix in women undergoing gynecologic surgery is the prevention of future appendicitis, which could require an emergent surgery. This could be especially helpful in populations who may have decreased ability to identify or complain of classic peritoneal symptoms (such as the mentally disabled or neurologically impaired) and in patients who have extensive abdominal adhesive disease or who are at risk of developing severe adhesions. It may also be beneficial in ruling out the appendix as an etiology for unexplained chronic pain and in removing a vulnerable structure in women who are planning to undergo radiation or chemotherapy.

The lifetime risk of acute appendicitis is estimated at 7%. Among these women, the risk of an emergent appendectomy is 23%. It is more common in younger patients, with the greatest incidence in those ages 10 to 19. After age 50, the incidence decreases to 2% to 3%; however, acute appendicitis in this age group is typically more complicated, resulting in a higher mortality rate. The risk of appendicitis-related complications, such as increased hospitalization, wound or pelvic infection, perforation, and death, can be as high as 50% to 60% in this older age group.

The advantages of removing a nondiseased appendix are balanced by the risk of appendectomy itself. Complications of appendectomy include postoperative infection, ileus, bowel leak/perforation, abdominal adhesions, bowel obstruction, bleeding, and death. It is difficult to estimate the overall complication rate in incidental appendectomies because of the heterogeneity among study populations and the varied risks associated with the concomitant surgical procedures. However, the morbidity is considered to be overall quite low at 3%. There is also the issue of the additional cost associated with what would otherwise be an unnecessary procedure.

When balancing the above factors, the current recommendations support elective coincidental appendectomy in patients undergoing benign gynecologic procedures who are under age 35. Patients between ages 35 and 50 may benefit also from incidental appendectomy if there are other concerning clinical circumstances, such as those listed above. Currently, there are no data to support elective appendectomy after age 50. If appendectomy is considered as a concomitant procedure, patients should be appropriately counseled regarding risks and benefits of this procedure.

BEST SURGICAL PRACTICES

- Acute appendicitis occurs in 7% of the population over a lifetime, resulting in the most commonly performed emergent surgical procedure for abdominal pain. Approximately 300,000 emergent appendectomies are performed annually in the United States. The majority of cases occur in young patients, usually under age 20. Overall mortality rate is low, less than 1%, due to appropriate detection and early treatment. However, in individuals over age 50, the risk of mortality from acute appendicitis and subsequent complications may be as high as 15%. Delayed diagnosis is the primary reason for increased mortality is this group.
- The most common presenting symptom of acute appendicitis is abdominal pain, which is present in more than 95% of patients with appendicitis. The pain can be associated with fever, nausea, vomiting, and anorexia. Acute appendicitis is diagnosed primarily by physical exam, although imaging and lab studies may be helpful to confirm the diagnosis. CT and US imaging have contributed to decreased rates of rupture and negative appendectomies. A pelvic and rectal exam should be included to rule out other gynecologic causes of acute abdominal pain.
- The standard treatment of appendicitis is appendectomy, which has been shown to be safe and effective. This can be accomplished via the open route or laparoscopically. Preoperative use of antibiotics is important to reduce morbidity and mortality, especially in the setting of appendiceal rupture. Postoperative antibiotics may be warranted, as well. An additional treatment option is CT or US-guided percutaneous drainage of an abdominal abscess, which manages the infection while awaiting an interval appendectomy.
- The advantages of open appendectomy are quick access to the abdominal cavity, the ability to run the bowel, a larger incision in which to manage a variety of surgical findings, and more universal acceptability as it is technically less complicated than is laparoscopic surgery. The advantages of laparoscopic appendectomy are decreased wound infection, less postoperative pain, shorter hospital stays, quicker return to normal activities, and the ability to visualize the entire abdominal cavity—which can be helpful in ruling out other causes of acute abdominal pain. Overall, the clinical differences between the two approaches are very small and usually come down to surgeon preference.
- Appendectomy is the most common nonobstetrical operation in the pregnant patient. In the setting of acute appendicitis, pregnancy itself exposes the patient to delayed diagnosis, risk of fetal effects and preterm birth, difficulties with surgery, and increased risk of postoperative complications. US and MRI are the imaging modalities of choice for the pregnant patient with suspected appendicitis. When appendicitis is diagnosed, or strongly suspected, then appendectomy must be performed, regardless of gestational age. Both open and laparoscopic routes are options in the pregnant patient, with the choice dependent on gestational age, stage of appendicitis, body habitus, preexisting abdominal scars, and surgeon preference.
- The appendix is a key component in the evaluation of chronic pelvic pain in women. Appendiceal endometriosis, chronic appendicitis, carcinoid tumors, and mucinous cystadenomas can all lead to chronic pelvic pain, with endometriosis being the most common in women. In patients with known pelvic endometriosis, the prevalence of appendiceal endometriosis has been reported to be up to 22%. The appendix should be evaluated during diagnostic laparoscopy. Appendectomy may be warranted in those patients with no other obvious source of pelvic pain and symptoms suspicious for appendix involvement.
- Elective coincidental appendectomy is the removal of an otherwise normal-appearing appendix during an unrelated surgical procedure. The appropriateness of this procedure is widely debated and should be evaluated on a case-by-case basis. In general, the current recommendations support elective coincidental appendectomy in patients undergoing benign gynecologic procedures who are under age 35. Patients between ages 35 and 50 may benefit also from incidental appendectomy. Currently, there are no data to support elective appendectomy after age 50.

BIBLIOGRAPHY

Addiss DG, Shaffer N, Fowler BS, et al. The epidemiology of appendicitis and appendectomy in the United States. *Am J Epidemiol* 1990;132:910.

Elective coincidental appendectomy. ACOG Committee Opinion No. 323. American College of Obstetricians and Gynecologists. *Obstet Gynecol* 2005;106:1141.

Baer JL, Reis RS, Arens RA. Appendicitis in pregnancy with changes in position and axis of the normal appendix in pregnancy. *J Am Med Assoc* 1932;16:1359.

Basaran A, Basaran MD. Diagnosis of acute appendicitis during pregnancy: a systematic review. *Obstet Gynecol Surv* 2009;64:481.

Burns RP, Cochran JL, Russel WL, et al. Appendicitis in mature patients. *Ann Surg* 1985;201:695.

Collins DC. A study of 50,000 specimens of the human vermiform appendix. *Surg Gynecol Obstet* 1955;101:437.

Curet MJ, Vogt DA, Schob O, et al. Effects of CO_2 pneumoperitoneum in pregnant ewes. *J Surg Res* 1996;63:339.

DeFrances CJ, Podgornik MN. 2004 National Hospital Discharge Survey. *Adv Data* 2006;371:1.

Dewhurst C, Beddy P, Pedrosa I. MRI evaluation of acute appendicitis in pregnancy. *J Magn Reson Imaging* 2013;37:566.

Doherty G, ed. *Current diagnosis and treatment: surgery*, 13th ed. New York: The McGraw-Hill Companies, Inc., 2010.

Doria AS, Moineddin R, Kellenberger CJ, et al. US or CT for diagnosis of appendicitis in children and adults? A meta-analysis. *Radiology* 2006;241:83.

Engstrom L, Fenyo G. Appendicectomy: assessment of stump invagination versus simple ligation: a prospective, randomized trial. *Br J Surg* 1985;72:971.

Farahnak M, Talaei-Khoei M, Gorouhi F, et al. The Alvarado score and antibiotics therapy as a corporate protocol versus conventional clinical management: randomized controlled pilot study of approach to acute appendicitis. *Am J Emerg Med* 2007;25:850.

Gasior AC, St. Peter SD, Knott EM, et al. National trends in approach and outcomes with appendicitis in children. *J Pediatr Surg* 2012;47:2264.

Gilo NB, Amini D, Landy HJ. Appendicitis and cholecystitis in pregnancy. *Clin Obstet Gynecol* 2009;52:586.

Gustofson R, Kim N, Liu S, et al. Endometriosis and the appendix: a case series and comprehensive review of the literature. *Fertil Steril* 2006;86:298.

Harris RS, Foster WG, Surrey MW, et al. Appendiceal disease in women with endometriosis and right lower quadrant pain. *J Am Assoc Gynecol Laparosc* 2001;8:536.

Jocko JA, Shenassa H, Singh SS. The role of appendectomy in gynaecologic surgery: a Canadian retrospective case series. *J Obstet Gynaecol Can* 2013;35:44.

Kraemer M, Ohmann C, Leppert R, et al. Macroscopic assessment of the appendix at diagnostic laparoscopy is reliable. *Surg Endosc* 2000;14:625.

VIII

Krajewski S, Brown J, Phang PT, et al. Impact of computed tomography of the abdomen on clinical outcomes in patients with acute right lower quadrant pain: a meta-analysis. *Can J Surg* 2011: 54:43.

Lowry S, Davidov T, Shiroff A. Appendicitis and appendiceal abscess. In: Fischer J, ed. *Fischer's mastery of surgery*, 6th ed. Philadelphia, PA: Lippincott Williams and Wilkins, 2012.

Malik AA, Bari SU. Conservative management of acute appendicitis. *J Gastrointest Surg* 2009;13:966.

Miloudi N, Brahem M, Ben Abid S, et al. Acute appendicitis in pregnancy: specific features of diagnosis and treatment. *J Visc Surg* 2012;149:e275.

Mourad J, Elliott J, Erickson L, et al. Appendicitis in pregnancy: new information that contradicts long-held clinical beliefs. *Am J Obstet Gynecol* 2000;182:1027.

Nezhat C, Berger G, Nezhat F, et al., ed. *Endometriosis: Advanced Management and Surgical Techniques*. Springer-Verlag, 1995.

Nguyen NT, Zainabadi K, Mavandadi S, et al. Trends in utilization and outcomes of laparoscopic versus open appendectomy. *Am J Surg* 2004;188:813.

Pelosi MA, Pelosi III MA. Laparoscopic appendectomy using a single umbilical puncture (minilaparoscopy). *J Reprod Med* 1992; 37:588.

Prystowsky JB, Pugh CM, Nagle AP. Current problems in surgery: appendicitis. *Curr Probl Surg* 2005;42:688.

Redwine DB. Ovarian endometriosis: a marker for more extensive pelvic and intestinal disease. *Fertil Steril* 1999;72:310.

Salom EM, Schey D, Penalver M, et al. The safety of incidental appendectomy at the time of abdominal hysterectomy. *Am J Obstet Gynecol* 2003;189:1563.

Sauerland S, Jaschinski T, Neugebauer EA. Laparoscopic versus open surgery for suspected appendicitis. *Cochrane Database Syst Rev* 2010;10.

Sauerland S, Lefering R, Neugebauer EA. Laparoscopic versus open surgery for suspected appendicitis. *Cochrane Database Syst Rev* 2004;4.

Semm K. Endoscopic appendectomy. *Endoscopy* 1983;15:59.

Silvestri MT, Pettker CM, Brousseau C, et al. Morbidity of appendectomy and cholecystectomy in pregnant and nonpregnant women. *Obstet Gynecol* 2011;118:1261.

Smith GV. Endometrioma: a clinical and pathologic study of 159 cases treated at the clinic of the free hospital for women, Brookline, Massachusetts. *Am J Obstet Gynecol* 1929;17:806.

Snyder TE, Selanders JR. Incidental appendectomy: yes or no? A retrospective case study and review of the literature. *Infect Dis Obstet Gynecol* 1998;6:30.

Soni L. Appendectomy. In: Hoballah JJ, Scott-Conner CE, eds. *Operative dictations in general and vascular surgery*, 2nd ed. New York: Springer Science + Business Media, 2011:184.

St Peter SD, Adibe OO, Juang D, et al. Single incision versus standard 3-port laparoscopic appendectomy: a prospective randomized trial. *Ann Surg* 2011;254:586.

Styrud J, Eriksson S, Nilsson I, et al. Appendectomy versus antibiotic treatment in acute appendicitis: a prospective multicenter randomized controlled trial. *World J Surg* 2006;30:1033.

Tsoulfas G. Laparoscopic appendectomy. In: Hoballah JJ, Scott-Conner CE, eds. *Operative dictations in general and vascular surgery*, 2nd ed. New York: Springer Science + Business Media, 2011:189.

Van Sonnenberg E, Wittich GR, Casola G, et al. Periappendiceal abscesses: percutaneous drainage. *Radiology* 1987;15:59.

Wei PL, Keller JJ, Liang HH, et al. Acute appendicitis and adverse pregnancy outcomes: a nationwide population-based study. *J Gastrointest Surg* 2012;16:1204.

Wie HJ, Lee JH, Kyung MS, et al. Is incidental appendectomy necessary in women with ovarian endometrioma? *Aust N Z J Obstet Gynaecol* 2008;48:107.

Wilasrusmee C, Sukrat B, McEvoy M, et al. Systematic review and meta-analysis of safety of laparoscopic versus open appendicectomy for suspected appendicitis in pregnancy. *Br J Surg* 2012; 99:1470.

Wray CJ, Kao LS, Millas SG, et al. Acute appendicitis: controversies in diagnosis and management. *Curr Probl Surg* 2013;50:54.

CHAPTER 47
Intestinal Surgery for the Gynecologic Surgeon

Mitchel Hoffman and Emmanuel Zervos

DEFINITIONS

Bubble test—Transanal instillation of air into the submersed and proximally compressed rectum for the purpose of looking for a hole or an anastomotic gap.

Closed loop obstruction—Anatomic state wherein a segment of bowel is excluded from the fecal stream due to malignancy, adhesions, or a surgically induced state.

Complicated diverticulitis—Refers to the presence of a perforation, obstruction, abscess, or fistula. Approximately 25% of patients diagnosed with diverticulitis for the first time present with complicated diverticulitis, and nearly all of these cases require surgery.

Cytoreduction—Refers to surgical reduction of the metastatic tumor load in the context of surgery for ovarian cancer.

Diversion—Indicates preclusion of passage of stool to the portion of the intestinal tract distal to the stoma in an ileostomy or colostomy.

Enteric fistula—Epithelialized tract from a portion of the intestine to the skin or mucosa of another organ.

Enterolysis—Division of adhesions involving the intestinal tract.

Enterostomal therapist—Specialist who provides education and assistance to patients who are planned for or have undergone a stoma.

Enterotomy—Hole or laceration in the wall of the intestine.

Hartmann pouch—Healed segment of retained rectosigmoid colon following sigmoid resection with end colostomy.

Inanition—Condition of exhaustion due to starvation.

Laplace law—Explanation for the propensity of the cecum to be the first site of colonic perforation due to dilatation from distal colonic obstruction. The law (T = PR) directly correlates tension (T) to the radius (R) and internal pressure (P) of the bowel.

Lembert sutures—Series of sutures incorporating only the serosa and muscular layers of any portion of the GI tract and designed to reinforce and relieve tension on mucosal suture lines.

Malecot catheter, mushroom catheter—Rubber catheter ranging in size from 6 to 38 French with a mushroom-shaped tip ideally suited to drain large spaces that communicate with the skin through considerably smaller tracts.

Mucous fistula—Portion of defunctionalized bowel exteriorized to a stoma for the purpose of drainage and avoidance of an intestinal mucocele.

Obstipation—Severe constipation, usually due to intestinal obstruction.

Pelvic exenteration—Operation undertaken for pelvic malignancy in which the bladder, vagina, and uterus (anterior); vagina, uterus, and rectum (posterior); or all four organs (complete) are removed.

Percutaneous endoscopic gastrostomy (PEG)—Percutaneous placement of a gastrostomy tube under gastroscopic guidance without laparotomy.

Proctosigmoiditis—Inflammation of the sigmoid colon and/or rectum.

Rectal stump—Segment of rectum remaining after a rectosigmoid resection.

Short bowel syndrome—Any clinical circumstance wherein the inherent small bowel provides insufficient absorptive capacity to maintain a noncatabolic state.

Tenesmus—Urge to defecate, despite empty colon or bladder.

Uncomplicated diverticulitis—Diverticulitis without the complications noted above and accounts for 75% of diverticulitis cases. The majority of cases respond to medical therapy, although up to 30% require surgery.

INTRODUCTION

The female pelvic cavity is a confined space occupied by the female genitalia, the lower urinary tract, and the rectosigmoid colon. Anatomically, these structures are intimately associated. Other portions of the intestinal tract may occupy the pelvis as well, such as the cecum, appendix, and/or small intestine. It is not surprising, therefore, that gynecologic diseases and the complications resulting from their treatment often involve the urinary tract, the intestinal tract, or both. Similarly, diseases of the urinary and intestinal tract may often mimic or influence manifestations of gynecologic disease.

The complete pelvic surgeon must have medical and surgical expertise in the management of specific types of intestinal disorders. With any type of operation, the abdominal surgeon must be prepared for the eventuality of intestinal injury. For the gynecologic oncologist, common indications for intestinal surgery include resection of tumor and bowel obstruction. Oncologists also perform exenterative surgery, urinary diversion, fistula repair, and surgery for severe radiation damage to the bowel. Pelvic reconstructive surgeons are called on to repair rectal prolapse. Bowel resection is occasionally indicated for infiltrating endometriosis. When operating for presumed

gynecologic pathology, the pelvic surgeon occasionally discovers a primary bowel disorder that must be managed surgically.

The purpose of this chapter is to provide the pelvic surgeon with basic information necessary for the surgical management of the more common intestinal problems encountered in the management of presumed gynecologic disorders and complications of their treatment.

ANATOMY

Knowledge of the anatomy of the gastrointestinal tract is essential for the performance of intestinal surgery and management of complex pelvic pathology. The relevant anatomy is reviewed here.

Stomach

The stomach is the uppermost organ of the gastrointestinal tract, residing completely in the abdominal cavity. The intraabdominal esophagus ranges from 3 to 6 cm in length under normal anatomic conditions. It is located in the left upper quadrant of the peritoneal cavity. The stomach is composed of the cardia, the portion immediately surrounding the gastroesophageal junction and the largest portion of the stomach; the fundus, the upward extension of the stomach toward the dome of the diaphragm on the left side; the body; and the antrum, the portion of the stomach between the incisura and the pylorus. The incisura is a notched portion of the stomach along the lesser curvature. Being a derivative of the foregut, the stomach receives its arterial blood supply from the celiac trunk, the lower thoracic aorta, and collaterals arising from the superior mesenteric artery (SMA) (Fig. 47.1).

Small Intestine

The small intestine averages 21 feet in length. From the pylorus of the stomach, the duodenum curves retroperitoneally to the ligament of Treitz, left of the second lumbar vertebrae. In the left upper quadrant of the peritoneal cavity, the intestine then

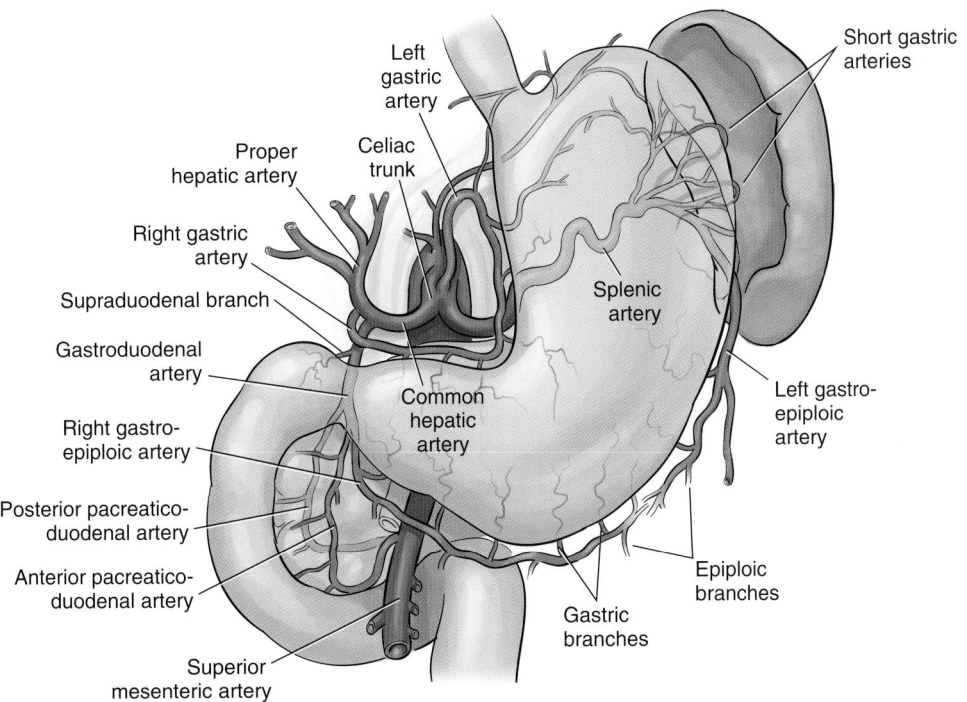

FIGURE 47.1 Blood supply of the stomach.

VIII

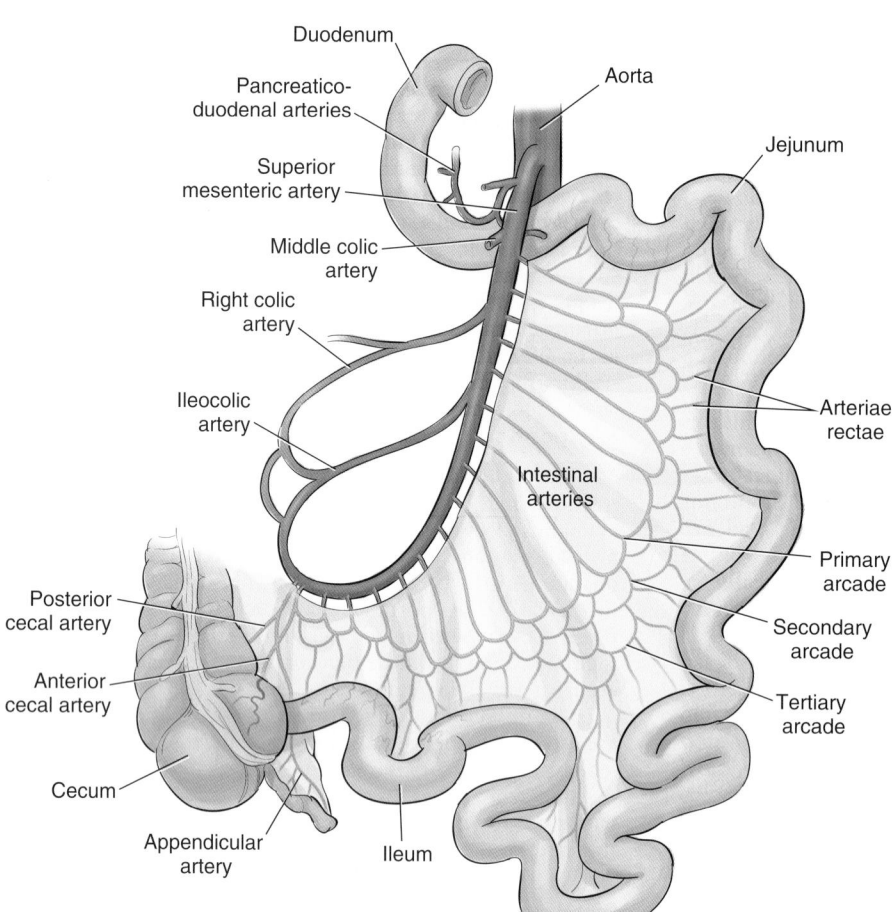

FIGURE 47.2 Blood supply of the jejunum and ileum.

becomes intraperitoneal as the jejunum, which is approximately 8 feet in length. An arbitrary transition to the ileum occurs, which is approximately 12 feet in length and terminates at the ileocecal junction in the right lower quadrant of the peritoneal cavity. Clinically, the jejunum is slightly thicker and greater in diameter, more vascular, and of deeper color.

The blood supply of the jejunum and ileum is derived from the SMA (**Fig. 47.2**). There is a progression of arcades from the intestinal branches that are single in the jejunum and increase to four of five in the ileum. The mesentery of the small intestine is fan shaped and is positioned obliquely over the posterior abdominal wall. From its body attachments at the ligament of Treitz, the mesentery travels to the right iliac fossa.

Large Intestine

The large intestine extends from the cecum to the anus and is approximately 5 feet in length. Beginning at the base of the appendix and merging in the rectum, the external muscle layer of the colon is arranged in three longitudinal bands known as taenia. The colon also has small projections of peritonealized fat, known as appendices epiploicae.

The blood supply to the right colon (**Fig. 47.3**) and the left colon (**Fig. 47.4**) are derived from the superior and inferior mesenteric arteries, which form a rich collateral network within the mesentery as the arc of Riolan (proximal branches) and the marginal artery of Drummond (distal branches).

The appendix arises near the base of the cecum distal to the ileocecal junction. From the cecum in the right lower quadrant, the partially peritonealized ascending colon extends cephalad

to the hepatic flexure. The second portion of the duodenum is intimate with the hepatic flexure, and care must be taken when mobilizing the flexure or resecting this part of the colon. Similarly, the right ureter is also intimately associated with the appendix and ileocecum and should be identified when mobilizing this portion of the colon.

The transverse colon is the longest and most mobile colonic segment, extending from the hepatic to the splenic flexure. It is further attached to the stomach by the gastrocolic ligament (greater omentum), which is intimate with the transverse mesocolon and ventral surface of the colon. Careful separation of the gastrocolic ligament gains access to the lesser sac and is necessary for complete omentectomy. Again, care must be taken when mobilizing this portion of the colon, as excessive traction on the splenic flexure can cause downward tension on the splenocolic ligaments and thus lead to tears in the splenic capsule.

The partially peritonealized descending colon extends from the splenic flexure to the sigmoid colon. The upper descending mesocolon is intimate with the kidney, which is close to the proper plane of dissection as this part of the colon is mobilized. The anastomotic blood supply to the splenic flexure is less robust, is frequently referred to as the watershed area, and may be prone to compromise during dissection.

At the pelvic brim, the descending colon becomes the completely peritonealized and mobile sigmoid colon. The sigmoid mesentery (with its root at the inferior mesenteric artery [IMA]) is generous and extends to the posterior cul-de-sac. This is the rectosigmoid colon, and the blood supply transitions to the lateral sides of the rectum.

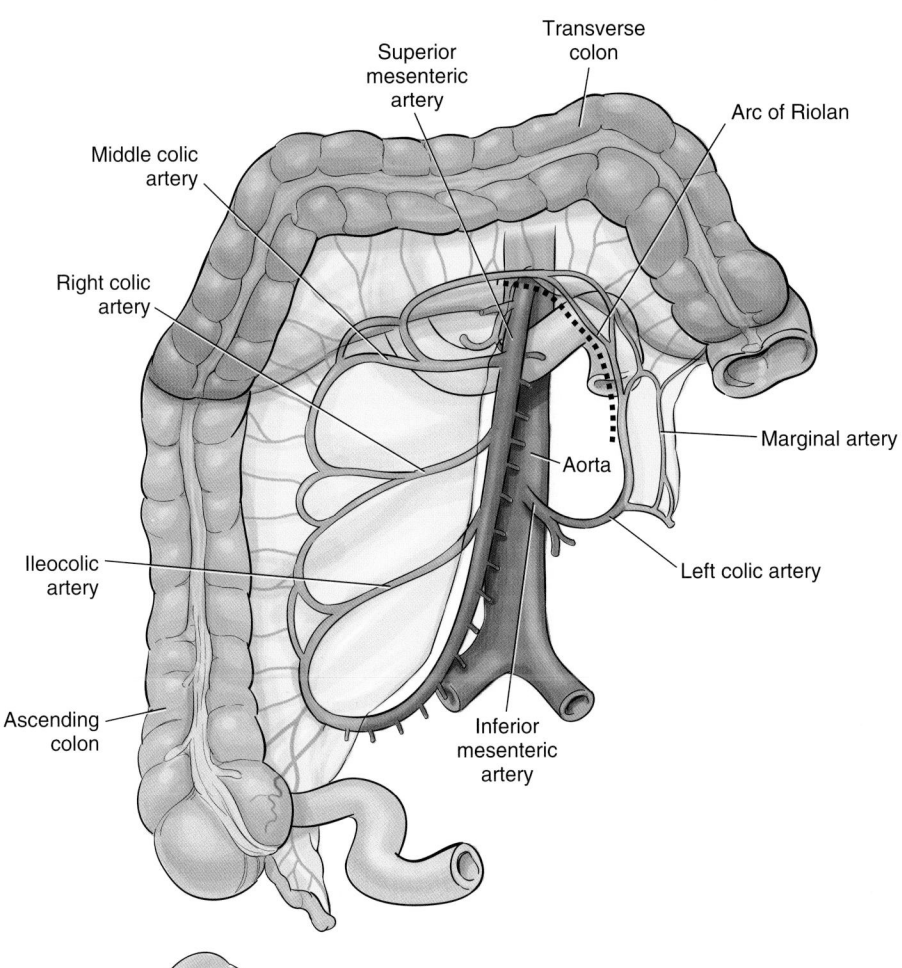

FIGURE 47.3 Blood supply of the right and transverse colon.

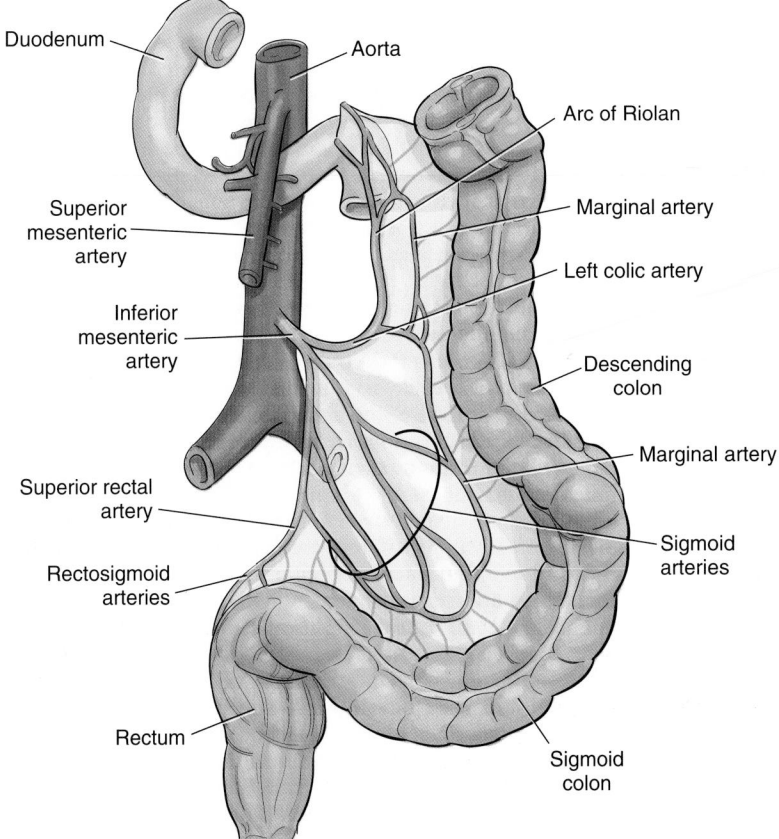

FIGURE 47.4 Blood supply of the left colon.

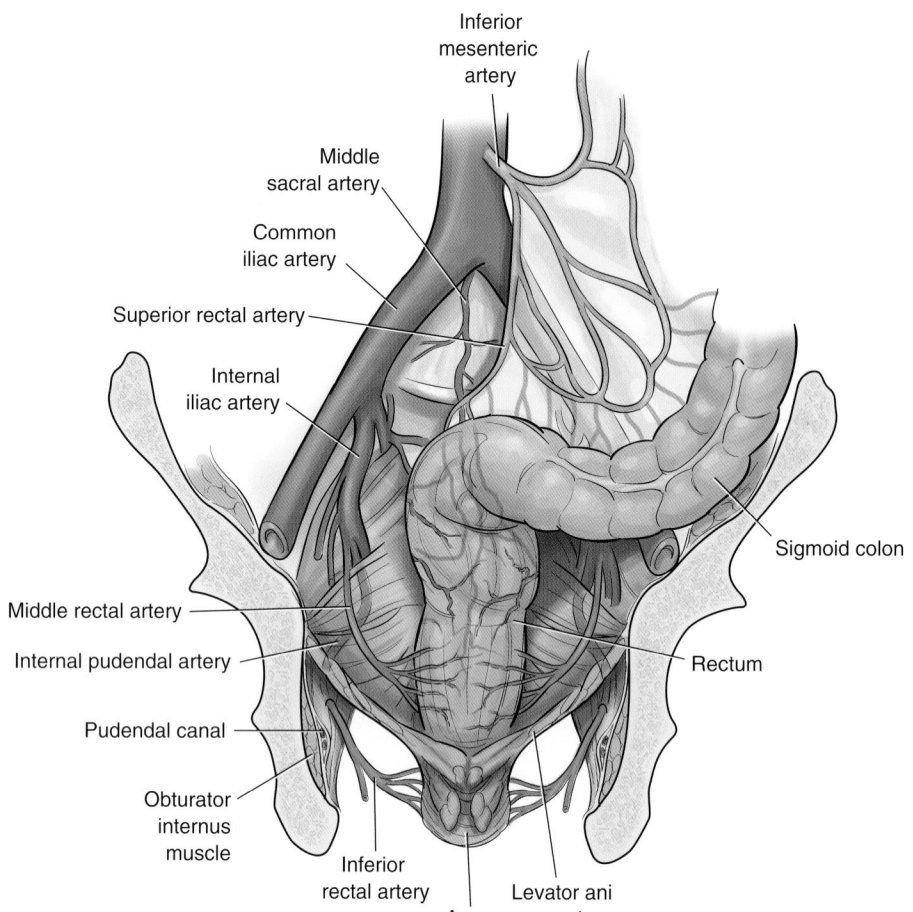

Inferior
mesenteric
artery

Middle
sacral artery

Common
iliac artery

Superior rectal artery

Internal
iliac artery

Sigmoid colon

Middle rectal artery

Internal pudendal artery

Rectum

Pudendal canal

Obturator
internus
muscle

Inferior
rectal artery

Anus

Levator ani
muscle

FIGURE 47.5 Blood supply of the rectum.

The rectum follows the curve of the sacrum, increasing in size to form the ampulla (i.e., fecal reservoir) just above the levator ani. The anorectal angle is formed here. Ventrally, the rectal wall is invested with a delicate layer of connective tissue known as "Denonvilliers" fascia. This fascial layer extends from the base of the cul-de-sac to the perineal body, separating the rectum from the lower two-thirds of the posterior vaginal wall. During cephalad mobilization of an infiltrating cul-de-sac tumor, division of this fascia is useful for mobilizing the tumor and gaining additional rectal length before transection. The blood supply of the rectum is derived from the terminal branches of the IMA and branches of the internal iliac arteries (Fig. 47.5). There are vast anastomoses between these vessels along the rectal wall.

INDICATIONS

Enterolysis

Adhesions in the peritoneal cavity commonly occur in patients who have undergone prior surgery or have experienced an inflammatory process such as endometriosis or salpingo-oophoritis. Such adhesions frequently involve the intestinal tract and may lead to obstruction, obstipation, or pain. Bowel adhesions may interfere with access to the pelvis during surgery and/or may involve pelvic structures with which the gynecologic surgeon is concerned. Any surgeon who operates in the peritoneal cavity must be competent in intraperitoneal adhesiolysis.

It is important for the surgeon approaching adhesiolysis to have an understanding of the likely cause of the adhesions and to know what operations the patient has previously undergone. The approach to intestinal adhesions is modified by factors such as prior radiotherapy, known inflammatory bowel disease, prior intestinal resection (with potential risk for short gut syndrome), and/or the presence of carcinomatosis.

In a patient with normal intestinal function and intestinal adhesions that will not interfere with the planned operation, lysis of such adhesions may not be indicated. In the setting of small bowel obstruction due to peritoneal carcinomatosis, examination of the entire small bowel is necessary to ensure that downstream adhesion is not overlooked, as a transition point may not be present in the setting of more proximal obstruction.

When adhesiolysis is indicated, some general principles should be followed. Some adhesions are well exposed with clear lines for separation. Dividing these adhesions first will help further restore normal anatomy and improve exposure to remaining adhesions. To the extent possible, define the direction of involved bowel loops before embarking on separation. Use gentle traction–countertraction to define lines of adhesion and to facilitate separation while avoiding traction injury and serosal tears. When segments of the intestine are adhered tightly, use sharp dissection. In general, as adhesions become denser, their separation requires progressively sharper instrumentation. When known or suspected intestinal injury occurs, control any gross contamination with bowel clamps or sutures, and tag these areas for later inspection or repair. When partial enterolysis fails to address adhesions posing a risk for intestinal obstruction, these adhesions must also be divided. It is critical to define a fixed

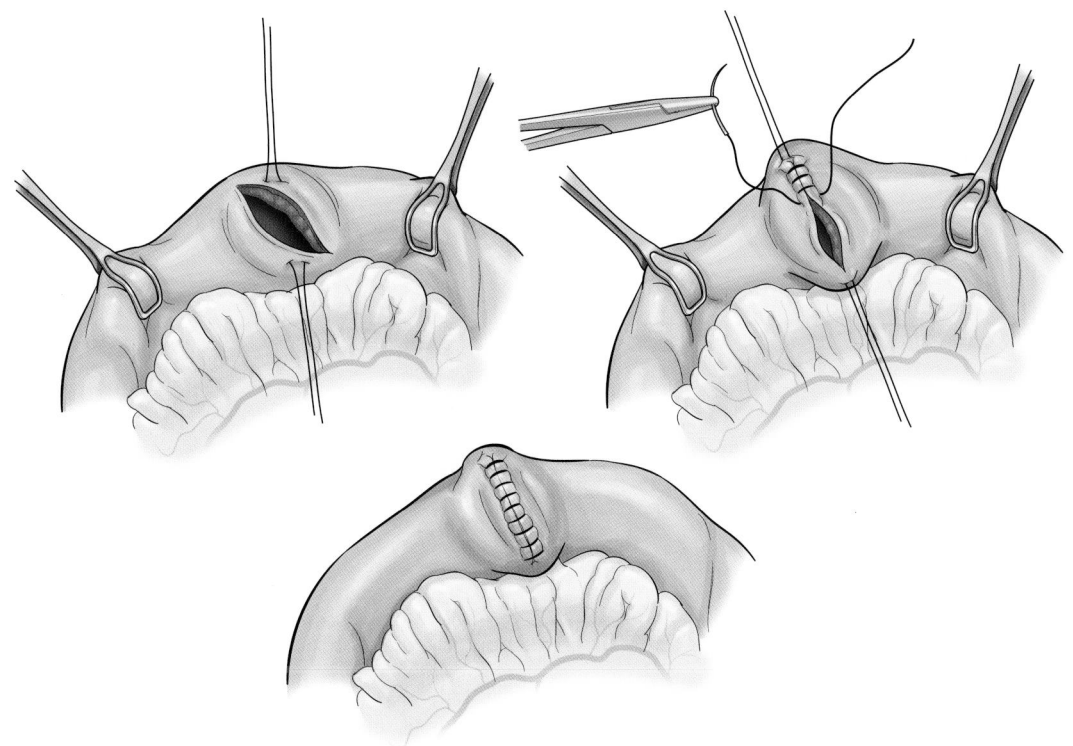

FIGURE 47.6 Repair of a simple enterotomy.

point—either at the ligament of Treitz (moving forward) or at the ileocecal valve (moving backward)—to ensure complete adhesiolysis.

Incidental Injury

In addition to the intimate anatomic relationship between the female genital tract and the rectosigmoid colon, intestinal adhesions in the pelvis are common. The widespread use of laparoscopy in gynecologic surgery places other portions of the intestinal tract at risk. During gynecologic surgery, occasional injury to the intestinal tract can be expected. Certain disease processes or operations may increase the likelihood of injury, such as obliteration of the posterior cul-de-sac (by endometriosis, salpingo-oophoritis, or malignancy), radical pelvic surgery, and extensive enterolysis. Most injuries will consist of a simple seromuscular tear or full-thickness laceration, which is closed with one or two layers of suture. More significant injuries, such as multiple enterotomies within a short distance of each other, require bowel resection.

Management of thermal bowel injury is highly individualized according to the surgeon's impression of the extent of damage. Blanched, contracted tissue should be considered nonviable. There may be at least several millimeters of less apparent damage beyond the apparent injury. A limited, superficial cautery burn witnessed by the surgeon generally requires no treatment. If concern exists, the area may be oversewn with inverting seromuscular sutures. More substantial thermal damage requires at least seromuscular resection (including a normal-appearing margin) and repair.

Full-thickness injury of the small bowel should be repaired perpendicular to the lumen to avoid constriction (Fig. 47.6). This is less important when closing a colotomy, since the lumen is larger.

Cytoreduction

Most women who develop ovarian cancer present with intra-abdominal metastases. Following a combination of radical surgery and chemotherapy, clinical remission is achieved for a large percentage of these women, who can subsequently enjoy long-term survival. Cytoreductive surgery for ovarian cancer appears to improve survival only when no residual tumor (or a minimal volume residual tumor) is left behind. To achieve optimal clearance of tumor, a large percentage of women require procedures that extend beyond simply the removal of gynecologic organs; the most common of these is colon resection.

In recent published series and as shown in Tables 47.1 and 47.2, more than 33% of women with ovarian cancer

TABLE 47.1 Primary Cytoreduction; % Colon Resection		
	N	**COLON**
Scarabelli et al. (2000)	238	66
Obermair et al. (2001)	456	65
Jaeger et al. (2001)	194	104
Hoffman et al. (2005)	458	137
Aletti et al. (2006)	294	57
Chi et al. (2009)	210	73
	1,850	502 (37%)

VIII

TABLE 47.2 Secondary Cytoreduction: % Colon Resection

	TOTAL *N*	# COLON RESECTION
Eisenkop et al. (2000)	106	46 (43)
Scarabelli et al. (2001)	149	32 (2)
Tay et al. (2002)	46	11 (24)
Zang et al. (2004)	117	39 (33)
Chi et al. (2006)	153	48 (31)
Tebes et al. (2007)	85	51 (60)
	656	227 (35)

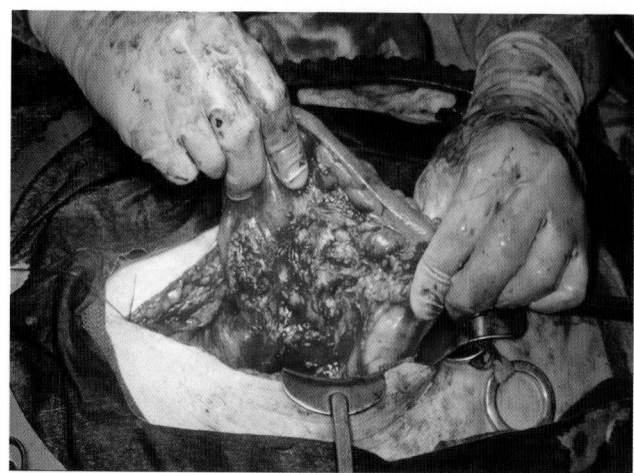

FIGURE 47.7 Extensive tumor infiltration of the sigmoid mesentery.

underwent colon resection as part of their primary (Table 47.1) or secondary (Table 47.2) cytoreductive operation. Based on proximity alone, the rectosigmoid colon is the segment of bowel most frequently resected during cytoreductive surgery for ovarian cancer (Fig. 47.7; Table 47.3). In such cases, the internal genitalia, rectosigmoid colon, and cul-de-sac peritoneum become agglutinated as a tumor mass. Original descriptions of radical cytoreductive surgery for ovarian cancer, dating back to the 1960s, were in fact surgical techniques designed to resect such tumors en bloc. In recent series of such operations, nearly all women underwent primary colorectal anastomosis without a protective ostomy, with an average leak/fistula rate of 2.6%, and a mortality rate of 0.8% (Table 47.4).

Colon resection is central to ovarian cancer cytoreduction due to its frequency of involvement (over 50% in some recent series), technical considerations, and complications of resection. It is therefore not surprising that the rectosigmoid colon is the most frequent segment of the bowel resected during cytoreductive surgery. However, as seen in Table 47.3, other portions of the colon may also become involved with disease to the point of requiring resection.

The high incidence of bulky omental metastasis readily explains growth onto the transverse colon and/or its mesentery (Fig. 47.8). Omentectomy en bloc with transverse colectomy is a straightforward operation. Such metastases may extend to involve the splenic hilum, the greater curvature of the stomach, and, less frequently, the tail of the pancreas.

TABLE 47.3 Segments of Bowel Resected for Primary Cytoreduction

	N	RECTOSIGMOID	SMALL BOWEL	LEFT HEMICOLECTOMY	RIGHT HEMICOLECTOMY	TRANSVERSE COLECTOMY	SUBTOTAL COLECTOMY
Tamussino (2001)	n.a.	117	64	0	13	14	0
Gilette-Clover et al. (2001)	105	75	27	5	17	25	0
Bristow (2003)	31	31	9[a]	[b]	3	2	0
Hoffman (2005)	144	99	9	4	35[c]	10	5
Mourton (2005)	70	75	1	0	11	2	0
Estes (2006)	48	23	16	0	4[d]	11	0
Peiretti (2010)	?	148	15	8	26[e]	8	0

[a]Ileocecal and small bowel resections were combined.
[b]Right and left hemicolectomies were combined.
[c]Twenty-six were ileocecal resections.
[d]Two cecum and two ascending colon.
[e]Seventeen were ileocecal resection.

TABLE 47.4 Primary Cytoreduction

	RECTOSIGMOID COLECTOMY	PROTECTIVE OSTOMY	OTHER BOWEL RESECTION	LEAK/FISTULA	OPERATIVE MORTALITY
Spirtos et al. (2000)	212	44 (40)	60	4	3
Scarabelli et al. (2000)	66	0	Excluded	0	0
Obermair et al. (2001)	65	38 (25)	NG	2	1
Tamussino et al. (2001)	117	35 (NG)	NG	1	NG
Gillette-Clover et al. (2001)	75	46 (15)	31	NG	NG
Clayton et al. (2002)	129	5 (NG)	43	3	4
Bristow et al. (2003)	31	0	14	1	0
Hoffman et al. (2005)	99	2 (2)	63	1	0
Mourton et al. (2005)	70	12 (11)	14	1	1
Aletti et al. (2006)	57	3 (3)	NG	1	0
Richardson et al. (2006)	115	Excluded	NG	10	NG
Park et al. (2006)	46	3 (NG)	5	2	0
Peiretti et al. (2012)	238	7 (NG)	81	7	0
	1,320		31%	2.6%	0.7%

Values in "( )" indicates number of ostomies reversed.
NG, not given.

Complete cytoreduction of such disease requires extensive left upper quadrant resection (Fig. 47.9).

Due to its location in the pelvis, it is not surprising that the ileocecum is the second most frequent portion of the bowel to become extensively involved with ovarian cancer (Table 47.2). Inasmuch as possible, resection of such tumors is carried out en bloc with the pelvic tumor. Reconstruction generally consists of an ileoascending colonic anastomosis (Fig. 47.10A, B). More extensive involvement may require a right hemicolectomy; the same is true of rectosigmoid involvement (left hemicolectomy).

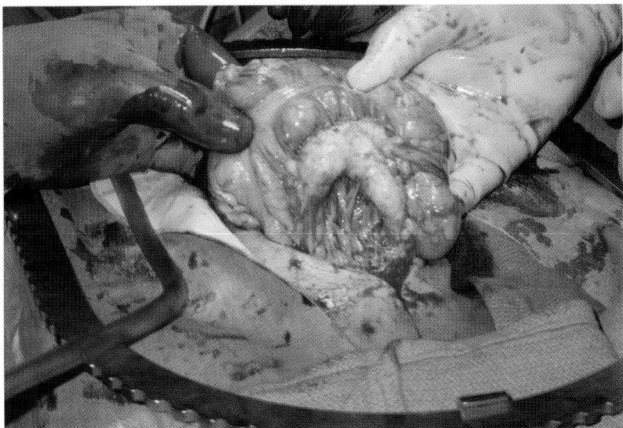

FIGURE 47.8 Tumor encasing the mesentery and growing onto the wall of the transverse colon.

Because of the haphazard and often widespread intra-abdominal distribution of ovarian cancer metastases, multiple bowel segments may become involved in a single patient. In the authors' experience, the most frequent manifestation has been extensive tumor involving both the rectosigmoid colon and ileocecum. Resection of these two sites leaves the patient with the majority of the colon, although restoration does require two anastomoses.

When metastatic ovarian cancer involves the transverse colon and separately involves either the rectosigmoid colon or ileocecum, surgical management is less straightforward. The segments may be excised separately, followed by two bowel anastomoses; alternatively, an en bloc resection can be performed, which then requires only a single ileocolic or colo-rectal anastomosis. Factors to be taken into account when considering these two options include length of normal colon that can be saved, integrity of blood supply to the two anastomoses, technical ability to restore bowel continuity with each option, tension on the anastomosis, quality of bowel preparation, condition of the colon (particularly of the left side), length of the small bowel remaining, and overall condition of the patient.

The authors prefer to perform en bloc resection with a single restorative anastomosis. Less frequently, there is extensive multifocal involvement of the colon. Intervening segments of colon might be saved in some women, but this may require three colon anastomoses. Subtotal colectomy with an ileostomy, ileoproctostomy, or cecoproctostomy are all reasonable alternatives. Defecatory function is acceptable as long as at least 12 cm of rectosigmoid colon and the full length of

VIII

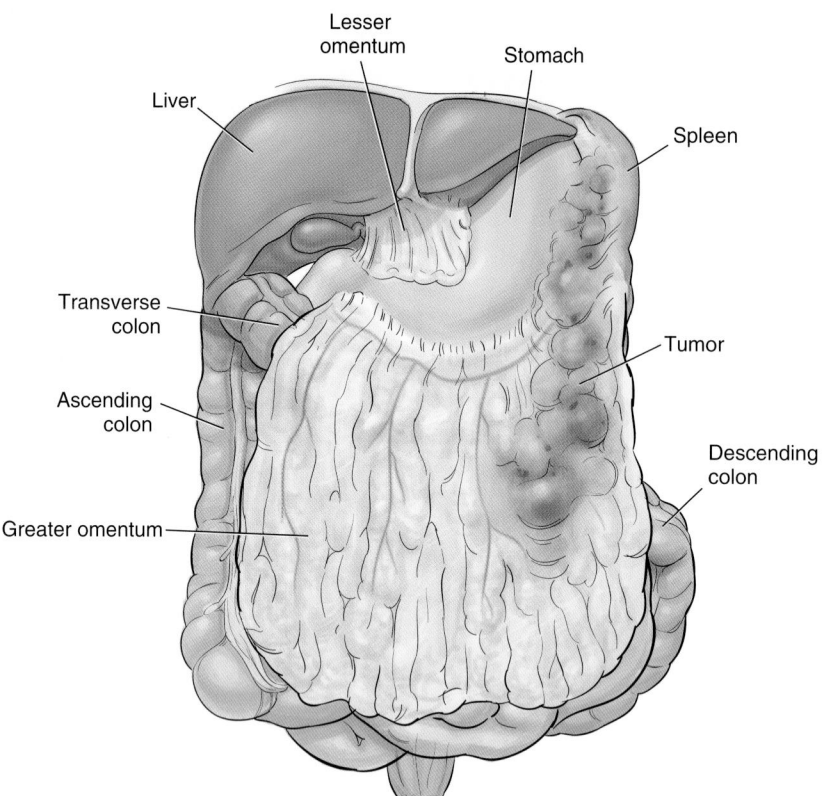

FIGURE 47.9 Metastatic omental tumor mass extending in the left upper quadrant to involve the splenic hilum and stomach.

the small bowel remain. With a shorter rectal segment, many authors advocate creation of an ileal pouch for anastomosis to the rectum, in an attempt to augment the reservoir capacity and minimize bowel frequency.

Endometriosis

Endometriosis occasionally involves the bowel, especially when severe. The most common sites of involvement are located in the pelvis, including the appendix, rectosigmoid

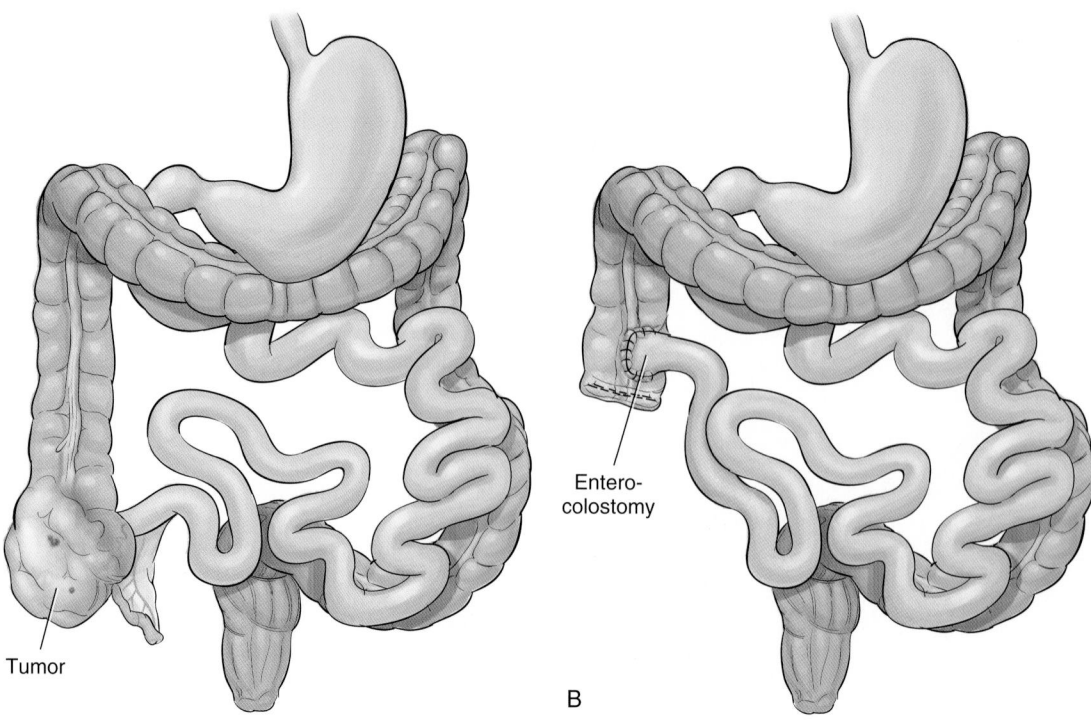

FIGURE 47.10 **A:** Ovarian cancer involving cecum. **B:** Right hemicolectomy with ileo-ascending enterocolostomy.

colon, cecum, and terminal ileum. Appendiceal endometriosis is generally an incidental finding not clinically significant. The most important potential consequence of bowel involvement is obstruction, which is more likely to occur in the small intestine. Other clinically significant consequences include pain (from dyschezia, tenesmus, dyspareunia, or nonspecific pelvic, or rectal), cyclic rectal bleeding, and nonspecific bowel symptoms. Further, the fibrotic mass effect and symptoms of bowel endometriosis may create the suspicion of malignancy.

Asymptomatic endometriosis of the bowel does not require surgical treatment. A trial of medical management is warranted for symptomatic disease but is not effective against large, fibrotic lesions. A small percentage of patients require bowel resection for endometriosis. Indications for bowel resection include obstruction, suspicion of malignancy, or other severe symptoms. A common scenario requiring bowel resection involves extensive endometriosis in the posterior cul-de-sac, including the anterior wall of the rectosigmoid colon. When focal, resection can be limited to a portion of the anterior rectal wall. With larger and more extensive involvement, segmental resection is necessary.

In patients with a known history of endometriosis and prior abdominal surgery, deposits of endometriosis may manifest in the abdominal wall in and around the prior incision. These implants are often confused with soft tissue tumors, especially when the interpreting radiologist is unaware of the patient's past medical or surgical history.

Bowel Obstruction

The gynecologic surgeon must be familiar with the management of bowel obstruction. In women who have undergone prior surgery or have experienced an extensive inflammatory process (e.g., infection, endometriosis), small bowel obstruction may develop secondary to surgically induced adhesions or internal hernia formation. When persistent obstruction is secondary to adhesions, simple adhesiolysis may resolve the problem. Occasionally, however, resection of a nonviable portion of the bowel is required.

The gynecologic oncologist must manage bowel obstruction in a variety of settings. As previously described, epithelial ovarian cancer has a propensity toward intra-abdominal spread and may present with bowel obstruction. When the disease recurs and progresses, it is especially common for the patient to develop intestinal obstruction. Although other gynecologic malignancies may also cause bowel obstruction secondary to intra-abdominal carcinomatosis, ovarian cancer is by far the most common risk factor. Small intestinal obstruction is most common, but colonic obstruction or both can also occur (Fig. 47.11).

The prognosis for patients with small intestinal and colonic obstruction is extremely poor, and decisions regarding surgical intervention must be carefully considered. A recent analysis of patients with malignant bowel obstruction due to ovarian cancer undergoing surgical intervention found symptomatic improvement in 88% of patients at 30 days and 61% at 60 days with median survival just over 6 months. Endoscopic intervention (with palliative, decompressive procedures) yielded much less durable relief of symptoms at just over 2 months. The same authors reviewed 141 patients undergoing surgical or endoscopic procedures for symptoms of malignant bowel obstruction of all types; this review showed that the presence of carcinomatosis, ascites, or multifocal obstruction predicted the application of decision to pursue palliative decompression (percutaneous endoscopic gastrostomy [PEG], G-tube, or stoma) rather than resection.

Regardless of the origin of malignant bowel obstruction, a thorough discussion must be embarked on with patients and

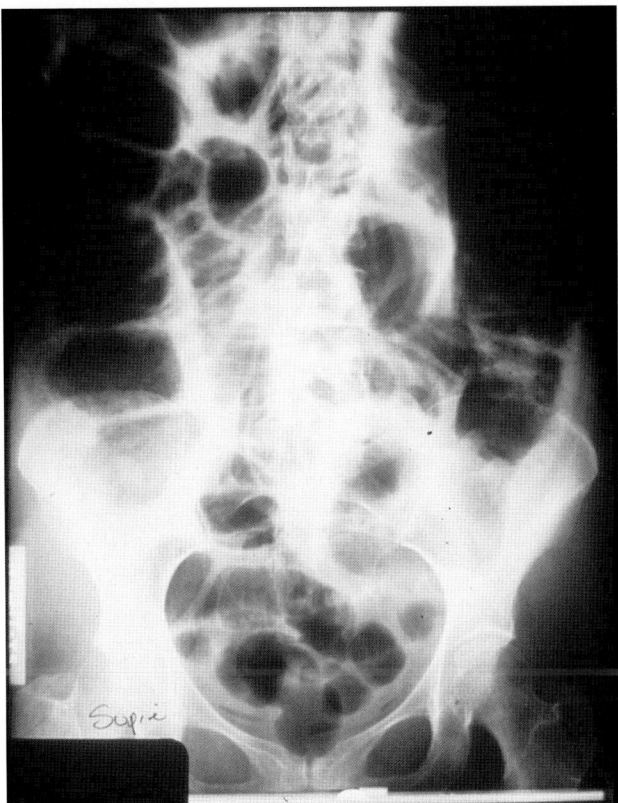

FIGURE 47.11 Abdominal plain film showing small and large bowel obstruction.

their families regarding goals and objectives of the proposed intervention, ensuring to ensure that each party understands the implications of aggressive surgical management—and the potential for extended recovery—in the setting of limited life expectancy.

Where there is an occurrence of extensive ascites, bulky intra-abdominal tumor, or an ileus-type pattern, or when the patient is malnourished (albumin <3 g/dL) or in generally in poor condition, surgical management of the obstruction is unlikely to be beneficial. A gastrostomy tube may provide substantial relief and free the patient from the discomfort of a nasogastric tube. In most instances, a gastrostomy tube may be placed percutaneously. Some women with left colon obstruction may be palliated with an endoscopically placed, expandable metallic stent. Select patients with advanced ovarian cancer and persistent obstruction do appear to benefit from surgical intervention. Due to extensive carcinomatosis, the intra-abdominal anatomy in these patients may be difficult to establish. The unobstructed proximal small bowel is freed to the extent possible, and a simple bypass to the proximal colon is carried out. In the presence of large bowel obstruction, a proximal diverting ostomy will generally be necessary. Even in the presence of obvious small bowel obstruction, whenever possible, the large bowel should be evaluated preoperatively for concomitant obstruction. Gastrografin enema performed prior to exploration for malignant small bowel obstruction provides assurance that resected or bypassed small bowel obstruction will not be undermined by existing or impending downstream colonic obstruction.

Small bowel obstruction following radiotherapy for a gynecologic malignancy requires a more calculated approach. These obstructions typically occur in the terminal ileum, although coexistent rectosigmoid colon injury is not uncommon. As such,

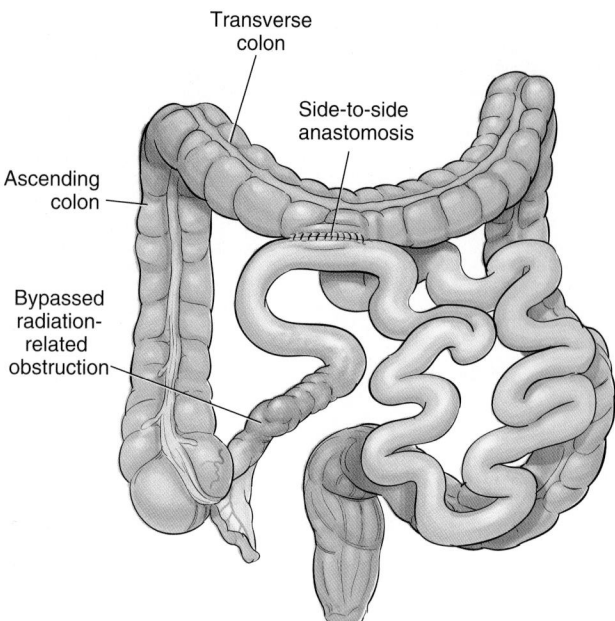

FIGURE 47.12 Simple side-to-side anastomosis of proximal small bowel to transverse colon in order to bypass radiation-related obstruction of the terminal ileum.

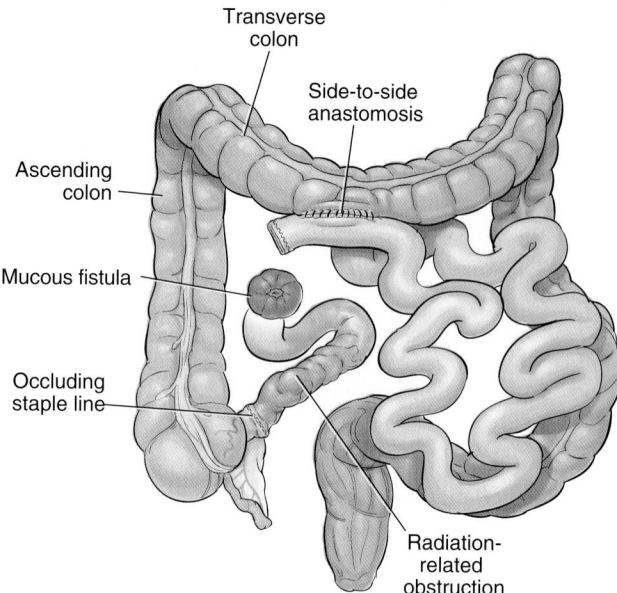

FIGURE 47.13 Enterocolostomy that both bypasses and diverts the fecal stream from the obstructed ileum.

both areas should be evaluated prior to surgical intervention. Surgical management of radiation-related small bowel obstruction remains controversial. Some experts recommend bypass of the obstruction while others believe the damaged bowel should be resected with primary reanastomosis. Simple bypass involves a side-to-side anastomosis of the proximal uninvolved small bowel to a relatively nonirradiated portion of the colon (Fig. 47.12). This is the fastest and least complicated surgical intervention. Advantages include the avoidance of extensive dissection of matted loops of the bowel—which dissection presents a potential for injury—in the resultant raw, previously irradiated pelvis. The side-to-side anastomosis ensures a good blood supply, avoids the need for a mucous fistula, and may allow the remainder of the bowel to provide some absorptive capacity in cases of partial obstruction; this is especially important when there is a short afferent limb. It also minimizes the risk of injury to other organs or structures, such as the ureter or vascular system. Overall, the results of simple bypass for these patients are reasonably good.

If the fecal stream is incompletely diverted, there is the potential for development of blind loops and/or fistulization of the remaining damaged and potentially necrotic bowel. Certain individuals may be at increased risk for subsequent fistulization, including those who have received greater than 50 Gray to the pelvis, are thin or elderly, or have arteriosclerosis, hypertension, or diabetes and those who have had prior pelvic surgery, chemotherapy (i.e., doxorubicin or actinomycin D), or pelvic inflammatory disease. An end-to-side or end-to-end enterocolostomy without resection and with one or two mucous fistulae is an alternative to simple bypass (Fig. 47.13). The main advantage is complete diversion of the fecal stream from the damaged segment and thus avoidance of subsequent fistulization from this area. This type of procedure is often used to manage a postirradiation enterovaginal fistula. Bypass with isolation for management of radiation-related obstruction has not been carefully evaluated separately from simple bypass.

Resection with anastomosis involves removal of all diseased intestine and anastomosis of minimally radiated bowel

(Fig. 47.14) and prevents the development of a mucous fistula. This is an often extensive and time-consuming surgery that frequently leaves the remaining bowel exposed to a raw, irradiated pelvis. Other potential disadvantages of resection include a less optimal blood supply at the anastomosis; the functional maintenance of portions of the bowel that have been dissected out (many experts resect all of this bowel) and, though not obstructed, are still radiated and potentially damaged subclinically (e.g., blood supply, enterotomies, aperistaltic); and the injury of other structures during dissection, such as bladder, colon, ureter, and major blood vessels.

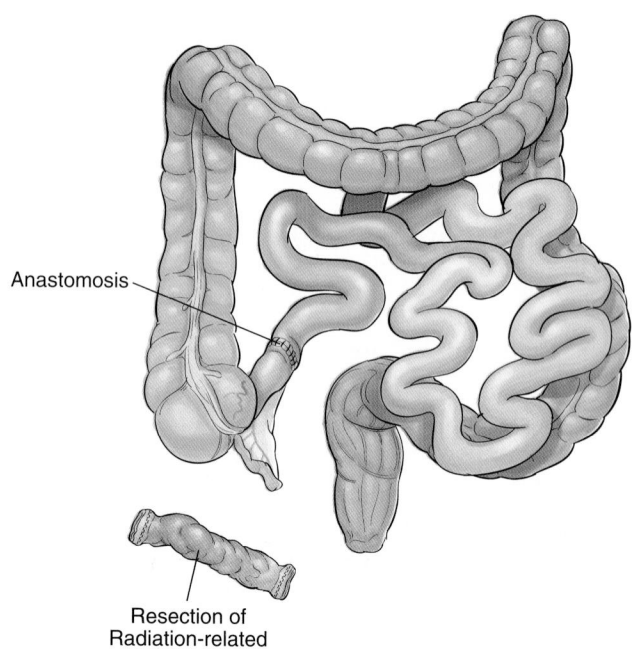

FIGURE 47.14 Resection of obstructed, damaged bowel with anastomosis of small bowel to unirradiated transverse colon.

The surgical approach to a patient with radiation-related small bowel obstruction must be individualized. If the overall condition of the patient is poor or there is recurrent disease, the most expeditious and least complicated procedure (i.e., simple bypass) should be carried out. If there is potential impending necrosis of the involved bowel, there are multiple injuries to the bowel as a result of dissection, or the involved bowel is a simple loop that is not densely adherent, resection with end-to-end enterocolostomy is preferred. Isolation bypass may still be applicable in some of these cases. Matted loops of bowel in the irradiated pelvis should be left in place as long as a reasonable length of proximal small bowel can be bypassed to nonirradiated proximal colon. It is preferable to avoid resection, but the bypassed bowel should be diverted from the fecal stream in the event that further necrosis with potential fistulization should develop.

Colon resection secondary to benign gynecologic disease is infrequent. Gynecologic malignancy, especially ovarian cancer, may encase and partially obstruct the sigmoid or transverse colon. When such disease is surgically resected, the decision for left colon anastomosis is individualized. Radiation-related stricture of the rectosigmoid colon is discussed below. Rarely does endometriosis cause partial obstruction of the rectosigmoid colon.

Fistulae

The common sources of an intestinal fistula include anastomotic failure, occult operative injury, incorporation into wound closure, inflammatory bowel disease, tumor erosion into adjacent bowel (e.g., enterovaginal), radiation necrosis of the bowel wall, an exposed and/or compromised bowel following fascial dehiscence, or any combination of these factors. In the general surgery literature, the majority of fistulae communicate with the skin and can arise from any portion of the gastrointestinal tract. The reported overall mortality rate is between 5% and 20%, with most deaths resulting from uncontrolled sepsis. The mortality rate is significantly enhanced in the setting of small bowel fistulae, inflammatory bowel disease, cancer, or previous abdominal radiation.

Enteric fistulae occurring in gynecologic cancer patients encompass a much different population. The majority of patients have active intra-abdominal cancer, prior extensive radiotherapy, or both. Most fistulae develop, at least in part, as a consequence of these factors. A large percentage of the fistulae in these patients communicate with the vagina (Fig. 47.15), and the majority arise from the terminal ileum or rectosigmoid colon.

A leaking small bowel anastomosis may form a communication with the abdominal wall or vagina, resulting in an enterocutaneous or enterovaginal fistula. During the process of fistulization, intra-abdominal leakage of bowel contents may result in peritonitis or abscess formation, and in some cases there may be continued intraperitoneal leakage. Uncontrolled sepsis in these patients is the major factor associated with mortality. In the presence of active malignancy or prior radiation, these complications are more likely to occur and more difficult to detect.

More proximal small bowel fistulae cause other types of difficulties and, fortunately, are less commonly seen in the gynecologic cancer patient. Jejunal fistulae have a high output of caustic succus that is corrosive to the skin and results in substantial loss of fluids and electrolytes. As fistulae become more proximal, total parenteral nutrition (TPN)—and its associated complications and expense—becomes less a matter of preference and more a matter of necessity. In some cases, however, the distal small bowel may be intubated with a catheter or feeding tube to allow for nutritional support/supplementation as the fistula contracts and heals.

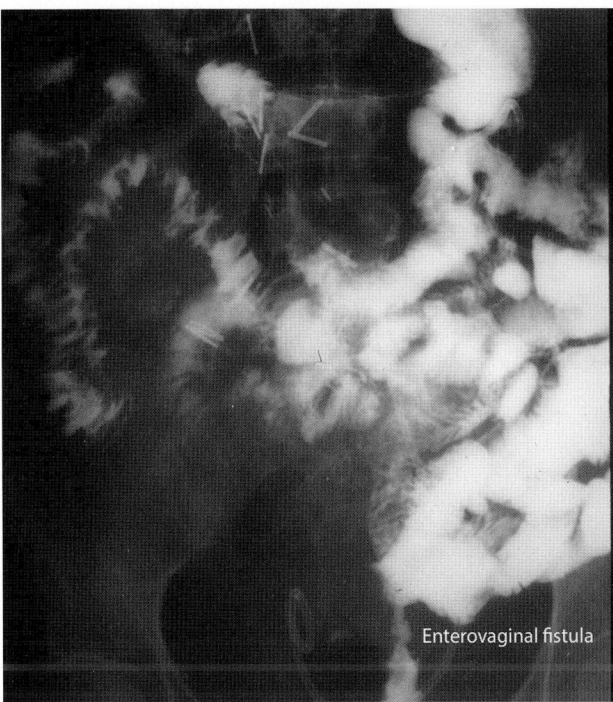

FIGURE 47.15 Contrast study demonstrating enterovaginal fistula. Note that the contrast passes from the distal small bowel into the vagina in the center lower area of this radiograph.

Initial management of the patient with a small bowel fistula consists of bowel rest with nasogastric suction, fluid resuscitation, electrolyte replacement, local management of the fistula output to prevent skin erosion, and control of sepsis. The extent of intra-abdominal contamination requiring laparotomy, washout, and drainage must be assessed either radiographically or by physical exam, specifically eliciting signs of peritonitis, such as rigidity, guarding, or rebound tenderness. In the setting of a contained leak, sepsis may resolve with bowel rest and antibiotics but in some cases will require drainage of an abscess and/or prompt proximal diversion.

TPN is often used to enable complete bowel rest in patients whose fistulae have a high probability of spontaneous closure (i.e., long tract, incompletely diverting, absence of radiation injury, or distal obstruction). With TPN, the overall condition of the patient improves, and time can be allowed for the inflammatory reaction of the bowel and peritoneal cavity to subside. After sepsis and local wound issues are addressed, oral or enteral feeding can be reinstituted.

Once sepsis is controlled, spontaneous closure of the fistula is reported to occur in 30% to 60% of cases, and nearly all spontaneous closures occur within 4 weeks. During that time, placement of a gastrostomy tube may be considered as a replacement for the nasogastric tube if necessary. After the patient has been initially stabilized, a thorough radiologic evaluation of the fistula and the remaining small and large bowel is undertaken. An early attempt at closure of a postoperative fistula is associated with a low likelihood of success and a high rate of morbidity. The use of somatostatin (or octreotide) has been shown in some series to shorten the interval to spontaneous closure, improve the spontaneous closure rate, and reduce gastrointestinal secretions through the fistula. A recent meta-analysis comprising 14 randomized controlled trials supported early use of somatostatin or its analogues in increasing both the likelihood and rate of fistulae closure.

VIII

In certain clinical situations, spontaneous closure is unlikely to occur, and indeed, the majority of fistulae in gynecologic cancer patients will not close spontaneously. These situations include intestinal obstruction distal to the fistula, malignancy at the fistula site, fistula location in a previously irradiated field, the presence of a foreign body, epithelialization of the fistula tract, and a fistula related to inflammatory bowel disease. The mnemonic F.R.I.E.N.D.S. is often used to remember factors that prevent fistulae from closing spontaneously: foreign body, radiation, inflammation, epithelialization, neoplasm, distal obstruction, and short (≤2 cm) tract fistulae.

In patients with fistulae that have not closed spontaneously, operative intervention should be postponed as long as the patient is doing well. If spontaneous closure has not occurred after 4 to 5 weeks of stabilization, then surgery will be eventually required to restore continuity. The actual point at which decision regarding when closure should be attempted surgically is dependent on a number of factors, including the patient's remaining life expectancy, nutritional state, overall medical condition, and his or her ability to manage the fistula as is.

Surgical management of a small bowel fistula must be highly individualized. Occasionally, it is possible to excise the fistula opening from the bowel and close the defect in layers or to resect the involved segment and perform an end-to-end anastomosis (EEA). However, small bowel fistulae to the vagina encountered in gynecologic cancer patients must often be bypassed, leaving the irradiated or tumor-involved adherent loops of bowel in the pelvis. As with the case of obstruction, the proximal uninvolved small bowel is followed as far as possible, avoiding dissection of densely adherent loops from the pelvis. At this point, the small bowel is divided and anastomosed to a relatively nonirradiated portion of the large intestine. This should be a functional EEA so as to completely exclude the fistula from the fecal stream. Mucus fistulae should be utilized whenever the risk of closed loop obstruction exists.

As a consequence of advancing pelvic malignancy, prior extensive pelvic radiotherapy (possibly combined with the effects of prior extensive pelvic surgery), or a combination of these factors, occasionally develops between the bowel and the bladder. The first concern is to stabilize the patient and control sepsis, which may be more difficult due to involvement of the urinary tract. After short-term stabilization, surgical intervention will be required.

For relatively simple cases of small bowel involvement, the fistulized loop is resected. Repair of the bladder is individualized. It is less preferable to bypass the fecal stream due to the persistent ill-effects of mucus or partially contaminated drainage into the bladder. Usually, management of a sigmoidovesical fistula will require a diverting colostomy, at least temporarily. In more complicated cases of fistula development between the bowel and bladder—and especially when there is evident involvement of the bladder by radiation necrosis or tumor, or when there is persistent sepsis, bypass, or diversion of both the intestinal and urinary tracts will be necessary. The mortality rate for such cases is high.

The other type of fistula commonly encountered in gynecologic patients arises from the sigmoid colon to the vagina or from the rectum to the vagina. Such a fistula may develop as a complication of surgery (delayed leak from a partial or segmental resection or from an inadvertent injury) or radiation therapy. A postmenopausal woman presenting with a sigmoidovaginal fistula most likely has ruptured diverticulitis. Women may develop an intestinal fistula to the vagina as a result of inflammatory bowel disease, or as a consequence of advanced colorectal cancer, although the latter is uncommon. In gynecologic cancer patients, a sigmoidovaginal fistula may be related to the malignancy, occurring often as a result of or associated with distal obstruction. A large percentage of these cases is due to radiation injury or perhaps to a combination of factors. After short-term stabilization, a diverting or end (if permanent) colostomy is performed.

Severe Radiation Injury of the Rectosigmoid Colon

Severe proctosigmoiditis develops in a small percentage of patients following pelvic radiotherapy for gynecologic cancer. Abdominal cramping, diarrhea, and/or bleeding may result. With medical management, some of these symptoms improve over time. However, if progressive or left unattended to, the injury may progress to perforation or a fistula. As previously discussed, the area of injury may be mapped out with the use of contrast studies through the normal GI tract and fistula and with endoscopy. Resection is performed accordingly, and in some cases, colorectal continuity can be reestablished. A diverting colostomy is advisable until it is certain that the anastomosis has healed (i.e., at least 6 months).

Radiation stricture of the rectosigmoid colon may also develop, causing obstruction (Fig. 47.16) and necessitating surgical intervention. The area of involvement should be mapped out preoperatively with radiologic and endoscopic studies. When feasible, this portion of the large bowel may be resected and anastomosed. The anastomosis should be wrapped with transposed omentum when available. Proximal diversion is strongly considered. The colon anastomosis is reevaluated 6 months postoperatively, and if healing is satisfactory, the ostomy is taken down.

As in the case of severe radiation sigmoiditis, the patient with a radiation-induced sigmoidovaginal fistula can sometimes undergo resection and colorectal anastomosis in hopes of eventually restoring bowel continuity. Some radiation-induced rectovaginal fistulae can eventually be surgically closed. Boronow et al. described local repair of such fistulae after a period of diversion. Park described resection of the rectum beyond the fistula (and the region of severe radiation damage) with transanal anastomosis of the colon to the anus.

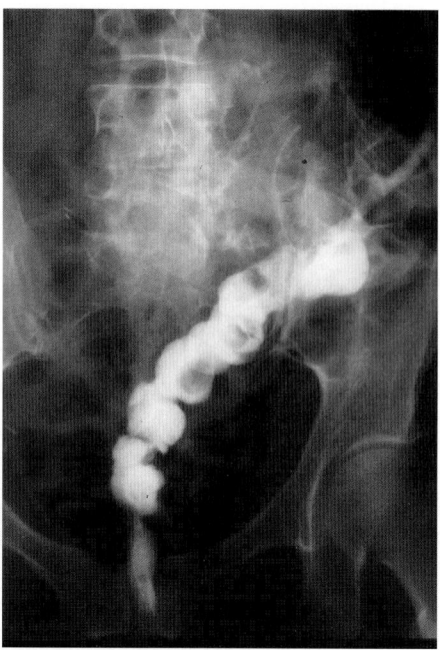

FIGURE 47.16 Contrast study of a symptomatic radiated patient, demonstrating stricture of the rectosigmoid colon.

Bricker described the technique of folding the rectosigmoid colon over itself to cover the fistula with anastomosis of the colon to the top of the loop.

Perforated Bowel

Perforated bowel with intraperitoneal leakage is infrequently encountered in gynecologic and nongynecologic cancer patients. The complication may develop as a result of radiation-induced necrosis (usually of the terminal ileum or sigmoid colon), leakage from an intestinal anastomosis or occult operative injury, or bowel ischemia related to obstruction. When perforated bowel with intraperitoneal leakage is due to radiation injury, diagnosis is often delayed, and the mortality rate is high.

Surgery is performed on an emergent basis. If the perforation is highly localized and walled off, resection or exclusionary bypass of the small bowel may be considered. In general, however, proximal exteriorization should be carried out. The peritoneal cavity should be thoroughly lavaged with an antibiotic solution. Several months of stabilization should elapse to allow the inflammatory reaction of the bowel and peritoneal cavity to resolve before considering an attempt at reestablishment of bowel continuity.

Exenteration

Pelvic exenteration is occasionally performed for recurrent or persistent gynecologic cancer in the central pelvis and is covered in Chapter 54. Diversion or reconstruction of the urinary and/or intestinal tract is necessary in these patients, requiring one or more surgical procedures involving the bowel. The majority of these patients have received prior radiotherapy, which further complicates treatment. For purposes of urinary tract reconstruction, a portion of the bowel is isolated from the fecal stream and intestinal continuity is reestablished. In the case of an ileal conduit performed in a previously radiated patient, it is recommended that the anastomosis occur between the ileum and the nonirradiated transverse colon to ensure better healing.

When the rectum or anus must be removed, a permanent colostomy is performed. When a portion of the rectum can be preserved, it may be possible to perform a colorectal (i.e., coloanal) anastomosis. Strong consideration is given to proximal diversion. Even when continuity cannot be restored, it may be preferable in some cases to leave a very short rectal stump to avoid potential morbidity of a perineal wound.

Urinary Tract Reconstruction

Urinary diversion and bladder reconstruction utilize intestine that has been isolated from the fecal stream. These procedures are covered in detail in Chapter 24. Another infrequent use for intestine in urinary tract reconstruction is ureteral substitution, generally done with a portion of ileum.

Vaginal Reconstruction

One of the myriad types of vaginal reconstruction in gynecologic patients is intestinal substitution. There are few reports on this type of neovagina in the gynecologic cancer patient, and the results obtained are unclear. After pelvic resection, a portion of the sigmoid colon or ileum is diverted from the fecal stream. In exenterative surgery, this should be coordinated with other necessary intestinal components to minimize the number of anastomoses. The intestinal segment with its blood supply is mobilized so that one end may be anastomosed to the introitus or vaginal stump. The other end is closed to form a pouch.

PRIMARY INTESTINAL DISEASE

Diverticulitis

Acute diverticulitis can mimic benign adnexal pathology, such as torsion, ovarian cysts, abscesses, or malignant pathology of either gynecologic or colorectal origin. Perhaps the most useful means of distinguishing diverticulitis from these diagnoses is a history of radiographically or endoscopically diagnosed diverticular disease or a prior acute episode resulting in emergency department presentation or inpatient hospitalization. In patients without a diagnosis of diverticular disease, arriving at the correct diagnosis may be difficult, especially in the absence of absolute indications for exploration (e.g., free intra-abdominal perforation, uncontrollable hemorrhage, or obstruction). In these cases, the diagnosis relies on the combined efforts of an astute radiologist and clinician, with an abdominopelvic computed tomography (CT) scan being the most useful diagnostic maneuver.

In most cases, pericolonic inflammation, abscess, or colonic wall thickening in association with left lower quadrant pain and normal-appearing ovaries and uterus is sufficient to establish a diagnosis of diverticulitis. Based on CT findings, diverticulitis can then be subcategorized into complicated or uncomplicated diverticulitis. Nonoperative therapy through bowel rest and antibiotics is successful in 70% to 100% of patients with uncomplicated diverticulitis. A CT scan demonstrating uncomplicated diverticulitis is shown in **Figure 47.17**. More recently, prospective randomized data have brought the routine use of antibiotics in uncomplicated diverticulitis into question. Complicated diverticulitis—as manifested by obstruction, abscess, perforation, or fistula—may be managed with percutaneous drainage with a low threshold for surgical exploration in the setting of progressive peritonitis or in high-risk patients (i.e., older, deconditioned, or immunocompromised patients).

Distinguishing diverticulitis from colorectal malignancy in both complicated and uncomplicated diverticulitis is critical and can be challenging. Missing or delaying the latter diagnosis may have devastating consequences for the patient and, as soon as clinically feasible, a limited endoscopic evaluation should be undertaken to rule out a mucosal-based lesion. This can be safely undertaken as early as 2 to 6 weeks after the acute inflammatory phase has resolved (normal white blood cell count, afebrile, resolved left lower quadrant pain, and

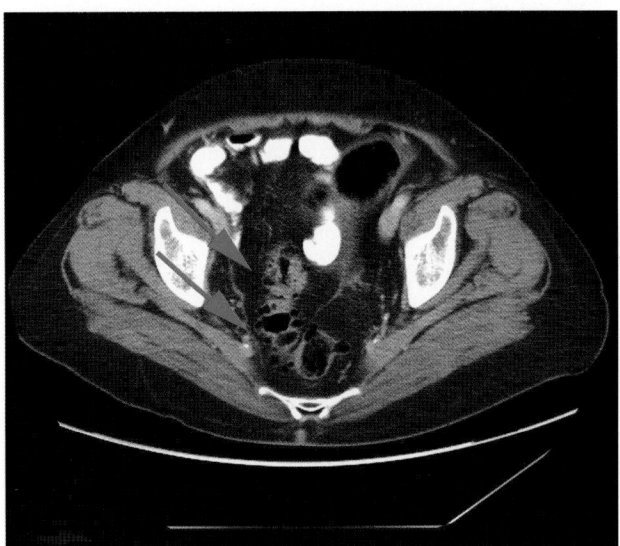

FIGURE 47.17 CT scan showing acute, uncomplicated diverticulitis.

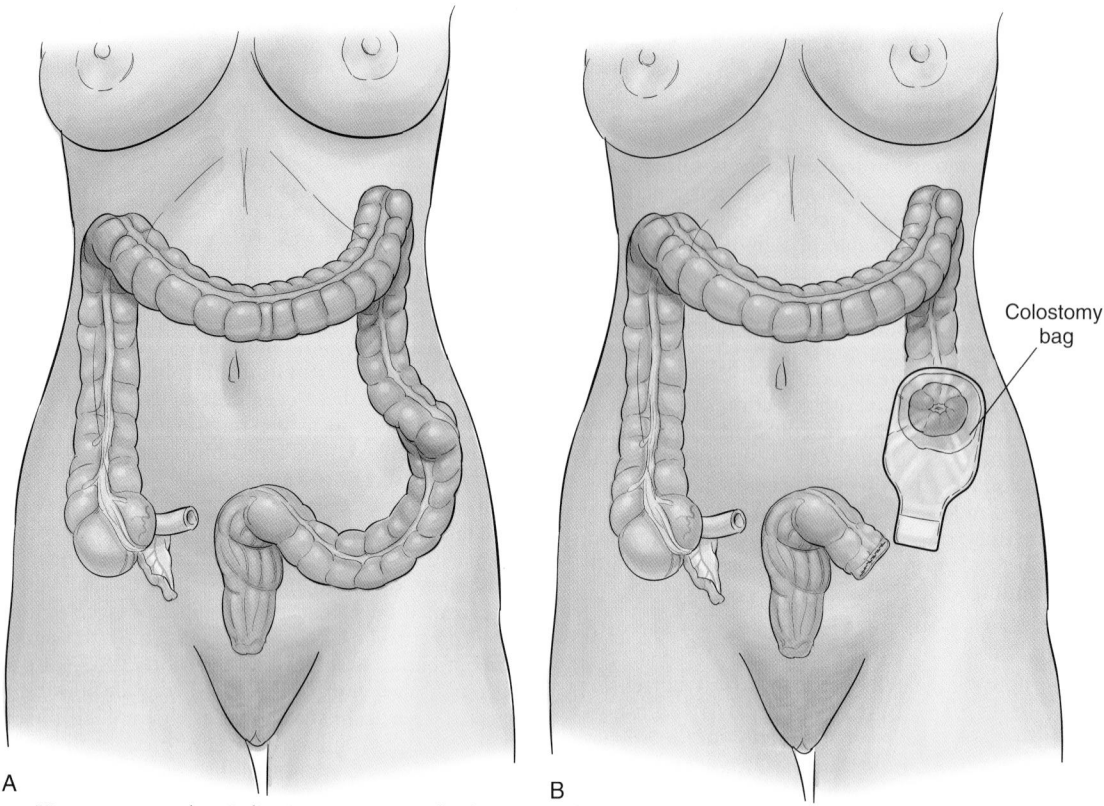

FIGURE 47.18 Hartmann procedure indicating resection, end colostomy, and rectal pouch (**A, B**).

resumption of normal bowel activity). At initial presentation, if the suspicion for cancer is high, then surgical exploration with Hartmann procedure (i.e., resection, end colostomy, rectal pouch) is the safest and most effective diagnostic and therapeutic intervention (Fig. 47.18).

Acute Appendicitis

Due to the profound overlap in presenting symptoms, age, and prodrome illness in a patient, acute appendicitis is the gastrointestinal diagnosis most difficult to distinguish from gynecologic pathology. Pregnancy, especially in the second and third trimesters, may further confound the diagnosis as the gravid uterus displaces not only the appendix but also the focal point of pain. Delayed diagnosis of appendicitis due to pregnancy is a source of significant added morbidity. Although female patients are slightly less likely to develop acute appendicitis than are males, the high prevalence of this disease in the third decade of life continues to make this a diagnostic challenge.

The classic presentation consists of three fundamental components: periumbilical pain migrating to the right lower quadrant, anorexia, and nausea/vomiting. Most surgeons trained prior to the CT-scan era relied heavily on the presence of fever and/or leukocytosis to establish the diagnosis of appendicitis. More recently, several scoring systems have been established that assign a relative numeric value to those presenting signs and symptoms most predictive of appendicitis. These scoring systems are designed to avoid axial imaging in patients with a high probability of acute appendicitis based on clinical presentation alone.

The Alvarado score is the most popular of these scoring systems and takes into account leukocytosis (2 points), iliac fossa tenderness (2 points), migratory pain, anorexia, nausea/vomiting, rebound pain, and fever (all 1 point). A high Alvarado score (≥7) generally supports exploration without

further diagnostic studies, while lower scores, especially in diagnostically challenging subgroups (e.g., children younger than 3 years, adults older than 60 years, and pregnant women in the second and third trimesters) supports further diagnostic imaging such as CT scan. In one recent review in 71 patients with appendicitis and 167 patients with alternative diagnoses, CT findings consistent with appendicitis identified enlarged appendix (93% sensitive/92% specific), appendiceal wall thickening (66% sensitive/96% specific), periappendiceal fat stranding (87% sensitive/74% specific), and appendiceal wall enhancement (75% sensitive/85% specific).

Ultrasound is similarly useful in establishing the diagnosis with sensitivity, specificity, and positive and negative predictive value all as high as 99% in some series. Sonographic findings consistent with appendicitis include diameter greater than 6 mm, noncompressibility, presence of appendicolith, periappendiceal fat changes, or nonvisualization of the appendix (i.e., negative finding). In patients whose diagnosis remains uncertain despite all imaging modalities, early engagement of the general surgery team for serial abdominal exam is essential.

Meckel Diverticulum

Meckel diverticulum is a relatively common diagnosis occurring in 1% to 2% of adult patients in autopsy studies. Since the majority of patients with Meckel diverticulum are asymptomatic, the disorder is most commonly diagnosed as an incidental finding during celiotomy for other intra-abdominal pathology. Meckel diverticulum represents a remnant of the vitelline yolk duct and usually occurs within 2 feet of the ileocecal valve along the antimesenteric border of the ileum (Fig. 47.19). Most Meckel diverticula are lined by small bowel mucosa, but as many as 20% of patients have ectopic gastric or pancreatic tissue in the lining that causes symptoms of bleeding or pain. In addition to bleeding,

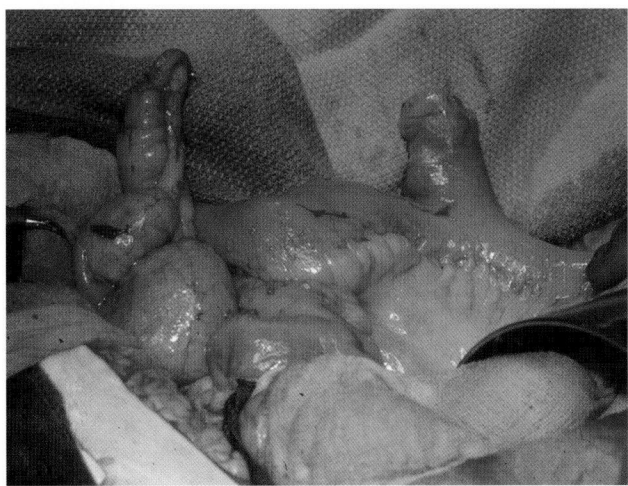

FIGURE 47.19 Appendix with metastatic implants, Meckel diverticulum.

patients with Meckel diverticulum may obstruct or develop diverticulitis. Symptomatic diverticula should be resected, while those found incidentally in adult patients may be safely observed and should not be resected; the likelihood of a Meckel diverticulum becoming symptomatic during adulthood is less than 2%. Resection should be undertaken in patients being explored for abdominal pain or gastrointestinal hemorrhage who demonstrate no other intra-abdominal pathology. In cases where the diverticulum is lined by gastric or pancreatic mucosa and bleeding in the adjacent ileum has occurred, complete resection of the segment of ileum bearing the diverticulum is necessary.

Volvulus/Intussusception

Spontaneous small intestinal volvulus and intussusception are rare diagnoses in adult patients, usually presenting as a bowel obstruction. Radiographic findings may be subtle; as such, patients are often definitively diagnosed during celiotomy for nonspecific obstruction. Small bowel intussusception rarely occurs spontaneously in adult patients; rather, it is a manifestation of some type of lead point within the lumen, such as a small bowel or extrinsic compression from adjacent pathology or obstructive processes.

Occasionally, a radiologist may suggest the diagnosis based on the presence of CT findings consistent with internal hernia (e.g., dilated small bowel loops ending in a mass or mesenteric twist). As more women (and men) undergo surgical weight loss procedures, the incidence of internal hernias and small bowel volvulus is increasing. These hernias occur through newly created spaces, including the mesenteric defect of the jejunojejunostomy, the defect between the transverse mesocolon and the Roux limb mesentery commonly known as Petersen defect, and the mesocolic defect through which the Roux limb is passed (Fig. 47.20). As with any other obstructive process, volvulus and hernia commonly present as pain, obstipation, and abdominal distention.

Colonic volvulus most commonly presents as a sudden onset of abdominal pain, distention, and obstipation (sometimes accompanied by nausea and vomiting), and may occur in the cecum or the sigmoid colon. Care must be taken to distinguish cecal volvulus from sigmoid volvulus, as subtle differences in diagnosis and management exist.

Cecal volvulus accounts for 10% to 40% of colonic volvuli and can be more difficult to diagnose radiographically than sigmoid volvulus, due to its varied findings on plain films. In general, cecal volvulus manifests as a dilated cecum, with the long axis extending from the right lower quadrant to the midepigastrium

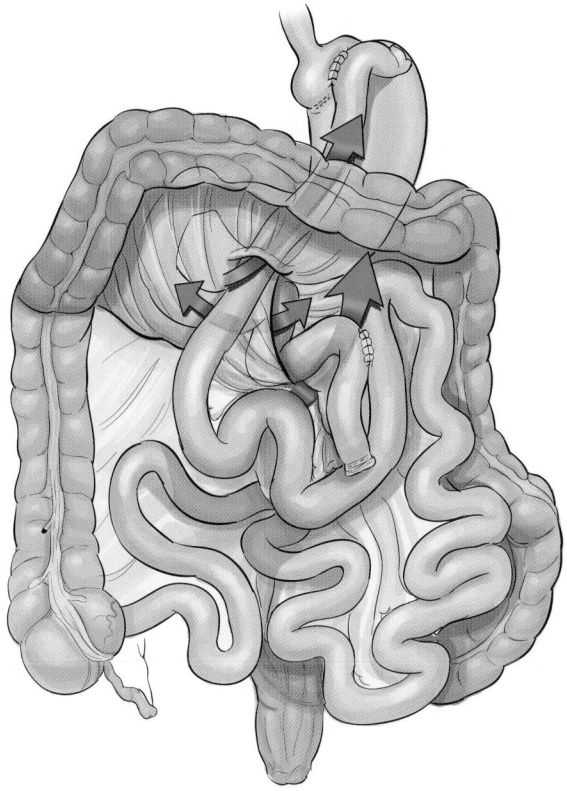

FIGURE 47.20 Internal herniation following jejunojejunostomy.

and decompressed distal colon. It is frequently associated with small bowel dilatation as well. Cecal volvulus can be decompressed endoscopically but has a recurrence rate as high as 75%. Surgical management is therefore recommended. Retrospective series have shown ileocecectomy to be more effective than less invasive maneuvers such as cecostomy or cecopexy.

Sigmoid volvulus is the most common colonic volvulus. Whereas cecal volvulus can be distinguished by the long axis extending to the midepigastrium from the right lower quadrant, sigmoid volvulus demonstrates dilated large bowel with the long axis extending from the left lower quadrant to the midepigastrium or to the right upper quadrant. The classic radiographic finding is known as the coffee bean sign, where the apex of the bean originates in the right upper quadrant (Fig. 47.21A, B).

Flexible sigmoidoscopy is both diagnostic and therapeutic, with immediate relief of obstruction manifested by a rush of fecal material, which can soil the naïve endoscopist. High-risk patients responding to nonsurgical therapy on their first presentation may be safely observed; however, recurrence rates have been reported in up to 61% of patients at a median of 31 days. As such, recurrent sigmoid volvulus is a strong indication for sigmoid colectomy.

Pelvic Malignancy

The origin of advanced pelvic malignancy may be impossible to establish without immunohistochemical analysis of tissue obtained by open, percutaneous, endoscopic, transvaginal, or cystoscopic procedures. Cancers of colorectal origin typically express CK20 and CDX2 and may be associated with elevated serum CEA levels. Pelvic tumors of gynecologic origin typically express CD7, CA-125, estrogen/progesterone receptors (i.e., endometrioid tumors), and WT1 (i.e., serous ovarian tumors,); these pelvic tumors are additionally associated with

VIII

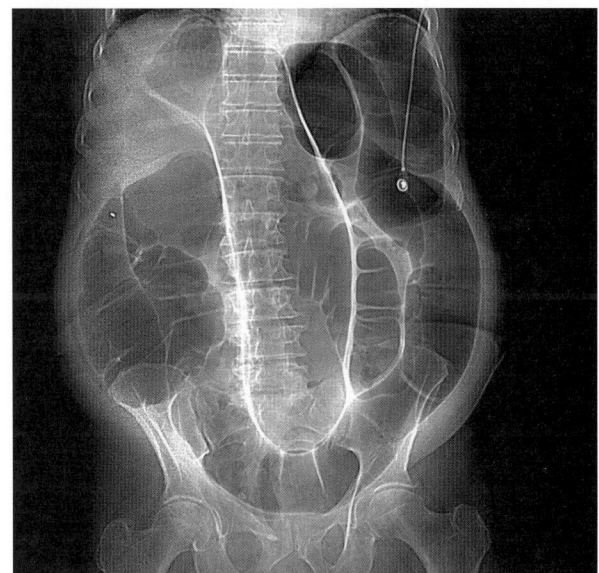

A

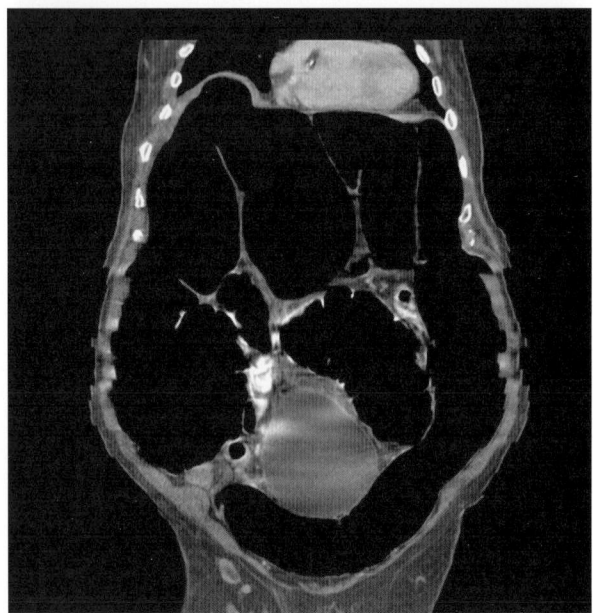

B

FIGURE 47.21 A and B: The classic radiographic "coffee bean" sign of a sigmoid volvulus with the apex of the bean originating in the right upper quadrant.

elevated serum CA-125 and/or CA 27-29. Absence of CK20 and CEA strongly favors gynecologic primary.

The origin of advanced pelvic malignancy is of critical importance in determining neoadjuvant chemotherapy strategy. Pelvic malignancy involving multiple organ sites should be palliated with diversion of the fecal and urinary stream (when completely obstructed) and chemoradiotherapy utilized to downstage. In those patients who manifest tumor shrinkage or downstaging with neoadjuvant treatment, multivisceral resection including anterior, posterior, or complete pelvic exenteration may be indicated for long-term palliation or even cure.

Colorectal Cancer

In addition to rectosigmoid cancer locally, advanced ileocecal and appendiceal cancer may manifest as a pelvic process. At the level of the pelvic brim, it is not uncommon for

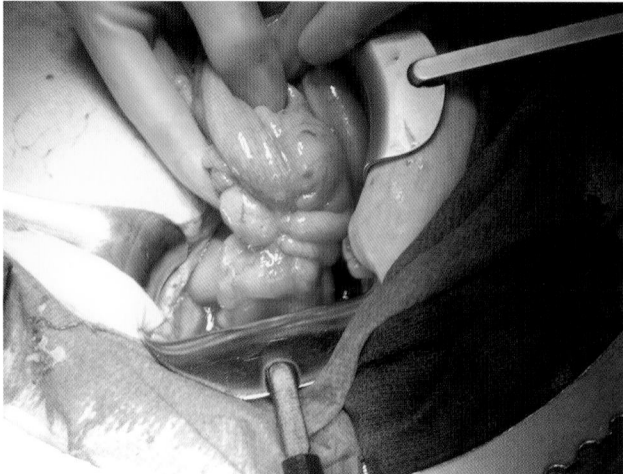

FIGURE 47.22 Obstructing "apple core" carcinoma of the sigmoid colon.

the sigmoid flexure and the ileocecum to abut one another, thereby creating a potential that T4 lesions (i.e., the extension of primary tumor into surrounding organs) arising from either site may require en bloc resection of the rectosigmoid and right colon as they fall or are pulled into the pelvis. This necessitates two anastomoses: an ileocolostomy and a coloproctostomy. In the absence of obstruction, this is an acceptable approach.

Obstructive pathology (as manifested by the inability to adequately prepare the colon and/or a significant size discrepancy between the anastomosed segments) mandates resection with ileostomy and mucus fistula or ileocolostomy and end colostomy with rectal pouch. Occasionally, patients with obstructing upper rectal and sigmoid cancers (Fig. 47.22) can have limited (i.e., liquid diet only) continuity restored with endoscopic stents to facilitate preoperative colonic decompression and preparation, thereby alleviating the need for temporary colostomy (Fig. 47.23). A recent

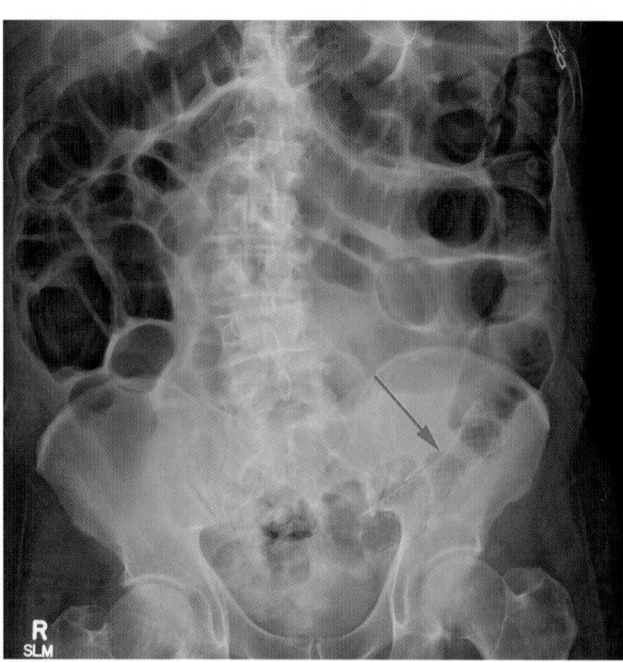

FIGURE 47.23 Decompressive stent in patient with near-complete sigmoid obstruction.

prospective study in 182 patients with obstructing cancers of the rectosigmoid or descending in the left side of the colon reported successful stent placement in 98%. Subsequently, 94% of 150 patients undergoing elective resection avoided colostomy.

As surgeons have become increasingly specialized in colorectal and pelvic malignancy, the technique of total mesorectal excision first described by Heald in 1986 has become the de facto standard of care for rectal cancer. Heald originally described the technique—as "the painstaking downward development of the avascular plane between visceral structures (rectum and mesorectum) and somatic structures (autonomic nerve plexuses; sympathetic above and parasympathetic below)." This technique not only yielded superior lymph node harvest but significantly lowered patient incidence of pelvic recurrence (3% to 7%) and improved long-term survival (80%). Total mesorectal excision may now be accomplished sharply or with thermal energy devices.

Pelvic recurrence of rectal cancer is a devastating manifestation of suboptimally resected primary rectal tumors or nodal recurrence. In either event, opportunities for curative reresection are limited and usually involve limited (e.g., anterior or posterior) or complete exenteration. Factors limiting this reresection—one of the most invasive of all cancer interventions—are pelvic sidewall and sacral (above S3) involvement of the tumor. Sacrectomy below the level of S3 may be accomplished while still maintaining stability of the pelvis and is usually undertaken with the assistance of neurosurgery or orthopedic spinal surgeons.

Rectal Prolapse

Rectal prolapse (**Fig. 47.24**) shares similar pathophysiology with prolapse of the uterus and bladder. It can result from progressive weakening or stretching of the mesocolon of

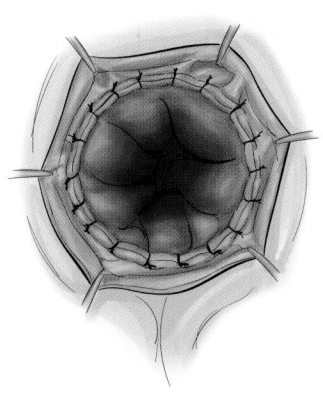

FIGURE 47.24 Rectal prolapse.

rectosigmoid and can eventually lead to prolapse. This process may be exacerbated in patients with redundant sigmoid colon and chronic constipation. In contrast to uterine or bladder prolapse, definitive surgical therapy for rectal prolapse involves either rectopexy or resection of the prolapsed segment with an open or laparoscopic approach and primary reanastomosis with or without rectopexy.

Since rectal prolapse most commonly occurs in elderly patients—oftentimes deconditioned patients with medical comorbidities—the morbidity and mortality of this intervention for a benign process is high. As such, many patients are either forced to live with their prolapse or to undergo "less invasive" intervention, such as the Altemeier procedure (**Fig. 47.25**). Undertaken in a manner similar to a vaginal hysterectomy, the Altemeier procedure involves delivery of the prolapsed segment through the rectum with resection and primary coloanal anastomosis.

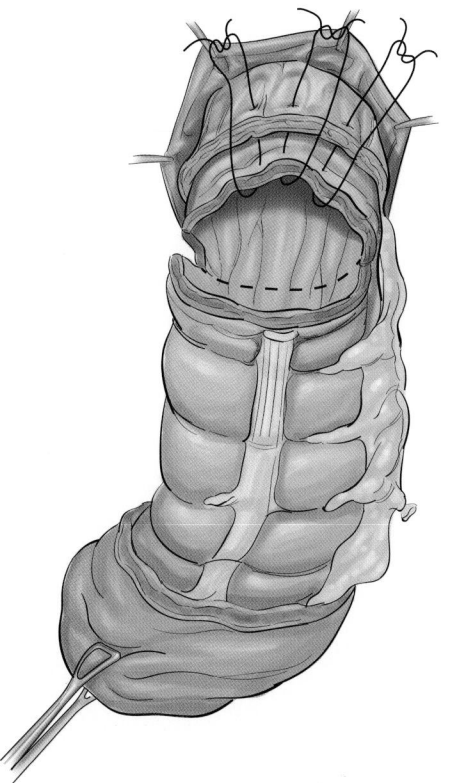

FIGURE 47.25 Altemeier procedure.

Most series of this ostensibly less invasive intervention report complications commensurate with those of open laparotomy; in the laparoscopic era, the technique has been supplanted by minimally invasive approaches. A recent review of the American College of Surgeons Quality Improvement Program (NSQIP) database demonstrated in 685 patients decreased length of stay and decreased incidence of surgical site infections (SSIs) with a trend toward decreased morbidity in patients managed with laparoscopic versus open rectopexy or sigmoidectomy and rectopexy.

Ogilvie Syndrome

Ogilvie syndrome, also known as acute colonic pseudo-obstruction, presents with abdominal distention, nausea, vomiting, and diarrhea. Plain radiographs demonstrate dilated cecum and right colon (Fig. 47.26). Ogilvie syndrome rarely occurs spontaneously and is rather associated with an underlying medical condition in over 90% of cases. Such conditions may include (in decreasing prevalence) trauma, sepsis, cardiac disease, gynecologic disease, recent abdominopelvic surgery, neurologic conditions, orthopedic surgery, and miscellaneous medical/surgical conditions.

Ogilvie syndrome can be differentiated from mechanical bowel obstruction and toxic megacolon with the use of CT scan or Gastrografin enema. Treatment initially consists of conservative measures (e.g., NPO, IVF, NG, electrolyte replacement) followed by neostigmine if after 24 to 48 hours if there is no resolution. Neostigmine, administered at a dose of 2 mg IV, results in rapid resolution (range 3 to 30 minutes) in 80% to 90% of patients. Patients with underlying asthma, recent myocardial infarction, or those who are actively taking beta-blockers should be approached with caution, as severe bradycardia can result with the use of Neostigmine. Atropine should be readily available, and patients should receive continuous ECG monitoring for at least 30 minutes following neostigmine therapy.

In patients who fail to respond to conservative or medical management, colonic decompression achieved either endoscopically or with rectal tube should be pursued, especially as the colonic diameter approaches 12 cm (beyond which Laplace's law predicts a high likelihood of spontaneous perforation). Surgical decompression is rarely required and is reserved for refractory patients at high risk for colonic perforation or for immunocompromised or neutropenic patients in whom colonic perforation would be catastrophic.

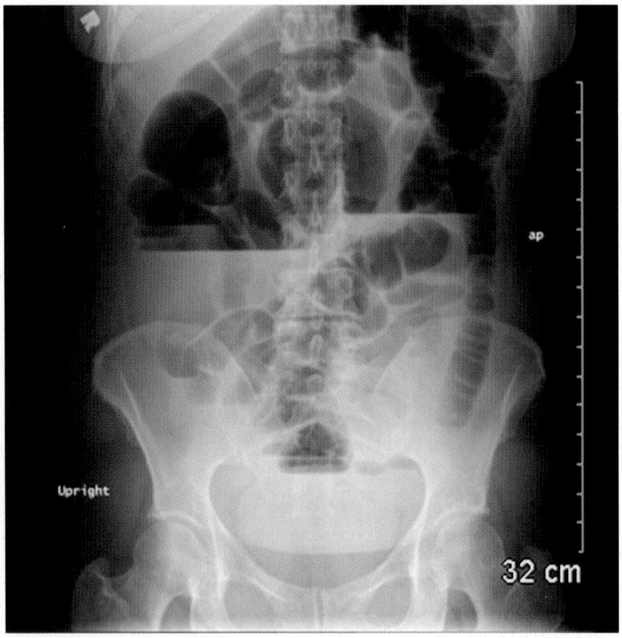

Gastrointestinal Stromal Tumors

Gastrointestinal stromal tumors (GISTs) are spindle cell tumors arising from the muscular layers of the stomach (75%), duodenum (12%), and small bowel (9%). As such, they have typical appearance on axial imaging (Fig. 47.27) and oftentimes no mucosal abnormality on endoscopic exam; a bulge is frequently the only endoscopic finding. GIST tumors can also infrequently arise from the esophagus and colorectum. Most GIST tumors stain positive for cKIT (80%), which is a defining characteristic. A smaller (5% to 7%) percentage of these tumors stain positive for platelet-derived growth factor receptor alpha, and the remainder are wild type.

Primary resection represents the mainstay of treatment for nonmetastatic GIST tumors isolated to a single organ. Prognosis after resection is based on size and mitotic rate. In general, primarily resected tumors less than 5 cm in size with fewer than 10 mitoses per high-power field have low risk of recurrence; they seldom require adjuvant chemotherapy with imatinib (Gleevec). Bulky, locally invasive (i.e., multiorgan) or metastatic tumors that cannot be completely resected are best treated preoperatively with imatinib to downstage, followed by resection if possible. High-risk and incompletely resected tumors should all be treated with imatinib in the adjuvant setting.

Inflammatory Bowel Disease

Crohn disease and ulcerative colitis represent distinct pathologic disease states easily confused by nonspecialists. Terminal ileitis is a catchall diagnosis for anything presenting as inflammation in the right lower quadrant. In the absence of malignancy or chemotherapy-induced neutropenia, terminal ileitis is a common manifestation of Crohn disease or, occasionally, of ulcerative colitis that spills into the terminal ileum. Even more confounding is the distinction of Crohn disease

FIGURE 47.26 Postoperative radiograph of a patient with Ogilvie syndrome demonstrating dilation of entire colon.

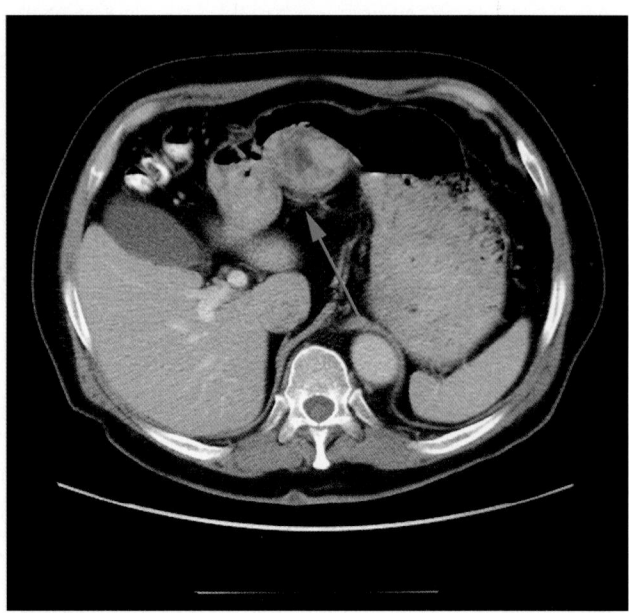

FIGURE 47.27 CT of GIST tumor.

from ulcerative colitis, resulting in the diagnosis of nonspecific colitis. Unfortunately, the cause of terminal ileitis can be a difficult diagnosis to establish based on gross or endoscopic findings, due to the relative inaccessibility of this portion of the GI tract. A skilled endoscopist may, however, reach the terminal ileum with the colonoscope to obtain tissue for histologic assessment.

The pathologic distinction between Crohn disease and ulcerative colitis requires integration of both the histologic and gross findings. Crohn disease manifests as a transmural process with epithelioid granulomas and fissuring ulcers, while ulcerative colitis is confined to the mucosa with crypt abscesses and absence of granulomas. Grossly, proper categorization of the acutely inflamed colon will aid in ultimately arriving at the correct histologic diagnosis and may aid intraoperative decision making. Crohn disease manifests with a skip lesion and fat creeping around the antimesenteric portions of the affected intestine (Fig. 47.28), while ulcerative colitis begins in the rectum and moves proximally in a continuous manner.

In the absence of obstruction, abscess, or nutritionally significant internal fistulae, Crohn disease is a medical illness that occurs primarily in adolescents and young adults. Ulcerative colitis is a surgical illness with significant malignant potential. While it is possible for ulcerative colitis to remain quiescent for prolonged periods of time, the chronic inflammatory state associated with it 10 years after initial diagnosis leads to malignant degeneration of the involved segments at a rate of 0.5% to 1% per year. Twenty percent of patients with ulcerative colitis eventually undergo surgical resection to manage symptoms and mitigate cancer risk.

Toxic megacolon, an extreme manifestation of ulcerative colitis, is defined by pancolonic distention, bleeding with associated leukocytosis, and constitutional symptoms. This is a life-threatening emergency that demands expeditious surgical intervention. When inflammatory bowel disease is suspected or encountered during otherwise routine gynecologic assessment or as an incidental intraoperative finding, long-term medical and surgical management is most appropriately undertaken by gastroenterologists or surgeons specializing in this area.

Hemorrhoids

Hemorrhoids are one of the most common diagnoses seen by general surgeons. External hemorrhoids occur outside of the

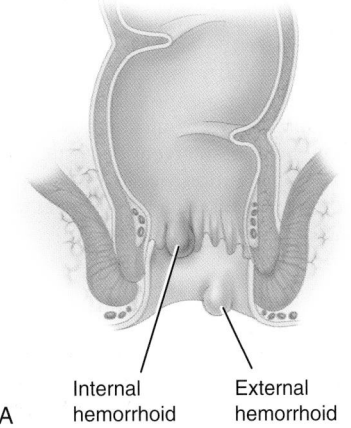
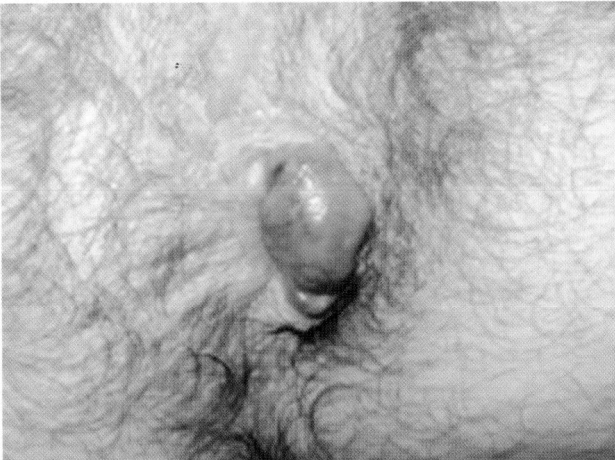

A   Internal hemorrhoid   External hemorrhoid

B

FIGURE 47.29 A: Types of internal hemorrhoids. **B:** Thrombosed hemorrhoid.

dentate (or pectinate) line, while internal hemorrhoids occur proximal to it. Internal hemorrhoids are further categorized as those that spontaneously reduce, those that reduce with digital aid, and those that are irreducible (Fig. 47.29A). In the absence of the latter subtype or extreme symptoms (e.g., pain, rupture, tenesmus), most hemorrhoids are managed medically. The mainstay of medical treatment is stool softeners and local anti-inflammatory agents.

Thrombosed hemorrhoids present with extreme pain, frequently bringing the patient to the emergency department (Fig. 47.29B). An acutely thrombosed hemorrhoid causing pain may be immediately relieved with incision and drainage. Unfortunately, this does not prevent recurrence, and whenever possible, hemorrhoidectomy is the preferred treatment. The ubiquity of hemorrhoid clinics in this country and the multitude of treatment options, including excisional, stapled, and ablative intervention, are a testament to the pervasive nature of this diagnosis and the absence of any one defined superior method of treatment.

PREOPERATIVE PREPARATION

Consent

When planning a major gynecologic operation, the likelihood of an intestinal resection and/or an ostomy can frequently be anticipated. Informed consent for this must be obtained from

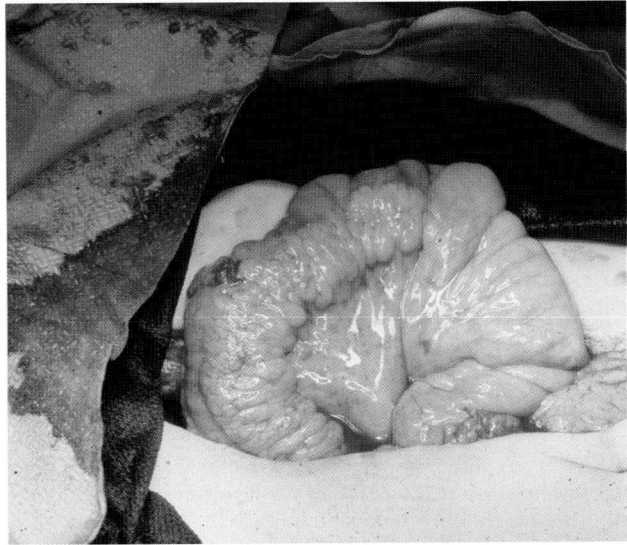

FIGURE 47.28 Crohn disease of the terminal ileum.

VIII

the patient, especially in regard to a potential or likely stoma. In the event that the patient adamantly refuses consent for a stoma, the physician must respect the patient's wishes but should make her aware of the possibility that this may compromise the benefits and goals of the operation. In situations where any otherwise-curative procedure would be precluded by a patient's refusal for stoma, surgical intervention should be avoided, as the benefit of such intervention would be negated by any residual cancer except in certain settings, such as carcinoid tumor or mucosal melanoma of the anorectum.

Planning for a Stoma

Any pelvic surgeon must develop the knowledge and judgment necessary to properly place intestinal stomas. A working knowledge of stomal management is also important. However, an enterostomal therapist is very helpful in the care of these patients.

Preoperatively, an enterostomal therapist can provide the patient with information and reassurance, better preparing her for a stoma postoperatively. The preoperative stoma therapy consult also serves to reinforce the inevitability of fecal diversion. The enterostomal therapist can also suggest optimal sites for stoma placement, though the surgeon must ultimately make this decision based on patient-specific and intraoperative factors.

The surgeon can anticipate, to some extent, the quadrant(s) of the abdomen where a stoma or stomas are likely to be placed. The abdomen is carefully inspected in the supine, sitting, and standing positions, with the surgeon noting the presence of any abdominal wall folds that could interfere with the application of the stomal appliance. Ideally, the stoma site is within the boundaries of the rectus muscle, with at least 3 inches of flat skin around the stoma and good visibility for the patient. A lower abdominal stoma (e.g., ileostomy or end sigmoid colostomy) is placed somewhere between the umbilicus and the anterior superior iliac spine, whereas an upper abdominal stoma is placed lateral to the umbilicus or somewhere between the umbilicus and the rib cage, as in a transverse colostomy (**Fig. 47.30**). The stoma must be kept far enough from bony prominences and the belt line to avoid interference with appliance application. Potential stomal sites are marked, and in the operating room prior to scrubbing the abdomen, the mark is preserved using a scratch or an intradermal injection of dye.

Nutrition

Preoperatively, it is important to assess the nutrition of a patient undergoing major surgery. The nutritional status of the majority of patients will be reasonably good. A few women will benefit from intensive preoperative nutritional support; many of these women can be identified during initial history, physical examinations. Examples of those likely to be severely malnourished at presentation include elderly patients, patients with advanced ovarian cancer, recent history of significant (>10%) weight loss, prolonged anorexia, generalized weakness and inanition, end-stage liver disease, and slowly developing bowel obstruction. Physical examination findings, including anthropometric measurements, laboratory values, and skin tests, are used to corroborate the presence of severe malnutrition.

The decision to intervene preoperatively with nutritional support is based on a number of factors. Mild to moderately malnourished patients are unlikely to benefit. When surgery is needed on an urgent basis, there will not be adequate time for meaningful preoperative nutritional support. Severely malnourished patients who are to undergo very extensive

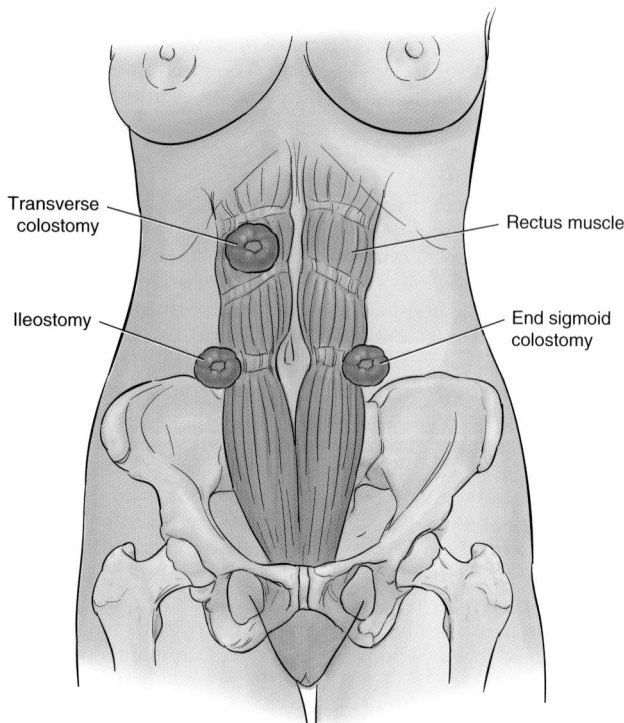

FIGURE 47.30 Placement of intestinal stomas in the abdominal wall.

surgery or are elderly are more likely to benefit from this support. The major complication rate of patients undergoing intestinal surgery may be reduced by intensive preoperative nutritional support.

When the decision is made to administer preoperative nutritional support, the surgeon must individualize the use of enteral and parenteral routes. A period of 7 to 14 days of hyperalimentation has been recommended as the time frame necessary to provide optimal benefit. Nutritional support is continued postoperatively for an appropriate period of time. Hospitalized patients with malignant bowel obstruction will benefit most from TPN, while malnourished patients with normal GI function should be replenished with nasogastric or nasoduodenal supplements that can be administered in the outpatient setting. Nasogastric supplementation has the advantage of bolus feeding every 4 to 6 hours and does not require a feeding pump. Nasoduodenal feeding minimizes the risk of aspiration, especially in patients with delayed gastric emptying, but requires more home resources.

Bowel preparation

Routine use of mechanical bowel preparation (MBP) for colonic resection has become a matter of controversy in recent years. This is due to the paucity of data that support reduced postoperative complications, from rare but significant complications associated with MBP and from overall patient discomfort with the procedure. A recently published review of 14 randomized controlled trials and 8 meta-analyses analyzing the efficacy of MBP in patients undergoing elective colorectal surgery showed no difference in postoperative infectious complication rates. The utility of MBP in low anterior resection is neither supported nor refuted by this review, and its use in this setting is at the discretion of the operating surgeon. Other studies, though, show that combining MBP with oral antibiotics does reduce risk of postoperative complications.

A recent review of the Veterans Affairs Surgical Quality Improvement program comprising 9,940 patients undergoing elective colectomy—while showing no difference in SSI in patients receiving MBP only versus no preparation—did demonstrate a 67% decrease in SSI for patients receiving oral antibiotics alone. A 57% decrease in SSI was noted in patients receiving oral antibiotics and MBP. The authors conclude that the data strongly support the use of preoperative oral antibiotics, while the benefits of antibiotic administration in conjunction with MBP remain uncertain.

Preoperatively, the likelihood of intestinal colonic surgery and subsequent necessity of bowel preparation must be assessed. Proper bowel preparation will reduce the risk of fecal spillage into the peritoneal cavity, infectious morbidity, anastomotic leak rate, and the need for colostomy. Bowel preparation has two components, mechanical and antibiotic. Mechanical preparation is aimed at clearing the majority of fecal material. Antibiotic prophylaxis is used to protect surgical sites from colonic flora.

Currently, there are two alternative methods of MBP: whole gut lavage and the traditional multiday cathartics and enemas. The traditional method generally takes about 3 days, during which the diet is restricted to clear liquids, and the patient ingests multiple doses of a cathartic, such as magnesium citrate. The diet may be supplemented with elemental nutrients to help maintain the patient's nutritional status. Toward the latter half of this regimen, several rounds of enemas are given.

The whole gut lavage method is done the day before surgery with a commercially available preparation of polyethylene glycol and a balanced electrolyte solution. Ranges of 1 to 4 L/hour have been recommended for lavage to extend over a 3- to 4-hour period. If the lavage cannot be tolerated orally, it may be administered via a nasogastric tube. Metoclopramide has been recommended by some to improve the tolerance and passage of the lavage.

The advantages of the lavage method are minimal alterations in fluid and electrolyte balance (it is nonosmotic), maintenance of weight and nutrition, simplicity, and the convenience of 1-day administration. The disadvantages are intolerance and/or the requirement of a nasogastric tube in some patients. The lavage method should not be used in patients who may have a bowel obstruction. In patients with partial obstruction of the colon or rectum, as is often encountered with advanced ovarian cancer, a 3-day cathartic-enema mechanical preparation or slow lavage is more appropriate. Studies comparing the 3-day cathartic-enema and whole gut lavage methods have demonstrated similar efficacy.

Antibiotic prophylaxis for colonic surgery consists of intravenous administration of antibiotics effective against the gram-negative (i.e., *Escherichia coli*) and anaerobic (i.e., *Bacteroides fragilis*) colonic bacteria, such as *Klebsiella* and *Enterococcus*. The effect of these antibiotics on the colonic bacterial flora is probably negligible, their aim being to provide antibiotic concentrations in blood and tissue to deal with fecal spillage.

Bowel Obstruction

Preoperative preparation of the patient with bowel obstruction begins with optimization of fluid and electrolyte balance and with gastrointestinal decompression. A nasogastric tube is placed and connected to low, intermittent suction, and the likelihood of ischemia or necrosis of the bowel wall is assessed. As previously discussed, bowel obstruction in gynecologic cancer patients tends to occur in the context of certain clinical scenarios. Some patients will be candidates for aggressive surgical management as deemed necessary (i.e., adhesion-related), while others will not (i.e., advanced recurrent intra-abdominal malignancy). When a patient has a small bowel obstruction thought to be amenable to surgical management and when there is evidence of compromise of the bowel, surgery proceeds promptly after initial correction of hypovolemia. Broad-spectrum antibiotics should also be initiated in these patients. However, most gynecologic cancer patients who develop small bowel obstruction will not require prompt surgical intervention, and many patients deserve an attempt at conservative management in the hope that the obstruction will resolve.

In addition to hydration and nasogastric suction, passage of a long intestinal tube into the small bowel may be beneficial. After passing into the jejunum, the tube is connected to low intermittent suction and allowed to continue to pass, hopefully to the point of the obstruction. The long tube will decompress the small bowel more effectively, which may improve the chances for the obstruction to resolve and will improve the condition of the proximal small bowel, should surgery be necessary. TPN may also be advisable on an individualized basis. After initial stabilization, radiologic studies should be performed to evaluate the possibility of coexisting large bowel obstruction. With large bowel obstruction, surgical intervention will be necessary.

During the period of conservative management, if the patient develops any signs of compromised bowel, surgery must proceed. If, however, the patient remains stable and the bowel decompresses well, there is no urgency in the situation. The patient can be maintained on TPN while allowing 5 to 10 days for the condition of the bowel to improve and a chance for the obstruction to resolve. If the bowel does not decompress by 48 to 72 hours, then surgery should proceed.

OPERATIVE TECHNIQUES

This section deals with descriptions of actual surgical techniques. It is not meant to be an exhaustive review of methods or techniques, but rather is designed to convey basic principles and techniques commonly used in the management of the intestinal tract as it relates to gynecologic patients.

Gastrostomy Tube Placement

For palliation, a gastrostomy tube can most often be placed percutaneously with either fluoroscopic or gastroscopic guidance. If the procedure is an isolated open one, the operation may be performed through an upper midline, or through a left subcostal or transverse epigastric incision that incorporates the tube. When there is extensive bulky intra-abdominal carcinomatosis, the surgeon should attempt to make the incision over a relatively free space in the region of the stomach.

To gain exposure, the inferior border of the stomach is grasped with Babcock clamps (avoiding injury to the gastroepiploic vessels), and with gentle traction the fundus is brought into the operative field. A site for the gastrostomy is selected in the distal fundus midway between the two curvatures and is grasped with another Babcock clamp. A purse-string suture of 0 chromic catgut is placed around the clamp and held (**Fig. 47.31A**). If there is carcinomatosis, inflammatory reaction of the peritoneal surfaces, or other concerns about healing, silk sutures should be used. A second purse-string suture is used at this point or after the tube is in place, designed to imbricate the gastrostomy. A 28-French Malecot catheter or 24-French MIC tube is brought through a separate stab wound in the abdominal wall at a selected site several centimeters from the incision (**Fig. 47.31B**). The stomach should easily reach the abdominal wall at the chosen site.

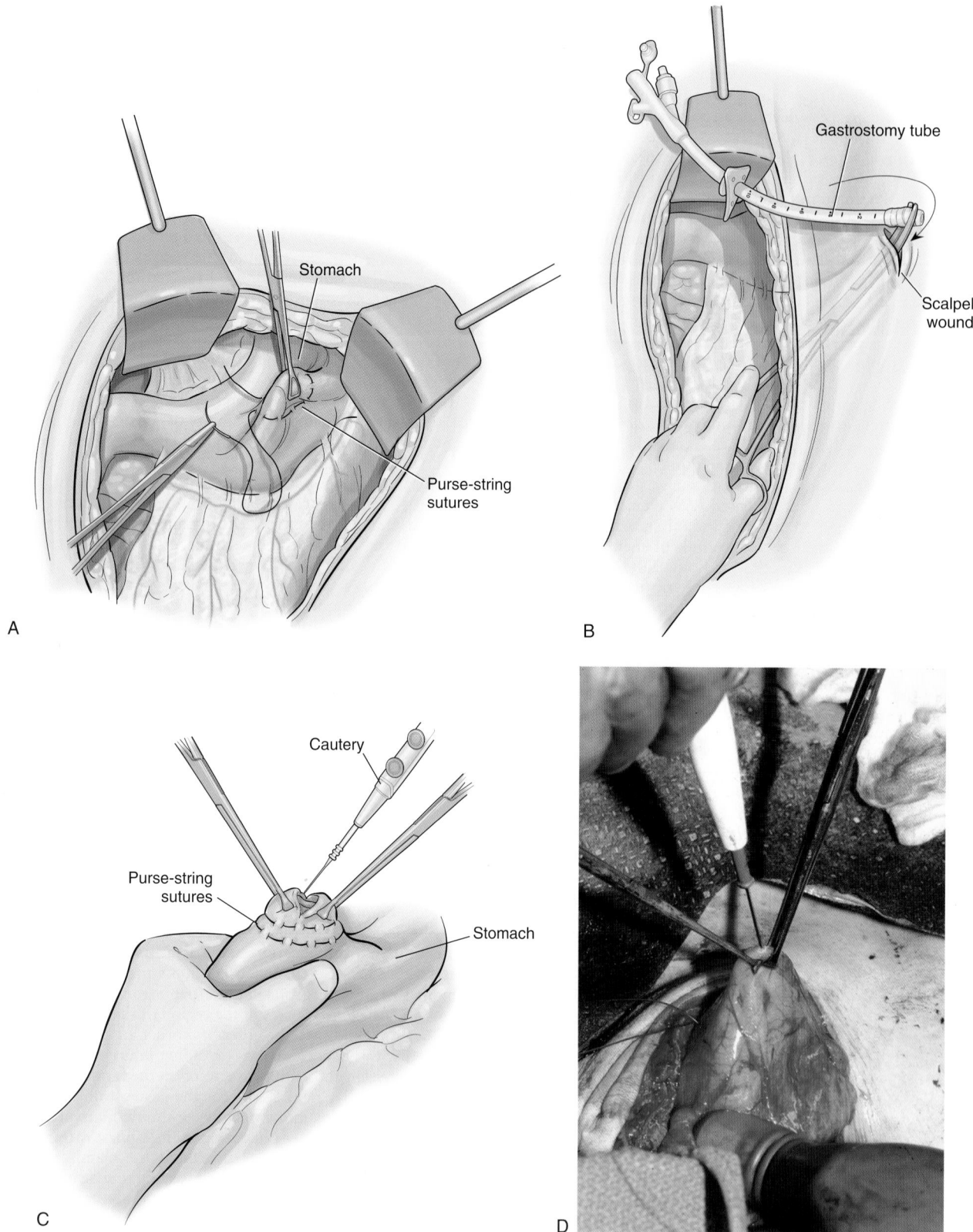

FIGURE 47.31 **A:** Purse-string suture being placed into stomach wall around selected site for gastrostomy. **B:** Gastrostomy tube being pulled through abdominal wall incision at selected skin site. **C and D:** Small opening being made in stomach within purse-string sutures.

Within the purse-string suture, the gastrostomy is carefully made with cautery between two Allis clamps and the tube is placed into the stomach, directed distally (Fig. 47.31C, D). The balloon (MIC tube) is inflated and the inner purse-string suture is tied. The second purse-string suture is tied while carefully manipulating the tube and stomach to allow imbrication of the first purse-string suture and the folding of a short segment of the stomach wall around the tube. This is done to reduce the risk of leakage of gastric contents.

The stomach is then secured to the anterior abdominal wall with interrupted 2-0 silk sutures placed around the gastrostomy site. These are tied while traction is applied to the tube, which draws the balloon against the abdominal wall. The tube is secured to the skin with sutures through the MIC apparatus. The tube is irrigated with saline and aspirated of gastric contents to confirm position and patency.

Bowel Resection

This operation begins with careful planning for the resection and anastomosis, followed by mobilization of the involved portion or portions of the bowel. The bowel portions to be anastomosed must be healthy, have adequate blood supply, and approximate one another without tension.

The blood supply of the small bowel is based on the SMASMA, with branches extending through a widely fanned out mesentery. In the mesentery, the arterial branches form anastomosing primary and secondary arcades, with the terminal arcades supplying small parallel vessels (vasa recta) that extend to the bowel. Resection of a segment of small bowel must preserve an adequate arterial arcade, including the vasa recta, to supply the remaining divided ends of bowel. Small bowel resection in gynecologic cancer patients generally does not necessitate associated wide resection of the mesentery. Accordingly, resection of the mesentery should be as conservative as possible.

Following mobilization of the bowel, the remainder of the operative field is carefully isolated from contamination with moist packs. At the points of planned bowel division, a hemostat is placed through an avascular area of the mesentery immediately under the bowel wall. Along the planned mesenteric resection, the peritoneum on both sides is divided. The mesentery is then hemostatically divided. A linear gastrointestinal stapler or noncrushing bowel clamps are placed across the bowel, directed toward the mesentery, and slightly angulated to give a mesenteric advantage. The angulation avoids an ischemic corner of bowel and creates a slightly larger EEA. The bowel is divided by the GIA stapler or between bowel clamps (Fig. 47.32).

Colon resection is carried out utilizing similar principles. Depending on the segment, mobilization of the colon involves incision of the peritoneal attachments laterally and caudally, separation from the omentum, and division of the hepatic and/or splenic flexures (Fig. 47.33A, B). As previously described, the blood supply of the colon is derived from branches of the superior and inferior mesenteric arteries. These branches feed an anastomosing marginal artery, which extends from the ileocecal valve to the sigmoid colon (Figs. 47.3 and 47.4). From the marginal artery, vasa recta extend to the colon. With resection of the colon, the marginal artery and vasa recta supplying the two remaining ends must be preserved. As with small bowel resection, wide resection of the mesentery with the colon is generally not necessary in gynecologic cancer patients. The exception is rectosigmoid colon, the mesentery of which is often extensively infiltrated in cases of ovarian cancer. In resection for primary colonic malignancy, the rule of thumb is to extend the mesenteric resection to the first-named vessel proximal and distal to the site of pathology.

Rectosigmoidectomy in the context of extensive gynecologic disease is more difficult. It is one of the more common segments of the bowel that the gynecologic oncologist must resect. Removal of this portion of the bowel in gynecologic cancer patients is sometimes done as an isolated procedure (e.g., because of complications from radiation therapy) but is more often done in concert with an extensive pelvic resection for tumor. In most instances, the majority of the rectum

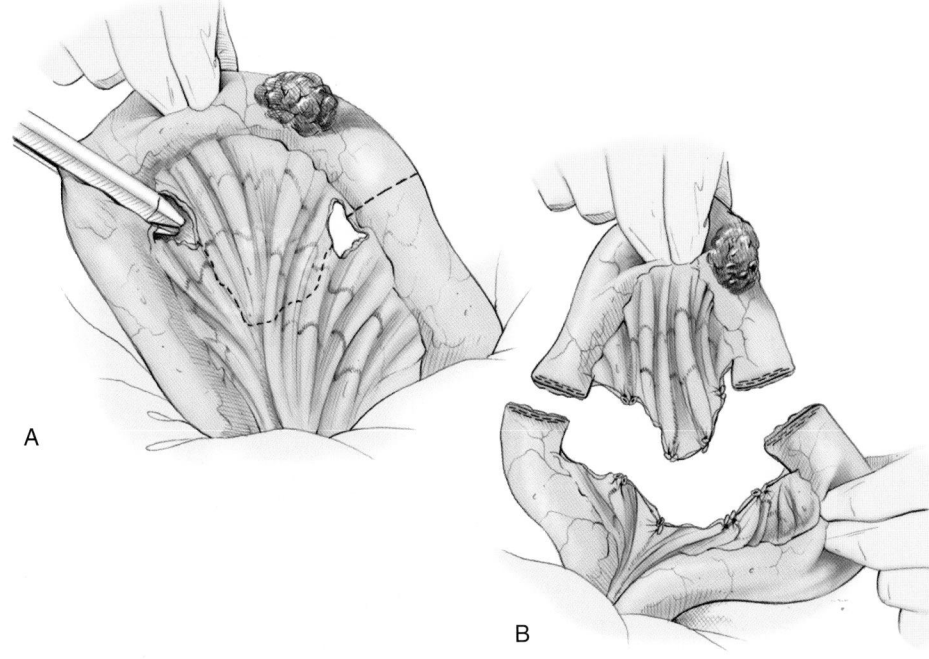

A

B

FIGURE 47.32 Planned resection of small bowel, dividing intestine with a gastrointestinal stapler (**A, B**).

VIII

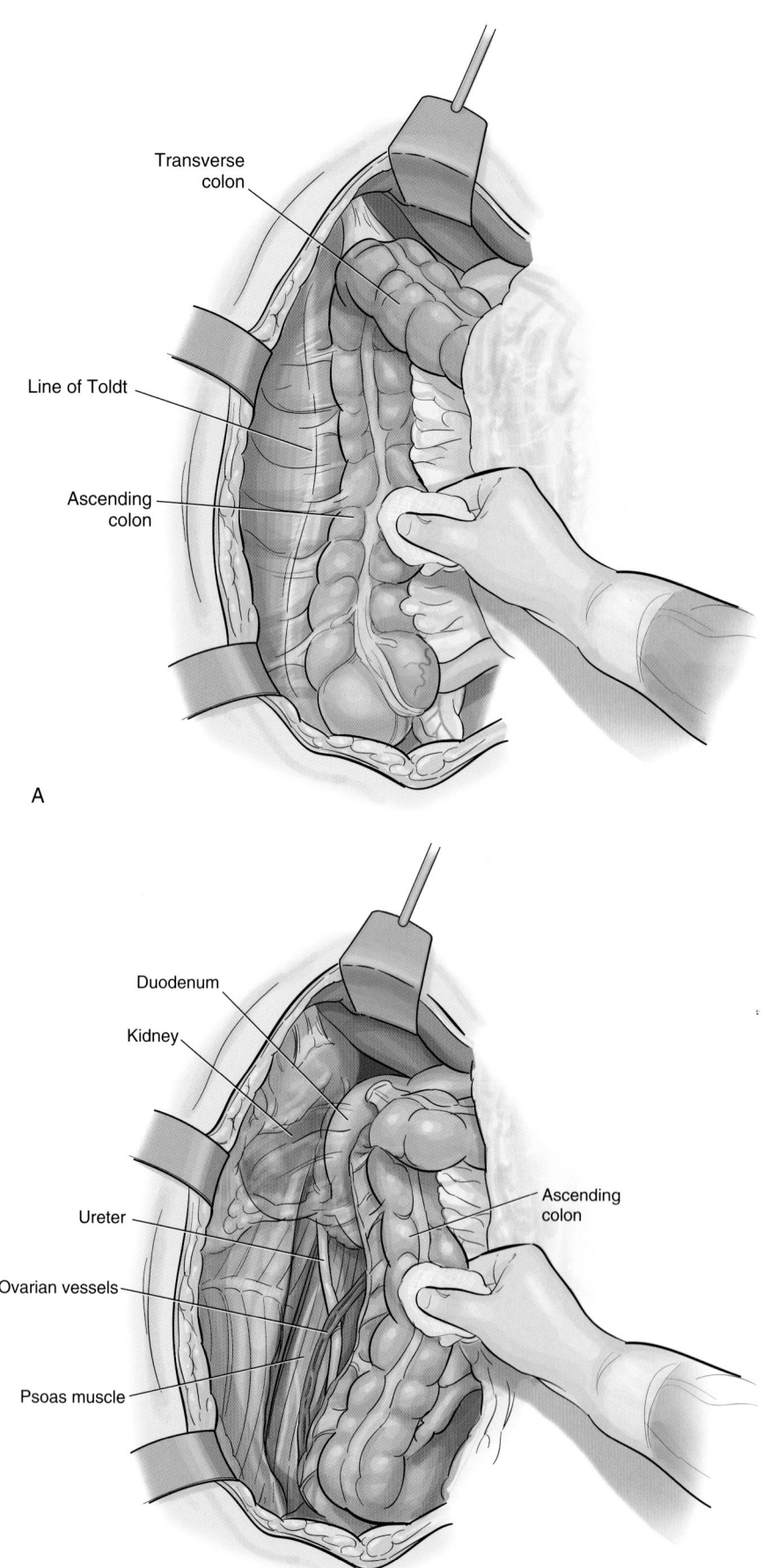

A

B

FIGURE 47.33 A: Division of the hepatic flexure. **B:** Together with division of the lateral peritoneal, retroperitoneal (duodenum), and omental attachments, this mobilizes the right and proximal transverse colon.

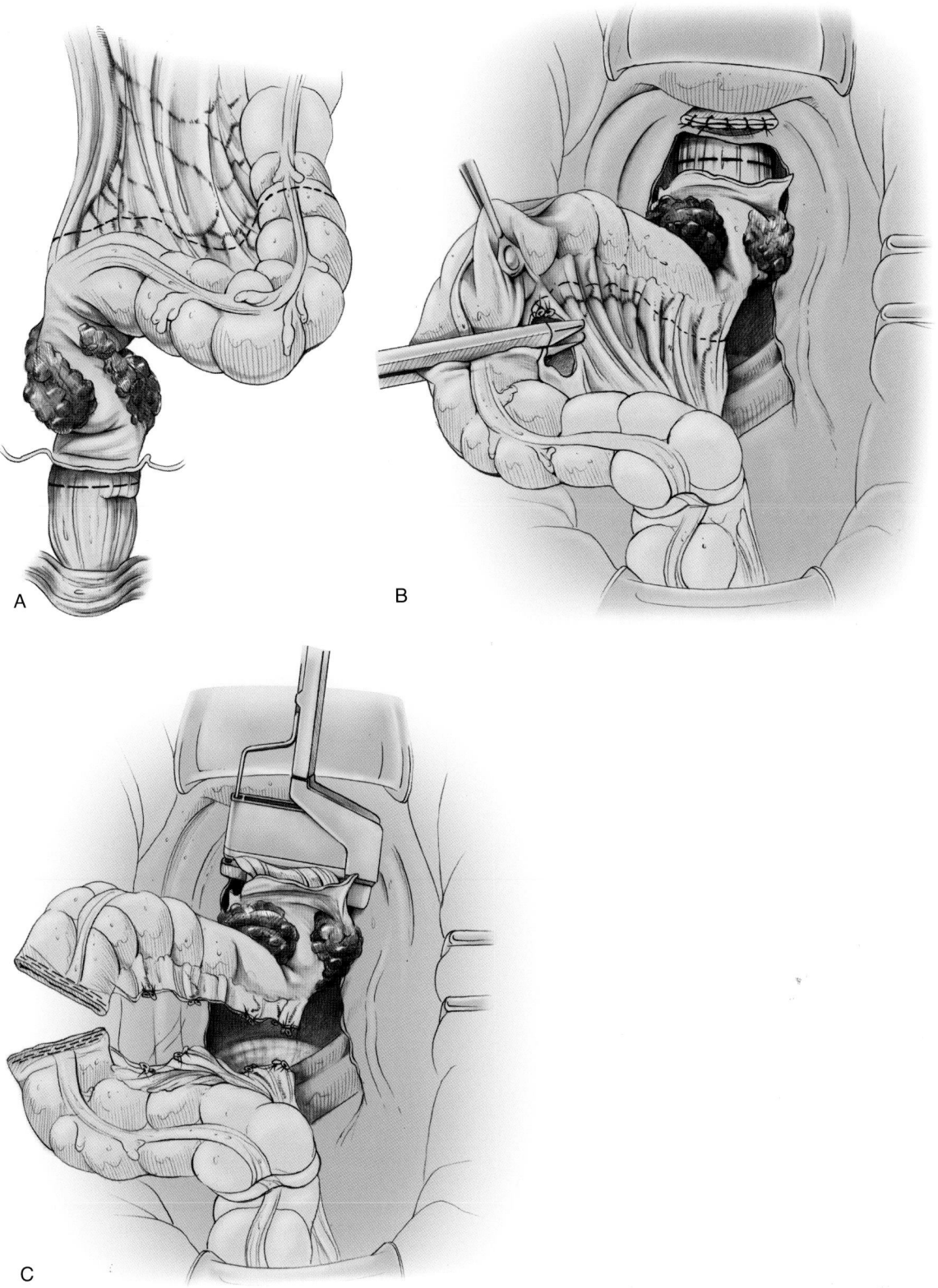

FIGURE 47.34 A and **B:** Division of the sigmoid colon cephalad to the tumor as one of the preliminary steps to extensive pelvic resection. The line of pelvic peritoneal incision is dictated by tumor extent. All of the pelvic peritoneum extending across the infundibulopelvic ligaments and the posterior cul-de-sac is resected en bloc with the rectosigmoid colon (**C**). In some cases, all of the pelvic peritoneum must be removed, requiring additional dissection of the lower urinary tract.

VIII

may be preserved and an immediate anastomosis carried out. In other situations, the nature of the disease process or other factors prohibits an anastomosis and a permanent colostomy is performed. Finally, some cases—usually by virtue of tumor extent—require resection of the entire rectum and anus.

As mentioned previously, the blood supply to the sigmoid colon and upper rectum is based on the IMA that branches through the sigmoid mesentery. The remainder of the anorectum receives blood through the internal iliac artery. The midrectum receives blood by the middle hemorrhoidal artery; the blood reaches the rectum in an anterior–lateral fashion and through the lateral rectal stalks, which are also the major support structures of the rectum to the levator ani. These stalks must be ligated to achieve mobilization of the midrectum. The region of the rectosigmoid junction was previously thought to

have a rather tenuous blood supply. However, arteriographic studies have documented rich collateral circulation with anastomoses between the middle and superior rectal arteries, and modern surgical experience with this region bears that out.

Resection of the rectosigmoid colon generally begins with division of the sigmoid colon at a selected site, followed by complete division of the sigmoid colon mesentery cephalad to the tumor infiltration (**Fig. 47.34A, B**). At the base of the mesentery is the superior rectal artery; this is also ligated. It is important to safely retract the ureters prior to this. During mobilization of the specimen, the pararectal spaces should be opened carefully—but widely—down to the levator muscles. Further mobilization is achieved by incision of the posterior pelvic peritoneum from the points of the completed mesenteric dissection anteriorly to meet the remainder of the

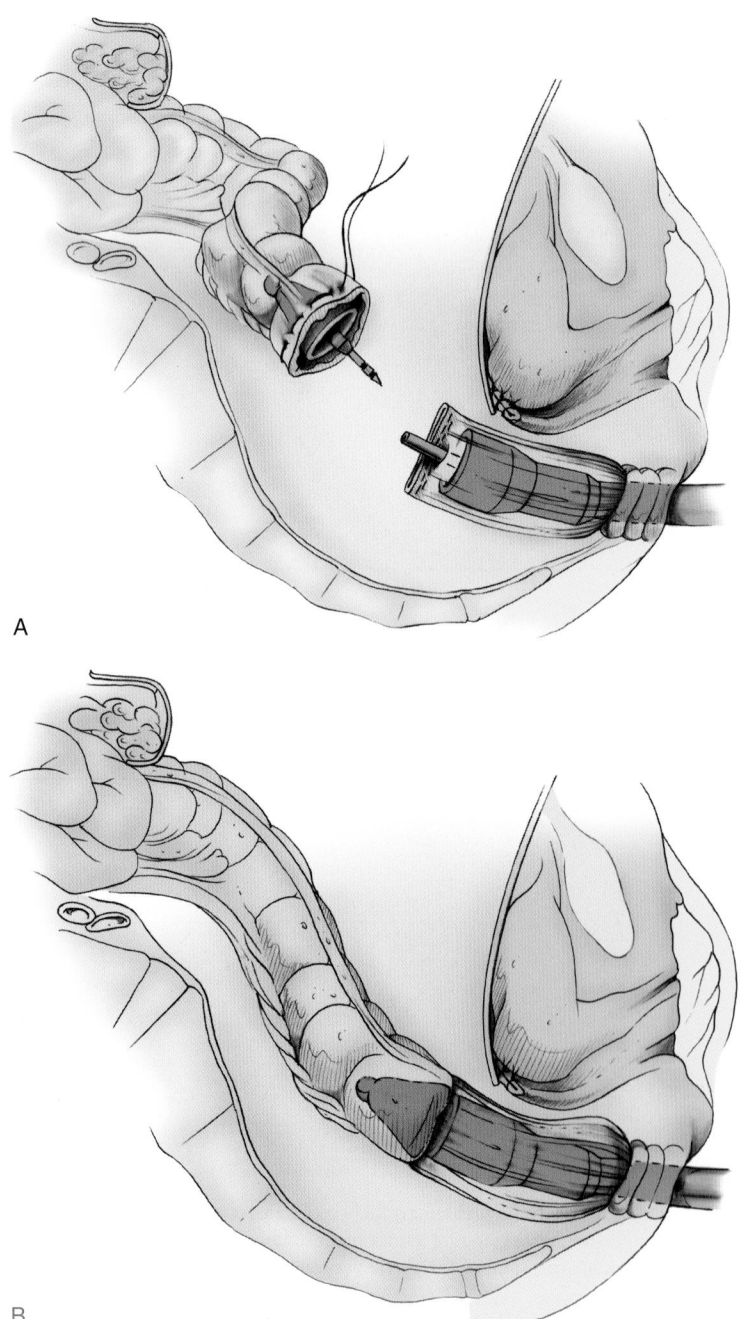

A

B

FIGURE 47.35 End-to-end rectosigmoid staple anastomosis. **A:** A purse-string suture holds the anvil and spike within the sigmoid lumen. The EEA stapler is inserted transanally. Clockwise rotation of the central wing nut advances the sharp trocar to pierce the apex of the rectal stump. In this illustration, the trocar has been removed, and the hollow center shaft of the EEA remains in place. **B:** The spike and hollow center shaft are locked into position. Further rotation of the EEA central wing nut brings the sigmoid and rectum into direct opposition. The stapler is fired to deliver dual circular staple rows as the knife transects the central tissue core to complete the anastomosis.

pelvic dissection (often dictated by peritoneal tumor extent). The rectum is carefully freed from the presacral space all the way to the levator muscles if necessary. Depending on the additional pelvic resections being performed (e.g., hysterectomy, exenteration, etc.), the rectovaginal space may be developed and additional vascular/supportive structures will need to be divided.

When the distal aspect of the dissection has been reached, the pelvic specimen is mobilized such that the only remaining attachment is the rectum. This portion of the rectum should be mobilized for anastomosis prior to resection if possible. At the planned level of transection, the fat around the rectum is cleaned. A stapler, automatic purse-stringer or right-angled bowel clamp is placed across the rectum at this level, and transection is completed against the instrument. Immediately following resection, it is our habit to irrigate the pelvis with antibiotic solution, particularly if any stool has spilled. Transanal irrigation of the rectal stump is done at this time.

Colorectal Anastomosis with a Circular Stapler

Anastomosis of the colon to the rectum is difficult, due to the rectum being recessed within the pelvic cavity, particularly when the remaining rectal stump is short. Anastomosis is greatly facilitated by a circular stapler. If the rectum was transected with a stapler, the only additional preparation is to clear the fat from the area where the anastomosis will take place.

During surgery, the colon should be mobilized so that the end will reach the rectum without tension. Excessive mobilization from the mesentery will compromise the blood supply. By transilluminating the sigmoid mesentery, the surgeon may see that proximal portions may be divided while still leaving adequate blood supply to the end of the colon. Incising the lateral peritoneal, avascular retroperitoneal, and splenic flexure attachments will achieve additional mobility. Infrequently, the IMA must be divided. The end of the colon is opened and irrigated if necessary. It is the authors' habit to irrigate the rectal stump transanally.

Sizers are then used to determine which stapler is appropriate. The largest stapler that the colon will comfortably accommodate should be used in order to avoid anastomotic stenosis. A size 28 or 31 instrument can be used in most instances. A purse-string suture with 2-0 monofilament is placed along the edge of the proximal colon. The separated anvil of the stapler is placed into the open end of the colon, and the purse-string is secured around the shaft. The stapler (with completely withdrawn trocar) is then introduced transanally. Directed into the proper position by the abdominal and perineal surgeons working together, the trocar is advanced through the rectal staple line; a small incision may be made into the middle of the staple line to facilitate this. The anvil shafts are then connected (**Fig. 47.35A, B**).

The stapler is closed while applying gentle, inward pressure to ensure that the colon stays aligned and does not fall into the stapling device. The instrument is fired, creating an inverted circular anastomosis with staggered rows of metal staples, while simultaneously cutting from the staple line the portions of the two bowel ends within the instrument. While the instrument is still in place, it can be used for careful manipulation in order to place seromuscular imbricating sutures or other sutures designed to protect the suture line. These sutures should not be tied until after the instrument is removed and the anastomosis tested.

The stapler is then opened and removed transanally again with gentle inward pressure to allow complete separation of the anvil from the staple line. Allis clamps or sutures are used to facilitate retrieval of the instrument past the anastomosis.

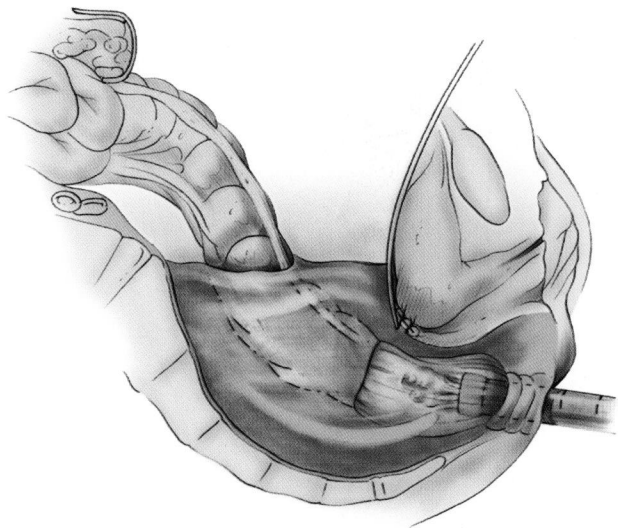

FIGURE 47.36 Testing the anastomotic integrity. The pelvis is filled with sterile crystalloid. The descending colon is manually occluded as air is insufflated via a rigid sigmoidoscope to create pressure across the anastomosis. Holding the anastomosis under water, it is examined for the air bubbles that would suggest an anastomotic leak.

The instrument is completely opened and separated, and the two pieces of removed tissue are inspected. There should be two complete mucosal rings. The pelvis is then irrigated with antibiotic solution; a small amount of antibiotic is left in the pelvis just over the top of the anastomosis. The rectum is then filled with air, and the anastomosis is inspected for leaks (i.e., bubble test) (**Fig. 47.36**). Any leak is closed with suture.

Endoscopic inspection of the anastomosis for hemostasis is also recommended by some authors. If omentum is available, it is transposed into the pelvis and wrapped completely around the anastomosis. The role of prophylactic drains in these patients is unclear.

If the colorectal anastomosis will be low (within 6 to 8 cm from the anal verge), consideration should be given to replacement of the rectal reservoir with a colonic J-pouch (**Fig. 47.37**).

Open Hand-Sewn Anastomosis

The technique illustrated in **Figure 47.38** is an EEA. However, this circular technique is easily adaptable to an end-to-side or side-to-side anastomosis. The technique used is identical for the large and small bowel. Some surgeons, particularly in the past, have preferred a closed technique of anastomosis to reduce contamination by bowel contents. This technique is done by first aligning the two bowel ends being held by noncrushing clamps and then placing interrupted anastomosing seromuscular sutures across the clamps. The sutures are pulled tight as the clamps are removed and then immediately tied. This technique is considered by some to be cumbersome and less accurate than the open or stapled anastomosis.

To begin the anastomosis, the ends of the bowel are approximated and aligned by an assistant. Using 3-0 silk (or delayed absorbable suture) Lembert sutures, a row of seromuscular stitches placed 3 to 4 mm apart and 4 to 5 mm from the edges of the bowel are placed to create a back row. If bowel clamps were used, these are left in place and used for alignment and manipulation during placement of this back row. If staples were used, these are also initially left in place. The first and last back row stitches are held long with hemostats for purposes of orientation and alignment.

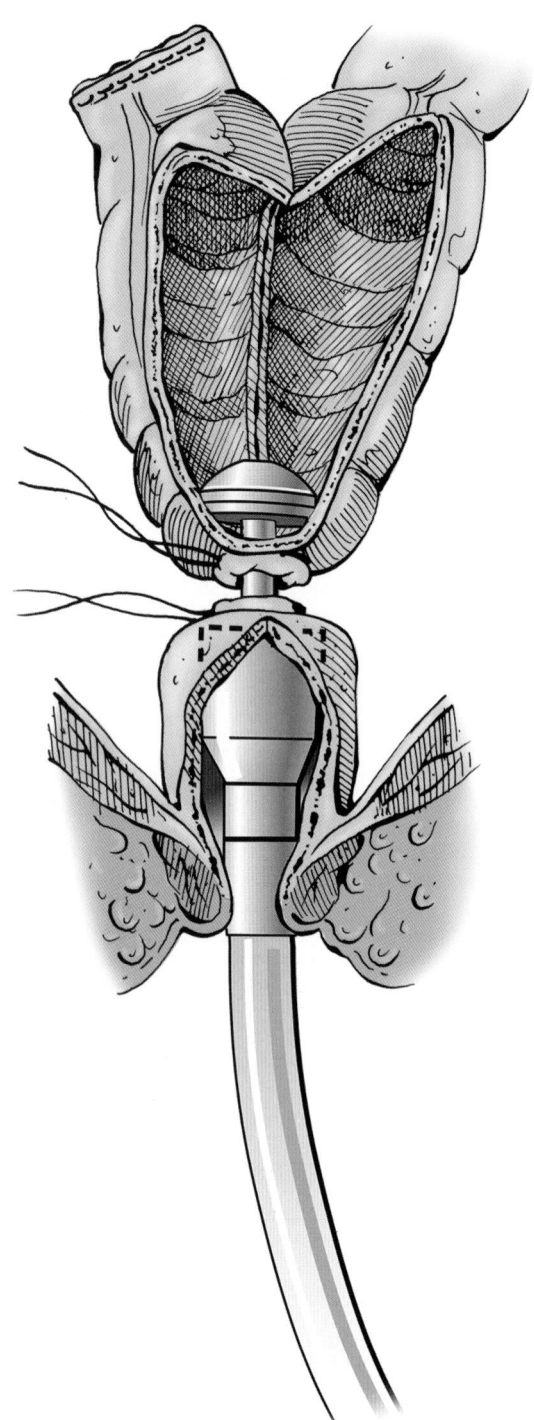

FIGURE 47.37 Rectal J-pouch coloproctostomy.

Padded or rubber-shod bowel clamps are placed several inches from the bowel ends in order to occlude the lumens and thereby prevent spillage of bowel contents. The clamps on the bowel ends are then removed, or the staple lines are excised, and the open portions of the bowel are emptied. The bowel walls approximated by the posterior row of seromuscular sutures will also have been inverted by these sutures.

Using 3-0 chromic or delayed absorbable monofilament suture, the full thickness of the two inverted bowel walls are sutured together to form an inner layer (Fig. 47.38A–C). The sutures should be about 3 mm apart using a running or interrupted technique. If a running technique is used, sutures should be placed slightly closer than 3 mm apart to help prevent stenosis.

The anastomosis proceeds by continuing the inner layer until it is completed. As the inner suture line continues beyond the inverted posterior row, it is desirable to continue to invert the bowel edges into the lumen, while at the same time suturing through all layers. With a running technique, this is best accomplished using Connell stitches. Using an interrupted technique, the edges may be inverted by taking a slightly larger bite of the bowel wall relative to a small bite of mucosa. The outer layer of interrupted Lembert sutures is then completed (Fig. 47.38D, E); a carefully performed single layer is acceptable as well. The occluding bowel clamps are then removed and the anastomosis palpated for adequacy. Finally, the mesenteric defect is carefully closed, avoiding injury or ligation of blood vessels. A hand-sewn side-to-side anastomosis is shown in Figure 47.39A, B.

Anastomosis with a Linear Stapler

Stapled bowel anastomoses are comparable to that of hand-sewn anastomosis with regard to leak and anastomotic stricture rate. Advantages include reduced operative time and relative simplicity. Disadvantages include cost, requirement of a more mobilized bowel, and a theoretically higher potential for stricture. The technique illustrated in Figure 47.40 is a functional EEA. As with the hand-sewn method, this technique is easily adaptable to end-to-side and side-to-side anastomoses. The stapler simultaneously places two rows of staggered staples side by side and cuts between them.

To begin the anastomosis, the two ends of bowel are aligned in a side-to-side fashion. Along the borders of the mesenteries, the bowel walls are aligned with interrupted 3-0 silk seromuscular sutures for a length of approximately 6 to 10 cm. The suture at the end of the bowel is held with a hemostat for the purpose of orientation.

As before, occluding clamps are placed to reduce contamination. If the resection was done with staplers, antimesenteric corners of the staple lines should be excised to accommodate the forks of the stapler (Fig. 47.40A). One fork is inserted fully into each lumen; care must be taken to ensure that the bowel ends are aligned evenly and that their mesenteries are clear (Fig. 47.40B, C). The instrument is then carefully closed and fired, creating an anastomosis. Before opening the instrument, a few seromuscular stitches may be placed to imbricate and take tension off of the anterior row of staples. The stapler is then opened in situ, and prior to removal the staple line is carefully inspected for bleeding (Fig. 47.40D). Bleeding sites may be sutured or carefully cauterized. The remaining common opening is then closed with sutures or a stapler (Fig. 47.40E, F). The additional staple line may also be imbricated with Lembert sutures. The occluding bowel clumps are removed, and the anastomosis is palpated for adequacy. A side-to-side anastomosis is performed in a similar manner.

Ileostomy

Depending on the situation, an ileostomy may be formed from the end of the transected functional ileum (end ileostomy) or from a loop of ileum. The main role of a loop ileostomy is temporary diversion. If an isolated procedure, an ileostomy can sometimes be done through a small right lower quadrant incision or with laparoscopy.

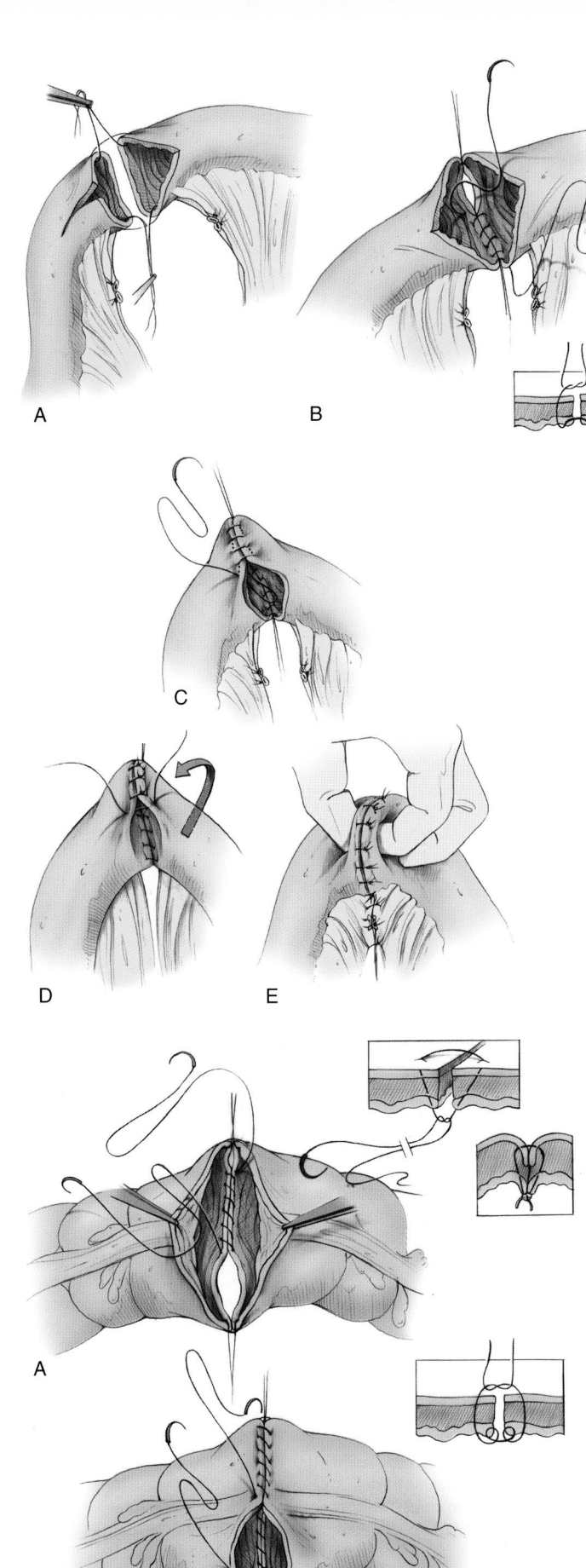

FIGURE 47.38 End-to-end hand-seven double-layer small bowel anastomosis. **A:** The bowel segments are aligned end to end and secured by stay sutures placed midway between the mesenteric and antimesenteric borders. Each luminal diameter is increased via a linear incision along the antimesenteric border (Cheatle slit). **B:** The inner running layer is started on the mesenteric (posterior) bowel edges. A double-arm needle facilitates bidirectional sewing as the closure continues around the corners onto the antimesenteric (anterior) edges. **Inset:** Conventional inner layer inverting technique. **C:** The anterior inner layer is completed with a continuous over-and-over or Connell suture (as shown). **D:** The bowel is rotated 180 degrees to expose the posterior wall. Interrupted seromuscular 3-0 silk sutures are placed to finish the posterior outer layer. **E:** The bowel is rotated back into its normal alignment, and the anterior outer layer is closed with interrupted silk sutures. The mesenteric defect is reapproximated, and the adequacy of the lumen is assessed.

FIGURE 47.39 End-to-end hand-sewn single-layer colon anastomosis. **A:** The bowel edges are brought together, and their alignment is stabilized with stay sutures. Sewing is started on the mucosal surfaces of the posterior bowel edges. A double-arm suture enables bidirectional sewing in a continuous fashion. **Insets:** The needle enters near the transected mucosal edge and passes obliquely through the bowel wall to exit 5 mm from the serosal edge. The needle is passed through the adjoining segment in the same oblique fashion, which inverts the tissue edges as the running suture is secured. **B:** Suturing is continued around the corners onto the anterior edges, which are closed from the serosal side. **Inset:** Alternative method of single-layer closure known as the Gambee technique, which results in end-to-end opposition of the tissue edges without puckering the mucosa.

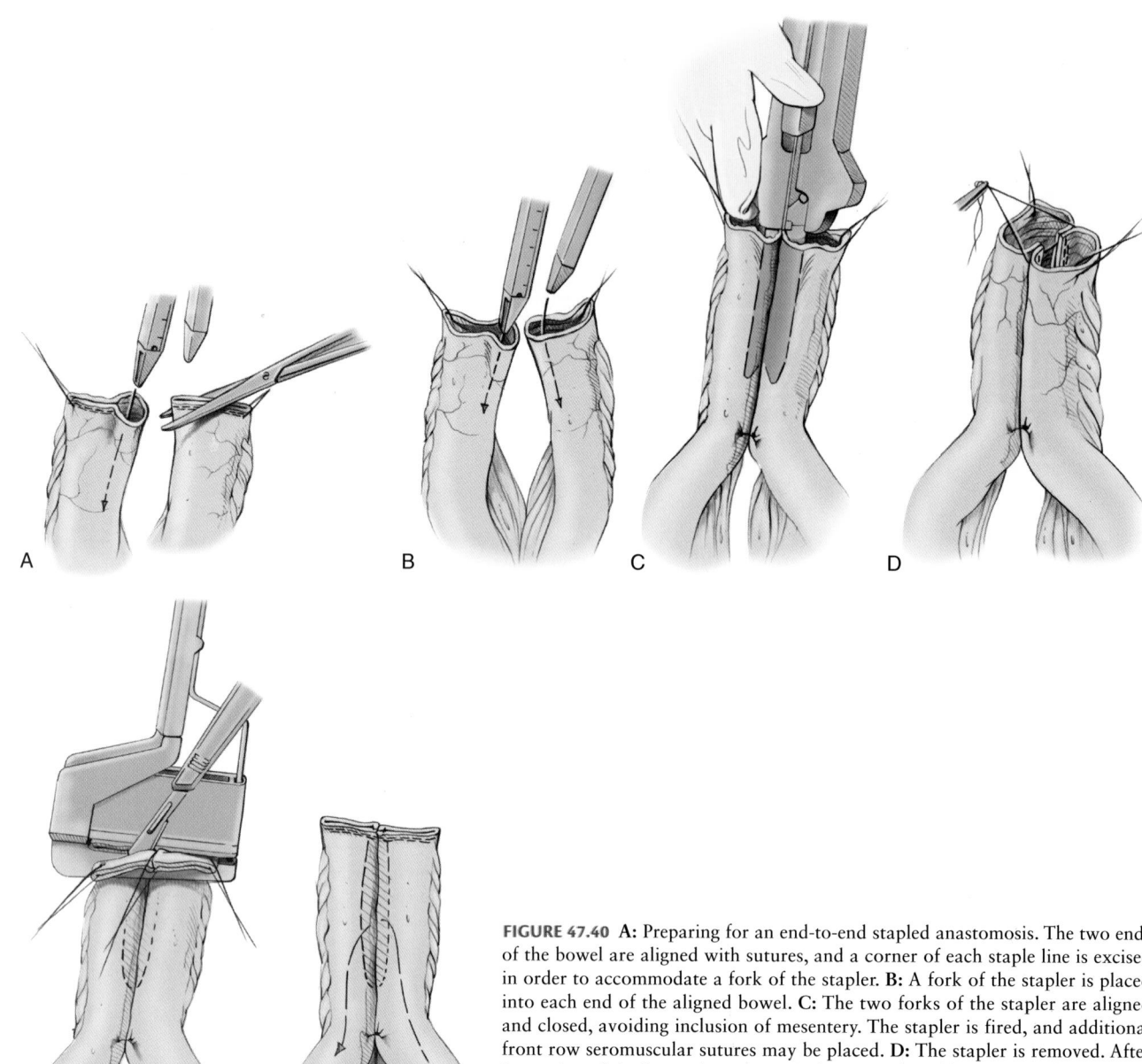

FIGURE 47.40 A: Preparing for an end-to-end stapled anastomosis. The two ends of the bowel are aligned with sutures, and a corner of each staple line is excised in order to accommodate a fork of the stapler. **B:** A fork of the stapler is placed into each end of the aligned bowel. **C:** The two forks of the stapler are aligned and closed, avoiding inclusion of mesentery. The stapler is fired, and additional front row seromuscular sutures may be placed. **D:** The stapler is removed. After inspection of the internal anastomosis for patency and hemostasis, the open end (which accommodated the stapler and is now common) is held closed and aligned with sutures or a series of Allis clamps. **E and F:** A stapler is placed underneath the Allis clamps across the common opening and fired. This closes the opening and completes the anastomosis.

The technique of end ileostomy is relatively straightforward. The mesentery is carefully mobilized so that the end of the ileum may be brought through the right lower quadrant with adequate blood supply. A site is chosen and a circular, quarter-sized segment of skin and underlying fat is excised. The fascia is exposed, and a cruciate incision is made (Fig. 47.41A), followed by completion of the incision into the peritoneal cavity. The entire opening should be large enough to accommodate the end of the ileum without compromising the mesentery. The ileum is brought up through the opening with a Babcock clamp until it extends approximately 6 cm above the skin without tension (Fig. 47.41B). The bowel wall is then secured to the peritoneum with interrupted 2-0 silk sutures. The ileostomy is matured after closing the abdomen and isolating the abdominal incision with an occlusive dressing to

avoid soilage (Fig. 47.41C). The maturation should create a protruding nipple-like stoma (as described by Brooke), which directs the liquid bowel contents directly into the appliance bag. If circumstances dictate that the transected end of the defunctionalized ileum should be exteriorized as a mucous fistula, this may be brought out at a separate site as a small, flat stoma or with the functional end as a modified loop ileostomy.

A loop ileostomy is brought through a similar opening in the right lower quadrant of the abdominal wall. The loop is delivered with a Babcock clamp until it protrudes approximately 5 cm above the skin, at which level it is secured to the fascia with interrupted 2-0 delayed absorbable sutures and to the peritoneum with interrupted 2-0 silk sutures. A supporting bridge is generally not necessary. After closing the abdomen, the ostomy is matured by making a transverse incision

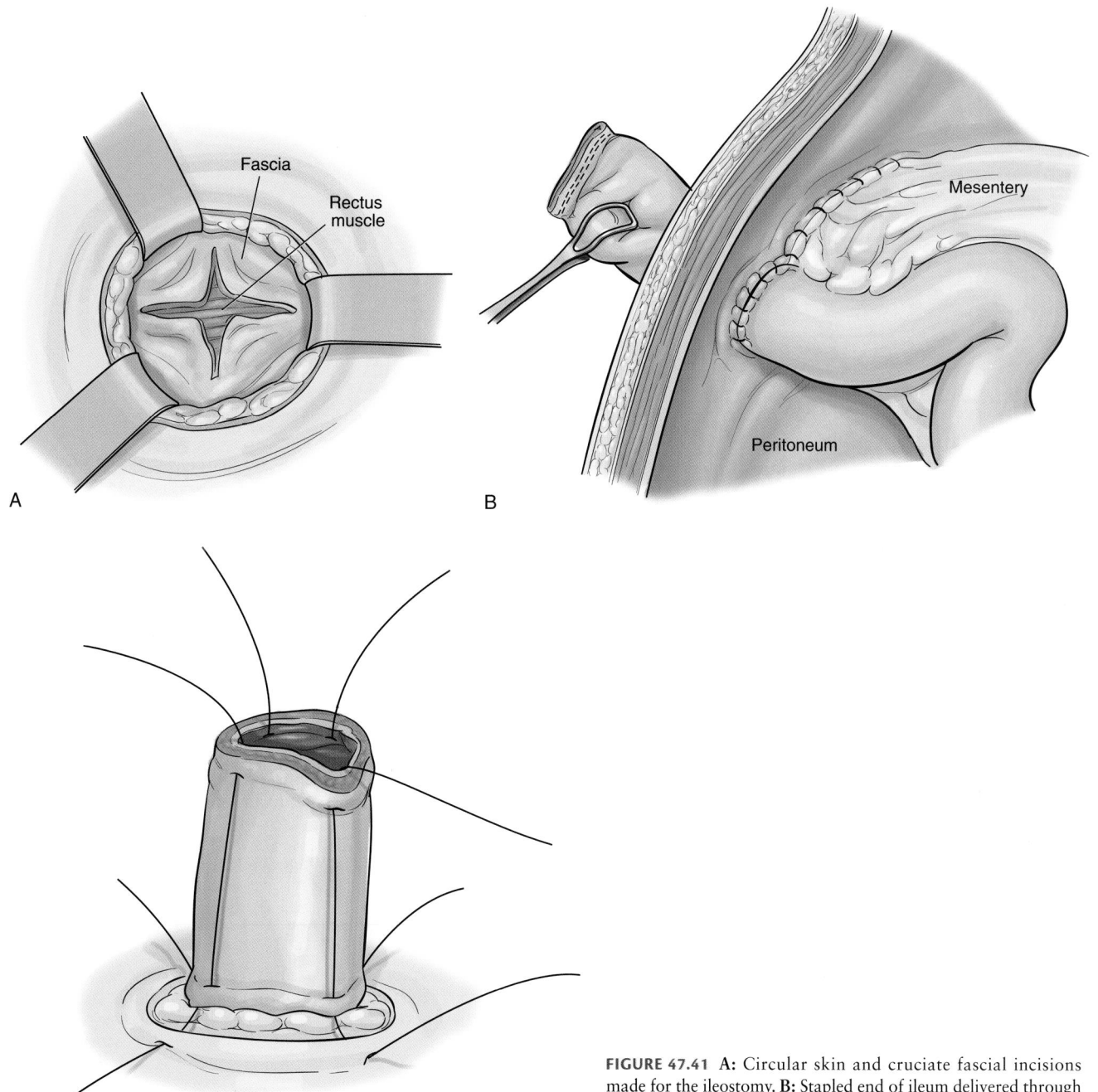

FIGURE 47.41 A: Circular skin and cruciate fascial incisions made for the ileostomy. **B:** Stapled end of ileum delivered through the ostomy incision. **C:** Creation of the protruding, nipple-like ileostomy stoma.

across the efferent limb just above the skin (Fig. 47.42A). The efferent opening is sutured to the skin with interrupted 2-0 sutures. The functional end is then matured in a protruding fashion in the manner described with the end ileostomy (Fig. 47.42B).

Colostomy

A colostomy may be formed either from the transected end of the colon (usually sigmoid or end descending) or from a loop of colon (usually transverse). The main role of a loop colostomy is temporary diversion. Most end colostomies are intended to be permanent. In certain situations, a colostomy may also be performed as an isolated procedure laparoscopically or through a small incision placed over the anticipated location of that part of the colon.

A transverse loop colostomy is brought through a circular incision in the right or left upper quadrant. A mobile portion of the transverse colon is selected, to come through the chosen site of the abdominal wall. To accomplish this, it is occasionally necessary to take down the hepatic and/or splenic flexure. This portion of the colon is separated from the omentum and to a limited extent is cleared of fat. A defect is made in the mesentery and a Penrose drain passed through and held. The loop of colon is then delivered through the ostomy incision until it protrudes approximately 5 cm above the skin (Fig. 47.43).

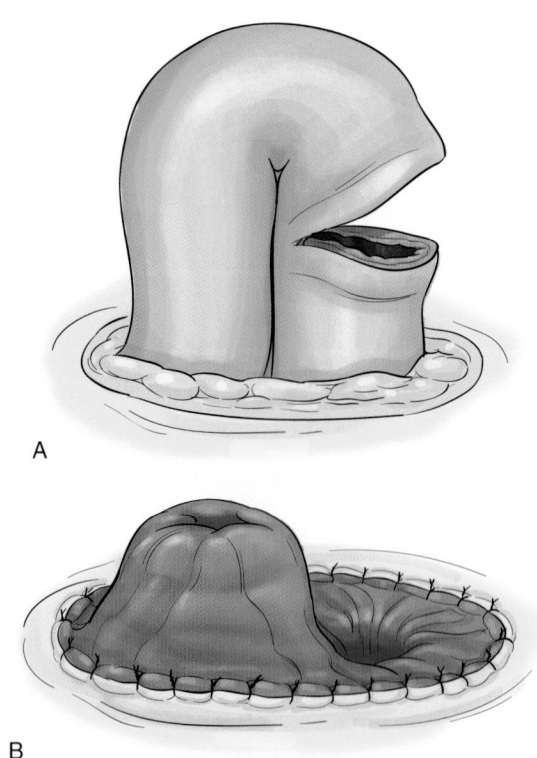

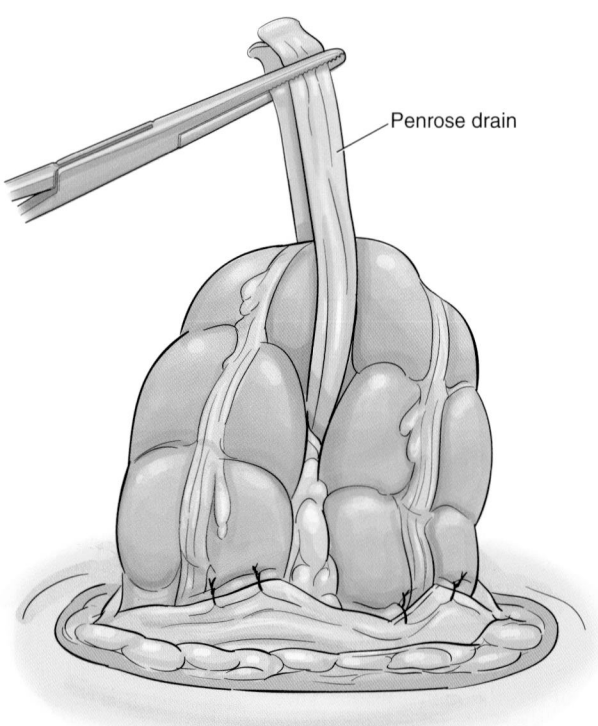

FIGURE 47.42 A: Bowel incision for loop ileostomy. Length is maintained on the functional side so that it can be matured as a protruding stoma. **B:** Maturation of the loop ileostomy.

FIGURE 47.43 Loop of colon delivered through the ostomy incision by a Penrose drain through the mesentery.

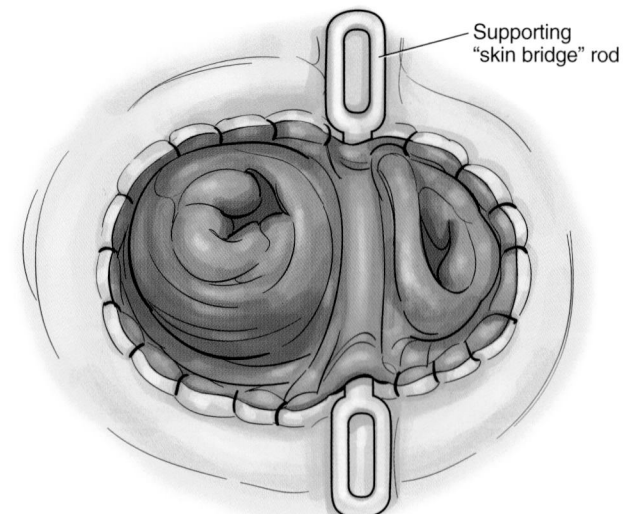

FIGURE 47.44 The Penrose drain has been replaced by a supporting skin bridge rod. The loop has been partially divided and matured into a colostomy in a manner similar to that described for ileostomy.

A plastic bar is then placed through the mesenteric defect across the skin to ensure maintenance of colostomy elevation and complete diversion of stool (Fig. 47.44).

An end sigmoid or descending colostomy is placed at a selected site in the left lower quadrant. This portion of the colon is adequately mobilized and the end is cleared of fat. With a Babcock clamp, the end is then delivered through the ostomy incision until it extends approximately 3 to 5 cm above the skin. In order to reduce complications, consideration may be given to tunneling a permanent end sigmoid colostomy extraperitoneally before bringing the end through the ostomy incision. After closure of the abdomen, the colostomy is matured as described for the end ileostomy (Fig. 47.45). With the expectation of solid stool, the end sigmoid colostomy need only protrude 1 to 2 cm.

Loop Ostomy Closure

Takedown of a loop ileostomy or colostomy is done using a similar technique and can generally be accomplished through a peristomal incision. An elliptical incision is made, which includes a margin of skin along the stomal edges (Fig. 47.46). The loop is then freed to the fascia and separated from the fascial ring. If necessary, a small ring of fascia may be excised to safely free the loop. The loop is separated from the peritoneum and nearby adhesions until it is freely mobile for closure and replacement into the peritoneal cavity. Depending on the circumstances, the surgeon may elect to simply excise the stomal margin and close the anterior intestinal wall defect transversely, insert a linear stapler through the two ends of the colon and close the transverse colostomy with a stapler or sutures, or resect the stoma and perform an EEA.

End Colostomy Takedown

This description is restricted to takedown of an end sigmoid colostomy with anastomosis to the rectal stump. Such a situation is infrequently encountered in patients with benign or malignant gynecologic nonpathology.

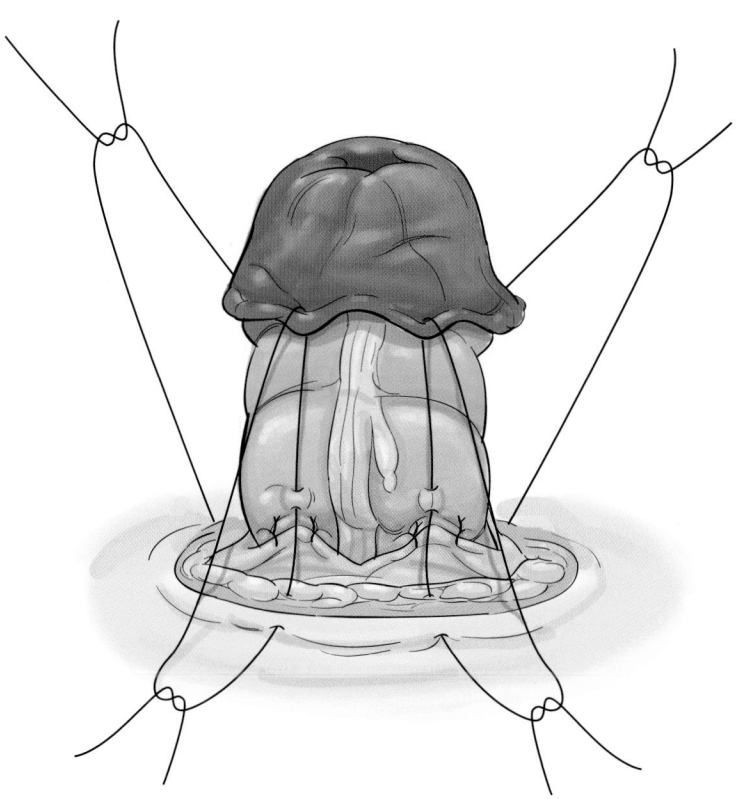

FIGURE 47.45 Sutures placed for maturation of the end colostomy that will protrude in a manner similar to that described for the end ileostomy.

Prior to preparation of the abdomen, the stoma is closed with a purse-string suture or with a running monofilament suture to approximate the skin edges surrounding the stoma in a linear fashion. Alternatively, a large-bore catheter may be placed to occlude the stoma, drain the colon, and aid in identification of the intraperitoneal colon segment. The abdomen is opened through the previous incision, and adhesions are taken down. The colostomy is mobilized by making an elliptical incision around the skin and freeing the colon from the fascia and peritoneum. Alternatively and if length allows, the colon may be transected with a stapler just under the abdominal wall; the stoma is excised separately. The end is prepared

for anastomosis and sized, and the purse-string suture is placed. The rectal stump is mobilized only so far as to define an apex that allows proper placement of the stapler. From this point, the procedure is identical to that of the colorectal anastomosis previously described using the circular stapler, with the exception that the trocar simply penetrates the apex of the rectal stump.

POSTOPERATIVE CARE AND COMPLICATIONS

Patients who have undergone intestinal surgery are maintained at bowel rest until return of bowel function, or until diet is cautiously advanced at the discretion of the surgeon. Maintenance of a nasogastric tube for 24 hours or longer postoperatively may be associated with an increased risk of respiratory complications and causes discomfort to the patient. The benefit of the nasogastric tube is unclear but is utilized at the discretion of the surgeon. In theory, the tube helps to keep the intestinal tract somewhat decompressed, which may protect the anastomosis and reduce the time to return of bowel function and which will guard against aspiration until gastrointestinal function returns. As previously discussed, when slow return of bowel function or the need for prolonged bowel rest is anticipated intraoperatively, it is reasonable to place a gastrostomy tube. Most of the tubes used for this purpose are not sump tubes and are best placed to allow postoperative gravity drainage. In general, a gastrostomy tube should not be removed before the 10th day to ensure that the intestine has become well adhered to the anterior abdominal wall.

When the patient is severely malnourished, is anticipated to have slow return of bowel function, needs prolonged bowel

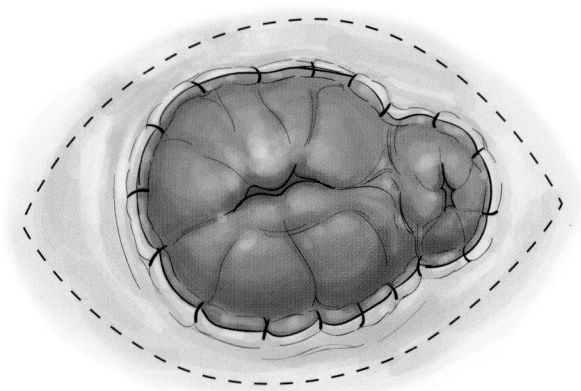

FIGURE 47.46 Peristomal incision in preparation for closure of a loop colostomy.

VIII

rest (more than 55 to 77 days), or has undergone very extensive surgery (e.g., exenteration), TPN is begun or reinstituted as soon as the patient is stabilized postoperatively. This should be anticipated so that a central venous catheter may be placed intraoperatively.

Wound Management

Wound infection rates following intestinal surgery are generally in the range of 5% to 10%, but this complication is much more likely to occur in some settings than in others. Wound infection is more likely to develop if the bowel (particularly the colon or obstructed small bowel) has been opened or if a colostomy has been constructed. Wounds that have been extensively contaminated with stool should undergo delayed primary closure. All of these wounds require vigilant surveillance for infection, which tends to appear 7 to 14 days postoperatively. Other major risk factors for wound infection, such as obesity and poorly controlled diabetes, must be considered as well.

Enterostomy Tubes

Significant gastrostomy-related complications occur in approximately 5% of patients. Lapses in technique are the most important factors related to these complications. Early complications include dislodgement, hemorrhage, gastric or esophageal perforation, gastric prolapse through the opening, pressure necrosis of the gastric wall, and subphrenic abscess. Accidental removal of the tube within the first week poses a risk of intraperitoneal leakage, and reoperation is required if signs of peritonitis develop. If the tip of a large-bore catheter or a balloon migrates to the pylorus, it can cause gastric outlet obstruction. After being in place for several weeks, leakage may develop around the tube. This will usually resolve with replacement of the tube, which is done readily in the office. When a gastrostomy is placed for early postoperative management, our practice is to send the patient home with the tube plugged and remove it in the office 2 to 3 weeks later. If nausea or vomiting due to chemotherapy is anticipated early in the postoperative period, the tube may be opened to gravity on an as-needed basis.

The use of PEG tubes has been associated with the same low rate of complications as with the use of a surgically placed gastrostomy tube. Significant complications have also been reported with jejunostomy and needle jejunostomy, including hemorrhage, intestinal obstruction, and intraperitoneal leakage. As with a gastrostomy, technique is the most important factor related to these complications.

Small Bowel Anastomosis

Complications specifically related to small bowel resection and anastomosis include anastomotic leak with its attendant sequelae—hemorrhage, stricture, internal herniation, folate or vitamin B_{12} deficiency, and short bowel syndrome. The chief concern regarding complications in the immediate postoperative period is the possibility for the occurrence of an anastomotic leak. This is a potentially devastating occurrence that may lead to sepsis and death. The leak can be contained with resultant intra-abdominal abscess, fistulae formation, or both. Management of enteric fistulae was previously discussed. Certain factors increase the likelihood of an anastomotic leak including prior radiotherapy, carcinomatosis, severe malnutrition, peritonitis or intra-abdominal sepsis, and poor condition of the bowel, such as marked dilation or extensive inflammatory reaction. Following a small bowel anastomosis or enterocolostomy, oral intake is restricted until return of bowel function. In the presence of the above risk factors (especially

prior radiotherapy), TPN should be started or reinstituted and bowel rest maintained for a minimum of 7 to 10 days.

If a long tube was passed into the intestine preoperatively, it should be maintained at low intermittent suction following surgery. By keeping the bowel decompressed, the tube may protect the anastomosis. In addition, the tube acts as a stent and may prevent recurrent small bowel obstruction. The tube itself is partially obstructing, is uncomfortable, and may produce complications; it should be removed once bowel function begins to return or once the period of planned bowel rest is completed. These tubes have been associated with intussusception, especially upon removal. This complication is best prevented by gradual removal of the tube, topping as resistance is encountered.

Recurrent or persistent small bowel obstruction related to extensive dense adhesions is an uncommon occurrence that frustrates the patient and the surgeon and appears at the time to be an unsolvable dilemma. Although investigations continue, there is no proven available method for preventing redevelopment of the adhesions. Rather, described operative techniques for managing such patients have consisted of attempts to control the pattern in which the bowel adhesions form, such that there are smooth, gradual, nonobstructing turns in the small bowel. Plication of the small bowel and mesentery upon itself in smooth, gradual loops was described by Nobel in 1937. This method, considered outdated for the most part, has been associated with significant bowel dysfunction and morbidity.

Transmesenteric plication, introduced by Childs and Phillips in 1960, appears to yield improved results. A modification of the Nobel procedure, this technique involves placement of transmesenteric mattress sutures with a long needle in such a manner so as to fold the bowel into gentle, back and forth curves. There is the potential for mesenteric vascular injury with hematoma and/or bowel ischemia with this method. Currently, the main approach to patients with primary or recurrent small bowel obstruction related to complex adhesions consists of complete adhesiolysis alone or together with internal bowel stenting.

The value of decompression with adhesiolysis is unclear, but it is the authors' practice to perform retrograde decompression concomitantly. In such cases, the authors place a gastrostomy tube for management in the event that the obstruction fails to open up. When adhesive small bowel obstruction fails to resolve postoperatively or develops subsequent to very extensive surgery, patients should remain on TPN and bowel rest for at least several weeks prior to considering reoperation, provided that the condition is nonacute. Early reoperation on such patients may prove difficult and morbid due to an intense inflammatory reaction with edema and friability involving the bowel and peritoneal cavity.

Significant postoperative hemorrhage from a bowel anastomosis is an uncommon occurrence. It usually occurs early and has been related to intestinal stapler malfunction. As previously discussed, this complication is best prevented by careful inspection of the staple lines following removal of the stapling instrument.

After extensive small bowel resection, functional capacity of the intestine may be markedly reduced, resulting in a number of problems for the patient. The ability of the patient to adapt and maintain homeostasis with the remaining small intestine is dependent on several factors, including the length and specific segment of remaining bowel, the presence of an ileocecal valve and length of intact colon, the age of the patient (minimal intestinal adaptation after age 65), and hormonal factors. Significant problems occur when fewer than 5 to 10 feet of functional small bowel remain, including severe diarrhea, dehydration, perianal or stoma excoriation, electrolyte imbalance, and malnutrition. Over several months, adaptation of the preserved intestine occurs, with variable improvement in diarrhea and malabsorption depending on the previously cited factors.

Gastric hypersecretion is another recognized phenomenon in these patients; it may result in gastrointestinal ulceration, but the problem is transient and best managed with proton pump inhibitors. Cimetidene (an H2 blocker) has been found effective in correcting malabsorption in patients with short bowel syndrome or those with exceptionally high ileostomy outputs (>1.5 L/day). Somatostatin (and ocreotide) has been of limited benefit in the management of severe diarrhea in these patients. Other complications that may develop in patients with short bowel syndrome include cholelithiasis and nephrolithiasis. At the time of surgery, if fewer than 3 feet of small bowel segment is preserved, especially in the absence of an intact ileocecal valve and colon, consideration should be given to bringing the segment out as a stoma to improve patient comfort and dietary freedom.

In patients expected to be long-term survivors dependent on TPN, another consideration is prophylactic cholecystectomy. Following surgery, intestinal adaptation is dependent on stimulation by luminal nutrients. Maintenance of the patient with TPN should be supplemented as much as possible with oral/enteral feeding. Depending on the length of remaining functional bowel, supplementation may vary widely from vitamins only to complete reliance on TPN. Investigational surgical techniques for the management of patients with short bowel syndrome include intestinal valves and sphincters, interposition of an antiperistaltic segment of intestine, colon interposition, recirculating loops and pouches, intestinal pacing, intestinal tapering and lengthening, new intestinal mucosa growth, and intestinal transplantation.

Colorectal Anastomosis

Postoperatively, oral intake should be restricted until gastrointestinal function returns (a minimum of 5 to 7 days) and until there is no sign of an anastomotic leak. Routine nasogastric suction is not necessary but should be maintained in complicated cases. Patients at increased risk for an anastomotic leak from malnutrition, diabetes, heavy tobacco use, severe vascular disease, prior irradiation, and severe blood loss/shock should be kept at complete bowel rest and on TPN for at least 10 days. Once the patient is on solid food, a bulk-forming agent should be added to the diet.

Anastomotic leak is the most serious complication of colorectal anastomosis, with a reported incidence in approximately 5% of patients and an associated mortality ranging from 10% to 30% of patients. Depending on the level of the anastomosis and the length of time since surgery, the leakage may present as diffuse peritonitis and sepsis (if leak occurs within the first 48 hours), localized peritonitis, abscess, or a rectovaginal fistula. If there is clinical uncertainty about a leakage, then a gentle Gastrografin enema should be performed. Feculent or purulent drainage may be noted from a pelvic drain. A pelvic drain positioned away from the anastomosis and placed at the time of surgery is generally removed after 24 to 48 hours. If a clinically occult or localized small leakage is noted and the patient is otherwise well, the drain should be left in place and the patient placed on bowel rest and TPN in hopes of spontaneous healing. Most clinically evident anastomotic leaks require prompt laparotomy (emergent if the patient has peritonitis) with resection of the anastomosis, proximal colostomy, irrigation of the abdomen, and closure and/or wide drainage of the rectal stump.

Anastomotic stenosis occurs in 1% to 10% of patients undergoing colorectal anastomosis. As with anastomotic leakage, the likelihood of this complication occurring may be much higher in patients who have undergone full pelvic radiotherapy for carcinoma of the cervix. In patients who have a protective colostomy, it is particularly important to evaluate the anastomosis for the presence of stenosis prior to taking the colostomy down. After healing, some anastomotic strictures can be successfully dilated.

Postoperative bleeding from the anastomosis is uncommon in the absence of a bleeding diathesis. The diagnosis may be difficult to make and should not be aggressively pursued unless the bleeding is significant. If the bleeding persists, hemostatic agents administered through an arterial catheter can be considered, although this may result in ischemia at the site of the anastomosis. If the anastomosis was to the anus, an attempt should be made at suture ligation transanally. In the presence of significant bleeding not amenable to the above approaches, a laparotomy will be necessary.

Like all extensive pelvic operations, surgery involving the colorectum carries the risk of ureteral injury that may be recognized during the postoperative period.

Following colorectal resection, a Foley catheter should be left in place for a minimum of 55 days. If there has been an associated extensive pelvic resection under the bladder for gynecologic malignancy or dissection under a previously radiated bladder, the catheter should be maintained for at least 3 to 4 weeks. As with extensive radical hysterectomy, bladder dysfunction is to be expected after extensive pelvic resection.

Following colorectal anastomosis, the patient may experience problems with rectal function including incontinence, tenesmus, and frequency of defecation. These difficulties are more likely to occur with anastomoses to the distal rectum and particularly those below the anorectal angle. Medical management of such patients generally consists of diet modification and constipating agents (including narcotics). As long as a reasonable rectal stump length was maintained, these problems will largely resolve within 6 months in a majority of patients.

Intestinal Stomas

Postoperative care begins in the operating room, where the surgeon must take responsibility for proper placement of the initial ostomy appliance so that contamination of the incisions and the psychological effects that early leakage can cause are avoided. The initial bag should be transparent so that the stoma can be checked for viability. Once the patient begins to recover from surgery, postoperative teaching about the stoma begins. Along with continued emotional support, this includes information about the anatomy of the stoma and its function, potential complications, and detailed aspects of day-to-day care. As with preoperative teaching, an enterostomal therapist is a valuable resource who should continue patient involvement intermittently on a long-term basis.

A comprehensive discussion of ostomy care is beyond the scope of this chapter, but specific areas to be addressed with the patient include peristomal skin care, diet, activities, odor, and emotional support. Some patients with an end-descending or sigmoid colostomy are candidates for routine irrigation that may allow predictability of bowel movements and better control over odor and gas. A few experimental techniques and devices aimed at producing a continent colostomy have been described or are available; however, results are variable, and it appears that their use should be individualized.

Complications of ileostomy and colostomy are similar. Many gynecologic oncology patients undergoing ileostomy

VIII

have advanced malignancy and will not be subject to late complications. One complication unique to ileostomy is food bolus impaction, which occurs close to the stoma. This situation may be difficult to differentiate from mechanical small bowel obstruction. In either case, the initial management consists of bowel rest with nasogastric suction and intravenous fluids. The ileostomy is then gently irrigated in an attempt to dislodge the impaction. A windsock enema may be applied to allow gentle irrigation using gravity of an impacted small or large bowel stoma. Other common ostomy-related complications include peristomal wound infection, peristomal skin problems, site choice problems, ischemia, retraction, stenosis, prolapse, peristomal hernia, and carcinomatous involvement.

Peristomal skin problems include contact dermatitis, fungal dermatitis, and hyperplasia. Attention to appliance application and removal, avoidance of leakage, and meticulous skin care can help avoid and resolve most of these problems. An improperly placed stoma will make appliance placement and general stomal care more difficult for the patient and can contribute to the above skin problems.

Ischemia of the ostomy is more likely to occur with a descending colostomy and usually develops in the early postoperative period. The stoma must be closely monitored during the first 24 hours, and if it appears dusky or black the extent of ischemia must be evaluated. This may be done by placing a test tube into the stoma (Fig. 47.47) and shining a penlight inside of it. If the level of involvement is superficial, then it is best managed by local wound care with later revision as necessary. Recession of the stoma and/or stenosis are potential consequences of ischemia. Frank stomal necrosis requires close monitoring and exploration if peritoneal signs develop.

Significant retraction of the stoma is more common with colostomies and occurs in approximately 3% of cases. With a retracted stoma, leakage under the stomal appliance is much more likely. Revision can usually be accomplished locally by freeing the stoma completely so that it can be elevated, secured to the fascia, and resutured to the skin in a rosebud fashion.

Significant stomal stenosis may be a consequence of ischemia or infection, or may result from a too-small skin or fascial opening. This complication occurs in approximately 3% of colostomy patients. Initial gentle dilation may resolve the problem, but persistent stenosis requires revision. Local revision with excision of the constricting scar tissue is the best approach.

Stomal prolapse (Fig. 47.48) develops as a consequence of a too-large fascial opening and more commonly involves the proximal limb of a transverse loop colostomy. This complication occurs in approximately 3% of colostomy patients. Local revision with resection of the redundant colon, closure of the fascial defect, and fixation to the fascia is usually successful. If the colostomy is temporary, then the prolapse may be managed conservatively.

A peristomal hernia develops in approximately 4% of patients after colostomy and is also a result of a too-large fascial opening. The hernia is repaired by excision of the sac and closure of the fascial defect (with mesh if necessary), although relocation of the stoma is sometimes necessary.

Carcinomatous replacement of the stoma occasionally occurs in patients with advanced intra-abdominal malignancy. Resection and relocation of the stoma is ideal but often not feasible. Local radiotherapy may also be considered. Patients face difficulty with odor, pain, and control of ostomy effluent and tumor discharge.

Ostomy Closure

Many significant complications that occur after colostomy closure in gynecologic cancer patients are related to the extensively radiated and/or extensively resected colorectal area that has been protected. Complications specifically related to closure of a loop ileostomy or colostomy are similar to those of other bowel anastomoses. These include wound infection (12%), anastomotic leak or fecal fistula (6%), anastomotic stricture or obstruction (2%), and incisional hernia (6%).

Factors that have been related to the complication rate of colostomy closure include patient age, timing of operation, underlying pathologic abnormality, type and site of colostomy, presence of steroid dependence, moderate to severe malnutrition (albumin <3.0), use of oral preoperative antibiotics, method of closure, and experience of the surgeon. Timing of closure is controversial, but should be delayed until the condition of the patient is optimal, especially when there has been an inflammatory process of the colon or peritoneal cavity or when the colon has been radiated. Closure of an end colostomy to a Hartmann pouch has been simplified by the use of a

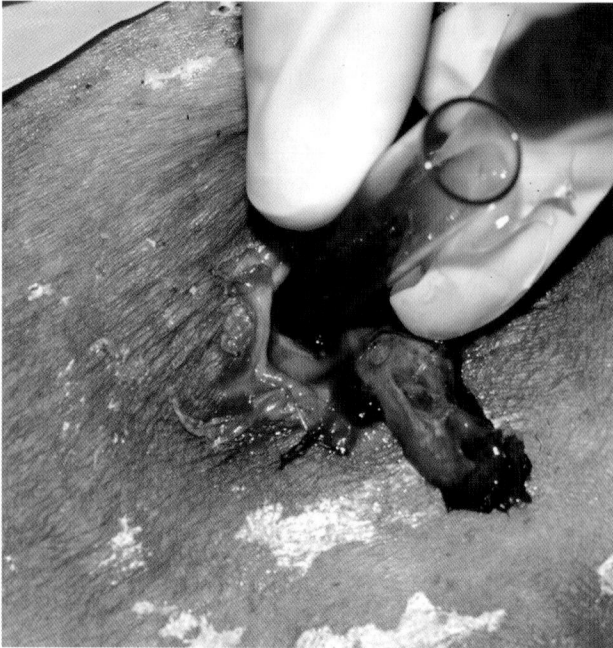

FIGURE 47.47 Examination of the lumen of a necrotic stoma with a test tube.

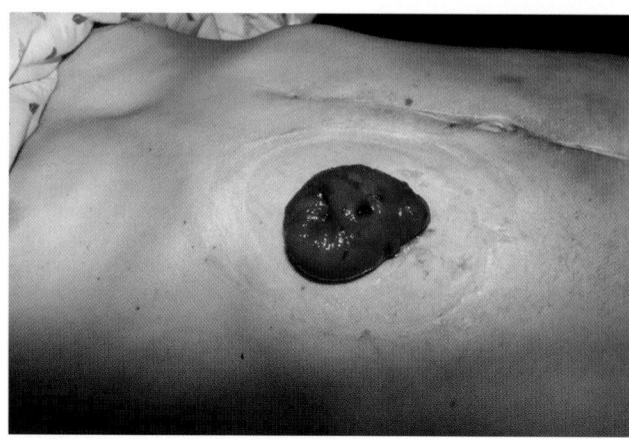

FIGURE 47.48 Prolapsed loop colostomy.

stapling device; the closure-related complication rate is probably not significantly greater than that of a transverse loop colostomy. However, closure of a transverse loop colostomy is simpler and does not require laparotomy.

BEST SURGICAL PRACTICES

- The pelvic surgeon must have medical and surgical expertise in the management of specific types of intestinal disorders. With any type of abdominal operation, the surgeon must be prepared for the eventuality of intestinal injury.
- When operating for presumed gynecologic pathology, the pelvic surgeon occasionally discovers a primary bowel disorder that must be managed surgically.
- Knowledge of the anatomy of the intestinal tract is necessary for the performance of intestinal surgery and management of complex pelvic pathology.
- Bowel adhesions may interfere with access to the pelvis during surgery and/or may involve pelvic structures with which the gynecologic surgeon is concerned. Any surgeon who operates in the peritoneal cavity must be competent in intraperitoneal adhesiolysis.
- In a patient with normal intestinal function and intestinal adhesions that will not interfere with the planned operation, lysis of such adhesions is not indicated.
- Management of thermal bowel injury is highly individualized according to the perceived extent of damage. Blanched, contracted tissue should be considered nonviable. There may be at least several millimeters of less apparent damage beyond the apparent injury.
- Laceration of the small bowel should be repaired perpendicular to the lumen to avoid constriction.
- In order to achieve optimal clearance of tumor, a large percentage of patients require extended procedures, the most common of these being colon resection.
- Likely a result of its location in the pelvis, the rectosigmoid colon is the bowel segment most frequently resected during cytoreductive surgery for ovarian cancer.
- The most important potential consequence of bowel involvement by endometriosis is obstruction, which is more likely to occur in the small intestine. Asymptomatic endometriosis of the bowel does not require surgical treatment.
- For a patient with recurrent ovarian cancer and bowel obstruction, the presence of extensive ascites, bulky intra-abdominal tumor, an ileus-type pattern, or generally poor condition indicates that surgical management of the obstruction is unlikely to be of benefit.
- The surgical approach to a patient with radiation-related small bowel obstruction must be individualized. If the overall condition of the patient is poor or there is recurrent disease, the fastest and least complicated procedure (i.e., simple bypass) should be carried out. If there is apparent impending necrosis of the involved bowel, multiple injuries to the bowel have occurred during dissection, or the involved bowel is a simple loop that is not densely adherent, resection with end-to-end enterocolostomy is preferred. Isolation bypass may still be applicable in some of these cases. Matted loops of bowel in the irradiated pelvis should be left in place as long as a reasonable length of proximal small bowel can be bypassed to nonirradiated proximal colon.
- A leaking small bowel anastomosis may form a communication to the abdominal wall or vagina resulting in an enterocutaneous or enterovaginal fistula. During the process of fistulization, intra-abdominal leakage of bowel contents may result in peritonitis or abscess formation,

and in some cases there may be continued intraperitoneal leakage. Uncontrolled sepsis in these patients is the major factor associated with mortality.
- Initial management of the patient with a small bowel fistula consists of bowel rest with nasogastric suction, fluid and electrolyte resuscitation, local management of the fistula output to prevent skin erosion, control of sepsis, and institution of TPN.
- Perforated bowel with intraperitoneal leakage is infrequently encountered in gynecologic and nongynecologic cancer patients. The complication may develop as a result of radiation-induced necrosis (usually of the terminal ileum or sigmoid colon), leakage from an intestinal anastomosis or occult operative injury, or bowel ischemia related to obstruction. Surgery is performed on an emergent basis.
- During conservative management of small bowel obstruction, if the patient develops any signs of compromised bowel, surgery must proceed. If, however, the patient remains stable and the bowel decompresses well, there is no urgency to the situation. The patient can be maintained on TPN while allowing 5 to10 days for the condition of the bowel to improve and a chance for the obstruction to resolve. If the bowel does not decompress by 48 to 72 hours, surgery should proceed.
- The operative approach to bowel resection begins with careful planning of resection and anastomosis followed by mobilization of the involved portion or portions of the bowel. The bowel to be anastomosed must be healthy, have an adequate blood supply, and appose without tension.
- Significant gastrostomy-related complications occur in approximately 5% of patients. Careful attention to technique is the most important factor related to these complications.
- Following anastomosis of the small bowel, the chief complication of concern in the immediate postoperative period is an anastomotic leak. This is a potentially devastating occurrence that may lead to sepsis and death.
- After extensive small bowel resection, functional capacity of the intestine may be markedly reduced, resulting in a number of problems for the patient. Significant problems occur when less than 5 to 10 feet of functional small bowel remain, including severe diarrhea, dehydration, perianal or stoma excoriation, electrolyte imbalance, and malnutrition.
- Anastomotic leak is the most serious complication of colorectal anastomosis, with a reported incidence of approximately 5% and an associated mortality ranging from 10% to 30%.
- Following placement of an abdominal wall stoma, postoperative care begins in the operating room where the surgeon must take responsibility for proper placement of the ostomy appliance. This is important so that contamination of the incisions and psychological effects that early leakage will cause are avoided.

BIBLIOGRAPHY

Abrams BL, Alsikafi FH, Waterman NG. Colostomy—new look at morbidity and mortality. *Am Surg* 1979;45:462.

Addiss DG, Shaffer N, Fowler BS, et al. The epidemiology of appendicitis and appendectomy in the United-States. *Am J Epidemiol* 1990;132:910.

Adelson, MD, Kasowitz MH. Percutaneous endoscopic drainage gastrostomy in the treatment of gastrointestinal obstruction from intraperitoneal malignancy. *Obstet Gynecol* 1993;81:467.

VIII

Adloff M, Arnaud JP, Beehary S. Stapled vs sutured colorectal anastomosis. *Arch Surg* 1980;115:1436 [in English].

Adloff M, Arnaud JP, Thibaud D, et al. Facilitating low colorectal anastomosis—preliminary-results. *Am J Surg* 1986;151:286 [in English].

Aletti GD, Podratz KC, Jones MB, et al. Role of rectosigmoidectomy and stripping of pelvic peritoneum in outcomes of patients with advanced ovarian cancer. *J Am Coll Surg* 2006;203:521 [in English].

Alvarado A. A practical score for the early diagnosis of acute appendicitis. *Ann Emerg Med* 1986;15:557 [in English].

Anderberg B, Enblad P, Sjodahl R, et al. The EEA-stapling device in anterior resection for carcinoma of the rectum. Technique and early recurrences. *Acta Chir Scand* 1983;149:99 [in English].

Antonsen HK, Kronborg O. Early complications after low anterior resection for rectal-cancer using the EEA stapling device—a prospective trial. *Dis Colon Rectum* 1987;30:579 [in English].

Baggish M. Major laparoscopic complications: a review in two parts. *J Gynecol Surg* 1981;28:315.

Bahadursingh AM, Longo WE. Colovaginal fistulas. Etiology and management. *J Reprod Med* 2003;48:489.

Bailey HR, Ott MT, Hartendorp P. Aggressive surgical management for advanced colorectal endometriosis. *Dis Colon Rectum* 1994;37:747.

Baker JW. A historical overview of surgical decompression in advanced intestinal-obstruction. *Surg Gynecol Obstet* 1984;158:593 [in English].

Baker JW. Stitchless plication for recurring obstruction of the small bowel. *Am J Surg* 1968;116:316 [in English].

Barber HR, Brunschwig A. Pelvic exenteration for locally advanced and recurrent ovarian cancer. Review of 22 cases. *Surgery* 1965; 58:935.

Bauer JJ, Gelernt IM, Salky BA, et al. Is routine postoperative nasogastric decompression really necessary. *Ann Surg* 1985;201: 233 [in English].

Beart RW, Kelly KA. Randomized prospective evaluation of the EEA stapler for colorectal anastomoses. *Am J Surg* 1981;141: 143 [in English].

Beck DE, DiPalma JA. A new oral lavage solution vs cathartics and enema method for preoperative colonic cleansing. *Arch Surg* 1991;126:552.

Belli L, Beati CA, Frangi M, et al. Outcome of patients with rectal cancer treated by stapled anterior resection. *Br J Surg* 1988; 75:422.

Bernard D, Morgan S, Tasse D, et al. Preliminary results of coloanal anastomosis. *Dis Colon Rectum* 1989;32:580.

Berne TV, Griffith CN, Hill J, et al. Colostomy wound closure. *Arch Surg* 1985;120:957.

Blamey SL, Lee PW. A comparison of circular stapling devices in colorectal anastomoses. *Br J Surg* 1982;69:19.

Boman-Sandelin K, Fenyo G. Construction and closure of the transverse loop colostomy. *Dis Colon Rectum* 1985;28:772.

Boronow RC. Management of radiation-induced vaginal fistulas. *Am J Obstet Gynecol* 1971;110:1.

Bozzetti F, Nava M, Bufalino R, et al. Early local complications following colostomy closure in cancer patients. *Dis Colon Rectum* 1983;26:25.

Brennan SS, Pickford IR, Evans M, et al. Staples or sutures for colonic anastomoses—a controlled clinical trial. *Br J Surg* 1982;69:722.

Bricker EM, Johnston WD. Repair of postirradiation rectovaginal fistula and stricture. *Surg Gynecol Obstet* 1979;148:499.

Brightwell NL, McFee AS, Aust JB. Bowel obstruction and the long tube stent. *Arch Surg* 1977;112:505.

Bristol JB, Williamson RC. Postoperative adaptation of the small intestine. *World J Surg* 1985;9:825.

Bristow RE, del Carmen MG, Kaufman HS, et al. Radical oophorectomy with primary stapled colorectal anastomosis for resection of locally advanced epithelial ovarian cancer. *J Am Coll Surg* 2003;197:565.

Bristow RE, Peiretti M, Zanagnolo V, et al. Transverse colectomy in ovarian cancer surgical cytoreduction: operative technique and clinical outcome. *Gynecol Oncol* 2008;109:364.

Brodman RF, Brodman HR. Staple suturing of the colon above the peritoneal reflection. *Arch Surg* 1981;116:191.

Brooke BN. The management of an ileostomy—including its complications. *Lancet* 1952;263:102 [in English].

Brown AA, Gasson JE, Brown RA. Experience with the EEA stapler in carcinoma of the lower rectum. *S Afr Med J* 1981;59:258.

Burger RA, Riedmiller H, Knapstein PG, et al. Ileocecal vaginal construction. *Am J Obstet Gynecol* 1989;161:162.

Burke ER, Welvaart K. Complications of stapled anastomoses in anterior resection for rectal carcinoma: colorectal anastomosis versus coloanal anastomosis. *J Surg Oncol* 1990;45:180.

Burns FJ. Complications of colostomy. *Dis Colon Rectum* 1970; 13:448.

Buzby GP. Perioperative total parenteral-nutrition in surgical patients. *N Engl J Med* 1991;325:525 [in English].

Caceres A, Zhou Q, Lasonos A, et al. Colorectal stents for palliation of large-bowel obstructions in recurrent gynecologic cancer: an updated series. *Gynecol Oncol* 2008;108:482 [in English].

Cade D, Gallagher P, Schofield PF, et al. Complications of anterior resection of the rectum using the EEA stapling device. *Br J Surg* 1981;68:339.

Cannon JA, Altom LK, Deierhoi RJ, et al. Preoperative oral antibiotics reduce surgical site infection following elective colorectal resections. *Dis Colon Rectum* 2012;55:1160 [in English].

Chabok A, Pahlman L, Hjern F, et al., AVOD Study Group. Randomized clinical trial of antibiotics in acute uncomplicated diverticulitis. *Br J Surg* 2012;99:532 [in English].

Chapman C, Bosscher J, Remmenga S, et al. A technique for managing terminally ill ovarian carcinoma patients. *Gynecol Oncol* 1991;41:88.

Chi DS, Eisenhauer EL, Lang J, et al. What is the optimal goal of primary cytoreductive surgery for bulky stage IIIC epithelial ovarian carcinoma (EOC)? *Gynecol Oncol* 2006;103:559.

Chi DS, Eisenhauer EL, Zivanovic O, et al. Improved progression-free and overall survival in advanced ovarian cancer as a result of a change in surgical paradigm. *Gynecol Oncol* 2009;114:26.

Chi DS, Franklin CC, Levine DA, et al. Improved optimal cytoreduction rates for stages IIIC and IV epithelial ovarian, fallopian tube, and primary peritoneal cancer: a change in surgical approach. *Gynecol Oncol* 2004;94:650.

Chi DS, McCaughty K, Diaz JP, et al. Guidelines and selection criteria for secondary cytoreductive surgery in patients with recurrent, platinum-sensitive epithelial ovarian carcinoma. *Cancer* 2006;106:1933.

Chi DS, Phaeton R, Miner TJ, et al. A prospective outcomes analysis of palliative procedures performed for malignant intestinal obstruction due to recurrent ovarian cancer. *Oncologist* 2009; 14:835.

Childs WA, Phillips RB. Experience with intestinal plication and a proposed modification. *Ann Surg* 1960;152:258.

Chilimindris CP, Stonesifer GL Jr. Complications associated with the baker tube jejunostomy. *Am Surg* 1978;44:707.

Choi D, Park H, Lee YR, et al. The most useful findings for diagnosing acute appendicitis on contrast-enhanced helical CT. *Acta Radiol* 2003;44:574 [in English].

Clague MB, Heald RJ. Achievement of stomal continence in one-third of colostomies by use of a new disposable plug. *Surg Gynecol Obstet* 1990;170:390.

Clarke-Pearson DL, Chin NO, DeLong ER, et al. Surgical management of intestinal obstruction in ovarian cancer. I. Clinical features, postoperative complications, and survival. *Gynecol Oncol* 1987;26:11.

Clarke-Pearson DL, DeLong ER, Chin N, et al., Intestinal obstruction in patients with ovarian cancer. Variables associated with surgical complications and survival. *Arch Surg* 1988;123:42.

Clayton RD, Obermair A, Hammond IG, et al. The Western Australian experience of the use of en bloc resection of ovarian cancer with concomitant rectosigmoid colectomy. *Gynecol Oncol* 2002; 84:53.

Close MB, Christensen NM. Transmesenteric small bowel plication or intraluminal tube stenting. Indications and contraindications. *Am J Surg* 1979;138:89.

Copeland EM, Macfayden BV Jr, Dudrick SJ. Intravenous hyperalimentation in cancer patients. *J Surg Res* 1974;16:241.

Crowson WN, Wilson CS. An experimental study of the effects of drains on colon anastomoses. *Am Surg* 1973;39:597.

Curtin JP, Burt LL. Successful treatment of small intestine fistula with somatostatin analog. *Gynecol Oncol* 1990;39:225.

Dalal KM, Gollub MJ, Miner TJ, et al. Management of patients with malignant bowel obstruction and stage IV colorectal cancer. *J Palliat Med* 2011;14:822.

DeCosse JJ, Rhodes RS, Wentz WB, et al. The natural history and management of radiation induced injury of the gastrointestinal tract. *Ann Surg* 1969;170:369.

Deitel M, To TB. Major intestinal complications of radiotherapy. Management and nutrition. *Arch Surg* 1987;122:1421.

Delgado G. Use of the automatic stapler in urinary conduit diversions and pelvic exenterations. *Gynecol Oncol* 1980;10:93.

Demetriades D, Pezikis A, Melissas J, et al. Factors influencing the morbidity of colostomy closure. *Am J Surg* 1988;155:594.

Didolkar MS, Reed WP, Elias EG, et al. A prospective randomized study of sutured versus stapled bowel anastomoses in patients with cancer. *Cancer* 1986;57:456.

Doberneck RC. Revision and closure of the colostomy. *Surg Clin North Am* 1991;71:193.

Dorricott NJ, Baddeley RM, Keighley MR, et al. Complications of rectal anastomoses with end-to-end anastomosis (EEA) stapling instrument. Clinical and radiological leak rates and some practical hints. *Ann R Coll Surg Engl* 1982;64:171.

Edlich RF, Rogers W, Kasper G, et al. Studies in the management of the contaminated wound. I. Optimal time for closure of contaminated open wounds. II. Comparison of resistance to infection of open and closed wounds during healing. *Am J Surg* 1969;117:323.

Eisenkop SM, Friedman RL, Spirtos NM. The role of secondary cytoreductive surgery in the treatment of patients with recurrent epithelial ovarian carcinoma. *Cancer* 2000;88:144.

Eisenkop SM, Spirtos NM. Procedures required to accomplish complete cytoreduction of ovarian cancer: is there a correlation with biological aggressiveness and survival? *Gynecol Oncol* 2001;82:435.

Eskicioglu C, Forbes SS, Fenech DS, et al.; Best Practice Gen Surg Comm. Preoperative bowel preparation for patients undergoing elective colorectal surgery: a clinical practice guideline endorsed by the Canadian Society of Colon and Rectal Surgeons. *Can J Surg* 2010;53:385 [in English].

Estes JM, Leath CA III, Straughn JM Jr, et al. Bowel resection at the time of primary debulking for epithelial ovarian carcinoma: outcomes in patients treated with platinum and taxane-based chemotherapy. *J Am Coll Surg* 2006;203:527.

Fasth S, Hulten L, Fazio VW. Loop ileostomy—a superior diverting stoma in colorectal surgery. *World J Surg* 1984;8:401 [in English].

Fazio VW, Jagelman DG, Lavery IC, et al. Evaluation of the proximate-ILS circular stapler. A prospective study. *Ann Surg* 1985;201:108.

Fedele L, Bianchi S, Zanconato G, et al. Long-term follow-up after conservative surgery for rectovaginal endometriosis. *Am J Obstet Gynecol* 2004;190:1020.

Fedele L, Bianchi S, Zanconato G, et al. Is rectovaginal endometriosis a progressive disease? *Am J Obstet Gynecol* 2004;191:1539.

Fegiz G, Angelini L, Bezzi M. Rectal cancer: restorative surgery with the EEA stapling device. *Int Surg* 1983;68:13.

Feinberg SM, Parker F, Cohen Z, et al. The double stapling technique for low anterior resection of rectal carcinoma. *Dis Colon Rectum* 1986;29:885.

Fernandes JR, Seymour RJ, Suissa S. Bowel obstruction in patients with ovarian cancer: a search for prognostic factors. *Am J Obstet Gynecol* 1988;158:244.

Feuer DJ, Broadley KE, Shepherd JH, et al. Systematic review of surgery in malignant bowel obstruction in advanced gynecological and gastrointestinal cancer. The Systematic Review Steering Committee. *Gynecol Oncol* 1999;75:313.

Feuer DJ, Broadley KE, Shepherd JH, et al. Surgery for the resolution of symptoms in malignant bowel obstruction in advanced gynaecological and gastrointestinal cancer. *Cochrane Database Syst Rev* 2000;CD002764.

Fischer MG. Bleeding from stapler anastomosis. *Am J Surg* 1976;131:745.

Foutch PG, Haynes WC, Bellapravalu S, et al. Percutaneous endoscopic gastrostomy (PEG)—a new procedure comes of age. *J Clin Gastroenterol* 1986;8:10 [in English].

Freund HR, Raniel J, Muggia-Sulam M. Factors affecting the morbidity of colostomy closure: a retrospective study. *Dis Colon Rectum* 1982;25:712.

Freundt I, Toolenaar TA, Huikeshoven FJ, et al. Long-term psychosexual and psychosocial performance of patients with a sigmoid neovagina. *Am J Obstet Gynecol* 1993;169:1210.

Friis J, Hjortrup A, Nielsen OV. Sphincter-saving resection of the rectum using the EEA autostapler. *Acta Chir Scand* 1982;148:379.

Galland RB, Spencer J. Surgical aspects of radiation injury to the intestine. *Br J Surg* 1979;66:135.

Gillette-Cloven N, Burger RA, Monk BJ, et al. Bowel resection at the time of primary cytoreduction for epithelial ovarian cancer. *J Am Coll Surg* 2001;193:626.

Goligher JC. The use of circular staplers for the construction of colorectal anastomoses after anterior resection. In: Denecke HG, ed. *Colorectal surgery*. Springer-Verlag, 1982:107.

Greene HG. Loop colostomy. Bar versus rod. *Dis Colon Rectum* 1971;14:308.

Griffen FD, Knight CD. Stapling technique for primary and secondary rectal anastomoses. *Surg Clin North Am* 1984;64:579.

Griffen FD, Knight CD, Whitaker JM, et al. The double stapling technique for low anterior resection—results, modifications, and observations. *Ann Surg* 1990;211:745 [in English].

Hatch KD, Shingleton HM, Potter ME, et al. Low rectal resection and anastomosis at the time of pelvic exenteration. *Gynecol Oncol* 1988;31:262.

Haun JL, Thompson JS. Comparison of needle catheter versus standard tube jejunostomy. *Am Surg* 1985;51:466.

Heald RJ. Towards fewer colostomies—the impact of circular stapling devices on the surgery of rectal cancer in a district hospital. *Br J Surg* 1980;67:198.

Heald RJ, Leicester RJ. The low stapled anastomosis. *Dis Colon Rectum* 1981;24:437.

Heald RJ, Ryall RDH. Recurrence and survival after total mesorectal excision for rectal-cancer. *Lancet* 1986;1:1479 [in English].

Helm W, Rowe PH. Rectal anastomosis with the EEA stapling instrument. *Ann R Coll Surg Engl* 1982;64:356.

Hewitt J, Reeve J, Rigby J, et al. Whole-gut irrigation in preparation for large-bowel surgery. *Lancet* 1973;2:337.

Hill GL. Massive enterectomy: indications and management. *World J Surg* 1985;9:833.

Hines JR, Harris GD. Colostomy and colostomy closure. *Surg Clin North Am* 1977;57:1379 [in English].

Hoffman MS, Barton DP, Gates J, et al. Complications of colostomy performed on gynecologic cancer patients. *Gynecol Oncol* 1992;44:231.

Hoffman MS, Cardosi RJ, Lemert R, et al. Stamm gastrostomy for postoperative gastric decompression in gynecologic oncology patients. *Gynecol Oncol* 2001;82:360.

Hoffman MS, Fiorica JV, Cavanagh D. Palliative gastro-intestinal diversion via minilaparotomy in gynecologic cancer patients. *J Gynecol Tech* 1997;3:107.

Hoffman MS, Gleeson NC, Finan MA, et al. Palliative intestinal surgery for patients with carcinoma of the cervix. *J Gynecol Surg* 1994;10:63 [in English].

Hoffman MS, Gleeson N, Diebel D, et al. Colostomy closure on a gynecologic oncology service. *Gynecol Oncol* 1993;49:299.

Hoffman MS, Griffin D, Tebes S, et al. Sites of bowel resected to achieve optimal ovarian cancer cytoreduction: implications regarding surgical management. *Am J Obstet Gynecol* 2005;193:582.

Hoffman MS, Lynch CM, Gleeson NC, et al. Colorectal anastomosis on a gynecologic oncology service. *Gynecol Oncol* 1994;55:60.

Hoffman MS, Roberts WS, Fiorica JV, et al. Severe radiation injury to the sigmoid colon. *J Gynecol Surg* 1996;12:191 [in English].

Hoffman MS, Tebes SJ, Sayer RA, et al. Extended cytoreduction of intra-abdominal metastatic ovarian cancer in the left upper quadrant utilizing en bloc resection. *Am J Obstet Gynecol* 2007;197:209 e1.

VIII

Hoffman MS, Zervose E. Colon resection for ovarian cancer: intraoperative decisions. *Gynecol Oncol* 2008;111:S56.

Hopkins MP, Roberts JA, Morley GW. Outpatient management of small bowel obstruction in terminal ovarian cancer. *J Reprod Med* 1987;32:827.

Hoskins WJ, Burke TW, Weiser EB, et al. Right hemicolectomy and ileal resection with primary reanastomosis for irradiation injury of the terminal ileum. *Gynecol Oncol* 1987;26:215.

Howard L, Heaphey LL, Timchalk M. A review of the current national status of home parenteral and enteral nutrition from the provider and consumer perspective. *JPEN J Parenter Enteral Nutr* 1986;10:416.

Hudson CN. A radical operation for fixed ovarian tumours. *J Obstet Gynaecol Br Commonw* 1968;75:1155.

Isbister WH, Beasley SW, Dowle CS. The EEA stapler—a Wellington experience. *Coloproctology* 1983;6:323.

Jaeger W, Ackermann S, Kessler H, et al. The effect of bowel resection on survival in advanced epithelial ovarian cancer. *Gynecol Oncol* 2001;83:286.

Jimenez-Perez J, Casellas J, Garcia-Cano J, et al. Colonic stenting as a bridge to surgery in malignant large-bowel obstruction: a report from two large multinational registries. *Am J Gastroenterol* 2011; 106:2174 [in English].

Julian TB, Ravitch MM. Evaluation of the safety of end-to-end (EEA) stapling anastomoses across linear stapled closures. *Surg Clin North Am* 1984;64:567.

Kalogera E, Dowdy SC, Mariani A, et al. Utility of closed suction pelvic drains at time of large bowel resection for ovarian cancer. *Gynecol Oncol* 2012;126:391.

Kavanagh D, Neary P, Dodd JD, et al. Diagnosis and treatment of enterovesical fistulae. *Colorectal Dis* 2005;7:286.

Kennedy HL, Rothenberger DA, Goldberg SM, et al. Colocolostomy and coloproctostomy utilizing the circular intraluminal stapling devices. *Dis Colon Rectum* 1983;26:145.

Khubchandani IT, Trimpi HD, Sheets JA, et al. The magnetic stoma device: a continent colostomy. *Dis Colon Rectum* 1981; 24:344.

Kirkegaard P, Christiansen J, Hjortrup A. Anterior resection for mid-rectal cancer with the EEA stapling instrument. *Am J Surg* 1980;140:312.

Kirkegaard P, Luke M, Rasmussen JG, et al. Closure of terminal and loop colostomy. *Dis Colon Rectum* 1982;25:567 [in English].

Knight CD, Griffen FD. Techniques of low rectal reconstruction. *Curr Probl Surg* 1983;20:387.

Kolomainen DF, Barton DP. Surgical management of bowel obstruction in gynaecological malignancies. *Curr Opin Support Palliat Care* 2011;5:55.

Krebs HB, Goplerud DR. Mechanical intestinal obstruction in patients with gynecologic disease: a review of 368 patients. *Am J Obstet Gynecol* 1987;157:577.

Krebs H-B, Goperlud DR. Surgical management of bowel obstruction in advanced ovarian carcinoma. *Obstet Gynecol* 1983;61:327.

Krebs HB, Helmkamp BF. Management of intestinal obstruction in ovarian cancer. *Oncology (Williston Park)* 1989;3:25.

Kucukmetin A, Naik R, Galaal K, et al. Palliative surgery versus medical management for bowel obstruction in ovarian cancer. *Cochrane Database Syst Rev* 2010;CD007792.

Kumar SS. Tube gastrostomy. A routine adjunct in major abdominal operations. *Am Surg* 1985;51(4):201.

Laitinen S, Huttunen R, Stahlberg M, et al. Experiences with the EEA stapling instrument for colorectal anastomosis. *Ann Chir Gynaecol* 1980;69:102 [in English].

Larsen E, Pories WJ. Frequency of wound complications after surgery for small bowel obstruction. *Am J Surg* 1971;122:384.

Larson JE, Podczaski ES, Manetta A, et al. Bowel obstruction in patients with ovarian carcinoma: analysis of prognostic factors. *Gynecol Oncol* 1989;35:61.

Lee YM, Law WL, Chu KW, et al. Emergency surgery for obstructing colorectal cancers: a comparison between right-sided and left-sided lesions. *J Am Coll Surg* 2001;192:719.

Lee YTN. A simple technic for fixing loop colostomy. *Am J Surg* 1968;116:138 [in English].

Leff EI, Hoexter B, Labow SB, et al. The EEA stapler in low colorectal anastomoses: initial experience. *Dis Colon Rectum* 1982; 25:704.

Leitman IM, Sullivan JD, Brams D, et al. Multivariate analysis of morbidity and mortality from the initial surgical management of obstructing carcinoma of the colon. *Surg Gynecol Obstet* 1992;174:513.

Levenback C, Gershenson DM, McGehee R, et al. Enterovesical fistula following radiotherapy for gynecologic cancer. *Gynecol Oncol* 1994;52:296 [in English].

Lillemoe KD, Brigham RA, Harmon JW, et al. Surgical management of small-bowel radiation enteritis. *Arch Surg* 1983;118:905 [in English].

Madiba TE, Thomson SR. The management of cecal volvulus. *Dis Colon Rectum* 2002;45:264 [in English].

Magruder JT, Efron JE, Wick EC, et al. Laparoscopic rectopexy for rectal prolapse to reduce surgical-site infections and length of stay. *World J Surg* 2013;37:1110.

Malone JM Jr., Koonce T, Larson DM, et al. Palliation of small bowel obstruction by percutaneous gastrostomy in patients with progressive ovarian carcinoma. *Obstet Gynecol* 1986;68:431.

Manji N, Bistrian BR, Mascioli EA, et al. Gallstone disease in patients with severe short bowel syndrome dependent on parenteral nutrition. *JPEN J Parenter Enteral Nutr* 1989;13:461.

Martinez-Mora J, Isnard R, Castellvi A, et al. Neovagina in vaginal agenesis: surgical methods and long-term results. *J Pediatr Surg* 1992;27:10.

McGinn FP, Gartell PC, Clifford PC, et al. Staples or sutures for low colorectal anastomoses: a prospective randomized trial. *Br J Surg* 1985;72:603.

McGregor JR, O'Dwyer PJ. The surgical management of obstruction and perforation of the left colon. *Surg Gynecol Obstet* 1993;177:203.

Micha JP, Goldstein BH, Rettenmaier MA, et al. Cecal pelvic transposition following total pelvic exenteration. *Gynecol Oncol* 2004;94:589.

Miles RM, Greene RS. Review of colostomy in a community hospital. *Am Surg* 1983;49:182.

Mileski WJ, Joehl RJ, Rege RV, et al. Treatment of anastomotic leakage following low anterior colon resection. *Arch Surg* 1988; 123:968.

Mileski WJ, Rege RV, Joehl RJ, et al. Rates of morbidity and mortality after closure of loop and end colostomy. *Surg Gynecol Obstet* 1990;171:17.

Miller G, Boman J, Shrier I, et al. Small-bowel obstruction secondary to malignant disease: an 11-year audit. *Can J Surg* 2000;43:353.

Mirelman D, Corman ML, Veidenheimer MC, et al. Colostomies—indications and contraindications: Lahey clinic experience, 1963–1974. *Dis Colon Rectum* 1978;21:172.

Mitchell C, Garrahy P, Peake P. Postoperative respiratory morbidity: identification and risk factors. *Aust N Z J Surg* 1982;52:203.

Mitchell WH, Kovalcik PH, Cross GH. Complications of colostomy closure. *Dis Colon Rectum* 1978;21:180.

Montesani C, De Milito R, Chiappalone S, et al. Critical evaluation of the anastomoses in large bowel surgery: experience gained in 533 cases. *Hepatogastroenterology* 1992;39:304 [in English].

Mourton SM, Temple LK, Abu-Rustum NR, et al. Morbidity of rectosigmoid resection and primary anastomosis in patients undergoing primary cytoreductive surgery for advanced epithelial ovarian cancer. *Gynecol Oncol* 2005;99:608.

Mullen JL. Consequences of malnutrition in the surgical patient. *Surg Clin North Am* 1981;61:465 [in English].

Muller JM, Brenner U, Dienst C, et al. Preoperative parenteral feeding in patients with gastrointestinal carcinoma. *Lancet* 1982; 1:68.

Nightingale JMD, Walker ER, Burnham WR, et al. Short bowel syndrome. *Digestion* 1990;45:77 [in English].

Noble TB. Plication of the small intestine as prophylaxis against adhesions. *Am J Surg* 1937;35:41.

Obermair A, Hagenauer S, Tamandl D, et al. Safety and efficacy of low anterior en bloc resection as part of cytoreductive surgery for patients with ovarian cancer. *Gynecol Oncol* 2001;83:115 [in English].

Orr JW Jr, Shingleton HM. Importance of nutritional assessment and support in surgical and cancer patients. *J Reprod Med* 1984;29:635.

Osborne MP, Sizer J, Frederick PL, et al. Massive bowel resection and gastric hypersecretion. Its mechanism and a plan for clinical study and management. *Am J Surg* 1967;114:393.

Palmer JA, Bush RS. Radiation injuries to the bowel associated with the treatment of carcinoma of the cervix. *Surgery* 1976;80:458.

Papa MZ, Karni T, Koller M, et al. Avoiding diarrhea after subtotal colectomy with primary anastomosis in the treatment of colon cancer. *J Am Coll Surg* 1997;184:269.

Park JY, Seo SS, Kang S, et al. The benefits of low anterior en bloc resection as part of cytoreductive surgery for advanced primary and recurrent epithelial ovarian cancer patients outweigh morbidity concerns. *Gynecol Oncol* 2006;103:977 [in English].

Parks AG, Allen CL, Frank JD, et al. A method of treating post-irradiation rectovaginal fistulas. *Br J Surg* 1978;65:417.

Parks SE, Hastings PR. Complications of colostomy closure. *Am J Surg* 1985;149:672.

Parrish RA, Cohen J. Temporary tube gastrostomy. *Am Surg* 1972;38:168.

Pearl RK, Prasad ML, Orsay CP, et al. Early local complications from intestinal stomas. *Arch Surg* 1985;120:1145 [in English].

Peiretti M, Bristow RE, Zapardiel I, et al. Rectosigmoid resection at the time of primary cytoreduction for advanced ovarian cancer. A multi-center analysis of surgical and oncological outcomes. *Gynecol Oncol* 2012;126:220.

Peiretti M, Zanagnolo V, Aletti GD, et al. Role of maximal primary cytoreductive surgery in patients with advanced epithelial ovarian and tubal cancer: surgical and oncological outcomes. Single institution experience. *Gynecol Oncol* 2010;119:259.

Pittman DM, Smith LE. Complications of colostomy closure. *Dis Colon Rectum* 1985;28:836.

Piver MS, Barlow JJ, Lele SB, et al. Survival after ovarian cancer induced intestinal obstruction. *Gynecol Oncol* 1982;13:44.

Polglase AL, Cunningham IG, Hughes ES, et al. Initial clinical experience with the EEA stapler. *Aust N Z J Surg* 1982;52:71.

Pollock AV, Playforth MJ, Evans M. Preoperative lavage of the obstructed left colon to allow safe primary anastomosis. *Dis Colon Rectum* 1987;30:171.

Porter JA, Salvati EP, Rubin RJ, et al. Complications of colostomies. *Dis Colon Rectum* 1989;32:299 [in English].

Pothuri B, Montemarano M, Gerardi M, et al. Percutaneous endoscopic gastrostomy tube placement in patients with malignant bowel obstruction due to ovarian carcinoma. *Gynecol Oncol* 2005;96:330.

Pothuri B, Vaidya A, Aghajanian C, et al. Palliative surgery for bowel obstruction in recurrent ovarian cancer: an updated series. *Gynecol Oncol* 2003;89:306.

Poticha SM. A new technic for loop colostomy with use of a plastic bridge. *Am J Surg* 1974;127:620.

Prager E. The continent colostomy. *Dis Colon Rectum* 1984;27:235 [in English].

Prystowsky JB, Stryker SJ, Ujiki GT, et al. Gastrointestinal endometriosis. Incidence and indications for resection. *Arch Surg* 1988;123:855.

Pullan JM. Massive intestinal resection. *Proc R Soc Med* 1959;52:31.

Purdum PP III, Kirby DF. Short-bowel syndrome: a review of the role of nutrition support. *JPEN J Parenter Enteral Nutr* 1991;15:93.

Raahave D, Bulow S, Jakobsen BH, et al. Whole bowel irrigation: a bacteriologic assessment. *Infect Surg* 1986;12.

Rahbour G, Siddiqui MR, Ullah MR, et al. A meta-analysis of outcomes following use of somatostatin and its analogues for the management of enterocutaneous fistulas. *Ann Surg* 2012;256:946.

Rath KS, Loseth D, Muscarella P, et al. Outcomes following percutaneous upper gastrointestinal decompressive tube placement for malignant bowel obstruction in ovarian cancer. *Gynecol Oncol* 2013;129:103.

Ravitch MM. Varieties of stapled anastomoses in rectal resection. *Surg Clin North Am* 1984;64:543.

Reber HA, Roberts C, Way LW, et al. Management of external gastrointestinal fistulas. *Ann Surg* 1978;188:460 [in English].

Redmond P, Ambos M, Berliner L, et al. Iatrogenic intussusception: a complication of long intestinal tubes. *Am J Gastroenterol* 1982;77:39.

Reiling RB, Reiling WA Jr, Bernie WA, et al. Prospective controlled study of gastrointestinal stapled anastomoses. *Am J Surg* 1980;139:147.

Resnick SD, Burstein AE, Viner YL. Use of the stapler in anterior resection for cancer of the rectosigmoid. *Isr J Med Sci* 1983;19:128.

Richardson DL, Mariani A, Cliby WA. Risk factors for anastomotic leak after recto-sigmoid resection for ovarian cancer. *Gynecol Oncol* 2006;103:667.

Rubin SC, Hoskins WJ, Benjamin I, et al. Palliative surgery for intestinal obstruction in advanced ovarian cancer. *Gynecol Oncol* 1989;34:16.

Salani R, Zahurak ML, Santillan A, et al. Survival impact of multiple bowel resections in patients undergoing primary cytoreductive surgery for advanced ovarian cancer: a case–control study. *Gynecol Oncol* 2007;107:495.

Scarabelli C, Gallo A, Carbone A. Secondary cytoreductive surgery for patients with recurrent epithelial ovarian carcinoma. *Gynecol Oncol* 2001;83:504.

Scarabelli C, Gallo A, Franceschi S, et al. Primary cytoreductive surgery with rectosigmoid colon resection for patients with advanced epithelial ovarian carcinoma. *Cancer* 2000;88:389.

Schecter WP, Hirshberg A, Chang DS, et al. Enteric fistulas: principles of management. *J Am Coll Surg* 2009;209:484.

Scher KS, Scott-Conner C, Jones CW, et al. A comparison of stapled and sutured anastomoses in colonic operations. *Surg Gynecol Obstet* 1982;155:489.

Schmidt E. The continent colostomy. *World J Surg* 1982;6:805.

Schmitt EH III, Symmonds RE. Surgical treatment of radiation induced injuries of the intestine. *Surg Gynecol Obstet* 1981;153:896.

Schneider W, Nguyen-Thanh P, Dralle H, et al. Ileal J-pouch vaginoplasty reconstruction of a physiologic vagina with an ileal J-pouch (Vol 200, Pg 694.E1, 2009). *Am J Obstet Gynecol* 2009;201 [in English].

Scribner BH, Cole JJ, Christopher TG, et al. Long-term total parenteral nutrition. The concept of an artificial gut. *JAMA* 1970;212:457.

Sehapaya S, Mcnatt M, Carter HG, et al. Continuous sump-suction drainage of pelvis after low anterior resection—reappraisal. *Dis Colon Rectum* 1973;16:485 [in English].

Shafer KE, Cohen AC, Wiebke EA. Novel approach to surgical repair of enterovaginal fistula in the irradiated pelvis. *Plast Reconstr Surg* 2012;130:385e.

Shellito PC, Malt RA. Tube gastrostomy. Techniques and complications. *Ann Surg* 1985;201:180.

Silberman H, Granson M, Fong G, et al. Management of external gastrointestinal fistulas with glucose and lipids. *Surg Gynecol Obstet* 1980;150:856.

Silver DF, Zgheib NB. Extended left colon resections as part of complete cytoreduction for ovarian cancer: tips and considerations. *Gynecol Oncol* 2009;114:427.

Simchen E, Shapiro M, Sacks TG, et al. Determinants of wound-infection after colon surgery. *Ann Surg* 1984;199:260 [in English].

Smale BF, Mullen JL, Buzby GP, et al. The efficacy of nutritional assessment and support in cancer surgery. *Cancer* 1981;47:2375.

Smith DH, Pierce VK, Lewis JL Jr. Enteric fistulas encountered on a gynecologic oncology service from 1969 through 1980. *Surg Gynecol Obstet* 1984;158:71.

Smith GK, Farris JM. Re-evaluation of temporary gastrostomy as a substitute for nasogastric suction. *Am J Surg* 1961;102:168 [in English].

Smith JP. Complications related to the radiated gastrointestinal tract. In: Delgado G, Smith JP, eds. *Management of complications in gynecologic oncology*. New York: John Wiley & Sons, 1982:103.

Smith JP, Golden PE, Rutledge FN. *The surgical management of intestinal injuries following irradiation for carcinoma of the cervix, in cancer of the uterus and ovary.* University of Texas M.D. Anderson Hospital and Tumor Institute at Houston, Yearbook Medical Publishers Inc., 1969:241.

VIII

Smith ST, Seski JC, Copeland LJ, et al. Surgical management of irradiation-induced small bowel damage. *Obstet Gynecol* 1985; 65:563.

Soeters PB, Ebeid AM, Fischer JE. Review of 404 patients with gastrointestinal fistulas. Impact of parenteral nutrition. *Ann Surg* 1979;190:189.

Song YJ, Lim MC, Kang S, et al. Total colectomy as part of primary cytoreductive surgery in advanced Mullerian cancer. *Gynecol Oncol* 2009;114:183.

Spiliotis J, Briand D, Gouttebel MC, et al. Treatment of fistulas of the gastrointestinal-tract with total parenteral-nutrition and octreotide in patients with carcinoma. *Surg Gynecol Obstet* 1993;176:575 [in English].

Spirtos NM, Eisenkop SM, Schlaerth JB, et al. Second-look laparotomy after modified posterior exenteration: patterns of persistence and recurrence in patients with stage III and stage IV ovarian cancer. *Am J Obstet Gynecol* 2000;182:1321.

Steiger E, Srp F. Morbidity and mortality related to home parenteral nutrition in patients with gut failure. *Am J Surg* 1983; 145:102.

Swan RW, Fowler WC Jr, Boronow RC. Surgical management of radiation injury to the small intestine. *Surg Gynecol Obstet* 1976;142:325.

Tamussino KF, Lim PC, Webb MJ, et al. Gastrointestinal surgery in patients with ovarian cancer. *Gynecol Oncol* 2001;80:79.

Tan SG, Nambiar R, Rauff A, et al. Primary resection and anastomosis in obstructed descending colon due to cancer. *Arch Surg* 1991;126:748.

Tay EH, Grant PT, Gebski V, et al. Secondary cytoreduction surgery for recurrent epithelial ovarian cancer—in reply. *Obstet Gynecol* 2002;100:1360 [in English].

Tchervenkov CI, Gordon PH. Simple techniques of enlarging the diameter of the bowel lumen for the performance of end-to-end anastomoses using the EEA stapler. *Dis Colon Rectum* 1984;27:630 [in English].

Tebes SJ, Cardosi RJ, Hoffman MS. Colorectal resection and reanastamosis in ovarian cancer patients with rectosigmoid obstruction. *Gynecol Oncol* 2006;101:S138.

Tebes SJ, Sayer RA, Palmer JM, et al. Cytoreductive surgery for patients with recurrent epithelial ovarian carcinoma. *Gynecol Oncol* 2007;106:482.

Thomas RJ. The response of patients with fistulas of the gastrointestinal tract to parenteral nutrition. *Surg Gynecol Obstet* 1981; 153:77.

Thompson JS. Strategies for preserving intestinal length in the short-bowel syndrome. *Dis Colon Rectum* 1987;30:208.

Thompson JS. Surgical considerations in the short bowel syndrome. *Surg Gynecol Obstet* 1993;176:89.

Tomasdelavega JE, Banner BF, Haklin MF, et al. Effect of cimetidine on intestinal adaptation following massive resection of the small-intestine. *Surg Gynecol Obstet* 1983;156:41 [in English].

Tominaga K, Maetani I, Sato K, et al. Favorable long-term clinical outcome of uncovered D-weave stent placement as definitive palliative treatment for malignant colorectal obstruction. *Dis Colon Rectum* 2012;55:983.

Tsai MS, Liang JT. Surgery is justified in patients with bowel obstruction due to radiation therapy. *J Gastrointest Surg* 2006; 10:575.

Tunca JC, Buchler DA, Mack EA, et al. The management of ovarian-cancer-caused bowel obstruction. *Gynecol Oncol* 1981;12: 186 [in English].

Turina M, Mulhall AM, Mahid SS, et al. Frequency and surgical management of chronic complications related to pelvic radiation. *Arch Surg* 2008;143:46.

Tuson JR, Everett WG. A retrospective study of colostomies, leaks and strictures after colorectal anastomosis. *Int J Colorectal Dis* 1990;5:44.

Van Ooijen B, van der Burg ME, Planting AS, et al. Surgical treatment or gastric drainage only for intestinal obstruction in patients with carcinoma of the ovary or peritoneal carcinomatosis of other origin. *Surg Gynecol Obstet* 1993;176:469.

Vanek VW, Al-Salti M. Acute pseudo-obstruction of the colon (Ogilvie's syndrome). An analysis of 400 cases. *Dis Colon Rectum* 1986;29:203.

Varnell J, Pemberton LB. Risk factors in colostomy closure. *Surgery* 1981;89:683.

Vezeridis M, Evans JT, Mittelman A, et al. EEA stapler in low anterior anastomosis. *Dis Colon Rectum* 1982;25:364.

Wassner JD, Yohai E, Heimlich HJ. Complications associated with the use of gastrointestinal stapling devices. *Surgery* 1977;82:395.

Weigelt JA, Snyder WH III, Norman JL. Complications and results of 160 baker tube plications. *Am J Surg* 1980;140:810.

Wheeless CR Jr. Small bowel bypass for complications related to pelvic malignancy. *Obstet Gynecol* 1973;42:661.

Whittaker M, Goligher JC. A comparison of the results of extraperitoneal and intraperitoneal techniques for construction of terminal iliac colostomies. *Dis Colon Rectum* 1976;19:342.

Williams NS, Johnston D. Prospective controlled trial comparing colostomy irrigation with spontaneous-action method. *Br Med J* 1980;281:107.

Williams NS, Nasmyth DG, Jones D, et al. De-functioning stomas: a prospective controlled trial comparing loop ileostomy with loop transverse colostomy. *Br J Surg* 1986;73:566.

Winkler MJ, Volpe PA. Loop transverse colostomy. The case against. *Dis Colon Rectum* 1982;25:321.

Wolff BG, Beart RW Jr, Dozois RR, et al. A new bowel preparation for elective colon and rectal surgery. A prospective, randomized clinical trial. *Arch Surg* 1988;123:895.

Yassaie O, Thompson-Fawcett M, Rossaak J. Management of sigmoid volvulus: is early surgery justifiable? *ANZ J Surg* 2013;83:74 [in English].

Zang RY, Li ZT, Tang J, et al. Secondary cytoreductive surgery for patients with relapsed epithelial ovarian carcinoma: who benefits? *Cancer* 2004;100:1152.

Zani A, Eaton S, Rees CM, et al. Incidentally detected Meckel diverticulum—to resect or not to resect? *Ann Surg* 2008;247: 276 [in English].

Zannini G, Renda A, Lepore R, et al. Mechanical anterior resection for carcinoma of the midrectum—long-term results. *Int Surg* 1987;72:18 [in English].

Zera RT, Bubrick MP, Sternquist JC, et al. Enterocutaneous fistulas—effects of total parenteral-nutrition and surgery. *Dis Colon Rectum* 1983;26:109 [in English].

CHAPTER 48
Nongynecologic Conditions Encountered by the Gynecologic Surgeon

Kellie L. Mathis and William A. Cliby

DEFINITIONS

Hartmann procedure—Resection of the diseased colon (usually for diverticulitis) with end colostomy and oversewn rectal stump.

Mechanical bowel preparation—Vigorous oral preoperative cleansing of the bowel most commonly with balanced electrolyte solutions.

Phlegmon—An inflammatory mass with ill-defined borders; often precedes a defined abscess.

INTRODUCTION

In the majority of patients proceeding to the operating room for surgery in the pelvis, an accurate diagnosis has been made preoperatively. Advances in imaging should reduce the number of unanticipated findings intraoperatively for the pelvic surgeon. But, occasionally, the gynecologic surgeon will encounter an unexpected finding in the abdomen or pelvis intraoperatively arising from outside of the reproductive tract. This is commonly a problem in obese patients and elderly patients with atypical or ill-defined pelvic pathology and requires methodical consideration of the differential diagnosis preoperatively to appropriately triage and plan for these unanticipated findings. We discuss the most common nongynecologic findings in this chapter.

PREOPERATIVE EVALUATION

A thorough history and physical exam is absolutely critical. This should include presenting symptoms and past medical history as well as family history. The examination should include a thorough pelvic exam as well as a digital rectal examination. If the patient has any gastrointestinal complaints, a fecal occult blood test should be performed as well. Perianal abnormalities such as fistulae, atypical fissures, and large skin tags should raise the suspicion of Crohn disease.

If the patient complains of abdominal pain, low-grade fevers, changes in bowel habit, or blood in the stool, then a complete gastrointestinal workup should precede surgery. This may require endoscopy as well as computed tomography (CT) imaging. CT enterography should be ordered when there is a concern for small-bowel disorders. Patients suspected of having gynecologic infections and possible tuboovarian abscesses should be screened for sexually transmitted diseases.

If the patient has urinary symptoms, a urinalysis and culture should be done. If there is evidence of hematuria and/or bacteria, the patient should be treated for a urinary tract infection and reevaluation done to confirm clearance. If hematuria persists, further urinary workup should be considered to evaluate the upper urinary tracts as well as rule out intrinsic bladder pathology. This may include CT imaging, cystoscopy, or renal ultrasound.

PREOPERATIVE PREPARATION

The most important preoperative consideration is to make an accurate diagnosis or when not possible to define the differential diagnosis so the appropriate surgical expertise can be involved in the case. If there is any uncertainty about the diagnosis, an extensive discussion with the patient and informed consent about possible findings and interventions should occur. If there is any suspicion that intestinal surgery may be necessary, then the patient should be informed that a protective ostomy may also be necessary, and the abdomen should be marked preoperatively by a wound ostomy nurse. Emerging evidence suggests that postoperative complications are less common when a wound ostomy nurse sees, marks, and educates the patient preoperatively. Other subspecialists should meet and counsel the patient as appropriate. Other principles of safe surgery should be followed, including ensuring adequate nutritional and hydration status. Mechanical bowel preparation is no longer recommended or necessary for safe intestinal surgery. If the surgeon anticipates possible left-sided colon resection, and most commonly for pelvic pathology where pelvic colon involvement is always a possibility, we recommend that the patient be given two tap water enemas upon admission on the morning of surgery. The rectum should also be irrigated with dilute Betadine just before prepping the abdomen and perineum.

INTRAOPERATIVE FINDINGS AND MANAGEMENT

The patient should be placed in the modified lithotomy position, and a sterile Foley catheter should be placed. Appropriate antibiotics timed correctly should be given, and in most cases, venous thromboembolism prophylaxis would be recommended according to current standards of care. Ureteral stents should be considered, especially in the setting of multiply recurrent surgeries and large pelvic masses. Consider a minimally invasive approach (laparoscopic/robotic) to perform the operation, or in cases of uncertain etiology, a diagnostic laparoscopy can be performed to aid in the diagnosis or incision planning or to determine if triage to a higher-level care center is necessary. If an open approach is followed, careful placement of the abdominal incision is essential to ensure that the upper abdomen can be reached if necessary; a midline incision is preferred, particularly when the diagnosis is uncertain. Adhesiolysis should be performed first if necessary followed by a full abdominal exploration. Self-retaining retractors should be placed to minimize the risk of neurologic injury, particularly femoral nerve injuries, and avoid undue tension on the abdominal muscles. If the small intestine is uninvolved, then it should be packed away into upper abdomen. Generally, the patient is put in the Trendelenburg position, and the pelvis should then be assessed.

We now consider some of the nongynecologic pathology that may be encountered in the abdomen and pelvis.

GASTROINTESTINAL DISORDERS

Appendicitis

If appendicitis is in the differential diagnosis preoperatively, laparoscopy should be performed. A 12-mm Hasson trocar should be placed at the umbilicus with two additional 5-mm trocars in the suprapubic midline and left lower quadrant. The patient should be positioned with the right side up. If the appendix is grossly inflamed and dilated in the absence of other pathology, the appendix should be removed. The appendix should be gently grasped with a Babcock clamp. The mesoappendix can be transected using hemostatic clips or vessel-sealing device or with an endoscopic linear stapler. A stapler should be used to transect the appendix at the base of the cecum. The specimen can then be pulled through the umbilicus in a bag or glove to avoid wound contamination. If there is gross purulence due to perforation, the area should be copiously irrigated with saline prior to closure. If a phlegmon is encountered in the right lower quadrant and the cecum is involved, it is reasonable to abort the procedure and treat the appendicitis with intravenous antibiotics and percutaneous drainage if an abscess develops. Surgery in this setting is associated with higher morbidity. If an organized abscess is seen, placement of a drain at the time of surgery is suggested; in the case of a phlegmon, no drain is recommended.

Diverticular Disease

Diverticulosis is common among Americans, with prevalence rates up to 45%. Diverticulitis is inflammation of the diverticulum, usually occurring in the sigmoid colon, and it is generally managed nonoperatively. Uncomplicated diverticulitis accounts for 75% of all cases and is initially treated with bowel

VIII

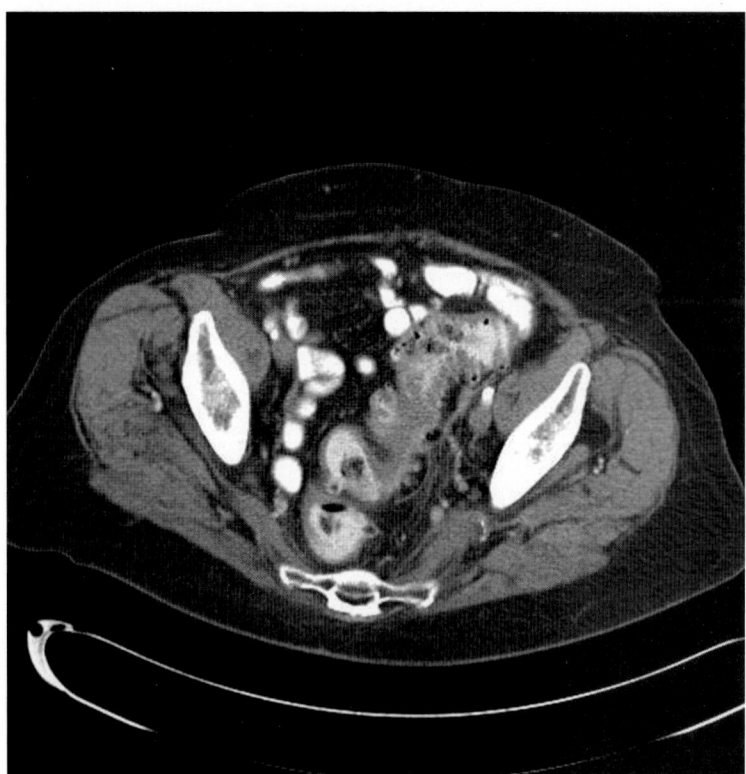

FIGURE 48.1 Uncomplicated sigmoid diverticulitis.

rest, antibiotics, and possible hospitalization (Fig. 48.1). Only when the attacks become recurrent and frequent enough to affect lifestyle is elective sigmoid resection entertained. Complicated diverticulitis (presence of abscess, perforation, fistula, or stricture) generally requires surgery (Figs. 48.2 to 48.4).

These cases often present to, or are referred to, a gynecologist because pain localizes to the pelvis and imaging demonstrates a pelvic mass, so a high index of suspicion is required when evaluating patients with preoperative gastrointestinal symptoms or systemic signs of infectious etiologies. When a

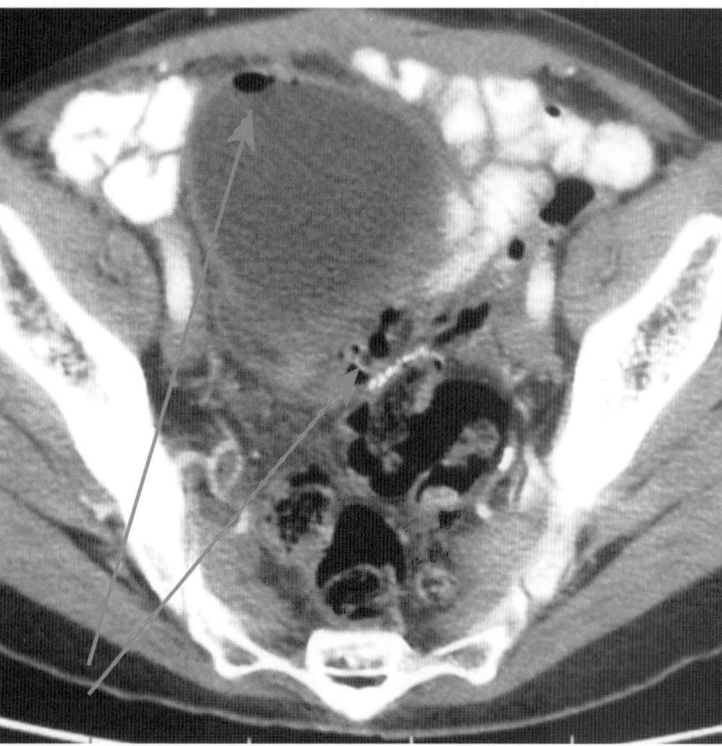

FIGURE 48.2 Sigmoid diverticular disease with colovesical fistula (note pericolic gas and gas in bladder [*arrows*]).

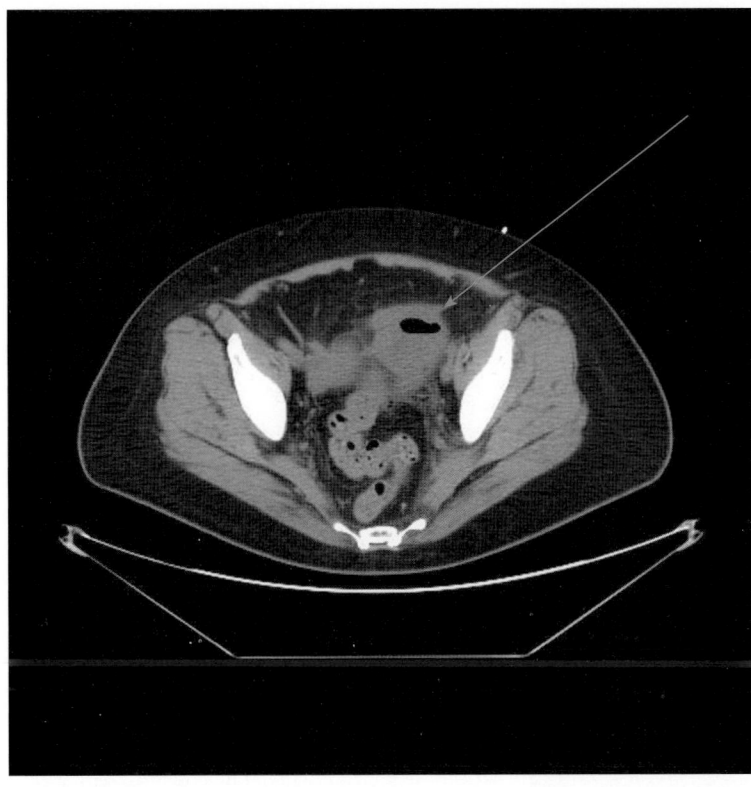

FIGURE 48.3 Complicated diverticulitis versus tuboovarian abscess (*arrow*).

contained abscess is seen on CT imaging, percutaneous drainage is attempted (Fig. 48.5). Surgery is ideally performed a few weeks after drain removal in an effort to avoid an end or diverting stoma. Patients with an acute perforation will present with an acute abdomen and require emergency surgery (Fig. 48.6).

If inactive diverticulosis is found intraoperatively, it should be ignored. Diverticulosis is common, and the majority of

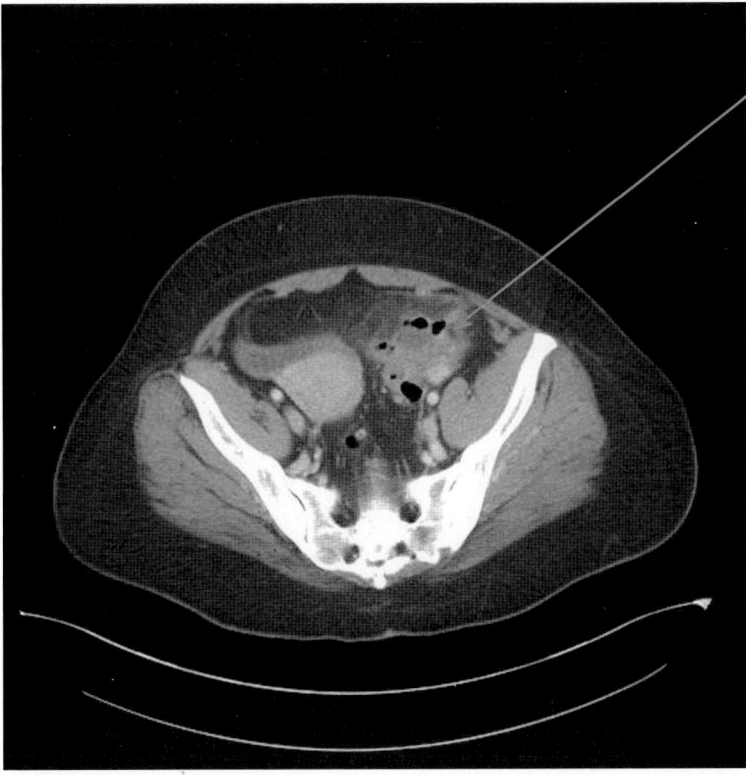

FIGURE 48.4 Perforated diverticulitis with abscess involving left adnexa (*arrow*).

VIII

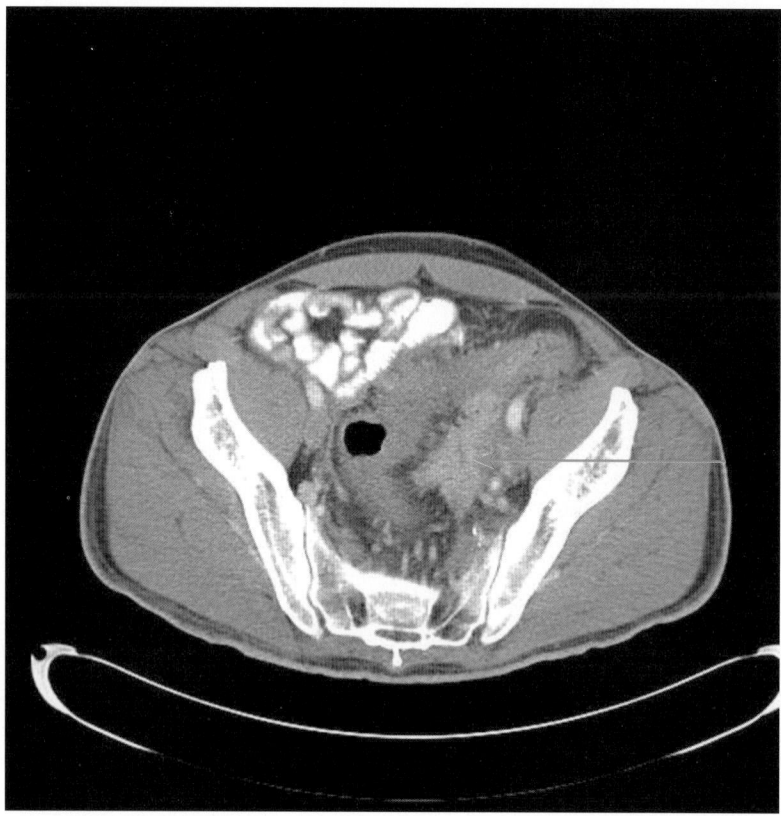

FIGURE 48.5 Acute sigmoid diverticulitis with a contained abscess (*arrow*).

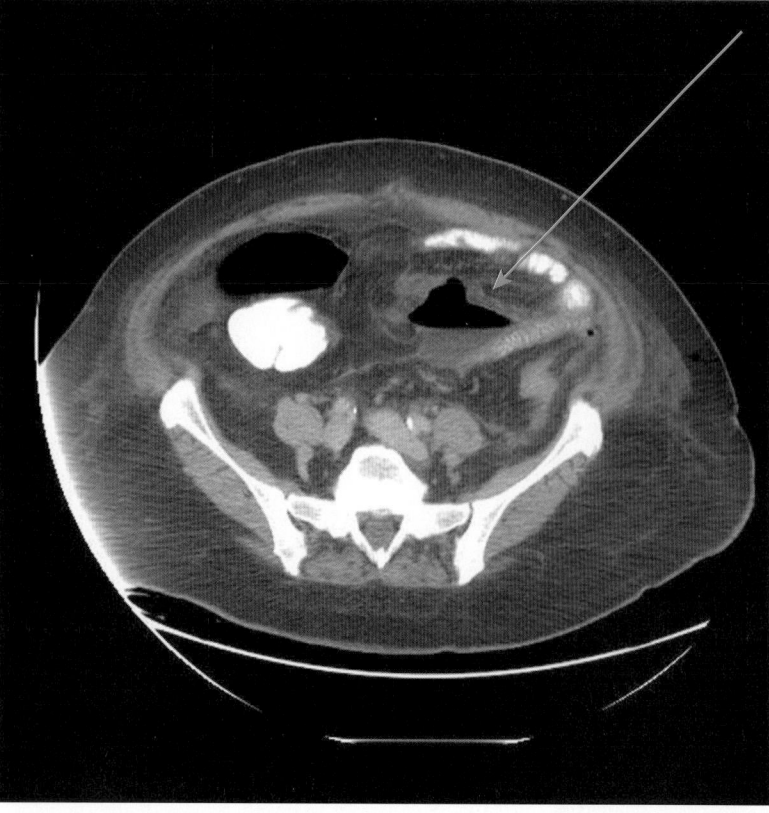

FIGURE 48.6 Acute diverticulitis with noncontained perforation (*arrow*).

patients will never require resection. If the patient has acute diverticulitis or chronic smoldering diverticulitis, it is reasonable to consider a sigmoid resection. The technique of sigmoid resection is outlined in the Steps in the Procedure box.

STEPS IN THE PROCEDURE

Sigmoid Resection for Diverticulitis

- Retract the sigmoid colon medially and separate the colon from the white line of Toldt and Gerota fascia. Identify and protect the left ureter and ovarian vessels.

- Mobilization of the splenic flexure may be necessary if there is not a natural redundancy in the colon.

- Divide the mesentery to the sigmoid colon, staying close to the bowel wall. This is done with right angle clamps and ligatures in the open technique and with a vessel-sealing device in the laparoscopic technique.

- Identify and transect the upper rectum with a TA stapler.

- Identify and transect the descending colon. Secure the anvil of the circular stapler into the proximal lumen with a purse-string suture.

- Perform a tension-free end-to-end stapled anastomosis using a circular stapler.

In order to avoid recurrence of diverticulitis, it is critical that the surgeon resects the entire sigmoid colon and perform the anastomosis between the soft and nonedematous descending colon and the upper rectum. It is not necessary to resect all of the diverticula from the proximal colon. Mobilization

of the splenic flexure may be required to perform an anastomosis without tension. If the setting of significant inflammation around the new connection, it is prudent to consider a temporary proximal diversion. If the tissue quality is poor (due to inflammation, edema, size mismatch, etc.), a Hartmann procedure is the safest approach.

Diverticulitis with an abscess involving the adnexa can sometimes be mistaken for a tuboovarian abscess, and this should always be in the differential diagnosis of a pelvic mass in the older female patient. In such cases, moderate elevation of CA-125 is common secondary to inflammation, which can further complicate the diagnostic challenge.

Colorectal Cancer

Cancers of the colon are common with over 100,000 new diagnoses in the United States every year. Ninety percent of colon cancers occur after the age of 50, but they can occur in every age group. Surgical resection is the primary treatment colon and rectal cancer. If a cancer of the colon is unexpectedly encountered intraoperatively, a decision should be made as to whether to proceed with bowel resection immediately or close the abdomen and perform the definitive surgery at a later date. If an operating surgeon experienced in oncologic colon resections is immediately available, then resection and primary anastomosis can be done. As stated before, mechanical bowel preparation is not necessary, but enemas are generally given preoperatively to empty the colon of the bulk of the stool for a left-sided resection. The most frequent tumors unexpectedly encountered by the gynecologic surgeon are cecal (**Figs. 48.7** and **48.8**) or rectosigmoid in location. Due to locations, these can often be mistaken for an adnexal mass. Techniques for each are described in the "Steps in the Procedure" boxes. The liver and peritoneal surfaces should be closely inspected for metastatic lesions prior to closure of the abdomen.

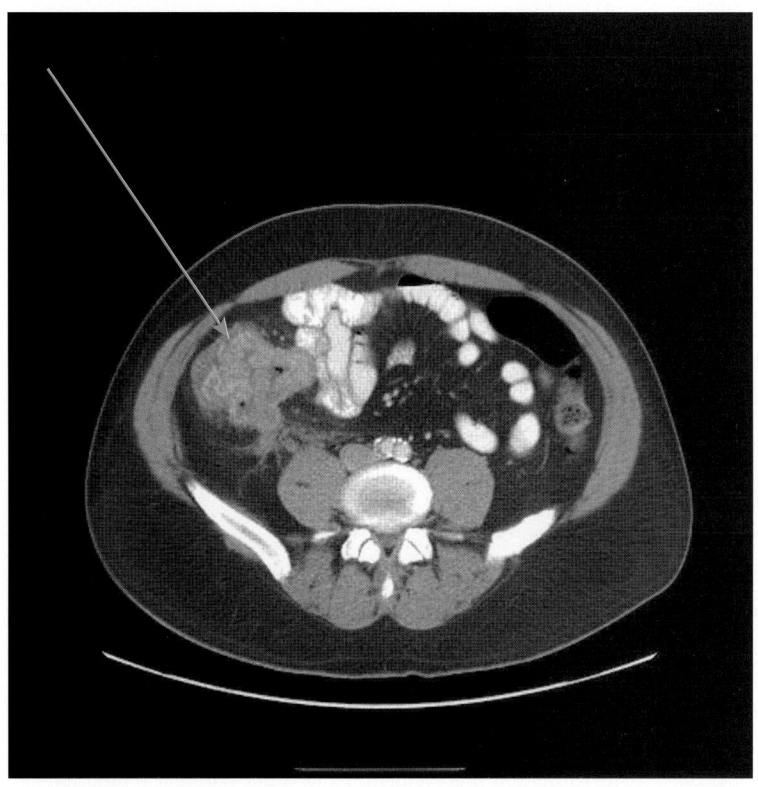

FIGURE 48.7 Advanced cecal cancer (*arrow*).

VIII

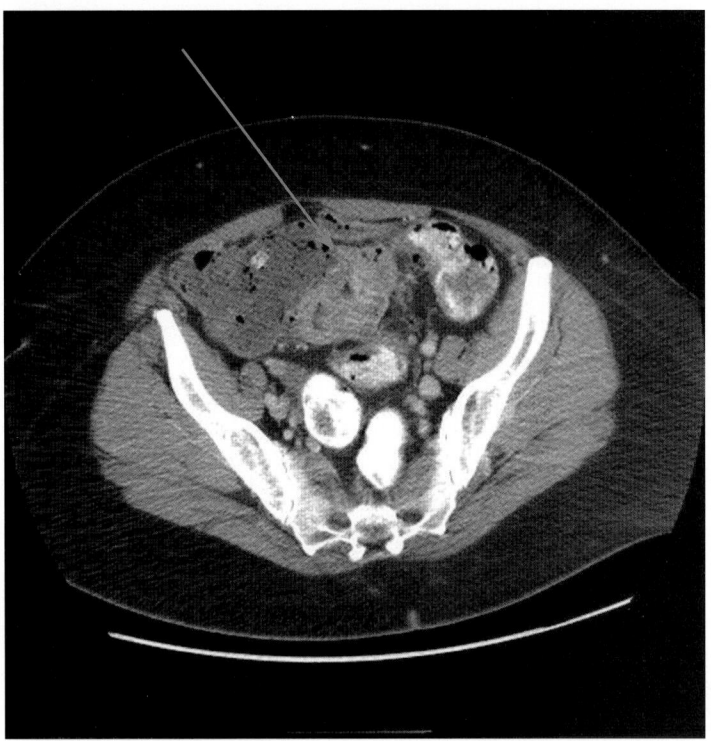

FIGURE 48.8 Large cecal cancer with local invasion into the sigmoid colon (*arrow*).

STEPS IN THE PROCEDURE

Right Colectomy Technique for Cecal Cancer

- Explore for resectability (omentum, peritoneum, liver, duodenum, superior mesenteric vessels).

- Retract the colon medially and separate the colon from the white line of Toldt and Gerota fascia. Identify and protect the ureter, gonadal vessels, and duodenum.

- Dissect the gastrocolic ligament to complete the mobilization of the hepatic flexure.

- Identify the appropriate vessels. Divide the ileocolic, right colic, and right branch of the middle colic vessels near their origins.

- Complete the mesenteric dissection. There is an expectation that at least 12 lymph nodes (LNs) are harvested because of a known survival advantage associated with increasing number of LNs.

- Wait for the demarcation of the bowel after vessel ligation, and then transect the terminal ileum and the transverse colon.

- Perform a side-to-side anastomosis using either a stapled or hand-sewn technique.

STEPS IN THE PROCEDURE

Sigmoid Colectomy Technique for Cancer

- Explore for resectability (omentum, peritoneum, liver).

- Retract the colon medially and separate the colon from the white line of Toldt and Gerota fascia. Identify and protect the left ureter and gonadal vessels.

- Mobilization of the splenic flexure may be necessary if there is no redundancy in the colon.

- Identify the appropriate vessels. Divide the inferior mesenteric vessels just beyond the takeoff of the left colic vessels and divide the sigmoidal branches.

- Complete the mesenteric dissection. There is an expectation that at least 12 LNs are harvested because of a known survival advantage associated with increasing number of LNs.

- Wait for demarcation of the bowel after vessel ligation to ensure adequate perfusion to the bowel outside the planned lines of resection.

- Identify and transect the upper rectum with a TA stapler.

- Identify and transect the descending colon. Secure the anvil of the circular stapler into the proximal lumen with a purse-string suture.

- Perform a tension-free end-to-end stapled anastomosis using a circular EEA stapler.

If a rectal mass concerning for cancer is encountered unexpectedly, it is best to close the abdomen and perform a thorough workup and staging. The management of rectal cancer is stage dependent with many patients benefiting from neoadjuvant chemoradiotherapy (Fig. 48.9).

Crohn Disease

Crohn disease is a chronic recurring inflammatory disorder that can affect the entire gastrointestinal tract. The most common site of midgut involvement is the ileum. There is a bimodal age distribution, with the first peak occurring in the second and

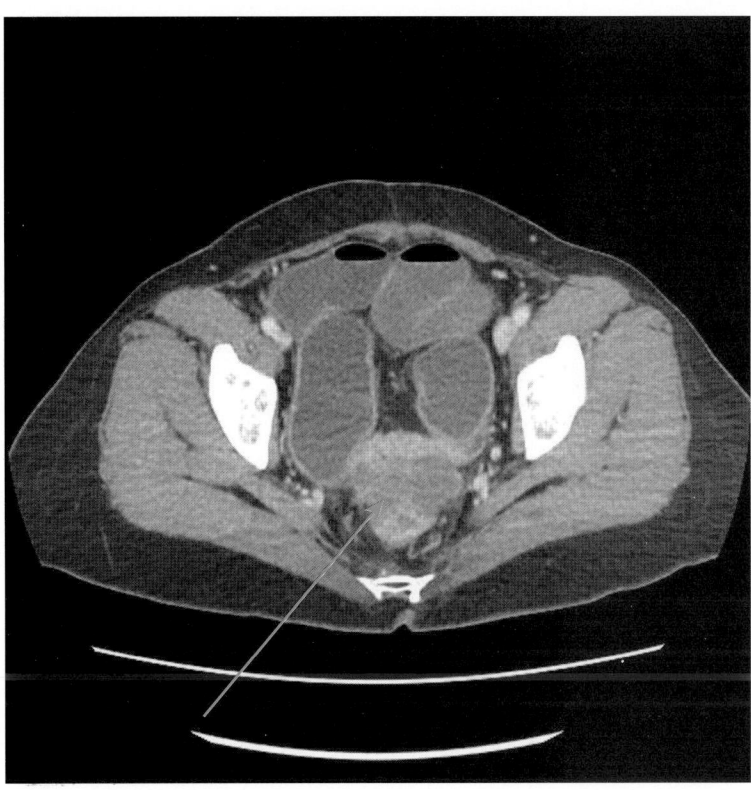

FIGURE 48.9 Recurrent rectal cancer with associated small-bowel obstruction (*arrow*).

third decades and the second peak occurring in the elderly. Symptoms are often vague and include chronic abdominal and pelvic pain. Patients can present with bowel obstructions from fibrotic strictures in the small and large bowel (**Fig. 48.10**). They can also suffer from intra-abdominal and pelvic fistulizing disease or abscess formation (**Fig. 48.11**). The diagnosis is usually made preoperatively by endoscopic findings in the case of colitis (ulcerations, pseudopolyps, skip lesions, granulomas, etc.) and by axial imaging with CT or magnetic resonance (MR) enterography in the setting of small-bowel disease. Surgery is

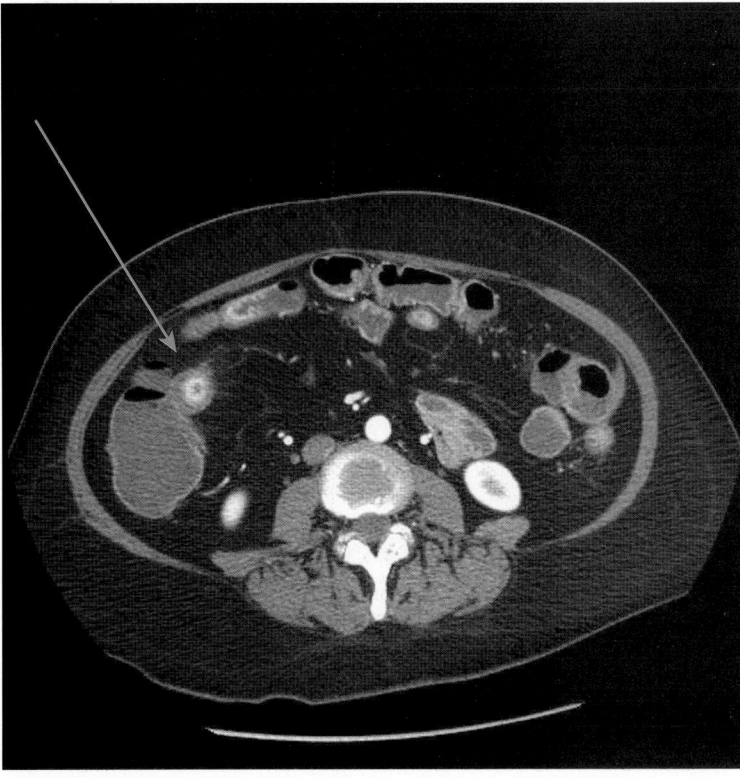

FIGURE 48.10 Stricturing disease in the terminal ileum in Crohn disease (*arrow*).

VIII

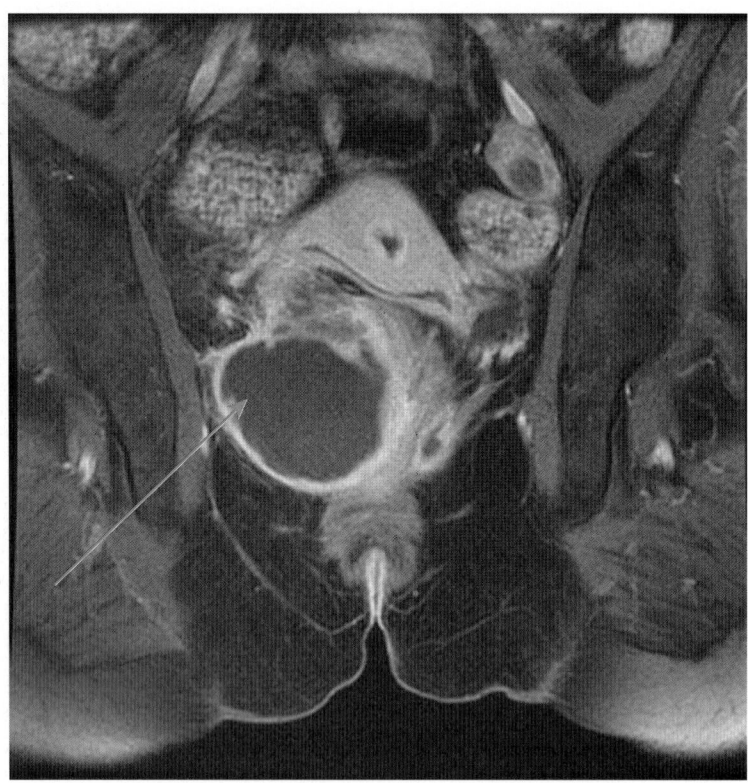

FIGURE 48.11 MR enterography showing a supralevator pelvic abscess in a patient with Crohn disease (*arrow*).

not curative and is, therefore, avoided until the patient develops medical intractability or failure to thrive. Intraoperatively, the surgeon may find inflammation of the ileum and cecum with the classic "creeping fat" along the antimesenteric side of the bowel. If this is found, it is best to close the abdomen and refer to gastroenterology for consideration of medical treatments. However, if the inflammation is associated with a proximal obstruction, a surgeon with experience treating inflammatory bowel disease should assist with ileocecal resection to grossly negative margins or stricturoplasty. If a contained abscess is found preoperatively, percutaneous drainage is preferred over surgical drainage. And if a phlegmon is encountered in the OR, conservative measures should be taken to avoid the risk of short-gut syndrome. Intestinal bypass procedures are not recommended due to the risk of blind loop syndrome and malignancy in the bypassed segment.

Carcinoid Tumors

Carcinoids are neuroendocrine tumors and may be found in the GI tract, lungs, and kidneys. Carcinoid tumors are the most common neoplasms of the appendix; they are usually asymptomatic but a common incidental finding at the time of pelvic surgery (**Figs. 48.12** and **48.13**). When a small mass at the tip of the appendix is found, a formal appendectomy as described earlier is appropriate. If the carcinoid is greater than 2 cm or located at the base of the appendix, a right hemicolectomy would ideally be performed. Carcinoids of the small intestine can be associated with extensive mesenteric lymphadenopathy and a small-bowel resection with careful mesenteric dissection is required. The liver should also be evaluated for evidence of metastases. Given the benefits of a systemic workup prior to extensive surgery, we would generally recommend a minimal initial procedure (e.g., appendectomy) in cases where an unexpected finding is encountered to allow a more complete workup and resection at a later date with appropriate expertise.

Meckel Diverticulum

Meckel diverticulum is the most common congenital abnormality of the GI tract and results from failure of the omphalomesenteric/vitelline duct to be obliterated. It is most commonly located in the ileum within 2 feet of the ileocecal valve and appears as an outpouching of the bowel at the antimesenteric border (**Fig. 48.14**). If a Meckel's is encountered, it should be palpated. If there are any masses palpable within the lumen of the Meckel's, our practice is to resect. A linear TA stapler can often be used to transect the base of the Meckel's, taking care not to narrow the lumen of the small intestine. If there is a concern of narrowing with a diverticulectomy, then a small-bowel resection with a two-layer hand-sewn end-to-end closure is preferred.

Small-Bowel Lymphoma

Surgery is not generally first-line therapy for this broad group of tumors, so a specialist should be consulted to determine if the patient should be closed or resection performed (**Fig. 48.15**). Generally, an excisional biopsy of an involved mesenteric LN is preferable over smaller biopsy or fine-needle aspiration to allow accurate pathologic diagnosis and subtyping of lymphomas. Lymphoma may also present as a retroperitoneal mass and should be considered in the differential of pelvic lymphadenopathy as management would be medical after appropriate biopsy.

Small-Bowel Adenocarcinoma

Localized adenocarcinomas of the small bowel are treated with resection of the primary tumor and the draining mesentery. Adjuvant therapy is often given, but no survival advantage has been shown. In patients with carcinomatosis, debulking therapy and intraperitoneal chemotherapy have been described.

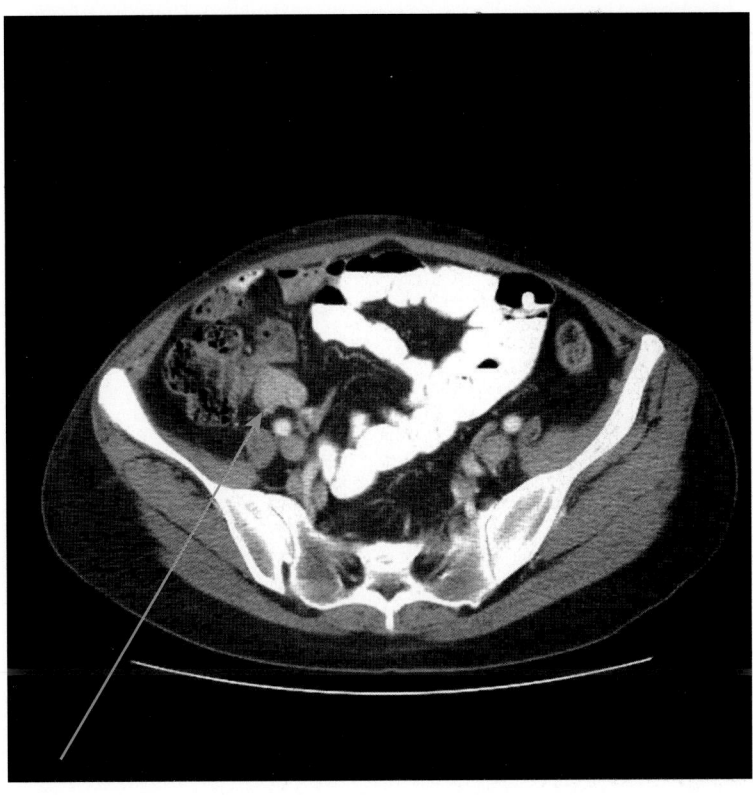

FIGURE 48.12 Appendiceal carcinoid tumor (*arrow*).

Intussusception

Intussusception refers to the invagination of a part of the intestine into itself, essentially an "internal prolapse." If this is identified in the operating room in an adult patient, the surgeon should search for a lesion (polyp, malignancy, Meckel's) that may be acting as a lead point. If a lead point is seen, a small-bowel resection should be performed. Preoperative CT scan will often show a "target sign." Colonic intussusception is caused by cancer until proven otherwise.

Gastrointestinal Stromal Tumors

Gastrointestinal stromal tumors (GISTs) are tumors of the GI tract characterized by a mutation in the KIT protooncogene. These tumors are often hemorrhagic and involving the antimesenteric portion of the small bowel (Fig. 48.16). Because of the small-bowel mobility, they often drape down into the pelvis and present as pelvic masses easily confused with adnexal tumors on exam and imaging. At laparoscopic assessment, this mobility can allow the tumor and small bowel to retract into the upper abdomen in association with steep Trendelenburg position. The surgeon should be aware of this possibility if no pelvic tumor is found. Absence of a pelvic mass previously demonstrated on exam or imaging should prompt a thorough evaluation of the remainder of the abdomen. Segmental bowel resection is the preferred surgical approach. The mesenteric dissection is minimized as LN metastasis is rare. Tyrosine kinase inhibitors are given in selected patients (unresectable disease, primary tumor >3 cm, high mitotic rate) in the adjuvant setting with improvement in recurrence rate. They have also been used in the neoadjuvant setting with success.

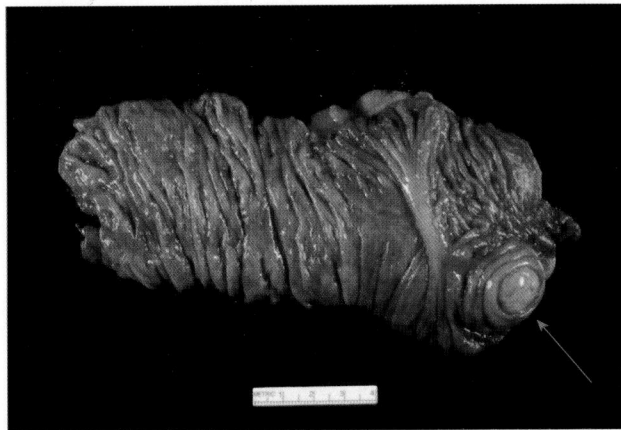

FIGURE 48.13 Right hemicolectomy for appendiceal carcinoid tumor (*arrow*).

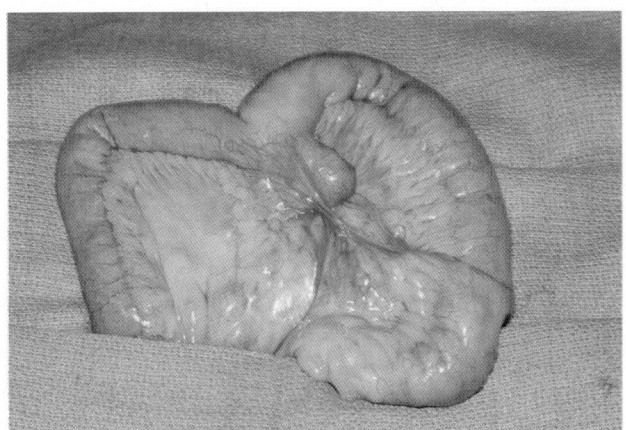

FIGURE 48.14 Meckel diverticulum with recent diverticulitis.

VIII

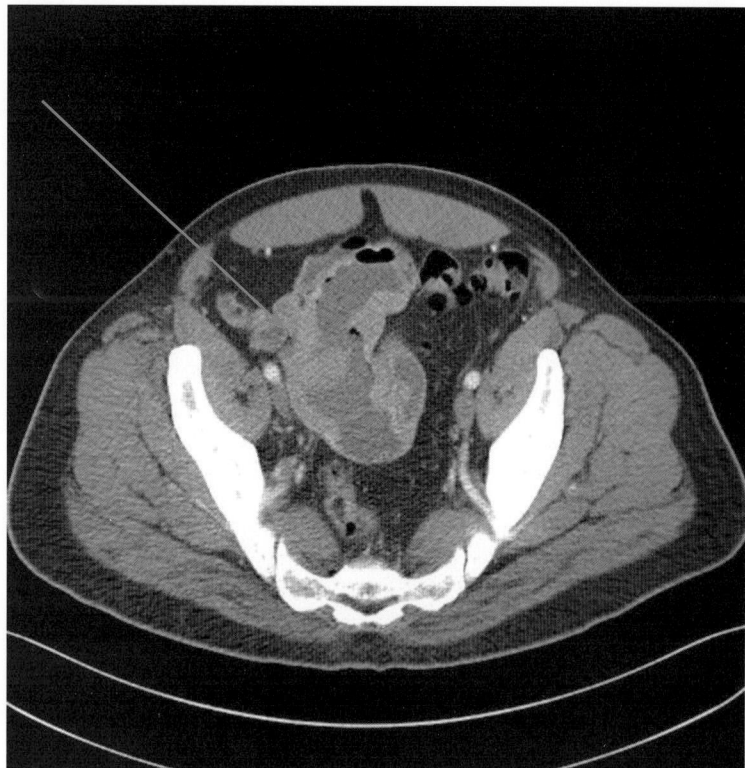

FIGURE 48.15 Large ileal lymphoma (*arrow*).

Epithelial Tumors of Appendiceal Origin

This includes a spectrum of lesions from mucoceles (**Fig. 48.17**) to pseudomyxoma peritonei (PMP). It is not possible to differentiate a benign mucocele from a cystadenocarcinoma by imaging, so we recommend performing an appendectomy if a cystic lesion is identified in the appendix. If a malignancy is identified, a right hemicolectomy should follow. It is critical that the appendix be handled with care; if a mucocele is ruptured (either spontaneously or iatrogenically), neoplastic

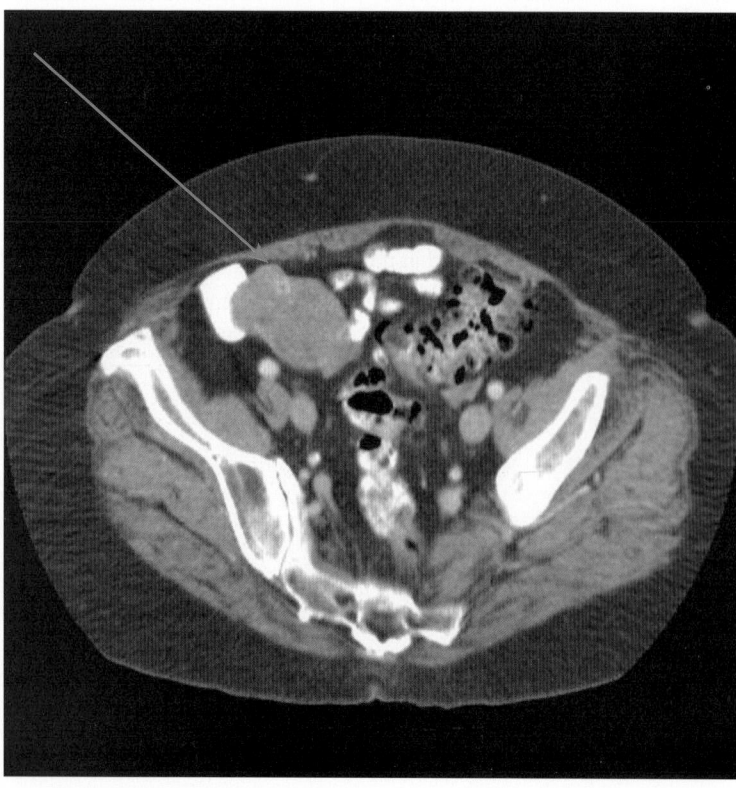

FIGURE 48.16 Terminal ileal GIST, axial view (*arrow*).

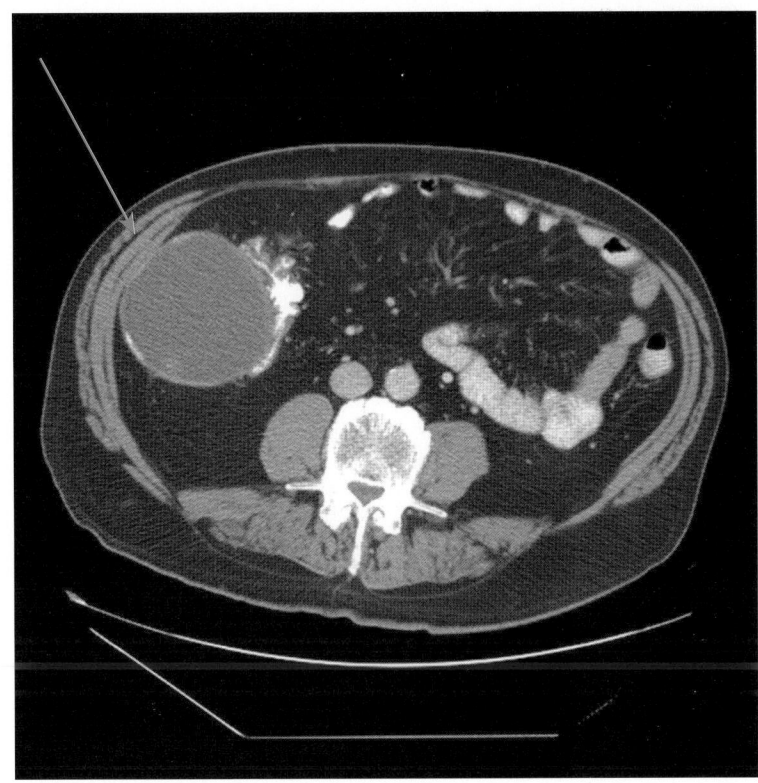

FIGURE 48.17 Mucocele of the appendix (*arrow*).

cells can be spread to the peritoneum. This could result in PMP. Treatment of PMP is surgical debulking with or without adjuvant therapy. Five-year survival is up to 75%, but recurrence is expected. PMP patients do benefit from aggressive surgical debulking and intraperitoneal chemotherapy, and this procedure should be performed only in experienced treatment centers. As an aside, when mucinous ovarian tumors are resected, the appendix should be carefully inspected as synchronous or metastatic lesions from appendix to ovary are common.

Fistulae

Fistulae from the small bowel to small bowel, small bowel to colon, small bowel to bladder, or small bowel to vagina should raise concern for Crohn disease, malignancy, or complications from prior surgery and/or radiation. Fistulae from the sigmoid colon to the bladder or vagina could be associated with any of the previous diagnoses as well as diverticulitis. The fistula should be treated according to the suspected cause. If malignancy is suspected, an en bloc resection is required. If the fistula is associated with an inflammatory or infectious disease, it is generally safe to finger fracture the organs apart, resect the segment of offending bowel, and repair the recipient side of the fistula.

UROLOGIC DISORDERS

Congenital

Pelvic kidney occurs in approximately 1 in 10,000 live births in the United States and can occur as a result of failure of migration of one kidney during embryogenesis or fusion of one pole of each kidney, which can result in a horseshoe kidney. When the fusion occurs at the lower poles, two ureters will be present. Extra care must be taken to identify and protect the ureters and the vascular supply to the pelvic kidney during any dissection. With current imaging modalities, these anatomic variants of ectopic kidneys should rarely present a diagnostic challenge in a case of a pelvic mass, excepting emergency cases. However, in a benign gynecologic procedure done for anatomic indications such as pelvic organ prolapse, imaging may often be omitted. It is paramount that the surgeon considers the possibility of ectopic kidney should a retroperitoneal mass be noted intraoperatively to avoid catastrophic iatrogenic injury.

Urologic Malignancies

Bladder cancer is the most common malignancy of the urinary tract and is most often urothelial in origin. Surgical treatment varies widely from transurethral resection with intravesical bacillus Calmette-Guerin (BCG) immunotherapy to radical cystectomy. Primary malignancy of the ureter is usually urothelial in origin, and in up to half of the patients, a synchronous bladder cancer will be present. Nephroureterectomy is the gold standard surgical procedure for localized disease. Extensive lymphadenectomy is controversial. Both bladder and ureteral cancers are best managed by an urologist, and incidental findings should prompt immediate referral to a urologic oncologist (Fig. 48.18).

Nephrolithiasis

Small stones (<4 mm) will usually pass spontaneously and stones greater than 10 mm in diameter are unlikely to pass. Stones that lead to urinary sepsis are treated with antibiotics and appropriate drainage (stenting or percutaneous nephrostomy). Most of these stones will then require lithotripsy or endoscopic removal after clearance of any associated infection. An urologist should be consulted for any obstructing stones found incidentally in the operating room.

VIII

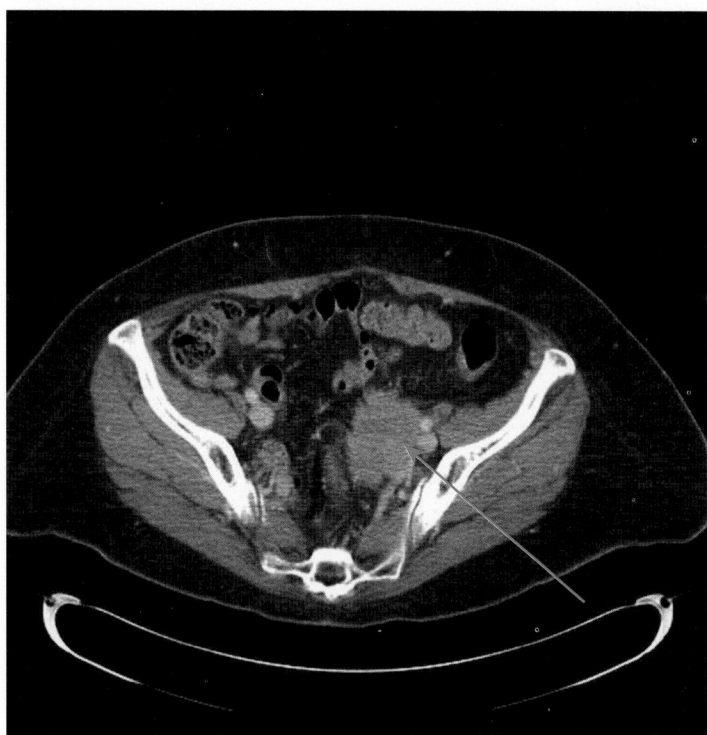

FIGURE 48.18 Urothelial cancer presenting as a pelvic mass (*arrow*).

VASCULAR NEOPLASMS

Angiomyxoma

Aggressive angiomyxoma is an uncommon hypervascular soft tissue tumor that is usually seen in the pelvis and perineum (Fig. 48.19). They often present as a perineal bulge or mass palpated on pelvic exam that is in the ischiorectal fossa. It is classified as a benign lesion as they rarely metastasize, but they are usually large and locally aggressive. Surgical resection is the treatment of choice, but local recurrence is very common (70% at 2 years). Complete resection is critical to minimize risk of recurrence and often requires a combined abdominal and perineal approach.

Hemangiopericytoma

Malignant hemangiopericytoma is a rare vascular tumor that may arise from small venules or capillaries of any

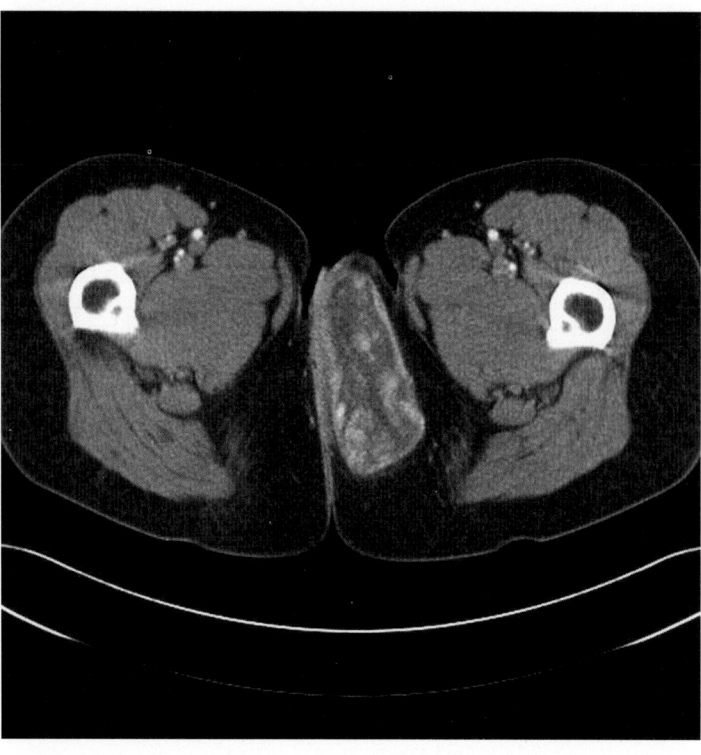

FIGURE 48.19 Angiomyxoma (*arrow*).

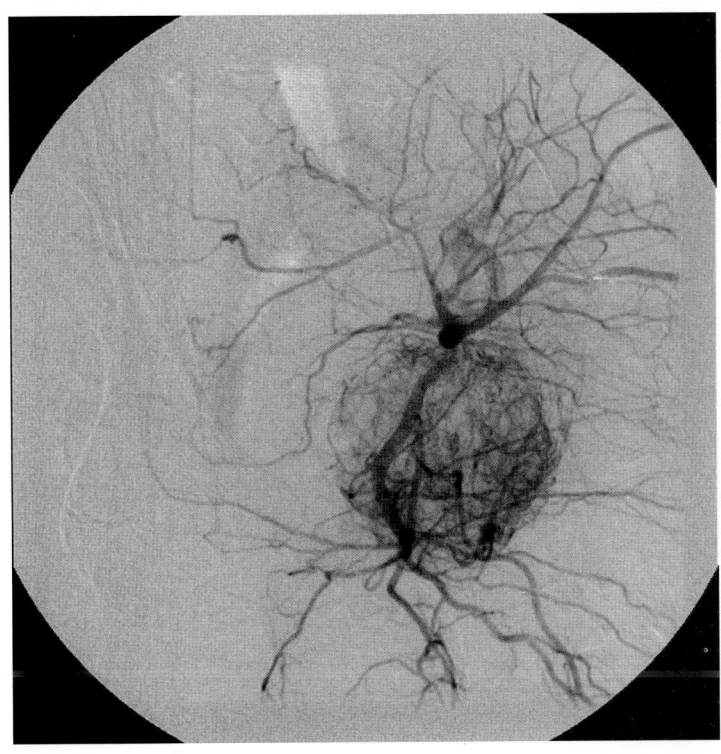

FIGURE 48.20 Hemangiopericytoma, vascularity appreciated on angiography.

structure. They are often found in the abdomen and/or pelvis and may be misdiagnosed preoperatively as an ovarian neoplasm. Surgery is first-line therapy, and use of adjuvant chemotherapy and radiation is described. Because of the vascularity, preoperative embolization of feeding vessels is often recommended to decrease the risk of catastrophic blood loss (Fig. 48.20).

PRESACRAL TUMORS

Many congenital, benign, and malignant lesions can originate in the retrorectal or presacral space, and they are often asymptomatic. As these masses enlarge, they may cause nonspecific symptoms from displacing or invading other structures (Figs. 48.21 and 48.22). Many of these lesions will be

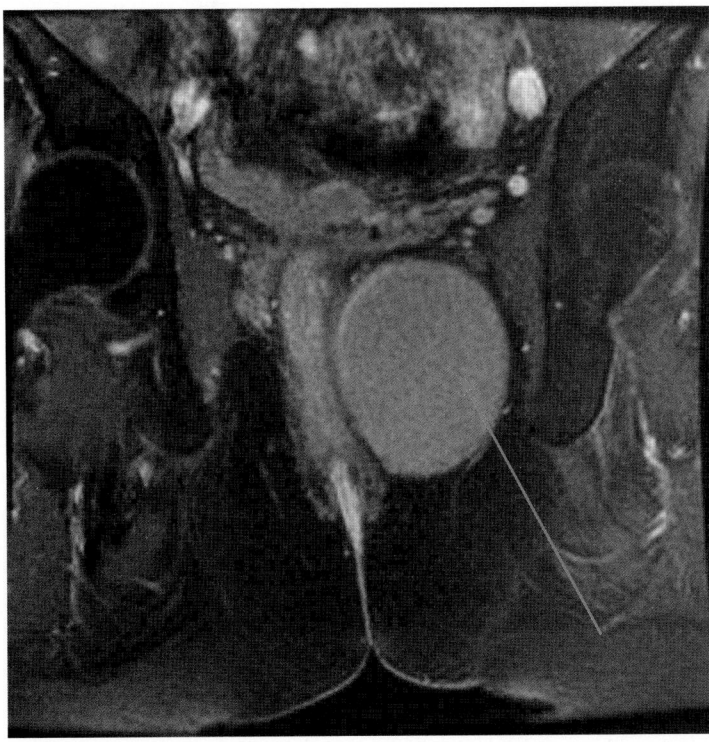

FIGURE 48.21 Large tailgut cyst displacing the rectum laterally (*arrow*).

VIII

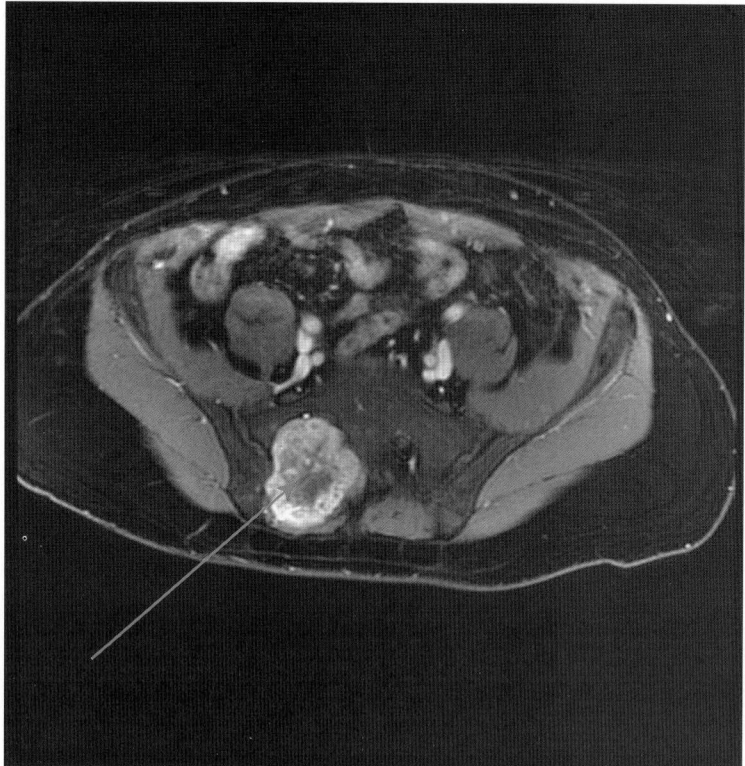

FIGURE 48.22 Pelvic schwannoma.

appreciated during the digital rectal examination and close inspection of the perineum, including the paracoccygeal region, during the preoperative physical examination. Careful inspection on exam and imaging will reveal a location that is atypical for most gynecologic processes as it will be far posterior in the pelvis, often retrorectal as opposed to disease in the cul-de-sac originating from the adnexa or+ uterus. There is typically limited mobility and fixation to the posterior pelvis. Congenital cystic lesions include developmental cysts, epidermoid and dermoid cysts, duplication cysts, and tailgut cysts. Tailgut cysts can harbor malignancy in up to 25% of cases. Meningoceles and meningomyeloceles are caused by herniation of the dural sac through a defect in the anterior sacrum. The sacrum of patients with meningoceles is abnormal with a "scimitar sign," which can be seen on a preoperative plain x-ray. Biopsy of a meningocele could result in fatal meningitis.

Solid lesions in the presacral space include teratomas and chordomas. Teratomas can be solid, cystic, or heterogeneous. They are usually benign, but malignant degeneration is common in adults. Chordomas are the most common malignancy of this region and are locally invasive with high recurrence rates despite radical resection.

As a general rule, if any of these lesions associated with the spine or fixed posteriorly are found incidentally, they should not be resected. Biopsies also should not be performed without consulting first with an expert in the field. Biopsies, if necessary, can usually be obtained percutaneously. These lesions all require specific preoperative workups and multidisciplinary approaches to their surgical management.

SUMMARY

With the availability of modern imaging, it is rare to proceed to the operating room without a narrow differential diagnosis. Gynecologic surgeons should be aware of the most common nongynecologic findings in the pelvis and lower abdomen and should prepare the patient and obtain an operative consent prior to the planned surgery which includes potential bowel resections and stomas.

BEST SURGICAL PRACTICES

- Consider broad differential preoperatively, and try to anticipate nongynecologic causes for a pelvic mass. Preoperative imaging and appropriate workup are essential.
- Establish functional close working relationships with nongynecologic surgical disciplines in your institution. This facilitates communication and availability for pre- and intraoperative consultations in emergent situations.
- If the diagnosis is uncertain, consider preoperative preparation with stents, bowel enemas, stoma markings, and appropriate consent.
- Assess the entire abdomen and pelvis, running the intestine from the ligament of Treitz to the rectosigmoid junction. This affects the choice of incision.
- Consult the expert when in doubt.
- Do not biopsy or attempt resection of any retroperitoneal mass.

BIBLIOGRAPHY

AUA and WOCN Society joint position statement on the value of preoperative stoma marking for patients undergoing creation of an incontinent urostomy. *J Wound Ostomy Continence Nurs* 2009;36:267.

Benn PL, Wolff BG, Ilstrup DM. Level of anastomosis and recurrent colonic diverticulitis. *Am J Surg* 1986;151:269.

Bergh P, Kindblom LG, Gunterberg B, et al. Prognostic factors in chordoma of the sacrum and mobile spine: a study of 39 patients. *Cancer* 2000;88:2122.

Chang GJ, Rodriguez-Bigas MA, Skibber JM, et al. Lymph node evaluation and survival after curative resection of colon cancer: systematic review. *J Natl Cancer Inst* 2007;99:433.

Connor SJ, Hanna GB, Frizelle FA. Appendiceal tumors: retrospective clinicopathologic analysis of appendiceal tumors from 7,970 appendectomies. *Dis Colon Rectum* 1998;41:75.

Dematteo RP, Ballman KV, Antonescu CR, et al. Adjuvant imatinib mesylate after resection of localised, primary gastrointestinal stromal tumour: a randomised, double-blind, placebo-controlled trial. *Lancet* 2009;373:1097.

Doyon C, Sideris L, Leblanc G, et al. Prolonged therapy with imatinib mesylate before surgery for advanced gastrointestinal stromal tumor results of a phase II trial. *Int J Surg Oncol* 2012;2012: 761576.

Eskicioglu C, Forbes SS, Fenech DS, et al. Preoperative bowel preparation for patients undergoing elective colorectal surgery: a clinical practice guideline endorsed by the Canadian Society of Colon and Rectal Surgeons. *Can J Surg* 2010;53:385.

Fanning J, Valea FA. Perioperative bowel management for gynecologic surgery. *Am J Obstet Gynecol* 2011;205:309.

Fazio VW, Marchetti F, Church M, et al. Effect of resection margins on the recurrence of Crohn's disease in the small bowel. A randomized controlled trial. *Ann Surg* 1996;224:563.

Fleshman JW. Pyogenic complications of Crohn's disease, evaluation, and management. *J Gastrointest Surg* 2008;12:2160.

Geerts WH, Bergqvist D, Pineo GF, et al. Prevention of venous thromboembolism: American College of Chest Physicians Evidence-Based Clinical Practice Guidelines (8th Edition). *Chest* 2008; 133:381S.

Golder WA. The "creeping fat sign"-really diagnostic for Crohn's disease? *Int J Colorectal Dis* 2009;24:1.

Gorospe EC. Adult intussusception presenting with target sign. *Scientific World Journal* 2008;8:1154.

Halfdanarson TR, McWilliams RR, Donohue JH, et al. A single-institution experience with 491 cases of small bowel adenocarcinoma. *Am J Surg* 2010;199:797.

Hinson FL, Ambrose NS. Pseudomyxoma peritonei. *Br J Surg* 1998;85:1332.

Hughes LE. Postmortem survey of diverticular disease of the colon. I. Diverticulosis and diverticulitis. *Gut* 1969;10:336.

Jacks SP, Hundley JC, Shen P, et al. Cytoreductive surgery and intraperitoneal hyperthermic chemotherapy for peritoneal carcinomatosis from small bowel adenocarcinoma. *J Surg Oncol* 2005;91:112.

Jensen MD, Nathan T, Rafaelsen SR, et al. Ileoscopy reduces the need for small bowel imaging in suspected Crohn's disease. *Dan Med J* 2012;59:A4491.

Lahat G, Madewell JE, Anaya DA, et al. Computed tomography scan-driven selection of treatment for retroperitoneal liposarcoma histologic subtypes. *Cancer* 2009;115:1081.

Lo NS, Sarr MG. Mucinous cystadenocarcinoma of the appendix. The controversy persists: a review. *Hepatogastroenterology* 2003;50:432.

Lughezzani G, Sun M, Perrotte P, et al. Should bladder cuff excision remain the standard of care at nephroureterectomy in patients with urothelial carcinoma of the renal pelvis? A population-based study. *Eur Urol* 2010;57:956.

Lughezzani G, Jeldres C, Isbarn H, et al. A critical appraisal of the value of lymph node dissection at nephroureterectomy for upper tract urothelial carcinoma. *Urology* 2010;75:118.

Mathis KL, Dozois EJ, Grewal MS, et al. Malignant risk and surgical outcomes of presacral tailgut cysts. *Br J Surg* 2010;97:575.

Miettinen M, Majidi M, Lasota J. Pathology and diagnostic criteria of gastrointestinal stromal tumors (GISTs): a review. *Eur J Cancer* 2002;38:S39.

Moertel CG, Weiland LH, Nagorney DM, et al. Carcinoid tumor of the appendix: treatment and prognosis. *N Engl J Med* 1987;317:1699.

Neale JA. Retrorectal tumors. *Clin Colon Rectal Surg* 2011;24:149.

Nguyen DL, Sandborn WJ, Loftus EV Jr, et al. Similar outcomes of surgical and medical treatment of intra-abdominal abscesses in patients with Crohn's disease. *Clin Gastroenterol Hepatol* 2012;10:400.

Oliak D, Yamini D, Udani VM, et al. Initial nonoperative management for periappendiceal abscess. *Dis Colon Rectum* 2001;44:936.

Olgac S, Mazumdar M, Dalbagni G, et al. Urothelial carcinoma of the renal pelvis: a clinicopathologic study of 130 cases. *Am J Surg Pathol* 2004;28:1545.

Person B, Ifargan R, Lachter J, et al. The impact of preoperative stoma site marking on the incidence of complications, quality of life, and patient's independence. *Dis Colon Rectum* 2012;55:783.

Dozois E, Herreros Marcos M. Presacral tumors. In: Wolff BG, Fleshman JW, Beck DE, et al., eds. *The ASCRS textbook of colon and rectal surgery*. New York: Springer, 2007:501.

Rafferty J, Shellito P, Hyman NH, et al. Practice parameters for sigmoid diverticulitis. *Dis Colon Rectum* 2006;49:939.

Roka YB, Koirala R, Bajracharya A, et al. Giant sacrococcygeal teratoma in an adult: case report. *Br J Neurosurg* 2009;23:628.

Rutledge RH, Alexander JW. Primary appendiceal malignancies: rare but important. *Surgery* 1992;111:244.

Sagar J, Kumar V, Shah DK. Meckel's diverticulum: a systematic review. *J R Soc Med* 2006;99:501.

Schulman J, Edmonds LD, McClearn AB, et al. Surveillance for and comparison of birth defect prevalences in two geographic areas— United States, 1983–88. *MMWR CDC Surveill Summ* 1993;42:1.

Siegel R, Naishadham D, Jemal A. Cancer statistics, 2013. *CA Cancer J Clin* 2013;63:11.

Smith HO, Worrell RV, Smith AY, et al. Aggressive angiomyxoma of the female pelvis and perineum: review of the literature. *Gynecol Oncol* 1991;42:79.

Sonnenberg A. Age distribution of IBD hospitalization. *Inflamm Bowel Dis* 2010;16:452.

Stocchi L, Wolff BG, Larson DR, et al. Surgical treatment of appendiceal mucocele. *Arch Surg* 2003;138:585.

Thaler K, Baig MK, Berho M, et al. Determinants of recurrence after sigmoid resection for uncomplicated diverticulitis. *Dis Colon Rectum* 2003;46:385.

VIII

CHAPTER 49
Malignancies of the Vulva

Mitchel S. Hoffman and Xiaomang B. Stickles

DEFINITIONS

Lymphoscintigraphy—A nuclear medicine study examining the distribution of uptake of radiocolloid (injected peritumorally) into the lymphatic system.

Modified radical vulvectomy—Radical removal of the portion of the vulva containing the tumor with approximately a 2-cm margin.

Neoadjuvant therapy—Therapy given prior to definitive surgical treatment, usually with the intention to decrease the required radicality of surgical resection.

Radical vulvectomy—Removal of the vulvar soft tissue. The lateral borders are the labiocrural folds. The anterior border is located in the mons pubis. The posterior border is across the perineal body. The medial borders are within the vestibule.

Sentinel lymph node—The concept of a sentinel lymph node in the context of malignancy relies on the presumption that this lymph node(s) is the initial site of metastatic disease and that the histology of the sentinel lymph node reflects the histology of the rest of the lymph nodes in the basin.

Superficial inguinal lymphadenectomy—Removal of the inguinal lymph nodes superficial to the cribriform fascia, mainly associated with the great saphenous and superficial epigastric veins.

INTRODUCTION

Carcinoma of the vulva is an uncommon malignancy accounting for only 2% of all female genital malignancies. It is predominantly a disease of older women. In this country as a whole, the steady increase in life expectancy has brought carcinoma of the vulva into a place of more importance among gynecologic malignancies. The predominant histologic type is squamous cell carcinoma, which accounts for about 90% of the tumors in most series. This malignancy metastasizes primarily through the lymphatic system in an orderly manner through the superficial inguinal, deep inguinal, and pelvic lymph nodes.

During the first half of the 20th century, the absolute 5-year survival rate for carcinoma of the vulva was 15%. During the late 19th and early 20th centuries, principles of surgical oncology were developed and put into clinical practice. The application of these surgical principles to the treatment of vulvar cancer resulted in a significant improvement in survival. The survival of patients with invasive squamous cell carcinoma of the vulva is dependent on a number of histopathologic factors, but it most closely relates to the pathologic status of the inguinal lymph nodes. Until the early 1980s, patients with invasive carcinoma of the vulva were routinely treated with radical vulvectomy and bilateral inguinofemoral and pelvic lymphadenectomy. Accumulation of data on vulvar cancer during the mid- to late 20th century led to earlier diagnosis and a better understanding of the nature and modes of spread of this disease. Especially over the past several decades, treatment of this malignancy has undergone a number of significant modifications resulting in less radical surgery with good survival rates and significantly better quality of life for women with this malignancy.

This chapter first reviews the epidemiology, clinical characteristics, staging, and prognostic factors for invasive carcinoma of the vulva. The broad spectrum of treatment of this disease is then reviewed with an emphasis on the surgical treatment. Finally, histologic variants of vulvar malignancy and their treatment are discussed individually.

EPIDEMIOLOGY

Invasive squamous cell carcinoma of the vulva is typically a disease of postmenopausal women, with a median age at diagnosis of about 65 years (Fig. 49.1). However, the age range is wide, and there appears to be an increasing incidence in younger women. This has been mainly attributed to infection with the human papillomavirus (HPV), which accounts for approximately 60% of vulvar squamous cell carcinoma. HPV subtypes 18 and 33 account for about half of HPV-associated vulvar cancers. HPV does not appear to play as significant of a role in the pathogenesis of invasive squamous cell carcinoma of the vulva in older women, who frequently have coexisting lichen sclerosis. In the older population, vulvar carcinoma commonly arises from a background of chronic inflammation without evidence of HPV involvement. Other sexually transmitted factors that have been epidemiologically associated with vulvar cancer are the granulomatous venereal diseases, especially in countries where these are prevalent.

It is to yet to be determined what effect the implementation of HPV vaccination will have on the incidence of vulvar squamous cell carcinoma. The full impact will likely not be known for many decades as vulvar carcinoma is most common in older women.

Vulvar carcinoma in situ (Fig. 49.2), like cervical carcinoma in situ, is considered a precursor to invasive disease, although the risk of progression appears to be lower. Although Jones and Rowan found in 7 of 8 women with untreated vulvar intraepithelial neoplasia (VIN) that invasive cancer developed within 8 years, three other studies found progression rates of 5% to 16%. In a recent systematic review of 3,322 published patients, 8 of 88 untreated women with VIN 3 progressed to invasive cancer in 12 to 96 months. In a large review, 3.2% of women treated with partial or total vulvectomy for VIN were found to have occult invasive cancer. However, several selected series showed higher rates of 16% to 22%. The risk

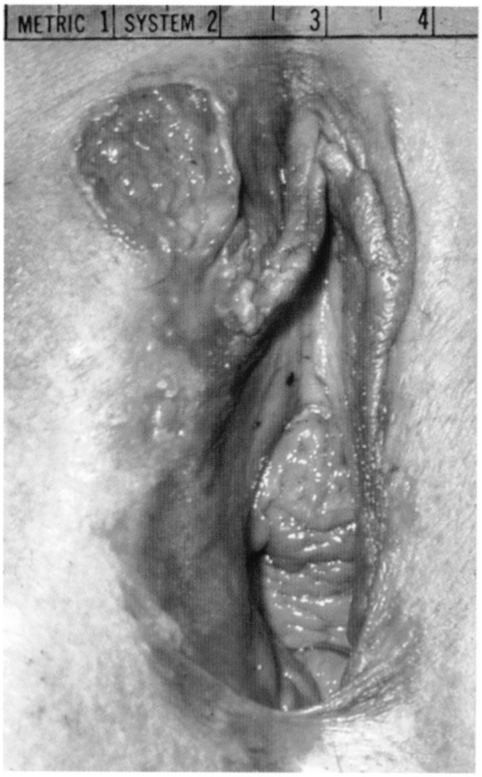

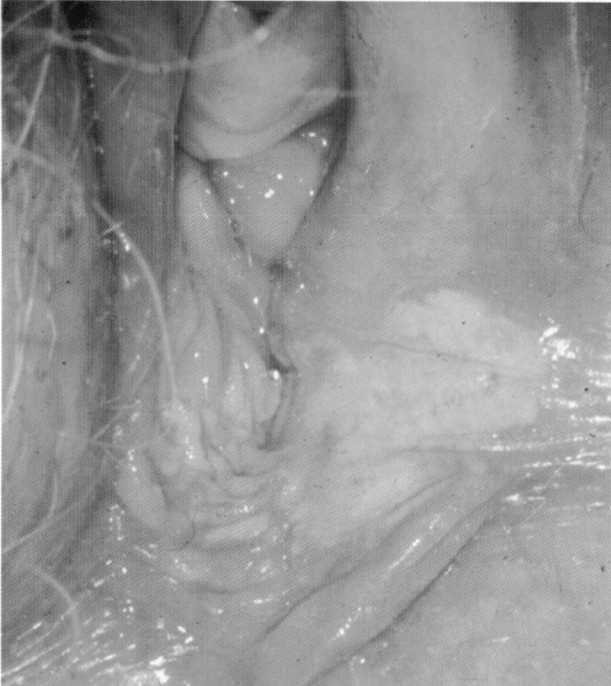

FIGURE 49.1 Invasive squamous cell carcinoma of the vulva. This is a 1.8-cm ulcerative lesion on the right anterior vulva.

for invasive cancer may be greater with perianal location, increased age, immunosuppression, and previous radiotherapy.

Vulvar carcinoma in situ tends to be multifocal with a lower risk of invasive cancer in younger women, but it tends to be unifocal with a higher risk of invasive disease in older women. Most patients with VIN 3 should be treated, and long-term follow-up is mandatory. Although progression of VIN from grade 1 to grades 2 and 3 has been demonstrated, in the absence of atypical changes, other vulvar epithelial abnormalities do not appear to have significant precancerous potential. Patients who have cervical neoplasia are at increased risk for developing vulvar neoplasia and vice versa. This so-called field phenomenon should heighten the physician's surveillance for the development of other lesions once a lower genital tract neoplasm occurs.

Hypertension and diabetes mellitus are common in patients with invasive vulvar cancer, but this may simply be related to the elderly population affected. The association of vulvar cancer with obesity is unclear. There does not appear to be any significant association with parity or race. Smoking is associated with an increased risk of vulvar cancer. One group that does appear to be at particular increased risk for the development of invasive vulvar cancer is chronically immunosuppressed women.

CLINICAL PRESENTATION

The most common initial symptom of vulvar cancer is pruritus, which may be of long duration. Vulvar pain, discharge, and bleeding are less commonly reported. The patient often becomes aware of a lesion on her vulva; but because of the superficial nature of the lesion, delay in seeking medical help is common. Physician delay has also been commonly reported, often related to prolonged empiric medical treatment before a biopsy is done.

Invasive squamous cell carcinoma of the vulva may present as an exophytic, cauliflower-like lesion or it may have an ulcerative appearance (**Fig. 49.3**). It involves the labia majora in about two thirds of patients. The remaining tumors involve the clitoris, labia minora, posterior fourchette, and perineum. These cancers can be exophytic, ulcerating, or flat. Rarely, a patient may present with erosive tumor growth from the groin nodes if symptoms have been ignored for long periods of time.

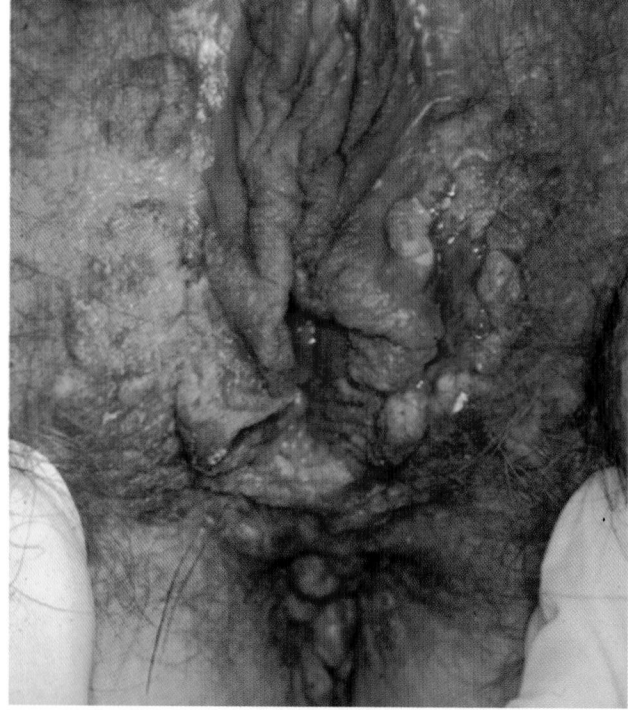

FIGURE 49.2 Carcinoma in situ of the vulva. Vulvar intraepithelial lesions can be white, brown, or red.

FIGURE 49.3 Invasive carcinoma of the left vulva with extensive associated carcinoma in situ involving both labia.

HISTOLOGY

Squamous cell carcinoma accounts for about 90% of the invasive vulvar malignancies. Melanoma is the second most common histologic type, accounting for 5% to 10% of vulvar cancers. Some of the less common vulvar malignancies include Bartholin gland carcinoma (either adenocarcinoma or squamous carcinoma), basal cell carcinoma, verrucous carcinoma, invasive Paget disease, and sarcomas.

PRETREATMENT INVESTIGATION

Biopsy

The relative rarity of vulvar cancer and the general lack of awareness of typical signs and symptoms, even by medical professionals, frequently lead to a delay in diagnosis. These observations underscore the need for patient and physician education with regard to the early diagnosis of carcinoma of the vulva. Therefore, biopsy of any questionable vulvar lesion prior to empiric treatment is warranted. Vulvar biopsy is a simple procedure that can be done in the office under local anesthesia. Biopsy technique is demonstrated in Chapter 23 (Fig. 23.1).

Preoperative Clinical Evaluation

Patients with carcinoma of the vulva are generally elderly and often have coexisting medical problems. A thorough preoperative evaluation by internal medicine and anesthesiology consultants should be requested when appropriate. As previously discussed, these women have an increased incidence of cervical and vaginal neoplasia, indicating the importance of a careful pelvic examination and Pap test screening.

Imaging Studies

Beyond physical examination and a chest radiograph, routine studies to rule out metastases are generally not indicated except in the presence of locally advanced disease. Cystoscopy, intravenous pyelography, or proctoscopy (or all three) is indicated if it appears that locally advanced cancer may involve the bladder, urethra, or rectum. Magnetic resonance imaging (MRI) or computed tomography (CT) may help to determine resectability and treatment planning. When a locally advanced tumor or inguinal lymph node enlargement is noted, CT scan of the groins, pelvis, and abdomen is suggested. This aids in determining the resectability of the tumor and metastases, extension to the pelvic lymph nodes, and

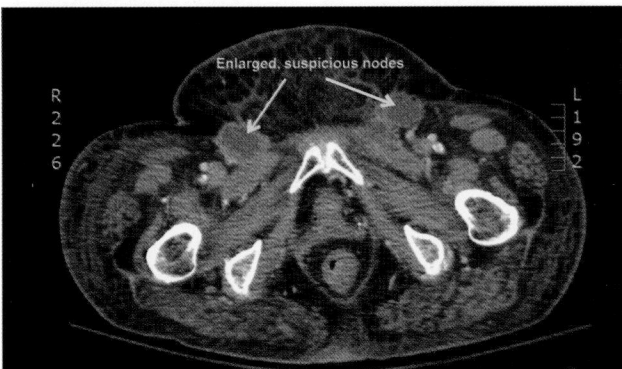

FIGURE 49.4 Computerized tomography (CT) image of the inguinal area showing enlarged lymph nodes typical for metastatic cancer (*arrows*).

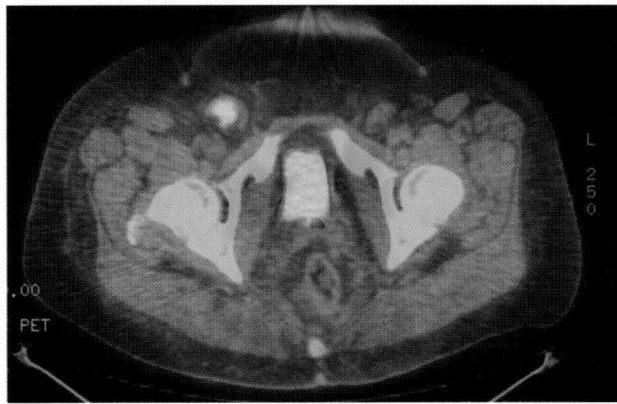

FIGURE 49.5 Positron emission tomography (PET) of the groin areas showing significantly increased FGD uptake in bilateral nodes very typical of metastatic cancer (same patient as in **Fig. 49.4**).

distant metastases (**Fig. 49.4**). Increasingly, positron emission tomography (PET) has been utilized to evaluate the presence or absence of metastatic disease, though scant data exist to support its use in vulvar cancer (**Fig. 49.5**). In a small series of 15 patients reported by Cohn and colleagues, the sensitivity of PET in detection of pathologically confirmed groin metastasis was 67% and specificity was 95%. Another recent analysis by Kamran et al. showed a sensitivity of only 50% and specificity and positive predictive value of 100%. Larger studies validating its utility are lacking. Due to limited sensitivity, omission of lymphadenectomy should not be based on PET results alone.

STAGING

Route of Spread

Squamous cell carcinoma of the vulva can spread by local extension to involve the vagina, urethra, anus, or pubic bone. Metastasis is primarily via the lymphatic system, but hematologic spread is also possible. The lymphatics of the labia communicate to the inguinal lymph nodes. The lymphatics of the perianal area drain in a similar manner, but lesions that involve the vagina, anus, or rectovaginal septum can drain directly into the pelvic lymph nodes. Although there are channels that interconnect the clitoris to the deep pelvic nodes, it appears that they are of minimal clinical significance. The lymphatics of the vulva are numerous and tend to cross the midline. The regional lymph nodes include the superficial inguinal nodes, the deep inguinal–femoral nodes, and the pelvic lymph nodes. The superficial inguinal lymph nodes are the primary nodal group of the vulva. Depending on the location of the primary carcinoma, one or two of these superficial inguinal nodes is the first site of metastatic spread. This node is referred to as the *sentinel lymph node*. Because of the predictably orderly progression of lymph node metastases in vulvar cancer, involvement of the deeper femoral lymph nodes or the pelvic nodes is very infrequent if the sentinel node(s) is uninvolved. These superficial inguinal lymph nodes drain through the cribriform fascia to the femoral lymph nodes. Drainage from here is under the inguinal ligament into the pelvic lymph nodes. The pelvic lymph nodes are virtually never positive in the absence of inguinofemoral lymph node metastases. The invasion of lymph node metastases roughly correlates with the size of the primary tumor.

IX

TABLE 49.1 2009 FIGO Staging System for Vulvar Cancer

STAGE	EXTENT
IA	Lesion ≤2 cm and stromal invasion ≤1 mm, confined to vulva or perineum, no nodal metastasis
IB	Lesion >2 cm or stromal invasion >1 mm, confined to vulva or perineum, no nodal metastasis
II	Tumor of any size with extension to adjacent perineal structures (one-third lower urethra, vagina, or anus), no nodal metastasis
III	Tumor of any size with or without extension to adjacent perineal structures with positive inguinofemoral lymph nodes
IIIA	(i) With one lymph node metastasis (≥5 mm) (ii) One to two lymph node metastasis (<5 mm)
IIIB	(i) With two or more lymph node metastasis (≥5 mm) (ii) With three or more lymph node metastasis (<5 mm)
IIIC	With positive nodes with extracapsular spread
IVA	(i) Upper urethral and/or vaginal mucosa, bladder mucosa, rectal mucosa, or fixed to pelvic bone (ii) Fixed or ulcerated inguinofemoral lymph nodes
IVB	Distant metastasis, including pelvic lymph nodes

FIGO Staging System

In 1979, the International Federation of Gynecology and Obstetrics (FIGO) approved a clinical classification for invasive squamous cell carcinoma of the vulva. This was based on an analysis of tumor (T) by size and location; node (N) status by palpation; distant metastases (M) as assessed by physical examination; endoscopic evaluation of the bladder or rectum, or both; and radiologic investigation. Most patients with invasive carcinoma of the vulva are treated surgically, and it was recognized that the clinical evaluation of inguinal lymph node metastases was often inaccurate. Therefore, in 1988, FIGO approved a surgical staging system. This staging system has undergone several revisions over the years as new surgical pathologic findings have been correlated with outcome. The most recent FIGO staging classification adopted in 2009 is shown in Table 49.1.

Stage I is divided into stages IA and IB because primary tumors less than 2 cm in diameter with very superficial invasion have a very low incidence of lymph node involvement and these patients have an excellent prognosis. However, a number of patients with small tumors have been reported with metastatic disease, which emphasizes the importance of surgical staging whenever possible (Table 49.2).

In the FIGO staging revision of 2009, the involvement of lower one third of the urethra, vagina, or anus was downgraded from stage III to stage II. Stage III was subdivided to reflect the prognostic significance of both the number and extent of lymph node involvement.

With increasing use of sentinel lymph node biopsy for staging and improvements in anesthetic techniques and perioperative care, it is rare today that a patient cannot be surgically staged, but the old clinical staging system should be used with appropriate notation in such patients.

TABLE 49.2 Tumors with Invasion of Less Than 1 mm with Nodal Disease, Either at Diagnosis or Recurrence

INVESTIGATOR	PATIENT AGE	TUMOR SIZE (CM)	TUMOR GRADE	TUMOR DEPTH (MM)	CAPILLARY OR LYMPHATIC SPACE INVOLVEMENT	MONTHS TO DIAGNOSIS OF NODAL DISEASE	STATUS
Sedlis (1987)	61	2.5	4[a]	1		0	NA
Atamdede (1989)	75	1	1	0.72	No	13	AWD
van der Valden (1992)	84	1	3	0.3	No	20	DOD
Kelley (1992)	52	NA	NA	<1	NA	31	A at 27 mo
Stehman (1992)	57	2	3	0.6	NA	26	A at 35 mo
Thangavelu (2006)	64	NA	2	<1	No	3	DOD
	51	NA	1	0.9	No	36	DOD
Volgger (1997)	39	0.3	1	<1	No	4	DOD
Iyibozkurt (2010)	62	2	NA	<1	NA	27	DOD

[a]GOG grading system.
NA, not available; AWD, alive with disease; DOD, dead of disease; A, alive.

PROGNOSTIC FACTORS

Primary Tumor Characteristics

Primary tumor factors that appear to have prognostic importance include tumor diameter, depth of invasion or tumor thickness, tumor differentiation, lymph–vascular space involvement, and surgical margin status. Tumor involvement of the distal urethra, vagina, or perineum is also an adverse prognostic factor. Sedlis and colleagues reported on a Gynecologic Oncology Group (GOG) study of 272 patients with early vulvar cancer less than or equal to 5 mm in tumor thickness. They found that histologic grade, capillary-like space involvement, tumor thickness, and clitoral or perineal location were all significant predictors of groin node metastases. A subsequent GOG study reported by Homesley and associates on 588 evaluable patients with invasive carcinoma found lymph–vascular space involvement, tumor differentiation, age, and tumor thickness to be significant independent risk factors for groin node metastases. Factors that predicted an increased risk of local recurrence included margin status, large tumor size, and deep invasion. Tumor extending to less than 8 mm from surgical margin was associated with an increased risk of recurrence.

A few histologic variants of squamous cell carcinoma have been associated with a more favorable prognosis, including verrucous carcinoma (discussed later), warty carcinoma, carcinoma in situ with early stromal invasion, and keratoacanthoma.

Lymph Node Status

The status of the groin nodes is clearly the most important prognostic factor for patients with invasive squamous cell carcinoma of the vulva. This disease has a relatively low propensity for distant metastases. Recurrences tend to be local or regional, and even unremitting disease tends to remain locoregional for long periods of time.

The overall 5-year survival rate for all treated patients is about 60%, with a corrected 5-year survival rate of about 70%. In the GOG study previously mentioned, 65.5% of the patients had negative groin nodes and 34.5% had positive nodes; this is consistent with other reports in the literature. In this large surgically treated series, the survival rate was 90.9% for patients with negative lymph nodes and 57.7% for patients with lymph node metastasis. When the pelvic lymph nodes are known to be positive, the survival rate decreases to about 20%. Figure 49.6 shows the survival of patients with squamous cell carcinoma of the vulva staged with the older FIGO staging classification. No large studies have reported long-term results with the 2009 staging.

Metastatic involvement of multiple lymph nodes further decrease the prognosis that was recognized in the 2009 FIGO staging system, which subdivided stage III disease depending on the number of nodes involved and the size of the metastatic deposits. Several studies have shown that when only one lymph node is involved, survival is still quite good. However, survival decreases drastically with metastases to three or more

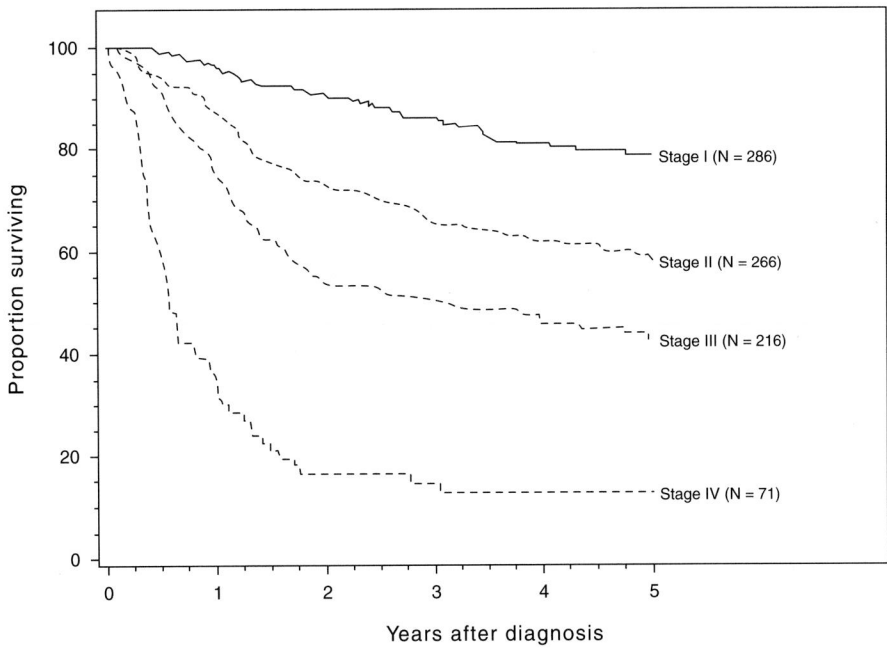

Stage	Patients (n)	Mean age (yr)	Overall survival (%) at					Hazards ratio[a] (95% CI)
			1 year	2 years	3 years	4 years	5 years	
I	286	64.0	96.4	90.4	86.1	80.7	78.5	Reference
II	266	69.7	87.6	73.2	65.9	62.0	58.8	1.9 (1.4–2.7)
III	216	69.3	74.7	53.8	50.2	45.9	43.2	3.3 (2.4–4.7)
IV	71	71.8	35.3	16.9	15.2	13.0	13.0	12.4 (8.3–18.5)

[a] Hazards ratio and 95% Confidence Intervals obtained from a Cox model adjusted for age, stage and country.

FIGURE 49.6 Survival curves for patients with squamous cell carcinoma of the vulva related to FIGO stage. These patients were treated from 1999 through 2001 and were staged according to the FIGO staging system of 1996. (Reprinted from Beller U, Benedet JL, Creasman WT, et al. Carcinoma of the vagina: 26th Annual report on the results of treatment in gynecological cancer. *Int J Gynecol Obstet* 2006;95:S29–S42, with permission. Copyright © 2006 International Federation of Gynecology and Obstetrics. Published by Elsevier Ireland Ltd. All rights reserved.)

IX

nodes or with bilateral nodal involvement. On the basis of limited data from a few studies, it appears that large nodal diameter, extensive nodal replacement, and especially extracapsular extension of a lymph node metastasis are adverse prognostic factors. In a report by Origoni and colleagues in 1992 that was based on 53 vulvar cancer patients with groin node metastases, the survival rate varied from 90.9% when the diameter of the metastasis was less than 5 mm to 20% when it was larger than 15 mm, and from 85.7% to 25% when the metastases were intracapsular and extracapsular, respectively. Especially important are the data from the 19 patients in that study with a single positive node. For these patients, the 5-year cancer-related survival rate was 90% when the metastasis diameter was less than 5 mm versus 37.5% when it was 15 mm, and 85.7% when the metastasis was intracapsular versus 20% when it was extracapsular. Results from a study by Paladini and associates were similar; they reported that patients with intracapsular metastases tended to have recurrence at distant sites, whereas patients with extracapsular nodal disease were more likely to have local or groin recurrence.

TREATMENT OF INVASIVE SQUAMOUS CELL CARCINOMA OF THE VULVA

Historical Perspective

In the 1940s, Taussig and Way reported favorable outcomes in carcinoma of the vulva after radical vulvectomy with bilateral inguinal lymphadenectomy performed by en bloc excision. This radical procedure then became the standard therapy applied to most patients. It involved radical removal of the entire vulva, the mons pubis, the inguinofemoral lymph nodes, and often the pelvic lymph nodes. The large surgical defect thus created was generally closed under tension with a high subsequent breakdown rate, significant postoperative morbidity, and marked disfigurement of the genital area. Important concerns with this approach for the treatment of vulvar cancer led to a number of modifications, especially over the past 25 years (Fig. 49.7). Some of these concerns include the high rate and the severity of wound complications and the psychosexual effects of radical removal of the vulvar tissues. Other potential problems related

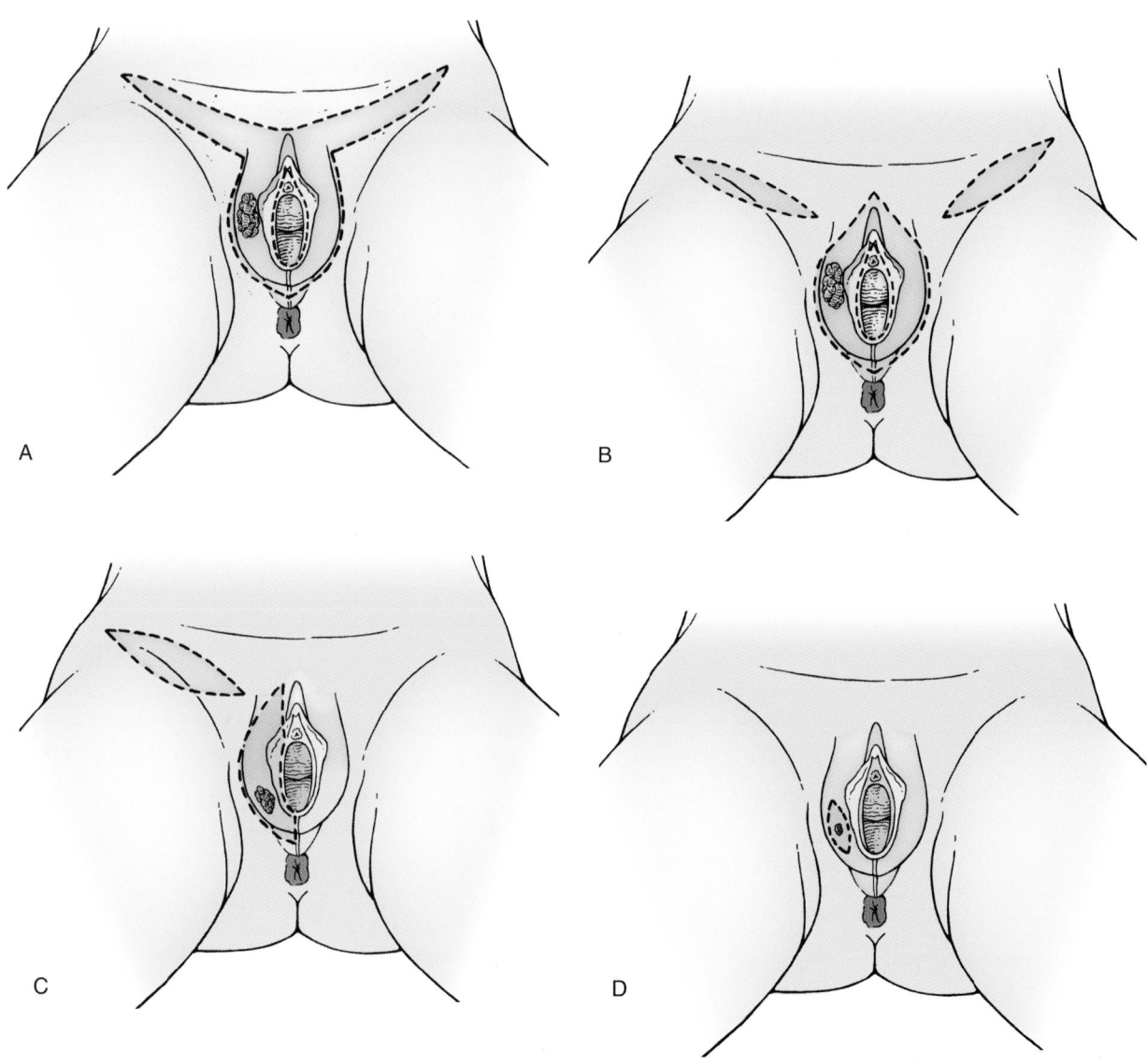

FIGURE 49.7 Modification in regional lymph node management. **A:** En bloc removal. **B:** Radical vulvectomy with bilateral inguinal–femoral lymphadenectomy through three separate incisions. **C:** Unilateral lymphadenectomy for a well-lateralized lesion. **D:** Early lesion with omission of lymphadenectomy.

to the en bloc radical resection include urinary or fecal incontinence and vaginal prolapse. The "one-size-fits-all" approach of treating all patients with the same radical vulvectomy and inguinal–femoral lymphadenectomy resulted in overtreatment of many patients and undertreatment of some with inadequate attention to local margin and the risk of lymph node metastasis. The following section provides a more individualized approach based on current literature and extensive surgical experience.

Primary Surgery: Selection of Appropriate Primary Operation

Appropriate Candidates for Primary Surgery

Certain tumor characteristics may preclude an otherwise medically fit patient from undergoing primary surgery. Proximity to important functional structures such as the urethra, clitoris, and anal sphincter must be considered. If adequate surgical margins cannot be obtained without sacrificing such a structure, neoadjuvant treatment with radiation and/or chemotherapy should be considered. Very large primary tumors may leave a large defect after primary resection, which may prove challenging to close. These patients may be candidates for neoadjuvant radiation plus chemotherapy to shrink the size of the primary cancer before surgical resection. The patient's ability to tolerate a radical resection must also be taken into consideration. Some elderly patients or those with significant comorbidities who may not recover from a radical resection would tolerate a more limited resection after neoadjuvant treatment.

Types of Incisions

The most important modification to the classic en bloc excision came after Hacker and colleagues and DiSaia and associates reported that separation of the vulvar and groin incisions resulted in a significant reduction in wound morbidity (**Fig. 49.7B**). The report by Hacker and colleagues in 1981 consisted of 100 patients in whom three separate incisions were used to perform the bilateral inguinofemoral lymphadenectomy and radical vulvectomy, leaving a bridge of tissue between the incisions and sparing the mons pubis. Major groin wound breakdown occurred in 14 patients, which was a considerable reduction from the 50% or higher groin wound breakdown rate generally seen with the en bloc excision. In this report, there were no isolated recurrences in either the groin or the inguinal skin bridge. There were two recurrences in the inguinal skin bridge associated with other recurrence sites; both patients originally had positive inguinal lymph nodes. In addition to these two patients, there have been other isolated reports of inguinal skin bridge recurrence. However, this still appears to be a rare event. Some authors believe that in the presence of advanced disease or grossly positive inguinal lymph nodes, an en bloc excision of the tumor and the lymph nodes is still the best approach. En bloc excision is certainly warranted at times to obtain an adequate resection of the malignancy.

Modified Radical and Radical Vulvectomy

Modified radical vulvectomy is an ambiguously defined operation that generally refers to radical removal of the portion of the vulva containing the tumor (**Fig. 49.8**). In recent

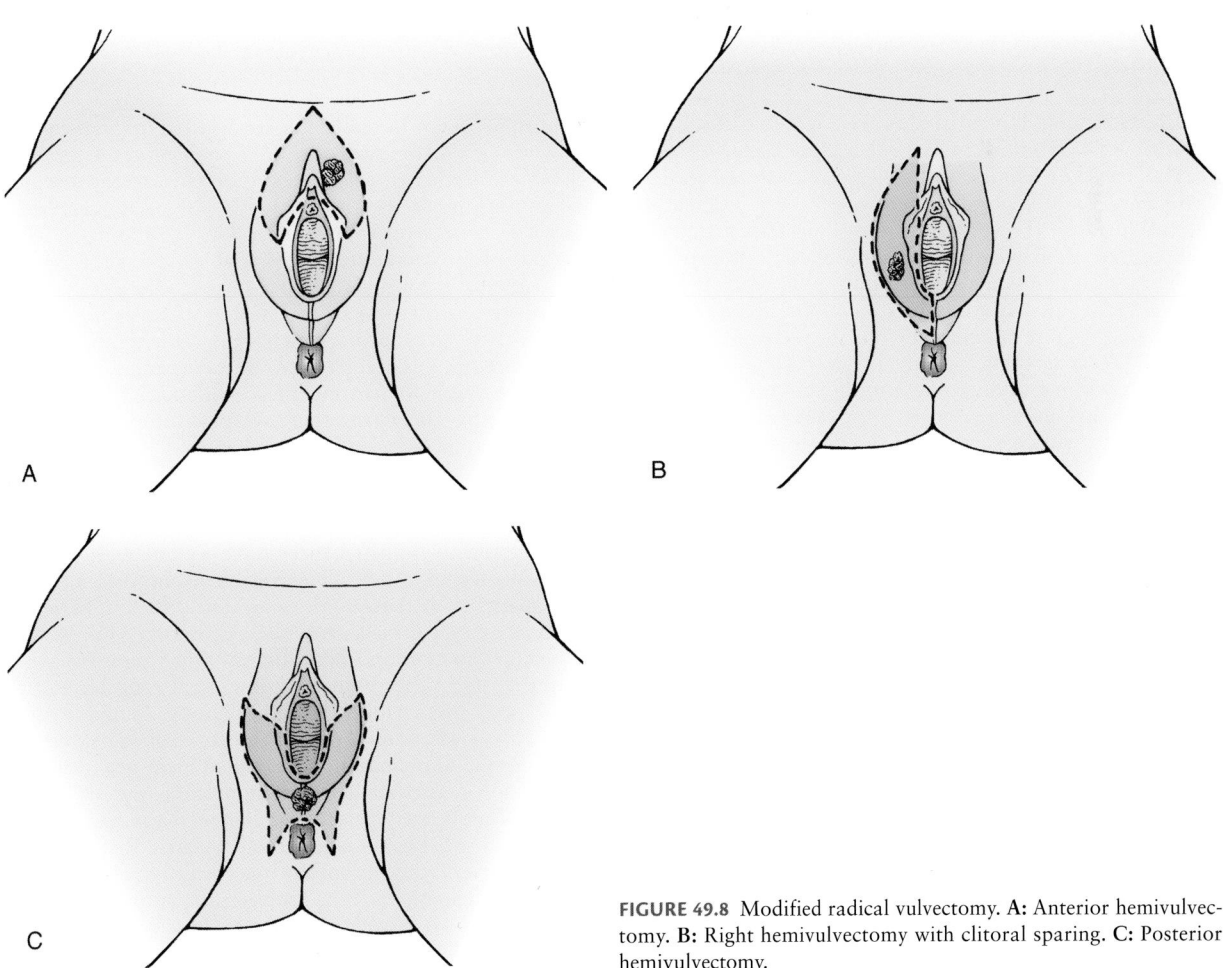

FIGURE 49.8 Modified radical vulvectomy. **A:** Anterior hemivulvectomy. **B:** Right hemivulvectomy with clitoral sparing. **C:** Posterior hemivulvectomy.

IX

years, the extent of the radical vulvectomy has been modified to emphasize wide excision of the primary cancer with adequate skin and deep margins but not necessarily radically resecting the entire (uninvolved) vulva. Recommendations have included 1- to 3-cm skin margins for well-localized, unifocal lesions and to the depth of the inferior fascia of the urogenital diaphragm. The main type of morbidity relating to increasing the radicality of vulvectomy is subsequent sexual dysfunction and disfigurement. Modification of the surgical resection or the use of neoadjuvant chemoradiation should be considered to avoid compromising the function of the anus or urethra. In a 1979 study, DiSaia and colleagues reported complete preservation of sexual function in 17 of 18 patients who underwent wide local excision for early invasive tumors. They also reported that preservation of the mons pubis as well as the major portion of the superior aspect of the vulva resulted in an appreciably more satisfactory cosmetic result.

The chief concerns with decreasing the radicality of vulvectomy are the possibility of an increased risk of local recurrence and later an increased risk of a second primary vulvar cancer. Hacker and colleagues have demonstrated that the extent of the vulvectomy can be decreased as long as careful attention to the margins is observed. They compared radical vulvectomy (56 patients) with wide local excision (28 patients) in the treatment of superficially invasive squamous cell carcinoma of the vulva. The local recurrence rate was identical, 4% in both groups. A later review by Hacker and van der Velden of literature regarding patients with vulvar cancer 2 cm or less in diameter showed a local invasive recurrence rate of 7.2% for 165 patients treated with radical local excision versus 6.3% for 365 patients treated with radical vulvectomy. In a comparative study reported by Hoffman, 45 patients underwent radical vulvectomy and 45 patients were treated with modified radical vulvectomy. The local recurrence rates were 2.2% and 4.4%, respectively. Several additional studies have reported excellent local control with a modified radical vulvectomy (Table 49.3).

In a GOG study, Stehman and colleagues analyzed recurrences following modified radical hemivulvectomy. The mean time to "relapse" on the vulva was 43.4 months, and 11 of 18 patients had recurrence on the contralateral side from the primary lesion. This suggests a second cancer rather than a true local recurrence. A study by de Hullu and associates also reported a significant number of late recurrences following modified radical vulvectomy. From these results, it is apparent that women undergoing a modified vulvar operation for cancer are at increased risk for later development of a new primary vulvar tumor and require long-term close follow-up.

It appears reasonable to conclude that modified radical vulvectomy is an efficacious treatment for well-localized invasive squamous cell carcinoma of the vulva. Attention should be focused on obtaining a 2-cm gross margin around the tumor while sparing as much vulvar tissue as possible. Most patients with squamous cell carcinoma of the vulva are candidates for a modified radical vulvectomy via a separate incision from the groin lymphadenectomy. A few patients, however, by virtue of disease extent, require a traditional radical vulvectomy with radical resection of the entire vulva. Whatever the vulvar phase of the operation is called, the aim should be to excise the tumor with a 2-cm gross margin.

Because of tumor proximity, it is occasionally necessary to remove a portion of the urethra to obtain an adequate resection of a vulvar carcinoma. Although several authors have stated that removal of the outer urethra does not result in significant problems with incontinence, there are no substantial

TABLE 49.3 Modified Radical Vulvectomy Literature: Local Recurrence			
INVESTIGATOR	NO. OF PATIENTS	LOCAL RECURRENCE (%)	MINIMUM FOLLOW-UP (MONTHS)
Di Saia (1979)	18	0	7
Hacker (1984)	28	1 (4%)	24
Burrell (1988)	28	0	16
Berman (1989)	50	4 (8%)	12
Sutton (1991)	56	7 (13%)	1
Stehman (1992)	121	10 (8%)	36
Hoffman (1992)	45	1 (2%)	12
Lin (1992)	12	2 (17%)	24
Andrews (1994)	28	2 (7%)	12
Burke (1995)	76	9 (12)	NA
de Hullu (2002)	85	7 (8%)	NA
Arvas (2005)	40	17 (43%)	NA
Total	**587**	**60 (10%)**	

confirming data. In one small study, Reid and colleagues did find urinary incontinence to be a problem after resection of the distal urethra or even an excision close to the urethra. If a portion of the urethra is resected, a Foley catheter should be left in place (carefully taped to the leg) for about 1 week postoperatively to facilitate healing and to splint the urethra. A surgical anti-incontinence procedure should also be strongly considered at the time of resection, especially if there is any preoperative stress urinary incontinence or if more than 1 cm of the urethra has to be removed. Increasingly, consideration has been given to treating these patients with neoadjuvant radiotherapy and chemotherapy to minimize or avoid urethral resection.

There is scant literature concerning the local management of vulvar cancer with perianal involvement (Fig. 49.9). However, we have noted that about one third of our patients who are referred for vulvar cancer have lesions with perianal or anal involvement. The chief problems in the management of patients with these tumors are the difficulty in obtaining adequate surgical margins while attempting to preserve anal sphincter function and deciding on which patients would be better treated either with a more radical excision and colostomy or with neoadjuvant radiotherapy. In our experience with vulvar carcinoma, partial resection of the external anal sphincter in combination with radical local resection of perianal tissue is associated with a significant rate of subsequent fecal incontinence. Careful sphincter reapproximation and levator muscle plication are done in an effort to minimize incontinence. Other important measures include good bowel preparation preoperatively, prophylactic antibiotics, and careful postoperative bowel management. In addition, we have had

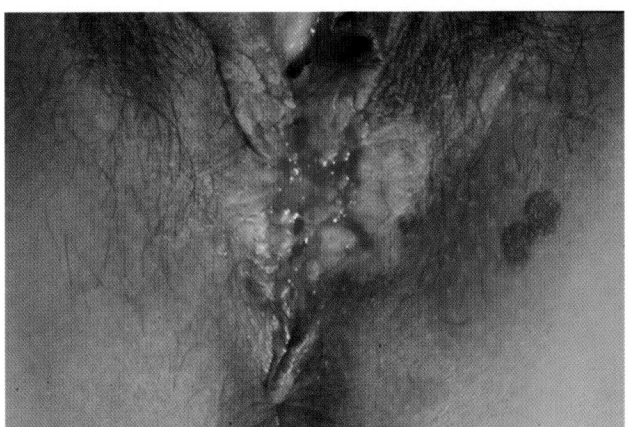

FIGURE 49.9 Invasive squamous cell carcinoma involving the perineum and perianal skin. Note the pigmented lesions of carcinoma in situ adjacent to the ulcerated invasive cancer.

good results with the use of cutaneous rhomboid flaps in the reconstruction of the perineum and perianal area. These flaps allow for reconstruction of a perineal body, they bring tissue with a good blood supply into the area that promotes healing, and they allow closure of the wound without tension on the anus. However, if there is concern that these functional structures would be sacrificed in order to obtain margins, strong consideration should be given to neoadjuvant treatment as discussed later in the chapter.

Regional Lymph Nodes

It should be kept in mind that certain vulvar cancers, by virtue of their anatomic extent, may have access to lymphatics that bypass the groins. These include tumors that extensively involve the anus (particularly the anal canal or its surrounding tissue), the rectovaginal septum, the vagina above the lower third, and the proximal urethra. However, for the vast majority of vulvar cancers, the primary metastatic pathway is via the inguinal lymph nodes.

Sentinel Lymph Node Dissection

A large number of reports have been published over the past 25 years on sentinel lymph node detection in various cancers. The concept relies on the presumption that the sentinel lymph node is the initial site of metastatic disease and that lack of metastatic involvement of the sentinel lymph node reflects an absence of metastasis in the rest of the lymph nodes in the basin. Lymphatic mapping is the standard of care in the United States for the surgical treatment of patients with clinically early-stage melanoma and breast cancer.

In the case of invasive squamous cell carcinoma of the vulva, interest in sentinel lymph node was driven by the high incidence and significant morbidity of complications following full inguinal–femoral lymphadenectomy. Though the incidence of groin wound complications has been reduced by separate incisions, it still may occur in up to 30% of patients, and the risk is increased by patient comorbidities and adjuvant chemotherapy or radiation. Therefore, the use of a lesser surgical procedure such as sentinel lymph node dissection is particularly relevant to vulvar cancer.

The concept of sentinel lymph node dissection applies well to vulvar cancer as the tumor location is easily accessible to injection of both radiocolloid and blue dye, and the lymphatic drainage is predictable for most tumors. With lymphatic

mapping, the pathologist has only a few lymph nodes to examine, allowing a more detailed examination. Techniques such as serial sectioning, immunohistochemical staining, and reverse transcriptase–polymerase chain reaction analysis can be applied, increasing the sensitivity of the examination and allowing the detection of micrometastases.

When using the combined technique for vulvar cancer patients, lymphatic mapping is nearly always successful in identifying sentinel lymph nodes (Fig. 49.10). Further, the false-negative rate (based on standard pathology) is very low. A meta-analysis by Hassanzade and colleagues showed that pooled sensitivity of 27 studies was 92% and a negative predictive value of 97%. A phase III trial by the GOG including tumors from 2 to 6 cm showed a sensitivity of 92.1% and a negative predictive value of 97.4% when a combination of blue dye and radiocolloid was used. Another multiinstitutional observational study by van der Zee et al. revealed a sensitivity of 94.1% and negative predictive value of 97.1%. A full inguinal–femoral lymph node dissection is reserved for those patients in which the sentinel node is positive or has not been successfully identified.

Sentinel lymph node mapping is a promising method to substantially reduce the morbidity of inguinal lymphadenectomy. It is widely used in the management of vulvar cancer today. However, many unanswered questions remain, including who the best candidates are for the technique, the role of frozen section, the role of immunohistochemistry, the role of lymphoscintigraphy, the reliability of an isolated lymphoscintigraphy-directed unilateral negative sentinel node with a midline lesion, the role of ultrasound, management of a patient with a microscopically positive sentinel lymph node, the incidence of "skip" metastases, the reliability of lymphatic mapping after prior excisional biopsy, and the optimal lymphatic mapping methodology for vulvar cancer patients.

Modifications on the Extent of Inguinal–Femoral Lymphadenectomy

Various modifications on the extent of lymphadenectomy have been examined. Before the introduction of sentinel lymph node biopsies, a technique involving limited resection of the inguinal lymph nodes in the management of superficially invasive vulvar cancer was reported by DiSaia and coworkers in 1979. The dissection they described is aimed at removal of the superficial lymph nodes above the cribriform fascia, mainly associated with the great saphenous and superficial epigastric veins. These lymph nodes were sent for frozen section analysis. If results were positive, a complete bilateral inguinofemoral lymphadenectomy was performed. In the 1979 study, DiSaia and colleagues also reported 79 cases of invasive squamous cell carcinoma of the vulva treated with radical vulvectomy and bilateral inguinal–femoral lymphadenectomy. In these cases, it was noted that the deep femoral lymph nodes were never positive in the absence of positive superficial inguinal lymph nodes. The purpose of a superficial dissection only is to reduce the morbidity of the groin lymphadenectomy. The dissection is less radical and resulted in only one groin breakdown in the 18 patients in the series of DiSaia and associates. The series was updated in 1989, and they reported no groin recurrences in 50 patients, 42 of whom had been followed for a median of 36 months.

A GOG study specifically studied the issue of superficial inguinal lymphadenectomy in patients with early carcinoma of the vulva. The study group included clinical stage I patients with tumor invasion of 5 mm or less and no capillary or lymphatic space involvement. A modified radical vulvectomy

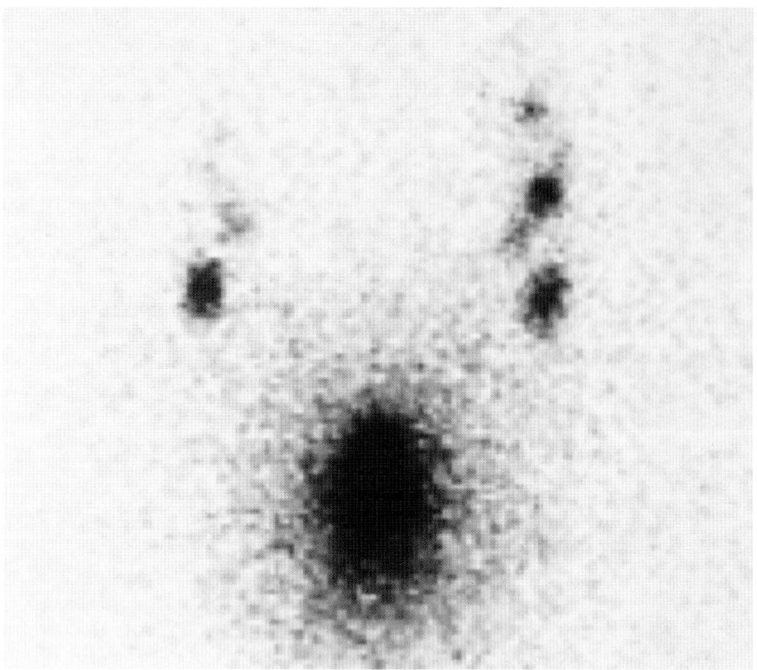
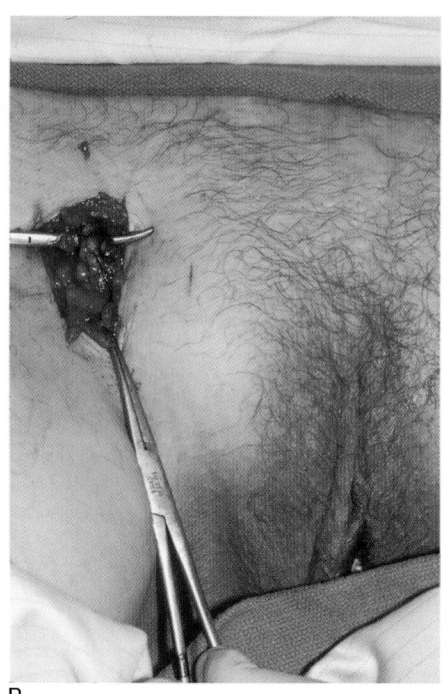

A   B

FIGURE 49.10 **A:** Preoperative lymphoscintigram 60 minutes after intralesional injection of technetium-99. **B:** Intraoperative blue node blue sentinel node in the right groin after injection of isosulfan blue dye into the primary vulvar cancer.

and ipsilateral superficial inguinal lymphadenectomy were performed, and 121 patients were evaluable. These were compared with a historical control group in the GOG registry who had undergone radical vulvectomy with bilateral inguinofemoral lymphadenectomy. Nine patients in this study, or 7.3%, experienced groin recurrences versus no recurrence in the control group. Six of the groin recurrences were in the ipsilateral groin, and 5 of the 9 patients died of the recurrent vulvar cancer. The interpretation from this study was that superficial inguinal lymphadenectomy may not be adequate treatment even for early vulvar carcinoma. However, in a number of patients in this study, the tumors approached the midline; there is evidence that more medial tumors may have direct drainage to the deep inguinal lymph nodes. Another area of concern in this study is the high percentage of poorly differentiated tumors—almost twice as many as in the control group. Six of the nine groin recurrences in this study were from the poorly differentiated tumors. Whether poorly differentiated tumors are more likely to metastasize to deep inguinal or contralateral inguinal lymph nodes deserves further study. Subsequent additional retrospective data from large cancer centers also report a 5% to 10% incidence of groin relapse in patients with negative nodes from superficial inguinal lymphadenectomy.

The technique of superficial lymphadenectomy of the inguinal nodes above the cribriform fascia has been largely replaced by sentinel lymph node biopsy, but the occurrences of groin recurrences after apparently negative superficial nodes in these studies remains concerning.

The benefit of sparing versus sacrificing the saphenous vein remains unclear. Various studies have found conflicting results on the reduction of the incidence of lymphedema. A randomized trial by the GOG showed that application of fibrin sealant at time of lymphadenectomy also did not reduce the incidence of lymphedema.

Unilateral Groin Lymphadenectomy Unilateral lymphadenectomy only on the side of a unilateral vulvar tumor has been another modification of surgical treatment that has been used for selected patients (Fig. 49.11). In 1981, Iversen reported on 53 women with unilateral tumors and lymph node metastases. Eighty-three percent of these patients had only one positive ipsilateral node, 15% had bilateral positive nodes, and one patient had contralateral positive lymph nodes only. Other retrospective studies have confirmed these results. It has been the opinion of a number of authors that capillary or lymphatic space involvement by tumor may increase the

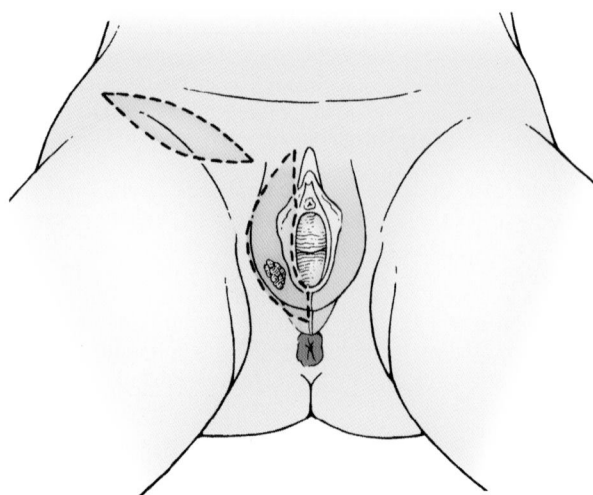

FIGURE 49.11 Unilateral lymphadenectomy in a patient with a focal right-sided small vulvar primary.

risk of contralateral nodal metastases. Patients with tumors approaching the midline or involving more medial structures (perineum, clitoral hood or clitoris, vagina, and labia minora) are at increased risk for contralateral lymph node metastases. The issue of unilateral groin lymphadenectomy was studied to some extent in 1992 by Stehman and associates in a GOG study. Patients with early disease and negative ipsilateral superficial inguinal lymph nodes were treated with ipsilateral superficial inguinal lymphadenectomy and a modified radical vulvectomy. A few patients in this study did have a bilateral inguinal lymphadenectomy because of midline involvement. A total of 121 patients were in the study, and 3 experienced contralateral inguinal lymph node recurrences. The vulvar lesions of these 3 patients ranged from 0.6 to 2.5 mm in depth of invasion, and all were poorly differentiated. Although lesion location was not given for these 3 cases, a large percentage of patients included in this study had lesions approaching the midline, as defined by involvement of the labia minora. Tumors with capillary or lymphatic space involvement were excluded from this study.

At present, unilateral inguinal–femoral lymphadenectomy appears to be a reasonable approach in a patient with a well-lateralized early tumor that is well differentiated, with no capillary or lymphatic space involvement and with negative ipsilateral inguinal lymph nodes.

Pelvic Lymphadenectomy During the late 1970s and early 1980s, several studies were published showing that carcinoma of the vulva metastasizes to the inguinofemoral lymph nodes before spreading to the pelvic lymph nodes. Extension of the groin lymphadenectomy to include removal of the pelvic lymph nodes continued to be performed in selected patients with positive inguinofemoral lymph nodes. A number of studies also showed that the 5-year survival rate of vulvar cancer patients with positive pelvic lymph nodes is less than 20%. A 1986 study by the GOG directed by Homesley compared pelvic lymph node dissection with groin and pelvic radiotherapy in patients with positive inguinofemoral lymph nodes. The study included 114 patients and showed no difference in morbidity between the two treatment arms and a better 2-year survival rate in the radiotherapy group (68% vs. 54%). The improved survival was seen in those patients with suspicious or grossly positive lymph nodes or those with more than one positive groin lymph node. There was no evidence that groin radiation therapy was beneficial to those patients with occult metastases and only one positive groin node. Review of the pattern of recurrence in that study suggested that adjuvant radiation was more effective largely because groin recurrences were reduced. The value of removing positive pelvic lymph nodes before radiotherapy is unknown. Pelvic lymphadenectomy is now rarely indicated in the treatment of vulvar cancer.

Omitting Groin Dissection for Superficial Disease Extensive data support the contention that a subset of early vulvar carcinomas (carefully studied pathologically) can be identified that have an extremely low risk of nodal involvement. In a GOG study reported by Sedlis and associates, a subgroup (63 of 272) of patients with early disease was identified as having a zero incidence of lymph node metastases. This subset included nonmidline tumors with no capillary or lymphatic space involvement that were well differentiated or were grade 2 and limited to 2 mm in thickness. Other factors that have been studied for the purpose of identifying a low-risk group include tumor volume (which does not appear to have received further attention since Wilkinson's report in 1985), tumors that

are largely carcinoma in situ with very early stromal invasion and with a pushing rather than an infiltrative pattern, tumor diameter, squamous cell type, the presence of an inflammatory response, and tumor ploidy.

There seems to be general agreement that the patients for whom it would be most reasonable to omit the lymphadenectomy are those with tumor invasion less than or equal to 1 mm and less than 2 cm in diameter. However, certain tumors with less than 1 mm of invasion should still be considered for lymphadenectomy. As reported in the literature, three of nine patients with nodal disease or nodal recurrence in association with tumor invasion less than or equal to 1 mm had poorly differentiated cancers (Table 49.2). Thus, women with suspicious lymph nodes, poorly differentiated tumors, tumors with capillary or lymphatic space involvement, and perhaps those with multiple foci or broad areas of invasion or aneuploidy should still undergo lymphadenectomy. It is important to remember that even with superficial invasion, metastases to the nodes do occur. In the report by Sedlis and colleagues of 272 patients with invasion of 5 mm or less, the groin nodes were positive in approximately 20%.

Operative Technique

Radical Vulvectomy

With the classic en bloc resection, the inguinal specimens are mobilized toward the vulva as just described (Fig. 49.12). This operation is rarely employed now due to its morbidity and data on favorable oncologic outcomes with less radical surgery. From the point of completion of the inferior inguinal dissections, incisions are continued down along the labiocrural folds on each side and across the perineum, where they meet. A medial mucosal incision is made along the introitus extending through the anterior vestibule and around the urethral meatus.

When radical vulvectomy is performed through a separate vulvar incision, the same labiocrural, posterior, and mucosal

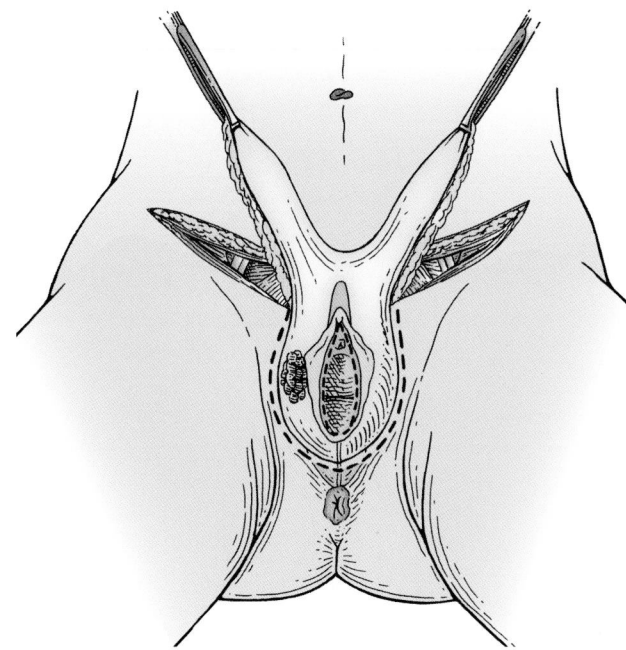

FIGURE 49.12 Classic en bloc resection of the vulva and inguinal–femoral nodes through one interconnected incision.

incisions are used, and the same vulvar tissue is excised (Fig. 49.13A). The superior incision extends from the top of the labiocrural folds as an inverted V, with the point above the base of the clitoris. As previously discussed, a variable amount of superior tissue (i.e., mons pubis) is removed, depending on the location and size of the lesion.

The radical vulvectomy incisions may be modified somewhat depending on the location and extent of the tumor and the condition of the remaining uninvolved vulvar skin. The surgeon should attempt to attain at least a 2-cm margin of normal-appearing skin or mucosa around the tumor. To accomplish this, it may be necessary to excise a portion of the vagina,

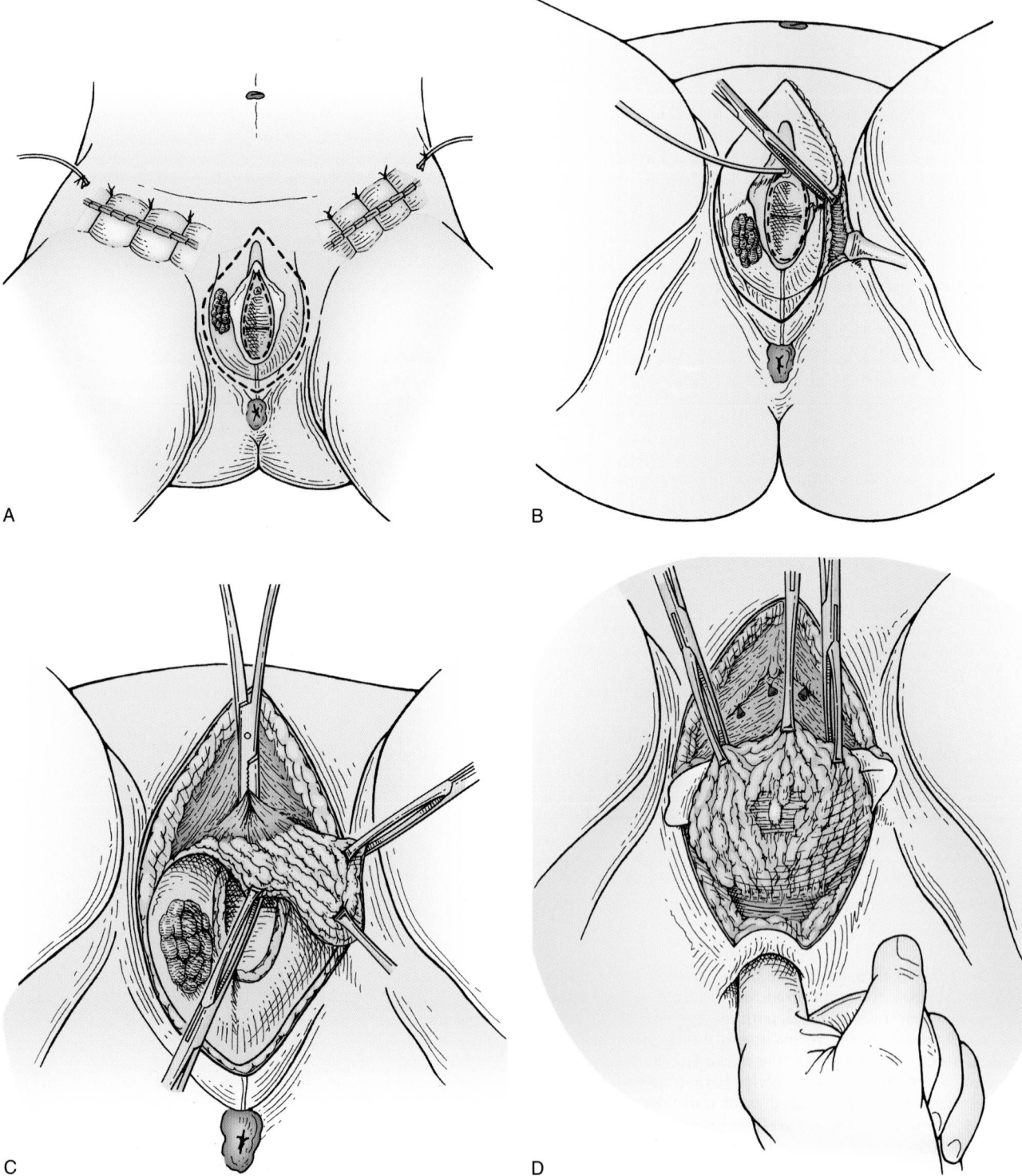

FIGURE 49.13 Radical vulvectomy with bilateral inguinal lymphadenectomy done through three separate incisions. **A:** Bilateral inguinofemoral lymphadenectomy through separate incisions is completed. Separate incision for radical vulvectomy is marked. **B:** Labiocrural incisions are extended to deep fascia of the urogenital diaphragm. **C:** Dissection proceeds dorsally off of the pubic bone. The vascular base of the clitoris is clamped, followed by transection and ligation. **D:** Perineal body and posterior vulvar tissues are dissected away from the anus.

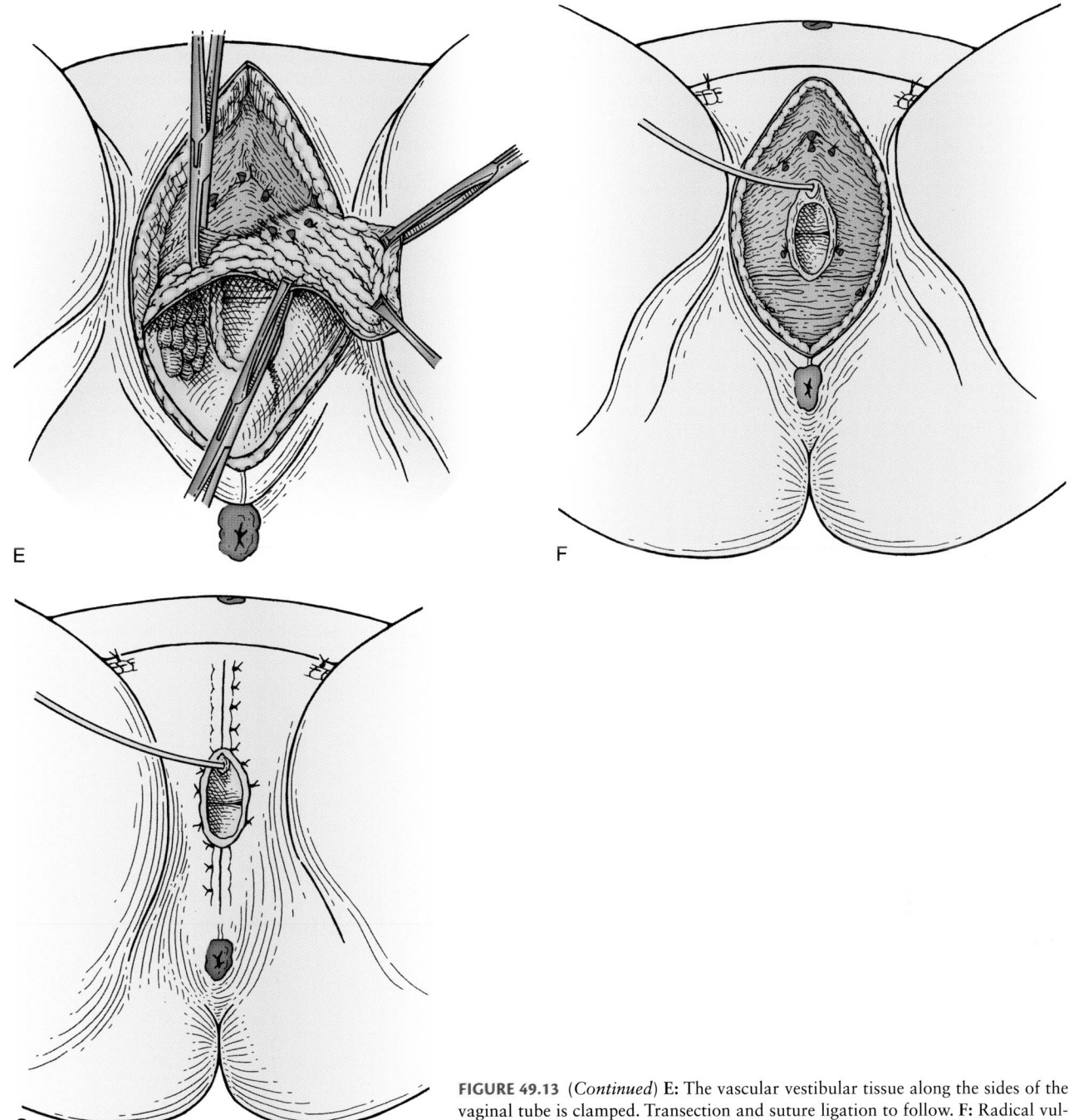

FIGURE 49.13 (*Continued*) **E:** The vascular vestibular tissue along the sides of the vaginal tube is clamped. Transection and suture ligation to follow. **F:** Radical vulvectomy resection is completed. **G:** Closure of the vulvar wound is completed.

anus, or distal urethra. For an anterior lesion, it is reasonable to spare the perineal body; but for a posterior lesion, it is important to incorporate radical resection of this area. For a lesion (especially superficial) in proximity to the urethral meatus or anus, it is reasonable to limit the margin of resection to 1 cm (but not less) to preserve these structures and their function.

The labiocrural incisions are extended to the lateral margins of the deep fascia of the urogenital diaphragm (**Fig. 49.13B**). The internal pudendal vessels are ligated as they are encountered entering the vulva at about the 4 o'clock and 8 o'clock positions. Superiorly, the specimen is dissected off the pubic periosteum and adductor fascia. The vascular base of the clitoris is clamped and transected, and a transfixion suture ligature is placed (**Fig. 49.13C**). If deemed necessary, the attachment of the

ischiocavernosus muscles can also be transected at this level. Dissection of the superior portion of the vulva off of the pubic bone and adductor fascia is completed and joined, in the midline, to the transvestibular mucosal incision above the urethra. Inferiorly, a variable portion of the perineum (and in some cases the anus) is dissected upward and cephalad toward the vaginal incision (**Fig. 49.13D**). Care is taken as the vaginal incision is approached above the perineum to avoid injury to the anal canal. Using the index finger or a large Kelly clamp, the surgeon separates the vaginal tube bluntly from the underlying soft tissue cephalad to the vestibular structures. The mucosal incision is then completed, separating the vagina (with the urethra) from the specimen. This dissection can be facilitated by splitting the specimen in the midline anteriorly or posteriorly. The remainder of the dissection off the underlying deep fascia of the urogenital diaphragm is completed. Clamps and transfixion suture ligatures of no. 0 or 2-0 polyglactin are used during transection of the tissue along the side of the vaginal tube in the region of the vestibular bulbs (**Fig. 49.13E**).

After removal of the specimen, the wounds are copiously irrigated with antibiotic solution, and hemostasis is secured (**Fig. 49.13F**). After en bloc resection, the superior abdominal wall flap and the groin and vulvar thigh flaps are further mobilized as necessary to achieve closure of the wounds without tension. Any ischemic-appearing skin is excised. It is very useful, especially if there is an element of vaginal relaxation, to mobilize the lower vagina to facilitate wound closure. Any pelvic relaxation defects (i.e., cystocele, rectocele, loss of the posterior urethrovesical angle) are repaired at this time. To the extent that it is necessary or possible, the perineal body is also reinforced or reconstructed at this time.

The vulvar wound and the perineal area are closed with vertical mattress 2-0 delayed absorbable sutures (**Fig. 49.13G**). Depending on the amount of tissue that has been removed, the superior portion of an en bloc wound may be difficult to close.

When done through a separate incision, closure of the vulvar wound is under much less tension, again because of preservation of the inguinal skin bridges. Careful attention must be paid to closure of the periurethral area. The urethra should be secured on a straight course without tension. A hood of skin above the urethra is also avoided because this can obstruct the path of the urinary stream and cause spraying.

Modified Radical Vulvectomy

As previously discussed, it is reasonable in most patients to manage the vulvar lesion locally with a modified radical vulvectomy. This operation consists of radical removal of the portion of the vulva containing the tumor and any skin, which is involved with high-grade VIN. It is performed with the techniques described earlier except that the excision is basically limited to removal of that particular part of the vulva. The lateral and deep tumor margins are not compromised by this operation. After the surgeon carefully demarcates a 2-cm radius of normal skin or mucosa around the tumor, an encompassing incision is designed that will readily close and be as cosmetically acceptable as possible (**Fig. 49.14**).

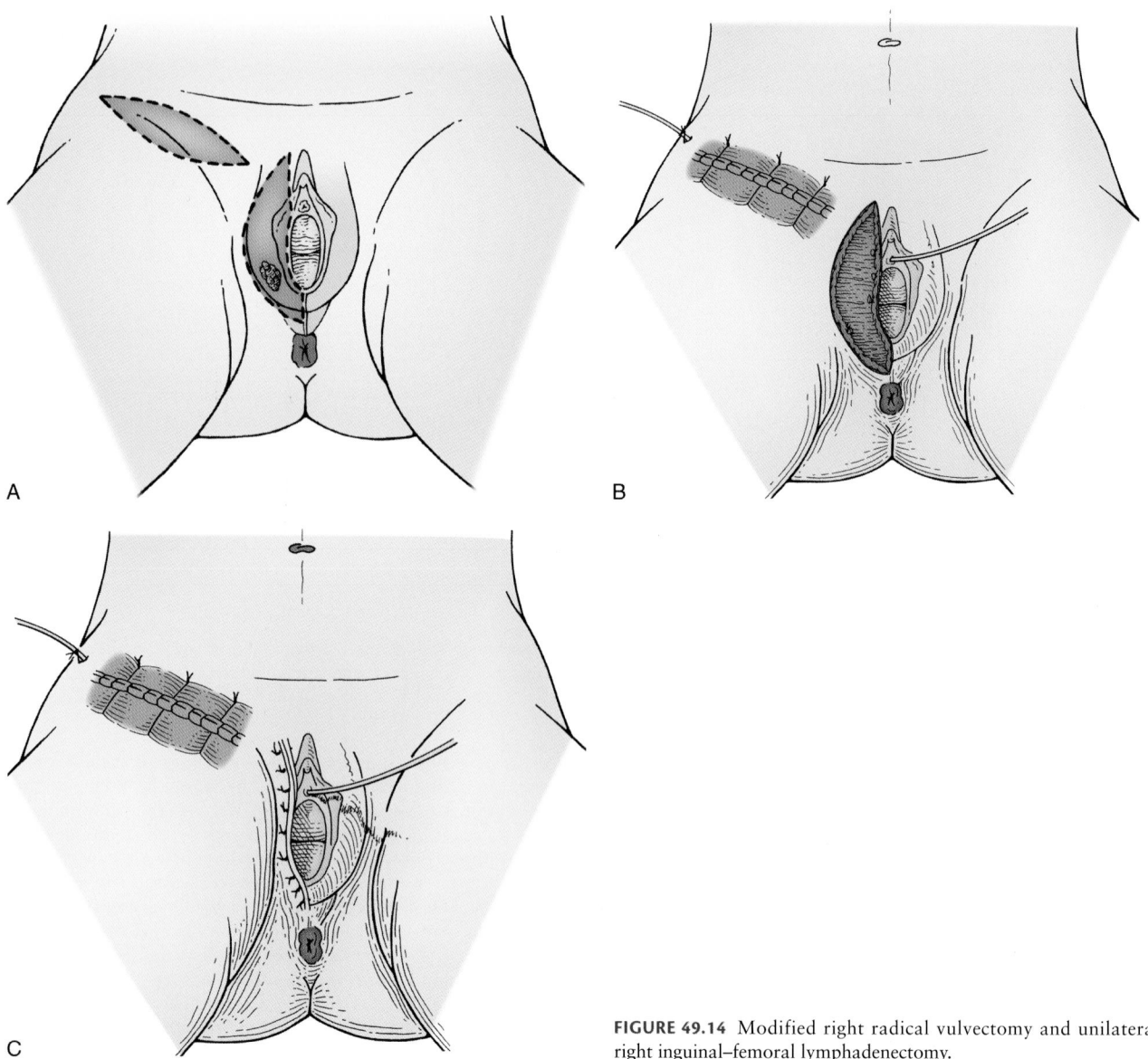

FIGURE 49.14 Modified right radical vulvectomy and unilateral right inguinal–femoral lymphadenectomy.

Lymphadenectomy

Sentinel Lymph Node Dissection
Sentinel lymph node detection is currently accomplished using two methods of lymphatic mapping: blue dye and radiocolloid. One to two milliliters of isosulfan blue dye (Lymphazurin) is injected superficially around the periphery of the primary tumor, and the blue-dyed lymphatic channels are followed. An incision is made over the anticipated location, and the dyed lymph node or nodes that have been stained by accumulating the blue dye are removed. Alternatively, the periphery of the tumor is injected with 400 mCi of technetium-labeled sulfur colloid 2 to 4 hours before surgery. A preoperative technetium scan (lymphoscintigraphy) is done, which may be helpful in confirming lymph node uptake, localization of target lymph nodes, unilateral versus bilateral lymphatic drainage, and identification of the unusual case of predominant drainage to pelvic lymph nodes. An intraoperative gamma counter is used to identify one or more sentinel lymph nodes (Fig. 49.15). The removed lymph nodes are checked with the gamma counter, and complete removal is assured when the radioactivity in the inguinal area returns to background levels. In practice, the two techniques are complementary and are frequently used together. The removed nodes are sent for frozen section, and the small skin incision in the groin is closed with absorbable sutures. Drains are not required. If the frozen section is negative, no further lymphadenectomy is required. However, if metastatic disease is detected, a complete inguinal–femoral lymphadenectomy is indicated.

Inguinal–Femoral Lymphadenectomy
An incision is made starting about 2 to 4 cm medial and about 2 cm caudal to the anterior superior iliac spine. The incision gradually curves downward just above the superior border of the inguinal ligament medially to the inguinal ring or about 2 cm below and 2 cm medial to the pubic tubercle. Unless there is a large clitoral lesion or palpably suspicious nodes, the mons pubis is spared, and separate incisions with a skin bridge are made as illustrated in Figure 49.16. For anterior lesions, such as those involving the clitoris, a portion of the mons pubis is included in the resection and the lymphadenectomy on one or both sides may be done en bloc with the radical vulvectomy as illustrated in Figure 49.12. From the lateral points, caudal incisions are carried medially so as to excise a strip of skin (optional) 2 to

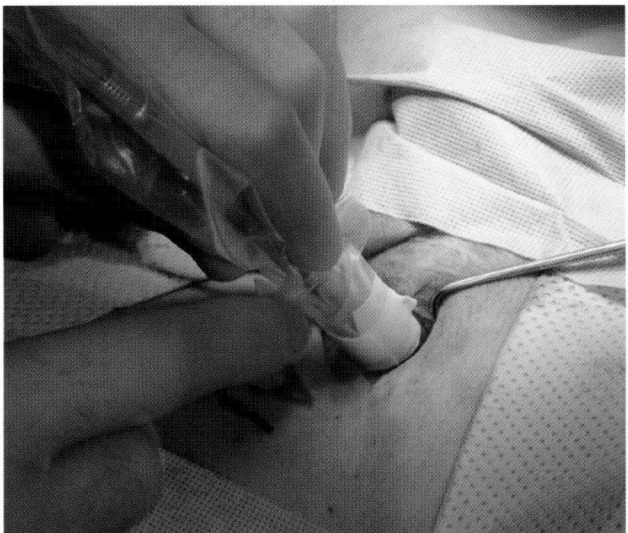

FIGURE 49.15 Intraoperative use of the gamma probe to identify the radioactive sentinel node.

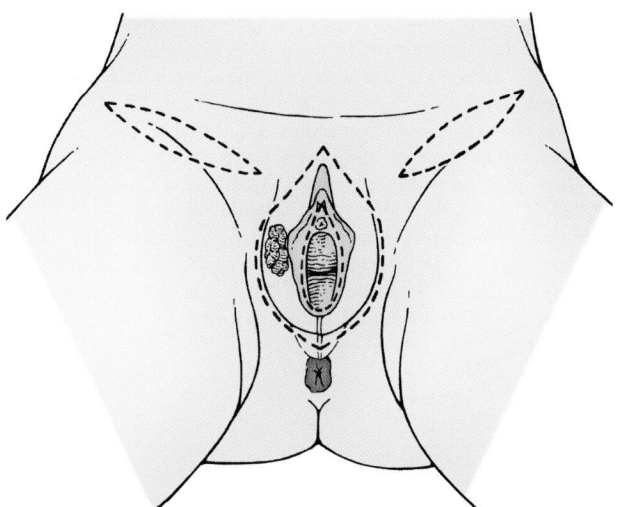

FIGURE 49.16 Separate incisions for bilateral lymphadenectomy done with a radical vulvectomy.

4 cm in width. Excising an ellipse of the skin may reduce the likelihood of skin necrosis and facilitate more complete dissection of the groin. This incision is designed to extend from just below the fossa ovalis (this can generally be identified clinically as the area just medial to the femoral pulsation in the groin) to the top of the labiocrural fold above a point just medial to the external inguinal ring. In the presence of grossly positive inguinal lymph nodes, a wider resection of both the groin skin and fat is necessary to help ensure adequate tumor clearance. The separate groin skin incision may also be done vertically (with the leg), centered across the fossa ovalis, and about halfway between the femoral artery and pubic tubercle.

Leaving a layer of subcutaneous tissue with the skin, the superior incision is undermined so that the lymph node–bearing adipose tissue above the inguinal ligament and around the superficial circumflex iliac, as well as the superficial epigastric vessels, are included with the resection. These vessels are ligated or electrocoagulated as they are encountered. The superior dissection over the groin area is carried down to the superior border of the inguinal ligament (Fig. 49.17A and B). The midline aspect of the superior flap can be mobilized off the pubic bone and rectus fascia at this point to facilitate later closure of the wound without tension. Dissection of the block of inguinal tissue is carried inferiorly off of the inguinal ligament. The lateral corner is dissected medially off of the sartorius fascia. The inferior flap of the lower incision is also mobilized, especially medially, and the saphenous vein is identified as it enters the region of the femoral triangle (Fig. 49.17C). Accessory saphenous veins can also be seen entering this area. If it is to be sacrificed, the long saphenous vein is isolated and ligated with a free-tie and a transfixion ligature of 2-0 polyglactin (Vicryl). The vein with its surrounding block of lymph node–bearing tissue is dissected superiorly off of the sartorius and adductor fascia. Dissection of the block of inguinal tissue is continued from the three sides toward the fossa ovalis. As this area is approached, the overlying cribriform fascia is recognized, and the femoral artery pulsation can be palpated in the lateral aspect. En bloc dissection continues and includes the contents of the fossa ovalis (Fig. 49.17D). The area under the fascia lateral to the femoral artery should be left undisturbed as the femoral nerve lies lateral. There are no lymph nodes of consequence here, and avoidance of this area prevents injury to the femoral nerve and possibly reduces subsequent

IX

lymphedema. Rather, resection of the cribriform fascia begins over the area of femoral pulsation, exposing the underlying femoral vessels. A few small branches of the femoral nerve are sacrificed during this dissection. The sheath of the femoral artery is incised along its anteromedial aspect from somewhere between the base of the fossa ovalis and the apex of the femoral triangle to its emergence from under the inguinal ligament. Branches, such as the external pudendal artery, are ligated as they are encountered. There is no purpose in dissecting under the artery or between the femoral artery and vein. Rather, the dissection that has been performed over the top of the artery is continued over the top of the vein, mobilizing the specimen

to the medial aspect of the femoral vein. During this process, the saphenofemoral venous junction is identified, ligated with a 2-0 silk free-tie followed by a suture ligature for security, and transected, thus removing several centimeters of the saphenous vein with the specimen (Fig. 49.17E).

An alternative method, as long as there are no adherent suspicious lymph nodes, is to dissect the saphenous vein free of the specimen so that it can be preserved, potentially reducing the risk of subsequent lymphedema. Complete dissection of the space medial to the vein is important because this is where most of the femoral groin nodes are located. The specimen is freed from the femoral vein medially, from the inguinal

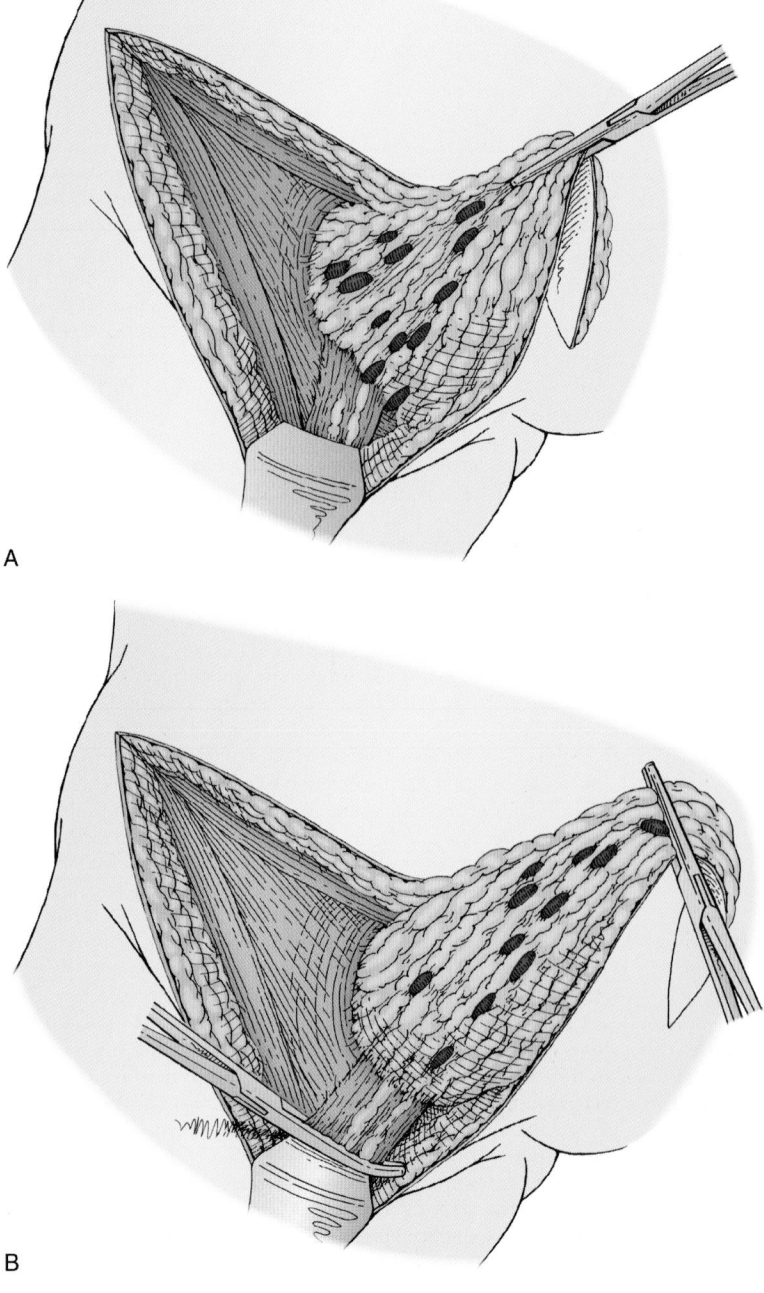

A

B

FIGURE 49.17 A: Inguinal–femoral lymphadenectomy. The corner of the groin specimen is dissected up from lateral to medially off the sartorius muscle. The lateral portion of fossa ovalis and cribriform fascia are exposed. **B:** The block of lymph node–bearing tissue has been mobilized, and the fatty lymphatic tissue overlying the saphenous vein is clamped.

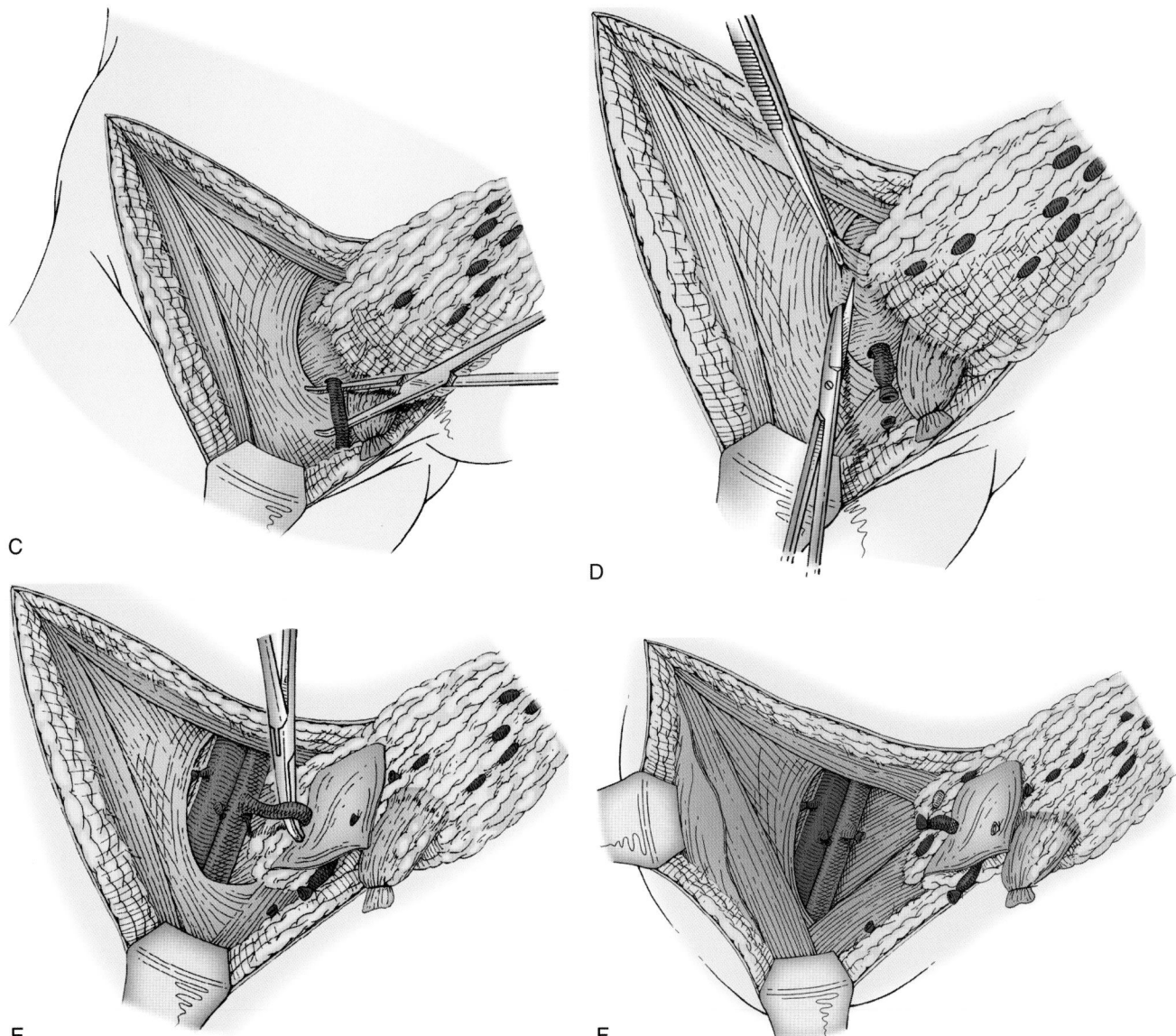

C

D

E

F

FIGURE 49.17 (*Continued*) **C:** The saphenous vein is identified, isolated, clamped, and divided near its entrance into the femoral triangle. **D:** Dissection of the femoral lymph nodes beginning with the separation of the cribriform fascia and the contents of the fossa ovalis from the anterior aspect of the femoral artery. **E:** The groin specimen containing the fatty nodal tissue above the cribriform fascia and the femoral nodes below the cribriform fascia are reflected medially exposing the femoral vessels and the insertion of the saphenous vein. **F:** The saphenous vein has been divided and ligated. The nodal tissue bundle is then completely excised and removed. The femoral triangle has been cleared of all nodal tissue.

ligament superiorly, and from the underlying pectineal fascia. Dissection is continued toward and off of the adductor longus fascia until the labiocrural fold is reached (Fig. 49.17F).

To protect the exposed femoral vessels in the event of subsequent wound breakdown, the sartorius muscle can be transposed over them at this point. Alternatively, the vessels can be covered by a variety of other materials or simple approximation of musculofascial tissues. To accomplish sartorius transposition, the muscle is divided with cautery at its tendinous attachment to the anterior superior iliac spine. The proximal end of the muscle is then mobilized and transposed so that it covers the femoral vessels. It is sutured at this location to the inguinal ligament and pectineal fascia with 0 polyglactin (Fig. 49.18). We have largely discontinued the practice of transposing the sartorius muscles because of the improved healing of these wounds and less radical dissection.

If a superficial inguinal lymphadenectomy has been chosen (also generally done through separate incisions), the same general dissection is done except that the cribriform fascia and underlying femoral lymph node–bearing tissue are left intact. All lymph nodes around the saphenofemoral junction should be included, and any prominent deeper lymph nodes medial to the femoral vein should also be removed. In the absence of clinical suspicion, the only lymph nodes of concern deep to the cribriform fascia are those medial to the femoral vein. There is unlikely to be a significant increase in morbidity by extending the dissection to include removal of these femoral lymph nodes.

If a prominent femoral lymph node can be identified at the most superior aspect of the dissection in the space just medial to the femoral vein (Cloquet node or node of Rosenmüller), this can be used as a sentinel lymph node when evaluating the

IX

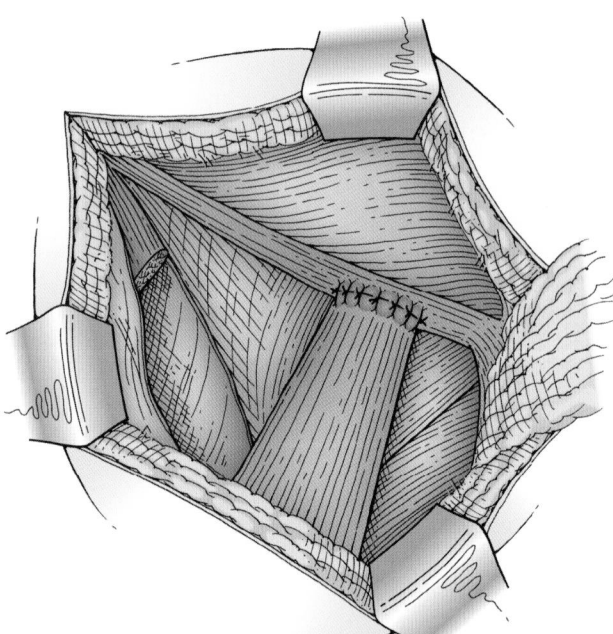

FIGURE 49.18 The transposed sartorius muscle.

risk of pelvic lymph node metastases. When such a lymph node is positive, a search may be made for further nodes above this by carrying the dissection up along the femoral artery under the inguinal ligament or the patient may be treated with pelvic radiation postoperatively.

Soft, active suction drains are placed in each groin and are brought out through separate stab wounds superolaterally. The lymphadenectomy site is copiously irrigated. When there is anticipated tension in the closure, the groin wound may be approximated with a large mass closure using no. 2 polypropylene vertical mattress retention sutures (Fig. 49.19A). Three to five sutures are placed on each side. Each suture starts several centimeters from the edge of the superior flap, with a bite then taken of the underlying inguinal ligament. This is designed to close the dead space under the superior flap. Under the inferior flap, a bite of sartorius, adductor, or pectineal fascia is taken (with care taken to avoid injury to the femoral vessels and nerve), followed by placement of the suture from inside to out through the inferior flap several centimeters from the edge. Again, this is designed to close the dead space of the inferior flap and, once pulled together, to close the dead space of the midline wound. Going back from inferior to superior, a small bite of each skin edge is then taken, which is designed to approximate these edges. The sutures are not tied until all have been placed. The sutures are tied somewhat loosely, with only enough tension to bring the wound together (Fig. 49.19B). The skin is further closed with staples (Fig. 49.19C). When there has been less extensive dissection, the groin wound may be closed with 2-0 polyglycolic acid suture, approximating first the dead space with interrupted sutures and then the skin with vertical mattress or subcuticular sutures. En bloc groin incisions are closed in an identical manner, but this is delayed until completion of the entire resection. With separate incisions, the medial aspects of the groin wounds are under much less tension and are easily closed because of preservation of the inguinal skin bridge. Separation of the groin and vulvar wounds and especially closure without tension are the factors thought to be largely responsible for the reduced wound complications seen with the three-incision technique.

Vulvar Reconstruction

After radical resection for carcinoma of the vulva, the wounds can generally be closed primarily. This is greatly facilitated when the incisions are modified somewhat (as with sparing of the mons pubis) and especially when separate groin incisions are used. When an extensive resection is necessary, it may not be possible to close the wound primarily or at least not without considerable tension. This is often the case after resection of a recurrent tumor, where previous radical surgery has already left a paucity of tissue. If the area was treated previously with radiotherapy, then closure may be difficult because of the lack of elasticity of the fibrotic tissue and because of radiation-induced healing impairment. Under these various circumstances, closure of the incisions and healing can be facilitated by a variety of reconstructive procedures. Other potential benefits of such reconstruction include maintenance of anal, urethral, and sexual function and a more cosmetically acceptable result. However, packing the wound open is sometimes the best option, and healing by secondary intention is usually quite satisfactory.

Closure of groin and vulvar wounds using reconstructive techniques involves moving a block of expendable tissue (with its blood supply intact) from some nearby site into the deficient area. The mobilized block of tissue is commonly referred to as a flap. Flaps are classified according to what layers of tissue they include and according to their blood supply. The types of flaps that have been useful in reconstruction of the vulva and groin are full-thickness skin (random and arterial based), fasciocutaneous, and myocutaneous flaps. Some flaps remain completely attached at their base and are rotated into the defect, whereas others are partially separated from the base and are transposed as an island of tissue.

Full-Thickness Skin Flaps
A full-thickness skin flap involves rotating an adjacent block of skin with its underlying subcutaneous tissue into the defect. The flap is mobilized from the donor site but remains attached at its base; through this base travels the arterial and venous circulation. The blood supply of the flap may be random, or it may depend on a specifically planned arterial source. A random flap relies on the many small musculocutaneous perforating vessels that are retained through the base. For this reason, the subcutaneous layer must be kept thick, and the length of the flap should not be much greater than the width of the base (1 to 1.5 times greater). This is the type of flap most commonly used for reconstruction of a radical vulvectomy wound. The healing of such flaps is less reliable in patients with impaired wound healing ability, such as those with diabetes, heavy tobacco users, those with vascular disease, and patients who have previously received radiation therapy to the region.

A few specific arterial-based full-thickness skin flaps, sometimes called axial flaps, have been used for reconstruction in vulvar cancer patients. Arterial sources of these flaps have included the internal pudendal, circumflex iliac, superficial circumflex iliac, superficial inferior epigastric, superficial branch of the deep external pudendal, and superficial external pudendal arteries. With some of these arterial flaps, the deep fascia must be carefully mobilized with the subcutaneous tissue to maintain an adequate blood supply. The main advantage of an arterial flap, because of the good arterial blood supply, is that it can be considerably longer than a random flap. However, these flaps are technically more difficult to construct and have a low margin for error in terms of compromising blood supply.

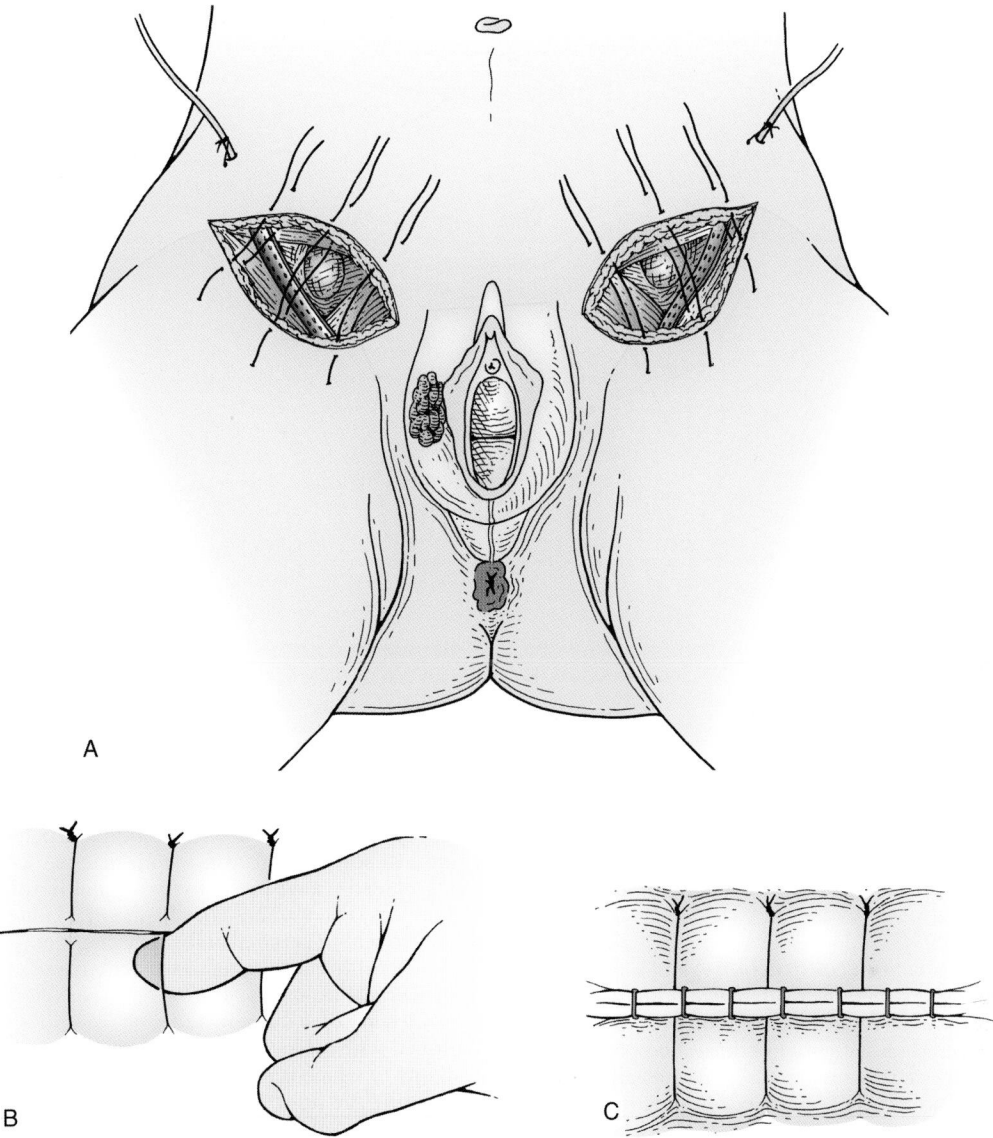

FIGURE 49.19 A: Large block closure of separate groin incisions with vertical mattress sutures. Note the lateral/superior placement of the suction drains. **B:** The mattress sutures are tied somewhat loosely. **C:** The skin closure is completed with staples.

Fasciocutaneous Flap Full-thickness skin flaps that include the deep fascia off the underlying muscle are known as fasciocutaneous flaps. These are more reliable than random cutaneous flaps because the preserved fascial layer provides additional musculocutaneous perforating vessels along its length. A fasciocutaneous flap can also be relatively long and is transposable as an island of tissue. Some fasciocutaneous flaps have a designated arterial blood supply. Locally useful fasciocutaneous flaps include the pudendal thigh, superior medial thigh, inferior gluteal, and island groin flaps.

Myocutaneous Flap A myocutaneous flap makes use of an expendable muscle with its intact overlying fascia and cutaneous tissue. The use of these flaps for vulvovaginal reconstruction began after the 1976 report by McCraw and colleagues. A substantial blood supply is preserved through a narrow pedicle connected to the muscle, which allows the flap to be transposed as an island with a wide arc of rotation. Another advantage of a myocutaneous flap is its capacity to bring tissue into the defect that has a blood supply separate and independent from that of the operative site. This makes these flaps particularly valuable in the reconstruction of heavily radiated tissues. These flaps are also somewhat bulky and have the ability to fill a large tissue defect. The main disadvantage of myocutaneous flaps is that they are technically demanding, and the viability of these flaps is somewhat tenuous.

The difficulties resulting from a large wound created by an extensive radical vulvectomy with bilateral inguinofemoral lymphadenectomy were previously discussed. Reconstruction of large vulvar wounds with bilateral tensor fasciae latae (TFL) myocutaneous flaps has been reported. The TFL originates from the anterior superior iliac spine. It inserts into the fascia lata and is supplied by the lateral femoral circumflex artery. The base is just lateral to the groin wound, into which the flap is directly rotated. The flaps are easily made long enough to reach and close the often large area created by resection of the mons pubis and anterior vulva. A TFL myocutaneous flap is also useful for reconstruction of the groin after extensive resection for recurrent disease (Fig. 49.20).

IX

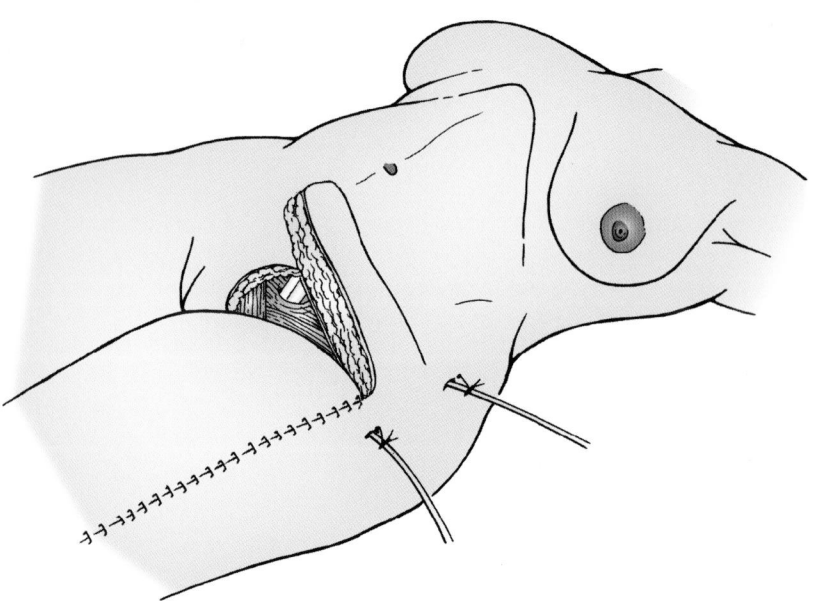

FIGURE 49.20 Tensor fasciae latae flap being rotated from the thigh to close a large groin wound.

The rectus abdominis myocutaneous flap, based on the inferior epigastric artery, is also useful for reconstruction of a large groin defect. The block of tissue based on this muscle is taken from the abdominal wall, and the muscle is divided at the superior border of the flap. The island of cutaneous tissue is completely mobilized with its carefully preserved attachment to the muscle, and this is further mobilized inferiorly. This allows the island flap to rotate down easily into the groin (or vulva) through a generous subcutaneous tunnel. The rectus abdominis myocutaneous flap is also suitable for the reconstruction of large vulvar wounds (Fig. 49.21).

Other Considerations in Reconstruction Flaps are particularly useful in the reconstruction of vulvar wounds after radical resection of cancer involving the perineal or perianal tissues. Such a resection removes the entire perineal body as well as portions of the superficial muscles and leaves a large defect that is difficult to close (Fig. 49.22A). Poor healing of this area

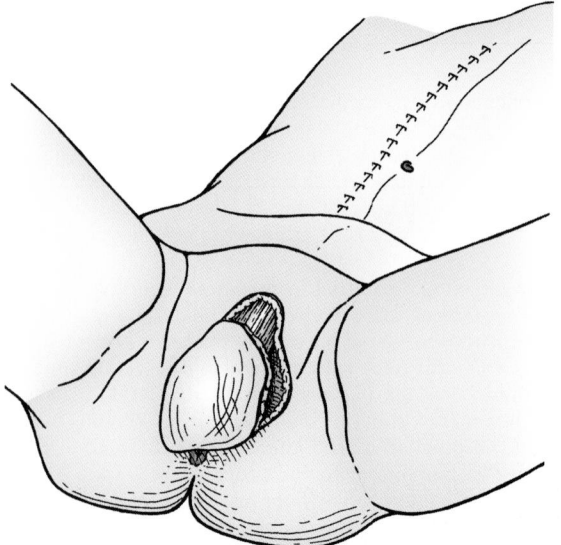

FIGURE 49.21 Rectus abdominis myocutaneous flap is brought through a subcutaneous tunnel to close a large perineal wound.

may significantly compromise both anal and coital function. The use of flaps for such a defect allows closure without tension and brings tissue with a good blood supply into the area, which promotes healing and helps recreate a perineal body. Preventing tension on the anal apparatus helps promote healing of its associated reconstructed musculature and helps preserve its function. Reconstruction of a perineal body separates the vagina from fecal contamination and helps create a smooth and less scarred platform for intercourse. For reconstruction of such defects, we prefer to use local, full-thickness rhomboid skin flaps (Fig. 49.22B–D). Closure of a larger defect involving the perineal or perianal and vulvar areas may be better accomplished with gluteal thigh fasciocutaneous, gluteus maximus myocutaneous, or gracilis myocutaneous flaps.

Closure of a heavily radiated wound should be accomplished with a block of relatively unradiated tissue, the blood supply to which is unlikely to have been significantly compromised by the prior treatment. In general, myocutaneous flaps are better for this purpose.

Many other flaps have been reported to be useful for groin and vulvar reconstruction and may be used depending on the individual situation and preference of the surgeon.

Postoperative Care

Vulvar Wound Care

After closure, silver sulfadiazine (Silvadene, Hoechst Marion Roussel) cream is applied to the perineal wound, and a light dressing is placed. In the recovery room, ice is applied to the vulvar wound, and this is continued off and on for 48 to 72 hours. Depending on the degree of perineal or perianal resection, several days of bowel rest may be indicated, with or without a constipating agent, followed by a stool softener. On postoperative day 3 or 4, the patient is started on a regimen of cleansing the vulvar wound with a showerhead, followed immediately by complete drying of the area with a hair dryer on the cool air setting. This is done three times a day and as needed (i.e., after a liquid bowel movement) and is continued until the wounds are healed. If moisture in the wound is a problem despite this regimen, other useful measures include placing a roll of gauze between the legs and against the wound between washings, increasing the frequency of washings, not wearing

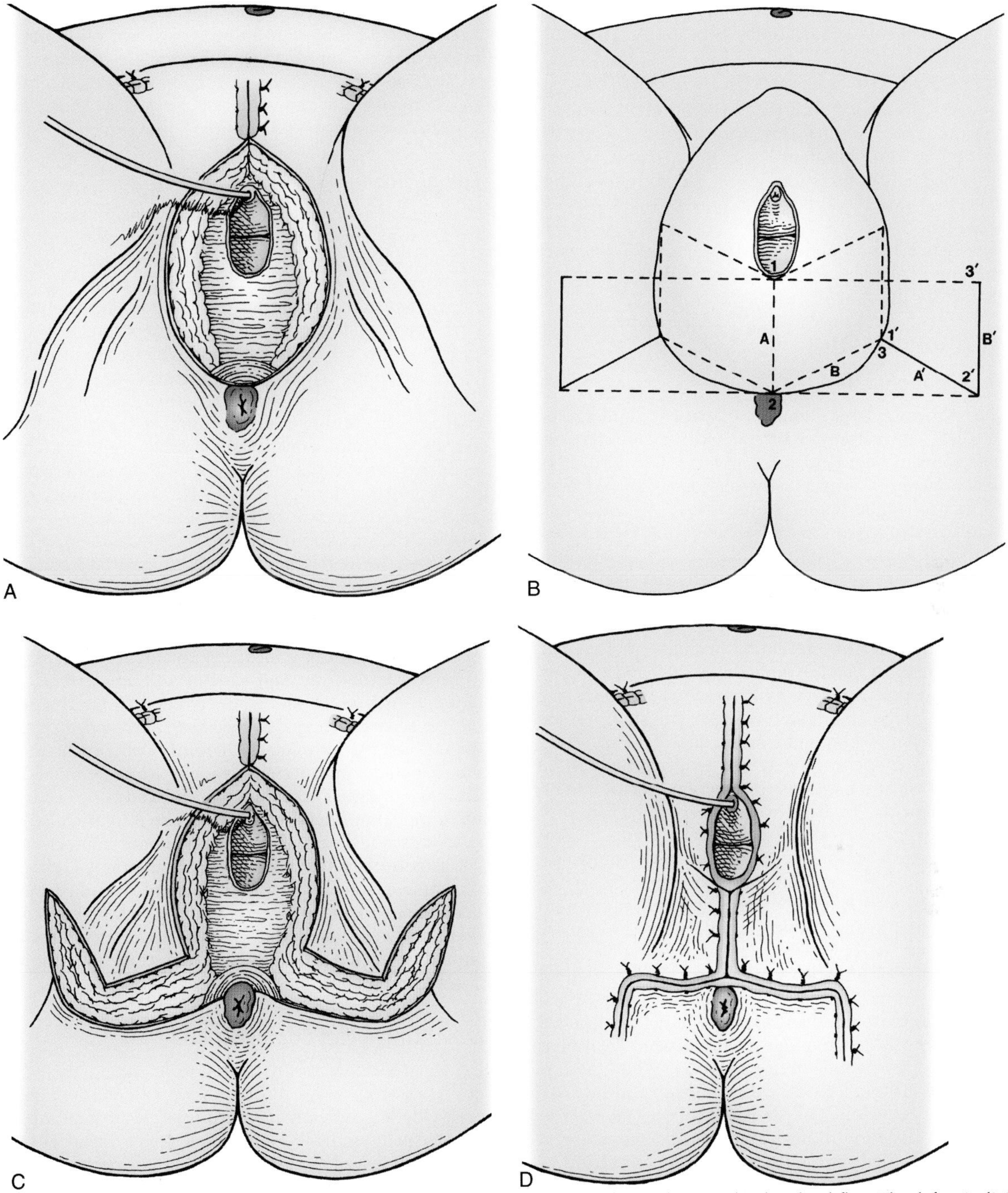

FIGURE 49.22 A: Large posterior perineal defect that may be difficult to close primarily. **B:** Planning the rhomboid flap. The defect is divided into two rhomboids. Measurements *A* and *B* are made and marked on the skin of the thigh (*A′* and *B′*). After the flap is mobilized, *1′* will be located at the posterior vaginal introitus (1) and *2′* at the anterior anus (2). **C:** The bilateral rhomboid flaps are developed. **D:** The flaps have been rotated, and the posterior perineal defect is closed.

an undergarment, and applying a heat lamp to the area three times a day between washings. All of these efforts are aimed at keeping this normally warm and moist area clean and dry, which reduces the risk of infection and promotes healing. Intermittently leaving the legs slightly apart to air (the immodest position) is also beneficial. The patient should also avoid sitting on the healing wound.

If the vulvar wound is left open, postoperative management is the same except that silver sulfadiazine cream is applied after

each showerhead, blow-drying until there is good granulation tissue formation. In addition, these women are seen more frequently in the office to ensure good wound care and healing.

The patient is usually immobilized for at least 24 hours after a radical resection. Venous thromboembolic prophylaxis is necessary until the patient is ambulating. If the wounds are closed under tension, ambulation is restricted for 3 to 5 days, and the patient is instructed to avoid leg abduction when getting into and out of bed. A no. 18 Foley catheter is left in place for 3 to 5 days until the patient is easily ambulatory to act as a stent and divert urine while the urethra is healing.

Groin Care and Drains

A closed-suction drain such as a Jackson-Pratt or Blake drain is placed in the groin wounds. Drains are removed when the output has decreased to 30 mL or less per day to prevent lymphocyst formation. Compression boots are continued during this time, and care is taken to avoid marked femoral vein compression.

Especially when lymph node dissection has been extensive or radiotherapy is planned, long-term use of fitted graduated compression stockings may be beneficial.

Surgical Complications

Groin Complications

In published series of large numbers of patients undergoing en bloc radical vulvectomy with bilateral inguinofemoral lymphadenectomy, a high percentage (overall about 50%) of significant wound breakdown in the inguinal sites has been reported. Extensive undermining of the skin, fluid collections in the wound, and infection are all contributing factors, but the main problem is the considerable tension placed on these wounds during closure. The single most effective method of reducing groin wound breakdown (to around 20%) has been the use of separate incisions, as previously discussed. Suggested but unproven methods of prevention include prophylactic antibiotics, attempts to ligate lymphatic vessels, and prophylactic suction drainage. Modifying the resection by preserving the mons pubis, minimizing undermining of the skin, leaving a layer of fat with the skin, and excising any dark or dusky skin at the end of the operation may also reduce groin wound complications. With more extensive resection, plastic reconstruction (such as with TFL flaps) is also likely to be helpful.

Management of groin wound breakdown is similar to that of other wounds, with debridement and wet-to-dry dressings. During debridement, the surgeon must be cognizant of the femoral vessels. If infection has completely cleared, the wound is clean, and the tissues are pliable, secondary closure may be attempted.

About 10% to 20% of patients develop a clinically evident fluid collection (seroma or lymphocyst) in the groin. When such fluid collections are small and asymptomatic, they should be left alone. The most commonly recommended treatment has been repeated aspirations until resolution. When there is infection, prompt hospitalization with drainage and intravenous antibiotics is necessary. For persistent collections, we prefer reinstitution of suction drainage combined with pressure. Sclerotherapy is another option. If the problem is recalcitrant, the best course of action is to open and pack the cavity.

Femoral nerve injury is a rare but potentially debilitating complication of inguinofemoral lymphadenectomy. Not uncommonly, a few sensory branches are sacrificed, resulting in numbness or paresthesia of the anterior thigh. However, surgical injury of a major portion of the nerve lateral to the artery results in significant and potentially permanent difficulty with ambulation. As previously discussed, this complication is prevented by avoiding dissection on the lateral side of the femoral artery.

In the past, large series of patients undergoing en bloc radical vulvectomy with bilateral inguinofemoral lymphadenectomy reported a 1% to 2% incidence of severe postoperative hemorrhage from femoral vessel rupture. This was related to the extensive wound breakdown that occurred in a high percentage of these patients, with associated infection and necrosis involving the exposed and denuded femoral vessel walls. Coverage of the vessels by transposition of the sartorius muscle largely prevented this complication. With the use of separate incisions as well as other techniques that have reduced groin wound breakdown, and with avoidance of vessel skeletonization, postoperative femoral vessel rupture is now exceedingly rare.

Lymphedema

After groin node dissection, it is not uncommon for a patient to develop some degree of lower extremity edema. It is most often transient or mild but persists chronically as a significant problem in about 10% of patients. Factors that have been implicated as contributing to this complication include the performance of a pelvic lymphadenectomy, groin or pelvic radiotherapy, major groin wound breakdown, postoperative lower extremity lymphangitis, sartorius muscle transposition, and preoperative lymphangiography. Suggested methods for reducing this problem include limiting the groin dissection to the sentinel lymph nodes when feasible, confining femoral lymphadenectomy to the medial side of the femoral vein, preserving the fascia lata, avoiding pelvic lymphadenectomy, using adjuvant radiotherapy in a more tailored and selective manner, sparing the saphenous vein, wearing fitted support stockings prophylactically for the first 6 months to 1 year after surgery, using a low-dose prophylactic antibiotic to prevent lower extremity lymphangitis, and treating lymphangitis promptly with antibiotics when it occurs. Management of lymphedema begins with patient education, avoidance of trauma to the affected leg, and meticulous skin and nail care. Constricting clothing or jewelry should be avoided. A treatment program with a physical therapist specifically trained in lymphedema management is particularly helpful. Components of management include intermittent leg elevation, manual lymphatic drainage (massage) combined with bandaging, a carefully tailored moderate exercise program, carefully fitted compression stockings, and a carefully fitted pneumatic compression device. There is no effective pharmacologic therapy, and lymphangioplasty remains investigational. Some lymphedema patients occasionally develop lymphangitis, which presents with fever, pain, and redness of the involved extremity. This condition should be treated promptly with an intravenous antibiotic that covers streptococci.

Other Urogenital Complications

Urinary tract infection is common in these patients and generally resolves with antibiotics or catheter removal. However, elderly women sometimes tolerate urosepsis poorly and become profoundly ill. A diligent search for urinary tract infection, treatment of the infection, and removal of the Foley catheter as soon as is practical are important measures in these patients.

Osteitis pubis and osteomyelitis are rare complications that may not become symptomatic until several weeks after radical vulvectomy. The patient reports pain over the pubic bone and difficulty with ambulation, which may become chronic and debilitating. This complication is more likely to develop if the periosteum is traumatized, although this is not always avoidable. Extensive use of the cautery on the periosteum should be avoided. The mainstay of treatment is bed rest and nonsteroidal anti-inflammatory drugs. Even more rarely, frank osteomyelitis of the pubic bone develops. This is a serious condition that requires debridement and drainage of the bone, along with prolonged antibiotic therapy.

Rarely, a rectovaginal fistula develops days to weeks after radical vulvectomy. Prevention of this complication is based on preoperative evacuation of the colon, careful surgical dissection of this area, and prompt recognition of rectal entry. Surgical repair of the fistula is carried out once the area has healed and regained its elasticity.

During follow-up of radical vulvectomy patients, it is not uncommon to discover pelvic relaxation (cystocele or rectocele). This may be related to resection of the perineal body with the attendant loss of its support functions or it may simply be a result of aging. If the patient's medical condition and extent of cancer surgery permit, any stress urinary incontinence or defects in vaginal support should be repaired at the time of radical vulvectomy because they are likely to worsen subsequently.

Spraying or misdirection of the urinary stream is related to poor alignment of the urethra, a hood of periclitoral tissue obstructing the path of the urinary stream, or asymmetry created by a hemivulvectomy. Digital manipulation or the use of an applied collection or directing device is useful, but in some cases, minor surgical revision may offer the best solution.

Rarely, after inguinofemoral lymphadenectomy, a femoral or inguinal hernia develops. When a hernia or any apparent weakness of the femoral or inguinal canal is noted at the time of surgery, it should be repaired at that time. Avoiding incision of the inguinal ligament is also important in the prevention of this complication.

Sexual Function

More studies on sexual function and sexuality after vulvar surgery have been done recently. Generally, the capacity for intercourse remains. However, patients experience a marked sense of disfigurement and a reduction in genital sensitivity, and depression related to negative body image is also seen. A decrease in desire and relationship dissatisfaction are also common in women treated with radical vulvectomy. Dyspareunia can occur as a result of stenosis or scar tissue, and these problems may be surgically treatable. Some patients remain orgasmic. There is evidence to suggest that a modified radical vulvectomy, especially with preservation of the anterior vulvar structures, helps maintain sexual function. It does seem reasonable to assume that sparing of as much normal vulvar tissue as possible is less likely to produce sexual dysfunction and a sense of disfigurement than is radical resection.

Postoperative Adjuvant Treatment

This section deals with adjuvant therapy following radical or modified radical vulvectomy with inguinofemoral lymphadenectomy. Postoperatively, the only adjuvant therapy that appears to be of value is radiotherapy often given together with chemotherapy (see below). This can consist of radiotherapy to the local area of primary tumor resection, to the groins, to the pelvic nodal areas, or to all three. Postoperative radiotherapy administered to the remaining vulvar tissues is rarely indicated but may be considered when an extensive tumor has been resected with positive or close margins that cannot be readily excised further. As discussed later, this type of therapy may be particularly indicated in some Bartholin cancers because they are sometimes difficult to resect widely because of their deep-seated location.

Postoperative adjuvant radiotherapy has been used primarily in patients with metastases to the groin lymph nodes. Substantial data now exist regarding the prognosis and recurrence pattern in these patients. Because vulvar cancer has a recurrence pattern that tends to remain largely locoregional, its use for patients at high risk of recurrence is rational. There are further data to substantiate the benefit of radiotherapy in this setting. When a patient has metastases limited to microscopic involvement of one or perhaps two unilateral groin lymph nodes, the incidence of groin recurrence and pelvic lymph node metastases is very low, the overall prognosis is still reasonably good, and the benefit of postoperative radiotherapy is not great. If, however, there is gross replacement or extracapsular involvement of a lymph node, or involvement of three or more lymph nodes, the risk of groin recurrence and pelvic nodal metastases is substantial and the benefit of adjuvant postoperative radiotherapy is much more evident. A head-to-head comparison of pelvic lymphadenectomy alone versus adjuvant groin and pelvic radiotherapy showed a decrease in recurrence and increase in survival in the radiation group. When such treatment is anticipated, placement of metal clips to localize metastatic sites may aid the radiation oncologist in treatment planning.

Postoperative adjuvant chemotherapy has not been extensively studied, but it is unlikely to be of substantial benefit with use of the currently available agents.

Special Management Techniques

Concurrent Chemoradiotherapy

Combined chemoradiotherapy with or without resection has been used increasingly over the past few decades with promising results in squamous cell carcinomas of several different primary sites. This approach has been particularly successful in the treatment of squamous cell carcinoma of the anus. This type of carcinoma may be somewhat analogous to carcinoma of the vulva in terms of location and, in some instances, preservation of the anus.

The most commonly used chemotherapeutic agents are 5-fluorouracil, mitomycin-C, and cisplatin. Most data have been accumulated over the past 20 years with the use of regimens similar to those used at other sites. There have been no trials of head-to-head comparison between chemoradiotherapy and radiotherapy alone for primary treatment of vulvar cancer. A single trial by Raffeto et al. of 20 cases of recurrent vulvar cancer using both modalities showed only 20% long-term survival in the entire cohort. The addition of cisplatin to radiotherapy in vulvar cancer is largely extrapolated from the literature on cervical cancer. Results suggest a high rate of local control for locally advanced or recurrent disease (Table 49.4). However, an increase in the degree of local morbidity is seen with this type of therapy. Most of these patients develop a moderate amount of mucositis in the vulvovaginal area. This leads to dysuria and generalized pelvic and perineal discomfort. An indwelling catheter (suprapubic in some cases) and the use of various perianal and rectal preparations help ease the discomfort, although treatment interruption is necessary at times. A GOG trial of chemoradiotherapy with cisplatin and gemcitabine in as primary treatment for locally advanced vulvar cancer is ongoing.

Primary or Neoadjuvant Radiotherapy

The role of radiotherapy in the treatment of this malignancy remains unclear. In our experience, teletherapy combined with interstitial needles for locally advanced carcinoma of the vulva appears to be effective but associated with extensive morbidity. With the use of more modern treatment techniques and better definition of the optimal delivery of radiotherapy to the vulva, the role of this modality has been expanded. A modified course of radiotherapy used in combination with other treatment modalities appears to be more efficacious than radiotherapy alone in the treatment of this disease. Combined treatment modalities for this disease present an important form of

IX

TABLE 49.4 Results of Chemoradiotherapy with and without Resection

INVESTIGATOR	RADIOTHERAPY (Gy)	STAGE	CHEMOTHERAPY	SURGERY	PATIENTS WITH LOCAL CONTROL (%)	SEVERE COMPLICATIONS (%)	FOLLOW-UP (MONTHS)
Kalra (1981)	⁶⁰Co (30)	III	Mit-C, 5FU, bleo	RV, GND	1/1 (100%)	0	NA
Iversen (1982)	Meg (30–40)	Inoperable, recurrent	Bleo	2 RV, GND	4/15 (26%)	40	1–4
Nori (1983)	Meg (34–58)	III, IV, recurrent	Metronidazole	1 vulvectomy	5/6 (83%)	0	1–3
Levin (1986)	Meg (18–45)	T3N1-T4N0	Mit-C, 5FU	4 RV	5/5 (100%)	17	1–25
Lovett (1987)	Meg (40 ± implant)	III, IV	Cisplatin, 5FU	NA	1/2 (50%)	NA	10
Evans (1988)	Meg (20–64 ± implant)	NA	Mit-C, 5FU	NA	4/4 (100%)	NA	18
Thomas (1989)	Meg (40–64)	Recurrent	5FU ± Mit-C	5 LE	7/9 (77%)	9	5–43
Whitaker (1990)	Meg (25–45)	III, IV, recurrent	Mit-C, 5FU	2 RV	3/12 (25%)	25	6–9
Carson (1990)	Meg (45–50)	III, IV, recurrent	5FU, Mit-C, cisplatin	4 RV, 3 LE	6/8 (75%)	12.5	NA
Podczaski (1990)	Meg (51 + hyperthermia)	IV	5FU, cisplatin	RV	1/1 (100%)	0	8
Berek (1991)	Meg (44–50)	III, IV	Cisplatin, 5FU	3 RV, 1 PE	10/12 (83%)	0	7–60
Russel (1992)	Meg (46–78)	III, IV	5 FU ± cisplatin	1 RV	20/25 (80%)	8	2–52
Scheistroen (1993)	Meg (9–45)	III, IV	bleo	4 RV	6/20 (30%)	30	7–60
Koh (1993)	Meg (34–70)	III, IV, recurrent	5FU	9 LE, 2 RV, 1 PE	11/20 (55%)	5	14–75
Sebag-Montefiore (1994)	Meg (45–50)	III, IV, recurrent	Mit-C, 5FU	8 RV	17/32 (53%)	11	3–40

Study	Radiation	Stage	Chemotherapy	Surgery	Response	Toxicity	Range
Whalen (1995)	Meg (45–50 ± implant)	II, III	Mit-C, 5FU	6 LE	14/19 (74%)	0	11–72
Eifel (1995)	Meg (40–50)	Recurrent, T4N3	Cisplatin, 5 FU	6 LE, 1 RV, 1 PE, 3 GND	4/12 (33%)	17	17–37
Lupi (1996)	Meg (NA)	Recurrent, T4N2	Mit-C, 5FU	18 RV, 11LE, 29 GND	25/31 (80%)	20	22–90
Landoni (1996)	Meg (54)	II, III, IV, recurrent	Mit-C, 5FU	39 RV, 30 GND	47/58 (82%)	20	4–48
Cunningham (1997)	Meg (50–65)	III, IV	Cisplatin, 5FU	NA	9/14 (64%)	23	7–81
Moore (1998)	Meg (41–50)	III, IV	Cisplatin, 5FU	24 LE, 24 RV, 2 PE	60/71 (84%)	21	22–72
Montana (2000)	Meg (47)	N2/N3 nodes	Cisplatin, 5FU	34 LE, 37 GND	28/38 (74%)	47	56–89
Mulayim (2004)	Meg (45–62)	T3, T3N1	Mit-C, 5FU	None	5/6 (83%)	17	13–74
Beriwal (2008)	IMRT (42.8–46.4)	II, III, IVA	Cisplatin + 5FU	NA	13/18 (72%)	0	2–60
Mak (2011)	Meg (22–75)	II, III, IVA	Cisplatin, 5FU, Mit-C, carboplatin, paclitaxel	9 MRV, 28 RV, 7 WLE	26/44 (60%)	20	4–166
Moore (2012)	IMRT (57.6)	T3, T4	Cisplatin	34 GND, 13 RV	31/58 (53%)	131 grades 3 and 4[a] events, 1 treatment-related death	Median 24.8

[a]CTCAE v. 2.
Mit-C, mitomycin-C; 5FU, 5-fluorouracil; bleo, bleomycin; RV, radical vulvectomy; GND, inguinal lymphadenectomy; Meg, megavoltage; LE, local excision; PE, pelvic exenteration; NA, not available; IMRT, intensity-modulated radiotherapy.

management. Especially in patients with locally unresectable disease, initial treatment with external radiation therapy combined with chemotherapy appears to be the most reasonable approach. With the guidance of imaging and perhaps random biopsies, an additional treatment course could be planned. Careful planning of how much surgery may be necessary or how much volume needs additional radiation therapy may contribute to an overall decrease in morbidity in these patients.

Starting with the work of Boronow and others, data confirm that megavoltage radiotherapy can cause marked regression of even locally advanced vulvar carcinoma to the point at which a more limited resection can be undertaken (often with an improved resection margin) with sparing of organ function and improved quality of life. In an update of his study in 1987, Boronow reported that, of 48 bladders and 48 rectums at risk, 1 bladder and 2 rectums were lost because of local failure, and 1 bladder and 1 rectum were lost because of radiation injury. The report did not mention other types of bladder or bowel morbidity. Of 40 patients who underwent vulvectomy, 17 contained no identifiable residual cancer. There were no reported problems with wound healing. Similar results have been reported in other studies (Table 49.5). In these studies, survival with locally advanced disease so far has been comparable to that with ultra-radical surgery. Again, the optimal radiotherapeutic techniques for such treatment are not well defined. Boronow's group generally used a combination of external beam radiation and intracavitary brachytherapy, delivering a mean vaginal surface maximum dose of 86.26 Gy. His group and others have also used preoperative external beam therapy only, generally delivering a dose of about 50 Gy to the whole pelvis, including the vulva and groins. Surgery has generally been performed 2 to 6 weeks after completion of radiotherapy. Boronow and associates reported 42.5% of vulvectomy specimens and Hacker and colleagues reported 4 of 7 (57%) vulvectomy specimens to be negative for residual tumor.

Management of the regional lymph nodes in the context of combined treatment modalities has been variable and, by necessity, highly individualized.

Complications of Radiotherapy

Acute skin changes are seen almost universally in patients undergoing radiotherapy to the vulva and groin regions. A meta-analysis showed that moist desquamation was the most common complication in patients undergoing radiotherapy to the vulva and groin, and a GOG trial found that half cutaneous complications were severe (grades 3 and 4). Careful skin care, treatment of any associated infection, and even breaks in treatment are sometimes necessary. Adjuvant radiotherapy to the groin also increases the risk of lymphedema, as described in the previous section. Preoperative radiotherapy also increases the risk of surgical complications including necrosis, wound breakdown, abscess, and hematoma. Long-term complications are usually due to radiation fibrosis, which causes loss of tissue elasticity leading to contracture. This is the case in radiation-related urethral stricture, which may require repeated dilation. When the radiation field is extended into the pelvis, there is also the added risk of cystitis and proctitis.

Neoadjuvant Chemotherapy

A large number of pilot studies have reported on the use of neoadjuvant chemotherapy (NACT) in cervical cancer. The planned course of chemotherapy has been followed by surgery, radiotherapy, or both. Reported response rates have been high, and preliminary results with NACT followed by radical surgery are somewhat encouraging.

TABLE 49.5 Neoadjuvant Radiotherapy for Carcinoma of the Vulva

INVESTIGATOR	NO. OF PATIENTS	STAGE	SURVIVAL RATE (%)	SURVIVAL	SEVERE COMPLICATIONS (%)
Boronow (1987)	48	III, IV, recurrent	72	4–168 mo	23
Acosta (1978)	14	II, III	71	2 mo–8 y	14
Jafari (1981)	4	II–III	100	4–5 y	0
Hacker (1984)	8	IV	62.5	15 mo–10 y	12
Carlino (1984)	6	II–III	66.6	15 mo	NA
Fairey (1985)	7	I–IV	86	13 mo–3 y	14
Pao (1988)	2	I, III	100	1–2 y	0
Rotmensch (1990)	16	III, IV	45	12–72 mo	4
Zhang (1992)	51	III, IV	60.8	NA	NA
Perez (1993)[a]	16	T1–T4	50	NA	25
Balat (2000)	76	II, III, IV, recurrent	58	NA	NA
Landrum (2008)	33	III, IV	75	NA	NA

[a]Definitive radiotherapy without surgery.

TABLE 49.6 Neoadjuvant Chemotherapy for Locally Advanced Vulvar Cancer

INVESTIGATOR	NO. OF PATIENTS	STAGE	CHEMOTHERAPY AGENTS	RESPONSE RATE[a] (%)	SURVIVAL[b]
Shimizu (1990)	1	IV	Bleo, vinc, Mit-C, cisplatin	1 (100%)	100%
Durant (1990)	28	"Inoperable,"[c] recurrent	Bleo, MTX, CCNU	18 (64%)	NA
Benedetti-Panici (1993)	21	IVA	Cisplatin, bleo, MTX	Vulvar 2 (10%), nodal 14 (67%)	23%
Wagenaar (2001)	25	III, IV, recurrent	Bleo, MTX, CCNU	14 (56%)	12%
Geisler (2006)	13	IVA	Cisplatin, 5FU	10 (77%)	70%
Aragona (2012)	33	NA	Cisplatin, bleo, 5FU, paclitaxel, vinc	30 (90.9%)	NA
Raspagliesi (2014)	10	II, III, IV	Paclitaxel, ifos, cisplatin	8 (50%)	55%

[a]Response rate defined as partial + complete response excludes stable disease.
[b]Survival reported at the end of study period.
[c]Inoperable at time of diagnosis determined by treating surgeon.
Bleo, bleomycin; Mit-C, mitomycin-C; vinc, vincristine; MTX, methotrexate; NA, not available.

In 1993, Benedetti-Panici and colleagues reported the results of a pilot study using NACT followed by surgery in patients with locally advanced carcinoma of the vulva. Twenty-one patients with FIGO stage IVA (clinical) were treated. Chemotherapy consisted of cisplatin, bleomycin, and methotrexate plus citrovorum factor rescue. Local control was achieved in 12 of 21 (57%) of the patients (3 to 37 months), and the 3-year corrected survival rate was 24%. The study just discussed does not demonstrate any benefit of NACT over standard treatment approaches. Two European cooperative studies that used bleomycin, methotrexate, and CCNU and included patients with recurrent disease reported similar results. Response rates vary highly according to chemotherapy regimens used, as is survival (Table 49.6). It is difficult to draw any rational conclusion on the utility of NACT based on these limited data.

Ultra-Radical Surgery

Ultra-radical surgery has been used for patients with clinically resectable vulvar lesions and has generally consisted of a radical vulvar operation extended to include the anorectum and/or the lower urinary tract. This has included resection of bone in a few reports. Inguinofemoral and pelvic lymphadenectomies are usually performed as well.

In some cases, resection can be limited to partial removal of the urethra, anus, or anterior rectal wall. Subsequent incontinence may occur, but this can be prevented to some degree by reconstructive efforts. Reid and associates reported problems with urinary incontinence in 4 of 4 patients who underwent resection of 1 to 1.5 cm of the distal urethra and in 2 of 14 patients who underwent resection within 1 cm of the urethra for carcinoma of the vulva. The value of urethral reconstruction in this setting is uncertain, but it would seem worthwhile. Three recent studies have reported preservation of anal continence after partial sphincter resection and reconstruction for posteriorly located carcinoma of the vulva.

The cumulative literature from 1970 to 2014 includes 227 vulvar cancer "exenteration" patients (Table 49.7). The postoperative mortality rate ranges from 0% to 31%, with a mean of about 5%. The cumulative disease-free survival rate for these patients is 45%. In those series that have included an analysis, the survival has correlated well with the status of the regional lymph nodes. Most studies have not differentiated inguinal and pelvic lymph nodes. There have been very few survivors with positive nodes, either in our series or elsewhere. Some series also suggest that lymphovascular space invasion is an adverse prognostic factor. Although not well addressed in the literature, there is also significant physical and psychological morbidity resulting from these operations as a result of the extensive nature of the surgery and the need for a permanent colostomy and/or urostomy. Neoadjuvant chemoradiotherapy has lead to a decrease in such extensive surgery. Its use is now largely reserved for those patients with locally advanced disease who have previously received radiotherapy to the region.

Conclusion

The management of locally advanced vulvar cancer continues to evolve as reports of small series of these patients accumulate. Considering the relative paucity of data and the rarity and heterogeneity of these tumors, no clear-cut management guidelines can be constructed. It seems reasonable to individualize the management of these patients, carefully considering all of the various treatment modalities available.

POSTTREATMENT SURVEILLANCE

Following completion of treatment for vulvar cancer, long-term follow-up is warranted. It is reasonable to examine these women at least every 6 months for the first 5 years and annually thereafter. Some women are at higher risk for recurrence or have ongoing problems, and more frequent office visits may be warranted.

TABLE 49.7 Postoperative Mortality and Survival of Patients with Advanced Vulvar Cancer Treated by Exenteration

INVESTIGATOR	NO. OF PATIENTS	POSTOPERATIVE MORTALITY	NO. OF DISEASE-FREE SURVIVORS (FOLLOW-UP PERIOD)
Rutledge (1970)	13	0	10 (3 y)
Thornton (1973)	12	1	4 (7 mo–9.5 y)
Kaplan (1975)	9	1	4 (5+ y)
Krupp (1975)	13	2	3 (1.5–15 y)
Adams (1979)	5	1	2 (10–41 mo)
Benedet (1979)	5	0	1 (5+ y)
Phillips (1981)	12	1	5 (52–153 mo)
Cavanagh (1982)	13	1	5 (5+ y)
King (1989)	7	0	3 (9 mo–18 y)
Hopkins (1992)	19	0	10 (5 y)
Grimshaw (1991)	23	0	15 (4–146 mo)
Miller (1992)	21	0	9 (5 y)
Hoffman (1993)	11	0	6 (30–84 mo)
Miller (1995)	21	0	7
Forner (2012)	27	0	15 (6–123 mo)
Chiantera (2014)	16	5	4
Total	227	12 (5.3%)	103 (45%)

Follow-up is directed at early detection of recurrence (or later, a new primary vulvar tumor), identification and management of treatment-related complications, and surveillance for associated malignancies. As previously discussed, it is only with local recurrence of vulvar cancer that there is a reasonable expectation for effective salvage treatment.

Approximately 10% to 15% of women treated for vulvar cancer will develop an isolated local recurrence or a subsequent new primary vulvar tumor, well more than half of whom receive effective salvage therapy. During follow-up visits, attention is directed at careful inspection and palpation of the vulvovaginal area and groins. Annual cervical or vaginal cuff cytology is also recommended. Patients are encouraged to do self-examinations and promptly report new symptoms or lesions.

RECURRENT DISEASE

About 15% to 40% of patients with squamous cell carcinoma of the vulva develop recurrence after treatment. As discussed previously, the incidence of recurrence is influenced by a number of factors, most importantly the original stage of the disease, but also the depth of invasion, and the regional lymph node status. For patients with recurrent squamous cell carcinoma of the vulva, the site of recurrence is the strongest predictor of outcome. Only with an isolated local recurrence is there a reasonable expectation of successful salvage therapy (Table 49.8).

The most common site of recurrence is on the vulva. About 70% of recurrences have a local component, and 55% to 90% of these are isolated local recurrences. This is more likely to occur in the patient with negative lymph nodes at initial treatment. Certain factors predispose the patient to develop local recurrence, including a close resection margin (<1 cm), deep invasion, and a large tumor size. When a patient develops an isolated local recurrence, the reported salvage rate ranges from 40% to 80%. Treatment depends on the individual situation. When feasible, radical resection is performed. Otherwise, the best approach is probably preoperative radiotherapy with or without chemotherapy followed by resection.

The presence of inguinal nodal metastases, especially when multiple, bilateral, or extracapsular spread is seen, predisposes the patient to recurrence within the groin or pelvis and systemically. The prognosis for a patient with regional or systemic recurrence is poor. Regional recurrences do not lend themselves well to salvage resection. Radiotherapy is not very effective against grossly recurrent disease, and there is no effective systemic therapy. A small percentage of patients with groin recurrence can be salvaged with resection followed by radiotherapy.

Distant recurrence carries a dismal prognosis, as vulvar carcinoma is not very responsive to available chemotherapeutic agents. Currently used chemotherapy regiments are largely based on those used for metastatic squamous cell carcinoma of the cervix, with platinum plus a taxane as first line.

IX

TABLE 49.8 Vulvar Cancer Recurrence Site and Salvage Rate

INVESTIGATOR	NO. OF PATIENTS	LOCAL RECURRENCE ONLY	GROIN ± LOCAL	PELVIS ± LOCAL
Buchler (1979)	27	13/18 (72%)	0/7	1/2
Podrat (1982)	59	15/30 (50%)	NA	NA
Simonsen (1984)	41	11/29 (38%)	1/12	None
Prempre (1984)[a]	21	6/12 (50%)	2/5	0/4
Hopkins (1990)	34	19/24 (79%)	0/10	None
Tilmans (1992)	40	9/17 (53%)	2/12	1/11
Piura (1993)	73	24/39 (61%)	NA	NA
Stehman (1996)	37	13/21 (62%)	0/12	None
Maggino (2000)	187	56/94 (60%)	8/33	0/10
Landrum (2008)	63	7/12 (58%)	3/12	2/12
Total	582	173/296 (58%)	16/103 (15%)	4/39 (10%)

[a]All patients treated with radiotherapy *only*.

Response rates are generally less than 20%. Even those patients who respond to chemotherapy have a relatively short progression-free interval. Palliative care referral should be considered for patients with progressive disease or those who are not candidates for chemotherapy.

UNUSUAL VULVAR TUMORS

Vulvar Melanoma

Melanoma is the second most common histologic type of malignancy of the vulva but only accounts for about 10% of all vulvar cancers (Fig. 49.23). This lesion occurs predominantly in white women in the seventh decade, and although the vulva covers only 1% to 2% of the body surface, vulvar melanoma accounts for 3% to 5% of malignant melanomas in women. The most common presenting symptoms are bleeding, a lump or changing mole, and pruritus or irritation. In a small percentage of patients, there is a family history of melanoma. Melanoma of the vulva is uncommon, so most of the literature on the subject consists of retrospective studies of small numbers of patients. However, the behavior of vulvar melanoma appears to be very similar to that of cutaneous melanomas in general.

Therefore, the treatment of vulvar melanoma is individualized based on clinical–pathologic factors, including melanoma microstaging, and modeled using experience derived from cutaneous melanomas in other skin sites.

What Do We Know about Cutaneous Melanoma?

Important areas of information that can be extrapolated from the general melanoma literature include individualization of management based primarily on microstaging, determination of what constitutes an adequate margin of resection, and definition of which groups of patients might benefit from an elective regional lymph node dissection.

Clark classification has historically been used extensively for the microstaging of melanomas, with division into five levels of invasion. More recently, Breslow classification—based

on millimeters of invasion from the upper granular layer of the epidermis to the deepest point of invasion—has become widely used. According to Breslow staging classification, tumor confined to a depth of 0.76 mm or less is generally within the epidermis and behaves as carcinoma in situ. It is generally agreed that melanomas less than 0.76 mm in thickness are associated

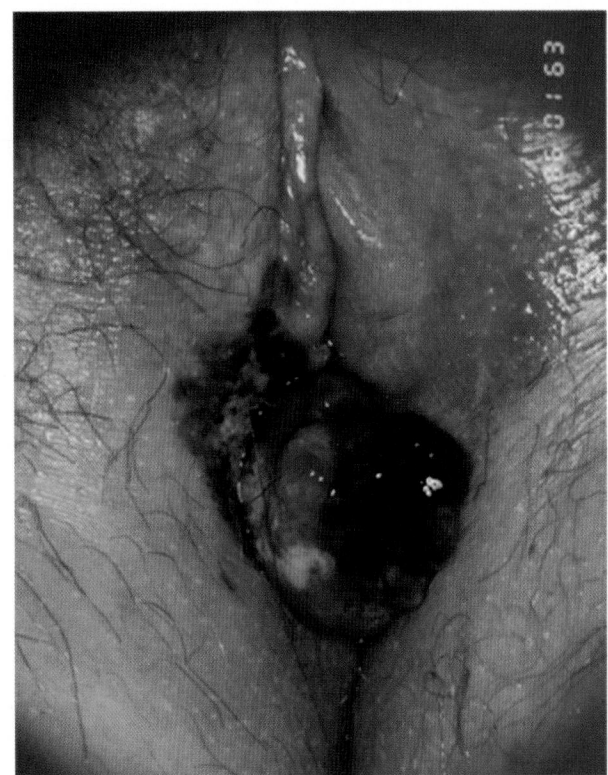

FIGURE 49.23 Large vulvar melanoma.

IX

with a very low risk of lymph node metastases, and elective regional lymph node dissection is not indicated in this group. The dominant prognostic factors for regional spread of melanoma include the number or percentage of metastatic lymph nodes, macroscopic versus microscopic metastases, and the presence of clinical or microscopic satellites around a primary tumor. In patients with distant metastases, the site of metastases, the number of metastatic sites, and an elevated serum lactate dehydrogenase (LDH) level are most predictive of poor survival. In the 2009 revision of AJCC melanoma staging system, tumor mitotic rate was added due to its significant association with survival outcomes.

Vulvar Melanoma

When a vulvar melanoma is suspected, as with any vulvar lesion, the diagnosis is best confirmed by biopsy. Workup of the patient with a clinically localized vulvar melanoma consists of a careful history and physical examination, a serum LDH level, and PET scan for evaluation of possible metastatic disease.

As with squamous cell carcinoma, the main modification in the local management of vulvar melanomas has been to tailor the resection to the individual lesion. A GOG trial demonstrated that centralized vulvar melanomas have a higher risk of nodal metastasis and are associated with a worse prognosis. For most women with vulva melanoma treatment of the primary lesion consists of a wide or radical local excision. For apparently localized lesions amenable to local removal, margin size should probably be that which is appropriate for a cutaneous melanoma, based on the depth of invasion of the melanoma as determined from the biopsy. For melanomas less than 1 mm in thickness, a margin of 1 cm is considered adequate. For those 1 to 4 mm, a 2-cm margin should be obtained. The excision should contain all layers of skin and subcutaneous fatty tissue. As with vulvar tumors in general, the excision must be tailored to the local vulvar anatomy. The frequent encroachment on midline vulvar structures by the melanoma creates difficulty in obtaining adequate margins while avoiding compromise of urinary or bowel function. Because of the propensity for early hematogenous spread in patients with deeply invasive tumors, ultra-radical resection is rarely, if ever, indicated.

Groin nodal metastasis is an important prognostic factor. Inguinal–femoral lymphadenectomy is not generally recommended for very superficial or deeply invasive vulvar melanoma. Nodal metastases are rarely found in lesions with less than 0.76-mm invasion, and systemic disease is usually present in women with a depth of invasion greater than 4 mm. In melanomas with depth of invasion between 0.76 and 4 mm, the data are unclear, but many experts now recommend sentinel lymph node biopsies for staging and prognostic information. There appears to be no therapeutic benefit from inguinal lymphadenectomy, although excision of isolated, enlarged, and suspicious nodes may be palliative. The overall incidence of lymph node metastases in vulvar melanoma patients is reported to be around 30%. If, during follow-up, isolated metastases appear in a previously undissected groin, they should be excised.

Local recurrence after resection of vulvar melanoma is reported to occur in about one third of patients, and the prognosis for these women is poor. Local tumor control and survival are reduced with more central and deeply invasive tumors. The presence of lymph node metastases also carries a poor prognosis, as previously mentioned. Management of cutaneous melanoma continues to evolve, and effective immunotherapy with BRAF inhibitors has been reported in patients with BRAF mutations. Following surgery, patients with vulvar melanoma should be referred to medical oncologists who specialize in melanoma treatment.

Extramammary Paget Disease

Paget disease is classified, according to location, as mammary or extramammary disease. The original lesion described by Paget is a skin (nipple and areola) lesion related to an underlying invasive ductal adenocarcinoma. Extramammary Paget disease most commonly involves the anogenital region, appearing as a patchy, reddish and whitish, velvety, and eczematous lesion (Fig. 49.24). Patients with Paget disease of the vulva are usually white, postmenopausal women who report localized itching and burning.

Paget disease of the vulva is of apocrine origin and is confined to the epithelium in most cases. However, invasive disease is present in about 15% to 25% of cases, either as a result of direct invasion through the basement membrane or, less commonly, because of the presence of an underlying apocrine gland adenocarcinoma. As with all vulvar lesions, biopsy is essential to the accurate diagnosis. Histologically, intraepithelial Paget disease appears as large, pale cells, often in nests at the tips of the rete ridges (Fig. 49.25). The cells are often seen infiltrating upward in the epithelium, which is hyperkeratotic. The Paget cells can be located within any of the skin adnexa.

Vulvar Paget disease occurs with other malignancies in about 25% of patients; the most common of these is breast carcinoma. Other commonly associated malignancies are basal cell, rectal, and genitourinary carcinomas. When Paget disease involves the anus, there is a very high incidence of coexisting rectal cancer. Part of the preoperative workup should be directed at screening for these malignancies. Wilkinson and Brown proposed a classification of vulvar Paget disease as primary or secondary (involvement of the vulvar skin by a noncutaneous internal neoplasm). They subclassified primary disease according to the presence of invasive cancer and subclassified secondary disease according to tumor origin. They report that secondary vulvar Paget disease is always intraepithelial.

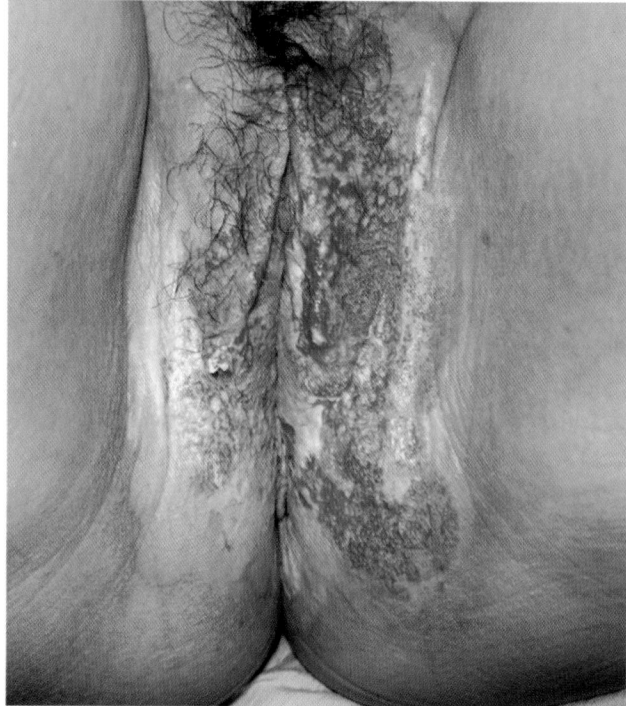

FIGURE 49.24 Extensive Paget disease of the vulva in a 47-year-old woman. This lesion is so severe and so extensive a total vulvectomy with careful histology is necessary to rule out an associated invasive cancer.

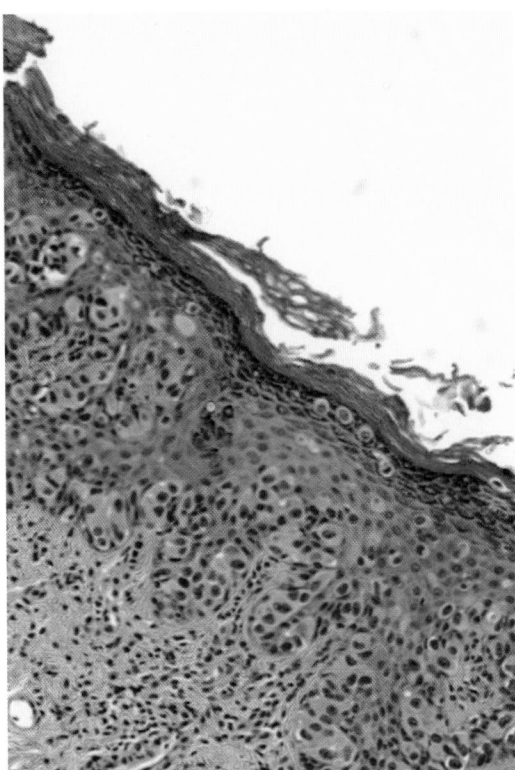

FIGURE 49.25 Histology of Paget disease. Extensive parakeratosis with nests of Paget cells infiltrating the stroma. (Photograph courtesy of Dr. Mokhtar Desouki, Vanderbilt University.)

When a patient is diagnosed with Paget disease of the vulva, the area of involvement should be carefully inspected and palpated to detect any masses or induration, which might be suspicious for invasive cancer. If the disease clinically appears to be intraepithelial, a wide local excision is performed, including a small amount of subcutaneous tissue. A well-known characteristic of intraepithelial Paget disease is histologic extension far beyond that which is clinically apparent. Intraoperative assessment of margins with frozen sections may be helpful. Multiple biopsies around the proposed margins of resection can also be done preoperatively or sent for frozen section in the initial phase of the resection to help guide to extent of the skin removed. Mohs micrographic surgery and fluorescein dye with ultraviolet light have also been used. Colposcopy and toluidine blue staining are not helpful, according to Friedrich and colleagues.

When intraepithelial Paget disease extends far beyond that which is clinically apparent, very extensive excision may be necessary to obtain clear margins. Experienced clinical judgment taking into account the short- and long-term morbidity related to the proposed extensive resection, the patient's age and lifestyle, other comorbidities, and the likelihood of symptomatic recurrence should be included in the discussion and decision about the extent of surgical resection. Primary closure of extensive vulvar excisions is desirable but may not be possible. Reported means of dealing with such cases include skin grafting and laser vaporization of the occult disease (guided by peripheral biopsies). There are a few reports of Paget disease recurring within a skin graft. Topical 5-fluorouracil, imiquimod or bleomycin, administered either preoperatively or postoperatively, has also been used to treat the clinically negative disease with positive margins. If it appears that excision of persistently positive margins may prevent primary closure, it is not unreasonable to close the wound and follow the patient closely.

After excision of intraepithelial Paget disease of the vulva, local recurrence develops in about one third of patients. Because of the difficulty of accurately evaluating the margin status due to the very irregular borders of Paget disease, recurrences are frequently seen in patients with a reportedly "negative" margin. Multiple recurrences over a prolonged period of time are common, and long-term follow-up is required. In some studies, recurrence risk has been correlated with excisional margin status, but it also has been pointed out that the initial disease in some cases is multifocal. Of particular concern are a few reports of patients whose recurrent lesions eventually became invasive. Whether such instances are preventable by diligently eradicating the full histologic extent of the disease is not known.

When vulvar Paget disease is found to contain an invasive component, the treatment is radical surgery, as for squamous cell carcinoma. Overall, these patients have a high incidence of inguinal lymph node metastases with an associated poor prognosis. The role of adjuvant therapy in these patients is unclear.

Verrucous Carcinoma

Verrucous carcinoma of the vulva is a rare variant of squamous cell carcinoma, accounting for less than 1% of vulvar carcinomas. This tumor was first described in the oral cavity by Ackerman in 1948 and most commonly occurs in the oral cavity, larynx, and anogenital region. The mean age of the women diagnosed with this malignancy of the vulva is about 50 years. The reported tumors have ranged from 1 to 10 cm in maximum diameter and appear as a slow-growing, cauliflower-like tumor. Characteristically, verrucous cancers have well-demarcated borders that are pushing rather than infiltrating. Verrucous carcinoma can be confused with condyloma (Fig. 49.26); when

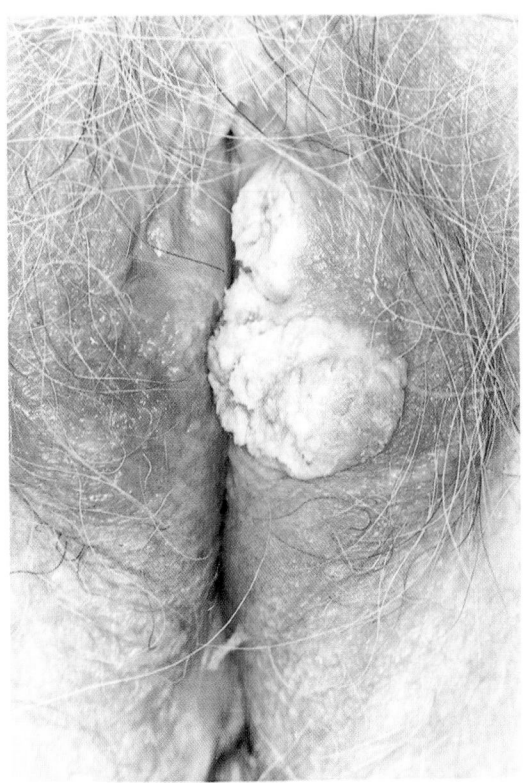

FIGURE 49.26 Verrucous carcinoma of the left vulva in an 83-year-old woman.

an apparent condyloma (especially when large and in an older woman) does not respond to the usual conservative measures, suspicion should be raised for a verrucous carcinoma. About one third of patients with vulvar verrucous carcinoma have a history of genital warts, and HPV has been detected in some lesions, the most common type being HPV-6.

The diagnosis of verrucous carcinoma requires a large (preferably excisional) biopsy that must include the base of the lesion. Verrucous carcinoma can also be confused with so-called warty carcinoma, another variant of well-differentiated squamous cell carcinoma that tends to remain in situ or superficially infiltrating. Differentiation of these two entities is not of great importance because both have a very low incidence of metastases, and treatment is essentially the same.

Verrucous carcinoma is rarely associated with metastatic disease, and many of the reports of such spread have shown histologic evidence of nests of squamous cell carcinoma invading the stroma beneath the tumor. Some authors have suggested that if areas of distinct invasion are found beneath a verrucous lesion, the behavior may be more aggressive, and treatment should be more radical. Inflammatory enlargement of the inguinal lymph nodes has been a frequently reported finding with verrucous carcinoma of the vulva.

It is generally agreed that the main treatment of verrucous carcinoma of the vulva is excision with free margins. How radical this resection should be is unclear, but local recurrences have not been uncommon. Local lesions have had a good initial response to radiation therapy but a high rate of subsequent recurrence and about a 30% incidence of anaplastic transformation with associated aggressive behavior. The few reported cases of metastatic verrucous carcinoma of the genital tract have followed radiotherapy. However, many tumors have been successfully treated with a combination of surgery and radiotherapy; when a tumor is locally advanced, this seems to be a reasonable treatment. Inguinal lymphadenectomy may be indicated in patients with large tumors; in patients with persistence or recurrence of disease, especially after radiotherapy; and in patients with infiltrating cancer beyond very early invasion below the verrucous tumor. Biopsy specimens may be obtained of enlarged lymph nodes thought to be inflammatory.

Verrucous carcinoma of the vulva has been associated with second malignant tumors, most commonly of the cervix, breast, and anogenital skin. Although verrucous carcinoma of the genital tract is a slow-growing tumor that rarely metastasizes, a 1988 review by Andersen and Sorensen reported that 26.1% of the patients with this type of carcinoma had died of disease.

Bartholin Gland Carcinoma

A malignancy can arise from the Bartholin gland or duct. The most common histology is adenocarcinoma, but squamous cell carcinoma is not uncommon. Other much rarer histologic types include transitional cell carcinoma, mixed carcinoma, and sarcoma. Bartholin carcinoma accounts for only 1% to 2% of vulvar malignancies, and, in some cases, a Bartholin origin is not clear-cut. Several criteria have been described to define a primary Bartholin malignancy, including anatomic position consistent with a Bartholin tumor, intact overlying skin, areas of apparent transition from normal to neoplastic elements, involvement of areas of the Bartholin gland with an origin histologically compatible with the gland, and no evidence of any other primary cancer. Although some of these criteria may not be met in an individual case, the tumor should at least be in a location consistent with a Bartholin tumor. As with the other rare types of vulvar malignancy, the available information on Bartholin malignancy is derived from retrospective studies of small series of patients.

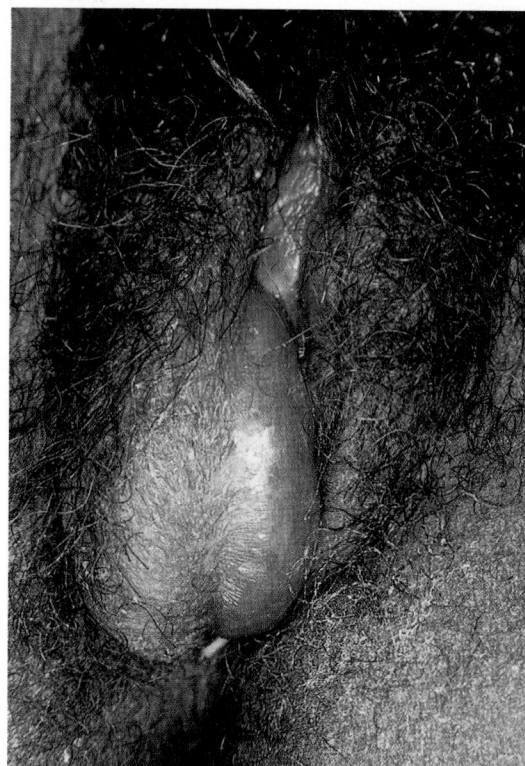

FIGURE 49.27 Large right labial cyst in the Bartholin gland. Excisional biopsy is needed to make a definitive diagnosis.

Diagnosis

Bartholin carcinoma should be suspected when a mass is noted in the region of the Bartholin gland, particularly in a woman older than 40 years of age (Fig. 49.27). The average age at diagnosis is about 50 years, but there is a wide age range. Many studies report a significant delay in diagnosis, attributed both to the deep-seated location of the tumor and to frequent misdiagnosis and treatment as a Bartholin abscess. When a woman presents with a Bartholin mass, biopsy or excision should be considered if she is older than 40 years of age, if the mass is suspicious, or when an apparently benign process does not resolve promptly with conservative therapy.

Treatment

Because of their deep location in the vulva, Bartholin malignancies tend to invade the ischiorectal fossa, close to the anorectum, or close to the pubic ramus (or all three) before they are diagnosed. These cancers also can erode through the overlying skin. As with other vulvar cancers, surgical resection should be aimed at adequate resection of the tumor. Radical excision with an adequate margin tends to be more difficult with Bartholin malignancies due to their deeper location. Depending on the tumor extent, local resection must consist of at least a radical hemivulvectomy, but it may need to include removal of portions of vagina, levator ani, ischiorectal fat, perineal body, anal sphincter, anorectum, pubic bone, or all of these. In locally advanced but respectable cases, exenterative surgery or multimodality therapy may be necessary.

Due to the difficulty in obtaining an adequate local resection, Copeland and associates reported improved local control with the administration of adjuvant postoperative radiotherapy. This is especially appropriate in the presence of close or positive margins. However, external radiotherapy alone should not be expected to control gross residual disease.

At the time of diagnosis, inguinal lymph node metastases are present in about half of patients with a Bartholin carcinoma. This propensity for lymphatic spread has been attributed to the frequent delay in diagnosis and the more advanced local extent of these tumors. The pattern of lymphatic spread is the same as that for other vulvar malignancies, primarily to the ipsilateral inguinofemoral lymph nodes. There are not enough data on which to base a reasonable estimate of the risk of metastases to the contralateral groin nodes. As with other vulvar cancers, if positive nodes are found, dissection of the opposite groin or radiotherapy to the inguinal and pelvic nodal basins, or both, may be warranted. Inguinal lymphadenectomy in these patients appears to be both prognostic and therapeutic.

Local, regional, and distant recurrences are common with Bartholin malignancies, and overall survival rate is lower than that for carcinoma of the vulva in general. Copeland and associates reported on a series of 36 patients with this cancer. The local recurrence rate was 2 of 12 (17%) for patients treated with hemivulvectomy (with or without radiotherapy) and 5 of 24 (21%) for patients treated with radical total vulvectomy.

Basal Cell Carcinoma

Although basal cell carcinoma is the most common malignancy of the skin, basal cell carcinoma of the vulva is a rarely reported tumor. Approximately 250 cases have been reported in the literature, and basal cell carcinoma constitutes 2% to 3% of vulvar cancers. The cause is unknown, but there is frequently a history of chronic vulvar irritation. This lesion shares many features with vulvar squamous cell carcinoma. The average age of patients at diagnosis is 65 years, and there is a predilection for white women. Common symptoms include chronic pruritus vulvae and the presence of a mass. As with squamous cell carcinomas, many authors have repeatedly reported a delay in diagnosis. Most basal cell carcinomas occur on the labia majora and, less commonly, on the labia minora, urethral meatus, and prepuce of the clitoris. The gross appearance is variable. Tumor size has ranged from 0.2 to 13 cm in greatest diameter, averaging 1.5 to 2 cm. There are also reports of multifocal lesions.

Treatment

Most authorities agree that the treatment of choice for vulvar basal cell carcinoma is wide local excision including a generous amount of underlying subcutaneous tissue. For a multifocal lesion, complete vulvectomy may be appropriate. Even when surgical resection margins are positive, local recurrence is not guaranteed. Mulvany and colleagues reported only three recurrences in 10 patients with a positive resection margin. If a malignant squamous component is present, however, then treatment is the same as that for invasive squamous cell carcinoma of the vulva as outlined above. There is little information available on the use of radiotherapy or chemotherapy in the treatment of primary or metastatic basal cell carcinoma of the vulva, but there is one report of a locally advanced lesion that had a complete response to radiotherapy. Close follow-up is essential, because the local recurrence rate has been reported to be 10% to 30%.

Prognosis

The overall prognosis for patients with vulvar basal cell carcinoma is good, but exact figures are difficult to ascertain. In a review by Breen and colleagues, there was a 5-year survival rate of about 64%. However, they were unable to find documentation for a single death directly related to recurrent or residual basal cell carcinoma. Rather, they attributed the deaths to other age-related illnesses and complications of overzealous therapy.

The prognosis for the rare metastatic basal cell carcinoma of the vulva is even more difficult to predict. Sworn and coworkers concluded that the prognosis is similar to that for basal cell carcinoma at other skin sites. With basal cell carcinoma elsewhere on the skin, the mean survival after discovery of metastatic disease has been reported to be 10 to 14 months. However, Conway and Hugo reported prolonged survival if only regional lymph nodes are involved.

Sarcomas

Primary sarcoma constitutes 1% to 3% of all vulvar malignancies. The literature consists of case reports and small series of patients, often with very limited follow-up. In addition, this is a heterogeneous group because of the variety of histologic types and their associated differences in behavior. Hence, the natural history and appropriate treatment of these tumors have not been well defined.

Leiomyosarcoma

The most common histologic type of primary vulvar sarcoma is leiomyosarcoma. Most of these patients are in the age range of 40 to 50 years, but a few are younger. At least four cases of pregnant women with leiomyosarcoma have been reported. According to the descriptions, most patients present with an enlarging mass in the labia majora or Bartholin region. Like tumors at other sites, smooth muscle tumors of the vulva appear to have a range of appearances and behavior, from benign to malignant. Tavassoli and Norris reported 32 smooth muscle tumors of the vulva and attempted to delineate the histologic features that might relate to prognosis. They believed that their analysis was impeded by small numbers of patients in subgroups and by varied adequacy of excision. According to their results, prognosis was best predicted by three main determinants (size, tumor contour, and mitotic activity). Neoplasms greater than 5 cm that have infiltrating margins and five or more mitotic figures per 10 high-power fields are likely to recur unless controlled by total excision. It was also determined that lesions larger than 5 cm with infiltrative margins and prominent mitotic activity have a more aggressive behavior as the number of mitotic figures increases. The significance of mitotic activity could not be fully evaluated because of the small number of cases with intermediate grades of mitotic activity and because of other factors. The degree of cellular atypism did not correlate well with the mitotic activity or with recurrence. In 1996, Nielsen and colleagues proposed similar prognostic criteria but included cytologic atypia. In keeping with a range of behaviors, according to the available reports, vulvar leiomyosarcomas may do well with adequate excision, may follow a slowly progressive course, or may rapidly progress to fatality. Local recurrences are common, and several authors have recommended early radical excision of these tumors to improve treatment results.

As with the other genital tract sarcomas, there is a propensity for hematogenous metastases that may develop early. From the few studies reporting long-term follow-up, it appears that only about half of these patients are 5-year survivors. Information regarding the propensity of these tumors to metastasize to the regional lymph nodes and the prognostic and therapeutic value of inguinal lymphadenectomy is scant. On the basis of general knowledge of the behavior of these types of sarcomas,

IX

the regional lymph nodes are probably at minimal risk with a low-grade tumor. In patients with high-grade tumors, removal of regional lymph nodes is probably of prognostic value only, although control of disease in the groin may have palliative value. In a fit patient with a high-risk but apparently localized tumor, inguinal lymphadenectomy seems reasonable. Radiotherapy has been used in only a few cases with mixed results. Postoperative adjuvant radiotherapy to the pelvis (including the perineum) may be worthwhile in selected cases to improve local control. As with other genital tract leiomyosarcomas, chemotherapy has been of limited palliative benefit.

Other Sarcomas

At least 100 cases of *aggressive angiomyxoma* involving the female pelvis or perineum, or both, have been described. Vulvar tumors often present as a pedunculated soft tissue mass. Most patients are aged 30 to 40. A few cases during pregnancy have been reported. It is an unusual tumor derived from fibroblasts or myofibroblasts with nuclei that have no atypical features or mitotic activity. The tumor appears to be locally invasive and spreads by direct extension only. Local recurrences are common, although there have been no reported deaths attributable to this tumor. The mainstay of treatment is wide excision both primarily and for recurrences. Response to gonadotropin-releasing hormone has been reported.

Other histologic types of sarcomas arising in the vulva have been described. These include DermatoFibroSarcoma Protuberans (DFSP), proximal epithelioid sarcoma, malignant fibrous histiocytoma, and variants of fibrosarcoma. Theses tumors vary widely in their aggressiveness and metastatic potential, but size of the primary tumor and mitotic activity seem to be important prognostic characteristics. Wide local excision with as much margin as possible is indicated, and additional surgery, radiation, or chemotherapy may be desirable based on the histology of the primary tumor, margin status, and metastatic workup.

Although sarcomas constitute only a small percentage of vulvar malignancies in general, they account for most vulvar cancers in children and young women. Overall, pediatric vulvovaginal *rhabdomyosarcoma* has a good prognosis and greatly reduced treatment morbidity because of the efficacy of combined treatment modalities (especially chemotherapy and brachytherapy). Radical surgery is no longer indicated in young patients with rhabdomyosarcoma. Rhabdomyosarcoma arising in older women and other histologic variants of rhabdomyosarcoma may not be so responsive to chemotherapy.

Isolated reports of a variety of other types of sarcomas arising in the vulva have been published. Treatment of these various sarcomas must be individualized according to the scant literature available, the potential aggressiveness of the malignancy as suggested by the pathologist, and the individual situation.

Merkel Cell Carcinoma

Merkel cell carcinomas are small cell (neuroendocrine) tumors of the skin that occur most commonly in sun-exposed areas (head, neck, and extremities) and behave in an aggressive manner. This malignancy was first described in 1972 by Toker. At least 15 cases of vulvar origin have been reported. The ages of these patients ranged from 28 to 79 years, and the tumors occurred in all regions of the vulva (four in the Bartholin gland). When originating from the vulva, Merkel cell carcinoma has behaved in a highly aggressive manner (even more so than Merkel cell tumors in general), with 11 patients having regional lymph node metastases. At least 8 developed distant metastases and died within 30 months of diagnosis. Surgery

and radiotherapy appear to be of value for local control only, and as yet, no effective systemic treatment exists. As in the treatment of small cell carcinoma of the lung, etoposide and cisplatin have been used for a few cases of Merkel cell carcinoma, with good responses. Three of the vulvar cases were treated with this regimen. Two progressed, and one had a partial response of very short duration.

Miscellaneous Tumors

Adenoid Cystic Carcinoma

Adenoid cystic carcinoma accounts for up to 15% of Bartholin gland carcinomas. As seen with electron microscopy, the tumor contains gland-like lumens filled with eosinophilic material derived from basement membrane, so it is of squamous cell origin. The behavior of this rare malignancy appears to be different from that of other Bartholin and vulvar cancers and to be similar to that of adenoid cystic carcinomas arising from other sites, such as the salivary gland. These vulvar tumors have a high local recurrence rate and a propensity for hematogenous metastases usually developing subsequent to local recurrence. Both local recurrences and metastases can be slowly progressive over a period of years but are not very responsive to radiotherapy or chemotherapy. In view of the difficulty in obtaining adequate surgical margins with Bartholin malignancies in general, and the high local recurrence rate and uncertain sensitivity to radiotherapy with adenoid cystic carcinoma in particular, a concerted effort to obtain at least 2-cm margins should be made when resecting this tumor. However, from the 65 cases reported, margin status did not seem to significantly impact recurrence risk. Postoperative adjuvant radiotherapy for close or positive margins did appear to be of possible benefit. From the scant information available, inguinal lymph node metastases occur less frequently with this tumor and have all been ipsilateral. The prognostic and therapeutic value of lymphadenectomy in these patients remains to be defined. The role of adjuvant postoperative chemotherapy for this malignancy also deserves further study.

Supernumerary Mammary Adenocarcinoma

Ectopic breast tissue in the vulva is very rare, but there are at least 26 cases of mammary-type adenocarcinoma arising in the vulvar location have been reported since 1872. These patients ranged in age from 49 to 81 years, and many patients present with an asymptomatic vulvar nodule. The labia majora was the location in 65% of patients according to a review by Abbott et al. Only one of the patients had evidence of primary breast cancer, but rather than representing metastatic disease, the vulvar lesion appeared to be primary from ectopic tissue. The diagnosis of vulvar mammary adenocarcinoma is based primarily on the histologic pattern of the vulvar tumor. Other criteria can include the finding of adjacent normal mammary glandular elements (one case of adjacent in situ malignancy), the presence of estrogen or progesterone receptor positivity, positivity for common breast markers, and ruling out an origin from skin appendages.

One of the reported patients died of disease without treatment 1 month after diagnosis. The patient with coexistent primary breast carcinoma died of widespread metastatic (including cerebral) disease 22 months after the diagnosis. Reports suggest that these tumors follow the same progression and dissemination routes as typical breast cancers via the lymphatics to the inguinofemoral nodes and hematogenously. Given that these tumors are histologically identical to primary breast cancers, most authors advocate application of standard breast cancer adjuvant treatments such as radiation, tamoxifen, and aromatase inhibitors.

BEST SURGICAL PRACTICES

- Prognostic factors
  - The dominant prognostic factor for invasive squamous cell carcinoma of the vulva is the status of the inguino-femoral lymph nodes.
  - Primary tumor factors that appear to have prognostic importance include depth of invasion or tumor thickness, tumor diameter, tumor differentiation, lymph–vascular space involvement, and margin status at resection.
- Pretreatment investigation
  - A biopsy confirming the presence of invasive cancer is necessary before any therapy. Because of the frequent advanced age and coexisting medical problems typical of women with vulvar cancer, a thorough preoperative evaluation by internal medicine and anesthesiology consultants should be considered. PET scanning is increasingly used to evaluate patients for evidence of metastatic disease, but it may not be sufficiently sensitive to justify omission of lymphadenectomy if the scan is negative.
- Treatment of invasive squamous cell carcinoma of the vulva
  - *Unilateral groin lymphadenectomy.* Limiting inguino-femoral lymphadenectomy to the ipsilateral side appears to be a reasonable approach in a patient with a well-lateralized early tumor that is well differentiated, with no lymph–vascular space involvement, and with negative ipsilateral inguinal lymph nodes.
  - *Sentinel lymph node identification.* An increasing body of evidence indicates that lymphatic mapping with a combination of isosulfan blue dye and technetium-labeled sulfur colloid followed by sentinel lymph node dissection is applicable to a large percentage of women with early invasive squamous cell carcinoma of the vulva. Injection of both substances increase the chance of sentinel node identification compared to either alone. Inguinal–femoral lymphadenectomy can be omitted if the sentinel node(s) are negative for metastatic cancer.
  - *Pelvic lymphadenectomy.* Pelvic lymphadenectomy is not indicated in most patients with vulvar cancer. Pelvic radiation therapy is usually administered in patients with positive groin nodes.
- Locally advanced vulvar cancer
  - About 30% to 40% of vulvar cancers are locally advanced. Current approaches to the treatment of locally advanced vulvar cancer include radiotherapy +/– chemotherapy, followed by surgical resection if there is sufficient response and the patient is a good surgical candidate. Ultra-radical surgery such as exenteration is largely reserved for those patients with recurrent disease and prior radiotherapy.
- Recurrent squamous cell carcinoma of the vulva
  - About 15% to 40% of patients with squamous cell carcinoma of the vulva develop recurrence after treatment. Only with an isolated local recurrence is there reasonable expectation of successful salvage therapy (preferably resection).
- Reconstructive techniques for the vulva and groin
  - When an extensive resection of a vulvar malignancy or a groin node metastasis is necessary, it may not be possible to close the wound primarily. Under these circumstances, closure of the incision and healing can be facilitated by a variety of reconstructive procedures. Leaving the wound open is another reasonable option.
- Uncommon histologic types
  - Melanoma, basal cell carcinoma, cancers of the Bartholin gland, invasive Paget disease, and other uncommon or rare vulvar tumors are often managed differently from squamous cell carcinoma. A biopsy of the lesion should identify these lesions to allow special treatment planning.

BIBLIOGRAPHY

Adelson MD, Miranda FR, Strumpf KB. Necrotizing fasciitis: a complication of squamous cell carcinoma of the vulva. *Gynecol Oncol* 1991;42:98.

Al-Ghamdi A, Freedman D, Miller D, et al. Vulvar squamous cell carcinoma in young women: a clinicopathologic study of 21 cases. *Gynecol Oncol* 2002;84:94.

Andersen ES, Sorensen IM. Verrucous carcinoma of the female genital tract: report of a case and review of the literature. *Gynecol Oncol* 1988;30:427.

Anderson BL. Sexual functioning complications in women with gynecologic cancer: outcomes and direction for prevention. *Cancer* 1987;60:2123.

Andreasson B, Nyboe J. Value of prognostic parameters in squamous cell carcinoma of the vulva. *Gynecol Oncol* 1985;22:341.

Andreasson B, Visfeldt J, Bock JE, et al. Value of four models for selecting patients for local excision of invasive squamous cell carcinoma of the vulva. *J Reprod Med* 1990;35:1041.

Andrews SJ, Williams BT, DePriest PD, et al. Therapeutic implications of lymph nodal spread in lateral T1 and T2 squamous cell carcinoma of the vulva. *Gynecol Oncol* 1994;55:41.

Ansink AC, Sie-Go DM, van der Velden J, et al. Identification of sentinel lymph nodes in vulvar carcinoma patients with the aid of a patent blue V injection. *Cancer* 1999;86:652.

Ansink A, van der Velden J. Surgical interventions for early squamous cell carcinoma of the vulva (Cochrane Review). In: *The Cochrane Library*, Issue 4. Oxford, UK: Update Software; 2002.

Anthony JP, Mathes SJ, Hoffman WY. Immediate flap coverage in the treatment of large surgical defects after tumor resection. *Surg Gynecol Obstet* 1993;176:355.

Aragona AM, Cuneo NA, Soderini AH, et al. An analysis of reported independent prognostic factors for survival in squamous cell carcinoma of the vulva: is tumor size significance being underrated? *Gynecol Oncol* 2014;132:643.

Ayhan A, Tuncer R, Tuncer ZS, et al. Risk factors for groin node metastasis in squamous carcinoma of the vulva: a multivariate analysis of 39 cases. *Eur J Obstet Gynecol Reprod Biol* 1993;48:33.

Baachi CE, Goldfogel GA, Greer BE, et al. Paget's disease and melanoma of the vulva. *Gynecol Oncol* 1992;46:216.

Bachrendtz H, Einhorn N, Pettersson F, et al. Paget's disease of the vulva: the Radiumhemmet series 1975–1990. *Int J Gynecol Cancer* 1994;4:1.

Bailey CL, Sankey HZ, Donovan JT, et al. Primary breast cancer of the vulva. *Gynecol Oncol* 1993;50:379.

Baird WL, Hester TR, Nahai F, et al. Management of perineal wounds following abdominoperineal resection with inferior gluteal flaps. *Arch Surg* 1990;125:1486.

Balat O, Edwards C, Delclos L. Complications following combined surgery (radical vulvectomy versus wide local excision) and radiotherapy for the treatment of carcinoma of the vulva: report of 73 patients. *Eur J Gynaecol Oncol* 2000;21(5):501.

Balch CM, Buzaid AC, Soong SJ, et al. Final version of the American Joint Committee on cancer staging system for cutaneous melanoma. *J Clin Oncol* 2001;19:3635.

Balch CM, Soong S-J, Milton GW, et al. A comparison of prognostic factors and surgical results in 1,786 patients with localized (stage 1) melanoma treated in Alabama, USA, and New South Wales, Australia. *Ann Surg* 1982;196:677.

Balch CM, Urist MM, Karakousis CP, et al. Efficacy of 2-cm surgical margins for intermediate-thickness melanomas (1 to 4 mm): results of a multi-institutional randomized surgical trial. *Ann Surg* 1993;218:262.

Ballon SC, Lamb EJ. Separate inguinal incisions in the treatment of carcinoma of the vulva. *Surg Gynecol Obstet* 1975;140:81.

Barnhill DR, Boling R, Nobles W, et al. Vulvar dermatofibrosarcoma protuberans. *Gynecol Oncol* 1988;30:149.

Barnhill DR, Hoskins WJ, Metz P. Use of the rhomboid flap after partial vulvectomy. *Obstet Gynecol* 1983;62:444.

Barton DP, Hoffman MS, Roberts WS, et al. Use of local flaps in the preservation of fecal continence following resection of perianal neoplasias. *Int J Gynecol Cancer* 1992;3:318.

Beller U, Quinn MA, Benedet JL, et al. Carcinoma of the vulva. FIGO 26th Annual Report on the Results of Treatment in Gynecological Cancer. *Int J Gynecol Obstet* 2006;95(Suppl 1):S7–S27.

IX

Benedet JL, Miller DM, Ehlen TG, et al. Basal cell carcinoma of the vulva: clinical features and treatment results in 28 patients. *Obstet Gynecol* 1997;90:765.

Benedetti-Panici P, Greggi S, Scambia G, et al. Cisplatin (P), bleomycin (B) and methotrexate (M) preoperative chemotherapy in locally advanced vulvar carcinoma. *Gynecol Oncol* 1993;50:49.

Ben-Izhak O, Levy R, Weill S, et al. Anorectal malignant melanoma: a clinicopathologic study, including immunohistochemistry and DNA flow cytometry. *Cancer* 1997;79:18.

Bergen S, DiSaia PJ, Liao SY, et al. Conservative management of extramammary Paget's disease of the vulva. *Gynecol Oncol* 1989;33:151.

Berman ML, Soper JT, Creasman WT, et al. Conservative surgical management of superficially invasive stage 1 vulvar carcinoma. *Gynecol Oncol* 1989;35:352.

Bjerregaard B, Andreasson B, Visfeldt J, et al. The significance of histology and morphometry in predicting lymph node metastases in patients with squamous cell carcinoma of the vulva. *Gynecol Oncol* 1993;50:323.

Bleicher RJ, Essner R, Foshag LJ, et al. Role of sentinel lymphadenectomy in thin invasive cutaneous melanomas. *J Clin Oncol* 2003;21:1326.

Boronow RC, Hickman BT, Reagan MT, et al. Combined therapy as an alternative to exenteration for locally advanced vulvovaginal cancer. II. Results, complications, and dosimetric and surgical considerations. *Am J Clin Oncol* 1987;10:171.

Bosquet JG, Magrina JF, Gaffey TA, et al. Long-term survival and disease recurrence in patients with primary squamous cell carcinoma of the vulva. *Gynecol Oncol* 2005;97:828.

Bottles K, Lacey CG, Goldberg J, et al. Merkel cell carcinoma of the vulva. *Obstet Gynecol* 1984;63:61S.

Bouma J, Dankert J. Recurrent acute leg cellulitis in patients after radical vulvectomy. *Gynecol Oncol* 1988;29:50.

Brand A, Covert A. Malignant rhabdoid tumor of the vulva: case report and review of the literature with emphasis on clinical management and outcome. *Gynecol Oncol* 2001;80:99.

Brooks JJ, LiVolsi VA. Liposarcoma presenting on the vulva. *Am J Obstet Gynecol* 1987;156:73.

Brunschwig A, Brockunier A Jr. Surgical treatment of squamous cell carcinoma of the vulva. *Obstet Gynecol* 1967;29:362.

Bryson SC, Dembo AJ, Colgan TJ, et al. Invasive squamous cell carcinoma of the vulva. Defining low and high risk groups for recurrence. *Int J Gynecol Cancer* 1991;1:25.

Burke TW, Levenback C, Coleman RL, et al. Surgical therapy of T1 and T2 vulvar carcinoma: further experience with radical wide excision and selective inguinal lymphadenectomy. *Gynecol Oncol* 1995;57:215.

Burke TW, Morris M, Levenback C, et al. Closure of complex vulvar defects using local rhomboid flaps. *Obstet Gynecol* 1994;84:1043.

Burke TW, Morris M, Roh RS, et al. Perineal reconstruction using single gracilis myocutaneous flaps. *Gynecol Oncol* 1995;57:221.

Burke TW, Stringer A, Gershenson DM, et al. Radical wide excision and selective inguinal node dissection for squamous cell carcinoma of the vulva. *Gynecol Oncol* 1990;38:328.

Burrell MO, Franklin EW III, Campion MJ, et al. The modified radical vulvectomy with groin dissection: an eight-year experience. *Am J Obstet Gynecol* 1988;159:715.

Cady B. Sentinel lymph node procedure in squamous cell carcinoma of the vulva. *J Clin Oncol* 2000;18(15):2795.

Cardosi RJ, Speights A, Fiorica JV, et al. Bartholin's gland carcinoma: a 15-year experience. *Gynecol Oncol* 2001;82:247.

Carlson JW, McGlennen RC, Gomez R, et al. Sebaceous carcinoma of the vulva: a case report and review of the literature. *Gynecol Oncol* 1996;60:489.

Carter J, Carlson J, Fowler J, et al. Invasive tumors in young women—a disease of the immunosuppressed? *Gynecol Oncol* 1993;51:307.

Cavanagh D, Fiorica J, Hoffman MS, et al. Invasive carcinoma of the vulva: changing trends in surgical management. *Am J Obstet Gynecol* 1990;163:1007.

Cavanagh D, Shepherd JH. The place of pelvic exenteration in the primary management of advanced carcinoma of the vulva. *Gynecol Oncol* 1982;13:318.

Chan JK, Sugiyama V, Tajalli TR, et al. Conservative clitoral preservation surgery in the treatment of vulvar squamous cell carcinoma. *Gynecol Oncol* 2004;95:152.

Collins CG, Lee FYL, Roman-Lopez JJ. Invasive carcinoma of the vulva with lymph node metastases. *Am J Obstet Gynecol* 1971;109:446.

Copeland LJ, Cleary K, Sneige N, et al. Neuroendocrine (Merkel cell) carcinoma of the vulva: a case report and review of the literature. *Gynecol Oncol* 1985;22:367.

Copeland LJ, Sneige N, Gershenson DM, et al. Bartholin gland carcinoma. *Obstet Gynecol* 1986;67:794.

Corney RH, Everett H, Howells A, et al. Psychosocial adjustment following major gynaecological surgery for carcinoma of the cervix and vulva. *J Psychosom Res* 1992;36:561.

Creasman WT, Phillips JL, Menck HR. The National Cancer Database Report on early stage invasive vulvar carcinoma. *Cancer* 1997;80:505.

Crum CP. Carcinoma of the vulva: epidemiology and pathogenesis. *Obstet Gynecol* 1992;79:448.

Cunningham MJ, Goyer RP, Gibbons SK, et al. Primary radiation, cisplatin, and 5-fluorouracil for advanced squamous carcinoma of the vulva. *Gynecol Oncol* 1997;66:258.

de Hullu JA, Oonk MHM, Ansink AC, et al. Pitfalls in the sentinel lymph nodes procedure in vulvar cancer. *Gynecol Oncol* 2004;94:10.

DeCesare SL, Fiorica JV, Roberts WS, et al. A pilot study utilizing intraoperative lymphoscintigraphy for identification of the sentinel lymph nodes in vulvar cancer. *Gynecol Oncol* 1997;66:425.

DiSaia PJ. Management of superficially invasive vulvar carcinoma. *Clin Obstet Gynecol* 1985;28:196.

Downs LS Jr, Ghosh K, Dusenbery KE, et al. Stage IV carcinoma of the Bartholin gland managed with primary chemoradiation. *Gynecol Oncol* 2002;87:210.

Eifel PJ, Morris M, Burke TW, et al. Prolonged continuous infusion cisplatin and 5-fluorouracil with radiation for locally advanced carcinoma of the vulva. *Gynecol Oncol* 1995;59:51.

Elit L, Hancock G, Carey M, et al. Comparing the morbidity of single versus separate incision surgical approaches to vulvar cancer. *J Gynecol Tech* 1999;5:147.

Elsandabesee D, Sharma B, Preston J, et al. Sclerotherapy with bleomycin for recurrent massive inguinal lymphoceles following partial vulvectomy and bilateral lymphadenectomy—case report and literature review. *Gynecol Oncol* 2004;92:716.

Fairey RN, Mackay PA, Benedet JL, et al. Radiation treatment of carcinoma of the vulva: 1950–1980. *Am J Obstet Gynecol* 1985;151:591.

Fanning J, Lambert L, Hale T, et al. Paget's disease of the vulva: prevalence of associated vulvar adenocarcinoma, invasive Paget's disease, and recurrence after surgical excision. *Am J Obstet Gynecol* 1999;180:24.

Farias-Eisner R, Cirisano FD, Grouse D, et al. Conservative and individualized surgery for early squamous carcinoma of the vulva: the treatment of choice for stage I and II (T1–2, N0–1, M0) disease. *Gynecol Oncol* 1994;53:55.

Fishman DA, Chambers SK, Schwartz PE, et al. Extramammary Paget's disease of the vulva. *Gynecol Oncol* 1995;56:266.

Flannelly GM, Foley ME, Lenehan PM, et al. En bloc radical vulvectomy and lymphadenectomy with modifications of separate groin incisions. *Obstet Gynecol* 1992;79:307.

Fons G, ter Rahe B, Sloof G, et al. Failure in the detection of the sentinel lymph node with a combined technique of radioactive tracer and blue dye in a patient with cancer of the vulva and a single positive lymph node. *Gynecol Oncol* 2004;92:981.

Frankman O, Kabulski Z, Nilsson B, et al. Prognostic factors in invasive squamous cell carcinoma of the vulva. *Int J Gynecol Obstet* 1991;36:219.

Frumovitz M, Ramirez PT, Tortolero-Luna G, et al. Characteristics of recurrence in patients who underwent lymphatic mapping for vulvar cancer. *Gynecol Oncol* 2004;92:205.

Ghamande SA, Kasznica J, Griffiths CT, et al. Mucinous adenocarcinomas of the vulva. *Gynecol Oncol* 1995;57:117.

Gil-Moreno A, Garcia-Jimenez A, Gonzalez-Bosquet J, et al. Merkel cell carcinoma of the vulva. *Gynecol Oncol* 1997;64:526.

Gleeson NC, Hoffman MS, Cavanagh D. Isolated skin bridge metastasis following modified radical vulvectomy and bilateral inguinofemoral lymphadenectomy. *Int J Gynecol Cancer* 1994;4:356.

Gleeson NC, Ruffolo EH, Hoffman MS, et al. Basal cell carcinoma of the vulva with groin node metastasis. *Gynecol Oncol* 1994;53:366.

Gordinier ME, Malpica A, Burke TW, et al. Groin recurrence in patients with vulvar cancer with negative nodes on superficial inguinal lymphadenectomy. *Gynecol Oncol* 2003;90:625.

Gould N, Kamelle S, Tillmanns T, et al. Predictors of complications after inguinal lymphadenectomy. *Gynecol Oncol* 2001;82:329.

Green TH Jr, Ulfelder H, Meigs JV. Epidermoid carcinoma of the vulva: an analysis of 238 cases. *Am J Obstet Gynecol* 1958;75:834.

Grimshaw RN, Murdoch JB, Monaghan JM. Radical vulvectomy and bilateral inguino-femoral lymphadenectomy through separate incisions: experience with 100 cases. *Int J Gynecol Cancer* 1993;3:18.

Hackera NF, Eifelb PJ, van der Velden J. Cancer of the vulva. FIGO Cancer Report 2012. *Int J Gynecol Obstet* 2012;119S2:S90–S96.

Hacker NF, van der Velden J. Conservative management of early vulvar cancer. *Cancer* 1993;71:1673.

Heaps JM, Fu YS, Montz FJ, et al. Surgical-pathologic variables predictive of local recurrence in squamous cell carcinoma of the vulva. *Gynecol Oncol* 1990;38:309.

Helm CW, Hatch K, Austin JM, et al. A matched comparison of single and triple incision techniques for surgical treatment of carcinoma of the vulva. *Gynecol Oncol* 1992;46:150.

Helm CW, Hatch KD, Partridge EE, et al. The rhomboid transposition flap for repair of the perineal defect after radical vulvar surgery. *Gynecol Oncol* 1993;50:164.

Herod JJ, Shafi MI, Rollason TP, et al. Vulvar intraepithelial neoplasia: long term follow-up of treated and untreated women. *BJOG* 1996;103:446.

Herod JJO, Shafi MI, Rollason TP, et al. Vulvar intraepithelial neoplasia with superficially invasive carcinoma of the vulva. *BJOG* 1996;103:453.

Hoffman MS, Cavanagh D, Roberts WS, et al. Ultraradical surgery for advanced carcinoma of the vulva: an update. *Int J Gynecol Cancer* 1993;3:369.

Hoffman MS, Gunasekaran S, Arango H, et al. Lateral microscopic extension of squamous cell carcinoma of the vulva. *Gynecol Oncol* 1999;73:72.

Hoffman MS, LaPolla JP, Roberts WS, et al. Use of local flaps for primary anal reconstruction following perianal resection for neoplasia. *Gynecol Oncol* 1990;36:348.

Hoffman MS, Mark JE, Cavanagh D. A management scheme for postoperative groin lymphocysts. *Gynecol Oncol* 1995;56:262.

Hoffman MS, Roberts WS, Finan MA, et al. A comparative study of radical vulvectomy and modified radical vulvectomy for the treatment of invasive squamous cell carcinoma of the vulva. *Gynecol Oncol* 1992;45:192.

Homesley HD, Bundy BN, Sedlis A, et al. Assessment of current International Federation of Gynecology and Obstetrics staging of vulvar carcinoma relative to prognostic factors for survival (a Gynecologic Oncology Group study). *Am J Obstet Gynecol* 1991;164:997.

Homesley HD, Bundy BN, Sedlis A, et al. Prognostic factors for groin node metastasis in squamous cell carcinoma of the vulva (a Gynecologic Oncology Group study). *Gynecol Oncol* 1993;49:279.

Homesley HD, Bundy BN, Sedlis A, et al. Radiation therapy versus pelvic node resection for carcinoma of the vulva with positive groin nodes. *Obstet Gynecol* 1986;68:733.

Hopkins MP, Reid GC, Morley GW. Radical vulvectomy; the decision for the incision. *Cancer* 1993;72:799.

Husseinzadeh N, Recinto C. Frequency of invasive cancer in surgically excised vulvar lesions with intraepithelial neoplasia (VIN 3). *Gynecol Oncol* 1999;73:119.

Hyde SE, Ansink AC, Burger MPM, et al. The impact of performance status on survival in patients of 80 years and older with vulvar cancer. *Gynecol Oncol* 2002;84:388.

International Society of Lymphology Executive Committee. Diagnosis and treatment of peripheral lymphedema. Consensus document of the International Society of Lymphology Executive Committee. *Lymphology* 1995;28:113.

Irvin WP, Cathro HP, Grosh WW, et al. Primary breast carcinoma of the vulva: a case report and literature review. *Gynecol Oncol* 1999;73:155.

Irvin WP Jr, Legallo RL, Stoler MH, et al. Vulvar melanoma: a retrospective analysis and literature review. *Gynecol Oncol* 2001;83:457.

Irvin W, Pelkey T, Rice L, et al. Endometrial stromal sarcoma of the vulva arising in extraovarian endometriosis: a case report and literature review. *Gynecol Oncol* 1998;71:313.

Jackson KS, Das N, Naik NDR, et al. Contralateral groin node metastasis following ipsilateral groin node dissection in vulval cancer: a case report. *Gynecol Oncol* 2003;89:529.

Jones RW, Baranyai J, Stables S. Trends in squamous cell carcinoma of the vulva: the influence of vulvar intraepithelial neoplasia. *Obstet Gynecol* 1997;90:448.

Jones RW, Rowan DM. Vulvar intraepithelial neoplasia III: a clinical study of the outcome in 113 cases with relation to the later development of invasive vulvar carcinoma. *Obstet Gynecol* 1994;84:741.

Judson PL, Jonson AL, Paley PJ, et al. A prospective, randomized study analyzing sartorius transposition following inguinal–femoral lymphadenectomy. *Gynecol Oncol* 2004;95:226.

Kelley JL III, Burke TW, Tornos C, et al. Minimally invasive vulvar carcinoma: an indication for conservative surgical therapy. *Gynecol Oncol* 1992;44:240.

Khoury-Collado F, Elliott KS, et al. Merkel cell carcinoma of the Bartholin's gland. *Gynecol Oncol* 2005;97:928.

Kirby TO, Rocconi RP, Numnum TM, et al. Outcomes of stage I/II vulvar cancer patients after negative superficial inguinal lymphadenectomy. *Gynecol Oncol* 2005;98:309.

Kirschner CV, Yordan EL, Geest KD, et al. Smoking, obesity, and survival in squamous cell carcinoma of the vulva. *Gynecol Oncol* 1995;56:79.

Klemm P, Marnitz S, Köhler C, et al. Clinical implication of laparoscopic pelvic lymphadenectomy in patients with vulvar cancer and positive groin nodes. *Gynecol Oncol* 2005;99:101.

Kodama S, Kaneko T, Saito M, et al. A clinicopathologic study of 30 patients with Paget's disease of the vulva. *Gynecol Oncol* 1995;56:63.

Koh W-J, Wallace J III, Greer BE, et al. Combined radiotherapy and chemotherapy in the management of local-regional advanced vulvar cancer. *Int J Radiat Oncol Biol Phys* 1993;26:809.

Krupp PJ, Bohm JW. Lymph gland metastases in invasive squamous cell cancer of the vulva. *Am J Obstet Gynecol* 1978;130:943.

Landoni F, Proserpio M, Maneo A, et al. Skin flap reconstruction of the perineal defect after radical vulvar surgery. *J Gynecol Surg* 1995;11:165.

Lataifeh I, Nascimento MC, Nicklin JL, et al. Patterns of recurrence and disease-free survival in advanced squamous cell carcinoma of the vulva. *Gynecol Oncol* 2004;95:701.

Lawton G, Rasque H, Ariyan S. Preservation of muscle fascia to decrease lymphedema after complete axillary and ilioinguinofemoral lymphadenectomy for melanoma. *J Am Coll Surg* 2002;195:339.

Leiserowitz GS, Russell AH, Kinney WK, et al. Prophylactic chemoradiation of inguinofemoral lymph nodes in patients with locally extensive vulvar cancer. *Gynecol Oncol* 1997;66:509.

Lens MB, Dawes M, Goodacre T, et al. Elective lymph node dissection in patients with melanoma: systemic review and meta-analysis of randomized controlled trials. *Arch Surg* 2002;137:458.

Levenback C, Coleman RL, Burke TW, et al. Intraoperative lymphatic mapping and sentinel node identification with blue dye in patients with vulvar cancer. *Gynecol Oncol* 2001;83:276.

Lewandowski G, O'Toole RV, Delgado G, et al. Carcinoma of the vulva: significance of surgical margin involvement in assessing prognosis. *J Reprod Med* 1989;34:884.

Lin JY, DuBeshter B, Angel C, et al. Morbidity and recurrence with modifications of radical vulvectomy and groin dissection. *Gynecol Oncol* 1992;47:80.

Loree TR, Hempling RE, Eltabbakh GH, et al. The inferior gluteal flap in the difficult vulvar and perineal reconstruction. *Gynecol Oncol* 1997;66:429.

Lupi G, Raspagliesi F, Zucali R, et al. Combined preoperative chemoradiotherapy followed by radical surgery in locally advanced vulvar carcinoma. *Cancer* 1996;77:1472.

Maggino T, Landoni F, Sartori E, et al. Patterns of recurrence in patients with squamous cell carcinoma of the vulva: a multicenter CTF study. *Cancer* 2000;89:116.

Magrina JF, Gonzalez-Bosquet J, Weaver AL, et al. Squamous cell carcinoma of the vulva stage 1A: long-term results. *Gynecol Oncol* 2000;76:24.

Malfetano JH, Piver MS, Tsukada Y, et al. Univariate and multivariate analyses of 5-year survival, recurrence, and inguinal node metastases in stage I and II vulvar carcinoma. *J Surg Oncol* 1985;30:124.

Marsden DE, Hacker NF. Urinary problems following simple and radical vulvectomy. *CME J Gynecol Oncol* 2002;7:61.

Massad LS, DeGeest K. Multimodality therapy for carcinoma of the Bartholin gland. *Gynecol Oncol* 1999;75:305.

Mazouni C, Morice P, Duvillard P, et al. Contralateral groin recurrence in patients with stage 1 Bartholin's gland squamous cell carcinoma and negative ipsilateral nodes: report on two cases and implications for lymphadenectomy. *Gynecol Oncol* 2004;94:843.

Mendenhall WM, Zlotecki RA, Scarborough MT. Dermatofibrosarcoma protuberans. *Cancer* 2004;101:2503.

Messing MJ, Gallup DG. Carcinoma of the vulva in young women. *Obstet Gynecol* 1995;86:51.

Microinvasive cancer of the vulva: report of the ISSVD Task Force. *J Reprod Med* 1984;29:454.

Miller B, Morris M, Levenback C, et al. Pelvic exenteration for primary and recurrent vulvar cancer. *Gynecol Oncol* 1995;58:202.

Modesitt SC, Waters AB, Walton L, et al. Vulvar intraepithelial neoplasia III: occult cancer and the impact of margin status on recurrence. *Obstet Gynecol* 1998;92:962.

Moore RG, DePasquale SE, Steinhoff MM, et al. Sentinel node identification and the ability to detect metastatic tumor to inguinal lymph nodes in squamous cell cancer of the vulva. *Gynecol Oncol* 2003;89:475.

Moore RG, Granai CO, Gajewski W, et al. Pathologic evaluation of inguinal sentinel lymph nodes in vulvar cancer patients: a comparison of immunohistochemical staining versus ultrastaging with hematoxylin and eosin staining. *Gynecol Oncol* 2003;91:378.

Moore RG, Steinhoff MM, Granai CO, et al. Vulvar epithelioid sarcoma in pregnancy. *Gynecol Oncol* 2002;85:218.

Morley GW. Infiltrative carcinoma of the vulva: results of surgical treatment. *Am J Obstet Gynecol* 1976;124:874.

Mulayim N, Silver DF, Ocal IT, et al. Vulvar basal cell carcinoma: two unusual presentations and review of the literature. *Gynecol Oncol* 2002;85:532.

Mulayim N, Silver DF, Schwartz PE, et al. Chemoradiation with 5-fluorouracil and mitomycin C in the treatment of vulvar squamous cell carcinoma. *Gynecol Oncol* 2004;93:659.

Nicklin JL, Hacker NF, Heintze SW, et al. An anatomical study of inguinal lymph node topography and clinical implications for the surgical management of vulvar cancer. *Int J Gynecol Cancer* 1995;5:128.

Nielsen GP, Rosenberg AE, Koerner FC, et al. Smooth-muscle tumors of the vulva: a clinicopathological study of 25 cases and review of the literature. *Am J Surg Pathol* 1996;20:779.

Oonk MHM, de Hullu JA, Hollema H, et al. The value of routine follow-up in patients treated for carcinoma of the vulva. *Cancer* 2003;98:2624.

Origoni M, Sideri M, Garsia S, et al. Prognostic value of pathological patterns of lymph node positivity in squamous cell carcinoma of the vulva stage III and IVA FIGO. *Gynecol Oncol* 1992;45:313.

Paley PJ, Johnson PR, Adcock LL, et al. The effect of sartorius transposition on wound morbidity following inguinal-femoral lymphadenectomy. *Gynecol Oncol* 1997;64:237.

Pao WM, Perez CA, Kuske RR, et al. Radiation therapy and conservation surgery for primary and recurrent carcinoma of the vulva: report of 40 patients and a review of the literature. *Int J Radiat Oncol Biol Phys* 1988;14: 1123.

Perez CA, Grigsby PW, Galakatos A, et al. Radiation therapy in management of carcinoma of the vulva with emphasis on conservation therapy. *Cancer* 1993;71:3707.

Pinto AP, Signorello LB, Crum CP, et al. Squamous cell carcinoma of the vulva in Brazil: prognostic importance of host and viral variables. *Gynecol Oncol* 1999;74:61.

Piura B, Masotina A, Murdoch J, et al. Recurrent squamous cell carcinoma of the vulva: a study of 73 cases. *Gynecol Oncol* 1993;48:189.

Podratz KC, Symmonds RE, Taylor WF, et al. Carcinoma of the vulva: analysis of treatment and survival. *Obstet Gynecol* 1983;61:63.

Potkul RK, Barnes WA, Barter JF, et al. Vulvar reconstruction using a mons pubis pedicle flap. *Gynecol Oncol* 1994;55:21.

Powless CA, Aletti GD, Bakkum-Gamez JN, et al. Risk factors for lymph node metastasis in apparent early-stage epithelial ovarian cancer: implications for surgical staging. *Gynecol Oncol* 2011;122(3):536–540.

Puig-Tintoré LM, Ordi J, Vidal-Sicart S, et al. Further data on the usefulness of sentinel lymph node identification and ultrastaging in vulvar squamous cell carcinoma. *Gynecol Oncol* 2003;88:29.

Ragnarsson-Olding BK, Kanter-Lewensohn LR, Lagerlof B, et al. Malignant melanoma of the vulva in a nationwide, 25-year study of 219 Swedish females: clinical observations and histopathologic features. *Cancer* 1999;86:1273.

Ragnarsson-Olding BK, Nilsson BR, Kanter-Lewensohn LR, et al. Malignant melanoma of the vulva in a nationwide, 25-year study of 219 Swedish females: predictors of survival. *Cancer* 1999;86:1285.

Reid R. Local and distant skin flaps in the reconstruction of vulvar deformities. *Am J Obstet Gynecol* 1997;177:1372.

Ribaldone R, Piantanida P, Surico D, et al. Aggressive angiomyxoma of the vulva. *Gynecol Oncol* 2004;95:724.

Rockson SG, Miller LT, Senie R, et al. Workgroup III: diagnosis and management of lymphedema. *Cancer* 1998;83:2882.

Rodriguez A, Isaac MA, Hidalgo E, et al. Villoglandular adenocarcinoma of the vulva. *Gynecol Oncol* 2001;83:409.

Rose PG, Tak WK, Reale FR, et al. Adenoid cystic carcinoma of the vulva: a radiosensitive tumor. *Gynecol Oncol* 1991;43:81.

Rosen C, Malmstrom H. Invasive cancer of the vulva. *Gynecol Oncol* 1997;65:213.

Rotmensch J, Rubin SJ, Sutton HG, et al. Preoperative radiotherapy followed by radical vulvectomy with inguinal lymphadenectomy for advanced vulvar carcinomas. *Gynecol Oncol* 1990;36:181.

Rouzier R, Haddad B, Dubernard G, et al. Inguinofemoral dissection for carcinoma of the vulva: effect of modifications of extent and technique on morbidity and survival. *J Am Coll Surg* 2003;196:442.

Rutledge F, Smith JP, Franklin EW. Carcinoma of the vulva. *Am J Obstet Gynecol* 1970;106:1117.

Rutledge FN, Mitchell MF, Munsell MF, et al. Prognostic indicators for invasive carcinoma of the vulva. *Gynecol Oncol* 1991;42:239.

Scheistroen M, Tropé C, Kaern J, et al. Malignant melanoma of the vulva FIGO stage 1: evaluation of prognostic factors in 43 patients with emphasis on DNA ploidy and surgical treatment. *Gynecol Oncol* 1996;61:253.

Scurry J, Brand A, Planner R, et al. Vulvar Merkel cell tumor with glandular and squamous differentiation. *Gynecol Oncol* 1996;62:292.

Sebag-Montefiore DJ, McLean C, Arnott SJ, et al. Treatment of advanced carcinoma of the vulva with chemoradiotherapy: can extensive surgery be avoided? *Int J Gynecol Cancer* 1994;4:150.

Selman TJ, Luesley DM, Acheson N, et al. A systematic review of the accuracy of diagnostic tests for inguinal lymph node status in vulvar cancer. *Gynecol Oncol* 2005;99:206.

Shepherd JH, Van Dam PA, Jobling TW, et al. The use of rectus abdominis myocutaneous flaps following excision of vulvar cancer. *BJOG* 1990;97:1020.

Siller BS, Alvarez RD, Conner WD, et al. T2/3 vulva cancer: a case-control study of triple incision versus en bloc radical vulvectomy and inguinal lymphadenectomy. *Gynecol Oncol* 1995;57:335.

Snijders-Keilholz T, Trimbos JB, Hermans J, et al. Management of vulvar carcinoma radiation toxicity, results and failure analysis in 44 patients (1980–1989). *Acta Obstet Gynecol Scand* 1993;72:668.

Soergel TM, Doering DL, O'Connor D. Metastatic dermatofibrosarcoma protuberans of the vulva. *Gynecol Oncol* 1998;71:320.

Soper JT, Elbendary AA, Hurteau JA, et al. Bulbocavernosus myocutaneous flap for perineal reconstruction. *J Gynecol Tech* 1996;2:141.

Stacy D, Burrell MO, Franklin EW III. Extramammary Paget's disease of the vulva and anus: use of intraoperative frozen-section margins. *Am J Obstet Gynecol* 1986;155:519.

Stehman FB, Bundy BN, Ball H, et al. Sites of failure and times to failure in carcinoma of the vulva treated conservatively: a Gynecologic Oncology Group study. *Am J Obstet Gynecol* 1996;174:1128.

Stehman FB, Bundy BN, Dvoretsky PM, et al. Early stage I carcinoma of the vulva treated with ipsilateral superficial inguinal lymphadenectomy and modified radical hemivulvectomy: a prospective study of the Gynecologic Oncology Group. *Obstet Gynecol* 1992;79:490.

Stehman FB, Bundy BN, Thomas G, et al. Groin dissection versus groin radiation in carcinoma of the vulva: a Gynecologic Oncology Group study. *Int J Radiat Oncol Biol Phys* 1992;24:389.

Tabbaa ZM, Gonzalez J, Sznurkowski JJ, et al. Impact of the new FIGO 2009 staging classification for vulvar cancer on prognosis and stage distribution. *Gynecol Oncol.* 2012 Oct;127(1):147–152.

Tamussino KF, Bader AA, Lax SF, et al. Groin recurrence after micrometastasis in a sentinel lymph node in a patient with vulvar cancer. *Gynecol Oncol* 2002;86:99.

Tateo A, Tateo S, Bernasconi C, et al. Use of V-Y flap for vulvar reconstruction. *Gynecol Oncol* 1996;62:203.

Tebes S, Cardosi R, Hoffman M. Paget's disease of the vulva. *Am J Obstet Gynecol* 2002;187:281.

Terada KY, Shimizu DM, Wong JH. Sentinel node dissection and ultrastaging in squamous cell cancer of the vulva. *Gynecol Oncol* 2000;76:40.

van der Velden J, van Lindert ACM, Lammes FB, et al. Extracapsular growth of lymph node metastases in squamous cell carcinoma of the vulva: the impact on recurrence and survival. *Cancer* 1995;75:2885.

Van der Zee AG, Oonk MH, De Hullu JA, et al. Sentinel lymph node dissection is safe in the treatment of early-stage vulvar cancer. *J Clin Oncol* 2008;26(6):884.

van Seters M, van Beurden M, de Craen AJM. Is the assumed natural history of vulvar intraepithelial neoplasia III based on enough evidence? A systematic review of 3322 published patients. *Gynecol Oncol* 2005;97:645.

Visco AG, Del Priore G. Postmenopausal Bartholin gland enlargement: a hospital-based cancer risk assessment. *Obstet Gynecol* 1996;87:286.

Wagenaar HC, Colombo N, Vergote I, et al. Bleomycin, methotrexate, and CCNU in locally advanced or recurrent, inoperable, squamous-cell carcinoma of the vulva: an EORTC Gynaecological Cancer Cooperative Group Study. *Gynecol Oncol* 2001;81:348.

Way S. The anatomy of the lymphatic drainage of the vulva and its influence on the radical operation for carcinoma. *Ann R Coll Surg Engl* 1948;3:187.

Way S, Benedet JL. Involvement of inguinal lymph nodes in carcinoma of the vulva. *Gynecol Oncol* 1973;1:119.

Weikel W, Hoffmann M, Steiner E, et al. Reconstructive surgery following resection of primary vulvar cancers. *Gynecol Oncol* 2005;99:92.

Wharton JT, Gallager S, Rutledge FN. Microinvasive carcinoma of the vulva. *Am J Obstet Gynecol* 1974;118:159.

Wheeless CR Jr, McGibbon B, Dorsey JH, et al. Gracilis myocutaneous flap in reconstruction of the vulva and female perineum. *Obstet Gynecol* 1979; 54:97.

Wilkinson EJ, Brown HM. Vulvar Paget disease of urothelial origin: a report of three cases and a proposed classification of vulvar Paget disease. *Hum Pathol* 2002;33:549.

Wilkinson EJ, Kneale B, Lynch PJ. Report of the ISSVD Terminology Committee. *J Reprod Med* 1986;31:973.

Zhang SH, Sood AK, Sorosky JI, et al. Preservation of the saphenous vein during inguinal lymphadenectomy decreases morbidity in patients with carcinoma of the vulva. *Cancer* 2000;89(7):1520.

CHAPTER 50
Cervical Cancer Precursors and Their Management

L. Stewart Massad

DEFINITIONS

The Bethesda System (TBS)—A classification system originally introduced in 1988 for grading cytologic abnormalities.

Cervical cytology—A diagnostic technique that involves microscopic examination of individual cells or cell clusters scraped, brushed, or washed from the surface of the cervix and stained with Papanicolaou stain. The nuclear characteristics and the nuclear–cytoplasmic ratio are used to diagnose the degree of cervical abnormality present. It is a common screening test for cervical cancer.

Cervical dysplasia—Dysplasia is a pathologic term to indicate noninvasive epithelial atypia that involves various degrees of the cervical epithelium. By convention, in *mild dysplasia*,

the nuclear atypia, mitoses, and cellular irregularity involve the lower one third of the squamous epithelium, moderate dysplasia the middle third, and *severe dysplasia* the upper third. Full-thickness dysplasia is termed *carcinoma in situ*.

Cervical intraepithelial neoplasia (CIN)—A cytologic and histologic classification of preinvasive cervical atypias or neoplastic changes. In general, CIN 1 = mild dysplasia, CIN 2 = moderate dysplasia, and CIN 3 = severe dysplasia/carcinoma in situ.

Colposcopy—A diagnostic technique involving visual inspection of the cervix and other areas of the lower genital tract with a low-power (3 to 15×) binocular scope. The surface contour, vascular pattern, and staining pattern of changes seen with dilute acetic acid and Lugol iodine reflect the severity and extent of cervical abnormality and help the clinician to select a location for biopsy confirmation.

Conization—Removal of the cervical transformation zone and part of the endocervix in a cone-shaped specimen. Traditionally performed with a scalpel, it also can be done with laser or wire loops.

Human papillomavirus—One of a family of protein-encapsulated DNA viruses, some of which are the necessary though not sufficient cause of cervical cancer. DNA sequence variations allow distinction of more than 150 genotypes.

Lower Anogenital Squamous Terminology (LAST)—A classification system introduced in 2011 for grading histologic abnormalities while incorporating the impact of papillomavirus infection on disease. Its two tiers mirror TBS terminology, including low- and high-grade squamous intraepithelial lesions. It includes provisions for molecular testing for equivocal lesions.

Loop electrosurgical excision procedure (LEEP)—Also called a large loop excision of the transformation zone (LLETZ). Cone biopsy performed with a thin wire electrosurgical loop electrode 1 to 2.5 cm, usually under local anesthesia.

Squamocolumnar junction (SCJ)—The junction between the squamous and columnar epithelium on the cervix. As columnar epithelium undergoes metaplasia to squamous epithelium on the cervical portion, the SCJ has a dynamic location.

Transformation zone—A colposcopic term for the area of metaplasia that is observed between the original prepubertal ("original SCJ"—lateral edge) and present squamocolumnar junction (medical edge).

Cervical cancer prevention has been very successful because of two important factors. First, preinvasive cervical changes that develop and progress slowly over years have been identified; second, relatively simple and inexpensive methods to detect and destroy these preinvasive cervical changes have been developed over the past 50 years. In recent years, the cause of these cervical changes has been identified as due to the human papillomavirus (HPV), and this has led to major changes in our understanding and management of both screening and treatment of cervical cancer precursors. Because of the sensitivity of screening tests, which rely on HPV detection and the fact that most women, even with high-risk HPV infection, will *not* progress to invasive cervical cancer, balancing the risk and costs of triage and treatment of these early cervical changes requires a thorough understanding of the natural history of these lesions and the risk and benefits of the triage and treatment options available.

EPIDEMIOLOGY AND ONCOGENESIS

In 1842, Rigoni-Stern noted that cervical cancer was found in married women, but was virtually absent in celibate women, such as Catholic nuns. Subsequent epidemiologic studies reported that number of sexual partners, early age at first sexual

IX

intercourse, low socioeconomic status, cigarette smoking, and early age at first pregnancy increased a woman's risk of cervical neoplasia. More recently, it has become clear that immunosuppression from any cause, including infection with human immunodeficiency virus and therapeutic immunosuppression after organ transplantation, is associated with an increased rate of cervical neoplasia. Oral contraceptive use has been reported to increase a woman's risk of cervical cancer, especially adenocarcinoma. Cellular changes on Pap smear described as "koilocytosis" have been recognized since the 1940s as correlates of cervical disease, but the human papillomavirus (HPV) was not identified as the etiologic agent in cervical oncogenesis until 1980 by zur Hausen. This discovery and the demonstration that HPV infection is the necessary though far from sufficient cause of cervical cancer won him the Nobel Prize in 2008.

The current understanding of the role of HPV in cervical oncogenesis is illustrated in **Figure 50.1**. The more than 150 types of HPV are members of a large family of encapsulated DNA viruses known as the *Papovaviridae*. Unlike many viruses that infect humans and that are serotyped by their surface antigens, the papillomaviruses are classified according to their DNA base-pair sequence. The degree of relatedness is determined by the degree of their DNA hybridization homology. HPVs are epitheliotropic viruses that infect virtually all surface epithelia, including the skin and mucous membranes. In addition to cervical cancer, they have been shown to cause significant proportions of vulvar, vaginal, anal, and oropharyngeal cancers and may contribute to malignancies at other sites.

The most prevalent anogenital HPVs can be divided into three groups that are predictive of their ability to produce neoplasia (**Table 50.1**). Low-risk HPV types are commonly associated with condylomas and cervical intraepithelial neoplasia (CIN) 1 and some CIN 2 s, but they almost never are associated with true precancer or cancer. HPV types 6 and 11 are responsible for approximately 90% of all condylomas of the lower genital tract. On the other hand, the anogenital HPV types with a high oncogenic risk are mainly types 16, 18, 31, 33, 35, 39, 45, 51, 52, 58, 59, and 68. HPVs in this risk group are overrepresented in high-grade lesions and cancers. HPV types 16 and 18 are highly oncogenic, accounting for two thirds of cancers and about half of precancers. The carcinogenicity of a few HPV types, such as 56, remains uncertain at this time.

TABLE 50.1 Anogenital HPV Types

Low-risk types	6, 11, 26, 40, 42, 43, 44, 53, 54, 61, 68, 72, 73, 81, 82
High-risk types	16, 18, 31, 33, 35, 39, 45, 51, 52, 56, 58, 59
Possible high-risk types	66

HPVs infect the cervix by entering basal cells following microtrauma to thin, immature portions of the transformation zone adjacent to the SCJ. Some 80% of sexually active adults appear to have been infected with HPV at some point. When a mitotically active epithelial cell is infected, the virus may remain in the cell in a form termed a *latent infection*. Latent infections can be detected only by molecular techniques and may be undetectable. In most women with an initial HPV infection, the infection clears spontaneously as a result of innate and cell-mediated immunologic host defense mechanisms. About half the women who test positive for HPV will test negative at 6 months later, about 70% will be negative at 12 months, and by 2 years only 8% to 20% continue to test positive. The highly oncogenic types 16 and 18 are more slowly cleared and more commonly persist compared with less oncogenic HPV types. Although women with transient infections may develop cervical epithelial abnormalities that result in abnormal Pap tests and even colposcopic abnormalities, these are usually low- or mid-grade lesions that often clear spontaneously. Approximately 50% of women with CIN 1 will resolve their lesions over 2 years without therapy. Among adolescents, with a more active immune defense system clearance rates approach 90%.

In some individuals, however, for reasons that are not well understood, the latent papillomavirus begins to replicate independent of the host cell cycle, and large numbers of complete virions are produced. This is referred to as a *productive viral infection*. These latent or productive viral infections may be clinically unrecognizable or may be associated with genital warts or CIN 1 or sometimes CIN 2, but they do not result in neoplastic transformation of the infected epithelial cells.

Transient Infection   Persistent HPV Infection

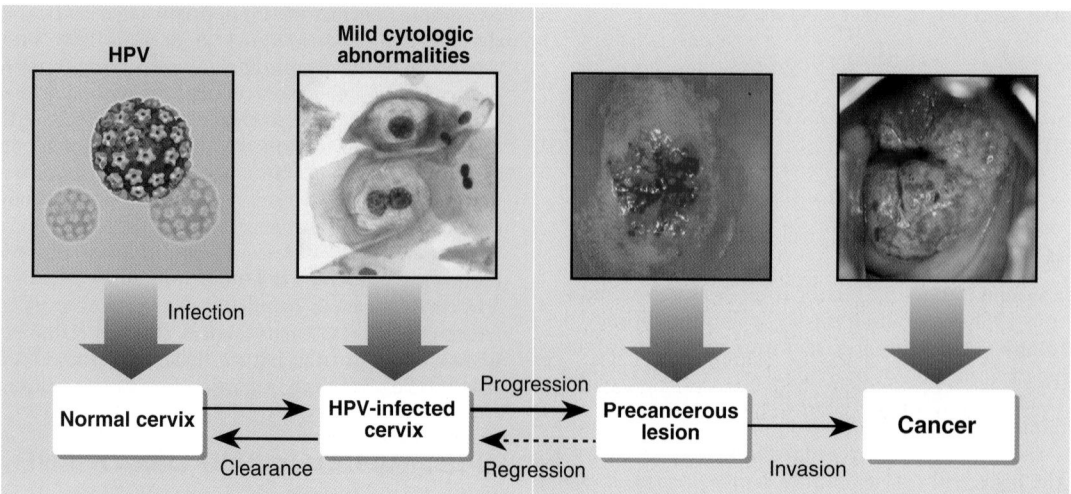

FIGURE 50.1 Natural history of cervical carcinogenesis. (From Schiffman M, Kjaer SK. Chapter 2: Natural history of anogenital HPV infection and neoplasia. *J Natl Cancer Inst Monogr* 2003;31:14–19. Reprinted with permission from the Journal of the National Cancer Institute Monographs. Copyright © 2003, Oxford University Press.)

In contrast to latent infections, some HPV infections are accompanied by alterations in the virus–host interaction critical to the transformation of normal epithelial cells to neoplastic cells. The key alteration seems to be the integration of the viral DNA into host chromosomes. Often, this is associated with loss of regulatory regions of the HPV genome and disruption of a host tumor suppressor gene. The E_7 protein binds to the pRB protein, which in turn triggers E_2F transcription factor and induces $p16^{ink4}$ expression, which leads to DNA synthesis and cell cycling. Other gene products employ host cell synthetic mechanisms to produce new viral DNA and viral proteins. These changes in cellular mechanisms would ordinarily lead to activation of epithelial cell p53 protein, an important protector of the normal cell cycle. However, the HPV E_6 protein targets p53 for proteolytic degradation, allowing oncogenic HPV types to bypass this key cellular control mechanism. Identification of E_6 and E_7 mRNA has been proposed as a more specific marker of epithelial cell transformation leading to cancer than simple HPV detection.

The likelihood of this oncogenic transformation after HPV infection varies by HPV type. In an analysis of HPV screening data of more than 20,000 women in the Portland, Oregon, area, Khan and colleagues found that women who had a negative Pap test and tested negative for any HPV had a less than 1% risk of developing CIN 3 within 10 years of follow-up. This contrasted sharply with women who had a negative Pap but who tested positive for HPV 16 on study entry; those women had a 17.3% risk of developing CIN 3 or a more severe lesion during the next 10 years. At least half of these women developed high-grade CIN within 24 months. For those who tested positive for other HPV types, the risk of developing CIN 3 was only 3%.

Although Rubin recognized "incipient carcinoma" in 1909, it was not until the 1950s that the preinvasive potential of *carcinoma in situ* of the cervix became generally accepted. In their 1952 publication, Galvin, Jones, and Te Linde described their observations of the natural history of carcinoma in situ. Their report confirmed and advanced previous studies by Cullen and by Pemberton and Smith. The concept of a clearly identifiable preinvasive neoplastic change in the cervical epithelium represented a major breakthrough in an understanding of the development and natural history of cervical cancer, but *carcinoma in situ* is clinically occult. Techniques such as the Schiller test with application of Lugol iodine and random four-quadrant biopsy proved imprecise in identifying women with *carcinoma in situ*, and many women with this diagnosis were treated with radical hysterectomy because of the uncertainty of the natural history of this diagnosis and of the risk of concomitant cancer. It was the parallel development of *cervical cytology* by George Papanicolaou and Herbert Trout in the United States after 1941 and of *colposcopy* by Hans Hinselmann in Germany after 1927 that provided techniques that rendered clinically useful the concept of a precancerous cervical lesion whose treatment would prevent the development of invasive cancer. Cytology allowed identification of women at risk, and colposcopy allowed clinicians to identify preinvasive lesions without conization, determine their extent, select sites for biopsy confirmation, and institute fertility-sparing therapy. These developments have led to a 70% reduction in cervical cancer deaths in the United States over the past 50 years. This chapter discusses how these preinvasive lesions evolve, how they can be diagnosed and distinguished from HPV-related lesions destined to clear, and how they can be treated.

TERMINOLOGY

Although *carcinoma in situ* became well recognized as a full-thickness epithelial change without stromal invasion, the terminology and clinical significance of adjacent, less-than-full-thickness atypia was uncertain. In 1956, Reagan and Hamonic introduced the term *dysplasia* to designate these cervical epithelial abnormalities that were characterized by cytologic atypia, increased mitotic activity, and loss of polarity, graded as *mild*, *moderate*, and *severe dysplasia*. The poor reproducibility of the distinction between CIS and severe dysplasia and the clear premalignant nature of the latter led Ralph Richart in 1969 to propound the concept of CIN. CIN 1, CIN 2, and CIN 3 were terms used to describe a continuum of disease, representing basaloid changes extending into the lower, middle, and upper thirds of the cervical epithelium with CIN 3 incorporating both CIS and severe dysplasia. Modification of the Bethesda cytologic and histologic grading was proposed by Darragh and colleagues in 2012. CIN 1 and other manifestations of HPV infection are labeled as *low-grade squamous intraepithelial lesions* (LSIL) and CIN 3 s a *high-grade squamous intraepithelial lesions* (HSIL). Since the histologic changes of CIN 2 are heterogenous, including both premalignant and spontaneously regressing lesions, this system encourages use of molecular tests, such as the HPV-related transformation marker $p16^{ink4}$, to assign mid-grade abnormalities to either the LSIL or HSIL categories. Although the Bethesda System terminology for reporting the results of cervical cytology has been accepted throughout the United States and is used in many other countries, other terminology and definitions are used in Great Britain, Germany, Australia, and other countries, which with different thresholds for colposcopy and treatment creates some difficulty in comparing study results across countries.

The original four- or five-step Papanicolaou cytologic classification, in which "class 1" was normal or benign and "class 5" was suspicious of invasive cancer; the World Health Organization classification of *mild, moderate, or severe dysplasia* and *carcinoma in situ*; and the Richart CIN terminal have been replaced in the United States by *the Bethesda system* (Table 50.2). Development of this consensus system was driven by several factors, including intraobserver variation and a lack of reproducibility. Multiple classification systems without common diagnostic criteria left clinicians unsure about appropriate management.

The Bethesda system was introduced in 1988 and subsequently updated and revised in 1991 and 2001. While cytology allows the identification of various infections and other nonneoplastic findings, the core of any report is the identification of epithelial cell abnormalities, either squamous or glandular. The Bethesda system combined HPV cytopathologic effects, often referred to as *koilocytosis*, with mild dysplasia or CIN 1 into a category called *low-grade squamous intraepithelial lesion* (LSIL). More significant lesions—including moderate and severe dysplasia and carcinoma in situ, or CIN 2 and 3—were combined into *high-grade squamous intraepithelial lesion* (HSIL). Pap tests with cellular abnormalities insufficient for definitive diagnosis of LSIL were categorized as *atypical squamous cells* (ASC). In 2001, these results were further subcategorized as *of undetermined significance* (ASC-US) or *cannot exclude high grade* (ASC-H). Glandular abnormalities less than cancer have been classified as *atypical glandular cells* (AGC), either *not otherwise specified* (AGC-NOS) or *favoring neoplasia*, and as *adenocarcinoma in situ* (AIS).

In the United States, a typical laboratory that processes cervical cytology from an average, generally low-risk population reports epithelial cell abnormalities in about 5% to 6% of patients. Usually, one half to two thirds of these abnormalities are ASC (2% to 4%), whereas 1% to 2% are LSIL and 0.5% to 1.0% are HSIL diagnoses, with about 0.5% glandular cell abnormalities. The ratio of ASC to SIL diagnoses should

---

TABLE 50.2 The Bethesda System of Cytologic Classification

The 2001 Bethesda System (Abridged)
SPECIMEN ADEQUACY
Satisfactory for evaluation (*note presence/absence of endocervical/transformation zone component*)
Unsatisfactory for evaluation … (*specify reason*)
   Specimen rejected/not processed (*specify reason*)
   Specimen processed and examined, but unsatisfactory for evaluation of epithelial abnormality because of (*specify reason*)

GENERAL CATEGORIZATION (OPTIONAL)
Negative for intraepithelial lesion or malignancy
Epithelial cell abnormality
Other

INTERPRETATION/RESULT

Negative for Intraepithelial Lesion or Malignancy
Organisms
   Trichomonas vaginalis
   Fungal organisms morphologically consistent with *Candida* species
   Shift in flora suggestive of bacterial vaginosis
   Bacteria morphologically consistent with *Actinomyces* species
   Cellular changes consistent with herpes simplex virus
Other nonneoplastic findings (*optional to report; list not comprehensive*)
   Reactive cellular changes associated with inflammation (includes typical repair), radiation, and intrauterine contraceptive device
   Glandular cells status posthysterectomy
   Atrophy

Epithelial Cell Abnormalities
Squamous cell
   Atypical squamous cells (ASC)
      Of undetermined significance (ASC-US)
      Cannot exclude HSIL (ASC-H)
   Low-grade squamous intraepithelial lesion (LSIL)
      Encompassing HPV/mild dysplasia/cervical CIN 1
   High-grade squamous intraepithelial lesion (HSIL)
      Encompassing moderate and severe dysplasia, carcinoma in situ, and CIN 2 and CIN 3
   Squamous cell carcinoma
Glandular cell
   Atypical glandular cells (AGC) (*specify endocervical, endometrial, or not otherwise specified*)
   Atypical glandular cells, favor neoplastic (*specify endocervical or not otherwise specified*)
   Endocervical AIS
   Adenocarcinoma

Other (*list not comprehensive*)
Endometrial cells in a woman ≥40 y of age
Automated Review and Ancillary Testing (Include as Appropriate)
Educational Notes and Suggestions (Optional)

---

be between 2:1 and 3:1 for most cytology laboratories, and roughly half of ASC-US and more than 80% of LSIL should test positive for high-risk HPV. Most cytology specimens are now processed using automated suspensions of exfoliated cells in liquid-based media (liquid-based cytology, LBC) rather than conventional Pap smears. LBC results in fewer unsatisfactory tests and has a greater yield but does not appear to be more sensitive in detecting true premalignant lesions compared to conventional Pap smears. An important advantage of LBC is the possibility of testing for HPV and other biomarkers from the same liquid-based specimen; women with ASC-US cytology who test negative for high-risk HPV types are at low risk for CIN.

The effectiveness of cytology screening has been demonstrated in organized national screening programs. In the United States, demonstration projects in the 1950s showed cytologic screening identified asymptomatic cancers. In Scandinavian countries, the introduction of national screening programs led to a dramatic decline in cervical cancer. However, screening may not be effective in women before ages 25 to 30. Most women who develop cervical cancer in countries with widespread screening availability have not had regular screening.

Despite its effectiveness in cervical cancer prevention programs, limitations to Papanicolaou test screening exist. A single Pap test has a sensitivity of only 50% to 60%. This means that a single test will not detect cervical lesions in many women. However, the slow progression of CIN before the development of an invasive cancer provides the opportunity for multiple screening cytologies over a period of years. So even with limited sensitivity, if three consecutive tests are negative, there is less than a 1% chance that the patient will have a high-grade cervical abnormality. Other screening problems include lesions that do not shed cells, do not transfer from the collecting device, or are not sampled by the clinician. Rarely, the slide preparation or staining is unsatisfactory. Another reason for screening failure is that cytotechnicians and cytopathologists may fail to identify abnormal cells or may misinterpret dysplastic cells as reactive or metaplastic. Glandular lesions are more commonly missed than squamous lesions. Women who are diagnosed with invasive cervical cancer after a reportedly "negative" Papanicolaou test often have abnormal cells on review of their slides that are few in number or obscured by blood or inflammatory changes. The threat of a lawsuit when cancer arises after cytology interpreted as negative may cause cytologists and cytopathologists to "overcall" an equivocal diagnosis and the gynecologist to recommend colposcopy and possibly cervical biopsy or even treatment in a patient with any hint of abnormality. This increases not only the anxiety and morbidity associated with cervical cancer screening but also the costs.

First popularized by Hinselmann in Germany, the *colposcope* is a magnifying instrument used to examine the cervix. With the colposcope, vascular changes and other epithelial patterns were recognized and correlated with cytologic and histologic changes. These early neoplastic changes were most prominent adjacent to the squamocolumnar junction (SCJ); this area was called the *transformation zone*, the area of the cervix that had undergone metaplasia from the prepubertal columnar epithelium to mature squamous epithelium. With time, colposcopic patterns associated with the developing stages of dysplasia and early invasive cancer were described. Adoption of colposcopy in North America was limited by cumbersome German terminology and the association of colposcopy with Nazi experimenters, including Hinselmann's associate Eduard Wirths. However, by the 1970s, colposcopy with directed biopsy had generally replaced cone biopsy as the triage test for women with cytologic abnormalities.

Following the announcement of the 2001 Bethesda System terminology for reporting the results of cervical cytology, the American Society of Colposcopy and Cervical Pathology has sponsored consensus conferences to develop and update management guidelines, expanding recommendations to cover results of cotesting. The guidelines are based on 5-year risk of CIN 3+ and prescribe similar management for problems with similar risks. They also incorporate cotesting into follow-up to improve sensitivity of surveillance for persistent or recurrent lesions, with longer intervals between follow-up tests to minimize the risk of identifying transient lesions. When cytology, colposcopy, and histology findings are discordant, expert review may be in order. Multiple biopsies minimize the likelihood of missing CIN 3+.

Once the importance of HPV in cervical oncogenesis had been demonstrated, other investigators suggested that a vaccine might prevent infection and perhaps even eliminate the HPVs in already infected individuals. Koutsky and colleagues tested immunization against HPV type 16 in a clinical trial, prospectively randomizing almost 2,400 young women who tested negative for HPV type 16 infection to three doses of a vaccine made from synthetic capsule protein or placebo. This and other trials showed that vaccinated HPV-naïve women develop essentially 100% immunity to targeted HPV types, with substantial reduction in subsequent CIN. Currently approved prophylactic HPV vaccines are targeted against L_1 capsid proteins and thus are HPV-type specific. The quadrivalent vaccine targets the high-risk HPV types 16 and 18, as well as low-risk types 6 and 11, while the bivalent vaccine targets only HPV 16 and 18. Minor side effects are common and include injection site pain and fever. Serious side effects are rare, but anaphylaxis and vagal reactions have been reported. Vaccines appear only prophylactic, with little or no effect on established infections. Multivalent and therapeutic vaccines are in development.

Screening for Cervical Neoplasia

The goal of cervical cancer prevention is the identification and destruction of precancer before the development of invasive disease that threatens life, health, and reproductive capacity. This must be balanced against the harms of screening, including stigmatization from the identification of HPV as a sexually transmitted infection, fear of cancer, and the potential for bleeding, local injury, and preterm delivery after treatment when lesions identified through screening are not destined to lead to cancer. For this reason, screening should not begin until age 21, since the risk of cancer in teens is negligible, and although precancers do occur earlier, they are unlikely to progress to invasion prior to detection in subsequent screening rounds. Similarly, cancer late in life is unlikely among women with long negative screening histories, so screening should cease in such women at age 65. The sensitivity of screening appears sufficient to allow 3-year intervals between Pap tests and 5-year intervals between Pap and HPV cotests. These screening recommendations were revised in 2013 (www.ASCCP.org).

A variety of devices have been devised for cervical sampling, including spatulas, brooms, and brushes. The spatula is rotated with gentle pressure twice around the cervix with the longer lobe in the os to enhance sampling. A broom is also rotated against the ectocervix. An endocervical brush is placed in the cervical canal with some bristles visible and rotated 90 to 180 degrees; deeper penetration and more vigorous rotation increase bleeding without improving cell collection. Cells should be transferred to slide or vial according to manufacturer's instructions; inadequate cell transfer may result in uninterpretable results.

Visual Inspection

Although colposcopy has been used instead of or in addition to cytology for cervical cancer screening in some areas of Europe and South America, it is time-consuming, requires well-trained clinicians, and is expensive. Simple visual inspection of the cervix after application of acetic acid (VIA) or Lugol iodine (VILI) has been studied in resource-poor settings for cervical cancer screening, alone or in combination with HPV testing. Areas of cervical dysplasia turn white after application of acetic acid and turn yellow after application of iodine. Inspection of the cervix using handheld low-power magnifying lenses can identify many lesions. Although these techniques have proved useful and cost-effective in resource poor settings, they are not appropriate for developed countries because of limited sensitivity and specificity. In most settings, VIA and VILI remain investigational.

Human Papillomavirus Testing

Primary HPV screening promises greater sensitivity but lower specificity than screening cytology. However, without longitudinal testing, HPV tests cannot distinguish the majority of women with transient infections from those few with persistent infections, which can progress to cancer. Current technology can identify DNA or mRNA from one or more high-risk HPV subtypes. Testing for low-risk HPV has no role in cervical cancer screening and should be discouraged. HPV testing can be automated and requires no interpretation, in contrast to the Pap test. These advantages must be weighed against its lack of specificity for high-grade lesions. Several approaches have been suggested to improve the specificity of HPV testing. Because the prevalence of HPV infection in most populations decreases around age 30, HPV screening should be more specific for cervical neoplasia in an older population. Despite promising studies conducted outside the United States, the appropriate triage test after a positive HPV screen is unclear. Recently, a type-specific HPV test for primary cervical cancer screening has been approved by the Federal Drug Administration for use in the United States. Experience with primary HPV testing for cervical cancer screening outside of a clinical study is limited. Cotesting that combines Pap and HPV testing increases sensitivity while preserving the familiarity of a Pap result is well suited for women 30 to 64 years of age. Since women with HPV types 16 and 18 are at increased risk for precancer, genotyping tests that identify these types can be used to identify women who need immediate assessment.

EVALUATION OF ABNORMAL SCREENING TESTS

Cytology

Collection of cervical cytology specimens depends on full visualization of the cervix, including the cervical os. This may require use of a variety of different specula. Graves specula, with their flared blades mirroring the vaginal fornices, are best adapted for reproductive age women. The straight blades of Pedersen specula are more suited to postmenopausal women or some young nulligravid women. After visual inspection confirms absence of gross lesions, cervical sampling is undertaken. A variety of different instruments are available, with little clinically meaningful difference among them in screening effectiveness. For spatulas and brooms, the instrument should be rotated at least twice. With the Ayre spatula, the longer lobe is placed within the endocervix. Cervical brushes, when employed, should not be inserted beyond the last bristles and should not be rotated more than 180 degrees to minimize bleeding. Samples should be place in liquid media according to manufacturers' instructions.

Colposcopy

The earliest and most severe epithelial changes on the cervix occur adjacent to the cervical SCJ. The location of the SCJ migrates inward during a woman's life. After vaginal acidification at puberty, columnar cells on the exocervix are transformed into squamous cells by a process called *metaplasia*. The area between the prepubertal and current SCJ where this metaplastic change has occurred is called the *transformation zone*. This epithelium can be recognized as a circumferential, pale white, translucent ring around the SCJ. These metaplastic cells are especially susceptible to coital trauma and HPV infection. As CIN develops, vascular changes occur, and these may be recognized as punctation or mosaic. If the lesion progresses, nonbranching vascular changes become visible. These atypical vessels have grossly abnormal architecture and are the colposcopic hallmarks of invasive cancer.

A standard colposcopic examination involves inspection of the cervix with both low- and high-power magnification after application of normal saline and then 3% to 5% acetic acid. Both optical and video colposcopes are available. The onset of acetowhitening peaks after 1 to 2 minutes, so some delay between acetic acid application and inspection is important. Low-grade lesions lose acetowhitening faster than high-grade lesions; repeated application of acetic acid may be required. After examination with the standard white light, a green filter may be used on the light source to increase the contrast of the red blood vessels and help clarify any vascular changes and the margins of acetowhite epithelium that may be present. Lugol iodine solution also may be used after inspection with acetic acid to clarify areas of dysplasia, metaplasia, or columnar epithelium. Manipulation with an endocervical speculum or cotton-tipped applicators may help to expose the SCJ and lesions within the endocervix. Large swabs may be needed to inspect the vaginal fornices, where low- and high-grade lesions may otherwise be hidden, especially when the cervix appears colposcopically normal.

Colposcopic terminology was updated by the International Federation for Cervical Pathology and Colposcopy in 2011. All of the squamous epithelium must be visualized for the examination to be *adequate* or satisfactory. An inadequate exam means that cancer cannot be excluded with confidence, and diagnostic excision is required when cancer risk. Once the adequacy of the examination has been evaluated, a careful systematic evaluation of the cervix and upper vagina is performed, concentrating on the *transformation zone* adjacent to the SCJ. Areas of white epithelium, punctation, and mosaic are noted. The severity of any lesions seen are graded based on the whiteness of the epithelium, the intercapillary distance in vascular lesions, the sharpness of the lesion border, and the surface contour (flat, ulcerated, or raised). Application of Lugol iodine can inform the grading of equivocal lesions, as normal epithelium stains dark brown, low-grade lesions are mottled yellow and brown, and high-grade lesions are yellow with sharp borders.

Traditionally, colposcopic grading was used to identify the most severely abnormal area or areas for a colposcopically directed biopsy. Lesions assessed as grade 1 (minor) have vascular changes such as mosaicism or punctation that are fine in caliber and are associated with thin acetowhite epithelium with irregular borders. Grade 2 (major) colposcopic lesions have denser, more long-lasting acetowhite epithelium in association with coarse vascular change and the presence of inner borders and ridging.

However, recent US studies have shown that while colposcopic grading reflects a true spectrum of disease, grading is imprecise and poorly reproducible, even among experts.

Colposcopic assessment may be more accurate in young women and those with larger lesions. With colposcopy alone, some high-grade lesions will be missed, and some low-grade lesions will be overcalled. For this reason, a histologic diagnosis based on one or more colposcopically directed cervical biopsies is the gold standard for determining the final diagnosis of the cervical lesion. Random biopsy of normal appearing areas of the cervix is not standard for US women with abnormal cytology, but achieving maximal sensitivity for precancer requires biopsy of all acetowhite areas. A recent prospective study by Wentzensen and colleagues showed improvement in colposcopic sensitivity for high-grade disease as biopsy number increased up to four, regardless of the level of colposcopist training, lesion size, or antecedent Pap grade.

Colposcopic biopsies are obtained using punch forceps, commonly Tischler or Kevorkian-Younge forceps. As colposcopists have embraced taking multiple biopsies, use of smaller biopsy forceps has increased to minimize pain. Unfortunately, local anesthetics and oral nonsteroidal analgesics are ineffective in decreasing pain.

Endocervical curettage can identify disease within the canal. However, it can be contaminated by inadvertent sampling of ectocervical lesions, and yield is low. It offers greatest benefit among older women with inadequate colposcopy exams and high-grade cytology. When indicated, endocervical curettage is undertaken with a Kevorkian curette, whose multiple sharp surfaces allow endocervical sampling with either a rotating in-and-out motion using the tip as a cutting edge or rotating lateral motion using the longer lateral blades of the curette. With either technique, the endocervical sample should include both tissue fragments adherent to the curette and those in the clot of mucus and blood developed by curettage. Some experts prefer vigorous sampling with an endocervical brush, with the sample submitted for histologic rather than cytologic analysis.

In 2007, the National Cancer Institute proposed risk-based concepts for cervical cancer screening prevention and the frequency of screening and the indications for treatment are based on the women's risk of cervical cancer or CIN 3. Since risk cannot be reduced to zero despite intensive screening, women with a low risk are observed at intervals. Long intervals are appropriate for women at lowest risk. For example, women with negative results on Pap and HPV testing and no prior abnormalities can be observed with repeat cotesting in 5 years. In contrast, women with CIN 2, women with CIN 3, and those with HPV-positive HSIL cytology merit treatment. Women with other results, such as those from biomarker or HPV genotyping tests, that raise risk for CIN 3 close to 50% also may merit immediate treatment. For women with intermediate risk, colposcopy with biopsy of all acetowhite areas allows triage to treatment or observation.

Using this risk-based concept, colposcopy is indicated for women with ASC-H, LSIL, HSIL, and AGC cytology. Women with ASC-US cytology should undergo colposcopy when ASC-US is persistent or associated with high-risk HPV infection. Colposcopy is also indicated when high-risk HPV persists or when HPV types 16 or 18 are found regardless of the cytologic diagnosis. Some evidence suggests that negative cytology and an abnormal molecular marker, such as p16[ink4a], may also be an indication for colposcopy. Colposcopy may be useful for the more detailed assessment of the nature and extent of visible cervical lesions. These general guidelines should be helpful in most cases, but there are many special situations—including the evaluation of young, pregnant, and postmenopausal women—in which alternative management plans may be more suitable. More detailed management guidelines are available on the American Society for Colposcopy and Cervical

Pathology Web site, www.asccp.org, where the most recent guidelines are available. Delay in colposcopy may allow regression of abnormalities, but is not recommended because of the risk for progression.

Abnormal Papanicolaou Results in Pregnancy

The goal of evaluation of the pregnant patient with CIN is to rule out invasive cancer, since CIN is unlikely to progress to cancer during pregnancy and treatments jeopardize both fetus and mother. CIN is not treated in pregnancy but is followed up until the postpartum period, when the patient is reevaluated and managed as indicated by the biopsy results and her social situation. The pregnant woman with significant cytologic abnormality generally is evaluated by colposcopic examination and directed biopsy, although colposcopic assessment of those with ASC-US and LSIL can be deferred until the woman is postpartum. During pregnancy, biopsy is advisable when high-grade colposcopic features are present, and it is acceptable for lesser colposcopic lesions. In clinics where biopsy was limited to women with colposcopic features of invasion, invasive cancers were missed. The pregnant cervix is quite vascular, especially in the last trimester, so a biopsy may bleed profusely, and cervical trauma can initiate uterine contractions. Use of mini-Tischler forceps minimizes bleeding. Multiple biopsies are usually not well tolerated. ECC is contraindicated in pregnancy, because of the risk of rupturing the membranes.

Rarely, diagnostic excision is required in pregnancy to rule out invasive cancer suspected cytologically, colposcopically, or on biopsy. This can be a difficult and potentially bloody procedure and should be undertaken by an experienced gynecologist only after all other avenues to rule out invasion have been exhausted. Because of bleeding risk, excisional procedures during pregnancy should be performed only in settings where transfusion is available, usually in an operating room. Placement of a circumferential suture near the cervicovaginal junction can evert the SCJ and minimize bleeding. When the goal is to identify deep invasion rather than to treat microinvasive cancer or CIN, the size of the excision can be limited to the colposcopically apparent lesion, and treatment of the remainder of the transformation zone can be deferred until after postpartum involution is complete. Because of the eversion of the transformation zone during pregnancy, deep cone-shaped excisions are usually unnecessary, and a "coin" biopsy that is shallow and flat may be more appropriate. Electrosurgical excision with a loop electrode or straight wire rather than knife conization during pregnancy may reduce blood loss.

MANAGEMENT OF CERVICAL INTRAEPITHELIAL NEOPLASIA

Although high-grade cervical neoplasia can regress, cervical treatments designed to destroy premalignant lesions in the transformation zone are standard for women at high risk. CIN 3 is recognized as true precancer, and CIN 2 is a mix of precancerous lesions and benign HPV infections. However, because the natural history of CIN 2 is difficult to predict with current technology, it has become the threshold for treatment. Despite low risk for cancer, CIN 1 also may be treated to speed reversion to normal epithelium and minimize the morbidity, inconvenience, and expense of repeated Pap tests and colposcopies, but only when it is persistent. Persistent HPV infection and atypical or low-grade cytology without CIN 2+ should not be treated, as the relevant HPV infection may not be in the transformation zone. Recent consensus suggests that when assessment indicates a risk of CIN 2+ of 50% or more, treatment is indicated. Within each cytologic grade, concomitant detection of high-risk HPV confers a higher risk of CIN 2+. Diagnostic excision is also indicated if there is a significant discrepancy between cytologic, colposcopic, and histologic findings, although review of these findings by experts may avoid overtreatment. Increased risk for later preterm delivery is a risk for all cervical therapies, in proportion to the amount of cervix destroyed, and in addition to risk of CIN, the patient's desire for future childbearing may influence treatment decisions. Regression of HPV-related disease is more common in younger women, and age may influence treatment decisions as well. For example, a 32-year-old mother of three with a tubal ligation and a two-quadrant CIN 2 lesion should probably be treated, whereas the same lesion in a 24-year-old unmarried nulligravida might well be watched in expectation of regression. The most recent treatment guidelines can be found on the Web site of the American Society for Colposcopy and Cervical Pathology, www.asccp.org.

Treatment Techniques

In general, treatment techniques can be divided into ablative and excisional. Ablative methods such as cryotherapy, CO_2 laser ablation, and electrocautery rely on an accurate colposcopically directed biopsy diagnosis to exclude invasive cancer because no tissue specimen is provided by the treatment procedure. For this reason, ablative treatments are contraindicated when endocervical curettings contain CIN, when colposcopic examination is inadequate, when the biopsy and cytology results are discordant, and when cancer is suspected on cytology, colposcopy, or biopsy. In these circumstances, diagnostic excisions using scalpel, laser, and electrosurgical needle or loop all provide a specimen, so these techniques are both diagnostic and therapeutic..

Cryotherapy

Cryosurgery is a destructive technique that was introduced to gynecologists in the late 1960s to treat CIN. It has since been superseded for many indications by office excisional techniques. The cryosurgical instruments use nitrous oxide or carbon dioxide as a refrigerant to lower the temperature of the tissue below $-22°C$. This produces cell death by intracellular and extracellular water crystallization. The refrigerant is applied to the cervix with a cryoprobe, which is covered with lubricant gel to enhance thermal transfer and placed in contact with the cervical epithelium. As the gas is circulated through the cryoprobe, it withdraws heat from the cervix until freezing temperatures occur. The cervix and cryoprobe generally reach a steady state after 3 to 5 minutes of freezing, at which time the amount of heat brought to the cervix by the vascular supply balances the amount of heat withdrawn from the cervix by the evaporating cryogenic gas. Many experts advise double-freeze cryotherapy, with a second freeze after a 5-minute thaw with the cryoprobe removed. Visible ice must extend at least 5 mm past the edge of the cryoprobe, and the cryoprobe must cover the transformation zone. This is best defined with acetic acid or Lugol iodine prior to applying the cryoprobe. The need for multiple probe placements to cover a large lesion is a relative contraindication to cryotherapy.

Patients treated with cryotherapy may experience minor cramping during the procedure, but otherwise the treatment is not painful, so anesthesia is not needed. During the 2 weeks after cryosurgery, about 20% of patients experience a profuse watery discharge that may require wearing a pad. Some patients experience light spotting, particularly 12 to 15 days after cryotherapy, when the eschar begins to separate from the treated area; pelvic rest through this period will minimize the

IX

risk of heavy bleeding. Infections, including endometritis or tuboovarian abscess, following cervical cryotherapy are rare but can occur, especially in women who already have a subclinical cervicitis.

Long-term complications of cryotherapy are minimal and consist principally of cervical stenosis in 1% to 4% of patients. Several studies have reported that there is no change in fertility and that pregnancy complications seldom occur, except in patients who have excessive cervical fibrosis and in whom cervical dystocia may be a problem. Postcryotherapeutic healing is generally completed within 12 weeks. Cryoprobes with deep endocervical extensions may lead to a higher rate of cervical stenosis. In many patients, the SCJ will not be visible after the cervix has healed following cryotherapy.

Carbon Dioxide Laser

The CO_2 laser is another useful treatment modality for the management of CIN lesions, most often for ablation. The CO_2 laser produces a high-intensity collimated light beam that can be focused with high-power density. Absorption of laser energy at the site of light impact results in flash boiling of cells, vaporizing the tissue. Increasing the power density and narrow focusing of the beam allows the CO_2 laser to cut tissue. Defocusing the laser beam to lower-power density results in coagulation rather than flash boiling. This can be used focally as a hemostatic technique, but inadequate power density results in serious stromal injury that may increase preterm delivery risk.

The CO_2 laser has the following advantages: it can be used for either cutting or ablation; therapy can be targeted individually, based on the extent of the transformation zone and the lesion being treated; the healing after laser surgery is rapid; and there are minimal side effects, including limited vaginal discharge. Because depth control is relatively straightforward, laser ablation is especially useful for lesions that extend onto the vaginal walls, where excisional treatments risk injury to bladder, rectum, and vasculature. Patients treated with the CO_2 laser generally have minimal cervical scarring and a lower stenosis rate than those treated with cryotherapy. Few obstetric complications have been reported after laser ablation, though deep laser conization like other techniques can predispose to preterm delivery. The major disadvantages of the laser are (a) its acquisition expense; (b) the time required to acquire and maintain laser skills, particularly for excisional laser conization; and, (c) the relatively high maintenance cost of the instrument. Use of the CO_2 laser for the management of CIN has decreased dramatically since the introduction of the loop electrosurgical excision procedure (LEEP).

To perform CO_2 laser ablation, the cervix is visualized after placement of a matte speculum with smoke evacuation tubing attached. Matte instruments are important, because their surfaces will scatter laser light that strikes them accidentally, dispersing the laser energy and reducing the risk for inadvertent injury. The perineum should be protected by draping with wet towels, and use of potentially flammable paper drapes avoided. The cervix is injected with a vasoconstrictive agent, either epinephrine as in local anesthetics or vasopressin. The cervix is visualized using a colposcope at 3 to 10× magnification. The laser is set to achieve a power density of 750 to 1,250 W/cm² by adjusting the input power and the spot size. Ablation is carried out to cover the entire transformation zone and any lateral lesion, as focused ablation is associated with a lower success rate. In the transformation zone, the depth of ablation should extend beyond the 5-mm depth of cervical glands or about 7 mm. Over the vagina, ablation should not extend beyond 2 mm. An endocervical button should be preserved to facilitate regrowth of cervical epithelium with minimal risk

of stenosis. This should not obstruct ablation of any visualized lesion, as ablation is only acceptable when the SCJ is fully visible. If bleeding occurs, rapid defocusing of the beam will allow coagulation, or suturing may be accomplished.

Laser conization can be done with the beam tightly focused. Tailored excision is done under colposcopic guidance using matte hooks to manipulate the specimen. Again, bleeding is controlled with rapid defocusing of the beam.

Loop Electrosurgical Excision

LEEP was introduced as the large loop excision of the transformation zone, by Prendeville, who modified a small electrosurgical wire loop biopsy instrument developed by Cartier. LEEP was introduced in North America in the early 1990s and rapidly became the procedure of choice for the management of CIN. Unless anatomy or anxiety contraindicate, it is done under local anesthesia as an outpatient procedure.

LEEP takes advantage of the properties of electrosurgical generators coupled with loop electrodes made with a thin stainless steel or tungsten wire to excise portions of the cervix (Fig. 50.2). In contrast to ablative procedures, LEEP provides a tissue specimen that is assessed for early invasive cancer and unsuspected AIS. Some 0.5% of cases diagnosed as CIN by colposcopy, punch biopsies, and ECC in fact have invasive cancer or AIS in the LEEP specimen.

LEEP begins with the insertion of an insulated speculum; the insulation prevents inadvertent contact with a live electrode from creating a vaginal epithelial injury or shock. The largest tolerable speculum is placed and is opened maximally both in the fornices and at the yoke. Obese women and those with vaginal laxity may benefit from insertion of a sidewall retractor prior to speculum placement, but some women are unable to tolerate placement of both. A local anesthetic with epinephrine is injected to reduce bleeding. This is used for its vasoconstrictive action, even if the patient is having general or regional anesthesia. The injection is made subepithelially, not into the deep stroma, and blanching of tissues should be apparent. Potocky needles allow precise subepithelial injection but

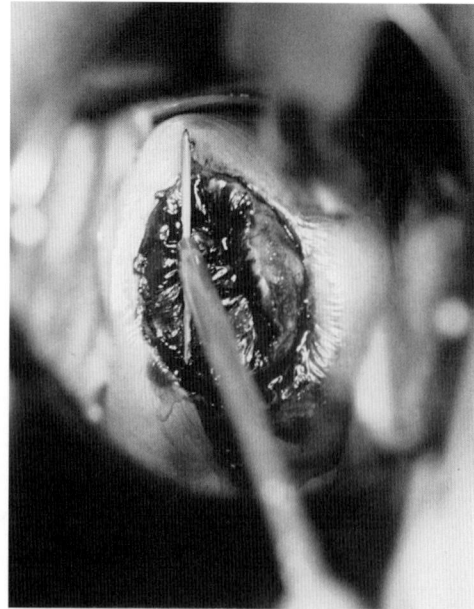

FIGURE 50.2 Loop electrosurgical excision procedure. Endosurgical loop is passed through the cervix from right to left. Note cut surface of cervical stroma from the 12-o'clock to the 6-o'clock position.

increase cost. Loops should be selected to excise the transformation zone, and excision should be accomplished under 3 to 10× colposcopic magnification after application of 3% to 5% acetic acid or Lugol iodine to ensure that all at-risk epithelium is excised. Power settings vary with the generator and should follow manufacturer's instructions. The LEEP electrode diameter is commonly 15 to 25 mm and is selected based on the size of the cervix and the extent of the transformation zone. Since CIN can extend into glands, the depth of the ectocervical excision should extend more than 5 mm beneath the surface, usually 7 to 8 mm. If the transformation zone is wide and cannot be removed intact with a single pass of the electrode, the first pass should encompass the cervical os. Because most high-grade disease will lie at or near the SCJ, every effort should be made to excise this area intact so that the histologic orientation of the tissue will not be damaged by physical or thermal injury. An intact, adequate specimen of the SCJ will allow the pathologist the best opportunity to correctly diagnose invasive disease and the measure depth of invasion if the basement membrane is breached. Additional lateral or anterior or posterior passes can be made to encompass the outer portions of the transformation zone. The central pass can be made from side to side or bottom to top; excision from top to bottom allows the partially excised specimen to fall forward, obstructing the operator's view and making completion of the posterior excision difficult. Edges should be beveled slightly to avoid sharp angles that cannot be fulgurated. Since loop electrodes cut by sparking that causes flash boiling of tissue, the electrode should be activated immediately prior to contacting the cervix, and the wire should be passed gently through the tissue with the insulated support just above the epithelium. Current should be maintained until excision is complete. Loss of current during the procedure stops the cutting wave of sparks and requires either reactivation of the electrode in place, with increased thermal artifact, or reinitiation of excision in the opposite direction, with potential for increased bleeding at the jagged edge where the two excisional passes meet. When the lesion extends into the endocervix, especially when colposcopy is inadequate, an additional, deeper, specimen ("top hat") with a 10 × 10-mm or 15 × 10-mm loop can excise a deeper area of the endocervical canal. This specimen should encompass tissue at least 5 mm lateral to the canal to include gland crypts. A postprocedure endocervical curettage can provide prognostic information, suggesting the presence or absence of residual CIN.

An alternative to LEEP is the cone biopsy excisor, a straight wire mounted on a right-angled base that is inserted into the endocervix and rotated. Indications and results are similar to LEEP. The cone biopsy excisor may be most appropriate for central and endocervical lesions and less suitable for lateral lesions or when there is anatomic asymmetry.

Once excision is complete, electrofulguration of the cautery bed should be carried out using a 5-mm cautery ball. Fulguration within the endocervical excision bed after top hat excision can be done with a 3-mm ball, but cautery near the endocervical canal should be kept to a minimum to allow eversion of endocervical epithelium with healing. A large swab may be useful in absorbing blood so cautery can be applied directly to the excision bed. Bleeding points can be controlled with direct coagulation rather than fulguration (contacting tissue rather than sparking onto it). Bleeding from the cervix can also be temporally controlled by clamping the cervical lip with a ring forceps. In some cases, suturing is required, either for control of brisk cervical bleeding or from vaginal lacerations that result from contact between an active wire and the vaginal wall. For those situations, the clinic should be equipped with a 12-inch needle holder, 12-inch toothed tissue forceps, and 0-gauge delayed absorbable suture on a 1-inch curved, taper-point needle, which should always be available in an outpatient area where LEEP is done. In rare cases, packing may be required. Monsel paste should be applied after hemostasis has been achieved.

Because LEEP is easy to learn, easy to teach, and relatively easy to perform, it can be used to treat patients with high-grade CIN without the disadvantages and greater cost of cold-knife or laser conization. The major advantage of LEEP over conventional cold-knife conization is that the procedure can be performed in the outpatient setting under colposcopic control. The advantage over outpatient ablative procedures is the fact that LEEP produces a tissue specimen of the entire transformation zone for pathologic examination. Invasive disease can be identified and excision margins evaluated. Women with positive margins can be managed with observation or reexcision; hysterectomy may be indicated when reexcision is not feasible and childbearing is complete. However, margins are less predictive for LEEP than for knife conization, especially when the specimen is removed in slices.

For LEEP to be used effectively, the extent of excision and the choice of electrodes must be tailored to the size and distribution of the lesion (Fig. 50.3). The use of extremely large

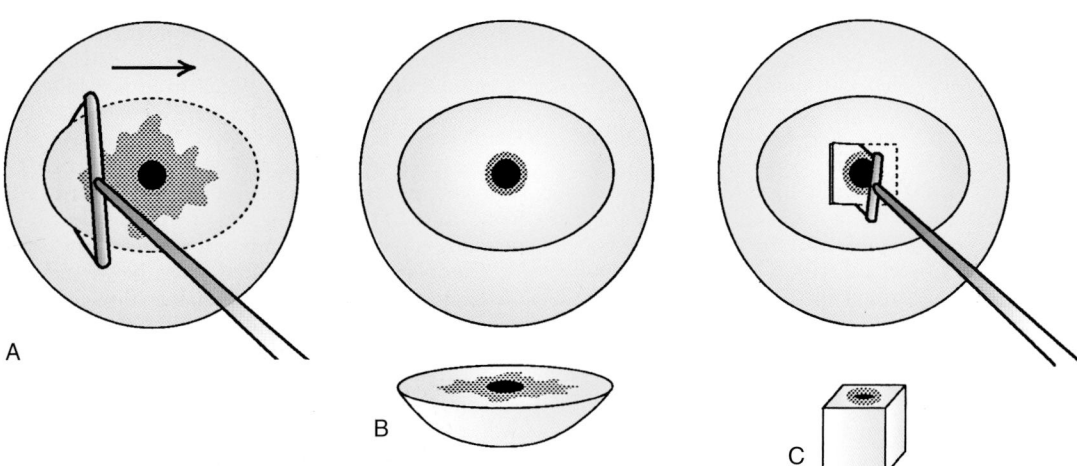

FIGURE 50.3 Diagram of approach to loop excision of small portion of lesion, which can be removed by a single pass (**A**) of the 2-cm × 7 to 8-mm loop. **B**: Note the shallow dish configuration of the removed tissue. If squamous epithelium remains in the canal, it can be removed by a second pass with a smaller loop (**C**).

IX

electrodes (e.g., 20 × 20 mm) may lead to inadvertent cervical amputation; injury to vaginal walls, rectum, and bladder; and significant obstetric morbidity. These large loops should be used only by those who have mastered more standard excision using loops 15 to 20 mm in width and 7 to 12 mm in depth. They are best suited for women with microinvasive squamous cell carcinoma in situ and AIS, when a large, intact specimen is needed to assess need for hysterectomy.

Infection in the cervix or an ascending endometritis, parametritis, or salpingitis can be seen following LEEP, but they are rare and usually represent a flare-up of an already existing subclinical infection. Long-term complications include cervical incompetence and cervical stenosis.

Although cervical incompetence leading to premature cervical dilation and delivery in subsequent pregnancies has been a well-known complication of traditional cold-knife cone biopsy for many years, the risk of pregnancy complications after LEEP was only recognized after 2000. LEEP appears to roughly double risk of preterm delivery, although most patients will deliver at term and most preterm deliveries occur between 34 and 36 weeks' gestation, with little long-term morbidity. Risk for preterm delivery appears related to greater depth and number of excisions, and commonly employed 20 mm by 7 or 8 mm excisions may have minimal impact. Women with cervical dysplasia have a higher incidence of prematurity than the general population, and some authors have suggested that the association of LEEP with preterm delivery reflects confounding. Prospective trials are unlikely, and prudence suggests that for fertile women LEEP should be undertaken only when the risk of precancer is substantial.

Because LEEP is a simple procedure that can be used for both diagnosis and treatment during a single office visit, its use has been recommended in the so-called "see-and-treat" mode. With this application, LEEP is performed for patients with HSIL cytology after colposcopic assessment for suitability and the absence of evident invasive cancer. The patient does not first have to undergo cervical biopsies and an ECC. This approach is especially valuable in clinics with high no show rates and is unsuitable for young women wishing to minimize risk to future pregnancies. It is not indicated for women with minor cytologic abnormalities or HPV infection with normal cytology.

Cervical Conization

Traditional cold-knife conization has been used successfully for generations to excise lesions that extend into the endocervical canal and to rule out invasive cancer. Hot cautery was used in the past to remove a cone-shaped piece of tissue from an inflamed, hypertrophic, chronically infected cervix. A standard surgical scalpel is more appropriate for the excision of CIN, and, thus, the term *cold knife* was introduced to differentiate these two procedures. Cone biopsies can be excised from the cervix using a sharply focused laser beam or an electrosurgical needle as well as a scalpel. The laser is more expensive and requires considerable operator experience to be used effectively. The electrosurgical wire is quite effective and hemostatic. Both techniques result in some thermal artifact, which may make interpretation of the surgical margins difficult. Cold-knife conization does not have that drawback, making it ideal when management depends on knowing whether the lesion excised extends to the margin of excision, as with endocervical glandular lesions and suspected microinvasion. The cone usually is performed in an operating room under anesthesia; thus, it is more expensive than outpatient excision.

Conization can be tailored to lesion location, with cone-shaped excisions for lesions encompassing both endo- and ectocervix, flattened "coin" biopsies for ectocervical lesions, and cylindrical excisions for endocervical lesions. Although most glandular lesions are located within a few millimeters of the SCJ, a cone biopsy for a glandular abnormality should extend deeply into the cervical canal. Colposcopic examination and Lugol iodine staining may help the surgeon determine the size and location of the lesion to be excised.

After a careful examination under anesthesia, a gentle vaginal prep is done. The cervix should not be scrubbed vigorously to avoid denuding the surface epithelium containing the intraepithelial lesion. To decrease blood loss, the cervix is injected with a vasoconstrictive agent, commonly a commercially available mixture of local anesthetic (lidocaine) with 1:100,000 epinephrine. Acute hypertension can be caused by this drug, and its use should be considered and discussed with the anesthesiologist. Approximately 1.5 to 2 mL is injected directly into the cervix, at 12, 2, 3, 6, 8, and 10 o'clock outside the planned incision line, for a total of 9 to 10 mL. Injection should cause some "ballooning" up and blanching of the cervix. Although deep lateral sutures in the side of the cervix at 3 and 9 o'clock have been said to decrease blood loss by ligating the descending branches of the uterine arteries, there is no evidence that this reduces bleeding with a cone biopsy. These sutures may assist in manipulation of the cervix.

The cervix is then re-stained with Lugol iodine to outline the lesion, and a scalpel is used to cut the cone. The cervix can be stabilized with a tenaculum placed high on the anterior lip away from the anticipated line of excision. Sometimes, two tenacula are better, or the lateral stay sutures described above may be used if the cervix is large or the vagina small. A pointed no. 11 scalpel blade is preferred, but a large no. 10 blade or a smaller no. 15 blade can be used. Some experts use an electrosurgical needle or thin pointed electrosurgical blade. As the cone is cut, the cervix is retracted to the opposite side to provide visibility at the base of the incision. Manipulations that may strip epithelium should be avoided. Once the incision has extended well into the cervical stroma, Allis clamps can be used to grasp the specimen's outer cut edges, and further traction will expose bands of fibrous stroma that can be cut to release the specimen. If possible, the cone should be symmetrical around the endocervical canal with the apex in the canal. It is desirable to remove the specimen intact and to mark it with a suture at 10 or 6 o'clock so that the pathologist can orient any positive margins or foci of invasive cancer.

There are several ways to manage the cone bed once the specimen has been removed. If bleeding is minimal, the cone bed may be cauterized and left open to granulate. This may result in a visible SCJ more frequently than if the bed is sutured. If this fails to control bleeding, the cone bed can be closed with a running locked suture placed from just lateral to the cone edge to deep in the cervical stroma by the canal. This is run circumferentially around the cervix. Finally, the classic Sturmdoff suture can be employed, as illustrated in **Figure 50.4**. The anterior and posterior cervical mucosa are pulled in to cover the cone defect. This is the most aesthetically pleasing closure, but in many cases, the SCJ cannot be seen after the cervix is healed.

Complications of cold-knife cone biopsy are similar to but perhaps somewhat more common than those with LEEP because the specimen is larger. Significant bleeding may occur in the first 24 hours or 10 to 21 days after surgery as the sutures dissolve. Five to 10% of patients will require reevaluation, packing, or suturing after cold-knife cone biopsy, and occasional patients will require transfusion. Cervical stenosis occurs in about 3% of patients. This is more common in postmenopausal women. The risk of premature labor and delivery caused by an excisional cone biopsy has already been discussed in the section on LEEP. The depth of the cone is related to the risk of premature labor.

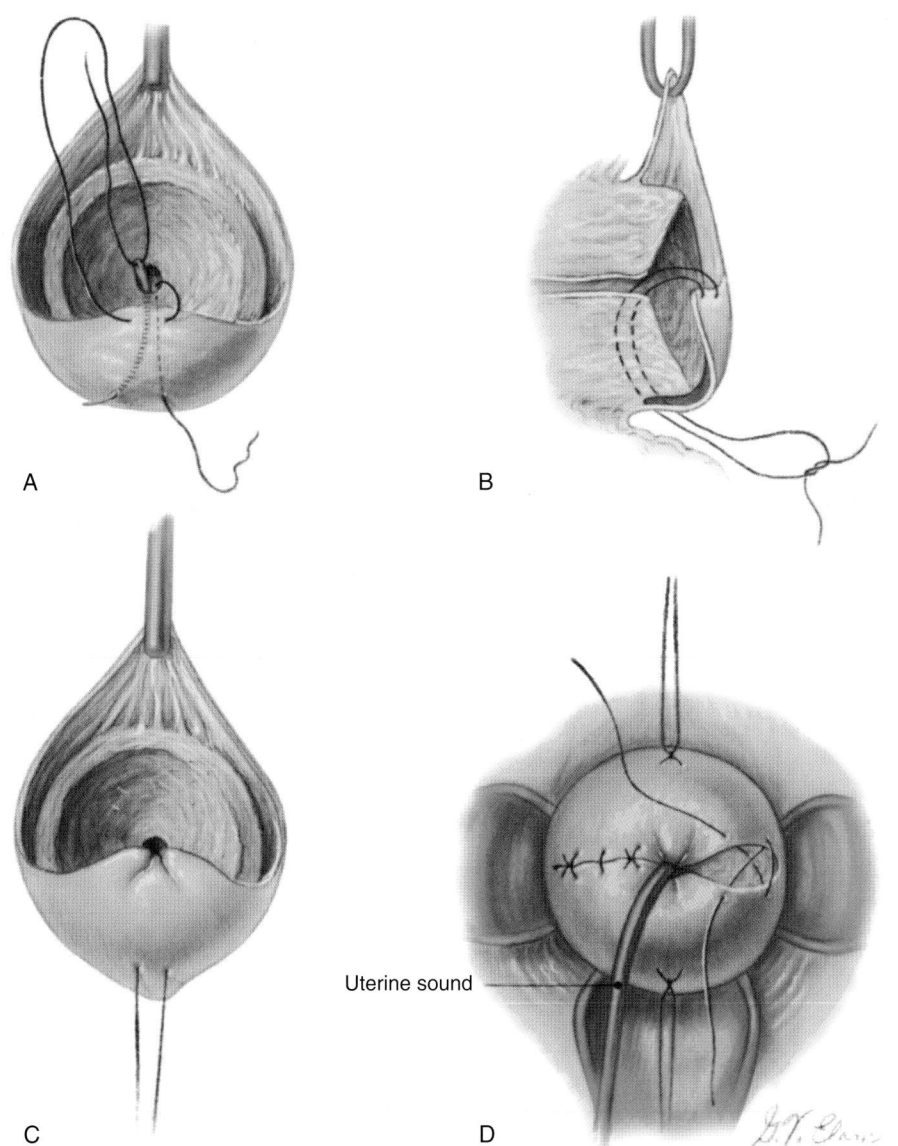

FIGURE 50.4 A: Mattress suture is placed as in Sturmdorf tracheloplasty. **B:** Method of action of suture in drawing the flap into the canal. **C:** The lower flap has been pulled into position. **D:** Anterior and posterior flaps have been drawn into the canal. Lateral mucosa wounds are being sutured.

Uterine sound

Posttreatment Outcomes and Assessment The overall "cure" rate for most cervical treatment is 90% to 95%. With all treatments, persistence is related to lesion size, lesion grade, and extension into the endocervical canal, but the incidence of persistent disease is related to the anatomy of the lesion. For excisional procedures, a positive excision margin predicts persistent CIN, although it does not appear independent of other factors. However, even with a histologically involved margin, immediate reexcision is not required unless invasive cancer is suspected above the excision line. Healing of the treatment bed often results in destruction of small areas of residual dysplasia. Women treated for CIN remain at risk for recurrence and cancer for at least 20 years and should be followed with cytology or Pap and HPV cotesting.

BEST SURGICAL PRACTICES

- The identification of a preinvasive lesion that precedes the development of invasive cancer of the cervix and development of screening tests and diagnostic procedures that allow the clinician to screen for, diagnose, and treat these

precursor lesions has greatly reduced the incidence of cervical cancer worldwide.
- Persistent cervical infection with certain genotypes (especially type 16 and 18) of human papillomaviruses (HPV) has been identified to be the cause of cervical cancer.
- Most HPV-related lesions will regress with relatively low potential for cancer. Risk-based management of women with screening abnormalities and cancer precursors allows clinicians to prevent most cervical cancers while minimizing cervical trauma and focusing resources on patients with greatest need.
- Colposcopy is indicated for most women with ASC-US cytology and associated HPV infection, as well as for most other women with abnormal cytology.
- Colposcopy identifies most precancers, but colposcopic grading cannot be used reliably to direct treatment, even in expert hands. Cervical biopsy is required. Up to four biopsies will result in increased accuracy of identifying a high-grade lesion. Endocervical curettage has relatively low yield but is indicated when colposcopy is inadequate.

IX

- Excision and ablation have similar cure rates, but ablation is contraindicated unless cancer has been excluded. Treatment is recommended for most women with CIN 2 or CIN 3, although pregnant women and those under age 25 with CIN 2 may be monitored. Deep excision can result in injury and can predispose to preterm delivery.
- LEEP begins with activation of the electrode before contacting tissue, and current flow should continue till excision is complete. Sharp angles in the incision bed make hemostasis difficult, so angles should be beveled or rounded. Fulguration provides hemostasis with minimal deep coagulation injury, although direct coagulation of active bleeding points is effective.
- Traditional cold-knife cone biopsy of the cervix or large loop excision should be used for women with suspected microinvasive cancer or glandular lesions. For these women, excision should provide a single large, deep specimen that can be well oriented and has a better chance for a clear margin.

BIBLIOGRAPHY

Agency for Health Care Policy and Research. *Evaluation of cervical cytology.* AHCPR Publication No. 99-E010. Rockville, MD: AHCPR, 1999.

Ayre JE. Diagnosis of preclinical cancer of the cervix. *JAMA* 1948;138:11–13.

Barron BA, Richart RM. A statistical model of the natural history of cervical carcinoma based on a prospective study of 557 cases. *J Natl Cancer Inst* 1968;41:1343.

Belinson J, Qiao YL, Pretorius R, et al. Shanxi Province Cervical Cancer Screening Study: a cross-sectional comparative trial of multiple techniques to detect cervical neoplasia. *Gynecol Oncol* 2001;83:3429.

Benedet JL, Matisic JP, Bertrand MA. An analysis of 84,244 patients from the British Columbia cytology-colposcopy program. *Gynecol Oncol* 2004;92:127–134.

Berkova Z, Kaufmann RH, Unger ER, et al. The effect of time interval between referral and colposcopy on detection of human papillomavirus DNA and on outcome of biopsy. *Am J Obstet Gynecol* 2003;188:932–937.

Boardman LA, Steinhoff MM, Shackelton R, et al. A randomized trial of the Fischer cone biopsy excisor and loop electrosurgical excision procedure. *Obstet Gynecol* 2004;104:745–750.

Bornstein J, Bentley J, Bosze P, et al. 2011 colposcopic terminology of the International Federation for Cervical Pathology and Colposcopy. *Obstet Gynecol* 2012;120:166–172.

Brown DR, Shew ML, Qadadri B, et al. A longitudinal study of genital human papillomavirus infection in a cohort of closely followed adolescent women. *J Infect Dis* 2005;1912:182.

Bruinsma F, Lumley J, Tan J, et al. Precancerous changes in the cervix and risk of subsequent preterm birth. *BJOG* 2007;114:70–80.

Burke L, Covell L, Antonioli D. Carbon dioxide laser therapy of cervical intraepithelial neoplasia: factors determining success rate. *Lasers Surg Med* 1980;1:113–122.

Burghardt E, Pickel H, Girardi F, eds. *Colposcopy-cervical pathology,* 3rd ed. Stuttgart, Germany: Thieme, 1998.

Cartier R, Cartier I. *Practical colposcopy,* 3rd ed. Paris, France: Laboratoire Cartier, 1993.

Castle PE, Gage JC, Wheeler CM, et al. The clinical meaning of a cervical intraepithelial neoplasia grade 1 biopsy. *Obstet Gynecol* 2011;118:1222–1229.

Castle PE, Glass AG, Rush BB, et al. Clinical human papillomavirus detection forecasts cervical cancer risk in women over 18 years of follow-up. *J Clin Oncol* 2012;30:3044–3050.

Castle PE, Schiffman M, Wheeler CM, et al. Evidence for frequent regression of cervical intraepithelial neoplasia-Grade 2. *Obstet Gynecol* 2009;113:18–25.

Castle PE, Sideri M, Jeronimo J, et al. Risk assessment to guide the prevention of cervical cancer. *Am J Obstet Gynecol* 2007;197:356. e1–356.e6.

Castle PE, Wacholder S, Lorincz AT, et al. A prospective study of high-grade cervical neoplasia risk among human papillomavirus-infected women. *J Natl Cancer Inst* 2002;94:1406–1414.

Chan BKS, Melnikow J, Slee CA, et al. Posttreatment human papillomavirus testing for recurrent cervical intraepithelial neoplasia: a systematic review. *Am J Obstet Gynecol* 2009;200:422.e1–422.e9.

Church L, Oliver L, Dobie S, et al. Analgesia for colposcopy: double-masked, randomized comparison of ibuprofen and benzocaine gel. *Obstet Gynecol* 2001;97:5–10.

Clavel C, Masure M, Bory JP, et al. Human papillomavirus testing in primary screening for the detection of high-grade cervical lesions: as study of 7932 women. *Br J Cancer* 2001;89:1616.

Clifford G, Franceschi S, Diaz M, et al. Chapter 3: HPV type-distribution in women with and without cervical neoplastic diseases. *Vaccine* 2006;24(suppl 3):S326–S344.

Coppleson M, Pixley E, Reid BL. *Colposcopy. A scientific and practical approach to the cervix in health and disease.* Springfield, IL: Thomas, 1971.

Creasman WT, Weed JC Jr, Curry SL, et al. Efficacy of cryosurgical treatment of severe cervical intraepithelial neoplasia. *Obstet Gynecol* 1973;41:501.

Cristoforoni PM, Gerbaldo DL, Philipson J, et al. Management of the abnormal Papanicolaou smear during pregnancy: lessons for quality improvement. *J Low Genit Tract Dis* 1999;4:225–230.

Cullen TS. *Cancer of the uterus.* Philadelphia, PA: W.B. Saunders, 1909.

Cuzick J, Mayrand MH, Ronco G, et al. New dimensions in cervical cancer screening. *Vaccine* 2006;24(suppl 3):90.

Mesher D, Szarewski A, Cadman L, et al. Long-term follow-up of cervical disease in women screened by cytology and HPV testing: results from the HART study. *Br J Cancer* 2010;102(9):1405–1410.

Denny L, Quinn M, Sankaranarayanan R. Screening for cervical cancer in developing countries. *Vaccine* 2006;24(suppl 3):71.

Dunn TS, Ginsburg V, Wolf D. Loop-cone cerclage in pregnancy: a 5-year review. *Gynecol Oncol* 2003;90:566–580.

Dunne EF, Unger ER, Sternberg M, et al. Prevalence of HPV infection among females in the United States. *JAMA* 2007;297:813–819.

Elfgren K, Kalantari M, Moberger B, et al. A population-based five-year follow-up study of cervical human papillomavirus infection. *Am J Obstet Gynecol* 2000;183:561–567.

Erickson CC, Everett BE, Graves LM, et al. Population screening for uterine cancer by vaginal cytology: preliminary summary of results of first examination of 108,000 women and second testing of 33,000 women. *JAMA* 1956;162:167–173.

Ferris DG, Litaker M; for the ALTS Group. Interobserver agreement for colposcopy quality control using digitized colposcopic images during the ALTS Trial. *J Low Genit Tract Dis* 2005;9:29–35.

Gage JC, Duggan MA, Nation JG, et al. Detection of cervical cancer and its precursors by endocervical curettage in 13,115 colposcopically guided biopsies. *Am J Obstet Gynecol* 2010;203:481.e1–481.e9.

Gage JC, Hanson VW, Abbey K, et al.; for the ASCUS LSIL Triage Study (ALTS) Group. Number of cervical biopsies and sensitivity of colposcopy. *Obstet Gynecol* 2006;108:264–272

Galvin GA, Jones HW Jr, Te Linde RW. Clinical relationship of carcinoma in situ and invasive carcinoma of the cervix. *JAMA* 1952;149:744.

Gram IT, Austin H, Stalsberg H. Cigarette smoking and the incidence of cervical intraepithelial neoplasia grade 3 and cancer of the cervix. *Am J Epidemiol* 1992;135:341.

Gram IT, Macaluso M, Stalsberg H. Incidence of cervical intraepithelial neoplasia grade III, and cancer of the cervix uteri following a negative Pap-smear in an opportunistic screening. *Acta Obstet Gynecol Scand* 1998;77:228.

Grohs HK, Husain OAN, eds. *Automated cervical cancer screening.* New York: Igaku-Shoin, 1994.

Gustafsson L, Ponten J, Zack M, et al. International incidence rates of invasive cervical cancer after introduction of cytological screening. *Cancer Causes Control* 1997;8:755–763.

Halioua B. The participation of Hans Hinselmann in medical experiments at Auschwitz. *J Low Genit Tract Dis* 2010;14:1–4.

Hinselmann H. *Colposcopy (with a section on colpophotography by A. Schmitt).* Wuppertal-Elberfeld, Germany: Girardet, 1955.

Ho GYF, Bierman R, Beardsley L. Natural history of cervicovaginal papillomavirus infection in young women. *N Engl J Med* 1998;338:423.

Jeronimo J, Massad LS, Castle PE, et al.; for the NIH-ASCCP Research Group. Interobserver agreement in the evaluation of digitized cervical images. *Obstet Gynecol* 2007;110:833–840.

Khan MJ, Castle PE, Lorincz AT, et al. The elevated 10-year risk of cervical precancer and cancer in women with human papillomavirus (HPV) type 16 or 18 and the possible utility of type-specific HPV testing in clinical practice. *J Natl Cancer Inst* 2005;97:1072.

Kinney WK, Manos MM, Hurley LB, et al. Where's the high-grade cervical neoplasia? The importance of minimally abnormal Papanicolaou diagnoses. *Obstet Gynecol* 1998;91:973.

Kitchener HC, Almonte M, Thomson C, et al. HPV testing in combination with liquid-based cytology in primary cervical screening (ARTISTIC): a randomized controlled trial. *Lancet Oncol* 2009;10:672–682.

Kiviat NB, Koutsky LA, Paavonen JA, et al. Prevalence of genital papillomavirus infection among women attending a college student health clinic or an STD clinic. *J Infect Dis* 1989;159:293–302.

Kjaer S, Hogdall E, Frederiksen K, et al. The absolute risk of cervical abnormalities in high-risk human papillomavirus-positive, cytologically normal women over a 10-year period. *Cancer Res* 2006;66:10630–10636.

Kolstad P, Klem V. Long-term follow-up of 1121 cases of carcinoma in situ. *Obstet Gynecol* 1979;48:125.

Kolstad P, Stafl A, eds. *Atlas of colposcopy.* Oslo, Bergen, Tromso: Scandinavian University Books, 1972.

Koutsky LA, Ault KA, Wheeler CM, et al. A controlled trial of a human papillomavirus type 16 vaccine. *N Engl J Med* 2002;347:1645.

Kyrgiou M, Koliopoulos P, Martin-Hirsch P, et al. Obstetric outcomes after conservative treatment for intraepithelial or early invasive cervical lesions: systematic review and meta-analysis. *Lancet* 2006;367.9509:489.

Luesley DM, Cullimore J, Redman CW, et al. Loop diathermy excision of the cervical transformation zone in patients with abnormal cervical smears. *BMJ* 1990;300:1690.

Massad LS, Jeronimo J, Schiffman M; for the NIH/ASCCP Research Group. Interobserver agreement in the assessment of components of colposcopic grading. *Obstet Gynecol* 2008;111:1279–1284.

McIndoe WA, McLean MR, Jones RW, et al. The invasive potential of carcinoma in situ of the cervix. *Obstet Gynecol* 1984;64:451.

Moscicki A-B, Palefsky J, Gonzales J, et al. Colposcopic and histologic findings and human papillomavirus (HPV) DNA test variability in young women positive for HPV DNA. *J Infect Dis* 1992;166:951.

Moscicki A-B, Ma Y, Wibbelsman C, et al. Rate of and risks for regression of cervical intraepithelial neoplasia 2 in adolescents and young women. *Obstet Gynecol* 2010;116:1373–1380.

Munoz N, Bosch FX, de Sanjose S, et al. Epidemiologic classification of human papillomavirus types associated with cervical cancer. *N Engl J Med* 2003;348:518.

Munoz N, Catellsague X, de Gonzalez AB, et al. HPV in the etiology of human cancer. *Vaccine* 2006;24(suppl 3):1.

Nanda K, McCrory D, Myers ER, et al. Accuracy of the Papanicolaou test in screening for and follow-up of cervical cytologic abnormalities: a systematic review. *Ann Intern Med* 2000;132:810.

Nuovo J, Melnikow J, Willan AR, et al. Treatment outcomes for squamous intraepithelial lesions. *Int J Gynecol Obstet* 2000;68:25.

Papanicolaou GN, Traut HF. Diagnostic value of vaginal smears in carcinoma of the uterus. *Am J Obstet Gynecol* 1941;42:193–206.

Prendiville W, Cullimore J, Norman S. Large loop excision of the transformation zone (LLETZ). A new method of management for women with cervical intraepithelial neoplasia. *BJOG* 1989;57:145.

Reagan JW, Hamonic MJ. The cellular pathology in carcinoma in situ: a cytohistopathological correlation. *Cancer* 1956;9:385.

Richart, RM. Natural history of cervical intraepithelial neoplasia. *Clin Obstet Gynecol* 1967;10:748–784.

Reid R, Scalzi P. Genital warts and cervical cancer. VII. An improved colposcopic index for differentiating benign papillomaviral infections from high-grade cervical intraepithelial neoplasia. *Am J Obstet Gynecol* 1985;153:611–618.

Rigoni-Stern D. Fatti statistici relativi alle malattie cancerose. *Gior Serv Progr Pathol Terap* 1842;2:507.

Rijkaart DC, Berkhof J, Rozendaal L, et al. Human papillomavirus testing for the detection of high-grade cervical intraepithelial neoplasia and cancer: final results of the PoBASCAM randomized controlled trial. *Lancet Oncol* 2012;13:78–88.

Rodriguez AC, Schiffman M, Herrero R, et al. Rapid clearance of human papillomavirus and implications for clinical focus on persistent infections. *J Natl Cancer Inst* 2008;100:513–517.

Russell J, Crothers BA, Kaplan KJ, et al. Current cervical screening technology considerations: liquid-based cytology and automated screening. *Clin Obstet Gynecol* 2005;48:108–119.

Rubin IC. Pathological diagnosis of incipient carcinoma of the uterus. *Am J Obstet Dis Women Child* 1910;62:668–676.

Sasieni P, Castanon A, Cuzick J. Effectiveness of cervical screening with age: population based case–control study of prospectively recorded data. *BMJ* 2009;339:b2968.

Saslow D, Solomon D, Lawson HW, et al.; for the ACS-ASCCP-ASCP Cervical Cancer Guideline Committee. American Cancer Society, American Society for Colposcopy and Cervical Pathology, and American Society for Clinical Pathology screening guidelines for the prevention and early detection of cervical cancer. *CA Cancer J Clin* 2012;62:147–172.

Scheffey LC, Lang WR, Tatarian G. An experimental program with colposcopy. *Am J Obstet Gynecol* 1955;70:876–888

Schiffman M, Herrero R, Hildesheim A, et al. HPV DNA testing in cervical cancer screening: results from women in a high-risk province of Costa Rica. *JAMA* 2000;283:87.

Schiffman M, Kjaer SK. Chapter 2: Natural history of anogenital HPV infection and neoplasia. *J Natl Cancer Inst Monogr* 2003;31:14–19.

Solomon D, Davey D, Kurman R, et al. The 2001 Bethesda System: terminology for reporting results of cervical cytology. *JAMA* 2002;287:2114.

Solomon D, Schiffman M, Tarone R. Comparison of three management strategies for patients with atypical squamous cells of undetermined significance: baseline results from a randomized trial. *J Natl Cancer Inst* 2001;93:293–299.

Stafl A, Mattingly RF. Colposcopic diagnosis of cervical neoplasia. *Obstet Gynecol* 1973;41:168–176.

Stoler MH, Vichnin MD, et al.; for the Future I, II and III Investigators. The accuracy of colposcopic biopsy: analyses from the placebo arm of the Gardasil clinical trials. *Int J Cancer* 2011;128:1354–1362.

Strander B, Andersson-Ellstrom A, Milsom I, et al. Long term risk of invasive cancer after treatment for cervical intraepithelial neoplasia grade 3: population based cohort study. *BMJ* 2007;335:1077

Townsend DE, Ostergard DR, Mishell DR, et al. Abnormal Papanicolaou smears: evaluation by colposcopy, biopsies, and endocervical curettage. *Am J Obstet Gynecol* 1970;180:429–434.

Trimble CL, Piantadosi S, Gravitt P, et al. Spontaneous regression of high-grade cervical dysplasia: effects of human papillomavirus type and HLA phenotype. *Clin Cancer Res* 2005;11:4717–1423.

Wallin KL, Wiklund F, Angstrom T, et al. Type-specific persistence of human papillomavirus DNA before the development of invasive cervical cancer. *N Engl J Med* 1999;341:1633–1638.

Weid GL. *Proceedings of the first International Congress on Exfoliative Cytology.* Philadelphia, PA: JB Lippincott, 1961.

Wentzensen N, Zuna RE, Sherman ME, et al. Accuracy of cervical specimens obtained for biomarker studies in women with CIN3. *Gynecol Oncol* 2009;115:493–496.

Werness BA, Levine AJ, Howley PM. Association of human papillomavirus types 16 and 18 proteins with p53. *Science* 1990;248:76.

Willet GD, Kurman RJ, Reid R. Correlation of the histological appearance of intraepithelial neoplasia of the cervix with human papillomavirus types. *Int J Gynecol Pathol* 1989;8:18.

Wright TC Jr, Stoler MH, Sharma A, et al.; ATHENA (Addressing THE Need for Advanced HPV Diagnostics) Study Group. Evaluation of HPV-16 and HPV-18 genotyping for the triage of women with high-risk HPV+cytology-negative results. *Am J Clin Pathol* 2011;136:578–586.

Wright TC Jr, Cox JT, Massad LW, et al. 2001 consensus guidelines for the management of women with cervical cytological abnormalities. *JAMA* 2002;287:2120.

Wright TC Jr, Denny L, Kuhn L, et al. HPV DNA testing of self-collected vaginal samples compared with cytologic screening to detect cervical cancer. *JAMA* 2000;283:81.

Wright TC, Ellerbrock TV, Chiasson MA, et al. Cervical intraepithelial neoplasia in women infected with human immunodeficiency virus: prevalence, risk factors, and validity of Papanicolaou smears. *Obstet Gynecol* 1994;84:591.

Wright TC Jr, Massad LS, Dunton CJ, et al. 2006 American Society for Colposcopy and Cervical Pathology-sponsored Consensus Conference. 2006 consensus guidelines for the management of women with abnormal cervical cancer screening tests. *Am J Obstet Gynecol* 2007;197:346–355.

Wright TC, Schiffman M, Solomon D, et al. Interim guidance for the use of human papillomavirus DNA testing as an adjunct to cervical cytology for screening. *Obstet Gynecol* 2004;103:304.

Aahm DM, Nindl I, Greinke C. Colposcopic appearance of cervical intraepithelial neoplasia is age dependent. *Am J Obstet Gynecol* 1998;179:1298–1304.

zur Hausen H. Human papillomaviruses and their possible role in squamous cell carcinomas. *Curr Top Microbiol Immunol* 1977;78:1.

zur Hausen H. Papillomaviruses and cancer: from basic studies to clinical application. *Nat Rev Cancer* 2002;2:342.

CHAPTER 51
Cancer of the Cervix

Nadeem R. Abu-Rustum, Laszlo Ungar, Kaled Alektiar, and Dennis S. Chi

DEFINITIONS

FIGO staging—The International Federation of Gynecology and Obstetrics (FIGO) has defined staging of gynecologic cancers for more than 50 years. The cancer stage defines the extent of disease at diagnosis before treatment. FIGO staging is used worldwide to compare clinical experience and results of treatment.

Lymphovascular space invasion (LVSI)—Small endothelial-lined vessels within the cervical stroma may be either lymphatic vessels or small capillaries. On histologic examination of a surgical specimen, tumor cells or clusters of tumor cells are sometimes seen in these vessels. Tumor invasion or involvement of these lymphovascular spaces is generally believed to increase the risk of nodal metastases and worsen prognosis.

Parametrium—Connective tissue lateral to the cervix and uterus within the broad ligament.

Pararectal space—The avascular space in the posterolateral pelvis. It is bounded medially by the rectum, laterally by the pelvic wall, posteriorly by the presacral fascia, and anteriorly by the broad ligament and cardinal ligament. During pelvic surgery, we commonly define the boundaries of the pararectal space as follows: laterally, the internal iliac system and medially, the ureter and mesoureter.

Paravesical space—The avascular space in the anterolateral pelvis is bounded by the bladder medially, the pelvic sidewall laterally, and the broad ligament and cardinal ligament posteriorly. During pelvic surgery, we define the paravesical space into two spaces—the lateral paravesical space components are bound laterally by the external iliac vessels and medially by the obliterated umbilical artery. The medial paravesical space is bound medially by the bladder and laterally by the obliterated umbilical ligament. Opening this medial paravesical space facilitates the identification of the uterine artery at its origin from the internal iliac vessel.

SEER database—The Surveillance, Epidemiology and End Results Database is managed by the U.S. National Cancer Institute. It collects data from population-based tumor registries around the country that represent a cross section of 23% of the population.

Sentinel lymph node—The sentinel node is the first node involved in lymphatic metastases from the primary cancer. The sentinel node concept holds that lymph node metastasis occurs in an orderly, stepwise progression so that if the first, or *sentinel node*, is negative, then the ensuing nodes are unlikely to be involved with metastatic cancer. Because cervical cancer is a midline tumor that may spread to either pelvic side and perhaps by more than one lymphatic pathway, these sentinel nodes are bilateral, and frequently, more than one node is identified on either side of the pelvis.

In the first half of the 20th century, more women died from cervical cancer in the United States than from any other cancer. With the introduction of the Papanicolaou (Pap) smear in the 1940s, the early detection and treatment of preinvasive disease became possible. Consequently, both the incidence and mortality rates due to invasive cervical cancer in the United States declined approximately 75% by the end of the 20th century. In the United States, approximately 11 to 12 thousand women will be diagnosed with new invasive cervical cancer annually. It is also estimated that approximately 3 to 4 thousand women will succumb to the disease annually. Based on these figures, cervical cancer currently ranks as the third most common female genital tract malignancy in the United States (behind uterine corpus and ovarian cancer).

Worldwide, however, the burden of this disease remains large, with estimates of 300–400 thousand new cases annually and approximately 200 thousand deaths per year. This makes cervical cancer not only the most common gynecologic malignancy but also the third most frequently diagnosed cancer in women (behind breast and colorectal cancer). In general terms, the disease is much more common in developing countries, with 80% of worldwide cases occurring in these areas. In developing countries, cervical cancer accounts for 15% of female malignancies, carrying a lifetime risk of approximately 3%. In contrast, the cervical cancer lifetime risk is approximately 1% in developed countries. The highest incidence rates are observed in Latin America, the Caribbean, sub-Saharan Africa, and Southern and Southeast Asia. This geographical disparity is often attributed to the presence or absence of effective screening and treatment programs, since epidemiologic and biologic studies have not shown significant differences in tumor biology in countries with high rates of cervical cancer.

STAGING OF CERVICAL CANCER

In 1937, the Health Organization of the League of Nations adopted a clinical classification system for cervical cancer, making it the first cancer to be classified so. In 1950, this classification was modified to include preinvasive (in situ) cervical cancer, which was designated stage 0. New recommendations for the clinical classification of carcinoma of the cervix were adopted by the General Assembly of the International Federation of Gynecology and Obstetrics (FIGO) in 1961, and several other modifications have been made since. The general use of this classification abroad and in the United States has been extremely helpful in reporting and comparing results of various modalities of therapy. Descriptions of the clinical stages in carcinoma of the cervix uteri as updated by FIGO in 2009 appear in Table 51.1 and Figure 51.1.

The major redefinition and refinements involve stage I disease. Microinvasive (stage IA) carcinoma has been subdivided into stage IA1 and IA2 based on the depth of cervical stromal invasion by carcinoma. Stage IB has been subdivided into stage IB1 and IB2 based on the size of the clinical lesion.

TABLE 51.1 Staging of Carcinoma of the Cervix Uteri (FIGO Committee on Gynecologic Oncology, 2009)

Stage I		The carcinoma is strictly confined to the cervix (extension to the corpus would be disregarded).
	IA	Invasive carcinoma that can be diagnosed only by microscopy, with deepest invasion ≤5 mm and largest extension ≥7 mm
		IA1	Measured stromal invasion of ≤3.0 mm in depth and extension of ≤7.0 mm
		IA2	Measured stromal invasion of >3.0 mm and not >5.0 mm, with an extension not >7.0 mm
	IB	Clinically visible lesions limited to the cervix uteri or preclinical cancers greater than stage IA[a]
		IB1	Clinically visible lesion ≤4.0 cm in greatest dimension
		IB2	Clinically visible lesion >4.0 cm in greatest dimension
Stage II		Cervical carcinoma invades beyond the uterus, but not to the pelvic wall or to the lower third of the vagina.
	IIA	Without parametrial invasion
		IIA1	Clinically visible lesion ≤4.0 cm in greatest dimension
		IIA2	Clinically visible lesion >4 cm in greatest dimension
	IIB	With obvious parametrial invasion
Stage III		The tumor extends to the pelvic wall and/or involves the lower third of the vagina and/or causes hydronephrosis or nonfunctioning kidney.[b]
	IIIA	Tumor involves the lower third of the vagina, with no extension to the pelvic wall.
	IIIB	Extension to the pelvic wall and/or hydronephrosis or nonfunctioning kidney
Stage IV		The carcinoma has extended beyond the true pelvis or has involved (biopsy proven) the mucosa of the bladder or rectum. A bullous edema, as such, does not permit a case to be allotted to stage IV.
	IVA	Spread to adjacent organs
	IVB	Spread to distant organs

[a]All macroscopically visible lesions—even with superficial invasion—are allotted to stage IB carcinomas. Invasion is limited to a measured stromal invasion with a maximal depth of 5.00 mm and a horizontal extension of not >7.00 mm. Depth of invasion should not be >5.00 mm taken from the base of the epithelium of the original tissue—superficial or glandular. The depth of invasion should always be reported in mm, even in those cases with "early (minimal) stromal invasion" (~1 mm).
The involvement of vascular/lymphatic spaces should not change the stage allotment.
[b]On rectal examination, there is no cancer-free space between the tumor and the pelvic wall. All cases with hydronephrosis or nonfunctioning kidney are included, unless they are known to be due to another cause.

HISTOPATHOLOGY

The principal histologic type of invasive cervical cancer, occurring in approximately 80% of cases, is the *squamous (epidermoid)* lesion. In 1923, Martzloff classified these squamous tumors into three main histologic subtypes and grades. Grade 1 tumors contain well-differentiated cells, keratin, and squamous pearls (Fig. 51.2A). Grade 2 tumors, the most common, are predominantly composed of transitional cells of the large cell nonkeratinizing type (Fig. 51.2B). Grade 3 tumors, the least common, are poorly differentiated small basal cell–type tumors (Fig. 51.2C). The classification of Martzloff did not prove to be clinically useful, mainly because biopsies taken from different areas of the same tumor often show different degrees of differentiation and different predominant cell types. Martzloff's work did inspire Broders, Wentz and Reagan, and others to continue to categorize the histologic types and degree of differentiation of squamous cell cervical

tumors and to study their clinical behavior and response to treatment. The histologic classification of squamous cell tumor types introduced in 1959 by Wentz and Reagan is sometimes used in pathology reports. However, Willen and coworkers were unable to confirm a predictive value for survival from the Wentz-Reagan classification. Similarly, most recent studies, including those by the Gynecologic Oncology Group (GOG), have shown that grading squamous carcinomas has little predictive value.

A rare form of squamous cell cancer of the cervix is a *verrucous carcinoma*. It is a very well-differentiated squamous cell carcinoma with extensive keratinization that usually presents as a large bulky tumor of the cervix and often is confused with giant condylomas, such as those seen on the vulva. There is a sharp line between the tumor and underlying cervical stroma. Verrucous carcinoma, like most cervical cancers, has been shown to be associated with human papillomavirus (HPV)

IX

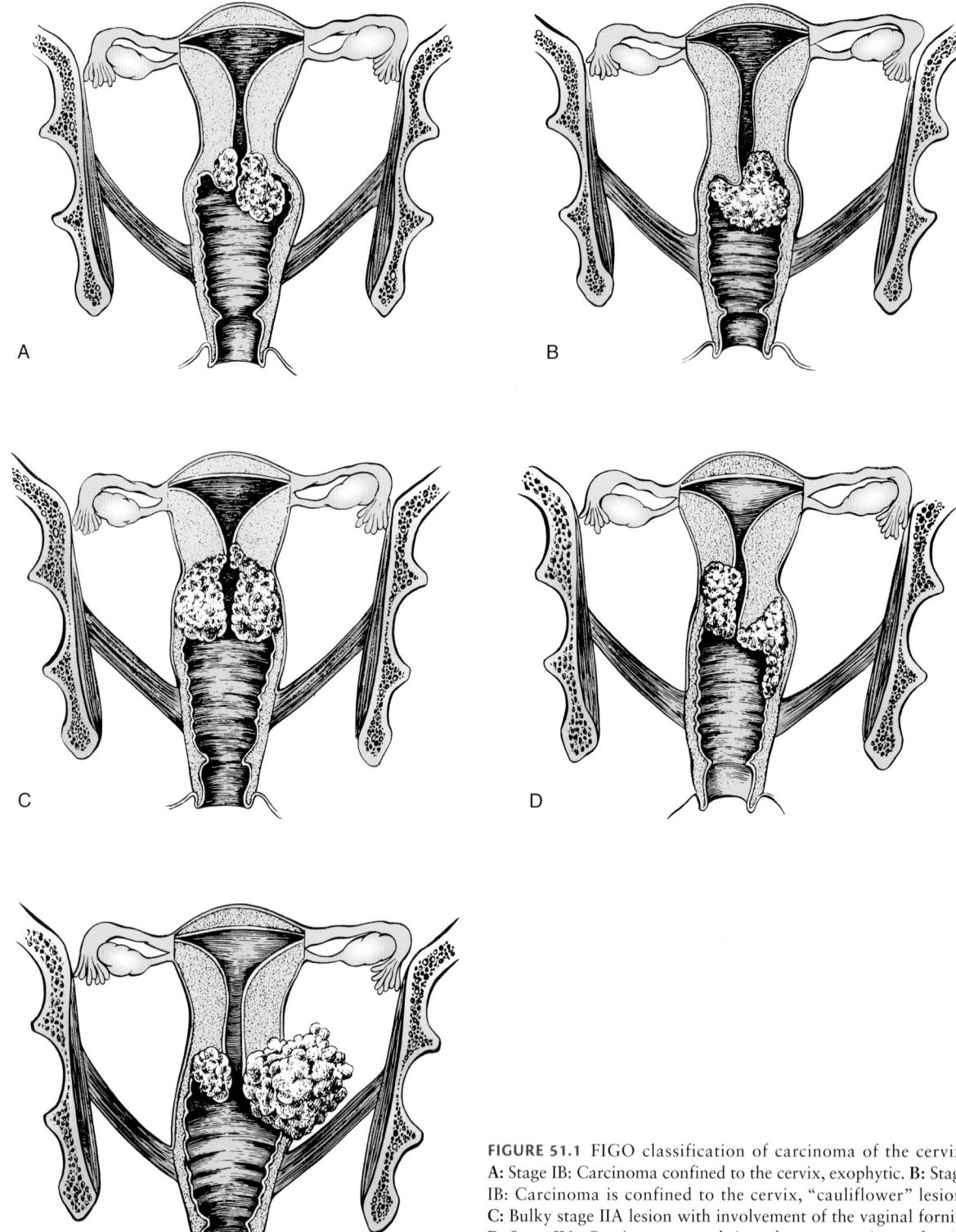

FIGURE 51.1 FIGO classification of carcinoma of the cervix.
A: Stage IB: Carcinoma confined to the cervix, exophytic. **B:** Stage
IB: Carcinoma is confined to the cervix, "cauliflower" lesion.
C: Bulky stage IIA lesion with involvement of the vaginal fornix.
D: Stage IIA: Carcinoma extends into the upper vagina or fornix.
E: Stage IIB: Carcinoma extends into the parametrium but does
not extend to the pelvic wall.

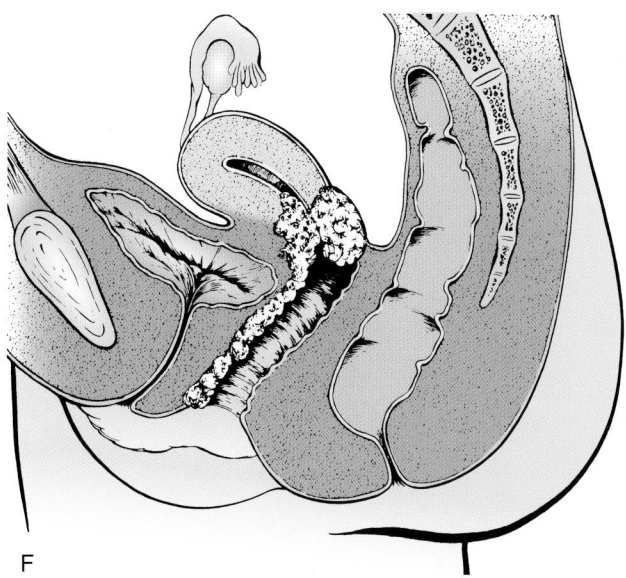

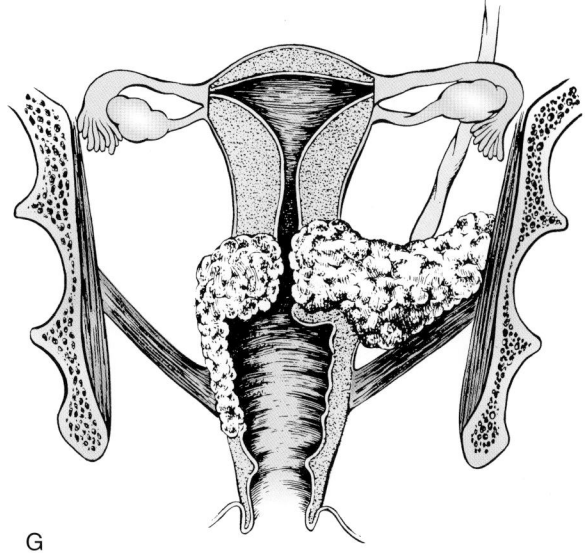

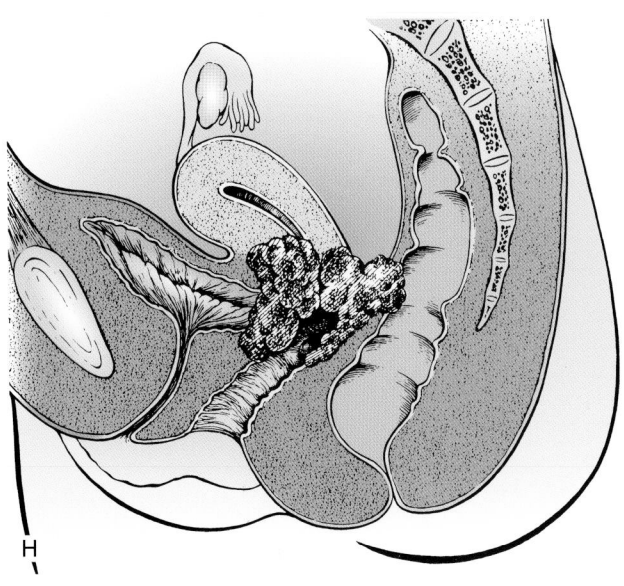

FIGURE 51.1 (*Continued*) **F:** Stage IIIA: Carcinoma involves the anterior vaginal wall, extending to the lower third. **G:** Stage IIIB: The parametrium is infiltrated, and the carcinoma extends to the pelvic wall. **H:** Stage IVA: The bladder base or rectum is involved.

infection. Although metastatic disease is rare, this tumor has been noted to become more virulent if treated with irradiation. Goldberger and coworkers reported an unusually aggressive verrucous carcinoma of the cervix. According to deJesus and coworkers, at least 49 cases of this tumor have been reported in the female genital tract, sometimes as verrucous carcinoma and sometimes as squamous papillary tumor.

Adenocarcinomas of the cervix are becoming more common, especially in younger women. In a review of the Surveillance, Epidemiology, and End Results (SEER) Cancer Incidence Public-Use database from 1973 to 1996, Smith and colleagues reported that although the age-adjusted incidence rates per 100,000 for all invasive cervical cancers and squamous cell cancers decreased by 37% and 42%, respectively, the rates for adenocarcinoma of the cervix increased by 29% during the study period. These results suggest that current screening practices may be insufficient in detecting a significant proportion of adenocarcinoma precursor lesions.

Approximately one half of cervical adenocarcinomas are exophytic, usually polypoid, or papillary; others diffusely enlarge or ulcerate the cervix. Approximately 15% of patients have no visible lesion because the epicenter of the carcinoma is within the endocervical canal. Even without visible signs or symptoms, the lesion may infiltrate deeply into the cervix. Drescher and colleagues reported a higher frequency of uterine corpus invasion and nodal metastasis in 26 patients with cervical adenocarcinoma compared with 139 cases of squamous cell carcinoma. More recent studies have reached contradictory conclusions regarding the prognostic significance of this histology compared to the squamous counterpart. In general, most practitioners would treat stage I cervical cancer of squamous or adeno histology in a similar manner, without much regard to the histology. This is drastically different from the approach to stage I small cell neuroendocrine tumors and other rare tumors, such as adenoma malignum, which tends to be much more lethal.

IX

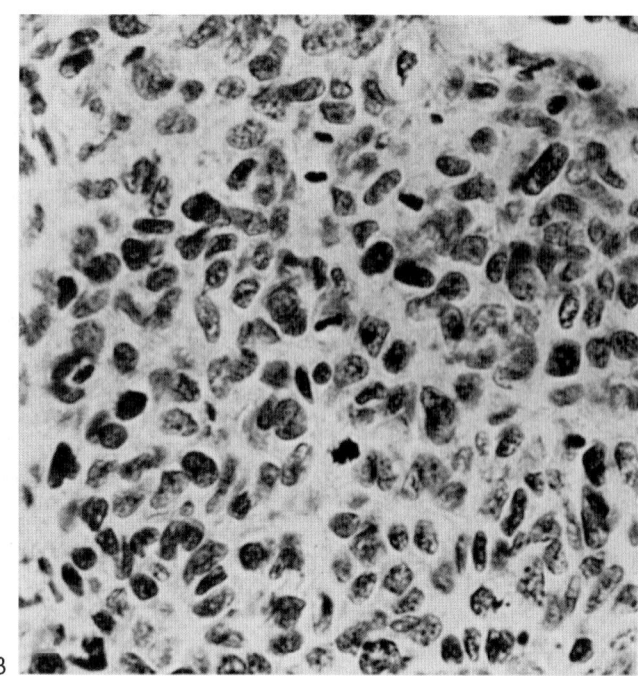

FIGURE 51.2 A: Grade 1: Well-differentiated epidermoid carcinoma of the cervix. High-power view of spinal cell type. The tumor cells contain abundant keratin that forms epithelial pearls. **B:** Grade 2: Moderately differentiated epidermoid carcinoma of the cervix, transitional cell type. The tumor cells are characterized by a moderate amount of cytoplasm but are without pearl formation. Extensive pleomorphism and mitosis are evident. The tumor is frequently classified as being of large cell, nonkeratinizing type. **C:** Grade 3: Poorly differentiated epidermoid carcinoma of the cervix, fat spindle or basal cell type. The tumor cells have little cytoplasm, numerous mitoses, and no keratin or epithelial pearls.

In addition to pure (endocervical) adenocarcinoma (Fig. 51.3), cervical adenocarcinomas can exhibit a variety of patterns and can be composed of diverse cell types. Other histologic patterns include *endometrioid, clear cell, serous, mesonephric,* and *adenoma malignum.* Different histologic patterns and cell types often appear in the same cervical tumor. Because mixtures are common, the designation of tumor type is based on the predominant component. In general, if a second histologic type constitutes 20% or more of the tumor, the lesion is designated as a *mixed cell type,* but pathologists also use various criteria to distinguish mixed lesions. Not infrequently, an adenocarcinoma and squamous cell carcinoma coexist in the same tumor, and these lesions are referred to as *adenosquamous carcinomas.* The so-called glassy cell adenocarcinoma of the cervix is rare and considered a variant of poorly differentiated adenosquamous carcinoma. It is known to be clinically

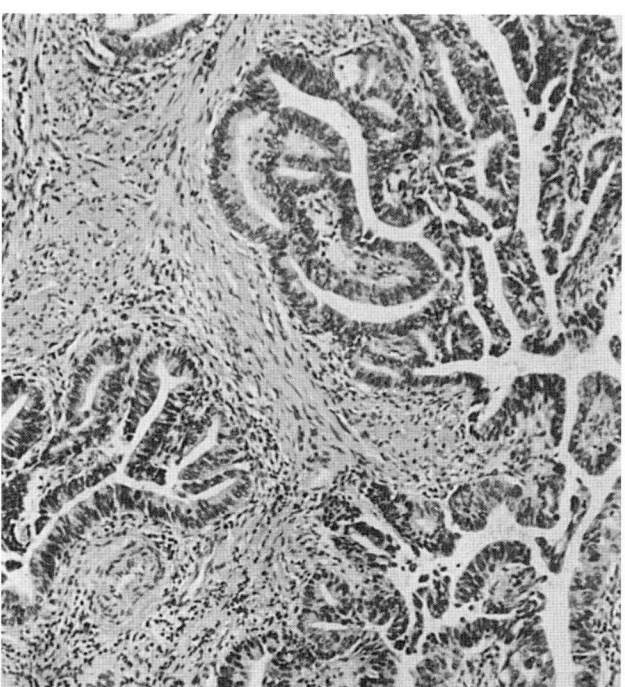

FIGURE 51.3 Adenocarcinoma of the cervix.

aggressive, with frequent early distant metastasis. *Clear cell adenocarcinoma* of the cervix can occur in the presence or absence of intrauterine exposure to diethylstilbestrol (DES). Saigo and coworkers found that the endometrioid pattern was associated with a more favorable prognosis than any was other histologic type of cervical adenocarcinoma; however, other authors believe that the subpatterns have no prognostic significance. DES-related neoplasia is rarely seen by most practitioners, but clear cell neoplasia of the cervix unrelated to DES is occasionally encountered.

The early classifications of squamous cell carcinoma of the cervix proposed by Martzloff and others divided these tumors into three categories: keratinizing squamous cell carcinoma, large cell nonkeratinizing squamous cell carcinoma, and small cell carcinoma. Over the years, however, it became apparent that the subgroup designated as *small cell carcinoma* was composed of a heterogeneous group of tumors, many of which displayed neuroendocrine differentiation. Recent changes in the nomenclature have led to the subdivision of these *neuroendocrine tumors* into four categories: carcinoid, atypical carcinoid, large cell neuroendocrine carcinoma, and small cell carcinoma. Typical carcinoid and atypical carcinoid tumors are rare in the cervix; therefore, their clinical and pathologic features have not been well characterized. Large cell neuroendocrine and small cell carcinomas are highly aggressive neoplasms, with a propensity to metastasize early and widely. Usual methods of therapy incorporate systemic chemotherapy to treat potential distant metastasis, even in apparent clinical stage I disease.

Various *cervical sarcomas* have been described by Rotmensch and coworkers. These tumors constitute less than 0.5% of all cervical cancers and include adenosarcomas, leiomyosarcomas, carcinosarcomas, and rhabdomyosarcomas. Melanoma may also develop in the cervix and upper vagina and is often highly lethal. It is extremely rare for a lymphoma to develop primarily in the cervix, but lymphoma in the cervix is more likely to represent evidence of generalized lymphomatous disease.

CLINICAL PRESENTATION

Invasive cervical cancer is more likely than are its intraepithelial precursors to cause symptoms such as *abnormal vaginal bleeding* (menorrhagia, metrorrhagia, postcoital bleeding, or postmenopausal bleeding) or discharge. Many patients describe a profuse and often malodorous discharge, especially when the disease is advanced. Thus, any patient with abnormal vaginal bleeding or discharge should have a pelvic examination, including a speculum examination with visualization of the cervix. Failure to examine and visualize the cervix in a patient with abnormal vaginal bleeding or discharge could result in failure to diagnose cervical cancer.

Pain is not a common symptom in patients with cervical cancer, unless the disease is locally advanced and has invaded the adjacent pelvic structures, including pelvic nerves. In more advanced stages, patients may report bladder and rectal symptoms. When the disease involves lumbosacral and sciatic nerve roots and the lateral pelvic sidewall, chronic pelvic pain radiating down the leg can be excruciating and indicative of advanced disease. Edema of the lower extremities likewise indicates tumor obstruction of lymphatic and/or venous drainage and is a sign of advanced disease. Palpable supraclavicular or inguinal adenopathy may indicate distant spread and should be evaluated to exclude nodal spread. Ascites is uncommon in cervical cancer. Peritoneal dissemination is uncommon in early stages and is highly lethal regardless of histologic subtype.

Unfortunately, the physician cannot rely on the presence of symptoms to lead to a diagnosis of early carcinoma of the cervix. Many women remain without symptoms for many months. Approximately one third of patients with advanced-stage (III or IV) disease report symptoms for less than 3 months. The only way to diagnose cervical cancer in the earliest possible stages is to routinely apply special diagnostic procedures to large groups of women with and without gynecologic symptoms. This means screening the adult female population with Pap smears and cervical HPV testing at set intervals.

Invasive cervical lesions can be exophytic, infiltrative, ulcerative, or occult. The size of the visible lesion on the cervix may correlate with the depth of stromal invasion, but exceptions do occur with superficial exophytic lesions (Fig. 51.4).

An everted exophytic carcinomatous growth may be friable. Bits of tissue may break off on the examining fingers. On inspection, the friable exophytic cancer shows a rough, granular bleeding surface that can be sloughing and infected, with a foul-smelling discharge.

A tumor that develops beneath the mucosa of the ectocervix and infiltrates the cervical stroma usually causes cervical enlargement (expansion). The surface of the cervix may still feel smooth, but the cervical consistency to palpation is firm, hard, or nodular. It is characteristic of cervical cancers that develop in the endocervical canal to cause cervical enlargement and a firm cervical consistency before breaking through the mucosa of the exocervix to cause a visible lesion on speculum exam. This also is characteristic of some cervical cancers that develop in postmenopausal women. In fact, it is possible, although uncommon, for a cervical cancer that is developing from an epicenter high in the endocervical canal to invade the parametrial tissue and even obstruct the ureters before causing a visible cervical lesion. An ulcerative lesion can look like a large punched-out ulcer, but more commonly, it is an irregular crater with a necrotic bleeding base and a foul-smelling discharge. The normal contour of the cervix is absent in these ulcerative cases, and complete loss of a significant portion of the ectocervix is common.

IX

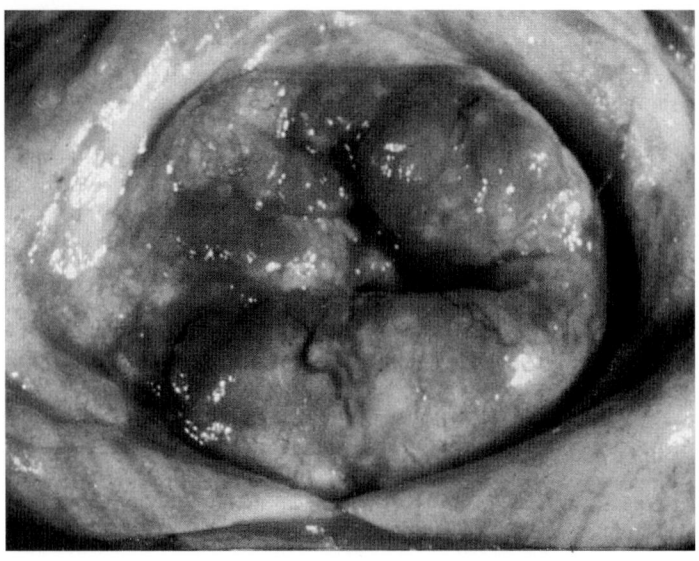

FIGURE 51.4 Squamous cell carcinoma, cervix uteri, FIGO stage IIA.

Any grossly visible lesion of the cervix should be considered suspicious for cancer, and biopsy should be performed. Good visualization with a speculum and adequate illumination are essential. A Pap smear can be performed, even though it can be less accurate in the presence of a grossly visible cervical lesion, but the main diagnostic procedure should be a biopsy.

Colposcopic examination is neither needed nor particularly effective for a gross cervical lesion but can be helpful when there is a small surface lesion to identify the most abnormal area for directed biopsies. The primary benefit of colposcopy is in visualizing noninvasive, precursor, or minimally invasive lesions that cannot be visualized without magnification.

Cervical biopsy techniques are discussed in another chapter. Biopsies can be undertaken with any of a number of special instruments: The Kevorkian (**Fig. 51.5**), Younge, or Gaylor biopsy forceps are particularly functional for taking an adequate biopsy specimen. It is important to obtain a sufficient specimen where frank stromal invasion can be demonstrated. Surgical conization under anesthesia is unnecessary when a grossly visible lesion is present. Iodine (Schiller) staining can be used to demarcate the vaginal margins of a neoplastic area from adjacent normal epithelium. All of these procedures, as well as the popular loop diathermy conizations (LEEP), can be done in the outpatient setting. It is rarely necessary to take the patient to the operating room to diagnose cervical cancer. If an anesthetic is deemed necessary for some other reason, a careful pelvic examination under anesthesia, biopsy of any vaginal lesions, cervical and uterine sounding, cystoscopy and

proctoscopy (if warranted), and even uterine curettage can be done; therefore, useful information to plan treatment can be obtained.

PROGNOSTIC FACTORS

Several factors have been reported to affect prognosis in cervical cancer. However, the most important determinant of prognosis remains FIGO clinical stage. Based on studies by Piver and colleagues, van Nagell and associates, Delgado and coworkers, and numerous others that have demonstrated the prognostic significance of depth of cervical stromal invasion (DSI) and clinical or histologic tumor size in early-stage disease, FIGO incorporated these factors into its current clinical staging system by subdividing stage I. The 5-year survival rates by stage as reported by FIGO are shown in Table 51.2.

In addition to FIGO stage, other reported prognostic factors include regional (pelvic) and distant (paraaortic) lymph node metastases, lymphovascular space invasion (LVSI), and select histologic subtypes, such as the small cell neuroendocrine tumors mentioned earlier.

Uterine corpus and endometrial cavity extension from primary cervical cancer was originally deemed a poor prognostic factor. The original League of Nations classification of 1937 included such lesions in the stage II category. Over the years, classification of the disease based on extension to the uterine corpus or endometrial cavity has gradually been discounted. These lesions, classified as stage IC in 1950, were included in

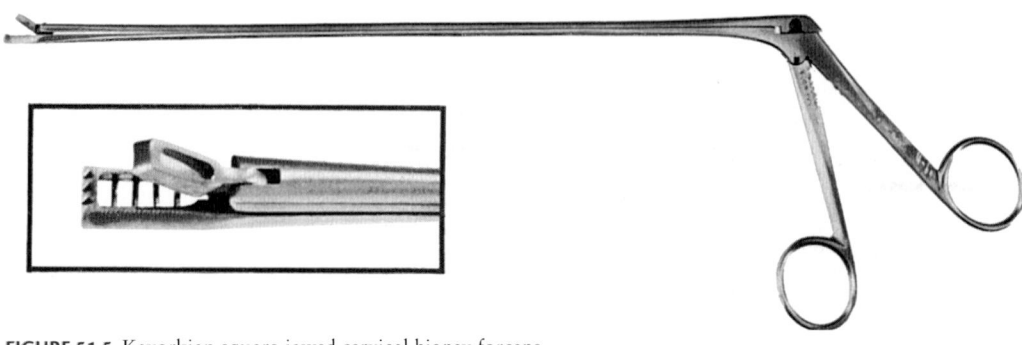

FIGURE 51.5 Kevorkian square-jawed cervical biopsy forceps.

TABLE 51.2 Five-Year Survival by Figo Stage

STAGE	NUMBER OF PATIENTS	5-YEAR SURVIVAL RATE (%)
Ia1	860	98.7
Ia2	227	95.9
IB1	2,530	88.0
IB2	950	78.8
IIA	881	68.8
IIB	2,375	64.7
IIIA	160	40.4
IIIB	1,949	43.3
IVA	245	19.5
IVB	189	15.0

From International Federation of Gynecology and Obstetrics.

the broad category of stage IB in 1961. Despite the change in classification, there is still some concern about patients whose tumor extends into the corpus of the uterus; this is of paramount importance in fertility-sparing radical trachelectomy cases. Evidence from Washington University reported by Perez and coworkers showed that tumor extension into the endometrial cavity lowers the 5-year survival rate of stage IB and IIA lesions by 10% to 20%. Lesions that involve the corpus also were found to have a twofold greater incidence of distant metastases compared with lesions without corpus extension. Similar observations have been reported by Prempree and coworkers from 82 cases of stage I and II disease with endometrial extension. The absolute 5-year cure rates of 68% for stage I and 62% for stage II disease with endometrial extension reflect the higher risk of metastases: 20% for

stage I cases and 24% for stage II cases. Such reports must be studied with consideration of the difficulty of establishing a diagnosis of endometrial extension by using microscopic study of endometrial curettage specimens. The curettage specimen is frequently contaminated by the cervical tumor, making it difficult to be certain about endometrial extension. Treatment planning is not altered by such observations, nor is a fractional curettage recommended as part of pretreatment evaluation.

Lymph node metastases, either regional (pelvic) or to higher-level (common iliac and paraaortic) lymph nodes, have proven to be one of the most reliable prognostic factors for patients with cervical cancer (Fig. 51.6). The frequency of metastases to pelvic lymph nodes is approximately 0% to 1% for patients with stage IA1, 7% to 9% for stage IA2, 12% to 20% for stage IB, 20% to 38% for stage IIA, 16% to 36% for stage IIB, and greater than 35% for stage III and IV disease. Historically, preoperative detection of positive pelvic and paraaortic lymph nodes was unreliable; however, with the advent of newer radiologic imaging techniques, such as positron emission tomography (PET) scan, radiologic imaging has significantly improved the detection of nodal metastasis. Nevertheless, detection of positive lymph nodes is best made by pathologic evaluation and more accurately determined when lymphadenectomy or sentinel lymph node (SLN) mapping is used in preoperative staging or treatment. Although Kolstad showed that when intraoperative lymphography is used, 15% to 25% more patients with stage IB disease are found to have positive regional lymph nodes, this technique is rarely used nowadays and is mostly of historical relevance. The development of cervical injection techniques for SLN mapping has become a more accepted strategy in conjunction with pelvic lymphadenectomy to map early cervical cancer and determine nodal status.

When patients with stage IB cervical cancer are primarily treated with radical hysterectomy and pelvic lymphadenectomy, the 5-year cure rate is approximately 90% if there are no lymph node metastases. However, if metastatic disease to lymph nodes is detected, the 5-year cure rate falls to approximately 65% to 80%. The number of positive nodes also influences prognosis. In a review of the literature before the current standard of postoperative concurrent chemoradiation therapy,

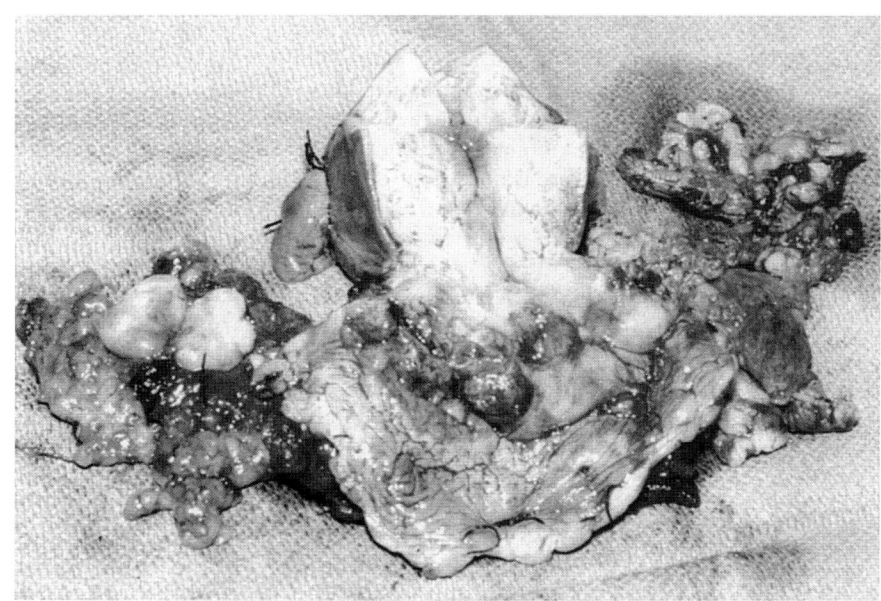

FIGURE 51.6 Squamous cell carcinoma, cervix uteri, FIGO stage IIA, with gross metastatic tumor in a right parametrial lymph node.

Hoskins reported an 83% survival rate for patients with stage IB and IIA disease who had negative lymph nodes at the time of radical hysterectomy and pelvic lymphadenectomy. The survival rate decreased to 57% in patients with one to two positive nodes and 31% in those with more than three positive nodes.

Metastatic disease to paraaortic lymph nodes occurs in 4% to 7% of patients with stage I disease, 15% to 20% with stage II disease, 25% to 30% with stage III disease, and 30% to 50% with stage IVA disease. Most studies confirm that metastasis to paraaortic nodes occurs more frequently when positive pelvic nodes also are present. The rarity of patients found to have isolated positive paraaortic nodes when pelvic nodes are negative raises the question: How well sampled and/or sectioned were the pelvic nodes? With more incorporation of SLN mapping and pathologic ultrastaging of pelvic nodes, it is likely that the incidence of isolated aortic nodal metastasis will be even less than previously reported. Even with extended-field radiation therapy, the 5-year survival rate for patients with metastases to the paraaortic nodes is only approximately 25% to 35%. Combined modality chemoradiation is a standard of care in many countries for node-positive cases. The addition of more chemotherapy after definitive chemoradiation has been investigated and is gaining popularity as a consolidation strategy in advanced cases.

Historically, tumor grade has been reported to affect prognosis. Early studies by Chung and coworkers and van Nagell and colleagues demonstrated a poorer prognosis among patients with poorly differentiated tumors. However, more recent studies by Zaino and the GOG have shown the grading of squamous tumors to be of little predictive value in cervical carcinoma. Shingleton and Orr reviewed nine publications that reported on 3,761 patients with predominantly squamous cell carcinoma. Twenty-eight different factors were evaluated for prognostic significance. *On multivariate analysis, tumor volume, lymph node metastasis, parametrial invasion, and LVSI were found to be significant independent prognostic factors, but patient age and tumor grade were not.*

On the other hand, tumor differentiation may have a significant prognostic role in adenocarcinoma of the cervix. Shingleton and Orr also reviewed eight studies of 577 patients with adenocarcinoma of the cervix. As with squamous cell carcinoma, the strongest independent prognostic variables were tumor size and nodal metastasis. However, unlike with squamous cell carcinoma, tumor grade appeared to have prognostic significance.

Several investigators, including Swan and Roddick, Wheeless and Graham, and Julian and coworkers, have drawn attention to the fact that when there is a mixture of adenocarcinomatous and squamous elements—so-called adenosquamous tumors—the prognosis is poor and the incidence of pelvic lymph node metastases is high. Histologic combinations should be considered when comparing the prognoses of adenocarcinoma and squamous cancers of the cervix. The literature is mixed on the overall issue of whether adenocarcinoma in general and adenosquamous cancers specifically are more virulent and less curable than are their squamous counterparts. Stehman and colleagues performed a multivariate analysis of prognostic variables for 626 patients with locally advanced cervical carcinoma treated with radiation therapy on three GOG protocols. Histologic cell type was not found to be a significant prognostic factor. A national pattern of care and evaluation study of the American College of Surgeons also failed to report statistically different 5-year survival rates for squamous and adenocarcinoma, regardless of type of therapy chosen.

In a landmark GOG prospective study of 645 patients with stage IB squamous cell carcinoma of the cervix treated with radical hysterectomy and pelvic lymphadenectomy, Delgado and colleagues identified three independent risk factors in relation to disease-free survival: the depth of invasion, the size of the tumor, and LVSI. The disease-free interval was 89% for patients without LVSI compared with 77% for those with LVSI. Although not all studies have found LVSI to be an independent prognostic factor, as stated, in a review of nine studies (including the study by Delgado et al.) of 3,761 patients, Shingleton and Orr found LVSI to be a significant independent prognostic factor on multivariate analysis. The incidence of LVSI in early-stage lesions varies widely, depending on multiple factors, including the number of sections of the cervix prepared, the depth of stromal invasion, and the interest of the examining pathologist. Observations from Austria and Germany indicate that there is considerable variation in the frequency with which LVSI is recognized by the pathologist. In a combined study of more than 1,000 patients at three different reference centers (Graz, Munich, and Erlangen), Burghardt and associates reported that the frequency with which LVSI was identified ranged from 9% in Munich, where only blood vessel involvement was so classified, to 43% in Graz, where it was classified as capillary-like space involvement. At the third center, Erlangen, the corresponding value was intermediate at 23%. Such variations in histopathologic criteria may well contribute to some of the controversy that exists regarding the prognostic significance of LVSI. LVSI in itself, although a risk factor for nodal metastasis, is not a contraindication to consider and offer fertility-sparing surgery, such as radical trachelectomy.

To this point, this discussion of prognostic factors has included only anatomic and morphologic factors. Peipert and associates emphasized that cancer, including cervical cancer, has both form and function. Accordingly, other clinical variables, such as the patient's symptoms, symptom severity, and comorbidity, affect the survival rate of patients with invasive cervical cancer. Unless these variables are suitably included such as in nomograms, prognostic estimates based on morphology alone are imprecise, and therapeutic evaluations can be misleading. According to Rutledge and associates, there is no consistent effect of age on survival rate in patients treated for cervical cancer. Younger patients with early-stage disease seemed to survive longer than did older patients, but the tendency reversed when disease was advanced.

PRETREATMENT EVALUATION AND STAGING

When a diagnosis of invasive cervical cancer has been established, the clinician should perform an evaluation of relevant pelvic organs to determine whether the tumor is confined to the cervix or has extended to the adjacent vagina, parametrium, bladder, ureters, or rectum. To determine clinical stage, a pelvic exam with palpation, inspection, and estimation of tumor involvement and measurements is allowed; in addition, a conization is also allowed as a staging tool in occult early-stage lesions. According to FIGO guidelines for clinical staging, diagnostic studies may include intravenous urography (IVU), cystoscopic examination of the bladder and urethra, a proctosigmoidoscopic study, a barium enema (BE), and in the case of early-stage disease, a colposcopic study of the vagina and the vaginal fornices. Colposcopic findings may be used for assigning a stage to the tumor (for instance, FIGO stage IIA), but the results must be confirmed by biopsy. Standard x-rays, such as a chest x-ray and routine bone films, are allowed for staging. Chest radiographs and electrocardiographic studies are also used to determine cardiopulmonary disease, particularly in the older patient. Advanced imaging modalities with pelvic MRI, computerized tomography (CT), and whole-body PET scan, although very useful to help triage treatment, are not available to the majority of women in developing nations.

When studies detect ureteral obstruction, a tumor is classified as a stage IIIB lesion, regardless of the size of the primary lesion. Ureteral obstruction, either hydronephrosis or nonfunction of the kidney, is well established as an indicator of poor prognosis, as recognized in the FIGO classification system. Retrograde pyelography can be performed after the ureteral obstruction is located for further evaluation, and stenting of the blocked ureter is frequently considered. Kidney function studies such as serum creatinine and creatinine clearance provide important baseline information before treatment; complete urinalysis is useful for detecting the presence of albumin or white and red blood cells and renal tubular casts. The majority of women with advanced cervical cancer will be candidates for chemotherapy, and maintaining good renal function is important in these patients.

In women with bulky or advanced-stage tumors, the bladder mucosa also should be inspected cystoscopically for possible bullous edema, which indicates lymphatic obstruction within the bladder wall. Evidence of tumor in the bladder must be confirmed by biopsy before the lesion can be classified as stage IVA. Urine cytology is usually not sufficient to make that diagnosis. Rectal mucosal lesions from cervical cancer are infrequent and also require a biopsy via proctosigmoidoscopy, because they can be related to an inflammatory or other neoplastic process rather than to the cervical tumor.

A pelvic examination must be performed as part of the staging process, and it may be necessary to have the patient completely relaxed by general anesthesia for a satisfactory exam. In as many as 20% of patients, the initial clinical classification of the disease based on office evaluation has been proven to be incorrect based on findings at the time of pelvic examination under anesthesia. Such an examination can reveal a more advanced stage of the disease than was originally found; additional biopsies (if indicated) or fractional curettage can be done, as well as colposcopy, cystoscopy, and proctosigmoidoscopy. In today's health care climate, however, the cost of a separate examination under anesthesia may need to be reserved for only the most problematic cases. Moreover, the advancements in pelvic MRI quality are giving gynecologic oncologists better information about the extent of locally advanced cervical neoplasia.

A main goal of tumor staging is to define prognostic groups, to enable clinicians to compare disease status, screening efficacy, treatment results, and other health care outcomes. The present form of the FIGO cervical cancer staging system is in principle a series of definitions of the most important prognostic features of cervical cancer, and it has been used in treatment protocols for generations. However, in the present form of the system, some of the stages do not refer to the presence or absence of paramount prognostic features that are recognized as definition criteria for lower (previous) stages. For example, stage IIA is defined as vaginal vault spread of the disease. Stage IIB does not contain information about the disease involvement of the vaginal vault (presence or absence of criteria for stage IIA), although extensive tumor spread to the vaginal vault seems to be at least as significant a prognostic factor as parametrium involvement (definition of stage IIB). Likewise, stage IIIB does not describe the presence or absence of a condition described in stage IIIA, although extensive tumor spread

to the lower parts of the vagina (criteria of stage IIIA) is indeed a severe prognostic sign that should be considered in treatment planning. Similar weaknesses of the staging system include the lack of tumor size description in stage IIB and upper stages. (This problem was recognized by the new staging system, which differentiates between stage IIA1 and IIA2.)

The introduction of a more complex system of stages might better define prognostic groups, but inevitably, it would be more difficult to use and would make it difficult to collect large enough patient cohorts in a given substage for research. However, considering these weaknesses of the FIGO staging, a descriptive combination of the FIGO stages might be used in daily practice. For example, a patient with a bulky tumor involving the vaginal vault, inner half of the parametrium with hydroureter, should be defined as stage IIIB disease (based upon the ureter compression). But the disease (prognosis) might be better defined by adding information about criteria of previous stages, stating, for example, this is stage IIIB disease, with features of stage IIA2 and IIB, that is, no lower vaginal invasion or pelvic sidewall invasion.

Using an extension or combination of findings from lower stages might help to better define prognostic groups, explain results, and create treatment suggestions for special conditions without the need for creating a completely new and more complex staging system.

Pretreatment pedal lymphangiography has been used in the past to detect pelvic and paraaortic lymph node metastases, but the procedure is tedious and associated with many false-negative and false-positive findings. When compared with lymphadenectomy, positive lymphangiograms have an accuracy rate of less than 75% and a false-negative rate as high as 50%. Furthermore, a lymphangiogram only detects metastatic lesions when the parenchyma of the lymph node has become distorted, by which time the lesions are macroscopic. The procedure is therefore not recommended for routine use in the pretreatment evaluation of cervical cancer patients and is mostly mentioned nowadays for historical value.

Surgical experience from pelvic lymphadenectomy has confirmed an error rate of 15% to 25% in the clinical staging of patients with stage IB or II lesions. In 10% to 30% of cases with stage II or III tumors, in addition to positive findings of occult pelvic lymph nodes, other metastases may be found in the paraaortic nodes. Unfortunately, pelvic examinations and clinical staging as defined by FIGO cannot detect such metastases. Consequently, there is a growing body of literature showing the superiority of cross-sectional imaging (CT, MRI, and PET) over clinical staging in delineating the extent of disease in patients with cervical cancer. As stated earlier, official FIGO guidelines do not incorporate the use of advanced imaging, such as PET and MRI, into the staging of cervical cancer. This is due to FIGO's determination to create guidelines with universally available staging methods so that staging can be a standardized means of communication between different institutions worldwide. However, as knowledge of prognostic factors and the value of cross-sectional imaging have accumulated, its use in treatment planning has increased despite the lack of change in the official FIGO clinical staging guidelines, and in developed countries, MRI and PET scans are frequently performed as a routine part of the workup and management of suspected advanced cervical cancer.

In a Patterns of Care Study conducted between 1978 and 1988, Montana et al. reported a decrease in the use of IVU (86% to 42%) and BE (58% to 32%) in the staging of cervical cancer patients. During the same time period, the use of CT scan increased from 6% to 70%. In another Patterns of Care Study in the United States recently reported by Amendola and colleagues, the use of lymphangiography, IVU, and BE had fallen to 1% in the pretreatment evaluation of patients with clinical FIGO stage IB1 or greater cervical cancer who were scheduled for surgery.

The greatest value of a CT scan in the pretreatment evaluation of patients with cervical cancer is in the assessment of advanced disease (stage IB2 and greater) and in the detection and biopsy of suspected lymph node metastasis and possible ureteral obstruction. The treatment plan for patients with locally advanced disease must be modified if retroperitoneal lymph node involvement and/or distant metastasis is discovered. A meta-analysis by Schneidler et al. reported a positive predictive value of 61% for CT scan in the pretreatment evaluation of nodal disease in cervical cancer. Moreover, in experienced hands, fine needle aspiration of retroperitoneal nodes with CT scan guidance has an accuracy rate of 80% to 95%. When the aspiration study unequivocally shows malignant cells, a surgical biopsy need not be performed. This information is most valuable in patients who have metastasis to the paraaortic nodes, because these patients would need the pelvic radiation fields extended to incorporate the involved region if there is no other evidence of distant metastasis. The use of laparoscopy and robotic surgery to "surgically stage" the paraaortic nodes is common in many practices, and pathologic evaluation of these nodes remains the most reliable strategy to exclude disease despite advances with imaging, such as PET scan. Recent studies have shown that even with a negative PET scan in the paraaortic region, a nodal dissection may identify a 10% to 15% nodal positivity on microscopic examination.

SURGICAL TREATMENT OF EARLY-STAGE CERVICAL CANCER

Based on the pretreatment evaluation of the patient, including the prognostic factors of tumor size, clinical stage of the disease, and risk of pelvic node metastases, a treatment schema can be developed for invasive cervical cancer, as shown in Table 51.3. Almost all patients are treated with either primary surgery or primary radiation therapy with concurrent chemotherapy. Some patients are appropriately treated with combinations of all three. The standard management of patients with early cervical carcinoma is surgical removal of the cervix and pelvic nodal evaluation. The extent of resection of the surrounding tissue depends on the stage, size of the lesion, and the depth of cervical stromal invasion.

Stage IA1 Disease

The exact definition of early-stage cervical cancer has been debated for several decades. This is illustrated by the fact that FIGO changed the definition of early-stage cervical cancer at least five times since 1960. In 2009, FIGO made its most recent revision to the stage IA cervical cancer staging system. After an extensive evaluation of the data in the literature, as well as seeking advice from specialty societies and individuals worldwide, FIGO changed the definition of stage IA1 disease to lesions that invade the cervical stroma ≤3 mm in depth and ≤7 mm in width. Stage IA2 includes patients with >3 mm but <5 mm invasion and ≤7 mm lateral extent.

In an exhaustive review of the literature, Ostor identified 31 studies spanning the years 1976 to 1993 that reported on 3,598 patients with squamous cell carcinoma of the cervix and ≤3 mm stromal invasion. Although not all patients had lymph nodes removed as part of their treatment, the calculated incidence of lymph node metastasis in this group of patients was less than 1%.

TABLE 51.3 General Treatment Schema for Invasive Cervical Carcinoma[a]

DISEASE STAGE	TREATMENT
Stage IA1	Simple hysterectomy, abdominal or vaginal, or cervical conization If there is LVI, consider sentinel node mapping or pelvic lymphadenectomy
Stages IA2[b], IB1, and nonbulky IIA	Radical (type C)[c] hysterectomy or trachelectomy,[d] bilateral pelvic lymphadenectomy (consider sentinel node mapping) with postoperative irradiation, ±concurrent chemotherapy in selected high-risk patients
Stages IB2 and bulky IIA[e]	Full external and intracavitary pelvic irradiation with concurrent chemotherapy (±extrafascial hysterectomy) or radical abdominal hysterectomy and pelvic (±periaortic lymphadenectomy)
Stages IIB to IVA[f]	Full external and intracavitary pelvic irradiation with concurrent chemotherapy
Stage IVB	Palliative chemotherapy

[a]For individual patients, recommendations for treatment can vary, depending on the clinical circumstances.
[b]Some authorities recommend modified (type B) radical hysterectomy, bilateral pelvic lymphadenectomy for stage IA2 disease.
[c]Refer to Figure 51.7.
[d]In highly selected cases.
[e]Some authorities recommend simple hysterectomy in addition to radiation/chemotherapy for stage IB2 and bulky stage IIA disease.
[f]A patient with a stage IVA lesion that extends only in the anterior or posterior direction may be a candidate for pelvic exenteration.

Diagnosis

Microinvasive carcinoma cannot be diagnosed from a punch biopsy because adjacent areas may contain more advanced tumor; conization is required for definitive diagnosis in this situation. The accuracy of the diagnosis depends on the adequacy of the cone and the adequacy of the pathologic examination of the cone. The entire cone should be blocked so that an adequate number of histologic sections can be taken from each block. If the diagnosis is still not ascertainable, more sections should be made. Although some experts can obtain a large tissue specimen with negative margins using loop electrosurgical excision techniques for a satisfactory diagnosis of microinvasive cancer, a traditional cold-knife cone biopsy in the operating room under anesthesia is often preferable. This is thoroughly discussed in another chapter.

Treatment

In 1996, the National Institutes of Health (NIH) invited an international panel of experts to develop a consensus conference statement on cervical cancer. After an extensive literature review and presentation of the scientific evidence, they concluded that patients who have squamous cell carcinoma of the cervix with ≤3 mm stromal invasion and negative conization margins have virtually a 100% cure rate when treated with simple hysterectomy or conization alone. However, for patients treated by conization alone, both the internal conization margin and the postconization endocervical curettage must be negative for cancer and dysplasia, because the risk of residual invasive cancer is significantly increased if either the margin or the curettage is positive. The definition of a negative margin remains debatable, and whether no tumor at the inked margin is sufficient versus a 1- to 3-mm tumor-free margin remains to be determined, but it is preferable to have a non-fragmented specimen for evaluation of margins. The choice of therapy should also be influenced by the patient's desire to maintain fertility. Although LVSI generally is considered to be an adverse prognostic factor in cervical cancer, its prognostic significance in stage IA1 disease is uncertain. Because of this uncertainty, some clinicians suggested that the presence of LVSI in stage IA1 disease might be more appropriately treated with radical hysterectomy and pelvic lymphadenectomy. SLN mapping is gaining increasing credibility in early-stage cervical cancer, and stage IA1 cases with LVSI are reasonable candidates for SLN injection and mapping as a strategy to evaluate pelvic nodes.

Recurrence in the vaginal vault may be the result of failing to accurately define the extent of the lesion and the presence of involvement of adjacent vaginal mucosa. This usually can be prevented with a careful colposcopic examination before hysterectomy. If vaginal fornices are involved, partial vaginectomy may be easier to perform with hysterectomy if the operation is done vaginally (**Fig. 51.7**). Alternatively, if the woman is not a good surgical candidate, radiation therapy (usually in the form of brachytherapy alone) can be selected.

Increased infection morbidity has been reported with intracavitary irradiation of a recently coned cervix. The cervix must be allowed to heal completely before intracervical irradiation. The survival rates for microinvasive disease (all treatments) should reach 98% to 99% if patients are adequately studied and properly treated.

Several studies of microinvasive adenocarcinoma of the cervix have been done. Webb and colleagues recently reviewed the SEER public-use database to identify 131 cases of cervical adenocarcinoma with 3-mm or less stromal invasion. Fifty patients had a radical hysterectomy and pelvic lymph node dissection, and none were found to have lymph node metastasis. Furthermore, there were no deaths among the 54 patients treated with simple hysterectomy alone. Others have reported a 0% rate of lymph node metastasis with depths of stromal invasion of up to 5 and 12 mm. However, bilateral pelvic lymph node metastases have been reported with as little as 2.5 mm of stromal invasion. Furthermore, Elliot and associates reported a case of lymph node metastasis with cervical adenocarcinoma with less than 1-mm invasion and a second case of recurrence and death after radical hysterectomy and pelvic lymphadenectomy in a patient with 1.8 mm of stromal invasion. From a clinical standpoint, stage IA1 adenocarcinoma is treated similarly to its squamous counterpart, except gynecologic pathology consultation is highly recommended in all cases of early cervical cancer to accurately determine the diagnosis and stage and to identify any LVSI. In summary, stage IA1 disease is highly curable with conization or trachelectomy or hysterectomy. The need to evaluate pelvic lymph nodes is appropriate to consider in women with LVSI or if higher stage is suspected and may be accomplished with SLN mapping or pelvic lymphadenectomy. Parametrectomy

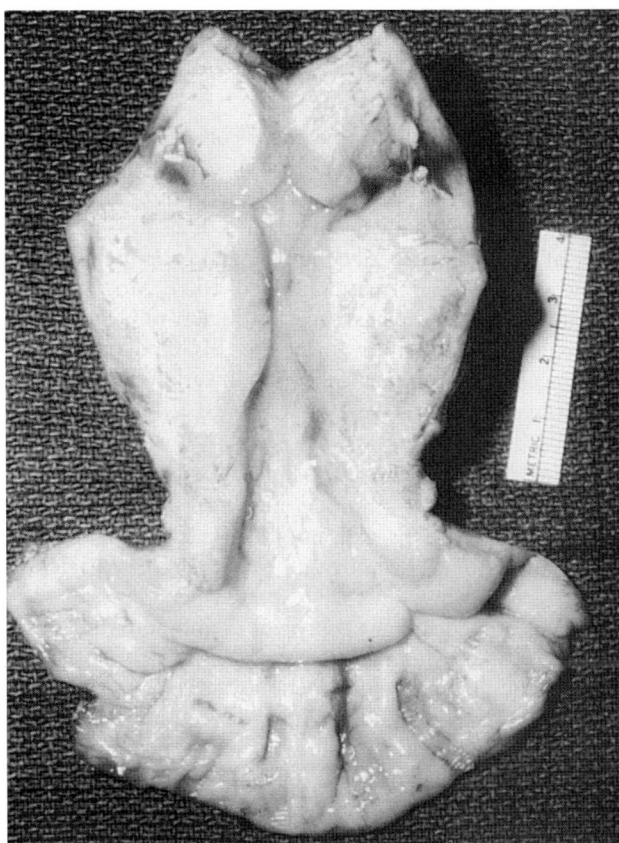

FIGURE 51.7 Vaginal hysterectomy and partial vaginectomy specimen from a patient with squamous cell carcinoma, cervix uteri, FIGO stage IA1, with extension to adjacent vaginal fornix. Note uniform width of vaginal cuff.

is being decreasingly utilized in true stage IA1 disease, and fertility-sparing surgery has become a standard of care with favorable oncologic and obstetrical outcomes in many women with early-stage cervical cancer.

If simple hysterectomy is subsequently chosen as the definitive surgical treatment after a conization, the hysterectomy should be done within 48 hours of the conization or delayed until the cervix has healed, usually about 6 weeks later. If the hysterectomy is done after 48 hours and before the cervix has healed, the risk of postoperative infectious morbidity is increased. However, a radical abdominal hysterectomy and bilateral pelvic lymphadenectomy can be done at almost any time after cervical conization, even before the cervix is completely healed. The reason for this difference is not clear, but may be related to the fact that indurated and possibly infected paracervical and parametrial tissue is actually removed when a radical hysterectomy is done.

Stages IA2, IB1, and Nonbulky (≤4 cm) IIA Disease

The recommended treatment by the NIH Consensus Conference for patients with stage IA2 disease is primary radical or modified radical hysterectomy with bilateral pelvic lymphadenectomy or primary radiation therapy, because the risk of nodal metastases is 4% to 10% in these patients. Again, the diagnosis of both stage IA1 and IA2 diseases should be based

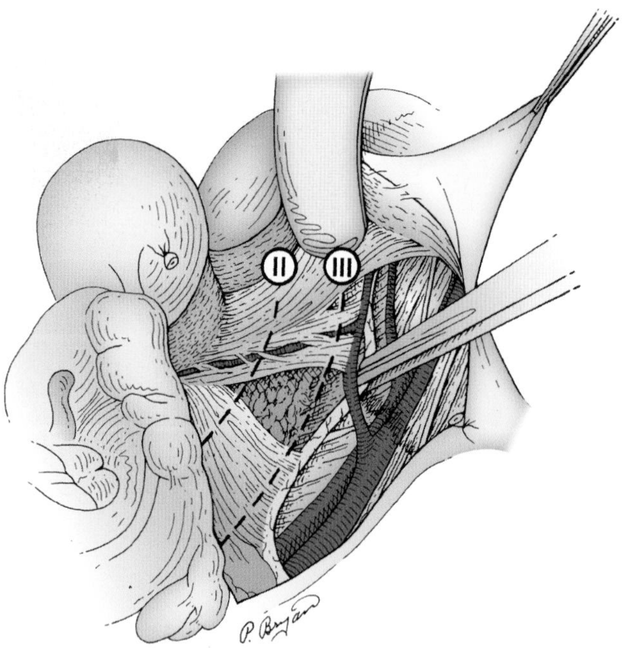

FIGURE 51.8 The cardinal ligament is excised medially in women with microscopic lesions (class II operation) or laterally in those with larger-volume lesions (class III operation). (Modified from Piver MS, Rutledge F, Smith JP. Five classes of extended hysterectomy for women with cervical cancer. *Obstet Gynecol* 1974;44:265, with permission.)

on microscopic examination of removed tissue, preferably a conization or large loop excision specimen, which must include the entire lesion. For stage IA2 disease, the depth of invasion should not be more than 5 mm taken from the base of the epithelium, either surface or glandular, from which

it originates. The second dimension, the horizontal spread, must not exceed 7 mm. Vascular space involvement, either venous or lymphatic, should not alter the staging but should be specifically recorded. The remaining stage I cases should be allotted to stage IB. All grossly visible lesions are defined as stage IB.

For stage IA2 disease, standard treatment is a type C1 (class III) nerve-sparing radical hysterectomy with bilateral pelvic lymphadenectomy; however, some authors recommend a type B (class II) modified radical hysterectomy (Fig. 51.8). The type B, or class II, hysterectomy removes the medial half of the cardinal and uterosacral ligaments, ligating the uterine artery at the ureter. This more conservative operation has been used by some authors in the past 3 decades to excise small primary tumors while reducing the partial bladder denervation associated with the complete excision of the cardinal and uterosacral ligaments required for a type C, or class III, hysterectomy. Five-year survival rates of 97% to 98% have been reported for patients with small cervical lesions treated with a type B, class II, hysterectomy. The role of the class II modified radical hysterectomy was recently evaluated in a randomized, prospective study reported by Landoni and colleagues. Two hundred forty-three patients with FIGO stages IB and IIA were randomized to either class II or III hysterectomy. The recurrence-free and overall survivals were similar between the two groups. Patients treated with type II radical hysterectomy had a statistically significant reduction in operative time and postoperative morbidity, particularly bladder dysfunction. However, given the relatively high cure rate for early cervical cancer treated by radical hysterectomy, larger trials are necessary to prove equivalence in survival between the two types of hysterectomy. As stated by Rose, larger trials are required before we can accept these results as the new standard of care. The estimated extent of tissue resection in surgical procedures for early cervical cancer is summarized in Table 51.4.

TABLE 51.4 Comparison of Extent of Resection for Surgical Procedures to Treat Early-Stage Cervical Cancer

TISSUE	CERVICAL CONIZATION	TOTAL ABDOMINAL/ VAGINAL HYSTERECTOMY	MODIFIED RADICAL HYSTERECTOMY (TYPE B)	RADICAL ABDOMINAL HYSTERECTOMY (TYPE C)	RADICAL VAGINAL TRACHELECTOMY (TYPE B)	RADICAL VAGINAL HYSTERECTOMY (TYPE C)
Cervix uteri	Partially removed	Completely removed	Completely removed	Completely removed	Majority removed	Completely removed
Corpus uteri	Preserved	Completely removed	Completely removed	Completely removed	Preserved removed	Completely removed
Ovaries and tubes	Preserved	Preserved	Preserved	Preserved	Preserved	Preserved
Parametria and paracolpos	Preserved	Preserved	Removed at level of ureter	Removed lateral to ureter	Partially removed	Removed at level of ureter
Uterine vessels	Preserved	Ligated at level of cervical internal os	Ligated at level of ureter	Ligated at origin from hypogastric vessels	Descending cervicovaginal branch ligated	Ligated at level of ureter
Uterosacral ligaments	Preserved	Ligated at uterus	Divided midway to rectum	Divided near rectum	Partially removed	Partially removed
Vaginal cuff	Preserved	None removed	1–2 cm removed	≥2 cm removed	1–2 cm removed	≥2 cm removed

RADICAL HYSTERECTOMY

Historical Points in the Development of Radical Surgery for Cervical Cancer

Radical hysterectomy for cervical cancer was performed by John Clark while still a resident trainee at the Johns Hopkins Hospital in Baltimore in 1895; however, earlier reports describe the radical hysterectomy performed in 1888 by the Czech surgeon Pavlik. The procedure is linked in perpetuity to Wertheim of Vienna, who reported his series of 500 cases of radical extended abdominal hysterectomy and partial lymphadenectomy performed from 1898 until 1911. Despite the skill and enthusiasm of Wertheim, Schauta (who developed the vaginal radical hysterectomy in 1901), Okabayashi, and others, radical pelvic surgery was fraught with significant operative morbidity and mortality. Therefore, the introduction of radium brought irradiation to the forefront of primary treatment for carcinoma of the cervix for the next several decades.

In the United States, Joe V. Meigs reintroduced radical hysterectomy as the treatment of choice, publishing a series of 344 cases in 1945. Until formalization of training fellowships in gynecologic oncology in the early 1970s, many outstanding gynecologic surgeons in the United States (Parsons, Ulfelder, Green, and many others) made important contributions and modifications to the radical surgical approach that have markedly decreased complications while preserving the cure rate. Proficient performance of the radical hysterectomy remains a benchmark of the gynecologic oncology surgeon.

Patient Selection for Radical Hysterectomy

Simple hysterectomy is not adequate treatment for stage IB cervical cancer. In 1943, Jones and Jones reported a 5-year survival rate of only 41.6% in patients who had been treated for stage I cervical cancer with simple hysterectomy only. Such poor results also have been reported by Schmidt and others. When more than FIGO stage IA1 invasive cervical cancer is a surprise finding in a simple hysterectomy specimen, additional therapy—usually radiation therapy with or without chemotherapy—should be given postoperatively. Suggested indications for radical abdominal hysterectomy are summarized in Table 51.5.

Although radical hysterectomy and pelvic lymphadenectomy occasionally are used to treat patients with adenocarcinoma of the endometrium with involvement of the cervical stroma (stage IIB) and, rarely, patients who have a small cervical cancer that persists or recurs in the cervix after primary radiation therapy, in this chapter, emphasis is given to the use of the operation as primary treatment for invasive cervical cancer.

In most institutions, the majority of patients with stages IA2, IB1, and nonbulky IIA cervical cancer are offered radical abdominal hysterectomy and bilateral pelvic lymphadenectomy as primary treatment.

Patients with bulky stage IB disease (currently FIGO stage IB2) have traditionally been treated with radical hysterectomy and bilateral pelvic lymphadenectomy or primary radiation therapy, with equivalent survivals. However, patients with these larger lesions treated surgically have a very high risk of having lymph node metastasis or close resection margins or local tumors risk factors, such as deep stromal invasion with LVSI, which are often reasons for postoperative pelvic radiation treatment. Landoni and colleagues performed a randomized trial of radical hysterectomy and pelvic lymphadenectomy versus pelvic radiation therapy for stage IB to IIA

TABLE 51.5 Indication for Radical Abdominal Hysterectomy	
INDICATION	**EXTENT OF DISEASE**
Invasive cervical cancer	Stage IA1 with lymphvascular invasion Stage IA2 Stage IB1 Stage IB2 (selected) Stage IIA (selected)
Invasive vaginal cancer	Stage I–II (limited to upper one third of vagina, usually involving posterior vaginal fornix)
Endometrial carcinoma	Clinical stage IIB (gross cervical invasion)
Persistent or recurrent cervical cancer after radiotherapy	Clinically limited to cervix or proximal vaginal fornix

cervical cancer. Patients randomized to the surgery arm who had pathologic risk factors, such as lymph node metastasis, received adjuvant radiation therapy. Of the 55 patients with tumors greater than 4 cm, 46 (84%) required postoperative irradiation. The disease-free and overall survival rates for these patients treated with surgery and radiation therapy were the same as those for patients with bulky tumors treated with radiation therapy alone; however, the combination therapy significantly increased morbidity. Subsequently, a randomized trial performed by the GOG has demonstrated the benefit of the addition of cisplatin chemotherapy to pelvic radiation followed by extrafascial hysterectomy in this group of patients. Therefore, many experts feel that patients with FIGO stage IB2 and bulky IIA cervical cancer are best treated with concomitant cisplatin chemotherapy and radiation therapy with or without completion extrafascial hysterectomy.

In the United States, patients with stage IIB invasive cervical cancer usually are excluded from primary treatment with surgery. They are usually treated with concomitant radiation therapy and chemotherapy. However, it should be noted that select stage IIB cases have traditionally been considered in some countries (Japan, Germany, Hungary, and other European countries) as an indication for primary radical hysterectomy. Recent studies from Japan demonstrated equal overall survival with a favorable quality-of-life outcome of radical hysterectomy compared to primary chemoradiotherapy in this stage of the disease. The question about radical hysterectomy indication in select stage IIB patients cannot be considered resolved; thus, although radical hysterectomy treatment of stage IIB cervical cancer is not suggested in this book, it should be considered as an acceptable alternative concept in the appropriate hands and clinical setup.

The clinical significance of parametrial involvement dates to the early studies of Kundrat and Sampson. Kundrat, working in Wertheim's clinic, studied more than 21,000 serial microscopic sections of the parametrium, finding that the parametrium of one or both sides was involved in 44 of 80 patients. In a similar study at the Johns Hopkins Hospital, Sampson pointed out that the parametrium could feel indurated and yet show no evidence of cancer. Also, the parametrium can feel normal and yet contain cancer. Sampson emphasized that only

IX

by the microscope can the surgeon exclude cancer involvement of the parametrium. More recently, Inoue and Okumura found parametrial extension in 7% of stage IB patients and in only 34% of stage IIB patients. Burghardt and Pickel found true parametrial involvement in only 19% of stage IIB patients. Matsuyama and coworkers found no parametrial cancer in 58% of stage IIB patients. These studies were based on careful examination of microscopic sections and reemphasize the difficulty of being certain about parametrial extension from pelvic examination alone, emphasizing the shortcomings of a clinical staging system. Inoue and Okumura studied 628 operative specimens from patients treated with radical hysterectomy and lymphadenectomy and found that parametrial extension is an important factor in the number of positive lymph nodes found and in patient survival. If there is suspicion of spread into the parametrial tissues by examination, CT scan, or MRI scan, it is reasonable to offer radiation therapy with concomitant chemotherapy as primary treatment (despite the fact that the official FIGO stage should remain unchanged).

The major point to be emphasized is that the gynecologic surgeon should not attempt to treat a patient with a large cervical tumor with primary radical surgery unless there is reasonable assurance that the operation will result in the complete removal of the central tumor with an adequate margin of tumor-free tissue around it. The surgeon should not operate on patients with the idea that radiation therapy with or without chemotherapy can be used postoperatively to eliminate residual fragments of tumor tissue after incomplete resection. Such patients usually are better treated with concurrent pelvic radiation and chemotherapy from the beginning.

Primary radical surgical treatment is not contraindicated in any histologic type of cervical cancer. Shingleton and coworkers have suggested that the survival of patients with stage I adenocarcinoma of the cervix is better with surgery than with irradiation. Patients with stage I adenosquamous cancer, clear cell cancer, and undifferentiated adenocarcinoma have a poorer prognosis, regardless of the method of treatment chosen, and therefore are often considered for adjuvant radiation therapy and/or chemotherapy after primary surgery.

Patients considered for radical hysterectomy must be acceptable candidates for an operation and free of serious medical problems that contraindicate extensive surgery. In former years, some institutions limited radical surgery as primary treatment to premenopausal women so that ovarian function might be conserved. As experience has accumulated, it has become apparent that the operation is also well tolerated by older women. In a study of 45 women aged 65 years and older with cervical cancer, Fuchtner and associates concluded that age alone should not be a contraindication to extensive hysterectomy in the elderly patient with American Society of Anesthesiologists physical status I to III. Kinney and coworkers reported their experience with the Wertheim operation in a geriatric population. Thirty-eight selected women between 65 and 89 years of age (median age, 69 years) were compared with 320 patients younger than age 65. The survival rates were almost identical in the two groups. Perioperative morbidity was minimally increased in the geriatric group. Geisler recently compared the outcomes after radical hysterectomy and pelvic lymphadenectomy of 62 patients older than age 65 to 124 matched controls age 50 or younger. Even using this relatively younger cohort for comparison, there were no significant differences in operative mortality or morbidity. However, to achieve such excellent results in older women, Kinney and coworkers pointed out that "meticulous surgical technique, high-quality ancillary services, and support from internal medicine and anesthesia services" are required. Such extended supportive care is not available in every hospital.

Extreme morbid obesity presents especially difficult technical problems when radical surgery is chosen for primary treatment. Not only is the performance of the operation more challenging and possibly less satisfactory, but also there may be an increased risk of wound complications, postoperative infection, intraoperative hemorrhage, pulmonary embolus, pulmonary atelectasis, and anesthesia-related and other problems. Unfortunately, primary treatment with radiation therapy with or without chemotherapy also is frequently less than satisfactory in extremely morbid obese patients. The introduction of robotic minimally invasive surgery may play a role in treating select obese women with early cervical cancer, avoiding the need for laparotomy.

Studies by Soisson and Levrant compared outcomes after radical hysterectomy for cervical cancer in obese versus nonobese women. They found that survival was not compromised, and the incidence of serious complications was not increased in obese patients. However, in obese women, the authors reported that the operative technique is more difficult, the procedure lasts longer, and the surgery is associated with greater blood loss. Cohn and colleagues recently reported their results with radical hysterectomy for cervical cancer in 46 obese women. The median body mass index was 36 kg/m², and the median weight was 95 kg. Nine patients (20%) experienced postoperative morbidity, mostly related to wound complications. No patient developed a fistula. Massi and associates have reported that the Schauta-Amreich vaginal hysterectomy can be used as an alternative to the radical abdominal hysterectomy in the presence of obesity or elevated surgical risks.

According to Shingleton, primary treatment with radical surgery paradoxically also can be riskier in very thin patients because of a higher incidence of fistula. It is speculated that easy exposure and lack of excess fatty tissue in these patients may result in removing essential vasculature around the ureters and bladder, resulting in ischemic necrosis. A thin patient has less fat around the pelvic vessels and in the lymph fields; thus, the surgeon should be satisfied to remove less tissue in an operation that will still be adequate in a thin patient.

The management of the *pregnant patient* diagnosed with invasive cervical carcinoma is more challenging. First, a decision must be made to either save the pregnancy or treat the cancer. Pregnancy is not a contraindication to primary treatment of stage IB or IIA carcinoma of the cervix with radical surgery (**Fig. 51.9**). In 1974, Sall and coworkers reported on 29 patients with stage IB carcinoma of the cervix in pregnancy treated with radical hysterectomy and pelvic lymphadenectomy. At the time of publication, 28 patients were alive and well, and 23 patients had been followed for more than 5 years. There were no fistulae or major complications. Others have confirmed 5-year survival rates of 85% to 95% for patients treated with radical surgery for stage IB cervical cancer in pregnancy. Funnell and associates, operating on 17 pregnant patients, suggested that the associated pregnancy changes facilitated the surgical dissection. Sood and colleagues performed a case–control study comparing the outcomes after radical hysterectomy and pelvic lymphadenectomy for 26 pregnant versus 26 nonpregnant patients. Operative times and postoperative complication rates were similar between the two groups. There was a statistically significant increase in blood loss at the time of surgery for pregnant patients; however, there was no difference in the frequency of blood transfusion. Eleven patients underwent surgical treatment in the third trimester of pregnancy, with a mean planned delay in therapy of 16 weeks. None of the patients with the planned delay in therapy developed recurrent disease. The authors concluded that surgical management of early cervical cancer is safe during pregnancy. In select obstetric patients who desire to maintain

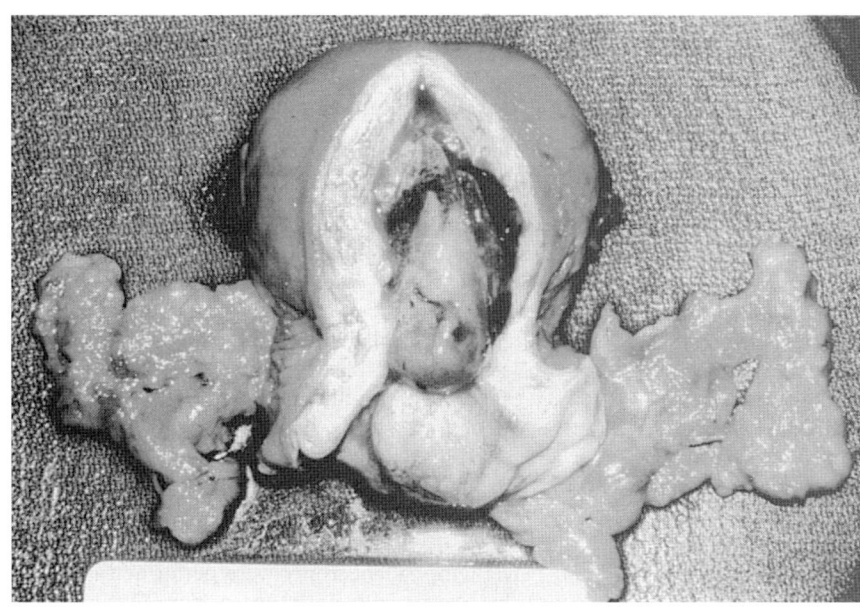

FIGURE 51.9 Squamous cell carcinoma, cervix uteri, FIGO stage IB with intrauterine pregnancy, 16 weeks (lymphadenectomy specimen not included).

their pregnancies, Sood and colleagues agreed with the conclusions of Greer and coworkers that planned delay in therapy to increase the likelihood of fetal maturity is safe for early-stage I squamous cell cancers diagnosed in the late second and early third trimester. All other patients should be treated promptly in an attempt to cure the cancer.

Finally, based on data from Orr, Chapman, and others, extensive parametrectomy and pelvic lymphadenectomy appear to be appropriate management for selected patients found to have *unexpected invasive cancer of the cervix on pathologic examination of a uterus removed for benign conditions.* Low morbidity rates and acceptable rates of long-term disease-free survival have been reported. However, pelvic irradiation is usually recommended for these patients.

Advantages of Radical Surgery as Primary Treatment for Invasive Cervical Cancer

The most important considerations in choosing a method of therapy for any cancer are, first, effectiveness of the treatment in curing the disease and, second, mortality and morbidity rates associated with the treatment plan. For the indications listed previously, the cure rates of primary radiation therapy and primary extensive surgery are about equal. The modern mortality rates also are about equal. Both modalities of therapy have a list of complications unique to each that seem about equal. There are, however, important major and minor advantages of primary radical surgery over irradiation for early-stage disease, some of which are discussed in the following sections.

Accurate Evaluation of Extent of Disease

The findings at operation and from careful pathologic examination of the surgical specimen can be immensely helpful in selecting high-risk patients for adjuvant postoperative radiation therapy, chemotherapy, or both. Most patients with FIGO stages IA2, IB1, and nonbulky IIA disease are not found to have high-risk factors and thus are spared the potential morbidity associated with whole pelvic radiation therapy. Furthermore, the findings at operation and careful pathologic examination of the surgical specimen can be helpful in determining prognosis and in identifying patients at greatest risk for persistence or recurrence of disease. Such high-risk patients may require additional therapy.

In addition to an accurate assessment of the extent of the cervical cancer, primary surgical treatment allows for discovery of other intra-abdominal incidental conditions and diseases entirely unrelated to the cancer. Ovarian malignancies, pelvic tuberculosis, sigmoid diverticulitis, cholelithiasis, and other diseases and conditions may be encountered at the time of operation.

Preservation of Ovarian Function

When primary radiation therapy with or without chemotherapy is used to treat invasive cervical cancer in premenopausal women, premature loss of ovarian function is an unfortunate and inevitable result. When primary surgery is used instead, the function of normal ovaries can be conserved. Sutton and associates analyzed the incidence of ovarian metastasis for 991 patients with stage IB carcinoma of the cervix treated with radical hysterectomy and pelvic lymphadenectomy on a prospective GOG protocol. Ovarian spread was found in 4 of 770 patients (0.5%) with squamous cell carcinoma and in 2 of 121 patients (1.7%) with adenocarcinoma. The difference was not statistically significant. All six patients with ovarian metastases had other evidence of extracervical disease. This study confirmed that ovarian metastasis is rare in patients with stage IB cervical cancer and extremely rare in the absence of other evidence of extracervical disease.

Although the incidence of ovarian metastasis is slightly higher in women with adenocarcinoma of the cervix as compared with squamous cell carcinoma, ovarian conservation should still be considered, especially in young women. Brand and Berek reported no ovarian metastases in more than 60 patients with adenocarcinoma of the cervix treated with radical surgery. Angel and associates found no ovarian metastases in 41 patients with adenocarcinoma of the cervix who underwent oophorectomy. Greer and coworkers treated 55 patients with stage IB adenocarcinoma of the cervix with radical hysterectomy and pelvic lymphadenectomy. Ninety-one percent had ovarian preservation, and there was no evidence that this contributed to tumor recurrence. Hopkins and coworkers found that the best cumulative 5-year survival rate (93%) with cervical adenocarcinoma was in patients treated by radical hysterectomy without bilateral salpingo-oophorectomy and concluded that "ovarian conservation seems to be an acceptable alternative to bilateral salpingo-oophorectomy" in young patients.

Some authors have advocated transposing the ovaries into the paracolic gutters at the time of radical hysterectomy in premenopausal women to protect the ovaries from radiation damage should postoperative pelvic radiation therapy be needed. The technique used for ovarian transposition was described by Husseinzadeh and coworkers. However, in the series reported by Chambers and coworkers, there was a threefold increase in symptomatic benign ovarian cyst formation with lateral ovarian transposition compared with those who did not have their ovaries transposed. Furthermore, Anderson and coworkers reported that only 4 of 24 patients (17%) who had ovarian transposition retained ovarian function after postoperative radiation therapy. Moreover, after transposition, 17.6% of patients required surgical treatment for ovarian-associated pain or cysts. These data raise the question of whether paracolic gutter transposition actually achieves its goal of protecting the ovaries.

Sexual Function

Studies of the effect of surgical and radiation treatment for cervical carcinoma on sexual function have been published by Seibel and coworkers from Emory University and by others. Among patients treated with radiation, there are decreases in sexual enjoyment, ability to attain orgasm, frequency of intercourse, and desire for intercourse. Marked alterations can be seen and felt in the upper vagina and paravaginal tissues. The vagina usually is shorter from stenosis. The upper vagina is less pliable. Tissues are fixed and firm. The vaginal mucosa is thin, smooth, and dry, with a tendency to split and bleed with slight trauma. Some of these changes are made more pronounced in young women because of hypoestrogenism from radiation-induced premature menopause. They are not completely reversed by intravaginal or oral administration of estrogen. Such functional and anatomic changes are not seen nearly as frequently in patients treated with primary extensive surgery. Even if the vagina has been surgically shortened by several centimeters with primary surgery, it remains soft, pliable, moist, and functional. Unfortunately, in women who undergo postoperative adjuvant pelvic irradiation, some of these characteristics are lost.

Fewer Late Complications

Late complications after treatment for cervical cancer are rarely seen after primary radical surgery. They occur more often when patients are treated with primary radiation therapy. Because of the gradual and progressive obliterative endarteritis produced by irradiating tissue, complications resulting from ischemic changes (e.g., cystitis, proctitis, enteritis, colpocleisis, pyelonephritis) can be seen many years after radiation treatment. Late onset of complications after primary radical hysterectomy and pelvic lymphadenectomy are unusual. These points are especially important when selecting a method of primary treatment for young women.

Psychological Benefits

There are probably important psychological benefits of primary treatment with radical surgery compared with radiation therapy. Most patients prefer to have the tumor removed and are especially encouraged when the surgeon can report that "the cancer is out" and that no evidence of metastatic disease was found at operation. Radiation therapy carries an unfortunate connotation in some patients who feel that it is the treatment of last resort, that the tumor is still there (albeit treated), or that irradiation will cause other cancers. All gynecologic surgeons have heard the disappointment patients express when they are told that they cannot be treated with an operation. Some patients continue to request an operation even after they have completed radiation therapy. It is paramount to council patients thoroughly and outline the many advantages modern radiation therapy may provide in select cases.

Justification for Pelvic Lymphadenectomy

Historically, there was competition between gynecologic surgeons who advocated radical vaginal hysterectomy without lymphadenectomy and those who advocated radical abdominal hysterectomy with lymphadenectomy. The advocates of extensive vaginal hysterectomy without lymphadenectomy (the Schauta-Amreich-Navratil operation) argued that their patients had fewer postoperative complications (especially urinary fistulae), a lower operative mortality rate, and a cure rate that was almost equal to that achieved by an abdominal operation that included lymphadenectomy. Furthermore, they pointed out that pelvic lymphadenectomy is an incomplete operation, at best, in that the removal of all pelvic lymph nodes that can possibly be involved with metastatic tumor is technically not feasible in many cases. This is especially important for those inferior gluteal nodes that are located in the region of the ischial spine, as pointed out by Reiffenstuhl. However, even Navratil stated in 1965 that "indications for the Schauta operation must take the lymph node problem into account." Later, he performed extraperitoneal pelvic lymphadenectomy with the Schauta operation in all stage I and II cases that were locally advanced, as did Mitra, the Indian gynecologist who performed the pelvic node dissection through a bilateral extraperitoneal abdominal incision after radical vaginal hysterectomy.

In recent years, the operative mortality and complication rates in patients who have undergone radical abdominal hysterectomy and bilateral pelvic lymphadenectomy have significantly decreased. Operative mortality and fistulae occur in less than 1% and approximately 2% of patients, respectively. Therefore, one purported disadvantage of radical hysterectomy (high morbidity) has essentially been removed, and the surgeon can concentrate on the question of whether lymphadenectomy adds anything to the possibility of cure. If a pelvic lymphadenectomy is not done in patients who have a radical hysterectomy for cervical cancer, at least 15% to 20% of patients (those with positive nodes) will be inadequately treated for their disease (unless perhaps all patients receive postoperative pelvic irradiation). In our judgment, it is better to do a pelvic lymphadenectomy in all eligible patients and then give postoperative radiation therapy selectively than to avoid a lymphadenectomy and give postoperative radiation therapy to all patients.

It is the opinion of some that pelvic lymphadenectomy is of no value in those 80% to 90% of patients who have negative lymph nodes. We believe that lymphadenectomy is helpful in achieving an adequate central dissection around the cervical tumor, the most important part of the operation. This is especially true of that part of the lymphadenectomy that involves removal of tissue from around the hypogastric vessels, from the obturator fossa, and from the lower presacral region. Admittedly, dissection of lymph nodes from the common iliac vessels and from the paraaortic region does not add to the completeness of the central dissection. Removal of these and other nodes, however, is helpful in prognosis and in identifying patients at greater risk for persistent disease who might receive adjuvant postoperative radiation therapy to the pelvis and perhaps to extended fields along the aorta. Although we seldom dissect and remove the highest paraaortic lymph nodes, we do remove the lower paraaortic nodes around and just above the aortic bifurcation. If pelvic lymph nodes involved with tumor are found during the operation, a concerted effort is made to do a more complete paraaortic dissection. Although it is possible for paraaortic nodes to be directly involved without involvement of pelvic nodes, this is rare. For the group of patients who usually would be chosen for treatment with primary radical surgery, routine extensive paraaortic lymph node dissection would not result in a therapeutic benefit very often. Podczaski and coworkers found positive paraaortic lymph nodes in 7 of 52 patients (13.4%) with stage IB and IIA disease. Twenty-eight of the 52 patients, however, had bulky tumors greater than 5 cm in greatest diameter. Currently, such patients are considered by many gynecologic oncologists not to be appropriate candidates for treatment with primary radical surgery. Patsner and coworkers performed paraaortic lymph node sampling in patients with small (tumor ≤3 cm) stage IB cervical cancer. Only 2 of the 125 patients who underwent radical hysterectomy, bilateral pelvic lymphadenectomy, and paraaortic node sampling had metastases to the paraaortic nodes. No patient had gross paraaortic nodal involvement, and both patients with microscopic paraaortic nodal metastases had grossly positive pelvic nodal involvement. These investigators recommended that paraaortic sampling in patients with small stage IB cervical tumors be restricted to patients with suspicious or positive pelvic or paraaortic nodes. The paraaortic region should be carefully palpated and any enlarged or firm nodes removed, but the gynecologic surgeon should be aware of the added morbidity associated with comprehensive paraaortic lymphadenectomy.

A study reported by Downey and colleagues provides indirect evidence that postoperative pelvic irradiation is more effective in controlling disease after pelvic lymphadenectomy has removed clinically positive lymph nodes that contain metastatic tumor. The amount of irradiation required to eliminate tumor in lymph nodes is directly related to the volume of tumor present (Table 51.6). Thus, removing the larger nodes involved with tumor increases the probability of control of tumor with irradiation. Patients in this study who underwent resection of large positive pelvic nodes followed by postoperative extended-field irradiation had a surprisingly high 5-year recurrence-free survival rate of 51%. The advantages of surgical debulking of positive lymph nodes also were discussed by Potish and coworkers in a later study from the same center. No patient with unresectable pelvic nodes survived 5 years. In 84% (49/58) of cases with grossly positive pelvic nodes, the nodes were able to be debulked. The 5-year actuarial relapse-free survival rates were the same for patients with only microscopically involved pelvic node metastases (56%) and for patients with grossly involved but surgically resected pelvic node metastases (57%). All patients with positive pelvic nodes received postoperative irradiation to the pelvis and paraaortic nodes. These authors believe that surgical debulking of grossly involved pelvic lymph nodes to microscopic residual disease may improve the chance of control with postoperative irradiation.

TABLE 51.6	Squamous Cell Carcinoma of the Cervix: Dose–Tumor–Volume Relation[a]	
TUMOR VOLUME (CM)	**DOSE (GY)**	
<2	50	
2	60	
2–4	70	
4–6	75–89	
6	80–100	

[a]Average radiation dose required to obtain 90% control in area treated.
From Shingleton HM, Orr JW. *Cancer of the cervix: Diagnosis and treatment.* New York, NY: Churchill Livingstone, 1987:174, with permission of Elsevier.

PERTINENT PELVIC ANATOMY ARTERIAL AND VENOUS ANATOMY

Although the lower portions of the aorta and vena cava are frequently incorporated into the operative field of the pelvic lymphadenectomy, the major operative dissection includes the common iliac, external iliac, and hypogastric (also known as the internal iliac) arteries and veins and their various branches and tributaries. The abdominal aorta emerges through the aortic hiatus of the diaphragm at the lower border of the last thoracic vertebra and descends along the ventral surface of the vertebral column, where it bifurcates into the left and right common iliac arteries at the fourth lumbar vertebra (Fig. 51.10). This is an important anatomic landmark because the bifurcation at L4 lies directly beneath the umbilicus in most cases. Therefore, an abdominal midline incision that provides surgical exposure to the lower aorta needs to be extended somewhat above the umbilicus. The right common iliac artery crosses the upper portion of the left common iliac vein at the aortic bifurcation. This segment of the venous drainage of the left side of the pelvis

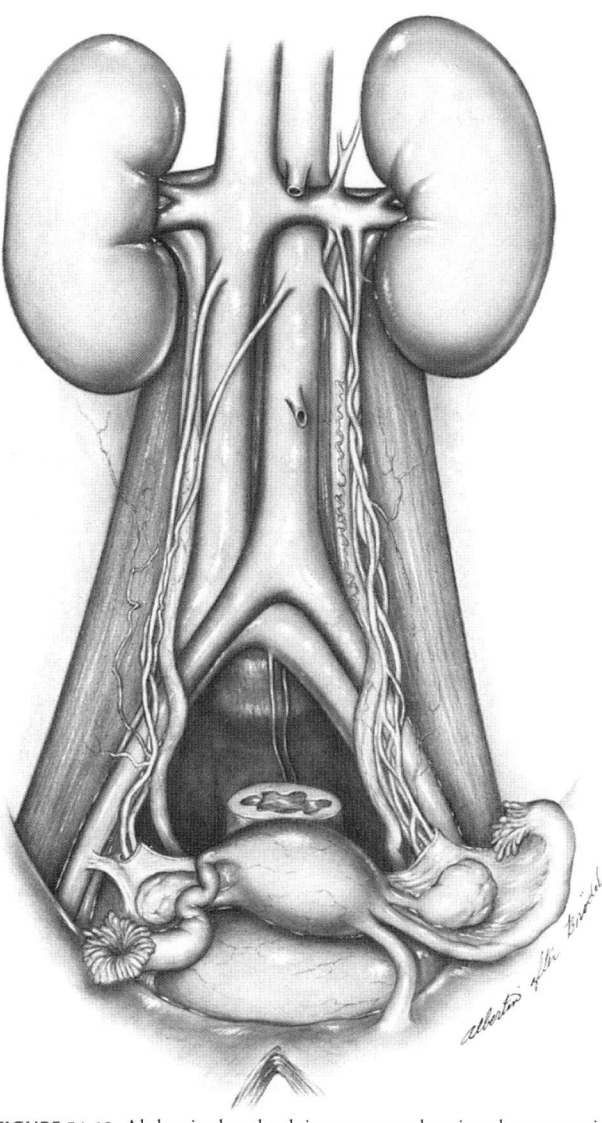

FIGURE 51.10 Abdominal and pelvic anatomy, showing the anatomic relations of the aorta, vena cava, iliac vessels, and ureters. Note the arteriovenous crossing of the right common iliac artery and the left iliac vein.

IX

joins with the right common iliac vein to form the vena cava, which lies directly along the right side of the aorta and on the right lateral side of the bodies of the lumbar vertebrae in its retroperitoneal course through the abdomen.

Both common iliac arteries continue along the medial border of the psoas muscle to the pelvic brim, where they divide into external iliac and hypogastric vessels. As shown in **Figure 51.10**, this important vascular division marks the site where the ureters enter the pelvis from the abdomen, usually overlying the terminal end of the common iliac artery on the left and commonly crossing the actual bifurcation of the artery on the right. Both external iliac arteries pass beneath the inguinal ligament to proceed into the leg as the femoral artery. The external iliac artery makes no direct vascular contribution to the pelvis, although there is a fairly consistent arterial branch to the ureter from the midportion of the common iliac artery.

The external iliac vein emerges from beneath the inguinal ligament, where it courses along the lateral pelvic brim on the medial side of the artery until it reaches the proximal segment. Here, the vein passes directly beneath the artery at the bifurcation of the common iliac artery and then passes along the lateral side of the upper half of the artery. It then joins the left common iliac vein to become the inferior vena cava at the fifth lumbar vertebra. In dissecting the lymph nodes along the external iliac vessels, these anatomic landmarks are important to avoid trauma to the wall of the vein as it deviates from the medial to the lateral side of the arterial tree.

The hypogastric artery provides the major blood supply to the pelvic viscera. For descriptive purposes, it is conveniently divided into an anterior and a posterior division. The important branches of the hypogastric artery are shown in **Figures 51.11** and **51.12**.

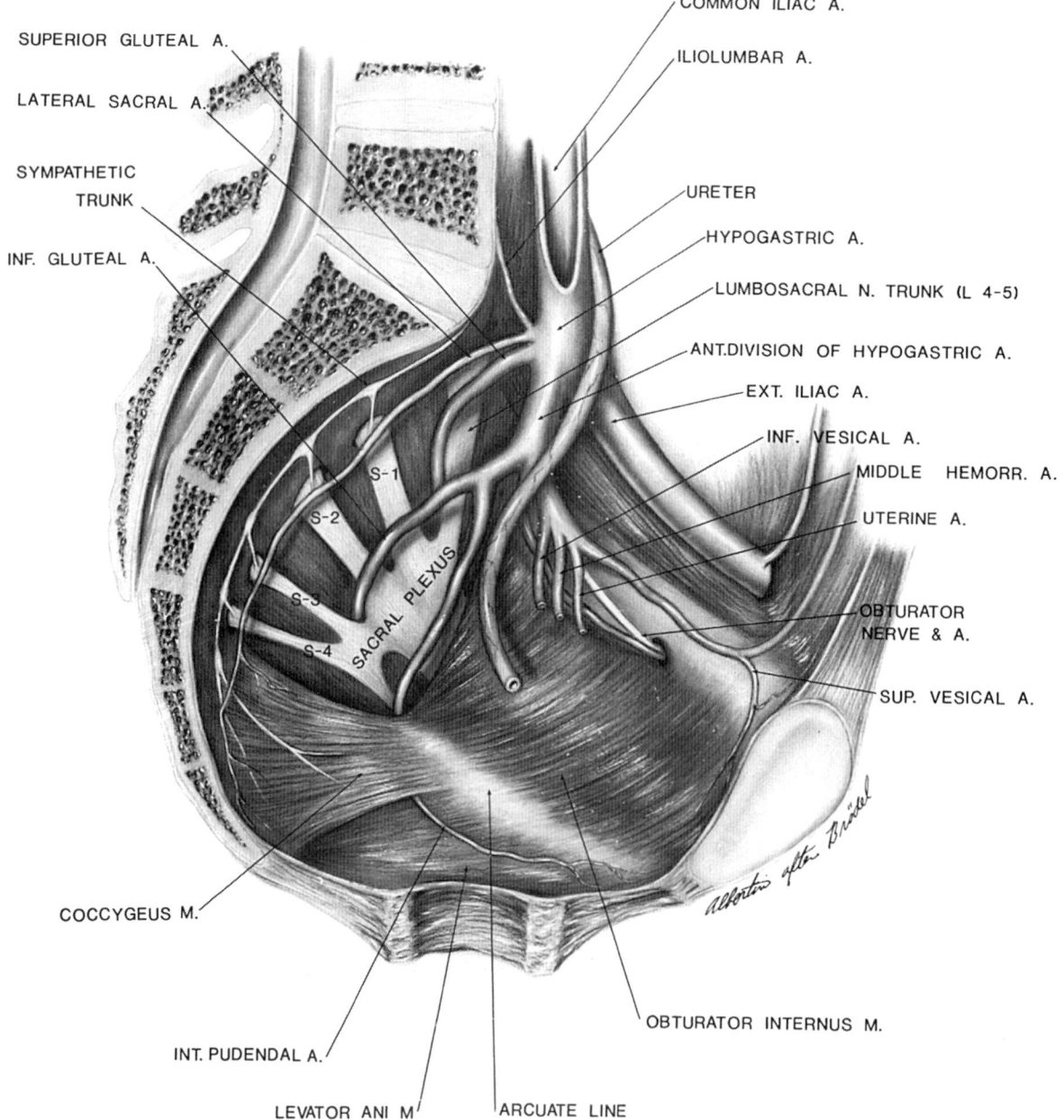

FIGURE 51.11 Anatomy of the arterial blood supply to the female pelvis showing relations of pelvic musculature, divisions of hypogastric artery, and lumbosacral and sacral nerve plexuses. Note that the anterior division of the hypogastric artery provides the blood supply to the pelvic viscera.

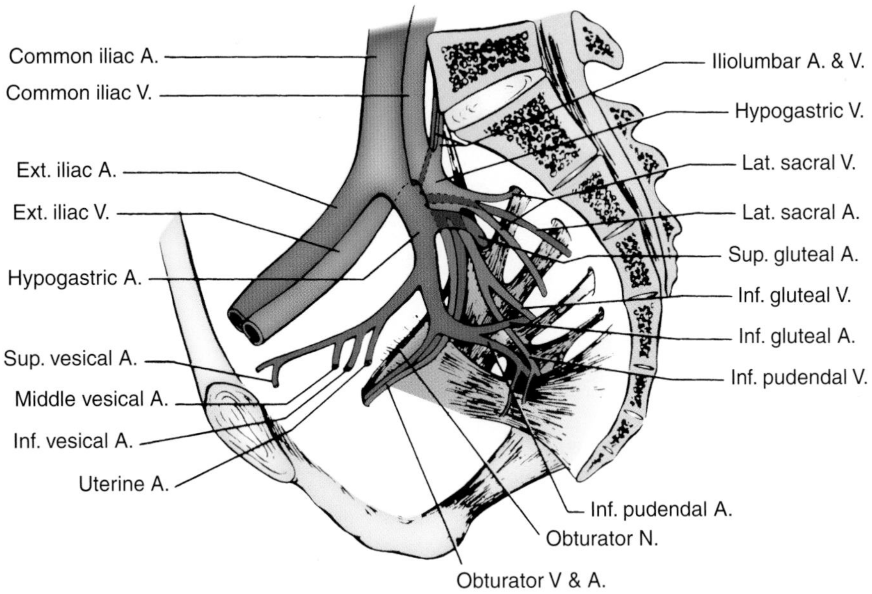

FIGURE 51.12 Anatomy of hypogastric vein. (From Thompson JD. Extensive hysterectomy and bilateral pelvic lymphadenectomy. In: Coppleson M, ed. *Gynecologic oncology*, 2nd ed. New York, NY: Churchill Livingstone, 1992, with permission.)

A fairly consistent arterial branch to the ureter arises from the hypogastric artery near the common iliac bifurcation. This vessel passes medially to the ureter and should be preserved, if possible, during the dissection of the hypogastric vessels. The posterior division of the hypogastric artery continues beneath the coccygeus muscle through the ischiorectal fossa, where it becomes the internal pudendal artery to supply the perineum and vulva.

The major blood supply to the pelvic viscera is derived from the anterior division of the hypogastric artery. **Figure 51.11** shows the anterior division, which gives off the uterine artery before continuing along the posterolateral pelvic wall to supply the superior and inferior vesical branches to the bladder. The anterior division then continues as the obliterated umbilical artery as it passes cephalad along the inferior surface of the rectus muscle to the umbilicus. In dissecting along the hypogastric artery in a caudad direction, the uterine artery is the first vessel encountered; it emanates from the medial side of the vessel. Passing more inferiorly and medially is the middle hemorrhoidal artery, which supplies a major segment of the rectum and communicates with the superior hemorrhoidal (from the inferior mesenteric) and the inferior hemorrhoidal (from the internal pudendal) arteries.

The hypogastric vein and its tributaries course along the pelvic floor and medial side of the artery to drain the pelvis in close relation to the arterial blood supply. Its extensive anatomic variations and its location along the pelvic sidewall and floor place these tortuous, thin-walled veins in a precarious and vulnerable position for trauma during deep dissection of the pelvis. As shown in **Figure 51.12**, the delicate tributaries of the trunk of the hypogastric vein extend into sacral foramina and pass beneath nerve fibers and muscles within the pelvis, so that their visualization during the dissection of the pelvis frequently is obscured. The continuation of the hypogastric vein, in association with the artery, beneath the coccygeus muscle is a frequent site of bleeding when dissection is undertaken along the pelvic floor. When this occurs, it is difficult to identify the vessel because it retracts beneath the margins of the muscle.

The profuse collateral blood supply to the ureter is an important anatomic safeguard that protects its pelvic segment from ischemic necrosis as a result of radical hysterectomy (Fig. 51.13). The ureter has the advantage of a multiple-source blood supply. This favorable collateral circulation permits interruption of small arteries and veins deep in the pelvis during extensive dissection of the base of the broad ligament without producing a significant incidence of ischemic necrosis and fistula formation. The freely anastomosing arterial and venous network that courses along the longitudinal surface of the ureter in its adventitial layer is supplied in its superior segment by branches from the renal and ovarian arteries. The middle segment of the ureter derives its blood supply directly from aortic branches and from a vessel from the common iliac artery. As the ureter enters the pelvis and courses along the lateral pelvic wall, it receives arterial branches from the uterine, vaginal, middle hemorrhoidal, and vesical arteries. As it approaches the trigone of the bladder, it has a rich arteriovenous collateral circulation from the arterial branches to the vagina and base of the bladder. Protection of this important vascular network is important for the integrity of the terminal ureter during extensive dissection of the cardinal ligament. Preservation of the lateral aspect of the posterior segment of the vesicouterine ligament has been recommended to ensure adequate vascularity to the terminal segment of the ureter, but we have encountered no difficulty in removing this tissue and have no hesitation in doing so to enhance the adequacy of the central dissection.

Lymphatic Anatomy

The lymphatic drainage of the pelvis follows the course of the arterial and venous blood supply. Although there are multiple variations in the lymphatic anatomy of the pelvis, in general, lateral, superior, medial, and inferior lymph nodes and communicating lymphatic channels surround the common iliac, external iliac, and hypogastric vessels. One of the important pathways of the pelvic nodes and thin-walled lymphatics that drain the upper vagina, cervix, and uterus courses along the posterior aspect of the endopelvic fascia. Here, the pelvic nodes pass through the uterosacral ligament area and terminate in lymph nodes along the lateral aspect of the sacrum. These nodes communicate freely with lymphatic channels from the bifurcation of the common iliac artery near the lateral sacral and ischiosacral fossae. These can be difficult nodes to resect because they are closely attached to the thin-walled tributaries of the hypogastric vein. In dissecting the nodes from the

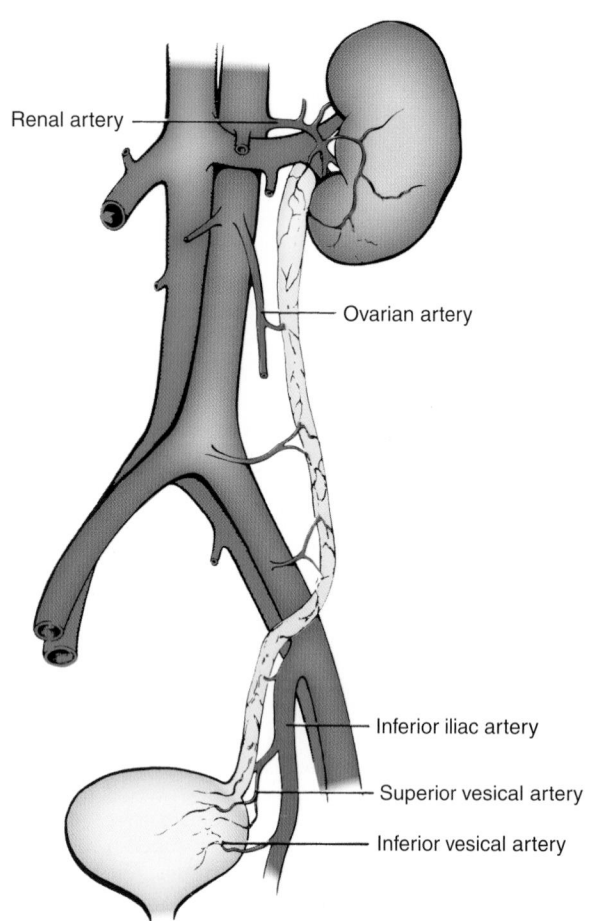

FIGURE 51.13 Blood supply of the ureter showing multiple sources of collateral arterial circulation.

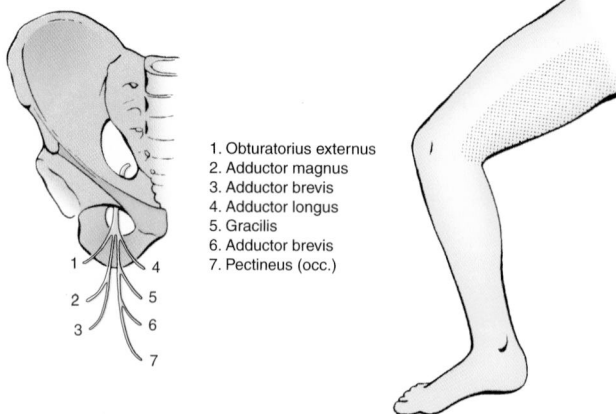

1. Obturatorius externus
2. Adductor magnus
3. Adductor brevis
4. Adductor longus
5. Gracilis
6. Adductor brevis
7. Pectineus (occ.)

FIGURE 51.14 Obturator nerve (L2 through L4): motor and sensory innervation.

bifurcation of the common iliac vessels, care must be taken to avoid injury to the hypogastric vein, which extends from beneath the artery on the medial side in this area.

The most direct lymphatic drainage of the cervix and upper vagina is through the lateral parametrium (cardinal ligament) to the hypogastric and obturator lymphatics. Because of the presence of obscure obturator veins and multiple venous tributaries from the hypogastric vein along the pelvic floor, the obturator dissection can be associated with troublesome venous bleeding. Injury also can occur to the obturator nerve, which arises from the anterior division of the second, third, and fourth lumbar nerves; enters the pelvis through the psoas muscle; and runs along the lateral pelvic wall in the obturator fossa to exit the pelvis through the obturator foramen along with the obturator vessels. It is a motor nerve to the adductor muscles of the thigh and is the only motor nerve that arises from the lumbar plexus without innervating any of the pelvic structures. Damage to the obturator nerve produces not only motor impairment to the adductor muscles but also sensory loss along the medial aspect of the thigh (**Fig. 51.14**). Deep dissection posterior to the obturator nerve can be complicated by bleeding from the tributaries of the hypogastric and obturator veins, so dissection in this area must be done with great care, using clips or vessel sealers on the small vessels and compression for troublesome venous bleeding.

Reiffenstuhl, in his classic study of the lymphatics of the female genital organs, described efferent lymph channels from the cervix to the interiliac lymph nodes, the lateral and

medial external iliac lymph nodes, the lateral and medial common iliac lymph nodes, the sacral lymph nodes, the subaortic lymph nodes, the aortic lymph nodes, the superior gluteal lymph nodes, the inferior gluteal lymph nodes, and the rectal lymph nodes. Of these, the inferior gluteal nodes are not technically possible to remove with the standard approach. This is because the nodes lie around the ischial spine in proximity to the inferior gluteal artery and pudendal artery and nerve. An imposing network of veins also surrounds the inferior gluteal nodes. They are thin walled, easy to damage, difficult to expose, and difficult to control when damaged. Reiffenstuhl's concepts of the lymphatic drainage of the cervix are partially shown in **Figure 51.15**.

Sentinel lymph node studies in women with cervical cancer are also adding greatly to our knowledge of the lymphatic drainage in vivo (**Fig. 51.16A**), and identification of SLNs with blue dye (**Fig. 51.16B**), fluorescent indocyanine green (ICG) (**Fig. 51.16C**), and technetium injections is feasible, with very low morbidity. These SLNs can be submitted for ultrastaging with immunohistochemistry staining and may help in the postoperative management of cases. Further evaluation and validation of SLN techniques is leading many investigators to recommend the routine use of SLN with pelvic nodal dissection and even consider an SLN algorithm as a comprehensive strategy to evaluate nodal metastasis. Recent studies have strongly suggested that SLN identification can potentially replace complete pelvic lymphadenectomy in select early-stage (I) cervical cancer. The SLN algorithm may help reduce the total operative time as well as some perioperative complications and long-term complications, such as postoperative leg lymphedema, which is occasionally seen in patients undergoing pelvic lymphadenectomy. The most common injection sites for SLN mapping are shown in **Figure 51.16D**.

EVOLUTION OF THE CLASSIFICATION SYSTEMS OF RADICAL HYSTERECTOMY AND PELVIC LYMPHADENECTOMY

There are several variations of hysterectomy used in the management of cervical carcinoma. The description of the five classes of hysterectomy by Piver and colleagues has found general acceptance and was used for many years. The first three classes are used in the primary treatment of cervical carcinoma, whereas the last two classes are generally reserved for patients

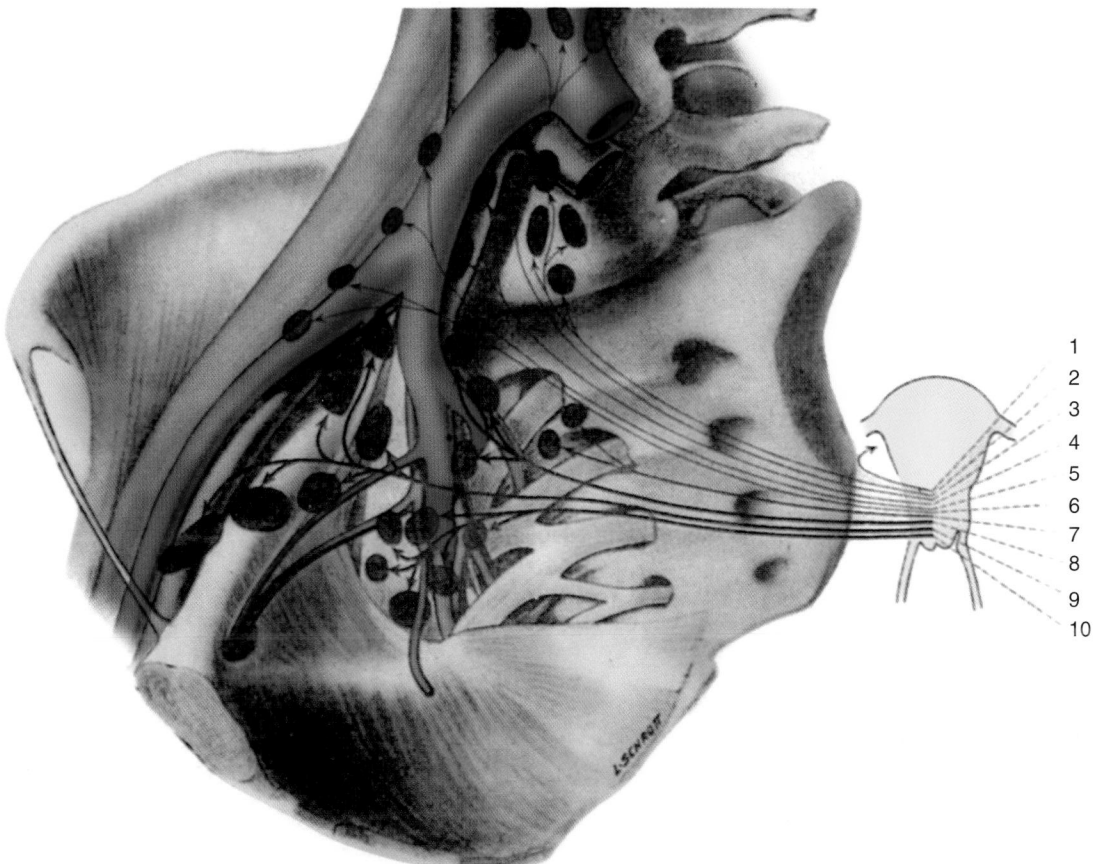

FIGURE 51.15 The regional lymph node stations of the uterine cervix. Channels 8, 9, and 10 (indicated by especially heavy lines) lead to those regional lymph node stations most frequently reached by the efferent lymph vessels of the cervix. Nonetheless, it is necessary to remember that carcinoma cells also can reach the pelvic lymph nodes by way of channels 1 through 7, without previous interruption, to (*1*) rectal, (*2*) subaortic (promontorial), (*3*) aortic, (*4*) medial common iliac, (*5*) lateral common iliac, (*6*) lateral external iliac, (*7*) sacral, (*8*) superior gluteal, (*9*) interiliac, and (*10*) inferior gluteal lymph nodes. (From Reiffenstuhl G. *The lymphatics of the female genital organs*. Philadelphia, PA: JB Lippincott, 1964, with permission.)

with recurrent disease. The class I hysterectomy is a simple extrafascial total hysterectomy. It is used as primary treatment for stage IA1 disease and after concurrent chemotherapy and radiation therapy for stage IB2 and bulky stage IIA cervical carcinoma. The class II hysterectomy (Fig. 51.8), also known as a modified radical hysterectomy, removes a more generous vaginal cuff, ligates the uterine artery on the medial side of the ureter (but does not dissect the ureter from the vesicouterine ligament), and removes the inner one third to one half of the cardinal ligament. As previously stated, some authors recommend the performance of the class II hysterectomy for stage IA2 cervical carcinoma. The class III operation is the classic Meigs procedure, with removal of all of the parametrium and paravaginal tissue in addition to the pelvic lymph nodes (Fig. 51.8). A more extensive procedure is performed in the class IV radical hysterectomy, in which the ureter is completely dissected from the cardinal and vesicouterine ligaments, the superior vesical artery is sacrificed, and three fourths of the vagina is removed, as well as the uterus and parametria, along with a complete lymphadenectomy. A far more extensive procedure is done with the class V radical hysterectomy, in which the terminal ureter or a segment of the bladder or rectum is removed along with the uterus, parametria, adnexa, and pelvic lymph nodes.

Although many techniques emphasize a more or less extensive dissection in one phase of the operation or another, the management of the parametria and the dissection of the pelvic lymph nodes appear relatively uniform. Because the most serious complication of this procedure is related to ureteral fistulae and stenosis, many modifications have been undertaken to ensure an adequate blood supply to the terminal ureter. We agree that the terminal ureter must have a good blood supply and believe that this can be accomplished without jeopardizing the adequacy of the central dissection. The classic radical hysterectomy with wide resection of the parametrium, dissection of the terminal ureter from the vesicouterine ligament, and wide resection of the uterosacral ligaments, upper 2 to 3 cm of vagina, and paravaginal tissues, along with a thorough pelvic lymphadenectomy, is the traditional procedure that is used in our institution.

The major focus of the operation is the adequacy of the central dissection. The central cervical tumor must be removed with an adequate margin of uninvolved normal tissue around it. This is the most crucial point in the success of the operation and has been emphasized by many of the famous pelvic surgeons of former years, especially Parsons and Navratil. The central dissection can be facilitated by developing the pelvic spaces and using proper planes for dissection. Correct

IX

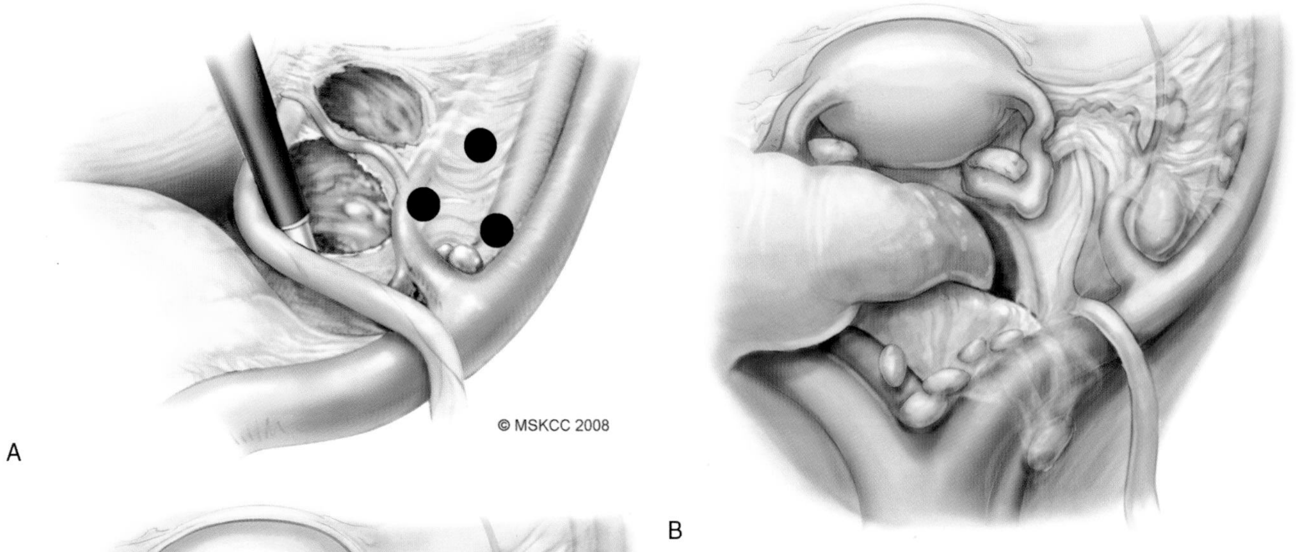

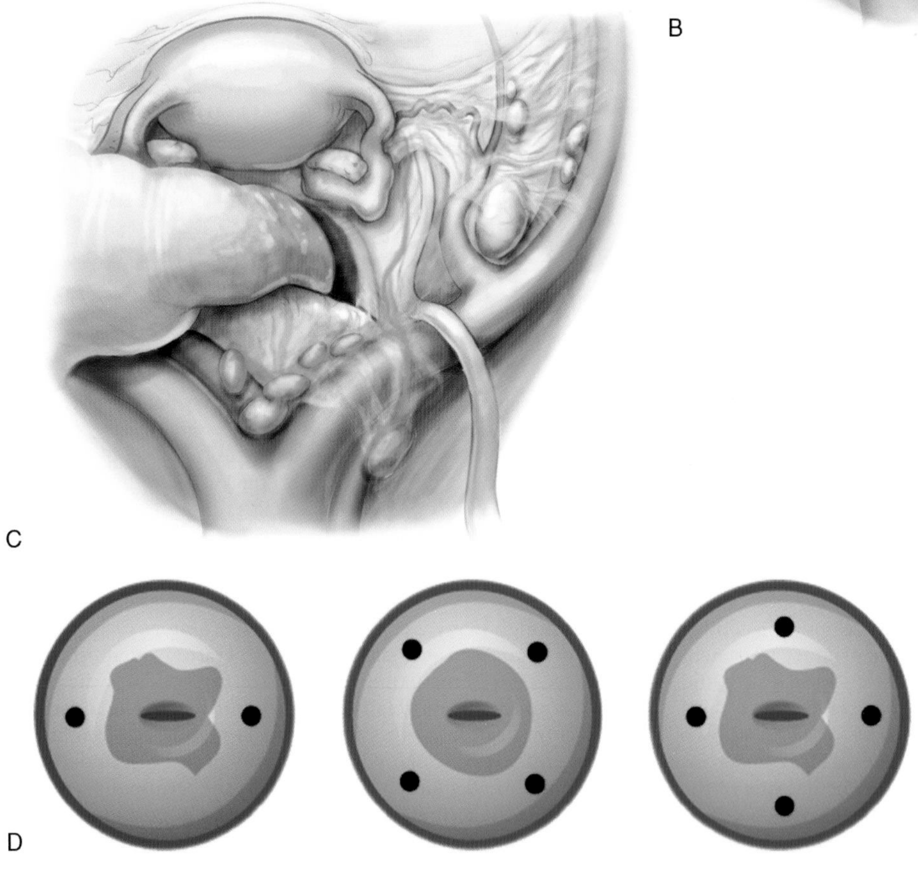

A

© MSKCC 2008

B

C

D

dissection along natural rather than artificial connective tissue planes and correct development of the pelvic spaces (paravesical, pararectal, vesicocervical, and rectovaginal) avoid unnecessary injury to pelvic vessels, keep blood loss to a minimum, and facilitate an adequate central dissection (Fig. 51.17). The central dissection also is facilitated by a complete removal of the contents of the obturator fossa (except the obturator nerve) so that branches of the hypogastric artery and vein in the cardinal ligament are clearly visible and can be dissected away from their attachments to the lateral pelvic sidewall.

The importance of an adequate central dissection also was emphasized by Girardi and coworkers. By studying surgical specimens processed according to the giant-section technique of Burghardt and Pickel, parametrial lymph nodes were found in 280 (78%) of the 359 surgical specimens from radical hysterectomies. Metastases to parametrial nodes were found in 63 (22.5%) of these 280 specimens. The lymphatic drainage from the cervix to the pelvic lymph nodes runs through the parametrium, and deposits of tumor often are found there. An adequate central dissection must include removal of a wide margin of parametrial tissue around the central tumor and total removal of the parametria from the bladder, the rectum, and the lateral pelvic wall because positive lymph nodes can be found in the lateral as well as medial parametrium.

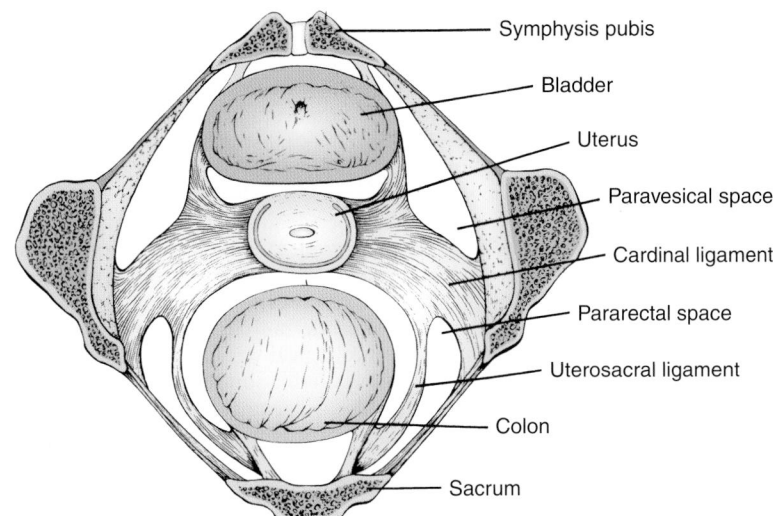

Symphysis pubis

Bladder

Uterus

Paravesical space

Cardinal ligament

Pararectal space

Uterosacral ligament

Colon

Sacrum

FIGURE 51.17 Cross section of pelvis showing paravesical and pararectal space. The base of the broad ligament (cardinal ligament) extends to the lateral pelvic wall and contains the major lymphatics draining the cervix.

When a large vaginal cuff must be removed because of a bulky cervical tumor or involvement of adjacent vaginal mucosa, starting the operation from below may facilitate the central dissection. Sometimes, a bulky lesion is excised and fulgurated transvaginally. The formation of the vaginal cuff is done in a manner similar to that in the Schauta-Amreich procedure. The vaginal incision is made around the entire circumference of the vagina, mobilizing the vaginal cuff from paravaginal tissue. Further dissection into the paravesical space, vesicocervical space, and rectovaginal space from below may be easier than from above.

Superior to the midcommon iliac arteries and in the paraaortic region, lymph nodes are sampled in selected patients (usually stage IB1 and IIA). A special effort is made to remove any nodes that look or feel suspicious. The paraaortic lymph nodes then are sent for frozen section analysis. Approximately 5% to 10% of stage IB patients have paraaortic lymph node metastasis. Metastasis to the paraaortic lymph nodes is considered by many gynecologic oncologists as a contraindication to radical hysterectomy. These patients are currently being treated with extended-field radiation therapy with concurrent chemotherapy.

In recent years, Querlu and Morrow suggested a modernization of the classic classification system, with a main emphasis on the role of a nerve-sparing radical hysterectomy (type C1) and on three-dimensional topography of radical pelvic surgery. Simply put, a type B resection is equivalent to a class II hysterectomy, a type C1 resection is equivalent to a class III hysterectomy with nerve sparing, and a class C2 hysterectomy is equivalent to a more radical class III operation with disregard to hypogastric and pelvic splanchnic nerves.

RADICAL ABDOMINAL HYSTERECTOMY SURGICAL TECHNIQUE

Preoperative Evaluation and Preparation

After the initial history and physical examination have indicated the possibility of primary treatment with radical hysterectomy and pelvic lymphadenectomy, the usual preoperative evaluation common before any extensive operation is indicated. We also recommend a chest x-ray to screen for cardiac or pulmonary disease as well as the very low risk of pulmonary metastases.

Contrary to the frequent practice of doing all possible tests on every patient, it is our practice to be selective and to do only those tests and procedures that are expected to yield useful information. It is not necessary (and indeed may be inappropriate) to subject every patient to a long list of preoperative procedures that are expensive and exhausting and have little, if any, expectation of providing useful information. Indeed, it is most unfortunate when a test or procedure yields questionable or suspicious findings that require one or more additional studies that, after delay, discomfort, and expense, turn out to be negative or even perhaps nondiagnostic. Good judgment from an experienced clinician is usually the most helpful.

A young, healthy patient with a small cervical lesion requires an admission history and physical examination, chest radiograph and routine laboratory studies, and anesthesia consultation. If the patient is older, has medical complications, or has a larger or undifferentiated cervical lesion, the preoperative workup and preparation may be more involved and thorough. Although an intravenous pyelogram provides good visualization of the course and number of ureters, if radiologic evaluation of the abdomen and pelvis is being considered, most surgeons obtain a CT scan of the abdomen and pelvis with contrast, which also shows the course and number of ureters and also may provide additional information about nodal or other metastases. However, because of the uncertainty of enlarged nodes on CT scan, patients with clinical stage IB1 disease and enlarged pelvic nodes on CT scan would not make us cancel the surgical approach in favor of radiation therapy. These nodes need to be evaluated further, possibly with a surgical resection, biopsy, or PET scan.

Larger lesions or those more likely to have metastases may be investigated by pelvic and abdominal CT scan or magnetic resonance scans, but we have rarely found those to be helpful in women with small cervical cancers. They may be most helpful when the clinician is undecided regarding whether primary surgery or radiation is the best management option—a clean, normal study may be reassuring that primary surgery is the way to go, whereas suspicious, enlarged nodes in a woman with a 4-cm cervical lesion help make the decision to recommend radiation. Likewise, cystoscopy or proctoscopy is rarely indicated or helpful in the preoperative evaluation of early-stage cervical cancer. As much as possible

IX

should be done on an outpatient basis before admission to the hospital.

Bowel Preparation

In our institution, patients are asked to start a liquid diet 24 hours before surgery. They also are given a mechanical bowel preparation if significant peritoneal adhesions are anticipated or there is a history of previous major pelvic surgery or radiation. An intestinal tube for suction is not necessary.

Positioning and Incision

Multiple approaches to performing a radical abdominal hysterectomy and bilateral pelvic lymphadenectomy have been described. The traditional transperitoneal approach has been used in our institution for many years, with satisfactory results. The transverse Maylard or Cherney incision is used by some, whereas others prefer midline incisions. Orr and Scribner have reported shorter hospital stays when a Pfannenstiel incision is used. Currie has presented and published a technique using a transverse cosmetic incision with vertical fascial entry for selected patients.

After anesthesia is induced, some surgeons prefer that the patient be placed comfortably in stirrups, with the buttocks brought to the edge of the "broken" table. Pneumatic compression devices are placed on both lower extremities, and the knees are separated approximately 90 degrees. The thighs are elevated only 15 to 20 degrees relative to the abdomen. Care is taken to avoid pressure on the peroneal nerves in the legs. Proponents of this position claim several advantages. There is less strain on the patient's lumbosacral spine when the thighs are slightly flexed. This is especially important for patients with lumbosacral back problems. It is possible to have a second assistant stand at the foot of the table between the patient's legs. His or her participation in the operation is greatly facilitated by being closer to the operative field. Finally, in this position, the urethral orifice, vaginal introitus, and anal orifice are all available for instrumentation in case this is necessary to clarify anatomy.

After the patient is positioned on the operating table, a careful rectovaginal–abdominal pelvic examination is done. This can be followed by cystoscopy or proctosigmoidoscopy if desired. If hair needs to be removed, it is preferable to use an electric hair trimmer rather than a razor. The skin is prepared from the rib margin to the midthigh, with special attention given to the umbilicus, perineum, and vagina. The patient is draped, a transurethral Foley catheter is inserted into the bladder, and the operation is begun. If an SLN injection is planned, the injection is done at the time of exam under anesthesia just before the patient is prepped and draped.

When operating abdominally, the exposure achieved depends on the choice of incision, the method of retracting, the placement and intensity of overhead lights, and the participation of willing and skillful assistants. Suction should be available to keep the field dry. Dry sponges are likely more traumatic to delicate serosal surfaces and other tissues. It usually is possible (and always desirable) to keep the number of clamps in the operative field to an absolute minimum. If the field is cluttered with clamps, the operator cannot see well to operate. There is sometimes a tendency for gynecologic surgeons to use instruments that are too short. Pedicle clamps, tissue forceps, dissecting scissors, needle holders, and all other instruments must be longer when operating deep in the pelvis and when operating on obese patients. The handles of the instruments must come all the way out and above the level of the incision so that they do not interfere with the operator's vision.

Evaluation at Laparotomy

As stated, the operation is initiated through a low-transverse (Maylard, Cherney, Pfannenstiel) or low midline incision; the same exploratory strategy should apply if a minimally invasive approach is being utilized. In most patients, the umbilicus identifies the location of the bifurcation of the aorta; therefore, extension of the incision approximately 2 to 3 cm above the umbilicus is recommended for adequate exposure of this area if a lower midline incision is used. The midline incision is protected by a moist pack beneath each arm of the self-retaining retractor to avoid excessive compression of the epigastric vessels that course beneath the rectus muscles. In case of a lengthy operative procedure, the mechanical retractors are released at periodic intervals to improve circulation through the abdominal musculature. The bladder is decompressed by an indwelling catheter throughout the procedure to facilitate exposure and maintain an accurate record of urine output.

Before initiating the pelvic procedure, the abdominal viscera and parietal peritoneum of the abdominal cavity are evaluated meticulously for possible evidence of metastatic tumor. The superior and inferior surfaces of the liver are carefully palpated, as is the region of the celiac plexus. The undersurface of the diaphragm is particularly vulnerable to metastases, especially the right hemidiaphragm, where the paraaortic lymphatics pass from the abdominal cavity into the mediastinum. The mesentery of the large and small bowel and the serosal surface of the bowel along with the omentum should be examined carefully for evidence of metastatic tumor. The kidneys are examined, and the retroperitoneal space along the aorta and vena cava is palpated assiduously because these are the major sites of extrapelvic spread of cervical cancer. It is well known that 15% or more of paraaortic node metastases are occult; therefore, even the most unsuspecting node should be removed and evaluated histologically by frozen section study for possible metastatic tumor. If there is histopathologic evidence of unsuspected, metastatic tumor in a paraaortic lymph node, we generally do not proceed with a radical hysterectomy, and the operation is abandoned. These patients are currently being treated with concurrent chemotherapy and extended-field radiation therapy.

Peritoneal washings for cytologic examination usually are not obtained because the yield is low and the prognostic significance is undetermined.

At this point in the procedure, any adhesions in the pelvis are lysed, and the intestines are placed in the upper abdomen and held there with moist packs. A suitable self-retaining retractor can be used. If Bookwalter, Turner-Warwick, or Balfour retractor is used in a lower midline incision, care must be taken to avoid compression of the femoral nerves by the lateral blades.

An evaluation of the extent of the pelvic tumor is undertaken at this time by examining the course of the lymphatic drainage of the pelvis, which is carefully palpated along the pelvic vessels. When enlarged or clinically suspicious nodes are found, they are removed and immediately sent for frozen section study while further evaluation of the pelvis is undertaken. The paravesical and pararectal spaces are important anatomic landmarks. When developed, they provide an opportunity for thorough exploration of the intervening base of the broad ligament (Fig. 51.17). Tumor can extend into the base of the broad ligament without detection of anatomic evidence of disease before operation. This step, therefore, is a safeguard in determining the possible extension of tumor beyond the cervix and into the immediate paracervical tissues. When there is evidence of extracervical disease, we may abandon the surgical procedure unless there is clear evidence that the disease can be removed cleanly. In either case, full pelvic irradiation is indicated. Certainly, the lateral pelvic wall must be free of tumor. When the central tumor is clearly resectable, we do not hesitate to complete the operation, even if there is evidence of metastatic disease in the pelvic lymph nodes.

A decision must be made about conservation or removal of the tubes and ovaries before the pelvic planes and spaces are developed. If normal ovaries are conserved in premenopausal patients, the tubes usually may be removed. After the round ligaments are clamped, cut, and ligated, the utero-ovarian ligaments and medial fallopian tubes are clamped and doubly ligated. The infundibulopelvic ligaments are carefully mobilized, and the adnexal organs are packed out of the operative field with the intestines.

Development of Paravesical Space

The anterior leaf of the broad ligament forms the roof of the *paravesical space* and blends with the bladder peritoneum medially and the parietal peritoneum laterally. This deep fossa beneath the peritoneal covering is composed of loose connective tissue and fat. It occupies the area between the bladder and the retropubic space medially, with the pelvic sidewall and obturator muscle forming the lateral boundaries. The superior boundary is formed by the cardinal ligament, whereas the floor is composed of the levator ani muscle. After clamping and ligating the round ligament about midway along its course, the anterior leaf of the broad ligament is opened in an inferior direction, passing well into the pelvis before diverting the incision medially to reflect the bladder peritoneum from the lower uterine segment (**Fig. 51.18A**). The paravesical space can be entered without difficulty with gentle digital pressure, making

certain that the dissection is initiated between the external iliac vein laterally and the obliterated hypogastric artery (lateral umbilical ligament) medially. The dissection is carried all the way down to the levator ani muscle (**Fig. 51.18B**). There are no major blood vessels in this potential space, although occasionally, an aberrant obturator vessel emerges from the inferior epigastric artery and courses along the posterior aspect of the pubic bone to the obturator space. With gentle digital dissection, the pelvic floor can be palpated and the posterior aspect of the space can be identified, including the anterior margin of the cardinal ligament.

Development of Pararectal Space

The *pararectal space* lies beneath the pelvic peritoneum and extends between the cardinal ligament laterally and the uterosacral ligament medially. It can be entered by extending the incision in the anterior leaf of the broad ligament in a cephalic direction along the lateral margin of the infundibulopelvic ligament (**Fig. 51.19A**). By retracting the infundibulopelvic ligament and displacing the uterus medially, the uterosacral ligament is placed on a stretch, and the pararectal space is widened. Dissection of this space is much more precarious than that of the paravesical space. Unskilled dissection in this area frequently is associated with troublesome bleeding. The medial border of the fossa is bounded by the uterosacral ligament and rectum, and the lateral border is formed superiorly by the piriformis muscle and inferiorly by the levator muscle. The sacrum forms the posterior margin of the space, and the ureter is attached to the peritoneum along the roof of the space before entering the medial aspect of the cardinal ligament. The hypogastric artery and vein are located in the deeper aspect of the pararectal space along the levator ani muscle.

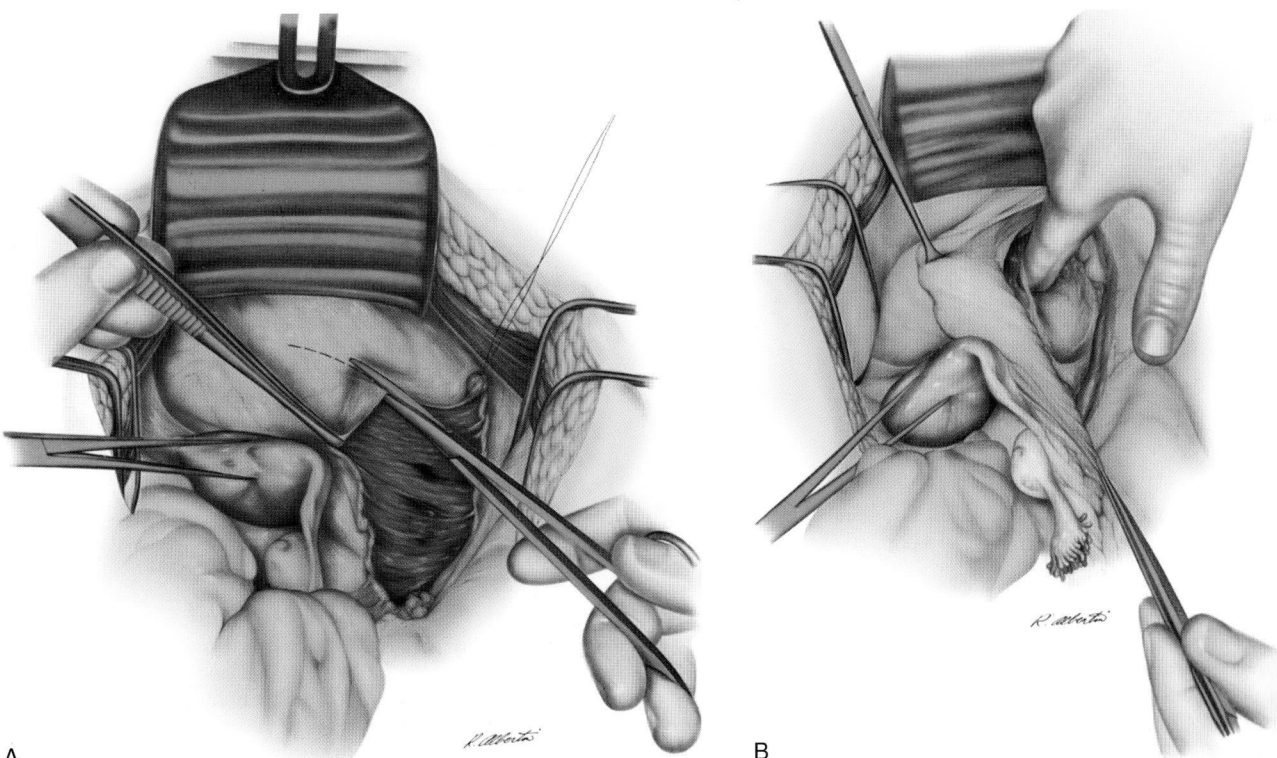

A   B

FIGURE 51.18 A: Opening the anterior leaf of the broad ligament after ligation of the right round ligament and infundibulopelvic ligament. **B:** Development of paravesical space.

IX

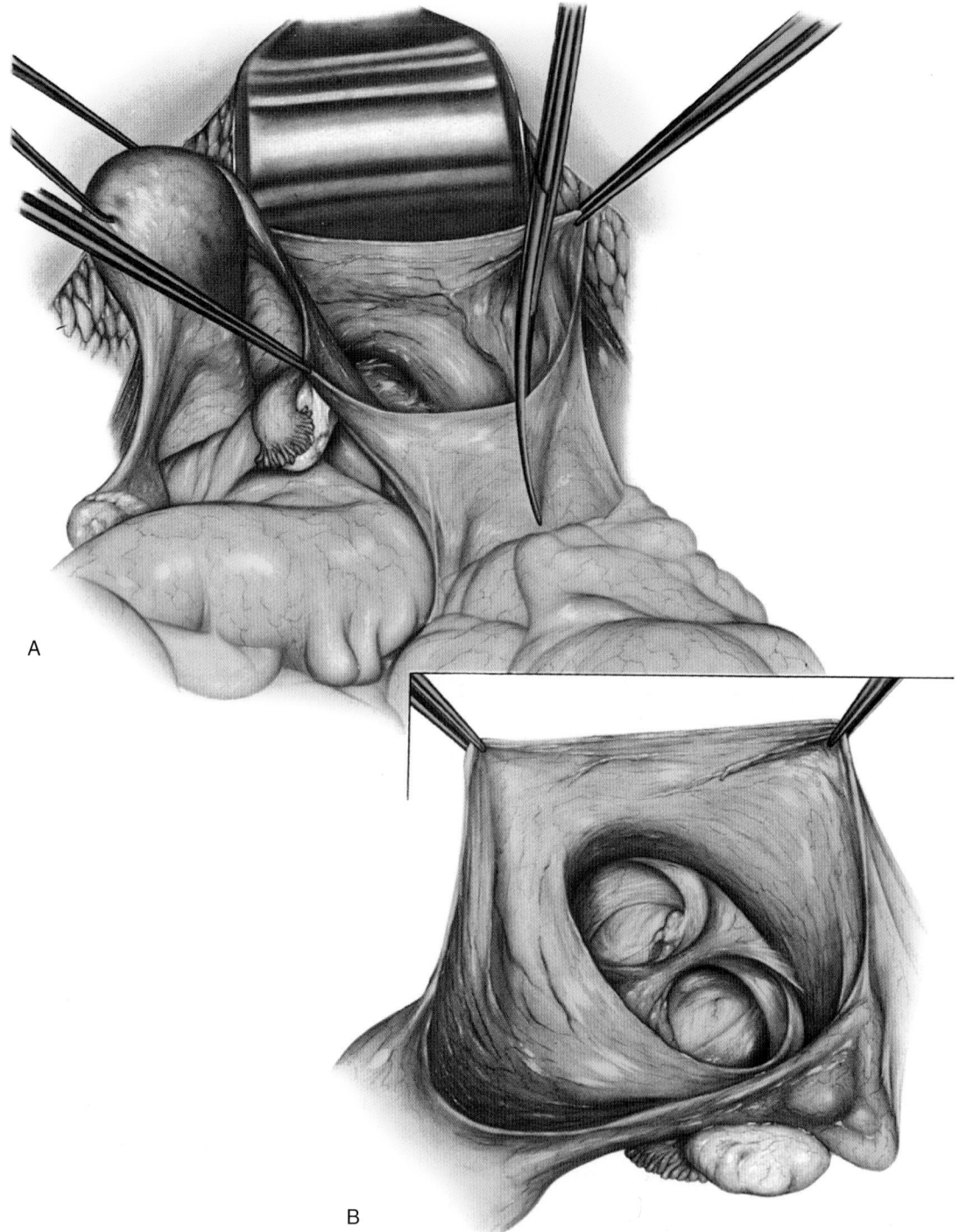

FIGURE 51.19 A: Extending the incision in the anterior leaf of the broad ligament in a cephalic direction along the lateral margin of the right infundibulopelvic ligament. **B:** Paravesical and pararectal fossae, with intervening base of broad ligament attached to pelvic floor and lateral pelvic wall.

The cardinal ligament forms the caudal and lateral borders of this important area. Entry into the pararectal space must be made cautiously (Fig. 51.19A) with medial displacement of the ureter and its attached peritoneum. A point between the ureter, which is attached to the medial leaf of peritoneum, and the hypogastric artery is selected. Blunt dissection should be used in this area, and careful handling of tissue is imperative to avoid unnecessary damage to small veins deep in this fossa. When the examining finger reaches the pelvic floor and levator

ani muscle, the fossa narrows, and care must be taken to avoid damage to the lateral sacral and hemorrhoidal vessels. The dissection is carried vertically downward for a short distance. The further development of the space then changes to an inferior and caudad direction lateral to the rectum. If the development of the space is difficult, it should be delayed until a later time in the operation. When the paravesical and pararectal spaces have been dissected (Fig. 51.19B), the pelvic floor and cardinal ligament easily can be identified and palpated. In the absence of demonstrable tumor extension, the case is considered operable, and the lymph node dissection is initiated at this time.

Pelvic Lymphadenectomy

If an SLN mapping is planned, the SLNs are removed first. Dissection of the lymphatic tissue along the iliac vessels can begin in the region of the bifurcation of the common iliac artery and extended superiorly to the bifurcation of the aorta and inferiorly to the inguinal ligament and deep circumflex iliac vein, or it can begin at another point along the course of the iliac vessels. The opening of the posterior peritoneal leaf of the broad ligament must be extended to the area of the pelvic brim, where the ureter is easily identified as it enters the pelvis at the bifurcation of the common iliac artery. This dissection is made easier if the infundibulopelvic ligament has been ligated and divided; however, the ligament and ovarian vessels can be retracted medially if the adnexa are preserved. The ovary and tube also can be detached from the uterine corpus and gently tucked beneath the retractor above. In dissecting the presacral area in the angle of the bifurcation of the aorta, care must be taken to avoid bleeding from the middle sacral vessels as well as from the proximal

part of the left external iliac vein, which courses through this retroperitoneal space. It is best to occlude the middle sacral vessels with smaller vascular clips as they are identified, and if traumatized, the venous bleeding can be controlled with positive pressure against the sacrum and with vascular clips. The lymphatic tissue along the common iliac vessels is removed by sharp dissection with the points of the Metzenbaum scissors directed upward, while special care is taken to avoid trauma to the ureter (Fig. 51.20). The ureter is reflected medially during the dissection of the common iliac vessels and left attached to the parietal peritoneum to maintain its blood supply.

It is important to remove the loose areolar tissue and fascial sheath from the iliac vessels; however, to avoid trauma to the intima or wall of the vessels (particularly the veins), the surgeon should not attempt to skeletonize the pelvic vessels to the point of producing a pearl-white vascular tree. If there is tumor in the adventitia of the vessel wall, the patient probably will not be cured by this procedure; consequently, such compulsive surgical efforts produce far more complications than benefits. It is important to rotate the vessels medially and laterally with a vein retractor during the dissection of the common and external iliac trunks to obtain the posterior

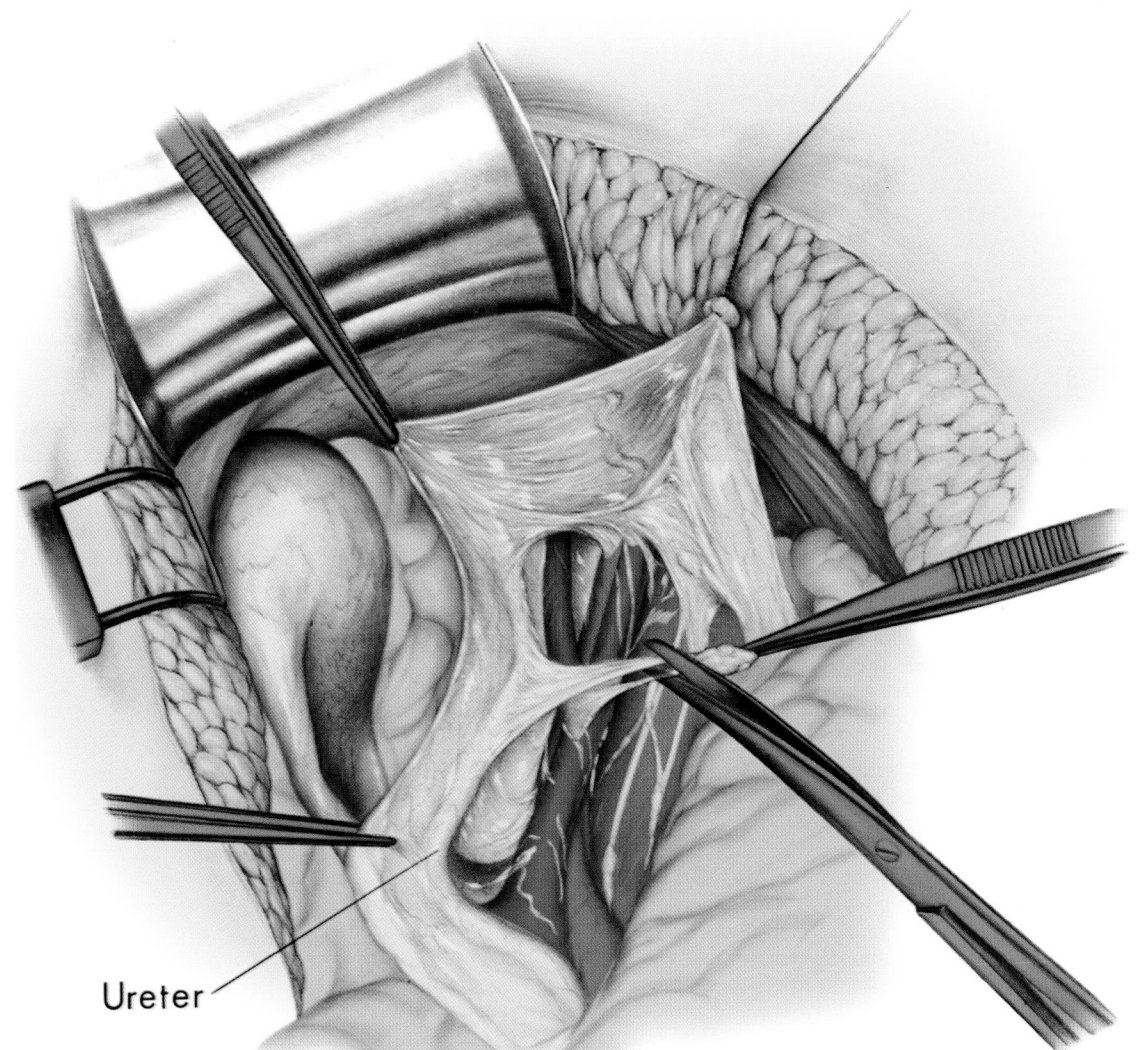

Ureter

FIGURE 51.20 Pelvic lymphadenectomy with dissection of right common iliac vessels and their branches, including the external iliac and hypogastric arteries and veins. Note attachment of ureter to parietal peritoneum. The genitofemoral nerve courses along the psoas muscle.

lymphatic chain behind the vessels along the psoas muscle. The genitofemoral nerve, which is seen lateral to the external iliac vessels, should be preserved, if possible, because damage to this peripheral nerve occasionally produces postoperative discomfort in the groin and medial aspect of the thigh.

The external iliac vessels are carefully dissected down to the point where the deep circumflex iliac vein crosses over the external iliac artery. At this point, care must be taken to avoid injury to the inferior epigastric artery and vein, which arise from the anterior and medial side of the iliac vessels and course along the anterior peritoneum onto the lower abdominal wall. Removal of the distal external iliac or circumflex iliac nodes cephalad to the Cloquet node likely increases the risk of leg lymphedema. The surgeon also must be cognizant of the anomalous obturator artery and vein, which can arise from the lower portion of the external iliac or inferior epigastric vessels and course over the pelvic sidewall into the obturator space. If accidentally traumatized, they should be ligated at their point of origin from the artery or vein. To avoid bleeding in the obturator space, these vessels are frequently occluded with small vascular clips as they pass through the obturator space, regardless of their origin. Clips also can be used to occlude the lymphatic channels coming into the pelvis from the leg.

The obturator space is entered by reflecting the external iliac vessels medially away from the psoas muscle and freeing the areolar tissue that lies directly between these vessels and the lateral pelvic wall (Fig. 51.21A), usually with blunt dissection. Once the space has been entered and the adjacent tissue cleaned from the external iliac vessels, the artery and vein are released and gently retracted laterally with a vein retractor, and the obturator space is clearly exposed. The lymphatic and areolar tissue are dissected from the obturator space to the region of the pelvic floor, with particular care taken to avoid trauma to the obturator nerve and vessels (Fig. 51.21B). The dissection is continued by removing all of the nodes below the bifurcation of the iliac vessels, including the hypogastric nodes and the nodes in the obturator fossa. A lymph node may be encountered in the angle formed by the external iliac and hypogastric arteries and must be carefully dissected out, avoiding trauma to the adjacent hypogastric vein.

Retraction of the common iliac artery and vein medially exposes a group of lymph nodes that should be removed carefully. These lymph nodes are the lateral common iliac nodes. There is danger of venous bleeding in this area. When this area has been cleared, the surgeon can see the obturator nerve entering the obturator fossa through the body of the psoas muscle. The nerve roots of the lumbosacral plexus also are exposed. Particular care must be exercised in the dissection of the lateral sacral and sacroiliac plexus, just medial to the hypogastric artery and vein, near their origin. The rich arcade of small arteries and veins increases the risk of bleeding in this area. When the vessels retract into the sacral foramen, control of bleeding becomes difficult.

The obturator artery can be identified as it courses along the lateral pelvic wall adjacent to the obturator nerve. The nerve, artery, and vein advance toward the obturator foramen, through which they leave the pelvis. Care must be taken to avoid trauma to all of the structures, particularly the obturator veins, which have a rich anastomotic network against the lateral pelvic wall and communicate freely with the adjacent hypogastric veins. It is best to ligate or clip the obturator vessels, but if uncontrolled bleeding occurs in this area, hemostasis is best obtained by packing the space tightly with a hot pack and providing adequate time for a fibrin clot to develop. If excessive bleeding occurs on one side of the pelvis, dissection can continue on the opposite side in the interim after pressure packing.

Dissection of Hypogastric Artery, Uterine Artery, Bladder, and Ureter

The hypogastric artery is dissected with identification of the visceral branches of the anterior trunk, which include the uterine; superior, middle, and inferior vesical; vaginal; and middle hemorrhoidal arteries. The anterior division of the hypogastric artery continues along the paravesical fossa to become the obliterated lateral umbilical ligament beneath the anterior abdominal wall. If the superior vesical artery is damaged, it can be ligated without serious compromise to the blood supply of the bladder. At this point, we ligate the uterine artery at its origin from the hypogastric artery. Some authors believe that a more adequate central dissection is achieved by ligating the anterior division of the hypogastric artery just distal to the point of origin of its posterior division rather than ligating the uterine artery individually. Whichever vessel is chosen, after double ligation, the distal branches traversing the cardinal ligament are removed with the specimen. No attempt is made to remove the hypogastric vein. The other, adjacent veins should be ligated to avoid brisk bleeding in this area.

The bladder then is reflected off the lower uterine segment by incising the bladder peritoneum from its attachment to the uterus. The fascial adhesions of the base of the bladder are released from the cervix and upper vagina by electrocautery or sharp scissors dissection, and the vesicocervical space is developed inferiorly and laterally. The ureter tunnels between the anterior fascial bundles of the base of the broad ligament, commonly called the vesicouterine ligament. This fascial tunnel is carefully opened by sliding the Metzenbaum scissors or an Adson right angle clamp, with concave surface pointed upward, along the anterior and medial surface of the ureter, and by gently spreading the blades, as shown in Figure 51.22A. The uterine artery and vein course along the fascial roof of this ligament. As shown in Figure 51.22B, the anterior sheath of the vesicouterine ligament is opened by doubly clamping and incising this tissue. Each of the fascial bundles is suture ligated for control of bleeding, and the ureter is dissected free of its attachment to the posterior leaf of the vesicouterine ligament. As with the pelvic vessels, care must be taken to prevent damage to the adventitia and muscular wall of the ureter, which contain nutrient vessels from the collateral circulation. In the event that the blood supply to the ureter is compromised by thrombosis or trauma to the veins, fistula formation is a serious and frequent complication. The ureter is gently retracted with an umbilical tape or vein retractor. If forceps are used to handle the ureter, they should gently grasp only the adventitia.

Dissection of Cardinal Ligament

The base of the broad ligament (the cardinal ligament) then can be excised from its attachment at the lateral pelvic wall. The technique of clamping and ligating the vascular cardinal ligament varies, depending on the circumstances. Sometimes, part of the ligament can be included in a single clamp. Sometimes, it is better to ligate or clip individual vessels. The ligament is excised with sharp scissors dissection and ligated with 2-0 delayed absorbable suture. A series of clamps are placed until the dissection is completed to the pelvic floor and along the paravaginal tissues (Fig. 51.23). If serious bleeding occurs in this region owing to trauma to the pelvic floor veins, hemostatic control is best obtained by firm packing of the pelvis and shifting the dissection temporarily to the opposite side.

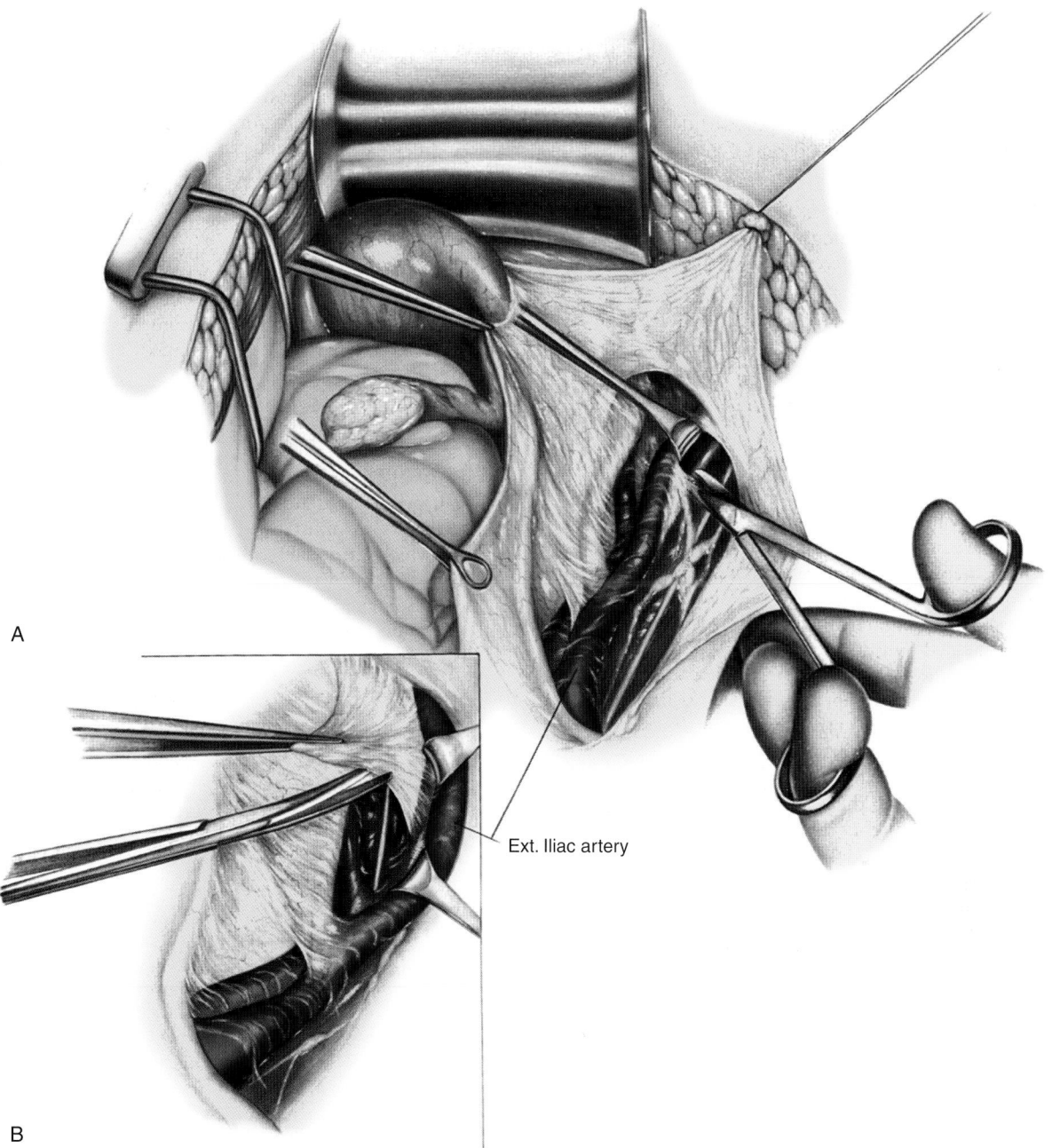

Ext. Iliac artery

FIGURE 51.21 A: Entry into obturator space by medial reflection of external iliac vessels. **B:** Dissection of obturator fossa, demonstrating obturator nerve with areolar tissue attached superiorly to external iliac vessels.

The uterosacral ligaments originate from a posterolateral position on the cervix, where they are thickest, and run posteriorly to the anterolateral aspect of the rectum. As the ligaments approach the rectum, they broaden so that they have a wider attachment to the rectum than to the cervix. The uterosacral ligaments are stretched by sharply drawing the uterus forward. The peritoneal reflection of the cul-de-sac of Douglas then is incised, leaving a small segment of peritoneum attached to the anterior surface of the rectum. Care must be taken to avoid injury to the ureters, which are attached to the peritoneum just lateral to the uterosacral ligament (Fig. 51.24A). The rectovaginal space is opened by sharp

scissors dissection and deepened by blunt and sharp dissection (Fig. 51.24B). This procedure separates the posterior reflection of the endopelvic fascia from the lateral wall of the rectum, which includes the more superficial uterosacral ligaments. The entire fascial bundle of the uterosacral ligament is identified, clamped as far posteriorly and close to the anterior rectal wall as possible, and cut and ligated (Fig. 51.24C). No attempt is made to divide the attachments to the sacrum. Using modern vessel-sealing devices to transect both the cardinal and uterosacral ligaments is advocated by some authors to significantly reduce operating time and blood loss, without any adverse effects on complication or tumor recurrence

IX

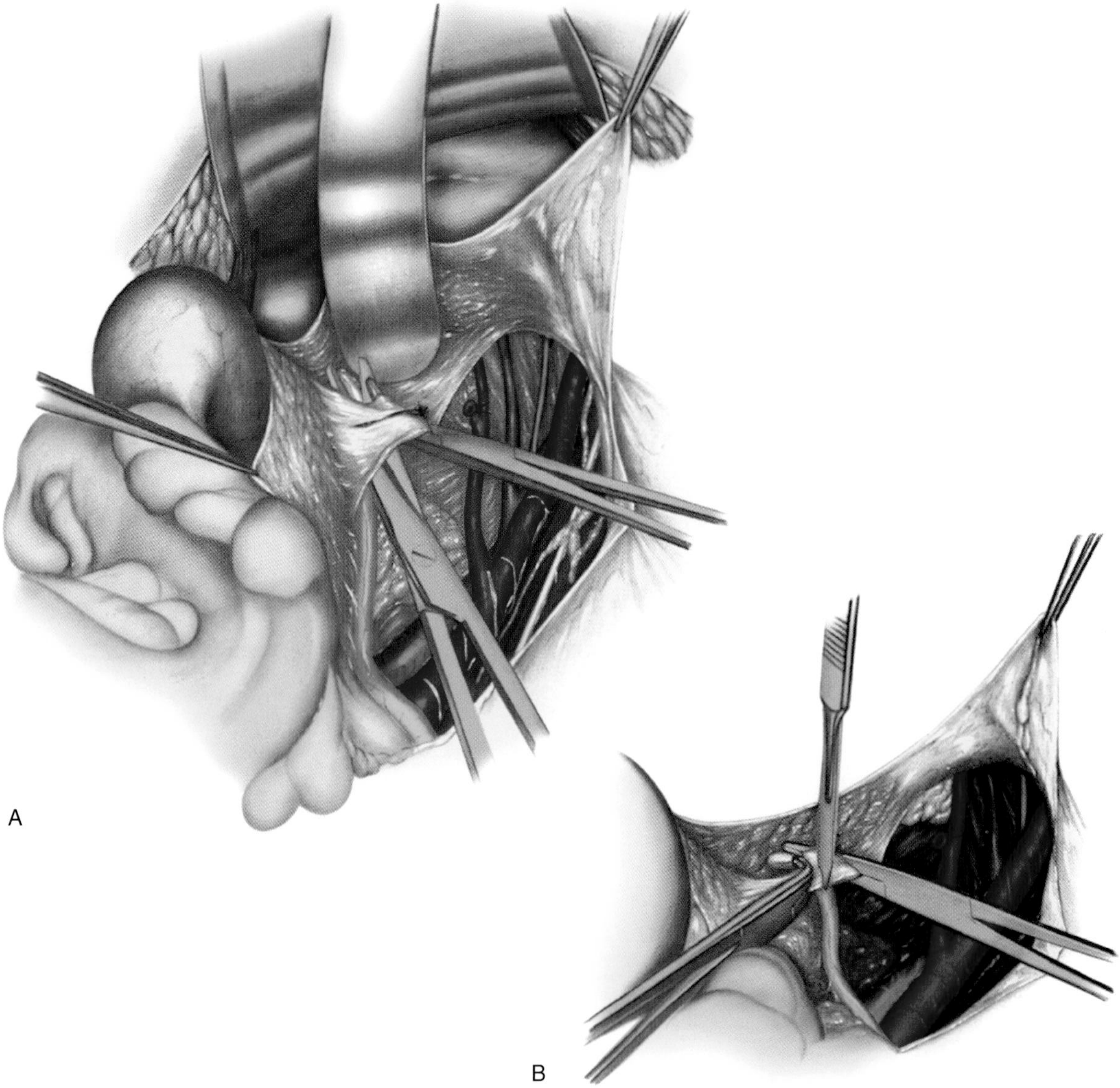

FIGURE 51.22 A: Metzenbaum scissors inserted above the ureter in the vesicouterine ligament or ureteral tunnel of the broad ligament. Note ligated uterine artery in anterior fascial sheath of tunnel. **B:** Roof of tunnel is opened between clamps.

rates. Continuation of this plane of dissection along the posterior endopelvic fascia frees the posterior aspect of the cervix from the pelvic floor. Trimbos and colleagues have described a "nerve-sparing" radical hysterectomy that involves a less radical dissection of the uterosacral ligament, which reduces the incidence of bladder dysfunction, without compromising cure rates.

It is important to dissect the paravaginal fascia to obtain all of the microlymphatic channels that communicate between the cervix and upper vagina (Fig. 51.25). The bladder then is dissected further from the upper portion of the vagina by sharp and blunt dissection, making certain to avoid trauma to the blood supply of this organ. It is important, therefore, that sharp dissection, rather than blunt trauma, be used to free the base of the bladder from the anterior vagina to avoid forceful tearing of the blood vessels and musculature of the bladder. When the specimen is ready to be removed, a long right-angled Wertheim clamp is placed across the vagina below the cervix (not shown) to avoid gross spillage of tumor

cells into the pelvis. The specimen then is removed by dividing the vagina above clamps placed on the lateral vaginal angles (Fig. 51.26).

Closure

The vaginal angles are suture ligated separately to secure hemostasis, and then the remaining cuff is closed in an anteroposterior direction using a continuous or interrupted 2-0 or no. 0 absorbable suture. No additional attempt is made to support the vaginal vault because all of the fascial support of the uterus and vagina has been removed. The remaining vagina, which has been shortened by about 2 to 3 cm, is well supported by its attachments to the levator ani muscles and urogenital diaphragm and mainly by the effects of postoperative fibrosis during the healing phase.

At the end of the procedure, some surgeons place suction catheters in the obturator fossae and along the lateral pelvic walls and bring them out through stab wounds in the lower

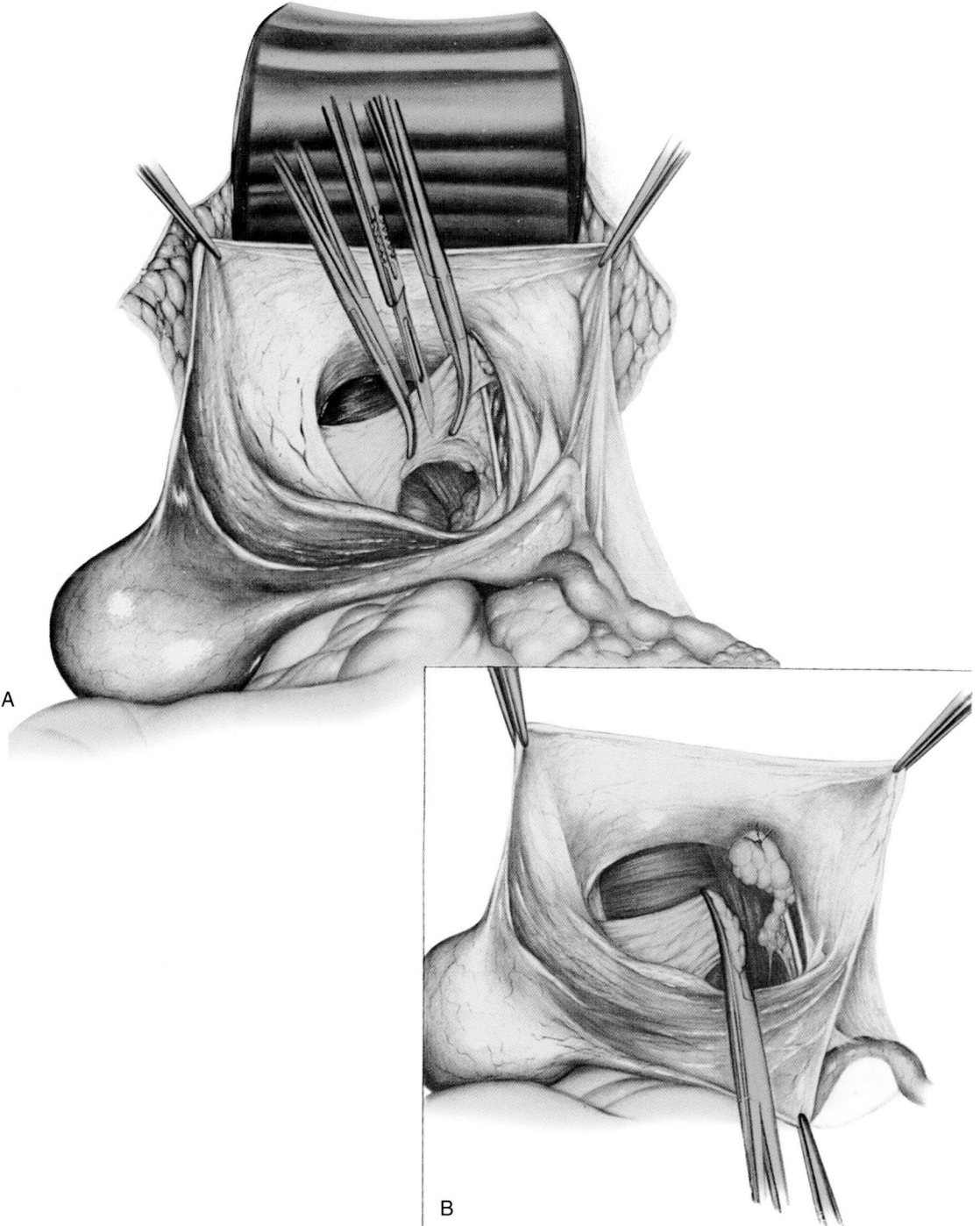

FIGURE 51.23 A: Clamping and incision of lateral portion of cardinal ligament adjacent to the lateral pelvic wall. **B:** Excised ligament showing pelvic floor and levator muscles. Dissected obturator nerve is seen in obturator space.

abdomen. After the abdomen is closed, these catheters are connected to intermittent, low-suction drainage units. Traditionally, these drains were thought to be effective in preventing pelvic infection and fistula and lymphocyst formation. However, recent retrospective and prospective studies have demonstrated that the incidence of these complications is minimal and the same whether or not drains are used. Therefore, many gynecologic oncologists no longer routinely use pelvic drains.

No attempt is made to suspend the ureters to the hypogastric artery, as suggested by Green and coworkers, or to place the terminal ureter on the inside of the peritoneal surface, as recommended by Novak. Furthermore, there appears to be no benefit to reperitonizing the pelvis as described by Symmonds and Pratt.

If the ovaries are to be transposed out of the pelvis, a tunnel is dissected beneath the peritoneum laterally and superiorly toward each lateral gutter. An incision in the peritoneum

IX

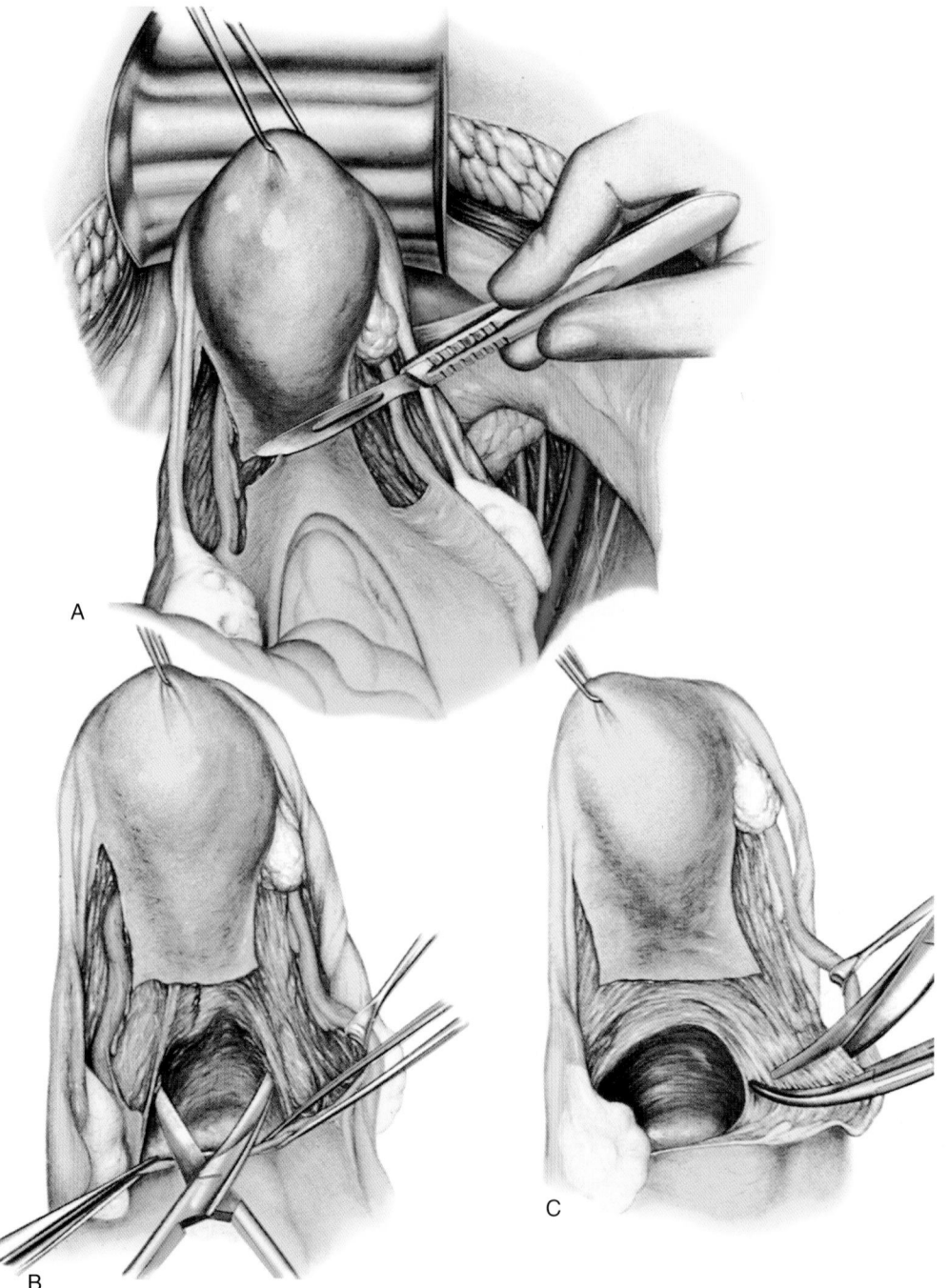

FIGURE 51.24 A: Cutting the cul-de-sac peritoneum as it reflects onto the rectum. Ureters course laterally, devoid of peritoneum. **B:** Dissection of the rectovaginal septum with development of rectal stalks (uterosacral ligaments). **C:** Clamping the uterosacral ligament. The ureter is gently retracted to avoid trauma.

is made as high as possible at the top of the tunnel. The adnexal structures are guided through the tunnel and through the incision at the top of the tunnel, making absolutely certain that the ovarian vessels in the infundibulopelvic ligament are not twisted. Permanent suture material is used to suture the tubo-ovarian pedicle as high as possible to the peritoneum and underlying muscle. Two large metal clips also are placed across the pedicle to later identify the location of the ovaries with an abdominal radiograph. This ovarian suspension is done when there is a reasonable chance that a patient will need postoperative pelvic irradiation, and recent studies suggest that at minimum, the ovary should be placed 1.5 cm cephalad to the iliac crest cased on planar radiology films (**Figs. 51.27** and **51.28**). In most operations, however, the tubes and ovaries can be left in their natural positions in the pelvis. If the ovary is to be transposed, it is reasonable to remove the tube and fimbriae; this may decrease the formation of future benign and malignant tubal disease and likely has limited compromise in the vascular perfusion to the remaining ovary.

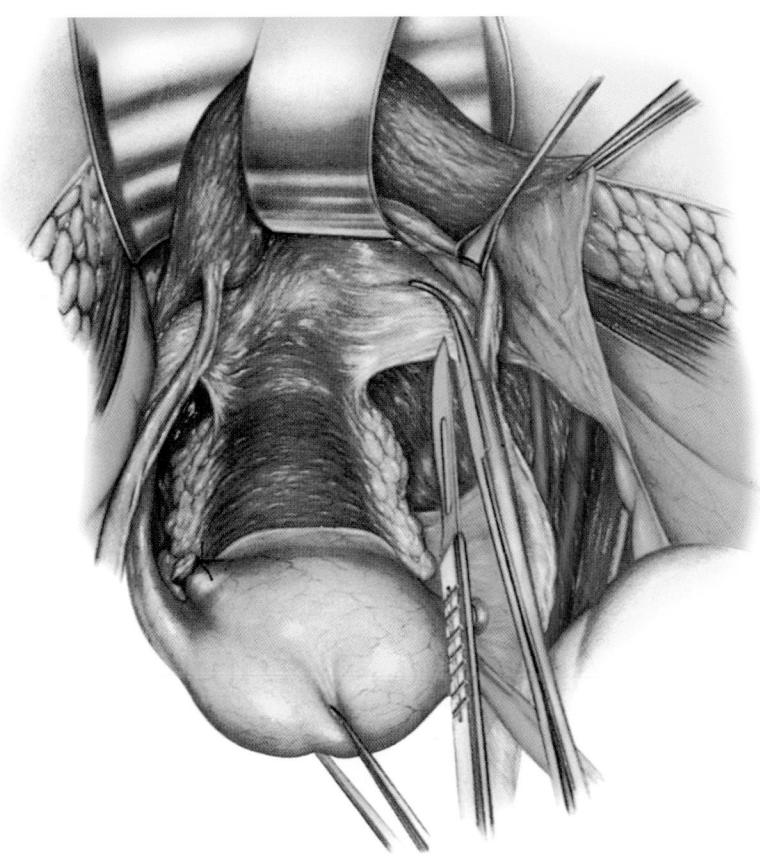

FIGURE 51.25 Dissection and retraction of bladder and terminal ureter from vagina and excision of the paravaginal fascia from the lateral pelvic wall.

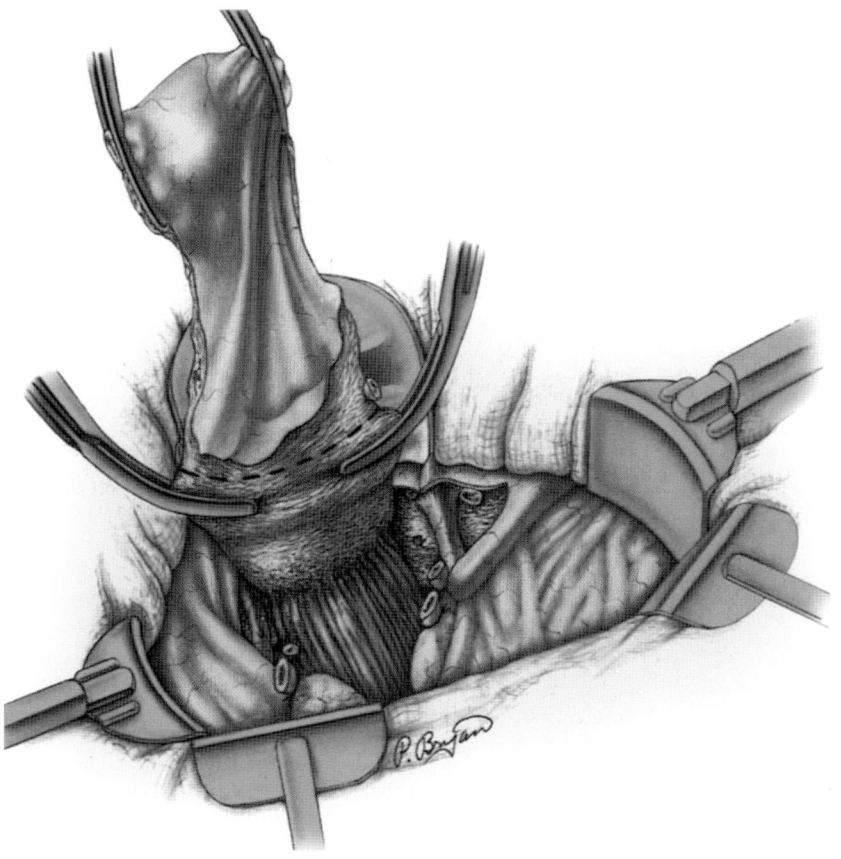

FIGURE 51.26 After clamping and ligating paravaginal tissue laterally, an incision is made in the vagina several centimeters below the cervix.

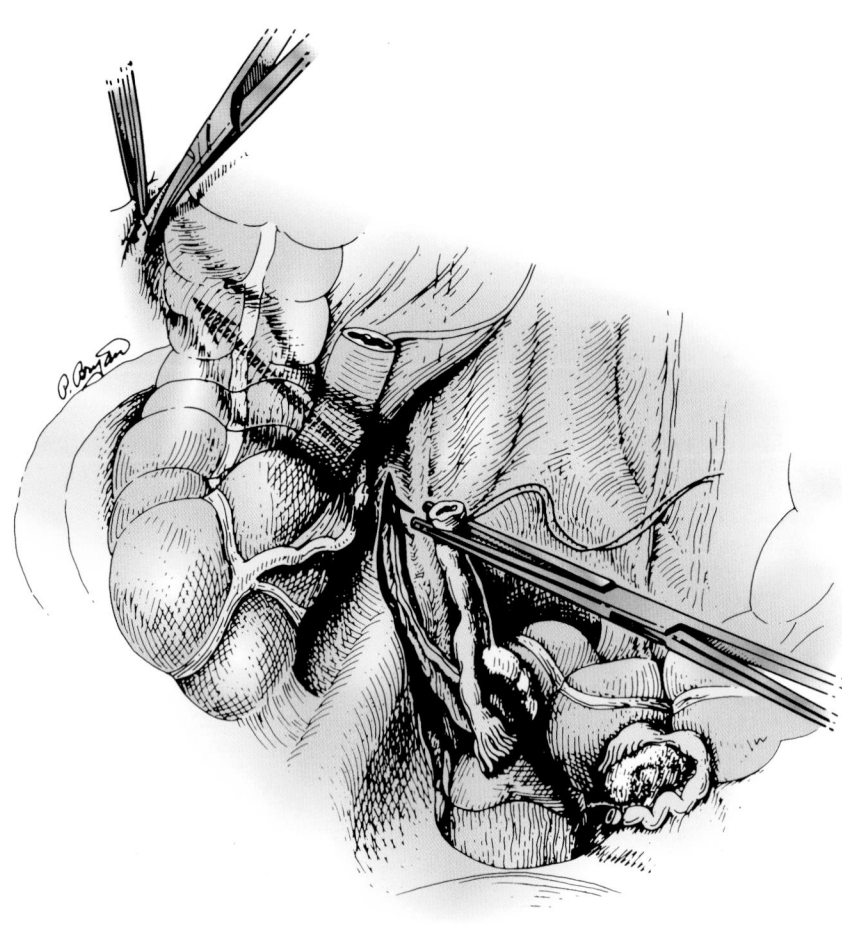

FIGURE 51.27 If the ovaries are to be suspended, a tunnel can be made under the peritoneum and the cecum on the right. The tube and ovary are guided through the tunnel to the new position in the right colic gutter above the pelvis.

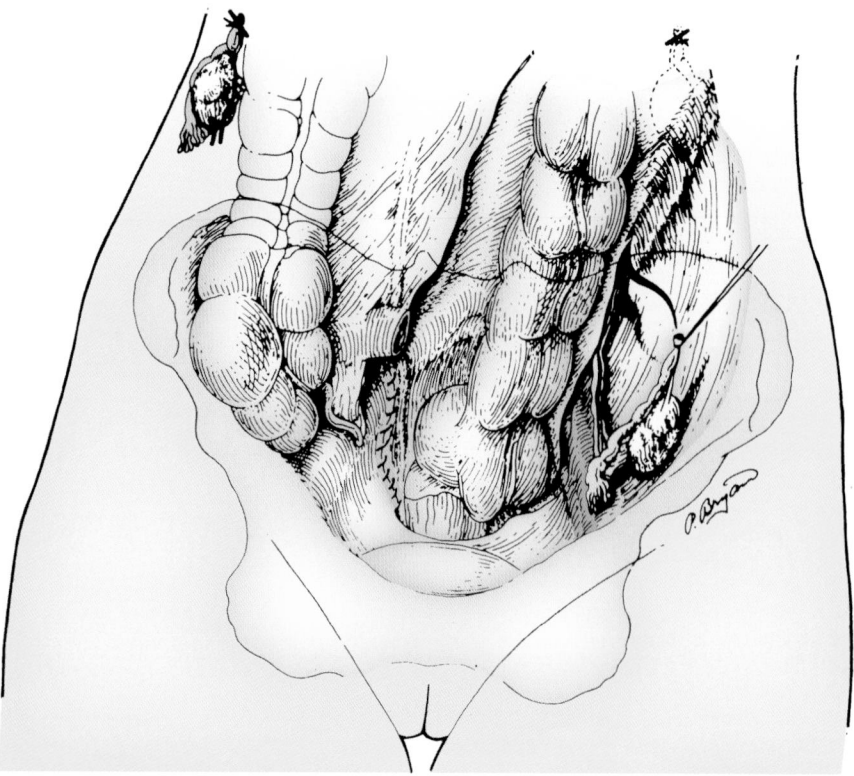

FIGURE 51.28 A similar procedure can be performed on the left. The ovarian vessels should not be twisted. Metal clips are placed on the pedicles to allow later identification with abdominal radiograph.

FERTILITY-SPARING RADICAL ABDOMINAL TRACHELECTOMY

Historically, the recommended surgical treatment for a stage IA2–IB1 cervical cancer is a total radical hysterectomy and pelvic lymphadenectomy. This operation is very effective at treating early-stage cervical cancer; however, infertility is one of the serious and inevitable consequences of treatment. Partial radical organ resection has been accepted in many solid tumors, such as partial gastrectomy, nephrectomy, pneumonectomy, and colectomy to treat malignancies affecting these organs. In gynecologic oncology, partial organ resection with radical abdominal or vaginal trachelectomy and pelvic lymph node dissection are relatively new techniques used in women with early cervical cancer who wish to retain fertility (Table 51.7). This operation and technique are to be distinguished from the radical abdominal trachelectomy, which is occasionally used for resection of retained cervical stump malignancy following a previous supracervical hysterectomy in the setting in which fertility preservation is not an issue. The first reports of abdominal trachelectomy came from Europe in the 1950s by two separate gynecologists—F. Novak and E. Aburel; however, it is the work of D. Dargent in radical vaginal trachelectomy in the early 1990s that revived interest in the abdominal approach, with several investigators, namely, the Budapest team lead by L. Ungar, who started routinely performing the abdominal operation in adult women in 1997. The operation also appeared suited for pediatric cases with cervical cancer in whom the vaginal approach was not feasible; this approach was pioneered by a combined effort of the gynecology and pediatric surgery teams at Memorial Sloan Kettering Cancer Center in New York in 2004.

Technique

A laparotomy and a bilateral complete pelvic lymphadenectomy are performed in a similar manner to a radical abdominal hysterectomy. The limits of nodal dissection are the deep circumflex iliac vein caudally and the proximal common iliac artery cephalad. Any suspicious lymph nodes are sent for frozen section analysis. It is our intent to abandon a fertility-sparing approach if positive lymph nodes are identified. SLN biopsy following a structured algorithm is also a reasonable option and may allow for pathologic ultrastaging of these SLNs. The removal of paraaortic nodes is also considered for select lesions stage IB1 or greater.

TABLE 51.7 Summary of Series Describing Fertility-Sparing Radical Abdominal Trachelectomy

AUTHOR	N[a]	AGE (YEARS)[b]	STAGE	EBL (ML)	COMPLICATIONS	LIVEBIRTHS[a]	RECURRENCE
Smith et al. (1997)	1		IB				
Rodriguez et al. (2001)	3	26.3	IA1–IA2	417	1 abscess	1	0
Palfalvi (2003)	1		IB1			1	
Del Priore et al. (2004)	1	28	IB1				Pelvic at 6 mo
Ungar et al. (2005)	33	30.5	IA2–IB2		6% amenorrhea	2	0, median follow-up, 47 mo
Abu-Rustum et al. (2005)	2	7	IB1		0	0	0
Ungar et al. (2006)	91	30.7	IA2–IB2	656	4.8% amenorrhea	6	2.4%
Cibula et al. (2005)	3		IA2–IB1	350–3,500	1 ileus 1 bladder atony		
Bader et al. (2005)	1	34	IB1			0	1
Abu-Rustum et al. (2006)	5	36	IB1	280	1 needed completion hysterectomy for positive margin	0	0
Li et al. (2011)	62[c]	29.5	IA1–IB1	362	2 infected pelvic lymphocysts 5 cervical stenoses	1	0
Wethington et al. (2012)	101	31	IA1–IB2		12 cervical stenoses 4 lymphocele 4 ileus	16	4

[a]Some patients may be reported more than once.
[b]Mean when calculated.
[c]Three pediatric cases
EBL, estimated blood loss.

IX

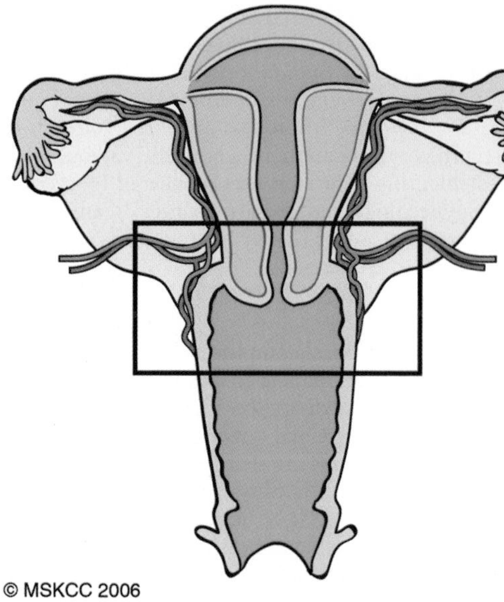

© MSKCC 2006

FIGURE 51.29 Diagrammatic representation of the tissue renewed at radical abdominal trachelectomy.

The intent of the radical abdominal trachelectomy is to resect the cervix, upper 1 to 2 cm of the vagina, parametrium, and paracolpos in a similar manner to a type C1 nerve-sparing radical abdominal hysterectomy while preserving the uterine fundus or corpus (**Figs. 51.29** and **51.30**).

The procedure is begun by developing the paravesical and pararectal spaces and dissecting the bladder caudal to the midvagina. The round ligaments are divided (some surgeons preserve the round ligaments), and large Kelly clamps are placed on the medial round ligaments to manipulate the uterus. Care is taken not to destroy the cornu or the utero-ovarian pedicles. The infundibulopelvic ligaments, with ovarian blood supply,

are kept intact. Care is also taken not to injure the fallopian tubes or disrupt the utero-ovarian ligament.

The uterine vessels are then ligated and divided at their origin from the hypogastric vessels. The parametria and paracolpos with uterine vessels are mobilized medially with the specimen, and a complete ureterolysis is performed similar to a type C1 radical abdominal hysterectomy. The posterior cul-de-sac peritoneum is incised and the uterosacral ligament divided; similarly, the parametria and paracolpos are divided. Using a vaginal cylinder (Apple Medical Corporation; Marlborough, MA), the desired length of vaginectomy is performed, and the specimen is completely separated from the vagina and placed in the midpelvis, keeping its attachment to the utero-ovarian ligaments.

The lower uterine segment is then estimated, and clamps are placed at the level of the internal os (**Fig. 51.31**). Using a knife, the radical trachelectomy is completed by separating the fundus from the isthmus or upper endocervix at approximately 5 mm below the level of the internal os, if possible (**Figs. 51.32** and **51.33**).

The uterine fundus with preserved attachments to the utero-ovarian ligaments, placed in the superior part of the pelvis, and the specimen, consisting of radical trachelectomy and parametria with suture marking the vaginal cuff at 12 o'clock, are sent for frozen section evaluation of its endocervical margin. The uterine fundus is inspected, and curettage of the endometrial cavity is performed as well as a shave disc margin on the remaining cervical tissue, which is sent for frozen section analysis (**Fig. 51.34**). This is performed to ensure that the reconstructed uterus to the vagina is disease free. A frozen section analysis is also obtained on the distal vaginal margin, if clinically indicated.

If all frozen sections tested are benign and at least a 5-mm clear margin is obtained on the endocervical edge, a permanent cerclage with no. 0 Ethibond or no. 0 GoreTex suture (knot tied posteriorly) may be placed before the reconstruction (**Fig. 51.35**). Some surgeons do not recommend cerclage. The uterus is then reattached to the upper vagina with six to eight no. 2-0 absorbable sutures (**Figs. 51.36–51.38**).

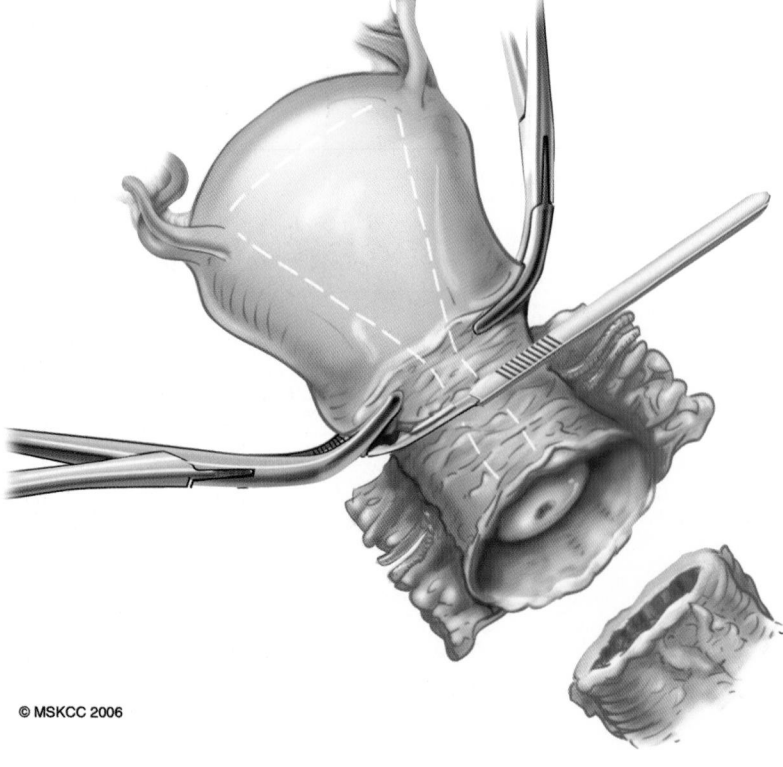

© MSKCC 2006

FIGURE 51.30 The intent of the radical abdominal trachelectomy is to resect the cervix, upper 1 to 2 cm of the vagina, parametrium, and paracolpos in a similar manner to a type III radical abdominal hysterectomy but sparing the uterine corpus.

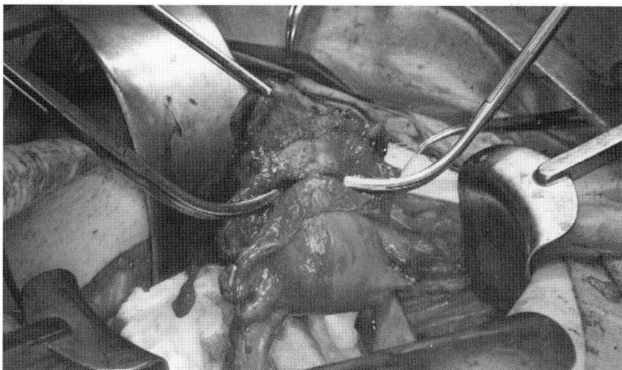

FIGURE 51.31 The uterus is separated from the vagina and remains attached to the adnexa and utero-ovarian vessels.

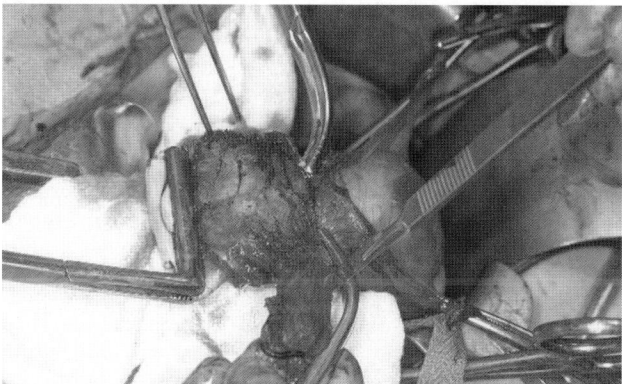

FIGURE 51.32 The radical abdominal trachelectomy incision is done at or just below the internal os, ideally preserving 5 mm or so of upper endocervix.

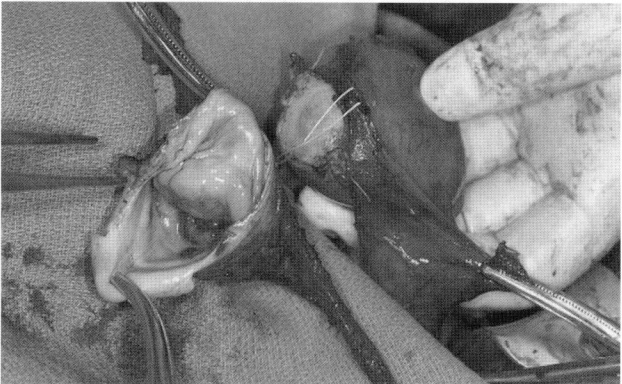

FIGURE 51.33 Radical abdominal trachelectomy: The cervical tissue and parametria are separated from the fundus.

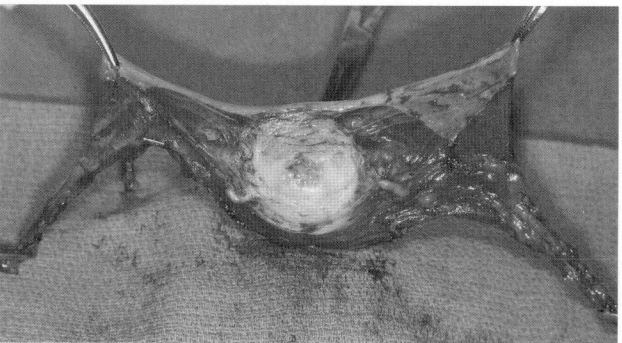

FIGURE 51.34 Radical abdominal trachelectomy specimen showing endocervical margin and uterine vessels with parametria. Endometrial and upper endocervical curettage as well as a shave margin on the remaining uterine tissue is sent for frozen section analysis before reconstruction.

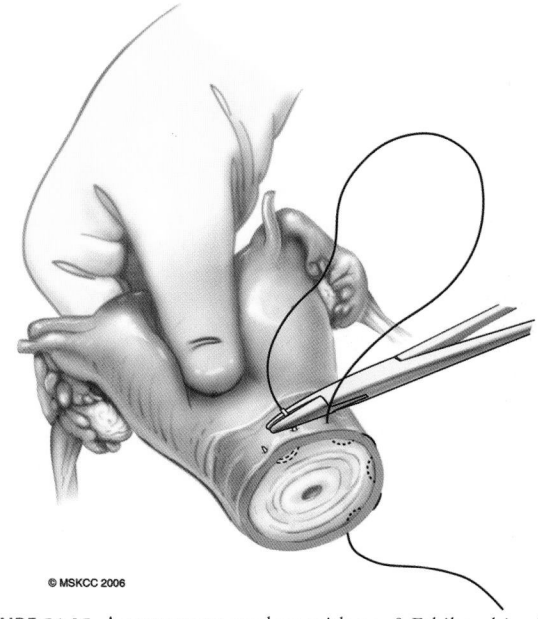

© MSKCC 2006

FIGURE 51.35 A permanent cerclage with no. 0 Ethibond is placed and the knot tied posteriorly.

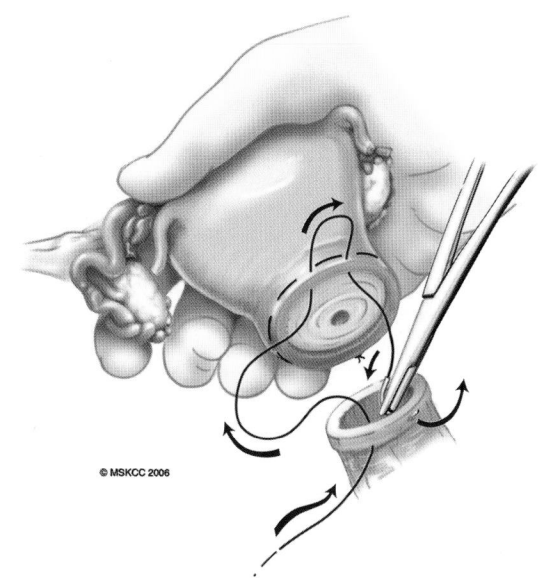

© MSKCC 2006

FIGURE 51.36 Reconstruction of the uterine corpus to upper vagina after the cerclage is placed.

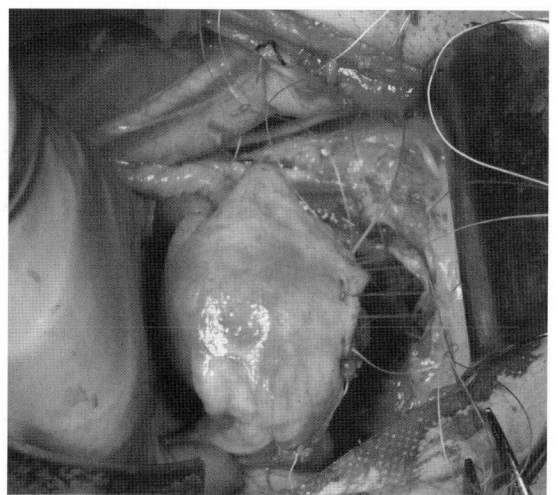

FIGURE 51.37 The uterine fundus is reattached to the vaginal apex with six to eight interrupted no. 2-0 absorbable sutures.

IX

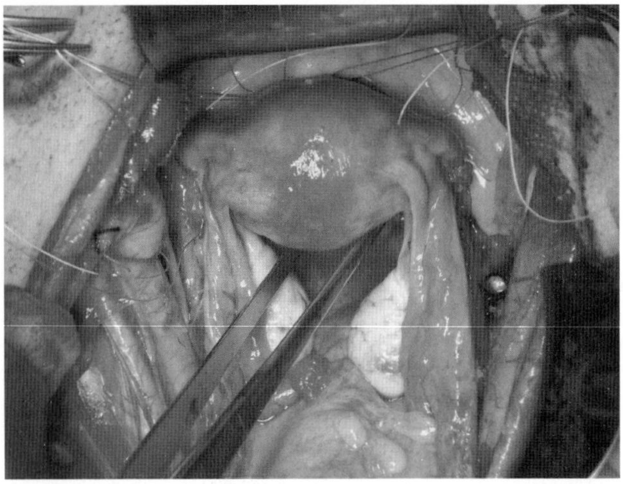

FIGURE 51.38 The reconstructed fundus with remaining blood supply from the intact utero-ovarian ligaments: uterine serosa without evidence of fundal ischemia.

No drains are placed. Standard antibiotic prophylaxis and routine postoperative care is prescribed. We do not routinely place a stent or IUD into the uterus, but some investigators suggest it may help reduce the risk of postoperative stenosis; however, neocervical stenosis can occur beyond 6 weeks postsurgery, and such short-term devices used in the immediate post-op weeks are unlikely to affect that outcome. Use of vaginal dilators starting at 6 weeks post-op may help reduce the extent of upper vaginal agglutination around the neocervix.

An alternative approach to performing the operation, similar to what Aburel described, is to separate the fundus from the cervix before the colpotomy, pack the fundus with the intact utero-ovarian blood supply in the upper pelvis, place retraction clamps on the cervix, and perform the radical trachelectomy. The role of cystourethroscopy with bilateral temporary ureteral catheterization is optional.

LAPAROSCOPICALLY ASSISTED RADICAL VAGINAL HYSTERECTOMY (SCHAUTA)

History

The "extended" hysterectomy performed vaginally for the treatment of cervical cancer was invented by Schauta in Austria in 1901. A few years earlier, in 1898, also in Austria, Wertheim had reported on the abdominal extended hysterectomy. The mortality and morbidity of the Wertheim method was initially much higher, but it had the advantage of including a pelvic lymphadenectomy, which is now appreciated as an important and necessary part of the procedure. Because the initial Schauta operation did not include the lymph node assessment, it gradually became less popular. In 1959, Mitra combined the Schauta operation with a retroperitoneal approach for the pelvic lymphadenectomy. This was a clever idea, but it did not gain a lot of acceptance because it necessitated bilateral flank incisions. More recently, in 1987, Dargent revived the Schauta operation by combining it with laparoscopic surgery, allowing thorough and complete pelvic lymphadenectomy. The Schauta operation preceded by a laparoscopic pelvic lymphadenectomy is thus a perfect example of the recent trend toward minimally invasive surgery in gynecologic oncology.

Technique

Laparoscopic Part of the Surgery

Pelvic Lymphadenectomy The procedure begins with a complete laparoscopic pelvic lymphadenectomy using a 4-trocar technique, as detailed in the laparoscopic surgical staging section below. In the future, if SLN mapping proves acceptable to gynecologic oncologists, the extent of the lymphadenectomy may be further minimized to the removal of only the SLNs.

Division of the Uterine Artery Caudally to the crossing point of the uterine artery, an opening is created bluntly just under the superior vesical artery, which is then retracted laterally in such a way that the uterine vessels lie between the two openings created. Once the uterine artery is divided, the stump can be retracted medially and freed gently from the ureter. This will facilitate the dissection of the uterine artery vaginally. Of note, several collaterals of the uterine artery are frequently encountered and should be clipped, excised, or cauterized individually to avoid bleeding. The vaginal branch of the uterine artery is also frequently seen appearing under the excised uterine artery. It can be divided now or later during the vaginal excision of the parametrial tissue. Lastly, the uterine veins are usually located under the artery and again should be managed individually. On occasion, uterine veins cross over the ureter and can be the source of bleeding during the vaginal part of the surgery.

Vaginal Part of the Surgery

The vaginal part of the surgery can be divided into five steps: (a) vaginal cuff preparation, (b) anterior phase (opening of the vesicouterine space and paravesical space and mobilization and dissection of the ureter), (c) posterior phase (opening of the cul-de-sac and pararectal space and excision of the paracolpos), (d) lateral phase (excision of the parametrium), and (e) excision of the specimen and closure.

Vaginal Cuff Preparation Because the radical vaginal hysterectomy is primarily offered to women with cervical lesions less than 3 cm, it is rarely necessary to remove more than 1 cm of vaginal mucosa. A rim of vaginal mucosa is delineated circumferentially clockwise around the cervix with six to eight straight Kocher clamps placed at regular intervals, about 1 cm below the cervix (**Fig. 51.39**).

To reduce bleeding from the edges of the vaginal mucosa, a 10- to 20-mL solution of xylocaine 1% mixed with epinephrine 1:100,000 is injected between each Kocher clamp, and then a circumferential incision is made with the scalpel just above the Kocher clamp (**Fig. 51.40**). The anterior and posterior edges of the vaginal mucosa are grasped with four to six Chrobak clamps to completely cover the cervix.

Anterior Phase (Described for the Patient's Right Side)

OPENING OF THE VESICOUTERINE SPACE While pulling the specimen slightly downward with the Chrobak clamps, a single-tooth forceps is used to hold and retract the anterior vaginal mucosa, which usually creates a triangular fold indicating where to cut (**Fig. 51.41**). The vesicouterine space is opened with Metzenbaum scissors held perpendicular to the cervix in the midline to avoid bleeding from the bladder pillars laterally. The space is further defined and stretched by gentle dissection with the index finger. Care is taken not to enter the anterior peritoneum as in a simple vaginal hysterectomy as

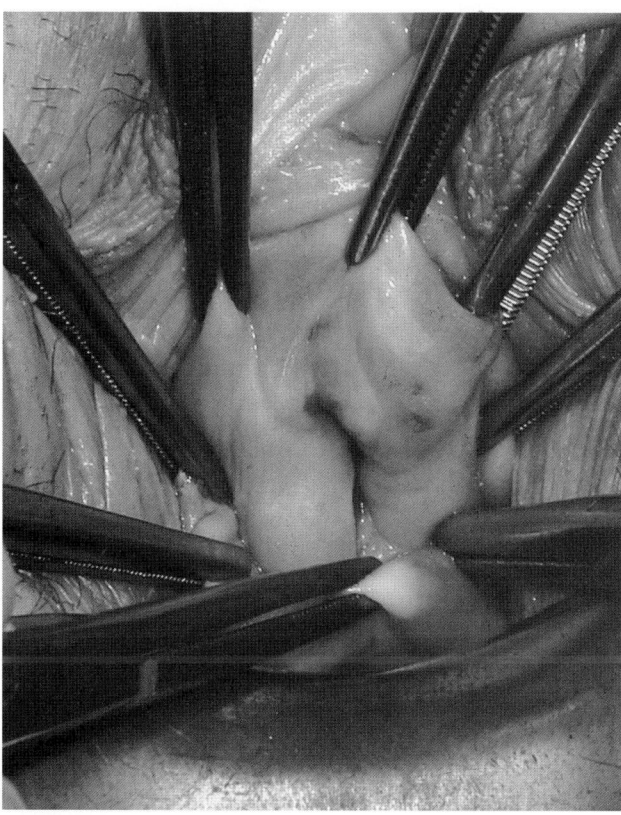

FIGURE 51.39 A vaginal cuff is prepared to remove about 1 to 2 cm of vaginal mucosa.

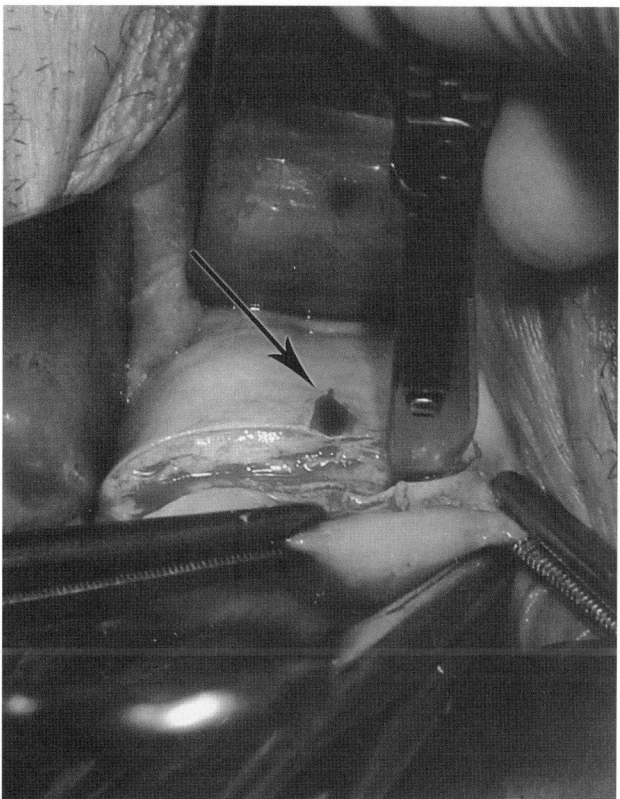

FIGURE 51.40 Section of the anterior vaginal mucosa, with the 12-o'clock mark (*arrow*).

it makes identification of the bladder base and ureters more difficult. If entered correctly, the space should be avascular, and the anterior surface of the endocervix and isthmus should be easily identified without resistance. If resistance is encountered, it usually means that the plane of dissection is either too posterior and that the surgeon is digging into the endocervix, or too anterior, which carries a risk of damage to the bladder. For that reason, the bladder base should be carefully delineated. In patients who have had a recent conization, there may be substantial fibrosis and scarring between the cervix and the bladder base. The opening of the vesicouterine space may be particularly difficult in those cases. In such situations, a metal bladder catheter introduced in the urethra may be used to locate the bladder base and facilitate its mobilization. Once clearly identified, the vesicouterine space is stretched upward with a narrow Deaver retractor, showing the intact peritoneum (**Fig. 51.42**).

OPENING OF THE PARAVESICAL SPACE To open the right paravesical space, the Chrobak clamps are slightly pulled toward the patient's right side. Straight Kocher clamps are placed onto the vaginal mucosa at 11 and 9 o'clock and stretched out (this is where the 12-o'clock mark made earlier is useful). This maneuver defines a triangle formed by the bladder pillars, the vaginal mucosa, and the Chrobak clamps. An areolar opening is seen just medial and slightly anterior to the 9-o'clock clamp, indicating where to enter to define the paravesical space. The space is blindly entered by opening and closing Metzenbaum scissors, with the tips pointing upward and outward in an oblique axis. If entered correctly, the space should be avascular and the scissors should slide inside easily. Once entered, the space is widened by rotating

the scissors under the pubic bone in a semicircular, rotating motion to the patient's left side. A small Breisky retractor is then placed in the space. This step is unquestionably the most "scary" part of the procedure as it is a blind maneuver. Having defined the paravesical space laparoscopically facilitates the entry of the scissors.

IDENTIFICATION AND MOBILIZATION OF THE URETER To palpate the ureter, the Chrobak clamps are pulled to the left of the patient, and the surgeon's right index finger is placed in the vesicouterine space while a Breisky retractor (or the back of the scissors) is placed in the right paravesical space. By pulling down and "rubbing" the finger against the Breisky retractor, the "click" of the ureter rolling under the finger should be heard and felt. This maneuver orients the surgeon as to the location of the ureter in relation to the bladder pillars. Next, with the Breisky retractor placed in the right paravesical space and the narrow Deaver retractor placed in the vesicouterine space, the bladder pillars are clearly identified. The knee of the ureter is normally located on the lateral aspect of the bladder pillars (**Fig. 51.43**).

Once the ureter has been precisely located by palpation, the bladder pillars are excised midway between the bladder base and the endocervix. (Bipolar scissors are useful to decrease bleeding from the bladder pillars.) With the scissors, the medial and lateral pillars of the bladder pillars should be separated first before cutting (**Fig. 51.44**). The most proximal fibers of the pillars can then be excised, and normally, the knee of the ureter should appear anteriorly. At that point, a Babcock clamp is extremely useful to grab the ureter to allow a good traction on it and to constantly keep it under direct visualization. Once the ureter is clearly identified, the medial and lateral

IX

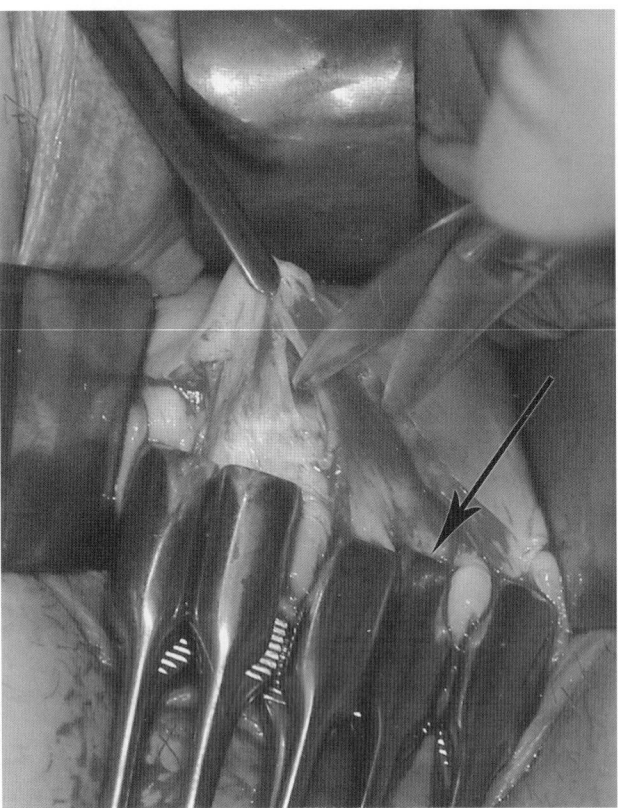

FIGURE 51.41 Opening of the vesicouterine space, with the Chrobak clamps pulling the vaginal cuff.

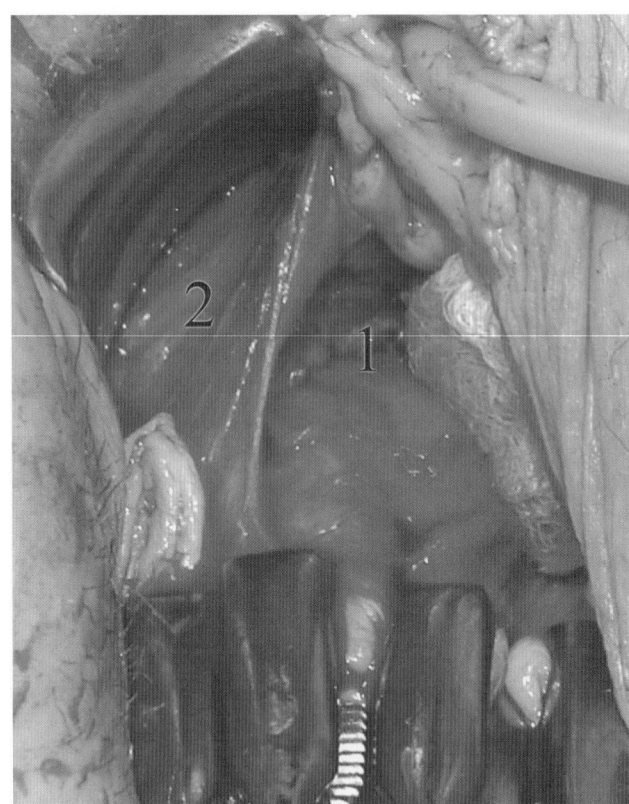

FIGURE 51.43 The right bladder pillars separate the vesicouterine (*1*) and the right paravesical (*2*) spaces.

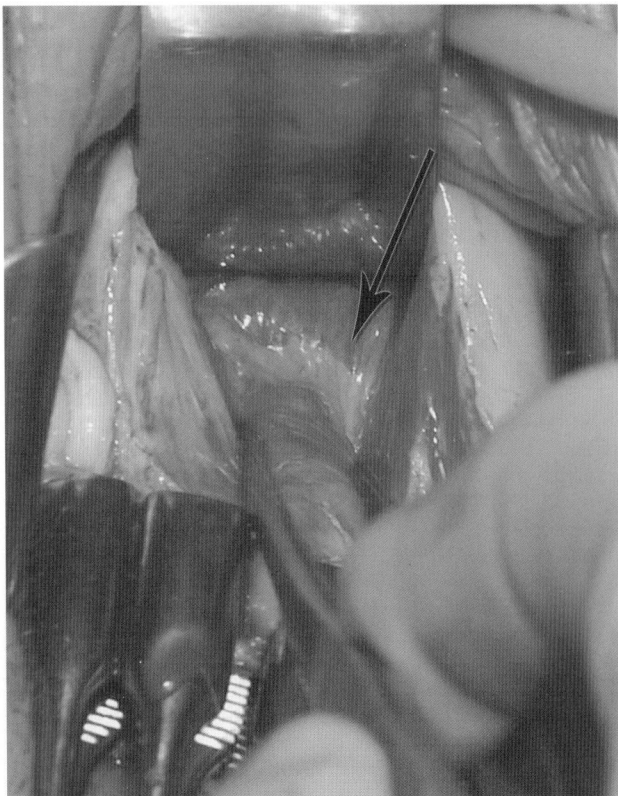

FIGURE 51.42 The vesicovaginal space is open, showing the intact peritoneum (*arrow*).

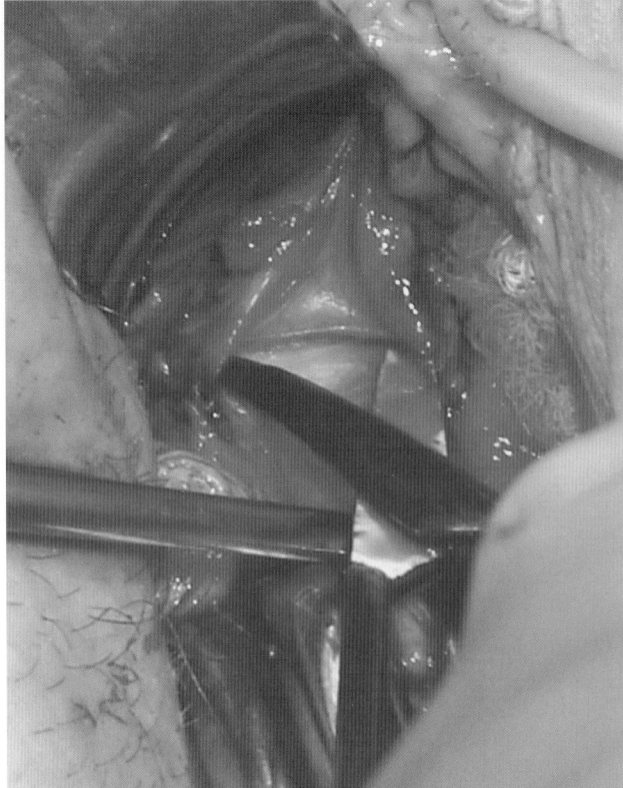

FIGURE 51.44 The ureter is localized by opening the bladder pillars.

bladder pillars are safely excised. If the ureter is not seen unequivocally, it should be palpated again to relocate its position before cutting the pillars.

DISSECTION OF THE URETER Once the ureter is clearly identified and placed under traction with a Babcock clamp, it is possible to dissect the ureter. (It is easier if part of the unroofing has been done laparoscopically.) The uterine vessels are usually seen just under the knee of the ureter (**Fig. 51.45**). With a Kelly clamp, the vessels are pulled down from under the ureter, while at the same time, Metzenbaum scissors are used to free the filmy attachments and allow mobilization of the ureter upward. The uterine artery can be drawn completely into the operative field along with the clips (if they have been used laparoscopically to divide the uterine artery).

Posterior Phase (Described for the Patient's Right Side)
OPENING OF THE CUL-DE-SAC Chrobak clamps are sharply angulated anteriorly, and the posterior cul-de-sac is opened using Metzenbaum scissors as for a simple vaginal hysterectomy. Once entered, the space is stretched laterally to allow placement of a retractor.

OPENING OF THE PARARECTAL SPACE AND EXCISION OF THE UTEROSACRAL LIGAMENTS Using Metzenbaum scissors, the pararectal space is defined by opening a space just lateral to the peritoneal folds of the uterosacral ligaments. The medial or rectouterine fibers of the uterosacral ligaments are separated and excised.

EXCISION OF THE PARACOLPOS To complete the posterior phase preparation, the paracolpos is excised. The paracolpos is the inferior border of the parametrium. With the Chrobak clamps rotated to the left, the paracolpos is clamped just medial to the vaginal mucosa, excised, and ligated.

Lateral Phase (Excision of the Parametrium) Before clamping the parametrium, the paravesical space and the ureter should be relocated. The space is verified by palpation with the finger, and a Breisky retractor is replaced in the paravesical space. The ureter should be readily visible and placed under traction with a Babcock clamp. While the Chrobak clamps are pulled and rotated to the patient's left side, a curved Heaney clamp is placed proximally on the parametrium, and then a second clamp is placed higher and more lateral to obtain wider parametrium. The second Heaney clamp should be placed at the contact of the knee of the ureter, which can be further dissected if needed (**Fig. 51.46**). The parametrial tissue is excised and ligated.

Once completed on the other side, the uterus can now be tilted backward and should only be held by the ovarian ligaments (if the adnexae are preserved) or by residual peritoneal attachments. These can be clamped, excised, and ligated. The specimen is removed (**Fig. 51.47**).

Closure In general, an attempt is made to include the anterior and posterior pelvic peritoneum along with the vaginal mucosa. Interrupted figures-of-eight of Vicryl 2-0 sutures are used for the closure, starting with the lateral angles. No drains are left in place, except for the Foley catheter.

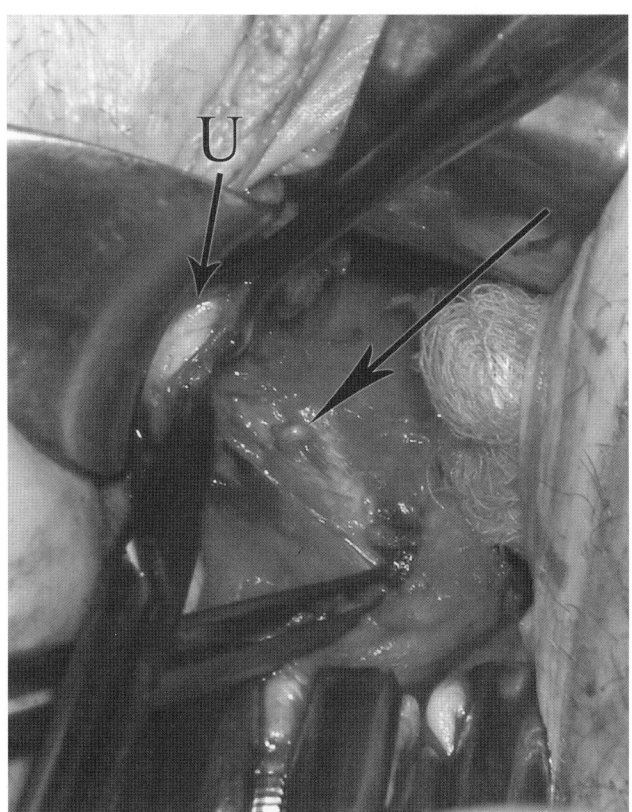

FIGURE 51.45 After dissection of the ureter (*U*), the uterine vessels are seen underneath (*arrow*).

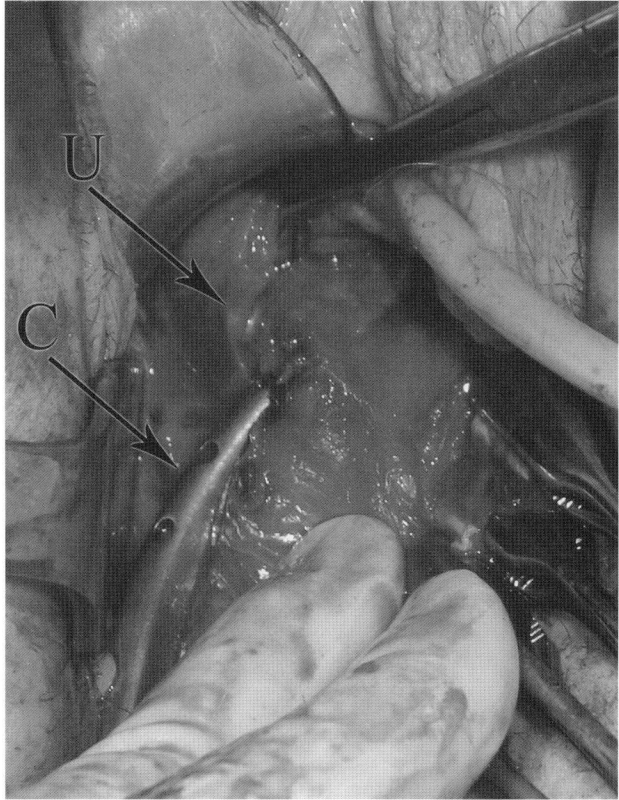

FIGURE 51.46 A clamp (*C*) has been applied to the right parametrium, very close to the ureter (*U*).

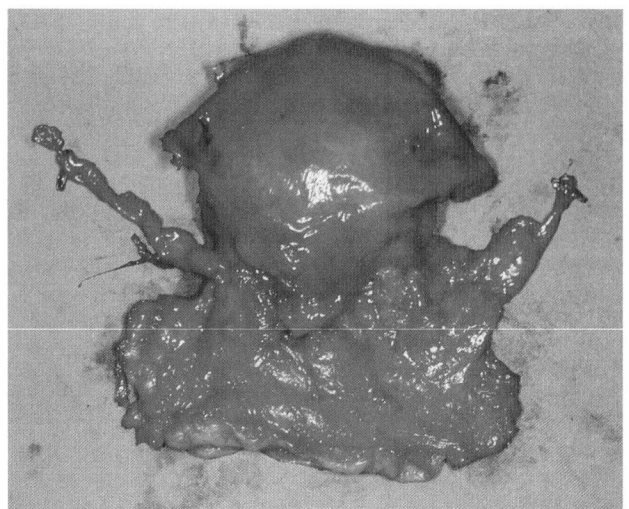

FIGURE 51.47 Specimen with parametrium and uterine arteries.

Results

Over the last two decades, data have been accumulating in the literature to indicate that the laparoscopically assisted radical vaginal hysterectomy is a safe procedure, with an overall low morbidity rate. Several studies—including those of Jackson and associates, Malur and colleagues, Nam and coworkers, Renaud and associates, Roy and colleagues, and Steed and coworkers—compared laparotomy versus laparoscopically assisted vaginal route. In general, the data suggest that the operative time is longer for the laparoscopically assisted vaginal group, but blood loss, transfusion rate, and hospital stay are significantly lower. The lymph node yield is similar between the two groups. Malur even reported a higher lymph node count in the laparoscopically assisted vaginal group. The intraoperative complication rate appears to be higher in the laparoscopically assisted vaginal group, probably related in part to the initial learning curve. In the study by Steed and coworkers, most of the complications were related to bladder and ureteral injuries. However, postoperative complications, such as wound infection and bleeding, tend to be higher in the laparotomy group. Jackson and associates reported the incidence of bladder and bowel dysfunction to be less in the laparoscopically assisted vaginal group, whereas Steed and coworkers found the opposite. Renaud and associates reported that the conversion rate to laparotomy is low. Importantly, there does not appear to be a statistically significant difference in recurrence rate and overall survival, suggesting that the radicality of the vaginal approach is adequate. However, Nam and coworkers noted a higher recurrence rate in the laparoscopically assisted vaginal group in patients with larger tumor volume and concluded that the vaginal approach should be restricted to patients with small tumor (<2 cm).

For larger-sized lesions, Possover and colleagues and Querleu have described a technique to provide extended radicality comparable to that of a type III radical hysterectomy with the idea that it may reduce long-term lateropelvic recurrences. However, the more radical the hysterectomy, the more side effects on bladder and bowel function. In recent years, attention has been paid to this matter, and laparoscopic nerve-sparing surgical techniques have been developed by Querleu and associates to reduce these side effects. However, this extensive paracervical and parametrial dissection is of limited value in patients with small lesions (measuring <2 cm), as the risk of lateropelvic recurrence is low.

LAPAROSCOPICALLY ASSISTED RADICAL VAGINAL TRACHELECTOMY (DARGENT PROCEDURE)

History

In 1987, Dargent proposed a modification of the Schauta-Amreich radical vaginal hysterectomy to preserve the body of the uterus and thus the reproductive function. The procedure, the radical vaginal trachelectomy, today known as the *Dargent procedure*, implies the removal of the cervix along with the proximal portion of the parametrium and is preceded by a complete laparoscopic pelvic lymph node dissection. After nearly three decades, the accumulating experience worldwide summarized by Plante and coworkers suggests that the oncologic outcomes with this conservative procedure are comparable to those obtained following a radical hysterectomy for similarly sized lesions. Obstetrical outcomes are also very encouraging.

Indications

Eligibility criteria for this conservative procedure were initially proposed by Roy and Plante in 1998 and, for the most part, have remained unchanged.

1. Desire to preserve fertility
2. No clinical evidence of impaired fertility (relative contraindication)
3. Lesion size lesser or equal to 2 cm
4. FIGO stage IA1 with presence of vascular space invasion, IA2 and IB1
5. Squamous cell or adenocarcinoma
6. No involvement of the upper endocervical canal as determined by colposcopy or MRI
7. No metastasis to regional lymph nodes

The procedure can be offered to women older than age 40, understanding that the fertility potential is obviously reduced, or to women who already have children, as they may wish to have more children in the future. Sonoda and colleagues reviewed the Memorial Sloan Kettering Cancer Center experience over the course of 10 years and noted that 43% of their patients who underwent a radical hysterectomy for early-stage cervical cancer were younger than 40 years old; of those, 48% would have met the eligibility criteria for a radical trachelectomy. Therefore, a substantial proportion of young women with cervical cancer are potential candidates for this fertility preservation alternative.

Technique

The technique described in this chapter is based on the original technique developed by D. Dargent with modifications by M. Roy. The laparoscopic part of the procedure is identical to that of the Schauta, except that the uterine arteries are obviously not excised. The first three steps of the vaginal part of the surgery are also identical to the Schauta operation (vaginal cuff preparation, anterior phase, and posterior phase). The initial part of the lateral phase—that is, excision of the parametrium—is also identical; however, only the descending branch of the uterine artery is excised. The excision of the trachelectomy specimen and closure also differ from the Schauta operation and will be detailed here.

Lateral Phase (Described for the Patient's Left Side)

Ligation of the Cervicovaginal Artery As opposed to the Schauta operation, in which the uterine artery is clamped at

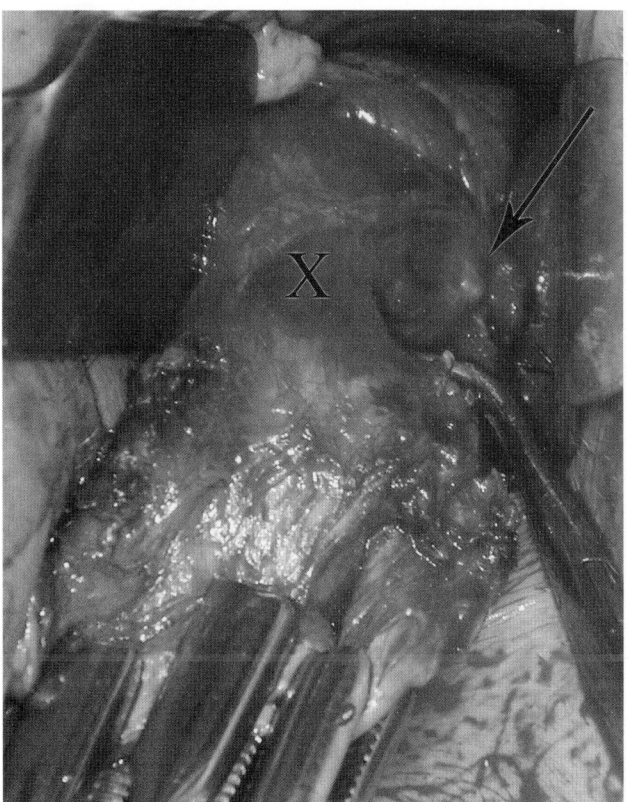

FIGURE 51.48 A clamp is applied just under the arch of the left uterine artery (*arrow*). The uterine isthmic area is visible (*X*).

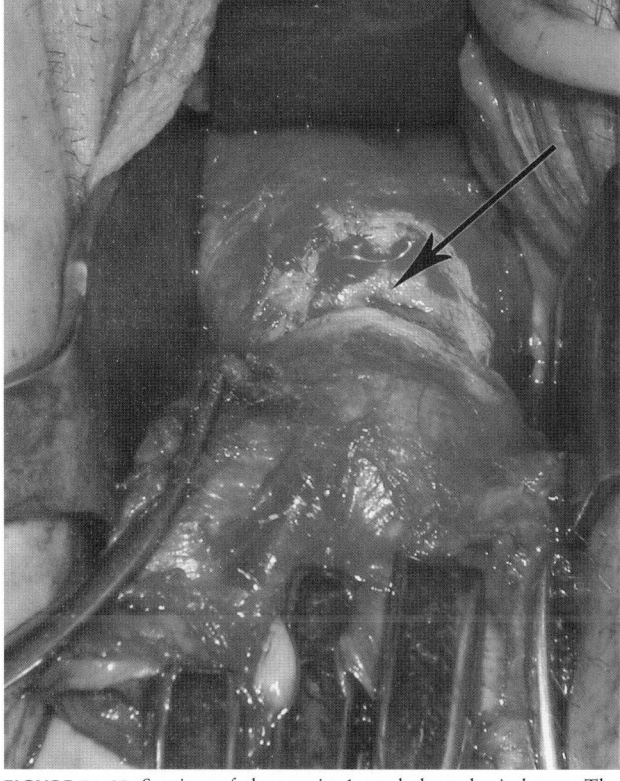

FIGURE 51.49 Section of the cervix 1 cm below the isthmus. The endocervical canal is visible (*arrow*).

its origin, pulled down, and unroofed from under the ureter, the cross of the uterine artery is actually preserved in the case of a trachelectomy to maintain optimal vascularization of the uterus in the event of a future pregnancy. Therefore, only the cervicovaginal or descending branch of the uterine artery is excised. So, after precise localization of the isthmus and the cross of the uterine artery, the cervicovaginal artery is clamped with a right angle clamp placed at 90 degrees and directly applied to the isthmus (**Fig. 51.48**); then it is sectioned and ligated.

Excision of the Specimen and Closure The uterine isthmus and endocervix are precisely located by palpating the uterus anteriorly and posteriorly. The cervix is amputated with a scalpel held perpendicular to the specimen about 1 cm distal to the isthmus (**Fig. 51.49**). As the specimen is excised, the cervical os appears gradually, and the anterior lip can be grasped with a straight Kocher clamp. Care is taken not to angulate the scalpel to avoid removing too much cervix posteriorly. The specimen is completely excised in one piece to facilitate the pathologic evaluation of the margins.

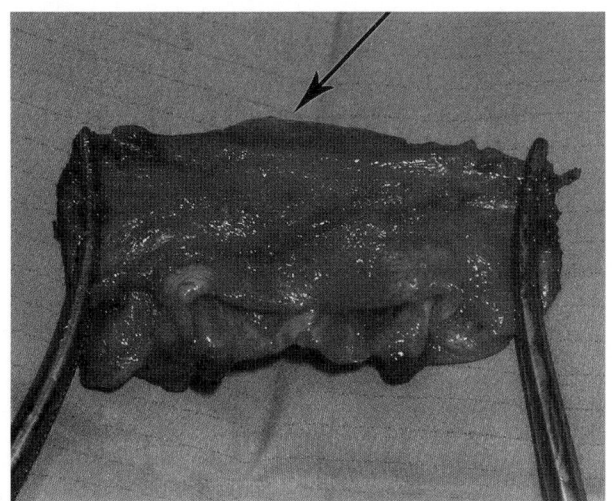

A

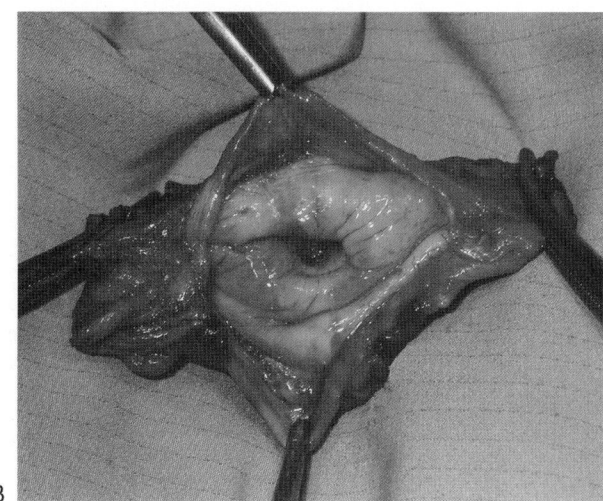

B

FIGURE 51.50 A, B: The specimen with its parametrium. The superior endocervical canal is shown (*arrow*).

IX

Ideally, the specimen should be at least 1 to 2 cm wide, with 1 cm of vaginal mucosa and 1 to 2 cm of parametrium (**Fig. 51.50A, B**). When there is no clinical evidence of residual tumor, a frozen section analysis is not performed. The specimen is kept intact for final analysis and will be processed as a cone specimen. However, in patients with a visible lesion, the trachelectomy specimen is sent for immediate frozen section analysis to assess the level of the tumor in relation to the endocervical resection margin. At least 8 to 10 mm of tumor-free tissue should be obtained between the level of the tumor and the endocervical resection margin; otherwise, additional endocervix should be removed or the trachelectomy should be completed by a radical vaginal hysterectomy (Schauta). It is thus extremely important to ask the pathologist to do a frozen section analysis of the cervix with a section made longitudinally from the ectocervix to the endocervix to evaluate the distance between the most cephalad edge of the tumor and the endocervical resection margin. A permanent cerclage is placed at the level of the isthmus using a nonresorbable Prolene or Ethibond 0 suture starting posteriorly at 6 o'clock to have the knot lying posteriorly. The sutures should not be placed too deeply into the cervical stroma, as the cerclage can eventually erode into the endocervical canal and be expelled. When tying the cerclage knot, a uterine probe can be placed in the cervical os to avoid tightening the knot too much, as this may cause cervical stenosis (**Fig. 51.51**).

The Dargent procedure is completed by reapproximating the edges of the vaginal mucosa to the new exocervix. This is accomplished with interrupted figures-of-eight sutures of 2-0 Vicryl. It is easier to begin with the sutures at 12 and 6 o'clock first. The lateral sutures are then placed separately to include

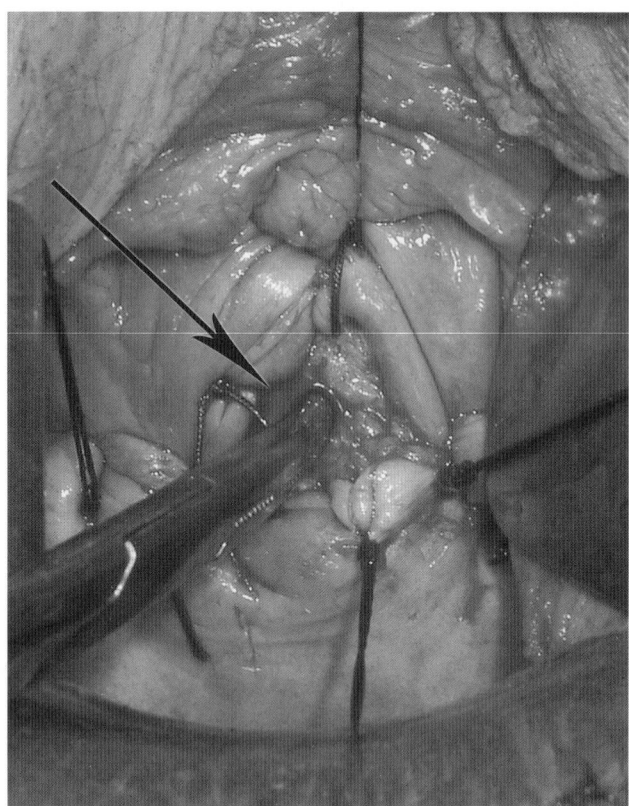

FIGURE 51.52 Suturing the vaginal mucosa to the cervical stroma. A clamp (*arrow*) indicates the endocervical canal.

the anterior and posterior vaginal mucosa only. Although easy to do, the closure of the vaginal mucosa is an extremely important step of the procedure, and care should be taken not to bury the cervical opening into folds of redundant vaginal mucosa (**Fig. 51.52**). The new exocervix should remain accessible for monitoring with colposcopic examination and cytology.

At the end of the trachelectomy procedure, laparoscopy is performed to verify hemostasis in the pelvis and the integrity of the pelvic structures. No drains or packings are left.

Oncologic Outcome of Radical Trachelectomy

Data are accumulating worldwide indicating that the oncologic outcome following the radical trachelectomy is comparable to the outcome following a radical hysterectomy for similar-sized lesions. It should also be emphasized that adenocarcinoma histology and the presence of LVSI are NOT contraindications to offer or consider a fertility-sparing approach. Indeed, several large series consistently report a large percentage of adenocarcinoma cases with LVSI and a recurrence rate of less than 4% and a death rate of less than 2% (**Table 51.8**). Plante and colleagues have noted that the size of the lesion (≥2 cm) and the presence of LVSI seem to be the most important risk factors for recurrences. The recent work of Hertel and coworkers also suggests that adenocarcinomas may carry a higher risk of recurrence, but this is not uniformly agreed upon.

Morice and associates noted unusual sites of recurrences, such as in the vesicovaginal septum and in the bladder, which suggests that very meticulous surgical technique should be observed to avoid entering the wrong planes of dissection and

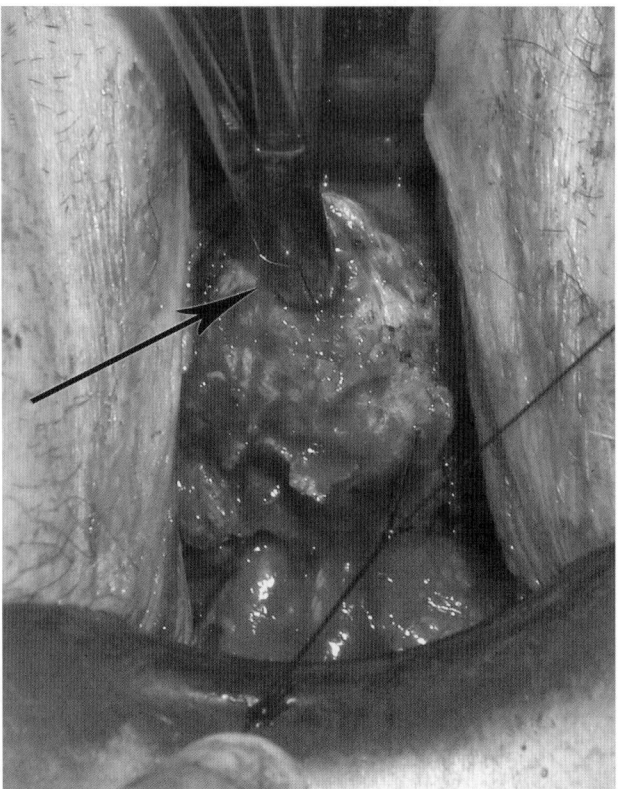

FIGURE 51.51 A cerclage is put in place and ligated posteriorly with a dilator (*arrow*) in the cervical canal.

TABLE 51.8 Oncologic Outcome Postradical Trachelectomy

AUTHORS	NUMBER	RECURRENCES	DEATHS
Plante and Roy	100	2 (2.0%)[a]	1 (1.0%)
Covens and Steed	121	7 (5.8%)	4 (3.3%)
Shepherd et al.	112	3 (2.7%)	2 (1.8%)
Hertel et al.	100	4 (4.0%)	2 (2.0%)
Dargent and Mathevet	95	4 (4.2%)[a]	3 (3.1%)
Ungar et al.[b]	91	2 (2.2%)	0
Diaz	40	1 (2.5%)	1 (2.5%)
Wethington	101	4 (4%)	0
Total	760	27 (3.5%)	13 (1.7%)

[a]Excluding one case of neuroendocrine tumor.
[b]Abdominal radical trachelectomy.

potentially disseminating tumor cells at the time of the procedure. Piketty recently reported a recurrence in the ovary in a patient with an adenocarcinoma. Few recurrences have been reported on the residual cervix itself. The first, which occurred nearly 7 years following the initial surgery, was reported by Bali. It is unclear, however, whether it was a recurrence or a new primary. The other was reported by Bader and coworkers; it occurred 6 months after an abdominal trachelectomy and was picked up on a routine Pap smear. A radical hysterectomy was performed and disclosed a 3-mm recurrence (or persistence) in the cervix.

Ungar and associates and del Priore and colleagues reported two recurrences following the abdominal radical trachelectomy procedure, and both were in patients with bulky lesions: One had a 3.8-cm lesion, and she recurred within 4 months of the surgery with a 6-cm lesion; the other had a 5-cm glassy-cell adenocarcinoma and recurred 14 months after surgery. Strict selection criteria are extremely important to lower the risk of recurrences. Further experience will determine if the abdominal radical trachelectomy is safe in bulky lesions. Another alternative for patients with larger lesions is the use of neoadjuvant chemotherapy to reduce the size of the tumor followed by a fertility-preserving radical trachelectomy. Plante and coworkers have recently published their preliminary experience with three cases. All have had a complete pathologic response to the chemotherapy with no residual cancer in the surgical specimen. Obviously, this approach is currently experimental, but it has potential merits and deserves further investigation.

Shepherd recommends regular follow-ups after trachelectomy, including a colposcopic examination, cytology, and rectovaginal examination every 3 to 4 months for the first 2 to 3 years, every 6 months for the next 2 years, and yearly thereafter. Unfortunately, colposcopy and cytologies are frequently unsatisfactory after trachelectomy because the squamous columnar junction is often not visualized and the cytology frequently contains only squamous cells. Conversely, atypical glandular cells from the lower uterine segment are commonly picked up on the smear and misinterpreted as suspicious for recurrence. Singh and coworkers reported their experience with nearly 200 smears posttrachelectomy and concluded that a high proportion of the smears were unsatisfactory; 2% of the smears were reported as suspicious and, in fact, represented atypical endometrial cells, but two patients recurred and retrospectively had abnormal smears long before the recurrence was diagnosed. Reports of cytology posttrachelectomy should thus be interpreted with caution. Shepherd and coworkers recommend the use of an endocervical cytobrush for the cytology and an MRI at 6, 12, and 24 months postsurgery. The superb work by Sahdev and associates emphasizes the fact that radiologists interpreting those MRIs should be very well aware of the anatomical changes posttrachelectomy, as some of the changes may be misinterpreted as cancer recurrences.

Obstetric Outcome

The collected data on obstetric outcome are also very promising. As seen in Table 51.9, there have been hundreds of pregnancies reported from the same groups of investigators, mostly with the vaginal but increasingly with the abdominal approach. In general, the rate of first-trimester miscarriage does not seem to be higher than in the general population, at approximately 16%. It is interesting to note that even though women undergoing a radical trachelectomy do so to preserve their fertility, there is a surprising 4% rate of elective pregnancy termination. The rate of second-trimester losses is higher than in the general population (8%). Overall, 66% to 75% of all pregnancies reach the third trimester. Of those, approximately 15% will end with significant prematurity at less than 32 weeks of gestation. Luckily, less than 10% will deliver before 28 weeks, when most of the severe neonatal morbidities and mortalities occur. Of note, multiple pregnancies appear to be at a particularly high risk of severe prematurity posttrachelectomy, and this should be taken into consideration when discussing in vitro fertilization in patients with infertility. Overall, 85% of the pregnancies reaching the third trimester will evolve normally beyond 32 weeks, and the majority will actually deliver at term (>37 weeks of gestation). The work of Klemm and colleagues suggests that there is no evidence that birth weight of newborns delivered from women who had a trachelectomy is lower. They showed that the vascular flow to the uterine artery before and after vaginal trachelectomy is well preserved.

The etiology of the second-trimester losses and the preterm deliveries is considered mechanical and/or infectious. Indeed, the short cervix probably does not offer as much support to the lower uterine segment. As the uterus enlarges and gets heavier, the cervix is more likely to dilate prematurely. However, the main etiology is felt to be infectious. Indeed, the shortened cervix after the trachelectomy procedure seems to prevent the formation of an efficacious mucus plug. The mucus plug is thought to play an important role as a physiologic barrier between the vaginal flora and the membranes to prevent ascending infections. Hence, the subclinical chorioamnionitis is thought to be responsible for the premature rupture of membranes and premature labor. Plante and associates proposed some guidelines for the follow-up of these high-risk pregnancies. A consultation with a specialist in fetal–maternal medicine is recommended. The value of prophylactic antibiotic coverage—as well as steroid injections to accelerate fetal lung maturity near term—is unclear, although Shepherd and colleagues strongly recommend it. The work of Berghella and coworkers showed that serial transvaginal ultrasound is the best modality for the follow-up of cervical length in the general obstetric

IX

TABLE 51.9 Obstetrical Outcome Post–Radical Trachelectomy

AUTHOR	PREGANCY	T-1[a] MISCARRIAGE	TAB[b]	T-2 MISCARRIAGE	T-3 DELIVERY	DELIVERY <32 WK	DELIVERY >32 WK
Plante and Roy	59	10 (16%)	3 (4%)	2 (5%)	44 (75%)	3 (7%)	41 (93%)
Dargent and Mathevet	56	11 (18%)[c]	3 (5%)	8 (14%)	34 (61%)	5 (15%)	29 (85%)
Shepherd et al.	52	15 (29%)	2 (4%)	7 (13%)	28 (54%)	7 (25%)	21 (75%)
Covens and Bernardini	45	8 (16%)	0	3 (7%)	34 (77%)	6 (18%)[d]	28 (82%)
Hertel et al.[e]	14	1 (7%)	2 (14%)	0	11 (78%)	3 (27%)	8 (73%)
Ungar et al.[f]	10	4 (40%)	0	0	6 (60%)	1 (17%)	5 (83%)
Kim et al.	27	1 (4%)	3 (11%)	3 (12%)	20 (74%)	0	20 (100%)
Total	263	50 (19%)	13 (5%)	23 (9%)	177 (67%)	25 (14%)	152 (86%)

[a]T-1, first trimester; T-2, second trimester; T-3, third trimester.
[b]TAB, therapeutic abortions.
[c]Includes two ectopic.
[d]Includes 6 sets of twins.
[e]Personal communication, April 2006.
[f]Abdominal radical trachelectomy.

population and has been used in the follow-up of pregnant women posttrachelectomy. If the pregnancy evolves normally, delivery is planned at 38 to 39 weeks of gestation. Because of the permanent cerclage, women should be delivered by elective cesarean section.

Outcomes of pregnancy following an abdominal trachelectomy also appear promising. Although the numbers are smaller, Ungar and coworkers reported 10 pregnancies, with results comparable to pregnancies after the vaginal approach. There was concern that ligating the uterine arteries at the time of the procedure might have an impact on the vascularization of the uterus and potentially lead to intrauterine growth retardation. So far, the data seem reassuring in that regard, particularly after a recent publication by Wethington of an international series of abdominal trachelectomy with robust fertility outcomes, similar to those of the vaginal approach.

Conclusion

Based on the collected data available, the radical trachelectomy truly offers a valuable alternative to young women with small, early-stage cervical cancer who wish to preserve their fertility. Oncologic outcomes are comparable to standard radical hysterectomy for similar-sized lesions, and the complication rate is low. Pregnancies are possible after this procedure, and overall obstetrical outcome is good despite the rate of second-trimester loss and premature delivery. In the last three decades, there has been a tremendous shift toward minimally invasive surgical techniques in gynecologic oncology. Laparoscopic, robotic, and radical vaginal/abdominal fertility-sparing surgeries have revolutionized the surgical management of cervical cancer. The radical trachelectomy (Dargent operation) is unquestionably the most important surgical development in the treatment of early-stage cervical

cancer in the last century. Importantly, in 2013, the NCCN cervical cancer management guidelines began dedicating a full panel for the surgical treatment options of women with stage IA1–IB1 cervical cancer who wish to preserve fertility and included a conization or trachelectomy as a standard of care in select women.

TOTAL LAPAROSCOPIC AND ROBOTIC RADICAL HYSTERECTOMY WITH LYMPHADENECTOMY

Laparoscopic radical hysterectomy with pelvic and aortic lymph node dissection was first reported by Nezhat in 1992. This technically challenging procedure initially was received with caution by gynecologic oncologists who have used the abdominal radical hysterectomy as the traditional approach for decades. So far, there have not been any reported randomized trials to compare these two surgical approaches; however, such a trial is currently ongoing, and there have been hundreds of reported cases worldwide, with encouraging results. Well-recognized, pioneer work was undertaken by Spirtos and associates, who described 78 consecutive patients, all with early cervical cancer and a Quetelet body mass index less than 35, who underwent the procedure. In all, 94% of the procedures were completed laparoscopically, with an average operative time of 205 minutes and an average blood loss of 225 mL, with only one patient (1.3%) requiring transfusion. There was one ureterovaginal fistula documented. The average lymph node count was 34, with 11.5% of patients having positive lymph nodes. Three patients (3.8%) had close or positive surgical margins, and 5.1% recurred with a minimum of 3 years of follow-up. Table 51.10 summarizes reports on laparoscopic radical hysterectomy with pelvic and aortic lymphadenectomy.

IX

TABLE 51.10 Summary of Initial Reports on Laparoscopic Radical Hysterectomy and Lymphadenectomy

AUTHOR	N[a]	PLN	ORT (MIN)	EBL (ML)	LOS (DAYS)	COMPLICATIONS	RECURRENCES
Nezhat et al. (1992, 1993)	7	22	315	30–250	2.1	None	None
Sedlacek et al. (1994, 1995)	14	16	420	334	5.5	1 VVF, 1 ureteral injury	—
Ting (1994)	4	8	330–480	150–500	—	None	—
Osterzenski (1996)	6	—	280	—	2–6	1 hydronephrosis	—
Spirtos et al. (1996)	10	18.3	253	300	3.2	None	—
Kim and Moon (1998)	18	22	363	619	—	None	—
Hsieh et al. (1998)	8	—	—		6.5	None	1 distant
Spirtos (2002)	78	23.8	205	250	2.9	1.3% transfusion, 3 cystotomies, 1 UVF, 1 DVT 5 conversions	8 (10.3%)
Lee (2002)	12	19.2	235	428	6.8	2 transfusion	None at 1 y
Lin (2003)	10	—	—	250	4.1	None	—
Obemair (2003)	55	—	210	200	5	3 vascular, 1 nerve, 1 fistula	None
Pomel (2003)	50	13.2	258	—	7.5	1 bladder fistula, 1 ureter stenosis	5-y survival 96%
Abu-Rustum (2003)	19	25.5	371	301	4.5	1 transfusion, 2 conversion, 1 fever	None
Gil-Moreno (2005)	27	19.1	—	400	5	—	None

[a]Some patients may be reported more than once.
N, number of patients; PLN, mean pelvic lymph nodes; ORT, mean operating room time; EBL, mean estimated blood loss; LOS, mean hospital stay; VVF, vesicovaginal fistula; UVF, ureterovaginal fistula; DVT, deep venous thrombosis.

Total Laparoscopic or Robotic Radical Hysterectomy

One technique of the laparoscopic radical hysterectomy is well described by Spirtos and associates and Chen and colleagues. The laparoscopic approach uses different surgical instruments and techniques than the classic approach to accomplish the same procedure performed via laparotomy. The technique of laparoscopic radical hysterectomy described in this section relies on the use of the monopolar electrosurgical devices and vessel-sealing instruments or bipolar traditional graspers. The robotic platform brought much improvement in ergonomics and visualization and helped popularize the use of laparoscopy in radical hysterectomy, but the energy sources and technology remain similar to the laparoscopic counterpart and all pneumoperitoneum-based surgery. Four to six trocars are needed, with the camera near the umbilical site. The retroperitoneum is opened and the round ligaments coagulated. The paravesical and pararectal spaces are developed with monopolar devices, and the ureter is clearly identified. Resection of the adnexa is managed on an individual basis as per the open approach. The uterine artery is identified after developing the pararectal and paravesical spaces, and the umbilical ligament is isolated. The uterine artery and vein are sealed and divided. The bladder flap is then developed. The posterior cul-de-sac peritoneum is incised and the rectouterine ligaments exposed. The ureter is then unroofed from the parametria by placing medial traction on the stapled uterine artery stump, and the bladder is dissected further inferiorly. The uterosacral/rectouterine ligaments are divided, and the ureter is retracted laterally to resect the desired length of parametria. Anterior colpotomy is performed at the desired vaginal length. A vaginal probe facilitates stretching the vagina for easier incision. The remaining parametria and paracolpos are resected with monopolar devices. The specimen is removed vaginally with a single-tooth tenaculum, and the vaginal cuff is closed laparoscopically with endoscopic sutures. The placement of ureteral catheters or stents to facilitate ureteric manipulation is optional. The pelvic and aortic lymphadenectomy is performed, as described. Pelvic drains usually are not necessary, and a suprapubic catheter is optional.

IX

LAPAROSCOPIC SURGICAL STAGING

Currently available clinical staging methods and imaging studies are not completely accurate in the detection of pelvic and aortic lymph node metastasis from cervical cancer, and pathologic evaluation of retroperitoneal lymph nodes remains the gold standard for establishing metastasis. In addition, identifying retroperitoneal nodal metastasis may alter the overall therapeutic approach and affect the patient's prognosis.

Laparoscopic surgical staging with pelvic and aortic lymph node dissection for cervical cancer was initially reported by Querleu in France. Since that initial report, many investigators have adopted the laparoscopic pretreatment surgical approach and continue to modify the technical details of the procedure. It is well established at this point that transperitoneal or extraperitoneal laparoscopic pelvic and aortic lymph node dissection for cervical cancer, in experienced hands, is feasible, yields similar results as the open approach, and is associated with low morbidity. Furthermore, this approach may provide valuable information that is not available using clinical staging techniques. Computed tomography was able to detect retroperitoneal nodal metastasis in only 17% to 57% of cervical cancer patients staged laparoscopically. Table 51.11 summarizes selected reports on laparoscopic pelvic and aortic lymph node dissection in the management of stage I to IV cervical cancer.

Laparoscopic Surgical Staging Technique

The technique of laparoscopic surgical staging continues to evolve as experience with this minimally invasive approach increases; the introduction of the robotic approach has added to this evolution, although the principles of this procedure are similar to those of the laparoscopic approach, except whether the nodes are approached transperitoneally or extraperitoneally. Therefore, these are the two main approaches: the transperitoneal approach and the extraperitoneal approach (popularized by Querleu and Dargent from France). For the transperitoneal approach, four laparoscopic trocars usually are needed (Fig. 51.53): 10-mm trocars in the umbilical and suprapubic regions and 5-mm trocars just medial to the iliac crest on each side. For the aortic nodal dissection, the laparoscope is placed in the suprapubic region, and the monitors are moved cephalad. For the pelvic lymphadenectomy, the laparoscope is placed in the umbilical region, and the monitors are placed caudal. A variety of endoscopic tools may be used with similar results. The selection usually is based on the surgeon's preference and experience. Both monopolar and bipolar currents are available, and a wide variety of endoscopic dissecting instruments, clip appliers, and specimen retrieval devices are available. A retroperitoneal nodal dissection may be satisfactorily completed in the majority of cases with the aid of a tissue grasper and an endoscopic clip applier or vessel-sealing device.

TABLE 51.11 Summary of Pretreatment Laparoscopic Pelvic and Aortic Lymph Node Dissection in the Management of Stage I to IV Cervical Cancer

AUTHOR	N	STAGE	PLN (% +)	PAN (% +)	ORT	HD	COMPLICATIONS
Querleu (1991)	39	IB–IIB	8.7 (12.8%)	—	90	1	3 minor
Childers (1993)	18	IB–IVA	31.4 (both) (33.3%)	(6.2%)	75–175	1.5	Not significant
Fowler (1993)	12	IB	23.5 (16.7%)	6.5 (0%)	373 With laparotomy	7.4 With laparotomy	2 minor
Su (1995)	38	—	15	—	77	—	1 vascular 1 Ureteral
Recio (1996)	12	IB2	18 (25%)	7 (0%)	176	1	Not significant
Chu (1997)	67	IA2–IIIB	26.7 (12.8%)	8 (35.7%)	93	2	1 vascular
Possover (1998)	26	IIB–IIIB	15.3 (11.5%)	6.8 (7.7%)	162	3.2	1 vascular
Vidaurreta (1999)	84	IB2–IV	18.5 (45.2%)	—	108	1–2	1 vascular
Schlaerth (1999)	40	IA–IIA	32.1	12.1	—	—	—
Querleu (2000)	53	≥IB2	With common iliac	20.7 (32%)	126	1–2	1 ureteral
Altgassen (2000)	108	IA1–IVB	21–24.3	5.1–10.6	Aortic: 35–73 Pelvic: 61–70	—	3 vascular
11 reports	497	I–IV	9–32 (24%–25%)	6–21 (19%–20%)	120	1–2	1%–2% vascular 0.4% ureteral

HD, mean hospital stay in days; N, number of patients; ORT, mean operating room time in minutes; PAN, mean aortic lymph nodes; PLN, mean pelvic lymph nodes.

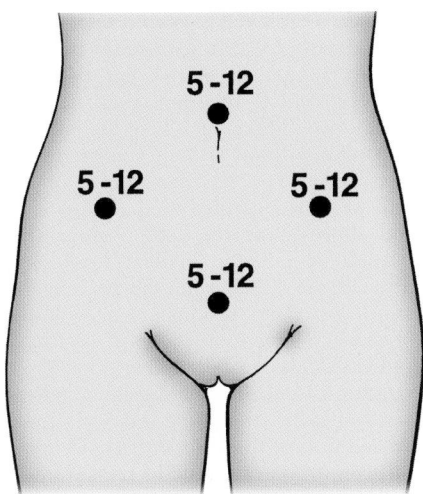

FIGURE 51.53 The transperitoneal minimally invasive approach for laparoscopic surgical staging. Four laparoscopic trocars usually are needed. (Figure © MSKCC, 2002.)

The right aortic nodal tissue is approached via a retroperitoneal incision over the right common iliac artery. The right ureter and ovarian vessels are identified, and the nodal tissue over the inferior vena cava is removed. The left aortic nodal tissue may be approached via the same incision. The inferior mesenteric artery, left ureter, and left ovarian vessels are identified, and the nodal tissue over the left aortic region is removed.

Dissection above the inferior mesenteric artery to include the infrarenal nodal regions may be accomplished through a similar approach, and a left-sided laparoscopic suprarenal retrocrural paraaortic lymphadenectomy in advanced cervical cancer has been described, but the resection of infrarenal aortic nodes using the transperitoneal approach is technically challenging, particularly in obese patients. Robotics may improve on the popularization of paraaortic minimally invasive lymphadenectomy.

PATHOLOGIC EXAMINATION OF THE OPERATIVE SPECIMEN

Considerable useful information about the extent of the disease can be obtained by a careful pathologic examination of the operative specimen. This is helpful in determining prognosis but is also absolutely essential to the identification of patients at greater risk for persistent disease so that additional therapy and close surveillance can be provided. Even though the operator may be fatigued at the end of the operation, in cases where there is a major critical decision based on the specimen, the surgeon should consider accompanying the specimen to the pathology laboratory, where it can be examined with the pathologist before it is placed in fixative and sectioned. Another alternative is to call the pathologist to the operating room for a joint examination of the specimen while the surgical incisions are being closed. The gynecologic surgeon then can indicate worrisome parts of the specimen; such information assists the pathologist in taking sections. Critical margins of dissection can be pointed out and stained with India ink so that they can be seen on microscopic slides. The primary cervical tumor should be measured as accurately as possible so that at least an estimate of its size and volume can be recorded. Numerous microscopic sections of the cervix with adjacent vaginal cuff; lower uterine segment; and paravaginal,

paracervical, and parametrial tissue should be examined to show the cell type, degree of differentiation, depth of stromal invasion, and presence or absence of invasion of lymphatic and vascular spaces. It is important to know not only the depth of invasion but also the thickness of the uninvolved fibromuscular stroma of the cervix, as pointed out by Kishi and coworkers. These authors found that the nodal metastasis and 5-year cancer death rates were 7% and 8%, respectively, in patients with uninvolved fibromuscular stroma thickness greater than 3 mm, and 37% and 26%, respectively, in patients with thickness less than 3 mm. Furthermore, the GOG has demonstrated that the percentage of invasion of tumor into the cervical stroma is an independent prognostic factor and is used to help determine the need for postoperative adjuvant treatment.

Unfortunately, the exquisite giant section technique of pathologic examination used by Burghardt and coworkers is not available in any US pathology laboratory. These authors measured ratio of tumor size to the size of the cervix. The incidence of lymph node involvement increased with tumor size, reaching a maximum of 68.3% in the group with a ratio from 70% to 80% of cervical anatomic involvement. Surprisingly, direct spread into the parametrium seldom was found, even when large tumors were found to occupy the entire cervix. This finding is contrary to that of Bleker and coworkers, who found 16.8% unrecognized parametrial tumor involvement in patients with stage IB and IIA lesions. The 5-year survival rate fell with parametrial involvement.

Thorough examination of the lymphadenectomy specimens must be done. Tumor metastasis to lymph nodes affects patient survival adversely and is an indication for postoperative adjuvant therapy. In patients with positive nodes, the pathologic examination should report whether the metastatic disease is microscopic or macroscopic, single or multiple, and unilateral or bilateral. The location of lymph nodes positive for tumor also should be reported because the prognosis is especially poor in patients with positive common iliac or paraaortic nodes. The usual standard technique of pathologic examination of lymphadenectomy specimens involves removal of visible and palpable nodes from fatty tissue, with bisection of each node for microscopic examination. This standard technique may not be adequate for an accurate assessment of lymph node metastases. A significant increase in positive findings can be obtained if special pathologic examination techniques are used, as demonstrated by To and coworkers, Ahrens and Tschoke, and Wilkinson and Hause. With their technique of dissection of lymph nodes at multiple levels before paraffin embedding, To and coworkers showed that 9% of patients originally reported to have negative nodes actually had positive nodes.

An accurate assessment of the extent of disease by a careful pathology examination of the operative specimen is imperative in deciding whether additional treatment is needed. Indeed, it is such an important component in the surgical management of patients with cervical cancer that these patients should be operated on only in hospitals where such expert specimen evaluation is available.

POSTOPERATIVE COMPLICATIONS

Bladder

Neurogenic Dysfunction

A non–nerve-sparing radical hysterectomy substantially denervates the bladder and upper urethra; the more extensive the dissection, the greater the degree of interference with their function. Therefore, a type C1 nerve-sparing resection has been popularized. Parasympathetic and sympathetic nerve fibers to and from the bladder and urethra are removed, along with paracervical, paravaginal, cardinal ligament tissues and pelvic lymph nodes. All patients have some degree of bladder dysfunction; the incidence of significant bladder dysfunction can be as high as 50%.

Studies have demonstrated that the bladder initially can be hypertonic, with decreased bladder capacity, increased resting pressure, and increased residual urine volume. Many patients have difficulty initiating micturition and experience a loss of sensation of bladder fullness. Using sensitive urodynamic instrumentation, Scotti and coworkers found a variety of abnormalities, including obstructive voiding patterns, immediate and delayed loss of compliance, sensory losses, and genuine stress incontinence. Some patients had complete absence of bladder contractions during voiding. Although these findings are quite compelling, Lin and associates recently reported normal preoperative urodynamic findings in only 17% of 210 patients with cervical cancer scheduled to undergo radical hysterectomy.

Mundy and Sasaki and coworkers have suggested that the posterior part of the cardinal ligament (pars nervosa) contains the major part of the parasympathetic and sympathetic nerve supply to the bladder and urethra and that its removal is responsible for postoperative bladder dysfunction. Sasaki and coworkers demonstrated that removal of the anterior cardinal ligament (pars vasculosa) with preservation of the pars nervosa reduces the incidence of postoperative bladder dysfunction. The work of Kadar and coworkers and that of Asmussen and Ulmsten suggests that the nerve supply to the bladder and urethra can be spared without compromising the necessary extensive dissection and tissue removal around the central disease, thus sparing many patients the loss of urethrovesical function. Kuwabara and colleagues recently reported a decrease in bladder dysfunction by using a technique of intraoperative electrical stimulation to identify and preserve the vesical nerve branches. These nerve-sparing modifications have not been widely adopted by gynecologic oncologists in the United States because of a concern that this same cardinal ligament tissue also carries lymphatic channels draining the cervix and should be removed in a complete central dissection. However, Trimbos and colleagues, from the Netherlands, reported no increase in recurrence or decreased survival in a series of patients treated with nerve-sparing radical hysterectomy.

Techniques of managing the postoperative bladder have varied widely. Duration of catheter drainage, suprapubic versus transurethral drainage, the value of self-catheterization, and the value of cystometric studies have all been debated, as described by Bandy and coworkers. These authors also found that patients receiving postoperative adjunctive pelvic radiation had significantly more contracted and unstable bladders than patients treated with surgery alone. Proper management of the bladder in the first several weeks after operation is essential to avoid overdistension. The duration of postoperative bladder catheterization has decreased in recent years. Chamberlin and investigators reported a contemporary median indwelling catheter duration of 6 days compared with 30 days in historical controls, with no increase in complication rates.

Although some clinicians leave an indwelling catheter or suprapubic tube in place 2 to 3 weeks, we prefer continuous transurethral catheter drainage until 7 days after surgery. Early postoperative intravenous pyelography (IVP) in the absence of intraoperative urinary tract injury or clinical symptoms suggestive of injury is not indicated; moreover, an abnormal early IVP is not predictive of subsequent urinary tract dysfunction.

When the catheter is removed, postvoid residuals are checked with a bladder ultrasound scan (transurethral catheterization also can be used). If the postvoid residual volume is below 50 to 75 mL and the volume of urine spontaneously voided is greater than the postvoid residual, then the patient is allowed to leave the hospital without an indwelling catheter. She must be thoroughly schooled in the importance of not allowing her bladder to become overdistended. Allowing the bladder to overdistend, especially in the early postoperative recovery period, can result in a flaccid bladder from stretching and decompensation of the detrusor muscle, prolongation of bladder dysfunction with high residual urine volumes, and the likelihood of urinary infections. Patients who have unacceptable postvoid residuals are best managed with intermittent self-catheterization or prolonged indwelling catheter drainage for several weeks before attempting removal. If a serious episode of overdistension of the bladder ever occurs, continuous indwelling catheter drainage should be reinstituted, sometimes for 1 to 2 weeks, with the hope that permanent impairment of bladder function can be avoided. Urinary tract infections can occur in conjunction with bladder dysfunction and should be looked for with periodic urinalysis and culture and treated with appropriate antibiotics. Patients should be encouraged to maintain a urine output above 2,000 mL per day to avoid urinary tract infection.

In most patients, a satisfactory voiding pattern can be established within several months. Urodynamic studies, however, can show some evidence of slight and persistent chronic bladder dysfunction for several years. Fraser stated that 20% of his patients continued to report changes in bladder sensation 5 to 15 years after operation. In many patients who have had properly performed radical hysterectomy and pelvic lymphadenectomy, it is inevitable that bladder function will never be completely normal again. With proper postoperative bladder care and rehabilitation, however, function should be satisfactory in most patients at the end of the first year. According to Fishman and coworkers, 35% of patients continued to express unhappiness at the extent and effect of their postoperative urinary dysfunction.

Vesicovaginal Fistula

In the absence of prior pelvic irradiation, bladder ischemia and vesicovaginal fistula are infrequent complications of this procedure. Vesicovaginal fistulae occur in less than 1% of patients (Table 51.12). Nearly one third of urinary tract fistulae following surgery heal spontaneously, compared with none if adjuvant radiation therapy is given. The management of vesicovaginal fistulae is discussed in Chapter 39.

Ureter

Clark, working at the Johns Hopkins Hospital, published one of the first descriptions of radical hysterectomy for cervical cancer in 1895. Sampson, working in the same institution during the same time, recognized that injury to the ureter was the most serious problem associated with primary radical surgery for this disease. His publications on ureteral anatomy and blood supply and the relation between the ureter and gynecologic disease are classic and pertinent today. Devascularization and ischemic necrosis of the wall of the terminal ureter has proven to be one of the more serious complications of this operation. Wertheim found this complication to be one of the more serious sequelae. In Meigs's clinic, there was a 12.5% significant ureteral complication rate, including an 8.5% incidence of ureterovaginal fistulae and a 4% incidence of ureteral stricture.

TABLE 51.12 Urinary Fistulae in Nonirradiated Patients Treated by Radical Abdominal Hysterectomy

INVESTIGATORS	NUMBER OF PATIENTS	URETERAL FISTULA (%)	VESICAL FISTULA (%)
Kaser et al. (1973)	717	3.3	0.6
Park et al. (1973)	156	0	0
Hoskins et al. (1976)	224	1.3	0.45
Morley and Seski (1976)	208	4.8	0.5
Sail et al. (1979)	349	2.0	0.8
Webb and Symmonds (1979)	423	1.4	0.7
Benedet et al. (1980)	241	1.2	0.4
Langley et al. (1980)	284	5.6	1.4
Lerner et al. (1980)	108	0.9	0
Bostofte et al. (1981)	479	3.8	1.4
Powell et al. (1981)	135	1.5	0
Zander et al. (1981)	1,092	1.4	0.3
Gitsch et al. (1984)	187	0.5	NS
Shingleton (1985)	444	1.4	0.23
Artman et al. (1987)	153	1.3	1.3
Larson et al. (1987)	233	0.8	NS
Ralph et al. (1988)	320	1.9	2.5
Lee et al. (1989)	954	1.2	1.2
Kenter et al. (1989)	213	3.3	3.3
Burghardt et al. (1989)	325	2.5	2.8
Massi et al. (1993)	228	0.9	0.4
Total	7,473	2.0	0.9

NS, no sample.
From Shingleton HM, Orr JW. *Cancer of the cervix: Diagnosis and treatment.* New York, NY: Churchill Livingstone, 1987:174, with permission of Elsevier.

For many years, gynecologic surgeons have attempted to lower the rate of ureteral complications with special techniques. Novak, from Yugoslavia, reduced the incidence of ureteral fistulae to 2% after primary radical surgery by placing the dissected pelvic ureter on the inside (peritoneal surface) of the pelvic peritoneum and by preserving the lateral mesentery to the terminal ureter. Green and coworkers suggested that the terminal ureter should be lifted out of the accumulated fluid in the retroperitoneal space by suturing it to the obliterated hypogastric artery. Ohkawa developed a procedure that attempted to elevate and isolate the ureter from the infected retroperitoneal fluid and also to develop a new blood supply to the terminal ureter by placing it in a peritoneal envelope from the pelvic brim to the bladder. Blythe and coworkers compared this technique with simple retroperitoneal suction drainage first advised by Symmonds and Pratt. They found that ureteral obstruction and ureterovaginal fistulae occurred twice as often and that the operative time was extended 45 minutes to 1 hour with the Ohkawa technique. More recently, Patsner and others have recommended the routine use of the omental J-flap (omentopexy) at the conclusion of radical hysterectomy and pelvic lymphadenectomy as an effective means of minimizing urinary tract fistulae.

Given a normal unirradiated ureter, we believe that the incidence of ureteral fistulae and permanent stenosis can be kept below 1% with meticulous intraoperative management of the ureter by a technically skillful operator who can prevent vascular trauma to the periureteral sheath and injury to the muscularis of the ureter.

Some temporary postoperative changes in ureteral function are an almost inevitable result of radical hysterectomy, as pointed out by Gal and Buchsbaum. Using special static and cinefluoroscopic IVP techniques, these authors found ureteral dilation in 87% of patients in the first week after surgery. In most cases, by 6 weeks after surgery, the dilation had regressed and the pyelograms had returned to normal. Peristalsis was altered in the distal ureter, which appeared as a rigid conduit during the first postoperative week. Peristalsis had returned 1 month later. These changes may explain the increased frequency of urinary tract infections after radical hysterectomy, and the possibility of permanent ureteral stenosis if radiation, serious infection, or lymphocyst formation is superimposed.

Table 51.12 shows the frequency of urinary fistulae in a collected series of 7,473 nonirradiated patients treated by radical hysterectomy as compiled by Shingleton and Orr. The management of ureterovaginal fistulae is discussed in Chapter 39.

Lymphocyst Formation

Traditionally, a closed system of constant suction was placed in the retroperitoneal spaces on each side at the end of the procedure. These drains were thought to be effective for reducing the risk of pelvic infection, fistula, and lymphocyst formation. However, recent retrospective and prospective studies have demonstrated that the incidence of these complications is not decreased in patients who have retroperitoneal drains placed compared with those who do not. Furthermore, the drains may actually increase infectious complications. Therefore, we do not routinely place drains in the retroperitoneal spaces.

Whether drains are placed or not, a small percentage of patients will develop lymphocysts. A lymphocyst becomes obvious by symptoms and examination in the weeks after radical hysterectomy and pelvic lymphadenectomy. It may be small and asymptomatic. Most patients with large lymphocysts report lower abdominal discomfort on the same side with radiation to the back, hip, or thigh. Some edema of the lower extremity on the same side may be present and mistaken for postoperative chronic lymphedema due to nodal dissection, but it is more likely due to acute pressure obstruction of lymphatics with the large sidewall lymphocyst and may improve after cyst drainage. Evidence of ureteral obstruction may be found on IVP or CT urogram.

Small lymphocysts that do not cause ureteral obstruction can be observed without treatment. Large symptomatic lymphocysts and those that cause ureteral obstruction should be aspirated. CT-directed needle aspiration can be done with local anesthesia and repeated as needed. The fluid should be submitted for cytologic examination and culture. It is seldom necessary to perform open drainage of a lymphocyst. Mann and coworkers reported successful sclerosis of a recurrent lymphocyst by injection of a solution of tetracycline. Others have used povidone–iodine sclerosis.

Infection

Historically, patients were treated with antibiotics only if postoperative infection occurred. However, antibiotic prophylaxis has been associated with decreased febrile morbidity and decreased rates of serious infection in women undergoing radical abdominal hysterectomy. Furthermore, Orr and colleagues have demonstrated that a single dose of prophylactic antibiotic is as effective as a multiple-dose regimen and lessens patient exposure and cost. Thus, the prophylactic use of broad-spectrum antibiotics with both aerobic and anaerobic coverage has proved to be a useful addition to the surgical armamentarium.

We initiate single-agent broad-spectrum antibiotic coverage immediately before surgery. The administration of the drug is timed to allow adequate distribution before incision. During an extended operation, if the antibiotic given has a short half-life, a second dose is administered.

When secondary infection occurs despite the use of prophylactic antibiotics, the appropriate cultures are obtained, and bacteria-specific antibiotic therapy is chosen.

Venous Thrombosis and Pulmonary Embolus

Patients who undergo radical pelvic surgery fulfill the components of Virchow's triad and are at high risk for the development of venous thrombosis of the lower extremities and thromboembolic phenomena. Factors such as postoperative alteration of blood coagulation, trauma to the vein wall, and venous stasis are recognizable features of this type of surgery. In particular, pelvic lymphadenectomy invariably produces some trauma to the vein wall during the mobilization of the vessel and resection of the adherent lymphatic tissue. One of the biologic effects of radical surgery is the occurrence of local tissue necrosis during healing. This results in the release of tissue thromboplastin into the circulation, which contributes to venous thrombosis by acceleration of the clotting mechanism. The release of thromboplastin from the intima of the vein wall also provides an excellent nidus for the formation of fibrin, particularly in an area of the venous system where there is alteration in venous flow with stagnation of blood. This is frequently seen behind the valves of the veins of the lower extremity, where silent thrombosis is common. Prolonged immobilization of the lower extremities during a lengthy operative procedure is responsible for intraoperative venous stasis and clot formation. There is evidence to document that postoperative thrombosis of the lower extremity is a result of the surgical procedure in more than 50% of cases. The prevention, diagnosis, and treatment of venous thromboembolic events are extensively discussed in another chapter.

Efforts to decrease the frequency of this complication initially used prophylactic low-dose heparin, 5,000 U subcutaneously, three times daily, beginning 2 hours before surgery, and given every 8 hours thereafter for the subsequent 5 postoperative days. By using perioperative heparin alone, the incidence of deep vein thrombosis in a study by Kakkar and associates was decreased from 24.6% in the untreated control group to 7.7% in the heparin-treated group of surgical cases. More impressive was the observation in a subsequent study by the same investigators that 16 patients in the control group, compared with only 2 patients in the heparin-treated group, were found on autopsy study to have died of acute, massive pulmonary embolism.

We use intermittent pneumatic calf compression beginning in the operating room and continuing whenever the patient is in bed until she is discharged. These compression boots are used not only in our patients undergoing radical hysterectomy but in all our patients undergoing major gynecologic surgical procedures. In very high-risk patients, we add prophylactic low molecular weight heparin.

Approximately 3% to 5% of patients with occult venous thrombosis of the lower extremities develop pulmonary emboli. Unfortunately, more than half of the cases of fatal pulmonary embolism occur in patients with silent venous thrombosis and without any clinical evidence of this complication before the acute pulmonary catastrophe. When evidence of venous thrombosis of the lower extremity is verified, full anti-coagulation therapy is required for prevention of pulmonary embolism. However, the decision about how soon after radical surgery it is safe to fully anticoagulate a patient may be very difficult. In the rare case that a pulmonary embolus occurs after full anticoagulation has been achieved, it is necessary to prevent further migration of clot to the lung by either inferior vena cava ligation or the use of an intracaval Silastic umbrella. These complications are rare, but the sinister effects of thromboembolism must be carefully evaluated on a daily basis, and a high index of suspicion needs to be maintained in this high-risk group of patients.

Hemorrhage

Intraoperative and postoperative pelvic hemorrhages also are discussed in another chapter.

Intraoperative Bleeding

Despite the surgeon's adequate technical skills and careful dissection, serious hemorrhage can suddenly appear, especially during retroperitoneal dissections on the lateral pelvic sidewalls and around the sacrum. When it happens, it is hoped that the operative field will not be cluttered with clamps; exposure, lighting, and suction will be adequate; the patient's condition will be stable; and anesthesia will be sufficient to maintain good relaxation. If the bleeding vessel cannot be clamped quickly, the simplest and most effective method of controlling the bleeding is provided by pressure applied by the index finger of the gloved hand. With cessation of bleeding, the operative site can be cleared of accumulated blood by suctioning, exposure of the area can be improved, and the surgeon can gain a few moments to evaluate the situation and choose the best possible course of action. Arterial bleeding is easy to identify and control with clips, clamps, or ligatures. The difficult problem with hemorrhage in the pelvis comes from lacerations of deep pelvic veins that are fragile, tortuous, distended, sometimes hidden or retracted from view, and sometimes held open by attachment of the vein wall to surrounding tissue. Blood returning through the lacerated vein can come from multiple sources unavailable for ligation. Placing clamps or sutures blindly is dangerous and can even make the problem worse. Sometimes, digital pressure for at least 5 minutes is the most effective procedure to control venous bleeding. Sometimes, additional careful dissection in the area is required to free the vessel above and below the bleeding point to allow more precise clipping or suture ligation. A cardinal rule in dissecting in the pelvis is to avoid creating a deep hole, the bottom of which cannot be exposed in case a deep vein is lacerated. This is the reason that dissection of the pararectal space, for instance, should not be forced if it does not develop easily.

Whenever an extensive pelvic dissection is anticipated, preparations should be made in advance in case severe intraoperative bleeding is suddenly encountered. Adequate quantities of blood should be available to replace lost volume. More blood should be requested in advance of its need, if possible. A responsible member of the operating team or anesthesia team should be assigned the task of monitoring blood loss, blood replacement, and urine output. When bleeding is profuse, in the excitement of the moment, it is possible to lose count of the number of units of whole blood, blood components, crystalloids, and other fluids that have been given and how much blood has been lost. A dependable route for administering blood must be maintained. Without it, rapid blood replacement is not possible. If massive hemorrhage occurs or if even a possibility of its occurrence exists, a Swan-Ganz or similar catheter should be placed for better monitoring of physiologic functions and blood replacement. In extreme cases in which no other vessels are available for rapid intraoperative blood volume replacement, transfusions can be given under pressure directly into the common iliac artery, with the needle pointed in the direction of the heart.

The most frequent site of troublesome intraoperative bleeding during radical hysterectomy occurs from the pelvic floor veins in the dissection of the cardinal ligament and the hypogastric vessels. The collateral venous circulation of the hypogastric veins is an ever-present source of potential hemorrhage owing to difficulty in identification of these vessels as they course among muscle bundles and fascial planes on the pelvic floor. The pararectal fossa, cardinal ligament, and presacral and paraaortic areas are frequent sites of venous bleeding. Therefore, meticulous dissection is important to avoid these complications. When venous bleeding does occur, it can be difficult to identify the site of the lacerated vein. In these circumstances, it is important to use compression of the pelvic floor veins by either a sponge stick or finger held in place for several minutes or to use an abdominal pack placed firmly against the site of bleeding for a similar length of time. In these cases, it is advisable to keep pressure on the vein until full control of the bleeding has been established, in the meantime dissecting in other places in the pelvis. Only when the wall of a major pelvic vein has been severely traumatized and has retracted out of the operative field is there a serious problem in reestablishing hemostasis. In contrast to arterial bleeding, hemorrhage from deep pelvic veins is seldom improved by hypogastric artery ligation, owing to the extensive collateral venous circulation to the pelvis from the lower extremity and vena cava. It occasionally is beneficial to ligate the anterior division of both hypogastric arteries to determine whether interruption of the major arterial blood supply to the pelvis can reduce the venous bleeding. When more extensive trauma to the wall of the external or common iliac vein has occurred, it is necessary to place vascular clamps above and below the area of injury and to repair the defect with fine vascular sutures.

Postoperative Hemorrhage

This condition is a rare complication of radical pelvic surgery. Because all of the blood supply to the pelvis has been skeletonized as part of the operative procedure, it is exceedingly rare for secondary hemorrhage to occur unless there has been uncontrolled bleeding at the completion of the operation. In these cases, the pelvis usually is packed with multiple gauze packs, with one end exteriorized through the open vagina. Tamponade of the pelvis by means of an umbrella or parachute gauze pack and external ring (see Chapter 19) has been advocated by some when there is persistent venous oozing in the pelvis at the completion of the operation. Pelvic packs should be advanced within 24 to 48 hours and removed shortly thereafter to avoid ascending infection from the vagina.

In certain cases of postoperative hemorrhage, selective embolization by invasive radiographic techniques can prevent reoperation.

Neuropathies

Nerve injury with radical hysterectomy was reviewed by Hoffman and coworkers, who reported its infrequent occurrence. The most important injuries are to the femoral, obturator,

IX

peroneal, sciatic, genitofemoral, ilioinguinal, iliohypogastric, lateral femoral cutaneous, and pudendal nerves. Awareness of the anatomic location of these nerves in the operative field, careful surgical technique in dissection and securing hemostasis, careful placement of self-retaining retractors, and careful positioning of patients in stirrups prevent most nerve injuries. Fortunately, most nerve injuries are not associated with serious or permanent disability.

However, injury to the obturator nerve can lead to difficulty with adduction of the lower extremity. Obturator nerve injuries are the most common neurologic injuries, and they occur most frequently during the removal of the obturator lymph nodes from the obturator fossa. If the nerve is transected, it should be repaired as described by Vasilev.

Rectum

Although much less frequently reported than bladder dysfunction, both acute and chronic rectal dysfunction may occur following radical hysterectomy. The rectal dysfunction is characterized by difficulty with defecation and loss of defecation urge and constipation. Barnes and associates reported that postoperative anorectal manometry studies were abnormal in all patients studied, suggesting disruption of the spinal reflex arcs controlling rectal emptying, possibly secondary to partial denervation of the rectum. Nerve-sparing radical surgery will hopefully abbreviate and reduce the burden of this complication. Dietary fiber modifications and rectal stimulation with suppositories over several weeks or months are effective in addressing these problems.

ADJUVANT THERAPY IN CONJUNCTION WITH RADICAL SURGERY

Postoperative Pelvic Irradiation

External beam radiation therapy is used in the postoperative period as an adjunct to radical abdominal hysterectomy and bilateral pelvic lymphadenectomy in selected cases. It is given selectively to patients considered to be at high risk for persistent disease based on operative findings and careful study of the surgical specimens. Previously, if only one or two lymph nodes showed micrometastases, postoperative irradiation may not have been given. However, when several nodes are involved, the risk of persistent disease is greater, and postoperative irradiation is usually given; it can be extended as high as T12 if proximal common iliac or paraaortic nodes are involved with metastatic disease. However, nodal metastasis is not the only risk factor for recurrence, and other local tumor-related factors may be indicators of high-risk tumors that may warrant adjuvant radiation therapy.

Sedlis and associates—in a GOG randomized trial of pelvic radiation therapy versus no further therapy in selected patients with stage IB carcinoma of the cervix with negative lymph nodes after radical hysterectomy and pelvic lymphadenectomy—evaluated the benefits and risk of adjuvant pelvic radiation therapy aimed at reducing recurrence in this group of patients. In this study, 277 eligible patients were entered with at least two of the following tumor-related risk factors: greater than one-third stromal invasion, capillary lymphatic space involvement, or large clinical tumor diameter. Table 51.13 summarizes the eligibility criteria: Of the 277 patients, 137 were randomized to pelvic radiation therapy and 140 to no further treatment. Twenty-one patients (15%) in the radiation therapy group and 39 (28%) in the

TABLE 51.13 Eligibility Criteria for Radiation Therapy after Radical Hysterectomy in Node-Negative Patients (Sedlis Criteria)

CLVI	STROMAL INVASION	TUMOR SIZE (CM)
+	Deep one third	Any
+	Middle one third	≥2
+	Superficial one third	≥5
−	Middle or deep one third	≥4

From Sedlis A, Bundy BN, Rotman MZ, et al. A randomized trial of pelvic radiation therapy versus no further therapy in selected patients with stage IB carcinoma of the cervix after radical hysterectomy and pelvic lymph adenectomy: a Gynecologic Oncology Group Study. *Gynecol Oncol* 1999;73:177–183, with permission.

no-further-treatment group had a cancer recurrence, 18 and 27 of which were vaginal/pelvic, respectively. Life table analysis indicated a statistically significant (47%) reduction in risk of recurrence (relative risk = 0.53, $p = 0.008$, one tail) among the radiation therapy group, with recurrence-free rates at 2 years of 88% versus 79% for the radiation therapy and no-further-treatment groups, respectively. Toxicity was generally acceptable, with severe or life-threatening urologic adverse effects occurring in four (3.1%) in the radiation therapy group and two (1.4%) in the control group. The authors concluded that adjuvant pelvic radiation therapy following radical surgery in selected women with stage IB cervical cancer reduces the number of recurrences at the cost of 6% grade 3 and 4 adverse events versus 2.1% in the control group.

Many physicians use these data to identify node-negative patients with local cervical risk factors following radical hysterectomy and pelvic lymphadenectomy to prescribe adjuvant radiation therapy.

If invasive cervical cancer is unexpectedly found after a simple hysterectomy has been done, postoperative pelvic radiation therapy is recommended. Survival rates in these patients have improved with the advent of megavoltage irradiation, as reported by Andras and coworkers, Davy and coworkers, and Papavasilou and coworkers. Heller and coworkers reported 35 patients with invasive cervical carcinoma discovered in uteri removed for benign conditions. All patients received postoperative radiation therapy; patients with presumed stage IB disease had a corrected 5-year survival rate of 78%, and those with presumed stage IIB disease had a corrected 5-year survival rate of 67%.

Postoperative Adjuvant Chemoradiation

After radical surgery in high-risk, early-stage cancer of the cervix, Peters and colleagues reported a phase III trial of adjunctive concurrent chemotherapy and pelvic radiation therapy compared with pelvic radiation therapy alone. In all, 243 assessable patients with clinical stage IA (2), IB, and IIA carcinoma of the cervix, initially treated with radical hysterectomy and pelvic lymphadenectomy, and who had positive pelvic lymph nodes and/or positive margins and/or microscopic involvement of the parametrium were evaluated. Patients were randomized to receive platinum-based chemoradiation or radiation only. Patients in each group received 49.3-Gy radiation therapy in 29 fractions to a standard pelvic field. Chemotherapy consisted of cisplatin 70 mg/m² and a 96-hour infusion of fluorouracil 1,000 mg/m² day every 3 weeks for four cycles, with the first and second cycles given concurrent to radiation therapy.

Progression-free and overall survivals were significantly better in women receiving chemoradiation. The projected progression-free survival at 4 years was 63% with radiation therapy alone and 80% with chemoradiation. The projected overall survival rate at 4 years was 71% with adjuvant radiation therapy and 81% with adjuvant chemoradiation. However, grade 3 and 4 hematologic and gastrointestinal toxicity were more frequent in the chemoradiation group.

The authors concluded that the addition of concurrent cisplatin-based chemotherapy to radiation significantly improves progression-free and overall survival for high-risk, early-stage patients who undergo radical hysterectomy and pelvic lymphadenectomy for carcinoma of the cervix and are found to have positive pelvic lymph nodes and/or positive margins and/or microscopic involvement of the parametrium. Although the data from this study are compelling, use of this regimen should be undertaken only with understanding of the toxicities encountered.

The data from this randomized trial and the Sedlis trial currently provide practical guidelines for eligibility of patients for adjuvant chemoradiation following primary radical hysterectomy or trachelectomy and pelvic lymphadenectomy.

Postoperative Extended-Field Irradiation or Chemoradiation

In selected cases, with multiple positive pelvic nodes, metastasis to common iliac nodes, or aortic nodal metastasis, patients are treated with pelvic and extended-field radiation to include the paraaortic lymph chain. To numerous previous studies can be added two studies from Japan that describe the results of paraaortic nodal irradiation in the treatment of cervical cancer. Inoue and Morita (1988) administered extended-field radiation after extensive surgery to 76 patients with aortic nodal metastases. Two patients developed severe intestinal complications that required reoperation. Postoperative extended-field irradiation improved the survival rate of patients with four or more positive nodes from 39% to 69% as well as the survival rate of patients with unresectable nodes from 0% to 44%. The authors concluded that postoperative extended-field irradiation can control the distant spread by way of lymphatic routes and can increase the survival time of patients. In addition, 86 patients with cervical cancer were treated with paraaortic nodal irradiation by Horii and coworkers (1988). None of the patients developed severe complications from the treatment. Based on their selection criteria for paraaortic nodal irradiation, the authors found a statistically significant improvement in the prognosis for the treated group.

In 1987, Jones reported on a collected series of 332 patients with paraaortic lymph node metastases who received extended-field radiation. Twenty-six percent were long-term survivors. Although it is true that most patients with positive paraaortic lymph nodes die of their disease (probably because systemic disease is already present), it also is clear that some patients are curable with extended-field radiation or chemoradiation, especially if the nodes are involved with only microscopic disease. The surgeon must anticipate a 10% incidence of enteric complications even with doses limited to 5,000 cGy. Again, micrometastatic disease is more likely to be

eradicated by a dose of paraaortic radiation that can be tolerated by the patient. Patients with paraaortic nodes that contain a large volume of tumor are not likely to be cured, even with a dose of paraaortic radiation that exceeds 5,000 cGy, unless the bulky nodes are excised before the irradiation.

Extended-field chemoradiation also may be used. The GOG reported on a multicenter trial of chemoradiation therapy to evaluate the feasibility of extended-field radiation therapy with 5-fluorouracil (5-FU) and cisplatin and to determine the progression-free interval, overall survival, and recurrence sites in patients with biopsy-confirmed paraaortic node metastases from cervical carcinoma. In all, 86 evaluable stage I to IV patients with aortic metastases were reported. Radiation therapy doses were 4,500 cGy to paraaortic nodes, and concomitant chemotherapy consisted of 5-FU 1,000 mg/m² per day for 96 hours and cisplatin 50 mg/m² in weeks 1 and 5.

Initial sites of recurrence were pelvis alone, 20.9%; distant metastases only, 31.4%; and pelvic plus distant metastases, 10.5%. The 3-year overall and progression-free survival rates were 39% and 34%, respectively, for the entire group. Overall survival was stage I, 50%; stage II, 39%; and stage III/IVA, 38%.

GOG grade 3 and 4 acute toxicity was gastrointestinal (18.6%) and hematologic (15.1%). Late morbidity actuarial risk of 14% at 4 years primarily involved the rectum. The authors concluded that extended-field radiation therapy with 5-FU and cisplatin chemotherapy was feasible in a multicenter clinical trial, that a progression-free survival of 33% at 3 years suggests that a proportion of patients achieve control of advanced pelvic disease, and that not all patients with paraaortic metastases have systemic disease. This points to the importance of assessment and treatment of paraaortic metastases.

Adjuvant Postoperative Chemotherapy

Few studies of adjuvant chemotherapy following radical hysterectomy have been done. Wertheim et al. from Memorial Sloan Kettering Cancer Center in 1985 reported on a pilot study of adjuvant chemotherapy with cisplatin and bleomycin and pelvic radiation therapy in patients with cervical cancer at high risk of recurrence after radical hysterectomy and pelvic lymphadenectomy.

The continuous disease-free survival rate for the 32 evaluable patients was 84% at a median follow-up time of 28 months. In addition, the complications of this treatment program were not significantly greater than those observed in prior studies using the combination of surgery and adjuvant radiation therapy without chemotherapy. When compared with the results from historical controls in a large series of similar patients at the same institution, the results in this pilot study were encouraging and appeared to justify a randomized prospective clinical trial.

Two randomized trials have attempted to clarify the role of adjuvant postoperative chemotherapy. In 1992, Tattersall and colleagues reported a randomized trial comparing standard pelvic radiation therapy versus three cycles of combination chemotherapy with cisplatin, vinblastine, and bleomycin followed by pelvic radiation therapy. No difference in disease-free or overall survival emerged between the two treatment groups. Relapse was more common in patients with nonsquamous tumors (44%) and in those with metastases in several pelvic lymph nodes.

In 1996, Curtin et al. from MSKCC reported on a prospective multicenter randomized phase III trial of adjuvant chemotherapy versus chemotherapy plus pelvic irradiation for high-risk stage IB to IIA cervical cancer patients after radical hysterectomy and pelvic lymphadenectomy. The objective was to compare the clinical efficacy of adjuvant chemotherapy alone versus chemotherapy plus whole pelvic radiation therapy on recurrence rates, patterns of recurrence, and survival of patients after radical hysterectomy and pelvic lymphadenectomy for cervical cancer at high risk for recurrence.

Risk factors included deep cervical invasion, tumor greater than 4 cm, parametrial involvement, nonsquamous histology, and/or pelvic lymph node metastasis. Chemotherapy consisted of cisplatin and bleomycin alone or in combination with whole pelvic radiation therapy. Eighty-nine patients were entered, 19 had recurrences, and 16 died. Nine of 44 (20%) patients receiving chemotherapy alone recurred compared with 10 of 45 (22%) patients receiving chemotherapy and radiation ($p =$ NS). Patterns of recurrence were statistically similar between the two treatment arms, even among the subgroup of patients with more than three risk factors. In addition, both regimens were well tolerated. The authors concluded that recurrence rates and patterns of recurrences (local, regional, or distant) were not influenced by the addition of radiation therapy.

However, in view of the more recent randomized trial of adjuvant chemoradiation, most high-risk patients with nodal metastasis will probably be offered adjuvant platinum-based chemoradiation. Whether weekly cisplatin or other platinum-based regimes are the optimal choice remains to be determined.

FOLLOW-UP AFTER RADICAL SURGERY FOR CERVICAL CANCER

Despite carefully planned and executed radical surgery for early-stage cervical cancer, 5% to 20% of patients in various series show evidence of recurrent or persistent tumor. About half occur in the first year after treatment. Almost all occur within the first 3 years. Few occur later. Recurrences many years later are extremely rare after primary surgical treatment and are more likely to be seen in patients treated with primary radiation therapy.

Persistent or recurrent disease after primary radical surgery may represent incomplete resection of the central tumor undetected at operation or by the pathologist's examination of the surgical specimen. Microscopic metastatic involvement of lymph nodes may be undetected by incomplete pathologic examination, or these nodes may be left behind by incomplete lymphadenectomy. Viable tumor cells in small numbers may escape by way of lymphatics or vascular channels to distant sites and overcome host resistance. Probably in as many as 10% of patients with persistent disease, recurrence may result from continued growth of unrecognized intraperitoneal spread of tumor.

After the immediate postoperative recovery is completed, patients are scheduled for regular follow-up examinations, which vary depending on circumstances. Patients who are at greater risk for recurrence should be followed especially closely at frequent intervals. These usually are the same patients who have been given postoperative therapy, including patients with metastatic disease in lymph nodes and/or parametria, close surgical margins, large-volume cervical tumors, deep cervical stromal invasion, and lymphatic and/or vascular channel involvement. The frequency of examination varies somewhat from patient to patient. Most patients are seen every 3 to 6 months during the first 3 years after primary treatment, every 6 months during the 4th and

5th years, and annually thereafter. Patients are instructed to immediately report unusual signs or symptoms (e.g., vaginal bleeding or discharge, leg swelling or discomfort, discomfort in the pelvis, difficulty with urination or defecation, enlarged neck or groin nodes). Krebs and coworkers, however, reported that 25% of their patients did not have symptoms when persistent disease was diagnosed. In the study reported by Larson and coworkers, 37% did not have symptoms.

A follow-up examination should include palpation of the neck for enlarged lymph nodes, abdominal and leg examination, and a speculum and bimanual rectovaginal pelvic examination. A vaginal cytology smear is performed with each visit. Computed tomography or MRI scan of the abdomen and pelvis, PET scan, proctosigmoidoscopy, cystoscopy, and biopsy (needle, punch, or both) of any suspicious lesions may be required, depending on the patient's symptoms and examination findings. These special diagnostic procedures are not done routinely as part of postoperative follow-up surveillance in patients without symptoms. Positive findings are rare, unless the patient has symptoms. For example, IVP seldom shows ureteral obstruction in a patient who does not also have symptoms of persistent pelvic sidewall disease and is, therefore, not routinely done at specific intervals. It is in the patient's best interest to have follow-up examinations done in the same center in which her treatment was administered. Findings at each visit must be compared with previous information all the way back to her original presentation.

Soisson and coworkers reported a comparison of symptoms, physical examination, and vaginal cytology in the detection of recurrent cervical carcinoma after radical hysterectomy. The study group consisted of 203 women with stage IB and IIA cervical cancer followed at the Duke University Medical Center. Thirty-one (15%) patients developed recurrence. For the detection of recurrent tumor, vaginal cytology had a sensitivity and specificity of 13% and 100%, pelvic or general physical examination 58% and 96%, and the presence of suspicious symptoms 71% and 95%, respectively. Ninety-four percent of all patients with recurrent tumor had at least one abnormal surveillance index. Another Duke study by Weber and associates found that MRI correctly demonstrated the extent of recurrence in 18 of 21 cases.

Regular pelvic examinations and vaginal cytology smears may detect a central pelvic recurrence early. This can be a great advantage. Just as it is important to detect the original cancer in the earliest stage possible so that the patient can have the best possible chance of cure, it also is important to detect persistent disease at the earliest possible moment for the same reason. For example, Jobsen and coworkers reported on the use of radiation therapy to treat local–regional recurrence of carcinoma of the cervix after primary surgery. The overall 5-year survival rate was 44%. Response to radiation therapy was strongly correlated with tumor volume, providing additional supportive evidence to the idea that persistent disease should be diagnosed as early as possible and, it is hoped, when the volume of persistent tumor is still small and responsive.

Patients with recurrent or persistent cancer of the uterine cervix after initial radiation therapy can have radical surgery provided the disease is limited and judged to be surgically resectable. Usually, some type of pelvic exenteration is required to resect the recurrent tumor with negative margins. In carefully selected patients with centrally recurrent disease, 5-year survivals of 40% to 60% have been reported. Pelvic exenteration is discussed in another chapter.

Tumor ulceration in the upper vagina can produce vaginal discharge and spotting, a palpable tumor mass, and induration and nodularity of tissue extending to the pelvic sidewalls. Pain may not be present unless the tumor involves nerve roots. Symptoms related to urination and defecation can result from pressure, infection, or tumor involvement of the bladder and rectum. Either unilateral or bilateral edema of the lower extremities or unilateral or bilateral hydroureter and hydronephrosis can be an ominous sign of persistent disease, but these also can be the result of a combination of the effects of radical surgery and postoperative irradiation. When initially diagnosed, recurrences are central in about one fourth of patients, involve the pelvic sidewall in one fourth, and involve distant sites in one fourth; the remaining one fourth of patients have multiple sites of involvement.

Approximately 20% to 25% of patients with recurrence after primary radical surgery still can be cured. The best chance of cure is in patients who had no postoperative radiation treatment and no metastatic disease to pelvic lymph nodes and in whom persistent disease is limited to the central pelvis. A combination of total pelvic irradiation plus vaginal brachytherapy can be effective in controlling the disease. The addition of concurrent platinum-based chemotherapy also should be considered.

Chemotherapy can be given for palliation when there is evidence of unresectable persistent disease in the pelvis in patients who have already received postoperative pelvic radiation or when there is metastatic disease in distant sites.

Because recurrence or persistence of cervical cancer after treatment is difficult but important to detect as early as possible, attempts have been made to use a serum marker that would monitor the course of the disease. Kato and Torigoe isolated a squamous cell carcinoma antigen from cervical carcinoma tissue. A squamous cell carcinoma antigen radioimmunoassay kit developed by Abbott Laboratories (Abbott Park, IL) has been tested, but the role of this antigen in the follow-up of patients with cervical carcinoma is yet to be determined.

Although the early detection of persistence is the primary purpose of and justification for follow-up visits, assessment of urinary tract function also is important. Particular attention should be paid to bladder function and maintaining a satisfactory voiding pattern. Urinary tract infection should be diagnosed and treated promptly. If ureteral stenosis impairs renal function, early intervention can be successful in avoiding nephrectomy. This is more likely to be seen in patients who receive a combination of radical surgery and irradiation as primary treatment.

Rehabilitation of sexual function after surgical therapy for cervical cancer usually is easily done by the patient and her partner but is more difficult if the vagina and paravaginal tissues have received heavy doses of radiation or if the patient has lost ovarian function as a result of treatment. The gynecologic surgeon should inquire about sexual problems and should give advice and permission when needed. Counseling, including instruction in the technique of alternative means of sexual gratification, may be needed. If ovarian function has been lost as a result of treatment, estrogen replacement therapy should be provided, even though symptoms of hypoestrogenism are not present. If normal ovaries were conserved, their function should be monitored with periodic follicle-stimulating hormone and estrogen levels so that estrogen replacement can be discussed when ovaries cease functioning in future years. There may be other contraindications to estrogen replacement therapy in patients treated for cervical cancer, but a history of treatment for cervical cancer is not one of them.

And finally, patients who have been treated for cervical cancer are at greater risk for developing other primary cancers at different sites, especially if their treatment included irradiation. Detection of other primary cancers should be part of posttreatment follow-up. This subject has been studied by Hoffman and coworkers, Buchler, and others. Axelrod and coworkers reported that 3.9% of patients with invasive cervical cancer had second primaries. In 1987, Arneson and Kao reported that 61 new primary cancers were detected among 718 patients with invasive cervical cancer who had been studied from 1955 to 1979.

RADIATION THERAPY

Although radical hysterectomy is generally recommended for women with early-stage cervical cancer who can tolerate the surgery, women with stage IIB or more advanced disease are usually treated with radiation therapy. Radiation is also appropriate for women who are poor surgical candidates because of medical conditions or age.

Ionizing radiation can destroy tumor and cure cancer effectively. Radiation therapy for cervical cancer is usually delivered by two techniques. *Intracavitary therapy* or *brachytherapy* is administered by placing a radioactive element—such as radium, cesium, or iridium—in close contact with the tumor. This produces a very effective, high-dose local treatment, but the dose rate delivered falls off very sharply as the distance away from the radioactive source increases. This is called "the inverse square law." The radiation dose delivered to a given point is equal to 1 divided by the square of the distance away from the radiation source (dose = $1/\text{distance}^2$). Because of the rapid decrease in the dose, it is necessary to treat potential pelvic lymph node metastases and large primary cervical cancer with *external beam radiation*. This type of radiation was originally produced by modified diagnostic x-ray machines, but now, special high-energy linear accelerators or betatrons are used. These machines are capable of delivering a uniform dose of radiation across the whole pelvis or even an extended field to include the paraaortic lymph nodes.

The use of radiation for the treatment of cervical cancer followed very shortly after the discovery of radium by Marie and Pierre Curie. Beginning in 1903, several methods of intracavitary therapy were developed, including the Stockholm technique from the Radiumhemmet; the Paris technique, designed at the Curie Foundation; and the Manchester technique from England. The Stockholm radium technique consisted of high-intensity central irradiation, repeated two or three times within 3 weeks, whereas the Paris technique used low-intensity central irradiation, continuously delivered over 1 week. The Manchester technique, derived from the Paris method, used low-dosage rates that required at least two separate intracervical insertions of radiation sources. Other radioactive elements, including cesium and iridium, have replaced radium in central brachytherapy for cervical cancer.

The traditional brachytherapy systems for cervical cancer have been low-dose-rate systems delivering 0.4 to 2 Gy per hour, and typical implants have been of 24- to 72-hour durations. More recently, high-dose-rate systems have been employed capable of delivering dose rates of more than 0.2 Gy per minute, thereby allowing treatments of only a few minutes' duration and adaptable to the outpatient—rather than the inpatient—setting. A comparison of 5-year survival rates of the two systems by clinical stage documents the usefulness of the newer system (**Table 51.14**).

TABLE 51.14 5-Year Survival Rates of Patients with Stage I Cancer of the Cervix by Treatment Modality

INVESTIGATORS	NUMBER OF PATIENTS	5-YEAR SURVIVAL RATE (%)
SURGERY		
Morley and Seski (1976)	149	91.3
Zander et al. (1981)	747	84.5
Noguchi (1987)	191	85.3
Barber (1988)	273	78.8
Carenza (1988)	105	85.7
Fuller et al. (1989)	285	86.0
Kentler (1989)	178	87.0
Lee (1989)	237	86.1
Monaghan (1990)	494	83.0
Hopkins (1991)	213	89.0
Alvarez (1991)	401	85.0
Burghardt (1992)	443	83.4
Massi (1993)	211	75.8
Total	3,526	84.2
RADIOTHERAPY		
Madowski et al. (1962)	442	81.3
Kottmeier (1964)	611	89.5
Crawford et al. (1965)	63	46.0
Masubuchi et al. (1969)	152	88.2
Marcial (1970)	41	87.0
Neinminen and Pollanen (1970)	77	70.0
Fletcher (1971)	549	91.5
Newton (1975)	61	74.0
Einhorn (1975)	60	88.0
Petersson (1987)	160	76.9
Total	2,196	85.1

TABLE 51.15 Comparison of Outcomes with High Dose Rate (HDR) versus Low-Dose Rate (LDR) Brachytherapy for Cervical Cancer (5-Year Actuarial Survival Rates

ENDPOINT	STAGE	LDR GROUP	HDR GROUP	*p*-VALUE
Overall survival	I	83%	80%	0.77
	II	78%	71%	0.30
	III	46%	36%	0.04
Disease-free survival	I	83%	82%	0.80
	II	82%	71%	0.12
	III	49%	37%	0.03
Local control	I	92%	91%	0.92
	II	87%	75%	0.09
	III	58%	50%	0.19

Reprinted from Ferrigno R, Nishimoto IN, Novaes PE, et al. Comparison of low and high dose rate brachytherapy in the treatment of uterine cervix cancer. Retrospective analysis of two sequential series. *Int J Radiat Oncol Biol Phys* 2005;62(4): 1108–1116, with permission. Copyright © 2005 Elsevier Inc. All rights reserved.

With the establishment of the roentgen as a defined unit of radiation exposure (Stockholm, 1921), it became possible to measure the quantity of irradiation delivered to the tumor. Although many clinicians are most familiar with the dosing measure of rads, modern therapy is calculated in grays (Gy) [1 Gy = 100 rads; 1 centigray (1 cGy) = 1 rad]. High-energy, external beam radiation sources, ranging to 25 mV for the betatron and linear accelerator, have significantly reduced the complication rates after radiation therapy and have improved the cure rates. An intracavitary pelvic dosage derived from the gamma rays of radium or cesium is complementary to the megavoltage external beam irradiation to ensure tumoricidal dosages to the cervix, broad ligaments, and lateral pelvic walls. Extended fields of external radiation can deliver therapy to common iliac and aortic nodal tissues.

The balance between enough radiation to destroy the tumor and too much radiation (which results in damage to adjacent normal tissues such as the bladder, vagina, or rectum) is sometimes difficult to achieve. It requires using the correct combination of brachytherapy with external radiation therapy. Treatment planning has been enormously improved in recent years because of the integration of imaging techniques (such as CT scanners) with computer programs that can calculate the dose to the tumor volume and adjacent normal tissues, which helps the radiation oncologist maximize the tumor dose while minimizing the damage to nearby organs.

Survival rates of irradiation and primary surgery can be compared by analyzing the reports from patients treated for stage I cervical cancer. Patients treated by irradiation have an average 5-year survival rate essentially identical to the survival rate for those who undergo radical surgery (Table 51.15).

In the United States, radical hysterectomy generally is recommended for women with stage IA2 and IB1 cervical cancer who are good operative risks, especially if they are premenopausal. Women with larger tumors and those who are at risk for surgical complications generally are referred for radiation therapy.

SUMMARY

Many improvements have been made in the operative technique of the radical hysterectomy and lymphadenectomy since its original description. The incidence of complications after this procedure has decreased during the past 75 years, and the survival rates have increased. The operation has achieved its peak of clinical usefulness during this period and is now considered the principal method of treatment of early invasive carcinoma of the cervix. Among the better surgical institutions, the meticulous execution of this operative procedure has reduced the incidence of complications to an acceptable and infrequent occurrence. In medical centers in which the operation is performed well, the 5-year cure rate for stage IB1 carcinoma of the cervix is greater than 90%. Newer laparoscopic approaches are gaining acceptance, with comparable cure rates and the potential to retain fertility in carefully selected patients. Radical trachelectomy has proven safe and effective for selected patients with stage I tumors who wish to preserve their fertility.

Comparative studies with primary radiation therapy have demonstrated an equal cure rate with primary radical surgery in the treatment of early-stage disease. However, the complications of irradiation are more difficult to manage than are those of primary surgery. In young women, when preservation of ovarian function is important, primary surgery is a preferable choice of treatment.

The major limiting factor in the long-term surgical cure of cervical cancer is related to the spread of the disease at the time of initiation of treatment. Historically, in cases in which pelvic lymph nodes were positive for metastatic tumor, the 5-year cure rate was reduced to approximately 60%. However, numerous recently reported prospective, randomized trials have demonstrated the benefit of concurrent chemotherapy and radiation therapy in various settings. In the management of high-risk patients after radical hysterectomy and pelvic lymphadenectomy, including those with positive nodes, the reported 4-year disease-free survival is 80%.

It is important to understand that it is the individual surgical expertise that offers the highest cure rate and lowest incidence of complications to the patient with invasive carcinoma of the cervix. One of the greatest errors in clinical judgment is made by the gynecologist who attempts a radical hysterectomy and pelvic lymph node dissection without adequate surgical training and experience. Unless the pelvic surgeon is performing this type of surgery regularly in a well-staffed medical center with trained assistants, he or she would be well advised to refer the patient to an established cancer center. From the patient's point of view, the initial treatment, whether primary surgery or irradiation, provides the best chance for long-term cure of this disease. It would be to her advantage to have the treatment conducted in the most expert hands because secondary treatment for recurrent disease offers only limited potential long-term cure.

BEST SURGICAL PRACTICES

- Invasive cancer of the cervix is predominantly of squamous histology. Adenocarcinoma is increasingly common in many practices and now accounts for up to 20% to 50% of the lesions in some series. Adenosquamous, clear cell, and small cell neuroendocrine histology are seen infrequently. Tumor grade in squamous lesions is not prognostically significant, but grade may be important in adenocarcinoma lesions.
- Although most women with early-stage cancer are asymptomatic, patients with larger tumors may have vaginal discharge, vaginal bleeding (especially postcoital bleeding), and eventually pelvic or low back or hip pain. Leg edema and ureteral obstruction are signs of advanced disease.
- A careful and thorough staging workup should be done after a diagnosis is made. This evaluation of the extent of disease is very important for treatment planning and prognosis. FIGO staging should be used, but the metastatic workup should not be limited by FIGO's restrictive guidelines. MRI and PET scans provide very important information to guide treatment even though they are not part of the FIGO staging system.
- Patients with microinvasion (stage IA1) are generally treated with cone biopsy or simple hysterectomy. Patients with stage IA2 disease should be treated by radical hysterectomy or trachelectomy with pelvic lymphadenectomy. Most of these patients can be adequately treated by a modified radical hysterectomy (type B), but women with larger tumors and LVSI may benefit from a traditional (type C1) radical hysterectomy. Expert gynecologic pathology review is essential for correct diagnosis.
- In the United States, most women with stage IB1 and stage IIA cervical cancer are treated with radical surgery. Women with larger, higher-stage tumors are usually treated with radiation therapy plus adjuvant chemotherapy. Women who are poor surgical risks are also usually treated with radiation ± chemotherapy. The main advantage of surgery compared with radiation is the preservation of ovarian function, which is most advantageous in younger patients. There is also less risk of upper vaginal stenosis and dyspareunia following surgery. Bladder and rectal dysfunction and, rarely, fistulae occur with both surgery and radiation. Surgical complications tend to occur in the perioperative period, whereas complications and side effects from radiation are often delayed and long lasting.
- Radical surgery for cervical cancer requires training, experience, and good ancillary support. This means well-trained operating room personnel; surgical assistants, and anesthesia staff, as well as adequate radiology, intensive care, and consulting physicians need to be a regular part of the patient care team.
- In a radical hysterectomy for stage IB cervical cancer, we do not routinely do a paraaortic lymphadenectomy, but any suspicious nodes are removed and sent for frozen section. The surgical procedure is usually abandoned if aortic lymph node metastases are identified.
- Radical hysterectomy for cervical cancer can be done using the classic abdominal approach, a vaginal approach (Schauta), or a total laparoscopic or robotic approach. There are advantages and disadvantages to each of these techniques, but overall survival appears to be similar. The basic technique is the same.
- Fertility-sparing radical trachelectomy with lymphadenectomy has become a standard of care in many practices. Women with stage IA and early IB1 tumors who wish to preserve fertility have been treated successfully, and the cure rates are comparable to radical hysterectomy. SLN mapping techniques for operable stage I cervical cancer are gaining popularity worldwide and have become a standard of care in many practices.

BIBLIOGRAPHY

Abu-Rustum NR, Gemignani M, Moore K, et al. Total laparoscopic radical hysterectomy with pelvic lymphadenectomy using the argon beam coagulator: pilot data and comparison to laparotomy. *Gynecol Oncol* 2003;91:402.

Abu-Rustum NR, Hoskins WJ. Radical abdominal hysterectomy. *Surg Clin North Am* 2001;81(4):815.

Abu-Rustum NR, Lee S, Correa A, et al. Compliance with and acute hematologic toxic effects of chemoradiation in indigent women with cervical cancer. *Gynecol Oncol* 2001;81(1):88.

Abu-Rustum NR, Lee S, Massad LS. Screening for HIV infection in indigent women with newly diagnosed cervical cancer. *J Acquir Immune Defic Syndr* 2001;27(1):95.

Abu-Rustum NR, Lee S, Massad LS. Topotecan for recurrent cervical cancer after platinum-based therapy. *Int J Gynecol Cancer* 2000;10(4):285.

Abu-Rustum NR, Neubauer N, Sonoda Y, et al. Surgical and pathologic outcomes of fertility-sparing radical abdominal trachelectomy for FIGO stage IB1 cervical cancer. *Gynecol Oncol* 2008;111(2):261.

Abu-Rustum NR, Rajbhandari D, Glusman S, et al. Acute lower extremity paralysis following radiation therapy for cervical cancer. *Gynecol Oncol* 1999;75(1):152.

Abu-Rustum NR, Sonoda Y. Fertility-sparing surgery in early-stage cervical cancer: indications and applications. *J Natl Compr Canc Netw* 2010;8(12):1435.

Abu-Rustum NR, Sonoda Y, Black D, et al. Fertility-sparing radical abdominal trachelectomy for cervical carcinoma: technique and review of the literature. *Gynecol Oncol* 2006;103:1083.

IX

Abu-Rustum NR, Sonoda Y, Black D, et al. Cystoscopic temporary ureteral catheterization during radical vaginal and abdominal trachelectomy. *Gynecol Oncol* 2006;103(2):729.

Abu-Rustum NR, Su W, Levine DA, et al. Pediatric radical abdominal trachelectomy for cervical clear cell carcinoma: a novel surgical approach. *Gynecol Oncol* 2005;97:296.

Abu-Rustum NR, Tal MN, Delair D, et al. Radical abdominal trachelectomy for stage IB1 cervical cancer at 15-week gestation. *Gynecol Oncol* 2010;116(1):151.

Ahrens CA, Tschoke S. Lvmphknotenbefunde nach Wertheim Meigscher operation. *Geburtshilfe Frauenheilkd* 1961;21:219.

Albores-Saavedra J, Gersell D, Gilks CB, et al. Terminology of endocrine tumors of the uterine cervix: results of a workshop sponsored by the College of American Pathologists and the National Cancer Institute. *Arch Pathol Lab Med* 1997;121:34.

Alexander-Sefre F, Chee N, Spencer C, et al. Surgical morbidity associated with radical trachelectomy and radical hysterectomy. *Gynecol Oncol* 2006;101:450.

Altgassen C, Possover M, Krause N, et al. Establishing a new technique of laparoscopic pelvic and paraaortic lymphadenectomy. *Obstet Gynecol* 2000;95(3):348.

Alvarez RD, Potter ME, Soong S-J, et al. Rationale for using pathologic tumor dimensions and nodal status to sub-classify treated stage IB cervical cancer patients. *Gynecol Oncol* 1991;43:108.

Amendola MA, Hricak H, Mitchell DG, et al. Utilization of diagnostic studies in the pretreatment evaluation of invasive cervical cancer in the United States: results of intergroup protocol ACRIN 6651/GOG 183. *J Clin Oncol* 2005;23(30):7454.

Anderson B, LaPolla J, Turner D, et al. Ovarian transposition in cervical cancer. *Gynecol Oncol* 1993;40:206.

Andras EJ, Hetcher EH, Rutledge F. Radiotherapy of carcinoma of the cervix following simple hysterectomy. *Am J Obstet Gynecol* 1973;115(5):647–655.

Angel C, DuBeshter B, Lin JY. Clinical presentation and management of stage 1 cervical adenocarcinoma: a 25-year experience. *Gynecol Oncol* 1992;44:71.

Bader AA, Tamussino KF, Moinfar F, et al. Isolated recurrence at the residual uterine cervix after abdominal radical trachelectomy for early cervical cancer. *Gynecol Oncol* 2005;99:785.

Balega J, Michael H, Hurteau JA, et al. The risk of nodal metastasis in early adenocarcinoma of the uterine cervix [Abstract]. *Gynecol Oncol* 2000;76:235.

Bandy LC, Clarke-Pearson DL, Soper JT, et al. Long-term effects on bladder function of radical hysterectomy with and without postoperative radiation. *Gynecol Oncol* 1987;26:160.

Barber HRK. Cervical cancer: pelvic and paraaortic lymph nodes sampling and its consequences. *Baillieres Clin Obstet Gynaecol* 1988;2:768.

Barnes W, Waggoner S, Delgado G, et al. Manometric characterization of rectal dysfunction following radical hysterectomy. *Gynecol Oncol* 1991;42:116.

Behbakht K, Abu-Rustum NR, Lee S, et al. Characteristics and survival of cervical cancer patients managed at adjacent urban public and university medical centers. *Gynecol Oncol* 2001;81(1):40.

Beller U, Abu-Rustum NR. Cervical cancer after HPV vaccination. *Obstet Gynecol* 2009;113(2 Pt 2):550.

Bellomi M, Bonomo G, Landoni F, et al. Accuracy of computed tomography and magnetic resonance imaging in the detection of lymph node involvement in cervix carcinoma. *Eur Radiol* 2005;15:2469.

Benedet JL, Anderson GH. Stage IA carcinoma of the cervix revisited. *Obstet Gynecol* 1996;87:1052.

Benedet JL, Odicino F, Maisonneuve P, et al. Carcinoma of the cervix uteri. *Int J Gynaecol Obstet* 2003;83:41.

Berman ML, Keys H, Creasman W, et al. Survival and patterns of recurrence in cervical cancer metastatic to periaortic lymph nodes: a Gynecologic Oncology Group study. *Gynecol Oncol* 1984;19:8.

Bernardini M, Barrett J, Seaward G, et al. Pregnancy outcome in patients post radical trachelectomy. *Am J Obstet Gynecol* 2003;189:1378.

Bleker OP, Ketting BW, van Wayjen-Eecen B, et al. The significance of microscopic involvement of the parametrium and or pelvic lymph nodes in cervical cancer stages IB and IIA. *Gynecol Oncol* 1983;6:56.

Blythe JG, Hodel KA, Wahl TP. A comparison between peritoneal sheathing of the ureters (Ohkawa technique) and retroperitoneal pelvic suction drainage in the prevention of ureteral damage during radical abdominal hysterectomy. *Gynecol Oncol* 1988;30:222.

Bonney V. The results of 500 cases of Wertheim's operation for carcinoma of the cervix. *J Obstet Gynaecol Br Emp* 1941;48:421.

Brewer CA, Chan J, Kurosaki T, et al. Radical hysterectomy with the endoscopic stapler. *Gynecol Oncol* 1998;71:50.

Broders AC. The grading of carcinoma. *Minn Med* 1925;8:726.

Buchsbaum HJ. Extrapelvic lymph node metastases in cervical carcinoma. *Am J Obstet Gynecol* 1979;133:814.

Buller RE, Tamir IL, DiSaia PJ, et al. Early evaluation of the urinary tract following radical hysterectomy: structure and function relationships. *Obstet Gynecol* 1991;78:840.

Burghardt E, Baltzer J, Tulusan AH, et al. Results of surgical treatment of 1028 cervical cancers studied with volumetry. *Cancer* 1992;70:648.

Burghardt E, Pickel H, Haas J, et al. Prognostic factors and operative treatment of stages IB to IIB cervical cancer. *Am J Obstet Gynecol* 1987;156:988.

Carter J, Raviv L, Sonoda Y, et al. Recovery issues of fertility-preserving surgery in patients with early-stage cervical cancer and a model for survivorship: the physician checklist. *Int J Gynecol Cancer* 2011;21(1):106.

Carter J, Rowland K, Chi D, et al. Gynecologic cancer treatment and the impact of cancer-related infertility. *Gynecol Oncol* 2005;97:90.

Carter J, Sonoda Y, Abu-Rustum NR. Reproductive concerns of women treated with radical trachelectomy for cervical cancer. *Gynecol Oncol* 2007;105(1):13.

Carter J, Sonoda Y, Baser RE, et al. A 2-year prospective study assessing the emotional, sexual, and quality of life concerns of women undergoing radical trachelectomy versus radical hysterectomy for treatment of early-stage cervical cancer. *Gynecol Oncol* 2010;119(2):358.

Carter J, Sonoda Y, Chi DS, et al. Radical trachelectomy for cervical cancer: postoperative physical and emotional adjustment concerns. *Gynecol Oncol* 2008;111(1):151.

Chamberlin DH, Hopkins MP, Roberts JA, et al. The effects of early removal of indwelling urinary catheter after radical hysterectomy. *Gynecol Oncol* 1991;43:98.

Chambers SK, Chambers JT, Holm C, et al. Sequelae of lateral ovarian transposition in unirradiated cervical cancer patients. *Gynecol Oncol* 1990;39:155.

Chapman JA, Mannel RS, DiSaia PJ, et al. Surgical treatment of unexpected invasive cervical cancer found at total hysterectomy. *Obstet Gynecol* 1992;80:931.

Chen MD, Spirtos NM, Lim PC. Laparoscopic radical hysterectomy. *CME J Gynecol Oncol* 2001;1:110.

Chi DS. Laparoscopy in gynecologic malignancies. *Oncology (Huntington)* 1999;13(6):773.

Childers JM, Hatch K, Surwit EA. The role of laparoscopic lymphadenectomy in the management of cervical carcinoma. *Gynecol Oncol* 1992;47(1):38.

Chu KK, Chang SD, Chen FP, et al. Laparoscopic surgical staging in cervical cancer—preliminary experience among Chinese. *Gynecol Oncol* 1997;64(1):49.

Cibula D, Abu-Rustum NR. Pelvic lymphadenectomy in cervical cancer-surgical anatomy and proposal for a new classification system. *Gynecol Oncol* 2010;116(1):33.

Cibula D, Abu-Rustum NR, Benedetti-Panici P, et al. New classification system of radical hysterectomy: emphasis on a three-dimensional anatomic template for parametrial resection. *Gynecol Oncol* 2011;122(2):264.

Cibula D, Abu-Rustum NR, Dusek L, et al. Prognostic significance of low volume sentinel lymph node disease in early-stage cervical cancer. *Gynecol Oncol* 2012;124(3):496.

Cibula D, Abu-Rustum NR, Dusek L, et al. Bilateral ultrastaging of sentinel lymph node in cervical cancer: Lowering the false-negative rate and improving the detection of micrometastasis. *Gynecol Oncol* 2012;127(3):462.

Cibula D, Ungar L, Svarovsky J, et al. Abdominal radical trachelectomy-technique and experience. *Ceska Gynekol* 2005;70:117.

Clark JG. A more radical method of performing hysterectomy for cancer of the uterus. *Bull Johns Hopkins Hosp* 1895;6:120.

Clarke-Pearson DL, Jelovsek FR, Creasman WT. Thromboembolism complicating surgery for cervical and uterine malignancy: incidence, risk factors, and prophylaxis. *Obstet Gynecol* 1983;61:87.

Clarke-Pearson DL, Synan IS, Dodge R, et al. A randomized trial of low-dose heparin and intermittent pneumatic calf compression for the prevention of deep venous thrombosis after gynecologic oncology surgery. *Am J Obstet Gynecol* 1993;168:1146.

Cohn DE, Swisher EM, Herzog TJ, et al. Radical hysterectomy for cervical cancer in obese women. *Obstet Gynecol* 2000;96:727.

Cormier B, Diaz JP, Shih K, et al. Establishing a sentinel lymph node mapping algorithm for the treatment of early cervical cancer. *Gynecol Oncol* 2011;122(2):275.

Corney RH, Crowther ME, Everett H, et al. Psychosexual dysfunction in women with gynaecological cancer following radical pelvic surgery. *BJOG* 1993;100:73.

Covens A. Preserving fertility in early cervical cancer with radical trachelectomy. *Contemp Obstet Gynecol* 2003;48:46.

Covens A, Shaw P, Murphy J, et al. Is radical trachelectomy a safe alternative to radical hysterectomy for patients with stage IA-B carcinoma of the cervix? *Cancer* 1999;86(11):2273.

Creasman WT. New gynecologic cancer staging [editorial]. *Gynecol Oncol* 1995;58:157.

Creasman WT, Zaino RJ, Major FJ, et al. Early invasive carcinoma of the cervix (3 to 5 mm invasion): risk factors and prognosis. A Gynecologic Oncology Group study. *Am J Obstet Gynecol* 1998;178:62.

Currie JL. *A cosmetically-pleasing transverse incision for pelvic surgery.* ACOG Film Library, 1996.

Curtin JP, Hoskins WJ, Venkatraman ES, et al. Adjuvant chemotherapy versus chemotherapy plus pelvic irradiation for high-risk cervical cancer patients after radical hysterectomy and pelvic lymphadenectomy (RH-PLND): a randomized phase III trial. *Gynecol Oncol* 1996;61(1):3.

Dargent D. A new future for Schauta's operation through pre-surgical retroperitoneal pelviscopy. *Eur J Gynecol Oncol* 1987;8:292.

Dargent D. Using radical trachelectomy to preserve fertility in early invasive cervical cancer. *Contemp Ob/Gyn* 2000;45:23.

Dargent D, Ansquer Y, Mathevet P. Technical development and results of left extraperitoneal laparoscopic paraaortic lymphadenectomy for cervical cancer. *Gynecol Oncol* 2000;77(1):87.

Dargent D, Brun JL, Roy M. La trachtomie rgie (T.E.). Une alternative hysterectomy radicale dans le traitement des cancers infiltrants doppler la face externe du col utn. *J Obstet Gynecol* 1994;2:292.

Dargent D, Brun JL, Roy M, et al. Pregnancies following radical trachelectomy for invasive cervical cancer [Abstract]. *Gynecol Oncol* 1994;52:105.

Dargent D, Franzosi F, Ansquer Y, et al. Extended trachelectomy relapse: plea for patient involvement in the medical decision. *Bull Cancer* 2002;89:1027.

Dargent D, Martin X, Sacchetoni A, et al. Laparoscopic vaginal radical trachelectomy: a treatment to preserve the fertility of cervical carcinoma patients. *Cancer* 2000;88(8):1877.

Dargent D, Mathevet P. Schauta's vaginal hysterectomy combined with laparoscopic lymphadenectomy. *Baillieres Clin Obstet Gynaecol* 1995;9(4):691.

Dary M, Bentzen H, Jahren R. Simple hysterectomy in the presence of invasive cervical cancer. *Acta Obstet Gynecol Scand* 1977;56(2):105–108.

Delgado G, Bundy BN, Zaino R, et al. Prospective surgical-pathological study of disease-free interval in patients with stage IB squamous cell carcinoma of the cervix: a Gynecologic Oncology Group study. *Gynecol Oncol* 1990;38:352.

Del Priore G, Ungar L, Richard Smith J, et al. Regarding "First case of a centropelvic recurrence after radical trachelectomy: literature review and implications for the preoperative selection of patients" [Letter]. *Gynecol Oncol* 2004;95:414.

Diaz JP, Gemignani ML, Pandit-Taskar N, et al. Sentinel lymph node biopsy in the management of early-stage cervical carcinoma. *Gynecol Oncol* 2011;120(3):347.

Diaz JP, Sonoda Y, Leitao MM, et al. Oncologic outcome of fertility-sparing radical trachelectomy versus radical hysterectomy for stage IB1 cervical carcinoma. *Gynecol Oncol* 2008;111(2):255.

Downey GO, Potish RA, Adcock LL, et al. Pretreatment surgical staging in cervical carcinoma: therapeutic efficacy of pelvic lymph node resection. *Am J Obstet Gynecol* 1989;160:1055.

Drescher CW, Hopkins MP, Roberts JA. Comparison of the pattern of metastatic spread of squamous cell cancer and adenocarcinoma of the uterine cervix. *Gynecol Oncol* 1989;33:340.

Eifel PJ, Burke TW, Morris M, et al. Adenocarcinoma as an independent risk factor for disease recurrence in patients with stage IB cervical carcinoma. *Gynecol Oncol* 1995;59:38.

Einstein MH, Park KJ, Sonoda Y, et al. Radical vaginal versus abdominal trachelectomy for stage IB1 cervical cancer: a comparison of surgical and pathologic outcomes. *Gynecol Oncol* 2009;112(1):73.

Elliott P, Coppleson M, Russell P, et al. Early invasive (FIGO stage IA) carcinoma of the uterine cervix: a clinico-pathologic study of 475 cases. *Int J Gynecol Cancer* 2000;10:42.

Ellsworth LR, Allen HH, Nisker JA. Ovarian function after radical hysterectomy for stage IB carcinoma of the cervix. *Am J Obstet Gynecol* 1983;145:185.

Estape R, Angioli R, Wagman F, et al. Significance of intraperitoneal cytology in patients undergoing radical hysterectomy. *Gynecol Oncol* 1998;68:169.

Fanning J, Kraus K. Surgical stapling technique for radical hysterectomy: survival, recurrence, and late complications. *Gynecol Oncol* 2000;79:281.

Feratovic R, Lewin SN, Sonoda Y, et al. Cytologic findings after fertility-sparing radical trachelectomy. *Cancer* 2008;114(1):1.

Fernando JN, Moskovic E, Fryatt I, et al. Is there a role for lymphography in the management of early-stage carcinoma of the cervix? *Br J Radiol* 1994;67:1052.

Folkert MR, Shih KK, Abu-Rustum NR, et al. Postoperative pelvic intensity-modulated radiotherapy and concurrent chemotherapy in intermediate- and high-risk cervical cancer. *Gynecol Oncol* 2013;128(2):288.

Fowler JM, Carter JR, Carlson JW, et al. Lymph node yield from laparoscopic lymphadenectomy in cervical cancer: a comparative study. *Gynecol Oncol* 1993;51(2):187.

Franchi M, Ghezzi F, Zanaboni F, et al. Nonclosure of peritoneum at radical abdominal hysterectomy and pelvic node dissection: a randomized study. *Obstet Gynecol* 1997;90:622.

Freund WA. Method of complete removal of the uterus. *Am J Obstet Gynecol* 1879;7:200.

Fuchtner C, Manetta A, Walker JL, et al. Radical hysterectomy in the elderly patient: analysis of morbidity. *Am J Obstet Gynecol* 1992;166:593.

Fuller AF Jr, Elliott N, Kosloff C, et al. Determinants of increased risk for recurrence in patients undergoing radical hysterectomy for stage IB and IIA carcinoma of the cervix. *Gynecol Oncol* 1989;33:34.

Gallion HH, van Nagell JR Jr, Donaldson ES, et al. Combined radiation therapy and extrafascial hysterectomy in the treatment of stage IB barrel-shaped cervical cancer. *Cancer* 1985;56:262.

Gallup DG, Jordan GH, Talledo OE. Extraperitoneal lymph node dissections with use of a midline incision on patients with female genital cancer. *Am J Obstet Gynecol* 1986;155:559.

Geisler JP, Geisler HE. Radical hysterectomy in the elderly female: a comparison to patients age 50 or younger. *Gynecol Oncol* 2001;80:258.

Gilks CB, Young RH, Gersell D, et al. Large cell neuroendocrine carcinoma of the uterine cervix: a clinicopathologic study of 12 cases. *Am J Surg Pathol* 1997;21:905.

Gilliland JD, Spies JB, Brown SB, et al. Lymphoceles: percutaneous treatment with povidone-iodine sclerosis. *Radiology* 1989;171:227.

Girardi F, Lichtenegger W, Tamussino K, et al. The importance of parametrial lymph nodes in the treatment of cervical cancer. *Gynecol Oncol* 1989;34:206.

Green TH Jr, Meigs JV, Ulfelder H, et al. Urologic complications of radical Wertheim hysterectomy: incidence, etiology, management and prevention. *Obstet Gynecol* 1962;20:293.

Greer BE, Easterling TR, McLennan DA, et al. Fetal and maternal considerations in the management of stage I-B cervical cancer during pregnancy. *Gynecol Oncol* 1989;34:61.

Greer BE, Figge DC, Tamimi HK, et al. Stage IB adenocarcinoma of the cervix treated by radical hysterectomy and pelvic lymph node dissection. *Am J Obstet Gynecol* 1989;160:1509.

IX

Griffenberg L, Morris M, Atkinson N, et al. The effect of dietary fiber on bowel function following radical hysterectomy. *Gynecol Oncol* 1997;66:417.

Hatch KD, Hallum AV III, Nour M. New surgical approaches to treatment of cervical cancer. *J Natl Cancer Inst Monogr* 1996;21:71.

Heller PB, Barnhill DR, Mayer AR, et al. Cervical carcinoma found incidentally in a uterus removed for benign indications. *Obstet Gynecol* 1986;67(2):187–190.

Hertel H, Kohler C, Hillemanns P, et al. Radical vaginal trachelectomy (RVT) combined with laparoscopic pelvic lymphadenectomy: prospective multicenter study of 100 patients with early cervical cancer. *Gynecol Oncol* 2006;103:506–511.

Hoffman MS, Parsons M, Gunasekaran S, et al. Distal external iliac lymph nodes in early cervical cancer. *Obstet Gynecol* 1999;94:391.

Hoffman MS, Roberts WS, Cavanagh D. Neuropathies associated with radical pelvic surgery for gynecologic cancer. *Gynecol Oncol* 1988;31:462.

Hoffman MS, Roberts WS, Cavanagh D. Second pelvic malignancies following radiation therapy for cervical cancer. *Obstet Gynecol Surv* 1985;40:611.

Hopkins MP, Morley GW. The prognosis and management of cervical cancer associated with pregnancy. *Obstet Gynecol* 1992;80:9.

Hopkins MP, Schmidt RW, Roberts JA, et al. The prognosis and treatment of stage adenocarcinoma of the cervix. *Obstet Gynecol* 1988;72:915.

Horii T, Mitsumoto T, Noda K. Significance of paraaortic node irradiation in the treatment of cervical cancer. *Gynecol Oncol* 1988;31:371.

Hoskins WJ. Prognostic factors for risk of recurrence in stages IB and IIA cervical cancer. *Baillieres Clin Obstet Gynecol* 1988;2:817.

Hsieh YY, Lin WC, Chang CC, et al. Laparoscopic radical hysterectomy with low paraaortic, subaortic and pelvic lymphadenectomy: results of short-term follow-up. *J Reprod Med* 1998;43(6):528.

Jackson KS, Das N, Naik R, et al. Laparoscopically assisted radical vaginal hysterectomy vs. radical abdominal hysterectomy for cervical cancer: a match controlled stud. *Gynecol Oncol* 2004;95:655.

Jensen JK, Lucci JA, DiSaia PH, et al. To drain or not to drain: a retrospective study of closed-suction drainage following radical hysterectomy with pelvic lymphadenectomy. *Gynecol Oncol* 1993;512:46.

Jones HW, Jones GES. Panhysterectomy versus irradiation in early cancer of the cervix. *JAMA* 1943;122:930.

Jones WB. Surgical approaches for advanced or recurrent cancer of the cervix. *Cancer* 1987;60:2094.

Kadar N. Laparoscopic vaginal radical hysterectomy: an operative technique and its evolution. *Gynaecol Endosc* 1994;3:109.

Kayton ML, Wexler LH, Lewin SN, et al. Pediatric radical abdominal trachelectomy for anaplastic embryonal rhabdomyosarcoma of the uterine cervix: an alternative to radical hysterectomy. *J Pediatr Surg* 2009;44(4):862.

Keys HM, Bundy BN, Stehman FB, et al. Cisplatin, radiation, and adjuvant hysterectomy compared with radiation and adjuvant hysterectomy for bulky stage IB cervical carcinoma. *N Engl J Med* 1999;340:1154.

Khoury-Collado F, Bowes RJ, Jhamb N, et al. Unexpected long-term survival without evidence of disease after salvage chemotherapy for recurrent metastatic cervical cancer: a case series. *Gynecol Oncol* 2007;105(3):823.

Kilgore LC, Soong S-J, Gore H, et al. Analysis of prognostic features in adenocarcinoma of the cervix. *Gynecol Oncol* 1988;31:137.

Kim CH, Abu-Rustum NR, Chi DS, et al. Reproductive outcomes of patients undergoing radical trachelectomy for early-stage cervical cancer. *Gynecol Oncol* 2012;125(3):585.

Kim DH, Moon JS. Laparoscopic radical hysterectomy with pelvic lymphadenectomy for early, invasive cervical carcinoma. *J Am Assoc Gynecol Laparosc* 1998;5(4):411.

Kim SH, Choi BI, Han JK, et al. Preoperative staging of uterine cervical carcinoma: comparison of CT and MR imaging in 99 patients. *J Comput Assist Tomogr* 1993;17:633.

Kinney WK, Egorshin EV, Podratz KC. Wertheim hysterectomy in the geriatric population. *Gynecol Oncol* 1988;31:227.

Klemm P, Tozzi R, Kohler C, et al. Does radical trachelectomy influence uterine blood supply? *Gynecol Oncol* 2005;96:283.

Koh WJ, Greer BE, Abu-Rustum NR, et al. Cervical cancer. *J Natl Compr Canc Netw* 2013;11(3):320.

Kolstad P. Follow-up study of 232 patients with stage Ia1 and 411 patients with stage Ia2 squamous cell carcinoma of the cervix (microinvasive carcinoma). *Gynecol Oncol* 1989;33:265.

Kurman RJ, Norris HJ, Wilkinson F. *Atlas of tumor pathology, tumors of the cervix, vagina, and vulva, third series, fascicle 4*. Washington, DC: Armed Forces Institute of Pathology, 1992.

Kuwabara Y, Suzuki M, Hashimoto M, et al. New method to prevent bladder dysfunction after radical hysterectomy for uterine cervical cancer. *J Obstet Gynaecol Res* 2000;26:1.

Lagasse LD, Creasman WT, Shingleton HM, et al. Results and complications of operative staging in cervical cancer: experience of the Gynecologic Oncology Group. *Gynecol Oncol* 1980;9:90.

Landoni F, Maneo A, Cormio G, et al. Class II versus class III radical hysterectomy in stage IB-IIA cervical cancer: a prospective randomized study. *Gynecol Oncol* 2001;80:3.

Larson DM, Copeland LJ, Malone JM Jr, et al. Diagnosis of recurrent cervical carcinoma after radical hysterectomy. *Obstet Gynecol* 1988;71:6.

Larson DM, Malone JM Jr, Copeland LJ, et al. Ureteral assessment after radical hysterectomy. *Obstet Gynecol* 1987;69:612.

Latzko W, Schiffmann J. Klinisches and anatomisches zur radikaloperation des gebarmutterkrebses. *Zentralbl Gynakol* 1919;43:715.

Levrant SG, Fruchter RG, Maiman M. Radical hysterectomy for cervical cancer: morbidity and survival in relation to weight and age. *Gynecol Oncol* 1992;45:317.

Lin HH, Yu HJ, Sheu BC, et al. Importance of urodynamic study before radical hysterectomy for cervical cancer. *Gynecol Oncol* 2001;81:270.

Look KY, Brunetto VL, Clarke-Pearson DL, et al. An analysis of cell type in patients with surgically staged IB carcinoma of the cervix: a Gynecologic Oncology Group study. *Gynecol Oncol* 1996;63:304.

Lopes AD, Hall JR, Monaghan JM. Drainage following radical hysterectomy and pelvic lymphadenectomy: dogma or need? *Obstet Gynecol* 1995;86:960.

Lovecchio JL, Averette HE, Donato D, et al. Five-year survival of patients with periaortic nodal metastasis in clinical stage IB and IIA cervical cancer. *Gynecol Oncol* 1989;34:43.

Malur S, Possover M, Schneider A. Laparoscopically assisted radical vaginal versus radical abdominal hysterectomy type II in patients with cervical cancer. *Surg Endosc* 2001;15:289.

Mann WJ, Vogel F, Patsner B, et al. Management of lymphocysts after radical gynecologic surgery. *Gynecol Oncol* 1989;33:248.

Martzloff KH. Carcinoma of the cervix uteri: a pathological and clinical study with particular reference to the relative malignancy of the neoplastic process as indicated by the predominant type of cancer cell. *Bull Johns Hopkins Hosp* 1923;34:141.

Massad LS, Calvello CA, Gilkey SH, et al. Assessing disease extent in women with bulky or clinically evident metastatic cervical cancer: yield of pretreatment studies. *Gynecol Oncol* 2000;76:383.

Massad LS, Cejtin HE, Abu-Rustum NR. Presentation and screening history of indigent women with cervical cancer: implications for prevention. *J Lower Genital Tract Dis* 2000;4(4):208.

Massi G, Savino L, Susini T. Schauta-Amreich vaginal hysterectomy and Wertheim-Meigs abdominal hysterectomy in the treatment of cervical cancer: a retrospective analysis. *Am J Obstet Gynecol* 1993;168:928.

Mathevet P, Laszlo de Kaszon E, Dargent D. Fertility preservation in early cervical cancer. *Gynecol Obstet Fertil* 2003;31:706.

Maxwell GL, Synan I, Dodge R, et al. A prospective randomized comparison of pneumatic compression and low-molecular-weight heparin in the postoperative prophylaxis of gynecologic oncology patients [Abstract]. *Gynecol Oncol* 2001;80:284.

McCall ML, Keaty EC, Thompson JD. Conservation of ovarian tissue in the treatment of carcinoma of the cervix with radical surgery. *Am J Obstet Gynecol* 1958;75:590.

McIntyre JF, Eifel PJ, Levenback C, et al. Ureteral stricture as a late complication of radiotherapy for stage IB carcinoma of the uterine cervix. *Cancer* 1995;75:836.

Meigs JV. The Wertheim operation for carcinoma of the cervix. *Am J Obstet Gynecol* 1945;49:542.

Mitra S. Radikale vaginale hysterektomie and extraperitoneale lymphadenektomie bei rvixkrebs. *Zentralbl Gynakol* 1951;73:574.

Mitra S. Extraperitoneal lymphadenectomy and radical vaginal hysterectomy for cancer of the cervix (Mitra technique). *Am J Obstet Gynecol* 1959;78:191.

Montana GS, Hanlon AL, Brickner TJ, et al. Carcinoma of the cervix: patterns of care studies; review of 1978, 1983 and 1988–1989 surveys. *Int J Radiat Oncol Biol Phys* 1995;32:1481.

Moore DH, Fowler WC, Walton LA, et al. Morbidity of lymph node sampling in cancers of the uterine corpus and cervix. *Obstet Gynecol* 1989;74:180.

Morice P, Dargent D, Haie-Meder C, et al. First case of a centropelvic recurrence after radical trachelectomy: literature review and implications for the preoperative selection of patients. *Gynecol Oncol* 2004;92:1002.

Morris M, Eifel PJ, Lu J, et al. Pelvic radiation with concurrent chemotherapy versus pelvic and paraaortic radiation for high-risk cervical cancer: a randomized radiation therapy oncology group clinical trial. *N Engl J Med* 1999;340:1137.

Morris PC, Haugen J, Anderson B, et al. The significance of peritoneal cytology in stage IB cervical cancer. *Obstet Gynecol* 1992;80:196.

Morrow CP. Panel report: is pelvic radiation beneficial in the postoperative management of stage IB squamous-cell carcinoma of the cervix with pelvic node metastases treated by radical hysterectomy and pelvic lymphadenectomy? *Gynecol Oncol* 1980;10:105.

Nagarsheth NP, Maxwell GL, Bentley RC, et al. Bilateral pelvic lymph node metastases in a case of FIGO stage IA1 adenocarcinoma of the cervix. *Gynecol Oncol* 2000;77:467.

Nahhas WA, Abt AB, Mortel R. Stage IB glassy cell carcinoma of the cervix with ovarian metastases. *Gynecol Oncol* 1977;5:87.

Nam JH, Kim JH, Kim DY, et al. Comparative study of laparoscopico-vaginal radical hysterectomy and abdominal radical hysterectomy in patients with early cervical cancer. *Gynecol Oncol* 2004;92:277.

Navratil E. Indications and results of the vaginal and abdominal radical operation in the treatment of carcinoma of the cervix. *J Int Coll Surg* 1965;43:82.

Nezhat CR, Nezhat FR, Burrell MO, et al. Laparoscopic radical hysterectomy and laparoscopically assisted vaginal radical hysterectomy with pelvic and paraaortic node dissection. *J Gynecol Surg* 1993;9(2):105.

Nori D, Valentine E, Hilaris BS. The role of paraaortic node irradiation in the treatment of cancer of the cervix. *Int J Radiat Oncol Biol Phys* 1985;11:1469.

Okabayashi H. Radical abdominal hysterectomy for cancer of the cervix uteri. *Surg Gynecol Obstet* 1921;33:335.

Orr JW Jr, Orr PJ, Bolen DD, et al. Radical hysterectomy: does the type of incision matter? *Am J Obstet Gynecol* 1995;173:399.

Ostor AG. Pandora's box or Ariadne's thread? Definition and prognostic significance of microinvasion in the uterine cervix. Squamous lesions. *Pathol Ann* 1995;30:103.

Ostor AG, Rome R, Zuinn M. Microinvasive adenocarcinoma of the cervix: a clinicopathologic study of 77 women. *Obstet Gynecol* 1997;89:88.

Owens S, Roberts WS, Fiorica JV, et al. Ovarian management at the time of radical hysterectomy for cancer of the cervix. *Gynecol Oncol* 1989;35:349.

Pandit-Taskar N, Gemignani ML, Lyall A, et al. Single photon emission computed tomography SPECT-CT improves sentinel node detection and localization in cervical and uterine malignancy. *Gynecol Oncol* 2010;117(1):59.

Papavasiliou C, Yiogarakis D, Pappas J, et al. Treatment of cervical carcinoma by total hysterectomy and postoperative external irradiation. *Int J Radiat Oncol Biol Phys* 1980;6(7):871–874.

Park KJ, Soslow RA, Sonoda Y, et al. Frozen-section evaluation of cervical adenocarcinoma at time of radical trachelectomy: pathologic pitfalls and the application of an objective scoring system. *Gynecol Oncol* 2008;110(3):316.

Patsner B. Closed-suction drainage versus no drainage following radical abdominal hysterectomy with pelvic lymphadenectomy for stage IB cervical cancer. *Gynecol Oncol* 1995;57:232.

Patsner B. Radical abdominal hysterectomy using the ENDO-GIA stapler: a report of 150 cases and literature review. *Eur J Gynaecol Oncol* 1998;19:215.

Patsner B, Hackett TE. Use of the omental J-flap for prevention of postoperative complications following radical abdominal hysterectomy: report of 140 cases and review of the literature. *Gynecol Oncol* 1997;65:405.

Patsner B, Sedlacek TV, Lovecchio JL. Paraaortic node sampling in small (3-cm or less) stage IB invasive cervical cancer. *Gynecol Oncol* 1992;44:53.

Pavlik K. O extirpaci cele dèlohy a casti vaziva Panvichnio. *Casopis Lekaru Ceskych* 1889;18:28.

Peipert JF, Wells CK, Schwartz PE, et al. Prognostic value of clinical variables in invasive cervical cancer. *Obstet Gynecol* 1994;84:746.

Peters WA III, Liu PY, Barrett RJ II, et al. Concurrent chemotherapy and pelvic radiation therapy compared with pelvic radiation therapy alone as adjuvant therapy after radical surgery in high-risk early-stage cancer of the cervix. *J Clin Oncol* 2000;18(8):1606.

Piver MS, Rutledge F, Smith JP. Five classes of extended hysterectomy for women with cervical cancer. *Obstet Gynecol* 1974;44:265.

Plante M, Lau S, Brydon L, et al. Neoadjuvant chemotherapy followed by vaginal radical trachelectomy in bulky stage IB1 cervical cancer: case report. *Gynecol Oncol* 2006;101:367.

Plante M, Renaud MC, Harel F, et al. Vaginal radical trachelectomy: an oncologically safe fertility-preserving surgery. An updated series of 72 cases and review of the literature. *Gynecol Oncol* 2004;94:614.

Plante M, Renaud MC, Hoskins IA, et al. Vaginal radical trachelectomy: a valuable fertility-preserving option in the management of early-stage cervical cancer. A series of 50 pregnancies and review of the literature. *Gynecol Oncol* 2005;98:3.

Plante M, Renaud MC, Roy M. Sentinel node evaluation in gynecologic cancer. *Oncology* 2004;18:75.

Plante M, Roy M. Radical trachelectomy. *Oper Tech Gynecol Surg* 1997;3(3):187.

Possover M, Krause N, Drahonovsky J, et al. Left-sided suprarenal retrocrural paraaortic lymphadenectomy in advanced cervical cancer by laparoscopy. *Gynecol Oncol* 1998;71(2):219.

Possover M, Krause N, Kuhne-Heid R, et al. Laparoscopic assistance for extended radicality of radical vaginal hysterectomy: description of a technique. *Gynecol Oncol* 1998;70:94.

Possover M, Krause N, Plaul K, et al. Laparoscopic paraaortic and pelvic lymphadenectomy: experience with 150 patients and review of the literature. *Gynecol Oncol* 1998;71(1):19.

Potish RA, Downey GO, Adcock LL, et al. The role of surgical debulking in cancer of the uterine cervix. *Int J Radiat Oncol Biol Phys* 1989;17:979.

Querleu D. Laparoscopically assisted radical vaginal hysterectomy. *Gynecol Oncol* 1993;51(2):248.

Querleu D, Dargent D, Ansquer Y, et al. Extraperitoneal endosurgical aortic and common iliac dissection in the staging of bulky or advanced cervical carcinomas. *Cancer* 2000;88(8):1883.

Querleu D, Leblanc E, Cartron G, et al. Audit of preoperative and early complications of laparoscopic lymph node dissection in 1000 gynecologic cancer patients. *Am J Obstet Gynecol* 2006; 195:1287.

Querleu D, Leblanc E, Castelain B. Laparoscopic pelvic lymphadenectomy in the staging of early carcinoma of the cervix. *Am J Obstet Gynecol* 1991;164(2):579.

Querleu D, Narducci F, Poulard V, et al. Modified radical vaginal hysterectomy with or without laparoscopic nerve-sparing dissection: a comparative study. *Gynecol Oncol* 2002;85:154.

Ralph G, Tamussino K, Lichtenegger W. Urological complications after radical hysterectomy with or without radiotherapy for cervical cancer. *Arch Gynecol Obstet* 1990;248:61.

Recio FO, Piver MS, Hempling RE. Pretreatment transperitoneal laparoscopic staging pelvic and paraaortic lymphadenectomy in large (≥5 cm) stage IB2 cervical carcinoma: report of a pilot study. *Gynecol Oncol* 1996;63(3):333.

Reiffenstuhl G. *The lymphatics of the female genital organs.* Philadelphia, PA: JB Lippincott, 1964.

Renaud MC, Plante M, Roy M. Combined laparoscopic and vaginal radical surgery in cervical cancer. *Gynecol Oncol* 2000;79(1):59.

Rodriguez M, Guimares O, Rose PG. Radical abdominal trachelectomy and pelvic lymphadenectomy with uterine conservation and subsequent pregnancy in the treatment of early invasive cervical cancer. *Am J Obstet Gynecol* 2001;185:370.

IX

Rose PG. Type II radical hysterectomy: evaluating its role in cervical cancer [Editorial]. *Gynecol Oncol* 2001;80:1.

Rose PG, Bundy BN, Watkins EB, et al. Concurrent cisplatin-based radiotherapy and chemotherapy for locally advanced cervical cancer. *N Engl J Med* 1999;340:1144.

Rose PG, Lappas T. Analysis of cost effectiveness of concurrent cisplatin-based chemoradiation in cervical cancer: implications from five randomized trials. *Gynecol Oncol* 2000;78:3.

Roy M, Plante M. Pregnancies after radical vaginal trachelectomy for early-stage cervical cancer. *Am J Obstet Gynecol* 1998;179(6):1491.

Roy M, Plante M, Renaud MC, et al. Vaginal radical hysterectomy versus abdominal radical hysterectomy in the treatment of early-stage cervical cancer. *Gynecol Oncol* 1996;62(3):336.

Russell AH, Anderson M, Walter J, et al. The integration of computed tomography and magnetic resonance imaging in treatment planning for gynecologic cancer. *Clin Obstet Gynecol* 1992;35:55.

Rutledge FN, Fletcher GH, MacDonald RJ. Pelvic lymphadenectomy as an adjunct to radiation therapy in treatment for cancer of the cervix. *Am J Roentgenol Radium Ther Nucl Med* 1965;93:607.

Rutledge FN, Mitchell MF, Munsell M, et al. Youth as a prognostic factor in carcinoma of the cervix: a matched analysis. *Gynecol Oncol* 1992;44:123.

Sahdev A, Jones J, Shepherd JH, et al. MR imaging appearances of the female pelvis after trachelectomy. *Radiographics* 2005;25:41.

Sampson JA. A careful study of the parametrium in twenty-seven cases of carcinoma cervices uteri and its clinical significance. *Am J Obstet* 1906;54:433.

Sandadi S, Tanner EJ, Khoury-Collado F, et al. Radical surgery with individualized postoperative radiation for stage IB cervical cancer: oncologic outcomes and severe complications. *Int J Gynecol Cancer* 2013;23(3):553.

Sardi J, Vidaurreta J, Bermudez A, et al. Laparoscopically assisted Schauta operation: learning experience at the Gynecologic Oncology Unit, Buenos Aires University Hospital. *Gynecol Oncol* 1999;75(3):361.

Schellhas HF. Extraperitoneal paraaortic node sampling in small stage IB invasive cervical cancer. *Gynecol Oncol* 1992;44:53.

Schneider A, Possover M, Kamprath S, et al. Laparoscopy-assisted radical vaginal hysterectomy modified according to Schauta-Stoeckel. *Obstet Gynecol* 1996;88(6):1057.

Schuchardt K. Ein neue Methode der Gebärmutter Exstirpation. *Zbl Chir* 1893;20:1121.

Schneidler J, Hricak H, Yu KK, et al. Radiologic evaluation of lymph nodes in patients with cervical cancer: meta analysis. *JAMA* 1997;278:1096.

Scotti RJ, Bergman A, Bhatia NN, et al. Urodynamic changes in urethrovesical function after radical hysterectomy. *Obstet Gynecol* 1986;68:111.

Sedlacek TV, Campion MJ, Reich H, et al. Laparoscopic radical hysterectomy: a feasibility study [Abstract]. *Gynecol Oncol* 1995;56:126.

Sedlis A, Bundy BN, Rotman MZ, et al. A randomized trial of pelvic radiation therapy versus no further therapy in selected patients with stage IB carcinoma of the cervix after radical hysterectomy and pelvic lymphadenectomy: a Gynecologic Oncology Group Study. *Gynecol Oncol* 1999;73(2):177.

Seibel MM, Freeman MG, Graves WL. The effect of surgical and radiation treatment for cervical carcinoma on sexual function. *South Med J* 1982;75:1195.

Sheets EE, Berman ML, Hrountas CK, et al. Surgically treated, early stage neuroendocrine small-cell cervical carcinoma. *Obstet Gynecol* 1988;71:10.

Shepherd JH, Crawford RA, Oram DH. Radical trachelectomy: a way to preserve fertility in the treatment of early cervical cancer. *BJOG* 1998;105(8):912.

Shepherd JH, Mould T, Oram DH. Radical trachelectomy in early stage carcinoma of the cervix: outcome as judged by recurrence and fertility rates. *BJOG* 2001;108(8):882.

Shepherd JH, Spencer C, Herod J, et al. Radical vaginal trachelectomy as a fertility-sparing procedure in women with early-stage cervical cancer-cumulative pregnancy rate in a series of 123 women. *BJOG* 2006;113:719.

Shih KK, Folkert MR, Kollmeier MA, et al. Pelvic insufficiency fractures in patients with cervical and endometrial cancer treated with postoperative pelvic radiation. *Gynecol Oncol* 2013;128(3):540.

Shingleton HM, Bell MC, Fremgen A, et al. Is there really a difference in survival of women with early stage squamous cell carcinoma, adenocarcinoma and adenosquamous cell carcinoma of the cervix? *Cancer* 1995;76:1948.

Shingleton HM, Orr JW, eds. *Cancer of the cervix*. Philadelphia, PA: JB Lippincott, 1995.

Shingleton HM, Soong SJ, Gelder MS, et al. Clinical and histopathologic factors predicting recurrence and survival after pelvic exenteration for cancer of the cervix. *Obstet Gynecol* 1989;73:1027.

Sidebotham EL, DeLair D, Comerci JT, et al. Pediatric radical abdominal trachelectomy for solitary fibrous tumor of the uterine cervix. *Gynecol Oncol* 2009;115(2):302.

Singh N, Titmuss E, Aleong JC, et al. A review of post-trachelectomy isthmic and vaginal smear cytology. *Cytopathology* 2004;15:97.

Smith HO, Tiffany MF, Qualls CR, et al. The rising incidence of adenocarcinoma relative to squamous cell carcinoma of the uterine cervix in the United States—a 24-year population-based study. *Gynecol Oncol* 2000;78:97.

Smith JR, Boyle DC, Corless DJ, et al. Abdominal radical trachelectomy: a new surgical technique for the conservative management of cervical carcinoma. *BJOG* 1997;104:1196.

Soisson AP, Geszler G, Soper JT, et al. A comparison of symptomatology, physical examination, and vaginal cytology in the detection of recurrent cervical carcinoma after radical hysterectomy. *Obstet Gynecol* 1990;76:106.

Soisson AP, Soper JT, Berchuck A, et al. Radical hysterectomy in obese women. *Obstet Gynecol* 1992;80:940.

Sonoda Y, Abu-Rustum NR, Gemignani ML, et al. A fertility-sparing alternative to radical hysterectomy: how many patients may be eligible? *Gynecol Oncol* 2004;95:534.

Sonoda Y, Chi DS, Carter J, et al. Initial experience with Dargent's operation: the radical vaginal trachelectomy. *Gynecol Oncol* 2008;108(1):214.

Sood AK, Sorosky JI, Krogman S, et al. Surgical management of cervical cancer complicating pregnancy: a case–control study. *Gynecol Oncol* 1996;63:294.

Spirtos NM, Eisenkop SM, Schlaerth JB, et al. Laparoscopic radical hysterectomy (type III) with aortic and pelvic lymphadenectomy: surgical morbidity and intermediate-term follow-up [Abstract]. *Gynecol Oncol* 2000;76:232.

Spirtos NM, Schlaerth JB, Kimball RE, et al. Laparoscopic radical hysterectomy (type III) with aortic and pelvic lymphadenectomy. *Am J Obstet Gynecol* 1996;174(6):1763.

Spirtos NM, Schlaerth JB, Spirtos TW, et al. Laparoscopic bilateral pelvic and paraaortic lymph node sampling: an evolving technique. *Am J Obstet Gynecol* 1995;173(1):105.

Stallworthy J. Radical surgery following radiation treatment for cervical carcinoma. *Ann R Coll Surg Engl* 1964;34:161.

Steed H, Covens A. Radical vaginal trachelectomy and laparoscopic pelvic lymphadenectomy for preservation of fertility. *Postgrad Obstet Gynecol* 2003;23:1.

Steed H, Rosen B, Murphy J, et al. A comparison of laparoscopic-assisted radical vaginal hysterectomy and radical abdominal hysterectomy in the treatment of cervical cancer. *Gynecol Oncol* 2004;93:588.

Stehman FB, Bundy BN, DiSaia PJ, et al. Carcinoma of the cervix treated with radiation therapy I: a multi-variate analysis of prognostic variables in the gynecologic oncology group. *Cancer* 1991;67:2776.

Stryker JA, Mortel R. Survival following extended field irradiation in carcinoma of cervix metastatic to paraaortic lymph nodes. *Gynecol Oncol* 2000;79:399.

Su TH, Wang KG, Yang YC, et al. Laparoscopic paraaortic lymph node sampling in the staging of invasive cervical carcinoma: including a comparative study of 21 laparotomy cases. *Int J Gynaecol Obstet* 1995;49(3):311.

Sutton G, Bundy B, Delgado G, et al. Ovarian metastases in stage IB carcinoma of the cervix. *Am J Obstet Gynecol* 1992;166:50.

Symmonds RE, Pratt JH. Prevention of fistulas and lymphocysts in radical hysterectomy: preliminary report of a new technique. *Obstet Gynecol* 1961;17:57.

Tattersall MH, Ramirez C, Coppleson M. A randomized trial of adjuvant chemotherapy after radical hysterectomy in stage Ib-IIa cervical cancer patients with pelvic lymph node metastases. *Gynecol Oncol* 1992;46(2):176.

Trimbos JB, Franchi M, Zanaboni F, et al. "State of the art" of radical hysterectomy: current practice in European oncology centers. *Eur J Cancer* 2004;40:375.

Trimbos JB, Maas CP, Deruiter MC, et al. A nerve-sparing radical hysterectomy: guidelines and feasibility in Western patients. *Int J Gynecol Cancer* 2001;11:180.

Underwood PB Jr, Lutz MH, Smoak DL. Ureteral injury following irradiation therapy for carcinoma of the cervix. *Obstet Gynecol* 1977;49:663.

Ungar L, Palfalvi L, Hogg R, et al. Abdominal radical trachelectomy: a fertility-preserving option for women with early cervical cancer. *BJOG* 2005;112:366.

Ungar L, Palfalvi L, Smith JR, et al. Update on and long term follow-up of 91 abdominal radical trachelectomies [Abstract]. *Gynecol Oncol* 2006;101:S20.

van Nagell JR Jr, Donaldson ES, Parker JC, et al. The prognostic significance of pelvic lymph node morphology in carcinoma of the uterine cervix. *Cancer* 1977;39:2624.

Varia MA, Bundy BN, Deppe G, et al. Cervical carcinoma metastatic to paraaortic nodes: extended field radiation therapy with concomitant 5-fluorouracil and cisplatin chemotherapy: a Gynecologic Oncology Group study. *Int J Radiat Oncol Biol Phys* 1998;42(5):1015.

Vasilev SA. Obturator nerve injury: a review of management options. *Gynecol Oncol* 1994;53:152.

Vidaurreta J, Bermudez A, di Paola G, et al. Laparoscopic staging in locally advanced cervical carcinoma: a new possible philosophy? *Gynecol Oncol* 1999;75(3):366.

Wagenaar HC, Trimbos JB, Postema S et al. Tumor diameter and volume assessed by magnetic resonance imaging in the prediction of outcome for invasive cervical cancer. *Gynecol Oncol* 2001;82:474.

Weber TM, Sostman HD, Spirtzer CE, et al. Cervical carcinoma: determination of current tumor extent versus radiation changes with MR imaging. *Radiology* 1995;194:135.

Weiser EB, Bundy BN, Hoskins WJ, et al. Extraperitoneal versus transperitoneal selective paraaortic lymphadenectomy in the pretreatment surgical staging of advanced cervical carcinoma (Gynecologic Oncology Group Study). *Gynecol Oncol* 1989;33:283.

Wentz WB, Reagan JW. Survival in cervical cancer with respect to cell type. *Cancer* 1959;12:384.

Wertheim E. *Die erweiterte abdominale operation bei carcinoma colli uteri (auf grund von 500 fallen)*. Berlin, Germany: Urban, 1911.

Wertheim E. Discussion on the diagnosis and treatment of carcinoma of the uterus. *BMJ* 1905;2:689.

Wertheim E. The extended abdominal operation for carcinoma of the cervix. *Am J Obstet Gynecol* 1912;66:169.

Wertheim E. Zur frag der radikaloperation beim uteruskrebs. *Arch Gynakol* 1900;61:627.

Wertheim MS, Hakes TB, Daghestani AN, et al. A pilot study of adjuvant therapy in patients with cervical cancer and pelvic lymphadenectomy. *J Clin Oncol* 1985;3(7):912.

Wethington SL, Cibula D, Duska LR, et al. An international series on abdominal radical trachelectomy: 101 patients and 28 pregnancies. *Int J Gynecol Cancer* 2012;22(7):1251.

Whitney CW, Sause W, Bundy BN, et al. Randomized comparison of fluorouracil plus cisplatin versus hydroxyurea as an adjunct to radiation therapy in stage IIB-IVA carcinoma of the cervix with negative paraaortic lymph nodes: a Gynecologic Oncology Group and Southwest Oncology Group study. *J Clin Oncol* 1999;17:1339.

Wilkinson EJ, Hause L. Probability in lymph node sectioning. *Cancer* 1974;33:1269.

Zaino RJ, Ward S, Delgado G, et al. Histopathologic predictors of the behavior of surgically treated stage IB squamous cell carcinoma of the cervix: a GOG study. *Cancer* 1990;69:1750.

Zivanovic O, Alektiar KM, Sonoda Y, et al. Treatment patterns of FIGO Stage IB2 cervical cancer: a single-institution experience of radical hysterectomy with individualized postoperative therapy and definitive radiation therapy. *Gynecol Oncol* 2008;111(2):265.

CHAPTER 52
Endometrial Cancer

Marta Ann Crispens

INTRODUCTION

The management of endometrial cancer has changed significantly over the last 40 to 50 years. During the 1970s, endometrial cancer was clinically staged. Patients with early-stage disease were treated with preoperative packing of the endometrial cavity with radiation sources, Heyman capsules, followed by hysterectomy. In 1988, the International Federation of Gynecology and Obstetrics (FIGO) approved a surgical staging system for endometrial cancer. This acknowledged the shift to surgery as primary therapy, with pelvic radiotherapy being used postoperatively as adjuvant therapy for women at increased risk for recurrence. The FIGO staging system for endometrial cancer was again revised in 2009 to reflect our improved understanding of the prognostic factors for this disease. The role of lymphadenectomy and postoperative radiotherapy in the treatment of patients with endometrial cancer remains controversial. Laparoscopic surgery, particularly robotic-assisted laparoscopy, is becoming more important in the treatment of this disease.

In 1983, JV Bokhman described two pathogenetic types of endometrial cancer. Type I tumors account for approximately 90% of endometrial cancers and are associated with exposure to unopposed estrogen from either internal or external sources. They are typically of endometrioid pathology, low grade, diagnosed at early stage, and have an excellent prognosis. Type II tumors are high grade and often have papillary serous or clear cell pathology. They tend to be diagnosed at a later stage, but have a poor prognosis even if diagnosed at an early stage. There is a clear difference in the molecular biology of these tumors. Type I tumors may be associated with a number of genetic changes, including microsatellite instability (20% to 45%), inactivation of the PTEN tumor suppressor gene (57% to 83%), PIK3CA mutation (up to 50%), PIK3R1 mutation (20% to 40%), EGFR overexpression (38% to 46%), E-cadherin loss (6% to 57%), mutational activation of the K-ras oncogene (22% to 43%), BAF250a loss (29% to 39%), and gain of function mutation of the β-catenin gene (14% to 47%). Type II tumors are characterized by aneuploidy. Overall, 9% to 54% of type II tumors exhibit inactivating mutations of p53 gene locus. However, in serous endometrial cancers, over 90% demonstrate p53 inactivation. Type II endometrial cancers may show other mutations, such as PIK3CA (30%), PIK3CA amplification (45%), HER2 amplification (17% to 50%), EGFR overexpression (35% to 56%), E-cadherin loss (41% to 87%), and BAF250 loss (18% to 26%).

EPIDEMIOLOGY

According to American Cancer Society (ACS) estimates, endometrial cancer remains the most common of the gynecologic malignancies in the United States, with 52,630 new cases anticipated in 2014. This makes it the fourth most common cancer occurring in women, behind only breast, lung, and colorectal cancer. It is estimated that there will be 8,590 deaths

TABLE 52.1 Stage and Survival of Endometrial Cancer

STAGE	PATIENTS	5-YR SURVIVAL
I	70%	89.6%
II	13%	78.3%
III	14%	61.9%
IV	3%	21.1%

TABLE 52.2 FIGO Staging of Carcinoma of the Corpus Uteri, 2009

Stage I	Tumor Confined to the Corpus Uteri
IA	No or less than half myometrial invasion
IB	Invasion equal to or more than half of the myometrium
Stage II	Tumor invades cervical stroma, but does not extend beyond the uterus
Stage III	Local and/or regional spread of tumor
IIIA	Tumor invades the serosa of the corpus uteri and/or adnexa
IIIB	Vaginal and/or parametrial involvement
IIIC	Metastases to pelvic and/or paraaortic lymph nodes
IIIC1	Positive pelvic lymph nodes
IIIC2	Positive paraaortic lymph nodes with or without positive pelvic lymph nodes
Stage IV	Tumor invades bladder and/or bowel mucosa and/or distant metastases
IVA	Tumor invasion of bladder and/or bowel mucosa
IVB	Distant metastases, including intra-abdominal metastases and/or inguinal lymph nodes

Positive cytology has to be reported separately without changing the stage.

Histopathology: Degree of Differentiation
Grade 1	5% or less of a solid growth pattern
Grade 2	6%–50% of a solid growth pattern
Grade 3	More than 50% of a solid growth pattern

Notable nuclear atypia, inappropriate for the architectural grade, raises the grade of a grade 1 or grade 2 tumor by 1.

Uterine papillary serous carcinomas and clear cell carcinomas of the endometrium are always high-grade tumors, by definition.

due to endometrial cancer in the year 2014. That most women with newly diagnosed endometrial cancer can expect a good prognosis is due to the fact that endometrial cancer is usually diagnosed at an early stage, when it is readily treatable with surgery alone. However, there remain a few patients with endometrial cancer who present with high-risk histologic subtypes or advanced stage disease, in whom the prognosis is more guarded. Table 52.1 shows the stage distribution and survival of patients diagnosed with endometrial cancer from 1999 to 2001, as reported in the 26th annual FIGO report.

The 2009 FIGO staging system for endometrial cancer as described by Pecorelli et al. is shown in Table 52.2. Tumor grade and depth of myometrial invasion are important prognostic features for endometrial cancer. In the 1988 surgical staging system, tumors confined to the uterine corpus had been divided into three groups: (a) those with no invasion, (b) those with less than 50% myometrial invasion, and (c) those with greater than 50% myometrial invasion. Because FIGO data demonstrated no significant difference in 5-year survival between patients with grade 1 or grade 2 tumor without myometrial invasion as compared to patients with grade 1 or grade 2 tumor with less than 50% myometrial invasion, these two groups were combined.

The 2009 FIGO staging system for endometrial cancer no longer upstages a patient for extension to the endocervical glands. Stage II tumors are now defined as those that invade the cervical stroma. Tumors involving the endocervical glands only are classified as stage I and subdivided according to the depth of myometrial invasion.

The 1988 FIGO staging system had defined patients with positive peritoneal washings as having stage IIIA disease. Positive peritoneal washings are associated with a worse prognosis only in patients with other adverse prognostic features. The presence of malignant cells in the peritoneal washings has been demonstrated not to be an independent adverse prognostic variable. Thus, it has been removed from the staging system. Peritoneal washings should still be performed and reported on every patient with endometrial cancer. Extension to the parametrium has been added to vaginal metastases in stage IIIB.

Stage IIIC previously encompassed metastases to the pelvic and/or paraaortic lymph nodes. Many studies suggest a worse prognosis with spread to the paraaortic lymph nodes. Thus, stage IIIC has been subdivided into IIIC1, pelvic lymph node involvement only, and stage IIIC2, paraaortic lymph node involvement with or without pelvic lymph node involvement.

Uterine sarcomas account for less than 10% of all uterine cancers. The more common histologic types of uterine sarcoma include leiomyosarcoma, endometrial stromal sarcoma, high-grade undifferentiated sarcoma, and adenosarcoma. Prior to the revision of the FIGO staging system in 2009, uterine sarcomas had been staged using the same staging system as endometrial cancers. However, uterine sarcomas and endometrial cancers have significantly different patterns of spread and prognostic features. In the revised 2009 staging system, FIGO introduced a separate staging system for uterine sarcomas (Table 52.3). Carcinosarcoma, also known as malignant mixed müllerian tumor, was previously classified as a sarcoma but is now understood to be a poorly differentiated endometrial carcinoma. Therefore, malignant mixed müllerian tumors are staged according to endometrial cancer staging system.

TABLE 52.3 FIGO Staging of Uterine Sarcomas, 2009

Leiomyosarcomas and ESS[a]
Stage definition
  I Tumor limited to uterus
    IA ≤5 cm
    IB >5 cm
  II Tumor extends beyond the uterus, within the pelvis
    IIA Adnexal involvement
    IIB Involvement of other pelvic tissues
  III Tumor invades abdominal tissues (not just protruding into the abdomen)
    IIIA 1 site
    IIIB >1 site
    IIIC Metastases to pelvic and/or paraaortic lymph nodes
  IV Tumor with
    IVA Bladder and/or rectum invasion
    IVB Distant metastases

Adenosarcomas
Stage definition
  I Tumor limited to uterus
    IA Tumor limited to endometrium/endocervix with no myometrial invasion
    IB ≤ half myometrial invasion
    IC > half myometrial invasion
  II Tumor extends beyond the uterus, within the pelvis.
    IIA Adnexal involvement
    IIB Involvement of other pelvic tissues
  III Tumor invades abdominal tissues (not just protruding into the abdomen).
    IIIA 1 site
    IIIB >1 site
    IIIC Metastases to pelvic and/or paraaortic lymph nodes
  IV Tumor with
    IVA Bladder and/or rectum invasion
    IVB Distant metastases

Carcinosarcomas
Carcinosarcomas should be staged as carcinomas of the endometrium.

[a]Note: Simultaneous endometrial stromal sarcomas of the uterine corpus and ovary/pelvis in association with ovarian/pelvic endometriosis should be classified as independent primary tumors.

TABLE 52.4 Risk Factors for the Development of Endometrial Cancer

Increased risk
Increasing age
Residence in North America or Northern Europe
Higher socioeconomic status
Higher level of education
White race
Nulliparity
Infertility
Menstrual irregularities
Early menarche
Late menopause
Treatment with unopposed estrogen
Tamoxifen use
Anovulatory disorders, such as polycystic ovarian syndrome
Estrogen-producing tumors, such as granulosa-theca cell tumors
Obesity
Hypertension
Diabetes
High fat diet
Hereditary nonpolyposis colon cancer syndrome

Decreased risk
Oral contraceptive use
Nonmedicated plastic or copper IUD use
Consumption of some phytoestrogens, such as isoflavones and lignans
Diet rich in fruits, vegetables, and fiber
Physical activity
Cigarette smoking

RISK FACTORS

There are no clear risk factors for type II endometrial cancers. Type I endometrial cancers are usually related to exposure to unopposed estrogen, whether exogenous or endogenous. Risk factors for type I tumors are summarized in Table 52.4. Endometrial cancer incidence increases with age, until about 70 years, when rates begin to decline. Living in North America or Northern Europe is associated with an increased risk of endometrial cancer.

Reproductive factors are associated with an increased risk of endometrial cancer. Endometrial cancer risk is increased in women who are nulliparous or infertile or have menstrual irregularities. Early onset of menarche or late age at menopause is also associated with an increased risk of endometrial cancer.

Exogenous exposure, such as estrogen replacement therapy, has been shown to be associated with an increased risk of endometrial cancer in a number of studies. A meta-analysis

that combined data from both case–control and cohort studies found a 2.3-fold increased risk of endometrial cancer among women who had ever used estrogen replacement therapy as compared to never users. The risk increases with increasing estrogen dose and increasing duration of estrogen use. In the same meta-analysis noted above, the relative risk of developing endometrial cancer rose to 9.5 among women who had used estrogen replacement therapy for 10 or more years as compared to never users. The risk can be reduced by the concurrent use of cyclic or continuous progestin.

The use of tamoxifen by postmenopausal women for the prevention or treatment of breast cancer is associated with an approximately twofold increased risk of endometrial cancer as well as an increased risk of uterine sarcoma. However, this small increased risk of uterine cancer is outweighed by the survival benefit of tamoxifen use among women with breast cancer. As compared to other endometrial cancers, tamoxifen-related endometrial cancers are not associated with an increased incidence of adverse prognostic features. Although tamoxifen acts as a weak estrogen in the postmenopausal endometrium, it has predominantly antiestrogenic effects in the premenopausal endometrium. Thus, there is no increased risk of endometrial cancers among premenopausal women using tamoxifen. The use of aromatase inhibitors for the treatment of breast cancer has not been associated with an increased risk of endometrial cancer.

Patient metabolic factors such as obesity are associated with an increased risk of endometrial cancer and an increased risk of mortality from the disease. Weiderpass et al. found that as compared to women of normal body mass index (BMI), women with a BMI of 30 to 33.99 had a threefold increased risk of endometrial cancer that rose to a sixfold increased risk among women with a BMI greater than 34. In the Million Women Study, the relative risk of developing endometrial cancer was 2.73 and the relative risk of dying of endometrial cancer was 2.28 among women with a BMI ≥ 30 as compared to women with a normal BMI. Likewise, in a large prospective study of the effect of obesity on the risk of death from cancer, Calle et al. found that the relative risk of death from endometrial cancer was increased over sixfold among women with a BMI ≥ 40 as compared to those with a normal.

In the past, the increased risk of endometrial cancer among obese women has been attributed to increased levels of unopposed estrogen due to peripheral conversion of androgen to estrogen by the aromatase enzyme in adipose tissue. More recently, the roles of proinflammatory adipokines, which are cytokines produced in the adipose tissues, and of insulin and insulin-like growth factor on stimulating endometrial cancer development have begun to be elucidated.

The ovaries may be a source of unopposed estrogen in women with anovulatory disorders, such as polycystic ovarian syndrome (PCOS). In a retrospective study of 128 women with endometrial cancer, Pillay and colleagues found that among women less than 50 years old, PCOS was significantly more prevalent among women with endometrial cancer than among normal controls. They observed no relationship between PCOS and endometrial cancer in postmenopausal women.

Fearnley et al. conducted a case–control study of the incidence of endometrial cancer in 156 women with PCOS as compared to 398 controls. They identified a statistically significant fourfold increased risk of endometrial cancer among women with PCOS. After controlling for BMI, the difference in endometrial cancer risk did not remain significant. Therefore, some experts contend that PCOS, per se, is not a risk factor for endometrial cancer. They emphasize that women with PCOS have multiple other risk factors for endometrial cancer, including chronic anovulation, centripetal obesity, and diabetes. Premenopausal women with PCOS should be counseled on the risk of endometrial cancer and the importance of maintaining regular withdrawal bleeding cycles. The optimal treatment regimen is unknown (ACOG Practice Bulletin 108). Estrogen-producing tumors, such as granulosa cell tumors of the ovary, may be another source of endogenous, unopposed estrogen, and endometrial hyperplasia or cancer is common in women with estrogen-producing tumors.

The risk of endometrial cancer is increased in patients with diabetes. This risk is further increased in obese diabetic patients. Similarly, the risk of endometrial cancer is increased in patients with metabolic syndrome. Of the components of the metabolic syndrome, elevated BMI is the factor most strongly associated with endometrial cancer risk.

Factors that decrease exposure to unopposed estrogens decrease the risk of endometrial cancer. The Cancer and Steroid Hormone Study demonstrated that 12 months of oral contraceptive use decreased the risk of endometrial cancer by 40%, and the effect persisted for at least 15 years after the cessation of use. A large, Chinese case–control study demonstrated a 50% decrease in the risk of endometrial cancer after 3 years of oral contraceptive use.

Smoking also decreases the risk of endometrial cancer. The exact mechanism is unknown. It may be due to alterations in sex hormone metabolism, a reduction in body weight among smokers, or an earlier age at menopause among smokers. Obviously, the overall detrimental health effects of smoking far outweigh any benefit related to decreased endometrial cancer risk.

A number of studies have suggested a protective effect of IUD use on the risk of endometrial cancer. Tao's large case–control study of 2,416 women in Shanghai, China, demonstrated an approximately 50% reduction in the risk of endometrial cancer among women who had ever used an intrauterine device (IUD). The type of IUD was not specified. Case–control studies by Castellsague in patients using unspecified type of IUDs and by Hill in patients using nonhormonal IUDs demonstrated a similar approximately 50% decreased risk of endometrial cancer in IUD users as compared to nonusers.

Gardner et al. conducted a randomized controlled trial of levonorgestrel IUD versus observation in 122 postmenopausal women with breast cancer who were being treated with tamoxifen. The mean follow-up time was 26 months, range 14 to 36 months. They were able to demonstrate benign endometrial changes and a decrease in the development of endometrial polyps in the IUD users as compared to nonusers. This study was unable to assess the effect of IUD use on the development of endometrial cancer. Nor could this study assess the safety of levonorgestrel-containing IUD use in women with breast cancer.

Endometrial cancer is one of the components of the Lynch syndrome. This autosomal, dominant cancer risk syndrome is caused by inactivation of one of several genes involved in DNA mismatch repair. A personal and/or family history of colon, endometrial, ovarian, ureteral, or small-bowel malignancy should prompt the clinician to consider referral of the patient for genetic counseling and possible genetic testing. Diagnosis of an endometrial or ovarian cancer often triggers the identification of a family with Lynch syndrome.

The lifetime risk of endometrial cancer in women with Lynch syndrome is 40% to 60%. Patients with Lynch syndrome may consider chemoprevention with OCPs, although there are no clear data to support this approach. A woman with Lynch syndrome may consider increased surveillance with annual endometrial biopsy beginning at age 30 to 35, although there is no definitive evidence to support this approach. Patients should be counseled to promptly report and be evaluated for any abnormal uterine bleeding. Risk-reducing surgery with hysterectomy and bilateral salpingo-oophorectomy (BSO), performed after the completion of childbearing, has been demonstrated to reduce the risk of endometrial cancer in patients with Lynch syndrome.

PROGNOSTIC FEATURES

The prognostic features for endometrial cancer have been well defined (Table 52.5). These include age, race, FIGO stage, tumor grade, histologic subtype, depth of myometrial invasion, cervical or adnexal involvement, positive peritoneal cytology, metastasis to pelvic or paraaortic lymph nodes, and presence of lymphovascular space invasion.

Among women with stage I endometrial cancer, risk factors that adversely affect survival include increasing age, grade 2 to 3 histology, the presence of lymphovascular space invasion, and invasion to the outer third of the myometrium. Using these factors, patients with "*high-intermediate risk*" for recurrence can be identified. These patients have an approximately 27% chance of recurrence at 48 months. The GOG defines high-intermediate risk endometrial cancer as (a) any age with greater than or equal to 3 or more risk factors; (b) age greater than or equal to 50 but less than 70 with greater than or equal to 2 or more risk factors, and (c) age greater than or equal to 70 with greater than or equal to 1 or more risk factors (Keys). Many experts suggest that these are the patients who should be targeted for surgical staging and/or postoperative adjuvant therapy.

TABLE 52.5 Prognostic Features for Endometrial Cancer

Race
FIGO stage
Depth of myometrial invasion[a]
Tumor grade[a]
Histologic subtype[a]
Cervical involvement
Adnexal involvement
Positive pelvic washings
Metastases to the pelvic or paraaortic lymph nodes
Lymphovascular space invasion
DNA aneuploidy

[a]Denotes prognostic features that are most important in patients with endometrial cancers confined to the uterus.

SCREENING FOR ENDOMETRIAL CANCER

The ACS guidelines for the early detection of cancer recommend that for average-risk, asymptomatic individuals, endometrial cancer screening should consist of education of women at the time of menopause regarding the risks and symptoms of endometrial cancer. Women should be strongly encouraged to report any unexpected bleeding or spotting to their physician.

Even women at increased risk for endometrial cancer due to a history of unopposed estrogen therapy, tamoxifen use, late menopause, nulliparity, infertility, anovulation, obesity, diabetes, or hypertension do not benefit from routine screening for endometrial cancer, beyond the reporting of symptoms. The ACS recommends that women at high risk for endometrial cancer, such as women known or at substantial risk to be a carrier of a Lynch syndrome mutation, should be offered annual screening with endometrial biopsy by the age of 35, in addition to being informed about the symptoms of endometrial cancer. Patients should be counseled regarding the potential benefits, risks, and limitations of endometrial cancer screening. These recommendations are based on expert opinion. There is no current evidence that this approach will result in earlier diagnosis or improved outcomes for these women.

EVALUATION OF THE SYMPTOMATIC PATIENT

Abnormal uterine bleeding is the most common presenting symptom of endometrial cancer. In a review of the pathologic findings among women with postmenopausal bleeding, Gredmark and colleagues found that the risk of adenomatous endometrial hyperplasia or cancer in a woman with postmenopausal bleeding is approximately 18%. The risk of malignancy increased with increasing age, with the peak incidence of endometrial cancer occurring in women between 65 and 69 years of age. The most common cause of postmenopausal bleeding was endometrial atrophy, which was identified in 50% of the patients. All patients with postmenopausal bleeding should undergo evaluation for possible endometrial cancer.

Endometrial cancer can also occur in premenopausal women and may present with heavy or irregular vaginal bleeding. The American Congress of Obstetricians and Gynecologists recommends that any women aged 45 or older with abnormal bleeding should have endometrial sampling performed. Younger women with risk factors for endometrial cancer, such as obesity or anovulation, who have failed hormonal treatment, or who have persistent abnormal uterine bleeding should also undergo endometrial sampling. A 25-year-old woman who experienced menarche at age 12, is obese, and has PCOS will already have experienced more than 10 years of exposure to unopposed estrogen.

There are several options for the evaluation of a woman with postmenopausal bleeding. The ACOG Committee Opinion on the assessment of postmenopausal bleeding recommends either transvaginal pelvic ultrasonography or office endometrial biopsy as the initial approach, but not both together (**Fig. 52.1**).

Transvaginal pelvic ultrasound to evaluate the endometrial stripe thickness is one of the options for primary evaluation of postmenopausal bleeding. Several meta-analyses have been published evaluating the use of transvaginal pelvic ultrasound in the triage of women with postmenopausal bleeding. The most referenced meta-analysis, performed by Smith-Bindman et al., evaluated 35 studies performed between 1966 and 1996 that included 5,892 patients. Women with a pretest probability of cancer of 10% had only a 1% risk of having cancer following a transvaginal ultrasound result showing 5 mm or less endometrial stripe.

Gupta et al. performed a subsequent meta-analysis that assessed 57 studies in 9,031 postmenopausal women. Only four studies using a cutoff of less than or equal to 5 mm were of adequate quality to be included in the analysis. They found that among women with an endometrial stripe thickness of 5 mm or less, the risk of endometrial cancer was approximately 2.5%.

Timmermans et al. performed a meta-analysis using original datasets from 13 studies including 2,896 patients. They calculated receiver operating characteristic curves of endometrial thickness. The commonly used cutoff values of 4 and 5 mm were found to have a sensitivity to detect endometrial cancer of 95% and 90%, respectively. These authors recommend the use of a 3-mm cutoff value, which yielded a sensitivity of 98% for the detection of endometrial cancer.

ACOG recommends that endometrial sampling is not required in a patient with postmenopausal bleeding and an endometrial stripe thickness of less than or equal to 4 mm. If the

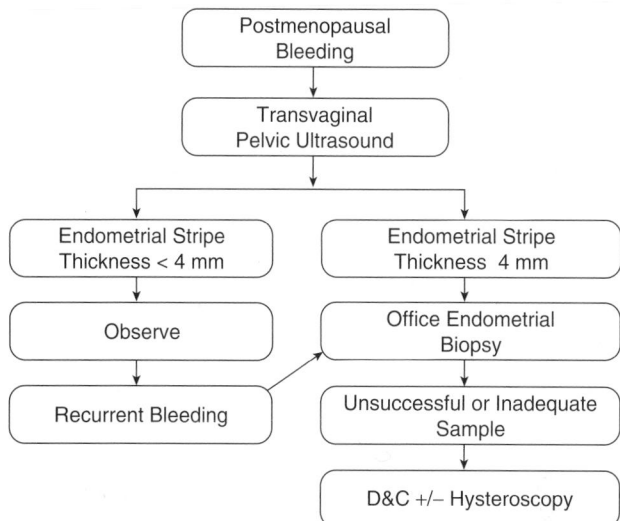

FIGURE 52.1 Algorithm for the evaluation of postmenopausal bleeding. (Adapted from Moodley M, Roberts C. Clinical pathway for the evaluation of postmenopausal bleeding with an emphasis on endometrial cancer detection. *J Obstet and Gynaecol* 2004;24:736–741, with permission. Copyright © 2004, Informa Healthcare.)

endometrial stripe thickness is greater than 4 mm or if the endometrial stripe thickness cannot be assessed, then further evaluation with endometrial biopsy, sonohysterography to rule out endometrial polyps or submucosal fibroids, or office hysteroscopy is indicated.

Another option for the initial evaluation of postmenopausal vaginal bleeding is to proceed directly to office endometrial biopsy. This is typically accomplished with a Pipelle instrument, which is a disposable plastic catheter that can be placed through the cervix into the endometrial cavity for the aspiration of endometrial cells. Its use occasionally may require the placement of a single-toothed tenaculum on the cervix for countertraction or gentle cervical dilatation.

In a meta-analysis comparing endometrial sampling techniques, the Pipelle was found to be the most accurate. Among postmenopausal women, the sensitivity for the detection of atypical endometrial hyperplasia was 81% and for the detection of endometrial cancer was 99.6%. The sensitivity of the device for the detection of endometrial cancer among premenopausal women was 91%. The specificity of the Pipelle device for the diagnosis of endometrial hyperplasia or malignancy was 98%.

Up to 54% of patients will have failure of endometrial sampling. Farrell and coworkers have reported a 20% incidence of uterine pathology after an "insufficient" endometrial biopsy, with 3% of these patients having malignancy. These patients may be further evaluated with transvaginal pelvic ultrasound. If the stripe thickness is ≤4 mm, then the risk of malignancy is low (Farrell).

Dilatation and curettage (D&C) in the operating room is considered the "gold standard" for endometrial sampling. However, even D&C fails to sample the entire endometrial cavity. Stock and Kanbour performed prehysterectomy D&Cs and found that in approximately 60% of patients, less than half of the endometrium had been sampled. There are limited data regarding the sensitivity and specificity of D&C for the diagnosis of endometrial hyperplasia and malignancy. Women with persistent postmenopausal bleeding despite a negative prior workup should undergo reevaluation.

Both Pipelle endometrial biopsy and D&C are limited for the evaluation of focal endometrial lesions. Studies differ as to whether adding hysteroscopy may improve the diagnostic accuracy of D&C. Patients with endometrial cancer who undergo hysteroscopy are more likely to have positive pelvic peritoneal washings than those who do not undergo hysteroscopy, which may be due to insufflation of the uterus with fluid during hysteroscopy. There is currently no evidence that this results in an increased risk of recurrence or decreased survival. This conclusion is limited by the small number of patients with recurrent disease and short follow-up intervals.

ENDOMETRIAL HYPERPLASIA

Endometrial hyperplasia is a proliferation or overgrowth of the endometrium caused by exposure to unopposed estrogen. Kurman et al. further classified endometrial hyperplasia into four groups, simple hyperplasia with and without atypia and complex hyperplasia with or without atypia. Simple hyperplasia is characterized by an increase in the number of endometrial glands, which may be dilated with little crowding or may have irregular outline and exhibit crowding. Complex hyperplasia is characterized by glands with irregular outline that demonstrate marked structural complexity and back-to-back crowding. Atypical hyperplasias demonstrate cytologic atypia and loss of cellular polarity. These criteria were adopted by the World Health Organization for the classification of endometrial hyperplasia in 1994.

More recently, Muter and colleagues have introduced a two-tier system for the classification of premalignant lesions of the endometrium, the endometrial intraepithelial neoplasia system. This system uses morphometric analysis to differentiate between monoclonal, premalignant lesions as compared to polyclonal and not premalignant lesions. In this system, the lesion must exceed 1 mm, the area of glands exceeds that of the stroma, and the cytology differs between the architecturally crowded focus and the background endometrial glands. Cytologic atypia is associated with an increased risk of progression to endometrial cancer. In Kurmans's series of 170 women with endometrial hyperplasia not treated with progesterone, progression to cancer occurred in 1% of patients with simple hyperplasia without atypia, 3% of patients with complex hyperplasia without atypia, 8% of patients with simple hyperplasia with atypia, and 29% of patients with complex hyperplasia with atypia during a mean follow-up time of 13.4 years. In another study by Horn et al., among women with complex hyperplasia without atypia, only 2% progressed to cancer and 10.5% progressed to complex atypical endometrial hyperplasia. Among women with complex hyperplasia without atypia treated with progestin therapy, 128 of 208 (61.5%) regressed. Progression to cancer occurred in 58 of 112 women (52%) with complex atypical hyperplasia. Of the seven patients with complex atypical endometrial hyperplasia treated with progestins, four had persistent disease and three progressed to cancer.

Endometrial hyperplasias without atypia are typically treated with some form of progestin therapy. Common regimens include medroxyprogesterone acetate 10 to 20 mg daily or cyclically for 14 days per month, depot medroxyprogesterone 150 mg intramuscularly every 3 months, megestrol acetate 40 to 160 mg daily, or the levonorgestrel-containing IUD (Trimble).

Complex atypical hyperplasia of the endometrium is a premalignant condition, which is typically treated with hysterectomy with or without BSO. Approximately 40% of women with complex atypical endometrial hyperplasia diagnosed by biopsy will have the finding of endometrial cancer in the hysterectomy specimen. The risk of change in diagnosis from hyperplasia to cancer may be slightly higher with preoperative Pipelle endometrial biopsy (46%) than with D&C (27%).

Progestin therapy can be considered for women with complex atypical endometrial hyperplasia or in selected women with grade 1 endometrial cancer who are either poor operative candidates or who wish to retain their fertility. Gunderson and colleagues performed a systematic review of 45 published studies including a total of 391 women, 111 with complex atypical endometrial hyperplasia and 280 with grade 1 endometrioid adenocarcinoma of the endometrium who were treated with progestin therapy. The median age of the patients was 31.7 years in trials for which patient age was reported. Median follow-up was 39 months. The most common progestins used were medroxyprogesterone in 49%, megestrol acetate in 25%, and levonorgestrel-containing IUD in 19%. The complete response rate was 65.8% in women with complex atypical endometrial hyperplasia and 48.2% in women with endometrial cancer. The median time to complete response was 6 months. Recurrence was diagnosed in 23.2% of women with hyperplasia and 35.4% of women with cancer. There were 117 live births among the 391 women in this study.

Before progestin therapy is considered in a young woman with complex atypical endometrial hyperplasia or grade 1 endometrial cancer who is attempting to retain her fertility, a thorough evaluation of the endometrial cancer by D&C should be performed. If endometrial cancer is confirmed, then transvaginal pelvic ultrasound and magnetic resonance imaging (MRI) of the pelvis should be performed to rule out myometrial invasion and any ovarian pathology. Chest x-ray or chest computed tomography (CT) with CT of the abdomen and pelvis should be performed to evaluate for the possibility of metastatic disease. Patients with hyperplasia or cancer who are being treated with progestins should have endometrial sampling every 3 months to evaluate response to therapy. They should be extensively counseled regarding the risks of this approach. There is a case report describing progression to grade 2 endometrioid adenocarcinoma of the endometrium metastatic to the lymph nodes in a 40-year-old patient with complex atypical hyperplasia who was treated with progestin.

SURGICAL STAGING AND TREATMENT

Rationale

Endometrial cancer is surgically staged and treated. The procedure includes thorough exploration of the peritoneal contents, pelvic washings, hysterectomy, and BSO. The role of bilateral pelvic and paraaortic lymph node dissection remains controversial. Laparotomy has been the principle surgical approach to hysterectomy and staging for endometrial cancer. Laparoscopy and robotically assisted laparoscopy are increasingly being used for endometrial cancer surgery. Since laparoscopic hysterectomy and lymph node dissection techniques are discussed in detail elsewhere in this text, the discussion below will focus on open techniques.

Type I endometrial cancers have three main patterns of spread, by direct extension, to regional lymph nodes, and hematogenously. The most common mechanism of spread for type I endometrial cancer is by direct extension, invading into the myometrium or by extension to the adjacent cervix. Hematogenous metastasis tends to occur late in the course of the disease. Type II endometrial cancers, particularly uterine papillary serous carcinomas, may also metastasize within the peritoneal cavity, similar to ovarian carcinomas.

Endometrial carcinoma spreads through three separate lymphatic pathways: Paracervical and parametrial lymphatics drain to the pelvic lymph nodes, ovarian lymphatics drain to the paraaortic lymph nodes, and round ligament lymphatics drain to the inguinal lymph nodes (Fig. 52.2). The lymphatic drainage of the uterine fundus and cervix directs most of the metastases to the pelvic lymph nodes. Although the paraaortic lymph nodes may be primary metastatic sites via spread through the infundibulopelvic ligament lymphatics, it is rare for an endometrial cancer patient to have isolated paraaortic lymph node metastases without concomitant pelvic lymph node metastases. The incidence of isolated paraaortic lymph node metastases is approximately 1% to 1.5%.

Performance of pelvic and paraaortic lymphadenectomy for the staging of endometrial cancer remains controversial. Kilgore and colleagues retrospective study suggested that lymphadenectomy might have a therapeutic effect for patients with endometrial cancer. They evaluated the outcomes of 649 patients surgically managed for endometrial cancer. In this study, 212 patients had pelvic lymph nodes sampled from at least 4 separate sites (multiple-site lymph node sampling), 205 patients had pelvic lymph nodes sampled from fewer than 4 sites (limited-site lymph node sampling), and 208 patients had no pelvic lymph nodes sampled. Patients undergoing multiple-site lymph node sampling had a survival of approximately 85%, whereas patients in whom pelvic lymph nodes were not sampled had a survival of approximately 65%, a statistically significant difference (P = 0.0027). This survival advantage for patients with multiple-site lymph node sampling

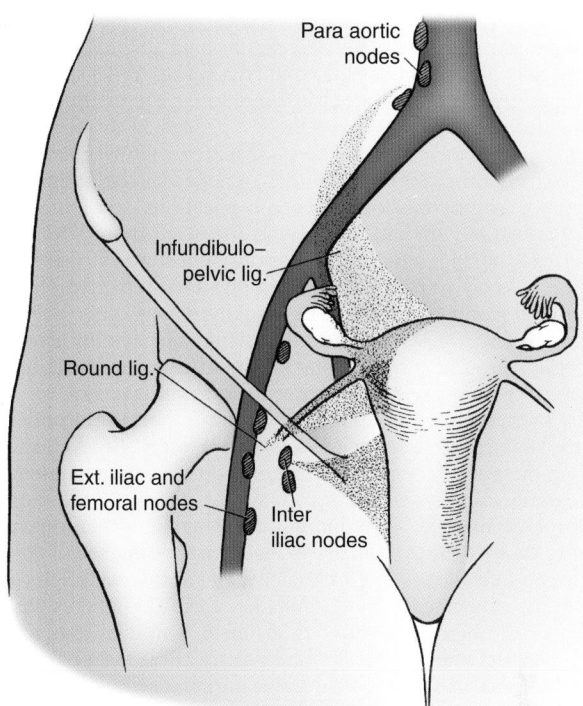

FIGURE 52.2 Lymphatic pathways of tumor spread of endometrial carcinoma to pelvic and extrapelvic nodes.

persisted even in a subgroup analysis of patients treated with postoperative whole pelvic radiotherapy.

There have been two prospective randomized trials assessing the therapeutic value of pelvic lymphadenectomy in patients with apparent stage I endometrial cancer. The ASTEC trial enrolled 1,408 patients at 85 centers in 4 countries. Median follow-up was 37 months. Patients were randomized to "standard surgery" with hysterectomy, BSO, washings, and palpation of the paraaortic lymph nodes versus standard surgery with pelvic lymphadenectomy. Postoperatively, patients were enrolled in a second randomized trial of postoperative radiotherapy versus no radiotherapy based on uterine findings. The overall morbidity was low, but patients in the lymphadenectomy group were more likely to develop lower extremity lymphedema. The authors reported that there was no difference in overall or recurrence-free survival in patients who did not undergo pelvic lymphadenectomy versus those who did.

This trial has been extensively criticized. Although the patients were randomized, there was an excess of patients with adverse prognostic features in the lymphadenectomy arm, including 10% more patients in the lymphadenectomy arm having deep myometrial invasion. The lymph node sampling itself was inadequate, with a median of only nine nodes being recovered. The Gynecologic Oncology Group Surgical Procedures Manual, revised January 2010, requires a minimum of four nodes from each side for an adequate pelvic lymph node dissection. The performance of paraaortic lymph node dissection was left to the discretion of the surgeon. Since the randomization to postoperative external beam radiotherapy was based on uterine factors and not the presence of metastases to the pelvic lymph nodes, approximately half of those who might have benefited the most from pelvic radiotherapy, those with lymph node metastases, did not receive it.

CONSORT was a phase III randomized trial of routine lymphadenectomy versus no lymphadenectomy in women with apparent stage I endometrial cancer who were undergoing standard surgery with hysterectomy and BSO. Paraaortic lymph node sampling was left to the discretion of the surgeon. Postoperative therapy was at the discretion of the treating physician, but was similar between the two groups. In this trial, the pelvic lymph node dissection was adequate by GOG standards with a median of 30 lymph nodes removed in the lymphadenectomy group. Intraoperative complications were similar. Patients in the lymphadenectomy group were more likely to experience postoperative complications, which was largely due to an excess of lymphedema and lymphoceles in the lymphadenectomy group. These authors also found no difference in overall or disease-free survival in the lymphadenectomy group. However, they did conclude that systematic lymphadenectomy significantly improved the accuracy of surgical staging.

In assessing the preceding studies, it is important to understand the purpose of staging. According to the SEER Web site, among the purposes of cancer staging is to "adequately assess the extent of cancer in order to treat the disease in the most appropriate manner." The findings of a staging evaluation are used to direct therapy in order to maximize the chance of cure while minimizing the risk of toxicity. Using this paradigm, it may be appropriate to omit lymphadenectomy in patients with grade 1 endometrial cancer confined to the endometrium who have essentially no risk of lymph node metastases. In patients with high-intermediate risk disease, surgical staging may be useful to identify those patients with lymph node metastases who may benefit from radiotherapy, while avoiding short- and long-term radiotherapy toxicity in women who can be confirmed to have negative lymph nodes.

Ben-Shachar and coworkers evaluated the impact of routine surgical staging on the treatment of 181 women with a preoperative diagnosis of grade 1 endometrioid adenocarcinoma of the endometrium. Surgical staging was performed in 82% of cases and was omitted only when the disease was apparently confined to the endometrium and the surgical risk was high. High-risk uterine features, including greater than one-half myometrial invasion, grade 3 tumors, high-risk histologic variants, and/or cervical extension were identified in 26% of patients. Lymph node metastases were identified in 3.9% of patients. Overall, the findings of the surgical staging procedure significantly impacted postoperative treatment decisions in 29% of patients, including 12% of patients who were determined to need adjuvant therapy and 17% of patients who were able to forego external beam whole pelvic radiotherapy or chemotherapy. The incidence of severe surgical complications in the surgically staged group was 3.2%.

Preoperative Assessment and Preparation

As noted above, many patients with endometrial cancer may be older and have multiple medical comorbidities. Thus, preoperative preparation is important. All patients should have a thorough history and physical examination. The history should assess the length and severity of the patient's bleeding or other presenting complaint. It should also assess for symptoms of metastatic disease, such as abdominal or pelvic pain, changes in bowel or bladder function, lower extremity pain or swelling, abdominal bloating, early satiety, shortness of breath, or cough. Previous medical history and symptoms suggestive of occult cardiopulmonary disease or other medical illnesses should be ascertained. Careful attention should be paid to the family history, as endometrial cancer may develop before colon cancer in up to half of women with Lynch syndrome.

The physical examination should focus on assessment for supraclavicular and inguinal lymphadenopathy, abdominal distension or fluid wave suggestive of ascites, abdominal masses, and lower extremity edema. On pelvic examination, close attention should be paid to possible vaginal, cervical, or parametrial extension of disease. Uterine size and mobility, the presence of adnexal masses, and cul-de-sac nodularity should be assessed.

Basic laboratory evaluation should include a hematocrit and type and screen. Ca-125 testing is not indicated, except in patients with uterine papillary serous carcinoma. A chest x-ray should be performed both to rule out lung metastases and to evaluate for concurrent pulmonary disease. An electrocardiogram will be needed in most patients for preoperative assessment for potential cardiac disease. Extensive preoperative radiographic assessment for metastatic disease with CT, MRI, or positron emission tomography is not indicated, unless the history or physical examination or uterine histology is suggestive of distant disease. This would be most likely to occur in patients with uterine papillary serous or clear cell carcinomas. Other preoperative testing should be performed as dictated by the patient's history and physical findings and may include complete blood count, electrolytes, and assessment of hepatic and renal function. For patients with multiple medical comorbidities, preoperative cardiac, pulmonary, or other medical consultations may be necessary. In such patients, preoperative consultation with the anesthesiologist may also be of benefit.

Once a patient has completed her preoperative evaluation and has been cleared for surgery, she should be recounseled regarding her options for therapy, including surgical therapy; primary pelvic radiotherapy, which is usually reserved for patients who are not good candidates for surgery; and no therapy. Patients should be thoroughly counseled on the indications, risks, and benefits of surgery, that there is no guarantee as to outcome, and that further therapy in the form of additional surgery, chemotherapy, or radiotherapy may be necessary. The patient and her family should be given the opportunity to have all of their questions answered. Patient understanding should be confirmed by having her perform teach-back. Written informed consent should be obtained.

Standard preoperative antibiotic prophylaxis for hysterectomy should be employed, typically with cefazolin 1 to 2 g intravenously administered within 60 minutes prior to incision. For patients with penicillin allergy, clindamycin plus gentamicin or a quinolone or aztreonam or metronidazole plus gentamicin or a quinolone are acceptable alternatives.

Deep vein thrombosis occurs in 15% to 40% of patient undergoing major gynecologic surgery who do not receive thromboprophylaxis. High-risk features for thromboembolism in patients undergoing gynecologic surgery include patients older than 40 years with any of the following: history of prior deep venous thrombosis or pulmonary embolism, varicose veins, infection, malignancy, estrogen therapy, obesity, or prolonged surgery. All patients undergoing surgery for endometrial cancer should receive thromboembolism prophylaxis with low-dose heparin 5,000 units every 8 hours subcutaneously, low molecular weight heparin with enoxaparin 40 mg daily subcutaneously, or dalteparin 5,000 units daily subcutaneously or pneumatic compression devices. Double prophylaxis with pneumatic compression devices and either low-dose heparin or low molecular weight heparin should be considered for patients at highest risk. This would include patients older than 60 years with a history of prior venous thromboembolism, cancer, or hypercoagulable state. In these patients, consideration should also be given to continuing pharmacologic prophylaxis for 2 to 4 weeks after discharge.

Surgical Technique—Laparotomy

Prior to taking the patient to the operating room, the patient should confirm the surgical site (abdomen), and this should be marked according to hospital protocol. Once in the operating room, a time-out is performed as per hospital protocol to ensure the correct patient and procedure. After the induction of anesthesia, the patient should be positioned for surgery. Some surgeons prefer the supine position for hysterectomy. It does avoid the risk of neurologic injury that can rarely occur with lithotomy position in Allen stirrups. Many gynecologic oncologists will place the patient in the lithotomy position due to the ready access to the paraaortic lymph nodes that can be achieved with the surgeon between the patient's legs.

The abdomen is usually opened through a vertical midline lower abdominal incision. This is preferable to a low transverse incision, such as a Pfannenstiel incision, because it allows for better access to the paraaortic lymph nodes. In morbidly obese patients, a paramedian or high transverse incision is sometimes used to keep the incision out of the pannus and reduce the risk of infection. Occasionally, panniculectomy in conjunction with hysterectomy may be performed.

On entering the abdominal cavity, *peritoneal washings are obtained*. The operator washes the pelvic organs with 50 to 100 mL of saline. The fluid is gently agitated, then aspirated from the posterior cul-de-sac, mixed with heparin, and submitted for cytologic evaluation.

Next, the *peritoneal cavity is carefully explored*. The approach to abdominal exploration should be systematic. Explore the pelvis last, so as not to be distracted by findings there. Facilitate the exploration of the upper abdomen by having the assistant elevate the anterior abdominal wall at the apex of the incision using a large Richardson retractor. The omentum is brought into the field and carefully examined for metastatic implants. The upper abdominal contents, including the anterior surface of the stomach, the surface of the liver, and the gallbladder, can be visualized. Starting on the right, the operator's hand is used to palpate the peritoneum of the anterior abdominal wall and the paracolic gutter. As the hand moves posteriorly, the kidney can be palpated. Then, palpate the gallbladder, right lobe of the liver, and right hemidiaphragm. The operator then explores the left upper abdomen, including the left diaphragm, left lobe of the liver, spleen, and stomach, including the pylorus. Finally, follow the left anterior abdominal wall and paracolic gutter inferiorly back to the pelvis, palpating the left kidney in the process. At this point, the cecum is identified and the appendix can be examined. The small bowel is run from the ileocecal valve to the ligament of Treitz. With the bowel on the surface of the abdomen, palpation of the retroperitoneum is facilitated. Start superiorly with the pancreas and continue inferiorly to palpate the paraaortic lymph nodes. Continue the nodal palpation to the pelvic lymph nodes bilaterally. The small bowel is returned to the abdomen. The large bowel is run in situ. Finally, while retracting the small bowel into the upper abdomen, the pelvis is carefully explored. Assess the pelvic peritoneum, with careful attention to the cul-de-sac peritoneum, for implants. Note the size and mobility of the uterus. Assess the ovaries and fallopian tubes for any masses or implants.

Once the peritoneal exploration is completed, a self-retaining retractor can be placed and the bowel can be packed into the upper abdomen with the assistance of moist laparotomy sponges. This is assisted with the use of gentle Trendelenburg positioning. Care must be taken with the use of a self-retaining retractor to keep the blades off of the psoas muscles in order to avoid injury to the femoral nerves.

Hysterectomy with BSO is begun by grasping the uterine cornua bilaterally with long Kelley or similar clamps, occluding the fallopian tubes. This allows for manipulation of the uterus during the hysterectomy, while preventing efflux of malignant cells via the tubes during the course of the procedure. A tenaculum, Leahy, or other perforating clamps should not be placed on the uterine fundus in order to avoid contamination of the field by malignant cells from the interior of the uterus.

On either side, the round ligament is ligated and transected. The pelvic sidewall peritoneum is then incised approximately 1 cm lateral and parallel to the infundibulopelvic ligament. The retroperitoneal space can be bluntly dissected to reveal the course of the ureter through the pelvis. The ureter lies on the medial peritoneal leaf. Its identification is facilitated by the use of the suction tip in one hand and the back of a DeBakey pickup in the other. These instruments can be used to gently separate the loose areolar tissue in the retroperitoneum by dissecting in the plane medial and parallel to the iliac vessels. The ureter is at its most superficial, and therefore easiest to identify, as it crosses the bifurcation of the common iliac artery at the pelvic brim. A common mistake is to look for the ureter deep in the pelvis, where it can be confused with the superior vesicle artery. A helpful anatomic point is that the superior vesicle artery will be seen to rise out of the retroperitoneum as it is followed distally, while the ureter will tend to course more deeply in the retroperitoneum as it is followed distally. Positive identification of the ureter is achieved by visualizing its distinct peristalsis. When palpated between the operator's fingers, it gives a "popping" sensation, like a rubber band.

Once the ureter has been clearly identified, the infundibulopelvic ligament can be identified coursing anterior and parallel. It should be isolated by making a window in the posterior leaf of the broad ligament between the infundibulopelvic ligament and the ureter. Ideally, this should be performed under direct visualization so as to avoid injury to the vessels within or to the ureter. The infundibulopelvic ligament is doubly clamped using Haney clamps, transected and doubly ligated with a free tie and transfixion suture. The application of the free tie first compresses the vessels within the infundibulopelvic ligament, preventing the formation of a hematoma when the transfixion suture is placed. Thus, the transfixion suture must be placed through the infundibulopelvic ligament distal to the free tie. The utero-ovarian ligament is skeletonized back to the uterus. The adnexa should not be amputated unless there is an adnexal mass preventing access to the pelvis. This is to prevent spillage of tumor cells into the peritoneal cavity. The adnexa can be suspended off of the Kelley clamp on either uterine cornua in order to keep them out of the way during the hysterectomy.

The anterior leaves of the broad ligament and the vesicouterine peritoneum are incised, and the bladder can be dissected sharply off of the lower uterine segment and cervix. Identify the correct incision line by elevating the vesicouterine peritoneum at either end. A line of loose areolar tissue will become apparent as the air enters the vesicouterine space. If the initial incision is made inferior to this, then the bladder may be injured. If the initial incision is made superior to this, along the line where the vesicouterine peritoneum actually invests into the uterine serosa, then the plane of dissection will tend to be intrafascial instead of in the vesicouterine/vesicocervical space. Blunt dissection of the bladder should be avoided due to the risk of injury to the bladder. The operator should attempt to keep the dissection in the fine areolar tissue between the bladder and the cervix. If there is difficulty with the bladder dissection, the bladder can be dissected down just far enough

IX

to allow the uterine artery pedicles to be taken. After the initial pedicles are taken, the bladder dissection often becomes easier. The bladder flap is advanced through the course of the hysterectomy, as necessary. Be sure that the bladder has been taken down onto the vagina sufficiently to allow the placement of clamps below the cervix and to allow for the placement of suture to close the vaginal cuff.

The uterine arteries are now skeletonized to isolate the vessels. If possible, the pedicles on both sides are clamped before either pedicle is cut simultaneously, obviating the need to place a back clamp. The uterine artery pedicle is clamped with a Haney clamp, placing the tip perpendicular to the cervix. The pedicle is transected on the clamp with curved scissors and then ligated. Straight Ballentine clamps are then used to clamp serially down the cardinal ligaments bilaterally. Each pedicle should be approximately 1 to 1.5 cm in length. Smaller pedicles allow for the ureter to effectively fall away with each bite and allow for better hemostasis. In taking the uterine artery and cardinal ligament pedicles, the clamp should be placed just against the cervix and not "rolled off" of the cervix. The practice of "rolling" the clamp off of the cervix may cause the lateral cervix to be caught in the clamp, with risk of leaving residual cervix. Be sure that each clamp is placed medial to the last pedicle, so as to not clamp the ureter. The uterosacral ligaments can be clamped, cut, and ligated separately. Often, this is best done with a curved Haney clamp.

When the cervicovaginal junction is reached, either a right-angled Zeppelin clamp or a curved Haney clamp, depending upon the size of the cervix and vagina, is used to clamp across the upper vagina from either side, approximately 1 cm below the cervix. The specimen, consisting of uterus, cervix, bilateral fallopian tubes, and bilateral ovaries, is now amputated with curved scissors. A figure-of-eight suture is placed through the vaginal apex between the two clamps and held, in order to decrease contamination of the peritoneal cavity with the contents of the vagina and to decrease bleeding. The lateral pedicles are sutured with Haney sutures, and the suture in the middle of the vagina is tied. Any remaining open vagina is closed with figure-of-eight sutures. The pelvis is copiously irrigated and hemostasis is assured. The pelvis should be carefully examined to be sure that there has been no injury to the surrounding pelvic organs, particularly the bladder, rectum, and ureters.

As an alternative to the traditional clamp, cut, tie technique of hysterectomy, surgical energy sources, such as bipolar cautery or harmonic scalpel, can be used to take the surgical pedicles. These modalities are more commonly employed for laparoscopic than for open hysterectomy. A popular instrument in gynecologic surgery uses a high-power current, low-voltage system that melts collagen and elastin, leading to fusion of vessels and obliteration of the vessel lumen and can fuse vessels measuring 2 to 7 mm. This system measures tissue impedance to determine when the tissue has been adequately cauterized.

Bipolar vessel sealing using the system described above for the performance of abdominal hysterectomy has been evaluated in two randomized trials. In a study of 88 patients, Aydin et al. observed that for abdominal hysterectomies performed for uterine fibroids more than 14 weeks in size, the use of bipolar cautery was associated with a significantly reduced operative time as compared to conventional suture technique, 109.9 minutes versus 124.8 minutes. There was no difference in postoperative hemoglobin reduction, hospital stay, postoperative pain, or complication rate. Hagen and colleagues found no difference in operative time, blood loss, or complications with the use of a bipolar vessel-sealing device as compared to conventional suture technique in a randomized trial of 30 women undergoing total abdominal or supracervical

hysterectomy. There have been no randomized trials assessing the use of the harmonic scalpel for the performance of abdominal hysterectomy.

The choice of conventional suture technique versus the use of surgical energy should importantly include the surgeon's understanding and level of comfort with the use of the particular surgical energy source to be used. There is a risk of collateral thermal damage with the use of surgical energy. Finally, the cost of the instrument to be used as compared to any cost savings related to decreased operating time should be considered. There are no published data that assess cost issues associated with the use of surgical energy for open hysterectomy.

Once the hysterectomy has been completed, attention can now be turned to the *pelvic and paraaortic lymphadenectomy*. The bowel will need to be packed to the opposite side of the dissection. The peritoneum should be incised superiorly along the white line of Toldt. The colon can then be mobilized bluntly anteriorly and medially. The paravesical space can be opened by bluntly dissecting the bladder off of the pubic ramis, staying lateral to the superior vesicle artery. The pararectal space is opened by bluntly dissecting between the ureter and hypogastric artery.

The colon and ureter can be retracted with a large Deaver retractor, which should be oriented toward the contralateral shoulder. Sharp dissection with Metzenbaum scissors with hemoclips for hemostasis, electrocautery, or harmonic scalpel can be used to excise the fatty, lymph node-bearing tissues in the pelvis. This should include the tissues anterior and medial to the common iliac artery, anterior and medial to the external iliac artery, medial to the external iliac vein, and anterior to the hypogastric artery, extending distally along the superior vesicle artery. The external iliac vein is retracted anteriorly with a vein retractor. Blunt dissection is performed within the obturator space in order to reveal the course of the obturator nerve, often using the suction tip. The lymph nodes anterior to the obturator nerve are removed. The superior margin of the resection is the mid–common iliac artery. The inferior margin of the dissection is the point at which the circumflex iliac vein crosses over the external iliac artery. The lateral margin of the resection is the psoas muscle. The medial margin of the resection is the ureter.

The left paraaortic lymph node dissection is extended from the level of the mid–common iliac artery superiorly along the lateral aspect of the aorta. Care must be taken not to extend the dissection too far posteriorly, where the lumbar arteries arise from the aorta. On the right, the paraaortic lymph node dissection is performed superiorly, along the anterior surface of the inferior vena cava. Small, perforating vessels are numerous on both sides, so careful hemostasis as the dissection proceeds is important.

The incidence of isolated paraaortic lymph node metastases in the absence of pelvic lymph node metastases has traditionally been estimated at 1% to 1.5%. Thus, many authors define the superior margin of the paraaortic lymph node dissection as the level of the takeoff of the inferior mesenteric artery from the aorta. However, investigators at the Mayo Clinic reported that among 63 patients undergoing pelvic and paraaortic lymphadenectomy, 16% had isolated paraaortic lymph node metastases. Among all patients with metastases to the paraaortic lymph nodes, 77% were found to have disease superior to the inferior mesenteric artery. Additionally, studies of sentinel lymph node assessment after the injection of dye into the midline of the uterine fundus demonstrate a sentinel lymph node in the paraaortic region in over half of patients. Thus, other surgeons perform paraaortic lymphadenectomy to the level of the renal vessels.

The role of sentinel lymph node mapping in the treatment of endometrial cancer is currently being evaluated. It is based on the concept that the lymphatic drainage from a tumor occurs in a specific pattern. If the first draining node, or sentinel lymph node, is negative for tumor, then there should be no spread of disease to lymph nodes distal to that node. By limiting the extent of the lymph node dissection, side effects, such as lymphedema, should be minimized.

The optimal technique for sentinel lymph node biopsy in uterine cancer has yet to be defined. Strategies include cervical injection, subserosal uterine injection in the area of the tumor, hysteroscopic injection directly into the tumor, and transvaginal ultrasound-guided injection into the tumor. Injection is performed using technetium 99 and/or a colored dye, such as methylene blue or isosulfan blue. The procedure can also be performed using indocyanine green, which is visualized during laparoscopy using a near-infrared camera. To maximize the detection of micrometastatic disease, the pathologic evaluation of negative lymph nodes may include immunohistochemistry for cytokeratin. The prognostic significance of micrometastases detected by immunohistochemistry is unclear. When performing a sentinel lymph node dissection, all identified sentinel lymph nodes and any suspicious lymph nodes are removed. If no sentinel lymph nodes are identified, then a full pelvic lymph node dissection should be performed on that side. In this algorithm, paraaortic lymph node dissection is left to the discretion of the surgeon.

STEPS IN THE PROCEDURE

Endometrial Cancer

- Open the abdomen through an incision sufficient to perform pelvic and paraaortic lymph node dissection, if necessary.
- Obtain pelvic washings.
- Perform systematic exploration of the peritoneal cavity and retroperitoneum.
- Grasp the bilateral uterine cornua with clamps, occluding the fallopian tubes and maintaining upward traction on the uterus throughout the hysterectomy.
- Ligate and transect the round ligament on one side, and then extend the peritoneal incision superiorly, 1 cm lateral and parallel to the infundibulopelvic ligament.
- Bluntly open the retroperitoneal space to identify the course of the ureter through the pelvis.
- Isolate, doubly clamp, and transect the infundibulopelvic ligament, being sure to exclude the ureter from the clamps. Doubly secure the infundibulopelvic ligament with a free tie and transfixion suture.
- Repeat steps 5 through 7 on the opposite side.
- Incise the anterior leaves of the broad ligament and vesicouterine peritoneum, and then dissect the bladder off of the lower uterine segment, cervix, and upper vagina.
- Skeletonize, clamp, transect, and ligate the uterine vessels on either side at the level of the isthmus.
- Serially clamp, transect, and ligate the cardinal and uterosacral ligaments.

- After being sure that the bladder is well down, place clamps from either side across the upper vagina about 1 cm distal to the cervix, and then amputate the specimen.
- Frozen section is performed to assess grade and depth of invasion to determine the need for lymph node dissection.
- Incise the peritoneum on one side superiorly along the white line of Toldt, and then bluntly mobilize the colon anteriorly and medially.
- Bluntly open the paravesical and pararectal spaces.
- Retract the colon and ureter toward the contralateral shoulder to expose the bifurcation of the common iliac artery.
- Excise the fatty, lymph node-bearing tissues from the mid–common iliac artery proximally to the deep circumflex iliac vein distally and from the medial aspect of the psoas muscle laterally to the ureter medially. Extend the dissection into the obturator space, anterior to the obturator nerve. This will remove the tissues anterior and medial to the distal common iliac artery, anterior and medial to the external iliac artery, medial to the external iliac vein, and anterior to the internal iliac artery and extending distally along the superior vesical artery.
- Repeat steps 14 through 17 on the opposite side.
- On the left, extend the dissection laterally along the proximally common iliac artery and distal aorta to the level of the inferior mesenteric artery to complete the left paraaortic lymph node dissection.
- On the right, extend the dissection over the anterior surface of the inferior vena cava to the level of the inferior mesenteric artery to complete the right paraaortic lymph node dissection.
- Obtain hemostasis and carefully assess for any previously unrecognized operative injuries.
- Perform abdominal closure.

The use of cervical injection has been questioned, as studies have demonstrated that with dye injection into the midline uterine fundus, sentinel lymph nodes can be identified in the paraaortic lymph nodes between the inferior mesenteric artery and renal artery in over 50% of patients. With cervical injection of dye, only 5% of sentinel lymph nodes were identified along the aorta. Cervical injection for sentinel lymph node sampling is currently undergoing validation trials to confirm its accuracy.

Special Situations

Uterine papillary serous carcinomas behave in a manner similar to ovarian cancers, demonstrating spread within the peritoneal cavity even when the primary tumor is confined to the endometrium. Goff et al. evaluated the patterns of spread in patients with noninvasive uterine papillary serous carcinomas and found that with complete surgical staging, 36% of patients were found to have lymph node metastases and

43% of patients were found to have intraperitoneal metastases. Chan et al. found that 25% of patients with noninvasive uterine papillary serous carcinomas had occult omental disease. Thus, *staging of patients with uterine papillary serous carcinoma* should include hysterectomy with BSO, peritoneal washings and biopsies, bilateral pelvic and paraaortic lymph node dissection, and omentectomy, as is typically performed for ovarian cancer.

For patients with *stage IIB endometrial cancers with a bulky cervix*, there is a risk of parametrial extension, as for primary cervical carcinomas. Further, it can sometimes be difficult to distinguish between a primary endometrial adenocarcinoma with extension to the cervix versus a primary cervical adenocarcinoma that may extend into the lower uterine segment or above. Pelvic MRI can be helpful in making this distinction (He).

The literature regarding *treatment of patients with stage II endometrial cancers* must be evaluated carefully. Patients with endometrial cancer extending into the cervical stroma may be treated similarly to cervical cancer patients with a radical hysterectomy and pelvic and paraaortic lymphadenectomy if they are good surgical candidates. Five-year survival rates of 90% to 93% have been reported for this treatment strategy. The alternative is to treat these patients with preoperative external beam whole pelvic radiotherapy and intracavitary brachytherapy followed by completion hysterectomy with BSO. Completion hysterectomy is necessary, as radiotherapy is not as effective in treating disease in the uterine corpus as in the uterine cervix. Reisinger and colleagues reported a 5-year actuarial survival of 82% in patients with endometrioid histology treated with this strategy. Patients with high-risk histologic subtypes had only a 38% 5-year actuarial survival, with a high incidence of recurrence in the upper abdomen.

In *patients with stage III or IV endometrial cancers*, tumor debulking may be of benefit. Goff et al. reported on 47 patients with stage IV endometrial cancer. Overall median survival for these patients was 12 months. Among those patients who underwent successful cytoreduction, overall median survival was 18 months as compared to 8 months among patients who did not undergo surgery. Similarly, Chi et al. showed that among 55 patients with stage IV endometrial cancer, overall median survival was 31 months for those whose disease could be optimally cytoreduced to less than or equal to 2-cm residual disease, 12 months for those whose disease was suboptimally cytoreduced, and 3 months for those whose disease was unresectable.

Lambrou et al. also evaluated the efficacy and safety of cytoreductive surgery in patients with stage III and IV endometrial cancer. They excluded patients with uterine papillary serous carcinomas and clear cell carcinomas. They found that optimal cytoreduction to less than or equal to 2-cm maximal residual disease was possible in 72% of their patients. Overall median survival was 17.8 months for patients undergoing optimal cytoreduction and only 6.7 months for patients who could not be optimally cytoreduced. Further, they observed that the proportion of patients having major postoperative complications was actually higher among patients who were suboptimally cytoreduced as compared to those who were not, 37.5% versus 7.25%, respectively.

Bristow and coworkers evaluated the survival benefit of lymph node debulking among patients with stage IIIC endometrial cancer. All patients had macroscopic spread to pelvic lymph nodes, and approximately 50% had macroscopic involvement of the paraaortic lymph nodes. Disease-specific survival was 37.5 months among patients whose involved lymph nodes could be completely resected as compared to

8.8 months among patients whose involved lymph nodes could not be completely resected.

A retrospective analysis of 248 patients presenting with surgical stage IV endometrial cancer by Eto et al. assessed the effect of resection of intra-abdominal disease on survival in patients with and without extra-abdominal disease. Among the 93 patients with extra-abdominal disease, the most common site was lung. The extra-abdominal disease was completely resected in only 13. Complete resection of intra-abdominal disease was associated with a median overall survival of 48 months as compared with 23 months in women with ≤1-cm residual disease and 14 months in women with greater than 1-cm residual disease. Even among women with residual extra-abdominal disease, there was a survival advantage associated with complete resection of the intra-abdominal disease. Other factors associated with an improved survival were better performance status, endometrioid pathology, low grade, and receiving postoperative therapy. In this study, there was no difference in survival between women treated with chemotherapy alone, radiotherapy alone, or combined chemoradiation therapy.

In a meta-analysis of 14 retrospective cohort studies that included 672 women with metastatic or recurrent endometrial cancer, Barlin et al. observed that optimal cytoreduction to no gross residual disease was associated with a statistically significant 9.3-month improvement in overall survival for every 10% increase in the rate of optimal cytoreduction. Receipt of postoperative radiotherapy was associated with a statistically significant improvement in survival, while being treated with chemotherapy postoperatively actually had a statistically significant adverse effect on survival. The authors suggest that this may be due to suboptimally debulked patients having been more likely treated with chemotherapy rather than radiotherapy.

Role of Laparoscopy

The use of laparoscopy and particularly robotic-assisted laparoscopy has been increasing over time. Wright et al. reviewed the SEER-Medicare Database from 1997 to 2005. They identified 8,545 patients 65 years of age or older who had undergone surgery for stage I endometrial cancer. Overall, 8,018 (93.8%) underwent laparotomy while only 527 (6.2%) underwent laparoscopy. There was a clear increase in the use of laparoscopy over time, with only 3.9% of surgeries being performed via laparoscopy in 1997 as compared to 8.5% in 2005. Patient-specific factors that were associated with a greater likelihood of laparoscopic surgery included more recent year of diagnosis, younger age, white race, fewer comorbidities, higher socioeconomic status, lower tumor grade and stage, and residence in a metropolitan area. Physician-specific factors that were associated with greater likelihood of performing laparoscopy included being trained in the United States, specializing in gynecologic oncology, being at an academic institution, and later year of graduation. In a recent study evaluating hospital discharge data from the Florida Agency for Healthcare Administration, Yu reviewed data on 2,247 patients treated for endometrial cancer from October 2008 to December 2009. In this cohort, 61% of the surgeries were performed by laparotomy, 10% by conventional laparoscopy, and 29% by robotic-assisted laparoscopy.

The GOG conducted a prospective randomized trial of laparoscopy (*n* = 1,696) versus laparotomy (*n* = 920) for the treatment of stage I to IIA endometrial cancer (Lap2). Patients in both groups underwent hysterectomy, BSO, pelvic peritoneal cytology, and pelvic and paraaortic lymph node lymphadenectomy. In this study, Walker et al. reported that 434 (25.8%)

patients had their surgery converted from laparoscopy to laparotomy. Laparoscopy was associated with a longer operative time (median 204 minutes vs. 130 minutes, $P < 0.001$)), but a similar rate of intraoperative complications. Laparoscopy was associated with fewer moderate-to-severe postoperative complications (14% vs. 21%, $P < 0.0001$). Patients undergoing laparoscopy were significantly less likely to be hospitalized for more than 2 days (52% vs. 94%, $P < 0.0001$). Importantly, in a follow-up study reported in 2012, Walker and colleagues reported that although the estimated 3-year recurrence rate was 1.14% higher in the laparoscopy group as compared to the laparotomy group, the estimated 5-year survival was identical in both arms at 89.8%.

Patients undergoing laparoscopy demonstrated improved quality of life over several parameters during the first 6 weeks post-op as compared to patients undergoing laparotomy. These differences had largely disappeared by 6 months, except for better body image in the laparoscopy group. There was a modest improvement in time to return to work among patients undergoing laparoscopy. In an Australian trial comparing total laparoscopic hysterectomy to total abdominal hysterectomy (TAH) for the treatment of stage I endometrial cancer, there was overall a significantly greater improvement in quality of life at 6 weeks and 6 months as compared to baseline among women undergoing laparoscopic surgery.

Galaal et al. performed a meta-analysis of 8 randomized controlled trials, including 3,644 women, comparing conventional laparoscopic surgery to laparotomy for the treatment of early-stage endometrial cancer. Not all trials could be assessed for all parameters. Women undergoing laparoscopy were found to have a significantly decreased blood loss and significantly fewer severe postoperative complications than women undergoing laparotomy. There was no difference in the rates of perioperative death, need for blood transfusion, or injury to the urinary tract, bowel, or vascular structures. Importantly, there was no difference in the risk of death from disease or recurrence among women undergoing laparoscopic surgery and compared to laparotomy.

Gynecologic oncologists have rapidly adopted robotically assisted laparoscopy for the performance of endometrial cancer surgery. Potential benefits over conventional laparoscopy include greater dexterity, three-dimensional vision, elimination of the counterintuitive movement of conventional laparoscopy, and improved ergonomics. The lack of tactile sensation for the surgeon may be a potential disadvantage as compared to open or conventional laparoscopic surgery. Both robotically assisted and conventional laparoscopy have a long learning curve.

A number of studies have compared outcomes of robotically assisted with conventional laparoscopy for the treatment of early-stage endometrial cancer. They consistently demonstrate that the two approaches have comparable complication rates with patients undergoing robotic surgery having a decreased blood loss, shorter hospital stay, and decreased risk of conversion to laparotomy as compared to patients undergoing conventional laparoscopy. These studies are small, nonrandomized retrospective reviews written by high-volume, experienced laparoscopic surgeons. Although the data are premature, with median follow-up of 20.7 to 31 months, recurrence risk and survival appear comparable to historical data for women treated for endometrial cancer by laparotomy or conventional laparoscopy.

The robotic surgical platform is highly complex and requires the use of specialized, disposable instruments. A significant issue with the rapid adoption of this technology without evidence of significant superiority over existing technologies is cost. Studies evaluating the cost of robotic surgery in US

dollars have consistently demonstrated that it is a more expensive approach than is laparoscopy or in some studies even laparotomy, despite the longer hospital stay. Bell and colleagues compared the cost of endometrial cancer staging performed by laparotomy with a cost of $12,943.60 versus conventional laparoscopy at a cost of $7,569.80 versus robotically assisted laparoscopy at a cost of $8,212.0. They concluded that there was no significant difference in cost of conventional and robotic laparoscopy. However, a difference of over $1,000 per case adds significantly to the overall health care budget when considering that approximately 50,000 new cases of endometrial cancer are diagnosed in the United States each year.

Wright et al. used the perspective database to perform a comparaative effectiveness analysis of robotic versus laparoscopic hysterectomy for endometrial cancer, analyzing data from 2,463 women. There was no difference in complication rates between the two groups. The mean cost of robotic hysterectomy was $10,618 versus $8,996 for conventional laparoscopic hysterectomy. They observed that patients were more likely to be treated with robotically assisted laparoscopic hysterectomy if they were treated in a larger, nonteaching hospital located outside the northeastern United States. African Americans, patients with no insurance, and women living in rural areas were more likely to undergo surgery via conventional laparoscopy.

Although some authors have suggested that conventional or robotic laparoscopy, rather than laparotomy, should be considered the standard surgical approach for endometrial cancer, it is important to keep in mind that laparotomy and laparoscopy are only methods of abdominal entry. The surgical management of early-stage endometrial cancer should include hysterectomy, BSO, pelvic and paraaortic lymph node dissection in intermediate risk and above patients, and pelvic washings. The surgeon must choose the approach that allows him or her to best care for the patient with the least risk of complications. Although for certain surgeons this may be either conventional or robotic laparoscopy, there are many surgeons for whom laparotomy remains the best and safest approach. On the other hand, *it is incumbent on all surgeons to continue to advance our skills throughout our surgical careers, so that we may provide the most effective, safest, and financially responsible surgical management for our patients.* The best approach to the surgical treatment of endometrial cancer is likely only to continue to evolve with the introduction of new surgical technologies.

RADIATION THERAPY

At the present time, radiation therapy is rarely used as the primary or sole treatment modality for women with endometrial cancer. The goal of postoperative radiotherapy in patients with endometrial cancer is to treat the pelvic lymph node beds with external beam whole pelvic radiotherapy and upper vagina with vaginal vault brachytherapy. This has been demonstrated to decrease the risk of local recurrence, but not to improve survival. With the increasing use of surgical staging with pelvic and paraaortic lymph node dissection in the United States, the use of adjuvant pelvic radiotherapy has decreased.

The PORTEC-1 trial was a randomized trial of postoperative radiotherapy versus observation in 714 patients with stage IB, grade 2 or 3 and IC, grade 1 or 2 endometrial cancer who had undergone hysterectomy with BSO. These patients had not undergone lymph node dissection. At 10 years, Creutzberg et al. reported that the pelvic failure rate was 5% in the patients who received pelvic radiotherapy and 14% among controls, which was statistically significantly different. However, there was no statistically significant difference in survival, with an overall survival of 66% among patients who received pelvic radiotherapy and 73% among controls. There is general agreement that patients with low-risk endometrial cancers, stage IA or IB, grade 1 or 2, require no additional treatment postoperatively.

The role of pelvic radiotherapy in patients with high-intermediate risk endometrial cancer, as previously defined above, is less clear. In the PORTEC-2 trial, 427 patients with high-intermediate risk stage I or IIA endometrial carcinoma were randomized to postoperative treatment with external beam whole pelvic radiotherapy versus vaginal cuff brachytherapy. The primary outcome was vaginal cuff recurrence. Median follow-up was 45 months. Nout and colleagues found there was no difference in the rates of vaginal cuff recurrence or in overall or disease-free survival. There was significantly less acute grade 1 to 2 gastrointestinal toxicity in the vaginal brachytherapy group. The authors concluded that vaginal cuff brachytherapy should be the treatment of choice in patients with high-intermediate risk endometrial cancer.

Both the PORTEC trials have been criticized because comprehensive surgical staging with pelvic and paraaortic lymphadenectomy was not performed. Treatment was based on uterine findings only. Straughn and colleagues performed a retrospective review of 613 patients with stage I endometrial cancer who had undergone comprehensive surgical staging. Among 325 patients with stage IB disease, 321 did not receive pelvic radiotherapy. Fifteen (5%) of these patients recurred. All nine local recurrences were salvaged. There were 77 patients with stage IC disease, of whom 53 (69%) did not receive pelvic radiotherapy. Four (8%) patients recurred, and three of them were salvaged. For all stage I patients, the 5-year disease-free survival was 93% and overall survival was 98%. These authors concluded that pelvic radiotherapy is not needed in patients who have undergone comprehensive surgical staging because of the low risk of recurrence and high salvage rate with subsequent therapy.

In a follow-up to this study in 2003, Straughn et al. subsequently evaluated an expanded cohort of 220 patients with stage IC endometrial cancer. Ninety-nine (45%) patients were treated with radiotherapy, with external beam whole pelvic, vaginal cuff brachytherapy, or both, and 121 (55%) patients were observed. There was no statistically significant difference in the recurrence rate between the two groups. The overall 5-year survival was 92% for the patients who received radiotherapy and 90% for those who were observed. There was noted to be an improved 5-year disease-free survival of 93% among the radiated patients as compared to 75% among those who were observed. The overall salvage rate for patients who recurred was 64%.

In a separate report from the PORTEC-1 trial, there were 99 evaluable patients with stage IC, grade 3 endometrial cancers. All of these patients were treated with pelvic radiotherapy. The 5-year overall survival for this group was 58%, which is significantly lower than that found by Straughn et al. among patients with stage IC disease. It is important to remember that patients in the PORTEC-1 trial did not undergo pelvic and paraaortic lymph node dissection. The difference in survival noted is likely largely due to upstaging of patients with microscopic lymph node metastases in the Straughn series. However, it is important to note that the use of pelvic radiotherapy in the PORTEC-1 trial did not salvage these unstaged patients. Because of the higher risk of recurrence among patients with stage IC disease, particularly those with grade 3 disease, these patients are often considered for adjuvant postoperative radiotherapy, even after complete surgical staging.

Pelvic radiotherapy does carry a significant risk of complications. Among the patients randomized to whole pelvic radiotherapy in the PORTEC-1 trial, Creutzberg et al. reported 3% of patients had serious (grade 3 or 4) acute toxicity and over 20% had mild symptoms during treatment. In long-term follow-up, at a median of 13.3 years, patients treated with pelvic radiotherapy as compared to those who were not had increased incidence of urinary incontinence, diarrhea, and fecal leakage with resultant increased limitation in daily activities. Patients treated with pelvic radiotherapy also had an increased incidence of second malignancy with an observed versus expected ratio of 1.6 for patients receiving external beam radiotherapy and 1.2 for patients receiving no additional therapy as compared to a matched control population.

Patients with pelvic and/or paraaortic lymph node metastases are usually treated with postoperative radiotherapy directed to the involved nodal basins. Nelson et al. reported a 5-year disease-free survival rate of 72% for patients with pelvic lymph node metastases treated with pelvic or whole abdominal radiotherapy. Rose et al. demonstrated improved survival for patients with paraaortic lymph node metastases who were treated with paraaortic radiotherapy as compared to those who were not treated with paraaortic radiation.

Patients with stage I or II endometrial cancers who are not surgical candidates due to medical comorbidities are sometimes treated with primary pelvic radiotherapy. Fishman et al. reviewed experience at Yale from 1975 to 1992, 3.5% of all patients with stage I or II endometrial cancer were deemed medically inoperable and treated with pelvic radiotherapy alone. The 5-year disease-specific survival rate for inoperable patients with stage I disease was 80%, which was significantly less than that for operable patients at 98%. Notably, the overall 5-year survival of medically inoperable patients was only 30%, as compared to 88% for operable patients, demonstrating that many of these patients succumb to their intercurrent medical illnesses. Another treatment option for selected medically ill patients is vaginal hysterectomy.

Radiotherapy can be used successfully for *the treatment of vaginal cuff recurrence.* Huh et al. evaluated the outcomes of 69 women with stage I endometrial cancer who had been treated with hysterectomy, BSO, and pelvic (±paraaortic) lymph node dissection who had an isolated vaginal cuff recurrence. Treatment was whole pelvic radiotherapy with vaginal cuff brachytherapy in 62 (90%) and brachytherapy alone in 2 (3%). Treatment information was unavailable for five patients. Among these women, 81% achieved remission and the overall 5-year survival rate was 75%. Given the excellent outcomes for these patients, the authors questioned the use of adjuvant radiotherapy, either external beam whole pelvic or cuff brachytherapy, in women with surgical stage I endometrioid adenocarcinomas of the endometrium, citing benefits of decreased cost, decreased complication rates, and potential impact on quality of life.

SYSTEMIC THERAPY

Patients with advanced or recurrent endometrial cancer are often treated with *cytotoxic chemotherapy.* A recent GOG trial has demonstrated that for patients with stage III or IV endometrial cancer, chemotherapy with doxorubicin and cisplatin is superior to whole abdominal radiotherapy. Based on the findings of this trial, some authorities have advocated for the use of systemic chemotherapy rather than pelvic and paraaortic radiotherapy in patients with node-positive disease. However, a retrospective review of 71 patients treated for stage IIIC endometrial adenocarcinoma demonstrated a higher rate of local–regional recurrence in patients treated without regional radiotherapy. Some authors advocate for "sandwich" therapy in node-positive and other high-risk patients, with chemotherapy followed for regional radiotherapy followed by additional chemotherapy.

RTOG 9708 was a phase 2 study to assess the feasibility, safety, toxicity, and patterns of recurrence of external beam radiotherapy with concurrent cisplatin chemotherapy followed by four cycles of cisplatin and paclitaxel chemotherapy for patients with high-risk endometrial cancer. The trial included patients with grade 2 or 3 endometrial adenocarcinoma with greater than 50% myometrial invasion, cervical stromal invasion, or pelvic-confined extrauterine disease. Overall survival and disease-free survival at 4 years were 85% and 81%, respectively. For patients with stage III disease, 4-year overall survival was 77% and disease-free survival was 72%. The regimen was well tolerated. This approach is currently being further evaluated in an RTOG trial comparing volume-directed radiation therapy with concurrent cisplatin chemotherapy followed by four cycles of paclitaxel and carboplatin chemotherapy with six cycles of carboplatin and paclitaxel chemotherapy in patients with stage III or IVA endometrial carcinoma or patients with stage I or II serous or clear cell endometrial carcinoma and positive cytology. Endometrial cancer patients with recurrent disease or distant metastases outside of the pelvis are usually treated with paclitaxel and carboplatin chemotherapy.

Hormonal therapy is also an option for patients with advanced stage disease. Both progestins and tamoxifen have been used. A recent study by Fiorica et al. demonstrated a median overall survival of 14 months in patients with advanced endometrial cancer treated with an alternating regimen of megestrol acetate and tamoxifen. Hormonal therapy tends to work best in patients with grade 1 endometrioid adenocarcinomas, which express estrogen and progesterone receptors. The major side effect of hormonal therapy is thromboembolic disease.

INCIDENTAL DIAGNOSIS OF ENDOMETRIAL CANCER AT HYSTERECTOMY

For patients who undergo hysterectomy and have the unexpected diagnosis of endometrial cancer, there are three options: observation, reoperation for staging, or pelvic radiotherapy. Treatment decisions need to be individualized and will depend on the risk of nodal or extrauterine spread, which may be estimated from the tumor grade, depth of invasion, and evidence of lymphadenopathy on CT of the abdomen and pelvis. The patient's medical status and her willingness to undergo further surgery or radiotherapy should also be taken into account. Consultation with a gynecologic oncologist is strongly considered.

POSTTREATMENT SURVEILLANCE

The appropriate follow-up for any malignancy is dependent upon the pattern of recurrence. This will differ somewhat for type I and type II endometrial cancers. Aalders et al. evaluated 379 patients with recurrent endometrial cancer seen at the Norwegian Radium Hospital between 1960 and 1976. Local recurrence was observed in 50%, distant recurrence was observed in 29%, and both local and distant recurrence was observed in 21%. Patients who had received postoperative pelvic radiotherapy were much less likely to recur in the pelvis. One third of patients were diagnosed with recurrence within 1 year after the completion of therapy, and two thirds of patients were diagnosed with recurrence within 3 years.

There is no single, accepted follow-up strategy for patients with endometrial cancer. Physicians have often recommended routine follow-up visits at 3- to 6-month intervals with vaginal cytology at each visit and an annual chest radiograph. However, recent studies by multiple groups have demonstrated that this surveillance protocol is neither clinically nor cost-effective. These studies demonstrate that 60% to 75% of patients are symptomatic at the time of recurrence. Most patients with curable recurrences had vaginal bleeding from a vaginal lesion. Curable asymptomatic recurrences were uncommonly detected by routine screening.

Cooper et al. reported that among women with endometrial cancer, 430 Pap tests were required to detect one asymptomatic vaginal recurrence at an additional cost of $15,142 per asymptomatic recurrence detected. Berchuck and colleagues found that the salvage rate for patients with vaginal recurrences diagnosed by vaginal cytology alone was no different than that for women with a visible lesion. They also observed that no patient with an isolated pulmonary recurrence diagnosed by chest radiograph was salvaged. In a similar study from Canada by Shumsky et al., no isolated vaginal recurrence was diagnosed by Pap test alone. Similar to the Duke study, no patient with pulmonary metastases diagnosed by chest x-ray was cured.

Despite the limited ability of routine follow-up to improve the outcomes of women with recurrent endometrial cancer, both patients and their physicians continue to favor some form of posttreatment surveillance. As emphasized by Berchuck, continued regular follow-up for some period of time with normal periodic exams is likely to provide some psychological reassurance to the patient. The focus should be on evaluation for complications of treatment and detection of vaginal recurrences, since most of these patients can be salvaged. Effective therapy is typically not available for patients who recur at distant sites.

Given these observations, routine surveillance for patients with endometrial cancer should include education of patients regarding the symptoms of recurrence, particularly vaginal bleeding, abdominopelvic or back pain, leg swelling, abdominal bloating, cough, or shortness of breath. Symptomatic patients should be instructed to report promptly for evaluation. The recent ACOG Practice Bulletin on the Management of Endometrial Cancer suggests that women with endometrial cancer could be seen in follow-up every 3 to 4 months for 2 to 3 years, then every 6 months. Berchuck recommends biannual follow-up visits. Most authors agree that patients can return to routine annual well-woman care after 5 years. Each visit should include a thorough review of systems to evaluate for symptoms of recurrence and a focused physical exam, including lymph node survey, abdominal examination, and pelvic examination with speculum exam, bimanual exam, and rectovaginal exam. Routine surveillance with Pap testing and chest radiographs cannot currently be recommended. Other studies should be obtained as dictated by the findings of the patient's history and physical examination.

Certain groups may require modifications of this follow-up scheme. For example, patients with uterine papillary serous carcinoma are often followed with serial Ca-125 determinations, similarly to patients with ovarian cancer. They are much more likely than patients with type I endometrial cancers to recur with peritoneal carcinomatosis. Patients who have been treated with radiation and/or chemotherapy may need more intensive follow-up to monitor for long-term complications of therapy. Again, there are no data to suggest that more intensive follow-up results in improved salvage rates.

IX

UTERINE SARCOMAS

Uterine sarcomas are rare tumors that account for only about 3% of all uterine malignancies. The most common are leiomyosarcomas, which are cancers arising from the smooth muscle of the myometrium. In a large study using population-based databases in the Nordic countries, the incidence of leiomyosarcoma was estimated at 0.3 per 100,000 (incidence of endometrial stromal sarcomas [ESSs] 0.4 per 100,000).

Pathologically, leiomyosarcomas are differentiated from various forms of benign leiomyomas and from smooth muscle tumors of uncertain malignant potential by high mitotic rate with 10 or more mitoses per 10 high-power fields, nuclear atypia, and the presence of tumor cell necrosis. These are very aggressive tumors that commonly metastasize hematogenously. In a review of data from the Norwegian Cancer Registry from 1970 to 2000, the 5-year survival for stage I disease (by the 1988 FIGO classification) was 51% and for stage II disease was 25%. All patients with metastatic disease outside of the pelvis died within 5 years. Prognostic features for patients with stage I disease included tumor size and mitotic index.

Uterine leiomyosarcomas are typically treated with hysterectomy with resection of intraabdominal disease, if present. Removal of the ovaries has not been shown to affect survival. Thus, ovarian preservation can be considered in premenopausal women. Lymph node dissection is commonly not performed due to the low risk of lymph node metastasis. Postoperative adjuvant pelvic radiotherapy has been shown to improve local control, but not disease-free or overall survival in patients with stage I or II disease. The role of adjuvant chemotherapy is unclear. There is currently no proof that it improves survival. However, it is often offered to patients because of the high risk of distant recurrence. Treatment is usually with gemcitabine and docetaxel. There is an ongoing phase III trial, GOG 277, which compares postoperative adjuvant chemotherapy to observation for patients with early-stage leiomyosarcoma. Advanced or recurrent disease may be treated with surgical resection or radiotherapy for localized disease or with chemotherapy.

Uterine leiomyosarcoma diagnosed after uterine morcellation for presumed benign disease represents a special case that has received considerable attention recently in both the professional literature and the lay press. The incidence of leiomyosarcoma in hysterectomy or myomectomy specimens of presumed leiomyomata is unclear. The FDA Safety Communication regarding the use of laparoscopic uterine power morcellation estimates this risk as 1 in 350 women. Other studies have estimated the risk to be between 1 in 500 and 1 in 1,000. In a study of 58 patients with an incidental pathologic diagnosis of leiomyosarcoma, those undergoing uterine morcellation ($n = 19$) had an increased risk of abdominal/pelvic recurrence ($P = 0.001$) and a significantly shorter median recurrence-free survival (10.8 months vs. 39.6 months, $P = 0.002$) as compared to those undergoing TAH ($n = 39$). It is not possible to reliably differentiate between leiomyomata and leiomyosarcoma preoperatively. However, every reasonable effort should be made to rule out cervical or endometrial cancer prior to performing a uterine morcellation. Patients considering any surgical procedure should be fully counseled on the risks, benefits, and alternatives to the procedure being proposed.

ESSs are low-grade tumors that rarely metastasize distantly, but may be locally invasive. Late recurrences after 5 years may occur. Treatment is typically hysterectomy. These are hormonally sensitive tumors, and there are conflicting data regarding the effect of BSO on survival. Metastatic or recurrent disease is often treated with progestins or aromatase inhibitors. Tamoxifen should not be used, as it may stimulate the growth of these tumors.

Undifferentiated endometrial sarcomas (previously high-grade ESSs) are rare and aggressive tumors. Treatment is hysterectomy with BSO. The role of adjuvant therapy is unclear. Pelvic radiotherapy may improve local control, but not survival. Most patients die within 2 years of diagnosis.

Adenosarcomas are another rare form of uterine sarcoma. These are low-grade tumors with benign epithelial component and malignant stromal component. The prognosis is generally good, unless there is myometrial invasion or sarcomatous overgrowth. The treatment is hysterectomy with BSO.

FUTURE DIRECTIONS

As with all malignancies, the future will see increasing use of molecular staging to identify patients at risk for recurrence. This should allow for greater individualization of therapy. The GOG is currently conducting a molecular staging study in endometrial cancer. Laparoscopic and robotic surgical techniques will continue to evolve. Complete lymphadenectomy may decrease in importance, if sentinel lymph node techniques can be developed, as in melanoma and breast cancer. Chemotherapy is likely to play an increasing role in the therapy of advanced stage and recurrent disease.

BIBLIOGRAPHY

Aalders JG, Abeler V, Kolstad P. Recurrent adenocarcinoma of the endometrium: a clinical and histopathological study of 379 patients. *Gynecol Oncol* 1984;17:85–103.

Abaid LN, Rettenmaier MA, Brown JV III. Sequential chemotherapy and radiotherapy as sandwich therapy for the treatment of high risk endometrial cancer. *J Gynecol Oncol* 2012;23:22–27.

Abeler VM, Royne O, Thorensen S, et al. Uterine sarcomas in Norway. A histopathological and prognostic survey of a total population from 1970 to 2000 including 419 patients. *Histopathology* 2009;54:355–364.

Abu-Rustum NR, Gomez JD, Alektiar KM. The incidence of isolated paraaortic nodal metastases in surgically staged endometrial cancer patients with negative pelvic lymph nodes. *Gynecol Oncol* 2009;115:236–238.

Abu-Rustum NR. Sentinel lymph node mapping for endometrial cancer: a modern approach to surgical staging. *J Natl Compr Canc Netw* 2014;12:288–297.

ACOG Committee on Gynecologic Practice. Committee Opinion number 440: the role of transvaginal ultrasonography in the evaluation of postmenopausal bleeding. *Obstet Gynecol* 2009;114:409–411.

ACOG Committee on Practice Bulletins—Gynecology. ACOG Committee Opinion number 108: polycystic ovary syndrome. *Obstet Gynecol* 2009;114:936–949.

ACOG Committee on Practice Bulletins—Gynecology. ACOG practice bulletin number 104: antibiotic prophylaxis for gynecologic procedures. *Obstet Gynecol* 2009;113:1180–1189.

ACOG Committee on Practice Bulletins—Gynecology. ACOG practice bulletin number 84: prevention of deep venous thrombosis and pulmonary embolism. *Obstet Gynecol* 2007;110:429–440.

ACOG Committee on Practice Bulletins—Gynecology. Practice bulletin number 128: diagnosis of abnormal uterine bleeding in reproductive-aged women. *Obstet Gynecol* 2012;120:197–206.

Amant F, Moerman P, Neven P, et al. Endometrial cancer. *Lancet* 2005;366:491–505.

Amir E, Seruga B, Niraula S, et al. Toxicity of adjuvant endocrine therapy in postmenopausal breast cancer patients: a systematic review and meta-analysis. *J Natl Cancer Inst* 2011;103:1299–1309.

Assikis VJ, Jordan VC. Gynecologic effects of tamoxifen and the association with endometrial carcinoma. *Int J Gynaecol Obstet* 1995;49:241–257.

Aydin C, Yildiz A, Kasap B, et al. Efficacy of electrosurgical bipolar vessel sealing for abdominal hysterectomy with uterine myomas more than 14 weeks in size: a randomized controlled trial. *Gynecol Obstet Invest* 2012;73:326–329.

Ayhan A, Taskiran C, Celik C, et al. The long-term survival of women with surgical stage II endometrioid type endometrial cancer. *Gynecol Oncol* 2004;93:9–13.

Ballester M, Dubernard G, Lecuru F, et al. Detection rate and diagnostic accuracy of sentinel-node biopsy in early stage endometrial cancer: a prospective multicentre study (SENTI-ENDO). *Lancet Oncol* 2011;12:469–476.

Barakat RR, Wong G, Curtin JP, et al. Tamoxifen use in breast cancer patients who subsequently develop corpus cancer is not associated with a higher incidence of adverse histologic features. *Gynecol Oncol* 1994;55:164–168.

Barlin JN, Puri I, Bristow RE. Cytoreductive surgery for advanced or recurrent endometrial cancer: a meta-analysis. *Gynecol Oncol* 2010;118:14–18.

Bedner R, Rzopka-Gorska I. Hysteroscopy with directed biopsy versus dilatation and curettage for the diagnosis of endometrial hyperplasia and cancer in perimenopausal women. *Eur J Gynaecol Oncol* 2007;28:400–402.

Bell MC, Torgerson J, Seshadri-Kreaden U, et al. Comparison of outcomes and cost for endometrial cancer staging via traditional laparotomy, standard laparoscopy and robotic techniques. *Gynecol Oncol* 2008;111:407–411.

Ben-Arie A, Tamir S, Dubnik S, et al. Does hysteroscopy affect prognosis in apparent early-stage endometrial cancer? *Int J Gynecol Cancer* 2008;18:813–819.

Ben-Shachar I, Pavelka J, Cohn DE, et al. Surgical staging for patients presenting with grade 1 endometrial carcinoma. *Obstet Gynecol* 2005;105:487–493.

Ben-Yehuda OM, Kim YB, Leuchler RS. Does hysteroscopy improve upon the sensitivity of dilatation and curettage in the diagnosis of endometrial hyperplasia or carcinoma? *Gynecol Oncol* 1998;68:4–7.

Beral V, Bull D, Reeves G, et al. Endometrial cancer and hormone-replacement therapy in the Million Women Study. *Lancet* 2005;365:1543–1551.

Berretta R, Merisio C, Melpignano M, et al. Vaginal versus abdominal hysterectomy in endometrial cancer: a retrospective study in a selective population. *Int J Gynecol Cancer* 2008;18:797–802.

Blakely T, Barendregt JJ, Foster RH, et al. The association of active smoking with multiple cancers: national census-cancer registry cohorts with quantitative bias analysis. *Cancer Causes Control* 2013;24:1243–1255.

Boggess JF, Gehrig PA, Cantrell L, et al. A comparative study of 3 surgical methods for hysterectomy with staging for endometrial cancer: robotic assistance, laparoscopy, laparotomy. *Am J Obstet Gynecol* 2008;199:360.e1–360.e9.

Bokhman JV. Two pathogenetic types of endometrial carcinoma. *Gynecol Oncol* 1983;15:10–17.

Boronow RC, Morrow CP, Creasman WT, et al. Surgical staging in endometrial cancer: clinical-pathologic findings of a prospective study. *Obstet Gynecol* 1984;63:825–832.

Brinton LA, Berman ML, Mortel R, et al. Reproductive, menstrual, and medical risk factors for endometrial cancer: results from a case–control study. *Am J Obstet Gynecol* 1992;167:1317–1325.

Bristow RE, Zahurak ML, Alexander CJ, et al. FIGO stage IIIC endometrial carcinoma: resection of macroscopic nodal disease and other determinants of survival. *Int J Gynecol Cancer* 2003;13:664–672.

Brudie LA, Backes FJ, Ahmad S. Analysis of recurrence and survival for women with uterine malignancies undergoing robotic surgery. *Gynecol Oncol* 2013;128:309–315.

Buda A, Guerra L, Signorelli M. Regarding: "Pathologic ultrastaging improves micrometastasis detection in sentinel lymph nodes during endometrial cancer staging." *Int J Gynecol Cancer* 2014;24:964–965.

Buijs CB, Willemse PHB, de Vries EGE, et al. Effect of tamoxifen on the endometrium and menstrual cycle of premenopausal breast cancer patients. *Int J Gynecol Cancer* 2009;19:677–681.

Burchuck A, Anspach C, Evans AC, et al. Postsurgical surveillance of patients with FIGO stage I/II endometrial adenocarcinoma. *Gynecol Oncol* 1995;59:20–24.

Calle EE, Rodriguez C, Walker-Thurmond K, et al. Overweight, obesity, and mortality from cancer in a prospectively studied cohort of US adults. *N Engl J Med* 2003;348:1625–1638.

Cancer and Steroid Hormone Study Group. Combination oral contraceptive use and the risk of endometrial cancer. The Cancer and Steroid Hormone Study of the Centers for Disease Control and the National Institute of Child Health and Human Development. *JAMA* 1987;257:796–800.

Cardenas-Goicoechea J, Soto E, Chuang L, et al. Integration of robotics into two established programs of minimally invasive surgery for endometrial cancer appears to decrease surgical complications. *J Gynecol Oncol* 2013;24:21–28.

Castellsague X, Thompson WD, Dubrow R. Intrauterine contraception and the risk of endometrial cancer. *Int J Cancer* 1993;54:911–916.

Chan JK, Loizzi V, Youssef M, et al. Significance of comprehensive surgical staging in noninvasive papillary serous carcinoma of the endometrium. *Gynecol Oncol* 2003;90:181–185.

Chi DS, Welshinger M, Venkatraman ES, et al. The role of surgical cytoreduction in stage IV endometrial carcinoma. *Gynecol Oncol* 1997;67:56–60.

Cooper AL, Dornfeld-Finke JM, Banks HW, et al. Is cytologic screening an effective surveillance method for detection of vaginal recurrence of uterine cancer? *Obstet Gynecol* 2006;107(1):71–76.

Cornelison TL, Trimble EL, Kosary CL. SEER date, corpus uteri cancer: treatment trends versus survival for FIGO stage II, 1988–1994. *Gynecol Oncol* 1999;74:350–355.

Coronado PJ, Herraiz MA, Magrina JF, et al. Comparison of perioperative outcomes and cost of robotic-assisted laparoscopy, laparoscopy, and laparotomy for endometrial cancer. *Eur J Obstet Gynecol Reprod Biol* 2012;165:289–294.

Cramer DW. The epidemiology of endometrial and ovarian cancer. *Hematol Oncol Clin North Am* 2012;26:1–12.

Creasman W. Revised FIGO staging for carcinoma of the endometrium. *Int J Gynecol Obstet* 2009;105:109.

Creasman WT, Morrow CP, Bundy BN, et al. Surgical pathologic spread patterns of endometrial cancer. A Gynecologic Oncology Group Study. *Cancer* 1987;60:2035–2041.

Creasman WT, Mutch D, Herzog TJ. ASTEC lymphadenectomy and radiation therapy studies. Are conclusions valid? *Gynecol Oncol* 2010;116:293–294.

Creasman WT, Odicino F, Maisonneuve P, et al. Carcinoma of the corpus uteri. *Int J Gynaecol Obstet* 2006;95(suppl 1):S105–S143.

Creutzberg CL, Nout RA, Lybeert ML, et al.; PORTEC Study Group. Fifteen-year radiotherapy outcomes of the randomized PORTEC-1 trial for endometrial cancer. *Int J Radiat Oncol Biol Phys* 2011;81:e631–e638.

Creutzberg CL, van Putten WLJ, Koper PC, et al. The morbidity of treatment for patients with stage I endometrial cancer: results from a randomized trial. *Int J Radiat Oncol Biol Phys* 2001;51:1246–1255.

Creutzberg CL, van Putten WLJ, Koper PCM, et al. Surgery and postoperative radiotherapy versus surgery alone for patients with stage-1 endometrial carcinoma: multicentre randomised trial. *Lancet* 2000;355:1404–1411.

Creutzberg CL, van Putten WL, Wariam-Rodenhuis CC, et al. Outcome of high-risk stage IC, grade 3, compared with stage I endometrial carcinoma patients: the Postoperative Radiation in Endometrial Carcinoma Trial. *J Clin Oncol* 2004;22:1234–1241.

Dahhan T, Fons G, Buist MR, et al. The efficacy of hormonal treatment for residual or recurrent low-grade endometrial stromal sarcoma. A retrospective study. *Eur J Obstet Gynecol Reprod Biol* 2009;144:80–84.

D'Angelo E, Prat J. Uterine sarcomas: a review. *Gynecol Oncol* 2010;116:131–139.

Dargent DF. Laparoscopic surgery in gynecologic oncology. *Surg Clin North Am* 2001;81:949–964.

Demirkiran F, Yavuz E, Erenel H. Which is the best technique for endometrial sampling? Aspiration (pipelle) versus dilatation and curettage (D&C). *Arch Gynecol Obstet* 2012;286:1277–1282.

Dijkhuizen FPHLJ, Mol BWJ, Brolmann HAM, et al. The accuracy of endometrial sampling in the diagnosis of patients with endometrial carcinoma and hyperplasia: a meta-analysis. *Cancer* 2000;89:1765–1772.

Early Breast Cancer Trialists' Collaborative Group. Tamoxifen for early breast cancer: an overview of the randomized trials. *Lancet* 1998;351:1451–1467.

Esposito K, Chiodini P, Capuano A, et al. Metabolic syndrome and endometrial cancer: a meta-analysis. *Endocrine* 2014;45:28–36.

Eto T, Saito T, Kasamatsu T, et al. Clinicopathological prognostic factors and the role of cytoreduction in surgical stage IVb endometrial cancer: a retrospective multi-institutional analysis of 248 patients in Japan. *Gynecol Oncol* 2012;127:338–344.

Farrell T, Jones N, Owen P, et al. The significance of an "insufficient" Pipelle sample in the investigation of postmenopausal bleeding. *Acta Obstet Gynecol Scand* 1999;78:810–812.

Fearnley EJ, Marquart L, Spurdle AB, et al. Polycystic ovary syndrome increases the risk of endometrial cancer in women aged less than 50 years: an Australian case–control study. *Cancer Causes Control* 2010;21:2303–2308.

Feng W, Hua K, Gudlauqsson E, et al. Prognostic indicators in WHO 2003 low-grade endometrial stromal sarcoma. *Histopathology* 2013;62:675–687.

Fiorca JV, Brunetto V, Hanjani P, et al.; Gynecologic Oncology Group study. Phase II trial of alternating courses of megestrol acetate and tamoxifen in advanced endometrial carcinoma: a Gynecologic Oncology Group study. *Gynecol Oncol* 2004;92:10–14.

Fisher B, Costantino JP, Redmond CK, et al. Endometrial cancer in tamoxifen-treated breast cancer patients: findings from the National Surgical Adjuvant Breast and Bowel Project (NSABP) B-14. *J Natl Cancer Inst* 1994;86:527–537.

Fishman DA, Roberts KB, Chambers JT, et al. Radiation therapy as exclusive treatment for medically inoperable patients with stage I and II endometrioid carcinoma of the endometrium. *Gynecol Oncol* 1996;61:189–196.

Friberg E, Orsini N, Matzoros CS, et al. Diabetes mellitus and risk of endometrial cancer: a meta-analysis. *Diabetologia* 2007;50:1365–1374.

Frumovitz M, Coleman RC, Soliman PT, et al. A case for caution in the pursuit of the sentinel node in women with endometrial carcinoma. *Gynecol Oncol* 2014;132:275–279.

Galaal K, Bryant A, Fisher AD, et al. Laparoscopy versus laparotomy for the management of early stage endometrial cancer. *Cochrane Database Syst Rev* 2012;9:CD006655.

Gardner FJ, Konje JC, Bell SC, et al. Prevention of tamoxifen induced endometrial polyps using a levonorgestrel releasing intrauterine system long-term follow-up of a randomized control trial. *Gynecol Oncol* 2009;114:452–456.

Gehrig PA, Cantrell LA, Shafer A, et al. What is the optimal minimally invasive surgical procedure for endometrial cancer staging in the obese and morbidly obese woman? *Gynecol Oncol* 2008;111:41–45.

Geller MA, Ivy J, Dusenbery KE. A single institution experience using sequential multi-modality adjuvant chemotherapy and radiation in the "sandwich" method for high risk endometrial carcinoma. *Gynecol Oncol* 2010;118:19–23.

George S, Barysauskas C, Serrano C, et al. Retrospective cohort study evaluating the impact of intraperitoneal morcellation on outcomes of localized uterine leiomyosarcoma. *Cancer* 2014 120:3154–3158.

Goff BA, Goodman A, Muntz HG, et al. Surgical stage IV endometrial carcinoma: a study of 47 cases. *Gynecol Oncol* 1994;52:237–240.

Goff BA, Kato D, Schmidt RA, et al. Uterine papillary serous carcinoma: patterns of metastatic spread. *Gynecol Oncol* 1994;54:264–268.

Grady D, Gebretsadik T, Kerlikowske K, et al. Hormone replacement therapy and endometrial cancer risk: a meta-analysis. *Obstet Gynecol* 1995;85:304–313.

Gredmark T, Kvint S, Havel G, et al. Histopathological findings in women with postmenopausal bleeding. *BJOG* 1995;102:133–136.

Greven K, Winter K, Underhill K, et al. Final analysis of RTOG 9708: adjuvant postoperative irradiation combined with cisplatin/paclitaxel chemotherapy following surgery for patients with high-risk endometrial cancer. *Gynecol Oncol* 2006;103:155–159.

Gunderson CC, Fader AN, Carson KA, et al. Oncologic and reproductive outcomes in women with endometrial hyperplasia and grade 1 adenocarcinoma: a systematic review. *Gynecol Oncol* 2012;125;477–482.

Gupta JK, Chien PF, Voit D, et al. Ultrasonographic endometrial thickness for diagnosing endometrial pathology in women with postmenopausal bleeding: a meta-analysis. *Acta Obstet Gynecol Scand* 2002;81:799–816.

Hagen B, Eriksson N, Sundset M. Randomized controlled trial of LigaSure versus conventional suture ligature for abdominal hysterectomy. *BJOG* 2005;112:968–970.

Hardiman P, Pillay OC, Atiomo W. Polycystic ovary syndrome and endometrial carcinoma [published erratum appears in *Lancet* 2003;362:1082]. *Lancet* 2003;361:1810–1812.

He H, Bhosale P, Wei W, et al. MRI is highly specific in determining primary cervical versus endometrial cancer when biopsy results are inconclusive. *Clin Radiol* 2013;68:1107–1113.

Hensley ML, Ishill N, Soslow R, et al. Adjuvant gemcitabine plus docetaxel for completely resected stages I–IV high grade uterine leiomyosarcoma: results of a prospective study. *Gynecol Oncol* 2009;112:563–567.

Hill DA, Weiss NS, Voigt LF, et al. Endometrial cancer in relation to intra-uterine device use. *Int J Cancer* 1997;70:278–281.

Holub Z, Jabor A, Bartos P, et al. Laparoscopic surgery in women with endometrial cancer: the learning curve. *Eur J Obstet Gynecol Reprod Biol* 2003;107:195–200.

Horn L-C, Schnurrbusch U, Bilek K, et al. Risk of progression in complex and atypical endometrial hyperplasia: clinicopathologic analysis in cases with and without progesterone treatment. *Int J Gynecol Cancer* 2004;14:348–353.

Hubacher D, Grimes DA. Noncontraceptive health benefits of intrauterine devices: as systematic review. *Obstet Gynecol Surv* 2002;57: 120–128.

Huh WK, Straughn JM Jr, Mariani A, et al. Salvage of isolated vaginal recurrences in women with surgical stage I endometrial cancer: a multiinstitutional experience. *Int J Gynecol Cancer* 2007;17:886–889.

Janda M, Gebski V, Brand A, et al. Quality of life after total laparoscopic hysterectomy versus total abdominal hysterectomy for stage I endometrial cancer (LACE): a randomised trial. *Lancet Oncol* 2010;11:772–780.

Jones HW III, Carlson JW. *Staging of gynecologic malignancies handbook*, 3rd ed. Chicago, IL: SGO, 2010.

Kapp DS, Shin JY, Chan JK. Prognostic factors and survival in 1396 patients with uterine leiomyosarcomas; emphasis on impact of lymphadenectomy and oophorectomy. *Cancer* 2008;112:820–830.

Karageorgi A, Hankinson SE, Kraft P, et al. Reproductive factors and postmenopausal hormone use in relation to endometrial cancer risk in the Nurses' Health Study cohort 1976–2004. *Int J Cancer* 2010;126:208–216.

Kasamatusu T, Onda T, Katsumata N, et al. Prognostic significance of positive peritoneal cytology in endometrial carcinoma confined to the uterus. *Br J Cancer* 2003;88:245–250.

Kazandi M, Okmen F, Ergenoglu AM. Comparison of the success of histopathological diagnosis with dilatation-curettage and Pipelle endometrial sampling. *J Obstet Gynaecol* 2012;32:790–794.

Keys HM, Roberts JA, Brunetto VL, et al. A phase III trial of surgery with or without adjunctive external pelvic radiation therapy in intermediate risk endometrial adenocarcinoma; a Gynecologic Oncology Group study. *Gynecol Oncol* 2004;92:744–751.

Kilgore JE, Jackson AL, Ko EM, et al. Recurrence-free and 5-year survival following robotic-assisted surgical staging for endometrial carcinoma. *Gynecol Oncol* 2013;129:49–53.

Kilgore LC, Partridge EE, Alvarez RD, et al. Adenocarcinoma of the endometrium: survival comparisons of patients with and without pelvic node sampling. *Gynecol Oncol* 1995;56:29–33.

Kim CH, Soslow RA, Park KJ, et al. Pathologic ultrastaging improves micrometastasis detection in sentinel lymph nodes during endometrial cancer staging. *Int J Gynecol Cancer*. 2013;23(5):964–970.

Kim HS, Song YS. International Federation of Gynecology and Obstetrics (FIGO) staging system revised: what should be considered critically for gynecologic cancer? *J Gynecol Oncol* 2009;20:135–136.

Kitchener H, Swart AM, Qian Q, et al.; ASTEC study group. Efficacy of systematic pelvic lymphadenectomy in endometrial cancer (MRC ASTEC trial): a randomised study. *Lancet* 2009;373:125–136.

Klopp AH, Jhingran A, Ramondetta L, et al. Node-positive adenocarcinoma of the endometrium: outcome and patterns of recurrence with and without external beam irradiation. *Gynecol Oncol* 2009:115:6–11.

Koh WJ, Greer BE, Abu-Rustum NR, et al. Uterine neoplasms, version 1.2014. *J Natl Compr Canc Netw* 2014;12:248–280.

Koivisto-Korander R, Martinsen JI, Weiderpass E, et al. Incidence of uterine leiomyosarcoma and endometrial stromal sarcoma in Nordic countries: results from NORDCAN and NOCCA databases. *Maturitas* 2012;72:56–60.

Kornblith AB, Huang HQ, Walker JL, et al. Quality of life of patients with endometrial cancer undergoing laparoscopic International Federation of Gynecology and Obstetrics staging compared with laparotomy: a Gynecologic Oncology Group study. *J Clin Oncol* 2009;27:5337–5342.

Kosary CL. FIGO stage, histology, histologic grade, age, and race as prognostic factors in determining survival for cancers of the female gynaecological system: an analysis of 1973–87 SEER cases of cancers of the endometrium, cervix, ovary, vulva, and vagina. *Semin Surg Oncol* 1994;10:31–46.

Kurman RJ, Kaminski PF, Norris HJ. The behavior of endometrial hyperplasia. A long-term study of "untreated" hyperplasia in 170 patients. *Cancer* 1985;56:403–412.

Lai GY, Park, Y, Hartge P, et al. The association between self-reported diabetes and cancer incidence in the NIH-AARP Diet and Health Study. *J Clin Endocrinol Metab* 2013;98:E497–E502.

Lambrou NC, Gomez-Marin O, Mirhashemi R, et al. Optimal surgical cytoreduction in patients with stage III and stage IV endometrial carcinoma: a study of morbidity and survival. *Gynecol Oncol* 2004;93:653–658.

Leibsohn S, d'Ablaing G, Mishell DR Jr, et al. Leiomyosarcoma in a series of hysterectomies performed for presumed uterine leiomyosarcomas. *Am J Obstet Gynecol* 1990;162:968–974.

Leitao MM Jr, Han G, Lee LX. Complex atypical hyperplasia of the uterus: characteristics and prediction of underlying carcinoma risk. *Am J Obstet Gynecol* 2010;203:349–346.

Lenihan JP Jr, Kovanda C, Seshadri-Kreaden U. What is the learning curve for robotic assisted gynecologic surgery? *J Minim Invasive Gynecol* 2008;15:589–594.

Li AJ, Giuntoli RL II, Drake R, et al. Ovarian preservation in stage I low-grade endometrial stromal sarcomas. *Obstet Gynecol* 2005;106:1304–1308.

Lim PC, Kang E, Park do H. A comparative detail analysis of the learning curve and surgical outcome for robotic hysterectomy with lymphadenectomy versus laparoscopic hysterectomy with lymphadenectomy in treatment of endometrial cancer: a case-matched controlled study of the first one hundred twenty two patients. *Gynecol Oncol* 2011;120:413–418.

Lu KH, Dinh M, Kohlmann W, et al. Gynecologic cancer as a "sentinel cancer" for women with hereditary nonpolyposis colorectal cancer syndrome. *Obstet Gynecol* 2005;105:569–574.

Mansell H, Hertig AT. Granulosa-theca cell tumors and endometrial carcinoma; a study of their relationship and a survey of 80 cases. *Obstet Gynecol* 1955;6:385–394.

Mariani A, Dowdy SC, Cliby WA. Prospective assessment of lymphatic dissemination in endometrial cancer: a paradigm shift in surgical staging. *Gynecol Oncol* 2008;109:11–18.

McCluggage WG. Malignant biphasic uterine tumours: carcinosarcomas or metaplastic carcinomas. *J Clin Pathol* 2002;55:321–325.

Meyer LA, Broadus RR, Lu KH. Endometrial cancer and Lynch syndrome: clinical and pathologic considerations. *Cancer Control* 2009;16:14–22.

Miller D, Filiaci V, Fleming G, et al. Randomized phase III noninferiority trial of first line chemotherapy for metastatic or recurrent endometrial carcinoma: A Gynecologic Oncology Group study. *Gynecol Oncol* 2012;125:771.

Morrow CP, Bundy BN, Kurman RJ, et al. Relationship between surgical-pathological risk factors and outcome in clinical stage I and II carcinoma of the endometrium: a Gynecologic Oncology Group study. *Gynecol Oncol* 1991;40:55–65.

Mutch DG. The new FIGO staging system for cancers of the vulva, cervix, endometrium, and sarcomas. *Gynecol Oncol* 2009;115:325–328.

Mutter GL, Baak JPA, Crum CP, et al. Endometrial precancer diagnosis by histopathology, clonal analysis, and computerized morphometry. *J Pathol* 2000;190:462–469.

Naumann RW. The role of lymphadenectomy in endometrial cancer: Was the ASTEC trial doomed by design and are we destined to repeat that mistake? *Gynecol Oncol* 2012;126:5–11.

Nelson G, Randall M, Sutton G, et al. FIGO stage IIIC endometrial carcinoma with metastases confined to pelvic lymph nodes: analysis of treatment outcomes, prognostic variables, and failure patterns following adjuvant radiation therapy. *Gynecol Oncol* 1999;75:211–214.

Nout RA, Smit VTHBM, Putter H. Vaginal brachytherapy versus pelvic external beam radiotherapy for patients with endometrial cancer of high-intermediate risk (PORTEC-2): an open-label, non-inferiority, randomised trial. *Lancet* 2010;375:816–823.

Nout RA, van de Poll-Franse LV, Lybeers MLM, et al. Long-term outcome and quality of life of patients with endometrial carcinoma treated with or without pelvic radiotherapy in the Post Operative Radiation Therapy in Endometrial Carcinoma 1 (PORTC-1) trial. *J Clin Oncol* 2011;29:1692–1700.

Obermair A, Geramou M, Gucer F, et al. Impact of hysteroscopy on disease-free survival in clinically stage I endometrial cancer patients. *Int J Gynecol Cancer* 2000;10:275–279.

Organisation for Research and Treatment of Cancer Gynaecological Cancer Group. Phase III randomized study to evaluate the role of adjuvant pelvic radiotherapy in the treatment of uterine sarcomas stages I and II: an European Organisation for Research and Treatment of Cancer Gynaecological Cancer Group Study (protocol 55874). *Eur J Cancer* 2008;44:808–818.

Panici PB, Basile S, Maneschi F, et al. Systematic pelvic lymphadenectomy vs no lymphadenectomy in early-stage endometrial carcinoma: randomized clinical trial. *J Natl Cancer Inst* 2008;100: 1707–1716.

Parslov M, Lidegaard O, Klintorp S, et al. Risk factors among young women with endometrial cancer: a Danish case–control study. *Am J Obstet Gynecol* 2000;182:23–29.

Pecorelli S. Revised FIGO staging of carcinoma of the vulva, cervix, endometrium. *Int J Gynaecol Obstet* 2009;105:103–104.

Pillay OC, Te Fong LF, Crow JC, et al. The association between polycystic ovaries and endometrial cancer. *Hum Reprod* 2006;21: 924–929.

Pink D, Lindner T, Mrozek A, et al. Harm or benefit of hormonal treatment in metastatic low-grade endometrial stromal sarcoma: single center experience with 10 cases and review of the literature. *Gynecol Oncol* 2006;101:464–469.

Polyzos NP, Mauri D, Tsioras S. Intraperitoneal dissemination of endometrial cancer cells after hysteroscopy: a systematic review and meta-analysis. *Int J Gynecol Cancer* 2010;20:261–267.

Randall ME, Filiaci VL, Muss H, et al.; Gynecologic Oncology Group study. Randomized phase III trial of whole abdominal irradiation versus doxorubicin and cisplatin chemotherapy in advanced endometrial carcinoma: a Gynecologic Oncology Group Study. *J Clin Oncol* 2006;24:36–44.

Reed NS, Mangioni C, Malmstrom H, et al.; European Organisation for Research and Treatment of Cancer Gynaecological Cancer Group. Phase III randomized study to evaluate the role of adjuvant pelvic radiotherapy in the treatment of uterine sarcomas stages I and II: an European Organisation for Research and Treatment of Cancer Gynaecological Cancer Group Study (protocol 55874). *Eur J Cancer* 2008;44:808–818.

Reeves GK, Pirie K, Beral V, et al. Cancer incidence and mortality in relation to body mass index in the Million Women Study: cohort study. *BMJ* 2007;335:1134–1145.

Reisinger AS, Staros EB, Feld R, et al. Preoperative radiation therapy in clinical stage II endometrial cancer. *Gynecol Oncol* 1992;45:174–178.

Rose PG, Cha SD, Tak WK, et al. Radiation therapy for surgically proven para-aortic node metastasis in endometrial cancer. *Int J Radiat Oncol Biol Phys* 1992;24:229–233.

Rubatt JM, Slomovitz BM, Burke TW, et al. Development of metastatic endometrioid adenocarcinoma while on progestin therapy for endometrial hyperplasia. *Gynecol Oncol* 2005;99:472–476.

Sainz de la Cuesta R, Espinosa JA, Crespo E, et al. Does fluid hysteroscopy increase the stage or worsen the prognosis in patients with endometrial cancer: a randomized controlled trial. *Eur J Obstet Gynecol Reprod Biol* 2004;115:211–215.

Schmandt RE, Iglesias DA, Co NN, et al. Understanding obesity and endometrial cancer risk: opportunities for prevention. *Am J Obstet Gynecol* 2011;205:518–525.

Schmeler KM, Lynch HT, Chen LM, et al. Prophylactic surgery to reduce the risk of gynecologic cancers in the Lynch syndrome. *N Engl J Med* 2006;19:261–269.

Seamon LG, Cohn DE, Henretta MS, et al. Minimally invasive comprehensive surgical staging for endometrial cancer: robotics or laparoscopy? *Gynecol Oncol* 2009;113:36–41.

IX

SEER Training Modules, *Purpose of Staging*. U.S. National Institutes of Health, National Cancer Institute. August 14, 2013. http://training.seer.cancer.gov/staging/intro/purpose.html/

Shah JP, Bryant CS, Kumar S, et al. Lymphadenectomy and ovarian preservation in low-grade endometrial stromal sarcoma. *Obstet Gynecol* 2008;112:1102–1108.

Shumsky AG, Stuart GC, Brasher PM, et al. An evaluation of routine follow-up of patients treated for endometrial cancer. *Gynecol Oncol* 1994;55:229–233.

Siegel R, Ma J, Zou Z, et al. Cancer statistics, 2014. *CA Cancer J Clin* 2014;64:9–29.

Smith RA, Brooks D, Cokkinides V, et al. Cancer screening in the United States, 2013. A review of current American Cancer Society Guidelines, current issues in cancer screening, and new guidance on cervical cancer screening and lung cancer screening. *Cancer J Clin* 2013;63:87–105.

Smith-Bindman R, Kerlikowske K, Feldstein VA, et al. Endovaginal ultrasound to exclude endometrial cancer and other endometrial abnormalities. *JAMA* 1998;280:1510–1517.

Society of Gynecologic Oncologists. SGO Position Statement: Morcellation. December 2013. https://www.sgo.org/newsroom/position-statements-2/morcellation/

Solima E, Martinelli F, Ditto A, et al. Diagnostic accuracy of sentinel node in endometrial cancer by using hysteroscopic injection of radiolabeled tracer. *Gynecol Oncol* 2012:126:419–423.

Stock RJ, Kanbour A. Prehysterectomy curettage. *Obstet Gynecol* 1975;45:537–541.

Straughn JM Jr, Huh WK, Kelly FJ, et al. Conservative management of stage I endometrial carcinoma after surgical staging. *Gynecol Oncol* 2001;84:194–200.

Straughn JM Jr, Huh WK, Orr JW, et al. Stage IC adenocarcinoma of the endometrium: survival comparisons of surgically staged patients with and without adjuvant therapy. *Gynecol Oncol* 2003;89:295–300.

Takamizawa S, Minakami H, Usui R, et al. Risk of complications and uterine malignancies in women undergoing hysterectomy for presumed leiomyomas. *Gynecol Obstet Invest* 1999;48:193–196.

Tew W, Spriggs D, Aghajanian CA. Adjuvant gemcitabine plus docetaxel for completely the endometrium. *Gynecol Oncol* 1996;61:189–196.

Toleda G, Oliva E. Smooth muscle tumors of the uterus: a practical approach. *Arch Pathol Lab Med* 2008;132:595–605.

Takeshima N, Nishida H, Tabata T, et al. Positive peritoneal cytology in endometrial cancer: enhancement of other prognostic indicators. *Gynecol Oncol* 2001;82:470–473.

Tao MH, Xu WH, Zheng W, et al. Oral contraceptive and IUD use and endometrial cancer: a population based case–control study in Shanghai, China. *Int J Cancer* 2006;119:2142–2147.

Timmermans A, Opmeer BC, Khan KS, et al. Endometrial thickness measurement for detecting endometrial cancer in women with postmenopausal bleeding. *Obstet Gynecol* 2010;116:160–167.

Toleda G, Oliva E. Smooth muscle tumors of the uterus: a practical approach. *Arch Pathol Lab Med* 2008;132:595–605.

Trimble CL, Kauderer J, Zaino R, et al. Concurrent endometrial carcinoma in women with a biopsy diagnosis of atypical endometrial hyperplasia: a Gynecologic Oncology Group study. *Cancer* 2006;106:812–819.

Trimble CL, Method M, Leitao M, et al. Management of endometrial precancers. *Obstet Gynecol* 2012;120:1160–1175.

U.S. Food and Drug Administration. Laparoscopic uterine power morcellation in hysterectomy and myomectomy: FDA safety communication. Last Updated June 3, 2014. http://www.fda.gov/medicaldevices/safety/alertandnotices/ucm39357.

Viswanathan AN, Feskanich D, De Vivo I, et al. Smoking and the risk of endometrial cancer: results from the Nurses' Health Study. *Int J Cancer* 2005;114:996–1001.

Walker JL, Piedmonte MR, Spirtos NM, et al. Laparoscopy compared with laparotomy for comprehensive surgical staging of uterine cancer: Gynecologic Oncology Group Study LAP2. *J Clin Oncol* 2009;27:5331–5336.

Walker JL, Piedemonte MR, Spirtos NM, et al. Recurrence and survival after random assignment to laparoscopy versus laparotomy for comprehensive surgical staging of uterine cancer: Gynecologic Oncology Group LAP2 Study. *J Clin Oncol* 2012;30:695–700.

Weiderpass E, Adami HO, Baron JA, et al. Risk of endometrial cancer following estrogen replacement with and without progestins. *J Natl Cancer Inst* 1999;91:1131–1137.

Weiderpass E, Persson I, Adami HO, et al. Body size in different periods of life, diabetes mellitus, hypertension and risk of postmenopausal endometrial cancer. *Cancer Causes Control* 2000;11:185–192.

Weigelt B, Banerjee S. Molecular targets and targeted therapeutics in endometrial cancer. *Curr Opin Oncol* 2012;24:554–563.

Wickerham DL, Fisher B, Wolmark N, et al. Association of tamoxifen and uterine sarcoma. *J Clin Oncol* 2002;20:2758–2760.

Wilson EB. The evolution of robotic general surgery. *Scand J Surg* 2009;98:125–129.

Woelk JL, Casiano ER, Weaver AL, et al. The learning curve of robotic hysterectomy. *Obstet Gynecol* 2013;121:87–95.

Wright JD, Burke WM, Wilde ET. Comparative effectiveness of robotic versus laparoscopic hysterectomy for endometrial cancer. *J Clin Oncol* 2012;30:783–791.

Wright JD, Neugut AI, Wilde ET, et al. Use and benefits of laparoscopic hysterectomy for stage I endometrial cancer among medicare beneficiaries. *J Oncol Pract* 2012;8:e89–e99.

Yoon A, Park JY, Park JY, et al. Prognostic factors and outcomes in endometrial stromal sarcoma with the 2009 FIGO staging system: a multicenter review of 114 cases. *Gynecol Oncol* 2014;132(1):70–75.

Yu X, Lum D, Kiet TK, et al. Utilization of and charges for robotic versus laparoscopic versus open surgery for endometrial cancer. *J Surg Oncol* 2013;107;653–658.

CHAPTER 53
Ovarian Cancer

Pedro T. Ramirez and David M. Gershenson

DEFINITIONS

Intraperitoneal chemotherapy—Cytotoxic chemotherapy given intraperitoneally rather than intravenously. This is usually given via an intraperitoneal catheter in patients who have undergone optimal cytoreductive surgery.

Neoadjuvant chemotherapy—Chemotherapy given before definitive surgery to chemically debulk cancer with the intention of making future surgical efforts more successful and less complicated. Usually, several cycles of chemotherapy are given to women with advanced ovarian cancer who are poor surgical candidates because of their medical condition or perhaps the extent of disease. At the start of therapy, surgical debulking is planned if there is a response to chemotherapy, although surgery may not occur if the patient does not respond to chemotherapy or her medical condition fails to improve.

Optimal cytoreduction—Survival is related to the volume of residual cancer after initial surgery. It is preferable to remove as much tumor as possible. The definition of *optimal cytoreduction* has continued to change over the years and currently means surgical debulking so that the largest residual tumor mass is less than 1 cm in diameter.

Ovarian cancer is the leading cause of death from gynecologic malignancies in the United States. For 2014, the American Cancer Society estimates that approximately 21,980 new cases of ovarian cancer will be detected and nearly 14,270 women will die from the disease. The lifetime risk for ovarian cancer in

American women without a family history of the disease is 1 in 70 (1.4%). Because early ovarian cancer produces few specific symptoms, most women present with advanced-stage disease for which the cost of treatment is high and the prognosis poor. Approximately 90% of malignant ovarian tumors in adults are of epithelial origin followed by sex cord–stromal tumors (6%) and germ-cell tumors (3%). Good surgery is a blend of good judgment and sound surgical technique. Much of this chapter is devoted to the natural history and results of various surgical and other treatment approaches for ovarian cancer. This background information provides the surgeon with the basis for clinical decision making concerning patient selection, choice of the right operation, and postoperative treatment recommendations. The operative techniques involved in surgery for ovarian cancer are illustrated in many of the other chapters in this text.

INCIDENCE AND RISK FACTORS

The incidence of ovarian cancer is highest in Sweden (19.6/ 100,000) and the United States (15.4/100,000) and lowest in Japan (10.1/100,000). In the United States, ovarian cancer incidence rates are highest in Caucasian women, intermediate in African American women, and lowest in Native American women.

Factors associated with an increase in ovarian cancer risk are age, nulliparity, and a family history of the disease. Ovarian cancer is rare before the age of 40, increases steadily thereafter, and peaks at ages 65 to 75. Parity is the most important nongenetic factor affecting risk for ovarian cancer (Table 53.1). Whittemore and colleagues analyzed 12 case–control studies in the United States and reported a significant risk reduction for ovarian cancer with each term pregnancy (odds ratio [OR] = 0.47). The risk of ovarian cancer decreased progressively with increasing numbers of pregnancies. Similarly, the use of oral contraceptives has been shown to reduce the risk of ovarian cancer. Ovarian cancer risk decreases approximately 11% per year of oral contraceptive use to a maximum of 46% after 5 years of use. These observations have led to the theory of "incessant ovulation" in the etiology of ovarian cancer. According to this theory, risk for epithelial ovarian cancer is related directly to the number of uninterrupted ovulatory cycles. With ovulation, the surface epithelium is ruptured and then undergoes rapid proliferation and repair. At the time of ovulation, there is invagination of the surface epithelium into the underlying stroma forming inclusion cysts. The epithelium lining these inclusion cysts then undergoes neoplastic transformation under the influence of oncogenic factors. The observation that early age of menarche and late menopause are associated with an increase in ovarian cancer risk is consistent with this theory, because both increase the number of ovulatory cycles.

A second theory of ovarian carcinogenesis is the retrograde menstruation hypothesis. According to this hypothesis, retrograde transportation of carcinogens from the uterus and lower genital tract through the fallopian tube to the ovary occurs at the time of menstruation. The protective effect of oral contraceptives is consistent with this hypothesis because their use has been associated with a reduction in menstrual blood loss, thus with decreased retrograde menstruation. Conversely, the observed increase in ovarian cancer risk associated with hormone replacement therapy (Table 53.1) may be mediated through the periods of abnormal uterine bleeding that occur with many hormonal regimens. This hypothesis is also supported by the known decrease in ovarian cancer risk in women who have undergone tubal ligation or hysterectomy, because

TABLE 53.1 Risk Factors for Ovarian Cancer

FACTOR	ODDS RATIO
Parity[a]	
Nulliparous	1
Parous	0.47
Oral contraceptive use[b]	
Never	1
2–5 y	0.73
Estrogen use[b]	
Never	1[c]
Ever	1.4
Clomid use[d]	
No	1
Yes	2.3
Tubal ligation[a]	
No	1
Yes	0.59
Hysterectomy[a]	
No	1
Yes	0.66
Talc use[e]	
No	1
Yes	1.5
Breast-feeding[a]	
No	1
Yes	0.73
Family history[f]	
1 first-degree relative with ovarian cancer	3.1
>2 first-degree relatives with ovarian cancer	4.6

[a]Whittemore AS, Harris R, Itnyre J. Collaborative Ovarian Cancer Group: characteristics relating to ovarian cancer risk, collaborative analysis of 12 U.S. case–control studies. II. Invasive epithelial ovarian cancers in white women. *Am J Epidemiol* 1992;136:1184.
[b]Riman T, Dickman PW, Nilsson S, et al. Hormone replacement therapy and the risk of invasive epithelial ovarian cancer in Swedish women. *J Natl Cancer Inst* 2002;94:497.
[c]Not significant.
[d]Rossing MA, Daling JR, Weiss NS, et al. Ovarian tumors in a cohort of infertile women. *N Engl J Med* 1994;331:771.
[e]Cook LS, Kamb ML, Weiss NS. Perineal powder exposure and risk of ovarian cancer. *Am J Epidemiol* 1997;145:459.
[f]Kerlikowske K, Brown JS, Grady DG. Should women with familial ovarian cancer undergo prophylactic oophorectomy? *Obstet Gynecol* 1992;80:700.

these procedures prevent the ascent of potential oncogenic factors from the lower genital tract to the ovary.

A final hypothesis concerning the genesis of ovarian cancer is that exposure of ovarian epithelium to persistently high levels of pituitary gonadotropins results in neoplastic transformation. Follicle-stimulating hormone (FSH) has been shown to promote the growth of epithelial ovarian cancer cells in vitro, and this effect can be blocked by luteinizing hormone (LH). A corollary to this hypothesis is that elevated circulating gonadotropin levels promote estrogen biosynthesis in the ovarian stroma, which, in turn, causes abnormal proliferation of the adjacent epithelium. Breast-feeding, which has been reported to lower the risk of ovarian cancer, is associated with reduced serum concentrations of LH and estradiol. Pregnancy and the use of oral contraceptives presumably lower the risk of ovarian cancer by inhibiting pituitary secretion of gonadotropins. This theory also receives support from the observed increased risk of ovarian cancer in women taking fertility drugs because these drugs stimulate ovulation by increasing levels of FSH, particularly in the follicular phase of the cycle.

Perhaps the most important risk factor for epithelial ovarian cancer is a family history of the disease. The estimated odds ratio for the development of ovarian cancer in a woman with one first-degree relative who has ovarian cancer is 3.1 (95% CI = 2.1 to 4.5). This risk increases even further (OR 4.6 CI = 1.1 to 18.4) in a woman with two or more primary or secondary relatives who have ovarian cancer. These odds ratios translate to a lifetime risk for ovarian cancer of approximately 5% in a woman with one first-degree relative who has the disease and 7% in a woman with two or more relatives with the disease. It should be mentioned, however, that familial ovarian cancers make up a relatively small proportion of total ovarian cancer cases. Only 5% to 10% of ovarian cancer patients report having a positive family history of the disease.

Three familial ovarian cancer syndromes have been described: Hereditary breast–ovarian cancer syndrome (HBOC), hereditary site-specific ovarian cancer syndrome (HSSOC), and hereditary nonpolyposis colon cancer syndrome (HNPCC). HBOC, the most common of the familial syndromes, is characterized by multiple cases of early-onset (<50 years of age) breast and ovarian cancers. This syndrome accounts for 75% to 90% of all hereditary ovarian cancer cases. HSSOC is manifested only by an increase in cases of early-onset ovarian cancer and makes up about 5% of hereditary ovarian cancers. Women with HSSOC are often younger and more commonly have tumors with serous histology than do women with sporadic ovarian cancer. HNPCC, or Lynch syndrome type II, is characterized by a predominance of early-onset proximal colon cancer in association with cancers of the endometrium and ovary. HNPCC is often confirmed by a mutation in one of several mismatch repair genes, in particular MLH1, MSH2, and MSH6. The estimated lifetime risk of ovarian cancer in women with HNPCC is 10% to 12%. These three familial ovarian cancer syndromes are inherited by autosomal dominant transmission through either maternal or paternal lineage. Therefore, the children of an affected parent have a 50% risk of inheriting the genetic abnormality.

Germline mutations in the BRCA1 or BRCA2 gene appear to account for most hereditary ovarian cancers. BRCA1 was identified in 1994 and is located on the long (q) arm of chromosome 17. BRCA1 is thought to be a tumor suppressor because the normal copy of BRCA1 is always deleted in ovarian cancers that arise in women who inherit a mutant BRCA1 gene. It is estimated that germline mutations in BRCA1 are responsible for 80% to 90% of hereditary ovarian cancers. BRCA2 was identified in 1995 and is located on the long (q) arm of chromosome 13. In a recent report from the Breast Cancer Linkage Consortium, BRCA1 mutations were identified in 81% of ovarian cancer families, whereas BRCA2 mutations were detected in 14% of those families. Penetrance is variable (range 10% to 50%) from one individual to another, and it is estimated that the lifetime risk of ovarian cancer is approximately 39% in BRCA1 carriers and 11% in BRCA2 carriers.

SIGNS AND SYMPTOMS

Although most reports indicate that patients with early-stage ovarian cancer have few symptoms, a recent national survey of 1,725 ovarian cancer patients provides evidence that many of these patients actually had symptoms that they or their primary health providers ignored. The most common symptoms of patients with stage I or II ovarian cancer were abdominal bloating or pain, indigestion, urinary frequency, and constipation. Because many of these symptoms are nonspecific, patients were unaware that they could be associated with ovarian cancer. As a result, 22% of patients ignored their symptoms entirely, and 30% reported that the wrong diagnosis was made. A pelvic examination was performed in only two thirds of patients, and 45% had a delay in diagnosis of more than 3 months. Patients with advanced disease commonly reported abdominal swelling, fatigue, and weight loss. In a subsequent study, four target symptoms were significantly more common in ovarian cancer patients before diagnosis than in age-matched control patients. These symptoms included abdominal pain (frequency 30%, OR 6), abdominal swelling (frequency 16.5%, OR 30), gastrointestinal (GI) symptoms (frequency 8.5%, OR 2.3), and pelvic pain (frequency 5.4%, OR 4.3). These observations emphasize the need for patient and physician education concerning the possible relationship of rather nonspecific abdominal symptoms to ovarian cancer. A high index of suspicion, coupled with pelvic ultrasound and CA-125 testing, may lead to the earlier diagnosis of ovarian cancer in selected patients with these symptoms. Routine yearly pelvic examination has not been shown to increase the diagnosis of early-stage ovarian cancer.

Although vaginal bleeding is not commonly associated with ovarian cancer, it may be present in patients with metastatic involvement of the uterus. Likewise, endometrial hyperplasia and abnormal uterine bleeding can be caused by excess estrogen production from an ovarian stromal tumor. Ovarian cancer must be considered in a patient who presents with a pelvic mass and shortness of breath. A malignant pleural effusion from metastatic ovarian cancer is more common on the right side and is usually associated with dullness to percussion and decreased breath sounds. Finally, any patient with a clinically detected pelvic tumor on pelvic examination should undergo careful palpation of both groins to rule out inguinal lymphadenopathy secondary to metastatic disease.

PREOPERATIVE EVALUATION

Before operative intervention, each patient should undergo a thorough evaluation designed to determine the anatomic location, size, and morphology of the ovarian tumor, as well as possible sites of metastases. In addition, her general medical condition and ability to undergo a major surgical procedure should be established. All patients should undergo routine hematologic and biochemical testing. A computed tomography (CT) scan provides valuable information concerning cardiac size, as well as the presence of pulmonary metastases or a pleural effusion. Positron emission tomography (PET) scans may be more sensitive, but their value in the preoperative assessment of primary ovarian cancer has not been proven.

CT scanning with contrast may identify ureteral obstruction, retroperitoneal lymphadenopathy, omental disease, and peritoneal metastases. In a patient with ascites but no ovarian tumor, liver function studies should be performed to exclude cirrhosis or liver disease. Rarely, the presence of right heart failure and hepatic congestion will cause ascites. Paracentesis may be useful in a patient who presents with ascites and

TABLE 53.2 Serum Markers in Ovarian Cancer

TUMOR HISTOLOGY	SERUM MARKER
Epithelial ovarian cancer	CA-125
Mucinous cystadenocarcinoma	CEA
Endodermal sinus tumor	AFP
Embryonal cell carcinoma	hCG, AFP
Choriocarcinoma	hCG
Dysgerminoma	LDH-1, LDH-2
Granulosa cell tumor	Inhibin

AFP, alpha-fetoprotein; CEA, carcinoembryonic antigen; hCG, human chorionic gonadotropin; LDH, lactate dehydrogenase.

no evidence of an ovarian abnormality. The characteristics of malignant cells present in ascitic fluid may help identify the primary site of intra-abdominal malignancy. An electrocardiogram is indicated in all women older than age 40 or in a patient with specific signs or symptoms of cardiac disease.

Common sites of nongynecologic cancer that spreads to the ovary include gastric malignancy, colonic carcinoma, and breast carcinoma. A careful history and physical examinations should arouse suspicion of other possible primary malignancies. Any such possibilities should be evaluated with appropriate ongoing studies and diagnostic evaluation, possibly including colonoscopy, upper GI endoscopy, and/or mammography. A biopsy of a suspicious finding or easily accessible lymph node may clarify the diagnosis.

Finally, serum markers should be obtained according to the age and clinical findings of each patient. Serum CA-125 and CEA often are elevated in patients with epithelial ovarian cancer, whereas serum alpha-fetoprotein, human chorionic gonadotropin, or lactate dehydrogenase is more commonly increased in younger women with germ-cell ovarian malignancies. Serum inhibin is the most reliable marker in patients with ovarian granulosa cell tumors. The specific marker associated with each type of ovarian cancer is illustrated in Table 53.2. It is important to obtain a baseline serum marker value before surgery so that it can be used to monitor response to therapy.

PATTERNS OF SPREAD

Ovarian cancer spreads by (a) direct extension and exfoliation of tumor cells into the peritoneal cavity, (b) lymphatic metastases to regional and paraaortic lymph nodes, and (c) hematogenous dissemination (Fig. 53.1). The specific pattern of spread depends on the stage, cell type, and histologic differentiation of the tumor.

The earliest method of spread in epithelial ovarian cancer is by exfoliation of tumor cells from the ovarian surface. These cells migrate with the circulation of peritoneal fluid along the surfaces of the pelvic and mesenteric peritoneum. They also are carried cephalad in the paracolic spaces to the omentum and undersurface of the diaphragm. Spread to the right lung occurs through the transdiaphragmatic lymphatics in the right hemidiaphragm, often producing a right pleural effusion. Surface spread to the peritoneal surfaces of the bowel and bladder is a common finding in advanced-stage ovarian cancer, but involvement of the bowel lumen or bladder mucosa is rare.

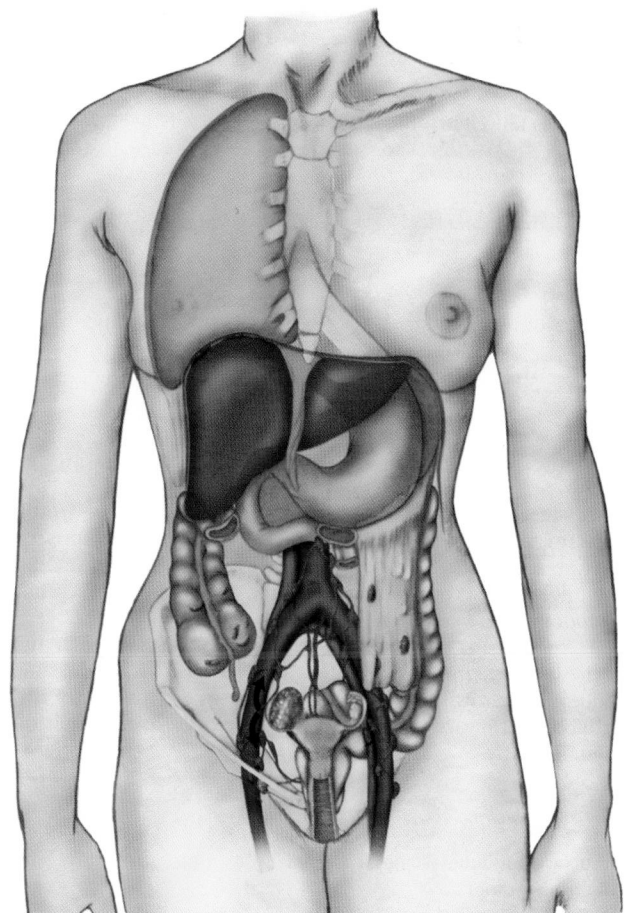

FIGURE 53.1 Patterns of spread of ovarian cancer.

Lymphatic drainage from the ovary follows two pathways. The first involves lateral spread through the broad ligament to the pelvic lymph nodes. In patients with advanced-stage disease, there may be retrograde dissemination via the lymphatics of this pathway to the round ligament to the inguinal lymph nodes. The second pathway of efferent lymphatic drainage follows the ovarian vein to the paracaval and paraaortic lymph nodes. Metastatic spread of ovarian cancer to lymph nodes is well documented even in early-stage disease (Table 53.3) and confirms that there may be separate pathways of dissemination to the pelvic and paraaortic lymph nodes. Cass and coworkers, for example, reported that 14 of 96 patients (15%) with disease visibly confined to one ovary had microscopic lymph node metastases. All 14 patients with nodal spread had poorly differentiated tumors. Isolated ipsilateral lymph node metastases occurred in five patients, and isolated contralateral lymph node metastases occurred in three patients. Pelvic lymph nodes were involved in six patients, paraaortic lymph nodes in five patients, and both in three patients. As expected, the frequency of lymph node metastases is related to stage of disease, cell type, and histologic differentiation of the tumor. Chen and Lee, for example, reported that the frequency of pelvic lymph node metastases increased from 9% in patients with clinically apparent stage I ovarian cancer to 33% in patients with stage IV disease. Similarly, the frequency of paraaortic lymph node involvement increased from 18% in patients with clinically apparent stage I disease to 67% in patients with stage IV disease. These findings are similar to those of Burghardt and colleagues, who noted lymph node metastases in 74% of patients

TABLE 53.3 Lymph Nodal Metastases in Patients with Clinically Apparent Stage I Epithelial Ovarian Cancer

AUTHOR	PATIENTS	PELVIC LYMPH NODE METASTASES	PARAAORTIC LYMPH NODE METASTASES
Onda et al. (1996)	30	6 (18%)	5 (15%)
Carnino et al. (1997)	47	1 (4%)	0 (0%)
Burghardt et al. (1991)	20	3 (15%)	1 (5%)
Sakai et al. (1997)	46	1 (2%)	1 (2%)
Chen and Lee (1983)	11	1 (9%)	2 (18%)
Li et al. (2000)	91	9 (10%)	8 (9%)
Total	245	21 (9%)	17 (7%)

with stage III or IV ovarian cancer. The incidence of lymph node metastases increased from 20% in well-differentiated ovarian cancers to 65% in poorly differentiated tumors and was higher in serous ovarian malignancies than in mucinous or endometrioid cancers.

Hematogenous spread of ovarian cancer to the parenchyma of the liver or lung is fortunately quite rare (<5%) at the time of initial diagnosis, but may occur, particularly in poorly differentiated tumors that become refractory to combination chemotherapy.

EXAMINATION OF OVARIAN TUMOR SPECIMENS AND HISTOLOGIC CLASSIFICATION

Ovarian tumor specimens should be described, fixed, and sectioned according to the guidelines established by the College of American Pathologists (CAP). Tumors should be classified histologically according to the World Health Organization classification and nomenclature of ovarian tumors (Table 53.4).

TABLE 53.4 World Health Organization Histological Classification of Ovarian Tumors

Surface epithelial–stromal tumors
Serous tumors
  Malignant
    Adenocarcinoma
    Surface papillary adenocarcinoma
    Adenocarcinofibroma (malignant adenofibroma)
  Borderline tumor
    Papillary cystic tumor
    Surface papillary tumor
    Adenofibroma, cystadenofibroma
  Benign
    Cystadenoma
    Surface papilloma
    Adenofibroma and cystadenofibroma
Mucinous tumors
  Malignant
    Adenocarcinoma
    Adenocarcinofibroma (malignant adenofibroma)
  Borderline tumor
    Intestinal type
    Endocervical-like
  Benign
    Cystadenoma
    Adenofibroma and cystadenofibroma
  Mucinous cystic tumor with mural nodules
  Mucinous cystic tumor with pseudomyxoma
    peritonei
Endometrioid tumors, including variants with squamous
  differentiation
  Malignant
    Adenocarcinoma, not otherwise specified
    Adenocarcinofibroma (malignant adenofibroma)
    Malignant mullerian mixed tumor (carcinosarcoma)
    Adenosarcoma
    Endometrioid stromal sarcoma (low grade)
    Undifferentiated ovarian sarcoma

  Borderline tumor
    Cystic tumor
    Adenofibroma and cystadenofibroma
  Benign
    Cystadenoma
    Adenofibroma and cystadenofibroma
Clear cell tumors
  Malignant
    Adenocarcinoma
    Adenocarcinofibroma (malignant adenofibroma)
  Borderline tumor
    Cystic tumor
    Adenofibroma and cystadenofibroma
  Benign
    Cystadenofibroma
    Adenofibroma and cystadenofibroma
Transitional cell tumors
  Malignant
    Transitional cell tumor (non-Brenner type)
    Malignant Brenner tumor
  Borderline
    Brenner tumor
      Proliferating variant
  Benign
    Brenner tumor
      Metaplastic variant
Squamous cell tumors
    Squamous cell carcinoma
    Epidermoid cyst
Mixed epithelial tumors (specify components)
    Malignant
    Borderline
    Benign
Undifferentiated and unclassified tumors
    Undifferentiated carcinoma
    Adenocarcinoma, not otherwise specified

TABLE 53.4 World Health Organization Histological Classification of Ovarian Tumors (*Continued*)

Sex cord–stromal tumors
Granulosa–stromal cell tumors
  Granulosa cell tumor group
    Adult granulosa cell tumor
    Juvenile granulosa cell tumor
  Thecoma–fibroma group
    Thecoma, not otherwise specified
      Typical
    Luteinized
    Fibroma
    Cellular fibroma
    Fibrosarcoma
    Stromal tumor with mixed sex cord elements
    Sclerosing stromal tumor
    Signet-ring stromal tumor
    Unclassified (fibrothecoma)
Sertoli-stromal cell tumors
  Sertoli-Leydig cell tumor group (androblastomas)
    Well differentiated
    Of intermediate differentiation
      Variant with heterologous elements (specify type)
    Poorly differentiated (sarcomatoid)
      Variant with heterologous elements (specify type)
    Retiform
      Variant with heterologous elements (specify type)
  Sertoli cell tumor
  Stromal-Leydig cell tumor
  Sex cord–stromal tumors of mixed or unclassified cell types
    Sex cord tumor with annular tubules
    Gynandroblastoma (specify components)
    Sex cord–stromal tumor, unclassified
  Steroid cell tumors
    Stromal luteoma
    Leydig cell tumor group
      Hilus cell tumor
      Leydig cell tumor, nonhilar type
      Leydig cell tumor, not otherwise specified
    Steroid cell tumor, not otherwise specified
      Well differentiated
      Malignant
Germ-cell tumors
Primitive germ-cell tumors
  Dysgerminoma
  Yolk sac tumor
    Polyvesicular vitelline tumor
    Glandular variant
    Hepatoid variant
  Embryonal carcinoma
  Polyembryoma
  Nongestational choriocarcinoma
  Mixed germ-cell tumor (specify components)
Biphasic or triphasic teratoma
  Immature teratoma
  Mature teratoma
    Solid
    Cystic
      Dermoid cyst
    Fetiform teratoma (homunculus)
  Monodermal teratoma and somatic-type tumors
    associated with dermoid cysts
    Thyroid tumor group
      Struma ovarii
        Benign
        Malignant (specify type)

    Carcinoid group
      Insular
      Trabecular
      Mucinous
      Strumal carcinoid
      Mixed
    Neuroectodermal tumor group
      Ependymoma
      Primitive neuroectodermal tumor
      Medulloepithelioma
      Glioblastoma multiforme
      Others
    Carcinoma group
      Squamous cell carcinoma
      Adenocarcinoma
      Others
    Melanocytic group
      Malignant melanoma
      Melanocytic nevus
    Sarcoma group (specify type)
    Sebaceous tumor group
      Sebaceous adenoma
      Sebaceous carcinoma
    Primary-type tumor group
    Retinal anlage tumor group
    Others
Germ-cell sex cord–stromal tumors
  Gonadoblastoma
    Variant with malignant germ-cell tumor
  Mixed germ-cell/sex cord–stromal tumor
    Variant with malignant germ-cell tumor
Tumors of the rete ovarii
  Adenocarcinoma
  Adenoma
  Cystadenoma
  Cystadenofibroma
Miscellaneous tumors
  Small-cell carcinoma, hypercalcemic type
  Small-cell carcinoma, pulmonary type
  Large-cell neuroendocrine carcinoma
  Hepatoid carcinoma
  Primary ovarian mesothelioma
  Wilms tumor
  Gestational choriocarcinoma
  Hydatidiform mole
  Adenoid cystic carcinoma
  Basal cell tumor
  Ovarian wolffian tumor
  Paraganglioma
  Myxoma
  Soft tissue tumors not specific to the ovary
  Others
Tumorlike conditions
  Luteoma of pregnancy
  Stromal hyperthecosis
  Stromal hyperplasia
  Fibromatosis
  Massive ovarian edema
  Others
Lymphoid and hematopoietic tumors
  Malignant lymphoma (specify type)
  Leukemia (specify type)
  Plasmacytoma
Secondary tumors

IX

Although there are numerous grading systems for ovarian cancers that use both architectural and nuclear features, it is recommended that four grades be used, with grade 4 (undifferentiated) applied to tumors with minimal or no differentiation. Recommendations concerning the use of special staining techniques or flow cytometry in establishing the correct histologic diagnosis of ovarian tumors are made in the CAP report. Immunohistochemical staining of ovarian tumors for cytokeratin 7 (CK7) and cytokeratin 20 (CK20) is helpful in differentiating primary mucinous ovarian carcinoma from colorectal adenocarcinoma that has metastasized to the ovary. Colorectal adenocarcinomas usually stain positively for CK20 and negatively for CK7. In contrast, ovarian carcinomas usually stain negatively for CK20 and positively for CK7.

PRIMARY SURGERY

Patterns of Care in Ovarian Cancer Surgery

All patients with suspected ovarian cancer should be referred to a gynecologic oncologist for evaluation and possible surgery. Unfortunately, in both Europe and the United States (where most of the outcomes studies have been conducted), too high a proportion of women with ovarian cancer are receiving substandard care. The role of comprehensive staging, particularly pelvic and paraaortic lymphadenectomy, in patients with early-stage ovarian cancer has been a topic of wide discussion, primarily because many women with early-stage disease are inadequately staged and because surgeons with the expertise to perform a lymphadenectomy are not always involved with the initial surgery. A study by Goff et al. (2006) that evaluated patterns of surgical care across the United States revealed that among women with early-stage disease, 21.4% underwent an oophorectomy with or without a hysterectomy but without any additional staging or debulking procedure and 47% did not have nodal sampling. Carney and associates found that less than 50% of ovarian cancer patients in Utah were cared for by a gynecologic oncologist. In addition, they also noted that care by a gynecologic oncologist was associated with a survival advantage. In the Maryland study, Bristow and coworkers found that the majority of ovarian cancer patients in Maryland were undergoing primary surgery in low-volume settings.

In patients with early-stage disease, lymphadenectomy, in addition to providing prognostic information, may have therapeutic value. Chan et al. evaluated 6,686 women diagnosed with clinical stage I ovarian cancer to estimate the survival impact of lymphadenectomy. The authors found that lymphadenectomy was associated with improved 5-year disease-specific survival. In addition, the extent of lymphadenectomy was significantly associated with the 5-year disease-specific survival rate (0 nodes sampled, 87%; fewer than 10 nodes sampled, 92%; and 10 or more nodes sampled, 94%; $P < 0.001$). In a study of the SEER program database from 1991 and 1996, Harlan and colleagues found that comparing the two treatment periods, the majority of women with early-stage ovarian cancer did not receive guideline therapy in both periods, although the rate was improved in the 1996 cohort. For women with advanced-stage ovarian cancer, there was a higher rate of guideline therapy use but no improvement between 1991 and 1996—62.6% versus 62.3%. The totality of this information clearly underscores the need for improvement in patterns of referral.

Early-Stage Ovarian Cancer

Comprehensive Surgical Staging

> **STEPS IN THE PROCEDURE**
>
> **Comprehensive Staging of Early Disease (Laparoscopy)**
> - Entry into abdominal cavity and inspection of pelvic and peritoneal cavity
> - Cytology obtained
> - Affected ovary isolated by identification of infundibulopelvic ligament
> - Ureter identified and isolated
> - Infundibulopelvic ligament cauterized and transected
> - Utero-ovarian ligament cauterized and transected
> - Ovary placed in endoscopic bag intact and removed through largest trocar site assuring no spilling of ovarian tissue
> - Frozen section obtained and if consistent with cancer, then formal staging performed
> - Omental biopsy performed by coagulation and transection of dessicated tissue
> - Pelvic and paraaortic lymph node dissection is performed bilaterally.
> - Multiple peritoneal biopsies performed including both paracolic gutters, pelvic peritoneal surfaces bilaterally, and diaphragm peritoneum

Ovarian cancer is staged according to the International Federation of Gynecology and Obstetrics (FIGO) staging system (Table 53.5). The official FIGO staging for ovarian cancer was extensively changed in 2012 and has been recently published. Staging is based on a thorough surgical evaluation of the possible metastatic spread of the cancer and histologic evaluation of the primary ovarian lesion. It is too early to know if substaging of stage IC or IIIA will be reliable prognostic characteristics in general, nonresearch settings. Should preoperative evaluation suggest an area of extra-abdominal or intrahepatic metastasis, fine needle aspiration or needle biopsy of this lesion should be performed. Because ovarian cancer frequently spreads to upper abdominal structures, a vertical midline abdominal incision is recommended. This incision should be extended high enough to remove the primary ovarian tumor and to evaluate the stomach, omentum, liver, and undersurface of the diaphragm. Rupture of a cystic ovarian malignancy is associated with a poorer prognosis, so the incision should be sufficient to allow excision of the primary tumor with its capsule intact. Once the abdomen has been opened, the following steps should be performed for adequate surgical staging (Table 53.6):

1. The volume of ascitic fluid should be recorded, and a minimum of 25 mL should be sent for cytologic evaluation.
2. In the absence of ascites, separate saline washings should be obtained from the (a) pelvic cul-de-sac, (b) right paracolic space, (c) left paracolic space, and (d) undersurface of each hemidiaphragm. Approximately 100 mL of saline should be instilled in each of these areas, recovered, and sent for cytologic evaluation.

TABLE 53.5 FIGO Ovarian Cancer Staging (January 01, 2014)

STAGE I: Tumor confined to ovaries

OLD		NEW	
IA	Tumor limited to 1 ovary, capsule intact, no tumor on surface, negative washings/ascites	IA	Tumor limited to 1 ovary, capsule intact, no tumor on surface, negative washings
IB	Tumor involves both ovaries	IB	Tumor involves both ovaries otherwise like IA
IC	Tumor involves 1 or both ovaries with any of the following: capsule rupture, tumor on surface, positive washings/ascites	IC	*Tumor limited to 1 or both ovaries*
		IC1	*Surgical spill*
		IC2	*Capsule rupture before surgery or tumor on ovarian surface*
		IC3	*Malignant cells in the ascites or peritoneal washings*

STAGE II: Tumor involves 1 or both ovaries with pelvic extension (below the pelvic brim) or primary peritoneal cancer

OLD		NEW	
IIA	Extension and/or implant on uterus and/or fallopian tubes	IIA	Extension and/or implant on uterus and/or fallopian tubes
IIB	Extension to other pelvic intraperitoneal tissues	IIB	Extension to other pelvic intraperitoneal tissues
IIC[a]	IIA or IIB with positive washings/ascites		

STAGE III: Tumor involves 1 or both ovaries with cytologically or histologically confirmed spread to the peritoneum outside the pelvis and/or metastasis to the retroperitoneal lymph nodes

OLD		NEW		
IIIA	Microscopic metastasis beyond the pelvis	*IIIA (Positive retroperitoneal lymph nodes and/or microscopic metastasis beyond the pelvis)*		
		IIIA1	*Positive retroperitoneal lymph nodes only*	
			IIIA1(i)	*Metastasis ≤ 10 mm*
			IIIA1(ii)	*Metastasis > 10 mm*
		IIIA2	*Microscopic, extrapelvic (above the brim) peritoneal involvement ± positive retroperitoneal lymph nodes*	
IIIB	Macroscopic, extrapelvic, peritoneal metastasis ≤2 cm in greatest dimension	*IIIB*	*Macroscopic, extrapelvic, peritoneal metastasis ≤2 cm ± positive retroperitoneal lymph nodes. Includes extension to capsule of liver/spleen*	
IIIC	Macroscopic, extrapelvic, peritoneal metastasis >2 cm in greatest dimension and/or regional lymph node metastasis	*IIIC*	*Macroscopic, extrapelvic, peritoneal metastasis >2 cm ± positive retroperitoneal lymph nodes. Includes extension to capsule of liver/spleen*	

STAGE IV: Distant metastasis excluding peritoneal metastasis

OLD		NEW	
IV	Distant metastasis excluding peritoneal metastasis. Includes hepatic parenchymal metastasis.	*IVA*	*Pleural effusion with positive cytology*
		IVB	*Hepatic and/or splenic parenchymal metastasis, metastasis to extra-abdominal organs (including inguinal lymph nodes and lymph nodes outside of the abdominal cavity)*

[a]*Old stage IIC has been eliminated.*
Other major recommendations are as follows:
• Histologic type including grading should be designated at staging.
• Primary site (ovary, fallopian tube, or peritoneum) should be designated where possible.
• Tumors that may otherwise qualify for stage I but involved with dense adhesions justify upgrading to stage II if tumor cells are histologically proven to be present in the adhesions.

TABLE 53.6 Surgical Staging of Apparent Early-Stage Ovarian Cancer

Vertical midline incision
Evacuation of ascites or multiple cytologic washings
Complete abdominal inspection and palpation
Resection of ovaries, fallopian tubes, and uterus[a]
Omentectomy
Random peritoneal biopsies
Retroperitoneal lymph node sampling

[a]Exceptions may be made in selected patients who wish to preserve fertility.

TABLE 53.7 Criteria for Potential Fertility-Sparing Surgery in Ovarian Cancer Patients

Patient desirous of preserving fertility
Patient and family consent and agree to close follow-up
No evidence of dysgenetic gonads
Specific situations
  Any unilateral malignant germ-cell tumor
  Any unilateral sex cord–stromal tumor
  Any unilateral borderline tumor
  Stage IA invasive epithelial tumor

3. The ovarian tumor should be inspected, with particular attention to the presence of papillary excrescences on the surface or rupture of the capsule. The contralateral ovary and uterus should be examined for the presence of metastatic tumor. The pathways of ovarian tumor should be removed and sent for frozen section examination. Removal of the opposite ovary and/or uterus is dependent on several factors and is discussed on the following pages.

4. Careful inspection and palpation of the peritoneal surfaces and intra-abdominal viscera should be performed. This evaluation should be approached in a systematic fashion, beginning with the peritoneum of the cul-de-sac and small bowel mesentery. Inspection should continue with the ascending colon, liver, omentum, undersurface of the right and left hemidiaphragms, and stomach. Finally, the transverse colon, spleen, descending colon, and bladder peritoneum should be evaluated.

5. All areas suspicious for malignancy should be biopsied. In the absence of visible disease, biopsies should be taken of the cul-de-sac peritoneum, bladder peritoneum, both lateral pelvic walls, paracolic peritoneum bilaterally, and undersurface of the right hemidiaphragm. An infracolic omentectomy should be performed in patients with epithelial ovarian cancer and an omental wedge biopsy taken in patients with germ-cell or stromal tumors. Appendectomy should be performed in all patients with mucinous epithelial cancers involving the ovary. Primary appendiceal cancers, although rare, commonly spread to the ovaries and usually require right hemicolectomy as part of initial surgical staging.

6. As has been mentioned, ovarian cancer commonly spreads to both pelvic and paraaortic lymph nodes. Some patients with early-stage ovarian cancer have paraaortic lymph node metastases in the absence of pelvic lymph node spread. Therefore, these lymph node groups should be sampled separately in all patients. It is important that sampling include lymph nodes on the opposite side of the primary ovarian tumor, because isolated contralateral spread has been reported. In the setting of advanced-stage disease, prospective randomized trials reviewed by Panici et al. have shown that routine lymphadenectomy is not associated with a higher survival rate; however, it is associated with an improvement in the disease-free interval.

7. Finally, it should be emphasized that operative findings present at the time of staging must be carefully documented. Prognosis is related to the site and volume of metastatic tumor, as well as the amount of residual disease remaining after surgical debulking. Important data concerning the location and size of tumor metastases are often lost if the details concerning operative staging are not recorded.

Fertility-Sparing Surgery

Although the majority of ovarian malignancies occur in older women for whom bilateral salpingo-oophorectomy and hysterectomy are standard treatment, a significant subset of patients is young and can be managed more conservatively (Table 53.7). Conservative management is used here to denote surgery that preserves reproductive potential without compromising curability. With some exceptions, such a strategy may be applicable for women younger than 40 years who wish to bear children.

When contemplating surgery on a young patient with a suspected ovarian malignancy, it is important to discuss with her all possible operative findings and procedures and the long-term implications of the various options. If the patient is a child, the parents need to clearly understand this information. In most instances, young patients have their initial surgery done outside major university hospitals or cancer centers. Common errors in surgical management include incomplete surgical staging and unnecessary bilateral salpingo-oophorectomy. In addition, some patients are mismanaged because of an error in the pathologic diagnosis of a rare ovarian neoplasm.

The optimal candidate for conservative surgical management is a young patient who has stage IA disease. If, on initial inspection, the suspected cancer is confined to one ovary, then unilateral salpingo-oophorectomy is appropriate. If the mass is thought to be benign, then ovarian cystectomy may be preferable. The specimen should be sent for frozen section examination. If malignancy is diagnosed, then appropriate staging biopsies should be performed, as discussed. If the contralateral ovary appears normal, it is recommended that it not be biopsied to avoid potential infertility caused by peritoneal adhesions or ovarian failure.

One should not rely too heavily on frozen section examination in making the decision to perform a hysterectomy and bilateral salpingo-oophorectomy. If the histologic diagnosis is in question, it is always preferable to wait for permanent section results for a young patient, even if this requires a repeat surgery.

The advent of in vitro fertilization technology has been a significant impact on intraoperative management. Previously, convention dictated that if a bilateral salpingo-oophorectomy is necessary, a hysterectomy should also be performed. However, current technology for donor oocyte transfer and hormonal support allows a woman without ovaries to sustain an intrauterine pregnancy. Similarly, if the uterus and one ovary are resected because of tumor involvement, current techniques allow retrieval of oocytes from the patient's remaining ovary, in vitro fertilization with sperm from her male partner, and implantation of the embryo into a surrogate's uterus. Therefore, traditional guidelines concerning surgical management of ovarian cancer may no longer be applicable in selected young patients.

Approximately 50% to 70% of *malignant germ-cell tumors* are stage I. Except for dysgerminoma, in which the incidence of bilaterality is 10% to 15%, bilateral ovarian tumors are exceedingly rare. Such a finding almost always signifies advanced disease with metastatic spread from one ovary to the other or a mixed germ-cell tumor with a dysgerminoma component. Benign cystic teratoma is associated with malignant germ-cell tumors in 5% to 10% of cases and may occur in one or both ovaries. Therefore, *unilateral salpingo-oophorectomy—preserving the contralateral ovary and uterus—combined with surgical staging can be performed in most patients with malignant germ-cell tumors, even many with advanced-stage disease.* If the contralateral ovary is enlarged, most likely it represents a benign cystic teratoma that can be managed with an ovarian cystectomy only. With the exception of stage IA pure dysgerminoma or stage IA, grade 1 immature teratoma, patients with germ-cell tumors require postoperative chemotherapy consisting of the combination of bleomycin, etoposide, and cisplatin (BEP). Several series have documented normal reproductive function in at least 80% of patients as well as pregnancies following fertility-sparing surgery and chemotherapy.

In the past few years, some investigators have advocated the practice of surgery alone for other categories of malignant germ-cell tumors, including stage IA, grade 2 and 3 immature teratomas, and stage IA yolk sac tumors. Such an approach, however, should be taken with caution; many experts would still consider it experimental. Nevertheless, there is a trend toward careful observation following surgery alone for most patients with stage I malignant ovarian germ-cell tumors. The Children's Oncology Group is currently conducting a clinical trial that includes postoperative surveillance for patients with stage I disease. Chemotherapy is initiated only for serum tumor marker elevation.

Most *sex cord–stromal tumors* are confined to the ovary. Stage I accounts for greater than 50% (in some series as high as 100%) of granulosa cell tumors. More than 90% of Sertoli-Leydig cell tumors are stage IA. Bilaterality occurs in less than 5% of cases with either tumor type. *Therefore, optimal surgical management of most patients with stromal tumors consists of unilateral adnexectomy.* There does not appear to be a role for lymphadenectomy in patients with sex cord–stromal tumors. A study by Brown et al. evaluated 262 patients with sex cord–stromal tumors. Of these, 111 patients underwent a complete or partial staging procedure. None of the patients had evidence of positive nodes. The authors also noted that of the 117 patients whose disease eventually recurred, 6 patients (5.1%) had nodal metastases at the time of recurrence. Endometrial biopsy or curettage also should be performed in any young patient whose uterus is preserved because 5% to 15% of patients with granulosa cell tumors develop endometrial cancer or hyperplasia. Postoperative therapy may be indicated for patients with metastatic disease or for selected patients with stage I disease (e.g., poorly differentiated Sertoli-Leydig cell tumor or granulosa cell tumor with rupture). The most commonly used regimens in this setting include either BEP or the combination of paclitaxel and carboplatin.

Approximately 10% to 15% of all ovarian neoplasms are of the *borderline or low malignant potential* classification. Although they were first described more than 70 years ago, only in the last few years have we begun to fully appreciate their biologic behavior. Approximately 33% to 60% of serous borderline tumors are limited to one ovary. Extraovarian spread is noted in approximately 20% to 30% of cases. Approximately 80% to 90% of mucinous borderline tumors are confined to one ovary. Both endometrioid and clear cell

borderline tumors are almost always stage I, and the vast majority is unilateral. *For patients with borderline tumors seemingly confined to one ovary, appropriate surgical management includes unilateral salpingo-oophorectomy with surgical staging.* The use of ovarian cystectomy instead of unilateral adnexectomy also has been reported, although some patients treated in this manner require repeat surgery for a recurrence of tumor in the same or opposite ovary. If bilateral borderline tumors are present, portions of one or both ovaries may be preserved with ovarian cystectomy, if feasible. Whatever the surgical approach, reported 5-year survival rates for patients with stage I borderline tumors treated with surgery alone are 95% or better.

For patients with borderline tumors and peritoneal implants, the optimal management remains controversial. However, surgical excision is the mainstay of treatment. After frozen section confirmation of borderline tumor, an effort should be made to resect all gross disease. In addition, staging biopsies of peritoneal surfaces and lymph nodes are indicated, as are cytologic washings. However, there is no consensus regarding the extent of surgical staging required, particularly with regard to the need for lymphadenectomy. A recent study was conducted to evaluate the prognostic value of lymph node involvement for borderline tumors. This was a retrospective study on 49 patients at a single institution, and a broader analysis was also performed on 1,503 patients obtained from the Surveillance, Epidemiology and End Results (SEER) database. The authors concluded that lymph node involvement does not appear as a prognosis factor in patients with advanced-stage borderline tumors. Even in the face of metastatic disease, a normal contralateral ovary may be preserved in young patients. In patients with advanced-stage serous disease, the incidence of bilateral tumors is approximately 75%. There are several reports detailing successful pregnancies following treatment in patients with borderline ovarian tumors.

The relapse risk for patients with peritoneal implants is related to the type: noninvasive versus invasive. For patients with noninvasive peritoneal implants, the lifetime risk is estimated to be at least 20%. For those with invasive peritoneal implants, the lifetime risk of relapse is estimated to be at least 50%. Consequently, postoperative platinum-based chemotherapy is recommended for the latter diagnosis by many groups. However, no study has demonstrated a survival benefit related to postoperative chemotherapy.

Invasive epithelial tumors account for approximately 70% of all ovarian malignancies. Despite the low overall survival rate associated with these tumors, selected young patients with stage I disease can be treated conservatively. The major factors that influence the selection process are histologic grade and bilaterality, in addition to stage. Serous tumors are bilateral in about 50% of cases. The incidence of bilaterality for mucinous tumors varies widely in reported series from as low as 5% to as high as 50%, but probably is no greater than 10% to 20%. Approximately 30% to 50% of endometrioid and clear cell cancers are bilateral.

Several reports have detailed the reproductive outcomes of women with early-stage invasive epithelial ovarian cancer following treatment with fertility-sparing surgery with or without chemotherapy. A multiinstitutional study in the United States evaluated the recurrence rate, survival, and pregnancy outcome in patients with stage IA and IC invasive epithelial ovarian cancer treated with unilateral adnexectomy. Fifty-two patients with stage I epithelial ovarian cancer treated from 1965 to 2000 at eight participating institutions were identified. Cell type was distributed as follows: mucinous, 25; serous, 10; endometrioid, 10; clear cell, 5; and mixed, 2.

IX

A total of 20 patients received adjuvant chemotherapy. The median duration of follow-up was 68 months. Five patients developed tumor recurrence 8 to 78 months after initial surgery. Sites of recurrence were as follows: contralateral ovary, 3; peritoneum, 1; and lung, 1. At the time of publication, 50 patients were alive without evidence of disease and 2 had died of disease 13 and 97 months after initial treatment. Twenty-four patients attempted pregnancy and 17 (71%) conceived. Of these, 17 patients had 26 term deliveries (no congenital anomalies noted) and 5 spontaneous abortions. The authors concluded that the long-term survival of patients with stage IA and IC epithelial ovarian cancer treated with unilateral adnexectomy is excellent.

Adjuvant Therapy

To begin making decisions about which patients might benefit from postoperative or adjuvant therapy, one must categorize them based on risk of relapse. The risk of relapse is approximately 1% for patients with stage I borderline ovarian tumors; thus, adjuvant therapy is not recommended.

For women with stage IA or IB *sex cord–stromal tumors*, no adjuvant therapy is recommended because of the low risk of relapse. For those with stage IC disease, however, the level of risk remains uncertain; some studies suggest that tumor rupture or the presence of ascites is prognostic, whereas others do not. For patients with high-risk *early-stage sex cord–stromal tumors* (stage IC or II), there is no standard postoperative treatment. The most commonly used regimens include the combination of bleomycin, etoposide, and cisplatin (BEP) or the combination of paclitaxel and carboplatin.

For several years, the dogma has dictated that all patients with early-stage malignant ovarian *germ-cell tumors*, except those with stage IA dysgerminoma or stage IA, grade 1 immature teratoma, require postoperative chemotherapy. Standard therapy since the 1980s has been the BEP combination. However, over the past few years, a number of groups have reported provocative results with the strategy of surveillance following primary surgery for patients with stage IA of all subtypes. In considering this strategy, the critical issue is ultimate outcome. Of course, if surveillance is successful, one can avoid the myriad acute effects of chemotherapy as well as the risk of significant late effects, such as secondary leukemia or premature ovarian failure. Even if there is a moderate relapse risk necessitating chemotherapy, if one can avoid chemotherapy in a significant proportion of patients and in addition salvage those who relapse, such management will be deemed successful. On the other hand, if very many of those who relapse ultimately succumb to their disease, it will most certainly not become part of standard practice. Where the threshold lies on the latter remains unresolved.

Bonazzi et al. conducted a prospective study of 22 patients with stage I or II, grade 1 or 2, immature teratoma of the ovary who were treated with surgery alone. Two patients relapsed—one with stage IA, grade 2 and the other with stage IC, grade 2. Both were salvaged with surgery that revealed only grade 0 immature teratoma. Dark et al. reported on 24 patients who underwent surveillance after surgery for stage IA malignant ovarian germ-cell tumors. Nine had dysgerminoma (which most already would observe), nine had immature teratoma, and six had yolk sac tumors, with or without immature teratoma. Eight patients—three with grade 2 immature teratoma, three with dysgerminoma, and two with contralateral dysgerminoma (presumably second primary tumor)—required subsequent chemotherapy. After a median follow-up of 6.8 years, all but one patient are alive and in remission. In a follow-up report from the Charing Cross/Mt. Vernon group in the United Kingdom, which apparently included those reported earlier, 37 patients with stage I malignant ovarian germ-cell tumors underwent surveillance. However, one patient had a squamous carcinoma arising in a mature cystic teratoma, which, in our opinion, is a completely different entity. The other 36 patients included 3 with grade 0 immature teratoma (which would never require chemotherapy unless thought to represent a growing teratoma syndrome), 9 dysgerminomas, 1 embryonal carcinoma, 15 immature teratomas, 6 yolk sac tumors, and 2 with mixed germ-cell tumors. Of these 36 patients, 11 (31%) relapsed—1 with mature teratoma (which may represent growing teratoma syndrome), 2 with dysgerminoma (although 1 was a second primary in the contralateral ovary), 4 with immature teratoma, 2 with mixed germ-cell tumors, and 1 each with yolk sac tumor and embryonal carcinoma. Two of the 11 patients died. One had grade 2 immature teratoma and became pregnant. She was diagnosed 13 months after diagnosis and died of a pulmonary embolus during chemotherapy. The second patient had grade 3 immature teratoma. She relapsed 3 months after diagnosis and subsequently died after secondary surgery and multiple lines of chemotherapy.

Mitchell et al. reported nine patients with stage I malignant ovarian germ-cell tumors—six with immature teratoma and three with mixed germ-cell tumors, all of whom had yolk sac tumor elements. At the time of the report, only one patient had relapsed. She had immature teratoma of unknown grade and relapsed 8 months after a unilateral salpingo-oophorectomy, but her parents refused further therapy. Cushing et al. described 44 patients with completely resected immature teratoma (31 pure and 13 with yolk sac tumor) treated with surgery alone. With a median follow-up of 4.2 years, one patient with a mixed germ-cell tumor relapsed at 18 weeks, as indicated by a rising alpha-fetoprotein, and was salvaged with four cycles of BEP. At the time of the report, she was disease free at 57 months after completing chemotherapy.

Most recently, Mangili et al. reported 28 patients with stage I pure immature teratoma of whom 19 were treated with surgery alone. Of these 19 patients, 9 had grade 1 disease, 8 had grade 2, and 2 had grade 3 disease. Four patients (21%) relapsed—two with mature teratoma and two with immature teratoma. The two with mature teratoma recurrence were treated with secondary cytoreductive surgery, and the two with immature teratoma were treated with secondary surgery followed by BEP chemotherapy. All were salvaged.

The Children's Oncology Group (COG) is currently studying the treatment strategy of surgery plus surveillance in children with stage I malignant ovarian germ-cell tumors. If the findings appear to be promising, further study will be required in adult patients.

For patients with early-stage *epithelial ovarian cancer*, most experts currently accept a classification system of low and high risk (Table 53.8). Within the stage I category, histologic grade is the most powerful predictor of outcome. Patients with well-differentiated or grade 1 tumors have an excellent prognosis, with a 5-year survival rate of more than 90%. On the other hand, the 5-year survival rates for patients with grade 2 or 3 tumors are approximately 75% to 80% and 50% to 60%, respectively. Other factors that have been found to have prognostic significance include large-volume ascites, dense adherence, and clear cell histology. Although older studies suggested that capsular rupture or excrescences may be associated with a worsened prognosis, more recent studies have found no independent influence of these features on prognosis. However, the issue of the influence of tumor rupture on prognosis remains controversial.

TABLE 53.8 Early-Stage Epithelial Ovarian Cancer Risk Groups

LOW RISK	HIGH RISK
Stage IA or IB, grade 1 and 2	Stage IA or IB, grade 3
	Stage IC
	Tumor on external surface
	Ruptured capsule
	Ascites or positive peritoneal washing
	All stage II

Therefore, *low-risk early-stage epithelial ovarian cancer includes patients with the following factors: (a) stage IA or IB (intact capsule, no tumor excrescences, and no malignant ascites or negative peritoneal cytology) and (b) grade 1 or 2 disease. The standard treatment for this group of patients is surgery alone, and the 5-year survival is at least 95%.* A controversy about whether grade 2 belongs in the low- or high-risk category remains unresolved; it is compounded by the lack of uniformity of grading systems.

High-risk early-stage epithelial ovarian cancer includes those patients with the following factors: (a) stages IC (ruptured capsule, tumor excrescences, positive peritoneal cytology, or malignant ascites) to II, (b) grade 3 disease, or (c) clear cell histology. In some classification systems, dense adherence is also included in the high-risk category; however, in the view of many experts, this designation is simply a surrogate for stage II disease. This high-risk subset is thought to have a relapse risk in the range of 40% to 50% and is the focus of adjuvant therapy trials.

Persistent problems with incomplete surgical staging and interobserver variability in assigning histologic grade lead one to the realization that more objective and reliable methods would be desirable for assessment of risk in early-stage ovarian cancer. Currently, there is no universally accepted prognostic molecular biomarker. There are, however, reports of several potential biomarkers. Among these are DNA ploidy, computerized morphometry, Ki-67, p53, and HER2/neu. Although none of the markers studied yet qualifies as prognostic, as technology advances, future studies will most certainly identify reliable biomarkers. Because there is no universal histologic grading system for epithelial ovarian cancer, investigators at M.D. Anderson Cancer Center recently reported a two-tier grading system for invasive serous carcinomas that emphasizes nuclear atypia rather than architecture, with mitotic count as a secondary feature. There is mounting evidence, both from genomic/molecular studies and clinical reports, supporting this low-grade/high-grade model.

Platinum-based chemotherapy has emerged as the standard treatment for patients with *early-stage epithelial ovarian cancer.* Bolis et al. reported the results of two multicenter trials conducted by the Gruppo Italiano Collaborativo in Oncologia Ginecologica. A total of 271 patients were included in these 2 trials. Trial 1 compared single-agent cisplatin with observation in patients with stage IA and IB, grade 2 or 3. Trial 2 compared single-agent cisplatin with intraperitoneal chromic phosphate in patients with stages IA, grade 2; IB, grade 2; and IC disease. In both trials, although the cisplatin groups had a better disease-free survival, overall survival was not significantly different compared with the other arm. One possible explanation for these finding is that patients in the nonchemotherapy arm crossed over to cisplatin at time of relapse.

The Gynecologic Oncology Group (GOG) reported a randomized trial of cisplatin plus cyclophosphamide for three cycles versus intraperitoneal chromic phosphate in patients with high-risk early-stage ovarian cancer. With 204 evaluable patients randomized, relapse-free rates were 77% for the chemotherapy arm and 66% for the P[32] arm. After adjusting for stage and histologic grade, the group receiving chemotherapy had a 29% decrement in estimated relapse. Chemotherapy was recommended as standard adjuvant therapy for this subset of patients because of the superior progression-free survival (PFS) and the late bowel toxicity associated with P[32].

In a subsequent GOG trial, Bell and colleagues compared three versus six cycles of paclitaxel/carboplatin for patients with high-risk early-stage epithelial ovarian cancer. Although the recurrence rate associated with six cycles was 24% lower, the study was powered for a 50% or greater reduction in recurrence rate for six cycles. In addition, there was no difference in overall survival between the arms. In a recently completed GOG trial for early-stage disease, all patients initially received three cycles of paclitaxel/carboplatin and then were randomized between observation and 26 weekly doses of paclitaxel. Results of this trial are not yet available.

Two large European cooperative group trials in early-stage ovarian cancer were combined for analysis. Both the International Collaborative Ovarian Neoplasm 1 (ICON1) trial and the European Organisation for Research and Treatment of Cancer Collaborators—Adjuvant ChemoTherapy in Ovarian Neoplasm (EORTC-ACTION) trial randomized patients with early-stage epithelial ovarian cancer following surgery to observation versus platinum-based chemotherapy. Both overall survival and recurrence-free survival at 5 years were superior in the chemotherapy arm (82% vs. 74% and 76% vs. 65%, respectively).

A follow-up GOG study (GOG 0175) addressed the role of maintenance therapy in early-stage epithelial ovarian cancer. In this trial, women were randomized to three cycles of paclitaxel and carboplatin followed by either surveillance or low-dose weekly paclitaxel for 24 doses. The authors concluded that maintenance paclitaxel following standard paclitaxel/carboplatin provided no significant increase in relapse-free interval.

Advanced-Stage Ovarian Cancer

Primary Cytoreductive Surgery—Rationale

STEPS IN THE PROCEDURE

Primary Cytoreductive Surgery—Advanced Disease

- Midline abdominal incision is performed from pubic symphysis to xiphoid.

- Ascites is drained from all quadrants of the abdomen and pelvis.

- Supracolic omentectomy is performed extending from hepatic flexure to splenic flexure of transverse colon.

- Resection of pelvic tumor including total hysterectomy and bilateral salpingo-oophorectomy and any grossly visible tumor.

- When pelvic tumor involves the distal large bowel, a rectosigmoid resection with anastomosis is performed.

- When disease is present in the small bowel, a resection of the involved segment of the small bowel is performed.

IX

- Splenectomy performed when there is evidence of capsular or parenchymal disease.
- Diaphragmatic stripping or resection is performed when the diaphragm is either superficially involved with tumor or when there is penetration of tumor through the diaphragm.
- Partial hepatectomy or distal pancreatectomy is performed when segments of the liver or distal pancreas are involved with tumor.

Cytoreductive or debulking surgery refers to a surgical procedure for which the goal is to reduce the amount of tumor to a residual of less than 1 cm maximum diameter in a patient with metastatic ovarian cancer. Early studies suggested a relationship between the completeness of the surgery or the amount of residual tumor and survival. In a landmark paper, Griffiths demonstrated an inverse relationship between residual tumor diameter and survival; patients having residual disease less than 1.5 cm in diameter had a significantly improved survival compared with patients with bulky residual disease. Subsequent reports have confirmed these findings. As our philosophy about cytoreductive surgery has evolved, *optimal debulking* has come to denote minimal residual disease ≤1 cm in greatest diameter; *suboptimal debulking* denotes bulky residual disease greater than 1 cm in diameter. Chi et al. analyzed survival by diameter of residual disease to determine the optimal goal of primary tumor reduction for patients with stage IIIC epithelial ovarian cancer. The median overall survival durations by diameter of residual disease in each of the five categories were as follows: no gross residual disease, 106 months; 0.5 cm or less, 66 months; 0.6 to 1 cm, 48 months; 1 to 2 cm, 33 months; and greater than 2 cm, 34 months. Defining the extent of residual disease when dealing with tumor plaques on the peritoneal surfaces remains problematic. Furthermore, there is most certainly a lack of precision in measuring residual disease. The same group of investigators also published a study seeking to determine the survival impact of adding extensive upper abdominal surgical tumor reduction to standard surgical techniques in patients with advanced ovarian cancer. Extensive upper abdominal surgery was defined as diaphragm peritonectomy/resection, resection of parenchymal liver or porta hepatis disease, and/or splenectomy with or without distal pancreatectomy. They concluded that the addition of extensive upper abdominal tumor reduction was associated with improved survival in patients with stages IIIC to IV epithelial ovarian cancer. Interestingly, the rate of major surgical complications and the length of hospitalization were not significantly different between these patients and patients who did not undergo extensive upper abdominal tumor reduction. However, operative time and estimated blood loss were greater in the group of patients who underwent extensive upper abdominal surgery (264 minutes vs. 174 minutes, 880 mL vs. 460 mL, respectively; $P < 0.001$ for both).

Cytoreductive surgery, of course, must be considered not in a vacuum but rather in the context of responsiveness of residual tumor to postoperative therapies. Both radiotherapy and chemotherapy trials have shown a higher response rate in patients with minimal residual disease. These observations are supported by basic studies that suggest that larger tumor masses have poorly perfused anoxic areas that are not accessible to cytotoxic agents. Furthermore, larger tumors may have a greater proportion of cells in the resting phase. These nonproliferating cells may be less sensitive to cytotoxic agents. Skipper espoused the fractional cell kill hypothesis, stating that the ability of chemotherapeutic agents to eradicate cancer cells depends on both the dose of drug and the number of cells present. A given dose of drug kills a constant fraction of cells with each exposure. However, certain factors—such as cell repair mechanisms, tumor heterogeneity, the fraction of cells in G0 phase, and the development of drug resistance—serve to counteract this process. Goldie and Coldman have shown that tumor cells have an intrinsic spontaneous mutation rate; larger tumors that go untreated for an extended period theoretically have a greater probability of containing cell populations resistant to anticancer agents. Therefore, even though patients with advanced ovarian cancer may undergo optimal debulking, the small residual tumor masses may still contain drug-resistant cells that preclude ultimate cure.

Several reports have described the accomplishment of optimal cytoreductive surgery in a high percentage of patients. The morbidity and mortality associated with cytoreductive surgery also have been analyzed. These studies generally reflect an operative mortality rate of less than 2%, a mean operating time of 3 to 5 hours, and a mean blood loss of approximately 500 to 1,500 mL. There is a wide range of postoperative complications, the most common of which are infection, hemorrhage (at times requiring reexploration), prolonged ileus, and cardiopulmonary problems. The primary question concerning the efficacy of primary cytoreductive surgery is whether improved survival is related more to the biology of the tumor or the skill and aggressiveness of the surgeon. In other words, are those tumors that can be debulked optimally also tumors that are less invasive, less infiltrative, and more indolent? Earlier studies did not suggest that this was the case. They demonstrated that patients who required extensive surgery to achieve minimal residual disease and those who had minimal disease at the outset had similar survival rates. More recent studies, however, suggest that patients with de novo minimal disease have a superior prognosis to those who are debulked to minimal disease with aggressive debulking surgery. These findings support the concept of the prognostic influence of substage categories within the FIGO stage III classification. Unfortunately, there are no randomized studies to resolve important issues in this area. Studies indicate that optimal cytoreductive surgery may confer a survival advantage, even for patients with stage IV ovarian cancer. Four large retrospective reports noted that patients with stage IV disease who were optimally cytoreduced had a statistically superior survival to patients who were suboptimally cytoreduced (Table 53.9).

Technique

Exploration The patient is placed in either the supine or semilithotomy, depending on the likelihood of a rectosigmoid resection. A vertical midline incision is employed and extended cephalad to the level of the xiphoid. On entering the abdomen, the initial steps outlined under surgical staging are followed. After evacuation of ascites, if present, and inspection and palpation, the size of the primary tumors(s) and size and extent of metastatic deposits should be noted.

During this initial phase of the operation, the surgeon must make an assessment of the feasibility of cytoreductive surgery. In a typical patient with advanced disease, the omentum may be totally replaced by tumor, and the pelvis may be filled with tumor, making it difficult or impossible for the surgeon to distinguish normal pelvic structures. Findings that may initially dissuade the surgeon from proceeding with aggressive tumor resection include extensive parenchymal hepatic involvement, diaphragmatic involvement with extension to the pleural cavity, extensive

TABLE 53.9 Effect of Debulking on Survival in Stage IV Ovarian Cancer

FIRST AUTHOR	YEAR	SURGICAL RESULT	PATIENTS	OPTIMAL	MEDIAN SURVIVAL	P
Curtin	1997	Optimal (<2 cm) Suboptimal	41 51	45%	40 18	0.01
Liu	1997	Optimal (<2 cm) Suboptimal	14 33	30%	37 17	0.02
Munkarah	1997	Optimal (<2 cm) Suboptimal	31 61	34%	25 15	0.02
Bristow	1999	Optimal (≤1 cm) Suboptimal	25 59	30%	38 10	0.0004

infiltration of the small intestinal mesentery, or bulky nodal disease above the renal vessels. On the other hand, even if minimal residual disease cannot be achieved, debulking of omental and pelvic masses may relieve production of ascites, reduce pressure on adjacent organs, and allow the patient increased comfort, at least temporarily. Moreover, intestinal resection still may be indicated for relief of impending or true obstruction.

Omentectomy It is our preference to perform an omentectomy before focusing on the pelvis if the omentum is largely or completely replaced by tumor. If the omental tumor is adherent to the parietal peritoneum of the anterior abdominal wall, the pelvic structures, or loops of small intestine, it should be dissected from these structures. Once

the omentum is mobilized and lifted cephalad, a dissection plane is developed between it and the serosa of the transverse colon, extending the dissection laterally in both directions (Fig. 53.2A). If the supracolic omentum is heavily involved with tumor and densely adherent to the transverse colon, it also may be necessary to establish a plane between the greater curvature of the stomach and the omentum by ligating the right and left gastroepiploic arteries and the individual gastric branches (Fig. 53.2B). Entrance into the lesser sac allows traction on the greater curvature of the stomach and facilitates exposure and transection of the gastric branches of the gastroepiploic arch. Occasionally, omental tumor may also involve the spleen or splenic hilum, necessitating splenectomy (see "Splenectomy").

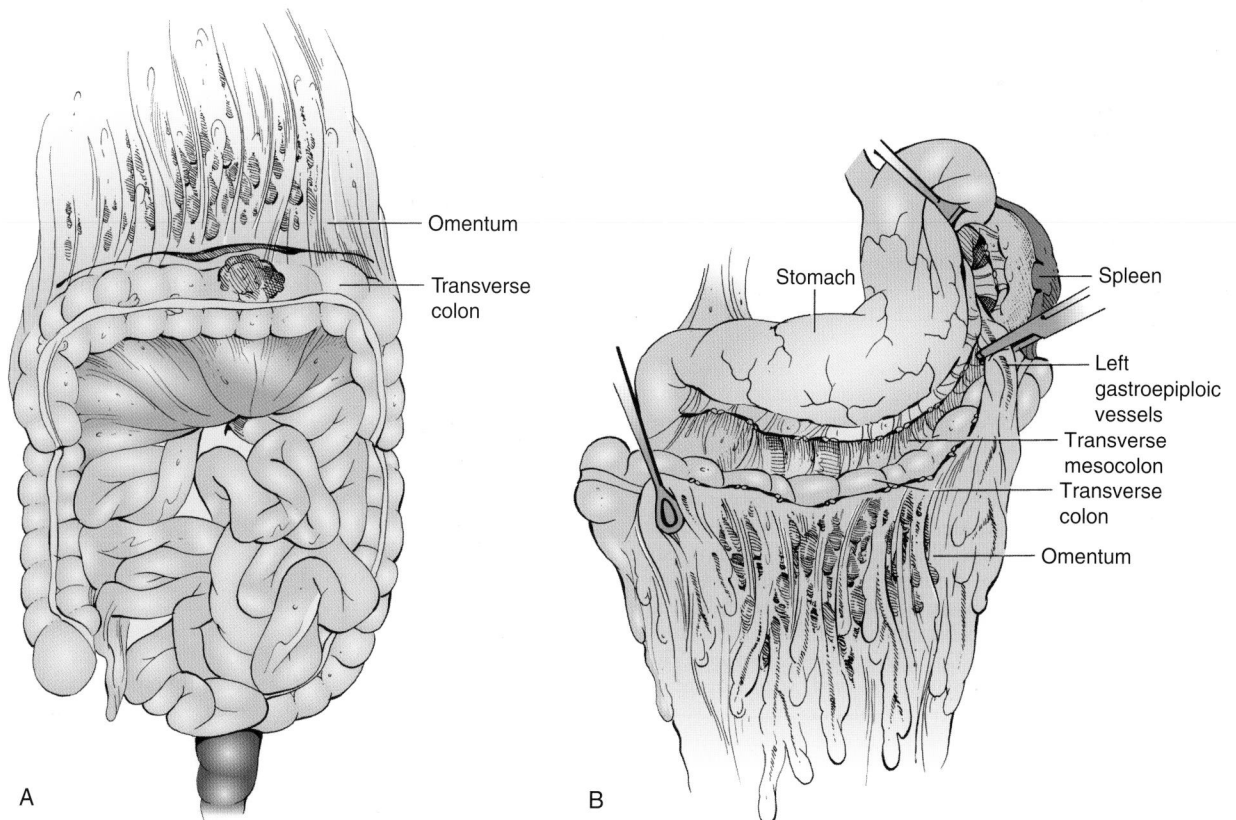

FIGURE 53.2 A: Omentectomy. Avascular dissection plane between omentum with metastatic ovarian tumor and transverse colon. **B:** Omentectomy. Dissection of omentum with tumor from stomach with ligation of gastric branches.

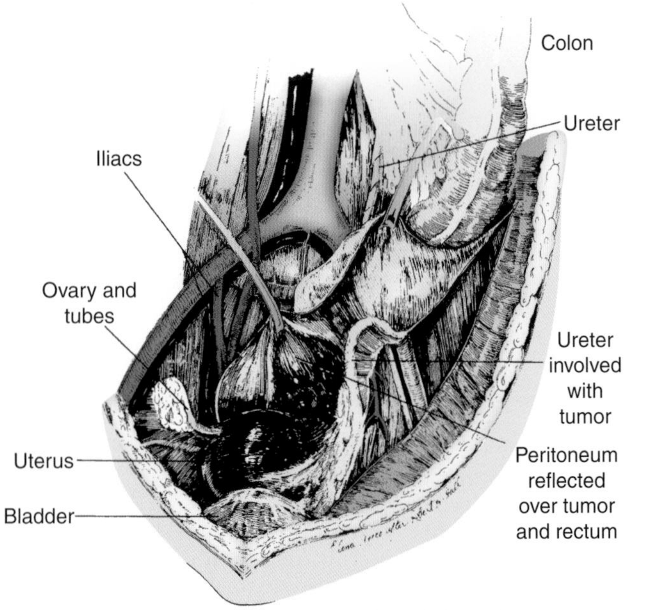

FIGURE 53.3 Retroperitoneal approach with lateral peritoneum incised, demonstrating the proximity of the left ovarian tumor to major pelvic vessels, the ureter, and the rectum.

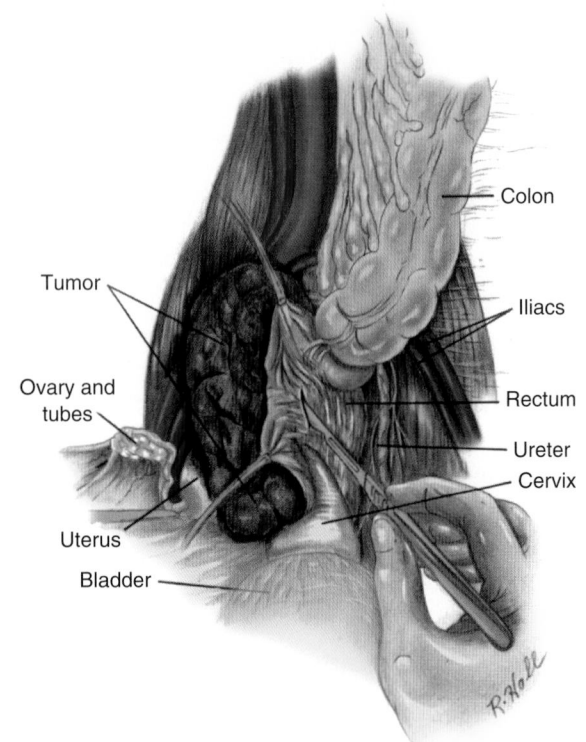

FIGURE 53.4 In the retroperitoneal approach, the proximity of the left ovarian tumor to the rectum is visualized before it is decided whether the tumor can be safely dissected from the rectum or resection of the rectosigmoid colon is required.

Resection of Pelvic Tumor Any adhesions of small intestine or cecum to the pelvic structures should be lysed. A self-retaining retractor then may be inserted and the bowel packed for adequate exposure. We consider that one of the most effective retractors for adequate exposure during a tumor reductive surgery is the Thompson retractor (Thompson Surgical Instruments, Traverse City, MI). If normal pelvic spaces and planes are obliterated by tumor, then the retroperitoneal approach is preferred (Fig. 53.3). The lateral pelvic peritoneum is incised, and the incision is carried cephalad and caudad. As part of this maneuver, the round ligament is identified and ligated as well. The retroperitoneal space is thus entered and the structures—ureter, iliac vessels, and ovarian vessels—identified by using both sharp and blunt dissection. A suction tip is ideal for dissecting areolar tissue planes if used properly. Next, the ovarian vessels are ligated. The identical procedure is performed on the opposite side of the pelvis, and the tumor mass(es) is (are) mobilized medially.

If the ureters are densely adherent to the pelvic tumor, the surgeon may need to dissect them free, in some instances along the entire length of the pelvic portion of the ureter to the ureterovesical junction. In addition, the surgeon must establish a dissection plane between the sigmoid colon and the uterus and ovaries. This portion of the procedure may take considerable effort if this plane is obliterated by tumor. On the other hand, if the surgeon determines that such dissection is not feasible or that the wall of the colon is heavily infiltrated with tumor, resection of the rectosigmoid colon may be indicated (Fig. 53.4). Resection of the pelvic portion of the colon allows the surgeon access to the avascular retrorectal space. The uterus is dissected from the bladder as well. It is extremely rare for ovarian cancer to involve the bladder mucosa at the time of primary surgery, but the vesicouterine peritoneum may be heavily infiltrated. In such cases, resection of this area may be necessary, occasionally in conjunction with a partial cystectomy (see "Resection of the Urinary Tract"). Hysterectomy is then performed, the vagina is entered, and the mass is removed en bloc. In some instances, it may be necessary to ligate the uterine vessels at their origin rather than near the uterus if tumor is extensive in this area. Also, supracervical hysterectomy may be advisable if there is extensive unresectable tumor in the cul-de-sac.

Resection of Rectosigmoid Colon A rectosigmoid resection may be performed in approximately 10% of patients during primary debulking (Fig. 53.5). The decision to perform this procedure depends on several factors, including the presence or absence of rectosigmoid obstruction, the amount of tumor infiltration of the lower colon and its contiguity with the ovarian tumor(s), and the probability that such a procedure will render the patient "optimally debulked." Occasionally, a patient will limit the surgeon's intraoperative decision-making ability by refusing to consent to possible colostomy. In our experience, resection of the rectosigmoid colon almost always can be accomplished with consequent minimal residual disease in the pelvis; the limiting factor in achieving optimal cytoreduction, however, may be unresectable bulky residual tumor in the upper abdomen or retroperitoneum. In such cases, palliative resection in the absence of obstruction is not recommended. If a rectosigmoid colon resection is performed, in most cases the colon can be reanastomosed using either a suture technique or the end-to-end anastomosis (EEA) stapler (Chapter 47). For patients who undergo a reanastomosis, a protective hepatic flexure transverse loop colostomy or loop ileostomy protects the anastomosis for those who have received pelvic radiotherapy, those with unprepared colon, or those whose anastomosis is judged to be suboptimal. Occasionally, a colostomy with a Hartmann pouch is necessary.

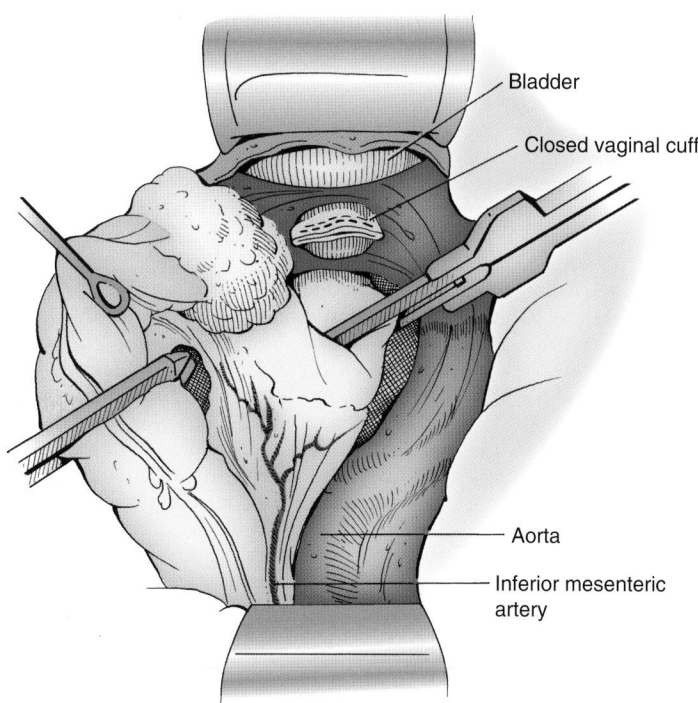

Bladder

Closed vaginal cuff

Aorta

Inferior mesenteric
artery

FIGURE 53.5 Resection of rectosigmoid colon involved with
ovarian cancer. The uterus and bilateral ovarian tumors have
already been removed. After mobilization of the specimen and
ligation of mesenteric vessels, transection is performed using gastrointestinal anastomotic stapling devices (or reticulating stapler
for distal transection), and remainder of mesentery is ligated.
Usually, reanastomosis using EEA stapler can be accomplished.

A recent study by Peiretti et al. evaluated 238 patients
who underwent rectosigmoid resection at the time of primary
cytoreductive surgery to determine morbidity and overall survival. The investigators found that complete cytoreduction
was achieved in 41% of the cases. The complications associated with rectosigmoid resection were anastomotic leakage in
3% of patients and pelvic abscess in 3.7%. The median overall survival among patients with complete cytoreduction was
72 months compared with 42 months among the rest of
patients ($P = 0.002$).

Small Intestinal Resection Although the small intestine is
a common site of metastasis, both to the serosa and the mesentery, extensive tumor involvement is an uncommon finding at primary surgery. If the small intestine is extensively
involved with tumor, it is usually in the terminal ileum.
Occasionally, small intestinal obstruction, either partial or
complete, is present at diagnosis. As noted, complete surgical
staging includes careful examination of the entire length of
the small intestine from the ligament of Treitz to the cecum.
If, on exploration, loops of small intestine are adherent to
the pelvic tumor, omental tumor, or other loops of intestine, then these adhesions should be lysed. Indications for
small intestinal resection include obstruction or impending
obstruction by tumor infiltrating the serosa and muscularis of a segment or a nonobstructing extensive lesion of the
small intestine for which resection would result in minimal
residual disease.

If the lesion involves the very terminal portion of the ileum,
an ileocolectomy with resection of the cecum and portion of
ascending colon adjacent to the small intestine may be necessary. Care should be taken to avoid the presence of tumor at
the points of reanastomosis. The reanastomosis may be performed using either the suture or the stapling technique. In our
experience and in the literature, small intestinal resection is
indicated in approximately 5% to 10% of primary operations
for ovarian cancer.

Resection of the Urinary Tract Indications for ureteral resection or partial cystectomy are uncommon during cytoreductive
surgery for ovarian cancer. If ureteral obstruction is noted preoperatively, it is almost always a result of ureteral compression rather than tumor infiltration. Although adherence of the
ureter(s) to masses of ovarian cancer is not an unusual finding,
the surgeon can almost always separate the ureter from the
tumor using sharp dissection. If the distal ureter is resected
as part of cytoreductive surgery, it usually can be reimplanted
into the bladder. More commonly, the ureter may be injured
during the course of debulking surgery. Depending on the site
of injury, a primary reanastomosis, transureteroureterostomy,
or ureteroneocystostomy may be indicated. In a report by
Berek and associates, 16 of 848 patients (2%) underwent partial ureteral resection. Five patients had transureteroureterostomy, two had reanastomosis, and four had urinary diversion.
Twelve of the operations were part of primary cytoreductive surgery, and four were part of secondary surgery. Nine
of these 16 patients had evidence of ureteral obstruction on
preoperative intravenous pyelograms. A recent study by Ang
et al. reported on 442 patients who underwent laparotomy
for advanced ovarian cancer. Of these, a total of 14 patients
underwent prophylactic stent placement. The investigators
found that there were no ureteric complications during the
postoperative period. Optimal cytoreduction rate in this study
was 88%.

On the other hand, tumor involvement of the peritoneum
overlying the urinary bladder is not an uncommon finding
during primary cytoreductive surgery. Occasionally, a partial
cystectomy may be necessary to achieve optimal cytoreduction. In the series of Berek and associates, eight patients had a
partial cystectomy for advanced ovarian cancer. Reconstruction necessitated ureteral reimplantation in two patients and
an ileal conduit in one patient. If a partial cystotomy is indicated, we prefer a simple closure with two layers of chromic
catgut suture, the inner layer as a continuous running suture
and the outer layer as interrupted sutures.

IX

In our experience, it is exceedingly rare to find involvement of the bladder mucosa with ovarian cancer at initial diagnosis. Such patients usually report hematuria in association with obvious massive disease. The definitive diagnosis can be made easily by preoperative cystoscopy.

Splenectomy Splenectomy is indicated occasionally during primary cytoreductive surgery. Various series report the incidence of splenectomy during primary cytoreductive surgery in 5% to 11% of cases of advanced ovarian cancer. Most commonly, the hilum of the spleen is involved with ovarian cancer in association with extensive omental involvement. Rarely, isolated splenic capsular involvement or even splenic parenchymal involvement may be found. In addition to tumor debulking, splenectomy also may be indicated during cytoreductive surgery because of a traction injury with avulsion of the splenic capsule during omentectomy or mobilization of the splenic flexure of the colon in association with descending colostomy or reanastomosis after rectosigmoid colon resection.

In a report from M.D. Anderson Cancer Center, Morris and colleagues reported on 23 patients for whom the procedure was performed as part of cytoreductive surgery for advanced ovarian cancer. Splenectomy was planned preoperatively in only three of these patients. Seven patients had parenchymal involvement by tumor, 11 had capsular disease, and 5 had no pathologic involvement by tumor. Magtibay et al. evaluated 112 patients who underwent splenectomy as part of primary or secondary cytoreductive surgery. They found that the most common indications for splenectomy were direct metastatic involvement (46%), facilitation of an en bloc resection of perisplenic disease (41%), and intraoperative trauma (13%).

In that same study, the authors found that 65% of patients had hilar involvement, 52% capsular involvement, and 16% parenchymal metastases. Interestingly, patients with disease directly involving the splenic parenchyma did not have a worse prognosis than patients with disease involving the splenic hilum or capsule. In another study by Tanner et al., the investigators evaluated the significance of parenchymal splenic metastasis in patients with advanced ovarian cancer, fallopian tube cancer, and primary peritoneal cancer. A total of 576 patients were identified, and of these, 97 patients underwent splenectomy. Optimal cytoreduction was performed in 74.7% of these patients. Parenchymal disease was identified in 20.6% of patients. In the subset of patients undergoing splenectomy, overall survival was lower for patients with parenchymal splenic metastases versus those without parenchymal disease (28.5 months vs. 51.2 months, $P = 0.004$).

The methods of performing splenectomy during cytoreductive surgery may vary depending on the circumstances. Under controlled conditions (no uncontrolled hemorrhage), the surgeon may prefer to incise the gastrosplenic ligament, gain access to the lesser sac, and identify and ligate the splenic vessels as they run along the superior border of the pancreas (Fig. 53.6). The spleen then can be mobilized by transecting its attachments to the colon, the left kidney, and the diaphragm. If hemorrhage is occurring or access to the lesser sac is limited by the distribution of tumor, the surgeon may prefer to first mobilize the spleen by dividing its peritoneal attachments while compressing the splenic vessels and then ligate the splenic vessels using a posterior approach. The spleen is rotated anteriorly and medially in this technique.

Complications associated with splenectomy include hemorrhage, infection, thromboembolic phenomena, left-sided

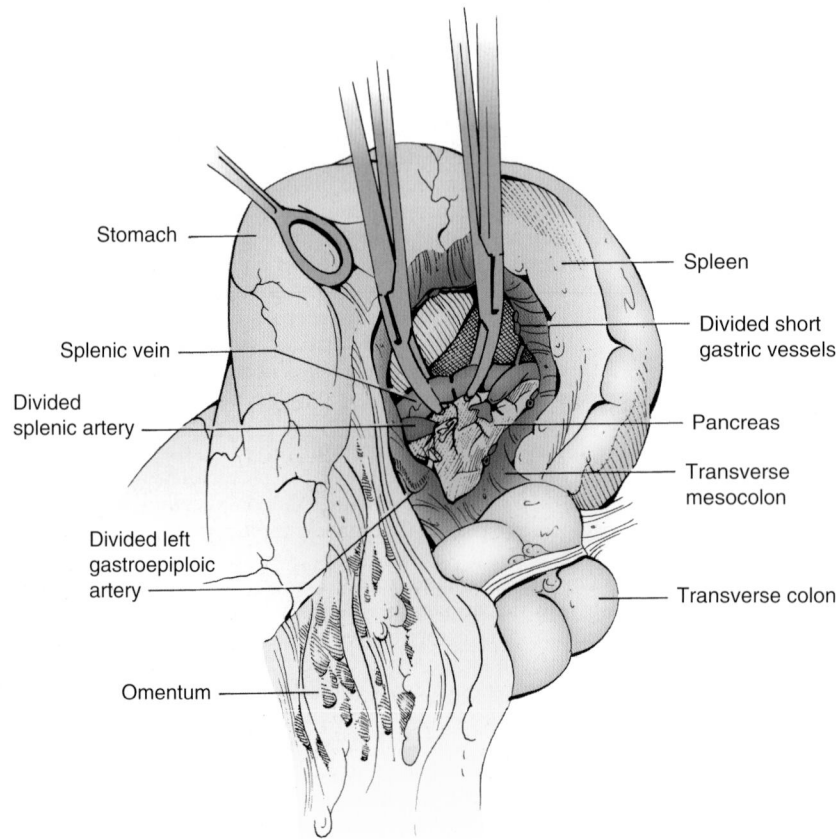

Stomach

Splenic vein

Divided splenic artery

Divided left gastroepiploic artery

Omentum

Spleen

Divided short gastric vessels

Pancreas

Transverse mesocolon

Transverse colon

FIGURE 53.6 Splenectomy. Transection of splenic artery and vein along the superior border of the pancreas after access is gained to lesser sac with transection of gastrosplenic ligament.

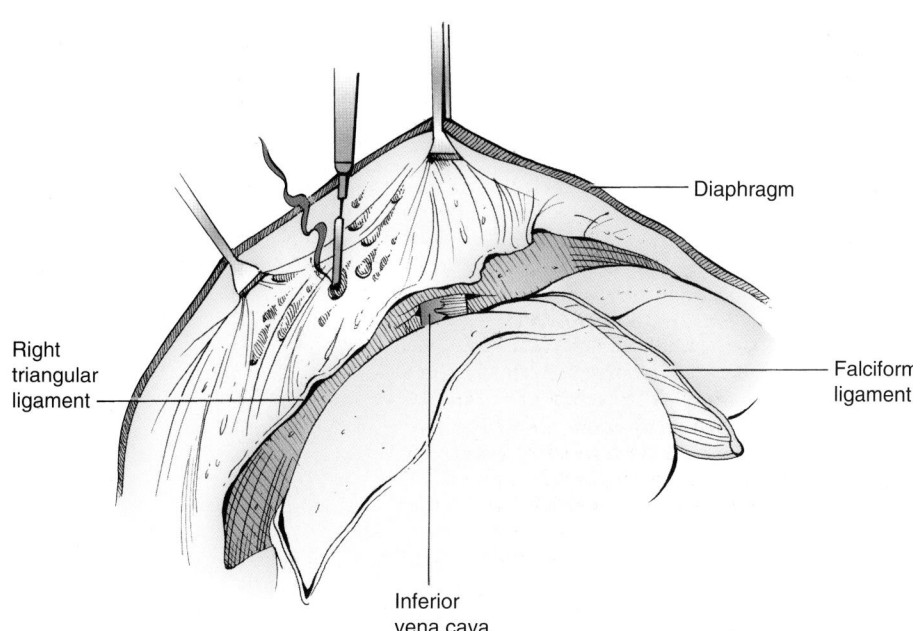

FIGURE 53.7 Ablation of subdiaphragmatic tumor implants with cautery after mobilization of liver. Sharp dissection, argon beam coagulator, or Cavitron ultrasonic surgical aspirator also may be used for the same purpose.

atelectasis or pneumonia, injury to the tail of the pancreas (with resultant pancreatic pseudocyst), or injury to the stomach (with resultant gastric fistula). Because of the risk of severe infection following splenectomy, the patient should receive perioperative antibiotic coverage and should be vaccinated with polyvalent pneumococcal, quadrivalent meningococcal, and Haemophilus influenzae vaccines.

Resection of Diaphragmatic Tumor Several reports have described experience with resection of diaphragmatic metastatic deposits in patients with advanced ovarian cancer. To gain access to the diaphragmatic surfaces, the abdominal incision is extended to just below the xiphoid process, and the liver is mobilized by transecting the entire falciform ligament and the coronary and triangular ligaments. After it is adequately exposed, the diaphragmatic tumor may be resected by stripping the peritoneum from the diaphragmatic muscle using sharp dissection with either Metzenbaum scissors or electrocautery (Fig. 53.7). The anesthesiologist should be notified if the pleural cavity is entered. Defects in the diaphragm may be closed with interrupted sutures. If a large defect cannot be closed primarily or can be closed only under tension, then the defect may be closed using synthetic mesh. If the pleural cavity is entered, then a thoracostomy tube should be placed.

Possible complications associated with resection of diaphragmatic tumor include pneumothorax, hemorrhage from the phrenic arteries, infection, injury to the pericardial sac, and injury to such structures as the lung, the vena cava, or the phrenic nerves.

In a review of the Mayo Clinic experience, Aletti and associates found that for the subgroup of 181 patients with ovarian cancer metastatic to the diaphragm, those who underwent diaphragm surgery had improved 5-year overall survival compared with those who did not (53% vs. 15%). In another recent study of 262 patients with stages IIIC to IV epithelial ovarian cancer, Eisenhauer and colleagues found that patients requiring extensive upper abdominal procedures to achieve optimal debulking demonstrated a similar initial response, PFS, and overall survival to patients optimally debulked by standard surgical techniques. A recent study by Zapardiel et al.

examined the value of peritoneal stripping versus full-thickness diaphragmatic resection. A total of 112 cases were identified; among them, 79 underwent diaphragmatic stripping and 33 underwent full-thickness resection. Larger residual tumors (mean, 5.1 mm vs. 1.6 mm; respectively; $P < 0.01$) were observed in the stripping group. Higher postoperative pleural effusion rates (63.6% vs. 37.9%, $P = 0.01$), but no differences in the remaining complications, were observed in the full-thickness resection group. After a mean of 31 months of follow-up, disease-free survival rates were 28% in the stripping group and 39.4% in the resection group ($P = 0.04$). No significant differences were observed for overall survival.

Resection of Retroperitoneal Lymph Nodes The initial retroperitoneal approach for cytoreductive surgery exposes the node-bearing areas. Lymph nodes are sampled as part of the staging technique, and every effort is extended to remove suspicious retroperitoneal nodes when the peritoneal cavity has been cleared of disease (Fig. 53.8). Whether systematic removal of retroperitoneal lymph nodes should be part of optimal cytoreductive surgery had been a topic of debate for many years. Recently, the issue of systematic aortic and pelvic lymphadenectomy has come more to the forefront. Eisenkop and Spirtos reported on 100 patients with stage IIC to IV epithelial ovarian cancer who underwent a retroperitoneal lymph node dissection at the time of primary cytoreductive surgery. Sixty-six percent had positive lymph nodes. Five were microscopically positive, and 61 were macroscopically positive, of which 19 (31%) were positive by palpation, 16 (26%) were positive by inspection, and 26 (43%) were positive by dissection. On the other hand, there were 39 patients with negative or only microscopically positive nodes, and 15 of these patients (39%) were thought to have clinically positive nodes by the operating surgeon. The authors concluded that a significant proportion of patients had macroscopically positive lymph nodes that were detectable only after a dissection was in progress, and clinical impression of lymph node status was unreliable.

Morice and colleagues reported on 276 women with epithelial ovarian cancer who underwent systematic bilateral pelvic and paraaortic lymphadenectomy. The overall frequency

IX

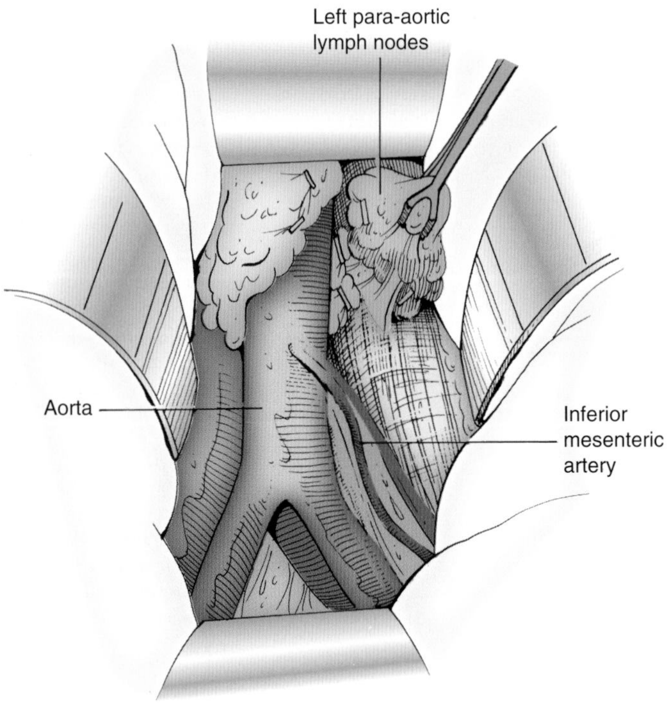

Left para-aortic
lymph nodes

Aorta

Inferior
mesenteric
artery

FIGURE 53.8 Retroperitoneal dissection of paraaortic lymph nodes involved with metastatic ovarian cancer.

of lymph node involvement was 44%. Pelvic and paraaortic lymph nodes were involved 30% and 40% of the time, respectively. In patients with apparent stage IA, IB, and IC disease, the rates of nodal involvement were 13%, 33%, and 38%, respectively.

A recent prospective randomized trial by Benedetti-Panici et al. showed that systematic lymphadenectomy improves PFS but not overall survival in women with optimally debulked advanced ovarian cancer. In addition, the median operating time was longer (300 minutes vs. 210 minutes, $P < 0.001$), and the percentage of patients requiring blood transfusions was higher (72% vs. 59%, $P = 0.006$) in the systematic lymphadenectomy arm.

For patients with malignant germ-cell tumors, especially dysgerminoma, the advantages of debulking metastatic retroperitoneal nodes are even less apparent, because these tumors are generally much more sensitive to chemotherapy than are other ovarian tumors.

Until further information becomes available, it is probably reasonable to consider debulking enlarged retroperitoneal nodes if peritoneal metastases can be cytoreduced optimally, if there is no fixation to blood vessels, and if the surgeon believes that the procedure can be successfully accomplished without undue risk.

Role of Minimally Invasive Surgery in Ovarian Cancer

At present, the role of laparoscopy in the management of ovarian cancer is evolving. There are several clinical settings in which the potential for this surgical modality has been investigated: (a) primary surgery for early-stage ovarian cancer, (b) restaging of unstaged ovarian cancer, (c) primary cytoreductive surgery for advanced-stage ovarian cancer, (d) assessment of resectability, (e) intraperitoneal catheter placement, (f) second-look surgery, and (g) secondary cytoreductive surgery.

Chi and colleagues compared 20 patients who underwent surgical staging via a laparoscopic approach with 30 patients who underwent surgical staging via laparotomy for ovarian or fallopian tube cancer. They found no differences in body mass index, omental specimen size, and number of resected lymph nodes. The estimated blood loss and hospital stay were lower for laparoscopy patients, but operating time was longer. LeBlanc and associates performed laparoscopic restaging in 53 patients—42 early after initial surgery for ovarian or fallopian tube cancer and 11 for second-look surgery after primary chemotherapy. Of the 42 early restaging procedures, 41 were completed successfully. An average of 20 paraaortic lymph nodes and 14 pelvic lymph nodes were removed in these procedures. Complications included a hematoma from an inferior epigastric artery injury and two lymphocysts. Eight patients were upstaged: two patients to stage IIA, two patients to stage IIIA, and four patients to stage IIIC. In addition, Lecuru and coworkers found no difference in survival between patients who underwent surgical staging for stage I epithelial ovarian cancer by either laparoscopy, laparotomy, or laparoscopy converted to laparotomy.

For patients with apparent advanced-stage ovarian cancer, laparoscopic evaluation has been investigated in the context of assessment of resectability. Two recent studies have described this approach. Fagotti and colleagues employed laparoscopy in 64 patients with suspected advanced ovarian cancer before laparotomy for primary cytoreduction. The overall accuracy rate of laparoscopy in predicting optimal cytoreduction was 90%. In a study by Angioli and associates, 87 patients with suspected advanced ovarian cancer underwent diagnostic laparoscopy. Of the 53 (61%) patients who were judged to be operable, 96% were optimally debulked. The question of whether laparoscopy is a useful tool in determining which patients are ideal for attempt at cytoreduction has never been addressed in a well-conducted and powered study. Currently, a prospective randomized trial is being conducted in Europe where patients with advanced ovarian cancer (stage IIIC) will undergo laparoscopic assessment of tumor volume and then proceed with an attempt at cytoreduction versus neoadjuvant chemotherapy. This trial is known as the SCORPION trial (Surgical Complications Related to Primary or Interval Debulking in Ovarian Neoplasm).

One of the primary concerns regarding the use of laparoscopic surgery in the management of ovarian cancer has been spread of the cancer, particularly port site metastasis. Ramirez and coworkers estimated the rate of port site metastasis in patients undergoing laparoscopy for gynecologic malignancies as 1% to 2%. Vergote and colleagues reported 173 patients with advanced ovarian cancer who underwent diagnostic laparoscopy. Seventy-one patients underwent complete excision of port sites at the time of primary cytoreductive surgery. Thirty (17%) patients subsequently developed port site metastases. However, only 8 (5%) of these were clinically diagnosed, whereas 22 (31%) were diagnosed on pathologic examination of resected port sites. All of the port site metastases resolved during primary chemotherapy, and prognosis was not worsened by this finding.

Therefore, the role of laparoscopy is evolving. At present, the most useful settings for this approach appear to be primary surgery for apparent early-stage disease, restaging of apparent early-stage disease that is unstaged before referral, and assessment of resectability in patients with advanced-stage disease to determine whether primary cytoreductive surgery or neoadjuvant chemotherapy and interval debulking is preferable.

More recently, there is increasing enthusiasm for the use of robotic surgery in the management of patients with gynecologic malignancies. The use of such technology in patients with ovarian cancer has been limited. Magrina et al. performed a retrospective case–control analysis of 25 patients undergoing primary surgical debulking with the robotic approach, compared to 27 patients treated by laparoscopy and 119 patients treated by laparotomy. Sixty to seventy-five percent of patients had stage III to IV disease in the robotic and laparoscopy groups, respectively. Patients were subdivided according to extent of surgery and number of procedures required to achieve adequate cytoreduction. There was a significant increase in mean operative time among the robotics cohort (315 minutes), compared to laparoscopy (254 minutes) or laparotomy (261 minutes; $P = 0.009$). However, the robotics group had less blood loss and shortest mean hospital stay compared to laparoscopy or laparotomy. Complete debulking was achieved in 84% of patients in the robotic group, 93% in the laparoscopy group, and 56% in the laparotomy group ($P < 0.001$). There was no difference in overall survival among the three groups. These data, however, must be analyzed carefully due to the retrospective nature of the study and patient selection bias.

Primary Chemotherapy for Advanced Ovarian Cancer

For patients with advanced-stage *malignant ovarian germ-cell tumors*, the standard regimen for patients who require chemotherapy is the BEP (bleomycin, etoposide, and platinum) regimen. The optimal number of cycles remains unknown, but for these patients with a potentially greater tumor burden than those with early-stage disease, four to six cycles may be required in some instances. Generally, administering two cycles following normalization of serum tumor markers may be a reasonable guide, although there are no definitive studies to support this practice. Currently, the GOG and COG (Canadian Oncology Group) are in the process of developing an international trial for pediatric and adult patients with intermediate-risk and high-risk malignant germ-cell tumors.

For patients with advanced-stage *sex cord–stromal tumors*, platinum-based combination chemotherapy is generally recommended. As noted, the BEP combination regimen and the combination of paclitaxel/carboplatin are the most popular regimens in the United States. The GOG is currently conducting a randomized phase II study of BEP versus paclitaxel/carboplatin in women with newly diagnosed advanced-stage and recurrent chemo-naïve ovarian sex cord–stromal tumors.

For advanced-stage *epithelial ovarian cancer*, the combination of cisplatin and cyclophosphamide was the standard postoperative regimen throughout most of the 1980s and until the mid-1990s. Subsequently, GOG initiated a randomized trial comparing the standard regimen of cyclophosphamide/cisplatin with the combination of paclitaxel/cisplatin in patients with suboptimally debulked advanced epithelial ovarian cancer. The findings of this study revealed a significant outcome advantage for the paclitaxel/cisplatin regimen in terms of PFS and overall survival. A subsequent similar study conducted by a European consortium confirmed the results of the GOG study.

Based on the results of several randomized clinical trials demonstrating equivalence of carboplatin to cisplatin in ovarian cancer, paclitaxel/carboplatin became the standard and remains so to the present.

Vasey and colleagues conducted a phase III trial of docetaxel/carboplatin versus paclitaxel/carboplatin as first-line chemotherapy for stage IC to IV epithelial ovarian cancer and peritoneal cancer. A total of 1,077 patients were enrolled in the study. Although there were no differences in PFS or overall survival between the two groups, the docetaxel/carboplatin regimen was associated with significantly less neurotoxicity but more myelotoxicity.

Variations on the Paclitaxel/Carboplatin Backbone

Several different strategies have been studied to improve the efficacy of taxane/platinum-based chemotherapy. The overarching concept is that agents with nonoverlapping cross-resistance mechanisms or alternative mechanisms of action may be complementary and may result in an enhanced therapeutic index.

The Addition of a Third Agent The Gynecologic Cancer InterGroup reported the results of a phase III trial in advanced ovarian cancer (GOG 0182). This was a five-arm study that introduced three new drugs into first-line therapy as either three-drug combinations or sequential doublets, including liposomal doxorubicin, topotecan, and gemcitabine. The results indicated that no regimen demonstrated superiority to the control arm of paclitaxel/carboplatin.

The Addition of Antiangiogenic Agents Two clinical trials—GOG 218 and ICON7—studied the role of bevacizumab added to the taxane/platinum backbone for women with advanced epithelial ovarian cancer. GOG 218 included two experimental arms with bevacizumab; one arm also administered bevacizumab as a maintenance agent for 16 cycles following primary chemotherapy, and the other experimental arm administered only placebo in maintenance. There was a PFS benefit in women who received bevacizumab with chemotherapy and as maintenance compared with the other two arms. However, neither bevacizumab arm demonstrated a survival advantage over chemotherapy alone. ICON7 was a 2-arm trial in which bevacizumab was administered with chemotherapy and then as maintenance versus chemotherapy alone. Similar to GOG 218, PFS was improved in the bevacizumab arm but with no survival advantage. Two subsequent phase III GOG trials—GOG 252 and GOG 262—involve the

IX

addition of bevacizumab to chemotherapy. GOG 252 is also testing intraperitoneal versus intravenous chemotherapy, and GOG 262 is testing the question of dose-dense paclitaxel as well. Both of these trials have completed accrual, but no results are yet available. Several other antiangiogenic agents are under study in either the primary or recurrent settings, including aflibercept, AMG 386, BIBF 1120, cediranib, pazopanib, sunitinib, and sorafenib.

Dose-Dense Paclitaxel Dose-dense paclitaxel has also gained considerable attention recently based on the positive results of a trial conducted by the Japanese Gynecologic Oncology Group. In this trial, 631 patients with stage II to IV epithelial ovarian cancer were randomized to 6 cycles of standard paclitaxel (180 mg/m^2 over 3 hours) plus carboplatin (AUC = 6) every 21 days or dose-dense paclitaxel (80 mg/m^2 over 1 hour) given on days 1, 8, and 15 plus carboplatin (AUC = 6) given on day 1 every 21 days. PFS was significantly better in the dose-dense group (28 months vs. 17.2 months), and overall survival at 3 years was higher in the dose-dense group (72% vs. 65%). GOG protocol 0262 (described above) is also testing the dose-dense strategy.

Intraperitoneal Chemotherapy Intraperitoneal chemotherapy also has been studied as primary treatment for patients with optimally cytoreduced advanced epithelial ovarian cancer. With the recent publication of GOG 172, three GOG studies have now demonstrated the benefits of intraperitoneal chemotherapy over intravenous chemotherapy in the treatment of this subgroup. In an intergroup study, the first such trial, 654 patients with less than 2-cm residual disease were randomized to receive intravenous cisplatin/cyclophosphamide versus intraperitoneal cisplatin plus intravenous cyclophosphamide. The median survival was significantly longer in the group receiving intraperitoneal cisplatin (49 months) than in the group receiving intravenous cisplatin (41 months). In addition, toxicity was worse in the intravenous group. The second GOG intraperitoneal study used intravenous versus intraperitoneal cisplatin as part of initial therapy. Patients on the intraperitoneal arm received an initial two cycles of moderate-dose systemic carboplatin. The results of that study showed a significant improvement in PFS for the intraperitoneal arm but only a borderline effect on overall survival. Because of significant design flaws associated with each of these GOG studies, the role of intraperitoneal chemotherapy in the management of advanced ovarian cancer remained unclear.

In the most definitive trial to date, Armstrong and associates conducted a phase III trial comparing intravenous paclitaxel plus cisplatin versus intravenous paclitaxel and intraperitoneal cisplatin, with intraperitoneal paclitaxel on day 8. The median overall survival was significantly better for the intraperitoneal chemotherapy arm: 66 versus 50 months ($P = 0.03$). However, short-term quality of life and toxicity—principally fatigue, hematologic, GI, metabolic, and neurologic—were significantly worse in the intraperitoneal arm. Furthermore, only 42% of patients in the intraperitoneal chemotherapy arm were able to complete all six cycles of planned treatment. Nevertheless, this study has generated much renewed enthusiasm for the intraperitoneal chemotherapy approach, as well as controversy. GOG 0252 tested intraperitoneal chemotherapy versus intravenous chemotherapy using a modified GOG 172 regimen as well as a second intraperitoneal regimen including paclitaxel and carboplatin. All arms also included bevacizumab. The results of this trial should be available within the next several months.

Neoadjuvant Chemotherapy and Interval Cytoreductive Surgery

Over the past 2 decades, the concept of neoadjuvant chemotherapy followed by interval debulking (as a primary cytoreductive procedure after a few cycles of chemotherapy) has emerged. This approach began to be reported in the late 1970s for certain subsets of patients, patients who were referred to an oncologist after a surgical or nonsurgical biopsy or patients who initially were poor surgical candidates because of a debilitated state related to massive effusions or comorbid conditions. However, this approach has been proposed as a potential alternative for all patients with advanced epithelial ovarian cancer or for certain subsets, such as those predicted to be suboptimally resected. The potential advantage of such an approach is to operate on a patient with an improved nutritional status, a smaller tumor burden, and superior perioperative risk.

Although several studies have explored the concept of a surrogate marker of unresectability of advanced ovarian cancer, as evidenced by the outcome of bulky residual disease, this issue remains unresolved. If accurate, such a strategy could potentially avoid a suboptimal debulking surgical procedure with the associated morbidity. The principal focus has been on preoperative serum CA-125 or CT appearance of disease. Unfortunately, to date, neither has been accurate enough to be incorporated into standard care. Diagnostic laparoscopy has also been investigated as a tool for assessing respectability; this approach may ultimately prove to be the most practical and accurate method, but further study is indicated.

A number of retrospective series have reported the feasibility of neoadjuvant chemotherapy and interval debulking. Clinical observations from these reports indicate the following: (a) a high proportion (70% to 80%) of patients treated with neoadjuvant chemotherapy have partial or complete responses before interval surgery; (b) a high proportion of patients so treated, possibly higher than with primary cytoreductive surgery, are optimally debulked with minimal residual disease; and (c) the surgical morbidity may be reduced compared with that associated with primary cytoreductive surgery.

A recent multi-institutional trial was conducted in Europe evaluating upfront debulking surgery versus neoadjuvant chemotherapy in patients with stage IIIC or IV epithelial ovarian cancer (EORTC 55971). In this trial by Vergote and associates, 670 patients with stage IIIC or IV epithelial ovarian carcinoma, fallopian tube carcinoma, or primary peritoneal carcinoma were randomly assigned to primary debulking surgery followed by platinum-based chemotherapy or to neoadjuvant platinum-based chemotherapy followed by debulking surgery (so-called interval debulking surgery). The largest residual tumor was 1 cm or less in diameter in 41.6% of patients after primary debulking and in 80.6% of patients after interval debulking. Postoperative rates of adverse effects and mortality tended to be higher after primary debulking than after interval debulking. The hazard ratio for death (intention-to-treat analysis) in the group assigned to neoadjuvant chemotherapy followed by interval debulking, as compared with the group assigned to primary debulking surgery followed by chemotherapy, was 0.98 (90% confidence interval [CI], 0.84 to 1.13; $P = 0.01$ for noninferiority), and the hazard ratio for progressive disease was 1.01 (90% CI, 0.89 to 1.15). Complete resection of all macroscopic disease (at primary or interval surgery) was the strongest independent variable in predicting overall survival. The authors of that study concluded that neoadjuvant chemotherapy followed by interval debulking surgery was not inferior to primary debulking surgery followed by chemotherapy as a treatment option for patients with bulky stage IIIC or IV ovarian carcinoma in this study.

MAINTENANCE THERAPY

Since 70% or more patients with advanced epithelial ovarian cancer ultimately develop disease recurrence, the strategy of maintenance or consolidation therapy after completion of primary chemotherapy has been studied. Several approaches to maintenance therapy have been tested, including hormonal therapy, vitamins, radiation therapy, chemotherapy, radioimmunoconjugates, immunotherapy, vaccines, gene therapy, biologic therapy, and complementary medicines. Unfortunately, all of these strategies have not improved overall survival. However, one trial demonstrated an improvement in PFS. Markman and colleagues studied whether 3 or 12 additional months of paclitaxel could affect time to progression in patients who had achieved a complete clinical response following primary treatment. This trial demonstrated a 7-month improvement in median PFS (28 months vs. 21 months; $P = 0.0035$). No effect on overall survival was observed. As noted above, a subsequent trial (GOG 218) reported an improved PFS in patients who continued maintenance bevacizumab versus placebo following primary chemotherapy plus bevacizumab but failed to demonstrate improved overall survival. Additional strategies are currently ongoing or planned. However, toxicity, cost, and potential adverse effects on tumor biology remain a challenge.

SECONDARY SURGERY

Secondary Cytoreductive Surgery

The term *secondary cytoreductive surgery* has no universal definition. It has been previously in multiple different settings; however, the term is currently most commonly used to refer to surgery done in patients who have developed recurrent disease after receiving primary therapy and experience a recurrence. Generally, most patients have had a prolonged disease-free interval off therapy.

Optimal candidates for such a procedure appear to be those who are platinum sensitive (>6-month disease-free interval from completion of upfront chemotherapy). To detect recurrences, the NCCN guidelines for epithelial ovarian cancer, fallopian tube cancer, and primary peritoneal cancer recommend follow-up visits every 2 to 4 months for the first 2 years, followed by 6-month intervals for the next 3 years. At each visit, physical examination and identification of the CA-125 level are recommended. Serial monitoring of serum CA-125 levels can be used as an indicator of ovarian cancer relapse. As shown by Rustin et al., such studies have a sensitivity of 79% to 95% and a positive predictive value of nearly 100%. CT is the most commonly used study to detect recurrent ovarian cancer. The sensitivity of this test is 40% to 93%.

Bristow et al. evaluated the utility of PET/CT imaging in identifying macroscopic (>1 cm) disease among ovarian cancer patients with clinically occult recurrent disease by conventional CT imaging. All patients in that study had to have a rising serum CA-125 level. The authors found that the overall accuracy of PET/CT in detecting recurrent ovarian cancer greater than 1 cm was 82%, with a sensitivity of 83% and a positive predictive value of 94%. In that study, no lesion smaller than 0.8 cm was identified by imaging.

The longer the interval between completion of primary chemotherapy and the time of recurrence, the better the outcome. Results of published studies on secondary cytoreduction for recurrent ovarian cancer are summarized in Table 53.10.

Chi and colleagues analyzed their experience with 153 evaluable patients who underwent secondary cytoreductive surgery for platinum-sensitive recurrent epithelial ovarian cancer. They confirmed previous observations that the longer

TABLE 53.10 Survival After Secondary Cytoreductive Surgery for Recurrent Epithelial Ovarian Cancer

STUDY	PATIENTS	MEDIAN SURVIVAL (MO)	SIGNIFICANCE
Morris et al. (1989)			
≤2 cm	17	18	$P = 0.2$
>2 cm	13	13	
Janicke et al. (1992)			
None	14	29	
≤2 cm	12	9	$P = 0.004$
>2 cm	4	8	
Segna et al. (1993)			
≤2 cm	61	27	$P = 0.0001$
>2 cm	39	9	
Vacarello et al. (1995)			
<0.5 cm	14	NR	$P < 0.0001$
>0.5 cm	24	23	
Eisenkop et al. (1995)			
Microscopic	87	44	$P = 0.007$
Macroscopic	19	19	
Gaducci et al. (2000)			
Microscopic	17	37	$P = 0.04$
Macroscopic	13	19	
Tay et al. (2002)			
None	30	38	
<1 cm	10	14.5	$P < 0.01$
>1 cm	6	11	
Zang et al. (2004)			
None	11	NR	
≤1 cm	61	26	$P < 0.0001$
>1 cm	45	14.5	
Pfisterer et al. (2005)			
Microscopic	133	45	$P < 0.0001$
Macroscopic	134	19	
Gungor et al. (2005)			
Microscopic	34	19	$P = 0.007$
Macroscopic	10	9	
Chi et al. (2006)			
≤0.5 cm	79	56	$P < 0.001$
>0.5 cm	73	27	
Harter et al. (2006)			
None	133	45	$P < 0.0001$
≤1 cm	69	20	
>1 cm	65	2	

NR, not reported.

the disease-free interval, the longer the survival time after secondary cytoreduction (30 months for disease-free interval of 6 to 12 months, 39 months for disease-free interval of 13 to 30 months, and 51 months for disease-free interval >30 months). For patients who had residual disease ≤0.5 cm, the median survival was 56 months compared with a median survival of 27 months for those patients with residual disease greater than 0.5 cm. The authors further devised a set of recommendations for selection of candidates for secondary cytoreductive surgery based on the disease-free interval, the number of recurrence sites, and evidence of carcinomatosis.

Bristow and colleagues conducted a meta-analysis to determine the effect of prognostic variables on overall postrecurrence survival time among patients with recurrent ovarian cancer undergoing cytoreductive surgery. In that study of 2,019 patients, the authors found that the only statistically significant variable independently associated with postrecurrence survival time was the proportion of patients undergoing complete (no gross residual disease) cytoreductive surgery ($P = 0.019$). After controlling for other factors, each 10% increase in the proportion of patients undergoing complete cytoreductive surgery was associated with a 3-month increase in median cohort survival time.

Currently, there is an ongoing trial conducted by the GOG (Protocol 213) that is evaluating the role of secondary cytoreduction in patients with recurrent platinum-sensitive epithelial ovarian cancer, fallopian tube cancer, and primary peritoneal cancer. In this trial, patients who are considered appropriate surgical candidates are randomized to either surgery or no surgery. A second randomization is then performed where patients undergo treatment with either combination of intravenous carboplatin and paclitaxel or intravenous carboplatin, paclitaxel, and bevacizumab followed by maintenance bevacizumab. It is estimated that 660 women will be needed to address the primary objectives of this study. Another similar prospective randomized trial in Europe is also underway evaluating the role of surgery in the recurrent setting in patients with platinum-sensitive recurrent ovarian cancer, fallopian tube cancer, or primary peritoneal cancer. The trial, known as the DESKTOP III trial, randomizes patients to surgery or no surgery followed by platinum-based chemotherapy.

Tertiary Cytoreductive Surgery

Several studies have examined the impact of a tertiary cytoreductive surgery on patient outcomes. Leitao et al. reviewed the outcomes of patients diagnosed with ovarian cancer who underwent a tertiary cytoreduction. They found that treatment-free interval before tertiary cytoreduction, the extent of residual disease after the procedure, and the time to first recurrence were significant prognostic factors. The median disease-specific survival was 15 months for patients with a treatment-free interval up to 12 months compared to 60.4 months for patients with a treatment-free interval of greater than 12 months ($P = 0.002$). The median disease-specific survival for patients with residual disease 0.5 cm or less was 36.3 months, compared to 10.6 months for patients with residual disease greater than 0.5 cm ($P < 0.0001$). In another study, Karam et al. sought to find predictors of optimal tertiary cytoreductive surgery. They found that 64% of patients underwent an optimal cytoreductive surgery and that tumor implants of less than 5 cm on preoperative imaging were the only predictor of achieving optimal cytoreductive surgery. It should be noted that 26% of patients experienced severe postoperative complications. It is important to recognize that the only available data on tertiary cytoreduction are from retrospective studies with a small cohort of patients.

The largest series published to date on this topic was recently reported by Fotopoulou et al. In that study, the investigators evaluated 406 patients who underwent tertiary cytoreductive surgery. Median time from first to second recurrence was

18 months (2 to 204 months). Median follow-up was 14 months (0 to 182 months), and median overall survival was 26 months (95% CI, 19.62 to 32.38 months). Median overall survival for patients without residual tumor versus any visible tumor remaining was 49 months (95 % CI, 42.5 to 56.4 months) versus 12 months (95% CI 9.3 to 14.7 months) ($P < 0.001$). A total of 224 patients (54.1%) underwent complete tumor resection. The most frequent tumor dissemination site was the pelvis (73%). Rates of major operative morbidity and 30-day mortality were 25.9% and 3.2%, respectively. Multivariate analysis identified platinum resistance, tumor residuals at secondary surgery, and peritoneal carcinomatosis to be of predictive significance for complete tumor resection, while tumor residuals at secondary and tertiary surgery, decreasing interval to second relapse, ascites, upper abdominal tumor involvement, and nonplatinum third-line chemotherapy significantly affected overall survival.

MANAGEMENT OF RECURRENT OVARIAN CANCER

As noted, approximately 70% of women with advanced epithelial ovarian cancer will recur after primary treatment. Although many of these women may have prolonged survival with contemporary management, few are cured. Because the therapy is largely palliative, efficacy must be balanced with toxicity. Choice of therapy is empirical, and patients with recurrent cancer typically receive multiple agents or regimens in sequence. Surgery, as discussed above, chemotherapy, hormonal therapy, radiotherapy, immunotherapy, and target agents are options.

When recurrence is initially diagnosed, patients are generally categorized as being platinum sensitive, platinum resistant, or platinum refractory. This classification is based on the duration from the completion of primary therapy until diagnosis of recurrence. Patients exhibiting a treatment-free interval of 6 months or longer are considered to be platinum sensitive. Those who recur in less than 6 months are classified as platinum resistant. And the worst prognosis group, platinum refractory, are those whose disease progresses during primary therapy.

Platinum-sensitive disease. Patients who are considered to be platinum sensitive have a relatively high probability of responding again to platinum-based chemotherapy. Based on the literature, options include paclitaxel/carboplatin, docetaxel/carboplatin, pegylated liposomal doxorubicin/carboplatin, or gemcitabine carboplatin. The choice of regimen is based on several factors, including any residual toxicity from primary therapy and potential side effects of each regimen. In general, all of these regimens appear to be roughly equivalent in terms of efficacy. In addition, bevacizumab may be added to any of these regimens.

In 2012, Aghajanian reported the results of the OCEANS trial, in which 484 women with platinum-sensitive ovarian cancer were randomized to either gemcitabine/carboplatin plus bevacizumab for 6 to 10 cycles followed by bevacizumab until progression versus gemcitabine/carboplatin plus placebo for 6 to 10 cycles followed by placebo until progression. Both the response rate (78.5% vs. 58.4%) and the median PFS (12.4 months vs. 8.4 months) were significantly improved for women receiving bevacizumab.

Platinum-resistant disease. For women with platinum-resistant disease, a nonplatinum agent is generally recommended. Options include pegylated liposomal doxorubicin, gemcitabine (with or without cisplatin), topotecan, docetaxel, weekly paclitaxel, or hormonal therapy (tamoxifen or aromatase inhibitors). In addition, bevacizumab with or without chemotherapy is an option. Patients who achieve stable disease or response are usually treated until disease progression or untoward toxicity occurs. While clinical trials are always recommended as an option in every disease setting, this group is particularly encouraged to consider trials, if available.

Platinum-refractory disease. This disease status is fortunately uncommon. However, the probability of response to any agent is low. These patients are also excellent candidates for clinical trials.

Novel therapeutics. Several promising novel drugs or targeted agents are currently under investigation in women with recurrent ovarian cancer. Several trials involving PARP (poly[ADP-ribose] polymerase) inhibitors have been reported, are ongoing, or are planned in the near future. Apparently, deficiency in BRCA1 or BRCA2 causes extreme sensitivity to the inhibition of PARP. PARP inhibition blocks repair of single-strand breaks. Although normal cells can bypass these lesions by using homologous recombination, this is not possible for BRCA-mutated cancer cells. Several different PARP inhibitors are currently under development.

Targeted therapies are also currently under investigation. However, none has yet been approved for ovarian cancer treatment. Genes within the PI3K/AKT and MAP kinase pathways have commanded the most attention based on early molecular investigations. For example, potential druggable targets for clear cell carcinoma of the ovary include *mTOR*, *PI3K*, *c-MET*, and *VEGF*. Based on the observations that low-grade serous carcinomas have a 5% frequency of *BRAF* mutations and a 20% to 40% frequency of *KRAS* mutations, the MAP kinase pathway is a major focus for therapeutics. In the initial phase II trial of the MEK inhibitor, selumetinib, for recurrent low-grade serous carcinoma, a promising response rate of 15% was observed. A number of subsequent MEK inhibitor trials for this subtype are planned in the near future.

Other novel agents under investigation include antifolate receptor antibodies, vaccines, various immunologic therapies, and drugs that may affect p53-mutated cancer cells, among others.

MANAGEMENT OF INTESTINAL OBSTRUCTION

Approximately 25% of ovarian cancer patients develop intestinal obstruction in the terminal phase of their illness. One of the major dilemmas facing the gynecologic oncologist is whether to operate on a patient with refractory ovarian cancer and an intestinal obstruction. Signs and symptoms of intestinal obstruction resulting from ovarian cancer include nausea and vomiting, abdominal cramping, abdominal distention, and progressive constipation. In patients who have only partial obstruction, these symptoms and findings may be episodic and more subtle. Routine abdominal x-ray may support the diagnosis. Dilatation of the small intestine and air fluid levels suggest involvement of the small bowel. Dilatation of the colon may characterize large-bowel obstruction. In patients with early, partial obstruction, the radiographic findings may be nonspecific. CT scan of the abdomen and pelvis is often useful given the fact that it may provide information regarding sites of obstruction and degree of carcinomatosis at the time of patient presentation.

Although intestinal obstruction in patients with ovarian cancer may be caused by adhesions, progressive tumor usually is the inciting factor. Of course, if the patient has received abdominopelvic radiotherapy, obstruction that is due to adhesions should be considered. In our experience, and that of others, however, most cases of intestinal obstruction in ovarian cancer patients who have received prior radiotherapy are related primarily to tumor progression. Surgical options may be offered to the patient depending on a number of factors that dictate the success of surgical management. These include the site of obstruction, the number of obstructions along the small or large bowel, the number of prior chemotherapies regimens, prior episodes of bowel obstruction, the nutritional status of the patient, and the overall functional status of the patient.

The site(s) of the obstruction may be solitary or multiple. In 5% to 10% of patients, there is simultaneous obstruction of the small and large bowel. Colon obstruction usually occurs in the area of the sigmoid colon because of growth of pelvic tumor and resultant extrinsic compression; occasionally, there may be obstruction of more proximal segments. Small-bowel obstruction is usually the result of adherence of loops of bowel by mesenteric or serosal tumor implants.

Once the appropriate evaluation is completed and the diagnosis of intestinal obstruction is made, the gynecologist should outline a plan of management. The decision of whether to operate or manage the patient nonoperatively is colored by the fact that surgery for patients with refractory ovarian cancer is associated with significant morbidity and mortality, the obstruction cannot be relieved in almost 20% of those undergoing surgery, and postoperative survival is disappointingly brief. In reported series, the serious complication rate has ranged from 28% to 49%, and the operative mortality rate is in the range of 12% to 16%. The median survival rate for patients who have undergone surgery is in the range of 3 to 5 months.

Although some investigators have used projected survival (usually >2 months) as a parameter to decide on type of management, such an indicator is too unpredictable. Pothuri et al. reviewed a series of patients undergoing surgery for intestinal obstruction due to recurrent ovarian cancer and found that the mean time from original diagnosis of ovarian cancer to obstruction was 2.8 years. Surgical correction (intestinal surgery performed for relief of obstruction) was attained in 84% of cases. Successful palliation (the ability to tolerate a regular or low-residue diet by 60 days after surgery) was achieved in 71% of cases. Major surgical morbidity was documented in 22% of patients. Interestingly, postoperative chemotherapy was administered in 79% of patients in whom surgical correction was possible. In addition, the median survival was 11.6 months in patients with successful palliation versus 3.9 months for all other patients. The authors noted that with respect to quality of life, it is important to consider that 56% of patients undergoing surgery for bowel obstruction had either a colostomy or permanent gastrostomy tube. Finally, the authors recommended that patients not be considered ideal surgical candidates if they have bulky carcinomatosis, rapidly progressive disease, multiple sites of obstruction, poor performance status, or heavy pretreatment with chemotherapy and radiation.

For initial management of a patient with small-bowel obstruction, we prefer the insertion of a nasogastric tube. In patients for whom no surgery is planned, a percutaneous gastrostomy is recommended. This procedure has resulted in excellent palliation for terminal-stage ovarian cancer patients, avoiding the discomfort of the nasogastric tube and allowing the patient to be easily cared for at home in most cases. With such a device, the patient may even continue to eat, although the nutritional benefit is essentially nil.

A recent study by Chi et al. evaluated outcomes data on patients undergoing palliative operative or endoscopic

IX

procedures for malignant bowel obstruction due to recurrent ovarian cancer. This report focused on patients with malignant bowel obstruction due to recurrent ovarian cancer. Procedures performed with an upper or lower GI endoscope were considered "endoscopic." All other cases were classified as "operative." Following the procedure, the presence or absence of symptoms was determined and followed over time. Palliative interventions were performed on 74 gynecologic oncology patients during the study period, of which 26 (35%) were for malignant GI obstruction due to recurrent ovarian cancer. The site of obstruction was small bowel in 14 (54%) cases and large bowel in 12 (46%) cases. Palliative procedures were operative in 14 (54%) patients and endoscopic in the other 12 (46%). Overall, symptomatic improvement or resolution within 30 days was achieved in 23 (88%) of 26 patients, with 1 (4%) postprocedure mortality. At 60 days, 10 (71%) of 14 patients who underwent operative procedures and 6 (50%) of 12 patients who had endoscopic procedures had symptom control. Median survival from the time of the palliative procedure was 191 days (range, 33 to 902) for those undergoing an operative procedure and 78 days (range, 18 to 284) for those undergoing an endoscopic procedure. The authors concluded that patients with malignant bowel obstructions due to recurrent ovarian cancer have a high likelihood of experiencing relief of symptoms with palliative procedures.

Optimal preoperative preparation is desirable if a patient is judged to be a suitable candidate for surgical intervention. For patients with complete colonic obstruction or perforation of the small or large intestine, a surgical emergency exists unless the patient is in such poor condition that such an intervention is not feasible. In emergency cases, the patient should be stabilized with intravenous fluids and antibiotics before surgery. Emergency surgery is rarely indicated for patients with a small intestinal obstruction. It is preferable to optimize the patient's condition with nasogastric tube decompression and rehydration. In addition, a barium enema is usually indicated to rule out a coexisting colonic obstruction. If the patient is malnourished, then intravenous hyperalimentation may be indicated preoperatively.

Colonic obstruction usually is treated by performing a colostomy. The selection of the site of colostomy depends on the area of obstruction and the ability to find an adequate bowel segment free of cancer. Most commonly, a transverse loop colostomy is indicated in the presence of a descending colon or sigmoid colon obstruction. There is increasing experience with the use of colonic stents as a substitute for colostomy. A study by Caceres et al. aimed to review the experience with colonic stent placement for patients presenting with a large-bowel obstruction due to recurrent gynecologic malignancy. Thirty-five patients were identified—25 patients had recurrent ovarian cancer, 7 patients had recurrent endometrial cancer, 2 patients had primary peritoneal carcinoma, and 1 patient had recurrent cervical cancer. The median age at the time of stent placement was 54 years (range, 21 to 79). The median length of the large-bowel obstruction was 6.5 cm (range, 1 to 20 cm). Six patients had a lumen of 1 to 2 mm before stent placement, while 29 patients had complete obstruction and needed balloon dilatation before deployment of the stent. Twenty-seven patients (77%) underwent successful stent placement and immediate decompression at the time of colorectal stent placement. Of the patients who had successful stent placement, 9 (33%) underwent additional surgery to relieve obstruction. Of the 27 patients who underwent successful stent placement, the median survival after placement was 7.7 months (95% CI, 3.19 to 11.9 months). The authors concluded that in the management of patients with large-bowel obstructions due

to recurrent gynecologic cancer, colonic stents appear to be a reasonable option that may enable patients to avoid major surgery.

A number of options are available for small-bowel obstruction, depending on the operative findings. Most commonly, there are multiple sites of obstruction in the terminal ileum, in which case an ileo-ascending colon bypass or ileo-transverse colon bypass is preferable. In such situations, it is usually both unwise and inappropriate to attempt resection and reanastomosis. If, on the other hand, there is an isolated area of obstruction, then a resection and reanastomosis may be indicated. The anastomosis may be either hand sewn using a two-layer technique or approximated with surgical staplers (Chapter 47). We generally prefer the latter because of the time-saving aspect. Frequently, there may be extensive tumor with multiple areas of obstruction, making both bypass and resection impossible. A tube gastrostomy, if possible, is indicated in such a situation. Procedures such as these are among the most demanding because of the meticulous, often tedious dissection required. Enterotomies are not uncommon and should be repaired as soon as they are identified. Complications of small intestinal procedures include wound infection, intraperitoneal abscess, sepsis, pneumonia, "blind loop syndrome," and enterocutaneous fistula.

BEST SURGICAL PRACTICES

- In the United States, more than 22,000 new cases of ovarian cancer are detected annually, and more than 16,000 women will die of the disease. The lifetime risk of ovarian cancer for a woman in the United States is 1/70. This risk increases to 5% in a woman with one first-degree relative who has ovarian cancer and to 7% if she has two or more relatives with the disease.
- Pelvic examination is inaccurate in assessing ovarian size and morphology, particularly in postmenopausal women and in women who are overweight. No ovarian cancer screening technique has been shown to be cost-effective to reduce the incidence or improve survival of ovarian cancer.
- Numerous studies have shown improved survival in both early- and advanced-stage ovarian cancer when the initial surgery has been done by a gynecologic oncologist. A careful evaluation of an adnexal mass using transvaginal ultrasound, serum CA-125, and, occasionally, supplemented by other imaging studies will usually identify the patient with a high risk of malignancy who should be referred for surgery by a gynecologic oncologist.
- Surgery for ovarian cancer includes both careful staging to document the extent of the disease and resection or debulking of the tumor. Careful attention to accurate and comprehensive staging is most important in early-stage disease, for which postoperative therapy decisions may depend on the findings and histopathologic diagnosis. In patients with advanced disease, maximum surgical debulking to less than 1-cm diameter of residual disease should be the goal.
- In some young women with ovarian cancer, fertility-sparing surgery is possible. In a woman with a lesion apparently confirmed to a single ovary (or rarely both ovaries) who desires future pregnancy, ovarian and uterine conservation should be discussed preoperatively. At surgery, a unilateral oophorectomy and careful staging should be done, but the opposite ovary should not be biopsied if it appears normal. If the diagnosis or staging findings are uncertain, it is best to close and await a final review of the permanent sections on the staging studies. Reoperation is preferable to unnecessary radicality in a young woman in whom fertility is a concern.

- In women with advanced ovarian cancer, optimal cytoreduction to less than 1-cm residual disease—ideally to microscopic residual—has clearly been shown to confer a survival advantage. This is true even in patients with stage IV disease. The techniques required to perform radical cytoreduction in ovarian cancer patients and the judgment to know when it is appropriate are a combination of skill and experience, and it is usually done by gynecologic oncologists operating in hospitals with good teams of anesthesiologists, consultants, and critical care experts.
- Laparoscopic and robotic surgery for ovarian cancer is currently limited to patients with apparent early-stage disease. Its role in the setting of advanced disease remains investigation.
- Postoperative chemotherapy is usually required for patients with ovarian cancer; in some cases, chemotherapy may be given before any definitive surgery. This is an important part of the management of ovarian cancer, but it is not addressed in this surgical textbook.
- Patients with recurrent ovarian cancer may benefit from secondary cytoreductive surgery if there is a disease-free interval greater than 6 months, there is isolated recurrent disease, and location and number of recurrences are predictive of complete cytoreduction.

BIBLIOGRAPHY

Adelson MD. Cytoreduction of diaphragmatic metastases using the Cavitron ultrasonic surgical aspirator. *Gynecol Oncol* 1991; 41:1220.

Adelson MD, Baggish MS, Seifer DB, et al. Cytoreduction of ovarian cancer with the Cavitron ultrasonic surgical aspirator. *Obstet Gynecol* 1988;72:140.

Aghajanian C, Blank SV, Goff BA, et al. OCEANS: a randomized, double-blind, placebo-controlled phase III trial of chemotherapy with or without bevacizumab in patients with platinum-sensitive recurrent epithelial ovarian, primary peritoneal, or fallopian tube cancer. *J Clin Oncol* 2012;30(17):2039–2045.

Alberts DS, Liu PY, Hannigan EV, et al. Intraperitoneal cisplatin plus intravenous cyclophosphamide versus intravenous cisplatin plus intravenous cyclophosphamide for stage III ovarian cancer. *N Engl J Med* 1996;335:1950.

Alberts DS, Liu PY, Wilczynski SP, et al. Randomized trial of pegylated liposomal doxorubicin (PLD) plus carboplatin versus carboplatin in platinum-sensitive (PS) patients with recurrent epithelial ovarian or peritoneal carcinoma after failure of initial platinum-based chemotherapy (Southwest Oncology Group Protocol S0200). *Gynecol Oncol* 2008;108(1):90–94.

Alcazar JL, Errasti T, Zornoza A, et al. Transvaginal color Doppler ultrasonography and CA-125 in suspicious adnexal masses. *Int J Gynecol Obstet* 1999;66:255.

Allen DG, Baak J, Belpomme D, et al. Advanced epithelial ovarian cancer: 1993 consensus statement. *Ann Oncol* 1993;4(suppl 4):S83.

Aletti GD, Dowdy SC, Podratz KC, et al. Surgical treatment of diaphragm disease correlates with improved survival in optimally debulked advanced stage ovarian cancer. *Gynecol Oncol* 2006;100:283.

American Cancer Society. *Cancer Facts and Figures*, 2006. Atlanta, GA: American Cancer Society, 2006.

Ang C, Naik R. The value of ureteric stents in debulking surgery for disseminated ovarian cancer. *Int J Gynecol Cancer* 2009; 19(5):978–980.

Angioli R, Palaia I, Zullo MA, et al. Diagnostic open laparoscopy in the management of advanced ovarian cancer. *Gynecol Oncol* 2006;100:455.

Armstrong DK, Bundy B, Wenzel L, et al. Intraperitoneal cisplatin and paclitaxel in ovarian cancer. *N Engl J Med* 2006;354:34.

Aure JC, Hoeg K, Kalstad P. Clinical and histologic studies of ovarian carcinoma: long-term follow-up of 990 cases. *Obstet Gynecol* 1971;37:1.

Ayhan A, Gultekin M, Taskiran C, et al. Routine appendectomy in epithelial ovarian carcinoma: is it necessary? *Obstet Gynecol* 2005;105:719.

Baggerly K, Morris J, Edmonson S, et al. Signal in noise: evaluating reported reproducibility of serum proteomic tests for ovarian cancer. *J Natl Cancer Inst* 2005;97:307.

Bailey CL, Ueland FR, Land GL, et al. Malignant potential of small cystic ovarian tumors in postmenopausal women. *Gynecol Oncol* 1998;69:3.

Barnhill DR, Kurman RJ, Brady MF, et al. Preliminary analysis of the behavior of stage I ovarian serous tumors of low malignant potential: a Gynecologic Oncology Group study. *J Clin Oncol* 1995;13:2752.

Bast RC, Klug TL, St. John ER, et al. A radioimmunoassay using a monoclonal antibody to monitor the course of epithelial ovarian cancer. *N Engl J Med* 1983;308:883.

Bast RC, Xu FJK, Yu YH, et al. CA-125: the past and the future. *Int J Biol Markers* 1998;13:179.

Bell J, Brady MF, Young RC, et al. Randomized phase III trial of three versus six cycles of adjuvant carboplatin and paclitaxel in early stage epithelial ovarian carcinoma: a Gynecologic Oncology Group study. *Gynecol Oncol* 2006;102:432.

Benedetti-Panici GS, Scambia G, Baiocchi G, et al. Technique and feasibility of radical paraaortic and pelvic lymphadenectomy for gynecologic malignancies: a prospective study. *Int J Gynecol Cancer* 1991;1:133.

Benedetti-Panici P, Maggioni A, Hacker N, et al. Systematic aortic and pelvic lymphadenectomy versus resection of bulky nodes only in optimally debulked advanced ovarian cancer: a randomized clinical trial. *J Natl Cancer Inst* 2005;97:560.

Berchuck A, Schildkraut JM, Marks JR, et al. Managing hereditary ovarian cancer risk. *Cancer* 1999;86(suppl):1697.

Berek JS, Griffiths CT, Leventhal J. Laparoscopy for second-look evaluation in ovarian cancer. *Obstet Gynecol* 1981;58:192.

Berek JS, Hacker NF, Lagasse LD, et al. Lower urinary tract resection as part of cytoreductive surgery for ovarian cancer. *Gynecol Oncol* 1982;13:87.

Berek JS, Hacker NF, Lagasse LD. Rectosigmoid colectomy and reanastomosis to facilitate resection of primary and recurrent gynecologic cancer. *Obstet Gynecol* 1984;64:715.

Berek JS, Hacker NF, Lagasse LD, et al. Survival of patients following secondary cytoreductive surgery in ovarian cancer. *Obstet Gynecol* 1983;61:189.

Bolis G, Colombo N, Pecorelli S, et al. Adjuvant treatment for early epithelial ovarian cancer: results of two randomised clinical trials comparing cisplatin to no further treatment or chromic phosphate (^{32}P). *Ann Oncol* 1995;6:887.

Bolis G, Scarfone G, Giardina G, et al. Carboplatin alone vs carboplatin plus epidoxorubicin as second-line therapy for cisplatin- or carboplatin-sensitive ovarian cancer. *Gynecol Oncol* 2001;81(1):3–9.

Bonazzi C, Peccatori F, Colombo N, et al. Pure ovarian immature teratoma, a unique and curable disease: 10 years' experience of 32 prospectively treated patients. *Obstet Gynecol* 1994;84:598.

Bookman MA, Brady MF, McGuire WP. Evaluation of new platinum-based treatment regimens in advanced-stage ovarian cancer: a phase III trial of the Gynecologic Cancer InterGroup. *J Clin Oncol* 2009;27:1419–1425.

Bostwick DG, Tazelaar HD, Ballon SC, et al. Ovarian epithelial tumors of borderline malignancy: a clinical and pathologic study of 109 cases. *Cancer* 1986;58:2052.

Brewer M, Gershenson DM, Herzog CE, et al. Outcome and reproductive function after chemotherapy for ovarian dysgerminoma. *J Clin Oncol* 1999;17:2670.

Bristow RE, Chi DS. Platinum-based neoadjuvant chemotherapy and interval surgical cytoreduction for advanced ovarian cancer: a meta-analysis. *Gynecol Oncol* 2006;103:1070.

Bristow RE, del Carmen MG, Pannu HK, et al. Clinically occult recurrent ovarian cancer: patient selection for secondary cytoreductive surgery using combined PET/CT. *Gynecol Oncol* 2003;90(3):519–528.

Bristow RE, Eisenhauer EL, Santillan A, et al. Delaying the primary surgical effort for advanced ovarian cancer: a systematic review of neoadjuvant chemotherapy and interval cytoreduction. *Gynecol Oncol* 2007;104:480.

IX

Bristow RE, Montz FJ. Complete surgical cytoreduction of advanced ovarian carcinoma using the argon beam coagulator. *Gynecol Oncol* 2001;83:39.

Bristow RE, Montz FJ, Lagasse LD, et al. Survival impact of surgical cytoreduction in Stage IV epithelial ovarian cancer. *Gynecol Oncol* 1999;72:278.

Bristow RE, Puri I, Chi DS. Cytoreductive surgery for recurrent ovarian cancer: a meta-analysis. *Gynecol Oncol* 2009;112(1):265–274.

Bristow RE, Zahurak ML, del Carmen MG, et al. Ovarian cancer surgery in Maryland: volume-based access to care. *Gynecol Oncol* 2004;93:353.

Brown J, Shvartsman H, Deavers M, et al. The activity of taxanes in the treatment of sex cord-stromal ovarian tumors. *J Clin Oncol* 2004;22:3517.

Brown J, Sood AK, Deavers MT, et al. Patterns of metastasis in sex cord-stromal tumors of the ovary: can routine staging lymphadenectomy be omitted? *Gynecol Oncol* 2009;113(1):86–90.

Burger RA, Brady MF, Bookman MA, et al. Incorporation of bevacizumab in the primary treatment of ovarian cancer. *N Engl J Med* 2011;365(26):2473–2483.

Burghardt E, Girardi F, Lahousen M, et al. Patterns of pelvic and paraaortic lymph node involvement in ovarian cancer. *Gynecol Oncol* 1991;40:103.

Burghardt E, Pickel H, Lahousen M, et al. Pelvic lymphadenectomy in operative treatment of ovarian cancer. *Am J Obstet Gynecol* 1986;155:15.

Caceres A, Zhou Q, Iasonos A, et al. Colorectal stents for palliation of large-bowel obstructions in recurrent gynecologic cancer: an updated series. *Gynecol Oncol* 2008;108(3):482–485.

Carlson KJ, Skates SJ, Singer D. Screening for ovarian cancer. *Ann Intern Med* 1994;121:124.

Carney ME, Lancaster JM, Ford C, et al. A population-based study of patterns of care for ovarian cancer: who is seen by a gynecologic oncologist and who is not? *Gynecol Oncol* 2002;84:36.

Carnino F, Fuda G, Ciccone G, et al. Significance of lymph node sampling in epithelial carcinoma of the ovary. *Gynecol Oncol* 1997;65:467.

Casagrande JT, Louie EW, Pike MC. Incessant ovulation and ovarian cancer. *Lancet* 1979;2:170.

Cass I, Li AJ, Runowicz CD, et al. Pattern of lymph node metastases in clinically unilateral stage I invasive epithelial ovarian carcinoma. *Gynecol Oncol* 2001;80:56.

Castaldo TW, Petrilli ES, Ballon SC, et al. Intestinal operations in patients with ovarian carcinoma. *Am J Obstet Gynecol* 1981;139:80.

Chambers S, Chambers J, Kohorn E, et al. Evaluation of the role of second-look surgery in ovarian cancer. *Obstet Gynecol* 1988;72:404.

Chan JK, Munro EG, Cheung MK, et al. Association of lymphadenectomy and survival in stage I ovarian cancer patients. *Obstet Gynecol* 2007;109(1):12–19.

Chang J, Fryatt I, Ponder B, et al. A matched control study of familial epithelial ovarian cancer: patient characteristics, response to chemotherapy and outcome. *Ann Oncol* 1995;6:80.

Chen SS, Bochner R. Assessment of morbidity and mortality in primary cytoreductive surgery for advanced ovarian carcinoma. *Gynecol Oncol* 1985;20:190.

Chen SS, Lee L. Incidence of paraaortic and pelvic lymph node metastases in epithelial carcinoma of the ovary. *Gynecol Oncol* 1983;15:95.

Chi DS, Abu-Rustum NR, Sonoda Y, et al. The safety and efficacy of laparoscopic surgical staging of apparent stage I ovarian and fallopian tube cancers. *Am J Obstet Gynecol* 2005;192:1614.

Chi DS, Eisenhauer EL, Lang J, et al. What is the optimal goal of primary cytoreductive surgery for bulky stage IIIC epithelial ovarian carcinoma (EOC)? *Gynecol Oncol* 2006;103(2):559–564.

Chi DS, McCaughty K, Diaz JP, et al. Guidelines and selection criteria for secondary cytoreductive surgery in patients with recurrent, platinum-sensitive epithelial ovarian carcinoma. *Cancer* 2006;106:1933.

Chi DS, Phaëton R, Miner TJ, et al. A prospective outcomes analysis of palliative procedures performed for malignant intestinal obstruction due to recurrent ovarian cancer. *Oncologist* 2009;14(8):835–839.

Clarke-Pearson D, Bandy L, Dudzinski M, et al. Computed tomography in evaluation of patients with ovarian carcinoma in complete clinical remission: correlation with surgical-pathologic findings. *JAMA* 1986;255:627.

Clarke-Pearson DL, Chin NO, DeLong ER, et al. Surgical management of intestinal obstruction in ovarian cancer. *Gynecol Oncol* 1987;26:11.

Clarke-Pearson DL, DeLong ER, Chin NE, et al. Surgical management of intestinal obstruction in ovarian cancer. II. Analysis of factors associated with complications and survival. *Arch Surg* 1988;123:42.

Clayton RD, Obermair A, Hammond IG, et al. The western Australian experience of the use of en bloc resection of ovarian cancer with concomitant rectosigmoid colectomy. *Gynecol Oncol* 2002;84:53.

Cook LS, Kamb ML, Weiss NS. Perineal powder exposure and risk of ovarian cancer. *Am J Epidemiol* 1997;145:459.

Copeland L, Gershenson DM. Ovarian cancer recurrences in patients with no macroscopic tumor at second-look laparotomy. *Obstet Gynecol* 1986;68:873.

Copeland L, Gershenson D, Wharton JT, et al. Microscopic disease at second-look laparotomy in advanced ovarian cancer. *Cancer* 1985;55:472.

Cramer DW, Welch WR. Determinants of ovarian cancer. Risk II. Inferences regarding pathogenesis. *J Natl Cancer Inst* 1983;71:717.

Creasman WT, Rutledge F. The prognostic value of peritoneal cytology in gynecologic malignant disease. *Am J Obstet Gynecol* 1971; 110:773.

Curtin JP, Malik R, Venkatraman ES, et al. Stage IV ovarian cancer: impact of surgical debulking. *Gynecol Oncol* 1997;64:9.

Cushing B, Giller R, Ablin A, et al. Surgical resection alone is effective treatment for ovarian immature teratoma in children and adolescents: a report of the Pediatric Oncology Group and the Children's Cancer Group. *Am J Obstet Gynecol* 1999;181:353–358.

Dark GG, Bower M, Newlands ES, et al. Surveillance policy for stage I ovarian germ cell tumors. *J Clin Oncol* 1997;15:620.

Dembo AJ, Davy D, Stenwig AE, et al. Prognostic factors in patients with stage I epithelial ovarian cancer. *Obstet Gynecol* 1990;75:263.

Deppe G, Malviya VK, Malone JM, et al. Debulking of pelvic and paraaortic lymph node metastases in ovarian cancer with the Cavitron ultrasonic surgical aspirator. *Obstet Gynecol* 1990;76:1140.

Deppe G, Zbella EA, Skogerson K, et al. The rare indication for splenectomy as part of cytoreductive surgery in ovarian cancer. *Gynecol Oncol* 1983;16:282.

DePriest DP, Banks ER, Powell DE, et al. Endometrioid carcinoma of the ovary and endometriosis: the association in postmenopausal women. *Gynecol Oncol* 1992;47:71.

DePriest P, Shenson D, Fried A, et al. Evaluation of CA-125 levels in differentiating malignant from benign tumors in patients with pelvic masses. *Obstet Gynecol* 1988;72:23.

DePriest P, Shenson D, Fried A, et al. A morphologic index based on sonographic findings in ovarian cancer. *Gynecol Oncol* 1993;51:7.

Di-Xia C, Schwartz PE, Xinguo L, et al. Evaluation of CA-125 levels in differentiating malignant from benign tumors in patients with pelvic masses. *Obstet Gynecol* 1988;72:23.

DuBois A, Lueck HJ, Meier W, et al. A randomized clinical trial of cisplatin/paclitaxel versus carboplatin/paclitaxel as first-line treatment of ovarian cancer. *J Natl Cancer Inst* 2003;95:1320.

Earle CC, Schrag D, Neville BA, et al. Effect of surgeon specialty on processes of care and outcomes for ovarian cancer patients. *J Natl Cancer Inst* 2006;98:172.

Easton DR, Bishop DT, Ford D. Genetic linkage analysis in familial breast and ovarian cancer: results in 214 families. The Breast Cancer Linkage Consortium. *Am J Hum Genet* 1993;52:678.

Einhorn N, Sjovak K, Knapp RC, et al. Prospective evaluations of serum CA-125 levels for early detection of ovarian cancer. *Obstet Gynecol* 1992;8:14.

Eisenhauer EL, Abu-Rustum NR, Sonoda Y, et al. The addition of extensive upper abdominal surgery to achieve optimal cytoreduction improves survival in patients with stages IIIC-IV epithelial ovarian cancer. *Gynecol Oncol* 2006;103:1083.

Eisenkop SM, Friedman RL, Wang H-J. Secondary cytoreductive surgery for recurrent ovarian cancer. *Cancer* 1995;76:1606.

Eisenkop SM, Spirtos NM. The clinical significance of occult macroscopically positive retroperitoneal nodes in patients with epithelial ovarian cancer. *Gynecol Oncol* 2001;82:143.

Fagotti A, Fanfani F, Ludovisi M, et al. Role of laparoscopy to assess the chance of optimal cytoreductive surgery in advanced ovarian cancer: a pilot study. *Gynecol Oncol* 2005;96:729.

Farley J, Brady WE, Vathipadiekal V, et al. Selumetinib in women with recurrent low-grade serous carcinoma of the ovary or peritoneum: an open-label, single-arm, phase 2 study. *Lancet* 2013;14:134–140.

Fathalla MF. Incessant ovulation: a factor in ovarian neoplasia? [Letter]. *Lancet* 1971;2:163.

Ferlay J, Bray P, Pisani P, et al. *Globocan 2002: cancer incidence mortality and prevalence worldwide.* IARC Cancer Base No. 5. Lyon, France: IARC Press, 2004.

Fiorica JV, Hoffman MS, LaPolla JP, et al. The management of diaphragmatic lesions in ovarian carcinoma. *Obstet Gynecol* 1989;74:927.

Fleischer AC, Cullinan JA, Kepple DM, et al. Conventional and color Doppler transvaginal sonography of pelvic masses: a comparison of relative histologic specificities. *J Ultrasound Med* 1993;12:705.

Ford D, Easton DF. The genetics of breast and ovarian cancer. *Br J Cancer* 1995;72:805.

Ford D, Easton DF, Stratton M, et al. Genetic heterogeneity and penetrance analysis of the BRCA1 and BRCA2 genes in breast cancer families. The Breast Cancer Linkage Consortium. *Am J Hum Genet* 1998;62:676.

Fotopoulou C, Zang R, Gultekin M, et al. Value of tertiary cytoreductive surgery in epithelial ovarian cancer: an international multicenter evaluation. *Ann Surg Oncol* 2013;20(4):1348–1354.

Friedman J, Weiss N. Second thoughts about second-look laparotomy in advanced ovarian cancer. *N Engl J Med* 1990;322:1079.

Gadducci A, Iacconi P, Cosio S, et al. Complete salvage surgical cytoreduction improves further survival of patients with late recurrent ovarian cancer. *Gynecol Oncol* 2000;79:344.

Gershenson DM. Conservative management of ovarian cancer. *Curr Probl Obstet Gynecol Fertil* 1994;27:165.

Gershenson DM. Management of early ovarian cancer: germ cell and sex cord-stromal tumors. *Gynecol Oncol* 1994;55:S62.

Gershenson DM. Update on malignant ovarian germ cell tumors. *Cancer* 1993;71:1581.

Gershenson DM, Copeland L, Del Junco G, et al. Second-look laparotomy in the management of malignant germ cell tumors of the ovary. *Obstet Gynecol* 1986;67:789.

Gershenson D, Copeland L, Wharton JT, et al. Prognosis of surgically determined complete responders in advanced ovarian cancer. *Cancer* 1985;55:1129.

Gershenson DM, Morris M, Burke TW, et al. Treatment of poor-prognosis sex cord-stromal tumors of the ovary with the combination of bleomycin, etoposide, and cis-platinum. *Obstet Gynecol* 1996;87:527.

Gershenson DM, Morris M, Cangir A, et al. Treatment of malignant germ cell tumors of the ovary with bleomycin, etoposide, and cis-platin. *J Clin Oncol* 1990;8:715.

Gershenson DM, Silva EG. Serous ovarian tumors of low malignant potential with peritoneal implants. *Cancer* 1990;65:578.

Gershenson DM, Silva EG, Levy L, et al. Ovarian serous borderline tumors with invasive peritoneal implants. *Cancer* 1998;82:1096.

Gershenson DM, Silva EG, Tortolero-Luna G, et al. Serous borderline tumors of the ovary with noninvasive peritoneal implants. *Cancer* 1998;83:2157.

Gertig DM, Hunter DJ, Cramer DW, et al. Ovarian carcinoma diagnosis: results of a national ovarian cancer survey. *Cancer* 2000;89:2068.

Gertig DM, Hunter DJ, Cramer DW, et al. Prospective study of talc use and ovarian cancer. *J Natl Cancer Inst* 2000;92:249.

Goff, BA, Mandel L, Muntz H, et al. Ovarian carcinoma diagnosis: results of a National Ovarian Cancer Survey. *Cancer* 2000;89:2068.

Goff BA, Matthews BJ, Wynn M, et al. Ovarian cancer: patterns of surgical care across the United States. *Gynecol Oncol* 2006;103:383.

Goldie JH, Coldman AJ. A mathematical model for relating the drug sensitivity of tumors to their spontaneous mutation rate. *Cancer Treat Rep* 1979;63:1727.

Gonzalez-Martin AJ, Calvo E, Bover I, et al. Randomized phase II trial of carboplatin versus paclitaxel and carboplatin in platinum-sensitive recurrent advanced ovarian carcinoma: a GEICO (Grupo Espanol de Investigacion en Cancer de Ovario) study. *Ann Oncol* 2005;16(5):749–755.

Greenlee RT, Murray T, Bolden S, et al. Cancer statistics 2000. *Cancer* 2000;50:7.

Griffiths CT, Parker LM, Fuller AF. Role of cytoreductive surgical treatment in the management of advanced ovarian cancer. *Cancer Treat Rep* 1979;63:235.

Gungor M, Ortac F, Arvas M, et al. The role of secondary cytoreductive surgery for recurrent ovarian cancer. *Gynecol Oncol* 2005;97:74.

Hacker NF, Berek JS, Lagasse LD, et al. Primary cytoreductive surgery for epithelial ovarian cancer. *Obstet Gynecol* 1983;61:413.

Hankinson SE. Prospective study of talc use and ovarian cancer. *J Natl Cancer Inst* 2000;92:249.

Hankinson SE, Colditz GA, Hunter DJ, et al. A quantitative assessment of oral contraceptive use and risk of ovarian cancer. *Obstet Gynecol* 1992;180:708.

Harlan LC, Clegg LX, Trimble EL. Trends in surgery and chemotherapy for women diagnosed with ovarian cancer in the United States. *J Clin Oncol* 2003;21:3488.

Hart WR, Norris HJ. Borderline and malignant mucinous tumors of the ovary: histologic criteria and clinical behavior. *Cancer* 1973;31:1031.

Harter P, du Bois A, Hahmann M, et al. Surgery in recurrent ovarian cancer: the Arbeitsgemeinschaft Gynaekologische OnKologie (AGO) DESKTOP OVAR trial. *Ann Surg Oncol* 2006;13:1702.

Hartge P, Hoover R, McGowan L, et al. Menopause and ovarian cancer. *Am J Epidemiol* 1988;127:990.

Heintz APM, Hacker NF, Berek JS, et al. Cytoreductive surgery in ovarian carcinoma: feasibility and morbidity. *Obstet Gynecol* 1986;67:783.

Henriksen R, Runa K, Wilander E, et al. Expression and prognostic significance of platelet-derived growth factor and its receptors in epithelial ovarian neoplasms. *Cancer Res* 1993;53:4550.

Ho AG, Beller U, Speyer J, et al. A reassessment of the role of second-look laparotomy in advanced ovarian cancer. *J Clin Oncol* 1987;5:1316.

Homesley HD, Bundy BN, Hurteau JA, et al. Bleomycin, etoposide, and cis-platinum combination therapy of ovarian granulosa cell tumors and other stromal malignancies: a Gynecologic Oncology Group study. *Gynecol Oncol* 1999;72:131.

Hoskins W, Bundy B, Thigpen J, et al. The influence of initial surgery on progression-free interval (PFI) and survival (S) in optimal (<1 cm) stage III epithelial ovarian cancer (EOC). Society of Gynecologic Oncologist Abstract. *Gynecol Oncol* 1992;45:76.

Hoskins WJ, Rubin SC, Dulaney E, et al. Influence of secondary cytoreduction at the time of second-look laparotomy on the survival of patients with epithelial ovarian carcinoma. *Gynecol Oncol* 1989;34:365.

Hunter J, Andrews S, van Nagell JR. Efficacy of a sonographic morphology index in identifying ovarian cancer: a multi-institutional investigation. *Gynecol Oncol* 1994;55:174.

Inciura A, Simavisius A, Juozaityte E, et al. Comparison of adjuvant and neoadjuvant chemotherapy in the management of advanced ovarian cancer: a retrospective study of 574 patients. *BMC Cancer* 2006;6:153.

International Collaborative Ovarian Neoplasm (ICON) Group. Paclitaxel plus carboplatin versus standard chemotherapy with either single-agent carboplatin or cyclophosphamide, doxorubicin, and cisplatin in women with ovarian cancer: the ICON3 randomized trial. *Lancet* 2002;360:505.

International Collaborative Ovarian Neoplasm 1 (ICON1) and European Organisation for Research and Treatment of Cancer Collaborators-Adjuvant Chemotherapy in Ovarian Neoplasms (EORTC-ACTION). International Collaborative Ovarian Neoplasm Trial 1 and Adjuvant Chemotherapy in Ovarian Neoplasm Trial: Two parallel randomized phase III trials of adjuvant chemotherapy in patients with early-stage ovarian carcinoma. *J Natl Cancer Inst* 2003;95:105.

International Federation of Gynecology and Obstetrics. FIGO staging for carcinoma of the ovary. In: Pecorelli S, ed. *Annual report on the results of treatment in gynecological cancer,* 24th ed. Milan, Italy: *J Epidemiol Biostat* (Italy) 2001;6(2).

International Federation of Gynecology and Obstetrics. FIGO staging for carcinoma of the ovary. In: Pettersson F, ed. *Annual report on the results of treatment in gynecological cancer,* 22nd ed. Stockholm, Sweden, 1997.

Jacob J, Gershenson DM, Morris M, et al. Neoadjuvant chemotherapy and interval debulking for advanced epithelial ovarian cancer. *Gynecol Oncol* 1991;42:146.

Jacobs I, Bast RC. The CA-125 tumour-associated antigen: a review of the literature. *Hum Reprod* 1989;4:1.

IX

Jacobs I, Davies AP, Bridges J, et al. Prevalence screening for ovarian cancer in postmenopausal women by CA-125 measurement and ultrasonography. *Br Med J* 1993;306:1030.

Janicke F, Holscher M, Kuhn W, et al. Radical surgical procedure improves survival time in patients with recurrent ovarian cancer. *Cancer* 1992;70:2129.

Joyeux H, Szawlowski A, Saint-Aubert B, et al. Aggressive regional surgery for advanced ovarian carcinoma. *Cancer* 1986;57:142.

Kapnick SJ, Griffiths CG, Finkler NJ. Occult pleural involvement in stage III ovarian carcinoma: role of diaphragm resection. *Gynecol Oncol* 1990;39:135.

Karam AK, Santillan A, Bristow RE, et al. Tertiary cytoreductive surgery in recurrent ovarian cancer: selection criteria and survival outcome. *Gynecol Oncol* 2007;104(2):377–380.

Katsumata N, Yasuda M, Takahashi F, et al. Dose-dense paclitaxel once a week in combination with carboplatin every 3 weeks for advanced ovarian cancer: a phase 3, open-label, randomised controlled trial. *Lancet* 2009;374:1331–1338.

Kaunitz AM. Oral contraceptive health benefits: perception versus reality. *Contraception* 1999;91:1131.

Kawai M, Kano K, Kikkawa F, et al. Transvaginal Doppler ultrasound with color flow imaging in the diagnosis of ovarian cancer. *Obstet Gynecol* 1992;79:163.

Kaye SB, Lubinski J, Matulonis U, et al. Phase II, open-label, randomized, multicenter study comparing the efficacy and safety of olaparib, a poly (ADP-ribose) polymerase inhibitor, and pegylated liposomal doxorubicin in patients with BRCA1 or BRCA2 mutations and recurrent ovarian cancer. *J Clin Oncol* 2012;30(4):372–379.

Kerlikowske K, Brown JS, Grady DG. Should women with familial ovarian cancer undergo prophylactic oophorectomy? *Obstet Gynecol* 1992;80:700.

Knapp RC, Friedman EA. Aortic lymph node metastases in early ovarian cancer. *Am J Obstet Gynecol* 1974;119:1013.

Koch M, Gaedke H, Jenkins H. Family history of ovarian cancer patients: a case control study. *Int J Epidemiol* 1989;18:782.

Kohler MF, Kerns BM, Humphrey PA, et al. Mutation and overexpression of p53 in early-stage epithelial ovarian cancer. *Obstet Gynecol* 1993;81:643.

Krebs HB, Goplerud DR. The role of intestinal intubation in obstruction of the small intestine due to carcinoma of the ovary. *Surg Gynecol Obstet* 1984;158:467.

Krebs HB, Goplerud DR. Surgical management of bowel obstruction in advanced ovarian carcinoma. *Obstet Gynecol* 1983;61:327.

Kryscio RJ. The efficacy of transvaginal sonographic screening in asymptomatic women at risk for ovarian cancer. *Gynecol Oncol* 2000;77:350.

Kryscio RJ, van Nagell JR. A morphologic index based on sonographic findings in ovarian cancer. *Gynecol Oncol* 1993;51:7.

Kurjak A, Kupesic S, Anic T, et al. Three dimensional ultrasound and power Doppler improve the diagnosis of ovarian lesions. *Gynecol Oncol* 2000;76:28.

Kurjak A, Predanic M. New scoring system for prediction of ovarian malignancy based on transvaginal color Doppler sonography. *J Ultrasound Med* 1992;11:631.

Kurjak A, Schulman H, Zalud I, et al. Transvaginal ultrasound color flow and Doppler waveform of the postmenopausal adnexal mass. *Obstet Gynecol* 1992;80:917.

Larson JE, Podczaski ES, Manetta A, et al. Bowel obstruction in patients with ovarian carcinoma: analysis of prognostic factors. *Gynecol Oncol* 1989;35:61.

Lawton FG, Luesley D, Redman C, et al. Feasibility and outcome of complete secondary tumor resection for patients with advanced ovarian cancer. *J Surg Oncol* 1990;45:14.

LeBlanc E, Querleu D, Narducci F, et al. Laparoscopic staging of early stage invasive adnexal tumors: a 10-year experience. *Gynecol Oncol* 2004;94:624.

Lecuru F, Desfeux P, Camatte S, et al. Impact of initial surgical access on staging and survival of patients with stage I ovarian cancer. *Int J Gynecol Cancer* 2006;16:87.

Ledermann J, Harter P, Gourley C, et al. Olaparib maintenance therapy in platinum-sensitive relapsed ovarian cancer. *N Engl J Med* 2012;366(15):1382–1392.

Leitao MM Jr, Kardos S, Barakat RR, et al. Tertiary cytoreduction in patients with recurrent ovarian carcinoma. *Gynecol Oncol* 2004;95(1):181–188.

Lele S, Piver MS. Interval laparoscopy as predictor of response to chemotherapy in ovarian carcinoma. *Obstet Gynecol* 1986;68:345.

Lesieur B, Kane A, Duvillard P, et al. Prognostic value of lymph node involvement in ovarian serous borderline tumors. *Am J Obstet Gynecol* 2011;204(5):438.e1–438.e7.

Levine D, Gossink B, Wolf SI, et al. Simple adnexal cysts: the natural history in postmenopausal women. *Radiology* 1992;184:653.

Lewis MR, Deavers MT, Silva EG, et al. Ovarian involvement by metastatic colorectal adenocarcinoma. *Am J Surg Pathol* 2006; 30:177.

Li A, Otero F, Funowica CD, et al. Pattern of lymph node metastases in apparent Stage IA invasive epithelial ovarian carcinomas. *Gynecol Oncol* 2000;76:239.

Liotta L, Kohn E, Pertricoin E. Clinical proteomics: personalized molecular medicine. *JAMA* 2001;286:2211.

Liu PC, Benjamin I, Morgan MA, et al. Effect of surgical debulking on survival in stage IV ovarian cancer. *Gynecol Oncol* 1997;64:4.

Low JJH, Perrin LC, Crandon J, et al. Conservative surgery to preserve ovarian function in patients with malignant ovarian germ cell tumors: a review of 74 cases. *Cancer* 2000;89:391.

Lu JL, Zheng Y, Yuan J, et al. Decreased luteinizing hormone receptor in RNA expression in human ovarian epithelial cancer. *Gynecol Oncol* 2000;79:158.

Luesley D, Chan K, Lawton F, et al. Survival after negative second-look laparotomy. *Eur J Surg Oncol* 1989;15:205.

Lund B, Jaconsen K, Rasch L, et al. Correlation of abdominal ultrasound and computed tomography scans with second- or third-look laparotomy in patients with ovarian carcinoma. *Gynecol Oncol* 1990;37:279.

Lund B, Williamson P. Prognostic factors for outcome of and survival after second-look laparotomy in patients with advanced ovarian carcinoma. *Obstet Gynecol* 1990;76:617.

Lynch HT, Harris RE, Guirgis HA, et al. Familial association of breast/ovarian carcinoma. *Cancer* 1978;41:1543.

Lynch HT, Lemon SJ, Karr B. Etiology natural history, management and molecular genetics of hereditary non-polyposis colorectal cancer (Lynch syndromes). *Cancer Epidemiol Biomarkers Prev* 1977;6:978.

Lynch HT, Watson P, Bewtra C. Hereditary ovarian cancer: heterogeneity in age at diagnosis. *Cancer* 1991;67:1460.

Magrina JF, Zanagnolo V, Noble BN, et al. Robotic approach for ovarian cancer: perioperative and survival results and comparison with laparoscopy and laparotomy. *Gynecol Oncol* 2011; 121(1):100–105.

Magtibay PM, Adams PB, Silverman MB, et al. Splenectomy as part of cytoreductive surgery in ovarian cancer. *Gynecol Oncol* 2006;102(2):369–374.

Malfetano JH. Splenectomy for optimal cytoreduction in ovarian cancer. *Gynecol Oncol* 1986;24:392.

Malkasian GD, Knapp RC, Zurawaski VR, et al. Preoperative evaluation of serum CA-125 levels in premenopausal and postmenopausal patients with pelvic masses: discrimination from malignant disease. *Am J Obstet Gynecol* 1988;159:341.

Malone JM, Koonce T, Larson DM, et al. Palliation of small bowel obstruction by percutaneous gastrostomy in patients with progressive ovarian carcinoma. *Obstet Gynecol* 1986;68:431.

Malpica A, Deavers M, Lu K, et al. Grading ovarian serous carcinoma using a two-tier system. *Am J Surg Pathol* 2004;28(4):496.

Mangili G, Scarfone G, Gadducci A, et al. Is adjuvant chemotherapy indicated in stage I pure immature ovarian teratoma (IT)? A multicentre Italian trial in ovarian cancer (MITO-9). *Gynecol Oncol* 2010;119:48–52.

Mann W, Patsner B, Cohen H, et al. Preoperative serum CA-125 levels in patients with surgical stage I invasive ovarian adenocarcinoma. *J Natl Cancer Inst* 1988;80:208.

Mannel RS, Brady MF, Kohn EC, et al. A randomized phase III trial of IV carboplatin and paclitaxel x 3 courses followed by observation versus weekly maintenance low-dose paclitaxel in patients with early-stage ovarian carcinoma: a Gynecologic Oncology Group study. *Gynecol Oncol* 2011;122:89–94.

Marina NM, Cushing B, Giller R, et al. Complete surgical excision is effective treatment for children with immature teratomas with or without malignant elements: a Pediatric Oncology Group/Children's Cancer Group intergroup study. *J Clin Oncol* 1999;17:2137.

Markman M, Bundy B, Alberts DS, et al. Phase III trial of standard-dose intravenous cisplatin plus paclitaxel versus moderately high-dose carboplatin followed by intravenous paclitaxel and intraperitoneal cisplatin in small-volume stage III ovarian carcinoma: an intergroup study of the Gynecologic Oncology Group, Southwestern Oncology Group, and Eastern Cooperative Oncology Group. *J Clin Oncol* 2001;19:1001.

Markman M, Liu PY, Wilczynski M, et al. Phase III randomized trial of 12 versus 3 months of maintenance paclitaxel in patients with advanced ovarian cancer after complete response to platinum and paclitaxel-based chemotherapy: A Southwest Oncology Group and Gynecologic Oncology Group Trial. *J Clin Oncol* 2003;21:2460–2465.

Marret H, Saugnet S, Giraudeau B, et al. Contrast-enhanced sonography helps in discrimination of benign from malignant adnexal masses. *J Ultrasound Med* 2004;23:1629.

Mazzeo F, Berliere M, Kerger J, et al. Neoadjuvant chemotherapy followed by surgery and adjuvant chemotherapy in patients with primarily unresectable, advanced-stage ovarian cancer. *Gynecol Oncol* 2003;90:163.

McGowan L, Lesher LP, Norris HJ, et al. Misstaging of ovarian cancer. *Obstet Gynecol* 1985;65:568.

McGuire WP, Hoskins WJ, Brady MF, et al. Cyclophosphamide and cis-platinum compared with paclitaxel and cisplatin in patients with stage III and stage IV ovarian cancer. *N Engl J Med* 1996;334:1.

McMahill HL, Calle EE, Koskinski AS, et al. Tubal ligation and fatal ovarian cancer in a large prospective cohort study. *Am J Epidemiol* 1997;145:349.

Miki Y, Swensen J, Shattuck-Eidens D, et al. A strong candidate for the breast ovarian cancer susceptibility gene BRCA1. *Science* 1994;266:66.

Miller D, Ballon S, Teng N, et al. A critical reassessment of second-look laparotomy in epithelial ovarian carcinoma. *Cancer* 1986;57:530.

Mitchell PL, Al-Nasiri N, A'Hern R, et al. Treatment of nondysgerminomatous ovarian germ cell tumors: An analysis of 69 cases. *Cancer* 1999;85:2232–2244.

Modesitt SC, Pavlik EJ, Ueland FR, et al. Risk of malignancy in unilocular ovarian cystic tumors less than 10 cm in diameter. *Obstet Gynecol* 2003;102:594.

Monga M, Carmichael JA, Shelley WE, et al. Surgery without adjuvant chemotherapy for early epithelial ovarian carcinoma after comprehensive surgical staging. *Gynecol Oncol* 1992;43:195.

Montz FJ, Schlaerth JB, Berek JS. Resection of diaphragmatic peritoneum and muscle: role in cytoreductive surgery for ovarian cancer. *Gynecol Oncol* 1989;35:338.

Morice P, Dubernard G, Rey A, et al. Results of interval debulking surgery compared with primary debulking surgery in advanced stage ovarian cancer. *J Am Coll Surg* 2003;197:955.

Morice P, Joulie F, Camatte S, et al. Lymph node involvement in epithelial ovarian cancer: analysis of 276 pelvic and paraaortic lymphadenectomies and surgical implications. *J Am Coll Surg* 2003;197:198.

Morice P, Wicart-Poque F, Rey A, et al. Results of conservative treatment in epithelial ovarian carcinoma. *Cancer* 2001;92:2412.

Morris M, Gershenson DM, Burke TW, et al. Splenectomy in gynecologic oncology: indications, complications, and technique. *Gynecol Oncol* 1991;43:118.

Morris RT, Gershenson DM, Silva EG, et al. Outcome and reproductive function after conservative surgery for borderline ovarian tumors. *Obstet Gynecol* 2000;95:541.

Morris M, Gershenson DM, Wharton JT. Secondary cytoreductive surgery in epithelial ovarian cancer: nonresponders to first-line therapy. *Gynecol Oncol* 1989;33:1.

Morris M, Gershenson DM, Wharton JT, et al. Secondary cytoreductive surgery for recurrent epithelial ovarian cancer. *Gynecol Oncol* 1989;34:334.

Morrow CP. An opinion in support of second-look surgery in ovarian cancer [Editorial]. *Gynecol Oncol* 2000;79:341.

Muggia FM, Braly PS, Brady MF, et al. Phase III randomized study of cis-platinum versus paclitaxel versus cis-platinum and paclitaxel in patients with suboptimal stage III or IV ovarian cancer: a Gynecologic Oncology Group study. *J Clin Oncol* 2000;18:106.

Munkarah AR, Hallum AV, Morris M, et al. Prognostic significance of residual disease in patients with stage IV epithelial ovarian cancer. *Gynecol Oncol* 1997;64:13.

Munkarah A, Levenback C, Wolf JK, et al. Secondary cytoreductive surgery for localized intra-abdominal recurrences in epithelial ovarian cancer. *Gynecol Oncol* 2001;81:237.

Muñoz KA, Harlan LC, Trimble EL. Patterns of care for women with ovarian cancer in the United States. *J Clin Oncol* 1997;15:3408.

Nelson BE, Rosenfeld AT, Schwartz PE. Preoperative abdominopelvic computed tomographic prediction of optimal cytoreduction in epithelial ovarian carcinoma. *J Clin Oncol* 1993;11:166.

Nelson HD, Huffman LH, Rongwei F, et al. Genetic risk assessment and BRCA mutation testing for breast and ovarian cancer susceptibility: systematic evidence review for the U.S. Preventive Services Task Force. *Ann Intern Med* 2005;143:362.

Onda T, Yoshikawa H, Yokota H, et al. Assessment of metastases to aortic and pelvic lymph nodes in epithelial ovarian carcinoma. *Cancer* 1996;78:803.

Ozols RF, Bundy BN, Greer BE, et al. Phase III trial of carboplatin and paclitaxel compared with cisplatin and paclitaxel in patients with optimally resected stage III ovarian cancer: a Gynecologic Oncology Group study. *J Clin Oncol* 2003;21:3194.

Parazzini F, Negri E, LaVecchia C, et al. Family history of reproductive cancers and ovarian cancer risk: an Italian case–control study. *Am J Epidemiol* 1992;135:35.

Park J-Y, Seo S-S, Kang S, et al. The benefits of low anterior en bloc resection as part of cytoreductive surgery for advanced primary and recurrent epithelial ovarian cancer patients outweigh morbidity concerns. *Gynecol Oncol* 2006;103:977.

Parmar MK, Ledermann JA, Colombo N, et al. Paclitaxel plus platinum-based chemotherapy versus conventional platinum-based chemotherapy in women with relapsed ovarian cancer: the ICON4/AGO-OVAR-2.2 trial. *Lancet* 2003;361:2099.

Partridge EE, Gunter B, Gelder M, et al. The validity and significance of substages in advanced ovarian carcinoma. *Gynecol Oncol* 1993;48:236.

Patterson DM, Murugaesu N, Holden L, et al. A review of the close surveillance policy for stage 1 female germ cell tumors of the ovary and other sites. *Int J Gynecol Cancer* 2008;18(1):43–50.

Pavlik EJ, DePriest PD, Gallion HH, et al. Ovarian volume related to age. *Gynecol Oncol* 2000;77:410.

Peiretti M, Bristow RE, Zapardiel IA, et al. Rectosigmoid resection at the time of primary cytoreduction for advanced ovarian cancer. A multi-center analysis of surgical and oncological outcomes. *Gynecol Oncol* 2012;126(2):220–223.

Perren TJ, Swart AM, Pfisterer J, et al. A phase 3 trial of bevacizumab in ovarian cancer. *N Engl J Med* 2011;365(26):2484–2496.

Petricoin EF, Ardekani AM, Hitt BA, et al. Use of proteomic patterns in serum to identify ovarian cancer. *Lancet* 2002;359:572.

Pfisterer J, Plante M, Vergote I, et al. Gemcitabine plus carboplatin compared with carboplatin in patients with platinum-sensitive recurrent ovarian cancer: an intergroup trial of the AGO-OVAR, the NCIC CTG, and the EORTC GCG. *J Clin Oncol* 2006;24(29):4699–4707.

Pfisterer J, Vergote I, Du Bois A, et al. Combination therapy with gemcitabine and carboplatin in recurrent ovarian cancer. *Int J Gynecol Cancer* 2005;15(suppl 1):36.

Piccart MJ, Bertelsen K, James K, et al. Randomized intergroup trial of cis-platinum-paclitaxel versus cis-platinum-cyclophosphamide in women with advanced epithelial ovarian cancer: three-year results. *J Natl Cancer Inst* 2000;92:699.

Plentl AA, Friedman EA. Lymphatics of the ovary. In: *Lymphatic system of the female genitalia*. Philadelphia, London, Toronto: Sanders, 1971:173.

Podratz K, Malkasian G, Hilton J, et al. Second-look laparotomy in ovarian cancer: evaluation of pathologic variables. *Am J Obstet Gynecol* 1985;152:230.

Podratz K, Malkasian G, Wieand H, et al. Recurrent disease after negative second-look laparotomy in stages III and IV ovarian carcinoma. *Gynecol Oncol* 1988;29:274.

IX

Podratz KC, Schwarz MF, Wieand HS, et al. Evaluation of treatment and survival after positive second-look laparotomy. *Gynecol Oncol* 1988;31:9.

Pothuri B, Vaidya A, Aghajanian C, et al. Palliative surgery for bowel obstruction in recurrent ovarian cancer:an updated series. *Gynecol Oncol* 2003;89:306–313.

Prat J; for the FIGO Committee on Gynecologic Oncology. Staging classification for cancer of the ovary, fallopian tube and peritoneum. *Int J Gynecol Obstet* 2014;124:1–5.

Pujade-Lauraine E, Wagner U, Aavall-Lundqvist E, et al. Pegylated liposomal Doxorubicin and Carboplatin compared with Paclitaxel and Carboplatin for patients with platinum-sensitive ovarian cancer in late relapse. *J Clin Oncol* 2010;28(20):3323–3329.

Puls LE, Powell DE, DePriest PD, et al. Transition from benign to malignant epithelium in mucinous and serous ovarian cystadenocarcinoma. *Gynecol Oncol* 1992;47:53.

Ramirez PT, Wolf JK, Levenback C. Laparoscopic port-site metastases: etiology and prevention. *Gynecol Oncol* 2003;91:179.

Ransohoff D. Lessons from controversy: ovarian cancer screening and serum proteomics. *J Natl Cancer Inst* 2005;97:315.

Reuter K, Griffin T, Hunter R. Comparison of abdominopelvic computed tomography results and findings at second-look laparotomy in ovarian carcinoma patients. *Cancer* 1989;63:1123.

Riman T, Dickman PW, Nilsson S, et al. Hormone replacement therapy and the risk of invasive epithelial ovarian cancer in Swedish women. *J Natl Cancer Inst* 2002;94:497.

Ripa R, Katballe N, Wikman FP, et al. Presymptomatic diagnosis using a deletion of a single codon in families with hereditary nonpolyposis colorectal cancer. *Mutat Res* 2005;570:89.

Risch HA. Hormonal etiology of epithelial ovarian cancer, with a hypothesis concerning the role of androgens and progesterone. *J Natl Cancer Inst* 1998;90:1774.

Risch HA, Marrett LD, Howe GR. Parity, contraception, infertility, and the risk of epithelial ovarian cancer. *Am J Epidemiol* 1994;146:585.

Roberts W, Hodel K, Rich W, et al. Second-look laparotomy in the management of gynecologic malignancy. *Gynecol Oncol* 1982;13:345.

Roman LD, Muderspac LI, Stein SM, et al. Pelvic examination, tumor marker level and gray-scale and Doppler sonography in the prediction of pelvic cancer. *Obstet Gynecol* 1997;89:493.

Rose PG, Nerenstone S, Brady MF, et al. Secondary surgical cytoreduction for advanced ovarian carcinoma. *N Engl J Med* 2004;351:2489.

Rossing MA, Daling JR, Weiss NS, et al. Ovarian tumors in a cohort of infertile women. *N Engl J Med* 1994;331:771.

Rubin S, Hoskins W, Hakes T, et al. Recurrence after negative second-look laparotomy for ovarian cancer: analysis of risk factors. *Am J Obstet Gynecol* 1988;159:1094.

Rubin S, Hoskins W, Saigo P. Update on prognostic factors for recurrence following negative second-look laparotomy in ovarian cancer patients treated with platinum-based chemotherapy. *Gynecol Oncol* 1991;42:137.

Rubin SC, Hoskins WJ, Benjamin I, et al. Palliative surgery for intestinal obstruction in advanced ovarian cancer. *Gynecol Oncol* 1989;34:16.

Rubin SC, Wong GYC, Curtin JP, et al. Platinum-based chemotherapy of high-risk stage I epithelial ovarian cancer following comprehensive surgical staging. *Obstet Gynecol* 1993;82:143.

Rustin GJ, Marples M, Nelstrop AE, et al. Use of CA-125 to define progression of ovarian cancer in patients with persistently elevated levels. *J Clin Oncol* 2001;19(20):4054–4057.

Sakai K, Kamura T, Hirakawa T, et al. Relationship between pelvic lymph node involvement and other disease sites in patients with ovarian cancer. *Gynecol Oncol* 1997;65:164.

Sassone AM, Timor-Tritsch I, Artner A, et al. Transvaginal sonographic characterization of ovarian disease: evaluation of a new scoring system to predict ovarian malignancy. *Obstet Gynecol* 1991;78:70.

Scarabelli C, Gallo A, Carbone A, et al. Secondary cytoreductive surgery for patients with recurrent epithelial ovarian carcinoma. *Gynecol Oncol* 2001;83:504.

Scarabelli C, Gallo A, Zarrelli A, et al. Systematic pelvic and para-aortic lymphadenectomy during cytoreductive surgery in advanced ovarian cancer: potential benefit on survival. *Gynecol Oncol* 1995;56:328.

Schilder JM, Thompson AM, DePriest PD, et al. Outcome of reproductive age women with stage IA or IC invasive epithelial ovarian cancer treated with fertility-sparing surgery. *Gynecol Oncol* 2002;87:1.

Schildkraut JM, Thompson WD. Familial ovarian cancer: a population-based case control study. *Am J Epidemiol* 1988;128:456.

Schneider VL, Schneider A, Reed KL, et al. Comparison of Doppler with two dimensional sonography and CA-125 for prediction of malignancy of pelvic masses. *Obstet Gynecol* 1993;81:983.

Schmeler K, Lynch HT, Chen LM, et al. Prophylactic surgery to reduce the risk of gynecologic cancers in the Lynch syndrome. *N Engl J Med* 2006;354:261.

Schwartz PE, Rutherford TJ, Chambers JT, et al. Neoadjuvant chemotherapy for advanced ovarian cancer: long-term survival. *Gynecol Oncol* 1999;72:93.

Scully RE, Henson DE, Nielsen ML, et al. Ovary. Reporting on cancer specimens: protocols and case summaries. In: CAP Cancer Committee. *Cancer protocol manual*. 1998:1.

Scully RE, Hensen DE, Nielson ML, et al. Practice protocol for the examination of specimens removed from patients with ovarian tumors. *Arch Pathol Lab Med* 1995;199:1012.

Segna RA, Dottino PR, Mandeli JP, et al. Secondary cytoreduction for ovarian cancer following cis-platinum therapy. *J Clin Oncol* 1993;11:434.

Sevelda P, Dittrich C, Salzer H. Prognostic value of the rupture of the capsule in stage I epithelial ovarian carcinoma. *Gynecol Oncol* 1989;35:321.

Skates SJ, Feng J, Yin-Hua Y, et al. Toward an optimal algorithm for ovarian cancer screening with longitudinal tumor markers. *Cancer* 1995;76:2004.

Skates SJ, Manon U, MacDonald N, et al. Calculations of the risk of ovarian cancer from serial CA-125 values for preclinical detection in postmenopausal women. *J Clin Oncol* 2003;21:206s.

Smith LH, Morris CR, Yasmeen S, et al. Ovarian cancer: can we make the clinical diagnosis earlier? *Cancer* 2005;104:1398.

Sonnendecker EW, Guidozzi F, Margolius KA. Splenectomy during primary maximal cytoreductive surgery for epithelial ovarian cancer. *Gynecol Oncol* 1989;35:301.

Soper JT, Couchman G, Berchuck A, et al. The role of partial sigmoid colectomy for debulking epithelial ovarian carcinoma. *Gynecol Oncol* 1991;41:239.

Stehman F, Calkins A, Wass J, et al. A comparison of findings at second-look laparotomy with preoperative computed tomography in patients with ovarian cancer. *Gynecol Oncol* 1988;29:37.

Stein S, Laifer-Narin S, Johnson MB, et al. Differentiation of benign and malignant adnexal masses: relative value of gray scale, color Doppler and spectral Doppler sonography. *AJR Am J Roentgenol* 1995;164:381.

Surwit E, Childers J, Atlas I, et al. Neoadjuvant chemotherapy for advanced ovarian cancer. *Int J Gynecol Cancer* 1996;6:356.

Tangir J, Zelterman D, Ma W, et al. Reproductive function after conservative surgery and chemotherapy for malignant germ cell tumors of the ovary. *Obstet Gynecol* 2003;101:251.

Tanner EJ, Long KC, Feffer JB, et al. Parenchymal splenic metastasis is an independent negative predictor of overall survival in advanced ovarian, fallopian tube, and primary peritoneal cancer. *Gynecol Oncol* 2013;128(1):28–33.

Tay E-H, Grant PT, Gebski V, et al. Secondary cytoreductive surgery for recurrent epithelial ovarian cancer. *Obstet Gynecol* 2002;99:1008.

Taylor JWK, Ramas I, Carter D, et al. Correlation of Doppler US tumor signals with neovascular morphologic features. *Radiology* 1988;166:157.

Tazelaar HD, Bostwick DG, Ballon SC, et al. Conservative treatment of borderline ovarian tumors. *Obstet Gynecol* 1985;66:417.

Tinelli R, Tinelli A, Tinelli FG, et al. Conservative surgery for borderline ovarian tumors: a review. *Gynecol Oncol* 2006;100:185.

Tingulstad S, Skjeldestad FE, Hagen B. The effect of centralization of primary surgery on survival in ovarian cancer patients. *Obstet Gynecol* 2003;102:499.

Topuz E, Aydiner A, Saip P, et al. Correlations of serum CA125 level and computerized tomography (CT) imaging with laparotomic findings following intraperitoneal chemotherapy in patients with ovarian cancer. *Eur J Gynaecol Oncol* 2000;21(6):599–602.

IX

Tortolero-Luna G, Mitchell MF. The epidemiology of ovarian cancer. *J Cell Biochem Suppl* 1995;13:200.

Trimbos JB, Schueler JA, van Lent M, et al. Reasons for incomplete surgical staging in early ovarian carcinoma. *Gynecol Oncol* 1990;37:374.

Ueland FR, DePriest PD, DeSimone CP, et al. The accuracy of examination under anesthesia and transvaginal sonography in evaluating ovarian size. *Gynecol Oncol* 2005;99:400.

Ueland FR, DePriest PD, Pavlik EJ, et al. Preoperative differentiation of malignant from benign ovarian tumors: the efficacy of morphology indexing and Doppler flow sonography. *Gynecol Oncol* 2003;91:46.

Vacarello L, Rubin SC, Vlamis V, et al. Cytoreductive surgery in ovarian carcinoma patients with a documented previously complete surgical response. *Gynecol Oncol* 1995;57:61.

Valentin L, Sladkevicius P, Marsal K. Limited contribution of Doppler velocimetry to the differential diagnosis of extra-uterine pelvic tumors. *Obstet Gynecol* 1994;83:425.

Van der Burg MEL, van Lent M, Buyse M, et al. The effect of debulking surgery after induction chemotherapy: on the prognosis in advanced epithelial ovarian cancer. *N Engl J Med* 1995;332:629.

van Nagell JR, DePriest PD, Reedy MB, et al. The efficacy of transvaginal sonographic screening in asymptomatic women at risk for ovarian cancer. *Gynecol Oncol* 2000;77:350.

van Nagell JR, Higgins RV, Donaldson ES, et al. Transvaginal sonography as a screening method for ovarian cancer: a report of the first 1000 cases screened. *Cancer* 1990;65:573.

Vasey PA, Jayson GC, Gordon A, et al. Phase III randomized trial of docetaxel-carboplatin versus paclitaxel-carboplatin as first-line chemotherapy for ovarian carcinoma. *J Natl Cancer Inst* 2004;96:1682.

Vergote IB, Kaern J, Abeler VM, et al. Analysis of prognostic factors in stage I epithelial ovarian cancer: importance of degree of differentiation and deoxyribonucleic acid ploidy in predicting relapse. *Am J Obstet Gynecol* 1993;169:40.

Vergote I, Marquette S, Amant F, et al. Port-site metastases after open laparoscopy: a study in 173 patients with advanced ovarian cancer. *Int J Gynecol Cancer* 2005;15:776.

Vergote I, Trope CG, Amant F, et al. Neoadjuvant chemotherapy or primary surgery in stage IIIC or IV ovarian cancer. *N Engl J Med* 2010;363:943–953.

Vergote IB, Vergote-De Vos LN, Abeler VM, et al. Randomized trial comparing cis-platinum with radioactive phosphorus or whole-abdomen irradiation as adjuvant treatment of ovarian cancer. *Cancer* 1992;69:741.

Walker JL, Armstrong DK, Huang HQ, et al. Intraperitoneal catheter outcomes in a phase III trial of intravenous versus intraperitoneal chemotherapy in optimal stage III ovarian and primary peritoneal cancer: a Gynecologic Oncology Group study. *Gynecol Oncol* 2006;100:27.

Whittemore AS, Gong G, Itnyre J. Prevalence and contribution of BRCA1 mutations in breast cancer and ovarian cancer: results from three U.S. population-based case–control studies of ovarian cancer. *Am J Hum Genet* 1997;60:496.

Whittemore AS, Harris R, Itnyre J. Collaborative Ovarian Cancer Group: characteristics relating to ovarian cancer risk, collaborative analysis of 12 U.S. case–control studies. II. Invasive epithelial ovarian cancers in white women. *Am J Epidemiol* 1992;136:1184.

Williams S, Blessing JA, Liao S, et al. Adjuvant therapy of ovarian germ cell tumors with cisplatin, etoposide, and bleomycin: a trial of the Gynecologic Oncology Group. *J Clin Oncol* 1994;12:701.

Williams SD, Blessing JA, DiSaia PJ, et al. Second-look laparotomy in ovarian germ cell tumors: the Gynecologic Oncology Group experience. *Gynecol Oncol* 1994;52:287.

Wiltshaw E, Raju KS, Dawson I. The role of cytoreductive surgery in advanced carcinoma of the ovary: an analysis of primary and second surgery. *BJOG* 1985;92:522.

Woods CH, Thompson EA. Transvaginal sonography as a screening method for ovarian cancer: a report of the first 1000 cases screened. *Cancer* 1990;65:573.

Wooster R, Bignell G, Lancaster J, et al. Identification of the breast cancer susceptibility gene BRCA2. *Nature* 1995;378:789.

World Health Organization. Histological classification of ovarian tumours. In: Tavassoli FA, Devilee P, eds. *Pathology and genetics: Tumors of the breast and female genital organs*. London, UK: Oxford University Press, 2003:114.

World Health Organization. Histological classification of ovarian tumors. In: Scully RE, Young RH, Clement PB, eds. *Atlas of tumor pathology, tumors of the ovary, maldeveloped gonads, fallopian tube and broad ligament*. Bethesda, MD: AFIP, 1998:28.

Wu P-C, Qu J-Y, Lang J-H, et al. Lymph node metastasis of ovarian cancer: a preliminary survey of 74 cases of lymphadenectomy. *Am J Obstet Gynecol* 1986;155:1103.

Young RC. A second look at second-look laparotomy [Editorial]. *J Clin Oncol* 1987;5:1311.

Young RC, Brady MF, Nieberg RM, et al. A randomized phase III trial of intraperitoneal ^{32}P or intravenous cyclophosphamide and cisplatin: a Gynecologic Oncology Group study. *J Clin Oncol* 2003;21:4350.

Young RC, Walton LA, Ellenberg SS, et al. Adjuvant therapy in stage I and II epithelial ovarian cancer: results of two prospective randomized trials. *N Engl J Med* 1990;322:1021.

Zanetta G, Bonazzi C, Cantu MG, et al. Survival and reproductive function after treatment of malignant germ cell ovarian tumors. *J Clin Oncol* 2001;19:1015.

Zanetta G, Chiari S, Rota S, et al. Conservative surgery for stage I ovarian carcinoma in women of childbearing age. *BJOG* 1997; 104:1030.

Zang R-Y, Li Z-T, Tang J, et al. Secondary cytoreductive surgery for patients with relapsed epithelial ovarian carcinoma: who benefits? *Cancer* 2004;100:1152.

Zapardiel I, Peiretti M, Zanagnolo V, et al. Diaphragmatic surgery during primary cytoreduction for advanced ovarian cancer: peritoneal stripping versus diaphragmatic resection. *Int J Gynecol Cancer* 2011;21(9):1698–1703.

CHAPTER 54
Pelvic Exenteration

Mario M. Leitao Jr and Richard R. Barakat

DEFINITIONS

Total pelvic exenteration—Removal of all pelvic organs, often en bloc, including removal of the uterus (if present), cervix (if present), bilateral adnexa (if present), bladder, possibly urethra, rectum, and possibly anus. This can be done in either a supralevator or infralevator fashion (see later definitions).

Anterior pelvic exenteration—Similar to total pelvic exenteration except that the rectum and anus are not removed. Additionally, the posterior aspect of the vagina may also be left in place.

Posterior pelvic exenteration—Similar to total pelvic exenteration except that the bladder and urethra are not removed. Additionally, the anterior aspect of the vagina may also be left in place.

Supralevator exenteration—Any of the above (total, anterior, or posterior) but the dissection and resection are limited to the pelvic contents above the levator muscles of the pelvis.

Translevator exenteration—Any of the above (total, anterior, or posterior) and the dissection and resection involve resection of a portion of the levator muscles with the contents traversing these muscles and including portions of the labia minora, and occasionally the labia majora, as well as surrounding tissues.

Wet colostomy—An end colostomy with the ureters placed into the colostomy resulting in drainage of both stool and urine. This is an old practice that was abandoned, but it has resurfaced with a recent modification.

IX

Noncontinent urinary conduit—A constant drainage system for the urinary stream most often involving insertion of the ureters into a portion of isolated small intestine that is then brought out to the abdomen.

Continent urinary conduit—A urinary drainage system in which the patient ultimately will self-catheterize and avoid a bag for constant drainage. Various types of these conduits exist.

INTRODUCTION

Dr. Alexander Brunschwig was the first to report on the complete excision of pelvic viscera for advanced cancer (i.e., pelvic exenteration) in 1948. He described this procedure as "the most radical surgical attack so far described for pelvic cancer and also [what] would appear to be the most radical of abdominal operations that have been carried out with some measure of consistency." The first operation was performed on December 12, 1946, at Memorial Hospital, which eventually became Memorial Sloan Kettering Cancer Center, in New York. Figures 54.1 and 54.2 are diagrams from Brunschwig's manuscript. This manuscript included 22 cases, 15 of which were recurrent cervical cancers, and follow-up was very short (maximum follow-up was 8 months). There were 5 (23%) perioperative mortalities and a total of 9 (41%) deaths within 8 months. Subsequent reports from the same institution of the same procedure in patients with ovarian and endometrial cancers described 5-year overall survival (OS) of 7% and 14%, respectively, with morbidities of over 60% and perioperative mortalities of 23%. In 1989, Lawhead and colleagues reported an updated series on mostly cervical cancer patients; the 5-year OS was 23%. These early reports suggested that the procedure had a perioperative mortality that was similar to the 5-year OS, at the cost of severe short-term and long-term morbidity

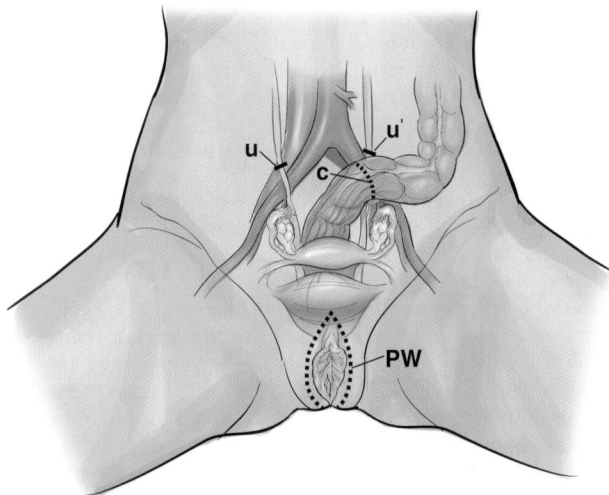

FIGURE 54.1 Levels of transection for a translevator total pelvic exenteration, as described by Dr. Alexander Brunschwig. "c" is the transection at the rectosigmoid junction. "u" and "u'" are the levels of transection of the ureters. "PW" is the perineal phase with transection of the vulva, perineum, and anus. This has remained the basic level of transection to date. However, portions of the labia and the entire clitoris can often be spared. (Reprinted from Brunschwig A. Complete excision of pelvic viscera for advanced carcinoma. *Cancer* 1948;1:177–183, with permission. Copyright © 1948 American Cancer Society.)

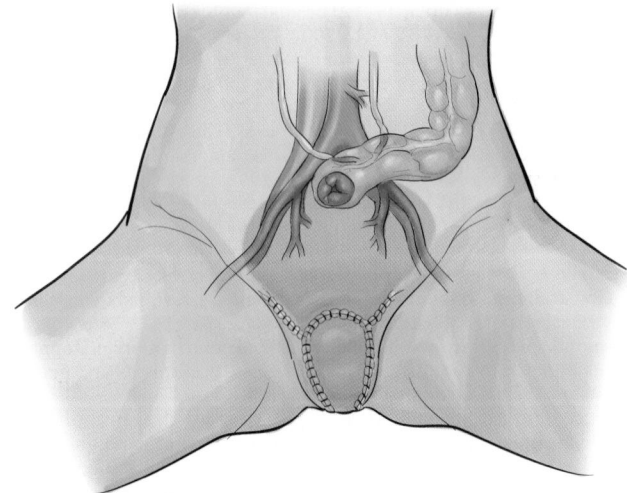

FIGURE 54.2 The end result of an exenteration as described in Dr. Alexander Brunschwig's original manuscript. The perineum is primarily closed without vaginal reconstruction, and a wet colostomy is noted. (Reprinted from Brunschwig A. Complete excision of pelvic viscera for advanced carcinoma. *Cancer* 1948;1:177–183, with permission. Copyright © 1948 American Cancer Society.)

as well as absence of vagina. Therefore, it fell out of favor and was infrequently performed for many years.

As surgical techniques and perioperative management improved over subsequent years, investigators began to report improving outcomes with decreasing perioperative mortalities. Additionally, publications after the year 2000 report continued decreases in perioperative mortality. These reports are described in greater detail later in the chapter. Pelvic exenteration is now felt to be a reasonable option in select cases, if performed by experienced surgeons. It can provide a chance at long-term cancer control and survival, but it remains a highly morbid procedure.

Pelvic exenterations can be modified based on the tumor size and location. There are multiple options for vaginal reconstruction as well as for different types of urinary system diversions separate from the fecal system. Permanent end colostomies are still required in the vast majority of cases, but in highly select situations, it may be possible to reconnect the large bowel and avoid a permanent colostomy. The indications for these pelvic exenterative procedures have also been expanded at certain institutions. More attention is also paid to sexual issues in these women as well as to overall quality of life after such extensive procedures. The most commonly performed exenteration is a total pelvic exenteration, followed by anterior, and then posterior (Table 54.1).

INDICATIONS AND PREOPERATIVE EVALUATIONS

The selection of patients suitable for a pelvic exenteration is highly complex and individualized. The most common indication is recurrent cervical carcinoma limited to the central pelvis in a patient who has received prior full-dose pelvic radiotherapy (Table 54.2). Exenteration is also considered in select cases of patients with recurrent endometrial, vulvar, or vaginal carcinomas. Uterine sarcomas are extremely rare. The majority of patients with these tumors will have extrapelvic sites of disease at the time of recurrence, in which case

TABLE 54.1 Types of Exenterations Performed in Published Series of Pelvic Exenteration for Gynecologic Malignancies

AUTHOR (REFERENCE)	YEAR OF PUBLICATION	STUDY YEARS	N	TYPE OF EXENTERATION		
				TOTAL	ANTERIOR	POSTERIOR
Brunschwig	1948	1946–1948	22	22	0	0
Barber	1968	1947–1963	36	22	14	0
Symmonds	1975	1950–1971	198	66	114	18
Rutledge	1977	1955–1976	296	176	85	35
Lawhead	1989	1972–1981	65	48	14	3
Shingleton	1989	1969–1986	143	78	63	2
Soper	1989	1970–1987	69	41	16	12
Morley	1989	1964–1984	100	69	13	18
Stanhope	1990	1977–1986	133	49	22	1
Robertson	1994	1974–1992	83	28	54	1
Morris	1996	1955–1988	20	10	9	1
Goldberg	1998	1954–1994	154	72	65	17
Barakat	1999	1947–1994	44	23	20	1
Berek	2005	1956–2011	75	46	23	6
Goldberg	2006	1987–2003	103	103	0	0
Ungar	2008	1993–2006	41	2	39	0
Fotopoulou	2010	2003–2009	47	32	12	3
Benn	2011	1990–2009	54	36	13	5
Forner	2011	1999–2010	35	16	17	2
Kaur	2012	1999–2010	36	27	5	3
Khoury-Collado	2012	1997–2001	21	14	6	1
Schmidt	2012	—	282	262	14	6
Yoo	2012	2001–2011	61	42	17	2
Baiocchi	2013	1982–2010	77	42	18	8
TOTAL			2,195	1,326 (60%)	653 (30%)	145 (10%)

exenterative procedures are contraindicated. However, in cases of pelvic-only recurrences in patients with uterine sarcomas, exenteration may be possible. Exenteration is most often only considered if radiation therapy has been already utilized in the past and no further radiation therapy is possible. Primary exenteration at the time of initial diagnosis, as well as in patients who have not undergone prior radiation, has been reported, but should be reserved for few select cases.

Exenteration was largely abandoned for patients with recurrent ovarian cancers after Barber and colleagues reported a dismal 5-year survival of 7%. However, this report was published in a time prior to effective systemic therapies. Total and/or anterior pelvic exenteration is still not a consideration in the vast majority of patients with newly diagnosed or recurrent ovarian cancers except in exceptional situations (e.g., palliation for a hemorrhaging pelvic tumor not amenable to other palliative measures). In general, palliation is rarely accepted as an indication for exenterative procedures. However, some form of supralevator posterior exenteration (i.e., "modified posterior exenteration"), as well as other bowel resections, are now routinely considered and performed in patients with newly diagnosed and recurrent ovarian cancers. These modified

TABLE 54.2 Primary Tumor Sites in the Published Series of Exenterations in Gynecologic Malignancies

AUTHOR (REFERENCE)	YEAR OF PUBLICATION	STUDY YEARS	PRIMARY TUMOR SITE							
			CERVIX	ENDOMETRIUM	UTERINE SARCOMA	VAGINA	VULVA	CANCER, NOS	OVARY	NON-GYN
Brunschwig	1948	1946–1948	15	1	1	1	2	1	0	1
Barber	1965	1947–1958	0	0	0	0	0	0	22	0
Barber	1968	1947–1963	0	36	0	0	0	0	0	0
Symmonds	1975	1950–1971	59	13	0	27	8	7	4	22
Rutledge	1977	1955–1976	195	8	0	37	14	0	0	20
Lawhead	1989	1972–1981	51	2	0	5	4	1	2	0
Shingleton	1989	1969–1986	143	0	0	0	0	0	0	0
Soper	1989	1970–1987	41	4	0	14	4	5	0	1
Morley	1989	1964–1984	66	4	4	13	12	0	1	0
Stanhope	1990	1977–1986	133	0	0	0	0	0	0	0
Robertson	1994	1974–1992	54	4	0	14	6	0	1	4
Morris	1996	1955–1988	0	20	0	0	0	0	0	0

IX

Goldberg	1998	1954–1994	109	13	0	15	9	2	4	2
Barakat	1999	1947–1994	0	44	0	0	0	0	0	0
Berek	2005	1956–2011	53	8	0	14	0	0	0	0
Goldberg	2006	1987–2003	95	2	0	0	1	0	0	5
Ungar	2008	1993–2006	41	0	0	0	0	0	0	0
Fotopoulou	2010	2003–2009	38	0	0	8	0	0	1	0
Benn	2011	1990–2009	40	0	0	5	9	0	0	0
McLean	2011	1990–2008	29	6	0	5	4	0	0	0
Forner	2011	1999–2010	35	0	0	0	0	0	0	0
Kaur	2012	1999–2010	18	9	0	8	0	0	1	0
Khoury-Collado	2012	1997–2001	0	17	4	0	0	0	0	0
Schmidt	2012	—	282	0	0	0	0	0	0	0
Yoo	2012	2001–2011	61	0	0	0	0	0	0	0
Baiocchi	2013	1982–2010	53	0	0	24	0	0	0	0
TOTAL[a]			1,611 (71%)	191 (8%)	9 (<1%)	190 (8%)	73 (3%)	16 (<1%)	36 (2%)	22 (<1%)

[a]Total number of cases (i.e., denominator) = 2,261.

posterior exenterations are not as extensive, and ovarian cancer outcomes are generally quite different from those of the other sites. We will not include these modified posterior exenteration procedures for ovarian cancer in the remainder of the chapter.

The first important step in the preoperative assessment is a thorough medical evaluation. Exenterations are highly morbid procedures, and patients must be deemed fit to undergo such an extensive surgery. Patient age is also an important consideration. Patients must be able to manage the multiple drains that are placed at the time of surgery and, ultimately, the permanent abdominal stomas that are created. An exenteration may not be a good option for a patient who has significant limitations in self-care. These procedures are also significantly body altering. Patients often are not quite prepared for, nor truly understand, the impact that this surgery will have on their bodies. It is our routine practice to have all patients who are being considered for an exenterative procedure undergo a formal psychological assessment to identify any potential underlying psychological pathology, assess their understanding of the proposed surgical procedure, prepare them for the sexual implications of the procedure, and provide guidance on coping methods. This consultation will also help the patient make more informed decisions regarding continent or noncontinent urinary diversions as well as vaginal reconstruction.

The ideal candidate for a pelvic exenteration is a patient with primary cervix or vaginal apex cancer who develops a small (<2 cm) central pelvic recurrence at the vaginal apex (or cervix if present) after definitive whole pelvic radiation. Patients with pelvic recurrence after radical hysterectomy are usually best treated with pelvic radiation. Patients should be evaluated by a radiation oncologist to determine whether all radiation options have been exhausted and also to discuss the possible use of intraoperative radiation therapy.

A "terrible triad" of symptoms has been described to be clinical contraindications to exenterative procedures. These include hydronephrosis, sciatic pain, and leg edema. These symptoms are felt to reflect lateral pelvic extension and/or involvement of the pelvic sidewall structures. Lateral extension of tumor is considered a contraindication to exenterative procedures by many. However, experienced centers have reported reasonable outcomes after exenterative and nonexenterative procedures in patients with laterally extended or pelvic sidewall–based recurrences. Laterally extended resections present unique challenges that require special procedures. It is beyond the scope of this chapter to describe the details of the surgical steps of such laterally extended resections, which often involve major vascular resections, major nerve resections, bony resections including sacrectomy, and/or sidewall musculature resection in addition to the other typical exenterative resection of pelvic viscera.

An absolute contraindication to exenteration is the presence of confirmed extrapelvic disease. It is imperative to rule out the presence of such distant disease as best as possible. Computed tomography (CT) or positron emission tomography (PET) scanning of the chest, abdomen, and pelvis must be routinely performed. Any suspicious findings must be thoroughly evaluated. Any easily accessible lesion, such as palpable adenopathy in the inguinal or supraclavicular regions, can be biopsied in the office. Assessment of most other lesions can be accomplished utilizing image-guided biopsies by interventional radiologists. Occasionally, a surgical procedure, such as diagnostic laparoscopy or mediastinoscopy, is needed to evaluate a suspicious lesion seen on CT or PET scanning. A pelvic magnetic resonance imaging (MRI) should also be considered as it will provide a more detailed anatomic view of the pelvic recurrence in relation to

surrounding structures. This could help in determining the extent of the exenteration.

Pelvic MRI is a valuable imaging modality in the preoperative assessment of resectability and surgical planning in patients considering exenteration. It is standard at our institution to obtain a preoperative pelvic MRI as we feel it most accurately details the extent of lateral, anterior, and posterior tumor involvement. However, few data exist specific to the value of pelvic MRI in these rare recurrent gynecologic malignancies eligible for exenteration. MRI has been reported to be a valuable tool in surgical planning for patients with locally advanced and recurrent colorectal cancers. Forner and colleagues reported less enthusiastic results in a series of 43 patients undergoing pelvic exenteration for gynecologic malignancies. The sensitivity, specificity, positive and negative predictive values for MRI, and complete resection were 85%, 52%, 60%, and 80%, respectively. This is a small single institution experience and may not reflect that at other institutions. Preoperative MRI should be considered, but surgeons must recognize the potential limitations of the correlation of MRI findings with intraoperative and final pathologic results. Pelvic MRI may not be entirely accurate for determining complete resection, but it will help in deciding whether a less than translevator total pelvic exenteration may be an option. It will also help in assessing cases that may require laterally extended resections.

The value of preoperative PET scanning is controversial. Many surgeons who perform exenteration will obtain a PET scan to assess for the presence of metastatic disease. It is unclear if routine PET imaging adds more value as compared to good-quality multidetector thin-slice CT scan. Husain and colleagues reported the results of a prospective trial assessing PET scan prior to pelvic exenteration. In four cases, CT or MRI failed to detect metastatic disease that was identified on PET scan and confirmed with pathologic sampling. The negative predictive value of PET scanning was 100%, meaning no metastatic disease was found at surgery in the setting of a normal PET scan. PET scanning did have some false-positive cases. Increased FDG uptake was noted in nine cases on PET scanning. Biopsies were performed in all nine cases, and only five (56%) were confirmed to have metastatic disease.

Combined PET/CT scanning has become more commonplace and is often ordered nowadays instead of separate CT and PET scans. A small retrospective series of 33 cases by Burger et al. reported some promising accuracy data on preoperative PET/CT scanning. However, none of the 33 cases had distant metastasis. False-positive nodal findings were noted in two cases. PET/CT imaging is useful and accurate in ruling out metastatic disease in these patients and should be considered (PET scanning if CT was already done). However, it is important to recognize the significant false-positive rate associated with this type of imaging. Before abandoning an attempt at exenteration, all suspicious metastatic lesions should be biopsied in order to confirm the presence of disease.

An exploratory minimally invasive surgical (MIS) procedure (i.e., laparoscopy) may also be useful in patients under evaluation for exenteration. Laparoscopic exploration can be done prior to the planned exenteration, or it could be performed the same day. Findings may aid with the decision of whether or not to proceed with the exenteration. The value of this is most likely greatest in centers in which MRI and PET/CT imaging are not easily available. Plante and Roy and Kohler et al. have reported that an exploratory laparoscopy can avoid an unnecessary laparotomy in nearly 50% of patients planned for exenteration due to findings of metastatic or unresectable disease. Both of these series did not utilize routine, nor current, imaging modalities such as PET scanning or the more modern stronger magnet MRI scanners.

SURGICAL TECHNIQUES

Preoperative Preparation

The obvious first step is an extensive, detailed discussion with the patient and the family regarding the planned procedure, what will be removed, the significant risk of morbidity, the body changes that will occur, the effects on sexuality, and the long-term outcomes. As mentioned previously, we would suggest that these patients be referred to a psychologist who has knowledge of exenterative procedures. This psychologist should perform a formal evaluation and any needed counseling and will provide the patient with resources for issues that may develop after surgery. A discussion is needed regarding patient desires for vaginal reconstruction and type of urinary diversion as well as regarding the potential for rectal reanastomosis versus end colostomy. Patients should be referred to stoma specialist for marking of the abdomen to assist in optimal positioning of the stoma.

Although routinely done in the past, admission to the hospital the day before surgery usually is unwarranted unless there is a significant medical concern that arises during standard preoperative outpatient medical and surgical evaluation and clearance processes. Any underlying medical comorbidities should be optimized. The role of preoperative bowel preparation is unclear. Multiple randomized trials in patients undergoing colorectal resections failed to demonstrate any advantage to mechanical bowel preparations, and some actually suggested a potential disadvantage to such preparations. Mechanical bowel preparation is likely unnecessary in patients who will not have a large bowel–based continent urinary diversion. Elimination of stool from the large intestine may ease the creation of a continent pouch, but this is highly surgeon dependent. Strong recommendations regarding routine bowel preparation prior to exenteration cannot be made. While there is no evidence-based reason for routine bowel preparation, some surgeons find that gross fecal contamination during the construction of a large bowel conduit is unappealing.

Patient positioning is standard low lithotomy using some form of Allen stirrups. Hair removal should be avoided. However, if absolutely necessary, then clippers, not razors, should

be used prior to scrubbing of the skin. Large-bore peripheral intravenous access should be placed, as well as some form of central venous access. This will be tremendously helpful in managing these patients during and after surgery. Standard antibiotic prophylaxis should be administered prior to skin incision. Combined thromboprophylaxis should be used as these patients are at the highest risk of venous thromboembolism. Sequential compression devices are placed prior to induction of anesthesia. Low molecular weight heparin (LMWH) is also administered prior to the start of the surgical procedure. Many would recommend that LMWH be continued for 4 weeks postoperatively.

Some gynecologic oncologists will be able to perform not only the exenteration but also most of the reconstructive procedures. However, these are long procedures and many centers take a team approach in which gynecologic oncologists work with colleagues from their group and possibly colleagues from other specialties as well to complete these cases. It is becoming more common for a gynecologic oncologist, plastic surgeon, urologist, and radiation oncologist all to be involved for various parts of the procedure. Teamwork and communication prior to, during, and after surgery are most important.

Initial Steps and Exploration

As described previously, surgeons first may choose to perform a laparoscopic evaluation to potentially avoid an unnecessary laparotomy. However, this is not routinely done in the setting of normal preoperative MRI and PET/CT scanning.

The abdomen is opened using a standard large vertical midline incision extending above the umbilicus. These procedures are not amenable to lower transverse abdominal incisions. The entire peritoneal cavity is closely inspected, and any suspicious lesions are sent for frozen section. A standard paraaortic nodal assessment is performed and frozen section also obtained. It is controversial as to whether to limit the paraaortic nodal assessment to the lower area below the inferior mesenteric artery or to carry this assessment up to the level of the renal veins. An exenteration should not be performed if there is confirmed disease outside the pelvis, including the paraaortic lymph nodes.

The retroperitoneal pelvic spaces can all be developed while awaiting frozen section results. The pararectal and paravesical spaces are developed first (**Fig. 54.3**). The pararectal

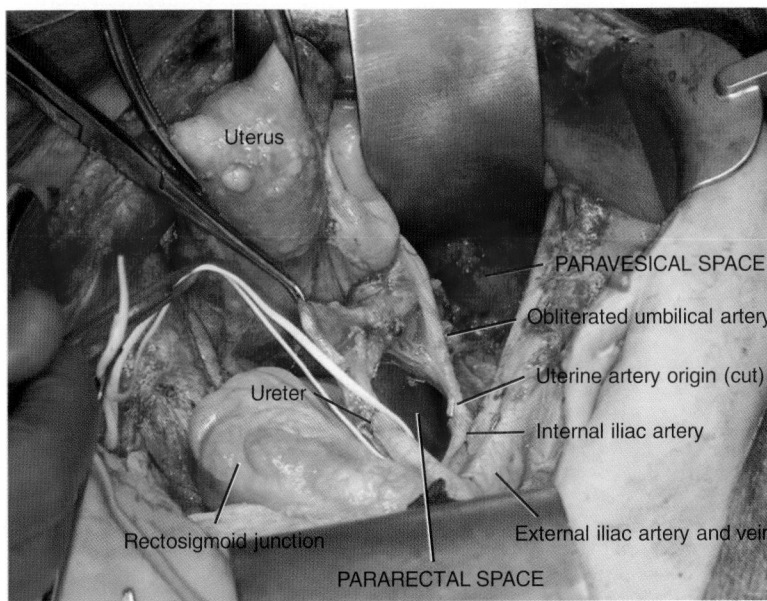

Uterus

PARAVESICAL SPACE

Obliterated umbilical artery

Uterine artery origin (cut)

Ureter

Internal iliac artery

Rectosigmoid junction

External iliac artery and vein

PARARECTAL SPACE

FIGURE 54.3 Developed paravesical and pararectal spaces of the right hemipelvis. These spaces are relatively avascular and often can be developed bluntly with some sharp dissection using cautery if needed. These spaces should be developed distally to the levator muscles of the pelvic diaphragm.

IX

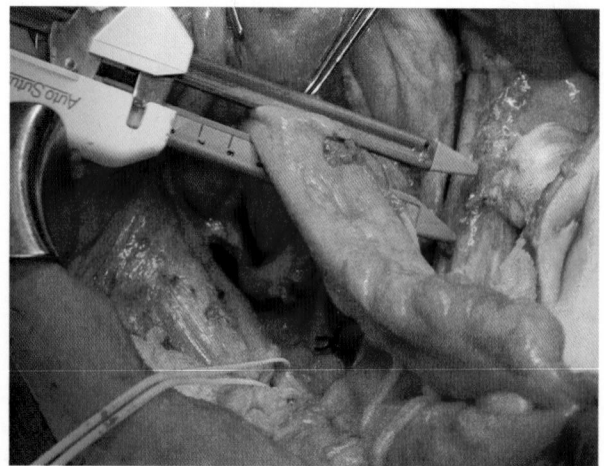

FIGURE 54.4 Space of Retzius. This is also an avascular space if developed correctly with blunt and sharp dissection using cautery. Care should be taken to not injure the venous plexus overlying the inferior aspect of the bladder and surrounding urethra (plexus of Santorini) in order to avoid excessive bleeding from this area. This dissection is carried distally to the level of the urogenital diaphragm.

space is delineated by the iliac vessels laterally, by the ureter medially, and by the uterine vessels anteriorly. The paravesical space is delineated by the iliac vessels and obturator muscle laterally, obliterated umbilical artery and bladder medially, and the pubic rami anteriorly. These two spaces are developed and lateral tumor extension can be assessed. The round ligament, if present, is ligated, and the paravesical space is carried forward and medially into the space of Retzius (**Fig. 54.4**). Dissection of these spaces is important in assessing resectability. *No major organs are transected until the result of all frozen section analyses are available and do not reveal disease, and dissection of the planes suggests a negative resection margin.* The above dissection and development of spaces should be performed regardless of whether a total, anterior, or posterior exenteration is planned. The decision to perform a total, anterior, or posterior exenteration is based on the tumor location and size and whether a negative margin resection is possible. These decisions can be made based on preoperative imaging and pelvic examination. However, the

final determination is made intraoperatively. All patients who are planned to undergo a less than total exenteration should be counseled and consented for a possible total exenteration if deemed necessary intraoperatively to achieve a negative margin resection.

Total Pelvic Exenteration

The rectum is then transected at the upper portion of the rectum or at the level of the rectosigmoid junction, depending on the location and size of the tumor. A mesenteric window is created just beneath the colonic wall. A stapler (GIA) is then used to transect the rectum, rectosigmoid, or sigmoid (**Fig. 54.5**). The mesentery is then divided straight back to the origin of the mesentery. This can be done in several ways. Most commonly, the peritoneum of the mesentery is scored with monopolar cautery. The mesenteric fat and vessels are then ligated and transected, most often with a vessel-sealing device. The proximal end of the transected colon is then retracted upward and out of the surgical field. The ureters are clipped with metal clips and transected with a scalpel or scissor above the level of prior pelvic radiation therapy field, which is often just at the pelvic inlet where they encounter the common iliac arteries (**Fig. 54.6**).

The lateral pelvic vessels are then sequentially secured and transected at the pelvic sidewalls all the way down to the levator muscles of the pelvis (**Fig. 54.7**). Again, this is facilitated with the use of any of the commercially available vessel-sealing devices. Stapling devices can also be considered but are now less commonly used. The internal iliac artery and vein can be ligated beyond their posterior divisions if needed to facilitate specimen resection and/or control pelvic bleeding. The rectal mesentery and vessels are secured at the level of the presacral fascia down to the planned level of rectal transection. Extreme caution is needed to not enter behind the presacral fascia. This will risk injury to the sacral veins, which are very difficult to control because they retract into the bony spaces of the sacrum. Various techniques can be used to control sacral bleeding if encountered. These include (a) use of a sterile thumbtack into the sacral foramina; (b) use of bone wax, which can be difficult to handle; and (c) use of commercially available hemostatic agents. A unique method to possibly control sacral hemorrhage is to place a small piece of abdominal wall muscle into the sacral foramina where the bleeding is coming from. Monopolar coagulation current

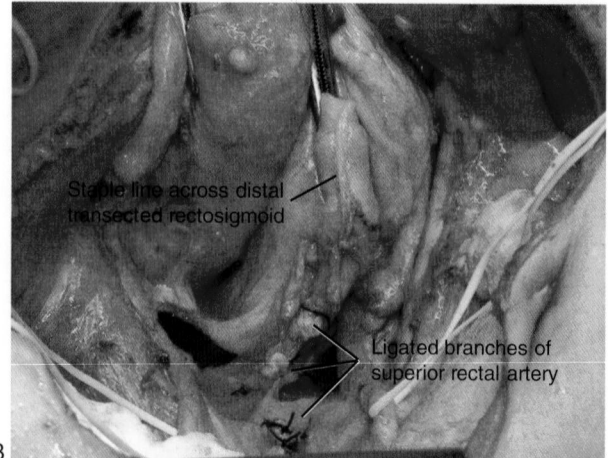

FIGURE 54.5 Rectosigmoid transection. A stapling device can be used to transect the rectum/rectosigmoid/sigmoid at the desired point (**A**). Branches of the superior rectal artery must be controlled either with standard suture techniques or using any of the available vessel-sealing devices (**B**).

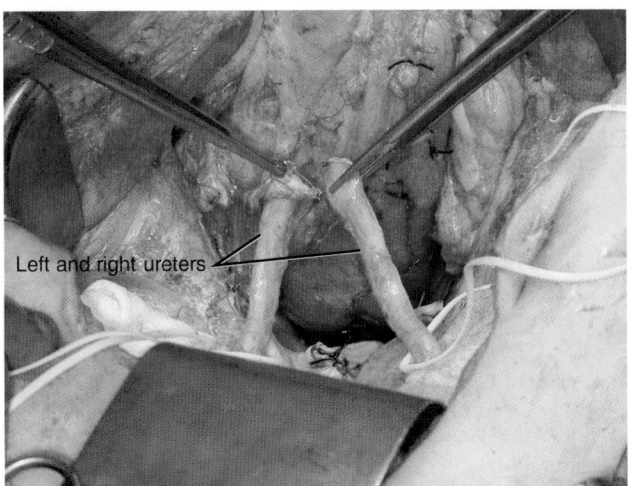

FIGURE 54.6 The ureters are clipped with metal clips and transected at or above the pelvic brim. The resulting hydronephrosis during the remainder of the procedure will facilitate the ureteral anastomosis to the conduit.

can then be applied to this piece of muscle to form a seal. Finally, in the rare situations in which all else fails to control pelvic/sacral hemorrhage, a pelvic pack (using multiple lap pads individually or a larger bag) can be compressed into the entire pelvis. The procedure is then terminated and the

patient taken to the recovery room with a plan to remove the pelvic packing the following day. Anteriorly, the space of Retzius is further developed down to the level of the levator muscles.

If a supralevator approach is planned, the urethra and vagina can be transected at the level of the levator muscles. This can be done with simple monopolar cautery. The distal rectal wall is isolated and transected with a stapling device. The en bloc specimen can then be delivered vaginally. If a translevator approach is planned, the levator muscles must be incised and the urethra, vagina, and rectum are not transected. A perineal approach is initiated just prior to or at the time that the levator muscles are approached abdominally. A line of transection is identified and encompasses the entire urethral meatus, labia minora, vaginal opening, and anus (Fig. 54.8). The labia majora and clitoris are generally spared unless involved by tumor. This line of transection can be made with a scalpel, but most often, it is done using monopolar cautery. The paravaginal and para-anal and para-rectal fatty tissue is then transected. Monopolar cautery may be used, but even so, this transection is often bloody. Currently available vessel-sealing devices can again be used for this portion of the procedure and will greatly facilitate this dissection and lessen bleeding. The perineal approach aims toward the coccyx, the levator muscles are transected at this level and circumferentially to encompass the entire specimen (Fig. 54.9), and the specimen is delivered through the large defect (Fig. 54.10).

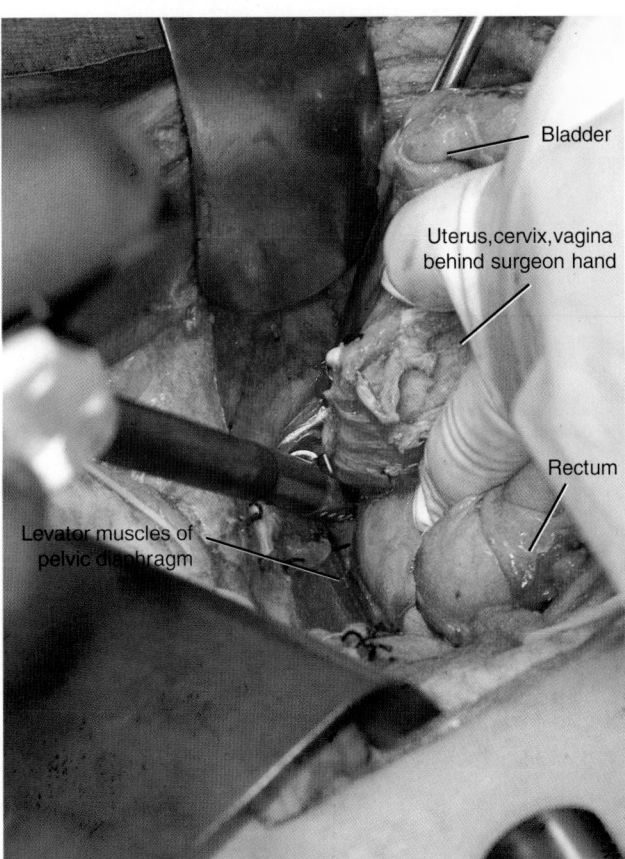

FIGURE 54.7 The lateral and posterior pelvic vessels and other pedicles are transected sequentially and circumferentially down to the level of the levator muscles. Here we see a stapling device being used, but any of the available vessel-sealing devices can be used to facilitate this dissection.

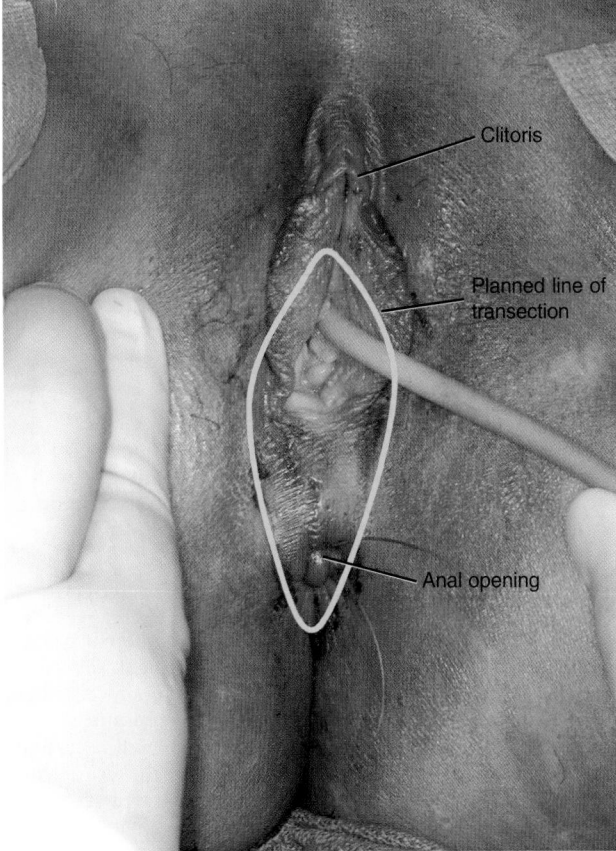

FIGURE 54.8 Planned line of perineal transection. The perineum is incised using monopolar cautery and encompasses the urethra, vaginal opening, and the anal opening. The labia majora and clitoris can often be spared.

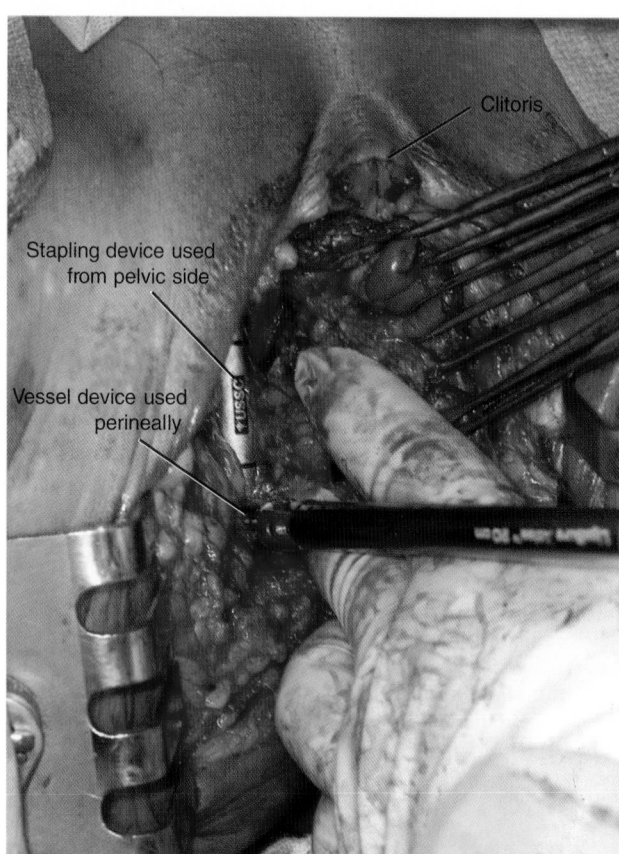

FIGURE 54.9 Completing the exenteration. The tissue lateral to the specimen is transected and secured using a vessel device circumferentially. The levator muscles are transected and, as seen here, approached jointly from the pelvic and perineal sides.

Anterior Pelvic Exenteration

Many of the steps for an anterior exenteration are the same as above except that the rectum is not resected. The posterior aspect of the vagina can sometimes be preserved as well and may help prevent development of rectal fistulae.

Posterior Pelvic Exenteration

As above, many of the steps are similar except that the bladder is preserved and the ureters are not cut. The anterior wall of the vagina also may be preserved and may help prevent development of urinary fistulae.

URINARY DIVERSION

The decision to perform a noncontinent or continent urinary diversion must be individualized. Noncontinent diversions are created from a portion of terminal ileum, and continent diversions are made with portions of the ileum and ascending/transverse colon. Noncontinent diversions will necessitate a permanent stoma bag on the abdomen as the urine freely empties from the stoma. A continent diversion will eventually allow for patient self-catheterization and eliminate a stomal bag. However, continent diversions are more complex and take much longer to create than a simpler noncontinent diversion. There are no best guidelines to help select between the two; often, it is left to the surgeon's experience and discretion.

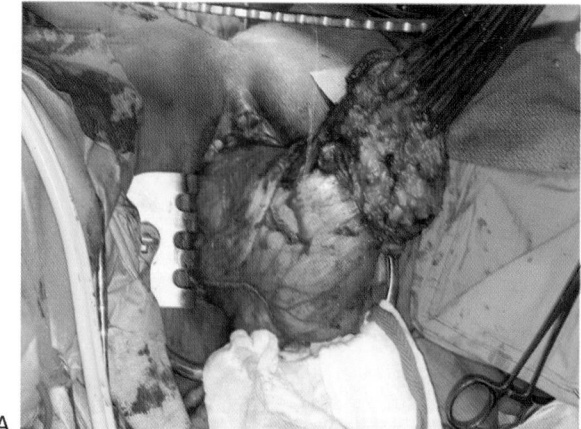

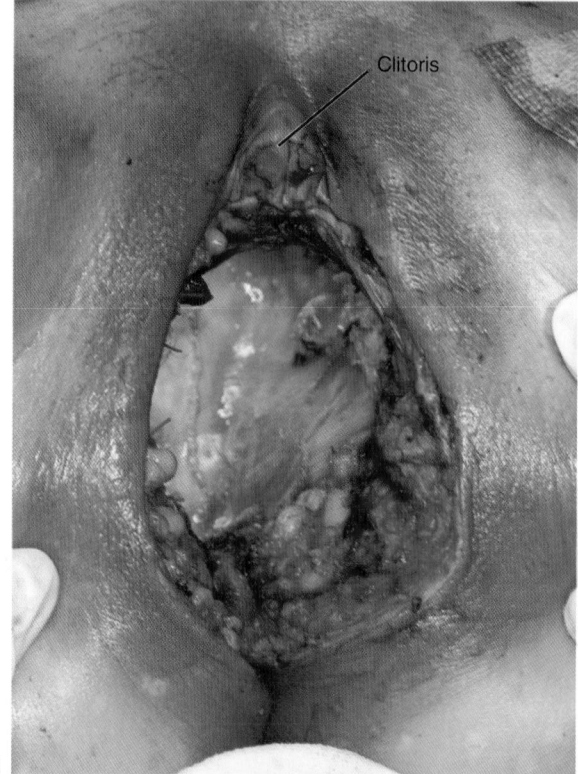

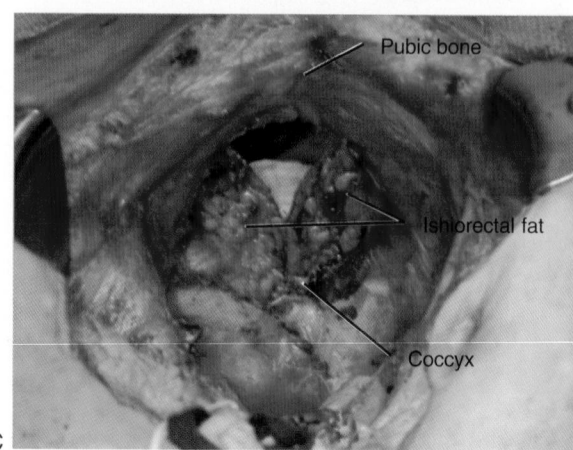

FIGURE 54.10 Removal of the en bloc specimen (**A**) with resultant defect seen from the perineal aspect (**B** and **C**).

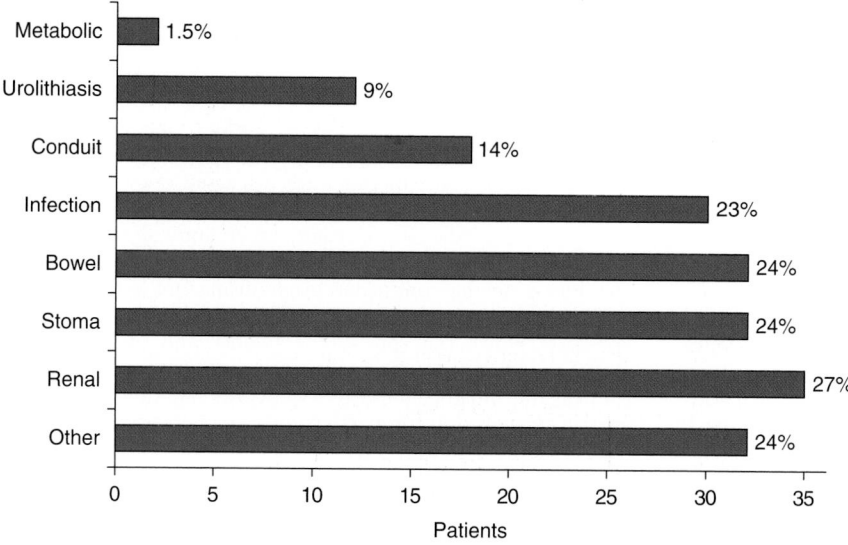

FIGURE 54.11 Types of long-term ileal conduit–related complications. (Reprinted from Madersbacher S, Schnidt J, Eberle JM, et al. Long-term outcome of ileal conduit diversion. *J Urol* 2003;169:985–990, with permission. Copyright © 2003, Elsevier.)

Generally speaking, noncontinent diversions may be a better option for patients in whom the ability to self-catheterize may be problematic, such as the elderly or those with physical limitations.

The noncontinent ileal conduit is easier to create than are the continent conduits, but it does result in a permanent bag on the abdomen for urinary drainage. The possibility of not needing an additional bag on the abdomen with a continent pouch is attractive to many patients. However, there are little data assessing complication rates or patient satisfaction between the two types of urinary conduits. Madersbacher and colleague reported on 131 patients who had an ileal conduit created at the time of cystectomy and had been followed for at least 5 years. They noted a total of 192 conduit-related complications among 87 (66%) patients, with a mean of 2.2 complications per patient. Figure 54.11 depicts the types of complications that developed. The most common stomal complications were parastomal herniae, stomal stenosis, and bleeding/irritation. Surgical intervention to correct a stomal complication was necessary in 15 patients. Bowel-related complications included bowel obstruction, diarrhea, and fistulae. Infectious complications were mostly urinary tract infections and pyelonephritis. Conduit complications were mostly anastomotic stricturing. A fair number of patients required surgical interventions to manage some of the complications that developed. The rate of complications continued to increase

with longer survival. Figure 54.12 illustrates the number of complications and the rate of patients experiencing complications based on the number of years since conduit creation. Complications developed in 45% of patients surviving 5 years and 94% of those surviving more than 15 years.

In a series of 100 patients undergoing exenteration for gynecologic malignancies, Forner and Lampe reported that continent pouch creation resulted in an increased median operating time of 97 minutes compared to cases in which an ileal conduit was done. The mean age of patients receiving a noncontinent diversion was 63 years, compared to 52 years for those in which a continent diversion was created. The overall complication rate was slightly higher with continent pouches (48% vs. 31%). Long-term, continent pouches were associated with more instances of urinary stone formation and more urinary tract infections. Similarly, Urh et al. noted a significantly higher rate of stone formation with continent pouches compared to ileal conduits (35% vs. 2%). However, they did not note an increased infectious risk with continent compared to noncontinent diversions. Continent diversions were also associated with greater rates of urostomy stricturing. In this series, noncontinent ileal diversions were preferentially performed in older patients and in those with multiple medical comorbidities. There was no difference between the two types of diversion with regard to anastomotic leaks or strictures, renal insufficiency, fistulae

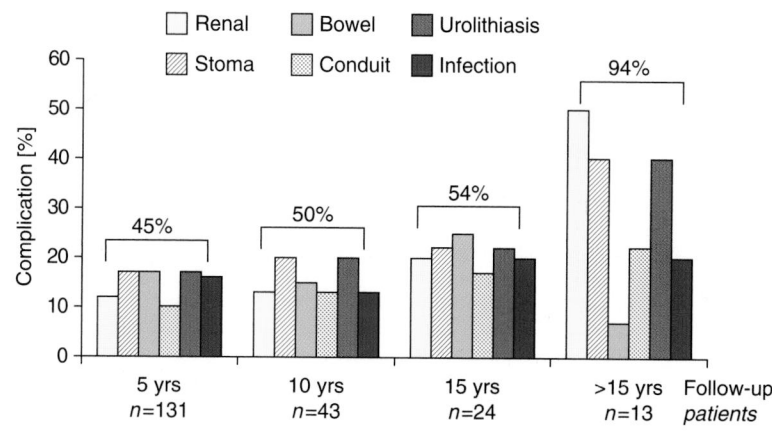

FIGURE 54.12 Rate of complications based on time from creation of ileal conduit. (Reprinted from Madersbacher S, Schnidt J, Eberle JM, et al. Long-term outcome of ileal conduit diversion. *J Urol* 2003;169: 985–990, with permission. Copyright © 2003, Elsevier.)

IX

formation, or reoperation to correct a conduit problem. It is important to note that planned continent diversions may not actually be continent. Up to a quarter of these continent diversions may ultimately be incontinent for various reasons, and difficulty catheterizing the stoma may be an issue in some patients. Overall, quality of life is quite similar between patients who have a continent diversion and those who have a noncontinent diversion.

Noncontinent Conduit Creation

A 15- to 25-cm portion of terminal ileum is identified and isolated 15 cm from the ileocecal valve. The length of ileum used is dependent on the length needed from the ureters to the skin. This portion of ileum that will become the ileal conduit is transected at either end. Various methods can be used, but most commonly, this is accomplished using a GIA stapling device. The small bowel can then be reanastomosed in a side-to-side fashion using a standard approach. The associated mesentery is preserved to maintain adequate blood supply. If needed for mobility, the mesenteric fat can be transected toward the base of the mesentery. The proximal end of the conduit will be the end that the ureters will be inserted into (i.e., the "butt" end), and the distal end will become the stoma. The ureters are trimmed so that the distal end is free of radiation effect. If the rectosigmoid has not be transected (i.e., an anterior exenteration), then the left ureter must be tunneled underneath the rectosigmoid through an avascular window in the posterior aspect of the mesentery. A site is chosen on either side of the proximal end of the conduit to ensure a tension-free anastomosis. This site is usually 2 to 3 cm from the staple line, and a 1-cm opening is created. Stents are used by most surgeons, although some feel they are unnecessary.

The distal (i.e., stomal) end of the ileal segment is opened by transecting the staple line. A long thin clamp, such as an Addison clamp, can be passed through this open stomal end and passed to the small ureteral opening at the proximal end. The stent is passed through this opening and out the stomal end and also passed retrograde into the renal pelvis. The ureter is spatulated for about 5 to 6 mm prior to inserting the stent. The ureteral anastomosis is then created using interrupted 3-0 or 4-0 absorbable sutures, such as Vicryl, and sutured to the serosa of the ileal conduit. Care should be taken not to place too many sutures, as doing so may lead to necrosis and stricturing. Tunneling of the ureter through the ileum has been reported, but this is not necessary. These steps are then repeated for the other ureter. The butt end of the conduit can then be secured to the fascia overlying the sacral promontory to prevent excessive motion of the conduit and avoid tension on the newly created anastomoses.

The distal (stomal) end of the conduit is then brought through a preselected site on the abdomen. The stoma is then created using a typical "rosebud" technique. Interrupted 2-0 or 3-0 absorbable sutures are used. A bite is taken through the skin and then brought through a portion of the ileal serosa, then passed through the entire end of the stomal opening. The knots are placed laterally on the skin. The ileal conduit can be sutured to the peritoneum just under the stomal opening. A large-bore catheter without a balloon can be placed through the stoma to maintain patency. This catheter, as well as the ureteral stents, can be secured to the skin with suture. The catheter can be removed 2 to 4 weeks postoperatively, and the ureteral stents can be removed 6 to 8 weeks postoperatively. A peritoneal drain is often placed in the vicinity of the ureteral anastomosis to assess for any urinary leakage in the postoperative period. This drain can be removed 1 to 2 weeks later if there are no signs of urinary leakage.

Continent Conduit Creation

Multiple types of continent diversions have been described. The details of some of these are discussed elsewhere in this textbook. The majority of these continent conduits use varying portions of the ileum, cecum, ascending colon, transverse colon, and, in some, the appendix. The two main types differ based on the continence mechanism. One type relies on pressure differentials between the stomal limb and the low-pressure pouch (i.e., pressure gradient), and the other type relies on a flap-valve mechanism for continence. In the United States, the most commonly used continent diversions after pelvic exenteration for gynecologic malignancies are the Indiana or Miami pouch. These have minor differences but are quite similar. In both, the appendix is removed if still present, the colonic portions are used to create the pouch, the ureters are anastomosed directly into the colonic pouch, and the ileal limb is plicated and becomes the catheterizable stoma. These pouches rely on the higher pressure in the ileal limb, compared to the low-pressure colonic urinary reservoir, to maintain continence. The flap-valve–based pouches use the appendix as the catheterizable stoma, which is hidden in the umbilicus using an appendiceal Mitronoff approach; various modifications exist. This type of pouch allows for the ureters to be anastomosed into the ileal limb as described above for the ileal conduit instead of directly into the colonic reservoir. Surgical details of Miami pouch are described in Chapter 55.

It is beyond the scope of this chapter to detail the steps of all the available types of continent urinary diversions. In general, a low-pressure urinary reservoir is created from the colonic segment that is isolated by detubularizing it and folding it upon itself. Ureteral stents are brought through the colonic reservoir and through the abdominal wall through separate stab wounds instead of through the stoma. For drainage, a large-bore catheter such as a Malecot is placed through the pouch and brought through another separate stab wound on the abdomen. This large-bore catheter allows for irrigation of the pouch, which will continue to secrete mucus for some period of time. A Foley catheter or red Robinson catheter is also placed through the catheterizable stoma to maintain patency. All of these catheters and stents are secured to the abdominal wall to help prevent them from being prematurely dislodged. A peritoneal drain is placed in the vicinity of the pouch to assess for postoperative urinary leakage. The drains, catheters, and stents are removed over time depending on postoperative healing, usually within 6 to 8 weeks.

The decision as to which type of continent urinary diversion to create will depend on surgeon preferences and experience as well as certain patient characteristics. There are advantages and disadvantages to pressure gradient and flap-valve diversions. Pressure gradient pouches are slightly less complex to create and are the only option, other than a noncontinent ileal conduit, for patients who do not have an appendix. The stoma in these diversions also tends to be easier to catheterize, but is placed on the abdomen; thus, there will be an additional stoma on the abdomen in patients who may also have an end colostomy. Flap-valve urinary diversions are slightly more technically challenging and require an intact appendix of sufficient length. However, the appendiceal stoma can be created at the base of the umbilicus, resulting in a "hidden" stoma. Another advantage of these appendiceal pouches is that the ileum is no longer the stoma and is used as a site to attach the ureters. This has the advantage of allowing the surgeon to make the ileal limb as long as needed to reach the ureters, thereby minimizing the additional ureterolysis needed when creating the other type of pouches in which the ureters have to be brought up to the urinary reservoir.

COLONIC DIVERSION

A permanent end colostomy is the most commonly performed colonic diversion and/or reconstruction. It is the only option in patients who undergo a translevator total or posterior exenteration. An end colostomy is relatively simple to create, and standard approaches are well described (Chapter 47). The transected end of the proximal colon is brought through the abdomen through a preselected site that is best located in the left lower quadrant just below the level of the umbilicus. The colostomy creation is often reserved for the end of the procedure just as the abdomen is planned to be closed. The staple line is excised. Absorbable (2-0 or 3-0) sutures are used to secure and mature the stoma. The mucosa is everted and approximated to the skin. Approximately four or five sutures are placed circumferentially and are passed through the skin, through the seromuscular layer approximately 2 to 3 cm below the level of the stoma, through the serosal edge of the stomal opening, and through approximately 1 to 2 cm of mucosa. The suture is then tied, everting the distal colonic mucosa.

Colorectal or coloanal anastomoses are generally discouraged in patients who have undergone a supralevator exenteration and have previously had their pelvis irradiated. The greatest concern is the high rate of anastomotic leak. Husain and colleagues noted that 7 of the 13 (54%) patients in whom a low rectal anastomosis was created without a diverting colostomy or ileostomy developed a rectal anastomotic leak. All required surgical intervention with creation of a permanent colostomy. One of these patients died of sepsis postoperatively. An additional 2 patients developed a rectovaginal fistula within 6 months, leaving only 4 (30%) of the 13 patients with intact bowel continuity. Depending on how one views these data, a low rectal anastomosis may or may not be a viable consideration. Similarly, Mirhashemi and colleagues noted a 35% rate of anastomotic leaks or fistulae in previously radiated patients irrespective of whether a protective stoma was created. The rate of anastomotic complications was only 8% in those who had not been previously irradiated. These findings have been confirmed by other investigators. In general, a permanent colostomy is preferred in patients who have been previously irradiated, whereas a colorectal anastomosis may be possible in those who have not been previously irradiated. A colorectal anastomosis may be considered in highly select, previously irradiated patients who are highly desirous of avoiding a colostomy. These patients must be well informed of the high rate of complications associated with reanastomosis and of the fact that there is a real possibility of ultimately requiring a permanent colostomy.

Wet Colostomy

The wet colostomy was the urinary and fecal diversion first used by Brunschwig (Fig. 54.2). In his original description, the ureters were inserted into the colon just proximal to the stoma. This was associated with a significant rate of ascending urinary tract infections, metabolic abnormalities, renal disease, and large amounts of foul-smelling watery output. This wet colostomy approach was abandoned in favor of separate urinary and fecal diversions as described above. In 1989, a new technique for a wet colostomy, using a double-barrel approach, was described by Carter et al. In this procedure, the rectosigmoid is transected as indicated for the exenterative procedure. Instead of bringing out the end of the transected colon to form an end colostomy, a loop colostomy is formed approximately 10 to 15 cm from the transected end (Fig. 54.13). The selected portion is pulled through the abdomen at the preselected site.

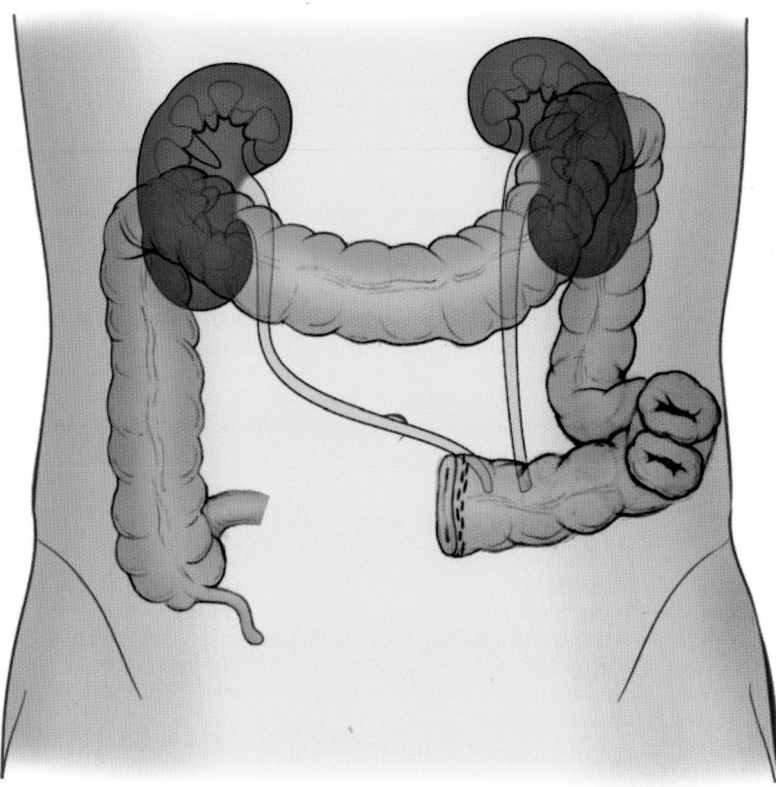

FIGURE 54.13 Double-barreled wet colostomy. (Reprinted from Chokshi RJ, Kuhrt MP, Schmidt C, et al. Single institution experience comparing double-barreled wet colostomy to ileal conduit for urinary and fecal diversion. *Urology* 2011;78:856–862, with permission. Copyright © 2011, Elsevier.)

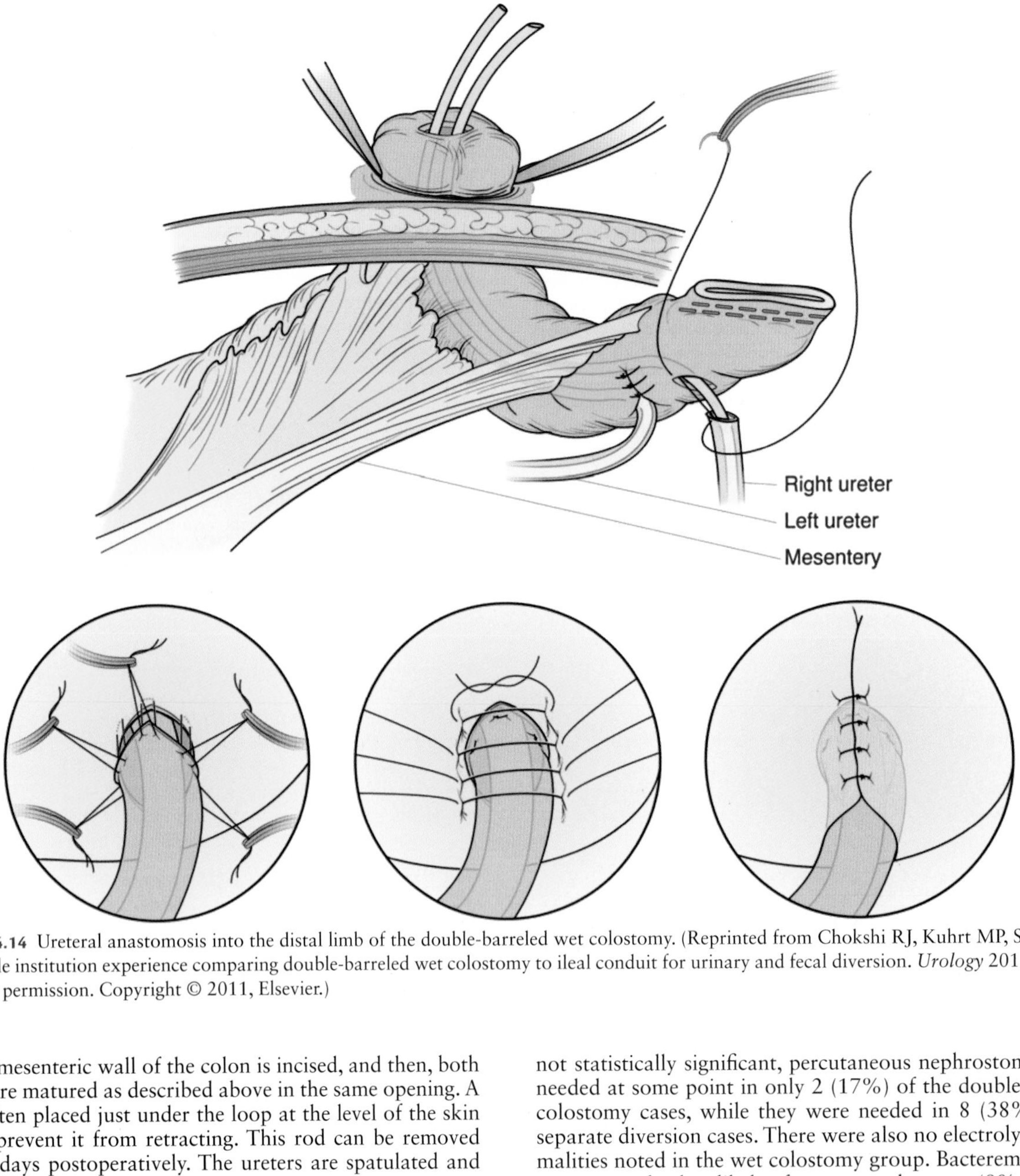

- Right ureter
- Left ureter
- Mesentery

FIGURE 54.14 Ureteral anastomosis into the distal limb of the double-barreled wet colostomy. (Reprinted from Chokshi RJ, Kuhrt MP, Schmidt C, et al. Single institution experience comparing double-barreled wet colostomy to ileal conduit for urinary and fecal diversion. *Urology* 2011;78:856–862, with permission. Copyright © 2011, Elsevier.)

The antimesenteric wall of the colon is incised, and then, both stomas are matured as described above in the same opening. A rod is often placed just under the loop at the level of the skin to help prevent it from retracting. This rod can be removed 7 to 10 days postoperatively. The ureters are spatulated and anastomosed into the distal limb of the wet colostomy in a similar manner as described above. The seromuscular layer can be imbricated over the ureteral anastomosis as shown in Figure 54.14, but this is controversial and not done by all surgeons. Ureteral stents are brought through the stoma.

Backes et al. reported their outcomes after a double-barreled wet colostomy compared to separate urinary and fecal diversions at the time of pelvic exenteration for recurrent gynecologic cancers previously irradiated. A double-barreled colostomy was performed in 12 patients, and separate diversions of various types were performed in 21 other cases. The median length of stay was significantly shorter after a double-barreled colostomy (14.5 days vs. 20 days; $P = 0.01$). Creation of a double-barreled colostomy also resulted in shorter operative times (627 minutes vs. 724 minutes; $P = 0.01$). There were no conduit or anastomotic leaks in the patients who had a double-barreled colostomy, compared to 6 (29%) patients in the other group who developed a leak ($P = 0.06$). Although

not statistically significant, percutaneous nephrostomies were needed at some point in only 2 (17%) of the double-barreled colostomy cases, while they were needed in 8 (38%) of the separate diversion cases. There were also no electrolyte abnormalities noted in the wet colostomy group. Bacteremia and/or sepsis was also less likely after a wet colostomy (8% vs. 48%; $P = 0.03$). These favorable outcomes were still seen when comparing wet colostomy to ileal conduits alone. It appears that a double-barreled wet colostomy may be a valuable technique for urinary diversion at the time of total pelvic exenteration.

PELVIC FLOOR RECONSTRUCTION

A multitude of techniques and approaches exist for reconstruction of the pelvic floor with or without neovagina creation. Some of these procedures are detailed in the following chapter. Although gynecologic oncologists introduced many of these techniques in pelvic surgery, these days, most of these reconstructive procedures are now often performed by our plastic surgery colleagues.

The optimal reconstruction in patients who do not wish to have a neovagina is unclear. The most simple method would be primary closure of the perineal defect alone. Some recommend placement of an omental J-flap in the pelvic defect to help ameliorate complications such as bowel obstructions, enterocutaneous fistulae, and perineal herniae seen after primary closure. However, the data are not consistent in demonstrating such a benefit. Myocutaneous flaps, mostly vertical rectus abdominis myocutaneous (VRAM) flaps, have also been suggested to be beneficial in closure of the large perineal/pelvic defects. This has not been confirmed, and Chokshi et al. found no difference in outcomes comparing VRAM flaps to primary closure.

Neovagina creation has been described using various methods including procedures that use the omentum, portions of the colon, various synthetic and allogenic grafts, or myocutaneous flaps. The gracilis myocutaneous neovagina has been the most commonly used technique for neovagina construction. VRAM-based neovagina creation has also been suggested to be a reasonable option. There are advantages and disadvantages to any type of pelvic reconstruction with or without neovagina creation. Because pelvic exenteration with neovagina construction is a relatively infrequent procedure, there are insufficient data to strongly support one method over another, and the choice of pelvic reconstruction remains individualized.

OUTCOMES AFTER PELVIC EXENTERATION

Morbidity and Mortality

Pelvic exenteration is a complex procedure with a significant risk of morbidity. These complex procedures should only be considered and offered at specialized centers that can provide the multidisciplinary and intense perioperative care that is required. Tables 54.3 and 54.4 summarize some of the reported perioperative outcomes and complications. These tables provide a general idea of the outcomes, but it is important to note that there is extensive heterogeneity in the manner in which perioperative outcomes and complications are captured, assessed, and reported between all the referenced articles. Pelvic exenterations are lengthy procedures associated with significant blood loss and a long postoperative length of stay. Many centers report median/mean operative times in excess of 6 hours, with some in excess of 9 hours. Multiple liters of blood loss can be expected. Even today, the length of hospital stays ranges from 2 to 4 weeks.

Perioperative mortality is also significant but has dramatically decreased over time (Table 54.3). The initial series of pelvic exenterations reported a perioperative mortality of 23%, but modern series report much lower rates of mortality ranging from 0% to 9%. The average perioperative mortality is 9% combining series published before 2000, compared to 3% in those published after 2000. This is likely a reflection of vast improvements in preoperative medical optimization of patients, improved surgical techniques often with subspecialized surgical teams, routine use of prophylactic antibiotics, improved intraoperative anesthetic management, and improved postoperative care in modern intensive care units. Despite a significant reduction in perioperative mortality, both mortality and morbidity are significant following pelvic exenteration, and careful and thorough preoperative informed consent for the patient and her family is important.

Perioperative complications can be expected to occur in at least half of all pelvic exenteration cases (Table 54.3). There is also a significant risk of requiring additional surgical procedures to correct some of these complications. The spectrum of complications is vast, and virtually any type of complication can occur (Table 54.4). Surgeons and centers must be aware of this and be able to appropriately handle and manage these complications. Infectious, wound-related complications, venous thrombosis and embolic events, fistulae, bowel obstruction/ileus, and renal/metabolic abnormalities account for the majority of complications that can occur both in the early and late (often much later) postoperative periods.

Because of the variation in the surgical procedure and patient comorbidities, there are no data to provide specific guidance for optimal postoperative care. However, there are some general principles that may optimize postoperative outcomes. Continuous gastric drainage with either a nasogastric or orogastric tube is discouraged as this can lead to an increased risk of pulmonary and other complications. Early ambulation is a key to improving recovery. Total parenteral nutrition is used so that a favorable metabolic state can be maintained during the immediate postoperative period and there is no urgency to resume oral feedings. Antibiotic prophylaxis beyond 24 hours of surgery should not be done unless there are signs or symptoms of an infectious process. Intravenous patient-controlled analgesic delivery systems have been useful at our institution.

Survival

OS was dismal in the early series of pelvic exenteration, with almost no patients surviving 5 years after the exenteration. However, this has dramatically changed, and series published since then report approximately 40% to 60% of patients surviving 5 years or more (Table 54.5). In highly select cases, pelvic exenteration is the only currently available therapeutic option that can provide any chance of long-term survival. Prognostic indicators of survival following pelvic exenteration have been evaluated, but data remain inconsistent. Tumor histology, lymphovascular space invasion, age, primary site, primary versus recurrent disease, tumor size, tumor grade, and BMI have not been shown to be reliable. The only prognostic factor that has been consistently associated with a significant improvement in OS has been a negative margin resection (R0). To offer the greatest chances of prolonged survival, the surgeon should attempt to evaluate the margins intraoperatively and make every effort to obtain a negative surgical margin.

Forner and Lampe found that pelvic nodal metastasis was associated with a worse outcome. However, multiple other series have not confirmed a worse outcome in the setting of pelvic or paraaortic nodal metastasis. Schmidt and colleagues noted a 5-year OS of 51% in patients with pelvic nodal metastasis, which was not statistically worse compared to those with negative nodes (5-year OS 67%). However, cases with paraaortic nodal metastasis had a 5-year OS of only 17%. Based on this evidence, most gynecologic oncologists will not proceed with an exenterative procedure if aortic nodal metastasis is identified, but may be willing to complete the surgery in the face of a single positive pelvic node.

MINIMALLY INVASIVE SURGICAL APPROACHES

Pelvic exenteration has traditionally been performed via a large vertical midline incision, and this remains the standard approach. Recent advances in MIS techniques have led some surgeons to consider exenterative procedures using laparoscopy with or without robotic/computer assistance. The first report of a successful laparoscopic total pelvic exenteration for recurrent gynecologic malignancy was published in 2003 by Pomel and colleagues. This was a supralevator total exenteration with en bloc resection of bladder, uterus, vagina, ovaries, and rectum using endoscopic stapling devices. The specimen was delivered through the resulting vulvar opening.

TABLE 54.3 Select Reported Perioperative Outcomes, Morbidity and Mortality after Pelvic Exenteration

AUTHOR (REFERENCE)	YEAR OF PUBLICATION	N	OPERATIVE TIME (MIN)[a]	EBL (CC)[a]	LOS (D)[a]	PERIOPERATIVE MORTALITY N (%)	NUMBER OF PATIENTS WITH COMPLICATION(S) N (%)	REOPERATION TO CORRECT COMPLICATION(S) N (%)
Brunschwig	1948	22	—	—	—	5 (23%)	—	—
Barber	1965	22	—	—	—	5 (23%)	—	—
Barber	1968	36	—	—	—	—	22 (61%)	10 (28%)
Symmonds	1975	198	—	—	—	16 (8%)	—	—
Rutledge	1977	296	—	—	—	40 (14%)	—	—
Lawhead	1989	65	—	—	—	6 (9%)	—	—
Shingleton	1989	143	—	—	—	9 (6%)	—	—
Soper	1989	69	500	3,500	26	5 (7%)	32 (46%)[b]	20 (29%)
Morley	1989	100	345	2,800	30	2 (2%)	49 (49%)	—
Stanhope	1990	133	—	—	—	3 (2%)	89 (67%)	—
Robertson	1994	83	150	—	22	3 (4%)	39 (47%)	—
Morris	1996	20	—	—	—	1 (5%)	12 (60%)	—
Goldberg	1998	154	—	—	—	22 (14%)	69 (45%)	—
Barakat	1999	44	240	3,138	33	7 (16%)	35 (80%)	—

	Year		EBL					
Berek	2005	75	466	23	2,510	3 (4%)	65 (87%)[b]	—
Goldberg	2006	103	—	—	—	1 (1%)	73 (71%)[b]	—
Ungar	2008	41	—	—	—	0 (0%)	—	9 (22%)
Fotopoulou	2010	47	325	29	—	4 (9%)	33 (70%)	14 (30%)
Benn	2011	54	—	10	1,000	0 (0%)	33 (61%)[b]	—
McLean	2011	44	544	15	2,497	1 (2%)	36 (82%)[b]	2 (5%)
Forner	2011	35	442	33	—	0 (0%)	24 (69%)	—
Kaur	2012	36	390	25	2,000	0 (0%)	21 (58%)[b]	14 (39%)
Khoury-Collado	2012	21	685	17	1,500	0 (0%)	13 (62%)[b]	5 (24%)
Schmidt	2012	282	—	—	—	14 (5%)	143 (51%)	21 (7%)
Yoo	2012	61	600	34	1,089	0 (0%)	27 (44%)	—
Baiocchi	2013	77	420	14	—	5 (6%)	43 (56%)[b]	10 (13%)
TOTAL						152/2,225 (7%)	858/1,474 (58%)	105/653 (16%)

[a]Most values are medians; some are means.
[b]Minimum number of cases that could be ascertained from manuscript. Likely much higher number in reality.
EBL, estimated blood loss; LOS, length of postoperative hospital stay.

IX

TABLE 54.4 Select Reported Types of Complications after Pelvic Exenteration

AUTHOR (REFERENCE)	YEAR OF PUBLICATION	N	INFECTIOUS[a]	WOUND RELATED[b]	VTE	GU/GI FISTULAE[c]	ANASTOMOTIC LEAKS[d]	BOWEL OBSTRUCTION OR ILEUS	OTHER CARDIAC[e]	OTHER RENAL[f]	OTHER
Brunschwig	1948	22	—	—	—	—	—	—	—	—	—
Barber	1965	22	—	—	—	—	—	—	—	—	—
Barber	1968	36	7	4	1	2	0	2	0	1	5
Symmonds	1975	198	22	44	14	33	0	23	0	86	21
Rutledge	1977	296	—	—	—	—	—	—	—	—	—
Lawhead	1989	65	52	1	2	6	0	4	8	4	6
Shingleton	1989	143	—	—	—	—	—	—	—	—	—
Soper	1989	69	14	8	5	27	0	3	1	13	5
Morley	1989	100	6	11	4	16	2	19	0	11	1
Stanhope	1990	133	—	—	—	—	—	—	—	—	—
Robertson	1994	83	6	20	8	2	0	4	0	0	15
Morris	1996	20	2	0	1	4	0	2	0	3	3
Goldberg	1998	154	19	20	5	12	9	11	0	7	18
Barakat	1999	44	7	4	1	7	0	4	2	7	7
Berek	2005	75	33	26	0	17	0	25	0	21	0

Study	Year	N									
Goldberg	2006	103	0	17	7	12	14	9	0	43	14
Ungar	2008	41	—	—	—	—	—	—	—	—	—
Fotopoulou	2010	47	0	3	0	0	17	4	0	0	13
Benn	2011	54	31	30	6	0	0	24	2	25	18
McLean	2011	44	14	15	0	0	0	8	0	0	0
Forner	2011	35	0	0	0	0	7	0	0	4	11
Kaur	2012	36	3	10	0	6	0	3	0	5	35
Khoury–Collado	2012	21	—	—	—	—	—	—	—	—	—
Schmidt	2012	282	20	0	10	42	0	0	0	0	0
Yoo	2012	61	1	9	1	15	0	11	0	1	0
Baiocchi	2013	77	—	—	—	—	—	—	—	—	—
TOTAL[g]			237 (18%)	222 (16%)	65 (5%)	201 (15%)	49 (4%)	156 (12%)	13 (1%)	231 (17%)	172 (13%)

[a] Includes pelvic infections, intra-abdominal abscesses, surgical site infections, septicemia, bacteremia, sepsis, peritonitis, and pneumonia.
[b] Includes wound infections, eviscerations, dehiscences, separation, disruption, and perineal eviscerations.
[c] Includes enterocutaneous fistulae (abdominal or perineal), rectovaginal fistulae, vesicovaginal fistulae, and other complex fistulae.
[d] Includes colonic or ureteral anastomotic leaks.
[e] Includes congestive heart failure (?) and myocardial ischemia.
[f] Includes renal failure, urinary tract infections, pyelonephritis, urinary stones, urinary obstruction, and metabolic abnormalities.
[g] Denominator is the total number of complications listed in table (N = 1,346).
VTE, venous thromboembolic event; GU, genitourinary; GI, gastrointestinal.

TABLE 54.5 Overall Survival after Pelvic Exenterations Performed for Mostly Recurrent Gynecologic Malignancies

AUTHOR (REFERENCE)	STUDY YEARS	N	5-YEAR OS
Brunschwig	1946–1948	22	9 (41%) died within 8 mo[a]
Barber	1947–1958	22	7%
Barber	1947–1963	36	14%
Symmonds	1950–1971	198	32%
Rutledge	1955–1976	296	42%
Lawhead	1972–1981	65	23%
Shingleton	1969–1986	143	50%
Soper	1970–1987	69	48%
Morley	1964–1984	100	61%
Stanhope	1977–1986	133	46%
Robertson	1974–1992	83	41%
Morris	1955–1988	20	56%
Goldberg	1954–1994	154	24%
Barakat	1947–1994	44	Median 10.2 mo
Berek	1956–2011	75	54%
Goldberg	1987–2003	103	47%
Khoury-Collado	1997–2001	21	40%
Yoo	2001–2011	61	56%
Baiocchi	1982–2010	77	24%

[a]Short median follow-up of 1.75 mo.
OS, overall survival.

A coloanal anastomosis was performed perineally, and a protective, temporary loop ileostomy was matured through the left lower abdominal trocar site. An ileal conduit was performed extracorporally by extending the infraumbilical trocar site. The ileal conduit stoma was then matured through the right lower abdominal trocar site. The estimated blood loss (EBL) was 250 cc, and the operative time was 9 hours. The patient was discharged 16 days later. Ferron et al. reported their experience with five laparoscopically assisted vaginal pelvic exenterations. The umbilicus was used as the camera trocar site, and an additional four operative trocars were used. Urinary reconstructions were performed through a lateral 5-cm incision. Trocar sites were used to place stomas and bring out drains to the extent possible. No complications were noted in three (60%) of the five patients, and the other two patients developed a perineal and abdominal wall abscess only. Hospital stay ranged from 13 to 33 days.

A larger series of 16 consecutive laparoscopic anterior pelvic exenterations for recurrent gynecologic malignancies was reported by Puntambekar and colleagues in 2006. A total of five ports were used, and these were all supralevator anterior exenterations. Urinary diversion was created by implanting both ureters into the intact sigmoid colon and using stents to exiting through the anal canal. The average operative time was 240 minutes and EBL was 200 mL. Only three (19%) patients experienced a postoperative complication: partial small bowel obstruction (n = 2) and ureteric leak (n = 1). The mean postoperative stay was only 3.5 days. No long-term follow-up is available.

Martinez and colleagues reported their outcomes comparing 14 laparoscopic pelvic exenterations to 29 pelvic exenterations performed via laparotomy. All types of exenterative procedures were performed using both approaches. The median operative time was 13 minutes longer laparoscopically, and the median length of stays was similar (26.5 days vs. 28 days). Blood loss was significantly less using a laparoscopic approach, but overall complications were similar between laparoscopy and laparotomy. A few case series have been published using the robotically assisted surgical platform, including reports by Lambaudie et al. and Davis and colleagues.

MIS approaches have uniformly been shown to offer significant advantages for many other gynecologic procedures for both benign and malignant conditions. An MIS approach to perform an exenteration is interesting. However, only small series have been published and no short- or long-term follow-up is yet available. Ongoing refinement of MIS techniques hopefully will lead to further improvements in perioperative outcomes for these patients, but that remains to be determined.

BEST SURGICAL PRACTICES

- Pelvic exenteration is a complex surgical procedure that should be performed by experienced surgeons in centers familiar with this procedure and capable of offering the intense and complex perioperative care that is required.
- The important first step is the identification and adequate evaluation of appropriate candidates in whom exenteration may offer a benefit. Medical comorbidities and performance status must be carefully evaluated and optimized preoperatively. All efforts must be made to exclude extrapelvic metastasis, and exenteration must be abandoned if this is discovered. PET/CT scanning has been shown to be useful in this evaluation.
- The goal of exenteration should be a negative margin (R0) resection. We have found preoperative pelvic MRI to be helpful in this regard.
- The ideal candidate for exenteration is a patient with a recurrent gynecologic malignancy in the central pelvis measuring 2 cm or less who has been previously treated with primary radiation. However, because of reduction of morbidity and mortality, the indications for exenterative procedures have been tremendously expanded and can be considered in other settings.
- Pelvic exenteration requires a multidisciplinary approach involving a gynecologic oncologist, plastic surgeon, sometimes urologist, often a radiologist, radiation oncologist, and a psychologist. Intraoperatively, a multiteam approach will help reduce individual surgeon fatigue since these are long procedures.

- It is important to offer as much psychological evaluation, assessment, and assistance as possible since most patients cannot fully understand the consequences of the procedure they will be undergoing.
- The choice of urinary diversion is complex. Advantages and disadvantages exist for noncontinent and continent diversions. Similarly, various types of continent diversions exist, each with their own advantages and disadvantages.
- A wet colostomy had been largely abandoned, and separate urinary and fecal diversions have been thought to be superior. However, a recently described use of a novel double-barreled colostomy technique suggests that this may be a very reasonable method for a combined urinary and fecal diversion with comparable, or even improved, outcomes compared to the various separate techniques.
- The optimal method for pelvic defect reconstruction and neovagina creation remains to be determined. Multiple techniques exist, and the decisions must be individualized.

BIBLIOGRAPHY

Andikyan V, Khoury-Collado F, Sonoda Y, et al. Extended pelvic resections for recurrent or persistent uterine and cervical malignancies: an update on out of the box surgery. *Gynecol Oncol* 2012;125:404–408.

Angioli R, Panici PB, Mirhashemi R, et al. Continent urinary diversion and low colorectal anastomosis after pelvic exenteration. Quality of life and complication risk. *Crit Rev Oncol Hematol* 2003;48:281–285.

Backes FJ, Tierney BJ, Eisenhauer EL, et al. Complications after double-barreled wet colostomy compared to separate urinary and fecal diversion during pelvic exenteration: time to change back? *Gynecol Oncol* 2013;128:60–64.

Baiocchi G, Guimaraes GC, Faloppa CC, et al. Does histologic type correlate to outcome after pelvic exenteration for cervical and vaginal cancer? *Ann Surg Oncol* 2013;20:1694.

Barakat RR, Goldman NA, Patel DA, et al. Pelvic exenteration for recurrent endometrial cancer. *Gynecol Oncol* 1999;75:99–102.

Barber HRK, Brunschwig A. Pelvic exenteration for locally advanced and recurrent ovarian cancer. Review of 22 cases. *Surgery* 1965;58:935–937.

Barber HRK, Brunschwig A. Treatment and results of recurrent cancer of corpus uteri in patients receiving anterior and total pelvic exenteration, 1947–1963. *Cancer* 1968;22:949–955.

Benn T, Brooks RA, Zhang Q, et al. Pelvic exenteration in gynecologic oncology: a single institution study over 20 years. *Gynecol Oncol* 2011;122:14–18.

Berek JS, Howe C, Lagasse LD, et al. Pelvic exenteration for recurrent gynecologic malignancy: survival and morbidity analysis of the 45-year experience at UCLA. *Gynecol Oncol* 2005;99:153–159.

Berger JL, Westin SN, Fellman B, et al. Modified vertical rectus abdominis myocutaneous flap vaginal reconstruction: an analysis of surgical outcomes. *Gynecol Oncol* 2012;125:252–255.

Brunschwig A, Daniel W. Observations of the urinary tract four to seven years after total pelvic exenteration and wet colostomy. *Ann Surg* 1955;142:729–738.

Brunschwig A. Complete excision of pelvic viscera for advanced carcinoma. *Cancer* 1948;1:177–183.

Bucher P, Mermillod B, Gervaz P, et al. Mechanical bowel preparation for elective colorectal surgery: a meta-analysis. *Arch Surg* 2004;139:1359–1364.

Burger IA, Vargas HA, Donati OF, et al. The value of ¹⁸F-FDG PET/CT in recurrent gynecologic malignancies prior to pelvic exenteration. *Gynecol Oncol* 2013;129:586.

Carter MF, Dalton DP, Garnett JE. Simultaneous diversion of the urinary and fecal streams utilizing a single abdominal stoma: the double barreled wet colostomy. *J Urol* 1989;141:1189–1191.

Chokshi RJ, Kuhrt MP, Arrese D, et al. Reconstruction of total pelvic exenteration defects with rectus abdominis myocutaneous flaps versus primary closure. *Am J Surg* 2013;205:64–70.

Chokshi RJ, Kuhrt MP, Schmidt C, et al. Single institution experience comparing double-barreled wet colostomy to ileal conduit for urinary and fecal diversion. *Urology* 2011;78:856–862.

Creagh TA, Dixon L, Frizelle FA. Reconstruction with vertical rectus abdominus myocutaneous flap in advanced pelvic malignancy. *J Plast Reconstr Aesthet Surg* 2012;65:791–797.

Davis M, Adams S, Eun D, et al. Robotic-assisted laparoscopic exenteration in recurrent cervical cancer: robotics improved the surgical experience for 2 women with recurrent cervical cancer. *Am J Obstet Gynecol* 2010;202:663.e1.

Eisenkop SM, Nalick RH, Teng NN. Modified posterior exenteration for ovarian cancer. *Obstet Gynecol* 1991;78:879–885.

Ferron G, Querleu D, Martel P, et al. Laparoscopy-assisted vaginal pelvic exenteration. *Gynecol Oncol* 2006;100:551–555.

Forner DM, Lampe B. Exenteration as a primary treatment for locally advanced cervical cancer: long-term results and prognostic factors. *Am J Obstet Gynecol* 2011;205:148.e1–148.e6.

Forner DM, Lampe B. Ileal conduit and continent ileocecal pouch for patients undergoing pelvic exenteration: comparison of complications and quality of life. *Int J Gynecol Cancer* 2011;21:203–208.

Forner DM, Meyer A, Lampe B. Preoperative assessment of complete tumor resection by magnetic resonance imaging in patients undergoing pelvic exenteration. *Eur J Obstet Gynecol Reprod Biol* 2010;148:182–185.

Fotopoulou C, Neumann U, Kraetschell R, et al. Long-term clinical outcome of pelvic exenteration in patients with advanced gynecological malignancies. *J Surg Oncol* 2010;101:507–512.

Georgiou PA, Tekkis PP, Constantinides VA, et al. Diagnostic accuracy and value of magnetic resonance imaging (MRI) in planning exenterative pelvic surgery for advanced colorectal cancer. *Eur J Cancer* 2013;49:72–81.

Goldberg GL, Sukumvanich P, Einstein MH, et al. Total pelvic exenteration: the Albert Einstein College of Medicine/Montefiore Medical Center experience (1987 to 2003). *Gynecol Oncol* 2006;101:261–268.

Goldberg JM, Piver MS, Hempling RE, et al. Improvements in pelvic exenteration: factors responsible for reducing morbidity and mortality. *Ann Surg Oncol* 1998;5:399–406.

Hockel M, Horn L, Einenkel J. (Laterally) Extended endopelvic resection: surgical treatment of locally advanced and recurrent cancer of the uterine cervix and vagina based on ontogenetic anatomy. *Gynecol Oncol* 2012;127:297–302.

Houvenaeghel G, Gutowski M, Buttarelli M, et al. Modified posterior pelvic exenteration for ovarian cancer. *Int J Gynecol Cancer* 2009;19:968–973.

Husain A, Akhurst T, Larson S, et al. A prospective study of the accuracy of ¹⁸Fluorodeoxyglucose positron emission tomography (¹⁸FDG PET) in identifying sites of metastasis prior to pelvic exenteration. *Gynecol Oncol* 2007;106:177–180.

Husain A, Curtin J, Brown C, et al. Continent urinary diversion and low-rectal anastomosis in patients undergoing exenterative procedures for recurrent gynecologic malignancies. *Gynecol Oncol* 2000;78:208–211.

Jurado M, Alcazar JL, Baixauli J, et al. Low colorectal anastomosis after pelvic exenteration for gynecologic malignancies: risk factor analysis for leakage. *Int J Gynecol Cancer* 2011;21:397–402.

Jurado M, Alcazar JL, Martinez-Monge R. Resectability rates of previously irradiated recurrent cervical cancer (PIRCC) treated with pelvic exenteration: is still the clinical involvement of the pelvis wall a real contraindication? A twenty-year experience. *Gynecol Oncol* 2010;116:38–43.

Kaur M, Joniau S, D'Hoore A, et al. Pelvic exenterations for gynecological malignancies: a study of 36 cases. *Int J Gynecol Cancer* 2012;22:889–896.

Khoury-Collado F, Einstein MH, Bochner BH, et al. Pelvic exenteration with curative intent for recurrent uterine malignancies. *Gynecol Oncol* 2012;124:42–47.

Kohler C, Tozzi R, Possover M, et al. Explorative laparoscopy prior to exenterative surgery. *Gynecol Oncol* 2002;86:311–315.

Lambaudie E, Narducci F, Leblanc E, et al. Robotically-assisted laparoscopic anterior pelvic exenteration for recurrent cervical cancer: report of three first cases. *Gynecol Oncol* 2010;116:582–583.

Lawhead RA Jr, Clark DGC, Smith DH, et al. Pelvic exenteration for recurrent or persistent gynecologic malignancies: a 10-year review of the Memorial Sloan-Kettering Cancer Center experience (1972–1981). *Gynecol Oncol* 1989;33:279–282.

Madersbacher S, Schmidt J, Eberle JM, et al. Long-term outcome of ileal conduit diversion. *J Urol* 2003;169:985–990.

Martinez A, Filleron T, Vitse L, et al. Laparoscopic pelvic exenteration for gynaecological malignancy: is there any advantage? *Gynecol Oncol* 2011;120:374–379.

McLean KA, Zhang W, Dunsmoor-Su RF, et al. Pelvic exenteration in the age of modern chemoradiation. *Gynecol Oncol* 2011;121:131–134.

Mirhashemi R, Averette HE, Estape R, et al. Low colorectal anastomosis after radical pelvic surgery: a risk factor analysis. *Am J Obstet Gynecol* 2000;183:1375–1380.

Morley GW, Hopkins MP, Lindenauer SM, et al. Pelvic exenteration, University of Michigan: 100 patients at 5 years. *Obstet Gynecol* 1989;74:934–943.

Morris M, Alvarez RD, Kinney WK, et al. Treatment of recurrent adenocarcinoma of the endometrium with pelvic exenteration. *Gynecol Oncol* 1996;60:288–291.

Nelson RA, Butler CE. Surgical outcomes of VRAM versus thigh flaps for immediate reconstruction of pelvic and perineal cancer resection defects. *Plast Reconstr Surg* 2009;123:175–183.

O'Connell C, Mirhashemi R, Kassira N, et al. Formation of functional neovagina with vertical rectus abdominis musculocutaneous (VRAM) flap after total pelvic exenteration. *Ann Plast Surg* 2005;55:470–473.

Plante M, Roy M. Operative laparoscopy prior to a pelvic exenteration in patients with recurrent cervical cancer. *Gynecol Oncol* 1998;69:94–99.

Pomel C, Rouzier R, Pocard M, et al. Laparoscopic total pelvic exenteration for cervical cancer relapse. *Gynecol Oncol* 2003;91:616–618.

Puntambekar S, Kudchadkar RJ, Gurjar AM, et al. Laparoscopic pelvic exenteration for advanced pelvic cancers: a review of 16 cases. *Gynecol Oncol* 2006;102:513–516.

Robertson G, Lopes A, Beynon G, et al. Pelvic exenteration: a review of the Gateshead experience 1974–1992. *Br J Obstet Gynaecol* 1994;101:529–531.

Rutledge FN, Smith JP, Wharton JT, et al. Pelvic exenteration: analysis of 296 patients. *Am J Obstet Gynecol* 1977;129:881–892.

Schmidt A, Imesch P, Fink D, et al. Indications and long-term clinical outcomes in 282 patients with pelvic exenteration for advanced or recurrent cervical cancer. *Gynecol Oncol* 2012;125:604–609.

Shingleton HM, Soong S, Gelder MS, et al. Clinical and histopathologic factors predicting recurrence and survival after pelvic exenteration for cancer of the cervix. *Obstet Gynecol* 1989;73:1027–1034.

Slim K, Vicaut E, Launay-Savary M, et al. Updated systematic review and meta-analysis of randomized clinical trials on the role of mechanical bowel preparation before colorectal surgery. *Ann Surg* 2009;249:203–209.

Soper JT, Berchuck A, Creasman WT, et al. Pelvic exenteration: factors associated with major surgical morbidity. *Gynecol Oncol* 1989;35:93–98.

Stanhope CR, Webb MJ, Podratz KC. Pelvic exenteration for recurrent cervical cancer. *Clin Obstet Gynecol* 1990;33:897–909.

Symmonds RE, Pratt JH, Webb MJ. Exenterative operations: experience with 198 patients. *Am J Obstet Gynecol* 1975;121:907–918.

Ungar L, Palfalvi L, Novak Z. Primary pelvic exenteration in cervical cancer patients. *Gynecol Oncol* 2008;111:S9–S12.

Urh A, Soliman PT, Schmeler KM, et al. Postoperative outcomes after continent versus incontinent urinary diversion at the time of pelvic exenteration for gynecologic malignancies. *Gynecol Oncol* 2013;129(3):580–585. http://dx.doi.org/10.1016/j.ygyno.2013.02.024.

Vasilescu C, Tudor S, Popa M, et al. Entirely robotic total robotic exenteration. *Surg Laparosc Endosc Percutan Tech* 2011;21:e200–e202.

Yoo HJ, Lim MC, Seo S, et al. Pelvic exenteration for recurrent cervical cancer: ten-year experience at National Cancer Center in Korea. *J Gynecol Oncol* 2012;23:242–250.

INDEX

Note: Page numbers followed by f indicate figures and those followed by t indicate tables.